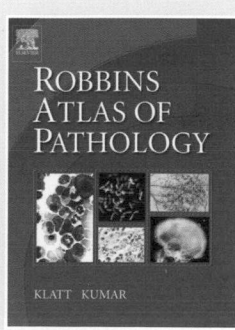

Robbins and Cotran

PATHOLOGIC BASIS OF DISEASE

Robbins and Cotran

PATHOLOGIC BASIS OF DISEASE

Seventh Edition

VINAY KUMAR, MBBS, MD, FRCPath
Alice Hogge and Arthur Baer Professor
Chairman, Department of Pathology
The University of Chicago, Pritzker School of Medicine
Chicago, Illinois

ABUL K. ABBAS, MBBS
Chair, Department of Pathology
University of California, San Francisco
San Francisco, California

NELSON FAUSTO, MD
Chairman, Department of Pathology
University of Washington School of Medicine
Seattle, Washington

With Illustrations by
James A. Perkins, MS, MFA

ELSEVIER
SAUNDERS

ELSEVIER
SAUNDERS
An Imprint of Elsevier

The Curtis Center
170 S Independence Mall W 300E
Philadelphia, Pennsylvania 19106

ROBBINS AND COTRAN PATHOLOGIC BASIS OF DISEASE, 7/E

NOTICE

Medicine is an ever-changing field. Standard safety precautions must be followed, but as new research and clinical experience broaden our knowledge, changes in treatment and drug therapy may become necessary or appropriate. Readers are advised to check the most current product information provided by the manufacturer of each drug to be administered to verify the recommended dose, the method and duration of administration, and contraindications. It is the responsibility of the treating physician, relying on experience and knowledge of the patient, to determine dosages and the best treatment for each individual patient. Neither the publisher nor the authors assume any liability for any injury and/or damage to persons or property arising from this publication.

Previous editions copyrighted 1999, 1994, 1989, 1984, 1979, 1974

Library of Congress Cataloging-in-Publication Data
Robbins and Cotran pathologic basis of disease.—7th ed./[edited by]
Vinay Kumar, Abul K. Abbas, Nelson Fausto ; with illustrations by James A. Perkins.
p. ; cm.
Rev. ed. of: Robbins pathologic basis of disease, 1999.
ISBN-13: 978-0-7216-0187-8 ISBN-10: 0-7216-0187-1
1. Pathology.
[DNLM: 1. Pathology. QZ 4 R6354 2004] I. Title: Pathologic basis of disease. II. Kumar, Vinay. III. Abbas, Abul K. IV. Fausto, Nelson. V. Robbins, Stanley L. (Stanley Leonard). VI. Cotran, Ramzi S. Robbins pathologic basis of disease.
RB111.R62 2004
616.07—dc22

2004046835

ISBN-13: 978-0-7216-0187-8
ISBN-10: 0-7216-0187-1
IE ISBN-13: 978-0-8089-2302-2
IE ISBN-10: 0-8089-2302-1

Publishing Director: William Schmitt
Managing Editor: Rebecca Gruliow
Design Manager: Ellen Zanolle

Printed in China

Last digit is the print number: 9 8 7 6 5 4

IN MEMORY OF

Dr. Stanley L. Robbins (1915–2003)

and

Dr. Ramzi S. Cotran (1932–2000)

Dear friends, respected colleagues, and dedicated teachers

They leave a legacy of excellence
that will enrich the lives of generations
of future physicians.

Contributors

Charles E. Alpers, MD
Professor of Pathology, Adjunct Professor of Medicine, University of Washington School of Medicine; Pathologist, University of Washington Medical Center, Seattle, WA

The Kidney

Douglas C. Anthony, MD, PhD
Professor and Chair, Department of Pathology and Anatomical Sciences, University of Missouri, Columbia, MO

Peripheral Nerve and Skeletal Muscle; The Central Nervous System

Jon C. Aster, MD, PhD
Associate Professor of Pathology, Harvard Medical School; Staff Pathologist, Brigham and Women's Hospital, Boston, MA

Red Blood Cell and Bleeding Disorders; Diseases of White Blood Cells, Lymph Nodes, Spleen, and Thymus

James M. Crawford, MD, PhD
Professor and Chair, Department of Pathology, Immunology and Laboratory Medicine, University of Florida College of Medicine; Professor and Chair, Shands Hospital at the University of Florida, Gainesville, FL

The Gastrointestinal Tract; Liver and Biliary Tract

Christopher P. Crum, MD
Professor of Pathology, Harvard Medical School; Director, Women's and Perinatal Pathology, Brigham and Women's Hospital, Boston, MA

The Female Genital Tract

Umberto De Girolami, MD
Professor of Pathology, Harvard Medical School, Boston; Director of Neuropathology, Brigham and Women's Hospital, Boston, MA

Peripheral Nerve and Skeletal Muscle; The Central Nervous System

Jonathan I. Epstein, MD
Professor of Pathology, Urology, and Oncology; The Rinehard Professor of Urologic Pathology, The Johns Hopkins University School of Medicine, Baltimore; Director of Surgical Pathology, The Johns Hopkins Hospital, Baltimore, MD

The Lower Urinary Tract and Male Genital System

Robert Folberg, MD
Frances B. Greever Professor and Head, Department of Pathology, University of Illinois at Chicago, Chicago, IL

The Eye

Matthew P. Frosch, MD, PhD
Assistant Professor of Pathology, Harvard Medical School Boston; Assistant Pathologist, C.S. Kubik Laboratory for Neuropathology, Massachusetts General Hospital, Boston, MA

Peripheral Nerve and Skeletal Muscle; The Central Nervous System

Ralph H. Hruban, MD
Professor of Pathology and Oncology, The Johns Hopkins University School of Medicine; Attending Pathologist, The Johns Hopkins Hospital, Baltimore, MD

The Pancreas

Aliya N. Husain, MBBS
Professor, Department of Pathology, Pritzker School of Medicine, University of Chicago, Chicago, IL

The Lung

Agnes B. Kane, MD, PhD
Professor and Chair, Department of Pathology and Laboratory Medicine, Brown University Medical School, Providence, RI

Environmental and Nutritional Pathology

Susan C. Lester, MD, PhD
Assistant Professor of Pathology, Harvard Medical School; Chief, Breast Pathology, Brigham and Women's Hospital, Boston, MA

The Breast

Mark W. Lingen, DDS, PhD
Associate Professor, Department of Pathology, University of Chicago, Chicago, IL

Head and Neck

Chen Liu, MD, PhD
Assistant Professor of Pathology, University of Florida College of Medicine, Gainesville, FL

The Gastrointestinal Tract

Anirban Maitra, MBBS
Assistant Professor, Department of Pathology, The Johns Hopkins University School of Medicine; Pathologist, The Johns Hopkins Hospital, Baltimore, MD

Diseases of Infancy and Childhood; The Endocrine System

Alexander J. McAdam, MD, PhD
Assistant Professor of Pathology, Harvard Medical School; Medical Director, Infectious Diseases Diagnostic Laboratory, Children's Hospital Boston, Boston, MA

Infectious Diseases

Martin C. Mihm, Jr., MD
Clinical Professor of Pathology, Harvard Medical School; Pathologist and Associate Dermatologist, Massachusetts General Hospital, Boston, MA

The Skin

Richard N. Mitchell, MD
Associate Professor, Department of Pathology, Harvard Medical School; Director, Human Pathology, Harvard-MIT Division of Health Sciences and Technology, Harvard Medical School; Staff Pathologist, Brigham and Women's Hospital, Boston, MA

Hemodynamic Disorders, Thromboembolic Disease, and Shock

George F. Murphy, MD
Professor of Pathology, Harvard Medical School; Director of Dermatopathology, Brigham and Women's Hospital, Boston, MA

The Skin

Andrew E. Rosenberg, MD
Associate Professor of Pathology, Harvard Medical School; Associate Pathologist, James Homer Wright Laboratories, Department of Pathology, Massachusetts General Hospital, Boston, MA

Bones, Joints, and Soft Tissue Tumors

Frederick J. Schoen, MD, PhD
Professor of Pathology and Health Sciences and Technology, Harvard Medical School; Director, Cardiac Pathology and Executive Vice Chairman, Department of Pathology, Brigham and Women's Hospital, Boston, MA

Blood Vessels; The Heart

Klaus Sellheyer, MD
Assistant Professor of Pathology, Thomas Jefferson University; Attending Dermatopathologist, Jefferson Medical College, Philadelphia, PA

The Skin

Arlene H. Sharpe, MD, PhD
Professor of Pathology, Harvard Medical School; Chief, Immunology Research Division, Department of Pathology, Brigham and Women's Hospital, Boston, MA

Infectious Diseases

Robb E. Wilentz, MD
Voluntary Faculty, Department of Dermatology, University of Miami School of Medicine; Laboratory Director, Division of Pathology, Skin and Cancer Associates, Miami, FL

The Pancreas

Preface

We launch the seventh edition of *Pathologic Basis of Disease* with mixed emotions, excitement and enthusiasm, as we enter the new millennium, tempered by sadness over the loss of our dear colleagues Drs. Stanley Robbins and Ramzi Cotran. To acknowledge their immeasurable and everlasting contribution to this text, the book is now renamed *Robbins and Cotran Pathologic Basis of Disease.*

This edition, like all previous ones, has been extensively revised, and some areas completely rewritten. Some of the more significant changes are as follows:

- Chapter 1 has been completely reorganized to include the entire spectrum of cellular responses to injury, from adaptations and sublethal injury to cell death. This was accomplished by combining the first two chapters of the sixth edition. We believe that this integrated and extensively revised chapter will allow a better understanding of cell injury, the most fundamental process in disease causation.
- Chapter 3, covering tissue repair and wound healing, has been extensively revised to include new and exciting information in stem cell biology and the emerging field of regenerative medicine.
- Chapter 8, dealing with infectious diseases, has been organized taxonomically with emphasis on mechanisms of tissue injury by different categories of infectious agents. While examples of infections by prototypic microorganisms have been retained, most of the organ-specific infectious diseases have been moved to later chapters where other diseases of the organ are described.
- Discussion of diabetes mellitus has been moved from the chapter on pancreatic diseases to the chapter on endocrine disorders, where it blends more logically with other hormonal diseases.
- Discussions of the lower urinary tract and the male genital system have been combined and grouped into a single chapter in recognition of the fact that there is overlap in diseases and diagnostic considerations.
- A new feature best described as "boxes" has been introduced in selected chapters. For boxes, we have selected topics at the cutting edge of science that are worthy of a more detailed presentation than is essential for a student textbook. In doing so, we hope that we have presented the excitement of the topic without encumbering the body of the text with details that may appear overwhelming to the beginning reader.
- The chapter on ocular diseases has been rewritten and reorganized to facilitate an understanding of ophthalmic pathology by the non-specialist.
- In addition to the revision and reorganization of the text, there have been significant changes in illustrations. Many new photographs and schematics have been added and a large number of the older "gems" have been enhanced by digital technology. Thus we hope that even the veterans of the Robbins Pathology titles who have seen many previous editions of the book will find the color illustrations more sparkling and fresh. Approximately 50 new pages of illustrations have been added.

In the 5 years since the previous edition, spectacular advances, including the completion of the human genome project, have occurred. Whenever appropriate we have blended the new discoveries into the discussion of pathogenesis and pathophysiology, yet never losing sight that the "state of the art" has little value if it does not enhance the understanding of disease mechanisms. As in the past, we have not avoided discussions of "unsolved" problems because of our belief that many who read the text might be encouraged to embark on a path of discovery.

Despite the changes outlined above and extensive revisions, our goals remain essentially the same.

- To integrate into the discussion of pathologic processes and disorders the newest established information available—morphologic and molecular.
- To organize the presentations into logical and uniform approaches, thereby facilitating readability, comprehension, and learning.
- To maintain a reasonable size of the book, and yet to provide adequate discussion of the significant lesions, processes, and disorders, allotting space in proportion to their clinical and biologic importance.
- To place great emphasis on clarity of writing and good usage of language in the recognition that struggling to comprehend is time-consuming and wearisome and gets in the way of the learning process.
- To make this first and foremost a student text—used by students throughout their 4 years of medical school and into their residencies—but, at the same time, to provide sufficient detail and depth to meet the needs of more advanced readers.

We have been repeatedly told by the readers that one of the features they value most in this book is its up-to-dateness. We have strived to maintain such timeliness by providing references from recent literature, many published in 2003 and some from the early part of 2004. However, older classics have also been retained to provide original source material for advanced readers.

With this edition, we also move into the digital age: the text will be available online to those who own the print version. This online access gives the reader the ability to search across the entire text, bookmark passages, add personal notes, use PubMed to view references, and many other exciting features, including timely updates. In addition, included in the text is a CD-ROM of case studies, previously available separately as the Interactive Case Study Companion developed by one of us (VK) in collaboration with Herb Hagler, PhD, and Nancy Schneider, MD, PhD, at the University of Texas, Southwestern Medical School in Dallas. This will enhance and reinforce learning by challenging students to apply their knowledge in solving clinical cases. A virtual microscope feature enables the viewing of selected images at various powers.

This edition is also marked by the addition of two new "seasoned" coauthors. All three of us have reviewed, critiqued, and edited each chapter to ensure uniformity of style and flow that have been the hallmarks of the text. Together, we hope that we have succeeded in bringing to the reader the excitement of the study of disease mechanisms and the desire to learn more than what can be offered in any textbook.

VK
AKA
NF

Acknowledgments

The authors are grateful to a large number of individuals who have contributed in many ways toward the completion of this textbook.

First and foremost, all three of us offer our tributes and gratitude to two stalwarts of American pathology, Dr. Stanley Robbins and Dr. Ramzi Cotran. Their passion for excellence and uncompromising standards have made this book what it is. While neither of the two will see this edition in its completed form, their stamp on *Pathologic Basis of Disease* is indelible. Second, we thank our contributing authors for their commitment to this textbook. Many are veterans of previous editions; others are new to the seventh edition. All are acknowledged in the Table of Contents. Their names lend authority to this book, for which we are grateful.

Many colleagues have enhanced the text by reading various chapters and providing helpful critiques in their area of expertise. They include (at the University of Chicago): Drs. Todd Kroll, Michelle LeBeau, Olaf Schneewind, Josephine Morello, Megan McNerney, Fred Wondisford, Aliya Husain, Jonathan Miller, Julian Solway, John Hart, Amy Noffsinger, Thomas Krausz, Raminder Kumar, Joanne Yocum, Christopher Weber, Elizabeth McNally, and Manny Utset; (at the University of California at San Francisco): Drs. Steve Gitelman, Jonathan Lin, David Wofsy, Patrick Treseler, Mark Anderson, and Aaron Tward; (at the University of Washington, Seattle): Drs. Zsolt Argenyi, Peter Beyers, Ann DeLancey, Charles Murry, Thomas Norwood, Brian Rubin, Paul Swanson, Melissa Upton, and Mathew Yeh. Dr. David Walker, at the University of Texas Medical Branch at Galveston provided a thorough critique of the chapter on infectious disease. Dr. Lora Hendrick Ellenson at Cornell University (Weill Medical College) provided a critique of the chapter on the female genital tract. Dr. Arlene Herzberg and Kelly McGuigan provided help with the chapter on skin diseases.

Special thanks are owed to Dr. Henry Sanchez at the University of California at San Francisco for his painstaking review and revision of the older color illustrations and for his magic touch in enhancing them digitally. Their freshness will be obvious to the readers. Many colleagues provided photographic gems from their collection. They are individually acknowledged in the text.

Our administrative staff needs to be acknowledged since they maintain order in the chaotic lives of the authors and have willingly chipped in when needed for multiple tasks relating to the text. At the University of Chicago, they include Ms. Vera Davis and Ms. Ruthie Cornelius; at The University of California at San Francisco, Ms. Ana Narvaez; and at the University of Washington, Seattle, Ms. Catherine Alexander, Steven Berard, Carlton Kim, Ms. Genevieve Thomas, and Ms. Vicki Tolbert. Ms. Beverly Shackelford at the University of Texas at Dallas, who has helped one of us (VK) for 21 years, deserves special mention since she coordinated the submission of all manuscripts, proofread many of them, and maintained liaison with the contributors and publisher. Without her dedication to this book and her meticulous attention to detail, our task would have been much more difficult. Most of the graphic art in this book was created by Mr. James Perkins, Assistant Professor of Medical Illustration at Rochester Institute of Technology. His ability to convert complex ideas into simple and aesthetically pleasing sketches has considerably enhanced this book.

Many individuals associated with our publisher, Elsevier (under the imprint of W.B. Saunders), need our special thanks. Outstanding among them is Ellen Sklar, Production Editor, supervising the production of this book. Her understanding of the needs of the authors and the complexity of publishing a textbook went a long way in making our lives less complicated. Mr. William Schmitt, Publishing Director of Medical Textbooks, has always been our cheerleader and is now a dear friend. Our thanks also go to Managing Editor Rebecca Gruliow and Design Manager Ellen Zanolle at Elsevier. Undoubtedly there are many other "heroes" who may have been left out unwittingly—to them we say "thank you" and tender apologies for not acknowledging you individually.

Efforts of this magnitude take a heavy toll on the families of the authors. We thank our spouses Raminder Kumar, Ann Abbas, and Ann DeLancey for their patience, love, and support of this venture, and for their tolerance of our absences.

Finally, Vinay Kumar wishes to express his deep appreciation to Drs. Abul Abbas and Nelson Fausto for joining the team, and together we salute each other for shared vision and dedication to medical education. Despite differences in our vantage points, opinions, and individual styles, our common goal made this an exciting and rewarding partnership.

VK
AA
NF

Contents

Contributors vii
Preface ix
Acknowledgments xi

UNIT I General Pathology

CHAPTER 1
Cellular Adaptations, Cell Injury, and Cell Death 3

CHAPTER 2
Acute and Chronic Inflammation 47

CHAPTER 3
Tissue Renewal and Repair: Regeneration, Healing, and Fibrosis 87

CHAPTER 4
Hemodynamic Disorders, Thromboembolic Disease, and Shock 119
Richard N. Mitchell

CHAPTER 5
Genetic Disorders 145

CHAPTER 6
Diseases of Immunity 193
Abul K. Abbas

CHAPTER 7
Neoplasia 269

CHAPTER 8
Infectious Diseases 343
Alexander J. McAdam • Arlene H. Sharpe

CHAPTER 9
Environmental and Nutritional Pathology 415
Agnes B. Kane • Vinay Kumar

CHAPTER 10
Diseases of Infancy and Childhood 469
Anirban Maitra • Vinay Kumar

UNIT II Diseases of Organ Systems

CHAPTER 11
Blood Vessels 511
Frederick J. Schoen

CHAPTER 12
The Heart 555
Frederick J. Schoen

CHAPTER 13
Red Blood Cell and Bleeding Disorders 619
Jon C. Aster

CHAPTER 14
Diseases of White Blood Cells, Lymph Nodes, Spleen, and Thymus 661
Jon C. Aster

CHAPTER 15
The Lung 711
Aliya N. Husain • Vinay Kumar

CHAPTER 16
Head and Neck 773
Mark W. Lingen • Vinay Kumar

CHAPTER 17
The Gastrointestinal Tract 797
Chen Liu • James M. Crawford

CHAPTER 18
Liver and Biliary Tract 877
James M. Crawford

CHAPTER 19
The Pancreas 939
Ralph H. Hruban • Robb E. Wilentz

CHAPTER 20
The Kidney 955
Charles E. Alpers

CHAPTER 21
The Lower Urinary Tract and Male Genital System 1023
Jonathan I. Epstein

CHAPTER 22
The Female Genital Tract 1059
Christopher P. Crum

CHAPTER 23
The Breast 1119
Susan C. Lester

CHAPTER 24
The Endocrine System 1155
Anirban Maitra • Abul K. Abbas

CHAPTER 25
The Skin 1227
George F. Murphy • Klaus Sellheyer • Martin C. Mihm, Jr.

CHAPTER 26
Bones, Joints, and Soft Tissue Tumors 1273
Andrew E. Rosenberg

CHAPTER 27
Peripheral Nerve and Skeletal Muscle 1325
Douglas C. Anthony • Matthew P. Frosch • Umberto De Girolami

CHAPTER 28
The Central Nervous System 1347
Matthew P. Frosch • Douglas C. Anthony • Umberto De Girolami

CHAPTER 29
The Eye 1421
Robert Folberg

Index 1449

UNIT I

General Pathology

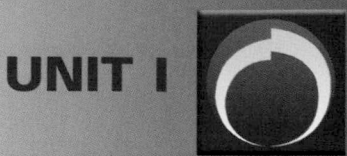

CHAPTER 1

Cellular Adaptations, Cell Injury, and Cell Death

INTRODUCTION TO PATHOLOGY

OVERVIEW: CELLULAR RESPONSES TO STRESS AND NOXIOUS STIMULI

CELLULAR ADAPTATIONS OF GROWTH AND DIFFERENTIATION

Hyperplasia

Physiologic Hyperplasia

Pathologic Hyperplasia

Hypertrophy

Atrophy

Metaplasia

OVERVIEW OF CELL INJURY AND CELL DEATH

CAUSES OF CELL INJURY

MECHANISMS OF CELL INJURY

Depletion of ATP

Mitochondrial Damage

Influx of Intracellular Calcium and Loss of Calcium Homeostasis

Accumulation of Oxygen-Derived Free Radicals (Oxidative Stress)

Defects in Membrane Permeability

REVERSIBLE AND IRREVERSIBLE CELL INJURY

MORPHOLOGY OF CELL INJURY AND NECROSIS

Reversible Injury

Necrosis

EXAMPLES OF CELL INJURY AND NECROSIS

Ischemic and Hypoxic Injury

Ischemia–Reperfusion Injury

Chemical Injury

APOPTOSIS

Causes of Apoptosis

Apoptosis in Physiologic Situations

Apoptosis in Pathologic Conditions

Biochemical Features of Apoptosis

Mechanisms of Apoptosis

Examples of Apoptosis

SUBCELLULAR RESPONSES TO INJURY

Lysosomal Catabolism

Induction (Hypertrophy) of Smooth Endoplasmic Reticulum

Mitochondrial Alterations

Cytoskeletal Abnormalities

INTRACELLULAR ACCUMULATIONS

Lipids

Steatosis (Fatty Change)

Cholesterol and Cholesterol Esters

Proteins

Hyaline Change

Glycogen

Pigments

PATHOLOGIC CALCIFICATION

Dystrophic Calcification

Metastatic Calcification

CELLULAR AGING

Introduction to Pathology

Pathology is literally the study *(logos)* of suffering *(pathos)*. More specifically, it is a bridging discipline involving both basic science and clinical practice and is devoted to the study of the structural and functional changes in cells, tissues, and organs that underlie disease. By the use of molecular, microbiologic, immunologic, and morphologic techniques, pathology attempts to explain the whys and wherefores of the signs and symptoms manifested by patients while providing a sound foundation for rational clinical care and therapy.

Traditionally, the study of pathology is divided into general pathology and special, or systemic, pathology. The former is concerned with the basic reactions of cells and tissues to abnormal stimuli that underlie all diseases. The latter examines the specific responses of specialized organs and tissues to more or less well-defined stimuli. In this book, we first cover the principles of general pathology and then proceed to specific disease processes as they affect particular organs or systems.

The four aspects of a disease process that form the core of pathology are its cause *(etiology)*, the mechanisms of its development *(pathogenesis)*, the structural alterations induced in the cells and organs of the body *(morphologic changes)*, and the functional consequences of the morphologic changes *(clinical significance)*.

Etiology or Cause. The concept that certain abnormal symptoms or diseases are "caused" is as ancient as recorded history. For the Arcadians (2500 BC), if someone became ill, it was the patient's own fault (for having sinned) or the makings of outside agents, such as bad smells, cold, evil spirits, or gods.[1] In modern terms, there are two major classes of etiologic factors: intrinsic or genetic, and acquired (e.g., infectious, nutritional, chemical, physical). The concept, however, of one etiologic agent for one disease — developed from the study of infections or single-gene disorders — is no longer sufficient. Genetic factors are clearly involved in some of the common environmentally induced maladies, such as atherosclerosis and cancer, and the environment may also have profound influences on certain genetic diseases. Knowledge or discovery of the primary cause remains the backbone on which a diagnosis can be made, a disease understood, or a treatment developed.

Pathogenesis. Pathogenesis refers to the sequence of events in the response of cells or tissues to the etiologic agent, from the initial stimulus to the ultimate expression of the disease. The study of pathogenesis remains one of the main domains of pathology. Even when the initial infectious or molecular cause is known, it is many steps removed from the expression of the disease. For example, to understand cystic fibrosis is to know not only the defective gene and gene product, but also the biochemical, immunologic, and morphologic events leading to the formation of cysts and fibrosis in the lung, pancreas, and other organs. Indeed, as we shall see throughout the book, the molecular revolution has already identified mutant genes underlying a great number of diseases, and the entire human genome has been mapped. Nevertheless, the functions of the encoded proteins and how mutations induce disease are often still obscure. Because of technologic advances, it is becoming increasingly feasible to link specific molecular abnormalities to disease manifestations and to use this knowledge to design new therapeutic approaches. For these reasons, the study of pathogenesis has never been more exciting scientifically or more relevant to medicine.

Morphologic Changes. The morphologic changes refer to the structural alterations in cells or tissues that are either characteristic of the disease or diagnostic of the etiologic process. The practice of diagnostic pathology is devoted to identifying the nature and progression of disease by studying morphologic changes in tissues and chemical alterations in patients. More recently, the limitations of morphology for diagnosing diseases have become increasingly evident, and the field of diagnostic pathology has expanded to encompass molecular biologic and immunologic approaches for analyzing disease states. Nowhere is this more striking than in the study of tumors — breast cancers and tumors of lymphocytes that look morphologically identical may have widely different courses, therapeutic responses, and prognosis. Molecular analysis by techniques such as DNA microarrays has begun to reveal genetic differences that bear on the behavior of the tumors. Increasingly, such techniques are being used to extend and even supplant traditional morphologic methods.

Functional Derangements and Clinical Manifestations. The nature of the morphologic changes and their distribution in different organs or tissues influence normal function and determine the clinical features (symptoms and signs), course, and prognosis of the disease.

Virtually all forms of organ injury start with molecular or structural alterations in cells, a concept first put forth in the nineteenth century by Rudolf Virchow, known as the father of modern pathology. We therefore begin our consideration of pathology with the study of the origins, molecular mechanisms, and structural changes of cell injury. Yet different cells in tissues constantly interact with each other, and an elaborate system of *extracellular matrix* is necessary for the integrity of organs. Cell–cell and cell–matrix interactions contribute significantly to the response to injury, leading collectively to *tissue and organ injury*, which are as important as cell injury in defining the morphologic and clinical patterns of disease.

Overview: Cellular Responses to Stress and Noxious Stimuli

The normal cell is confined to a fairly narrow range of function and structure by its genetic programs of metabolism, differentiation, and specialization; by constraints of neighboring cells; and by the availability of metabolic substrates. It is nevertheless able to handle normal physiologic demands, maintaining a steady state called *homeostasis*. More severe physiologic stresses and some pathologic stimuli may bring about a number of physiologic and morphologic *cellular adaptations*, during which new but altered steady states are achieved, preserving the viability of the cell and modulating its function as it responds to such stimuli (Fig. 1–1 and Table 1–1). The adaptive response may consist of an increase in the number of cells, called *hyperplasia*, or an increase in the sizes of individual cells, called *hypertrophy*. Conversely, *atrophy* is an adaptive response in which there is a decrease in the size and function of cells.

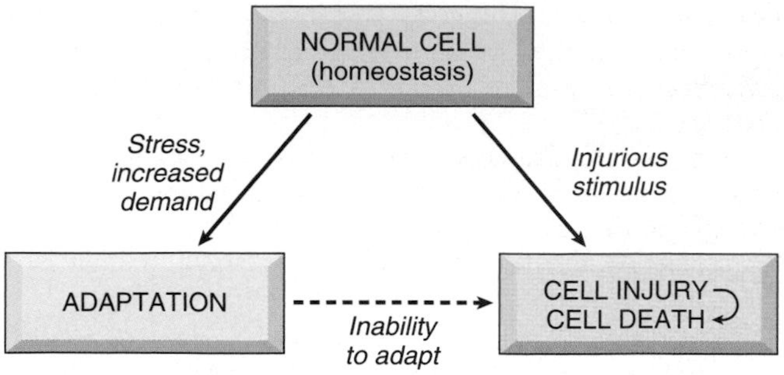

FIGURE 1–1 Stages in the cellular response to stress and injurious stimuli.

If the limits of adaptive response to a stimulus are exceeded, or in certain instances when the cell is exposed to an injurious agent or stress, a sequence of events follows that is loosely termed *cell injury*. Cell injury is *reversible* up to a certain point, but if the stimulus persists or is severe enough from the beginning, the cell reaches a "point of no return" and suffers *irreversible* cell injury and ultimately *cell death*. *Adaptation*, *reversible injury*, and *cell death* can be considered stages of progressive impairment of the cell's normal function and structure (see Fig. 1–1). For instance, in response to increased hemodynamic loads, the heart muscle first becomes enlarged, a form of adaptation. If the blood supply to the myocardium is insufficient to cope with the demand, the muscle becomes reversibly injured and finally undergoes cell death (Fig. 1–2).

Cell death, the ultimate result of cell injury, is one of the most crucial events in the evolution of disease of any tissue or organ. It results from diverse causes, including ischemia (lack of blood flow), infection, toxins, and immune reactions. In addition, cell death is a normal and essential part of embryogenesis, the development of organs, and the maintenance of homeostasis, and is the aim of cancer therapy. There are two principal patterns of cell death, necrosis and apoptosis. *Necrosis* is the type of cell death that occurs after such abnormal stresses as ischemia and chemical injury, and it is always pathologic. *Apoptosis* occurs when a cell dies through activation of an internally controlled suicide program. It is designed to eliminate unwanted cells during embryogenesis and in various physiologic processes, such as involution of hormone-responsive tissues upon withdrawal of the hormone. It also occurs in certain pathologic conditions, when cells are damaged beyond repair, and especially if the damage affects the cell's nuclear DNA. We will return to a detailed discussion of these pathways of cell death later in the chapter.

Stresses of different types may induce changes in cells and tissues other than adaptations, cell injury, and death (see Table 1–1). Cells that are exposed to sublethal or chronic stimuli may not be damaged but may show a variety of *subcellular alterations*. Metabolic derangements in cells may be associated with *intracellular accumulations* of a number of substances, including proteins, lipids, and carbohydrates. Calcium is often deposited at sites of cell death, resulting in *pathologic calcification*. Finally, *cell aging* is also accompanied by characteristic morphologic and functional changes.

In this chapter, we discuss first how cells adapt to stresses, and then the causes, mechanisms, and consequences of the various forms of acute cell damage, including cell injury and cell death. We conclude with subcellular alterations induced by sublethal stimuli, intracellular accumulations, pathologic calcification, and cell aging.

Cellular Adaptations of Growth and Differentiation

Cells respond to increased demand and external stimulation by *hyperplasia* or *hypertrophy*, and they respond to reduced supply of nutrients and growth factors by *atrophy*. In some situations, cells change from one type to another, a process called *metaplasia*. There are numerous molecular mechanisms for cellular adaptations. Some adaptations are induced by direct stimulation of cells by factors produced by the responding cells themselves or by other cells in the environment. Others are due to activation of various cell surface receptors and downstream signaling pathways. Adaptations may be associated with the induction of new protein synthesis by the target cells, as in the response of muscle cells to increased physical demand, and the induction of cellular proliferation, as in responses of the endometrium to estrogens. Adaptations can also involve a switch by cells from producing one type of proteins to another or markedly overproducing one protein; such is the case in cells producing various types of collagens and extracellular matrix proteins in chronic inflammation and fibrosis (Chapters 2 and 3).

TABLE 1–1 Cellular Responses to Injury

Nature and Severity of Injurious Stimulus	Cellular Response
Altered physiologic stimuli: • Increased demand, increased trophic stimulation (e.g. growth factors, hormones) • Decreased nutrients, stimulation • Chronic irritation (chemical or physical)	**Cellular adaptations:** • Hyperplasia, hypertrophy • Atrophy • Metaplasia
Reduced oxygen supply; chemical injury; microbial infection • Acute and self-limited • Progessive and severe (including DNA damage) • Mild chronic injury	**Cell injury:** • Acute reversible injury • Irreversible injury → cell death Necrosis Apoptosis • Subcellular alterations in various organelles
Metabolic alterations, genetic or acquired	**Intracellular accumulations; calcifications**
Prolonged life span with cumulative sublethal injury	**Cellular aging**

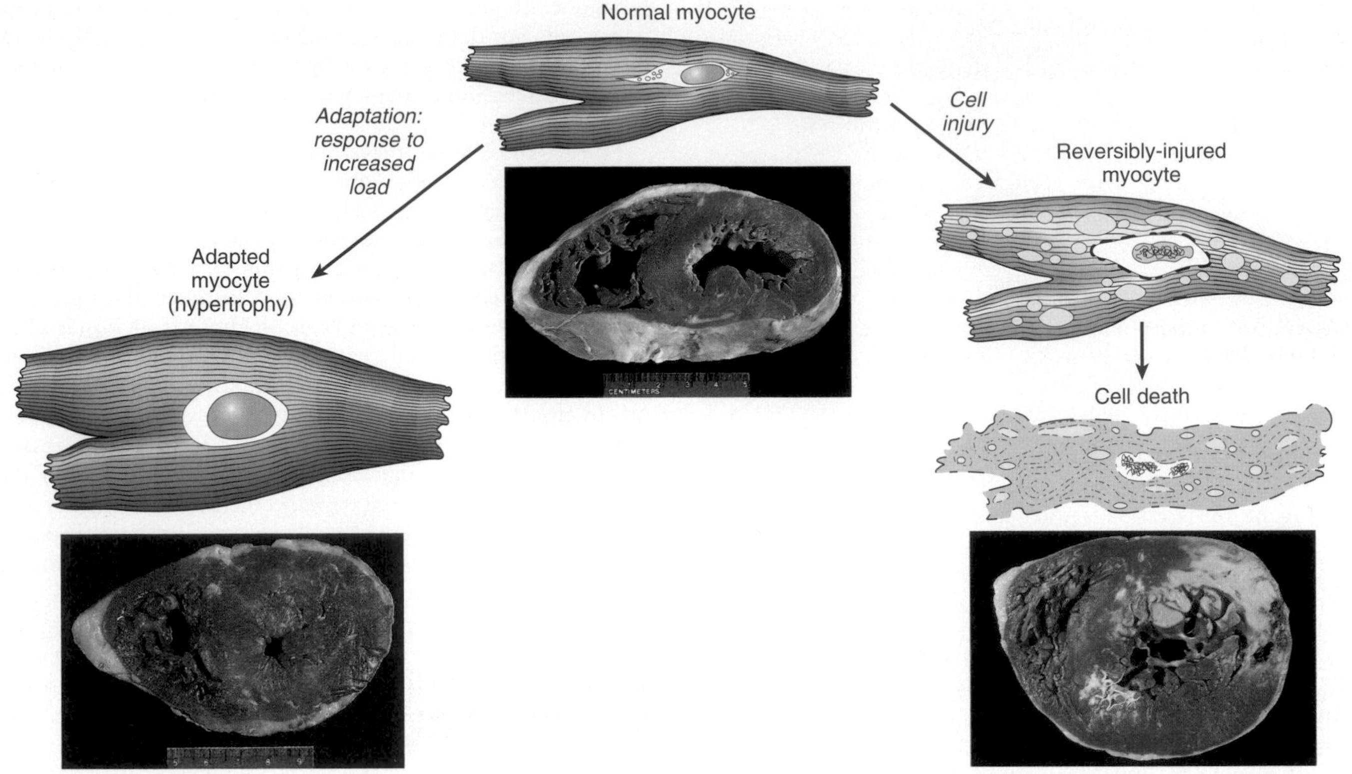

FIGURE 1–2 The relationships between normal, adapted, reversibly injured, and dead myocardial cells. The cellular adaptation depicted here is hypertrophy, and the type of cell death is ischemic necrosis. In reversibly injured myocardium, generally effects are only functional, without any readily apparent gross or even microscopic changes. In the example of myocardial hypertrophy, the left ventricular wall is more than 2 cm in thickness (normal is 1 to 1.5 cm). In the specimen showing necrosis, the transmural light area in the posterolateral left ventricle represents an acute myocardial infarction. All three transverse sections have been stained with triphenyltetrazolium chloride, an enzyme substrate that colors viable myocardium magenta. Failure to stain is due to enzyme leakage after cell death.

HYPERPLASIA

Hyperplasia is an increase in the number of cells in an organ or tissue, usually resulting in increased volume of the organ or tissue. Although hyperplasia and hypertrophy are two distinct processes, frequently both occur together, and they may be triggered by the same external stimulus. For instance, hormone-induced growth in the uterus involves both increased numbers of smooth muscle and epithelial cells and the enlargement of these cells. Hyperplasia takes place if the cellular population is capable of synthesizing DNA, thus permitting mitotic division; by contrast, hypertrophy involves cell enlargement without cell division. Hyperplasia can be physiologic or pathologic.

Physiologic Hyperplasia

Physiologic hyperplasia can be divided into: (1) *hormonal hyperplasia*, which increases the functional capacity of a tissue when needed, and (2) *compensatory hyperplasia*, which increases tissue mass after damage or partial resection. Hormonal hyperplasia is best exemplified by the proliferation of the glandular epithelium of the female breast at puberty and during pregnancy and the physiologic hyperplasia that occurs in the pregnant uterus. The classical illustration of compensatory hyperplasia comes from the myth of Prometheus, which shows that the ancient Greeks recognized the capacity of the liver to regenerate. As punishment for having stolen the secret of fire from the gods, Prometheus was chained to a mountain, and his liver was devoured daily by a vulture, only to regenerate anew every night.[1] The experimental model of partial hepatectomy has been especially useful in examining the mechanisms that stimulate proliferation of residual liver cells and regeneration of the liver (Chapter 3). Similar mechanisms are likely involved in other situations when remaining tissue grows to make up for partial tissue loss (e.g., after unilateral nephrectomy, when the remaining kidney undergoes compensatory hyperplasia).

Mechanisms of Hyperplasia. Hyperplasia is generally caused by increased local production of growth factors, increased levels of growth factor receptors on the responding cells, or activation of particular intracellular signaling pathways. All these changes lead to production of transcription factors that turn on many cellular genes, including genes encoding growth factors, receptors for growth factors, and cell cycle regulators, and the net result is cellular proliferation.[2] In hormonal hyperplasia, the hormones may themselves act as growth factors and trigger the transcription of various cellular genes. The source of growth factors in compensatory hyperplasia and the stimuli for the production of these growth factors are less well defined. The increase in tissue mass after some types of cell loss is achieved not only by proliferation of the remaining cells but also by the development of new cells from *stem cells*.[3,4] For instance, in the liver, intrahepatic stem cells do not play a major role in the hyperplasia that occurs after hepatectomy but they may participate in regeneration after certain forms of liver injury, such as chronic hepatitis, in which the proliferative capacity of hepatocytes is compromised. Recent data from clinical observations and experimental studies have demonstrated that the bone marrow contains stem cells that may be able to give rise to many types of differentiated, specialized cell types, including some liver cells.[5] These observations highlight the plasticity of adult stem cells and raise the potential of repopulating damaged tissues with bone marrow-derived stem cells. We will return to a discussion of stem cells, their biology, and their clinical relevance in Chapter 3.

Pathologic Hyperplasia

Most forms of pathologic hyperplasia are caused by excessive hormonal stimulation or growth factors acting on target cells. Endometrial hyperplasia is an example of abnormal hormone-induced hyperplasia. After a normal menstrual period, there is a rapid burst of proliferative activity that is stimulated by pituitary hormones and ovarian estrogen. It is brought to a halt by the rising levels of progesterone, usually about 10 to 14 days before the anticipated menstrual period. In some instances, however, the balance between estrogen and progesterone is disturbed. This results in absolute or relative increases in the amount of estrogen, with consequent hyperplasia of the endometrial glands. This form of hyperplasia is a common cause of abnormal menstrual bleeding. Benign prostatic hyperplasia is another common example of pathologic hyperplasia induced by responses to hormones, in this case, androgens. Although these forms of hyperplasia are abnormal, the process remains controlled, because the hyperplasia regresses if the hormonal stimulation is eliminated. As is discussed in Chapter 7, it is this response to normal regulatory control mechanisms that distinguishes benign pathologic hyperplasias from cancer, in which the growth control mechanisms become defective. *Pathologic hyperplasia, however, constitutes a fertile soil in which cancerous proliferation may eventually arise.* Thus, patients with hyperplasia of the endometrium are at increased risk for developing endometrial cancer (Chapter 22).

Hyperplasia is also an important response of connective tissue cells in wound healing, in which proliferating fibroblasts and blood vessels aid in repair (Chapter 3). Under these circumstances, growth factors are responsible for the hyperplasia. Stimulation by growth factors is also involved in the hyperplasia that is associated with certain *viral infections*, such as papillomaviruses, which cause skin warts and a number of mucosal lesions composed of masses of hyperplastic epithelium.

HYPERTROPHY

Hypertrophy refers to an increase in the size of cells, resulting in an increase in the size of the organ. Thus, the hypertrophied organ has no new cells, just larger cells. The increased size of the cells is due not to cellular swelling but to the synthesis of more structural components. As mentioned above, cells capable of division may respond to stress by undergoing both hyperplasia and hypertrophy, whereas in *nondividing cells* (e.g., myocardial fibers), hypertrophy occurs. Nuclei in hypertrophied cells may have a higher DNA content than in normal cells, probably because the cells arrest in the cell cycle without undergoing mitosis.

Hypertrophy can be *physiologic* or *pathologic* and is caused by increased functional demand or by specific hormonal stimulation. The striated muscle cells in both the heart and the skeletal muscles are capable of tremendous hypertrophy, perhaps because they cannot adequately adapt to increased metabolic demands by mitotic division and production of more cells to share the work. The most common stimulus for hypertrophy of muscle is increased workload. For example, the bulging muscles of bodybuilders engaged in "pumping iron" result from an increase in size of the individual muscle fibers in response to increased demand. The workload is thus shared by a greater mass of cellular components, and each muscle fiber is spared excess work and so escapes injury. The enlarged muscle cell achieves a new equilibrium, permitting it to function at a higher level of activity. In the heart, the stimulus for hypertrophy is usually *chronic hemodynamic overload*, resulting from either hypertension or faulty valves. Synthesis of more proteins and filaments occurs, achieving a balance between the demand and the cell's functional capacity. The greater number of myofilaments per cell permits an increased workload with a level of metabolic activity per unit volume of cell not different from that borne by the normal cell.

The massive physiologic growth of the uterus during pregnancy is a good example of hormone-induced increase in the size of an organ that results from both hypertrophy and hyperplasia (Fig. 1–3*A*). The cellular hypertrophy is stimulated by estrogenic hormones acting on smooth muscle estrogen receptors, eventually resulting in increased synthesis of smooth muscle proteins and an increase in cell size (Fig. 1–3*B*). Similarly, prolactin and estrogen cause hypertrophy of the breasts during lactation. These are examples of physiologic hypertrophy induced by hormonal stimulation.

Although the traditional view of cardiac and skeletal muscle is that these tissues are incapable of proliferation and, therefore, their enlargement is entirely a result of hypertrophy, recent data suggest that even these cell types are capable of limited proliferation as well as repopulation from precursors.[6] This view emphasizes the concept, mentioned earlier, that hyperplasia and hypertrophy often occur concomitantly during the responses of tissues and organs to increased stress and cell loss.

Mechanisms of Hypertrophy. Much of our understanding of hypertrophy is based on studies of the heart. The mechanisms of cardiac muscle hypertrophy involve many signal transduction pathways, leading to the induction of a number of genes, which in turn stimulate synthesis of numerous cellular proteins (Fig. 1–4).[7,8] The genes that are induced during hypertrophy include those encoding transcription factors (such as c-*fos*, c-*jun*); growth factors (TGF-β, insulin-like growth factor-1 [IGF-1], fibroblast growth factor); and vasoactive agents (α-adrenergic agonists, endothelin-1, and angiotensin II). These factors are discussed in detail in Chapter 3. There may also be a switch of contractile proteins from adult to fetal or neonatal forms. For example, during muscle hypertrophy, the α-myosin heavy chain is replaced by the β form of the myosin heavy chain, which leads to

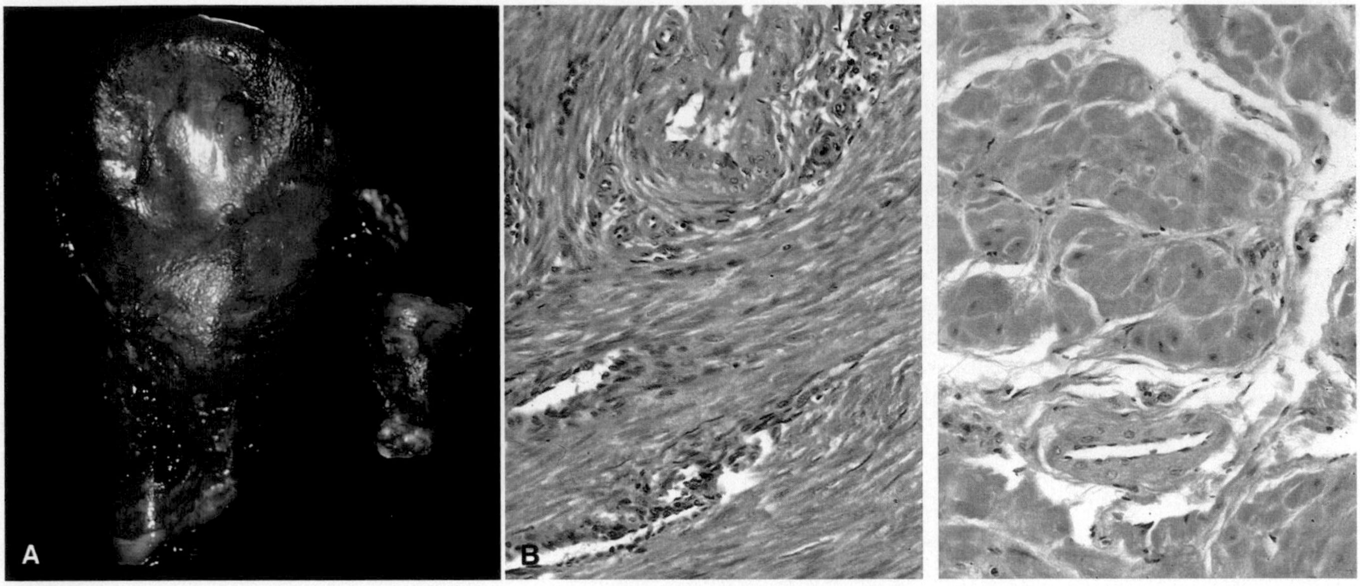

FIGURE 1–3 Physiologic hypertrophy of the uterus during pregnancy. *A,* Gross appearance of a normal uterus *(right)* and a gravid uterus (removed for postpartum bleeding) *(left)*. *B,* Small spindle-shaped uterine smooth muscle cells from a normal uterus *(left)* compared with large plump cells in gravid uterus *(right)*.

decreased myosin adenosine triphosphatase (ATPase) activity and a slower, more energetically economical contraction. In addition, some genes that are expressed only during early development are re-expressed in hypertrophic cells, and the products of these genes participate in the cellular response to stress. For example, in the embryonic heart, the gene for atrial natriuretic factor (ANF) is expressed in both the atrium and the ventricle. After birth, ventricular expression of the gene is down-regulated. Cardiac hypertrophy, however, is associated with reinduction of ANF gene expression.[9] ANF is a peptide hormone that causes salt secretion by the kidney, decreases blood volume and pressure, and therefore serves to reduce hemodynamic load.

What are the triggers for hypertrophy and for these changes in gene expression? In the heart, there are at least two groups of signals: *mechanical triggers*, such as stretch, and *trophic triggers*, such as polypeptide growth factors (IGF-1) and vasoactive agents (angiotensin II, α-adrenergic agonists). Current models suggest that growth factors or vasoactive agents produced by cardiac nonmuscle cells or by myocytes themselves in response to hemodynamic stress stimulate the expression of various genes, leading to myocyte hypertrophy. The size of

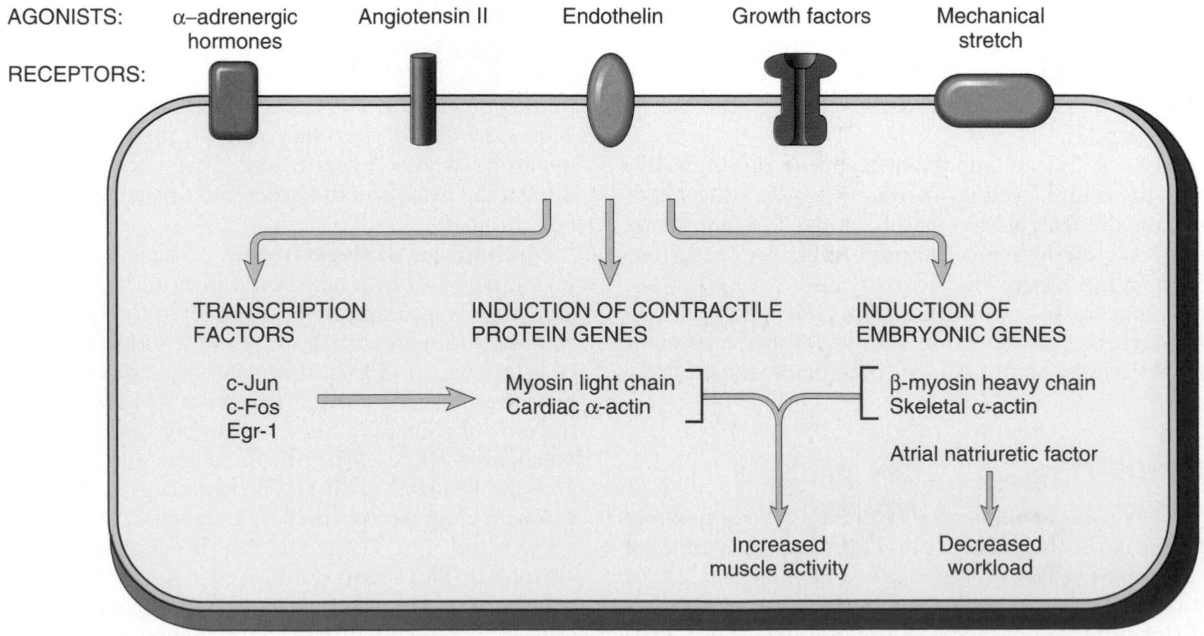

FIGURE 1–4 Changes in the expression of selected genes and proteins during myocardial hypertrophy.

cells is regulated by nutrients and environmental cues and involves several signal transduction pathways that are being unraveled.[10]

Whatever the exact mechanism of cardiac hypertrophy, it eventually reaches a limit beyond which enlargement of muscle mass is no longer able to compensate for the increased burden, and cardiac failure ensues. At this stage, a number of *degenerative* changes occur in the myocardial fibers, of which the most important are lysis and loss of myofibrillar contractile elements. Myocyte death can occur by either apoptosis or necrosis.[11] The limiting factors for continued hypertrophy and the causes of the cardiac dysfunction are poorly understood; they may be due to limitation of the vascular supply to the enlarged fibers, diminished oxidative capabilities of mitochondria, alterations in protein synthesis and degradation, or cytoskeletal alterations.

ATROPHY

Shrinkage in the size of the cell by loss of cell substance is known as atrophy. It represents a form of adaptive response and may culminate in cell death. When a sufficient number of cells are involved, the entire tissue or organ diminishes in size, or becomes atrophic. Atrophy can be physiologic or pathologic. *Physiologic atrophy* is common during early development. Some embryonic structures, such as the notochord and thyroglossal duct, undergo atrophy during fetal development. The uterus decreases in size shortly after parturition, and this is a form of physiologic atrophy. *Pathologic atrophy* depends on the underlying cause and can be local or generalized. The common causes of atrophy are the following:

- *Decreased workload (atrophy of disuse).* When a broken limb is immobilized in a plaster cast or when a patient is restricted to complete bed rest, skeletal muscle atrophy rapidly ensues. The initial rapid decrease in cell size is reversible once activity is resumed. With more prolonged disuse, skeletal muscle fibers decrease in number as well as in size; this atrophy can be accompanied by increased bone resorption, leading to osteoporosis of disuse.
- *Loss of innervation (denervation atrophy).* Normal function of skeletal muscle is dependent on its nerve supply. Damage to the nerves leads to rapid atrophy of the muscle fibers supplied by those nerves (Chapter 27).
- *Diminished blood supply.* A decrease in blood supply (ischemia) to a tissue as a result of arterial occlusive disease results in atrophy of tissue owing to progressive cell loss. In late adult life, the brain undergoes progressive atrophy, presumably as atherosclerosis narrows its blood supply (Fig. 1–5).
- *Inadequate nutrition.* Profound protein-calorie malnutrition (marasmus) is associated with the use of skeletal muscle as a source of energy after other reserves such as adipose stores have been depleted. This results in marked muscle wasting *(cachexia)*. Cachexia is also seen in patients with chronic inflammatory diseases and cancer. In the former, chronic overproduction of the inflammatory cytokine tumor necrosis factor (TNF) is thought to be responsible for appetite suppression and muscle atrophy.
- *Loss of endocrine stimulation.* Many endocrine glands, the breast, and the reproductive organs are dependent on endocrine stimulation for normal metabolism and function. The loss of estrogen stimulation after menopause results in physiologic atrophy of the endometrium, vaginal epithelium, and breast.
- *Aging (senile atrophy).* The aging process is associated with cell loss, typically seen in tissues containing permanent cells, particularly the brain and heart.
- *Pressure.* Tissue compression for any length of time can cause atrophy. An enlarging benign tumor can cause atrophy in the surrounding compressed tissues. Atrophy in this setting is probably the result of ischemic changes caused by compromise of the blood supply to those tissues by the expanding mass.

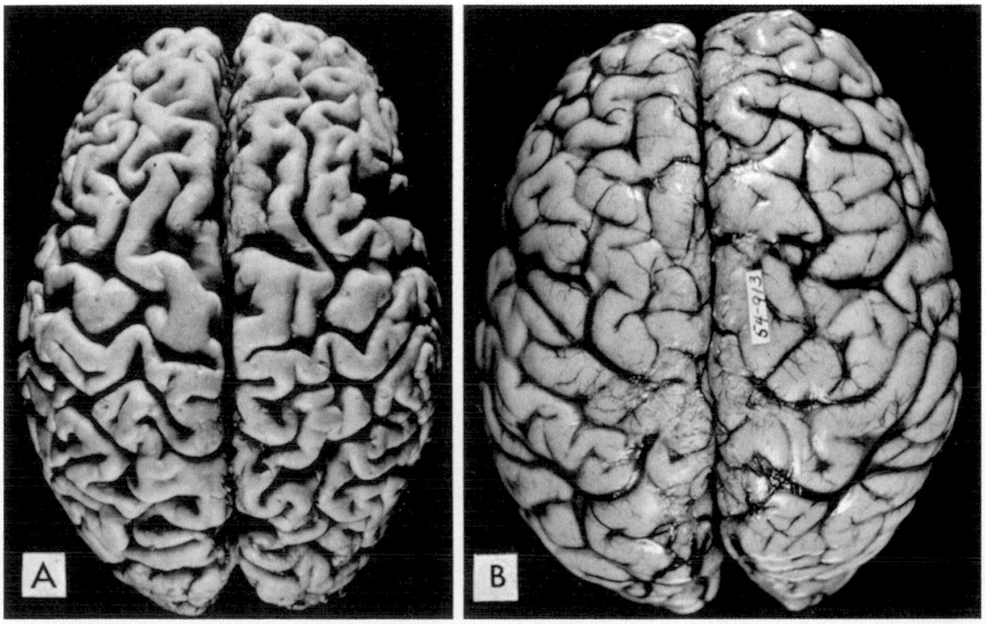

FIGURE 1–5 *A,* Atrophy of the brain in an 82-year-old male with atherosclerotic disease. Atrophy of the brain is due to aging and reduced blood supply. The meninges have been stripped. *B,* Normal brain of a 36-year-old male. Note that loss of brain substance narrows the gyri and widens the sulci.

The fundamental cellular changes associated with atrophy are identical in all of these settings, representing a retreat by the cells to a smaller size at which survival is still possible. Atrophy results from a reduction in the structural components of the cell. In atrophic muscle, the cells contain fewer mitochondria and myofilaments and a reduced amount of endoplasmic reticulum. By bringing into balance cell volume and lower levels of blood supply, nutrition, or trophic stimulation, a new equilibrium is achieved. *Although atrophic cells may have diminished function, they are not dead.* However, atrophy may progress to the point at which cells are injured and die. In ischemic tissues, if the blood supply is inadequate even to maintain the life of shrunken cells, injury and cell death may supervene. Furthermore, apoptosis may be induced by the same signals that cause atrophy and thus may contribute to loss of organ mass. For example, apoptosis contributes to the regression of endocrine organs after hormone withdrawal.

Mechanisms of Atrophy. The biochemical mechanisms responsible for atrophy are incompletely understood but are likely to affect the balance between protein synthesis and degradation. Increased protein degradation probably plays a key role in atrophy. Mammalian cells contain multiple proteolytic systems that serve distinct functions. *Lysosomes* contain acid hydrolases (e.g., cathepsins) and other enzymes that degrade endocytosed proteins from the extracellular environment and the cell surface as well as some cellular components. The *ubiquitin-proteasome pathway* is responsible for the degradation of many cytosolic and nuclear proteins.[12] Proteins to be degraded by this process are first conjugated to ubiquitin and then degraded within a large cytoplasmic proteolytic organelle called the *proteasome.* This pathway is thought to be responsible for the accelerated proteolysis seen in a variety of catabolic conditions, including cancer cachexia. Hormones, particularly glucocorticoids and thyroid hormone, stimulate proteasome-mediated protein degradation; insulin opposes these actions. Additionally, cytokines, such as tumor necrosis factor (TNF), are capable of increasing muscle proteolysis by way of this mechanism.

In many situations, atrophy is also accompanied by marked increases in the number of *autophagic vacuoles.* These are membrane-bound vacuoles within the cell that contain fragments of cell components (e.g., mitochondria, endoplasmic reticulum) that are destined for destruction and into which the lysosomes discharge their hydrolytic contents. The cellular components are then digested. Some of the cell debris within the autophagic vacuole may resist digestion and persist as membrane-bound residual bodies that may remain as a sarcophagus in the cytoplasm. An example of such *residual bodies* is the *lipofuscin granules,* discussed later in the chapter. When present in sufficient amounts, they impart a brown discoloration to the tissue *(brown atrophy).*

METAPLASIA

Metaplasia is a reversible change in which one adult cell type (epithelial or mesenchymal) is replaced by another adult cell type.[13] It may represent an adaptive substitution of cells that are sensitive to stress by cell types better able to withstand the adverse environment.

The most common epithelial metaplasia is *columnar* to *squamous* (Fig. 1–6*A*), as occurs in the respiratory tract in response to chronic irritation. In the habitual cigarette smoker, the normal ciliated columnar epithelial cells of the trachea and bronchi are often replaced focally or widely by stratified squamous epithelial cells. Stones in the excretory ducts of the salivary glands, pancreas, or bile ducts may cause replacement of the normal secretory columnar epithelium by nonfunctioning stratified squamous epithelium. A deficiency of vitamin A (retinoic acid) induces squamous metaplasia in the respiratory epithelium, and vitamin A excess suppresses keratinization (Chapter 9). In all these instances, the more rugged stratified squamous epithelium is able to survive under circumstances in which the more fragile specialized columnar epithelium most likely would have succumbed. Although the metaplastic squamous cells in the respiratory tract, for example, are capable of surviving, an important protective mechanism—mucus secretion—is lost. Thus, epithelial metaplasia is a two-edged sword and, in most circumstances, represents an undesirable change. Moreover, *the influences that predispose to metaplasia, if persistent, may induce malignant transformation in metaplastic epithelium.* Thus, the common form of cancer in the respiratory tract is composed of squamous cells, which arise in areas of metaplasia of the normal columnar epithelium into squamous epithelium.

Metaplasia from squamous to columnar type may also occur, as in *Barrett esophagus,* in which the esophageal squamous epithelium is replaced by intestinal-like columnar cells under the influence of refluxed gastric acid (Fig. 1–6*B*). Cancers may arise in these areas, and these are typically glandular (adeno)carcinomas (Chapter 17).

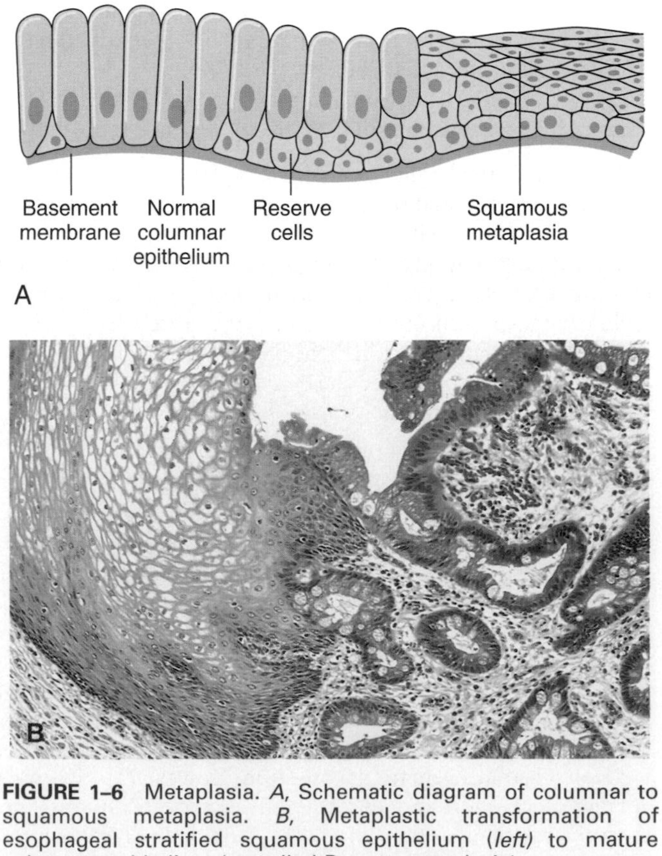

FIGURE 1–6 Metaplasia. *A,* Schematic diagram of columnar to squamous metaplasia. *B,* Metaplastic transformation of esophageal stratified squamous epithelium *(left)* to mature columnar epithelium (so-called Barrett metaplasia).

Connective tissue metaplasia is the formation of cartilage, bone, or adipose tissue (mesenchymal tissues) in tissues that normally do not contain these elements. For example, bone formation in muscle, designated *myositis ossificans*, occasionally occurs after bone fracture. This type of metaplasia is less clearly seen as an adaptive response.

Mechanisms of Metaplasia. Metaplasia does not result from a change in the phenotype of a differentiated cell type; instead it is the result of a reprogramming of stem cells that are known to exist in normal tissues, or of undifferentiated mesenchymal cells present in connective tissue. In a metaplastic change, these precursor cells differentiate along a new pathway. The differentiation of stem cells to a particular lineage is brought about by signals generated by cytokines, growth factors, and extracellular matrix components in the cell's environment. Tissue-specific and differentiation genes are involved in the process, and an increasing number of these are being identified.[14] For example, bone morphogenetic proteins, members of the TGF-β superfamily, induce chondrogenic or osteogenic expression in stem cells while suppressing differentiation into muscle or fat.[15] These growth factors, acting as external triggers, then induce specific transcription factors that lead the cascade of phenotype-specific genes toward a fully differentiated cell. How these normal pathways run amok to cause metaplasia is unclear in most instances. In the case of vitamin A deficiency or excess, it is known that retinoic acid regulates cell growth, differentiation, and tissue patterning and may thus influence the differentiation pathway of stem cells.[16] Certain *cytostatic* drugs cause a disruption of DNA methylation patterns and can transform mesenchymal cells from one type (fibroblast) to another (muscle, cartilage).

Overview of Cell Injury and Cell Death

As stated at the beginning of the chapter, cell injury results when cells are stressed so severely that they are no longer able to adapt or when cells are exposed to inherently damaging agents. Injury may progress through a reversible stage and culminate in cell death (Fig. 1–7). An overview of the morphologic changes in cell injury is shown in Figure 1–8. The biochemical alterations and the associated morphologic abnormalities are described later, under "Mechanisms of Cell Injury." These alterations may be divided into the following stages:

- *Reversible cell injury.* Initially, injury is manifested as functional and morphologic changes that are reversible if the damaging stimulus is removed. The hallmarks of reversible injury are reduced oxidative phosphorylation, adenosine triphosphate (ATP) depletion, and cellular swelling caused by changes in ion concentrations and water influx.
- *Irreversible injury and cell death.* With continuing damage, the injury becomes irreversible, at which time the cell cannot recover. Is there a critical biochemical event (the "lethal hit") responsible for the point of no return? There are no clear answers to this question. However, as discussed later, in ischemic tissues such as the myocardium, certain structural changes (e.g., amorphous densities in mitochondria, indicative of severe mitochondrial damage) and functional changes (e.g., loss of membrane permeability) are indicative of cells that have suffered irreversible injury.

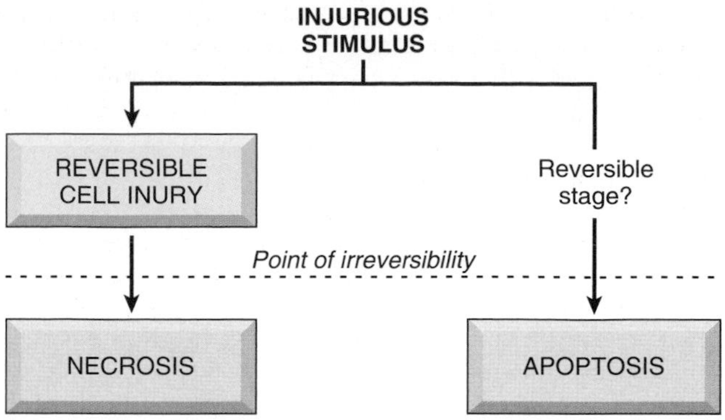

FIGURE 1–7 Stages in the evolution of cell injury and death.

Irreversibly injured cells invariably undergo morphologic changes that are recognized as cell death. There are two types of cell death, necrosis and apoptosis, which differ in their morphology, mechanisms, and roles in disease and physiology (Fig. 1–9 and Table 1–2). When damage to membranes is severe, lysosomal enzymes enter the cytoplasm and digest the cell, and cellular contents leak out, resulting in *necrosis.* Some noxious stimuli, especially those that damage DNA, induce another type of death, *apoptosis*, which is characterized by nuclear dissolution without complete loss of membrane integrity. *Whereas necrosis is always a pathologic process, apoptosis serves many normal functions and is not necessarily associated with cell injury.* Although we emphasize the distinctions between necrosis and apoptosis, there may be some overlaps and common mechanisms between these two pathways. In addition, at least some types of stimuli may induce either apoptosis or necrosis, depending on the intensity and duration of the stimulus, the rapidity of the death process, and the biochemical derangements induced in the injured cell. The mechanisms and significance of these two death pathways are discussed later in the chapter.

In the following sections, we will discuss the causes and mechanisms of cell injury. We first describe the sequence of events in cell injury and its common end point, necrosis, and discuss selected illustrative examples of cell injury and necrosis. We conclude with a discussion of the unique pattern of cell death represented by apoptosis.

Causes of Cell Injury

The causes of cell injury range from the external gross physical violence of an automobile accident to internal endogenous causes, such as a subtle genetic mutation causing lack of a vital enzyme that impairs normal metabolic function. Most injurious stimuli can be grouped into the following broad categories.

Oxygen Deprivation. *Hypoxia* is a deficiency of oxygen, which causes cell injury by reducing aerobic oxidative respiration. Hypoxia is an extremely important and common cause of cell injury and cell death. It should be distinguished from *ischemia*, which is a loss of blood supply from impeded arterial flow or reduced venous drainage in a tissue. Ischemia

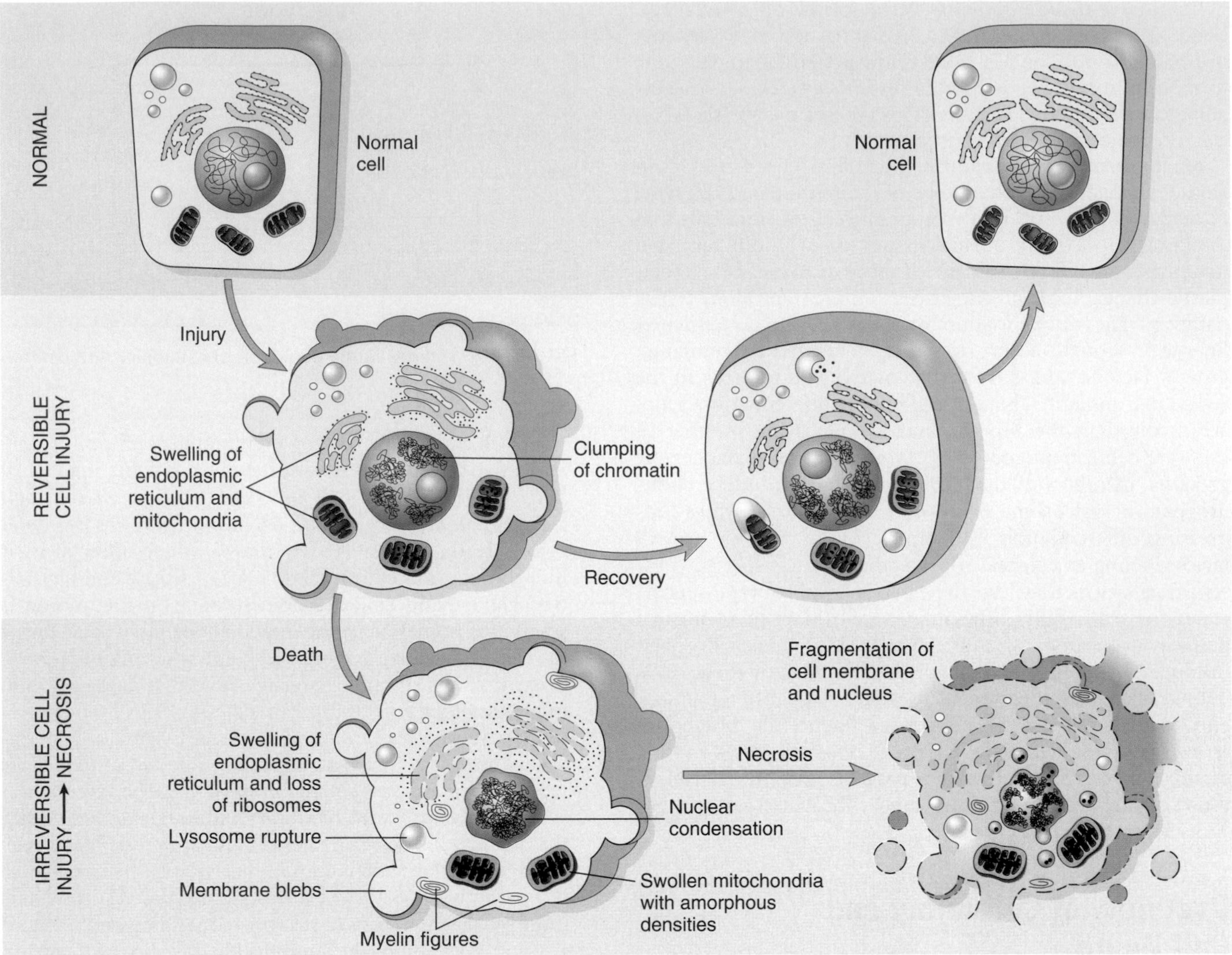

FIGURE 1–8 Schematic representation of a normal cell and the changes in reversible and irreversible cell injury. Depicted are morphologic changes, which are described in the following pages and shown in electron micrographs in Figure 1–17. Reversible injury is characterized by generalized swelling of the cell and its organelles; blebbing of the plasma membrane; detachment of ribosomes from the endoplasmic reticulum; and clumping of nuclear chromatin. Transition to irreversible injury is characterized by increasing swelling of the cell; swelling and disruption of lysosomes; presence of large amorphous densities in swollen mitochondria; disruption of cellular membranes; and profound nuclear changes. The latter include nuclear condensation (pyknosis), followed by fragmentation (karyorrhexis) and dissolution of the nucleus (karyolysis). Laminated structures (myelin figures) derived from damaged membranes of organelles and the plasma membrane first appear during the reversible stage and become more pronounced in irreversibly damaged cells. The mechanisms underlying these changes are discussed in the text that follows.

compromises the supply not only of oxygen, but also of metabolic substrates, including glucose (normally provided by flowing blood). Therefore, ischemic tissues are injured more rapidly and severely than are hypoxic tissues. One cause of hypoxia is inadequate oxygenation of the blood due to cardiorespiratory failure. Loss of the oxygen-carrying capacity of the blood, as in anemia or carbon monoxide poisoning (producing a stable carbon monoxyhemoglobin that blocks oxygen carriage), is a less frequent cause of oxygen deprivation that results in significant injury. Depending on the severity of the hypoxic state, cells may adapt, undergo injury, or die. For example, if the femoral artery is narrowed, the skeletal muscle cells of the leg may shrink in size (atrophy). This reduction in cell mass achieves a balance between metabolic needs and the available oxygen supply. More severe hypoxia induces injury and cell death.

Physical Agents. Physical agents capable of causing cell injury include mechanical trauma, extremes of temperature (burns and deep cold), sudden changes in atmospheric pressure, radiation, and electric shock (Chapter 9).

Chemical Agents and Drugs. The list of chemicals that may produce cell injury defies compilation. Simple chemicals such as glucose or salt in hypertonic concentrations may cause cell injury directly or by deranging electrolyte homeostasis of cells. Even oxygen, in high concentrations, is severely toxic. Trace amounts of agents known as *poisons*, such as arsenic, cyanide, or mercuric salts, may destroy sufficient numbers of cells within minutes to hours to cause death. Other substances,

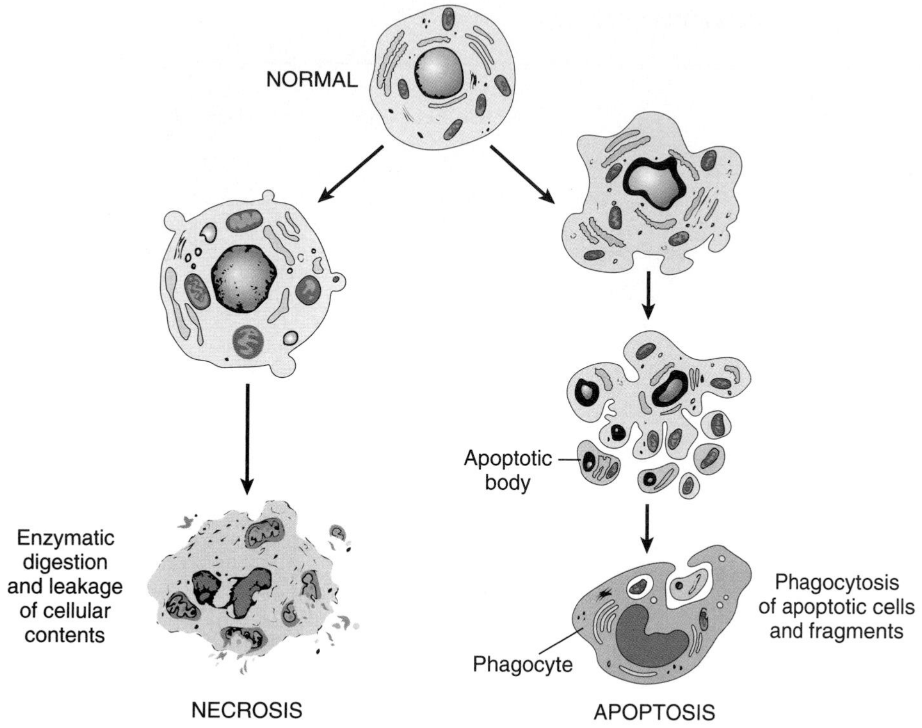

FIGURE 1–9 The sequential ultrastructural changes seen in necrosis *(left)* and apoptosis *(right)*. In apoptosis, the initial changes consist of nuclear chromatin condensation and fragmentation, followed by cytoplasmic budding and phagocytosis of the extruded apoptotic bodies. Signs of cytoplasmic blebs, and digestion and leakage of cellular components. (Adapted from Walker NI, et al: Patterns of cell death. Methods Archiv Exp Pathol 13:18–32, 1988. Reproduced with permission of S. Karger AG, Basel.)

TABLE 1–2 Features of Necrosis and Apoptosis

Feature	Necrosis	Apoptosis
Cell size	Enlarged (swelling)	Reduced (shrinkage)
Nucleus	Pyknosis → karyorrhexis → karyolysis	Fragmentation into nucleosome size fragments
Plasma membrane	Disrupted	Intact; altered structure, especially orientation of lipids
Cellular contents	Enzymatic digestion; may leak out of cell	Intact; may be released in apoptotic bodies
Adjacent inflammation	Frequent	No
Physiologic or pathologic role	Invariably pathologic (culmination of irreversible cell injury)	Often physiologic, means of eliminating unwanted cells; may be pathologic after some forms of cell injury, especially DNA damage

however, are our daily companions: environmental and air pollutants, insecticides, and herbicides; industrial and occupational hazards, such as carbon monoxide and asbestos; social stimuli, such as alcohol and narcotic drugs; and the ever-increasing variety of therapeutic drugs.

Infectious Agents. These agents range from the submicroscopic viruses to the large tapeworms. In between are the rickettsiae, bacteria, fungi, and higher forms of parasites. The ways by which this heterogeneous group of biologic agents cause injury are diverse and are discussed in Chapter 8.

Immunologic Reactions. Although the immune system serves an essential function in defense against infectious pathogens, immune reactions may, in fact, cause cell injury. The anaphylactic reaction to a foreign protein or a drug is a prime example, and reactions to endogenous self-antigens are responsible for a number of autoimmune diseases (Chapter 6).

Genetic Derangements. Genetic defects as causes of cell injury are of major interest to scientists and physicians today (Chapter 5). The genetic injury may result in a defect as severe as the congenital malformations associated with Down syndrome, caused by a chromosomal abnormality, or as subtle as the decreased life of red blood cells caused by a single amino acid substitution in hemoglobin S in sickle cell anemia. The many inborn errors of metabolism arising from enzymatic abnormalities, usually an enzyme lack, are excellent examples of cell damage due to subtle alterations at the level of DNA. Variations in the genetic makeup can also influence the susceptibility of cells to injury by chemicals and other environmental insults.

Nutritional Imbalances. Nutritional imbalances continue to be major causes of cell injury. Protein-calorie deficiencies cause an appalling number of deaths, chiefly among underprivileged populations. Deficiencies of specific vitamins are found throughout the world (Chapter 9). Nutritional problems can be self-imposed, as in anorexia nervosa or self-induced starvation. Ironically, nutritional excesses have also become important causes of cell injury. Excesses of lipids predispose to atherosclerosis, and obesity is a manifestation of the overloading of some cells in the body with fats. Atherosclerosis is virtually endemic in the United States, and obesity is rampant. In addition to the problems of undernutrition and overnutrition, the composition of the diet makes a significant

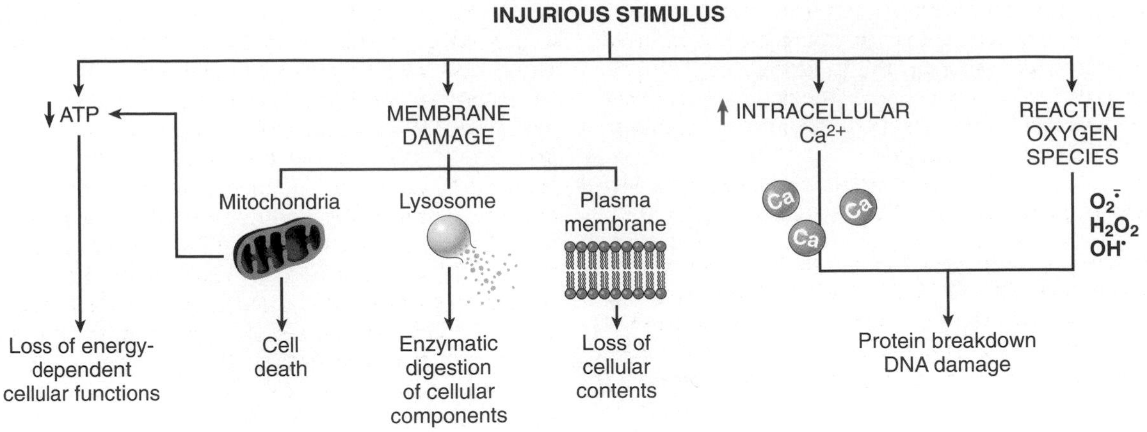

FIGURE 1–10 Cellular and biochemical sites of damage in cell injury.

contribution to a number of diseases. Metabolic diseases such as diabetes also cause severe cell injury.

Mechanisms of Cell Injury

The biochemical mechanisms responsible for cell injury are complex. There are, however, a number of principles that are relevant to most forms of cell injury:

- *The cellular response to injurious stimuli depends on the type of injury, its duration, and its severity.* Thus, small doses of a chemical toxin or brief periods of ischemia may induce reversible injury, whereas large doses of the same toxin or more prolonged ischemia might result either in instantaneous cell death or in slow, irreversible injury leading in time to cell death.
- *The consequences of cell injury depend on the type, state, and adaptability of the injured cell.* The cell's nutritional and hormonal status and its metabolic needs are important in its response to injury. How vulnerable is a cell, for example, to loss of blood supply and hypoxia? The striated muscle cell in the leg can be placed entirely at rest when it is deprived of its blood supply; not so the striated muscle of the heart. Exposure of two individuals to identical concentrations of a toxin, such as carbon tetrachloride, may produce no effect in one and cell death in the other. This may be due to genetic variations affecting the amount and activity of hepatic enzymes that convert carbon tetrachloride to toxic byproducts (Chapter 9). With the complete mapping of the human genome, there is great interest in identifying genetic polymorphisms that affect the cell's response to injurious agents.
- *Cell injury results from functional and biochemical abnormalities in one or more of several essential cellular components* (Fig. 1–10). The most important targets of injurious stimuli are: (1) aerobic respiration involving mitochondrial oxidative phosphorylation and production of ATP; (2) the integrity of cell membranes, on which the ionic and osmotic homeostasis of the cell and its organelles depends; (3) protein synthesis; (4) the cytoskeleton; and (5) the integrity of the genetic apparatus of the cell.

In the following section, we describe each of the biochemical mechanisms that are responsible for cell injury induced by different stimuli. It should be noted that with most stimuli, multiple mechanisms contribute to injury, and in the case of many injurious stimuli, the actual biochemical locus of injury remains unknown.

DEPLETION OF ATP

ATP depletion and decreased ATP synthesis are frequently associated with both hypoxic and chemical (toxic) injury (Fig. 1–11). High-energy phosphate in the form of ATP is required for many synthetic and degradative processes within the cell. These include membrane transport, protein synthesis, lipogenesis, and the deacylation–reacylation reactions necessary for phospholipid turnover. ATP is produced in two ways. The major pathway in mammalian cells is *oxidative phosphorylation* of adenosine diphosphate, in a reaction that results in reduction of oxygen by the electron transfer system of mito-

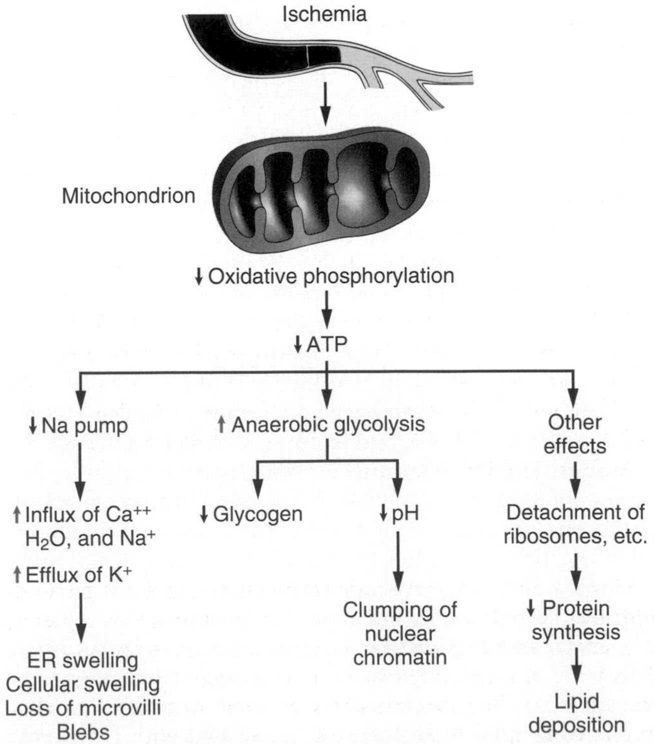

FIGURE 1–11 Functional and morphologic consequences of decreased intracellular ATP during cell injury.

chondria. The second is the *glycolytic pathway*, which can generate ATP in the absence of oxygen using glucose derived either from body fluids or from the hydrolysis of glycogen. Thus, tissues with greater glycolytic capacity (e.g., liver) have an advantage when ATP levels are falling because of inhibition of oxidative metabolism by injury.

Depletion of ATP to <5% to 10% of normal levels has widespread effects on many critical cellular systems:

- The activity of the *plasma membrane energy-dependent sodium pump* (ouabain-sensitive Na^+, K^+-ATPase) is reduced. Failure of this active transport system, due to diminished ATP concentration and enhanced ATPase activity, causes sodium to accumulate intracellularly and potassium to diffuse out of the cell. The net gain of solute is accompanied by isosmotic gain of water, causing *cell swelling*, and dilation of the endoplasmic reticulum (see Fig. 1–8).
- *Cellular energy metabolism is altered.* If the supply of oxygen to cells is reduced, as in ischemia, oxidative phosphorylation ceases and cells rely on glycolysis for energy production. This switch to anaerobic metabolism is controlled by energy pathway metabolites acting on glycolytic enzymes. The decrease in cellular ATP and associated increase in adenosine monophosphate stimulate phosphofructokinase and phosphorylase activities. These result in an increased rate of *anaerobic glycolysis* designed to maintain the cell's energy sources by generating ATP through metabolism of glucose derived from glycogen. As a consequence, *glycogen stores are rapidly depleted.* Glycolysis results in the accumulation of *lactic acid* and inorganic phosphates from the hydrolysis of phosphate esters. This reduces the intracellular pH, resulting in decreased activity of many cellular enzymes.
- Failure of the Ca^{2+} pump leads to influx of Ca^{2+}, with damaging effects on numerous cellular components, described below.
- With prolonged or worsening depletion of ATP, structural disruption of the protein synthetic apparatus occurs, manifested as detachment of ribosomes from the rough endoplasmic reticulum and dissociation of polysomes into monosomes, with a consequent *reduction in protein synthesis.* Ultimately, there is irreversible damage to mitochondrial and lysosomal membranes, and the cell undergoes necrosis (see Fig. 1–8).
- In cells deprived of oxygen or glucose, proteins may become misfolded, and misfolded proteins trigger a cellular reaction called the *unfolded protein response* that may lead to cell injury and even death. This process is described later in the chapter. Protein misfolding is also seen in cells exposed to stress, such as heat, and when proteins are damaged by enzymes (such as Ca^{2+}-responsive enzymes, described below) and free radicals.

MITOCHONDRIAL DAMAGE

Mitochondria are important targets for virtually all types of injurious stimuli, including hypoxia and toxins. Cell injury is frequently accompanied by morphologic changes in mitochondria. Mitochondria can be damaged by increases of cytosolic Ca^{2+}, by oxidative stress, by breakdown of phospholipids through the phospholipase A_2 and sphingomyelin pathways, and by lipid breakdown products derived therefrom, such as free fatty acids and ceramide. Mitochondrial damage often results in the formation of a high-conductance channel, the so-called mitochondrial permeability transition, in the inner mitochondrial membrane (Fig. 1–12).[17] Although reversible in its early stages, this nonselective pore becomes permanent if the inciting stimuli persist, precluding maintenance of mitochondrial proton motive force, or potential. Because maintenance of membrane potential is critical for mitochondrial oxidative phosphorylation, it follows that irreversible mitochondrial permeability transition is a deathblow to the cell. Mitochondrial damage can also be associated with leakage of cytochrome *c* into the cytosol. Because cytochrome *c* is an integral component of the electron transport chain and can trigger apoptotic death pathways in the cytosol (see later), this pathologic event is also likely to be a key determinant of cell death.

INFLUX OF INTRACELLULAR CALCIUM AND LOSS OF CALCIUM HOMEOSTASIS

Calcium ions are important mediators of cell injury.[18] Cytosolic free calcium is maintained at extremely low concentrations (<0.1 μmol) compared with extracellular levels of 1.3 mmol, and most intracellular calcium is sequestered in mitochondria and endoplasmic reticulum. Such gradients are modulated by membrane-associated, energy-dependent Ca^{2+}, Mg^{2+}-ATPases. Ischemia and certain toxins cause an early increase in cytosolic calcium concentration, owing to the net influx of Ca^{2+} across the plasma membrane and the release of Ca^{2+} from mitochondria and endoplasmic reticulum (Fig. 1–13). Sustained rises in intracellular Ca^{2+} subsequently result from nonspecific increases in membrane permeability. Increased Ca^{2+} in turn activates a number of enzymes, with potential deleterious cellular effects. The enzymes known to be activated by calcium include *ATPases* (thereby hastening ATP depletion), *phospholipases* (which cause membrane

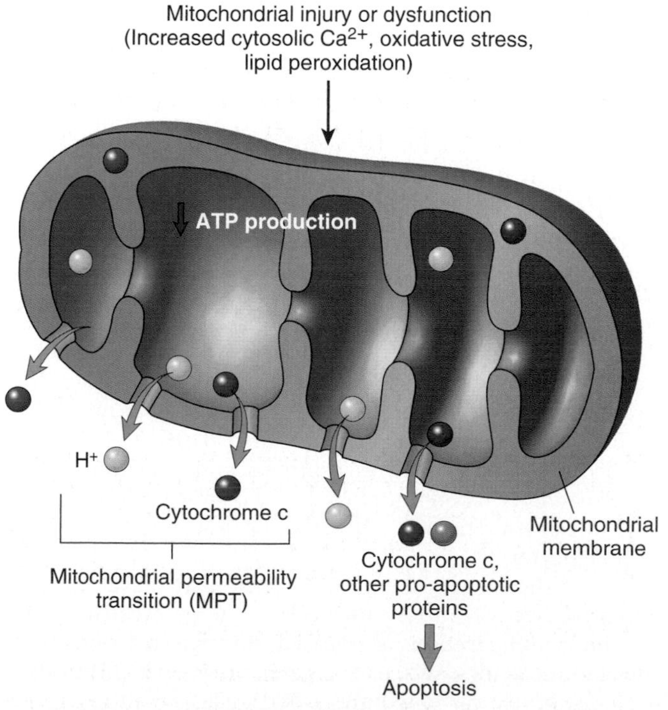

FIGURE 1–12 Mitochondrial dysfunction in cell injury.

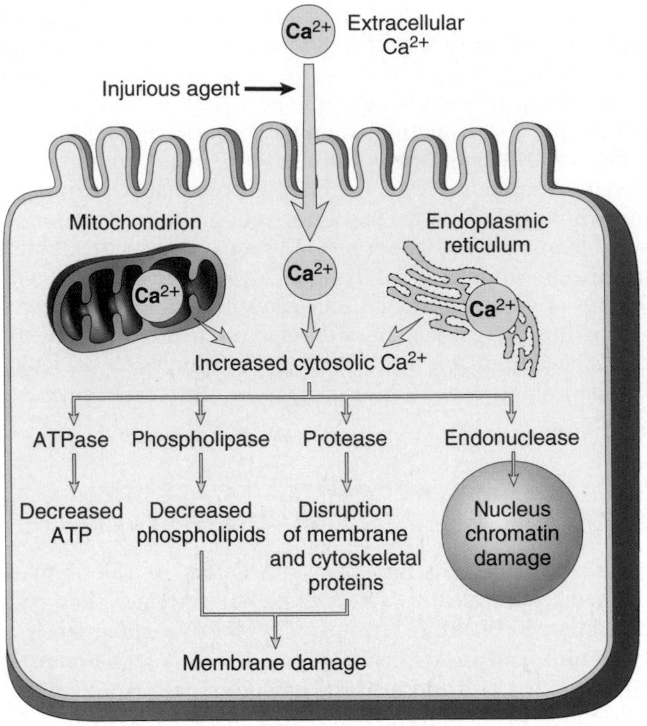

FIGURE 1–13 Sources and consequences of increased cytosolic calcium in cell injury. ATP, adenosine triphosphate.

damage), *proteases* (which break down both membrane and cytoskeletal proteins), and *endonucleases* (which are responsible for DNA and chromatin fragmentation). Increased intracellular Ca^{2+} levels also result in increased mitochondrial permeability and the induction of apoptosis.[18–20] Although cell injury often results in increased intracellular calcium and this in turn mediates a variety of deleterious effects, including cell death, loss of calcium homeostasis is not always a proximal event in irreversible cell injury.

ACCUMULATION OF OXYGEN-DERIVED FREE RADICALS (OXIDATIVE STRESS)

Cells generate energy by reducing molecular oxygen to water. During this process, small amounts of partially reduced reactive oxygen forms are produced as an unavoidable byproduct of mitochondrial respiration. Some of these forms are free radicals that can damage lipids, proteins, and nucleic acids. They are referred to as *reactive oxygen species*. Cells have defense systems to prevent injury caused by these products. An imbalance between free radical-generating and radical-scavenging systems results in *oxidative stress*, a condition that has been associated with the cell injury seen in many pathologic conditions. Free radical–mediated damage contributes to such varied processes as chemical and radiation injury, ischemia–reperfusion injury (induced by restoration of blood flow in ischemic tissue), cellular aging, and microbial killing by phagocytes.[21–24]

Free radicals are chemical species that have a single unpaired electron in an outer orbit. Energy created by this unstable configuration is released through reactions with adjacent molecules, such as inorganic or organic chemicals—proteins, lipids, carbohydrates—particularly with key molecules in membranes and nucleic acids. Moreover, free radicals initiate autocatalytic reactions, whereby molecules with which they react are themselves converted into free radicals to propagate the chain of damage.

Free radicals may be *initiated* within cells in several ways (Fig. 1–14):

- *Absorption of radiant energy* (e.g., ultraviolet light, x-rays). For example, ionizing radiation can hydrolyze water into hydroxyl (OH) and hydrogen (H) free radicals.
- *Enzymatic metabolism of exogenous chemicals or drugs* (e.g., carbon tetrachloride [CCl_4] can generate CCl_3, described later in this chapter).
- *The reduction-oxidation reactions that occur during normal metabolic processes.* During normal respiration, molecular oxygen is sequentially reduced by the addition of four electrons to generate water. Such conversion occurs by oxidative enzymes in the endoplasmic reticulum, cytosol, mitochondria, peroxisomes, and lysosomes. In this process, small amounts of toxic intermediates are produced; these include superoxide anion radical (O_2^-), hydrogen peroxide (H_2O_2), and hydroxyl ions (OH). Rapid bursts of superoxide production occur in activated polymorphonuclear leukocytes during inflammation. This occurs by a precisely controlled reaction in a plasma membrane multiprotein complex that uses NADPH oxidase for the redox reaction (Chapter 2). In addition, some intracellular oxidases (such as xanthine oxidase) generate superoxide radicals as a consequence of their activity.
- *Transition metals* such as iron and copper donate or accept free electrons during intracellular reactions and catalyze free radical formation, as in the Fenton reaction ($H_2O_2 + Fe^{2+} \rightarrow Fe^{3+} + OH + OH^-$). Because most of the intracellular free iron is in the ferric (Fe^{3+}) state, it must be first reduced to the ferrous (Fe^{2+}) form to participate in the Fenton reaction. This reduction can be enhanced by superoxide, and thus sources of iron and superoxide are required for maximal oxidative cell damage.
- *Nitric oxide* (NO), an important chemical mediator generated by endothelial cells, macrophages, neurons, and other cell types (Chapter 2), can act as a free radical and can also be converted to highly reactive peroxynitrite anion ($ONOO^-$) as well as NO_2 and NO_3^-.

The effects of these reactive species are wide-ranging, but three reactions are particularly relevant to cell injury (see Fig. 1–14):

- *Lipid peroxidation of membranes.* Free radicals in the presence of oxygen may cause peroxidation of lipids within plasma and organellar membranes. Oxidative damage is initiated when the double bonds in unsaturated fatty acids of membrane lipids are attacked by oxygen-derived free radicals, particularly by OH. The lipid–free radical interactions yield peroxides, which are themselves unstable and reactive, and an autocatalytic chain reaction ensues (called *propagation*), which can result in extensive membrane, organellar, and cellular damage. Other more favorable termination options take place when the free radical is captured by a scavenger, such as vitamin E, embedded in the cell membrane.
- *Oxidative modification of proteins.* Free radicals promote oxidation of amino acid residue side chains, formation of protein-protein cross-linkages (e.g., disulfide bonds), and

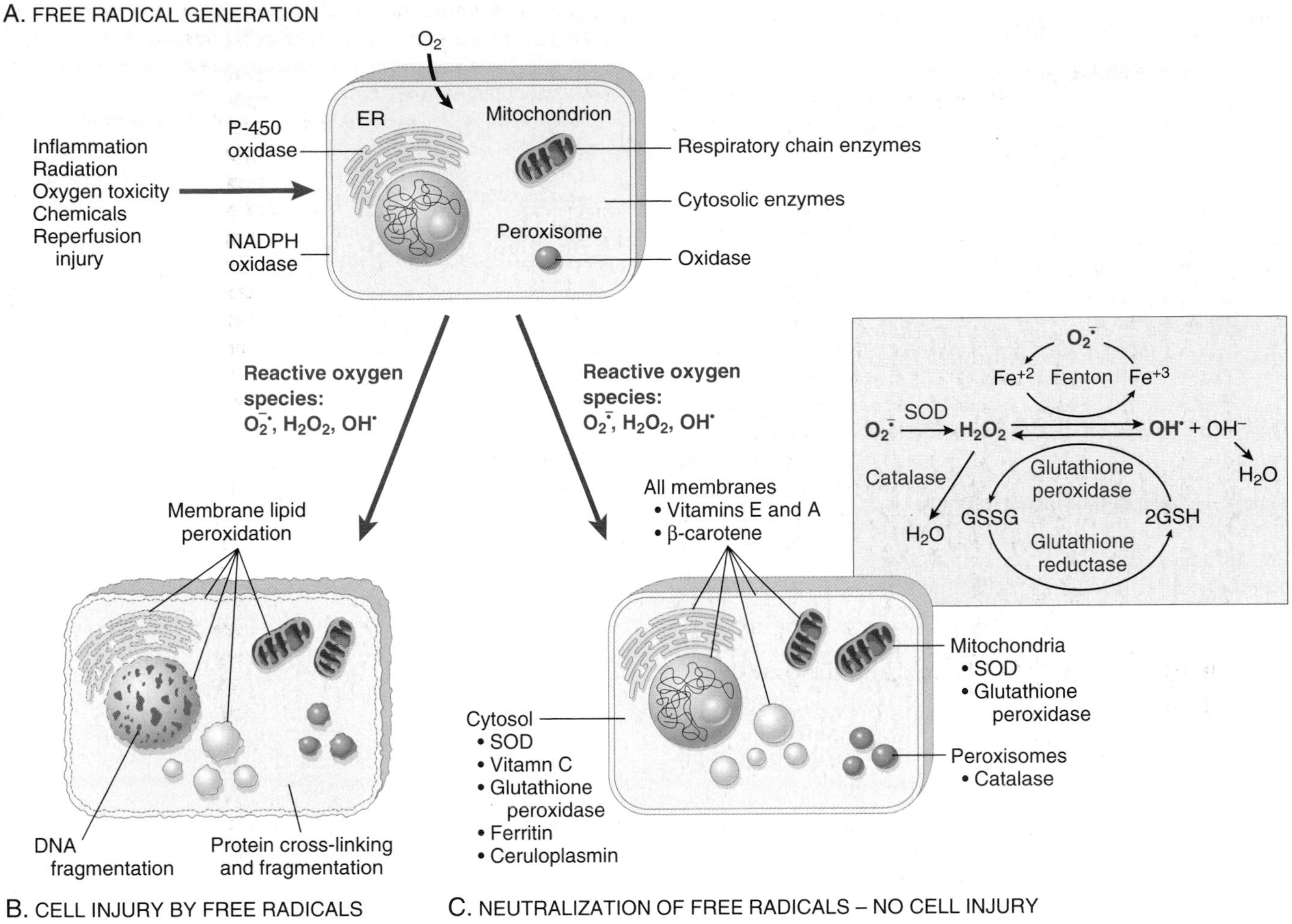

FIGURE 1–14 The role of reactive oxygen species in cell injury. O_2 is converted to superoxide (O_2^-) by oxidative enzymes in the endoplasmic reticulum (ER), mitochondria, plasma membrane, peroxisomes, and cytosol. O_2^- is converted to H_2O_2 by dismutation and thence to OH by the Cu^{2+}/Fe^{2+}-catalyzed Fenton reaction. H_2O_2 is also derived directly from oxidases in peroxisomes. Not shown is another potentially injurious radical, singlet oxygen. Resultant free radical damage to lipid (peroxidation), proteins, and DNA leads to various forms of cell injury. Note that superoxide catalyzes the reduction of Fe^{3+} to Fe^{2+}, thus enhancing OH generation by the Fenton reaction. The major antioxidant enzymes are superoxide dismutase (SOD), catalase, and glutathione peroxidase. GSH, reduced glutathione; GSSG, oxidized glutathione; NADPH, reduced form of nicotinamide adenine dinucleotide phosphate.

oxidation of the protein backbone, resulting in protein fragmentation. Oxidative modification enhances degradation of critical proteins by the multicatalytic proteasome complex, raising havoc throughout the cell.

- *Lesions in DNA*. Reactions with thymine in nuclear and mitochondrial DNA produce single-stranded breaks in DNA. This DNA damage has been implicated in cell aging (discussed later in this chapter) and in malignant transformation of cells (Chapter 7).

Cells have developed multiple mechanisms to remove free radicals and thereby minimize injury. Free radicals are inherently unstable and generally decay spontaneously. Superoxide, for example, is unstable and decays (dismutates) spontaneously into oxygen and hydrogen peroxide in the presence of water. There are, however, several nonenzymatic and enzymatic systems that contribute to inactivation of free radical reactions (see Fig. 1–14). These include the following:

- *Antioxidants* either block the initiation of free radical formation or inactivate (e.g., scavenge) free radicals and terminate radical damage. Examples are the lipid-soluble vitamins E and A as well as ascorbic acid and glutathione in the cytosol.
- As we have seen, *iron* and *copper* can catalyze the formation of reactive oxygen species. The levels of these reactive forms are minimized by binding of the ions to storage and transport proteins (e.g., transferrin, ferritin, lactoferrin, and ceruloplasmin), thereby minimizing OH formation.
- A series of *enzymes* acts as free radical–scavenging systems and break down hydrogen peroxide and superoxide anion. These enzymes are located near the sites of generation of these oxidants and include the following:
  - *Catalase,* present in peroxisomes, which decomposes H_2O_2 ($2\ H_2O_2 \rightarrow O_2 + 2\ H_2O$).
  - *Superoxide dismutases* are found in many cell types and convert superoxide to H_2O_2 ($2\ O_2^- + 2\ H \rightarrow H_2O_2 + O_2$).[23] This group includes both manganese–superoxide dismutase, which is localized in mitochondria, and copper-zinc–superoxide dismutase, which is found in the cytosol.

- *Glutathione peroxidase* also protects against injury by catalyzing free radical breakdown ($H_2O_2 + 2\ GSH \rightarrow GSSG$ [glutathione homodimer] $+ 2\ H_2O$, or $2\ OH + 2\ GSH \rightarrow GSSG + 2\ H_2O$). The intracellular ratio of oxidized glutathione (GSSG) to reduced glutathione (GSH) is a reflection of the oxidative state of the cell and is an important aspect of the cell's ability to detoxify reactive oxygen species.

In many pathologic processes, the final effects induced by free radicals depend on the net balance between free radical formation and termination. As stated earlier, free radicals are thought to be involved in many pathologic and physiologic processes, to be mentioned throughout this book.

DEFECTS IN MEMBRANE PERMEABILITY

Early loss of selective membrane permeability leading ultimately to overt membrane damage is a consistent feature of most forms of cell injury. Membrane damage may affect the mitochondria, the plasma membrane, and other cellular membranes. In ischemic cells, membrane defects may be the result of a series of events involving ATP depletion and calcium-modulated activation of phospholipases (see below). The plasma membrane, however, can also be damaged directly by certain bacterial toxins, viral proteins, lytic complement components, and a variety of physical and chemical agents. Several biochemical mechanisms may contribute to membrane damage (Fig. 1–15):

- *Mitochondrial dysfunction*. Defective mitochondrial function results in decreased phospholipid synthesis, which affects all cellular membranes, including the mitochondria themselves. At the same time, increase of cytosolic calcium associated with ATP depletion results in increased uptake of Ca^{2+} into the mitochondria, activating phospholipases and leading to breakdown of phospholipids. The net result is depletion of phospholipids from the mitochondria and other cellular membranes, and accumulation of free fatty acids. In the mitochondria, these changes cause permeability defects, such as the mitochondrial permeability transition,[17,26] leading to progresive cell injury (see Fig. 1–12).
- *Loss of membrane phospholipids*. Severe cell injury is associated with a decrease in the content of membrane phospholipids, because of degradation likely due to activation of endogenous phospholipases by increased levels of cytosolic calcium.[26] Phospholipid loss can also occur secondary to decreased ATP-dependent reacylation or diminished de novo synthesis of phospholipids.
- *Cytoskeletal abnormalities*. Cytoskeletal filaments serve as anchors connecting the plasma membrane to the cell interior. Activation of proteases by increased cytosolic calcium may cause damage to elements of the cytoskeleton. In the presence of cell swelling, this damage results, particularly in myocardial cells, in detachment of the cell membrane from the cytoskeleton, rendering it susceptible to stretching and rupture.
- *Reactive oxygen species*. Partially reduced oxygen free radicals cause injury to cell membranes and other cell constituents, by mechanisms that were discussed earlier.
- *Lipid breakdown products*. These include unesterified free fatty acids, acyl carnitine, and lysophospholipids, catabolic products that are known to accumulate in injured cells as a result of phospholipid degradation. They have a detergent effect on membranes. They also either insert into the lipid bilayer of the membrane or exchange with membrane phospholipids, potentially causing changes in permeability and electrophysiologic alterations.[17]

Damage to mitochondrial membranes has consequences that were described above. Plasma membrane damage results in loss of osmotic balance and influx of fluids and ions, as well as loss of proteins, enzymes, coenzymes, and ribonucleic acids. The cells may also leak metabolites, which are vital for the reconstitution of ATP, thus further depleting net intracellular high-energy phosphates. *Injury to lysosomal membranes results in leakage of their enzymes into the cytoplasm and activation of these enzymes.* Lysosomes contain RNases, DNases, proteases,

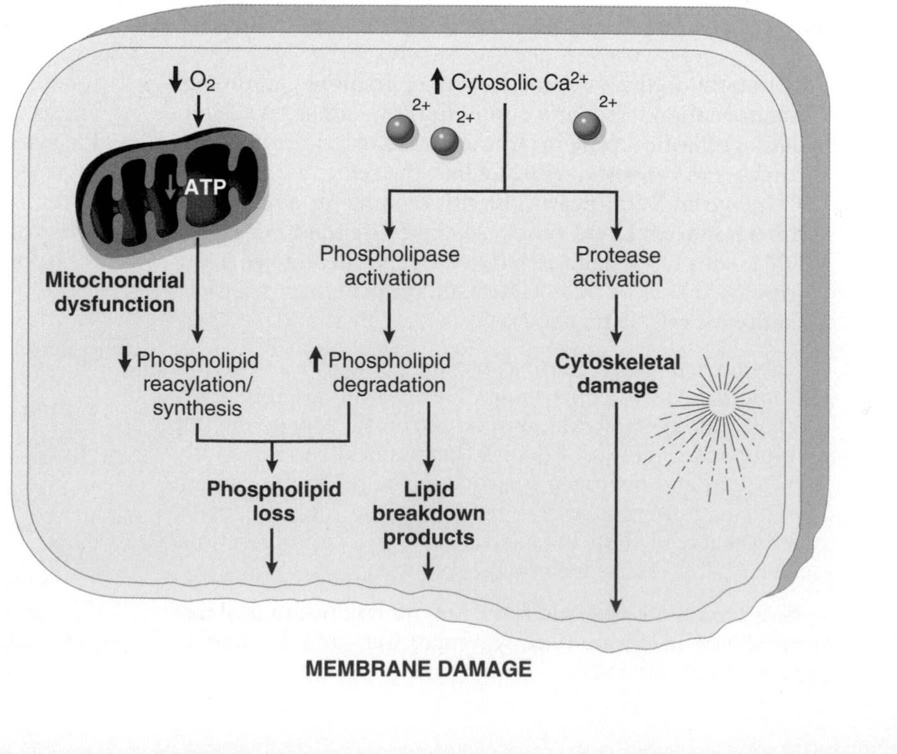

FIGURE 1–15 Mechanisms of membrane damage in cell injury. Decreased O_2 and increased cytosolic Ca^{2+} are typically seen in ischemia but may accompany other forms of cell injury. Reactive oxygen species, which are often produced on reperfusion of ischemic tissues, also cause membrane damage (not shown).

phosphatases, glucosidases, and cathepsins. Activation of these enzymes leads to enzymatic digestion of cell components, resulting in loss of ribonucleoprotein, deoxyribonucleoprotein, and glycogen, and the cells die by necrosis.

Reversible and Irreversible Cell Injury

Up to this point, we have focused on the causes and general biochemical mechanisms of cell injury. In this section, we will turn our attention to the pathways underlying the sequence of events whereby *reversible injury becomes irreversible*, leading to *cell death*, principally *necrosis*.

As discussed previously, the earliest changes associated with various forms of cell injury are decreased generation of ATP, loss of cell membrane integrity, defects in protein synthesis, cytoskeletal damage, and DNA damage. Within limits, the cell can compensate for these derangements and, if the injurious stimulus abates, will return to normalcy. Persistent or excessive injury, however, causes cells to pass the threshold into *irreversible injury* (see Fig. 1–8). This is associated with extensive damage to all cellular membranes, swelling of lysosomes, and vacuolization of mitochondria with reduced capacity to generate ATP. Extracellular calcium enters the cell and intracellular calcium stores are released, resulting in the activation of enzymes that can catabolize membranes, proteins, ATP, and nucleic acids. Following this, there is continued loss of proteins, essential coenzymes, and ribonucleic acids from the hyperpermeable plasma membrane, with cells leaking metabolites vital for the reconstitution of ATP and further depleting intracellular high-energy phosphates.

The molecular mechanisms connecting most forms of cell injury to ultimate cell death have proved elusive, for several reasons. First, there are clearly many ways to injure a cell, not all of them invariably fatal. Second, the numerous macromolecules, enzymes, and organelles within the cell are so closely interdependent that it is difficult to distinguish a primary injury from secondary (and not necessarily relevant) ripple effects. Third, the "point of no return," at which irreversible damage has occurred, is still largely undetermined; thus, we have no precise cut-off point to establish cause and effect. Finally, there is probably no single common final pathway by which cells die. It is, therefore, difficult to define the stage beyond which the cell is irretrievably doomed to destruction. And when does the cell actually die? Two phenomena consistently characterize irreversibility. *The first is the inability to reverse mitochondrial dysfunction* (lack of oxidative phosphorylation and ATP generation) even after resolution of the original injury. *The second is the development of profound disturbances in membrane function.* As mentioned earlier, injury to the lysosomal membranes results in leakage of their enzymes into the cytoplasm; the acid hydrolases are activated in the reduced intracellular pH of the ischemic cell and degrade cytoplasmic and nuclear components. This dissolution of the injured cell is characteristic of *necrosis*, one of the recognized patterns of cell death. There is also widespread leakage of potentially destructive cellular enzymes into the extracellular space, with damage to adjacent tissues and a host response (Chapter 2). Whatever the mechanism(s) of membrane damage, the end result is a massive leak of intracellular materials and a massive influx of calcium, with the consequences described above.

It is worth noting that leakage of intracellular proteins across the degraded cell membrane into the peripheral circulation provides a means of detecting tissue-specific cellular injury and death using blood serum samples. Cardiac muscle, for example, contains a specific isoform of the enzyme creatine kinase and of the contractile protein troponin; liver (and specifically bile duct epithelium) contains a temperature-resistant isoform of the enzyme alkaline phosphatase; and hepatocytes contain transaminases. Irreversible injury and cell death in these tissues are consequently reflected in increased levels of such proteins in the blood.

Morphology of Cell Injury and Necrosis

Cells undergo sequential biochemical and morphologic changes as they are progressively injured and ultimately die by necrosis. All stresses and noxious influences exert their effects first at the molecular or biochemical level. There is a time lag between the stress and the morphologic changes of cell injury or death; the duration of this delay may vary with the sensitivity of the methods used to detect these changes (Fig. 1–16). With histochemical or ultrastructural techniques, changes may be seen in minutes to hours after ischemic injury; however, it may take considerably longer (hours to days) before changes can be seen by light microscopy or on gross examination. As would be expected, the morphologic manifestations of necrosis take more time to develop than those of reversible damage. For example, cell swelling is a reversible morphologic change, and this may occur in a matter of minutes. Unmistakable light microscopic changes of cell death, however, do not occur in the myocardium until 4 to 12 hours after total ischemia, yet we know that irreversible injury occurs within 20 to 60 minutes.

Reversible Injury

Two patterns of reversible cell injury can be recognized under the light microscope: *cellular swelling* and *fatty change*.

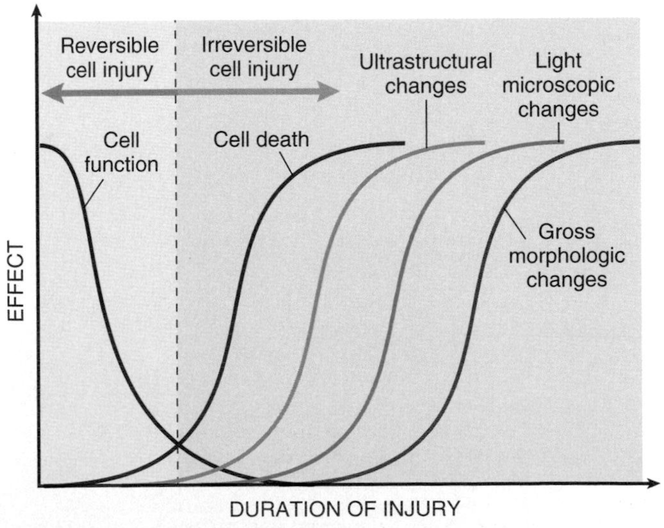

FIGURE 1–16 Timing of biochemical and morphologic changes in cell injury.

Cellular swelling appears whenever cells are incapable of maintaining ionic and fluid homeostasis and is the result of loss of function of plasma membrane energy-dependent ion pumps. Fatty change occurs in hypoxic injury and various forms of toxic or metabolic injury. It is manifested by the appearance of small or large lipid vacuoles in the cytoplasm and occurs in hypoxic and various forms of toxic injury. It is principally encountered in cells involved in and dependent on fat metabolism, such as the hepatocyte and myocardial cell. The mechanisms of fatty change are discussed in more detail later in the chapter.

Morphology. Cellular swelling is the first manifestation of almost all forms of injury to cells. It is a difficult morphologic change to appreciate with the light microscope; it may be more apparent at the level of the whole organ. When it affects many cells in an organ, it causes some pallor, increased turgor, and increase in weight of the organ. On microscopic examination, small clear vacuoles may be seen within the cytoplasm; these represent distended and pinched-off segments of the endoplasmic reticulum. This pattern of nonlethal injury is sometimes called hydropic change or vacuolar degeneration. Swelling of cells is reversible.

The ultrastructural changes of reversible cell injury (Fig. 1–17) include:

1. **plasma membrane alterations,** such as blebbing, blunting, and distortion of microvilli; creation of myelin figures; and loosening of intercellular attachments
2. **mitochondrial changes,** including swelling, rarefaction, and the appearance of small phospholipid-rich amorphous densities
3. **dilation of the endoplasmic reticulum,** with detachment and disaggregation of polysomes
4. **nuclear alterations,** with disaggregation of granular and fibrillar elements.

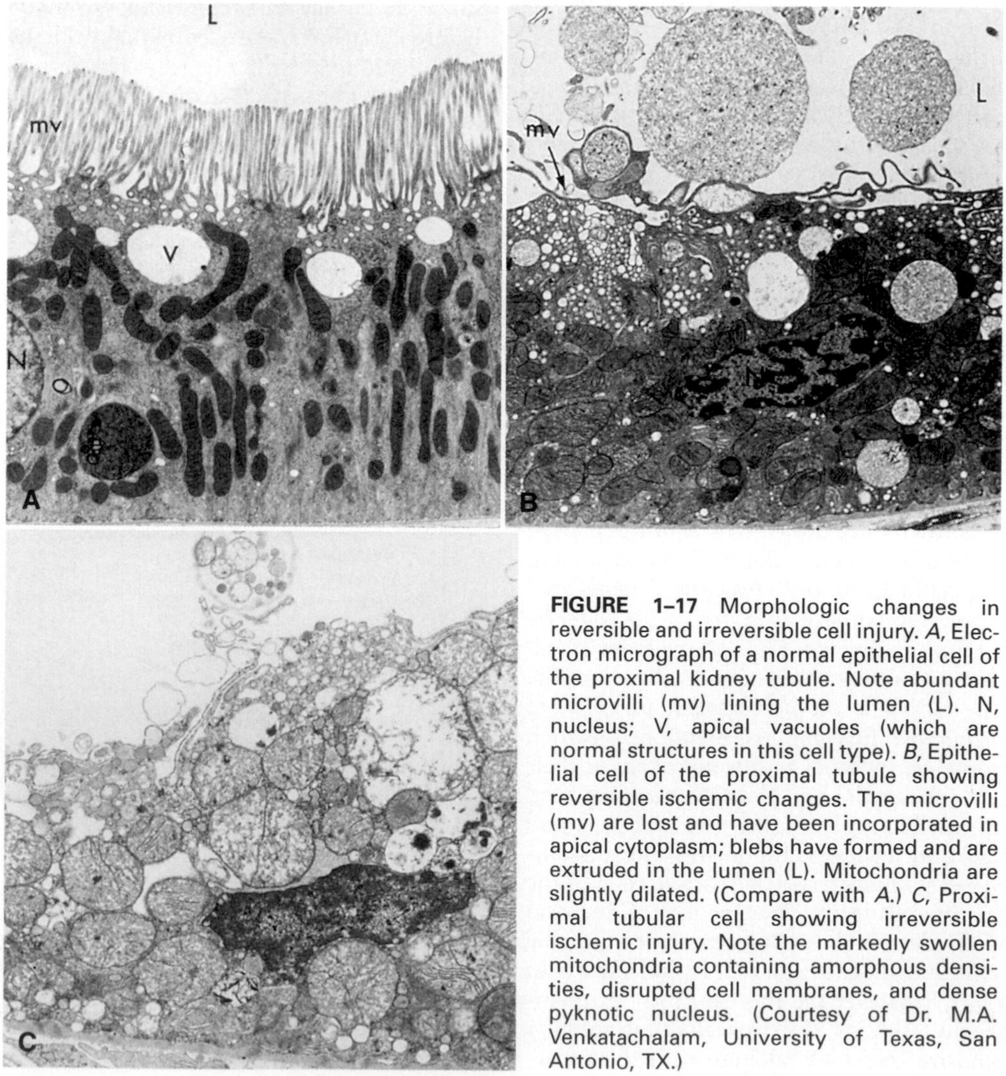

FIGURE 1–17 Morphologic changes in reversible and irreversible cell injury. *A,* Electron micrograph of a normal epithelial cell of the proximal kidney tubule. Note abundant microvilli (mv) lining the lumen (L). N, nucleus; V, apical vacuoles (which are normal structures in this cell type). *B,* Epithelial cell of the proximal tubule showing reversible ischemic changes. The microvilli (mv) are lost and have been incorporated in apical cytoplasm; blebs have formed and are extruded in the lumen (L). Mitochondria are slightly dilated. (Compare with *A.*) *C,* Proximal tubular cell showing irreversible ischemic injury. Note the markedly swollen mitochondria containing amorphous densities, disrupted cell membranes, and dense pyknotic nucleus. (Courtesy of Dr. M.A. Venkatachalam, University of Texas, San Antonio, TX.)

Necrosis

Necrosis refers to a spectrum of morphologic changes that follow cell death in living tissue, largely resulting from the progressive degradative action of enzymes on the lethally injured cell (cells placed immediately in fixative are dead but not necrotic). As commonly used, necrosis is the gross and histologic correlate of cell death occurring in the setting of irreversible exogenous injury. Necrotic cells are unable to maintain membrane integrity and their contents often leak out. This may elicit inflammation in the surrounding tissue.

The morphologic appearance of necrosis is the result of denaturation of intracellular proteins and enzymatic digestion of the cell. The enzymes are derived either from the lysosomes of the dead cells themselves, in which case the enzymatic digestion is referred to as *autolysis*, or from the lysosomes of immigrant leukocytes, during inflammatory reactions. These processes require hours to develop, and so there would be no detectable changes in cells if, for example, a myocardial infarct caused sudden death. The only telling evidence might be occlusion of a coronary artery. The earliest histologic evidence of myocardial necrosis does not become manifest until 4 to 12 hours later, but cardiac-specific enzymes and proteins that are released from necrotic muscle can be detected in the blood as early as 2 hours after myocardial cell death.

Morphology. Necrotic cells show **increased eosinophilia** attributable in part to loss of the normal basophilia imparted by the RNA in the cytoplasm and in part to the increased binding of eosin to denatured intracytoplasmic proteins (Fig. 1–18). The necrotic cell may have a more glassy homogeneous appearance than that of normal cells, mainly as a result of the loss of glycogen particles. When enzymes have digested the cytoplasmic organelles, the cytoplasm becomes vacuolated and appears moth-eaten. Finally, calcification of the dead cells may occur. Dead cells may ultimately be replaced by large, whorled phospholipid masses called **myelin figures.** These phospholipid precipitates are then either phagocytosed by other cells or further degraded into fatty acids; calcification of such fatty acid residues results in the generation of calcium soaps. By electron microscopy, necrotic cells are characterized by overt discontinuities in plasma and organelle membranes, marked dilation of mitochondria with the appearance of large amorphous densities, intracytoplasmic myelin figures, amorphous osmiophilic debris, and aggregates of fluffy material probably representing denatured protein (see Fig. 1–17*C*).

Nuclear changes appear in the form of one of three patterns, all due to nonspecific breakdown of DNA (see Figs. 1–8 and 1–17*C*). The basophilia of the chromatin may fade **(karyolysis)**, a change that presumably reflects DNase activity. A second pattern (also seen in apoptotic cell death) is **pyknosis,** characterized by nuclear shrinkage and increased basophilia. Here the DNA apparently condenses into a solid, shrunken basophilic mass. In the third pattern, known as **karyorrhexis,** the pyknotic or partially pyknotic nucleus undergoes fragmentation. With the passage of time (a day or two), the nucleus in the necrotic cell totally disappears.

Once the necrotic cells have undergone the early alterations described, the mass of necrotic cells may have several morphologic patterns. Although the terms are somewhat outmoded, they are routinely used and their meanings are understood by both pathologists and clinicians. When denaturation is the primary pattern, **coagulative necrosis** develops. In the instance of dominant enzyme digestion, the result is **liquefactive necrosis;** in special circumstances, **caseous necrosis** and **fat necrosis** may occur.

Coagulative necrosis implies preservation of the basic outline of the coagulated cell for a span of at least some days (Fig. 1–19*A*). The affected tissues exhibit a firm texture. Presumably, the injury or the subsequent increasing intracellular acidosis denatures not only structural proteins but also enzymes and so blocks the proteolysis of the cell. The myocardial infarct is an excellent example in which acidophilic, coagulated, anucleate cells may persist for weeks. Ultimately, the necrotic myocardial cells are removed by fragmentation and phagocytosis of the cellular debris by scavenger leukocytes and by the action of proteolytic lysosomal enzymes brought in by the immigrant white cells. The process of coagulative

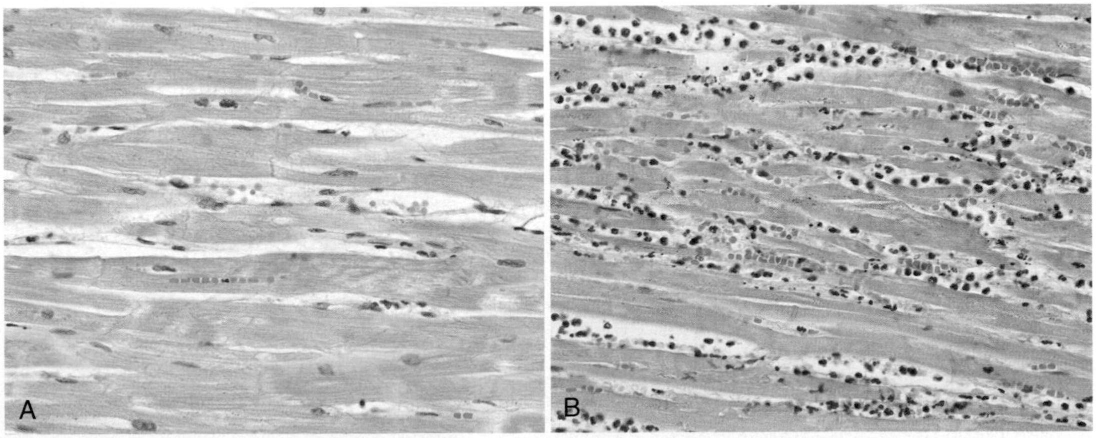

FIGURE 1–18 Ischemic necrosis of the myocardium. *A,* Normal myocardium. *B,* Myocardium with coagulation necrosis (upper two thirds of figure), showing strongly eosinophilic anucleate myocardial fibers. Leukocytes in the interstitium are an early reaction to necrotic muscle. Compare with *A* and with normal fibers in the lower part of the figure.

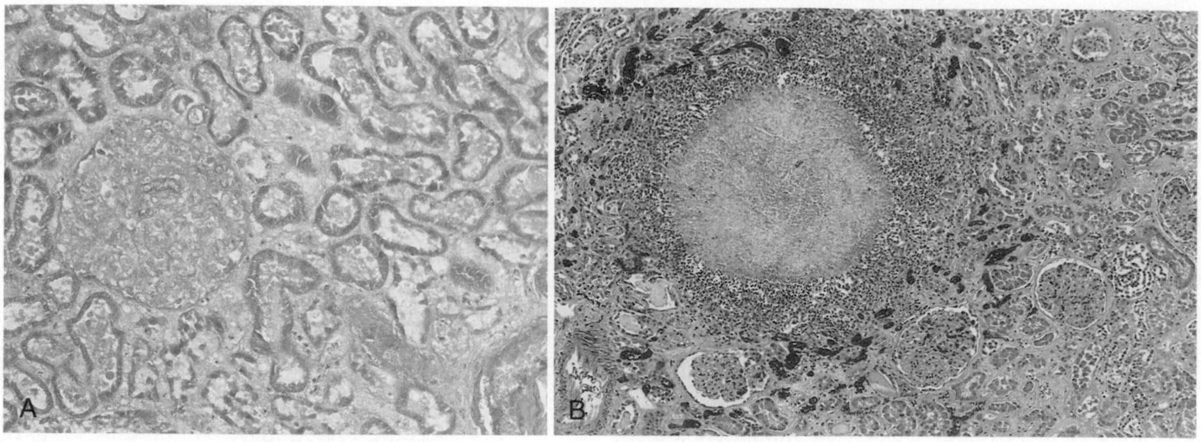

FIGURE 1–19 Coagulative and liquefactive necrosis. *A,* Kidney infarct exhibiting coagulative necrosis, with loss of nuclei and clumping of cytoplasm but with preservation of basic outlines of glomerular and tubular architecture. *B,* A focus of liquefactive necrosis in the kidney caused by fungal infection. The focus is filled with white cells and cellular debris, creating a renal abscess that obliterates the normal architecture.

necrosis, with preservation of the general tissue architecture, is characteristic of hypoxic death of cells in all tissues except the brain.

Liquefactive necrosis is characteristic of focal bacterial or, occasionally, fungal infections, because microbes stimulate the accumulation of inflammatory cells (Fig. 1–19*B*). For obscure reasons, hypoxic death of cells within the central nervous system often evokes liquefactive necrosis. Whatever the pathogenesis, liquefaction completely digests the dead cells. The end result is transformation of the tissue into a liquid viscous mass. If the process was initiated by acute inflammation (Chapter 2), the material is frequently creamy yellow because of the presence of dead white cells and is called *pus.* Although **gangrenous necrosis** is not a distinctive pattern of cell death, the term is still commonly used in surgical clinical practice. It is usually applied to a limb, generally the lower leg, that has lost its blood supply and has undergone coagulation necrosis. When bacterial infection is superimposed, coagulative necrosis is modified by the liquefactive action of the bacteria and the attracted leukocytes (so-called **wet gangrene**).

Caseous necrosis, a distinctive form of coagulative necrosis, is encountered most often in foci of tuberculous infection (Chapter 8). The term caseous is derived from the cheesy white gross appearance of the area of necrosis (Fig. 1–20). On microscopic examination, the necrotic focus appears as amorphous granular debris seemingly composed of fragmented, coagulated cells and amorphous granular debris enclosed within a distinctive inflammatory border known as a granulomatous reaction (Chapter 2). Unlike coagulative necrosis, the tissue architecture is completely obliterated.

Fat necrosis is a term that is well fixed in medical parlance but does not in reality denote a specific pattern of necrosis. Rather, it is descriptive of focal areas of fat destruction, typically occurring as a result of release of activated pancreatic lipases into the substance of the pancreas and the peritoneal cavity. This occurs in the calamitous abdominal emergency known as acute pancreatitis (Chapter 19). In this disorder, activated pancreatic enzymes escape from acinar cells and ducts, the activated enzymes liquefy fat cell membranes, and the activated lipases split the triglyceride esters contained within fat cells. The released fatty acids combine with calcium to produce grossly visible chalky white areas (fat saponification), which enable the surgeon and the pathologist to identify the lesions (Fig. 1–21). On histologic examination, the necrosis takes the form of foci of shadowy outlines of necrotic fat cells, with basophilic calcium deposits, surrounded by an inflammatory reaction.

Ultimately, in the living patient, most necrotic cells and their debris disappear by a combined process of enzymatic digestion and fragmentation, followed by phagocytosis of the particulate debris by leukocytes. If necrotic cells and cellular debris are not promptly destroyed and reabsorbed, they tend to attract calcium salts and other minerals and to become calcified. This phenomenon, called *dystrophic calcification*, is considered later in the chapter.

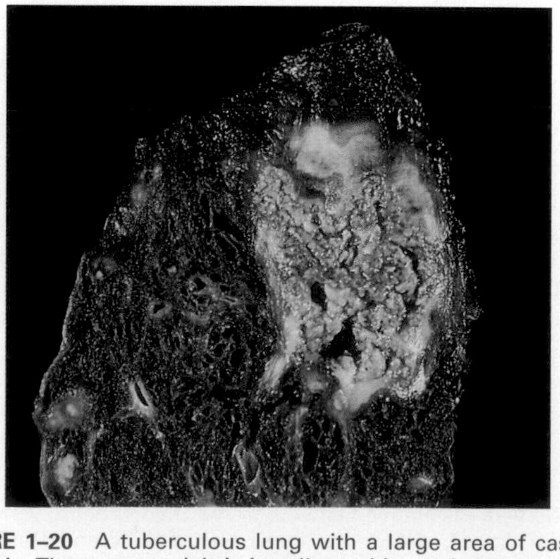

FIGURE 1–20 A tuberculous lung with a large area of caseous necrosis. The caseous debris is yellow-white and cheesy.

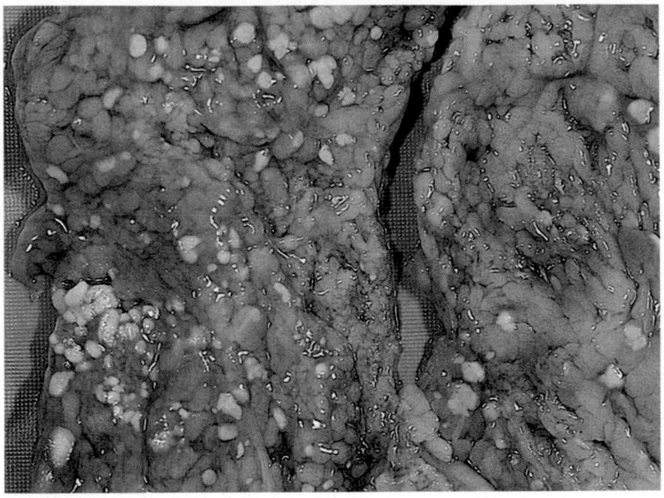

FIGURE 1–21 Foci of fat necrosis with saponification in the mesentery. The areas of white chalky deposits represent calcium soap formation at sites of lipid breakdown.

Examples of Cell Injury and Necrosis

Having briefly reviewed the general causes, mechanisms, and morphology of cell injury and necrotic cell death, we now describe some common forms of cell injury, namely ischemic and hypoxic injury, and some types of toxic injury. Although apoptosis contributes to cell death in some of these conditions, it has many unique features and is therefore discussed later in the chapter.

ISCHEMIC AND HYPOXIC INJURY

This is the most common type of cell injury in clinical medicine and has been studied extensively in humans, in experimental animals, and in culture systems.[27–29] Reasonable scenarios concerning the mechanisms underlying the morphologic changes have emerged. Hypoxia refers to any state of reduced oxygen availability. It may be caused by reduced amounts or saturation of hemoglobin. Ischemia, on the other hand, is brought about by reduced blood flow, usually as a consequence of a mechanical obstruction in the arterial system but sometimes as a result of a catastrophic fall in blood pressure or loss of blood. In contrast to hypoxia, during which glycolytic energy production can continue, ischemia compromises the delivery of substrates for glycolysis. Thus, in ischemic tissues, anaerobic energy generation stops after glycolytic substrates are exhausted, or glycolytic function becomes inhibited by the accumulation of metabolites that would have been removed otherwise by blood flow. For this reason, *ischemia tends to injure tissues faster than does hypoxia.*

Types of Ischemic Injury. Ischemic injury is the most common clinical expression of cell injury by oxygen deprivation. The most useful models for studying ischemic injury involve complete occlusion of one of the end-arteries to an organ (e.g., a coronary artery) and examination of the tissue (e.g., cardiac muscle) in areas supplied by the artery. Complex pathologic changes occur in diverse cellular systems during ischemia. Up to a certain point, for a duration that varies among different types of cells, the injury is amenable to repair, and the affected cells can recover if oxygen and metabolic substrates are again made available by restoration of blood flow. With further extension of the ischemic duration, cell structure continues to deteriorate, owing to relentless progression of ongoing injury mechanisms. With time, the energetic machinery of the cell—the mitochondrial oxidative powerhouse and the glycolytic pathway—becomes irreparably damaged, and restoration of blood flow (reperfusion) cannot rescue the damaged cell. Even if the cellular energetic machinery were to remain intact, irreparable damage to the genome or to cellular membranes will ensure a lethal outcome regardless of reperfusion. This irreversible injury is usually manifested as *necrosis*, but apoptosis may also play a role.

Under certain circumstances, when blood flow is restored to cells that have been previously made ischemic but have not died, injury is often paradoxically exacerbated and proceeds at an accelerated pace. As a consequence, reperfused tissues may sustain *loss of cells in addition to cells that are irreversibly damaged at the end of ischemia.* This is a clinically important process that contributes to net tissue damage during myocardial and cerebral infarction, as described in Chapters 12 and 28. This so-called *ischemia–reperfusion injury* (discussed later) is particularly significant because appropriate medical treatment can decrease the fraction of cells that may otherwise be destined to die in the "area at risk."

Mechanisms of Ischemic Cell Injury. The sequence of events following hypoxia was described earlier and is summarized in Figure 1–22.[28,29] Briefly, as the oxygen tension within the cell decreases, there is loss of oxidative phosphorylation and decreased generation of ATP. The depletion of ATP results in failure of the sodium pump, with loss of potassium, influx of sodium and water, and cell swelling. There is progressive loss of glycogen and decreased protein synthesis. There may be severe functional consequences at this stage. For instance, heart muscle ceases to contract within 60 seconds of coronary occlusion. Note, however, that loss of contractility does not mean cell death. If hypoxia continues, worsening ATP depletion causes further morphologic deterioration. The cytoskeleton disperses, resulting in the loss of ultrastructural features such as microvilli and the formation of "blebs" at the cell surface (see Fig. 1–17). "Myelin figures," derived from plasma as well as organellar membranes, may be seen within the cytoplasm or extracellularly. They are thought to result from dissociation of lipoproteins with unmasking of phosphatide groups, promoting the uptake and intercalation of water between the lamellar stacks of membranes. At this time, the mitochondria are usually swollen, owing to loss of volume control by these organelles; the endoplasmic reticulum remains dilated; and the entire cell is markedly swollen, with increased concentrations of water, sodium, and chloride and a decreased concentration of potassium. *If oxygen is restored, all of these disturbances are reversible.*

If ischemia persists, irreversible injury and necrosis ensue. Irreversible injury is associated morphologically with severe swelling of mitochondria, extensive damage to plasma membranes, and swelling of lysosomes (see Fig. 1–17*C*). Large, flocculent, amorphous densities develop in the mitochondrial matrix. In the myocardium, these are indications of irreversible injury and can be seen as early as 30 to 40 minutes after ischemia. Massive influx of calcium into the cell then occurs, particularly if the ischemic zone is reperfused. Death

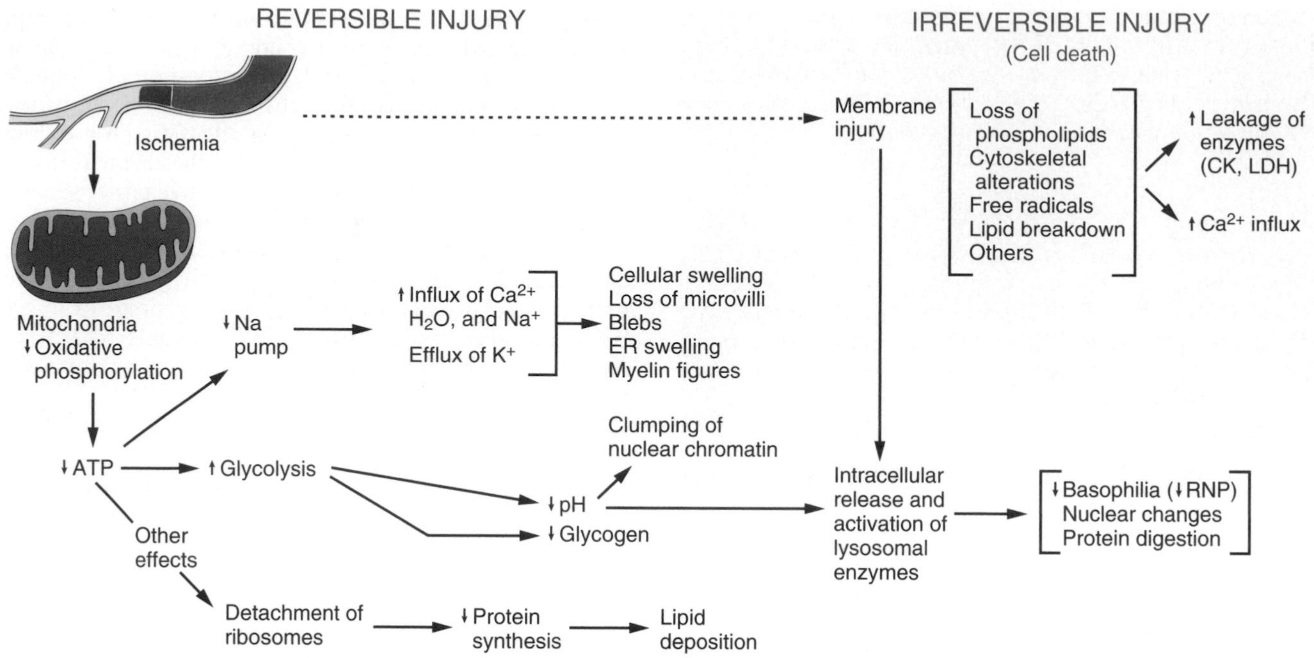

FIGURE 1–22 Postulated sequence of events in reversible and irreversible ischemic cell injury. Note that although reduced oxidative phosphorylation and ATP levels have a central role, ischemia can cause direct membrane damage. ER, endoplasmic reticulum; CK, creatine kinase; LDH, lactate dehydrogenase; RNP, ribonucleoprotein.

is mainly by necrosis, but apoptosis also contributes; the apoptotic pathway is activated probably by release of pro-apoptotic molecules from leaky mitochondria. After death, cell components are progressively degraded, and there is widespread leakage of cellular enzymes into the extracellular space and, conversely, entry of extracellular macromolecules from the interstitial space into the dying cells. Finally, the dead cell may become replaced by large masses composed of phospholipids in the form of myelin figures. These are then either phagocytosed by other cells or degraded further into fatty acids. *Calcification* of such fatty acid residues may occur with the formation of calcium soaps.

As we mentioned previously, leakage of intracellular enzymes and other proteins across the abnormally permeable plasma membrane and into the plasma provides important clinical parameters of cell death. For example, elevated serum levels of cardiac muscle creatine kinase MB and troponin are valuable clinical indicators of myocardial infarction, an area of cell death in heart muscle (Chapter 12).

ISCHEMIA–REPERFUSION INJURY

Restoration of blood flow to ischemic tissues can result in recovery of cells if they are reversibly injured, or not affect the outcome if irreversible cell damage has occurred. However, depending on the intensity and duration of the ischemic insult, variable numbers of cells may proceed to die *after* blood flow resumes, by necrosis as well as by apoptosis.[30] The affected tissues often show neutrophilic infiltrates. As noted earlier, this ischemia–reperfusion injury is a clinically important process in such conditions as myocardial infarction and stroke and may be amenable to therapeutic interventions.

How does reperfusion injury occur? The likely answer is that *new damaging processes* are set in motion during reperfusion, causing the death of cells that might have recovered otherwise.[31,32] Several mechanisms have been proposed:

- New damage may be initiated during reoxygenation by increased generation of *oxygen free radicals* from parenchymal and endothelial cells and from infiltrating leukocytes.[31,33] Superoxide anions can be produced in reperfused tissue as a result of incomplete and vicarious reduction of oxygen by damaged mitochondria or because of the action of oxidases derived from leukocytes, endothelial cells, or parenchymal cells.[32] Cellular antioxidant defense mechanisms may also be compromised by ischemia, favoring the accumulation of radicals. Free radical scavengers may be of therapeutic benefit.
- Reactive oxygen species can further promote the *mitochondrial permeability transition*, referred to earlier, which, when it occurs, precludes mitochondrial energization and cellular ATP recovery and leads to cell death.[25]
- Ischemic injury is associated with *inflammation* as a result of the production of cytokines and increased expression of adhesion molecules by hypoxic parenchymal and endothelial cells.[31,33] These agents recruit circulating polymorphonuclear leukocytes to reperfused tissue; the ensuing inflammation causes additional injury (Chapter 2). The importance of neutrophil influx in reperfusion injury has been demonstrated by experimental studies that have used anti-inflammatory interventions, such as antibodies to cytokines or adhesion molecules, to reduce the extent of the injury.[30,32]
- Recent data suggest that activation of the *complement pathway* may contribute to ischemia–reperfusion injury.[34] The complement system is involved in host defense and is an important mechanism of immune injury (Chapter 6). Some IgM antibodies have a propensity to deposit in

ischemic tissues, for unknown reasons, and when blood flow is resumed, complement proteins bind to the antibodies, are activated, and cause cell injury and inflammation. Knockout mice lacking several complement proteins are resistant to this type of injury.[35]

CHEMICAL INJURY

The mechanisms by which chemicals, certain drugs, and toxins produce injury are described in greater detail in Chapter 9 in the discussion of environmental disease. Here we will describe two forms of chemically induced injury as examples of the sequence of events leading to cell death.

Chemicals induce cell injury by one of two general mechanisms:[36]

- Some chemicals can act *directly* by combining with some critical molecular component or cellular organelle. For example, in *mercuric chloride poisoning*, mercury binds to the sulfhydryl groups of the cell membrane and other proteins, causing increased membrane permeability and inhibition of ATPase-dependent transport. In such instances, the greatest damage is usually to the cells that use, absorb, excrete, or concentrate the chemicals — in the case of mercuric chloride, the cells of the gastrointestinal tract and kidney (Chapter 9). *Cyanide* poisons mitochondrial cytochrome oxidase and blocks oxidative phosphorylation. Many antineoplastic chemotherapeutic agents and antibiotic drugs also induce cell damage by direct cytotoxic effects.
- Most other chemicals are not biologically active but must be converted to reactive toxic metabolites, which then act on target cells. This modification is usually accomplished by the P-450 mixed function oxidases in the smooth endoplasmic reticulum of the liver and other organs.[37,38] Although these metabolites might cause membrane damage and cell injury by *direct covalent binding* to membrane protein and lipids, by far the most important mechanism of membrane injury involves the formation of *reactive free radicals* and subsequent lipid peroxidation.

The diverse mechanisms of chemical injury are well illustrated by carbon tetrachloride and acetaminophen. *Carbon tetrachloride* (CCl_4) was once used widely in the dry-cleaning industry.[39] The toxic effect of CCl_4 is due to its conversion by P-450 to the *highly reactive toxic free radical* CCl_3 ($CCl_4 + e \rightarrow CCl_3 + Cl^-$) (Fig. 1–23). The free radicals produced locally cause autooxidation of the polyenoic fatty acids present within the membrane phospholipids. There, oxidative decomposition of the lipid is initiated, and organic peroxides are formed after reacting with oxygen (lipid peroxidation). This *reaction is autocatalytic* in that new radicals are formed from the peroxide radicals themselves. Thus, rapid breakdown of the structure and function of the endoplasmic reticulum is due to decomposition of the lipid. It is no surprise, therefore, that *CCl_4-induced liver cell injury is both severe and extremely rapid in onset.* Within less than 30 minutes, there is a decline in hepatic protein synthesis; within 2 hours, there is swelling of smooth endoplasmic reticulum and dissociation of ribosomes from the rough endoplasmic reticulum. Lipid export from the hepatocytes is reduced owing to their inability to synthesize apoprotein to complex with triglycerides and thereby facilitate

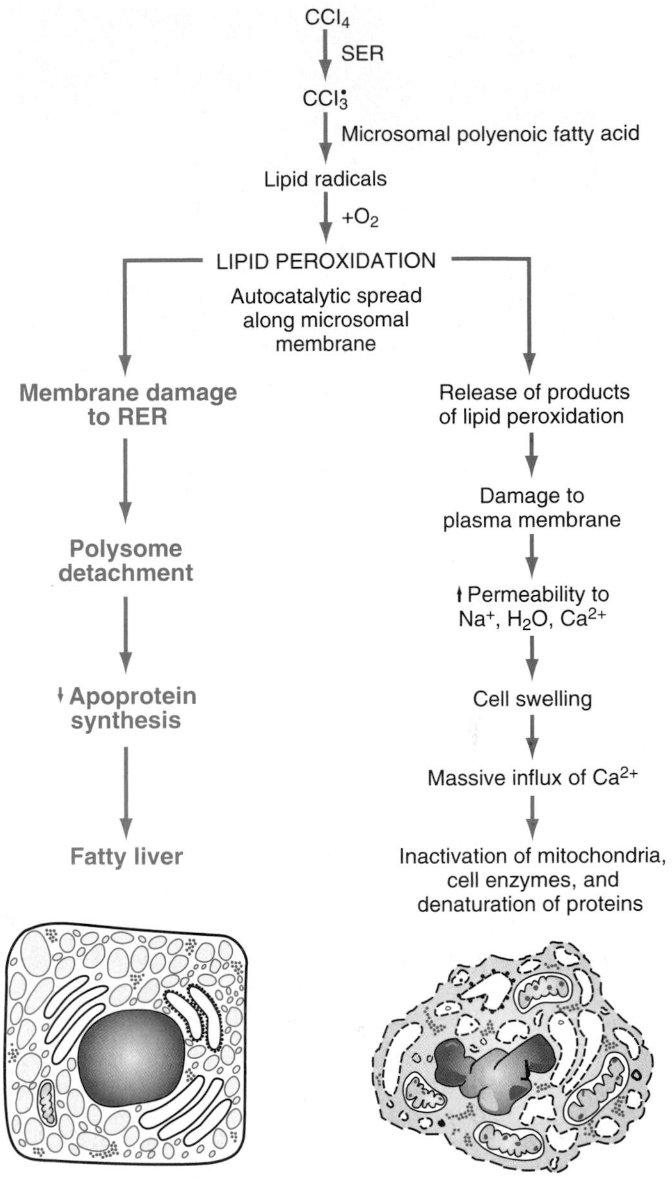

FIGURE 1–23 Sequence of events leading to fatty change and cell necrosis in carbon tetrachloride (CCl_4) toxicity. RER, rough endoplasmic reticulum; SER, smooth endoplasmic reticulum.

lipoprotein secretion. The result is the fatty liver of CCl_4 poisoning (Fig. 1–24). (Fatty liver is discussed later in the chapter.) Mitochondrial injury then occurs, and this is followed by progressive swelling of the cells due to increased permeability of the plasma membrane. Plasma membrane damage is thought to be caused by relatively stable fatty aldehydes, which are produced by lipid peroxidation in the smooth endoplasmic reticulum but are able to act at distant sites. This is followed by massive influx of calcium and cell death (see Fig. 1–23).

Acetaminophen (Tylenol), a commonly used analgesic drug, is detoxified in the liver through sulfation and glucuronidation, and small amounts are converted by cytochrome P-450–catalyzed oxidation to an electrophilic, highly toxic metabolite.[40] This metabolite itself is detoxified by interaction with GSH. When large doses of the drug are ingested, GSH is depleted, and thus the toxic metabolites accumulate in the cell,

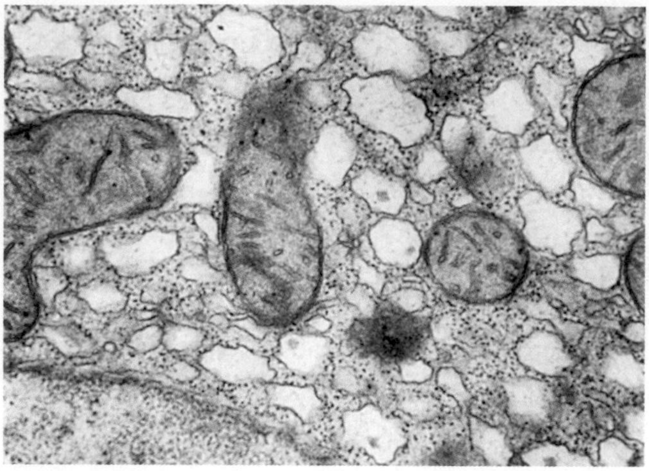

FIGURE 1–24 Rat liver cell 4 hours after carbon tetrachloride intoxication, with swelling of endoplasmic reticulum and shedding of ribosomes. At this stage, mitochondria are unaltered. (Courtesy of Dr. O. Iseri, University of Maryland, Baltimore, MD.)

destroy nucleophilic macromolecules, and covalently bind proteins and nucleic acids. The decrease in GSH concentration, coupled with covalent binding of toxic metabolites, increases drug toxicity, resulting in massive liver cell necrosis, usually 3 to 5 days after the ingestion of toxic doses. This hepatotoxicity correlates with lipid peroxidation and can be reduced by administration of antioxidants, suggesting that the oxidative damage may be more important than covalent binding in the ultimate toxicity of the drug.[41]

Apoptosis

Apoptosis is a pathway of cell death that is induced by a tightly regulated intracellular program in which cells destined to die activate enzymes that degrade the cells' own nuclear DNA and nuclear and cytoplasmic proteins. The cell's plasma membrane remains intact, but its structure is altered in such a way that the apoptotic cell becomes an avid target for phagocytosis. The dead cell is rapidly cleared, before its contents have leaked out, and therefore cell death by this pathway does not elicit an inflammatory reaction in the host. Thus, apoptosis is fundamentally different from necrosis, which is characterized by loss of membrane integrity, enzymatic digestion of cells, and frequently a host reaction (see Fig. 1–9 and Table 1–2). However, apoptosis and necrosis sometimes coexist, and they may share some common features and mechanisms.

CAUSES OF APOPTOSIS

Apoptosis was initially recognized in 1972 by its distinctive morphology and named after the Greek designation for "falling off."[42] It occurs normally in many situations, and serves to eliminate unwanted or potentially harmful cells and cells that have outlived their usefulness. It is also a pathologic event when cells are damaged beyond repair, especially when the damage affects the cell's DNA; in these situations, the irreparably damaged cell is eliminated. Apoptosis is responsible for numerous physiologic, adaptive, and pathologic events, listed next.

Apoptosis in Physiologic Situations

Death by apoptosis is a normal phenomenon that serves to eliminate cells that are no longer needed, as, for example, during development, and to maintain a steady number of various cell populations in tissues. It is important in the following physiologic situations:

- *The programmed destruction of cells during embryogenesis*, including implantation, organogenesis, developmental involution, and metamorphosis. The term "programmed cell death" was originally coined to denote death of specific cell types at defined times during development.[43] Apoptosis is a generic term for this pattern of cell death, regardless of the context, but it is often used interchangeably with "programmed cell death."
- *Hormone-dependent involution in the adult*, such as endometrial cell breakdown during the menstrual cycle, ovarian follicular atresia in the menopause, the regression of the lactating breast after weaning, and prostatic atrophy after castration.
- *Cell deletion in proliferating cell populations*, such as intestinal crypt epithelia, in order to maintain a constant number.
- Death of host cells that have served their useful purpose, such as neutrophils in an *acute inflammatory response*, and lymphocytes at the end of an *immune response*. In these situations, cells undergo apoptosis because they are deprived of necessary survival signals, such as growth factors.
- *Elimination of potentially harmful self-reactive lymphocytes*, either before or after they have completed their maturation (Chapter 6).
- *Cell death induced by cytotoxic T cells*, a defense mechanism against viruses and tumors that serves to eliminate virus-infected and neoplastic cells. The same mechanism is responsible for cellular rejection of transplants (Chapter 6).

Apoptosis in Pathologic Conditions

Death by apoptosis is also responsible for loss of cells in a variety of pathologic states:

- *Cell death produced by a variety of injurious stimuli.* For instance, radiation and cytotoxic anticancer drugs damage DNA, and if repair mechanisms cannot cope with the injury the cell kills itself by apoptosis. In these situations, elimination of the cell may be a better alternative than risking mutations and translocations in the damaged DNA, which may result in malignant transformation. These injurious stimuli, as well as heat and hypoxia, can induce apoptosis if the insult is mild, but large doses of the same stimuli result in necrotic cell death. Endoplasmic reticulum (ER) stress, which is induced by the accumulation of unfolded proteins, also triggers apoptotic death of cells (described later in the chapter).
- *Cell injury in certain viral diseases*, such as viral hepatitis, in which loss of infected cells is largely because of apoptotic death.
- *Pathologic atrophy in parenchymal organs after duct obstruction*, such as occurs in the pancreas, parotid gland, and kidney.
- *Cell death in tumors*, most frequently during regression but also in actively growing tumors.

- As we mentioned earlier, even in situations in which cell death is mainly by necrosis, the pathway of apoptosis may contribute. For instance, injurious stimuli that cause increased mitochondrial permeability trigger apoptosis.

Before the mechanisms of apoptosis are discussed, we describe the morphologic and biochemical characteristics of this process.

Morphology. The following morphologic features, some best seen with the electron microscope, characterize cells undergoing apoptosis (Fig. 1–25).

- **Cell shrinkage.** The cell is smaller in size; the cytoplasm is dense; and the organelles, although relatively normal, are more tightly packed.
- **Chromatin condensation.** This is the most characteristic feature of apoptosis. The chromatin aggregates peripherally, under the nuclear membrane, into dense masses of various shapes and sizes. The nucleus itself may break up, producing two or more fragments.
- **Formation of cytoplasmic blebs and apoptotic bodies.** The apoptotic cell first shows extensive surface blebbing, then undergoes fragmentation into membrane-bound apoptotic bodies composed of cytoplasm and tightly packed organelles, with or without nuclear fragments.
- **Phagocytosis of apoptotic cells or cell bodies, usually by macrophages.** The apoptotic bodies are rapidly degraded within lysosomes, and the adjacent healthy cells migrate or proliferate to replace the space occupied by the now deleted apoptotic cell.

Plasma membranes are thought to remain intact during apoptosis, until the last stages, when they become permeable to normally retained solutes. This classical description is accurate with respect to apoptosis during physiologic conditions such as embryogenesis and deletion of immune cells. However, forms of cell death with features of necrosis as well as of apoptosis are not uncommon after injurious stimuli.[44] Under such conditions, the severity, rather than the specificity, of stimulus determines the form in which death is expressed. If necrotic features are predominant, early plasma membrane damage occurs, and cell swelling, rather than shrinkage, is seen.

On histologic examination, in tissues stained with hematoxylin and eosin, apoptosis involves single cells or small clusters of cells. The apoptotic cell appears as a round or oval mass of intensely eosinophilic cytoplasm with dense nuclear chromatin fragments (Fig. 1–26). Because the cell shrinkage and formation of apoptotic bodies are rapid and the fragments are quickly phagocytosed, considerable apoptosis may occur in tissues before it becomes apparent in histologic sections. In addition, apoptosis—in contrast to necrosis—does not elicit inflammation, making it more difficult to detect histologically.

BIOCHEMICAL FEATURES OF APOPTOSIS

Apoptotic cells usually exhibit a distinctive constellation of biochemical modifications that underlie the structural changes described above. Some of these features may be seen in necrotic cells also, but other alterations are more specific.

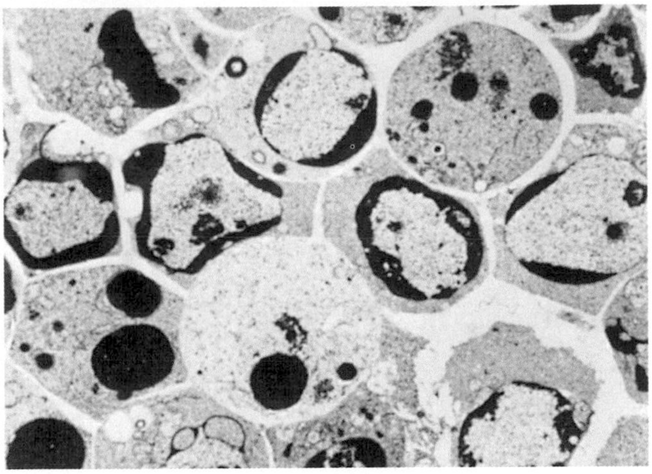

FIGURE 1–25 Ultrastructural features of apoptosis. Some nuclear fragments show peripheral crescents of compacted chromatin, whereas others are uniformly dense. (From Kerr JFR, Harmon BV: Definition and incidence of apoptosis: a historical perspective. In Tomei LD, Cope FO (eds): Apoptosis: The Molecular Basis of Cell Death. Cold Spring Harbor, NY, Cold Spring Harbor Laboratory Press, 1991, pp 5–29.)

Protein Cleavage. A specific feature of apoptosis is protein hydrolysis involving the activation of several members of a family of cysteine proteases named *caspases*.[45] Many caspases are present in normal cells as inactive pro-enzymes, and they need to be activated to induce apoptosis. Active caspases cleave many vital cellular proteins, such as lamins, and thus break up the nuclear scaffold and cytoskeleton; in addition, caspases activate DNAses, which degrade nuclear DNA. These changes underlie the nuclear and cytoplasmic structural alterations seen in apoptotic cells.

DNA Breakdown. Apoptotic cells exhibit a characteristic breakdown of DNA into large 50- to 300-kilobase pieces.[46] Subsequently, there is internucleosomal cleavage of DNA into oligonucleosomes, in multiples of 180 to 200 base pairs, by Ca^{2+}- and Mg^{2+}-dependent endonucleases. The fragments may be visualized by agarose gel electrophoresis as DNA ladders (Fig. 1–27). Endonuclease activity also forms the basis for detecting cell death by cytochemical techniques that recognize double-stranded breaks of DNA.[47] However, internucleosomal DNA cleavage is not specific for apoptosis. A "smeared" pattern of DNA fragmentation is thought to be indicative of necrosis, but this may be a late autolytic phenomenon, and typical DNA ladders may be seen in necrotic cells as well.[47]

Phagocytic Recognition. Apoptotic cells express phosphatidylserine in the outer layers of their plasma membranes, the phospholipid having "flipped" out from the inner layers. (Because of these changes, apoptotic cells can be identified by binding of special dyes, such as Annexin V.) In some types of apoptosis, thrombospondin, an adhesive glycoprotein, is also expressed on the surfaces of apoptotic bodies, and other proteins secreted by phagocytes may bind to apoptotic cells and opsonize the cells for phagocytosis.[48] These alterations permit the early recognition of dead cells by macrophages, resulting in phagocytosis without the release of proinflammatory cellular components.[49] In this way, the apoptotic response dis-

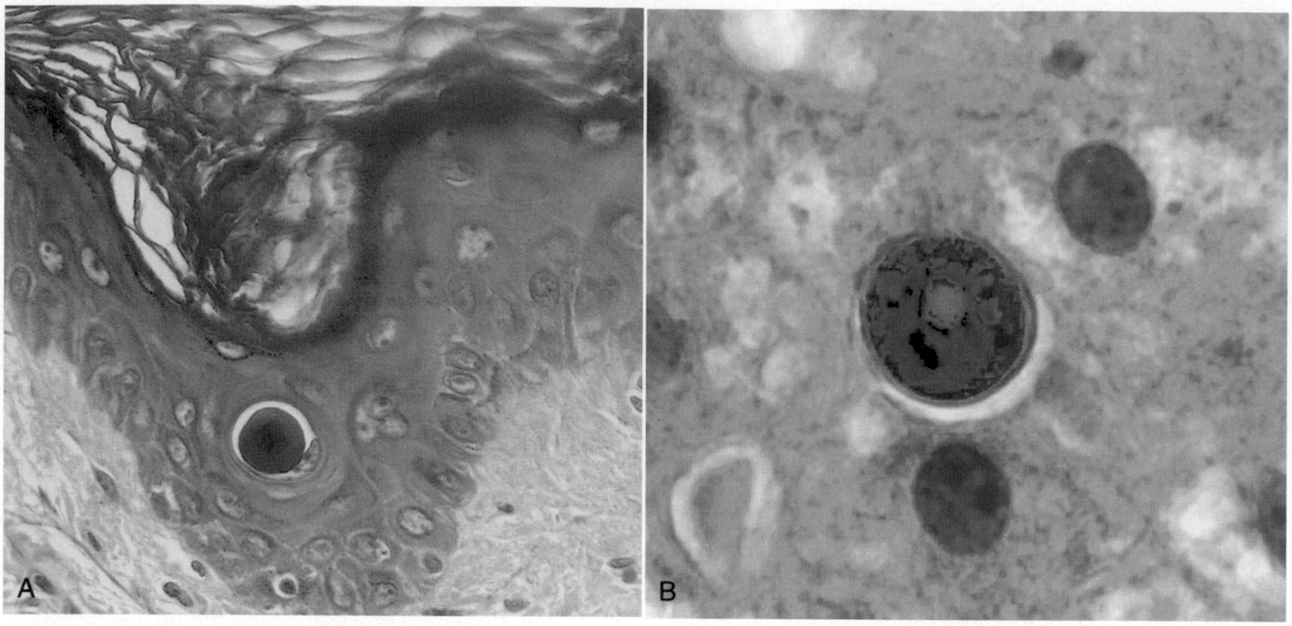

FIGURE 1–26 *A,* Apoptosis of epidermal cells in an immune-mediated reaction. The apoptotic cells are visible in the epidermis with intensely eosinophilic cytoplasm and small, dense nuclei. H&E stain. (Courtesy of Dr. Scott Granter, Brigham and Women's Hospital, Boston, MA.) *B,* High power of apoptotic cell in liver in immune-mediated hepatic cell injury. (Courtesy of Dr. Dhanpat Jain, Yale University, New Haven, CT.)

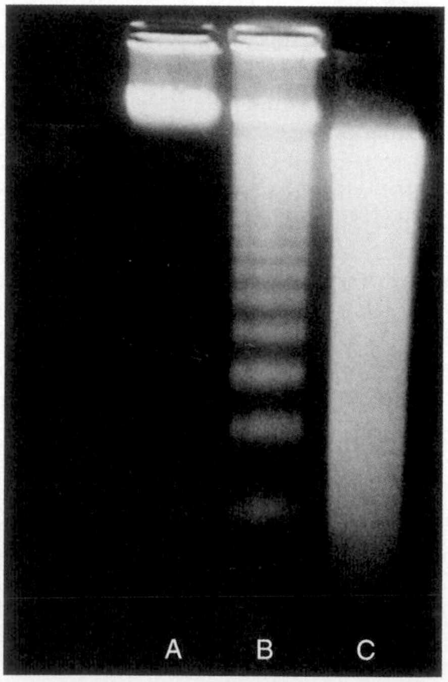

FIGURE 1–27 Agarose gel electrophoresis of DNA extracted from culture cells. Ethidium bromide stain; photographed under ultraviolet illumination. *Lane A,* Control culture. *Lane B,* Culture of cells exposed to heat showing extensive apoptosis; note ladder pattern of DNA fragments, which represent multiples of oligonucleosomes. *Lane C,* Culture showing massive necrosis; note diffuse smearing of DNA. The ladder pattern is produced by enzymatic cleavage of nuclear DNA into nucleosome-sized fragments, usually multiples of 180–200 base pairs. *These patterns are characteristic of but not specific for apoptosis and necrosis, respectively.* (From Kerr JFR, Harmon BV: Definition and incidence of apoptosis: a historical perspective. In Tomei LD, Cope FO [eds]: Apoptosis: The Molecular Basis of Cell Death. Cold Spring Harbor, NY, Cold Spring Harbor Laboratory Press, 1991, p 13.)

poses of cells with minimal compromise to the surrounding tissue.

MECHANISMS OF APOPTOSIS

Apoptosis is induced by a cascade of molecular events that may be initiated in distinct ways and culminate in the activation of caspases (Fig. 1–28).[45] Because too much or too little apoptosis is thought to underlie many diseases, such as degenerative diseases and cancer, there is great interest in elucidating the mechanisms of this form of cell death. Tremendous progress has been made in our understanding of apoptosis. One of the remarkable facts to emerge is that the basic mechanisms of apoptosis are conserved in all metazoans.[50] In fact, some of the major breakthroughs came from observations made in the nematode *Caenorhabditis elegans*, whose development proceeds by a highly reproducible, programmed pattern of cell growth followed by cell death. Studies of mutant worms have allowed the identification of specific genes (called *ced* genes, for *ce*ll *d*eath abnormal) that initiate or inhibit apoptosis and for which there are defined mammalian homologues.

The process of apoptosis may be divided into an initiation phase, during which caspases become catalytically active, and an execution phase, during which these enzymes act to cause cell death. Initiation of apoptosis occurs principally by signals from two distinct but convergent pathways — the extrinsic, or receptor-initiated, pathway and the intrinsic, or mitochondrial, pathway. Both pathways converge to activate caspases. We will describe these two pathways separately because they involve largely distinct molecular interactions, but it is important to remember that they may be interconnected at numerous steps.

The Extrinsic (Death Receptor–Initiated) Pathway. This pathway is initiated by engagement of cell surface death recep-

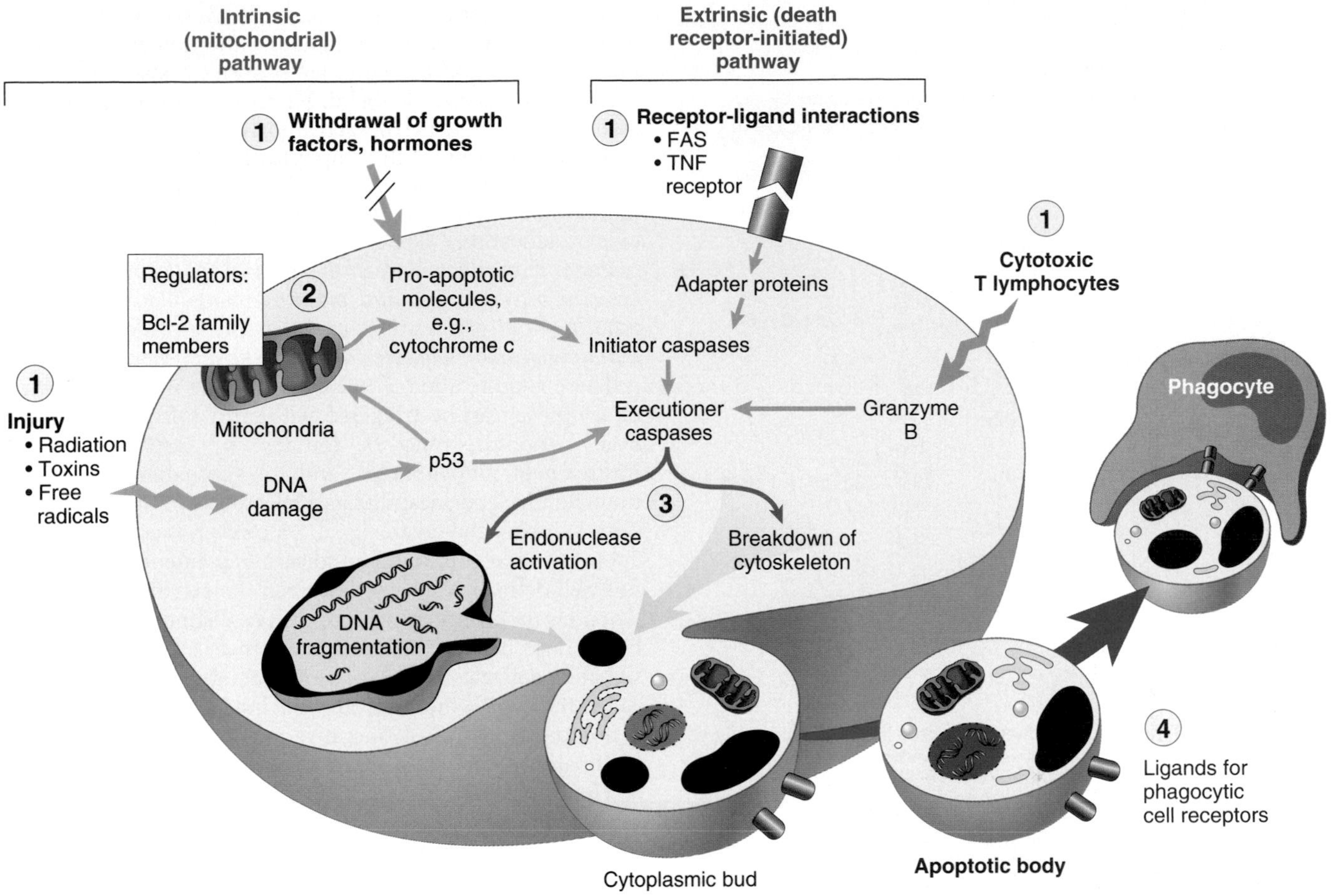

FIGURE 1–28 Mechanisms of apoptosis. Labeled (1) are some of the major inducers of apoptosis. These include specific death ligands (tumor necrosis factor [TNF] and Fas ligand), withdrawal of growth factors or hormones, and injurious agents (e.g., radiation). Some stimuli (such as cytotoxic cells) directly activate execution caspases *(right).* Others act by way of adapter proteins and initiator caspases, or by mitochondrial events involving cytochrome *c.* (2) Control and regulation are influenced by members of the Bcl-2 family of proteins, which can either inhibit or promote the cell's death. (3) Executioner caspases activate latent cytoplasmic endonucleases and proteases that degrade nuclear and cytoskeletal proteins. This results in a cascade of intracellular degradation, including fragmentation of nuclear chromatin and breakdown of the cytoskeleton. (4) The end result is formation of apoptotic bodies containing intracellular organelles and other cytosolic components; these bodies also express new ligands for binding and uptake by phagocytic cells.

tors on a variety of cells.[51] Death receptors are members of the tumor necrosis factor receptor family that contain a cytoplasmic domain involved in protein-protein interactions that is called the *death domain* because it is essential for delivering apoptotic signals. (Some TNF receptor family members do not contain cytoplasmic death domains; their role in triggering apoptosis is much less established). The best-known death receptors are the type 1 TNF receptor (TNFR1) and a related protein called Fas (CD95), but several others have been described. The mechanism of apoptosis induced by these death receptors is well illustrated by Fas (Fig. 1–29). When Fas is cross-linked by its ligand, membrane-bound Fas ligand (FasL), three or more molecules of Fas come together, and their cytoplasmic death domains form a binding site for an adapter protein that also contains a death domain and is called FADD (*F*as-*a*ssociated *d*eath *d*omain). FADD that is attached to the death receptors in turn binds an inactive form of caspase-8 (and, in humans, caspase-10), again via a death domain. Multiple pro-caspase-8 molecules are thus brought into proximity, and they cleave one another to generate active caspase-8. The enzyme then triggers a cascade of caspase activation by cleaving and thereby activating other pro-caspases, and the active enzymes mediate the execution phase of apoptosis (discussed below). This pathway of apoptosis can be inhibited by a protein called FLIP, which binds to pro-caspase-8 but cannot cleave and activate the enzyme because it lacks enzymatic activity.[52] Some viruses and normal cells produce FLIP and use this inhibitor to protect infected and normal cells from Fas-mediated apoptosis. The sphingolipid ceramide has been implicated as an intermediate between death receptors and caspase activation, but the role of this pathway is unclear and remains controversial.[53]

The Intrinsic (Mitochondrial) Pathway. This pathway of apoptosis is the result of increased mitochondrial permeability and release of pro-apoptotic molecules into the cytoplasm, without a role for death receptors.[54,55] Growth factors and other survival signals stimulate the production of anti-apoptotic members of the Bcl-2 family of proteins.[56] This family is named after Bcl-2, which was identified as an oncogene in a B cell lymphoma and is homologous to the *C. elegans* protein, Ced-9. There are more than 20 proteins in this family, all of which function to regulate apoptosis; the two main anti-apoptotic ones are Bcl-2 and Bcl-x. These anti-apoptotic proteins normally reside in mitochondrial membranes and the cyto-

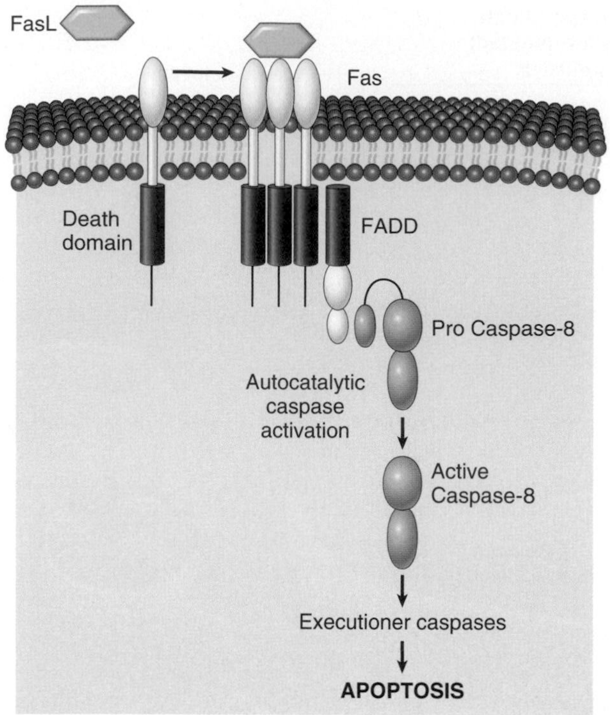

FIGURE 1–29 The extrinsic (death receptor-initiated) pathway of apoptosis, illustrated by the events following Fas engagement (see text).

plasm. When cells are deprived of survival signals or subjected to stress, Bcl-2 and/or Bcl-x are lost from the mitochondrial membrane and are replaced by pro-apoptotic members of the family, such as Bak, Bax, and Bim. When Bcl-2/Bcl-x levels decrease, the permeability of the mitochondrial membrane increases, and several proteins that can activate the caspase cascade leak out (Fig. 1–30). One of these proteins is cytochrome *c*, well known for its role in mitochondrial respiration. In the cytosol, cytochrome *c* binds to a protein called Apaf-1 (apoptosis activating factor-1, homologous to Ced-4 in *C. elegans*), and the complex activates caspase-9.[57] (Bcl-2 and Bcl-x may also directly inhibit Apaf-1 activation, and their loss from cells may permit activation of Apaf-1). Other mitochondrial proteins, such as apoptosis inducing factor (AIF), enter the cytoplasm, where they bind to and neutralize various inhibitors of apoptosis, whose normal function is to block caspase activation.[58] The net result is the initiation of a caspase cascade. Thus, *the essence of this intrinsic pathway is a balance between pro-apoptotic and protective molecules that regulate mitochondrial permeability and the release of death inducers that are normally sequestered within the mitochondria.*

There is quite a lot of evidence that the intrinsic pathway of apoptosis can be triggered without a role for mitochondria.[59] Apoptosis may be initiated by caspase activation upstream of mitochondria, and the subsequent increase in mitochondrial permeability and release of pro-apoptotic molecules amplify the death signal.[46] However, these pathways of apoptosis involving mitochondria-independent initiation are not well defined. We have described the extrinsic and intrinsic pathways for initiating apoptosis as distinct, but there may be overlaps between them. For instance, in hepatocytes, Fas signaling activates a pro-apoptotic member of the Bcl family called Bid, which then activates the mitochondrial pathway. It is not known if such cooperative interactions between apoptosis pathways are active in most other cell types.

The Execution Phase. This final phase of apoptosis is mediated by a proteolytic cascade, toward which the various initiating mechanisms converge. The proteases that mediate the execution phase are highly conserved across species and belong to the caspase family, as previously mentioned. They are mammalian homologues of the *ced-3* gene in *C. elegans*.[44] The term *caspase* is based on two properties of this family of enzymes: the "c" refers to a cysteine protease (i.e., an enzyme with cysteine in its active site), and "aspase" refers to the unique ability of these enzymes to cleave after aspartic acid residues.[60] The caspase family, now including more than 10

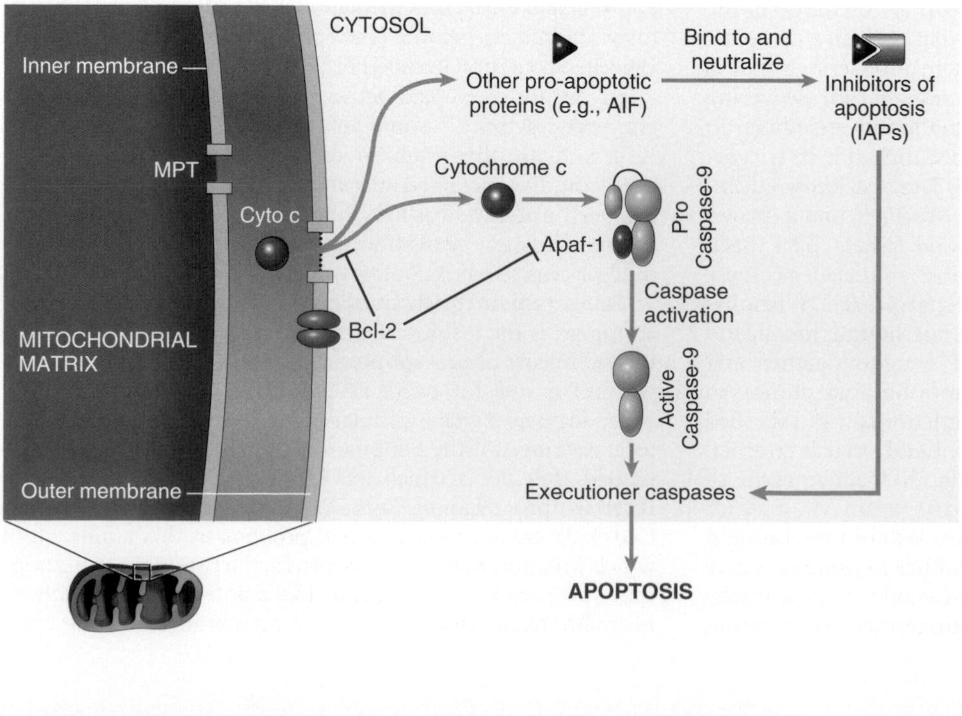

FIGURE 1–30 The intrinsic (mitochondrial) pathway of apoptosis. Death agonists cause changes in the inner mitochondrial membrane, resulting in the mitochondrial permeability transition (MPT) and release of cytochrome *c* and other pro-apoptotic proteins into the cytosol, which activate caspases (see text).

members, can be divided functionally into two basic groups—initiator and executioner—depending on the order in which they are activated during apoptosis.[60] Initiator caspases, as we have seen, include caspase-8 and caspase-9. Several caspases, including caspase-3 and caspase-6, serve as executioners.

Like many proteases, caspases exist as inactive pro-enzymes, or zymogens, and must undergo an activating cleavage for apoptosis to be initiated. Caspases have their own cleavage sites that can be hydrolyzed not only by other caspases but also autocatalytically. After an initiator caspase is cleaved to generate its active form, the enzymatic death program is set in motion by rapid and sequential activation of other caspases. Executioner caspases act on many cellular components. They cleave cytoskeletal and nuclear matrix proteins and thus disrupt the cytoskeleton and lead to breakdown of the nucleus.[60] In the nucleus, the targets of caspase activation include proteins involved in transcription, DNA replication, and DNA repair. In particular, caspase-3 activation converts a cytoplasmic DNase into an active form by cleaving an inhibitor of the enzyme; this DNase induces the characteristic internucleosomal cleavage of DNA, described earlier.

Removal of Dead Cells. At early stages of apoptosis, dying cells secrete soluble factors that recruit phagocytes.[61] This facilitates prompt clearance of apoptotic cells before they undergo secondary necrosis and release their cellular contents (which can result in inflammation). As already alluded to, apoptotic cells and their fragments have marker molecules on their surfaces, which facilitates early recognition by adjacent cells or phagocytes for phagocytic uptake and disposal. Numerous macrophage receptors have been shown to be involved in the binding and engulfment of apoptotic cells. In addition, macrophages can also secrete substances that bind specifically to apoptotic but not live cells and opsonize these cells for phagocytosis. In contrast to markers on apoptotic cells, viable cells appear to prevent their own engulfment by macrophages through expression of certain surface molecules (such as CD31). This process of phagocytosis of apoptotic cells is so efficient that dead cells disappear without leaving a trace, and inflammation is virtually absent.

EXAMPLES OF APOPTOSIS

The signals that induce apoptosis include *lack of growth factor or hormone*, *specific engagement of death receptors*, and particular *injurious agents*. Although the classic example of apoptosis has been programmed death of cells during embryogenesis, we still do not know what triggers apoptosis in this situation. However, many other well-defined examples of apoptosis are known.

Apoptosis After Growth Factor Deprivation. Hormone-sensitive cells deprived of the relevant hormone, lymphocytes that are not stimulated by antigens and cytokines, and neurons deprived of nerve growth factor die by apoptosis.[62] In all these situations, apoptosis is triggered by the intrinsic (mitochondrial) pathway and is attributable to an excess of pro-apoptotic members of the Bcl family relative to anti-apoptotic members.

DNA Damage–Mediated Apoptosis. Exposure of cells to radiation or chemotherapeutic agents induces apoptosis by a mechanism that is initiated by DNA damage (genotoxic stress) and that involves the tumor-suppressor gene *p53*.[63] p53 accumulates when DNA is damaged and arrests the cell cycle (at the G_1 phase) to allow time for repair (Chapter 7). However, if the DNA repair process fails, p53 triggers apoptosis. When p53 is mutated or absent (as it is in certain cancers), it is incapable of inducing apoptosis and it favors cell survival. Thus, p53 seems to serve as a critical "life or death" switch in the case of genotoxic stress. The mechanism by which p53 triggers the distal death effector machinery—the caspases—is complex but seems to involve its well-characterized function in transcriptional activation. Among the proteins whose production is stimulated by p53 are several pro-apoptotic members of the Bcl family, notably Bax and Bak, as well as Apaf-1, mentioned earlier. These proteins activate caspases and cause apoptosis.

Apoptosis Induced by Tumor Necrosis Factor Family of Receptors. As discussed above, the cell surface receptor Fas (CD95) induces apoptosis when it is engaged by Fas ligand (FasL or CD95L), which is produced by cells of the immune system. This system is important in the elimination of lymphocytes that recognize self-antigens, and mutations in Fas or FasL result in autoimmune diseases in humans and mice (Chapter 6).[64]

The cytokine TNF is an important mediator of the inflammatory reaction (Chapter 2), but it is also capable of inducing apoptosis. (The name "tumor necrosis factor" arose not because the cytokine kills tumor cells directly, but because it induces thrombosis of tumor blood vessels, resulting in ischemic death of the tumor.) The binding of TNF to TNFR1 leads to association of the receptor with the adapter protein TRADD (*T*NF *r*eceptor-*a*ssociated *d*eath *d*omain containing protein). TRADD in turn binds to FADD and leads to apoptosis through caspase activation, as with Fas–FasL interactions.[52] The major functions of TNF, however, are mediated not by inducing apoptosis but by activation of the important transcription factor nuclear factor-κB (NF-κB). TNF-mediated signals accomplish this by stimulating degradation of the inhibitor of NF-κB (IκB).[65] The NF-κB/IκB transcriptional regulatory system is important for cell survival and, as we shall see in Chapter 2, for a number of inflammatory responses. Since TNF can induce cell death and promote cell survival, what determines this yin and yang of its action? The answer is unclear, but it probably depends on which adapter protein attaches to the TNF receptor after binding of the cytokine. TRADD and FADD favor apoptosis, and other adapter proteins, called TRAFs (TNF receptor associated factors) favor NF-κB activation and survival.

Cytotoxic T-Lymphocyte–Mediated Apoptosis. Cytotoxic T lymphocytes (CTLs) recognize foreign antigens presented on the surface of infected host cells (Chapter 6). On recognition, CTLs secrete *perforin*, a transmembrane pore-forming molecule, which allows entry of the CTL granule serine protease called *granzyme B*. Granzyme B has the ability to cleave proteins at aspartate residues and is able to activate a variety of cellular caspases.[66] *In this way, the CTL kills target cells through bypassing the upstream signaling events and directly induces the effector phase of apoptosis.* CTLs also express FasL on their surfaces and kill target cells by ligation of Fas receptors, as described earlier.

Dysregulated apoptosis ("too little or too much") has been postulated to explain components of a wide range of diseases.[67] In essence, two groups of disorders may result from such dysregulation:

- *Disorders associated with defective apoptosis and increased cell survival.* Here, an inappropriately low rate of apoptosis may prolong the survival or reduce the turnover of abnormal cells. These accumulated cells can give rise to: (1) *cancers*, especially tumors with *p53* mutations, or hormone-dependent tumors, such as breast, prostate, or ovarian cancers (Chapter 7); and (2) *autoimmune disorders*, which could arise if autoreactive lymphocytes are not eliminated after encounter with self antigens (Chapter 6).
- *Disorders associated with increased apoptosis and excessive cell death.* These diseases are characterized by a marked loss of normal or protective cells and include: (1) *neurodegenerative diseases*, manifested by loss of specific sets of neurons, such as in the spinal muscular atrophies (Chapter 27); (2) *ischemic injury*, as in myocardial infarction (Chapter 12) and stroke (Chapter 28); and (3) *death of virus-infected cells*, in many viral infections (Chapter 8).

Subcellular Responses to Injury

To this point in the chapter, the focus has been on the cell as a unit. Certain conditions, however, are associated with distinctive alterations in cell organelles or the cytoskeleton. Some of these alterations coexist with those described for acute lethal injury; others represent more chronic forms of cell injury; still others are adaptive responses that serve to maintain homeostasis. Here we touch on only some of the more common or interesting of these reactions.

LYSOSOMAL CATABOLISM

Primary lysosomes are membrane-bound intracellular organelles that contain a variety of hydrolytic enzymes, including acid phosphatase, glucuronidase, sulfatase, ribonuclease, and collagenase. These enzymes are synthesized in the rough endoplasmic reticulum and then packaged into vesicles in the Golgi apparatus. Primary lysosomes fuse with membrane-bound vacuoles that contain material to be digested, forming *secondary lysosomes* or *phagolysosomes*. Lysosomes are involved in the breakdown of phagocytosed material in one of two ways: heterophagy and autophagy (Fig. 1–31).

- **Heterophagy.** Heterophagy is the process of lysosomal digestion of materials ingested from the extracellular environment. Extracellular materials are taken up by cells through the general process of *endocytosis*. Uptake of particulate matter is known as *phagocytosis*; uptake of soluble smaller macromolecules is called *pinocytosis*. Extracellular materials are endocytosed into vacuoles (endosomes or phagosomes), which eventually fuse with lysosomes to form phagolysosomes, where the engulfed material is digested. Heterophagy is most common in the "professional" phagocytes, such as neutrophils and macrophages, although it may also occur in other cell types. Examples of heterophagocytosis include the uptake and digestion of bacteria by neutrophils and the removal of apoptotic cells by macrophages.
- **Autophagy.** Autophagy refers to lysosomal digestion of the cell's own components. In this process, intracellular organelles and portions of cytosol are first sequestered from the cytoplasm in an *autophagic vacuole* formed from ribosome-free regions of the rough endoplasmic reticulum. The vacuole fuses with lysosomes or Golgi elements to form an *autophagolysosome*.[68,69] Autophagy is a common phenomenon involved in the removal of damaged organelles during cell injury and the cellular remodeling of differentiation, and it is particularly pronounced in cells undergoing atrophy induced by nutrient deprivation or hormonal involution.

The enzymes in lysosomes are capable of degrading most proteins and carbohydrates, but some lipids remain undigested. Lysosomes with undigested debris may persist within cells as *residual bodies* or may be extruded. *Lipofuscin pigment* granules represent undigested material derived from intracel-

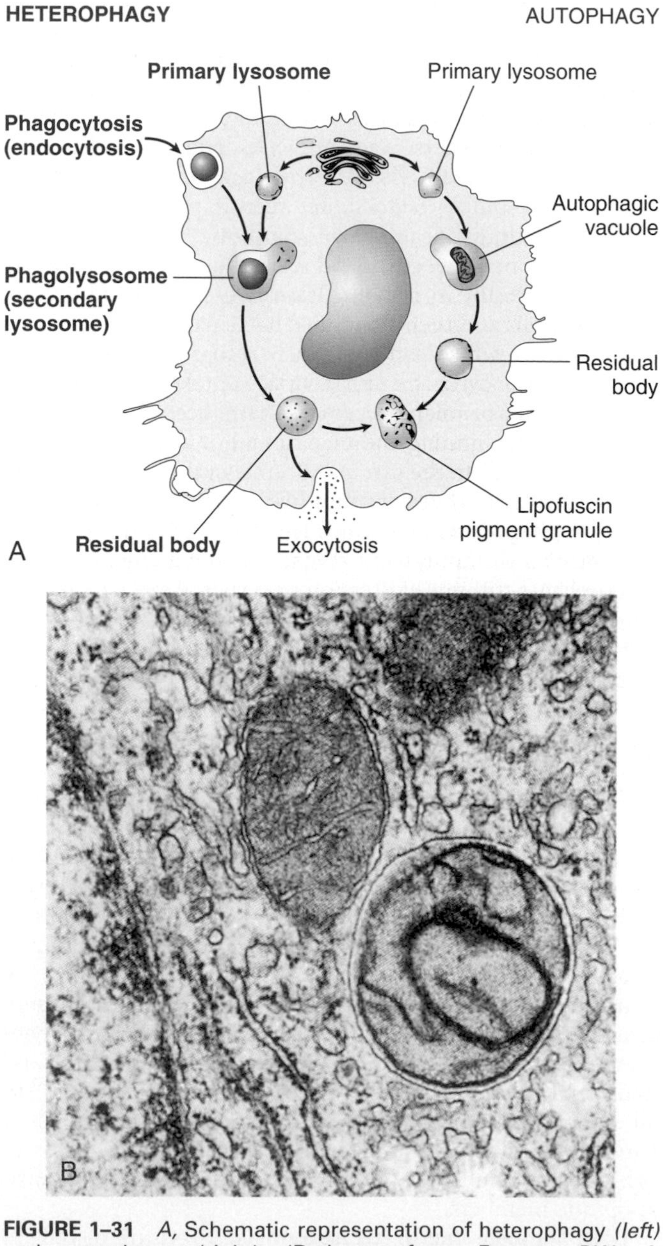

FIGURE 1–31 *A,* Schematic representation of heterophagy *(left)* and autophagy *(right).* (Redrawn from Fawcett DW: A Textbook of Histology, 11th ed. Philadelphia, WB Saunders, 1986, p 17.) *B,* Electron micrograph of an autophagolysosome containing a degenerating mitochondrion and amorphous material.

lular lipid peroxidation. Certain indigestible pigments, such as carbon particles inhaled from the atmosphere or inoculated pigment in tattoos, can persist in phagolysosomes of macrophages for decades.

Lysosomes are also repositories where cells sequester abnormal substances that cannot be completely metabolized. Hereditary *lysosomal storage disorders*, caused by deficiencies of enzymes that degrade various macromolecules, result in the accumulation of abnormal amounts of these compounds in the lysosomes of cells all over the body, particularly neurons, leading to severe abnormalities (Chapter 5). Certain drugs can disturb lysosomal function and cause *acquired or drug-induced (iatrogenic) lysosomal diseases*. Drugs in this group include chloroquine, an antimalarial agent that raises the internal pH of the lysosome, thus inactivating its enzymes. By inhibiting lysosomal enzymes, chloroquine reduces tissue damage in inflammatory reactions, which are mediated in part by enzymes released from leukocytes; this action is the basis of the use of the drug in autoimmune diseases like rheumatoid arthritis. The same inhibition of enzymes, however, can result in abnormal accumulation of glycogen and phospholipids in lysosomes, causing toxic myopathy.

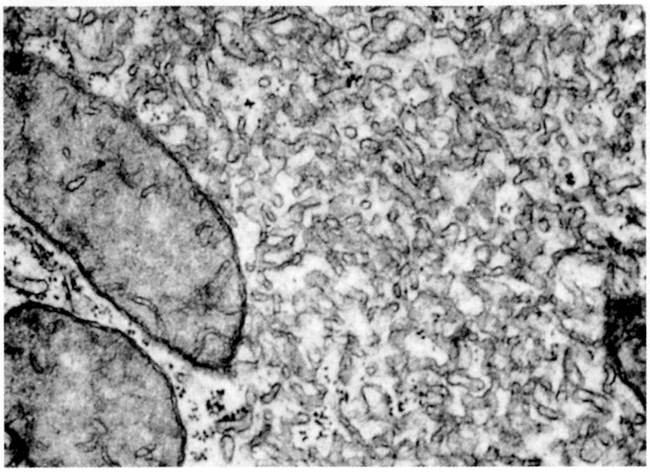

FIGURE 1–32 Electron micrograph of liver from phenobarbital-treated rat showing marked increase in smooth endoplasmic reticulum. (From Jones AL, Fawcett DW: Hypertrophy of the agranular endoplasmic reticulum in hamster liver induced by Phenobarbital. J Histochem Cytochem 14:215, 1966. Courtesy of Dr. Fawcett.)

INDUCTION (HYPERTROPHY) OF SMOOTH ENDOPLASMIC RETICULUM

The smooth ER is involved in the metabolism of various chemicals, and cells exposed to these chemicals show hypertrophy of the ER as an adaptive response that may have important functional consequences. Protracted use of barbiturates leads to a state of tolerance, with a decrease in the effects of the drug and the need to use increasing doses. Patients are said to have "adapted" to the medication. This adaptation is due to increased volume (hypertrophy) of the smooth ER of hepatocytes, which metabolizes the drug (Fig. 1–32). Barbiturates are modified in the liver by oxidative demethylation, which involves the P-450 mixed function oxidase system found in the smooth ER. The role of these enzyme modifications is to increase the solubility of a variety of compounds (e.g., alcohol, steroids, eicosanoids, and carcinogens as well as insecticides and other environmental pollutants) and thereby facilitate their secretion.[37] Although this is often thought of as "detoxification," many compounds are rendered *more* injurious by P-450 modification. In addition, the products formed by this oxidative metabolism include reactive oxygen species, which can cause injury of the cell. With prolonged use, the barbiturates (and many other agents) stimulate the synthesis of more enzymes, as well as more smooth ER. In this manner, the cell is better able to modify the drugs and adapt to its altered environment. Cells adapted to one drug have increased capacity to metabolize other compounds handled by the system. Thus, if patients taking phenobarbital for epilepsy increase their alcohol intake they may have subtherapeutic levels of the antiseizure medication because of induction of smooth ER in response to the alcohol.

MITOCHONDRIAL ALTERATIONS

We have seen that mitochondrial dysfunction plays an important role in cell injury and apoptosis. In addition, various alterations in the number, size, and shape of mitochondria occur in some pathologic conditions. For example, in cell hypertrophy and atrophy, there is an increase and decrease, respectively, in the number of mitochondria in cells. Mitochondria may assume extremely large and abnormal shapes (megamitochondria), as can be seen in the liver in alcoholic liver disease and in certain nutritional deficiencies (Fig. 1–33). Abnormalities of mitochondria are now recognized as the basis of many genetic diseases[70] (Chapter 5). In certain inherited metabolic diseases of skeletal muscle, the *mitochondrial myopathies*, defects in mitochondrial metabolism are associated with increased numbers of mitochondria that are often unusually large, have abnormal cristae, and contain crystalloids (Chapter 27). In addition, certain benign tumors found in salivary glands, thyroid, parathyroids, and kidneys consist of cells (sometimes called "oncocytes") with abundant enlarged mitochondria, giving the cell a distinctly eosinophilic appearance.

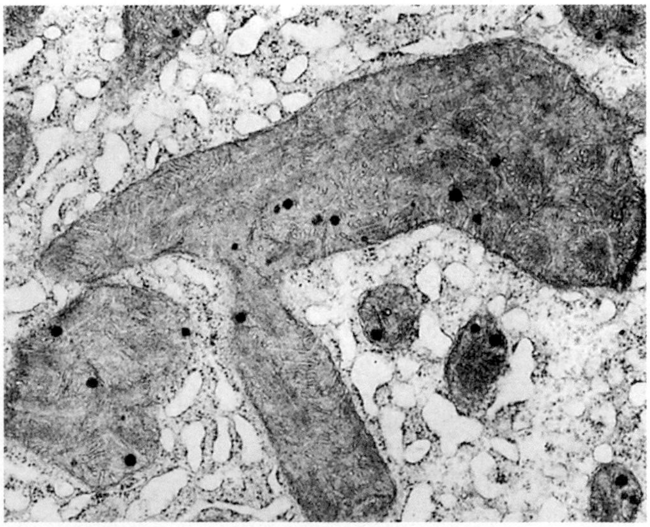

FIGURE 1–33 Enlarged, abnormally shaped mitochondria from the liver of a patient with alcoholic cirrhosis. Note also crystalline formations in the mitochondria.

CYTOSKELETAL ABNORMALITIES

Abnormalities of the cytoskeleton underlie a variety of pathologic states. The *cytoskeleton* consists of microtubules (20 to 25 nm in diameter), thin actin filaments (6 to 8 nm), thick myosin filaments (15 nm), and various classes of intermediate filaments (10 nm). Several other nonpolymerized and nonfilamentous forms of contractile proteins also exist. Cytoskeletal abnormalities may be reflected by: (1) defects in cell function, such as cell locomotion and intracellular organelle movements, and (2) in some instances by intracellular accumulations of fibrillar material. Only a few examples are cited.

- *Thin filaments.* Thin filaments are composed of actin, myosin, and their associated regulatory proteins.[71] Functioning thin filaments are essential for various stages of leukocyte movement or the ability of such cells to perform phagocytosis adequately. Some drugs and toxins target actin filaments and thus affect these processes. For example, cytochalasin B prevents polymerization of actin filaments, and phalloidin, a toxin of the mushroom *Amanita phalloides*, also binds actin filaments.
- *Microtubules.* Defects in the organization of microtubules can inhibit sperm motility, causing male sterility, and can immobilize the cilia of respiratory epithelium, causing interference with the ability of this epithelium to clear inhaled bacteria, leading to bronchiectasis (Kartagener's syndrome, or the *immotile cilia syndrome*; Chapter 15). Microtubules, like microfilaments, are essential for leukocyte migration and phagocytosis. Drugs such as colchicine bind to tubulin and prevent the assembly of microtubules. The drug is used in acute attacks of gout to prevent leukocyte migration and phagocytosis in response to deposition of urate crystals. Microtubules are an essential component of the mitotic spindle, which is required for cell division. Drugs that bind to microtubules (e.g., vinca alkaloids) can be antiproliferative and therefore act as antitumor agents.
- *Intermediate filaments.* These components provide a flexible intracellular scaffold that organizes the cytoplasm and resists forces applied to the cell.[72] The intermediate filaments are divided into five classes, including keratin filaments (characteristic of epithelial cells), neurofilaments (neurons), desmin filaments (muscle cells), vimentin filaments (connective tissue cells), and glial filaments (astrocytes). Accumulations of keratin filaments and neurofilaments are associated with certain types of cell injury. For example, the *Mallory body*, or "alcoholic hyalin," is an eosinophilic intracytoplasmic inclusion in liver cells that is characteristic of alcoholic liver disease,[73] although it can be present in other conditions. Such inclusions are composed predominantly of *keratin* intermediate filaments (Fig. 1–34). In the nervous system, neurofilaments are present in the axon, where they provide structural support. The *neurofibrillary tangle* found in the brain in Alzheimer's disease contains microtubule-associated proteins and neurofilaments, a reflection of a disrupted neuronal cytoskeleton (Chapter 28). Mutations in intermediate filament genes cause multiple human disorders, including myopathies, neurologic diseases, and skin diseases.

Much of the emphasis on the functions of the cytoskeleton has been on its mechanical role, in maintaining cellular architecture and in cell attachment and locomotion. It has recently been appreciated that *cytoskeletal proteins are linked to many cellular receptors*, such as lymphocyte receptors for antigens, and are active participants in signal transduction by these receptors (Chapter 3). Therefore, defects in the links between receptors and cytoskeletal proteins may affect many cellular responses. The *Wiskott-Aldrich syndrome* is an inherited disease characterized by eczema, platelet abnormalities, and immune deficiency. The protein that is mutated in this disease is involved in linking lymphocyte antigen receptors (and perhaps other receptors) to the cytoskeleton, and defects in the protein interfere with diverse cellular responses (Chapter 6).[74]

Intracellular Accumulations

One of the manifestations of metabolic derangements in cells is the intracellular accumulation of abnormal amounts of various substances. The stockpiled substances fall into three categories: (1) a *normal cellular constituent* accumulated in excess, such as water, lipids, proteins, and carbohydrates; (2)

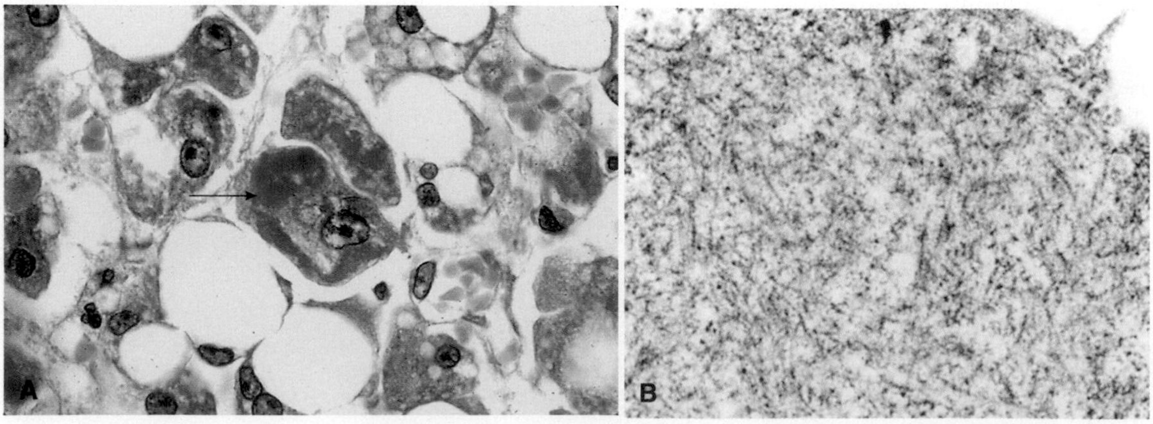

FIGURE 1–34 *A,* The liver of alcohol abuse (chronic alcoholism). Hyaline inclusions in the hepatic parenchymal cell in the center appear as eosinophilic networks disposed about the nuclei *(arrow)*. *B,* Electron micrograph of alcoholic hyalin. The material is composed of intermediate (prekeratin) filaments and an amorphous matrix.

an *abnormal substance,* either exogenous, such as a mineral or products of infectious agents, or endogenous, such as a product of abnormal synthesis or metabolism; and (3) a *pigment.* These substances may accumulate either transiently or permanently, and they may be harmless to the cells, but on occasion they are severely toxic. The substance may be located in either the cytoplasm (frequently within phagolysosomes) or the nucleus. In some instances, the cell may be producing the abnormal substance, and in others it may be merely storing products of pathologic processes occurring elsewhere in the body.

Many processes result in abnormal intracellular accumulations, but most accumulations are attributable to three types of abnormalities (Fig. 1–35).

1. *A normal endogenous substance is produced at a normal or increased rate, but the rate of metabolism is inadequate to remove it.* An example of this type of process is fatty change in the liver because of intracellular accumulation of triglycerides (see later). Another is the appearance of reabsorption protein droplets in renal tubules because of increased leakage of protein from the glomerulus.
2. *A normal or abnormal endogenous substance accumulates because of genetic or acquired defects in the metabolism, packaging, transport, or secretion of these substances.* One example is the group of conditions caused by genetic defects of specific enzymes involved in the metabolism of lipid and carbohydrates resulting in intracellular deposition of these substances, largely in lysosomes. These so-called storage diseases are discussed in Chapter 5. Another is alpha$_1$-antitrypsin deficiency, in which a single amino acid substitution in the enzyme results in defects in protein folding and accumulation of the enzyme in the endoplasmic reticulum of the liver in the form of globular eosinophilic inclusions (see later and Chapter 18).
3. *An abnormal exogenous substance is deposited and accumulates* because the cell has neither the enzymatic machinery to degrade the substance nor the ability to transport it to other sites. Accumulations of carbon particles and such nonmetabolizable chemicals as silica particles are examples of this type of alteration.

Whatever the nature and origin of the intracellular accumulation, it implies the storage of some product by individual cells. If the overload is due to a systemic derangement and can be brought under control, the accumulation is reversible. In genetic storage diseases, accumulation is progressive, and the cells may become so overloaded as to cause secondary injury, leading in some instances to death of the tissue and the patient.

LIPIDS

All major classes of lipids can accumulate in cells: triglycerides, cholesterol/cholesterol esters, and phospholipids. Phospholipids are components of the myelin figures found in necrotic cells. In addition, abnormal complexes of lipids and carbohydrates accumulate in the lysosomal storage diseases (Chapter 5). Here we concentrate on triglyceride and cholesterol accumulations.

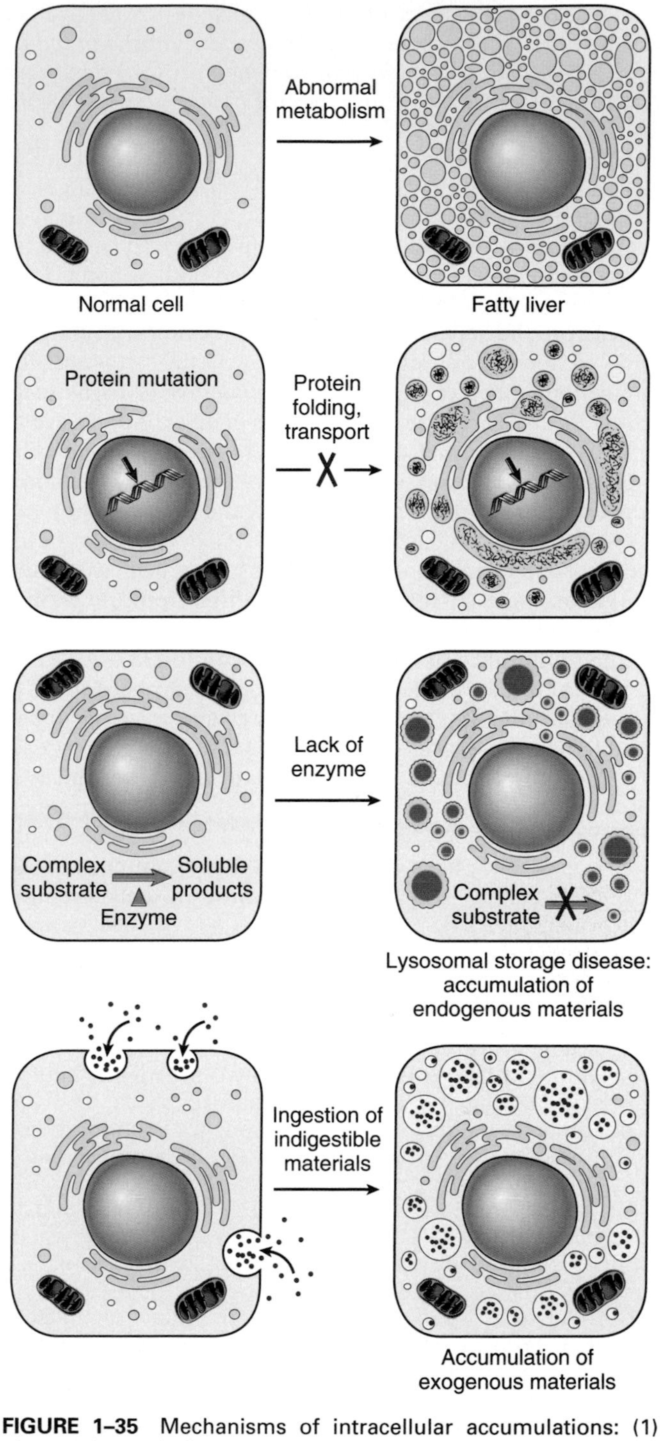

FIGURE 1–35 Mechanisms of intracellular accumulations: (1) abnormal metabolism, as in fatty change in the liver; (2) mutations causing alterations in protein folding and transport, as in alpha$_1$-antitrypsin deficiency; (3) deficiency of critical enzymes that prevent breakdown of substrates that accumulate in lysosomes, as in lysosomal storage diseases; and (4) inability to degrade phagocytosed particles, as in hemosiderosis and carbon pigment accumulation.

Steatosis (Fatty Change)

The terms *steatosis* and *fatty change* describe abnormal accumulations of triglycerides within parenchymal cells. Fatty change is often seen in the liver because it is the major organ involved in fat metabolism, but it also occurs in heart, muscle, and kidney. The causes of steatosis include toxins, protein malnutrition, diabetes mellitus, obesity, and anoxia. *In industrialized nations, by far the most common cause of significant fatty change in the liver (fatty liver) is alcohol abuse* (Chapter 18).[75]

Different mechanisms account for triglyceride accumulation in the liver. Free fatty acids from adipose tissue or ingested food are normally transported into hepatocytes. In the liver, they are esterified to triglycerides, converted into cholesterol or phospholipids, or oxidized to ketone bodies. Some fatty acids are synthesized from acetate as well. Release of triglycerides from the hepatocytes requires association with apoproteins to form lipoproteins, which may then traverse the circulation (Chapter 4). *Excess accumulation of triglycerides within the liver may result from defects in any one of the events in the sequence from fatty acid entry to lipoprotein exit* (Fig. 1–36*A*). A number of such defects are induced by alcohol, a hepatotoxin that alters mitochondrial and microsomal functions. CCl_4 and protein malnutrition act by decreasing synthesis of apoproteins. Anoxia inhibits fatty acid oxidation. Starvation increases fatty acid mobilization from the peripheral stores.

The significance of fatty change depends on the cause and severity of the accumulation. When mild, it may have no effect on cellular function. More severe fatty change may impair cellular function, typically when some vital intracellular process is also impaired (e.g., in CCl_4 poisoning). As a severe form of injury, fatty change may be a harbinger of cell death. In recent years, nonalcoholic steatohepatitis and nonalcoholic fatty liver disease have been recognized as fairly common disease entities that may lead to cirrhosis and even hepatocellular cancer (Chapter 18).

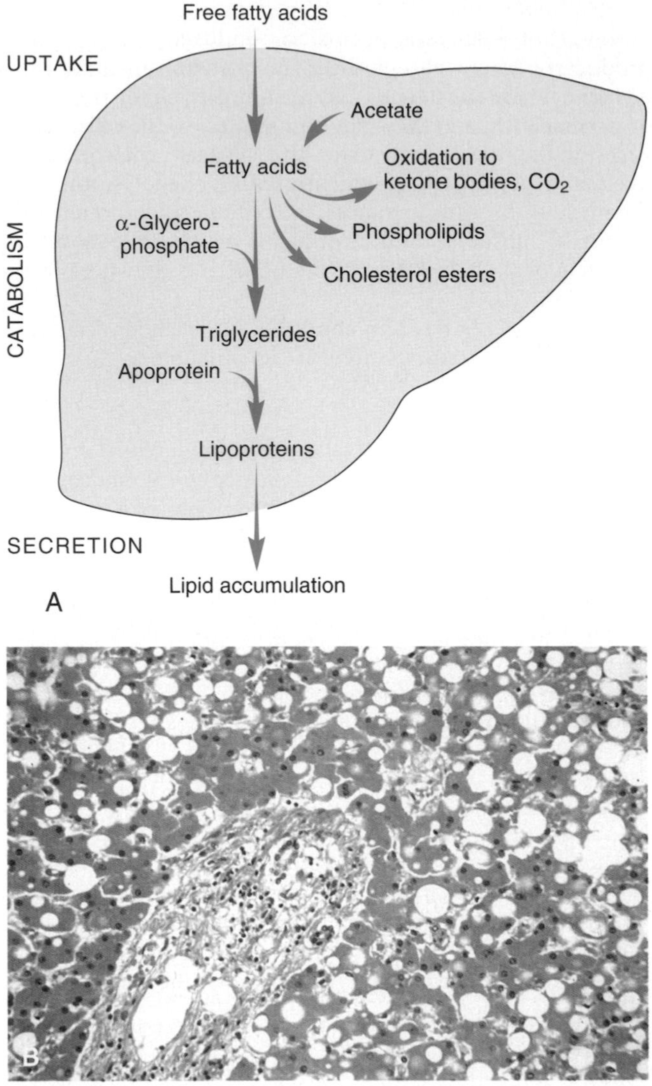

FIGURE 1–36 Fatty liver. *A*, Schematic diagram of the possible mechanisms leading to accumulation of triglycerides in fatty liver. Defects in any of the steps of uptake, catabolism, or secretion can result in lipid accumulation. *B*, High-power detail of fatty change of the liver. In most cells, the well-preserved nucleus is squeezed into the displaced rim of cytoplasm about the fat vacuole. (*B*, Courtesy of Dr. James Crawford, Department of Pathology, Yale University School of Medicine, New Haven, CT.)

Morphology. Fatty change is most often seen in the liver and heart. In all organs, fatty change appears as clear vacuoles within parenchymal cells. Intracellular accumulations of water or polysaccharides (e.g., glycogen) may also produce clear vacuoles, and it becomes necessary to resort to special techniques to distinguish these three types of clear vacuoles. The identification of lipids requires the avoidance of fat solvents commonly used in paraffin embedding for routine hematoxylin and eosin stains. To identify the fat, it is necessary to prepare frozen tissue sections of either fresh or aqueous formalin-fixed tissues. The sections may then be stained with Sudan IV or Oil Red-O, both of which impart an orange-red color to the contained lipids. The periodic acid-Schiff (PAS) reaction is commonly employed to identify glycogen, although it is by no means specific. When neither fat nor polysaccharide can be demonstrated within a clear vacuole, it is presumed to contain water or fluid with a low protein content.

Liver. In the liver, mild fatty change may not affect the gross appearance. With progressive accumulation, the organ enlarges and becomes increasingly yellow until, in extreme instances, the liver may weigh 3 to 6 kg and be transformed into a bright yellow, soft, greasy organ.

Fatty change begins with the development of minute, membrane-bound inclusions (liposomes) closely applied to the endoplasmic reticulum. Fatty change is first seen by light microscopy as small vacuoles in the cytoplasm around the nucleus. As the process progresses, the vacuoles coalesce, creating cleared spaces that displace the nucleus to the periphery of the cell (Fig. 1–36*B*). Occasionally, contiguous cells rupture, and the enclosed fat globules coalesce, producing so-called fatty cysts.

Heart. Lipid is found in cardiac muscle in the form of small droplets, occurring in two patterns. In one, prolonged moderate hypoxia, such as that produced by profound anemia, causes intracellular deposits of fat, which create grossly apparent bands of yellowed myocardium alternating with bands of darker, red-brown, uninvolved myocardium **(tigered effect)**. The other pattern of hypoxia is produced by more profound hypoxia or by some forms of myocarditis (e.g., diphtheria) and shows more uniformly affected myocytes.

Cholesterol and Cholesterol Esters

The cellular metabolism of cholesterol (discussed in detail in Chapter 5) is tightly regulated such that most cells use cholesterol for the synthesis of cell membranes without intracellular accumulation of cholesterol or cholesterol esters. Accumulations, however, manifested histologically by intracellular vacuoles, are seen in several pathologic processes.

- *Atherosclerosis.* In atherosclerotic plaques, smooth muscle cells and macrophages within the intimal layer of the aorta and large arteries are filled with lipid vacuoles, most of which are made up of cholesterol and cholesterol esters. Such cells have a foamy appearance (foam cells), and aggregates of them in the intima produce the yellow cholesterol-laden atheromas characteristic of this serious disorder. Some of these fat-laden cells rupture, releasing lipids into the extracellular space. The mechanisms of cholesterol accumulation in both cell types in atherosclerosis are discussed in detail in Chapter 11. The extracellular cholesterol esters may crystallize in the shape of long needles, producing quite distinctive clefts in tissue sections.
- *Xanthomas.* Intracellular accumulation of cholesterol within macrophages is also characteristic of acquired and hereditary hyperlipidemic states. Clusters of foamy cells are found in the subepithelial connective tissue of the skin and in tendons, producing tumorous masses known as xanthomas.
- *Inflammation and necrosis.* Foamy macrophages are frequently found at sites of cell injury and inflammation, owing to phagocytosis of cholesterol from the membranes of injured cells, including parenchymal cells, leukocytes, and erythrocytes. Phospholipids and myelin figures are also found in inflammatory foci. When abundant, the cholesterol-laden macrophages impart a yellowish discoloration to such inflammatory foci.
- *Cholesterolosis.* This refers to the focal accumulations of cholesterol-laden macrophages in the lamina propria of the gallbladder (Fig. 1–37). The mechanism of accumulation is unknown.
- *Niemann-Pick disease, type C.* In this lysosomal storage disease, an enzyme involved in cholesterol trafficking is mutated, and hence cholesterol accumulates in multiple organs (Chapter 5).

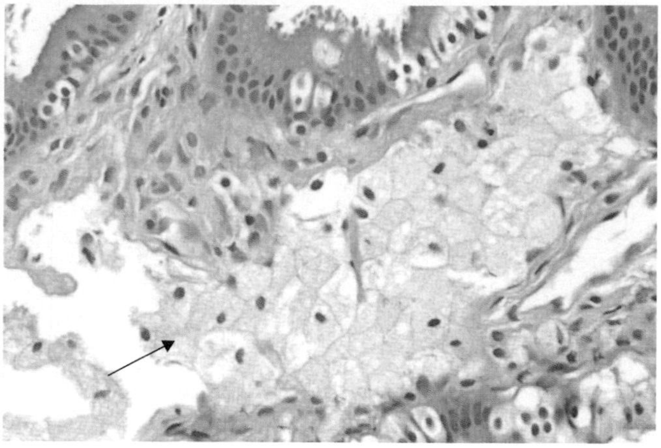

FIGURE 1–37 Cholesterolosis. Cholesterol-laden macrophages (foam cells) from a focus of gallbladder cholesterolosis (*arrow*). (Courtesy of Dr. Matthew Yeh, University of Washington, Seattle, WA.)

PROTEINS

Intracellular accumulations of proteins usually appear as rounded, eosinophilic droplets, vacuoles, or aggregates in the cytoplasm. By electron microscopy, they can be amorphous, fibrillar, or crystalline in appearance. In some disorders, such as certain forms of amyloidosis, abnormal proteins deposit primarily in the extracellular space (Chapter 6).

Excesses of proteins within the cells sufficient to cause morphologically visible accumulation have diverse causes.

- *Reabsorption droplets in proximal renal tubules* are seen in renal diseases associated with protein loss in the urine (proteinuria). In the kidney, small amounts of protein filtered through the glomerulus are normally reabsorbed by pinocytosis in the proximal tubule. In disorders with heavy protein leakage across the glomerular filter, there is increased reabsorption of the protein into vesicles. These vesicles fuse with lysosomes to produce phagolysosomes, which appear as pink hyaline droplets within the cytoplasm of the tubular cell (Fig. 1–38). The process is reversible; if the proteinuria diminishes, the protein droplets are metabolized and disappear.
- A second cause is synthesis of excessive amounts of normal secretory protein, as occurs in certain plasma cells engaged in active synthesis of immunoglobulins. The ER becomes hugely distended, producing large, homogeneous eosinophilic inclusions called *Russell bodies.*
- *Defects in protein folding* may underlie some of these depositions in a variety of unrelated diseases.[76] Nascent polypeptide chains of proteins, made on ribosomes, are ultimately arranged into either α helices or β sheets, and the proper configuration of these arrangements (protein folding) is critical to the individual protein's function and its transport into cell organelles.[77] In the process of folding, partially folded intermediates arise, and these may form intracellular aggregates among themselves or by entangling other proteins. Under normal conditions, however, these intermediates are stabilized by a number of molecular chaperones, which interact with proteins directly.[78] Chaperones aid in proper folding and in transport across the ER, Golgi complex, and beyond (Fig. 1–39). Some chaperones are synthesized constitutively and affect normal intracellular protein trafficking, whereas others

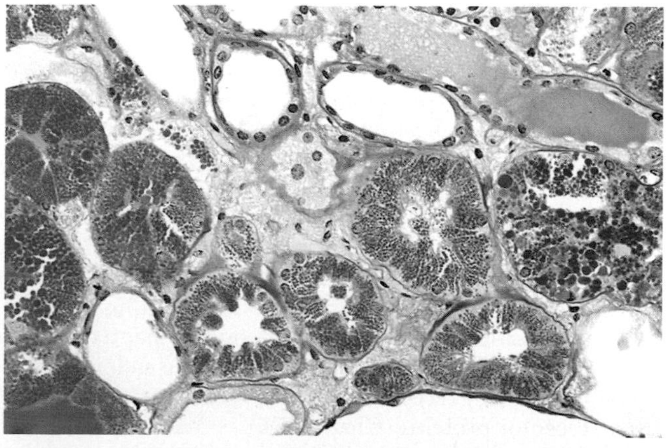

FIGURE 1–38 Protein reabsorption droplets in the renal tubular epithelium. (Courtesy of Dr. Helmut Rennke, Department of Pathology, Brigham and Women's Hospital, Boston, MA.)

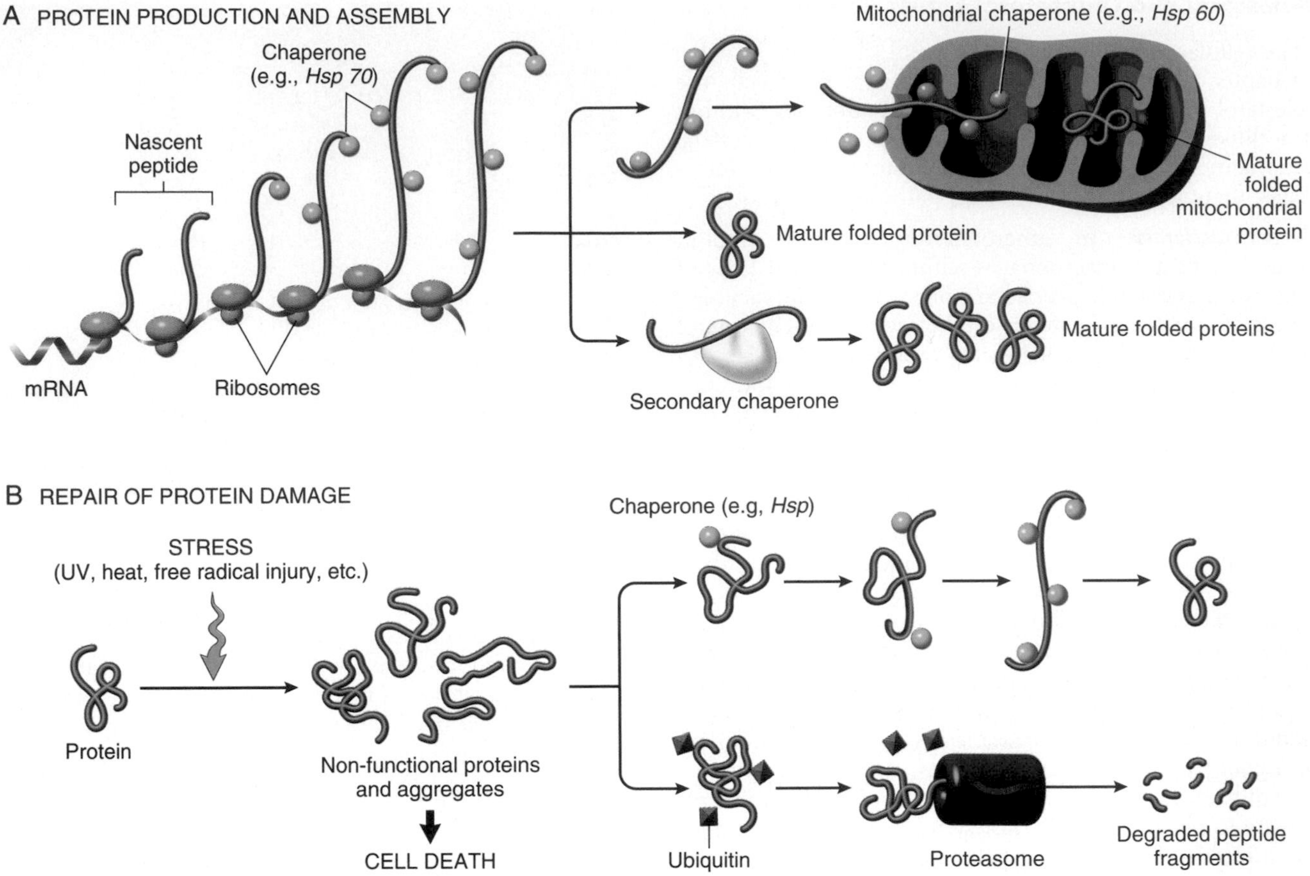

FIGURE 1–39 Mechanisms of protein folding and the role of chaperones. *A,* Chaperones, such as heat shock proteins (Hsp), protect unfolded or partially folded protein from degradation and guide proteins into organelles. *B,* Chaperones repair misfolded proteins; when this process is ineffective, proteins are targeted for degradation in the proteasome, and if misfolded proteins accumulate they trigger apoptosis.

are induced by stress, such as heat (heat-shock proteins, e.g., hsp70, hsp90), and "rescue" shock-stressed proteins from misfolding. If the folding process is not successful, the chaperones facilitate degradation of the damaged protein. This degradative process often involves ubiquitin (also a heat-shock protein), which is added to the abnormal protein and marks it for degradation by the proteasome complex. There are several mechanisms by which protein folding defects can cause intracellular accumulations or result in disease.

- *Defective intracellular transport and secretion of critical proteins.* In *α_1-antitrypsin deficiency*, mutations in the protein significantly slow folding, resulting in the build-up of partially folded intermediates, which aggregate in the ER of the liver and are not secreted. The resultant deficiency of the circulating enzyme causes emphysema (Chapter 15). In *cystic fibrosis,* mutation delays dissociation of a chloride channel protein from one of its chaperones, resulting in abnormal folding and loss of function (Chapter 10). In *familial hypercholesterolemia*, mutations in low-density lipoprotein receptors interfere with proper folding of receptor proteins (Chapter 5).
- *ER stress induced by unfolded and misfolded proteins.* Unfolded or misfolded proteins accumulate in the ER and trigger a number of cellular responses, collectively called the *unfolded protein response.*[79–81] The unfolded protein response is mediated by several proteins that reside in and span the ER membrane. The luminal domains of these proteins sense perturbations in protein folding, and the cytoplasmic domains activate signaling pathways that reduce the levels of misfolded proteins in the cell, by increasing the production of chaperones and slowing down protein translation. Paradoxically, the activation of the unfolded protein response also leads to cell death by activating caspases, particularly an ER-resident caspase called caspase-12. Thus, misfolded proteins initially trigger the cytoprotective function of this response, but if these abnormal proteins persist, the pro-apoptotic cytotoxic functions take over. Aggregation of abnormally folded proteins, caused by genetic mutations, aging, or unknown environmental factors, is now recognized as a feature of a number of neurodegenerative diseases, including Alzheimer's, Huntington's, and Parkinson's diseases (Chapter 28), and possibly type II diabetes. Deprivation of glucose and oxygen, and stress such as heat, also result in protein misfolding and trigger the unfolded protein response, culminating in cell injury and death.

- *Aggregation of abnormal proteins.* Abnormal or misfolded proteins may deposit in tissues and interfere with normal functions. The deposits can be intracellular, extracellular, or both, and there is accumulating evidence that the aggregates may either directly or indirectly cause the pathologic changes. Certain forms of *amyloidosis* (Chapter 6) fall in this category of diseases. These disorders are sometimes called *proteinopathies* or *protein-aggregation diseases.*

HYALINE CHANGE

The term *hyaline* usually refers to an alteration within cells or in the extracellular space, which gives a homogeneous, glassy, pink appearance in routine histologic sections stained with hematoxylin and eosin. It is widely used as a descriptive histologic term rather than a specific marker for cell injury. This tinctorial change is produced by a variety of alterations and does not represent a specific pattern of accumulation. Intracellular accumulations of protein, described earlier (reabsorption droplets, Russell bodies, Mallory alcoholic hyalin), are examples of intracellular hyaline deposits.

Extracellular hyalin has been somewhat more difficult to analyze. Collagenous fibrous tissue in old scars may appear hyalinized, but the physiochemical mechanism underlying this change is not clear. In long-standing hypertension and diabetes mellitus, the walls of arterioles, especially in the kidney, become hyalinized, owing to extravasated plasma protein and deposition of basement membrane material.

GLYCOGEN

Glycogen is a readily available energy store that is present in the cytoplasm. Excessive intracellular deposits of glycogen are seen in patients with an abnormality in either glucose or glycogen metabolism. Whatever the clinical setting, the glycogen masses appear as clear vacuoles within the cytoplasm. Glycogen is best preserved in nonaqueous fixatives; for its localization, tissues are best fixed in absolute alcohol. Staining with Best carmine or the periodic acid schiff (PAS) reaction imparts a rose-to-violet color to the glycogen, and diastase digestion of a parallel section before staining serves as a further control by hydrolyzing the glycogen.

Diabetes mellitus is the prime example of a disorder of glucose metabolism. In this disease, glycogen is found in the epithelial cells of the distal portions of the proximal convoluted tubules and sometimes in the descending loop of Henle, as well as within liver cells, β cells of the islets of Langerhans, and heart muscle cells.

Glycogen also accumulates within the cells in a group of closely related disorders, all genetic, collectively referred to as the *glycogen storage diseases*, or *glycogenoses* (Chapter 5). In these diseases, enzymatic defects in the synthesis or breakdown of glycogen result in massive accumulation, with secondary injury and cell death.

PIGMENTS

Pigments are colored substances, some of which are normal constituents of cells (e.g., melanin), whereas others are abnormal and collect in cells only under special circumstances. Pigments can be exogenous, coming from outside the body, or endogenous, synthesized within the body itself.

Exogenous Pigments. The most common *exogenous pigment* is *carbon* or coal dust, which is a ubiquitous air pollutant of urban life. When inhaled, it is picked up by macrophages within the alveoli and is then transported through lymphatic channels to the regional lymph nodes in the tracheobronchial region. Accumulations of this pigment blacken the tissues of the lungs *(anthracosis)* and the involved lymph nodes. In coal miners, the aggregates of carbon dust may induce a fibroblastic reaction or even emphysema and thus cause a serious lung disease known as *coal worker's pneumoconiosis* (Chapter 15). *Tattooing* is a form of localized, exogenous pigmentation of the skin. The pigments inoculated are phagocytosed by dermal macrophages, in which they reside for the remainder of the life of the embellished (sometimes with embarrassing consequences for the bearer of the tattoo!). The pigments do not usually evoke any inflammatory response.

Endogenous Pigments. *Lipofuscin* is an insoluble pigment, also known as lipochrome and wear-and-tear or aging pigment. Lipofuscin is composed of polymers of lipids and phospholipids complexed with protein, suggesting that it is derived through lipid peroxidation of polyunsaturated lipids of subcellular membranes. Lipofuscin is not injurious to the cell or its functions. Its importance lies in its being the telltale sign of free radical injury and lipid peroxidation. The term is derived from the Latin (*fuscus* = brown), thus brown lipid. In tissue sections, it appears as a yellow-brown, finely granular intracytoplasmic, often perinuclear pigment (Fig. 1–40). It is seen in cells undergoing slow, regressive changes and is particularly prominent in the liver and heart of aging patients or patients with severe malnutrition and cancer cachexia. On electron microscopy, the granules are highly electron dense, often have membranous structures in their midst, and are usually in a perinuclear location.

Melanin, derived from the Greek (*melas* = black), is an endogenous, non-hemoglobin-derived, brown-black pigment formed when the enzyme tyrosinase catalyzes the oxidation of tyrosine to dihydroxyphenylalanine in melanocytes. It is discussed further in Chapter 25. For all practical purposes, melanin is the *only endogenous brown-black pigment.* The only other that could be considered in this category is homogentisic acid, a black pigment that occurs in patients with *alkaptonuria*, a rare metabolic disease. Here the pigment is deposited in the skin, connective tissue, and cartilage, and the pigmentation is known as *ochronosis* (Chapter 5).

Hemosiderin is a hemoglobin-derived, golden yellow-to-brown, granular or crystalline pigment in which form iron is stored in cells. Iron metabolism and the synthesis of ferritin and hemosiderin are considered in detail in Chapter 13. Iron is normally carried by specific transport proteins, transferrins. In cells, it is stored in association with a protein, apoferritin, to form ferritin micelles. Ferritin is a constituent of most cell types. *When there is a local or systemic excess of iron, ferritin forms hemosiderin granules*, which are easily seen with the light microscope (Fig. 1–41). Thus, hemosiderin pigment represents aggregates of ferritin micelles. Under normal conditions, small amounts of hemosiderin can be seen in the mononuclear phagocytes of the bone marrow, spleen, and liver, all actively engaged in red cell breakdown.

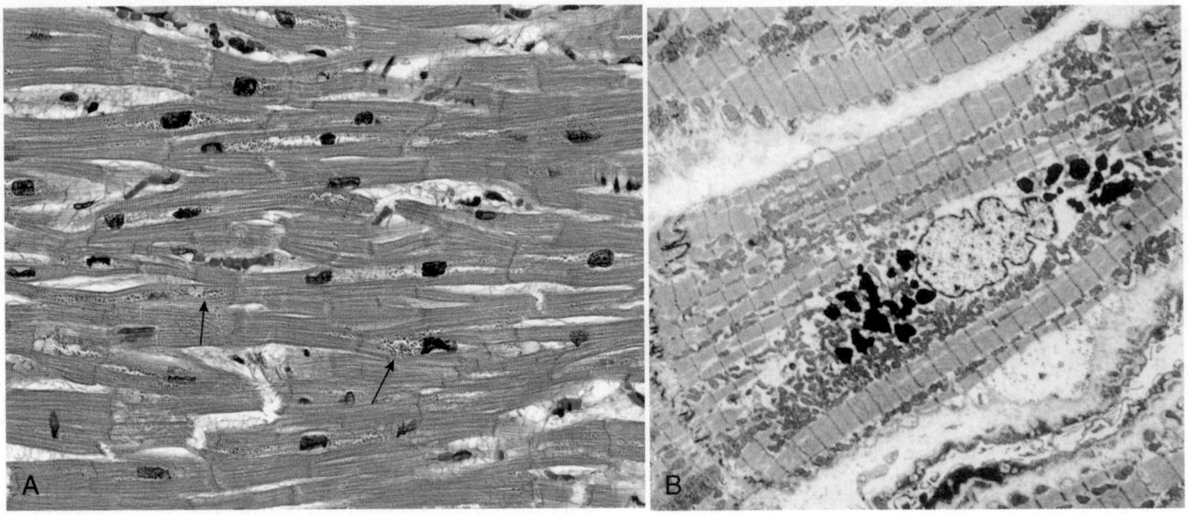

FIGURE 1–40 Lipofuscin granules in a cardiac myocyte as shown by *A,* light microscopy (deposits indicated by *arrows*), and *B,* electron microscopy (note the perinuclear, intralysosomal location).

Excesses of iron cause hemosiderin to accumulate within cells, either as a localized process or as a systemic derangement. *Local excesses* of iron and hemosiderin result from gross hemorrhages or the myriad minute hemorrhages that accompany severe vascular congestion. The best example of localized hemosiderosis is the common bruise. After local hemorrhage, the area is at first red-blue. With lysis of the erythrocytes, the hemoglobin eventually undergoes transformation to hemosiderin. Macrophages take part in this process by phagocytiosing the red cell debris, and then lysosomal enzymes eventually convert the hemoglobin, through a sequence of pigments, into hemosiderin. The play of colors through which the bruise passes reflects these transformations. The original red-blue color of hemoglobin is transformed to varying shades of green-blue, comprising the local formation of biliverdin (green bile), then bilirubin (red bile), and thereafter the iron moiety of hemoglobin is deposited as golden yellow hemosiderin.

Whenever there are causes for *systemic overload of iron,* hemosiderin is deposited in many organs and tissues, a condition called *hemosiderosis.* It is seen with: (1) increased absorption of dietary iron, (2) impaired use of iron, (3) hemolytic anemias, and (4) transfusions because the transfused red cells constitute an exogenous load of iron. These conditions are discussed in Chapter 18.

Morphology. Iron pigment appears as a coarse, golden, granular pigment lying within the cell's cytoplasm. When the basic cause is the localized breakdown of red cells, the pigmentation is found at first in the phagocytes in the area. In systemic hemosiderosis, it is found at first in the mononuclear phagocytes of the liver, bone marrow, spleen, and lymph nodes and in scattered macrophages throughout other organs such as the skin, pancreas, and kidneys. With progressive accumulation, parenchymal cells throughout the body (principally in the liver, pancreas, heart, and endocrine organs) become pigmented. Iron can be visualized in tissues by the Prussian blue histochemical reaction, in which colorless potassium ferrocyanide is converted by iron to blue-black ferric ferrocyanide (Fig. 1–41*B*).

In most instances of systemic hemosiderosis, the pigment does not damage the parenchymal cells or

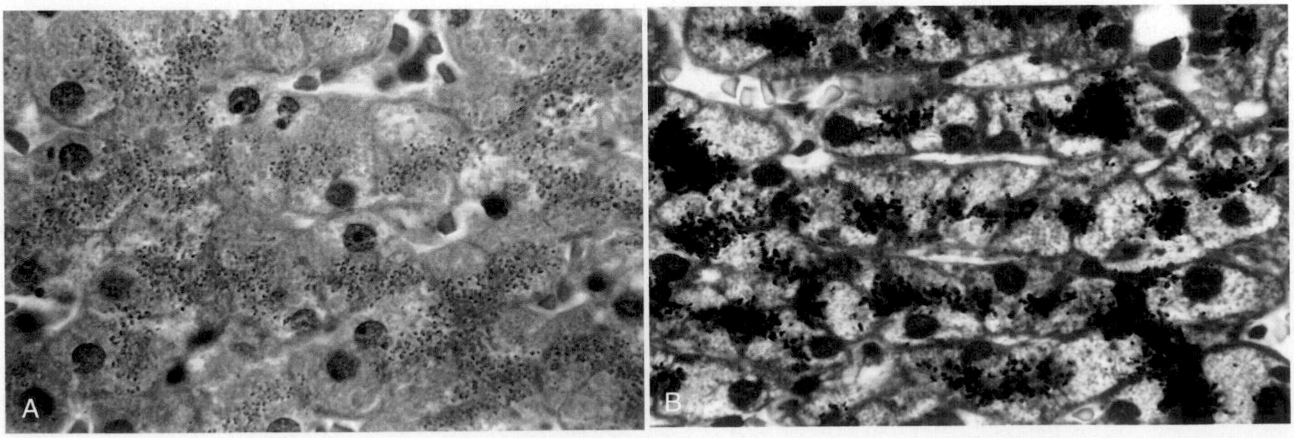

FIGURE 1–41 Hemosiderin granules in liver cells. *A,* H&E section showing golden-brown, finely granular pigment. *B,* Prussian blue reaction, specific for iron.

impair organ function. The more extreme accumulation of iron, however, in a disease called **hemochromatosis,** is associated with liver, heart, and pancreatic damage, resulting in liver fibrosis, heart failure, and diabetes mellitus (Chapter 18).

Bilirubin is the normal major pigment found in bile. It is derived from hemoglobin but contains no iron. Its normal formation and excretion are vital to health, and jaundice is a common clinical disorder caused by excesses of this pigment within cells and tissues. Bilirubin metabolism and jaundice are discussed in Chapter 18.

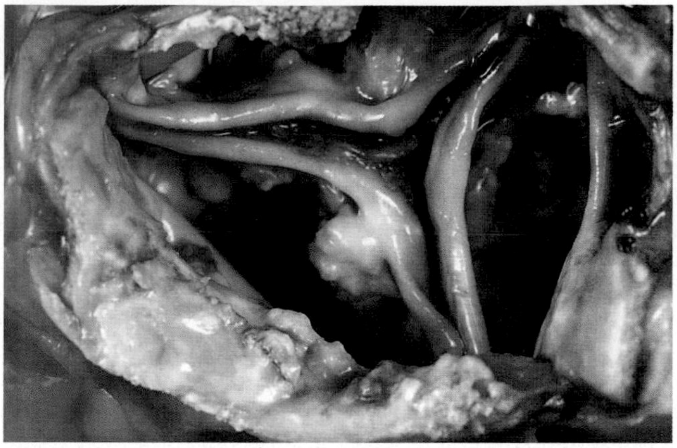

FIGURE 1–42 View looking down onto the unopened aortic valve in a heart with calcific aortic stenosis. The semilunar cusps are thickened and fibrotic. Behind each cusp are seen irregular masses of piled-up dystrophic calcification.

Pathologic Calcification

Pathologic calcification is the abnormal tissue deposition of calcium salts, together with smaller amounts of iron, magnesium, and other mineral salts. It is a common process occurring in a variety of pathologic conditions. There are two forms of pathologic calcification. When the deposition occurs locally in dying tissues, it is known as *dystrophic calcification*; it occurs despite normal serum levels of calcium and in the absence of derangements in calcium metabolism. In contrast, the deposition of calcium salts in otherwise normal tissues is known as *metastatic calcification*, and it almost always results from hypercalcemia secondary to some disturbance in calcium metabolism.

DYSTROPHIC CALCIFICATION

Dystrophic calcification is encountered in areas of necrosis, whether they are of coagulative, caseous, or liquefactive type, and in foci of enzymatic necrosis of fat. Calcification is almost inevitable in the atheromas of advanced atherosclerosis. It also commonly develops in aging or damaged heart valves, further hampering their function (Fig. 1–42). Whatever the site of deposition, the calcium salts appear macroscopically as fine, white granules or clumps, often felt as gritty deposits. Sometimes a tuberculous lymph node is virtually converted to stone.

Morphology. Histologically, with the usual hematoxylin and eosin stain, the calcium salts have a basophilic, amorphous granular, sometimes clumped, appearance. They can be intracellular, extracellular, or in both locations. In the course of time, **heterotopic** bone may be formed in the focus of calcification. On occasion, single necrotic cells may constitute seed crystals that become encrusted by the mineral deposits. The progressive acquisition of outer layers may create lamellated configurations, called **psammoma bodies** because of their resemblance to grains of sand. Some types of papillary cancers (e.g., thyroid) are apt to develop psammoma bodies. Strange concretions emerge when calcium iron salts gather about long slender spicules of asbestos in the lung, creating exotic, beaded dumbbell forms.

Pathogenesis. In the pathogenesis of dystrophic calcification, the final common pathway is the formation of crystalline calcium phosphate mineral in the form of an apatite similar to the hydroxyapatite of bone. The process has two major phases: *initiation* (or nucleation) and *propagation*; both can occur intracellularly and extracellularly. Initiation of *intracellular calcification* occurs in the *mitochondria* of dead or dying cells that accumulate calcium. Initiators of *extracellular dystrophic calcification* include phospholipids found in membrane-bound *vesicles* about 200 nm in diameter; in cartilage and bone, they are known as *matrix vesicles,* and in pathologic calcification, they are derived from degenerating or aging cells. It is thought that calcium is concentrated in these vesicles by a process of membrane-facilitated calcification, which has several steps: (1) calcium ion binds to the phospholipids present in the vesicle membrane, (2) phosphatases associated with the membrane generate phosphate groups, which bind to the calcium, (3) the cycle of calcium and phosphate binding is repeated, raising the local concentrations and producing a deposit near the membrane, and (4) a structural change occurs in the arrangement of calcium and phosphate groups, generating a microcrystal, which can then propagate and perforate the membrane. Propagation of crystal formation depends on the concentration of Ca^{2+} and PO_4 and the presence of inhibitors and other proteins in the extracellular space, such as the connective tissue matrix proteins.

Although dystrophic calcification may be simply a telltale sign of previous cell injury, it is often a cause of organ dysfunction. Such is the case in calcific valvular disease and atherosclerosis, as becomes clear in further discussion of these diseases.

METASTATIC CALCIFICATION

Metastatic calcification may occur in normal tissues whenever there is hypercalcemia. Hypercalcemia also accentuates dystrophic calcification. There are four principal causes of hypercalcemia: (1) increased secretion of parathyroid hormone (PTH) with subsequent bone resorption, as in hyperparathyroidism due to parathyroid tumors, and ectopic secretion of PTH-related protein by malignant tumors (Chapter 7); (2) *destruction of bone tissue*, occurring with primary tumors of bone marrow (e.g., multiple myeloma, leukemia) or diffuse skeletal metastasis (e.g., breast cancer), accelerated bone turnover (e.g., Paget disease), or immobilization; (3) *vitamin D–related disorders*, including vitamin D intoxication, sarcoidosis (in which macrophages activate a vitamin D precursor), and idiopathic hypercalcemia of infancy (Williams syndrome), characterized by abnormal sensitivity to vitamin D; and (4) *renal failure*, which causes retention of phosphate, leading to secondary hyperparathyroidism. Less common causes include aluminum intoxication, which occurs in patients on chronic renal dialysis, and milk-alkali syndrome, which is due to excessive ingestion of calcium and absorbable antacids such as milk or calcium carbonate.

Metastatic calcification may occur widely throughout the body but principally affects the interstitial tissues of the gastric mucosa, kidneys, lungs, systemic arteries, and pulmonary veins. Although quite different in location, all of these tissues *lose acid* and therefore have an internal alkaline compartment that predisposes them to metastatic calcification. In all these sites, the calcium salts morphologically resemble those described in dystrophic calcification. Thus, they may occur as noncrystalline amorphous deposits or, at other times, as hydroxyapatite crystals.

Usually, the mineral salts cause no clinical dysfunction, but, on occasion, massive involvement of the lungs produces remarkable x-ray films and respiratory deficits. Massive deposits in the kidney (nephrocalcinosis) may in time cause renal damage (Chapter 20).

Cellular Aging

Shakespeare probably characterized aging best in his elegant description of the seven ages of man. It begins at the moment of conception, involves the differentiation and maturation of the organism and its cells, at some variable point in time leads to the progressive loss of functional capacity characteristic of senescence, and ends in death.

With age, there are physiologic and structural alterations in almost all organ systems. Aging in individuals is affected to a great extent by genetic factors, diet, social conditions, and occurrence of age-related diseases, such as atherosclerosis, diabetes, and osteoarthritis. In addition, there is good evidence that aging-induced alterations in cells are an important component of the aging of the organism. Here we discuss cellular aging because it could represent the progressive accumulation over the years of sublethal injury that may lead to cell death or at least to the diminished capacity of the cell to respond to injury.

Cellular aging is the result of a progressive decline in the proliferative capacity and life span of cells and the effects of continuous exposure to exogenous influences that result in the progressive accumulation of cellular and molecular damage (Fig. 1–43). These processes are reviewed next.

Structural and Biochemical Changes with Cellular Aging. A number of cell functions decline progressively with age. Oxidative phosphorylation by mitochondria is reduced, as is synthesis of nucleic acids and structural and enzymatic proteins, cell receptors, and transcription factors. Senescent cells have a decreased capacity for uptake of nutrients and for repair of chromosomal damage. The morphologic alterations in aging cells include irregular and abnormally lobed nuclei, pleomorphic vacuolated mitochondria, decreased endoplasmic reticulum, and distorted Golgi apparatus. Concomitantly, there is a steady accumulation of the pigment lipofuscin, which, as we have seen, represents a product of lipid peroxidation and evidence of *oxidative damage; advanced glycation end products*, which result from nonenzymatic glycosylation and are capable of cross-linking adjacent proteins; and the accumulation of *abnormally folded proteins*. The role of oxidative damage is discussed later. Advanced glycation end products are important in the pathogenesis of diabetes mellitus and are discussed in Chapter 24, but they may also participate in aging. For example, age-related glycosylation of lens proteins may underlie senile cataracts. The nature of abnormally folded proteins was discussed earlier in the chapter.

Replicative Senescence. The concept that cells have a limited capacity for replication was developed from a simple experimental model for aging. Normal human fibroblasts, when placed in tissue culture, have limited division potential.[82] Cells from children undergo more rounds of replication than cells from older people (Fig. 1–44). In contrast, cells from patients with *Werner syndrome*, a rare disease characterized by premature aging, have a markedly reduced in vitro life span. After a fixed number of divisions, all cells become arrested in a terminally nondividing state, known as *cellular senescence*. Many changes in gene expression occur during cellular aging, but a key question is which of these are causes and which are effects of cellular senescence.[83] For example, some of the proteins that inhibit progression of the cell growth cycle

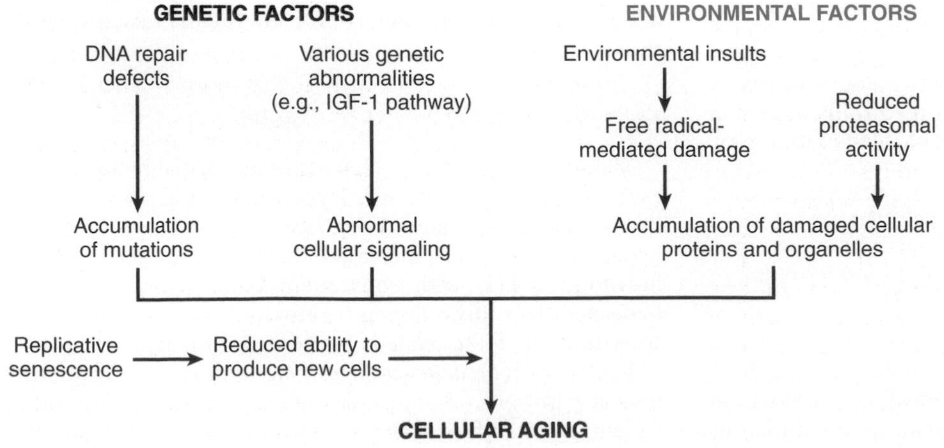

FIGURE 1–43 Mechanisms of cellular aging. Genetic factors and environmental insults combine to produce the cellular abnormalities characteristic of aging.

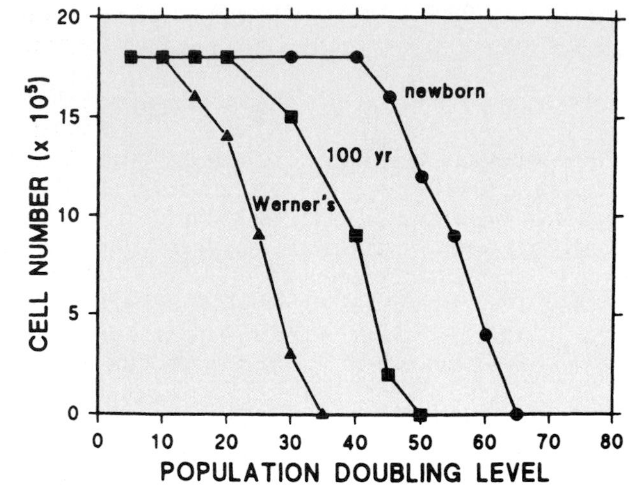

FIGURE 1–44 Finite population doublings of primary human fibroblasts derived from a newborn, a 100-year-old person, and a 20-year-old patient with Werner's syndrome. The ability of cells to grow to a confluent monolayer decreases with increasing population-doubling levels. (From Dice JF: Cellular and molecular mechanisms of aging. Physiol Rev 73:150, 1993.)

(as detailed in Chapter 7)—such as the products of the cyclin-dependent kinase inhibitor genes (e.g., *p21*)—are overexpressed in senescent cells.

How dividing cells can *count* their divisions is under intensive investigation. One likely mechanism is that with each cell division, there is *incomplete replication of chromosome ends (telomere shortening), which ultimately results in cell cycle arrest. Telomeres* are short repeated sequences of DNA (TTAGGG) present at the linear ends of chromosomes that are important for ensuring the complete replication of chromosome ends and protecting chromosomal termini from fusion and degradation.[84,85]

When somatic cells replicate, a small section of the telomere is not duplicated, and telomeres become progressively shortened. As the telomeres become shorter, the ends of chromosomes cannot be protected and are seen as broken DNA, which signals cell cycle arrest. The lengths of the telomeres are normally maintained by nucleotide addition mediated by an enzyme called *telomerase*. Telomerase is a specialized RNA–protein complex that uses its own RNA as a template for adding nucleotides to the ends of chromosomes (Fig. 1–45). The activity of telomerase is repressed by regulatory proteins, which restrict telomere elongation, thus providing a length sensing mechanism. Telomerase activity is expressed in germ cells and is present at low levels in stem cells, but it is usually absent in most somatic tissues. Therefore, as cells age, their telomeres become shorter, and they exit the cell cycle, resulting in an inability to generate new cells to replace damaged ones. Conversely, in immortal cancer cells, telomerase is reactivated, and telomeres are not shortened, suggesting that telomere elongation might be an important—possibly essential—step in tumor formation.[85] Despite such alluring observations, however, the relationship of telomerase activity and telomeric length to aging and cancer still needs to be fully established.[86]

Genes That Influence the Aging Process. Studies in *Drosophila, C. elegans,* and mice are leading to the discovery of genes that influence the aging process.[87] One interesting set of genes involves the insulin/insulin growth factor-1 pathway. Decreased signaling through the IGF-1 receptor as a result of decreased caloric intake, or mutations in the receptor, result in prolonged life span in *C. elegans*. The signals downstream of the IGF-1 receptor involve a number of kinases and may lead to the silencing of particular genes, thus promoting aging. Analyses of humans with premature aging are also establishing the fundamental concept that aging is not a random process but is regulated by specific genes, receptors, and signals.[88]

Accumulation of Metabolic and Genetic Damage. In addition to the importance of timing and a genetic clock, cellular life span may also be determined by the balance between cellular damage resulting from *metabolic events* occurring within the cell and counteracting molecular responses that can repair the damage. Smaller animals have generally shorter life spans and faster metabolic rates, suggesting that the life span of a species is limited by fixed total metabolic consumption over a lifetime.[89] One group of products of normal metabolism are reactive oxygen species. As we have seen, these byproducts of oxidative phosphorylation cause covalent modifications of proteins, lipids, and nucleic acids. The amount of oxidative damage, which increases as an organism ages, may be an important component of senescence, and the accumulation of lipofuscin in aging cells is seen as the telltale sign of such damage. Consistent with this proposal are the following observations: (1) variation in longevity among different species is inversely correlated with the rates of mitochondrial generation of superoxide anion radical, and (2) overexpression of the antioxidative enzymes superoxide dismutase (SOD) and catalase extends life span in transgenic forms of *Drosophila*. Thus, part of the mechanism that times aging may be the cumulative damage that is generated by toxic byproducts of metabolism, such as oxygen radicals. Increased oxidative damage could result from repeated environmental exposure to such influences as ionizing radiation, progressive reduction of antioxidant defense mechanisms (e.g., vitamin E, glutathione peroxidase), or both.

A number of protective responses counterbalance progressive damage in cells, and an important one is the recognition and repair of damaged DNA.[90] Although most DNA damage is repaired by endogenous DNA repair enzymes, some persists and accumulates as cells age. Several lines of evidence point to the importance of DNA repair in the aging process. Patients with *Werner syndrome* show premature aging, and the defective gene product is a DNA helicase — a protein involved in DNA replication and repair and other functions requiring DNA unwinding.[91] A defect in this enzyme causes rapid accumulation of chromosomal damage that mimics the injury that normally accumulates during cellular aging. Genetic instability in somatic cells is also characteristic of other disorders in which patients display some of the manifestations of aging at an increased rate, such as *ataxia-telangiectasia*, in which the mutated gene encodes a protein involved in repairing double strand breaks in DNA (Chapter 7). Studies of mutants of budding yeast and *C. elegans* show that life span is increased if responses to DNA damage are enhanced. Thus, the balance between cumulative metabolic damage and the response to that damage could determine the rate at which we age. In this scenario, aging can be delayed by decreasing the accumulation of damage or by increasing the response to that damage.

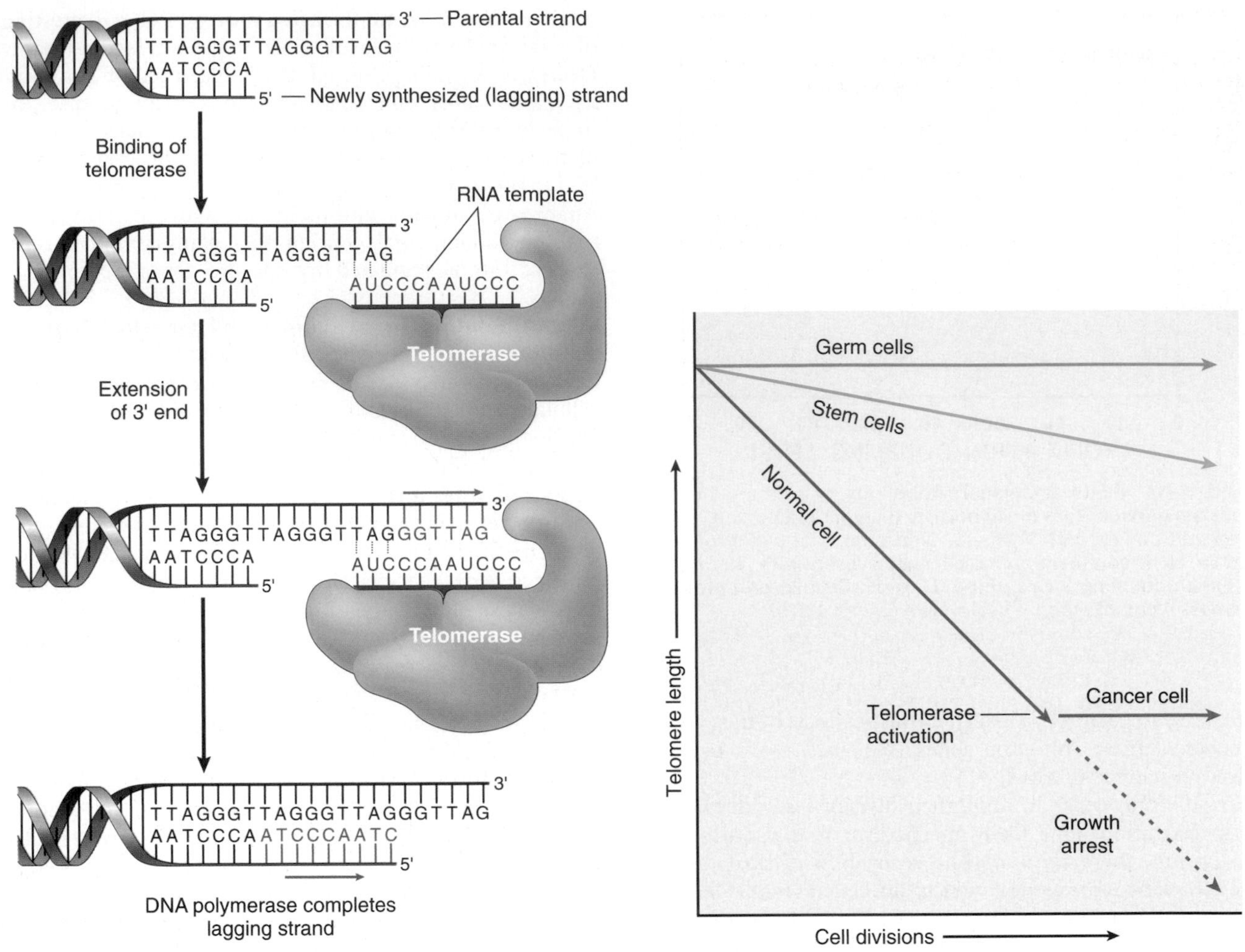

FIGURE 1–45 The role of telomeres and telomerase in replicative senescence of cells. *A,* Telomerase directs RNA template-dependent DNA synthesis, in which nucleotides are added to one strand at the end of a chromosome. The lagging strand is presumably filled in by DNA polymerase α. The RNA sequence in the telomerase is different in different species. (Modified from Alberts BR, et al: Molecular Biology of the Cell, 2002, Garland Science, New York.) *B,* Telomere–telomerase hypothesis and proliferative capacity. Telomere length is plotted against the number of cell divisions. In normal somatic cells, there is no telomerase activity, and telomeres progressively shorten with increasing cell divisions until growth arrest, or senescence, occurs. Germ cells and stem cells both contain active telomerase, but only the germ cells have sufficient levels of the enzyme to stabilize telomere length completely. Telomerase activation in cancer cells inactivates the teleomeric clock that limits the proliferative capacity of normal somatic cells. (Modified and redrawn with permission from Holt SE, et al.: Refining the telomer–telomerase hypothesis of aging and cancer. Nature Biotech 14:836, 1996. Copyright 1996, Macmillan Magazines Limited.)

Not only damaged DNA but damaged cellular organelles also accumulate as cells age. In part, this may be the result of declining function of the proteasome, the proteolytic machine that serves to eliminate abnormal and unwanted intracellular proteins.[92]

In conclusion, it should be apparent that the various forms of cellular derangements and adaptations described in this chapter cover a wide spectrum, ranging from adaptations in cell size, growth, and function; to the reversible and irreversible forms of acute cell injury; to the regulated type of cell death represented by apoptosis; to the pathologic alterations in cell organelles; and to the less ominous forms of intracellular accumulations, including pigmentations. Reference is made to all these alterations throughout this book because all organ injury and ultimately all clinical disease arise from derangements in cell structure and function.

REFERENCES

1. Majno G: The Healing Hand: Man and Wound in the Ancient World. Cambridge: Harvard University Press, 1975, p 43.
2. Taub R: Transcriptional control of liver regeneration. FASEB J 10:413, 1997.
3. Thorgeirsson SS: Hepatic stem cells in liver regeneration. FASEB J 10:1249, 1996.
4. Forbes S, et al: Hepatic stem cells. J Pathol 197:510, 2002.
5. Korbling M, Estrovz Z: Adult stem cells for tissue repair: a new therapeutic concept? New Eng J Med 349:570, 2003.
6. Anversa P, Nadal-Ginard B: Myocyte renewal and ventricular remodeling. Nature 415:240, 2002.
7. Molkentin JD, Dorn GW: Cytoplasmic signaling pathways that regulate cardiac hypertrophy. Annu Rev Physiol 63:391, 2001.
8. MacLellan WR, Schneider MD: Genetic dissection of cardiac growth control pathways. Annu Rev Physiol 62:289, 2000.
9. Saito Y, et al: Augmented expression of atrial natriuretic polypeptide gene in ventricle of human failing heart. J Clin Invest 83:298, 1989.
10. Kozma SC, Thomas G: Regulation of cell size in growth, development and human disease: PI3K, PKB and S6K. Bioessays 24:65, 2002.

11. Anversa P, et al: Myocyte death in heart failure. Curr Opin Cardiol 11:245, 1996.
12. Glickman MH, Ciechanover A: The ubiquitin–proteasome proteolytic pathway: destruction for the sake of construction. Physiol Rev 82:373, 2002.
13. Lugo M, Putong PB: Metaplasia: an overview. Arch Pathol Lab Med 108:185, 1984.
14. Tosh D, Slack JM: How cells change their phenotype. Nat Rev Mol Cell Biol 3:187, 2002.
15. Reddi HA: BMPs: actions in flesh and bone. Nat Med 3:837, 1997.
16. Ross SA, McCaffrey PJ, Drager UC, DeLuca LM: Retinoids in embryonal development. Physiol Rev 80:1021, 2000.
17. Newmeyer DD, Ferguson-Miller S: Mitochondria: releasing power for life and unleashing the machineries of death. Cell 112:481, 2003.
18. Trump BF, Berezesky I: The reactions of cells to lethal injury: oncosis and necrosis—the role of calcium. In Lockshin RA (ed): When Cells Die—A Comprehensive Evaluation of Apoptosis and Programmed Cell Death. New York: Wiley-Liss, 1998, p 57.
19. Orrenius S, Zhivotovsky B, Nicotera P: Regulation of cell death: the calcium-apoptosis link. Nat Rev Mol Cell Biol 4:552, 2003.
20. Paschen W: Role of calcium in neuronal cell injury: which subcellular compartment is involved? Brain Res Bull 53:409, 2000.
21. Droge W: Free radicals in the physiological control of cell function. Physiol Rev 82:47, 2002.
22. Hensley K, Robinson KA, Gabbita SP, Salsman S, Floyd RA: Reactive oxygen species, cell signaling, and cell injury. Free Radic Biol Med 28:1456, 2000.
23. Salvemini D, Cuzzocrea S: Superoxide, superoxide dismutase and ischemic injury. Curr Opin Investig Drugs 3:886, 2002.
24. Li C, Jackson RM: Reactive species mechanisms of cellular hypoxia-reoxygenation injury. Am J Physiol Cell Physiol 282:C227, 2002.
25. Mitch WE, Goldberg AE: Mechanisms of muscle wasting: the role of the ubiquitin–proteosome pathway. N Engl J Med 335:1897, 1996.
26. Kim JS, He L, Lemasters JJ: Mitochondrial permeability transition: a common pathway to necrosis and apoptosis. Biochem Biophys Res Commun 304:463, 2003.
27. Trump BF, et al: Cell injury and cell death: apoptosis, oncosis, and necrosis. In Acosta D (ed): Cardiovascular Toxicology, 3rd ed. London and New York: Taylor & Francis, 2001, p 105.
28. Sheridan AM, Bonventre JV: Cell biology and molecular mechanisms of injury in ischemic acute renal failure. Curr Opin Nephral Hypertens 9:427, 2000.
29. Hou ST, McManus JP: Molecular mechanisms of cerebral ischemia-induced neuronal death. Int Rev Cytol 221:93, 2002.
30. Daemen MARC, De Vries B, Buurman WA: Apoptosis and inflammation in renal reperfusion injury. Transplantation 73:1693, 2002.
31. Anaya-Prado R, et al: Ischemia/reperfusion injury. J Surg Res 105:248, 2002.
32. Kaminski KA, et al: Oxidative stress and neutrophil activation — the two keystones of ischemia/reperfusion injury. Int J Cardiol 86:41, 2002.
33. Thiagarajan RR, et al: The role of leukocyte and endothelial adhesion molecules in ischemia–reperfusion injury. Thromb Haemost 78:310, 1997.
34. Riedemann NC, Ward PA: Complement in ischemia reperfusion injury. Am J Pathol 162:363, 2003.
35. Weiser MR, et al: Reperfusion injury of ischemic skeletal muscle is mediated by natural antibody and complement. J Exp Med 183:2343, 1996.
36. Snyder JW: Mechanisms of toxic cell injury. Clin Lab Med 10:311, 1990.
37. Coon MJ, et al: Cytochrome P450: peroxidative reactions of diversozymes. FASEB J 10:428, 1996.
38. Gonzalez FJ: The use of gene knockout mice to unravel the mechanisms of toxicity and chemical carcinogenesis. Toxicol Lett 120:199, 2001.
39. Plaa GL: Chlorinated methanes and liver injury: highlights of the past 50 years. Annu Rev Pharmacol Toxicol 40:42, 2000.
40. Jaeschke H, et al: Mechanisms of hepatotoxicity. Toxicol Sci 65:166, 2002.
41. Cohen SD, Khairallah EA: Selective protein arylation and acetaminophen-induced hepatotoxicity. Drug Metab Rev 29:59, 1997.
42. Kerr JF, et al: Apoptosis: a basic biological phenomenon with wide-ranging implications in tissue kinetics. Br J Cancer 26:239, 1972.
43. Metzstein MM, Stanfield GM, Horvitz HR: Genetics of programmed cell death in *C. elegans:* past, present and future. Trends Genet 14:410, 1998.
44. Wyllie AH: Apoptosis: an overview. Br Med Bull 53:451, 1997.
45. Strasser A, O'Connor L, Dixit VM: Apoptosis signaling. Annu Rev Biochem 69:217, 2000.
46. Vaux D, Silke J: Mammalian mitochondrial IAP-binding proteins. Biochem Biophys Res Commun 203:449, 2003.
47. McCarthy NJ, Evan GI: Methods for detecting and quantifying apoptosis. Curr Top Dev Biol 36:259, 1998.
48. Hanayama R, et al: Identification of a factor that links apoptotic cells to phagocytes. Nature 417:182, 2002.
49. Savill J, Fadok V: Corpse clearing defines the meaning of cell death. Nature 407:784, 2000.
50. Vaux DL, Strasser A: The molecular biology of apoptosis. Proc Natl Acad Sci U S A 93:2239, 1996.
51. Wallach D, et al: Tumor necrosis factor receptor and Fas signaling mechanisms. Annu Rev Immunol 17:331, 1999.
52. Thome M, Tschopp J: Regulation of lymphocyte proliferation and death by FLIP. Nat Rev Immunol 1:50, 2001.
53. Van Blitterswijk WJ, et al: Ceramide: second messenger or modulator of membrane structure and dynamics? Biochem J 369:199, 2003.
54. Scorrano L, Korsmeyer SJ: Mechanisms of cytochrome release by proapoptotic BCL-2 family members. Biochem Biophys Res Commun 304:437, 2003.
55. Ravagnan L, Roumier T, Kroemer G: Mitochondria, the killer organelles and their weapons. J Cell Physiol 192:131, 2002.
56. Cory S, Adams JM: The Bcl2 family: regulators of the cellular life-or-death switch. Nature Rev Cancer 2:647, 2002.
57. Reed JC: Cytochrome *c:* can't live with it — can't live without it. Cell 91:559, 1997.
58. Salvesen GS, Duckett CS: IAP proteins: blocking the road to death's door. Nature Rev Mol Cell Biol 3:401, 2002.
59. Joza N, Kroemer G, Penninger JM: Genetic analysis of the mammalian cell death machinery. Trends Genet 18:142, 2002.
60. Salvesen GS, Dixit VM: Caspases: intracellular signaling by proteolysis. Cell 91:443, 1997.
61. Ravichandran KS: "Recruitment signals" from apoptotic cells: invitation to a quiet meal. Cell 113:817, 2003.
62. Rathmell JC, Thompson CB: Pathways of apoptosis in lymphocyte development, homeostasis, and disease. Cell 109:S97, 2002.
63. Vousden KH, Lu X: Live or let die: the cell's response to p53. Nature Rev Cancer 2:594, 2002.
64. Siegel RM, et al: The multifaceted role of Fas signaling in immune cell homeostasis and autoimmunity. Nat Immunol 1:469, 2000.
65. Locksley RM, Killeen N, Lenardo MJ: The TNF and TNF receptor superfamilies: integrating mammalian biology. Cell 104:487, 2001.
66. Russell JH, Ley TJ: Lymphocyte-mediated cytotoxicity. Annu Rev Immunol 20:323, 2002.
67. Webb SJ, et al: Apoptosis. An overview of the process and its relevance in disease. Adv Pharmacol 41:1, 1997.
68. Dunn WA: Studies on the mechanisms of autophagy. J Cell Biol 110:1923, 1990.
69. Klionsky DJ, Emr SD: Autophagy as a regulated pathway of cellular degradation. Science 290:1717, 2000.
70. Di Mauro S, Schon EA: Mitochondrial respiratory-chain diseases. New Engl J Med 348:2656, 2003.
71. Mermall V, et al: Unconventional myosins in cell movement, membrane traffic and signal transduction. Science 279:527, 1998.
72. Fuchs E, Cleveland DW: A structural scaffolding of intermediate filaments in health and disease. Science 279:514, 1998.
73. Denk H, Stumptner C, Zatloukal K: Mallory bodies revisited. J Hepatol 32:689, 2000.
74. Snapper SB, Rosen FS: The Wiskott-Aldrich syndrome protein (WASP): roles in signaling and cytoskeletal organization. Annu Rev Immunol 17:905, 1999.
75. Lee RJ: Fatty change and steatohepatitis. In Lee RJ (ed): Diagnostic Liver Pathology. St. Louis: Mosby-Year Book, 1994, p 167.
76. Soto C: Protein misfolding and disease; protein refolding and therapy. FEBS Lett 498:204, 2001.
77. Horwich A: Protein aggregation in disease: a role for folding intermediates forming specific multimeric interactions. J Clin Invest 110:1221, 2002.
78. Hartl FU, Hayer-Hartl M: Molecular chaperones in the cytosol: from nascent chain to folded protein. Science 295:1852, 2002.
79. Kaufman RJ: Orchestrating the unfolded protein response in health and disease. J Clin Invest 110:1389, 2002.
80. Patil C, Walter P: Intracellular signaling from the endoplasmic reticulum to the nucleus: the unfolded protein response in yeast and mammals. Curr Opin Cell Biol 13:349, 2001.

81. Ma Y, Hendershot LM: The unfolding tale of the unfolded protein response. Cell 107:827, 2001.
82. Hayflick L, Moorhead PS: The serial cultivation of human diploid cell strains. Exp Cell Res 25:585, 1961.
83. Smith JR, Pereira-Smith OM: Replicative senescence: implications for in vivo aging and tumor suppression. Science 273:63, 1996.
84. Blackburn EH: Switching and signaling at the telomere. Cell 106:661, 2001.
85. Wong JMY, Collins K: Telomere maintenance and disease. Lancet 362:983, 2003.
86. Stewart SA, Weinberg RA: Senescence: does it all happen at the ends? Oncogene 21:627, 2002.
87. Guarente L, Kenyon C: Genetic pathways that regulate ageing in model organisms. Nature 408:255, 2000.
88. Martin GM, Oshima J: Lessons from human progeroid syndromes. Nature 408:263, 2000.
89. Finkel T, Holbrook NJ: Oxidants, oxidative stress, and the biology of ageing. Nature 408:239, 2000.
90. Gilchrest BA, Bohr VA: Aging processes, DNA damage, and repair. FASEB J 11:322, 1997.
91. Bohr VA: Human premature aging syndromes and genomic instability. Mech Ageing Dev 123:987, 2002.
92. Carrard G, et al: Impairment of proteasome structure and function in aging. Int J Biochem Cell Biol 34:1461, 2002.

CHAPTER 2

Acute and Chronic Inflammation

GENERAL FEATURES OF INFLAMMATION

HISTORICAL HIGHLIGHTS

ACUTE INFLAMMATION

Stimuli for Acute Inflammation

Vascular Changes

Changes in Vascular Flow and Caliber

Increased Vascular Permeability (Vascular Leakage)

Cellular Events: Leukocyte Extravasation and Phagocytosis

Leukocyte Adhesion and Transmigration

Chemotaxis

Leukocyte Activation

Phagocytosis

Release of Leukocyte Products and Leukocyte-Induced Tissue Injury

Defects in Leukocyte Function

Termination of the Acute Inflammatory Response

CHEMICAL MEDIATORS OF INFLAMMATION

Vasoactive Amines

Histamine

Serotonin

Plasma Proteins

Complement System

Kinin System

Clotting System

Arachidonic Acid Metabolites: Prostaglandins, Leukotrienes, and Lipoxins

Platelet-Activating Factor

Cytokines and Chemokines

Tumor Necrosis Factor and Interleukin-1

Chemokines

Nitric Oxide

Lysosomal Constituents of Leukocytes

Oxygen-Derived Free Radicals

Neuropeptides

Other Mediators

Summary of Chemical Mediators of Acute Inflammation

OUTCOMES OF ACUTE INFLAMMATION

MORPHOLOGIC PATTERNS OF ACUTE INFLAMMATION

Serous Inflammation

Fibrinous Inflammation

Suppurative or Purulent Inflammation

Ulcers

SUMMARY OF ACUTE INFLAMMATION

CHRONIC INFLAMMATION

Causes of Chronic Inflammation

Morphologic Features

Mononuclear Cell Infiltration

Other Cells in Chronic Inflammation

Granulomatous Inflammation

Lymphatics in Inflammation

SYSTEMIC EFFECTS OF INFLAMMATION

CONSEQUENCES OF DEFECTIVE OR EXCESSIVE INFLAMMATION

General Features of Inflammation

In Chapter 1, we saw how various exogenous and endogenous stimuli can cause cell injury. In vascularized tissues, these same stimuli also provoke a host response called *inflammation. Inflammation is a complex reaction to injurious agents such as microbes and damaged, usually necrotic, cells that consists of vascular responses, migration and activation of leukocytes, and systemic reactions.* Invertebrates with no vascular system, and even single-celled organisms, are able to get rid of injurious agents such as microbes by a variety of mechanisms. These mechanisms include entrapment and phagocytosis of the offending agent, sometimes by specialized cells (hemocytes), and neutralization of noxious stimuli by hypertrophy of the host cell or one of its organelles. These cellular reactions have been retained through evolution, and the more potent defensive reaction of inflammation has been added in higher species. The unique feature of the inflammatory process is the *reaction of blood vessels, leading to the accumulation of fluid and leukocytes in extravascular tissues.*

The inflammatory response is closely intertwined with the process of repair. Inflammation serves to destroy, dilute, or wall off the injurious agent, and it sets into motion a series of events that try to heal and reconstitute the damaged tissue. Repair begins during the early phases of inflammation but reaches completion usually after the injurious influence has been neutralized. During repair, the injured tissue is replaced through *regeneration* of native parenchymal cells, by filling of the defect with fibrous tissue *(scarring)* or, most commonly, by a combination of these two processes.

Inflammation is fundamentally a protective response, the ultimate goal of which is to rid the organism of both the initial cause of cell injury (e.g., microbes, toxins) and the consequences of such injury (e.g., necrotic cells and tissues). Without inflammation, infections would go unchecked, wounds would never heal, and injured organs might remain permanent festering sores. *Inflammation and repair may be potentially harmful, however.* Inflammatory reactions, for example, underlie common chronic diseases, such as rheumatoid arthritis, atherosclerosis, and lung fibrosis, as well as life-threatening hypersensitivity reactions to insect bites, drugs, and toxins. Repair by fibrosis may lead to disfiguring scars or fibrous bands that cause intestinal obstruction or limit the mobility of joints. For this reason, our pharmacies abound with anti-inflammatory drugs, which ideally would control the harmful sequelae of inflammation yet not interfere with its beneficial effects.

The inflammatory response consists of two main components, a vascular reaction and a cellular reaction. Many tissues and cells are involved in these reactions, including the fluid and proteins of plasma, circulating cells, blood vessels, and cellular and extracellular constituents of connective tissue (Fig. 2–1). The circulating cells include *neutrophils, monocytes, eosinophils, lymphocytes, basophils,* and *platelets.* The connective tissue cells are the *mast cells,* which intimately surround *blood vessels;* the connective tissue *fibroblasts;* resident *macrophages;* and *lymphocytes.* The extracellular matrix, as described in Chapter 3, consists of the structural fibrous proteins *(collagen, elastin),* adhesive glycoproteins *(fibronectin, laminin, nonfibrillar collagen, tenascin,* and others), and proteoglycans. The basement membrane is a specialized compo-

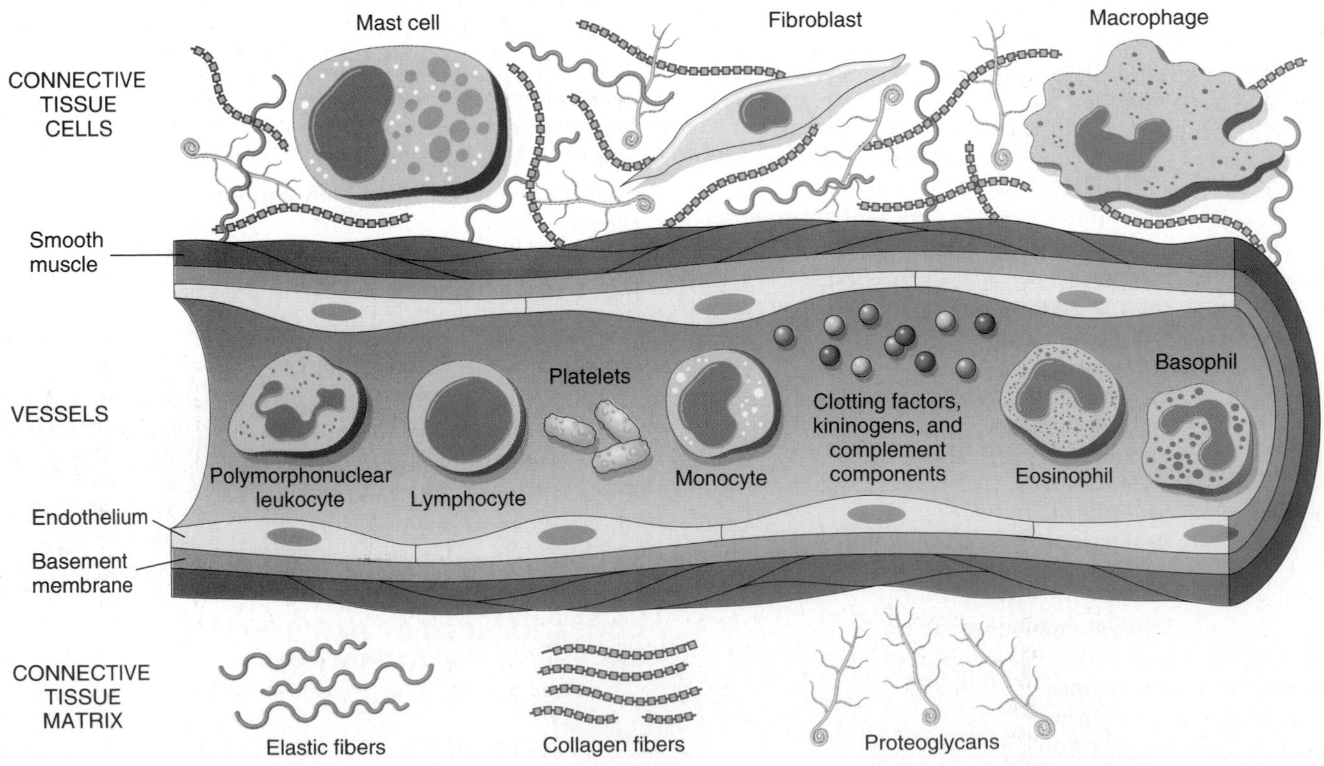

FIGURE 2–1 The components of acute and chronic inflammatory responses: circulating cells and proteins, cells of blood vessels, and cells and proteins of the extracellular matrix.

nent of the extracellular matrix consisting of adhesive glycoproteins and proteoglycans.

Inflammation is divided into acute and chronic patterns. *Acute inflammation* is rapid in onset (seconds or minutes) and is of relatively short duration, lasting for minutes, several hours, or a few days; its main characteristics are the exudation of fluid and plasma proteins (edema) and the emigration of leukocytes, predominantly neutrophils. *Chronic inflammation* is of longer duration and is associated histologically with the presence of lymphocytes and macrophages, the proliferation of blood vessels, fibrosis, and tissue necrosis. Many factors modify the course and morphologic appearance of both acute and chronic inflammation, and these will become apparent later in this chapter.

The vascular and cellular reactions of both acute and chronic inflammation are mediated by chemical factors that are derived from plasma proteins or cells and are produced in response to or activated by the inflammatory stimulus. Such mediators, acting singly, in combinations, or in sequence, then amplify the inflammatory response and influence its evolution. Necrotic cells or tissues themselves—whatever the cause of cell death—can also trigger the elaboration of inflammatory mediators. Such is the case with the acute inflammation after myocardial infarction.

Inflammation is terminated when the offending agent is eliminated and the secreted mediators are broken down or dissipated. In addition, there are active anti-inflammatory mechanisms that serve to control the response and prevent it from causing excessive damage to the host.

This chapter first describes the sequence of events in acute inflammation as well as the structural and molecular mechanisms underlying them, and then reviews the mediators that initiate these events. This is followed by a discussion of the major features of chronic inflammation. Inflammation has a rich history, intimately linked to the history of wars, the migrations of populations, and infections,[1] and we first touch on some of the historical highlights in our understanding of this fascinating process.[2,3]

Historical Highlights

Although clinical features of inflammation were described in an Egyptian papyrus (dated around 3000 BC), Celsus, a Roman writer of the first century AD, first listed the four cardinal signs of inflammation: *rubor, tumor, calor*, and *dolor* (redness, swelling, heat, and pain). These signs are typically more prominent in acute inflammation than in chronic inflammation. A fifth clinical sign, loss of function *(functio laesa)*, was later added by Virchow. In 1793, the Scottish surgeon John Hunter noted what is now considered an obvious fact: that inflammation is not a disease but a nonspecific response that has a *salutary* effect on its host.[4] Julius Cohnheim (1839–1884) first used the microscope to observe inflamed blood vessels in thin, transparent membranes, such as in the mesentery and tongue of the frog. Noting the initial changes in blood flow, the subsequent edema caused by increased vascular permeability, and the characteristic leukocyte emigration, he wrote descriptions of inflammation that can hardly be improved on.[5]

In the 1880s, the Russian biologist Elie Metchnikoff discovered the process of *phagocytosis* by observing the ingestion of rose thorns by amebocytes of starfish larvae and of bacteria by mammalian leukocytes.[6] He concluded that the purpose of inflammation was to bring phagocytic cells to the injured area to engulf invading bacteria. At that time, Metchnikoff contradicted the prevailing theory that the purpose of inflammation was to bring in factors from the serum to neutralize the infectious agents. It soon became clear that both cells (phagocytes) and serum factors (antibodies) were critical for defense against microorganisms, and in recognition of this, Metchnikoff and Paul Ehrlich (who developed the humoral theory of immunity) shared the Nobel Prize in 1908.

To these names must be added that of Sir Thomas Lewis, who, on the basis of simple experiments studying the inflammatory response in skin, established the concept that *chemical substances, such as histamine locally induced by injury, mediate the vascular changes of inflammation.* This fundamental concept underlies the important discoveries of chemical mediators of inflammation and the use of anti-inflammatory agents in clinical medicine.

Acute Inflammation

Acute inflammation is a rapid response to an injurious agent that serves to deliver mediators of host defense—leukocytes and plasma proteins—to the site of injury. Acute inflammation has three major components: (1) *alterations in vascular caliber that lead to an increase in blood flow*; (2) *structural changes in the microvasculature that permit plasma proteins and leukocytes to leave the circulation*; and (3) *emigration of the leukocytes* from the microcirculation, *their accumulation* in the focus of injury, *and their activation* to eliminate the offending agent (Fig. 2–2).

Certain terms must be defined before specific features of inflammation are described. The escape of fluid, proteins, and blood cells from the vascular system into the interstitial tissue or body cavities is known as *exudation*. An *exudate* is an inflammatory extravascular fluid that has a high protein concentration, cellular debris, and a specific gravity above 1.020. It implies significant alteration in the normal permeability of small blood vessels in the area of injury. In contrast, a *transudate* is a fluid with low protein content (most of which is albumin) and a specific gravity of less than 1.012. It is essentially an ultrafiltrate of blood plasma that results from osmotic or hydrostatic imbalance across the vessel wall without an increase in vascular permeability. *Edema* denotes an excess of fluid in the interstitial or serous cavities; it can be either an exudate or a transudate. *Pus*, a *purulent* exudate, is an inflammatory exudate rich in leukocytes (mostly neutrophils), the debris of dead cells and, in many cases, microbes.

STIMULI FOR ACUTE INFLAMMATION

Acute inflammatory reactions are triggered by a variety of stimuli:

- Infections (bacterial, viral, parasitic) and microbial toxins
- Trauma (blunt and penetrating)
- Physical and chemical agents (thermal injury, e.g., burns or frostbite; irradiation; some environmental chemicals)

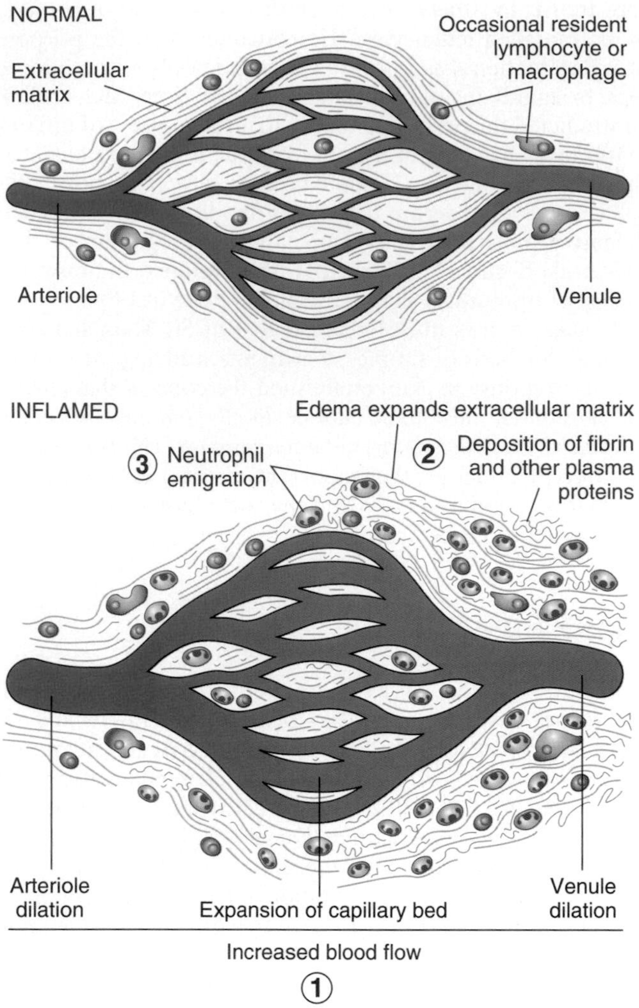

FIGURE 2–2 The major local manifestations of acute inflammation, compared to normal. (1) Vascular dilation and increased blood flow (causing erythema and warmth), (2) extravasation and deposition of plasma fluid and proteins (edema), and (3) leukocyte emigration and accumulation in the site of injury.

- Tissue necrosis (from any cause)
- Foreign bodies (splinters, dirt, sutures)
- Immune reactions (also called hypersensitivity reactions)

Each of these stimuli may induce reactions with some distinctive features, but all inflammatory reactions share the same basic features. We first describe the characteristic reactions of acute inflammation, and then the chemical mediators responsible for these reactions.

VASCULAR CHANGES

Since the two major mechanisms of host defense against microbes—antibodies and leukocytes—are normally carried in the bloodstream, it is not surprising that vascular phenomena play a major role in acute inflammation. Normally, plasma proteins and circulating cells are sequestered inside the vessels and move in the direction of flow. In inflammation, blood vessels undergo a series of changes that are designed to maximize the movement of plasma proteins and circulating cells out of the circulation and into the site of injury or infection.

Changes in Vascular Flow and Caliber

Changes in vascular flow and caliber begin early after injury and develop at varying rates depending on the severity of the injury. The changes occur in the following order:

- *Vasodilation* is one of the earliest manifestations of acute inflammation; sometimes, it follows a transient constriction of arterioles, lasting a few seconds. Vasodilation first involves the arterioles and then results in opening of new capillary beds in the area. Thus comes about *increased blood flow*, which is the cause of the heat and the redness (see Fig. 2–2). *Vasodilation is induced by the action of several mediators, notably histamine and nitric oxide, on vascular smooth muscle*; these mediators are described later in the chapter.
- Vasodilation is quickly followed by *increased permeability of the microvasculature*, with the outpouring of protein-rich fluid into the extravascular tissues; this process is described in detail below.
- The loss of fluid results in concentration of red cells in small vessels and increased viscosity of the blood, reflected by the presence of dilated small vessels packed with red cells and slower blood flow, a condition termed *stasis*. With mild stimuli, stasis may not become apparent until 15 to 30 minutes have elapsed, whereas with severe injury, stasis may occur in a few minutes.
- As stasis develops, leukocytes, principally neutrophils, accumulate along the vascular endothelium. Leukocytes then stick to the endothelium, and soon afterward they migrate through the vascular wall into the interstitial tissue, in processes that are described later.

Increased Vascular Permeability (Vascular Leakage)

A hallmark of acute inflammation is increased vascular permeability leading to the escape of a protein-rich fluid (exudate) into the extravascular tissue. The loss of protein from the plasma reduces the intravascular osmotic pressure and increases the osmotic pressure of the interstitial fluid. Together with the increased hydrostatic pressure owing to increased blood flow through the dilated vessels, this leads to a marked *outflow* of fluid and its accumulation in the interstitial tissue (Fig. 2–3). The net increase of extravascular fluid results in *edema.*

Normal fluid exchange and microvascular permeability are critically dependent on an intact endothelium. How then does the endothelium become leaky in inflammation? The following mechanisms have been proposed (Fig. 2–4):

- *Formation of endothelial gaps in venules.*[7,8] This is the most common mechanism of vascular leakage and is elicited by histamine, bradykinin, leukotrienes, the neuropeptide substance P, and many other classes of chemical mediators. It occurs rapidly after exposure to the mediator and is usually reversible and short-lived (15 to 30 minutes); it is thus known as the *immediate transient response. Classically, this type of leakage affects venules 20 to 60 μm in diameter*, leaving capillaries and arterioles unaffected[9]

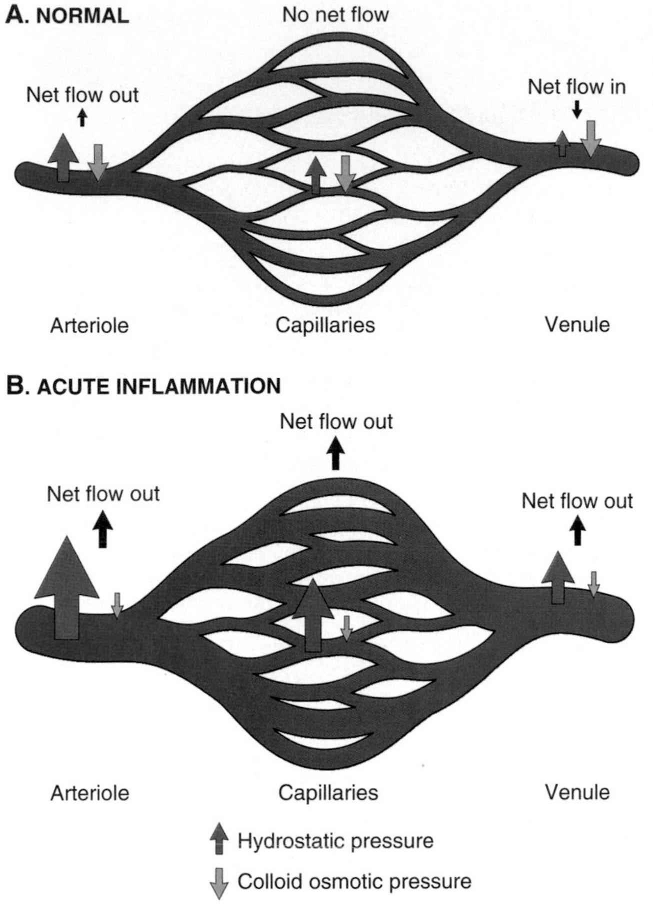

FIGURE 2–3 Blood pressure and plasma colloid osmotic forces in normal and inflamed microcirculation. *A,* Normal hydrostatic pressure (*red arrows*) is about 32 mm Hg at the arterial end of a capillary bed and 12 mm Hg at the venous end; the mean colloid osmotic pressure of tissues is approximately 25 mm Hg (*green arrows*), which is equal to the mean capillary pressure. Although fluid tends to leave the precapillary arteriole, it is returned in equal amounts via the postcapillary venule, so that the net flow (*black arrows*) in or out is zero. *B,* Acute inflammation. Arteriole pressure is increased to 50 mm Hg, the mean capillary pressure is increased because of arteriolar dilation, and the venous pressure increases to approximately 30 mm Hg. At the same time, osmotic pressure is reduced (averaging 20 mm Hg) because of protein leakage across the venule. The net result is an excess of extravasated fluid.

(Fig. 2–5). The precise reason for this restriction to venules is uncertain; it may be because there is a greater density of receptors for the mediators in venular endothelium. Parenthetically, many of the later leukocyte events in inflammation—adhesion and emigration—also occur predominantly in the venules in most organs. Binding of mediators, such as histamine, to their receptors on endothelial cells activates intracellular signaling pathways that lead to phosphorylation of contractile and cytoskeletal proteins, such as myosin.[10,11] These proteins contract, leading to *contraction of the endothelial cells* and separation of intercellular junctions. Thus, the gaps in the venular endothelium are largely intercellular or close to the intercellular junctions. Cytokines such as interleukin-1 (IL-1), tumor necrosis factor (TNF), and interferon-γ (IFN-γ) also increase vascu-

Gaps due to endothelial contraction

- Venules
- Vasoactive mediators (histamine, leukotrienes, etc.)
- Most common
- Fast and short-lived (minutes)

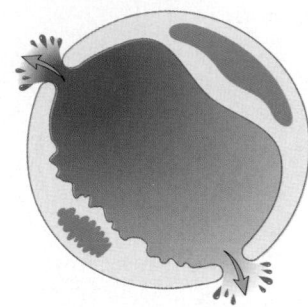

Direct injury

- Arterioles, capillaries, and venules
- Toxins, burns, chemicals
- Fast and may be long-lived (hours to days)

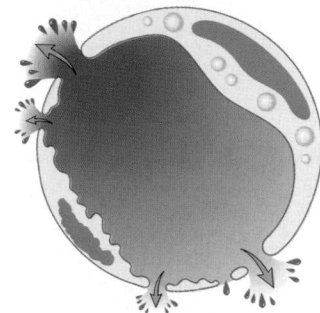

Leukocyte-dependent injury

- Mostly venules
- Pulmonary capillaries
- Late response
- Long-lived (hours)

Increased transcytosis

- Venules
- Vascular endothelium–derived growth factor

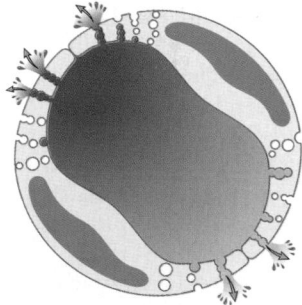

New blood vessel formation

- Sites of angiogenesis
- Persists until intercellular junctions form

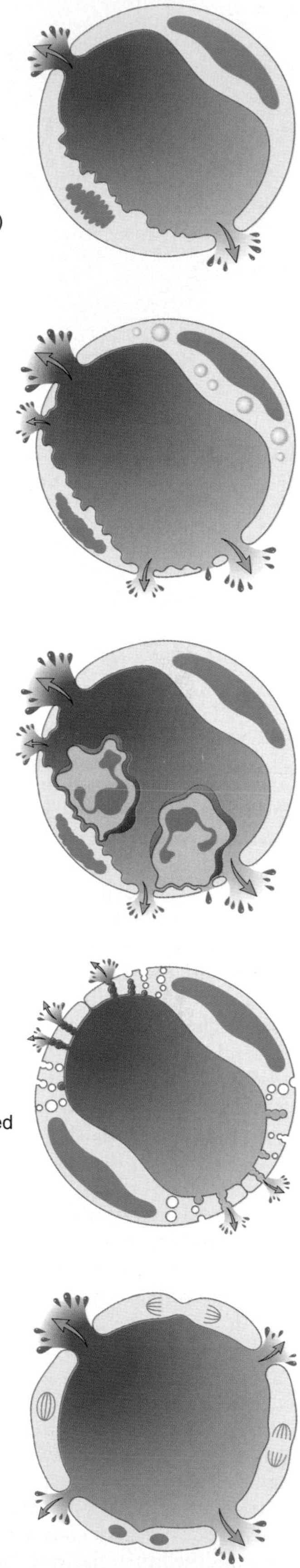

FIGURE 2–4 Diagrammatic representation of five mechanisms of increased vascular permeability in inflammation (see text).

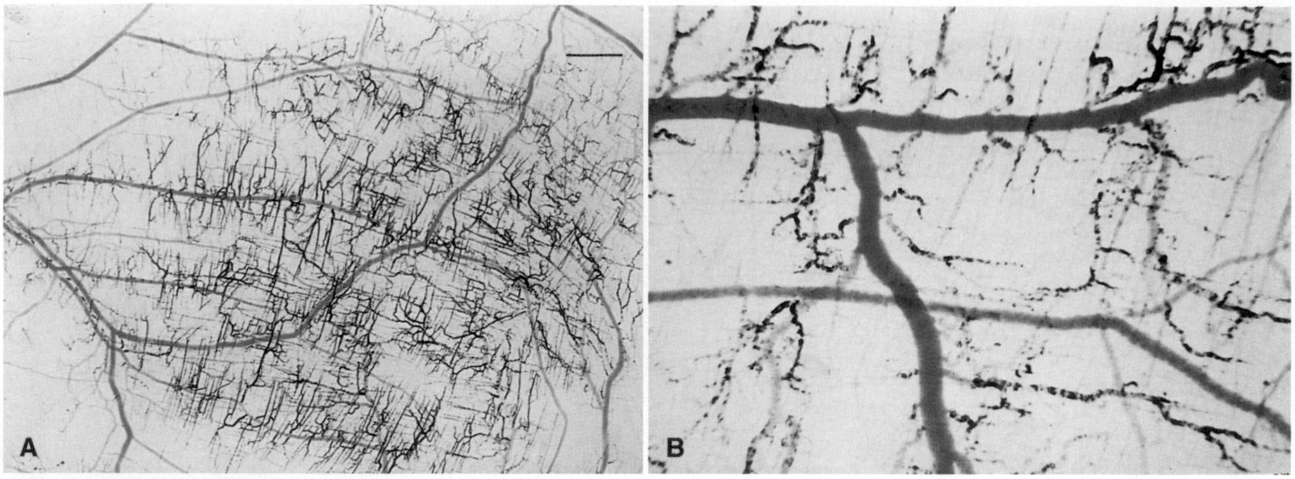

FIGURE 2–5 Vascular leakage induced by chemical mediators. *A,* This is a fixed and cleared preparation of a rat cremaster muscle examined unstained by transillumination. One hour before sacrifice, bradykinin was injected over this muscle, and colloidal carbon was given intravenously. Plasma, loaded with carbon, escaped, but most of the carbon particles were retained by the basement membrane of the leaking vessels, with the result that these became "labeled" black. Note that not all the vessels leak—only the venules. In *B,* a higher power, the capillary network is faintly visible in the background. (Courtesy of Dr. Guido Majno, University of Massachusetts Medical School, Worcester, MA.)

lar permeability by inducing a structural reorganization of the cytoskeleton, such that the endothelial cells retract from one another. In contrast to the histamine effect, the cytokine-induced response is somewhat delayed (4 to 6 hours) and long-lived (24 hours or more).

- *Direct endothelial injury, resulting in endothelial cell necrosis and detachment.*[12] This effect is usually encountered in necrotizing injuries and is due to direct damage to the endothelium by the injurious stimulus, as, for example, in severe burns or lytic bacterial infections. Neutrophils that adhere to the endothelium (discussed below) may also injure the endothelial cells. In most instances, leakage starts immediately after injury and is sustained at a high level for several hours until the damaged vessels are thrombosed or repaired. The reaction is known as the *immediate sustained response. All levels of the microcirculation are affected, including venules, capillaries, and arterioles.* Endothelial cell detachment is often associated with platelet adhesion and thrombosis.
- *Delayed prolonged leakage.* This is a curious but relatively common type of increased permeability that *begins after a delay of 2 to 12 hours, lasts for several hours or even days, and involves venules as well as capillaries.* Such leakage is caused, for example, by mild to moderate thermal injury, x-radiation or ultraviolet radiation, and certain bacterial toxins. Late-appearing sunburn is a good example of a delayed reaction. The mechanism of such leakage is unclear. It may result from the direct effect of the injurious agent, leading to delayed endothelial cell damage (perhaps by apoptosis), or the effect of cytokines causing endothelial retraction, as described earlier.
- *Leukocyte-mediated endothelial injury.* Leukocytes adhere to endothelium relatively early in inflammation. As discussed later, such leukocytes may be activated in the process, releasing toxic oxygen species and proteolytic enzymes, which then cause endothelial injury or detachment, resulting in increased permeability. In acute inflammation, this form of injury is largely restricted to vascular sites, such as venules and pulmonary and glomerular capillaries, where leukocytes adhere for prolonged periods to the endothelium.[12]
- *Increased transcytosis* across the endothelial cytoplasm. Transcytosis occurs across channels consisting of clusters of interconnected, uncoated vesicles and vacuoles called the *vesiculovacuolar organelle,* many of which are located close to intercellular junctions. Certain factors, for example, vascular endothelial growth factor (VEGF) (Chapter 3), appear to cause vascular leakage by increasing the number and perhaps the size of these channels.[13] It has been claimed that this is also a mechanism of increased permeability induced by histamine and most chemical mediators.
- *Leakage from new blood vessels.* As described in Chapter 3, during repair, endothelial cells proliferate and form new blood vessels, a process called *angiogenesis.* New vessel sprouts remain leaky until the endothelial cells mature and form intercellular junctions. In addition, certain factors that cause angiogenesis (e.g., VEGF) also increase vascular permeability,[14] and endothelial cells in foci of angiogenesis have increased density of receptors for vasoactive mediators, including histamine, substance P, and VEGF.[15] All these factors account for the edema that is characteristic of the early phases of healing that follow inflammation (Chapter 3).

Although these mechanisms are separable, all may play a role in response to one stimulus. For example, at different stages of a thermal burn, leakage results from chemically mediated endothelial contraction, direct and leukocyte-dependent endothelial injury, and regenerating capillaries when the injury begins to heal. The vascular leakage induced by all these mechanisms accounts for the life-threatening loss of fluid in severely burned patients.

In summary, *in acute inflammation, fluid loss from vessels with increased permeability occurs in distinct phases*: (1) an immediate transient response lasting for 30 minutes or less, mediated mainly by the actions of histamine and leukotrienes on endothelium; (2) a delayed response starting at about 2 hours and lasting for about 8 hours, mediated by kinins, complement products, and other factors; and (3) a prolonged response that is most noticeable after direct endothelial injury, for example, after burns.

CELLULAR EVENTS: LEUKOCYTE EXTRAVASATION AND PHAGOCYTOSIS

A critical function of inflammation is to deliver leukocytes to the site of injury and to activate the leukocytes to perform their normal functions in host defense. Leukocytes ingest offending agents, kill bacteria and other microbes, and get rid of necrotic tissue and foreign substances. A price that is paid for the defensive potency of leukocytes is that they may induce tissue damage and prolong inflammation, since the leukocyte products that destroy microbes and necrotic tissues can also injure normal host tissues.

The sequence of events in the journey of leukocytes from the vessel lumen to the interstitial tissue, called extravasation, can be divided into the following steps[16] (Fig. 2–6):

1. In the lumen: margination, rolling, and adhesion to endothelium. Vascular endothelium normally does not bind circulating cells or impede their passage. In inflammation, the endothelium has to be activated to permit it to bind leukocytes, as a prelude to their exit from the blood vessels.
2. Transmigration across the endothelium (also called diapedesis)
3. Migration in interstitial tissues toward a chemotactic stimulus

In normally flowing blood in venules, erythrocytes are confined to a central axial column, displacing the leukocytes toward the wall of the vessel. Because blood flow slows early in inflammation (stasis), hemodynamic conditions change (wall shear stress decreases), and more white cells assume a peripheral position along the endothelial surface. This process of leukocyte accumulation is called *margination*. Subsequently, individual and then rows of leukocytes tumble slowly along the endothelium and adhere transiently (a process called *rolling*), finally coming to rest at some point where they adhere firmly (resembling pebbles over which a stream runs without disturbing them). In time, the endothelium can be virtually lined by white cells, an appearance called *pavementing*. After firm adhesion, leukocytes insert pseudopods into the junctions between the endothelial cells, squeeze through interendothelial junctions, and assume a position between the endothelial cell and the basement membrane. Eventually, they traverse the basement membrane and escape into the extravascular space. Neutrophils, monocytes, lymphocytes, eosinophils, and basophils all use the same pathway to migrate from the blood into tissues. We now examine the molecular mechanisms of each of the steps.

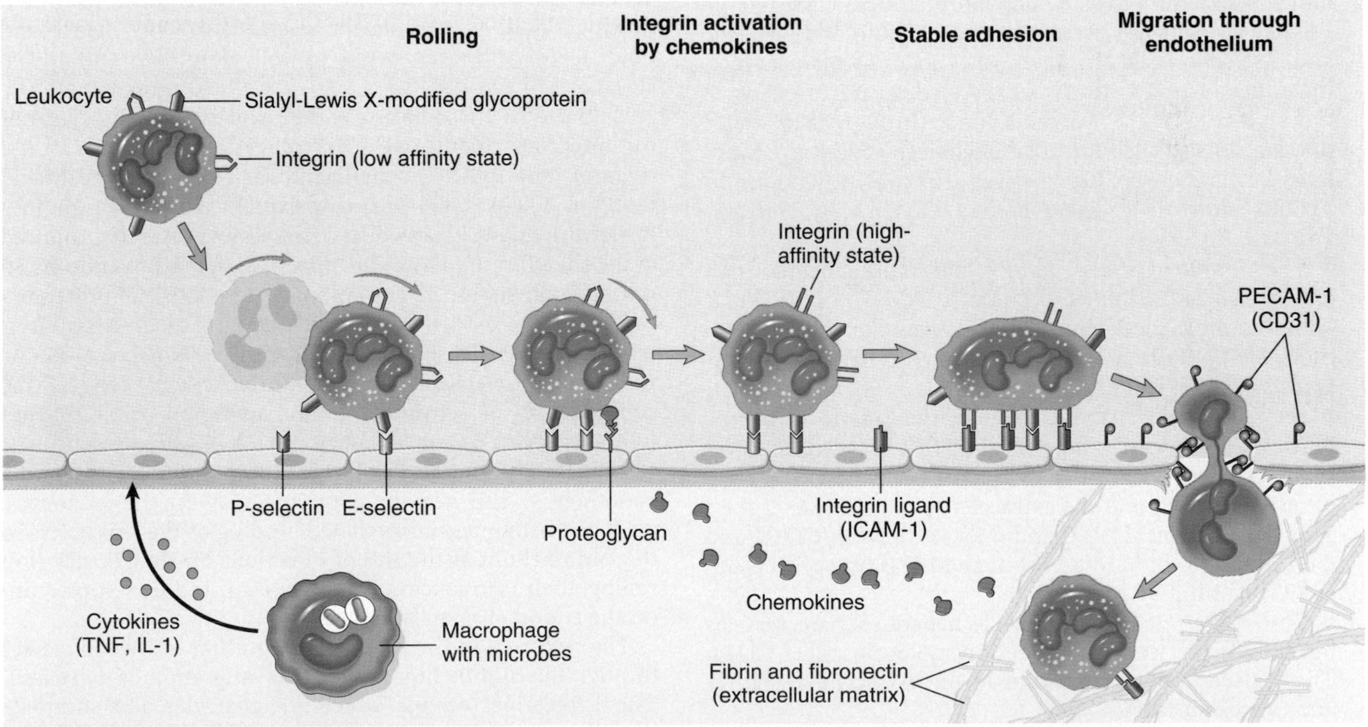

FIGURE 2–6 The multistep process of leukocyte migration through blood vessels, shown here for neutrophils. The leukocytes first roll, then become activated and adhere to endothelium, then transmigrate across the endothelium, pierce the basement membrane, and migrate toward chemoattractants emanating from the source of injury. Different molecules play predominant roles in different steps of this process—selectins in rolling; chemokines in activating the neutrophils to increase avidity of integrins (in green); integrins in firm adhesion; and CD31 (PECAM-1) in transmigration.

TABLE 2–1 Endothelial/Leukocyte Adhesion Molecules

Endothelial Molecule	Leukocyte Receptor	Major Role
P-selectin	Sialyl-Lewis X PSGL-1	Rolling (neutrophils, monocytes, lymphocytes)
E-selectin	Sialyl-Lewis X	Rolling, adhesion to activated endothelium (neutrophils, monocytes, T cells)
ICAM-1	CD11/CD18 (integrins) (LFA-1, Mac-1)	Adhesion, arrest, transmigration (all leukocytes)
VCAM-1	$\alpha 4\beta 1$ (VLA4) (integrins) $\alpha 4\beta 7$ (LPAM-1)	Adhesion (eosinophils, monocytes, lymphocytes)
GlyCam-1	L-selectin	Lymphocyte homing to high endothelial venules
CD31 (PECAM)	CD31	Leukocyte migration through endothelium

*ICAM-1, VCAM-1, and CD31 belong to the immunoglobulin family of proteins; PSGL-1, P-selectin glycoprotein ligand 1.

Leukocyte Adhesion and Transmigration

Leukocyte adhesion and transmigration are regulated largely by the binding of complementary adhesion molecules on the leukocyte and endothelial surfaces, and chemical mediators—chemoattractants and certain cytokines—affect these processes by modulating the surface expression or avidity of such adhesion molecules.[16,17] The adhesion receptors involved belong to four molecular families—the *selectins*, the *immunoglobulin superfamily*, the *integrins*, and *mucin-like glycoproteins*. The most important of these are listed in Table 2–1.

- *Selectins*, so called because they are characterized by an extracellular N-terminal domain related to sugar-binding mammalian lectins, consist of E-selectin (CD62E, previously known as ELAM-1), which is confined to endothelium; P-selectin (CD62P, previously called GMP140 or PADGEM), which is present in endothelium and platelets; and L-selectin (CD62L, previously known by many names, including LAM-1), which is expressed on most leukocyte types (Box 2–1).[18,19] Selectins bind, through their lectin domain, to sialylated forms of oligosaccharides (e.g., sialylated Lewis X), which themselves are covalently bound to various *mucin-like glycoproteins* (GlyCAM-1, PSGL-1, ESL-1, and CD34).
- The *immunoglobulin family* molecules include two endothelial adhesion molecules: ICAM-1 (intercellular adhesion molecule 1) and VCAM-1 (vascular cell adhesion molecule 1). Both these molecules serve as ligands for integrins found on leukocytes.
- *Integrins* are transmembrane heterodimeric glycoproteins, made up of α and β chains, that are expressed on many cell types and bind to ligands on endothelial cells, other leukocytes, and the extracellular matrix (Box 2–1).[20] The β_2 integrins LFA-1 and Mac-1 (CD11a/CD18 and CD11b/CD18) bind to ICAM-1, and the β_1 integrins (such as VLA-4) bind VCAM-1.
- *Mucin-like glycoproteins*, such as heparan sulfate, serve as ligands for the leukocyte adhesion molecule called CD44. These glycoproteins are found in the extracellular matrix and on cell surfaces.

The recruitment of leukocytes to sites of injury and infection is a multistep process involving attachment of circulating leukocytes to endothelial cells and their migration through the endothelium (see Fig. 2–6). The first events are the induction of adhesion molecules on endothelial cells, by a number of mechanisms (Fig. 2–7). Mediators such as histamine, thrombin, and platelet activating factor (PAF) stimulate the redistribution of P-selectin from its normal intracellular stores in granules (Weibel-Palade bodies) to the cell surface. Resident tissue macrophages, mast cells, and endothelial cells respond to injurious agents by secreting the cytokines TNF, IL-1, and chemokines (chemoattractant cytokines). (Cytokines are described in more detail below and in Chapter 6.) TNF and IL-1 act on the endothelial cells of postcapillary venules adjacent to the infection and induce the expression of several adhesion molecules. Within 1 to 2 hours, the endothelial cells begin to express E-selectin. Leukocytes express at the tips of their microvilli carbohydrate ligands for the selectins, which bind to the endothelial selectins. These are low-affinity interactions with a fast off-rate, and they are easily disrupted by the flowing blood. As a result, the bound leukocytes detach and bind again, and thus begin to roll along the endothelial surface.

TNF and IL-1 also induce endothelial expression of ligands for integrins, mainly VCAM-1 (the ligand for the VLA-4 integrin) and ICAM-1 (the ligand for the LFA-1 and Mac-1 integrins). Leukocytes normally express these integrins in a low-affinity state. Meanwhile, chemokines that were produced at the site of injury enter the blood vessel, bind to endothelial cell heparan sulfate glycosaminoglycans (labeled "proteoglycan" in Figure 2–6), and are displayed at high concentrations on the endothelial surface.[21] These chemokines act on the rolling leukocytes and activate the leukocytes. One of the consequences of activation is the conversion of VLA-4 and LFA-1 integrins on the leukocytes to a high-affinity state. The combination of induced expression of integrin ligands on the endothelium and activation of integrins on the leukocytes results in firm integrin-mediated binding of the leukocytes to the endothelium at the site of infection. The leukocytes stop rolling, their cytoskeleton is reorganized, and they spread out on the endothelial surface.

The next step in the process is migration of the leukocytes through the endothelium, called transmigration or *diapedesis*. Chemokines act on the adherent leukocytes and stimulate the cells to migrate through interendothelial spaces toward the chemical concentration gradient, that is, toward the site of injury or infection. Certain homophilic adhesion molecules (i.e., adhesion molecules that bind to each other) present in the intercellular junction of endothelium are involved in

Box 2–1 Selectins and Integrins: Adhesion Molecules Involved in the Inflammatory Response

The specific (nonrandom) adhesion of cells to other cells or to extracellular matrices is a basic component of cell migration and recognition and underlies many biologic processes, including embryogenesis, tissue repair, and immune and inflammatory responses. It is, therefore, not surprising that many different genes have evolved that encode proteins with specific adhesive functions. Two families of adhesive proteins that are especially important in inflammation are the *selectins* and the *integrins.*

Selectins

The selectins are a family of three closely related proteins that differ in their cellular distribution but all function in adhesion of leukocytes to endothelial cells. All selectins are single-chain transmembrane glycoproteins with an amino terminus that is related to carbohydrate-binding proteins known as C-type lectins. Like other C-type lectins, ligand binding by selectins is calcium-dependent (hence the name C-type). The binding of selectins to their ligands has a fast on rate but also has a fast off rate and is of low affinity; this property allows selectins to mediate initial attachment and subsequent rolling of leukocytes on endothelium in the face of flowing blood.

L-selectin, or CD62L, is expressed on lymphocytes and other leukocytes. It serves as a homing receptor for lymphocytes to enter lymph nodes by binding to high endothelial venules (HEVs). It also serves to bind neutrophils to cytokine-activated endothelial cells at sites of inflammation. L-selectin is located on the tips of microvillus projections of leukocytes, facilitating its interaction with ligands on endothelium. At least three endothelial cell ligands can bind L-selectin—glycan–bearing cell adhesion molecule-1 (GlyCAM-1), a secreted proteoglycan found on HEVs of lymph node; mucosal addressin cell adhesion molecule-1 (MadCAM-1), expressed on endothelial cells in gut-associated lymphoid tissues; and CD34, a proteoglycan on endothelial cells (and bone marrow cells). The protein backbones of all these ligands are modified by specific carbohydrates, which are the molecules actually recognized by the selectin.

E-selectin, or CD62E, previously known as endothelial leukocyte adhesion molecule-1 (ELAM-1), is expressed only on cytokine-activated endothelial cells, hence the designation E. E-selectin recognizes complex sialylated carbohydrate groups related to the Lewis X or Lewis A family found on various surface proteins of granulocytes, monocytes, and previously activated effector and memory T cells. E-selectin is important in the homing of effector and memory T cells to some peripheral sites of inflammation, particularly in the skin. Endothelial cell expression of E-selectin is a hallmark of acute cytokine-mediated inflammation, and antibodies to E-selectin can block leukocyte accumulation in vivo.

P-selectin (CD62P) was first identified in the secretory granules of platelets, hence the designation P. It has since been found in secretory granules of endothelial cells, called Weibel-Palade bodies. When endothelial cells or platelets are stimulated, P-selectin is translocated within minutes to the cell surface. On reaching the cell surface, P-selectin mediates binding of neutrophils, T lymphocytes, and monocytes. The complex carbohydrate ligands recognized by P-selectin appear similar to those recognized by E-selectin.

The essential physiologic roles of selectins have been reinforced by studies of gene knockout mice. L-selectin–deficient mice have small, poorly formed lymph nodes with few T cells. Mice lacking either E-selectin or P-selectin have only mild defects in leukocyte recruitment, suggesting that these two molecules are functionally redundant. Double knockout mice lacking both E-selectin and P-selectin have significantly impaired leukocyte recruitment and increased susceptibility to infections. Humans who lack one of the enzymes needed to express the carbohydrate ligands for E-selectin and P-selectin on neutrophils have similar problems, resulting in a syndrome called leukocyte adhesion deficiency-2 (LAD-2) (see text).

Integrins

The integrin superfamily consists of about 30 structurally homologous proteins that promote cell–cell or cell–matrix interactions. The name of this family of proteins derives from the hypothesis that they coordinate (i.e., "integrate") signals from extracellular ligands with cytoskeleton-dependent motility, shape change, and phagocytic responses.

All integrins are heterodimeric cell surface proteins composed of two noncovalently linked polypeptide chains, α and β. The extracellular domains of the two chains bind to various ligands, including extracellular matrix glycoproteins, activated complement components, and proteins on the surfaces of other cells. Several integrins bind to Arg-Gly-Asp (RGD) sequences in the fibronectin and vitronectin molecules. The cytoplasmic domains of the integrins interact with cytoskeletal components (including vinculin, talin, actin, α-actinin, and tropomyosin).

Three integrin subfamilies were originally defined on the basis of which of three β subunits were used to form the heterodimers. More recently, five additional β chains have been identified.

The β_1-containing integrins are also called VLA molecules, referring to "very late activation" molecules, because $\alpha_1\beta_1$ and $\alpha_2\beta_1$ were first shown to be expressed on T cells 2 to 4 weeks after repetitive stimulation in vitro. In fact, other VLA integrins are constitutively expressed on some leukocytes and rapidly induced on others. The β_1 integrins are also called CD49a-hCD29, CD49a-h referring to different α chains (α_1-α_8) and CD29 referring to the common β_1 subunit. Most of the β_1 integrins are widely expressed on leukocytes and other cells and mediate attachment of cells to extracellular matrices. VLA-4 ($\alpha_4\beta_1$) is expressed only on leukocytes and can mediate attachment of these cells to endothelium by interacting with vascular cell adhesion molecule-1 (VCAM-1). VLA-4 is one of the principal surface proteins that mediate homing of lymphocytes to endothelium at peripheral sites of inflammation.

The β_2 integrins are also called CD11a-cCD18, or the leukocyte function-associated antigen-1 (LFA-1) family, CD11a-c referring to different α chains and CD18 to the common β_2 subunit. LFA-1 (CD11aCD18) plays an important role in the adhesion of lymphocytes and other leukocytes with other cells, such as antigen-presenting cells and vascular endothelium. Other members of the family include CD11bCD18 (Mac-1 or CR3) and CD11cCD18 (p150,95 or CR4), which mediate leukocyte attachment to endothelial cells and subsequent extravasation. CD11bCD18 also functions as a fibrinogen receptor and as a complement receptor on phagocytic cells, binding particles opsonized with a by-product of complement activation called the inactivated C3b (iC3b) fragment.

The other integrins are expressed on platelets and other cell types, and bind to extracellular matrix proteins as well as proteins involved in coagulation.

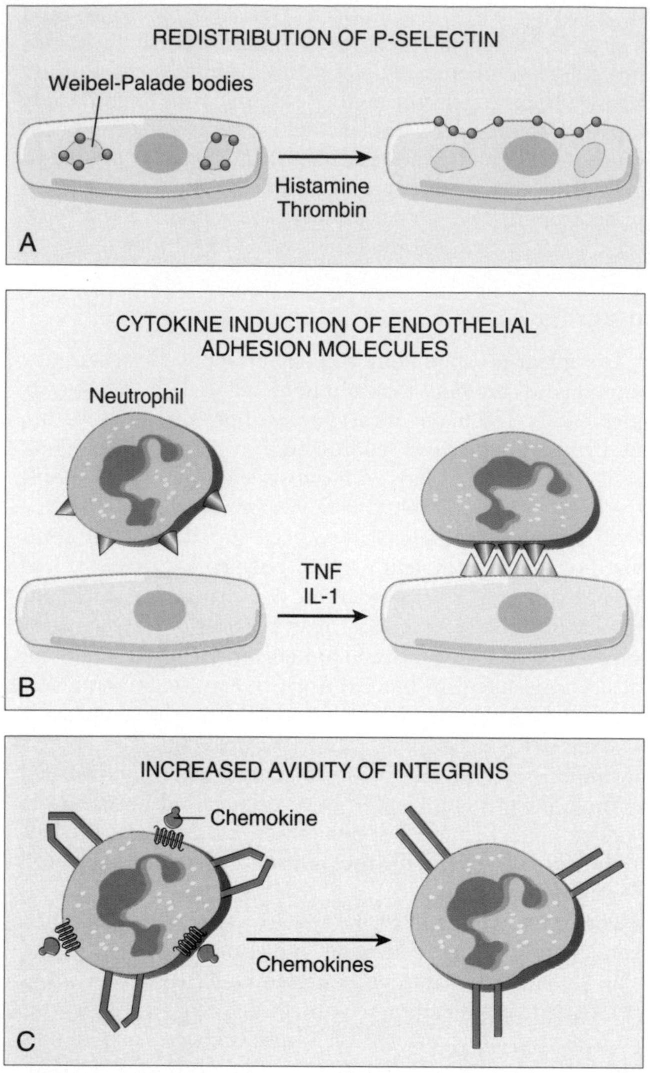

FIGURE 2–7 Regulation of endothelial and leukocyte adhesion molecules. *A*, Redistribution of P-selectin. *B*, Cytokine activation of endothelium. *C*, Increased binding avidity of integrins (see text).

the migration of leukocytes. One of these molecules is a member of the immunoglobulin superfamily called PECAM-1 (platelet endothelial cell adhesion molecule) or CD31.[22] *Leukocyte diapedesis, similar to increased vascular permeability, occurs predominantly in the venules* (except in the lungs, where it also occurs in capillaries). After traversing the endothelium, leukocytes are transiently retarded in their journey by the continuous basement membrane of the venules, but eventually the cells pierce the basement membrane, probably by secreting collagenases. The net result of this process is that leukocytes rapidly accumulate where they are needed.

Once leukocytes enter the extravascular connective tissue, they are able to adhere to the extracellular matrix by virtue of β_1 integrins and CD44 binding to matrix proteins. Thus, the leukocytes are retained at the site where they are needed.

The most telling proof of the importance of adhesion molecules is the existence of genetic deficiencies in the leukocyte adhesion proteins, which result in impaired leukocyte adhesion and recurrent bacterial infections.[23,24] In *leukocyte adhesion deficiency type 1* (LAD1), patients have a defect in the biosynthesis of the β_2 chain shared by the LFA-1 and Mac-1 integrins. *Leukocyte adhesion deficiency type 2* (LAD2) is caused by the absence of sialyl-Lewis X, the fucose-containing ligand for E-selectin, owing to a defect in a fucosyl transferase, the enzyme that attaches fucose moieties to protein backbones. In addition, antibodies to adhesion molecules abrogate leukocyte extravasation in experimental models of acute inflammation, and gene knockout mice deficient in these molecules show defects in leukocyte adhesion and extravasation.[23,25]

The type of emigrating leukocyte varies with the age of the inflammatory response and with the type of stimulus. In most forms of acute inflammation, *neutrophils predominate in the inflammatory infiltrate during the first 6 to 24 hours, then are replaced by monocytes in 24 to 48 hours* (Fig. 2–8). Several reasons account for this sequence—neutrophils are more numerous in the blood, they respond more rapidly to chemokines, and they may attach more firmly to the adhesion molecules that are rapidly induced on endothelial cells, such as P- and E-selectins. In addition, after entering tissues, neutrophils are short-lived; they undergo apoptosis and disappear after 24 to 48 hours, whereas monocytes survive longer. There are exceptions to this pattern of cellular exudation, however. In certain infections—for example, those produced by *Pseudomonas* organisms—neutrophils predominate over 2 to 4 days; in viral infections, lymphocytes may be the first cells to arrive; in some hypersensitivity reactions, eosinophilic granulocytes may be the main cell type.

Chemotaxis

After extravasation, leukocytes emigrate in tissues toward the site of injury by a process called *chemotaxis*, defined most simply as locomotion oriented along a chemical gradient. All granulocytes, monocytes and, to a lesser extent, lymphocytes respond to chemotactic stimuli with varying rates of speed. Both exogenous and endogenous substances can act as chemoattractants. The most common *exogenous* agents are *bacterial products.* Some of these are peptides that possess an *N*-formyl-methionine terminal amino acid. Others are lipid in nature. *Endogenous* chemoattractants, which are detailed later, include several chemical mediators: (1) *components of the complement system, particularly C5a*; (2) *products of the lipoxygenase pathway, mainly leukotriene B_4 (LTB_4)*; and (3) *cytokines*, particularly those of the chemokine family (e.g., IL-8).

How does the leukocyte sense the chemotactic agents, and how do these substances induce directed cell movement? Although not all the answers are known, several important steps and second messengers are recognized.[26,27] All the chemotactic agents mentioned above bind to specific seven-transmembrane G-protein–coupled receptors (GPCRs) on the surface of leukocytes. Signals initiated from these receptors result in recruitment of G-proteins and activation of several effector molecules, including phospholipase C (PLCγ) and phosphoinositol-3 kinase (PI3K), as well as protein tyrosine kinases. (The general steps in these signal transduction pathways are described in Chapter 3.) PLCγ and PI3K act on membrane inositol phospholipids to generate lipid second messengers that increase cytosolic calcium and activate small

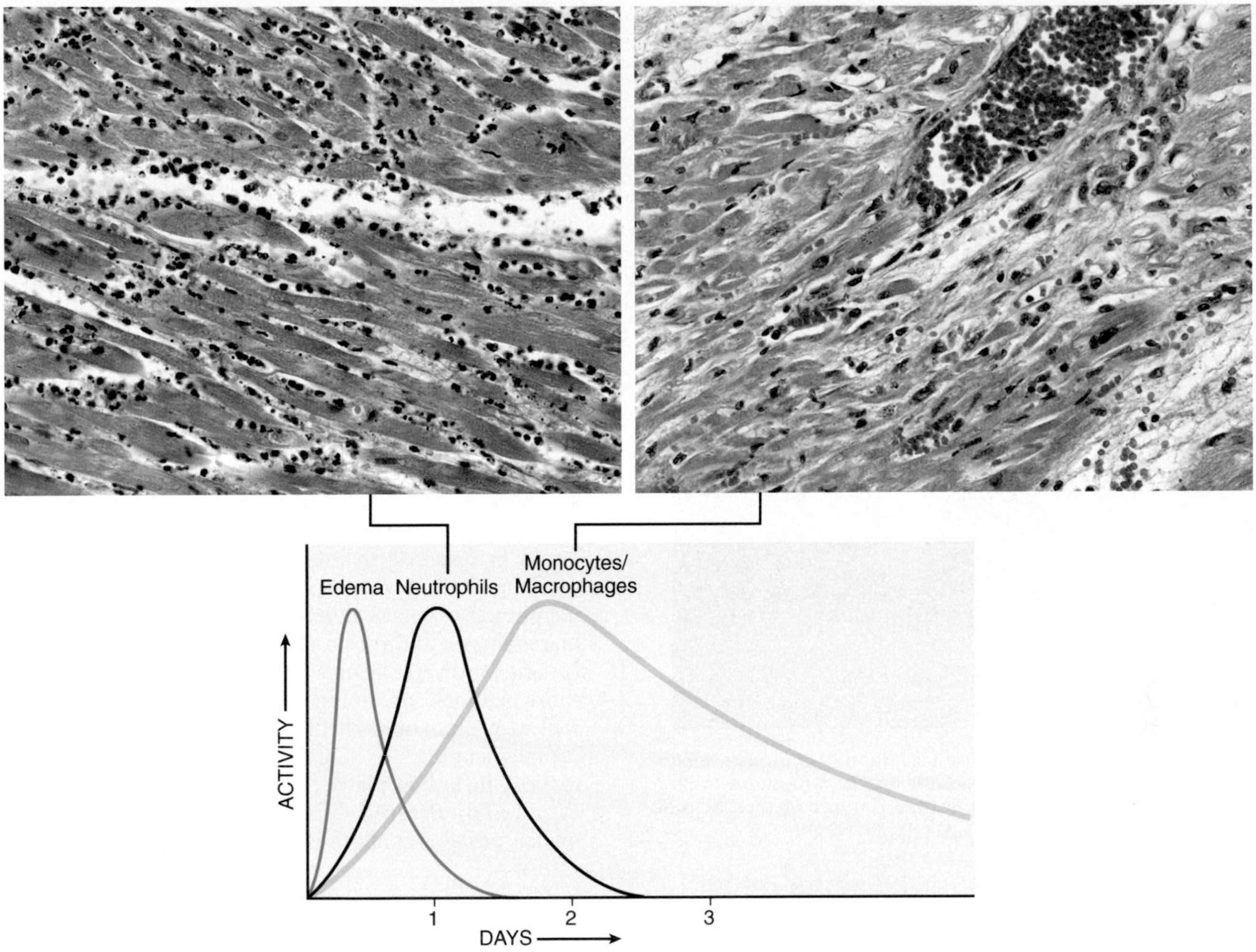

FIGURE 2–8 Schematic and histologic sequence of events following acute injury. The photomicrographs are representative of the early (neutrophilic) (*left*) and later (mononuclear) cellular infiltrates (*right*) of infarcted myocardium. The kinetics of edema and cellular infiltration are approximations. For sake of simplicity, edema is shown as an acute transient response, although secondary waves of delayed edema and neutrophil infiltration can also occur.

GTPases of the Rac/Rho/cdc42 family as well as numerous kinases. The GTPases induce polymerization of actin, resulting in increased amounts of polymerized actin at the leading edge of the cell. The leukocyte moves by extending filopodia that pull the back of the cell in the direction of extension, much as an automobile with front-wheel drive is pulled by the wheels in front (Fig. 2–9). Actin reorganization may also occur at the trailing edge of the cell. Locomotion involves rapid assembly of actin monomers into linear polymers at the filopodium's leading edge, followed by cross-linking of filaments, and disassembly of such filaments away from the leading edge.[28,29] A number of actin-regulating proteins, such as *filamin, gelsolin, profilin*, and *calmodulin*, interact with actin and myosin in the filopodium to produce contraction.

Leukocyte Activation

Microbes, products of necrotic cells, antigen-antibody complexes, and cytokines, including chemotactic factors, induce a number of responses in leukocytes that are part of the defensive functions of the leukocytes (neutrophils and monocytes/macrophages) and are referred to under the rubric of *leukocyte activation* (Fig. 2–10). Activation results from several signaling pathways that are triggered in leukocytes, resulting in increases in cytosolic Ca^{2+} and activation of enzymes such as protein kinase C and phospholipase A_2. The functional responses that are induced on leukocyte activation include the following:

- *Production of arachidonic acid metabolites* from phospholipids, as a result of activation of phospholipase A_2 by increased intracellular calcium and other signals.
- *Degranulation and secretion of lysosomal enzymes and activation of the oxidative burst* (discussed below under phagocytosis).
- *Secretion of cytokines*, which amplify and regulate inflammatory reactions. Activated macrophages are the chief source of the cytokines that are involved in inflammation, but mast cells and other leukocytes may contribute.
- *Modulation of leukocyte adhesion molecules.* As stated earlier, different cytokines cause increased endothelial expression of adhesion molecules and increased avidity of leukocyte integrins, allowing firm adhesion of activated neutrophils to endothelium.

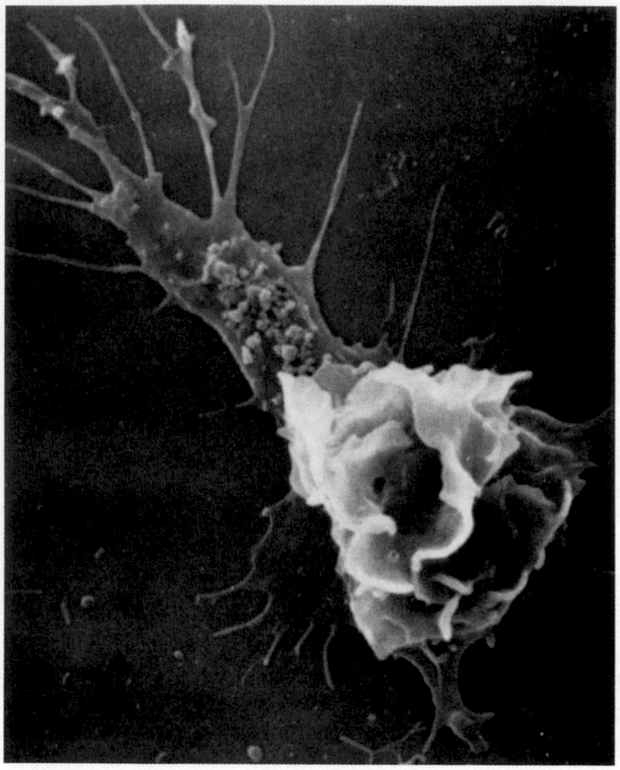

FIGURE 2–9 Scanning electron micrograph of a moving leukocyte in culture showing a filopodium (*upper left*) and a trailing tail. (Courtesy of Dr. Morris J. Karnovsky, Harvard Medical School, Boston, MA.)

Leukocytes express a number of surface receptors that are involved in their activation (see Fig. 2–10). These receptors include the following:

- *Toll-like receptors (TLRs)*, which are homologous to a *Drosophila* protein called Toll, function to activate leukocytes in response to different types and components of microbes. To date, 10 mammalian TLRs have been identified, and each appears to be required for responses to different classes of infectious pathogens (Chapter 6, Box 6–1). Different TLRs play essential roles in cellular responses to bacterial lipopolysaccharide (LPS, or endotoxin), other bacterial proteoglycans, and unmethylated CpG nucleotides, all of which are found only in bacteria, as well as double-stranded RNA, which is produced only by some viruses. These receptors function by receptor-associated kinases to stimulate the production of microbicidal substances and cytokines in the leukocytes.
- *Different seven-transmembrane G-protein–coupled receptors* recognize microbes and some mediators that are produced in response to infections and tissue injury. These receptors have a conserved structure with seven transmembrane α-helical domains; are found on neutrophils, macrophages, and most other types of leukocytes; and are specific for diverse ligands. Receptors of this class recognize short peptides containing *N*-formylmethionyl residues, as well as chemokines, chemotactic breakdown products of complement such as C5a, and lipid mediators of inflammation, including platelet-activating factor, prostaglandin E, and LTB_4. Because all bacterial proteins and few mammalian proteins (only those synthesized within mitochon-

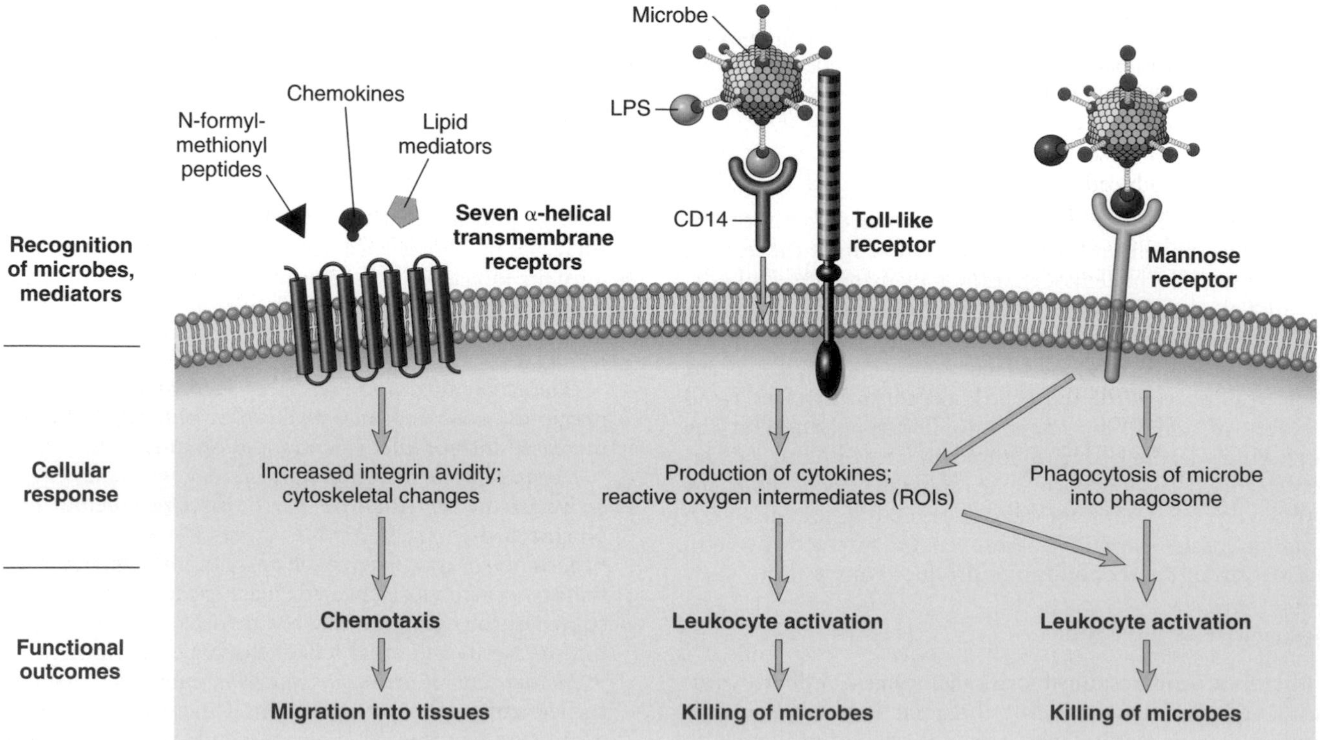

FIGURE 2–10 Leukocyte activation. Different classes of cell surface receptors of leukocytes recognize different stimuli. The receptors initiate responses that mediate the functions of the leukocytes. Only some receptors are depicted (see text for details).

dria) are initiated by *N*-formylmethionine, this receptor allows neutrophils to detect and respond to bacterial proteins. Binding of ligands, such as microbial products and chemokines, to the G-protein–coupled receptors induces migration of the cells from the blood through the endothelium and production of microbicidal substances by activation of the respiratory burst. In a resting cell, the receptor-associated G-proteins form a stable inactive complex containing guanosine diphosphate (GDP) bound to Gα subunits. Occupancy of the receptor by ligand results in an exchange of GTP for GDP. The GTP-bound form of the G-protein activates numerous cellular enzymes, including an isoform of phosphatidylinositol-specific phospholipase C that functions to degrade inositol phospholipids and ultimately to increase intracellular Ca^{2+} and activate protein kinase C. The G-proteins also stimulate cytoskeletal changes, resulting in increased cell motility.

- Phagocytes express *receptors for cytokines* that are produced during immune responses. One of the most important of these cytokines is IFN-γ, which is secreted by natural killer (NK) cells during innate immune responses and by antigen-activated T lymphocytes during adaptive immune responses. IFN-γ is the major macrophage-activating cytokine.
- *Receptors for opsonins* promote phagocytosis of microbes coated with various proteins and deliver signals that activate the phagocytes. The process of coating a particle, such as a microbe, to target it for phagocytosis is called *opsonization*, and substances that do this are *opsonins*. These substances include antibodies, complement proteins, and lectins. One of the most efficient systems for opsonizing particles is coating the particles with IgG antibodies, which are termed specific opsonins and are recognized by the high-affinity Fcγ receptor of phagocytes, called FcγRI (see Chapter 6). Components of the complement system, especially fragments of the complement protein C3, are also potent opsonins, because these fragments bind to microbes and phagocytes express a receptor, called the type 1 complement receptor (CR1), that recognizes breakdown products of C3 (discussed later). These complement fragments are produced when complement is activated by either the classical (antibody-dependent) or the alternative (antibody-independent) pathway. Many bacteria can activate the alternative pathway and produce complement proteins that efficiently opsonize the bacteria in the absence of antibody molecules. A number of plasma proteins, including mannose-binding lectin (MBL), fibronectin, fibrinogen, and C-reactive protein, can coat microbes and are recognized by receptors on phagocytes. For example, a macrophage cell surface receptor called the C1q receptor binds microbes opsonized with plasma MBL, and integrins bind fibrinogen-coated particles.

Phagocytosis

Phagocytosis and the release of enzymes by neutrophils and macrophages are responsible for eliminating the injurious agents and thus constitute two of the major benefits derived from the accumulation of leukocytes at the inflammatory focus. Phagocytosis involves three distinct but interrelated steps (Fig. 2–11*A*): (1) *recognition* and *attachment* of the particle to be ingested by the leukocyte; (2) its *engulfment*, with subsequent formation of a phagocytic vacuole; and (3) *killing* or *degradation* of the ingested material.[30]

Recognition and Attachment. Although neutrophils and macrophages can engulf bacteria or extraneous matter (e.g., latex beads) without attachment to specific receptors, typically the phagocytosis of microbes and dead cells is initiated by recognition of the particles by receptors expressed on the leukocyte surface. *Mannose receptors* and *scavenger receptors* are two important receptors that function to bind and ingest microbes. The mannose receptor is a macrophage lectin that binds terminal mannose and fucose residues of glycoproteins and glycolipids. These sugars are typically part of molecules found on microbial cell walls, whereas mammalian glycoproteins and glycolipids contain terminal sialic acid or *N*-acetylgalactosamine. Therefore, the macrophage mannose receptor recognizes microbes and not host cells. Scavenger receptors were originally defined as molecules that bind and mediate endocytosis of oxidized or acetylated low-density lipoprotein (LDL) particles that can no longer interact with the conventional LDL receptor. Macrophage scavenger receptors bind a variety of microbes in addition to modified LDL particles. Macrophage integrins, notably Mac-1 (CD11b/CD18), may also bind microbes for phagocytosis.

The efficiency of phagocytosis is greatly enhanced when microbes are opsonized by specific proteins (opsonins) for which the phagocytes express high-affinity receptors. As described above, the major opsonins are IgG antibodies, the C3b breakdown product of complement, and certain plasma lectins, notably MBL, all of which are recognized by specific receptors on leukocytes.

Engulfment. Binding of a particle to phagocytic leukocyte receptors initiates the process of active phagocytosis of the particle. During engulfment, extensions of the cytoplasm (pseudopods) flow around the particle to be engulfed, eventually resulting in complete enclosure of the particle within a phagosome created by the plasma membrane of the cell. The limiting membrane of this phagocytic vacuole then fuses with the limiting membrane of a lysosomal granule, resulting in discharge of the granule's contents into the phagolysosome (see Fig. 2–11*A*). During this process, the neutrophil and the monocyte become progressively degranulated.

The process of phagocytosis is complex and involves the integration of many receptor-initiated signals with the coordinated orchestration of membrane remodeling and cytoskeletal changes.[30] Phagocytosis is dependent on polymerization of actin filaments; it is, therefore, not surprising that the signals that trigger phagocytosis are many of the same that are involved in chemotaxis. (In contrast, fluid phase pinocytosis and receptor-mediated endocytosis of small particles involve internalization into clathrin-coated pits and vesicles and are not dependent on the actin cytoskeleton.)

Killing and Degradation. The ultimate step in the elimination of infectious agents and necrotic cells is their killing and degradation within neutrophils and macrophages, which occur most efficiently after activation of the phagocytes.[30] *Microbial killing is accomplished largely by oxygen-dependent mechanisms* (Fig. 2–11*B*).[31] Phagocytosis stimulates a burst in oxygen consumption, glycogenolysis, increased glucose oxidation via the hexose-monophosphate shunt, and production of *reactive oxygen intermediates (ROIs*, also called reactive oxygen sepecies*)*.

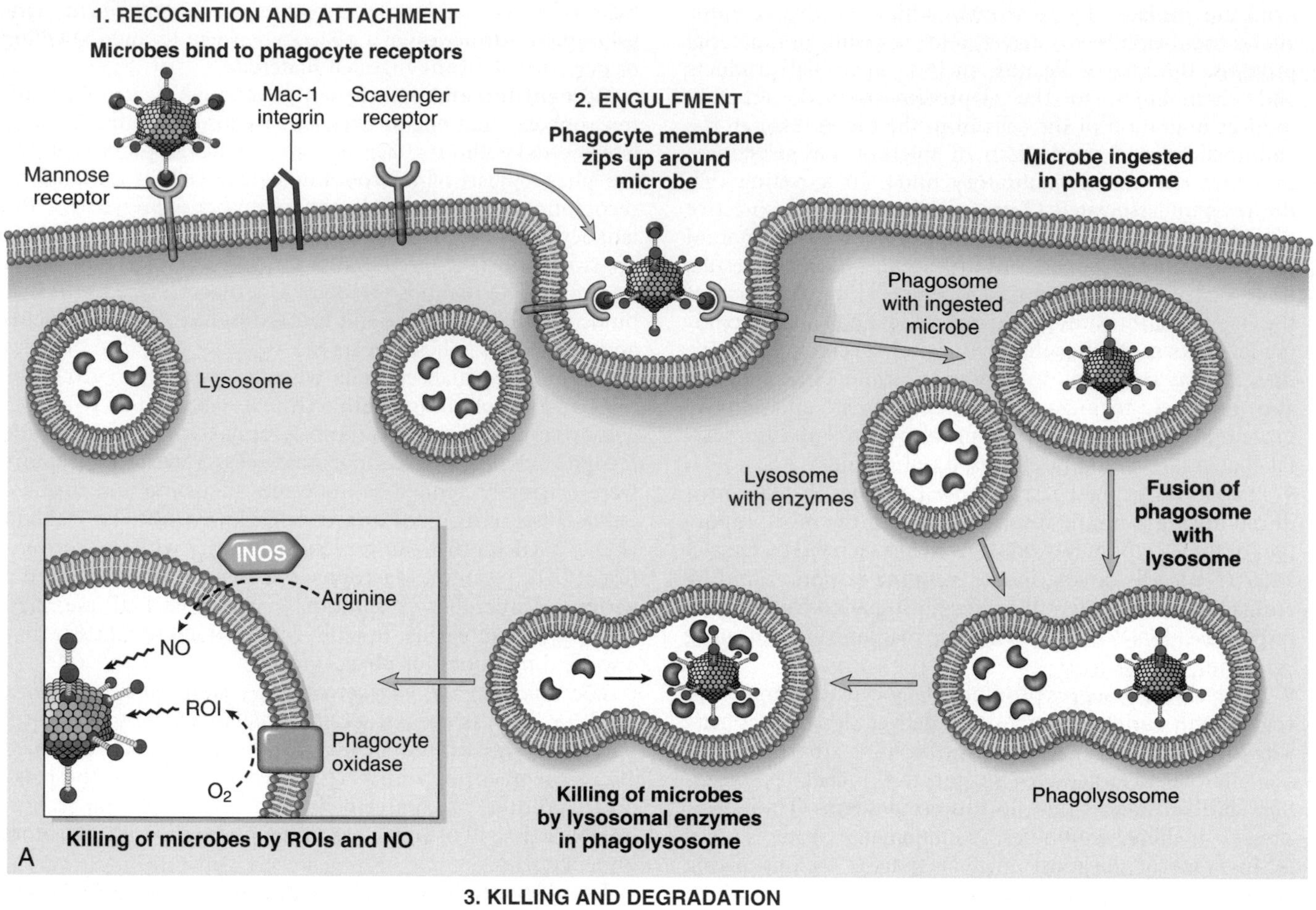

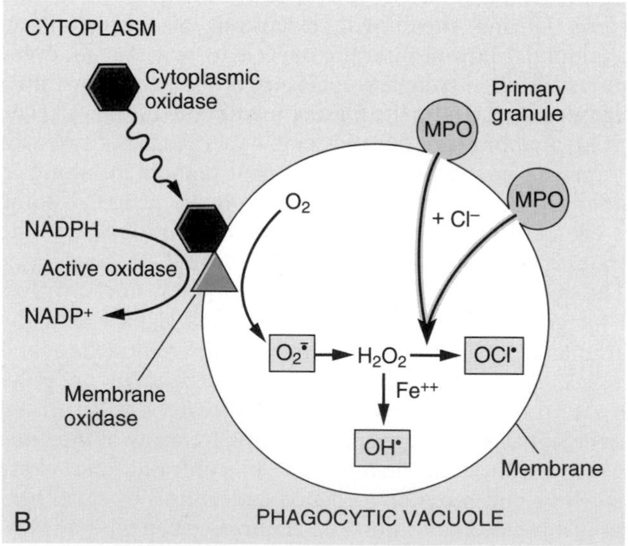

FIGURE 2–11 *A,* Phagocytosis of a particle (e.g., bacterium) involves attachment and binding of Fc and C3b to receptors on the leukocyte membrane, engulfment, and fusion of lysosomes with phagocytic vacuoles, followed by destruction of ingested particles within the phagolysosomes. Note that during phagocytosis, granule contents may be released into extracellular tissues. *B,* Production of microbicidal reactive oxygen intermediates within phagocytic vesicles.

The generation of reactive oxygen intermediates is due to the rapid activation of an oxidase (NADPH oxidase), which oxidizes NADPH (reduced nicotinamide-adenine dinucleotide phosphate) and, in the process, reduces oxygen to superoxide anion ($O_2^{\bar{\cdot}}$). Superoxide is then converted into hydrogen peroxide (H_2O_2), mostly by spontaneous dismutation. Hydrogen peroxide can also be further reduced to the highly reactive hydroxyl radical (OH). Most of the H_2O_2 is eventually broken down by catalase into H_2O and O_2, and some is destroyed by the action of glutathione oxidase. This process and its regulation were described in detail in Chapter 1.

NADPH oxidase is an enzyme complex consisting of at least seven proteins.[32] In resting neutrophils, different NADPH oxidase protein components are located in the plasma membrane and the cytoplasm. In response to activating stimuli, the cytosolic protein components translocate to the plasma membrane or phagosomal membrane, where they assemble and form the functional enzyme complex (see Fig. 2–11*B*). Thus, the *reactive oxygen intermediates are produced within the lysosome* where the ingested substances are segregated, and the cell's own organelles are protected from the harmful effects of the ROIs. A similar enzyme system generates reactive nitrogen intermediates, notably nitric oxide, which also helps to kill microbes.

The H_2O_2 generated by the NADPH oxidase system is generally not able to efficiently kill microbes by itself. However, the azurophilic granules of neutrophils contain the enzyme *myeloperoxidase* (MPO), which, in the presence of a halide such as Cl^-, converts H_2O_2 to hypochlorite (HOCl). The latter is a potent antimicrobial agent that destroys microbes by *halogenation* (in which the halide is bound covalently to cellular constituents) or by oxidation of proteins and lipids (lipid peroxidation).[33] *The H_2O_2-MPO-halide system is the most efficient bactericidal system in neutrophils.* MPO-deficient leukocytes are capable of killing bacteria (albeit more slowly than normal cells), by virtue of the formation of superoxide, hydroxyl radicals, and singlet-oxygen.

Bacterial killing can also occur by *oxygen-independent mechanisms*, through the action of substances in leukocyte granules.[34] These include *bactericidal permeability increasing protein* (BPI), a highly cationic granule-associated protein that causes phospholipase activation, phospholipid degradation, and increased permeability in the outer membrane of the microorganisms; *lysozyme*, which hydrolyzes the muramic acid-*N*-acetyl-glucosamine bond, found in the glycopeptide coat of all bacteria; *lactoferrin*, an iron-binding protein present in specific granules; *major basic protein*, a cationic protein of eosinophils, which has limited bactericidal activity but is cytotoxic to many parasites; and *defensins*, cationic arginine-rich granule peptides that are cytotoxic to microbes (and certain mammalian cells).[35] In addition, neutrophil granules contain many *enzymes*, such as elastase, that also contribute to microbial killing (discussed later in the chapter).

After killing, acid hydrolases, which are normally stored in lysosomes, degrade the microbes within phagolysosomes. The pH of the phagolysosome drops to between 4 and 5 after phagocytosis, this being the optimal pH for the action of these enzymes.

Release of Leukocyte Products and Leukocyte-Induced Tissue Injury

During activation and phagocytosis, leukocytes release microbicidal and other products not only within the phagolysosome but also into the extracellular space. The most important of these substances in neutrophils and macrophages are *lysosomal enzymes*, present in the granules; *reactive oxygen intermediates*; and *products of arachidonic acid metabolism*, including prostaglandins and leukotrienes. These products are capable of causing endothelial injury and tissue damage and may thus amplify the effects of the initial injurious agent. Products of monocytes/macrophages and other leukocyte types have additional potentially harmful products, which are described in the discussion of chronic inflammation. Thus, if persistent and unchecked, the leukocyte infiltrate itself becomes the offender,[36] and leukocyte-dependent tissue injury underlies many acute and chronic human diseases (Table 2–2). This fact becomes evident in the discussion of specific disorders throughout this book.

Regulated secretion of lysosomal proteins is a peculiarity of leukocytes and other hematopoietic cells. (Recall that in most secretory cells, the proteins that are secreted are not stored within lysosomes.) The contents of lysosomal granules are secreted by leukocytes into the extracellular milieu by diverse mechanisms. Release may occur if the phagocytic vacuole remains transiently open to the outside before complete closure of the phagolysosome *(regurgitation during feeding)*. If cells are exposed to potentially ingestible materials, such as immune complexes deposited on immovable flat surfaces (e.g., glomerular basement membrane), attachment of leukocytes to the immune complexes triggers leukocyte activation, but the fixed immune complexes cannot be phagocytosed, and lysosomal enzymes are released into the medium *(frustrated phagocytosis)*. *Cytotoxic release* occurs after phagocytosis of potentially membranolytic substances, such as urate crystals, which damage the membrane of the phagolysosome. In addition, there is some evidence that proteins in certain granules, particularly the specific (secondary) granules of neutrophils, may be directly secreted by *exocytosis*.[37,38]

After phagocytosis, neutrophils rapidly undergo *apoptotic cell death* and are ingested by macrophages.

Defects in Leukocyte Function

From the preceding discussion, it is obvious that leukocytes play a central role in host defense. Not surprisingly, therefore, defects in leukocyte function, both genetic and acquired, lead to increased vulnerability to infections (Table 2–3). Impairments of virtually every phase of leukocyte function—from adherence to vascular endothelium to microbicidal activity—have been identified, and the existence of clinical genetic deficiencies in each of the critical steps in the process has been described. These include the following:

- *Defects in leukocyte adhesion.* We previously mentioned the genetic deficiencies in leukocyte adhesion molecules (LAD types 1 and 2). LAD 1 is characterized by recurrent bacterial infections and impaired wound healing. LAD 2 is clinically milder than LAD 1 but is also characterized by recurrent bacterial infections.
- *Defects in phagolysosome function.* One such disorder is *Chédiak-Higashi syndrome*, an autosomal recessive condi-

TABLE 2–2 Clinical Examples of Leukocyte-Induced Injury

Acute	Chronic
Acute respiratory distress syndrome	Arthritis
Acute transplant rejection	Asthma
Asthma	Atherosclerosis
Glomerulonephritis	Chronic lung disease
Reperfusion injury	Chronic rejection
Septic shock	
Vasculitis	

TABLE 2–3 Defects in Leukocyte Functions

Disease	Defect
Genetic	
Leukocyte adhesion deficiency 1	β chain of CD11/CD18 integrins
Leukocyte adhesion deficiency 2	Fucosyl transferase required for synthesis of sialylated oligosaccharide (receptor for selectin)
Chronic granulomatous disease	Decreased oxidative burst
X-linked	NADPH oxidase (membrane component)
Autosomal recessive	NADPH oxidase (cytoplasmic components)
Myeloperoxidase deficiency	Absent MPO–H_2O_2 system
Chédiak-Higashi syndrome	Protein involved in organelle membrane docking and fusion
Acquired	
Thermal injury, diabetes, malignancy, sepsis, immunodeficiencies	Chemotaxis
Hemodialysis, diabetes mellitus	Adhesion
Leukemia, anemia, sepsis, diabetes, neonates, malnutrition	Phagocytosis and microbicidal activity

Data from Gallin JI: Disorders of phagocytic cells. In Gallin JI, et al (eds): Inflammation: Basic Principles and Clinical Correlates, 2nd ed. New York, Raven Press, 1992, pp 860, 861.

tion characterized by neutropenia (decreased numbers of neutrophils), defective degranulation, and delayed microbial killing. The neutrophils (and other leukocytes) have *giant granules*, which can be readily seen in peripheral blood smears and which are thought to result from aberrant organelle fusion.[39] In this syndrome, there is reduced transfer of lysosomal enzymes to phagocytic vacuoles in phagocytes (causing susceptibility to infections) and abnormalities in melanocytes (leading to albinism), cells of the nervous system (associated with nerve defects), and platelets (generating bleeding disorders). The gene associated with this disorder encodes a large cytosolic protein that is apparently involved in vesicular traffic but whose precise function is not yet known. The secretion of granule proteins by cytotoxic T cells is also affected, accounting for part of the immunodeficiency seen in the disorder.

- *Defects in microbicidal activity.* The importance of oxygen-dependent bactericidal mechanisms is shown by the existence of a group of congenital disorders with defects in bacterial killing called *chronic granulomatous disease*, which render patients susceptible to recurrent bacterial infection. Chronic granulomatous disease results from *inherited defects in the genes encoding several components of NADPH oxidase*, which generates superoxide. The most common variants are an *X-linked defect* in one of the plasma membrane-bound components (gp91phox) and *autosomal recessive* defects in the genes encoding two of the cytoplasmic components (p47phox and p67phox).[40,41]
- Clinically, the most frequent cause of leukocyte defects is *bone marrow suppression*, leading to reduced production of leukocytes. This is seen following therapies for cancer (radiation and chemotherapy) and when the marrow space is compromised by tumor metastases to bone.

Although we have emphasized the role of leukocytes recruited from the circulation in the acute inflammatory response, *cells resident in tissues also serve important functions in initiating acute inflammation*. The two most important of these cell types are *mast cells* and tissue *macrophages*. Mast cells react to physical trauma, breakdown products of complement, microbial products, and neuropeptides. The cells release histamine, leukotrienes, enzymes, and many cytokines (including TNF, IL-1, and chemokines), all of which contribute to inflammation. The functions of mast cells are discussed in more detail in Chapter 6. Macrophages recognize microbial products and secrete most of the cytokines important in acute inflammation. These cells are stationed in tissues to rapidly recognize potentially injurious stimuli and initiate the host defense reaction.

TERMINATION OF THE ACUTE INFLAMMATORY RESPONSE

It is predictable that such a powerful system of host defense, with its inherent capacity to cause tissue damage, needs tight controls to minimize the damage. In part, inflammation declines simply because the mediators of inflammation have short half-lives, are degraded after their release, and are produced in quick bursts, only as long as the stimulus persists. In addition as inflammation develops, the process also triggers a variety of stop signals that serve to actively terminate the reaction.[42] These active mechanisms include a switch in the production of pro-inflammatory leukotrienes to anti-inflammatory lipoxins from arachidonic acid (described below); the liberation of an anti-inflammatory cytokine, transforming growth factor-β (TGF-β), from macrophages and other cells; and neural impulses (cholinergic discharge) that inhibit the production of TNF in macrophages.[43] There are, in addition, many other controls whose existence is suspected from the phenotypes of mice in which genes encoding putative regulatory molecules have been knocked out—these mice develop uncontrolled inflammation, but precisely how the regulation works normally is not yet defined.[42] Not surprisingly, there is great interest in defining the molecular basis of the brakes on inflammation, since this knowledge could be used to design powerful anti-inflammatory drugs.

Chemical Mediators of Inflammation

Having described the events in acute inflammation, we can now turn to a discussion of the chemical mediators that are responsible for the events. Many mediators have been identified, and how they function in a coordinated manner is still not fully understood. Here we review general principles and highlight some of the major mediators (Fig. 2–12).

- *Mediators originate either from plasma or from cells.* Plasma-derived mediators (e.g., complement proteins, kinins) are present in plasma in *precursor forms that must be activated*, usually by a series of proteolytic cleavages, to acquire their biologic properties. Cell-derived mediators are normally *sequestered in intracellular granules* that need to be secreted (e.g., histamine in mast cell granules) or are *synthesized de novo* (e.g., prostaglandins, cytokines) in response to a stimulus. The major cellular sources are platelets, neutrophils, monocytes/macrophages, and mast cells, but mesenchymal cells (endothelium, smooth muscle, fibroblasts) and most epithelia can also be induced to elaborate some of the mediators.
- *The production of active mediators is triggered by microbial products or by host proteins, such as the proteins of the complement, kinin, and coagulation systems, that are themselves activated by microbes and damaged tissues.*
- Most mediators perform their biologic activity by initially *binding to specific receptors on target cells.* Some, however, have direct enzymatic activity (e.g., lysosomal proteases) or mediate oxidative damage (e.g., reactive oxygen and nitrogen intermediates).
- *One mediator can stimulate the release of other mediators by target cells themselves.* These secondary mediators may be identical or similar to the initial mediators but may also have opposing activities. They provide mechanisms for amplifying—or in certain instances counteracting—the initial mediator action.
- Mediators can act on one or few target cell types, have diverse targets, or may even have differing effects on different types of cells.
- *Once activated and released from the cell, most of these mediators are short-lived.* They quickly decay (e.g., arachidonic acid metabolites) or are inactivated by enzymes (e.g., kininase inactivates bradykinin), or they are otherwise scavenged (e.g., antioxidants scavenge toxic oxygen metabolites) or inhibited (e.g., complement regulatory proteins break up and degrade activated complement components). There is thus a system of checks and balances in the regulation of mediator actions.
- Most mediators have the potential to cause harmful effects.

We now discuss some of the more important mediators of acute inflammation.

VASOACTIVE AMINES

The two amines, histamine and serotonin, are especially important because they are present in preformed stores in cells and are therefore among the first mediators to be released during inflammation.

Histamine

Histamine is widely distributed in tissues, the richest source being the mast cells that are normally present in the connective tissue adjacent to blood vessels (Fig. 2–13). It is also found in blood basophils and platelets. Preformed histamine is present in mast cell granules and is released by mast cell degranulation in response to a variety of stimuli: (1) physical injury such as trauma, cold, or heat; (2) immune reactions involving binding of antibodies to mast cells (Chapter 6);

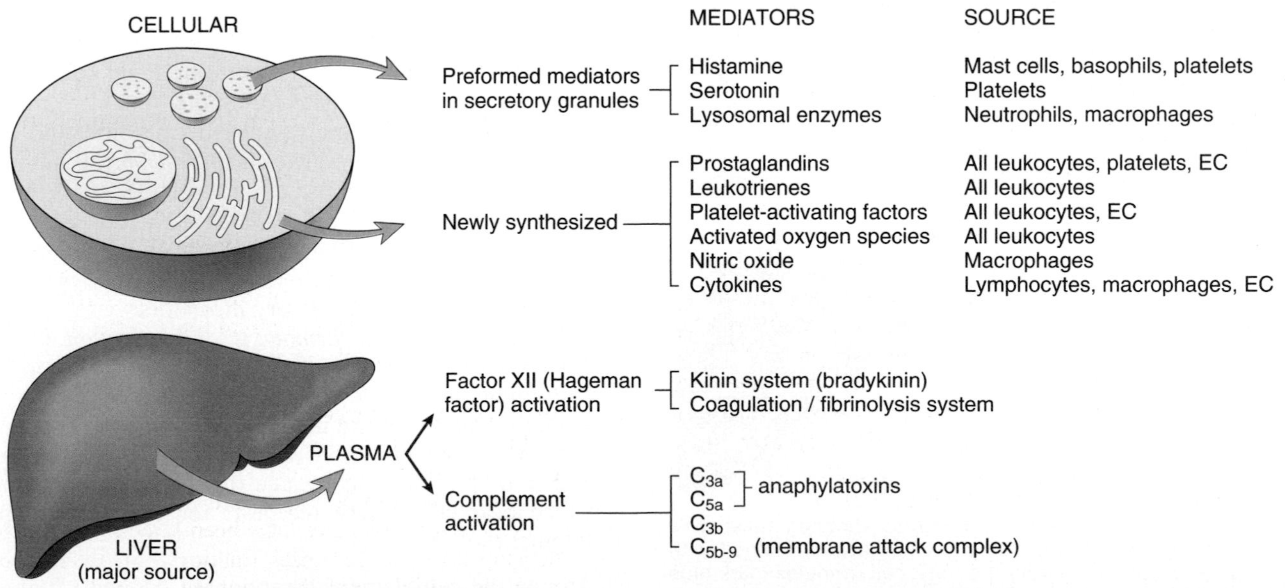

FIGURE 2–12 Chemical mediators of inflammation. EC, endothelial cells.

(3) fragments of complement called *anaphylatoxins* (C3a and C5a); (4) histamine-releasing proteins derived from leukocytes; (5) neuropeptides (e.g., substance P); and (6) cytokines (IL-1, IL-8).

In humans, histamine causes dilation of the arterioles and increases the permeability of venules (it, however, *constricts* large arteries). It is considered to be the principal mediator of the immediate transient phase of increased vascular permeability, causing venular gaps, as we have seen. It acts on the microcirculation mainly via binding to H_1 receptors on endothelial cells.[44]

Serotonin

Serotonin (5-hydroxytryptamine) is a preformed vasoactive mediator with actions similar to those of histamine. It is present in platelets and enterochromaffin cells, and in mast cells in rodents but not humans.

Release of serotonin (and histamine) from *platelets* is stimulated when platelets aggregate after contact with collagen, thrombin, adenosine diphosphate (ADP), and antigen-antibody complexes. Platelet aggregation and release are also stimulated by platelet activating factors (PAF) derived from mast cells during IgE-mediated reactions. In this way, the platelet release reaction results in increased permeability during immunologic reactions. As discussed later, PAF itself has many inflammatory properties.

PLASMA PROTEINS

A variety of phenomena in the inflammatory response are mediated by plasma proteins that belong to three interrelated systems, the complement, kinin, and clotting systems.

Complement System

The complement system consists of 20 component proteins (and their cleavage products), which are found in greatest concentration in plasma. This system functions in both innate and adaptive immunity for defense against microbial agents.[45] In the process of complement activation, a number of complement components are elaborated that cause increased vascular permeability, chemotaxis, and opsonization. The activation and regulation of the complement system are described in Box 2–2, and the main features and functions of complement are shown in Figure 2–14 and are outlined below.

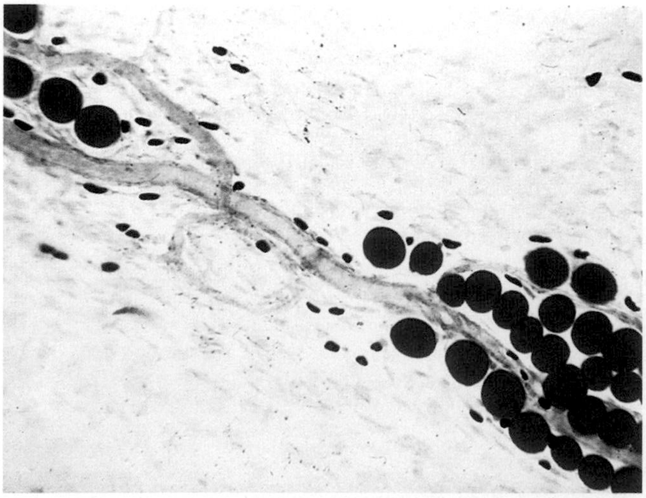

FIGURE 2–13 A flat spread of omentum showing mast cells around blood vessels and in the interstitial tissue. Stained with metachromatic stain to identify the mast cell granules (dark blue or purple). The red structures are fat globules stained with fat stain. (Courtesy of Dr. G. Majno, University of Massachusetts Medical School, Worcester, MA.)

Complement proteins are present as inactive forms in plasma and are numbered C1 through C9. Many of these proteins are activated to become proteolytic enzymes that degrade other complement proteins, thus forming a cascade capable of tremendous enzymatic amplification. The critical step in the elaboration of the biologic functions of complement is the activation of the third (and most abundant) component, C3. Cleavage of C3 can occur by one of three pathways: the *classical pathway,* which is triggered by fixation of C1 to antibody (IgM or IgG) combined with antigen; the *alternative pathway,* which can be triggered by microbial surface molecules (e.g., endotoxin, or LPS), complex polysaccharides, cobra venom, and other substances, in the absence of antibody; and the *lectin pathway,* in which plasma mannose-binding lectin binds to carbohydrates on microbes and directly activates C1. Whichever pathway is involved in the early steps of complement activation, they all lead to the formation of an active enzyme called the *C3 convertase,* which splits C3 into two functionally distinct fragments, C3a and C3b. C3a is released and C3b becomes covalently attached to the cell or molecule where complement is being activated. C3b then binds to the previously generated fragments to form *C5 convertase,* which cleaves C5 to release C5a. The remaining C5b binds the late components (C6–C9), culminating in the formation of the membrane attack complex (MAC, composed of multiple C9 molecules).

The biologic functions of the complement system fall into two general categories: cell lysis by the MAC, and the effects of proteolytic fragments of complement. Complement-derived factors mediate a variety of phenomena in acute inflammation:

- *Vascular phenomena. C3a, C5a,* and, to a lesser extent, *C4a* are split products of the corresponding complement components that stimulate histamine release from mast cells and thereby increase vascular permeability and cause vasodilation. They are called *anaphylatoxins* because they have effects similar to those of mast cell mediators that are involved in the reaction called *anaphylaxis* (Chapter 6). C5a also activates the lipoxygenase pathway of arachidonic acid (AA) metabolism in neutrophils and monocytes, causing further release of inflammatory mediators.
- *Leukocyte adhesion, chemotaxis, and activation. C5a* is a powerful chemotactic agent for neutrophils, monocytes, eosinophils, and basophils.
- *Phagocytosis. C3b* and its cleavage product *iC3b* (inactive C3b), when fixed to the bacterial cell wall, act as opsonins and favor phagocytosis by neutrophils and macrophages, which bear cell surface receptors for these complement fragments.

Among the complement components, C3 and C5 are the most important inflammatory mediators. In addition to the mechanisms already discussed, *C3 and C5 can be activated by*

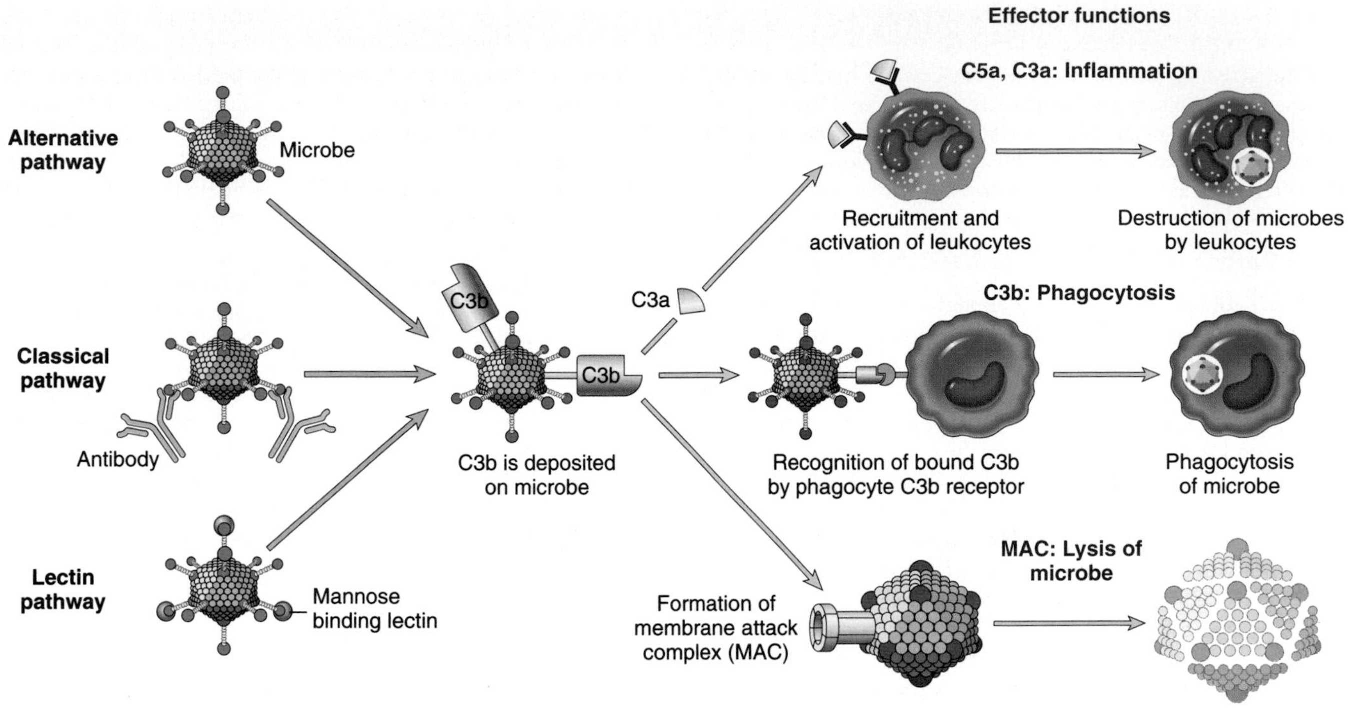

FIGURE 2–14 The activation and functions of the complement system. Activation of complement by different pathways leads to cleavage of C3. The functions of the complement system are mediated by breakdown products of C3 and other complement proteins, and by the membrane attack complex (MAC). The steps in the activation and regulation of complement are described in Box 2–2.

several proteolytic enzymes present within the inflammatory exudate. These include plasmin and lysosomal enzymes released from neutrophils (discussed later in this chapter). Thus, the chemotactic effect of complement and the complement-activating effects of neutrophils can set up a self-perpetuating cycle of neutrophil emigration.

The *activation of complement is tightly controlled by cell-associated and circulating regulatory proteins.*[46] The presence of these inhibitors in host cell membranes protects the host from inappropriate damage during protective reactions against microbes. These regulatory mechanisms are described in Box 2–2.

Kinin System

The kinin system generates vasoactive peptides from plasma proteins, called *kininogens,* by the action of specific proteases called *kallikreins.*[47,48] Activation of the kinin system results in the release of the vasoactive nonapeptide *bradykinin. Bradykinin increases vascular permeability and causes contraction of smooth muscle, dilation of blood vessels, and pain when injected into the skin.* These effects are similar to those of histamine. The cascade that eventually produces kinins is shown in Figure 2–15. It is triggered by activation of Hageman factor (factor XII of the intrinsic clotting pathway; see later) upon contact with negatively charged surfaces, such as collagen and basement membranes. A fragment of factor XII (prekallikrein activator, or factor XIIa) is produced, and this converts plasma *prekallikrein* into an active proteolytic form, the enzyme *kallikrein.* The latter cleaves a plasma glycoprotein precursor, *high-molecular-weight kininogen,* to produce *bradykinin.* High-molecular-weight kininogen also acts as a cofactor or catalyst in the activation of Hageman factor. The action of bradykinin is short-lived because it is quickly inactivated by an enzyme called *kininase.* Any remaining kinin is inactivated during passage of plasma through the lung by angiotensin-converting enzyme. *Kallikrein itself is a potent activator of Hageman factor, allowing for autocatalytic amplification of the initial stimulus.* Kallikrein has chemotactic activity, and it also directly converts C5 to the chemoattractant product C5a.

Clotting System

The clotting system and inflammation are intimately connected processes. The clotting system is divided into two pathways that converge, culminating in the activation of thrombin and the formation of fibrin (see Fig. 2–15 and Chapter 4). The intrinsic clotting pathway is a series of plasma proteins that can be activated by Hageman factor (factor XII), a protein synthesized by the liver that circulates in an inactive form until it encounters collagen or basement membrane or activated platelets (as occurs at the site of endothelial injury). Factor XII then undergoes a conformational change (becoming factor XIIa), exposing an active serine center that can subsequently cleave protein substrates and activate a variety of mediator systems (see later).

The protease thrombin provides the main link between the coagulation system and inflammation. Activation of the clotting system results in the activation of thrombin (factor IIa) from precursor prothrombin (factor II), by a series of reactions that are detailed in Chapter 4. Thrombin is the enzyme that cleaves circulating soluble fibrinogen to generate an insoluble fibrin clot and is the major coagulation protease. It binds to receptors that are called *protease-activated*

Box 2–2 The Complement System in Health and Disease

The activation of the complement cascade may be divided into early and late steps. In the early steps, three different pathways lead to the proteolytic cleavage of C3. In the late steps, all three pathways converge, and the major breakdown product of C3, C3b, activates a series of other complement components.

The Early Steps of Complement Activation

The pathways of early complement activation are the following (see Figure): The *classical pathway* is triggered by fixation of C1 to antibody (IgM or IgG) that has combined with antigen, and proteolysis of C2 and C4, and subsequent formation of a C4b2b complex that functions as a C3 convertase. The *alternative pathway* can be triggered by microbial surface molecules (e.g., endotoxin, or LPS), complex polysaccharides, and cobra venom. It involves a distinct set of plasma components (properdin, and factors B and D). In this pathway, the spontaneous cleavage of C3 that occurs normally is enhanced and stabilized by a complex of C3b and a breakdown product of Factor B called Bb; the C3bBb complex is a C3 convertase. In the *lectin pathway*, mannose-binding lectin, a plasma collectin, binds to carbohydrate-containing proteins on bacteria and viruses and directly activates C1; the remaining steps are as in the classical pathway. The C3 convertases break down C3 into C3b, which remains attached to the surface where complement is activated, and a smaller C3a fragment that diffuses away.

The Late Steps of Complement Activation

The C3b that is generated by any of the pathways binds to the C3 convertase and produces a C5 convertase, which cleaves C5. C5b remains attached to the complex and forms a substrate for the subsequent binding of the C6–C9 components. Polymerized C9 forms a channel in lipid membranes, called the *membrane attack complex,* which allows fluid and ions to enter and causes cell lysis.

Regulation of Complement Activation

To prevent inappropriate activation of complement and to limit its activation even when appropriate, mammals express many regulatory proteins. (These proteins are generally absent from microbes, which explains why complement is activated by and functions against microbes.) Complement activation can be controlled at several steps:

- *Regulation of C3 and C5 convertases.* Since the formation of C3 convertase and the generation of C3b are the central features of all complement pathways, it is not surprising that many of the regulatory proteins are directed at controlling these activities. These regulators function by enhancing the dissociation (decay acceleration) of the convertase complex (e.g., decay-accelerating factor [DAF]) or by proteolytically cleaving C3b (e.g., factor I).
- *Binding of active complement components* by specific proteins in the plasma. The first step in the classical pathway, which is triggered by C1 binding to an immune complex, is blocked by a plasma protein called *C1 inhibitor* (C1INH). C1INH interferes with the enzymatic activity of two of the proteins in the C1 complex. Excessive complement activation is also prevented by a number of proteins that act to inhibit MAC formation (e.g., CD59, also called *membrane inhibitor of reactive lysis*).

Disorders of the Complement System

Defects in complement proteins may result in increased susceptibility to infections, or to pathologic activation if the deficiencies affect regulatory proteins. Inherited deficiencies of

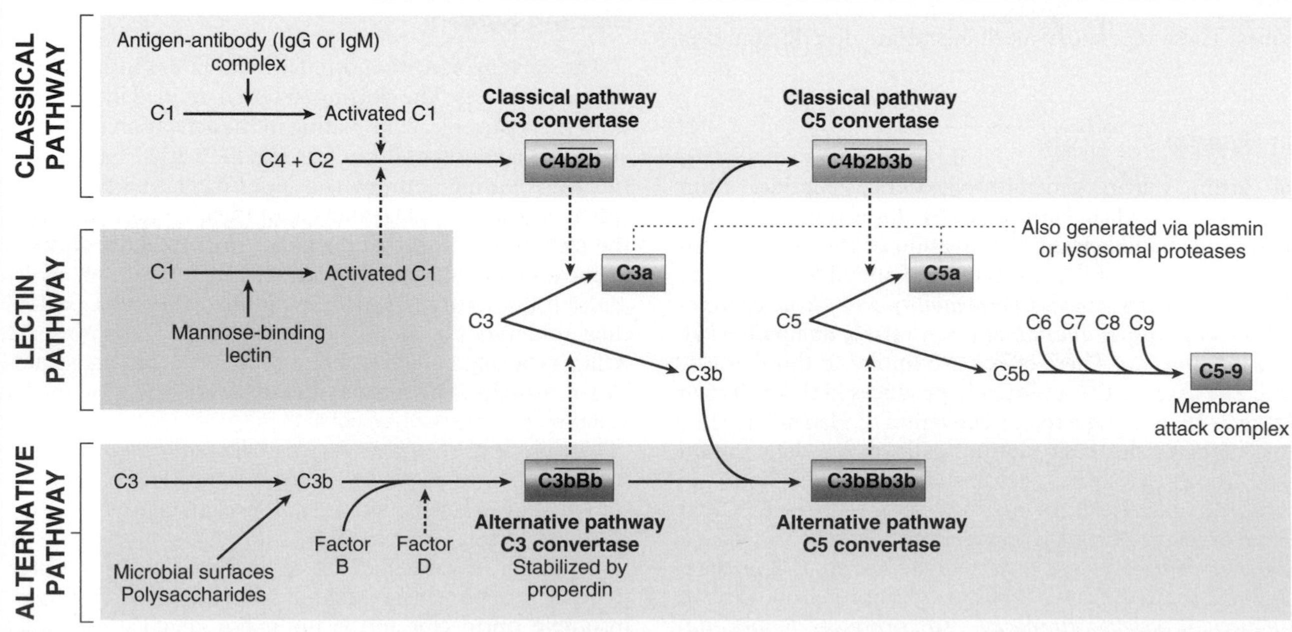

many complement proteins have been described in humans. Deficiency of C3 results in increased susceptibility to infections that is fatal unless treated. Deficiencies of the alternative pathway proteins are also associated with defective resistance to infections. Paradoxically, deficiencies of C2 and C4 are associated with autoimmune diseases, notably systemic lupus erythematosus, probably because of a failure to clear immune complexes that are formed. Deficiencies of the late components of complement result in defective formation of the MAC. For unknown reasons, the only infections these patients appear to suffer from are by *Neisseria* organisms.

Genetic deficiencies of complement regulatory proteins are also the cause of significant diseases. For example, *paroxysmal nocturnal hemoglobinuria* is a disease caused by mutations in the gene encoding the enzyme required to synthesize phosphatidylinositol linkages for membrane proteins. As a result, cells show defective expression of phosphatidylinositol-linked membrane proteins, including DAF and CD59, and the result is uncontrolled complement activation on these cells. Paroxysmal nocturnal hemoglobinuria is characterized by recurrent bouts of intravascular hemolysis resulting from complement-mediated lysis of red blood cells, leading to chronic hemolytic anemia (Chapter 13). Deficiency of C1 inhibitor (C1INH) is associated with the syndrome of *hereditary angioneurotic edema*, characterized by episodic edema accumulation in the skin and extremities as well as in the laryngeal and intestinal mucosa, provoked by emotional stress or trauma. In patients with this disorder, activation of C1 by immune complexes is not properly controlled, and increased breakdown of C4 and C2 occurs. The mediators of edema formation in patients with the disease include a proteolytic fragment of C2, called C2 kinin, and bradykinin. C1INH is an inhibitor of other plasma serine proteases besides C1, including kallikrein and coagulation factor XII, and both activated kallikrein and factor XII can promote increased formation of bradykinin.

receptors (PARs) because they bind multiple trypsin-like serine proteases in addition to thrombin.[49] These receptors are seven-transmembrane G protein–coupled receptors that are expressed on platelets, endothelial and smooth muscle cells, and many other cell types. Engagement of the so-called type 1 receptor (PAR-1) by proteases, particularly thrombin, triggers several responses that induce inflammation. They include mobilization of P-selectin, production of chemokines, and expression of endothelial adhesion molecules for leukocyte integrins; induction of cyclooxygenase-2 and production of

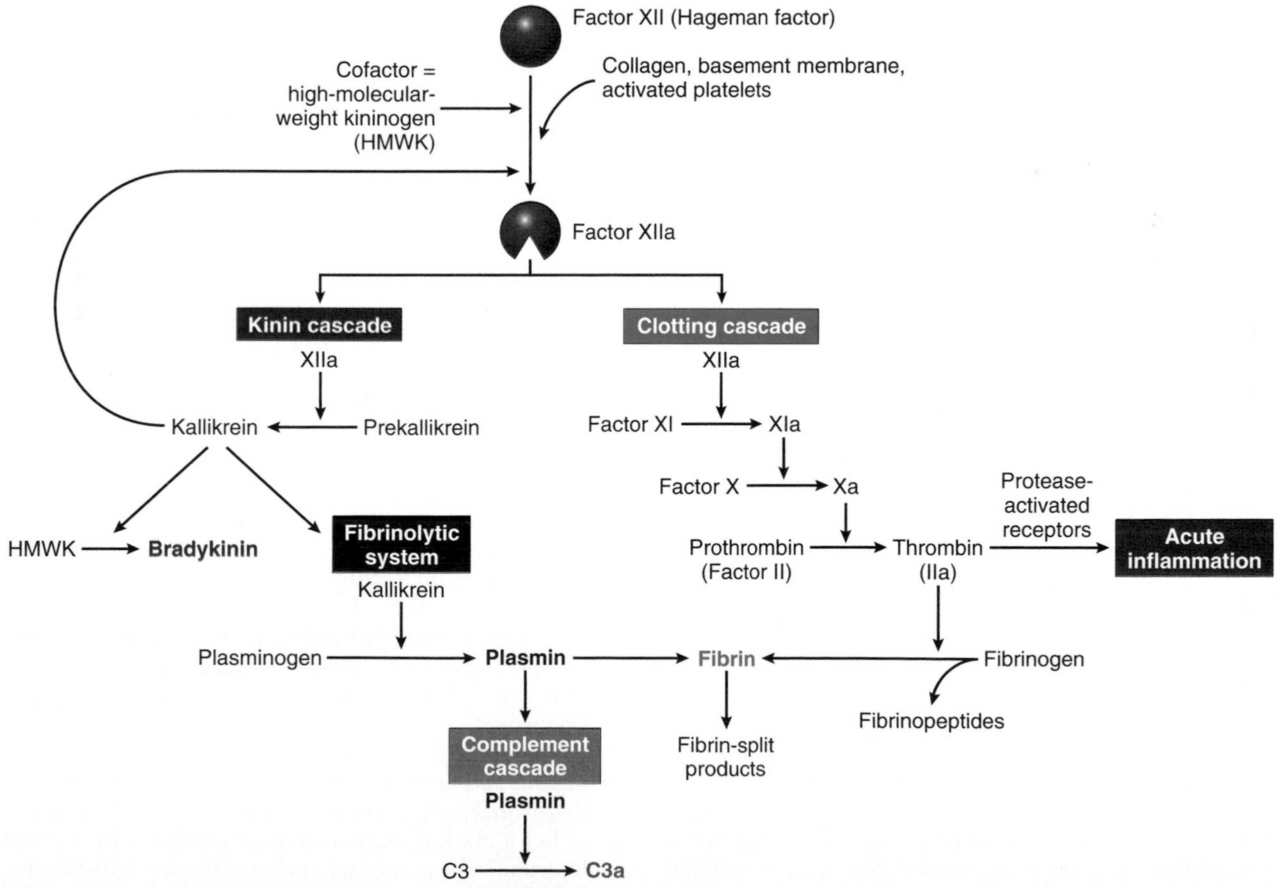

FIGURE 2–15 Interrelationships between the four plasma mediator systems triggered by activation of factor XII (Hageman factor). Note that thrombin induces inflammation by binding to protease-activated receptors (principally PAR-1) on platelets, endothelium, smooth muscle cells, and other cells.

prostaglandins; production of PAF and nitric oxide; and changes in endothelial shape.[50] As we have seen, these responses promote the recruitment of leukocytes and many other reactions of inflammation.

At the same time that factor XIIa is inducing clotting, it can also activate the *fibrinolytic system.* This cascade counterbalances clotting by cleaving fibrin, thereby solubilizing the fibrin clot. The fibrinolytic system contributes to the vascular phenomena of inflammation in several ways. Plasminogen activator (released from endothelium, leukocytes, and other tissues) cleaves plasminogen, a plasma protein that binds to the evolving fibrin clot to generate *plasmin,* a multifunctional protease. Plasmin is important in lysing fibrin clots, but in the context of inflammation it also cleaves C3 to produce C3 fragments, and it degrades fibrin to form *fibrin split products,* which may have permeability-inducing properties. Plasmin can also activate Hageman factor, which can trigger multiple cascades (see Fig. 2–15), amplifying the response.

From this discussion of the plasma proteases activated by the kinin, complement, and clotting systems, a few general conclusions can be drawn:

- *Bradykinin, C3a, and C5a (*as mediators of increased vascular permeability*); C5a (*as the mediator of chemotaxis*);* and *thrombin* (which has effects on endothelial and many other cell types) are likely to be the most important in vivo.
- *C3a* and *C5a* can be generated by several types of reactions: (1) immunologic reactions, involving antibodies and complement (the classical pathway); (2) activation of the alternative or lectin complement pathways by microbes, in the absence of antibodies; and (3) agents not directly related to immune responses, such as plasmin, kallikrein, and some serine proteases found in normal tissue.
- *Activated Hageman factor (factor XIIa)* initiates four systems involved in the inflammatory response: (1) the *kinin system,* which produces vasoactive kinins; (2) the *clotting system,* which induces formation of thrombin, fibrinopeptides, and factor X, which have inflammatory properties; (3) the *fibrinolytic system,* which produces plasmin and degrades the fibrin; and (4) the *complement system,* which produces anaphylatoxins. Some of the products of this initiation—particularly kallikrein—can, by feedback, activate Hageman factor, resulting in profound amplification of the effects of the initial contact.

It should be evident from the preceding that *coagulation and inflammation are tightly linked.* Acute inflammation, by activating or damaging the endothelium, can trigger coagulation and induce thrombus formation (Chapter 4). Conversely, the coagulation cascade induces inflammation, primarily via the actions of thrombin.

ARACHIDONIC ACID METABOLITES: PROSTAGLANDINS, LEUKOTRIENES, AND LIPOXINS

When cells are activated by diverse stimuli, their membrane lipids are rapidly remodeled to generate biologically active lipid mediators that serve as intracellular or extracellular signals to affect a variety of biologic processes, including inflammation and hemostasis. These lipid mediators are thought of as *autocoids,* or short-range hormones that are formed rapidly, exert their effects locally, and then either decay spontaneously or are destroyed enzymatically.[51]

Arachidonic acid (AA) is a 20-carbon polyunsaturated fatty acid (5,8,11,14-eicosatetraenoic acid) that is derived from dietary sources or by conversion from the essential fatty acid *linoleic acid.* It does not occur free in the cell but is normally esterified in membrane phospholipids. It is released from membrane phospholipids through the action of cellular phospholipases (e.g., phospholipase A_2), which may be activated by mechanical, chemical, and physical stimuli or by other mediators (e.g., C5a). The biochemical signals involved in the activation of phospholipase A_2 include an increase in cytoplasmic Ca^{2+} and activation of various kinases in response to external stimuli.[52] AA metabolites, also called *eicosanoids,* are synthesized by two major classes of enzymes: cyclooxygenases (prostaglandins and thromboxanes) and lipoxygenases (leukotrienes and lipoxins) (Fig. 2–16). Eicosanoids bind to G protein–coupled receptors on many cell types and can mediate virtually every step of inflammation (Table 2–4). They can be found in inflammatory exudates, and their synthesis is increased at sites of inflammation. Structurally distinct agents that suppress cyclooxygenase activity (aspirin, nonsteroidal anti-inflammatory drugs [NSAIDs], and COX-2 inhibitors[53]) reduce inflammation in vivo.

The cyclooxygenases and lipoxygenase produce different mediators from the AA precursor.

- The *cyclooxgenase pathway,* initiated by two different enzymes (the constitutively expressed COX-1 and the inducible enzyme COX-2), leads to the generation of *prostaglandins.* Prostaglandins are divided into series based on structural features as coded by a letter (PGD, PGE, PGF, PGG, and PGH) and a subscript numeral (e.g., 1, 2), which indicates the number of double bonds in the compound. The most important ones in inflammation are PGE_2, PGD_2, $PGF_{2\alpha}$, PGI_2 (prostacyclin), and TxA_2 (thromboxane), each of which is derived by the action of a specific enzyme on an intermediate in the pathway. Some of these enzymes have restricted tissue distribution. For example, platelets contain the enzyme thromboxane synthetase, and hence TxA_2 is the major product in these cells. TxA_2, a potent platelet-aggregating agent and vasoconstrictor, is itself unstable and rapidly converted to its inactive form TxB_2. Vascular endothelium lacks thromboxane synthetase but possesses prostacyclin synthetase, which leads to the formation of prostacyclin (PGI_2) and its stable end product $PGF_{1\alpha}$. Prostacyclin is a vasodilator, a potent inhibitor of platelet aggregation, and also markedly potentiates the permeability-increasing and chemotactic effects of other mediators. A thromboxane–prostacyclin imbalance has been implicated as an early event in thrombus formation in coronary and cerebral blood vessels. The opposing roles of TxA_2 and PGI_2 in hemostasis are further discussed in Chapter 4.

  The prostaglandins are also involved in the pathogenesis of *pain* and *fever* in inflammation. PGE_2 is hyperalgesic in that it makes the skin hypersensitive to painful stimuli. It causes a marked increase in pain produced by intradermal injection of suboptimal concentrations of histamine and bradykinin and is involved in cytokine-induced fever during infections (described later). PGD_2 is the major metabolite of the cyclooxygenase pathway in mast cells;

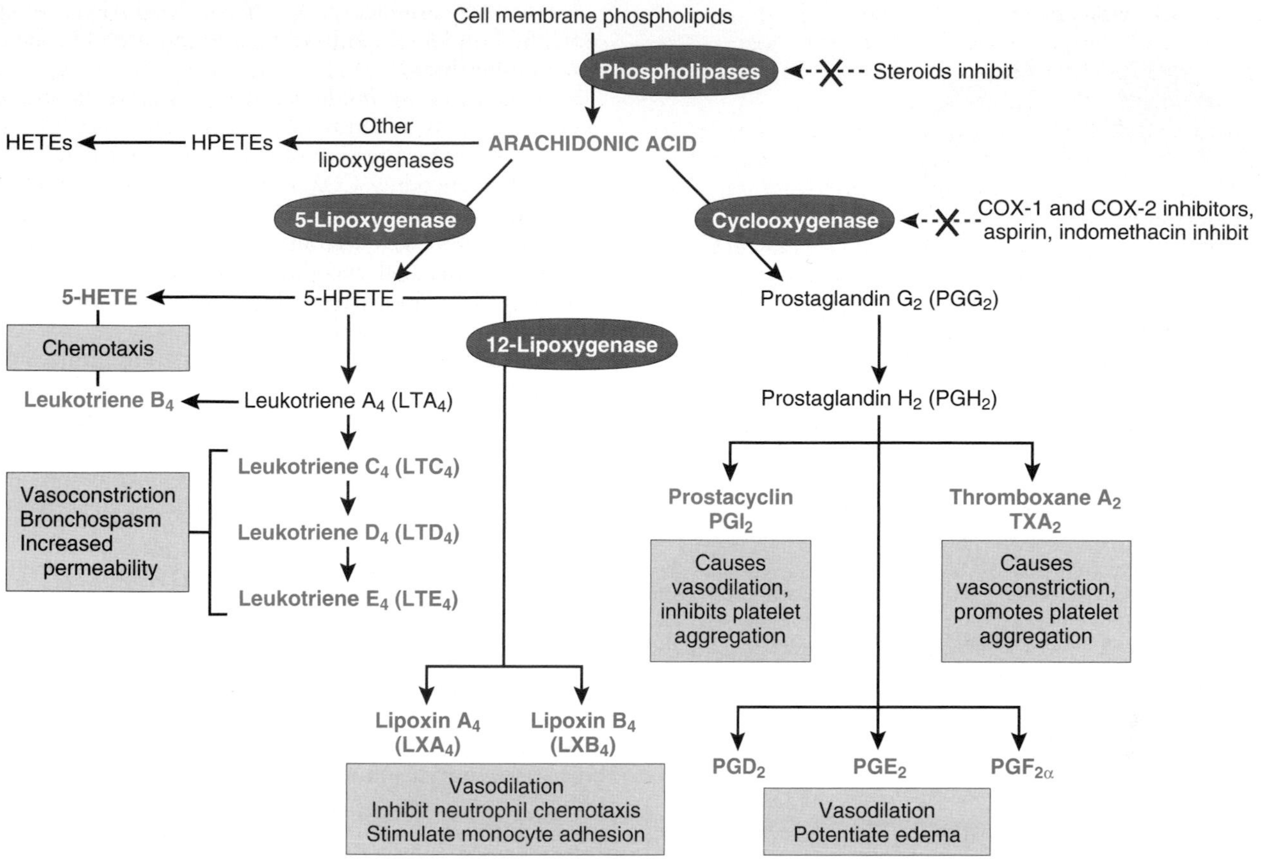

FIGURE 2–16 Generation of arachidonic acid metabolites and their roles in inflammation. The molecular targets of action of some anti-inflammatory drugs are indicated by a red X. COX, cyclooxygenase; HETE, hydroxyeicosatetraenoic acid; HPETE, hydroperoxyeicosatetraenoic acid.

along with PGE_2 and $PGF_{2\alpha}$ (which are more widely distributed), it causes vasodilation and increases the permeability of postcapillary venules, thus potentiating edema formation.

There has been great interest in the COX-2 enzyme because it is induced by a variety of inflammatory stimuli and is absent in most tissues under normal "resting" conditions. COX-1, by contrast, is produced in response to inflammatory stimuli and is also constitutively expressed in most tissues. This difference has led to the notion that *COX-1 is responsible for the production of prostaglandins that are involved in inflammation but also serve a homeostatic function* (e.g., fluid and electrolyte balance in the kidneys, cytoprotection in the gastrointestinal tract). In contrast, *COX-2 stimulates the production of the prostaglandins that are involved in inflammatory reactions.*

- In the *lipoxygenase pathway,* the initial products are generated by three different lipoxygenases, which are present in only a few types of cells. 5-lipoxygenase (5-LO) is the predominant enzyme in neutrophils. The main product, 5-HETE, which is chemotactic for neutrophils, is converted into a family of compounds collectively called *leukotrienes.* *LTB_4* is a potent chemotactic agent and activator of neutrophil functional responses, such as aggregation and adhesion of leukocytes to venular endothelium, generation of oxygen free radicals, and release of lysosomal enzymes. The cysteinyl-containing leukotrienes C_4, D_4, and E_4 (*LTC_4, LTD_4,* and *LTE_4*) cause intense vasoconstriction, bronchospasm, and increased vascular permeability. The vascular leakage, as with histamine, is restricted to venules. Leukotrienes are several orders of magnitude more potent than histamine in increasing vascular permeability and causing bronchospasm. Leukotrienes mediate their actions by binding to cysteiny leukotreine 1 (CysLT1) and CysLT2 receptors. They are important in the pathogenesis of bronchial asthma.

TABLE 2–4 Inflammatory Actions of Eicosanoids

Action	Metabolite
Vasoconstriction	Thromboxane A_2, leukotrienes C_4, D_4, E_4
Vasodilation	PGI_2, PGE_1, PGE_2, PGD_2
Increased vascular permeability	Leukotrienes C_4, D_4, E_4
Chemotaxis, leukocyte adhesion	Leukotriene B_4, HETE, lipoxins

- *Lipoxins* are a recent addition to the family of bioactive products generated from AA, and transcellular biosynthetic mechanisms (involving two cell populations) are key to their production. Leukocytes, particularly neutrophils, produce intermediates in lipoxin synthesis, and these are converted to lipoxins by platelets interacting with the leukocytes. Lipoxins A_4 and B_4 (LXA_4, LXB_4) are generated by the action of platelet 12-lipoxygenase on neutrophil-derived LTA_4 (Fig. 2–17). Cell–cell contact enhances transcellular metabolism, and blocking adhesion inhibits lipoxin

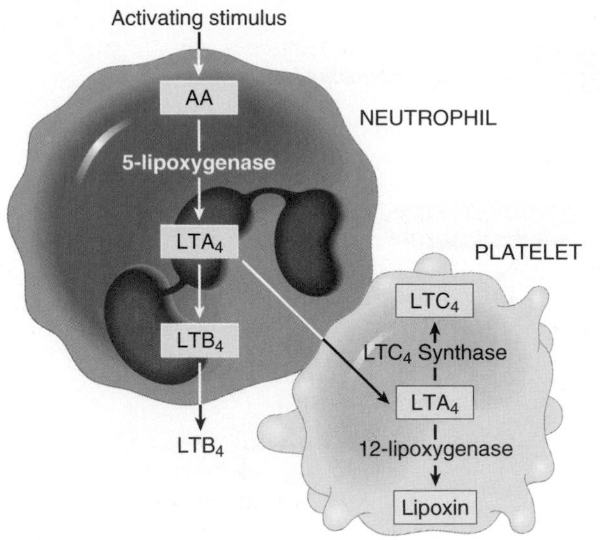

FIGURE 2–17 Biosynthesis of leukotrienes and lipoxins by cell–cell interaction. Activated neutrophils generate LTB_4 from arachidonic acid-derived LTA_4 by the action of 5-lipoxygenase, but they do not possess LTC_4-synthase activity and consequently do not produce LTC_4. In contrast, platelets cannot form LTC_4 from endogenous substrates, but they can generate LTC_4 and lipoxins from neutrophil-derived LTA_4. (Courtesy of Dr. C. Serhan, Brigham and Women's Hospital, Boston, MA.)

production. *The principal actions of lipoxins are to inhibit leukocyte recruitment and the cellular components of inflammation.* They inhibit neutrophil chemotaxis and adhesion to endothelium.[55] There is an inverse relationship between the amount of lipoxin and leukotrienes formed, suggesting that the lipoxins may be endogenous negative regulators of leukotriene action and may thus play a role in the resolution of inflammation.

- A new class of arachidonic acid-derived mediators, called *resolvins,* have been identified in experimental animals treated with aspirin.[54] These mediators inhibit leukocyte recruitment and activation, in part by inhibiting the production of cytokines. Thus, the anti-inflammatory activity of aspirin is likely attributable to its ability to inhibit cyclooxygenases (see below) and, perhaps, to stimulate the production of resolvins.

Anti-inflammatory therapy can be directed at many targets along the eicosanoid biosynthetic pathways:

- *Cyclooxygenase inhibitors* include aspirin and other nonsteroidal anti-inflammatory drugs (*NSAIDs*), such as indomethacin. They function by inhibiting prostaglandin synthesis; aspirin does this by irreversibly acetylating and inhibiting cyclooxygenase. *COX-2 inhibitors* are a newer class of these drugs. The finding that COX-2 is inducibly expressed only in response to inflammatory stimuli was the impetus for developing antagonists against this enzyme to reduce inflammation without interfering with the physiologic functions of AA metabolites. COX-2 inhibitors are now widely used as anti-inflammatory drugs and generally produce less toxicity than the older COX-1 inhibitors.[53]
- *Lipoxygenase inhibitors.* 5-lipoxygenase is not affected by NSAIDs, and many new inhibitors of this enzyme pathway have been developed. Pharmacologic agents that inhibit leukotriene production or block leukotriene receptors (CysLT1 and CysLT2) have been found useful in the treatment of asthma.
- *Broad-spectrum inhibitors* include *glucocorticoids.* These powerful anti-inflammatory agents may act by down-regulating the expression of specific target genes, including the genes encoding COX-2, phospholipase A_2, proinflammatory cytokines (such as IL-1 and TNF), and nitric oxide synthase (iNOS) (see later). Glucocorticoids also up-regulate genes that encode potent anti-inflammatory proteins, such as lipocortin 1. Lipocortin 1 inhibits release of AA from membrane phospholipids.[56]
- Another approach to manipulating inflammatory responses has been to modify the intake and content of dietary lipids by increasing the consumption of *fish oil.* The basis for this approach is that fish oil fatty acids serve as poor substrates for conversion to active metabolites by both the cyclooxygenase and the lipoxygenase pathways.[57]

PLATELET-ACTIVATING FACTOR (PAF)

PAF is another bioactive phospholipid-derived mediator.[58] Its name comes from its initial discovery as a factor derived from antigen-stimulated, IgE-sensitized basophils that causes platelet aggregation, but it is now known to have multiple inflammatory effects. Chemically, PAF is acetyl-glyceryl-ether-phosphorylcholine (AGEPC), a phospholipid with a typical glycerol backbone, a long-chain fatty acid in the A position, an unusually short chain substituent in the B location, and a phosphatidylcholine moiety.

PAF mediates its effects via a single G-protein–coupled receptor, and its effects are regulated by a family of inactivating PAF acetylhydrolases. A variety of cell types, including platelets, basophils (and mast cells), neutrophils, monocytes/macrophages, and endothelial cells, can elaborate PAF, in both secreted and cell-bound forms. In addition to platelet stimulation, PAF causes vasoconstriction and bronchoconstriction, and at extremely low concentrations it induces vasodilation and increased venular permeability with a potency 100 to 10,000 times greater than that of histamine. PAF also causes increased leukocyte adhesion to endothelium (by enhancing integrin-mediated leukocyte binding), chemotaxis, degranulation, and the oxidative burst. Thus, PAF can elicit most of the cardinal features of inflammation. PAF also boosts the synthesis of other mediators, particularly eicosanoids, by leukocytes and other cells. A role for PAF in vivo is supported by the ability of synthetic PAF receptor antagonists to inhibit inflammation in some experimental models. There are as yet no drugs approved for clinical use that function as specific PAF antagonists.

CYTOKINES AND CHEMOKINES

Cytokines are proteins produced by many cell types (principally activated lymphocytes and macrophages, but also endothelium, epithelium, and connective tissue cells) that modulate the functions of other cell types. Long known to be involved in cellular immune responses, these products have additional effects that play important roles in both acute and chronic inflammation. They are discussed in detail in Chapter 6. Here we review the properties of cytokines that are involved in acute inflammation.

Tumor Necrosis Factor and Interleukin-1

TNF and IL-1 are two of the major cytokines that mediate inflammation. They are produced mainly by activated macrophages. A cytokine resembling TNF, called *lymphotoxin* (previously called TNF-β, to distinguish it from TNF, which was called TNF-α), is produced by activated T lymphocytes, and IL-1 may be produced by many other cell types as well. The secretion of TNF and IL-1 can be stimulated by endotoxin and other microbial products, immune complexes, physical injury, and a variety of inflammatory stimuli. Their most important actions in inflammation are their effects on endothelium, leukocytes, and fibroblasts, and induction of systemic acute-phase reactions (Fig. 2–18). In endothelium, they induce a spectrum of changes—mostly regulated at the level of gene transcription—referred to as *endothelial activation*.[59] In particular, they induce the synthesis of endothelial adhesion molecules and chemical mediators, including other cytokines, chemokines, growth factors, eicosanoids, and nitric oxide (NO); production of enzymes associated with matrix remodeling; and increases in the surface thrombogenicity of the endothelium.[60] TNF also induces *priming* of neutrophils, leading to augmented responses of these cells to other mediators.

IL-1 and TNF (as well as IL-6) induce the systemic *acute-phase responses* associated with infection or injury. Features of these systemic responses include fever, loss of appetite, slow-wave sleep, the release of neutrophils into the circulation, the release of corticotropin and corticosteroids and, particularly with regard to TNF, the hemodynamic effects of septic shock—hypotension, decreased vascular resistance, increased heart rate, and decreased blood pH (described in Chapter 4). TNF also regulates body mass by promoting lipid and protein mobilization and by suppressing appetite. Sustained production of TNF contributes to cachexia, a pathologic state characterized by weight loss and anorexia that accompanies some infections and neoplastic diseases.[61]

Chemokines

Chemokines are a family of small (8 to 10 kD) proteins that act primarily as chemoattractants for specific types of leukocytes.[62–65] About 40 different chemokines and 20 different receptors for chemokines have been identified. They are classified into four major groups, according to the arrangement of the conserved cysteine (C) residues in the mature proteins:

- *C-X-C chemokines* (also called α chemokines) have one amino acid residue separating the first two conserved cysteine residues. The C-X-C chemokines act primarily on neutrophils. *IL-8* is typical of this group. It is secreted by activated macrophages, endothelial cells, and other cell types and causes activation and chemotaxis of neutrophils, with limited activity on monocytes and eosinophils. Its most important inducers are microbial products and other cytokines, mainly IL-1 and TNF.
- *C-C chemokines* (also called β chemokines) have the first two conserved cysteine residues adjacent. The C-C chemokines, which include *monocyte chemoattractant protein* (MCP-1), *eotaxin, macrophage inflammatory protein-1α* (MIP-1α), and *RANTES* (regulated and normal T cell expressed and secreted), generally attract monocytes, eosinophils, basophils, and lymphocytes but not neutrophils. Although most of the chemokines in this class have overlapping properties, eotaxin selectively recruits eosinophils.

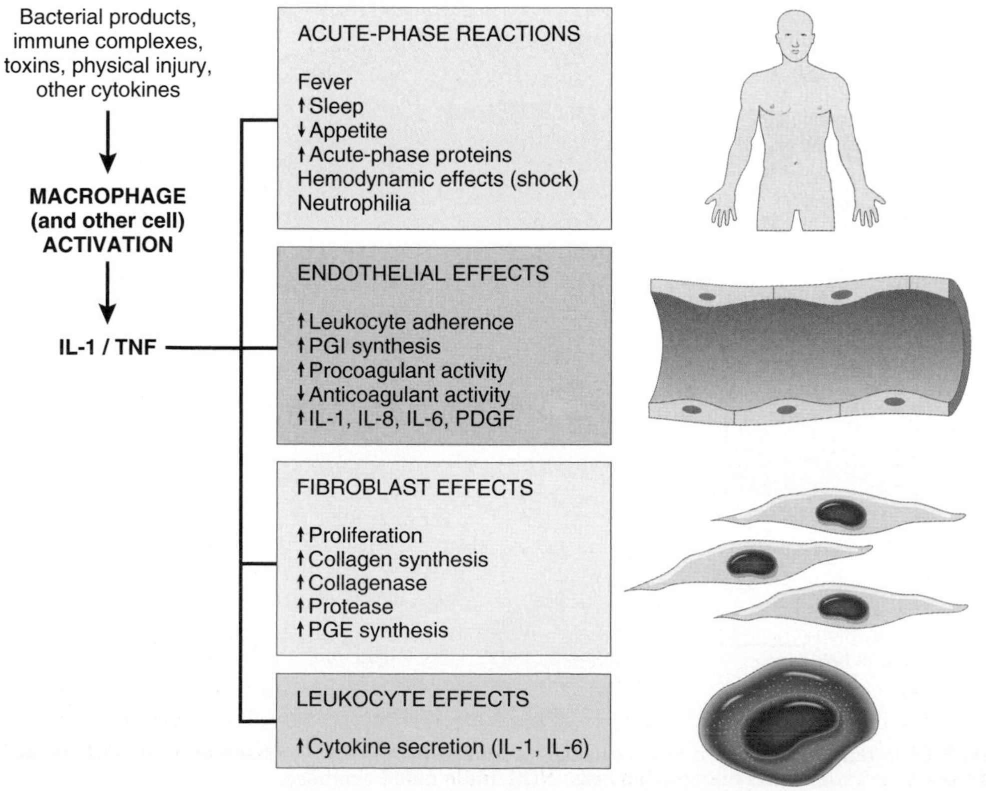

FIGURE 2–18 Major effects of interleukin-1 (IL-1) and tumor necrosis factor (TNF) in inflammation.

- *C chemokines* (also called γ chemokines) lack two (the first and third) of the four conserved cysteines. The C chemokines (e.g., lymphotactin) are relatively specific for lymphocytes.
- *CX_3C chemokines* contain three amino acids between the two cysteines. The only known member of this class is called *fractalkine*. This chemokine exists in two forms: the cell surface–bound protein can be induced on endothelial cells by inflammatory cytokines and promotes strong adhesion of monocytes and T cells, and a soluble form, derived by proteolysis of the membrane-bound protein, has potent chemoattractant activity for the same cells.

Chemokines mediate their activities by binding to seven transmembrane G-protein–coupled receptors. These receptors (called CXCR or CCR, for C-X-C or C-C chemokine receptors) usually exhibit overlapping ligand specificities, and leukocytes generally express more than one receptor type. As discussed in Chapter 6, certain chemokine receptors (CXCR-4, CCR-5) act as coreceptors for a viral envelope glycoprotein of human immunodeficiency virus (HIV-1) and are thus involved in binding and entry of the virus into cells.

Chemokines stimulate leukocyte recruitment in inflammation and control the normal migration of cells through various tissues.[21] Some chemokines are produced transiently in response to inflammatory stimuli and promote the recruitment of leukocytes to the sites of inflammation. Other chemokines are produced constitutively in tissues and function in organogenesis to organize different cell types in different anatomic regions of the tissues. In both situations, chemokines may be displayed at high concentrations attached to proteoglycans on the surface of endothelial cells and in the extracellular matrix.

NITRIC OXIDE (NO)

NO, a pleiotropic mediator of inflammation, was discovered as a factor released from endothelial cells that caused vasodilation by relaxing vascular smooth muscle and was therefore called endothelium-derived relaxing factor.[65] NO is a soluble gas that is produced not only by endothelial cells, but also by macrophages and some neurons in the brain. NO acts in a paracrine manner on target cells through induction of cyclic guanosine monophosphate (GMP), which, in turn, initiates a series of intracellular events leading to a response, such as the relaxation of vascular smooth muscle cells. Since the in vivo half-life of NO is only seconds, the gas acts only on cells in close proximity to where it is produced.

NO is synthesized from L-arginine by the enzyme nitric oxide synthase (NOS).[66] There are three different types of NOS—endothelial (eNOS), neuronal (nNOS), and inducible (iNOS) (Fig. 2–19)—which exhibit two patterns of expression. eNOS and nNOS are *constitutively* expressed at low levels and can be activated rapidly by an increase in cytoplasmic calcium ions. Influx of calcium into cells leads to a rapid production of NO. iNOS, in contrast, is *induced* when macrophages and other cells are activated by cytokines (e.g., TNF, IFN-γ) or other agents.

NO plays an important role in the vascular and cellular components of inflammatory responses.[65] NO is a potent *vasodilator* by virtue of its actions on vascular smooth muscle. In addition, NO reduces platelet aggregation and adhesion (Chapter 4), inhibits several features of mast cell–induced

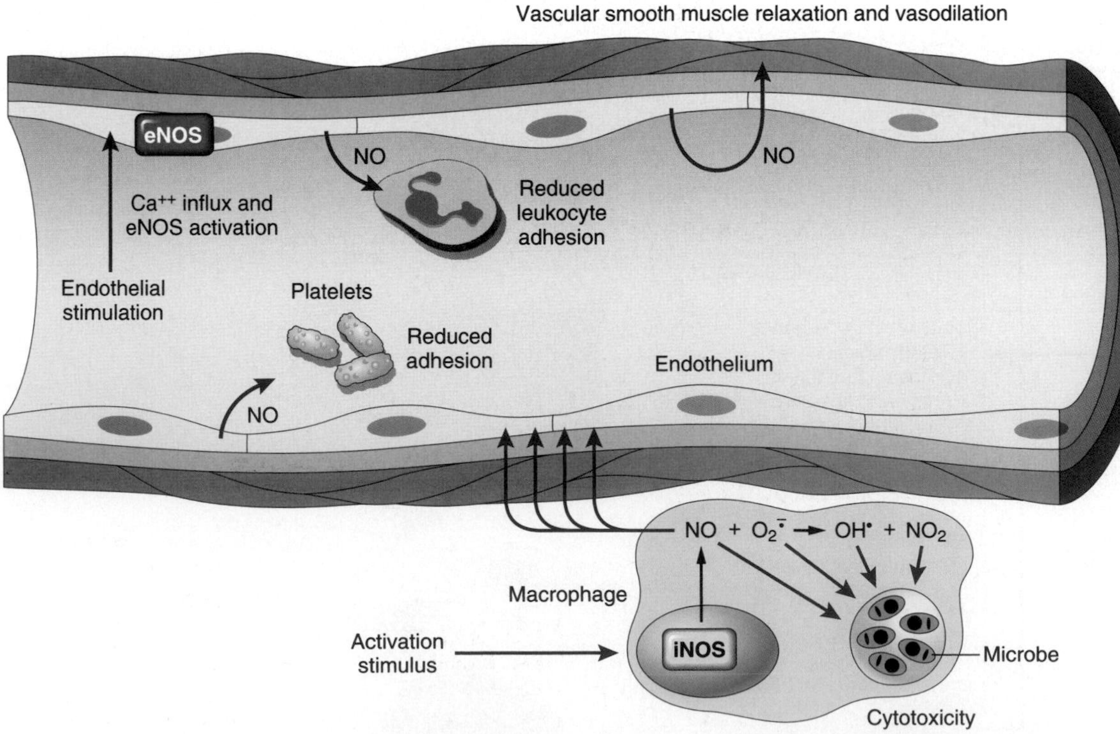

FIGURE 2–19 Functions of nitric oxide (NO) in blood vessels and macrophages, produced by two NO synthase enzymes. NO causes vasodilation, and NO free radicals are toxic to microbial and mammalian cells. NOS, nitric oxide synthase.

inflammation, and serves as an endogenous regulator of leukocyte recruitment. Blocking NO production under normal conditions promotes leukocyte rolling and adhesion in postcapillary venules, and delivery of exogenous NO reduces leukocyte recruitment. *Thus, production of NO is an endogenous compensatory mechanism that reduces inflammatory responses.*[67] Abnormalities in endothelial production of NO occur in atherosclerosis, diabetes, and hypertension (Chapter 11).

NO and its derivatives are microbicidal, and thus NO is also a mediator of host defense against infection.[31] Evidence supporting the importance of this antimicrobial activity of NO includes the following: (1) reactive nitrogen intermediates derived from NO possess antimicrobial activity; (2) interactions occur between NO and reactive oxygen intermediates, leading to the formation of multiple antimicrobial metabolites; (3) production of NO is increased during host responses to infection; and (4) genetic inactivation of iNOS enhances microbial replication in experimental animal models. High levels of NO production by a variety of cells appear to limit the replication of bacteria, helminths, protozoa, and viruses (as well as tumor cells).

LYSOSOMAL CONSTITUENTS OF LEUKOCYTES

Neutrophils and monocytes contain lysosomal granules, which, when released, may contribute to the inflammatory response. Neutrophils have two main types of granules (Fig. 2–20). The smaller *specific* (or secondary) granules contain lysozyme, collagenase, gelatinase, lactoferrin, plasminogen activator, histaminase, and alkaline phosphatase. The large *azurophil* (or primary) granules contain myeloperoxidase, bactericidal factors (lysozyme, defensins), acid hydrolases, and a variety of neutral proteases (elastase, cathepsin G, nonspecific collagenases, proteinase 3).[68] Both types of granules can empty into phagocytic vacuoles that form around engulfed material, or the granule contents can be released into the extracellular space. The specific granules are secreted extracellularly more readily and by lower concentrations of agonists, whereas the potentially more destructive azurophil granules release their contents primarily within the phagosome and require high levels of agonists to be released extracellularly.

Different granule enzymes serve different functions. *Acid proteases* degrade bacteria and debris *within the phagolysosomes,* in which an acid pH is readily reached. *Neutral proteases* are capable of degrading various *extracellular components.* These enzymes can attack collagen, basement membrane, fibrin, elastin, and cartilage, resulting in the tissue destruction that accompanies inflammatory processes. Neutral proteases can also cleave C3 and C5 directly, releasing anaphylatoxins, and release a kinin-like peptide from kininogen. Neutrophil elastase has been shown to degrade virulence factors of bacteria and thus combat bacterial infections.[69] *Monocytes* and *macrophages* also contain acid hydrolases, collagenase, elastase, phospholipase, and plasminogen activator. These may be particularly active in chronic inflammatory reactions.

Because of the destructive effects of lysosomal enzymes, the initial leukocytic infiltration, if unchecked, can potentiate further increases in vascular permeability and tissue damage. These harmful proteases, however, are held in check by a system of *antiproteases* in the serum and tissue fluids. Foremost among these is α_1-antitrypsin, which is the major inhibitor of neutrophil elastase. A deficiency of these inhibitors may lead to sustained action of leukocyte proteases, as is the case in patients with α_1-antitrypsin deficiency (Chapter 15). α_2-Macroglobulin is another antiprotease found in serum and various secretions.

OXYGEN-DERIVED FREE RADICALS

Oxygen-derived free radicals may be released extracellularly from leukocytes after exposure to microbes, chemokines, and immune complexes, or following a phagocytic challenge.[68] Their production is dependent, as we have seen, on the activation of the NADPH oxidative system. Superoxide anion ($O_2^{\bar{\cdot}}$), hydrogen peroxide (H_2O_2), and hydroxyl radical (OH) are the major species produced within the cell, and these metabolites can combine with NO to form other reactive nitrogen intermediates.[70] Extracellular release of low levels of these potent mediators can increase the expression of chemokines (e.g., IL-8), cytokines, and endothelial leukocyte adhesion molecules, amplifying the cascade that elicits the inflammatory response.[71] As mentioned earlier, the physiologic function of these reactive oxygen intermediates is to destroy phagocytosed microbes. At higher levels, release of

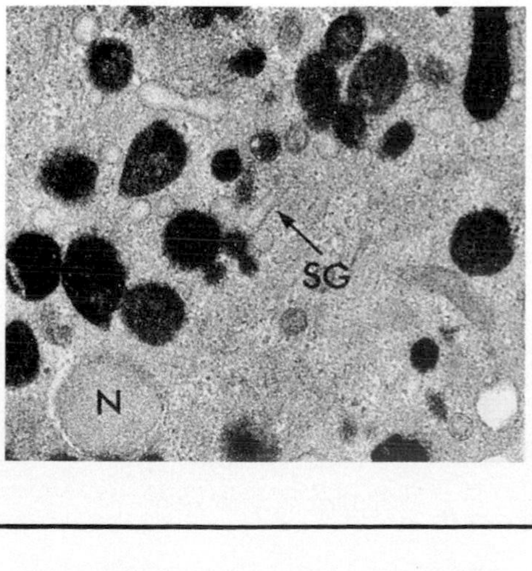

SPECIFIC GRANULES
- Lactoferrin
- Lysozyme
- Alkaline phosphatase
- Type IV collagenase
- Leukocyte adhesion molecules
- Plasminogen activation
- Phospholipase A_2

AZUROPHIL GRANULES
- Myeloperoxidase
- Lysozyme←Bactericidal factors
- Cationic proteins
- Acid hydrolases
- Elastase
- Nonspecific collagenase
- BPI
- Defensins
- Cathepsin G
- Phospholipase A_2

FIGURE 2–20 Ultrastructure and contents of neutrophil granules, stained for peroxidase activity. The large peroxidase-containing granules are the azurophil granules; the smaller peroxidase-negative ones are the specific granules (SG). N, portion of nucleus; BPI, bactericidal permeability increasing protein.

these potent mediators can be *damaging* to the host. They are implicated in the following responses:

- *Endothelial cell damage, with resultant increased vascular permeability*. Adherent neutrophils, when activated, not only produce their own toxic species, but also stimulate xanthine oxidation in endothelial cells themselves, thus elaborating more superoxide.
- *Inactivation of antiproteases*, such as α_1-antitrypsin. This leads to unopposed protease activity, with increased destruction of extracellular matrix.
- *Injury to other cell types* (parenchymal cells, red blood cells).

Serum, tissue fluids, and host cells possess *antioxidant mechanisms* that protect against these potentially harmful oxygen-derived radicals. These antioxidants were discussed in Chapter 1; they include: (1) the copper-containing serum protein *ceruloplasmin*; (2) the iron-free fraction of serum, *transferrin*; (3) the enzyme *superoxide dismutase,* which is found or can be activated in a variety of cell types; (4) the enzyme *catalase,* which detoxifies H_2O_2; and (5) *glutathione peroxidase,* another powerful H_2O_2 detoxifier.

Thus, the influence of oxygen-derived free radicals in any given inflammatory reaction depends on the *balance* between the production and the inactivation of these metabolites by cells and tissues.

NEUROPEPTIDES

Neuropeptides, similar to the vasoactive amines and the eicosanoids previously discussed, play a role in the initiation and propagation of an inflammatory response. The small peptides, such as *substance P* and neurokinin A, belong to a family of tachykinin neuropeptides produced in the central and peripheral nervous systems.[72] Nerve fibers containing substance P are prominent in the lung and gastrointestinal tract. Substance P has many biologic functions, including the transmission of pain signals, regulation of blood pressure, stimulation of secretion by endocrine cells, and increasing vascular permeability.[73] Sensory neurons appear to produce other pro-inflammatory molecules, which are thought to link the sensing of dangerous stimuli to the development of protective host responses.[74]

OTHER MEDIATORS

The mediators described above account for inflammatory reactions to microbes, toxins, and many types of injury, but may not explain why inflammation develops in some specific situations. Recent studies are providing clues about the mechanisms of inflammation in two frequently encountered pathologic conditions.

- *Response to hypoxia.* In Chapter 1 we described the role of hypoxia in causing cell injury and necrosis. Hypoxia by itself is also an inducer of the inflammatory response. This response is mediated largely by a protein called hypoxia-induced factor 1α, which is produced by cells deprived of oxygen and activates many genes involved in inflammation, including VEGF, which increases vascular permeability.[75]
- *Response to necrotic cells.* Although it has been known for many years that necrotic cells elicit inflammatory reactions that serve to eliminate these cells, the molecular basis of this reaction has been largely unknown. One participant may be uric acid, which is a product of DNA breakdown, and crystallizes when present at sufficiently high concentrations in extracellular tissues. Uric acid crystals stimulate inflammation and subsequent immune response.[76] This pro-inflammatory action of uric acid is the basis of the disease gout, in which excessive amounts of uric acid are produced and crystals deposit in joints and other tissues.

SUMMARY OF CHEMICAL MEDIATORS OF ACUTE INFLAMMATION

Table 2–5 summarizes the major actions of the principal mediators. When Lewis discovered the role of histamine in

TABLE 2–5 Summary of Mediators of Acute Inflammation

		Action		
Mediator	**Source**	***Vascular Leakage***	***Chemotaxis***	***Other***
Histamine and serotonin	Mast cells, platelets	+	–	
Bradykinin	Plasma substrate	+	–	Pain
C3a	Plasma protein via liver	+	–	Opsonic fragment (C3b)
C5a	Macrophages	+	+	Leukocyte adhesion, activation
Prostaglandins	Mast cells, from membrane phospholipids	Potentiate other mediators	–	Vasodilation, pain, fever
Leukotriene B_4	Leukocytes	–	+	Leukocyte adhesion, activation
Leukotriene C_4, D_4, E_4	Leukocytes, mast cells	+	–	Bronchoconstriction, vasoconstriction
Oxygen metabolites	Leukocytes	+	–	Endothelial damage, tissue damage
PAF	Leukocytes, mast cells	+	+	Bronchoconstriction, leukocyte priming
IL-1 and TNF	Macrophages, other	–	+	Acute-phase reactions, endothelial activation
Chemokines	Leukocytes, others	–	+	Leukocyte activation
Nitric oxide	Macrophages, endothelium	+	+	Vasodilation, cytotoxicity

inflammation, one mediator was thought to be enough. Now, we are wallowing in them! Yet, from this menu of substances we can emphasize a few mediators that may be particularly relevant in vivo (Table 2–6). Vasodilation, an early event in inflammation, is caused by histamine, prostaglandins, and nitric oxide. Increased vascular permeability is caused by histamine; the anaphylatoxins (C3a and C5a); the kinins; leukotrienes C, D, and E; PAF; and substance P. For chemotaxis, the most likely contributors are complement fragment C5a, lipoxygenase products (LTB_4), and chemokines. Prostaglandins play an important role in vasodilation, pain, and fever, and in potentiating edema. IL-1 and TNF are critical for endothelial–leukocyte interactions and subsequent leukocyte recruitment, and for the production of acute-phase reactants. Lysosomal products and oxygen-derived radicals are the most likely candidates responsible for the ensuing tissue destruction. NO is involved in vasodilation and also causes tissue damage.

Outcomes of Acute Inflammation

The discussion of mediators completes the description of the basic, relatively uniform pattern of the inflammatory reaction encountered in most injuries. Although hemodynamic, permeability, and leukocyte changes have been described sequentially and may be initiated in this order, all these phenomena may be concurrent in the fully evolved reaction to injury. As might be expected, many variables may modify this basic process, including the nature and intensity of the injury,

TABLE 2–6 Role of Mediators in Different Reactions of Inflammation

Vasodilation	Prostaglandins Nitric oxide Histamine
Increased vascular permeability	Vasoactive amines C3a and C5a (through liberating amines) Bradykinin Leukotrienes C_4, D_4, E_4 PAF Substance P
Chemotaxis, leukocyte recruitment and activation	C5a Leukotriene B_4 Chemokines IL-1, TNF Bacterial products
Fever	IL-1, TNF Prostaglandins
Pain	Prostaglandins Bradykinin
Tissue damage	Neutrophil and macrophage lysosomal enzymes Oxygen metabolites Nitric oxide

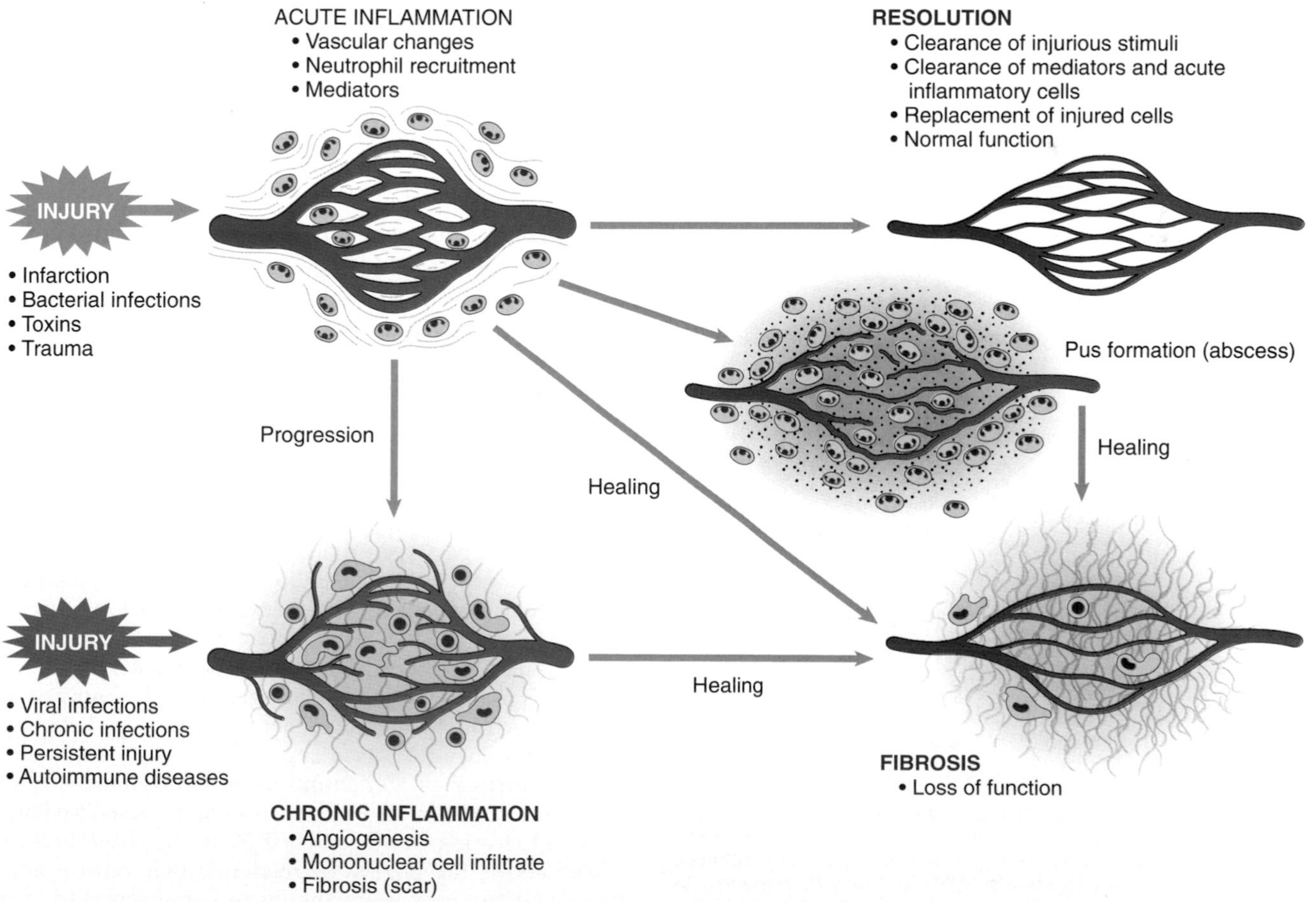

FIGURE 2–21 Outcomes of acute inflammation: resolution, healing by fibrosis, or chronic inflammation (see text).

the site and tissue affected, and the responsiveness of the host. In general, however, *acute inflammation may have one of three outcomes* (Fig. 2–21):

1. *Complete resolution.* In a perfect world, all inflammatory reactions, once they have succeeded in neutralizing and eliminating the injurious stimulus, should end with restoration of the site of acute inflammation to normal. This is called *resolution* and is the usual outcome when the injury is limited or short-lived or when there has been little tissue destruction and the damaged parenchymal cells can regenerate. Resolution involves neutralization or spontaneous decay of the chemical mediators, with subsequent return of normal vascular permeability, cessation of leukocytic infiltration, death (largely by apoptosis) of neutrophils, and finally removal of edema fluid and protein, leukocytes, foreign agents, and necrotic debris from the site (Fig. 2–22). Lymphatics and phagocytes play a role in these events, as described later in this Chapter and in Chapter 3.
2. *Healing by connective tissue replacement (fibrosis).* This occurs after substantial tissue destruction, when the inflammatory injury involves tissues that are incapable of regeneration, or when there is abundant fibrin exudation. When the fibrinous exudate in tissue or serous cavities (pleura, peritoneum) cannot be adequately cleared, connective tissue grows into the area of exudate, converting it into a mass of fibrous tissue—a process also called *organization.* In many pyogenic infections there may be intense neutrophil infiltration and liquefaction of tissues, leading to pus formation. The destroyed tissue is resorbed and eventually replaced by fibrosis.
3. Progression of the tissue response to *chronic inflammation* (discussed below). This may follow acute inflammation, or the response may be chronic almost from the onset. Acute to chronic transition occurs when the acute inflammatory response cannot be resolved, owing either to the persistence of the injurious agent or to some interference with the normal process of healing. For example, bacterial infection of the lung may begin as a focus of acute inflammation (pneumonia), but its failure to resolve may lead to extensive tissue destruction and formation of a cavity in which the inflammation continues to smolder, leading eventually to a chronic lung abscess. Another example of chronic inflammation with a persisting stimulus is peptic ulcer of the duodenum or stomach. Peptic ulcers may persist for months or years and, as discussed below, are manifested by both acute and chronic inflammatory reactions.

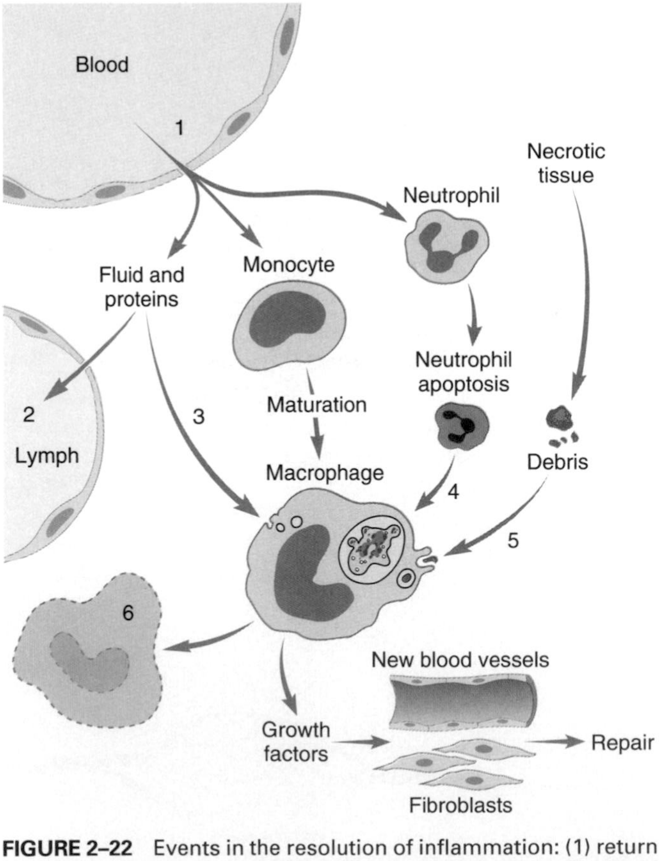

FIGURE 2–22 Events in the resolution of inflammation: (1) return to normal vascular permeability; (2) drainage of edema fluid and proteins into lymphatics or (3) by pinocytosis into macrophages; (4) phagocytosis of apoptotic neutrophils and (5) phagocytosis of necrotic debris; and (6) disposal of macrophages. Macrophages also produce growth factors that initiate the subsequent process of repair. Note the central role of macrophages in resolution. (Modified from Haslett C, Henson PM: In Clark R, Henson PM (eds): The Molecular and Cellular Biology of Wound Repair. New York, Plenum Press, 1996.)

Morphologic Patterns of Acute Inflammation

Although all acute inflammatory reactions are characterized by vascular changes and leukocyte infiltration, the severity of the reaction, its specific cause, and the particular tissue and site involved introduce morphologic variations in the basic patterns. Several types of inflammation are recognized, which vary in their morphology and clinical correlates.

SEROUS INFLAMMATION

Serous inflammation is marked by the outpouring of a thin fluid that, depending on the size of injury, is derived from either the plasma or the secretions of mesothelial cells lining the peritoneal, pleural, and pericardial cavities (called *effusion*). The skin blister resulting from a burn or viral infection represents a large accumulation of serous fluid, either within or immediately beneath the epidermis of the skin (Fig. 2–23).

FIBRINOUS INFLAMMATION

With more severe injuries and the resulting greater vascular permeability, larger molecules such as fibrinogen pass the vascular barrier, and fibrin is formed and deposited in the extracellular space. A fibrinous exudate develops when the vascular leaks are large enough or there is a procoagulant stimulus in the interstitium (e.g., cancer cells). A fibrinous exudate is characteristic of inflammation in the lining of body cavities, such as the meninges, pericardium (Fig. 2–24*A*), and pleura. Histologically, fibrin appears as an eosinophilic meshwork of threads or sometimes as an amorphous coagulum (Fig. 2–24*B*). Fibrinous exudates may be removed by fibrinolysis and clearing of other debris by macrophages. As mentioned above, the process of *resolution* may restore normal tissue structure, but when the fibrin is not removed, it may stimulate the ingrowth of fibroblasts and blood vessels and

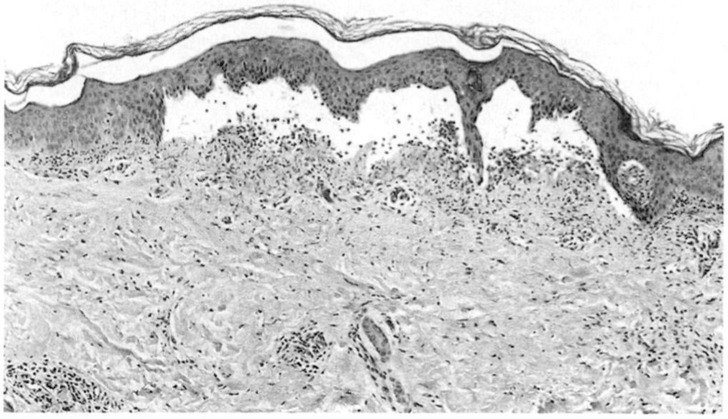

FIGURE 2–23 Serous inflammation. Low-power view of a cross-section of a skin blister showing the epidermis separated from the dermis by a focal collection of serous effusion.

thus lead to scarring. Conversion of the fibrinous exudate to scar tissue (*organization*) within the pericardial sac leads either to opaque fibrous thickening of the pericardium and epicardium in the area of exudation or, more often, to the development of fibrous strands that reduce and may even obliterate the pericardial space.

SUPPURATIVE OR PURULENT INFLAMMATION

Suppurative or purulent inflammation is characterized by the production of large amounts of pus or purulent exudate consisting of neutrophils, necrotic cells, and edema fluid. Certain bacteria (e.g., staphylococci) produce this localized suppuration and are therefore referred to as *pyogenic* (pus-producing) bacteria. A common example of an acute suppurative inflammation is acute appendicitis. *Abscesses are localized collections of purulent inflammatory tissue* caused by suppuration buried in a tissue, an organ, or a confined space. They are produced by deep seeding of pyogenic bacteria into a tissue (Fig. 2–25). Abscesses have a central region that appears as a mass of necrotic leukocytes and tissue cells. There is usually a zone of preserved neutrophils around this necrotic focus, and outside this region vascular dilation and parenchymal and fibroblastic proliferation occur, indicating the beginning of repair. In time, the abscess may become walled off and ultimately replaced by connective tissue.

ULCERS

An ulcer is a local defect, or excavation, of the surface of an organ or tissue that is produced by the sloughing (shedding) of inflammatory necrotic tissue (Fig. 2–26). Ulceration can occur only when tissue necrosis and resultant inflammation exist on or near a surface. It is most commonly encountered in: (1) inflammatory necrosis of the mucosa of the mouth, stomach, intestines, or genitourinary tract; and (2) subcutaneous inflammation of the lower extremities in older persons who have circulatory disturbances that predispose to extensive necrosis.

Ulcerations are best exemplified by peptic ulcer of the stomach or duodenum, in which acute and chronic inflammation coexist. During the acute stage, there is intense polymorphonuclear infiltration and vascular dilation in the margins of the defect. With chronicity, the margins and base of the ulcer develop fibroblastic proliferation, scarring, and the accumulation of lymphocytes, macrophages, and plasma cells.

Summary of Acute Inflammation

Now that we have described the components, mediators, and pathologic manifestations of acute inflammatory responses, it is useful to summarize the sequence of events in a typical response of this type. When a host encounters an injurious agent, such as an infectious microbe or dead cells, phagocytes that reside in all tissues try to get rid of these agents. At the same time, phagocytes and other host cells react to the presence of the foreign or abnormal substance by liberating cytokines, lipid messengers, and the various other mediators of inflammation. Some of these mediators act on endothelial cells in the vicinity and promote the efflux of plasma and the recruitment of circulating leukocytes to the

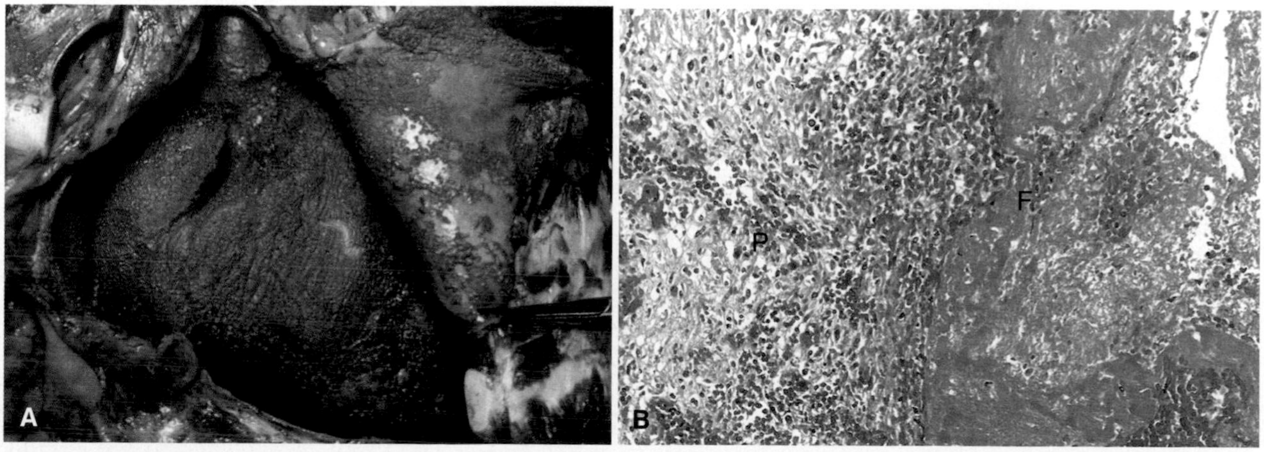

FIGURE 2–24 Fibrinous pericarditis. *A,* Deposits of fibrin on the pericardium. *B,* A pink meshwork of fibrin exudate (F) overlies the pericardial surface (P).

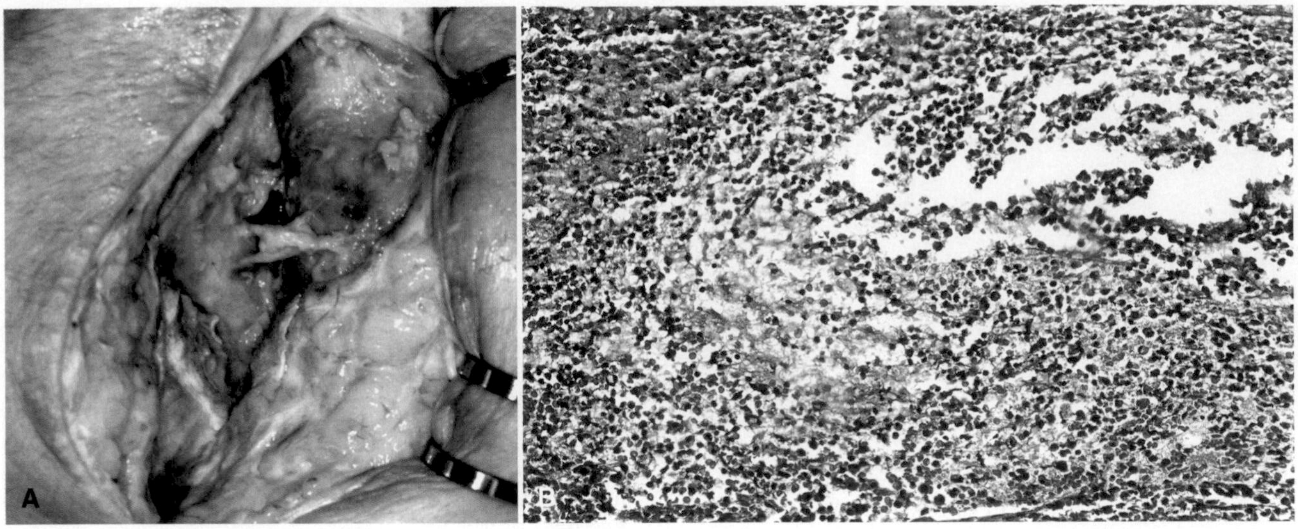

FIGURE 2–25 Suppurative inflammation. *A,* A subcutaneous bacterial abscess with collections of pus. *B,* The abscess contains neutrophils, edema fluid, and cellular debris.

site where the offending agent is located. The recruited leukocytes are activated by the injurious agent and by locally produced mediators, and the activated leukocytes try to remove the offending agent by phagocytosis. As the injurious agent is eliminated and anti-inflammatory mechanisms become active, the process subsides and the host returns to a normal state of health. If the injurious agent cannot be quickly eliminated, the result may be chronic inflammation.

The different components of the inflammatory response are mediated by different signals and serve distinct (and overlapping) functions. The vascular phenomena of acute inflammation are characterized by increased blood flow to the injured area, resulting mainly from arteriolar dilation and opening of capillary beds induced by mediators such as histamine. Increased vascular permeability results in the accumulation of protein-rich extravascular fluid, which forms the exudate. Plasma proteins leave the vessels, most commonly through widened interendothelial cell junctions of the venules. The redness *(rubor)*, warmth *(calor)*, and swelling *(tumor)* of acute inflammation are caused by the increased blood flow and edema. Circulating leukocytes, initially predominantly neutrophils, adhere to the endothelium via adhesion molecules, transmigrate across the endothelium, and migrate to the site of injury under the influence of chemotactic agents. Leukocytes that are activated by the offending agent and by endogenous mediators may release toxic metabolites and proteases extracellularly, causing tissue damage. During the damage, and in part as a result of the liberation of prostaglandins, neuropeptides, and cytokines, one of the local symptoms is pain (*dolor*).

Chronic Inflammation

Although difficult to define precisely, *chronic inflammation* is considered to be *inflammation of prolonged duration* (weeks or months) *in which active inflammation, tissue destruction, and attempts at repair are proceeding simultaneously.* Although it may follow acute inflammation, as described earlier, chronic inflammation frequently begins insidiously, as a low-grade,

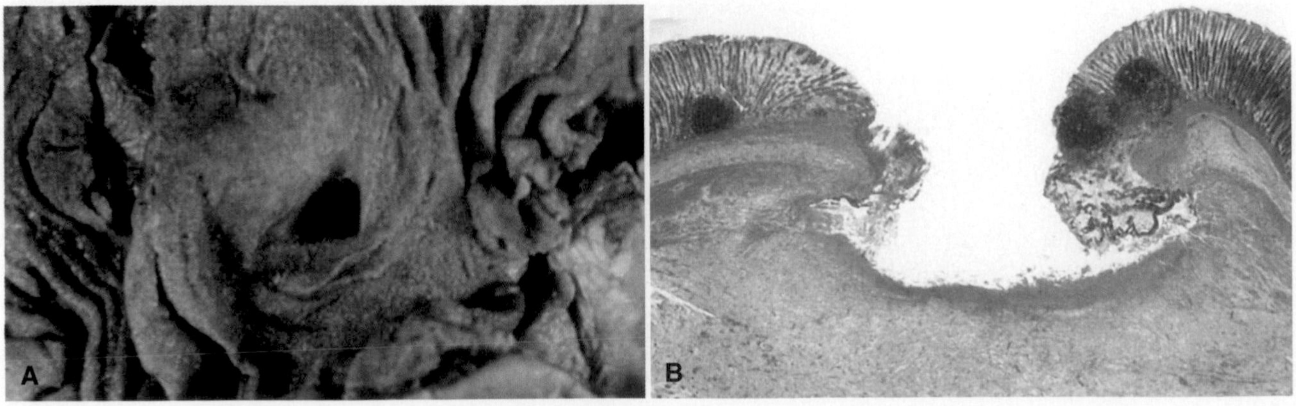

FIGURE 2–26 The morphology of an ulcer. *A,* A chronic duodenal ulcer. *B,* Low-power cross-section of a duodenal ulcer crater with an acute inflammatory exudate in the base.

smoldering, often asymptomatic response. This latter type of chronic inflammation is the cause of tissue damage in some of the most common and disabling human diseases, such as rheumatoid arthritis, atherosclerosis, tuberculosis, and chronic lung diseases.

CAUSES OF CHRONIC INFLAMMATION

Chronic inflammation arises in the following settings:

- *Persistent infections* by certain microorganisms, such as tubercle bacilli, *Treponema pallidum* (the causative organism of syphilis), and certain viruses, fungi, and parasites. These organisms are of low toxicity and evoke an immune reaction called *delayed type hypersensitivity* (Chapter 6). The inflammatory response sometimes takes a specific pattern called a *granulomatous reaction* (discussed later).
- *Prolonged exposure to potentially toxic agents, either exogenous or endogenous.* An example of an exogenous agent is particulate silica, a nondegradable inanimate material that, when inhaled for prolonged periods, results in an inflammatory lung disease called *silicosis* (Chapter 15). *Atherosclerosis* (Chapter 11) is thought to be a chronic inflammatory process of the arterial wall induced, at least in part, by endogenous toxic plasma lipid components.
- *Autoimmunity.* Under certain conditions, immune reactions develop against the individual's own tissues, leading to *autoimmune diseases* (Chapter 6). In these diseases, autoantigens evoke a self-perpetuating immune reaction that results in chronic tissue damage and inflammation. Immune reactions play an important role in several common chronic inflammatory diseases, such as rheumatoid arthritis and lupus erythematosus.

MORPHOLOGIC FEATURES

In contrast to acute inflammation, which is manifested by vascular changes, edema, and predominantly neutrophilic infiltration, *chronic inflammation is characterized by:*

- *Infiltration with mononuclear cells,* which include macrophages, lymphocytes, and plasma cells.
- *Tissue destruction,* induced by the persistent offending agent or by the inflammatory cells.
- Attempts at *healing by connective tissue replacement of damaged tissue,* accomplished by proliferation of small blood vessels (*angiogenesis*) and, in particular, *fibrosis.*[77]

Because angiogenesis and fibrosis are also components of wound healing and repair, they are discussed more fully in Chapter 3.

MONONUCLEAR CELL INFILTRATION

The *macrophage* is the dominant cellular player in chronic inflammation, and we begin our discussion with a brief review of its biology. *Macrophages* are one component of the *mononuclear phagocyte system* (Fig. 2–27). The mononuclear phagocyte system (sometimes called reticuloendothelial system) consists of closely related cells of bone marrow origin, including blood monocytes and tissue macrophages. The latter are diffusely scattered in the connective tissue or located in organs such as the liver (Kupffer cells), spleen and lymph nodes (sinus histiocytes), and lungs (alveolar macrophages). Mononuclear phagocytes arise from a common precursor in the bone marrow, which gives rise to blood monocytes. From the blood, monocytes migrate into various tissues and differentiate into macrophages. The half-life of blood monocytes is

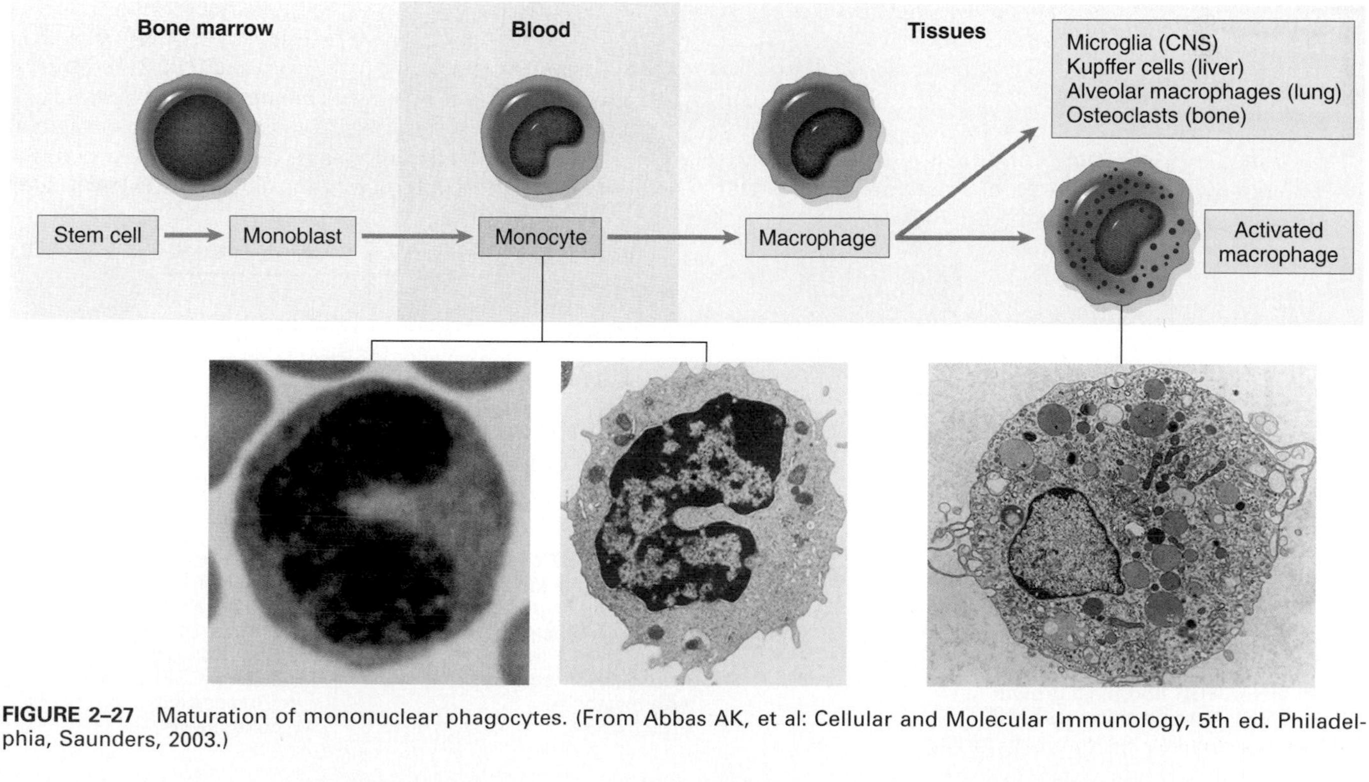

FIGURE 2–27 Maturation of mononuclear phagocytes. (From Abbas AK, et al: Cellular and Molecular Immunology, 5th ed. Philadelphia, Saunders, 2003.)

about 1 day, whereas the life span of tissue macrophages is several months or years. The journey from bone marrow stem cell to tissue macrophage is regulated by a variety of growth and differentiation factors, cytokines, adhesion molecules, and cellular interactions.

As discussed previously, monocytes begin to emigrate into extravascular tissues quite early in acute inflammation, and within 48 hours they may constitute the predominant cell type. Extravasation of monocytes is governed by the same factors that are involved in neutrophil emigration, that is, adhesion molecules and chemical mediators with chemotactic and activating properties. When the monocyte reaches the extravascular tissue, it undergoes transformation into a larger phagocytic cell, the *macrophage.* Macrophages may be *activated* by a variety of stimuli, including cytokines (e.g., IFN-γ) secreted by sensitized T lymphocytes and by NK cells, bacterial endotoxins, and other chemical mediators (Fig. 2–28). Activation results in increased cell size, increased levels of lysosomal enzymes, more active metabolism, and greater ability to phagocytose and kill ingested microbes. *Activated macrophages secrete a wide variety of biologically active products* that, if unchecked, result in the tissue injury and fibrosis characteristic of chronic inflammation (Fig. 2–29).

In short-lived inflammation, if the irritant is eliminated, macrophages eventually disappear (either dying off or making their way into the lymphatics and lymph nodes). In chronic inflammation, macrophage accumulation persists, and is mediated by different mechanisms (Fig. 2–30):

1. *Recruitment of monocytes from the circulation,* which results from the expression of adhesion molecules and chemotactic factors.[78] Most of the macrophages present in a focus of chronic inflammation are recruited from circulating monocytes. The process of monocyte recruitment is fundamentally similar to the recruitment of neutrophils, described earlier (see Fig. 2–6). Chemotactic stimuli for monocytes include chemokines produced by activated macrophages, lymphocytes, and other cell types (e.g., MCP-1); C5a; growth factors such as platelet-derived growth factor and transforming growth factor-α (TGF-α); fragments from the breakdown of collagen and fibronectin; and fibrinopeptides. Each of these may play a role under given circumstances; for example, chemokines are major stimuli for macrophage accumulation in delayed-hypersensitivity immune reactions.
2. *Local proliferation of macrophages* after their emigration from the bloodstream. Once thought to be an unusual event, macrophage proliferation is now known to occur prominently in some chronic inflammatory lesions, such as atheromatous plaques (Chapter 11).
3. *Immobilization of macrophages* within the site of inflammation. Certain cytokines and oxidized lipids (Chapter 11) can cause such immobilization.

The products of activated macrophages serve to eliminate injurious agents such as microbes and to initiate the process of repair, and are responsible for much of the tissue injury in

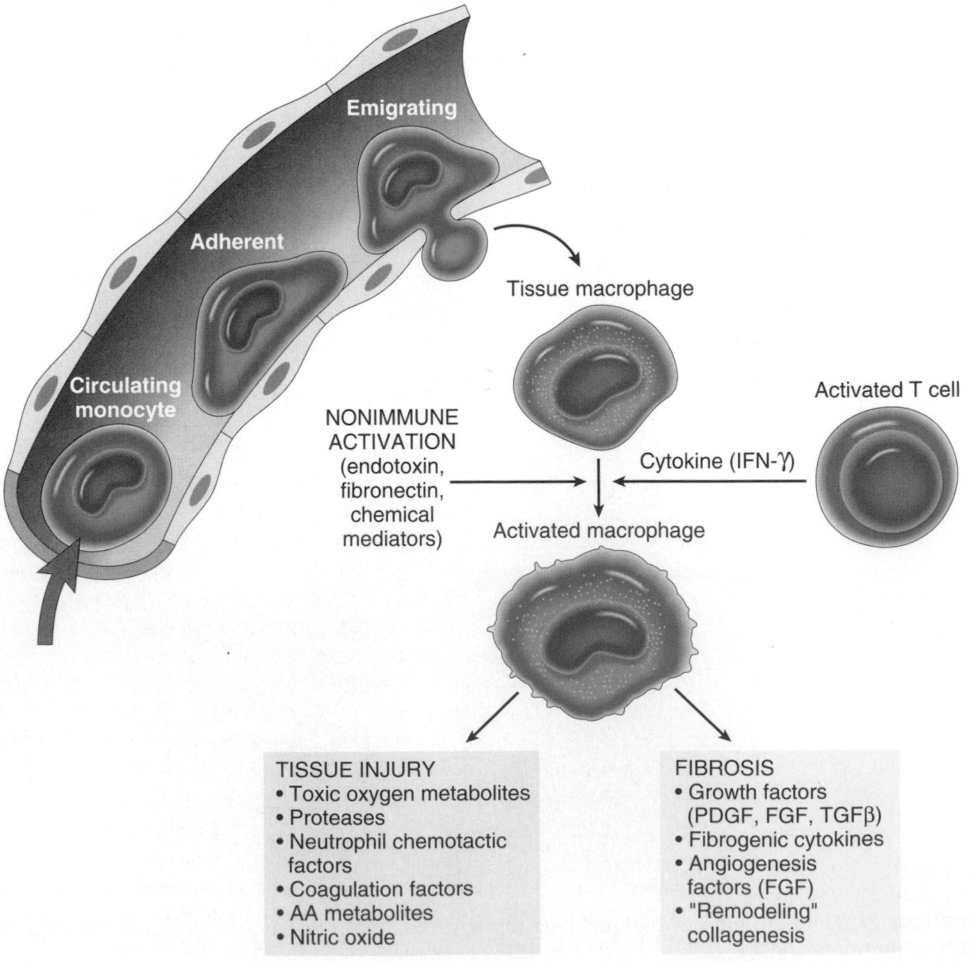

FIGURE 2–28 The roles of activated macrophages in chronic inflammation. Macrophages are activated by cytokines from immune-activated T cells (particularly IFN-γ) or by nonimmunologic stimuli such as endotoxin. The products made by activated macrophages that cause tissue injury and fibrosis are indicated. AA, arachidonic acid; PDGF, platelet-derived growth factor; FGF, fibroblast growth factor; TGFβ, transforming growth factor β.

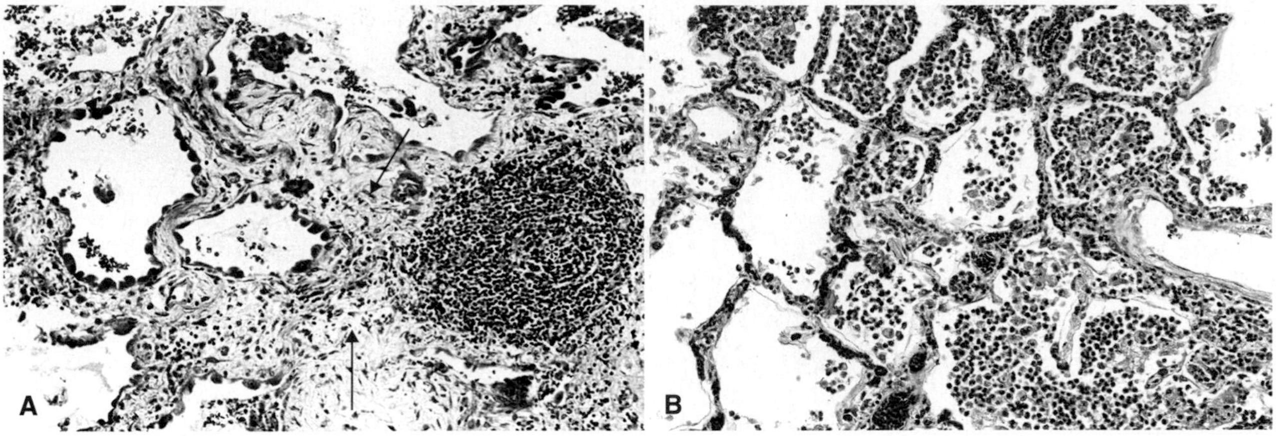

FIGURE 2–29 *A*, Chronic inflammation in the lung, showing all three characteristic histologic features: (1) collection of chronic inflammatory cells (*), (2) destruction of parenchyma (normal alveoli are replaced by spaces lined by cuboidal epithelium, *arrowheads*), and (3) replacement by connective tissue (fibrosis, *arrows*). *B*, By contrast, in acute inflammation of the lung (acute bronchopneumonia), neutrophils fill the alveolar spaces and blood vessels are congested.

chronic inflammation. Some of these products are toxic to microbes and host cells (e.g., reactive oxygen and nitrogen intermediates) or extracellular matrix (proteases); some cause influx of other cell types (e.g., cytokines, chemotactic factors); and still others cause fibroblast proliferation, collagen deposition, and angiogenesis (e.g., growth factors). This impressive arsenal of mediators makes macrophages powerful allies in the body's defense against unwanted invaders, but the same weaponry can also induce considerable tissue destruction when macrophages are inappropriately activated. Thus, *tissue destruction is one of the hallmarks of chronic inflammation.*

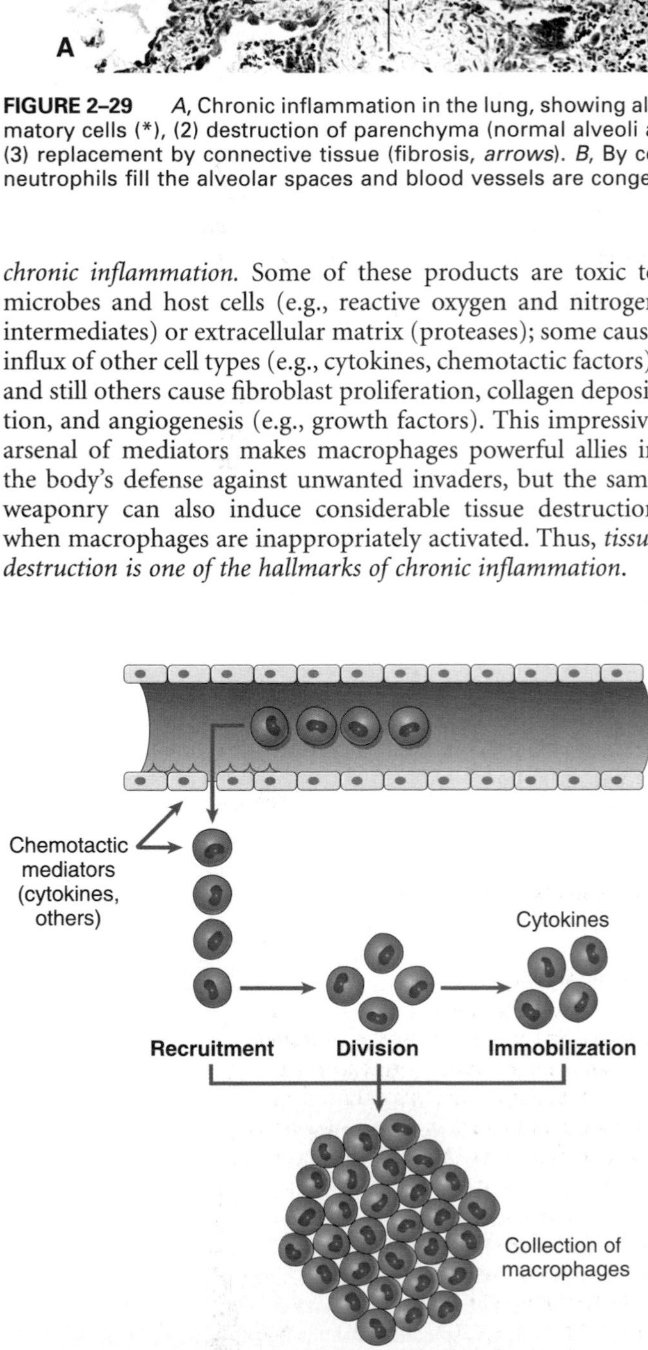

FIGURE 2–30 Mechanisms of macrophage accumulation in tissues. The most important is continued recruitment from the microcirculation. (Adapted from Ryan G, Majno G: Inflammation. Kalamazoo, MI, Upjohn, 1977.)

A variety of substances in addition to the products of macrophages may contribute to tissue damage in chronic inflammation. Necrotic tissue itself can perpetuate the inflammatory cascade through the activation of kinin, coagulation, complement and fibrinolytic systems, the release of mediators from leukocytes responding to the necrotic tissue, and liberation of substances like uric acid from dying cells. In cellular immune reactions, T lymphocytes may directly kill cells (see Chapter 6). Thus, ongoing tissue destruction can activate the inflammatory cascade by diverse mechanisms, so that features of both acute and chronic inflammation may coexist in certain circumstances.

OTHER CELLS IN CHRONIC INFLAMMATION

Other cell types present in chronic inflammation include lymphocytes, plasma cells, eosinophils, and mast cells:

- *Lymphocytes* are mobilized in both antibody-mediated and cell-mediated immune reactions and even in nonimmune inflammation. Antigen-stimulated (effector and memory) lymphocytes of different types (T, B) use various adhesion molecule pairs (predominantly the integrins and their ligands) and chemokines to migrate into inflammatory sites. Cytokines from activated macrophages, mainly TNF, IL-1, and chemokines, promote leukocyte recruitment, setting the stage for persistence of the inflammatory response.

Lymphocytes and macrophages interact in a bidirectional way, and these reactions play an important role in chronic inflammation (Fig. 2–31). Macrophages display antigens to T cells, and produce membrane molecules (costimulators) and cytokines (notably IL-12) that stimulate T-cell responses (Chapter 6). Activated T lymphocytes produce cytokines, and one of these, IFN-γ, is a major activator of macrophages. *Plasma cells* develop from activated B lymphocytes and produce antibody directed either against persistent antigen in the inflammatory site or against altered tissue components. In some strong chronic inflammatory reactions, the accumulation of lymphocytes, antigen-presenting cells, and

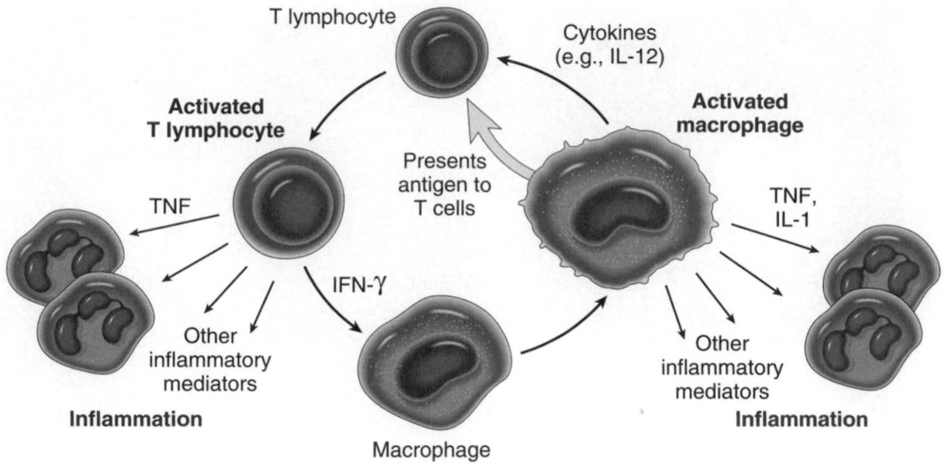

FIGURE 2–31 Macrophage–lymphocyte interactions in chronic inflammation. Activated lymphocytes and macrophages influence each other and also release inflammatory mediators that affect other cells.

plasma cells may assume the morphologic features of lymphoid organs, particularly lymph nodes, even containing well-formed germinal centers. This pattern of *lymphoid organogenesis* is often seen in the synovium of patients with long-standing rheumatoid arthritis.

- *Eosinophils* are abundant in immune reactions mediated by IgE and in parasitic infections (Fig. 2–32). The recruitment of eosinophils involves extravasation from the blood and their migration into tissue by processes similar to those for other leukocytes. One of the chemokines that is especially important for eosinophil recruitment is eotaxin. Eosinophils have granules that contain *major basic protein*, a highly cationic protein that is toxic to parasites but also causes lysis of mammalian epithelial cells. They may thus be of benefit in controlling parasitic infections but they contribute to tissue damage in immune reactions (Chapter 6).[79]
- *Mast cells* are widely distributed in connective tissues and participate in both acute and persistent inflammatory reactions. Mast cells express on their surface the receptor that binds the Fc portion of IgE antibody (FcεRI). In acute reactions, IgE antibodies bound to the cells' Fc receptors specifically recognize antigen, and the cells degranulate and release mediators, such as histamine and products of AA oxidation (Chapter 6). This type of response occurs during anaphylactic reactions to foods, insect venom, or drugs, frequently with catastrophic results. When properly regulated, this response can benefit the host. Mast cells are also present in chronic inflammatory reactions, and may produce cytokines that contribute to fibrosis.

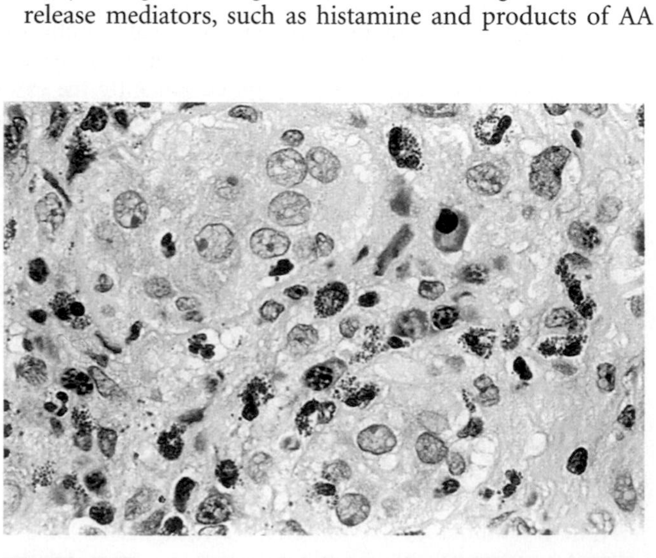

FIGURE 2–32 A focus of inflammation showing numerous eosinophils.

Although neutrophils are characteristic of acute inflammation, many forms of chronic inflammation, lasting for months, continue to show large numbers of neutrophils, induced either by persistent microbes or by mediators produced by macrophages and T lymphocytes. In chronic bacterial infection of bone (osteomyelitis), a neutrophilic exudate can persist for many months. Neutrophils are also important in the chronic damage induced in lungs by smoking and other irritant stimuli (Chapter 15).

GRANULOMATOUS INFLAMMATION

Granulomatous inflammation is a distinctive pattern of chronic inflammatory reaction characterized by focal accumulations of activated macrophages, which often develop an epithelial-like (epithelioid) appearance. It is encountered in a limited number of immunologically mediated, infectious and some noninfectious conditions. Its genesis is firmly linked to immune reactions and thus is described in more detail in Chapter 6. Tuberculosis is the prototype of the granulomatous diseases, but sarcoidosis, cat-scratch disease, lymphogranuloma inguinale, leprosy, brucellosis, syphilis, some mycotic infections, berylliosis, and reactions of irritant lipids are also included (Table 2–7). Recognition of the granulomatous pattern in a biopsy specimen is important because of the limited number of possible conditions that cause it and the significance of the diagnoses associated with the lesions.

A granuloma is a focus of chronic inflammation consisting of a microscopic aggregation of macrophages that are transformed into epithelium-like cells surrounded by a collar of mononuclear leukocytes, principally lymphocytes and occasionally plasma cells. In the usual hematoxylin and eosin stained tissue sections, the epithelioid cells have a pale pink granular cytoplasm with indistinct cell boundaries, often appearing to merge into one another. The nucleus is less dense than that of a lymphocyte, is oval or elongate, and may show folding of the nuclear membrane. Older granulomas develop an enclosing rim of

TABLE 2–7 Examples of Diseases with Granulomatous Inflammations

Disease	Cause	Tissue Reaction
Tuberculosis	*Mycobacterium tuberculosis*	Noncaseating tubercle (granuloma prototype): a focus of epithelioid cells, rimmed by fibroblasts, lymphocytes, histiocytes, occasional Langhans giant cell; caseating tubercle: central amorphous granular debris, loss of all cellular detail; acid-fast bacilli
Leprosy	*Mycobacterium leprae*	Acid-fast bacilli in macrophages; non-caseating granulomas
Syphilis	*Treponema pallidum*	Gumma: microscopic to grossly visible lesion, enclosing wall of histiocytes; plasma cell infiltrate; central cells are necrotic without loss of cellular outline
Cat-scratch disease	Gram-negative bacillus	Rounded or stellate granuloma containing central granular debris and recognizable neutrophils; giant cells uncommon

fibroblasts and connective tissue. Frequently, epithelioid cells fuse to form *giant cells* in the periphery or sometimes in the center of granulomas. These giant cells may attain diameters of 40 to 50 μm. They have a large mass of cytoplasm containing 20 or more small nuclei arranged either peripherally (Langhans-type giant cell) or haphazardly (foreign body-type giant cell) (Fig. 2–33). There is no known functional difference between these two types of giant cells, a fact that does not deter students from remembering the morphologic differences!

There are two types of granulomas, which differ in their pathogenesis. *Foreign body granulomas* are incited by relatively inert foreign bodies. Typically, foreign body granulomas form when material such as talc (associated with intravenous drug abuse) (Chapter 9), sutures, or other fibers are large enough to preclude phagocytosis by a single macrophage and do not incite any specific inflammatory or immune response. Epithelioid cells and giant cells form and are apposed to the surface and encompass the foreign body. The foreign material can usually be identified in the center of the granuloma, particularly if viewed with polarized light, in which it appears refractile.

Immune granulomas are caused by insoluble particles, typically microbes, that are capable of inducing a cell-mediated immune response (Chapter 6). This type of immune response does not necessarily produce granulomas but it does so when

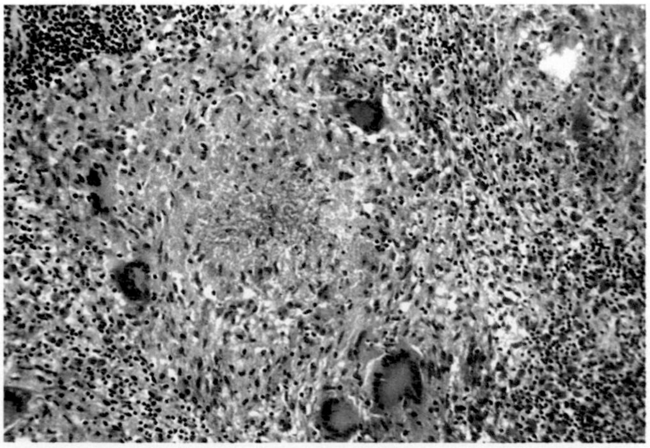

FIGURE 2–33 Typical tuberculous granuloma showing an area of central necrosis, epithelioid cells, multiple Langhans-type giant cells, and lymphocytes.

the inciting agent is poorly degradable or particulate. In these responses, macrophages engulf the foreign material and process and present some of it to appropriate T lymphocytes, causing them to become activated. The responding T cells produce cytokines, such as IL-2, which activates other T cells, perpetuating the response, and IFN-γ, which is important in activating macrophages and transforming them into epithelioid cells and multinucleate giant cells.

The prototype of the immune granuloma is that caused by the bacillus of tuberculosis. In this disease, the granuloma is referred to as a *tubercle* and is *classically characterized by the presence of central caseous necrosis* (see Fig. 2–33). In contrast, caseous necrosis is rare in other granulomatous diseases. The morphologic patterns in the various granulomatous diseases may be sufficiently different to allow reasonably accurate diagnosis by an experienced pathologist (see Table 2–7); however, there are so many atypical presentations that it is always necessary to identify the specific etiologic agent by special stains for organisms (e.g., acid-fast stains for tubercle bacilli), by culture methods (e.g., in tuberculosis and fungal diseases), by molecular techniques (e.g., the polymerase chain reaction in tuberculosis), and by serologic studies (e.g., in syphilis). In sarcoidosis, the etiologic agent is unknown (Chapter 15).

LYMPHATICS IN INFLAMMATION

The system of lymphatics and lymph nodes filters and polices the extravascular fluids. Together with the mononuclear phagocyte system, it represents a secondary line of defense that is called into play whenever a local inflammatory reaction fails to contain and neutralize an external agent, such as a microbe.

Lymphatics are delicate channels that are difficult to visualize in ordinary tissue sections because they readily collapse. They are lined by continuous, thin endothelium with loose, overlapping cell junctions; scant basement membrane; and no muscular support except in the larger ducts. In inflammation lymph flow is increased and helps drain the edema fluid from the extravascular space. Because the junctions of lymphatics are loose, lymphatic fluid eventually equilibrates with extravascular fluid. Not only fluid, but also leukocytes and cell debris may find their way into lymph. Valves are present in collecting lymphatics, allowing lymph content to flow only proximally. Delicate fibrils, attached at right angles to the walls of the lymphatic vessel, extend into the adjacent tissues and serve to maintain patency of the lymphatic channels.

In severe injuries, the drainage may transport the offending agent, be it chemical or microbial. The lymphatics may become secondarily inflamed *(lymphangitis)*, as may the draining lymph nodes *(lymphadenitis)*. Therefore, it is not uncommon in infections of the hand, for example, to observe red streaks along the entire arm up to the axilla following the course of the lymphatic channels, accompanied by painful enlargement of the axillary lymph nodes. The nodal enlargement is usually caused by hyperplasia of the lymphoid follicles as well as by hyperplasia of the phagocytic cells lining the sinuses of the lymph nodes. This constellation of nodal histologic changes is termed *reactive*, or *inflammatory, lymphadenitis* (Chapter 14).

The system of lymph nodes sometimes contains the spread of the infection, but in severe infections the organisms gain access to the vascular circulation, thus inducing a *bacteremia*. The phagocytic cells of the liver, spleen, and bone marrow constitute the next line of defense, but in massive infections, bacteria seed distant tissues of the body. The heart valves, meninges, kidneys, and joints are favored sites of implantation for blood-borne organisms, and when this happens endocarditis, meningitis, renal abscesses, and septic arthritis may develop.

Systemic Effects of Inflammation

Anyone who has suffered a severe sore throat or a respiratory infection has experienced the systemic manifestations of acute inflammation. The systemic changes associated with inflammation, especially in patients who have infections, are collectively called the *acute phase response*, or the systemic inflammatory response syndrome (SIRS).[80] These changes are reactions to cytokines whose production is stimulated by bacterial products such as LPS and by other inflammatory stimuli. The acute phase response consists of several clinical and pathologic changes:

- *Fever*, characterized by an elevation of body temperature, usually by 1° to 4°C, is one of the most prominent manifestations of the acute phase response, especially when inflammation is associated with infection. Fever is produced in response to substances called *pyrogens* that act by stimulating prostaglandin synthesis in the vascular and perivascular cells of the hypothalamus. Bacterial products, such as LPS (called *exogenous pyrogens*), stimulate leukocytes to release cytokines such as IL-1 and TNF (called *endogenous pyrogens*) that increase the enzymes (cyclooxygenases) that convert AA into prostaglandins.[81,82] In the hypothalamus, the prostaglandins, especially PGE_2, stimulate the production of neurotransmitters such as cyclic AMP, which function to reset the temperature set-point at a higher level. NSAIDs, including aspirin, reduce fever by inhibiting cyclooxygenase and thus blocking prostaglandin synthesis. An elevated body temperature has been shown to help amphibians ward off microbial infections, and it is assumed that fever does the same for mammals, although the mechanism is unknown. One hypothesis is that fever may induce heat shock proteins that enhance lymphocyte responses to microbial antigens.
- *Acute-phase proteins* are plasma proteins, mostly synthesized in the liver, whose plasma concentrations may increase several hundred-fold as part of the response to inflammatory stimuli.[83] Three of the best-known examples of these proteins are C-reactive protein (CRP), fibrinogen, and serum amyloid A protein (SAA). Synthesis of these molecules by hepatocytes is upregulated by cytokines, especially IL-6 (for CRP and fibrinogen) and IL-1 or TNF (for SAA). Many acute-phase proteins, such as CRP and SAA, bind to microbial cell walls, and they may act as opsonins and fix complement. They also bind chromatin, possibly aiding in the clearing of necrotic cell nuclei. During the acute phase response, serum amyloid A protein replaces apolipoprotein A, a component of high-density lipoprotein particles. This may alter the targeting of high-density lipoproteins from liver cells to macrophages, which can utilize these particles as a source of energy-producing lipids. The rise in fibrinogen causes erythrocytes to form stacks (rouleaux) that sediment more rapidly at unit gravity than do individual erythrocytes. This is the basis for measuring the *erythrocyte sedimentation rate (ESR)* as a simple test for the systemic inflammatory response, caused by any number of stimuli, including LPS. Acute-phase proteins have beneficial effects during acute inflammation, but as we shall see (Chapter 6), prolonged production of these proteins (especially SAA) causes *secondary amyloidosis* in chronic inflammation. Elevated serum levels of CRP are now used as a marker for increased risk of myocardial infarction in patients with coronary artery disease.[84] It is believed that inflammation involving atherosclerotic plaques in the coronary arteries may predispose to thrombosis and subsequent infarction, and CRP is produced during inflammation. On this basis, anti-inflammatory agents are being tested in patients to reduce the risk of myocardial infarction.
- *Leukocytosis* is a common feature of inflammatory reactions, especially those induced by bacterial infection. The leukocyte count usually climbs to 15,000 or 20,000 cells/μl, but sometimes it may reach extraordinarily high levels of 40,000 to 100,000 cells/μl. These extreme elevations are referred to as *leukemoid reactions* because they are similar to the white cell counts obtained in leukemia. The leukocytosis occurs initially because of *accelerated release* of cells from the bone marrow postmitotic reserve pool (caused by cytokines, including IL-1 and TNF) and is therefore associated with a rise in the number of more immature neutrophils in the blood *(shift to the left)*. Prolonged infection also induces proliferation of precursors in the bone marrow, caused by increased production of colony stimulating factors (CSFs). Thus, the bone marrow output of leukocytes is increased to compensate for the loss of these cells in the inflammatory reaction. (See also the discussion of leukocytosis in Chapter 14.) *Neutrophilia* refers to an increase in the blood neutrophil count. Most bacterial infections induce *neutrophilia*. Viral infections such as infectious mononucleosis, mumps, and German measles produce a leukocytosis by virtue of an absolute increase in the number of lymphocytes (*lymphocytosis*). In an additional group of disorders, which includes bronchial asthma, hay fever, and parasitic infestations, there is an absolute increase in the number of eosinophils, creating an *eosinophilia*. Certain infections (typhoid fever and infections caused by viruses, rickettsiae, and certain protozoa) are associated with a decreased number of circulating white cells *(leukopenia)*. Leukopenia is also encountered in infections that overwhelm patients debilitated by disseminated cancer or rampant tuberculosis.

- Other manifestations of the acute phase response include increased pulse and blood pressure; decreased sweating, mainly because of redirection of blood flow from cutaneous to deep vascular beds, to minimize heat loss through the skin; rigors (shivering), chills (search for warmth), anorexia, somnolence, and malaise, probably because of the actions of cytokines on brain cells.
- In severe bacterial infections (*sepsis*), the large amounts of organisms and LPS in the blood stimulate the production of enormous quantities of several cytokines, notably TNF and IL-1.[85,86] As a result, circulating levels of these cytokines increase and the form of the host response changes. High levels of TNF cause disseminated intravascular coagulation (DIC). Thrombosis results from two simultaneous reactions: LPS and TNF induce tissue factor (TF) expression on endothelial cells, which initiates coagulation; the same agents inhibit natural anticoagulation mechanisms, by decreasing the expression of tissue factor pathway inhibitor (TFPI) and endothelial cell thrombomodulin. Cytokines cause liver injury and impaired liver function, resulting in a failure to maintain normal blood glucose levels due to a lack of gluconeogenesis from stored glycogen. Overproduction of NO by cytokine-activated cardiac myocytes and vascular smooth muscle cells leads to heart failure and loss of perfusion pressure, respectively, resulting in hemodynamic shock. The clinical triad of DIC, hypoglycemia, and cardiovascular failure is described as *septic shock*; it is discussed in more detail in Chapter 4. Multiple organs show inflammation and intravascular thrombosis, which can produce organ failure. Tissue injury in response to LPS can also result from the activation of neutrophils before they exit the vasculature, thus causing damage to endothelial cells and reduced blood flow. The lungs and liver are particularly susceptible to injury by neutrophils. Lung damage in the systemic inflammatory response, commonly called the *adult respiratory distress syndrome* (ARDS), results when neutrophil-mediated endothelial injury allows fluid to escape from the blood into the airspace (Chapter 15). The kidney and the bowel are also injured, largely due to reduced perfusion. This condition is often fatal.

Consequences of Defective or Excessive Inflammation

Now that we have described the process of inflammation and its outcomes, it is helpful to summarize the clinical and pathological consequences of too much or too little inflammation.

- *Defective inflammation* typically results in increased susceptibility to infections and delayed healing of wounds and tissue damage. The susceptibility to infections reflects the fundamental role of the inflammatory response in host defense, and is the reason why this response is a central component of the defense mechanisms that immunologists call *innate immunity* (Chapter 6). Delayed repair is because the inflammatory response is essential for clearing damaged tissues and debris, and provides the necessary stimulus to get the repair process started.
- *Excessive inflammation* is the basis of many categories of human disease. It is well established that allergies, in which individuals mount unregulated immune responses against commonly encountered environmental antigens, and autoimmune diseases, in which immune responses develop against normally tolerated self-antigens, are disorders in which the fundamental cause of tissue injury is inflammation (Chapter 6). But recent studies are pointing to an important role of inflammation in a wide variety of human diseases that are not primarily disorders of the immune system. These include cancer, atherosclerosis and ischemic heart disease, and some neurodegenerative diseases such as Alzheimer disease. In addition, prolonged inflammation and the fibrosis that accompanies it are responsible for much of the pathology in many chronic infectious, metabolic and other diseases. The specific diseases are discussed in relevant chapters later in the book. Since these disorders are some of the major scourges of mankind, it is not surprising that the normally protective inflammatory response is being called the "silent killer".

Although our discussion of the molecular and cellular events in acute and chronic inflammation is concluded, we still need to consider the changes induced by the body's attempts to heal the damage, the process of *repair.* As described next, in Chapter 3, the repair begins almost as soon as the inflammatory changes have started and involves several processes, including cell proliferation, differentiation, and extracellular matrix deposition.

REFERENCES

1. Diamond J: Guns, Germs and Steel: The Fates of Human Societies. WW Norton, New York.
2. Majno G: The Healing Hand: Man and Wound in the Ancient World. Cambridge, MA: Harvard University Press, 1975.
3. Weissman G: Inflammation: historical perspectives. In Gallin JI, et al (eds.): Inflammation: Basic Principles and Clinical Correlates. New York: Raven Press, 1992, p 5.
4. Hunter J: A Treatise of the Blood, Inflammation, and Gunshot Wounds, Vol. 1. London: J. Nicoli, 1794.
5. Cohnheim J: Lectures in General Pathology (Translated by AD McKee, from the second German edition, Vol 1). London: New Sydenham Society, 1889.
6. Heifets L: Centennial of Metchnikoff's discovery. J Reticuloendothel Soc 31:381, 1982.
7. Majno G, Palade GE: Studies on inflammation: I. the effect of histamine and serotonin on vascular permeability: an electron microscopic study. J Biophys Biochem Cytol 11:571, 1961.
8. McDonald DM, Thurston G, Baluk P: Endothelial gaps as sites for plasma leakage in inflammation. Microcirculation 6:7, 1999.
9. Majno G, et al: Studies on inflammation: II. the site of action of histamine and serotonin along the vascular tree: a topographic study. J Biophys Biochem Cytol 11:607, 1961.
10. Lampugnani MG, Dejana E: Interendothelial junctions: structure, signalling and functional roles. Curr Opin Cell Biol 9:674, 1997.
11. van Hinsbergh VW, van Nieuw Amerongen GP: Intracellular signalling involved in modulating human endothelial barrier function. J Anat 200:549, 2002.
12. Lentsch AB, Ward PA: Regulation of inflammatory vascular damage. J Pathol 190:343, 2000.
13. Dvorak AM, Feng D: The vesiculo-vacuolar organelle (VVO). A new endothelial cell permeability organelle. J Histochem Cytochem 49:419, 2001.
14. Ferrara N: Role of vascular endothelial growth factor in physiologic and pathologic angiogenesis: therapeutic implications. Semin Oncol 29:10, 2002.
15. Bates DO, et al: Regulation of microvascular permeability by vascular endothelial growth factors. J Anat 200:581, 2002.
16. Muller WA: Leukocyte–endothelial cell interactions in the inflammatory response. Lab Invest 82:521, 2002.

17. Luscinskas FW, et al: Leukocyte transendothelial migration: a junctional affair. Semin Immunol 14:105, 2002.
18. Gonzalez-Amaro R, Sanchez-Madrid F: Cell adhesion molecules: selectins and integrins. Crit Rev Immunol 19:389, 1999.
19. McEver RP: Selectins: lectins that initiate cell adhesion under flow. Curr Opin Cell Biol 14:581, 2002.
20. Hynes RO: Integrins: bidirectional, allosteric signaling machines. Cell 110:673, 2002.
21. Johnston B, Butcher EC: Chemokines in rapid leukocyte adhesion triggering and migration. Semin Immunol 14:83, 2002.
22. Muller WA: Migration of leukocytes across endothelial junctions: some concepts and controversies. Microcirculation 8:181, 2001.
23. Etzioni A, Doerschuk CM, Harlan JM: Of man and mouse: leukocyte and endothelial adhesion molecule deficiencies. Blood 94:3281, 1999.
24. Bunting M, et al: Leukocyte adhesion deficiency syndromes: adhesion and tethering defects involving beta 2 integrins and selectin ligands. Curr Opin Hematol 9:30, 2002.
25. Cotran RS, Mayadas TN: Endothelial adhesion molecules in health and disease. Pathol Biol 46:164, 1998.
26. Cicchetti G, Allen PG, Glogauer M: Chemotactic signaling pathways in neutrophils: from receptor to actin assembly. Crit Rev Oral Biol Med 13:220, 2002.
27. Jones GE: Cellular signaling in macrophage migration and chemotaxis. J Leukoc Biol 68:593, 2000.
28. Stossel TP, et al: Cell crawling two decades after Abercrombie. Biochem Soc Symp 65:267, 1999.
29. Rickert P, et al: Leukocytes navigate by compass: roles of PI3Kγ and its lipid products. Trends Cell Biol 10:466, 2000.
30. Underhill DM, Ozinsky A: Phagocytosis of microbes: complexity in action. Annu Rev Immunol 20:825, 2002.
31. Nathan C, Shiloh MU: Reactive oxygen and nitrogen intermediates in the relationship between mammalian hosts and microbial pathogens. Proc Natl Acad Sci U S A 97:8841, 2000.
32. Babior BM, Lambeth JD, Nauseef W: The neutrophil NADPH oxidase. Arch Biochem Biophys 397:342, 2002.
33. Hampton MB, Kettle AJ, Winterbourn CC: Inside the neutrophil phagosome: oxidants, myeloperoxidase, and bacterial killing. Blood 92:3007, 1998.
34. Risso A: Leukocyte antimicrobial peptides: multifunctional effector molecules of innate immunity. J Leukoc Biol 68:785, 2000.
35. Lehrer RI, Ganz T: Defensins of vertebrate animals. Curr Opin Immunol 14:96, 2002.
36. Jaeschke H, Smith CW: Mechanisms of neutrophil-induced parenchymal injury. J Leukoc Biol 61:647, 1997.
37. Tapper H: The secretion of preformed granules by neutrophils and macrophages. Curr Opin Immunol 59:613, 1996.
38. Stinchcombe JC, Griffiths GM: Regulated secretion from hemopoietic cells. J Cell Biol 147:1, 1999.
39. Ward DM, Shiflett SL, Kaplan J: Chediak-Higashi syndrome: a clinical and molecular view of a rare lysosomal storage disorder. Curr Mol Med 2:469, 2002.
40. Lekstrom-Himes JA, Gallin JI: Immunodeficiency diseases caused by defects in phagocytes. N Engl J Med 343:1703, 2000.
41. Goldblatt D, Thrasher AJ: Chronic granulomatous disease. Clin Exp Immunol 122:1, 2000.
42. Nathan CF: Points of control in inflammation. Nature 420:846, 2002.
43. Tracey KJ: The inflammatory reflex. Nature 420:853, 2002.
44. Repka-Ramirez MS, Baraniuk JN: Histamine in health and disease. Clin Allergy Immunol 17:1, 2002.
45. Barrington R, et al: The role of complement in inflammation and adaptive immunity. Immunol Rev 180:5, 2001.
46. Liszewski MK, et al: Control of the complement system. Adv Immunol 61:201, 1996.
47. Kaplan AP, et al: The intrinsic coagulation/kinin-forming cascade: assembly in plasma and cell surfaces in inflammation. Adv Immunol 66:225, 1997.
48. Couture R, et al: Kinin receptors in pain and inflammation. Eur J Pharmacol 429:161, 2001.
49. Coughlin S: Thrombin signalling and protease-activated receptors. Nature 407:258, 2000.
50. Coughlin SR, Camerer E: PARticipation in inflammation. J Clin Invest. 111:25, 2003.
51. Funk CD: Prostaglandins and leukotrienes: advances in eicosanoid biology. Science 294:1871, 2001.
52. Murakami M, Kudo I: Cellular arachidonate-releasing functions of various phospholipase A_2s. Adv Exp Med Biol 525:87, 2003.
53. Flower RJ: The development of COX2 inhibitors. Nat Rev Drug Discov 2:179, 2003.
54. Serhan CN, et al: Resolvins: a family of bioactive products of omega-3 fatty acid transformation circuits initiated by aspirin treatment that counter proinflammation signals. J Exp Med 196:1025, 2002.
55. Levy BD, Serhan CN: Polyisoprenyl phosphates: natural antiinflammatory lipid signals. Cell Mol Life Sci 59:729, 2002.
56. Buckingham JC, Flower RJ: Lipocortin 1: a second messenger of glucocorticoid action in the hypothalamo-pituitary-adrenocortical axis. Mol Med Today 62:438, 1997.
57. Serhan CN, Oliw E: Unorthodox routes to prostanoid formation: new twists in cyclooxygenase-initiated pathways. J Clin Invest 107:1481, 2001.
58. Prescott SM, et al: Platelet-activating factor and related lipid mediators. Annu Rev Biochem 69:419, 2000.
59. Mantovani A, Sozzani S, Introna M: Endothelial activation by cytokines. Ann NY Acad Sci 832:93, 1997.
60. Madge LA, Pober JS: TNF signaling in vascular endothelial cells. Exp Mol Pathol 70:317, 2001.
61. Argiles JM, et al: Journey from cachexia to obesity by TNF. FASEB J 11:743, 1997.
62. Rossi D, Zlotnik A: The biology of chemokines and their receptors. Annu Rev Immunol 18:217, 2000.
63. Zlotnik A, Yoshie O: Chemokines: a new classification system and their role in immunity. Immunity 12:121, 2000.
64. Yoshie O, Imai T,Nomiyama H: Chemokines in immunity. Adv Immunol. 78:57, 2001.
65. Furchgott RF, Zawadzki JV: The obligatory role of endothelial cells in the relaxation of arterial smooth muscle by acetylcholine. Nature 288:373, 1980.
66. Nathan C: Inducible nitric oxide synthase. J Clin Invest 100:2417, 1997.
67. Laroux FS, et al: Role of nitric oxide in inflammation. Acta Physiol Scand 173:113, 2001.
68. Borregaard N, Cowland JB: Granules of the human neutrophilic polymorphonuclear leukocyte. Blood 89:3503, 1997.
69. Belaaouaj A: Neutrophil elastase-mediated killing of bacteria: lessons from targeted mutagenesis. Microbes Infect 4:1259, 2002.
70. Beckman JS, Koppenol WH: Nitric oxide, superoxide, and peroxynitrite: the good, the bad, and the ugly. Am J Physiol 271:C1424, 1996.
71. Babior BM: Phagocyles and oxidative stress. Am J Med 109:33, 2003.
72. Severini C, et al: The tachykinin peptide family. Pharmacol Rev 54:285, 2002.
73. Harrison S, Geppetti P. Substance P. Int J Biochem Cell Biol 33:555, 2001.
74. Richardson JD, Vasko MR: Cellular mechanisms of neurogenic inflammation. J Pharmacol Exp Ther 302:839, 2002.
75. Cramer T, et al: HIF-1α is essential for myeloid cell-mediated inflammation. Cell 112:645, 2003.
76. Shi Y, Evans JE, Rock KL: Molecular identification of a danger signal that alerts the immune system to dying cells. Nature 425:516, 2003.
77. Majno G: Chronic inflammation: links with angiogenesis and wound healing. Am J Pathol 153:1035, 1998.
78. Luscinskas FW, Gimbrone MAJ: Endothelial-dependent mechanisms in chronic inflammatory leukocyte recruitment. Ann Rev Med 47:413, 1996.
79. Robinson DS, Kay AB, Wardlaw AJ: Eosinophils. Clin Allergy Immunol 16:43, 2002.
80. Suffredini AF, et al: New insights into the biology of the acute phase response. J Clin Immunol 19:203, 1999.
81. Dinarello CA: Cytokines as endogenous pyrogens. J Infect Dis 179 Suppl 2:S294, 1999.
82. Dinarello CA, Gatti S, Bartfai T: Fever: links with an ancient receptor. Curr Biol 9:R147, 1999.
83. Gabay C, Kushner I: Acute-phase proteins and other systemic responses to inflammation. N Engl J Med 340:448, 1999.
84. Ridker PM: Clinical application of C-reactive protein for cardiovascular disease detection and prevention. Circulation 107:363, 2003.
85. Cohen J: The immunopathogenesis of sepsis. Nature 420:885, 2002.
86. Hotchkiss RS, Karl IE: The pathophysiology and treatment of sepsis. N Engl J Med 348:138, 2003.

CHAPTER 3

Tissue Renewal and Repair: Regeneration, Healing, and Fibrosis

DEFINITIONS

CONTROL OF NORMAL CELL PROLIFERATION AND TISSUE GROWTH

Tissue-Proliferative Activity

Stem Cells

Embryonic Stem Cells (ES cells)
Adult Stem Cells
Role of Stem Cells in Tissue Homeostasis

Growth Factors

Signaling Mechanisms in Cell Growth

Overview of Receptors and Signal Transduction Pathways
Transcription Factors

Cell Cycle and the Regulation of Cell Replication

MECHANISMS OF TISSUE REGENERATION

Liver Regeneration

EXTRACELLULAR MATRIX (ECM) AND CELL–MATRIX INTERACTIONS

Collagen

Elastin, Fibrillin, and Elastic Fibers

Cell Adhesion Proteins

Proteoglycans and Hyaluronic Acid

REPAIR BY HEALING, SCAR FORMATION, AND FIBROSIS

Angiogenesis

Angiogenesis from Endothelial Precursor Cells
Angiogenesis from Pre-Existing Vessels
Growth Factors and Receptors Involved in Angiogenesis
ECM Proteins as Regulators of Angiogenesis

Scar Formation

Fibroblast Migration and Proliferation
ECM Deposition and Scar Formation
Tissue Remodeling

CUTANEOUS WOUND HEALING

Healing by First Intention (Wounds with Opposed Edges)

Healing by Second Intention (Wounds with Separated Edges)

Wound Strength

Local and Systemic Factors that Influence Wound Healing

Summary of Cutaneous Wound Healing

Complications in Cutaneous Wound Healing

FIBROSIS

OVERVIEW OF REPAIR RESPONSES AFTER INJURY AND INFLAMMATION

The body's ability to replace injured or dead cells and to repair tissues after inflammation is critical to survival. When injurious agents damage cells and tissues, the host responds by setting in motion a series of events that serve to eliminate these agents, contain the damage, and prepare the surviving cells for replication. The repair of tissue damage caused by surgical resection, wounds, and diverse types of chronic injury can be broadly separated into two processes, *regeneration* and *healing* (Fig. 3–1). Regeneration results in restitution of lost tissues; healing may restore original structures but involves collagen deposition and scar formation.

Definitions

The mechanisms of regeneration and healing will be discussed later in this chapter, but it is important from the outset to establish some important distinctions between these processes and to become familiar with terms used to describe them.

- *Regeneration* refers to growth of cells and tissues to replace lost structures, such as the growth of an amputated limb in amphibians.[1] In mammals, whole organs and complex tissues rarely regenerate after healing, and the term is usually applied to processes such as liver and kidney growth after, respectively, partial hepatectomy and unilateral nephrectomy. These processes consist of compensatory growth rather than true regeneration. Regardless, the term regeneration is well established and is used throughout this book. Tissues with high proliferative capacity, such as the hematopoietic system and the epithelia of the skin and gastrointestinal tract, renew themselves continuously and can regenerate after injury, as long as the stem cells of these tissues are not destroyed.
- *Healing* is usually a tissue response (1) to a wound (commonly in the skin), (2) to inflammatory processes in internal organs, or (3) to cell necrosis in organs incapable of regeneration.[2] In this broad definition, one should also include conditions such as atherosclerosis, considered to be

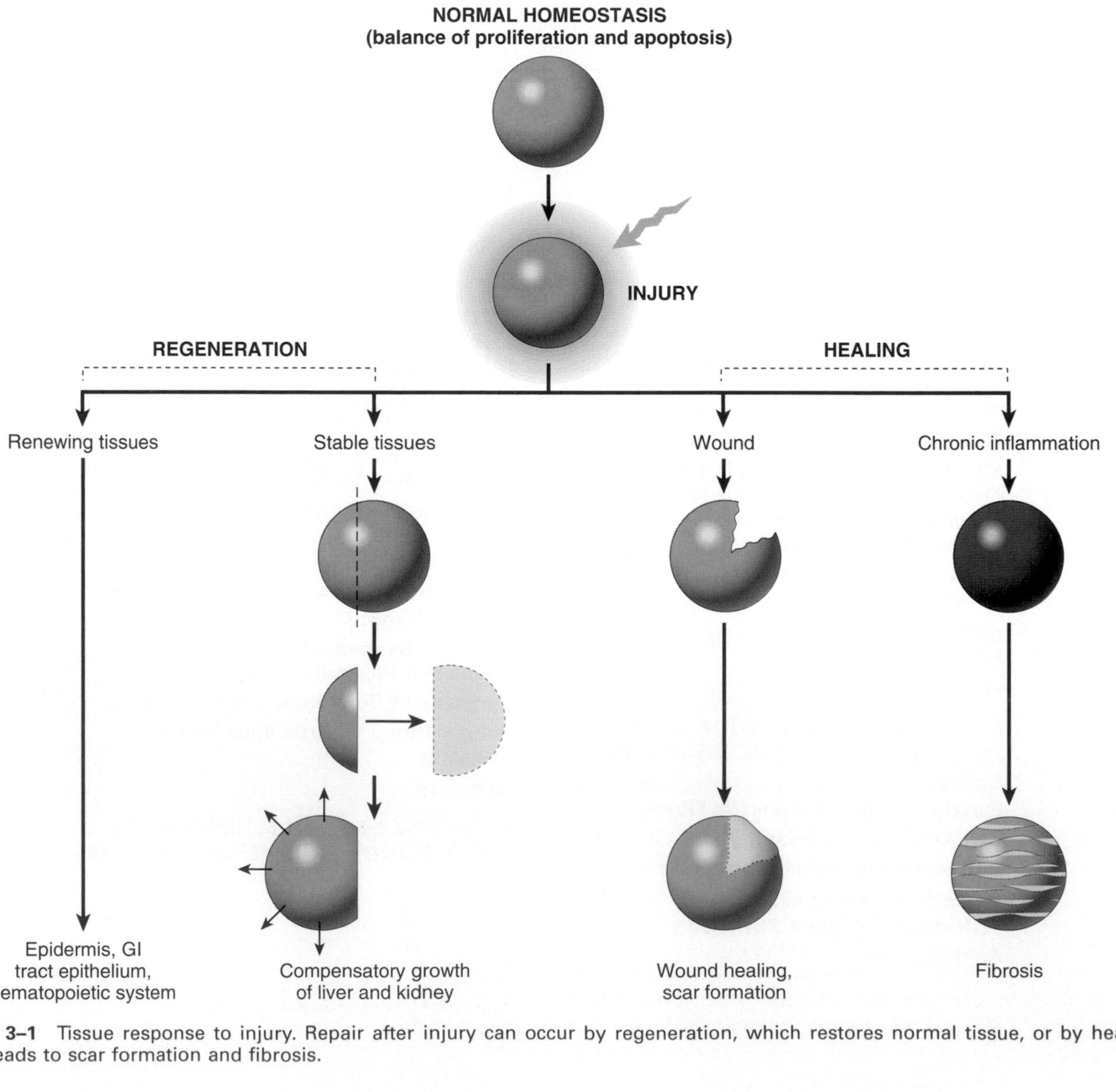

FIGURE 3–1 Tissue response to injury. Repair after injury can occur by regeneration, which restores normal tissue, or by healing, which leads to scar formation and fibrosis.

an attempt to heal injury of the arterial wall. Healing consists of variable proportions of two distinct processes—regeneration, and the laying down of fibrous tissue, or *scar formation*. Superficial wounds, such as a cutaneous wound that only damages the epithelium, can heal by epithelial regeneration. Incisional and excisional skin wounds that damage the dermis heal through the formation of a collagen scar. Scarring also occurs in the myocardium after infarction, as the original tissue is not reconstituted and is replaced by collagen (see Chapter 12). Inflammatory conditions of the pleura, peritoneum, and pericardium often heal through scar formation, creating adhesions between the visceral and parietal layers of these tissues. The development of a dense, fibrous scar in the pericardium can lead to a serious condition called *constrictive pericarditis*, discussed in Chapter 12. Persistent, chronic injury and inflammation can also lead to scarring in internal organs, as occurs in stomach ulcers caused by chronic infection with *Helicobacter pylori* (see Chapter 17). Extensive fibrosis is also present in cirrhosis of the liver and in some forms of coal- and silica-induced lung disease. In parenchymal organs, the replacement of inflammatory infiltrates by granulation tissue (described later) and ultimately fibrosis is called *organization.*

Regeneration requires an intact connective tissue scaffold. By contrast, healing with scar formation occurs if the extracellular matrix (ECM) framework is damaged, causing alterations of the tissue architecture. An example that clearly illustrates this point is the difference in the outcome of liver injury after a single large dose of a toxic chemical such as carbon tetrachloride (Chapter 1) or the application of multiple, small doses of the compound.[3] Acute injury caused by a high dose of the chemical kills more than 50% of hepatocytes. Nevertheless, it is followed by complete regeneration, because the injury does not damage the scaffold of reticular fibers that constitute the framework of the hepatic lobules. In contrast, multiple applications of the chemical in small doses disrupt ECM components, and the repair is by fibrosis. ECM scaffolds are essential for wound healing because they provide the framework for cell migration and maintain the correct cell polarity for the re-assembly of multilayer structures. Furthermore, cells in the ECM (fibroblasts, macrophages, and other cell types) are the source of agents that are critical for tissue repair.

Repair processes are critical for the maintenance of normal structure and function and survival of the organism. The healing of skin wounds and various other conditions mentioned above are just the most common examples of repair processes. However, in healthy tissues, repair, in the form of regeneration or healing, occurs after practically any insult that causes tissue destruction. In this chapter, we first review the proliferative capacity of tissues and the role of stem cells in maintaining tissue homeostasis. This is followed by an overview of growth factors and cell-signaling mechanisms, a brief introduction to the cell cycle and its main regulatory steps, and a discussion of liver regeneration as a model of organ regeneration. We then consider the important interactions between cells and the ECM, discuss healing and fibrosis, and provide clinical examples, both normal and pathologic, of these conditions.

Control of Normal Cell Proliferation and Tissue Growth

In adult tissues, the size of cell populations is determined by the rates of cell proliferation, differentiation, and death by apoptosis. Figure 3–2 depicts these relationships and shows that increased cell numbers may result from either increased proliferation or decreased cell death. *Apoptosis* is a physiologic process required for tissue homeostasis, but it can also be induced by a variety of pathologic stimuli[4] (see Chapter 1). The impact of *differentiation* depends on the circumstance under which it occurs. Myocytes and neurons are considered *terminally differentiated cells*; that is, they are at an end stage of differentiation and are not capable of replicating. In some adult tissues, such as liver and kidney, differentiated cells are normally quiescent but are able to proliferate when needed. In proliferative tissues such as the bone marrow and the multilayered epithelia of the skin and gut, the mature cells are terminally differentiated, short-lived, and incapable of replication, but they may be replaced by new cells arising from *stem cells*. Thus, in such tissues there is a homeostatic equilibrium between the proliferation of stem cells, their differentiation, and death of mature (differentiated) cells.

Cell proliferation can be stimulated by physiologic and pathologic conditions. The proliferation of endometrial cells under estrogen stimulation during the menstrual cycle and the thyroid-stimulating hormone–mediated replication of cells of the thyroid that enlarges the gland during pregnancy are examples of physiologic proliferation. Many pathologic conditions such as injury, cell death, and mechanical alterations

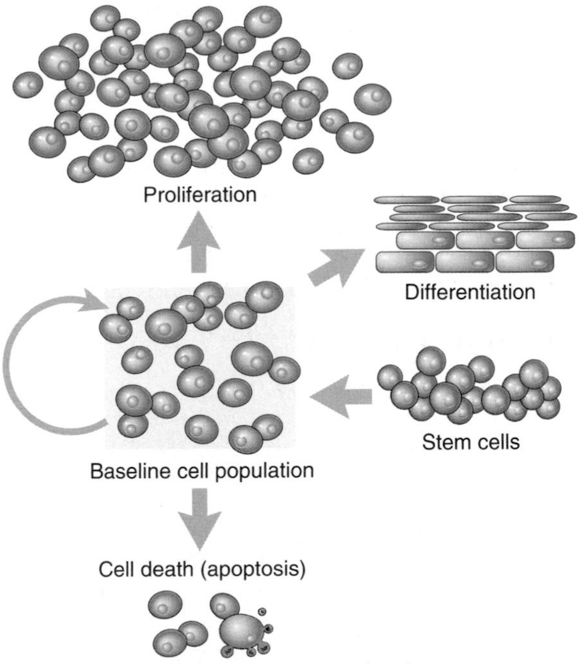

FIGURE 3–2 Mechanisms regulating cell populations. Cell numbers can be altered by increased or decreased rates of stem cell input, by cell death due to apoptosis, or by changes in the rates of proliferation or differentiation. (Modified from McCarthy NJ et al: Apoptosis in the development of the immune system: growth factors, clonal selection and bcl-2. Cancer Metastasis Rev 11:157, 1992.)

of tissues also stimulate cell proliferation. Physiologic stimuli may become excessive, creating pathologic conditions such as nodular prostatic hyperplasia resulting from dihydrotestosterone stimulation (Chapter 21) and the development of nodular goiters in the thyroid as a consequence of increased serum levels of thyroid-stimulating hormone (Chapter 24). Cell proliferation is largely controlled by signals (soluble or contact-dependent) from the microenvironment which either stimulate or inhibit cell proliferation. An excess of stimulators or a deficiency of inhibitors leads to net growth and, in the case of cancer, uncontrolled growth.[5] Although accelerated growth can be accomplished by shortening the cell cycle, the most important mechanism of growth is the conversion of resting or quiescent cells into proliferating cells by making the cells enter the cell cycle. Both the recruitment of quiescent cells into the cycle and cell-cycle progression require stimulatory signals to overcome the physiologic inhibition of cell proliferation.

TISSUE-PROLIFERATIVE ACTIVITY

The cell cycle consists of G_1 (presynthetic), *S* (DNA synthesis), G_2 (premitotic), and *M* (mitotic) phases (Fig. 3–3). Quiescent cells are in a physiologic state called G_0. Tissues may be composed primarily of quiescent cells in G_0, but most mature tissues contain some combination of continuously dividing cells, terminally differentiated cells, stem cells, and quiescent cells that occasionally enter into the cell cycle. Stem cells have special properties, which are described later. The tissues of the body are divided into three groups on the basis of their proliferative activity.

- In *continuously dividing tissues* (also called *labile* tissues) cells proliferate throughout life, replacing those that are destroyed. These tissues include surface epithelia, such as stratified squamous surfaces of the skin, oral cavity, vagina, and cervix; the lining mucosa of all the excretory ducts of the glands of the body (e.g., salivary glands, pancreas, biliary tract); the columnar epithelium of the gastrointestinal tract and uterus; the transitional epithelium of the urinary tract, and cells of the bone marrow and hematopoietic tissues. In most of these tissues, mature cells are derived from *stem cells,* which have an unlimited capacity to proliferate and whose progeny may undergo various streams of differentiation (discussed in more detail below).
- *Quiescent* (or *stable*) *tissues* normally have a low level of replication; however, cells from these tissues can undergo rapid division in response to stimuli and are thus capable of reconstituting the tissue of origin. They are considered to be in the G_0 stage of the cell cycle but can be stimulated to enter G_1. In this category are the parenchymal cells of liver, kidneys, and pancreas; mesenchymal cells, such as fibroblasts and smooth muscle; vascular endothelial cells; and resting lymphocytes and other leukocytes. The regen-

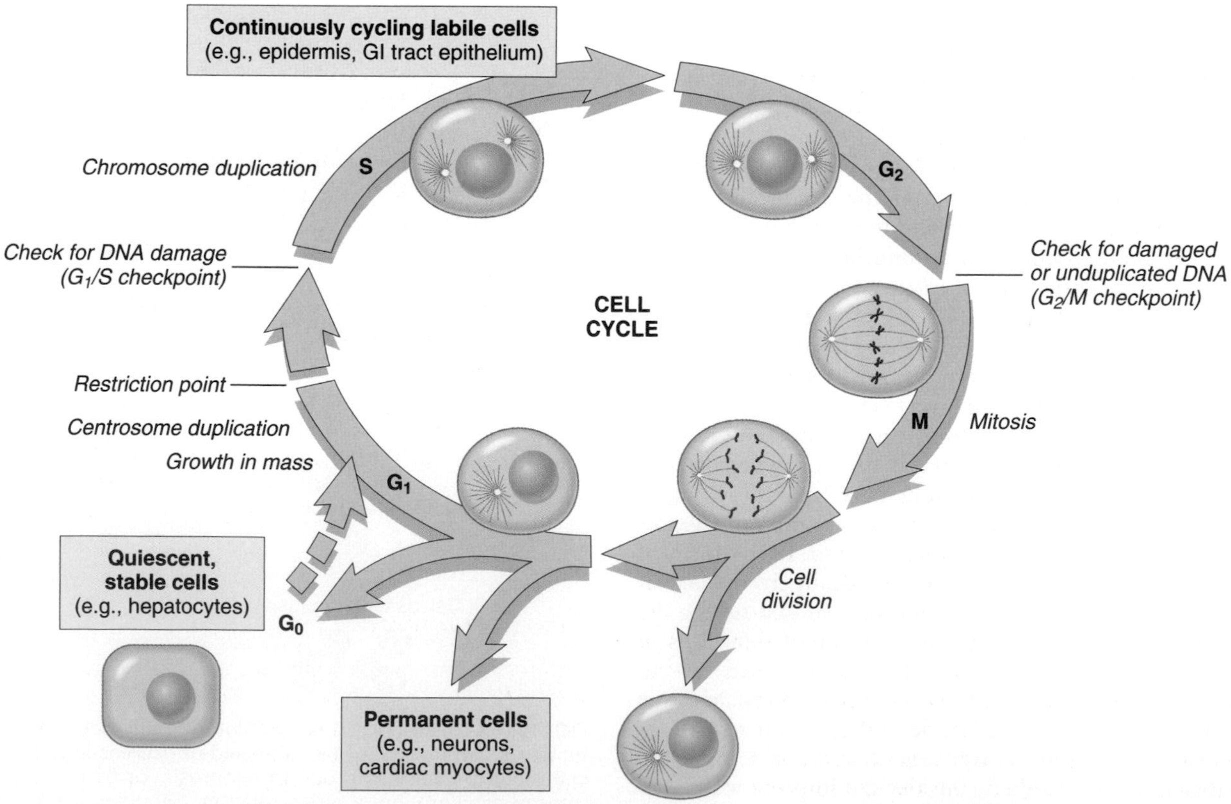

FIGURE 3–3 Cell-cycle landmarks. The figure shows the cell-cycle phases (G_0, G_1, G_2, S, and M), the location of the G_1 restriction point, and the G_1/S and G_2/M cell-cycle checkpoints. Cells from labile tissues such as the epidermis and the gastrointestinal tract may cycle continuously; stable cells such as hepatocytes are quiescent but can enter the cell cycle; permanent cells such as neurons and cardiac myocytes have lost the capacity to proliferate. (Modified from Pollard TD and Earnshaw WC: Cell Biology. Philadelphia, Saunders, 2002.)

erative capacity of stable cells is best exemplified by the ability of the liver to regenerate after partial hepatectomy and after acute chemical injury. Fibroblasts, endothelial cells, smooth muscle cells, chondrocytes, and osteocytes are quiescent in adult mammals but proliferate in response to injury. Fibroblasts in particular proliferate widely, constituting the connective tissue response to inflammation discussed later in this chapter.

- *Nondividing (permanent) tissues* contain cells that have left the cell cycle and cannot undergo mitotic division in postnatal life. To this group belong neurons and skeletal and cardiac muscle cells. If *neurons* in the central nervous system are destroyed, the tissue is generally replaced by the proliferation of the central nervous system supportive elements, the glial cells. However, recent results demonstrate that neurogenesis from stem cells may occur in adult brains (see below). Although mature skeletal muscle cells do not divide, *skeletal muscle* does have some regenerative capacity, through the differentiation of the *satellite cells* that are attached to the endomysial sheaths. If the ends of severed muscle fibers are closely juxtaposed, muscle regeneration in mammals can be excellent, but this is a condition that can rarely be attained under practical conditions. *Cardiac muscle* has very limited, if any, regenerative capacity, and a large injury to the heart muscle, as may occur in myocardial infarction, is followed by scar formation.

STEM CELLS

Stem cell research is one of the most exciting topics in modern-day biomedical investigation and stands at the core of a new field called *regenerative medicine*.[6,7] The enthusiasm about stem cell research derives both from data that challenge well-established biological concepts and from the hope that stem cells may one day be used to repair injury in human tissues, including heart, brain, and skeletal muscle.[8–10]

Stem cells are characterized by their prolonged self-renewal capacity and by their asymmetric replication. Asymmetric replication describes a special property of stem cells; that is, in every cell division, one of the cells retains its self-renewing capacity while the other enters a differentiation pathway and is converted to a mature, nondividing population.[11] This concept has, however, been modified to postulate that asymmetry exists within a whole population of stem cells rather than in every single stem cell division. Thus within a group of stem cells some self replicate and others differentiate. Stem cells were first identified as pluripotent cells in embryos, and these were called *embryonic stem cells*. It is now clear that stem cells are also present in many tissues in adult animals and contribute to the maintenance of tissue homeostasis.

In recent years, much effort has been devoted to the isolation and phenotypic characterization of stem cells. Although the development of specific markers to recognize stem cells is an ongoing challenge, a series of new observations have revolutionized and energized stem cell research. Among these are: (1) the identification of stem cells and their niches in various tissues, including the brain, which has been considered a permanent quiescent organ; (2) the recognition that stem cells from various tissues and particularly from the bone marrow may have broad developmental plasticity; and (3) the realization that some stem cells present in tissues of humans and mice may be similar to embryonic stem cells.

We start our discussion of stem cells with a brief consideration of embryonic stem cells, and then move on to adult stem cells and their role in regeneration and repair.

Embryonic Stem Cells (ES)

Embryos contain pluripotent ES cells, which can give rise to all the tissues of the human body. Such cells can be isolated from normal blastocysts, the structures formed at about the 32-cell stage during embryonic development.[12] ES cells can be maintained in culture as undifferentiated cell lines or induced to differentiate into many different lineages.[13,14] The pluripotency of ES cells may be related to the expression of unique transcription factors in these cells, such as a recently described homeobox protein called Nanog (named after Tir na n'Og, the Celtic land of the ever-young).[15] Recent studies also implicate the Wnt-β-catenin signaling (Chapter 7) in maintaining pluripotency.[15a]

ES cells have had an enormous impact on biology and medicine:

- ES cells have been used to study the specific signals and differentiation steps required for the development of many tissues.
- They have made possible the production of *knockout mice*. To produce these mice, a specific gene is inactivated or deleted from cultured ES cells. These cells are injected into blastocysts, which are then implanted into the uterus of a surrogate mother. The genetically modified implanted blastocysts develop into full embryos, as long as the gene defect does not cause embryonic lethality. Techniques for the genetic manipulation of ES cells have greatly expanded in scope to produce gene deficiencies that are specific for a single tissue and "conditional gene deficiencies," that is, gene deficiencies that can be turned on and off in adult animals. Knockout mice have become widely used models for the experimental study of human disease and provide essential information about gene function in vivo.
- ES cells may, in the future, be used to *repopulate damaged organs*, such as the liver after hepatocyte necrosis and the myocardium after infarction. The generation of some specific cell types from cultured ES cells has already been achieved. Insulin-producing pancreatic cells and nerve cells produced in these cultures have been implanted, respectively, in diabetic animals and in mice with neurologic defects. Although the effectiveness of these procedures for human diseases is still unknown, there is an intense debate about the ethical issues associated with this type of therapy, which is known as *therapeutic cloning*. The steps involved in therapeutic cloning using ES cells[16] are outlined in Figure 3–4.

Adult Stem Cells

Many tissues in adult animals have been shown to contain reservoirs of stem cells, which are called *adult stem cells*. Compared to ES cells, which are pluripotent, adult stem cells have a more restricted differentiation capacity and are usually lineage-specific. However, stem cell research may have come full circle, as stem cells with broad differentiation potential appear to exist in adult bone marrow and, perhaps, in other tissues as well. Stem cells located outside of the bone marrow as generally referred to as *tissue stem cells*.

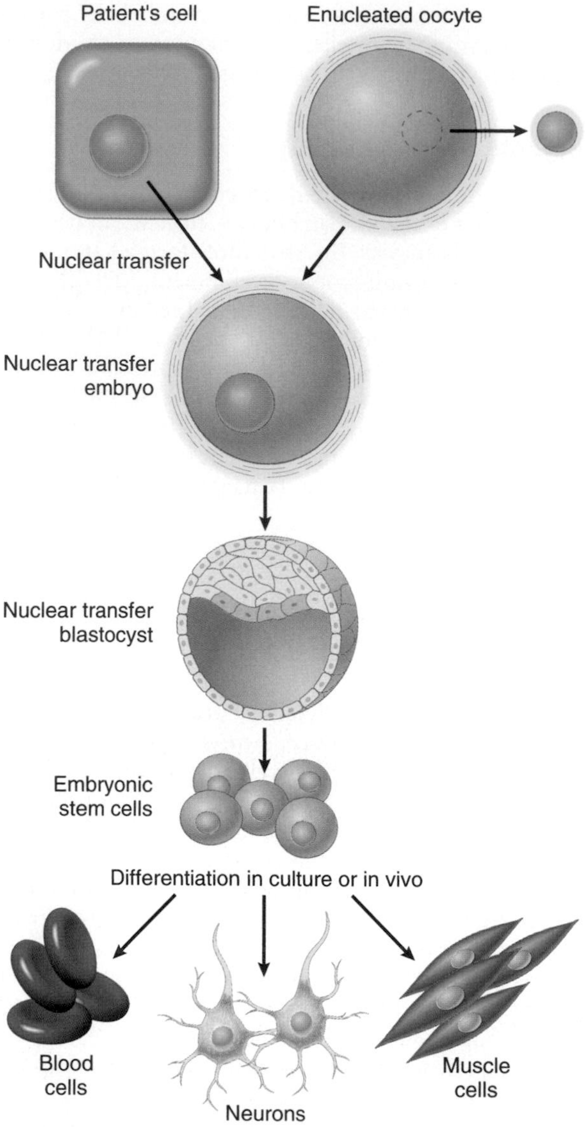

FIGURE 3–4 Steps involved in therapeutic cloning, using embryonic stem cells (ES cells) for cell therapy. The diploid nucleus of an adult cell from a patient is introduced into an enucleated oocyte. The oocyte is activated, and the zygote divides to become a blastocyst that contains the donor DNA. The blastocyst is dissociated to obtain ES. These cells are capable of differentiating into various tissues, either in culture or after transplantation into the donor. The goal of the procedure is to reconstitute or repopulate damaged organs of a patient, using the cells of the same patient to avoid immunologic rejection. (Modified from Hochedlinger K, Jaenisch R: Nuclear transplantation, embryonic stem cells, and the potential for cell therapy. N Engl J Med 349:275–286, 2003.)

Stem cells are located in sites called *niches*,[17] which differ among various tissues (Fig. 3–5). For instance, in the gastrointestinal tract,[18] they are located at the isthmus of stomach glands and at the base of the crypts of the colon (each colonic crypt is the clonal product of a single stem cell). Niches have been identified in other tissues, such as the bulge area of hair follicles and the limbus of the cornea.[19–21] We first consider bone marrow stem cells and then discuss stem cells located in other tissues (tissue stem cells).

Because of the easy accessibility of bone marrow and the need to replace hematopoietic cells in many clinical situations, there has been great interest in studying bone marrow stem cells. It is now recognized that the bone marrow contains *hematopoietic stem cells (HSCs)* as well as stromal cells capable of differentiation into various lineages. HSCs generate all of the blood cells and can reconstitute the bone marrow after depletion caused by disease or irradiation.[22,23] HSCs can be collected directly from the bone marrow, from umbilical cord blood, and from circulating blood of individuals receiving cytokines, such as granulocyte-macrophage colony-stimulating factor, which mobilizes HSCs. *Bone marrow stromal cells*, depending on the tissue environment, can generate chondrocytes, osteoblasts, adipocytes, myoblasts, and endothelial cell precursors (Fig. 3–6).

A remarkable observation about HSCs is that they may be capable of giving rise to neurons, hepatocytes, and other cell types. Adult bone marrow cells injected into mice can contribute, in variable proportions, to hepatocyte repopulation of injured livers and to muscle cell production in injured muscle.[24,25] When injected into the heart, a small proportion of these cells acquire a cardiac myoblast phenotype. In addition, there is some evidence that a small number of hepatocytes in transplanted livers, and cardiac myocytes in transplanted hearts,[26] may be derived from cells from the recipient's bone marrow. The vascular bed of these transplants contains a large proportion of endothelial cells generated from bone marrow stromal cells of the recipient. These results challenge the accepted wisdom that cells of adult organisms, including stem cells, are committed to the generation of restricted lineages, and suggest instead that stem cell differentiation programs are not fixed. A change in stem cell differentiation from one cell type to another is called *transdifferentiation* (Fig. 3–7), and the multiplicity of stem cell differentiation options is known as *developmental plasticity*.[6,7] More recent studies have raised questions about the plasticity of HSCs.[27,28] In some situations, transplanted HSCs fuse with host cells and transfer genetic material to them, thus giving the false appearance of having transdifferentiated with generation of new cells in the host.[29,30] The relative contribution of true transdifferentiation or cell fusion to the development of various mature cell types from HSC is unclear at present. Also, although HSC may be able to replace cells in damaged tissues, they do not appear to play a role in the maintenance of these tissues under physiologic conditions (steady state).[27] Perhaps the generation of tissue cells from HSCs occurs only at sites of injury, where the response to injury recruits stem cells from the bone marrow for local tissue repopulation. It is also possible that the main contribution of bone marrow–derived cells to the repair of non-hematopoietic tissues is not the generation of cells for these tissues. Instead, stem cells may produce growth factors and cytokines that act on the cells of the tissue to which they migrate, promoting injury repair and cell replication.

The adult bone marrow also harbors a heterogeneous population of stem cells, which appear to have very broad developmental capabilities.[31] These cells, called *multipotent adult progenitor cells*, or *MAPCs*, have been isolated from postnatal human and rodent bone marrow. They proliferate in culture without senescence, and can differentiate into mesodermal, endodermal, and neuroectodermal cell types. Interestingly, MAPCs are not confined to the bone marrow. They have been isolated from muscle, brain, and skin, and, similar to bone marrow MAPCs, can be made to differentiate into endothelium, neurons, hepatocytes and other cell types.[32,33] MAPCs

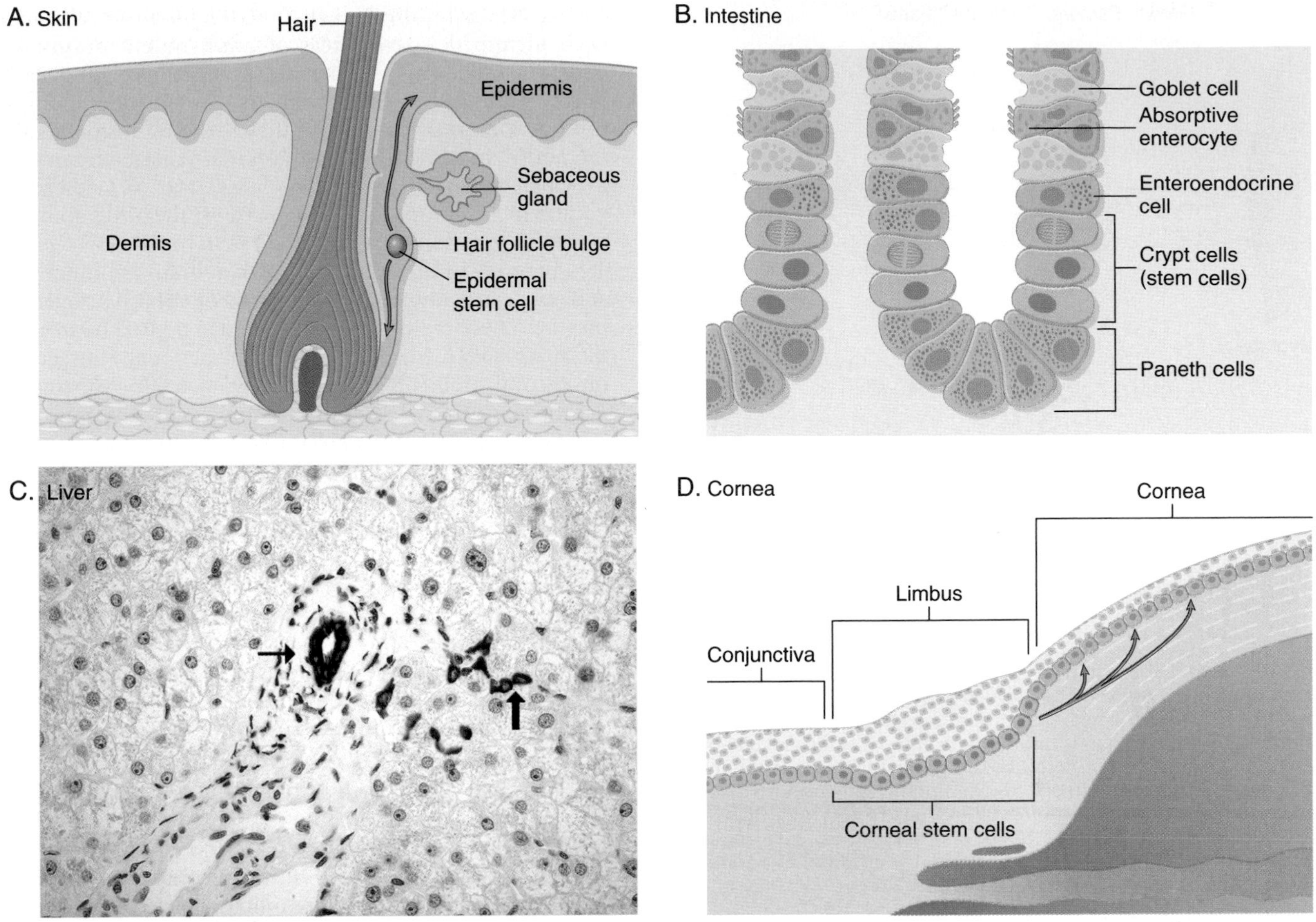

FIGURE 3–5 Stem-cell niches in various tissues. *A,* Epidermal stem cells located in the bulge area of the hair follicle serve as a stem cells for the hair follicle and the epidermis. *B,* Intestinal stem cells are located at the base of a colon crypt, above Paneth cells. *C,* Liver stem cells (commonly known as oval cells) are located in the canals of Hering *(thick arrow),* structures that connect bile ductules *(thin arrow)* with parenchymal hepatocytes (bile duct and Hering canals are stained for cytokeratin 7; courtesy of Tania Roskams, M.D., University of Leuven). *D,* Corneal stem cells are located in the limbus region, between the conjunctiva and the cornea. (Courtesy of T-T Sun, New York University, New York, NY.)

isolated from bone marrow, muscle, and brain have very similar gene expression profiles, suggesting that they may have a common origin. It has been proposed that *MAPCs constitute a population of stem cells derived from, or closely related to, ES cells*[32] (i.e., they may be the adult counterparts of ES cells). If this view is correct, what has been referred to as "transdifferentiation" and "plasticity" of stem cells in adult tissues may actually represent the process of differentiation of multipotent ES-like cells into specific lineages.[34] Indeed, mouse bone marrow MAPCs, injected into blastocysts, contribute to all somatic cell types, a demonstration of their pluripotency.[31] It is not known whether a single type of adult bone marrow stem cell is capable of generating all tissue lineages or if, alternatively, there are multiple types of bone marrow stem cells, each committed to differentiate into a specific tissue or a group of related tissues.[7]

Role of Stem Cells in Tissue Homeostasis

In addition to bone marrow cells that may migrate to various tissues after injury, adult stem cells reside permanently in most organs. These cells (known as *tissue stem cells*) can generate the mature cells of the organs in which they reside. However, their differentiation commitment can change when they are transplanted into a different tissue. Below we briefly discuss the role of stem cells in liver, brain, muscle and renewing epithelium.

■ *Liver.* After many years of debate, it is now recognized that the liver contains stem cells in the *canals of Hering* (Fig. 3–5*C*), the junction between the biliary ductular system and parenchymal hepatocytes (Chapter 18). Cells located in this niche can give rise to a population of precursor cells known as *oval cells*, which are bipotential progenitors, capable of differentiating into hepatocytes and biliary cells.[35] In contrast to stem cells in proliferating tissues, liver stem cells function as a secondary or reserve compartment activated only when hepatocyte proliferation is blocked. In hepatic growth processes such as liver regeneration after partial hepatectomy (discussed later in this chapter), and in liver growth after most types of acute necrotizing injury, hepatocytes themselves readily replicate and the stem cell compartment is not activated. On the other hand, oval cell proliferation and differentiation are prominent in the livers

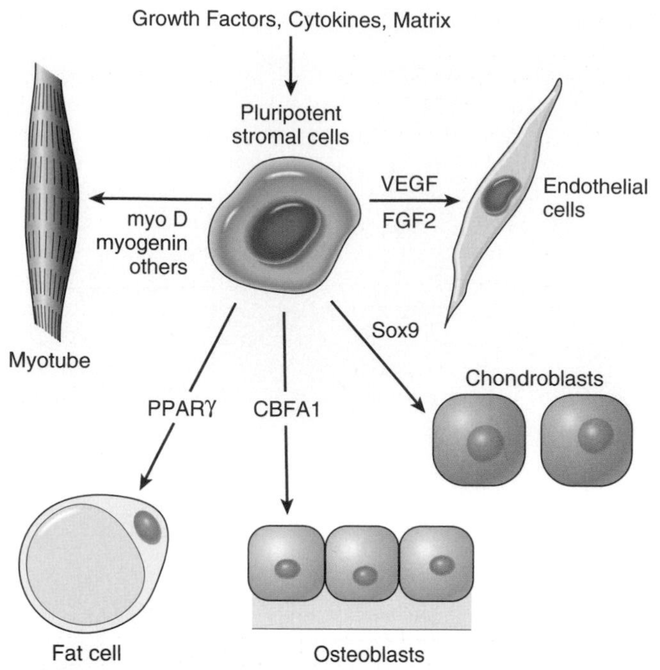

FIGURE 3–6 Differentiation pathways for pluripotent bone marrow stromal cells. Activation of key regulatory proteins by growth factors, cytokines, or matrix components leads to commitment of stem cells to differentiate into specific cellular lineages. Differentiation of myotubes requires the combined action of several factors (e.g., myoD, myogenin); fat cells require PPARγ, the osteogenic lineage requires CBFA1 (also known as RUNX2), cartilage formation requires Sox9, and endothelial cells require VEGF and FGF-2. (Adapted and redrawn from Rodan GA, Harada S: The missing bone. Cell 89:677, 1997.)

of patients recovering from fulminant hepatic failure, in liver carcinogenesis, and in some cases of chronic hepatitis and advanced liver cirrhosis, situations in which hepatocyte proliferation may be slow or blocked.[36]

- *Brain.* The brain is the prototype of a nonproliferative tissue in mammals. However, the long established dogma that no new neurons are generated in the brain of normal adult mammals is now known to be incorrect, because neurogenesis does occur in some areas of the adult brain. *Neural stem cells* (also known as *neural precursor cells*) have been identified in two areas of adult rodent brains, the olfactory bulb, and the dentate gyrus of the hippocampus.[37–39] The intermediate filament protein *nestin* can be used as a marker to identify these cells by histochemical methods.[40] In some species of birds, particularly in canaries, in which neurogenesis in adult brains was first described, vocal center neurogenesis is required for the bird's ability to sing. The question arises whether, as in birds, newly generated neurons in the adult mammalian brain are functional and, more broadly, what the purpose of adult neurogenesis may be. There is now proof that newly minted neurons in the mammalian hippocampus are functionally integrated into neural circuits.[41] However, it remains to be shown that neurogenesis in the adult brain increases "brain power" or improves the ability to sing!
- *Skeletal and cardiac muscle.* In contrast to hepatocytes, myocytes of skeletal muscle do not divide, even after injury. Growth and regeneration of injured skeletal muscle occur instead by replication of *satellite cells.*[42] These cells, located beneath the myocyte basal lamina, constitute a reserve pool of stem cells that can generate differentiated myocytes after injury. Placed in different tissue environments, satellite cells can be osteogenic and adipogenic. Stem cells have not been found in cardiac muscle, although it has been proposed that the heart may contain progenitor-like cells.[43]
- *Renewal of epithelial tissue.* Self-renewing epithelia contain stem cells, highly proliferative intermediate cells that constitute an amplifying compartment, and cells at various stages of differentiation. Terminally differentiated cells do not divide and are continuously lost at the external surface of the epithelium. After injury, self-renewing epithelia reconstitute themselves by following three nonmutually exclusive strategies: (1) increasing the number of actively dividing stem cells, (2) increasing the number of replications of cells in the amplifying compartment, and (3) decreasing the cell-cycle time for cell replication.

We will return to the role of stem cells in tissue homeostasis later in this chapter as we discuss the processes of regeneration and healing. Key to such processes is the regulation of cell proliferation, which is maintained under strict physiologic control. Cell proliferation is typically initiated by the

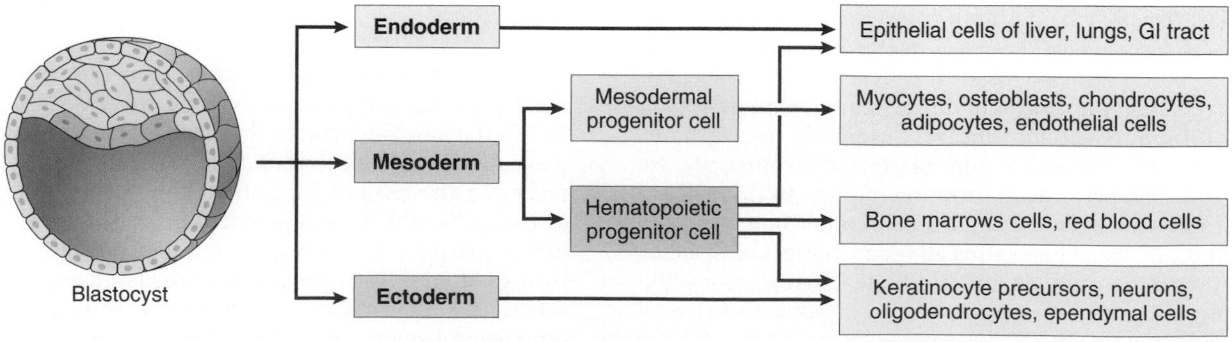

FIGURE 3–7 Differentiation of embryonic cells and generation of tissue cells by bone marrow precursors. During embryonic development the three germ layers—endoderm, mesoderm, and ectoderm—are formed, generating all tissues of the body. Adult stem cells localized in organs derived from these layers produce cells that are specific for the organs at which they reside. However, some adult bone marrow stem cells, in addition to producing the blood lineages (mesodermal derived), can also generate cells for tissues that originated from the endoderm and ectoderm (indicated by the *red lines*). (Modified from Korbling M, Estrov Z: Adult stem cells for tissue repair—a new theropeutic concept? N Engl J Med 349:570–582, 2003.)

action of growth factors. In the following sections we first describe various growth factors and then examine the main cell signaling mechanisms and cell-cycle events that regulate cell proliferation.

GROWTH FACTORS

There is a large number of known polypeptide growth factors, some of which act on many cell types, and others have restricted cellular targets. In addition to stimulating cell proliferation, growth factors may also have effects on cell locomotion, contractility, differentiation, and angiogenesis, activities that may be as important as their growth-promoting effects. Table 3–1 lists some of the most important growth factors involved in tissue regeneration and repair. Here we review only those that have major roles in these processes. Other growth factors are alluded to in various sections of the book.

Epidermal Growth Factor (EGF) and Transforming Growth Factor-α (TGF-α). These two factors belong to the EGF family and share a common receptor. EGF was discovered by its ability to cause precocious tooth eruption and eyelid opening in newborn mice. EGF is mitogenic for a variety of epithelial cells, hepatocytes, and fibroblasts. It is widely distributed in tissue secretions and fluids, such as sweat, saliva, urine, and intestinal contents. In healing wounds of the skin, EGF is produced by keratinocytes, macrophages, and other inflammatory cells that migrate into the area. EGF binds to a receptor (EGFR) with intrinsic tyrosine kinase activity, triggering the signal transduction events described later. TGF-α was originally extracted from sarcoma

TABLE 3–1 Growth Factors and Cytokines Involved in Regeneration and Wound Healing

Cytokine	Symbol	Source	Functions
Epidermal growth factor	EGF	Platelets, macrophages, saliva, urine, milk, plasma	Mitogenic for keratinocytes and fibroblasts; stimulates keratinocyte migration and granulation tissue formation
Transforming growth factor alpha	TGF-α	Macrophages, T lymphocytes, keratinocytes, and many tissues	Similar to EGF; stimulates replication of hepatocytes and certain epithelial cells
Hepatocyte growth factor/scatter factor	HGF	Mesenchymal cells	Enhances proliferation of epithelial and endothelial cells, and of hepatocytes; increases cell motility
Vascular endothelial cell growth factor (isoforms A, B, C, D)	VEGF	Mesenchymal cells	Increases vascular permeability; mitogenic for endothelial cells (see Table 3–3)
Platelet-derived growth factor (isoforms A, B, C, D)	PDGF	Platelets, macrophages, endothelial cells, keratinocytes, smooth muscle cells	Chemotactic for PMNs, marcrophages, fibroblasts, and smooth muscle cells; activates PMNs, macrophages, and fibroblasts; mitogenic for fibroblasts, endothelial cells, and smooth muscle cells; stimulates production of MMPs, fibronectin, and HA; stimulates angiogenesis and wound contraction; remodeling; inhibits platelet aggregation; regulates integrin expression
Fibroblast growth factor-1 (acidic), -2 (basic) and family	FGF	Macrophages, mast cells, T lymphocytes, endothelial cells, fibroblasts, and many tissues	Chemotactic for fibroblasts; mitogenic for fibroblasts and keratinocytes; stimulates keratinocyte migration, angiogenesis, fam wound contraction and matrix deposition
Transforming growth factor beta (isoforms 1, 2, 3); other members of the family are BMP and activin	TGF-β	Platelets, T lymphocytes, macrophages, endothelial cells, keratinocytes, smooth muscle cells, fibroblasts	Chemotactic for PMNs, macrophages, lymphocytes, fibroblasts, and smooth muscle cells; stimulates TIMP synthesis, keratinocyte migration, angiogenesis, and fibroplasia; inhibits production of MMPs and keratinocyte proliferation; regulates integrin expression and other cytokines; induces TGF-β production
Keratinocyte growth factor (also called FGF-7)	KGF	Fibroblasts	Stimulates keratinocyte migration, proliferation, and differentiation
Insulin-like growth factor-1	IGF-1	Macrophages, fibroblasts and other cells	Stimulates synthesis of sulfated proteoglycans, collagen, keratinocyte migration, and fibroblast proliferation; endocrine effects similar to growth hormone
Tumor necrosis factor	TNF	Macrophages, mast cells, T lymphocytes	Activates macrophages; regulates other cytokines; multiple functions
Interleukins	IL-1, etc.	Macrophages, mast cells, keratinocytes, lymphocytes, and many tissues	Many functions. Some examples: chemotactic for PMNs (IL-1) and fibroblasts (IL-4), stimulation of MMP-1 synthesis (IL-1), angiogenesis (IL-8), TIMP synthesis (IL-6); regulation of other cytokines
Interferons	IFN-α, etc.	Lymphocytes and fibroblasts	Activates macrophages; inhibits fibroblast proliferation and synthesis of MMPs; regulates other cytokines

BMP, bone morphogenetic proteins; PMNs, polymorphonuclear leukocytes; MMPs, matrix metalloproteinases; HA, hyaluronic acid; TIMP, tissue inhibitor of matrix metalloproteinase.

Modified from Schwartz SI: *Principles of Surgery*, McGraw Hill, New York, 1999.

virus–transformed cells and is involved in epithelial cell proliferation in embryos and adults and malignant transformation of normal cells to cancer. TGF-α has homology with EGF, binds to EGFR, and produces most of the biologic activities of EGF. The "EGF receptor" is actually a family of membrane tyrosine kinase receptors that respond to EGF, TGF-α, and other ligands of the EGF family.[44] The main EGFR is referred to as EGFR1, or ERB B1. The ERB B2 receptor (also known as HER-2/Neu) has received great attention because it is overexpressed in breast cancers and is a therapeutic target.

Hepatocyte Growth Factor (HGF). HGF was originally isolated from platelets and serum. Subsequent studies demonstrated that it is identical to a previously identified growth factor known as *scatter factor* (HGF is also referred to as HGF/scatter factor). It has mitogenic effects in most epithelial cells, including hepatocytes and cells of the biliary epithelium in the liver, and epithelial cells of the lungs, mammary gland, skin, and other tissues.[45] Besides its mitogenic effects, HGF acts as a morphogen in embryonic development and promotes cell scattering and migration. This factor is produced by fibroblasts, endothelial cells, and liver nonparenchymal cells. The receptor for HGF is the product of the proto-oncogene c-*MET,* which is frequently overexpressed in human tumors. HGF signaling is required for survival during embryonic development, as demonstrated by the lethality of knockout mice lacking c-*MET*.

Vascular Endothelial Growth Factor (VEGF). VEGF is a family of peptides that includes VEGF-A (referred throughout as VEGF), VEGF-B, VEGF-C, VEGF-D, and placental growth factor. VEGF is a potent inducer of blood vessel formation in early development *(vasculogenesis)* and has a central role in the growth of new blood vessels *(angiogenesis)* in adults (see Table 3–3).[46] It promotes angiogenesis in tumors, chronic inflammation, and healing of wounds. Mice that lack a single allele of the gene (heterozygous VEGF knockout mice) die during embryonic development with defective vasculogenesis and hematopoiesis. VEGF family members signal through three tyrosine kinase receptors: VEGFR-1, VEGFR-2, and VEGFR-3. VEGFR-2 is located in endothelial cells and is the main receptor for the vasculogenic and angiogenic effects of VEGF. The role of VEGFR-1 is less well understood, but it may facilitate the mobilization of endothelial stem cells and has a role in inflammation. VEGF-C and VEGF-D bind to VEGFR-3 and act on lymphatic endothelial cells to induce the production of lymphatic vessels (lymphangiogenesis). VEGF-B binds exclusively to VEGFR-1. It is not required for vasculogenesis or angiogenesis, but may play a role in maintenance of myocardial function.

Platelet-Derived Growth Factor (PDGF). PDGF is a family of several closely related proteins, each consisting of two chains designated *A* and *B*. All three isoforms of PDGF (AA, AB, and BB) are secreted and are biologically active. Recently, two new isoforms—PDGF-C and PDGF-D—have been identified. PDGF isoforms exert their effects by binding to two cell-surface receptors, designated PDGFR α and β, which have different ligand specificities.[47] PDGF is stored in platelet α granules and is released on platelet activation. It can also be produced by a variety of other cells, including activated macrophages, endothelial cells, smooth muscle cells, and many tumor cells. PDGF causes migration and proliferation of fibroblasts, smooth muscle cells, and monocytes, as demonstrated by defects in these functions in mice deficient in either the A or the B chain of PDGF. It also participates in the activation of hepatic stellate cells in the initial steps of liver fibrosis (Chapter 18).

Fibroblast Growth Factor (FGF). This is a family of growth factors containing more than 15 members, of which acidic FGF (aFGF, or FGF-1) and basic FGF (bFGF, or FGF-2) are the best characterized. FGF-1 and FGF-2 are made by a variety of cells. Released FGFs associate with heparan sulfate in the ECM, which can serve as a reservoir for storing inactive factors. FGFs are recognized by a family of cell-surface receptors that have intrinsic tyrosine kinase activity. A large number of functions are attributed to FGFs, including the following:

- *New blood vessel formation (angiogenesis):* FGF-2, in particular, has the ability to induce the steps necessary for new blood vessel formation both in vivo and in vitro (see below).
- *Wound repair:* FGFs participate in macrophage, fibroblast, and endothelial cell migration in damaged tissues and migration of epithelium to form new epidermis.
- *Development:* FGFs play a role in skeletal muscle development and in lung maturation. For example, FGF-6 and its receptor induce myoblast proliferation and suppress myocyte differentiation, providing a supply of proliferating myocytes. FGF-2 is also thought to be involved in the generation of angioblasts during embryogenesis. FGF-1 and FGF-2 are involved in the specification of the liver from endodermal cells.[48]
- *Hematopoiesis:* FGFs have been implicated in the differentiation of specific lineages of blood cells and development of bone marrow stroma.

TGF-β and Related Growth Factors. TGF-β belongs to a family of homologous polypeptides that includes three TGF-β isoforms (TGF-β1, TGF-β2, TGF-β3) and factors with wide-ranging functions, such as bone morphogenetic proteins (BMPs), activins, inhibins, and mullerian inhibiting substance.[49] TGF-β1 has the most widespread distribution in mammals and will be referred to as TGF-β. It is a homodimeric protein produced by a variety of different cell types, including platelets, endothelial cells, lymphocytes, and macrophages. Native TGF-βs are synthesized as precursor proteins, which are secreted and then proteolytically cleaved to yield the biologically active growth factor and a second *latent* component. Active TGF-β binds to two cell surface receptors (types I and II) with serine/threonine kinase activity and triggers the phosphorylation of cytoplasmic transcription factors called *Smads.*[50] TGF-β first binds to a type II receptor, which then forms a complex with a type I receptor, leading to the phosphorylation of Smad 2 and 3. Phosphorylated Smad2 and 3 form heterodimers with Smad4, which enter the nucleus and associate with other DNA-binding proteins to activate or inhibit gene transcription. TGF-β has multiple and often opposing effects depending on the tissue and the type of injury. Agents that have multiple effects are called pleiotropic; because of the large diversity of TGF-β effects, it has been said that TGF-β is pleiotropic with a vengeance.

- *TGF-β is a growth inhibitor for most epithelial cell types and for leukocytes.*[51] It blocks the cell cycle by increasing the expression of cell-cycle inhibitors of the Cip/Kip and INK4/ARF families (see Chapter 7). Loss of TGF-β receptors frequently occurs in human tumors, providing a proliferative advantage to tumor cells.

- The effects of TGF-β on mesenchymal cells depend on concentration and culture conditions, it generally *stimulates the proliferation of fibroblasts and smooth muscle cells.*
- *TGF-β is a potent fibrogenic agent* that stimulates fibroblast chemotaxis, enhances the production of collagen, fibronectin, and proteoglycans. It inhibits collagen degradation by decreasing matrix proteases and increasing protease inhibitor activities. TGF-β is involved in the development of fibrosis in a variety of chronic inflammatory conditions particularly in the lungs, kidney, and liver.
- *TGF-β has a strong anti-inflammatory effect.* Knockout mice lacking the *TGF-β1* gene have widespread inflammation and abundant lymphocyte proliferation, presumably because of unregulated T-cell proliferation and macrophage activation.

Cytokines. Cytokines have important functions as mediators of inflammation and immune responses (Chapter 6). Some of these proteins can be placed into the larger functional group of polypeptide growth factors because they have growth-promoting activities for a variety of cells. These are discussed in the appropriate chapters.

SIGNALING MECHANISMS IN CELL GROWTH

All growth factors function by binding to specific receptors, which deliver signals to the target cells. These signals have two general effects: (1) they stimulate the transcription of many genes that were silent in the resting cells, and (2) several of these genes regulate the entry of the cells into the cell cycle and their passage through the various stages of the cell cycle. In this section we review the process of receptor-initiated signal transduction as it applies to growth factors and signaling molecules in general, and their role in regulating the cell cycle.

Cell proliferation is a tightly regulated process that involves a large number of molecules and interrelated pathways. The first event that initiates cell proliferation is, usually, the binding of a signaling molecule, the *ligand,* to a specific cell *receptor.* As we shall see, typical ligands are growth factors and proteins of the ECM. We describe different classes of receptor molecules and the pathways by which receptor activation initiates a cascade of events leading to expression of specific genes. We end this section with brief comments about transcription factors.

Based on the source of the ligand and the location of its receptors—in the same, adjacent, or distant cells—three general modes of signaling, named *autocrine, paracrine*, and *endocrine*, can be distinguished (Fig. 3–8).

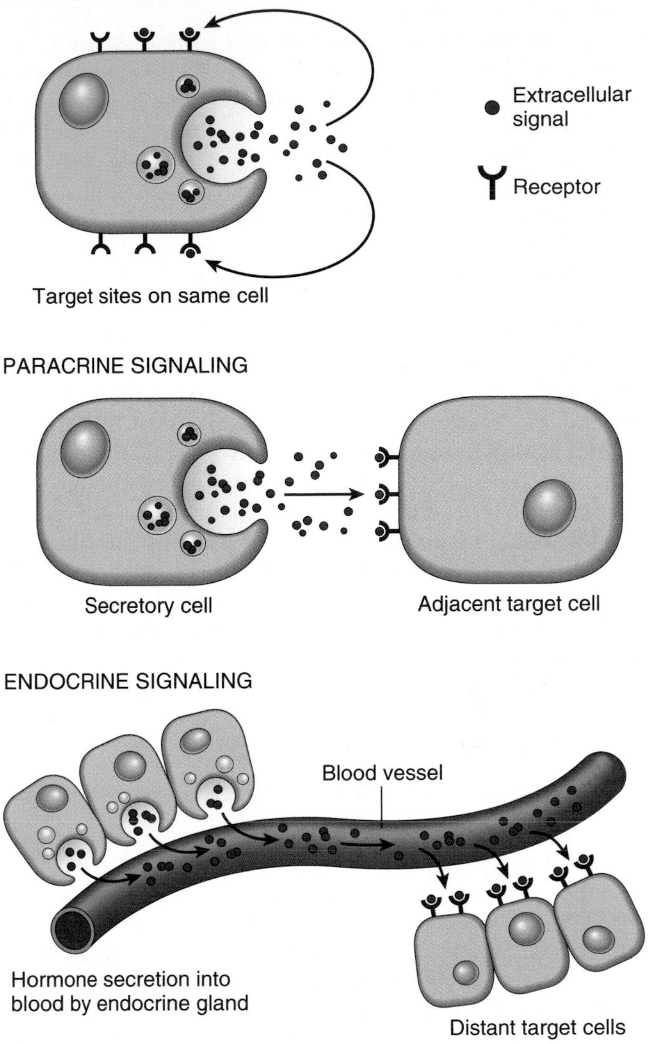

FIGURE 3–8 General patterns of intercellular signaling demonstrating autocrine, paracrine, and endocrine signaling (see text). (Modified from Lodish H, et al. [eds]: Molecular Cell Biology, 3rd ed. New York, WH Freeman, 1995, p. 855. © 1995 by Scientific American Books. Used with permission of WH Freeman and Company.)

- *Autocrine signaling:* Cells respond to the signaling molecules that they themselves secrete, thus establishing an *autocrine loop.* Several polypeptide growth factors and cytokines act in this manner. Autocrine growth regulation plays a role in liver regeneration, proliferation of antigen-stimulated lymphocytes, and the growth of some tumors. Tumors frequently overproduce growth factors and their receptors, thus stimulating their own proliferation through an autocrine loop.
- *Paracrine signaling:* One cell type produces the ligand, which then acts on adjacent target cells that express the appropriate receptors. The responding cells are in close proximity to the ligand-producing cell and are generally of a different type. Paracrine stimulation is common in connective tissue repair of healing wounds, in which a factor produced by one cell type (e.g., a macrophage) has its growth effect on adjacent cells (e.g., a fibroblast). Paracrine signaling is also necessary for hepatocyte replication during liver regeneration (see below). A special type of paracrine signaling, called *juxtacrine*, occurs when the signaling molecule (e.g., tumor necrosis factor, TGF-α, and heparin-binding epidermal growth factor) is anchored in the cell membrane and binds a receptor in the plasma membrane of another cell. In this type of signaling, receptor–ligand

interaction is dependent on and promotes cell–cell adhesion.

- *Endocrine signaling:* Hormones are synthesized by cells of endocrine organs and act on target cells distant from their site of synthesis, being usually carried by the blood. Growth factors may also circulate and act at distant sites, as is the case for HGF. Several cytokines, such as those associated with the systemic aspects of inflammation discussed in Chapter 2, also act as endocrine agents.

Overview of Receptors and Signal Transduction Pathways

The binding of a ligand to its receptor triggers a series of events by which extracellular signals are transduced into the cell and modulate changes in gene expression. A common form of ligand–receptor interaction involves the dimerization or trimerization of receptor molecules; single receptor molecules can also transduce signals but usually do so after recruiting and attaching cytoplasmic adapter proteins. Receptors are generally located on the surface of the target cell but can also be found in the cytoplasm or nucleus. A receptor protein has binding specificity for particular ligands, and the resulting receptor–ligand complex may initiate specific or multiple cellular responses.

Although the field of signal transduction is vast and beyond our scope, it is useful to summarize the properties of the major types of receptors and how they deliver signals to the cell interior (Fig. 3–9). This is pertinent not only to an understanding of normal cell growth, but also for the understanding of the molecular basis of cancer (Chapter 7).

- *Receptors with intrinsic tyrosine kinase activity.* The ligands for receptors with tyrosine kinase activity include most growth factors such as EGF (epidermal growth factor), TGF-α (transforming growth factor-α), HGF (hepatocyte growth factor/scatter factor), PDGF (platelet-derived growth factor), VEGF (vascular endothelial growth factor), FGF (fibroblast growth factor), c-KIT ligand, and insulin. Receptors belonging to this family have an extracellular ligand-binding domain, a transmembrane region, and a cytoplasmic tail that has intrinsic tyrosine kinase activity. Binding of the ligand induces *dimerization of the receptor*, tyrosine phosphorylation, and activation of the receptor tyrosine kinase[52,53] (Fig. 3–10). The active kinase then phosphorylates, and thereby activates, many downstream *effector molecules* (molecules that mediate the effects of receptor engagement with a ligand). Phosphorylated residues in the receptor also serve as docking sites for adapter molecules that bind effector molecules. Effector

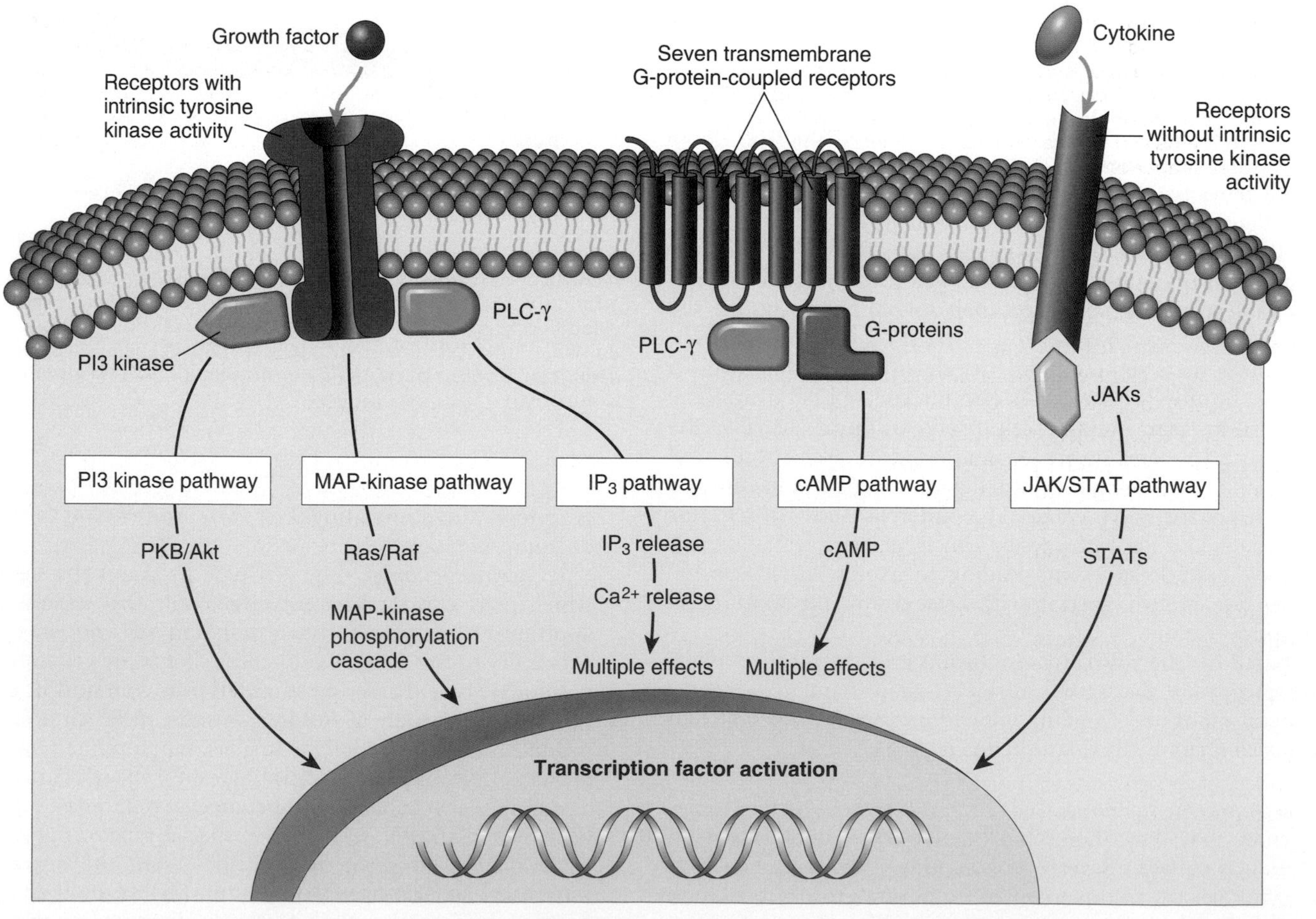

FIGURE 3–9 Examples of signal transduction systems that require cell-surface receptors. Shown are receptors with intrinsic tyrosine kinase activity, seven transmembrane G-protein–coupled receptors, and receptors without intrinsic tyrosine kinase activity. The figure also shows important signaling pathways transduced by the activation of these receptors through ligand binding.

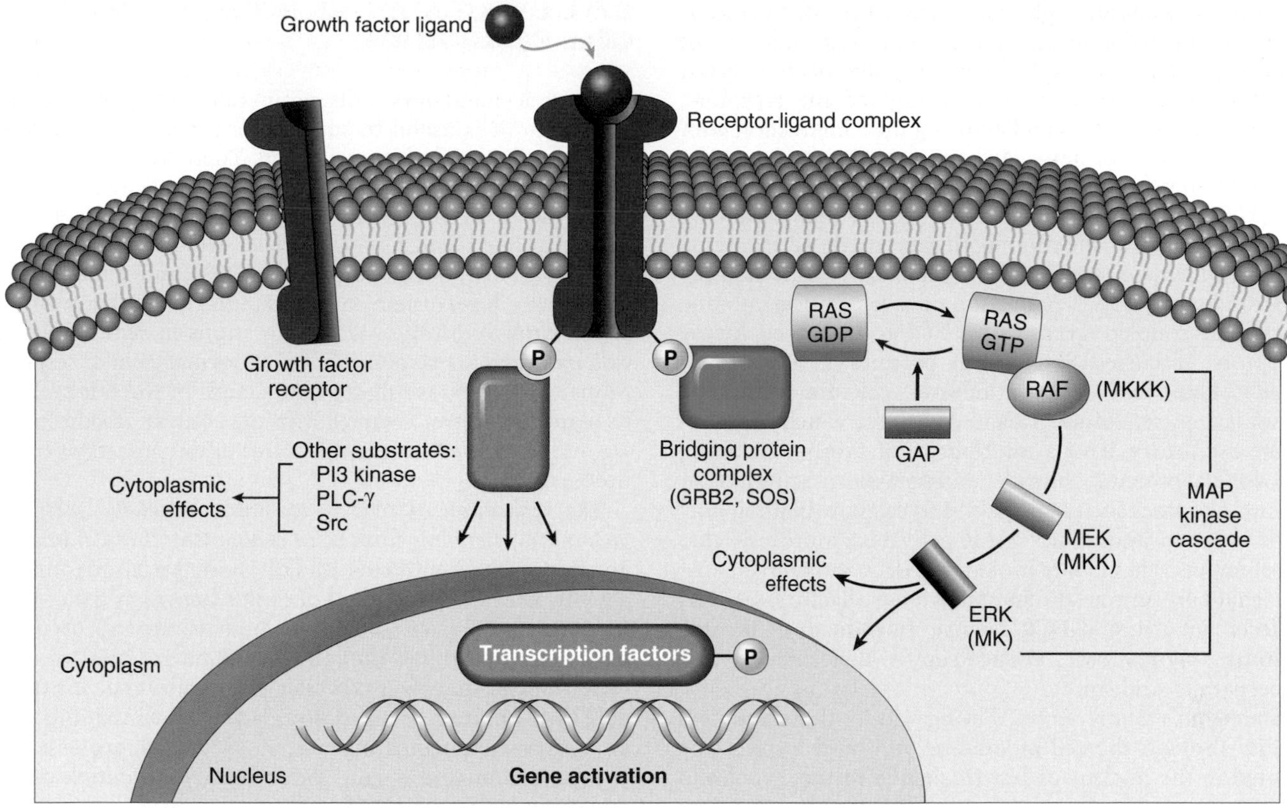

FIGURE 3–10 Signaling from tyrosine kinase receptors. Binding of the growth factor (ligand) causes receptor dimerization and autophosphorylation of tyrosine residues. Attachment of adapter (or bridging) proteins (e.g., GRB2 and SOS) couples the receptor to inactive RAS. Cycling of RAS between its inactive and active forms is regulated by GAP. Activated RAS interacts with and activates RAF (also known as MAP kinase kinase kinase). This kinase then phosphorylates a component of the MAP kinase signaling pathway, MEK (also known as MAP kinase kinase), which then phosphorylates ERK (MAP kinase). Activated MAP kinase phosphorylates other cytoplasmic proteins and nuclear transcription factors, generating cellular responses. The phosphorylated tyrosine kinase receptor can also bind other components, such as PI-3 kinase, which activates distinct signaling systems.

molecules include *phospholipase Cγ* (PLCγ) and PI-3 kinase (Fig. 3–9).[54] PLCγ catalyzes the breakdown of membrane inositol phospholipids into two products—inositol triphosphate (IP_3), which functions to increase concentrations of another important effector molecule, calcium; and diacylglycerol, which activates the serine-threonine kinase protein kinase C (PKC), which in turn activates various transcription factors. PI-3 kinase phosphorylates a membrane phospholipid, generating products that activate the kinase Akt (also referred to as protein kinase B). Akt is involved in cell proliferation and in inhibition of apoptosis and is a key intermediate in the insulin signal transduction pathway mediated by PI-3K[55] (see Chapter 24). As mentioned above, phosphorylated residues in the receptor also function as docking sites for adapter proteins that are capable of binding other effector proteins. A prototypical adapter protein is GRB-2, which binds a GTP:GDP exchange factor called SOS. SOS acts on the GTP-binding (G) protein RAS and catalyzes the formation of RAS-GTP, which triggers the mitogen-activated protein kinase (MAP kinase) cascade (see Fig. 3–10). Active MAP kinases stimulate the synthesis and phosphorylation of transcription factors, such as FOS and JUN. The transcription factors activated by these various signaling cascades in turn stimulate the production of growth factors, receptors for growth factors, and proteins that directly control the entry of cells into the cell cycle.[56] Defects in receptor tyrosine kinase pathways are found in many human diseases, including cancer (Chapter 7), type 2 diabetes (Chapter 25), and atherosclerosis (Chapter 11).

- *Receptors lacking intrinsic tyrosine kinase activity that recruit kinases.* Ligands for these receptors include many cytokines, such as interleukin-2 (IL-2), IL-3, and other interleukins; interferons α, β, and γ; erythropoietin; granulocyte colony-stimulating factor; growth hormone; and prolactin. These receptors transmit extracellular signals to the nucleus by activating members of the JAK (Janus kinase) family of proteins (Fig. 3–9).[57] The JAKs link the receptors with and activate cytoplasmic transcription factors called STATs (signal transducers and activation of transcription), which directly shuttle into the nucleus and activate gene transcription.[58] Cytokine receptors can also activate other signaling pathways, such as the MAP kinase pathways already mentioned.
- *Seven transmembrane G-protein–coupled receptors (GPCRs).* These receptors were so named because they contain seven transmembrane α-helices (Fig. 3–9).[59] They constitute the largest family of plasma membrane receptors (more than 1500 receptors of this class have been identified) and transmit signals into the cell through trimeric GTP-binding proteins *(G-proteins).* A large number of ligands signal through this type of receptor.[60] They include vasopressin, serotonin, histamine, epinephrine and norepi-

nephrine, calcitonin, glucagon, parathyroid hormone, corticotropin, rhodopsin, and an enormous number of common pharmaceutical drugs. Binding of the ligand induces changes in the conformation of the receptors, causing their activation and allowing their interaction with many different G-proteins. Activation of G-proteins occurs by the exchange of GDP, present in the inactive protein, with GTP, in the active protein. Among the many branches of this signal transduction pathway are those involving *calcium and adenosine 3′, 5′-cyclic monophosphate (cAMP) as second messengers.*[61] Activation of seven transmembrane G-protein–coupled receptors (as well as of tyrosine kinase receptors, discussed above) can produce inositol 1,4,5-triphosphate *(IP_3)*, which releases calcium from the endoplasmic reticulum. Calcium signals, which are generally oscillatory, have a multiplicity of targets, including cytoskeletal proteins, chloride- and potassium-activated ion pumps, enzymes such as calpain, and calcium-binding proteins such as calmodulin.[62] cAMP activates a more restricted set of targets that include protein kinase A and cAMP-gated ion channels, important in vision and olfactory sensing. Defects involving GPCR signal transduction include retinitis pigmentosa, corticotropin deficiencies, and hyperparathyroidism.[63]

- *Steroid hormone receptors.* The ligands for these receptors diffuse through the cell membrane and bind to receptors located in the nucleus or less frequently in the cytoplasm. Receptors of this family are transcription factors that bind a ligand and activate transcription.[64] The estrogen receptor, important in breast cancers, is localized in the cytoplasm.[65] In addition to steroid hormones, other ligands that bind to members of this receptor family include thyroid hormone, vitamin D, and retinoids. A group of receptors belonging to this family are called peroxisome proliferator-activated receptors (PPARs).[66] They are involved in a broad range of responses that include cell differentiation and adipogenesis (Chapter 24).

Transcription Factors

Many of the signal transduction systems used by growth factors transfer information to the nucleus and modulate gene transcription through the activity of *transcription factors.* Among the transcription factors that regulate cell proliferation are products of several growth promoting genes, such as c-*MYC* and c-*JUN,* and of cell-cycle inhibiting genes, such as *p53.*[67] Transcription factors have a modular design and contain domains for DNA binding and for transcriptional regulation. The DNA-binding domain permits binding to short sequence motifs of DNA, which may be unique to a particular target gene or may be present in many genes. In general, cellular events requiring rapid responses do not rely on new synthesis of transcription factors but depend on post-translational modifications that cause transcription factor activation and migration into the nucleus. These modifications include heterodimerization (for instance, dimerization of the products of the proto-oncogenes c-*FOS* and c-*JUN* to form the transcription factor activator protein-1 [AP-1],[68] which is activated by MAP kinase signaling pathways), phosphorylation of available factors (STATs in the JAK/STAT pathway), and release of inhibition to permit nuclear migration (NFκB).

CELL CYCLE AND THE REGULATION OF CELL REPLICATION

To understand how cells proliferate during regeneration and repair, it is useful to summarize the key features of the normal cell cycle and its regulation. There has been an explosion of knowledge about the molecular events involved in cell proliferation. In part this has been driven by the discovery that cellular genes called *proto-oncogenes* are directly involved in the regulation of normal cell proliferation, and defects in these genes can convert them into *oncogenes,* which contribute to cancer growth. More broadly, alterations in signal transduction pathways are responsible for abnormal cellular responses in many diseases. We discuss the details of the cell cycle and its abnormalities in Chapter 7, in the context of cancer. Here we summarize some salient features of the process of cellular proliferation.

The replication of cells is generally stimulated by growth factors or by signaling from ECM components through integrins. To achieve DNA replication and division, the cell goes through a highly controlled sequence of events known as the cell cycle (see Fig. 3–3). Each cell-cycle phase is dependent on the proper activation and completion of the previous one. The cycle will stop at a place at which an essential gene function is deficient. Because of its central role in maintaining tissue homeostasis and regulating physiologic growth processes such as regeneration and repair, *the cell cycle has multiple controls and redundancies, particularly during the transition between the G_1 and S phases.*[69–71] These controls include both activators and inhibitors, as well as checkpoint mechanisms.

To enter the cycle, quiescent cells first must go through the transition from G_0 to G_1, the first decision step, which functions as a gateway to the cell cycle. This transition involves the transcriptional activation of a large set of genes, including various proto-oncogenes and genes required for ribosome synthesis and protein translation. Cells can enter G_1 either from G_0 (quiescent cells) or after completing mitosis (continuously replicating cells). Cells that have entered G_1 progress through the cycle and reach a critical stage at the G_1/S transition, known as a *restriction point,* a rate-limiting step for replication (see Fig. 3–3). By passing this restriction point, normal cells become irreversibly committed to DNA replication. *Progression through the cell cycle, and particularly the G_1/S transition, is tightly regulated by proteins called cyclins and associated enzymes called cyclin-dependent kinases (CDKs).*[72] CDKs acquire catalytic activity by binding to and forming complexes with the cyclins. Activated CDKs in these complexes drive the cell cycle by phosphorylating proteins that are critical for cell cycle transitions. One such protein is the retinoblastoma susceptibility (RB) protein, which normally prevents cells from replicating by forming a tight, inactive complex with the transcription factor E2F. Phosphorylation of RB releases it, allowing E2F to become active and stimulate transcription of genes whose products drive cells through the cycle. Other cyclins are involved in the G_2/M transition (see Chapter 7). Many growth factors stimulate the production of cyclins.

The activity of cyclin-CDK complexes is tightly regulated by inhibitors, which are called *CDK inhibitors.* Some growth factors shut off production of these inhibitors. Embedded in the cell cycle are surveillance mechanisms that are geared primarily at sensing damage to DNA and chromosomes.[73,74] These quality control checks are called *checkpoints,* and they ensure that cells with damaged DNA or chromosomes do not complete replication. The G_1/S checkpoint checks the integrity of DNA before replication, whereas the G_2/M checkpoint checks DNA after replication and monitors whether the cell can safely enter mitosis. Checkpoint activation delays the cell cycle and triggers DNA repair mechanisms. If DNA damage is too severe to be repaired, the cells are eliminated by apoptosis, primarily through p53-dependent mechanisms. Checkpoint defects allow the replication of cells with DNA strand breaks and chromosome abnormalities that may cause tissue alterations and neoplasia (Chapter 7).

Mechanisms of Tissue Regeneration

Urodele amphibians such as the newt can regenerate their tails, limbs, lens, retina, jaws and even a large portion of the heart.[75] This remarkable regenerative capacity has been attributed to two main factors: (1) the capacity of quiescent cells such as cardiac myotubes to reenter the cell cycle, and (2) efficient differentiation of stem cells in the area of injury. Such capacity for regeneration of whole tissues and organs has been lost in mammals.[76] Most of the processes that are referred to as regeneration in mammalian organs are actually compensatory growth processes that involve cell hypertrophy and hyperplasia. They restore the functional capacity of an organ without necessarily reconstituting its original anatomy. The inadequacy of true regeneration in mammals has been attributed to the rapid fibroproliferative response and scar formation after wounding.[1,75]

In this section, we have chosen liver regeneration to illustrate the mechanisms of compensatory hyperplasia because this process has been studied in detail and has important biological and clinical aspects. Other organs, including kidney, pancreas, adrenal glands, thyroid, and the lungs of very young animals, are also capable of compensatory growth, although they display it in less dramatic form than the liver. Because new nephrons cannot be generated in the adult kidney, the growth of the contralateral kidney after unilateral inephrectomy involves nephron hypertrophy and some replication of proximal tubule cells. The pancreas has a limited capacity to regenerate its exocrine components and islets. Regeneration of pancreatic beta cells involves stem cell differentiation or the transdifferentiation of pancreatic ductal cells.[77,78] By contrast, regeneration of the liver after partial hepatectomy involves the replication of mature cells without stem cell participation.

LIVER REGENERATION

In rodents, removal of approximately 70% of the liver (partial hepatectomy) elicits a growth response known as *liver regeneration*.[3,79] The portions of the liver that remain after partial hepatectomy constitute an intact "mini-liver" that rapidly expands and reaches the mass of the original liver in 10 to 14 days (Fig. 3–11). The human liver also has a remarkable capacity to regenerate, as demonstrated by its growth after partial hepatectomy, performed for tumor resection or for living-donor hepatic transplantation (Fig. 3–12). *Restoration of liver mass is achieved without the regrowth of the lobes that were resected at the operation* (see Figs. 3–11 and 3–12). Instead, growth occurs by enlargement of the lobes that remain after the operation, a process known as *compensatory growth*. Thus, the end-point of liver regeneration after partial hepatectomy is the restitution of functional mass rather than form.

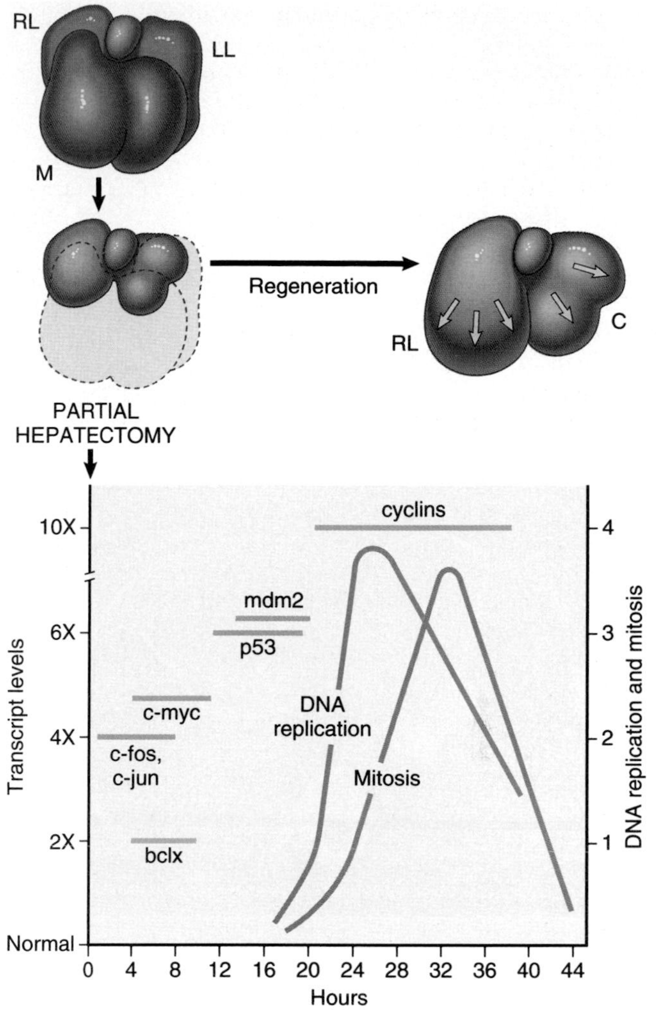

FIGURE 3–11 Liver regeneration after partial hepatectomy. *Upper panel,* The lobes of the liver of a rat are shown (M, median; RL and LL, right and left lateral lobes; C, caudate lobe). Partial hepatectomy removes two thirds of the liver (median and left lateral lobes), and only the right lateral and caudate lobes remain. After 3 weeks, the right lateral and caudate lobes enlarge to reach a mass equivalent to that of the original liver. Note that there is no regrowth of the median and left lateral lobes removed after partial hepatectomy. (From Goss RJ: Regeneration versus repair. In Cohen IK, Diegelman RF, Lindblad WJ (eds): Wound Healing. Biochemical and Clinical Aspects. Philadelphia, W. B. Saunders Co., 1992, pp. 20–39.) *Lower panel,* Timing of hepatocyte DNA replication, hepatocyte mitosis, and expression of messenger RNAs during liver regeneration. DNA replication is shown as the incorporation of tritiated thymidine $\times 10^{-4}$ *(right-side scale).* Mitosis presented as the percentage of hepatocytes undergoing mitosis *(right-side scale).* The expression of some of the many mRNAs in the regenerating rat liver is presented as fold elevation above normal *(left-side scale).* Expression of the proto-oncogenes c-*fos,* c-*jun,* and c-*myc* corresponds to the immediate early gene phase of gene expression during liver regeneration.

Almost all hepatocytes replicate during liver regeneration after partial hepatectomy. Because hepatocytes are quiescent cells, it takes them several hours to enter the cell cycle, progress through G_1, and reach the S phase of DNA replication (see Fig. 3–11). The wave of hepatocyte replication is synchronized and

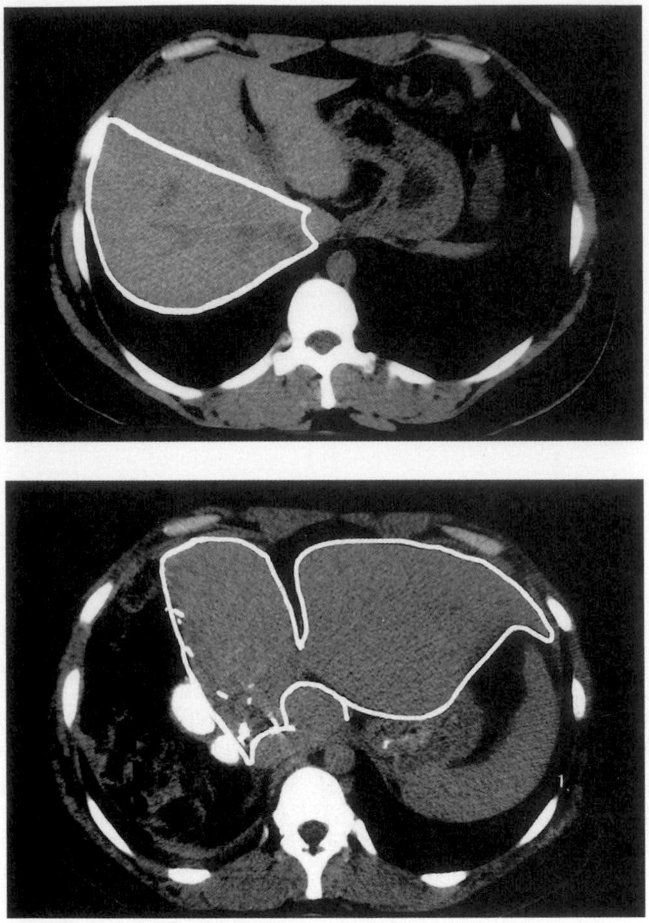

FIGURE 3–12 Regeneration of human liver. Computed tomography (CT) scans of the donor liver in living-donor hepatic transplantation. *Upper panel,* The liver of the donor before the operation. The right lobe, which will be used as a transplant, is outlined. *Lower panel,* A scan of the liver 1 week after performance of partial hepatectomy to remove the right lobe. Note the great enlargement of the left lobe (outlined in the panel) without regrowth of the right lobe (Courtesy of R. Troisi, M.D. Ghent University city; reproduced in part from Fausto; Liver Regeneration. In Arias, et al: The Liver: Biology and Pathobiology, 4th ed. Philadelphia, Lippincott Williams & Wilkins, 2001.)

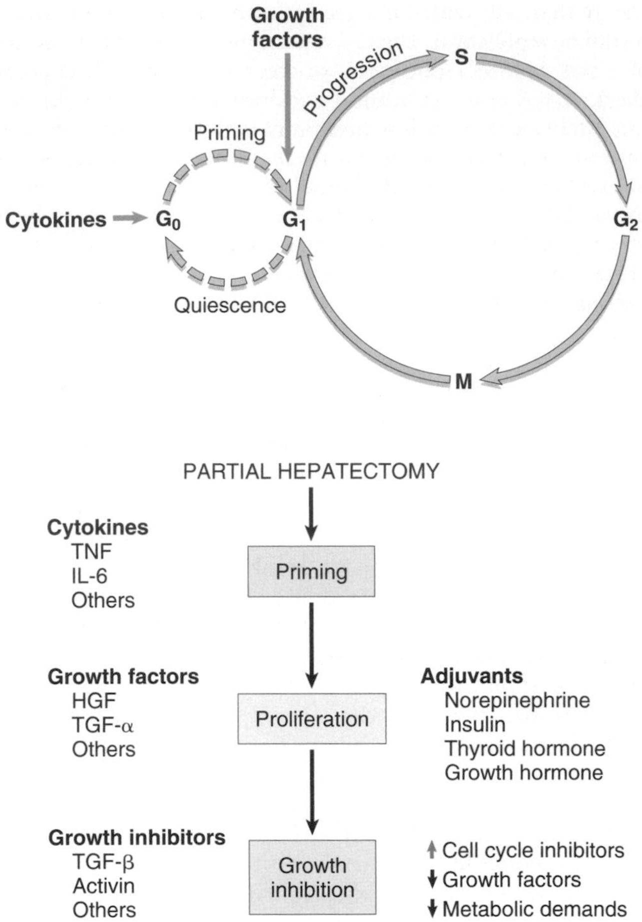

FIGURE 3–13 Priming and cell-cycle progression in hepatocyte replication during liver regeneration. Quiescent hepatocytes become competent to enter the cell cycle through a priming phase mostly mediated by the cytokines TNF and IL-6 *(upper panel).* Growth factors, mainly HGF and TGF-α, act on primed hepatocytes to make them progress through the cell cycle and undergo DNA replication *(lower panel).* Norepinephrine, insulin, thyroid hormone, and growth hormone act as adjuvants for liver regeneration. The factors that determine the termination of cell replication are not known but are likely to involve cell cycle inhibitors, shut-off of growth factor production, and decreased metabolic demand on the liver.

is followed by synchronous replication of nonparenchymal cells (Kupffer cells, endothelial cells, and stellate cells).

There is substantial evidence that hepatocyte proliferation in the regenerating liver is triggered by the combined actions of cytokines and polypeptide growth factors (Fig. 3–13). With the exception of the autocrine activity of TGF-α, hepatocyte replication is strictly dependent on paracrine effects of growth factors and cytokines produced by hepatic nonparenchymal cells. There are two major restriction points for hepatocyte replication: the G_0/G_1 transition, bringing quiescent cells into the cell cycle, and the G_1/S transition needed for passage through the late G_1 restriction point. Gene expression in the regenerating liver proceeds in phases, starting with the immediate early gene response, which is a transient response that corresponds to the G_0/G_1 transition.[80] More than 70 genes are activated during this response, including the proto-oncogenes c-*FOS* and c-*JUN*, which dimerize to form the AP-1 transcription factor, c-*MYC*, which encodes a transcription factor that activates many different genes, and other transcription factors, such as NFκB, STAT-3, and C/EBP. After the immediate early gene response, multiple genes are sequentially activated. As hepatocytes progress through the G_1 phase of the cell cycle, other genes, such as the anti-apoptotic gene *Bcl-X*, are expressed. Progression from G_1 to S starts with the formation of the cyclin D–CDK4 complex and phosphorylation of one component of the RB protein family. This is followed by activation of the cyclin E–CDK2 complex, after which replication becomes autonomous.

The cytokines TNF and IL-6 are implicated in the G_0/G_1 transition, and the growth factors HGF and TGF-α are involved in cell-cycle progression after the cells reach G_1 (see Fig. 3–13). It has been demonstrated that TNF provides a priming signal to the remnant hepatic cells after partial hepatectomy and that this signal is necessary for the full mitogenic effect of growth factors. While the infusion of HGF or TGF-α directly into the portal circulation causes only a very small proliferative response in normal livers, an injection of TNF given at the start of growth factor infusion greatly enhances hepatocyte proliferation. Priming signals activate several signal transduction pathways as a necessary prelude to cellular proliferation. They may also activate surface and extracellular metalloproteinases, causing the release of matrix-associated HGF, and convert inactive, membrane-bound TGF-α into an active growth factor. Certain hormones, such as norepinephrine, whose blood level increases after hepatectomy, as well as insulin and thyroid hormone, may function as adjuvants for cell proliferation.[81]

Although much has been learned about the steps that regulate hepatocyte replication, there is little information about the mechanisms that link the increased metabolic work after partial hepatectomy with the cell proliferation that follows. Similarly, the mechanisms of growth cessation have not been established. Hepatocytes replicate once or twice during regeneration and then return to quiescence in a strictly regulated sequence of events. Growth inhibitors, such as TGF-β and activins, may be involved in terminating hepatocyte replication, but there is no clear understanding of their mode of action. Intrahepatic stem cells do not play a role in the compensatory growth that occurs after partial hepatectomy and there is no evidence for hepatocyte generation from bone marrow–derived cells during this process. However, some endothelial cells in the regenerating liver may originate from the bone marrow.

Extracellular Matrix (ECM) and Cell–Matrix Interactions

In the previous sections we examined some of the important features of growth factor–induced signaling and cell proliferation. Cells grow, move, and differentiate in intimate contact with macromolecules outside the cell that constitute the ECM. There is overwhelming evidence that the matrix critically influences these cell functions. This section discusses those aspects of ECM structure and function that are most relevant to regeneration, healing, and fibrosis.

The ECM is secreted locally and assembles into a network in the spaces surrounding cells (Fig. 3–14). It forms a significant proportion of the volume of any tissue. The ECM serves many functions. For example, matrix proteins sequester water that provides turgor to soft tissues and minerals that give rigidity to skeletal tissues. They also function as a reservoir for growth factors controlling cell proliferation. ECM is important for cell-to-cell interactions and provides a substratum for cells to adhere, migrate, and proliferate, directly modulating cell form and function. Synthesis and degradation of ECM accompanies morphogenesis, wound healing, and chronic fibrotic processes, as well as tumor invasion and metastasis.

Three groups of macromolecules, which are often physically associated, constitute the ECM: (1) *fibrous structural proteins*, such as the collagens and elastins; (2) a diverse group of *adhesive glycoproteins*; and (3) *proteoglycans and hyaluronic acid*. These macromolecules are present in intercellular junctions and cell surfaces and may assemble into two general organizations: *interstitial matrix* and *basement membrane (BM)*. The interstitial matrix is present in spaces between epithelial, endothelial, and smooth muscle cells and in connective tissue. It consists of fibrillar and nonfibrillar collagen, elastin, fibronectin, proteoglycans, hyaluronate, and other components. BMs are produced by epithelial and mesenchymal cells and are closely associated with the cell surface. They consist of a network of amorphous nonfibrillar collagen (mostly type IV), laminin, heparan sulfate, proteoglycan, and other glycoproteins.[82]

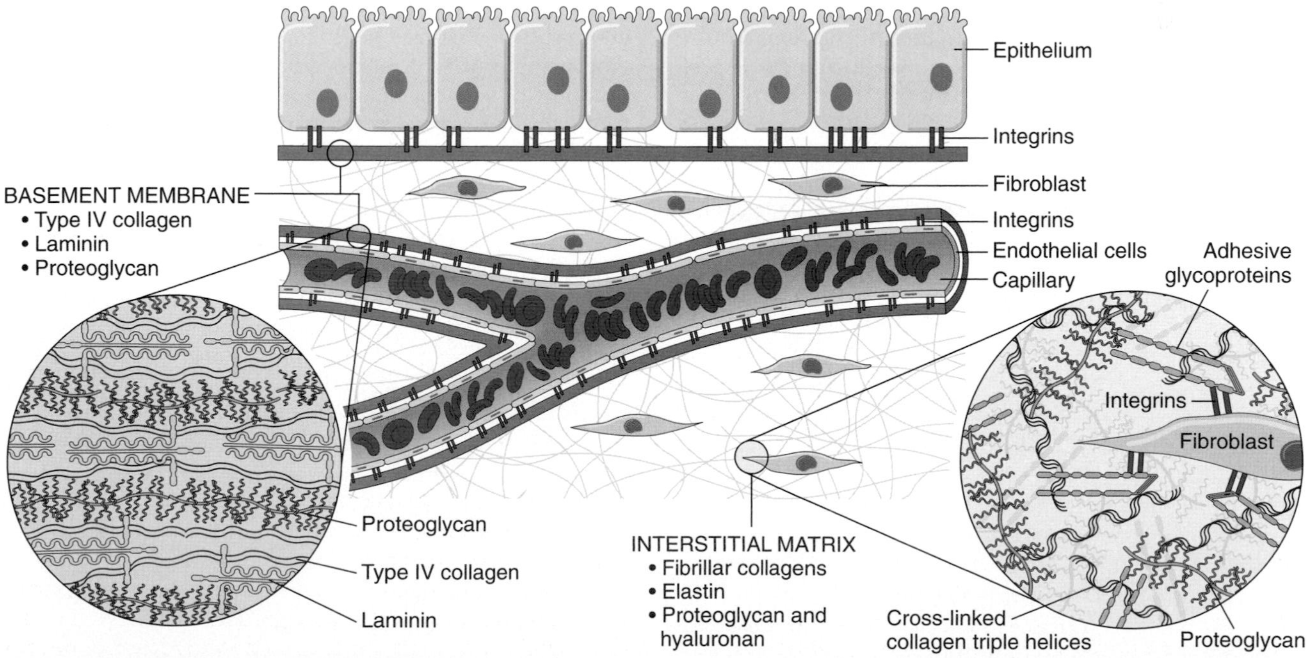

FIGURE 3–14 Major components of the extracellular matrix (ECM), including collagens, proteoglycans, and adhesive glycoproteins. Both epithelial and mesenchymal cells (e.g., fibroblasts) interact with ECM via integrins. To simplify the diagram, many ECM components (e.g., elastin, fibrillin, hyaluronan, syndecan) are not included.

COLLAGEN

Collagen is the most common protein in the animal world, providing the extracellular framework for all multicellular organisms. Without collagen, a human being would be reduced to a clump of cells, interconnected by a few neurons. The *collagens* are composed of a triple helix of three polypeptide α chains, having a gly-x-y repeating sequence. Currently 27 different types of collagens encoded by 41 genes dispersed on at least 14 chromosomes are known[83] (Table 3–2). Types I, II, III and V, and XI are the *interstitial* or *fibrillar collagens* and the most abundant. Type IV is nonfibrillar (forms sheets instead of fibrils) and is the main component of the BM, together with laminin. Other collagens may form meshworks and may function as anchors in epidermal–dermal junctions, cartilage, and blood vessel wall.[83]

Fibrillar collagen is synthesized from procollagen, a precursor molecule derived from preprocollagen, which is transcribed from collagen genes. After hydroxylation of proline and lysine residues and lysine glycosylation, three procollagen chains align in phase to form the triple helix (Fig. 3–15). Procollagen is secreted from the cell and cleaved by proteases to form the basic unit of the fibrils. Collagen fibril formation is associated with the oxidation of specific lysine and hydroxylysine residues by the extracellular enzyme lysyl oxidase. This results in *cross-linking* between the chains of adjacent molecules, thus stabilizing the array that is characteristic of collagen. Cross-linking is a major contributor to the tensile strength of collagen. *Vitamin C is required for the hydroxylation of procollagen*, a requirement that explains the inadequate wound healing in scurvy (Chapter 9). Genetic defects in collagen production (see Table 3–2) cause many inherited syndromes, including various forms of the Ehlers-Danlos syndrome and osteogenesis imperfecta[84] (Chapters 5 and 26).

ELASTIN, FIBRILLIN, AND ELASTIC FIBERS

Tissues such as blood vessels, skin, uterus, and lung require elasticity for their function. Although tensile strength is provided by the proteins of the collagen family, the ability of these tissues to recoil is provided by elastic fibers.[85] These fibers can stretch to several times their length and then return to their original size after release of the tension. Morphologically, elastic fibers consist of a central core made of elastin, surrounded by a peripheral network of microfibrils. Substantial amounts of elastin are found in the walls of large blood vessels, such as the aorta, and in the uterus, skin, and ligaments. The peripheral microfibrillar network that surrounds the core consists largely of *fibrillin*, a 350-kD secreted glycoprotein, which associates either with itself or with other components of the ECM. The microfibrils serve as scaffolding for deposition of elastin and the assembly of elastic fibers. Inherited defects in fibrillin[86] result in formation of abnormal elastic fibers in a fairly common familial disorder, Marfan syndrome, manifested by changes in the cardiovascular system (aortic dissection) and the skeleton (Chapter 5).

CELL ADHESION PROTEINS

Most adhesion proteins, also called CAMs (cell adhesion molecules), can be classified into four main families: immunoglobulin family CAMs, cadherins, integrins, and selectins. These proteins are located in the cell membrane, where they function as receptors, or they are stored in the cytoplasm. As receptors, CAMs can bind to similar or different molecules in other cells, providing for interaction between the same cells (homotypic interaction) or different cell types (heterotypic interaction). Cadherins are generally involved in calcium-dependent homotypic interactions, while immunoglobulin family CAMs, because of the types of ligands they can bind, participate in both homotypic and heterotypic cell-to-cell interactions. The integrins have broader ligand specificity and are responsible for many events involving cell adhesion.[87,88]

Integrins bind both to matrix proteins such as fibronectin and laminin, mediating adhesiveness between cells and ECM, as well as to adhesive proteins in other cells, establishing cell-to-cell contacts (see Box 2–1, Chapter 2). *Fibronectin* is a large protein that binds to many molecules, such as collagen, fibrin, proteoglycans, and cell-surface receptors. It consists of two glycoprotein chains, held together by disulfide bonds. Fibronectin mRNA has two splice forms, giving rise to tissue fibronectin and plasma fibronectin. The tissue fibronectin forms fibrillar aggregates at wound healing sites. The plasma form binds to fibrin, forming the provisional blood clot that

TABLE 3–2 Main Types of Collagens, Tissue Distribution, and Genetic Disorders

Collagen Type	Tissue Distribution	Genetic Disorders
Fibrillar Collagens		
I	Ubiquitous in hard and soft tissues	Osteogenesis Imperfecta Ehlers-Danlos syndrome—arthrochalasias type
II	Cartilage, intervertebral disk, vitreous	Achondrogenesis type II, spondyloepiphyseal dysplasia syndrome
III	Hollow organs, soft tissues	Vascular Ehlers-Danlos syndrome
V	Soft tissues, blood vessels	Classical Ehlers-Danlos syndrome
XI	Cartilage, vitreous	Stickler syndrome
Basement Membrane Collagens		
IV	Basement membranes	Alport syndrome
Other Collagens		
VI	Ubiquitous in microfibrils	Bethlem myopathy
VII	Anchoring fibrils at dermal-epidermal junctions	Dystrophic epidermolysis bullosa
IX	Cartilage, intervertebral disks	Multiple epiphyseal dysplasias
XVII	Transmembrane collagen in epidermal cells	Benign atrophic generalized epidermolysis bullosa
XV and XVIII	Endostatin-forming collagens, endothelial cells	Knobloch syndrome (type XVIII collagen)

Courtesy of Dr. Peter H. Byers, Department of Pathology, University of Washington, Seattle, WA

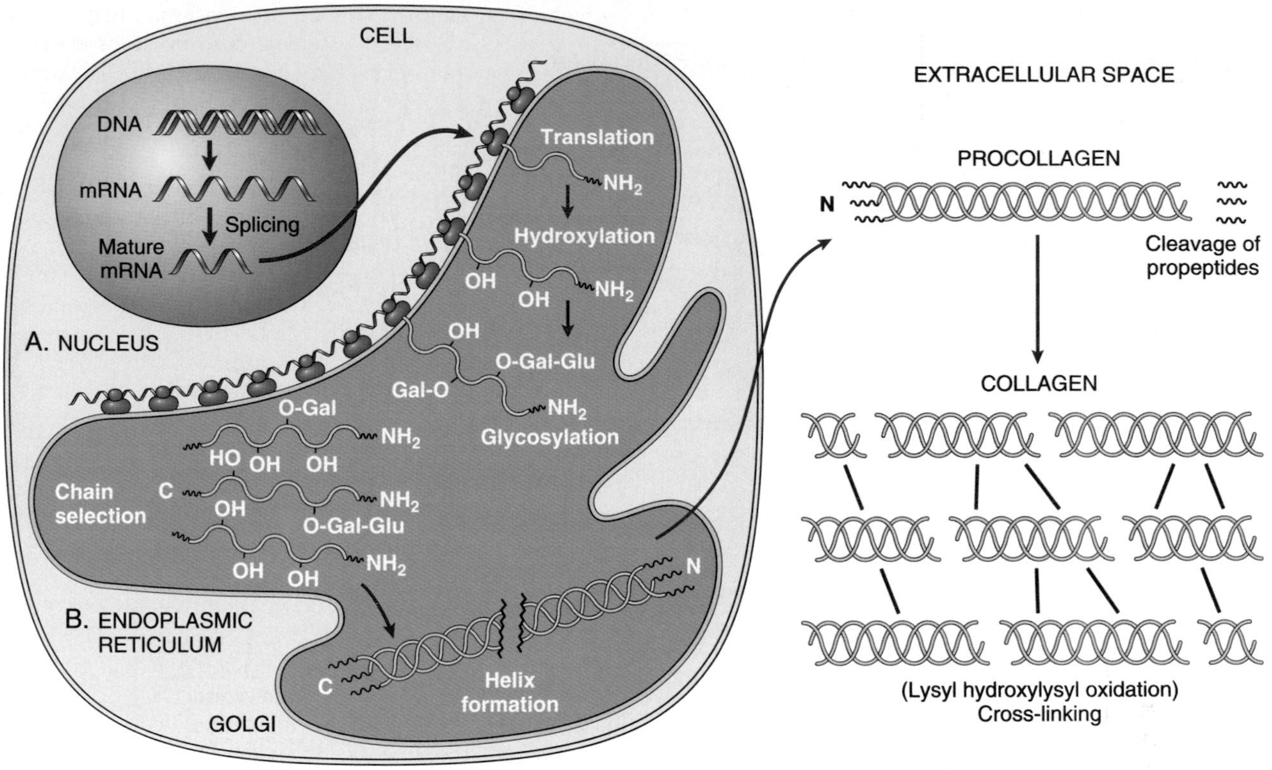

FIGURE 3–15 Steps in collagen synthesis (see text).

fills the space created by a wound, and serves as a substratum for ECM deposition. *Laminin* is the most abundant glycoprotein in the basement membrane and has binding domains for both ECM and cell-surface receptors. In the BM, polymers of laminin and collagen type IV form tightly bound networks. Laminin can also mediate the attachment of cells to connective tissue substrates.

Cadherins and integrins link the cell surface with the cytoskeleton through their binding to actin and intermediate filaments. These linkages, particularly for the integrins, provide a mechanism for the transmission of mechanical force and the activation of intracellular signal transduction pathways that respond to these forces. Ligand binding to integrins causes clustering of the receptors in the cell membrane and formation of *focal adhesion* complexes. The cytoskeletal proteins that colocalize with integrins at the cell focal adhesion complex include talin, vinculin, and paxillin. The integrin–cytoskeleton complexes function as activated receptors and trigger signal transduction pathways, which include the MAP kinase, PKC, and PI-3 kinase pathways. Not only is there functional overlap between integrin and growth factor receptors, but integrins and growth factor receptors interact ("cross-talk") to transmit environmental signals to the cell, which regulate cell proliferation, apoptosis, and differentiation (Fig. 3–16). Integrins and selectins are discussed in more detail in Box 2–1, Chapter 2.

The name *cadherin* is derived from the term "calcium-dependent adherence protein." This family contains almost 90 members, which, as mentioned, participate in interaction between cells of the same type. These interactions connect the plasma membrane of adjacent cells, forming two types of cell junctions called (1) *zonula adherens*, small, spotlike junctions located near the apical surface of epithelial cells; and (2) *desmosomes*, stronger and more extensive junctions, present in epithelial and muscle cells. Linkage of cadherins with the cytoskeleton occurs through two classes of *catenins.* β-catenin links cadherins with α-catenin, which, in turn, connects to actin, thus completing the connection with the cytoskeleton. Cell-to-cell interactions mediated by cadherins and catenins play a major role in regulating cell motility, proliferation, and differentiation and account for the inhibition of cell proliferation that occurs when cultured normal cells contact each other ("contact inhibition").

Free β-catenin can act independently of cadherins, functioning as a regulator of nuclear transcription factors in the *Wnt signaling pathway* described in Chapter 7. Mutation and altered expression of the β-catenin pathway is of major importance for cancer development, particularly in gastrointestinal and liver cancers (see Chapter 7).

In addition to the four families of adhesive proteins described above, some other secreted adhesion molecules may be mentioned because of their potential role in disease processes: (1) *SPARC* (secreted protein acidic and rich in cysteine), also known as *osteonectin*, contributes to tissue remodeling in response to injury, and functions as an angiogenesis inhibitor;[89] (2) the *thrombospondins*, a family of large multifunctional proteins, some of which, similar to SPARC, also inhibit angiogenesis; (3) *osteopontin*, which regulates calcification, and can also function as a mediator of leukocyte migration by serving as a ligand for the CD44 receptor[90] (see below); and (4) the *tenascin* family, which consist of large multimeric proteins involved in morphogenesis and cell adhesion.

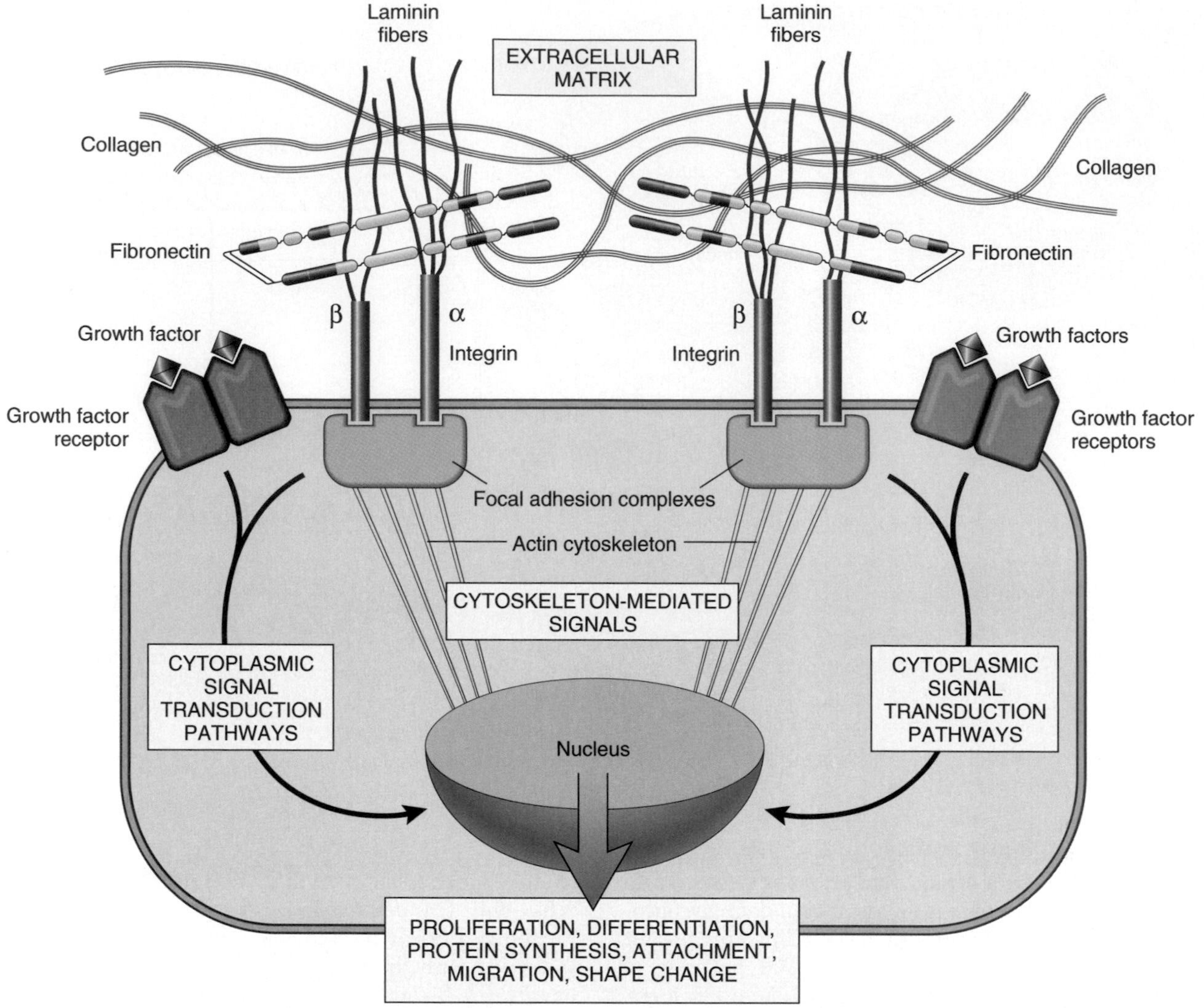

FIGURE 3–16 Mechanisms by which ECM (e.g., fibronectin and laminin) and growth factors can influence cell growth, motility, differentiation, and protein synthesis. Integrins bind ECM components and interact with the cytoskeleton at focal adhesion complexes (protein aggregates that include vinculin, α-actin, and talin). This can initiate the production of intracellular messengers or can directly mediate nuclear signals. Cell-surface receptors for growth factors may activate signal transduction pathways that overlap with those activated by integrins. Collectively, these are integrated by the cell to yield various responses, including changes in cell growth, locomotion, and differentiation.

PROTEOGLYCANS AND HYALURONIC ACID

Proteoglycans and hyaluronic acid (HA, hyaluronan or hyaluronate) make up the third type of component in the ECM, besides the fibrous structural proteins and cell adhesion proteins. *Proteoglycans* consist of a core protein linked to one or more polysaccharides called *glycosaminoglycans* (GAGs).[91] These are long repeating polymers of specific disaccharides in which one (or both) contains a sulfate residue. Proteoglycans are remarkable in their diversity. A specific ECM may contain several different core proteins, each containing different GAGs. Proteoglycans are named according to the structure of their principal repeating disaccharide. Some of the most common are heparan sulfate, chondroitin sulfate, and dermatan sulfate. They have diverse roles in regulating connective tissue structure and permeability. Proteoglycans can also be integral membrane proteins and, through their binding to other proteins and fibroblast growth factor, act as modulators of cell growth and differentiation.

HA is a polysaccharide of the GAG family found in the ECM of many tissues.[92] It is a huge molecule that consists of many repeats of a simple disaccharide stretched end-to-end. It binds a large amount of water, forming a viscous hydrated gel that gives connective tissue the ability to resist compression forces. HA helps provide resilience and lubrication to many types of connective tissue, notably for the cartilage in joints. HA is also found in the matrix of migrating and proliferating cells, where it inhibits cell-to-cell adhesion and facilitates cell motility. CD44,[93] a surface glycoprotein expressed by leukocytes, binds HA. Through such binding, T cells may be retained in tissues and remain bound to endothelium at sites of inflammation.

Repair by Healing, Scar Formation, and Fibrosis

As we have seen, regeneration involves the restitution of tissue components identical to those removed or killed. By contrast, healing is a fibroproliferative response that "patches" rather than restores a tissue.[2] It is a complex but orderly phenomenon involving a number of processes:

- Induction of an inflammatory process in response to the initial injury, with removal of damaged and dead tissue
- Proliferation and migration of parenchymal and connective tissue cells
- Formation of new blood vessels (angiogenesis) and granulation tissue
- Synthesis of ECM proteins and collagen deposition
- Tissue remodeling
- Wound contraction
- Acquisition of wound strength

Not all of these events occur in every repair reaction. The repair process is influenced by many factors, including:

- The tissue environment and the extent of tissue damage
- The intensity and duration of the stimulus
- Conditions that inhibit repair, such as the presence of foreign bodies or inadequate blood supply,
- Various diseases that inhibit repair (diabetes in particular), and treatment with steroids.

Regardless of these factors, the process of tissue repair has some basic general features. We first summarize these features and then discuss the components of the repair process.

- The goal of the repair process is to restore the tissue to its original state. The inflammatory reaction set in motion by the injury contains the damage, eliminates the damaging stimulus, removes injured tissue, and initiates the deposition of ECM components in the area of injury.
- Some tissues can be completely reconstituted after injury, such as the repair of bone after a fracture or the regeneration of the surface epithelium in a cutaneous wound. For tissues that are incapable of regeneration, repair is accomplished by connective tissue deposition, producing a *scar.* This term is most often used in connection to *wound healing* in the skin, but it is also used to describe the replacement of parenchymal cells by connective tissue, as in the heart after myocardial infarction.
- If damage persists, inflammation becomes chronic, and tissue damage and repair may occur concurrently. Connective tissue deposition in these conditions is usually referred to as *fibrosis.* In the broader sense, the term fibrosis applies to any abnormal deposition of connective tissue, regardless of cause.

Repair begins early in inflammation. Sometimes as early as 24 hours after injury, if resolution has not occurred, fibroblasts and vascular endothelial cells begin proliferating to form a specialized type of tissue that is the hallmark of healing, called *granulation tissue.* The term derives from its pink, soft, granular appearance on the surface of wounds, but it is the histologic features that are characteristic: *the formation of new small blood vessels (angiogenesis) and the proliferation of fibroblasts* (Fig. 3–17). These new vessels are leaky, allowing the passage of proteins and red cells into the extravascular space. *Thus, new granulation tissue is often edematous.* We next discuss mechanisms of angiogenesis and scar formation, the main components of the healing process.

ANGIOGENESIS

Blood vessels are assembled during embryonic development by *vasculogenesis,* in which a primitive vascular network is established from endothelial cell precursors called *angioblasts.* The process of blood vessel formation in adults is known as *angiogenesis* or *neovascularization* and, until recently, has been thought to depend on the branching and extension of adjacent blood vessels (Fig. 3–18). Recent work has demonstrated that angiogenesis can also occur by recruitment of endothelial progenitor cells (EPCs) from the bone marrow (see Fig. 3–18). Angiogenesis is critical to chronic inflammation and fibrosis, to tumor growth, and to the vascularization of ischemic tissues. Therefore, great efforts have

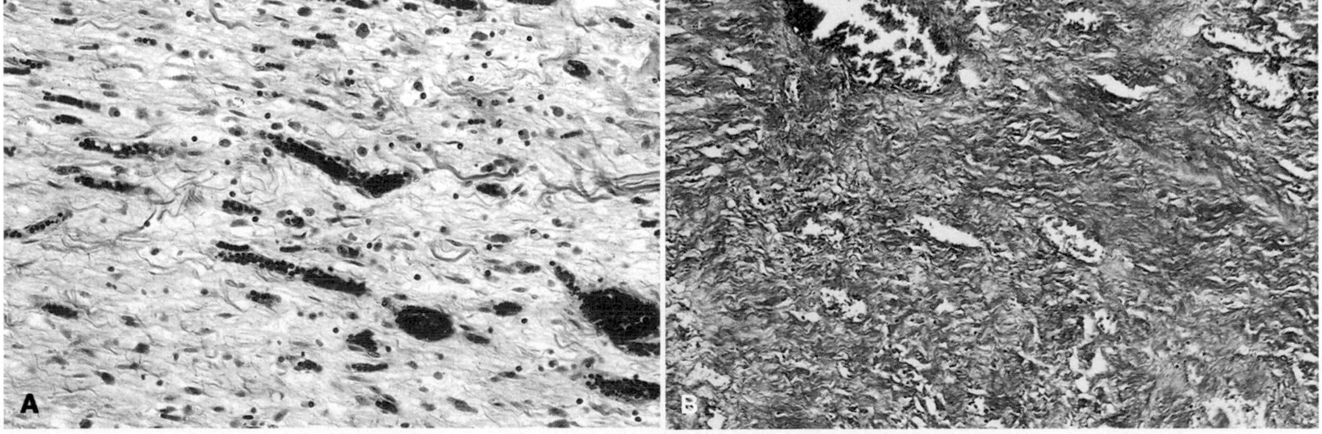

FIGURE 3–17 *A,* Granulation tissue showing numerous blood vessels, edema, and a loose ECM containing occasional inflammatory cells. This is a trichrome stain that stains collagen blue; minimal mature collagen can be seen at this point. *B,* Trichrome stain of mature scar, showing dense collagen, with only scattered vascular channels.

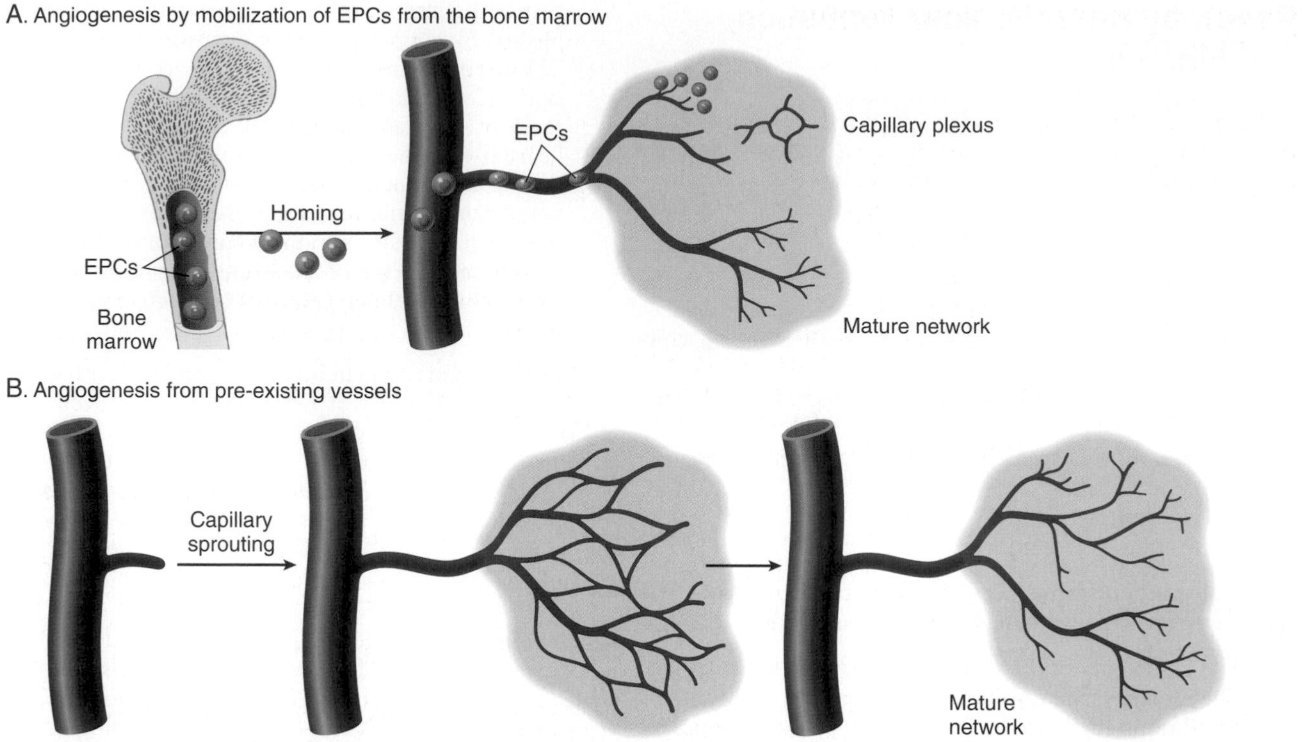

FIGURE 3–18 Angiogenesis by mobilization of endothelial precursor cells (EPCs) from the bone marrow and from pre-existing vessels (capillary growth). EPCs are mobilized from the bone marrow and may migrate to a site of injury or tumor growth *(upper panel)*. The homing mechanisms have not yet been defined. At these sites, EPCs differentiate and form a mature network by linking with existing vessels. In angiogenesis from pre-existing vessels, endothelial cells from these vessels become motile and proliferate to form capillary sprouts *(lower panel)*. Regardless of the initiating mechanism, vessel maturation (stabilization) involves the recruitment of pericytes and smooth muscle cells to form the periendothelial layer. (Modified from Conway EM, Collen D, Carmeliet P: Molecular mechanisms of blood vessel growth. Cardiovasc Res 49:507, 2001.)

been made to understand the mechanisms of angiogenesis and to explore potential therapeutic effects of agents that are proangiogenic (increase blood vessels when needed) and antiangiogenic (block pathologic angiogenesis).[46,94]

Angiogenesis from Endothelial Precursor Cells

The formation of the hematopoietic and vascular systems is closely linked during embryonic development.[95] The two systems share a common precursor, the hemangioblast, which can generate hematopoietic stem cells and angioblasts, the cells that give rise to the vascular system. Angioblasts proliferate, migrate to peripheral sites, and differentiate into endothelial cells that form arteries, veins, and lymphatics.[96,97] They also can generate pericytes and smooth muscle cells of the vessel wall (periendothelial cells). It has now been established that angioblast-like cells called EPCs are stored in the bone marrow of adult organisms[98] and can be recruited into tissues to initiate angiogenesis (see Fig. 3–18). The nature of the homing mechanism is uncertain. Marrow-derived circulating angioblasts, or EPCs in adults, express markers of hematopoietic stem cells[95] as well as endothelial-specific markers such as vascular endothelial-cadherin, E-selectin, and the Tie2 receptor (see below). EPCs participate in the replacement of lost endothelial cells, in the re-endothelization of vascular implants, and in neovascularization of ischemic organs, cutaneous wounds, and tumors. It has been proposed that the number of circulating EPCs may influence vascular function and determine the risk of cardiovascular diseases.[99]

Angiogenesis from Pre-Existing Vessels

In this type of angiogenesis, there is vasodilation and increased permeability of the existing vessels, degradation of ECM, and migration of endothelial cells. The major steps are listed below.

- Vasodilation in response to nitric oxide and VEGF-induced increased permeability of the pre-existing vessel
- Proteolytic degradation of the BM of the parent vessel by metalloproteinases and disruption of cell-to-cell contact between endothelial cells of the vessel by plasminogen activator[100]
- Migration of endothelial cells toward the angiogenic stimulus
- Proliferation of endothelial cells, just behind the leading front of migrating cells
- Maturation of endothelial cells, which includes inhibition of growth and remodeling into capillary tubes[101]
- Recruitment of periendothelial cells (including pericytes for small capillaries and vascular smooth muscle cells for larger vessels) to support the endothelial tubes and form the mature vessel.

Growth Factors and Receptors Involved in Angiogenesis

Many growth factors exhibit angiogenic activity, but most evidence points to a special role for *VEGF* (Table 3–3) and the *angiopoietins* in embryonic vasculogenesis and adult angiogenesis.[95,102] As mentioned earlier, VEGF is secreted by many mesenchymal and stromal cells, but VEGFR-2, a tyrosine kinase receptor that is the most important in angiogenesis, is largely restricted to endothelial cells and their precursors. Models for angiogenesis[94,95] generated from endothelial cell precursors and from the growth of pre-existing vessels are shown in Figure 3–18. In angiogenesis involving endothelial cell precursors, VEGF, acting through VEGFR-2, stimulates the mobilization of endothelial cell precursors from the bone marrow and enhances the proliferation and differentiation of these cells at the site of angiogenesis. Endothelial cells derived from these progenitors initially form a delicate capillary plexus that evolves into a mature capillary network. In angiogenesis originating from pre-existing local vessels, VEGF stimulates both proliferation and motility of endothelial cells, thus initiating the sprouting of new capillaries. Endothelial cell proliferation, differentiation, and migration can also be enhanced by FGF-2.

Regardless of the process that leads to capillary formation, newly formed vessels are fragile and need to become "stabilized." Stabilization requires the recruitment of pericytes and smooth muscle cells and the deposition of ECM proteins. *Angiopoietins 1 and 2 (Ang1 and Ang2)*, PDGF, and TGF-β participate in the stabilization process. Ang1 interacts with a receptor on endothelial cells called *Tie2* to recruit periendothelial cells. PDGF participates in the recruitment of smooth muscle cells, while TGF-β stabilizes newly formed vessels by enhancing the production of ECM proteins.[101] The Ang1/Tie2 interaction mediates vessel maturation from simple endothelial tubes into more elaborate vascular structures and helps maintain endothelial quiescence. Ang2, in contrast, also interacting with Tie2, has the opposite effect, loosening endothelial cells such that they become either more responsive to stimulation by growth factors such as VEGF or, in the absence of VEGF, more responsive to inhibitors of angiogenesis. A telling proof of the importance of these molecules is the existence of a genetic disorder caused by mutations in *Tie2* that is characterized by venous malformations.[103] Both physiologic and pathologic angiogenesis can be influenced by agents or conditions that stimulate VEGF expression, such as certain cytokines and growth factors (e.g., TGF-β, PDGF, TGF-α) and, notably, tissue hypoxia, which has long been associated with angiogenesis (see Table 3–3).

Despite the diversity of factors that may participate at various steps in angiogenesis, VEGF emerges as the most important growth factor in adult tissues undergoing physiologic angiogenesis (e.g., proliferating endometrium) as well as pathologic angiogenesis seen in chronic inflammation, wound healing, tumors, and diabetic retinopathy.

ECM Proteins as Regulators of Angiogenesis

A key component of angiogenesis is the motility and directed migration of endothelial cells, required for the formation of new blood vessels. These processes are controlled by several classes of proteins, including (1) *integrins*, especially $\alpha_v\beta_3$, which is critical for the formation and maintenance of newly formed blood vessels,[104] (2) *matricellular proteins*, including thrombospondin 1, SPARC, and tenascin C, which destabilize cell–matrix interactions and therefore promote angiogenesis,[105] and (3) *proteinases*, such as the plasminogen activators and *matrix metalloproteinases*, which are important in tissue remodeling during endothelial invasion. Additionally, these proteinases cleave extracellular proteins, releasing matrix-bound growth factors such as VEGF and FGF-2 that stimulate angiogenesis. Proteinases can also release inhibitors such as endostatin, a small fragment of collagen that inhibits endothelial proliferation and angiogenesis.[106] $\alpha_V\beta_3$ integrin expression in endothelial cells is stimulated by hypoxia. This integrin has multiple effects on angiogenesis: it directly interacts with a metalloproteinase (MMP-2, discussed below), it binds to and regulates the activity of VEGFR-2, and it mediates adhesion to ECM components such as fibronectin, thrombospondin, and osteopontin.[104]

TABLE 3–3 Vascular Endothelial Growth Factor (VEGF)

Proteins	Family members: VEGF (VEGF-A), VEGF-B, VEGF-C, VEGF-D Dimeric glycoprotein with multiple isoforms Targeted mutations in VEGF result in defective vasculogenesis and angiogenesis
Production	Expressed at low levels in a variety of adult tissues and at higher levels in a few sites, such as podocytes in the glomerulus and cardiac myocytes
Inducing Agents	Hypoxia TGF-β PDGF TGF-α
Receptors	VEGFR-1 VEGFR-2 (restricted to endothelial cells) VEGFR-3 (lymphatic endothelial cells) Targeted mutations in the receptors result in lack of vasculogenesis
Functions	Promotes angiogenesis Increases vascular permeability Stimulates endothelial cell migration Stimulates endothelial cell proliferation VEGF-C selectively induces hyperplasia of lymphatic vasculature Up-regulates endothelial expression of plasminogen activator, plasminogen activator inhibitor-1, tissue factor, and interstitial collagenase

SCAR FORMATION

Growth factors and cytokines released at the site of injury induce fibroblast proliferation and migration into the granulation tissue framework of new blood vessels and loose ECM that initially forms at the repair site. We discuss three processes that participate in the formation of a scar: (1) *emigration and proliferation of fibroblasts in the site of injury*, (2) *deposition of ECM*, and (3) *tissue remodeling*.

Fibroblast Migration and Proliferation

Granulation tissue contains numerous newly formed blood vessels. As discussed previously, VEGF promotes angiogenesis but is also responsible for a marked increase in vascular permeability (VEGF was first named vascular permeability factor).[107] The latter activity leads to exudation and deposition of plasma proteins, such as fibrinogen and plasma fibronectin, in the ECM and provides a provisional stroma for fibroblast and endothelial cell ingrowth. *Migration* of fibroblasts to the site of injury and their subsequent *proliferation* are triggered by multiple growth factors, including TGF-β, PDGF, EGF, FGF, and the cytokines IL-1 and TNF (see Table 3–5). The sources of these growth factors and cytokines include platelets, a variety of inflammatory cells (notably macrophages), and activated endothelium. Macrophages are important cellular constituents of granulation tissue, clearing extracellular debris, fibrin, and other foreign material at the site of repair. These cells also elaborate TGF-β, PDGF, and FGF and therefore promote fibroblast migration and proliferation.[108] If the appropriate chemotactic stimuli are present, mast cells, eosinophils, and lymphocytes may also accumulate. Each of these cells can contribute directly or indirectly to fibroblast migration and proliferation. Of the growth factors involved in inflammatory fibrosis, TGF-β appears to be the most important because of the multitude of effects that favor fibrous tissue deposition. TGF-β is produced by most of the cells in granulation tissue and causes *fibroblast migration and proliferation, increased synthesis of collagen and fibronectin, and decreased degradation of ECM by metalloproteinases* (discussed later). TGF-β is also chemotactic for monocytes and causes angiogenesis in vivo, possibly by inducing macrophage influx. TGF-β expression is increased in tissues in a number of chronic fibrotic diseases in humans and experimental animals.

ECM Deposition and Scar Formation

As repair continues, the number of proliferating endothelial cells and fibroblasts decreases. Fibroblasts progressively deposit increased amounts of ECM. Fibrillar collagens form a major portion of the connective tissue in repair sites and are important for the development of strength in healing wounds. As described later in the discussion of cutaneous wound healing, collagen synthesis by fibroblasts begins within 3 to 5 days after injury and continues for several weeks, depending on the size of wound. Many of the same growth factors that regulate fibroblast proliferation also stimulate ECM synthesis (see Table 3–4). For example, collagen synthesis is enhanced by several factors, including growth factors (PDGF, FGF, TGF-β) and cytokines (IL-1, IL-13), which are secreted by leukocytes and fibroblasts in healing wounds. *Net collagen accumulation, however, depends not only on increased collagen synthesis but also on decreased degradation.* Ultimately, the granulation tissue scaffolding is converted into a scar composed of spindle-shaped fibroblasts, dense collagen, fragments of elastic tissue, and other ECM components. As the scar matures, vascular regression continues, eventually transforming the richly vascularized granulation tissue into a pale, avascular scar.

Tissue Remodeling

The replacement of granulation tissue with a scar involves transitions in the composition of the ECM. Some of the growth factors that stimulate synthesis of collagen and other connective tissue molecules also modulate the synthesis and activation of metalloproteinases, enzymes that degrade these ECM components. The balance between ECM synthesis and degradation results in *remodeling* of the connective tissue framework—an important feature of both chronic inflammation and wound repair.

Degradation of collagen and other ECM proteins is achieved by a family of matrix metalloproteinases (MMPs), which are dependent on zinc ions for their activity[109,110] (Fig. 3–19). This

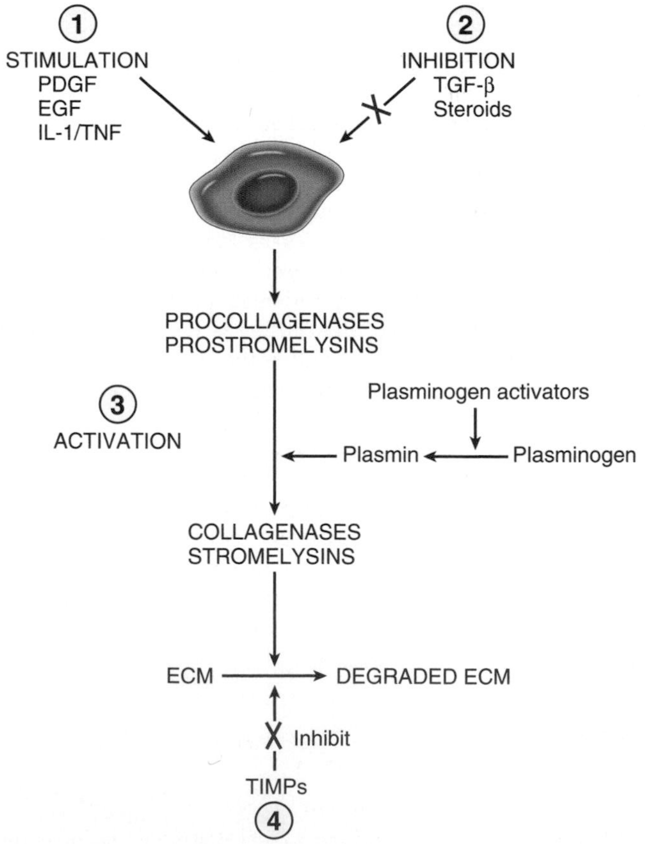

FIGURE 3–19 Matrix metalloproteinase regulation. Four mechanisms are shown: (1) regulation of synthesis by growth factors or cytokines, (2) inhibition of synthesis by corticosteroids or TGF-β, (3) regulation of the activation of the secreted but inactive precursors, and (4) blockage of the enzymes by specific tissue inhibitors of metalloproteinase (TIMPs). (Modified from Matrisian LM: Metalloproteinases and their inhibitors in matrix remodeling. Trends Genet 6:122, 1990, with permission from Elsevier Science.)

family of enzymes, which includes more than 20 members, has in common a 180-residue zinc-protease domain. (MMPs should be distinguished from neutrophil elastase, cathepsin G, kinins, plasmin, and other important proteolytic enzymes, which also degrade ECM components—these are *serine proteinases*, not metalloenzymes). MMPs include *interstitial collagenases* (MMP-1, 2, and 3), which cleave the fibrillar collagen types I, II, and III; *gelatinases (MMP-2 and 9)*, which degrade amorphous collagen as well as fibronectin; *stromelysins (MMP-3, 10, and 11)*, which act on a variety of ECM components, including proteoglycans, laminin, fibronectin, and amorphous collagens; and the family of *membrane-bound MMP*, surface-associated proteinases described below. MMPs are synthesized as propeptides that require proteolytic cleavage for activation. They are produced by several cell types (fibroblasts, macrophages, neutrophils, synovial cells, and some epithelial cells). Their secretion is induced by certain stimuli, including growth factors (PDGF, FGF), cytokines (IL-1, TNF), phagocytosis, and physical stress, and is inhibited by TGF-β and steroids. Collagenases cleave collagen under physiologic conditions, cutting the triple helix into two unequal fragments, which are then susceptible to digestion by other proteinases. As might be expected, collagenolytic activity is regulated. Collagenases are synthesized as a latent precursor (procollagenase) that is activated by chemicals, such as free radicals produced during the oxidative burst of leukocytes and proteinases (plasmin). Once formed, activated collagenases are rapidly inhibited by a family of specific *tissue inhibitors of metalloproteinases (TIMPs)*, which are produced by most mesenchymal cells, thus preventing uncontrolled action of these proteases (see Fig. 3–19). Collagenases and their inhibitors have been shown to be spatially and temporally regulated in healing wounds. They are essential in the debridement of injured sites and in the remodeling of connective tissue necessary to repair the defect.

A large and important family of enzymes related to MMPs is called ADAM (disintegrin and metalloproteinase-domain family). ADAMs are anchored to the plasma membrane and, through their proteolytic activity, cleave and release extracellular domains of cell-surface proteins,[111] such as the precursor forms of TNF and TGF-α. ADAM-17 (also known as TACE, for TNF-converting enzyme) cleaves the precursors of both of these molecules, producing active factors that can be released or remain anchored to the cell membrane. ADAM-17 deficiency in mice causes embryonic or neonatal lethality associated with pulmonary hypoplasia. Members of the ADAM family are also involved in the pathogenesis of bronchial asthma (Chapter 15), and thrombotic microangiopathies (Chapter 13).

Cutaneous Wound Healing

We discuss wound healing in the skin to illustrate general principles of repair that apply to most tissues. Although most skin lesions heal efficiently, the end product may not be functionally perfect. Epidermal appendages do not regenerate, and there remains a connective tissue scar in place of the mechanically efficient meshwork of collagen in the unwounded dermis. In very superficial wounds, the epithelium is reconstituted and there may be little scar formation.[112] In marked contrast with wound healing in adults, fetal cutaneous wounds heal without scar formation, up to mid-gestation age in some animals.[113] These wounds show little inflammation and practically no fibrosis, probably because of the differential expression of TGF-β isoforms that are less fibrogenic than TGF-β1.

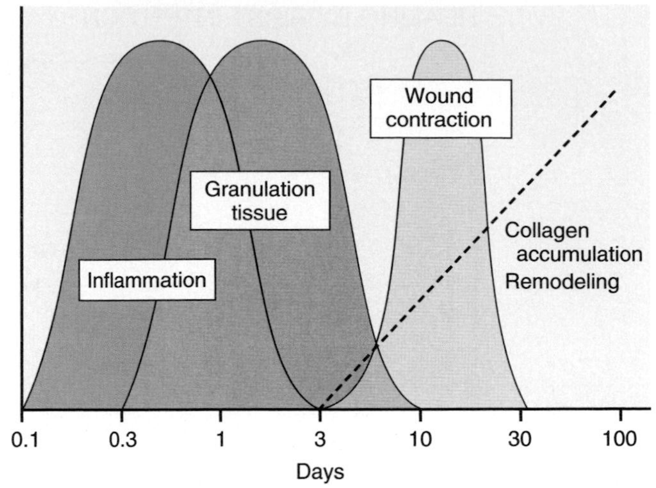

FIGURE 3–20 Phases of wound healing. (Modified from Clark RAF: Wound repair. In Clark RAF (ed): The molecular and cellular biology of wound repair, 2nd ed, New York, Plenum Press, 1996, p. 3.)

Cutaneous wound healing is generally divided into three phases: (1) inflammation (early and late); (2) granulation tissue formation and reepithelialization; and (3) wound contraction, ECM deposition, and remodeling (Fig. 3–20). These phases overlap, and their separation is somewhat arbitrary. Nevertheless, they help understand the sequence of events in wound healing. As already indicated, wound healing is a fibroproliferative response that is mediated through growth factors and cytokines. Growth factors and cytokines involved in cutaneous wound healing and their effects are listed in Table 3–1. Table 3–4 lists the main growth factors and cytokines affecting various steps in wound healing.[114–116]

Skin wounds are classically described to heal by primary or secondary intention. As will be discussed below, this distinction is based on the nature of the wound rather than the healing process itself.

HEALING BY FIRST INTENTION (WOUNDS WITH OPPOSED EDGES)

The least complicated example of wound repair is the healing of a clean, uninfected surgical incision approximated by surgical sutures (Fig. 3–21). Such healing is referred to as

TABLE 3–4 Growth Factors and Cytokines Affecting Various Steps in Wound Healing

Monocyte chemotaxis	PDGF, FGF, TGF-β
Fibroblast migration	PDGF, EGF, FGF, TGF-β, TNF, IL-1
Fibroblast proliferation	PDGF, EGF, FGF, TNF
Angiogenesis	VEGF, Ang, FGF
Collagen synthesis	TGF-β, PDGF
Collagenase secretion	PDGF, FGF, EGF, TNF, TGF-β inhibits

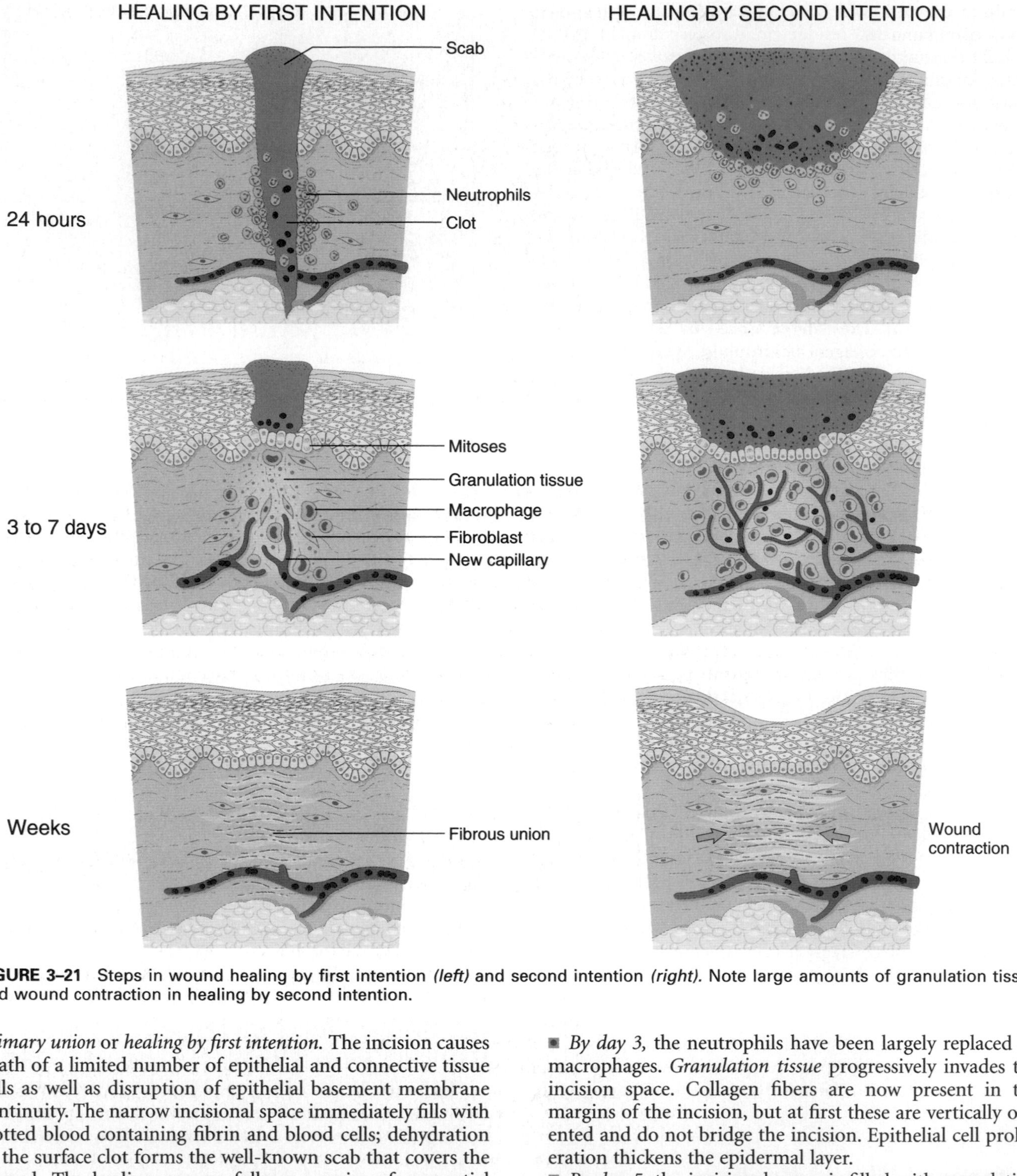

FIGURE 3–21 Steps in wound healing by first intention *(left)* and second intention *(right).* Note large amounts of granulation tissue and wound contraction in healing by second intention.

primary union or *healing by first intention.* The incision causes death of a limited number of epithelial and connective tissue cells as well as disruption of epithelial basement membrane continuity. The narrow incisional space immediately fills with clotted blood containing fibrin and blood cells; dehydration of the surface clot forms the well-known scab that covers the wound. The healing process follows a series of sequential steps:

- *Within 24 hours,* neutrophils appear at the margins of the incision, moving toward the fibrin clot. In 24 to 48 hours, spurs of epithelial cells move from the wound edges (with little cell proliferation) along the cut margins of the dermis, depositing basement membrane components as they move.[114] They fuse in the midline beneath the surface scab, producing a continuous but thin epithelial layer that closes the wound.
- *By day 3,* the neutrophils have been largely replaced by macrophages. *Granulation tissue* progressively invades the incision space. Collagen fibers are now present in the margins of the incision, but at first these are vertically oriented and do not bridge the incision. Epithelial cell proliferation thickens the epidermal layer.
- *By day 5,* the incisional space is filled with granulation tissue. Neovascularization is maximal. Collagen fibrils become more abundant and begin to bridge the incision. The epidermis recovers its normal thickness, and differentiation of surface cells yields a mature epidermal architecture with surface keratinization.
- *During the second week,* there is continued accumulation of collagen and proliferation of fibroblasts. The leukocytic infiltrate, edema, and increased vascularity have largely disappeared. At this time, the long process of blanching begins, accomplished by the increased accumulation of collagen

within the incisional scar, accompanied by regression of vascular channels.

- *By the end of the first month*, the scar is made up of a cellular connective tissue devoid of inflammatory infiltrate, covered now by intact epidermis. The dermal appendages that have been destroyed in the line of the incision are permanently lost. Tensile strength of the wound increases thereafter, but it may take months for the wounded area to obtain its maximal strength.

HEALING BY SECOND INTENTION (WOUNDS WITH SEPARATED EDGES)

When there is more extensive loss of cells and tissue, as in surface wounds that create large defects, the reparative process is more complicated. Regeneration of parenchymal cells cannot completely restore the original architecture, and hence abundant granulation tissue grows in from the margin to complete the repair. This form of healing is referred to as *secondary union* or *healing by second intention* (see Figs. 3–21 and 3–22). Secondary healing differs from primary healing in several respects:

- Inevitably, large tissue defects generate a larger fibrin clot that fills the defect and more necrotic debris and exudate that must be removed. Consequently the *inflammatory reaction is more intense.*
- *Much larger amounts of granulation tissue are formed.*
- Perhaps the feature that most clearly differentiates primary from secondary healing is the phenomenon of *wound contraction*, which occurs in large surface wounds. Large defects in the skin of a rabbit are reduced in approximately 6 weeks, to 5% to 10% of their original size, largely by contraction. The initial steps of wound contraction involve the formation of a network of actin-containing fibroblasts at the edge of the wound. Permanent wound contraction requires the action of *myofibroblasts*—altered fibroblasts that have the ultrastructural characteristics of smooth muscle cells.[118] Contraction of these cells at the wound site decreases the gap between the dermal edges of the wound.
- Substantial scar formation and thinning of the epidermis.

WOUND STRENGTH

How long does it take for a skin wound to achieve its maximal strength, and what substances contribute to this strength? When sutures are removed, usually at the end of the first week, wound strength is approximately 10% that of unwounded skin, but strength increases rapidly over the next 4 weeks. This rate of increase then slows at approximately the

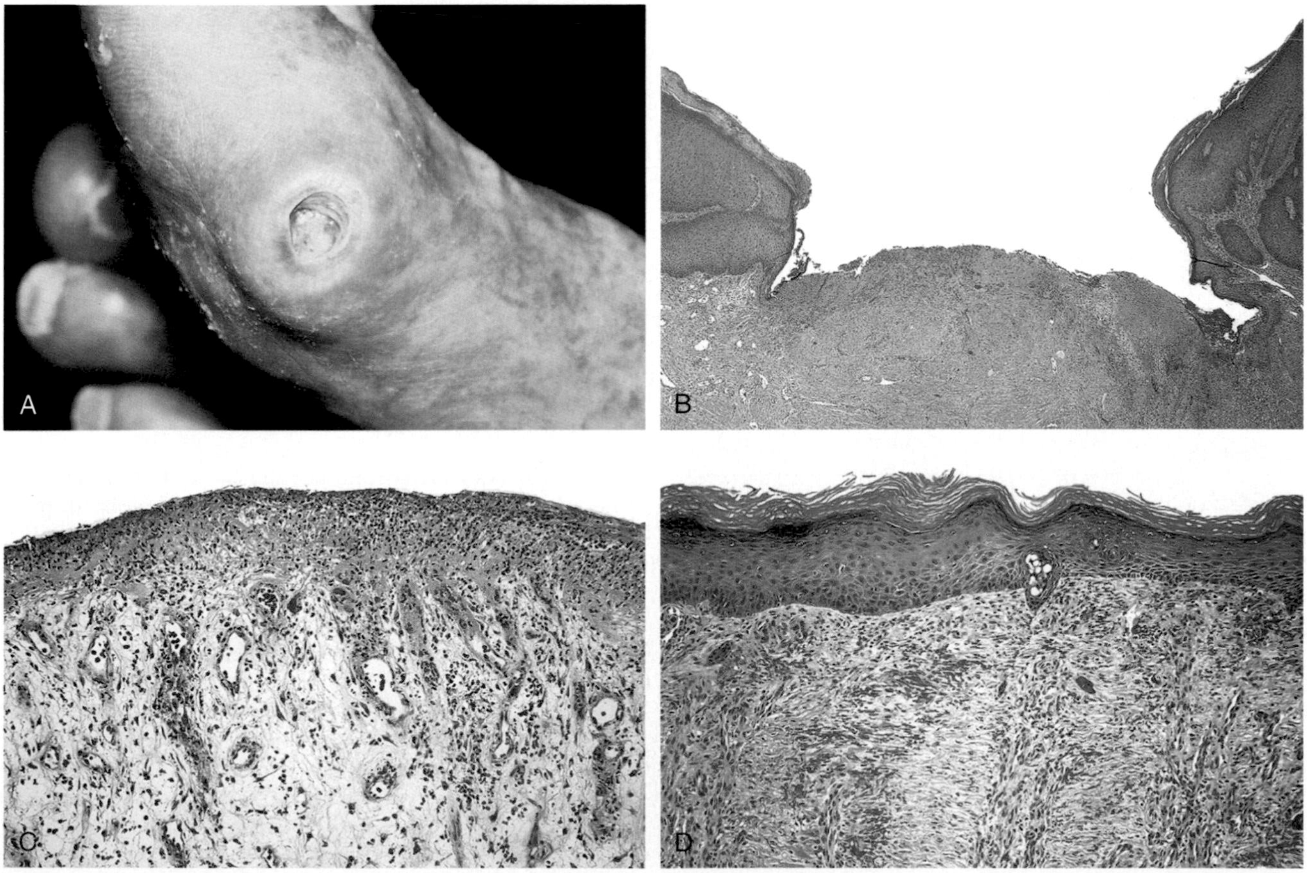

FIGURE 3–22 Healing of skin ulcers. *A,* Pressure ulcer of the skin, commonly found in diabetic patients. The histology slides show *B,* a skin ulcer with a large gap between the edges of the lesion; *C,* a thin layer of epidermal reepithelialization and extensive granulation tissue formation in the dermis; and *D,* continuing reepithelialization of the epidermis and wound contraction. (Courtesy of Z. Argenyi, M.D., University of Washington.)

third month after the original incision, and reaches a plateau at about 70% to 80% of the tensile strength of unwounded skin, a condition that may persist for life. The recovery of tensile strength results from the excess of collagen synthesis over collagen degradation during the first 2 months of healing, and, at later times, from structural modifications of collagen fibers (cross-linking, increased fiber size) after collagen synthesis ceases.[119]

LOCAL AND SYSTEMIC FACTORS THAT INFLUENCE WOUND HEALING

We have discussed the usual manifestations of repair and reviewed the orderly healing of wounds in healthy persons. Healing is modified by a number of known influences and some unknown ones, frequently impairing the quality and adequacy of both inflammation and repair. These influences include both *systemic and local host factors* (Table 3–5). Systemic factors include the following:

- *Nutrition* has profound effects on wound healing. Protein deficiency, for example, and particularly vitamin C deficiency, inhibit collagen synthesis and retard healing.
- *Metabolic status* can change wound healing. Diabetes mellitus, for example, is associated with delayed healing, as a consequence of the microangiopathy that is a frequent feature of this disease (Chapter 24).
- *Circulatory status* can modulate wound healing. *Inadequate blood supply*, usually caused by arteriosclerosis or venous abnormalities (e.g. varicose veins) that retard venous drainage, also impair healing.
- *Hormones*, such as *glucocorticoids*, have well-documented anti-inflammatory effects that influence various components of inflammation. These agents also inhibit collagen synthesis.

Local factors that influence healing include the following:

- *Infection* is the single most important cause of delay in healing because it results in persistent tissue injury and inflammation.
- *Mechanical factors*, such as early motion of wounds, can delay healing, by compressing blood vessels and separating the edges of the wound.
- *Foreign bodies*, such as unnecessary sutures or fragments of steel, glass, or even bone, constitute impediments to healing.
- *Size, location, and type of wound influence healing.* Wounds in richly vascularized areas, such as the face, heal faster than those in poorly vascularized ones, such as the foot. As we have discussed, small incisional injuries heal faster and with less scar formation than large excisional wounds or wounds caused by blunt trauma.

TABLE 3–5 Factors That Retard Wound Healing

Local Factors	
Blood supply	Mechanical stress
Denervation	Necrotic tissue
Local infection	Protection (dressings)
Foreign body	Surgical techniques
Hematoma	Type of tissue
Systemic Factors	
Age	Malnutrition
Anemia	Obesity
Drugs (steroids, cytotoxic medications, intensive antibiotic therapy)	Systemic infection
	Temperature
	Trauma, hypovolemia, and hypoxia
Genetic disorders (osteogenesis imperfecta, Ehlers-Danlos syndromes, Marfan syndrome)	Uremia
	Vitamin deficiency (vitamin C)
Hormones	Trace metal deficiency (zinc, copper)
Diabetes	
Malignant disease	

Adapted from Schwartz SI: Principles of Surgery. New York, McGraw Hill, 1999.

SUMMARY OF CUTANEOUS WOUND HEALING

Various stages in the healing of an ulcer of the skin are shown in Figure 3–22. The healing wound, as a prototype of tissue repair, is a dynamic and changing process. The early phase is one of inflammation, followed by formation of granulation tissue and subsequent tissue remodeling and scarring. Simple cutaneous incisional wounds heal by first intention. Large cutaneous wounds heal by second intention, generating a significant amount of scar tissue. Different mechanisms occurring at different times trigger the release of chemical signals that modulate the orderly migration, proliferation, and differentiation of cells and the synthesis and degradation of ECM proteins. These proteins, in turn, directly affect cellular events and modulate cell responsiveness to soluble growth factors. The magic behind the precise orchestration of these events under normal conditions remains beyond our grasp. It almost certainly lies in the regulation of specific soluble and membrane-anchored mediators and their receptors on particular cells, cell–matrix interactions, and the effect of physical factors, including ECM remodeling forces generated by changes in cell shape.

COMPLICATIONS IN CUTANEOUS WOUND HEALING

Complications in wound healing can arise from abnormalities in any of the basic components of the repair process. These aberrations can be grouped into three general categories: (1) *deficient scar formation*, (2) *excessive formation of the repair components*, and (3) *formation of contractures.*

Inadequate formation of granulation tissue or assembly of a scar can lead to two types of complications: *wound dehiscence* and *ulceration.* Dehiscence or rupture of a wound is most common after abdominal surgery and is due to increased abdominal pressure. This mechanical stress on the abdominal wound can be generated by vomiting, coughing, or ileus. Wounds can ulcerate because of inadequate vascularization during healing. For example, lower extremity wounds in individuals with atherosclerotic peripheral vascular disease typically ulcerate (Chapter 11). Nonhealing wounds also form in areas devoid of sensation. These neuropathic ulcers are occasionally seen in patients with diabetic peripheral neuropathy (Chapters 24 and 27).

Excessive formation of the components of the repair process can also complicate wound healing. Aberrations of growth may occur even in what may begin initially as normal wound healing. The accumulation of excessive amounts of collagen may give rise to a raised scar known as a *hypertrophic scar*; if the scar tissue grows beyond the boundaries of the original wound and does not regress, it is called a *keloid* (Fig. 3–23). Keloid formation appears to be an individual predisposition, and for unknown reasons this aberration is somewhat more common in African-Americans. The mechanisms of keloid formation are still unknown. Another deviation in wound healing is the formation of excessive amounts of granulation tissue, which protrudes above the level of the surrounding skin and blocks re-epithelialization. This has been called *exuberant granulation* (or, with more literary fervor, *proud flesh*). Excessive granulation must be removed by cautery or surgical excision to permit restoration of the continuity of the epithelium. Finally (fortunately rarely), incisional scars or traumatic injuries may be followed by exuberant proliferation of fibroblasts and other connective tissue elements that may, in fact, recur after excision. Called *desmoids*, or *aggressive fibromatoses*, these lie in the interface between benign proliferations and malignant (though low-grade) tumors. The line between the benign hyperplasias characteristic of repair and neoplasia is frequently finely drawn (Chapter 7).

Contraction in the size of a wound is an important part of the normal healing process. An exaggeration of this process is called a *contracture* and results in deformities of the wound and the surrounding tissues. Contractures are particularly prone to develop on the palms, the soles, and the anterior aspect of the thorax. Contractures are commonly seen after serious burns and can compromise the movement of joints. Impaired wound contraction occurs in stromelysin-1 (MMP3)—deficient mice, suggesting that proteolysis by this metalloproteinase is required for the assembly of fibroblasts containing actin filaments, needed for the contraction of early wounds.[120]

Fibrosis

The mechanisms underlying the formation of a cutaneous scar—cell proliferation, cell–cell interactions, cell–matrix interactions, and ECM deposition—are similar to those that occur in the fibrosis associated with chronic inflammatory diseases such as rheumatoid arthritis, lung fibrosis, and hepatic cirrhosis. In contrast to orderly wound healing, however, these diseases are associated with persistence of the initial stimuli for fibrosis or the development of immune and autoimmune reactions (Fig. 3–24). In such reactions, lymphocyte–monocyte interactions sustain the synthesis and secretion of growth factors and fibrogenic cytokines, proteolytic enzymes, and other biologically active molecules. Collagen degradation by collagenases, for example, which is important in the normal remodeling of healing wounds, causes much of the joint destruction in rheumatoid arthritis (Chapter 26). In liver cirrhosis caused by chronic alcoholism or infection with hepatitis B or C viruses, hepatic stellate cells are activated and produce collagen. The deposition of collagen in the liver parenchyma and the changes in the structure of sinusoids caused by deposition of ECM components greatly alter liver structure and function, leading to cirrhosis (Chapter 18). Fibrosis is a hallmark of the chronic interstitial lung diseases known as pneumoconiosis, caused by the inhalation of mineral dusts (discussed in Chapter 15). In such conditions, which are usually the consequence of inhalation of coal, asbestos or silica, macrophages play an important role in fibrogenesis. These cells became activated by engulfing mineral particles and secrete cytokines and growth factors that promote fibrosis. A common cause of organ fibrosis is ionizing radiation, used for cancer treatment. Delayed fibrosis may occur in the lungs, gastrointestinal tract, kidney, and other organs after radiation therapy (see Chapter 9). In chronic pancreatitis, repeated bouts of acute pancreatic inflammation lead to loss of pancreatic acinar cells and replacement by fibrous tissue (Chapter 19).

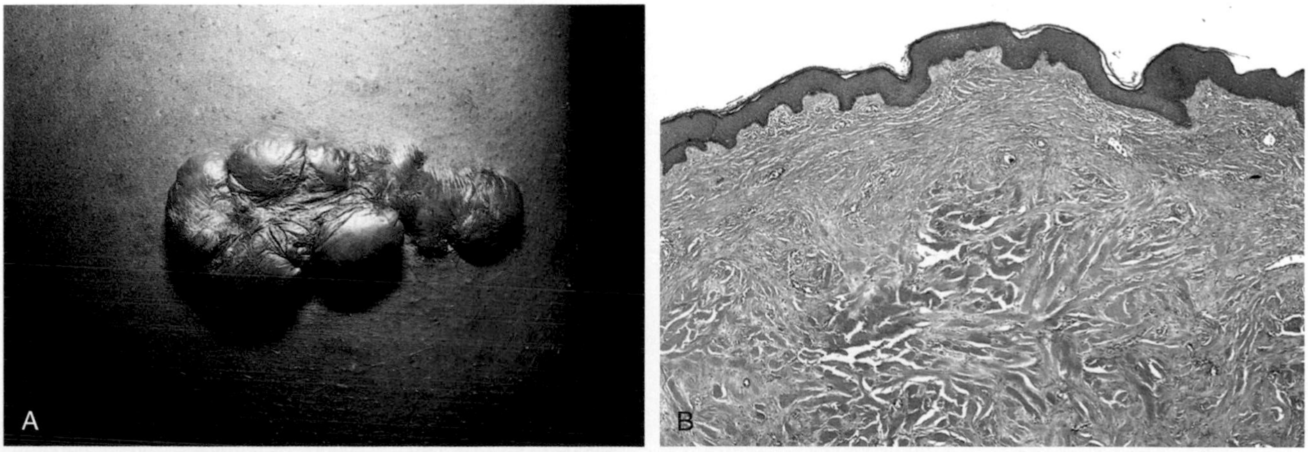

FIGURE 3–23 *A*, Keloid. Excess collagen deposition in the skin forming a raised scar known as keloid. (From Murphy GF, Herzberg AJ: Atlas of Dermatopathology. Philadelphia, Saunders, W.B. 1996, p. 219.) *B*, Note the thick connective tissue deposition in the dermis. (Slide courtesy of Z. Argenyi, M.D., University of Washington, Seattle, WA.)

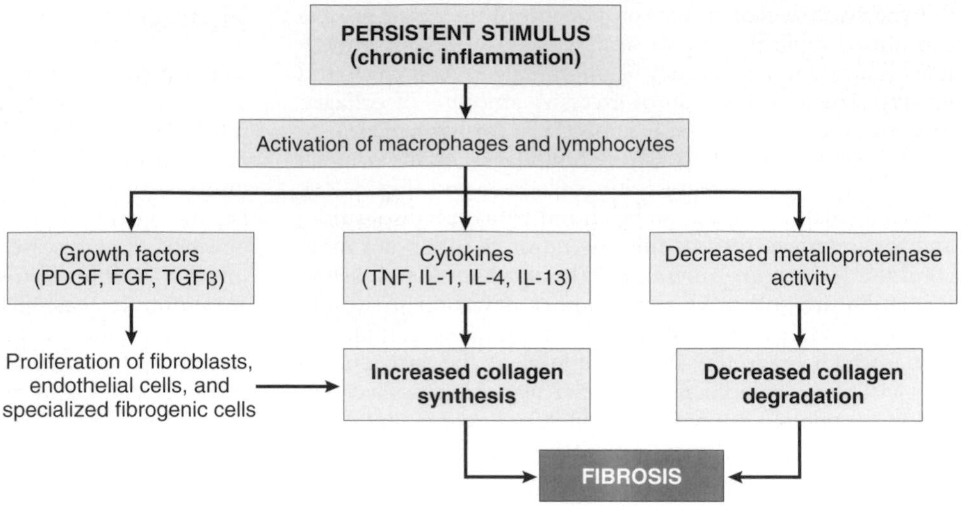

FIGURE 3–24 Development of fibrosis in chronic inflammation. The persistent stimulus of chronic inflammation activates macrophages and lymphocytes, leading to the production of growth factors and cytokines, which increase the synthesis of collagen. Deposition of collagen is enhanced by decreased activity of metalloproteinases.

Overview of Repair Responses After Injury and Inflammation

This concludes the discussion, begun in Chapter 1, of cellular and tissue injury, the reaction to such injury by inflammation (Chapter 2), and the tissue repair events underlying regeneration, healing, and fibrosis. At this point, a backward look may help relate the multitude of outcomes in various forms of injury (Fig. 3–25). Not all injuries result in permanent damage; some are resolved with almost perfect return of normal structure and function. As we have seen, the liver can regenerate after partial resection or acute necrotic injury, and superficial skin wounds heal with complete restitution of normal structures. Restitution may even occur in some types of inflammatory conditions such as lobar pneumonia, in which the abundant inflammatory exudate is resorbed. More often, however, the injury and inflammatory response may become organized with formation of granulation tissue (e.g., in fibrinous pericarditis and peritonitis) and scarring. Although it is functionally imperfect, scarring provides a permanent patch that permits the residual parenchyma to more or less continue functioning. Sometimes, however, the scar itself is so large or so situated that it may cause permanent dysfunction, as in a healed myocardial infarct. In this case, the fibrous tissue not only represents a loss of preexisting contractile muscle, but also constitutes a permanent burden to the overworked residual muscle. In chronic inflammation, persistent injury commonly results in tissue destruction and scarring, as for instance in liver cirrhosis, chronic pancreatitis, and the pneumoconioses. The processes of inflammation and repair underscore the remarkable capacity of the human body to restore itself, far surpassing any device conceived by humans.

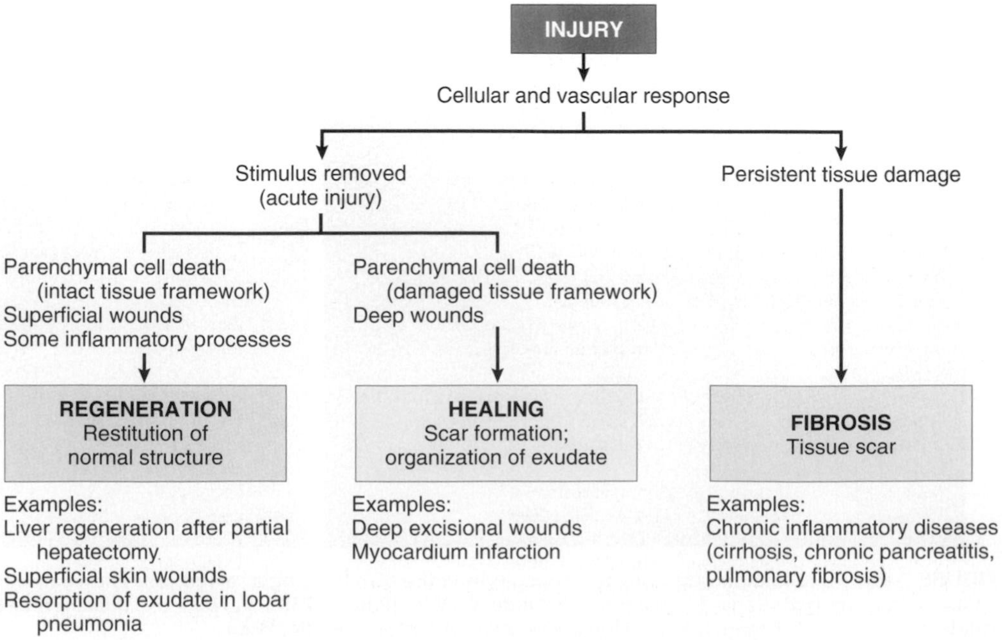

FIGURE 3–25 Repair responses after injury and inflammation. Repair after acute injury has several outcomes, including normal tissue restitution and healing with scar formation. Healing in chronic injury involves scar formation and fibrosis (see text).

REFERENCES

1. Goss RJ: Regeneration versus repair. In Cohen IK, Diegelman RF, Lindblad WJ (eds): Wound Healing. Biochemical and Clinical Aspects. Philadelphia, W.B. Saunders, 1992, pp 20–39.
2. Clark RAF: Wound repair. In Clark RAF (ed): The Molecular and Cellular Biology of Wound Repair, 2nd ed. New York, Plenum Press, 1996, pp 3–50.
3. Fausto N: Liver regeneration, in Arias I. M., et al (eds): The Liver: Biology and Pathobiology, 4th ed. Philadelphia, Lippicott, Williams & Wilkins, 2001, pp 591–610.
4. Mullauer L, et al: Mutations in apoptosis genes: a pathogenetic factor for human disease. Mutat Res 488:211, 2001.
5. Hanahan D, Weinberg RA: The hallmarks of cancer. Cell 100:57, 2000.
6. Rosenthal N: Prometheus's vulture and the stem-cell promise. N Engl J Med 349:267, 2003.
7. Korbling M, Estrov Z: Adult stem cells for tissue repair—a new therapeutic concept? N Engl J Med 349:570, 2003.
8. Weissman IL, Anderson DJ, Gage F: Stem and progenitor cells: origins, phenotypes, lineage commitments, and transdifferentiations. Annu Rev Cell Dev Biol 17:387, 2001.
9. Tsai RY, Kittappa R, McKay RD: Plasticity, niches, and the use of stem cells. Dev Cell 2:707, 2002.
10. Fuchs E, Segre JA: Stem cells: a new lease on life. Cell 100:143–155, 2000.
11. Weissman I: Stem cells: units of development, units of regeneration, and units in evolution. Cell 100:157, 2000.
12. Martin GR: Isolation of a pluripotent cell line from early mouse embryos cultured in medium conditioned by teratocarcinoma stem cells. Proc Natl Acad Sci USA 78:7634, 1981.
13. Hadjantonakis A, Papaioannou V: The stem cells of early embryos. Differentiation 68:159, 2001.
14. Murray P, Edgar D: The regulation of embryonic stem cell differentiation by leukaemia inhibitory factor (LIF). Differentiation 68:227, 2001.
15. Cavaleri F, Scholer HR: Nanog: a new recruit to the embryonic stem cell orchestra. Cell 113:551, 2003.

15a. Sato N, et al: Maintenance of pluripotency in human and mouse embryonic stem cells through activation of Wnt signaling by a pharmacological GSK-3-specific inhibitor. Nature Med 10:55, 2004.

16. Hochedlinger K, Jaenisch R: Nuclear transplantation, embryonic stem cells, and the potential for cell therapy. N Engl J Med 349:275, 2003.
17. Watt FM, Hogan BL: Out of Eden: stem cells and their niches. Science 287:1427, 2000.
18. Marshman E, Booth C, Potten CS: The intestinal epithelial stem cell. Bioessays 24:91, 2002.
19. Lavker RM, Sun TT: Epidermal stem cells: properties, markers, and location. Proc Natl Acad Sci USA 97:13473, 2000.
20. Alonso L, Fuchs E: Stem cells in the skin: waste not, Wnt not. Genes Dev 17:1189, 2003.
21. Tseng SCG, Sun-T-T: Stem cells: ocular surface maintenance. In Brightbill FS (ed): Corneal Surgery: Theory, Techniques and Tissue, 3rd ed. New York, Mosby, 1999, pp 9–18.
22. Verfaillie CM: Hematopoietic stem cells for transplantation. Nat Immunol 3:314, 2002.
23. Orkin SH, Morrison SJ: Stem-cell competition. Nature 418:25, 2002.
24. Lagasse E, et al: Purified hematopoietic stem cells can differentiate into hepatocytes in vivo. Nat Med 6:1229, 2000.
25. LaBarge MA, Blau HM: Biological progression from adult bone marrow to mononucleate muscle stem cell to multinucleate muscle fiber in response to injury. Cell 111:589, 2002.
26. Laflamme MA, et al: Evidence for cardiomyocyte repopulation by extracardiac progenitors in transplanted human hearts. Circ Res 90:634, 2002.
27. Wagers AJ, et al: Little evidence for developmental plasticity of adult hematopoietic stem cells. Science 297:2256, 2002.
28. Lemischka I: A few thoughts about the plasticity of stem cells. Exp Hematol 30:848, 2002.
29. Wang X, et al: Cell fusion is the principal source of bone-marrow–derived hepatocytes. Nature 422:897, 2003.
30. Vassilopoulos G, Wang PR, Russell DW: Transplanted bone marrow regenerates liver by cell fusion. Nature 24:901, 2003.
31. Jiang Y, et al: Pluripotency of mesenchymal stem cells derived from adult marrow. Nature 418:41, 2002.
32. Jiang Y, et al: Multipotent progenitor cells can be isolated from postnatal murine bone marrow, muscle, and brain. Exp Hematol 30:896, 2002.
33. Toma JG, et al: Isolation of multipotent adult stem cells from the dermis of mammalian skin. Nat Cell Biol 3:778, 2001.
34. Dorshkind K: Stem cells and lineage plasticity: the challenge to existing paradigms. Immunol Rev 187:5, 2002.
35. Fausto N, Campbell JS: The role of hepatocytes and oval cells in liver regeneration and repopulation. Mech Dev 120:117, 2003.
36. Libbrecht L, Roskams T: Hepatic progenitor cells in human liver diseases. Semin Cell Dev Biol 13:389, 2002.
37. Taupin P, Gage FH: Adult neurogenesis and neural stem cells of the central nervous system in mammals. J Neurosci Res 69:745, 2002.
38. Lois C, Alvarez-Buylla A: Proliferating subventricular zone cells in the adult mammalian forebrain can differentiate into neurons and glia. Virology 90:2074, 1993.
39. Pagano SF, et al: Isolation and characterization of neural stem cells from the adult human olfactory bulb. Stem Cells 18:295, 2000.
40. Panchision DM, McKay RD: The control of neural stem cells by morphogenic signals. Curr Opin Genet Dev 12:478, 2002.
41. van Praag H, et al: Functional neurogenesis in the adult hippocampus. 415:1030, 2002.
42. Zammit P, Beauchamp J: The skeletal muscle satellite cell: stem cell or son of stem cell? Differentiation 68:193, 2001.
43. Urbanek K, et al: Intense myocyte formation from cardiac stem cells in human cardiac hypertrophy. Proc Natl Acad Sci USA, 100:10440, 2003.
44. Carpenter G: The EGF receptor: a nexus for trafficking and signaling. Bioessays 22:697–707, 2000.
45. Zarnegar R, DeFrances MC, Michalopoulos GK: Hepatocyte growth factor: its role in hepatic growth and pathobiology. In Arias IM, et al (eds): The Liver: Biology and Pathobiology, 4th ed. Philadelphia, Lippincott, Williams & Wilkins, 2001, pp 611–629.
46. Ferrara N, Gerber HP, LeCouter J: The biology of VEGF and its receptors. Nat Med 9:669, 2003.
47. Heldin CH, Eriksson U, Ostman A: New members of the platelet-derived growth factor family of mitogens. Arch Biochem Biophys 398:284, 2002.
48. Zaret KS: Hepatocyte differentiation: from the endoderm and beyond. Curr Opin Genet Dev 11:568, 2001.
49. Massague J: How cells read TGF-β signals. Nature 1:169, 2000.
50. Attisano L, Wrana JL: Signal transduction by the TGF-β superfamily. Science 296:1646, 2002.
51. Moustakas A, et al: Mechanisms of TGF-β signaling in regulation of cell growth and differentiation. Immunol Lett 82:85, 2002.
52. Chang L, Karin M: Mammalian MAP kinase signalling cascades. Nature 410:37, 2001.
53. Garrington TP, Johnson GL: Organization and regulation of mitogen-activated protein kinase signaling pathways. Curr Opin Cell Biol 11:211, 1999.
54. Cantley LC: The phosphoinositide 3-kinase pathway. Science 296:1655, 2002.
55. Lawlor MA, Alessi DR: PKB/Akt: a key mediator of cell proliferation, survival and insulin responses? J Cell Sci 114:2903, 2001.
56. Wilkinson MG, Millar JB: Control of the eukaryotic cell cycle by MAP kinase signaling pathways. FASEB J 14:2147, 2000.
57. Aaronson DS, Horvath CM: A road map for those who don't know JAK-STAT. Science 296:1653, 2002.
58. Levy DE, Darnell JEJ: Stats: transcriptional control and biological impact. Nat Rev Mol Cell Biol 3:651, 2002.
59. Neves SR, Ram PT, Iyengar R: G protein pathways. Science 296:1636, 2002.
60. Pierce KL, Premont RT, Lefkowitz RJ: Seven-transmembrane receptors. Nat Rev Mol Cell Biol 3:639, 2002.
61. Berridge MJ, Lipp P, Bootman MD: The versatility and universality of calcium signalling. Nat Rev Mol Cell Biol 1:11, 2000.
62. Bootman MD, Berridge MJ, Roderick HL: Calcium signalling: more messengers, more channels, more complexity. Curr Biol 12:R563, 2002.
63. Farfel Z, Bourne HR, Iiri T: The expanding spectrum of G protein diseases. N Engl J Med 340:1012, 1999.
64. Beato M, Klug J: Steroid hormone receptors: an update. Hum Reprod Update 6:225, 2000.
65. McDonnell DP, Norris JD: Connections and regulation of the human estrogen receptor. Science 296:1642, 2002.

66. Qi C, Zhu Y, Reddy JK: Peroxisome proliferator–activated receptors, coactivators, and downstream targets. Cell Biochem Biophys 32:187, 2000.
67. Ryan KM, Phillips AC, Vousden KH: Regulation and function of the p53 tumor suppressor protein. Curr Opin Cell Biol 13:332, 2001.
68. Shaulian E, Karin M: AP-1 as a regulator of cell life and death. Nat Cell Biol 4:E131, 2002.
69. Lundberg AS, Weinberg RA: Control of the cell cycle and apoptosis. Eur J Cancer 35:1886, 1999.
70. Pietenpol JA, Stewart ZA: Cell cycle checkpoint signaling: cell cycle arrest versus apoptosis. Toxicology 181–182:475, 2002.
71. Agami R, Bernards R: Convergence of mitogenic and DNA damage signaling in the G_1 phase of the cell cycle. Cancer Lett 177:111, 2002.
72. Ekholm SV, Reed SI: Regulation of G_1 cyclin-dependent kinases in the mammalian cell cycle. Curr Opin Cell Biol 12:676, 2000.
73. Bartek J, Lukas J: Mammalian G_1- and S-phase checkpoints in response to DNA damage. Curr Opin Cell Biol 13:738, 2001.
74. Walworth NC: Cell-cycle checkpoint kinases: checking in on the cell cycle. Curr Opin Cell Biol 12:697, 2000.
75. Brockes JP, Kumar A: Plasticity and reprogramming of differentiated cells in amphibian regeneration. Nat Rev Mol Cell Biol 3:566, 2002.
76. Tanaka EM: Regeneration: if they can do it, why can't we? Cell 113:559, 2003.
77. Bonner-Weir S: Life and death of the pancreatic beta cells. Trends Endocrinol Metab 11:375, 2000.
78. Kritzik MR, et al: Transcription factor expression during pancreatic islet regeneration. Mol Cell Endocrinol 164:99, 2000.
79. Fausto N: Liver regeneration. J Hepatol 32:19, 2000.
80. Su AI, et al: Gene expression during the priming phase of liver regeneration after partial hepatectomy in mice. Proc Natl Acad Sci USA 99:11181, 2002.
81. Michalopoulos GK, DeFrances MC: Liver regeneration. Science 276:60, 1997.
82. Sanes JR: The basement membrane/basal lamina of skeletal muscle. J Biol Chem 278:12601, 2003.
83. Byers PH: Disorders of collagen biosynthesis and structure. In Scriver CR, et al (eds): The Metabolic & Molecular Basis of Inherited Disease. New York, McGraw-Hill, 2001, pp. 5241–5249.
84. Myllyharju J, Kivirikko KI: Collagens and collagen-related diseases. Ann Med 33:7, 2001.
85. Milewicz DM, Urban Z, Boyd C: Genetic disorders of the elastic fiber system. Matrix Biol 19:471, 2000.
86. Robinson PN, Booms P: The molecular pathogenesis of the Marfan syndrome. Cell Mol Life Sci 58:1698, 2001.
87. Hynes R: Integrins: bidirectional, allosteric signaling machines. Cell 110:673, 2002.
88. Stupack DG, Cheresh DA: Get a ligand, get a life: integrins, signaling and cell survival. J Cell Sci 115:3729, 2002.
89. Bradshaw AD, Sage EH: SPARC, a matricellular protein that functions in cellular differentiation and tissue response to injury. J Clin Invest 107:1049, 2001.
90. Sodek J, et al: Novel functions of the matricellular proteins osteopontin and osteonectin/SPARC. Connect Tissue Res 43:308, 2002.
91. Sugahara K, Kitagawa H: Recent advances in the study of the biosynthesis and functions of sulfated glycosaminoglycans. Curr Opin Struct Biol 10:518, 2000.
92. Toole BP, Wight TN, Tammi MI: Hyaluronan–cell interactions in cancer and vascular disease. J Biol Chem 277:4593, 2002.
93. Ponta H, Sherman L, Herrlich PA: CD44: from adhesion molecules to signalling regulators. Nat Rev Mol Cell Biol 4:33, 2003.
94. Carmeliet P: Angiogenesis in health and disease. Nat Med 9:653, 2003.
95. Conway EM, Collen D, Carmeliet P: Molecular mechanisms of blood vessel growth. Cardiovasc Res 49:507, 2001.
96. Kubo H, Alitalo K: The bloody fate of endothelial stem cells. Genes Dev 17:322, 2003.
97. Rafii S, et al: Contribution of marrow-derived progenitors to vascular and cardiac regeneration. Semin Cell Dev Biol 13:61, 2002.
98. Reyes M, et al: Origin of endothelial progenitors in human postnatal bone marrow. J Clin Invest 109:337, 2002.
99. Hill JM, et al: Circulating endothelial progenitor cells, vascular function, and cardiovascular risk. N Engl J Med 348:593, 2003.
100. Blasi F, Carmeliet P: uPAR: a versatile signalling orchestrator. Nat Rev Mol Cell Biol 3:932, 2002.
101. Jain RK: Molecular regulation of vessel maturation. Nat Med 9:685, 2003.
102. Folkman J: Role of angiogenesis in tumor growth and metastasis. Semin Oncol 29:15, 2002.
103. Vikkula M, Boon LM, Mulliken JB: Molecular genetics of vascular malformations. Matrix Biol 20:327, 2001.
104. Iivanainen E, Kahari VM, Heino J, et al: Endothelial cell–matrix interactions. Microsc Res Tech 60:13, 2003.
105. Bornstein P, Sage EH: Matricellular proteins: extracellular modulators of cell function. Curr Opin Cell Biol 14:608, 2002.
106. O'Reilly MS, et al: Endostatin: an endogenous inhibitor of angiogenesis and tumor growth. Cell 88:277, 1997.
107. Dvorak HF: VPF/VEGF and the angiogenic response. Semin Perinatol 24:75, 2000.
108. Schnaper HW, et al: TGF-β signal transduction and mesangial cell fibrogenesis. Am J Physiol Renal Physiol 284:F243, 2003.
109. McCawley LJ, Matrisian LM: Matrix metalloproteinases: they're not just for matrix anymore! Curr Opin Cell Biol 13:534, 2001.
110. Vu TH, Werb Z: Matrix metalloproteinases: effectors of development and normal physiology. Genes Dev 14:2123, 2000.
111. Kheradmand F, Werb Z: Shedding light on sheddases: role in growth and development. Bioessays 24:8, 2002.
112. O'Kane S: Wound remodelling and scarring. J Wound Care 11:296, 2002.
113. McCallion RL, Ferguson MWJ: Fetal wound healing and the development of antiscarring therapies for adult wound healing. In Clark RAF (ed): The Molecular and Cellular Biology of Wound Repair, 2nd ed. New York, Plenum Press, 1996, pp 561–600.
114. Werner S, Grose R: Regulation of wound healing by growth factors and cytokines. Physicl Rev 83:835–870, 2003.
115. Cross KJ, Mustoe TA: Growth factors in wound healing. Surg Clin North Am 83:531–545, vi, 2003.
116. Henry G, Garner WL: Inflammatory mediators in wound healing. Surg Clin North Am 83:483–507, 2003.
117. Yates S, Rayner TE: Transcription factor activation in response to cutaneous injury: role of AP-1 in reepithelialization. Wound Repair Regen 10:5, 2002.
118. Serini G, Gabbiani G: Mechanisms of myofibroblast activity and phenotypic modulation. Exp Cell Res 250:273, 1999.
119. Tomasek JJ, et al: Myofibroblasts and mechano-regulation of connective tissue remodelling. Nat Rev Mol Cell Biol 3:349, 2002.
120. Bullard KM, et al: Impaired wound contraction in stromelysin-1–deficient mice. Ann Surg 230:260, 1999.

CHAPTER 4

Hemodynamic Disorders, Thromboembolic Disease, and Shock

Richard N. Mitchell, MD, PhD*

EDEMA

HYPEREMIA AND CONGESTION

HEMORRHAGE

HEMOSTASIS AND THROMBOSIS

Normal Hemostasis

Endothelium

Platelets

Coagulation Cascade

Thrombosis

Disseminated Intravascular Coagulation (DIC)

EMBOLISM

Pulmonary Thromboembolism

Systemic Thromboembolism

Fat Embolism

Air Embolism

Amniotic Fluid Embolism

INFARCTION

SHOCK

Pathogenesis of Septic Shock

The health of cells and organs critically depends on an unbroken circulation to deliver oxygen and nutrients and to remove wastes. However, the well-being of tissues also requires normal fluid balance; abnormalities in vascular permeability or hemostasis can result in injury even in the setting of an intact blood supply. This chapter will describe major disturbances involving hemodynamics and the maintenance of blood flow, including edema, hemorrhage, thrombosis, embolism, infarction, and shock. *Normal fluid homeostasis encompasses maintenance of vessel wall integrity as well as intravascular pressure and osmolarity within certain physiologic ranges.* Changes in vascular volume, pressure, or protein content, or alterations in endothelial function, all affect the net movement of water across the vascular wall. Such water extravasation into the interstitial spaces is called *edema* and has different manifestations depending on its location. In the lower extremities, edema mainly causes swelling; in the lungs, edema causes water to fill alveoli, leading to difficulty in breathing. *Normal fluid homeostasis also means maintaining blood as a liquid until such time as injury necessitates clot formation.* Clotting at inappropriate sites *(thrombosis)* or migration of clots *(embolism)* obstructs blood flow to tissues and leads to cell death *(infarction)*. Conversely, inability to clot after vascular injury results in *hemorrhage*; local bleeding can compromise regional tissue perfusion, while more extensive hemorrhage can result in hypotension *(shock)* and death.

Some of the failures of fluid homeostasis reflect a *primary* pathology in a discrete vascular bed (e.g., hemorrhage due to local trauma) or in systemic coagulation (thrombosis due to hypercoagulability disorders); others may represent a

*The contributions of the late Dr. Ramzi Cotran to this chapter in previous editions are gratefully acknowledged.

secondary manifestation of some other disease process. Thus, pulmonary edema due to increased hydrostatic pressure may be a terminal complication of ischemic or valvular heart disease. Similarly, shock may be the fatal sequela of infection. Overall, disturbances in normal blood flow are major sources of human morbidity and mortality; thrombosis, embolism, and infarction underlie three of the most important causes of pathology in Western society—myocardial infarction, pulmonary embolism, and cerebrovascular accident (stroke). Thus, the hemodynamic disorders described in this chapter are important in a wide spectrum of human disease.

Edema

Approximately 60% of lean body weight is water; two thirds of this water is intracellular, and the remainder is found in the extracellular space, mostly as interstitial fluid (only about 5% of total body water is in blood plasma). The term *edema* signifies increased fluid in the interstitial tissue spaces. In addition, depending on the site, fluid collections in the different body cavities are variously designated *hydrothorax, hydropericardium,* and *hydroperitoneum* (the last is more commonly called *ascites*). *Anasarca* is a severe and generalized edema with profound subcutaneous tissue swelling.

Table 4–1 lists the pathophysiologic categories of edema. The mechanisms of inflammatory edema are largely related to local increases in vascular permeability and are discussed in Chapter 2. The *noninflammatory causes of edema* are described in further detail below. Because of increased vascular permeability, inflammatory edema is a protein-rich *exudate*, with a specific gravity usually over 1.020. Conversely, the edema fluid occurring in hydrodynamic derangements is typically a protein-poor *transudate*, with a specific gravity below 1.012.

In general, the opposing effects of vascular hydrostatic pressure and plasma colloid osmotic pressure are the major factors that govern movement of fluid between vascular and interstitial spaces. Normally the exit of fluid into the interstitium from the arteriolar end of the microcirculation is nearly balanced by inflow at the venular end; a small residuum of excess interstitial fluid is drained by the lymphatics. *Either increased capillary pressure or diminished colloid osmotic pressure can result in increased interstitial fluid* (Fig. 4–1). As extravascular fluid accumulates, the increased tissue hydrostatic pressure and plasma colloid osmotic pressure eventually achieve a new equilibrium, and water reenters the venules. Any excess interstitial edema fluid is typically removed by lymphatic drainage, ultimately returning to the bloodstream via the thoracic duct (see Fig. 4–1); clearly, lymphatic obstruction (e.g., due to scarring or tumor) will also impair fluid drainage and result in edema. Finally, a primary retention of sodium (and its obligatory associated water) in renal disease also leads to edema.

Increased Hydrostatic Pressure. *Local increases* in hydrostatic pressure may result from impaired venous outflow. For example, *deep venous thrombosis* in the lower extremities leads to edema, which is restricted to the affected leg. *Generalized increases* in venous pressure, with resulting systemic edema, occur most commonly in *congestive heart failure* (Chapter 12) affecting right ventricular cardiac function.

TABLE 4–1 Pathophysiologic Categories of Edema

Increased Hydrostatic Pressure
Impaired venous return
Congestive heart failure
Constrictive pericarditis
Ascites (liver cirrhosis)
Venous obstruction or compression
Thrombosis
External pressure (e.g., mass)
Lower extremity inactivity with prolonged dependency
Arteriolar dilation
Heat
Neurohumoral dysregulation
Reduced Plasma Osmotic Pressure (Hypoproteinemia)
Protein-losing glomerulopathies (nephrotic syndrome)
Liver cirrhosis (ascites)
Malnutrition
Protein-losing gastroenteropathy
Lymphatic Obstruction
Inflammatory
Neoplastic
Postsurgical
Postirradiation
Sodium Retention
Excessive salt intake with renal insufficiency
Increased tubular reabsorption of sodium
Renal hypoperfusion
Increased renin-angiotensin-aldosterone secretion
Inflammation
Acute inflammation
Chronic inflammation
Angiogenesis

Modified from Leaf A, Cotran RS: Renal Pathophysiology, 3rd ed., New York, Oxford University Press, 1985, p 146. Used by permission of Oxford Press, Inc.

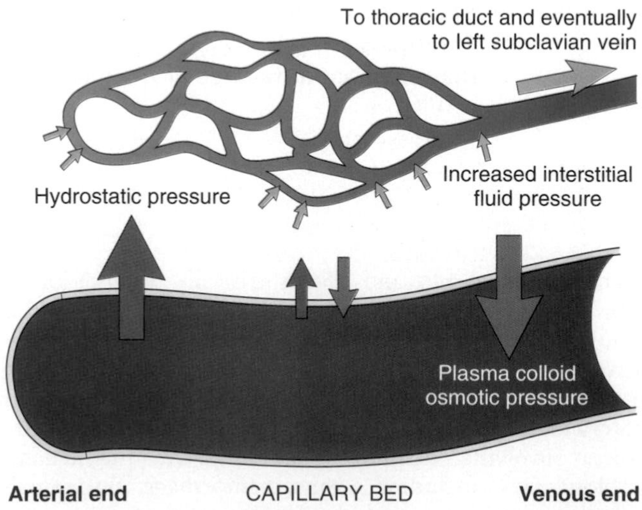

FIGURE 4–1 Factors affecting fluid balance across capillary walls. Capillary hydrostatic and osmotic forces are normally balanced so that there is no *net* loss or gain of fluid across the capillary bed. However, *increased* hydrostatic pressure or *diminished* plasma osmotic pressure leads to a net accumulation of extravascular fluid *(edema).* As the interstitial fluid pressure increases, tissue lymphatics remove much of the excess volume, eventually returning it to the circulation via the thoracic duct. If the ability of the lymphatics to drain tissue is exceeded, persistent tissue edema results.

Although increased venous hydrostatic pressure is important, the pathogenesis of cardiac edema is more complex (Fig. 4–2). Congestive heart failure is associated with reduced cardiac output and, therefore, reduced renal perfusion. Renal hypoperfusion, in turn, triggers the renin-angiotensin-aldosterone axis, inducing sodium and water retention by the kidneys *(secondary aldosteronism)*. This process is putatively designed to increase intravascular volume and thereby improve cardiac output (via the Frank-Starling law) with restoration of normal renal perfusion. If the failing heart cannot increase cardiac output, however, the extra fluid load results only in increased venous pressure and eventually edema.[1] Unless cardiac output is restored or renal water retention is reduced (e.g., by salt restriction, diuretics, or aldosterone antagonists), a cycle of renal fluid retention and worsening edema ensues. Although discussed here in the context of edema in congestive heart failure, salt restriction, diuretics, and aldosterone antagonists may also be used to manage generalized edema arising from a variety of other causes.

Reduced Plasma Osmotic Pressure. Reduced plasma osmotic pressure can result from excessive loss or reduced synthesis of albumin, the serum protein most responsible for maintaining colloid osmotic pressure. An important cause of albumin loss is the *nephrotic syndrome* (Chapter 20), characterized by a leaky glomerular capillary wall and generalized edema. Reduced albumin synthesis occurs in the setting of diffuse liver pathology (e.g., cirrhosis, Chapter 18) or as a consequence of protein malnutrition (Chapter 9). In each case, reduced plasma osmotic pressure leads to a net movement of fluid into the interstitial tissues and a resultant plasma volume contraction. Predictably, with reduced intravascular volume, renal hypoperfusion with secondary aldosteronism follows. The retained salt and water cannot correct the plasma volume deficit because the primary defect of low serum proteins persists. As with congestive heart failure, edema precipitated by *hypoproteinemia* is exacerbated by secondary salt and fluid retention.

Lymphatic Obstruction. Impaired lymphatic drainage and consequent *lymphedema* is usually localized; it can result from inflammatory or neoplastic obstruction. For example, the parasitic infection *filariasis* often causes massive lymphatic and lymph node fibrosis in the inguinal region. The resulting edema of the external genitalia and lower limbs is so extreme that it is called *elephantiasis*. Cancer of the breast may be treated by removal or irradiation (or both) of the breast and the associated axillary lymph nodes. The resection of the lymphatic channels as well as scarring related to the surgery and radiation can result in severe edema of the arm. In carcinoma of the breast, infiltration and obstruction of superficial lym-

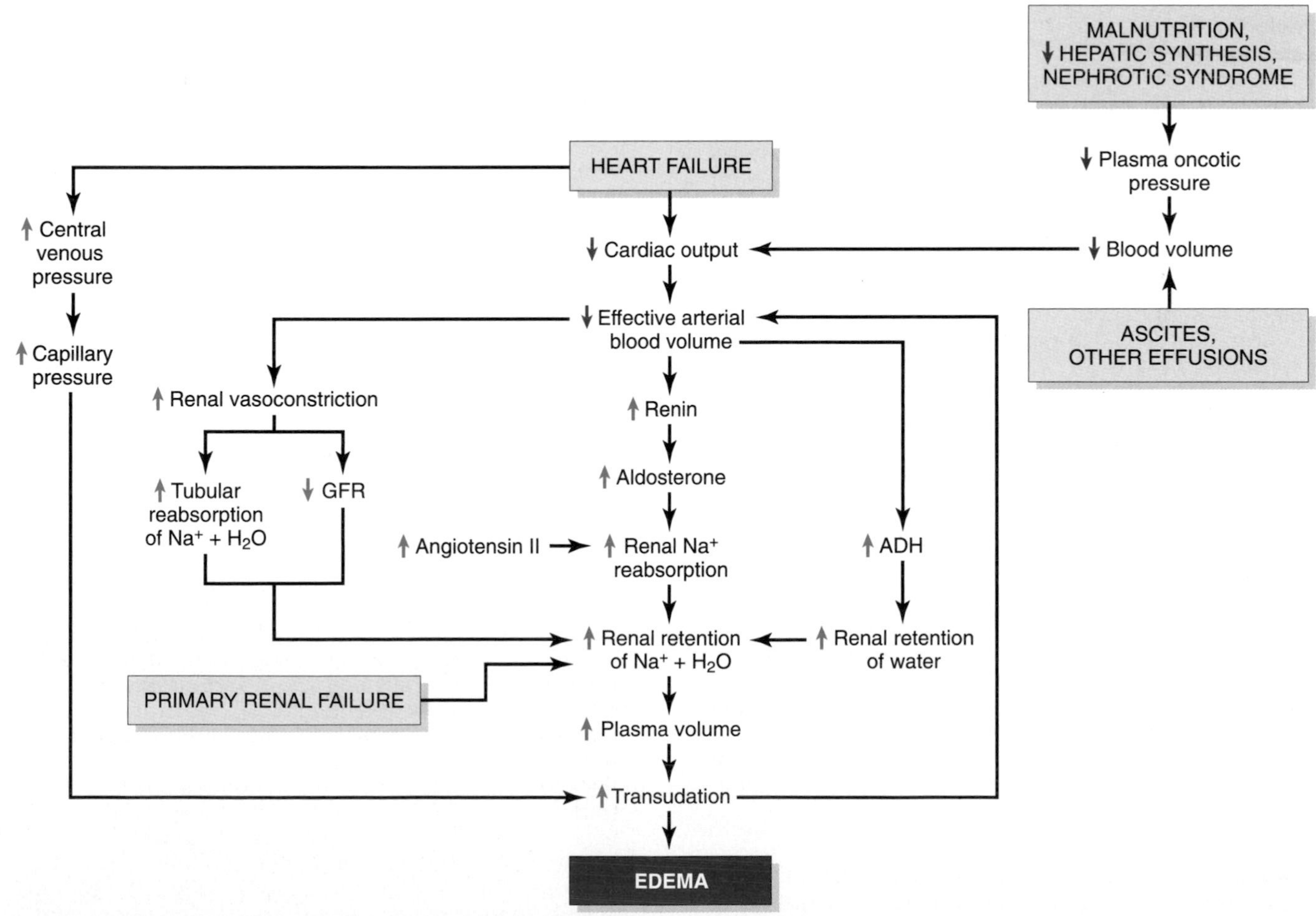

FIGURE 4–2 Sequence of events leading to systemic edema due to primary heart failure, primary renal failure, or reduced plasma osmotic pressure (as in malnutrition, diminished hepatic protein synthesis, or loss of protein owing to the nephrotic syndrome). ADH, antidiuretic hormone; GFR, glomerular filtration rate.

phatics can cause edema of the overlying skin, giving rise to the so-called peau d'orange (orange peel) appearance. Such a finely pitted appearance results from an accentuation of depressions in the skin at the site of hair follicles.

Sodium and Water Retention. Sodium and water retention are clearly contributory factors in several forms of edema; however, salt retention may also be a primary cause of edema. Increased salt, with the obligate accompanying water, causes both increased hydrostatic pressure (owing to expansion of the intravascular fluid volume) and diminished vascular colloid osmotic pressure. Salt (and water) retention may occur with any acute reduction of renal function, including *glomerulonephritis* and *acute renal failure* (Chapter 20).

Morphology. Edema is most easily recognized grossly; microscopically, edema fluid generally manifests only as subtle cell swelling, with clearing and separation of the extracellular matrix elements. Although any organ or tissue in the body may be involved, edema is most commonly encountered in subcutaneous tissues, the lungs, and the brain. Severe, generalized edema is called **anasarca**.

Subcutaneous edema may have different distributions depending on the cause. It can be diffuse, or it may be relatively more conspicuous at the sites of highest hydrostatic pressures. In the latter case, the edema distribution is typically influenced by gravity and is termed **dependent. Edema of the dependent parts of the body** (e.g., the legs when standing, the sacrum when recumbent) **is a prominent feature of congestive heart failure, particularly of the right ventricle.** Edema as a result of **renal dysfunction** or **nephrotic syndrome** is generally more severe than cardiac edema and **affects all parts of the body equally.** It may, however, initially manifest itself in tissues with a loose connective tissue matrix, such as the eyelids; thus, **periorbital edema** is a characteristic finding in severe renal disease. Finger pressure over substantially edematous subcutaneous tissue displaces the interstitial fluid and leaves a finger-shaped depression, so-called **pitting edema.**

Pulmonary edema is a common clinical problem (Chapter 15) most typically seen in the setting of left ventricular failure but also occurring in renal failure, acute respiratory distress syndrome (Chapter 15), pulmonary infections, and hypersensitivity reactions. The lungs are two to three times their normal weight, and sectioning reveals frothy, blood-tinged fluid representing a mixture of air, edema fluid, and extravasated red blood cells.

Edema of the brain may be localized (e.g., owing to abscess or neoplasm) or may be generalized, as in encephalitis, hypertensive crises, or obstruction to the brain's venous outflow. Trauma may result in local or generalized edema depending on the nature and extent of the injury. With generalized edema, the brain is grossly swollen, with narrowed sulci and distended gyri, showing signs of flattening against the unyielding skull (Chapter 28).

Clinical Correlation. Effects of edema may range from merely annoying to fatal. Subcutaneous tissue edema in cardiac or renal failure is important primarily because it signals underlying disease; however, when significant, it can also impair wound healing or the clearance of infection. Pulmonary edema can cause death by interfering with normal ventilatory function. Not only does fluid collect in the alveolar septa around capillaries and impede oxygen diffusion, but edema fluid in the alveolar spaces also creates a favorable environment for bacterial infection. Brain edema is serious and can be rapidly fatal; if severe, brain substance can *herniate* (extrude) through, for example, the foramen magnum, or the brain stem vascular supply can be compressed. Either condition can injure the medullary centers and cause death (Chapter 28).

Hyperemia and Congestion

The terms *hyperemia* and *congestion* both indicate a local increased volume of blood in a particular tissue. *Hyperemia* is an *active process* resulting from augmented tissue inflow because of arteriolar dilation, as in skeletal muscle during exercise or at sites of inflammation. The affected tissue is redder because of the engorgement of vessels with oxygenated blood. *Congestion* is a *passive process* resulting from impaired outflow from a tissue. It may occur systemically, as in cardiac failure, or it may be local, resulting from an isolated venous obstruction. The tissue has a blue-red color *(cyanosis)*, particularly as worsening congestion leads to accumulation of deoxygenated hemoglobin in the affected tissues (Fig. 4–3).

Congestion and edema commonly occur together, primarily since capillary bed congestion can result in edema due to increased fluid transudation. In long-standing congestion, called *chronic passive congestion,* the stasis of poorly oxygenated blood also causes chronic hypoxia, which can result in parenchymal cell degeneration or death, sometimes with microscopic scarring. Capillary rupture at these sites of chronic congestion may also cause small foci of hemorrhage; breakdown and phagocytosis of the red cell debris can eventually result in small clusters of hemosiderin-laden macrophages.

Morphology. The cut surfaces of hyperemic or congested tissues are hemorrhagic and wet. Microscopically, **acute pulmonary congestion** is characterized by alveolar capillaries engorged with blood; there may be associated alveolar septal edema and/or focal intra-alveolar hemorrhage. In **chronic pulmonary congestion**, the septa are thickened and fibrotic, and the alveolar spaces may contain numerous hemosiderin-laden macrophages **(heart failure cells).** In **acute hepatic congestion**, the central vein and sinusoids are distended with blood, and there may even be central hepatocyte degeneration; the periportal hepatocytes, better oxygenated because of their proximity to hepatic arterioles, experience less severe hypoxia and may only develop fatty change. In **chronic passive congestion of the liver**, the central regions of the hepatic lobules are grossly red-brown and slightly depressed (owing to a loss of cells) and are accentuated against the surrounding zones of uncongested tan liver **(nutmeg liver)** (Fig. 4–4*A*). Microscopically, there is evidence of centrilobular necrosis with loss of hepatocytes dropout and hemorrhage, including hemosiderin-laden macrophages (Fig. 4–4*B*). In severe, long-standing hepatic congestion (most commonly associated with heart failure), there may even be grossly evident hepatic fibrosis (cardiac cirrhosis).

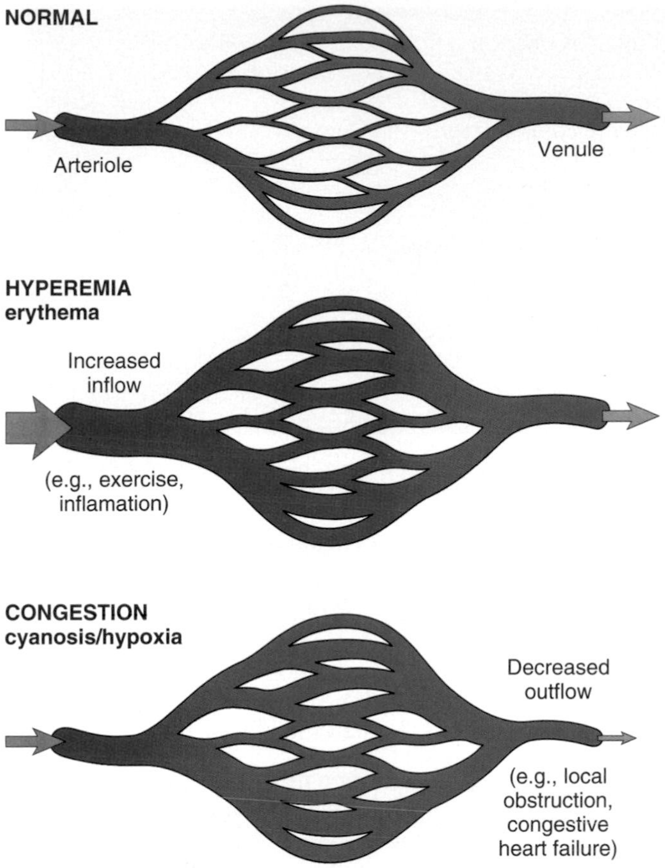

FIGURE 4–3 Hyperemia versus congestion. In both cases there is an increased volume and pressure of blood in a given tissue with associated capillary dilation and a potential for fluid extravasation. In hyperemia, increased inflow leads to engorgement with oxygenated blood, resulting in *erythema*. In congestion, diminished outflow leads to a capillary bed swollen with deoxygenated venous blood and resulting in *cyanosis*.

Because the central portion of the hepatic lobule is the last to receive blood, centrilobular necrosis can also occur whenever there is reduced hepatic blood flow (including shock from any cause); there need not be previous hepatic congestion.

Hemorrhage

Hemorrhage generally indicates extravasation of blood due to vessel rupture. As described previously, capillary bleeding can occur under conditions of chronic congestion, and an increased tendency to hemorrhage from usually insignificant injury is seen in a wide variety of clinical disorders collectively called *hemorrhagic diatheses* (Chapter 13). However, rupture of a large artery or vein is almost always due to vascular injury, including trauma, atherosclerosis, or inflammatory or neoplastic erosion of the vessel wall. Hemorrhage may be manifested in a variety of patterns, depending on the size, extent, and location of bleeding.

- Hemorrhage may be external or may be enclosed within a tissue; accumulation of blood within tissue is referred to as a *hematoma*. Hematomas may be relatively insignificant (a bruise) or may be sufficiently large as to be fatal (e.g., a massive retroperitoneal hematoma resulting from rupture of a dissecting aortic aneurysm; Chapter 11).
- Minute 1- to 2-mm hemorrhages into skin, mucous membranes, or serosal surfaces are denoted as *petechiae* (Fig. 4–5*A*) and are typically associated with locally increased intravascular pressure, low platelet counts *(thrombocytopenia)*, defective platelet function (as in uremia), or clotting factor deficits.
- Slightly larger (≥3 mm) hemorrhages are called *purpura*. These may be associated with many of the same disorders that cause petechiae and may also occur secondary to trauma, vascular inflammation *(vasculitis)*, or increased vascular fragility (e.g., in amyloidosis).
- Larger (>1 to 2 cm) subcutaneous hematomas (i.e., bruises) are called *ecchymoses* and are characteristically seen after trauma but may be exacerbated by any of the aforementioned conditions. The erythrocytes in these local hemorrhages are degraded and phagocytosed by macrophages; the hemoglobin (red-blue color) is then enzymatically converted into bilirubin (blue-green color) and eventually into hemosiderin (gold-brown color), accounting for the characteristic color changes in a hematoma.
- Large accumulations of blood in one or another of the body cavities are called *hemothorax, hemopericardium, hemoperitoneum*, or *hemarthrosis* (in joints). Patients with

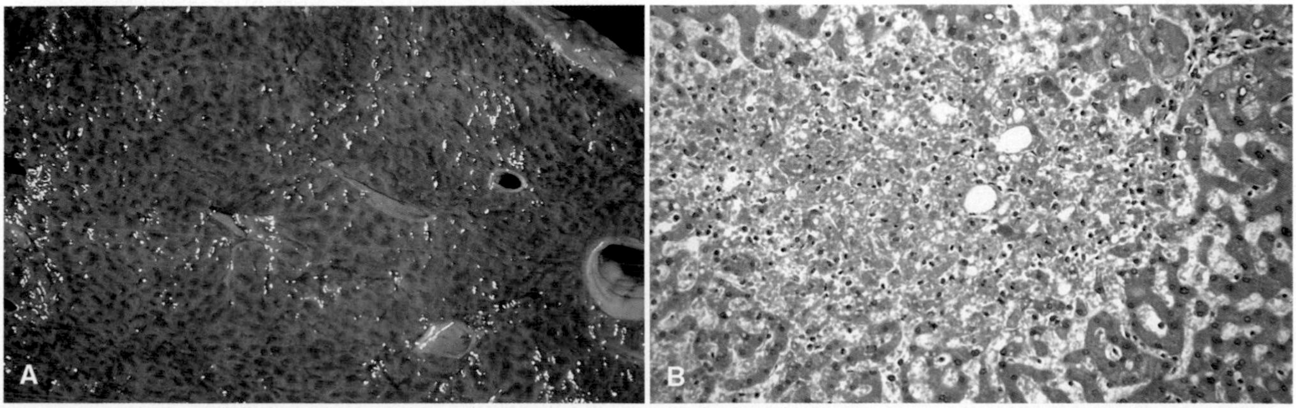

FIGURE 4–4 Liver with chronic passive congestion and hemorrhagic necrosis. *A*, Central areas are red and slightly depressed compared with the surrounding tan viable parenchyma, forming the so-called "nutmeg liver" pattern. *B*, Centrilobular necrosis with degenerating hepatocytes, hemorrhage, and sparse acute inflammation. (Courtesy of Dr. James Crawford, Department of Pathology, University of Florida, Gainesville, FL.)

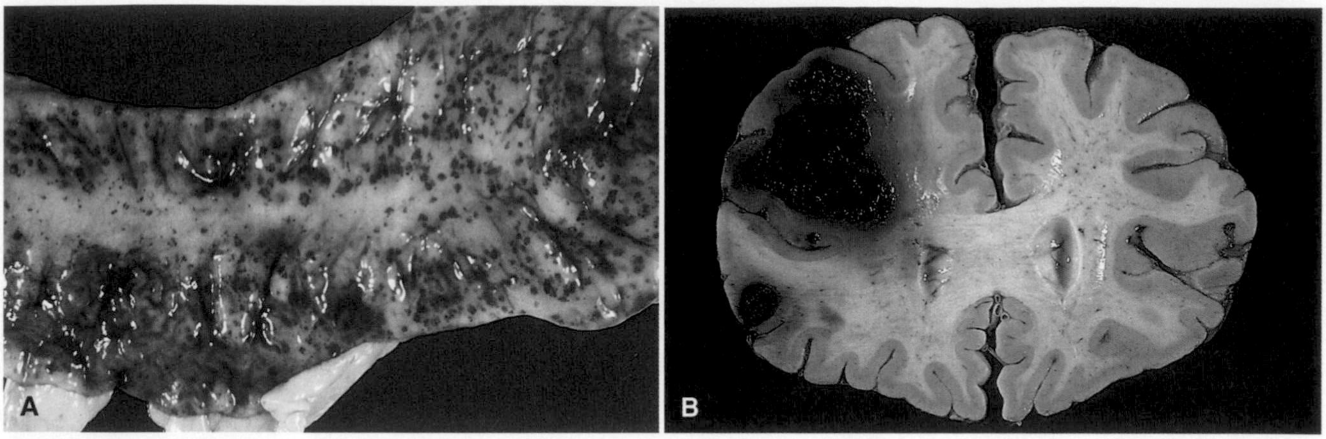

FIGURE 4–5 *A*, Punctate petechial hemorrhages of the colonic mucosa, seen here as a consequence of thrombocytopenia. *B*, Fatal intracerebral bleed. Even relatively inconsequential volumes of hemorrhage in a critical location, or into a closed space (such as the cranium), can have fatal outcomes.

extensive hemorrhage occasionally develop jaundice from the massive breakdown of red cells and systemic release of bilirubin.

The clinical significance of hemorrhage depends on the volume and rate of bleeding. Rapid loss of up to 20% of the blood volume or slow losses of even larger amounts may have little impact in healthy adults; greater losses, however, may result in *hemorrhagic (hypovolemic) shock* (discussed later). The site of hemorrhage is also important; bleeding that would be trivial in the subcutaneous tissues may cause death if located in the brain (Fig. 4–5*B*) because the skull is unyielding and bleeding there can result in increased intracranial pressure and herniation (Chapter 28). Finally, loss of iron and subsequent iron-deficiency anemia become a consideration in chronic or recurrent external blood loss (e.g., peptic ulcer or menstrual bleeding). In contrast, when red cells are retained, as in hemorrhage into body cavities or tissues, the iron can be reused for hemoglobin synthesis.

Hemostasis and Thrombosis

Normal hemostasis is the result of a set of well-regulated processes that accomplish two important functions: (1) They maintain blood in a fluid, clot-free state in normal vessels; and (2) They are poised to induce a *rapid and localized hemostatic plug* at a site of vascular injury. The pathologic opposite to hemostasis is *thrombosis;* it can be considered an inappropriate activation of normal hemostatic processes, such as the formation of a blood clot *(thrombus)* in uninjured vasculature or thrombotic occlusion of a vessel after relatively minor injury. Both hemostasis and thrombosis are regulated by three general components—the *vascular wall, platelets*, and the *coagulation cascade.* The following discussion begins with normal hemostasis and concludes with a description of the components that regulate normal coagulation processes.

NORMAL HEMOSTASIS

The general sequence of events in hemostasis at the site of vascular injury is shown in Figure 4–6.[2,3]

- After initial injury, there is a brief period of arteriolar vasoconstriction, largely attributable to *reflex neurogenic mechanisms* and augmented by the local secretion of factors such as *endothelin* (a potent endothelium-derived vasoconstrictor). The effect is transient, however, and bleeding would resume if not for activation of the platelet and coagulation systems (see Fig. 4–6*A*).
- Endothelial injury exposes highly thrombogenic subendothelial extracellular matrix (ECM), which allows platelets to adhere and become *activated,* that is, undergo a shape change and release secretory granules. Within minutes, the secreted products have recruited additional platelets *(aggregation)* to form a *hemostatic plug*; this is the process of *primary hemostasis* (see Fig. 4–6*B*).
- *Tissue factor*, a membrane-bound procoagulant factor synthesized by endothelium, is also exposed at the site of injury. It acts in conjunction with the secreted platelet factors to activate the coagulation cascade, culminating in the activation of *thrombin.* In turn, thrombin converts circulating soluble fibrinogen to insoluble *fibrin*, resulting in local fibrin deposition. Thrombin also induces further platelet recruitment and granule release. This sequence, *secondary hemostasis*, takes longer than the initial platelet plug (see Fig. 4–6*C*).
- Polymerized fibrin and platelet aggregates form a solid, *permanent plug* to prevent any further hemorrhage. At this stage, counterregulatory mechanisms (e.g., *tissue plasminogen activator {t-PA}*) are set into motion to limit the hemostatic plug to the site of injury (see Fig. 4–6*D*).

The following sections discuss the roles of endothelium, platelets, and the coagulation cascade in greater detail.

Endothelium

Endothelial cells modulate several—and frequently opposing—aspects of normal hemostasis. On the one hand, the normal flow of liquid blood is maintained by endothelial antiplatelet, anticoagulant, and fibrinolytic properties. On the other hand, after injury or activation, endothelium exhibits several *procoagulant* activities (Fig. 4–7). Endothelium may be activated by infectious agents, hemodynamic factors, plasma

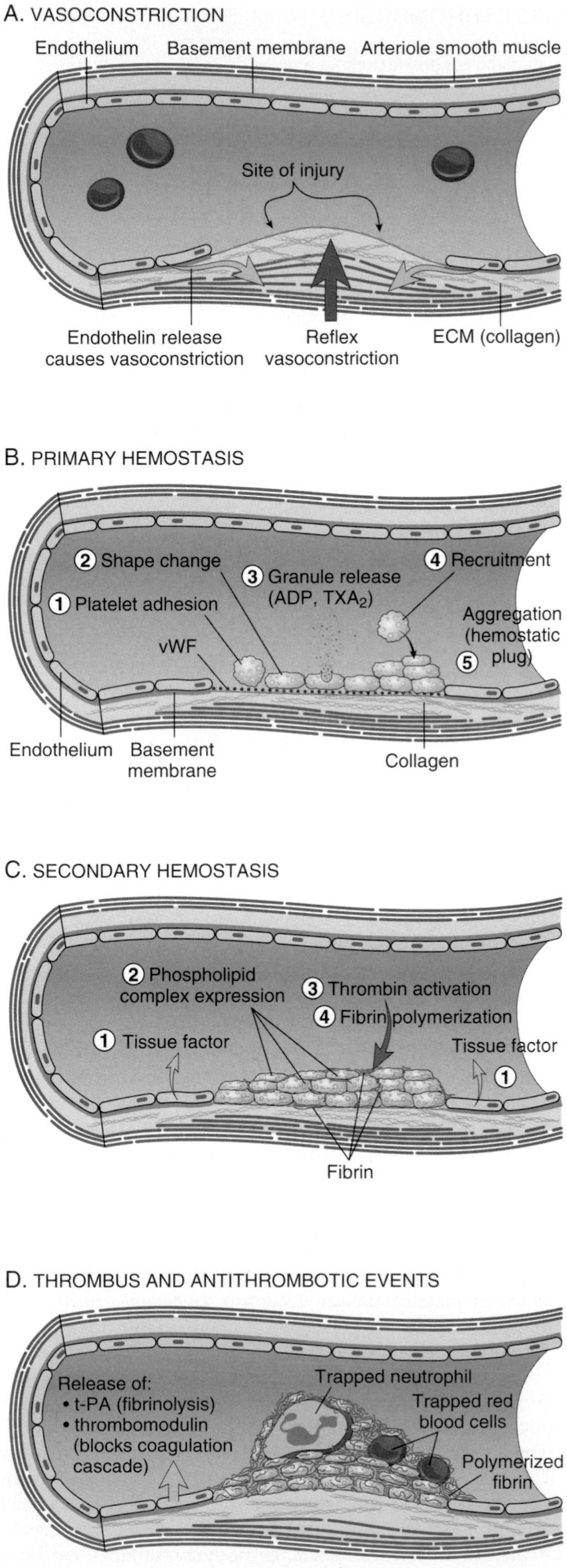

FIGURE 4–6 Diagrammatic representation of the normal hemostatic process. *A,* After vascular injury, local neurohumoral factors induce a transient vasoconstriction. *B,* Platelets adhere to exposed extracellular matrix (ECM) via von Willebrand factor (vWF) and are activated, undergoing a shape change and granule release; released adenosine diphosphate (ADP) and thromboxane A_2 (TxA_2) lead to further platelet aggregation to form the primary hemostatic plug. *C,* Local activation of the coagulation cascade (involving tissue factor and platelet phospholipids) results in fibrin polymerization, "cementing" the platelets into a definitive secondary hemostatic plug. *D,* Counter-regulatory mechanisms, such as release of tissue type plasminogen activator (t-PA) (fibrinolytic) and thrombomodulin (interfering with the coagulation cascade), limit the hemostatic process to the site of injury.

mediators, and, most significantly, cytokines (Chapters 2 and 6). The balance between endothelial antithrombotic and prothrombotic activities critically determines whether thrombus formation, propagation, or dissolution occurs.[4-6]

Antithrombotic Properties

Under most circumstances, endothelial cells maintain an environment conducive to liquid blood flow by mechanisms that block platelet adhesion and aggregation, interfere with the coagulation cascade, and actively lyse blood clots.

- *Antiplatelet effects.*[5] An intact endothelium prevents platelets and plasma coagulation factors from meeting the highly thrombogenic subendothelial ECM. Nonactivated platelets do not adhere to the endothelium, a property intrinsic to endothelial plasma membrane. Moreover, even if platelets are activated after focal endothelial injury, they are inhibited from adhering to the surrounding uninjured endothelium by endothelial prostacyclin (PGI_2) and nitric oxide (Chapter 2). Both mediators are potent vasodilators and inhibitors of platelet aggregation; their synthesis by endothelial cells is stimulated by a number of factors (e.g., thrombin and various cytokines) produced during coagulation. Endothelial cells also express adenosine diphosphatase, which degrades ADP and thereby contributes to the inhibition of platelet aggregation (see below).
- *Anticoagulant effects.* These effects are mediated by membrane-associated heparin-like molecules and by thrombomodulin, a specific thrombin receptor (see Fig. 4–7). The *heparin-like molecules* act indirectly; they are cofactors that interact with *antithrombin III* to inactivate thrombin, factor Xa, and several other coagulation factors (see below). *Thrombomodulin* also acts indirectly; it binds to thrombin, converting it from a procoagulant to an anticoagulant capable of activating *protein C.* Activated protein C, in turn, inhibits clotting by proteolytic cleavage of factors Va and VIIIa; it requires protein S, synthesized by endothelial cells, as a cofactor.[7] Endothelium is also a major synthetic source for *tissue factor pathway inhibitor,* a cell-surface protein that complexes and inhibits activated tissue factor–factor VIIa and factor Xa molecules.[8]
- *Fibrinolytic effects.* Endothelial cells synthesize *tissue-type plasminogen activator (t-PA),* promoting fibrinolytic activity to clear fibrin deposits from endothelial surfaces (see Fig. 4–6*D*).[9]

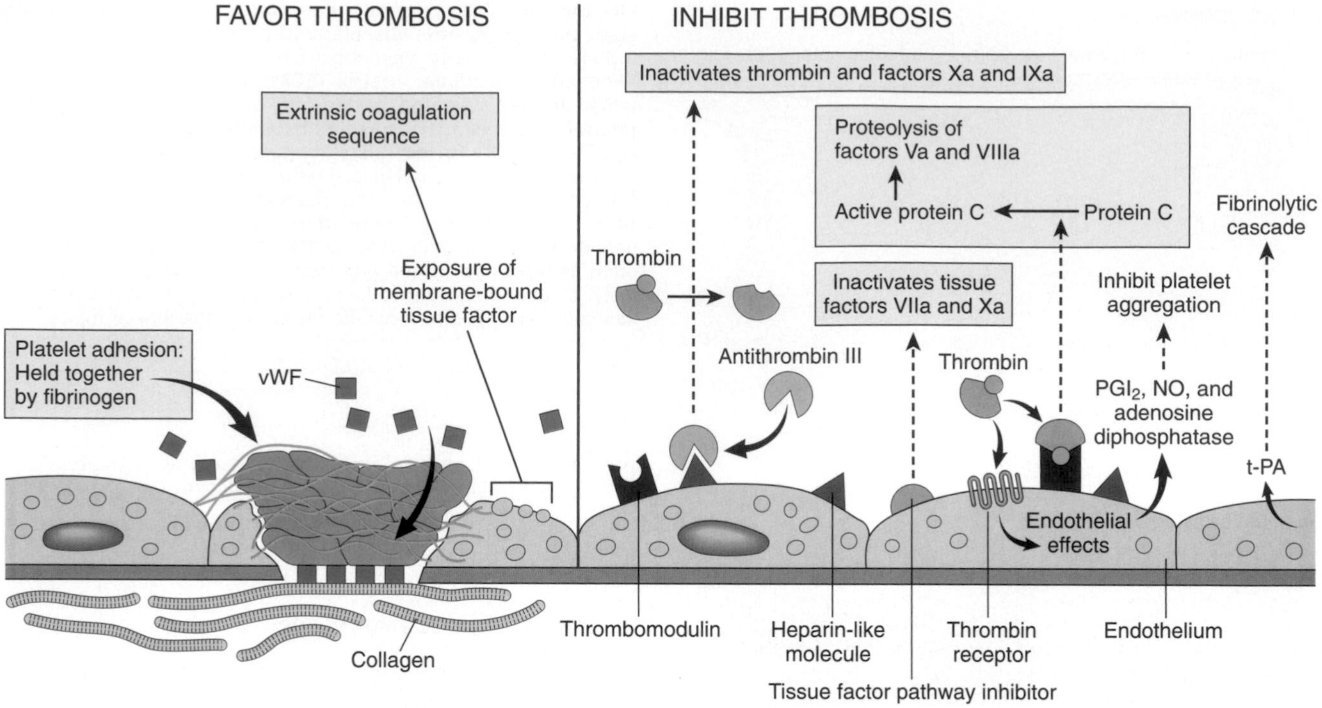

FIGURE 4–7 Schematic illustration of some of the pro- and anticoagulant activities of endothelial cells. Not shown are the pro- and antifibrinolytic properties. vWF, von Willebrand factor; PGI_2, prostacyclin; NO, nitric oxide; t-PA, tissue plasminogen activator. Thrombin receptor is referred to as protease activated receptor (PAR; see text).

Prothrombotic Properties

While endothelium normally limits blood clotting, it can also become prothrombotic, with activities that affect platelets, coagulation proteins, and the fibrinolytic system.

- *Platelet effects.* Recall that endothelial injury leads to adhesion of platelets to the underlying extracellular matrix; this is facilitated by endothelial production of *von Willebrand factor (vWF),* an essential cofactor for platelet binding to collagen and other surfaces.[10] It should be noted that vWF is a product of normal endothelium; it is not specifically synthesized after endothelial injury.
- *Procoagulant effects.* Endothelial cells are also induced by bacterial endotoxin or by cytokines (e.g., tumor necrosis factor [TNF] or interleukin-1 [IL-1]) to synthesize *tissue factor,* which, as we will see, activates the extrinsic clotting cascade.[11] By binding activated factors IXa and Xa, endothelial cells further augment the catalytic activities of these coagulation factors (see below).
- *Antifibrinolytic effects.* Endothelial cells also secrete inhibitors of plasminogen activator (PAIs), which depress fibrinolysis (not shown in Fig. 4–7).[12]

In summary, intact endothelial cells serve primarily to inhibit platelet adherence and blood clotting. Injury or activation of endothelial cells, however, results in a procoagulant phenotype that augments local clot formation.

Platelets

Platelets play a central role in normal hemostasis.[13] When circulating, they are membrane-bound smooth discs expressing a number of glycoprotein receptors of the integrin family on their surfaces. Platelets contain two specific types of granules. *Alpha granules* express the adhesion molecule P-selectin on their membranes (Chapter 2) and contain fibrinogen, fibronectin, factors V and VIII, platelet factor 4 (a heparin-binding chemokine), platelet-derived growth factor, and transforming growth factor-β. The other granules are *dense bodies*, or *δ granules*, which contain adenine nucleotides (ADP and adenosine triphosphate [ATP]), ionized calcium, histamine, serotonin, and epinephrine.

After vascular injury, platelets encounter ECM constituents that are normally sequestered beneath an intact endothelium; these include collagen (most important), proteoglycans, fibronectin, and other adhesive glycoproteins. On contact with ECM, platelets undergo three general reactions: (1) adhesion and shape change; (2) secretion (release reaction); and (3) aggregation (see Fig. 4–6*B*).

- *Platelet adhesion* to extracellular matrix is mediated largely via interactions with vWF, which acts as a bridge between platelet surface receptors (e.g., glycoprotein Ib, complexed with serum factors V and IX) and exposed collagen (Fig. 4–8). Although platelets can also adhere to other components of the ECM (e.g., fibronectin), vWF–glycoprotein Ib associations are the only interactions sufficiently strong to overcome the high shear forces of flowing blood. Thus, genetic deficiencies of vWF (von Willebrand disease; Chapter 13) or of its glycoprotein Ib (GpIb) receptor (Bernard-Soulier syndrome) result in defective platelet adhesion and bleeding disorders.
- *Secretion (release reaction)* of the contents of both granule types occurs soon after adhesion. The process is ini-

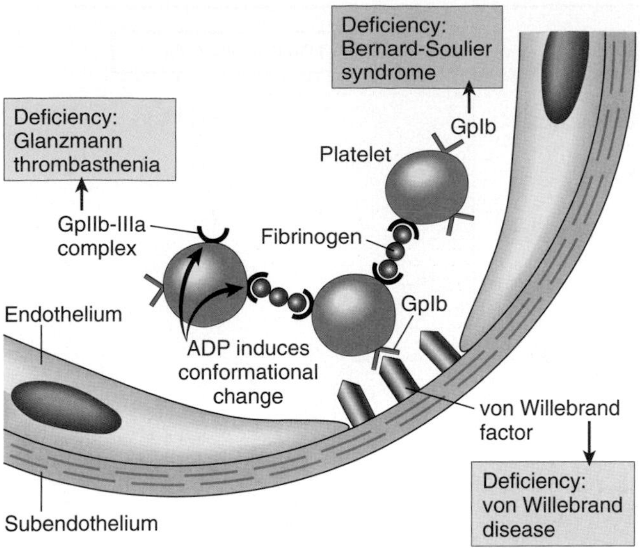

FIGURE 4–8 Platelet adhesion and aggregation. von Willebrand factor functions as an adhesion bridge between subendothelial collagen and the GpIb platelet receptor complex (the functional complex is composed of GpIb in association with factors V and IX). Aggregation involves linking platelets via fibrinogen bridges bound to the platelet GpIIb-IIIa receptors.

tiated by the binding of agonists to platelet surface receptors followed by an intracellular protein phosphorylation cascade. The release of the dense body contents is especially important because calcium is required in the coagulation cascade, and ADP is a potent mediator of *platelet aggregation* (platelets adhering to other platelets; see below). ADP also augments further ADP release from other platelets. Finally, platelet activation leads to the surface expression of *phospholipid complexes*, which provide critical nucleation and binding sites for calcium and coagulation factors in the *intrinsic clotting pathway*[14] (see below).

- *Platelet aggregation* follows adhesion and secretion. Besides ADP, the vasoconstrictor thromboxane A_2 (TxA_2) (Chapter 2), secreted by platelets, is also an important stimulus for platelet aggregation. ADP and TxA_2 set up an autocatalytic reaction leading to build-up of an enlarging platelet aggregate, the primary hemostatic plug. This primary aggregation is reversible, but with activation of the coagulation cascade, thrombin is generated. Thrombin binds to a platelet surface receptor (PARs, see later) and, along with ADP and TxA_2, causes further aggregation. This is followed by *platelet contraction*, creating an irreversibly fused mass of platelets *(viscous metamorphosis)* constituting the definitive *secondary hemostatic plug*. At the same time, thrombin converts fibrinogen to *fibrin* within and about the platelet plug, essentially cementing the platelets in place (see below). Thrombin is thus central in the formation of thrombi (Fig. 4–6C) and, as such, is a major target for therapeutic modulation of the thrombotic process.[15]

Noncleaved *fibrinogen* is also an important cofactor in platelet aggregation. ADP activation of platelets induces a conformational change of the platelet surface GpIIb-IIIa receptors so that they can bind fibrinogen. Fibrinogen then acts to connect multiple platelets together to form large aggregates (see Fig. 4–8). The importance of these interactions is demonstrated by the bleeding disorder seen in patients with congenitally deficient or inactive GpIIb-IIIa *(Glanzmann thrombasthenia)*.[16] Recent therapeutic advances have also taken advantage of this interaction; small molecular weight GpIIb-IIIa inhibitors are being increasingly employed as potent anticoagulants and to prevent thrombosis following vascular procedures (e.g., angioplasty).[17]

It is worth reiterating that the endothelium-derived PGI_2 is a potent vasodilator and inhibits platelet aggregation, whereas the platelet-derived TxA_2 is a potent vasoconstrictor and activates platelet aggregation (see also Chapter 2). The interplay of PGI_2 and TxA_2 constitutes an exquisitely balanced mechanism for modulating human platelet function: In the normal state, it prevents intravascular platelet aggregation, but after endothelial injury, it favors the formation of hemostatic plugs. The clinical utility of aspirin in patients at risk for coronary thrombosis—aspirin irreversibly acetylates and inactivates cyclooxygenase—is largely due to its ability to block TxA_2 synthesis. Nitric oxide, similar to PGI_2, also acts as a vasodilator and inhibitor of platelet aggregation (see Fig. 4–7).

Both erythrocytes and leukocytes are also found in hemostatic plugs; leukocytes adhere to platelets via the adhesion molecule P-selectin and to endothelium using a number of adhesion receptors (Chapter 2); they contribute to the inflammatory response that accompanies thrombosis. Thrombin also directly stimulates neutrophil and monocyte adhesion and generates chemotactic *fibrin split products* from the cleavage of fibrinogen.

The series of platelet events can be summarized as follows (see Fig. 4–6):

- *Platelets adhere to ECM at sites of endothelial injury and become activated.*
- *On activation, they secrete granule products (e.g., ADP) and synthesize TxA_2.*
- *Platelets also expose phospholipid complexes that are important in the intrinsic coagulation pathway.*
- *Injured or activated endothelial cells expose tissue factor, which triggers the extrinsic coagulation cascade.*
- *Released ADP stimulates the formation of a primary hemostatic plug, which is eventually converted (via ADP, thrombin, and TxA_2) into a larger, definitive, secondary plug.*
- *Fibrin deposition stabilizes and anchors the aggregated platelets.*

Coagulation Cascade

The coagulation cascade constitutes the third component of the hemostatic process and is a major contributor to thrombosis. The pathways are schematically presented in Figure 4–9; only general principles are discussed.[2,3,18]

The coagulation cascade is essentially a series of enzymatic conversions, turning inactive proenzymes into activated enzymes and culminating in the formation of thrombin. Thrombin then converts the soluble plasma protein *fibrinogen* precursor into the insoluble fibrous protein *fibrin.*

Each reaction in the pathway results from the assembly of a complex composed of an *enzyme* (activated coagulation factor), a *substrate* (proenzyme form of coagulation factor),

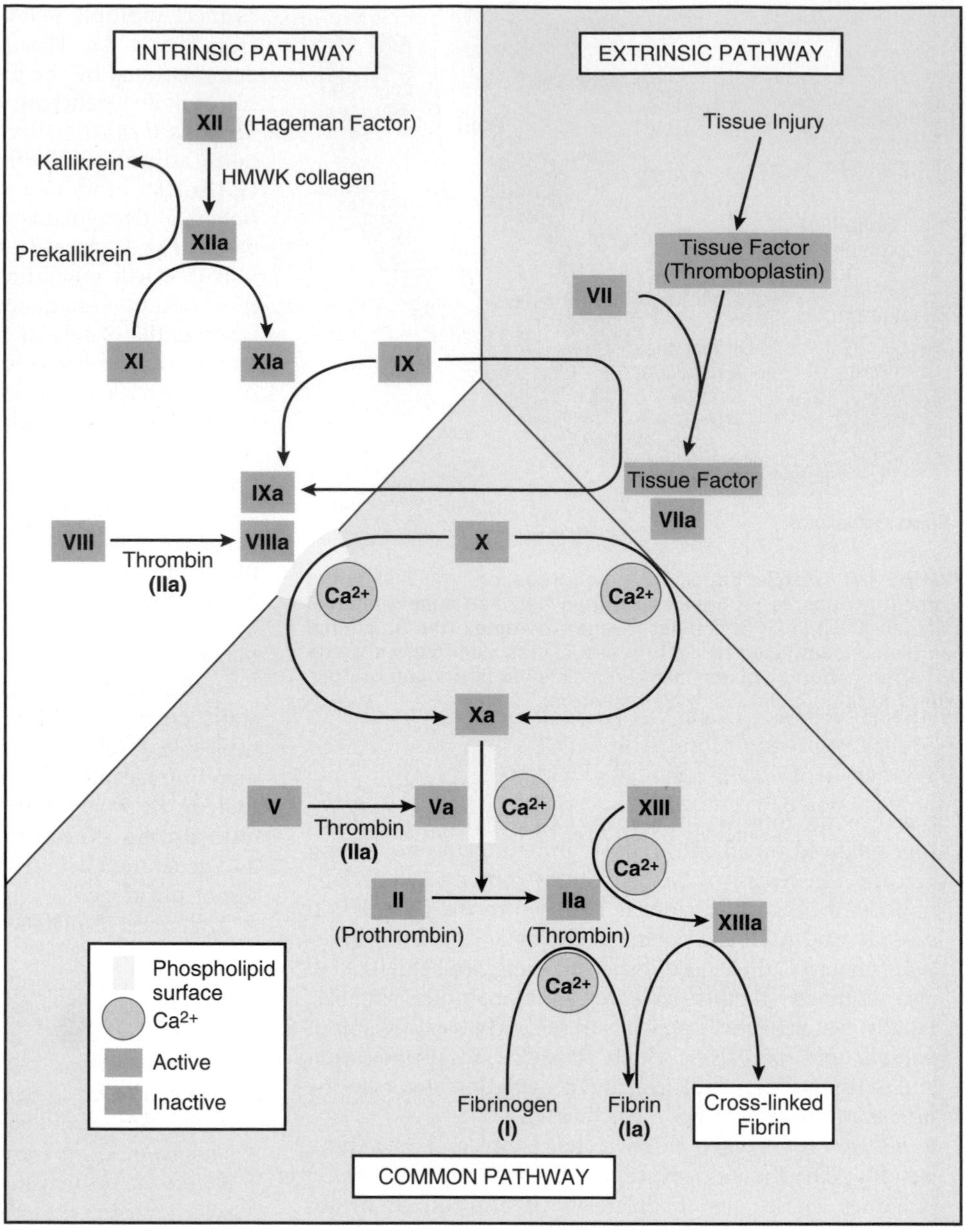

FIGURE 4–9 The coagulation cascade. Note the common link between the intrinsic and extrinsic pathways at the level of factor IX activation. Factors in red boxes represent inactive molecules; activated factors are indicated with a lower case "a" and a green box. PL, phospholipid surface; HMWK, high-molecular-weight kininogen. Not shown are the anticoagulant inhibitory pathways (see Figs. 4–7 and 4–12).

and a *cofactor* (reaction accelerator). These components are typically assembled on a *phospholipid complex* and held together by *calcium ions.* Thus, clotting tends to remain localized to sites where such assembly can occur (e.g., on the surface of activated platelets or endothelium).[3] Two such reactions, the sequential conversion of factor X to Xa and then II (prothrombin) to IIa (thrombin), are illustrated in Figure 4–10.

Traditionally, the blood coagulation scheme has been divided into *extrinsic* and *intrinsic* pathways, converging where factor X is activated (see Fig. 4–9). The intrinsic pathway may be initiated in vitro by the activation of Hageman factor (factor XII), while the extrinsic pathway is activated by *tissue factor,* a cellular lipoprotein exposed at sites of tissue injury.[8,19] However, such a division is mainly an artifact of in vitro testing; there are, in fact, interconnections between the two pathways. For example, a tissue factor–factor VIIa complex also activates factor IX in the *intrinsic pathway* (see Fig. 4–9).

In addition to catalyzing the final steps in the coagulation cascade, thrombin also exerts a wide variety of effects on the local vasculature and inflammation; it even actively participates in limiting the extent of the hemostatic process (Fig. 4–11). Most of these effects are induced via binding to a family of protease-activated receptors (PARs) that belong to the seven-transmembrane G-protein–coupled receptor family[20] (see Fig. 4–7). The mechanism of receptor activation involves clipping the extracellular end of the thrombin receptor via the proteolytic activity of thrombin. This generates a tethered peptide, which then binds to the rest of the receptor and

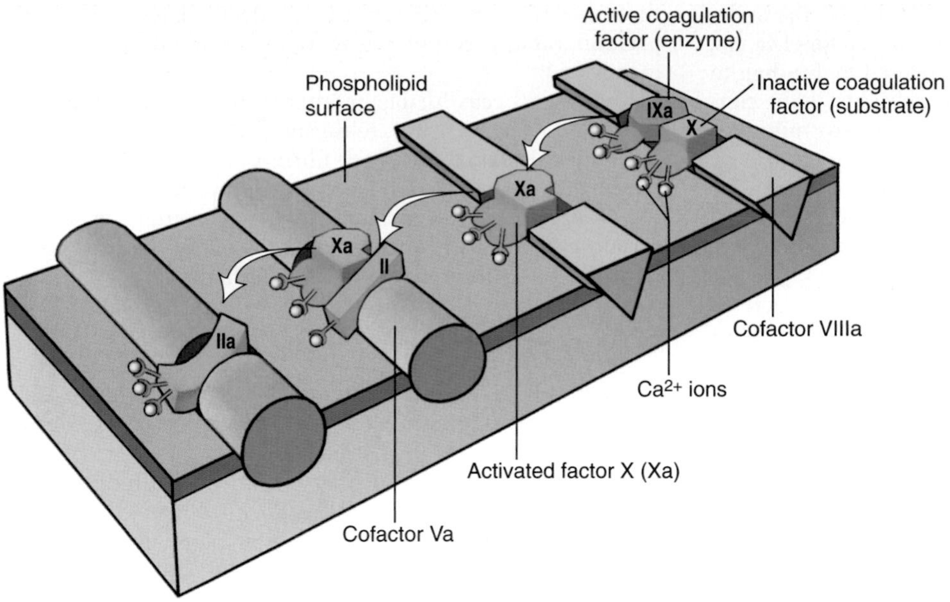

FIGURE 4–10 Schematic illustration of the conversion of factor X to factor Xa, which in turn converts factor II (prothrombin) to factor IIa (thrombin). The initial reaction complex consists of an enzyme (factor IXa), a substrate (factor X), and a reaction accelerator (factor VIIIa), which are assembled on the phospholipid surface of platelets. Calcium ions hold the assembled components together and are essential for reaction. Activated factor Xa then becomes the enzyme part of the second adjacent complex in the coagulation cascade, converting the prothrombin substrate (II) to thrombin (IIa), with the cooperation of the reaction accelerator factor Va. (Modified from Mann KG: Clin Lab Med 4:217, 1984.)

causes the conformational changes necessary to activate the associated G-protein. Thus, the interaction of thrombin and its receptor is essentially a catalytic process, which explains the impressive potency of even relatively small numbers of activated thrombin molecules in eliciting downstream effects.

Once activated, the coagulation cascade must be restricted to the local site of vascular injury to prevent clotting of the entire vascular tree. Besides restricting factor activation to sites of exposed phospholipids, clotting is also regulated by three types of natural anticoagulants:

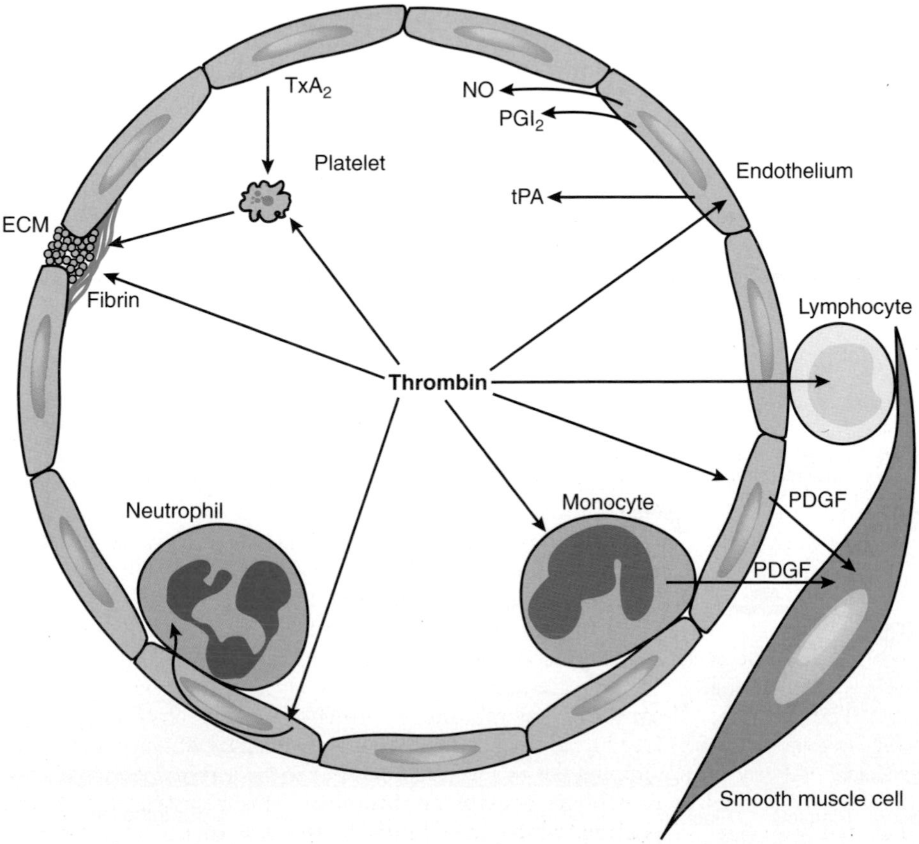

FIGURE 4–11 The central roles of thrombin in hemostasis and cellular activation. In addition to a critical function in generating cross-linked fibrin (via cleavage of fibrinogen to fibrin and activation of factor XIII), thrombin also directly induces platelet aggregation and secretion (e.g., of TxA_2). Thrombin also activates endothelium to generate leukocyte adhesion molecules and a variety of fibrinolytic (t-PA), vasoactive (NO, PGI_2), or cytokine (PDGF) mediators. Likewise, mononuclear inflammatory cells may be activated by the direct actions of thrombin. ECM, extracellular matrix; NO, nitric oxide; PDGF, platelet-derived growth factor; PGI_2, prostacyclin; TxA_2, thromboxane A_2; t-PA, tissue type plasminogen activator. See Fig. 4–7 for additional anticoagulant modulators of thrombin activity, such as antithrombin III and thrombomodulin. (Modified with permission from Shaun Coughlin, MD, PhD, Cardiovascular Research Institute, University of California at San Francisco.)

- *Antithrombins* (e.g., antithrombin III) inhibit the activity of thrombin and other serine proteases—factors IXa, Xa, XIa, and XIIa. Antithrombin III is activated by binding to heparin-like molecules on endothelial cells; hence the clinical usefulness of administering heparin to minimize thrombosis (see Fig. 4–7).
- *Proteins C and S,* two vitamin K–dependent proteins, are characterized by their ability to inactivate factors Va and VIIIa. The activation of protein C by thrombomodulin was described earlier (see Fig. 4–7).
- *Tissue factor pathway inhibitor (TFPI),* a protein secreted by endothelium (and other cell types), complexes to factor Xa and to tissue factor-VIIa and inactivates them to rapidly limit coagulation[21] (see Fig. 4–7).

Besides inducing coagulation, activation of the clotting cascade also sets into motion a *fibrinolytic cascade* that limits the size of the final clot. This is primarily accomplished by the generation of *plasmin.* Plasmin is derived from enzymatic breakdown of its inactive circulating precursor *plasminogen,* either by a factor XII-dependent pathway (see Chapter 2) or by two distinct types of plasminogen activators (PAs; Fig. 4–12). The first is the *urokinase-like PA (u-PA),* present in plasma and various tissues and capable of activating plasminogen in the fluid phase. Plasmin, in turn, converts the inactive pro-urokinase precursor to the active u-PA molecule, thus creating an amplification loop. The second, and physiologically the most important, kind of PA is the *tissue-type PA;* t-PA is synthesized principally by endothelial cells and is most active when attached to fibrin. The affinity for fibrin makes t-PA a much more useful therapeutic reagent, because it targets the fibrinolytic enzymatic activity to sites of recent clotting.[9] Plasminogen can also be activated by the bacterial product streptokinase, which may have some significance in certain bacterial infections. Plasmin breaks down fibrin and interferes with its polymerization (Fig. 4–12). The resulting *fibrin split products* (FSPs or so-called *fibrin degradation products*) can also act as weak anticoagulants. Elevated levels of FSPs (the fibrin split product characteristically measured by clinical laboratories is the fibrin *D-dimer*) are helpful in diagnosing abnormal thrombotic states, such as disseminated intravascular coagulation (DIC), deep venous thrombosis, or pulmonary thromboembolism (described in detail later). Any free plasmin rapidly complexes to α_2-plasmin inhibitor and is inactivated.

Endothelial cells further modulate the coagulation/anticoagulation balance by releasing plasminogen activator inhibitors (PAIs); these block fibrinolysis by inhibiting t-PA binding to fibrin and confer an overall procoagulant effect (see Fig. 4–12). The PAIs are increased by thrombin as well as certain cytokines and probably play a role in the intravascular thrombosis accompanying severe inflammation.[12]

THROMBOSIS

Having discussed the components of normal hemostasis, we now turn our attention to the dysregulation that underlies pathologic thrombus formation.

Pathogenesis. Three primary influences predispose to thrombus formation, the so-called *Virchow triad*: (1) endothelial injury; (2) stasis or turbulence of blood flow; and (3) blood hypercoagulability (Fig. 4–13).

Endothelial Injury. This is the dominant influence; endothelial injury by itself can lead to thrombosis. It is particularly important for thrombus formation occurring in the heart or in the arterial circulation, where the normally high flow rates might otherwise hamper clotting by preventing platelet adhesion or diluting coagulation factors. Thus, thrombus formation within the cardiac chambers (e.g., following endocardial injury due to myocardial infarction), over ulcerated plaques in atherosclerotic arteries, or at sites of traumatic or inflammatory vascular injury *(vasculitis)* is largely due to endothelial injury. Clearly, physical loss of endothelium will lead to exposure of subendothelial ECM, adhesion of platelets, release of tissue factor, and local depletion of PGI_2 and PAs. *However, it is important to note that endothelium need not be denuded or physically disrupted to contribute to the development of thrombosis; any perturbation in the dynamic balance of the pro- and antithrombotic effects of endothelium can influence local clotting events* (see Fig. 4–7). Thus, dysfunctional endothelium may elaborate greater amounts of procoagulant factors (e.g., platelet adhesion molecules, tissue factor, PAI) or may synthesize less anticoagulant effectors (e.g., thrombomodulin, PGI_2, t-PA). Significant endothelial dysfunction (in

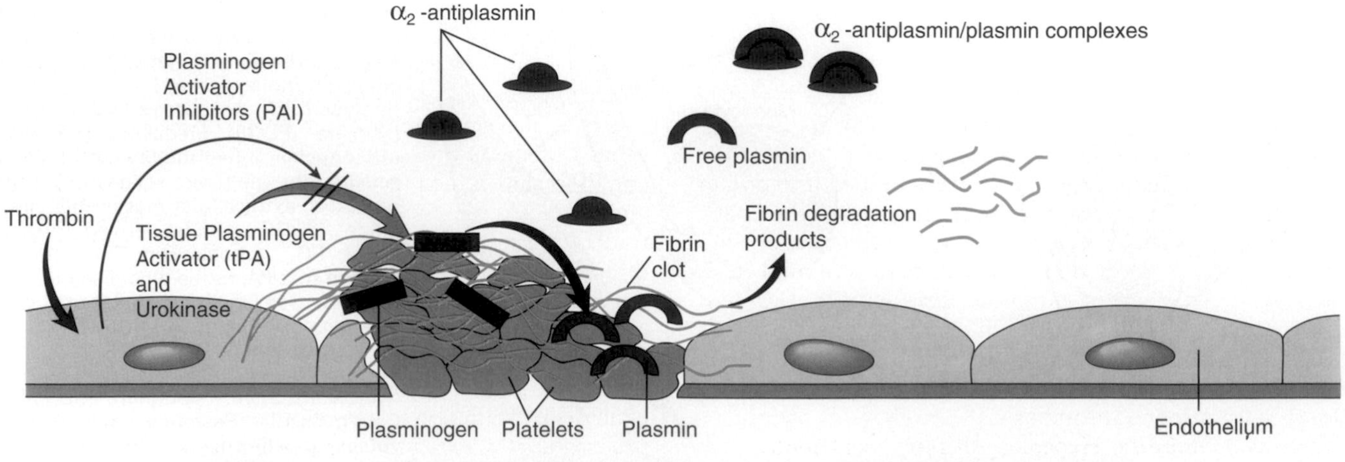

FIGURE 4–12 The fibrinolytic system, illustrating the plasminogen activators and inhibitors.

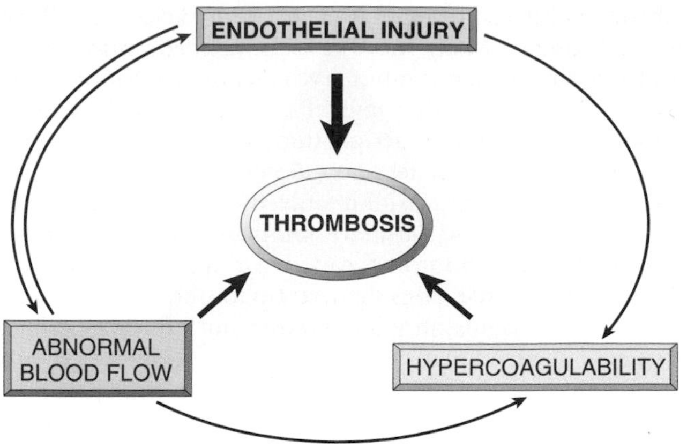

FIGURE 4–13 Virchow triad in thrombosis. Endothelial integrity is the single most important factor. Note that injury to endothelial cells can affect local blood flow and/or coagulability; abnormal blood flow (stasis or turbulence) can, in turn, cause endothelial injury. The elements of the triad may act independently or may combine to cause thrombus formation.

the absence of endothelial cell loss) may occur due to the hemodynamic stresses of hypertension, turbulent flow over scarred valves, or bacterial endotoxins. Even relatively subtle influences, such as homocystinuria, hypercholesterolemia, radiation, or products absorbed from cigarette smoke may initiate endothelial injury.

Alterations in Normal Blood Flow. *Turbulence* contributes to arterial and cardiac thrombosis by causing endothelial injury or dysfunction as well as by forming countercurrents and local pockets of stasis; *stasis* is a major factor in the development of venous thrombi.[5,22] Normal blood flow is *laminar* such that the platelets flow centrally in the vessel lumen, separated from the endothelium by a slower-moving clear zone of plasma. Stasis and turbulence therefore (1) disrupt laminar flow and bring platelets into contact with the endothelium; (2) prevent dilution of activated clotting factors by fresh flowing blood; (3) retard the inflow of clotting factor inhibitors and permit the build-up of thrombi; and (4) promote endothelial cell activation, predisposing to local thrombosis, leukocyte adhesion, and a variety of other endothelial cell effects.[23]

Turbulence and stasis clearly contribute to thrombosis in a number of clinical settings. Ulcerated atherosclerotic plaques not only expose subendothelial ECM, but are also sources of turbulence. Abnormal aortic and arterial dilations called *aneurysms* cause local stasis and are favored sites of thrombosis (Chapter 12). Myocardial infarctions not only have associated endothelial injury, but also have regions of noncontractile myocardium, adding an element of stasis in the formation of mural thrombi. Mitral valve stenosis (e.g., after rheumatic heart disease) results in left atrial dilation. In conjunction with atrial fibrillation, a dilated atrium is a site of profound stasis and a prime location for thrombus development. *Hyperviscosity syndromes* (such as polycythemia; Chapter 13) cause small vessel stasis; the deformed red cells in *sickle cell anemia* (Chapter 13) cause vascular occlusions, with the resulting stasis predisposing to thrombosis.

Hypercoagulability. Hypercoagulability contributes less frequently to thrombotic states but is nevertheless an important component in the equation. It is loosely defined as any alteration of the coagulation pathways that predisposes to thrombosis. The causes of hypercoagulability may be *primary* (genetic) and *secondary* (acquired) disorders (Table 4–2).[24,25]

Of the inherited causes of hypercoagulability, mutations in the factor V gene and prothrombin gene are the most common. Approximately 2% to 15% of Caucasians carry a specific factor V mutation (called the *Leiden mutation,* after the city in the Netherlands where it was discovered), substituting a glutamine for the normal arginine residue at position 506 and rendering the protein resistant to cleavage by protein C. Such resistance to protein C-mediated inactivation of factor Va promotes unchecked coagulation (see Fig. 4–7). Among patients with recurrent deep venous thrombosis, the carrier frequency is considerably higher, approaching 60% in some series.

A single nucleotide change (G to A transition) in the 3′-untranslated region of the *prothrombin gene* is a fairly common allele (1% to 2% of the population) that is associated with elevated prothrombin levels and an almost threefold increased risk of venous thromboses.[27,28] Elevated levels of *homocysteine* contribute to arterial and venous thrombosis and indeed to the development of atherosclerosis, as is discussed in Chapter 11. This effect is most likely due to inhibition of antithrombin III and endothelial thrombomodulin.[26] Hyperhomocystenemia may be inherited or acquired. Homozygosity for the C677T mutation in the methyltetrahydrofolate reductase gene causes mild homocystenemia in 5% to 15% of white and East Asian populations, thus matching the frequency of factor V Leiden. However, the relationship between the C677T mutation and thrombosis is less well established.[24] In addition to these well characterized point mutations, polymorphisms in coagulant factor genes also appear to impart an increased risk of venous thrombosis.[29] Other, less common, primary hypercoagulable states include inherited deficiencies of anticoagulants such as antithrombin III, protein C, or protein S; affected individuals typically present with venous thrombosis and recurrent thromboembolism in adolescence or early adult life.

Although individually these inherited disorders are uncommon, collectively they are significant for two reasons. First, the mutations underlying these inherited thrombophilias may be co-inherited, and the effect of having two mutations on the risk of thrombosis is much more than additive.[24] Second, those with such mutations have a much higher risk than normal individuals of developing venous thrombosis when acquired causes of hypercoagulability, such as pregnancy, are also present. *Inherited causes of hypercoagulability must be considered in patients under the age of 50 who present with thrombosis in the absence of any acquired predisposition.*

Unlike these uncommon hereditary disorders, the pathogenesis of the *acquired thrombotic diatheses* in a number of common clinical settings (see Table 4–2) is more complicated and multifactorial. In some situations (e.g., cardiac failure or trauma), factors such as stasis or vascular injury may be most important. In other cases (e.g., oral contraceptive use and the hyperestrogenic state of pregnancy), hypercoagulability may be partly caused by increased hepatic synthesis of many coagulation factors and reduced synthesis of antithrombin III;[30] heterozygosity for factor V Leiden may also be an underlying contributory component. In disseminated cancers, release of procoagulant tumor products predisposes to thrombosis.[31,32] The hypercoagulability seen with advancing age may be due

TABLE 4–2 Hypercoagulable States

Primary (Genetic)	
Common	
	Mutation in factor V gene (factor V Leiden)
	Mutation in prothrombin gene
	Mutation in methyltetrahydrofolate gene
Rare	
	Antithrombin III deficiency
	Protein C deficiency
	Protein S deficiency
Very rare	
	Fibrinolysis defects
Secondary (Acquired)	
High risk for thrombosis	
	Prolonged bed rest or immobilization
	Myocardial infarction
	Atrial fibrillation
	Tissue damage (surgery, fracture, burns)
	Cancer
	Prosthetic cardiac valves
	Disseminated intravascular coagulation
	Heparin-induced thrombocytopenia
	Antiphospholipid antibody syndrome (lupus anticoagulant syndrome)
Lower risk for thrombosis	
	Cardiomyopathy
	Nephrotic syndrome
	Hyperestrogenic states (pregnancy)
	Oral contraceptive use
	Sickle cell anemia
	Smoking

to increased susceptibility to platelet aggregation and reduced PGI_2 release by endothelium. Smoking and obesity promote hypercoagulability by unknown mechanisms.

Among the acquired causes of thrombotic diatheses, the so-called *heparin-induced thrombocytopenia syndrome* and *antiphospholipid antibody syndrome* (previously called the *lupus anticoagulant syndrome*) deserve special mention.

Heparin-induced thrombocytopenia syndrome.[33,34] Seen in upward of 5% of the population, this syndrome occurs when administration of unfractionated heparin (for purposes of therapeutic anticoagulation) induces formation of antibodies that bind to molecular complexes of heparin and platelet factor 4 membrane protein. This antibody can also bind to similar complexes present on platelet and endothelial surfaces; the result is platelet activation, endothelial injury, and a prothrombotic state. To reduce this problem, specially manufactured low-molecular-weight heparin preparations—which retain anticoagulant activity but do not interact with platelets—are used. These have the additional benefit of a prolonged serum half-life.

Antiphospholipid antibody syndrome.[35,36] This syndrome has protean clinical presentations, including multiple thromboses; the clinical manifestations are associated with high titers of circulating antibodies directed against anionic phospholipids (e.g., cardiolipin) or, more accurately, against plasma protein epitopes that are unveiled by binding to such phospholipids (e.g., prothrombin). Patients with anticardiolipin antibodies also have a false-positive serologic test for syphilis because the antigen in the standard tests is embedded in cardiolipin. In vitro these antibodies interfere with the assembly of phospholipid complexes and thus inhibit coagulation. However, in vivo, the antibodies induce a *hypercoagulable* state.

Patients with antiphospholipid antibody syndrome fall into two categories. Many have a well-defined autoimmune disease, such as systemic lupus erythematosus (Chapter 6) and have *secondary antiphospholipid syndrome* (such patients previously carried the designation of *lupus anticoagulant syndrome*). The remainder show no evidence of other autoimmune disorder and exhibit only the manifestations of a hypercoagulable state *(primary antiphospholipid syndrome)*. Occasionally the syndrome can occur in association with certain drugs or infections. How antiphospholipid antibodies lead to hypercoagulability is not clear, but possible explanations include direct platelet activation, inhibition of PGI_2 production by endothelial cells, or interference with protein C synthesis or activity. Although antiphospholipid antibodies are associated with thrombotic diatheses, they have also been identified in 5% to 15% of apparently normal individuals and may therefore be necessary but not sufficient to cause full-blown antiphospholipid antibody syndrome.

Individuals with the antiphospholipid antibody syndrome present with an extreme variety of clinical manifestations; these are typically characterized by *recurrent venous* or *arterial thrombi* but also include *repeated miscarriages, cardiac valvular vegetations*, or *thrombocytopenia.*[37] Venous thromboses occur most commonly in deep leg veins, but renal, hepatic, and retinal veins are also susceptible. Arterial thromboses typically occur in the cerebral circulation, but coronary, mesenteric, and renal arterial occlusions have also been described. Depending on the vascular bed involved, the clinical presentations can vary from pulmonary embolism (due to a lower extremity venous thrombus), to pulmonary hypertension (from recurrent subclinical pulmonary emboli), to stroke, bowel infarction, or renovascular hypertension. Fetal loss is attributable to antibody-mediated inhibition of t-PA activity necessary for trophoblastic invasion of the uterus. Antiphospholipid antibody syndrome is also a cause of renal microangiopathy, resulting in renal failure owing to multiple capillary and arterial thromboses (Chapter 20). Patients with antiphospholipid antibody syndrome are at increased risk of a fatal event (upward of 7% in one series of patients with lupus erythematosus, particularly with arterial thromboses or thrombocytopenia). Current treatment includes anticoagulation therapy (aspirin, heparin, and warfarin) and immunosuppression in refractory cases.[35,37,38]

Morphology. Thrombi may develop anywhere in the cardiovascular system: within the cardiac chambers; on valve cusps; or in arteries, veins, or capillaries. They are of variable size and shape, depending on the site of origin and the circumstances leading to their development. Arterial or cardiac thrombi usually begin at a site of endothelial injury (e.g., atherosclerotic plaque) or turbulence (vessel bifurcation); venous thrombi characteristically occur in sites of stasis. An area of attachment to the underlying vessel or heart wall, frequently firmest at the point of origin, is characteristic of all thromboses. Arterial thrombi tend to grow in a retrograde direction from the point of attachment, whereas venous thrombi extend in the direction of blood flow (i.e., toward the heart). The propagating tail may not be well attached and, particularly in veins, is prone to fragmentation, creating an **embolus**.

When formed in the heart or aorta, thrombi may have grossly (and microscopically) apparent laminations, called **lines of Zahn**; these are produced by alternating pale layers of platelets admixed with some fibrin and darker layers containing more red cells. Lines of Zahn are significant only in that they imply thrombosis at a site of blood flow; in veins or in smaller arteries, the laminations are typically not as apparent, and, in fact, thrombi formed in the sluggish flow of venous blood usually resemble statically coagulated blood (similar to blood clotted in a test tube). Nevertheless, careful evaluation generally reveals irregular, somewhat ill-defined laminations.

When arterial thrombi arise in heart chambers or in the aortic lumen, they usually adhere to the wall of the underlying structure and are termed **mural thrombi**. Abnormal myocardial contraction (arrhythmias, dilated cardiomyopathy, or myocardial infarction) leads to cardiac mural thrombi (Fig. 4–14*A*), while ulcerated atherosclerotic plaque and aneurysmal dilation are the precursors of aortic thrombus formation (Fig. 4–14*B*).

Arterial thrombi are usually **occlusive**; the most common sites, in descending order, are coronary, cerebral, and femoral arteries. The thrombus is usually superimposed on an atherosclerotic plaque, although other forms of vascular injury (vasculitis, trauma) may be involved. The thrombi are typically firmly adherent to the injured arterial wall and are gray-white and friable, composed of a tangled mesh of platelets, fibrin, erythrocytes, and degenerating leukocytes.

Venous thrombosis, or **phlebothrombosis**, is almost invariably occlusive; the thrombus often creates a long cast of the vein lumen. Because these thrombi form in a relatively static environment, they tend to contain more enmeshed erythrocytes and are therefore known as **red**, or **stasis, thrombi**. Phlebothrombosis most commonly affects the veins of the lower extremities (90% of cases). Less commonly, venous thrombi may develop in the upper extremities, periprostatic plexus, or the ovarian and periuterine veins; under special circumstances, they may be found in the dural sinuses, the portal vein, or the hepatic vein. At autopsy, postmortem clots may be confused for venous thrombi. Postmortem clots are gelatinous with a dark red dependent portion where red cells have settled by gravity and a yellow *chicken fat* supernatant resembling melted and clotted chicken fat; they are usually not attached to the underlying wall. In contrast, red thrombi are firmer, almost always have a point of attachment, and on transection reveal vague strands of pale gray fibrin.

Under special circumstances, thrombi may form on heart valves. Bacterial or fungal blood-borne infections may establish a foothold, leading to valve damage and the development of large thrombotic masses, or **vegetations** (**infective endocarditis**; Chapter 12). Sterile vegetations can also develop on noninfected valves in patients with hypercoagulable states, so-called **nonbacterial thrombotic endocarditis** (Chapter 12). Less commonly, noninfective, **verrucous (Libman-Sacks) endocarditis** attributable to elevated levels of circulating immune complexes may occur in patients with systemic lupus erythematosus (Chapter 6).

Fate of the Thrombus. If a patient survives the immediate effects of a thrombotic vascular obstruction, thrombi undergo some combination of the following four events in the ensuing days to weeks (Fig. 4–15):

- *Propagation.* The thrombus may accumulate more platelets and fibrin (propagate), eventually leading to vessel obstruction.
- *Embolization.* Thrombi may dislodge and travel to other sites in the vasculature.
- *Dissolution.* Thrombi may be removed by fibrinolytic activity.
- *Organization and recanalization.* Thrombi may induce inflammation and fibrosis *(organization)* and may eventually become *recanalized*; that is, may reestablish vascular flow, or may be incorporated into a thickened vascular wall.

Propagation and embolization are discussed further below. As for dissolution, activation of the fibrinolytic pathways can lead to rapid shrinkage and even total lysis of *recent* thrombi. With older thrombi, extensive fibrin polymerization renders the thrombus substantially more resistant to proteolysis, and

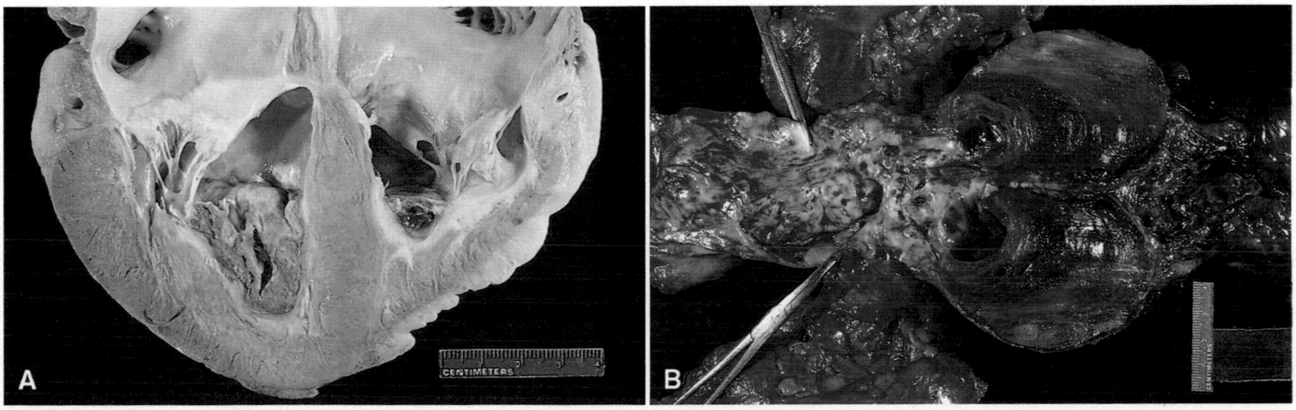

FIGURE 4–14 Mural thrombi. *A*, Thrombus in the left and right ventricular apices, overlying a white fibrous scar. *B*, Laminated thrombus in a dilated abdominal aortic aneurysm.

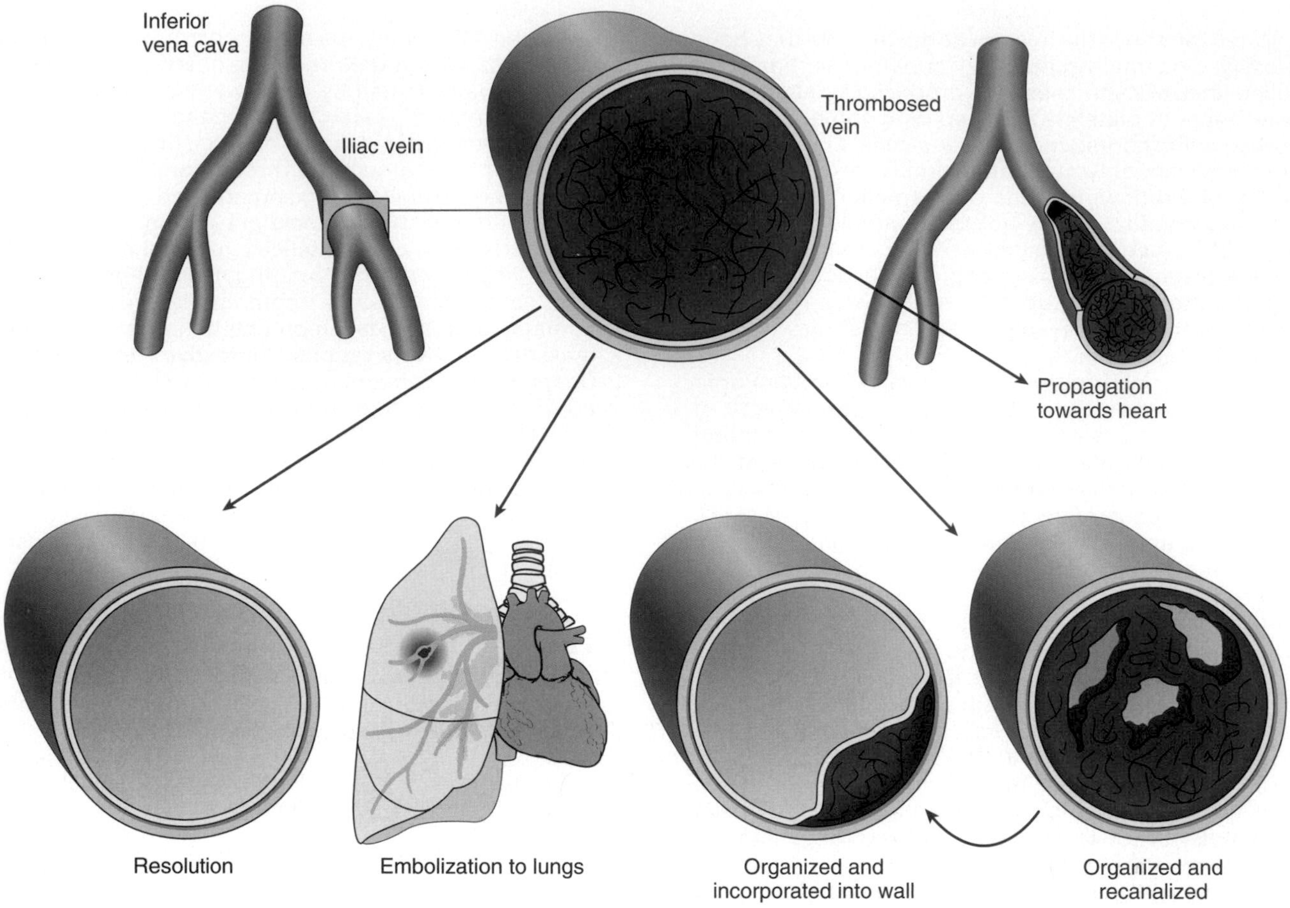

FIGURE 4–15 Potential outcomes of venous thrombosis.

lysis is ineffectual. This is important because therapeutic infusions of fibrinolytic agents such as t-PA (e.g., for pulmonary thromboemboli or coronary thrombosis) are likely to be effective for only a short time after thrombi form.

Older thrombi tend to become *organized.* This refers to the ingrowth of endothelial cells, smooth muscle cells, and fibroblasts into the fibrin-rich thrombus. In time, capillary channels are formed, which may anastomose to create conduits from one end of the thrombus to the other, re-establishing, to a limited extent, the continuity of the original lumen. Although the channels may not successfully restore significant flow to many obstructed vessels, such *recanalization* can potentially convert the thrombus into a vascularized mass of connective tissue (Fig. 4–16). With time and contraction of the mesenchymal cells (and particularly for smaller thrombi), the connective tissue may be incorporated as a subendothelial swelling of the vessel wall; eventually, only a fibrous lump may remain to mark the original thrombus site. Occasionally, instead of organizing, the center of a thrombus undergoes enzymatic digestion, presumably as a result of the release of lysosomal enzymes from trapped leukocytes and platelets. This is particularly likely in large thrombi within aneurysmal dilations or the cardiac chambers. If bacterial seeding occurs, such a degraded thrombus is an ideal culture medium, resulting, for example, in a so-called *mycotic aneurysm* (Chapter 11).

Clinical Correlations. Thrombi are significant because *they cause obstruction of arteries and veins,* and *they are possible sources of emboli.* The significance of each depends on where the thrombus occurs. Thus, while venous thrombi may cause congestion and edema in vascular beds distal to an obstruction, a far graver consequence is that they may embolize to the lungs, causing death. Conversely, although arterial thrombi can embolize, their role in vascular obstruction at critical sites (e.g., coronary arteries resulting in myocardial infarction) is much more important.

Venous Thrombosis (Phlebothrombosis). The great preponderance of venous thrombi occur in either the superficial or the deep veins of the leg.[39] Superficial venous thrombi usually occur in the saphenous system, particularly when there are varicosities. Such thrombi may cause local congestion, and swelling, pain, and tenderness along the course of the involved vein but rarely embolize. Nevertheless, the local edema and impaired venous drainage do predispose the involved overlying skin to infections from slight trauma and to the development of *varicose ulcers. Deep thrombi in the larger leg veins at or above the knee* (e.g., popliteal, femoral, and iliac veins) are more serious because they may embolize. Although they may cause local pain and distal edema, the venous obstruction may be rapidly offset by collateral bypass channels. Consequently, deep vein thromboses are entirely asymptomatic in approximately 50% of

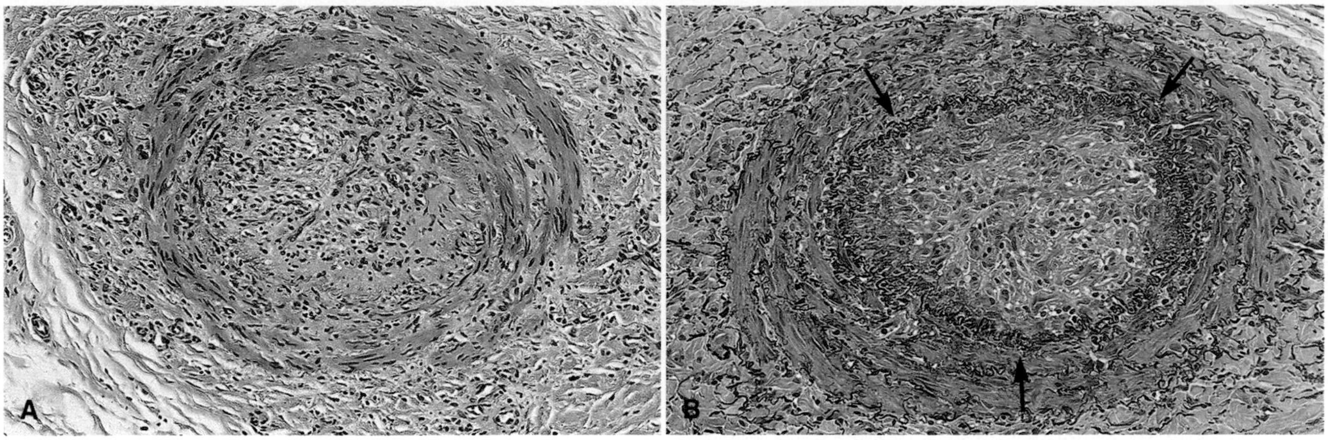

FIGURE 4–16 Low-power view of a thrombosed artery. *A,* H&E-stained section. *B,* Stain for elastic tissue. The original lumen is delineated by the internal elastic lamina *(arrows)* and is totally filled with organized thrombus, now punctuated by a number of small recanalized channels.

affected patients and are recognized only in retrospect after they have embolized.

Deep venous thrombosis may occur with stasis and in a variety of hypercoagulable states as described earlier (Table 4–2). Cardiac failure is an obvious reason for stasis in the venous circulation. Trauma, surgery, and burns usually result in reduced physical activity, injury to vessels, release of procoagulant substances from tissues, and/or reduced t-PA activity. Many factors act in concert to predispose to thrombosis in the puerperal and postpartum states. Besides the potential for amniotic fluid infusion into the circulation at the time of delivery, late pregnancy and the postpartum period are also associated with hypercoagulability. Tumor-associated procoagulant release is largely responsible for the increased risk of thromboembolic phenomena seen in disseminated cancers, so-called *migratory thrombophlebitis* or *Trousseau syndrome.* Regardless of the specific clinical setting, advanced age, bed rest, and immobilization increase the risk of deep venous thrombosis, particularly in those who have inherited susceptibility states (Table 4–2); reduced physical activity diminishes the milking action of muscles in the lower leg and so slows venous return.

Arterial and Cardiac Thrombosis. *Atherosclerosis* is a major initiator of thromboses, related to the associated abnormal vascular flow and loss of endothelial integrity (see Fig. 4–14*B*). Cardiac mural thrombi can arise in the setting of myocardial infarction related to dyskinetic contraction of the myocardium as well as damage to the adjacent endocardium (see Fig. 4–14*A*). *Rheumatic heart disease* may result in atrial mural thrombi due to mitral valve stenosis, followed by left atrial dilation; concurrent atrial fibrillation augments atrial blood stasis. In addition to the local obstructive consequences, cardiac and arterial (in particular, aortic) mural thrombi can also embolize peripherally. Virtually any tissue may be affected, but the brain, kidneys, and spleen are prime targets because of their large flow volume.

While we clearly understand a number of conditions that predispose to thrombosis, the phenomenon remains somewhat unpredictable. It continues to occur at a distressingly high frequency in healthy, ambulatory individuals without apparent provocation or underlying pathology.

DISSEMINATED INTRAVASCULAR COAGULATION (DIC)

A variety of disorders ranging from obstetric complications to advanced malignancy may be complicated by DIC, the sudden or insidious onset of widespread fibrin thrombi in the microcirculation. Although these thrombi are not usually visible on gross inspection, they are readily apparent microscopically and can cause diffuse circulatory insufficiency, particularly in the brain, lungs, heart, and kidneys. With the development of the multiple thrombi, there is a rapid concurrent consumption of platelets and coagulation proteins (hence the synonym *consumption coagulopathy*); at the same time, fibrinolytic mechanisms are activated, and as a result an initially thrombotic disorder can evolve into a serious bleeding disorder. *It should be emphasized that DIC is not a primary disease but rather a potential complication of any condition associated with widespread activation of thrombin.*[40] It is discussed in greater detail along with other bleeding diatheses in Chapter 13.

Embolism

An embolus is a detached intravascular solid, liquid, or gaseous mass that is carried by the blood to a site distant from its point of origin. Almost all emboli represent some part of a dislodged thrombus, hence the commonly used term *thromboembolism.* Rare forms of emboli include droplets of fat, bubbles of air or nitrogen, atherosclerotic debris *(cholesterol emboli),* tumor fragments, bits of bone marrow, or even foreign bodies such as bullets. However, unless otherwise specified, an embolism should be considered to be thrombotic in origin. Inevitably, emboli lodge in vessels too small to permit further passage, resulting in partial or complete vascular occlusion. The potential consequence of such thromboembolic events is the ischemic necrosis of distal tissue, known as *infarction.* Depending on the site of origin, emboli may lodge anywhere in the vascular tree; the clinical outcomes are best understood from the standpoint of whether emboli lodge in the pulmonary or systemic circulations.

PULMONARY THROMBOEMBOLISM

Pulmonary embolism has an incidence of 20 to 25 per 100,000 hospitalized patients.[41,42] Although the rate of fatal pulmonary emboli (as assessed at autopsy) has declined from 6% to 2% over the last quarter century,[43] pulmonary embolism still causes about 200,000 deaths per year in the United States. In more than 95% of instances, venous emboli originate from deep leg vein thrombi above the level of the knee as described previously. They are carried through progressively larger channels and usually pass through the right side of the heart into the pulmonary vasculature. Depending on the size of the embolus, it may occlude the main pulmonary artery, impact across the bifurcation *(saddle embolus)*, or pass out into the smaller, branching arterioles (Fig. 4–17). Frequently, there are multiple emboli, perhaps sequentially or as a shower of smaller emboli from a single large mass; in general, *the patient who has had one pulmonary embolus is at high risk of having more.* Rarely, an embolus may pass through an interatrial or interventricular defect to gain access to the systemic circulation *(paradoxical embolism)*. A more complete discussion of pulmonary emboli is presented in Chapter 15; an overview is offered here.[43,44]

- Most pulmonary emboli (60% to 80%) are clinically silent because they are small. With time, they undergo organization and are incorporated into the vascular wall (see Fig. 4–14); in some cases, organization of the thromboembolus leaves behind a delicate, bridging fibrous *web.*
- Sudden death, right heart failure *(cor pulmonale)*, or cardiovascular collapse occurs when 60% or more of the pulmonary circulation is obstructed with emboli.
- Embolic obstruction of medium-sized arteries may result in pulmonary hemorrhage but usually does not cause pulmonary infarction because of the dual blood flow into the area from the bronchial circulation. A similar embolus in the setting of left-sided cardiac failure (i.e., with sluggish bronchial artery flow), however, may result in a large infarct.
- Embolic obstruction of small end-arteriolar pulmonary branches usually does result in associated infarction.
- Multiple emboli over time may cause pulmonary hypertension with right heart failure.

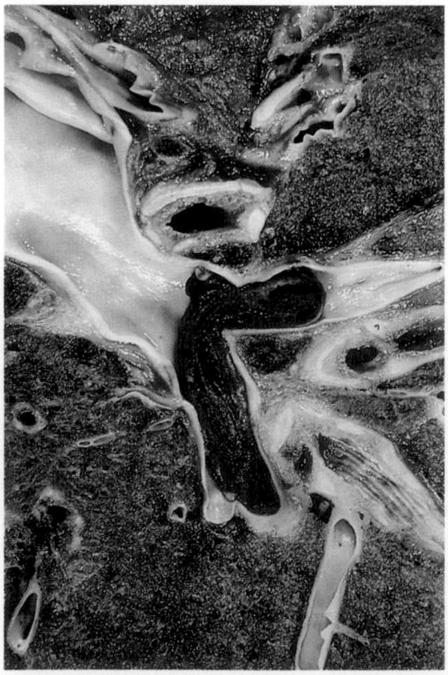

FIGURE 4–17 Large embolus derived from a lower extremity deep venous thrombosis and now impacted in a pulmonary artery branch.

SYSTEMIC THROMBOEMBOLISM

Systemic thromboembolism refers to emboli traveling within the arterial circulation. Most (80%) arise from intracardiac mural thrombi, two thirds of which are associated with left ventricular wall infarcts and another quarter with dilated and fibrillating left atria (e.g., secondary to mitral valve disease; Chapter 12). The remainder originate from aortic aneurysms, thrombi on ulcerated atherosclerotic plaques, or fragmentation of a valvular vegetation (Chapter 12), with a small fraction due to *paradoxical emboli*; 10% to 15% of systemic emboli are of unknown origin. In contrast to venous emboli, which tend to lodge primarily in one vascular bed (the lung), arterial emboli can travel to a wide variety of sites; the point of arrest depends on the source of the thromboembolus and the volume of blood flow through the downstream tissues. The major sites for arteriolar embolization are the lower extremities (75%) and the brain (10%), with the intestines, kidneys, spleen, and upper extremities involved to a lesser extent. The consequences of systemic emboli depend on the extent of collateral vascular supply in the affected tissue, the tissue's vulnerability to ischemia, and the caliber of the vessel occluded; in general, arterial emboli cause infarction of tissues downstream of the obstructed vessel.

FAT EMBOLISM

Microscopic fat globules may be found in the circulation after fractures of long bones (which have fatty marrow) or, rarely, in the setting of soft tissue trauma and burns. Presumably the fat is released by marrow or adipose tissue injury and enters the circulation by rupture of the marrow vascular sinusoids or of venules. Although traumatic fat embolism occurs in some 90% of individuals with severe skeletal injuries (Fig. 4–18), less than 10% of such patients have any clinical findings. *Fat embolism syndrome is characterized by pulmonary insufficiency, neurologic symptoms, anemia, and thrombocytopenia.* Symptoms typically begin 1 to 3 days after injury, with sudden onset of tachypnea, dyspnea, and tachycardia. Neurologic symptoms include irritability and restlessness, with progression to delirium or coma. Patients may present with thrombocytopenia, presumably caused by platelets adhering to the myriad fat globules and being removed from the circulation; anemia may result as a consequence of erythrocyte aggregation and hemolysis. A diffuse petechial rash in nondependent areas (related to rapid onset of thrombocytopenia) is seen in 20% to 50% of cases and is useful in establishing a diagnosis. In its full-blown form, the syndrome is fatal in up to 10% of cases.

The pathogenesis of fat emboli syndrome probably involves both mechanical obstruction and biochemical injury.[45,46] Microemboli of neutral fat cause occlusion of the pulmonary and cerebral microvasculature, aggravated by local platelet

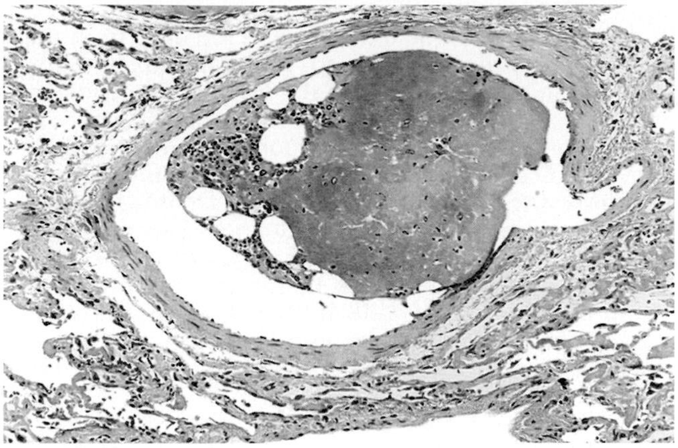

FIGURE 4–18 Bone marrow embolus in the pulmonary circulation. The cleared vacuoles represent marrow fat that is now impacted in a distal vessel along with the cellular hematopoietic precursors.

and erythrocyte aggregation; this is further exacerbated by release of free fatty acids from the fat globules, causing local toxic injury to endothelium. Platelet activation and recruitment of granulocytes (with free radical, protease, and eicosanoid release; Chapter 2) complete the vascular assault. Because lipids are dissolved out of tissue preparations by the solvents routinely used in paraffin embedding, the microscopic demonstration of fat microglobules (i.e., in the absence of accompanying marrow) typically requires specialized techniques, including frozen sections and fat stains.

AIR EMBOLISM

Gas bubbles within the circulation can obstruct vascular flow (and cause distal ischemic injury) almost as readily as thrombotic masses can. Air may enter the circulation during obstetric procedures or as a consequence of chest wall injury. Generally, in excess of 100 cc is required to have a clinical effect; the bubbles act like physical obstructions and may coalesce to form frothy masses sufficiently large to occlude major vessels.[47,48]

A particular form of gas embolism, called *decompression sickness*, occurs when individuals are exposed to sudden changes in atmospheric pressure.[49,50] Scuba and deep sea divers, underwater construction workers, and individuals in unpressurized aircraft in rapid ascent are all at risk. When air is breathed at high pressure (e.g., during a deep sea dive), increased amounts of gas (particularly nitrogen) become dissolved in the blood and tissues. If the diver then ascends (depressurizes) too rapidly, the nitrogen expands in the tissues and bubbles out of solution in the blood to form gas emboli.

The rapid formation of gas bubbles within skeletal muscles and supporting tissues in and about joints is responsible for the painful condition called *the bends* (so named in the 1880s because afflicted individuals characteristically arched their backs in a manner reminiscent of a then popular women's fashion called the *Grecian Bend*). Gas emboli may also induce focal ischemia in a number of tissues, including brain and heart. In the lungs, edema, hemorrhages, and focal atelectasis or emphysema may appear, leading to respiratory distress, the so-called *chokes*. Treatment of gas embolism requires placing the individual in a compression chamber where the barometric pressure may be raised, thus forcing the gas bubbles back into solution. Subsequent slow decompression theoretically permits gradual resorption and exhalation of the gases so that obstructive bubbles do not re-form.

A more chronic form of decompression sickness is called *caisson disease* (named for the pressurized vessels used in the construction of the base of the Brooklyn Bridge in New York; workers digging in these vessels suffered both acute and chronic forms of decompression sickness). In caisson disease, persistence of gas emboli in the skeletal system leads to multiple foci of ischemic necrosis; the more common sites are the heads of the femurs, tibia, and humeri.

AMNIOTIC FLUID EMBOLISM

Amniotic fluid embolism is a grave but fortunately uncommon complication of labor and the immediate postpartum period (1 in 50,000 deliveries). It has a mortality rate of 20% to 40%, and as other obstetric complications (e.g., eclampsia, pulmonary embolism) have been better managed, amniotic fluid embolism has become an important cause of maternal mortality. The onset is characterized by sudden severe dyspnea, cyanosis, and hypotensive shock, followed by seizures and coma. If the patient survives the initial crisis, pulmonary edema typically develops, along with (in half the patients) DIC, owing to release of thrombogenic substances from amniotic fluid.[51,52]

The underlying cause is the infusion of amniotic fluid or fetal tissue into the maternal circulation via a tear in the placental membranes or rupture of uterine veins. The classic findings are therefore the presence in the pulmonary microcirculation of squamous cells shed from fetal skin, lanugo hair, fat from vernix caseosa, and mucin derived from the fetal respiratory or gastrointestinal tract. There is also marked pulmonary edema and changes of *diffuse alveolar damage* (Chapter 15) as well as systemic fibrin thrombi indicative of DIC.

Infarction

An infarct is an area of ischemic necrosis caused by occlusion of either the arterial supply or the venous drainage in a particular tissue. Infarction involving different organs is a common and extremely important cause of clinical illness. In the United States, more than half of all deaths are caused by cardiovascular disease, and most of these are attributable to myocardial or cerebral infarction. Pulmonary infarction is a common complication in a number of clinical settings, bowel infarction is frequently fatal, and ischemic necrosis of the extremities (gangrene) is a serious problem in the diabetic population.

Nearly 99% of all infarcts result from thrombotic or embolic events, and almost all result from arterial occlusion. Occasionally, infarction may also be caused by other mechanisms, such as local vasospasm, expansion of an atheroma owing to hemorrhage within a plaque, or extrinsic compression of a vessel (e.g., by tumor). Other uncommon causes include twisting of the vessels (e.g., in testicular torsion or bowel volvulus), compression of the blood supply by edema or by entrapment in a hernia sac, or traumatic rupture of the blood supply. Although venous thrombosis may cause infarction, it more often merely induces venous obstruction and congestion. Usually, bypass channels rapidly open after the thrombosis, providing some outflow from the area, which, in turn, improves the arterial inflow. Infarcts caused by venous thrombosis are more likely in organs with a single venous outflow channel, such as the testis and ovary.

Morphology. Infarcts are classified on the basis of their color (reflecting the amount of hemorrhage) and the presence or absence of microbial infection. Therefore, infarcts may be either **red (hemorrhagic)** or **white (anemic)** and may be either **septic** or **bland**.

- *Red (hemorrhagic) infarcts* occur (1) with venous occlusions (such as in ovarian torsion); (2) in loose tissues (such as lung), which allow blood to collect in the infarcted zone; (3) in tissues with dual circulations (e.g., lung and small intestine), permitting flow of blood from the unobstructed vessel into the necrotic zone (obviously such perfusion is not sufficient to rescue the ischemic tissues); (4) in tissues that were previously congested because of sluggish venous outflow; and (5) when flow is re-established to a site of previous arterial occlusion and necrosis (e.g., following fragmentation of an occlusive embolus or angioplasty of a thrombotic lesion) (Fig. 4–19*A*).
- *White (anemic) infarcts* occur with arterial occlusions in solid organs with end–arterial circulation (such as heart, spleen, and kidney), where the solidity of the tissue limits the amount of hemorrhage that can seep into the area of ischemic necrosis from adjoining capillary beds (Fig. 4–19*B*).

Most infarcts tend to be wedge-shaped, with the occluded vessel at the apex and the periphery of the organ forming the base (see Fig. 4–19 *A* and *B*); when the base is a serosal surface, there is often an overlying fibrinous exudate. The lateral margins may be irregular, reflecting the pattern of vascular supply from adjacent vessels. At the outset, all infarcts are poorly defined and slightly hemorrhagic. The margins of both types of infarcts tend to become better defined with time by a narrow rim of hyperemia attributable to inflammation at the edge of the lesion.

In solid organs, the extravasated red cells from the limited hemorrhage are lysed. The released hemoglobin remains in the tissue in the form of hemosiderin within macrophages; this can microscopically identify sites of previous infarction but does not grossly impart any significant color to the tissue. White infarcts resulting from arterial occlusions typically become progressively more pale and sharply defined with time (see Fig. 4–19*B*). By comparison, in spongy organs the hemorrhage is too extensive to permit the lesion ever to become pale (see Fig. 4–19*A*). Over the course of a few days, it does, however, become more firm and brown, as the extensive bleeding progressively degrades into hemosiderin pigment.

The dominant histologic characteristic of infarction is **ischemic coagulative necrosis** (Chapter 1). It is important to recall that if the vascular occlusion has occurred shortly (minutes to hours) before the death of the patient, no demonstrable histologic changes may be evident; if the patient survives even 12 to 18 hours, the only change present may be hemorrhage.

An inflammatory response begins to develop along the margins of infarcts within a few hours and is usually well defined within 1 or 2 days. Inflammation at these sites is incited by the necrotic material; given sufficient time, there is gradual degradation of the dead tissue with phagocytosis of the cellular debris by neutrophils and macrophages. Eventually the inflammatory response is followed by a reparative response beginning in the preserved margins (Chapter 2). In stable or labile tissues, some parenchymal regeneration may occur at the periphery where the underlying stromal architecture has been spared. However, most infarcts are ultimately replaced by **scar tissue** (Fig. 4–20). The brain is an exception to these generalizations; as with all other causes of cell death, ischemic injury in the central nervous system results in **liquefactive necrosis** (Chapter 1).

Septic infarctions may develop when embolization occurs by fragmentation of a bacterial vegetation from a heart valve or when microbes seed an area of necrotic tissue. In these cases, the infarct is converted into an **abscess**, with a correspondingly greater inflammatory response (Chapter 2). The eventual sequence of organization, however, follows the pattern already described.

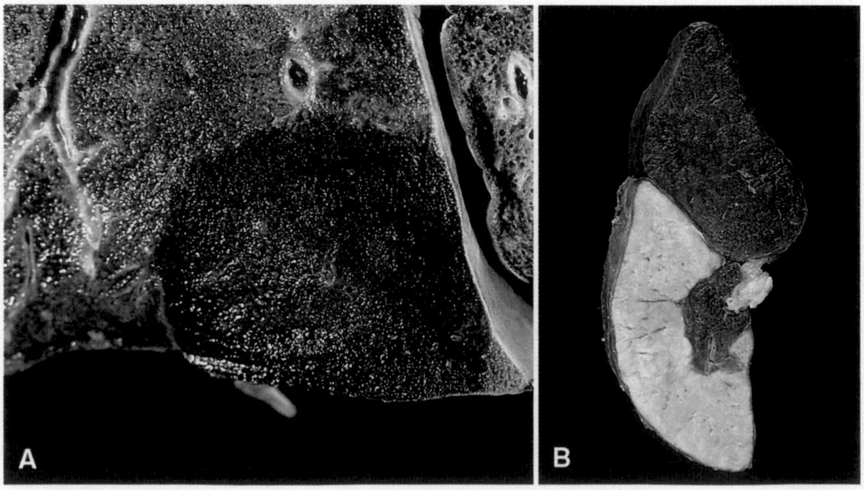

FIGURE 4–19 Examples of infarcts. *A*, Hemorrhagic, roughly wedge-shaped pulmonary infarct. *B*, Sharply demarcated white infarct in the spleen.

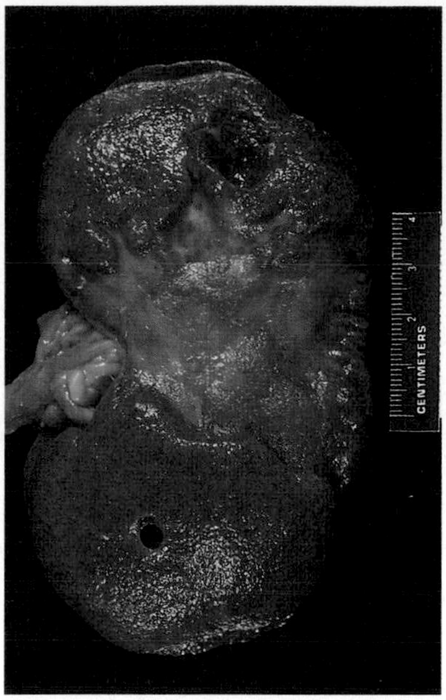

FIGURE 4–20 Remote kidney infarct, now replaced by a large fibrotic cortical scar.

Clinical Correlations: Factors That Influence Development of an Infarct. The consequences of a vascular occlusion can range from no or minimal effect, all the way up to death of a tissue or even the individual. *The major determinants include:* (1) *the nature of the vascular supply*; (2) *the rate of development of the occlusion*; (3) *the vulnerability of a given tissue to hypoxia*; and (4) *the blood oxygen content.*

- *Nature of the vascular supply.* The availability of an alternative blood supply is the most important factor in determining whether occlusion of a vessel will cause damage. Lungs, for example, have a dual pulmonary and bronchial artery blood supply; thus, obstruction of a small pulmonary arteriole does not cause infarction in an otherwise healthy individual with an intact bronchial circulation. Similarly, the liver, with its dual hepatic artery and portal vein circulation, and the hand and forearm, with their dual radial and ulnar arterial supply, are all relatively insensitive to infarction. In contrast, renal and splenic circulations are end-arterial, and obstruction of such vessels generally causes infarction.
- *Rate of development of occlusion.* Slowly developing occlusions are less likely to cause infarction because they provide time for the development of alternative perfusion pathways. For example, small interarteriolar anastomoses—normally with minimal functional flow—interconnect the three major coronary arteries in the heart. If one of the coronaries is only slowly occluded (i.e., by an encroaching atherosclerotic plaque), flow within this *collateral circulation* may increase sufficiently to prevent infarction, even though the major coronary artery is eventually occluded.
- *Vulnerability to hypoxia.* The susceptibility of a tissue to hypoxia influences the likelihood of infarction. Neurons undergo irreversible damage when deprived of their blood supply for only 3 to 4 minutes. Myocardial cells, although hardier than neurons, are also quite sensitive and die after only 20 to 30 minutes of ischemia. In contrast, fibroblasts within myocardium remain viable even after many hours of ischemia (Chapter 12).
- *Oxygen content of blood.* The partial pressure of oxygen in blood also determines the outcome of vascular occlusion. Partial flow obstruction of a small vessel in an anemic or cyanotic patient might lead to tissue infarction, whereas it would be without effect under conditions of normal oxygen tension. In this way, congestive heart failure, with *compromised flow and ventilation,* could cause infarction in the setting of an otherwise inconsequential blockage.

Shock

Shock, or *cardiovascular collapse,* is the final common pathway for a number of potentially lethal clinical events, including severe hemorrhage, extensive trauma or burns, large myocardial infarction, massive pulmonary embolism, and microbial sepsis. Regardless of the underlying pathology, *shock gives rise to systemic hypoperfusion caused by reduction either in cardiac output or in the effective circulating blood volume.* The end results are *hypotension, followed by impaired tissue perfusion and cellular hypoxia.* Although the hypoxic and metabolic effects of hypoperfusion initially cause only reversible cellular injury, persistence of shock eventually causes irreversible tissue injury and can culminate in the death of the patient.

Shock may be grouped into three general categories (Table 4–3). The mechanisms underlying cardiogenic and hypovolemic shock are fairly straightforward, essentially involving *low cardiac output.* Septic shock, by comparison, is substantially more complicated and is discussed in further detail below.

- *Cardiogenic shock* results from myocardial pump failure. This may be caused by intrinsic myocardial damage (infarction), ventricular arrhythmias, extrinsic compression (cardiac tamponade; Chapter 12), or outflow obstruction (e.g., pulmonary embolism).
- *Hypovolemic shock* results from loss of blood or plasma volume. This may be caused by hemorrhage, fluid loss from severe burns, or trauma.
- *Septic shock* is caused by systemic microbial infection. Most commonly, this occurs in the setting of gram-negative infections *(endotoxic shock),* but it can also occur with gram-positive and fungal infections.

Less commonly, shock may occur in the setting of anesthetic accident or spinal cord injury *(neurogenic shock),* owing to loss of vascular tone and peripheral pooling of blood. *Anaphylactic shock,* initiated by a generalized IgE-mediated hypersensitivity response, is associated with systemic vasodilation and increased vascular permeability (Chapter 6). In these instances, widespread vasodilation causes a sudden increase in the vascular bed capacitance, which is not adequately filled by the normal circulating blood volume. Thus, hypotension, tissue hypoperfusion, and cellular anoxia result.

PATHOGENESIS OF SEPTIC SHOCK

Septic shock, with a 25% to 50% mortality rate, ranks first among the causes of mortality in intensive care units and is

TABLE 4–3 Three Major Types of Shock

Type of Shock	Clinical Examples	Principal Mechanisms
Cardiogenic		
	Myocardial infarction Ventricular rupture Arrhythmia Cardiac tamponade Pulmonary embolism	Failure of myocardial pump owing to intrinsic myocardial damage, extrinsic pressure, or obstruction to outflow
Hypovolemic		
	Hemorrhage Fluid loss, e.g., vomiting, diarrhea, burns, or trauma	Inadequate blood or plasma volume
Septic		
	Overwhelming microbial infections Endotoxic shock Gram-positive septicemia Fungal sepsis Superantigens	Peripheral vasodilation and pooling of blood; endothelial activation/injury; leukocyte-induced damage; disseminated intravascular coagulation; activation of cytokine cascades

estimated to account for over 200,000 deaths annually in the United States.[53] Moreover, the reported incidence of sepsis syndromes has increased dramatically in the past two decades, owing to improved life support for high-risk patients, increasing use of invasive procedures, and growing numbers of immunocompromised hosts (secondary to chemotherapy, immunosuppression, or human immunodeficiency virus infection). Septic shock results from spread and expansion of an initially localized infection (e.g., abscess, peritonitis, pneumonia) into the bloodstream.

Most cases of septic shock (approximately 70%) are caused by endotoxin-producing gram-negative bacilli (Chapter 8), hence the term *endotoxic shock.* Endotoxins are bacterial wall lipopolysaccharides (LPSs) that are released when the cell walls are degraded (e.g., in an inflammatory response). LPS consists of a toxic fatty acid *(lipid A)* core and a complex polysaccharide coat (including O antigens) unique to each bacterial species. Analogous molecules in the walls of gram-positive bacteria and fungi can also elicit septic shock.

All of the cellular and resultant hemodynamic effects of septic shock may be reproduced by injection of LPS alone. Free LPS attaches to a circulating LPS-binding protein, and the complex then binds to a cell-surface receptor (called CD14), followed by binding of the LPS to a signal-transducing protein called *mammalian Toll-like receptor protein 4* (TLR-4). (Toll is a *Drosophila* protein involved in fly development; a variety of molecules with homology to Toll [i.e., "Toll-like"] participate in innate immune responses to different microbial components; see Box 6–1, Chapter 6.) Signals from TLR-4 can then directly activate vascular wall cells and leukocytes or initiate a cascade of cytokine mediators, which propagates the pathologic state.[54,55] Engagement of TLR-4 on endothelial cells can lead directly to down-regulation of natural anticoagulation mechanisms, including diminished synthesis of tissue factor pathway inhibitor (TFPI) and thrombomodulin. Engagement of the receptor on monocytes and macrophages (even at doses of LPS as minute as 10 picograms/ml) causes profound mononuclear cell activation with the subsequent production of potent effector cytokines such as IL-1 and TNF (Chapter 6). Presumably, this series of responses helps to isolate organisms and to trigger elements of the innate immune system to efficiently eradicate invading microbes. Unfortunately, depending on the dosage and numbers of macrophages that are activated, the secondary effects of LPS release can also cause severe pathologic changes, including fatal shock.

- At low doses, LPS predominantly serves to activate monocytes and macrophages, with effects intended to enhance their ability to eliminate invading bacteria. LPS can also directly activate complement, which likewise contributes to local bacterial eradication. The mononuclear phagocytes respond to LPS by producing cytokines, mainly TNF, IL-1, IL-6, and chemokines. TNF and IL-1 both act on endothelial cells to stimulate the expression of adhesion molecules (Chapter 2; Fig. 4–21) and the production of other cytokines and chemokines. Thus, the initial release of LPS results in a circumscribed cytokine cascade doubtless intended to enhance the *local* acute inflammatory response and improve clearance of the infection.
- With moderately severe infections, and therefore with higher levels of LPS (and a consequent augmentation of the cytokine cascade), cytokine-induced secondary effectors (e.g., nitric oxide; Chapter 2) become significant. In addition, systemic effects of the cytokines such as TNF and IL-1 may begin to be seen; these include fever and increased synthesis of acute phase reactants (Chapter 2; Fig. 4–21). LPS at higher doses also results in diminished endothelial cell production of thrombomodulin and TFPI, tipping the coagulation cascade toward thrombosis.
- Finally, at still higher levels of LPS, the syndrome of septic shock supervenes (Fig. 4–22); the same cytokines and secondary mediators, now at high levels, result in:
  - Systemic vasodilation (hypotension)
  - Diminished myocardial contractility
  - Widespread endothelial injury and activation, causing systemic leukocyte adhesion and pulmonary alveolar capillary damage (*acute respiratory distress syndrome*; Chapter 15)
  - Activation of the coagulation system, culminating in DIC

The hypoperfusion resulting from the combined effects of widespread vasodilation, myocardial pump failure, and DIC induces *multiorgan system failure* affecting the liver, kidneys,

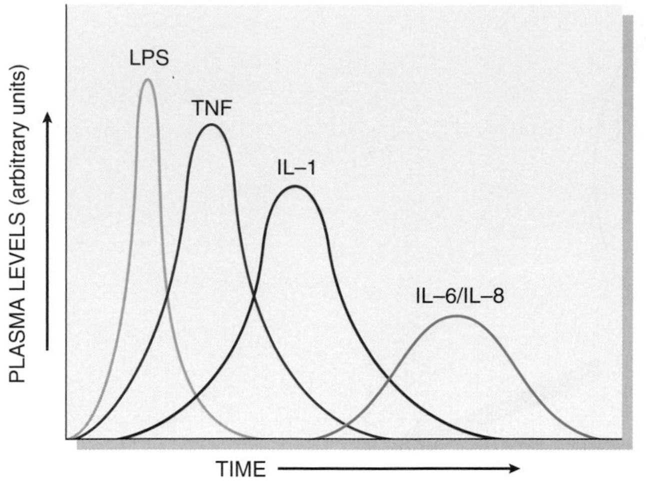

FIGURE 4–21 Cytokine cascade in sepsis. After release of lipopolysaccharide (LPS) from invading gram-negative microorganisms, there are successive waves of tumor necrosis factor (TNF), interleukin-1 (IL-1), and IL-6 secretion. (Modified from Abbas AK, et al: Cellular and Molecular Immunology, 4th ed. Philadelphia, WB Saunders, 2000.)

and central nervous system, among others.[56,57] Unless the underlying infection (and LPS overload) is rapidly brought under control, the patient usually dies. Of note, mice lacking LPS-binding protein, CD14, or the mammalian TLR-4 are protected against the effects of LPS. Clinical efforts to take advantage of these insights and induce pharmacologic blockade of the same pathways (e.g., soluble CD14 or antibodies to LPS-binding protein) have yet to bear fruit. Antibodies or antagonists to IL-1 or TNF (or their receptors), or pharmacologic inhibitors of various other secondary mediators (e.g., nitric oxide or prostaglandins) have some efficacy in animal models of septic shock, but they have not shown significant clinical benefit in human disease.[54,56,58] Indeed such failure of "anti-inflammatory" therapy in human shock has caused some investigators to challenge the model presented here (see Fig. 4–22). Instead, it has been argued that in later stages, sepsis is associated with a state of immunosuppression (rather than uncontrolled inflammation).[59] These observations may dictate different forms of therapy, but this remains to be tested.

An interesting group of bacterial proteins called *superantigens* also cause syndromes similar to septic shock. These include *toxic shock syndrome toxin-1*, produced by staphylococci and responsible for the *toxic shock syndrome.* Superantigens are polyclonal T-lymphocyte activators that induce systemic inflammatory cytokine cascades similar to those occurring downstream in septic shock.[60,61] Their actions can result in a variety of clinical manifestations ranging from a diffuse rash to vasodilation, hypotension, and death.[62,63]

Stages of Shock. Shock is a progressive disorder that, if uncorrected, leads to death. Unless the insult is massive and rapidly lethal (e.g., a massive hemorrhage from a ruptured aortic aneurysm), shock tends to evolve through three general (albeit somewhat artificial) phases. A brief discussion here can help to integrate the sequential pathophysiologic and clinical events in the progression of shock. These have been documented most clearly in hypovolemic shock but are common to other forms as well:

An initial *nonprogressive phase* during which reflex compensatory mechanisms are activated and perfusion of vital organs is maintained

A *progressive stage* characterized by tissue hypoperfusion and onset of worsening circulatory and metabolic imbalances, including acidosis

An *irreversible stage* that sets in after the body has incurred cellular and tissue injury so severe that even if the hemodynamic defects are corrected, survival is not possible.

In the early nonprogressive phase of shock, a variety of *neurohumoral mechanisms* help maintain cardiac output and blood pressure. These include baroreceptor reflexes, release of catecholamines, activation of the renin-angiotensin axis, antidiuretic hormone release, and generalized sympathetic stimulation. The net effect is *tachycardia, peripheral vasoconstriction, and renal conservation of fluid.* Cutaneous vasoconstriction, for example, is responsible for the characteristic coolness and pallor of skin in well-developed shock (although septic shock may initially cause cutaneous *vasodilation* and thus present with warm, flushed skin). Coronary and cerebral vessels are less sensitive to this compensatory sympathetic response and thus maintain relatively normal caliber, blood flow, and oxygen delivery to their respective vital organs.

If the underlying causes are not corrected, shock passes imperceptibly to the progressive phase, during which there is widespread tissue hypoxia. In the setting of persistent oxygen deficit, intracellular aerobic respiration is replaced by anaerobic glycolysis with excessive production of lactic acid. The resultant metabolic *lactic acidosis lowers the tissue pH and blunts the vasomotor response*; arterioles dilate, and blood begins to pool in the microcirculation. Peripheral pooling not only worsens the cardiac output, but also puts endothelial cells at risk for developing anoxic injury with subsequent DIC. With widespread tissue hypoxia, vital organs are affected and begin to fail; *clinically the patient may become confused, and the urine output declines.*

Unless there is intervention, the process eventually enters an irreversible stage. Widespread cell injury is reflected in lysosomal enzyme leakage, further aggravating the shock state. Myocardial contractile function worsens in part because of nitric oxide synthesis. If ischemic bowel allows intestinal flora to enter the circulation, endotoxic shock may be superimposed. At this point, the patient has complete renal shutdown owing to acute tubular necrosis (Chapter 20), and despite heroic measures, the downward clinical spiral almost inevitably culminates in death.

Morphology. The cellular and tissue changes induced by shock are essentially those of hypoxic injury (Chapter 1); since shock is characterized by **failure of multiple organ systems,** the cellular changes may appear in any tissue. Nevertheless, they are particularly evident in brain, heart, lungs, kidneys, adrenals, and gastrointestinal tract.

The **brain** may develop so-called ischemic encephalopathy, discussed in Chapter 28. The **heart** may undergo focal or widespread coagulation necrosis or

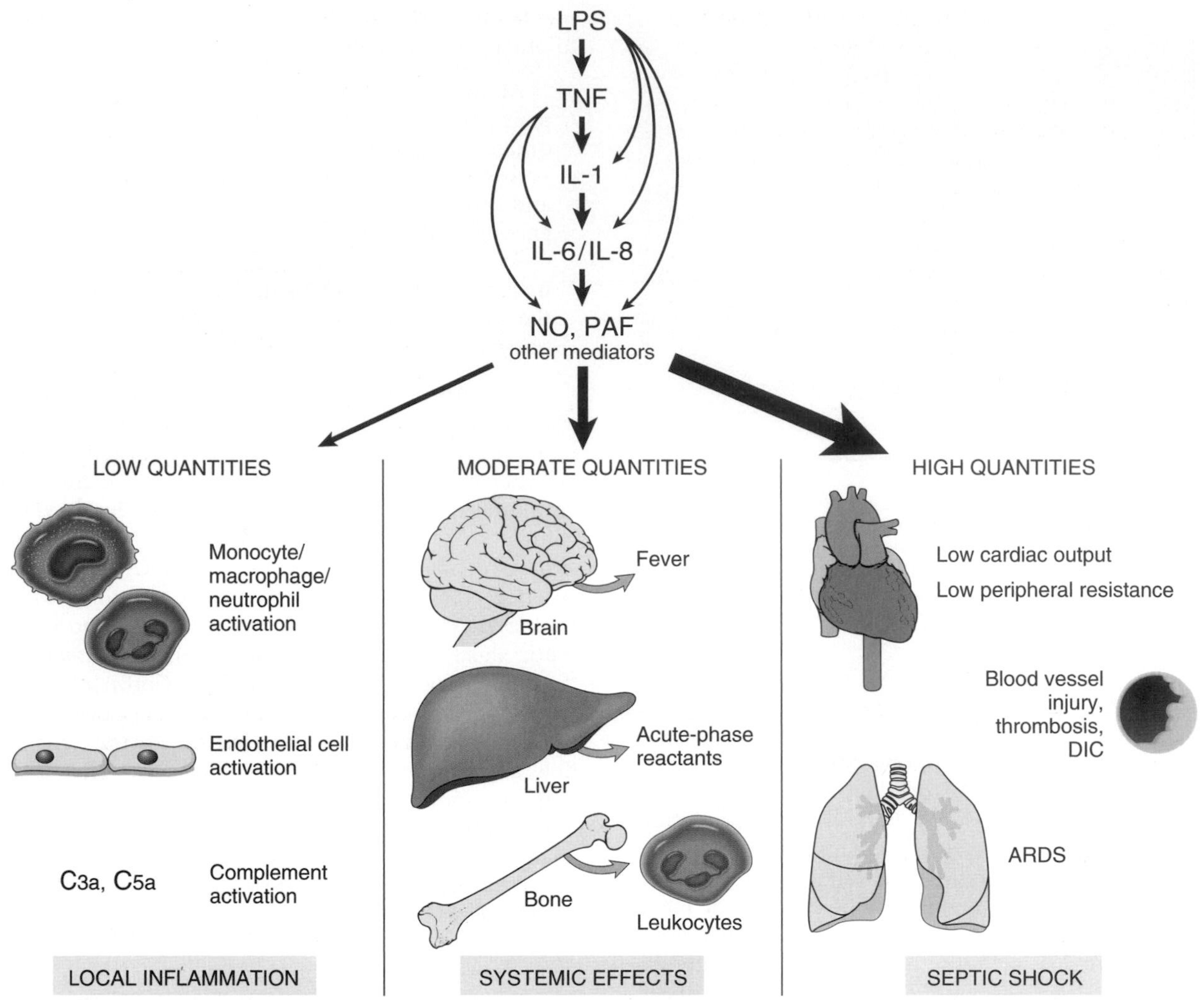

FIGURE 4–22 Effects of lipopolysaccharide (LPS) and secondarily induced effector molecules. LPS initiates the cytokine cascade described in Figure 4–21; in addition, LPS and the various factors can directly stimulate downstream cytokine production, as indicated. Secondary effectors that become important include nitric oxide (NO) and platelet-activating factor (PAF). At low levels, only local inflammatory effects are seen. With moderate levels, more systemic events occur in addition to the local vascular effects. At high concentrations, the syndrome of septic shock is seen. DIC, disseminated intravascular coagulation; ARDS, adult respiratory distress syndrome. (Modified from Abbas AK, et al: Cellular and Molecular Immunology, 4th ed. Philadelphia, WB Saunders, 2000.)

may exhibit subendocardial hemorrhage and/or **contraction band necrosis** (Chapter 12). Although the cardiac changes are not diagnostic of shock (they may also be seen in the setting of cardiac reperfusion after irreversible injury, or after administration of catecholamines), they are usually much more extensive in the setting of shock. The **kidneys** typically exhibit extensive tubular ischemic injury (**acute tubular necrosis**; Chapter 20), therefore oliguria, anuria, and electrolyte disturbances constitute major clinical problems. The **lungs** are seldom affected in pure hypovolemic shock because they are resistant to hypoxic injury. When shock is caused by bacterial sepsis or trauma, however, changes of diffuse alveolar damage (Chapter 15) may appear, the so-called **shock lung**. The **adrenal** changes in shock are those seen in all forms of stress; essentially, there is cortical cell lipid depletion. This does not reflect adrenal exhaustion but rather conversion of the relatively inactive vacuolated cells to metabolically active cells that utilize stored lipids for the synthesis of steroids. The **gastrointestinal tract** may suffer patchy mucosal hemorrhages and necroses, referred to as **hemorrhagic enteropathy**. The **liver** may develop fatty change and, with severe perfusion deficits, central hemorrhagic necrosis (Chapter 18).

With the exception of neuronal and myocyte loss, virtually all of these tissue changes may revert to normal if the patient survives. Unfortunately, most patients with irreversible changes owing to severe shock succumb before the tissues can recover.

Clinical Course. The clinical manifestations depend on the precipitating insult. In hypovolemic and cardiogenic shock, *the patient presents with hypotension; a weak, rapid pulse; tachypnea; and cool, clammy, cyanotic skin.* In septic shock, however, *the skin may initially be warm and flushed because of peripheral vasodilation.* The original threat to life stems from the underlying catastrophe that precipitated the shock state (e.g., myocardial infarct, severe hemorrhage, or uncontrolled bacterial infection). Rapidly, however, the cardiac, cerebral, and pulmonary changes secondary to the shock state materially worsen the problem. Eventually, electrolyte disturbances and metabolic acidosis also exacerbate the situation. If the patient survives the initial complications, he or she enters *a second phase dominated by renal insufficiency* and marked by a progressive fall in urine output as well as severe fluid and electrolyte imbalances.

The prognosis varies with the origin of shock and its duration. Thus, 80% to 90% of young, otherwise healthy patients with hypovolemic shock survive with appropriate management, whereas cardiogenic shock associated with extensive myocardial infarction and gram-negative shock carry mortality rates of up to 75%, even with the best care currently available.

REFERENCES

1. Schrier R, Abraham W: Hormones and hemodynamics in heart failure. N Engl J Med 341:577, 1999.
2. Bick R, Murano G: Physiology of hemostasis. Clin Lab Med 14:677, 1994.
3. Hoffman M, Monroe DR: A cell-based model of hemostasis. Thromb Haemost 85:958, 2001.
4. Gross P, Aird W: The endothelium and thrombosis. Semin Thromb Hemost 26:463, 2000.
5. Pearson J: Endothelial cell function and thrombosis. Best Pract Res Clin Haematol 12:329, 1999.
6. Michiels C: Endothelial cell functions. J Cell Physiol 196:430, 2003.
7. Esmon C: Protein C anticoagulant pathway and its role in controlling microvascular thrombosis and inflammation. Crit Care Med 29 (Suppl 7):S48, 2001.
8. Kato H: Regulation of functions of vascular wall cells by tissue factor pathway inhibitor: basic and clinical aspects. Arterioscler Thromb Vasc Biol 22:539, 2002.
9. Lijnen H, Collen D: Endothelium in hemostasis and thrombosis. Prog Cardiovasc Dis 39:343, 1997.
10. Denis C: Molecular and cellular biology of von Willebrand factor. Int J Hematol 75:3, 2002.
11. Doshi S, Marmur J: Evolving role of tissue factor and its pathway inhibitor. Crit Care Med 30 (5 Suppl):S241, 2002.
12. Binder B, et al: Plasminogen activator inhibitor 1: physiological and pathophysiological roles. News Physiol Sci 17:56, 2002.
13. Bouchard B, Tracy P: Platelets, leukocytes, and coagulation. Curr Opin Hematol 9:263, 2001.
14. Heemskerk JW, Bevers EM, Lindhout T: Platelet activation and blood coagulation. Thromb Hemost 88:186, 2002.
15. Mann KG, Butenas S, Brummel K: The dynamics of thrombin formation. Atheroscler Throm Vasc Biol 23:17, 2003.
16. Caen J, Rosa J: Platelet–vessel wall interaction: from bedside to molecules. Thromb Haemost 74:18, 1995.
17. Casserly I, Topol E: Glycoprotein IIb/IIIa antagonists - from bench to practice. Cell Mol Life Sci 59:478, 2002.
18. Norris LA: Blood coagulation. Best Pract Res Clin Obstet Gynaecol 17:369, 2003.
19. Semeraro N, Colucci M: Tissue factor in health and disease. Thromb Haemost 78:759, 1997.
20. Coughlin SR, Camerer E: PARticipation in inflammation. J Clin Invest 111:25, 2003.
21. Galino P: The inhibitor of tissue factor: factor VII pathway. Thromb Res 106:V257, 2002.
22. Pearson T, LaCava J, Weil H: Epidemiology of thrombotic-hemostatic factors and their associations with cardiovascular disease. Am J Clin Nutr 65 (Suppl 5):1674S, 1997.
23. Wootton D, Ku D: Fluid mechanics of vascular systems, diseases, and thrombosis. Annu Rev Biomed Eng 1:299, 1999.
24. Emmerich J et al: Combined effect of factor V Leiden and prothrombin 20210A on risk of venous thromboembolism—pooled analysis of 8 case-control studies including 2310 cases and 3204 controls. Study group for pooled analysis in venous thromboelmbolism. Thromb Haemost 86:809, 2001.
25. Thomas R: Hypercoagulability syndromes. Arch Intern Med 161:2433, 2001.
26. Harpel P, Zhang X, Borth W: Homocysteine and hemostasis: pathogenic mechanisms predisposing to thrombosis. J Nutr 126 (Suppl 4):1285S, 1996.
27. Poort S, et al: A common genetic variation in the 3'-untranslated region of the prothrombin gene is associated with elevated plasma prothrombin levels and an increase in venous thrombosis. Blood 88:3698, 1996.
28. Vicente V, et al: The prothrombin gene variant 20210A in venous and arterial thromboembolism. Haematologica 84:356, 1999.
29. Kottke-Marchant K: Genetic polymorphisms associated with venous and arterial thrombosis: an overview. Arch Pathol Lab Med 126:295, 2002.
30. Rosendaal F, Helmerhorst F, Vandenbroucke J: Oral contraceptives, hormone replacement therapy and thrombosis. Thromb Haemost 86:112, 2001.
31. Caine GJ, et al: The hypercoagulable state of malignancy: pathogenesis and current debate. Neoplasia 4:465, 2002.
32. Lip G, Chin B, Blann A: Cancer and the prothrombotic state. Lancet Oncol 3:27, 2002.
33. Januzzi JJ, Jang I: Fundamental concepts in the pathobiology of heparin-induced thrombocytopenia. J Thromb Thrombolysis 10 (Suppl 1):7, 2000.
34. Chong B: Heparin-induced thrombocytopenia. J Thromb Hemost 7:1472, 2003.
35. Rand JH: The antiphospholipid syndrome. Ann Rev Med 54:409, 2003.
36. Honley JG: Antiphospholipid syndrome: an overview. CMAJ 168:1675, 2003.
37. Alving B: Diagnosis and management of patients with the antiphospholipid syndrome. J Thromb Thrombolysis 12:89, 2001.
38. Shapiro S: The lupus anticoagulant/antiphospholipid syndrome. Ann Rev Med 47:533, 1996.
39. Becattini C, Agnelli G: Pathogenesis of venous thromboembolism. Curr Opin Pulmon Med 8:300, 2002.
40. Bick R: Disseminated intravascular coagulation: a review of etiology, pathophysiology, diagnosis, and management: guidelines for care. Clin Appl Thromb Hemost 8:1, 2002.
41. Perrier A: Noninvasive diagnosis of pulmonary embolism. Haematologica 82:328, 1997.
42. Perrier A, Bounameaux H: Diagnosis of pulmonary embolism in outpatients by sequential noninvasive tools. Semin Thromb Hemost 27:25, 2001.
43. Heit J: Venous thromboembolism epidemiology: implications for prevention and management. Semin Thromb Hemost 28 (Suppl 2):3, 2002.
44. Goldhaber S: Pulmonary embolism. N Engl J Med 339:93, 1998.
45. Mellor A, Soni N: Fat embolism. Anaesthesia 56:145, 2001.
46. Parisi DM, Koval K, Egol K: Fat embolism syndrome. Am J Orthop 31:507, 2002.
47. Dudney T, Elliot C: Pulmonary embolism from amniotic fluid, fat, and air. Prog Cardiovasc Dis 36:447, 1994.
48. King M, Harmon K: Unusual forms of pulmonary embolism. Clin Chest Med 15:561, 1994.
49. Madsen J, Hink J, Hyldegaard O: Diving physiology and pathophysiology. Clin Physiol 14:597, 1994.
50. Neuman T: Arterial gas embolism and decompression sickness. News Physiol Sci 17:77, 2002.
51. Davies S: Amniotic fluid embolus: a review of the literature. Can J Anaesth 48:88, 2001.
52. Locksmith GJ: Amniotic fluid embolism. Obstet Gynecol Clin 26:435, 1999.
53. Angus D, et al: Epidemiology of severe sepsis in the United States: Analysis of incidence, outcome, and associated costs of care. Crit Care Med 29:1303–1310, 2001.
54. Van Amersfoort ES, VanBerkel TJ, Kuiper J: Receptors, mediators, and mechanisms involved in bacterial sepsis and septic shock. Clin Microbiol Rev 16:379, 2003.
55. Opal S, Huber C: Bench-to-bedside review: Toll-like receptors and their role in septic shock. Crit Care 6:125, 2002.
56. Glauser M: Pathophysiologic basis of sepsis: considerations for future strategies of intervention. Crit Care Med 28 (9 Suppl):S4, 2000.
57. Hardaway R, Williams C, Vasquez Y: Disseminated intravascular coagulation in sepsis. Semin Thromb Hemost 27:577, 2001.

58. Natanson C: Anti-inflammatory therapies to treat sepsis and septic shock: a reassessment. Crit Care Med 25:1095, 1997.
59. Hotchkiss RS, Karl IE: Medical progress: the pathophysiology and treatment of sepsis. N Engl J Med 348:138, 2003.
60. Johnson H, Torres B, Soos J: Superantigens: structure and relevance to human disease. Proc Soc Exp Biol Med 212:99, 1996.
61. Llewelyn M, Cohen J: Superantigens: microbial agents that corrupt immunity. Lancet Infect Dis 2:156, 2002.
62. Stevens D: The toxic shock syndromes. Infect Dis Clin North Am 10:727, 1996.
63. Torres B, Johnson H: Modulation of disease by superantigens. Cur Opin Immunol 10:465, 1998.

CHAPTER 5

Genetic Disorders

MUTATIONS

MENDELIAN DISORDERS

Transmission Patterns of Single-Gene Disorders
Autosomal Dominant Disorders
Autosomal Recessive Disorders
X-Linked Disorders

Biochemical and Molecular Basis of Single-Gene (Mendelian) Disorders
Enzyme Defects and Their Consequences
Defects in Receptors and Transport Systems
Alterations in Structure, Function, or Quantity of Nonenzyme Proteins
Genetically Determined Adverse Reactions to Drugs

Disorders Associated with Defects in Structural Proteins
Marfan Syndrome
Ehlers-Danlos Syndromes

Disorders Associated with Defects in Receptor Proteins
Familial Hypercholesterolemia

Disorders Associated with Defects in Enzymes
Lysosomal Storage Diseases
Glycogen Storage Diseases (Glycogenoses)
Alkaptonuria (Ochronosis)

Disorders Associated with Defects in Proteins That Regulate Cell Growth
Neurofibromatosis: Types 1 and 2

DISORDERS WITH MULTIFACTORIAL INHERITANCE

NORMAL KARYOTYPE

CYTOGENETIC DISORDERS

Cytogenetic Disorders Involving Autosomes
Trisomy 21 (Down Syndrome)
Other Trisomies
Chromosome 22q11.2 Deletion Syndrome

Cytogenetic Disorders Involving Sex Chromosomes
Klinefelter Syndrome
Turner Syndrome
Hermaphroditism and Pseudohermaphroditism

SINGLE-GENE DISORDERS WITH NONCLASSIC INHERITANCE

Triplet-Repeat Mutations—Fragile-X Syndrome
Other Diseases with Unstable Nucleotide Repeats

Mutations in Mitochondrial Genes — Leber Hereditary Optic Neuropathy

Genomic Imprinting
Prader-Willi Syndrome and Angelman Syndrome

Gonadal Mosaicism

MOLECULAR DIAGNOSIS

DIAGNOSIS OF GENETIC DISEASES

Direct Gene Diagnosis

Indirect DNA Diagnosis: Linkage Analysis

Genetic disorders are far more common than is widely appreciated. The lifetime frequency of genetic diseases is estimated to be 670 per 1000.[1] Included in this figure are not only the "classic" genetic disorders but also cancer and cardiovascular diseases, the two most common causes of death in the Western world. Both of these have major genetic components. Cardiovascular diseases, such as atherosclerosis and hypertension, result from complex interactions of genes and environment, and most cancers are now known to result from an accumulation of mutations in somatic cells (Chapter 7).

The genetic diseases encountered in medical practice represent only the tip of the iceberg, that is, those with less extreme genotypic errors permitting full embryonic development and live birth. It is estimated that 50% of spontaneous abortuses during the early months of gestation have a demonstrable chromosomal abnormality; there are, in addition, numerous smaller detectable errors and many others still beyond our range of identification. About 1% of all newborn infants possess a gross chromosomal abnormality, and approximately 5% of individuals under age 25 develop a serious disease with a significant genetic component. How many more mutations remain hidden?

The draft sequence of the human genome is complete and much has been learned about the "genetic architecture" of humans. Some of what has been revealed was quite unexpected.[2] For example, we now know that less than 2% of the human genome codes for proteins, whereas more than one half represents blocks of repetitive nucleotide codes whose functions remain mysterious. What was totally unexpected was that humans have a mere 30,000 genes rather than the 100,000 predicted only recently. Quite remarkably, this figure is not much greater than that of the mustard plant, with 26,000 genes! However, it is also known that by alternative splicing, 30,000 genes can give rise to greater than 100,000 proteins. In addition, very recent studies indicate that fully formed proteins can be sliced and stitched together to give rise to peptides that could not have been predicted from the structure of the gene.[2a] Humans are not so poor, after all. With the completion of the human genome project, a new term, called *genomics*, has been added to the medical vocabulary. Whereas genetics is the study of single or a few genes and their phenotypic effects, genomics is the study of all the genes in the genome and their interactions. DNA microarray analysis of tumors (Chapter 7) is an excellent example of genomics in current clinical use.[3] However, the most important contribution of genomics to human health will be in the unraveling of complex multifactorial diseases (discussed later) that arise from the interaction of multiple genes with environmental factors.[4]

Another surprising revelation from the recent progress in genomics is that, on average, any two individuals share 99.9% of their DNA sequences. Thus, the remarkable diversity of humans is encoded in about 0.1% of our DNA. The secrets to disease predisposition and response to environmental agents and drugs must therefore reside within these variable regions. Although small as compared to the total nucleotide sequences, this 0.1% represents about 3 million base pairs. The most common form of DNA variations in the human genome is the single nucleotide polymorphism (SNP). Typically, the SNPs are biallelic (i.e., only two choices exist at a given site within the population), and they may occur anywhere in the genome—within exons, introns, or intergenic regions. Less than 1% of SNPs occur in coding regions. These could of course alter the gene product and give rise to a disease. Much more commonly, however, the SNP is just a marker that is co-inherited with a disease-causing gene, due to physical proximity. Another way of expressing this is to say that the SNP and the genetic factor are in linkage disequilibrium. Much effort is ongoing to make SNP maps of the human genome so that we can decipher genetic determinants of disease.[5] Just as genomics involves the study of all the DNA sequences, *proteomics* concerns itself with the measurement of all proteins expressed in a cell or tissue. Currently, progress in proteomics is lagging behind genomics, because the methodology to identify hundreds of distinct proteins simultaneously is not fully developed, but much effort continues.

Although genomics and proteomics are revealing a treasure-trove of information, our ability to organize and mine such a vast array of data is not yet fully developed. To simultaneously analyze patterns of expression involving thousands of genes and proteins has required the parallel development of computer-based techniques that can manage vast collections of data. In response to this, an exciting new discipline called *bioinformatics* has sprouted. This has involved biologists, computer scientists, physicists, and mathematicians, a true example of a multidisciplinary approach in modern medical practice.[6]

Much of the progress in medical genetics has resulted from the spectacular advances in molecular biology, involving recombinant DNA technology. The details of these techniques are well known and are not repeated here. Some examples, however, of the impact of recombinant DNA technology on medicine are worthy of attention.

- *Molecular basis of human disease:* Two general strategies have been used to isolate and characterize involved genes (Fig. 5–1). The *functional cloning*, or *classic*, approach has been successfully used to study a variety of inborn errors of metabolism, such as phenylketonuria and disorders of hemoglobin synthesis. Common to these genetic diseases is knowledge of the abnormal gene product and the corresponding protein. When the affected protein is known, a variety of methods can be employed to isolate the normal gene, to clone it, and ultimately to determine the molecular changes that affect the gene in patients with the disorder. Because in many common single-gene disorders, such as cystic fibrosis, there was no clue to the nature of the defective gene product, an alternative strategy called *positional cloning*, or the "candidate gene," approach had to be employed. This strategy initially ignores the biochemical clues from the phenotype and relies instead on mapping the disease phenotype to a particular chromosome location. This mapping is accomplished if the disease is associated with a distinctive cytogenetic change (e.g., fragile-X syndrome) or by linkage analysis. In the latter, the approximate location of the gene is determined by linkage to known "marker genes" or SNPs that are in close proximity to the disease locus. Once the region in which the mutant gene lies has been localized within reasonably narrow limits, the next step is to clone several pieces of DNA from the relevant segment of the genome. Expression of the cloned DNA in vitro, followed by identification of the protein products, can then be used to identify the aberrant protein encoded by the mutant genes. This approach has been used successfully in several diseases, such as cystic fibrosis, neurofibromatosis, Duchenne muscular dystrophy (a hereditary disorder characterized by progressive muscle weakness), polycystic

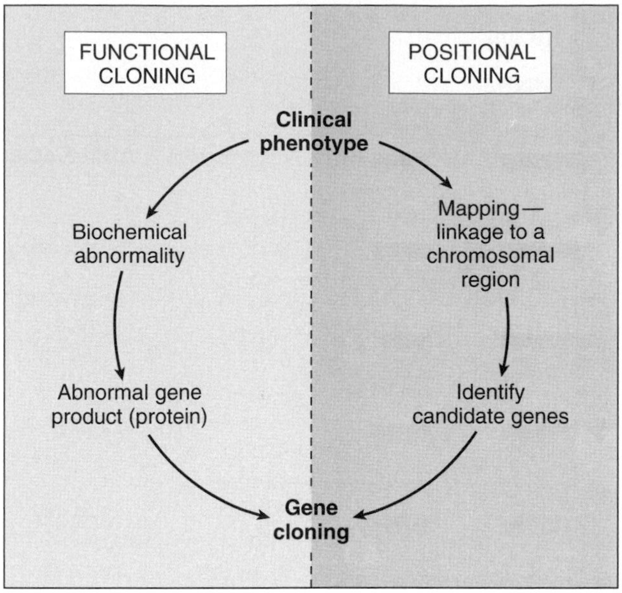

FIGURE 5–1 Schematic illustration of the strategies employed in functional and positional cloning. Functional cloning begins with relating the clinical phenotype to biochemical-protein abnormalities, followed by isolation of the mutant gene. Positional cloning, also called candidate gene approach, begins by mapping and cloning the disease gene by linkage analysis, without any knowledge of the gene product. Identification of the gene product and the mechanism by which it produces the disease follow the isolation of the mutant gene.

kidney disease, and Huntington disease. In addition to this step-by-step approach to cloning single genes, cDNA microarray analysis allows simultaneous detection of thousands of genes and their RNA products. When normal and diseased tissues are analyzed in this fashion, changes in the expression levels of multiple genes can be detected, thus providing a more comprehensive profile of genetic alterations in diseased tissues.

- *Production of human biologically active agents:* An array of ultrapure biologically active agents can now be produced in virtually unlimited quantities by inserting the requisite gene into bacteria or other suitable cells in tissue culture. Some examples of genetically engineered products already in clinical use include soluble TNF receptor for blocking TNF in treatment of rheumatoid arthritis, tissue plasminogen activator for the treatment of thrombotic states, growth hormone for the treatment of deficiency states, erythropoietin to reverse several types of anemia, and myeloid growth and differentiation factors (granulocyte-macrophage colony-stimulating factor, granulocyte colony-stimulating factor) to enhance production of monocytes and neutrophils in states of poor marrow function.
- *Gene therapy:* The goal of treating genetic diseases by transfer of somatic cells transfected with the normal gene, although simple in concept, has yet to succeed on a large scale. Problems include designing appropriate vectors to carry the gene and unexpected complications resulting from random insertion of the normal gene in the host genome. In recent well-publicized cases, gene therapy in patients with x-linked SCID (severe combined immunodeficiency, Chapter 6) who lack the common γ chain of cytokine receptors had to be put on hold because the transduced gene inserted next to a host gene that controls proliferation of cells. The resulting dysregulation gave rise to T-cell leukemia in the patient.
- *Disease diagnosis:* Molecular probes are proving to be extremely useful in the diagnosis of both genetic and nongenetic (e.g., infectious) diseases. The diagnostic applications of recombinant DNA technology are detailed at the end of this chapter.

With this background of developments in human genetics, we can turn next to the time-honored classification of human diseases into three categories: (1) those environmentally determined, (2) those genetically determined, and (3) those in which both environmental and genetic factors play a role. Obesity might appear to be representative of the first category; however, even here, with the discovery of genes that control satiety and energy metabolism (Chapter 9), it is evident that overnutrition—and all disorders to a greater or lesser degree—is conditioned by the genotype. Into the third category just mentioned fall many of the important diseases of humans, such as peptic ulcer, diabetes mellitus, atherosclerosis, schizophrenia, autoimmune disorders, and most cancers, in which clearly both nature and nurture play significant roles.

It is beyond the scope of this book to review normal human genetics. It is beneficial to review some fundamental concepts that have bearing on the understanding of genetic diseases. First, however, we clarify several commonly used terms—*hereditary, familial,* and *congenital.* Hereditary disorders, by definition, are derived from one's parents and are transmitted in the germ line through the generations and therefore are familial. The term *congenital* simply implies "born with." Some congenital diseases are not genetic; for example, congenital syphilis. Not all genetic diseases are congenital; patients with Huntington disease, for example, begin to manifest their condition only after their twenties or thirties.

Mutations

A *mutation* may be defined as a permanent change in the DNA. Mutations that affect germ cells are transmitted to the progeny and may give rise to inherited diseases. Mutations that arise in somatic cells understandably do not cause hereditary diseases but are important in the genesis of cancers and some congenital malformations.

Based on the extent of genetic change, mutations may be classified into three categories.[7] *Genome mutations* involve loss or gain of whole chromosomes, giving rise to monosomy or trisomy. *Chromosome mutations* result from rearrangement of genetic material and give rise to visible structural changes in the chromosome. Mutations involving changes in the number or structure of chromosomes are transmitted only infrequently because most are incompatible with survival. The vast majority of mutations associated with hereditary diseases are submicroscopic *gene mutations.* These may result in partial or complete deletion of a gene or, more often, affect a single base. For example, a single nucleotide base may be *substituted* by a different base, resulting in a *point mutation* (Fig. 5–2). Less commonly, one or two base pairs may be *inserted* into or *deleted* from the DNA, leading to alterations in the reading frame of the DNA strand; hence these are referred to as *frameshift* mutations (Figs. 5–3 and 5–4). The consequences

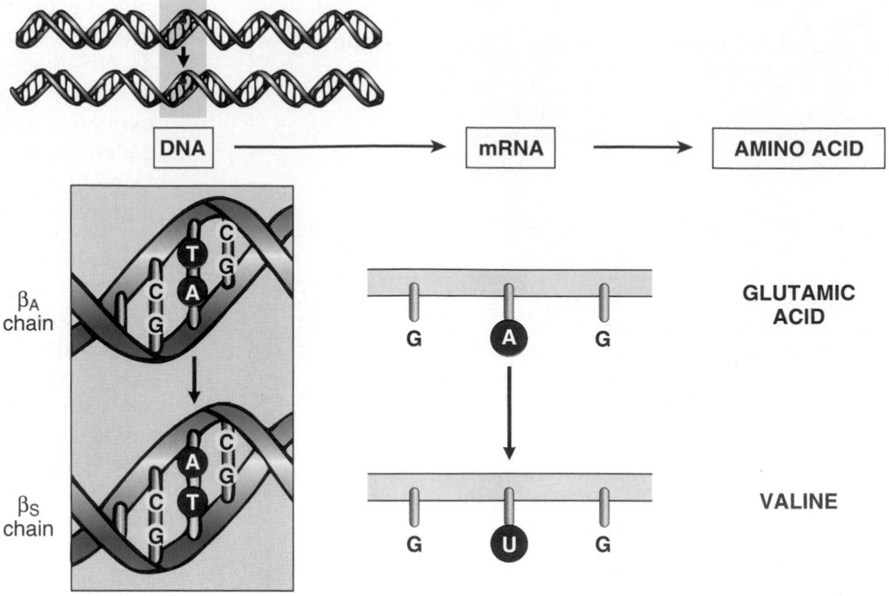

FIGURE 5–2 Schematic illustration of a point mutation resulting from a single base pair change in the DNA. In the example shown, a CTC to CAC change alters the meaning of the genetic code (GAG to GUG in the opposite strand), leading to replacement of glutamic acid by valine in the polypeptide chain. This change, affecting the sixth amino acid of the normal β-globin (β_A) chain, converts it to sickle β-globin (β_S).

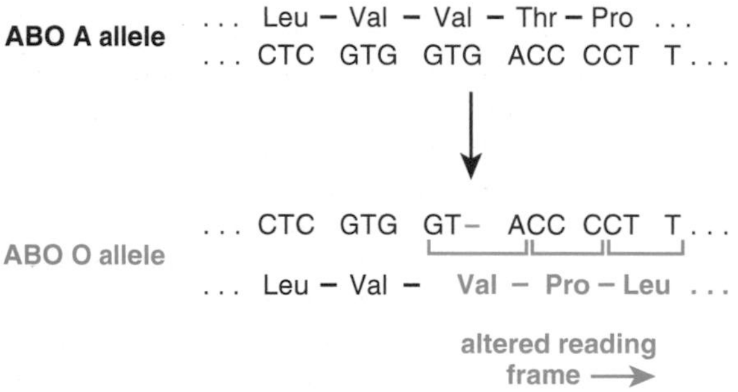

FIGURE 5–3 Single-base deletion at the ABO (glycosyltransferase) locus, leading to a frameshift mutation responsible for the O allele. (From Thompson MW, et al: Thompson and Thompson Genetics in Medicine, 5th ed. Philadelphia, WB Saunders, 1991, p 134.)

of mutations are varied, depending on several factors, including the type of mutation and the genomic site affected by it. Details of specific mutations and their effects are discussed along with the relevant disorders throughout this text. Here we briefly review some general principles relating to the effects of gene mutations.[2]

- *Point mutations within coding sequences:* A point mutation (single base substitution) may alter the code in a triplet of bases and lead to the replacement of one amino acid by another in the gene product. Because these mutations alter the meaning of the genetic code, they are often termed *missense mutations.* If the substituted amino acid causes little change in the function of the protein, the mutation is called a "conservative" missense mutation. On the other hand, a "nonconservative" missense mutation replaces the normal amino acid with a very different one. An excellent example of this type is the sickle mutation affecting the β-globin chain of hemoglobin (Chapter 13). Here the nucleotide triplet CTC (or GAG in messenger RNA [mRNA]), which codes for glutamic acid, is changed to CAC (or GUG in mRNA), which codes for valine (see Fig. 5–2). This single amino acid substitution alters the physicochemical properties of hemoglobin, giving rise to sickle cell anemia. Besides producing an amino acid substitution, a point mutation may change an amino acid codon to a chain terminator, or *stop codon (nonsense mutation).* Taking again the example of β-globin, a point mutation affecting the codon for glutamine (CAG) creates a stop codon (UAG) if U is substituted for C (Fig. 5–5). This change leads to premature termination of β-globin gene translation, and the resulting short peptide is rapidly degraded. The affected individuals lack β-globin chains and develop a severe form of anemia called β^0-thalassemia (Chapter 13).
- *Mutations within noncoding sequences:* Deleterious effects may also result from mutations that do not involve the exons. As is well known, transcription of DNA is initiated

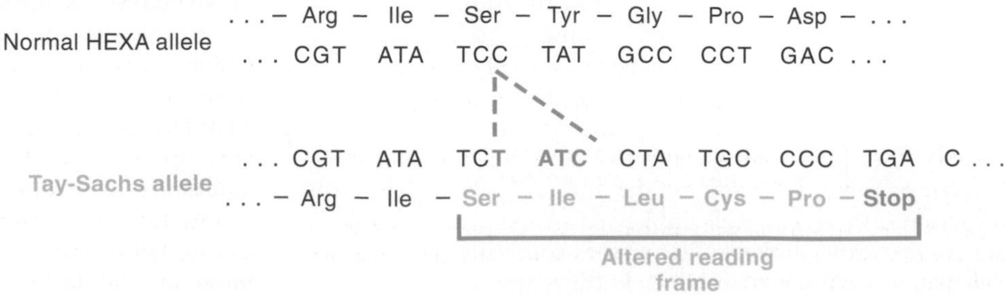

FIGURE 5–4 Four-base insertion in the hexosaminidase A gene in Tay-Sachs disease, leading to a frameshift mutation. This mutation is the major cause of Tay-Sachs disease in Ashkenazi Jews. (From Nussbaum, RL, et al: Thompson and Thompson Genetics in Medicine, 6th ed. Philadelphia, WB Saunders, 2001, p. 212.)

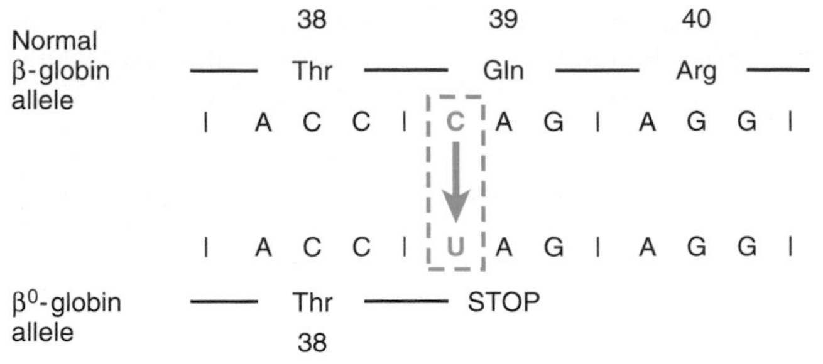

FIGURE 5–5 Point mutation leading to premature chain termination. Partial mRNA sequence of the β-globin chain of hemoglobin showing codons for amino acids 38 to 40. A point mutation (C→U) in codon 39 changes glutamine (Gln) codon to a stop codon, and hence protein synthesis stops at the 38th amino acid.

and regulated by promoter and enhancer sequences that are found downstream or upstream of the gene. Point mutations or deletions involving these regulatory sequences may interfere with binding of transcription factors and thus lead to a marked reduction in or total lack of transcription. Such is the case in certain forms of hereditary hemolytic anemias. In addition, point mutations within introns lead to defective splicing of intervening sequences. This, in turn, interferes with normal processing of the initial mRNA transcripts and results in a failure to form mature mRNA transcripts. Therefore, translation cannot take place, and the gene product is not synthesized.

- *Deletions and insertions:* Small deletions or insertions involving the coding sequence lead to alterations in the reading frame of the DNA strand; hence, they are referred to as *frameshift mutations* (see Figs. 5–3 and 5–4). If the number of base pairs involved is three or a multiple of three, frameshift does not occur (Fig. 5–6); instead an abnormal protein missing one or more amino acids is synthesized.
- *Trinucleotide repeat mutations:* Trinucleotide repeat mutations belong to a special category because these mutations are characterized by amplification of a sequence of three nucleotides. Although the specific nucleotide sequence that undergoes amplification differs in various disorders, almost all affected sequences share the nucleotides guanine (G) and cytosine (C). For example, in fragile-X syndrome, prototypical of this category of disorders, there are 250 to 4000 tandem repeats of the sequence CGG within a gene called *FMR-1*. In normal populations, the number of repeats is small, averaging 29. Such expansions of the trinucleotide sequences prevent normal expression of the *FMR-1* gene, thus giving rise to mental retardation. Another distinguishing feature of trinucleotide repeat mutations is that they are dynamic (i.e., the degree of amplification increases during gametogenesis). These features, discussed in greater detail later, influence the pattern of inheritance and the phenotypic manifestations of the diseases caused by this class of mutations.

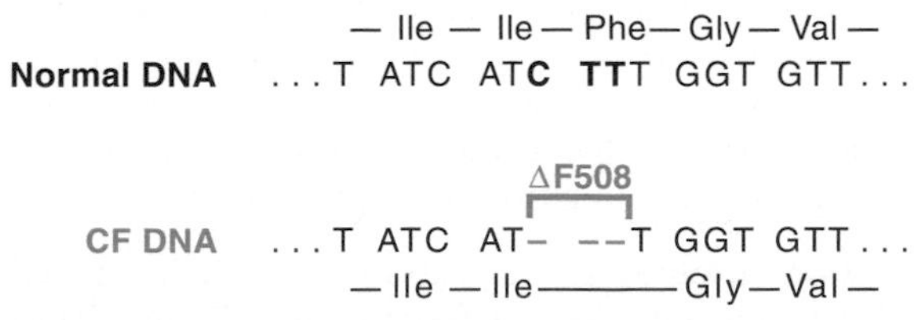

FIGURE 5–6 Three-base deletion in the common cystic fibrosis (CF) allele results in synthesis of a protein that is missing amino acid 508 (phenylalanine). Because the deletion is a multiple of three, this is not a frameshift mutation. (From Thompson MW, et al: Thompson and Thompson Genetics in Medicine, 5th ed. Philadelphia, WB Saunders, 1991, p. 135.)

To summarize, mutations can interfere with protein synthesis at various levels. Transcription may be suppressed with gene deletions and point mutations involving promoter sequences. Abnormal mRNA processing may result from mutations affecting introns or splice junctions or both. Translation is affected if a stop codon (chain termination mutation) is created within an exon. Finally, some point mutations may lead to the formation of an abnormal protein without impairing any step in protein synthesis.

In closing, it should be noted that, uncommonly, mutations may be protective. As will be discussed in Chapter 6, the human immunodeficiency virus (HIV) uses a chemokine receptor, CCR5, to enter cells; a deletion in the *CCR5* gene thus protects from HIV infection.

Against this background, we now turn our attention to the three major categories of genetic disorders: (1) disorders related to mutant genes of large effect, (2) diseases with multifactorial inheritance, and (3) chromosomal disorders. The first category includes many relatively uncommon conditions, such as storage disorders and inborn errors of metabolism, all resulting from single-gene mutations of large effect. Because most of these follow the classic mendelian patterns of inheritance, they are also referred to as *mendelian disorders.* The second category includes some of the most common diseases of humans, such as hypertension and diabetes mellitus. They are called *multifactorial* because they are influenced by both genetic and environmental factors. The genetic component involves the additive result of multiple genes of small effect; the environmental contribution may be small or large, and in some cases, it is required for the expression of disease. The third category includes diseases that result from genomic or chromosomal mutations and are therefore associated with numerical or structural changes in chromosomes.

To these three well-known categories must be added a heterogeneous group of *single-gene disorders with nonclassic patterns of inheritance.* This group includes disorders resulting from triplet repeat mutations, those arising from mutations in mitochondrial DNA, and those in which the transmission is influenced by genomic imprinting or gonadal mosaicism. Diseases within this group are caused by mutations in single genes, but they do not follow the mendelian pattern of inheritance. These are discussed later in this chapter.

Mendelian Disorders

All mendelian disorders are the result of expressed mutations in single genes of large effect. It is not necessary to detail Mendel's laws here, as every student in biology, and possibly every garden pea, has learned about them at an early age. Only some comments of medical relevance are made.

The number of mendelian disorders known has grown to monumental proportions. It is estimated that every individual is a carrier of five to eight deleterious genes. Most of these are recessive and therefore do not have serious phenotypic effects. About 80% to 85% of these mutations are familial. The remainder represent new mutations acquired de novo by an affected individual.

Some autosomal mutations produce partial expression in the heterozygote and full expression in the homozygote. Sickle cell anemia is caused by substitution of normal hemoglobin (HbA) by hemoglobin S (HbS). When an individual is homozygous for the mutant gene, all the hemoglobin is of the abnormal, HbS, type, and even with normal saturation of oxygen, the disorder is fully expressed (i.e., sickling deformity of all red cells and hemolytic anemia). In the heterozygote, only a proportion of the hemoglobin is HbS (the remainder being HbA), and therefore red cell sickling and possibly hemolysis occur only when there is exposure to lowered oxygen tension. This is referred to as the *sickle cell trait* to differentiate it from full-blown sickle cell anemia.

Although gene expression is usually described as dominant or recessive, in some cases, both of the alleles of a gene pair may be fully expressed in the heterozygote—a condition called *codominance.* Histocompatibility and blood group antigens are good examples of codominant inheritance.

A single mutant gene may lead to many end effects, termed *pleiotropism*; conversely, mutations at several genetic loci may produce the same trait *(genetic heterogeneity).* Sickle cell anemia may serve as an example of pleiotropism. In this hereditary disorder, not only does the point mutation in the gene give rise to HbS, which predisposes the red cells to hemolysis, but also the abnormal red cells tend to cause a logjam in small vessels, inducing, for example, splenic fibrosis, organ infarcts, and bone changes. The numerous differing end-organ derangements are all related to the primary defect in hemoglobin synthesis. On the other hand, profound childhood deafness, an apparently homogeneous clinical entity, results from any of 16 different types of autosomal recessive mutations. Recognition of genetic heterogeneity not only is important in genetic counseling but also is relevant in the understanding of the pathogenesis of some common disorders, such as diabetes mellitus.

Finally, it should be noted that not all nucleotide changes produce genes that cause disease. When such a DNA change occurs in at least 1% of the population, it is called a *polymorphism.* SNPs, the most common form of polymorphism, were described earlier in this chapter.

TRANSMISSION PATTERNS OF SINGLE-GENE DISORDERS

Mutations involving single genes typically follow one of three patterns of inheritance: autosomal dominant, autosomal recessive, and X-linked. The general rules that govern the transmission of single-gene disorders are well known and are not repeated here. Only a few salient features are summarized.[8] Single-gene disorders with nonclassic patterns of inheritance are described later.

Autosomal Dominant Disorders

Autosomal dominant disorders are manifested in the heterozygous state, so at least one parent of an index case is usually affected; both males and females are affected, and both can transmit the condition. When an affected person marries an unaffected one, every child has one chance in two of having the disease. In addition to these basic rules, autosomal dominant conditions are characterized by the following:

- With every autosomal dominant disorder, some patients do not have affected parents. Such patients owe their disorder to new mutations involving either the egg or the sperm from which they were derived. Their siblings are neither affected nor at increased risk for developing the disease. The proportion of patients who develop the disease as a result of a new mutation is related to the effect of the disease on reproductive capability. If a disease markedly reduces reproductive fitness, most cases would be expected to result from new mutations. Many new mutations seem to occur in germ cells of relatively older fathers.
- Clinical features can be modified by reduced penetrance and variable expressivity. Some individuals inherit the mutant gene but are phenotypically normal. This is referred to as *reduced penetrance.* Penetrance is expressed in mathematical terms: Thus, 50% penetrance indicates that 50% of those who carry the gene express the trait. In contrast to penetrance, if a trait is seen in all individuals carrying the mutant gene but is expressed differently among individuals, the phenomenon is called *variable expressivity.* For example, manifestations of neurofibromatosis type 1 range from brownish spots on the skin to multiple skin tumors and skeletal deformities. The mechanisms underlying reduced penetrance and variable expressivity are not fully understood, but they most likely result from effects of other genes or environmental factors that modify the phenotypic expression of the mutant allele. For example, the phenotype of a patient with sickle cell anemia (resulting from mutation at the β-globin locus) is influenced by the genotype at the α-globin locus because the latter influences the total amount of hemoglobin made (Chapter 13). The influence of environmental factors is exemplified by familial hypercholesterolemia. The expression of the disease in the form of atherosclerosis is conditioned by the dietary intake of lipids.
- In many conditions, the age at onset is delayed: symptoms and signs do not appear until adulthood (as in Huntington disease).

The biochemical mechanisms of autosomal dominant disorders are best considered in the context of the nature of the mutation and the type of protein affected. Most mutations lead to the reduced production of a gene product or give rise to an inactive protein. The effect of such *loss of function mutations* depends on the nature of the protein affected. If the mutation affects an enzyme protein, the heterozygotes are usually normal. Because up to 50% loss of enzyme activity can be compensated for, mutation in genes that encode enzyme proteins do not manifest an autosomal dominant pattern of inheritance. By contrast, two major categories of nonenzyme proteins are affected in autosomal dominant disorders:

1. Those involved in regulation of complex metabolic pathways that are subject to feedback inhibition: Membrane receptors such as the LDL receptor provide one such example; in familial hypercholesterolemia, discussed in detail later, a 50% loss of LDL receptors results in a secondary elevation of cholesterol that, in turn, predisposes to atherosclerosis in affected heterozygotes.

2. Key structural proteins, such as collagen and cytoskeletal elements of the red cell membrane (e.g., spectrin): The biochemical mechanisms by which a 50% reduction in the levels of such proteins results in an abnormal phenotype are not fully understood. In some cases, especially when the gene encodes one subunit of a multimeric protein, the product of the mutant allele can interfere with the assembly of a functionally normal multimer. For example, the collagen molecule is a trimer in which the three collagen chains are arranged in a helical configuration. Each of the three collagen chains in the helix must be normal for the assembly and stability of the collagen molecule. Even with a single mutant collagen chain, normal collagen trimers cannot be formed, and hence there is a marked deficiency of collagen. In this instance, the mutant allele is called *dominant negative* because it impairs the function of a normal allele. This effect is illustrated by some forms of osteogenesis imperfecta, characterized by marked deficiency of collagen and severe skeletal abnormalities (Chapter 26).

Less common than loss of function mutations are *gain of function* mutations. As the name indicates, in this type of mutation, the protein product of the mutant allele acquires properties not normally associated with the wild-type protein. The transmission of disorders produced by gain of function mutations is almost always autosomal dominant, as illustrated by Huntington disease (Chapter 28). In this disease, the trinucleotide repeat mutation affecting the Huntington gene (see later) gives rise to an abnormal protein. The mutant huntingtin protein is toxic to neurons, and hence even heterozygotes develop neurologic deficit.

To summarize, two types of mutations and two categories of proteins are involved in the pathogenesis of autosomal dominant diseases. The more common loss of function mutations affect regulatory proteins and subunits of mulitmeric proteins, the latter acting through a dominant negative effect. Gain of function mutations are less common; they endow normal proteins with toxic properties and hence affect the function of other proteins encoded by the mutant gene.

Table 5–1 lists common autosomal dominant disorders. Many are discussed more logically in other chapters. A few conditions not considered elsewhere are discussed later in this chapter to illustrate important genetic principles.

Autosomal Recessive Disorders

Autosomal recessive inheritance is the single largest category of mendelian disorders. Because autosomal recessive disorders result only when both alleles at a given gene locus are mutants, such disorders are characterized by the following features: (1) The trait does not usually affect the parents, but siblings may show the disease; (2) siblings have one chance in four of being affected (i.e., the recurrence risk is 25% for each birth); and (3) if the mutant gene occurs with a low frequency in the population, there is a strong likelihood that the proband is the product of a consanguineous marriage. In contrast to those of autosomal dominant diseases, the following features generally apply to most autosomal recessive disorders:

- The expression of the defect tends to be more uniform than in autosomal dominant disorders.
- Complete penetrance is common.
- Onset is frequently early in life.
- Although new mutations for recessive disorders do occur, they are rarely detected clinically. Since the individual with a new mutation is an asymptomatic heterozygote, several generations may pass before the descendants of such a person mate with other heterozygotes and produce affected offspring.
- In many cases, enzyme proteins are affected by a loss of function. In heterozygotes, equal amounts of normal and defective enzyme are synthesized. Usually the natural "margin of safety" ensures that cells with half their usual complement of the enzyme function normally.

Autosomal recessive disorders include almost all inborn errors of metabolism. The various consequences of enzyme deficiencies are discussed later. The more common of these conditions are listed in Table 5–2. Most are presented elsewhere; a few prototypes are discussed later in this chapter.

TABLE 5–1 Autosomal Dominant Disorders

System	Disorder
Nervous	Huntington disease Neurofibromatosis* Myotonic dystrophy Tuberous sclerosis
Urinary	Polycystic kidney disease
Gastrointestinal	Familial polyposis coli
Hematopoietic	Hereditary spherocytosis von Willebrand disease
Skeletal	Marfan syndrome* Ehlers-Danlos syndrome (some variants)* Osteogenesis imperfecta Achondroplasia
Metabolic	Familial hypercholesterolemia* Acute intermittent porphyria

*Discussed in this chapter. Other disorders listed are discussed in appropriate chapters of this book.

TABLE 5–2 Autosomal Recessive Disorders

System	Disorder
Metabolic	Cystic fibrosis Phenylketonuria Galactosemia Homocystinuria Lysosomal storage diseases* α_1-Antitrypsin deficiency Wilson disease Hemochromatosis Glycogen storage diseases*
Hematopoietic	Sickle cell anemia Thalassemias
Endocrine	Congenital adrenal hyperplasia
Skeletal	Ehlers-Danlos syndrome (some variants)* Alkaptonuria*
Nervous	Neurogenic muscular atrophies Friedreich ataxia Spinal muscular atrophy

*Discussed in this chapter. Many others are discussed elsewhere in the text.

X-Linked Disorders

All sex-linked disorders are X-linked, almost all X-linked recessive. Several genes are encoded in the "male-specific region of Y"; all of these are related to spermatogenesis.[9] Males with mutations affecting the Y-linked genes are usually infertile, and hence there is no Y-linked inheritance. As discussed later, a few additional genes with homologues on the X chromosome have been mapped to the Y chromosome, but no disorders resulting from mutations in such genes have been described.

X-linked recessive inheritance accounts for a small number of well-defined clinical conditions. The Y chromosome, for the most part, is not homologous to the X, and so mutant genes on the X are not paired with alleles on the Y. Thus, the male is said to be *hemizygous* for X-linked mutant genes, so these disorders are expressed in the male. Other features that characterize these disorders are as follows:

- An affected male does not transmit the disorder to his sons, but all daughters are carriers. Sons of heterozygous women have, of course, one chance in two of receiving the mutant gene.
- The heterozygous female usually does not express the full phenotypic change because of the paired normal allele. Because of the random inactivation of one of the X chromosomes in the female, however, females have a variable proportion of cells in which the mutant X chromosome is active. Thus, it is remotely possible for the normal allele to be inactivated in most cells, permitting full expression of heterozygous X-linked conditions in the female. Much more commonly, the normal allele is inactivated in only some of the cells, and thus the heterozygous female expresses the disorder partially. An illustrative condition is *glucose-6-phosphate dehydrogenase (G6PD) deficiency.* Transmitted on the X chromosome, this enzyme deficiency, which predisposes to red cell hemolysis in patients receiving certain types of drugs (Chapter 13), is expressed principally in males. In the female, a proportion of the red cells may be derived from marrow cells with inactivation of the normal allele. Such red cells are at the same risk for undergoing hemolysis as are the red cells in the hemizygous male. Thus, the female is not only a carrier of this trait, but also is susceptible to drug-induced hemolytic reactions. Because the proportion of defective red cells in heterozygous females depends on the random inactivation of one of the X chromosomes, however, the severity of the hemolytic reaction is almost always less in heterozygous women than in hemizygous men. Most of the X-linked conditions listed in Table 5–3 are covered elsewhere in the text.

There are only a few *X-linked dominant* conditions. They are caused by dominant disease alleles on the X chromosome. These disorders are transmitted by an affected heterozygous female to half her sons and half her daughters and by an affected male parent to all his daughters but none of his sons, if the female parent is unaffected. Vitamin D–resistant rickets is an example of this type of inheritance.

TABLE 5–3 X-Linked Recessive Disorders

System	Disease
Musculoskeletal	Duchenne muscular dystrophy
Blood	Hemophilia A and B Chronic granulomatous disease Glucose-6-phosphate dehydrogenase deficiency
Immune	Agammaglobulinemia Wiskott-Aldrich syndrome
Metabolic	Diabetes insipidus Lesch-Nyhan syndrome
Nervous	Fragile-X syndrome*

*Discussed in this chapter. Others discussed in appropriate chapters in the book.

BIOCHEMICAL AND MOLECULAR BASIS OF SINGLE-GENE (MENDELIAN) DISORDERS

Mendelian disorders result from alterations involving single genes. The genetic defect may lead to the formation of an abnormal protein or a reduction in the output of the gene product. As mentioned earlier, mutations may affect protein synthesis by affecting transcription, mRNA processing, or translation. The phenotypic effects of a mutation may result directly, from abnormalities in the protein encoded by the mutant gene, or indirectly, owing to interactions of the mutant protein with other normal proteins. For example, all forms of Ehlers-Danlos syndrome (EDS) are associated with abnormalities of collagen. In some forms (e.g., vascular type), there is a mutation in one of the collagen genes, whereas in others (e.g., kyphoscoliosis type), the collagen genes are normal, but there is a mutation in the gene that encodes lysyl hydroxylase, an enzyme essential for the cross-linking of collagen. In these patients, collagen weakness is secondary to a deficiency of lysyl hydroxylase.

Virtually any type of protein may be affected in single-gene disorders and by a variety of mechanisms (Table 5–4). To some extent, the pattern of inheritance of the disease is related to the kind of protein affected by the mutation, as was discussed earlier and is reiterated subsequently. For the purposes of this discussion, the mechanisms involved in single-gene disorders can be classified into four categories: (1) *enzyme defects and their consequences*; (2) *defects in membrane receptors and transport systems*; (3) *alterations in the structure, function, or quantity of nonenzyme proteins*; and (4) *mutations resulting in unusual reactions to drugs.*

Enzyme Defects and Their Consequences

Mutations may result in the synthesis of a defective enzyme with reduced activity or in a reduced amount of a normal enzyme. In either case, the consequence is a metabolic block. Figure 5–7 provides an example of an enzyme reaction in which the substrate is converted by intracellular enzymes, denoted as 1, 2, and 3, into an end product through intermediates 1 and 2. In this model, the final product exerts feedback control on enzyme 1. A minor pathway producing small quantities of M_1 and M_2 also exists. The biochemical consequences of an enzyme defect in such a reaction may lead to three major consequences:

1. *Accumulation of the substrate*, depending on the site of block, may be accompanied by accumulation of one or both intermediates. Moreover, an increased concentration of intermediate 2 may stimulate the minor pathway and thus

TABLE 5–4 Biochemical and Molecular Basis of Some Mendelian Disorders

Protein Type/Function	Example	Molecular Lesion	Disease
Enzyme	Phenylalanine hydroxylase	Splice site mutation: reduced amount	Phenylketonuria
	Hexosaminidase	Splice site mutation or frameshift mutation with stop codon: reduced amount	Tay-Sachs disease
	Adenosine deaminase	Point mutations: abnormal protein with reduced activity	Severe combined immunodeficiency
Enzyme Inhibitor	α_1-Antitrypsin	Missense mutations: impaired secretion from liver to serum	Emphysema and liver disease
Receptor	Low-density lipoprotein receptor	Deletions, point mutations: reduction of synthesis, transport to cell surface, or binding to low-density lipoprotein	Familial hypercholesterolemia
	Vitamin D receptor	Point mutations: failure of normal signaling	Vitamin D–resistant rickets
Transport			
Oxygen	Hemoglobin	Deletions: reduced amount	α-Thalassemia
		Defective mRNA processing: reduced amount	β-Thalassemia
		Point mutations: abnormal structure	Sickle cell anemia
Ions	Cystic fibrosis transmembrane conductance regulator	Deletions and other mutations	Cystic fibrosis
Structural			
Extracellular	Collagen	Deletions or point mutations cause reduced amount of normal collagen or normal amounts of mutant collagen	Osteogenesis imperfecta; Ehlers-Danlos syndromes
	Fibrillin	Missense mutations	Marfan syndrome
Cell membrane	Dystrophin	Deletion with reduced synthesis	Duchenne/Becker muscular dystrophy
	Spectrin, ankyrin, or protein 4.1	Heterogeneous	Hereditary spherocytosis
Hemostasis	Factor VIII	Deletions, insertions, nonsense mutations, and others: reduced synthesis or abnormal factor VIII	Hemophilia A
Growth Regulation	Rb protein	Deletions	Hereditary retinoblastoma
	Neurofibromin	Heterogeneous	Neurofibromatosis type 1

lead to an excess of M_1 and M_2. Under these conditions, tissue injury may result if the precursor, the intermediates, or the products of alternative minor pathways are toxic in high concentrations. For example, in galactosemia, the deficiency of galactose-1-phosphate uridyltransferase (Chapter 10) leads to the accumulation of galactose and consequent tissue damage. In phenylketonuria, a deficiency of phenylalanine hydroxylase (Chapter 10) results in the accumulation of phenylalanine. Excessive accumulation of complex substrates within the lysosomes as a result of deficiency of degradative enzymes is responsible for a group of diseases generally referred to as *lysosomal storage diseases.*

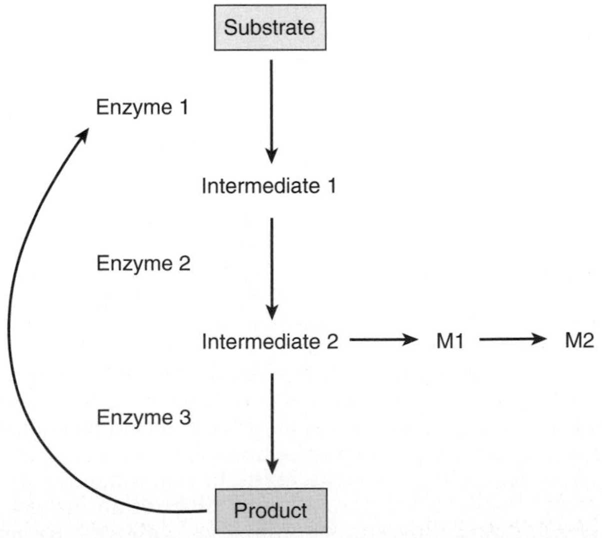

FIGURE 5–7 Scheme of a possible metabolic pathway in which a substrate is converted to an end product by a series of enzyme reactions. M1, M2, products of a minor pathway.

2. *An enzyme defect can lead to a metabolic block and a decreased amount of end product* that may be necessary for normal function. For example, a deficiency of melanin may result from lack of tyrosinase, which is necessary for the biosynthesis of melanin from its precursor, tyrosine. This results in the clinical condition called *albinism.* If the end product is a feedback inhibitor of the enzymes involved in the early reactions (in Fig. 5–7, it is shown that the product inhibits enzyme 1), the deficiency of the end product may permit overproduction of intermediates and their catabolic products, some of which may be injurious at high concentrations. A prime example of a disease with such an underlying mechanism is the Lesch-Nyhan syndrome (Chapter 26).

3. *Failure to inactivate a tissue-damaging substrate* is best exemplified by α_1-antitrypsin (α_1-AT) deficiency. Patients who have an inherited deficiency of serum α_1-AT are unable to inactivate neutrophil elastase in their lungs. Unchecked activity of this protease leads to destruction of elastin in the walls of lung alveoli, leading eventually to pulmonary emphysema (Chapter 15).

Defects in Receptors and Transport Systems

Many biologically active substances have to be actively transported across the cell membrane. This transport is generally achieved by one of two mechanisms—by receptor-mediated endocytosis or by a transport protein. A genetic defect in a receptor-mediated transport system is exemplified by familial hypercholesterolemia, in which reduced synthesis or function of low-density lipoprotein (LDL) receptors leads to defective transport of LDL into the cells and secondarily to excessive cholesterol synthesis by complex intermediary mechanisms. In cystic fibrosis, the transport system for chloride ions in exocrine glands, sweat ducts, lungs, and pancreas is defective. By mechanisms not fully understood, impaired chloride transport leads to serious injury to the lungs and pancreas (Chapter 10).

Alterations in Structure, Function, or Quantity of Nonenzyme Proteins

Genetic defects resulting in alterations of nonenzyme proteins often have widespread secondary effects, as exemplified by sickle cell disease. The hemoglobinopathies, sickle cell disease being one, all of which are characterized by defects in the structure of the globin molecule, best exemplify this category. In contrast to the hemoglobinopathies, the thalassemias result from mutations in globin genes that affect the amount of globin chains synthesized. Thalassemias are associated with reduced amounts of structurally normal α-globin or ß-globin chains (Chapter 13). Other examples of genetically defective structural proteins include collagen, spectrin, and dystrophin, giving rise to osteogenesis imperfecta (Chapter 26), hereditary spherocytosis (Chapter 13), and muscular dystrophies (Chapter 27), respectively.

Genetically Determined Adverse Reactions to Drugs

Certain genetically determined enzyme deficiencies are unmasked only after exposure of the affected individual to certain drugs. This special area of genetics, called *pharmacogenetics*, is of considerable clinical importance.[10] The classic example of drug-induced injury in the genetically susceptible individual is associated with a deficiency of the enzyme glucose-6-phosphate dehydrogenase (G6PD). Under normal conditions, G6PD deficiency does not result in disease, but on administration, for example, of the antimalarial drug primaquine, a severe hemolytic anemia results (Chapter 13). In recent years, an increasing number of polymorphisms of genes encoding drug-metabolizing enzymes, transporters, and receptors are being identified. In some cases these genetic factors have major impact on drug sensitivity and adverse reactions. It is expected that advances in pharmacogenetics will lead to patient-tailored therapy, or "personalized medicine."

With this overview of the biochemical basis of single gene disorders, we now consider selected examples grouped according to the underlying defect.

DISORDERS ASSOCIATED WITH DEFECTS IN STRUCTURAL PROTEINS

Several diseases caused by mutations in genes that encode structural proteins are listed in Table 5–4. Many are discussed elsewhere in the text. Only Marfan syndrome and Ehlers-Danlos syndromes are discussed here because they affect connective tissue and hence involve multiple organ systems.

Marfan Syndrome

Marfan syndrome is a disorder of the connective tissues of the body, manifested principally by changes in the skeleton, eyes, and cardiovascular system.[11] Its prevalence is estimated to be 1 in 5000. Approximately 70% to 85% of cases are familial and transmitted by autosomal dominant inheritance. The remainder are sporadic and arise from new mutations.

Pathogenesis. Marfan syndrome results from an inherited defect in an extracellular glycoprotein called *fibrillin-1*.[12] As alluded to in Chapter 3, fibrillin is the major component of microfibrils found in the extracellular matrix. These fibrils form a scaffolding on which tropoelastin is deposited to form elastic fibers. Although microfibrils are widely distributed in the body, they are particularly abundant in the aorta, ligaments, and ciliary zonules of the lens, where they support the lens; these tissues are prominently affected in Marfan syndrome.

Fibrillin occurs in two homologous forms, fibrillin-1 and fibrillin-2, encoded by two separate genes, *FBN1* and *FBN2*, mapped to chromosomes 15q21 and 5q3, respectively. Mutations of *FBN1* underlie Marfan syndrome; mutations of the related *FBN2* gene are less common, and they give rise to *congenital contractural arachnodactyly*, an autosomal dominant disorder characterized by skeletal abnormalities. Mutational analysis has revealed more than 500 distinct mutations of the *FBN1* gene in patients with Marfan syndrome. Most of these are missense mutations that give rise to abnormal fibrillin-1.[13] It is believed that in heterozygotes mutant fibrillin-1 disrupts the assembly of normal microfibrils, presumably by interacting with the products of the normal allele. This mechanism of action, as discussed previously, is called *dominant negative.*

Morphology. Skeletal abnormalities are the most striking feature of Marfan syndrome. Typically the patient is unusually tall with exceptionally long extremities and long, tapering fingers and toes. Because the lower segment of the body largely contributes the tall stature, the ratio of the upper segment (top of the head to the pubis) to the lower segment (top of pubic ramus to the floor) is significantly lower than the norm for age, race, and gender. The joint ligaments in the hands and feet are lax, suggesting that the patient is double-jointed; typically the thumb can be hyperextended back to the wrist. The head is commonly dolichocephalic (long-headed) with bossing of the frontal eminences and prominent supraorbital ridges. Because Abraham Lincoln possessed many of these physical characteristics, it is strongly suspected that he had Marfan syndrome. A variety of spinal deformities may appear, including kyphosis, scoliosis, or rotation or slipping of the dorsal or lumbar vertebrae. The chest is classically deformed, presenting either pectus excavatum (deeply depressed sternum) or a pigeon-breast deformity.

The **ocular changes** take many forms. Most characteristic is bilateral subluxation or dislocation (usually outward and upward) of the lens, referred to as **ectopia lentis**. This abnormality is so uncommon in persons who do not have this genetic disease that the finding of bilateral ectopia lentis should raise the suspicion of Marfan syndrome.

Cardiovascular lesions are the most life-threatening features of this disorder. The two most common lesions are mitral valve prolapse and, of greater importance, dilation of the ascending aorta owing to cystic medionecrosis. Histologically the changes in the media are virtually identical to those found in cystic medionecrosis not related to Marfan syndrome (see section on aortic dissection, Chapter 12). **Loss of medial support results in progressive dilation of the aortic valve ring and the root of the aorta, giving rise to severe aortic incompetence.** In addition, loss of fibrillin-1 from the adventia also likely contributes to aortic dilation. Weakening of the media predisposes to an intimal tear, which may initiate an intramural hematoma that cleaves the layers of the media to produce aortic dissection. After cleaving the aortic layers for considerable distances, sometimes back to the root of the aorta or down to the iliac arteries, the hemorrhage often ruptures through the aortic wall. Such a calamity is the cause of death in 30% to 45% of these individuals.

Although mitral valve lesions are more frequent, they are clinically less important than aortic lesions. Loss of connective tissue support in the mitral valve leaflets makes them soft and billowy, creating the so-called floppy valve (Chapter 12). Valvular lesions, along with lengthening of the chordae tendineae, frequently give rise to mitral regurgitation. Similar changes may affect the tricuspid and, rarely, the aortic valves. Echocardiography greatly enhances the ability to detect the cardiovascular abnormalities and is therefore extremely valuable in the diagnosis of Marfan syndrome. The great majority of deaths are caused by rupture of aortic dissections, followed in importance by cardiac failure.

Although the lesions just described typify Marfan syndrome, it must be emphasized that there is great variation in the clinical expression of this genetic disorder. Patients with prominent eye or cardiovascular changes may have few skeletal abnormalities, whereas others with striking changes in body habitus have no eye changes. Although variability in clinical expression may be seen within a family, interfamilial variability is much more common and extensive. Because of such variations, clinical diagnosis of Marfan syndrome must be based on major involvement of two of the four organ systems (skeletal, cardiovascular, ocular, and skin) and minor involvement of another organ.[14]

To account for the variable expression of the Marfan defect, it has been hypothesized that Marfan syndrome may be genetically heterogeneous. With one exception, however, all studies to date point to mutations in the *FBN1* gene, on chromosome 15q21.1, as the cause of this disease.[12] Thus, variable expressivity is best explained on the basis of allelic mutations within the same locus. Because so many different mutations of the *FBN1* gene have been detected in different Marfan families, direct gene diagnosis of this disorder is not feasible. Furthermore, it is now evident that all patients with *FBN1* mutations do not have the classic Marfan syndrome. Other manifestations include severe neonatal Marfan syndrome and isolated, or familial, thoracic aneurysms. Together, these disorders are sometimes called type 1 fibrillinopathies.

Ehlers-Danlos Syndromes

Ehlers-Danlos syndromes (EDS) comprise a clinically and genetically heterogeneous group of disorders that result from some defect in the synthesis or structure of fibrillar collagen.[15] Other disorders resulting from mutations affecting collagen synthesis include osteogenesis imperfecta (Chapter 26), Alport syndrome (Chapter 20), and epidermolysis bullosa (Chapter 25).

The mode of inheritance of EDS encompasses all three mendelian patterns. This should not be surprising because biosynthesis of collagen is a complex process that can be disturbed by genetic errors that may affect any one of the numerous structural collagen genes or enzymes necessary for post-transcriptional modifications of collagen. Because abnormalities of collagen are fundamental in the pathogenesis of EDS, collagen structure and synthesis should be reviewed (Chapter 3). As we see subsequently, to some extent the clinical heterogeneity and variable modes of transmission of EDS can be explained on the basis of the specific collagen type involved and the nature of the molecular defects.

On the basis of clinical and molecular characteristics, six variants of EDS have been recognized.[16] These are listed in Table 5–5. It is beyond the scope of this book to discuss each variant individually, and the interested reader is referred to several excellent reviews for such details.[17] Instead, we first summarize the important clinical features that are common to most variants and then correlate some of the clinical manifestations with the underlying molecular defects in collagen synthesis or structure.

As might be expected, tissues rich in collagen, such as skin, ligaments, and joints, are frequently involved in most variants of EDS. Because the abnormal collagen fibers lack adequate tensile strength, *skin is hyperextensible, and the joints are hypermobile.* These features permit grotesque contortions, such as bending the thumb backward to touch the forearm and bending the knee forward to create almost a right angle. It is believed that most contortionists have one of the EDS. A predisposition to joint dislocation, however, is one of the prices paid for this virtuosity. *The skin is extraordinarily stretchable, extremely fragile, and vulnerable to trauma.* Minor injuries produce gaping defects, and surgical repair or any surgical intervention is accomplished with great difficulty because of the lack of normal tensile strength. *The basic defect in connective tissue may lead to serious internal complications.* These include rupture of the colon and large arteries (vascular EDS), ocular fragility with rupture of cornea and retinal detachment (kyphoscoliosis EDS), and diaphragmatic hernia (classical EDS).

The biochemical and molecular bases of these abnormalities are known in several forms of EDS. These are described briefly because they offer some insights into the perplexing clinical heterogeneity of EDS. Perhaps the best characterized is the *kyphoscoliosis type, the most common autosomal recessive form of EDS.* It results from mutations in the gene encoding lysyl hydroxylase, an enzyme necessary for hydroxylation of lysine residues during collagen synthesis.[18] Affected patients have markedly reduced levels of this enzyme. Because hydroxylysine is essential for the cross-linking of collagen fibers, a

TABLE 5–5 Classification of Ehlers–Danlos Syndromes (EDS)

EDS Type*	Clinical Findings	Inheritance	Gene Defects
Classical (I/II)	Skin and joint hypermobility, atrophic scars, easy bruising	Autosomal dominant	COL5A1, COL5A2
Hypermobility (III)	Joint hypermobility, pain, dislocations	Autosomal dominant	Unknown
Vascular (IV)	Thin skin, arterial or uterine rupture, bruising, small joint hyperextensibility	Autosomal dominant	COL3A1
Kyphoscoliosis (VI)	Hypotonia, joint laxity, congenital scoliosis, ocular fragility	Autosomal recessive	Lysyl-hydroxylase
Arthrochalasia (VIIa,b)	Severe joint hypermobility, skin changes mild, scoliosis, bruising	Autosomal dominant	COL1A1, COL1A2
Dermatosparaxsis (VIIc)	Severe skin fragility, cutis laxa, bruising	Autosomal recessive	Procollagen *N*-peptidase

*EDS were previously classified by Roman numerals. Parentheses show previous numerical equivalents.

deficiency of lysyl hydroxylase results in the synthesis of collagen that lacks normal structural stability.

The *vascular type of EDS results from abnormalities of type III collagen.* This form is genetically heterogeneous because at least three distinct types of mutations affecting the *COL3A1* gene for collagen type III can give rise to this variant. Some affect the rate of synthesis of pro α1 (III) chains, others affect the secretion of type III procollagen, and still others lead to the synthesis of structurally abnormal type III collagen. Some mutant alleles behave as dominant negatives (see discussion under autosomal dominant disorders) and thus produce severe phenotypic effects. These molecular studies provide a rational basis for the pattern of transmission and clinical features that are characteristic of this variant. First, because vascular type EDS results from mutations involving a structural protein (rather than an enzyme protein), an autosomal dominant pattern of inheritance would be expected. Second, because blood vessels and intestines are known to be rich in collagen type III, an abnormality of this collagen is consistent with severe defects (e.g., spontaneous rupture) in these organs.

In two forms of EDS—arthrochalasia type and dermatosparaxis type—the fundamental defect is in the conversion of type I procollagen to collagen. This step in collagen synthesis involves cleavage of noncollagen peptides at the N-terminal and C-terminal of the procollagen molecule. This is accomplished by N-terminal–specific and C-terminal–specific peptidases. *The defect in the conversion of procollagen to collagen in the arthrocalasic type has been traced to mutations that affect one of the two type I collagen genes, COL1A1* and *COL1A2.* As a result, structurally abnormal pro α1 (I) or pro α2 (I) chains that resist cleavage of N-terminal peptides are formed. In patients with a single mutant allele, only 50% of the type I collagen chains are abnormal, but because these chains interfere with the formation of normal collagen helices, heterozygotes manifest the disease. By contrast, the related dermatosparaxis type is caused by mutations in the procollagen-N-peptidase genes, essential for the cleavage of collagens. In this case, the enzyme deficiency leads to an autosomal recessive form of inheritance.

Finally, the *classical type of EDS* is worthy of brief mention, since molecular analysis of the variant suggests that genes other than collagen genes may be involved in the pathogenesis of EDS. In 30% to 50% of these cases, mutations in the genes for type V collagen *(COL5A1* and *COL5A1)* have been detected. Surprisingly, despite a phenotype typical of EDS, no other collagen gene abnormalities have been found in these cases. This has led to the speculation that other proteins in the extracellular matrix, such as tenascin-X, may also be involved in regulating collagen synthesis.

To summarize, the common thread in EDS is some abnormality of collagen. These disorders, however, are extremely heterogeneous. At the molecular level, a variety of defects, varying from mutations involving structural genes for collagen to those involving enzymes that are responsible for post-transcriptional modifications of mRNA, have been detected. Such molecular heterogeneity results in the expression of EDS as a clinically heterogeneous disorder with several patterns of inheritance.

DISORDERS ASSOCIATED WITH DEFECTS IN RECEPTOR PROTEINS

Familial Hypercholesterolemia

Familial hypercholesterolemia is a "receptor disease" that is the consequence of a *mutation in the gene encoding the receptor for low density lipoprotein (LDL), which is involved in the transport and metabolism of cholesterol.* As a consequence of receptor abnormalities, there is a loss of feedback control and elevated levels of cholesterol that induce premature atherosclerosis, leading to a greatly increased risk of myocardial infarction.[19,20]

Familial hypercholesterolemia is possibly the most frequent mendelian disorder. Heterozygotes with one mutant gene, representing about 1 in 500 individuals, have from birth a twofold to threefold elevation of plasma cholesterol level, leading to tendinous xanthomas and premature atherosclerosis in adult life (Chapter 11). Homozygotes, having a double dose of the mutant gene, are much more severely affected and may have fivefold to sixfold elevations in plasma cholesterol levels. These individuals develop skin xanthomas and coronary, cerebral, and peripheral vascular atherosclerosis at an early age. Myocardial infarction may develop before age 20. Large-scale studies have found that familial hypercholesterolemia is present in 3% to 6% of survivors of myocardial infarction.

An understanding of this disorder requires that we briefly review the normal process of cholesterol metabolism and transport. Approximately 7% of the body's cholesterol circulates in the plasma, predominantly in the form of LDL. As might be expected, the level of plasma cholesterol is influenced by its synthesis and catabolism and the liver plays a crucial role in both these processes (Fig. 5–8). The first step in this complex sequence is the secretion of very-low-density lipoproteins (VLDL) by the liver into the bloodstream. VLDL particles are rich in triglycerides, although they do contain lesser amounts of cholesteryl esters. When a VLDL particle reaches the capillaries of adipose tissue or muscle, it is cleaved by lipoprotein lipase, a process that extracts most of the triglycerides. The resulting molecule, called *intermediate-density lipoprotein (IDL)*, is reduced in triglyceride content and enriched in cholesteryl esters, but it retains two of the three apoproteins (B-100 and E) present in the parent VLDL particle (see Fig. 5–8). After release from the capillary endothelium, the IDL particles have one of two fates. Approximately 50% of newly formed IDL is rapidly taken up by the liver through a receptor-mediated transport. The receptor responsible for the binding of IDL to liver cell membrane recognizes both apoprotein B-100 and apoprotein E. It is called the *LDL receptor*, however, because it is also involved in the hepatic clearance of LDL, as described later. In the liver cells,

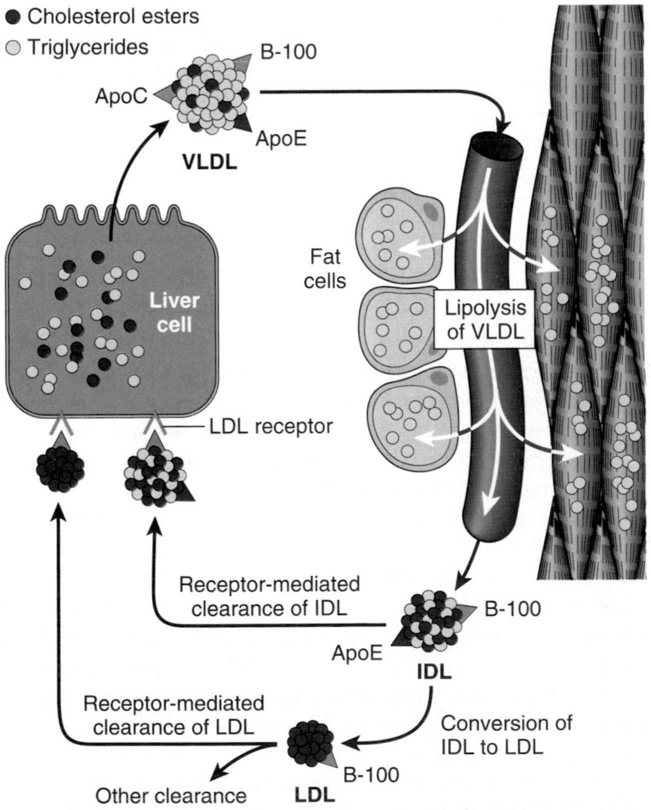

FIGURE 5–8 Schematic illustration of low-density lipoprotein (LDL) metabolism and the role of the liver in its synthesis and clearance. Lipolysis of very-low-density lipoprotein (VLDL) by lipoprotein lipase in the capillaries releases triglycerides, which are then stored in fat cells and used as a source of energy in skeletal muscles.

IDL is recycled to generate VLDL. The IDL particles not taken up by the liver are subjected to further metabolic processing that removes most of the remaining triglycerides and apoprotein E, yielding the cholesterol-rich LDL. *It should be emphasized that IDL is the immediate and major source of plasma LDL.* There appear to be two mechanisms for removal of LDL from plasma, one mediated by an LDL receptor and the other by a receptor for oxidized LDL (scavenger receptor), described later. Although many cell types, including fibroblasts, lymphocytes, smooth muscle cells, hepatocytes, and adrenocortical cells, possess high-affinity LDL receptors, approximately 70% of the plasma LDL appears to be cleared by the liver, using a relatively sophisticated transport process (Fig. 5–9). The first step involves binding of LDL to cell-surface receptors, which are clustered in specialized regions of the plasma membrane called *coated pits.* After binding, the coated pits containing the receptor-bound LDL are internalized by invagination to form coated vesicles, after which they migrate within the cell to fuse with the lysosomes. Here the LDL dissociates from the receptor, which is recycled to the surface. In the lysosomes, the LDL molecule is enzymatically degraded; the apoprotein part is hydrolyzed to amino acids, whereas the cholesteryl esters are broken down to free cholesterol. This free cholesterol, in turn, crosses the lysosomal membrane to enter the cytoplasm, where it is used for membrane synthesis and as a regulator of cholesterol homeostasis. Three separate processes are affected by the released intracellular cholesterol, as follows:

- Cholesterol *suppresses* cholesterol synthesis within the cell by inhibiting the activity of the enzyme 3-hydroxy-3-methylglutaryl coenzyme A (HMG CoA) reductase, which is the rate-limiting enzyme in the synthetic pathway.
- Cholesterol *activates* the enzyme acyl-coenzyme A:cholesterol acyltransferase, favoring esterification and storage of excess cholesterol.
- Cholesterol *suppresses* the synthesis of LDL receptors, thus protecting the cells from excessive accumulation of cholesterol.

As mentioned earlier, familial hypercholesterolemia results from mutations in the gene specifying the receptor for LDL. Heterozygotes with familial hypercholesterolemia possess only 50% of the normal number of high-affinity LDL receptors because they have only one normal gene. As a result of this defect in transport, the catabolism of LDL by the receptor-dependent pathways is impaired, and the plasma level of LDL increases approximately twofold. Homozygotes have virtually no normal LDL receptors in their cells and have much higher levels of circulating LDL. In addition to defective LDL clearance, both the homozygotes and heterozygotes have increased synthesis of LDL. The mechanism of increased synthesis that contributes to hypercholesterolemia also results from a lack of LDL receptors (see Fig. 5–8). Recall that IDL, the immediate precursor of plasma LDL, also uses hepatic LDL receptors (apoprotein B-100 and E receptors) for its transport into the liver. In familial hypercholesterolemia, impaired IDL transport into the liver secondarily diverts a greater proportion of plasma IDL into the precursor pool for plasma LDL.

The transport of LDL via the scavenger receptor appears to occur at least in part into the cells of the mononuclear phagocyte system. Monocytes and macrophages have receptors for

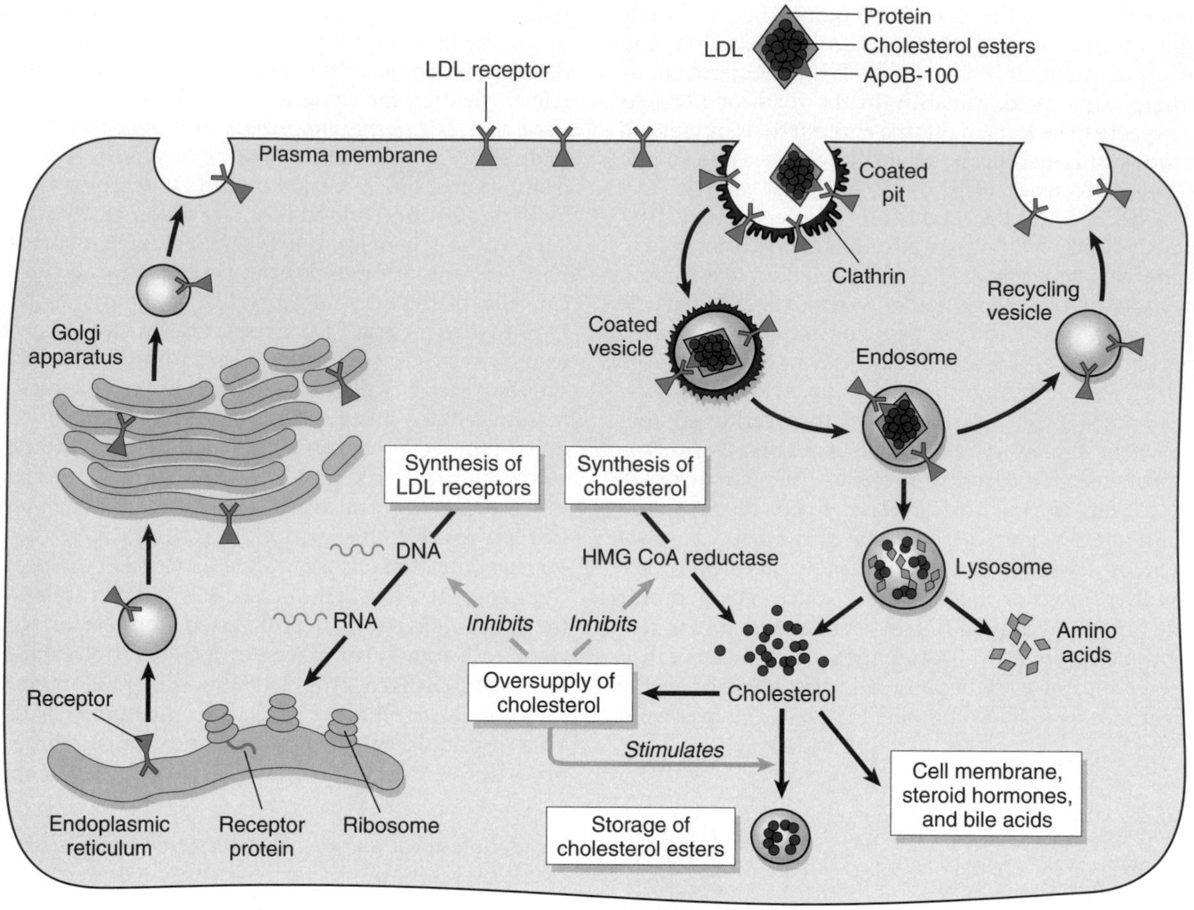

FIGURE 5–9 The LDL receptor pathway and regulation of cholesterol metabolism.

chemically altered (e.g., acetylated or oxidized) LDL. Normally the amount of LDL transported along this scavenger receptor pathway is less than that mediated by the LDL receptor-dependent mechanisms. In the face of hypercholesterolemia, however, there is a marked increase in the scavenger receptor-mediated traffic of LDL cholesterol into the cells of the mononuclear phagocyte system and possibly the vascular walls. This increase is responsible for the appearance of xanthomas and contributes to the pathogenesis of premature atherosclerosis.

The molecular genetics of familial hypercholesterolemia have proven to be extremely complex. The human LDL receptor gene, located on chromosome 19, is extremely large, with 18 exons and 5 domains that span a distance of about 45 kb. More than 900 mutations, including insertions, deletions, and missense and nonsense mutations, involving the LDL receptor gene have been identified. These can be classified into five groups (Fig. 5–10): *Class I mutations* are relatively uncommon, and they lead to a complete failure of synthesis of the receptor protein (null allele). *Class II mutations* are fairly common; they encode receptor proteins that accumulate in the endoplasmic reticulum because they cannot be transported to the Golgi complex. *Class III mutations* affect the LDL-binding domain of the receptor; the encoded proteins reach the cell surface but fail to bind LDL or do so poorly. *Class IV mutations* encode proteins that are synthesized and transported to the cell surface efficiently. They bind LDL normally, but they fail to localize in coated pits, and hence the bound LDL is not internalized. *Class V mutations* encode proteins that are expressed on the cell surface, can bind LDL, and can be internalized; however, the acid-dependent dissociation of the receptor and the bound LDL fails to occur. Such receptors are trapped in the endosome, where they are degraded, and hence they fail to recycle to the cell surface.

The discovery of the critical role of LDL receptors in cholesterol homeostasis has led to the rational design of drugs that lower plasma cholesterol by increasing the number of LDL receptors.[21] One strategy that has proven to be successful is based on the ability of certain drugs (statins) to suppress intracellular cholesterol synthesis by inhibiting the enzyme HMG CoA reductase. This, in turn, allows greater synthesis of LDL receptors (see Fig. 5–9). Efforts are also under way to develop gene therapy for this disorder.

DISORDERS ASSOCIATED WITH DEFECTS IN ENZYMES

Lysosomal Storage Diseases

Lysosomes are key components of the "intracellular digestive tract." They contain a battery of hydrolytic enzymes, which have two special properties. First, they can function in

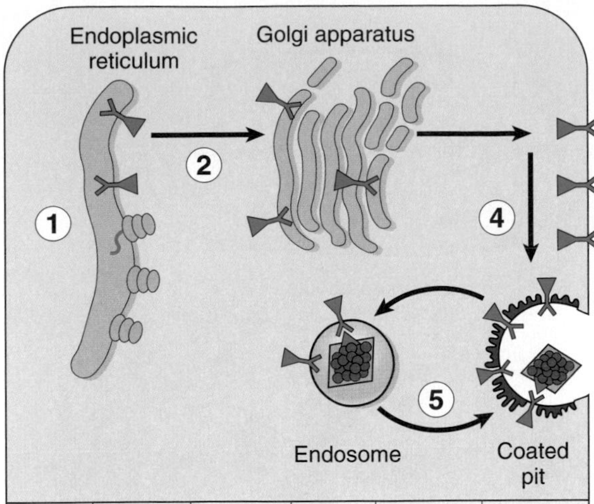

Mutation class	Synthesis	Transport	Binding	Clustering	Recycling
I	X				
II	→	X			
III	→	→	X		
IV	→	→	→	X	
V	→	→	→	→	X

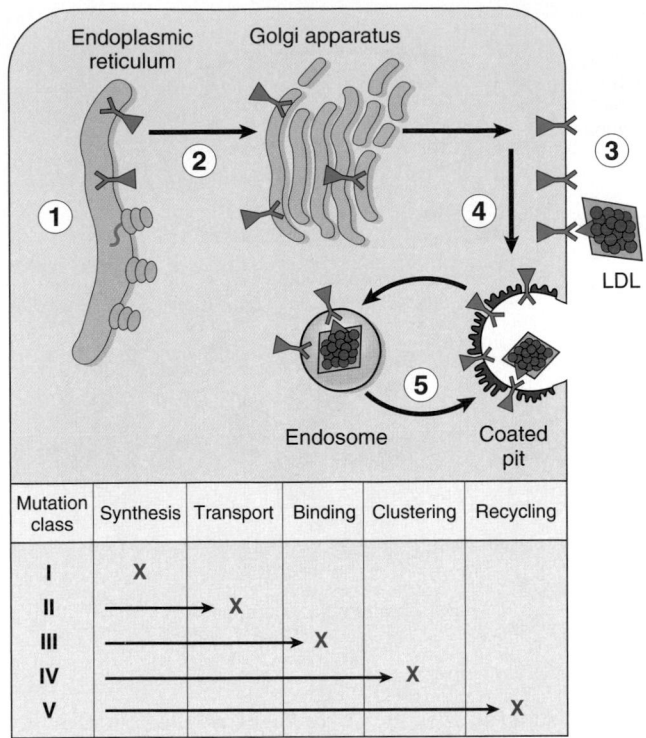

FIGURE 5–10 Classification of LDL receptor mutations based on abnormal function of the mutant protein. These mutations disrupt the receptor's synthesis in the endoplasmic reticulum, transport to the Golgi complex, binding of apoprotein ligands, clustering in coated pits, and recycling in endosomes. Each class is heterogeneous at the DNA level. (Modified with permission from Hobbs HH, et al: The LDL receptor locus in familial hypercholesterolemia: mutational analysis of a membrane protein. Annu Rev Genet 24:133–170, 1990. © 1990 by Annual Reviews.)

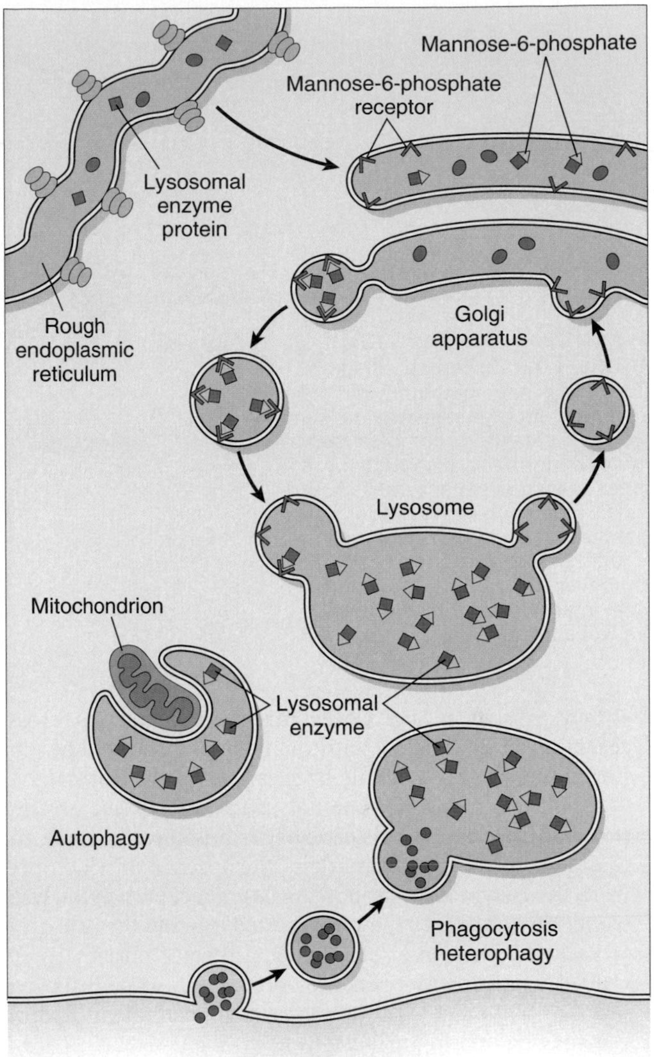

FIGURE 5–11 Synthesis and intracellular transport of lysosomal enzymes.

the acid milieu of the lysosomes. Second, these enzymes constitute a special category of secretory proteins that, in contrast to most others, are destined for secretion not into the extracellular fluids but into an intracellular organelle. This latter characteristic requires special processing within the Golgi apparatus, which is reviewed briefly. Similar to all other secretory proteins, lysosomal enzymes (or acid hydrolases, as they are sometimes called) are synthesized in the endoplasmic reticulum and transported to the Golgi apparatus. Within the Golgi complex, they undergo a variety of post-translational modifications, of which one is worthy of special note. This modification involves the attachment of terminal mannose-6-phosphate groups to some of the oligosaccharide side chains. The phosphorylated mannose residues may be viewed as an "address label" that is recognized by specific receptors found on the inner surface of the Golgi membrane. Lysosomal enzymes bind to these receptors and are thereby segregated from the numerous other secretory proteins within the Golgi. Subsequently, small transport vesicles containing the receptor-bound enzymes are pinched off from the Golgi and proceed to fuse with the lysosomes. Thus, the enzymes are targeted to their intracellular abode, and the vesicles are shuttled back to the Golgi (Fig. 5–11). As indicated later, genetically determined errors in this remarkable sorting mechanism may give rise to one form of lysosomal storage disease.

The lysosomal acid hydrolases catalyze the breakdown of a variety of complex macromolecules. These large molecules may be derived from the metabolic turnover of intracellular organelles (autophagy), or they may be acquired from outside the cells by phagocytosis (heterophagy). With an inherited deficiency of a functional lysosomal enzyme, catabolism of its substrate remains incomplete, leading to the accumulation of the partially degraded insoluble metabolite within the lysosomes. Stuffed with incompletely digested macromolecules, these organelles become large and numerous enough to interfere with normal cell functions, giving rise to the so-called *lysosomal storage disorders*[22] (Fig. 5–12). When this category of diseases was first discovered, it was thought that they resulted exclusively from mutations that led to reduced synthesis of lysosomal enzymes ("missing enzyme syndromes"). In the ensuing years, however, research focusing on the molecular pathology of lysosomal storage diseases has led to the discovery of several other defects.[23] Some of these are as follows:

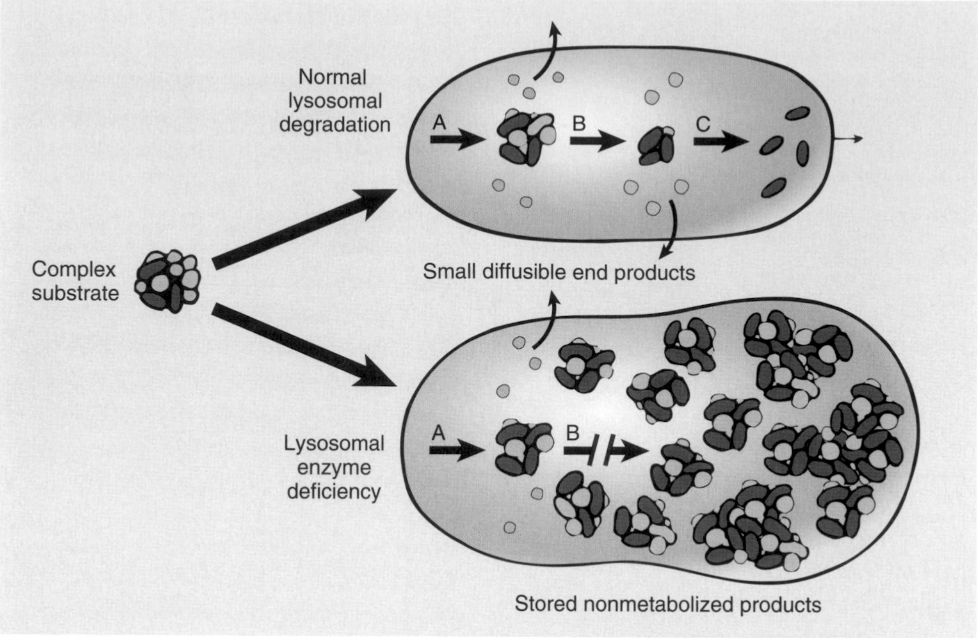

FIGURE 5–12 Schematic diagram illustrating the pathogenesis of lysosomal storage diseases. In the example shown, a complex substrate is normally degraded by a series of lysosomal enzymes (A, B, and C) into soluble end products. If there is a deficiency or malfunction of one of the enzymes (e.g., B), catabolism is incomplete and insoluble intermediates accumulate in the lysosomes.

- Synthesis of a catalytically inactive protein that cross-reacts immunologically with the normal enzyme. Thus, by immunoassays the enzyme levels appear to be normal.
- Defects in post-translational processing of the enzyme protein. Included in this category is a failure to attach the mannose-6-phosphate "marker," the absence of which prevents the enzyme from following its correct path to the lysosome. Instead the enzyme is secreted outside the cell.
- Lack of an enzyme activator or protector protein.
- Lack of a substrate activator protein. In some instances, proteins that react with the substrate to facilitate its hydrolysis may be missing or defective.
- Lack of a transport protein required for egress of the digested material from the lysosomes.

It should be evident, therefore, that lysosomal storage disorders can result from the lack of any protein essential for the normal function of lysosomes.

Several distinctive and separable conditions are included among the lysosomal storage diseases (Table 5–6). In general, the distribution of the stored material, and hence the organs affected, is determined by two interrelated factors: (1) the tissue where most of the material to be degraded is found and (2) the location where most of the degradation normally occurs. *For example, brain is rich in gangliosides, and hence defective hydrolysis of gangliosides, as occurs in GM_1 and GM_2 gangliosidoses, results primarily in storage within neurons and neurologic symptoms.* Defects in degradation of mucopolysaccharides affect virtually every organ because mucopolysaccharides are widely distributed in the body. Because cells of the mononuclear phagocyte system are especially rich in lysosomes and are involved in the degradation of a variety of substrates, organs rich in phagocytic cells, such as the spleen and liver, are frequently enlarged in several forms of lysosomal storage disorders. The ever-expanding number of lysosomal storage diseases can be divided into rational categories based on the biochemical nature of the accumulated metabolite, thus creating such subgroups as the *glycogenoses, sphingolipidoses (lipidoses), mucopolysaccharidoses (MPS),* and *mucolipidoses* (see Table 5–6). Only one among the many glycogenoses results from a lysosomal enzyme deficiency, and so this family of storage diseases is considered later. Only the most common disorders among the remaining groups are considered here.

Tay-Sachs Disease (GM_2 Gangliosidosis: Hexosaminidase α-Subunit Deficiency)

GM_2 gangliosidoses are a group of three lysosomal storage diseases caused by an inability to catabolize GM_2 gangliosides. Degradation of GM_2 gangliosides requires three polypeptides encoded by three separate loci (Fig. 5–13). The phenotypic effects of mutations affecting these genes are fairly similar because they result from accumulation of GM_2 gangliosides.[24] The underlying enzyme defect, however, is different for each. Tay-Sachs disease, the most common form of GM_2 gangliosidosis, results from mutations that affect the α-subunit locus on chromosome 15 and cause a severe deficiency of hexosaminidase A. This disease is especially prevalent among Jews, particularly among those of Eastern European (Ashkenazic) origin, in whom a carrier rate of 1 in 30 has been reported.

Morphology. The hexosaminidase A is absent from virtually all the tissues that have been examined, including leukocytes and plasma, and so GM_2 ganglioside accumulates in many tissues (e.g., heart, liver, spleen), but the **involvement of neurons in the central and autonomic nervous systems and retina dominates the clinical picture.** On histologic examination, the neurons are ballooned with cytoplasmic vacuoles, each of which constitutes a markedly distended lysosome filled with gangliosides (Fig. 5–14*A*). Stains for fat such as oil red O and Sudan black B are positive. With the electron microscope, several types

TABLE 5–6 Lysosomal Storage Diseases

Disease	Enzyme Deficiency	Major Accumulating Metabolites
Glycogenosis		
Type 2—Pompe disease	α-1,4-Glucosidase (lysosomal glucosidase)	Glycogen
Sphingolipidoses		
GM_1 gangliosidosis Type 1—infantile, generalized Type 2—juvenile	GM_1 ganglioside β-galactosidase	GM_1 ganglioside, galactose-containing oligosaccharides
GM_2 gangliosidosis		
Tay-Sachs disease	Hexosaminidase-α subunit	GM_2 ganglioside
Sandhoff disease	Hexosaminidase-β subunit	GM_2 ganglioside, globoside
GM_2 gangliosidosis, variant AB	Ganglioside activator protein	GM_2 ganglioside
Sulfatidoses		
Metachromatic leukodystrophy	Arylsulfatase A	Sulfatide
Multiple sulfatase deficiency	Arylsulfatases A, B, C; steroid sulfatase; iduronate sulfatase; heparan N-sulfatase	Sulfatide, steroid sulfate, heparan sulfate, dermatan sulfate
Krabbe disease	Galactosylceramidase	Galactocerebroside
Fabry disease	α-Galactosidase A	Ceramide trihexoside
Gaucher disease	Glucocerebrosidase	Glucocerebroside
Niemann-Pick disease: types A and B	Sphingomyelinase	Sphingomyelin
Mucopolysaccharidoses (MPS)		
MPS I H (Hurler)	α-L-Iduronidase	Dermatan sulfate, heparan sulfate
MPS II (Hunter)	L-Iduronosulfate sulfatase	
Mucolipidoses (ML)		
I-cell disease (ML II) and pseudo-Hurler polydystrophy	Deficiency of phosphorylating enzymes essential for the formation of mannose-6-phosphate recognition marker; acid hydrolases lacking the recognition marker cannot be targeted to the lysosomes but are secreted extracellularly	Mucopolysaccharide, glycolipid
Other Diseases of Complex Carbohydrates		
Fucosidosis	α-Fucosidase	Fucose-containing sphingolipids and glycoprotein fragments
Mannosidosis	α-Mannosidase	Mannose-containing oligosaccharides
Aspartylglycosaminuria	Aspartylglycosamine amide hydrolase	Aspartyl-2-deoxy-2-acetamido-glycosylamine
Other Lysosomal Storage Diseases		
Wolman disease	Acid lipase	Cholesterol esters, triglycerides
Acid phosphate deficiency	Lysosomal acid phosphatase	Phosphate esters

of cytoplasmic inclusions can be visualized, the most prominent being whorled configurations within lysosomes composed of onion-skin layers of membranes (Fig. 5–14*B*). In time, there is progressive destruction of neurons, proliferation of microglia, and accumulation of complex lipids in phagocytes within the brain substance. A similar process occurs in the cerebellum as well as in neurons throughout the basal ganglia, brain stem, spinal cord, and dorsal root ganglia and in the neurons of the autonomic nervous system. The ganglion cells in the retina are similarly swollen with GM_2 ganglioside, particularly at the margins of the macula. A **cherry-red spot** thus appears in the macula, representing accentuation of the normal color of the macular choroid contrasted with the pallor produced by the swollen ganglion cells in the remainder of the retina (Chapter 29). This finding is characteristic of Tay-Sachs disease and other storage disorders affecting the neurons.

Many alleles have been identified at the α-subunit locus, each associated with a variable degree of enzyme deficiency and hence with variable clinical manifestations. The affected infants appear normal at birth but begin to manifest signs and symptoms at about age 6 months. There is relentless motor and mental deterioration, beginning with motor incoordination, mental obtundation leading to muscular flaccidity, blindness, and increasing dementia. Sometime during the early course of the disease, the characteristic, but not pathognomonic, cherry-red spot appears in the macula of the eye grounds in almost all patients. Over the span of 1 or 2 years, a complete, pathetic vegetative state is reached, followed by death at age 2 to 3 years.

Antenatal diagnosis and carrier detection are possible by enzyme assays and DNA-based analysis.[25] The clinical features of the two other forms of GM_2 gangliosidosis (see Fig. 5–13), Sandhoff disease, resulting from β-subunit defect, and GM_2 activator deficiency, are similar to those of Tay-Sachs disease.

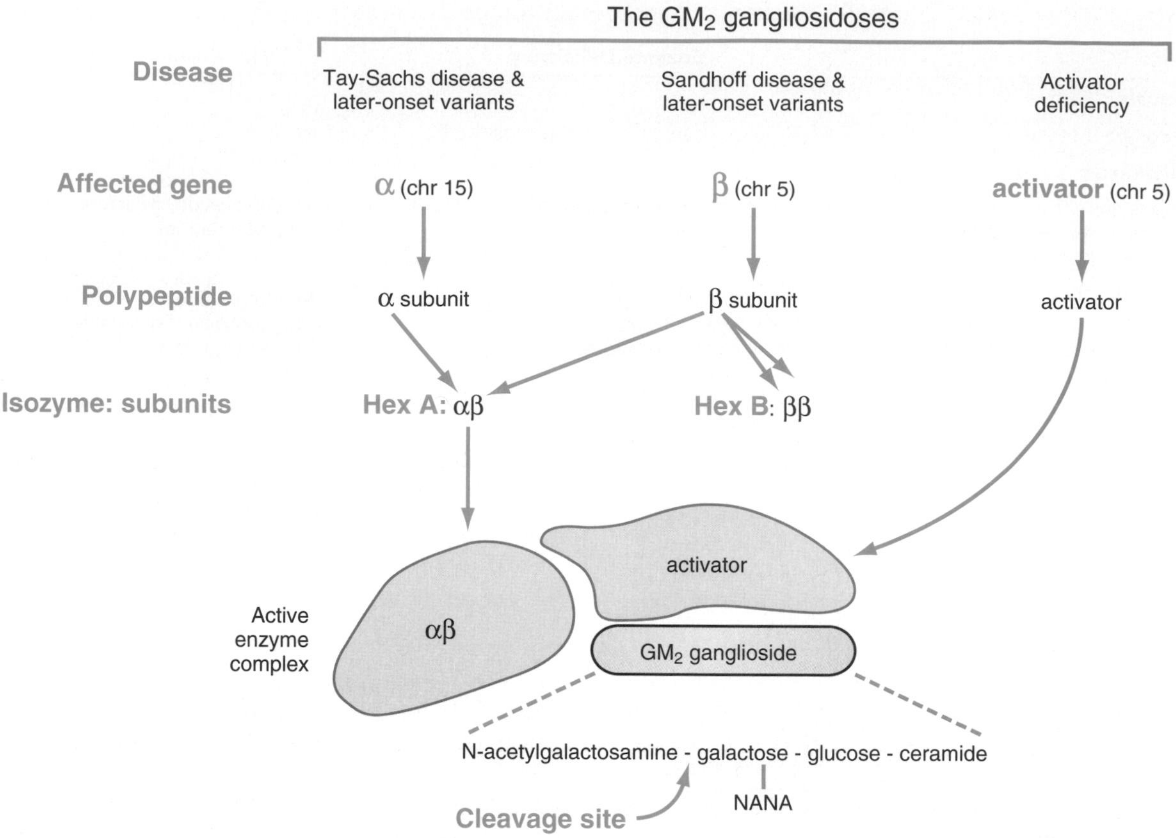

FIGURE 5–13 The three-gene system required for hexosaminidase A activity and the diseases that result from defects in each of the genes. The function of the activator protein is to bind the ganglioside substrate and present it to the enzyme. (Modified from Sandhoff K, et al: The GM_2 gangliosidoses. In Scriver CR, et al [eds]: The Metabolic Basis of Inherited Disease, 6th ed. New York, McGraw-Hill, 1989, p. 1824.)

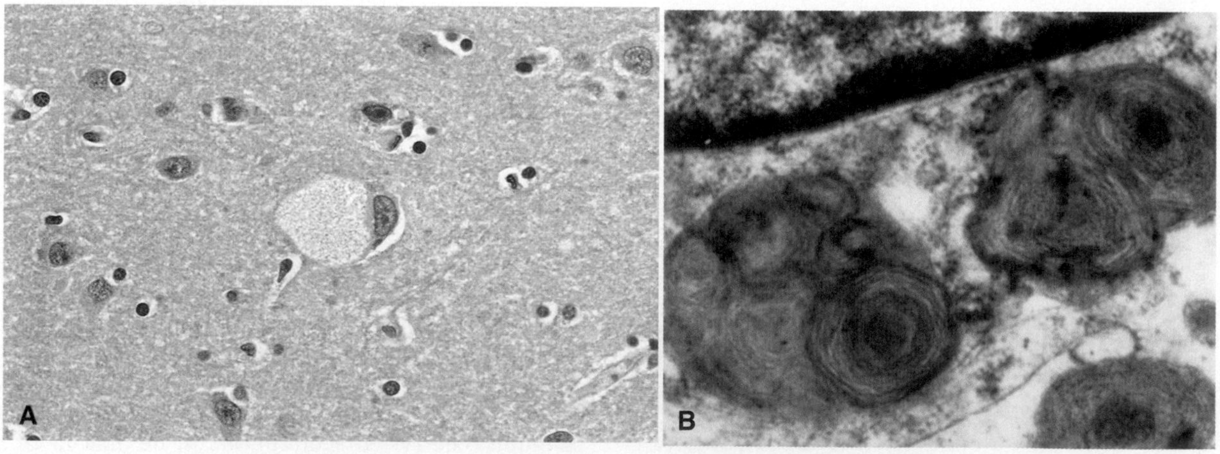

FIGURE 5–14 Ganglion cells in Tay-Sachs disease. *A,* Under the light microscope, a large neuron has obvious lipid vacuolation. (Courtesy of Dr. Arthur Weinberg, Department of Pathology, University of Texas Southwestern Medical Center, Dallas.) *B,* A portion of a neuron under the electron microscope shows prominent lysosomes with whorled configurations. Part of the nucleus is shown above. (Electron micrograph courtesy of Dr. Joe Rutledge, University of Texas Southwestern Medical Center, Dallas, TX.)

Niemann-Pick Disease: Types A and B

Niemann-Pick disease types A and B refers to two related disorders that are characterized by lysosomal accumulation of sphingomyelin resulting from an inherited deficiency of sphingomyelinase. In the past, these two conditions were grouped with an unrelated disorder, called *Niemann-Pick disease type C*, described separately below.[26] *Type A is the severe infantile form with extensive neurologic involvement, marked visceral accumulations of sphingomyelin, and progressive wasting and early death within the first 3 years of life.* To provide a perspective on the differences between the variants of Niemann-Pick disease, we need only point out that in type B, for example, patients have organomegaly but generally no central nervous system involvement. They usually survive into adulthood. As with Tay-Sachs disease, Niemann-Pick disease types A and B are common in Ashkenazi Jews.

Morphology. In the classic infantile type A variant, a missense mutation causes almost complete deficiency of sphingomyelinase. Sphingomyelin is a ubiquitous component of cellular (including organellar) membranes, and so the enzyme deficiency blocks degradation of the lipid, resulting in its progressive accumulation within lysosomes, particularly within cells of the mononuclear phagocyte system. Affected cells become enlarged, sometimes to 90 μm in diameter, secondary to the distention of lysosomes with sphingomyelin and cholesterol. Innumerable small vacuoles of relatively uniform size are created, imparting a foaminess to the cytoplasm (Fig. 5–15). In frozen sections of fresh tissue, the vacuoles stain for fat with Sudan black B and oil red O. Electron microscopy confirms that the vacuoles are engorged secondary lysosomes that often contain membranous cytoplasmic bodies resembling concentric lamellated myelin figures. Sometimes the lysosomal configurations take the form of parallel palisaded lamellae, creating so-called zebra bodies.

The lipid-laden phagocytic foam cells are widely distributed in the spleen, liver, lymph nodes, bone marrow, tonsils, gastrointestinal tract, and lungs. **The involvement of the spleen generally produces massive enlargement**, sometimes to 10 times its normal weight, but the hepatomegaly is usually not quite so striking. The lymph nodes are generally moderately to markedly enlarged throughout the body.

Involvement of the brain and eye deserves special mention. In the brain, the gyri are shrunken and the sulci widened. The neuronal involvement is diffuse, affecting all parts of the nervous system. Vacuolation and ballooning of neurons constitute the dominant histologic change, which in time leads to cell death and loss of brain substance. A retinal cherry-red spot similar to that seen in Tay-Sachs disease is present in about one third to one half of affected individuals. Its origin is similar to that described in Tay-Sachs disease except that the accumulated metabolite is sphingomyelin.

Clinical manifestations may be present at birth but almost invariably become evident by age 6 months. Infants typically have a protuberant abdomen because of the hepatosplenomegaly. Once the manifestations appear, they are followed by progressive failure to thrive, vomiting, fever, and generalized lymphadenopathy as well as progressive deterioration of psychomotor function. Death comes as a release, usually within the first or second year of life.

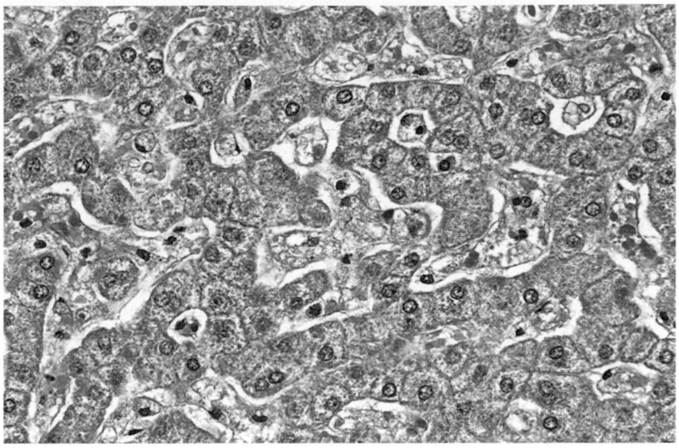

FIGURE 5–15 Niemann-Pick disease in liver. The hepatocytes and Kupffer cells have a foamy, vacuolated appearance owing to deposition of lipids. (Courtesy of Dr. Arthur Weinberg, Department of Pathology, University of Texas Southwestern Medical Center, Dallas, TX.)

The diagnosis is established by biochemical assays for sphingomyelinase activity in liver or bone marrow biopsy. The sphingomyelinase gene has been cloned, and hence individuals affected with types A and B as well as carriers can be detected by DNA analysis.

Nieman-Pick Disease: Type C (NPC)

Although discovered more recently as a distinct entity, this type is more common than types A and B combined. The affected gene, called *NPC-1*, encodes a protein involved in cholesterol trafficking;[27] therefore, in this disorder, cholesterol accumulates in the affected cells. In the brain, NPC-1 is present in astrocytic processes in close apposition to nerve terminals. With defective cholesterol trafficking, terminal axons and dendrites degenerate. NPC is clinically very heterogeneous. It may present with hydrops fetalis and stillbirth, as neonatal hepatitis, or as a chronic form characterized by progressive neurologic damage. Most common, however, is presentation in childhood, which is marked by ataxia, supranuclear palsy, psychomotor regression, hepatosplenomegaly, and dysarthria.

Gaucher Disease

Gaucher disease refers to a cluster of autosomal recessive disorders resulting from mutations in the gene encoding glucocerebrosidase.[28] This disease is the most common lysosomal storage disorder. The affected gene encodes glucocerebrosidase, an enzyme that normally cleaves the glucose residue from ceramide. As a result, glucocerebroside accumulates principally in the phagocytic cells of the body but in some forms also in the central nervous system. Glucocerebrosides are continually formed from the catabolism of glycolipids derived mainly from the cell membranes of senescent leukocytes and erythrocytes. Three clinical subtypes of Gaucher disease have been distinguished. The most common, accounting for 99% of cases, is called *type I*, or the chronic non-neuronopathic form. In this type, *storage of glucocerebrosides is limited to the mononuclear phagocytes throughout the body without involving the brain. Splenic and skeletal involvements dominate this pattern of the disease.* It is found principally in Jews of European stock. Patients with this disorder have reduced but detectable levels of glucocerebrosidase activity. Longevity is shortened but not markedly. *Type II,* or acute neuronopathic Gaucher disease, is the *infantile acute cerebral pattern. This infantile form has no predilection for Jews. In these patients, there is virtually no detectable glucocerebrosidase activity in the tissues.* Hepatosplenomegaly is also seen in this form of Gaucher disease, but the clinical picture is dominated by progressive central nervous system involvement, leading to death at an early age. A third pattern, type III, is sometimes distinguished, intermediate between types I and II. These patients are usually juveniles and have the systemic involvement characteristic of type I but have progressive central nervous system disease that usually begins in the teens or twenties. These specific patterns run within families, resulting from different allelic mutations in the structural gene for the enzyme.

Morphology. The glucocerebrosides accumulate in massive amounts within phagocytic cells throughout the body in all forms of Gaucher disease. The distended phagocytic cells, known as **Gaucher cells**, are found in the spleen, liver, bone marrow, lymph nodes, tonsils, thymus, and Peyer patches. Similar cells may be found in both the alveolar septa and the air spaces in the lung. In contrast to the lipid storage diseases already discussed, Gaucher cells rarely appear vacuolated but instead have a fibrillary type of cytoplasm likened to crumpled tissue paper (Fig. 5–16). Gaucher cells are often enlarged, sometimes up to 100 μm in diameter, and have one or more dark, eccentrically placed nuclei. Periodic acid–Schiff (PAS) staining is usually intensely positive. With the electron microscope, the fibrillary cytoplasm can be resolved as elongated, distended lysosomes, containing the stored lipid in stacks of bilayers.[29]

The accumulation of Gaucher cells produces a variety of gross anatomic changes. The spleen is enlarged in the type I variant, sometimes up to 10 kg. It may appear uniformly pale or have a mottled surface owing to focal accumulations of Gaucher cells. The lymphadenopathy is mild to moderate and is body-wide. The accumulations of Gaucher cells in the bone marrow may produce small focal areas of bone erosion or large, soft, gray tumorous masses that cause skeletal deformities or destroy sufficient bone to give rise to fractures. In patients with cerebral involvement, Gaucher cells are seen in the Virchow-Robin spaces, and arterioles are surrounded by swollen adventitial cells. There is no storage of lipids in the neurons, yet neurons appear shriveled and are progressively destroyed. It is suspected that the lipids that accumulate in the phagocytic cells around blood vessels are in some manner toxic to neural tissue.

The clinical course of Gaucher disease depends on the clinical subtype. In type I, symptoms and signs first appear in adult life and are related to splenomegaly or bone involvement. Most commonly, there is pancytopenia or thrombocytopenia secondary to hypersplenism. Pathologic fractures and bone pain occur if there has been extensive expansion of the marrow space. Although the disease is progressive in the adult, it is compatible with long life. In types II and III, central nervous system dysfunction, convulsions, and progressive mental deterioration dominate, although organs such as the liver, spleen, and lymph nodes are also affected.

The diagnosis of homozygotes can be made by measurement of glucocerebrosidase activity in peripheral blood leukocytes or in extracts of cultured skin fibroblasts. Because there is substantial overlap between the enzyme levels in normal individuals and heterozygotes, such assays are not reliable for carrier detection. In principle, detection of specific mutations can be used for detecting heterozygotes. Because more than 150 allelic mutations can cause Gaucher disease, however, it is not possible to use a single genetic test. Chitotriosidase, an enzyme synthesized by macrophages, is markedly elevated in patients with Gaucher disease. It is a reasonably specific

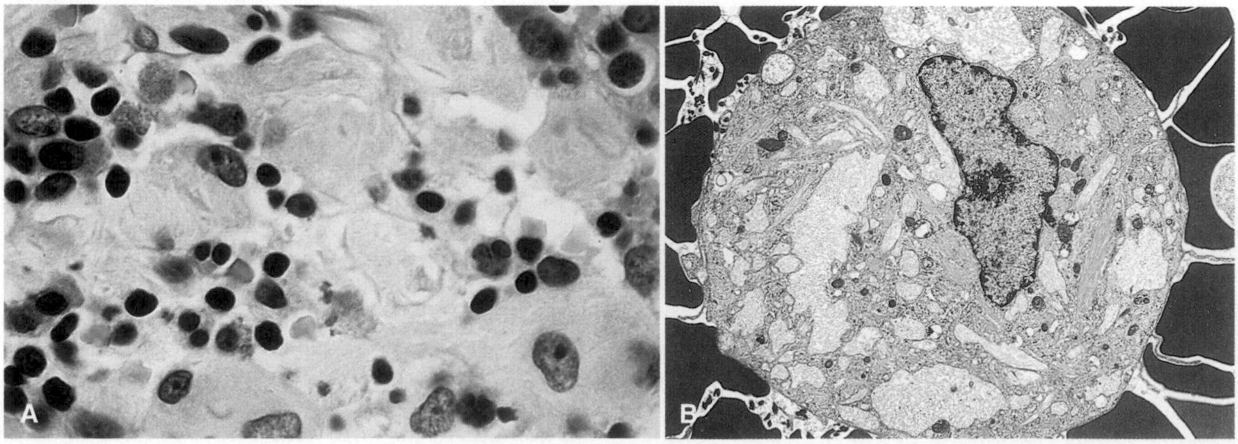

FIGURE 5–16 Gaucher disease involving the bone marrow. *A*, Gaucher cells with abundant lipid-laden granular cytoplasm. *B*, Electron micrograph of Gaucher cells with elongated distended lysosomes. (Courtesy of Dr. Matthew Fries, Department of Pathology, University of Texas Southwestern Medical Center, Dallas, TX.)

biomarker for Gaucher disease because levels are only slightly elevated in other disorders affecting macrophages.[30]

As with all lysosomal storage diseases, the treatment of Gaucher disease is difficult. Replacement therapy with recombinant enzymes is effective, and those with type I disease can expect normal life expectancy with enzyme replacement therapy. However, such therapy is extremely expensive. Because the fundamental defect resides in mononuclear phagocytic cells originating from marrow stem cells, bone marrow transplantation has been attempted. Attempts are also directed toward correction of the enzyme defect by transfer of the normal glucocerebrosidase gene into the patient's cells.

Mucopolysaccharidoses

The mucopolysaccharidoses (MPS) are a group of closely related syndromes that result from genetically determined deficiencies of lysosomal enzymes involved in the degradation of mucopolysaccharides (glycosaminoglycans). Chemically, mucopolysaccharides are long-chain complex carbohydrates that are linked with proteins to form proteoglycans. They are abundant in the ground substance of connective tissue. The glycosaminoglycans that accumulate in MPS are dermatan sulfate, heparan sulfate, keratan sulfate, and chondroitin sulfate.[31] The enzymes involved in the degradation of these molecules cleave terminal sugars from the polysaccharide chains disposed along a polypeptide or core protein. When there is a block in the removal of a terminal sugar, the remainder of the polysaccharide chain is not further degraded, and thus these chains accumulate within lysosomes in various tissues and organs of the body. Severe somatic and neurologic changes result.

Several clinical variants of MPS, classified numerically from MPS I to MPS VII, have been described, each resulting from the deficiency of one specific enzyme. All the MPS except one are inherited as autosomal recessive traits; the exception, called *Hunter syndrome*, is an X-linked recessive trait. Within a given group (e.g., MPS I, characterized by a deficiency of α-l-iduronidase), subgroups exist that result from different mutant alleles at the same genetic locus. Thus, the severity of enzyme deficiency and the clinical picture even within subgroups are often different.

In general, MPS are progressive disorders, characterized by involvement of multiple organs, including liver, spleen, heart, and blood vessels. Most are associated with *coarse facial features, clouding of the cornea, joint stiffness*, and *mental retardation*. Urinary excretion of the accumulated mucopolysaccharides is often increased.

Morphology. The accumulated mucopolysaccharides are generally found in mononuclear phagocytic cells, endothelial cells, intimal smooth muscle cells, and fibroblasts throughout the body. Common sites of involvement are thus the spleen, liver, bone marrow, lymph nodes, blood vessels, and heart.

Microscopically, affected cells are distended and have apparent clearing of the cytoplasm to create so-called balloon cells. The cleared cytoplasm can be resolved as numerous minute vacuoles, which, with the electron microscope, can be visualized as swollen lysosomes filled with a finely granular PAS-positive material that can be identified biochemically as mucopolysaccharide. Similar lysosomal changes are found in the neurons of those syndromes characterized by central nervous system involvement. In addition, however, some of the lysosomes in neurons are replaced by lamellated zebra bodies similar to those seen in Niemann-Pick disease. **Hepatosplenomegaly, skeletal deformities, valvular lesions, and subendothelial arterial deposits, particularly in the coronary arteries, and lesions in the brain, are common threads that run through all of the MPS.** In many of the more protracted syndromes, coronary subendothelial lesions lead to myocardial ischemia. Thus, myocardial infarction and cardiac decompensation are important causes of death.

Of the seven recognized variants, only two well-characterized syndromes are described briefly here. *Hurler syndrome*, also called MPS I H, results from a deficiency of α-l-iduronidase. It is one of the most severe forms of MPS. Affected children appear normal at birth but develop hepatosplenomegaly by age 6 to 24 months. Their growth is retarded, and, as in other forms of MPS, they develop coarse facial features and skeletal deformities. Death occurs by age 6 to 10 years and is often due to cardiovascular complications. *Hunter syndrome*, also called MPS II, differs from Hurler syndrome in mode of inheritance (X-linked), absence of corneal clouding, and milder clinical course.

Glycogen Storage Diseases (Glycogenoses)

A number of genetic syndromes have been identified that result from some metabolic defect in the synthesis or catabolism of glycogen. The best understood and most important category includes the *glycogen storage diseases*, resulting from a hereditary deficiency of one of the enzymes involved in the synthesis or sequential degradation of glycogen. Depending on the tissue or organ distribution of the specific enzyme in the normal state, *glycogen storage in these disorders may be limited to a few tissues, may be more widespread while not affecting all tissues, or may be systemic in distribution.*[32,33]

The significance of a specific enzyme deficiency is best understood from the perspective of the normal metabolism of glycogen (Fig. 5–17). As is well known, glycogen is a storage form of glucose. Glycogen synthesis begins with the conversion of glucose to glucose-6-phosphate by the action of a hexokinase (glucokinase). A phosphoglucomutase then transforms the glucose-6-phosphate to glucose-1-phosphate, which, in turn, is converted to uridine diphosphoglucose. A highly branched, large polymer is then built up (molecular weight, up to 100 million), containing up to 10,000 glucose molecules linked together by α-1,4-glucoside bonds. The glycogen chain and branches continue to be elongated by the addition of glucose molecules mediated by glycogen synthetases. During degradation, distinct phosphorylases in the liver and muscle split glucose-1-phosphate from the glycogen until about four glucose residues remain on each branch, leaving a branched oligosaccharide called *limit dextrin*. This can be further degraded only by the debranching enzyme. In addition to these major pathways, glycogen is also degraded in the lysosomes by acid maltase. If the lysosomes are deficient

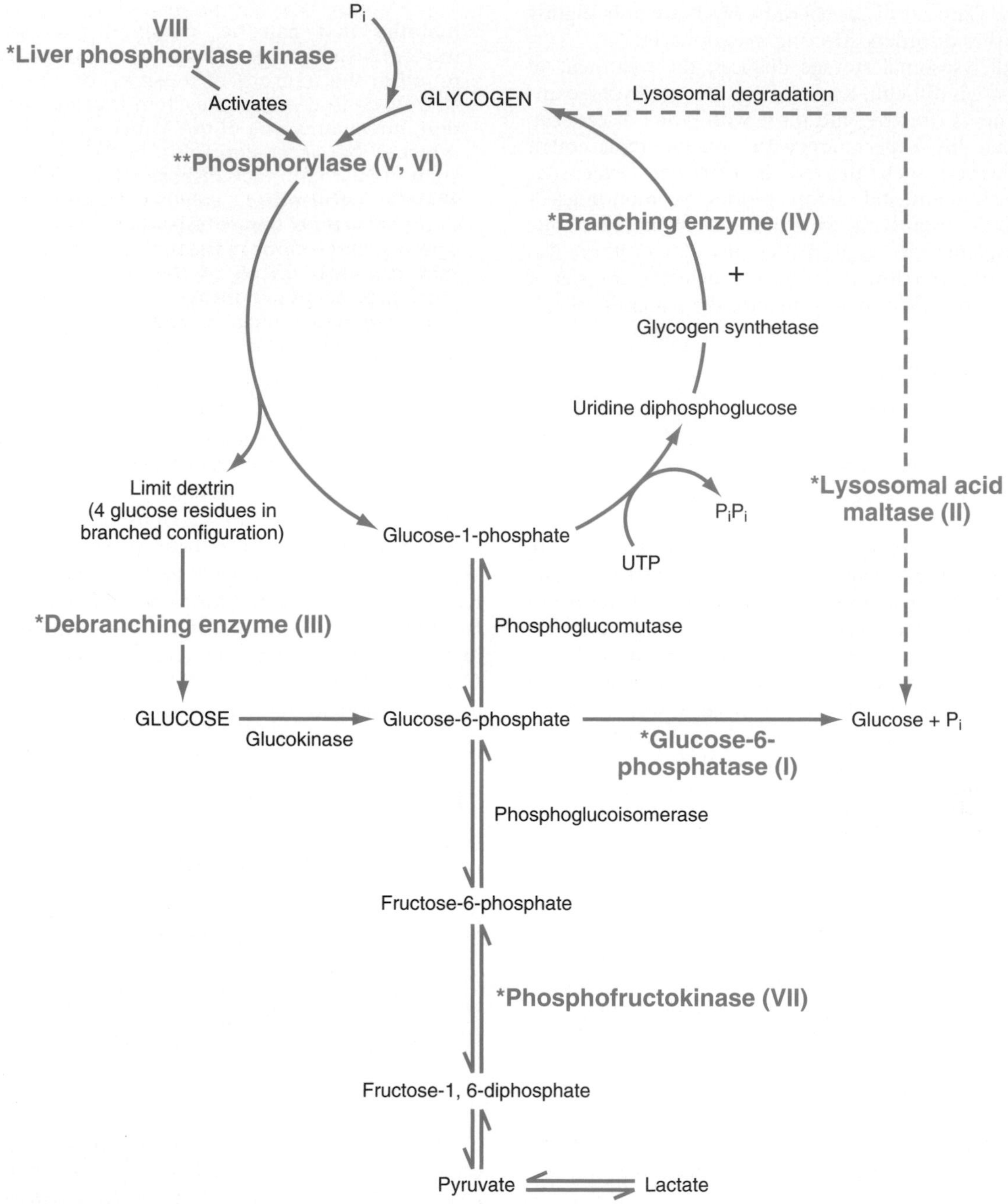

FIGURE 5–17 Pathways of glycogen metabolism. Asterisks mark the enzyme deficiencies associated with glycogen storage diseases. Roman numerals indicate the type of glycogen storage disease associated with the given enzyme deficiency. Types V and VI result from deficiencies of muscle and liver phosphorylases, respectively. (Modified from Hers H, et al: Glycogen storage diseases. In Scriver CR, et al [eds]: The Metabolic Basis of Inherited Disease, 6th ed. New York, McGraw-Hill, 1989, p. 425.)

in this enzyme, the glycogen contained within them is not accessible to degradation by cytoplasmic enzymes such as phosphorylases.

On the basis of specific enzyme deficiencies and the resultant clinical pictures, glycogenoses have traditionally been divided into a dozen or so syndromes designated by roman numerals, and the list continues to grow. Rather than describing each syndrome, we offer a more manageable classification that is based on the pathophysiology of these disorders.[34] According to this approach, glycogenoses can be divided into three major subgroups.

- *Hepatic forms:* As is well known, the liver is a key player in glycogen metabolism. It contains enzymes that synthesize glycogen for storage and ultimately break it down into free glucose, which is then released into the blood. An inherited deficiency of hepatic enzymes that are involved in glycogen metabolism therefore leads not only to the storage of glycogen in the liver, but also to a reduction in blood glucose level (hypoglycemia) (Fig. 5–18). Deficiency of the enzyme glucose-6-phosphatase (von Gierke disease, or type I glycogenosis) is a prime example of the hepatic-hypoglycemic form of glycogen storage disease (Table 5–7).

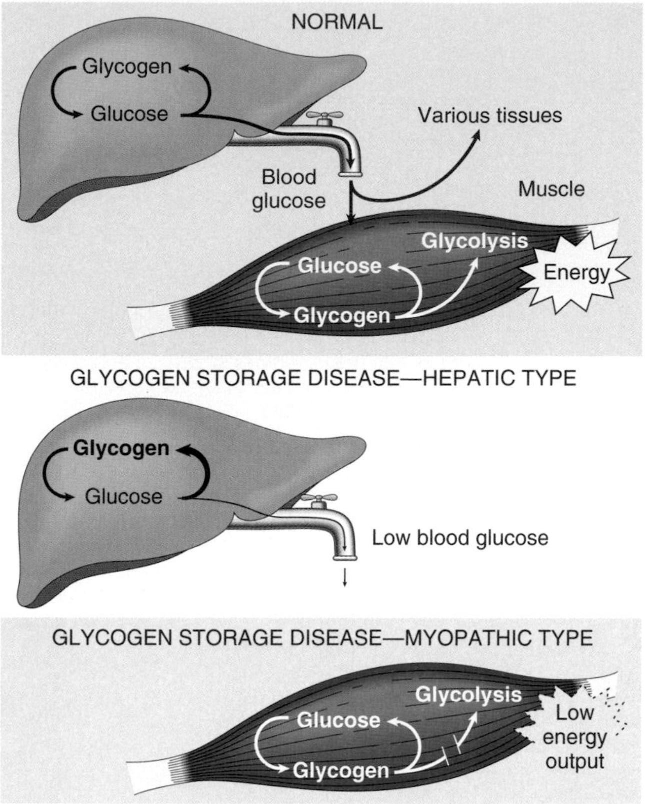

FIGURE 5–18 *Top,* Simplified schema of normal glycogen metabolism in the liver and skeletal muscles. *Middle,* Effects of an inherited deficiency of hepatic enzymes involved in glycogen metabolism. *Bottom,* Consequences of a genetic deficiency in the enzymes that metabolize glycogen in skeletal muscles.

Other examples include lack of liver phosphorylase and debranching enzyme, both involved in the breakdown of glycogen (see Fig. 5–17). In all of these cases, glycogen is stored in many organs, but the *hepatic enlargement and hypoglycemia dominate the clinical picture.*[35]

- *Myopathic forms:* In the striated muscles, as opposed to the liver, glycogen is used predominantly as a source of energy. This is derived by glycolysis, which leads ultimately to the formation of lactate (see Fig. 5–18). If the enzymes that fuel the glycolytic pathway are deficient, glycogen storage occurs in the muscles and is associated with muscular weakness owing to impaired energy production. Examples in this category include deficiencies of muscle phosphorylase (McArdle disease, or type V glycogenosis), muscle phosphofructokinase (type VII glycogen storage disease), and several others. *Typically, patients with the myopathic forms present with muscle cramps after exercise and a failure of exercise-induced rise in blood lactate levels owing to a block in glycolysis.*[36]
- Glycogen storage diseases associated with (1) deficiency of α-glucosidase (acid maltase) and (2) lack of branching enzyme do not fit into the hepatic or myopathic categories just described. They are associated with glycogen storage in many organs and death early in life. Acid maltase is a lysosomal enzyme, and hence its deficiency leads to lysosomal storage of glycogen (type II glycogenosis, or Pompe disease) in all organs, but cardiomegaly is most prominent (Fig. 5–19). Brancher glycogenosis (type IV) is associated with widespread deposition of an abnormal form of glycogen with detrimental effects on the brain, heart, skeletal muscles, and liver.

The principal features of some important examples from each of the aforementioned three categories are summarized in Table 5–7. Details of other forms may be found in specialized texts.[37]

Alkaptonuria (Ochronosis)

Alkaptonuria, the first human inborn error of metabolism to be discovered, was recognized by Garrod. It is an autosomal recessive disorder in which *the lack of homogentisic oxidase blocks the metabolism of phenylalanine-tyrosine at the level of homogentisic acid.* Thus, homogentisic acid accumulates in the body. A large amount is excreted, imparting a black color to

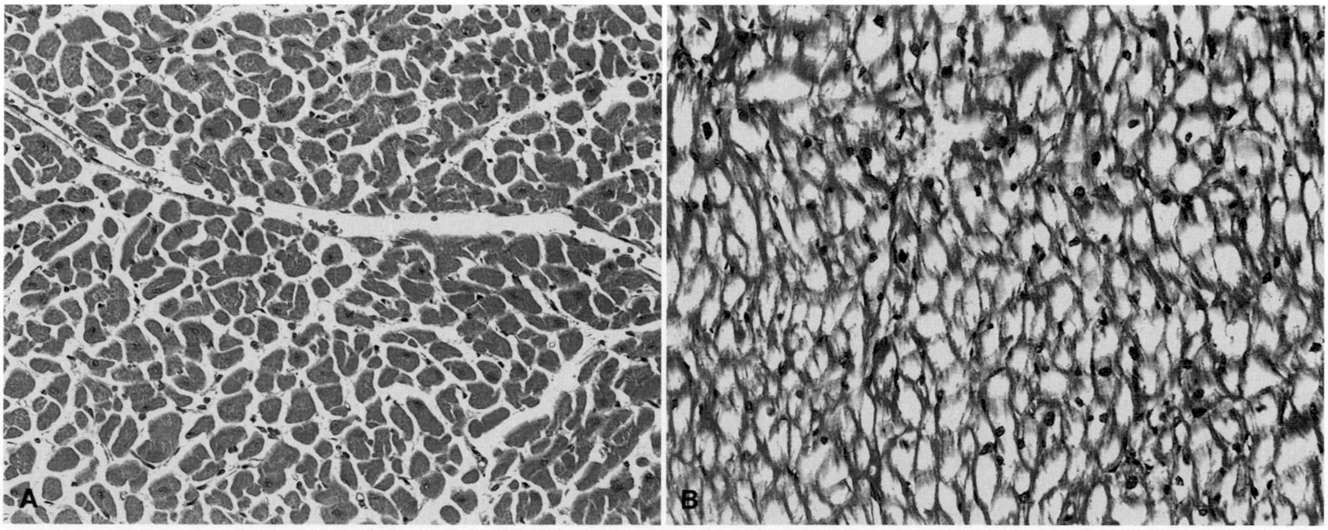

FIGURE 5–19 Pompe disease (glycogen storage disease type II). *A,* Normal myocardium with abundant eosinophilic cytoplasm. *B,* Patient with Pompe disease (same magnification) showing the myocardial fibers full of glycogen seen as clear spaces. (Courtesy of Dr. Trace Worrell, Department of Pathology, University of Texas Southwestern Medical Center, Dallas, TX.)

TABLE 5–7 Principal Subgroups of Glycogenoses

Clinicopathologic Category	Specific Type	Enzyme Deficiency	Morphologic Changes	Clinical Features
Hepatic Type	Hepatorenal—von Gierke disease (type I)	Glucose-6-phosphatase	Hepatomegaly—intracytoplasmic accumulations of glycogen and small amounts of lipid; intranuclear glycogen Renomegaly—intracytoplasmic accumulations of glycogen in cortical tubular epithelial cells	In untreated patients: failure to thrive, stunted growth, hepatomegaly, and renomegaly. Hypoglycemia due to failure of glucose mobilization, often leading to convulsions. Hyperlipidemia and hyperuricemia resulting from deranged glucose metabolism; many patients develop gout and skin xanthomas. Bleeding tendency due to platelet dysfunction. With treatment most survive and develop late complications, e.g., hepatic adenomas
Myopathic Type	McArdle syndrome (type V)	Muscle phosphorylase	Skeletal muscle only—accumulations of glycogen predominant in subsarcolemmal location	Painful cramps associated with strenuous exercise. Myoglobinuria occurs in 50% of cases. Onset in adulthood (>20 years). Muscular exercise fails to raise lactate level in venous blood. Serum creatine kinase always elevated. Compatible with normal longevity
Miscellaneous Types	Generalized glycogenosis—Pompe disease (type II)	Lysosomal glucosidase (acid maltase)	Mild hepatomegaly—ballooning of lysosomes with glycogen, creating lacy cytoplasmic pattern Cardiomegaly—glycogen within sarcoplasm as well as membrane-bound Skeletal muscle—similar to changes in heart	Massive cardiomegaly, muscle hypotonia, and cardiorespiratory failure within 2 years. A milder adult form with only skeletal muscle involvement, presenting with chronic myopathy

the urine if allowed to stand and undergo oxidation.[38] The gene encoding homogentisic oxidase, mapped to 3q21, was cloned in 1996,[39] 64 years after the initial description of the disease by Garrod.

Morphology. The retained homogentisic acid selectively binds to collagen in connective tissues, tendons, and cartilage, imparting to these tissues a blue-black pigmentation **(ochronosis)** most evident in the ears, nose, and cheeks. **The most serious consequences of ochronosis, however, stem from deposits of the pigment in the articular cartilages of the joints.** In some obscure manner, the pigmentation causes the cartilage to lose its normal resiliency and become brittle and fibrillated.[40] Wear-and-tear erosion of this abnormal cartilage leads to denudation of the subchondral bone, and often tiny fragments of the fibrillated cartilage are driven into the underlying bone, worsening the damage. The vertebral column, particularly the intervertebral disc, is the prime site of attack, but later the knees, shoulders, and hips may be affected. The small joints of the hands and feet are usually spared.

The metabolic defect is present from birth, but the degenerative arthropathy develops slowly and usually does not become clinically evident until the thirties. Although it is not life-threatening, it may be severely crippling. The disability may be as extreme as that encountered in the severe forms of osteoarthritis (Chapter 26) of the elderly, but in alkaptonuria the arthropathy occurs at a much earlier age.

DISORDERS ASSOCIATED WITH DEFECTS IN PROTEINS THAT REGULATE CELL GROWTH

Normal growth and differentiation of cells is regulated by two classes of genes: proto-oncogenes and tumor-suppressor genes, whose products promote or restrain cell growth (Chapter 7). It is now well established that mutations in these two classes of genes are important in the pathogenesis of tumors. In the vast majority of cases, cancer-causing mutations affect somatic cells and hence are not passed in the germ line. In approximately 5% of all cancers, however, mutations transmitted through the germ line contribute to the development of cancer. Most familial cancers are inherited in an autosomal dominant fashion, but a few recessive disorders have also been described. This subject is discussed in greater detail in Chapter 7. Here we provide an example of two common familial neoplasms.

Neurofibromatosis: Types 1 and 2

Neurofibromatoses comprise two autosomal dominant disorders, affecting approximately 100,000 people in the United States. They are referred to as *neurofibromatosis type 1* (previously called *von Recklinghausen disease*) and *neurofibromatosis type 2* (previously called *acoustic neurofibromatosis*). Although there is some overlap in clinical features, these two entities are genetically distinct.[41]

Neurofibromatosis type 1 is a relatively common disorder, with a frequency of almost 1 in 3000. Although approximately 50% of the patients have a definite family history consistent with autosomal dominant transmission, the remainder appear to represent new mutations. In familial cases, the expressivity of the disorder is extremely variable, but the penetrance is 100%. Neurofibromatosis type 1 has three major features: (1) *multiple neural tumors (neurofibromas) dispersed anywhere on or in the body*; (2) *numerous pigmented skin lesions, some of which are café au lait spots*; and (3) *pigmented iris hamartomas, also called Lisch nodules*. A bewildering assortment of other abnormalities (cited later) may accompany these cardinal manifestations.

Morphology. The neurofibromas arise within or are attached to nerve trunks anywhere in the skin, including the palms and soles, as well as in every conceivable internal site, including the cranial nerves. Three types of neurofibromas are found in individuals with neurofibromatosis type 1: cutaneous, subcutaneous, and plexiform. **Cutaneous**, or dermal, neurofibromas are soft, sessile, or pedunculated lesions that vary in number from a few to many hundreds. **Subcutaneous neurofibromas** grow just beneath the skin; they are firm, round masses that are often painful. The cutaneous and subcutaneous neurofibromas may be less than 1 cm in diameter; moderate-sized pedunculated lesions; or huge, multilobar pendulous masses, 20 cm or more in greatest diameter. The third variant, referred to as **plexiform neurofibroma**, diffusely involves subcutaneous tissue and contains numerous tortuous, thickened nerves; the overlying skin is frequently hyperpigmented. These may grow to massive proportions, causing striking enlargement of a limb or some other body part. Similar tumors may occur internally, and in general the deeply situated lesions tend to be large. Microscopically, neurofibromas reveal proliferation of all the elements in the peripheral nerve, including neurites, Schwann cells, and fibroblasts. Typically, these components are dispersed in a loose, disorderly pattern, often in a loose, myxoid stroma. Elongated, serpentine Schwann cells predominate, with their slender, spindle-shaped nuclei. The loose and disorderly architecture helps differentiate these neural tumors from schwannomas. The latter, composed entirely of Schwann cells, virtually never undergo malignant transformation, whereas plexiform neurofibromas become malignant in about 5% of patients with neurofibromatosis type 1.[42] Malignant transformation is most common in the large plexiform tumors attached to major nerve trunks of the neck or extremities. The superficial lesions, despite their size, rarely become malignant.

The cutaneous pigmentations, the second major component of this syndrome, are present in more than 90% of patients. Most commonly, they appear as light brown **café au lait** macules, with generally smooth borders, often located over nerve trunks. They are usually round to ovoid, with their long axes parallel to the underlying cutaneous nerve. Although normal individuals may have a few café au lait spots, it is a clinical maxim that when six or more spots greater than 1.5 cm in diameter are present in an adult, the patient is likely to have neurofibromatosis type 1.

Lisch nodules (pigmented hamartomas in the iris) are present in more than 94% of patients age 6 years or older. They do not produce any symptoms but are helpful in establishing the diagnosis.

A wide range of associated abnormalities has been reported in these patients. Perhaps most common (seen in 30% to 50% of patients) are skeletal lesions, which take a variety of forms, including (1) erosive defects owing to contiguity of neurofibromas to bone, (2) scoliosis, (3) intraosseous cystic lesions, (4) subperiosteal bone cysts, and (5) pseudoarthrosis of the tibia. Patients with neurofibromatosis type 1 have a twofold to fourfold greater risk of developing other tumors, especially Wilms tumors, rhabdomyosarcomas, meningiomas, optic gliomas, and pheochromocytomas. Affected children are at increased risk of developing chronic myeloid leukemia.

Although some patients with this condition have normal intelligence quotients (IQs), there is an unmistakable tendency for reduced intelligence. When neurofibromas arise within the gastrointestinal tract, intestinal obstruction or gastrointestinal bleeding may occur. Narrowing of a renal artery by a tumor may induce hypertension. Owing to variable expression of the gene, the range of clinical presentations is almost limitless, but ultimately the diagnosis rests on the concurrence of multiple café au lait spots and multiple skin tumors. The neurofibromatosis type 1 *(NF-1)* gene has been mapped to chromosome 17q11.2. It encodes a protein called *neurofibromin*, which down-regulates the function of the $p21^{Ras}$ oncoprotein (see section on oncogenes, Chapter 7). *NF-1* therefore belongs to the family of tumor-suppressor genes.

Neurofibromatosis type 2 is an autosomal dominant disorder in which patients develop a range of tumors, most commonly bilateral acoustic schwannomas and multiple meningiomas. Gliomas, typically ependymomas of the spinal cord, also occur in these patients. Many individuals with neurofibromatosis type 2 also have non-neoplastic lesions, which include nodular ingrowth of Schwann cells into the spinal cord (schwannosis), meningioangiomatosis (a proliferation of meningeal cells and blood vessels that grows into the brain), and glial hamartia (microscopic nodular collections of glial cells at abnormal locations, often in the superficial and deep layers of the cerebral cortex). Café au lait spots are present, but Lisch nodules in the iris are not found. This disorder is much less common than neurofibromatosis type 1, having a frequency of 1 in 40,000 to 50,000.

The *NF-2* gene, located on chromosome 22q12, is also a tumor-suppressor gene. As further discussed in Chapter 7, the product of the *NF-2* gene, called *merlin*, shows structural similarity to the ezrin, radixin, moesin (ERM) family of proteins. These cytoskeletal proteins interact with actin on the one hand and membrane proteins on the cell surface on the other hand. It is thought that *merlin* regulates contact inhibition and proliferation of Schwann cells.[43]

Disorders with Multifactorial Inheritance

As pointed out earlier, the multifactorial disorders result from the combined actions of environmental influences and two or more mutant genes having additive effects. The genetic component exerts a dosage effect—the greater the number of inherited deleterious genes, the more severe the expression of the disease. Because environmental factors significantly influence the expression of these genetic disorders, the term polygenic inheritance should not be used.

A number of normal phenotypic characteristics are governed by multifactorial inheritance, such as hair color, eye color, skin color, height, and intelligence. These characteristics exhibit a continuous variation in population groups, producing the standard bell-shaped curve of distribution. Environmental influences, however, significantly modify the phenotypic expression of multifactorial traits. For example, type II diabetes mellitus has many of the features of a multifactorial disorder. It is well recognized clinically that individuals often first manifest this disease after weight gain. Thus, obesity as well as other environmental influences unmasks the diabetic genetic trait. Nutritional influences may cause even monozygous twins to achieve different heights. The culturally deprived child cannot achieve his or her full intellectual capacity.

The following features characterize multifactorial inheritance. These have been established for the multifactorial inheritance of congenital malformations and, in all likelihood, obtain for other multifactorial diseases.[44]

- The risk of expressing a multifactorial disorder is conditioned by the number of mutant genes inherited. Thus, the risk is greater in siblings of patients having severe expressions of the disorder. For example, the risk of cleft lip in the siblings of an index case is 2.5% if the cleft lip is unilateral but 6% if it is bilateral. Similarly, the greater the number of affected relatives, the higher is the risk for other relatives.
- The rate of recurrence of the disorder (in the range of 2% to 7%) is the same for all first-degree relatives (i.e., parents, siblings, and offspring) of the affected individual. Thus, if parents have had one affected child, the risk that the next child will be affected is between 2% and 7%. Similarly, there is the same chance that one of the parents will be affected.
- The likelihood that both identical twins will be affected is significantly less than 100% but is much greater than the chance that both nonidentical twins will be affected. Experience has proven, for example, that the frequency of concordance for identical twins is in the range of 20% to 40%.
- The risk of recurrence of the phenotypic abnormality in subsequent pregnancies depends on the outcome in previous pregnancies. When one child is affected, there is up to a 7% chance that the next child will be affected, but after two affected siblings, the risk rises to about 9%.
- Expression of a multifactorial trait may be continuous (lack a distinct phenotype, e.g., height) or discontinuous (with a distinct phenotype, e.g., diabetes mellitus). In the latter, disease is expressed only when the combined influences of the genes and environment cross a certain threshold. In the case of diabetes, for example, the risk of phenotypic expression increases when the blood glucose levels go above a certain level.

Assigning a disease to this mode of inheritance must be done with caution. It depends on many factors but first on familial clustering and the exclusion of mendelian and chromosomal modes of transmission. A range of levels of severity of a disease is suggestive of multifactorial inheritance, but, as pointed out earlier, variable expressivity and reduced penetrance of single mutant genes may also account for this phenomenon. Because of these problems, sometimes it is difficult to distinguish between mendelian and multifactorial inheritance.

In contrast to the mendelian disorders, many of which are uncommon, the multifactorial group includes some of the most common ailments to which humans are heir (Table 5–8). Most of these disorders are described in appropriate chapters elsewhere in this book.

TABLE 5–8 Multifactorial Disorders

Disorder	Chapter
Cleft lip or cleft palate (or both)	Chapter 10
Congenital heart disease	Chapter 12
Coronary heart disease	Chapter 12
Hypertension	Chapter 11
Gout	Chapter 27
Diabetes mellitus	Chapter 24
Pyloric stenosis	Chapter 17

Normal Karyotype

As is well known, human somatic cells contain 46 chromosomes; these comprise 22 homologous pairs of autosomes and two sex chromosomes, XX in the female and XY in the male. The study of chromosomes—*karyotyping*—is the basic tool of the cytogeneticist. The usual procedure of producing a chromosome spread is to arrest mitosis in dividing cells in metaphase by the use of mitotic spindle inhibitors (e.g., colcemid) and then to stain the chromosomes. In a metaphase spread, the individual chromosomes take the form of two chromatids connected at the centromere. A karyotype is a standard arrangement of a photographed or imaged stained metaphase spread in which chromosome pairs are arranged in order of decreasing length.

A variety of staining methods that allow identification of each individual chromosome on the basis of a distinctive and reliable pattern of alternating light and dark bands along the length of the chromosome have been developed. The one most commonly employed uses a Giemsa stain and is hence called *G banding.* A normal male karyotype with G banding is illustrated in Figure 5–20. With G banding, approximately 400 to 800 bands per haploid set can be detected. The resolution obtained by banding techniques can be dramatically improved by obtaining the cells in prophase. The individual chromosomes appear markedly elongated, and up to 1500 bands per karyotype may be recognized. The use of these banding techniques permits certain identification of each chromosome as well as delineation of precise breakpoints and other subtle alterations, to be described later.

Before this discussion of the normal karyotype is concluded, reference must be made to commonly used cytogenetic terminology. Karyotypes are usually described using a shorthand system of notations. The following order is used: Total number of chromosomes is given first, followed by the sex chromosome complement, and finally the description of abnormalities in ascending numerical order. For example, a

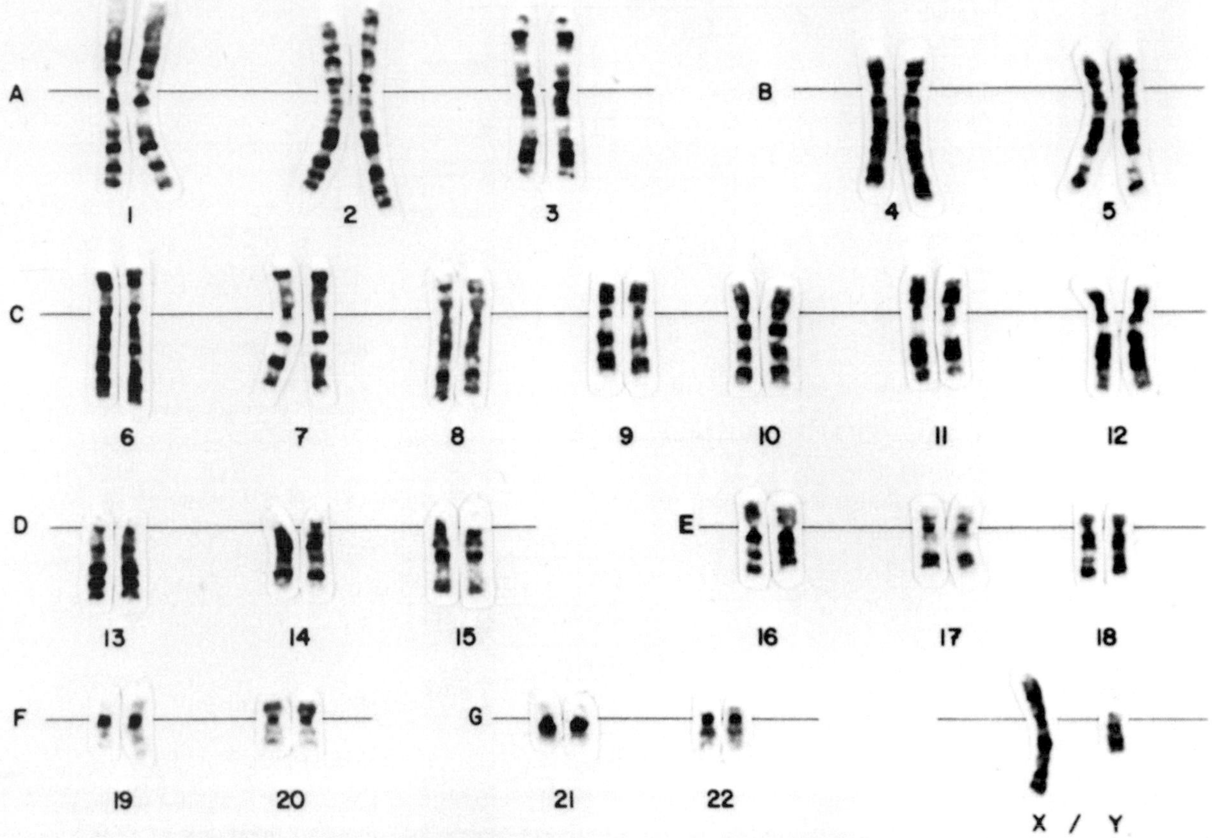

FIGURE 5–20 Normal male karyotype with G banding. (Courtesy of Dr. Nancy Schneider, Department of Pathology, University of Texas Southwestern Medical Center, Dallas, TX.)

male with trisomy 21 is designated *47,XY,+21*. Some of the notations denoting structural alterations of chromosomes are described along with the abnormalities in a later section. Here we should mention that the short arm of a chromosome is designated *p* (for petit), and the long arm is referred to as *q* (the next letter of alphabet). In a banded karyotype, each arm of the chromosome is divided into two or more regions by prominent bands. The regions are numbered (e.g., 1, 2, 3) from the centromere outward. Each region is further subdivided into bands and sub-bands, and these are ordered numerically as well (Fig. 5–21). Thus, the notation *Xp21.2* refers to a chromosomal segment located on the short arm of the X chromosome, in region 2, band 1, and sub-band 2.

Fluorescence in Situ Hybridization. Fluorescence in situ hybridization (FISH) has become an important adjunct to routine karyotyping and has greatly expanded the power of cytogenetic analysis.[45] A major limitation of karyotyping is that it is applicable only to cells that are dividing or can be induced to divide in vitro. This problem can be overcome with DNA probes that recognize chromosome-specific sequences. Such probes are labeled with fluorescent dyes and applied to interphase nuclei. The probe binds to its complementary sequence on the chromosome and thus labels the specific chromosome, which can then be visualized under a fluorescent microscope (Fig. 5–22). Thus, FISH can be used to enumerate chromosomes in interphase nuclei. The application of FISH is not limited to interphase nuclei, however. By using DNA probes that are specific for defined regions of the chromosomes, FISH can be used to demonstrate subtle microdeletions, complex translocations, and telomere alterations that are not readily detectable by routine karyotyping (Fig. 5–23). In addition to its diagnostic utility, FISH can also be used as a tool to physically map newly isolated genes of clinical interest. Novel DNA sequences are labeled with a fluorescent dye and then applied to a metaphase spread. The DNA binds to its complementary sequence and thus pinpoints the localization of the gene to a specific site. Chromosome painting is an extension of FISH, whereby whole chromosomes can be labeled with a series of fluorescent DNA probes that bind to multiple sites along a particular chromosome (Fig. 5–24). The number of chromosomes that can be *detected simultaneously* by chromosome painting is limited by the availability of fluorescent dyes that excite different wavelengths of visible light. Thus, chromosome painting has limited ability to visualize all 46 human chromosomes simultaneously. This hurdle has been overcome by the introduction of spectral karyotyping.[46] By using a combination of five fluorochromes and appropriate computer-generated signals, the entire human genome can be visualized (Fig. 5–25). So powerful is spectral karyotyping (SKY) that it might well be called "spectacular karyotyping."

Another recent FISH application directly compares the DNA content of differentially labeled normal and tumor cell

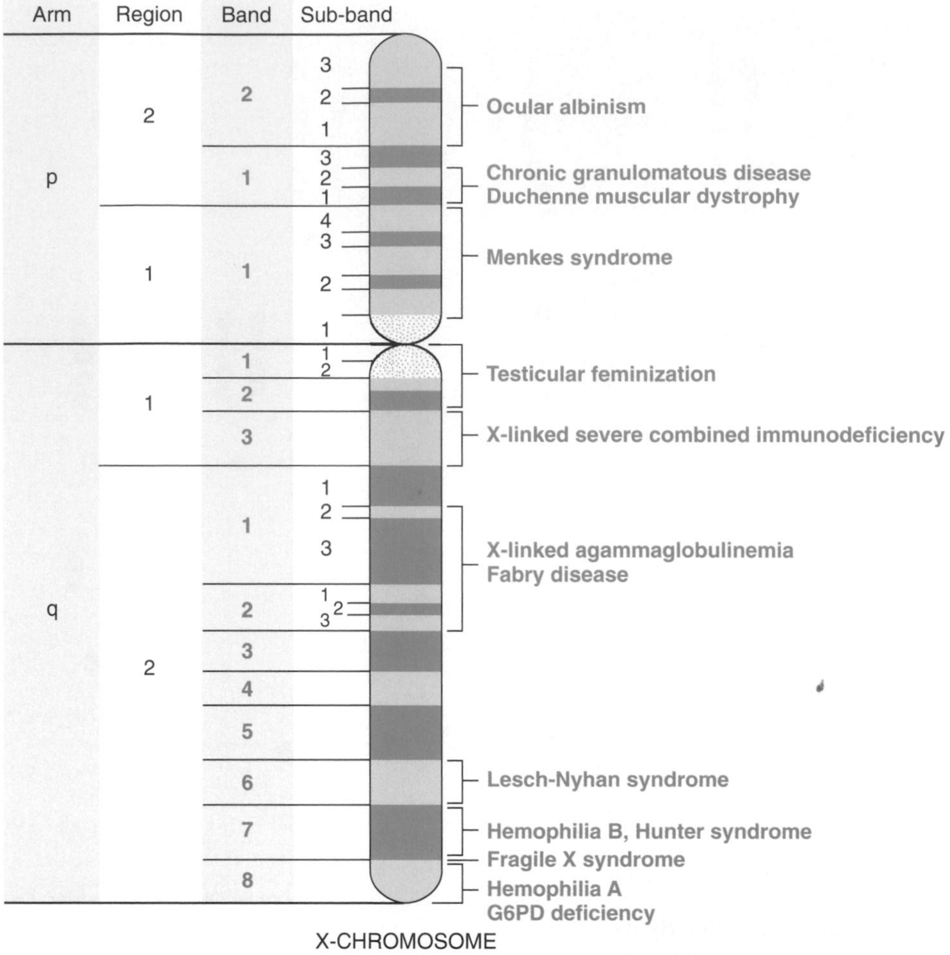

FIGURE 5–21 Details of banding pattern of the X chromosome (also called "idiogram"). Note the nomenclature of arms, regions, bands, and sub-bands. On the right side, the approximate locations of some genes that cause disease are indicated.

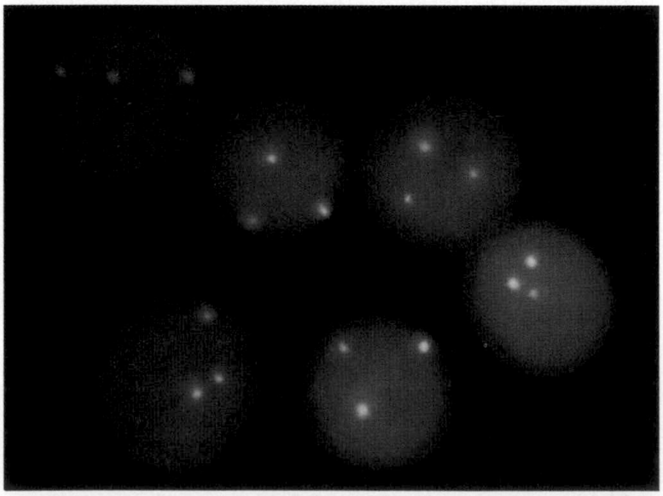

FIGURE 5–22 Fluorescence in situ hybridization (FISH). Interphase nuclei of a childhood hepatic cancer (hepatoblastoma) stained with a fluorescent DNA probe that hybridizes to chromosome 20. Under ultraviolet light, each nucleus reveals three bright yellow fluorescent dots, representing three copies of chromosome 20. Normal diploid cells *(not shown)* have two fluorescent dots. (Courtesy of Dr. Vijay Tonk, Department of Pathology, University of Texas Southwestern Medical Center, Dallas, TX.)

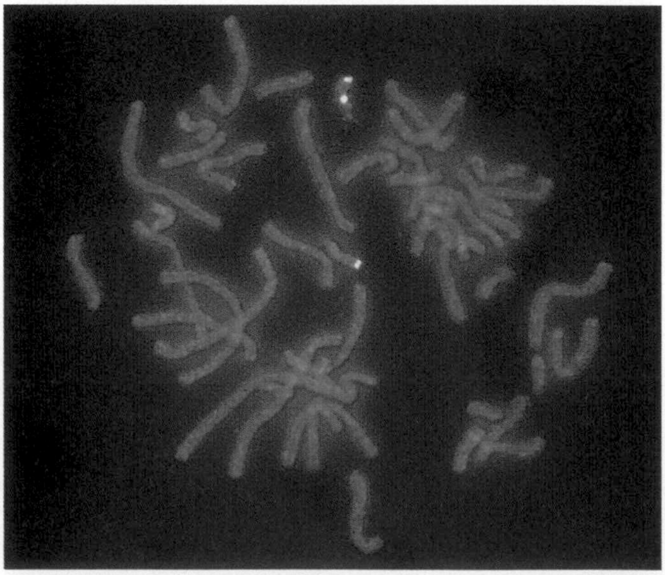

FIGURE 5–23 FISH. A metaphase spread in which two fluorescent probes, one for the terminal ends of chromosome 22 and the other for the D22S75 locus, which maps to chromosome 22, have been used. The terminal ends of the two chromosomes 22 have been labeled. One of the two chromosomes does not stain with the probe for the D22S75 locus, indicating a microdeletion in this region. This deletion gives rise to the 22q11.2 deletion syndrome. (Courtesy of Dr. Nancy Schneider, Department of Pathology, University of Texas Southwestern Medical Center, Dallas, TX.)

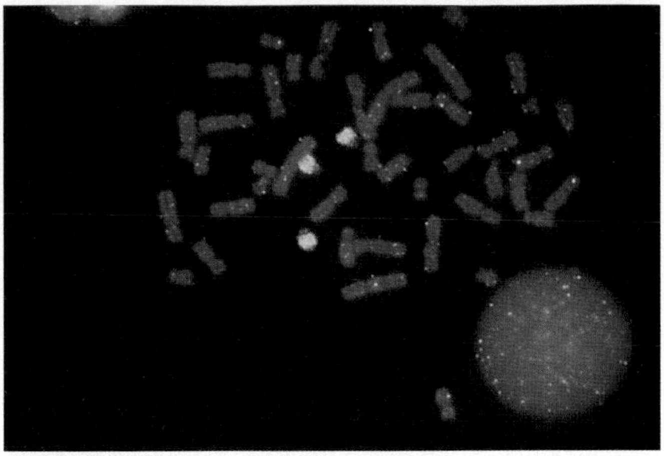

FIGURE 5–24 Chromosome painting with a library of chromosome 22–specific DNA probes. The presence of three fluorescent chromosomes indicates that the patient has trisomy 22. (Courtesy of Dr. Charleen M. Moore, The University of Texas Health Science Center at San Antonio, TX.)

populations by their co-hybridization to normal metaphase chromosome spreads (comparative genomic hybridization) or to a series of genomic DNA clones aligned on glass slides (array comparative genomic hybridization). In this manner, tumor-specific alterations in gene copy number can be ascertained.

Cytogenetic Disorders

The aberrations underlying cytogenetic disorders (chromosome mutations) may take the form of an abnormal number of chromosomes or alterations in the structure of one or more chromosomes. The normal chromosome complement is expressed as 46,XX for the female and 46,XY for the male. Any exact multiple of the haploid number is called *euploid.* If an error occurs in meiosis or mitosis, however, and a cell acquires a chromosome complement that is not an exact multiple of 23, it is referred to as *aneuploidy.* The usual causes for aneuploidy are *nondisjunction* and *anaphase lag.* The former occurs when a homologous pair of chromosomes fails to disjoin at the first meiotic division, or the two chromatids fail to separate either at the second meiotic division or in somatic cell divisions, resulting in two aneuploid cells. When nondisjunction occurs during gametogenesis, the gametes formed have either an extra chromosome (n+1) or one less chromosome (n−1). Fertilization of such gametes by normal gametes results in two types of zygotes—trisomic (2n+1) or monosomic (2n−1). In anaphase lag, one homologous chromosome in meiosis or one chromatid in mitosis lags behind and is left out of the cell nucleus. The result is one normal cell and one cell with monosomy. As seen subsequently, monosomy or trisomy involving the sex chromosomes, or even more bizarre aberrations, are compatible with life and are usually associated with variable degrees of phenotypic abnormalities. *Monosomy involving an autosome generally represents loss of too much genetic information to permit live birth or even embryogenesis, but a number of autosomal trisomies do permit survival.* With the exception of trisomy 21, all yield severely handicapped infants who almost invariably die at an early age.

Occasionally, *mitotic errors in early development give rise to two or more populations of cells in the same individual,* a condition referred to as *mosaicism.* Mosaicism can result from mitotic errors during the cleavage of the fertilized ovum or in somatic cells. Mosaicism affecting the sex chromosomes is relatively common. In the division of the fertilized ovum, an error may lead to one of the daughter cells receiving three sex chromosomes, whereas the other receives only one, yielding, for example, a 45,X/47,XXX mosaic. All descendent cells derived from each of these precursors thus have either a 47,XXX complement or a 45,X complement. Such a patient is a mosaic variant of Turner syndrome, with the extent of phenotypic expression dependent on the number and distribution of the 45,X cells. If the error occurs at a later cleavage, the mosaic has three populations of cells, with some possessing the normal 46,XX complement (i.e., 45,X/46,XX/47,XXX). Repeated mitotic errors may lead to many populations of cells.

Autosomal mosaicism appears to be much less common than that involving the sex chromosomes. An error in an early mitotic division affecting the autosomes usually leads to a nonviable mosaic with autosomal monosomy. Rarely, the loss of a nonviable cell line in embryogenesis is tolerated, yielding a mosaic (e.g., 46,XY/47,XY,+21). Such a patient is a trisomy 21 mosaic with variable expression of Down syndrome, depending on the proportion of cells expressing the trisomy.

A second category of chromosomal aberrations is associated with changes in the structure of chromosomes. To be visible by routine banding techniques, a fairly large amount of DNA (approximately 4 million base pairs), containing many genes, must be involved. The resolution is much higher with FISH. Structural changes in chromosomes usually result from chromosome breakage followed by loss or rearrangement of

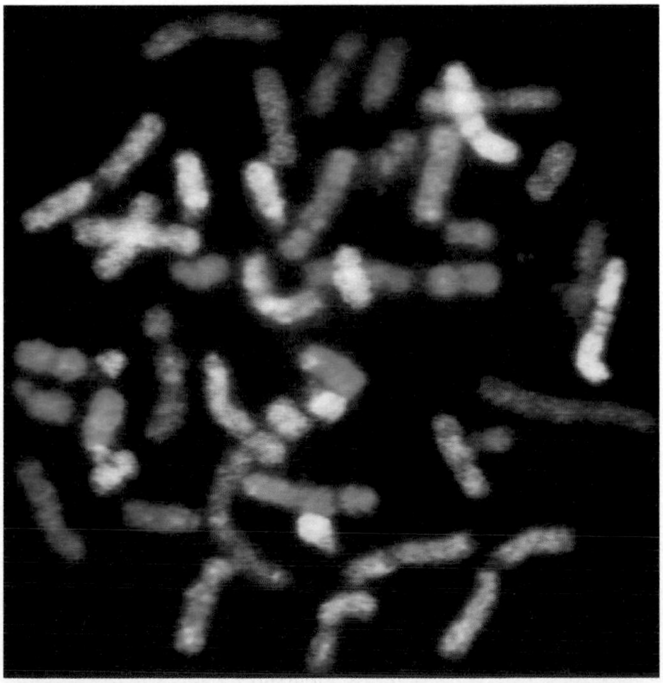

FIGURE 5–25 Spectral karyotype. (Courtesy of Dr. Janet D. Rowley, University of Chicago Pritzker Medical School, Chicago, IL.)

material. Such alterations occur spontaneously at a low rate that is increased by exposure to environmental mutagens, such as chemicals and ionizing radiation. In addition, several rare autosomal recessive genetic disorders—Fanconi anemia, Bloom syndrome, and ataxia-telangiectasia—are associated with such a high level of chromosomal instability that they are known as *chromosome-breakage syndromes.* As discussed later, in Chapter 7, there is a significantly increased risk of cancers in all these syndromes. In the following section, we briefly review the more common forms of alterations in chromosome structure and the notations used to signify them.

Deletion refers to loss of a portion of a chromosome (Fig. 5–26). Most deletions are interstitial, but terminal deletions may occur rarely. Interstitial deletions occur when there are two breaks within a chromosome arm, followed by loss of the chromosomal material between the breaks, and fusion of the broken ends. One can specify in which region(s) and at what bands the breaks have occurred. For example, *46,XY,del(16)(p11.2p13.1)* describes breakpoints in the short arm of chromosome 16 at 16p11.2 and 16p13.1 with loss of material between breaks. Terminal deletions result from a single break in a chromosome arm, producing a fragment with no centromere, which is then lost at the next cell division. The broken chromosome end is protected by acquiring telomeric sequences.

A *ring chromosome* is a special form of deletion. It is produced when a break occurs at both ends of a chromosome with fusion of the damaged ends (see Fig. 5–26). If significant genetic material is lost, phenotypic abnormalities result. This might be expressed as *46,XY,r(14).* Ring chromosomes do not behave normally in meiosis or mitosis and usually result in serious consequences.

Inversion refers to a rearrangement that involves two breaks within a single chromosome with inverted reincorporation of the segment (see Fig. 5–26). Such an inversion involving only one arm of the chromosome is known as *paracentric.* If the breaks are on opposite sides of the centromere, it is known as *pericentric.* Inversions are often perfectly compatible with normal development.

Isochromosome formation results when one arm of a chromosome is lost and the remaining arm is duplicated, resulting in a chromosome consisting of two short arms only or of two long arms (see Fig. 5–26). An isochromosome has morphologically identical genetic information in both arms. The most common isochromosome present in live births involves the long arm of the X and is designated *i(X)(q10).* The Xq isochromosome is associated with monosomy for genes on the short arm of X and with trisomy for genes on the long arm of X.

In a *translocation*, a segment of one chromosome is transferred to another (see Fig. 5–26). In one form, called *balanced reciprocal translocation*, there are single breaks in each of two chromosomes, with exchange of material. Such a translocation might not be disclosed without banding techniques. A balanced reciprocal translocation between the long arm of chromosome 2 and the short arm of chromosome 5 would be written *46,XX,t(2;5)(q31;p14).* This individual has 46 chromosomes with altered morphology of one of the chromosomes 2 and one of the chromosomes 5. Because there has been no loss of genetic material, the individual is likely to be phenotypically normal. A balanced translocation carrier, however, is at increased risk for producing abnormal gametes. For example, in the case cited above, a gamete containing one normal chromosome 2 and a translocated chromosome 5 may

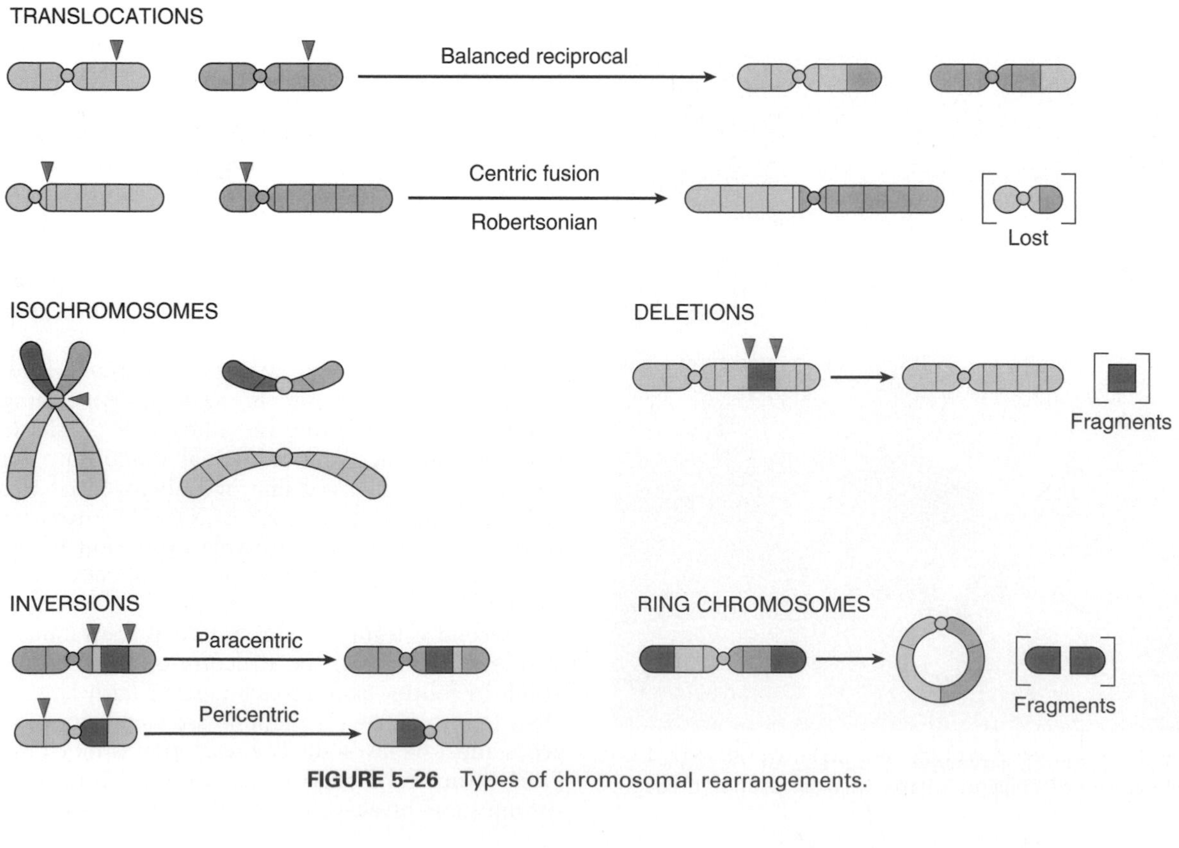

FIGURE 5–26 Types of chromosomal rearrangements.

be formed. Such a gamete would be unbalanced because it would not contain the normal complement of genetic material. Subsequent fertilization by a normal gamete would lead to the formation of an abnormal (unbalanced) zygote, resulting in spontaneous abortion or birth of a malformed child. The other important pattern of translocation is called a *robertsonian translocation* (or centric fusion), a translocation between two acrocentric chromosomes. Typically the breaks occur close to the centromeres of each chromosome. Transfer of the segments then leads to one very large chromosome and one extremely small one. Usually the small product is lost (see Fig. 5–26); however, because it carries only highly redundant genes (e.g., ribosomal RNA genes), this loss is compatible with a normal phenotype. Robertsonian translocation between two chromosomes is encountered in 1 in 1000 apparently normal individuals. The significance of this form of translocation also lies in the production of abnormal progeny, as discussed later with Down syndrome.

Many more numerical and structural aberrations are described in specialized texts, and the number of abnormal karyotypes encountered in genetic diseases increases with each passing month. As pointed out earlier, the clinically detected chromosome disorders represent only the "tip of the iceberg." It is estimated that approximately 7.5% of all conceptions have a chromosomal abnormality, most of which are not compatible with survival or live birth. Thus, chromosome abnormalities are identified in 50% of early spontaneous abortuses and in 5% of stillbirths and infants who die in the immediate postnatal period. Even in live-born infants, the frequency is approximately 0.5% to 1.0%. It is beyond the scope of this book to discuss most of the clinically recognizable chromosomal disorders. Hence, we focus attention on those few that are most common.

CYTOGENETIC DISORDERS INVOLVING AUTOSOMES

Trisomy 21 (Down Syndrome)

Down syndrome is the most common of the chromosomal disorders and is a *major cause of mental retardation*. In the United States, the incidence in newborns is about 1 in 700. Approximately 95% of affected individuals have trisomy 21, so their chromosome count is 47 (Fig. 5–27); most others have normal chromosome numbers, but the extra chromosomal material is present as a translocation. As mentioned

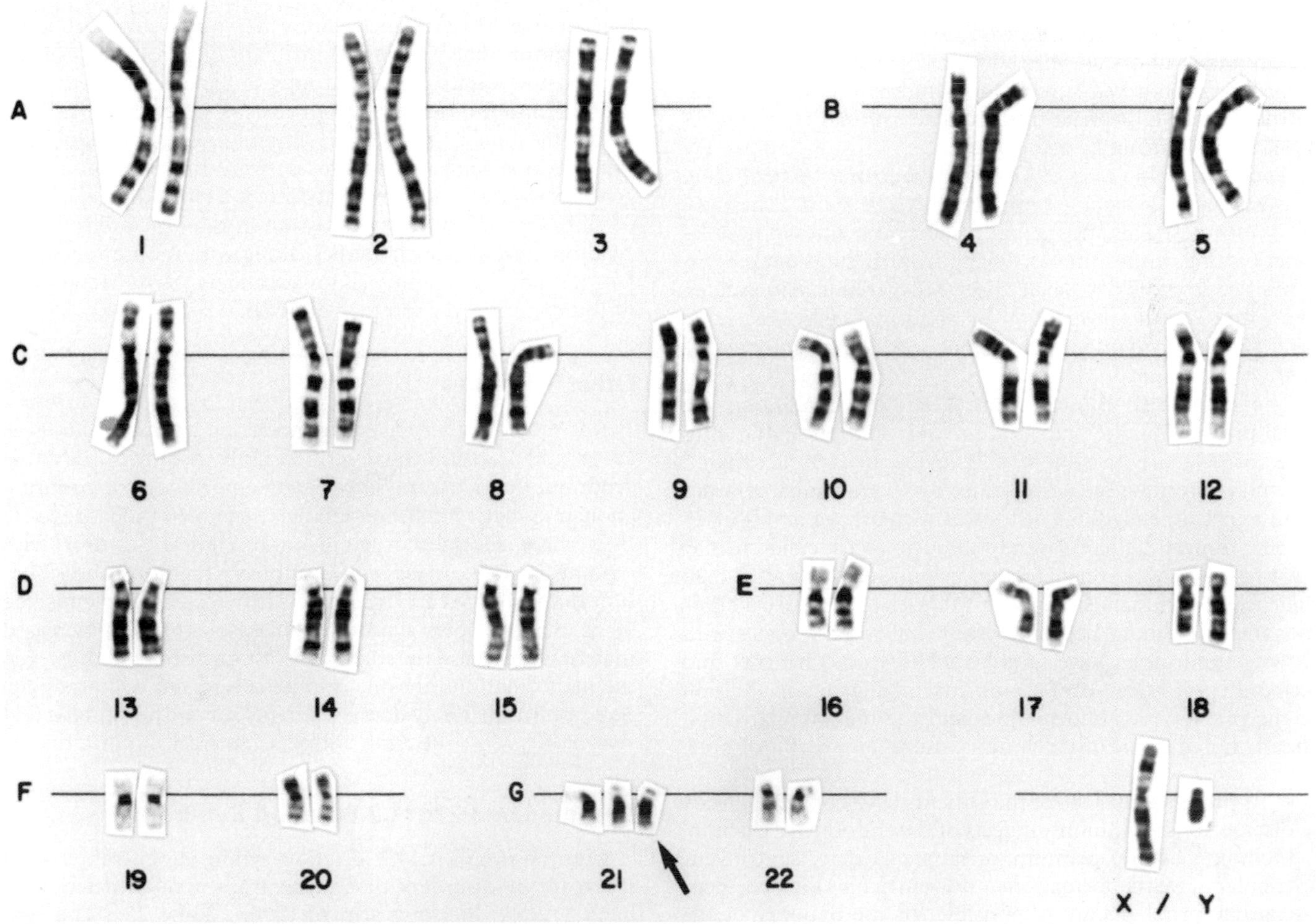

FIGURE 5–27 G banded karyotype of a male with trisomy 21. (Courtesy of Dr. Nancy Schneider, University of Texas Southwestern Medical Center, Dallas, TX.)

earlier, the most common cause of trisomy and therefore of Down syndrome is meiotic nondisjunction. The parents of such children have a normal karyotype and are normal in all respects.

Maternal age has a strong influence on the incidence of trisomy 21. It occurs once in 1550 live births in women under age 20, in contrast to 1 in 25 live births for mothers over age 45.[7] The correlation with maternal age suggests that in most cases the meiotic nondisjunction of chromosome 21 occurs in the ovum. Studies in which DNA polymorphisms were used to trace the parental origin of chromosome 21 have revealed that in 95% of the cases with trisomy 21 the extra chromosome is of maternal origin.[47] Although many hypotheses have been advanced, the reason for the increased susceptibility of the ovum to nondisjunction remains unknown.

In about 4% of all cases of Down syndrome, the extra chromosomal material derives from the presence of a robertsonian translocation of the long arm of chromosome 21 to another acrocentric chromosome (e.g., 22 or 14). Because the fertilized ovum already possesses two normal autosomes 21, the translocated material provides the same triple gene dosage as in trisomy 21. Such cases are frequently (but not always) familial, and the translocated chromosome is inherited from one of the parents (usually the mother), who is a carrier of a robertsonian translocation, for example, a mother with karyotype 45,XX,der(14;21)(q10;q10). Theoretically the carrier parent has a one in three chance of bearing a live child with Down syndrome; however, the observed frequency of affected children in such cases is much lower. The reasons for this discrepancy are not well understood. In those cases in which neither parent is a carrier of the translocation, the rearrangement occurs during gametogenesis.

Approximately 1% of Down syndrome patients are mosaics, usually having a mixture of cells with 46 and 47 chromosomes. This mosaicism results from mitotic nondisjunction of chromosome 21 during an early stage of embryogenesis. Symptoms in such cases are variable and milder, depending on the proportion of abnormal cells. Clearly, *in cases of translocation or mosaic Down syndrome, maternal age is of no importance.*

The diagnostic clinical features of this condition—flat facial profile, oblique palpebral fissures, and epicanthic folds (Fig. 5–28)—are usually readily evident, even at birth.[48] Down syndrome is a leading cause of severe mental retardation; approximately 80% of those afflicted have an IQ of 25 to 50. Ironically, these severely disadvantaged children may have a gentle, shy manner and may be more easily directed than their more fortunate siblings, not burdened with extra chromosomes. It should be pointed out that some mosaics with Down syndrome have mild phenotypic changes and may even have normal or near-normal intelligence. In addition to the phenotypic abnormalities and the mental retardation already noted, some other clinical features are worthy of note.

- Approximately 40% of the patients have congenital heart disease, most commonly defects of the endocardial cushion, including ostium primum, atrial septal defects, atrioventricular valve malformations, and ventricular septal defects. Cardiac problems are responsible for the majority of the deaths in infancy and early childhood. Several other congenital malformations, including atresias of the esophagus and small bowel, are also noted.[49]
- Children with trisomy 21 have a 10-fold to 20-fold increased risk of developing acute leukemia. Both acute lymphoblastic leukemias and acute myeloid leukemias occur. The latter, most commonly, is acute megakaryoblastic leukemia.
- Virtually all patients with trisomy 21 older than age 40 develop neuropathologic changes characteristic of Alzheimer disease, a degenerative disorder of the brain.[50]
- Patients with Down syndrome have abnormal immune responses that predispose them to serious infections, particularly of the lungs, and to thyroid autoimmunity. Although several abnormalities, affecting mainly T-cell subsets, have been reported, the cellular basis of immunologic disturbances is not clear.[51]

Despite all these problems, improved medical care has increased the longevity of patients with trisomy 21. Currently the median age at death is 47 years (up from 25 years in 1983).

Although the karyotype and clinical features of trisomy 21 have been known for decades, little is known about the molecular basis of Down syndrome. However, this situation should change rapidly, because the entire sequence of human chromosome 21 has been completed and approximately 300 genes have been found on this chromosome. Interestingly, there are several gene clusters that are predicted to participate in the same biologic pathway. For example, there are 16 genes that are involved in the mitochondrial energy pathway, several that are likely to influence central nervous system structure, and a group that is involved in folate metabolism. It is not known how each of these groups is related to Down syndrome. Until recently, it was not clear whether the extra copy of chromosome 21 *shuts down* certain genes due to abnormal feedback mechanisms or causes overexpression of critical genes. New studies suggest that there is a global up-regulation of chromosome 21 gene expression in the developing Down syndrome brain.[52] Such studies, along with mouse models of Down syndrome, augur well for advancing the understanding of this common yet complex disorder.

Other Trisomies

A variety of other trisomies, involving chromosomes 8, 9, 13, 18, and 22, have been described. Only trisomy 18 (Edwards syndrome) and trisomy 13 (Patau syndrome) are common enough to merit brief mention here. As noted in Figure 5–28, they share several karyotypic and clinical features with trisomy 21. Thus, most cases result from meiotic nondisjunction and therefore carry a complete extra copy of chromosome 18 or 13. As in Down syndrome, an association with increased maternal age is also noted. In contrast to trisomy 21, however, the malformations are much more severe and wide-ranging. As a result, only rarely do these infants survive beyond the first year of life. Most succumb within a few weeks to months.

Chromosome 22q11.2 Deletion Syndrome

Chromosome 22q11.2 deletion syndrome encompasses a spectrum of disorders that result from a small deletion of band 11.2 on the long arm of chromosome 22.[53] The syndrome is fairly common, occurring in up to 1 in 4000 births, but it is often missed due to variable clinical features. These include congenital heart defects, abnormalities of the palate,

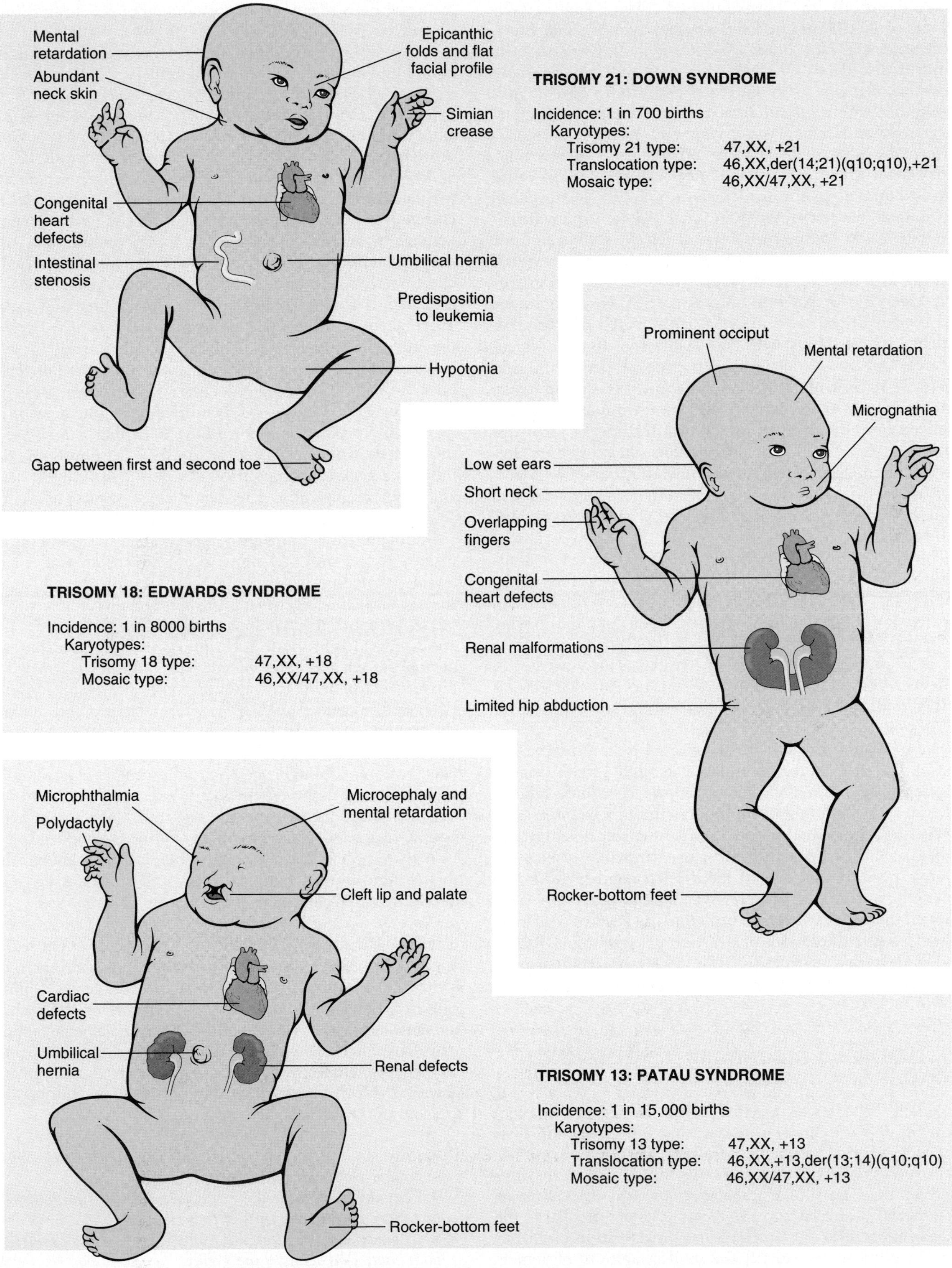
Mental retardation
Abundant neck skin
Epicanthic folds and flat facial profile
Simian crease
Congenital heart defects
Intestinal stenosis
Umbilical hernia
Predisposition to leukemia
Hypotonia
Gap between first and second toe
TRISOMY 21: DOWN SYNDROME
Incidence: 1 in 700 births
Karyotypes:
Trisomy 21 type: 47,XX, +21
Translocation type: 46,XX,der(14;21)(q10;q10),+21
Mosaic type: 46,XX/47,XX, +21
Prominent occiput
Mental retardation
Micrognathia
Low set ears
Short neck
Overlapping fingers
Congenital heart defects
Renal malformations
Limited hip abduction
Rocker-bottom feet
TRISOMY 18: EDWARDS SYNDROME
Incidence: 1 in 8000 births
Karyotypes:
Trisomy 18 type: 47,XX, +18
Mosaic type: 46,XX/47,XX, +18
Microphthalmia
Polydactyly
Microcephaly and mental retardation
Cleft lip and palate
Cardiac defects
Umbilical hernia
Renal defects
Rocker-bottom feet
TRISOMY 13: PATAU SYNDROME
Incidence: 1 in 15,000 births
Karyotypes:
Trisomy 13 type: 47,XX, +13
Translocation type: 46,XX,+13,der(13;14)(q10;q10)
Mosaic type: 46,XX/47,XX, +13

FIGURE 5–28 Clinical features and karyotypes of selected autosomal trisomies.

facial dysmorphism, developmental delay, and variable degrees of T-cell immunodeficiency and hypocalcemia. Previously, these clinical features were considered to represent two different disorders—*DiGeorge syndrome* and *velocardiofacial syndrome.* Patients with DiGeorge syndrome have thymic hypoplasia, with resultant T-cell immunodeficiency (Chapter 6), parathyroid hypoplasia giving rise to hypocalcemia, a variety of cardiac malformations affecting the outflow tract, and mild facial anomalies. The clinical features of the so-called velocardiofacial syndrome include facial dysmorphism (prominent nose, retrognathia), cleft palate, cardiovascular anomalies, and learning disabilities. Recent studies indicate that in addition to the numerous structural malformations, patients with the 22q11.2 deletion syndrome are at a particularly high risk for psychotic illnesses, such as schizophrenia and bipolar disorders.[54] In fact, it is estimated that approximately 25% of adults with this syndrome develop schizophrenia. Conversely, deletions of the region can be found in 2% to 3% of individuals with childhood-onset schizophrenia. Less frequently, these patients also have immunodeficiency. Until recently the overlapping clinical features of these two conditions (e.g., cardiac malformations, facial dysmorphology) were not appreciated; it was only after these two apparently unrelated syndromes were found to be associated with a similar cytogenetic abnormality that the clinical overlap came into focus.

The diagnosis of this condition may be suspected on clinical grounds but can be established only by detection of the deletion by FISH probes (see Fig. 5–23). By using this method, approximately 90% of those previously diagnosed as having DiGeorge syndrome and 60% of those with the velocardiofacial syndrome have a deletion of 22q11.2. Thirty percent of patients with conotruncal cardiac defects but no other features of this syndrome also reveal deletions of the same chromosomal region.

The molecular basis of this syndrome is not known. The size of the deleted region is large enough (approximately 1.5 megabases) to include many genes. The clinical heterogeneity, with predominant immunodeficiency in some cases (DiGeorge syndrome) and predominant dysmorphology and cardiac malformations in other cases, probably reflects the variable position and size of the deleted segment from this genetic region. Approximately 30 candidate genes have been mapped to the deleted region but none has been convincingly related to the causation of Di George syndrome. Recent studies have cast suspicion on *TBX1*, a T-box transcription factor that is involved in early development.[53]

CYTOGENETIC DISORDERS INVOLVING SEX CHROMOSOMES

Genetic diseases associated with karyotypic changes involving the sex chromosomes are far more common than those related to autosomal aberrations. Furthermore, imbalances (excess or loss) of sex chromosomes are much better tolerated than are similar imbalances of autosomes. In large part, this latitude relates to two factors that are peculiar to the sex chromosomes: (1) lyonization or inactivation of all but one X chromosome and (2) the modest amount of genetic material carried by the Y chromosome. We discuss these features briefly to aid our understanding of sex chromosomal disorders.

In 1961, Lyon[55] outlined the X-inactivation, or what is commonly known as the Lyon hypothesis. It states that (1) *only one of the X chromosomes is genetically active,* (2) *the other X of either maternal or paternal origin undergoes heteropyknosis and is rendered inactive,* (3) *inactivation of either the maternal or paternal X occurs at random among all the cells of the blastocyst on or about the 16th day of embryonic life,* and (4) *inactivation of the same X chromosome persists in all the cells derived from each precursor cell.* Thus, the great preponderance of normal females are in reality mosaics and have two populations of cells, one with an inactivated maternal X and the other with an inactivated paternal X. Herein lies the explanation of why females have the same dosage of X-linked active genes as have males. The inactive X can be seen in the interphase nucleus as a darkly staining small mass in contact with the nuclear membrane known as the *Barr body,* or *X chromatin.* The molecular basis of X inactivation is just beginning to be understood. It involves a unique gene called *Xist,* whose product is a noncoding RNA that is retained in the nucleus, where it "coats" the inactive X chromosome and initiates a gene-silencing process by chromatin modification and DNA methylation. The *Xist* allele is turned off in the active X.[56]

Although it was initially thought that all the genes on the inactive X are "shut off," more recent molecular studies have revealed that many genes escape X inactivation. Recent studies suggest that 21% of genes on Xp, and a smaller number (3%) on Xq, escape X inactivation. At least some of the genes that are expressed from both X chromosomes are important for normal growth and development. This notion is supported by the fact that patients with monosomy of the X chromosome (Turner syndrome: 45,X) have severe somatic and gonadal abnormalities. If a single dose of X-linked genes were sufficient, no detrimental effect would be expected in such cases. Furthermore, although one X chromosome is inactivated in all cells during embryogenesis, it is selectively reactivated in oogonia before the first meiotic division. Thus, it seems that both X chromosomes are required for normal oogenesis.

With respect to the Y chromosome, it is well known that this chromosome is both necessary and sufficient for male development. *Regardless of the number of X chromosomes, the presence of a single Y determines the male sex.* The gene that dictates testicular development (*Sry*: sex-determining region Y gene) has been located on its distal short arm. For quite some time, this was considered to be the only gene of significance on the Y chromosome. Recent studies of the Y chromosome, however, have yielded a rich harvest of gene families in the so-called "male-specific Y," or MSY region.[57] All of these are believed to be testes-specific genes involved in spermatogenesis. With this background, we review some features that are common to all sex chromosome disorders.

- *In general, they cause subtle, chronic problems relating to sexual development and fertility.*
- *They are often difficult to diagnose at birth, and many are first recognized at the time of puberty.*
- *In general, the higher the number of X chromosomes, in both male and female, the greater the likelihood of mental retardation.*

The most important disorders arising in aberrations of sex chromosomes are described briefly here.

Klinefelter Syndrome

Klinefelter syndrome is best defined as male hypogonadism that occurs when there are two or more X chromosomes and one or more Y chromosomes. It is one of the most frequent forms of genetic disease involving the sex chromosomes as well as one of the most common causes of hypogonadism in the male. The incidence of this condition is approximately 1 in 500 live male births.[58] It can rarely be diagnosed before puberty, particularly because the testicular abnormality does not develop before early puberty. Most patients have a distinctive body habitus with an increase in length between the soles and the pubic bone, which creates the appearance of an elongated body. Also characteristic are eunuchoid body habitus with abnormally long legs; small atrophic testes often associated with a small penis; and lack of such secondary male characteristics as deep voice, beard, and male distribution of pubic hair. Gynecomastia may be present. The mean IQ is somewhat lower than normal, but mental retardation is uncommon. This typical pattern is not seen in all cases, the only consistent finding being hypogonadism. Plasma gonadotropin levels, particularly follicle-stimulating hormone, are consistently elevated, whereas testosterone levels are variably reduced. Mean plasma estradiol levels are elevated by an as yet unknown mechanism. The ratio of estrogens and testosterone determines the degree of feminization in individual cases.

Klinefelter syndrome is the principal cause of reduced spermatogenesis and male infertility. In some patients, the testicular tubules are totally atrophied and replaced by pink, hyaline, collagenous ghosts. In others, apparently normal tubules are interspersed with atrophic tubules. In some patients, all tubules are primitive and appear embryonic, consisting of cords of cells that never developed a lumen or progressed to mature spermatogenesis. Leydig cells appear prominent, owing to the atrophy and crowding of tubules.

Patients with Klinefelter syndrome have several associated disorders such as breast cancer (20 times more common than in normal males), extragonadal germ cell tumors, and autoimmune diseases such as systemic lupus erythematosus (presumably related to low testosterone and high estrogen levels).

The classic pattern of Klinefelter syndrome is associated with a 47,XXY karyotype (82% of cases). This complement results from nondisjunction during the meiotic divisions in one of the parents. Maternal nondisjunction at the first meiotic division accounts for a little more than half of the cases. Most of the remaining result from nondisjunction during the first paternal meiotic division. There is no phenotypic difference between those who receive the extra X chromosome from their father and those who receive it from their mother. Maternal age is increased in the cases associated with errors in oogenesis. In addition to this classic karyotype, approximately 15% of patients with Klinefelter syndrome have been found to have a variety of mosaic patterns, most of them being 46,XY/47,XXY. Other patterns are 47,XXY/48,XXXY and variations on this theme. Rare individuals have also been found to possess 48,XXXY or 49,XXXXY karyotypes. Such polysomic X individuals have further physical abnormalities, including cryptorchidism, hypospadias, more severe hypoplasia of the testes, and skeletal changes, such as prognathism and radioulnar synostosis.

Turner Syndrome

Turner syndrome results from complete or partial monosomy of the X chromosome and is characterized primarily by hypogonadism in phenotypic females.[59] It is the most common sex chromosome abnormality in females, affecting about 1 in 2000 liveborn females.

With routine cytogenetic methods, three types of karyotypic abnormalities are seen in patients with Turner syndrome. Approximately 57% are missing an entire X chromosome, resulting in a 45,X karyotype. Of the remaining, approximately one third (approximately 14%) have structural abnormalities of the X chromosomes, and two thirds (approximately 29%) are mosaics. The net effect of structural abnormalities is to produce partial monosomy of the X chromosome. In order of frequency, the structural abnormalities of the X chromosome include (1) deletion of the small arm, resulting in the formation of an isochromosome of the long arm, 46,X,i(X)(q10); (2) deletion of portions of both long and short arms, resulting in the formation of a ring chromosome, 46,X,r(X); and (3) deletion of portions of the short or long arm, 46X,del(Xq) or 46X,del(Xp). The mosaic patients have a 45,X cell population along with one or more karyotypically normal or abnormal cell types. Examples of karyotypes that mosaic Turner females may have are the following: (1) 45,X/46,XX; (2) 45,X/46,XY; (3) 45,X/47,XXX; or (4) 45,X/46,X,i(X)(q10). Studies suggest that the prevalence of mosaicism in Turner syndrome may be much higher than the 30% detected by conventional cytogenetic studies. With the use of more sensitive techniques, including FISH and polymerase chain reaction (PCR), and analysis of more than one cell type (e.g., peripheral blood and fibroblasts), the prevalence of mosaic Turner syndrome increases to 75%.[60] Because 99% of 45,X conceptuses are nonviable, many authorities believe that there are no truly nonmosaic Turner syndrome patients. While this issue remains controversial, it is important to appreciate the karyotypic heterogeneity associated with Turner syndrome because it is responsible for significant variations in phenotype. In patients who are truly 45,X, or in whom the proportion of 45,X cells is high, the phenotypic changes are more severe than in those who have readily detectable mosaicism. The latter may have an almost normal appearance and may present only with primary amenorrhea. Similarly, those with a Y chromosome-containing population (e.g., 45,X/46,XY karyotype) may be at risk of developing a gonadal tumor (gonadoblastoma).

The most severely affected patients generally present during infancy with edema (owing to lymph stasis) of the dorsum of the hand and foot and sometimes *swelling of the nape of the neck.* The latter is related to markedly distended lymphatic channels, producing a so-called cystic hygroma (Chapter 10). As these infants develop, the swellings subside but often leave bilateral *neck webbing* and persistent looseness of skin on the back of the neck. *Congenital heart disease* is also common, particularly preductal coarctation of the aorta and bicuspid aortic valve. Cardiovascular abnormalities are the single most important cause of increased mortality in children with Turner syndrome.

The principal clinical features in the adolescent and adult are illustrated in Figure 5–29. At puberty, there is *failure to develop normal secondary sex characteristics.* The genitalia remain infantile, breast development is inadequate, and there is little pubic hair. The mental status of these patients is usually normal, but subtle defects in nonverbal, visual-spatial information processing have been noted. Of particular importance in establishing the diagnosis in the adult is the shortness of stature (rarely exceeding 150 cm in height) and the amenorrhea. *Turner syndrome is the single most important cause of primary amenorrhea*, accounting for approximately one third of the cases. For reasons not quite clear, approximately 50% of patients develop autoantibodies directed to the thyroid gland, and up to one half of these develop clinically manifest hypothyroidism. Equally mysterious is the presence of glucose intolerance, obesity, and insulin resistance in a minority of patients. The last mentioned is significant because therapy with growth hormone, commonly used in these patients, worsens insulin resistance.

The molecular pathogenesis of Turner syndrome is not completely understood, but studies have begun to shed some light.[61] As mentioned earlier, both X chromosomes are active during oogenesis and are essential for normal development of the ovaries. During normal fetal development, ovaries contain as many as 7 million oocytes. The oocytes gradually disappear so that by menarche their numbers have dwindled to a mere 400,000, and when menopause occurs fewer than 10,000 remain. In Turner syndrome, fetal ovaries develop normally early in embryogenesis, but the absence of the second X chromosome leads to an accelerated loss of oocytes, which is complete by age 2 years. In a sense, therefore, "menopause occurs before menarche," and the ovaries are reduced to atrophic fibrous strands, devoid of ova and follicles *(streak ovaries).* Because patients with Turner syndrome also have other (nongonadal) abnormalities, it follows that some genes for normal growth and development of somatic tissues must also reside on the X chromosome. Among the genes involved in the Turner phenotype is the short stature homeobox *(SHOX)* gene at Xp22.33. This is one of several genes that remain active in both X chromosomes, and it has a homologue on the short arm of the Y chromosome. Haploinsufficiency of this gene gives rise to short stature. Indeed, deletions of the *SHOX* gene are noted in 2% to 5% of otherwise normal children with short stature.[62] Several other candidate genes whose loss is likely to contribute to Turner syndrome are illustrated in Figure 5–30. The functions of many of these remain unknown. If some X-linked genes are required in diploid dosage for normal somatic development, then how do males develop normally with only one copy of the X chromosome? This apparent paradox has been resolved by the discovery of genes on the Y chromosome that are homologues of those X-linked genes that escape X-inactivation.

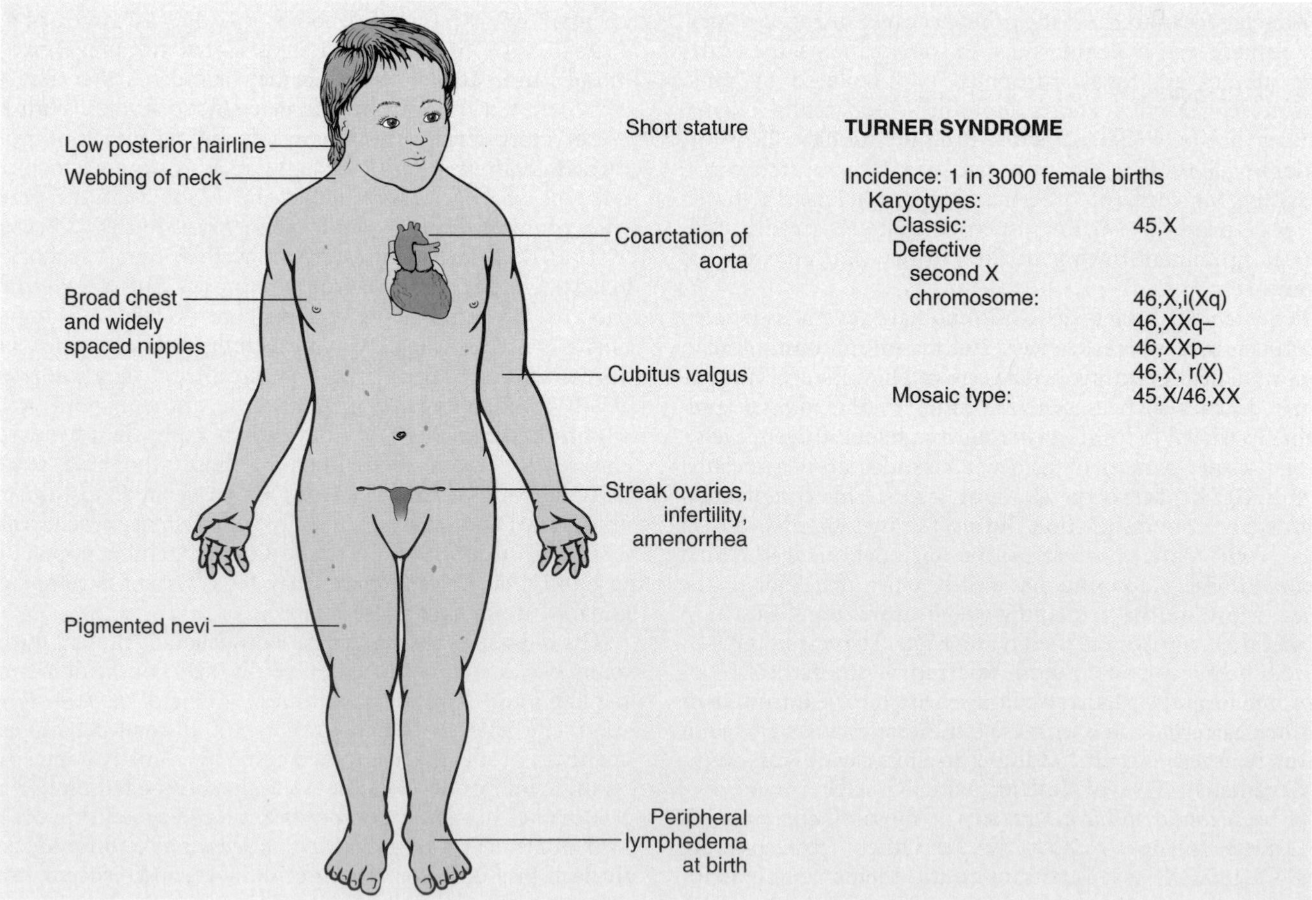

FIGURE 5–29 Clinical features and karyotypes of Turner syndrome.

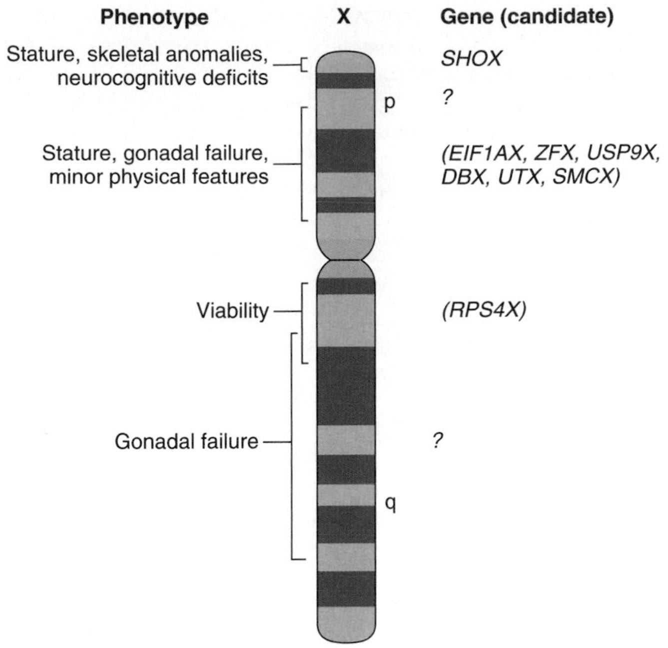

FIGURE 5–30 Turner syndrome critical regions and (candidate) genes. *SHOX*, short homeobox gene; *EIF1AX*, eukaryotic initiation factor 1A; *ZFX*, zinc finger X (transcription factor); *USP9X*, homologue of *Drosophila* gene involved in öogenesis; *DBX*, dead box polypeptide 3,X, a spermatogenesis gene; *UTX*, ubiquitously transcribed tetratricopeptide repeat gene, X chromosome; *SMCX*, homologue of the Y-encoded male antigen HY; *RPS4X* isoform of ribosomal protein S4 involved in lymphatic development. (Courtesy of Dr. Andrew Zinn, University of Texas Southwestern Medical School, Dallas, TX.)

Hermaphroditism and Pseudohermaphroditism

The problem of sexual ambiguity is exceedingly complex, and only limited observations are possible here; for more details, reference should be made to specialized texts.[63] It will be no surprise to medical students that the sex of an individual can be defined on several levels. *Genetic sex* is determined by the presence or absence of a Y chromosome. No matter how many X chromosomes are present, a single Y chromosome dictates testicular development and the genetic male gender. The initially indifferent gonads of both the male and the female embryos have an inherent tendency to feminize, unless influenced by Y chromosome-dependent masculinizing factors. *Gonadal sex* is based on the histologic characteristics of the gonads. *Ductal sex* depends on the presence of derivatives of the müllerian or wolffian ducts. *Phenotypic*, or *genital, sex* is based on the appearance of the external genitalia. Sexual ambiguity is present whenever there is disagreement among these various criteria for determining sex.

The term true hermaphrodite implies the presence of both ovarian and testicular tissue. In contrast, a pseudohermaphrodite represents a disagreement between the phenotypic and gonadal sex (i.e., a female pseudohermaphrodite has ovaries but male external genitalia; a male pseudohermaphrodite has testicular tissue but female-type genitalia).

True hermaphroditism, implying the presence of both ovarian and testicular tissue, is an extremely rare condition. In some cases, there is a testis on one side and an ovary on the other, whereas in other cases, there may be combined ovarian and testicular tissue, referred to as *ovotestes*. The karyotype is 46,XX in 50% of patients; of the remaining, most are mosaics with a 46,XX/46,XY karyotype. Only rarely is the chromosomal constitution 46,XY. The presence of testes implies that those with the 46,XX karyotype might possess Y chromosomal material, in particular, the *SRY* gene, which dictates testicular differentiation. Indeed, molecular analysis has revealed *SRY* gene expression in the ovotestis of 46,XX true hermaphrodites, indicating either cryptic chimerism localized to the gonads or possibly a Y-to-autosome translocation.[64]

Female pseudohermaphroditism is much less complex.[65] The genetic sex in all cases is XX, and the development of the gonads (ovaries) and internal genitalia is normal. Only the external genitalia are ambiguous or virilized. The basis of female pseudohermaphroditism is excessive and inappropriate exposure to androgenic steroids during the early part of gestation. Such steroids are most commonly derived from the fetal adrenal affected by congenital adrenal hyperplasia, which is transmitted as an autosomal recessive trait. Biosynthetic defects in the pathway of cortisol synthesis are present in these cases, which lead secondarily to excessive synthesis of androgenic steroids by the fetal adrenal cortex (Chapter 24).

Male pseudohermaphroditism represents the most complex of all disorders of sexual differentiation. These individuals possess a Y chromosome, and thus their gonads are exclusively testes, but the genital ducts or the external genitalia are incompletely differentiated along the male phenotype. Their external genitalia are either ambiguous or completely female. Male pseudohermaphroditism is extremely heterogeneous, with a multiplicity of causes. Common to all is defective virilization of the male embryo, which usually results from genetically determined defects in androgen synthesis or action or both. The most common form, called *complete androgen insensitivity syndrome (testicular feminization)*, results from mutations in the gene for the androgen receptor.[66] This gene is located at Xq11-Xq12, and hence this disorder is inherited as an X-linked recessive.

Single-Gene Disorders with Nonclassic Inheritance

It has become increasingly evident that transmission of certain single-gene disorders does not follow classic mendelian principles. This group of disorders can be classified into four categories:

- Diseases caused by triplet-repeat mutations
- Disorders caused by mutations in mitochondrial genes
- Disorders associated with genomic imprinting
- Disorders associated with gonadal mosaicism

Clinical and molecular features of some single-gene diseases that exemplify nonclassic patterns of inheritance are described next.

TRIPLET-REPEAT MUTATIONS—FRAGILE-X SYNDROME

Fragile-X syndrome is the prototype of diseases in which the mutation is characterized by a long repeating sequence of three nucleotides.[67] Although the specific nucleotide sequence that undergoes amplification differs in the twenty or so disorders included in this group, in most cases the affected sequences share the nucleotides guanine (G) and cytosine (C). In the ensuing discussion, we consider the clinical features and inheritance pattern of the fragile-X syndrome, to be followed by the causative molecular lesion. The remaining disorders in this group are discussed later, in this chapter and elsewhere in the book.

With a frequency of 1 in 1550 for affected males and 1 in 8000 for affected females, *fragile-X syndrome is the second most common genetic cause of mental retardation, after Down syndrome.* It is an X-linked disorder characterized by an inducible cytogenetic abnormality in the X chromosome and an unusual mutation within the familial mental retardation-1 (*FMR-1*) gene. The cytogenetic alteration is seen as a discontinuity of staining or as a constriction in the long arm of the X chromosome when cells are cultured in a folate-deficient medium. Because it appears that the chromosome is "broken" at this locale, it is referred to as a *fragile site* (Fig. 5–31). It should be noted that several other, in fact about 80, "fragile sites" have been found in the human genome.[68] Many, like the one seen in fragile-X syndrome, are folate sensitive, whereas others require different culture conditions. The significance of most fragile sites is unknown.

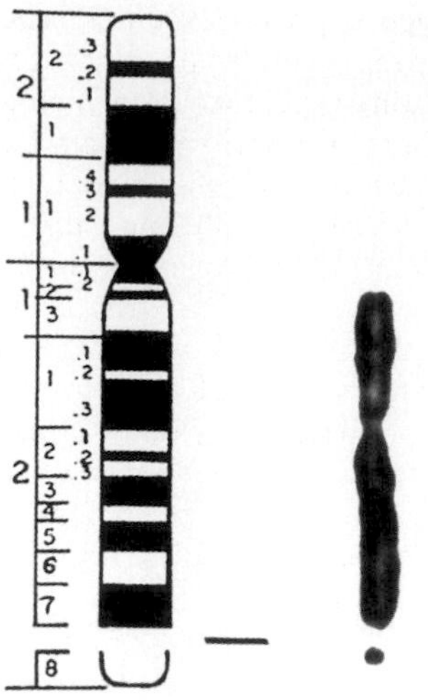

FIGURE 5–31 Fragile-X, seen as discontinuity of staining. (Courtesy of Dr. Patricia Howard-Peebles, University of Texas Southwestern Medical Center, Dallas, TX.)

In fragile-X syndrome, the affected males are *mentally retarded*, with an IQ in the range of 20 to 60. They express a characteristic physical phenotype that includes a *long face with a large mandible, large everted ears*, and *large testicles (macro-orchidism).* Hyperextensible joints, a high arched palate, and mitral valve prolapse noted in some patients mimic a connective tissue disorder. These and other physical abnormalities described in this condition, however, are not always present and, in some cases, are quite subtle. *The only distinctive feature that can be detected in at least 90% of postpubertal males with fragile-X syndrome is macro-orchidism.*[69]

As with all X-linked diseases, fragile-X syndrome affects males. Analysis of several pedigrees, however, reveals some patterns of transmission not typically associated with other X-linked recessive disorders (Fig. 5–32). These include the following:

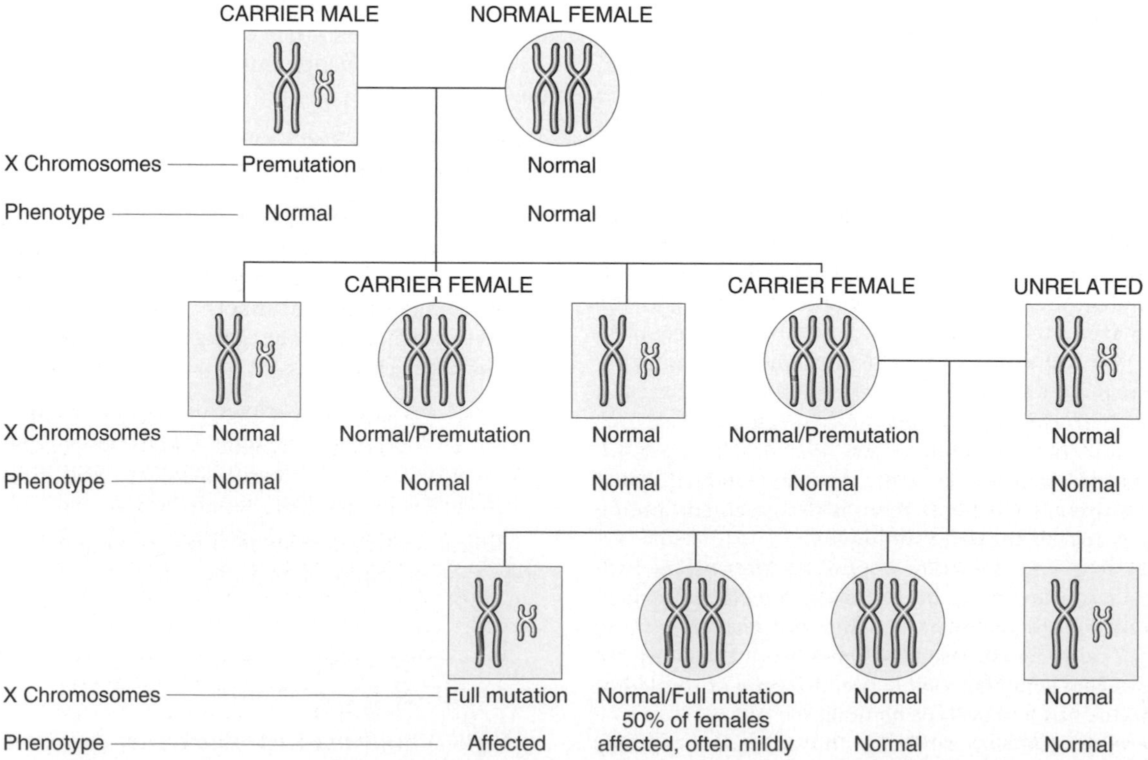

FIGURE 5–32 Fragile-X pedigree. Note that in the first generation all sons are normal and all females are carriers. During oogenesis in the carrier female, premutation expands to full mutation; hence in the next generation, all males who inherit the X with full mutation are affected. However, only 50% of females who inherit the full mutation are affected, and only mildly. (Courtesy of Dr. Nancy Schneider, Department of Pathology, University of Texas Southwestern Medical Center, Dallas, TX.)

- *Carrier males:* Approximately 20% of males who by pedigree analysis and by molecular tests are known to carry a fragile X mutation are clinically and cytogenetically normal. Because carrier males transmit the trait through all their daughters (phenotypically normal) to affected grandchildren, they are called *transmitting males.*
- *Affected females:* Approximately 50% of carrier females are affected (i.e., mentally retarded), a number much higher than that in other X-linked recessive disorders.
- *Risk of phenotypic effects:* Risk depends on the position of the individual in the pedigree. For example, brothers of transmitting males are at a 9% risk of having mental retardation, whereas grandsons of transmitting males incur a 40% risk. This positional risk is sometimes referred to as the Sherman paradox.
- *Anticipation:* This refers to the observation that clinical features of fragile-X syndrome worsen with each successive generation, as if the mutation becomes increasingly deleterious as it is transmitted from a man to his grandsons and great-grandsons.

These unusual patterns perplexed geneticists for years, but molecular studies have finally begun to unravel the complexities of this condition.[70,71] The first breakthrough came when linkage studies localized the mutation responsible for this disease to Xq27.3, within the cytogenetically abnormal region. Within this region lies the *FMR-1* gene, characterized by multiple tandem repeats of the nucleotide sequence CGG in its 5′ untranslated region. In the normal population, the number of CGG repeats is small, ranging from 10 to 55 (average, 29). The presence of clinical symptoms and a cytogenetically detectable fragile site seem related to the extent of amplification of the CGG repeats. Thus, normal transmitting males and carrier females carry 55 to 200 CGG repeats. Expansions of this size are called *premutations.* In contrast, affected individuals have an extremely large expansion of the repeat region (200 to 4000 repeats, or *full mutations*). Full mutations are believed to arise by further amplification of the CGG repeats seen in premutations. How this process takes place is quite peculiar. Carrier males transmit the repeats to their progeny with small changes in repeat number. When the premutation is passed on by a carrier female, however, there is a high probability of a dramatic amplification of the CGG repeats, leading to mental retardation in most male offspring and 50% of female offspring. Thus, *it appears that during the process of oogenesis, but not spermatogenesis, premutations can be converted to mutations by triplet-repeat amplification.* This explains the Sherman paradox; that is, the likelihood of mental retardation is much higher in grandsons than in brothers of transmitting males because grandsons incur the risk of inheriting a premutation from their grandfather that is amplified to a "full mutation" in their mothers' ova. By comparison, brothers of transmitting males, being "higher up" in the pedigree, are less likely to have a full mutation. These molecular details also provide a satisfactory explanation of anticipation—a phenomenon observed by clinical geneticists but not believed by molecular geneticists until triplet-repeat mutations were identified. Why only 50% of the females with full mutation are clinically affected is not clear. Presumably in those clinically affected, there is unfavorable lyonization (i.e., there is a higher frequency of cells in which the X chromosome carrying the mutation is active).

The molecular basis of mental retardation and other somatic manifestations is not entirely clear, but it is related to a loss of function of the familial mental retardation protein (FMRP). As mentioned earlier, the normal *FMR-1* gene contains up to 46 CGG repeats in its 5′ untranslated region. When the trinuleotide repeats in the *FMR-1* gene exceed approximately 230, the DNA of the entire 5′ region of the gene becomes abnormally methylated. Methylation also extends upstream into the promoter region of the gene, resulting in transcriptional suppression of *FMR-1.* The resulting absence of FMRP is believed to cause the phenotypic changes.

FMRP is a widely expressed cytoplasmic protein, most abundant in the brain and testis, the two organs most affected in this disease. The function of FMRP in the brain is beginning to be understood.[72] According to current thinking, within neurons, FMRP is transported from the cytoplasm to the nucleus, where it assembles into an mRNP complex, thereby binding specific RNA transcripts and proteins (Fig. 5–33). From here, the complexes are shuttled into the axon as well as the dendrites, close to synapses. It is at the synapses that the FMRP–mRNP complex seems to perform a key role in regulating the translation of specific mRNAs. Whether FMRP promotes or represses translation is not entirely clear and perhaps both occur with specific species of RNA. It is the absence of such FMRP-mediated regulation that interferes with synaptic transmission and ultimately causes mental retardation.

Although demonstration of an abnormal karyotype led to the identification of this disorder, PCR-based diagnosis is now the method of choice for diagnosis. With Southern blot analysis, distinction between premutations and mutations can be made prenatally as well as postnatally. Hence, this technique is valuable not only for establishing the diagnosis, but also for guiding genetic counseling. These techniques are described later.

Other Diseases with Unstable Nucleotide Repeats

The discovery in 1991 of expanding trinucleotide repeats as a cause of fragile-X syndrome was a landmark in human genetics. Since then, the origins of about 20 human diseases (Table 5–9) have been traced to a similar type of mutation,[73] and the number continues to grow. Some general principles that apply to these diseases are as follows:

- The causative mutations are associated with the expansion of a stretch of trinucleotides that usually share the nucleotides G and C. In all cases, the DNA is unstable, and mutations impair gene function by an expansion of the repeats. Above a certain threshold, the expansions impair gene function in various ways, discussed below.
- The proclivity to expand depends strongly on the sex of the transmitting parent. In the fragile-X syndrome, expansions occur during oogenesis, whereas in Huntington disease they occur during spermatogenesis.
- From a mechanistic standpoint, the mutations can be divided into two groups. In the first group of disorders, exemplified by fragile-X syndrome and myotonic dystrophy, the repeat expansions occur in noncoding regions, whereas in other disorders, such as Huntington disease, expansions occur in the exons (Fig. 5–34).

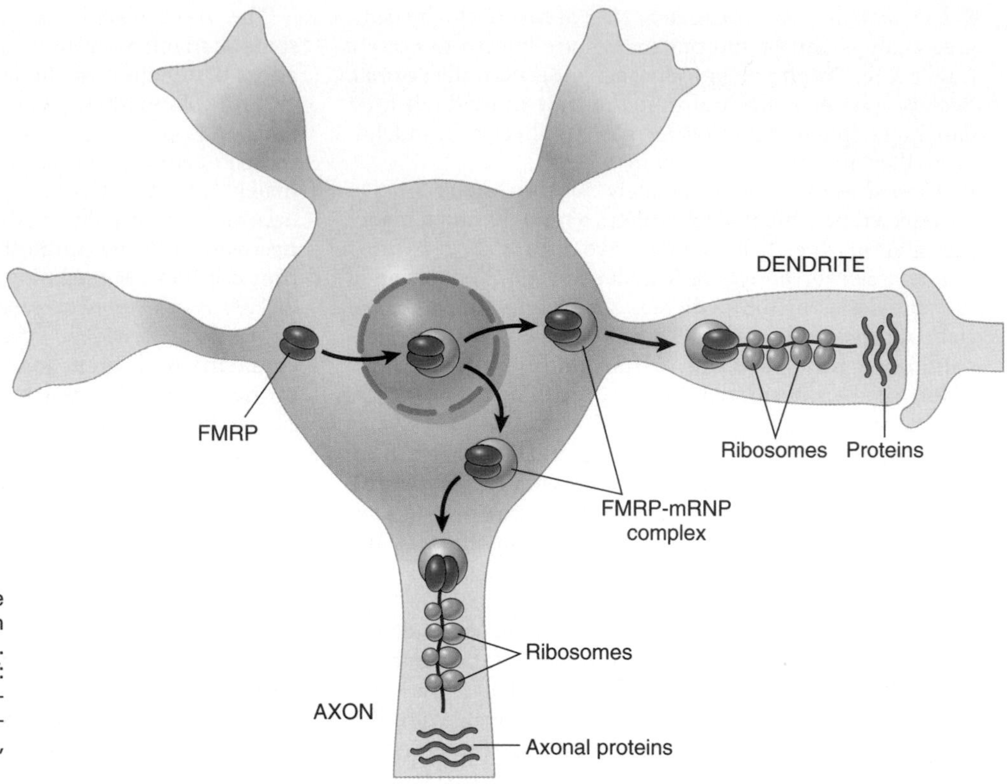

FIGURE 5–33 A model for the action of familial mental retardation protein (FMRP) in neurons. (Adapted from Hin P, Warren ST: New insights into fragile-X syndrome: from molecules to neurobehavior. Trends Biochem Sci 28:152, 2003.)

- The pathogenetic mechanisms underlying disorders caused by mutations that affect coding regions seem to be distinct from those in which the expansions affect noncoding regions. The former usually involve CAG repeats coding for polyglutamine tracts in the corresponding proteins. Such "polyglutamine diseases" are characterized by progressive neurodegeneration, typically striking in mid-life. Polyglutamine expansions lead to toxic gain of function, whereby the abnormal protein interferes with the function of the normal protein.[74] The abnormal proteins aggregate in the nucleus to produce inclusions. By contrast, when expansions affect noncoding regions, the resulting mutations are loss of function type, since protein synthesis (e.g., FMRP) is suppressed. Typically, such disorders affect many systems. Finally, many noncoding repeat disorders are characterized by a pool of intermediate-size expansions, or premutations, that expand to full mutations in germ cells.

TABLE 5–9 Summary of Trinucleotide Repeat Disorders

Disease	Gene	Locus	Protein	Repeat	Normal	Disease
Expansions Affecting Noncoding Regions						
Fragile-X syndrome	*FMRI(FRAXA)*	Xq27.3	FMR-1 protein (FMRP)	CGG	6–53	60–200 (pre) >230 (full)
Friedreich ataxia	*X25*	9q13–21.1	Frataxin	GAA	7–34	34–80 (pre) >100 (full)
Myotonic dystrophy	*DMPK*	19q13	Myotonic dystrophy protein kinase (DMPK)	CTG	5–37	50–thousands
Expansions Affecting Coding Regions						
Spinobulbar muscular atrophy (Kennedy disease)	*AR*	Xq13–21	Androgen receptor (AR)	CAG	9–36	38–62
Huntington disease	*HD*	4p16.3	Huntingtin	CAG	6–35	36–121
Dentatorubral-pallidoluysian atrophy (Haw River syndrome)	*DRPLA*	12p13.31	Atrophin-1	CAG	6–35	49–88
Spinocerebellar ataxia type 1	*SCA1*	6p23	Ataxin-1	CAG	6–44	39–82
Spinocerebellar ataxia type 2	*SCA2*	12q24.1	Ataxin-2	CAG	15–31	36–63
Spinocerebellar ataxia type 3 (Machado-Joseph disease)	*SCA3 (MJD1)*	14q32.1	Ataxin-3	CAG	12–40	55–84
Spinocerebellar ataxia type 6	*SCA6*	19p13	α_{1A}-Voltage-dependent calcium channel subunit	CAG	4–18	21–33
Spinocerebellar ataxia type 7	*SCA7*	3p12–13	Ataxin-7	CAG	4–35	37–306

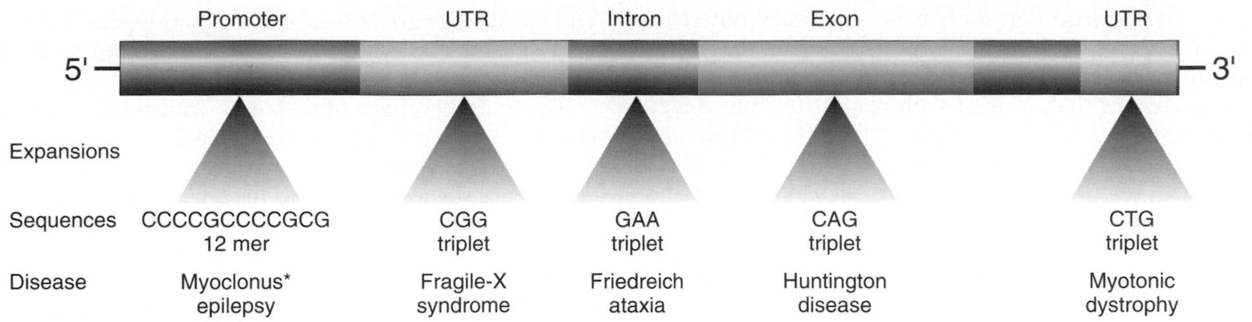

FIGURE 5–34 Sites of expansion and the affected sequence in selected diseases caused by nucleotide repeat mutations. UTR, untranslated region. *Although not strictly a trinucleotide repeat disease, progressive myoclonus epilepsy is caused, like others in this group, by a heritable DNA expansion. The expanded segment is in the promoter region of the gene.

MUTATIONS IN MITOCHONDRIAL GENES—LEBER HEREDITARY OPTIC NEUROPATHY

The vast majority of genes are located on chromosomes in the cell nucleus. Mendelian inheritance applies to such genes. There exist several mitochondrial genes, however, that are inherited in quite a different manner.[75] *A feature unique to mitochondrial DNA (mtDNA) is maternal inheritance.* This peculiarity results from the fact that ova contain mitochondria within their abundant cytoplasm, whereas spermatozoa contain few, if any, mitochondria. Hence, the mtDNA complement of the zygote is derived entirely from the ovum. Thus, mothers transmit mtDNA to all their offspring, male and female; however, daughters but not sons transmit the DNA further to their progeny (Fig. 5–35). Several other features apply to mitochondrial inheritance.[76,77] They are as follows:

- Human mtDNA contains 37 genes, of which 24 are needed for mtDNA translation and 13 encode subunits of the respiratory chain enzymes. Because mtDNA encodes enzymes involved in oxidative phosphorylation, mutations affecting these genes exert their deleterious effects primarily on the organs most dependent on oxidative phosphorylation. These include the central nervous system, skeletal muscle, cardiac muscle, liver, and kidneys.
- Each mitochondrion contains thousands of mtDNA molecules, and, typically, deleterious mutations of the mtDNA affect some but not all of these genes. Thus, tissues and, indeed, whole individuals may harbor both wild-type and mutant mtDNA, a situation called *heteroplasmy.* It should be evident that a minimum number of mutant mtDNA must be present in a cell or tissue before oxidative dysfunction gives rise to disease. This is called the "threshold effect." Not surprisingly, the threshold is reached most easily in the metabolically active tissues listed earlier.[78]
- During cell division, mitochondria and their contained DNA are randomly distributed to the daughter cells. Thus, when a cell containing normal and mutant mtDNA divides, the proportion of the normal and mutant mtDNA in daughter cells is extremely variable. Therefore, the expression of disorders resulting from mutations in mtDNA is quite variable.

Diseases associated with mitochondrial inheritance are rare and, as mentioned earlier, many of them affect the neuromuscular system. Leber hereditary optic neuropathy is a prototype of this disorder. It is described briefly. This is a neurodegenerative disease that manifests itself as progressive bilateral loss of central vision. Visual impairment is first noted between ages 15 and 35, and it leads, in due course, to blindness. Cardiac conduction defects and minor neurologic manifestations have also been observed in some families.[79]

GENOMIC IMPRINTING

As is well known, we all inherit two copies of each gene, carried on homologous maternal and paternal chromosomes.

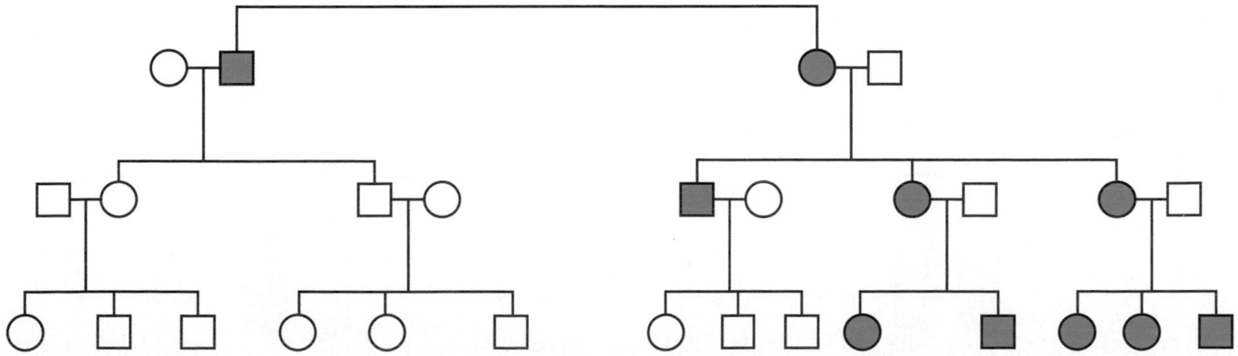

FIGURE 5–35 Pedigree of Leber hereditary optic neuropathy, a disorder caused by mutation in mitochondrial DNA. Note that all progeny of an affected male are normal, but all children, male and female, of the affected female manifest disease.

It is generally assumed that there is no functional difference between the genes derived from the mother or the father. Recent studies have challenged this notion, and there is accumulating evidence that, at least with respect to some genes, there are functional differences between the paternal gene and the maternal gene. These differences result from an epigenetic process, called *imprinting.* In most cases, *imprinting selectively inactivates either the maternal or paternal allele.* Thus, *maternal imprinting* refers to transcriptional silencing of the maternal allele, whereas *paternal imprinting* implies that the paternal allele is inactivated. Imprinting occurs in the ovum or the sperm, before fertilization, and then is stably transmitted to all somatic cells through mitosis.[80] As is often the case in medicine, genomic imprinting is best illustrated by considering two uncommon genetic disorders: Prader-Willi syndrome and Angelman syndrome.

Prader-Willi Syndrome and Angelman Syndrome

Prader-Willi syndrome is characterized by mental retardation, short stature, hypotonia, obesity, small hands and feet, and hypogonadism. In 65% to 70% of cases, an interstitial deletion of band q12 in the long arm of chromosome 15, del(15)(q11.2q13), can be detected.[81] *It is striking that in all cases the deletion affects the paternally derived chromosome 15.* In contrast with the Prader-Willi syndrome, patients with the phenotypically distinct Angelman syndrome are *born with a deletion of the same chromosomal region derived from their mothers.* Patients with Angelman syndrome are also mentally retarded, but in addition they present with ataxic gait, seizures, and inappropriate laughter. Because of their laughter and ataxia, they are also called "happy puppets."[82] A comparison of these two syndromes clearly demonstrates the *parent of origin* effects on gene function.

The molecular basis of these two syndromes can be understood in the context of imprinting (Fig. 5–36). It is believed that a gene or set of genes on maternal chromosome 15 is imprinted (and hence silenced), and thus the only functional allele(s) are provided by the paternal chromosome. When these are lost as a result of a deletion, the patient develops Prader-Willi syndrome. Conversely, a distinct gene that also maps to the same region of chromosome 15 is imprinted on the paternal chromosome. Only the maternally derived allele of this gene is normally active. Deletion of this maternal gene on chromosome 15 gives rise to the Angelman syndrome. Molecular studies of cytogenetically normal patients with the Prader-Willi syndrome (i.e. those without the deletion) have revealed that in most of these cases both of the structurally normal chromosome 15 are derived from the mother. Inheritance of both chromosomes of a pair from one parent is called *uniparental disomy.* The net effect is the same (i.e., the patient does not have a functional set of genes from the [nonimprinted] paternal chromosomes 15). Angelman syndrome, as might be expected, can also result from uniparental disomy of paternal chromosome 15.

The biochemical basis of imprinting is still not clear. Methylation of DNA is known to affect gene expression, and in many cases, imprinting is associated with differential patterns of DNA methylation. Other mechanisms include histone H4 deacetylation and methylation. Regardless of the mechanism, it is believed that the marking of paternal and maternal chromosomes occurs during gametogenesis, and thus it seems that from the moment of conception some chromosomes remember where they came from.

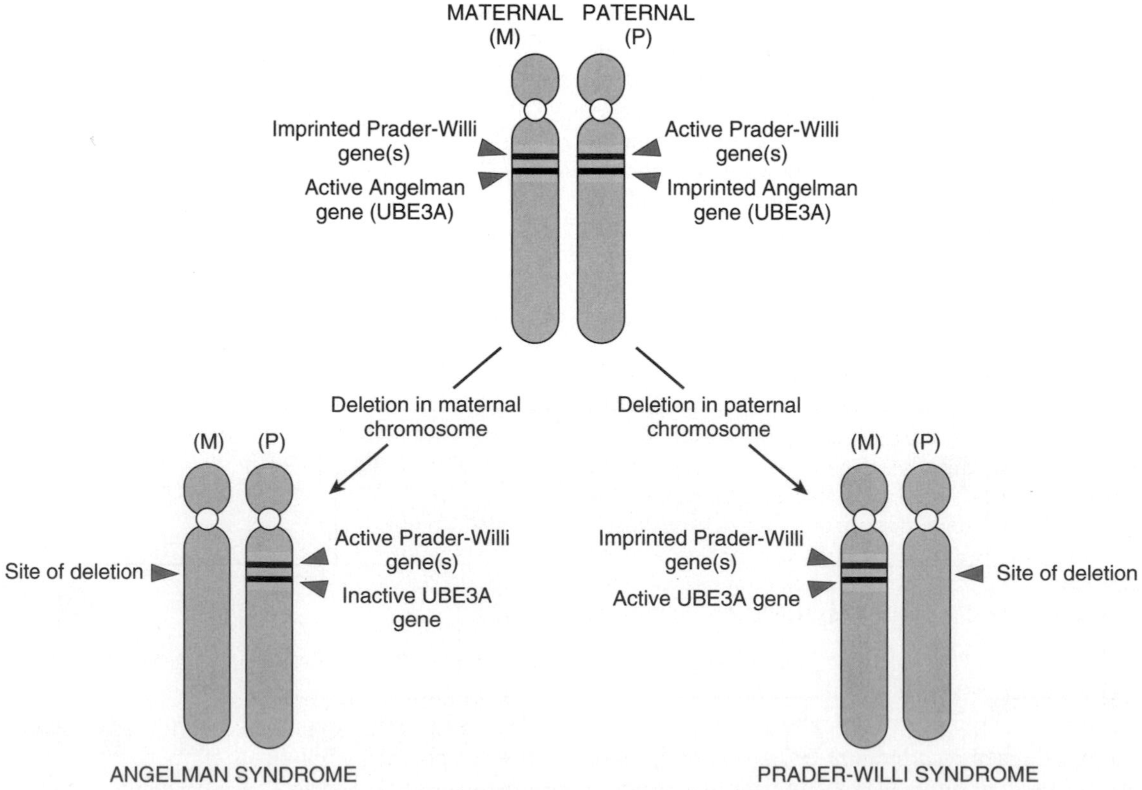

FIGURE 5–36 Diagrammatic representation of Prader-Willi and Angelman syndromes.

The molecular basis of these two imprinting disorders is now being unraveled. In the Angelman syndrome, the affected gene is a ubiquitin protein-ligase that has a role in the ubiquitin-proteosome proteolytic pathway. The gene, called *UBE3A,* maps within the 15q12 region, is imprinted on the paternal chromosome, and is expressed from the maternal allele primarily in specific regions of the normal brain. The imprinting is tissue-specific in that *UBE3A* is expressed from both alleles in most tissues. In approximately 10% of cases, Angelman syndrome occurs, not due to imprinting but due to a point mutation in the maternal allele, thus establishing a firm link between the *UBE3A* gene and Angelman syndrome. In contrast to Angelman syndrome, no single gene has been implicated in Prader-Willi syndrome. Instead, a series of genes located in the 15q11.2–13 interval (which are imprinted on the maternal chromosome and expressed from the paternal chromosome) are believed to be involved. These genes are being characterized.

The importance of imprinting is not restricted to rare chromosomal disorders. To date, about 30 human genes have been shown to have imprinted expression. Parent-of-origin effects have been identified in a variety of inherited diseases, such as Huntington disease and myotonic dystrophy and in tumorigenesis.[83] As discussed in Chapter 7, many cancers arise by loss of both copies of the so-called tumor-suppressor genes. This may occur by mutational inactivation of both alleles or alternatively by functional loss of one gene copy through transcriptional silencing via DNA methylation and the inactivation of the other copy by a mutation.

GONADAL MOSAICISM

It was mentioned earlier that with every autosomal dominant disorder some patients do not have affected parents. In such patients, the disorder results from a new mutation in the egg or the sperm from which they were derived; as such, their siblings are neither affected nor at increased risk of developing the disease. This is not always the case, however. In some autosomal dominant disorders, exemplified by osteogenesis imperfecta, phenotypically normal parents have more than one affected child. This clearly violates the laws of mendelian inheritance. Studies indicate that gonadal mosaicism may be responsible for such unusual pedigrees.[84] Gonadal mosaicism results from a mutation that occurs postzygotically during early (embryonic) development. If the mutation affects only cells destined to form the gonads, the gametes carry the mutation, but the somatic cells of the individual are completely normal. Such an individual is said to exhibit *germ line* or *gonadal mosaicism.* A phenotypically normal parent who has germ line mosaicism can transmit the disease-causing mutation to the offspring through the mutant gamete. Because the progenitor cells of the gametes carry the mutation, there is a definite possibility that more than one child of such a parent would be affected. Obviously the likelihood of such an occurrence depends on the proportion of germ cells carrying the mutation.

Molecular Diagnosis

Medical applications of recombinant DNA technology have come of age. With the completion of the human genome project, DNA probes can be powerful tools for the diagnosis of human disease, both genetic and acquired. Molecular diagnostic techniques have found application in virtually all areas of medicine. These include the following:

- Detection of inherited mutations that underlie the development of genetic diseases either prenatally or after birth
- Detection of acquired mutations that underlie the development of neoplasms
- Accurate diagnosis and classification of neoplasms, especially those that originate in the hematopoietic system
- Diagnosis of infectious diseases, including HIV disease
- Determination of relatedness and identity in transplantation, paternity testing, and forensic medicine.

In addition, future uses of molecular diagnosis will include detection of polymorphisms that influence disease susceptibility, as occurs, for example, in lung cancer. As described in Chapter 15, certain polymorphisms in the P-450 monooxygenase system predispose to cigarette smoke–induced lung cancer. Related to this is the field of pharmacogenomics, wherein certain polymorphisms dictate susceptibility to actions and adverse effects of drugs. Indeed, it is thought that with high throughput analysis, complete genetic profiles of individuals may allow presymptomatic diagnosis of all possible genetic diseases and the risk for environmentally induced disorders. Such powerful capacity has understandably spawned many concerns about confidentiality and ethical use of genetic information.[85]

In the next section, we briefly review the diagnostic applications of molecular techniques as they relate to genetic disorders.

Diagnosis of Genetic Diseases

Diagnosis of genetic diseases requires examination of genetic material (i.e., chromosomes and genes). Hence, two general methods are employed: cytogenetic analysis and molecular analysis. Cytogenetic analysis requires karyotyping.

Prenatal chromosome analysis should be offered to all patients who are at risk of cytogenetically abnormal progeny. It can be performed on cells obtained by amniocentesis, on chorionic villus biopsy, or on umbilical cord blood. Some important indications are the following:

- Advanced maternal age (>34 years) because of greater risk of trisomies
- A parent who is a carrier of a balanced reciprocal translocation, robertsonian translocation, or inversion (in these cases the gametes may be unbalanced, and hence the progeny would be at risk for chromosomal disorders)
- A parent with a previous child with a chromosomal abnormality
- A parent who is a carrier of an X-linked genetic disorder (to determine fetal sex).

Postnatal chromosome analysis is usually performed on peripheral blood lymphocytes. Indications are as follows:

- Multiple congenital anomalies
- Unexplained mental retardation or developmental delay
- Suspected aneuploidy (e.g., features of Down syndrome)
- Suspected unbalanced autosome (e.g., Prader-Willi syndrome)

- Suspected sex chromosomal abnormality (e.g., Turner syndrome)
- Suspected fragile-X syndrome
- Infertility (to rule out sex chromosomal abnormality)
- Multiple spontaneous abortions (to rule out the parents as carriers of balanced translocation; both partners should be evaluated).

Many genetic diseases are caused by subtle changes in individual genes that cannot be detected by karyotyping. Traditionally the diagnosis of single-gene disorders has depended on the identification of abnormal gene products (e.g., mutant hemoglobin or enzymes) or their clinical effects, such as anemia or mental retardation (e.g., phenylketonuria). Now it is possible to identify mutations at the level of DNA and offer gene diagnosis for several mendelian disorders. The use of recombinant DNA technology for the diagnosis of inherited diseases has several distinct advantages over other techniques:

- It is remarkably sensitive. The amount of DNA required for diagnosis by molecular hybridization techniques can be readily obtained from 100,000 cells. Furthermore, the use of PCR allows several millionfold amplification of DNA or RNA, making it possible to use as few as 100 cells or 1 cell for analysis. Tiny amounts of whole blood or even dried blood can supply sufficient DNA for PCR amplification.
- DNA-based tests are not dependent on a gene product that may be produced only in certain specialized cells (e.g., brain) or expression of a gene that may occur late in life. Because virtually all cells of the body of an affected individual contain the same DNA, each postzygotic cell carries the mutant gene.

These two features have profound implications for the prenatal diagnosis of genetic diseases because a sufficient number of cells can be obtained from a few milliliters of amniotic fluid or from a biopsy of chorionic villus that can be performed as early as the first trimester.

There are two distinct approaches to the diagnosis of single-gene diseases by recombinant DNA technology: direct detection of mutations and indirect detection based on linkage of the disease gene with a harmless "marker gene."

DIRECT GENE DIAGNOSIS

McKusick, an eminent geneticist, has appropriately called direct gene diagnosis the *diagnostic biopsy of the human genome.* Such diagnosis depends on the detection of an important qualitative change in the DNA. There are several methods of direct gene diagnosis, almost all based on PCR analysis, which involves exponential amplification of DNA from small quantities of starting material. If RNA is used as a substrate, it is first reverse transcribed to obtain cDNA and then amplified by PCR. This method is often abbreviated as RT-PCR.

- One technique relies on the fact that some mutations alter or destroy certain restriction sites on DNA; this occurs in the gene encoding factor V. This protein is involved in the coagulation pathway (Chapter 4), and a mutation affecting the factor V gene is the most common cause of inherited predisposition to thrombosis. Exon 10 of the factor V gene and the adjacent intron have two Mnl1 restriction sites. A G-to-A mutation within the exon destroys one of the two Mnl1 sites (Fig. 5–37). To detect the mutant gene, two primers that bind to the 3′ and 5′ prime ends of the normal sequence are designed. By using appropriate DNA polymerases and thermal cycling, the DNA between the primers is greatly amplified, producing millons of copies of the DNA between the two primer sites. The amplified normal DNA and patient's DNA are then digested with the Mnl1 enzyme. Under these conditions, the normal

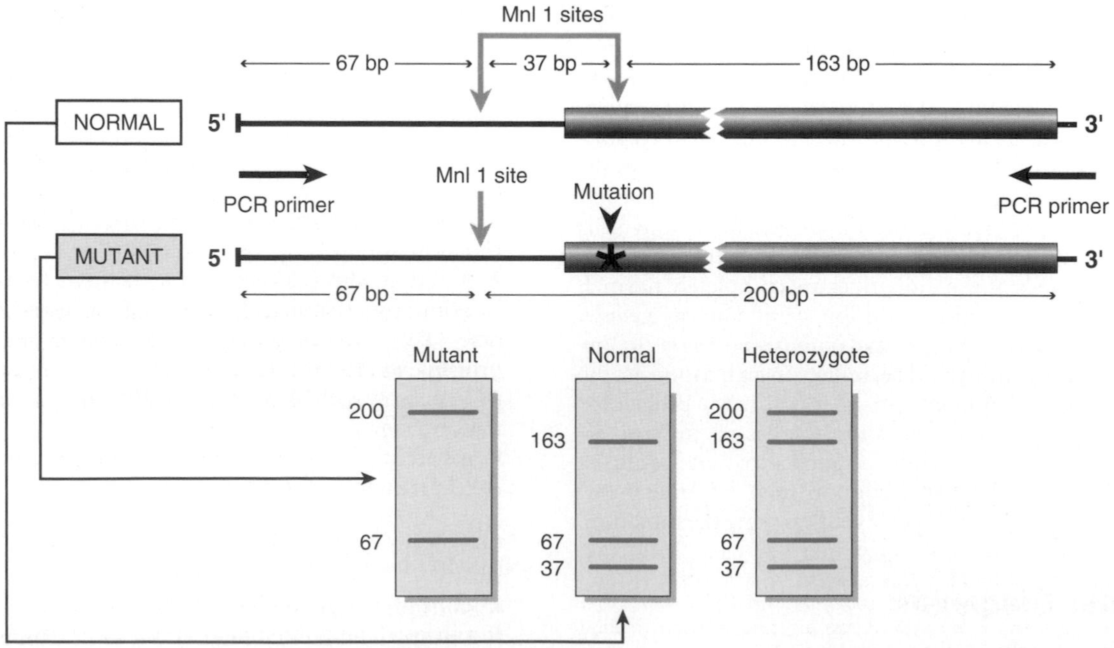

FIGURE 5–37 Direct gene diagnosis: detection of coagulation factor V mutation by polymerase chain reaction (PCR) analysis. A G→A substitution in an exon destroys one of the two Mnl1 restriction sites. The mutant allele therefore gives rise to two, rather than three, fragments by PCR analysis.

DNA yields three fragments (67 base pairs, 37 base pairs, and 163 base pairs long); by contrast, the patient's DNA yields only two products, an abnormal fragment that is 200 base pairs and a normal fragment that is 67 base pairs long. These DNA fragments can be readily resolved by polyacrylamide gel electrophoresis and then visualized after staining with ethidium bromide under ultraviolet light.

- Mutations that affect the length of DNA (e.g., deletions or expansions) can also be detected by PCR analysis. As discussed earlier, several diseases, such as the fragile-X syndrome, are associated with trinucleotide repeats. Figure 5–38 reveals how PCR analysis can be used to detect this mutation. Two primers that flank the region affected by trinucleotide repeats are used to amplify the intervening sequences. Because there are large differences in the number of repeats, the size of the PCR products obtained from the DNA of normal individuals, or those with premutation, is quite different. These size differences are revealed by differential migration of the amplified DNA products on a gel. Currently the full mutation cannot be detected by PCR analysis because the affected segment of DNA is too large for conventional PCR. In such cases, a Southern blot analysis of genomic DNA has to be performed.
- A variety of PCR-based technologies that use fluorophore indicators to detect the presence or absence of mutations in "real time" (i.e., during the exponential phase of DNA amplification) have become available. This has significantly reduced the time required for mutation detection by removing the restriction digestion and electrophoresis steps used in conventional PCR assays. One example of high-throughput mutation analysis is the molecular beacon technology. Molecular beacons are hairpin-shaped fluorescent oligonucleotide probes that fluoresce only on hybridization to target sequences (wild-type DNA). In the presence of nucleotide mismatch because of mutations, effective pairing does not occur and there is no fluorescence.

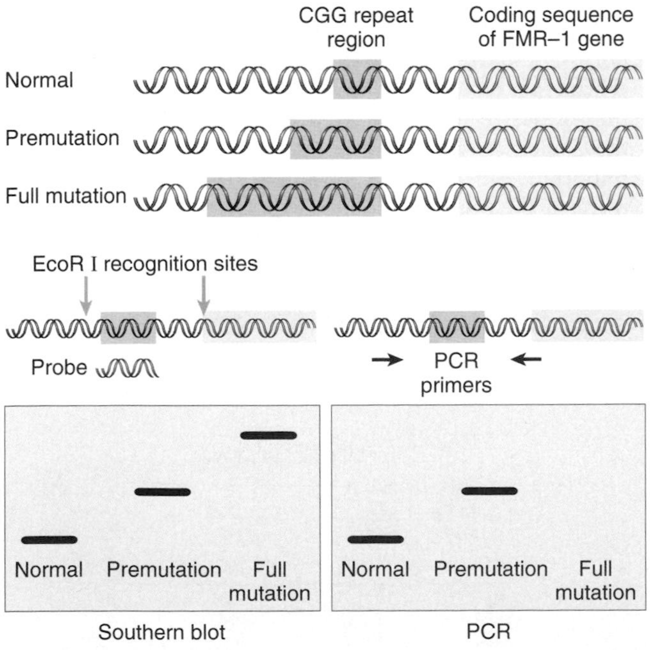

FIGURE 5–38 Diagnostic application of PCR and Southern blot analysis in fragile-X syndrome. With PCR, the differences in the size of CGG repeat between normal and premutation give rise to products of different sizes and mobility. With a full mutation, the region between the primers is too large to be amplified by conventional PCR. In Southern blot analysis the DNA is cut by enzymes that flank the CGG repeat region, and is then probed with a complementary DNA that binds to the affected part of the gene. A single small band is seen in normal males, a higher-molecular-weight band in males with premutation, and a very large (usually diffuse) band in those with the full mutation.

INDIRECT DNA DIAGNOSIS: LINKAGE ANALYSIS

Direct gene diagnosis is possible only if the mutant gene and its normal counterpart have been identified and cloned and their nucleotide sequences are known. In a large number of genetic diseases, including some that are relatively common, information about the gene sequence is lacking. Therefore, alternative strategies must be employed to track the mutant gene on the basis of its linkage to detectable genetic markers. In essence, one has to determine whether a given fetus or family member has inherited the same relevant chromosomal region(s) as a previously affected family member. It follows therefore that the success of such a strategy depends on the ability to distinguish the chromosome that carries the mutation from its normal homologous counterpart. This is accomplished by exploiting naturally occurring variations or polymorphisms in DNA sequences. Such polymorphisms can be grouped into two general categories: site polymorphisms and length polymorphisms.

- *Site polymorphisms* are also called *restriction fragment length polymorphisms (RFLPs)*. Examination of DNA from any two persons reveals variations in the DNA sequences involving approximately one nucleotide in every 200 to 500 base pair stretches. Most of these variations occur in noncoding regions of the DNA and are hence phenotypically silent; however, these single base pair changes may abolish or create recognition sites for restriction enzymes, thereby altering the length of DNA fragments produced after digestion with certain restriction enzymes. Using appropriate DNA probes that hybridize with sequences in the vicinity of the polymorphic sites, it is possible to detect the DNA fragments of different lengths by Southern blot analysis. To summarize, *RFLP* refers to variation in fragment length between individuals that results from DNA sequence polymorphisms.

With this background, we can discuss how RFLPs can be used in gene tracking. Figure 5–39 illustrates the principle of RFLP analysis. In this example of an autosomal recessive disease, both of the parents are heterozygote carriers and the children are normal, are carriers, or are affected. In the illustrated example, the normal chromosome (A) has two restriction sites, 7.6 kb apart, whereas chromosome B, which carries the mutant gene, has a DNA sequence polymorphism resulting in the creation of an additional (third) restriction site for the same enzyme. Note that the additional restriction site has not resulted from the mutation but from a naturally occurring polymorphism. When DNA from such an individual is digested with the appropriate restriction enzyme and probed with a cloned DNA fragment that hybridizes with a stretch of sequences between

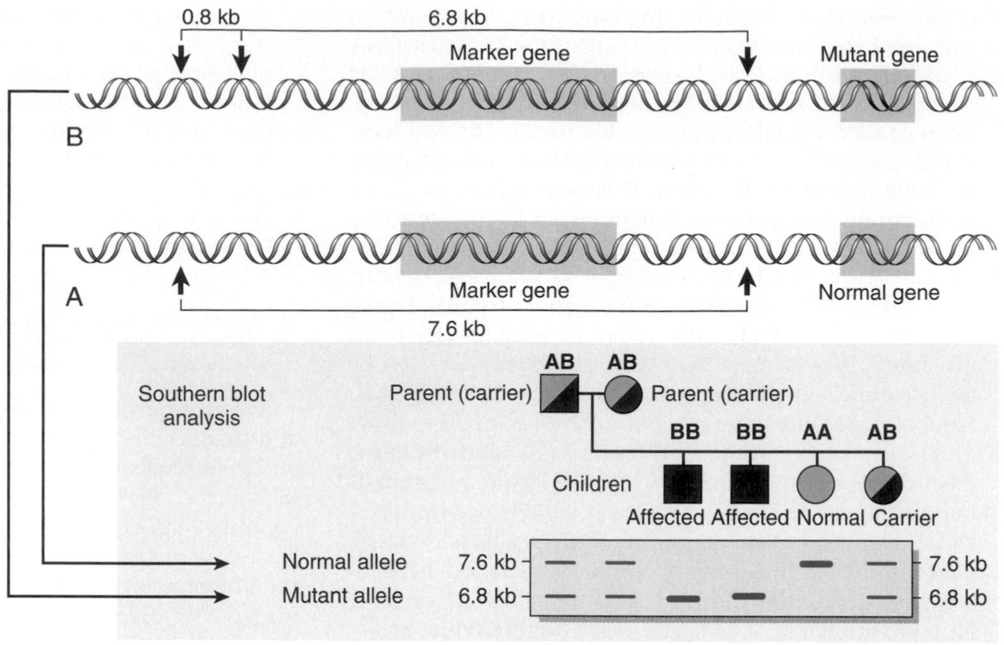

FIGURE 5–39 Schematic illustration of the principles underlying restriction fragment length polymorphism analysis in the diagnosis of genetic diseases.

the restriction sites, the normal chromosome yields a 7.6 kb band, whereas the other chromosome (carrying the mutant gene) produces a smaller, 6.8 kb, band. Thus, on Southern blot analysis, two bands are noted. It is possible by this technique to distinguish family members who have inherited both normal chromosomes from those who are heterozygous or homozygous for the mutant gene. PCR followed by digestion with the appropriate restriction enzyme and gel electrophoresis can also be used to detect RFLPs if the target DNA is of the size that can be amplified by conventional PCR.

- *Length polymorphisms:* Human DNA contains short repetitive sequences of noncoding DNA. Because the number of repeats affecting such sequences varies greatly between different individuals, the resulting length polymorphisms are quite useful for linkage analysis. These polymorphisms are often subdivided on the basis of their length into microsatellite repeats and minisatellite repeats. Microsatellites are usually less than 1 kb and are characterized by a repeat size of 2 to 6 base pairs. Minisatellite repeats, by comparison, are larger (1 to 3 kb), and the repeat motif is usually 15 to 70 base pairs. It is important to note that the number of repeats, both in microsatellites and minisatellites, is extremely variable within a given population, and hence these stretches of DNA can be used quite effectively to distinguish different chromosomes (Fig. 5–40*A*). Figure 5–40*B* illustrates how microsatellite polymorphisms can be used to track the inheritance of autosomal dominant polycystic kidney disease (PKD). In this case, allele C, which produces a larger PCR product than allele A or B, carries the disease-related gene. Hence all individuals who carry the C allele are affected. Microsatellites have assumed great importance in linkage studies and hence in the development of the human genome map. Currently, linkage to all human chromosomes can be identified by microsatellite polymorphisms.[86]

Single nucleotide polymorphisms (SNP) are a form of site polymorphism. As mentioned earlier, SNPs are the most common forms of polymorphisms in the human genome.

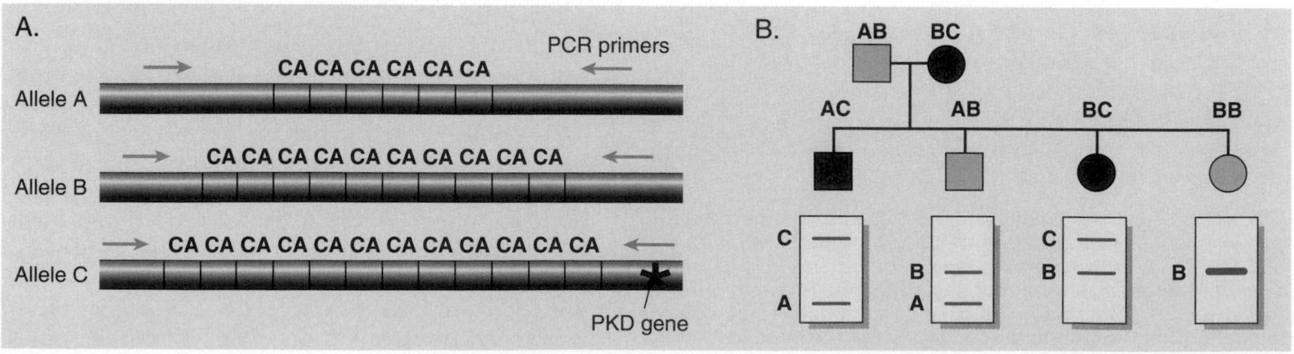

FIGURE 5–40 Schematic diagram of DNA polymorphisms resulting from a variable number of CA repeats. The three alleles produce PCR products of different sizes, thus identifying their origins from specific chromosomes. In the example depicted, allele C is linked to a mutation responsible for autosomal dominant polycystic kidney disease (PKD). Application of this to detect progeny carrying the disease gene is illustrated in one hypothetical pedigree.

They are found throughout the genome (e.g., in exons, introns, and regulatory sequences). SNPs serve both as a physical landmark within the genome and as a genetic marker whose transmission can be followed from parent to child. Because of their prevalence in the human genome and their stability, SNPs can be used in linkage analysis for identifying haplotypes associated with diseases, leading to gene discovery and mapping. In the last decade, SNPs have become the genetic marker of choice for the study for complex genetic traits. Population studies have found associations between specific SNPs and multifactorial diseases such as hypertension, heart disease, or diabetes. For example, certain polymorphisms within the *angiotensinogen* gene are associated with variations in resting blood pressures and a predisposition to hypertension. A move is under consideration to map all SNPs in the human genome, which would facilitate the eventual construction of "SNP chips" for genetic risk profiling of individuals.

Because in linkage studies the mutant gene itself is not identified, certain limitations listed below become apparent:

1. For diagnosis, several relevant family members must be available for testing. With an autosomal recessive disease, for example, a DNA sample from a previously affected child is necessary to determine the polymorphism pattern that is associated with the homozygous genotype.
2. Key family members must be heterozygous for the polymorphism (i.e., the two homologous chromosomes must be distinguishable for the polymorphic site). Because there can be only two variations of restriction sites (i.e., presence or absence of the restriction site), this is an important limitation of RFLPs. Microsatellite polymorphisms have multiple alleles and hence much greater chances of heterozygosity. These are therefore much more useful than restriction site polymorphism.
3. Normal exchange of chromosomal material between homologous chromosomes (recombination) during gametogenesis may lead to "separation" of the mutant gene from the polymorphism pattern with which it had been previously coinherited. This may lead to an erroneous genetic prediction in a subsequent pregnancy. Obviously the closer the linkage, the lower the degree of recombination and the lower the risk of a false test.

Molecular diagnosis by linkage analysis has been useful in the antenatal or presymptomatic diagnosis of disorders such as Huntington disease, cystic fibrosis, and adult polycystic kidney disease. In general, when a disease gene is identified and cloned, direct gene diagnosis becomes the method of choice. If the disease is caused by several different mutations in a given gene (e.g., fibrillin-1; see earlier), however, direct gene diagnosis is not feasible, and linkage analysis remains the preferred method.

REFERENCES

1. Rimoin DL, et al: Nature and frequency of genetic disease. In Rimoin DL, et al (eds): Emery and Rimoin's Principles and Practice of Medical Genetics, 3rd ed. New York, Churchill Livingstone, 1997, p 32.
2. Guttmacher AE, Collins FS: Genomic medicine—a primer. N Engl J Med 347:1512, 2002.

2a. Rammensee H-G: Protein surgery. Science 427:203, 2004.

3. Joos L, Eryuksel E, Brutsche MH: Functional genomics and gene microarrays—the use in research and clinical medicine. Swiss Med Wkly 133:31, 2003.
4. Botstein D, Risch N: Discovering genotypes underlying human phenotypes: past successes for mendelian disease, future approaches for complex disease. Nat Genet (Suppl) 33:228, 2003.
5. Taylor JG, et al: Using genetic variation to study human disease. Trends Mol Med 7:507, 2001.
6. Bayat A: Science, medicine, and the future: bioinformatics. BMJ 324:1018, 2002.
7. Nussbaum RL, McInnes RR, Willand HF: Thompson and Thompson Genetics in Medicine, 6th ed. Philadelphia, WB Saunders, 2001, p 79.
8. Ensenauer RE, et al: Primer on medical genomics. Part VIII: essentials of medical genetics for the practicing physician. Mayo Clin Proc 78:846, 2003.
9. Willard HF: Tales of the Y chromosome. Nature 423:810, 2003.
10. Ahar M, Lee VH: Pharmacogenomic considerations in drug delivery. Pharmacogenomics 4:443, 2003.
11. Pyeritz RE: Marfan syndrome and other disorders of fibrillin. In Rimoin DL, et al (eds): Emery and Rimoin's Principles and Practice of Medical Genetics, 3rd ed. New York, Churchill Livingstone, 1997, p 1027.
12. Collod-Beroud G, Boileau C: Marfan syndrome in the third Millennium. Eur J Hum Genet 10:673, 2002.
13. Robinson PN, et al: Mutations of FBN1 and genotype–phenotype correlations in Marfan syndrome and related fibrillinopathies. Hum Mut 20:153, 2002.
14. Robinson PN, Booms P: The molecular pathogenesis of the Marfan syndrome. Cell Mol Life Sci 58:1698, 2001.
15. Beighton P, et al: Ehlers-Danlos syndromes: revised nosology, Villefranche, 1997. Am J Med Genet 77:31, 1998.
16. Mao JR, Bristow J: The Ehlers-Danlos syndrome: on beyond collagens. J Clin Invest 07:1063, 2001.
17. Byers PH: Disorders of collagen biosynthesis and structure. In Scriver CR, et al (eds): The Metabolic and Molecular Basis of Inherited Disease, 7th ed. New York, McGraw-Hill Health Profession Division, 1995, p 4029.
18. Yeowell HN, Walker LC: Mutations in the lysyl hydroxylase 1 gene that result in enzyme deficiency and the clinical phenotype of Ehlers-Danlos syndrome type VI. Mol Genet Metab 71:212, 2000.
19. Goldstein JL, Brown MS: Molecular medicine. The cholesterol quartet. Science 292:1310, 2001.
20. Rader DJ, Cohen J, Hobbs HH: Monogenic hypercholesterolemia: new insights in pathogenesis and treatment. J Clin Invest 111:1795, 2003.
21. Illingworth DR, Sexton GJ: Hypocholesterolemic effects of mevinolin in patients with heterozygous familial hypercholesterolemia. J Clin Invest 74:1972, 1984.
22. Wraith JE: Lysosomal disorders. Semin Neonatol 7:75, 2002.
23. Tager JM: Inborn errors of cellular organelles: an overview. J Inherit Metab Dis 10 (Suppl 1):3, 1987.
24. Mahuran DJ: Biochemical consequences of mutations causing the GM_2 gangliosidoses. Biochim Biophys Acta 1455:105, 1999.
25. Triggs-Raine BL, et al: Screening for carriers of Tay-Sachs disease among Ashkenazi Jews: a comparison of DNA-based and enzyme-based tests. N Engl J Med 323:6, 1990.
26. Kolodny EH: Niemann-Pick disease. Curr Opin Hematol 7:48, 2000.
27. Ioannou YA: Multidrug permeases and subcellular cholesterol transport. Nat Rev Mol Cell Biol 2:657, 2001.
28. Elstein D, et al: Gaucher's disease. Lancet 358:324, 2001.
29. Lee RE, et al: Gaucher's disease: clinical, morphologic, and pathogenetic considerations. Pathol Annu 12:309, 1977.
30. Cox TM: Gaucher disease: understanding the molecular pathogenesis of sphingolipidoses. J Inherit Metab 24 (Suppl 2):106, 2001.
31. Spranger J: Mucopolysaccharidoses. In Rimoin DL, et al (eds): Emery and Rimoin's Principles and Practice of Medical Genetics, 3rd ed. New York, Churchill Livingstone, 1997, p 2071.
32. Wolfsdorf JI, Weinstein DA: Glycogen storage diseases. Rev Endocr Metab Disord 4:95, 2003.
33. DiMauro S, Lamperti C: Muscle glycogenoses. Muscle Nerve 24:984, 2001.
34. Chen Y-T: Glycogen storage diseases. In Fauci AS, et al (eds): Harrison's Principles of Internal Medicine, 14th ed. New York, McGraw-Hill, 1998, p 2176.
35. Lee PJ, Leonard JV: The hepatic glycogen storage diseases—problems beyond childhood. J Inherit Metab Dis 18:462, 1995.

36. Bartram C, et al: McArdle disease—muscle glycogen phosphorylase deficiency. Biochim Biophys Acta 1272:1, 1995.
37. Chen Y-T, Burchell A: Glycogen storage diseases. In Scriver CR, et al (eds): The Metabolic and Molecular Basis of Inherited Disease, 7th ed. New York, McGraw-Hill Health Profession Division, 1995, p 935.
38. Van Offel JF, et al: The clinical manifestations of ochronosis: a review. Acta Clin Belg 50:358, 1995.
39. Fernandez-Canon JM, et al: The molecular basis of alkaptonuria. Nat Genet 14:19, 1996.
40. Gaines JJ Jr: The pathology of alkaptonuric ochronosis. Hum Pathol 20:40, 1989.
41. Reynolds RM, et al: Von Recklinghausen's neurofibromatosis: neurofibromatosis type 1. Lancet 361:1552, 2003.
42. Ricardi VM, Eichner JE: Neurofibromatosis: Phenotype, Natural History and Pathogenesis. Baltimore, Johns Hopkins University Press, 1986, p 115.
43. Bretscher A, Edwards K, Fehon RG: ERM proteins and *merlin:* integrators at the cell cortex. Nat Rev Mol Cell Biol 3:586, 2002.
44. Nelson K, Holmes LB: Malformations due to presumed spontaneous mutations in newborn infants. N Engl J Med 320:19, 1989.
45. Pergament E: New molecular techniques for chromosome analysis. Baillieres Best Pract Res Clin Obstet Gynaecol 14:677, 2000.
46. Bayani JM, Squire JA: Applications of *SKY* in cancer cytogenetics. Cancer Invest 20:373, 2002.
47. Hassold T, Sherman S: Down syndrome: genetic recombination and the origin of the extra chromosome 21. Clin Genet 57:95, 2000.
48. Roizen NJ, Patterson D: Down's syndrome. Lancet 361:1281, 2003.
49. Kallen B, et al: Major congenital malformations in Down syndrome. Am J Med Genet 65:160, 1996.
50. Cork LC: Neuropathology of Down syndrome and Alzheimer disease. Am J Med Genet 7 (Suppl):282, 1990.
51. Ugazio AG, et al: Immunology of Down syndrome: a review. Am J Med Genet 7 (Suppl):204, 1990.
52. Mao R, et al: Global up-regulation of chromosome 21 gene expression in the developing Down syndrome brain. Genomics 81:457, 2003.
53. Yagi H, et al: Role of *TBX1* in human del22q11.2 syndrome. Lancet 362:1366, 2003.
54. Bassett AS, et al: The schizophrenia phenotype in 22q11 deletion syndrome. Am J Psychiatry 160:1580, 2003.
55. Lyon MF: X-chromosome inactivation and human genetic disease. Acta Paediatr 91(Suppl):107, 2002.
56. Plath K, et al: *Xist* RNA and the mechanism of X chromosome inactivation. Annu Rev Genet 36:233, 2002.
57. Hawley RS: The human Y chromosome: rumors of its death have been greatly exaggerated. Cell 113:825, 2003.
58. Smyth CM, Bremner WJ: Klinefelter syndrome. Arch Intern Med 158:1309, 1998.
59. Ranke MB, Saenger P: Turner's syndrome. Lancet 358:309, 2001.
60. Saeger P: Turner syndrome. N Engl J Med 335:1749, 1996.
61. Blaschke RJ, Rappold GA: *SHOX* in short stature syndromes. Horm Res 55 (Suppl 1):21, 2001.
62. Rappold GA, et al: Deletions of the homeobox gene *SHOX* (short stature homeobox) are an important cause of growth failure in children with short stature. J Clin Endocrinol Metab 87:1402, 2002.
63. McLauglin DT, Donahoe PK: Sex determination and differentiation. N Engl J Med 350:367, 2004.
64. Ortenberg J, et al: *SRY* gene expression in the ovotestes of XX true hermaphrodites. J Urol 167:1828, 2002.
65. Wiener JS: Insights into causes of sexual ambiguity. Curr Opin Urol 9:507, 1999.
66. Brinkmann AO: Molecular basis of androgen insensitivity. Mol Cell Endocrinol 179:105, 2001.
67. Cummings CJ, Zoghbi HY: Trinucleotide repeats: mechanisms and pathophysiology. Annu Rev Genomics Hum Genet 1:281, 2000.
68. Sutherland GR, Baker E: The clinical significance of fragile sites on human chromosomes. Clin Genet 58:157, 2000.
69. Maddalena A, et al: Fragile-X syndrome. In Rosenberg RN, et al (eds): The Molecular and Genetic Basis of Neurologic Diseases, 2nd ed. Boston, Butterworth & Heinemann, 1997, p 81.
70. Oostra BA: Functions of the fragile-X protein. Trends Mol Med 8:102, 2002.
71. Antar LN, Bassell GJ: Sunrise at the synapse: the FMRP mRNP shaping the synaptic interface. Neuron 37:555, 2003.
72. Jin P, Warren ST: New insights into fragile-X syndrome: from molecules to neurobehaviors. Trends Biochem Sci 28:152, 2003.
73. Mandel JL: Breaking the rule of three. Nature 386:767, 1997.
74. Fischbeck KH: Polyglutamine expansion neurodegenerative disease. Brain Res Bull 56:161, 2001.
75. Johns DR: The other human genome: mitochondrial DNA and disease. Nat Med 2:1065, 1996.
76. DiMauro S, Schon EA: Mitochondrial respiratory-chain diseases. N Engl J Med 348:2656, 2003.
77. DiMauro S, Schon EA: Mitochondrial DNA mutations in human disease. Am J Med Genet (Semin Med Genet) 106:18, 2001.
78. Rossignol R, et al: Mitochondrial threshold effects. Biochem J 370:751, 2003.
79. Man PY, Turnbull DM, Chinnery PF: Leber hereditary optic neuropathy. J Med Genet 39:162, 2002.
80. Hanel ML, Wevrick R: The role of genomic imprinting in human developmental disorders: lessons from Prader-Willi syndrome. Clin Genet 59:156, 2001.
81. Nicholls RD, Knepper JL: Genome organization, function, and imprinting in Prader-Willi and Angelman syndromes. Annu Rev Genomics Hum Genet 2:153, 2001.
82. Clayton-Smith J, Laan L: Angelman syndrome: a review of the clinical and genetic aspects. J Med Genet 40:87, 2003.
83. Squire J, Weksberg R: Genomic imprinting in tumors. Semin Cancer Biol 7:41, 1996.
84. Bernards A, Gusella JF: The importance of genetic mosaicism in human disease. N Engl J Med 331:1447, 1994.
85. Clayton EW: Ethical, legal, and social implications of genomic medicine. N Engl J Med 349:562, 2003.
86. Koreth J, et al: Microsatellites and PCR genomic analysis. J Pathol 178:239, 1996.

CHAPTER 6

Diseases of Immunity

Abul K. Abbas, MD

GENERAL FEATURES OF THE IMMUNE SYSTEM

Innate and Adaptive Immunity

Cells and Tissues of the Immune System

T Lymphocytes

B Lymphocytes

Macrophages

Dendritic Cells

Natural Killer Cells

Cytokines: Messenger Molecules of the Immune System

General Properties of Cytokines

Structure and Function of Histocompatibility Molecules

HLA and Disease Association

DISORDERS OF THE IMMUNE SYSTEM

Mechanisms of Hypersensitivity Reactions

Immediate (Type I) Hypersensitivity

Antibody-Mediated (Type II) Hypersensitivity

Immune Complex–Mediated (Type III) Hypersensitivity

Cell-Mediated (Type IV) Hypersensitivity

Transplant Rejection

Autoimmune Diseases

Immunologic Tolerance

Mechanisms of Autoimmune Diseases

Systemic Lupus Erythematosus

Rheumatoid Arthritis

Sjögren Syndrome

Systemic Sclerosis (Scleroderma)

Inflammatory Myopathies

Mixed Connective Tissue Disease

Polyarteritis Nodosa and Other Vasculitides

Immunologic Deficiency Syndromes

Primary Immunodeficiencies

Acquired Immunodeficiency Syndrome (AIDS)

Amyloidosis

General Features of the Immune System

Although vital to survival, the immune system is similar to the proverbial two-edged sword. On the one hand, immunodeficiency states render humans easy prey to infections and possibly tumors; on the other hand, a hyperactive immune system may cause fatal disease, as in the case of an overwhelming allergic reaction to the sting of a bee. In yet another series of derangements, the immune system may lose its normal capacity to distinguish self from non-self, resulting in immune reactions against one's own tissues and cells (*autoimmunity*). This chapter considers diseases caused by too little immunity as well as those resulting from too much immunologic reactivity. We also consider amyloidosis, a disease in which an abnormal protein, derived in some cases from fragments of immunoglobulins, is deposited in tissues. First, we review some advances in the understanding of innate and adaptive immunity and lymphocyte biology, then give a brief description of the histocompatibility genes because their products are relevant to several immunologically mediated diseases and to the rejection of transplants.

INNATE AND ADAPTIVE IMMUNITY

The physiologic function of the immune system is to protect individuals from infectious pathogens. The mechanisms that are responsible for this protection fall into two broad categories (Fig. 6–1). *Innate immunity* (also called natural, or native, immunity) refers to defense mechanisms that are present even before infection and have evolved to specifically recognize microbes and protect multicellular organisms against infections. *Adaptive immunity* (also called acquired, or specific, immunity) consists of mechanisms that are stimulated by (adapt to) microbes and are capable of also recognizing nonmicrobial substances, called *antigens*. Innate immunity is the first line of defense, because it is always ready to prevent and eradicate infections. Adaptive immunity develops later after exposure to microbes and is even more powerful in combating infections. By convention, the term "immune response" refers to adaptive immunity.

The major components of innate immunity are epithelial barriers that block entry of environmental microbes, phagocytic cells (mainly neutrophils and macrophages), natural killer (NK) cells, and several plasma proteins, including the proteins of the complement system. Phagocytes are recruited to sites of infection, resulting in inflammation (Chapter 2), and here the cells ingest the microbes and are then activated to destroy the ingested pathogens. Phagocytes recognize microbes by several membrane receptors. These include receptors for mannose residues and N-formyl methionine–containing peptides, which are produced by microbes but not by host cells, and a family of receptors that are homologous to a *Drosophila* protein called Toll.[1] Different Toll-like receptors (TLRs) are involved in responses to different microbial products[2] (Box 6–1). Upon recognition of the relevant microbial structure, the TLRs signal by a common pathway that leads to the activation of transcription factors, notably NF-κB (nuclear factor κB). NF-κB stimulates production of cytokines and several proteins that are responsible for the microbicidal activities of the phagocytes. Phagocytes internalize microbes into vesicles, where the microbes are destroyed by reactive oxygen and nitrogen intermediates and hydrolytic enzymes (see Chapter 2).

Complement proteins, which were described in Chapter 2, are some of the most important plasma proteins of the innate immune system. Recall that in innate immunity, the complement system is activated by binding to microbes using the alternative and lectin pathways; in adaptive immunity, it is activated by binding to antibodies using the classical pathway. Mammalian cells express regulatory proteins that prevent inappropriate complement activation. Other circulating proteins of innate immunity are mannose-binding lectin and C-reactive protein, both of which coat microbes for phagocytosis and complement activation. Lung surfactant is also a compo-

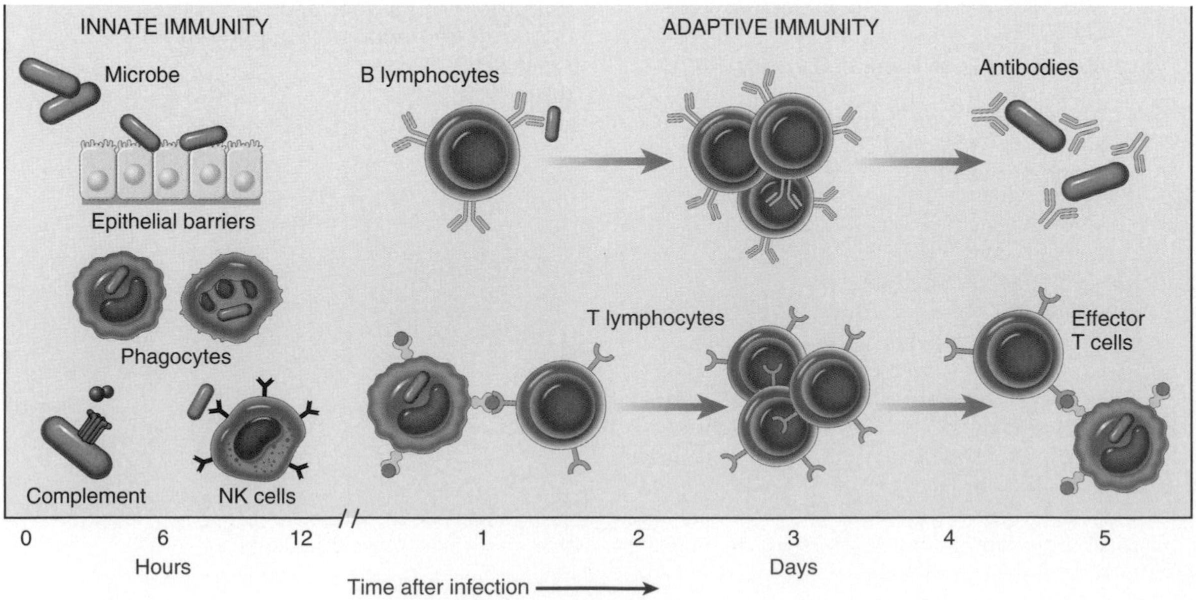

FIGURE 6–1 Innate and adaptive immunity. The principal mechanisms of innate immunity and adaptive immunity are shown.

Box 6–1 Toll-like Receptors

The Toll-like receptors (TLRs) are membrane proteins that recognize a variety of microbe-derived molecules and stimulate innate immune responses against the microbes. The first protein to be identified in this family was the *Drosophila* Toll protein, which is involved in establishing the dorsal-ventral axis during embryogenesis of the fly, as well as mediating antimicrobial responses. Ten different mammalian TLRs have been identified based on sequence homology to *Drosophila* Toll, and they are named TLR1–10. All these receptors contain leucine-rich repeats flanked by characteristic cysteine-rich motifs in their extracellular regions, and a conserved signaling domain in their cytoplasmic region that is also found in the cytoplasmic tails of the IL-1 and IL-18 receptors and is called the Toll/IL-1 receptor (TIR) domain. The TLRs are expressed on many different cell types that participate in innate immune responses, including macrophages, dendritic cells, neutrophils, NK cells, mucosal epithelial cells, and endothelial cells.

Mammalian TLRs are involved in responses to widely divergent types of molecules that are commonly expressed by microbial but not mammalian cells (see Figure). Some of the microbial products that stimulate TLRs include Gram-negative bacterial lipopolysaccharide (LPS), Gram-positive bacterial peptidoglycan, bacterial lipoproteins, the bacterial flagellar protein flagellin, heat shock protein 60, unmethylated CpG DNA motifs (found in many bacteria), and double-stranded RNA (found in RNA viruses). The specificity of TLRs for microbial products is dependent on associations between different TLRs and non-TLR adapter molecules. For instance, LPS first binds to soluble LPS-binding protein (LBP) in the blood or extracellular fluid, and this complex serves to facilitate LPS binding to CD14, which exists as both a soluble plasma protein and a glycophosphatidylinositol-linked membrane protein on most cells. Once LPS binds to CD14, LBP dissociates, and the LPS–CD14 complex physically associates with TLR4. An additional extracellular accessory protein, called MD2, also binds to the complex with CD14. LPS, CD14, and MD2 are all required for efficient LPS-induced signaling, but it is not yet clear if direct physical interaction of LPS with TLR4 is necessary.

Signaling by TLRs results in the activation of transcription factors, notably NF-κB (see Figure). Ligand binding to the TLR at the cell surface leads to recruitment of cytoplasmic signaling molecules, the first of which is the adapter protein MyD88. A kinase called IL-1 receptor associated kinase (IRAK) is recruited into the signaling complex. IRAK undergoes autophosphorylation, dissociates from MyD88, and activates another signaling molecule, called TNF-receptor (TNF-R) associated factor-6 (TRAF-6). TRAF-6 then activates the I-κB kinase cascade, leading to activation of the NF-κB transcription factor. In some cell types certain TLRs also engage other signaling pathways, such as the MAP kinase cascade, leading to activation of the AP-1 transcription factor. Some TLRs may use adapter proteins other than MyD88. The relative importance of these various pathways of TLR signaling, and the way the "choice" of pathways is made, are not well understood.

The genes that are expressed in response to TLR signaling encode proteins important in many different components of innate immune responses. These include inflammatory cytokines (TNF, IL-1, and IL-12), endothelial adhesion molecules (E-selectin), and proteins involved in microbial killing mechanisms (inducible nitric oxide synthase). The particular genes expressed will depend on the responding cell type.

A

TLR	Ligand	Microbial source
TLR2	Lipoproteins Peptidoglycan Zymosan LPS GPI anchor Lipoarabinomannan Phosphatidylinositol dimannoside	Bacteria Gram positive bacteria Fungi Leptospira Trypanosomes Mycobacteria Mycobacteria
TLR3	Double-stranded RNA	Viruses
TLR4	LPS HSF00	Gram negative bacteria Chlamydia
TLR5	Flagellin	Various bacteria
TLR6	CpG DNA	Bacteria, protozoans

B

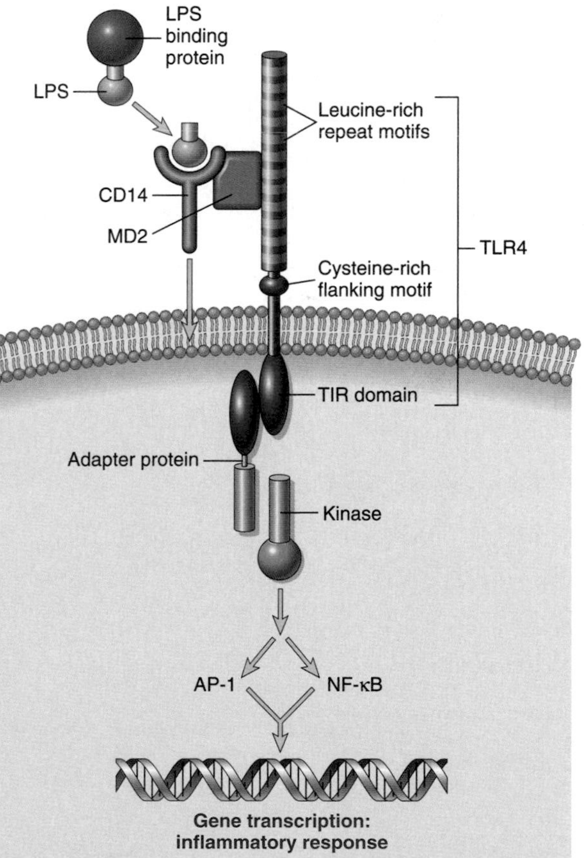

A, Different TLRs are involved in responses to different microbial products. *B,* Signaling by a prototypic TLR, TLR4, in response to bacterial LPS. An adapter protein links the TLR to a kinase, which activates transcription factors such as NF-κB and AP-1. TIR, Toll/IL-1 receptor domain.

nent of innate immunity, providing protection against inhaled microbes.

The adaptive immune system consists of lymphocytes and their products, including antibodies. The receptors of lymphocytes are much more diverse than those of the innate immune system, but lymphocytes are not inherently specific for microbes, and they are capable of recognizing a vast array of foreign substances. In the remainder of this introductory section we focus on lymphocytes and the reactions of the adaptive immune system.

CELLS AND TISSUES OF THE IMMUNE SYSTEM

There are two main types of adaptive immunity—cell-mediated (or cellular) immunity, which is responsible for defense against intracellular microbes, and humoral immunity, which protects against extracellular microbes and their toxins (Fig. 6–2). Cellular immunity is mediated by T (thymus-derived) lymphocytes, and humoral immunity is mediated by B (bone marrow–derived) lymphocytes and their secreted products, antibodies. All these mechanisms of adaptive immunity are capable of causing injury to the host and subsequent disease.

T Lymphocytes

T lymphocytes are generated from immature precursors in the thymus. Mature, naive T cells are found in the blood, where they constitute 60% to 70% of lymphocytes, and in T-cell zones of peripheral lymphoid organs, such as the paracortical areas of lymph nodes and periarteriolar sheaths of the spleen (Fig. 6–3). The segregation of naive T cells to these anatomic sites is because the cells express receptors for chemoattractant cytokines (chemokines) that are produced only in these regions of lymphoid organs.[3,4] Each T cell is genetically programmed to recognize a specific cell-bound antigen by means of an antigen-specific T-cell receptor (TCR).[5] In approximately 95% of T cells, the TCR consists of a disulfide-linked heterodimer made up of an α and a β polypeptide chain (Fig. 6–4), each having a variable (antigen-binding) and a constant region. The αβ TCR recognizes peptide antigens that are displayed by major histocompatibil-

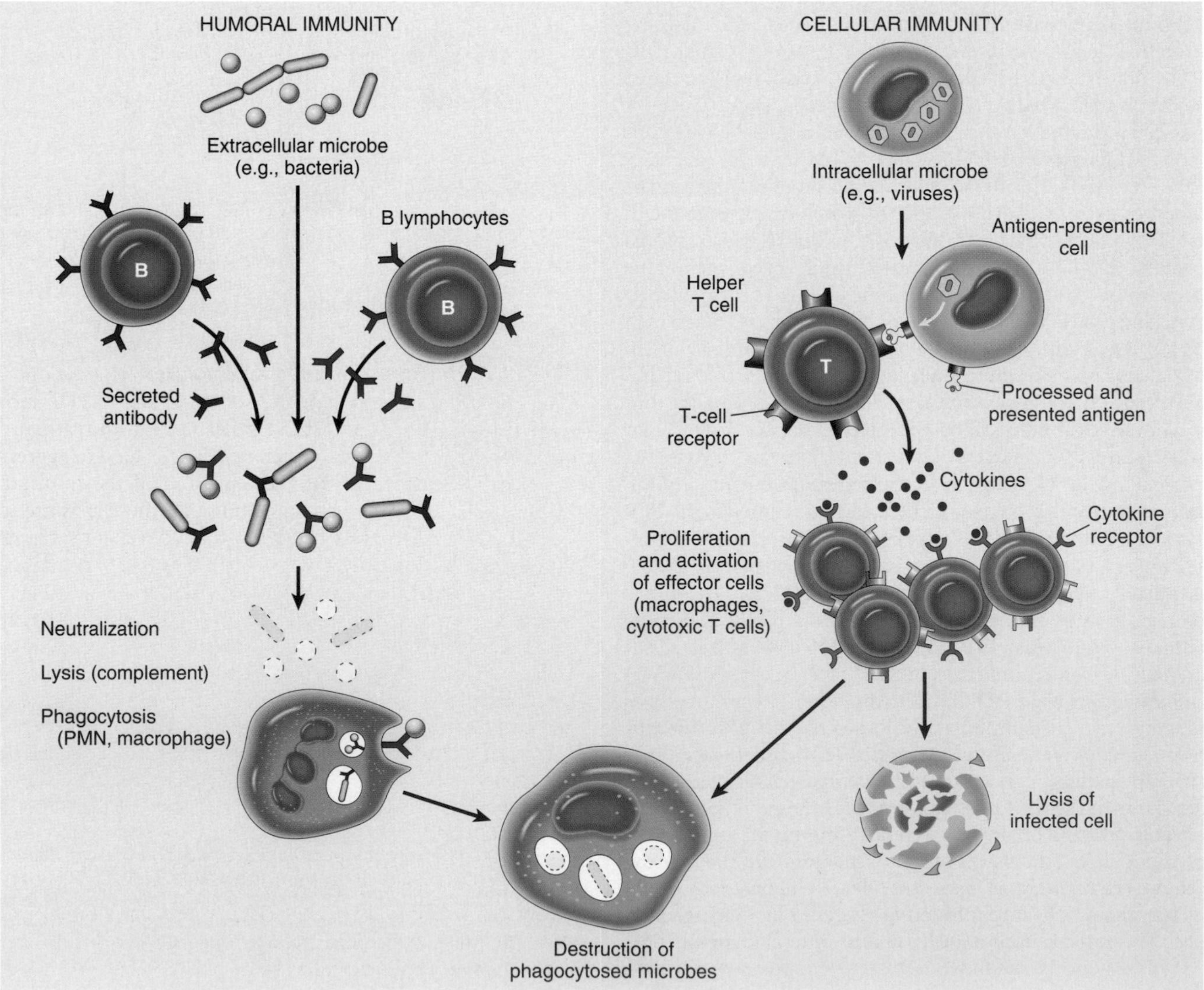

FIGURE 6–2 Humoral and cell-mediated immunity.

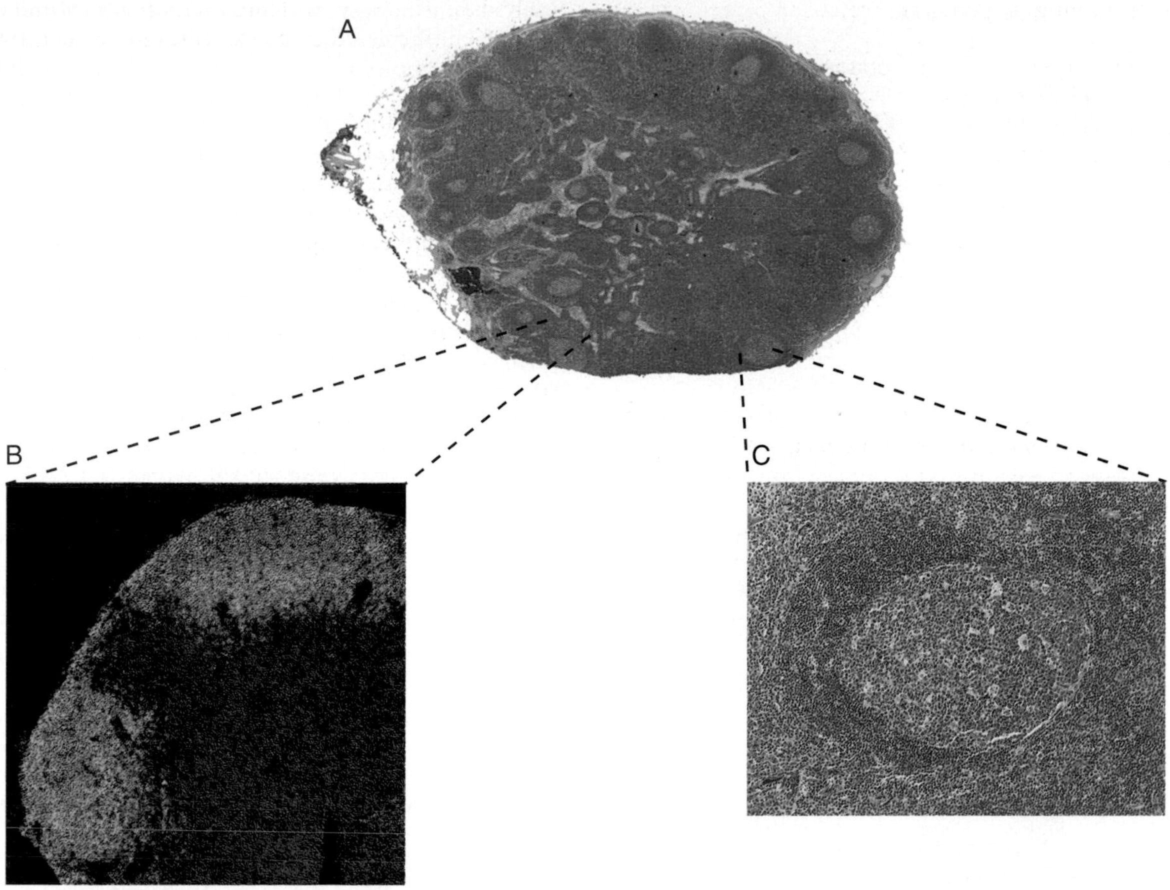

FIGURE 6–3 Histology of a lymph node. *A,* The organization of the lymph node, with an outer cortex containing follicles and an inner medulla. *B,* The location of B cells (stained green, using the immunofluorescence technique) and T cells (stained red) in a lymph node. *C,* A germinal center.

ity complex (MHC) molecules on the surfaces of antigen-presenting cells.[6] (The function of the MHC is described later.) T cells (in contrast to B cells) cannot be activated by soluble antigens; therefore, presentation of processed, membrane-bound antigens by antigen-presenting cells is required for induction of cell-mediated immunity. Each TCR is noncovalently linked to a cluster of five polypeptide chains, three of which form the CD3 molecular complex and two are a dimer of the ζ chain.[7] The CD3 and ζ proteins are invariant. They do not bind antigen but are involved in the transduction of signals into the T cell after the TCR has bound the antigen. T-cell receptors are capable of recognizing a very large number of peptides; each T cell expresses TCR molecules of one structure and specificity. TCR diversity is generated by somatic rearrangement of the genes that encode the TCR chains. As might be expected, every somatic cell has TCR genes from the germ line. Rearrangements of these genes occur only in T cells during their development in the thymus; hence the *presence of TCR gene rearrangements demonstrated by molecular analysis is a marker of T-lineage cells.* Such analyses are used in classification of lymphoid malignancies (Chapter 14). Furthermore, because each T cell has a unique DNA rearrangement (and hence a unique TCR), it is possible to distinguish polyclonal (non-neoplastic) T-cell proliferations from monoclonal (neoplastic) T-cell proliferations.

A minority of mature T cells express another type of TCR composed of γ and δ polypeptide chains.[8] The γδ TCR recognizes peptides, lipids, and small molecules, without a requirement for display by MHC proteins. γδ T cells tend to aggregate at epithelial surfaces, such as the mucosa of the respiratory and gastrointestinal tracts, suggesting that these cells are sentinels that protect against microbes that try to enter through these epithelia. However, the precise functions of γδ T cells are not known. Another small subset of T cells expresses markers that are found on natural killer (NK) cells; these cells are called NK-T cells. NK-T cells express a very limited diversity of TCRs, and they recognize glycolipids that are displayed by the MHC-like molecule CD1. The functions of NK-T cells are also not well defined.

In addition to CD3 and ζ proteins, T cells express a number of nonpolymorphic, function-associated molecules, also called accessory molecules, including CD4, CD8, CD2, integrins, and CD28. CD4 and CD8 are expressed on two mutually exclusive subsets of αβ T cells. CD4 is expressed on approximately 60% of mature CD3+ T cells, whereas CD8 is expressed on about 30% of T cells. These T-cell membrane-associated glycoproteins serve as coreceptors in T-cell activation. During antigen presentation, CD4 molecules bind to the nonpolymorphic portions of class II MHC molecules expressed on antigen-presenting cells (see Fig. 6–4). In con-

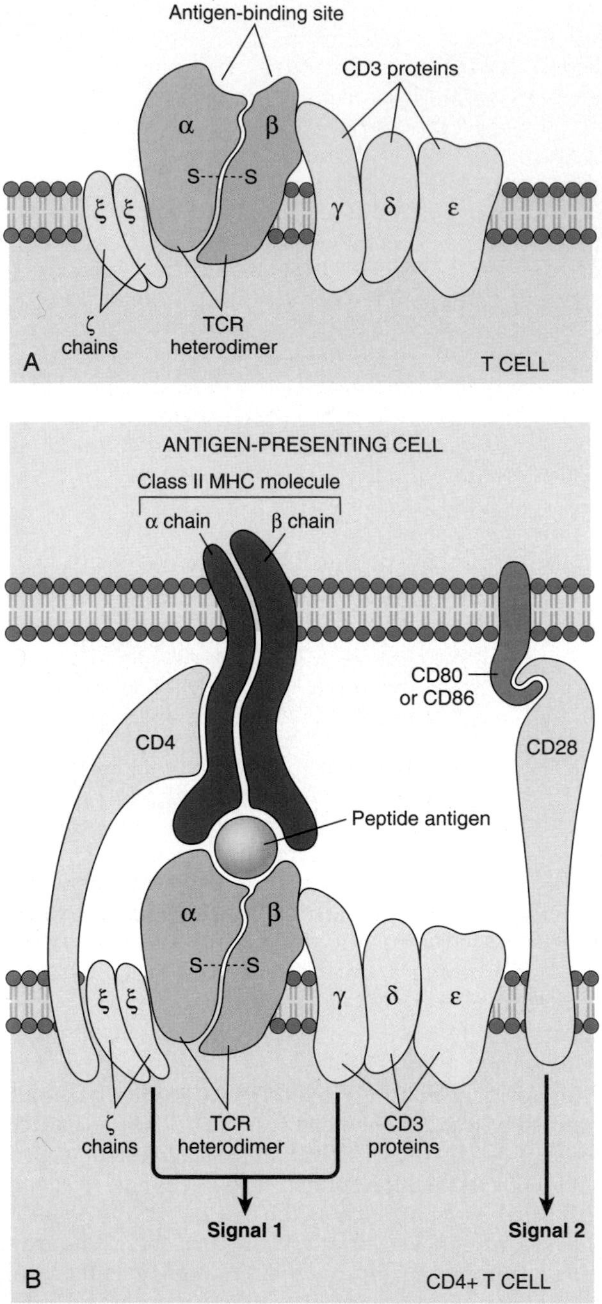

FIGURE 6–4 The T-cell receptor (TCR) complex. *A,* Schematic illustration of TCRα and TCRβ chains linked to the CD3 complex. *B,* Recognition of MHC-associated peptide displayed on an antigen-presenting cell (top) by the TCR. Note that the TCR-associated ζ chains and CD3 complex deliver signals (signal 1) upon antigen recognition, and CD28 delivers signals (signal 2) upon recognition of costimulators (B7 molecules).

trast, CD8 molecules bind to class I MHC molecules. CD4 and CD8 are required to initiate signals that activate T cells that recognize antigens. Because of this requirement for coreceptors, CD4+ helper T cells can recognize and respond to antigen only in the context of class II MHC molecules, whereas CD8+ cytotoxic T cells recognize cell-bound antigens only in association with class I MHC molecules. It is now well established that T cells need two signals for activation. Signal 1 is provided when the TCR is engaged by the appropriate MHC-bound antigen, and the coreceptors CD4 and CD8 bind to MHC molecules. Signal 2 is delivered by the interaction of the CD28 molecule on T cells with the costimulatory molecules B7-1 (CD80) and B7-2 (CD86) expressed on antigen-presenting cells (see Fig. 6–4). The importance of costimulation by this pathway is attested to by the fact that, in the absence of signal 2, the T cells fail to respond, undergo apoptosis, or become unreactive.[9] When T cells are activated by antigen and costimulators, they secrete locally acting proteins called *cytokines* (described below). Under the influence of a cytokine called interleukin-2 (IL-2), the T cells proliferate, thus generating a large number of antigen-specific lymphocytes. Some of these cells differentiate into effector cells, which perform the function of eliminating the antigen that started the response. Other activated cells differentiate into memory cells, which are long-lived and poised to respond rapidly to repeat encounters with the antigen.

CD4+ and CD8+ T cells perform distinct but somewhat overlapping effector functions.[10] The CD4+ T cell can be viewed as a master regulator—the conductor of a symphony orchestra, so to speak. By secreting cytokines, CD4+ T cells influence the function of virtually all other cells of the immune system, including other T cells, B cells, macrophages, and NK cells. The central role of CD4+ T cells is tragically illustrated when the human immunodeficiency virus cripples the immune system by selective destruction of this T-cell subset. In recent years, two functionally distinct populations of CD4+ helper cells have been recognized on the basis of the different cytokines they produce.[11] The T-helper-1 (T_H1) subset synthesizes and secretes IL-2 and interferon-γ (IFN-γ) but not IL-4 or IL-5, whereas T_H2 cells produce IL-4, IL-5 and IL-13 but not IL-2 or IFN-γ. This distinction is significant because the cytokines secreted by these subsets have different effects on other immune cells. The T_H1 subset is involved in facilitating delayed hypersensitivity, macrophage activation, and synthesis of opsonizing and complement-fixing antibodies, such as IgG2a in mice, all of which are actions of IFN-γ. The T_H2 subset aids in the synthesis of other classes of antibodies, notably IgE (mediated by IL-4 and IL-13) and in the activation of eosinophils (mediated by IL-5). CD8+ T cells function mainly as cytotoxic cells to kill other cells but, similar to CD4+ T cells, they can secrete cytokines, primarily of the T_H1 type.

B Lymphocytes

B lymphocytes develop from immature precursors in the bone marrow. Mature B cells constitute 10% to 20% of the circulating peripheral lymphocyte population and are also present in peripheral lymphoid tissues such as lymph nodes, spleen, or tonsils and extralymphatic organs such as the gastrointestinal tract. In lymph nodes, they are found in the superficial cortex. In the spleen, they are found in the white pulp. At both sites, they are aggregated in the form of lymphoid follicles, which on activation develop pale-staining germinal centers (see Fig. 6–3C). B cells are located in follicles, the B-cell zones of lymphoid organs, because the cells express receptors for a chemokine that is produced in follicles.[3,4]

B cells recognize antigen via the B-cell antigen receptor complex. Immunoglobulin M (IgM) and IgD, present on the surface of all naive B cells, constitute the antigen-binding component of the B-cell receptor complex (Fig. 6–5). As with

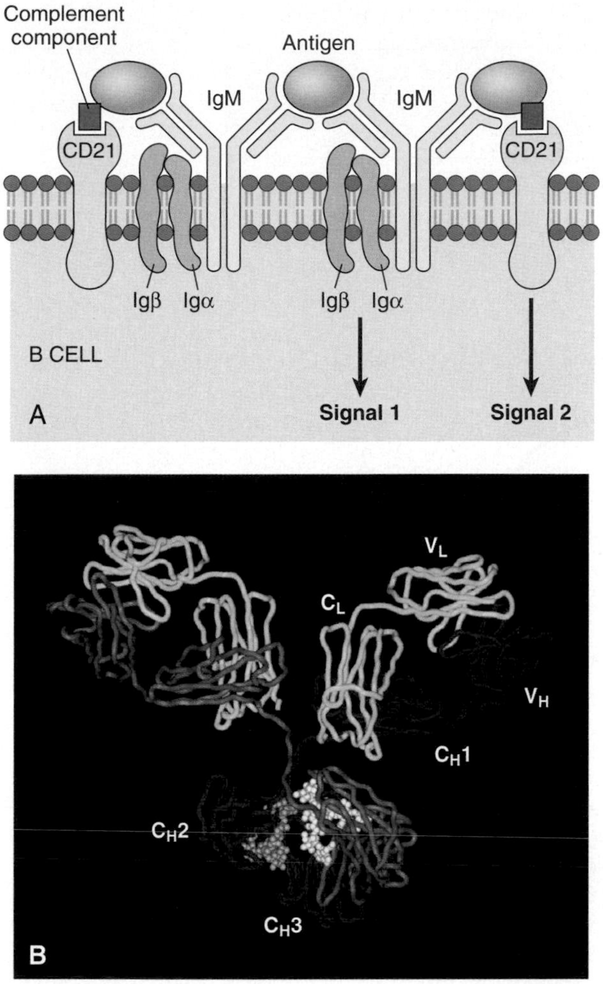

FIGURE 6–5 Structure of antibodies and the B-cell antigen receptor. *A,* The B-cell receptor complex composed of membrane IgM (or IgD, not shown) and the associated signaling proteins Igα and Igβ. CD21 is a receptor for a complement component that also promotes B-cell activation. *B,* Crystal structure of a secreted IgG molecule, showing the arrangement of the variable (V) and constant (C) regions of the heavy (H) and light (L) chains. (Courtesy of Dr. Alex McPherson, University of California, Irvine, CA.)

T cells, each B-cell receptor has unique antigen specificity, derived in part from somatic rearrangements of immunoglobulin genes. *Thus, the presence of rearranged immunoglobulin genes in a lymphoid cell is used as a molecular marker of B-lineage cells.* After antigenic stimulation, B cells form plasma cells that secrete immunoglobulins, which are the mediators of humoral immunity. In addition to membrane immunoglobulin, the B-cell antigen receptor complex contains a heterodimer of nonpolymorphic transmembrane proteins Igα and Igβ. Similar to the CD3 proteins of the TCR, Igα and Igβ do not bind antigen but are essential for signal transduction through the antigen receptor. B cells also express several other nonpolymorphic molecules that are essential for B-cell function. These include complement receptors, Fc receptors, and CD40. It is worthy of note that complement receptor-2 (CD21) is also the receptor for the Epstein-Barr virus (EBV), and hence EBV readily infects B cells.

B lymphocytes may be activated by protein and nonprotein antigens. The end result of B-cell activation is their differentiation into antibody-secreting cells, called plasma cells. Antibody-secreting cells reside in lymphoid organs and mucosal tissues, and some plasma cells may migrate to the bone marrow and live for many years in this tissue. Secreted antibodies enter mucosal secretions and the blood and are able to find, neutralize, and eliminate antigens. B-cell responses to protein antigens require help from CD4+ T cells.[12] Helper T cells activate B cells by engaging CD40, a member of the tumor necrosis factor (TNF)-receptor family, and by secreting cytokines. Activated helper T cells express CD40 ligand, which specifically binds to CD40 expressed on B cells.[13] This interaction is essential for B-cell maturation and secretion of IgG, IgA, and IgE antibodies. Patients with mutations in the CD40 ligand have an immunodeficiency disease called *X-linked hyper-IgM syndrome*, described later. Different cytokines stimulate B cells to produce different antibody classes, which perform distinct functions.

Macrophages

Macrophages are a part of the mononuclear phagocyte system; their origin, differentiation, and role in inflammation are discussed in Chapter 2. Here we need only to emphasize that macrophages play important roles both in the induction and in the effector phase of immune responses.

- Macrophages that have phagocytosed microbes and protein antigens process the antigens and present peptide fragments to T cells. Thus, macrophages are involved in the induction of cell-mediated immune responses.
- Macrophages are important effector cells in certain forms of cell-mediated immunity, such as the delayed hypersensitivity reaction. As mentioned earlier, macrophages are activated by cytokines, notably IFN-γ produced by the T_H1 subset of CD4+ cells. Such activation enhances the microbicidal properties of macrophages and augments their ability to kill tumor cells.
- Macrophages are also important in the effector phase of humoral immunity. As discussed in Chapter 2, macrophages phagocytose microbes that are opsonized (coated) by IgG or C3b.

Dendritic Cells

There are two types of cells with dendritic morphology that are functionally quite different. Both have numerous fine dendritic cytoplasmic processes, from which they derive their name. One type is called *interdigitating dendritic cells*, or just *dendritic cells*.[14,15] These cells are the most important antigen-presenting cells for initiating primary immune responses against protein antigens (Fig. 6–6). Several features of dendritic cells account for their key role in antigen presentation. First, these cells are located at the right place to capture antigens—under epithelia, the common site of entry of microbes and foreign antigens, and in the interstitia of all tissues, where antigens may be produced. Immature dendritic cells within the epidermis are called *Langerhans cells*. Second, dendritic cells express many receptors for capturing and responding to microbes (and other antigens), including TLRs and mannose receptors. Third, in response to microbes, dendritic cells express the same chemokine receptor as do naive T cells and are thus recruited to the T-cell zones of lymphoid organs,

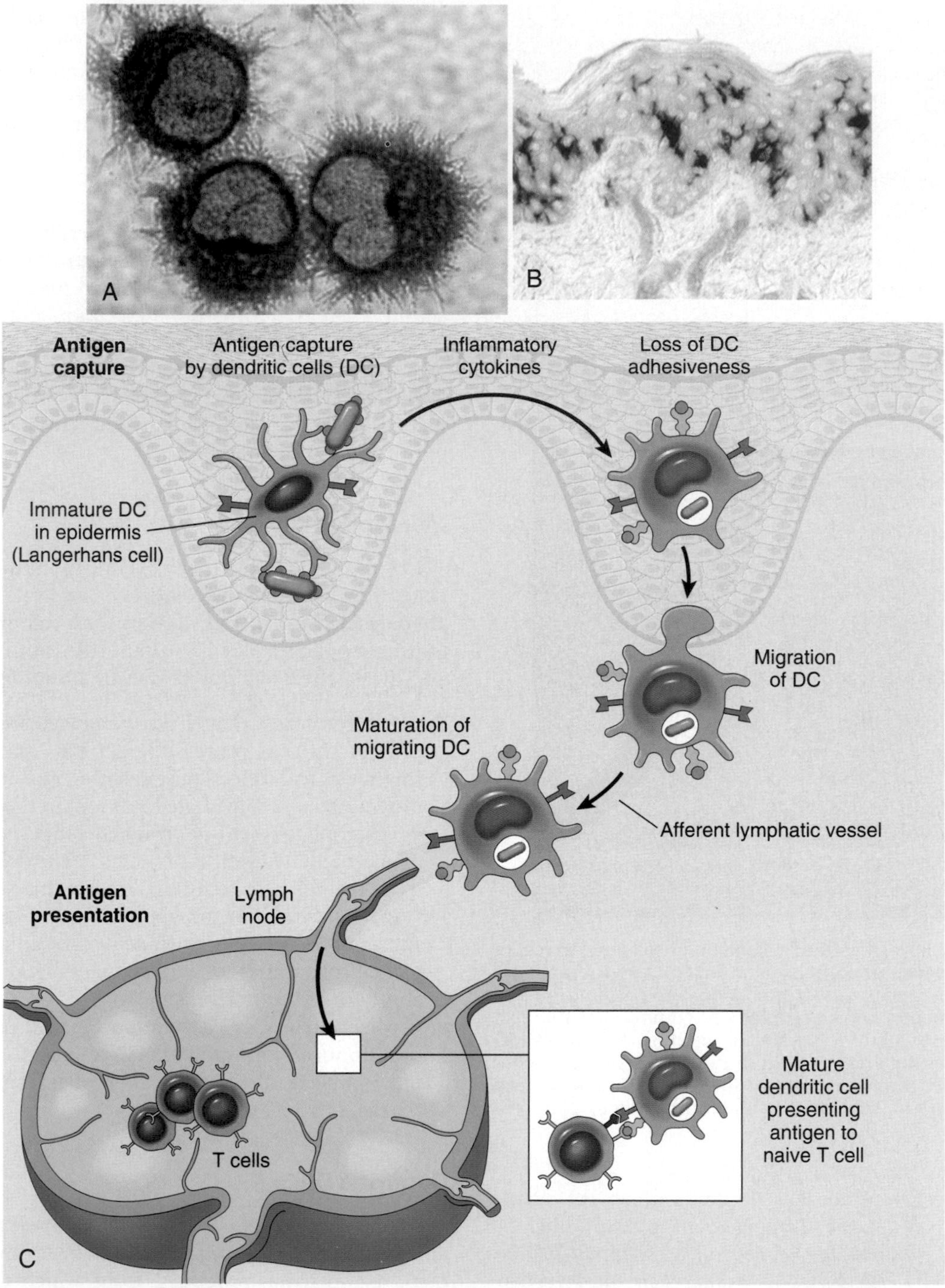

FIGURE 6–6 The morphology and functions of dendritic cells (DC). *A,* The morphology of cultured dendritic cells. (Courtesy of Dr. Y-J. Liu, M. D. Anderson Cancer Center, Houston.) *B,* The location of dendritic cells (Langerhans cells) in the epidermis. (Courtesy of Dr. Y-J. Liu, M. D. Anderson Cancer Center, Houston.) *C,* The role of dendritic cells in capturing microbial antigens from epithelia and transporting them to regional lymph nodes.

where they are ideally located to present antigens to recirculating T cells. Fourth, dendritic cells express high levels of MHC class II molecules as well as the costimulatory molecules B7-1 and B7-2. Thus, they possess all the machinery needed for presenting antigens to and activating CD4+ T cells.

The other type of cells with dendritic morphology is present in the germinal centers of lymphoid follicles in the spleen and lymph nodes and is hence called *follicular dendritic cells.* These cells bear Fc receptors for IgG and receptors for C3b and can trap antigen bound to antibodies or complement proteins. Such cells play a role in ongoing immune responses by presenting antigens to B cells and selecting the B cells that have the highest affinity for the antigen, thus improving the quality of the humoral immune response. Follicular dendritic cells also play a role in the pathogenesis of the acquired immunodeficiency syndrome (AIDS) and are discussed in this context later in the chapter.

Natural Killer Cells

NK cells make up approximately 10% to 15% of the peripheral blood lymphocytes and do not bear T-cell receptors or cell surface immunoglobulins. Morphologically, NK cells are somewhat larger than small lymphocytes, and they contain abundant azurophilic granules (Fig. 6–7). Hence, they are also called *large granular lymphocytes*. NK cells are endowed with an innate ability to kill a variety of tumor cells, virally infected cells, and some normal cells, without previous sensitization.[16] These cells are part of the innate immune system, and they may be the first line of defense against viral infections and, perhaps, some tumors. NK cells do not rearrange T-cell receptor genes and are CD3 negative. Two cell surface molecules, CD16 and CD56, are widely used to identify NK cells. CD16 is the Fc receptor for IgG and it endows NK cells with another function, the ability to lyse IgG-coated target cells. This phenomenon, known as *antibody-dependent cell-mediated cytotoxicity*, is described in greater detail later.

The functional activity of NK cells is regulated by a balance between signals from activating and inhibitory receptors. The activating receptors stimulate NK cell killing by recognizing ill-defined molecules on target cells, some of which may be viral products; the inhibitory receptors inhibit the activation of NK cells by recognition of self-class I MHC molecules. The class I MHC–recognizing inhibitory receptors on NK cells are aptly called killer inhibitory receptors. They are biochemically distinct from T-cell receptors. It is believed that NK cells are inhibited from killing normal cells because all nucleated normal cells express self-class I MHC molecules.[14] If virus infection or neoplastic transformation perturbs or reduces the expression of class I MHC molecules, inhibitory signals delivered to NK cells are interrupted, and lysis occurs (Fig. 6–8). However, merely the absence of inhibition is not sufficient for NK cell–mediated killing, and NK cell–mediated killing requires triggering of activating receptors in conjunction with release of inhibitory receptors. Several types of activating receptors have been discovered, including members of the NKG2D family and some Ig-like receptors. The NKG2D receptors recognize stress-induced proteins that are normally expressed by only a few cells in the gut epithelium but whose expression increases on many cells following viral infection or neoplastic transformation. Other activating receptors recognize viral proteins that are structurally similar to class I MHC molecules. Thus, NK cells are activated by contact with virus-infected and tumor cells, both of which often express reduced

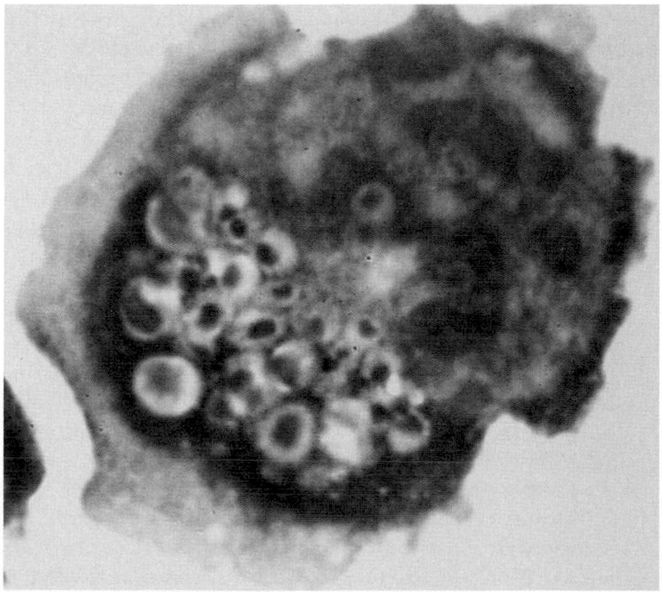

FIGURE 6–7 A highly activated natural killer cell with abundant cytoplasmic granules. (Courtesy of Dr. Noelle Williams, Department of Pathology, University of Texas Southwestern Medical School, Dallas, TX.)

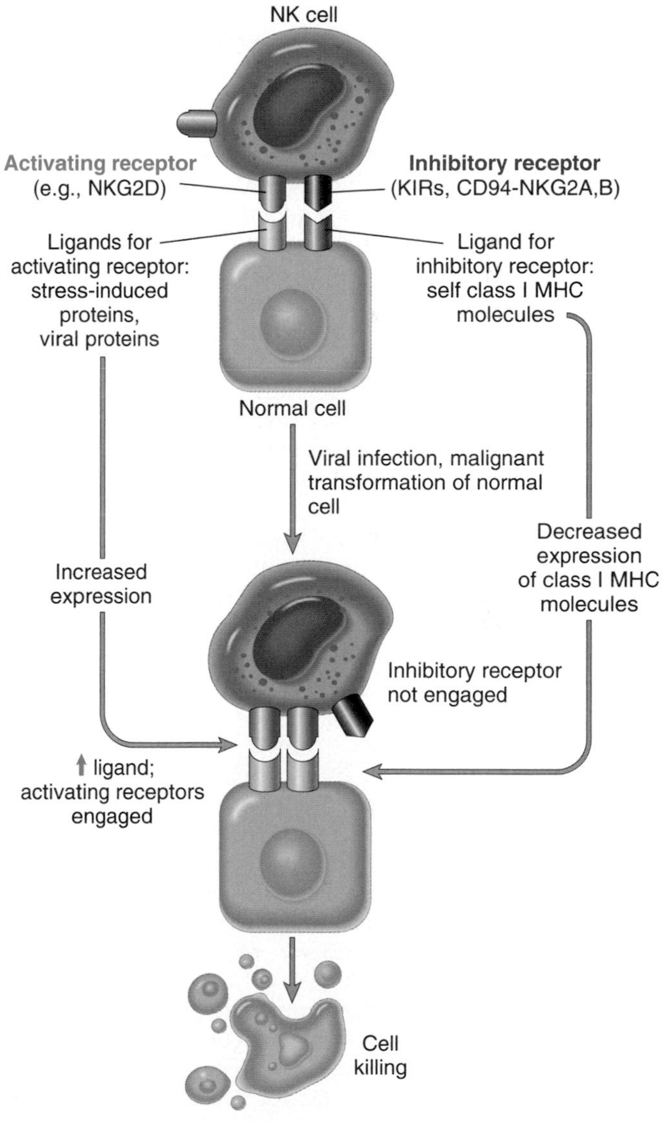

FIGURE 6–8 Schematic representation of NK-cell receptors and killing. NK cells express activating and inhibitory receptors; some examples of each are indicated. Normal cells are not killed because inhibitory signals from normal MHC class I molecules override activating signals. In tumor cells or virus-infected cells, there is increased expression of ligands for activating receptors, and reduced expression or alteration of MHC molecules, which interrupts the inhibitory signals, allowing activation of NK cells and lysis of target cells. KIR, killer cell Ig-like recepors.

levels of class I MHC molecules and therefore do not engage inhibitory receptors.

NK cells also secrete cytokines, such as IFN-γ, TNF, and granulocyte macrophage colony-stimulating factor (GM-CSF). IFN-γ activates macrophages to destroy ingested microbes, and thus NK cells provide early defense against intracellular microbial infections. IFN-γ also promotes the differentiation of naive CD4+ T-cells into T_H1 cells. Thus, activation of NK cells early in the immune response can favor induction of delayed hypersensitivity and secretion of opsonizing antibodies by promoting the development of T_H1 cells. The activity of NK cells is regulated by many cytokines, including IL-2, IL-15, and IL-12. IL-2 and IL-15 stimulate proliferation of NK cells, whereas IL-12 activates killing and secretion of IFN-γ.

CYTOKINES: MESSENGER MOLECULES OF THE IMMUNE SYSTEM

The induction and regulation of immune responses involve multiple interactions among lymphocytes, monocytes, inflammatory cells (e.g., neutrophils), and endothelial cells. Many such interactions depend on cell-to-cell contact; however, many interactions and effector functions are mediated by short-acting soluble mediators, called *cytokines.* This term includes the previously designated lymphokines (lymphocyte-derived), monokines (monocyte-derived), and several other polypeptides that regulate immunologic, inflammatory, and reparative host responses. Molecularly defined cytokines are called *interleukins*, implying that they mediate communications between leukocytes. Most cytokines have a wide spectrum of effects, and some are produced by several different cell types.

A large number of cytokines have been identified by molecular cloning, and the list continues to grow. Below we summarize the main cytokines whose functions are well established. It is convenient to classify these mediators into distinct functional classes, although many belong to multiple categories.

- Cytokines that mediate innate (natural) immunity. Included in this group are IL-1, TNF (tumor necrosis factor, also called TNF-α), type 1 interferons, and IL-6. Some cytokines, such as IL-12 and IFN-γ, are involved in both innate and adaptive immunity against intracellular microbes. Certain of these cytokines (e.g., the interferons) protect against viral infections, whereas others (e.g., IL-1 and TNF) promote leukocyte recruitment and acute inflammatory responses.
- Cytokines that regulate lymphocyte growth, activation, and differentiation. Within this category are IL-2, IL-4, IL-12, IL-15, and transforming growth factor-β (TGF-β). IL-2 is an important growth factor for T-cells, IL-4 stimulates differentiation to the T_H2 pathway and acts on B cells as well, IL-12 stimulates differentiation to the T_H1 pathway, and IL-15 stimulates the growth and activity of NK cells. Other cytokines in this group, such as IL-10 and TGF-β, down-regulate immune responses.
- Cytokines that activate inflammatory cells. In this category are IFN-γ, which activates macrophages; IL-5, which activates eosinophils; and TNF and lymphotoxin (also called TNF-β), which induce acute inflammation by acting on neutrophils and endothelial cells.
- Cytokines that affect leukocyte movement are also called *chemokines* (Chapter 2). Most fall into two structurally distinct subfamilies, referred to as C-C and C-X-C chemokines, on the basis of the position of cysteine (c) residues. The C-X-C chemokines are produced mainly by activated macrophages and tissue cells (e.g., endothelium), whereas the C-C chemokines are produced largely by T cells. Different chemokines recruit different types of leukocytes to sites of inflammation. Chemokines are also normally produced in tissues and are responsible for the anatomic localization of different cell types, for example, the location of T and B cells in distinct regions of lymphoid organs (see Fig. 6–3).
- Cytokines that stimulate hematopoiesis. Many cytokines derived from lymphocytes or stromal cells stimulate the growth and production of new blood cells by acting on hematopoietic progenitor cells. Several members of this family are called *colony-stimulating factors* (CSFs) because they were initially detected by their ability to promote the in vitro growth of hematopoietic cell colonies from the bone marrow. Some members of this group (e.g., GM-CSF and G-CSF) act on committed progenitor cells, whereas others, exemplified by stem cell factor (c-kit ligand), act on pluripotent stem cells.

General Properties of Cytokines

Although cytokines have many diverse actions, all of them share some important properties.

- Many individual cytokines are produced by several different cell types. For example, IL-1 can be produced by virtually any cell leukocytes, endothelial cells, and fibroblasts.
- The actions of cytokines are pleiotropic, meaning that any one cytokine may act on many cell types and mediate many effects. For example, IL-2, initially discovered as a T-cell growth factor, is known to affect the growth and differentiation of B cells and NK cells as well. Cytokines are also often redundant, meaning that different cytokines may stimulate the same or overlapping biologic responses.
- Cytokines induce their effects in three ways: (1) They act on the same cell that produces them (*autocrine* effect), such as occurs when IL-2 produced by antigen-stimulated T cells stimulates the growth of the same cells; (2) they affect other cells in their vicinity (*paracrine* effect), as occurs when IL-7 produced by bone marrow or thymic stromal cells promotes the maturation of B-cell progenitors in the marrow or T-cell precursors in the thymus, respectively; and (3) they affect many cells systemically (*endocrine* effect), the best examples in this category being IL-1 and TNF, which produce the systemic acute-phase response during inflammation.
- Cytokines mediate their effects by binding to specific high-affinity receptors on their target cells. For example, IL-2 activates T cells by binding to high-affinity IL-2 receptors (IL-2R). Blockade of the IL-2R by specific antireceptor monoclonal antibodies prevents T-cell activation. This observation is the basis for the use of anti-IL-2R antibodies to control undesirable T-cell activation, as in transplant rejection.

The knowledge gained about cytokines has practical therapeutic ramifications. First, by inhibiting cytokine production or action, it may be possible to control the harmful effects of inflammation or tissue-damaging immune reactions. Patients with rheumatoid arthritis often show dramatic responses to TNF antagonists, an elegant example of such therapy. Second, recombinant cytokines can be administered to enhance immunity against cancer or microbial infections (immunotherapy).

STRUCTURE AND FUNCTION OF HISTOCOMPATIBILITY MOLECULES

Although originally identified as antigens that evoke rejection of transplanted organs, histocompatibility molecules are now known to be extremely important for the induction and regulation of the immune response. *The principal physiologic function of the cell surface histocompatibility molecules is to bind peptide fragments of foreign proteins for presentation to antigen-specific T cells.* Recall that T cells (in contrast to B cells) can recognize only membrane-bound antigens, and hence histocompatibility molecules are critical to the induction of T-cell immunity. Here we summarize the salient features of human histocompatibility molecules, primarily to facilitate understanding of their role in rejection of organ transplants and in disease susceptibility.

In humans, the genes encoding the most important histocompatibility molecules are clustered on a small segment of chromosome 6, the *major histocompatibility complex*, or the *human leukocyte antigen* (HLA) complex in humans (Fig. 6–9), so named because MHC-encoded antigens were initially detected on leukocytes. The HLA system is highly polymorphic, meaning that there are many alleles of each MHC gene in the population and each individual inherits one (often unique) set of these alleles. This, as we see subsequently, constitutes a formidable barrier in organ transplantation.

On the basis of their chemical structure, tissue distribution, and function, the MHC gene products are classified into three categories. Class I and class II genes encode cell surface glycoproteins involved in antigen presentation. Class III genes encode components of the complement system (Chapter 2), and are not discussed in this section.

Class I MHC molecules are expressed on all nucleated cells and platelets. They are encoded by three closely linked loci, designated HLA-A, HLA-B, and HLA-C (see Fig. 6–9). Each of these molecules is a heterodimer, consisting of a polymorphic α, or heavy, chain (44-kD) linked noncovalently to a smaller (12-kD) nonpolymorphic peptide called *β_2-microglobulin*, which is not encoded within the MHC. The extracellular region of the heavy chain is divided into three domains: α_1, α_2, and α_3 (see Fig. 6–9). Crystal structure of class I molecules has revealed that the α_1 and α_2 domains form a cleft, or groove, where peptides bind to the MHC molecule.[17] Biochemical analyses of several different class I alleles have revealed that almost all polymorphic residues line the sides or the base of the peptide-binding groove. As a result, different

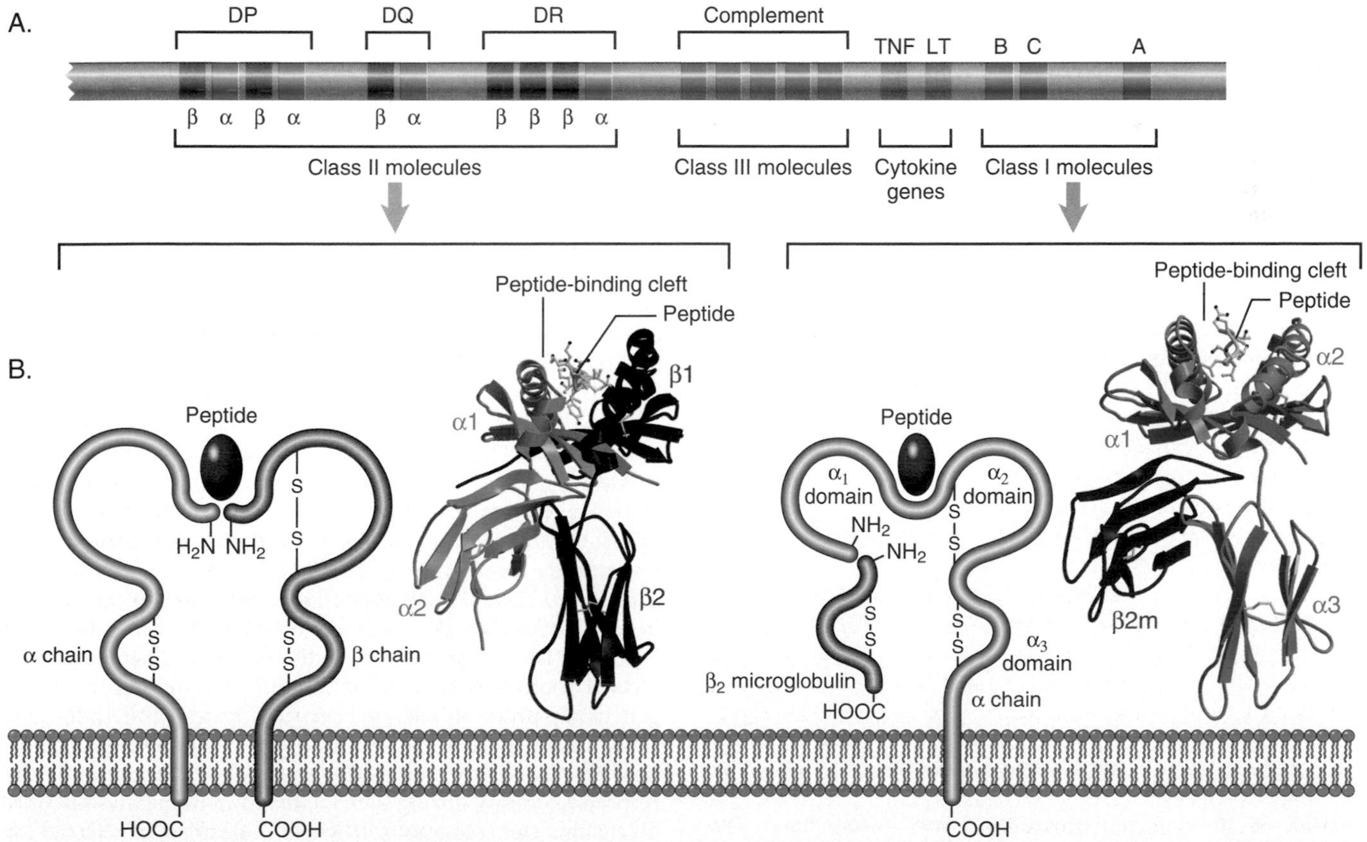

FIGURE 6–9 The HLA complex and the structure of HLA molecules. *A,* The location of genes in the HLA complex is shown. The sizes and distances between genes are not to scale. *B,* Schematic diagrams and crystal structures of class I and class II HLA molecules. (Crystal structures are courtesy of Dr. P. Bjorkman, California Institute of Technology, Pasadena, CA.)

class I alleles bind and display different peptide fragments. In general, class I MHC molecules bind and display peptides that are derived from proteins, such as viral antigens, synthesized within the cell. The generation of peptide fragments within the cells, and their association with MHC molecules and transport to the cell surface, is a complex process.[18] Involved in this sequence are proteolytic complexes (proteasomes), which digest antigenic proteins in the cytoplasm into short peptides, and transport proteins, which ferry peptide fragments from the cytoplasm to the endoplasmic reticulum. Within the endoplasmic reticulum, peptides bind to the antigen-binding cleft of newly synthesized class I heavy chains, which then associate with β_2-microglobulin to form a stable trimer that is transported to the cell surface for presentation to CD8+ cytotoxic T lymphocytes (Fig. 6–10). In this interaction, the TCR recognizes the MHC–peptide complex, and the CD8 molecule, acting as a coreceptor, binds to the nonpolymorphic α_3 domain of the class I heavy chain. CD8+ cytotoxic

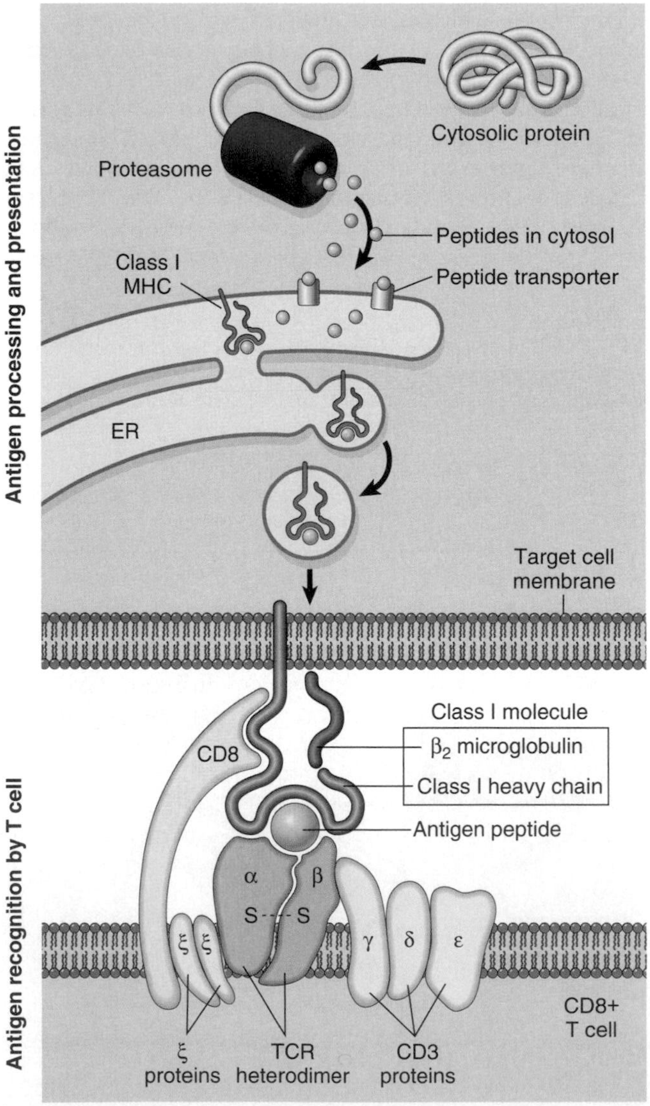

FIGURE 6–10 Antigen processing and recognition. The sequence of events in the processing of a cytoplasmic protein antigen and its display by class I MHC molecules are shown at the top. The recognition of this MHC-displayed peptide by a CD8+ T cell is shown at the bottom.

T cells can recognize viral (or other) peptides only if presented as a complex with self-class I antigens, and therefore CD8+ T cells are said to be *class I MHC–restricted.* In the eyes of T cells, self-MHC molecules are those that they "grew up with" during maturation within the thymus. Because one of the important functions of CD8+ T cells is to eliminate viruses, which may infect any nucleated cell, it makes good sense to have widespread expression of class I HLA molecules.

Class II MHC molecules are coded for in a region called *HLA-D*, which has three subregions: HLA-DP, HLA-DQ, and HLA-DR. Each class II molecule is a heterodimer consisting of a noncovalently associated α chain and β chain. Both chains are polymorphic, and each of the three HLA-D subregions encodes one α chain and one β chain (see Fig. 6–9). The extracellular portions of the α and β chains have two domains each: α_1, α_2 and β_1, β_2. Crystal structure of class II molecules has revealed that, similar to class I molecules, they have an antigen-binding cleft facing outward.[17] In contrast to class I molecules, however, the antigen-binding cleft is formed by an interaction of the α_1 and β_1 domains of both chains, and it is in this portion that most class II alleles differ. Thus, it seems that, as with class I molecules, polymorphism of class II molecules is associated with differential binding of antigenic peptides. The nature of peptides that bind to class II molecules is different from that of peptides that bind to class I molecules. In general, class II molecules present exogenous antigens (e.g., extracellular microbes, soluble proteins) that are first internalized and processed in the endosomes or lysosomes. Peptides resulting from proteolytic cleavage then associate with class II heterodimers that were assembled in the endoplasmic reticulum and transported into the vesicles. Finally, the peptide–MHC complex is transported to the cell surface, where it can be recognized by CD4+ helper T cells. In this interaction, the CD4 molecule acts as the coreceptor. Because CD4+ T cells can recognize antigens only in the context of self-class II molecules, they are referred to as *class II MHC–restricted.* In contrast to class I molecules, the tissue distribution of MHC class II molecules is largely restricted to antigen-presenting cells (macrophages, dendritic cells, and B cells). Expression of class II molecules can be induced on several other cell types, however, including endothelial cells and fibroblasts, by the action of IFN-γ.

MHC molecules play key roles in regulating T cell–mediated immune responses in two ways. First, because different antigenic peptides bind to different class II gene products, it follows that an individual mounts a vigorous immune response against an antigen only if he or she inherits the gene(s) for those class II molecule(s) that can bind the antigen and present it to helper T cells. The consequences of inheriting a given class II gene depend on the nature of the antigen bound by the class II molecule. For example, if the antigen is a peptide from ragweed pollen, the individual who expresses class II molecules capable of binding the antigen would be genetically prone to allergic reactions against pollen. In contrast, an inherited capacity to bind a bacterial peptide may provide resistance to disease by evoking a protective antibody response. Second, during their maturation in the thymus, only T cells that can recognize self-MHC molecules are selected for export to the periphery. Thus, the type of MHC molecules that T cells encounter during their development influences the reactivity of mature peripheral T cells.

HLA and Disease Association

A variety of diseases have been found to be associated with certain HLA alleles (Table 6–1).[17] The best known is the association between ankylosing spondylitis and HLA-B27; individuals who inherit this allele have a 90-fold greater chance (relative risk) of developing the disease than those who are negative for HLA-B27. The diseases that show association with the HLA locus can be broadly grouped into the following categories:

1. *Inflammatory diseases*, including ankylosing spondylitis and several postinfectious arthropathies, all associated with HLA-B27
2. *Inherited errors of metabolism*, such as 21-hydroxylase deficiency (HLA-BW47) and hereditary hemochromatosis (HLA-A)
3. *Autoimmune diseases*, including autoimmune endocrinopathies, associated mainly with alleles at the DR locus.

The mechanisms underlying these associations are not fully understood. In some cases (e.g., 21-hydroxylase deficiency), the linkage results from the fact that the relevant disease-associated gene, in this case the gene for 21-hydroxylase, maps within the HLA complex. Similarly, in hereditary hemochromatosis, a gene that is mutated, called *HFE*, maps within the HLA locus. *HFE* resembles MHC molecules structurally, but its function is not in the presentation of antigens to T cells but in the regulation of iron transport (Chapter 18). In the case of immunologically mediated disorders, it seems likely that the role of HLA class II molecules in regulating immune responsiveness may be relevant.

Disorders of the Immune System

Having reviewed some fundamentals of basic immunology, we can now turn to general features of immunologic tissue injury and immunopathology, and some specific immunologic diseases. Our discussion is divided into four broad headings:

- *Hypersensitivity reactions*, which give rise to immunologic injury in a variety of diseases, discussed throughout this book
- *Autoimmune diseases*, which are caused by immune reactions against self
- *Immunologic deficiency syndromes*, which result from genetically determined or acquired defects in some components of the normal immune system
- *Amyloidosis*, a poorly understood disorder having immunologic association.

TABLE 6–1 Association of HLA with Disease

Disease	HLA Allele	Relative Risk
Ankylosing spondylitis	B27	90
Postgonococcal arthritis	B27	14
Acute anterior uveitis	B27	14
Rheumatoid arthritis	DR4	4
Chronic active hepatitis	DR3	13
Primary Sjögren syndrome	DR3	9
Type-1 diabetes	DR3	5
	DR4	6
	DR3/DR4	20

MECHANISMS OF HYPERSENSITIVITY REACTIONS

Humans live in an environment teeming with substances capable of producing immunologic responses. Contact with antigen leads not only to induction of a protective immune response, but also to reactions that can be damaging to tissues. Exogenous antigens occur in dust, pollens, foods, drugs, microbiologic agents, chemicals, and many blood products used in clinical practice. The immune responses that may result from such exogenous antigens take a variety of forms, ranging from annoying but trivial discomforts, such as itching of the skin, to potentially fatal diseases, such as bronchial asthma. The various reactions produced are called *hypersensitivity reactions*, and tissue injury in these reactions may be caused by humoral or cell-mediated immune mechanisms.

Injurious immune reactions may be evoked not only by exogenous environmental antigens, but also by endogenous tissue antigens. Some of these immune reactions are triggered by homologous antigens that differ among individuals with different genetic backgrounds. Transfusion reactions and graft rejection are examples of immunologic disorders evoked by homologous antigens. Another category of disorders, those incited by self-, or autologous, antigens, constitutes the important group of autoimmune diseases (discussed later). These diseases arise because of the emergence of immune responses against self-antigens.

Hypersensitivity diseases can be classified on the basis of the immunologic mechanism that mediates the disease (Table 6–2). This classification is of value in distinguishing the manner in which the immune response ultimately causes tissue injury and disease, and the accompanying pathologic alterations. Prototypes of each of these immune mechanisms are presented in the subsequent sections.

- In *immediate hypersensitivity (type I hypersensitivity)*, the immune response releases vasoactive and spasmogenic substances that act on vessels and smooth muscle and proinflammatory cytokines that recruit inflammatory cells.
- In *antibody-mediated disorders (type II hypersensitivity)*, secreted antibodies participate directly in injury to cells by promoting their phagocytosis or lysis and injury to tissues by inducing inflammation. Antibodies may also interfere with cellular functions and cause disease without tissue injury.
- In *immune complex–mediated disorders (type III hypersensitivity)*, antibodies bind antigens and then induce inflammation directly or by activating complement. The leukocytes that are recruited (neutrophils and monocytes) produce tissue damage by release of lysosomal enzymes and generation of toxic free radicals.
- In *cell-mediated immune disorders (type IV hypersensitivity)*, sensitized T lymphocytes are the cause of the cellular and tissue injury.

Most hypersensitivity diseases show a genetic predisposition. Modern methods of mapping disease-associated suscep-

TABLE 6–2 Mechanisms of Immunologically Mediated Diseases

Type	Prototype Disorder	Immune Mechanisms	Pathologic Lesions
Immediate (type I) hypersensitivity	Anaphylaxis; allergies; bronchial asthma (atopic forms)	Production of IgE antibody → immediate release of vasoactive amines and other mediators from mast cells; recruitment of inflammatory cells (late-phase reaction)	Vascular dilation, edema, smooth muscle contraction, mucus production, inflammation
Antibody-mediated (type II) hypersensitivity	Autoimmune hemolytic anemia; Goodpasture syndrome	Production of IgG, IgM → binds to antigen on target cell or tissue → phagocytosis or lysis of target cell by activated complement or Fc receptors; recruitment of leukocytes	Cell lysis; inflammation
Immune complex–mediated (type III) hypersensitivity	Systemic lupus erythematosus; some forms of glomerulonephritis; serum sickness; Arthus reaction	Deposition of antigen–antibody complexes → complement activation → recruitment of leukocytes by complement products and Fc receptors → release of enzymes and other toxic molecules	Necrotizing vasculitis (fibrinoid necrosis); inflammation
Cell-mediated (type IV) hypersensitivity	Contact dermatitis; multiple sclerosis; type I, diabetes; transplant rejection; tuberculosis	Activated T lymphocytes → i) release of cytokines and macrophage activation; ii) T cell–mediated cytotoxicity	Perivascular cellular infiltrates; edema; cell destruction; granuloma formation

tibility genes are revealing the complex nature of these genetic influences. Many susceptibility loci have been identified in different diseases. Among the genes known to be associated with hypersensitivity diseases are MHC genes, but many non-MHC genes also play a role.

Immediate (Type I) Hypersensitivity

Immediate, or type I, hypersensitivity is a rapidly developing immunologic reaction occurring within minutes after the combination of an antigen with antibody bound to mast cells in individuals previously sensitized to the antigen.[20,21] These reactions are often called allergy, and the antigens that elicit them are allergens. Immediate hypersensitivity may occur as a systemic disorder or as a local reaction. The systemic reaction usually follows injection of an antigen to which the host has become sensitized. Often within minutes, a state of shock is produced, which is sometimes fatal. The nature of local reactions varies depending on the portal of entry of the allergen and may take the form of localized cutaneous swellings (skin allergy, hives), nasal and conjunctival discharge (allergic rhinitis and conjunctivitis), hay fever, bronchial asthma, or allergic gastroenteritis (food allergy). Many local type I hypersensitivity reactions have two well-defined phases (Fig. 6–11). The *immediate, or initial, response* is characterized by vasodilation, vascular leakage, and depending on the location, smooth muscle spasm or glandular secretions. These changes usually become evident within 5 to 30 minutes after exposure to an allergen and tend to subside in 60 minutes. In many instances (e.g., allergic rhinitis and bronchial asthma), a *second, late-phase* reaction sets in 2 to 24 hours later without additional exposure to antigen and may last for several days. This late-phase reaction is characterized by infiltration of tissues with eosinophils, neutrophils, basophils, monocytes, and CD4+ T cells as well as tissue destruction, typically in the form of mucosal epithelial cell damage.

Because mast cells are central to the development of immediate hypersensitivity, we first review some of their salient characteristics and then discuss the immune mechanisms that underlie this form of hypersensitivity.[22] *Mast cells* are bone

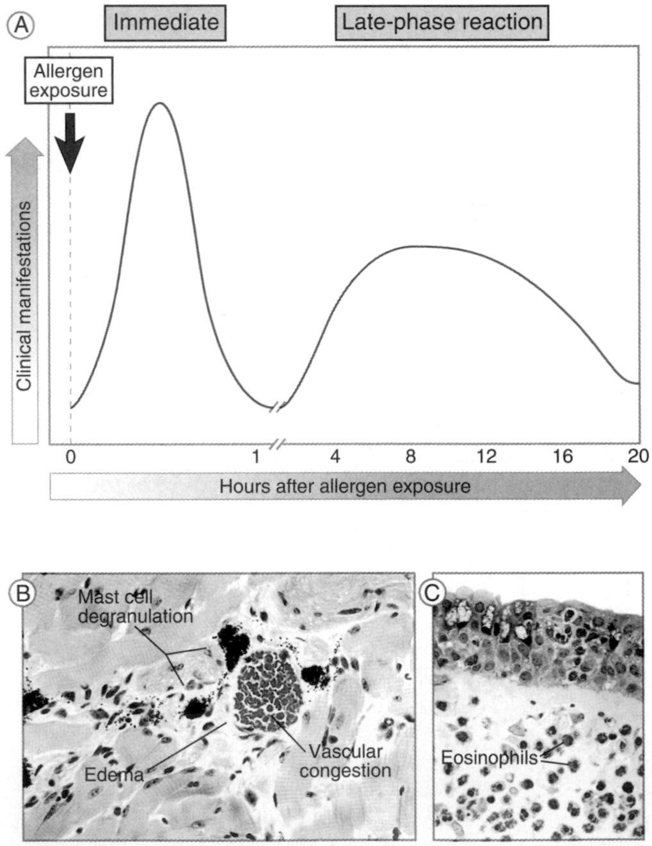

FIGURE 6–11 Immediate hypersensitivity. *A,* Kinetics of the immediate and late-phase reactions. The immediate vascular and smooth muscle reaction to allergen develops within minutes after challenge (allergen exposure in a previously sensitized individual), and the late-phase reaction develops 2 to 24 hours later. *B, C,* Morphology: The immediate reaction (*B*) is characterized by vasodilation, congestion, and edema, and the late phase reaction (*C*) is characterized by an inflammatory infiltrate rich in eosinophils, neutrophils, and T cells. (Courtesy of Dr. Daniel Friend, Department of Pathology, Brigham and Women's Hospital, Boston, MA.)

marrow–derived cells that are widely distributed in the tissues. They are found predominantly near blood vessels and nerves and in subepithelial sites, where local immediate hypersensitivity reactions tend to occur. Mast cells have cytoplasmic membrane-bound granules that contain a variety of biologically active mediators. In addition, mast-cell granules contain acidic proteoglycans that bind basic dyes such as toluidine blue. Because the stained granules often acquire a color that is different from that of the native dye, they are referred to as *metachromatic* granules. As is detailed next, mast cells (and basophils) are activated by the cross-linking of high-affinity IgE Fc receptors; in addition, mast cells may also be triggered by several other stimuli, such as complement components C5a and C3a (anaphylatoxins), both of which act by binding to their receptors on the mast-cell membrane. Other mast-cell secretagogues include macrophage-derived cytokines (e.g., IL-8), some drugs such as codeine and morphine, adenosine, mellitin (present in bee venom), and physical stimuli (e.g., heat, cold, sunlight). Basophils are similar to mast cells in many respects, including the presence of cell-surface IgE Fc receptors as well as cytoplasmic granules. In contrast to mast cells, however, basophils are not normally present in tissues but rather circulate in the blood in extremely small numbers. (Most allergic reactions occur in tissues, and the role of basophils in these reactions is not as well established as that of mast cells.) Similar to other granulocytes, basophils can be recruited to inflammatory sites.

Most immediate hypersensitivity reactions are mediated by IgE antibodies. IgE-secreting B cells differentiate from naive (membrane IgM and IgD-expressing) B cells, and this process is dependent on the activity of CD4+ helper T cells of the T_H2 type (Fig. 6–12). Hence, T_H2 cells are pivotal in the pathogen-

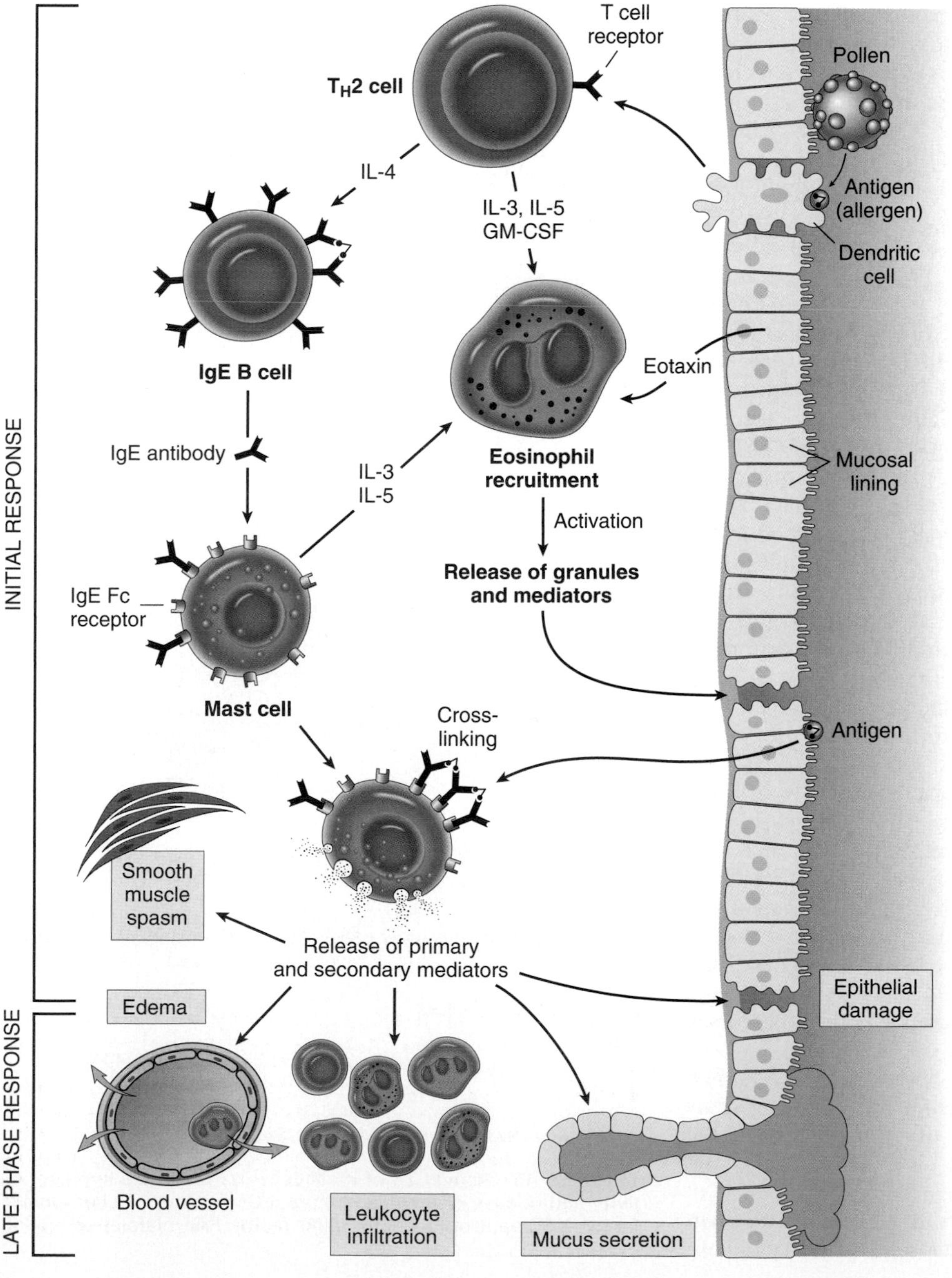

FIGURE 6–12 Pathogenesis of immediate (type I) hypersensitivity reaction. The late-phase reaction is dominated by leukocyte infiltration and tissue injury. T_H2, T-helper type 2 CD4 cells.

esis of type I hypersensitivity.[23] The first step in the synthesis of IgE is the presentation of the antigen to naive CD4+ helper T cells by dendritic cells that capture the antigen from its site of entry. In response to antigen and other stimuli, including cytokines produced at the local site,[24] the T cells differentiate into T_H2 cells. The newly minted T_H2 cells produce a cluster of cytokines upon subsequent encounter with the antigen; as we mentioned earlier, the signature cytokines of this subset are IL-4, IL-5, and IL-13. IL-4 is essential for turning on the IgE-producing B cells and for sustaining the development of T_H2 cells. IL-5 activates eosinophils, which, as we discuss subsequently, are important effectors of type I hypersensitivity. IL-13 promotes IgE production and acts on epithelial cells to stimulate mucus secretion. In addition, T_H2 cells and epithelial cells produce chemokines that attract more T_H2 cells, as well as eosinophils and occasionally basophils, to the reaction site.[23]

Mast cells and basophils express high-affinity receptors for the Fc portion of IgE, and therefore avidly bind IgE antibodies. When a mast cell, armed with cytophilic IgE antibodies, is re-exposed to the specific allergen, a series of reactions takes place, leading eventually to the release of a variety of powerful mediators responsible for the clinical expression of immediate hypersensitivity reactions. In the first step in this sequence, antigen (allergen) binds to the IgE antibodies previously attached to the mast cells. Multivalent antigens bind to more than one IgE molecule and thus cross-link adjacent IgE antibodies and the underlying IgE Fc receptors. The bridging of IgE molecules activates signal transduction pathways from the cytoplasmic portion of the IgE Fc receptors. These signals initiate two parallel and interdependent processes (Fig. 6–13)—one leading to mast cell degranulation with discharge of preformed (primary) mediators that are stored in the granules, and the other involving de novo synthesis and release of secondary mediators. These mediators are directly responsible for the initial, sometimes explosive, symptoms of immediate hypersensitivity, and they also set into motion the events that lead to the late-phase response.[20] In addition to inducing mediator release and production, signals from IgE Fc receptors promote the survival of mast cells and can enhance expression of the Fc receptor, providing an amplification mechanism.[25]

Primary Mediators. Primary mediators contained within mast-cell granules can be divided into three categories:

- *Biogenic amines.* The most important vasoactive amine is histamine. Histamine causes intense smooth muscle contraction, increased vascular permeability, and increased secretion by nasal, bronchial, and gastric glands.
- *Enzymes.* These are contained in the granule matrix and include neutral proteases (chymase, tryptase) and several acid hydrolases. The enzymes cause tissue damage and lead to the generation of kinins and activated components of complement (e.g., C3a) by acting on their precursor proteins.
- *Proteoglycans.* These include heparin, a well-known anticoagulant, and chondroitin sulfate. The proteoglycans serve to package and store the other mediators in the granules.

Secondary Mediators. Secondary mediators include two classes of compounds (1) lipid mediators and (2) cytokines. The *lipid mediators* are generated by sequential reactions in the mast-cell membranes that lead to activation of phospholipase A_2, an enzyme that acts on membrane phospholipids to yield *arachidonic acid.* This is the parent compound from which leukotrienes and prostaglandins are derived by the 5-lipoxygenase and cyclooxygenase pathways (Chapter 2).

- *Leukotrienes.* Leukotrienes C_4 and D_4 are the most potent vasoactive and spasmogenic agents known. On a molar basis, they are several thousand times more active than histamine in increasing vascular permeability and causing bronchial smooth muscle contraction. *Leukotriene B_4* is highly chemotactic for neutrophils, eosinophils, and monocytes.
- *Prostaglandin D_2.* This is the most abundant mediator derived by the cyclooxygenase pathway in mast cells. It causes intense bronchospasm as well as increased mucus secretion.
- *Platelet-activating factor (PAF).* PAF (Chapter 2) is produced by some mast-cell populations. It causes platelet aggregation, release of histamine, bronchospasm, increased vascular permeability, and vasodilation. In addition, it has important pro-inflammatory actions. PAF is chemotactic for neutrophils and eosinophils. At high concentrations, it activates the newly recruited inflammatory cells, causing them to aggregate and degranulate. Because of its ability to recruit and activate inflammatory cells, it is considered important in the initiation of the late-phase response. Although the production of PAF is also triggered by the

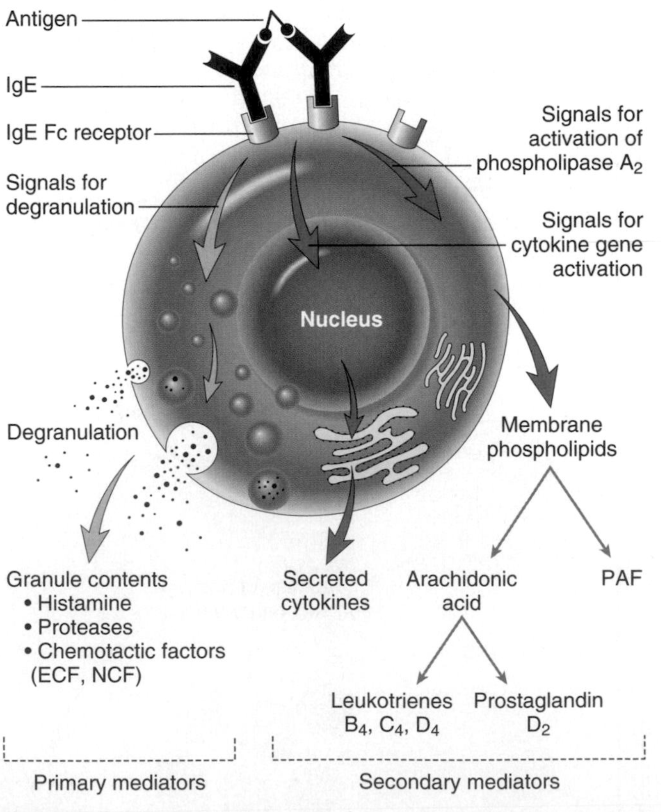

FIGURE 6–13 Activation of mast cells in immediate hypersensitivity and release of their mediators. ECF, eosinophil chemotactic factor; NCF, neutrophil chemotactic factor; PAF, platelet-activating factor.

activation of phospholipase A_2, it is not a product of arachidonic acid metabolism.

- *Cytokines.* Mast cells are sources of many cytokines, which play an important role in the late-phase reaction of immediate hypersensitivity because of their ability to recruit and activate inflammatory cells. The cytokines include TNF, IL-1, IL-3, IL-4, IL-5, IL-6, and GM-CSF, as well as chemokines, such as macrophage inflammatory protein (MIP)-1α and MIP-1β.[22] Mast cell–derived TNF and chemokines are important mediators of the inflammatory response seen at the site of allergic inflammation. Inflammatory cells that accumulate at the sites of type I hypersensitivity reactions are additional sources of cytokines and of histamine-releasing factors that cause further mast-cell degranulation.

The development of immediate hypersensitivity reactions is dependent on the coordinated actions of a variety of chemotactic, vasoactive, and spasmogenic compounds (Table 6–3). Some, such as histamine and leukotrienes, are released rapidly from sensitized mast cells and are responsible for the intense immediate reactions characterized by edema, mucus secretion, and smooth muscle spasm; others, exemplified by cytokines, set the stage for the late-phase response by recruiting additional leukocytes. Not only do these inflammatory cells release additional waves of mediators (including cytokines), but they also cause epithelial-cell damage. Epithelial cells themselves are not passive bystanders in this reaction; they can also produce soluble mediators, such as IL-6, IL-8, and GM-CSF.

Among the cells that are recruited in the late-phase reaction, *eosinophils* are particularly important.[26] They are recruited to sites of immediate hypersensitivity reactions by chemokines, such as eotaxin and others, that may be produced by epithelial cells under the influence of mediators such as TNF, T_H2 cells, and mast cells. The survival of eosinophils in tissues is favored by IL-3, IL-5, and GM-CSF, and IL-5 is the most potent eosinophil-activating cytokine known. These cytokines, as mentioned earlier, are derived from T_H2 cells and mast cells. The armamentarium of eosinophils is as extensive as that of mast cells, and in addition they produce major basic protein and eosinophil cationic protein, which are toxic to epithelial cells. Activated eosinophils and other leukocytes also produce leukotriene C_4 and PAF and directly activate mast cells to release mediators. Thus, *the recruited cells amplify and sustain the inflammatory response without additional exposure to the triggering antigen.* It is now believed that this late-phase inflammatory response is a major cause of symptoms in some type I hypersensitivity disorders, such as allergic asthma. Therefore, treatment of these diseases requires the use of broad-spectrum anti-inflammatory drugs, such as steroids.

A final point that should be mentioned in this general discussion of immediate hypersensitivity is that *susceptibility to these reactions is genetically determined.* The term *atopy* refers to a predisposition to develop localized immediate hypersensitivity reactions to a variety of inhaled and ingested allergens. Atopic individuals tend to have higher serum IgE levels, and more IL-4–producing T_H2 cells, compared with the general population. A positive family history of allergy is found in 50% of atopic individuals. The basis of familial predisposition is not clear, but studies in patients with asthma reveal linkage to several gene loci.[27] Candidate genes have been mapped to 5q31, where genes for the cytokines IL-3, IL-4, IL-5, IL-9, IL-13, and GM-CSF are located, consistent with the idea that these cytokines are involved in the reactions. Linkage has also been noted to 6p, close to the HLA complex, suggesting that the inheritance of certain HLA alleles permits reactivity to certain allergens. Another asthma-associated locus is on chromosome 11q13, the location of the gene encoding the β chain of the high-affinity IgE receptor, but many studies have failed to establish a linkage of atopy with the FcεRI β chain or even this chromosomal region.

To summarize, immediate (type I) hypersensitivity is a complex disorder resulting from an IgE-mediated triggering of mast cells and subsequent accumulation of inflammatory cells at sites of antigen deposition. These events are regulated in large part by the induction of T_H2-type helper T cells that promote synthesis of IgE and accumulation of inflammatory cells, particularly eosinophils. The clinical features result from release of mast-cell mediators as well as the accumulation of an eosinophil-rich inflammatory exudate. With this consideration of the basic mechanisms of type I hypersensitivity, we turn to some conditions that are important examples of IgE-mediated disease.

TABLE 6–3 Summary of the Action of Mast Cell Mediators in Immediate (Type I) Hypersensitivity

Action	Mediator
Vasodilation, increased vascular permeability	Histamine PAF Leukotrienes C_4, D_4, E_4 Neutral proteases that activate complement and kinins Prostaglandin D_2
Smooth muscle spasm	Leukotrienes C_4, D_4, E_4 Histamine Prostaglandins PAF
Cellular infiltration	Cytokines, e.g., TNF Leukotriene B_4 Eosinophil and neutrophil chemotactic factors (not defined biochemically) PAF

PAF, platelet-activating factor; TNF, tumor necrosis factor.

Systemic Anaphylaxis

Systemic anaphylaxis is characterized by vascular shock, widespread edema, and difficulty in breathing. In humans, systemic anaphylaxis may occur after administration of foreign proteins (e.g., antisera), hormones, enzymes, polysaccharides, and drugs (such as the antibiotic penicillin).[28] The severity of the disorder varies with the level of sensitization. Extremely small doses of antigen may trigger anaphylaxis, for example, the tiny amounts used in ordinary skin testing for various forms of allergies. Within minutes after exposure, itching, hives, and skin erythema appear, followed shortly thereafter by a striking contraction of respiratory bronchioles and respiratory distress. Laryngeal edema results in hoarseness. Vomiting, abdominal cramps, diarrhea, and laryngeal obstruction follow, and the patient may go into shock and even die within the hour. The risk of anaphylaxis must be borne in mind when certain therapeutic agents are administered. Although patients at risk can generally be identified by a previous history of some form of allergy, the absence of such a history does not preclude the possibility of an anaphylactic reaction.

Local Immediate Hypersensitivity Reactions

Local immediate hypersensitivity, or allergic, reactions are exemplified by so-called atopic allergy. About 10% of the population suffers from allergies involving localized reactions to common environmental allergens, such as pollen, animal dander, house dust, foods, and the like. Specific diseases include urticaria, angioedema, allergic rhinitis (hay fever), and some forms of asthma, all discussed elsewhere in this book. The familial predisposition to the development of this type of allergy has been mentioned earlier.

Antibody-Mediated (Type II) Hypersensitivity

Type II hypersensitivity is mediated by antibodies directed toward antigens present on cell surfaces or extracellular matrix. The antigenic determinants may be intrinsic to the cell membrane or matrix, or they may take the form of an exogenous antigen, such as a drug metabolite, that is adsorbed on a cell surface or matrix. In either case, the hypersensitivity reaction results from the binding of antibodies to normal or altered cell-surface antigens. Three different antibody-dependent mechanisms involved in this type of reaction are depicted in Figure 6–14 and described next. Most of these reactions involve the effector mechanisms that are used by antibodies, namely the complement system and phagocytes.

Opsonization and Complement- and Fc Receptor–Mediated Phagocytosis

The depletion of cells targeted by antibodies is, to a large extent, because the cells are coated (opsonized) with molecules that make them attractive for phagocytes. When antibodies are deposited on the surfaces of cells, they may activate the complement system (if the antibodies are of the IgM or IgG class). Complement activation generates byproducts, mainly C3b and C4b, which are deposited on the surfaces of the cells and recognized by phagocytes that express receptors for these proteins. In addition, cells opsonized by IgG antibodies are recognized by phagocyte Fc receptors, which are specific for the Fc portions of some IgG subclasses. The net result is the phagocytosis of the opsonized cells and their destruction (Fig. 6–14*A*). Complement activation on cells also leads to the formation of the membrane attack complex, which disrupts membrane integrity by "drilling holes" through the lipid bilayer, thereby causing osmotic lysis of the cells.

Antibody-mediated destruction of cells may occur by another process called *antibody-dependent cellular cytotoxicity (ADCC)*. This form of antibody-mediated cell injury does not involve fixation of complement but instead requires the cooperation of leukocytes. Cells that are coated with low concentrations of IgG antibody are killed by a variety of effector cells, which bind to the target by their receptors for the Fc fragment of IgG, and cell lysis proceeds without phagocytosis. ADCC may be mediated by monocytes, neutrophils, eosinophils, and NK cells. Although, in most instances, IgG antibodies are involved in ADCC, in certain cases (e.g., eosinophil-mediated cytotoxicity against parasites), IgE antibodies are used. The role of ADCC in hypersensitivity diseases is uncertain.

Clinically, antibody-mediated cell destruction and phagocytosis occur in the following situations: (1) *transfusion reactions*, in which cells from an incompatible donor react with and are opsonized by preformed antibody in the host; (2) *erythroblastosis fetalis*, in which there is an antigenic difference between the mother and the fetus, and antibodies (of the IgG class) from the mother cross the placenta and cause destruction of fetal red cells; (3) *autoimmune hemolytic anemia*, *agranulocytosis*, and *thrombocytopenia*, in which individuals produce antibodies to their own blood cells, which are then destroyed; and (4) *certain drug reactions*, in which antibodies are produced that react with the drug, which may be attached to the surface of erythrocytes or other cells.

Complement- and Fc Receptor–Mediated Inflammation

When antibodies deposit in extracellular tissues, such as basement membranes and matrix, the resultant injury is because of inflammation and not because of phagocytosis or lysis of cells. The deposited antibodies activate complement, generating byproducts, such as C5a (and to a lesser extent C4a and C3a), that recruit neutrophils and monocytes. The same cells also bind to the deposited antibodies via their Fc receptors. The leukocytes are activated, they release injurious substances, such as enzymes and reactive oxygen intermediates, and the result is damage to the tissues (Fig. 6–14*B*). It was once thought that complement was the major mediator of antibody-induced inflammation, but knockout mice lacking Fc receptors also show striking reduction in these reactions. It is now believed that inflammation in antibody-mediated (and immune complex–mediated) diseases is because of both complement and Fc receptor–dependent reactions.[29]

Antibody-mediated inflammation is the mechanism responsible for tissue injury in some forms of *glomerulonephritis*, *vascular rejection* in organ grafts, and other diseases (Table 6–4). As we shall discuss in more detail below, the same reaction is involved in immune complex–mediated diseases.

Antibody-Mediated Cellular Dysfunction

In some cases, antibodies directed against cell-surface receptors impair or dysregulate function without causing cell injury or inflammation. For example, in *myasthenia gravis*, antibodies reactive with acetylcholine receptors in the motor end-plates of skeletal muscles impair neuromuscular transmission and therefore cause muscle weakness (Fig. 6–14*C*). In *pemphigus vulgaris*, antibodies against desmosomes disrupt intercellular junctions in epidermis, leading to the formation of skin vesicles. The converse (i.e., antibody-mediated stimulation of cell function) is noted in *Graves disease*. In this disorder, antibodies against the thyroid-stimulating hormone receptor on thyroid epithelial cells stimulate the cells, resulting in hyperthyroidism.

Immune Complex–Mediated (Type III) Hypersensitivity

Antigen–antibody complexes produce tissue damage mainly by eliciting inflammation at the sites of deposition. The toxic

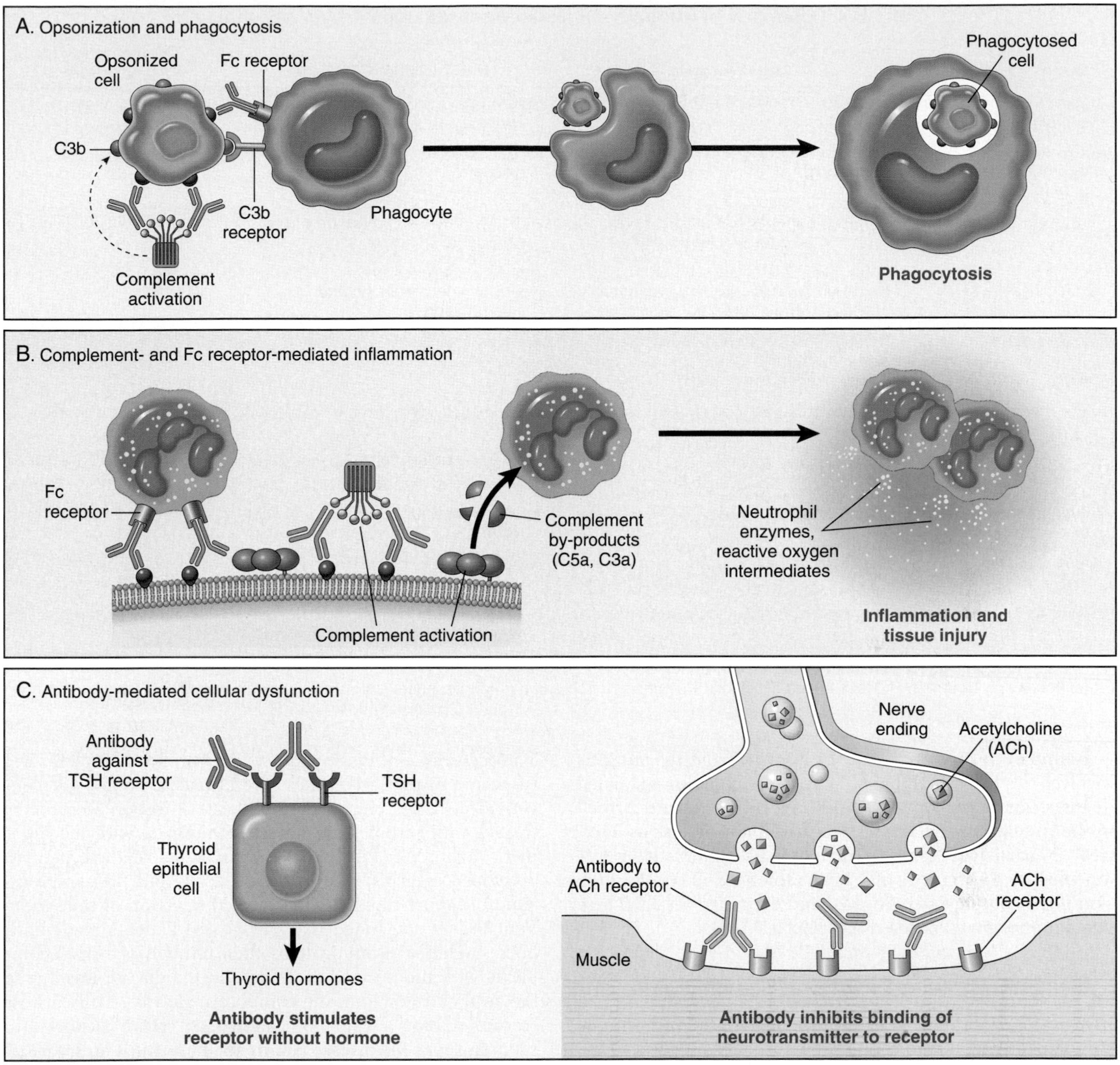

FIGURE 6–14 Schematic illustration of the three major mechanisms of antibody-mediated injury. *A,* Opsonization of cells by antibodies and complement components and ingestion by phagocytes. *B,* Inflammation induced by antibody binding to Fc receptors of leukocytes and by complement breakdown products. *C,* Antireceptor antibodies disturb the normal function of receptors. In these examples, antibodies against the thyroid stimulating hormone (TSH) receptor activate thyroid cells in Graves disease, and acetylcholine (ACh) receptor antibodies impair neuromuscular transmission in myasthenia gravis.

reaction is initiated when antigen combines with antibody within the circulation (circulating immune complexes) and these are deposited, typically in vessel walls, or the complexes are formed at extravascular sites where antigen may have been deposited previously (in situ immune complexes). Some forms of glomerulonephritis in which immune complexes are formed in situ after initial implantation of the antigen on the glomerular basement membrane are discussed in Chapter 20. *The mere formation of antigen–antibody complexes in the circulation does not imply the presence of disease*; immune complexes are formed during many immune responses and represent a normal mechanism of antigen removal. The factors that determine whether the immune complexes formed in circulation will be pathogenic are not fully understood, but some possible influences are discussed later.

Two general types of antigens cause immune complex-mediated injury: (1) The antigen may be *exogenous*, such as a foreign protein, a bacterium, or a virus; or (2) Under some circumstances, the individual can produce antibody against self-components—*endogenous antigens*. The latter can be circulating antigens present in the blood or, more commonly, antigenic components of one's own cells and tissues.

TABLE 6–4 Examples of Antibody-Mediated Diseases (Type II Hypersensitivity)

Disease	Target Antigen	Mechanisms of Disease	Clinicopathologic Manifestations
Autoimmune hemolytic anemia	Erythrocyte membrane proteins (Rh blood group antigens, I antigen)	Opsonization and phagocytosis of erythrocytes	Hemolysis, anemia
Autoimmune thrombocytopenic purpura	Platelet membrane proteins (gpIIb:IIIa intergrin)	Opsonization and phagocytosis of platelets	Bleeding
Pemphigus vulgaris	Proteins in intercellular junctions of epidermal cells (epidermal cadherin)	Antibody-mediated activation of proteases, disruption of intercellular adhesions	Skin vesicles (bullae)
Vasculitis caused by ANCA	Neutrophil granule proteins, presumably released from activated neutrophils	Neutrophil degranulation and inflammation	Vasculitis
Goodpasture syndrome	Noncollagenous protein in basement membranes of kidney glomeruli and lung alveoli	Complement- and Fc receptor–mediated inflammation	Nephritis, lung hemorrhage
Acute rheumatic fever	Streptococcal cell wall antigen; antibody cross-reacts with myocardial antigen	Inflammation, macrophage activation	Myocarditis, arthritis
Myasthenia gravis	Acetylcholine receptor	Antibody inhibits acetylcholine binding, down-modulates receptors	Muscle weakness, paralysis
Graves disease (hyperthyroidism)	TSH receptor	Antibody-mediated stimulation of TSH receptors	Hyperthyroidism
Insulin-resistant diabetes	Insulin receptor	Antibody inhibits binding of insulin	Hyperglycemia, ketoacidosis
Pernicious anemia	Intrinsic factor of gastric parietal cells	Neutralization of intrinsic factor, decreased absorption of vitamin B_{12}	Abnormal erythropoiesis, anemia

ANCA, antineutrophil cytoplasmic antibodies; TSH, thyroid-stimulating hormone.
From Abbas AK, Lichtman H: Cellular and Molecular Immunology. 5th edition. WB Saunders Company, Philadelphia, 2003.

Examples of immune complex disorders and the antigens involved are listed in Table 6–5. Immune complex–mediated diseases can be *generalized*, if immune complexes are formed in the circulation and are deposited in many organs, or *localized* to particular organs, such as the kidney (glomerulonephritis), joints (arthritis), or the small blood vessels of the skin if the complexes are formed and deposited locally. These two patterns are considered separately.

Systemic Immune Complex Disease

Acute serum sickness is the prototype of a systemic immune complex disease; it was at one time a frequent sequela to the administration of large amounts of foreign serum (e.g., immune serum from horses used for passive immunization.) The occurrence of diseases caused by immune complexes was suspected in the early 1900s by a physician named Clemens von Pirquet. Patients with diphtheria infection were being treated with serum from horses immunized with the diphtheria toxin. Von Pirquet noted that some of these patients developed arthritis, skin rash, and fever, and the symptoms appeared more rapidly with repeated injection of the serum. Von Pirquet concluded that the treated patients made antibodies to horse serum proteins, these antibodies formed complexes with the injected proteins, and the disease was due to the antibodies or immune complexes. He called this disease "serum disease"; it is now known as serum sickness. In modern times the disease is infrequent, but it is an informative model that has taught us a great deal about systemic immune complex disorders.

TABLE 6–5 Examples of Immune Complex–Mediated Diseases

Disease	Antigen Involved	Clinicopathologic Manifestations
Systemic lupus erythematosus	DNA, nucleoproteins, others	Nephritis, arthritis, vasculitis
Polyarteritis nodosa	Hepatitis B virus surface antigen (in some cases)	Vasculitis
Poststreptococcal glomerulonephritis	Streptococcal cell wall antigen(s); may be "planted" in glomerular basement membrane	Nephritis
Acute glomerulonephritis	Bacterial antigens *(Treponema)*; parasite antigens (malaria, schistosomes); tumor antigens	Nephritis
Reactive arthritis	Bacterial antigens *(Yersinia)*	Acute arthritis
Arthus reaction	Various foreign proteins	Cutaneous vasculitis
Serum sickness	Various proteins, e.g., foreign serum (anti-thymocyte globulin)	Arthritis, vasculitis, nephritis

For the sake of discussion, the pathogenesis of systemic immune complex disease can be divided into three phases: (1) formation of antigen–antibody complexes in the circulation; (2) deposition of the immune complexes in various tissues, thus initiating; and (3) an inflammatory reaction at the sites of immune complex deposition (Fig. 6–15). The *first phase* is initiated by the introduction of antigen, usually a protein, and its interaction with immunocompetent cells, resulting in the formation of antibodies approximately a week after the injection of the protein. These antibodies are secreted into the blood, where they react with the antigen still present in the circulation to form antigen-antibody complexes. In the *second phase*, the circulating antigen-antibody complexes are deposited in various tissues.

The factors that determine whether immune complex formation will lead to tissue deposition and disease are not fully understood, but two possible influences are the size of the immune complexes and the functional status of the mononuclear phagocyte system:

- Large complexes formed in great antibody excess are rapidly removed from the circulation by the mononuclear phagocyte system and are therefore relatively harmless. The most pathogenic complexes are of small or intermediate size (formed in slight antigen excess), which bind less avidly to phagocytic cells and therefore circulate longer.
- Because the mononuclear phagocyte system normally filters out the circulating immune complexes, its overload or intrinsic dysfunction increases the probability of persistence of immune complexes in circulation and tissue deposition.

In addition, several other factors, such as charge of the immune complexes (anionic versus cationic), valency of the antigen, avidity of the antibody, affinity of the antigen to various tissue components, three-dimensional (lattice) structure of the complexes, and hemodynamic factors, influence the tissue deposition of complexes. Because most of these influences have been investigated with reference to deposition of immune complexes in the glomeruli, they are discussed further in Chapter 20. In addition to the renal glomeruli, the favored sites of immune complex deposition are joints, skin, heart, serosal surfaces, and small blood vessels. For complexes to leave the microcirculation and deposit in the vessel wall, an increase in vascular permeability must occur. This is believed to occur when immune complexes bind to inflammatory cells through their Fc or C3b receptors and trigger release of vasoactive mediators as well as permeability-enhancing cytokines. Mast cells may also be involved in this phase of the reaction.

Once complexes are deposited in the tissues, they initiate an acute inflammatory reaction *(third phase)*. During this phase (approximately 10 days after antigen administration), clinical features such as fever, urticaria, arthralgias, lymph node enlargement, and proteinuria appear.

Wherever complexes deposit, the tissue damage is similar. Two mechanisms are believed to cause *inflammation* at the sites of deposition (Fig. 6–16): (1) activation of the complement cascade, and (2) activation of neutrophils and macrophages through their Fc receptors. As discussed in Chapter 2, *complement activation* promotes inflammation mainly by production of chemotactic factors, which direct the migration of polymorphonuclear leukocytes and monocytes

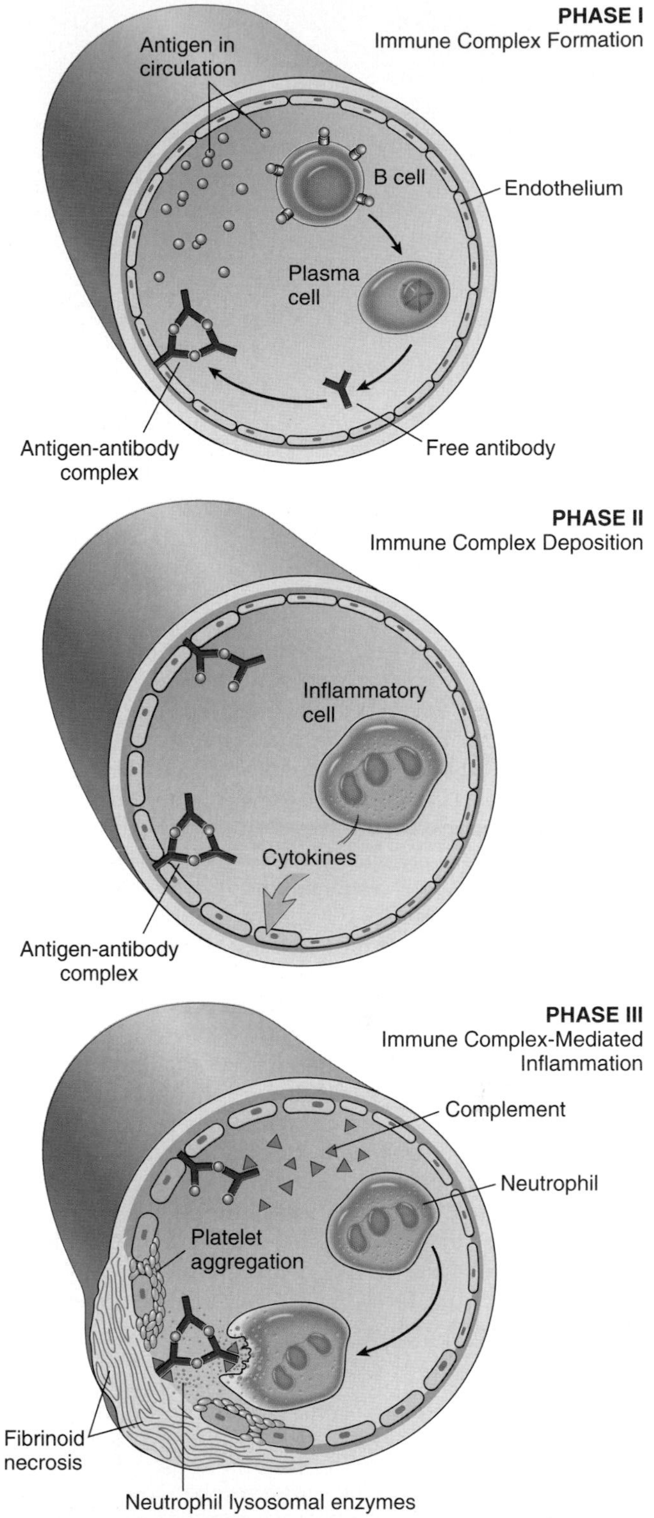

FIGURE 6–15 Schematic illustration of the three sequential phases in the induction of systemic immune complex–mediated disease (type III hypersensitivity).

(mainly C5a) and by release of anaphylatoxins (C3a and C5a), which increase vascular permeability.

The leukocytes that are drawn in by the chemotactic factors are activated by engagement of their C3b and Fc receptors by the immune complexes. This results in the release or genera-

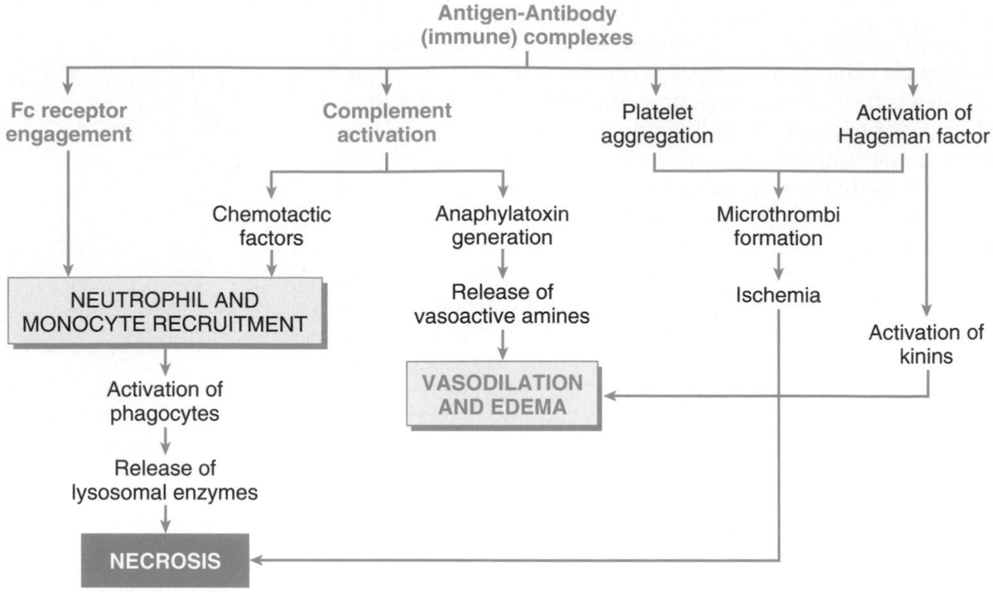

FIGURE 6–16 Pathogenesis of immune complex–mediated tissue injury. The morphologic consequences are depicted as boxed areas.

tion of a variety of pro-inflammatory substances, including prostaglandins, vasodilator peptides, and chemotactic substances, as well as several lysosomal enzymes, including proteases capable of digesting basement membrane, collagen, elastin, and cartilage. Tissue damage is also mediated by oxygen free radicals produced by activated neutrophils. Immune complexes have several other effects, including aggregation of platelets and activation of Hageman factor; both of these reactions augment the inflammatory process and initiate the formation of microthrombi. The resultant inflammatory lesion is termed *vasculitis* if it occurs in blood vessels, *glomerulonephritis* if it occurs in renal glomeruli, *arthritis* if it occurs in the joints, and so on.

It is clear from the foregoing that complement-fixing antibodies (i.e., IgG and IgM) and antibodies that bind to leukocyte Fc receptors (some subclasses of IgG) induce the pathologic lesions of immune complex disorders. Because IgA can activate complement by the alternative pathway, IgA-containing complexes may also induce tissue injury. The important role of complement in the pathogenesis of the tissue injury is supported by the observations that during the active phase of the disease, consumption of complement decreases the serum levels, and experimental depletion of complement greatly reduces the severity of the lesions.

Morphology. The morphologic consequences of immune complex injury are dominated by acute necrotizing vasculitis, with necrosis of the vessel wall and intense neutrophilic infiltration. The necrotic tissue and deposits of immune complexes, complement, and plasma protein produce a smudgy eosinophilic deposit that obscures the underlying cellular detail, an appearance termed **fibrinoid necrosis** (Fig. 6–17). When complexes are deposited in kidney glomeruli, the affected glomeruli are hypercellular because of swelling and proliferation of endothelial and mesangial cells, accompanied by neutrophilic and monocytic infiltration. **The complexes can be seen on immunofluorescence microscopy as granular lumpy deposits of immunoglobulin and complement** and on electron microscopy as electron-dense deposits along the glomerular basement membrane (see Figs. 6–33 and 6–34).

If the disease results from a single large exposure to antigen (e.g., acute serum sickness and perhaps acute poststreptococcal glomerulonephritis), the lesions tend to resolve, owing to catabolism of the immune complexes. A *chronic form of serum sickness* results from repeated or prolonged exposure to an antigen. Continuous antigenemia is necessary for the development of chronic immune complex disease because, as stated earlier, complexes in antigen excess are the ones most likely to be deposited in vascular beds. This occurs in several human diseases, such as systemic lupus erythematosus (SLE), which is associated with persistent antibody responses to autoantigens. In many diseases, however, the morphologic changes and other findings suggest immune complex deposition but the inciting antigens are unknown. Included in this category are membranous glomerulonephritis, many cases of polyarteritis nodosa, and several other vasculitides.

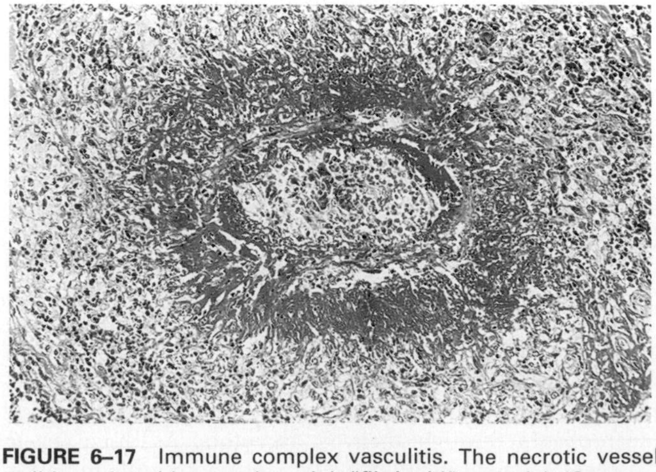

FIGURE 6–17 Immune complex vasculitis. The necrotic vessel wall is replaced by smudgy, pink "fibrinoid" material. (Courtesy of Dr. Trace Worrell, Department of Pathology, University of Texas Southwestern Medical School, Dallas, TX.)

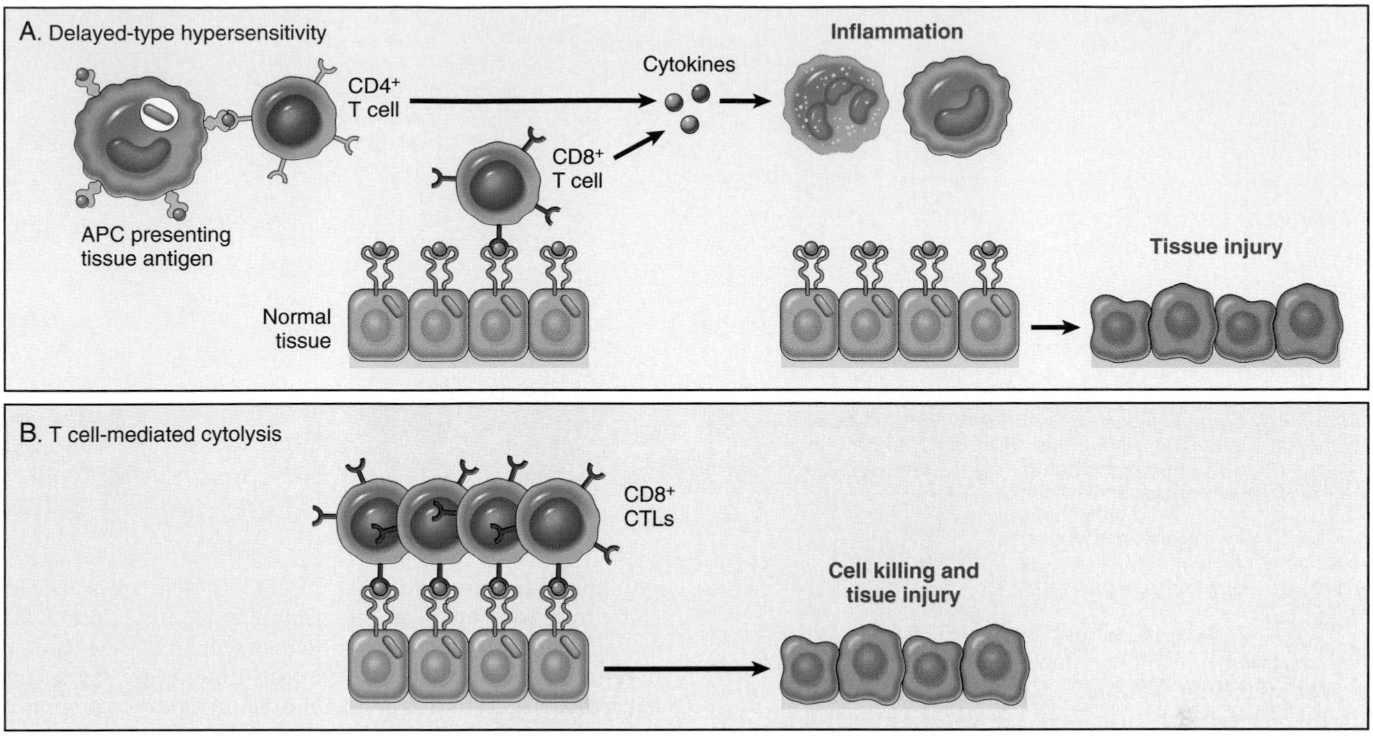

FIGURE 6–18 Mechanisms of T cell–mediated (type IV) hypersensitivity reactions. *A,* In delayed type hypersensitivity reactions, CD4+ T cells (and sometimes CD8+ cells) respond to tissue antigens by secreting cytokines that stimulate inflammation and activate phagocytes, leading to tissue injury. *B,* In some diseases, CD8+ cytolytic T lymphocytes (CTLs) directly kill tissue cells. APC, antigen-presenting cell.

Local Immune Complex Disease (Arthus Reaction)

The *Arthus reaction* is a localized area of tissue necrosis resulting from acute immune complex vasculitis, usually elicited in the skin. The reaction can be produced experimentally by intracutaneous injection of antigen in an immune animal having circulating antibodies against the antigen. As the antigen diffuses into the vascular wall, it binds the preformed antibody, and large immune complexes are formed locally, which precipitate in the vessel walls and trigger an inflammatory reaction. In contrast to IgE-mediated type I reactions, which appear immediately, the Arthus lesion develops over a few hours and reaches a peak 4 to 10 hours after injection, when it can be seen as an area of visible edema with severe hemorrhage followed occasionally by ulceration. Immunofluorescent stains reveal complement, immunoglobulins, and fibrinogen deposited in the vessel walls, usually the venules, and histologically the vessels show fibrinoid necrosis and inflammation (Fig. 6–17). Thrombi are formed in the vessels, resulting in local ischemic injury.

Cell-Mediated (Type IV) Hypersensitivity

The cell-mediated type of hypersensitivity is initiated by antigen-activated (sensitized) T lymphocytes. It includes the *delayed type hypersensitivity reactions* mediated by CD4+ T cells, and *direct cell cytotoxicity* mediated by CD8+ T cells (Fig. 6–18). It is the principal pattern of immunologic response not only to a variety of intracellular microbiologic agents, such as *Mycobacterium tuberculosis*, but also to many viruses, fungi, protozoa, and parasites. So-called contact skin sensitivity to chemical agents and graft rejection are other instances of cell-mediated reactions. In addition, many autoimmune diseases are now known to be caused by T cell–mediated reactions (Table 6–6). The two forms of T cell–mediated hypersensitivity are described next.

TABLE 6–6 Examples of T Cell–Mediated (Type IV) Hypersensitivity

Disease	Specificity of Pathogenic T Cells	Clinicopathologic Manifestations
Type 1 diabetes mellitus	Antigens of pancreatic islet β cells (insulin, glutamic acid decarboxylase, others)	Insulitis (chronic inflammation in islets), destruction of β cells; diabetes
Multiple sclerosis	Protein antigens in central nervous system myelin (myelin basic protein, proteolipid protein)	Demyelination in CNS with perivascular inflammation; paralysis, ocular lesions
Rheumatoid arthritis	Unknown antigen in joint synovium (type II collagen?); role of antibodies?	Chronic arthritis with inflammation, destruction of articular cartilage and bone
Peripheral neuropathy; Guillain-Barré syndrome?	Protein antigens of peripheral nerve myelin	Neuritis, paralysis

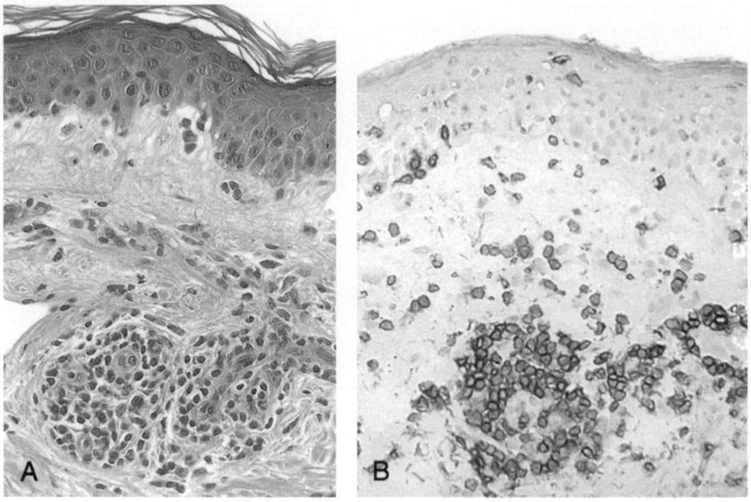

FIGURE 6–19 Delayed hypersensitivity in the skin. *A,* Perivascular infiltration by T cells and mononuclear phagocytes. *B,* Immunoperoxidase staining reveals a predominantly perivascular cellular infiltrate that marks positively with anti-CD4 antibodies. (Courtesy of Dr. Louis Picker, Department of Pathology, University of Texas Southwestern Medical School, Dallas, TX.)

Delayed Type Hypersensitivity

The classic example of delayed hypersensitivity is the *tuberculin reaction,* which is produced by the intracutaneous injection of tuberculin, a protein-lipopolysaccharide component of the tubercle bacillus. In a previously sensitized individual, reddening and induration of the site appear in 8 to 12 hours, reach a peak in 24 to 72 hours, and thereafter slowly subside. Morphologically, delayed type hypersensitivity is characterized by the accumulation of mononuclear cells around small veins and venules, producing a perivascular "cuffing" (Fig. 6–19). There is an associated increased microvascular permeability caused by mechanisms similar to those in other forms of inflammation (Chapter 2). Not unexpectedly, plasma proteins escape, giving rise to dermal edema and deposition of fibrin in the interstitium. The latter appears to be the main cause of induration, which is characteristic of delayed hypersensitivity skin lesions. In fully developed lesions, the lymphocyte-cuffed venules show marked endothelial hypertrophy and, in some cases, hyperplasia. Immunoperoxidase staining of the lesions reveals a preponderance of CD4+ (helper) T lymphocytes (see Fig. 6–19).

With certain persistent or nondegradable antigens, such as tubercle bacilli colonizing the lungs or other tissues, the initial perivascular lymphocytic infiltrate is replaced by macrophages over a period of 2 or 3 weeks. The accumulated macrophages often undergo a morphologic transformation into epithelium-like cells and are then referred to as *epithelioid cells.* A microscopic aggregation of epithelioid cells, usually surrounded by a collar of lymphocytes, is referred to as a *granuloma* (Fig. 6–20). This pattern of inflammation that is sometimes seen in type IV hypersensitivity is called *granulomatous inflammation* (Chapter 2).

The sequence of cellular events in delayed hypersensitivity can be exemplified by the tuberculin reaction. When an individual is first exposed to protein antigens of tubercle bacilli, naive CD4+ T cells recognize peptides derived from these antigens in association with class II molecules on the surface of antigen-presenting cells. This initial encounter drives the differentiation of naive CD4+ T cells to T_H1 cells. The induction of T_H1 cells is of central importance because the expression of delayed hypersensitivity depends in large part on the cytokines secreted by T_H1 cells. Why certain antigens preferentially induce the T_H1 response is not entirely clear, but the cytokine milieu in which naive CD4+ T cells are activated seems to be relevant,[9,24] as discussed subsequently. Some of the T_H1 cells enter the circulation and may remain in the memory pool of T cells for long periods, sometimes years. On intracutaneous injection of tuberculin in an individual previously exposed to tubercle bacilli, the memory T_H1 cells recognize the antigen displayed by antigen-presenting cells and are activated. These T_H1 cells secrete cytokines, mainly IFN-γ, which are responsible for the expression of delayed-type hypersensitivity (Fig. 6–21). Cytokines most relevant to this reaction and their actions are as follows:

- IL-12, a cytokine produced by macrophages and dendritic cells, is critical for the induction of the T_H1 response and hence delayed hypersensitivity. On initial encounter with a microbe, the macrophages and dendritic cells that are presenting microbial antigens secrete IL-12, which drives the differentiation of naive CD4+ helper cells to T_H1 cells. These, in turn, produce other cytokines, listed below. IL-12 is also a potent inducer of IFN-γ secretion by T cells and NK cells. IFN-γ further augments the differentiation of T_H1 cells.

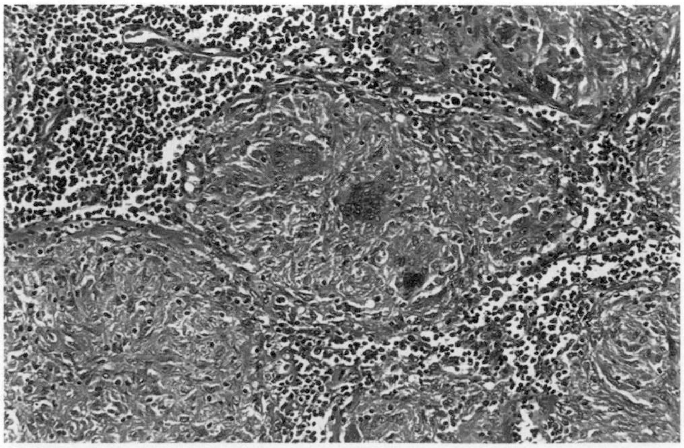

FIGURE 6–20 A section of a lymph node shows several granulomas, each made up of an aggregate of epithelioid cells and surrounded by lymphocytes. The granuloma in the center shows several multinucleate giant cells. (Courtesy of Dr. Trace Worrell, Department of Pathology, University of Texas Southwestern Medical School, Dallas, TX.)

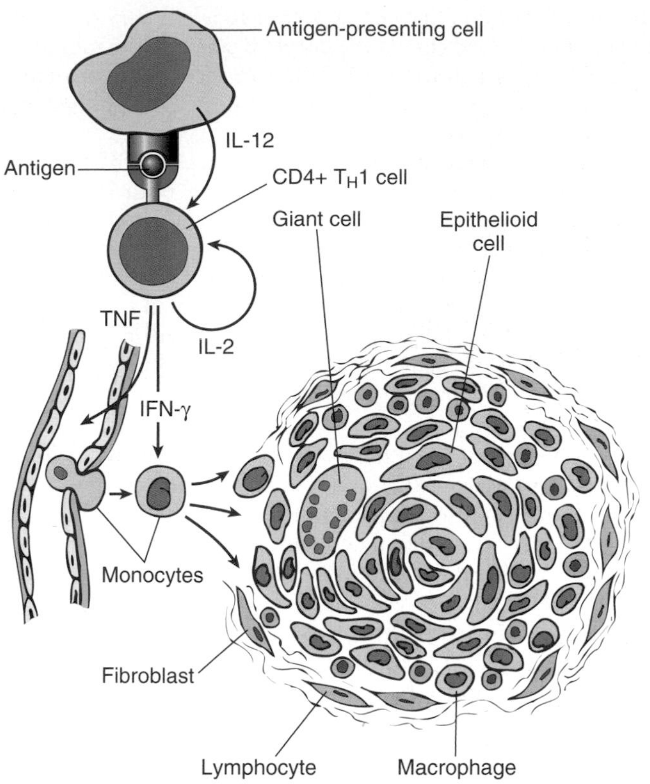

FIGURE 6–21 Schematic illustration of the events that give rise to the formation of granulomas in cell-mediated (type IV) hypersensitivity reactions. Note the role played by T cell–derived cytokines.

- IFN-γ has many effects and is the key mediator of delayed-type hypersensitivity. Most importantly, it is a powerful activator of macrophages. Activated macrophages are altered in several ways: their ability to phagocytose and kill microorganisms is markedly augmented; they express more class II molecules on the surface, thus facilitating further antigen presentation; they secrete several polypeptide growth factors, such as platelet-derived growth factor (PDGF), which stimulate fibroblast proliferation and augment collagen synthesis; they secrete TNF, IL-1, and chemokines, which promote inflammation; and they produce more IL-12, thereby amplifying the T_H1 response. Thus, activated macrophages serve to eliminate the offending antigen; if the activation is sustained, continued inflammation and, ultimately, fibrosis result.
- IL-2 causes autocrine and paracrine proliferation of T cells, which accumulate at sites of delayed hypersensitivity; included in this infiltrate are some antigen-specific CD4+ T_H1 cells and many more bystander T cells that are recruited to the site.
- TNF and lymphotoxin are two cytokines that exert important effects on endothelial cells: (1) increased secretion of prostacyclin, which, in turn, favors increased blood flow by causing local vasodilation; (2) increased expression of P-E-selectins (Chapter 2), adhesion molecules that promote attachment of the passing lymphocytes and monocytes; and (3) induction and secretion of chemokines such as IL-8. Together, all these changes in the endothelium facilitate the extravasation of lymphocytes and monocytes at the site of the delayed hypersensitivity reaction. The process by which T cells and monocytes exit the vasculature is generally similar to that described for neutrophils in Chapter 2. The steps in this process are initial rolling on the endothelium, followed by activation of integrins and firm adhesion and, ultimately, transmigration through the vessel wall.
- Chemokines produced by the T cells and macrophages recruit more leukocytes into the reaction site. This type of inflammation is sometimes called "immune inflammation."

T cell–mediated hypersensitivity is a major mechanism of defense against a variety of intracellular pathogens, including mycobacteria, fungi, and certain parasites, and is also involved in transplant rejection and tumor immunity. In addition to its beneficial, protective role, delayed type hypersensitivity can also be a cause of disease. *Contact dermatitis* is a common example of tissue injury resulting from delayed hypersensitivity. It may be evoked by coming in contact with urushiol, the antigenic component of poison ivy or poison oak, and manifests in the form of a vesicular dermatitis (Fig. 6–22). The basic mechanism is similar to that described for tuberculin sensitivity. On repeat exposure to the plants, the sensitized CD4+ cells of the T_H1 type first accumulate in the dermis, then migrate toward the antigen within the epidermis. Here they release cytokines that damage keratinocytes, causing separation of these cells and formation of an intraepidermal vesicle. Type I diabetes and multiple sclerosis are two diseases involving different organs in which tissue injury is caused by delayed type hypersensitivity reactions against autologous tissue antigens, mediated by the T_H1 type of CD4+ T cells. In these examples of T_H1-mediated autoimmune disease, there is some evidence that CD8+ cells may also be involved. In certain other forms of delayed hypersensitivity reactions, especially those that follow viral infections, cytokine-producing CD8+ cells may be the dominant effector cells.

T Cell–Mediated Cytotoxicity

In this variant of cell-mediated hypersensitivity, sensitized CD8+ T cells kill antigen-bearing target cells. Such effector cells are called *cytotoxic T lymphocytes* (CTLs). Tissue destruction by CTLs may be an important component of many T cell–mediated diseases. CTLs directed against cell surface histocompatibility antigens play an important role in graft rejec-

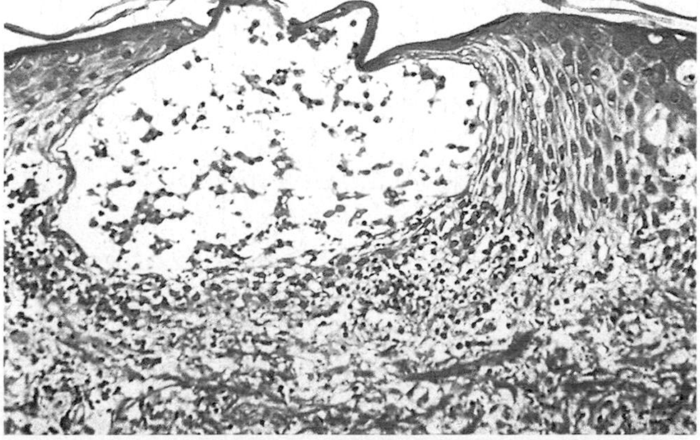

FIGURE 6–22 Contact dermatitis showing an epidermal blister (vesicle) with dermal and epidermal mononuclear infiltrates. (Courtesy of Dr. Louis Picker, Department of Pathology, University of Texas Southwestern Medical School, Dallas, TX.)

tion, to be discussed next. They also play a role in resistance to virus infections. In a virus-infected cell, viral peptides associate with the class I molecules within the cell, and the two are transported to the cell surface in the form of a complex that is recognized by the TCR of cytotoxic CD8+ T lymphocytes. The lysis of infected cells leads, in due course, to the elimination of the infection. It is believed that many tumor-associated antigens (Chapter 7) may also be similarly presented on the cell surface, and CTLs are therefore also involved in tumor immunity.

Much has been learned about the mechanisms by which CTLs kill their targets, and this knowledge may be of value in therapeutic modulation of T cell–mediated cytotoxicity in the settings of some autoimmune diseases. Two principal mechanisms of T cell-mediated damage have been discovered: (1) perforin-granzyme–dependent killing, and (2) Fas-Fas ligand–dependent killing.[30]

Perforins and granzymes are preformed mediators contained in the lysosome-like granules of CTLs. As its name indicates, *perforin* can perforate the plasma membranes of the target cells that are under attack by CD8+ lymphocytes. At first, CD8+ T cells come in close contact with the target cells; this is followed by polymerization of the released perforin molecules and their insertion into the target cell membranes, thus "drilling holes" into the membrane. The CTL granules contain proteases called *granzymes*, which are delivered into the target cells via the perforin-induced pores. Once within the cell, granzymes activate caspases, which induce apoptosis of the target cells (Chapter 1). In addition, the perforin pores allow water to enter the cells, thus causing osmotic lysis. Fas-dependent killing also induces apoptosis of the target cells but by a different mechanism. Activated CTLs express Fas ligand, a molecule with homology to TNF, that can bind to Fas expressed on target cells. This interaction leads to apoptosis by mechanisms discussed in Chapter 1.

Transplant Rejection

Transplant rejection is discussed here because it involves several of the immunologic reactions discussed earlier. A major barrier to transplantation is the process of *rejection*, in which the recipient's immune system recognizes the graft as being foreign and attacks it. One of the important goals of present-day immunologic research is successful transplantation of tissues in humans without rejection. Although the surgical expertise for the transplantation of skin, kidneys, heart, lungs, liver, spleen, bone marrow, and endocrine organs is now well in hand, it outpaces thus far the ability to confer on the recipient permanent acceptance of foreign grafts.

Mechanisms Involved in Rejection of Kidney Grafts

As stated above, graft rejection depends on recognition by the host of the grafted tissue as foreign. The antigens responsible for such rejection in humans are those of the HLA system. Because HLA genes are highly polymorphic, any two individuals (other than identical twins) will express some HLA proteins that are different. Thus, every individual will recognize some HLA molecules in another individual as foreign (allogeneic) and will react against these. This reaction is the basis of rejection of grafts from one individual to another. *Rejection is a complex process in which both cell-mediated immunity and circulating antibodies play a role*; moreover, the relative contributions of these two mechanisms to rejection vary among grafts and are often reflected in the histologic features of the rejected organs.

T Cell–Mediated Reactions. The critical role of T cells in transplant rejection has been documented both in humans and in experimental animals. T cell–mediated graft rejection is called *cellular rejection*, and it is induced by two mechanisms: destruction of graft cells by CD8+ CTLs and delayed hypersensitivity reactions triggered by activated CD4+ helper cells (Fig. 6–23). The recipient's T cells recognize antigens in the graft (the allogeneic antigens, or alloantigens) by two pathways, called *direct* and *indirect*.[31]

- In the *direct pathway*, T cells of the transplant recipient recognize allogeneic (donor) MHC molecules on the surface of an antigen-presenting cell in the graft (see Fig. 6–23). It is believed that dendritic cells carried in the donor organs are the most important immunogens because they not only richly express class I and II HLA molecules but also are endowed with costimulatory molecules (e.g., B7-1 and B7-2). The T cells of the host encounter the dendritic cells either within the grafted organ or after the dendritic cells migrate to the draining lymph nodes. Both the CD4+ and the CD8+ T cells of the transplant recipient are involved in this reaction. CD8+ T cells recognize class I HLA antigens and differentiate into mature CTLs. This process of CTL differentiation is complex and incompletely understood. It appears to be dependent on the release of cytokines, such as IL-2, from CD4+ helper cells and CD40 ligand on the helper cells activating antigen-presenting cells to promote the differentiation of CTLs. Once mature CTLs are generated, they kill the grafted tissue by mechanisms already discussed. The CD4+ helper T-cell subset is triggered into proliferation and differentiation into T_H1 effector cells by recognition of allogeneic class II molecules. As in delayed hypersensitivity reactions, cytokines secreted by the activated CD4+ T cells cause increased vascular permeability and local accumulation of mononuclear cells (lymphocytes and macrophages), and activate the macrophages, resulting in graft injury. The direct recognition of allogeneic MHC molecules seems paradoxical to the rules of self-MHC restriction: If T cells are normally restricted to recognizing foreign peptides displayed by self-MHC molecules, why should these T cells recognize foreign MHC? Such recognition has been explained by assuming that allogeneic MHC molecules, with their bound peptides, resemble, or mimic, the self-MHC–foreign peptide complexes that are recognized by self-MHC–restricted T cells. The structural basis of such mimicry is not entirely clear.
- In the so-called *indirect pathway* of allorecognition, recipient T lymphocytes recognize antigens of the graft donor after they are presented by the recipient's own antigen-presenting cells (see Fig. 6–23). This process involves the uptake and processing of MHC molecules from the grafted organ by host antigen-presenting cells. The peptides derived from the donor tissue are presented by the host's own MHC molecules, like any other foreign peptides. Thus, the indirect pathway is similar to the physiologic processing and presentation of other foreign (e.g., microbial) antigens. The indirect pathway generates CD4+ T cells that

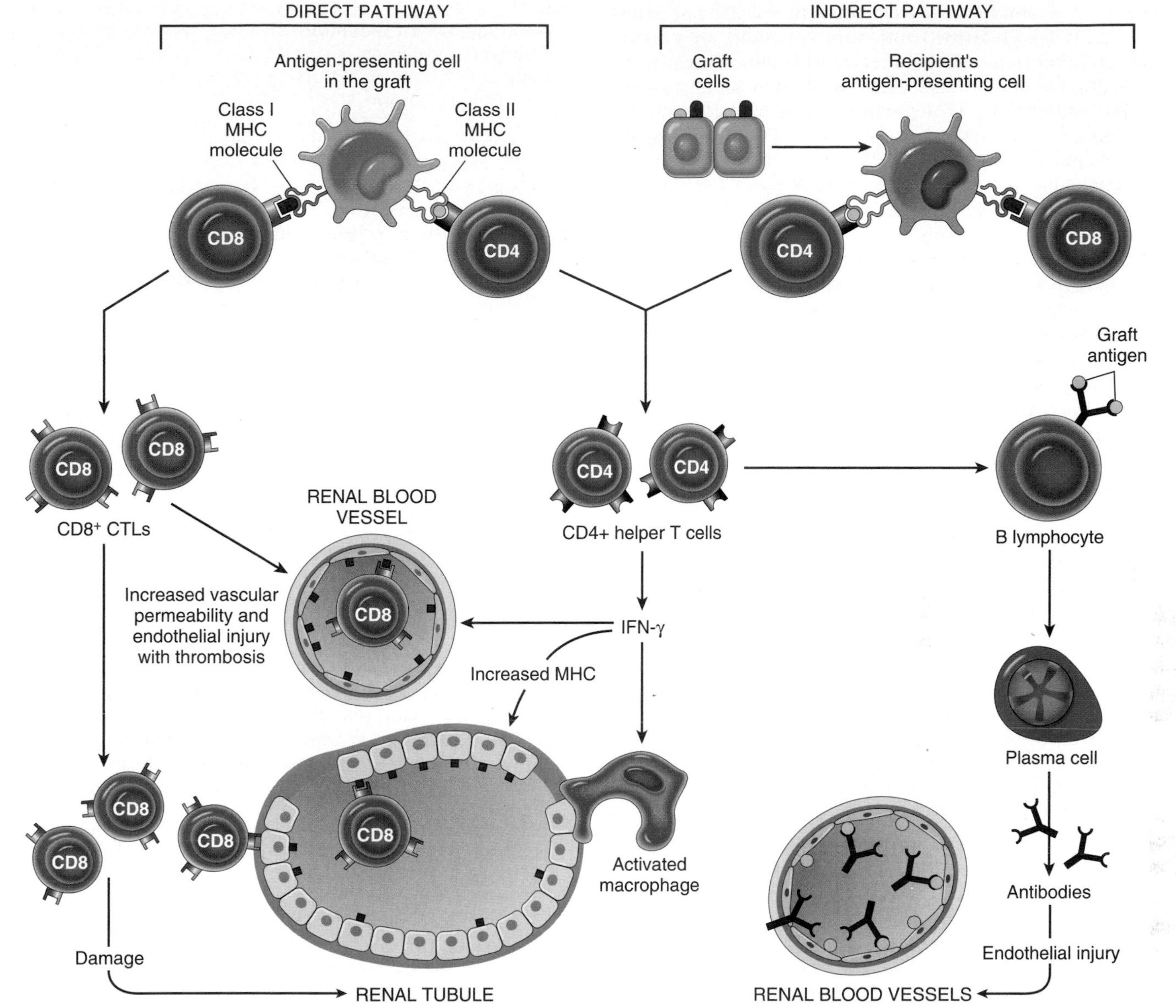

FIGURE 6–23 Schematic representation of the events that lead to the destruction of histoincompatible grafts. In the direct pathway, donor class I and class II antigens on antigen-presenting cells in the graft (along with B7 molecules, not shown) are recognized by CD8+ cytotoxic T cells and CD4+ helper T cells, respectively, of the host. CD4+ cells proliferate and produce cytokines that induce tissue damage by a local delayed hypersensitivity reaction and stimulate B cells and CD8+ T cells. CD8+ T cells responding to graft antigens differentiate into cytotoxic T lymphocytes that kill graft cells. In the indirect pathway, graft antigens are displayed by host APCs and activate CD4+ T cells, which damage the graft by a local delayed hypersensitivity reaction. The example shown is of a kidney allograft.

enter the graft and recognize graft antigens being displayed by host antigen-presenting cells that have also entered the graft, and the result is a delayed hypersensitivity type of reaction. However, CD8+ CTLs that may be generated by the indirect pathway cannot directly recognize or kill graft cells, because these CTLs recognize graft antigens presented by the host's antigen-presenting cells. Therefore, when T cells react to a graft by the indirect pathway, the principal mechanism of cellular rejection may be T-cell cytokine production and delayed hypersensitivity. It is postulated that the direct pathway is the major pathway in acute cellular rejection, whereas the indirect pathway is more important in chronic rejection. However, this separation is by no means absolute.

Antibody-Mediated Reactions. Although there is little doubt that T cells are pivotal in the rejection of organ transplants, antibodies evoked against alloantigens in the graft can also mediate rejection. This process is called *humoral rejection*, and it can take two forms. *Hyperacute rejection occurs when preformed antidonor antibodies are present in the circulation of the recipient.* Such antibodies may be present in a recipient who has already rejected a kidney transplant. Multiparous women who develop anti-HLA antibodies against paternal antigens shed from the fetus may also have preformed antibodies to grafts taken from their husbands or children, or even from unrelated individuals who share HLA alleles with the husbands. Prior blood transfusions can also lead to presensitization because platelets and white blood cells are rich in HLA antigens and donors and recipients are usually not HLA-identical. When preformed antidonor antibodies are present, rejection occurs immediately after transplantation because the circulating antibodies react with and deposit rapidly on the vascular endothelium of the grafted organ. Complement fixation occurs, resulting in thrombosis of vessels in the graft, and ischemic death of the graft. With the current practice of cross-matching, that is, testing recipient's serum for antibodies against donor's cells, hyperacute rejection is no longer a significant clinical problem.

In recipients not previously sensitized to transplantation antigens, exposure to the class I and class II HLA antigens of the donor may evoke antibodies, as depicted in Figure 6–23. The antibodies formed by the recipient may cause injury by several mechanisms, including complement-dependent cytotoxicity, inflammation, and antibody-dependent cell-mediated cytotoxicity. *The initial target of these antibodies in rejection appears to be the graft vasculature.* Thus, antibody-dependent, or *acute humoral rejection*, is usually manifested by a vasculitis, sometimes referred to as *rejection vasculitis.*

Morphology of Rejection Reactions. On the basis of the morphology and the underlying mechanism, **rejection reactions are classified as hyperacute, acute, and chronic.** The morphologic changes in these patterns are described below as they relate to renal transplants. Similar changes may occur in any other vascularized organ transplant.

Hyperacute Rejection. This form of rejection occurs within minutes or hours after transplantation and can sometimes be recognized by the surgeon just after the graft vasculature is anastomosed to the recipient's. In contrast to the nonrejecting kidney graft, which rapidly regains a normal pink coloration and normal tissue turgor and promptly excretes urine, a hyperacutely rejecting kidney rapidly becomes cyanotic, mottled, and flaccid and may excrete a mere few drops of bloody urine. Immunoglobulin and complement are deposited in the vessel wall, and electron microscopy discloses early endothelial injury together with fibrin–platelet thrombi. There is also a rapid accumulation of neutrophils within arterioles, glomeruli, and peritubular capillaries. **These early lesions point to an antigen-antibody reaction at the level of vascular endothelium.** Subsequently, these changes become diffuse and intense, the glomeruli undergo thrombotic occlusion of the capillaries, and fibrinoid necrosis occurs in arterial walls. The kidney cortex then undergoes outright infarction (necrosis), and such nonfunctioning kidneys have to be removed.

Acute Rejection. This may occur within days of transplantation in the untreated recipient or may appear suddenly months or even years later, after immunosuppression has been employed and terminated. As suggested earlier, acute graft rejection is a combined process in which both cellular and humoral tissue injuries contribute. In any one patient, one or the other mechanism may predominate. Histologically, humoral rejection is associated with vasculitis, whereas cellular rejection is marked by an interstitial mononuclear cell infiltrate.

Acute cellular rejection is most commonly seen within the initial months after transplantation and is heralded by an elevation of serum creatinine levels followed by clinical signs of renal failure. Histologically, there may be extensive interstitial mononuclear cell infiltration and edema as well as mild interstitial hemorrhage (Fig. 6–24*A*). As might be expected, immunoperoxidase staining reveals both CD4+ and CD8+ lymphocytes, and these cells express markers of activated T cells, such as the α chain of the IL-2 receptor. Glomerular and peritubular capillaries contain large numbers of mononuclear cells that may also invade the tubules, causing focal tubular necrosis (Fig. 6–24*B*). In addition to causing tubular damage, CD8+ cells may also injure vascular endothelial cells, causing a so-called *endothelitis.* This form of cell-mediated vascular damage is limited to the endothelium and is distinct from the antibody-mediated vasculitis described later. The affected vessels have swollen endothelial cells, and at places the lymphocytes can be seen between the endothelium and the vessel wall. The recognition of cellular rejection is important because, in the absence of an accompanying arteritis, patients promptly respond to immunosuppressive therapy. Cyclosporine, a widely used immunosuppressive drug, is also nephrotoxic, and hence the histologic changes resulting from cyclosporine may be superimposed.

Acute humoral rejection (rejection vasculitis) is mediated primarily by antidonor antibodies, and hence it is manifested mainly by damage to the blood vessels. This may take the form of necrotizing vasculitis with endothelial cell necrosis, neutrophilic infiltration, deposition of immunoglobulins, complement, and fibrin, and thrombosis. Such lesions are associated with extensive necrosis of the renal parenchyma. In many cases, the vasculitis is less acute and is characterized by marked thickening of the intima by proliferating fibroblasts, myocytes, and foamy macrophages (Fig. 6–25). The resultant narrowing of the arterioles may cause infarction or renal cortical atrophy. The proliferative vascular lesions mimic arteriosclerotic thickening and are believed to be caused by cytokines that cause growth of vascular smooth muscles.

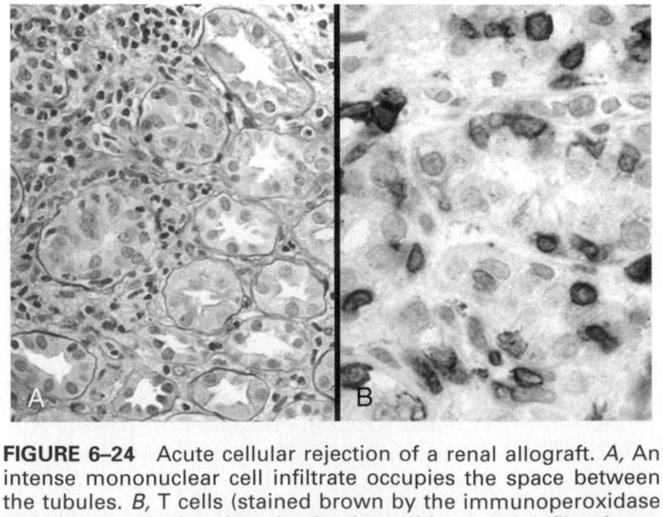

FIGURE 6–24 Acute cellular rejection of a renal allograft. *A,* An intense mononuclear cell infiltrate occupies the space between the tubules. *B,* T cells (stained brown by the immunoperoxidase technique) are abundant in the interstitium and infiltrating a tubule. (Courtesy of Dr. Robert Colvin, Department of Pathology, Massachusetts General Hospital, Boston, MA.)

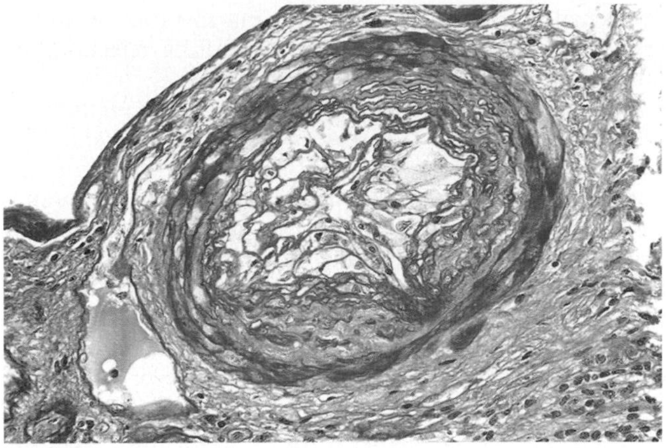

FIGURE 6–25 Antibody-mediated damage to the blood vessel in a renal allograft. The blood vessel is markedly thickened, and the lumen is obstructed by proliferating fibroblasts and foamy macrophages. (Courtesy of Dr. Ihsan Housini, Department of Pathology, University of Texas Southwestern Medical School, Dallas, TX.)

Chronic Rejection. In recent years, acute rejection has been significantly controlled by immunosuppressive therapy, and chronic rejection has emerged as an important cause of graft failure.[32] Patients with chronic rejection present clinically with a progressive rise in serum creatinine over a period of 4 to 6 months. Chronic rejection is dominated by vascular changes, interstitial fibrosis, and tubular atrophy with loss of renal parenchyma (Fig. 6–26). The **vascular changes** consist of dense, obliterative intimal fibrosis, principally in the cortical arteries. These vascular lesions result in renal ischemia, manifested by glomerular loss, interstitial fibrosis and tubular atrophy, and shrinkage of the renal parenchyma. The glomeruli may show duplication of basement membranes; this appearance is sometimes called chronic transplant glomerulopathy. Chronically rejecting kidneys usually have interstitial mononuclear cell infiltrates containing large numbers of plasma cells and numerous eosinophils.

Methods of Increasing Graft Survival

Because HLA antigens are the major targets of transplant rejection, minimizing the HLA disparity between the donor and the recipient would be expected to improve graft survival.[33] In the case of related donor kidney transplants, a beneficial effect of matching for class I HLA alleles has been observed. In cadaver renal transplants, matching for HLA class I antigens (HLA-A and HLA-B) has at best a modest effect on graft acceptance. Additional matching for class II antigens (HLA-DR) results in a definite improvement in graft survival. However, even HLA-matched unrelated donors are likely to differ from the host at one or more minor histocompatibility antigens. These antigens are formed by peptides derived from polymorphic proteins other than those encoded in the HLA complex. They evoke a weak or slower rejection reaction that, nevertheless, necessitates the use of immunosuppression.

Except in the case of identical twins, who are obviously matched for all possible histocompatibility antigens, *immunosuppressive therapy* is a practical necessity in all other donor-recipient combinations.[33] The mainstay of immunosuppression is the drug *cyclosporine*. Cyclosporine works by blocking activation of a transcription factor called nuclear factor of activated T cells, which is required for transcription of cytokine genes, in particular, the gene for IL-2. Additional drugs that are used to treat rejection include azathioprine (which inhibits leukocyte development from bone marrow precursors), steroids (which block inflammation), rapamycin and mycophenolate mofetil (both of which inhibit lymphocyte proliferation), and monoclonal anti–T-cell antibodies (e.g., monoclonal anti-CD3 and antibodies against the IL-2 receptor α chain, which block T-cell activation and may opsonize and help to eliminate the cells).

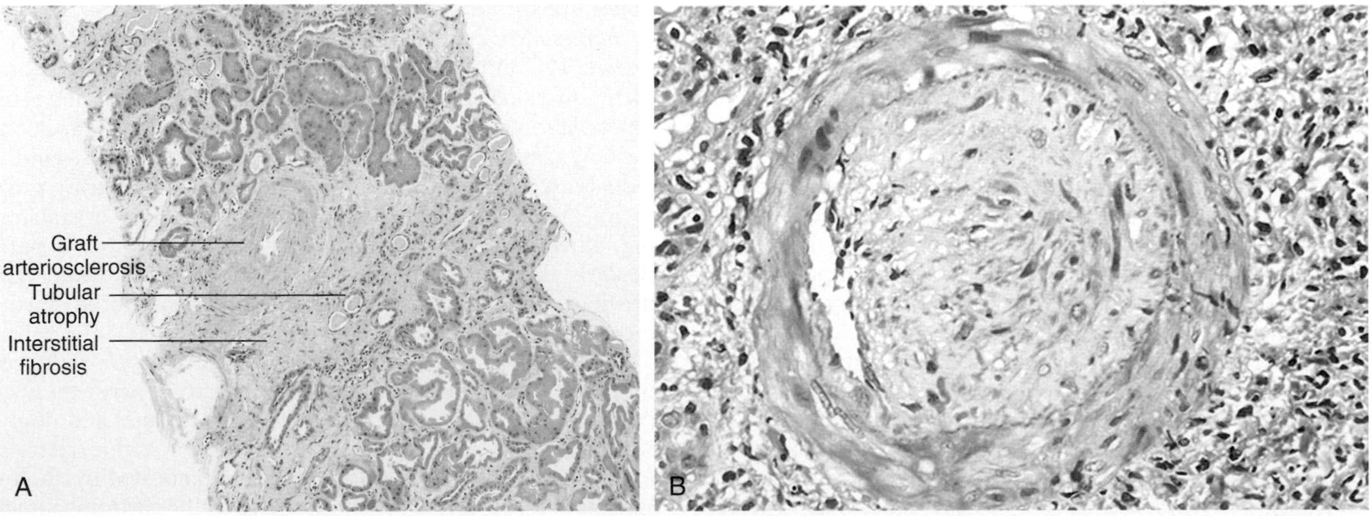

FIGURE 6–26 Chronic rejection in a kidney allograft. *A,* Changes in the kidney in chronic rejection. *B,* Graft arteriosclerosis. The vascular lumen is replaced by an accumulation of smooth muscle cells and connective tissue in the vessel intima. (Courtesy of Dr. Helmut Rennke, Department of Pathology, Brigham and Women's Hospital and Harvard Medical School, Boston, MA.)

Although immunosuppression has produced significant gains in terms of graft survival, immunosuppressive therapy carries its own risks. The price paid in the form of increased susceptibility to opportunistic fungal, viral, and other infections is not small. These patients are also at increased risk for developing EBV-induced lymphomas, human papillomavirus-induced squamous cell carcinomas, and Kaposi sarcoma (Chapter 11). To circumvent the untoward effects of immunosuppression, much effort is being devoted to induce donor-specific tolerance in host T cells.[33] One strategy being pursued in experimental animals is to prevent host T cells from receiving costimulatory signals from dendritic cells during the initial phase of sensitization. This can be accomplished by interrupting the interaction between the B7 molecules on the dendritic cells of the graft donor with the CD28 receptors on host T cells, as, for example, by administration of proteins that bind to B7 costimulators. This, as discussed earlier, interrupts the second signal for T-cell activation and renders the T cells anergic or induces their apoptosis. Antibodies that block CD40 ligand are also being tried; they presumably work by inhibiting humoral immune responses and CTL generation. In addition, giving donor cells to graft recipients may prevent reactions to the graft, perhaps because the donor inoculum contains cells, such as immature dendritic cells, that induce tolerance to the donor alloantigens. This approach may result in long-term *mixed chimerism*, in which the recipient lives with the injected donor cells. Such approaches are being tried in patients.

Transplantation of Other Solid Organs

In addition to the kidney, a variety of organs, such as the liver (Chapter 18), heart (Chapter 12), lungs, and pancreas, are also transplanted. Because patients in need of heart and liver transplants are severely ill, and because the transplanted heart or liver has to fit snugly into the space previously occupied by the host organ, the availability and size of the donor organ are of major importance, and take precedence over HLA match. Hence, HLA matching is not done in these cases. The rejection reaction against liver transplants is not as vigorous as might be expected from the degree of HLA disparity. The molecular basis of this "privilege" is not totally understood. Furthermore, with effective immunosuppression, the rejection reactions can be greatly reduced.

Transplantation of Hematopoietic Cells

Use of hematopoietic cell transplants for hematologic malignancies, certain nonhematologic cancers, aplastic anemias, and certain immunodeficiency states is increasing. Transplantation of genetically engineered hematopoietic stem cells is also likely to be useful for somatic cell gene therapy, and is being evaluated in some severe combined immunodeficiencies. Hematopoietic stem cells are usually obtained from the bone marrow but may also be harvested from peripheral blood after they are mobilized from the bone marrow by administration of hematopoietic growth factors. Several features distinguish bone marrow transplants from solid organ transplants. In most of the conditions in which bone marrow transplantation is indicated, the recipient is irradiated with lethal doses either to destroy the malignant cells (e.g., leukemias) or to create a graft bed (aplastic anemias). Three major problems arise in bone marrow transplantation: graft-versus-host (GVH) disease, transplant rejection, and immunodeficiency.

GVH disease occurs in any situation in which immunologically competent cells or their precursors are transplanted into immunologically crippled recipients, and the transferred cells recognize alloantigens in the host.[34] GVH disease occurs most commonly in the setting of allogeneic bone marrow transplantation but may also follow transplantation of solid organs rich in lymphoid cells (e.g., the liver) or transfusion of unirradiated blood.

Recipients of bone marrow transplants are immunodeficient because of either their primary disease or prior treatment of the disease with drugs or irradiation. When such recipients receive normal bone marrow cells from allogeneic donors, the immunocompetent T cells present in the donor marrow recognize the recipient's HLA antigens as *foreign* and react against them. Both CD4+ and CD8+ T cells recognize and attack host tissues. In clinical practice, GVH disease can be so severe that bone marrow transplants are done only between HLA-matched donor and recipient. However, it is possible that with conventional HLA typing, subtle molecular differences between donor and recipient HLA molecules are not picked up, and these may be enough to trigger GVH reactions. For this reason, DNA sequencing methods are now being used for molecular typing of HLA alleles. Furthermore, HLA matching will miss minor histocompatibility differences, and these may also be enough to induce GVH disease.

Acute GVH disease occurs within days to weeks after allogeneic bone marrow transplantation. Although any organ may be affected, the major clinical manifestations result from involvement of the *immune system and epithelia of the skin, liver, and intestines.* Involvement of skin in GVH disease is manifested by a generalized rash leading to desquamation in severe cases. Destruction of small bile ducts gives rise to jaundice, and mucosal ulceration of the gut results in bloody diarrhea. Despite considerable tissue damage, the affected tissues are not heavily infiltrated by lymphocytes. It is believed that in addition to direct cytotoxicity by CD8+ T cells, considerable damage is inflicted by cytokines released by the sensitized donor T cells.

Immunodeficiency is a frequent accompaniment of GVH disease. The immunodeficiency may be a result of prior treatment, myeloablative preparation for the graft, a delay in repopulation of the recipient's immune system, and attack on the host's immune cells by grafted lymphocytes. Affected individuals are profoundly immunosuppressed and are easy prey to infections. Although many different types of organisms may infect patients, infection with cytomegalovirus is particularly important. This usually results from activation of previously silent infection. Cytomegalovirus-induced pneumonitis can be a fatal complication.

Chronic GVH disease may follow the acute syndrome or may occur insidiously. These patients have extensive cutaneous injury, with destruction of skin appendages and fibrosis of the dermis. The changes may resemble systemic sclerosis (discussed later). Chronic liver disease manifested by cholestatic jaundice is also frequent. Damage to the gastrointestinal mucosa may cause esophageal strictures. The immune system is devastated, with involution of the thymus and depletion of lymphocytes in the lymph nodes. Not surprisingly, the patients experience recurrent and life-threatening infections. Some patients develop manifestations of autoimmunity, postulated to result from the grafted CD4+ helper T cells reacting with host B cells and stimulating these cells, some of which may be capable of producing autoantibodies.

Because GVH disease is mediated by T lymphocytes contained in the donor bone marrow, depletion of donor T cells before transfusion virtually eliminates the disease. This protocol, however, has proved to be a mixed blessing: GVH disease is ameliorated, but the incidence of graft failures and the recurrence of disease in leukemic patients increases. It seems that the multifaceted T cells not only mediate GVH disease but also are required for engraftment of the transplanted marrow stem cells and control of leukemic cells. The latter, called *graft-versus-leukemia* effect, can be quite dramatic. Deliberate induction of graft-versus-leukemia effect by infusion of allogeneic T cells is being tested in the treatment of chronic myelogenous leukemia if the patient relapses after bone marrow transplantation.

The mechanisms responsible for rejection of allogeneic bone marrow transplants are poorly understood. It seems to be mediated by NK cells and T cells that survive in the irradiated host. NK cells react against allogeneic stem cells because the latter are lacking self-MHC class I molecules and hence fail to deliver the inhibitory signal to NK cells.[35] There is great interest in exploiting the ability of NK cells to kill allogeneic hematopoietic cells for treating certain acute leukemias (another example of the graft-versus-leukemia effect).[36] The hope is that allogeneic NK cells will kill the tumor cells (because the NK cells will not see self-MHC molecules and will not be inhibited) but will not cause GVH reactions.

AUTOIMMUNE DISEASES

Immune reactions against *self-antigens*—autoimmunity—are an important cause of certain diseases in humans, estimated to affect at least 1% to 2% of the US population. A growing number of diseases have been attributed to autoimmunity (Table 6–7), but in many the evidence is not firm. Autoantibodies can be found in the serum of apparently normal individuals, particularly in older age groups. Furthermore, innocuous autoantibodies are also formed after damage to tissue and may serve a physiologic role in the removal of tissue breakdown products.

How, then, does one define *pathologic* autoimmunity? Ideally, at least three requirements should be met before a disorder is categorized as truly due to autoimmunity: (1) the presence of an autoimmune reaction; (2) evidence that such a reaction is not secondary to tissue damage, e.g., resulting from infection, but is of primary pathogenetic significance; and (3) the absence of another well-defined cause of the disease. Similarity with experimental models of proven autoimmunity is also often used to support this mechanism in human diseases.

Autoimmune disorders may result from tissue injury caused by T cells or antibodies that react against self-antigens. The autoimmune disorders form a spectrum, on one end of which are conditions in which the immune response is directed against a single organ or tissue, resulting in *organ-specific disease*, and on the other end are diseases in which the autoimmune reaction is against widespread antigens, resulting in *generalized* or *systemic disease*. Examples of organ-specific autoimmunity are type I diabetes mellitus, in which the autoreactive T cells and antibodies are specific for β cells of the pancreatic islets, and multiple sclerosis, in which autoreactive T cells react against central nervous system myelin. An example of systemic autoimmune disease is SLE, in which a diversity of antibodies directed against DNA, platelets, red cells, and protein-phospholipid complexes result in widespread lesions throughout the body. In the middle of the spectrum falls Goodpasture syndrome, in which antibodies to basement membranes of lung and kidney induce lesions in these organs.

TABLE 6–7 Autoimmune Diseases

Organ-Specific	Systemic
Hashimoto thyroiditis	Systemic lupus erythematosus
Autoimmune hemolytic anemia	Rheumatoid arthritis
Autoimmune atrophic gastritis of pernicious anemia	Sjögren syndrome
Multiple sclerosis	Reiter syndrome
Autoimmune orchitis	Inflammatory myopathies*
Goodpasture syndrome	Systemic sclerosis (scleroderma)*
Autoimmune thrombocytopenia	Polyarteritis nodosa*
Insulin-dependent diabetes mellitus	
Myasthenia gravis	
Graves disease	
Primary biliary cirrhosis*	
Autoimmune (chronic active) hepatitis*	
Ulcerative colitis*	

*The evidence supporting an autoimmune basis of these disorders is not strong.

It is obvious that autoimmunity results from the loss of self-tolerance, and the question arises as to how this happens. Before we look for answers to this question, we review the mechanisms of immunologic tolerance to self-antigens.

Immunologic Tolerance

Immunologic tolerance is a state in which the individual is incapable of developing an immune response to a specific antigen. Self-tolerance refers to lack of responsiveness to an individual's own antigens, and it underlies our ability to live in harmony with our cells and tissues. Several mechanisms, albeit not well understood, have been postulated to explain the tolerant state. They can be broadly classified into two groups: *central tolerance* and *peripheral tolerance.*[37–40] Each of these is considered briefly.

Central Tolerance. This refers to death (deletion) of self-reactive T- and B-lymphocyte clones during their maturation in the central lymphoid organs (the thymus for T cells and the bone marrow for B cells). Deletion of developing intrathymic T cells has been extensively investigated. Experiments with transgenic mice provide abundant evidence that T lymphocytes that bear receptors for self-antigens undergo apoptosis within the thymus during the process of T-cell maturation. It is proposed that many autologous protein antigens, including antigens thought to be restricted to peripheral tissues, are processed and presented by thymic antigen-presenting cells in association with self-MHC molecules.[37] A protein called AIRE (autoimmune regulator) is thought to stimulate expression of many "peripheral" self-antigens in the thymus and is thus critical for deletion of immature self-reactive T cells.[38] Mutations in the *AIRE* gene (either spontaneous in humans or created in knockout mice) are the cause of an autoimmune polyendocrinopathy (Chapter 24). The developing T cells that express high-affinity receptors for such self-antigens are *negatively selected*, or deleted, and therefore the peripheral T-cell pool is lacking or deficient in self-reactive cells (Fig. 6–27). What triggers apoptosis in self-reactive T-cell clones is not entirely clear. Some immature T cells that encounter self-antigens in the thymus develop into regulatory T cells, described below.

As with T cells, clonal deletion is also operative in B cells. When developing B cells encounter a membrane-bound antigen within the bone marrow, they undergo apoptosis.[41]

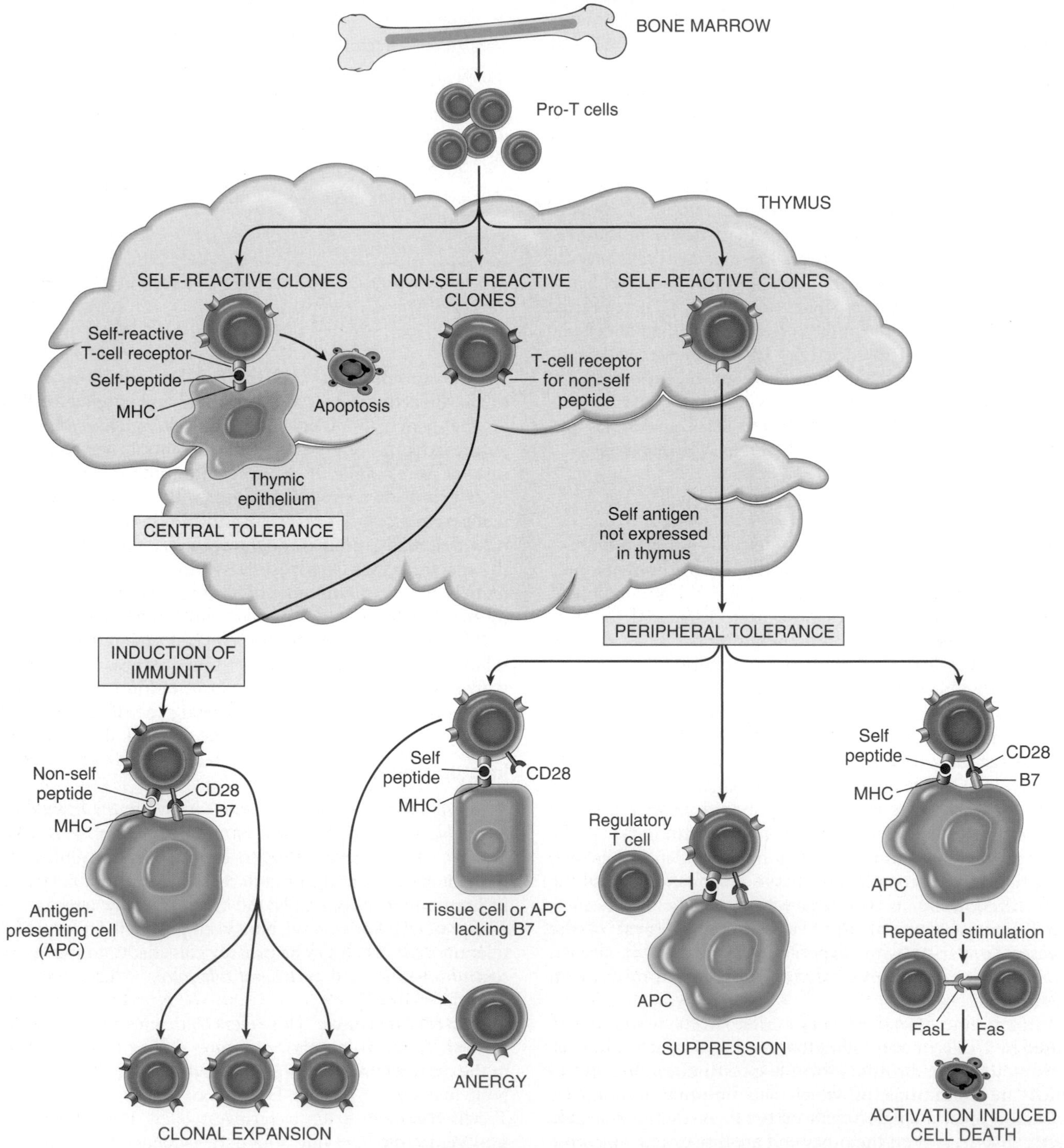

FIGURE 6–27 Schematic illustration of the mechanisms involved in central and peripheral tolerance. The principal mechanisms of tolerance in CD4+ T cells are shown. APC, antigen-presenting cell.

Clonal deletion of self-reactive lymphocytes, however, is far from perfect. Many self-antigens may not be present in the thymus, and hence T cells bearing receptors for such autoantigens escape into the periphery. There is similar "slippage" in the B-cell system as well. B cells that bear receptors for a variety of self-antigens, including thyroglobulin, collagen, and DNA, can be found in the peripheral blood of healthy individuals.

Peripheral tolerance. Those self-reactive T cells that escape intrathymic negative selection can inflict tissue injury unless they are deleted or muzzled in the peripheral tissues. Several "back-up" mechanisms that silence such potentially autoreactive T cells are known to exist.[39,40] They include the following:

1. *Anergy:* This refers to prolonged or irreversible functional inactivation of lymphocytes, induced by encounter with antigens under certain conditions.[42] We discussed earlier that activation of antigen-specific T cells requires two signals: recognition of peptide antigen in association with self-MHC molecules on the surface of antigen-presenting cells and a set of costimulatory signals ("second signals") provided by antigen-presenting cells. To initiate second signals, certain T cell–associated molecules, such as CD28, must bind to their ligands (the costimulators B7-1 and B7-2) on antigen-presenting cells. If the antigen is presented by cells that do not bear the costimulators, a negative signal is delivered, and the cell becomes anergic (Fig. 6–27). Once lymphocytes become anergic, they cannot be activated even if the relevant antigen is presented by competent antigen-presenting cells (e.g., dendritic cells) that can deliver costimulation. Because costimulatory molecules are not expressed or are weakly expressed on most normal tissues, the encounter between autoreactive T cells and their specific self-antigens may lead to anergy. In some situations, T cells that recognize self-antigens receive an inhibitory signal from a receptor called CTLA-4 that also binds to B7 molecules. Mice in which the gene for CTLA-4 is knocked out develop massive lymphproliferation and fatal multisystem autoimmune disease with T-cell infiltrates in tissues. Polymorphisms in the *CTLA-4* gene are associated with some autoimmune endocrine diseases in humans (Chapter 24). How T cells choose to use CD28 to recognize B7 molecules and be activated or CTLA-4 to recognize the same B7 molecules and become anergic is an intriguing question to which there are no clear answers. Anergy affects B cells in the tissues as well. It is believed that if B cells encounter antigen in the absence of specific helper T cells, the B cells become unable to respond to subsequent antigenic stimulation, and may be excluded from lymphoid follicles.
2. *Suppression by regulatory T cells:* Recent evidence, mostly from experiments in mice, has emphasized the role of a population of T cells called *regulatory T cells* in preventing immune reactions against self-antigens.[43] Regulatory T cells may develop in the thymus, as a result of recognition of self-antigens, or they may be induced in the periphery. The best-defined regulatory T cells are CD4+ cells that constitutively express CD25, the α chain of the IL-2 receptor, but some CD4+ cells lacking CD25 may serve the same function. The mechanisms by which these regulatory cells suppress immune responses are not fully defined. There is some evidence that peripheral suppression of autoreactivity may be mediated, in part, by the secretion of cytokines, such as IL-10 and TGF-β, which inhibit lymphocyte activation and effector functions. A transcription factor of the forkhead family, called Foxp3, is required for the development and function of CD4+ CD25+ regulatory T cells.[44] Mutations in Foxp3 result in severe autoimmunity in humans and mice; in humans, these mutations are the cause of an autoimmune disease called IPEX (for *I*mmune dysregulation, *P*olyendocrinopathy, *E*nteropathy, *X*-linked).
3. *Clonal deletion by activation-induced cell death:* CD4+ T cells that recognize self-antigens may receive signals that promote their death by apoptosis. This process has been called activation-induced cell death, because it is a consequence of T-cell activation. One mechanism of activation-induced death of CD4+ T cells involves the Fas-Fas ligand system.[45,46] Lymphocytes as well as many other cells express Fas (CD95), a member of the TNF-receptor family. FasL, a membrane protein that is structurally homologous to the cytokine TNF, is expressed mainly on activated T lymphocytes. The engagement of Fas by FasL induces apoptosis of activated T cells and may underlie the peripheral deletion of autoreactive T cells. It is believed that those self-antigens that are abundant in peripheral tissues cause repeated and persistent stimulation of self-antigen–specific T cells, leading eventually to their elimination via Fas-mediated apoptosis (Fig. 6–27). Self-reactive B cells may also be deleted by FasL on T cells engaging Fas on the B cells. The importance of this mechanism in the peripheral deletion of autoreactive lymphocytes is highlighted by two strains of mice that are natural "knockouts" of Fas or FasL. The so-called *lpr* mice have a mutation in the Fas gene, whereas the *gld* mice are born with defective FasL. Mice of both of these strains develop severe autoimmune disease resembling human SLE. (In contrast to SLE, however, these mice also suffer from generalized lymphoproliferation.) A small number of patients have also been identified with SLE-like autoimmunity and generalized lymphoproliferation associated with mutations in the *FAS* gene; this disease is called the autoimmune lymphoproliferative syndrome. Recently, another mechanism of activation-induced cell death has been proposed, again based on studies in mice.[47] It is postulated that if T cells recognize self-antigens, they may express a pro-apotic member of the BCL family, called BIM, and this protein inhibits the function of anti-apoptotic members of the family. The importance of this mechanism of cell death in self-tolerance is not established.
4. *Antigen sequestration:* Some antigens are hidden from the immune system because the tissues in which these antigens are located do not communicate with the blood and lymph. This is believed to be the case for the testis, eye, and brain, all of which are also called *immune-privileged sites* because it is difficult to induce immune responses to antigens in these sites. If the antigens of these tissues are released, for example, as a consequence of trauma or infection, the result may be an immune response that leads to prolonged tissue inflammation and injury. This is the postulated mechanism for post-traumatic orchitis and uveitis.

Prevention of autoimmunity is so vital to survival that several mechanisms have evolved to protect us from our "protectors." There is firm evidence in experimental animals for both central and peripheral mechanisms, but their relative importance in maintaining self-tolerance in humans is not established and may well vary with the nature of the autoantigen (e.g., abundance, expression in thymus).

Mechanisms of Autoimmune Diseases

Although it would be attractive to explain all autoimmune diseases by a single mechanism, it is now clear that there are a number of ways by which tolerance can be bypassed, thus terminating a previously unresponsive state to autoantigens.[48,49] More than one defect might be present in each disease, and the defects vary from one disorder to the other.

The development of autoimmunity is related to the inheritance of susceptibility genes, which may influence the maintenance of self-tolerance, and environmental triggers, particularly infections, which promote the activation of self-reactive lymphocytes (Fig. 6–28). These are discussed next.

Role of Susceptibility Genes. Most autoimmune diseases show a strong genetic predisposition.[50] Among the genes known to be associated with autoimmunity, the best defined are HLA genes. The concept of HLA association with diseases was mentioned earlier (Table 6–1). Despite the fact that this association has been well established for many years, the underlying mechanisms remain obscure. It is postulated that the presence of particular MHC alleles affects the negative selection of T cells in the thymus or the development of regulatory T cells, but there is little actual evidence for either possibility. It should be pointed out that many normal individuals inherit the MHC alleles that are disease-associated in patient populations, and normal MHC molecules are capable of presenting self-antigens. Therefore, the presence of particular MHC alleles is not, by itself, the cause of autoimmunity. In several autoimmune diseases, such as SLE and type I diabetes, many non-MHC genetic loci have been shown to be associated with autoimmunity. The story of SLE in a mouse model is particularly interesting—different susceptibility loci are believed to contribute to generalized B-cell activation, the production of anti-DNA autoantibodies, and the severity of nephritis.[51] A major limitation in these studies is that the susceptibility loci that have been identified so far usually span large segments of chromosome, and the actual disease-associated genes are not known. The relevant genes at such loci may be revealed by modern methods of gene mapping and the availability of genome sequence information.

In mice, mutations of several known genes result in autoimmunity, and many of these are instructive as far as pathogenetic mechanisms are concerned. The natural mouse mutants of Fas and FasL, which interfere with activation-induced cell death, and knockout mice lacking AIRE, the transcription factor involved in thymic expression of self-antigens, and CTLA-4, the inhibitory receptor involved in T-cell anergy, have been mentioned above. IL-2, which is a growth factor for T cells, is also required for the development and functions of regulatory T cells, and promotes Fas-mediated apoptosis if present for prolonged periods. Knockout mice lacking IL-2 or the α or β chain of the IL-2 receptor develop autoimmunity, with inflammatory bowel disease, anti-DNA antibodies, and autoimmune hemolytic anemia. In these mice, autoimmunity presumably results from a failure of suppression by regulatory T cells and a failure of activation-induced cell death, two of the mechanisms of peripheral tolerance.[52] B cells express an Fc receptor that recognizes IgG antibodies bound to antigens and shuts off further antibody production (a negative feedback mechanism). Knockout of this receptor results in autoimmunity, presumably because the B cells can no longer be controlled.[53] Mutations and polymorphisms in the Fas, AIRE, CTLA-4, and Foxp3 genes are also the cause of human autoimmune diseases, as we have mentioned previously. Although these examples teach us about the mechanisms of autoimmunity, it should be emphasized that *most human autoimmune disorders have complex, multigenic patterns of susceptibility and are not attributable to single gene mutations.*

Role of Infections. Many autoimmune diseases are associated with infections, and clinical flare-ups are often preceded by infectious prodromes. Two mechanisms have been postulated to explain the link between infections and autoimmunity (Fig. 6–29). First, infections may up-regulate the expression of costimulators on antigen-presenting cells. If these cells are presenting self-antigens, the result may be a breakdown of clonal anergy and activation of T cells specific for the self-antigens. Second, some microbes may express antigens that have the same amino acid sequences as self-antigens. Immune responses against the microbial antigens may result

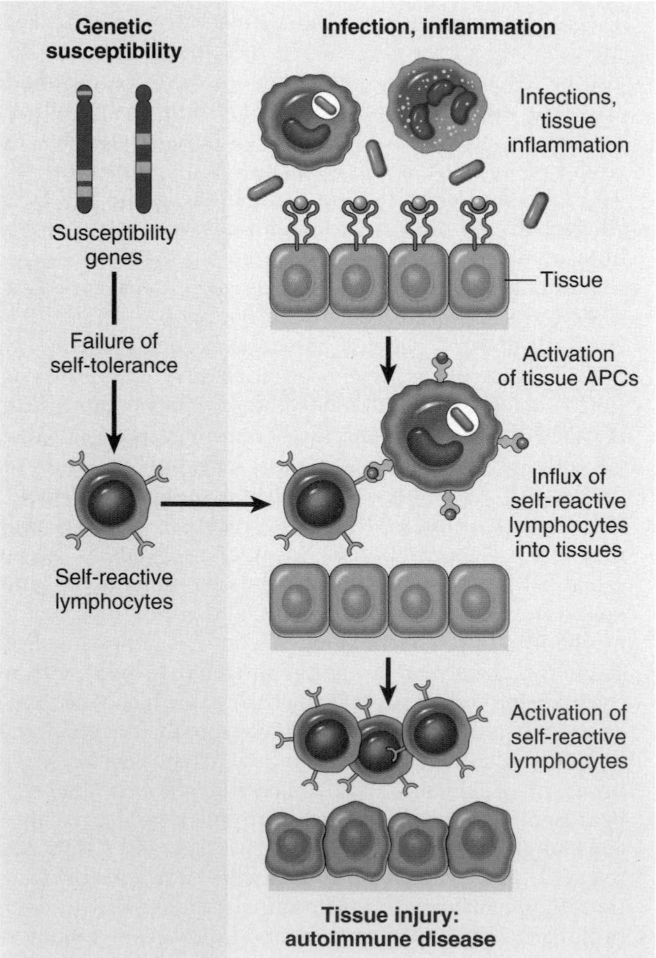

FIGURE 6–28 Pathogenesis of autoimmunity. Autoimmunity results from multiple factors, including susceptibility genes that may interfere with self-tolerance and environmental triggers (inflammation, other inflammatory stimuli) that promote lymphocyte entry into tissues, activation of lymphocytes, and tissue injury.

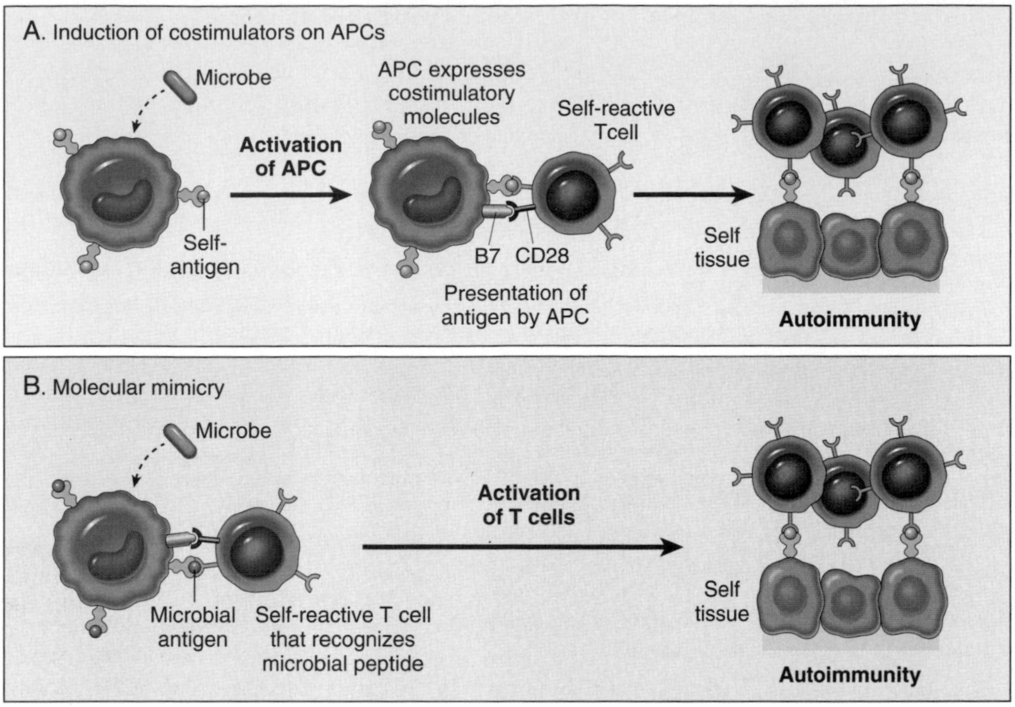

FIGURE 6–29 Role of infections in autoimmunity. Infections may promote activation of self-reactive lymphocytes by inducing the expression of costimulators (*A*), or microbial antigens may mimic self-antigens and activate self-reactive lymphocytes as a cross-reaction (*B*).

in the activation of self-reactive lymphocytes. This phenomenon is called *molecular mimicry*. A clear example of such mimicry is rheumatic heart disease, in which antibodies against streptococcal proteins cross-react with myocardial proteins and cause myocarditis (Chapter 12). But more subtle molecular mimicry may be involved in many other, classical autoimmune diseases.

Microbes may induce other abnormalities that promote autoimmune reactions. The tissue injury that is common in infections may release self-antigens and structurally alter self-antigens so that they are able to activate T cells that are not tolerant to these new, altered antigens. Infections may induce the production of cytokines that recruit lymphocytes, including potentially self-reactive lymphocytes, to sites of self-antigens.

Once an autoimmune disease has been induced, it tends to be progressive, sometimes with sporadic relapses and remissions, and the damage becomes inexorable. An important mechanism for the persistence and evolution of autoimmune disease is the phenomenon of *epitope spreading*. Infections, and even the initial autoimmune response, may release and damage self-antigens and expose epitopes of the antigens that are normally concealed from the immune system, or cryptic. The result is continuing activation of new lymphocytes that recognize these previously cryptic epitopes; since these epitopes were not expressed normally, the lymphocytes did not become tolerant to them. Thus, *regardless of the initial trigger of an autoimmune response, the progression and chronicity of the autoimmune response may be maintained by continued recruitment of autoreactive T cells that recognize normally cryptic self-determinants*. The induction of such autoreactive T cells is referred to as epitope spreading because the immune response "spreads" to determinants that were initially not recognized.[54]

With this background, we can proceed to discuss specific autoimmune diseases that illustrate the consequences of the loss of self-tolerance. As stated earlier, the autoimmune diseases of humans range from those in which the target is a single tissue, to those in which a host of self-antigens evoke a constellation of reactions against many organs and systems. In this chapter, we deal with autoimmune diseases that are primarily of a systemic nature, and we leave most single-tissue diseases to specific chapters throughout the book. For reference, however, Table 6–7 lists both systemic and organ-specific autoimmune disorders.

Systemic Lupus Erythematosus

SLE is the prototype of a multisystem disease of autoimmune origin, characterized by a bewildering array of autoantibodies, particularly antinuclear antibodies (ANAs). *Acute or insidious in its onset, it is a chronic, remitting and relapsing, often febrile illness characterized principally by injury to the skin, joints, kidney, and serosal membranes.* Virtually every other organ in the body, however, may also be affected. The clinical presentation of SLE is so variable that the American College of Rheumatology has established criteria for diagnosis of this disorder (Table 6–8). SLE is a fairly common disease, with a prevalence that may be as high as 1 in 2500 in certain populations.[55] Similar to many autoimmune diseases, SLE is predominantly a disease of women, with a frequency of 1 in 700 among women of childbearing age and a female-to-male ratio of 9 : 1. By comparison, the female-to-male ratio is only 2 : 1 for disease developing during childhood or after the age of 65. The disease is more common and severe in African-American women (1 in 245). Although SLE usually arises in the twenties and thirties, it may become manifest at any age, even in early childhood.

Etiology and Pathogenesis. The cause of SLE remains unknown, but the existence of a seemingly limitless number of antibodies in these patients against self-constituents indicates that the *fundamental defect in SLE is a failure of the*

TABLE 6–8 1997 Revised Criteria for Classification of Systemic Lupus Erythematosus*

Criterion	Definition
1. Malar rash	Fixed erythema, flat or raised, over the malar eminences
2. Discoid rash	Erythematous raised patches with adherent keratotic scaling and follicular plugging; atrophic scarring may occur
3. Photosensitivity	Skin rash as a result of exposure to UV light
4. Oral ulcers	Oral or nasopharyngeal ulceration, usually painless, observed by a physician
5. Arthritis	Nonerosive arthritis involving two or more peripheral joints, characterized by tenderness, swelling, or effusion
6. Serositis	Pleuritis—convincing history of pleuritic pain or rub heard by a physician or evidence of pleural effusion, or Pericarditis—documented by electrocardiogram or rub or evidence of pericardial effusion
7. Renal disorder	Persistent proteinuria >0.5 g/dl or >3+ if quantitation not performed, or Cellular casts—may be red blood cell, hemoglobin, granular, tubular, or mixed
8. Neurologic disorder	Seizures—in the absence of offending drugs or known metabolic derangements, e.g., uremia, ketoacidosis, or electrolyte imbalance, or Psychosis—in the absence of offending drugs or known metabolic derangements, e.g., uremia, ketoacidosis, or electrolyte imbalance
9. Hematologic disorder	Hemolytic anemia—with reticulocytosis, or Leukopenia—<4.0 × 10^9/L (4000/μl) total on two or more occasions, or Lymphopenia—<1.5 × 10^9/L (1500/μl) on two or more occasions, or Thrombocytopenia—<100 × 10^9/L (100 × 10^3/μl) in the absence of offending drugs
10. Immunologic disorder	Anti-ds DNA, anti-Sm, and/or antiphospholipid
11. Antinuclear antibody	An abnormal titer of antinuclear antibody by immunofluorescence or an equivalent assay at any point in time and in the absence of drugs known to be associated with drug-induced lupus syndrome

*The proposed classification is based on 11 criteria. For the purpose of identifying patients in clinical studies, a person is said to have systemic lupus erythematosus if any 4 or more of the 11 criteria are present, serially or simultaneously, during any interval of observation.

Data from Tan EM, et al: The revised criteria for the classification of systemic lupus erythematosus. Arthritis Rheum 25:1271, 1982; and Hochberg, MC: Updating the American College of Rheumatology revised criteria for the classification of systemic lupus erythematosus. Arthritis Rheum 40:1725, 1997.

mechanisms that maintain self-tolerance. Antibodies have been identified against an array of nuclear and cytoplasmic components of the cell that are neither organ nor species specific. In addition, a third group of antibodies is directed against cell-surface antigens of blood cells. Apart from their value in the diagnosis and management of patients with SLE, these antibodies are of major pathogenetic significance, as, for example, in the immune complex–mediated glomerulonephritis so typical of this disease.[56]

ANAs are directed against several nuclear antigens and can be grouped into four categories:[56] (1) antibodies to DNA, (2) antibodies to histones, (3) antibodies to nonhistone proteins bound to RNA, and (4) antibodies to nucleolar antigens. Table 6–9 lists several ANAs and their association with SLE as well as with other autoimmune diseases to be discussed later. Several techniques are used to detect ANAs. Clinically the most commonly used method is indirect immunofluorescence, which detects a variety of nuclear antigens, including DNA, RNA, and proteins (collectively called *generic ANAs*). The pattern of nuclear fluorescence suggests the type of antibody present in the patient's serum. Four basic patterns are recognized:

- *Homogeneous or diffuse nuclear staining* usually reflects antibodies to chromatin, histones and, occasionally, double-stranded DNA.
- *Rim or peripheral staining* patterns are most commonly indicative of antibodies to double-stranded DNA.
- *Speckled pattern* refers to the presence of uniform or variable-sized speckles. This is one of the most commonly observed patterns of fluorescence and therefore the least specific. It reflects the presence of antibodies to non-DNA nuclear constituents. Examples include Sm antigen, ribonucleoprotein, and SS-A and SS-B reactive antigens (Table 6–9).
- *Nucleolar pattern* refers to the presence of a few discrete spots of fluorescence within the nucleus and represents antibodies to nucleolar RNA. This pattern is reported most often in patients with systemic sclerosis.

The fluorescence patterns are not absolutely specific for the type of antibody, and because many autoantibodies may be present, combinations of patterns are frequent. *The immunofluorescence test for ANA is positive in virtually every patient with SLE; hence this test is sensitive, but it is not specific because patients with other autoimmune diseases also frequently score positive* (see Table 6–9). *Furthermore, approximately 5% to 15% of normal individuals have low titers of these antibodies.* The incidence increases with age.

Detection of antibodies to specific nuclear antigens requires specialized techniques. Of the numerous nuclear antigen–antibody systems,[57] some that are clinically useful are listed in Table 6–9. *Antibodies to double-stranded DNA and the so-called Smith (Sm) antigen are virtually diagnostic of SLE.*

There is some, albeit imperfect, correlation between the presence or absence of certain ANAs and clinical manifestations. For example, high titers of double-stranded DNA antibodies are usually associated with active renal disease. Conversely the risk of nephritis is low if anti–SS-B antibodies are present.[56]

TABLE 6–9 Antinuclear Antibodies in Various Autoimmune Diseases

		Disease, % Positive					
Nature of Antigen	**Antibody System**	***SLE***	***Drug-Induced LE***	***Systemic Sclerosis —Diffuse***	***Limited Scleroderma —CREST***	***Sjögren Syndrome***	***Inflammatory Myopathies***
Many nuclear antigens (DNA, RNA, proteins)	Generic ANA (indirect IF)	>95	>95	70–90	70–90	50–80	40–60
Native DNA	Anti–double-stranded DNA	[40–60]	<5	<5	<5	<5	<5
Histones	Antihistone	50–70	[>95]	<5	<5	<5	<5
Core proteins of small nuclear ribonucleoprotein particles (Smith antigen)	Anti-Sm	[20–30]	<5	<5	<5	<5	<5
Ribonucleoprotein (U1RNP)	Nuclear RNP	30–40	<5	15	10	<5	<5
RNP	SS-A(Ro)	30–50	<5	<5	<5	[70–95]	10
RNP	SS-B(La)	10–15	<5	<5	<5	[60–90]	<5
DNA topoisomerase I	Scl-70	<5	<5	[28–70]	10–18	<5	<5
Centromeric proteins	Anticentromere	<5	<5	22–36	[90]	<5	<5
Histidyl-t-RNA synthetase	Jo-1	<5	<5	<5	<5	<5	[25]

Boxed entries indicate high correlation.
SLE, systemic lupus erythematosus; LE, lupus erythematosus; ANA, antinuclear antibodies; RNP, ribonucleoprotein.

In addition to ANAs, lupus patients have a host of other autoantibodies. Some are directed against elements of the blood, such as red cells, platelets, and lymphocytes; others are directed against proteins complexed to phospholipids. In recent years, there has been much interest in these so-called antiphospholipid antibodies.[58] They are present in 40% to 50% of lupus patients. Although initially believed to be directed against anionic phospholipids, they are actually directed against epitopes of plasma proteins that are revealed when the proteins are complexed to phospholipids. A variety of protein substrates have been implicated, including prothrombin, annexin V, β_2-glycoprotein I, protein S, and protein C.[59] *Antibodies against the phospholipid–β_2-glycoprotein complex also bind to cardiolipin antigen, used in syphilis serology, and therefore lupus patients may have a false-positive test result for syphilis.* Some of these antibodies interfere with in vitro clotting tests, such as partial thromboplastin time. Therefore, these antibodies are sometimes referred to as *lupus anticoagulant.* Despite having a circulating anticoagulant that delays clotting in vitro, these patients have complications associated with a *hypercoagulable state.*[60] They have venous and arterial thromboses, which may be associated with recurrent spontaneous miscarriages and focal cerebral or ocular ischemia. This constellation of clinical features, in association with lupus, is referred to as the *secondary antiphospholipid antibody syndrome.* The pathogenesis of thrombosis in these patients is unknown; possible mechanisms are discussed in Chapter 4. Some patients develop these autoantibodies and the clinical syndrome without associated SLE. They are said to have the primary antiphospholipid syndrome (Chapter 4).

Given the presence of all these autoantibodies, we still know little about the mechanism of their emergence. Three converging lines of investigation hold center stage today: genetic predisposition, some nongenetic (environmental) factors, and a fundamental abnormality in the immune system.

Genetic Factors. SLE is a complex genetic trait with contribution from MHC and multiple non-MHC genes. Many lines of evidence support a genetic predisposition.[51,61]

- Family members of patients have an increased risk of developing SLE. Up to 20% of clinically unaffected first-degree relatives of SLE patients reveal autoantibodies and other immunoregulatory abnormalities.
- There is a higher rate of concordance (>20%) in monozygotic twins when compared with dizygotic twins (1% to 3%). Monozygotic twins who are discordant for SLE have similar patterns and titers of autoantibodies.[62] These data suggest that the genetic makeup regulates the formation of autoantibodies, but the expression of the disease (i.e., tissue injury) is influenced by non-genetic (possibly environmental) factors.
- Studies of HLA associations further support the concept that MHC genes regulate production of specific autoantibodies, rather than conferring a generalized predisposition to SLE. Specific alleles of the HLA-DQ locus have been linked to the production of anti–double-stranded DNA, anti-Sm, and antiphospholipid antibodies.
- Some lupus patients (approximately 6%) have inherited deficiencies of early complement components, such as C2, C4, or C1q. Lack of complement may impair removal of circulating immune complexes by the mononuclear phagocyte system, thus favoring tissue deposition. Knockout mice lacking C4 or certain complement receptors are also prone to develop lupus-like autoimmunity. Various mechanisms have been invoked, including failure to clear immune complexes and loss of B-cell self-tolerance. It has also been proposed that deficiency of C1q results in failure of phagocytic

clearance of apoptotic cells.[63] Such cells are produced normally, and if they are not cleared their nuclear components may elicit immune responses.

- In animal models of SLE, several non-MHC susceptibility loci have been identified. The best-known animal model is the (NZBxNZW)F1 mouse strain. In different versions of this strain, up to 20 loci are believed to be associated with the disease.[51]

Environmental Factors. There are many indications that, in addition to genetic factors, several *environmental* or nongenetic factors must be involved in the pathogenesis of SLE. The clearest example comes from the observation that *drugs* such as hydralazine, procainamide, and D-penicillamine can induce an SLE-like response in humans.[64] Exposure to *ultraviolet light* is another environmental factor that exacerbates the disease in many individuals. How ultraviolet light acts is not entirely clear, but it is suspected of modulating the immune response. For example, it induces keratinocytes to produce IL-1, a factor known to influence the immune response. In addition, UV irradiation may induce apoptosis in cells, and alter the DNA in such a way that it becomes immunogenic.[65] *Sex hormones* seem to exert an important influence on the occurrence and manifestations of SLE. During the reproductive years, the frequency of SLE is 10 times greater in women than in men, and exacerbation has been noted during normal menses and pregnancy.

Immunologic Factors. With all the immunologic findings in SLE patients, there can be little doubt that some fundamental derangement of the immune system is involved in the pathogenesis of SLE. Although a variety of immunologic abnormalities affecting both T cells and B cells have been detected in patients with SLE, it has been difficult to relate any one of them to the causation of this disease. For years, it had been thought that an intrinsic B-cell hyperactivity is fundamental to the pathogenesis of SLE. Polyclonal B-cell activation can be readily demonstrated in patients with SLE and in murine models of this disease. Molecular analyses of anti–double-stranded DNA antibodies, however, strongly suggest that pathogenic autoantibodies are not derived from polyclonally activated B cells. Instead, it appears that the production of tissue-damaging antibodies is driven by self-antigens and results from an antigen-specific helper T cell–dependent B-cell response with many characteristics of responses to foreign antigens.[66] These observations have shifted the onus of driving the autoimmune response squarely on helper T cells.[66a] Based on these findings, a model for the pathogenesis of SLE has been proposed (Fig. 6–30). Other contributing factors include defective clearance of apoptotic cells, mentioned above, and dysregulation of cytokines, notably interferons.[61] SLE is a heterogeneous disease, however, and as mentioned earlier, the production of different autoantibodies is regulated by distinct genetic factors. Hence, there may well be distinct immunoregulatory disturbances in patients with different genetic backgrounds and autoantibody profiles.[67]

Regardless of the exact sequence by which autoantibodies are formed, they are clearly the mediators of tissue injury. *Most of the visceral lesions are mediated by immune complexes (type III hypersensitivity).* DNA–anti-DNA complexes can be detected in the glomeruli and small blood vessels. Low levels of serum complement and granular deposits of complement

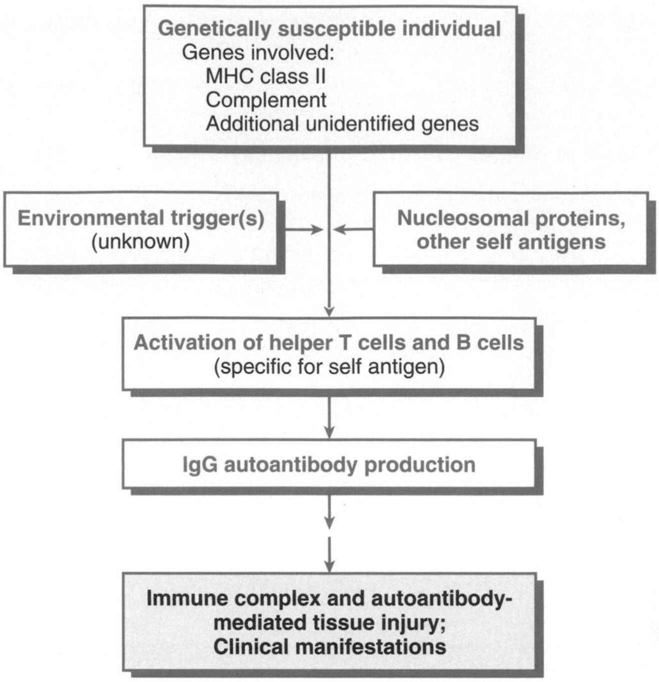

FIGURE 6–30 Model for the pathogenesis of systemic lupus erythematosus. (Modified from Kotzin BL: Systemic lupus erythematosus. Cell 65:303, 1996. Copyright 1996, Cell Press.)

and immunoglobulins in the glomeruli further support the immune complex nature of the disease. *Autoantibodies against red cells, white cells, and platelets opsonize these cells and promote their phagocytosis and lysis.* There is no evidence that ANAs, which are involved in immune complex formation, can penetrate intact cells. If cell nuclei are exposed, however, the ANAs can bind to them. In tissues, nuclei of damaged cells react with ANAs, lose their chromatin pattern, and become homogeneous, to produce so-called lupus erythematosus (LE) bodies or hematoxylin bodies. Related to this phenomenon is the LE cell, which is readily seen in vitro. The LE cell is any phagocytic leukocyte (neutrophil or macrophage) that has engulfed the denatured nucleus of an injured cell. The demonstration of LE cells in vitro was used in the past as a test for SLE. With new techniques for detection of ANAs, however, this test is now largely of historical interest. Sometimes LE cells are found in pericardial or pleural effusions in patients.

To summarize, SLE is a complex disorder of multifactorial origin resulting from interactions among genetic, hormonal, and environmental factors acting in concert to cause activation of helper T cells and B cells that results in the secretion of several species of autoantibodies. In this complex web, each factor may be necessary but not enough for the clinical expression of the disease; the relative importance of various factors may vary from individual to individual.

Morphology. The morphologic changes in SLE are extremely variable, as are the clinical manifestations and the course of the disease in individual patients. The constellation of clinical, serologic, and morphologic changes is essential for diagnosis (see Table 6–8). The frequency of individual organ involvement is shown in Table 6–10. The most characteristic

TABLE 6–10 Clinical and Pathologic Manifestations of Systemic Lupus Erythematosus

Clinical Manifestation	Prevalence in Patients, %
Hematologic	100
Arthritis	90
Skin	85
Fever	83
Fatigue	81
Weight loss	63
Renal	50
Central nervous system	50
Pleuritis	46
Myalgia	33
Pericarditis	25
Gastrointestinal	21
Raynaud phenomenon	20
Ocular	15
Peripheral neuropathy	14

lesions result from the deposition of immune complexes and are found in the blood vessels, kidneys, connective tissue, and skin.

An acute necrotizing vasculitis involving small arteries and arterioles may be present in any tissue.[68] The arteritis is characterized by fibrinoid deposits in the vessel walls. In chronic stages, vessels undergo fibrous thickening with luminal narrowing.

Kidney. The kidney is a frequent target of injury in SLE. The principal mechanism of injury is immune complex deposition in renal structures, including glomeruli, tubular and peritubular capillary basement membranes, and larger blood vessels. Other forms of injury may include a thrombotic process involving the glomerular capillaries and extraglomerular vasculature, thought to be caused by antiphospholipid antibodies.

A morphologic classification of the patterns of immune complex–mediated glomerular injury in SLE has proven to be clinically useful.[69] There are several versions of the World Health Organization (WHO) classification of lupus nephritis, but in all, five patterns are recognized: (1) minimal or no detectable abnormalities (class I), which is rare, seen in renal biopsies from less than 5% of SLE patients; (2) mesangial lupus glomerulonephritis (class II); (3) focal proliferative glomerulonephritis (class III); (4) diffuse proliferative glomerulonephritis (class IV); and (5) membranous glomerulonephritis (class V). None of these patterns is specific for lupus.

Mesangial lupus glomerulonephritis is characterized by mesangial cell proliferation and lack of involvement of glomerular capillary walls. It is seen in 10% to 25% of patients, most of whom have minimal clinical manifestations, such as mild hematuria or transient proteinuria. There is a slight to moderate increase in the intercapillary mesangial matrix as well as in the number of mesangial cells. Despite the mild histologic changes, **granular mesangial deposits of immunoglobulin and complement are always present**. Such deposits presumably reflect the earliest change because filtered immune complexes accumulate primarily in the mesangium. The other changes to be described are usually superimposed on the mesangial changes.

Focal proliferative glomerulonephritis is seen in 20% to 35% of patients. It is a focal lesion, affecting fewer than 50% of the glomeruli and generally only portions of each glomerulus. Typically, one or two tufts in an otherwise normal glomerulus exhibit swelling and proliferation of endothelial and mesangial cells, infiltration with neutrophils, and sometimes fibrinoid deposits and intracapillary thrombi (Fig. 6–31). Occasionally, affected glomeruli exhibit global injury. Focal lesions are associated with hematuria and proteinuria. In some patients, the nephritis progresses to diffuse proliferative disease.

Diffuse proliferative glomerulonephritis is the most serious of the renal lesions in SLE, occurring in 35% to 60% of patients who undergo biopsy. Anatomic changes are dominated by proliferation of endothelial, mesangial and, sometimes, epithelial cells (Fig. 6–32), producing in some cases epithelial crescents that fill the Bowman space (Chapter 20). The presence of fibrinoid necrosis, crescents, prominent infiltration by leukocytes, cell death as indicated by apoptotic bodies, and hyaline thrombi indicates active disease. Most or all glomeruli are involved in both kidneys, and the entire glomerulus is frequently affected. Patients with diffuse lesions are usually overtly symptomatic, showing microscopic or gross hematuria as well as proteinuria that is severe enough to cause the nephrotic syndrome in more than 50% of patients. Hypertension and mild to severe renal insufficiency are also common.

Membranous glomerulonephritis is a designation given to glomerular disease in which the principal histologic change consists of widespread thickening of the capillary walls. The lesions are similar to those encountered in idiopathic membranous glomerulonephritis, described more fully in Chapter 20. This type of lesion is seen in 10% to 15% of patients with

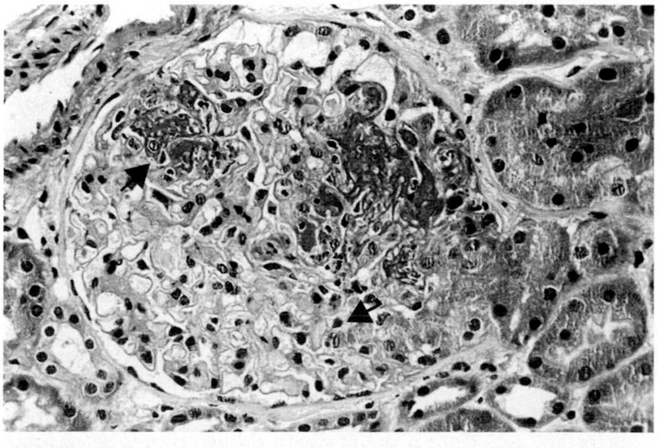

FIGURE 6–31 Lupus nephritis. There are two focal necrotizing lesions in the glomerulus *(arrowheads)*. (Courtesy of Dr. Helmut Rennke, Department of Pathology, Brigham and Women's Hospital, Boston, MA.)

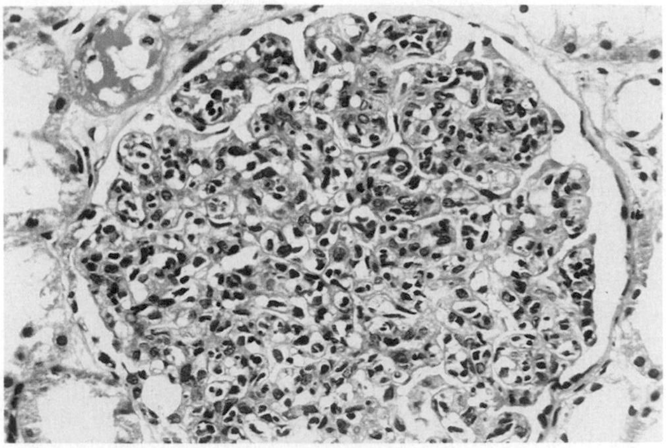

FIGURE 6–32 Lupus nephritis, diffuse proliferative type. Note the marked increase in cellularity throughout the glomerulus. (Courtesy of Dr. Helmut Rennke, Department of Pathology, Brigham and Women's Hospital, Boston, MA.)

SLE and is almost always accompanied by severe proteinuria with the nephrotic syndrome.

All of these glomerular lesions are thought to have the same general pathogenetic mechanism, that is, the deposition of immune complexes within the glomeruli. Some evidence indicates that the complexes are composed of DNA and anti-DNA antibodies, but other antigens such as histones have also been implicated. Some complexes are believed to form in situ (i.e., the DNA is deposited first on the basement membrane, followed by anti-DNA antibody), and others may deposit from the circulation, especially those located in subendothelial portions of the capillary walls. Granular deposits of immunoglobulin and complement are regularly present in the mesangium alone or along the entire basement membrane and sometimes massively throughout the entire glomerulus (Fig. 6–33). Why this same pathogenetic mechanism produces such different histologic lesions (and clinical manifestations) in different patients is not entirely clear.

Electron microscopy demonstrates electron-dense immune complexes that may be mesangial, intramembranous, subepithelial, or subendothelial in location. All histologic types show variable amounts of deposits in the mesangium. In membranous glomerulonephritis (class V), the deposits are predominantly between the basement membrane and the visceral epithelial cell (subepithelial), a location similar to that of deposits in other types of membranous nephropathy. Subendothelial deposits (between the endothelium and the basement membrane) are most commonly seen in the proliferative types (classes III and IV) (Fig. 6–34). When extensive and confluent, subendothelial deposits create a homogeneous thickening of the capillary wall, which can be seen by means of light microscopy as a **wire loop** lesion (Fig. 6–35). Such wire loops are often found in the diffuse proliferative type of glomerulonephritis (class IV) but can also be present in the focal (class III) and membranous (class V) types. They usually reflect active disease.

Changes in the **interstitium and tubules are also frequently present** in patients with SLE, especially in association with diffuse proliferative glomeru-

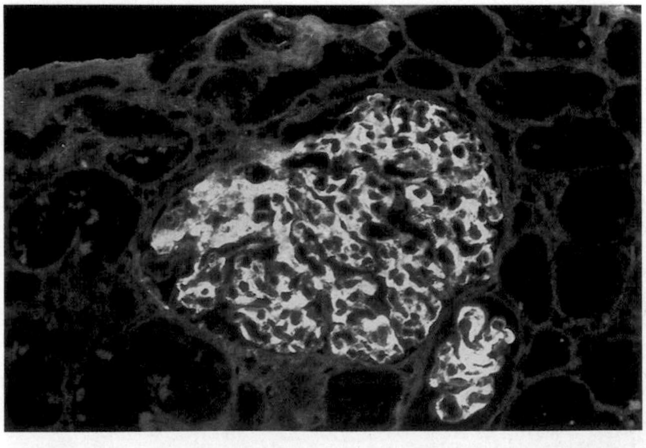

FIGURE 6–33 Immunofluorescence micrograph stained with fluorescent anti-IgG from a patient with diffuse proliferative lupus nephritis. One complete glomerulus and part of another one are seen. Note the mesangial and capillary wall deposits of IgG. (Courtesy of Dr. Helmut Rennke, Department of Pathology, Brigham and Women's Hospital, Boston, MA.)

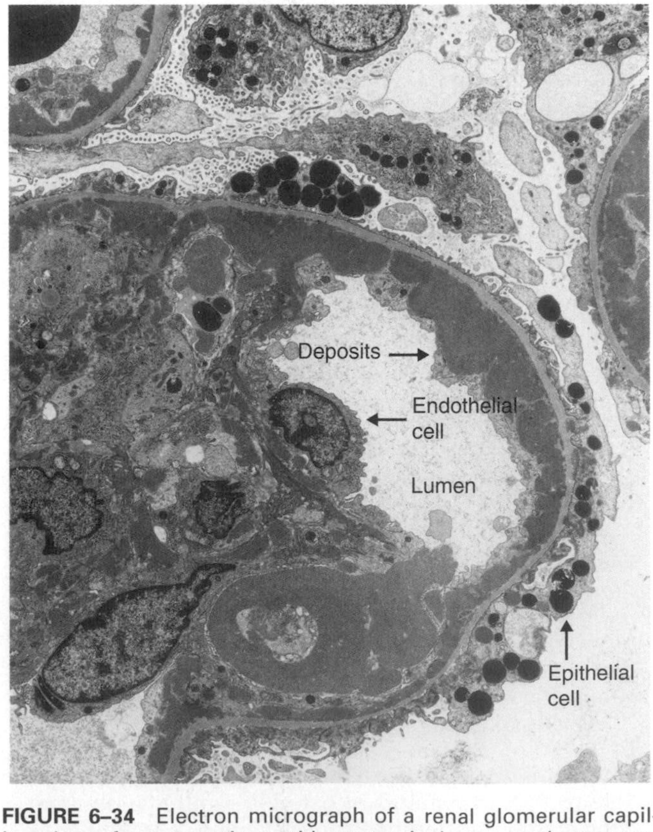

FIGURE 6–34 Electron micrograph of a renal glomerular capillary loop from a patient with systemic lupus erythematosus nephritis. Subendothelial dense deposits correspond to "wire loops" seen by light microscopy. Deposits are also present in the mesangium. (Courtesy of Dr. Jean Olson, Department of Pathology, University of California San Francisco, San Francisco, CA.)

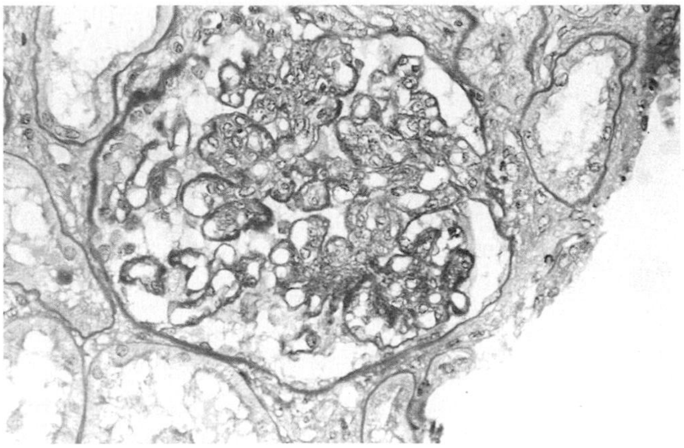

FIGURE 6–35 Lupus nephritis showing a glomerulus with several "wire loop" lesions representing extensive subendothelial deposits of immune complexes. (Periodic acid-Schiff [PAS] stain.) (Courtesy of Dr. Helmut Rennke, Department of Pathology, Brigham and Women's Hospital, Boston, MA.)

lonephritis. In a few cases, tubulointerstitial lesions may be the dominant abnormality. Granular deposits composed of immunoglobulin and complement similar to those seen in glomeruli are present in the tubular basement membranes in about 50% of patients with SLE, a pattern indicative of so-called tubular immune complex disease.

Skin. The skin is involved in the majority of patients. Characteristic erythema affects the facial butterfly area (bridge of the nose and cheeks) in approximately 50% of patients, but a similar rash may also be seen on the extremities and trunk. Urticaria, bullae, maculopapular lesions, and ulcerations also occur. **Exposure to sunlight incites or accentuates the erythema.** Histologically the involved areas show liquefactive degeneration of the basal layer of the epidermis together with edema at the dermal junction (Fig. 6–36). In the dermis, there is variable edema and perivascular mononuclear infiltrates. Vasculitis with fibrinoid necrosis of the vessels may be prominent. Immunofluorescence microscopy shows deposition of immunoglobulin and complement along the dermoepidermal junction (Fig. 6–36). Similar deposits may be present in uninvolved skin. The presence of immunoglobulin and complement at the dermoepidermal junction is not diagnostic of SLE because similar deposits are sometimes seen in the skin of patients with scleroderma or dermatomyositis.

Joints. Joint involvement is frequent, the typical lesion being a nonerosive synovitis with little deformity. The latter fact distinguishes this arthritis from that seen in rheumatoid disease. In the acute phases of arthritis in SLE, there is exudation of neutrophils and fibrin into the synovium and a perivascular mononuclear cell infiltrate in the subsynovial tissue.

Central Nervous System. The pathologic basis of central nervous system symptoms is not entirely clear. It has often been ascribed to acute vasculitis with resultant focal neurologic symptoms. However, histologic studies of the nervous system in patients

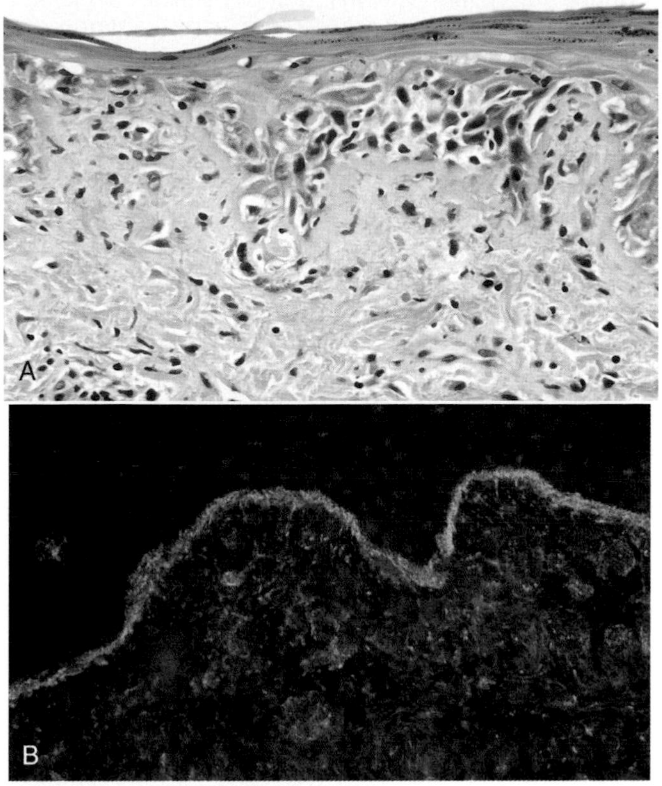

FIGURE 6–36 Systemic lupus erythematosus involving the skin. *A*, An H&E-stained section shows liquefactive degeneration of the basal layer of the epidermis and edema at the dermoepidermal junction. (Courtesy of Dr. Jag Bhawan, Boston University School of Medicine, Boston, MA.) *B*, An immunofluorescence micrograph stained for IgG reveals deposits of immunoglobulin along the dermal–epidermal junction. (Courtesy of Dr. Richard Sontheimer, Department of Dermatology, University of Texas Southwestern Medical School, Dallas, TX.)

with neuropsychiatric manifestations of SLE fail to reveal significant vasculitis. Instead, noninflammatory occlusion of small vessels by intimal proliferation is sometimes noticed. These changes are believed to result from damage to the endothelium by antiphospholipid antibodies. In addition, studies suggest that antibodies against a synaptic membrane protein may play a role in the pathogenesis of central nervous system symptoms.[70]

Pericarditis and Other Serosal Cavity Involvement. Inflammation of the serosal lining membranes may be acute, subacute, or chronic. During the acute phases, the mesothelial surfaces are sometimes covered with fibrinous exudate. Later they become thickened, opaque, and coated with a shaggy fibrous tissue that may lead to partial or total obliteration of the serosal cavity.

Cardiovascular system involvement is manifested primarily in the form of pericarditis. Symptomatic or asymptomatic pericardial involvement is present in the majority of patients. Myocarditis, manifested as nonspecific mononuclear cell infiltration, may also be present but is less common. It may cause resting tachycardia and electrocardiographic abnormalities.

Subtle or overt valvular abnormalities, detected readily by echocardiography, are fairly common in SLE. They affect mainly the mitral and aortic valves and are manifested as diffuse valve thickening that may be associated with dysfunction (stenosis or regurgitation).[71] Valvular endocarditis may occur, but it is clinically insignificant. In the era before the widespread use of steroids, so-called Libman-Sacks endocarditis was more common. This **nonbacterial verrucous endocarditis** takes the form of single or multiple irregular, 1- to 3-mm warty deposits on any valve in the heart, distinctively on either surface of the leaflets (i.e., on the surface exposed to the forward flow of the blood or on the underside of the leaflet) (Fig. 6–37). By comparison, the vegetations in infective endocarditis are considerably larger, and those in rheumatic heart disease (Chapter 12) are smaller and confined to the lines of closure of the valve leaflets.

An increasing number of patients have clinical evidence of coronary artery disease (angina, myocardial infarction) owing to coronary atherosclerosis. This complication is noted particularly in young patients with long-standing disease and especially in those who have been treated with corticosteroids. The pathogenesis of accelerated coronary atherosclerosis is unclear but is probably multifactorial. The traditional risk factors, including hypertension, obesity, and hyperlipidemia, are more common in patients with lupus than in control populations. In addition, immune complexes and antiphospholipid antibodies may deposit on the endothelium, causing damage and promoting atherosclerosis.

Spleen. The spleen may be moderately enlarged. Capsular thickening is common, as is follicular hyperplasia. Plasma cells are usually numerous in the pulp and can be shown to contain immunoglobulins of the IgG and IgM types by fluorescence microscopy. The central penicilliary arteries show thickening and perivascular fibrosis, producing so-called onion-skin lesions.

Lungs. Pleuritis and pleural effusions are the most common pulmonary manifestations, affecting almost 50% of patients. Less commonly, there is evidence of alveolar injury in the form of edema and hemorrhage. In some cases, there is chronic interstitial fibrosis. None of these changes is specific for SLE.

Other Organs and Tissues. Acute vasculitis may be seen in the portal tracts of the liver accompanied by lymphocytic infiltrates, creating nonspecific portal triaditis. LE, or hematoxylin, bodies in the bone marrow may be strongly indicative of SLE. Lymph nodes may be enlarged and contain hyperactive follicles as well as plasma cells, changes that are indicative of B-cell activation.

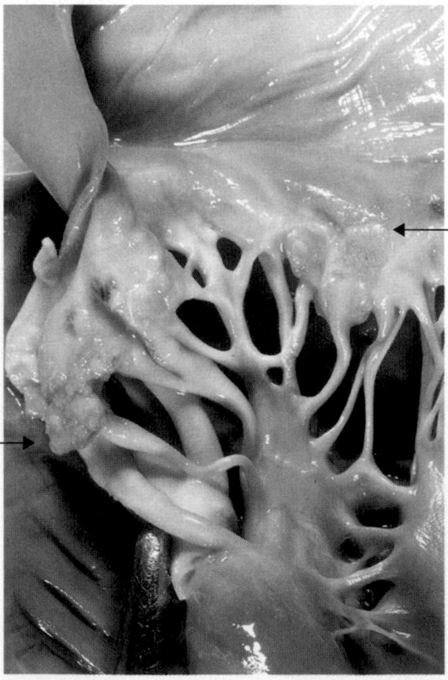

FIGURE 6–37 Libman-Sacks endocarditis of the mitral valve in lupus erythematosus. The vegetations attached to the margin of the thickened valve leaflet are indicated by *arrows*. (Courtesy of Dr. Fred Schoen, Department of Pathology, Brigham and Women's Hospital, Boston, MA.)

Clinical Course. It should be evident from Tables 6–8 and 6–10 that SLE is a multisystem disease, and it is highly variable in its clinical presentation. Typically, the patient is a young woman with some, but not necessarily all, of the following features: a butterfly rash over the face, fever, pain but no deformity in one or more peripheral joints (feet, ankles, knees, hips, fingers, wrists, elbows, shoulders), pleuritic chest pain, and photosensitivity. In many patients, however, the presentation of SLE is subtle and puzzling, taking forms such as a febrile illness of unknown origin, abnormal urinary findings, or joint disease masquerading as rheumatoid arthritis or rheumatic fever. ANAs can be found in virtually 100% of patients. ANAs, however, can also be found in patients with other autoimmune disorders (see Table 6–9). *As mentioned earlier, antibodies against double-stranded DNA and Sm antigen are virtually diagnostic of SLE.* A variety of clinical findings may point toward renal involvement, including hematuria, red cell casts, proteinuria and, in some cases, the classic nephrotic syndrome (Chapter 20). Laboratory evidence of some hematologic derangement is seen in virtually every case, but in some patients, anemia or thrombocytopenia may be the presenting manifestation as well as the dominant clinical problem. In still others, mental aberrations, including psychosis or convulsions, or coronary artery disease may be prominent clinical problems. Patients with SLE are also prone to infections, presumably because of their underlying immune dysfunction and treatment with immunosuppressive drugs.[72]

The course of the disease is variable and unpredictable. Rare acute cases result in death within weeks to months. More often, with appropriate therapy, the disease is characterized by flare-ups and remissions spanning a period of years or even decades. During acute flare-ups, increased formation of immune complexes and the accompanying complement activation often result in hypocomplementemia. Disease exacerbations are usually treated by corticosteroids or other immunosuppressant drugs. Even without therapy, in some patients, the disease may run a benign course with skin manifestations and mild hematuria for years. The outcome has improved significantly, and an approximately 90% 5-year and 80% 10-year survival can be expected. *The most common causes of death are renal failure and intercurrent infections.* Coronary artery disease is also becoming an important cause of death. Patients treated with steroids and immunosuppressive drugs incur the usual risks associated with such therapy.

As mentioned earlier, involvement of skin along with multisystem disease is fairly common in SLE. In addition, two syndromes have been recognized in which the cutaneous involvement is the most prominent or exclusive feature.

Chronic Discoid Lupus Erythematosus. Chronic discoid lupus erythematosus is a disease in which the skin manifestations may mimic SLE, but systemic manifestations are rare.[73,74] It is characterized by the presence of skin plaques showing varying degrees of edema, erythema, scaliness, follicular plugging, and skin atrophy surrounded by an elevated erythematous border. The face and scalp are usually affected, but widely disseminated lesions occasionally occur. The disease is usually confined to the skin, but 5% to 10% of patients with discoid lupus erythematosus develop multisystem manifestations after many years. Conversely, some patients with SLE may have prominent discoid lesions in the skin. Approximately 35% of patients show a positive ANA test, but *antibodies to double-stranded DNA are rarely present.* Immunofluorescence studies of skin biopsy specimens show the same deposition of immunoglobulin and C3 at the dermoepidermal junction that is seen in SLE.

Subacute Cutaneous Lupus Erythematosus. This condition also presents with predominant skin involvement and can be distinguished from chronic discoid lupus erythematosus by several criteria. The skin rash in this disease tends to be widespread, superficial, and nonscarring, although scarring lesions may occur in some patients. Most patients have mild systemic symptoms consistent with SLE. Furthermore, there is a strong association with antibodies to the SS-A antigen and with the HLA-DR3 genotype. Thus, the term *subacute cutaneous lupus erythematosus* seems to define a group intermediate between SLE and lupus erythematosus localized only to skin.[74]

Drug-Induced Lupus Erythematosus. A lupus erythematosus-like syndrome may develop in patients receiving a variety of drugs, including hydralazine (given for hypertension), procainamide, isoniazid, and D-penicillamine, to name only a few of the many therapeutic agents that have been implicated.[64] Many of these drugs are associated with the development of ANAs, but most patients do not have symptoms of lupus erythematosus. For example, 80% of patients receiving procainamide are positive for ANAs, but only one third of these manifest clinical symptoms, such as arthralgias, fever, and serositis. *Although multiple organs are affected, renal and central nervous system involvement is distinctly uncommon.* Compared with idiopathic SLE, there are serologic and genetic differences as well. Anti–double-stranded DNA antibodies are rare, but there is an *extremely high frequency of antihistone antibodies.* Persons with the HLA-DR4 allele are at a greater risk of developing lupus erythematosus after administration of hydralazine. The disease remits after withdrawal of the offending drug.

Rheumatoid Arthritis

Rheumatoid arthritis is a chronic inflammatory disease that affects primarily the joints, but may involve extra-articular tissues such as the skin, blood vessels, lungs, and heart. Abundant evidence supports the autoimmune nature of the disease. Because the principal manifestations of the disease are in the joints, it is discussed in Chapter 26.

Sjögren Syndrome

Sjögren syndrome is a chronic disease characterized by dry eyes (keratoconjunctivitis sicca) and dry mouth (xerostomia) resulting from immunologically mediated destruction of the lacrimal and salivary glands. It occurs as an isolated disorder (primary form), also known as the *sicca syndrome,* or more often in association with another autoimmune disease (secondary form). Among the associated disorders, rheumatoid arthritis is the most common, but some patients have SLE, polymyositis, scleroderma, vasculitis, mixed connective tissue disease, or thyroiditis.

Etiology and Pathogenesis. The characteristic decrease in tears and saliva (sicca syndrome) is the result of *lymphocytic infiltration* and fibrosis of the lacrimal and salivary glands.[75,76] The infiltrate contains predominantly activated CD4+ helper T cells and some B cells, including plasma cells that secrete antibody locally. About 75% of patients have rheumatoid factor regardless of whether coexisting rheumatoid arthritis is present or not. ANAs are detected in 50% to 80% of patients. A host of other organ-specific and non–organ-specific antibodies have also been identified. Most important, however, are antibodies directed against two ribonucleoprotein antigens, SS-A (Ro) and SS-B (La) (see Table 6–9), which can be detected in up to 90% of patients by highly sensitive techniques. These antibodies are thus considered serologic markers of the disease. Patients with high titers of antibodies to SS-A are more likely to have early disease onset, longer disease duration, and extraglandular manifestations, such as cutaneous vasculitis and nephritis.[77] These autoantibodies are also present in a smaller percentage of patients with SLE and hence are not diagnostic of Sjögren syndrome.

As with other autoimmune diseases, Sjögren syndrome shows some, albeit weak, association with certain HLA alleles. Studies of whites and blacks suggest linkage of the primary form with HLA-B8, HLA-DR3, and DRW52 as well as HLA-DQA1 and HLA-DQB1 loci; in patients with anti–SS-A or anti-SS-B antibodies, specific alleles of HLA-DQA1 and HLA-DQB1 are frequent. This suggests that, as in SLE, inheritance of certain class II molecules predisposes to the development of particular autoantibodies.[78]

Despite the plethora of autoantibodies, there is no evidence that they are the primary cause of tissue injury. Sjögren syndrome is in all likelihood initiated by CD4+ T cells. Molecular analysis of the T-cell receptors of the infiltrating CD4+ cells indicates that some of the T cells expand clonally, suggesting antigen-driven stimulation.[79] The nature of the autoantigen(s) recognized by these T cells is still mysterious. A cytoskeletal protein called α-fodrin is a candidate autoantigen,[80] but its role in disease development has not been established yet.

How autoimmune reactions are initiated is equally uncertain.[80a] Much attention has focused on viruses as potential etiologic agents.[81] There is some circumstantial evidence linking EBV, the perennial culprit, and hepatitis C virus to the causation of Sjögren syndrome. In addition, a small proportion of individuals infected with the human retrovirus human T-cell lymphotropic virus type 1 develop a clinical picture and pathologic changes virtually identical to those seen in Sjögren syndrome. Whether these viruses also play a role in the pathogenesis of Sjögren syndrome in patients who do not have other manifestations of such viral infection is not entirely clear. The mechanisms by which viruses can induce autoimmunity were discussed earlier.

Morphology. As mentioned earlier, lacrimal and salivary glands are the major targets of the disease, although other exocrine glands, including those lining the respiratory and gastrointestinal tracts and the vagina, may also be involved. The earliest histologic finding in both the major and the minor salivary glands is **periductal and perivascular lymphocytic infiltration**. Eventually the lymphocytic infiltrate becomes extensive (Fig. 6–38), and in the larger salivary glands, lymphoid follicles with germinal centers may be seen. The ductal lining epithelial cells may show hyperplasia, thus obstructing the ducts. Later, there is atrophy of the acini, fibrosis, and hyalinization; still later in the course, atrophy and replacement of parenchyma with fat are seen. In some cases, the lymphoid infiltrate may be so intense as to give the appearance of a lymphoma; however, the benign appearance of the lymphocytes, the heterogeneous population of cells, and the preservation of lobular architecture of the gland differentiate the lesions from those of lymphoma.

The lack of tears leads to drying of the corneal epithelium, which becomes inflamed, eroded, and ulcerated; the oral mucosa may atrophy, with inflammatory fissuring and ulceration; and dryness and crusting of the nose may lead to ulcerations and even perforation of the nasal septum. In approximately 25% of cases, extraglandular tissues, such as kidneys, lungs, skin, central nervous system, and muscles, are also involved. These are more common in patients with high titers of anti–SS-A antibodies. In contrast to SLE, glomerular lesions are extremely rare in Sjögren syndrome. Defects of tubular function, however, including renal tubular acidosis, uricosuria, and phosphaturia, are often seen and are associated histologically with **tubulointerstitial nephritis** (Chapter 20).

Clinical Manifestations. Sjögren syndrome occurs most commonly in older women, typically between ages 50 and 60.[82] As might be expected, symptoms result from inflammatory destruction of the exocrine glands. The keratoconjunctivitis produces blurring of vision, burning, and itching, and thick secretions accumulate in the conjunctival sac. The xerostomia results in difficulty in swallowing solid foods, a decrease in the ability to taste, cracks and fissures in the mouth, and dryness of the buccal mucosa. Parotid gland enlargement is present in half the patients; dryness of the nasal mucosa, epistaxis, recurrent bronchitis, and pneumonitis are other symptoms. Manifestations of extraglandular disease are seen in one third of patients and include synovitis, diffuse pulmonary fibrosis, and peripheral neuropathy. About 60% of patients have an accompanying autoimmune disorder, such as rheumatoid arthritis, and these patients also have the symptoms and signs of that disorder.

The combination of lacrimal and salivary gland inflammatory involvement was once called *Mikulicz disease.* The name has now been replaced, however, by *Mikulicz syndrome*, broadened to include lacrimal and salivary gland enlargement of whatever cause. Sarcoidosis, leukemia, lymphoma, and other tumors likewise produce Mikulicz syndrome. Thus, *biopsy of the lip (to examine minor salivary glands) is essential for the diagnosis of Sjögren syndrome.*

The lymph nodes of patients with Sjögren syndrome show not only enlargement, but also a pleomorphic infiltrate of cells with frequent mitoses. In the early stages of the disease, the B cells, responding presumably to several autoantigens, are polyclonal. Clear-cut non-Hodgkin lymphomas, however, mostly of the B-cell type, have developed in the salivary glands and lymph nodes in some patients, and it is believed that patients with Sjögren syndrome have an approximately 40-fold

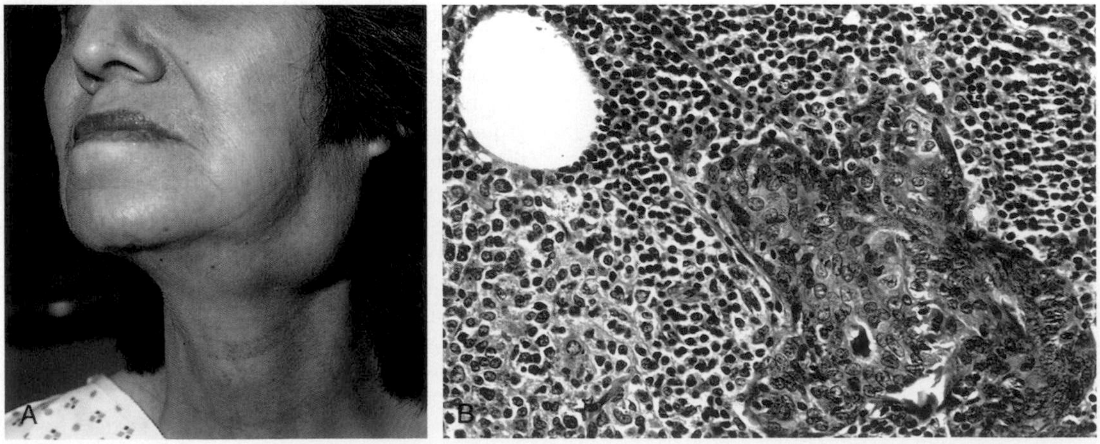

FIGURE 6–38 Sjögren syndrome. *A*, Enlargement of the salivary gland. (Courtesy of Dr. Richard Sontheimer, Department of Dermatology, University of Texas Southwestern Medical School, Dallas, TX.) *B*, Intense lymphocytic and plasma cell infiltration with ductal epithelial hyperplasia in a salivary gland. (Courtesy of Dr. Dennis Burns, Department of Pathology, University of Texas Southwestern Medical School, Dallas, TX.)

increased risk of developing lymphoid malignancies. Presumably, polyclonal B-cell activation within the glands and lymph nodes sets the stage for eventual emergence of a neoplastic, monoclonal B-cell population. These tumors are referred to as *marginal zone lymphomas* (Chapter 14).

Systemic Sclerosis (Scleroderma)

Systemic sclerosis is a chronic disease of unknown etiology characterized by abnormal accumulation of fibrous tissue in the skin and multiple organs. Although the term scleroderma is ingrained in the literature through common usage, this disease is better named systemic sclerosis because it is characterized by excessive fibrosis throughout the body. The skin is most commonly affected, but the gastrointestinal tract, kidneys, heart, muscles, and lungs also are frequently involved. In some patients, the disease appears to remain confined to the skin for many years, but in the majority, it progresses to visceral involvement with death from renal failure, cardiac failure, pulmonary insufficiency, or intestinal malabsorption. In recent years, the clinical heterogeneity of systemic sclerosis has been recognized by classifying the disease into two major categories: (1) *Diffuse scleroderma*, characterized by widespread skin involvement at onset, with rapid progression and early visceral involvement, and (2) *Limited scleroderma*, in which the skin involvement is often confined to fingers, forearms, and face. Visceral involvement occurs late; hence, the clinical course is relatively benign. Some patents with the limited disease also develop a combination of *c*alcinosis, *R*aynaud phenomenon, *e*sophageal dysmotility, *s*clerodactyly, and *t*elangiectasia, called the *CREST syndrome*. Several other variants and related conditions, such as eosinophilic fasciitis, are far less frequent and are not described here.

Etiology and Pathogenesis. The cause of systemic sclerosis is not known. *The likely trigger for excessive fibrosis is a combination of abnormal immune responses and vascular damage, resulting in local accumulation of growth factors that act on fibroblasts and stimulate collagen production* (Fig. 6–39).[83]

There is substantial evidence that abnormal immune responses play a role in the pathogenesis of systemic sclerosis. It is proposed that *CD4+ T cells responding to an as yet unidentified antigen accumulate in the skin and release cytokines that recruit and activate inflammatory cells*, including mast cells and macrophages. Although inflammatory infiltrates are typically sparse in the skin of patients with systemic sclerosis, activated CD4+ T cells can be found in many patients, and T_H2 cells have been isolated from the skin.[84] Molecular analysis of the antigen receptors of the infiltrating T cells suggests that the accumulated CD4+ cells are oligoclonal, and their expansion is antigen driven. In the skin and other affected tissues, the accumulated T cells and other inflammatory cells release a variety of mediators, such as histamine, heparin, IL-1, IL-2, IL-13, TNF, PDGF, and TGF-β. Several of these mediators, including TGF-β, IL-13, and PDGF, can stimulate transcription of genes that encode collagen and other extracellular matrix proteins (e.g., fibronectin) in fibroblasts.[85] Fibroblasts from patients may also be hyperresponsive to cytokines, such as TGF-β, and may respond by excessive collagen production. The possibility that immune system abnormalities contribute to the lesions of systemic sclerosis is further supported by the finding that several features of this disease (including the cuta-

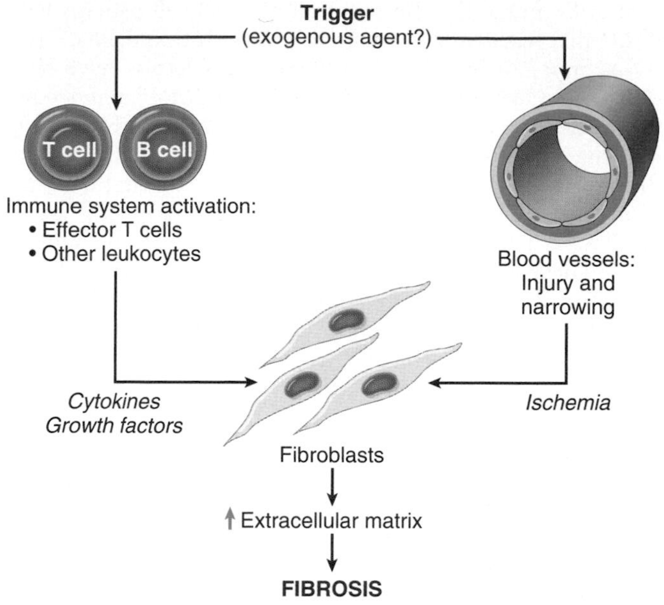

FIGURE 6–39 Schematic illustration of the possible mechanisms leading to systemic sclerosis.

neous sclerosis) are found in chronic GVH disease, a disorder that is known to result from activation of T cells.[84]

Microvascular disease is consistently present early in the course of systemic sclerosis. Intimal proliferation is evident in 100% of digital arteries of patients with systemic sclerosis. Capillary dilation with leaking, as well as destruction, is also common. Nailfold capillary loops are distorted early in the course of disease, and later they disappear. Thus, there is unmistakable morphologic evidence of microvascular injury. Telltale signs of endothelial injury (e.g., increased levels of von Willebrand factor) and increased platelet activation (increased percentage of circulating platelet aggregates) have also been noted. It is postulated that soluble mediators released by inflammatory cells inflict damage on microvascular endothelium. Some studies suggest that granzyme A, a protease released from activated CD8+ T cells, causes endothelial injury. Repeated cycles of endothelial injury followed by platelet aggregation lead to release of platelet factors (e.g., PDGF, TGF-β) that trigger periadventitial fibrosis. Activated or injured endothelial cells themselves may release PDGF and factors chemotactic for fibroblasts. Vascular smooth muscle cells also show abnormalities, such as increased expression of adrenergic receptors. Eventually, widespread narrowing of the microvasculature leads to ischemic injury and scarring. Whether endothelial injury can also be initiated by toxic effects of environmental triggers remains uncertain but cannot be definitively excluded.

Systemic sclerosis also has a genetic component, although no genes can be said to predispose to disease in an individual patient. Among the genetic loci implicated in the disease are HLA class II genes, as well as genes that may encode or regulate the production of proteins of the extracellular matrix, including fibrillin-1.[86]

Although T cell–mediated fibrogenesis and vascular injury are believed to be important in the pathogenesis of systemic sclerosis, there is abundant evidence for inappropriate activation of humoral immunity as well. Virtually all patients have ANAs that react with a variety of intranuclear antigens.[87] Two ANAs more or less unique to systemic sclerosis have been described. One of these, directed against *DNA topoisomerase* I (anti-Scl 70), is highly specific. Depending on the ethnic group and the assay, it is present in 28% to 70% of patients with diffuse systemic sclerosis. Patients who have this antibody are more likely to have pulmonary fibrosis and peripheral vascular disease. The other, an *anticentromere antibody*, is found in 22% to 36% of patients with limited systemic sclerosis.[87] The detection of anticentromere antibody is somewhat less specific for systemic sclerosis, being also found in 9% to 30% of patients with primary biliary cirrhosis. More importantly, the majority of those with the anticentromere antibody (including those with biliary cirrhosis) have the CREST syndrome. Hence this antibody, in contrast to the anti–DNA topoisomerase antibody, is restricted largely to patients with limited systemic sclerosis. It is rare to have both antibodies in the same patient.

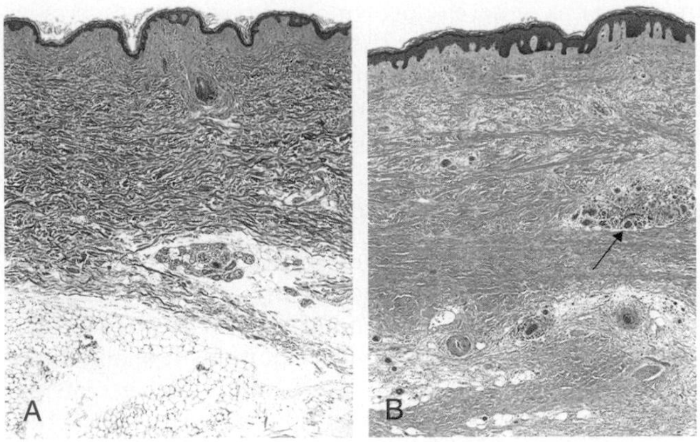

FIGURE 6–40 Systemic sclerosis. *A,* Normal skin. *B,* Skin biopsy from a patient with systemic sclerosis. Note the extensive deposition of dense collagen in the dermis with virtual absence of appendages (e.g. hair follicles) and foci of inflammation *(arrow).*

Morphology. Virtually all organs may be involved in systemic sclerosis.[88] Prominent changes occur in the skin, alimentary tract, musculoskeletal system, and kidney, but lesions also are often present in the blood vessels, heart, lungs, and peripheral nerves.

Skin. A great majority of patients have diffuse, sclerotic atrophy of the skin, which usually begins in the fingers and distal regions of the upper extremities and extends proximally to involve the upper arms, shoulders, neck, and face. In the early stages, affected skin areas are somewhat edematous and have a doughy consistency. Histologically, there are edema and perivascular infiltrates containing CD4+ T cells, together with swelling and degeneration of collagen fibers, which become eosinophilic. Capillaries and small arteries (150 to 500 μm in diameter) may show thickening of the basal lamina, endothelial cell damage, and partial occlusion. With progression, the edematous phase is replaced by progressive fibrosis of the dermis, which becomes tightly bound to the subcutaneous structures. There is marked increase of compact collagen in the dermis along with thinning of the epidermis, loss of rete pegs, atrophy of the dermal appendages, and hyaline thickening of the walls of dermal arterioles and capillaries (Fig. 6–40). Focal and sometimes diffuse subcutaneous calcifications may develop, especially in patients with the CREST syndrome. In advanced stages, the fingers take on a tapered, clawlike appearance with limitation of motion in the joints, and the face becomes a drawn mask. Loss of blood supply may lead to cutaneous ulcerations and to atrophic changes in the terminal phalanges (Fig. 6–41). Sometimes the tips of the fingers undergo autoamputation.

Alimentary Tract. The alimentary tract is affected in approximately 90% of patients. Progressive atrophy and collagenous fibrous replacement of the muscularis may develop at any level of the gut but are most severe in the esophagus. The lower two thirds of the esophagus often develops a rubber-hose inflexibility. The associated dysfunction of the lower esophageal sphincter gives rise to gastroesophageal reflux and its complications, including Barrett metaplasia (Chapter 17) and strictures. The mucosa is thinned and may be ulcerated, and there is excessive collagenization of the lamina propria and submucosa. Loss of villi and microvilli in the small bowel is the anatomic basis for the malabsorption syndrome sometimes encountered.

Musculoskeletal System. Inflammation of the synovium, associated with hypertrophy and hyperplasia of the synovial soft tissues, is common in the early stages; fibrosis later ensues. It is evident that these changes are closely reminiscent of rheumatoid arthritis, but joint destruction is not common in systemic sclerosis. In a small subset of patients (approximately 10%), inflammatory myositis indistinguishable from polymyositis may develop.

Kidneys. Renal abnormalities occur in two-thirds of patients with systemic sclerosis. The most prominent are those in the vessel walls. Interlobular arteries show intimal thickening as a result of deposition of mucinous or finely collagenous material, which stains histochemically for glycoprotein and acid

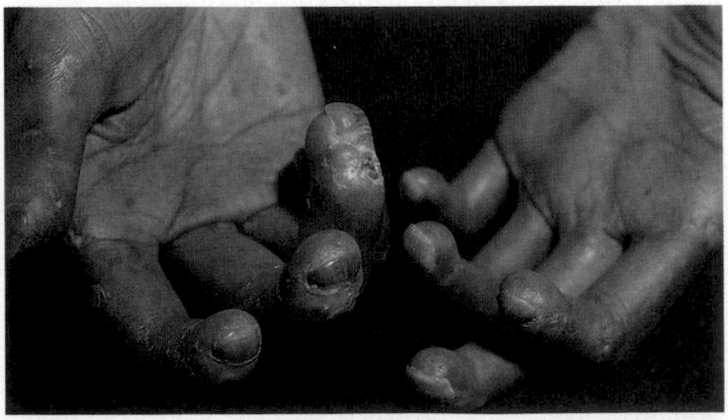

FIGURE 6–41 Advanced systemic sclerosis. The extensive subcutaneous fibrosis has virtually immobilized the fingers, creating a clawlike flexion deformity. Loss of blood supply has led to cutaneous ulcerations. (Courtesy of Dr. Richard Sontheimer, Department of Dermatology, University of Texas Southwestern Medical School, Dallas, TX.)

mucopolysaccharides. There is also concentric proliferation of intimal cells. These changes may resemble those seen in malignant hypertension, but in scleroderma the alterations are restricted to vessels 150 to 500 µm in diameter and are not always associated with hypertension. Hypertension, however, occurs in 30% of patients with scleroderma, and in 20% it takes an ominously rapid, downhill course (malignant hypertension). In hypertensive patients, vascular alterations are more pronounced and are often associated with fibrinoid necrosis involving the arterioles together with thrombosis and infarction. When this occurs, it becomes difficult to differentiate the lesions of scleroderma from those of other types of malignant hypertension (Chapter 20). Such patients often die of renal failure, which accounts for about 50% of deaths in patients with this disease. There are no specific glomerular changes.

Lungs. The lungs are involved in more than 50% of patients with systemic sclerosis. This involvement may manifest as pulmonary hypertension and interstitial fibrosis. Pulmonary hypertension with associated vascular changes may be noted, with or without coexistent pulmonary fibrosis. Pulmonary vasospasm, secondary to pulmonary vascular endothelial dysfunction, is considered important in the pathogenesis of pulmonary hypertension. Pulmonary fibrosis, when present, is indistinguishable from that seen in idiopathic pulmonary fibrosis (Chapter 15). Hence systemic sclerosis must be considered in the differential diagnosis of diffuse pulmonary interstitial disease as well as pulmonary hypertension.

Heart. Pericarditis with effusion and myocardial fibrosis, along with thickening of intramyocardial arterioles, occurs in one third of the patients. Clinical myocardial involvement, however, is less common.

Clinical Course. Systemic sclerosis is primarily a disease of women (female-to-male ratio, 3:1) with a peak incidence in the 50- to 60-year age group. It must be apparent from the described anatomic changes that systemic sclerosis shares many features with SLE, rheumatoid arthritis (Chapter 26), and polymyositis (Chapter 27). Its distinctive features are the striking cutaneous changes, notably skin thickening. Raynaud phenomenon, manifested as episodic vasoconstriction of the arteries and arterioles of the extremities, is seen in virtually all patients and precedes other symptoms in 70% of cases. Dysphagia attributable to esophageal fibrosis and its resultant hypomotility are present in more than 50% of patients. Eventually, destruction of the esophageal wall leads to atony and dilation, especially at its lower end. Abdominal pain, intestinal obstruction, or malabsorption syndrome with weight loss and anemia reflect involvement of the small intestine. Respiratory difficulties owing to the pulmonary fibrosis may result in right-sided cardiac dysfunction, and myocardial fibrosis may cause either arrhythmias or cardiac failure. Mild proteinuria occurs in up to 70% of patients, but rarely is the proteinuria so severe as to cause a nephrotic syndrome. The most ominous manifestation is malignant hypertension, with the subsequent development of fatal renal failure, but in its absence progression of the disease may be slow. The disease tends to be more severe in blacks, especially black women. As treatment of the renal crises has improved, pulmonary disease has become the major cause of death in systemic sclerosis.

As mentioned earlier, the CREST syndrome is seen in some patients with limited systemic sclerosis. It is characterized by *c*alcinosis, *R*aynaud phenomenon, *e*sophageal dysfunction, *s*clerodactyly, *t*elangiectasia, and the presence of anticentromere antibodies. Patients with the CREST syndrome have relatively limited involvement of skin, often confined to fingers, forearms, and face, and calcification of the subcutaneous tissues. Raynaud phenomenon and involvement of skin are the initial manifestations and often the only manifestations for several years. Involvement of the viscera, including esophageal lesions, pulmonary hypertension, and biliary cirrhosis, occurs late, and in general the patients live longer than those with systemic sclerosis with diffuse visceral involvement at the outset.

Inflammatory Myopathies

Inflammatory myopathies comprise an uncommon, heterogeneous group of disorders characterized by injury and inflammation of mainly the skeletal muscles, which are probably immunologically mediated. Three distinct disorders, *dermatomyositis*, *polymyositis*, and *inclusion-body myositis*, are included in this category. These may occur alone or with other immune-mediated diseases, particularly systemic sclerosis. These diseases are described in Chapter 27.

Mixed Connective Tissue Disease

The term *mixed connective tissue disease* is sometimes used to describe the disease seen in a group of patients who are identified clinically by the coexistence of features suggestive of SLE, polymyositis, rheumatoid arthritis, and systemic sclerosis, and *serologically by high titers of antibodies to RNP particle-containing U1 RNP*.[89] Two other factors have been considered important in lending distinctiveness to mixed connective tissue disease—the paucity of renal disease and an extremely good response to corticosteroids, both of which could be considered indicative of a good long-term prognosis.

Mixed connective tissue disease may present with arthritis, swelling of the hands, Raynaud phenomenon, abnormal esophageal motility, myositis, leukopenia and anemia, fever, lymphadenopathy, and hypergammaglobulinemia. These manifestations suggest SLE, polymyositis, and systemic sclerosis. Almost 85% of patients have lung involvement, which may be asymptomatic but may present as interstitial lung disease. Because of the overlapping clinical features, it has been suggested that mixed connective tissue disease is not a distinct disease but a heterogeneous mixture of subsets of SLE, systemic sclerosis, and polymyositis.[90] However, the presence of high titers of anti-U1 RNP antibodies, which is characteristic of the disease, may justify considering it a distinct entity.

Polyarteritis Nodosa and Other Vasculitides

Polyarteritis nodosa belongs to a group of diseases characterized by necrotizing inflammation of the walls of blood vessels and showing strong evidence of an immunologic pathogenetic mechanism.[91] The general term *noninfectious necrotizing vasculitis* differentiates these conditions from those due to direct infection of the blood vessel wall (such as occurs in the wall of an abscess) and serves to emphasize that any type of vessel may be involved—arteries, arterioles, veins, or capillaries.

Noninfectious necrotizing vasculitis is encountered in many clinical settings. A detailed classification and description of vasculitides is presented in Chapter 11, Blood Vessels, where the immunologic mechanisms are also discussed.

IMMUNOLOGIC DEFICIENCY SYNDROMES

Immunodeficiencies can be divided into the *primary immunodeficiency* disorders, which are almost always genetically determined, and *secondary immunodeficiency* states, which may arise as complications of infections; malnutrition; aging; or side effects of immunosuppression, irradiation, or chemotherapy for cancer and other autoimmune diseases. The primary immunodeficiency syndromes are experiments of nature that allow insights into the critical functions and complexities of the human immune system. Nowhere has the relevance of the individual components of the immune system been more distinctly shown than when genetically determined deficiencies of single components have given rise to distinctive disorders. Many of the important concepts of immunology either arose from or were confirmed by the study of clinical immunodeficiencies. Here we briefly discuss some of the more important primary immunodeficiencies, to be followed by a more detailed description of AIDS, the most devastating example of secondary immunodeficiency.

Primary Immunodeficiencies

Most primary immunodeficiency diseases are genetically determined and affect specific immunity (i.e., the humoral and cellular arms of adaptive immunity) or nonspecific host defense mechanisms mediated by complement proteins and cells such as phagocytes or NK cells (innate immunity). Defects in adaptive immunity are often subclassified on the basis of the primary component involved (i.e., B cells or T cells or both); however, in view of the extensive interactions between T and B lymphocytes, these distinctions are not clear-cut (Fig. 6–42). In particular, T-cell defects almost always lead to impaired antibody synthesis, and hence isolated deficiencies of T cells are often indistinguishable clinically from combined deficiencies of T and B cells. Although originally thought to be quite rare, some forms, such as IgA deficiency, are common, and collectively they are a significant health problem, especially in children. Most primary immunodeficiencies manifest themselves in infancy, between 6 months and 2 years of life, and they are detected because the affected infants are susceptible to recurrent infections. The nature of infecting organisms depends to some extent on the nature of the underlying defect, as summarized in Table 6–11. Detailed classification of the primary immunodeficiencies according to the suggested cellular defect may be found in the WHO report on immunodeficiency.[92] Defects of phagocytes were discussed in Chapter 2. Here we present selected examples of other immunodeficiencies. We begin with isolated defects in B cells, followed by a discussion of combined immunodeficiencies and defects in complement proteins. Finally, Wiskott-Aldrich syndrome, a complex disorder affecting lymphocytes as well as platelets, is presented. With rapid advances in genetic analyses, in the past ten years the mutations responsible for many primary immunodeficiencies have been identified.[93]

X-Linked Agammaglobulinemia of Bruton

X-linked agammaglobulinemia is one of the more common forms of primary immunodeficiency.[94] It is *characterized by the failure of B-cell precursors (pro-B cells and pre-B cells) to mature into B cells.* During normal B-cell maturation in the bone marrow, the immunoglobulin heavy-chain genes are rearranged first, followed by rearrangement of the light chain genes. In X-linked agammaglobulinemia, B-cell maturation stops after the rearrangement of heavy chain genes. Because light chains are not produced, the complete immunoglobulin molecule (which contains heavy and light chains) cannot be assembled and transported to the cell membrane. Free heavy chains can be found in the cytoplasm. This block in differentiation is due to mutations in a cytoplasmic tyrosine kinase, called *B-cell tyrosine kinase (Btk).*[95] Btk is a protein tyrosine kinase associated with the antigen receptor complex of pre-B and mature B cells. It is needed to transduce signals from the antigen receptor that are critical for driving maturation. When it is mutated, the pre-B cell receptor cannot deliver signals, and maturation stops at this stage. The *BTK* gene maps to the long arm of the X chromosome at Xq21.22.

TABLE 6–11 Examples of Infections in Immunodeficiencies

Pathogen Type	T-Cell Defect	B-Cell Defect	Granulocyte Defect	Complement Defect
Bacteria	Bacterial sepsis	Streptococci, staphylococci, *Haemophilus*	Staphylococci, *Pseudomonas*	Neisserial infections, other pyogenic bacterial infections
Viruses	Cytomegalovirus, Epstein-Barr virus, severe varicella, chronic infections with respiratory and intestinal viruses	Enteroviral encephalitis		
Fungi and parasites	*Candida, Pneumocystis carinii*	Severe intestinal giardiasis	*Candida, Nocardia, Aspergillus*	
Special features	Aggressive disease with opportunistic pathogens, failure to clear infections	Recurrent sinopulmonary infections, sepsis, chronic meningitis		

From Puck JM: Primary immunodeficiency diseases. JAMA 278:1835, 1997. Copyright 1997, American Medical Association.

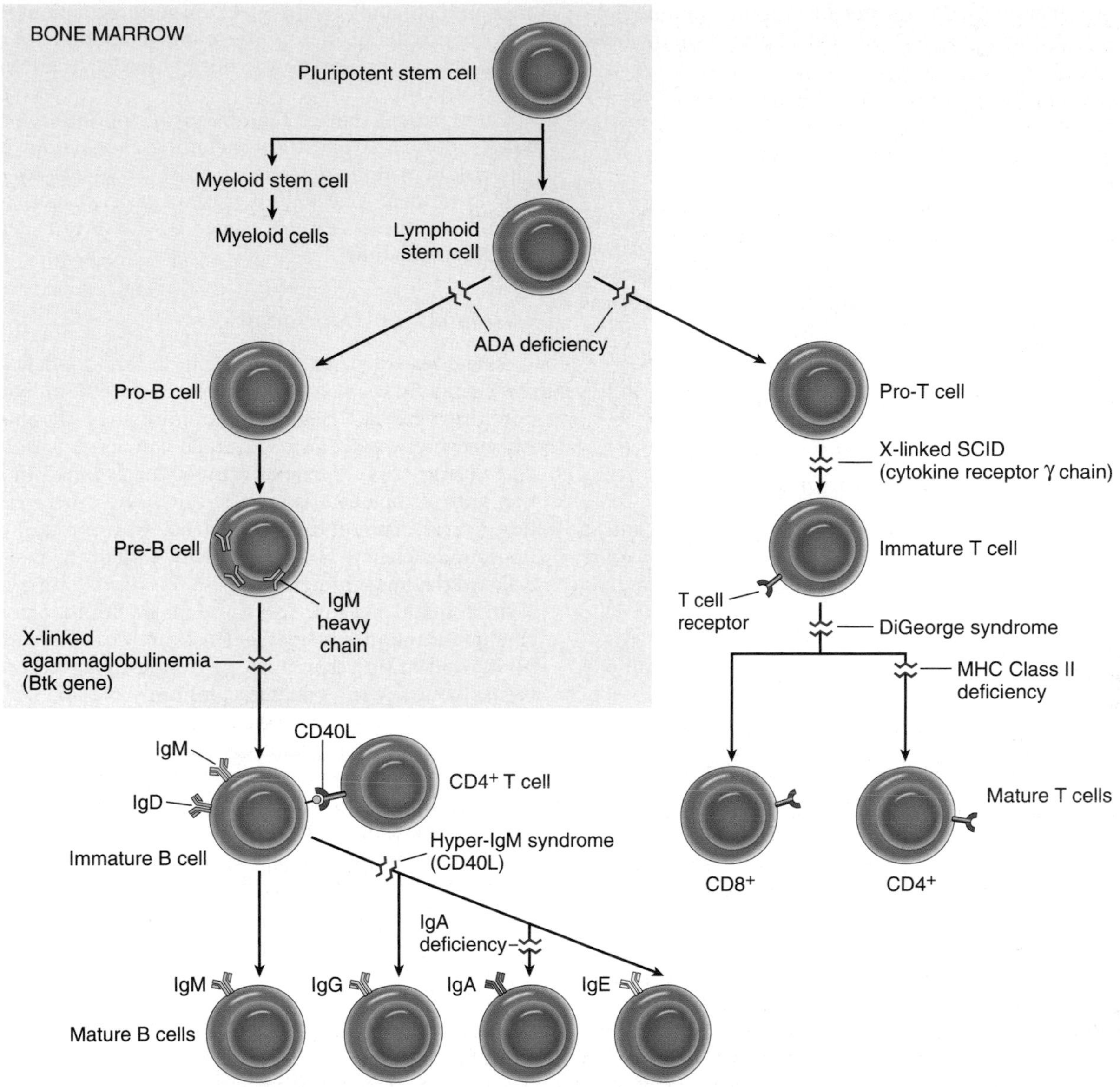

FIGURE 6–42 Scheme of lymphocyte development and sites of block in primary immunodeficiency diseases. The affected genes are indicated in parentheses for some of the disorders. ADA, adenosine deaminase; CD40L, CD40 ligand; SCID, severe combined immunodeficiency.

As an X-linked disease, this disorder is seen almost entirely in males, but sporadic cases have been described in females, possibly caused by mutations in some other gene. *The disease usually does not become apparent until about age 6 months, when maternal immunoglobulins are depleted.* In most cases, recurrent bacterial infections of the respiratory tract, such as acute and chronic pharyngitis, sinusitis, otitis media, bronchitis, and pneumonia, call attention to the underlying immune defect. Almost always the causative organisms are *Haemophilus influenzae*, *Streptococcus pneumoniae*, or *Staphylococcus aureus*. These organisms are normally opsonized by antibodies and cleared by phagocytosis. Because antibodies are important for neutralizing infectious viruses that are present in the bloodstream or mucosal secretions or being passed from cell to cell, these patients are also susceptible to certain viral infections, especially those caused by enteroviruses, such as echovirus, poliovirus, and coxsackievirus. These viruses infect the gastrointestinal tract, and from here they can disseminate to the nervous system via the blood. Thus, immunization with live poliovirus carries the risk of paralytic poliomyelitis, and echovirus can cause fatal encephalitis. For similar reasons, *Giardia lamblia*, an intestinal protozoon that is normally resisted by secreted IgA, causes persistent infections in these patients. In general, however, most viral, fungal, and protozoal infections are handled normally owing to intact T cell–mediated immunity. Approximately 35% of children develop arthritis that clears with restorative immunoglobulin therapy. This arthritis is believed to be infectious in origin, caused in some cases by *Mycoplasma* infection. The classic form of this disease has the following characteristics:

- B cells are absent or markedly decreased in the circulation, and the serum levels of all classes of immunoglobulins are depressed. Precursors of B cells that express the

B-lineage marker CD19 but not membrane immunoglobulin (pre-B cells) are found in normal numbers in the bone marrow.

- Germinal centers of lymph nodes, Peyer patches, the appendix, and tonsils are underdeveloped or rudimentary.
- Plasma cells are absent throughout the body.
- T cell–mediated reactions are entirely normal.

Paradoxically, autoimmune diseases, such as arthritis and dermatomyositis, occur with increased frequency in patients with this disease. The basis for this association is not known. The treatment of X-linked agammaglobulinemia is replacement therapy with immunoglobulins. In the past, most patients succumbed to infection in infancy or early childhood. Prophylactic intravenous immunoglobulin therapy allows most individuals to reach adulthood.

Common Variable Immunodeficiency

This relatively common but poorly defined derangement represents a heterogeneous group of disorders.[96] *The feature common to all patients is hypogammaglobulinemia, generally affecting all the antibody classes but sometimes only IgG.* The diagnosis of common variable immunodeficiency is based on exclusion of other well-defined causes of decreased antibody production.

As might be expected in a heterogeneous group of disorders, both sporadic and inherited forms of the disease occur. In familial forms, there is no single pattern of inheritance. Relatives of such patients have a high incidence of selective IgA deficiency (see later). These studies suggest that at least in some cases, selective IgA deficiency and common variable immunodeficiency may represent different expressions of a common genetic defect in antibody synthesis. The basis of immunoglobulin deficiency in common variable immunodeficiency is varied, but it is distinct from that in X-linked agammaglobulinemia. In contrast to the latter, most patients with common variable immunodeficiency have normal or near-normal numbers of B cells in the blood and lymphoid tissues. These B cells, however, are not able to differentiate into plasma cells.

The molecular basis of abnormal B-cell differentiation is not understood. According to some authorities, there is no evidence of any intrinsic B-cell defects. Rather, there are several different defects in the ability of T cells to send appropriate activation signals to B cells. According to others, some patients have intrinsic B-cell defects as well as abnormalities of T cell–mediated regulation of B cells.

The clinical manifestations of common variable immunodeficiency are caused by antibody deficiency, and hence they resemble those of X-linked agammaglobulinemia. Thus, the patients typically present with recurrent sinopulmonary pyogenic infections. In addition, about 20% of patients present with recurrent herpesvirus infections. Serious enterovirus infections causing meningoencephalitis may also occur. Patients are also prone to the development of persistent diarrhea caused by *G. lamblia.* In contrast to X-linked agammaglobulinemia, however, common variable immunodeficiency affects both sexes equally, and the onset of symptoms is later—in childhood or adolescence. Histologically the B-cell areas of the lymphoid tissues (i.e., lymphoid follicles in nodes, spleen, and gut) are hyperplastic. The enlargement of B-cell areas probably reflects defective immunoregulation, that is, B cells can proliferate in response to antigen but do not produce antibodies, and therefore the normal feedback inhibition by IgG is absent.

These patients have a high frequency of autoimmune diseases (approximately 20%), including rheumatoid arthritis. The risk of lymphoid malignancy is also increased, particularly in women. A 50-fold increase in gastric cancer has been noted. All these features suggest widespread defects in immunoregulation.

Isolated IgA Deficiency

Isolated IgA deficiency is a common immunodeficiency. In the United States, it occurs in about 1 in 600 individuals of European descent.[97] It is far less common in blacks and Asians. Affected individuals have extremely *low levels of both serum and secretory IgA.* It may be familial, or acquired in association with toxoplasmosis, measles, or some other viral infection. The association of IgA deficiency with common variable immunodeficiency was mentioned earlier. It is generally believed that most individuals with this disease are completely asymptomatic. Because IgA is the major immunoglobulin in external secretions, mucosal defenses are weakened, and infections occur in the respiratory, gastrointestinal, and urogenital tracts. Symptomatic patients commonly present with recurrent sinopulmonary infections and diarrhea. It is now apparent that some individuals previously classified as having selective IgA deficiency are also deficient in IgG_2 and IgG_4 subclasses of IgG. This group of patients is particularly prone to developing infections. In addition, IgA-deficient patients have a high frequency of respiratory tract allergy and a variety of autoimmune diseases, particularly SLE and rheumatoid arthritis. The basis of the increased frequency of autoimmune and allergic diseases is not known. Because secretory IgA normally acts as a mucosal barrier against foreign proteins and antigens, it could be speculated that the increased frequency of infections and increased absorption of foreign protein antigens trigger abnormal immune responses.

The basic defect in IgA deficiency is in the differentiation of naive B lymphocytes to IgA-producing cells. The molecular basis of this defect, however, is still unknown. In most patients, the number of IgA-positive B cells is normal, but only a few of these cells can be induced to differentiate into IgA plasma cells in vitro. Serum antibodies to IgA are found in approximately 40% of the patients. Whether this finding is of any etiologic significance is unclear, but it has important clinical implications. When transfused with blood containing normal IgA, some of these patients develop severe, even fatal, anaphylactic reactions, because the IgA behaves like a foreign antigen (since the patients do not produce it and are not tolerant to it).

Hyper-IgM Syndrome

Hyper-IgM syndrome was originally thought to be a B-cell disorder because the *affected patients make IgM antibodies but are deficient in their ability to produce IgG, IgA, and IgE antibodies.* It is now known that this is most frequently a T-cell disorder in which functionally abnormal T cells fail to induce B cells to make antibodies of isotypes other than IgM and to activate macrophages to eliminate intracellular microbes. To understand the molecular basis of this disorder, it is essential to review the mechanisms responsible for the formation of antibodies of different isotypes. Naive (unstimulated) B cells express IgM and IgD as membrane receptors for antigen. When these B cells are stimulated by antigens, IgM antibodies are produced first, and if the antigen is a protein this is followed by the sequential formation of IgG, IgA, and IgE antibodies. This orderly appearance of antibody isotypes during a normal immune response is called *isotype switching*. IgM-producing B cells turn on the transcription of genes that encode other immunoglobulin isotypes in response to cytokines and contact-mediated signals from CD4+ T cells. The contact-mediated signals are delivered by physical interaction between the CD40 molecule of B cells and CD40 ligand (CD40L) expressed on activated helper T cells. Thus, mutations in either CD40L or CD40 prevent the T cell–B cell interaction necessary for isotype switching, and the patients develop this type of immunodeficiency. IgM production continues because this isotype is produced mainly in response to nonprotein antigens (polysaccharides and lipids) and does not require T-cell help. Although the disease was identified on the basis of an antibody defect, patients also have defective cell-mediated immunity. The reason for this is that CD40L on helper T cells interacts with CD40 on macrophages and activates the macrophages to kill microbes, one of the central reactions of cellular immunity. CD40L–CD40 interactions are also involved in the development of CD8+ cytotoxic T lymphocytes, the other component of cell-mediated immunity.

In approximately 70% of the cases, the mutations affect the gene for CD40L, which maps to Xq26.[98,99] These patients have the X-linked form of the disease. In the remaining patients, the mutations affect CD40 or an enzyme called activation-induced deaminase, which is a DNA editing enzyme that is required for isotype switching but whose precise mechanism of action is not known.[99] The disease in these latter groups of patients is inherited in an autosomal recessive pattern.

Clinically, patients with the hyper-IgM syndrome present with recurrent pyogenic infections because the level of opsonizing IgG antibodies is low. In addition, they are also susceptible to pneumonia caused by the intracellular organism *Pneumocystis carinii*, because of the defect in cell-mediated immunity.

The serum of patients with this syndrome contains normal or elevated levels of IgM but no IgA or IgE and extremely low levels of IgG. The number of B and T cells is normal. Many of the IgM antibodies react with elements of blood, giving rise to autoimmune hemolytic anemia, thrombocytopenia, and neutropenia. In older patients, there may be uncontrolled proliferation of IgM-producing plasma cells with infiltrations of the gastrointestinal tract. Although the proliferating B cells are polyclonal, extensive infiltration may lead to death.

DiGeorge Syndrome (Thymic Hypoplasia)

DiGeorge syndrome is an example of a T-cell deficiency that results from failure of development of the third and fourth pharyngeal pouches. The latter give rise to the thymus, the parathyroids, some of the clear cells of the thyroid, and the ultimobranchial body. Thus, these patients have a variable loss of T cell–mediated immunity (owing to hypoplasia or lack of the thymus), tetany (owing to lack of the parathyroids), and congenital defects of the heart and great vessels. In addition, the appearance of the mouth, ears, and facies may be abnormal. Absence of cell-mediated immunity is reflected in low levels of circulating T lymphocytes and a poor defense against certain fungal and viral infections. Plasma cells are present in normal numbers in lymphoid tissues, but the T-cell zones of lymphoid organs—paracortical areas of the lymph nodes and the periarteriolar sheaths of the spleen—are depleted. Immunoglobulin levels may be normal or reduced, depending on the severity of the T-cell deficiency.

Patients with *partial* DiGeorge syndrome, who have an extremely small but histologically normal thymus, have also been recorded. T-cell function improves with age in these children, so that by 5 years of age, many have no detectable deficit. In those with a complete absence of thymus, transplantation of fetal thymus may be of benefit.

DiGeorge syndrome is not a familial disorder. It results from the deletion of a gene that maps to chromosome 22q11.[100] This deletion is seen in 90% of patients, and DiGeorge syndrome is now considered a component of the 22q11 deletion syndrome,[101] discussed in greater detail in Chapter 5. The specific gene believed to be mutated in DiGeorge syndrome is a member of the T-box family of transcription factors, which may be involved in development of the branchial arch and the great vessels. How this transcription factor influences development of these structures only is not known.

Severe Combined Immunodeficiency Diseases

Severe combined immunodeficiency disease (SCID) represents a constellation of genetically distinct syndromes, all having in common *defects in both humoral and cell-mediated immune responses*. Affected infants present with prominent thrush (oral candidiasis), extensive diaper rash, and failure to thrive. Some patients develop a morbilliform rash shortly after birth owing to transplacental transfer of maternal T cells that cause GVH disease. Patients with SCID are extremely susceptible to recurrent, severe infections by a wide range of pathogens, including *Candida albicans*, *P. carinii*, *Pseudomonas*, cytomegalovirus, varicella, and a whole host of bacteria. Without bone marrow transplantation, death occurs within the first year of life. Despite the common clinical manifestations, the underlying defects are quite different in different forms of SCID (Fig. 6–42) and in many cases unknown. The so-called classic form, initially described in Swiss infants and believed to result from a defect in the common lymphoid stem cell, is extremely uncommon. More commonly, the SCID defect resides in the T-cell compartment, with a secondary impairment of humoral immunity. The T-cell defects may occur at any stage of the T-cell differentiation and activation pathway.

The most common form, accounting for 50% to 60% of cases, is X-linked, and hence SCID is more common in boys than in girls. The genetic defect in the X-linked form is a *mutation in the common γ chain subunit (γc) of cytokine receptors*. This transmembrane protein is part of the signal-transducing components of the receptors for IL-2, IL-4, IL-7, IL-9, IL-11, and IL-15. The cytokine receptor that is mainly responsible for this defect is the receptor for IL-7, because IL-7 is required for the proliferation of lymphoid progenitors, particularly T-cell precursors (in humans). As a result of defective IL-7 receptor signaling, there is a profound defect in the earliest stages of lymphocyte development, especially T-cell development.[102,103] T-cell numbers are greatly reduced, and although B cells are normal in number, antibody synthesis is greatly impaired because of lack of T-cell help.

The remaining cases of SCID are inherited as autosomal recessives. The most common cause of autosomal recessive SCID is a *deficiency of the enzyme adenosine deaminase (ADA)*. Although the mechanisms by which ADA deficiency causes SCID are not entirely clear, it has been proposed that deficiency of ADA leads to accumulation of deoxyadenosine and its derivatives (e.g., deoxy-ATP), which are particularly toxic to immature lymphocytes,[104] especially those of T-cell lineage. Hence there may be a greater reduction in the number of T lymphocytes than of B lymphocytes.

Several other less common causes of autosomal recessive SCID have been discovered:[93]

- Mutations in recombinase-activating genes prevent the somatic gene rearrangements essential for the assembly of T-cell receptor and immunoglobulin genes. This blocks the development of T and B cells.
- An intracellular kinase called Jak3 is essential for signal transduction through the common cytokine receptor γ chain (which is mutated in X-linked SCID). Mutations of Jak3 therefore have the same effects as mutations in the γ chain.[103] The difference between these two forms of SCID is in their patterns of inheritance; Jak3 deficiency is an autosomal recessive disease.
- Mutations that impair the expression of class II MHC molecules prevent the development of CD4+ T cells. Class II MHC molecules present antigen to CD4+ T cells, and during T-cell development in the thymus, CD4+ T-cell development depends on interaction with MHC class II molecules expressed on thymic epithelium. CD4+ T cells are involved in cellular immunity and provide help to B cells, and hence MHC class II deficiency results in combined immunodeficiency. This disease is called the *bare lymphocyte syndrome*, and it is usually caused by mutations in transcription factors that are required for MHC class II gene expression.[105]

The histologic findings in SCID depend on the underlying defect. In the two most common forms (ADA deficiency and γc mutation), the thymus is small and devoid of lymphoid cells. In ADA-negative SCID, remnants of Hassall's corpuscles can be found, whereas in X-linked SCID, the thymus contains lobules of undifferentiated epithelial cells resembling fetal thymus.[106] In either case, other lymphoid tissues are hypoplastic as well, with marked depletion of T-cell areas and in some cases both T-cell and B-cell zones.

Currently, bone marrow transplantation is the mainstay of treatment, but X-linked SCID is the first human disease in which gene therapy has been successful.[107] The normal γc gene is expressed in bone marrow stem cells of patients using a retroviral vector, and the cells are transplanted back. The clinical experience is small, but some patients have shown reconstitution of their immune systems for over a year after therapy. A few patients receiving such treatments have developed leukemias, apparently because the retroviral genome integrated into a region of the cell's genome that carries a tumor suppressor gene. Because of this complication, currently gene therapy for X-linked SCID is on hold. Patients with ADA deficiency have also been treated with bone marrow transplantation and, more recently, with gene therapy. T cells harvested from the patient's peripheral blood are expanded in vitro, transfected with the ADA gene, then returned to the patient. This experimental form of therapy has met with some success.[108]

Immunodeficiency with Thrombocytopenia and Eczema (Wiskott-Aldrich Syndrome)

Wiskott-Aldrich syndrome has been deemed "curious," "enigmatic," or "confusing" because its immunologic defects are difficult to explain. *It is an X-linked recessive disease characterized by thrombocytopenia, eczema, and a marked vulnerability to recurrent infection, ending in early death.* The thymus is morphologically normal, at least early in the course of the disease, but there is progressive secondary depletion of T lymphocytes in the peripheral blood and in the T-cell zones (paracortical areas) of the lymph nodes, with variable loss of cellular immunity. Patients do not make antibodies to polysaccharide antigens, and the response to protein antigens is poor. IgM levels in the serum are low, but levels of IgG are usually normal. Paradoxically the levels of IgA and IgE are often elevated. Patients are also prone to developing malignant lymphomas. The Wiskott-Aldrich syndrome maps to Xp11.23, where the gene encoding *Wiskott-Aldrich syndrome protein (WASP)* is located.[109] This protein belongs to a family of proteins that are believed to link membrane receptors, such as antigen receptors, to cytoskeletal elements.[110] Thus, the WASP protein is involved in maintaining the integrity of the cytoskeleton as well as signal transduction. How this protein is responsible for normal lymphocyte and platelet function is unclear. The only treatment is bone marrow transplantation.

Genetic Deficiencies of the Complement System

The various components of the complement system play a critical role in inflammatory and immunologic responses. Hereditary deficiencies have been described for virtually all components of the complement system and two of the inhibitors.[111–113] A deficiency of C2 is the most common of all. With a deficiency of C2 or the other components of the classic pathway (i.e., C1 [C1q, r, or s] or C4), there is little or no increase in susceptibility to infections, but the dominant manifestation is an increased incidence of an SLE-like autoimmune disease. Presumably the alternative complement pathway is adequate for the control of most infections. The possible reasons for this association of complement deficiencies and SLE have been discussed earlier. Deficiency of components of the alternative pathway (properdin and factor D) is rare. It is associated with recurrent pyogenic infections. The C3 component of complement is required for both the classic and alternative pathways, and hence a deficiency of this protein gives rise to serious and recurrent pyogenic infections. There is also increased incidence of immune complex–mediated glomerulonephritis; in the absence of complement, immune complex-mediated inflammation is presumably caused by Fc receptor–dependent leukocyte activation. The terminal components of complement C5, 6, 7, 8, and 9 are required for the assembly of the membrane attack complex involved in the lysis of organisms. With a deficiency of these late-acting components, there is increased susceptibility to recurrent neisserial (gonococcal and meningococcal) infections, reflecting the importance of bacterial lysis in defense against *Neisseria*.

A deficiency of C1 inhibitor gives rise to *hereditary angioedema*. This autosomal dominant disorder is more common than complement deficiency states.[114] The C1 inhibitor is a protease inhibitor whose target enzymes are C1r and C1s of the complement cascade, factor XII of the coagulation pathway, and the kallikrein system. As discussed in Chapter 2, these pathways are closely linked, and their unregulated activation can give rise to vasoactive peptides such as bradykinin. Although the exact nature of the bioactive compound produced in hereditary angioedema is uncertain, these patients have episodes of edema affecting skin and mucosal surfaces such as the larynx and the gastrointestinal tract. This may result in life-threatening asphyxia or nausea, vomiting, and diarrhea after minor trauma or emotional stress. Acute attacks of hereditary angioedema can be treated with C1 inhibitor concentrates prepared from human plasma.

Deficiency of other complement regulatory proteins is the cause of paroxysmal nocturnal hemoglobinuria. In this disease, there are mutations in enzymes required for glycophosphatidyl inositol (GPI) linkages.[115] Many proteins are expressed on cell surfaces in a GPI-linked form; two of these are the complement regulatory proteins, decay accelerating factor and CD59. In the absence of these proteins, complement deposited on red cells is not controlled, resulting in hemolysis and hemoglobinuria. A more detailed discussion of the disease is in Chapter 13.

Acquired Immunodeficiency Syndrome (AIDS)

AIDS is a disease caused by the retrovirus human immunodeficiency virus (HIV) and characterized by profound immunosuppression that leads to opportunistic infections, secondary neoplasms, and neurologic manifestations. The magnitude of this modern plague is truly staggering. By the end of 2002, more than 900,000 cases of AIDS had been reported in the United States, where AIDS is the second leading cause of death in men between ages 25 and 44, and the third leading cause of death in women in this age group. Although initially recognized in the United States, AIDS is a global problem. By the year 2002, HIV had infected 60 million people worldwide, and nearly 20 million adults and children have died of the disease. There are now about 42 million people living with HIV/AIDS, of whom 70% are in Africa and 15% in Asia; the prevalence rate in adults in sub-Saharan Africa is over 8%. It is estimated that 5 million people were newly infected with HIV during 2002, and 3.1 million deaths were caused by AIDS in that year alone. AIDS has now been reported from more than 193 countries around the world, and the pool of HIV-infected persons in Africa and Asia is large and expanding. Because of the magnitude of the AIDS problem, there has been an explosion of research aimed at understanding HIV and its remarkable ability to cripple host defenses. So rapid is the growth of information on the molecular biology and immunology of HIV that any review of this rapidly changing field is destined to be out of date by the time it is published. It is with this realization that an attempt is made here to summarize the currently available data on the epidemiology, cause, pathogenesis, and clinical features of HIV infection.

Epidemiology

Epidemiologic studies in the United States have identified five groups of adults at risk for developing AIDS. The case distribution in these groups is as follows:

- *Homosexual or bisexual men* constitute by far the largest group, accounting for over 50% of the reported cases. This includes ~5% who were intravenous drug abusers as well. Transmission of AIDS in this category is on the decline: currently, about 42% of new cases can be attributed to male homosexual contacts.
- *Intravenous drug abusers* with no previous history of homosexuality are the next largest group, representing about 25% of infected individuals. They represent the majority of cases among heterosexuals.
- *Hemophiliacs*, especially those who received large amounts of factor VIII or factor IX concentrates before 1985, make up ~0.5% of all cases.
- *Recipients of blood and blood components* who are not hemophiliacs but who received transfusions of HIV-infected whole blood or components (e.g., platelets, plasma) account for ~1% of patients. (Organs obtained from HIV-infected donors can also transmit AIDS.)
- *Heterosexual contacts* of members of other high-risk groups (chiefly intravenous drug abusers) constitute ~10% of the patient population. About 33% of new cases are attributable to heterosexual contact.
- In approximately 6% of cases, the risk factors cannot be determined.

The epidemiology of AIDS is quite different in children under age 13. Close to 2% of all AIDS cases occur in this pediatric population, and worldwide over 800,000 new cases were reported in children in the year 2002. In this group, more than 90% have resulted from transmission of the virus from mother to child (discussed later). The remaining 10% are hemophiliacs and others who received blood or blood products before 1985.

It should be apparent from the preceding discussion that transmission of HIV occurs under conditions that facilitate exchange of blood or body fluids containing the virus or virus-infected cells. Hence the three major routes of transmission are *sexual contact, parenteral inoculation,* and *passage of the virus from infected mothers to their newborns.*

Sexual transmission is clearly the predominant mode of infection worldwide, accounting for over 75% of all cases of HIV transmission.[116] Because the majority of infected people in the United States are men who have sex with men, most sexual transmission has occurred among homosexual men. The virus is carried in the semen, both within the lymphocytes and in the cell-free state, and it enters the recipient's body through abrasions in rectal or oral mucosa or by direct contact with mucosal lining cells. Viral transmission occurs in two ways: (1) direct inoculation into the blood vessels breached by trauma, and (2) into dendritic cells or CD4+ cells within the mucosa. Heterosexual transmission, although initially of less numerical importance in the United States, is globally the most common mode by which HIV is spread. In the past few years, even in the United States, *the rate of increase of heterosexual transmission has outpaced transmission by other means.* Such spread is occurring most rapidly in female sex partners of male intravenous drug abusers. As such, the number of women with AIDS is rising rapidly. In contrast to the US experience, heterosexual transmission is the dominant mode of HIV infection in Asia and Africa.

In addition to male-to-male and male-to-female transmission, there is evidence supporting female-to-male transmission. HIV is present in vaginal secretions and cervical cells of infected women. In the United States, this form of heterosexual spread is approximately 20-fold less common than male-to-female transmission. By contrast, in Africa and parts of Asia, the risk of female-to-male transmission is much higher. This observation is believed to be attributable to the presence of concurrent sexually transmitted disease. All forms of sexual transmission of HIV are enhanced by coexisting sexually transmitted diseases, especially those associated with genital ulceration. In this regard, syphilis, chancroid, and herpes are particularly important. Other sexually transmitted diseases, including gonorrhea and chlamydia, are also cofactors for HIV transmission, perhaps because in these genital inflammatory states there is greater concentration of the virus and virus-containing cells in genital fluids, owing to increased numbers of inflammatory cells in the semen.

Parenteral transmission of HIV has occurred in three groups of individuals: intravenous drug abusers, hemophiliacs who received factor VIII concentrates, and random recipients of blood transfusion. Of these three, intravenous drug users constitute by far the largest group. Transmission occurs by sharing of needles, syringes, and other paraphernalia contaminated with HIV-containing blood. This group occupies a pivotal position in the AIDS epidemic because, especially in the US, it represents a link in the transmission of HIV to other adult populations through heterosexual activity.

Transmission of HIV by transfusion of blood or blood products, such as lyophilized factor VIII and factor IX concentrates, has been virtually eliminated. This fortunate outcome resulted from increasing use of recombinant factor VIII and from three public health measures: screening of donated blood and plasma for antibody to HIV, stringent purity criteria for factor VIII preparations, and screening of donors on the basis of history. However, an extremely small risk of acquiring AIDS through transfusion of seronegative blood persists because a recently infected individual may be antibody negative. Currently, this risk is estimated to be 1 per 2,000,000 units of blood transfused.[117] Because it is now possible to detect HIV-associated p24 antigens in the blood before the development of humoral antibodies, this small risk is likely to decrease even further.

As alluded to earlier, *mother-to-infant transmission* is the major cause of pediatric AIDS. Infected mothers can transmit the infection to their offspring by three routes: (1) in utero by transplacental spread; (2) during delivery through an infected birth canal; and (3) after birth by ingestion of breast milk. Of these, transmission during birth (intrapartum) and in the immediate period thereafter (peripartum) is considered to be the most common mode in the United States. The reported transmission rates vary from 7% to 49% in different parts of the world. In most North American locales, the rate for perinatal transmission was about 25% before the advent of antiretroviral therapy. Higher risk of transmission is associated with high maternal viral load and low CD4+ T-cell counts as well as chorioamnionitis. Currently, with antiretroviral therapy given to infected pregnant women in the United States, the mother-to-child transmission has been reduced to very low levels.[118]

Much concern has arisen in the lay public and among health care workers about spread of HIV infection outside the high-risk groups. Extensive studies indicate that *HIV infection cannot be transmitted by casual personal contact in the household, workplace, or school.* Spread by insect bites is virtually impossible. Regarding transmission of HIV infection to health care workers, an extremely small but definite risk seems to be present. Seroconversion has been documented after accidental needle-stick injury or exposure of nonintact skin to infected blood in laboratory accidents. After needle-stick accidents, the risk of seroconversion is believed to be about 0.3%,[119] and antiretroviral therapy given within 24 to 48 hours of a needle stick can reduce the risk of infection eightfold. By comparison, approximately 30% of those accidentally exposed to hepatitis B–infected blood become seropositive. Although much publicized and a cause of justifiable concern, the transmission of AIDS from an infected health care provider to a patient is extremely rare.

Etiology: The Properties of HIV

AIDS is caused by HIV, a nontransforming human retrovirus belonging to the lentivirus family. Included in this group are feline immunodeficiency virus, simian immunodeficiency virus, visna virus of sheep, bovine immunodeficiency virus, and the equine infectious anemia virus.

Two genetically different but related forms of HIV, called *HIV-1* and *HIV-2*, have been isolated from patients with AIDS. HIV-1 is the most common type associated with AIDS in the United States, Europe, and Central Africa, whereas HIV-2 causes a similar disease principally in West Africa and India. Although distinct, HIV-1 and HIV-2 share some antigens. Specific tests for HIV-2, however, are now available, and blood collected for transfusion is routinely screened for both HIV-1 and HIV-2 seropositivity. The ensuing discussion relates primarily to HIV-1 and diseases caused by it, but the information is generally applicable to HIV-2 as well.

Structure of HIV. Similar to most retroviruses, the HIV-1 virion is spherical and contains an electron-dense, cone-shaped core surrounded by a lipid envelope derived from the host cell membrane (Fig. 6–43). The virus core contains (1) the major capsid protein p24; (2) nucleocapsid protein p7/p9; (3) two copies of genomic RNA; and (4) the three viral enzymes (protease, reverse transcriptase, and integrase). p24 is the most readily detected viral antigen and, as such, is the target for the antibodies that are used for the diagnosis of HIV infection in the widely used enzyme-linked immunosorbent assay. The viral core is surrounded by a

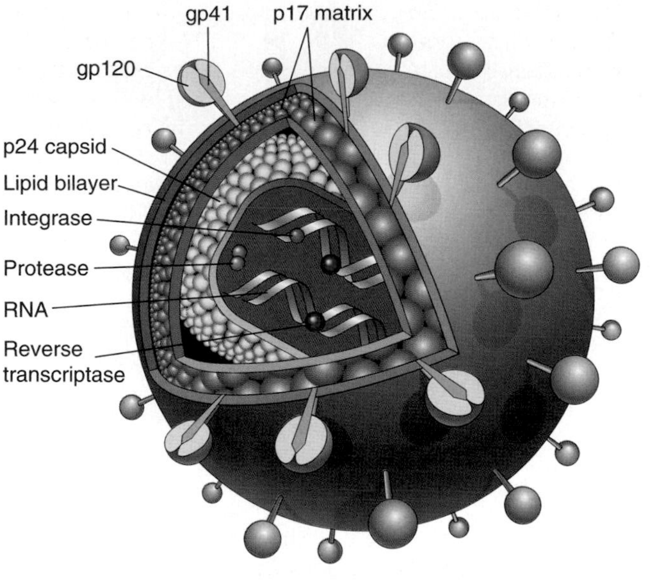
gp41
p17 matrix
gp120
p24 capsid
Lipid bilayer
Integrase
Protease
RNA
Reverse transcriptase

FIGURE 6–43 Schematic illustration of an HIV-1 virion. The viral particle is covered by a lipid bilayer that is derived from the host cell.

matrix protein called p17, which lies underneath the virion envelope. Studding the viral envelope are two viral glycoproteins, gp120 and gp41, which are critical for HIV infection of cells. The HIV-1 RNA genome contains the *gac*, *pol*, and *env* genes, which code for various viral proteins (Fig. 6–44). The products of the *gag* and *pol* genes are translated initially into large precursor proteins that must be cleaved by the viral protease to yield the mature proteins. The highly effective anti–HIV-1 protease inhibitor drugs prevent viral assembly by inhibiting the formation of mature viral proteins.

In addition to these three standard retroviral genes, HIV contains several other accessory genes, including *tat*, *rev*, *vif*, *nef*, *vpr*, and *vpu*, that regulate the synthesis and assembly of infectious viral particles and the pathogenicity of the virus.[120] For example, the product of the *TAT* (transactivator) gene, for example, is critical for virus replication. The Tat protein functions by causing a 1000-fold increase in the transcription of viral genes, thus it increases virus replication. The functions of other accessory proteins are indicated in Figure 6–44.

Molecular analysis of different HIV-1 isolates has revealed considerable variability in certain parts of their genome. Most variations are clustered in certain regions of the envelope glycoproteins. Because the humoral immune response against

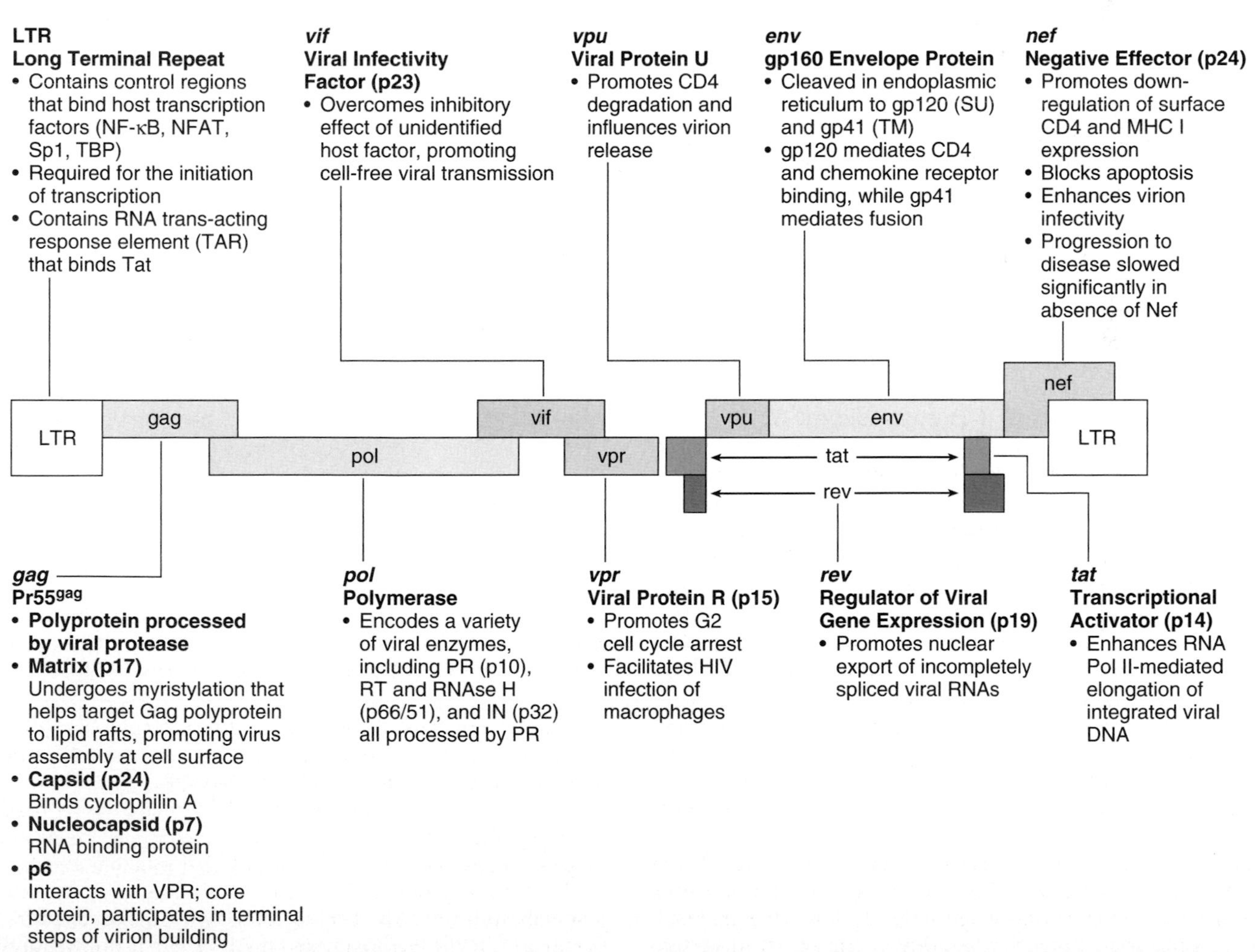
LTR
Long Terminal Repeat
• Contains control regions that bind host transcription factors (NF-κB, NFAT, Sp1, TBP)
• Required for the initiation of transcription
• Contains RNA trans-acting response element (TAR) that binds Tat
vif
Viral Infectivity Factor (p23)
• Overcomes inhibitory effect of unidentified host factor, promoting cell-free viral transmission
vpu
Viral Protein U
• Promotes CD4 degradation and influences virion release
env
gp160 Envelope Protein
• Cleaved in endoplasmic reticulum to gp120 (SU) and gp41 (TM)
• gp120 mediates CD4 and chemokine receptor binding, while gp41 mediates fusion
nef
Negative Effector (p24)
• Promotes down-regulation of surface CD4 and MHC I expression
• Blocks apoptosis
• Enhances virion infectivity
• Progression to disease slowed significantly in absence of Nef
LTR
gag
pol
vif
vpr
vpu
env
nef
tat
rev
LTR
gag
Pr55gag
• Polyprotein processed by viral protease
• Matrix (p17)
Undergoes myristylation that helps target Gag polyprotein to lipid rafts, promoting virus assembly at cell surface
• Capsid (p24)
Binds cyclophilin A
• Nucleocapsid (p7)
RNA binding protein
• p6
Interacts with VPR; core protein, participates in terminal steps of virion building
pol
Polymerase
• Encodes a variety of viral enzymes, including PR (p10), RT and RNAse H (p66/51), and IN (p32) all processed by PR
vpr
Viral Protein R (p15)
• Promotes G2 cell cycle arrest
• Facilitates HIV infection of macrophages
rev
Regulator of Viral Gene Expression (p19)
• Promotes nuclear export of incompletely spliced viral RNAs
tat
Transcriptional Activator (p14)
• Enhances RNA Pol II-mediated elongation of integrated viral DNA

FIGURE 6–44 HIV proviral genome. Several viral genes and their corresponding functions are illustrated. The genes outlined in red are unique to HIV; others are shared by all retroviruses.

HIV-1 is targeted against its envelope, such variability poses problems for the development of a single vaccine. On the basis of genetic analysis, HIV-1 can be divided into three subgroups, designated *M* (major), *O* (outlier), and *N* (neither *M* nor *O*). Group M viruses are the most common form worldwide, and they are further divided into several subtypes, or clades, designated A through K. Various subtypes differ in their geographic distribution; for example, subtype B is the most common form in western Europe and the United States, whereas subtype E is the most common clade in Thailand. Currently, clade C is the fastest-spreading clade worldwide, being present in India, Ethiopia, and Southern Africa.

Pathogenesis of HIV Infection and AIDS

While HIV can infect many tissues, *there are two major targets of HIV infection: the immune system and the central nervous system.* The effects of HIV infection on each of these two systems are discussed separately.

Profound immunosuppression, primarily affecting cell-mediated immunity, is the hallmark of AIDS. This results chiefly from infection of and a severe loss of CD4+ T cells as well as impairment in the function of surviving helper T cells.[121] As discussed later, macrophages and dendritic cells are also targets of HIV infection. HIV enters the body through mucosal tissues and blood and first infects T cells as well as dendritic cells and macrophages (Fig. 6–45). The infection becomes established in lymphoid tissues, where the virus may remain latent for long periods. Active viral replication is associated with more infection of cells and progression to AIDS. We first describe the mechanisms involved in viral entry into T cells and macrophages and the replicative cycle of the virus within cells. This is followed by a more detailed review of the interaction between HIV and its cellular targets.

Life Cycle of HIV. There is abundant evidence that the *CD4 molecule is a high-affinity receptor for HIV*. This explains the selective tropism of the virus for CD4+ T cells and other CD4+ cells, particularly monocytes/macrophages and dendritic cells. Binding to CD4 is not sufficient for infection, however. HIV gp120 must also bind to other cell surface molecules (coreceptors) for entry into the cell. Two chemokine receptors, CCR5 and CXCR4 (Chapter 2), serve this role.[122,123] HIV isolates can be distinguished by their use of these receptors: R5 strains use CCR5, X4 strains use CXCR4, and some strains (R5X4) are dual-tropic. Molecular details of the deadly handshake between HIV glycoproteins and their cell-surface receptors have been uncovered in elegant detail and are important to understand because they may provide the basis of anti-HIV therapy.

As illustrated in Figure 6–46, the HIV envelope contains two glycoproteins, surface gp120 that is noncovalently attached to transmembrane protein, gp41. *The initial step in infection is the binding of the gp120 envelope glycoprotein to CD4 molecules.* This binding leads to a conformational change that results in the formation of a new recognition site on gp120 for the coreceptors CCR5 or CXCR4. The next step involves conformational changes in gp41; these changes result in the insertion of a fusion peptide at the tip of gp41 into the cell membrane of the target cells (e.g., T cells or macrophages).[124] After fusion, the virus core containing the HIV genome enters the cytoplasm of the cell. Several lines of

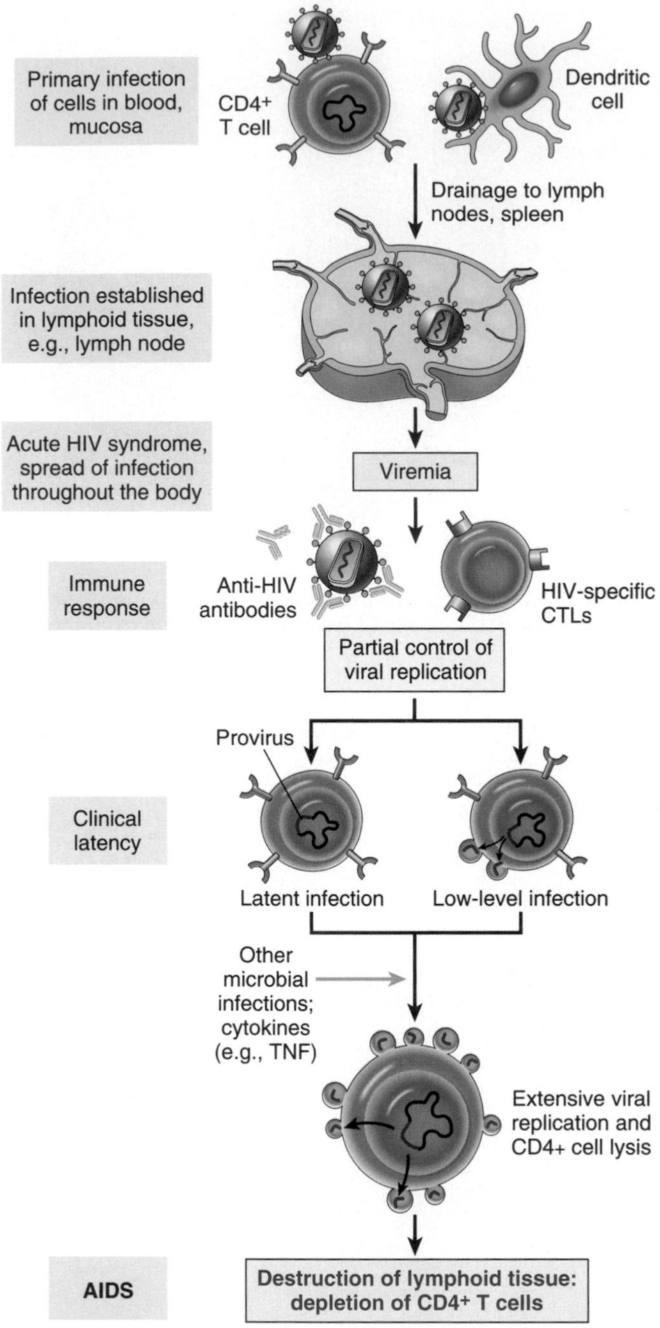

FIGURE 6–45 Pathogenesis of HIV-1 infection. Initially, HIV-1 infects T cells and macrophages directly or is carried to these cells by Langerhans cells. Viral replication in the regional lymph nodes leads to viremia and widespread seeding of lymphoid tissue. The viremia is controlled by the host immune response *(not shown)*, and the patient then enters a phase of clinical latency. During this phase, viral replication in both T cells and macrophages continues unabated, but there is some immune containment of virus *(not illustrated)*. There continues a gradual erosion of CD4+ cells by productive infection (or other mechanisms, *not shown*). Ultimately, CD4+ cell numbers decline, and the patient develops clinical symptoms of full-blown AIDS. Macrophages are also parasitized by the virus early; they are not lysed by HIV-1, and they may transport the virus to tissues, particularly the brain.

evidence indicate that binding of HIV to its coreceptors is important in the pathogenesis of AIDS. First, nonlymphoid cells engineered to express human CD4 cannot be infected with HIV unless one of the coreceptors is also expressed in these cells. Second, chemokines sterically hinder HIV infec-

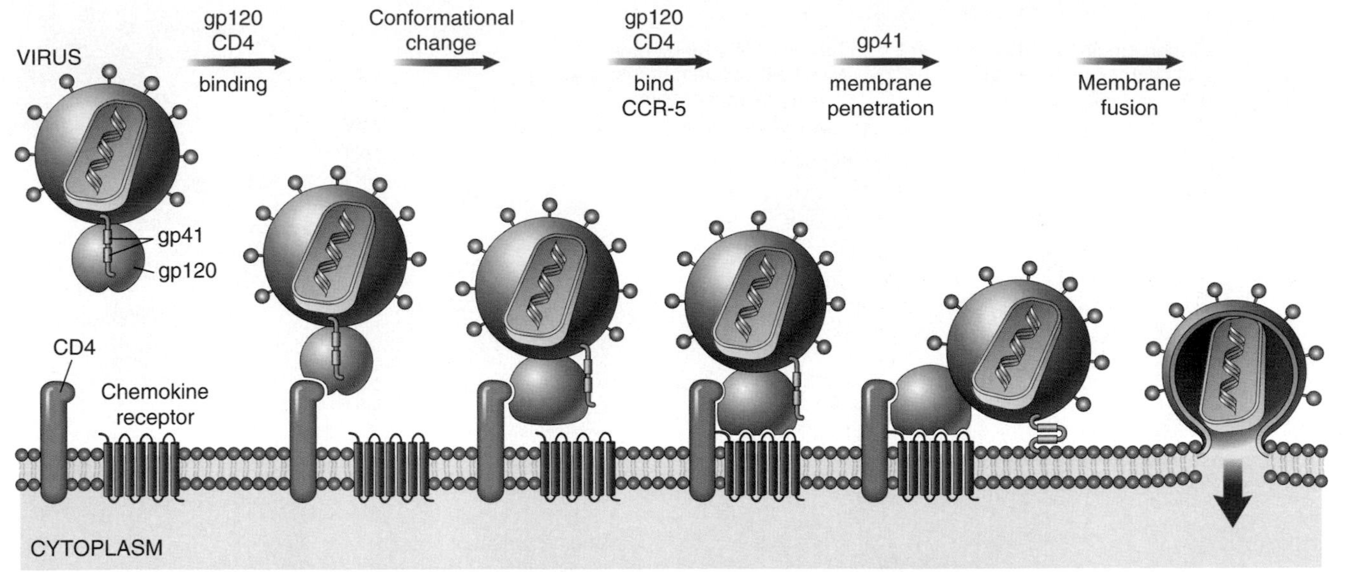

FIGURE 6–46 Mechanism of HIV entry into host cells. Interactions with CD4 and CCR5 coreceptor are illustrated. (Adapted with permission from Wain-Hobson S: HIV. One on one meets two. Nature 384:117, 1996. Copyright 1996, Macmillam Magazines Limited.)

tion of cells in culture by occupying their receptors. Thus, the level of chemokines in the microenvironment surrounding HIV and its target cells may influence the efficiency of viral infection in vivo. Third, individuals who inherit two defective copies of the CCR5 receptor gene are resistant to infection and the development of AIDS associated with R5 HIV isolates.[125] The frequency of those who are homozygous for the protective CCR5 mutation is about 1% in white Americans, whereas 18% to 20% of individuals are heterozygotes. The latter are not protected from AIDS, but the onset of their disease is somewhat delayed. Only rare homozygotes for the mutation have been found in African or East Asian populations.

The discovery of coreceptors for HIV infection has also solved previously puzzling observations of HIV tropism. It has been known for some time that HIV strains can be classified into two groups on the basis of their ability to infect macrophages and established CD4+ T-cell lines. Macrophage-tropic (M-tropic) strains, their name notwithstanding, can infect both monocytes/macrophages and freshly isolated peripheral blood T cells, but not in vitro propagated T-cell lines. By contrast, the T-cell line–tropic strains can infect only T cells, both freshly isolated and maintained in culture. This selectivity is based on coreceptor usage: M-tropic strains use CCR5, whereas T-tropic strains bind to CXCR4. Because CCR5 is expressed on both monocytes and T cells, they are susceptible to infection by M-tropic strains; CXCR4 is expressed on T cells but not on monocytes/macrophages, and hence T cells but not macrophages can be infected with T-tropic strains. Primary (freshly isolated) T cells express both CCR5 and CXCR4 and hence can be infected by either of the two viral types. In approximately 90% of cases, the R5 (M-tropic) type of HIV is the dominant virus found in the blood of acutely infected individuals and early in the course of infection. Over the course of infection, however, T-tropic viruses gradually accumulate; these are especially virulent and cause the final rapid phase of disease progression.[126] Because the ability to bind the coreceptors resides in the gp120 protein of the viral envelope, it follows that there must be molecular differences between the gp120 molecule of M-tropic and T-tropic HIV. Such is the case; further, it is thought that during the course of HIV infection M-tropic strains evolve into T-tropic strains, owing to mutations in genes that encode gp120. The resultant transition in the ability of the virus to bind CXCR4 but not CCR5 is probably important in the pathogenesis of AIDS because T-tropic (i.e., CXCR4-tropic) viruses are capable of infecting naive T cells and even thymic T-cell precursors and cause greater T-cell depletion and impairment. Whether M-tropic viruses are more efficient in transmission is not entirely clear. If this proves to be the case, there are two possible explanations. First, dendritic cells within the mucosal epithelium richly express CCR5 but do not express CXCR4, thus making them susceptible to infection by M-tropic viruses. Second, binding of M-tropic strains to CCR5 on T cells may signal these cells to make chemotactic factors for other T cells, thus increasing the population of potential targets in the vicinity of an infected T cell. Envelope glycoproteins of T-tropic viruses do not cause such activation of T-cell signals after binding to CXCR4.

Once internalized, the RNA genome of the virus undergoes reverse transcription, leading to formation of cDNA (proviral DNA) (Fig. 6–47). In quiescent T cells, HIV cDNA may remain in the cytoplasm in a linear episomal form. In dividing T cells, the cDNA circularizes, enters the nucleus and is then integrated into the host genome. After this integration, the provirus may remain locked into the chromosome for months or years, and hence the infection becomes latent. Alternatively, proviral DNA may be transcribed, with the formation of complete viral particles that bud from the cell membrane. Such productive infection, when associated with extensive viral budding, leads to cell death.

Completion of the viral life cycle in latently infected cells occurs only after cell activation, and in the case of most CD4+ T cells virus activation results in cell lysis. To understand the molecular basis of release from latency, we must briefly consider the events that are associated with activation of CD4+ helper T cells. It is well known that antigen-induced or

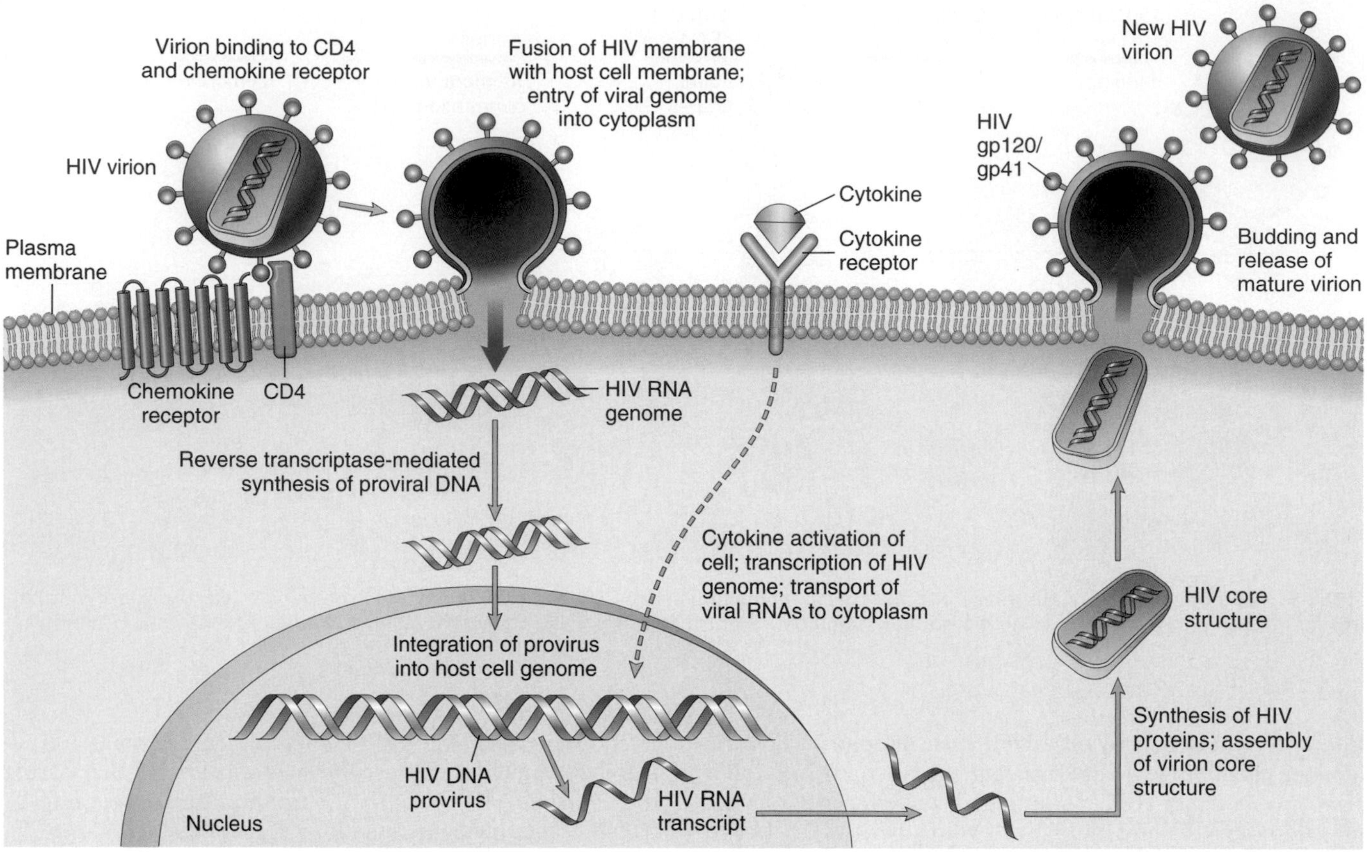

FIGURE 6–47 The life cycle of HIV. The steps from viral entry to production of infectious virions are illustrated.

mitogen-induced activation of T cells is associated with transcription of genes encoding the cytokine IL-2 and its receptor (IL-2R). At the molecular level, this is accomplished in part by the induction of the NF-κB transcription factor. In resting T cells, NF-κB is sequestered in the cytoplasm in a complex with members of the I-κB (inhibitor of κB) protein. Cellular activation by antigen or cytokines (e.g., TNF, IL-1, IL-2) induces cytoplasmic kinases that phosphorylate I-κB and target it for enzymatic degradation, thus releasing NF-κB and allowing it to translocate to the nucleus. In the nucleus, NF-κB binds to sequences (κB sites) within the promoter regions of several genes, including those of cytokines that are expressed in immunologically activated cells. The LTR sequences that flank the HIV genome also contain similar κB sites that can be triggered by the same nuclear regulatory factors.[127] Imagine now a latently infected CD4+ cell that encounters an environmental antigen. Induction of NF-κB in such a cell (a physiologic response) activates the transcription of HIV proviral DNA (a pathologic outcome) and leads ultimately to the production of virions and to cell lysis. Furthermore, TNF, a cytokine produced by activated macrophages, also stimulates NF-κB activity and thus leads to transcriptional activation of HIV-mRNA. The production of HIV-1 by macrophages is up-regulated by other pro-inflammatory cytokines, such as lymphotoxin, IFN-γ, IL-6, and GM-CSF, many of which are produced during a normal immune response. Anti-inflammatory cytokines, such as IL-10, inhibit HIV-1 replication by down-regulating the production of HIV-inducing cytokines. Thus, it seems that HIV thrives when the host macrophages and T cells are physiologically activated, an act that can be best described as "subversion from within." Such activation in vivo may result from antigenic stimulation by HIV itself or by other infecting microorganisms, such as cytomegalovirus, EBV, hepatitis B virus, and *M. tuberculosis*. The life style of most HIV-infected people in the United States places them at increased risk for recurrent exposure to other sexually transmitted diseases; in Africa, socioeconomic conditions probably impose a higher burden of chronic microbial infections. The multiple infections to which these patients are prone because of diminished helper T-cell function lead to increased production of pro-inflammatory cytokines, which, in turn, stimulate more HIV production, followed by infection and loss of additional CD4+ T cells. Thus, it is easy to visualize how in patients with AIDS a vicious cycle of cell destruction may be set up.

Mechanism of T-Cell Immunodeficiency in HIV Infection. *Productive infection of T cells and viral replication in infected cells is the major mechanism by which HIV causes lysis of CD4+ T cells.* Approximately 100 billion new viral particles are produced every day, and 1 to 2 billion CD4+ T cells die each day.[128] Early in the course of HIV infection, the immune system can replace the dying T cells, and hence the rate of CD4+ cell loss appears deceptively low. This masks the massive cell death occurring primarily in the lymphoid tissues. Later in the course of the disease, renewal of CD4+ T cells cannot keep up with the loss of these cells. Despite the relentless, and eventually profound, loss of CD4+ cells from the peripheral blood, however, there is a relative paucity of productively infected T cells in the circulation. These obser-

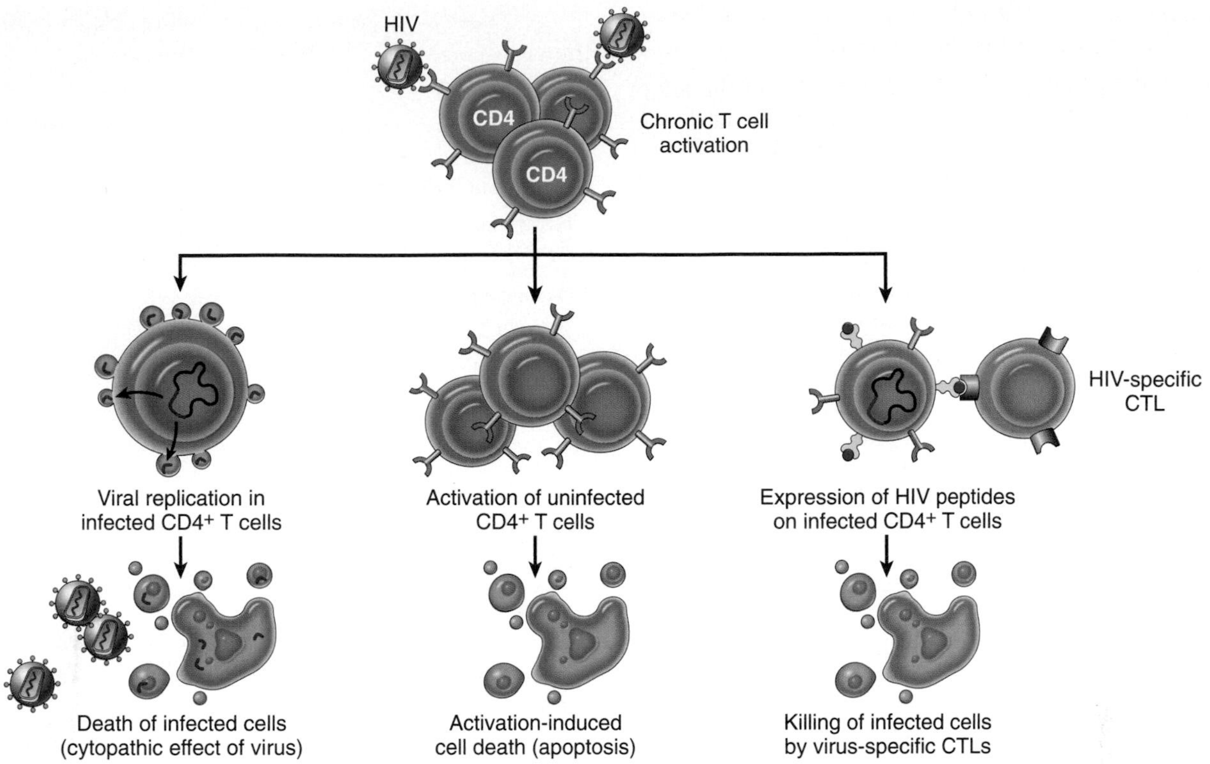

FIGURE 6–48 Mechanisms of CD4 cell loss in HIV infection.

vations have spawned many hypotheses (some described later) that attempt to explain the loss of CD4+ T cells by mechanisms other than direct cytolysis (Fig. 6–48).[130,131] It is now believed that *HIV can bring about the loss of T cells in several ways that do not involve a direct cytopathic effect of the virus.*

- Early in the course of disease, HIV colonizes the lymphoid organs (spleen, lymph nodes, tonsils). These, and not the peripheral blood, are reservoirs of infected cells. The virus may cause progressive destruction of the architecture and cellular composition of lymphoid tissues.
- Chronic activation of uninfected cells, responding to HIV itself or to infections that are common in patients, leads to apoptosis of these cells by the process of *activation-induced cell death.*[129–131] Thus, the numbers of CD4+ T cells that die are far greater than the numbers of infected cells. The molecular mechanism of this type of cell death is not known.
- Loss of immature precursors of CD4+ T cells, either by direct infection of thymic progenitor cells or by infection of accessory cells that secrete cytokines essential for CD4+ T-cell maturation. The idea that reduced production may underlie loss of CD4+ cells is supported by the observation that the telomeres of CD4+ cells from HIV-infected patients are not appreciably shorter than those of uninfected controls.[132] Because telomeres shorten every time a cell divides, the telomere length can provide an estimate of how many times a cell has divided over its lifetime (Chapter 1). With massive CD4+ cell death and compensatory cell proliferation, telomere length would be expected to have shortened.
- Fusion of infected and uninfected cells, with formation of syncytia (giant cells) (Fig. 6–49). In tissue culture, the gp120 expressed on productively infected cells binds to CD4 molecules on uninfected T cells, followed by cell fusion. Fused cells develop ballooning and usually die within a few hours. This property of syncytia formation is generally confined to the T-tropic X4 type of HIV-1. For this reason, this type is often referred to as syncytia-inducing (SI) virus, in contrast to the NSI R5 virus.
- Apoptosis of uninfected CD4+ T cells[133] by binding of soluble gp120 to the CD4 molecule, followed by activation through the T-cell receptor by antigens; such cross-linking of CD4 molecules and T-cell activation leads to aberrant signaling and activation of death pathways. CD8+ cytotoxic

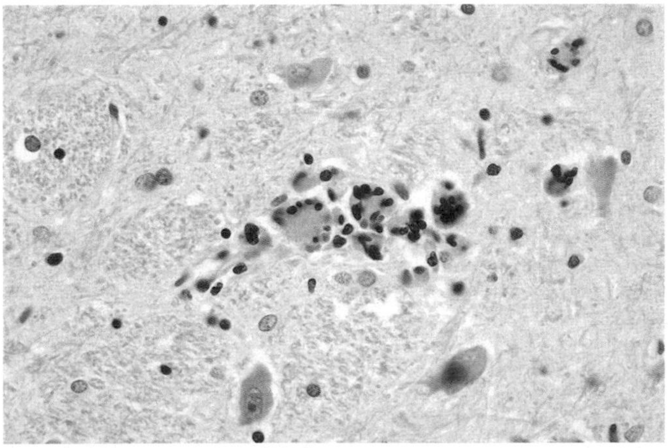

FIGURE 6–49 HIV infection showing the formation of giant cells in the brain. (Courtesy of Dr. Dennis Burns, Department of Pathology, University of Texas Southwestern Medical School, Dallas, TX.)

T lymphocytes may kill uninfected CD4+ T cells that are coated with gp120 released from infected cells.

Although marked reduction in CD4+ T cells, a hallmark of AIDS, can account for most of the immunodeficiency late in the course of HIV infection, there is compelling evidence for *qualitative defects in T cells that can be detected even in asymptomatic HIV-infected persons.* Reported defects include a reduction in antigen-induced T-cell proliferation, a decrease in T_H1 type responses relative to the T_H2 type, defects in intracellular signaling, and many more. The imbalance between the T_H1 and T_H2 responses results in profound deficiency in cell-mediated immunity, leading to increased susceptibility to infections by viruses and other intracellular microbes.[134] There is also a selective loss of the memory subset of CD4+ helper T cells early in the course of disease, possibly because memory T cells express higher levels of the HIV-1 coreceptor CCR5 and are the cells that are activated in response to HIV.[127] This observation explains the inability of peripheral blood T cells to be activated when challenged with common recall antigens.

Low-level chronic or latent infection of T cells (and macrophages, discussed below) is an important feature of HIV infection. Early in the course of this infection, only rare CD4+ T cells in the blood or lymph nodes express infectious virus, whereas in the lymph nodes, up to 30% can be demonstrated by polymerase chain reaction to harbor the HIV genome. It is widely believed that integrated provirus, without virus expression (latent infection), can remain in the cells for months to years. Even with potent antiviral therapy, which practically sterilizes the peripheral blood, latent virus lurks within the CD4+ cells (both T cells and macrophages) in the lymph nodes. According to some estimates, 0.05% of resting CD4+ T cells in the lymph nodes are latently infected. Because these CD4+ T cells are memory T cells, they are long-lived, with a life span of months to years, and thus provide a persistent reservoir of virus.[128]

CD4+ T cells play a pivotal role in regulating the immune response: they produce a plethora of cytokines, such as IL-2, IL-4, IL-5, IFN-γ, macrophage chemotactic factors, and hematopoietic growth factors (e.g., GM-CSF). Therefore, loss of this "master regulator" has ripple effects on virtually every other component of the immune system, as summarized in Table 6–12.

TABLE 6–12 Major Abnormalities of Immune Function in AIDS

Lymphopenia
Predominantly due to selective loss of the CD4+ helper-inducer T-cell subset; inversion of CD4 : CD8 ratio
Decreased T-Cell Function In Vivo
Preferential loss of memory T cells
Susceptibility to opportunistic infections
Susceptibility to neoplasms
Decreased delayed-type hypersensitivity
Altered T-Cell Function In Vitro
Decreased proliferative response to mitogens, alloantigens, and soluble antigens
Decreased specific cytotoxicity
Decreased helper function for pokeweed mitogen-induced B-cell immunoglobulin production
Decreased IL-2 and TFN-γ production
Polyclonal B-Cell Activation
Hypergammaglobulinemia and circulating immune complexes
Inability to mount de novo antibody response to a new antigen or vaccine
Refractoriness to the normal signals for B-cell activation in vitro
Altered Monocyte or Macrophage Functions
Decreased chemotaxis and phagocytosis
Decreased HLA class II antigen expression
Diminished capacity to present antigen to T cells
Increased spontaneous secretion of IL-1, TNF, IL-6

HIV Infection of Non-T Cells. In addition to infection and loss of CD4+ T cells, infection of monocytes and macrophages is also extremely important in the pathogenesis of HIV infection. Similar to T cells, the majority of the macrophages that are infected by HIV are found in the tissues and not in peripheral blood. In certain tissues, such as the lungs and brain, as many as 10% to 50% of macrophages are infected. Several aspects of HIV infection of macrophages need to be emphasized:

- Although cell division is required for replication of most retroviruses, HIV-1 can infect and multiply in terminally differentiated nondividing macrophages. This property of HIV-1 is dependent on the HIV-1 *vpr* gene. The Vpr protein allows nuclear targeting of the HIV preintegration complex through the nuclear pore.
- Infected macrophages bud relatively small amounts of virus from the cell surface, but these cells contain large numbers of virus particles often located exclusively in intracellular vacuoles. Despite the fact that macrophages allow viral replication, they are quite resistant to the cytopathic effects of HIV, in contrast to CD4+ T cells. Thus, macrophages may be reservoirs of infection.
- Macrophages, in all likelihood, act as gatekeepers of infection. Recall that in more than 90% of cases, acute HIV infection is characterized by predominantly circulating M-tropic strains. This finding suggests that the initial infection of macrophages or dendritic cells may be important in the pathogenesis of HIV disease.

HIV infection of macrophages has three important implications. First, monocytes and macrophages represent a veritable virus factory and reservoir, whose output remains largely protected from host defenses. Second, macrophages provide a safe vehicle for HIV to be transported to various parts of the body, including the nervous system. Third, in late stages of HIV infection, when the CD4+ T-cell numbers decline greatly, macrophages may be an important site of continued viral replication.[135]

In contrast to tissue macrophages, the number of monocytes in circulation infected by HIV is low, yet there are unexplained functional defects that have important consequences for host defense. These defects include impaired microbicidal activity, decreased chemotaxis, decreased secretion of IL-1, inappropriate secretion of TNF, and, most important, poor capacity to present antigens to T cells.

Studies have documented that, in addition to macrophages, two types of *dendritic cells* are also important targets for the initiation and maintenance of HIV infection: mucosal and follicular dendritic cells. It is thought that *mucosal dendritic cells are infected by the virus and transport it to regional lymph nodes*, where CD4+ T cells are infected.[136] Dendritic cells also express a lectin-like receptor that specifically binds HIV and displays it in an intact, infectious form to T cells, thus promoting infection of the T cells.[137] *Follicular dendritic cells in the germinal centers of lymph nodes are, similar to macrophages, important reservoirs of HIV.*[138] Although some follicular dendritic cells may be susceptible to HIV infection, most virus particles are found on the surface of their dendritic processes. Follicular dendritic cells have receptors for the Fc portion of immunoglobulins, and hence they trap HIV virions coated with anti-HIV antibodies. The antibody-coated virions localized to follicular dendritic cells retain the ability to infect CD4+ T cells as they traverse the intricate meshwork formed by the dendritic processes of the follicular dendritic cells. *To summarize, CD4+ T cells, macrophages, and follicular dendritic cells contained in the lymphoid tissues are the major sites of HIV infection and persistence.*

Although much attention has been focused on T cells, macrophages, and dendritic cells because they can be infected by HIV, patients with AIDS also display profound abnormalities of B-cell function. Paradoxically, these patients have hypergammaglobulinemia and circulating immune complexes owing to polyclonal B-cell activation. This may result from multiple interacting factors: reactivation of or re-infection with cytomegalovirus and EBV, both of which are polyclonal B-cell activators, can occur; gp41 itself can promote B-cell growth and differentiation; and HIV-infected macrophages produce increased amounts of IL-6, which stimulates proliferation of B cells. *Despite the presence of spontaneously activated B cells, patients with AIDS are unable to mount antibody responses to new antigens.* This could be due, in part, to lack of T-cell help, but antibody responses against T-independent antigens are also suppressed, and hence there may be other defects in B cells as well. Impaired humoral immunity renders these patients prey to disseminated infections caused by encapsulated bacteria, such as *S. pneumoniae* and *H. influenzae*, both of which require antibodies for effective opsonization and clearance.

Pathogenesis of Central Nervous System Involvement. The pathogenesis of neurologic manifestations deserves special mention because, in addition to the lymphoid system, the nervous system is a major target of HIV infection.[139,140] Macrophages and microglia, cells in the central nervous system that belong to the monocyte and macrophage lineage, are the predominant cell types in the brain that are infected with HIV. It is widely believed that HIV is carried into the brain by infected monocytes. In keeping with this, the HIV isolates from the brain are almost exclusively M-tropic. The mechanism of HIV-induced damage of the brain, however, remains obscure. Because neurons are not infected by HIV, and the extent of neuropathologic changes is often less than might be expected from the severity of neurologic symptoms, most workers believe that neurologic deficit is caused indirectly by viral products and by soluble factors produced by infected microglia. Included among the soluble factors are the usual culprits, such as IL-1, TNF, and IL-6. In addition, nitric oxide induced in neuronal cells by gp41 has been implicated. Direct damage of neurons by soluble HIV gp120 has also been postulated. According to some investigators, these diverse soluble neurotoxins act by triggering excessive entry of Ca^{2+} into the neurons through their action on glutamate-activated ion channels that regulate intracellular calcium.

Natural History of HIV Infection

The course of HIV infection can be best understood in terms of an interplay between HIV and the immune system. Three phases reflecting the dynamics of virus–host interaction can be recognized: (1) an acute retroviral syndrome; (2) a middle, chronic phase; and (3) full-blown AIDS (see Fig. 6–45; also Fig. 6–50).[141] We first present the cardinal features of the phases of HIV infection and their associated clinical syndromes then recount the sequential virologic and immunologic findings during the course of HIV infection.

The *acute retroviral syndrome* represents the initial or primary response of an immunocompetent adult to HIV infection.[142] It is characterized initially by a high level of virus production, viremia, and *widespread seeding of the lymphoid tissues.* The initial infection, however, is readily controlled by the development of an antiviral immune response. It is estimated that 40% to 90% of individuals who acquire a primary infection develop the viral syndrome 3 to 6 weeks after infection, and this resolves spontaneously in 2 to 4 weeks. Clinically, this phase is associated with a self-limited acute illness with nonspecific symptoms, including sore throat, myalgias, fever, rash, weight loss, and fatigue, resembling a flulike syndrome. Other clinical features, such as rash, cervical adenopathy, diarrhea, and vomiting, may also occur.

The middle *chronic phase* represents a stage of relative containment of the virus, associated with a period of clinical latency. The immune system is largely intact, but *there is continuous HIV replication, predominantly in the lymphoid tissues, which may last for several years.* Patients are either asymptomatic or develop persistent generalized lymphadenopathy. In addition, many patients have minor opportunistic infections, such as thrush and herpes zoster. Thrombocytopenia may also be noted (Chapter 13). Persistent lymphadenopathy with significant constitutional symptoms (fever, rash, fatigue) reflects the onset of immune system decompensation, escalation of viral replication, and onset of the *crisis* phase.

The final phase is *progression to AIDS.* It is characterized by a breakdown of host defense, a dramatic increase in plasma virus, and clinical disease. Typically the patient presents with long-lasting fever (>1 month), fatigue, weight loss, and diarrhea. After a variable period, serious opportunistic infections, secondary neoplasms, or clinical neurologic disease (grouped under the rubric *AIDS indicator diseases*, discussed below) supervene, and the patient is said to have developed AIDS.

In the absence of treatment, most but not all patients with HIV infection progress to AIDS after a chronic phase lasting from 7 to 10 years. Exceptions to this typical course are exemplified by long-term nonprogressors and by rapid progressors. Nonprogressors are defined as untreated HIV-1–infected individuals who remain asymptomatic for 10 years or more, with stable CD4+ counts and low levels of plasma viremia. In rapid progressors, the middle, chronic phase is telescoped to 2 to 3 years after primary infection. The possible basis for these variant outcomes is discussed later.

With this overview of the phases of HIV disease, we can consider some details of host-parasite relationships during the course of a typical HIV infection. The initial entry of the virus may be through a mucosal surface, as in sexual intercourse (via rectal or cervical mucosa) or via blood exposure (e.g., after intravenous drug use). From the mucosal portal, the virus is carried to the regional lymph nodes by dendritic cells.

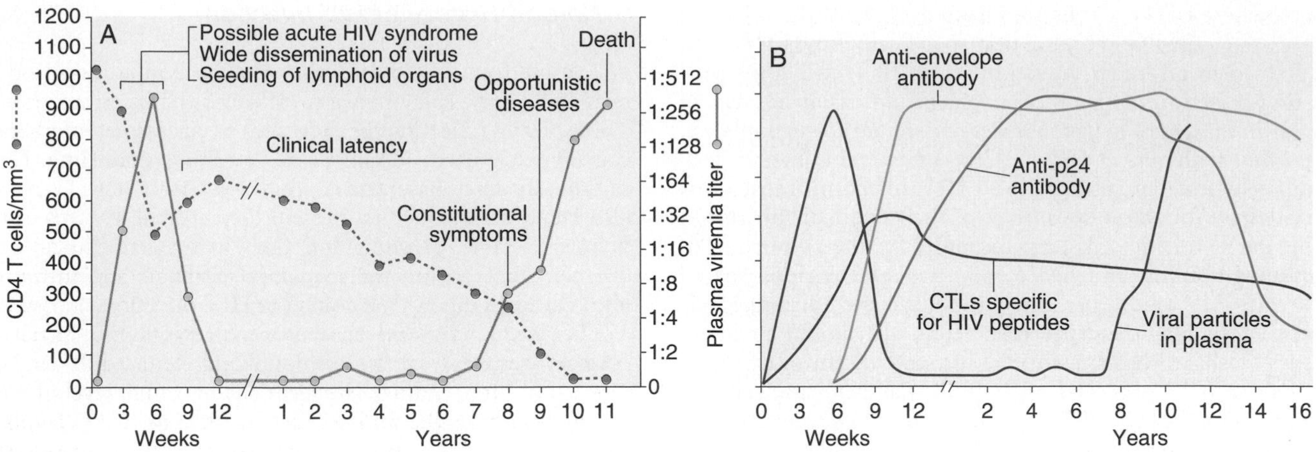

FIGURE 6–50 Typical course of HIV infection. *A,* During the early period after primary infection, there is widespread dissemination of virus and a sharp decrease in the number of CD4+ T cells in peripheral blood. An immune response to HIV ensues, with a decrease in viremia followed by a prolonged period of clinical latency. During this period, viral replication continues. The CD4+ T-cell count gradually decreases during the following years, until it reaches a critical level below which there is a substantial risk of opportunistic diseases. (Redrawn from Fauci AS, Lane HC: Human immunodeficiency virus disease: AIDS and related conditions. In Fauci AS, et al (eds): Harrison's Principles of Internal Medicine, 14th ed. New York, McGraw-Hill, 1997, p 1791.) *B,* Immune response to HIV infection. A cytolytic T lymphocyte (CTL) response to HIV is detectable by 2 to 3 weeks after the initial infection and peaks by 9 to 12 weeks. Marked expansion of virus-specific CD8+ T cell clones occurs during this time, and up to 10% of a patient's CTLs may be HIV specific at 12 weeks. The humoral immune response to HIV peaks at about 12 weeks.

Virus inoculated into the blood is rapidly cleared by the spleen and lymph nodes. Thus, with either mode of entry, the virus initially replicates in the lymphoid organs and then spills over into the blood. The patient now experiences the acute HIV syndrome described earlier. This phase is characterized initially by high levels of virus in plasma and an abrupt, sometimes severe, reduction in CD4+ T cells. During this period, HIV can be readily isolated from the blood, and there are high levels of HIV p24 antigen in serum. Soon, however, a virus-specific immune response develops, evidenced by seroconversion (usually within 3 to 7 weeks of presumed exposure) and, more importantly, by the development of virus-specific CD8+ cytotoxic T cells. *HIV-specific CD8+ T cells are detected in the blood at about the time viral titers begin to fall and are most likely responsible for the containment of HIV infection.*[143,144] As viral replication abates, CD4+ T cells return to near-normal numbers, signaling the end of the early acute phase. Although plasma viremia declines, there is widespread dissemination and seeding of the virus, especially in the lymphoid organs. With the formation of anti-HIV antibodies, antibody-coated virions are trapped by follicular dendritic cells in the germinal centers. As discussed earlier, both latent and replicating HIV can be found in CD4+ T cells and macrophages within the lymph nodes, and viral particles are readily detected on the surface of follicular dendritic cells.

The viral load at the end of the acute phase reflects the equilibrium reached between the virus and the host after the initial battle, and in a given patient it may remain fairly stable for several years. This level of steady-state viremia, or the viral "set-point," is a predictor of the rate of decline of CD4+ T cells, and therefore progression of HIV disease. In one study, only 8% of patients with a viral load of less than 4350 copies of viral mRNA/μL progressed to full-blown AIDS in 5 years, whereas 62% of those with a viral load of greater than 36,270 copies had developed AIDS in the same period.[145] From a practical standpoint, therefore, *the extent of viremia, measured as HIV-1 RNA, is a useful surrogate marker of HIV disease progression and is of clinical value in the management of people with HIV infection.* However, in patients treated with highly active antiretroviral therapy (HAART), clinical improvement is often greater than the decrease in plasma viremia, and it is generally accepted that viremia as well as the blood CD4+ T-cell count should be considered in the management.

Regardless of the viral burden, during the middle or chronic phase, there is a continuing battle between HIV and the host immune system. The CD8+ cytotoxic T-cell response remains activated, and extensive viral and CD4+ cell turnover continues. As emphasized earlier, however, because of the immense regenerative capacity of the immune system, a large proportion of the lost CD4+ cells is replenished. Thus, the decline in the CD4+ cell count in blood is modest. After an extended and variable period, there begins a gradual erosion of the CD4+ T cells. Concomitant with this loss of CD4+ T cells, host defenses begin to wane, and the proportion of the surviving CD4+ cells infected with HIV increases, as does the viral burden per CD4+ cell. Not unexpectedly, HIV spillover into the plasma increases. How HIV escapes immune control is not entirely clear, but several mechanisms have been proposed.[146–148] These include destruction of the CD4+ T cells that are critical for effective immunity, antigenic variation, and down-modulation of class I MHC molecules on infected cells so that viral antigens are not recognized by CD8+ CTLs.

Because the loss of immune containment is associated with declining CD4+ cell counts, the CDC classification of HIV infection stratifies patients into three categories on the basis of CD4+ cell counts: CD4+ greater than or equal to 500 cells/μL, 200 to 499 cells/μL, and fewer than 200 cells/μL (Table 6–13). For clinical management, blood CD4+ counts are perhaps the strongest indicator of disease progression.

It should be evident from our discussion that in each of the three phases of HIV infection, viral replication continues to occur. Even in the chronic phase, before the severe decline in

TABLE 6–13 CDC Classification Categories of HIV Infection

	CD4+ T-Cell Categories		
Clinical Categories	**1. ≥500/μL**	**2. 200–499/μL**	**3. ≤200/μL**
A. Asymptomatic, acute (primary) HIV, or persistent generalized lymphadenopathy	A1	A2	A3
B. Symptomatic, not A or C conditions	B1	B2	B3
C. AIDS indicator conditions: including constitutional disease, neurologic disease, or secondary infection or neoplasm			

Data from CDC. Centers for Disease Control and Prevention: 1993 revised classification system and expanded surveillance definition for AIDS among adolescents and adults. MMWR 41(RR-17):1, 1992.

CD4+ cell count and the development of AIDS, there is extensive turnover of the virus. In other words, *HIV infection lacks a phase of true microbiologic latency*, that is, a phase during which *all* the HIV is in the form of proviral DNA, and no cell is productively infected.

Before this discussion of the virus-host relationships is ended, some comments on those patients who are considered long-term nonprogressors are in order. Individuals in this group remain asymptomatic for long periods of time (10 years or more), have low levels of viremia, and have stable CD4+ cell counts. People with such an uncommon clinical course have attracted great attention in the hope that studying them may shed light on host and viral factors that influence disease progression. Studies to date suggest that this group is heterogeneous with respect to the factors that influence the course of the disease. In a small subset of nonprogressors, the infecting HIV had deletions or mutations in the *nef* gene, suggesting that Nef proteins are critical to disease progression. In most cases, the viral isolates do not show any qualitative abnormalities. In all cases, there is evidence of a vigorous anti-HIV immune response, but the immune correlates of protection are still unknown. Some of these patients have high levels of HIV-specific CD8+ cells, and these levels are maintained over the course of infection. It is not clear whether the robust CD8+ cell response is the cause or consequence of the slow progression. Further studies, it is hoped, will provide the answers to this and other questions critical to disease progression.

Clinical Features of AIDS

The clinical manifestations of HIV infection can be readily surmised from the foregoing discussion. They range from a mild acute illness to severe disease. Because the salient clinical features of the acute early and chronic middle phases of HIV infection were described earlier, here we summarize the clinical manifestations of the terminal phase, AIDS. At the outset it should be pointed out that the clinical manifestations and opportunistic infections associated with HIV infection may differ in different parts of the world. Typically, HIV-infected individuals in Africa show a more rapid progression of the disease and a shorter survival time than in other geographic areas. Importantly, the clinical course of the disease has been greatly modified by new anti-retroviral therapies, and many complications that were once devestating are now infrequent.

In the United States, the typical adult patient with AIDS presents with fever, weight loss, diarrhea, generalized lymphadenopathy, multiple opportunistic infections, neurologic disease and, in many cases, secondary neoplasms. The infections and neoplasms listed in Table 6–14 are included in the surveillance definition of AIDS.[149]

Opportunistic infections account for the majority of deaths in patients with AIDS. The actual frequency of infections varies in different regions of the world, and has been greatly reduced by the advent of HAART.[150] A brief summary of selected opportunistic infections is provided here. Extensive reviews on the subject are available.[151,152]

Approximately 15% to 30% of HIV-infected people develop pneumonia caused by the opportunistic fungus *P. carinii* (representing reactivation of a prior latent infection), despite prophylaxis. Prior to HAART, this infection was the presenting feature in about 20% of cases, but the incidence is much less in patients who respond to HAART. The risk of developing this infection is extremely high in individuals with fewer than 200 CD4+ cells/μL. Even in these patients there has been a substantial decline in the incidence of this infection because of effective prophylaxis.

An increasing number of patients present with an opportunistic infection other than *P. carinii* pneumonia. Among the most common pathogens are *Candida*, cytomegalovirus,

TABLE 6–14 AIDS-Defining Opportunistic Infections and Neoplasms Found in Patients with HIV Infection

INFECTIONS

Protozoal and Helminthic Infections

Cryptosporidiosis or isosporidiosis (enteritis)
Pneumocytosis (pneumonia or disseminated infection)
Toxoplasmosis (pneumonia or CNS infection)

Fungal Infections

Candidiasis (esophageal, tracheal, or pulmonary)
Cryptococcosis (CNS infection)
Coccidioidomycosis (disseminated)
Histoplasmosis (disseminated)

Bacterial Infections

Mycobacteriosis (atypical, e.g., *M. avium-intracellulare*, disseminated or extrapulmonary; *M. tuberculosis*, pulmonary or extrapulmonary)
Nocardiosis (pneumonia, meningitis, disseminated)
Salmonella infections, disseminated

Viral Infections

Cytomegalovirus (pulmonary, intestinal, retinitis, or CNS infections)
Herpes simplex virus (localized or disseminated)
Varicella-zoster virus (localized or disseminated)
Progressive multifocal leukoencephalopathy)

NEOPLASMS

Kaposi sarcoma
B-cell non-Hodgkin lymphomas
Primary lymphoma of the brain
Invasive cancer of uterine cervix

CNS, central nervous system.

atypical and typical mycobacteria, *Cryptococcus neoformans*, *Toxoplasma gondii*, *Cryptosporidium*, herpes simplex virus, papovaviruses, and *Histoplasma capsulatum*.

Candidiasis is the most common fungal infection in patients with AIDS. *Candida* infection of the oral cavity (thrush) and esophagus are the two most common clinical manifestations of candidiasis in HIV-infected patients. In asymptomatic HIV-infected individuals, oral candidiasis is a sign of immunologic decompensation, and it often heralds the transition to AIDS. Invasive candidiasis is not common in patients with AIDS, and it usually occurs when there is drug-induced neutropenia or use of indwelling catheters. *Cytomegalovirus* may cause disseminated disease, although, more commonly, it affects the eye and gastrointestinal tract. Chorioretinitis was seen in approximately 25% of patients pre-HAART, but this has decreased by over 50% after the intiation of HAART. Cytomegalovirus retinitis occurs almost exclusively in patients with CD4+ cell counts below 50/μl. Gastrointestinal disease, seen in 5% to 10% of cases, manifests as esophagitis and colitis, the latter associated with multiple mucosal ulcerations. Disseminated bacterial infection with *atypical mycobacteria* (mainly *M. avium-intracellulare*) also occurs late, in the setting of severe immunosuppression. Coincident with the AIDS epidemic, the incidence of tuberculosis has risen dramatically.[153] Worldwide, almost a third of all deaths in AIDS patients are attributable to tuberculosis; in the United states, about 5% of patients with AIDS develop active tuberculosis. Patients with AIDS have reactivation of latent pulmonary disease as well as outbreaks of primary infection. In contrast to infection with atypical mycobacteria, *M. tuberculosis* manifests itself early in the course of AIDS. As with tuberculosis in other settings, the infection may be confined to lungs or may involve multiple organs. The pattern of expression depends on the degree of immunosuppression; dissemination is more common in patients with very low CD4+ cell counts. Most worrisome are reports indicating that a growing number of isolates are resistant to multiple drugs.

Cryptococcosis occurs in about 10% of AIDS patients. Among fungal infections that prey on HIV-infected individuals, it is second only to candidiasis. As in other settings with immunosuppression, meningitis is the major clinical manifestation of cryptococcosis. In contrast to *Cryptococcus*, *T. gondii*, another frequent invader of the central nervous system in AIDS, causes encephalitis and is responsible for 50% of all mass lesions in the central nervous system. JC virus, a human papovavirus, is another important cause of central nervous system infections in HIV-infected patients. It causes progressive multifocal leukoencephalopathy (Chapter 28). *Herpes simplex virus infection* is manifested by mucocutaneous ulcerations involving the mouth, esophagus, external genitalia, and perianal region. *Persistent diarrhea*, so common in patients with AIDS, is often caused by infections with protozoans such as *Cryptosporidium*, *Isospora belli*, or microsporidia. These patients have chronic, profuse, watery diarrhea with massive fluid loss. Diarrhea may also result from infection with enteric bacteria, such as *Salmonella* and *Shigella*, as well as *M. avium-intracellulare*. Depressed humoral immunity renders AIDS patients susceptible to severe, recurrent bacterial pneumonias.

Patients with AIDS have a high incidence of certain tumors, especially *Kaposi sarcoma (KS)*, non-Hodgkin B-cell lymphoma, cervical cancer in women, and anal cancer in men.[154,155] It is estimated that 25% to 40% of HIV-infected individuals will eventually develop a malignancy. A common feature of these tumors is that they are all believed to be caused by oncogenic DNA viruses, that is, Kaposi sarcoma herpesvirus (Kaposi sarcoma), EBV (B-cell lymphoma), human papillomavirus (cervical and anal carcinoma). The increased risk of malignancy is thus mainly a consequence of increased susceptibility to infections by these viruses and decreased immunity against the tumors.

KS, a vascular tumor that is otherwise rare in the United States, is the most common neoplasm in patients with AIDS. The morphology of KS and its occurrence in patients not infected with HIV are discussed in Chapter 11. At the onset of the AIDS epidemic, up to 30% of infected homosexual or bisexual men had KS, but in recent years, with use of HAART there has been a marked decline in its incidence, from 15 cases per 1000 person years to less than 5 cases.

The lesions of KS are characterized by the proliferation of spindle-shaped cells that express markers of both endothelial (vascular or lymphatic) and smooth muscle lineages. There is also a profusion of slit-like vascular spaces, suggesting that the lesions may arise from primitive mesenchymal precursors of vascular channels. In addition, KS lesions display chronic inflammatory cell infiltrates. There is still some debate about whether the lesions represent an exuberant hyperplasia or a malignant neoplasm, but the weight of evidence favors the former. For instance, spindle cells in many KS lesions are polyclonal or oligoclonal, although more advanced lesions occasionally show monoclonality.[156] Moreover, spindle cells in many KS lesions are diploid, dependent on growth factors for their proliferation, and do not form tumors in immunodeficient mice.[157] When KS cells are implanted subcutaneously in such mice, they transiently induce slit-like new blood vessels and inflammatory infiltrates in the surrounding tissue; these elements recall features of human KS, but interestingly are of murine origin. When the human KS cells involute, these elements also regress. These observations suggest that KS pathogenesis involves a complex web of paracrine signaling interactions among different types of cells, no one of which is fully autonomous. One popular view envisions that spindle cells produce pro-inflammatory and angiogenic factors, recruiting the inflammatory and neovascular components of the lesion, while the latter components supply signals that aid in spindle cell survival or growth[157] (Fig. 6–51).

But what initiates this cycle of events? Clues to this came from the observation that not all HIV patients are at equal risk for KS development. AIDS-related KS is twenty times more frequent in individuals who acquire HIV by sexual routes compared to those who acquire it parenterally. This observation suggested that a sexually transmitted agent other than HIV might be implicated in KS etiology and prompted a search for new viruses in KS. This search yielded a novel herpesvirus, aptly labeled *KS herpesvirus* (KSHV), or *human herpesvirus 8*.[158] Epidemiologic studies strongly link KSHV to KS development. Infection is uncommon in the general population and strikingly increased in prevalence in groups in which KS is common. In individual patients, KSHV infection precedes KS development and is highly correlated with increased KS risk. KSHV DNA is found in virtually all KS lesions, including those that occur in HIV-negative populations. In the lesions, KSHV is strikingly localized to the spindle cells, which display predominantly latent infection.[159] Thus,

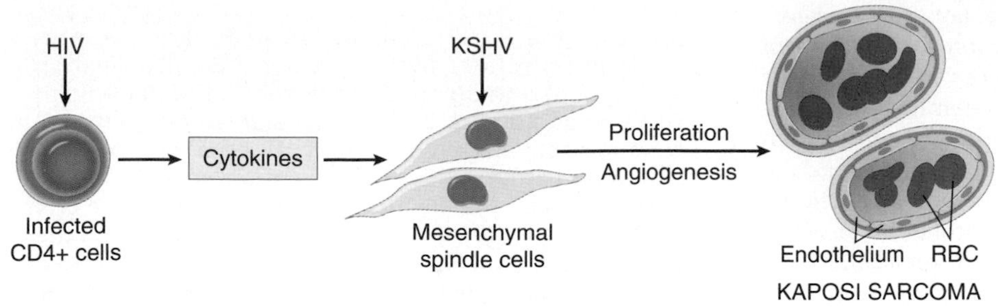

FIGURE 6–51 Proposed role of HIV, KSHV (HHV8), and cytokines in the pathogenesis of Kaposi sarcoma. Cytokines are produced by the mesenchymal cells infected by KSHV, or by HIV-infected CD4+ cells. B cells may also be infected by KSHV; their role in the disease is unclear.

KSHV is always present in patients with KS, and KS has not been reliably described to occur in its absence. However, KSHV infection, while necessary for KS development, is not sufficient, and additional cofactors are needed. In the AIDS-related form, that cofactor is clearly HIV. (The relevant cofactors for HIV-negative KS remain unknown.) Debate continues over exactly how HIV contributes to KS development. The simplest model is that HIV-mediated immune suppression allows widespread dissemination of KSHV in the host, allowing it to access more spindle cells and set them on the path to growth. Another idea is that HIV-infected T cells produce cytokines or other proteins that promote spindle cell proliferation and survival. None of these ideas, it should be noted, is mutually exclusive of the others.

Exactly how KSHV infection leads to KS is still unclear.[159] Like other herpesviruses, KSHV establishes latent infection, during which a number of proteins are produced with potential roles in stimulating spindle cell proliferation and preventing apoptosis. These include a viral homologue of cyclin D and several novel inhibitors of p53. Such proteins could give latently infected cells a growth advantage in vivo that would allow them to begin proliferating. But in addition to latent infection, a small subpopulation of cells in KS is undergoing lytic viral replication, with cell death and the release of viral progeny. The KSHV lytic cycle is remarkable for its production of numerous paracrine-signaling molecules, including viral homologues of IL-6 and several CC chemokines. The latter likely play prominent roles in eliciting the inflammatory infiltrates that are an important feature of KS. The contribution of viral IL-6 is not yet clear, though given the known role of its human homologue in B-cell proliferation it seems more likely to play a role in lymphoma development (see below). Another virally encoded lytic protein is a constitutively active G-protein–coupled receptor (vGPCR). This protein has attracted attention because its expression activates the release of vascular endothelial growth factor (VEGF), which can promote angiogenesis in the surrounding tissue. Interestingly, expression of vGPCR in transgenic mice leads to the development of neovascular spaces vaguely reminiscent of those in KS. Thus, there is ample reason to believe that both latent and lytic KSHV infection contribute to KS pathogenesis.

To summarize, KS is composed of mesenchymal (spindle) cells that form blood vessels; the proliferation of these cells is driven by a variety of cytokines and growth factors that are derived from the tumor cells themselves and from HIV-infected T cells. What triggers the outpouring of this mitogenic brew is not clear, but it is strongly linked to infection of the tumor cells by the KS-associated herpesvirus. Such infection can produce both a latent gene expression program linked to a cell-autonomous growth or survival advantage and a lytic infection that can produce paracrine mediators of inflammation and angiogenesis.

KSHV infection is not restricted to endothelial cells. The virus is related phylogenetically to the lymphotropic subfamily of herpesviruses (γ-herpesvirus); in keeping with this, its genome is found in B cells of infected subjects. In fact, KSHV infection is also linked to rare B-cell lymphomas in AIDS patients (primary effusion lymphoma) and to multicentric Castleman disease.

Clinically, AIDS-associated KS is quite different from the sporadic form (Chapter 11). In HIV-infected individuals, the tumor is generally widespread, affecting the skin, mucous membranes, gastrointestinal tract, lymph nodes, and lungs. These tumors also tend to be more aggressive than classic KS.

With prolonged survival, the number of AIDS patients who develop non-Hodgkin lymphoma has increased steadily. It is currently believed that approximately 6% of all patients with AIDS develop lymphoma during their lifetime. Thus, the risk of developing non-Hodgkin lymphoma is approximately 120-fold greater than in the general population. In contrast to KS, immunodeficiency is firmly implicated as the central predisposing factor. It appears that patients with CD4+ cell counts below 50/μL incur an extremely high risk.

AIDS-related lymphomas can be divided into three groups on the basis of their location: systemic, primary central nervous system, and body cavity–based lymphomas.[160] Systemic lymphomas involve lymph nodes as well as extranodal, visceral sites; they constitute 80% of all AIDS-related lymphomas. The central nervous system is the most common extranodal site affected, followed by the gastrointestinal tract and, less commonly, virtually any other location, including the orbit, salivary glands, and lungs. The vast majority of these lymphomas are aggressive B-cell tumors that present in an advanced stage (Chapter 14). In addition to being commonly involved by systemic non-Hodgkin lymphomas, the central nervous system is also the primary site of lymphomatous involvement in 20% of HIV-infected patients who develop lymphomas. Primary central nervous system lymphoma is 1000 times more common in patients with AIDS than in the general population. The third category of AIDS-related lymphomas is rare but has an unusual distribution. It grows exclusively in body cavities in the form of pleural, peritoneal, and pericardial effusions.

The pathogenesis of AIDS-associated B-cell lymphomas probably involves sustained polyclonal B-cell activation, followed by the emergence of monoclonal or oligoclonal B-cell populations.[161] It is believed that during the frenzy of proliferation, some clones undergo mutations or chromosomal translocations involving oncogenes or tumor suppressor genes, and subsequent neoplastic transformation (Chapter 7). There is morphologic evidence of B-cell activation in lymph nodes, and it is believed that such triggering of B cells is multifactorial.[160] Patients with AIDS have high levels of several cytokines, some of which, including IL-6, are growth factors for B cells. In addition, there seems to be a role for EBV, known to be a polyclonal mitogen for B cells. The EBV genome is found in approximately 50% of the systemic B-cell lymphomas and in virtually all lymphomas primary in the central nervous system. Other evidence of EBV infection includes oral hairy leukoplakia (white projections on the tongue), believed to result from EBV-driven squamous cell proliferation of the oral mucosa (Chapter 16). In cases in which molecular footprints of EBV infection cannot be detected, other viruses and microbes may initiate polyclonal B-cell proliferation. There is no evidence that HIV by itself is capable of causing neoplastic transformation. The rare body cavity–based B-cell lymphomas are uniformly associated with the presence of the KSHV genome, discussed earlier.

In addition to KS and lymphomas, patients with AIDS also have an increased occurrence of carcinoma of the uterine cervix and of anal cancer. This is most likely due to a high prevalence of human papillomavirus infection as a result of immunosuppression.[162] This virus is believed to be intimately associated with squamous cell carcinoma of the cervix and its precursor lesions, cervical dysplasia and carcinoma in situ (Chapters 7 and 22). Human papillomavirus–associated cervical dysplasia is ten times more common in HIV-infected women as compared with uninfected women attending family planning clinics. Hence it is recommended that gynecologic examination be part of a routine work-up of HIV-infected women.

Involvement of the central nervous system is a common and important manifestation of AIDS. *Ninety percent of patients demonstrate some form of neurologic involvement at autopsy, and 40% to 60% have clinically manifest neurologic dysfunction.* Importantly, in some patients, neurologic manifestations may be the sole or earliest presenting feature of HIV infection. In addition to opportunistic infections and neoplasms, several virally determined neuropathologic changes occur. These include a self-limited meningoencephalitis occurring at the time of seroconversion, aseptic meningitis, vacuolar myelopathy, peripheral neuropathies and, most commonly, a progressive encephalopathy designated clinically as the AIDS-dementia complex (Chapter 28).

Morphology. The anatomic changes in the tissues (with the exception of lesions in the brain) are neither specific nor diagnostic. In general, the pathologic features of AIDS include those of widespread opportunistic infections, KS, and lymphoid tumors. Most of these lesions are discussed elsewhere because they also occur in patients who do not have HIV infection. To appreciate the distinctive nature of lesions in the central nervous system, we discuss them in the context of other disorders affecting the brain. Here we concentrate on changes in the lymphoid organs.

Biopsy specimens from enlarged lymph nodes in the early stages of HIV infection reveal a **marked follicular hyperplasia.**[163] The enlarged follicles have irregular, sometimes serrated borders, and they are present not only in the cortex, but also in the medulla and may even extend outside the capsule. The mantle zones that surround the follicles are markedly attenuated, and hence the germinal centers seem to merge with the interfollicular area. These changes, affecting primarily the B-cell areas of the node, are the morphologic reflections of the polyclonal B-cell activation and hypergammaglobulinemia seen in patients with AIDS. In addition to B-cell expansion within germinal centers, activated monocytoid B cells are present within and around the sinusoids and trabecular blood vessels. Under the electron microscope and by in situ hybridization, HIV particles can be detected within the germinal centers. Here they seem to be concentrated on the villous processes of follicular dendritic cells, presumably trapped in the form of immune complexes. During the early phase of HIV infection, viral DNA can be found within the nuclei of CD4+ T cells located predominantly in the follicular mantle zone. With disease progression, the frenzy of B-cell proliferation subsides and gives way to a pattern of severe follicular involution. The follicles are depleted of cells, and the **organized network of follicular dendritic cells is disrupted.** The germinal centers may even become hyalinized. During this advanced stage, viral burden in the nodes is reduced, in part because of the disruption of the follicular dendritic cells. These "burnt-out" lymph nodes are atrophic and small and may harbor numerous opportunistic pathogens. Because of profound immunosuppression, the inflammatory response to infections both in the lymph nodes and at extranodal sites may be sparse or atypical. For example, mycobacteria may not evoke granuloma formation because CD4+ cells are deficient. In the empty-looking lymph nodes and in other organs, the presence of infectious agents may not be readily apparent without the application of special stains. As might be expected, lymphoid depletion is not confined to the nodes; in later stages of AIDS, the spleen and thymus also appear to be "wastelands."

Since the emergence of AIDS in 1981, the concerted efforts of epidemiologists, immunologists, and molecular biologists have resulted in spectacular advances in understanding this disorder. Despite all this progress, however, the prognosis of patients with AIDS remains dismal. Although the mortality rate has declined in the United States as a result of the use of potent combinations of antiretroviral drugs, the treated patients still carry viral DNA in their lymphoid tissues. In fact, there is compelling evidence that even treated patients who remain asymptomatic, with virtually undetectable plasma virus for years, develop active infection if they stop the treatment. Can there be a cure with persistent virus? Although a considerable effort has been mounted to develop a vaccine, many hurdles remain to be crossed before vaccine-based prophylaxis becomes a reality.[164,165] Molecular analyses have revealed an alarming degree of polymorphism in viral isolates from different patients; this renders the task of producing a vaccine remarkably difficult. This task is further complicated by the fact that the nature of the protective immune response is not yet fully understood. At present, therefore, prevention, effective public health measures and antiretroviral drugs remain the mainstay in the fight against AIDS.

AMYLOIDOSIS

Immunologic mechanisms are suspected of contributing to a large number of diseases in addition to those already

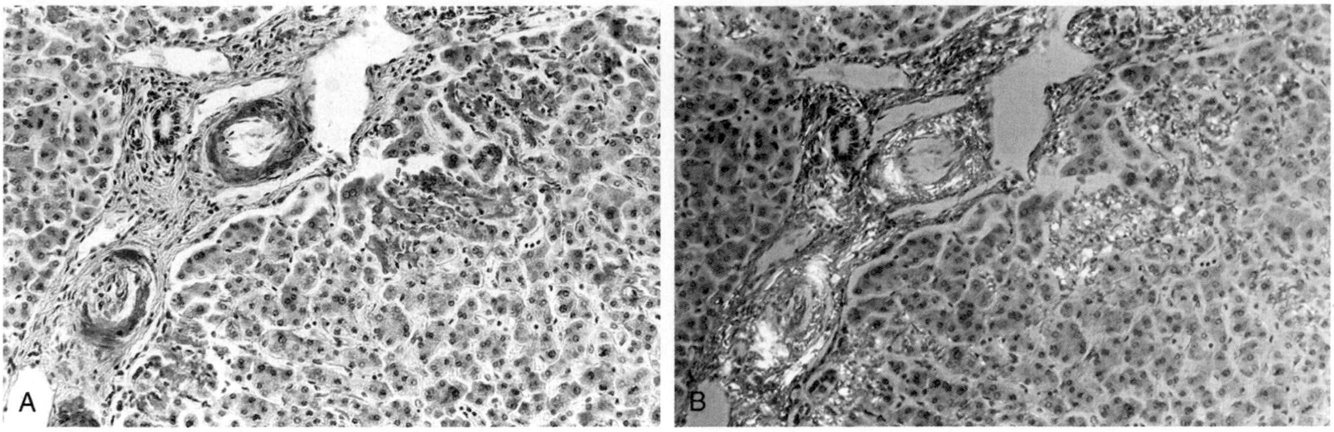

FIGURE 6–52 Amyloidosis. *A,* A section of the liver stained with Congo red reveals pink-red deposits of amyloid in the walls of blood vessels and along sinusoids. *B,* Note the yellow-green birefringence of the deposits when observed by polarizing microscope. (Courtesy of Dr. Trace Worrell and Sandy Hinton, Department of Pathology, University of Texas Southwestern Medical School, Dallas TX.)

described in this chapter. Some of the entities are discussed in the chapters dealing with individual organs and systems. Amyloidosis is described here because it is a systemic disease that may involve components of the immune system, although the pathogenesis of the disease is likely related to abnormal protein folding and there is no good evidence that it results from primary immunologic abnormalities.

Amyloid is a pathologic proteinaceous substance, deposited between cells in various tissues and organs of the body in a wide variety of clinical settings. Because amyloid deposition appears insidiously and sometimes mysteriously, its clinical recognition ultimately depends on morphologic identification of this distinctive substance in appropriate biopsy specimens. *With the light microscope and standard tissue stains, amyloid appears as an amorphous, eosinophilic, hyaline, extracellular substance that, with progressive accumulation, encroaches on and produces pressure atrophy of adjacent cells.* To differentiate amyloid from other hyaline deposits (e.g., collagen, fibrin), a variety of histochemical techniques, described later, are used. Perhaps most widely used is the Congo red stain, which under ordinary light imparts a pink or red color to tissue deposits, but far more dramatic and specific is the green birefringence of the stained amyloid when observed by polarizing microscopy (Fig. 6–52).

Despite the fact that all deposits have a uniform appearance and tinctorial characteristics, *it is quite clear that amyloid is not a chemically distinct entity.*[166,167] There are three major and several minor biochemical forms. These are deposited by several different pathogenetic mechanisms, and therefore amyloidosis *should not be considered a single disease; rather it is a group of diseases having in common the deposition of similar-appearing proteins.* At the heart of the morphologic uniformity is the remarkably uniform physical organization of amyloid protein, which we consider first. This is followed by a discussion of the chemical nature of amyloid.

Physical Nature of Amyloid. By electron microscopy, amyloid is seen to be made up largely of nonbranching fibrils of indefinite length and a diameter of approximately 7.5 to 10 nm. This electron microscopic structure is identical in all types of amyloidosis. X-ray crystallography and infrared spectroscopy demonstrate a characteristic cross–β-pleated sheet conformation (Fig. 6–53). This conformation is seen regardless of the clinical setting or chemical composition and is responsible for the distinctive staining and birefringence of Congo red–stained amyloid.

Chemical Nature of Amyloid. Approximately 95% of the amyloid material consists of fibril proteins, the remaining 5% being the P component and other glycoproteins. *Of the 15 biochemically distinct forms of amyloid proteins that have been identified, three are most common:* (1) *AL (amyloid light chain)* is derived from plasma cells and contains immunoglobulin light chains; (2) *AA (amyloid-associated)* is a unique nonimmunoglobulin protein synthesized by the liver; and (3) *Aβ amyloid* is found in the cerebral lesion of Alzheimer disease and is discussed in greater detail in Chapter 28.

The AL protein is made up of complete immunoglobulin light chains, the NH_2-terminal fragments of light chains, or both. Most of the AL proteins analyzed are composed of λ light chains or their fragments, but in some cases κ chains have been identified. As might be expected, the amyloid fibril protein of the AL type is produced by immunoglobulin-

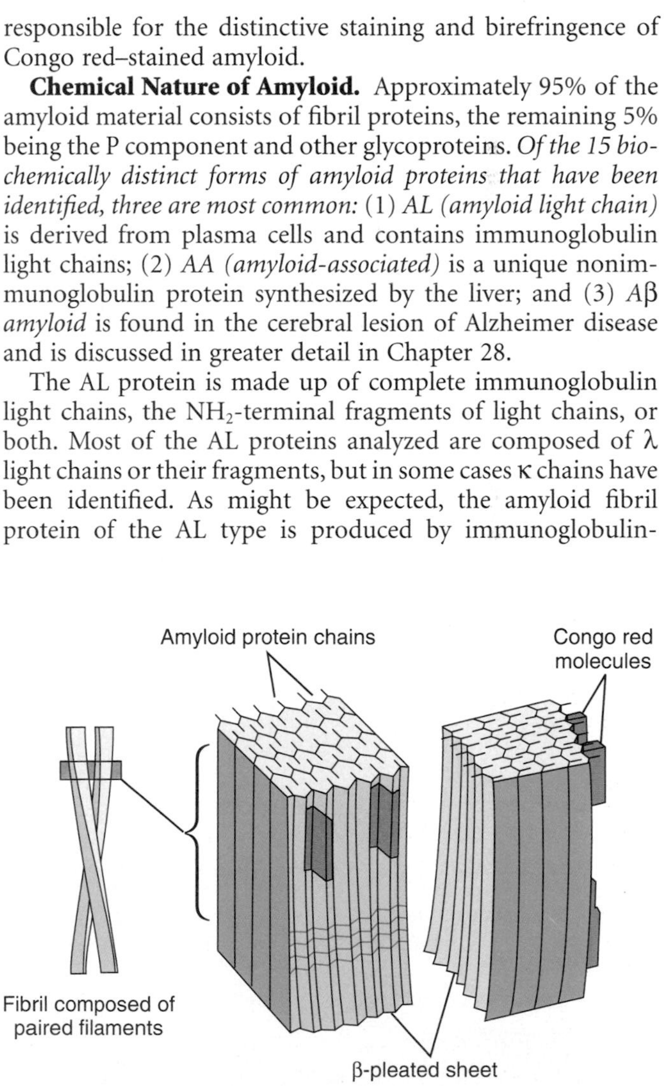

FIGURE 6–53 Structure of an amyloid fibril, depicting the β-pleated sheet structure and binding sites for the Congo red dye, which is used for diagnosis of amyloidosis. (Modified from Glenner GG: Amyloid deposit and amyloidosis. The β-fibrilloses. N Engl J Med 52:148, 1980. By permission of The New England Journal of Medicine.)

secreting cells, and their deposition is associated with some form of monoclonal B-cell proliferation.

The second major class of amyloid fibril protein (AA) does not have structural homology to immunoglobulins. It has a molecular weight of 8500 and consists of 76 amino acid residues. The AA protein is found in those clinical settings described as *secondary amyloidosis*. AA fibrils are derived from a larger (12,000 daltons) precursor in the serum called SAA (serum amyloid–associated) protein that is synthesized in the liver and circulates in association with the HDL3 subclass of lipoproteins.

Several other biochemically distinct proteins have been found in amyloid deposits in a variety of clinical settings.[166] Some of the more common ones are the following:

- *Transthyretin* (TTR) is a normal serum protein that binds and transports thyroxine and retinol, hence the name *trans-thy-retin. A mutant form of transthyretin (and its fragments) is deposited in a group of genetically determined disorders referred to as familial amyloid polyneuropathies.*[167] Several mutations have been identified in the transthyretin protein that contribute to its deposition in tissues in the form of amyloid. Transthyretin is also deposited in the heart of aged individuals (senile systemic amyloidosis), but in such cases the transthyretin molecule is structurally normal.
- *β_2-microglobulin*, a component of the MHC class I molecules and a normal serum protein, has been identified as the amyloid fibril subunit (Aβ_2m) in amyloidosis that complicates the course of patients on *long-term hemodialysis.* Aβ_2m fibers are structurally similar to normal β_2m protein.
- *β-amyloid protein* (Aβ), not to be confused with β_2-microglobulin, is a 4000-dalton peptide that constitutes the core of cerebral plaques found in Alzheimer disease as well as the amyloid deposited in walls of cerebral blood vessels in patients with Alzheimer disease. The Aβ protein is derived from a much larger transmembrane glycoprotein, called *amyloid precursor protein.*
- In a minority of cases of prion disease in the central nervous system, the misfolded *prion proteins* aggregate in the extracellular space and acquire the structural and staining characterstics of amyloid protein.[169] Therefore, prion diseases are sometimes considered examples of local amyloidosis.

In addition, other minor components are always present in amyloid. These include serum amyloid P component, proteoglycans, and highly sulfated glycosaminoglycans. Serum amyloid P protein may contribute to amyloid deposition by stabilizing the fibrils and decreasing their clearance.

Classification of Amyloidosis. According to devoted "amyloidologists," who congregate every few years to discuss their favorite protein, amyloid should be classified based on its constituent chemical fibrils into categories such as AL, AA, and ATTR and not based on clinical syndromes.[170] Because a given biochemical form of amyloid (e.g., AA) may be associated with amyloid deposition in diverse clinical settings, we follow a combined biochemical–clinical classification for our discussion (Table 6–15). Amyloid may be *systemic* (generalized), involving several organ systems, or it may be *localized*, when deposits are limited to a single organ, such as the heart. As should become evident, several different biochemical forms of amyloid are encompassed by such segregation.

On clinical grounds, the systemic, or generalized, pattern is subclassified into *primary amyloidosis*, when associated with some immunocyte dyscrasia, or *secondary amyloidosis*, when it occurs as a complication of an underlying chronic inflammatory or tissue destructive process. *Hereditary* or *familial amyloidosis* constitutes a separate, albeit heterogeneous group, with several distinctive patterns of organ involvement.

Immunocyte Dyscrasias with Amyloidosis (Primary Amyloidosis). Amyloid in this category is usually systemic in dis-

TABLE 6–15 Classification of Amyloidosis

Clinicopathologic Category	Associated Diseases	Major Fibril Protein	Chemically Related Precursor Protein
Systemic (Generalized) Amyloidosis			
Immunocyte dyscrasias with amyloidosis (primary amyloidosis)	Multiple myeloma and other monoclonal B-cell proliferations	AL	Immunoglobulin light chains, chiefly λ type
Reactive systemic amyloidosis (secondary amyloidosis)	Chronic inflammatory conditions	AA	SAA
Hemodialysis-associated amyloidosis	Chronic renal failure	Aβ_2m	β_2-microglobulin
Hereditary amyloidosis			
Familial Mediterranean fever	—	AA	SAA
Familial amyloidotic neuropathies (several types)	—	ATTR	Transthyretin
Systemic senile amyloidosis	—	ATTR	Transthyretin
Localized Amyloidosis			
Senile cerebral	Alzheimer disease	Aβ	APP
Endocrine			
Medullary carcinoma of thyroid	—	A Cal	Calcitonin
Islet of Langerhans	Type II diabetes	AIAPP	Islet amyloid peptide
Isolated atrial amyloidosis	—	AANF	Atrial natriuretic factor
Prion diseases	Various prion diseases of the CNS	Misfolded prion protein (PrP^{sc})	Normal prion protein PrP

tribution and is of the AL type. With approximately 1275 to 3200 new cases every year in the United States, this is the most common form of amyloidosis. In many of these cases, the patients have some form of plasma cell dyscrasia. Best defined is the occurrence of systemic amyloidosis in 5% to 15% of patients with multiple myeloma, a plasma-cell tumor characterized by multiple osteolytic lesions throughout the skeletal system (Chapter 14). The malignant B cells characteristically synthesize abnormal amounts of a single specific immunoglobulin (monoclonal gammopathy), producing an M (myeloma) protein spike on serum electrophoresis. In addition to the synthesis of whole immunoglobulin molecules, only the light chains (referred to as *Bence Jones protein*) of either the λ or the κ variety may be elaborated and found in the serum. By virtue of the small molecular size of the Bence Jones protein, it is frequently excreted in the urine. The amyloid deposits contain the same light chain protein. Almost all the patients with myeloma who develop amyloidosis have Bence Jones proteins in the serum or urine, or both, but a great majority of myeloma patients who have free light chains do not develop amyloidosis. Clearly, therefore, *the presence of Bence Jones proteins, although necessary, is by itself not enough to produce amyloidosis.* We discuss later the other factors, such as the type of light chain produced (*amyloidogenic potential*) and the subsequent handling (possibly degradation) that may have a bearing on whether Bence Jones proteins are deposited as amyloid.

The great majority of patients with AL amyloid do not have classic multiple myeloma or any other overt B-cell neoplasm; such cases have been traditionally classified as primary amyloidosis because their clinical features derive from the effects of amyloid deposition without any other associated disease. In virtually all such cases, however, monoclonal immunoglobulins or free light chains, or both, can be found in the serum or urine. Most of these patients also have a modest increase in the number of plasma cells in the bone marrow, which presumably secrete the precursors of AL protein. Clearly, these patients have an underlying B-cell dyscrasia in which production of an abnormal protein, rather than production of tumor masses, is the predominant manifestation. Recent studies have revealed chromosomal translocations in many of these patients, suggesting the presence of neoplastic clones.[171] Whether most of these clones would evolve into myeloma if the patients lived long enough can only be a matter for speculation.

Reactive Systemic Amyloidosis. The amyloid deposits in this pattern are systemic in distribution and are composed of AA protein. This category was previously referred to as *secondary amyloidosis* because it is secondary to an associated inflammatory condition. The feature common to most of the conditions associated with reactive systemic amyloidosis is protracted breakdown of cells resulting from a wide variety of infectious and noninfectious chronic inflammatory conditions. At one time, tuberculosis, bronchiectasis, and chronic osteomyelitis were the most important underlying conditions, but with the advent of effective antimicrobial chemotherapy, the importance of these conditions has diminished. More commonly now, reactive systemic amyloidosis complicates rheumatoid arthritis, other connective tissue disorders such as ankylosing spondylitis, and inflammatory bowel disease, particularly Crohn disease and ulcerative colitis. Among these, the most frequent associated condition is rheumatoid arthritis. Amyloidosis is reported to occur in approximately 3% of patients with rheumatoid arthritis and is clinically significant in one half of those affected. Heroine abusers who inject the drug subcutaneously also have a high occurrence rate of generalized AA amyloidosis. The chronic skin infections associated with "skin-popping" of narcotics seem to be responsible for amyloidosis in this group of patients. Reactive systemic amyloidosis may also occur in association with non–immunocyte-derived tumors, the two most common being renal cell carcinoma and Hodgkin disease.

Hemodialysis-Associated Amyloidosis. Patients on long-term hemodialysis for renal failure develop amyloidosis owing to deposition of β_2-microglobulin. This protein is present in high concentrations in the serum of patients with renal disease and is retained in circulation because it cannot be filtered through the cuprophane dialysis membranes. In some series, as many as 60% to 80% of the patients on long-term dialysis developed amyloid deposits in the synovium, joints, and tendon sheaths.

Heredofamilial Amyloidosis. A variety of familial forms of amyloidosis have been described. Most of them are rare and occur in limited geographic areas. The most common and best studied is an autosomal recessive condition called *familial Mediterranean fever.*[172] This is a febrile disorder of unknown cause characterized by attacks of fever accompanied by inflammation of serosal surfaces, including peritoneum, pleura, and synovial membrane. This disorder is encountered largely in individuals of Armenian, Sephardic Jewish, and Arabic origins. It is associated with widespread tissue involvement indistinguishable from reactive systemic amyloidosis. The amyloid fibril proteins are made up of AA proteins, suggesting that this form of amyloidosis is related to the recurrent bouts of inflammation that characterize this disease. The gene for familial Mediterranean fever has been cloned, and its product is called *pyrin* (for its relation to fever). Although its exact function is not known, it has been suggested that pyrin is responsible for regulating acute inflammation, presumably by inhibiting the function of neutrophils.[173] The relationship of this mutation to the disease is not understood.

In contrast to familial Mediterranean fever, a group of autosomal dominant familial disorders is characterized by deposition of amyloid predominantly in the nerves—peripheral and autonomic. These familial amyloidotic polyneuropathies have been described in different parts of the world. As mentioned previously, in all of these genetic disorders, the fibrils are made up of mutant transthyretins (ATTR).

Localized Amyloidosis. Sometimes, amyloid deposits are limited to a single organ or tissue without involvement of any other site in the body. The deposits may produce grossly detectable nodular masses or be evident only on microscopic examination. Nodular (tumor-forming) deposits of amyloid are most often encountered in the lung, larynx, skin, urinary bladder, tongue, and the region about the eye. Frequently, there are infiltrates of lymphocytes and plasma cells in the periphery of these amyloid masses, raising the question of whether the mononuclear infiltrate is a response to the deposition of amyloid or instead is responsible for it. At least in some cases, the amyloid consists of AL protein and may therefore represent a localized form of immunocyte-derived amyloid.

Endocrine Amyloid. Microscopic deposits of localized amyloid may be found in certain endocrine tumors, such as medullary carcinoma of the thyroid gland, islet tumors of the pancreas, pheochromocytomas, and undifferentiated carcinomas of the stomach, and in the islets of Langerhans in patients with type II diabetes mellitus. In these settings, the amyloidogenic proteins seem to be derived either from polypeptide hormones (e.g., medullary carcinoma) or from unique proteins (e.g., islet amyloid polypeptide).

Amyloid of Aging. Several well-documented forms of amyloid deposition occur with aging.[174] *Senile systemic amyloidosis* refers to the systemic deposition of amyloid in elderly patients (usually in their seventies and eighties). Because of the dominant involvement and related dysfunction of the heart, this form was previously called *senile cardiac amyloidosis.* Those who are symptomatic present with a restrictive cardiomyopathy and arrhythmias. The amyloid in this form is composed of the normal TTR molecule. In addition to the sporadic senile systemic amyloidosis, another form, affecting predominantly the heart, that results from the deposition of a mutant form of TTR has also been recognized. Approximately 4% of the black population in the United States is a carrier of the mutant allele, and cardiomyopathy has been identified in both homozygous and heterozygous patients. The precise prevalance of patients with this mutation who develop clinically manifest cardiac disease is not known.

Pathogenesis. *Amyloidosis results from abnormal folding of proteins, which are deposited as fibrils in extracellular tissues and disrupt normal function.* Misfolded proteins are often unstable and self-associate, ultimately leading to the formation of oligomers and fibrils that are deposited in tissues. The reason diverse conditions are associated with amyloidosis may be that each of these conditions results in excessive production of proteins that are prone to misfolding. The proteins that form amyloid fall into two general categories: (1) normal proteins that have an inherent tendency to fold improperly, associate and form fibrils, and do so when they are produced in increased amounts, and (2) mutant proteins that are structurally unstable and prone to misfolding and subsequent aggregation.[166,175]

Normally, misfolded proteins are degraded intracellularly in proteasomes, or extracellularly by macrophages. It appears that in amyloidosis, these quality control mechanisms fail so that too much of a misfolded protein accumulates outside cells.[166] This proposed mechanism may explain most forms of amyloidosis (Fig. 6–54). For instance, SAA is synthesized by the liver cells under the influence of cytokines such as IL-6 and IL-1 that are produced during inflammation; thus, long-standing inflammation leads to elevated SAA levels, and ultimately the AA form of amyloid deposits. However, increased production of SAA by itself is not sufficient for the deposition of amyloid. Elevation of serum SAA levels is common to inflammatory states but in most instances does not lead to amyloidosis. There are two possible explanations for this. According to one view, SAA is normally degraded to soluble end products by the action of monocyte-derived enzymes. Conceivably, individuals who develop amyloidosis have an enzyme defect that results in incomplete breakdown of SAA, thus generating insoluble AA molecules. Alternatively, a genetically determined structural abnormality in the SAA molecule itself renders it resistant to degradation by macrophages. In the case of immunocyte dyscrasias, there is an excess of immunoglobulin light chains, and amyloid can be derived by proteolysis of immunoglobulin light chains in vitro. Again, defective degradation has been invoked, and perhaps particular light chains are resistant to complete proteolysis. However, there are no sequence motifs peculiar to the immunoglobulin light chains found in amyloid deposits.

In familial amyloidosis the deposition of transthyretins as amyloid fibrils does not result from overproduction of transthyretins. It has been proposed that genetically detemined alterations of structure render the transthyretins prone to misfolding and aggregation, and resistant to proteolysis.

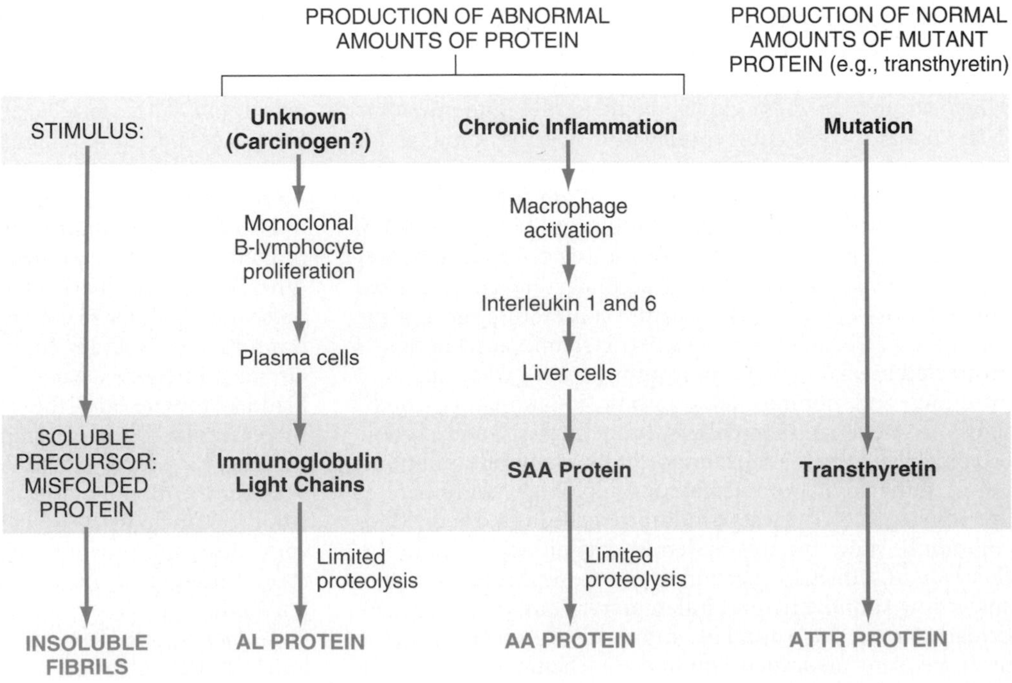

FIGURE 6–54 Proposed schema of the pathogenesis of the major forms of amyloid fibrils.

Morphology. There are no consistent or distinctive patterns of organ or tissue distribution of amyloid deposits in any of the categories cited. Nonetheless a few generalizations can be made. Amyloidosis secondary to chronic inflammatory disorders tends to yield the most severe systemic involvements. Kidneys, liver, spleen, lymph nodes, adrenals, and thyroid as well as many other tissues are classically involved. Although immunocyte-associated amyloidosis cannot reliably be distinguished from the secondary form by its organ distribution, more often it involves the heart, kidney, gastrointestinal tract, peripheral nerves, skin, and tongue.

Macroscopically the affected organs are often enlarged and firm and have a waxy appearance. If the deposits are sufficiently large, painting the cut surface with iodine imparts a yellow color that is transformed to blue violet after application of sulfuric acid.

As noted earlier, the histologic diagnosis of amyloid is based almost entirely on its staining characteristics. The most commonly used staining technique employs the dye **Congo red**, which under ordinary light imparts a pink or red color to amyloid deposits. Under polarized light, the Congo red–stained amyloid shows a green birefringence (see Fig. 6–52). This reaction is shared by all forms of amyloid and is due to the cross–β-pleated configuration of amyloid fibrils. Confirmation can be obtained by electron microscopy. AA, AL, and TTR amyloid can be distinguished in histologic sections by specific immunohistochemical staining. Because the pattern of organ involvement in different clinical forms of amyloidosis is variable, each of the major organ involvements is described separately.

Kidney. Amyloidosis of the kidney is the most common and potentially the most serious form of organ involvement. In most reported series of patients with amyloidosis, renal amyloidosis is the major cause of death. On gross inspection, the kidney may appear normal in size and color, or it may be enlarged. In advanced cases, it may be shrunken and contracted owing to vascular narrowing induced by the deposition of amyloid within arterial and arteriolar walls.

Histologically the amyloid is deposited primarily in the glomeruli, but the interstitial peritubular tissue, arteries, and arterioles are also affected. The glomerular deposits first appear as subtle thickenings of the mesangial matrix, accompanied usually by uneven widening of the basement membranes of the glomerular capillaries. In time, the mesangial depositions and the deposits along the basement membranes cause capillary narrowing and distortion of the glomerular vascular tuft. With progression of the glomerular amyloidosis, the capillary lumens are obliterated, and the obsolescent glomerulus is flooded by confluent masses or interlacing broad ribbons of amyloid (Fig. 6–55).

Spleen. Amyloidosis of the spleen may be inapparent grossly or may cause moderate to marked splenomegaly (up to 800 gm). For completely mysterious reasons, one of two patterns of deposition is seen. In one, the deposit is largely limited to the splenic follicles, producing tapioca-like granules on gross inspection, designated **sago spleen**. Histologically the entire follicle may be replaced in advanced cases. In the other pattern, the amyloid appears to spare the follicles and instead involves the walls of the splenic sinuses and connective tissue framework in the red pulp. Fusion of the early deposits gives rise to large, maplike areas of amyloidosis, creating what has been designated the **lardaceous spleen**.

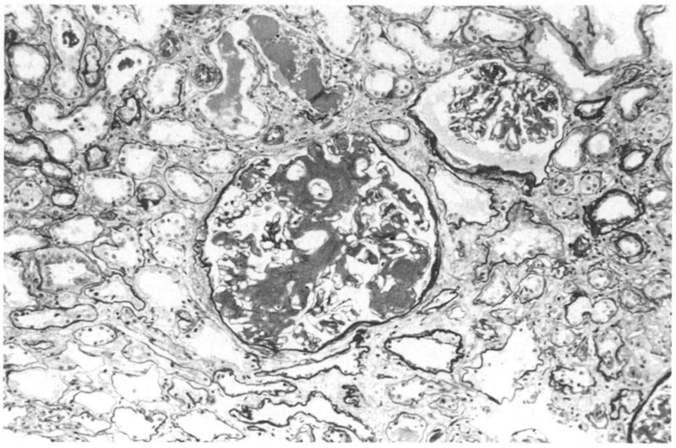

FIGURE 6–55 Amyloidosis of the kidney. The glomerular architecture is almost totally obliterated by the massive accumulation of amyloid.

Liver. The deposits may be inapparent grossly or may cause moderate to marked hepatomegaly. The amyloid appears first in the space of Disse and then progressively encroaches on adjacent hepatic parenchymal cells and sinusoids. In time, deformity, pressure atrophy, and disappearance of hepatocytes occur, causing total replacement of large areas of liver parenchyma. Vascular involvement and deposits in Kupffer cell are frequent. Normal liver function is usually preserved despite sometimes quite severe involvement of the liver.

Heart. Amyloidosis of the heart may occur in any form of systemic amyloidosis, much more commonly in persons with immunocyte-derived disease. It is also the major organ involved in senile systemic amyloidosis. The heart may be enlarged and firm, but more often it shows no significant changes on cross-section of the myocardium. Histologically the deposits begin in focal subendocardial accumulations and within the myocardium between the muscle fibers. Expansion of these myocardial deposits eventually causes pressure atrophy of myocardial fibers (Fig. 6–56). In most cases, the deposits are separated and widely distributed, but when they are subendocardial, the conduction system may be damaged, accounting for the electrocardiographic abnormalities noted in some patients.

Other Organs. Amyloidosis of other organs is generally encountered in systemic disease. The adrenals, thyroid, and pituitary are common sites of involvement. In the adrenals, the intercellular deposits begin adjacent to the basement membranes of the cortical cells, usually first in the zona glomerulosa. With progression, large sheets of amyloid may replace considerable amounts of the cortical parenchyma. Similar patterns are seen in the thyroid and pituitary. The gastrointestinal tract may be involved at any level, from the oral cavity (gingiva, tongue) to the anus. The early

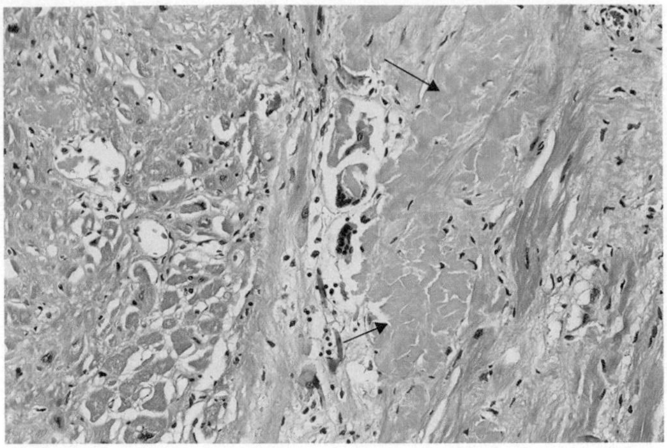

FIGURE 6–56 Cardiac amyloidosis. The atrophic myocardial fibers are separated by structureless, pink-staining amyloid *(arrows)*.

lesions mainly affect blood vessels but eventually extend to involve the adjacent areas of the submucosa, muscularis, and subserosa.

Nodular depositions in the tongue may cause macroglossia, giving rise to the designation **tumor-forming amyloid of the tongue**. The respiratory tract may be involved focally or diffusely from the larynx down to the smallest bronchioles. As mentioned earlier, a distinct chemical form of amyloid has been found in the brain of patients with Alzheimer disease. It involves so-called plaques as well as blood vessels (Chapter 28). Amyloidosis of peripheral and autonomic nerves is a feature of several familial amyloidotic neuropathies. Depositions of amyloid in patients on long-term hemodialysis are most prominent in the carpal ligament of the wrist, resulting in compression of the median nerve (carpal tunnel syndrome). These patients may also have extensive amyloid deposition in the joints.

Clinical Correlation. Amyloidosis may be found as an unsuspected anatomic change, having produced no clinical manifestations, or it may cause death. The symptoms depend on the magnitude of the deposits and on the particular sites or organs affected. Clinical manifestations at first are often entirely nonspecific, such as weakness, weight loss, lightheadedness, or syncope. Somewhat more specific findings appear later and most often relate to renal, cardiac, and gastrointestinal involvement.

Renal involvement gives rise to proteinuria and is an important cause of the nephrotic syndrome (Chapter 20). Progressive obliteration of glomeruli in advanced cases ultimately leads to renal failure and uremia. *Cardiac amyloidosis* may present as an insidious congestive heart failure. The most serious aspects of cardiac amyloidosis are conduction disturbances and arrhythmias, which may prove fatal. Occasionally, cardiac amyloidosis produces a restrictive pattern of cardiomyopathy and masquerades as chronic constrictive pericarditis (Chapter 12). *Gastrointestinal amyloidosis* may be entirely asymptomatic, or it may present in a variety of ways. Amyloidosis of the tongue may cause sufficient enlargement and inelasticity to hamper speech and swallowing. Depositions in the stomach and intestine may lead to malabsorption, diarrhea, and disturbances in digestion.

The diagnosis of amyloidosis depends on demonstration of amyloid deposits in tissues. The most common sites biopsied are the kidney, when renal manifestations are present, or rectal or gingival tissues in patients suspected of having systemic amyloidosis. Examination of abdominal fat aspirates stained with Congo red can also be used for the diagnosis of systemic amyloidosis. The test is quite specific, but its sensitivity is low.[176] In suspected cases of immunocyte-associated amyloidosis, serum and urine protein electrophoresis and immunoelectrophoresis should be performed. Bone marrow aspirates in such cases often show plasmacytosis, even in the absence of overt multiple myeloma. Scintigraphy with radiolabeled serum amyloid P (SAP) component is a rapid and specific test, since SAP binds to the amyloid deposits and reveals their presence.[177] It also gives a measure of the extent of amyloidosis, and can be used to follow patients undergoing treatment.

The prognosis for patients with generalized amyloidosis is poor. Those with immunocyte-derived amyloidosis (not including multiple myeloma) have a median survival of 2 years after diagnosis. Patients with myeloma-associated amyloidosis have a poorer prognosis. The outlook for patients with reactive systemic amyloidosis is somewhat better and depends to some extent on the control of the underlying condition. Resorption of amyloid after treatment of the associated condition has been reported, but this is a rare occurrence. New therapeutic strategies aimed at correcting protein misfolding and inhibiting fibrillogenesis are being developed.

REFERENCES

1. Janeway CA, Jr, Medzhitov R: Innate immune recognition. Annu Rev Immunol 20:197, 2002.
2. Takeda K, Kaisho T, Akira S: Toll-like receptors. Ann Rev Immunol 21:335, 2003.
3. Cyster JG: Chemokines and cell migration in secondary lymphoid organs. Science 286:2098, 1999.
4. Mebius RE: Organogenesis of lymphoid tissues. Nat Rev Immurol 3:292, 2003.
5. Davis MM, et al: Ligand recognition by alpha beta T cell receptors. Annu Rev Immunol 16:523, 1998.
6. Hennecke J, Wiley DC: T cell receptor–MHC interactions up close. Cell 104:1, 2001.
7. Weiss A: Structure and function of the T cell antigen receptor. J Clin Invest 86:1015, 1990.
8. Hayday AC: $\gamma\delta$ cells: a right time and a right place for a conserved third way of protection. Annu Rev Immunol 18:975, 2000.
9. Lenschow DJ, Walunas TL, Bluestone JA: CD28/B7 system of T cell costimulation. Annu Rev Immunol 14:233, 1996.
10. von Andrian UH, Mackay CR: T-cell function and migration. Two sides of the same coin. N Engl J Med 343:1020, 2000.
11. Abbas AK, et al: Functional diversity of helper T lymphocytes. Nature 383:787, 1996.
12. Clark EA, Ledbetter JA: How B and T cells talk to each other. Nature 367:425, 1994.
13. Clark LB, Foy TM, Noelle RJ: CD40 and its ligand. Adv Immunol 63:43, 1996.
14. Mellman I, Steinman RM: Dendritic cells: specialized and regulated antigen processing machines. Cell 106:255, 2001.
15. Banchereau J, et al: Immunobiology of dendritic cells. Annu Rev Immunol 18:767, 2000.
16. Cerwenka A, Lanier LL: Natural killer cells, viruses and cancer. Nat Rev Immunol 1:41, 2001.
17. Bjorkman PJ: MHC restriction in three dimensions: a view of T cell receptor/ligand interactions. Cell 89:167, 1997.

18. Germain RN: MHC-dependent antigen processing and peptide presentation: providing ligands for T lymphocyte activation. Cell 76:287, 1994.
19. Hammer J, Sturniolo T, Sinigaglia F: HLA class II peptide binding specificity and autoimmunity. Adv Immunol 66:67, 1997.
20. Kay AB: Allergy and allergic diseases. N Engl J Med 344:30, 109, 2001.
21. Gould HJ, et al.: The biology of IgE and the basis of allergic disease. Annu Rev Immunol 21:579, 2003.
22. Costa JJ, et al: The cells of the allergic response: mast cells, basophils, and eosinophils. JAMA 278:1815, 1997.
23. Romagnani S: Cytokines and chemoattractants in allergic inflammation. Mol Immunol 38:881, 2002.
24. Murphy KM, Reiner SL: The lineage decisions of helper T cells. Nat Rev Immunol 2:933, 2002.
25. Kawakami T, Galli SJ: Regulation of mast-cell and basophil function and survival by IgE. Nat Rev Immunol 2:773, 2002.
26. Robinson DS, Kay AB, Wardlaw AJ: Eosinophils. Clin Allergy Immunol 16:43, 2002.
27. Ono SJ: Molecular genetics of allergic diseases. Annu Rev Immunol 18:347, 2000.
28. Kemp SF, Lockey RF: Anaphylaxis: a review of causes and mechanisms. J Allergy Clin Immunol 110:341, 2002.
29. Baumann U, Schmidt RE: The role of Fc receptors and complement in autoimmunity. Adv Exp Med Biol 495:219, 2001.
30. Russell JH, Ley TJ: Lymphocyte-mediated cytotoxicity. Annu Rev Immunol 20:323, 2002.
31. Heeger PS: T-cell allorecognition and transplant rejection: a summary and update. Am J Transpl 3:525, 2003.
32. Libby P, Pober JS: Chronic rejection. Immunity 14:387, 2001.
33. Pascual M, et al: Strategies to improve long-term outcomes after renal transplantation. N Engl J Med 346:580, 2002.
34. Vogelsang GB, Lee L, Bensen-Kennedy DM: Pathogenesis and treatment of graft-versus-host disease after bone marrow transplant. Annu Rev Med 54:29, 2003.
35. Kumar V, et al: Role of murine NK cells and their receptors in hybrid resistance. Curr Opin Immunol 19:52, 1997.
36. Ruggeri L, et al: Effectiveness of donor natural killer cell reactivity in mismatched hematopoietic transplants. Science 295:2097, 2002.
37. Kyewski B, et al: Promiscuous gene expression and central T-cell tolerance: more than meets the eye. Trends Immunol 23:364, 2002.
38. Anderson MS, et al: Projection of an immunological self shadow within the thymus by the AIRE protein. Science 298:1395, 2002.
39. Van Parijs L, Abbas AK: Homeostasis and self-tolerance in the immune system: turning lymphocytes off. Science 280:243, 1998.
40. Walker LS, Abbas AK: The enemy within: keeping self-reactive T cells at bay in the periphery. Nat Rev Immunol 2:11, 2002.
41. Goodnow CC, et al: Self-tolerance checkpoints in B lymphocyte development. Adv Immunol 59:279, 1995.
42. Schwartz RH: T cell anergy. Ann Rev Immunol 21:305, 2003.
43. Shevach EM: CD4+ CD25+ suppressor T cells: more questions than answers. Nat Rev Immunol 2:389, 2002.
44. Ramsdell F: Foxp3 and natural regulatory T cells: key to a cell lineage? Immunity 19:165, 2003.
45. Siegel RM, et al: The multifaceted role of Fas signaling in immune cell homeostasis and autoimmunity. Nat Immunol 1:469, 2000.
46. Nagata S: Fas ligand-induced apoptosis. Annu Rev Genet 33:29, 1999.
47. Marsden VA, Strasser A: Control of apoptosis in the immune system. Ann Rev Immunol 21:71, 2003.
48. Marrack P, Kappler J, Kotzin BL: Autoimmune disease: why and where it occurs. Nat Med 7:899, 2001.
49. Kamradt T, Mitchison NA: Tolerance and autoimmunity. N Engl J Med 344:655, 2001.
50. Encinas JA, Kuchroo VK: Mapping and identification of autoimmunity genes. Curr Opin Immunol 12:691, 2000.
51. Wakeland EK, et al: Delineating the genetic basis of systemic lupus erythematosus. Immunity 15:397, 2001.
52. Nelson BH: Interleukin-2 signaling and the maintenance of self-tolerance. Curr Dir Autoimmun 5:92, 2002.
53. Ravetch JV, Bolland S: IgG Fc receptors. Annu Rev Immunol 19:275, 2001.
54. Vanderlugt CL, Miller SD: Epitope spreading in immune-mediated diseases: implications for immunotherapy. Nat Rev Immunol 2:85, 2002.
55. Ruiz-Irastorza G, et al: Systemic lupus erythematosus. Lancet 357:1027, 2001.
56. Hahn BH: Antibodies to DNA. New Engl J Med 338:1359, 1998.
57. Keren DF: Antinuclear antibody testing. Clin Lab Med 22:447, 2002.
58. Galli M, et al: Antiphospholipid antibodies: predictive value of laboratory tests. Thromb Hemost 78:75, 1997.
59. Arnout J: Antiphospholipid syndrome: diagnostic aspects of lupus anticoagulants. Thromb Haemost 86:83, 2001.
60. Levine JS, Branch DW, Rauch J: The anti-phospholipid syndrome. New Engl J Med 346:752, 2002.
61. Gaffney PM, Moser KL, Graham RR, Behrens TW: Recent advances in the genetics of systemic lupus erythematosus. Rheum Dis Clin North Am 28:111, 2003.
62. Criswell LA, Amos CI: Update on genetic risk factors for systemic lupus erythematosus and rheumatoid arthritis. Curr Opin Rheumatol 12:85, 2000.
63. Bolto M, Walport MJ: C1q, autoimmunity and apoptosis. Immunobiology 205:395, 2002.
64. Rubin RL: Etiology and mechanisms of drug-induced lupus. Curr Opin Rheumatol 11:357, 1999.
65. White S, Rosen A: Apoptosis in systemic lupus erythematosus. Curr Opin Rheumatol 15:557, 2003.
66. Shlomchik MJ, Craft JE, Mamula MJ: From T to B and back again: positive feedback in systemic autoimmune disease. Nat Rev Immunol 1:147, 2001.
66a. Nakken B, et al: T-helper cell tolerance to ubiquitous nuclear antigens. Scand J Immunol 58:478, 2003.
67. Tsao BP: The genetics of human systemic lupus erythematosus. Trends Immunol 24:595, 2003.
68. Belmart HM, Abramson SB: Pathology and pathogenesis of vascular injury in SLE. Arthritis Rheum 39:9, 1996.
69. Cameron JS: Lupus nephritis. J Am Soc Nephrol 10:413, 1999.
70. Moore PM, Lisak RP: Systemic lupus erythematosus: immunopathogenesis of neurologic dysfunction. Springer Semin Immunopathol 17:43, 1995.
71. Moder KG, Miller TD, Tazelaar HD: Cardiac involvement in systemic lupus erythematosus. Mayo Clin Proc 74:275, 1999.
72. Iliopoulos AG, Toskos GC: Immunopathogenesis and spectrum of infection in SLE. Semin Arthritis Rheum 25:318, 1996.
73. Donnelly AM, et al: Discoid lupus erythematosus. Australas J Dermatol 36:3, 1995.
74. Patel P, Werth V: Cutaneous lupus erythematosus: a review. Dermatol Clin 20:373, 2002.
75. Fox RI, Stern M, Michelson P: Update in Sjögren syndrome. Curr Opin Rheumatol 12:391, 2000.
76. Jonsson R, Haga HJ, Gordon TP: Current concepts on diagnosis, autoantibodies and therapy in Sjögren's syndrome. Scand J Rheumatol 29:341, 2000.
77. Hang LM, Nakamura RM: Current concepts and advances in clinical laboratory testing for autoimmune diseases. Crit Rev Clin Lab Sci 34:275, 1997.
78. Gordon TP, et al: Autoantibodies in primary Sjögren's syndrome: new insights into mechanisms of autoantibody diversification and disease pathogenesis. Autoimmunity 34:123, 2001.
79. Sumida T, et al: TCR in Sjögren syndrome. Br J Rheumatol 36:622, 1997.
80. Haneji N, et al: Identification of α-fodrin as a candidate autoantigen in primary Sjögren syndrome. Science 276:604, 1997.
80a. Hansen A, Lipsky PE, Domer T: New concepts in the pathogenesis of Sjogren syndrome: many questions, fewer answers. Curr Opin Rheumatol 15:556, 2003.
81. James JA, Harley JB, Scofield RH: Role of viruses in systemic lupus erythematosus and Sjögren syndrome. Curr Opin Rheumatol 13:370, 2001.
82. Manthorpe R, et al: Primary Sjögren syndrome: diagnostic criteria, clinical features, and disease activity. J Rheumatol 24 (suppl 50):8, 1997.
83. Kahaleh MB, LeRoy EC: Autoimmunity and vascular involvement in systemic sclerosis (SSc). Autoimmunity 31:195, 1999.
84. Scaletti C, et al: Microchimerism and systemic sclerosis. Int Arch Allergy Immunol 125:196, 2001.
85. Jimenez SA, et al: Pathogenesis of scleroderma: collagen. Rheum Dis Clin North Am 22:647, 1996.
86. Tan FK, Arnett FC: Genetic factors in the etiology of systemic sclerosis and Raynaud phenomenon. Curr Opin Rheumatol 12:511, 2000.
87. Harvey GR, McHugh NJ: Serologic abnormalities in systemic sclerosis. Curr Opin Rheumatol 11:495, 1999.

88. Mitchell H, et al: Scleroderma and related conditions. Med Clin North Am 81:129, 1997.
89. Hoffman RW, Greidinger EL: Mixed connective tissue disease. Curr Opin Rheumatol 12:386, 2000.
90. Smolen JS, Steiner G: Mixed connective tissue disease: to be or not to be? Arthritis Rheum 41:768, 1998.
91. Sneller MC, Fauci AS: Pathogenesis of vasculitis syndromes. Med Clin North Am 81:221, 1997.
92. Group WHOS: Primary immunodeficiency diseases. Clin Exp Immunol 109 (suppl):1, 1997.
93. Buckley RH: Primary immunodeficiency diseases: dissectors of the immune system. Immunobiol Rev 185:206, 2002.
94. Ochs HD, Smith CID: X-linked agammaglobulinemia: a clinical and molecular analysis. Medicine 75:287, 1996.
95. Satterthwaite AB, Witte ON: The role of Bruton's tyrosine kinase in B-cell development and function: a genetic perspective. Immunol Rev 175:120, 2000.
96. Spickett GP, et al: Common variable immunodeficiency: how many diseases? Immunol Today 18:325, 1997.
97. Burrows PD, Cooper MD: IgA deficiency. Adv Immunol 65:245, 1997.
98. Ramesh N, et al: The hyper-IgM (HIM) syndrome. Springer Semin Immunopathol 19:383, 1998.
99. Durandy A, Honjo T: Human genetic defects in class-switch recombination (hyper-IgM syndromes). Curr Opin Immunol 13:543, 2001.
100. Epstein JA: Developing models of DiGeorge syndrome. Trends Genet 17:S13, 2001.
101. McDermid HE, Morrow BE: Genomic disorders on 22q11. Am J Hum Genet 70:1077, 2002.
102. Sugamura K, et al: The interleukin-2 receptor gamma chain: its role in the multiple cytokine receptor complexes and T cell development in XSCID. Annu Rev Immunol 14:179, 1996.
103. Leonard WJ: Cytokines and immunodeficiency diseases. Nat Rev Immunol 1:200, 2001.
104. Resta R, Thompson LF: SCID: the role of adenosine deaminase deficiency. Immunol Today 18:371, 1997.
105. Reith W, Mach B: The bare lymphocyte syndrome and the regulation of MHC expression. Annu Rev Immunol 19:331, 2001.
106. Huber J, et al: Pathology of congenital immunodeficiencies. Semin Diagn Pathol 9:31, 1992.
107. Fischer A, Hacein-Bey S, Cavazzana-Calvo M: Gene therapy of severe combined immunodeficiencies. Nat Rev Immunol 2:615, 2002.
108. Parkman R, et al: Gene therapy for adenosine deaminase deficiency. Annu Rev Med 51:33, 2000.
109. Snapper SB, Rosen FS: The Wiskott-Aldrich syndrome protein (WASP): roles in signaling and cytoskeletal organization. Annu Rev Immunol 17:905, 1999.
110. Snapper SB, Rosen FS: A family of WASPs. N Engl J Med 348:350, 2003.
111. Walport MJ: Complement. First of two parts. N Engl J Med 344:1058, 2001.
112. Walport MJ: Complement. Second of two parts. N Engl J Med 344:1140, 2001.
113. Frank MM: Complement deficiencies. Pediatr Clin North Am 47:1339, 2000.
114. Carugati A, et al: C1-inhibitor deficiency and angioedema. Mol Immunol 38:161, 2001.
115. Rosse WF: New insights into paroxysmal nocturnal hemoglobinuria. Curr Opin Hematol 8:61, 2001.
116. Royce RA, et al: Sexual transmission of HIV. N Engl J Med 336:1072, 1997.
117. Goodnough LT, Shander A, Brecher ME: Transfusion medicine: looking to the future. Lancet 361:161, 2003.
118. Mofenson LM, McIntyre JA: Advances and research directions in the prevention of mother-to-child HIV-1 transmission. Lancet 355:2237, 2000.
119. Cardo DM, et al: A case control study of HIV seroconversion in health care workers after percutaneous exposure. N Engl J Med 337:1485, 1997.
120. Frankel AD, Young JA: HIV-1: fifteen proteins and an RNA. Annu Rev Biochem 67:1, 1998.
121. Letvin NL, Walker BD: Immunopathogenesis and immunotherapy in AIDS virus infections. Nat Med 9:861, 2003.
122. Berger EA, Murphy PM, Farber JM: Chemokine receptors as HIV-1 coreceptors: roles in viral entry, tropism, and disease. Annu Rev Immunol 17:657, 1999.
123. Littman DR: Chemokine receptors: keys to AIDS pathogenesis? Cell 93:677, 1998.
124. LaBranche CC, et al: HIV fusion and its inhibition. Antiviral Res 50:95, 2001.
125. O'Brien SJ, Moore JP: The effect of genetic variation in chemokines and their receptors on HIV transmission and progression to AIDS. Immunol Rev 177:99, 2000.
126. Kinter A, et al: Chemokines, cytokines and HIV: a complex network of interactions that influence HIV pathogenesis. Immunol Rev 177:88, 2000.
127. Greene WC, Peterlin BM: Charting HIV's remarkable voyage through the cell: Basic science as a passport to future therapy. Nat Med 8:673, 2002.
128. Haase AT: Population biology of HIV-1 infection: viral and CD4+ T cell demographics and dynamics in lymphatic tissues. Annu Rev Immunol 17:625, 1999.
129. Hazenberg MD, et al: T cell depletion in HIV-1 infection: how CD4+ T cells go out of stock. Nat Immunol 1:285, 2000.
130. McCune JM: The dynamics of CD4+ T-cell depletion in HIV disease. Nature 410:974, 2001.
131. Grossman Z, et al: CD4+ T-cell depletion in HIV infection: are we closer to understanding the cause? Nature Medicine 8:319, 2002.
132. Wolthers KC, et al: T cell telomere length in HIV-1 infection: no evidence for increased CD4+ T cell turnover. Science 274:1543, 1996.
133. Gougeor M-L: Apoptosis as an HIV strategy to escape immune attack. Nat Rev Immunol 3:392, 2003.
134. Shearer GM: HIV-induced immunopathogenesis. Immunity 9:587, 1998.
135. Blankson JN, Persaud D, Siliciano RF: The challenge of viral reservoirs in HIV-1 infection. Annu Rev Med 53:557, 2002.
136. Steinman RM, et al: The interaction of immunodeficiency viruses with dendritic cells. Curr Top Microbiol Immunol 276:1, 2003.
137. van Kooyk Y, Geijtenbeck TB: DC-SIGN: escape mechanisms for pathogens. Nat Rev Immunol 3:697, 2003.
138. Cohen OJ, et al: Studies on lymphoid tissue from HIV-infected individuals: implications for the design of therapeutic strategies. Springer Semin Immunopathol 18:305, 1997.
139. Power C, Johnson RT: Neuroimmune and neurovirological aspects of human immunodeficiency virus infection. Adv Virus Res 56:389, 2001.
140. Tardieu M, Boutet A: HIV-1 and the central nervous system. Curr Top Microbiol Immunol 265:183, 2002.
141. Stevenson M: HIV-1 pathogenesis. Nat Med 9:853, 2003.
142. Kahn JO, Walker BD: Acute human immunodeficiency virus type 1 infection. N Engl J Med 339:33, 1998.
143. McMichael AJ, Rowland-Jones SL: Cellular immune responses to HIV. Nature 410:980, 2001.
144. Gandhi RT, Walker BD: Immunologic control of HIV-1. Annu Rev Med 53:149, 2002.
145. Mellors JW, et al: Prognosis in HIV-1 infection predicted by the quantity of virus in plasma. Science 272:1167, 1996.
146. Piguet V, Trono D: Living in oblivion: HIV immune evasion. Semin Immunol 13:51, 2001.
147. Johnson WE, Desrosiers RC: Viral persistance: HIV's strategies of immune system evasion. Annu Rev Med 53:499, 2002.
148. Klenerman P, Wu Y, Phillips R: HIV: current opinion in escapology. Curr Opin Microbiol 5:408, 2002.
149. CDC: Centers for Disease Control and Prevention: 1993 revised classification system and expanded surveillance definition for AIDS among adolescents and adults. MMWR 41(RR-17):1, 1992.
150. Furrer H, Fux C: Opportunistic infections: an update. J HIV Ther 7:2, 2002.
151. Gold JWM, et al: Management of the HIV-infected patient: Part II. Med Clin North Am 81:299, 1997.
152. Kovacs JA, Masur H: Prophylaxis against opportunistic infections in patients with human immunodeficiency virus infection. N Engl J Med 342:1416, 2000.
153. Barnes PF, Lakey DL, Burman WJ: Tuberculosis in patients with HIV infection. Infect Dis Clin North Am 16:107, 2002.
154. Boshoff C, Weiss R: AIDS-related malignancies. Nat Rev Cancer 2:373, 2002.
155. Scadden DT: AIDS-related malignancies. Annu Rev Med 54:285, 2003.
156. Judde JG, Lacoste V, Briere J, et al: Monoclonality or oligoclonality of human herpesvirus 8 terminal repeat sequences in Kaposi's sarcoma and other diseases. J Natl Cancer Inst 92:729, 2000.
157. Ensoli B, et al: Biology of Kaposi's sarcoma. Eur J Cancer 37:1251, 2001.

158. Moore PS, Chang Y: Molecular virology of Kaposi's sarcoma-associated herpesvirus. Philos Trans R Soc Lond B Biol Sci 356:499, 2001.
159. Boshoff C: Coupling herpesvirus to angiogenesis. Nature 391:24, 1998.
160. Knowles DM, Pirog EC: Pathology of AIDS-related lymphomas and other AIDS-defining neoplasms. Eur J Cancer 37:1236, 2001.
161. Carbone A: Emerging pathways in the development of AIDS-related lymphomas. Lancet Oncology 4:22, 2003.
162. Shah KV: Human papillomavirus and anogenital cancers. N Engl J Med 337:1386, 1997.
163. Knowles DM: Immunodeficiency-associated lymphoproliferative disorders. Mod Pathol 12:200, 1999.
164. McMichael AJ, Hauke T: HIV vaccines 1983–2003. Nat Med 9:874, 2003.
165. Robinson HL: New hope for an AIDS vaccine. Nat Rev Immunol 2:239, 2002.
166. Pepys MB: Pathogenesis, diagnosis and treatment of systemic amyloidosis. Philos Trans R Soc Lond B Biol Sci 356:203, 2001.
167. Merlini G, Bellotti V: Molecular mechanisms of amyloidosis. New Engl J Med 349:583, 2003.
168. Plante-Bordeneuve V, Said G: Transthyretin related familial amyloid polyneuropathy. Curr Opin Neurol 13:569, 2000.
169. DeArmond SJ: Cerebral amyloidosis in prion diseases. Int J Exp Clin Invest 7:3, 2000.
170. Falk RH, Comenzo RL, Skinner M: The systemic amyloidoses. N Engl J Med 337:898, 1997.
171. Harrison CJ, et al: Translocations of 14q32 and deletions of 13q14 are common chromosomal abnormalities in systemic amyloidosis. Br J Haematol 117:427, 2002.
172. Drenth JP, van der Meer JW: Hereditary periodic fever. N Engl J Med 345:1748, 2001.
173. Touitou I: The spectrum of Familial Mediterranean Fever (FMF) mutations. Eur J Hum Genet 9:473, 2001.
174. Cornwell GG, et al: The age related amyloids: a growing family of unique biochemical substances. J Clin Pathol 48:984, 1995.
175. Dobson CM: Protein folding and its links with human disease. Biochem Soc Symp:1, 2001.
176. Guy CD, Jones CC: Abdominal fat pad aspiration biopsy for tissue confirmation of systemic amyloidosis: specificity, positive predictive value, and diagnostic pitfalls. Diagn Cytopathology 24:181, 2001.
177. Gilmore JD, et al: Amyloid load and clinical outcome in AA amyloidosis in relation to circulating concentration of serum amyloid A protein. Lancet 358:24, 2001.

CHAPTER 7

Neoplasia

DEFINITIONS

NOMENCLATURE

BIOLOGY OF TUMOR GROWTH: BENIGN AND MALIGNANT NEOPLASMS

Differentiation and Anaplasia

Rates of Growth

Cancer Stem Cells and Cancer Cell Lineages

Local Invasion

Metastasis

Pathways of Spread

EPIDEMIOLOGY

Cancer Incidence

Geographic and Environmental Factors

Age

Genetic Predisposition to Cancer

Nonhereditary Predisposing Conditions

MOLECULAR BASIS OF CANCER

Essential Alterations for Malignant Transformation

The Normal Cell Cycle

Self-Sufficiency in Growth Signals: Oncogenes

Protooncogenes, Oncogenes, and Oncoproteins

Insensitivity to Growth Inhibitory Signals: Tumor Suppressor Genes

Evasion of Apoptosis

DNA Repair Defects and Genomic Instability in Cancer Cells

Limitless Replicative Potential: Telomerase

Development of Sustained Angiogenesis

Invasion and Metastasis

Invasion of Extracellular Matrix

Vascular Dissemination and Homing of Tumor Cells

Molecular Genetics of Metastasis Development

Stromal Microenvironment and Carcinogenesis

Dysregulation of Cancer-Associated Genes

Chromosomal Changes

Gene Amplification

Epigenetic Changes

Molecular Profiles of Cancer Cells

MOLECULAR BASIS OF MULTISTEP CARCINOGENESIS

Tumor Progression and Heterogeneity

CARCINOGENIC AGENTS AND THEIR CELLULAR INTERACTIONS

Chemical Carcinogenesis

Steps Involved in Chemical Carcinogenesis

Initiation of Chemical Carcinogenesis

Promotion of Chemical Carcinogenesis

Carcinogenic Chemicals

Radiation Carcinogenesis

Ultraviolet Rays

Ionizing Radiation

Microbial Carcinogenesis

Oncogenic DNA Viruses

Oncogenic RNA Viruses

Helicobacter pylori

HOST DEFENSE AGAINST TUMORS—TUMOR IMMUNITY

Tumor Antigens

Antitumor Effector Mechanisms

Immune Surveillance

CLINICAL FEATURES OF TUMORS

Effects of Tumors on the Host

Local and Hormonal Effects

Cancer Cachexia

Paraneoplastic Syndromes

Grading and Staging of Tumors

Laboratory Diagnosis of Cancer

In the year 2000, there were 10 million new cases of cancer and 6 million cancer deaths worldwide.[1,2] In the United States each year, almost 1.5 million individuals learn for the first time that they have some type of cancer. Not included in these figures are more than 1 million new cases of the most common types of nonpigmented skin cancers and incipient, noninvasive cancers. Not only these noninvasive lesions but many invasive tumors as well can be cured. Nonetheless, according to American Cancer Society estimates, cancer caused approximately 556,000 deaths in 2003, corresponding to 1500 cancer deaths per day, accounting for about 23% of all deaths in the United States.[3] Some good news, however, has emerged: cancer mortality for both men and women in the United States declined during the last decade of the 20th century.[4] Thus, there has been progress, but the problem is still overwhelming. The discussion that follows deals with both benign tumors and cancers; the latter receive more attention. The focus is on the basic morphologic and biologic properties of tumors and on the present understanding of the molecular basis of carcinogenesis. We also discuss the interactions of the tumor with the host and the host response to tumors. Although the discussion of therapy is beyond the scope of this chapter, there are now dramatic improvements in therapeutic responses and 5-year survival rates with many forms of malignancy, notably the leukemias and lymphomas. A greater proportion of cancers is being cured or arrested today than ever before.

Definitions

Neoplasia literally means the process of "new growth," and a new growth is called a *neoplasm*. The term *tumor* was originally applied to the swelling caused by inflammation. Neoplasms also may induce swellings, but by long precedent, the non-neoplastic usage of *tumor* has passed into limbo; thus, the term is now equated with neoplasm. *Oncology* (Greek *oncos* = tumor) is the study of tumors or neoplasms. *Cancer is the common term for all malignant tumors.* Although the ancient origins of this term are somewhat uncertain, it probably derives from the Latin for crab, *cancer*—presumably because a cancer "adheres to any part that it seizes upon in an obstinate manner like the crab."

Although all physicians know what they mean when they use the term *neoplasm*, it has been surprisingly difficult to develop an accurate definition. The eminent British oncologist Willis[5] has come closest: "A neoplasm is an abnormal mass of tissue, the growth of which exceeds and is uncoordinated with that of the normal tissues and persists in the same excessive manner after cessation of the stimuli which evoked the change." We know that the persistence of tumors, even after the inciting stimulus is gone, results from *heritable genetic alterations that are passed down to the progeny of the tumor cells. These genetic changes allow excessive and unregulated proliferation that becomes autonomous (independent of physiologic growth stimuli),* although tumors generally remain dependent on the host for their nutrition and blood supply. As we shall discuss later, the entire population of cells within a tumor arises from a single cell that has incurred genetic change, and hence tumors are said to be *clonal*.

Nomenclature

All tumors, benign and malignant, have two basic components: (1) proliferating neoplastic cells that constitute their *parenchyma* and (2) supportive *stroma* made up of connective tissue and blood vessels. Although parenchymal cells represent the proliferating "cutting edge" of neoplasms and so determine their behavior and pathologic consequences, the growth and evolution of neoplasms are critically dependent on their stroma. An adequate stromal blood supply is requisite, and the stromal connective tissue provides the framework for the parenchyma. In addition, there is cross-talk between tumor cells and stromal cells that appears to directly influence the growth of tumors. In some tumors, the stromal support is scant and so the neoplasm is soft and fleshy. Sometimes the parenchymal cells stimulate the formation of an abundant collagenous stroma, referred to as *desmoplasia*. Some tumors—for example, some cancers of the female breast—are stony hard or *scirrhous*. The nomenclature of tumors is, however, based on the parenchymal component.

Benign Tumors. In general, benign tumors are designated by attaching the suffix *-oma* to the cell of origin. Tumors of mesenchymal cells generally follow this rule. For example, a benign tumor arising from fibroblastic cells is called a *fibroma*, a cartilaginous tumor is a *chondroma*, and a tumor of osteoblasts is an *osteoma*. In contrast, nomenclature of benign epithelial tumors is more complex. They are variously classified, some based on their cells of origin, others on microscopic architecture, and still others on their macroscopic patterns.

Adenoma is the term applied to a benign epithelial neoplasm that forms glandular patterns as well as to tumors derived from glands but not necessarily reproducing glandular patterns. On this basis, a benign epithelial neoplasm that arises from renal tubular cells growing in the form of numerous tightly clustered small glands would be termed an *adenoma*, as would a heterogeneous mass of adrenal cortical cells growing in no distinctive pattern. Benign epithelial neoplasms producing microscopically or macroscopically visible finger-like or warty projections from epithelial surfaces are referred to as *papillomas* (Fig. 7–1). Those that form large cystic masses, as in the ovary, are referred to as *cystadenomas*.

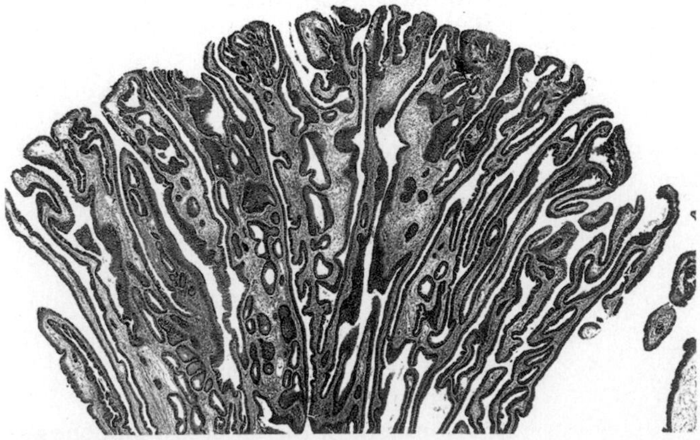

FIGURE 7–1 Papilloma of the colon with finger-like projections into the lumen. (Courtesy of Dr. Trace Worrell, University of Texas Southwestern Medical School, Dallas, TX.)

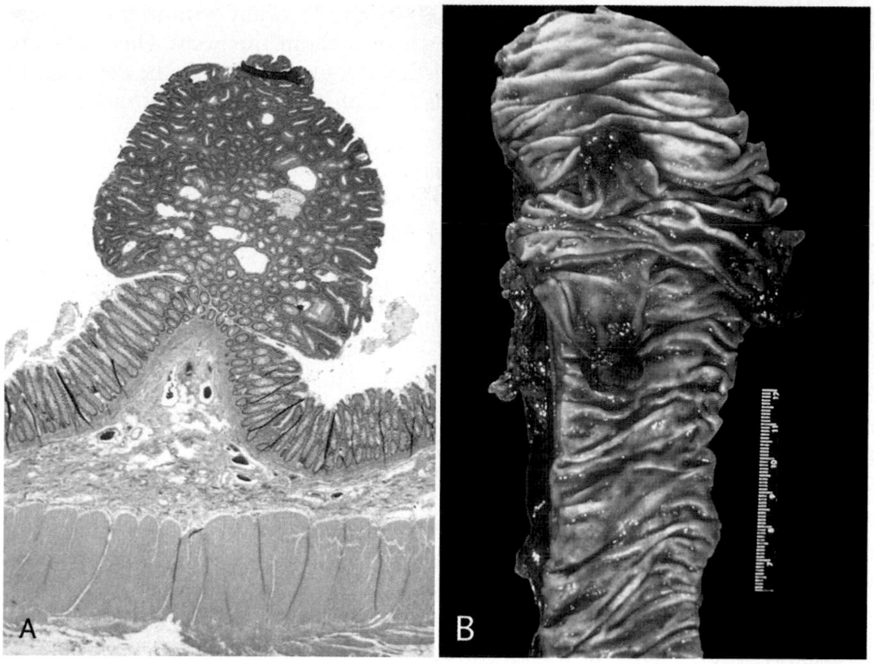

FIGURE 7–2 Colonic polyp. *A,* This benign glandular tumor (adenoma) is projecting into the colonic lumen and is attached to the mucosa by a distinct stalk. *B,* Gross appearance of several colonic polyps.

Some tumors produce papillary patterns that protrude into cystic spaces and are called *papillary cystadenomas.* When a neoplasm, benign or malignant, produces a macroscopically visible projection above a *mucosal* surface and projects, for example, into the gastric or colonic lumen, it is termed a *polyp* (Fig. 7–2). The term *polyp* is preferably restricted to benign tumors. Malignant polyps are better designated *polypoid cancers.*

Malignant Tumors. The nomenclature of malignant tumors essentially follows the same schema used for benign neoplasms, with certain additions. *Malignant tumors arising in mesenchymal tissue are usually called sarcomas* (Greek *sar* = fleshy) because they have little connective tissue stroma and so are fleshy (e.g., fibrosarcoma, liposarcoma, leiomyosarcoma for smooth muscle cancer, and rhabdomyosarcoma for a cancer that differentiates toward striated muscle). Malignant neoplasms of epithelial cell origin, derived from any of the three germ layers, are called *carcinomas.* Thus, cancer arising in the epidermis of ectodermal origin is a carcinoma, as is a cancer arising in the mesodermally derived cells of the renal tubules and the endodermally derived cells of the lining of the gastrointestinal tract. Carcinomas may be further qualified. One with a glandular growth pattern microscopically is termed an *adenocarcinoma,* and one producing recognizable squamous cells arising in any epithelium of the body is termed a *squamous cell carcinoma.* It is common practice to specify, when possible, the organ of origin (e.g., a renal cell adenocarcinoma or bronchogenic squamous cell carcinoma). Not infrequently, however, a cancer is composed of undifferentiated cells of unknown tissue origin, and must be designated merely as a poorly differentiated or undifferentiated malignant tumor.

In benign and in differentiated malignant neoplasms, the parenchymal cells bear a close resemblance to each other, as though all were derived from a single cell, as we know to be the case with cancers. Infrequently, divergent differentiation of a single line of parenchymal cells into another tissue creates what are called *mixed tumors.* The best example of this is the *mixed tumor of salivary gland origin.* These tumors contain epithelial components scattered within a myxoid stroma that sometimes contains islands of apparent cartilage or even bone (Fig. 7–3). All these elements, it is believed, arise from epithelial and myoepithelial cells of salivary gland origin; thus, the preferred designation of these neoplasms is *pleomorphic adenoma.* The great majority of neoplasms, even mixed tumors, are composed of cells representative of a single germ layer. *Teratomas,* in contrast, are made up of a variety of parenchymal cell types representative of more than one germ layer, usually all three. They arise from totipotent cells and so are principally encountered in the gonads; they occur rarely in sequestered primitive cell rests elsewhere. These totipotent cells differentiate along various germ lines, producing tissues

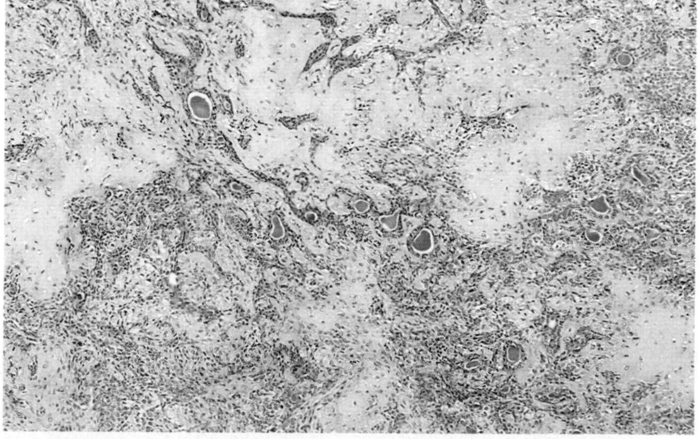

FIGURE 7–3 This mixed tumor of the parotid gland contains epithelial cells forming ducts and myxoid stroma that resembles cartilage. (Courtesy of Dr. Trace Worrell, University of Texas Southwestern Medical School, Dallas, TX.)

that can be identified, for example, as skin, muscle, fat, gut epithelium, tooth structures—indeed, any tissue of the body. A particularly common pattern is seen in the ovarian *cystic teratoma* (dermoid cyst), which differentiates principally along ectodermal lines to create a cystic tumor lined by skin replete with hair, sebaceous glands, and tooth structures (Fig. 7–4).

The nomenclature of the more common forms of neoplasia is presented in Table 7–1. It is evident from this compilation that there are some inappropriate but deeply entrenched usages. For generations, carcinomas of melanocytes have been called *melanomas,* although correctly they should be referred to as melanocarcinomas. Similarly, carcinomas of testicular origin are stubbornly called *seminomas,* and hepatocellular carcinomas are often called *hepatomas.* Other instances are encountered in which innocent designations belie ugly behavior. The converse is also true; ominous terms are applied to usually trivial lesions. An ectopic rest of normal tissue is sometimes called a *choristoma*—as, for example, a rest of adrenal cells under the kidney capsule. Occasionally a pancreatic nodular rest in the mucosa of the small intestine may mimic a neoplasm, providing some partial justification for the use of a term that implies a tumor. Aberrant differentiation may produce a mass of disorganized but mature specialized cells or tissue indigenous to the particular site, referred to as a *hamartoma.* Thus, a hamartoma in the lung may contain islands of cartilage, blood vessels, bronchial-type structures, and lymphoid tissue. Sometimes the lesion is purely cartilaginous or purely angiomatous. Although these might be considered neoplasms, the complete resemblance of the tissue to normal cartilage or blood vessels and the occasional admixture of other elements suggest that the lesions reflect anomalous development. In any event, the hamartoma is totally benign.

The nomenclature of tumors is important because specific designations have specific clinical implications, even among tumors arising from the same tissue. *Seminoma* is a form of testicular carcinoma that tends to spread to lymph nodes along the iliac arteries and aorta. Further, these tumors are extremely radiosensitive and can be eradicated by radiotherapy; thus, few patients with seminomas die of the neoplasm. By contrast, the embryonal carcinoma of the testis is not radiosensitive and tends to invade locally beyond the confines of the testis and spread throughout the body. There also are other varieties of testicular neoplasms, and so the designation *cancer of the testis* tells little of its clinical significance.

Biology of Tumor Growth: Benign and Malignant Neoplasms

The natural history of most malignant tumors can be divided into four phases: (1) malignant change in the target cell, referred to as transformation; (2) growth of the transformed cells; (3) local invasion; and (4) distant metastases. We discuss the molecular mechanisms underlying these phases later in the chapter. The differences between benign and malignant tumors correspond to these characteristics and are discussed under the headings of differentiation and anaplasia, rate of growth, local invasion, and metastasis. In the great majority of instances, a benign tumor may be distinguished from a malignant tumor with considerable confidence based on morphology; sometimes, however, a neoplasm defies categorization. Certain anatomic features may suggest innocence, whereas others point toward cancerous potential. Ultimately, morphologic diagnosis cannot predict the biologic behavior or clinical course of a neoplasm with absolute certainty. Occasionally, this prediction is confounded by a marked discrepancy between the morphologic appearance of a tumor and its behavior: An innocent face may mask an ugly nature. Such deception or ambiguity, however, is not the rule; in general, there are morphologic criteria by which benign and malignant tumors can be differentiated, and the behavior of the tumors can be predicted by these criteria.

DIFFERENTIATION AND ANAPLASIA

Differentiation refers to the extent to which neoplastic cells resemble comparable normal cells, both morphologically and functionally; lack of differentiation is called anaplasia. Well-differentiated tumors are composed of cells resembling the mature normal cells of the tissue of origin of the neoplasm (Fig. 7–5). Poorly differentiated or undifferentiated tumors

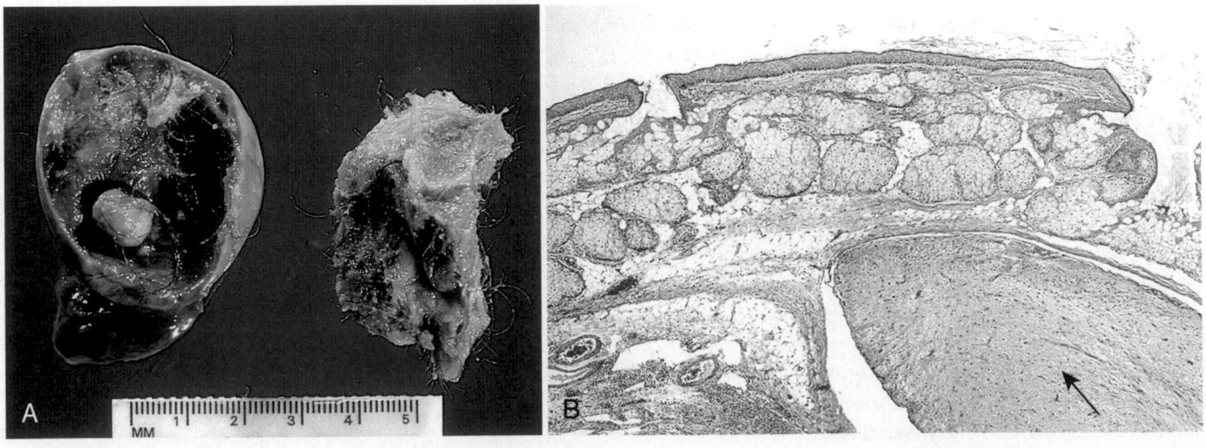

FIGURE 7–4 *A,* Gross appearance of an opened cystic teratoma of the ovary. Note the presence of hair, sebaceous material, and tooth. *B,* A microscopic view of a similar tumor shows skin, sebaceous glands, fat cells, and a tract of neural tissue *(arrow).*

TABLE 7–1 Nomenclature of Tumors

Tissue of Origin	Benign	Malignant
Composed of One Parenchymal Cell Type		
Tumors of mesenchymal origin		
Connective tissue and derivatives	Fibroma	Fibrosarcoma
	Lipoma	Liposarcoma
	Chondroma	Chondrosarcoma
	Osteoma	Osteogenic sarcoma
Endothelial and related tissues		
Blood vessels	Hemangioma	Angiosarcoma
Lymph vessels	Lymphangioma	Lymphangiosarcoma
Synovium		Synovial sarcoma
Mesothelium		Mesothelioma
Brain coverings	Meningioma	Invasive meningioma
Blood cells and related cells		
Hematopoietic cells		Leukemias
Lymphoid tissue		Lymphomas
Muscle		
Smooth	Leiomyoma	Leiomyosarcoma
Striated	Rhabdomyoma	Rhabdomyosarcoma
Tumors of epithelial origin		
Stratified squamous	Squamous cell papilloma	Squamous cell or epidermoid carcinoma
Basal cells of skin or adnexa		Basal cell carcinoma
Epithelial lining of glands or ducts	Adenoma	Adenocarcinoma
	Papilloma	Papillary carcinomas
	Cystadenoma	Cystadenocarcinoma
Respiratory passages	Bronchial adenoma	Bronchogenic carcinoma
Renal epithelium	Renal tubular adenoma	Renal cell carcinoma
Liver cells	Liver cell adenoma	Hepatocellular carcinoma
Urinary tract epithelium (transitional)	Transitional cell papilloma	Transitional cell carcinoma
Placental epithelium	Hydatidiform mole	Choriocarcinoma
Testicular epithelium (germ cells)		Seminoma
		Embryonal carcinoma
Tumors of melanocytes	Nevus	Malignant melanoma
More Than One Neoplastic Cell Type—Mixed Tumors, Usually Derived from One Germ Cell Layer		
Salivary glands	Pleomorphic adenoma (mixed tumor of salivary origin)	Malignant mixed tumor of salivary gland origin
Renal anlage		Wilms tumor
More Than One Neoplastic Cell Type Derived from More Than One Germ Cell Layer—Teratogenous		
Totipotential cells in gonads or in embryonic rests	Mature teratoma, dermoid cyst	Immature teratoma, teratocarcinoma

have primitive-appearing, unspecialized cells. In general, benign tumors are well differentiated (Fig. 7–6). The neoplastic cell in a benign smooth muscle tumor—a leiomyoma—so closely resembles the normal cell that it may be impossible to recognize it as a tumor by microscopic examination of individual cells. Only the massing of these cells into a nodule discloses the neoplastic nature of the lesion. One may get so close to the tree that one loses sight of the forest.

Malignant neoplasms, in contrast, range from well differentiated to undifferentiated. Malignant neoplasms composed of undifferentiated cells are said to be *anaplastic.* Lack of differentiation, or *anaplasia,* is considered a hallmark of malignant transformation. Anaplasia literally means "to form backward," implying a reversion from a high level of differentiation to a lower level. There is substantial evidence, however, that most cancers do not represent "reverse differentiation" of mature normal cells but, in fact, arise from stem cells that are present in all specialized tissues. The well-differentiated cancer (Fig. 7–7) evolves from maturation or specialization of undifferentiated cells as they proliferate, whereas the undifferentiated malignant tumor derives from proliferation without complete maturation of the transformed cells.

Lack of differentiation, or anaplasia, is marked by a number of morphologic changes.

- *Pleomorphism.* Both the cells and the nuclei characteristically display *pleomorphism*—variation in size and shape (Fig. 7–8). Cells may be found that are many times larger than their neighbors, and other cells may be extremely small and primitive appearing.

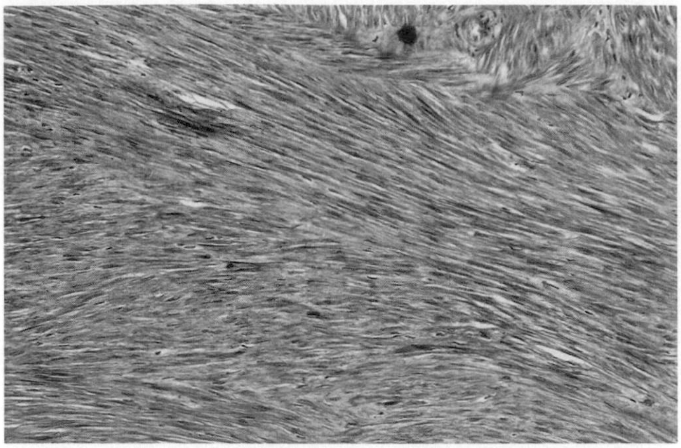

FIGURE 7–5 Leiomyoma of the uterus. This benign, well-differentiated tumor contains interlacing bundles of neoplastic smooth muscle cells that are virtually identical in appearance to normal smooth muscle cells in the myometrium.

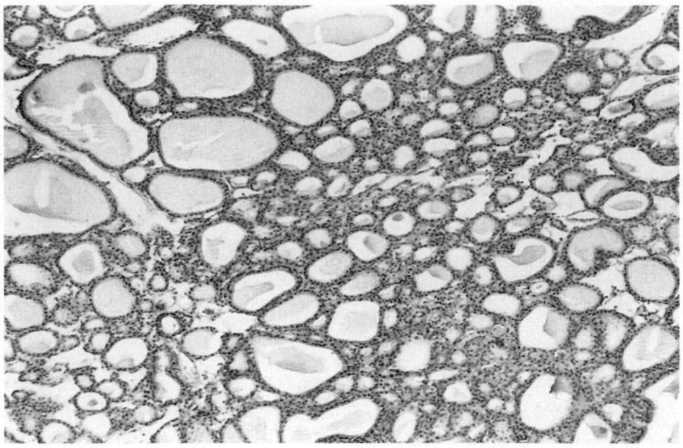

FIGURE 7–6 Benign tumor (adenoma) of the thyroid. Note the normal-looking (well-differentiated), colloid-filled thyroid follicles. (Courtesy of Dr. Trace Worrell, University of Texas Southwestern Medical School, Dallas, TX.)

- *Abnormal nuclear morphology.* Characteristically the nuclei contain an abundance of DNA and are extremely dark staining *(hyperchromatic).* The nuclei are disproportionately large for the cell, and the nucleus-to-cytoplasm ratio may approach 1:1 instead of the normal 1:4 or 1:6. The nuclear shape is very variable, and the chromatin is often coarsely clumped and distributed along the nuclear membrane. Large nucleoli are usually present in these nuclei.
- *Mitoses.* As compared with benign tumors and some well-differentiated malignant neoplasms, undifferentiated tumors usually possess large numbers of mitoses, reflecting the higher proliferative activity of the parenchymal cells. *The presence of mitoses, however, does not necessarily indicate that a tumor is malignant or that the tissue is neoplastic.* Many normal tissues exhibiting rapid turnover, such as bone marrow, have numerous mitoses, and non-neoplastic proliferations such as hyperplasias contain many cells in mitosis. More important as a morphologic feature of malignant neoplasia are atypical, bizarre mitotic figures, sometimes producing tripolar, quadripolar, or multipolar spindles (Fig. 7–9).
- *Loss of polarity.* In addition to the cytologic abnormalities, the *orientation of anaplastic cells is markedly disturbed (i.e., they lose normal polarity).* Sheets or large masses of tumor cells grow in an anarchic, disorganized fashion.
- *Other changes.* Another feature of anaplasia is the formation of *tumor giant cells,* some possessing only a single huge polymorphic nucleus and others having two or more nuclei. These giant cells are not to be confused with inflammatory Langhans or foreign body giant cells, which are derived from macrophages and contain many small, normal-appearing nuclei. In the cancer giant cell, the nuclei are hyperchromatic and large in relation to the cell. Although growing tumor cells obviously require a blood

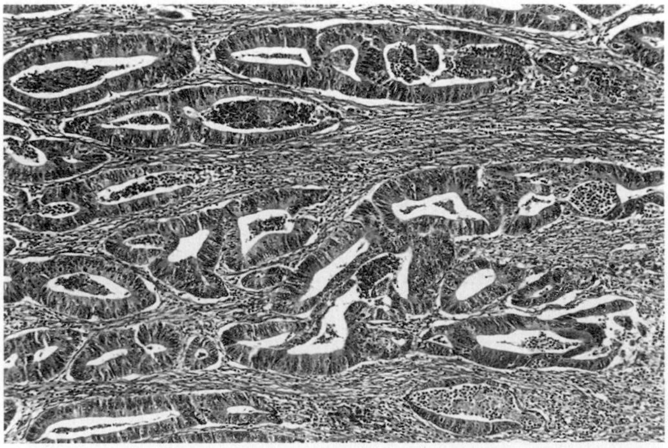

FIGURE 7–7 Malignant tumor (adenocarcinoma) of the colon. Note that compared with the well-formed and normal-looking glands characteristic of a benign tumor (see Fig. 7–6), the cancerous glands are irregular in shape and size and do not resemble the normal colonic glands. This tumor is considered differentiated because gland formation can be seen. The malignant glands have invaded the muscular layer of the colon. (Courtesy of Dr. Trace Worrell, University of Texas Southwestern Medical School, Dallas, TX.)

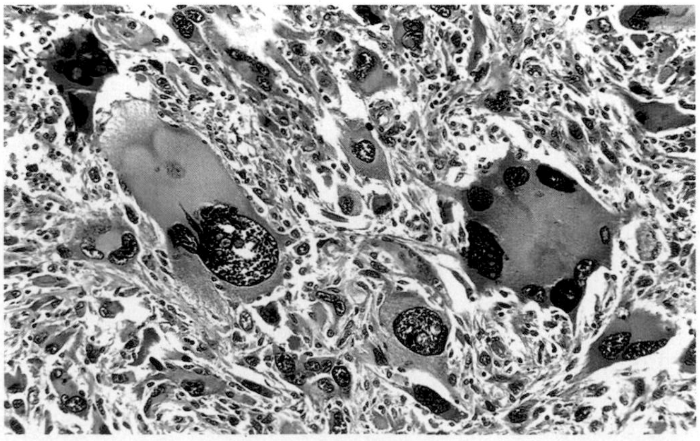

FIGURE 7–8 Anaplastic tumor of the skeletal muscle (rhabdomyosarcoma). Note the marked cellular and nuclear pleomorphism, hyperchromatic nuclei, and tumor giant cells. (Courtesy of Dr. Trace Worrell, University of Texas Southwestern Medical School, Dallas, TX.)

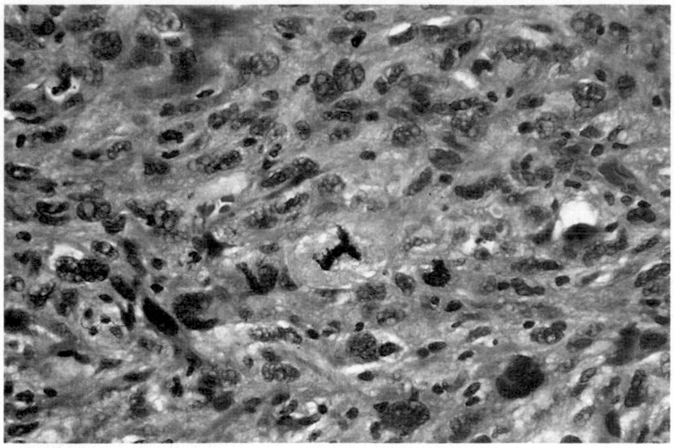

FIGURE 7–9 Anaplastic tumor showing cellular and nuclear variation in size and shape. The prominent cell in the center field has an abnormal tripolar spindle.

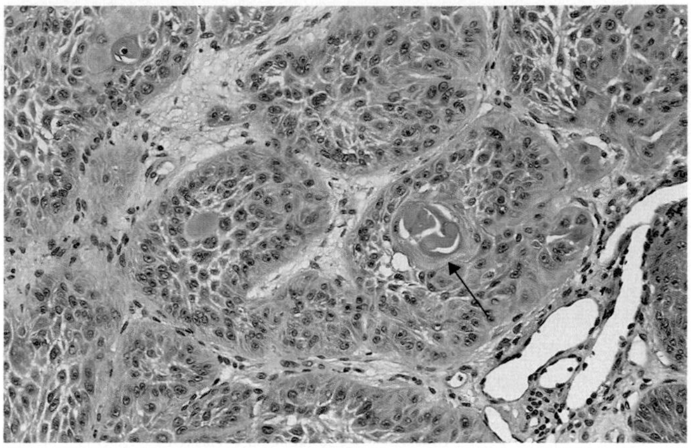

FIGURE 7–10 Well-differentiated squamous cell carcinoma of the skin. The tumor cells are strikingly similar to normal squamous epithelial cells, with intercellular bridges and nests of keratin pearls *(arrow)*. (Courtesy of Dr. Trace Worrell, University of Texas Southwestern Medical School, Dallas, TX.)

supply, often the vascular stroma is scant, and in many anaplastic tumors, large central areas undergo ischemic *necrosis.*

As mentioned, malignant tumors differ widely in the extent to which their morphologic appearance deviates from the norm. On one end of the spectrum are the extremely undifferentiated, anaplastic, tumors and at the other end are cancers that bear striking resemblance to their tissues of origin. Certain well-differentiated adenocarcinomas of the thyroid, for example, may form normal-appearing follicles, and some squamous cell carcinomas contain cells that do not differ cytologically from normal squamous epithelial cells (Fig. 7–10). Thus, the morphologic diagnosis of malignancy in well-differentiated tumors may sometimes be quite difficult. In between the two extremes lie tumors that are loosely referred to as *moderately well differentiated.*

Before we leave the subject of differentiation and anaplasia, we should discuss *dysplasia,* a term that literally means disordered growth. Dysplasia is encountered principally in epithelia, and it is characterized by a constellation of changes that include *a loss in the uniformity of the individual cells as well as a loss in their architectural orientation.* Dysplastic cells also exhibit considerable pleomorphism and often contain hyperchromatic nuclei that are abnormally large for the size of the cell. Mitotic figures are more abundant than usual, although almost invariably they conform to normal patterns. Frequently the mitoses appear in abnormal locations within the epithelium. Thus, in dysplastic stratified squamous epithelium, mitoses are not confined to the basal layers and may appear at all levels and even in surface cells. The architecture of the tissue may be disorderly. For example, the usual progressive maturation of tall cells in the basal layer to flattened squames on the surface may be lost and replaced by a scrambling of dark basal-appearing cells throughout the epithelium. When dysplastic changes are marked and involve the entire thickness of the epithelium, but the lesion remains confined to the normal tissue, it is considered a preinvasive neoplasm and is referred to as *carcinoma in situ* (Fig. 7–11). Once the tumor cells move beyond the normal confines, the tumor is said to be *invasive.* Dysplastic changes are often found adjacent to foci of invasive carcinoma, and in some situations, such as in long-term cigarette smokers and Barrett esophagus,

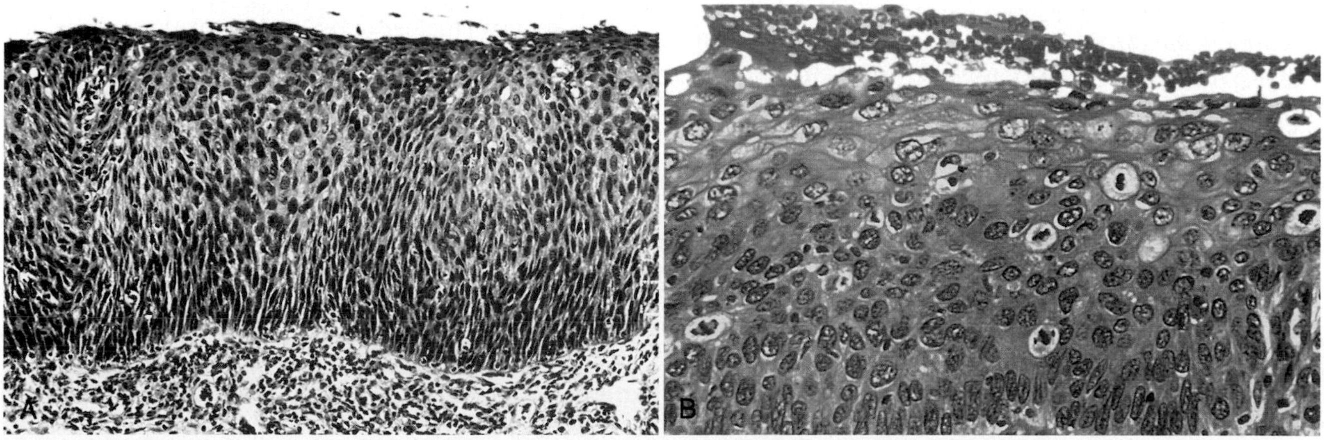

FIGURE 7–11 *A,* Carcinoma in situ. This low-power view shows that the entire thickness of the epithelium is replaced by atypical dysplastic cells. There is no orderly differentiation of squamous cells. The basement membrane is intact and there is no tumor in the subepithelial stroma. *B,* A high-power view of another region shows failure of normal differentiation, marked nuclear and cellular pleomorphism, and numerous mitotic figures extending toward the surface. The basement membrane *(below)* is not seen in this section.

severe epithelial dysplasia frequently antedates the appearance of cancer. However, *dysplasia does not necessarily progress to cancer.* Mild to moderate changes that do not involve the entire thickness of epithelium may be reversible, and with removal of the inciting causes, the epithelium may revert to normal.

As you might presume, the better the differentiation of the transformed cell, the more completely it retains the functional capabilities found in its normal counterparts. Thus, benign neoplasms and well-differentiated carcinomas of endocrine glands frequently elaborate the hormones characteristic of their origin. Increased levels of these hormones in the blood are used clinically to detect and follow such tumors. Well-differentiated squamous cell carcinomas of the epidermis elaborate keratin, just as well-differentiated hepatocellular carcinomas elaborate bile. Highly anaplastic undifferentiated cells, whatever their tissue of origin, lose their resemblance to the normal cells from which they have arisen. In some instances, new and unanticipated functions emerge. Some tumors may elaborate fetal proteins (antigens) not produced by comparable cells in the adult. Carcinomas of nonendocrine origin may produce a variety of hormones, often called ectopic hormones. For example, bronchogenic carcinomas may produce corticotropin, parathyroid-like hormone, insulin, and glucagons, as well as others. *Despite exceptions, the more rapidly growing and the more anaplastic a tumor, the less likely it is that there will be specialized functional activity. The cells in benign tumors are almost always well differentiated and resemble their normal cells of origin; the cells in cancer are more or less differentiated, but some loss of differentiation is always present.*

RATES OF GROWTH

A fundamental issue in tumor biology is to understand the factors that influence the growth rates of tumors and the role of these factors in clinical outcome and therapeutic responses. One can begin the consideration of tumor cell kinetics by asking the question: How long does it take to produce a clinically overt tumor mass? It can be readily calculated that the original transformed cell (approximately 10 µm in diameter) must undergo at least 30 population doublings to produce 10^9 cells (weighing approximately 1 gm), which is the smallest clinically detectable mass. In contrast, only 10 further doubling cycles are required to produce a tumor containing 10^{12} cells (weighing approximately 1 kg), which is usually the maximal size compatible with life (Fig. 7–12). These are minimal estimates, based on the assumption that all descendants of the transformed cell retain the ability to divide and that there is no loss of cells from the replicative pool. This concept of tumor as a "pathologic dynamo" is not entirely correct, as we discuss subsequently. Nevertheless, this calculation highlights an extremely important concept about tumor growth: *By the time a solid tumor is clinically detected, it has already completed a major portion of its life cycle.* This is a major impediment in the treatment of cancer, and underscores the need to develop diagnostic markers to detect early cancers.

The rate of growth of a tumor is determined by three main factors: the doubling time of tumor cells, the fraction of tumor cells that are in the replicative pool, and the rate at which cells are shed and lost in the growing lesion. Because cell-cycle controls are deranged in most tumors, tumor cells can be triggered into cycle more readily and without the usual restraints. The dividing cells, however, do not necessarily complete the cell cycle more rapidly than do normal cells. In reality, total cell-cycle time for many tumors is equal to or longer than that of corresponding normal cells. Thus, it can be safely concluded that growth of tumors is not commonly associated with a shortening of cell-cycle time.

The proportion of cells within the tumor population that are in the proliferative pool is referred to as the *growth fraction.* Clinical and experimental studies suggest that during the early, submicroscopic phase of tumor growth, the vast majority of transformed cells are in the proliferative pool (Fig. 7–13). As tumors continue to grow, cells leave the proliferative pool in ever-increasing numbers owing to shedding, lack of nutrients, or apoptosis; by differentiating; and by reversion to G_0. Most cells within cancers remain in the G_0 or G_1 phases. Thus, by the time a tumor is clinically detectable, most cells are not in the replicative pool. Even in some rapidly growing tumors, the growth fraction is only about 20% or less.

Ultimately the progressive growth of tumors and the rate at which they grow are determined by an *excess of cell production over cell loss.* In some tumors, especially those with a relatively high growth fraction, the imbalance is large, resulting in more rapid growth than in those in which cell production exceeds cell loss by only a small margin. Some leukemias and lymphomas and certain lung cancers (i.e., small cell carcinoma) have a relatively high growth fraction, and their clinical course is rapid. By comparison, many common tumors such as cancers of the colon and breast have low growth fractions, and cell production exceeds cell loss by only about 10%; they tend to grow at a much slower pace.

Several important conceptual and practical lessons can be learned from studies of tumor cell kinetics:

- Fast-growing tumors may have a high *cell turnover,* implying that rates of both proliferation and apoptosis are high. Obviously, for the tumor to grow, the rate of proliferation should exceed that of apoptosis.
- The growth fraction of tumor cells has a profound effect on their susceptibility to cancer chemotherapy. Because most anticancer agents act on cells that are in cycle, it is not difficult to imagine that a tumor that contains 5% of all cells in the replicative pool will be slow growing but relatively refractory to treatment with drugs that kill dividing cells. One strategy employed in the treatment of tumors with low growth fraction (e.g., cancer of colon and breast) is first to shift tumor cells from G_0 into the cell cycle. This can be accomplished by debulking the tumor with surgery or radiation. The surviving tumor cells tend to enter the cell cycle and thus become susceptible to drug therapy. Such considerations form the basis of combined modality treatment. Some aggressive tumors (such as certain lymphomas) that contain a large pool of dividing cells literally melt away with chemotherapy and cures may even be effected.

We can now return to the question posed earlier: How long does it take for one transformed cell to produce a clinically detectable tumor containing 10^9 cells? If every one of the daughter cells remained in cell cycle and no cells were shed or lost, we could anticipate the answer to be 90 days (30 population doublings, with a cell-cycle time of 3 days; see Fig. 7–12). In reality, *the latent period before which a tumor becomes clinically detectable is unpredictable but typically much longer than*

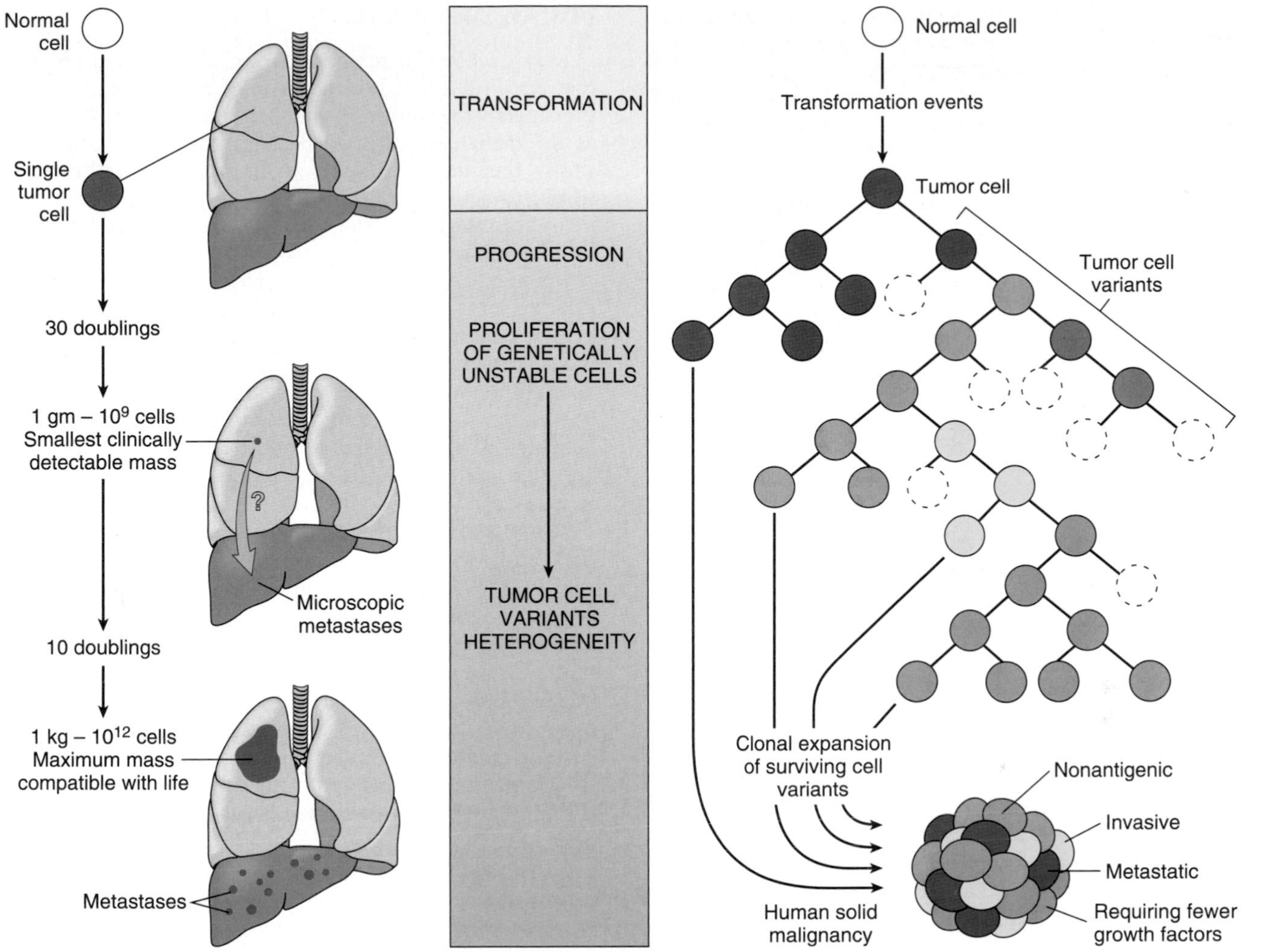

FIGURE 7–12 Biology of tumor growth. The left panel depicts minimal estimates of tumor cell doublings that precede the formation of a clinically detectable tumor mass. It is evident that by the time a solid tumor is detected, it has already completed a major portion of its life cycle as measured by cell doublings. The right panel illustrates clonal evolution of tumors and generation of tumor cell heterogeneity. New subclones arise from the descendants of the original transformed cell, and with progressive growth the tumor mass becomes enriched for those variants that are more adept at evading host defenses and are likely to be more aggressive. (Adapted from Tannock IF: Biology of tumor growth. Hosp Pract 18:81, 1983.)

90 days, up to many years for most solid tumors, emphasizing once again that human cancers are diagnosed only after they are fairly advanced in their life cycle. After they become clinically detectable, the average volume-doubling time for such common killers as cancer of the lung and colon is about 2 to 3 months. As might be anticipated from the discussion of the variables that affect growth rate, however, the range of doubling time values is extremely broad, varying from less than 1 month for some childhood cancers to more than 1 year for certain salivary gland tumors. Cancer is indeed an unpredictable disorder.

In general, *the growth rate of tumors is inversely correlated with their level of differentiation, and thus most malignant tumors grow more rapidly than do benign lesions.* There are, however, many exceptions to such an oversimplification. Some benign tumors have a higher growth rate than malignant tumors. Moreover, the rate of growth of benign as well as malignant neoplasms may not be constant over time. Factors such as hormonal stimulation, adequacy of blood supply, and unknown influences may affect their growth. For example, the growth of uterine leiomyomas (benign smooth muscle tumors) may change over time because of hormonal variations. Not infrequently, repeated clinical examination of women bearing such neoplasms over the span of decades discloses no significant increase in size. After menopause, the neoplasms may atrophy and may be replaced largely by collagenous, sometimes calcified, tissue. During pregnancy, leiomyomas frequently enter a growth spurt. Such changes reflect the responsiveness of the tumor cells to circulating levels of steroid hormones, particularly estrogens. Cancers show a wide range of growth. Some malignant tumors grow slowly for years and then suddenly increase in size, explosively disseminating to cause death within a few months of discovery. It is possible that such behavior results from the emergence of an aggressive subclone of transformed cells. At the other extreme are malignant neoplasms that grow more slowly than do benign tumors and may even enter periods of dormancy lasting for years. On occasion, cancers have been observed to decrease in size and even spontaneously disappear, but such "miracles" are rare enough that they remain curiosities.

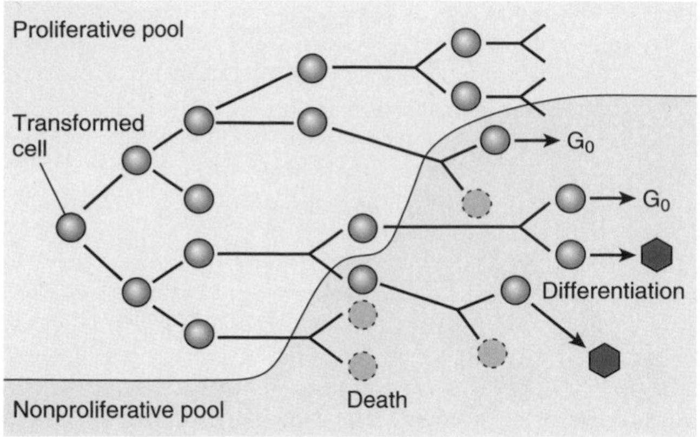

FIGURE 7–13 Schematic representation of tumor growth. As the cell population expands, a progressively higher percentage of tumor cells leaves the replicative pool by reversion to G_0, differentiation, and death.

CANCER STEM CELLS AND CANCER CELL LINEAGES

A clinically detectable tumor contains a heterogeneous population of cells, which originated from the clonal growth of the progeny of a single cell. Yet, it has been difficult to identify cancer stem cells, that is, the cells within a tumor that have the capacity to initiate and sustain the tumor.[6] Recently, cancer stem cells (called *tumor-initiating cells,* or *T-IC*) were identified in breast tumors and acute myeloid leukemia.[7,8] T-ICs constitute less than 2% of the cells in breast tumors and 0.1% to 1% of cells in acute myeloid leukemia.[9] To maintain their self-renewing capacity, leukemic T-ICs require the expression of the *BMI1* gene,[8,10] which represses the cell-cycle inhibitors p161NK4a and p14ARF (these inhibitors are discussed later in conjunction with the cell cycle). There is also strong experimental support for the idea that, in these leukemias, cancer stem cells are the initial targets for transformation.[9] These findings have important implications for cancer treatment aimed at the elimination of proliferating cells. Apparently, cancer stem cells, similar to their normal counterparts, have a low rate of replication. If this is the case, cancer therapies that may efficiently kill the replicating progeny of cancer stem cells would leave in place the cells capable of generating the tumor. Under these circumstances, tumors can easily recur after treatment. Whether such cancer stem cells exist in all tumors is not yet clear.

LOCAL INVASION

Nearly all benign tumors grow as cohesive expansile masses that remain localized to their site of origin and do not have the capacity to infiltrate, invade, or metastasize to distant sites, as do malignant tumors. Because they grow and expand slowly, they usually develop a rim of compressed connective tissue, sometimes called a fibrous *capsule,* which separates them from the host tissue. This capsule is derived largely from the stroma of the native tissue as the parenchymal cells atrophy under the pressure of expanding tumor. Such encapsulation does not prevent tumor growth, but it keeps the benign neoplasm as a discrete, readily palpable, and easily movable mass that can be surgically enucleated (Figs. 7–14 and 7–15). Although a well-defined cleavage plane exists around most benign tumors, in some it is lacking. Thus, hemangiomas (neoplasms composed of tangled blood vessels) are often unencapsulated and may appear to permeate the site in which they arise (commonly the dermis of the skin).

The growth of cancers is accompanied by progressive infiltration, invasion, and destruction of the surrounding tissue. In general, malignant tumors are poorly demarcated from the surrounding normal tissue, and a well-defined cleavage plane is lacking (Figs. 7–16 and 7–17). Slowly expanding malignant tumors, however, may develop an apparently enclosing fibrous capsule and may push along a broad front into adjacent normal structures. Histologic examination of such apparently encapsulated masses almost always shows rows of cells penetrating the margin and infiltrating the adjacent structures, a crablike pattern of growth that constitutes the popular image of cancer.

Most malignant tumors are obviously invasive and can be expected to penetrate the wall of the colon or uterus, for example, or fungate through the surface of the skin. They recognize no normal anatomic boundaries. Such invasiveness makes their surgical resection difficult, and even if the tumor appears well circumscribed, it is necessary to remove a considerable margin of apparently normal tissues adjacent to the infiltrative neoplasm. *Next to the development of metastases, invasiveness is the most reliable feature that differentiates malignant from benign tumors.* We noted earlier that some cancers

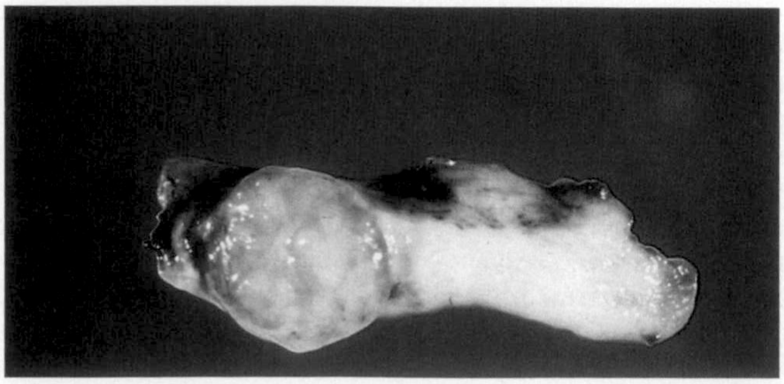

FIGURE 7–14 Fibroadenoma of the breast. The tan-colored, encapsulated small tumor is sharply demarcated from the whiter breast tissue.

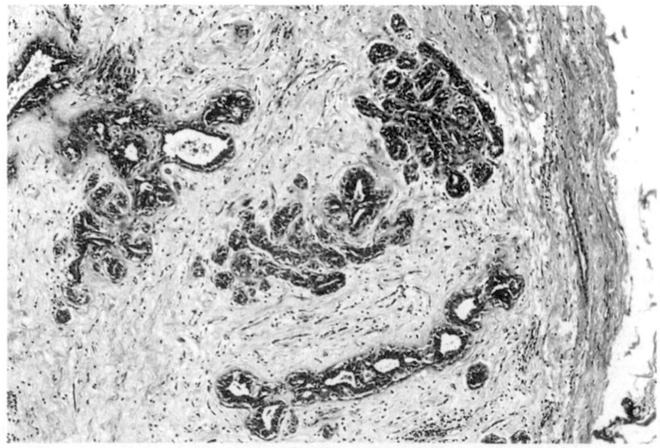

FIGURE 7–15 Microscopic view of fibroadenoma of the breast seen in Figure 7–14. The fibrous capsule (*right*) delimits the tumor from the surrounding tissue. (Courtesy of Dr. Trace Worrell, University of Texas Southwestern Medical School, Dallas, TX.)

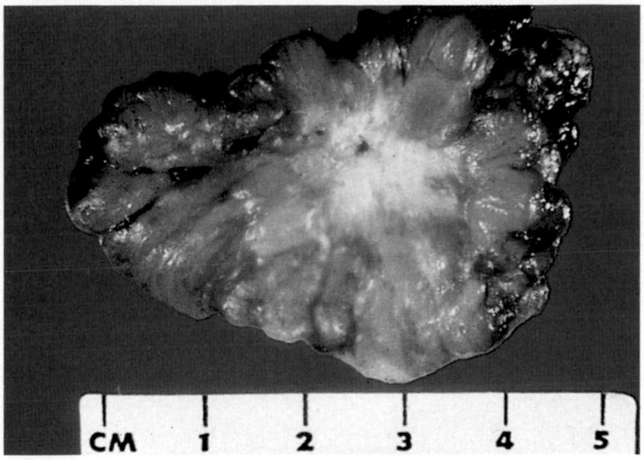

FIGURE 7–16 Cut section of an invasive ductal carcinoma of the breast. The lesion is retracted, infiltrating the surrounding breast substance, and would be stony hard on palpation.

seem to evolve from a preinvasive stage referred to as *carcinoma in situ.* This commonly occurs in tumors of the skin, breast, and certain other sites and is best illustrated by carcinoma of the uterine cervix (Chapter 23). *In situ epithelial cancers display the cytologic features of malignancy without invasion of the basement membrane.* They may be considered one step removed from invasive cancer; with time, most penetrate the basement membrane and invade the subepithelial stroma.

METASTASIS

Metastases are tumor implants discontinuous with the primary tumor. *Metastasis unequivocally marks a tumor as malignant because benign neoplasms do not metastasize.* The invasiveness of cancers permits them to penetrate into blood vessels, lymphatics, and body cavities, providing the opportunity for spread. *With few exceptions, all cancers can metastasize.* The major exceptions are most malignant neoplasms of the glial cells in the central nervous system, called *gliomas,* and basal cell carcinomas of the skin. Both are locally invasive forms of neoplasia (the latter being known in the older literature as *rodent ulcers* because of their invasive destructiveness), but they rarely metastasize. It is evident then that the properties of invasion and metastasis are separable. At the molecular level, however, invasion and metastases represent a continuum of changes.

In general, the more aggressive, the more rapidly growing, and the larger the primary neoplasm, the greater the likelihood that it will metastasize or already has metastasized. There are innumerable exceptions, however. Small, well-differentiated, slowly growing lesions sometimes metastasize widely; conversely, some rapidly growing, large lesions remain localized for years. No judgment can be made about the probability of metastasis from pathologic examination of the primary tumor. Many factors relating to both invader and host are involved.

Approximately 30% of newly diagnosed patients with solid tumors (excluding skin cancers other than melanomas) present with metastases. Metastatic spread strongly reduces the possibility of cure; hence, short of prevention of cancer, no achievement would confer greater benefit on patients than methods to block distant spread.

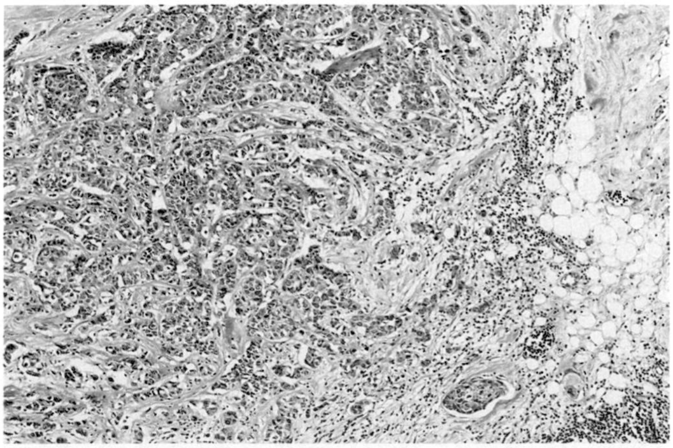

FIGURE 7–17 The microscopic view of the breast carcinoma seen in Figure 7–16 illustrates the invasion of breast stroma and fat by nests and cords of tumor cells (compare with fibroadenoma shown in Fig. 7–15). The absence of a well-defined capsule should be noted. (Courtesy of Dr. Trace Worrell, University of Texas Southwestern Medical School, Dallas, TX.)

Pathways of Spread

Dissemination of cancers may occur through one of three pathways: (1) direct seeding of body cavities or surfaces, (2) lymphatic spread, and (3) hematogenous spread. Although direct transplantation of tumor cells, as for example on surgical instruments, may theoretically occur, it is rare and we do not discuss this artificial mode of dissemination further. Each of the three major pathways is described separately.

Seeding of Body Cavities and Surfaces. Seeding of body cavities and surfaces may occur whenever a malignant neoplasm penetrates into a natural "open field." Most often involved is the peritoneal cavity (Fig. 7–18), but any other cavity—pleural, pericardial, subarachnoid, and joint space—may be affected. Such seeding is particularly characteristic of carcinomas arising in the ovaries, when, not infrequently, all peritoneal surfaces become coated with a heavy layer of cancerous glaze. Remarkably, the tumor cells may remain confined to the surface of the coated abdominal viscera without penetrating into the substance. Sometimes mucus-secreting appendiceal carcinomas fill the peritoneal cavity with a gelatinous neoplastic mass referred to as *pseudomyxoma peritonei.*

Lymphatic Spread. Transport through lymphatics is the most common pathway for the initial dissemination of carcinomas (Fig. 7–19), and sarcomas may also use this route. Tumors do not contain functional lymphatics, but lymphatic vessels located at the tumor margins are apparently sufficient for the lymphatic spread of tumor cells.[11] The emphasis on lymphatic spread for carcinomas and hematogenous spread for sarcomas is misleading because ultimately there are numerous interconnections between the vascular and the lymphatic systems. *The pattern of lymph node involvement follows the natural routes of lymphatic drainage.* Because carcinomas of the breast usually arise in the upper outer quadrants, they generally disseminate first to the axillary lymph nodes. Cancers of the inner quadrant may drain through lymphatics

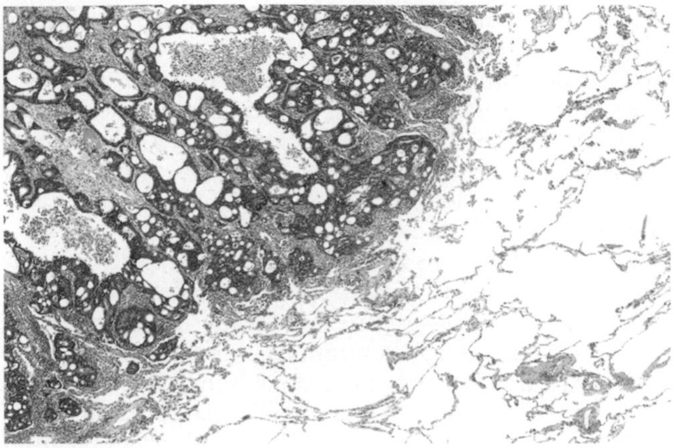

FIGURE 7–18 Colon carcinoma invading pericolonic adipose tissue. (Courtesy of Dr. Melissa Upton, University of Washington, Seattle, WA.)

to the nodes within the chest along the internal mammary arteries. Thereafter the infraclavicular and supraclavicular nodes may become involved. However, breast cancer is now considered to be a systemic disease even at the time of detection, and treatment is directed to both local control and the eradication of occult systemic micrometastases.[12] Carcinomas of the lung arising in the major respiratory passages metastasize first to the perihilar tracheobronchial and mediastinal nodes. Local lymph nodes, however, may be bypassed—"skip metastasis"—because of venous–lymphatic anastomoses or because inflammation or radiation has obliterated lymphatic channels.

In breast cancer, determining the involvement of axillary lymph nodes is very important for assessing the future course of the disease and for selecting suitable therapeutic strategies. Usually, lymphatic spread of breast cancers is assessed by performing a full axillary lymph node dissection. Because this procedure is associated with considerable surgical morbidity, *biopsy of sentinel nodes* is often used. A sentinel lymph node is defined as "the first node in a regional lymphatic basin that receives lymph flow from the primary tumor."[13] Sentinel node mapping can be done by injection of radiolabeled tracers or blue dyes, but the combination of these techniques provides the best results. Sentinel node identification has also been used for detecting the spread of melanomas, colon cancers, and other tumors.[13,14]

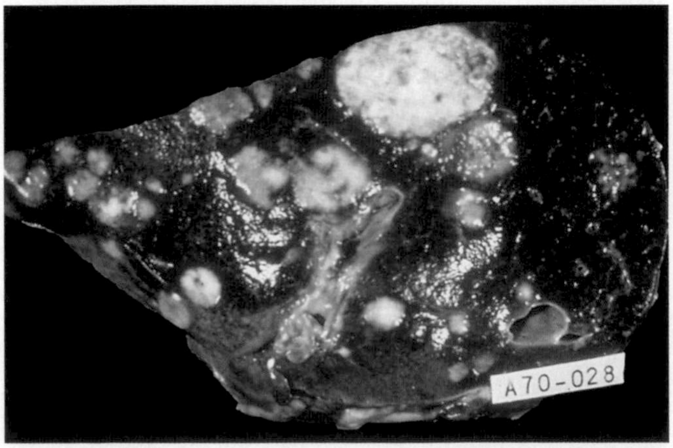

FIGURE 7–20 A liver studded with metastatic cancer.

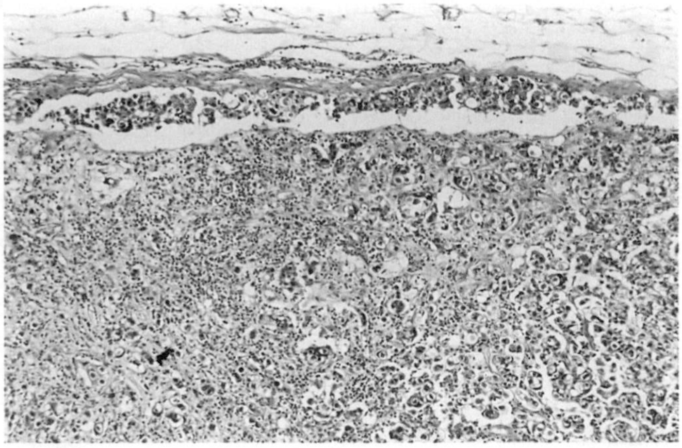

FIGURE 7–19 Axillary lymph node with metastatic breast carcinoma. The subcapsular sinus *(top)* is distended with tumor cells. Nests of tumor cells have also invaded the subcapsular cortex. (Courtesy of Dr. Trace Worrell, University of Texas Southwestern Medical School, Dallas, TX.)

In many cases, the regional nodes serve as effective barriers to further dissemination of the tumor, at least for a time. Conceivably the cells, after arrest within the node, may be destroyed by a tumor-specific immune response. Drainage of tumor cell debris or tumor antigens, or both, also induces reactive changes within nodes. Thus, enlargement of nodes may be caused by (1) the spread and growth of cancer cells or (2) reactive hyperplasia (Chapter 14). Therefore, *nodal enlargement in proximity to a cancer does not necessarily mean dissemination of the primary lesion.*

Hematogenous Spread. Hematogenous spread is typical of sarcomas but is also seen with carcinomas. Arteries, with their thicker walls, are less readily penetrated than are veins. Arterial spread may occur, however, when tumor cells pass through the pulmonary capillary beds or pulmonary arteriovenous shunts or when pulmonary metastases themselves give rise to additional tumor emboli. In such arterial spread, a number of factors condition the patterns of distribution of the metastases. With venous invasion, the blood-borne cells follow the venous flow draining the site of the neoplasm. Understandably the liver and lungs are most frequently involved secondarily in such hematogenous dissemination (Figs. 7–20 and 7–21). All portal area drainage flows to the

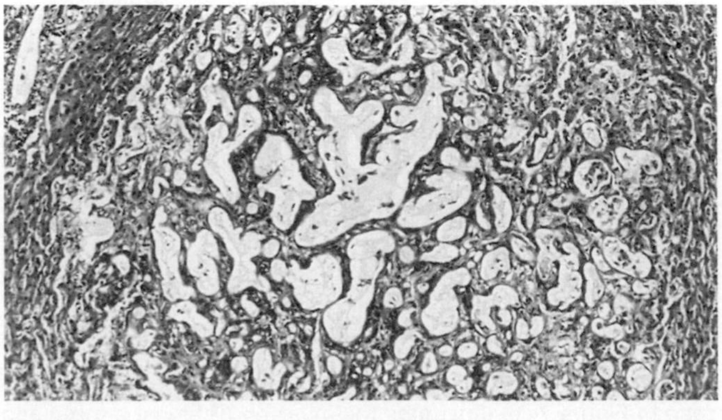

FIGURE 7–21 Microscopic view of liver metastasis. A pancreatic adenocarcinoma has formed a metastatic nodule in the liver. (Courtesy of Dr. Trace Worrell, University of Texas Southwestern Medical School, Dallax, TX.)

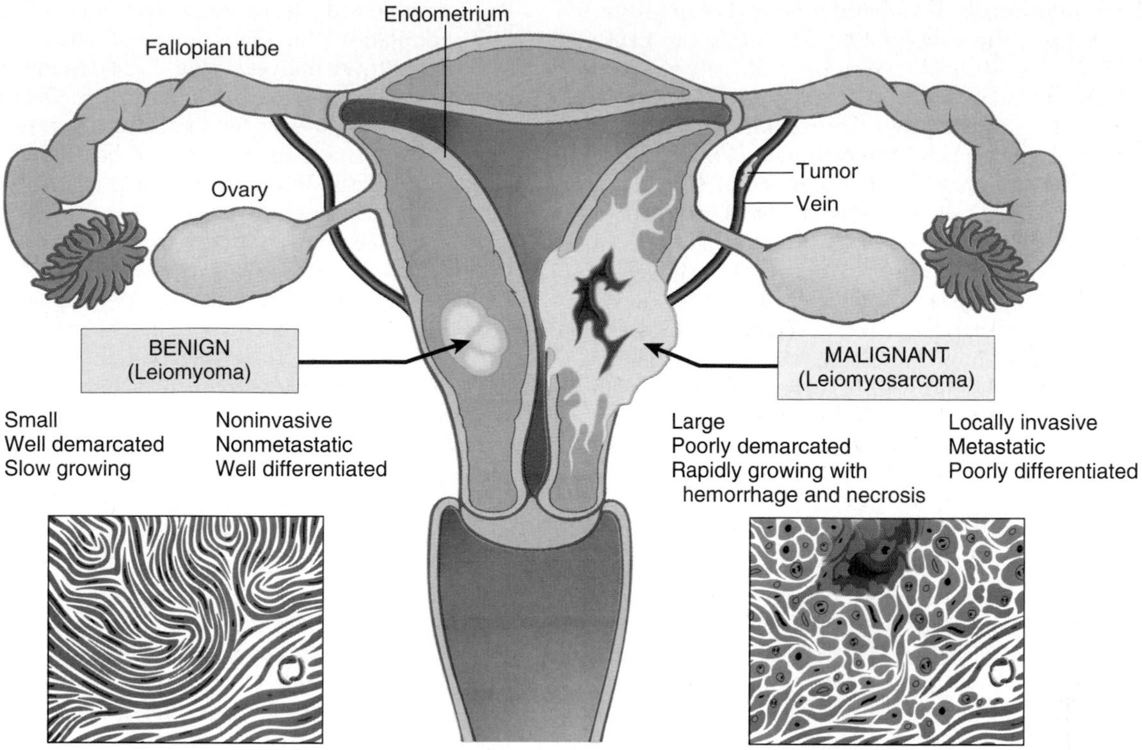

FIGURE 7–22 Comparison between a benign tumor of the myometrium (leiomyoma) and a malignant tumor of similar origin (leiomyosarcoma).

liver, and all caval blood flows to the lungs. Cancers arising in close proximity to the vertebral column often embolize through the paravertebral plexus, and this pathway is probably involved in the frequent vertebral metastases of carcinomas of the thyroid and prostate.

Certain cancers have a propensity for invasion of veins. Renal cell carcinoma often invades the branches of the renal vein and then the renal vein itself to grow in a snakelike fashion up the inferior vena cava, sometimes reaching the right side of the heart. Hepatocellular carcinomas often penetrate portal and hepatic radicles to grow within them into the main venous channels. Remarkably, such intravenous growth may not be accompanied by widespread dissemination. Histologic evidence of penetration of small vessels at the site of the primary neoplasm is obviously an ominous feature. Such changes, however, must be viewed guardedly because, for reasons discussed later, they do not indicate the inevitable development of metastases.

The distinguishing features of benign and malignant tumors discussed in this overview are summarized in Table 7–2 and Figure 7–22. With this background on the structure and behavior of neoplasms, we now discuss the origin of tumors, starting with insights gained from the epidemiology of cancer and followed by the molecular basis of carcinogenesis.

Epidemiology

Because cancer is a disorder of cell growth and behavior, its ultimate cause has to be defined at the cellular and subcellular levels. Study of cancer patterns in populations, however,

TABLE 7–2 Comparisons Between Benign and Malignant Tumors

Characteristics	Benign	Malignant
Differentiation/anaplasia	Well differentiated; structure may be typical of tissue of origin	Some lack of differentiation with anaplasia; structure is often atypical
Rate of growth	Usually progressive and slow; may come to a standstill or regress; mitotic figures are rare and normal	Erratic and may be slow to rapid; mitotic figures may be numerous and abnormal
Local invasion	Usually cohesive and expansile well-demarcated masses that do not invade or infiltrate surrounding normal tissues	Locally invasive, infiltrating the surrounding normal tissues; sometimes may be seemingly cohesive and expansile
Metastasis	Absent	Frequently present; the larger and more undifferentiated the primary, the more likely are metastases

can contribute substantially to knowledge about the origins of cancer. For example, the concept that chemicals can cause cancer arose from the astute observations of Sir Percival Pott, who related the increased incidence of scrotal cancer in chimney sweeps to chronic exposure to soot. Thus, major insights into the cause of cancer can be obtained by epidemiologic studies that relate particular environmental, hereditary, and cultural influences to the occurrence of malignant neoplasms. In addition, certain diseases associated with an increased risk of developing cancer can provide insights into the pathogenesis of malignancy. Therefore, in the following discussion, we first summarize the overall incidence of cancer to provide an insight into the magnitude of the cancer problem, and then review a number of factors relating to both the patient and the environment that influence predisposition to cancer.

CANCER INCIDENCE

In some measure, an individual's likelihood of developing a cancer is expressed by national incidence and mortality rates. For example, residents of the United States have about a one in five chance of dying of cancer. There were, it is estimated, about 556,000 deaths from cancer in 2003, representing 23% of all mortality,[3] a frequency surpassed only by deaths caused by cardiovascular diseases. These data do not include an additional 1 million, for the most part readily curable, nonmelanoma cancers of the skin and 100,000 cases of carcinoma in situ, largely of the uterine cervix but also of the breast. The major organ sites affected and the estimated frequency of cancer deaths are shown in Figure 7–23. The most common tumors in men are prostate, lung, and colorectal cancers. In women, cancers of the breast, lung, and colon and rectum are the most frequent. Cancers of the lung, female breast, prostate, and colon/rectum constitute more than 50% of cancer diagnoses and cancer deaths in the U.S. population.[15]

The age-adjusted death rates (number of deaths per 100,000 population) for many forms of cancer have significantly changed over the years (Fig. 7–24). Many of the long-term temporal comparisons are noteworthy. Over the past 50 years, the overall age-adjusted cancer death rate has significantly increased in men, whereas it has fallen slightly in women. The increase in men can be largely attributed to lung cancer. The improvement in women is mainly attributable to a significant decline in death rates from cancers of the uterus, stomach, liver, and most notably, carcinoma of the cervix, one of the most common forms of malignant neoplasia in women. Striking is the alarming increase in deaths from carcinoma of the lung in both sexes. In women, carcinomas of the breast occur about 2.5 times more frequently than those of the lung. Because of the large difference in the cure rates of these two cancers, however, lung cancer has become the leading cause of cancer deaths in women. The decline in the number of deaths caused by uterine, including cervical, cancer probably relates to earlier diagnosis and more cures made possible by the Papanicolaou (Pap) smear. The downward trend in deaths from stomach cancer has been attributed to a decrease in some dietary carcinogens, as a consequence of better food preservation or changes in dietary habits. Deaths from primary liver cancers, which declined between 1930 and 1970, have approximately doubled during the past 30 years.[16]

The most recent statistical data have brought some good news: the age-adjusted cancer death rates in the United States between 1990 and 2000 declined for both men and women.[4,15] For all types of cancers, the death rate declined 1.5% per year in males and 0.6% per year in females. Although race is strictly not a biologic categorization, it can define groups at risk for certain cancers.[17,18] The disparity in cancer mortality rates between white and black Americans persists, but African Americans had the largest decline in cancer mortality during the past decade. Hispanics living in the United States have a lower frequency of the most common tumors than the white

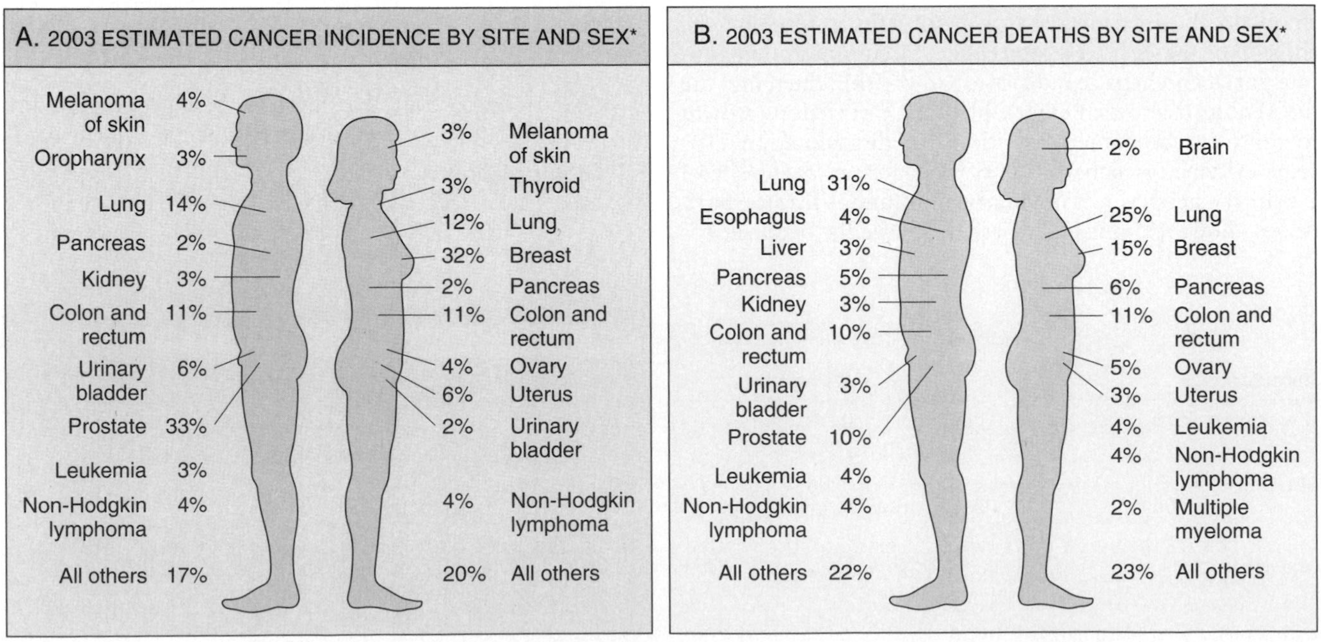

FIGURE 7–23 Cancer incidence and mortality by site and sex. Excludes basal cell and squamous cell skin cancers and in situ carcinomas, except urinary bladder. (Adapted from Jemal A, et al: Cancer statistics, 2003. CA Cancer J Clin 53:5, 2003.)

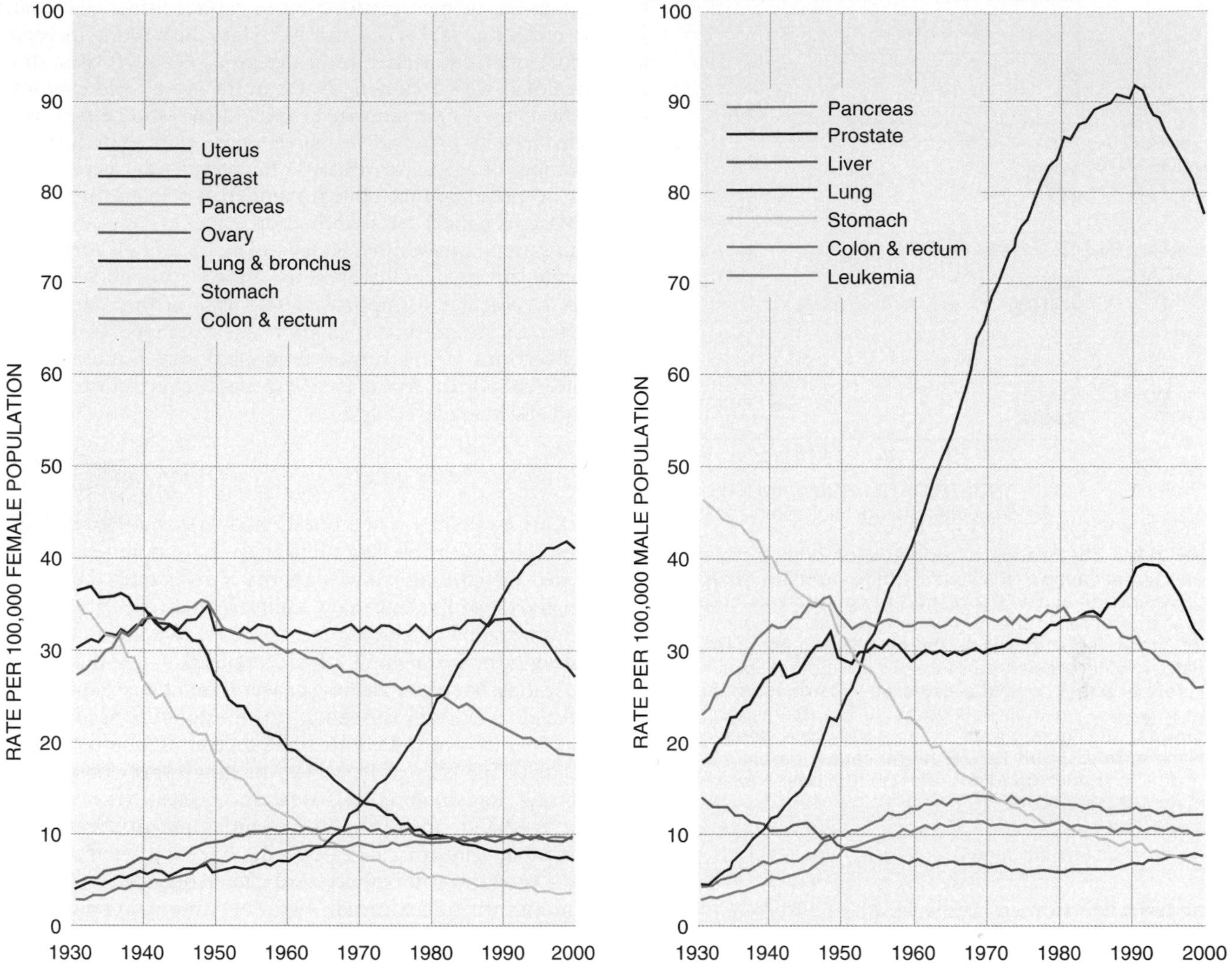

FIGURE 7–24 Age-adjusted cancer death rates for selected sites in the United States, adjusted for the 2000 U.S. population. (Adapted from Jemal A, et al: Cancer statistics, 2003. CA Cancer J Clin 53:5, 2003.)

non-Hispanic population but a higher incidence of tumors of the stomach, liver, uterine cervix, and gallbladder.[19] In contrast with the encouraging trends in cancer mortality in the overall population, the news is mixed regarding cancer incidence. During the past decade, it stabilized in males but increased at a rate of 0.3% per year in women.

GEOGRAPHIC AND ENVIRONMENTAL FACTORS

Remarkable differences can be found in the incidence and death rates of specific forms of cancer around the world.[1,2] For example, the death rate for stomach carcinoma in both men and women is seven to eight times higher in Japan than in the United States. In contrast, the death rate from carcinoma of the lung is slightly more than twice as great in the United States as in Japan, and in Belgium it is even higher than in the United States. Skin cancer deaths, largely caused by melanomas, are six times more frequent in New Zealand than in Iceland, which is probably attributable to differences in sun exposure. Although racial predispositions cannot be ruled out, it is generally believed that most of these geographic differences are the consequence of environmental influences. This is best brought out by comparing mortality rates for Japanese immigrants to the United States and Japanese born in the United States of immigrant parents (Nisei) with those of long-term residents of both countries. Figure 7–25 indicates that cancer mortality rates for first-generation Japanese immigrants are intermediate between those of natives of Japan and natives of California, and the two rates come closer with each passing generation. This points strongly to environmental and cultural factors rather than genetic predisposition. There is no paucity of environmental factors: they are found in the ambient environment, in the workplace, in food, and in personal practices.

The carcinogenicity of ultraviolet (UV) rays and many drugs is discussed in a later section. Asbestos, vinyl chloride, and 2-naphthylamine can serve as examples of occupational hazards, and many others are listed in Table 7–3; the risks may be incurred in lifestyle and personal exposures (e.g., dietary influences). Overall, mortality data indicate that the most overweight individuals in the U.S. population have a 52%

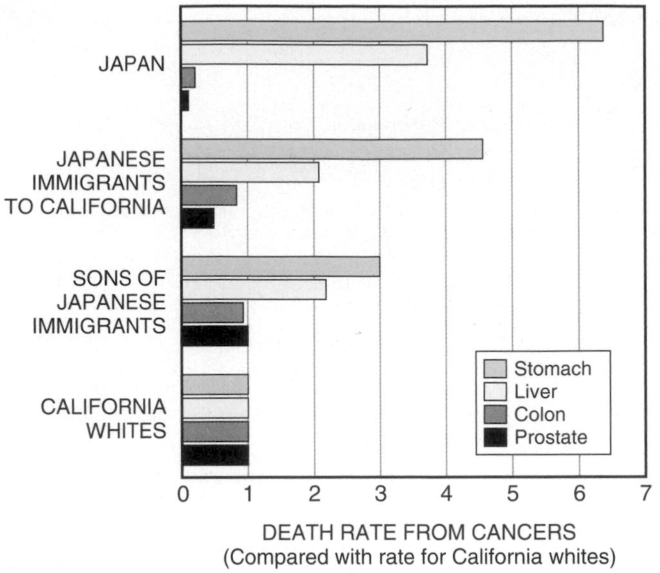

FIGURE 7–25 The change in incidence of various cancers with migration from Japan to the United States provides evidence that the occurrence of cancers is related to components of the environment that differ in the two countries. The incidence of each kind of cancer is expressed as the ratio of the death rate in the population being considered to that in a hypothetical population of California whites with the same age distribution; the death rates for whites are thus defined as 1. The death rates among immigrants and immigrants' sons tend consistently toward California norms. (From Cairns J: The cancer problem. In Readings from Scientific American—Cancer Biology. New York, WH Freeman, 1986, p. 13.)

(men) and 62% (women) higher death rate from cancer than do their slimmer counterparts. It has been estimated that overweight and obesity may account for approximately 14% of cancer deaths in men and 20% in women.[20] Alcohol abuse alone increases the risk of carcinomas of the oropharynx (excluding lip), larynx, and esophagus and, through the intermediation of alcoholic cirrhosis, carcinoma of the liver. Smoking, particularly of cigarettes, has been implicated in cancer of the mouth, pharynx, larynx, esophagus, pancreas, and bladder but most significantly, it is responsible for about 90% of lung cancer deaths (Chapter 9). Cigarette smoking has been called the single most important environmental factor contributing to premature death in the United States. Alcohol and tobacco together multiply the danger of incurring cancers in the upper aerodigestive tract. The risk of cervical cancer is linked to age at first intercourse and the number of sex partners. These associations point to a possible causal role for venereal transmission of cervical viral infections. It begins to appear that almost everything one does to gain a livelihood or for pleasure is fattening, immoral, illegal, or, even worse, oncogenic.

AGE

Age has an important influence on the likelihood of being afflicted with cancer. Most carcinomas occur in the later years of life (≥ 55 years). Cancer is the main cause of death among women aged 40 to 79 and among men aged 60 to 79. Each age group has its own predilection to certain forms of cancer, as is evident in Tables 7–4 and 7–5. Here the striking increase in mortality from cancer in the age group 60 to 79 years should be noted. The decline in deaths in the age 80 and over group reflects the lower number of individuals who reach this age. This trend is expected to change in the coming decade, as the number of aged individuals in the population increases. Also to be noted is that children under age 15 are not spared. Cancer accounts for slightly more than 10% of all deaths in this group in the United States and is second only to accidents. Acute leukemia and neoplasms of the central nervous system are responsible for approximately 60% of these deaths. The common neoplasms of infancy and childhood include neuroblastoma, Wilms tumor, retinoblastoma, acute leukemias, and rhabdomyosarcomas. These are discussed in Chapter 10 and elsewhere in the text.

GENETIC PREDISPOSITION TO CANCER

One frequently asked question is: "My mother and father both died of cancer. Does that mean I am doomed to get it?" Based on current knowledge, the answer must be carefully qualified.[21–23] Evidence now indicates that for a large number of cancer types, including the most common forms, there exist not only environmental influences but also hereditary predispositions. For example, lung cancer is in most instances clearly related to cigarette smoking, yet mortality from lung cancer has been shown to be four times greater among nonsmoking relatives (parents and siblings) of lung cancer patients than among nonsmoking relatives of controls (the effects of second-hand smoke may confound some of these results). Less than 10% of cancer patients have inherited mutations that predispose to cancer, and the frequency is even lower (around 0.1%) for certain types of tumors. Despite the low frequency, the recognition of inherited predisposition to cancer has had a major impact on the understanding of cancer pathogenesis. Moreover, genes that are causally associated with cancers that have a strong hereditary component are generally also involved in the much more common sporadic forms of the same tumor. Genetic predisposition to cancer can be divided into three categories (Table 7–6).

Autosomal Dominant Inherited Cancer Syndromes. Inherited cancer syndromes include several well-defined cancers in which inheritance of a single mutant gene greatly increases the risk of developing a tumor. The predisposition to these tumors shows an autosomal dominant pattern of inheritance. The inherited mutation is usually a point mutation occurring in a single allele of a tumor suppressor gene. The defect in the second allele occurs in somatic cells, generally as a consequence of chromosome deletion or recombination. Childhood *retinoblastoma* is the most striking example in this category. Approximately 40% of retinoblastomas are inherited. Carriers of a mutant of the *RB tumor suppressor gene* have a 10,000-fold increased risk of developing retinoblastoma, usually bilateral. They also have a greatly increased risk of developing a second cancer, particularly osteogenic sarcoma. Familial adenomatous polyposis is another hereditary disorder marked by an extraordinarily high risk of cancer. Individuals who inherit the autosomal dominant mutation of the adenomatous polyposis coli *(APC)* tumor suppressor gene have at birth or soon thereafter innumerable polypoid ade-

TABLE 7–3 Occupational Cancers

Agents or Groups of Agents	Human Cancer Site for Which Reasonable Evidence Is Available	Typical Use or Occurrence
Arsenic and arsenic compounds	Lung, skin, hemangiosarcoma	Byproduct of metal smelting. Component of alloys, electrical and semiconductor devices, medications and herbicides, fungicides, and animal dips
Asbestos	Lung, mesothelioma; gastrointestinal tract (esophagus, stomach, large intestine)	Formerly used for many applications because of fire, heat, and friction resistance; still found in existing construction as well as fire-resistant textiles, friction materials (i.e., brake linings), underlayment and roofing papers, and floor tiles
Benzene	Leukemia, Hodgkin lymphoma	Principal component of light oil. Although use as solvent is discouraged, many applications exist in printing and lithography, paint, rubber, dry cleaning, adhesives and coatings, and detergents. Formerly widely used as solvent and fumigant
Beryllium and beryllium compounds	Lung	Missile fuel and space vehicles. Hardener for lightweight metal alloys, particularly in aerospace applications and nuclear reactors
Cadmium and cadmium compounds	Prostate	Uses include yellow pigments and phosphors. Found in solders. Used in batteries and as alloy and in metal platings and coatings
Chromium compounds	Lung	Component of metal alloys, paints, pigments, and preservatives
Ethylene oxide	Leukemia	Ripening agent for fruits and nuts. Used in rocket propellant and chemical synthesis, in fumigants for foodstuffs and textiles, and in sterilants for hospital equipment
Nickel compounds	Nose, lung	Nickel plating. Component of ferrous alloys, ceramics, and batteries. Byproduct of stainless steel arc welding
Radon and its decay products	Lung	From decay of minerals containing uranium. Can be serious hazard in quarries and underground mines
Vinyl chloride	Angiosarcoma, liver	Refrigerant. Monomer for vinyl polymers. Adhesive for plastics. Formerly inert aerosol propellant in pressurized containers

Modified from Stellman JM, Stellman SD: Cancer and workplace. CA Cancer J Clin 46:70, 1996.

nomas of the colon and in virtually 100% of cases are fated to develop a carcinoma of the colon by age 50. Other autosomal dominant cancer syndromes are the Li-Fraumeni syndrome resulting from germ line mutations of the *p53* gene, multiple endocrine neoplasia types 1 and 2 (MEN-1 and MEN-2), and hereditary nonpolyposis colon cancer (*HNPCC*), a condition caused by inactivation of a mismatch repair gene (also listed below among repair defects).

There are several features that characterize inherited cancer syndromes:

- In each syndrome, tumors involve specific sites and tissues, although they may involve more than one site. For example, in MEN-2, caused by a mutation of the *RET* protooncogene, thyroid, parathyroid, and adrenals are involved. There is no increase in predisposition to cancers in general.
- Tumors within this group are often associated with a specific marker phenotype. For example, there may be multiple benign tumors in the affected tissue, as occurs in familial polyposis of the colon and in MEN. Sometimes, there are abnormalities in tissue that are not the target of transformation (e.g., Lisch nodules and café-au-lait spots in neurofibromatosis type 1; see Chapter 5).
- As in other autosomal dominant conditions, both incomplete penetrance and variable expressivity occur.

Defective DNA Repair Syndromes. Besides the dominantly inherited precancerous conditions, a group of cancer-predisposing conditions is collectively characterized by defects in DNA repair and resultant DNA instability. These conditions generally have an autosomal recessive pattern of inheritance. Included in this group are xeroderma pigmentosum, ataxia-telangectasia, and Bloom syndrome, all rare diseases characterized by genetic instability resulting from defects in DNA repair genes. Also included here is hereditary nonpolypoid colon cancer (HNPCC), an autosomal dominant condition caused by inactivation of a DNA mismatch repair gene.[24] HNPCC is the most common cancer predisposition syndrome, increasing the susceptibility to cancer in the colon and also in some other organs such as the small intestine, endometrium, and ovary (Chapter 17).

Familial Cancers. Besides the inherited syndromes of cancer susceptibility, cancer may occur at higher frequency in certain families without a clearly defined pattern of transmission. Virtually all the common types of cancers that occur sporadically have also been reported to occur in familial forms. Examples include carcinomas of colon, breast, ovary, and

TABLE 7–4 Reported Deaths for the Five Leading Cancer Types for Males by Age, US, 2000

All Ages	Under Age 20	Age 20–39	Age 40–59	Age 60–70	Age 80+
All cancers	*All cancers*	*All cancers*	*All cancers*	*All cancers*	*All cancers*
286,082	1298	4832	50,069	158,990	70,883
Lung and bronchus	Leukemia	Brain and ONS*	Lung and bronchus	Lung and bronchus	Lung and bronchus
90,415	430	626	15,827	57,470	16,626
Prostate	Brain and ONS*	Leukemia	Colon and rectum	Colon and rectum	Prostate
31,078	307	611	4801	15,420	15,630
Colon and rectum	Bones and joints	Lung and bronchus	Pancreas	Prostate	Colon and rectum
28,484	105	481	2929	14,428	7821
Pancreas	Endocrine system	Non-Hodgkin lymphoma	Esophagus	Pancreas	Urinary Bladder
14,238	104	444	2345	8179	3222
Non-Hodgkin lymphoma	Non-Hodgkin lymphoma	Colon and rectum	Liver	Non-Hodgkin lymphoma	Leukemia
11,812	79	431	2308	6107	3187

"All Cancers" excludes in situ carcinomas except urinary bladder. *ONS = other nervous system.
Source: US Mortality Public Use Data Tape, 2000, National Center for Health Statistics, Centers for Disease Control and Prevention, Hyattsville, MD 2002.

brain, as well as melanomas. *Features that characterize familial cancers include early age at onset, tumors arising in two or more close relatives of the index case, and sometimes, multiple or bilateral tumors.* Familial cancers are not associated with specific marker phenotypes. For example, in contrast to the familial adenomatous polyp syndrome, familial colonic cancers do not arise in pre-existing benign polyps. The transmission pattern of familial cancers is not clear. In general, siblings have a relative risk between two and three (two to three times greater than unrelated individuals). Segregation analyses of large families usually show that predisposition to the tumors is dominant, but multifactorial inheritance cannot be easily ruled out. It is likely that familial susceptibility to cancer may depend on multiple low-penetrance alleles, each contributing to only a small increase in the risk of tumor development. It has been estimated that 10% to 20% of patients with breast or ovarian cancer have a first- or second-degree relative with one of these tumors. Although two breast cancer susceptibility genes, named *BRCA1* and *BRCA2,* have been identified, mutation of these genes occurs in no more than 3% of breast cancers. Thus, mutations in *BRCA1* and *BRCA2* cannot account for the large proportion of familial breast cancers.[25] Changes in other genes, probably in low-penetrance susceptibility alleles, appear to be necessary for the development of these tumors. A similar situation occurs in familial melanomas, in which a mutation of the *p16INK4a* tumor suppressor gene has been identified. However, mutation in this gene accounts for only about 20% of familial melanoma kindreds, suggesting that other factors are involved in the familial predisposition.[26]

Interactions Between Genetic and Non-Genetic Factors. What can be said about the influence of heredity on the majority of malignant neoplasms? It could be argued that they are largely of environmental origin, but lack of family history does not preclude an inherited component. It is generally difficult to sort out the hereditary and acquired basis of a tumor because these factors often interact closely. The interaction between genetic and non-genetic factors is particularly complex when tumor development depends on the action of multiple contributory genes. Even in tumors with a well-defined inherited component, the risk of developing the tumor can be greatly influenced by non-genetic factors. For instance, breast cancer risk in female carriers of BRCA-1 or BRCA-2 mutations is almost three-fold higher for women born after 1940, compared to the risks for women born before that year.[27,28] Furthermore, the genotype can significantly influence the likelihood of developing environmentally induced cancers. Inherited variations (polymorphisms) of enzymes that metabolize procarcinogens to their active carcinogenic forms (see "Initiation of Carcinogenesis") can influence the susceptibility to cancer. Of interest in this regard are genes that encode the cytochrome P-450 enzymes. As discussed later under "Chemical Carcinogenesis," polymorphism at one of the P-450 loci confers inherited susceptibility to lung cancers in cigarette smokers. More such correlations are likely to be found.

NONHEREDITARY PREDISPOSING CONDITIONS

The only certain way of avoiding cancer is not to be born; to live is to incur the risk. The risk is greater than average, however, under many circumstances, as is evident from the predisposing influences discussed earlier. Certain clinical conditions are also important. Because cell replication is involved in neoplastic transformation, regenerative, hyperplastic, and dysplastic proliferations are fertile soil for the origin of a malignant tumor. There is a well-defined association between certain forms of endometrial hyperplasia and endometrial carcinoma and between cervical dysplasia and cervical carcinoma (Chapter 22). The bronchial mucosal metaplasia and dysplasia of habitual cigarette smokers are ominous

TABLE 7–5 Reported Deaths for the Five Leading Cancer Types for Females by Age, US, 2000

All Ages	Under Age 20	Age 20–39	Age 40–59	Age 60–70	Age 80+
All cancers	***All cancers***	***All cancers***	***All cancers***	***All cancers***	***All cancers***
267,009	973	5617	47,850	131,871	80,697
Lung and bronchus	Leukemia	Breast	Breast	Lung and bronchus	Lung and bronchus
65,016	302	1444	11,937	39,311	14,693
Breast	Brain and ONS*	Uterine cervix	Lung and bronchus	Breast	Colon and rectum
41,872	238	538	10,613	17,842	12,379
Colon and rectum	Endocrine system	Leukemia	Colon and rectum	Colon and rectum	Breast
28,950	82	452	3619	12,612	10,648
Pancreas	Bones and joints	Lung and bronchus	Ovary	Pancreas	Pancreas
15,094	76	397	3033	7825	5319
Ovary	Soft tissue	Brain and ONS*	Pancreas	Ovary	Non-Hodgkin lymphoma
14,060	69	354	1871	7217	4039

"All Cancers" excludes in situ carcinomas except urinary bladder. *ONS = other nervous system.
Source: US Mortality Public Use Data Tape, 2000, National Center for Health Statistics, Centers for Disease Control and Prevention, Hyattsville, MD, 2002.

antecedents of bronchogenic carcinoma. About 80% of hepatocellular carcinomas arise in cirrhotic livers, which are characterized by active parenchymal regeneration (Chapter 18).

Chronic Inflammation and Cancer. In 1863 Virchow proposed that *cancer develops at sites of chronic inflammation* and the potential relationships between cancer and inflammation have been studied since then.[29] This is exemplified by the increased risk of cancer development in patients affected by a variety of chronic inflammatory diseases of the gastrointestinal tract. These include ulcerative colitis, Crohn disease, *Helicobacter pylori* gastritis, viral hepatitis, and chronic pancreatitis. The precise mechanisms that link inflammation and cancer development have not been established.[30] Chronic inflammatory reactions may result in the production of cytokines, which stimulate the growth of transformed cells. In some cases, chronic inflammation may increase the pool of tissue stem cells, which become subject to the effect of mutagens. Interestingly, chronic inflammation may also directly promote genomic instability in cells through the production of reactive oxygen species (ROS), thus predisposing to malignant transformation. Whatever the precise mechanism, such a link may have practical implications. For instance, expression of the enzyme *cyclooxygenase-2 (COX-2)*, which converts arachidonic acid into prostaglandins (Chapter 2), is induced by inflammatory stimuli and is increased in colon cancers and other tumors.[31] The development of COX-2 inhibitors for cancer treatment is an active and promising area of research.[32]

Precancerous Conditions. Certain non-neoplastic disorders—*the chronic atrophic gastritis of pernicious anemia, solar keratosis of the skin, chronic ulcerative colitis, and leukoplakia of the oral cavity, vulva, and penis*—have such a well-defined association with cancer that they have been termed *precancerous conditions.* This designation is somewhat unfortunate because in the great majority of these lesions no malignant neoplasm emerges. Nonetheless, the term persists because it calls attention to the increased risk. Certain forms of benign neoplasia also constitute precancerous conditions. The villous adenoma of the colon, as it increases in size, develops cancerous change in up to 50% of cases. It might be asked: Is there not a risk with all benign neoplasms? Although some risk may be inherent, a large cumulative experience indicates that most benign neoplasms do not become cancerous. Nonetheless, numerous examples could be offered of cancers arising, albeit rarely, in benign tumors; for example, a leiomyosarcoma beginning in a leiomyoma, and carcinoma appearing in long-standing pleomorphic adenomas. Generalization is impossi-

TABLE 7–6 Inherited Predisposition to Cancer

Inherited Cancer Syndromes (Autosomal Dominant)

Gene	*Inherited Predisposition*
RB	Retinoblastoma
p53	Li-Fraumeni syndrome (various tumors)
p16INK4A	Melanoma
APC	Familial adenomatous polyposis/colon cancer
NF1, NF2	Neurofibromatosis 1 and 2
BRCA1, BRCA2	Breast and ovarian tumors
MEN1, RET	Multiple endocrine neoplasia 1 and 2
MSH2, MLH1, MSH6	Hereditary nonpolyposis colon cancer
PATCH	Nevoid basal cell carcinoma syndrome

Familial Cancers

Familial clustering of cases, but role of inherited predisposition not clear for each individual
- Breast cancer
- Ovarian cancer
- Pancreatic cancer

Inherited Autosomal Recessive Syndromes of Defective DNA Repair

- Xeroderma pigmentosum
- Ataxia-telangiectasia
- Bloom syndrome
- Fanconi anemia

ble because each type of benign neoplasm is associated with a particular level of risk ranging from virtually never to frequently. Only follow-up studies of large series of each neoplasm can establish the level of risk, and always the question remains: Did the cancer arise from a non-malignant cell in the benign tumor or did the benign tumor contain, from the outset, a silent or indolent malignant focus?

Molecular Basis of Cancer

The literature on the molecular basis of cancer continues to proliferate at such a rapid pace that it is easy to get lost in the growing forest of information. We list some fundamental principles before delving into the details of the molecular basis of cancer.

- *Nonlethal genetic damage lies at the heart of carcinogenesis.* Such genetic damage (or mutation) may be acquired by the action of environmental agents, such as chemicals, radiation, or viruses, or it may be inherited in the germ line. The term "environmental," used in this context, involves any acquired defect caused by exogenous agents or endogenous products of cell metabolism. Not all mutations, however, are "environmentally" induced. Some may be spontaneous and stochastic.
- *A tumor is formed by the clonal expansion of a single precursor cell that has incurred the genetic damage (i.e., tumors are monoclonal).* Clonality of tumors can be assessed in women who are heterozygous for polymorphic X-linked markers, such as the enzymes glucose-6-phosphate dehydrogenase (G6PD), iduronate-2-sulfatase and phosphoglycerate kinase. The principle underlying such an analysis is illustrated in Figure 7–26. The most commonly used method to determine tumor clonality involves the analysis of methylation patterns adjacent to the highly polymorphic locus of the human androgen receptor gene *(HUMARA)*.[33] The frequency of *HUMARA* polymorphism in the general population is more than 90%, so it is easy to establish clonality by showing that all the cells in a tumor express the same allele. For tumors with a specific translocation, such as in myeloid leukemias, the presence of the translocation can be used to assess clonality. Immunoglobulin receptor and T-cell receptor gene rearrangements serve as markers of clonality in B- and T-cell lymphomas, respectively.
- *Four classes of normal regulatory genes—the growth-promoting protooncogenes, the growth-inhibiting tumor suppressor genes, genes that regulate programmed cell death (apoptosis), and genes involved in DNA repair—are the principal targets of genetic damage.* Mutant alleles of protooncogenes are considered dominant because they transform cells despite the presence of a normal counterpart. In contrast, both normal alleles of the tumor suppressor genes must be damaged for transformation to occur, so this family of genes is sometimes referred to as *recessive oncogenes.* However, there are exceptions to this rule, and some tumor suppressor genes lose their suppressor activity when a single allele is lost or inactivated.[34] This loss of function of a recessive gene caused by damage of a single allele is called *haploinsufficiency.* Genes that regulate apoptosis may be dominant, as are protooncogenes, or they may behave as tumor suppressor genes.

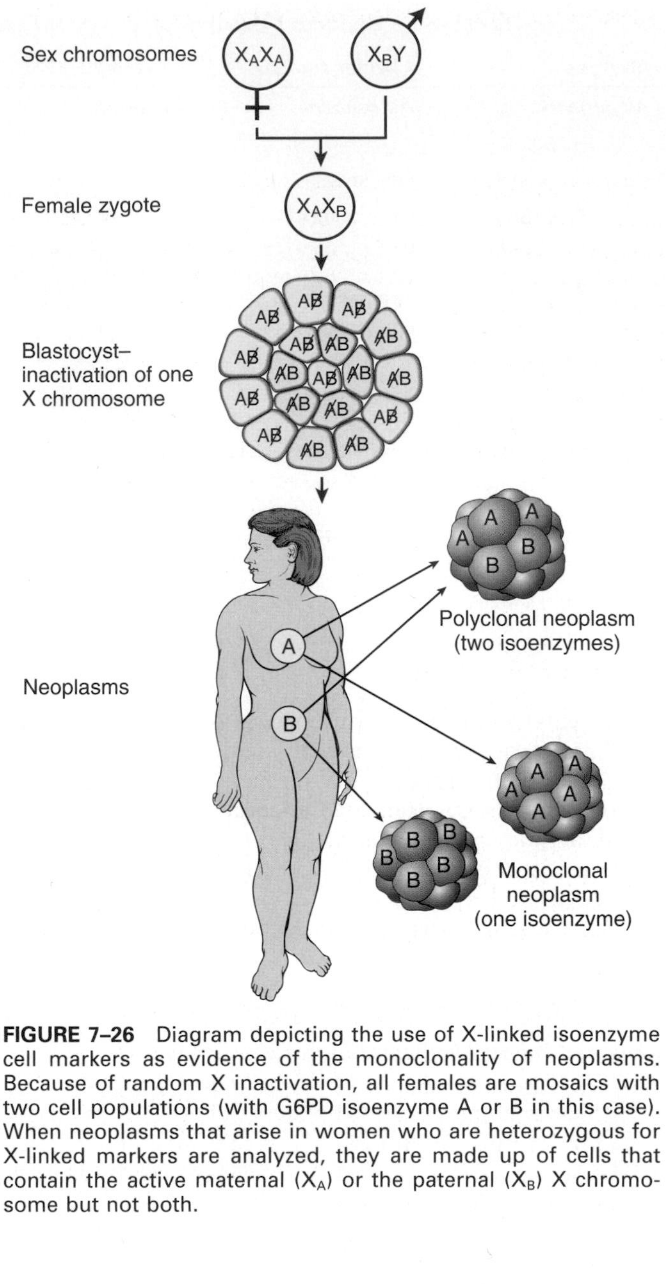

FIGURE 7–26 Diagram depicting the use of X-linked isoenzyme cell markers as evidence of the monoclonality of neoplasms. Because of random X inactivation, all females are mosaics with two cell populations (with G6PD isoenzyme A or B in this case). When neoplasms that arise in women who are heterozygous for X-linked markers are analyzed, they are made up of cells that contain the active maternal (X_A) or the paternal (X_B) X chromosome but not both.

- *DNA repair genes affect cell proliferation or survival indirectly by influencing the ability of the organism to repair nonlethal damage in other genes, including protooncogenes, tumor suppressor genes, and genes that regulate apoptosis.* A disability in the DNA repair genes can predispose to mutations in the genome and *hence to neoplastic transformation.* Such propensity to mutations is called a *mutator phenotype.*[35] With some exceptions, both alleles of DNA repair genes must be inactivated to induce such genomic instability; in this sense, DNA repair genes may also be considered as tumor suppressor genes.
- *Carcinogenesis is a multistep process at both the phenotypic and the genetic levels.* A malignant neoplasm has several phenotypic attributes, such as excessive growth, local invasiveness, and the ability to form distant metastases. These characteristics are acquired in a stepwise fashion, a phenomenon called *tumor progression.* At the molecular level, progression results from accumulation of genetic

lesions that in some instances are favored by defects in DNA repair.

ESSENTIAL ALTERATIONS FOR MALIGNANT TRANSFORMATION

With this overview we can now address in some detail the molecular pathogenesis of cancer and then discuss the carcinogenic agents that inflict genetic damage. Over the past two decades, hundreds of cancer-associated genes have been discovered. Some, such as *p53,* are commonly mutated; others, such as *c-ABL,* are affected only in certain leukemias. Each of the cancer genes has a specific function, the dysregulation of which contributes to the origin or progression of malignancy. It is traditional to describe cancer-causing genes on the basis of their presumed function. It is beneficial, however, to consider cancer-related genes in the context of *seven fundamental changes in cell physiology that together determine malignant phenotype.*[36] (Another important change for tumor development is *the escape from immunity and rejection.* This property is discussed later in this chapter.)

- *Self-sufficiency in growth signals*: Tumors have the capacity to proliferate without external stimuli, usually as a consequence of oncogene activation.
- *Insensitivity to growth-inhibitory signals*: Tumors may not respond to molecules that are inhibitory to the proliferation of normal cells such as transforming growth factor-β (TGF-β), and direct inhibitors of cyclin-dependent kinases.
- *Evasion of apoptosis*: Tumors may be resistant to programmed cell death, as a consequence of inactivation of *p53* or other changes.
- *Defects in DNA repair*: Tumors may fail to repair DNA damage caused by carcinogens or unregulated cellular proliferation.
- *Limitless replicative potential*: Tumor cells have unrestricted proliferative capacity, associated with maintenance of telomere length and function.
- *Sustained angiogenesis*: Tumors are not able to grow without formation of a vascular supply, which is induced by various factors, the most important being vascular endothelial growth factor (VEGF).
- *Ability to invade and metastasize*: Tumor metastases are the cause of the vast majority of cancer deaths and depend on processes that are intrinsic to the cell or are initiated by signals from the tissue environment.

Mutations in genes that regulate these cellular traits are seen in every cancer. However, the precise genetic pathways that give rise to these attributes differ between cancers, even within the same organ. It is widely believed that the occurrence of mutations in cancer-causing genes is conditioned by the robustness of the DNA repair machinery of the cell. When genes that normally sense and repair DNA damage are impaired or lost, the resultant genomic instability favors mutations in genes that regulate the other acquired capabilities of cancer cells. The main principles of the molecular basis of cancer are summarized in simplified form in Fig. 7–27.

In the following sections, we first discuss the molecular regulation of the normal cell cycle, since cell-cycle abnormalities are fundamental to cancer growth and many of the genes that cause cancer perturb the cell cycle. This is followed by discussion of the genes involved in each of the seven biologic alterations listed earlier. We end with a discussion of epigenetic changes and chromosomal abnormalities in cancer.

THE NORMAL CELL CYCLE

As discussed in Chapter 3, resting (nondividing) cells are in the G_0 stage of the cell cycle and need to be recruited into the G_1 stage and beyond in order to undergo replication (Fig. 3–3). *The orderly progression of cells through the various phases of cell cycle is orchestrated by cyclins and cyclin-dependent kinases (CDKs), and by their inhibitors.*[37–40] CDKs drive the cell cycle by phosphorylating critical target proteins that are required for progression of the cells to the next phase of the cell cycle. CDKs are expressed constitutively during the cell cycle but in an inactive form. They are activated by phosphorylation after binding to the family of proteins called cyclins.[37] By contrast with CDKs, cyclins are synthesized during specific phases of the cell cycle, and their function is to activate the CDKs. On completion of this task, cyclin levels decline rapidly (Fig. 7–28). More than 15 cyclins have been identified; cyclins D, E, A, and B appear sequentially during the cell cycle and bind to one or more CDKs.

Cyclin D and RB Phosphorylation. Cyclin D, the first cyclin to increase in the cell cycle, appears in mid G_1 but is no longer detectable in the S phase (see Fig. 7–28). There are three forms of cyclin D, named D1, D2, and D3, but to simplify matters, we will use the general term "cyclin D." Cyclin D, like other cyclins, is unstable and is degraded through the *ubiquitin–proteasome pathway* (Chapter 1). During the G_1 phase of the cell cycle, cyclin D binds to and activates CDK4, forming a *cyclin D–CDK4 complex* (Fig. 7–29). This complex has a critical role in the cell cycle by phosphorylating the retinoblastoma susceptibility protein (RB). *The phosphorylation of RB is a molecular ON-OFF switch for the cell cycle.*[38] In its hypophosphorylated state, RB prevents cells from replicating by forming a tight, inactive complex with the transcription factor E2F. (E2F is a family of transcription factors, referred to here as "E2F.") Phosphorylation of RB dissociates the complex and releases the inhibition on E2F transcriptional activity (see below). *Thus, phosphorylation of RB eliminates the main barrier to cell-cycle progression and promotes cell replication.*

The molecular basis of the RB braking action on the cell cycle has been unraveled in elegant detail.[38,39] Hypophosphorylated RB, present in quiescent cells (in G_0 or early G_1), binds to a protein complex that contains E2F and a subunit called DP1. The E2F/DP1/RB complex binds to promoters of E2F-responsive genes. Bound to the E2F/DP1/RB complex, such genes are silent because RB recruits histone deacetylase, an enzyme that causes compaction of chromatin and inhibition of transcription (Figs. 7–29 and 7–30). When quiescent cells are stimulated by growth factors, the concentrations of cyclins D and E go up, resulting in the activation of cyclin D–CDK4 and cyclin E–CDK2 at the G_1/S restriction point and causing phosphorylation of RB. Hyperphosphorylated RB dissociates from the complex, activating the transcription of E2F target genes that are essential for progression through the S phase. These include cyclin E, DNA polymerases, thymidine kinase, dihydrofolate reductase, and several others. During the M phase, the phosphate groups are removed from RB by cellular phosphatases, thus regenerating the hypophosphorylated form of RB.

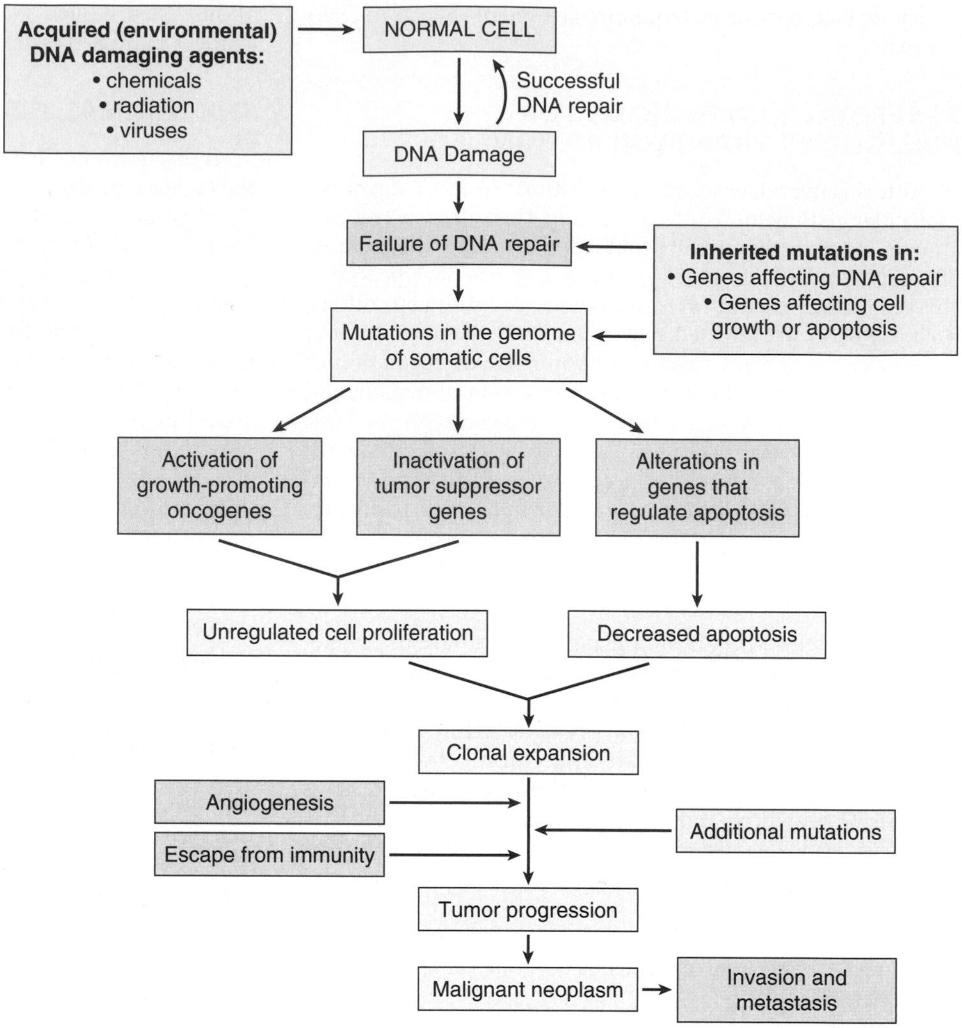

FIGURE 7–27 Flow chart depicting a simplified scheme of the molecular basis of cancer.

Cell-Cycle Progression Beyond the G_1/S Restriction Point. *Further progression through the S phase and the initiation of DNA replication involve the formation of an active complex between cyclin E and CDK2* (see Fig. 7–29). Activated E2F increases the transcription of cyclin E and of polymerases needed for DNA replication, thus stimulating DNA synthesis. The next decision point in the cell cycle is the G_2/M transition. This transition is initiated by the E2F-mediated transcription of cyclin A, which forms the cyclin A–CDK2 complex that regulates events at the mitotic prophase. The main mediator that propels the cell beyond prophase is the cyclin B–CDK1 complex, which is activated by a *protein phosphatase (Cdc 25)* and begins to accumulate in the nucleus in early prophase. Cyclin B–CDK1 activation causes the breakdown of the nuclear envelope and initiates mitosis. Complexes of CDKs with cyclins A (there are two cyclin A isoforms, A1 and A2; A2 is essential for the cell cycle) and B regulate some critical events at the G_2/M transition, such as the decrease in microtubule stability, the separation of centrosomes, and chromosome condensation. Exit from mitosis requires the inactivation of cyclin B–CDK1. Newly divided cells can then return to G_1 and initiate a new replicative cycle or go into quiescence. Recent data show that, in proliferating cells, cyclin E–CDK2 may be replaced in some of its functions by a complex between cyclin A2 and CDK1. However, the absence of both isoforms of cyclin E (E1 and E2) prevent quiescent cells from entering the cell cycle.[41]

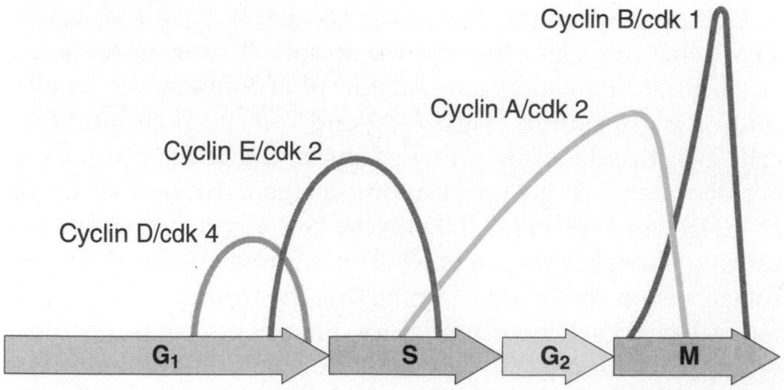

FIGURE 7–28 Expression of cyclin–cyclin-dependent kinase (CDK) complexes during the cell cycle. The phases of the cycle are indicated inside the arrows. (Modified from Pollard TD, Earnshaw WC: Cell Biology. Philadelphia, WB Saunders, 2002.)

Cell-Cycle Inhibitors. *The activity of cyclin–CDK complexes is tightly regulated by inhibitors, called CDK inhibitors.*[38–40] There are two main classes of CDK inhibitors: *the Cip/Kip and the INK4/ARF families* (see Fig. 7–29 and Table 7–7). These inhibitors function as tumor suppressors and are frequently altered in tumors (discussed below). The Cip/Kip family has

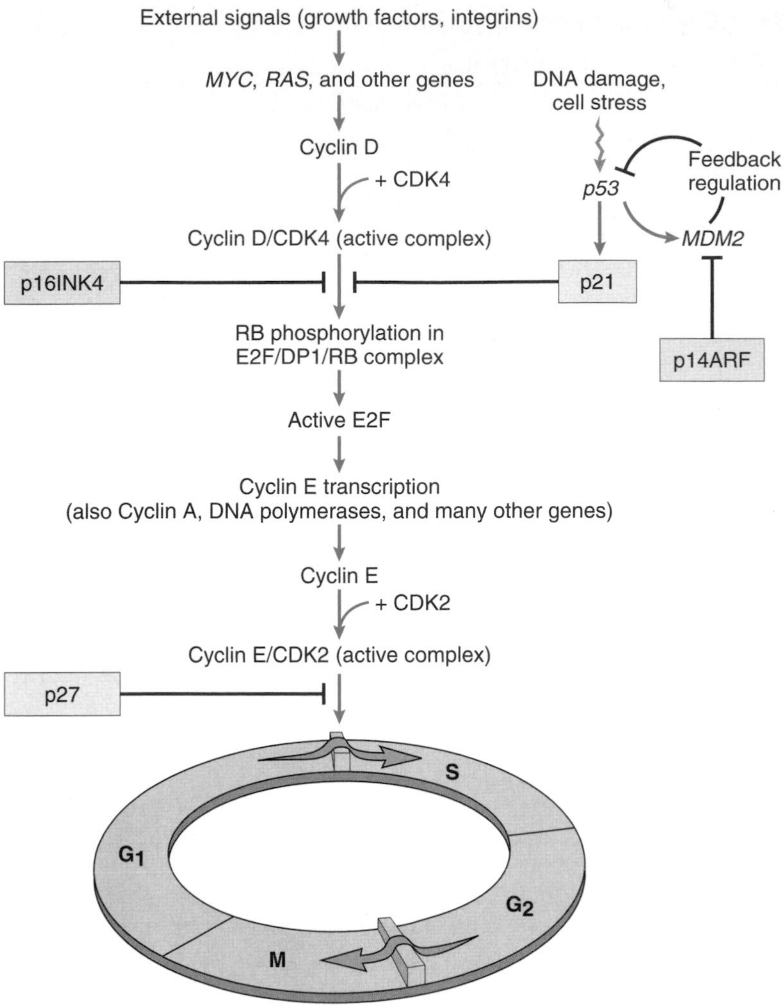

FIGURE 7–29 Schematic illustration of the role of cyclins, CDKs, and cyclin-dependent kinase inhibitors in regulating the G_1/S cell-cycle transition. External signals activate multiple signal transduction pathways, including those involving the *MYC* and *RAS* genes, which lead to synthesis and stabilization of cyclin D (there are several D cyclins, but, for simplification, we refer to them as "cyclin D"). Cyclin D binds to CDK4, forming a complex with enzymatic activity (cyclin D can also bind to CDK6, which appears to have a similar role as CDK4). The cyclin D–CDK4 complex phosphorylates RB, located in the E2F/DP1/RB complex in the nucleus, activating the transcriptional activity of E2F (E2F is a family of transcription factors, which we refer to as "E2F"), which leads to transcription of cyclin E, cyclin A and other proteins needed for the cell to go through the late G_1 restriction point. The cell cycle can be blocked by the Cip/Kip inhibitors p21 and p27 *(red boxes)* and the INK4A/ARF inhibitors p16INK4A and p14ARF *(green boxes).* Cell-cycle arrest in response to DNA damage and other cellular stresses is mediated through p53. The levels of p53 are under negative regulation by MDM2, through a feedback loop that is inhibited by p14ARF.

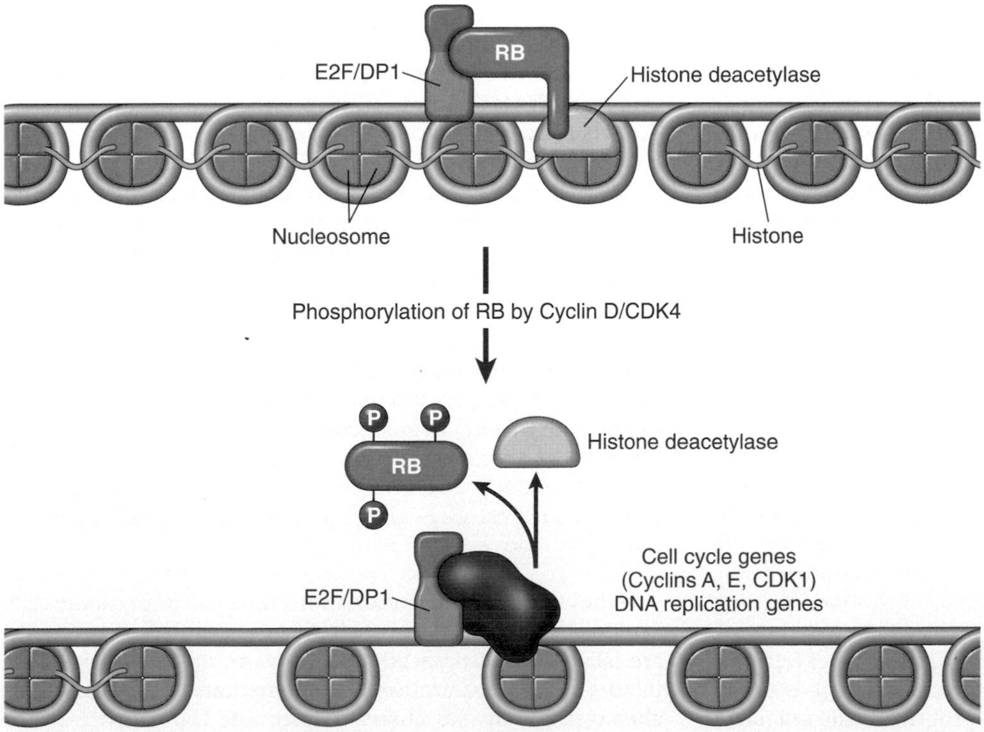

FIGURE 7–30 Mechanism of cell-cycle regulation by RB. In a resting cell, RB is a component of the E2F/DP1/RB complex, which represses gene transcription through the recruitment of histone deacetylase, an enzyme that alters the conformation of chromatin, making it more compact. Phosphorylation of RB by cyclin D–CDK4 removes histone deacetylase from chromatin, allowing the activation of E2F transcriptional activity (RB can also be phosphorylated by cyclin E–CDK2). E2F-mediated transcription of cyclins E and A, and of genes required for DNA replication, permit the passage through the G_1 restriction point. (Adapted from Pollard TD, Earnshaw WC: Cell Biology. Philadelphia, WB Saunders, 2002, p. 689.)

TABLE 7–7 Main Cell-Cycle Components and Their Inhibitors

Cell-Cycle Component	Main Function
Cyclin-Dependent Kinases	
• CDK4	Forms a complex with cyclin D. The complex phosphorylates RB, allowing the cell to progress through the G_1 restriction point.
• CDK2	Forms a complex with cyclin E in late G_1, which is involved in the G_1/S transition. Forms a complex with cyclin A at the S phase that facilitates the G_2/M transition.
• CDK1	Forms a complex with cyclin B, which acts on the G_2/M transition.
Inhibitors	
• Cip/Kip family: p21, p27	Block the cell cycle by binding to cyclin–CDK complexes. p21 is induced by the tumor suppressor *p53*. p27 responds to growth suppressors such as transforming growth factor-β.
• 1NK4/ARF family: p16INK4A, p14ARF	p16INK4a binds to cyclin D–CDK4 and promotes the inhibitory effects of RB. p14ARF increases p53 levels by inhibiting MDM2 activity.
Checkpoint Components	
• p53	Tumor suppressor altered in the majority of cancers; causes cell-cycle arrest and apoptosis. Acts mainly through p21 to cause cell-cycle arrest. Causes apoptosis by inducing the transcription of pro-apoptotic genes such as *BAX*. Levels of p53 are negatively regulated by MDM2 through a feedback loop. p53 is required for the G_1/S checkpoint and is a main component of the G_2/M checkpoint.
• Ataxia-telangiectasia mutated (*ATM*)	Activated by mechanisms that sense double stranded DNA breaks. Transmits signals to arrest the cell cycle after DNA damage. Acts through p53 in the G_1/S checkpoint. At the G_2/M checkpoint, it acts both through p53-dependent mechanisms and through the inactivation of CDC25 phosphatase, which disrupts the cyclin B–CDK1 complex. Component of a network of genes that include *BRCA1* and *BRCA2*, which link DNA damage with cell-cycle arrest and apoptosis.

three components, p21, p27, and p57, which bind to and inactivate the complexes formed between cyclins and CDKs. Transcriptional activation of p21 is under the control of *p53, a tumor suppressor gene that is mutated in a large proportion of human cancers.* The main role of p53 in the cell cycle is one of surveillance, triggering checkpoint controls that slow down or stop cell-cycle progression of damaged cells, or causes apoptosis. The human *INK4a/ARF* locus (a notation for "*in*hibitor of *k*inase *4*/*a*lternative *r*eading *f*rame") encodes two proteins, p16INK4a and p14ARF, which block the cell cycle and act as tumor suppressors. p16INK4a competes with cyclin D for binding to CDK4 and inhibits the ability of the cyclin D–CDK4 complex to phosphorylate RB, thus causing cell-cycle arrest at late G_1. It is frequently mutated or inactivated by hypermethylation (discussed later) in human cancers. The *INK4a* locus encodes a second gene product, p14ARF (p19ARF in mice), which acts on p53. p14ARF arises from an alternative reading of the *INK4a* gene, providing for an "economical" way to utilize gene-coding sequences.[42] Although both p16INK4a and p14ARF block the cell cycle, their targets are different; p16INK4a acts on cyclin D–CDK4, whereas p14ARF prevents p53 degradation.

Cell-Cycle Checkpoints. The cell cycle has its own internal controls, called *checkpoints*. There are two main checkpoints, one at the G_1/S transition and another at G_2/M.[43,44] The S phase is the point of no return in the cell cycle, and before a cell makes the final commitment to replicate, the G_1/S checkpoint checks for DNA damage. If DNA damage is present, the DNA repair machinery and mechanisms that arrest the cell cycle are put in motion. The delay in cell-cycle progression provides the time needed for DNA repair; if the damage is not repairable, apoptotic pathways are activated to kill the cell. Thus, the G_1/S checkpoint prevents the replication of cells that have defects in DNA, which would be perpetuated as mutations or chromosomal breaks in the progeny of the cell. DNA damaged after its replication can still be repaired as long as the chromatids have not separated. The G_2/M checkpoint monitors the completion of DNA replication and checks whether the cell can safely initiate mitosis and separate sister chromatids. This checkpoint is particularly important in cells exposed to ionizing radiation. Cells damaged by ionizing radiation activate the G_2/M checkpoint and arrest in G_2; defects in this checkpoint give rise to chromosomal abnormalities. To function properly, cell-cycle checkpoints require sensors of DNA damage, signal transducers, and effector molecules.[44] The sensors and transducers of DNA damage appear to be similar for the G_1/S and G_2/M checkpoints. They include, as sensors, proteins of the RAD family and ataxia telangiectasia mutated (ATM) and as transducers, the CHK kinase families. The checkpoint effector molecules differ, depending on the cell-cycle stage at which they act. In the G_1/S checkpoint, cell-cycle arrest is mostly mediated through p53, which induces the cell-cycle inhibitor p21. Arrest of the cell cycle by the G_2/M checkpoint involves both p53-dependent and independent mechanisms. *Defect in cell-cycle checkpoint components is a major cause of genetic instability in cancer cells.*

With this background on the cell cycle and its control, we now proceed to discuss the genes that determine the malignant phenotype. This discussion will take place in the context of the seven fundamental changes in cell physiology (listed earlier) that are the hallmarks of malignant cells.

SELF-SUFFICIENCY IN GROWTH SIGNALS: ONCOGENES

Genes that promote autonomous cell growth in cancer cells are called *oncogenes*, and their normal cellular counterparts are called *protooncogenes*. Protooncogenes are physiologic regulators of cell proliferation and differentiation; oncogenes are characterized by the ability to promote cell growth in the absence of normal mitogenic signals. Their products, called *oncoproteins,* resemble the normal products of protooncogenes with the exception that oncoproteins are devoid of important regulatory elements. Their production in the transformed cells becomes constitutive, that is, not dependent on growth factors or other external signals. To aid in the understanding of the nature and functions of oncoproteins, and their role in cancer, it is necessary to briefly mention the sequential steps that characterize normal cell proliferation. Under physiologic conditions, cell proliferation can be readily resolved into the following steps:

- The binding of a growth factor to its specific receptor generally located on the cell membrane
- Transient and limited activation of the growth factor receptor, which, in turn, activates several signal-transducing proteins on the inner leaflet of the plasma membrane
- Transmission of the transduced signal across the cytosol to the nucleus via second messengers or by signal transduction molecules that directly activate transcription
- Induction and activation of nuclear regulatory factors that initiate DNA transcription
- Entry and progression of the cell into the cell cycle, ultimately resulting in cell division

With this background, we can readily identify the strategies used by cancer cells to acquire self-sufficiency in growth signals. They can be grouped on the basis of their role in growth factor–mediated signal transduction cascades and cell-cycle regulation. We start with a description of oncogenes and their protein products, and how these were discovered.

Protooncogenes, Oncogenes, and Oncoproteins

As often happens in science, the discovery of protooncogenes was not straightforward. These cellular genes were first discovered in their mutated or "oncogenic" forms as "passengers" within the genome of *acute transforming retroviruses* by the 1989 Nobel laureates Harold Varmus and Michael Bishop. These retroviruses cause rapid induction of tumors in animals and can also transform animal cells in vitro. Molecular dissection of their genomes revealed the presence of unique transforming sequences (viral oncogenes [v-*onc*]) not found in the genomes of nontransforming retroviruses. Most surprisingly, molecular hybridization revealed that the v-*onc* sequences were almost identical to sequences found in normal cellular DNA. From this evolved the concept that during evolution, cellular oncogenes were *transduced* (captured) by the virus through a chance recombination with the DNA of a (normal) host cell that had been infected by the virus. Because they were discovered initially as *viral genes,* these protooncogenes were named after their viral homologues. Each v-*onc* is designated by a three-letter word that relates the oncogene to the virus from which it was isolated. Thus, the v-*onc* contained in *fe*line *s*arcoma virus is referred to as v-*FES,* whereas the oncogene in *si*mian *s*arcoma virus is called v-*SIS.* The corresponding protooncogenes are referred to as *FES* and *SIS,* dropping the prefix.

The viral oncogenes are not present in several cancer-causing RNA viruses. One such example is a group of so-called slow transforming viruses that cause leukemias in rodents after a long latent period. The mechanism by which they cause neoplastic transformation implicates protooncogenes. Molecular dissection of the cells transformed by these leukemia viruses revealed that the proviral DNA is always integrated (inserted) near a protooncogene. One consequence of proviral insertion near a protooncogene is to induce a structural change in the cellular gene, thus converting it into a cellular oncogene (c-*onc,* or *onc*). This mode of protooncogene activation is called *insertional mutagenesis.* Alternatively, strong retroviral promoters inserted in the vicinity of the protooncogenes lead to dysregulated expression of the cellular gene.

Although the study of transforming animal retroviruses provided the first glimpse of protooncogenes, these investigations did not explain the origin of human tumors, which (with rare exceptions) are not caused by infection with retroviruses. Hence the question was raised: Do nonviral tumors contain oncogenic DNA sequences? The answer was provided by experiments involving DNA-mediated gene transfer (DNA transfection). When DNA extracted from several different human tumors was transfected into mouse fibroblast cell lines in vitro, the recipient cells acquired some properties of neoplastic cells. The conclusion from such experiments was inescapable: DNA of spontaneously arising cancers contains oncogenic sequences, or oncogenes. One of the first oncogenic sequences detected in cancers was a mutated form of the *RAS* protooncogene. This protooncogene is the forbear of v-*oncs* contained in Harvey (H) and Kirsten (K) sarcoma viruses.

A large number of protooncogenes have been identified during the past 20 years, most of which do not have a viral counterpart. Protooncogenes have multiple roles, participating in cellular functions related to growth and proliferation. Proteins encoded by protooncogenes may function as growth factor ligands and receptors, signal transducers, transcription factors, and cell-cycle components (Fig. 7–31). Oncoproteins encoded by oncogenes generally serve similar functions as their normal counterparts (Table 7–8). However, because they are constitutively expressed, *oncoproteins endow the cell with self-sufficiency in growth.*[45]

To summarize, protooncogenes may be converted into cellular oncogenes (c-oncs) that are involved in tumor development. Two questions follow: (1) What are the functions of oncogene products, the oncoproteins? (2) How do the normally "civilized" protooncogenes turn into "enemies within"? These issues are discussed below.

Growth Factors. Many cancer cells develop growth self-sufficiency by acquiring the ability to synthesize the same growth factors to which they are responsive. The protooncogene *SIS,* which encodes the β chain of platelet-derived growth factor (PDGF), is overproduced in many tumors, especially low-grade astrocytomas and osteosarcomas. Furthermore, it appears that the same tumors also express receptors for PDGF and are hence responsive to autocrine stimulation. Although an autocrine loop is considered to be an important element in the pathogenesis of several tumors, in most instances the growth factor gene itself is not altered or mutated. More commonly, products of other oncogenes such as *RAS* (that lie along many signal transduction pathways) cause overexpression of growth factor genes, thus forcing the cells to secrete large amounts of growth factors, such as transforming growth factor-α (TGF-α). This growth factor is related to epidermal growth factor (EGF) and induces proliferation by binding to the EGF receptor. TGF-α is often

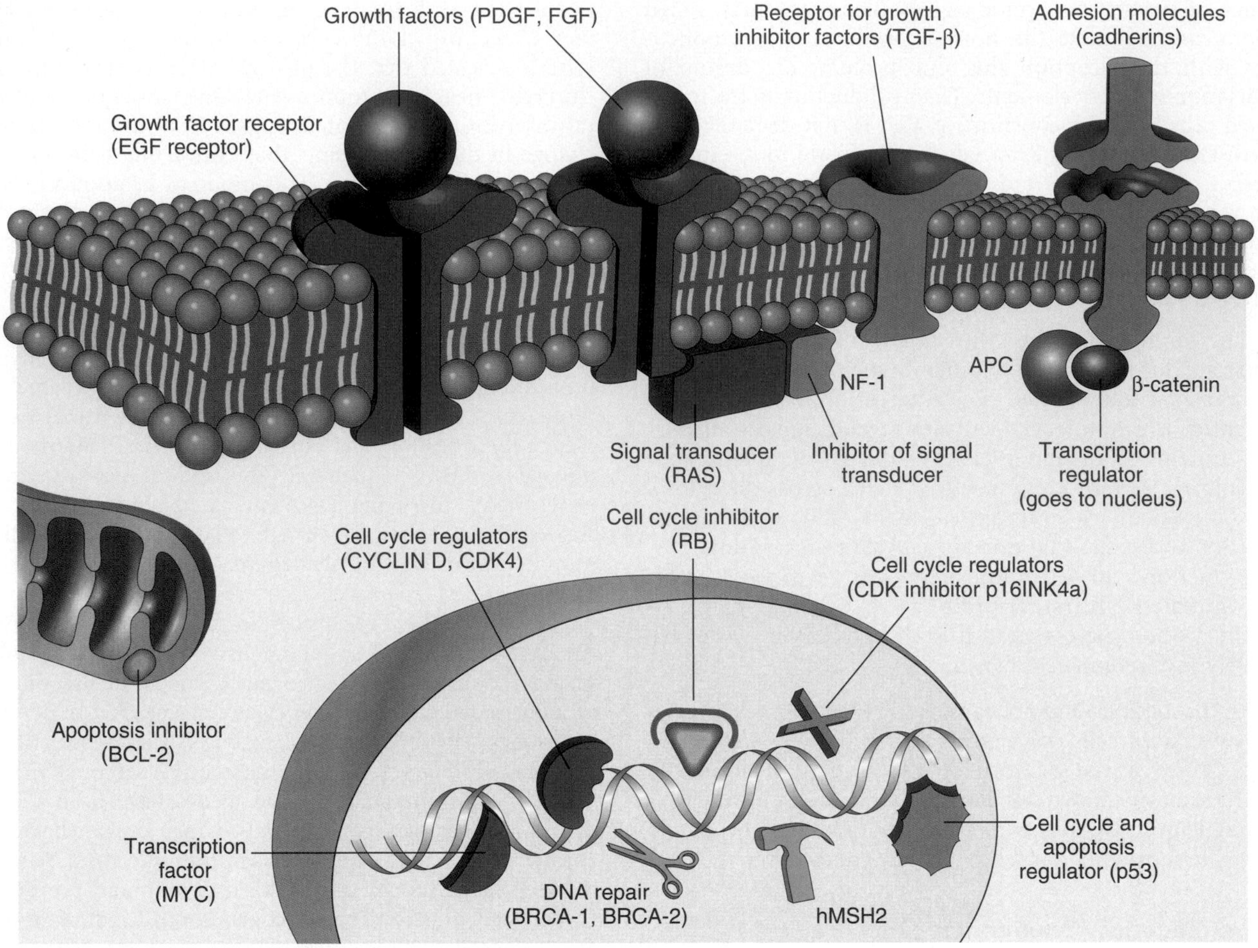

FIGURE 7–31 Subcellular localization and functions of major classes of cancer-associated genes. The protooncogenes are colored red, cancer suppressor genes blue, DNA repair genes green, and genes that regulate apoptosis purple.

detected in carcinomas such as astrocytomas that express high levels of EGF receptors.

In addition to *SIS*, a group of related oncogenes that encode homologues of fibroblast growth factors (FGFs) (e.g., *HST-1* and *INT-2*) is activated in several gastrointestinal and breast tumors; bFGF, a member of the fibroblast growth factor family, is expressed in human melanomas but not in normal melanocytes. Hepatocyte growth factor and its receptor c-MET are overexpressed in follicular carcinomas of the thyroid, constituting a growth-stimulatory autocrine loop. Small cell lung carcinomas produce bombesin-like peptides that stimulate their proliferation.

Despite extensive documentation of growth factor–mediated autocrine stimulation of transformed cells, increased growth factor production by itself is not sufficient for neoplastic transformation. Extensive cell proliferation, in all likelihood, contributes to the malignant phenotype by increasing the risk of spontaneous or induced mutations in the cell population.

Growth Factor Receptors. Several oncogenes that encode growth factor receptors have been found. To understand how mutations affect the function of these receptors, it should be recalled that several growth factor receptors are transmembrane proteins with an external ligand-binding domain and a cytoplasmic tyrosine kinase domain (Chapter 3). In the normal forms of these receptors, the kinase is *transiently* activated by binding of the specific growth factors, followed rapidly by receptor dimerization and tyrosine phosphorylation of several substrates that are a part of the signaling cascade. *The oncogenic versions of these receptors are associated with constitutive dimerization and activation without binding to the growth factor.* Hence, the mutant receptors deliver continuous mitogenic signals to the cell.

Growth factor receptors are activated in human tumors by several mechanisms. These include mutations, gene rearrangements, and overexpression. The *RET* protooncogene, a receptor tyrosine kinase, exemplifies oncogenic conversion via mutations and gene rearrangements.[46] The RET protein is a receptor for the glial cell line–derived neurotrophic factor and structurally related proteins that promote cell survival during neural development. RET is normally expressed in neuroendocrine cells, such as parafollicular C cells of the thyroid, adrenal medulla, and parathyroid cell precursors. Point mutations in the *RET* protooncogene are associated with dominantly inherited MEN types 2A and 2B and familial medullary thyroid carcinoma (Chapter 24). In MEN 2A, point mutations in the *RET* extracellular domain cause constitutive dimerization and activation, leading to medullary thyroid carcinomas and also adrenal and parathyroid tumors. In MEN 2B, point mutations in the *RET* cytoplasmic catalytic

TABLE 7–8 Selected Oncogenes, Their Mode of Activation, and Associated Human Tumors

Category	Protooncogene	Mode of Activation	Associated Human Tumor
Growth Factors			
PDGF-β chain	*SIS*	Overexpression	Astrocytoma Osteosarcoma
Fibroblast growth factors	*HST-1* *INT-2*	Overexpression Amplification	Stomach cancer Bladder cancer Breast cancer Melanoma
TGFα	TGFα	Overexpression	Astrocytomas Hepatocellular carcinomas
HGF	HGF	Overexpression	Thyroid cancer
Growth Factor Receptors			
EGF-receptor family	*ERB-B1 (ECFR)* *ERB-B2*	Overexpression Amplification	Squamous cell carcinomas of lung, gliomas Breast and ovarian cancers
CSF-1 receptor	*FMS*	Point mutation	Leukemia
Receptor for neurotrophic factors	*RET*	Point mutation	Multiple endocrine neoplasia 2A and B, familial medullary thyroid carcinomas
PDGF receptor	*PDGF-R*	Overexpression	Gliomas
Receptor for stem cell (steel) factor	*KIT*	Point mutation	Gastrointestinal stromal tumors and other soft tissue tumors
Proteins Involved in Signal Transduction			
GTP-binding	*K-RAS* *H-RAS* *N-RAS*	Point mutation Point mutation Point mutation	Colon, lung, and pancreatic tumors Bladder and kidney tumors Melanomas, hematologic malignancies
Nonreceptor tyrosine kinase	*ABL*	Translocation	Chronic myeloid leukemia Acute lymphoblastic leukemia
RAS signal transduction	*BRAF*	Point mutation	Melanomas
WNT signal transduction	*β-catenin*	Point mutation Overexpression	Hepatoblastomas, hepatocellular carcinoma
Nuclear Regulatory Proteins			
Transcriptional activators	*C-MYC* *N-MYC* *L-MYC*	Translocation Amplification Amplification	Burkitt lymphoma Neuroblastoma, small cell carcinoma of lung Small cell carcinoma of lung
Cell-Cycle Regulators			
Cyclins	*CYCLIN D* *CYCLIN E*	Translocation Amplification Overexpression	Mantle cell lymphoma Breast and esophageal cancers Breast cancer
Cyclin-dependent kinase	*CDK4*	Amplification or point mutation	Glioblastoma, melanoma, sarcoma

domain alter the substrate specificity of the tyrosine kinase and lead to thyroid and adrenal tumors but no involvement of the parathyroid. Complete loss of RET function results in Hirschsprung disease (Chapter 17), in which there is lack of development of intestinal nerve plexuses. In all these familial conditions, the affected individuals inherit the *RET* mutation in the germ line. Sporadic medullary carcinomas of the thyroid are associated with somatic rearrangements of the *RET* gene, generally similar to those found in MEN 2B.[46,47]

Oncogenic conversions by mutations and rearrangements have been found in other growth factor receptor genes. Point mutations that activate c-*FMS*, the gene encoding the colony-stimulating factor 1 (CSF-1) receptor, have been detected in myeloid leukemias. In certain chronic myelomonocytic leukemias with the t(12;9) translocation, the entire cytoplasmic domain of the PDGF receptor is fused with a segment of the ETS family transcription factor, resulting in permanent dimerization of the PDGF receptor.

Far more common than mutations of these protooncogenes is overexpression of normal forms of growth factor receptors. In sporadic papillary thyroid carcinomas, c-MET is overexpressed in almost every case.[48] In these tumors, increased expression of c-MET is not caused by gene mutation but results from enhanced transcription of the gene. In some tumors, increased receptor expression results from gene amplification, but in many cases, the molecular basis of increased receptor expression is not fully known. Two members of the EGF receptor family are most commonly involved. The normal form of *ERB B1*, the EGF receptor gene, usually referred to as *EGFR*, is overexpressed in up to 80% of squamous cell carcinomas of the lung, in 50% or more of high-grade astrocytomas called *glioblastomas* (Chapter 28), in 80% to 100% of head and neck tumors, and less commonly, in carcinomas of the urinary bladder and the gastrointestinal tract.[49,50] In contrast, the *ERB B2* gene (also called *HER 2/Neu*), the second member of the EGF receptor family, is amplified in approximately 25% of breast cancers and in human adenocarcinomas arising within the ovary, lung, stomach, and salivary glands.[51] Because the molecular alteration in *ERB B2* is specific for the cancer cells, new therapeutic agents consisting of monoclonal antibodies against ERB B2 have been developed and are currently in use clinically.[49,51] This type of therapy, directed to a specific alteration in the cancer cell, is called *targeted therapy*.[52] Another example of very successful targeted cancer therapy is the blockage of receptor tyrosine kinase activity of c-KIT in stromal tumors of the gastrointestinal tract.[53] In these tumors, a mutation in c-*KIT*, the gene encoding the receptor for stem cell factor (also known as *steel factor*), constitutively activates the receptor tyrosine kinase, independent of ligand binding.

Signal-Transducing Proteins. Several examples of oncoproteins that mimic the function of normal cytoplasmic signal-transducing proteins have been found. Most such proteins are strategically located on the inner leaflet of the plasma membrane, where they receive signals from outside the cell (e.g., by activation of growth factor receptors) and transmit them to the cell's nucleus. Biochemically, the signal-transducing proteins are heterogeneous. *The best and most well studied example of a signal-transducing oncoprotein is the RAS family of guanine triphosphate (GTP)-binding proteins (G proteins).*

The RAS Oncogene. The RAS proteins were discovered as products of viral oncogenes. *Point mutation of RAS family genes is the single most common abnormality of dominant oncogenes in human tumors.* Approximately 15% to 20% of all human tumors contain mutated versions of RAS proteins.[54] Several distinct mutations of *RAS* have been identified in cancer cells, all of which dramatically reduce the GTPase activity of the RAS proteins. The mutations generally involve codons 12, 59, or 61 of *HRAS*, *KRAS*, and *NRAS*. The frequency of such mutations varies with different tumors, but in some types it is very high. For example, 90% of pancreatic adenocarcinomas and cholangiocarcinomas contain a *RAS* point mutation, as do about 50% of colon, endometrial, and thyroid cancers and 30% of lung adenocarcinomas and myeloid leukemias.[55–57] In general, carcinomas (particularly from colon and pancreas) have mutations of *KRAS*, bladder tumors have *HRAS* mutations, and hematopoietic tumors bear *NRAS* mutations. *RAS* mutations are infrequent in certain other cancers, particularly those arising in the uterine cervix or breast.

Several studies indicate that RAS plays an important role in mitogenesis induced by growth factors. For example, blockade of RAS function by microinjection of specific antibodies blocks the proliferative response to EGF, PDGF, and CSF-1. Normal RAS proteins are tethered to the cytoplasmic aspect of the plasma membrane, and they flip back and forth between an activated, signal-transmitting form and an inactive, quiescent state. Recently it was found that these proteins may also be found in the endoplasmic reticulum and Golgi membranes, where they can be activated by growth factor binding to the plasma membrane, through a still-uncertain mechanism.[58] In the inactive state, RAS proteins bind guanosine diphosphate (GDP); when cells are stimulated by growth factors or other receptor–ligand interactions, RAS becomes activated by exchanging GDP for GTP (Fig. 7–32). Activated RAS, in turn, acts on the MAP kinase pathway by recruiting the cytosolic protein RAF-1. The MAP kinases so activated target nuclear transcription factors and thus promote mitogenesis. In normal cells, the activated signal-transmitting stage of the RAS protein is transient because its intrinsic GTPase activity hydrolyzes GTP to GDP, thereby returning RAS to its quiescent ground state (described below).

The orderly cycling of the RAS protein depends on two reactions: (1) nucleotide exchange (GDP by GTP), which activates RAS protein, and (2) GTP hydrolysis, which converts the GTP-bound, active RAS to the GDP-bound, inactive form. Both these processes are enzymatically regulated. The removal of GDP and its replacement by GTP during RAS activation are catalyzed by a family of guanine nucleotide–releasing proteins that are recruited to the cytosolic domain of activated growth factor receptors by adapter proteins. More importantly, the GTPase activity intrinsic to normal RAS proteins is dramatically accelerated by *GTPase-activating proteins (GAPs)*. These widely distributed proteins bind to the active RAS and augment its GTPase activity by more than 1000-fold, leading to rapid hydrolysis of GTP to GDP and termination of signal transduction. Thus, GAPs function as "brakes" that prevent uncontrolled RAS activity. The response to this braking action of GAPs seems to falter when mutations affect the *RAS* gene. *Mutant RAS proteins bind GAP, but their GTPase activity fails to be augmented.* Hence the mutant proteins are "trapped" in their excited GTP-bound form, causing, in turn, a pathologic activation of the mitogenic signaling pathway. The importance of GTPase activation in normal growth control is underscored by the fact that a disabling mutation of neurofibromin *(NF-1)*, a GTPase-activating protein, is also associated with neoplasia (see discussion of tumor suppressor genes below).

In addition to RAS, other members of the RAS signaling cascade (RAS/RAF/MAP kinase) may also be altered in cancer cells. Thus, mutations in *BRAF*, one of the members of the *RAF* family, have been detected in more than 60% of melanomas and in more than 80% of benign nevi.[59,60] This suggests that dysregulation of the RAS/RAF/MAP kinase pathway may be one of the initiating events in the development of melanomas, although it is not sufficient by itself to cause tumorigenesis.

Recent studies have revealed that, in addition to its role in transducing growth factor signals, RAS is also involved in regulation of the cell cycle. As described above, the passage of cells from G_1 to the S phase is modulated by cyclins and CDKs. RAS proteins can indirectly regulate the levels of cyclins by activating the MAP kinase pathway and the AP-1 transcription factor.

Because *RAS* is so frequently mutated in human cancers, much effort has been spent to develop anti-RAS modalities of targeted therapy. Several such strategies for cancer treatment are being evaluated. The specific targets include blockade of

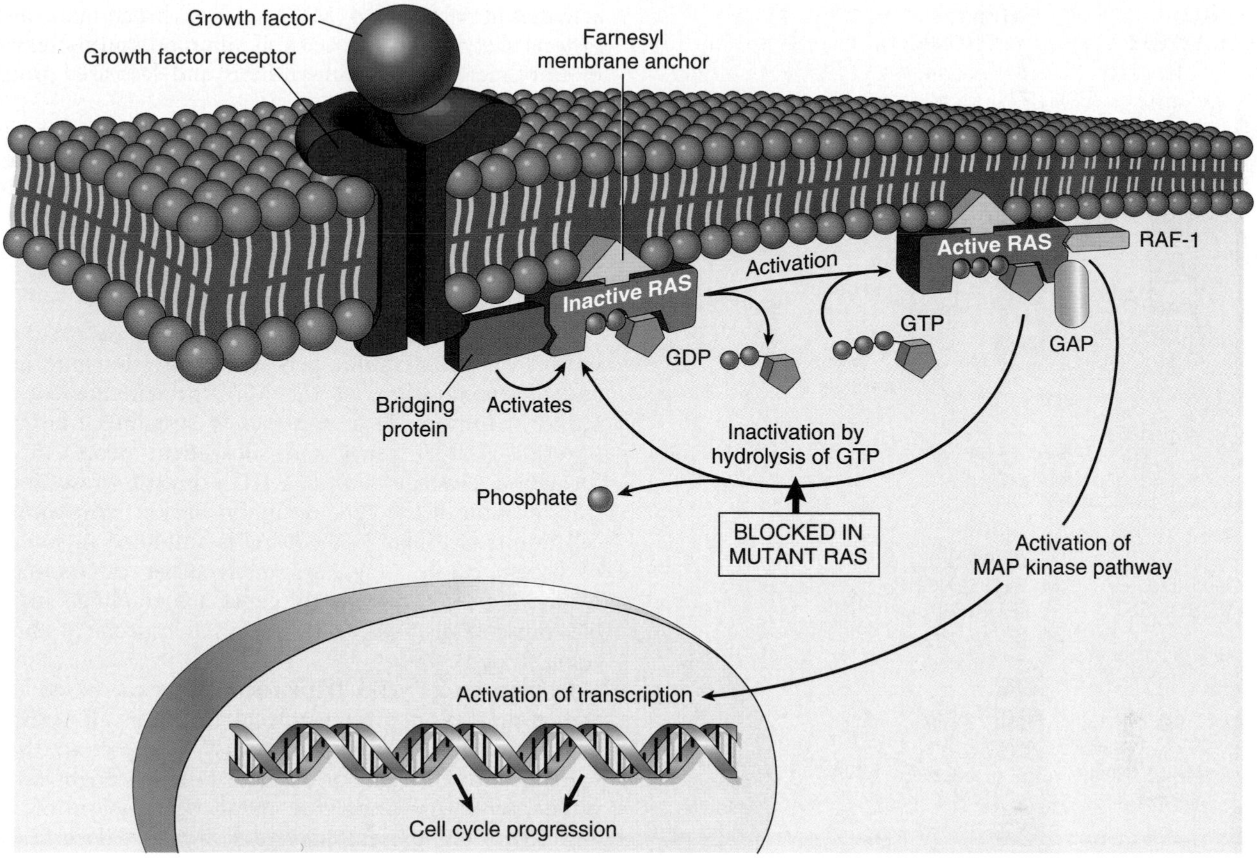

FIGURE 7–32 Model for action of *RAS* genes. When a normal cell is stimulated through a growth factor receptor, inactive (GDP-bound) RAS is activated to a GTP-bound state. Activated RAS recruits RAF and stimulates the MAP-kinase pathway to transmit growth-promoting signals to the nucleus. The mutant RAS protein is permanently activated because of inability to hydrolyze GTP, leading to continuous stimulation of cells without any external trigger. The anchoring of RAS to the cell membrane by the farnesyl moiety is essential for its action.

the association of RAS with the cell membrane, using inhibitors of farnesyl transferase (an enzyme that provides the bridge between RAS and the lipid components of the plasma membrane); blockade of downstream components of RAS signaling pathways (i.e., RAF and MAP kinase inhibitors); direct blockade of RAS; and blockade of signaling from the EGF receptor, to prevent the activation of RAS pathways. Unfortunately, none of these strategies has so far proven to be successful for clinical use.[61] Nevertheless, given the frequency of *RAS* mutations in human cancer and the importance of RAS in cell proliferation, efforts to disable this signaling pathway continue as a potential modality of cancer therapy.

Alterations in Nonreceptor Tyrosine Kinases. As discussed in Chapter 3, several nonreceptor-associated tyrosine kinases function in the signal transduction pathways that regulate cell growth. With the notable exception of c-*ABL*, however, they are rarely activated in human tumors. The ABL protooncogene product has tyrosine kinase activity, which is dampened by negative regulatory domains. In chronic myeloid leukemia and some acute lymphoblastic leukemias, however, this activity is unleashed because the c-*ABL* gene is translocated from its normal abode on chromosome 9 to chromosome 22 (Fig. 7–33), where it fuses with the *BCR* gene (see discussion of chromosomal translocations, later in this chapter). As a consequence of the fusion, c-*ABL* loses a region that controls tyrosine kinase activity.[62,63] Thus, the BCR-ABL protein, the product of the fusion gene, has potent and constitutive tyrosine kinase activity, which is critical to the oncogenic capacity of the gene. Treatment of chronic myeloid leukemia has been revolutionized by the development of *imatinib mesylate,* a "designer" drug that targets the BCR-ABL tyrosine kinase. It has low toxicity and high therapeutic efficacy.[52,62,63]

Transcription Factors. Signal transduction pathways generate transcriptional regulators that enter the nucleus and act on a large bank of responder genes. These genes orchestrate the cells' orderly entry and progression through the cell cycle, leading to DNA replication and cell division. Transcription factors contain specific amino acid sequences or motifs that allow them to bind DNA or to dimerize for DNA binding. Examples of such motifs include helix-loop-helix, leucine zipper, zinc-finger, and homeodomains. Many of these proteins bind DNA at specific sites from which they can activate or inhibit transcription of adjacent genes. Not surprisingly, therefore, mutations affecting genes that encode nuclear transcription factors are associated with malignant transformation.

A whole host of oncoproteins, including products of the *MYC, MYB,* the *JUN* family, and *FOS* oncogenes, is found in the nuclei of transformed cells. *Of these, MYC is most com-*

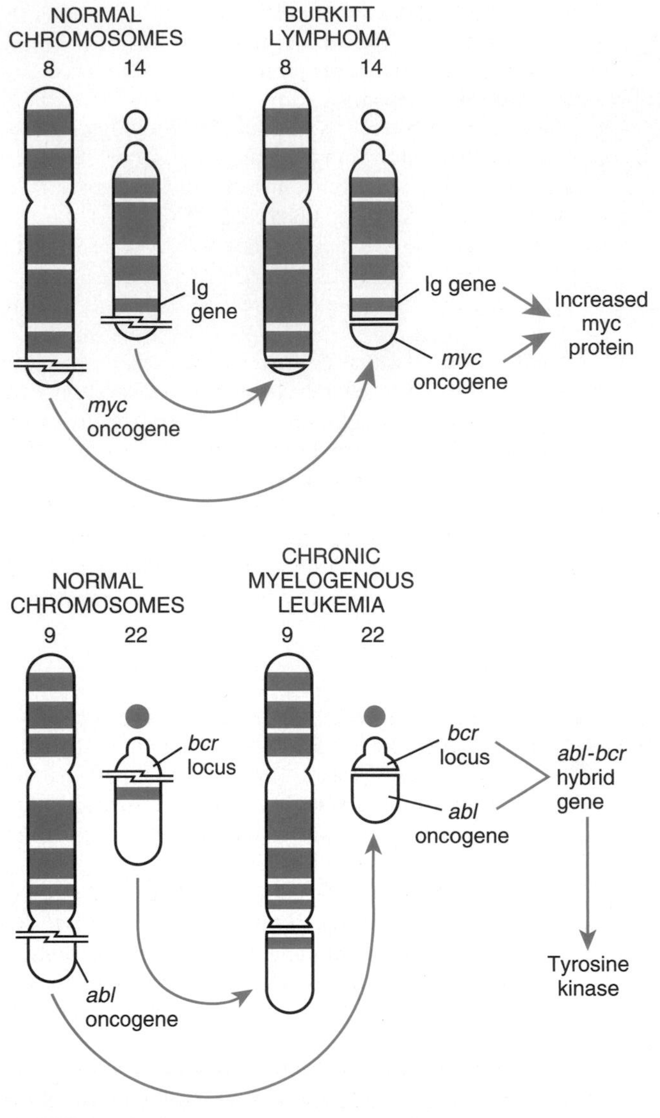

FIGURE 7–33 The chromosomal translocation and associated oncogenes in Burkitt lymphoma and chronic myelogenous leukemia.

monly involved in human tumors, and hence a brief overview of its function is warranted.

The MYC Oncogene. The *MYC* protooncogene is expressed in virtually all eukaryotic cells and belongs to the immediate early response genes, which are rapidly induced when quiescent cells receive a signal to divide (see discussion of liver regeneration in Chapter 3). After a transient increase of *MYC* mRNA, the expression declines to a basal level. The molecular basis of MYC function in cell replication is not entirely clear, but some general principles have emerged.[64,65] The MYC protein is rapidly translocated to the nucleus, sometimes as a dimer with another protein, called MAX. This heterodimer binds to DNA sequences in target genes and is a potent transcriptional activator. Some of its target genes, such as ornithine decarboxylase and cyclin D2, are known to be associated with cell proliferation. However, the range of activities attributed to MYC is very broad and includes histone acetylation, reduced cell adhesion and increased cell motility, increased protein synthesis, and decreased proteinase activity.[66]

While on one hand *MYC* activation is linked to proliferation, on the other hand, cells in culture undergo apoptosis if *MYC* activation occurs in the absence of survival signals (growth factors). The *MYC* protooncogene contains separate sequences that encode the growth promoting and apoptotic activities, but it is not clear whether MYC-induced apoptosis occurs in vivo.

In contrast to the regulated expression of *MYC* during normal cell proliferation, persistent expression, and in some cases overexpression, of the MYC protein are commonly found in tumors. This may lead to sustained transcription of critical target genes and subsequent neoplastic transformation. Dysregulation of *MYC* expression resulting from translocation of the gene occurs in Burkitt lymphoma, a B-cell tumor (see Fig. 7–33). *MYC* is amplified in some cases of breast, colon, lung, and many other carcinomas. The related N-*MYC* and L-*MYC* genes are amplified in neuroblastomas (Fig. 7–34) and small cell cancers of the lung, respectively.

Cyclins and Cyclin-Dependent Kinases. Based on our earlier discussion of the normal functions of cyclins and CDKs in cell-cycle control, it is easy to appreciate that dysregulation of the activity of these proteins might favor cell proliferation. Abnormalities in the expression of cyclins and CDKs are present in several human cancers. Indeed, mishaps affecting the expression of cyclin D or CDK4 seem to be a common event in neoplastic transformation. The cyclin D genes are overexpressed in many cancers, including those affecting the breast, esophagus, head and neck, and liver, and in a subset of lymphomas (mantle cell lymphomas), in which the *CYCLIN D1* gene is a component of a fusion gene created by chromosomal translocation (see below). Amplification of the *CDK4* gene occurs in sarcomas and glioblastomas. Cyclin E and its low-molecular-weight forms are overexpressed in breast cancers, and the level of expression correlates with disease progression and survival.[67]

INSENSITIVITY TO GROWTH INHIBITORY SIGNALS: TUMOR SUPPRESSOR GENES

The growth of cells has to be controlled by many external signals to maintain a steady state (homeostasis). Failure of growth inhibition is one of the fundamental alterations in the process of carcinogenesis. The proteins that apply brakes to cell proliferation are the products of *tumor suppressor genes* (Table 7–9). In a sense, the term "tumor suppressor genes" is a misnomer because the physiologic function of these genes is to regulate cell growth, not to prevent tumor formation.[68] Because the loss of function of these genes is a key event in many, possibly all, human tumors and because their discovery resulted from the study of tumors, the name tumor suppressor persists.

Similar to many discoveries in medicine, the tumor suppressor genes were discovered by studying rare diseases, in this case retinoblastoma, a tumor that affects about 1 in 20,000

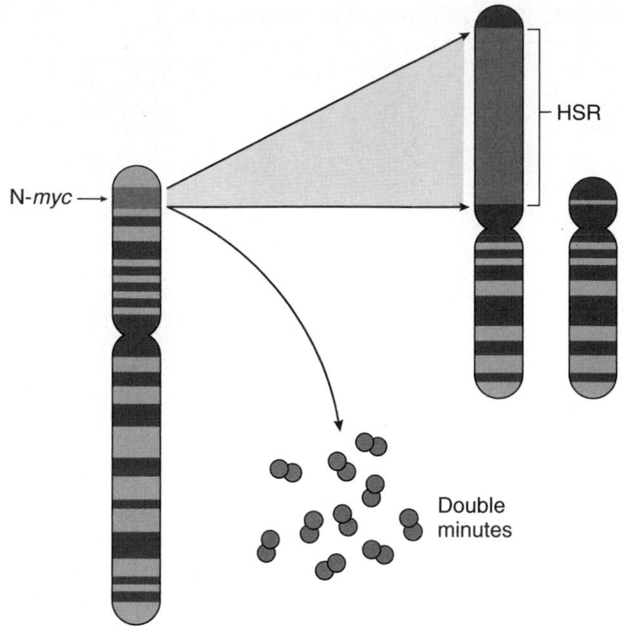

FIGURE 7–34 Amplification of the N-*MYC* gene in human neuroblastomas. The N-*MYC* gene, normally present on chromosome 2p, becomes amplified and is seen either as extra chromosomal double minutes or as a chromosomally integrated, homogeneous staining region. The integration involves other autosomes, such as 4, 9, or 13. (Modified from Brodeur GM: Molecular correlates of cytogenetic abnormalities in human cancer cells: implications for oncogene activation. In Brown EB (ed): Progress in Hematology, Vol 14. Orlando, FL, Grune & Stratton, 1986, pp. 229–256.)

infants and children. Approximately 60% of retinoblastomas are sporadic, and the remaining 40% are inherited, with the predisposition to develop the tumor being transmitted as an autosomal dominant trait. To explain the inherited and sporadic occurrence of an apparently identical tumor, Knudson proposed his now famous *"two-hit" hypothesis of oncogenesis.*[21,69] He suggested that in hereditary cases, one genetic change ("first hit") is inherited from an affected parent and is therefore present in all somatic cells of the body, whereas the second mutation ("second hit") occurs in one of the many retinal cells (which already carry the first mutation). In sporadic cases, however, both mutations (hits) occur somatically within a single retinal cell, whose progeny then form the tumor.

Retinoblastoma as a Paradigm for the Two-Hit Hypothesis of Oncogenesis. Knudson's hypothesis has been amply substantiated by cytogenetic and molecular studies with other tumor suppressor genes and can now be formulated in more precise terms, using retinoblastoma as a paradigm:

- The mutations required to produce retinoblastoma involve the *RB* gene, located on chromosome 13q14. In some cases, the genetic damage is large enough to be visible in the form of a deletion of 13q14.
- Both normal alleles of the *RB* locus must be inactivated (two hits) for the development of retinoblastoma (Fig. 7–35). In familial cases, children are born with one normal and one defective copy of the *RB* gene. They lose the intact copy in the retinoblasts through some form of somatic mutation (point mutation, interstitial deletion of 13q14, or even complete loss of the normal chromosome 13). In sporadic cases, both normal *RB* alleles are lost by somatic mutation in one of the retinoblasts. The end result is the same: A retinal cell that has lost both normal copies of the *RB* gene gives rise to cancer.
- Patients with familial retinoblastoma are also at greatly increased risk of developing osteosarcoma and some other soft tissue sarcomas. Furthermore, inactivation of the *RB* locus has been noted in several other tumors, including adenocarcinoma of the breast, small cell carcinoma of the lung, and bladder carcinoma. Most importantly, alterations in the "RB pathway," involving INK4a proteins, cyclin D-dependent kinases, and RB family proteins, are almost always present in cancer cells.[36]

At this point, we should clarify some terminology. A child carrying an inherited mutant *RB* allele in all somatic cells is perfectly normal (except for the increased risk of developing cancer). Because such a child is heterozygous at the *RB* locus, it implies that heterozygosity for the *RB* gene does not affect cell behavior. *Cancer develops when the cell becomes homozygous for the mutant allele or, put another way, when the cell loses heterozygosity for the normal RB gene (a condition known as LOH, for loss of heterozygosity). Because the RB gene is associated with cancer when both normal copies are lost, it is sometimes referred to as a recessive cancer gene.*

The *RB* gene stands as a paradigm for several other genes that act similarly. For example, one or more genes on the short arm of chromosome 11 play a role in the formation of Wilms tumor, hepatoblastoma, and rhabdomyosarcoma. The von Hippel Lindau *(VHL)* gene is a tumor suppressor gene that causes familial clear-cell renal carcinomas and is also involved in sporadic forms of the same tumor.[70] *Consistent and nonrandom LOH has provided important clues to the location of several tumor suppressor genes.*

The protein products of tumor suppressor genes are involved in cell-cycle control, the regulation of apoptosis, and many other activities critical for cell survival and growth. They may function as transcription factors, cell-cycle inhibitors, signal transduction molecules, cell surface receptors, and regulators of cellular responses to DNA damage. A list of selected tumor suppressor genes is provided in Table 7–9. In the following section we discuss the functions of the most important tumor suppressor genes, and how their defects contribute to carcinogenesis.

RB Gene. Much is known about the *RB* gene because this was the first tumor suppressor gene discovered.[68] RB protein, the product of the *RB* gene, is a nuclear phosphoprotein that plays a key role in regulating the cell cycle. It is expressed in every cell type examined; as we have already seen, RB exists in an active hypophosphorylated state in quiescent cells and an inactive hyperphosphorylated state in the G_1/S cell-cycle tran-

TABLE 7–9 Selected Tumor Suppressor Genes Involved in Human Neoplasms

Subcellular Location	Gene	Function	Tumors Associated with Somatic Mutations	Tumors Associated with Inherited Mutations
Cell surface	*TGF-β receptor*	Growth inhibition	Carcinomas of colon	Unknown
	E-cadherin	Cell adhesion	Carcinoma of stomach	Familial gastric cancer
Inner aspect of plasma membrane	*NF-1*	Inhibition of RAS signal transduction and of p21 cell-cycle inhibitor	Neuroblastomas	Neurofibromatosis type 1 and sarcomas
Cytoskeleton	*NF-2*	Cytoskeletal stability	Schwannomas and meningiomas	Neurofibromatosis type 2, acoustic schwannomas and meningiomas
Cytosol	*APC/β-catenin*	Inhibition of signal transduction	Carcinomas of stomach, colon, pancreas; melanoma	Familial adenomatous polyposis coli/colon cancer
	PTEN	PI-3 kinase signal transduction	Endometrial and prostate cancers	Unknown
	SMAD 2 and *SMAD 4*	TGF-β signal transduction	Colon, pancreas tumors	Unknown
Nucleus	*RB*	Regulation of cell cycle	Retinoblastoma; osteosarcoma carcinomas of breast, colon, lung	Retinoblastomas, osteosarcoma
	p53	Cell-cycle arrest and apoptosis in response to DNA damage	Most human cancers	Li-Fraumeni syndrome; multiple carcinomas and sarcomas
	WT-1	Nuclear transcription	Wilms tumor	Wilms tumor
	p16 (INK4a)	Regulation of cell cycle by inhibition of cyclin-dependent kinases	Pancreatic, breast, and esophageal cancers	Malignant melanoma
	BRCA-1 and *BRCA-2*	DNA repair	Unknown	Carcinomas of female breast and ovary; carcinomas of male breast
	KLF6	Transcription factor	Prostate	Unknown

sition (Fig. 7–36). When cells enter the S phase, they can continue to cell division independent of growth factors. It should be obvious from this discussion that if RB is absent (owing to gene deletions) or its ability to regulate E2F transcription factors is derailed, the molecular brakes on the cell cycle are released, and the cells move into the S phase followed by cell replication. The mutations of *RB* genes found in tumors are localized to a region of the *RB* protein, called the "*RB* pocket," that is involved in binding to E2F.

It was mentioned previously that germ-line loss or mutations of the *RB* gene predispose to occurrence of retinoblastomas and to a lesser extent osteosarcomas. Furthermore, somatically acquired mutations have been described in glioblastomas, small cell carcinomas of lung, breast cancers, and bladder carcinomas. Given the presence of RB in every cell and its importance in cell-cycle control, two questions arise: (1) Why do patients with germ line mutation of the *RB* locus develop mainly retinoblastomas? (2) Why are inactivating mutations of *RB* not much more common in human cancer? The basis for the occurrence of tumors restricted to the retina in patients who inherit one defective allele of *RB* is not fully understood, but some possible explanations have emerged from the study of mice with targeted disruption of the *RB* locus. For instance, *RB* mutation may be a critical initiating event for retinoblastomas but may be only an accessory factor for malignancies at other sites.

With respect to the second question (i.e., why the loss of *RB* is not more common in human tumors), the answer is much simpler: Mutations in other genes that control RB phosphorylation can mimic the effect of *RB* loss, and such genes are mutated in many cancers that may have normal *RB* genes. Thus, for example, mutational activation of cyclin D or CDK4 would favor cell proliferation by facilitating RB phosphorylation. As previously discussed, cyclin D is overexpressed in many tumors because of gene amplification or translocation. Mutational inactivation of CDK inhibitors would also drive the cell cycle by unregulated activation of cyclins and CDKs. Thus, *the emerging paradigm is that loss of normal cell-cycle control is central to malignant transformation and that at least one of four key regulators of the cell cycle (p16INK4a, CYCLIN D, CDK4, RB) is dysregulated in the vast majority of human cancers.*[38] In cells that harbor mutations in any one of these other genes, the function of RB is disrupted even if the *RB* gene itself is not mutated.[45]

Several other pathways of cell growth regulation, some to be discussed in more detail later, also converge on RB (Fig. 7–36):

- TGF-β induces inhibition of cellular proliferation. This effect of TGF-β is mediated, at least in part, by up-regulation of the CDK inhibitor p27.

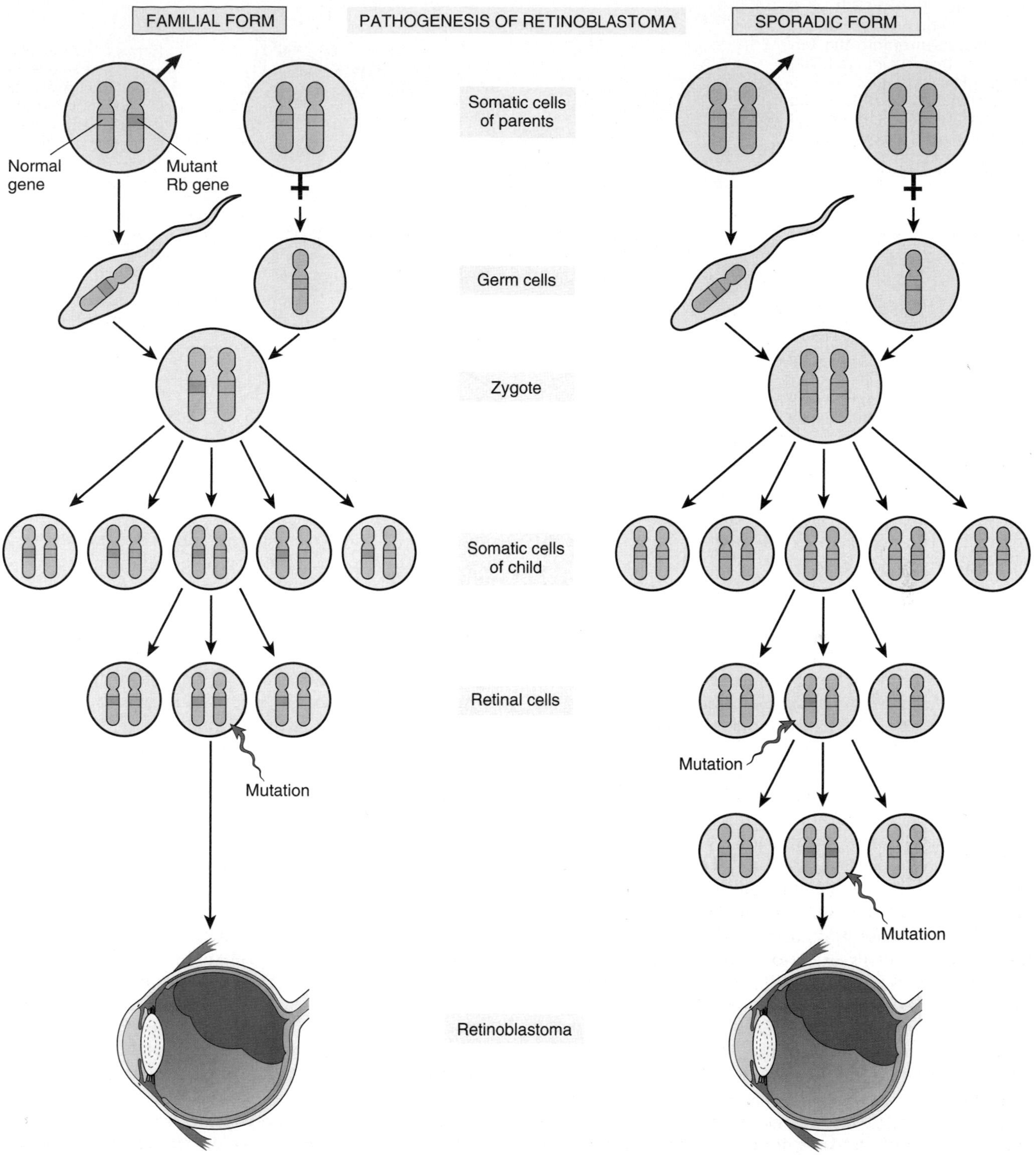

FIGURE 7–35 Pathogenesis of retinoblastoma. Two mutations of the *RB* locus on chromosome 13q14 lead to neoplastic proliferation of the retinal cells. In the familial form, all somatic cells inherit one mutant *RB* gene from a carrier parent. The second mutation affects the *Rb* locus in one of the retinal cells after birth. In the sporadic form, on the other hand, both mutations at the *RB* locus are acquired by the retinal cells after birth.

- The transforming proteins of several oncogenic animal and human DNA viruses seem to act, in part, by neutralizing the growth inhibitory activities of RB. In these cases, RB protein is functionally deleted by the binding of a viral protein and no longer acts as a cell-cycle inhibitor. Simian virus 40 and polyomavirus large T antigens, adenoviruses EIA protein, and human papillomavirus (HPV) E7 protein, all bind to the hypophosphorylated form of RB. The binding occurs in the same RB pocket that normally sequesters E2F transcription factors; in the case of HPV, the binding is particularly strong for viral types, such as HPV 16, which confer high risk for the development of

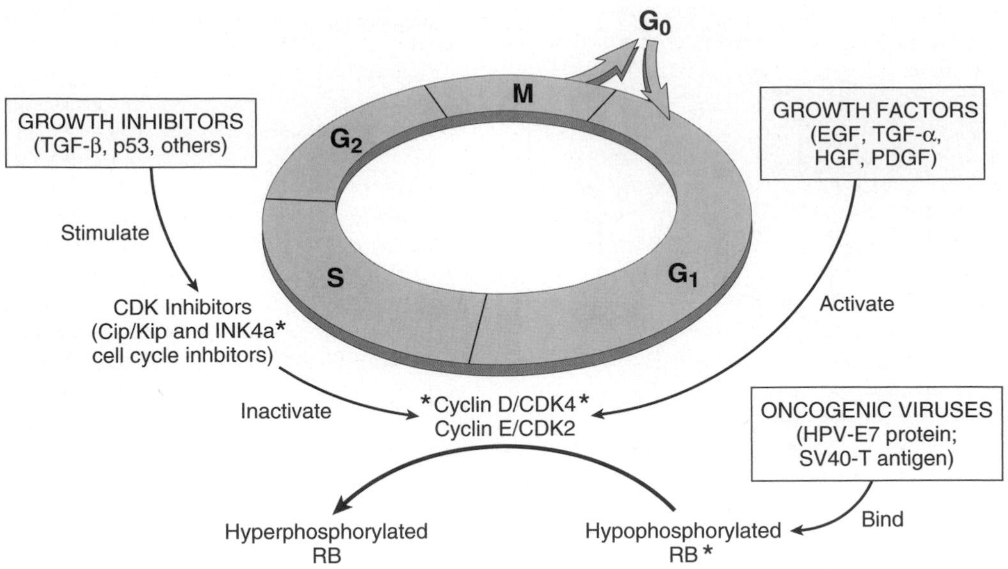

FIGURE 7–36 Role of RB as a cell-cycle regulator. Various growth factors promote the formation of the cyclin D–CDK4 complex. This complex (and to some extent cyclin E–CDK2) phosphorylates RB, changing it from an active (hypophosphorylated) to an inactive state (hyperphosphorylation). RB inactivation allows the cell to pass the G_1/S restriction point. Growth inhibitors such as TGF-β and *p53* and the Cip/Kip (e.g., p21, p57) and INK4a (p16INK4a and p19ARF) cell-cycle inhibitors prevent RB activation. Transforming proteins of oncogenic viruses bind hypophosphorylated RB and cause its functional inactivation. Virtually all cancers show dysregulation of the cell cycle by affecting the four genes marked by an asterisk.

cervical carcinomas. Thus, the RB protein, unable to bind the E2F transcription factors, is functionally deleted, and the transcription factors are free to cause cell-cycle progression.

- The *p53* tumor suppressor gene exerts its growth-inhibiting effects at least in part by up-regulating the synthesis of the CDK inhibitor p21 (see Figs. 7–29 and 7–36).

p53: Guardian of the Genome. The *p53* gene is located on chromosome 17p13.1, and it is the most common target for genetic alteration in human tumors.[71] *A little over 50% of human tumors contain mutations in this gene.* Homozygous loss of *p53* gene activity can occur in virtually every type of cancer, including carcinomas of the lung, colon, and breast—the three leading causes of cancer death.[72] In most cases, the inactivating mutations affect both *p53* alleles and are acquired in somatic cells (not inherited in the germ line). Less commonly, some individuals inherit one mutant *p53* allele. As with the *RB* gene, inheritance of one mutant allele predisposes individuals to develop malignant tumors because only one additional "hit" is needed to inactivate the second, normal allele. Such individuals, said to have the *Li-Fraumeni syndrome,* have a 25-fold greater chance of developing a malignant tumor by age 50 than the general population.[73] In contrast to patients who inherit a mutant *RB* allele, the spectrum of tumors that develop in patients with the Li-Fraumeni syndrome is quite varied; the most common types of tumors are sarcomas, breast cancer, leukemia, brain tumors, and carcinomas of the adrenal cortex. As compared with sporadic tumors, those that afflict patients with the Li-Fraumeni syndrome occur at a younger age, and a given individual may develop multiple primary tumors.[74]

The fact that *p53* mutations are common in a variety of human tumors suggests that the p53 protein functions as a critical gatekeeper against the formation of cancer. Indeed, it is evident that *p53* acts as a "*molecular policeman*" that prevents the propagation of genetically damaged cells. The p53 protein is a DNA-binding protein localized to the nucleus; when called into action, it functions primarily by controlling the transcription of several other genes. Approximately 80% of the *p53* point mutations present in human cancers are located in the DNA-binding domain of the protein. Mutated *p53* that does not bind to DNA, produces a defective protein (missense mutation) that blocks the activity of the normal protein. In addition to somatic and inherited mutations, p53 functions can be inactivated by other mechanisms. As with RB, the transforming proteins of several DNA viruses, including the E6 protein of HPV, can bind to and promote the degradation of p53. Another mechanism of p53 neutralization is via MDM2, a protein that normally inhibits the function of p53 by causing its degradation. MDM2 levels are increased in 33% of human sarcomas and in 50% of leukemias, thereby causing functional loss of p53 in these tumors.[75,76]

The major functional activities of the p53 protein are cell-cycle arrest and initiation of apoptosis in response to DNA damage. p53 is called in to apply emergency brakes when DNA is damaged by irradiation, UV light, or mutagenic chemicals and also in response to changes in cellular redox potential, hypoxia, senescence, and other stress conditions that may not directly damage DNA.[71] Following DNA damage, there is a rapid increase in p53 levels. At the same time, kinases such as DNA-dependent protein kinase and *ATM* (ataxia-telangectasia mutated) are activated in response to DNA damage. These enzymes phosphorylate p53, and the protein then unfolds, is able to bind to DNA, and becomes an active transcription factor (Fig. 7–37). p53 stimulates transcription of several genes that mediate cell-cycle arrest and apoptosis. p53-induced cell-cycle arrest occurs late in the G_1 phase and is caused by the p53-dependent transcription of the CDK inhibitor p21. Such a pause in cell cycling is welcome because it allows the cells enough time to repair the DNA damage inflicted by the mutagenic agent. Under physiologic conditions, p53 has a short half-life (about 20 minutes) because of ubiquitin-mediated proteolysis; hence, in contrast to RB, it does not police the normal cell cycle. p53 also helps in the repair process directly by inducing the transcription of *GADD45* (growth *a*rrest and *D*NA *d*amage), which encodes a protein involved in DNA repair. If the DNA damage is repaired successfully, quite ingeniously, p53 activates *MDM2,* whose product binds to and degrades p53, thus relieving the cell-cycle block (see Fig. 7–29). If during the pause in cell division the DNA damage cannot be successfully repaired, normal p53, perhaps as a last-ditch effort, sends the cell to the graveyard by inducing the activation of apoptosis-inducing genes, such as *BAX*. BAX, as we discuss later, binds to and antagonizes the apoptosis-inhibiting protein BCL-2; thus, *BAX* promotes cell death.

To summarize, p53 links cell damage with DNA repair, cell-cycle arrest, and apoptosis. In response to DNA damage, it is phosphorylated by genes that sense the damage and are involved in DNA repair. p53 assists in DNA repair by causing G_1 arrest and inducing DNA repair genes. A cell with damaged DNA that cannot be repaired is directed by p53 to undergo apoptosis (see Fig. 7–37). In view of these activities, p53 has been rightfully called a "guardian of the genome." With homozygous loss of p53, DNA damage goes unrepaired, mutations become fixed in dividing cells, and the cell turns onto a one-way street leading to malignant transformation.

The ability of *p53* to control apoptosis in response to DNA damage has important practical therapeutic implications. Radiation and chemotherapy, the two common modalities of cancer treatment, mediate their effects by inducing DNA damage and subsequent apoptosis. Tumors that retain normal *p53* are more likely to respond to such therapy than tumors that carry mutant alleles of the gene. Such is the case with testicular teratocarcinomas[77] and childhood acute lymphoblastic leukemias. By contrast, tumors such as lung cancers and colorectal cancers, which frequently carry *p53* mutations, are relatively resistant to chemotherapy and radiotherapy. Various therapeutic strategies aimed at increasing normal p53 activity in tumor cells that retain this type of activity or selectively killing cells defective in p53 function are being investigated. One type of strategy relies mostly on the modulation of MDM2 activity; a second uses modified adenoviruses that lyse cancer cells that lack p53 or p14ARF function.[38,78]

In closing this discussion of the *p53* gene, it should be pointed out that *p53* is actually a member of a multigene family.[79] The *p73* gene (dubbed the big brother of *p53*), another member of this family, is located on 1p36 and encodes a protein that has 60% homology to *p53*. It can cause cell-cycle arrest as well as apoptosis under appropriate conditions.[80] The newest member of the family is *p63*. It is likely that at least in some tissues, *p53* deficiency may be compensated by expression of the other genes of the same family.

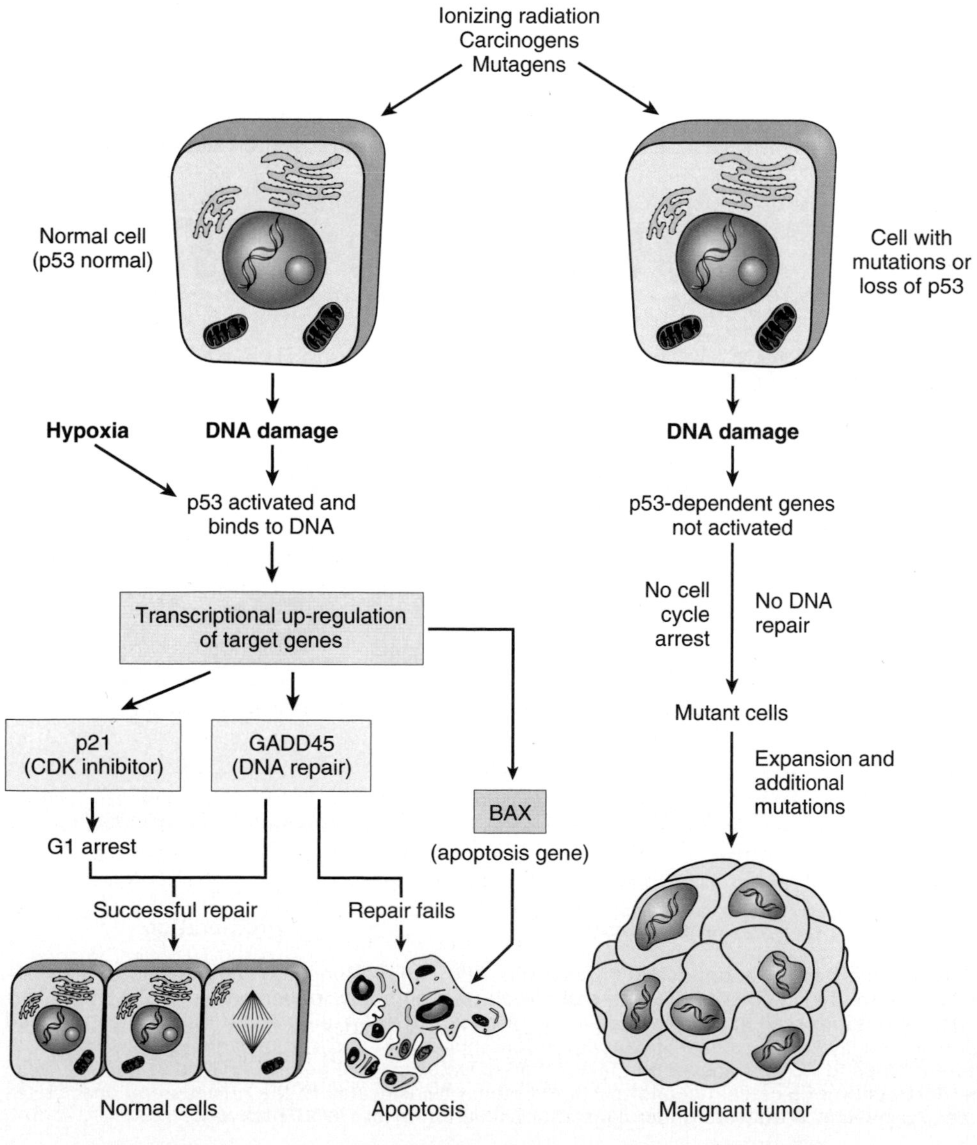

FIGURE 7–37 The role of *p53* in maintaining the integrity of the genome. Activation of normal *p53* by DNA-damaging agents or by hypoxia leads to cell-cycle arrest in G_1 and induction of DNA repair, by transcriptional up-regulation of the cyclin-dependent kinase inhibitor *p21,* and the *GADD45* genes, respectively. Successful repair of DNA allows cells to proceed with the cell cycle; if DNA repair fails, *p53*-induced activation of the *BAX* gene promotes apoptosis. In cells with loss or mutations of *p53,* DNA damage does not induce cell-cycle arrest or DNA repair, and hence genetically damaged cells proliferate, giving rise eventually to malignant neoplasms.

APC/β-Catenin Pathway. Down-regulation of growth-promoting signals is another potential area in which products of tumor suppressor genes may be operative. The products of the *APC* and *NF-1* genes fall into this category. Germ line mutations at the *APC* (5q21) and *NF-1* (17q11.2) loci are associated with benign tumors that are precursors of carcinomas that develop later.

In the case of the *APC* gene, all individuals born with one mutant allele develop thousands of adenomatous polyps in the colon during their teens or twenties (familial adenomatous polyposis; Chapter 17). Almost invariably, one or more of these polyps undergoes malignant transformation, giving rise to colon cancer. As with other tumor suppressor genes, both copies of the *APC* gene must be lost for tumor development. When this occurs, adenomas form. This conclusion is supported by the development of colon adenomas in mice with targeted disruption of *APC* genes in the colonic mucosa.[81] As discussed later, several additional mutations must occur for cancers to develop in adenomas. In addition to these tumors, which have a strong hereditary predisposition, 70% to 80% of nonfamilial colorectal carcinomas and sporadic adenomas also show homozygous loss of the *APC* gene, thus firmly implicating *APC* loss in the pathogenesis of colonic tumors.[56]

The molecular basis of *APC* action and the basis of its tumor suppressor activity have been learned by the study of homologous genes in the fruitfly *Drosophila* and the amphibian *Xenopus* (Fig. 7–38). APC is a component of the WNT signaling pathway, which has a major role in controlling cell fate, adhesion, and cell polarity during embryonic development. WNT signaling is also required for self-renewal of hematopoietic stem cells.[82] WNT signals through a family of cell-surface receptors called frizzled (FRZ), and stimulates several pathways, the central one involving β-catenin and APC.[83]

An important function of the APC protein is to down-regulate β-catenin. In the absence of WNT-signaling APC causes degradation of β-catenin, preventing its accumulation in the cytoplasm. It does so by forming a macromolecular complex with β-catenin, which results in the degradation of β-catenin. Inactivation of the *APC* gene disrupts the complex and increases the cellular levels of β-catenin, which, in turn, translocates to the nucleus.[84] Thus, with loss of APC the cell behaves as if it is under continuous WNT-signaling and there is an excess of free β-catenin. In the cell nucleus, β-catenin forms a complex with TCF, a transcription factor that up-regulates cellular proliferation by increasing the transcription of c-*MYC, CYCLIN D1,* and other genes. The importance of the APC/β-catenin signaling pathway in tumorigenesis is attested to by the fact that colon tumors may have normal *APC* genes but have mutations in β-catenin. Mutated β-catenin is not inhibited by APC and migrates into the nucleus. Dysregulation of the APC/β-catenin pathway is not restricted to colon cancers; mutations in β-catenin are present in more than 50% of hepatoblastomas and in approximately 20% of hepatocellular carcinomas.[85] As mentioned in Chapter 3, β-catenin binds to cytoplasmic E-cadherin, a cell-surface protein that maintains intercellular adhesiveness.

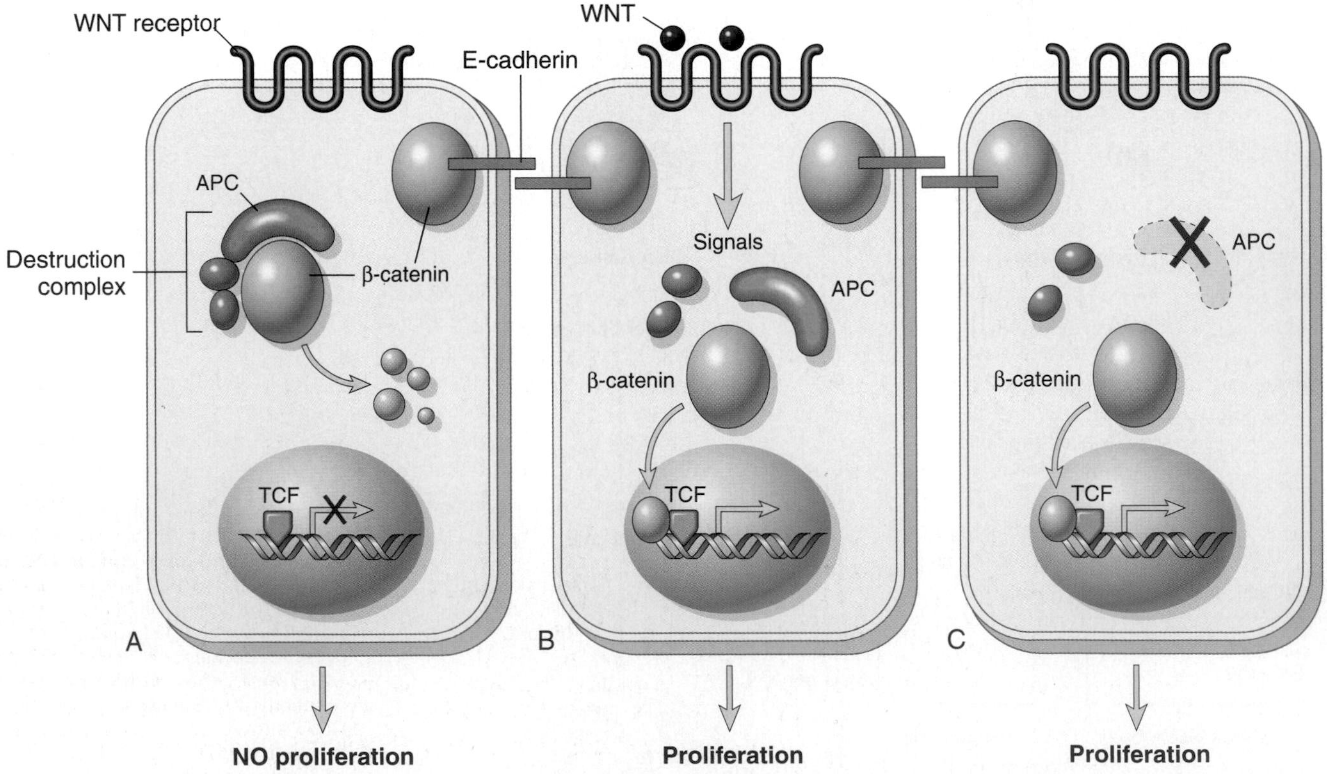

FIGURE 7–38 *A,* The role of APC in regulating the stability and function of β-catenin. APC and β-catenin are components of the WNT signaling pathway. In resting cells (not exposed to WNT), β-catenin forms a macromolecular complex containing the APC protein. This complex leads to the destruction of β-catenin, and intracellular levels of β-catenin are low. *B,* When cells are stimulated by secreted WNT molecules, the *destruction complex* is deactivated, β-catenin degradation does not occur, and cytoplasmic levels increase. β-catenin translocates to the nucleus, where it binds to TCF, a transcription factor that activates several genes involved in the cell cycle. *C,* When *APC* is mutated or absent, the destruction of β-catenin cannot occur. β-Catenin translocates to the nucleus and coactivates genes that promote the cell cycle, and cells behave as if they are under constant stimulation by the WNT pathway.

The reduced adhesiveness of cancer cells may result from defects in the cadherin–catenin axis. The cell adhesiveness effects of β-catenin are independent of its role as a transcription factor.

Other Genes That Function as Tumor Suppressors. There is little doubt that many more tumor suppressor genes remain to be discovered. Often, their location is suspected by the detection of consistent sites of *chromosomal deletions* or by analysis of *LOH*. Some of the tumor suppressor genes that are associated with well-defined clinical syndromes are briefly described below (see Table 7–9):

- **The *INK4a/ARF* locus.** Mutations of this locus have been found in about 20% of familial melanomas.[26] Among sporadic tumors, *p16INK4a* mutations are present in up to 50% of pancreatic adenocarcinomas and squamous cell carcinomas of the esophagus, and have also been detected in bladder, head, and neck tumors and in cholangiocarcinomas. Mutated alleles of *p16INK4a* present in these tumors have lost their capacity to block cyclin D–CDK4 activity and to prevent RB phosphorylation during the cell cycle. In some tumors, such as cervical cancer, *p16INK4a* is frequently inactivated by hypermethylation of the gene, without the presence of a mutation (see discussion of epigenetic changes).
- **The TGF-β pathway.** The gene encoding the type II TGF-β receptor is inactivated in 70% or more of colon cancers that develop in patients with HNPCC, in sporadic colon cancers with microsatellite instability (discussed in conjunction with DNA repair genes), and in gastric cancers that develop in HNPCC patients.[86] *SMAD4,* which encodes a component of the TGF-β growth-inhibitory signal transduction pathway, is inactivated in approximately 50% of pancreatic cancers, while mutations in *SMAD2*, another component of the pathway, are present in some colorectal tumors. Because of its association with pancreatic cancers, *SMAD4* was originally designated *DPC4, d*eleted in *p*ancreatic *c*ancer.[57, 87]
- ***NF-1* gene.** Individuals who inherit one mutant allele of the *NF-1* gene develop numerous benign neurofibromas as a result of inactivation of the second copy of the gene.[88] This condition is called *neurofibromatosis type 1* (Chapter 5). Some of the neurofibromas later develop into neurofibrosarcomas. Children with neurofibromatosis type 1 also are at increased risk of developing gliomas of the optic nerve. *Neurofibromin*, the protein product of the *NF-1* gene, regulates signal transduction through a RAS protein. Recall that RAS transmits growth-promoting signals and flips back and forth between GDP-binding (inactive) and GTP-binding (active) states. Neurofibromin is a member of a family of GTPase-activating proteins, which facilitate conversion of RAS from an active to an inactive state. With loss of NF-1 function, RAS is trapped in an active, signal-emitting state.
- ***NF-2* gene.** Germ line mutations in the *NF-2* gene predispose to the development of *neurofibromatosis type 2.*[89] As discussed in Chapter 5, patients with *NF-2* deficiency develop benign bilateral schwannomas of the acoustic nerve. In addition, somatic mutations affecting both alleles of *NF-2* have also been found in sporadic meningiomas and ependymomas. The product of the *NF-2* gene, called *merlin,* shows a great deal of homology with the red cell membrane cytoskeletal protein 4.1 (Chapter 13), and is related to the ERM (ezrin, radixin, and moesin) family of membrane cytoskeleton–associated proteins. Merlin binds, on one hand, to actin and, on the other hand, to CD44, a transmembrane protein that is involved in cell–matrix interactions (Chapter 3). Although the mechanism by which *NF2* deficiency leads to carcinogenesis is not known, cells lacking merlin are not capable of establishing stable cell-to-cell junctions and are insensitive to normal growth arrest signals generated by cell-to-cell contact.
- ***VHL.*** Germ line mutations of the von Hippel Lindau (*VHL*) gene on chromosome 3p are associated with hereditary renal cell cancers, pheochromocytomas, hemangioblastomas of the central nervous system, retinal angiomas, and renal cysts.[71] Mutations of the *VHL* gene have also been noted in sporadic renal cell cancers (Chapter 20). The VHL protein forms a complex that function as ubiquitin ligases. A main substrate for this activity is HIF-1 (hypoxia inducible transcription factor 1), which regulates several genes, including *VEGF* and *PDGF.* Lack of VHL activity prevents ubiquitination and degradation of HIF-1 and is associated with increased levels of angiogenic growth factors.
- ***PTEN.*** *P*hosphatase and *ten*sin homologue, deleted on chromosome 10 *(PTEN)* gene, mapped on chromosome 10q23, is frequently deleted in many human cancers but at particularly high frequency in endometrial carcinomas and glioblastomas.[90] PTEN activity causes cell-cycle arrest and apoptosis as well as inhibition of cell motility. It has been proposed that PTEN blocks the cell cycle by increasing the transcription of the p27 Cip/Kip cell-cycle inhibitor and stabilizing the protein.[90,91] With loss of PTEN, therefore, cells are released into the cell cycle.
- ***WT-1.*** The *WT-1* gene, located on chromosome 11p13, is associated with the development of *W*ilms *t*umor, a pediatric kidney cancer.[92] Both inherited and sporadic forms of Wilms tumor occur, and mutational inactivation of the *WT-1* locus has been seen in both forms. The WT-1 protein is a transcriptional activator of genes involved in renal and gonadal differentiation. It regulates the mesenchymal to epithelial transition that occurs in kidney development. Although not precisely known, it is likely that the tumorigenic effect of *WT-1* deficiency is intimately connected with the role of the gene in the differentiation of genitourinary tissues. Another Wilms gene, *WT-2,* located on 11p15, is associated with the Beckwith-Wiedeman syndrome (Chapter 10).
- ***Cadherins.*** These are a family of glycoproteins that act as glues between epithelial cells (Chapter 3). Loss of cadherins can favor the malignant phenotype by allowing easy disaggregation of cells, which can then invade locally or metastasize. Reduced cell-surface expression of E-cadherin has been noted in many types of cancers, including those that arise in the esophagus, colon, breast, ovary, and prostate.[93] Germ line mutations of the E-cadherin gene can predispose to familial gastric carcinoma, and mutation of the gene and decreased E-cadherin expression are present in a variable proportion of gastric cancers of the diffuse type. The molecular basis of reduced E-cadherin expression is varied. In a small proportion of cases, there are mutations in the E-cadherin gene (located on 16q); in other cancers,

E-cadherin expression is reduced as a secondary effect of mutations in β-catenin genes. β-catenins, as discussed earlier, bind to the intracellular portion of cadherins and stabilize their expression.

- ***KLF6.*** *KLF6* encodes a transcription factor that has many target genes, including *TGF-β* and *TGF-β* receptors. *KLF6* is mutated in more than 70% of primary prostate cancers. It has been proposed that *KLF6* inhibits cell proliferation by increasing the transcription of the Cip/Kip cell-cycle inhibitor p21, independent of p53. Mutation of the gene in tumor cells eliminates the cell-cycle–blocking activity of p21.[94]
- ***Patched (PTCH).*** *PTCH* is a tumor suppressor gene that encodes a cell-membrane protein (PATCHED), which functions as a receptor for a family of proteins called *Hedgehog.*[95] The Hedgehog/PATCHED pathway regulates several genes, including *TGF-β* and *PDGF-R.* Mutations in *PTCH* are responsible for Gorlin syndrome, an inherited condition also known as nevoid basal cell carcinoma syndrome (see Chapter 26). *PTCH* mutations are present in 20% to 50% of sporadic cases of basal cell carcinoma. About one half of such mutations are of the type caused by UV exposure.

EVASION OF APOPTOSIS

Just as cell growth is regulated by growth-promoting and growth-inhibiting genes, cell survival is conditioned by genes that promote and inhibit apoptosis. Therefore, the accumulation of neoplastic cells may occur not only by the activation of oncogenes or inactivation of tumor suppressor genes, but also by mutations in the genes that regulate apoptosis.[96–98] A large family of genes that regulate apoptosis has been identified in both normal and cancer cells. The main pathways of apoptosis were described in Chapter 1. Here we discuss the role of *BCL-2* in protecting tumor cells from apoptosis.

The discovery of *BCL-2,* the prototypic gene in this category, began with the observation that approximately 85% of B-cell lymphomas of the follicular type (Chapter 14) carry a characteristic t(14;18)(q32;q21) translocation, in which the *BCL-2* gene from 18q21 is translocated to the immunoglobulin heavy-chain locus on 14q32. (Recall that the immunoglobulin heavy-chain locus is also involved in translocation—of the *MYC* gene—in Burkitt lymphoma.) Removal of *BCL-2* from its normal controls leads to increased transcription and overexpression of the BCL-2 protein. As mentioned above and discussed in Chapter 1, BCL-2 protects cells from apoptosis by the mitochondrial pathway. Thus, there is a steady accumulation of B lymphocytes (the cells in which the translocation typically occurs as the immunoglobulin locus is open), resulting in lymphadenopathy and marrow infiltration. Because lymphomas that overexpress BCL-2 arise in large part from reduced cell death rather than explosive cell proliferation, they tend to be indolent (slow growing) compared with many other lymphomas. Supporting the role of *BCL-2* in lymphomagenesis is the observation that mice transgenic for *BCL-2* develop B-cell lymphomas. Not only is the function of *BCL-2* unusual among cancer-associated genes, but its location in the outer mitochondrial membrane is also different from that of most such genes.[99–100]

At least two other cancer-associated genes are also intimately connected with apoptosis: *p53* and *MYC.* The molecular mechanisms of cell death induced by these two intersect with the *BCL-2* pathways. As discussed, p53 increases the transcription of pro-apoptotic genes such as *BAX.* Lack of p53 activity, caused by mutations in *p53* or alterations in *INK4a* and *MDM2,* decreases transcription of the pro-apoptotic gene *BAX,* reduces apoptotic activity, and reduces the response to chemotherapy. Studies in mice show that *BAX* expression is required for the p53-induced apoptotic response. *BID,* another pro-apoptotic member of the *BCL-2* family, is also regulated by p53 and might enhance cell death in response to chemotherapy.[101] *MYC* and *BCL-2* may collaborate in tumorigenesis: *MYC* triggers proliferation, and *BCL-2* prevents cell death, even if growth factors become limiting. This is one of many examples in which two or more genes cooperate in giving rise to cancer. It should also be noted that normal cells require continuous survival signals as, for instance, signaling through the PI-3 kinase/AKT pathway, which prevents the activity of the apoptotic machinery. Lack of these signals can cause apoptosis, a condition known as "death by neglect."[98] AKT expression in cancer cells is often increased as a consequence of mutations in *AKT* or inactivating mutations in the *PTEN* tumor suppressor gene. These alterations increase the resistance of the cancer cell to apoptotic cell death.[102]

DNA REPAIR DEFECTS AND GENOMIC INSTABILITY IN CANCER CELLS

Humans literally swim in a sea of environmental carcinogens. Although exposure to naturally occurring DNA-damaging agents, such as ionizing radiation, sunlight, dietary carcinogens, and ROS generated by cell metabolism and oxidative stress, is common, cancer is a relatively rare outcome of such encounters. This fortunate state of affairs results from the ability of normal cells to repair DNA damage and thus prevent mutations in genes that regulate cell growth and apoptosis.[103] In addition to possible DNA damage from environmental agents, the DNA of normal dividing cells is susceptible to alterations resulting from errors that occur spontaneously during DNA replication. Such mistakes, if not repaired promptly, can also push the cells along the slippery slope of neoplastic transformation. The importance of DNA repair in maintaining the integrity of the genome is highlighted by several inherited disorders in which genes that encode proteins involved in DNA repair are defective. *Those born with such inherited mutations of DNA repair proteins are at a greatly increased risk of developing cancer. These conditions are known as genomic instability syndromes.* Moreover, defects in repair mechanisms are present in sporadic human cancers. *DNA repair genes themselves are not oncogenic, but their abnormalities allow mutations in other genes during the process of normal cell division.* Typically, genomic instability occurs when both copies of these genes are lost. Thus, in this respect they resemble tumor suppressor genes. Defects in three types of DNA repair systems, namely, *mismatch repair, nucleotide excision repair, and recombination repair*, are presented next.

Hereditary Nonpolyposis Cancer Syndrome. The role of DNA mismatch repair genes in predisposition to cancer is illustrated dramatically by the HNPCC syndrome.[104] This disorder is characterized by familial carcinomas of the colon affecting predominantly the cecum and proximal colon (Chapter 17). Although *mismatch errors* in DNA replication can occur in any dividing cell, carcinomas occur mainly in the proximal colon in those with HNPCC. In some families, there is also an associated increase in endometrial and ovarian cancers, but mysteriously, most other tissues are spared. In contrast to the carcinomas in patients with germ line *APC* mutations discussed earlier, the cancers in the HNPCC syndrome do not arise in adenomatous polyps.

When a strand of DNA is replicating, mismatch repair genes act as "spell checkers." Thus, for example, if there is an erroneous pairing of G with T, rather than the normal A with T, the mismatch repair proteins correct the defect. Without these proofreaders, errors slowly accumulate in several genes, including protooncogenes and tumor suppressor genes. Cells with such defects in DNA repair are said to have the *replication error phenotype,* which can be readily documented by examination of microsatellite sequences in the tumor cell DNA.[105] *Microsatellites* are tandem repeats of one to six nucleotides scattered throughout the genome (Chapter 5). Microsatellite sequences of an individual are fixed for life and are the same in every tissue. With errors in mismatch repair, there are expansions and contractions of these repeats in tumor cells, creating alleles not found in normal cells of the same patient. Such *microsatellite instability* is a hallmark of defective mismatch repair.[24] Of the various DNA mismatch repair genes, at least four are involved in the pathogenesis of HNPCC, but germ line mutations in the *MSH2* (2p16) and *MLH1* (3p21) genes each account for approximately 30% of cases. The remaining cases have mutations in *PMS, PMS2,* and other mismatch repair genes. Each affected individual inherits one defective copy of one of the several DNA mismatch repair genes and acquires the "second hit" in the colonic epithelial cells. Thus, DNA repair genes behave similarly to tumor suppressor genes in their mode of inheritance, but, in contrast to the classic tumor suppressor genes, they do not affect cell growth directly. Because mutations occur more readily and more rapidly in patients with HNPCC, the evolution of tumors occurs more rapidly, and hence patients develop colon cancers at a much younger age (<50 years) than those who do not have any defects in DNA repair.

Although HNPCC accounts for only 2% to 4% of all colonic cancers, microsatellite instability can be detected in about 15% of sporadic colon cancers. The growth-regulating genes that are mutated in patients with HNPCC have not yet been completely characterized but include the genes encoding TGF-β receptor II, the TCF component of the β-catenin pathway, *BAX,* and other oncogenes and tumor suppressor genes.[106] As discussed earlier, loss of TGF-β receptors nullifies the growth-inhibiting action of TGF-β, and mutations in the *BAX* gene dysregulate apoptosis.

Xeroderma Pigmentosum. Patients with *xeroderma pigmentosum,* another inherited disorder involving defective DNA repair genes, are at increased risk for the development of cancers of the skin when exposed to the UV rays contained in sunlight.[107] UV light causes cross-linking of pyrimidine residues, thus preventing normal DNA replication. Such DNA damage is repaired by the *nucleotide excision repair* (NER) pathway, which is discussed later in conjunction with the induction of carcinogenesis by UV rays. Several proteins and genes are involved in NER, and an inherited loss of any one can give rise to xeroderma pigmentosum.

Inherited Diseases with Defects in DNA Repair by Homologous Recombination. A group of autosomal recessive disorders, including *ataxia-telangiectasia, Bloom syndrome,* and *Fanconi anemia,* are characterized by hypersensitivity to other DNA-damaging agents, such as ionizing radiation (ataxia-telangiectasia and Bloom syndrome), or DNA cross-linking agents (Fanconi anemia). These syndromes include, in addition to predisposition to cancer, other features such as neural symptoms (ataxia-telangiectasia), anemia (Fanconi anemia), and developmental defects (Bloom syndrome).[108] Patients with Bloom syndrome have a predisposition to a very broad spectrum of tumors. The defective gene is located on chromosome 15 and encodes a helicase (*BLM* helicase), which participates in DNA repair by homologous recombination.[109]

Patients with *ataxia-telangiectasia* have a complex phenotype, characterized by gradual loss of Purkinje cells in the cerebellum that causes cerebellar ataxia, defective lymphocyte maturation and proliferation. These defects lead to immunodeficiency, acute sensitivity to ionizing radiation, and profound susceptibility to lymphoid malignancies. The disease is caused by mutation of the *ATM* gene, resulting in absence or almost complete loss of function of the protein. *ATM* encodes a protein kinase that senses DNA double-strand breaks, a type of damage caused by ionizing radiation and oxygen free radicals.[110] After such damage, the kinase activity of ATM is rapidly increased. ATM phosphorylates p53, leading to cell-cycle arrest in G_1 or apoptosis. In cells lacking the normal *ATM* genes, the p53-induced delay in the cell cycle does not occur, and hence the DNA-damaged cells continue to proliferate and are prone to transformation. There is much current interest in the *ATM* gene because it is estimated that approximately 1% of the population is heterozygous for this gene, and hence carriers. Although heterozygotes do not develop cancers, they are presumed to be at increased risk for radiation-induced DNA damage. It is therefore speculated that they may be at risk of developing cancers after exposure to doses of irradiation used in common radiologic procedures such as mammography.

***BRCA-1* and *BRCA-2* Genes.** *BRCA-1,* on chromosome 17q21, and *BRCA-2,* on chromosome 13q12-13, are two genes associated with the occurrence of breast and several other cancers[12] (Chapter 24). As with tumor suppressor genes, individuals who inherit mutations of *BRCA-1* or *BRCA-2* are highly susceptible to the development of breast cancer. With germ line mutations of the *BRCA-1* gene, there is, in addition, a substantially higher risk of epithelial ovarian cancers and a slightly increased risk of prostate and colon cancers. Likewise, mutations in the *BRCA-2* gene increase the risk of developing cancers of the ovary (although less than for *BRCA-1*) and of the male breast as well as other cancers such as melanomas and pancreatic tumors. Approximately 10% to 20% of breast cancers are familial; mutations in *BRCA-1* and *BRCA-2* account for 80% of the familial cases in families with multiple affected members but are present in less than 3% of all breast cancers.[25] Thus, in contrast to other tumor suppressor genes *(RB, p53, NF-1, VHL)* that are associated with heritable cancer syndromes, mutations in neither of the two *BRCA* genes are associated with the development of nonfamilial (sporadic) forms of breast cancer. Nevertheless, it is possible that alterations in the expression of genes related to *BRCA-1* and *BRCA-2* may be involved in non-hereditary breast cancer.[109a]

The functions of *BRCA-1* and *BRCA-2* are not completely defined. Protein products of both genes are localized to the nucleus and are believed to be involved in transcription regulation. *BRCA-1* is involved in the regulation of estrogen receptor activity and is also a co-activator of the androgen receptor.[22] Both *BRCA-1* and *BRCA-2* participate in the process of homologous recombination of DNA repair; they bind to *RAD51*, a gene involved in the repair of double-strand DNA breaks, and are also involved in chromatin remodeling (see below and Chapter 23). *BRCA-1* and *BRCA-2* have a close connection with components of the G_1/S checkpoint that delays the cell cycle to allow for repair of DNA damage. Given the many activities of *BRCA-1* and *BRCA-2*, there are multiple ways in which defects in these genes can increase the risk of development of breast and ovarian tumors, but a precise explanation of their role is not yet available.

There is now much evidence that cancer susceptibility genes, including those involved in breast cancer, are linked to a network of genes that participate in the repair of double-strand DNA breaks by homologous recombination[111,112] (Fig. 7–39). *ATM* and *CHEK2* (a protein kinase activated by DNA damage) phosphorylate *BRCA1* and *RAD51*, which co-localize at sites of DNA damage.[113] A Fanconi anemia complex of proteins also colocalizes at damage sites, and *BRCA2* was recently identified as the *FANCD1* gene, one of several genes involved in Fanconi anemia.[114] Thus *BRCA* genes may be mutated in Fanconi anemia and breast cancers, entirely different diseases that may have in common the genetic instability produced by deficiencies in homologous recombination DNA repair genes.[112] Another example of the linkages that exist between cancer susceptibility genes and DNA repair genes is the recent demonstration that *ATM* mutations are present at high frequency in individuals with a familial pattern of breast and ovarian tumors.[115]

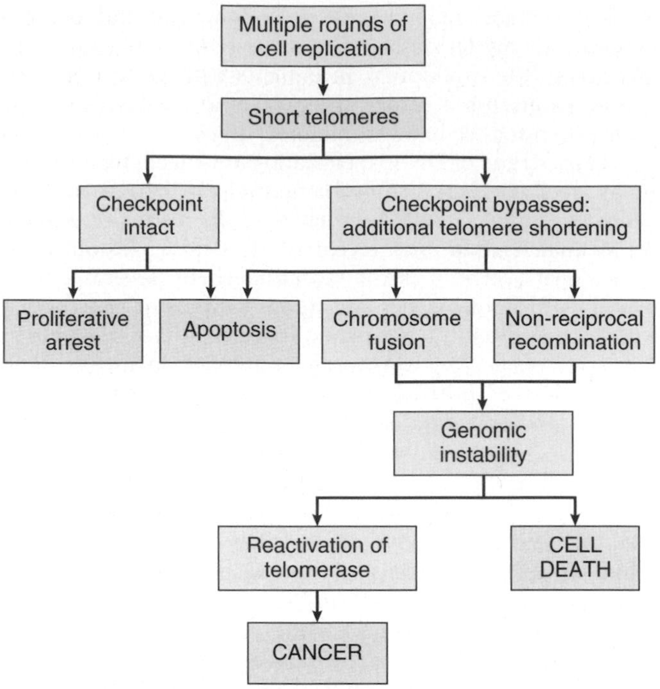

FIGURE 7–40 Cellular responses to telomere shortening. The figures show the responses of normal cells, which have intact cell-cycle checkpoints and of cells with checkpoint defects. (From Wong JMY, Collins K: Telomere maintenance and disease. Lancet 362:983, 2003.)

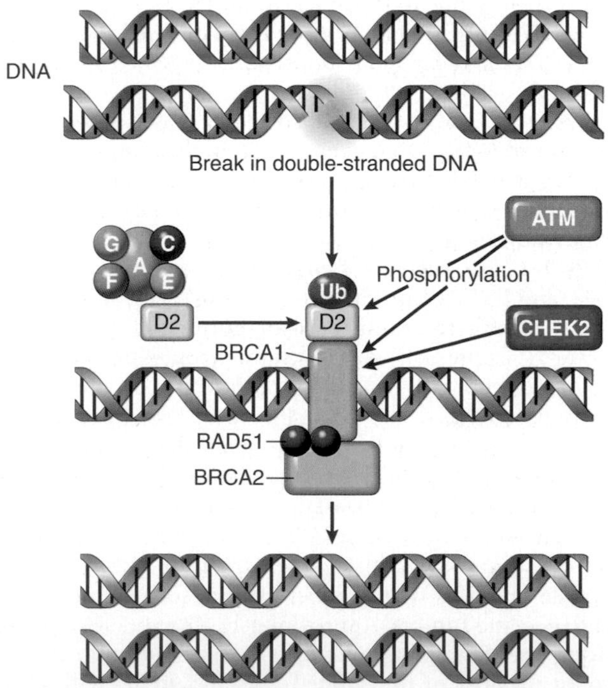

FIGURE 7–39 Interaction between cancer susceptibility genes and DNA repair. *ATM* (ataxia-telangiectasia mutated) senses a double-strand break in DNA, induced by agents such as ionizing radiation. *ATM* and *CHEK2* phosphorylate *BRCA1*, promoting its migration to the break site. The Fanconi's anemia protein complex (proteins A, C, E, F, G) triggers the ubiquitination and co-localization of the Fanconi protein D2 with *BRCA1* at the break site. *BRCA2* carries RAD51, an enzyme involved in DNA recombination repair, to the same site. BRCA1, BRCA2, and RAD51 repair the DNA break by an error-free recombination mechanism. RAD51 is a component of cell cycle check points. (Redrawn from Venkitaraman AR: A growing network of cancer-susceptibility genes. N Engl J Med 348:1917, 2003.)

LIMITLESS REPLICATIVE POTENTIAL: TELOMERASE

In the discussion of cellular aging (Chapter 1), it was pointed out that after a fixed number of divisions, normal cells become arrested in a terminally nondividing state known as *replicative senescence.* How normal cells can "count" their divisions is not known, but it has been noted that with each cell division there is some shortening of specialized structures, called *telomeres,* at the ends of chromosomes.[116] Once the telomeres are shortened beyond a certain point, the loss of telomere function leads to activation of *p53*-dependent cell-cycle checkpoints, causing proliferative arrest or apoptosis (Fig. 7–40). Thus, telomere shortening functions as a clock that counts cell divisions. In germ cells, telomere shortening is prevented by the sustained function of the enzyme *telom-*

erase, thus explaining the ability of these cells to self-replicate extensively. This enzyme is absent from most somatic cells, and hence they suffer progressive loss of telomeres. Introduction of telomerase into normal human cells causes considerable extension of their life span,[117] thus supporting the hypothesis that telomerase loss is causally associated with loss of replication ability. If loss of telomerase is the basis of the finite life span of cells, how do cancer cells continue to divide indefinitely? Cancer cells must find a way to prevent telomere shortening, and a mechanism that accomplishes this is the reactivation of telomerase activity. Indeed, telomerase activity has been detected in more than 90% of human tumors.[118] Telomerase may also act to promote tumorigenesis by mechanisms that do not depend on telomere length.[119] Thus, *telomerase activity and maintenance of telomere length are essential for the maintenance of replicative potential in cancer cells.* As mentioned above, in normal cells, short telomeres activate cell-cycle checkpoints that lead to cell-cycle arrest or apoptosis. However, transformed cells may have defects in cell-cycle checkpoints, allowing for critical telomere shortening in dividing cells. These cells may die by apoptosis or survive with chromosome defects that cause genomic instability (see Fig. 7–40). Reactivation of telomerase in cells with abnormal genomes confers an unlimited proliferative capacity to cells that have tumorigenic potential.

DEVELOPMENT OF SUSTAINED ANGIOGENESIS

Tumors stimulate the growth of host blood vessels, a process called *angiogenesis,* which is essential for supplying nutrients to the tumor. Even with genetic abnormalities that dysregulate growth and survival of individual cells, tumors cannot enlarge beyond 1 to 2 mm in diameter or thickness unless they are vascularized.[120] Presumably the 1- to 2-mm zone represents the maximal distance across which oxygen and nutrients can diffuse from blood vessels. Beyond this size, the tumor fails to enlarge without vascularization because of hypoxia-induced cell death. Neovascularization has a dual effect on tumor growth: perfusion supplies nutrients and oxygen, and newly formed endothelial cells stimulate the growth of adjacent tumor cells by secreting polypeptide growth factors such as insulin-like growth factors and PDGF.[121] Angiogenesis is a requisite not only for continued tumor growth, but also for metastasis. Without access to the vasculature, the tumor cells cannot readily spread to distant sites.

How do growing tumors develop a blood supply? Several studies indicate that tumors produce factors that are capable of triggering the entire series of events involved in the formation of new capillaries (Chapter 3). Tumor angiogenesis can occur by recruitment of endothelial cell precursors or by sprouting of existing capillaries, as in physiologic angiogenesis. However, tumor blood vessels differ from the normal vasculature by being tortuous and irregularly shaped (Fig. 7–41) and by being leaky. The leakiness is attributed largely to the increased production of VEGF.[122] In contrast to normal mature vessels, which are quiescent structures, tumor vessels may grow continuously. Tumor cells may, in some special cases, line structures that resemble capillaries, a phenomenon called *vasculogenic mimicry.*[123]

Tumor-associated angiogenic factors are produced by tumor cells or may be derived from inflammatory cells (e.g., macrophages) that infiltrate tumors. Of the dozen or so known tumor-associated angiogenic factors, the two most important are VEGF[124] and basic fibroblast growth factor (bFGF). VEGF is mostly produced by tumor cells but may also be made by cells of the tumor stroma. The mechanisms whereby bFGF and VEGF cause angiogenesis were discussed in Chapter 3. These two factors are commonly expressed in a wide variety of tumor cells, and elevated levels can be detected in the serum and urine of a significant fraction of cancer patients.

Experimental and clinical data indicate that early in their growth most human tumors do not induce angiogenesis. They exist in situ without developing a blood supply for months to years; then, some cells within the small tumor change to an angiogenic phenotype. This change is known as the *angiogenic switch.*[125] The molecular basis of the angiogenic switch is not entirely clear but may involve increased production of angiogenic factors or loss of angiogenesis inhibitors. In some cases, wild-type p53 inhibits angiogenesis by inducing the synthesis of the antiangiogenic molecule thrombospondin-1 and down-regulating the production of angiogenic factors such as VEGF and HIF-1, the hypoxia-inducible factor that stimulates VEGF transcription. With mutational inactivation of both *p53* alleles (common in many cancers), the levels of thrombospondin-1 drop precipitously, VEGF levels increase, and HIF-1 production is enhanced by tumor hypoxia, thus tilting the balance in favor of angiogenic factors.

Tumor cells not only produce angiogenic factors, but also induce anti-angiogenesis molecules. Tumor growth is thus controlled by the balance between angiogenic factors and those that inhibit angiogenesis.[126] Some anti-angiogenesis factors, such as thrombospondin-1, may be produced by the tumor cells themselves, whereas others, such as angiostatin, endostatin, and tumstatin, are produced in response to the tumor. These latter three potent angiogenesis inhibitors are derived by proteolytic cleavage of plasminogen (angiostatin) and of collagens (endostatin, tumstatin).

Because angiogenesis is critical for the growth and spread of tumors, much attention is focused on the use of angiogenesis inhibitors as adjuncts to other forms of therapy. Success has been achieved in treating several tumors in mice by administration of endostatin[120,126] and tumstatin. Endostatin is being tested for its effects on human tumors. Trials are also being conducted to test the antitumor effects of *antibodies to VEGF and VEGF-R2, and of small molecules that inhibit signal transduction through VEGF-R2.*[124,125]

INVASION AND METASTASIS

Invasion and metastasis are biologic hallmarks of malignant tumors. They are the major cause of cancer-related morbidity and mortality and hence are the subjects of intense scrutiny. For tumor cells to break loose from a primary mass, enter blood vessels or lymphatics, and produce a secondary growth at a distant site, they must go through a series of steps (summarized in Fig. 7–42). Each step in this sequence is subject to a multitude of influences; hence, at any point in the sequence the breakaway cell may not survive.[127]

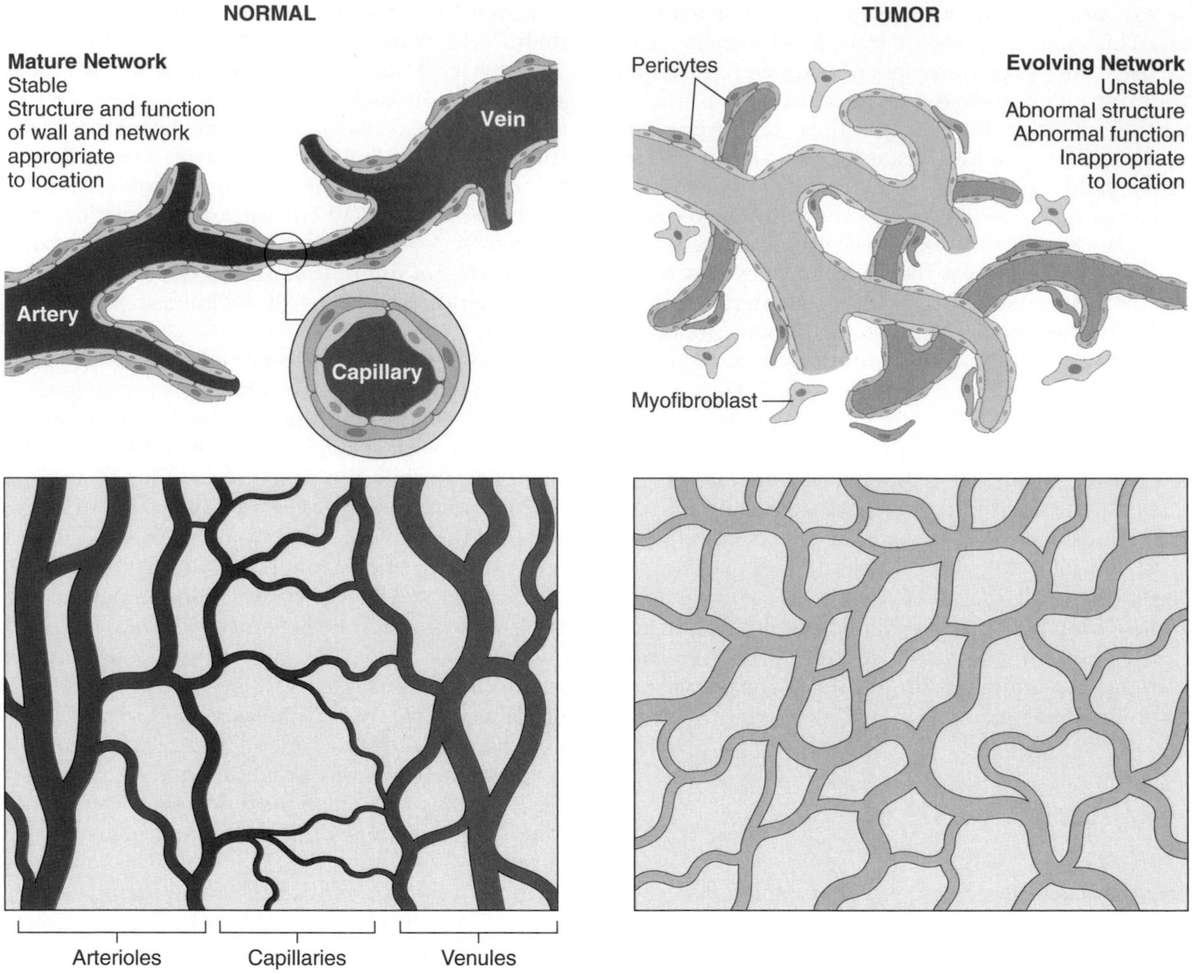

FIGURE 7–41 Tumor angiogenesis. Compared to normal blood vessels (left panels), tumor vessels are tortuous and irregularly shaped. The tumor vasculature *(upper right)* is formed from circulating endothelial precursor cells and existing host vessels (Chapter 3); myofibroblasts give rise to pericytes cells at the periphery of the vessels. By contrast to the stable vessel network of normal tissue, the networks formed by tumor vessels are unstable and leaky. Arterioles, capillaries, and veins are clearly distinguishable in the normal vasculature *(lower left)*; in the tumor the vessels are disorganized and not identifiable *(lower right)*. (Redrawn from Jain RK: Molecular regulation of vessel maturation. Nature Med 9:685, 2003; and McDonald DM, Choyke PL: Imaging of angiogenesis from microscope to clinic. Nature Med 9:713, 2003.)

Studies in mice reveal that although millions of cells are released into the circulation each day from a primary tumor, only a few metastases are produced. What then is the basis of the apparent inefficiency of this process? One prevalent view (Fig. 7–43*A*) is that certain tumor cell subclones possess the right combination of gene products to complete all the steps involved in metastasis. An alternative hypothesis is that metastasis is the result of multiple abnormalities that occur in many, perhaps most, cells of a primary tumor (Fig. 7–43*B* and *C*). Such abnormalities give the tumor a general predisposition for metastasis, which has been called a "metastasis signature."[128,129] This signature may involve not only properties intrinsic to the cancer cells, but also the characteristics of the stroma, such as the components of the stroma, the presence of infiltrating immune cells, and angiogenesis (Fig. 7–43*D*). A clear understanding of the origin of metastasis is of major importance for the management of cancer patients and the development of effective therapies to prevent tumor spread. For the purpose of this discussion, the metastatic cascade will be divided into two phases: (1) invasion of the extracellular matrix and (2) vascular dissemination and homing of tumor cells.

Invasion of Extracellular Matrix

The structural organization and function of normal tissues is to a great extent determined by interactions between cells and the extracellular matrix (ECM).[130] As we discussed in Chapter 3, tissues are organized into compartments separated from each other by two types of ECM: basement membrane and interstitial connective tissue. Although organized differently, each of these components of ECM is made up of collagens, glycoproteins, and proteoglycans. As shown in Figure 7–42, tumor cells must interact with the ECM at several stages in the metastatic cascade. A carcinoma must first breach the underlying basement membrane, then traverse the interstitial connective tissue, and ultimately gain access to the circulation by penetrating the vascular basement membrane. This cycle is repeated when tumor cell emboli extravasate at a distant site. *Invasion of the ECM is an active process that can be resolved into several steps* (Fig. 7–44):

- Detachment ("loosening up") of the tumor cells from each other
- Attachment to matrix components
- Degradation of ECM
- Migration of tumor cells

Normal cells are neatly glued to each other and their surroundings by a variety of adhesion molecules.[131] Of these, the cadherin family of transmembrane glycoproteins is of particular importance. E-cadherins mediate homotypic adhesions in epithelial tissue, thus serving to keep the epithelial cells together and to relay signals between the cells. In several epithelial tumors, including adenocarcinomas of the colon and breast, there is a down-regulation of E-cadherin expression. Presumably, this down-regulation reduces the ability of cells to adhere to each other and facilitates their detachment from the primary tumor and their advance into the surrounding tissues. E-cadherins are linked to the cytoskeleton by the *catenins,* proteins that lie under the plasma membrane (Fig. 7–38). The normal function of E-cadherin is dependent on its linkage to catenins. In some tumors, E-cadherin is normal, but its expression is reduced because of mutations in the gene for a catenin.

To penetrate the surrounding ECM, the tumor cells must first adhere to the matrix components. Epithelial cells of a tumor are separated from the stroma by a basement membrane. Thus, for tumor cells to penetrate the basement membrane, the membrane must be degraded and remodeled.[124] As this process occurs, components of the basement membrane send both positive and negative growth signals to tumor cells and have a major role in regulating angiogenesis. There is substantial evidence that receptor-mediated attachment of tumor cells to laminin and fibronectin is important for invasion and

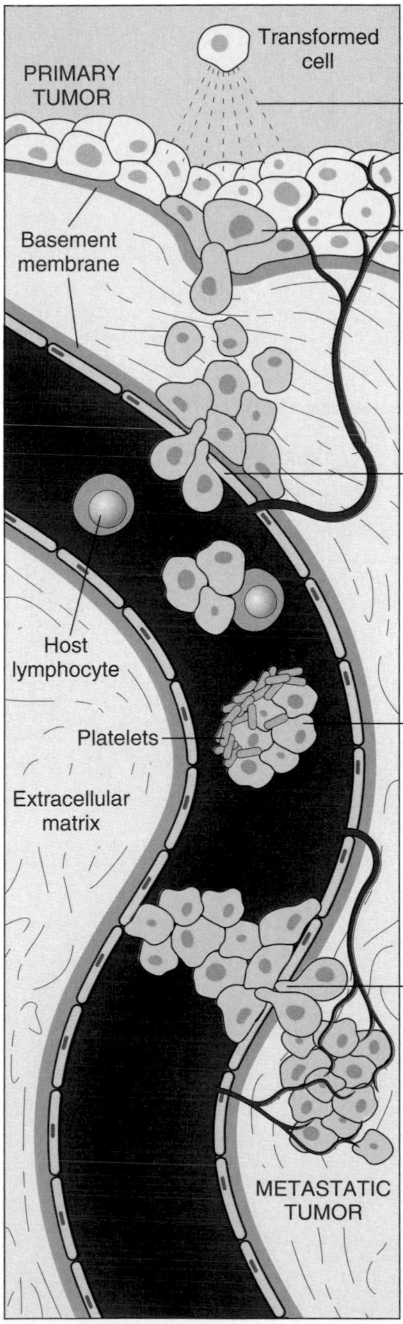

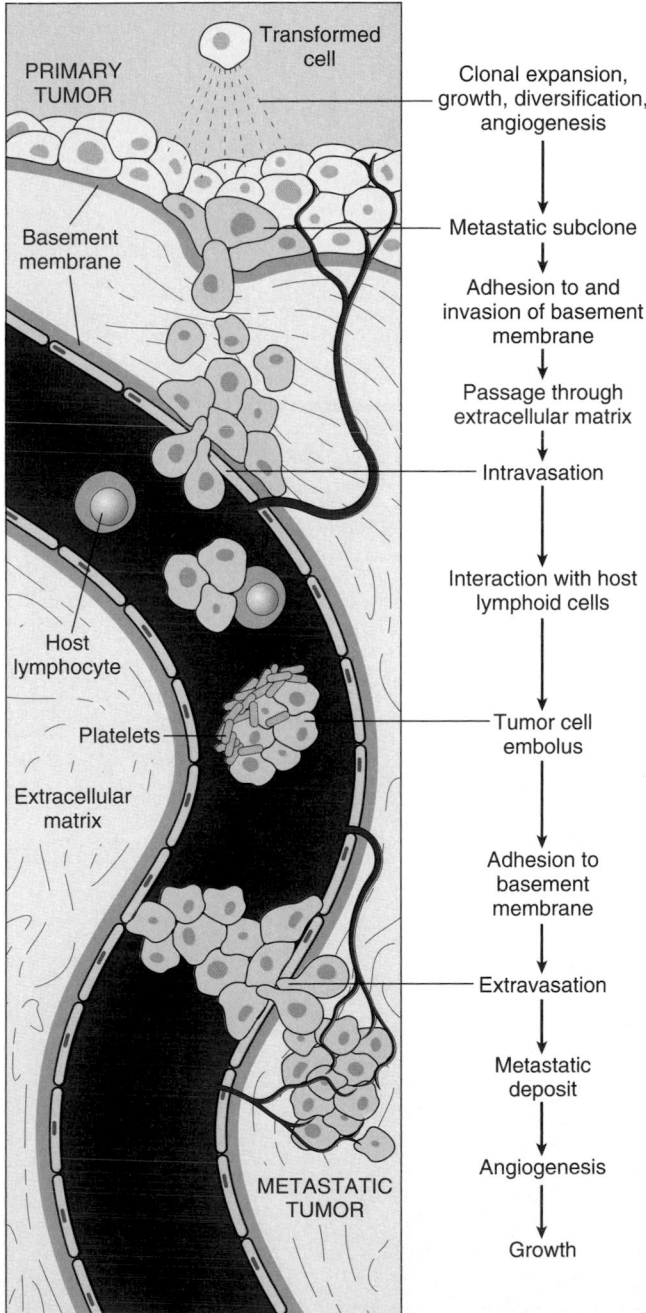

FIGURE 7–42 The metastatic cascade. Schematic illustration of the sequential steps involved in the hematogenous spread of a tumor.

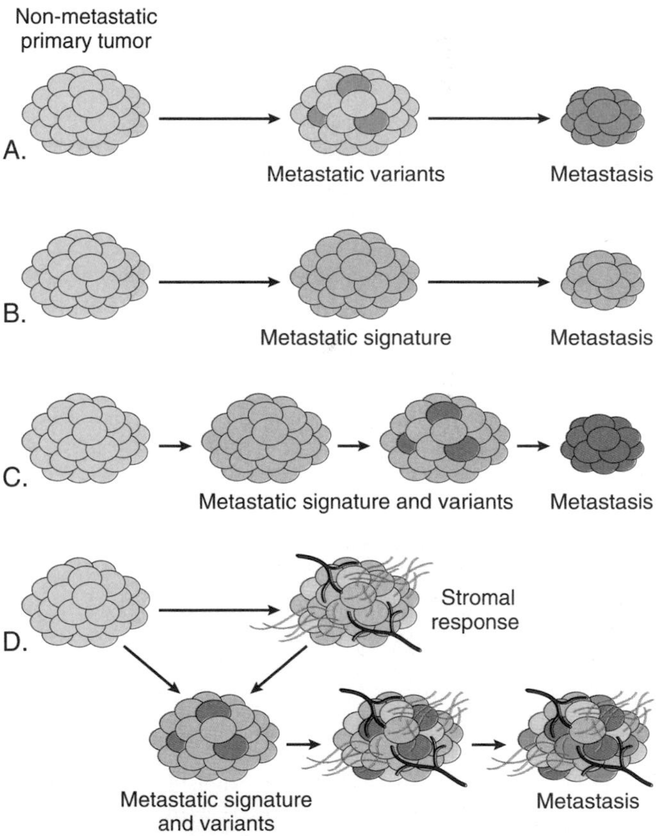

FIGURE 7–43 Mechanisms of metastasis development within a primary tumor. A nonmetastatic primary tumor is shown *(light blue)* on the left side of all diagrams. Four models are presented: *A,* Metastasis is caused by rare variant clones that develop in the primary tumor; *B,* Metastasis is caused by the gene expression pattern of most cells of the primary tumor, referred to as a metastatic signature; *C,* A combination of *A* and *B,* in which metastatic variants appear in a tumor with a metastatic gene signature; *D,* Metastasis development is greatly influenced by the tumor stroma, which may regulate angiogenesis, local invasiveness and resistance to immune elimination, allowing cells of the primary tumor, as in *C,* to become metastatic.

FIGURE 7–44 *A–D,* Schematic illustration of the sequence of events in the invasion of epithelial basement membranes by tumor cells. Tumor cells detach from each other because of reduced adhesiveness, and cells then attach to the basement membrane via the laminin receptors and secrete proteolytic enzymes, including type IV collagenase and plasminogen activator. Degradation of the basement membrane and tumor cell migration follow.

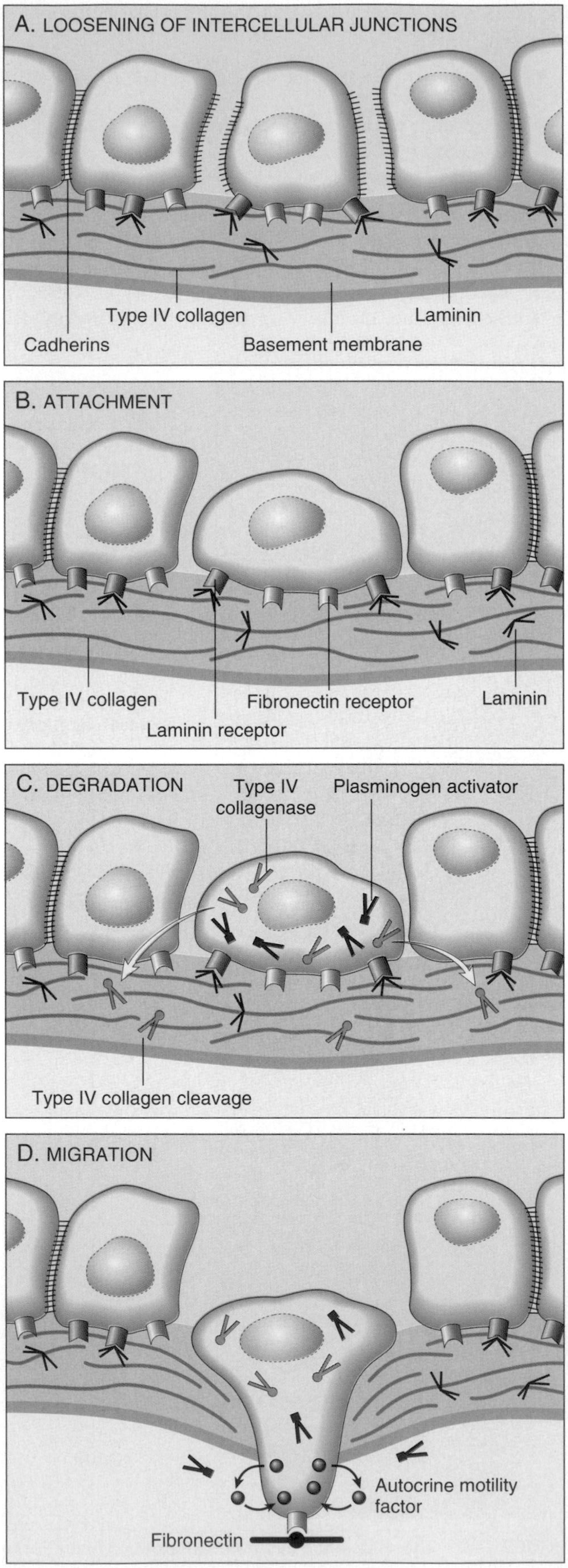

metastasis. Normal epithelial cells express high-affinity receptors (typically members of the integrin and immunoglobulin families of proteins) for basement membrane laminin that are polarized to their basal surface. In contrast, some carcinoma cells have many more receptors, and they are distributed all around the cell membrane. Moreover, there seems to be a correlation between the density of laminin receptors and invasiveness in cancers of the breast and colon. Tumor cells, like normal cells, also express integrins that serve as receptors for many components of the ECM, including fibronectin, laminin, collagen, and vitronectin. Neoplastic epithelial cells may express a higher amount of integrins and produce integrins that are not present in the corresponding normal tissue. As with laminin receptors, there seems to be a correlation between the expression of certain integrins (e.g., $\alpha_4\beta_1$ integrin on melanoma cells) and their ability to metastasize.

After attachment to the components of the basement membrane or interstitial ECM, tumor cells must create passageways for migration (Fig. 7–44). Invasion of the ECM is not merely due to passive growth pressure but requires active enzymatic degradation of the ECM components.[131] Tumor cells secrete proteolytic enzymes themselves or induce host cells (e.g., stromal fibroblasts and infiltrating macrophages) to elaborate proteases. The activity of these proteases is tightly regulated by antiproteases. At the invading edge of tumors, the balance between proteases and antiproteases is tilted in favor of proteases. Three classes of proteases have been identified: the serine, cysteine, and matrix metalloproteinases (MMPs). MMP9 and MMP2 are collagenases that cleave type IV collagen of epithelial and vascular basement membranes. There is compelling evidence[132] supporting the role of MMPs that degrade type IV collagen in tumor cell invasion:

- Several invasive carcinomas, melanomas, and sarcomas produce high levels of these collagenases.
- In situ lesions and adenomas of breast and colon express much less collagen IV–degrading collagenases than do invasive lesions. MMP expression is higher as tumors enlarge.
- Inhibition of collagenase activity by transfection with the gene for tissue inhibitors of metalloproteinases greatly reduces metastases in experimental animals. Thus, metalloproteinase inhibitors could be of value in the treatment of cancer. Synthetic compounds with such activity are being tested as therapeutic agents in certain forms of cancer.

While the most obvious effect of matrix destruction is to create a path for invasion by tumor cells, *cleavage products of matrix components, derived from collagen and proteoglycans, also have growth-promoting, angiogenic, and chemotactic activities.* The latter may promote the migration of tumor cells into the loosened ECM. MMPs are produced mostly by cells located in the tumor stroma, including cells of the immune system that migrate into this area. MMP9, and to a lesser extent MMP2, degrades collagen type IV and mobilizes VEGF that is sequestered in the basement membrane. Degradation of collagen IV also exposes normally cryptic domains of the protein, which serve as important signals for angiogenesis and cell interactions. Interestingly, collagen IV degradation in the basement membrane not only produces angiogenic stimuli, but also generates collagen fragments, such as endostatin and tumstatin, which are antiangiogenic. Thus, an important role of MMPs is to generate from the ECM, factors that promote angiogenesis, tumor growth, and tumor cell motility.[126] These factors counteract substances that inhibit angiogenesis, which are also produced by the partial digestion of basement membrane components.

Vascular Dissemination and Homing of Tumor Cells

Once in the circulation, tumor cells are particularly vulnerable to destruction by innate and adaptive immune defenses. The details of tumor immunity are considered later.

Within the circulation, tumor cells tend to aggregate in clumps. This is favored by homotypic adhesions among tumor cells as well as heterotypic adhesion between tumor cells and blood cells, particularly platelets (Fig. 7–42). Formation of platelet–tumor aggregates may enhance tumor cell survival and implantability. Arrest and extravasation of tumor emboli at distant sites involve adhesion to the endothelium, followed by egress through the basement membrane. Involved in these processes are adhesion molecules (integrins, laminin receptors) and proteolytic enzymes, discussed earlier. Of particular interest is the CD44 adhesion molecule, which is expressed on normal T lymphocytes and is used by these cells to migrate to selective sites in the lymphoid tissue. Such migration is accomplished by the binding of CD44 to hyaluronate on high endothelial venules, and overexpression of this molecule may favor metastatic spread. At the new site, tumor cells need to proliferate, develop a vascular supply, and evade the host defenses.[127]

The site at which circulating tumor cells leave the capillaries to form secondary deposits is related, in part, to the anatomic location of the primary tumor. Many observations, however, suggest that natural pathways of drainage do not wholly explain the distribution of metastases. For example, prostatic carcinoma preferentially spreads to bone, bronchogenic carcinomas tend to involve the adrenals and the brain, and neuroblastomas spread to the liver and bones. Such organ tropism may be related to the following mechanisms:

- Because the first step in extravasation is adhesion to the endothelium, tumor cells may have adhesion molecules whose ligands are expressed preferentially on the endothelial cells of the target organ. Indeed, it has been shown that the endothelial cells of the vascular beds of various tissues differ in their expression of ligands for adhesion molecules.[133]
- Chemokines have a very important role in determining the target tissues for metastasis. For instance, some breast cancer cells express the chemokine receptors CXCR4 and CCR7.[134] The chemokines that bind to these receptors are highly expressed in tissues to which breast cancers commonly metastasize. Blockage of the interaction between CXCR4 and its receptor decreases breast cancer metastasis to lymph nodes and lungs. Some target organs may liberate chemoattractants that tend to recruit tumor cells to the site. Examples include insulin-like growth factors I and II.
- In some cases, the target tissue may be an unpermissive environment—unfavorable soil, so to speak, for the growth of tumor seedlings. For example, although well vascularized, skeletal muscles are rarely the site of metastases.

While primary tumors at various sites have a preferential type of metastatic spread, the precise localization of metastases cannot be predicted with certainty for any form of cancer.

Molecular Genetics of Metastasis Development

Are there oncogenes or tumor suppressor genes that elicit metastases as their principal or sole contribution to tumorigenesis? This question is of more than academic interest because if altered forms of certain genes promote or suppress the metastatic phenotype, their detection in a primary tumor may have prognostic as well as therapeutic implications. Comparisons between genetic profiles of metastatic and nonmetastatic tumors have been used to search for candidate metastasis suppressor genes. At present, no single "metastasis gene" has been identified, with the exception of the membrane-cytoskeleton component ezrin, which appears to be necessary for metastases in rhabdomyoscarcoma and osteosarcoma.[135] Several genes have been proposed as suppressors of metastasis. They include *NM23* and the *KAI-1* and *KiSS* genes.[136] Much remains to be known.

STROMAL MICROENVIRONMENT AND CARCINOGENESIS

In the preceding sections, several examples of cross talk between the extracellular matrix and tumor cells were described. For example, cleavage of matrix components such as type IV collagen releases angiogenic factors (VEGF), and enzymatic degradation of laminin-5 by MMP-2 generates a proteolytic fragment that favors cancer cell motility. The ECM also stores growth factors in inactive forms, which are released by active matrix proteases. Such factors include PDGF, TGFβ, and b-FGF, which in turn affect the growth of tumor cells in a paracrine manner. In addition to these well-established interactions of tumor cells with stroma, there is emerging, tantalizing, evidence that stromal cells within the extracellular matrix can transmit oncogenic signals to tumor cells.[136a] This has been documented most extensively in experimental models of prostate and breast cancers. In prostate cancer, smooth muscle cells that normally lie adjacent to benign prostatic epithelium transform themselves into so called "carcinoma-associated fibroblasts," perhaps under the inductive influence of the tumor cells. These stromal cells acquire several altered properties such as enhanced collagen production and hyaluronate synthesis. But more interestingly, when isolated carcinoma-associated fibroblasts were recombined with immortalized, but non-tumorigenic, human prostate epithelial cells, the latter gave rise to poorly differentiated carcinomas in athymic mice. These carcinomas had multiple genetic abnormalities not present in the parent cell line, suggesting that the stroma can drive genetic changes that promote carcinogenesis. How such changes come about remains mysterious, as does their relevance to carcinogenesis in vivo. However, the results are sufficiently intriguing to merit attention since they suggest a novel form of cancer therapy that could be targeted to stromal cells.

DYSREGULATION OF CANCER-ASSOCIATED GENES

The genetic damage that activates oncogenes or inactivates tumor suppressor genes may be subtle (e.g., point mutations) or may involve segments of chromosomes and be large enough to be detected in a karyotype. Activation of oncogenes and loss of function of tumor suppressor genes by mutations were discussed earlier in this chapter. Here we discuss chromosomal abnormalities. We end this section by discussing the epigenic changes in cancer cells and global patterns of gene expression by cancer cells, known as *genetic profile or "signature."*

Chromosomal Changes

In certain neoplasms, karyotypic abnormalities are nonrandom and common. Specific chromosomal abnormalities have been identified in most leukemias and lymphomas and in an increasing number of nonhematopoietic tumors. In addition, whole chromosomes may be gained or lost. Although changes in chromosome number (aneuploidy) and structure are generally considered to be late phenomena in cancer progression, it has been suggested that aneuploidy and chromosomal instability may be initiating events in tumor growth.

The study of chromosomal changes in tumor cells is important on two accounts. First, molecular cloning of genes in the vicinity of chromosomal breakpoints or deletions has been extremely useful in identification of oncogenes (e.g., *BCL-2, ABL*) and tumor suppressor genes (e.g., *APC, RB*). Second, certain karyotypic abnormalities are specific enough to be of diagnostic value, and in some cases they are predictive of clinical course. The translocations associated with the *ABL* oncogene in chronic myeloid leukemia and with c-*MYC* in Burkitt lymphoma have been mentioned earlier, in conjunction with the discussion of molecular defects in cancer cells (see Fig. 7–32). Several other karyotype alterations in cancer cells are presented in the discussion of specific forms of neoplasia.

Two types of chromosomal rearrangements can activate protooncogenes—translocations and inversions. Chromosomal translocations are much more common (Table 7–10) and are discussed here. Translocations can activate protooncogenes in two ways:

- In lymphoid tumors, specific translocations result in overexpression of protooncogenes by removing them from their regulatory elements.
- In many hematopoietic tumors, the translocations allow normally unrelated sequences from two different chromosomes to recombine and form hybrid genes that encode growth-promoting chimeric proteins.

Overexpression of a protooncogene caused by translocation is best exemplified by Burkitt lymphoma. All such tumors carry one of three translocations, each involving chromosome 8q24, where the *MYC* gene has been mapped, as well as one of the three immunoglobulin gene–carrying chromosomes. At its normal locus, the expression of the *MYC* gene is tightly controlled; it is expressed only during certain stages of the cell cycle. In Burkitt lymphoma, the most common form of translocation results in the movement of the *MYC*–containing segment of chromosome 8 to chromosome 14q band 32 (Fig. 7–33), placing it close to the immunoglobulin heavy-chain (IgH) gene. The genetic notation for the translocation is t(8:14)(q24;q32). The molecular mechanisms of the translocation-associated activation of *MYC* are variable, as are the precise breakpoints within the gene. In most cases, the translocation causes mutations or loss of the regulatory sequences of the *MYC* gene. As the coding sequences remain intact, the gene is constitutively expressed at high levels. The gene may be translocated to the antigen receptor loci simply because these loci are accessible (i.e. in "open" chromatin) and active in developing lymphocytes. The invariable presence of the translocated *MYC* gene in Burkitt lymphomas attests to the importance of *MYC* overexpression in the pathogenesis of this tumor.

There are other examples of oncogenes translocated to antigen receptor loci in lymphoid tumors. As mentioned earlier, in mantle cell lymphoma, the *CYCLIN D1* gene on chromosome 11q13 is overexpressed by juxtaposition to the IgH locus on 14q32. In follicular lymphomas, a t(14;18)(q32;q21) translocation, the most common translocation in lymphoid malignancies, causes activation of the *BCL-2* gene. Not unexpectedly, all these tumors in which the immunoglobulin gene is involved are of B-cell origin. In an analogous situation, overexpression of several protooncogenes in T-cell tumors results from translocations of oncogenes into the T-cell antigen receptor locus. The affected oncogenes are diverse, but in most cases, as with *MYC,* they encode nuclear transcription factors.

The Philadelphia chromosome, characteristic of chronic myeloid leukemia and a subset of acute lymphoblastic leukemias, provides the prototypic example of an oncogene formed by *fusion of two separate genes.* In these cases, a reciprocal translocation between chromosomes 9 and 22 relo-

TABLE 7–10 Selected Examples of Oncogenes Activated by Translocation

Malignancy	Translocation	Affected Genes
Chronic myeloid leukemia	(9;22)(q34;q11)	Ab1 9q34 *bcr* 22q11
Acute leukemias (AML and ALL)	(4;11)(q21;q23)	AF4 4q21 <u>MLL</u> 11q23
	(6;11)(q27;q23)	AF6 6q27 <u>MLL</u> 11q23
Burkitt lymphoma	(8;14)(q24;q32)	c-*myc* 8q24 <u>IgH</u> 14q32
Mantle cell lymphoma	(11;14)(q13;q32)	Cyclin D 11q13 <u>IgH</u> 14q32
Follicular lymphoma	(14;18)(q32;q21)	<u>IgH</u> 14q32 *bcl*-2 18q21
T-cell acute lymphoblastic leukemia	(8;14)(q24;q11)	*c-myc* 8q24 <u>TCR-α</u> 14q11
	(10;14)(q24;q11)	*Hox* 11 10q24 <u>TCR-α</u> 14q11
Ewing sarcoma	(11;22)(q24;q12)	Fl-1 11q24 <u>EWS</u> 22q12

Underlined genes are involved in multiple translocations.
AML, acute myeloid leukemia; ALL, acute lymphoblastic leukemia.

cates a truncated portion of the protooncogene c-*ABL* (from chromosome 9) to the *BCR* (*b*reak point *c*luster *r*egion) on chromosome 22 (Fig. 7–33). The hybrid fusion gene *BCR-ABL* encodes a chimeric protein that has constitutive tyrosine kinase activity. As mentioned, BCR-ABL tyrosine kinase has served as a target for leukemia therapy, with remarkable success so far. Although the translocations are cytogenetically identical in chronic myeloid leukemia and acute lymphoblastic leukemias, they differ at the molecular level. In chronic myeloid leukemia, the chimeric protein has a molecular weight of 210 kD, whereas in the more aggressive acute leukemias, a 190-kD BCR-ABL fusion protein is formed.[62,63] The molecular pathways activated by the BCR-ABL protein are complex and not completely understood. It inhibits apoptosis, decreases the requirement for growth factors, binds to cytoskeleton components, decreases cell adhesion, and activates multiple pathways, including those of RAS, PI-3 kinase, and STATs (Chapter 3). BCR-ABL also acts on DNA repair and may cause genomic instability that contributes to the progression of the disease.

Transcription factors are often the partners in gene fusions occurring in cancer cells. For instance, the *MLL* (myeloid, lymphoid leukemia) gene on 11q23 is known to be involved in 25 different translocations with several different partner genes, some of which encode transcription factors (see Table 7–10). The *E*wing *S*arcoma (*EWS*) gene at 22q12 was first described in the t(11;22)(q24;12) reciprocal translocation present in Ewing sarcoma (a highly malignant tumor of children; Chapter 26) but may be translocated in other types of sarcomas. *EWS* is itself a transcription factor, and all of its partner genes analyzed so far also encode a transcription factor. In Ewing tumor, for example, the *EWS* gene fuses with the *FLI 1* gene; the resultant chimeric EWS-FLI 1 protein is a member of the ETS transcription factor family, which has transforming ability.

Gene Amplification

Activation of protooncogenes associated with overexpression of their products may result from reduplication and *amplification* of their DNA sequences. Such amplification may produce several hundred copies of the protooncogene in the tumor cell.[137] The amplified genes can be readily detected by molecular hybridization with appropriate DNA probes. In some cases, the amplified genes produce chromosomal changes that can be identified microscopically. Two mutually exclusive patterns are seen: multiple small, chromosome-like structures called *double minutes* (dms), and *homogeneous staining regions* (HSRs). The latter derive from the assembly of amplified genes into new chromosomes; because the regions containing amplified genes lack a normal banding pattern, they appear homogeneous in a G-banded karyotype (see Fig. 7–34). The most interesting cases of amplification involve N-*MYC* in neuroblastoma and *ERB B2* in breast cancers. N-*MYC* is amplified in 25% to 30% of neuroblastomas, and the amplification is associated with poor prognosis. In neuroblastomas with N-*MYC* amplification, the gene is present both in dms and HSRs. *ERB B2* amplification occurs in about 20% of breast cancers and may represent a distinct tumor phenotype. Amplification of C-*MYC*, L-*MYC*, and N-*MYC* correlates with disease progression in small cell cancer of the lung. Another gene frequently amplified is *CYCLIN D1* (breast carcinomas, head and neck carcinomas, and other squamous cell carcinomas).

Epigenetic Changes

It has become evident during the past few years that certain tumor suppressor genes may be inactivated not because of structural changes but because the gene *is silenced by hypermethylation of promoter sequences without a change in DNA base sequence.*[138] Such changes appear to be stably maintained through multiple rounds of cell division. Methylation takes place in CpG islands in DNA, but de novo methylation rarely occurs in normal tissues. However, methylation has been detected in various tumor suppressor genes in human cancers. They include *p14ARF* in colon and stomach cancers, *p16INK4a* in various types of cancers, *BRCA1* in breast cancer, *VHL* in renal cell carcinomas, and the *MLH1* mismatch repair gene in colorectal cancer.[139] Methylation also participates in the phenomenon called *genomic imprinting,* in which the maternal or paternal allele of a gene or chromosome is modified by methylation and is inactivated. The reverse phenomenon, that is, demethylation of an imprinted gene leading to its biallelic expression (loss of imprinting) can also occur in tumor cells.[140] Although the discussion of whether methylation of tumor suppressor genes has a causal role in cancer development continues, there has been great interest in developing potential therapeutic agents that act to demethylate DNA sequences in tumor suppressor genes. Recent data demonstrating that genomic hypomethylation causes chromosomal instability and induces tumors in mice greatly strengthens the notion that epigenetic changes may directly contribute to tumor development.[141]

Molecular Profiles of Cancer Cells

A new era in cancer research was initiated with the development of methods to measure the expression of thousands of genes in tumors and normal tissues. Among these new methods, the determination of RNA levels by microarray analysis has found wide application (Box 7–1). Currently, this method can measure RNA expression from virtually all known genes (Fig. 7–45). The expression profiles obtained from DNA microarray analysis are known as *gene expression signatures or molecular profiles.* The application of this technique to the study of breast cancers and leukemias has been particularly rewarding (see Box 7–1). It was recently found that there are breast cancer subtypes that can be identified by their molecular profiles and that the molecular signatures of some of these subtypes can help predict the course of the disease (see Box 23–1, Chapter 23).[142] Analysis of acute lymphoblastic leukemia by DNA microarrays has established the molecular signatures of prognostic subtypes and uncovered novel markers associated with these subtypes.[143]

Molecular Basis of Multistep Carcinogenesis

The notion that malignant tumors arise from a protracted sequence of events is supported by epidemiologic, experimental, and molecular studies. Many eons ago, before

Box 7–1. Gene Expression Profiles of Human Cancers. Microarrays and Proteomics

Until recently, studies of gene expression in tumors involved the analysis of individual genes. These studies have been revolutionized by the introduction of methods that can measure the expression of thousands of genes simultaneously.[208,209] The most common method for large-scale analysis of gene expression in use today is based on DNA microarray technology. In this method, DNA fragments, either cDNAs or oligonucleotides, are spotted on a glass slide or on some other solid support. As the techniques used for the spotting are similar to those employed to produce semiconductor chips for electronic products, the arrays are known as *"gene chips."* Chips can be purchased from commercial suppliers or produced in-house, and can contain more than 20,000 gene fragments. The fragments are typically obtained from complementary DNA (cDNA) libraries or sets of nucleotides from known and uncharacterized genes. The gene chip is then hybridized to "probes" prepared from tumor and control samples (the probes are usually cDNA copies of RNAs extracted from tumor and uninvolved tissues). Before hybridization to the chip, the probes are labeled with fluorochromes that emit different colors (e.g. red color for tumor RNA and green color for control RNA). After hybridization the chip is read using a laser scanner (Fig. 7–45); each spot on the array will be red (increased expression of a gene in the tumor), green (decreased expression in the tumor) or, if there is no difference in gene expression between the tumor and control sample, the spots will be either black or yellow (depending on the type of fluorescent scanning). Sophisticated software has been developed to measure the intensity of the fluorescence for each spot and produce data sets in which genes with similar expression patterns are clustered.[210] This method of analysis, called *hierarchical clustering,* groups together genes according to the similarity of their gene expression patterns. The software can be linked to large sequencing and array databases available through the Web. This allows appropriate gene identification and comparison between expression profiles from various sources. A major problem in the analysis of gene expression in tumors is the heterogeneity of the tissue. In addition to the heterogeneity between tumor cells, samples may contain variable amounts of stromal connective tissue, inflammatory infiltrates, and normal tissue cells. One way to overcome this problem is to obtain nearly pure tumor cells or small tumors free from associated tissues using *laser capture microdissection.* In this technique, the dissection of the tumor or cells is made under a microscope through a focused laser. The dissected material is then captured or "catapulted" into a small cap and processed for RNA and DNA isolation.

Gene expression profiling of tumors has multiple uses, and the number of publications using this technique has grown enormously during the past few years. Much of the work performed is not directed toward proving or disproving a proposed hypothesis. Gene expression analysis can be used to classify tumors; to predict metastatic potential, prognosis, and response to therapy; to reveal gene expression patterns that are dependent on the mutation of a single oncogene; and to analyze the effects of hormones and environmental agents on cancer development.[209] The applications of this technology keep expanding and being refined, but much has already been accomplished.[141,209–211] We mention only a few interesting examples. Profiling of cells from adult and pediatric T-cell acute lymphoblastic leukemia has identified the patterns of gene expression in leukemic blast cells and has accurately classified each prognostic subtype.[211] The work that has received the highest publicity involves gene expression profiling of breast cancers. In addition to identifying new subtypes of breast cancers, a 70-gene prognosis profile was established. Using this type of profile, it has been reported that: (1) the profile was a powerful predictor of disease prognosis for young patients; (2) it was particularly accurate for predicting metastasis during the first 5 years after diagnosis; and (3) prognosis determined by gene expression profiles correlated highly with histologic grade and estrogen receptor status but not with lymphatic spread of the tumor.[211] A more recent analysis has pooled together data gathered by different laboratories and has confirmed the identification of distinct subtypes of breast cancer.[142] Given all of these remarkable results, it is time to ask whether this technology is "ready for prime time"; that is, ready for day to day clinical applications. Things are moving very fast in this area, but before clinical applications are considered, many issues need to settled. Not only do larger trials need to be conducted to prove the reliability and accuracy of the analysis but also, just as important, the procedures for handling samples, performing the analyses, and reporting the data need to be standardized, so that data obtained in various laboratories can be compared.

Next on the horizon of molecular techniques for the global analysis of gene expression in cancers is *proteomics,* a technique used to obtain expression profiles of proteins contained in tissues, serum, or other body fluids. The original method consisted of the separation of proteins by 2-dimensional gel electrophoresis, followed by identification of individual proteins by mass spectrometry. A more recent technique, called *ICAT* (*i*sotope-*c*oding *a*ffinity *t*ags) does not rely on electrophoresis for protein separation. In ICAT, proteins in the test and control samples are labeled with light or heavy isotopes. The differentially labeled proteins are then identified and quantified by mass spectrometry. A variation of proteomic analysis has been used to obtain protein profiles in the blood of cancer patients without identification of individual proteins.[215]

The excitement created by the development of new techniques for the global molecular analysis of tumors has led some scientists to predict that the end of histopathology is in sight, and to consider existing approaches to tumor diagnosis as the equivalent of magical methods of divination. Indeed, it is hard to escape the excitement generated by the development of entirely new and powerful methods of molecular analysis. However, what lies ahead is not the replacement of one set of techniques by another. On the contrary, the most accurate diagnosis and prognosis of cancer will be arrived at by a combination of morphologic and molecular techniques.[208]

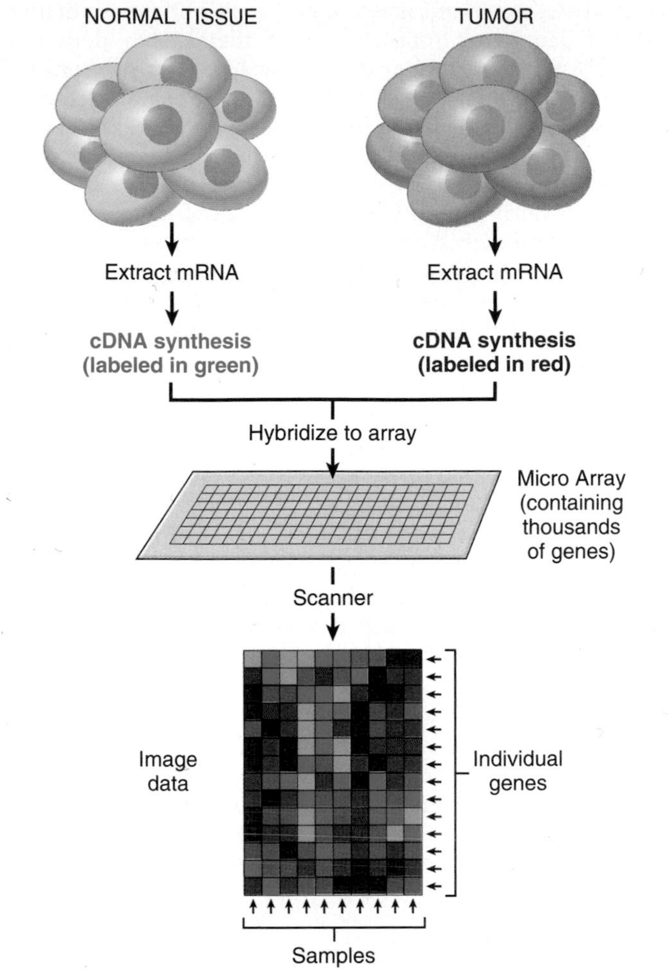

FIGURE 7–45 Schematic representation of the steps required for the analysis of global gene expression by DNA microarray. RNA is extracted from tumor and normal tissue. cDNA synthesized from each preparation is labeled with fluorescent dyes (in the example shown, normal tissue cDNA is labeled with a green dye; tumor cDNA is labeled with a red dye). The array consists of a solid support in which DNA fragments from many thousands of genes are spotted. The labeled cDNAs from tumor and normal tissue are combined and hybridized to the genes contained in the array. Hybridization signals are detected using a confocal laser scanner and downloaded to a computer for analysis (*red squares*, expression of the gene is higher in tumor; *green square*, expression of the gene is higher in normal tissue; *black squares*, no difference in the expression of the gene between tumor and normal tissue). In the display, the horizontal rows correspond to each gene contained in the array; each ventrical row corresponds to single samples.

oncogenes and tumor suppressor genes had infiltrated the scientific literature, cancer epidemiologists had suggested that the age-associated increase in cancers could best be explained by postulating that several sequential or concurrent cellular alterations were required for tumorigenesis. This idea received initial support from experimental models of chemical carcinogenesis in which the process of tumor formation could be divided into distinct steps, such as *initiation and promotion.* The study of oncogenes and tumor suppressor genes has provided a firm molecular footing for the concept of multistep carcinogenesis:[144]

- DNA transfection experiments revealed that no single oncogene can fully transform non-immortalized cells in vitro, but that such *cells can generally be transformed by combinations of oncogenes.* Such cooperation is required because each oncogene is specialized to induce part of the phenotype necessary for full transformation. For instance, the *RAS* oncogene induces cells to secrete growth factors and enables them to grow without anchorage to a normal substrate (anchorage independence), whereas the *MYC* oncogene renders cells more sensitive to growth factors and immortalizes cells. These two genes, acting in conjunction, can transform non-immortalized mouse fibroblasts in culture.
- *Most human cancers that have been analyzed reveal multiple genetic alterations involving activation of several oncogenes and loss of two or more tumor suppressor genes.* The prevalent view is that each of these alterations represents a crucial step in the progression from a normal cell to a malignant tumor. A dramatic example of incremental acquisition of the malignant phenotype is documented by the study of colon carcinoma.[145] These lesions evolve through a series of morphologically identifiable stages: colon epithelial hyperplasia, epithelial dysplasia, followed by formation of adenomas that progressively enlarge and ultimately undergo malignant transformation (Chapter 17). The proposed molecular correlates of this adenoma-carcinoma sequence are illustrated in Figure 7–46. According to this scheme, inactivation of the *APC* tumor suppressor gene occurs first, followed by activation of *RAS*, loss of genes on 18q (*SMAD2* and *SMAD4*), and ultimately, loss of *p53* and *TGF-β* receptor II genes.

Given that multiple mutations are essential for the development of cancer, one might ask whether the specific order of mutations is also important. In the case of colon cancer, *APC* inactivation is considered an important first step for carcino-

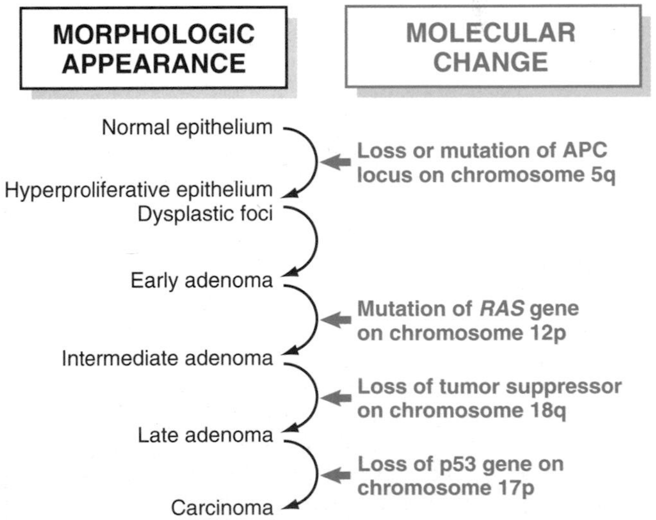

FIGURE 7–46 Molecular model for the evolution of colorectal cancers through the adenoma–carcinoma sequence. Although *APC* mutation is an early event and loss of *p53* occurs late in the process of tumorigenesis, the timing for the other changes may show variations. Note also that individual tumors may not have all of the changes listed. (Adapted from Vogelstein B, Kinzler KW: Colorectal tumors. In Vogelstein B, Kinzler KW: The Genetic Basis of Human Cancer. New York, McGraw-Hill, 2002, p. 583.)

genesis, and this mutation is present in the earliest neoplastic lesions (adenomas). Activation of *COX-2* and of EGF receptor are contributory factors to the initiation of these tumors.[56] Mice with targeted disruption of the *APC* gene develop multiple colonic adenomas; those with homozygous deletions of the *p53* gene develop tumors of many tissues but not colon carcinomas. This observation suggests that *p53* mutations play a role in the progression (but not initiation) of colonic cancer. Although the role of *APC* in colon cancer initiation is well established, there is some debate as to whether the other known genetic changes follow a defined temporal sequence. Unfortunately, few other cancers have been examined with the same degree of detail as colorectal tumors.

Gatekeeper and Caretaker Genes. Oncogenes and tumor suppressor genes directly control tumor growth by functioning, respectively, as accelerators and brakes for cellular proliferation. They are known as "gatekeeper" genes, which regulate entry of the cell into the tumorigenic path[45] (Fig. 7–47). Examples of this type of gene are the tumor suppressor genes associated with cancer susceptibility syndromes already discussed. For sporadic tumors, most evidence points to the dysregulation of two pathways involving tumor suppressor genes, with one or the other being defective in most tumors. These are the RB pathway involving INK4 proteins, cyclin D and its associated kinases, and RB itself (or members of the RB family); the other pathway is the p53 pathway that involves p14ARF, HDM2, and p53.

Genes that do not directly control tumor growth but affect genomic stability are called "caretaker" genes[45] (see Fig. 7–47). In this category are mismatch repair genes and other putative DNA repair genes. Inactivation of these genes does not promote tumor initiation directly. Instead, loss of caretaker genes results in increased mutation of all genes, including gatekeeper genes. Thus, in individuals with germ line mutations of caretaker genes (such as DNA mismatch repair genes), subsequent mutations in somatic cells, beyond the inactivation of the normal allele of the caretaker gene, are required for cancer initiation. By comparison, those who inherit one defective copy of a gatekeeper gene require only one more somatic event for cancer initiation. Thus, although individuals with germ line mutations of either the gatekeeper or caretaker genes are at a higher-than-normal risk of developing cancer, the relative risk is much greater in those born with a defective copy of a gatekeeper gene. It is also important to keep in mind that tumor suppressor genes may be silenced by epigenetic mechanisms and that mechanisms such as DNA hypermethylation are potentially reversible.

Mutator Phenotype. It has been proposed that defects in DNA repair are initiating events in tumorigenesis, leading to widespread mutagenesis and genetic instability.[35,146] These alterations would then generate cancer cells with a "mutator phenotype," that is, cells that are unusually susceptible to additional mutations. For this idea to be correct, it is necessary to demonstrate that such a phenotype (which by definition requires a very large number of mutational events per cell) occurs very early during cancer formation and is not a consequence of cancer progression. Much effort is being devoted to testing this hypothesis.

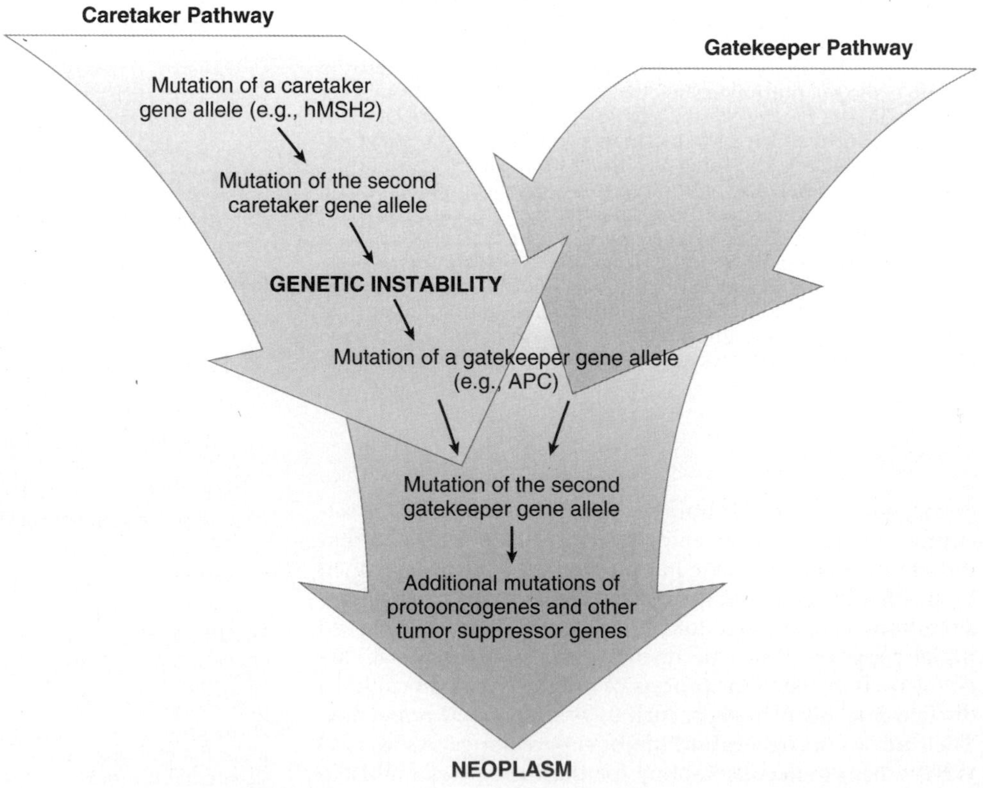

FIGURE 7–47 Schematic illustration of the pathways of malignancy initated by mutation of the gatekeeper genes (e.g., *APC, NF-1, RB*) or caretaker genes (e.g., *hMSH2, BRCA-1, BRCA-2*).

TUMOR PROGRESSION AND HETEROGENEITY

It is well established that over a period of time many tumors become more aggressive and acquire greater malignant potential. In some instances (e.g., colon cancer), there is an orderly evolution from preneoplastic lesions to benign tumors and, ultimately, invasive cancers. This phenomenon is referred to as tumor *progression.* Angiogenesis and changes in the tumor stroma are also components of tumor progression. Careful clinical and experimental studies reveal that increasing malignancy (e.g., accelerated growth, invasiveness, and ability to form distant metastases) is often acquired in an incremental fashion. *This biologic phenomenon is related to the sequential appearance of subpopulations of cells that differ with respect to several phenotypic attributes such as invasiveness, rate of growth, metastatic ability, karyotype, hormonal responsiveness, and susceptibility to antineoplastic drugs. Thus, despite the fact that most malignant tumors are monoclonal in origin, by the time they become clinically evident, their constituent cells are extremely heterogeneous.* At the molecular level, tumor progression and associated heterogeneity most likely result from multiple mutations that accumulate independently in different cells, thus generating subclones with different characteristics. However, tumor progression also depends on the tumor microenviroment and is greatly influenced by changes in the tumor stroma and angiogenesis, which may modulate the extent of cell proliferation, invasiveness, and metastatic potential.[130]

What predisposes the original transformed cell to additional genetic damage is not entirely clear. Transformed cells are genetically unstable. Such instability may result, for example, from the loss of *p53* or from inherited or acquired mutations in genes that regulate DNA repair. These and other unidentified factors render tumor cells prone to a high rate of random, spontaneous mutations during clonal expansion. Some of these mutations may be lethal; others may spur cell growth by affecting protooncogenes or tumor suppressor genes. Cells that are highly antigenic may be destroyed by host defenses, whereas those with reduced growth factor requirements are positively selected. *A growing tumor therefore tends to be enriched for those subclones that "beat the odds" and are adept at survival, growth, invasion, and metastases.*[147] Although progression is most obvious after a tumor is diagnosed, during the latent period many cell doublings occur (see Fig. 7–12), and hence *generation of heterogeneity begins well before the tumor is clinically evident.*

Carcinogenic Agents and Their Cellular Interactions

A large number of agents cause genetic damage and induce neoplastic transformation of cells. They include (1) chemical carcinogens, (2) radiant energy, and (3) oncogenic viruses and some other microbes. Radiant energy and some chemical carcinogens are documented causes of cancer in humans, and the evidence linking certain viruses to human cancers grows ever stronger. Each group of agents is considered separately, but several may act in concert or synergize the effects of others.

CHEMICAL CARCINOGENESIS

Although John Hill first called attention to the association of "immoderate use of snuff" and the development of "polypusses" (polyps), we owe largely to Sir Percival Pott our awareness of the potential carcinogenicity of chemical agents. In the 18th century Pott astutely related the increased incidence of scrotal skin cancer in chimney sweeps to chronic exposure to soot. A few years later, based on this observation, the Danish Chimney Sweeps Guild ruled that its members must bathe daily. Few public health measures since that time have so successfully controlled a form of cancer! Over the succeeding two centuries, hundreds of chemicals have been shown to transform cells in vitro and to be carcinogenic in animals. Some of the most potent (e.g., the polycyclic aromatic hydrocarbons) have been extracted from fossil fuels or are products of incomplete combustions. Some are synthetic products created by industry or for the study of chemical carcinogenesis. Some are naturally occurring components of plants and microbial organisms. Most important, a significant number (including, ironically, some medical drugs) have been strongly implicated in the causation of cancers in humans.

Steps Involved in Chemical Carcinogenesis

As discussed earlier, carcinogenesis is a multistep process. This is most readily demonstrated in experimental models of chemical carcinogenesis, in which the stages of initiation and progression during cancer development have been described.[148] The classic experiments that allowed the distinction between initiation and promotion were performed on mouse skin and are outlined in Figure 7–48. The following concepts relating to the initiation-promotion sequence have emerged from these experiments:

- Initiation results from exposure of cells to a sufficient dose of a carcinogenic agent (initiator); an initiated cell is altered, making it potentially capable of giving rise to a tumor (groups 2 and 3). *Initiation alone, however, is not sufficient for tumor formation* (group 1).
- *Initiation causes permanent DNA damage (mutations). It is therefore rapid and irreversible and has "memory."* This is illustrated by group 3, in which tumors were produced even if the application of the promoting agent was delayed for several months after a single application of the initiator.
- *Promoters can induce tumors in initiated cells, but they are nontumorigenic by themselves* (group 5). Furthermore, tumors do not result when the promoting agent is applied before, rather than after, the initiating agent (group 4). This indicates that, *in contrast to the effects of initiators, the cellular changes resulting from the application of promoters do not affect DNA directly and are reversible.* As discussed later, promoters enhance the proliferation of initiated cells, an effect that may contribute to the development of additional mutations in these cells. That the effects of promoters are reversible is further documented in group 6, in which tumors failed to develop in initiated cells if the time between multiple applications of the promoter was sufficiently extended.

Although the concepts of initiation and promotion have been derived largely from experiments involving induction of

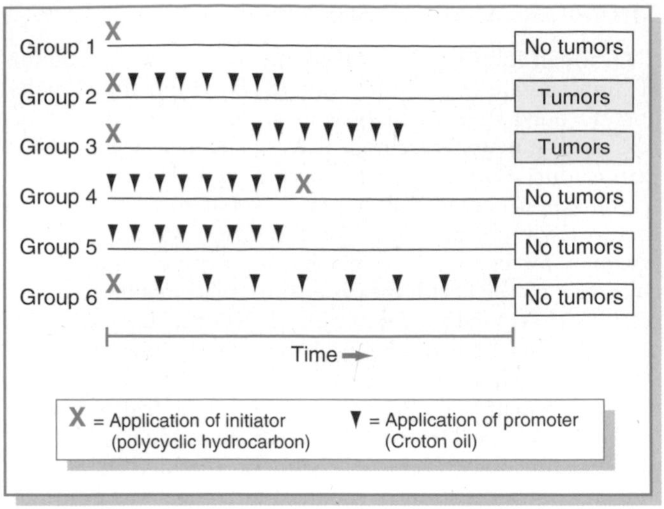

FIGURE 7–48 Experiments demonstrating the initiation and promotion phases of carcinogenesis in mice. Group 2: application of promoter repeated at twice-weekly intervals for several months. Group 3: application of promoter delayed for several months and then applied twice weekly. Group 6: promoter applied at monthly intervals.

skin cancer in mice, these stages are also discernible in the development of cancers of the liver, urinary bladder, breast, colon, and respiratory tract. With this brief overview of two major steps in carcinogenesis, we can examine initiation and promotion in more detail (see outline in Figure 7–49).

Initiation of Chemical Carcinogenesis

Chemicals that initiate carcinogenesis are extremely diverse in structure and include both natural and synthetic products (Table 7–11). They fall into one of two categories: (1) *direct-acting* compounds, which do not require chemical transformation for their carcinogenicity, and (2) *indirect-acting* compounds or *procarcinogens,* which require metabolic conversion in vivo to produce *ultimate carcinogens* capable of transforming cells. Most direct-acting and ultimate carcinogens have one property in common: *They are highly reactive electrophiles* (have electron-deficient atoms) *that can react with nucleophilic (electron-rich) sites in the cell.* These reactions are nonenzymatic and result in the formation of covalent adducts (addition products) between the chemical carcinogen and a nucleotide in DNA. The electrophilic reactions may attack several electron-rich sites in the target cells, including DNA, RNA, and proteins, thus sometimes producing lethal damage. In initiated cells, the interaction is obviously nonlethal, and, as expected, DNA is the primary target.

Metabolic Activation of Carcinogens. Except for the few direct-acting alkylating and acylating agents that are intrinsically electrophilic, most chemical carcinogens require metabolic activation for conversion into ultimate carcinogens (Fig. 7–49). Other metabolic pathways may lead to the inactivation (detoxification) of the procarcinogen or its derivatives. Thus, *the carcinogenic potency of a chemical is determined not only by the inherent reactivity of its electrophilic derivative but also by the balance between metabolic activation and inactivation reactions.*[149]

Most of the known carcinogens are metabolized by cytochrome P-450–dependent mono-oxygenases. The genes that encode these enzymes are quite polymorphic, and the activity and inducibility of these enzymes have been shown to vary among different individuals. Because these enzymes are essential for the activation of procarcinogens, the susceptibility to carcinogenesis is regulated in part by polymorphisms in the genes that encode these enzymes. A few examples suffice to illustrate this important concept. The product of the P-450 gene, *CYP1A1,* metabolizes polycyclic aromatic hydrocarbons such as benz(o)pyrene. Approximately 10% of the white population has a highly inducible form of this enzyme that is associated with an increased risk of lung cancer in smokers.[150] Light smokers with the susceptible genotype *CYP1A1* have a sevenfold higher risk of developing lung cancer compared with smokers without the permissive genotype. As another example, the enzyme glutathione-*S*-transferase, involved in the detoxification of polycyclic aromatic hydrocarbons, is also polymorphic; in about 50% of whites, this locus is entirely deleted, and hence these individuals incur a higher risk of lung and bladder cancer but only if exposed to tobacco smoke. Not all variations in the activation or detoxification of carcinogens are genetically determined. Age, sex, and nutritional status also determine the internal dose of toxicants produced and hence influence the risk of cancer development in a particular individual.[151]

Molecular Targets of Chemical Carcinogens. Because malignant transformation results from mutations that affect oncogenes, tumor suppressor genes, genes that regulate apoptosis, and genes involved in DNA repair, it comes as no surprise that the majority of initiating chemicals are mutagenic. Their mutagenic potential has been investigated, most commonly using the *Ames test,* which uses the ability of a chemical to induce mutations in the bacterium *Salmonella typhimurium.* The vast majority (70% to 90%) of known chemical carcinogens score positive in the Ames test.[152] Conversely, most but not all chemicals that are mutagenic in vitro are carcinogenic in vivo.

That DNA is the primary target for chemical carcinogens seems fairly well established, but there is no single or unique alteration that can be associated with initiation of chemical carcinogenesis. Nevertheless, the interaction of each chemical carcinogen with DNA is not completely random, and each class of carcinogens tends to produce a limited pattern of DNA damage. It should be emphasized that carcinogen-induced changes in DNA do not necessarily lead to initiation because most types of DNA damage can be repaired by cellular enzymes. Thus, environmentally induced insults to DNA are far more common than is the occurrence of cancer, as long as repair mechanisms are intact. This is illustrated by the rare hereditary disorder xeroderma pigmentosum, which is associated with a defect in DNA repair and a greatly increased vulnerability to skin cancers caused by UV light and some chemicals (see "Radiation Carcinogenesis").

The presence of certain types of DNA damage in human tumors can provide molecular clues to their causation. This is exemplified by the study of mutations in the *RAS* and *p53* genes. Although virtually any gene may be targeted by chemical carcinogens, *RAS* mutations are particularly common in several chemically induced tumors in rodents. Molecular analyses of mutant *RAS* genes isolated from such tumors reveal that the change in nucleotide sequence is precisely that

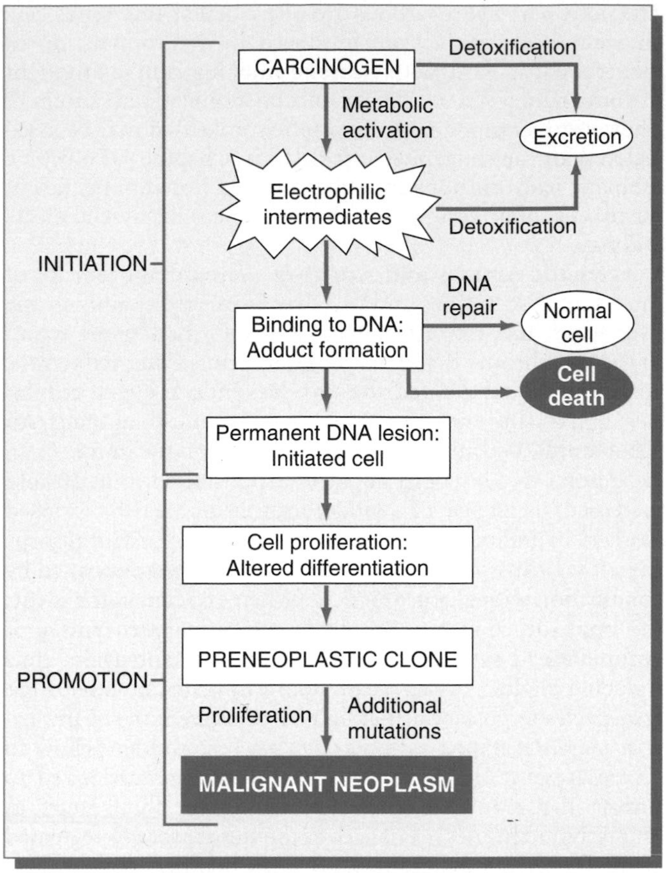

FIGURE 7–49 General schema of events in chemical carcinogenesis. Note that promoters cause clonal expansion of the initiated cell, thus producing a preneoplastic clone. Further proliferation induced by the promoter or other factors causes accumulation of additional mutations and emergence of a malignant tumor.

predicted from the known sites of reaction of the carcinogen with specific bases in DNA. Thus, it seems that each carcinogen produces a molecular "fingerprint" that can link specific chemicals with their mutational effects. A telling example of this phenomenon is provided by the study of *p53* mutations in hepatocellular carcinomas. In certain parts of China and Africa, hepatocellular carcinoma in patients with or without chronic infection with hepatitis B virus (HBV) is associated with the ingestion of the fungal metabolite aflatoxin B1. In other regions of China and in the rest of the world, hepatocellular carcinomas are associated with chronic infection with hepatitis B or C virus, without linkage to aflatoxin. In areas where aflatoxin B1 exposure is high, such as the Qidong province of China and The Gambia in Africa, *p53* mutations are present in most hepatocellular carcinomas, and 90% of more of these mutations are a characteristic G:C→T:A transversion in codon 249 (called *249^ser^ p53* mutation).[153] By contrast, *p53* mutations are much less frequent in liver tumors from areas where aflatoxin contamination of food is not a risk factor, and the *249^ser^* mutation is uncommon. This and other similar observations strongly support the notion that molecular fingerprinting of tumors can provide clues to the identity of initiating agents.

Initiated Cell. In the preceding sections, we noted that unrepaired alterations in the DNA are essential first steps in the process of initiation. *For the change to be heritable, the damaged DNA template must be replicated. Thus, for initiation to occur, carcinogen-altered cells must undergo at least one cycle of proliferation so that the change in DNA becomes fixed or permanent.* In the liver, many chemicals are activated to reactive electrophiles, yet most of them do not produce cancers unless the liver cells proliferate within 72 to 96 hours of the formation of DNA adducts. In tissues that are normally quiescent, the mitogenic stimulus may be provided by the carcinogen itself because many cells die owing to toxic effects of the carcinogenic chemical, thereby stimulating regeneration in the surviving cells. Alternatively, cell proliferation may be induced by concurrent exposure to biologic agents such as viruses and parasites, dietary factors, or hormonal influences.

Promotion of Chemical Carcinogenesis

It was mentioned earlier that initiation by itself is not sufficient for tumor formation (Fig. 7–49). The carcinogenicity of some chemicals is augmented by subsequent administration of *promoters* (such as phorbol esters, hormones, phenols, and drugs) that by themselves are nontumorigenic. Applica-

TABLE 7–11 Major Chemical Carcinogens

Direct-Acting Carcinogens
Alkylating Agents
β-Propiolactone
Dimethyl sulfate
Diepoxybutane
Anticancer drugs (cyclophosphamide, chlorambucil, nitrosoureas, and others)
Acylating Agents
1-Acetyl-imidazole
Dimethylcarbamyl chloride
Procarcinogens That Require Metabolic Activation
Polycyclic and Heterocyclic Aromatic Hydrocarbons
Benz(a)anthracene
Benzo(a)pyrene
Dibenz(a,h)anthracene
3-Methylcholanthrene
7,12-Dimethylbenz(a)anthracene
Aromatic Amines, Amides, Azo Dyes
2-Naphthylamine (β-naphthylamine)
Benzidine
2-Acetylaminofluorene
Dimethylaminoazobenzene (butter yellow)
Natural Plant and Microbial Products
Aflatoxin B_1
Griseofulvin
Cycasin
Safrole
Betel nuts
Others
Nitrosamine and amides
Vinyl chloride, nickel, chromium
Insecticides, fungicides
Polychlorinated biphenyls

tion of promoters leads to proliferation and clonal expansion of initiated (mutated) cells. Initiated cells respond differently to promoters than do normal cells and hence expand selectively. Such cells (especially after *RAS* activation) have reduced growth factor requirements and may also be less responsive to growth inhibitory signals in their extracellular milieu. Forced to proliferate, the initiated clone of cells suffers additional mutations, developing eventually into a malignant tumor. Thus, the process of tumor promotion includes multiple steps: proliferation of preneoplastic cells, malignant conversion, and eventually tumor progression, which depends on changes in tumor cells and the tumor stroma.

The initiation-promotion sequence of chemical carcinogenesis raises an important question: *Since promoters are not mutagenic, how do they contribute to tumorigenesis?* Although the effects of tumor promoters are pleiotropic, induction of cell proliferation is a sine qua non of tumor promotion. TPA (tetradecanoyl phorbol-13 acetate), a phorbol ester tumor promoter, is a powerful activator of protein kinase C (see Chapter 3), an enzyme that phosphorylates several substrates involved in signal transduction pathways, including those activated by growth factors. The promoting effect of phenobarbital in liver carcinogenesis has been linked to stimulation of cell proliferation associated with blockage of the TGF-β pathway.[154]

The concept that sustained cell proliferation increases the risk of mutagenesis and hence neoplastic transformation is also applicable to human carcinogenesis. For example, pathologic hyperplasia of the endometrium (Chapter 22) and increased regenerative activity that accompanies chronic liver cell injury (Chapter 18) are associated with the development of cancer in these organs.

Carcinogenic Chemicals

Before closing this discussion of chemical carcinogenesis, we briefly describe some initiators (see Table 7–11) and promoters of chemical carcinogenesis, with special emphasis on those that have been linked to cancer development in humans.[155]

Direct-Acting Alkylating Agents. These agents are activation independent, and in general they are weak carcinogens. Nonetheless, they are important because many therapeutic agents (e.g., cyclophosphamide, chlorambucil, busulfan, and melphalan) fall into this category. These are used as anticancer drugs but have been documented to induce lymphoid neoplasms, leukemia, and other forms of cancer. Some alkylating agents, such as cyclophosphamide, are also powerful immunosuppressive agents and are therefore used in treatment of immunologic disorders, including rheumatoid arthritis and Wegener granulomatosis. Although the risk of induced cancer with these agents is low, judicious use of them is indicated. Alkylating agents appear to exert their therapeutic effects by interacting with and damaging DNA, but it is precisely these actions that render them carcinogenic.

Polycyclic Aromatic Hydrocarbons. These agents represent some of the most potent carcinogens known. They require metabolic activation and can induce tumors in a wide variety of tissues and species. Painted on the skin, they cause skin cancers; injected subcutaneously, they induce sarcomas; introduced into a specific organ, they cause cancers locally. The polycyclic hydrocarbons are of particular interest as carcinogens because they are produced in the combustion of tobacco, particularly with cigarette smoking, and are thought to contribute to the causation of lung and bladder cancers.[156] The various components of cigarette smoke that may be associated with carcinogenicity are listed in Chapter 9. Polycyclic aromatic hydrocarbons are also produced from animal fats in the process of broiling meats and are present in smoked meats and fish.

Aromatic Amines and Azo Dyes. The carcinogenicity of most aromatic amines and azo dyes is exerted mainly in the liver, where the "ultimate carcinogen" is formed by the action of the cytochrome P-450 oxygenase systems. Thus, fed to rats, acetylaminofluorene and the azo dyes induce hepatocellular carcinomas (but not cancers of the gastrointestinal tract). An agent implicated in human cancers, β-naphthylamine, is an exception. In the past, it was responsible for a 50-fold increased incidence of bladder cancer in heavily exposed workers in aniline dye and rubber industries.[157] After absorption, it is hydroxylated into an active form, then detoxified by conjugation with glucuronic acid. When excreted in the urine, the nontoxic conjugate is split by the urinary enzyme glucuronidase to release the electrophilic reactant again, thus inducing bladder cancer. Regrettably, humans are one of the few species to possess urinary glucuronidase. Some of the azo dyes were developed as food coloring (e.g., butter yellow to give margarine the appearance of butter and scarlet red to impart the seductive coloration of certain foods such as maraschino cherries). These dyes are now federally regulated in the United States because of the fear that they may be dangerous to humans.

Naturally Occurring Carcinogens. Among the several known chemical carcinogens produced by plants and microorganisms, the potent hepatic carcinogen aflatoxin B1 is particularly important. This mycotoxin is produced by some strains of the fungus *Aspergillus flavus* that thrive on improperly stored corn, rice, and peanuts. A strong correlation has been found between the dietary level of this hepatocarcinogen and the incidence of hepatocellular carcinoma in some parts of Africa and China. As discussed earlier, the aflatoxin and HBV collaborate in the production of this form of neoplasia.

Nitrosamines and Amides. These carcinogens are of interest because of the possibility that they are formed in the gastrointestinal tract of humans and so may contribute to the induction of some forms of cancer, particularly gastric carcinoma. They are derived in the stomach from the reaction of nitrostable amines and nitrate used as a preservative, which is converted to nitrites by bacteria. Concerns about these agents have led many to shun processed food containing nitrate preservatives.

Miscellaneous Agents. Scores of other chemicals have been indicted as carcinogens. Only a few that represent important industrial hazards are listed in Table 7–3 and are briefly mentioned here. Occupational exposure to *asbestos* has been associated with an increased incidence of bronchogenic carcinomas, mesotheliomas, and gastrointestinal cancers, as discussed in Chapter 15. Concomitant cigarette smoking heightens the risk of bronchogenic carcinoma manyfold. *Vinyl chloride,* the monomer from which the polymer polyvinyl chloride is fabricated, was first identified as a carcinogen in animals, but investigations soon disclosed a scattered incidence of the extremely rare hemangiosarcoma of the liver among workers exposed to this chemical. *Chromium, nickel,* and other metals, when volatilized and inhaled in industrial environments, have caused cancer of the lung. Skin cancer associated with arsenic is also well established. Similarly, there is reasonable evidence that many insecticides, such as aldrin, dieldrin, and chlordane and the polychlorinated biphenyls, are carcinogenic in animals (Chapter 9).

Promoters of Chemical Carcinogenesis. Certain promoters may contribute to cancers in humans. It has been argued that promoters are at least as important as initiating chemicals in carcinogenesis because cells initiated by exposure to environmental carcinogens are innocuous unless subjected to repeated assault by promoters. Tumor promotion may occur after exposure to exogenous agents, such as cigarette smoke or viral infections, that cause tissue damage and reactive hyperplasia. Perhaps more serious, because they are difficult to control, are endogenous promoters such as hormones and bile salts. Hormones such as estrogens serve in animals as promoters of liver tumors. The prolonged use of diethylstilbestrol is implicated in the production of postmenopausal endometrial carcinoma and in the causation of vaginal cancer in offspring exposed in utero (Chapter 22). Intake of high levels of dietary fat has been associated with increased risk of colon cancer. This may be related to an increase in synthesis of bile acids, which have been shown to act as promoters in experimental models of colon cancer. Alcohol consumption increases the risk of development of cancers of the mouth, pharynx, and larynx by more than tenfold, probably by acting as a promoting agent (Chapter 9).

RADIATION CARCINOGENESIS

Radiant energy, whether in the form of the UV rays of sunlight or as ionizing electromagnetic and particulate radiation, can transform virtually all cell types in vitro and induce neoplasms in vivo in both humans and experimental animals. UV light is clearly implicated in the causation of skin cancers, and ionizing radiation exposure from medical or occupational exposure, nuclear plant accidents, and atomic bomb detonations have produced a variety of forms of malignant neoplasia. Although the contribution of radiation to the total human burden of cancer is probably small, the well-known latency of radiant energy and its cumulative effect require extremely long periods of observation and make it difficult to ascertain its full significance. An increased incidence of breast cancer has become apparent decades later among women exposed during childhood to the atomic bomb. The incidence peaked during 1988–1992 and then declined during the period 1993–1997.[158] Moreover, radiation's possible additive or synergistic effects with other potential carcinogenic influences add another dimension to the picture. The effects of UV light on DNA differ from those of ionizing radiation. The cellular and molecular effects of ionizing radiation are discussed in Chapter 9.

Ultraviolet Rays

There is ample evidence from epidemiologic studies that *UV rays* derived from the sun induce an increased incidence of squamous cell carcinoma, basal cell carcinoma, and possibly malignant melanoma of the skin.[159] The degree of risk depends on the type of UV rays, the intensity of exposure, and the quantity of light-absorbing "protective mantle" of melanin in the skin. Persons of European origin who have fair skin that repeatedly gets sunburned but stalwartly refuses to tan and who live in locales receiving a great deal of sunlight (e.g., Queensland, Australia, close to the equator) have among the highest incidence of skin cancers in the world. The UV portion of the solar spectrum can be divided into three wavelength ranges: UVA (320 to 400 nm), UVB (280 to 320 nm), and UVC (200 to 280 nm). Of these, UVB is believed to be responsible for the induction of cutaneous cancers. UVC, although a potent mutagen, is not considered significant because it is filtered out by the ozone shield around the earth (hence the concern about ozone depletion).

UV rays have a number of effects on cells, including inhibition of cell division, inactivation of enzymes, induction of mutations and, in sufficient dosage, death of cells. *The carcinogenicity of UVB light is attributed to its formation of pyrimidine dimers in DNA.* This type of DNA damage is repaired by the nucleotide excision repair (NER) pathway. There are five steps in NER: (1) recognition of the DNA lesion, (2) incision of the damaged strand on both sites of the lesion, (3) removal of the damaged nucleotide, (4) synthesis of a nucleotide patch, and (5) its ligation. In mammalian cells, the process may involve 30 or more proteins. It is postulated that with excessive sun exposure, the capacity of the NER pathway is overwhelmed; hence, some DNA damage remains unrepaired. This leads to large transcriptional errors and, in some instances, cancer. The importance of the NER pathway of DNA repair is most graphically illustrated by a study of patients with the hereditary disorder *xeroderma pigmentosum.* This autosomal recessive disorder is characterized by extreme photosensitivity, a 2000-fold increased risk of skin cancer in sun-exposed skin and, in some cases, neurologic abnormalities. The molecular basis of the degenerative changes in sun-exposed skin and occurrence of cutaneous tumors rests on an inherited inability to repair UV-induced DNA damage. Xeroderma pigmentosum is a genetically heterogeneous condition, with at least seven different variants. Each of these is caused by a mutation in one of several genes involved in NER.[160]

As with other carcinogens, UVB also causes mutations in oncogenes and tumor suppressor genes. In particular, mutant forms of the *RAS* and *p53* genes have been detected both in human skin cancers and in UVB-induced cancers in mice. These mutations occur mainly at dipyrimidine sequences within the DNA, thus implicating UVB-induced genetic damage in the causation of skin cancers. In animal models, *p53* mutations occur early after exposure to UVB, before the appearance of tumors.

Ionizing Radiation

Electromagnetic (x-rays, γ rays) and particulate (α particles, β particles, protons, neutrons) radiations are all carcinogenic. The evidence is so voluminous that a few examples suffice. Many of the pioneers in the development of X-rays developed skin cancers. Miners of radioactive elements in central Europe and the Rocky Mountain region of the United States have a tenfold increased incidence of lung cancers. Most telling is the follow-up of survivors of the atomic bombs dropped on

Hiroshima and Nagasaki. Initially, there was a marked increase in the incidence of leukemias—principally acute and chronic myelocytic leukemia—after an average latent period of about 7 years. Subsequently the incidence of many solid tumors with longer latent periods (e.g., breast, colon, thyroid, and lung) increased.

Residents of the Marshall Islands were exposed on one occasion to accidental fallout from a hydrogen bomb test that contained thyroid-seeking radioactive iodines. As many as 90% of the children under age 10 years on Rongelap Island developed thyroid nodules within 15 years, and about 5% of these nodules proved to be thyroid carcinomas. A marked increase in the incidence of thyroid cancer has also been noted in areas exposed to the fallout from the nuclear power plant accident in Chernobyl in 1986. In addition to approximately 30 deaths that occurred at the time of the accident, more than 2000 cases of thyroid cancers have been recorded in children living in the area.[161] Cytogenetic studies have detected an elevated frequency of chromosomal alterations in persons who did cleanup work at the power plant after the accident.[162] It is evident that radiant energy—whether absorbed in the pleasant form of sunlight, through the best intentions of a physician, or by tragic exposure to an atomic bomb blast or radiation released by nuclear plant accidents—has awesome carcinogenic potential. Even therapeutic irradiation has been documented to be carcinogenic. Thyroid cancers have developed in approximately 9% of those exposed during infancy and childhood to head and neck radiation. The previous practice of treating ankylosing spondylitis with therapeutic irradiation yielded a 10- to 12-fold increase in the incidence of leukemia years later.

In humans, there is a hierarchy of vulnerability of different tissues to radiation-induced cancers. Most frequent are the leukemias, except for chronic lymphocytic leukemia, which, for unknown reasons, almost never develops after radiation. Cancer of the thyroid follows closely but only in the young. In the intermediate category are cancers of the breast, lungs, and salivary glands. In contrast, skin, bone, and the gastrointestinal tract are relatively resistant to radiation-induced neoplasia, even though the gastrointestinal epithelial cells are vulnerable to the acute cell-killing effects of radiation, and the skin is in the pathway of all external radiation. Nonetheless, the physician dare not forget: practically *any* cell can be transformed into a cancer cell by sufficient exposure to radiant energy.

MICROBIAL CARCINOGENESIS

A large number of DNA and RNA viruses have proved to be oncogenic in a wide variety of animals, ranging from amphibia to primates, and the evidence grows stronger that certain forms of human cancer are of viral origin. In the following discussion, the better-characterized and most intensively studied human oncogenic viruses are presented first. This is followed by a brief account of the association between infection by the bacterium *Helicobacter pylori* and gastric tumors.

Oncogenic DNA Viruses

Several DNA viruses have been associated with the causation of cancer in animals.[163] Some, such as adenoviruses, cause tumors only in laboratory animals, whereas others, such as the bovine papillomaviruses, cause benign as well as malignant neoplasms in their natural hosts. Of the various human DNA viruses, four (papillomaviruses [HPV], Epstein-Barr virus [EBV], hepatitis B virus [HBV], and Kaposi sarcoma herpesvirus [KSHV]) are of particular interest because they have been implicated in the causation of human cancer. KSHV is discussed in Chapters 6 and 11. Although not a DNA virus, hepatitis C virus (HCV) is also associated with cancer. Before we discuss the role of these viruses in carcinogenesis, a few general comments relating to transformation by DNA viruses are offered:

- The genomes of oncogenic DNA viruses integrate into and form stable associations with the host cell genome. The virus is unable to complete its replicative cycle because the viral genes essential for completion of replication are interrupted during integration of viral DNA. Thus, the virus can remain in a latent state for years.
- Those viral genes that are transcribed early in the viral life cycle (early genes) are important for transformation, and are expressed in transformed cells.

Human Papillomavirus. Approximately 70 genetically distinct types of HPV have been identified. Some types (e.g., 1, 2, 4, and 7) cause benign squamous papillomas (warts) in humans. Human papillomaviruses have been implicated in the genesis of several cancers, particularly squamous cell carcinoma of the cervix and anogenital region, and in some cases, to the causation of oral and laryngeal cancers (Chapter 16).[164]

Epidemiologic studies suggest that carcinoma of the cervix is caused by a sexually transmitted agent, and HPV is the culprit. DNA sequences of HPV 16 and 18 and, less commonly, HPV 31, 33, 35, and 51 are found in approximately 85% of invasive squamous cell cancers and their presumed precursors (severe dysplasias and carcinoma in situ). In contrast to cervical cancers, genital warts with low malignant potential are associated with distinct HPV types, predominantly HPV 6 and HPV 11 ("low-risk" types).

Molecular analyses of HPV-associated carcinomas and benign genital warts reveal differences that may be pertinent to the transforming activity of these viruses. In benign warts and in preneoplastic lesions, the HPV genome is maintained in an episomal (nonintegrated) form, whereas in cancers, the viral DNA is usually integrated into the host cell genome. This suggests that integration of viral DNA is important in malignant transformation. Although the site of viral integration in host chromosomes is random (the viral DNA is found at different locations in different cancers), the pattern of integration is clonal; that is, the site of integration is identical within all cells of a given cancer. This would not occur if HPV were merely a passenger that infects cells after transformation. Furthermore, the viral DNA is interrupted at a fairly constant site in the process of integration: It is almost always within the E1/E2 open reading frame of the viral genome. Because the E2 region of the viral DNA normally represses the transcription of the E6 and E7 early viral genes, its interruption causes overexpression of the E6 and E7 proteins of HPV 16 and HPV 18. The oncogenic potential of HPV 16 and HPV 18 can be related to these two early viral gene products, which act in conjunction to immortalize and transform cells.[162,165] The replication of DNA viruses is dependent on the replication machinery of the host cells, and E6 and E7 act to overcome the activity of cell-cycle inhibitors (Fig. 7–50).[166] E6 binds to p53 and E7 binds to RB, inducing the degradation of these proteins. In addition, E7 can interfere with *p53* transcriptional activity and also inactivate *p21*. Thus, E6 and E7 block *p53* and *RB* cell cycle suppression pathways. The affinity of these viral proteins for the products of tumor suppressor genes differs depending on the oncogenic potential of HPV. E6 proteins derived from high-risk HPV (HPV 16, 18, and 31) inactivate p53 by enhancing its degradation through ubiquitin-dependent proteolysis.[167] E6 proteins of low-risk HPV (HPV 6 and 11) bind p53 with low affinity and have no effect on p53 stability. E7 proteins from high-risk HPV strongly bind to RB, disrupting the E2F/RB complex and promoting the degradation of RB. By contrast, E7 proteins from low-risk HPV have lower affinity for RB and have a weak capacity to transform cells. Thus, *E6 and E7 proteins of high-risk HPV disable two important tumor suppressor proteins that regulate the cell cycle.* In HPV-induced tumors, *p53* mutations are extremely uncommon, presumably because loss of *p53* function is accomplished by binding to the E6 oncoprotein. This binding not only blocks the inhibitory effect of p53 on the cell cycle but also interferes with p53 activation after DNA damage, a mechanism that allows DNA repair or elimination of cells with genomic damage. Moreover, E6 may have other effects independent of its binding of p53, such as the activation of telomerase and tyrosine kinases.[164]

The E6–p53 interaction may also offer some clues regarding risk factors for cervical cancer development in infected persons. Human *p53* is polymorphic at amino acid 72, encoding either a proline or arginine residue at that position. It turns out that the arginine-containing p53 at position 72 is much more susceptible to degradation by E6. The arginine form is found more frequently in infected individuals with cervical carcinomas than the overall population and may increase the risk for the development of cervical cancer.[168]

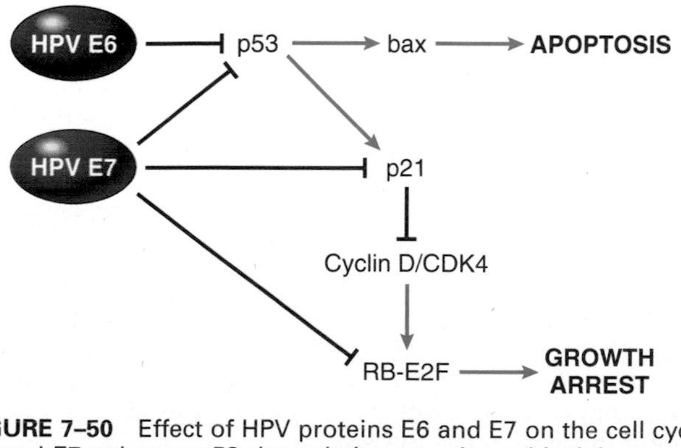

FIGURE 7–50 Effect of HPV proteins E6 and E7 on the cell cycle. E6 and E7 enhance p53 degradation, causing a block in apoptosis and decreased activity of the p21 cell cycle inhibitor. E7 associates with p21 and prevents its inhibition of the Cyclin/CDK4 complex; E7 can bind to RB, removing cell cycle restriction. The net effect of HPV E6 and E7 proteins is to block apoptosis and remove the restrains to cell proliferation (see Fig. 7–29). (Modified from Münger K, Howley PM: Human papillomavirus immortalization and transformation functions. Virus Research 89: 213–228, 2002.)

Although these observations implicate certain HPV types in the pathogenesis of human cancer, when human keratinocytes are transfected with DNA from HPV 16, 18, or 31 in vitro they are immortalized, but they do not form tumors in experimental animals. Cotransfection with a mutated *RAS* gene results in full malignant transformation. Thus, it seems most likely that infection with HPV acts as an initiating event and that additional somatic mutations are essential for malignant transformation. The occurrence of such changes is facilitated by cigarette smoking, coexisting microbial infections, dietary deficiencies, and hormonal changes, all of which have been implicated as cofactors in the pathogenesis of cervical cancers. A high proportion of women infected with HPV clear the infection by immunologic mechanisms, but the immune system factors that determine persistence of the virus have not been identified.

Epstein-Barr Virus. EBV, a member of the herpes family, has been implicated in the pathogenesis of four types of human tumors: the African form of Burkitt lymphoma; B-cell lymphomas in immunosuppressed individuals (particularly in those with human immunodeficiency virus infection and those undergoing immunosuppressive therapy after organ transplantation); some cases of Hodgkin lymphoma; and nasopharyngeal carcinomas.[169] These neoplasms are reviewed elsewhere in this book; therefore, only their association with EBV is discussed here.

EBV infects epithelial cells of the oropharynx and B lymphocytes. It gains entry into B cells via the CD21 molecule, which is expressed on all B cells. Within B lymphocytes, the linear genome of EBV circularizes to form an episome in the cell nucleus. The infection of B cells is latent; that is, there is no replication of the virus and the cells are not killed, but the latently infected B cells are immortalized and acquire the ability to propagate indefinitely in vitro. The molecular basis of B-cell immortalization by EBV is complex.[170] In contrast to HPV, there is no convincing evidence that tumor suppressor genes are targeted for inactivation by EBV. Instead, it appears that several viral genes dysregulate the normal proliferative and survival signals in latently infected cells. The latent membrane protein-1 (LMP-1) binds to and activates a signaling molecule that is normally activated by the CD40 receptor in B cells.[171] This receptor is the key recipient of helper T-cell signals, which are normally required for full B-cell responses (Chapter 6). Mimicking CD40, LMP-1 activates the NFκB and JAK/STAT signaling pathways and promotes B-cell survival and proliferation, all of which are helper T cell–induced responses that occur in the absence of T cells (or any other signals) in EBV-infected B cells. Thus, the virus has efficiently co-opted a normal pathway of B-cell activation in order to increase the number of cells it can infect and inhabit.[172] The importance of LMP-1 in mediating the effects of EBV is further highlighted by the observation that in transgenic mice, expression of LMP-1, under the control of the immunoglobulin promoter, increases the frequency of B-cell lymphomas.[169,173] The EBV-encoded *EBNA-2* gene transactivates several host genes, including *CYCLIN D* and members of the *SRC* family, promoting the transition of resting B cells from G_0 to G_1.[174] *EBNA-2* also activates the transcription of *LMP-1* and is a key regulator of viral gene expression. Thus, several viral genes collaborate to render B cells immortal.

Burkitt lymphoma is a neoplasm of B lymphocytes that is the most common childhood tumor in Central Africa and New Guinea. A morphologically identical lymphoma occurs sporadically throughout the world. The association between African Burkitt lymphoma and EBV is quite strong:

- More than 90% of African tumors carry the EBV genome.
- One hundred percent of the patients have elevated antibody titers against viral capsid antigens.
- Serum antibody titers against viral capsid antigens are correlated with the risk of developing the tumor.

Although these data strongly support the idea that EBV is intimately involved in the causation of Burkitt lymphoma, several other observations suggest that additional factors must also be involved. (1) EBV infection is not limited to the geographic locales where Burkitt lymphoma is found. EBV is a ubiquitous virus that asymptomatically infects almost all adults worldwide. (2) EBV is known to cause infectious mononucleosis, a self-limited disorder (Chapter 8) in which B cells are infected. (3) The EBV genome is found in only 15% to 20% of cases of Burkitt lymphoma outside Africa, but both the endemic (African) and the sporadic cases of Burkitt lymphoma have a t(8;14) or, less commonly, variant translocations that lead to dysregulated expression of the c-*MYC* oncogene. (4) Although EBV infection immortalizes B cells in vitro, these cells do not form tumors when injected into immunosuppressed mice in vivo. (5) There are significant differences in the patterns of viral gene expression in EBV-transformed (but not tumorigenic) B-cell lines and Burkitt lymphoma cells. For instance, the tumor cells do not express several viral-encoded membrane proteins targeted by host cytotoxic T cells.

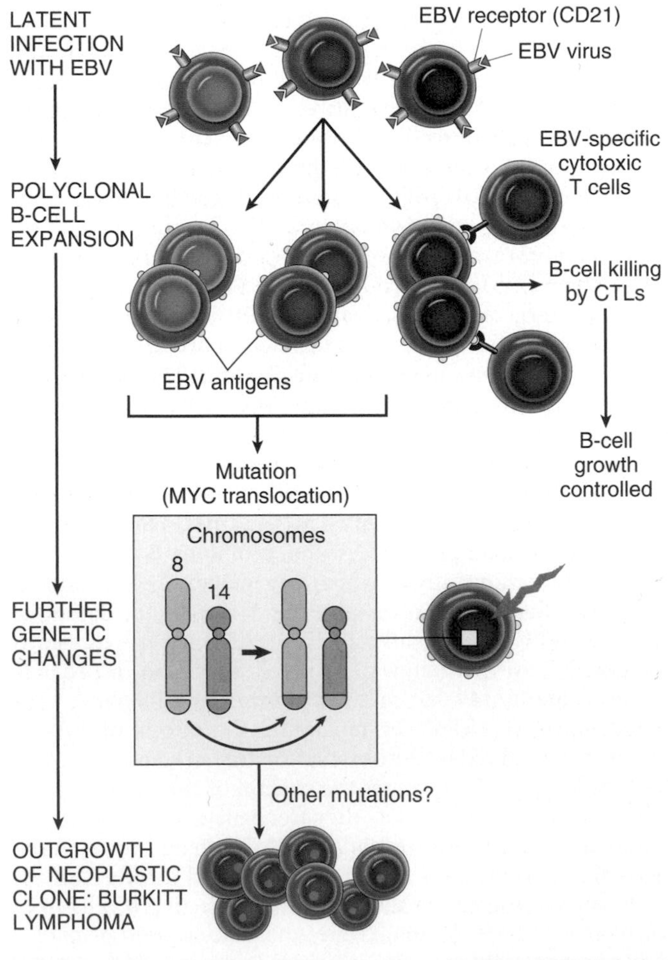

FIGURE 7–51 Schema depicting the possible evolution of Epstein-Barr virus (EBV)–induced Burkitt lymphoma.

It appears, therefore, that EBV serves as one factor in the multistep development of Burkitt lymphoma (Fig. 7–51).[175,176] In normal individuals, EBV infection is readily controlled by effective immune responses directed against viral antigens expressed on the cell membranes, and hence the vast majority of infected individuals remain asymptomatic or develop self-limited infectious mononucleosis. In regions of Africa where Burkitt lymphoma is endemic, poorly understood cofactors (e.g., chronic malaria) favor sustained proliferation of B cells immortalized by EBV. The actively dividing B-cell population is at increased risk for developing mutations, such as the t(8;14) translocation, that juxtapose *MYC* with one of the immunoglobulin gene loci. This provides growth advantage to the affected cell owing to activation of *MYC.* Approximately 80% of cases of Burkitt lymphoma carry this translocation, but all cases of the disease have reciprocal translocations that activate *MYC.* Overexpression of the *MYC* oncogene by itself is not sufficient for malignant transformation and most likely constitutes one of multiple steps in lymphomagenesis. EBV is not directly oncogenic, but by acting as a polyclonal B-cell mitogen, it sets the stage for the acquisition of the t(8;14) translocation and other mutations, which ultimately release the cells from normal growth regulation. Concurrent with these changes, viral genes may inhibit antigen presentation pathways, so that recognition by cytotoxic T lymphocytes is reduced. Tumor progression frequently involves mutations in *p53* or other defects affecting the p14ARF/MDM2/p53 pathway and inactivation of *p16INK4a* by deletion or hypermethylation.

The role played by the host immune response in controlling EBV-transformed B cells is illustrated dramatically by the occurrence of B-cell lymphomas in immunosuppressed patients. Some patients with acquired immunodeficiency syndrome (AIDS) and those who receive long-term immunosuppressive therapy for preventing allograft rejection present with multifocal B-cell tumors within lymphoid tissue or in the central nervous system. These tumors are polyclonal at the outset but can develop into monoclonal neoplasms. The expression of viral antigens such as LMP-1 remains high on these cells, and hence these tumors seem to represent the in vivo counterparts of the B-cell lines immortalized by EBV infection in vitro. That the growth of these EBV-driven cells is sensitive to immunologic control is evident from the observation that in some cases the tumors regress after relaxation of immunosuppressive therapy.

Nasopharyngeal carcinoma is the other tumor associated with EBV infection. This tumor is endemic in Southern China, in some parts of Africa, and in the Inuit population of the Arctic. In contrast to Burkitt lymphoma, 100% of nasopharyngeal carcinomas obtained from all parts of the world contain EBV DNA.[177] The viral integration in the host cells is clonal, thus ruling out the possibility that EBV infection occurred after tumor development. In addition, antibody titers to viral capsid antigens are greatly elevated, and in endemic areas patients develop IgA antibodies before the appearance of the tumor. The 100% correlation between EBV and nasopharyngeal carcinoma suggests that EBV plays a role in the genesis of this tumor, but (as with Burkitt tumor) the restricted geographic distribution indicates that genetic or environmental cofactors, or both, also contribute to tumor development.[177] The relationship of EBV to the pathogenesis of Hodgkin lymphoma is discussed in Chapter 14.

Hepatitis B Virus. Epidemiologic studies strongly suggest a close association between HBV infection and the occurrence of liver cancer (Chapter 18). HBV is endemic in countries of the Far East and Africa; correspondingly, these areas have the highest incidence of hepatocellular carcinoma. For example, in Taiwan, those who are infected with HBV have a greater than 200-fold increased risk of developing liver cancer compared with uninfected individuals in the same area.[178] Studies in experimental animals also support a role for HBV in the development of liver cancer. Although HBV infection is restricted to humans and chimpanzees, related hepadnaviruses cause hepatocellular cancers in woodchucks. Despite compelling epidemiologic and experimental evidence, the precise role of HBV in the causation of human liver cancer is not clear. In virtually all cases of HBV-related liver cell cancer, the viral DNA is integrated into the host cell genome and, as with HPV, the tumors are clonal with respect to these insertions. The HBV genome does not encode any oncoproteins, and it has been suggested that tumors could develop through insertional mutagenesis, a mechanism that was alluded to earlier. Despite the finding that in a few individual tumors the virus insertion site was adjacent to a protooncogene, in the vast majority of hepatocellular carcinomas, there is no consistent pattern of integration in the vicinity of known protooncogenes. It is likely therefore that the effect of HBV is indirect and possibly multifactorial:[179] (1) By causing chronic liver cell injury and accompanying regenerative hyperplasia, HBV expands the pool of cycling cells at risk for subsequent genetic changes. In the mitotically active liver cells, mutations may arise spontaneously or be inflicted by environmental agents, such as dietary aflatoxins. (2) HBV encodes a regulatory element called *HBx protein,* which disrupts normal growth control of infected liver cells by transcriptional activation of several growth-promoting genes, such as insulin-like growth factor II and receptors for insulin-like growth factor I. HBx binds to p53 and appears to interfere with its growth-suppressing activities.[153]

Although not a DNA virus, hepatitis C virus (HCV) is also strongly linked to the pathogenesis of hepatocellular carcinoma. As with HBV, the epidemiologic evidence of an association between hepatocellular carcinoma and HCV is compelling. The role of this virus in the pathogenesis of liver cancer seems to be related to its ability to cause chronic liver cell injury and inflammation that is accompanied by liver regeneration. Mitotically active hepatocytes, surrounded by an altered environment, are presumably prone to genetic instability and cancer development.

Oncogenic RNA Viruses

Although the study of animal retroviruses has provided spectacular insights into the molecular basis of cancer, only one human retrovirus, human T-cell leukemia virus type 1 (HTLV-1), is firmly implicated in the causation of cancer.

Human T-Cell Leukemia Virus Type 1. HTLV-1 is associated with a form of T-cell leukemia/lymphoma that is endemic in certain parts of Japan and the Caribbean basin but is found sporadically elsewhere, including the United States. Similar to the AIDS virus, HTLV-1 has tropism for CD4+ T cells, and hence this subset of T cells is the major target for neoplastic transformation. Human infection requires transmission of infected T cells via sexual intercourse, blood products, or breast-feeding. Leukemia develops in only 3% to 5% of the infected individuals after a long latent period of 40 to 60 years. In addition to leukemia, HTLV-1 is associated with a demyelinating neurologic disorder called *tropical spastic paraparesis* (Chapter 28) and possibly some forms of uveitis and arthritis in endemic areas.[180]

There is little doubt that HTLV-1 infection of T lymphocytes is necessary for leukemogenesis, but the molecular mechanisms of transformation are not entirely clear. In contrast to several murine retroviruses, HTLV-1 does not contain an oncogene, and no consistent integration next to a protooncogene has been discovered. In leukemic cells, however, viral integration shows a clonal pattern. The genomic structure of HTLV-1 reveals the *gag, pol, env*, and long terminal repeat (LTR) regions typical of other retroviruses, but, in contrast to other leukemia viruses, it contains another region, referred to as *tax.* It seems that the secrets of its transforming activity are locked in the *TAX* gene.[181] The product of this gene is essential for viral replication because it stimulates transcription of viral mRNA by acting on the 5′ LTR. It is now established that the TAX protein can also activate the transcription of several host cell genes involved in proliferation and differentiation of T cells. These include the immediate early gene c-*FOS*, genes encoding interleukin-2 (IL-2) and its receptor, and the gene for the myeloid growth factor granulocyte-macrophage colony-stimulating factor. In addition, TAX inactivates the cell-cycle inhibitor p16INK4a and enhances cyclin D activation, thus dysregulating the cell cycle. Another mechanism by which TAX can contribute to malignant transformation is through genomic instability. Recent data show that TAX interferes with DNA repair functions and inhibits ATM-mediated cell-cycle checkpoints activated by DNA damage.[182]

The main steps that lead to the development of adult T-cell leukemia/lymphoma may be summarized as follows. Infection by HTLV-1 causes the expansion of a nonmalignant polyclonal cell population through stimulatory effects of TAX on cell proliferation. The proliferating T cells are at increased risk of mutations and genomic instability induced by TAX. Eventually a monoclonal neoplastic T-cell population emerges from clonally expanding nonmalignant cells. The malignant cells replicate independent of IL-2 and contain molecular and chromosomal abnormalities.

Helicobacter pylori

There is much evidence linking gastric infection with the bacterium *H. pylori* to the causation of gastric carcinomas and gastric lymphomas.[183] This relationship, which is particularly strong for gastric lymphomas, has been established by epidemiologic studies as well as by detection of *H. pylori* infection in the great majority of tumors. Furthermore, treatment of *H. pylori* infection with antibiotics results in regression of the lymphoma in most cases. *H. pylori* is present in 90% of patients with chronic gastritis. In the great majority of infected persons, *H. pylori* infection causes no clinical consequences. However, in 20% to 30% of cases the infection leads to gastric ulcers, and in a smaller proportion of cases, gastric carcinomas, and gastric lymphomas may develop. The disease-causing strains contain a "pathogenicity island" containing the *CagA* (*c*ytotoxin *a*ssociated *g*ene *A*) gene and a secretory system, which injects the CagA protein into the host cells. Another gene associated with virulence is *VacA*, which encodes a vacuolating toxin that causes apoptosis. The infection is associated with gastric adenocarcinomas of the intestinal type (see Chapter 17) through a sequence that involves chronic gastritis, multifocal atrophy with lower gastric acid secretion, intestinal metaplasia, dysplasia, and carcinoma.

Gastric lymphomas arise in mucosa-associated lymphoid tissue (MALT); they sometimes are called *MALTomas*.[184] The B cells that give rise to these tumors normally reside in the marginal zones of lymphoid follicles; hence, the alternative name of *marginal zone lymphoma* (Chapter 14). It is thought that chronic infection with *H. pylori* leads to formation of lymphoid infiltrates in which B cells actively proliferate and may acquire genetic abnormalities, such as a t(11;18) translocation. Tumor growth is initially dependent on immune stimulation by *H. pylori*, but at later stages it no longer requires the presence of the bacterium.

Host Defense Against Tumors—Tumor Immunity

The idea that tumors are not entirely self and may be recognized by the immune system was conceived by Paul Ehrlich, who proposed that immune recognition of autologous tumor cells may be a positive mechanism capable of eliminating tumors. Subsequently, Lewis Thomas and Macfarlane Burnet formalized this concept by coining the term *immune surveillance,* which implies that a normal function of the immune system is to survey the body for emerging malignant cells and destroy them.[185,186] This idea has been supported by many observations—the occurrence of lymphocytic infiltrates around tumors and in lymph nodes draining sites of cancer; experimental results, mostly with transplanted tumors; the increased incidence of some cancers in immunodeficient individuals; and the direct demonstration of tumor-specific T cells and antibodies in patients. The fact that cancers occur in immunocompetent individuals suggests that immune surveillance is imperfect and often cannot control rapidly growing tumors; however, because some tumors escape such policing does not preclude the possibility that others may have been aborted.[187] The concept of tumor immune surveillance has recently been expanded to encompass not only the protective role of the immune system in tumor development, but also the effect of the immune system in selecting for tumor variants.[186,188] These variants have reduced immunogenicity and can more easily escape immunologic detection and rejection. The term *cancer immunoediting* is now being used to describe the effects of the immune system in preventing tumor formation and also in "sculpting" the immunogenic properties of tumors to select tumor cells that escape immune elimination.

In the following section we explore some of the important questions about tumor immunity: What is the nature of tumor antigens? What host effector systems may recognize tumor cells? Is antitumor immunity effective against spontaneous neoplasms? Can immune reactions against tumors be exploited for immunotherapy?

TUMOR ANTIGENS

Antigens that elicit an immune response have been demonstrated in many experimentally induced tumors and in some human cancers.[189] Initially, they were broadly classified into two categories based on their patterns of expression: *tumor-specific antigens,* which are present only on tumor cells and not on any normal cells, and *tumor-associated antigens,* which are present on tumor cells and also on some normal cells. This classification, however, is imperfect because many antigens thought to be tumor-specific turned out to be expressed by some normal cells as well. The modern classification of tumor antigens is based on their molecular structure and source.

The early attempts to purify and characterize tumor antigens were based on producing monoclonal antibodies specific for tumor cells and defining the antigens that these antibodies recognized. An important advance in the field was the development of techniques for identifying tumor antigens that were recognized by cytotoxic T lymphocytes (CTLs), because CTLs are the major immune defense mechanism against tumors. Recall that CTLs recognize peptides derived from cytoplasmic proteins that are displayed bound to class I major histocompatibility complex (MHC) molecules (Chapter 6). Below we describe the main classes of tumor antigens (Fig. 7–52).

Products of Mutated Oncogenes and Tumor Suppressor Genes. Neoplastic transformation, as we have discussed, results from genetic alterations, some of which may result in the expression of cell-surface antigens that are seen as nonself by the immune system.[190,191] The products of altered protooncogenes and tumor suppressor genes are synthesized in the cytoplasm of the tumor cells, and like any cytosolic protein, they may enter the class I MHC antigen processing pathway and be recognized by CD8+ T cells. In addition, these proteins may enter the class II antigen-processing pathway in antigen-presenting cells that have phagocytosed dead tumor cells, and thus be recognized by CD4+ T cells also. Because these altered proteins are not present in normal cells, they do not induce self-tolerance. Some cancer patients have circulating CD4+ and CD8+ T cells that can respond to the products of mutated oncogenes such as RAS, p53, and BCR-ABL proteins. In animals, immunization with mutated RAS or p53 proteins induces CTLs and rejection responses against tumors expressing these mutants. However, these proteins do not appear to be major targets of tumor-specific CTLs in most patients with a variety of tumors.

Products of Other Mutated Genes. Because of the genetic instability of tumor cells, many different genes may be mutated in these cells, including genes whose products are not related to the transformed phenotype and have no known function. Products of these mutated genes are potential tumor antigens. The tumor antigens that were discovered in transplanted carcinogen-induced tumors in animals, called tumor-specific transplantation antigens, are mutants of various host cellular proteins that are processed and presented in the form of peptide–class I MHC complexes capable of stimulating CTLs. These antigens are extremely diverse because the carcinogens that induce the tumors may randomly mutagenize virtually any host gene and the class I MHC antigen-presenting pathway can display peptides from any mutated cytosolic protein in each tumor. Mutated cellular proteins are found more frequently in chemical carcinogen- or radiation-induced animal tumors than in spontaneous human cancers, probably because chemical carcinogens and radiation mutagenize many cellular genes.

Overexpressed or Aberrantly Expressed Cellular Proteins. Tumor antigens may be normal cellular proteins that are abnormally expressed in tumor cells and elicit immune responses. One of the unexpected findings that has emerged from the search for tumor antigens in human tumors such as melanomas is that some tumor antigens are structurally normal proteins that are produced at low levels in normal cells and overexpressed in tumor cells. One such antigen is tyrosinase, an enzyme involved in melanin biosynthesis that is expressed only in normal melanocytes and melanomas.[192] T cells from melanoma patients recognize peptides derived from tyrosinase, raising the possibility that tyrosinase vaccines may stimulate such responses to melanomas; clinical trials with these vaccines are ongoing. On face value it is surprising that these patients are able to respond to a normal self-antigen. The likely explanation is that tyrosinase is normally produced in such small amounts and in so few cells that it is not recognized by the immune system and fails to induce tolerance.

Other tumor antigens may be derived from genes that are not expressed in normal tissues or are expressed only early during development (see below) and are dysregulated as a consequence of malignant transformation of a cell. The functions of the proteins encoded by these genes may be unknown, but they are not required for the malignant phenotype of the cells, and they are not mutated. Melanoma antigen *(MAGE)* genes, first isolated from human melanoma cells, encode cellular protein antigens recognized by melanoma-specific T cells derived from different melanoma-bearing patients. MAGE proteins are expressed in tumors in addition to melanomas, including carcinomas of the bladder, breast, skin, lung, and prostate and some sarcomas. In normal tissues, MAGE expression is restricted to the testis. Currently, at least 25 *MAGE* genes mapped to chromosome Xq have been identified in humans.[193] Because the MAGE antigens are shared by many different types of tumors, they are attractive targets for

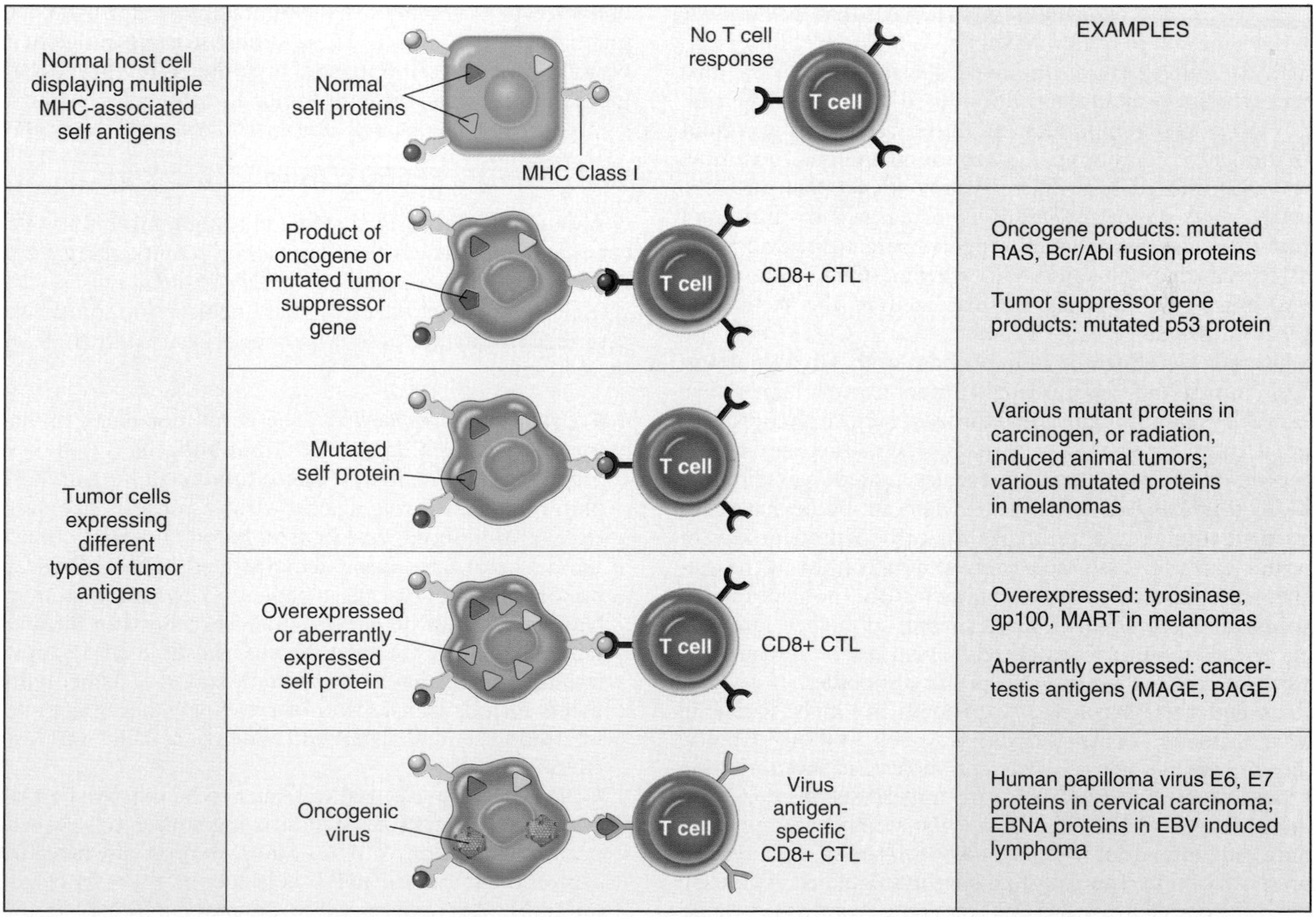

FIGURE 7–52 Tumor antigens recognized by CD8+ T cells. (Modified from Abbas AK, Lichtman AH: Cellular and Molecular Immunology, 5th ed. Philadelphia, WB Saunders, 2003.)

immunotherapy. Subsequent to identification of the *MAGE* genes, several other unrelated gene families have been identified that encode melanoma antigens recognized by T cells in melanoma patients, and these have been called *GAGE, BAGE,* and *RAGE.* Like the MAGE proteins, these other melanoma antigens are silent in most normal tissues except the testis, but they are expressed in a variety of malignant tumors. Because of their expression on cancers and in the testis, all these tumor antigens are now classified in the "cancer-testis antigen" family.

Tumor Antigens Produced by Oncogenic Viruses. As we have discussed, many viruses are associated with cancers. Not surprisingly, these viruses produce proteins that are recognized as foreign by the immune system. The most potent of these antigens are proteins produced by latent DNA viruses; examples in humans include HPV and EBV. There is abundant evidence that CTLs recognize antigens of these viruses and that a competent immune system plays a role in surveillance against virus-induced tumors because of its ability to recognize and kill virus-infected cells. In fact, the concept of immune surveillance against tumors is better established for DNA virus–induced tumors than for any other type of tumor.

Oncofetal Antigens. Oncofetal antigens are proteins that are expressed at high levels on cancer cells and in normal developing (fetal) but not adult tissues. It is believed that the genes encoding these proteins are silenced during development and are derepressed upon malignant transformation. Oncofetal antigens were identified with antibodies raised in other species, and their main importance is that they provide markers that aid in tumor diagnosis. As techniques for detecting these antigens have improved, it has become clear that their expression in adults is not limited to tumors. The proteins are increased in tissues and in the circulation in various inflammatory conditions and are found in small quantities even in normal tissues. There is no evidence that oncofetal antigens are important inducers or targets of antitumor immunity. The two most thoroughly characterized oncofetal antigens are carcinoembryonic antigen (CEA) and alphafetoprotein (AFP). These are discussed in the section on Tumor Markers.

Altered Cell-Surface Glycolipids and Glycoproteins. Most human and experimental tumors express higher than normal levels and/or abnormal forms of surface glycoproteins and glycolipids, which may be diagnostic markers and targets for therapy. These altered molecules include gangliosides, blood group antigens, and mucins. Many antibodies have been raised in animals that recognize the carbohydrate groups or peptide cores of these molecules. Although most of the epitopes recognized by these antibodies are not specifically expressed on tumors, they are present at higher levels on cancer cells than on normal cells. This class of antigens is a target for cancer therapy with specific antibodies.

Among the glycolipids expressed at high levels in melanomas are the gangliosides G_{M2}, G_{D2}, and G_{D3}. Clinical trials of anti-G_{M2} and anti-G_{D3} antibodies and immunization with vaccines containing G_{M2} are under way in melanoma patients. Mucins are high-molecular-weight glycoproteins containing numerous O-linked carbohydrate side chains on a core polypeptide. Tumors often have dysregulated expression of the enzymes that synthesize these carbohydrate side chains, which leads to the appearance of tumor-specific epitopes on the carbohydrate side chains or on the abnormally exposed polypeptide core. Several mucins have been the focus of diagnostic and therapeutic studies, including CA-125 and CA-19-9, expressed on ovarian carcinomas, and MUC-1, expressed on breast carcinomas. Unlike many mucins, MUC-1 is an integral membrane protein that is normally expressed only on the apical surface of breast ductal epithelium, a site that is relatively sequestered from the immune system. In ductal carcinomas of the breast, however, the molecule is expressed in an unpolarized fashion and contains new, tumor-specific carbohydrate and peptide epitopes detectable by mouse monoclonal antibodies. The peptide epitopes induce both antibody and T-cell responses in cancer patients and are therefore being considered as candidates for tumor vaccines.

Cell Type–Specific Differentiation Antigens. Tumors express molecules that are normally present on the cells of origin. These antigens are called *differentiation antigens* because they are specific for particular lineages or differentiation stages of various cell types. Their importance is as potential targets for immunotherapy and for identifying the tissue of origin of tumors. For example, lymphomas may be diagnosed as B cell–derived tumors by the detection of surface markers characteristic of this lineage, such as CD10 (previously called common acute lymphoblastic leukemia antigen, or CALLA) and CD20. Antibodies against these molecules are also used for tumor immunotherapy. The idiotypic determinants of the surface immunoglobulin of a clonal B-cell population are markers for that B-cell clone because all other B cells express different idiotypes. Therefore, the immunoglobulin idiotype is a highly specific tumor antigen for B-cell lymphomas and leukemias. These differentiation antigens are typically normal self-antigens, and therefore they do not induce immune responses in tumor-bearing hosts.

ANTITUMOR EFFECTOR MECHANISMS

Although both cell-mediated and humoral immunity have been demonstrated to have antitumor activity, *the principal mechanism of tumor immunity is killing of tumor cells by CD8+ CTLs.* The cellular effectors that mediate immunity were described in Chapter 6, so it is necessary here only to discuss them briefly:

- *Cytotoxic T lymphocytes:* The antitumor effect of cytotoxic T cells reacting against tumor antigens is well established in experimentally induced tumors. In humans, CTLs play a protective role against virus-associated neoplasms (e.g., EBV-induced Burkitt lymphoma and HPV-induced tumors) and have been demonstrated in the blood and tumor infiltrates of cancer patients. The tumor-specific T lymphocytes can be harvested and expanded in vitro and reinfused into the autologous host. Such adoptive immunotherapy has met with some success. Further refinements include transfection of cytokine genes into tumor-infiltrating lymphocytes to potentiate their antitumor effects.
- *Natural killer cells:* Natural killer (NK) cells are lymphocytes that are capable of destroying tumor cells without prior sensitization.[194] Also, many tumors down-regulate expression of class I MHC molecules as a way of evading immunity. As we discussed in Chapter 6, NK cells are particularly effective against cells with reduced MHC expression. After activation with IL-2, NK cells can lyse a wide

variety of human tumors in vitro. Adoptive immunotherapy with in vitro expanded and activated human NK cells has met with limited success. Although NK cells may provide the first line of defense against many tumors, their importance in defense against most spontaneously arising tumors remains unclear.

- *Macrophages:* Activated macrophages are effective at killing tumor cells in vitro. T cells and NK cells may collaborate with macrophages in antitumor reactivity because interferon-γ (IFN-γ), a cytokine produced by T cells and NK cells, is a potent activator of macrophages. These cells may kill tumors by mechanisms similar to those used to kill microbes, for example, production of reactive oxygen metabolites.
- *Antibodies:* Tumor-bearing hosts may produce antibodies against various tumor antigens. Antibodies may kill tumor cells by activating complement or by antibody-dependent cell-mediated cytotoxicity, in which Fc receptor–bearing macrophages or NK cells mediate the killing. However, the ability of antibodies to eliminate tumor cells has been demonstrated largely in vitro, and there is little evidence for effective humoral immunity against tumors.

IMMUNE SURVEILLANCE

Given the many potential antitumor mechanisms, is there any evidence that they operate in vivo to prevent emergence of neoplasms? The strongest argument for the existence of immune surveillance is the increased frequency of cancers in immunodeficient hosts. About 5% of persons with congenital immunodeficiencies develop cancers, about 200 times the prevalence in immunocompetent individuals. Immunosuppressed transplant recipients and patients with AIDS also have an increased incidence of malignancies. Most (but not all) of these neoplasms are lymphomas, often immunoblastic B-cell lymphomas. Particularly illustrative is the rare X-linked recessive immunodeficiency disorder termed *XLP (X-linked lymphoproliferative syndrome),* caused by mutations in the gene encoding an adapter protein *(SAP),* which participates in lymphocyte signaling pathways.[195] When boys affected by XLP develop an EBV infection, it does not take the usual self-limited form of infectious mononucleosis but, in the majority of cases, it evolves into a severe form of infectious mononucleosis. Approximately 25% of XLP patients develop malignant B-cell lymphomas.

Most cancers occur in persons who do not suffer from any overt immunodeficiency. It is evident then that *tumor cells must develop mechanisms to escape or evade the immune system* in immunocompetent hosts. Several such mechanisms may be operative (Fig. 7–53).

- *Selective outgrowth of antigen-negative variants:* During tumor progression, strongly immunogenic subclones may be eliminated.
- *Loss or reduced expression of MHC molecules:* Tumor cells may fail to express normal levels of HLA class I molecules, thereby escaping attack by cytotoxic T cells. Such cells, however, may trigger NK cells.
- *Lack of costimulation:* It may be recalled that sensitization of T cells requires two signals, one by foreign peptide presented by MHC molecules and the other by costimulatory molecules (Chapter 6); although tumor cells may express peptide antigens with class I molecules, they often do not express costimulatory molecules. This not only prevents sensitization, but also may render T cells anergic or, worse, cause them to undergo apoptosis. To bypass this problem, attempts are being made to immunize patients with autologous tumor cells that have been transfected with the gene for the costimulatory molecule B7-1. In another approach, autologous dendritic cells expanded in vitro and pulsed with tumor antigens (e.g., MAGE-1) are infused into cancer patients. Because dendritic cells express high levels of costimulatory molecules, it is expected that such immunization will stimulate antitumor T cells.
- *Immunosuppression:* Many oncogenic agents (e.g., chemicals and ionizing radiation) suppress host immune responses. Tumors or tumor products may also be immunosuppressive. For example, TGF-β, secreted by many tumors, is a potent immunosuppressant. In some cases, the immune response induced by the tumor (e.g., activation of regulatory T cells) may itself inhibit tumor immunity.
- *Antigen masking:* The cell-surface antigens of tumors may be hidden, or masked, from the immune system by glycocalyx molecules, such as sialic acid–containing mucopolysaccharides. This may be a consequence of the fact that tumor cells often express more of these glycocalyx molecules than normal cells do.
- *Apoptosis of cytotoxic T cells:* Some melanomas and hepatocellular carcinomas express Fas ligand. It has been postulated that these tumors kill Fas-expressing T lymphocytes that come in contact with them, thus eliminating tumor-specific T cells.[196]

Thus, it seems that there is no dearth of mechanisms by which tumor cells can outwit the host and thrive despite an intact immune system.

Although the increased occurrence of tumors in immunodeficient hosts supports the existence of immune surveillance, the strongest argument against the concept of immune surveillance also derives from the study of immunosuppressed patients. The most common forms of cancers in immunosuppressed and immunodeficient patients are lymphomas, notably immunoblastic B-cell lymphomas, which could be the consequence of abnormal lymphoproliferative responses to microbes such as EBV or to the various therapeutic agents administered to these patients. Significantly, an increased incidence of the most common forms of cancer—lung, breast, gastrointestinal tract—and multiple neoplasms might be anticipated in immunodeficient individuals, but it does not occur.

It is worth mentioning that although much of the focus in the field of tumor immunity has been on the mechanisms by which the host immune system defends against tumors, there is some recent evidence that, paradoxically, the immune system may promote the growth of tumors.[197] It is possible that activated lymphocytes and macrophages produce growth factors for tumor cells or enzymes, such as MMPs, that enhance tumor invasion. Harnessing the protective actions of

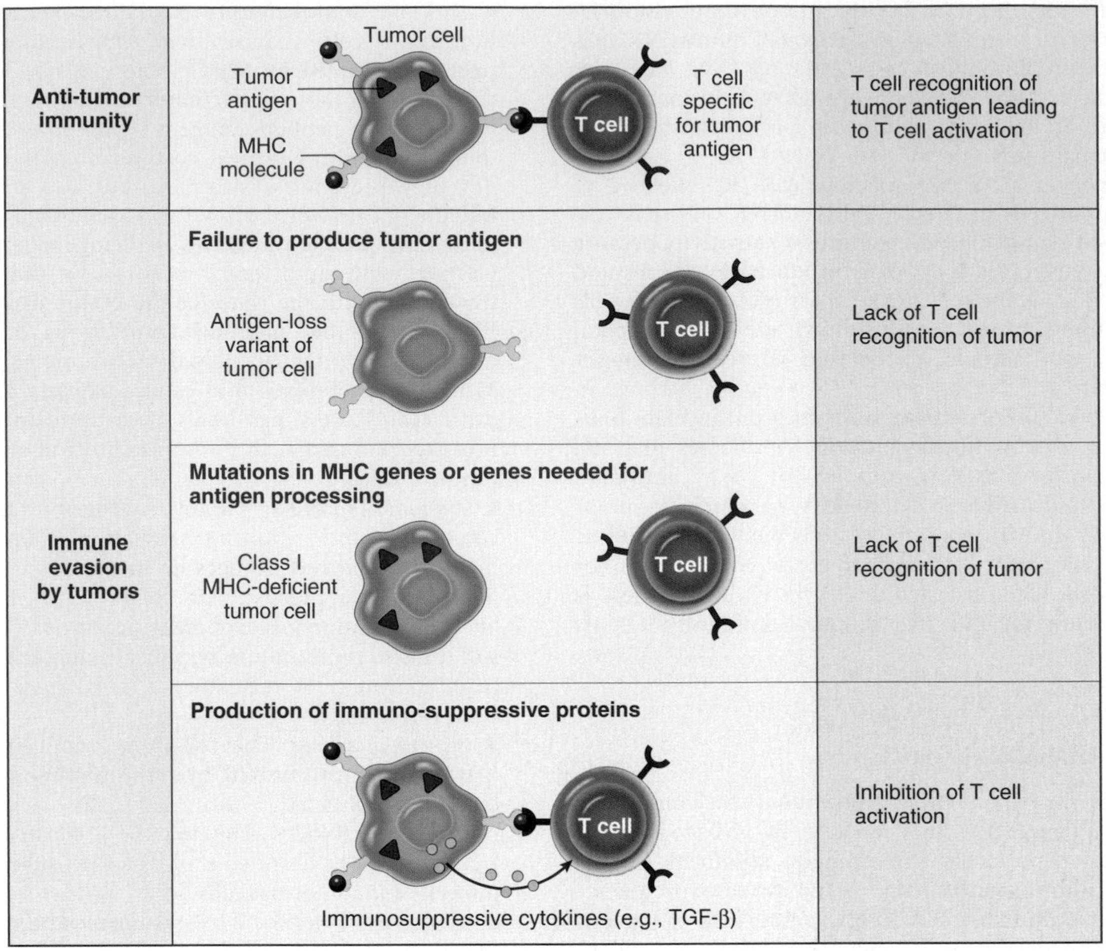

FIGURE 7–53 Mechanisms by which tumors evade the immune system. (Reprinted from Abbas AK, Lichtman AH: Cellular and Molecular Immunology, 5th ed. Philadelphia, WB Saunders, 2003.)

the immune system and abolishing its ability to increase tumor growth is obviously an important goal of immunologists and oncologists.

Clinical Features of Tumors

Neoplasms are essentially parasites. Some cause only trivial mischief, but others are catastrophic. All tumors, even benign ones, may cause morbidity and mortality. Moreover, every new growth requires careful appraisal lest it be cancerous. Differential diagnosis comes into sharpest focus with lumps in the female breast. Both cancers and many benign disorders of the female breast present as palpable masses. In fact, benign lesions are more common than cancers. Although clinical evaluation may suggest one or the other, the only unequivocally benign breast mass is the one that has been excised and anatomically diagnosed. This is equally true of all neoplasms. There are, however, instances when adherence to this dictum must be tempered by clinical judgment. Subcutaneous lipomas, for example, are quite common and readily recognized by their soft, yielding consistency. Unless they are uncomfortable, subject to trauma, or aesthetically disturbing, small lesions are often merely observed for significant increase in size. A few other examples might be cited, but it suffices that *with a few exceptions, all masses require anatomic evaluation.* Besides the concern that malignant neoplasms arouse, even benign ones may have many adverse effects. The sections that follow consider (1) the effects of a tumor on the host, (2) the grading and clinical staging of cancer, and (3) the laboratory diagnosis of neoplasms.

EFFECTS OF TUMORS ON THE HOST

Obviously, cancers are far more threatening to the host than benign tumors are. Nonetheless, both types of neoplasia may cause problems because of (1) location and impingement on adjacent structures, (2) functional activity such as hormone synthesis, (3) bleeding and secondary infections when they ulcerate through adjacent natural surfaces, and (4) initiation of acute symptoms caused by either rupture or infarction. Any metastasis has the potential to produce these same consequences. Cancers may also be responsible for cachexia (wasting) or paraneoplastic syndromes.

Local and Hormonal Effects

An example of disease related to critical location is the pituitary adenoma. Although the tumor is benign and possibly not producing hormones, expansile growth can destroy the remaining pituitary and thus lead to serious endocrinopathy. Cancers arising within or metastatic to an endocrine gland may cause an endocrine insufficiency by destroying the gland. Neoplasms in the gut, both benign and malignant, may cause obstruction as they enlarge. Infrequently, peristaltic movement telescopes the neoplasm and its affected segment into the downstream segment, producing an obstructing intussusception (Chapter 17).

Neoplasms arising in endocrine glands may produce manifestations by elaboration of hormones. Such functional activity is more typical of benign tumors than of cancers, which may be sufficiently undifferentiated to have lost such capability. A benign β-cell adenoma of the pancreatic islets less than 1 cm in diameter may produce sufficient insulin to cause fatal hypoglycemia. In addition, nonendocrine tumors may elaborate hormones or hormone-like products and give rise to paraneoplastic syndromes (discussed later). The erosive destructive growth of cancers or the expansile pressure of a benign tumor on any natural surface, such as the skin or mucosa of the gut, may cause ulcerations, secondary infections, and bleeding. Melena (blood in the stool) and hematuria, for example, are characteristic of neoplasms of the gut and urinary tract. Neoplasms, benign as well as malignant, may then cause problems in varied ways, but all are far less common than the cachexia of malignancy.

Cancer Cachexia

Patients with cancer commonly suffer progressive loss of body fat and lean body mass accompanied by profound weakness, anorexia, and anemia. This wasting syndrome is referred to as *cachexia.* The origins of cancer cachexia are obscure. There is little doubt, however, that cachexia is not caused by the nutritional demands of the tumor. Current evidence indicates that cachexia results from the action of soluble factors such as cytokines produced by the tumor and by the host in response to the tumor.

Clinically, anorexia is a common problem in patients with cancer, even in those who do not have mechanical obstruction caused by gastrointestinal tumors. Reduced food intake has been related to abnormalities in taste and central control of appetite, but reduced intake alone is not sufficient to explain the cachexia of malignancy. In patients with cancer, calorie expenditure often remains high, and basal metabolic rate is increased despite reduced food intake. By contrast, in starvation, there is an adaptational lowering of metabolic rate.[198] Furthermore, in cancer cachexia, there is equal loss of fat and muscle, whereas in starvation the muscle mass is relatively preserved at the expense of fat stores. The basis of these metabolic abnormalities is not fully understood. Many of the changes associated with cancer cachexia, including loss of appetite and alterations in fat metabolism, are mimicked by the administration of tumor necrosis factor (TNF) in experimental animals. It is suspected therefore that TNF produced by macrophages or possibly some tumor cells is a mediator of the wasting syndrome that accompanies cancer. Other cytokines, such as IL-1, IFN-γ, and leukemia inhibitory factor synergize with TNF. In addition to these cytokines, there is evidence for the existence of other soluble factors produced by tumors (such as the proteolysis-inducing factor PIF), which increase the catabolism of muscle and adipose tissue by acting directly on fat and muscle protein. Thus, several factors collaborate in contributing to malnutrition in cancer patients. Identification and neutralization of such factors may help ameliorate cancer cachexia.[186]

Paraneoplastic Syndromes

Symptom complexes in cancer-bearing patients that cannot readily be explained, either by the local or distant spread of the tumor or by the elaboration of hormones indigenous to the tissue from which the tumor arose, are known as *paraneoplastic syndromes.*[199] These occur in about 10% of patients with malignant disease. Despite their relative infrequency, paraneoplastic syndromes are important to recognize, for several reasons:

- They may represent the earliest manifestation of an occult neoplasm.
- In affected patients, they may represent significant clinical problems and may even be lethal.
- They may mimic metastatic disease and therefore confound treatment.

A classification of paraneoplastic syndromes and their presumed origins is presented in Table 7–12. A few comments on some of the more common and interesting syndromes follow.

The *endocrinopathies* are frequently encountered paraneoplastic syndromes.[200] Because the cancer cells are not of endocrine origin, the functional activity is referred to as *ectopic hormone production.* Cushing syndrome is the most common endocrinopathy. Approximately 50% of patients with this endocrinopathy have carcinoma of the lung, chiefly the small cell type. It is caused by excessive production of corticotropin or corticotropin-like peptides. The precursor of corticotropin is a large molecule known as pro-opiomelanocortin (POMC). Lung cancer patients with Cushing syndrome have elevated serum levels of POMC as well as of corticotropin. The former is not found in serum of patients with excess corticotropin produced by the pituitary.

Hypercalcemia is probably the most common paraneoplastic syndrome; overtly symptomatic hypercalcemia is most often related to some form of cancer rather than to hyperparathyroidism. Two general processes are involved in cancer-associated hypercalcemia: (1) osteolysis induced by cancer, whether primary in bone, such as multiple myeloma, or metastatic to bone from any primary lesion, and (2) the production of calcemic humoral substances by extraosseous neoplasms. *Hypercalcemia owing to skeletal metastases is not a paraneoplastic syndrome.*

Several humoral factors have been associated with paraneoplastic hypercalcemia of malignancy. Perhaps the most important is a molecule related to, but distinct from, parathyroid hormone (PTH). Parathyroid hormone–related protein (PTHRP) resembles the native hormone only in its amino terminus.[201] It has some biologic actions similar to those of PTH, and both hormones share a G-protein–coupled receptor, known as PTH/PTHRP receptor (often referred to as PTH-R or PTHRP-R). In contrast to PTH, PTHRP is produced by many normal tissues, including keratinocytes, muscles, bone, and ovary. The amounts produced by normal cells, however,

TABLE 7–12 Paraneoplastic Syndromes

Clinical Syndromes	Major Forms of Underlying Cancer	Causal Mechanism
Endocrinopathies		
Cushing syndrome	Small cell carcinoma of lung Pancreatic carcinoma Neural tumors	ACTH or ACTH-like substance
Syndrome of inappropriate antidiuretic hormone secretion	Small cell carcinoma of lung; intracranial neoplasms	Antidiuretic hormone or atrial natriuretic hormones
Hypercalcemia	Squamous cell carcinoma of lung Breast carcinoma Renal carcinoma Adult T-cell leukemia/lymphoma Ovarian carcinoma	Parathyroid hormone–related protein (PTHRP), TGF-α, TNF, IL-1
Hypoglycemia	Fibrosarcoma Other mesenchymal sarcomas Hepatocellular carcinoma	Insulin or insulin-like substance
Carcinoid syndrome	Bronchial adenoma (carcinoid) Pancreatic carcinoma Gastric carcinoma	Serotonin, bradykinin
Polycythemia	Renal carcinoma Cerebellar hemangioma Hepatocellular carcinoma	Erythropoietin
Nerve and Muscle Syndromes		
Myasthenia	Bronchogenic carcinoma	Immunologic
Disorders of the central and peripheral nervous systems	Breast carcinoma	
Dermatologic Disorders		
Acanthosis nigricans	Gastric carcinoma Lung carcinoma Uterine carcinoma	Immunologic; secretion of epidermal growth factor
Dermatomyositis	Bronchogenic, breast carcinoma	Immunologic
Osseous, Articular, and Soft Tissue Changes		
Hypertrophic osteoarthropathy and clubbing of the fingers	Bronchogenic carcinoma	Unknown
Vascular and Hematologic Changes		
Venous thrombosis (Trousseau phenomenon)	Pancreatic carcinoma Bronchogenic carcinoma Other cancers	Tumor products (mucins that activate clotting)
Nonbacterial thrombotic endocarditis	Advanced cancers	Hypercoagulability
Anemia	Thymic neoplasms	Unknown
Others		
Nephrotic syndrome	Various cancers	Tumor antigens, immune complexes

ACTH, adrenocorticotropic hormone; TGF, transforming growth factor; TNF, tumor necrosis factor; IL, interleukin.

are small. It is thought that PTHRP regulates calcium transport in the lactating breast and across the placenta. Tumors most often associated with paraneoplastic hypercalcemia are carcinomas of the breast, lung, kidney, and ovary. In breast cancers, PTHRP production is associated with osteolytic bone disease, bone metastasis, and humoral hypercalcemia. The most common lung neoplasm associated with hypercalcemia is the squamous cell bronchogenic carcinoma, rather than small cell cancer of the lung (more often associated with endocrinopathies). In addition to PTHRP, several other factors, such as IL-1, TGF-α, TNF, and dihydroxyvitamin D, have also been implicated in causing the hypercalcemia of malignancy.

The *neuromyopathic paraneoplastic syndromes* take diverse forms, such as peripheral neuropathies, cortical cerebellar degeneration, a polymyopathy resembling polymyositis, and a myasthenic syndrome similar to *myasthenia gravis.* The cause of these syndromes is poorly understood. In some cases, antibodies, presumably induced against tumor cells that cross-react with neuronal cells, have been detected. It is postulated that some neural antigens are ectopically expressed by visceral cancers. For some unknown reason, the immune system recognizes these antigens as foreign and mounts an immune response.

Acanthosis nigricans is characterized by gray-black patches of verrucous hyperkeratosis on the skin. This disorder occurs rarely as a genetically determined disease in juveniles or adults (Chapter 25). In addition, in about 50% of the cases, particularly in those over age 40, the appearance of such lesions is associated with some form of cancer. Sometimes the skin changes appear before discovery of the cancer.

Hypertrophic osteoarthropathy is encountered in 1% to 10% of patients with bronchogenic carcinomas. Rarely, other forms of cancer are involved. This disorder is characterized by (1) periosteal new bone formation, primarily at the distal ends of long bones, metatarsals, metacarpals, and proximal phalanges; (2) arthritis of the adjacent joints; and (3) clubbing of the digits. Although the osteoarthropathy is seldom seen in noncancer patients, clubbing of the fingertips may be encountered in liver diseases, diffuse lung disease, congenital cyanotic heart disease, ulcerative colitis, and other disorders. The cause of hypertrophic osteoarthropathy is unknown.

Several *vascular and hematologic manifestations* may appear in association with a variety of forms of cancer. As mentioned in the discussion of thrombosis (Chapter 4), *migratory thrombophlebitis* (Trousseau syndrome) may be encountered in association with deep-seated cancers, most often carcinomas of the pancreas or lung. Disseminated intravascular coagulation may complicate a diversity of clinical disorders (Chapter 13). Acute disseminated intravascular coagulation is most commonly associated with acute promyelocytic leukemia and prostatic adenocarcinoma. Bland, small, nonbacterial fibrinous vegetations sometimes form on the cardiac valve leaflets (more often on left-sided valves), particularly in patients with advanced mucin-secreting adenocarcinomas. These lesions, called *nonbacterial thrombotic endocarditis,* are described further in Chapter 12. The vegetations are potential sources of emboli that can further complicate the course of cancer.

GRADING AND STAGING OF TUMORS

Prognosis of the course of the disease and the determination of efficacy of various forms of cancer treatment require a high degree of similarity among the tumors being considered. Systems have been developed to express, at least in semiquantitative terms, the level of differentiation, or *grade,* and extent of spread of a cancer within the patient, or *stage,* as parameters of the clinical gravity of the disease.

Grading of a cancer is based on the degree of differentiation of the tumor cells and the number of mitoses within the tumor as presumed correlates of the neoplasm's aggressiveness. Thus, cancers are classified as grades I to IV with increasing anaplasia. Criteria for the individual grades vary with each form of neoplasia and so are not detailed here, but all attempt, in essence, to judge the extent to which the tumor cells resemble or fail to resemble their normal counterparts. Although histologic grading is useful, the correlation between histologic appearance and biologic behavior is less than perfect. In recognition of this problem and to avoid spurious quantification, it is common practice to characterize a particular neoplasm in descriptive terms, for example, well-differentiated, mucin-secreting adenocarcinoma of the stomach, or highly undifferentiated, retroperitoneal malignant tumor—probably sarcoma. In general, with a few exceptions, such as soft tissue sarcomas, grading of cancers has proved of less clinical value than has staging.

The staging of cancers is based on the size of the primary lesion, its extent of spread to regional lymph nodes, and the presence or absence of blood-borne metastases. Two major staging systems are currently in use, one developed by the Union Internationale Contre Cancer (UICC) and the other by the American Joint Committee (AJC) on Cancer Staging. The UICC employs a classification called the *TNM system—T* for primary tumor, *N* for regional lymph node involvement, and *M* for metastases. The TNM staging varies for each specific form of cancer, but there are general principles. With increasing size, the primary lesion is characterized as T1 to T4. T0 is added to indicate an in situ lesion. N0 would mean no nodal involvement, whereas N1 to N3 would denote involvement of an increasing number and range of nodes. M0 signifies no distant metastases, whereas M1 or sometimes M2 indicates the presence of blood-borne metastases and some judgment as to their number.

The AJC employs a somewhat different nomenclature and divides all cancers into stages 0 to IV, incorporating within each of these stages the size of the primary lesion as well as the presence of nodal spread and distant metastases. The staging systems and additional details are mentioned in appropriate chapters, in conjunction with the discussion of specific tumors. It merits emphasis here, however, that staging of neoplastic disease has assumed great importance in the selection of the best form of therapy for the patient. It bears repeating that *staging has proved to be of greater clinical value than grading.* In some cases, such as for lung cancers, staging has been greatly aided by imaging techniques such as *positron emission tomography.*[55]

LABORATORY DIAGNOSIS OF CANCER

Every year the approach to laboratory diagnosis of cancer becomes more complex, more sophisticated, and more specialized. For virtually every neoplasm mentioned in this text, the experts have characterized a number of subcategories; we must walk, however, before we can run. Each of the following sections attempts to present the state of the art, avoiding details of method.

Histologic and Cytologic Methods. The laboratory diagnosis of cancer is, in most instances, not difficult. The two ends of the benign–malignant spectrum pose no problems; however, in the middle lies a gray zone where one should tread cautiously. The focus here is on the roles of the clinician (often a surgeon) and the pathologist in facilitating the correct diagnosis.

Clinical data are invaluable for optimal pathologic diagnosis, but often clinicians tend to underestimate the value of the clinical data. Radiation changes in the skin or mucosa can be similar to those associated with cancer. Sections taken from a healing fracture can mimic an osteosarcoma. Moreover the laboratory evaluation of a lesion can be only as good as the specimen made available for examination. It must be adequate, representative, and properly preserved. Several sampling approaches are available: (1) excision or biopsy, (2) needle aspiration, and (3) cytologic smears. When excision of a small lesion is not possible, selection of an appropriate site for biopsy of a large mass requires awareness that the margins may not be representative and the center largely necrotic. Appropriate preservation of the specimen is obvious, yet it involves such actions as prompt immersion in a usual fixative (commonly formalin solution, but other fluids can be used), preservation of a portion in a special fixative (e.g., glutaraldehyde) for electron microscopy, or prompt refrigeration to permit optimal hormone, receptor, or other types of molecular analysis. Requesting "quick-frozen section" diagnosis is sometimes desirable, for example, in determining the nature of a mass lesion or in evaluating the margins of an excised cancer to ascertain that the entire neoplasm has been removed. This method permits histologic evaluation within minutes. In experienced, competent hands, frozen-section diagnosis is highly accurate, but there are particular instances in which the better histologic detail provided by the more time-consuming routine methods is needed—for example, when extremely radical surgery, such as the amputation of an extremity, may be indicated. Better to wait a day or two despite the drawbacks, than to perform inadequate or unnecessary surgery.

Fine-needle aspiration of tumors is another approach that is widely used. The procedure involves aspirating cells and attendant fluid with a small-bore needle, followed by cytologic examination of the stained smear. This method is used most commonly for the assessment of readily palpable lesions in sites such as the breast, thyroid, and lymph nodes. Modern imaging techniques enable the method to be extended to lesions in deep-seated structures, such as pelvic lymph nodes and pancreas. Fine-needle aspiration is less invasive and more rapidly performed than are needle biopsies. In experienced hands, it is an extremely reliable, rapid, and useful technique.

Cytologic (Pap) smears provide yet another method for the detection of cancer (Chapter 22). This approach is widely used for the discovery of carcinoma of the cervix, often at an in situ stage, but it is also used with many other forms of suspected malignancy, such as endometrial carcinoma, bronchogenic carcinoma, bladder and prostatic tumors, and gastric carcinomas; for the identification of tumor cells in abdominal, pleural, joint, and cerebrospinal fluids; and, less commonly, with other forms of neoplasia.

As pointed out earlier, cancer cells have lowered cohesiveness and exhibit a range of morphologic changes encompassed by the term *anaplasia*. Thus, shed cells can be evaluated for the features of anaplasia indicative of their origin in a cancer (Figs. 7–54 and 7–55). In contrast to the histologist's task, judgment here must be rendered based on the features of individual cells or, at most, a clump of a few cells, without the supporting evidence of architectural disarray, loss of orientation of one cell to another, and (perhaps most important) evidence of invasion. This method permits differentiation among normal, dysplastic, and cancerous cells and in addition permits the recognition of cellular changes characteristic of carcinoma in situ. The gratifying control of cervical cancer is the best testament to the value of the cytologic method.

Although histology and exfoliative cytology remain the most commonly used methods in the diagnosis of cancer, new techniques are being constantly added to the tools of the surgical pathologist. Some, such as immunohistochemistry, are already well established and widely used; others, including molecular methods, are rapidly finding their way into the "routine" category. Only some highlights of these diagnostic modalities are presented.

Immunohistochemistry. The availability of specific monoclonal antibodies has greatly facilitated the identification of cell products or surface markers. Some examples of the utility of immunohistochemistry in the diagnosis or management of malignant neoplasms follow.

- *Categorization of undifferentiated malignant tumors:* In many cases, malignant tumors of diverse origin resemble each other because of poor differentiation. These tumors are often quite difficult to distinguish on the basis of routine hematoxylin and eosin-stained tissue sections. For example,

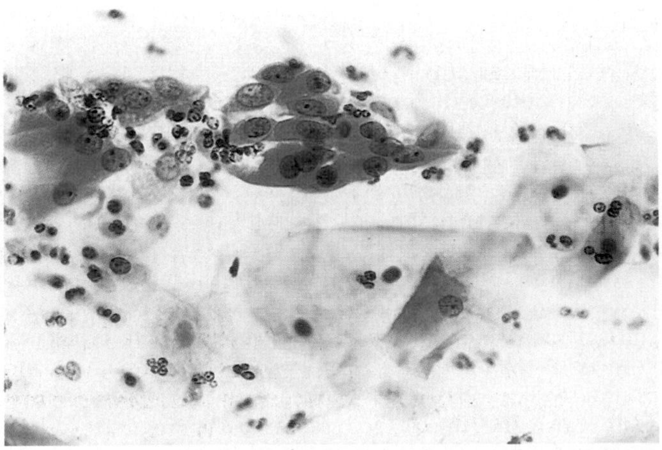

FIGURE 7–54 A normal cervicovaginal smear shows large, flattened squamous cells and groups of metaplastic cells; interspersed are some neutrophils. There are no malignant cells. (Courtesy of Dr. P.K. Gupta, University of Pennsylvania, Philadelphia, PA.)

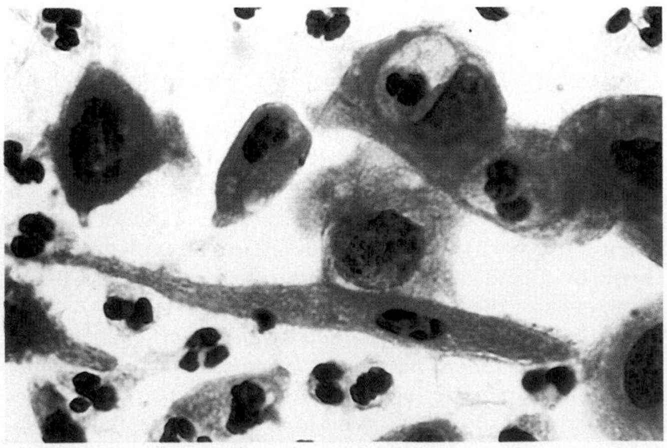

FIGURE 7–55 An abnormal cervicovaginal smear shows numerous malignant cells that have pleomorphic, hyperchromatic nuclei; interspersed are some normal polymorphonuclear leukocytes. (Courtesy of Dr. P.K. Gupta, University of Pennsylvania, Philadelphia, PA.)

certain anaplastic carcinomas, malignant lymphomas, melanomas, and sarcomas may look quite similar, but they must be accurately identified because their treatment and prognosis are different. Antibodies against intermediate filaments have proved to be of value in such cases because tumor cells often contain intermediate filaments characteristic of their cell of origin. For example, the presence of cytokeratins, detected by immunohistochemistry, points to an epithelial origin (carcinoma) (Fig. 7–56), whereas desmin is specific for neoplasms of muscle cell origin.

- *Categorization of leukemias and lymphomas:* Immunohistochemistry (in conjunction with immunofluorescence) has also proved useful in the identification and classification of tumors arising from T and B lymphocytes and from mononuclear-phagocytic cells. Monoclonal antibodies directed against various lymphohematopoietic cells are listed in Chapter 14.
- *Determination of site of origin of metastatic tumors:* Many cancer patients present with metastases. In some, the primary site is obvious or readily detected on the basis of clinical or radiologic features. In cases in which the origin of the tumor is obscure, immunohistochemical detection of tissue-specific or organ-specific antigens in a biopsy specimen of the metastatic deposit can lead to the identification of the tumor source. For example, prostate-specific antigen and thyroglobulin are markers of tumors of the prostate and thyroid, respectively.
- *Detection of molecules that have prognostic or therapeutic significance:* Immunohistochemical detection of hormone (estrogen/progesterone) receptors in breast cancer cells is of prognostic and therapeutic value because these cancers are susceptible to antiestrogen therapy (Chapter 23). In general, receptor-positive breast cancers have a better prognosis. Protein products of oncogenes such as *ERBB2* in breast cancers can also be detected by immunostaining. Breast cancers with overexpression of ERBB2 protein generally have a poor prognosis.

Molecular Diagnosis. Several molecular techniques—some established, others emerging—have been used for diagnosis and, in some cases, for predicting behavior of tumors.

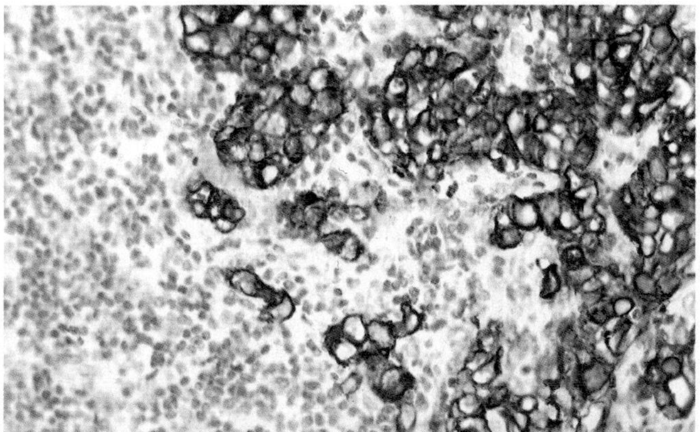

FIGURE 7–56 Anticytokeratin immunoperoxidase stain of a tumor of epithelial origin (carcinoma). (Courtesy of Dr. Melissa Upton, University of Washington, Seattle, WA.)

- *Diagnosis of malignant neoplasms:* Although molecular methods are not the primary modality of cancer diagnosis, they are of considerable value in selected cases. Molecular techniques are useful in differentiating benign (polyclonal) proliferations of T or B cells from malignant (monoclonal) proliferations. As discussed in Chapter 6, it is possible to identify monoclonal T-cell and B-cell proliferations on the basis of clonal rearrangement of their antigen receptor genes. Many hematopoietic neoplasms (leukemias and lymphomas) are associated with specific translocations that activate oncogenes. Detection of such translocations, usually by routine cytogenetic analysis or by FISH technique (Chapter 5), is often extremely helpful in diagnosis.[202] In some cases, molecular techniques can reveal translocations or other rearrangements, which may not be apparent by standard chromosome staining. Thus, for example, the detection of *BCR-ABL* transcripts by polymerase chain reaction (PCR) provides precise diagnosis of chronic myeloid leukemia, even in cases that appear to be negative by conventional karyotype analysis. Molecular detection of translocations is also of particular value in the diagnosis of certain sarcomas (Chapter 26) because chromosome preparations are often difficult to obtain from solid tumors. For example, many sarcomas of childhood, so-called round blue cell tumors (Chapter 10), can be difficult to distinguish from each other on the basis of morphology. However, the diagnosis of one such tumor, Ewing sarcoma [t(11;22)(q24;q12)] can be readily established using sensitive PCR-based assays for the specific translocations.[203] A molecular cytogenetic technique called *spectral karyotyping* has great sensitivity and allows the examination of all chromosomes in a single experiment.[204] This technique, which is based on 24-color chromosomal painting with a mixture of fluorochromes, can detect all types of chromosomal rearrangements in tumor cells, even very small translocations and insertions (Chapter 5; see Fig. 5–25). It can also detect the origin of unidentified chromosomes, called *marker chromosomes,* seen in many hematopoietic malignancies. Another available technique is *comparative genomic hybridization,* which is somewhat laborious and more frequently used in research laboratories. This technique allows the analysis of genome amplification and chromosomal gains and losses in tumor cells. It has been used to differentiate primary from metastatic carcinomas and to identify primary tumors of uncertain origin.[205]
- *Prognosis of malignant neoplasms:* Certain genetic alterations are associated with poor prognosis, and hence their detection allows stratification of patients for therapy. As an example, amplification of the N-*MYC* gene and deletions of 1p bode poorly for patients with neuroblastoma. These can be detected by routine cytogenetics and also by FISH or PCR assays. Oligodendrogliomas in which the only genomic abnormality is the loss of chromosomes 1p and 19q, respond well to therapy and are associated with long-term survival when compared to tumors with intact 1p and 19q but with EGF receptor amplification.[206]
- *Detection of minimal residual disease:* After treatment of patients with leukemia or lymphoma, the presence of minimal disease or the onset of relapse can be monitored by PCR-based amplification of unique nucleic acid sequences generated by the translocation. For example,

detection of *BCR-ABL* transcripts by PCR gives a measure of the residual leukemia cells in treated patients with chronic myeloid leukemia. Similarly, detection of specific K-*RAS* mutations in stool samples of patients previously treated for colon cancer can alert to the possible recurrence of the tumor. The clinical importance of minimal disease that is detected only by PCR remains to be established, and several studies addressing this issue are in progress.

- *Diagnosis of hereditary predisposition to cancer:* As was discussed earlier, germ line mutations in several tumor suppressor genes, including *BRCA1*, *BRCA2*, and the *RET* protooncogene, are associated with a high risk of developing specific cancers. Thus, detection of carriers of these mutations in family members of affected patients or in those at high risk of carrying the mutation has become important. Such analysis usually requires detection of a specific mutation (e.g., *RET* gene) or sequencing of the entire gene. The latter is necessitated when several different cancer-associated mutations are known to exist. Although the detection of mutations in such cases is relatively straightforward, the ethical issues surrounding such presymptomatic diagnosis are complex.
- *DNA microarray analysis and proteomics:* These methods are used to obtain gene expression signatures (molecular profiles) of cancer cells (see Box 7–1). DNA microarray techniques reveal the RNA expression from as many as 30,000 different genes using gene chip technology. This method has identified new subtypes with potential prognostic significance among breast cancers, acute lymphoblastic leukemias, and gliomas (see Box 7–1 and Chapter 23). An ever-increasing number of new tumor markers for human malignancies have also been identified with this technique. Proteomics determines the protein profiles of tumors. With the methods currently in use, protein profiles from about 3000 genes can be obtained.

Several other diagnostic applications of recombinant DNA technology are cited when discussing specific tumors. Validation of new markers for cancer diagnosis can be done on multiple tissue samples, using *tissue arrays.* In this technique, core samples are obtained from tissues embedded in a paraffin block and used to prepare a new block that may contain hundreds of tissue fragments. These multiple samples are then used to test the expression of potential tumor markers by immunohistochemical or in situ hybridization techniques.

Flow Cytometry. Flow cytometry can rapidly and quantitatively measure several individual cell characteristics, such as membrane antigens and the DNA content of tumor cells. Identification of cell-surface antigens by flow cytometry is widely used in the classification of leukemias and lymphomas (Chapter 14). Flow cytometric detection of ploidy is applied to specimens from a variety of sources, such as fresh-frozen surgical biopsy specimens (from which nuclei can be extracted), pleural or peritoneal effusions associated with cancer, bone marrow aspirations, and cells obtained by irrigation of the urinary bladder. A relationship between abnormal DNA content and prognosis is becoming apparent for a variety of malignancies. In general, aneuploidy seems to be associated with poorer prognosis in early-stage breast cancer, carcinoma of the urinary bladder, lung cancer, colorectal cancer, and prostate cancer.

Tumor Markers. Tumor markers are biochemical indicators of the presence of a tumor. They include cell-surface antigens, cytoplasmic proteins, enzymes, and hormones. In clinical practice, however, the term usually refers to a molecule that can be detected in plasma or other body fluids.[207] *Tumor markers cannot be construed as primary modalities for the diagnosis of cancer.* Their main utility in clinical medicine has been as a laboratory test to support the diagnosis. Some tumor markers are also of value in determining the response to therapy and in indicating relapse during the follow-up period.

A host of tumor markers have been described, and new ones are identified every year. Only a few have stood the test of time and proved to have clinical usefulness. The application of several markers, listed in Table 7–13, is considered in the discussion of specific forms of neoplasia in other chapters, so only two widely used examples suffice here.

CEA, normally produced in embryonic tissue of the gut, pancreas, and liver, is a complex glycoprotein that is elaborated by many different neoplasms. Depending on the serum level adopted as a significant elevation, it is variously reported to be positive in 60% to 90% of colorectal, 50% to 80% of pancreatic, and 25% to 50% of gastric and breast carcinomas. Much less consistently, elevated CEA has been described in other forms of cancer. CEA elevations have also been reported in many benign disorders, such as alcoholic cirrhosis, hepatitis, ulcerative colitis, Crohn disease, and others. Occasionally, levels of this antigen are elevated in apparently healthy smokers. Thus, *CEA assays lack both specificity and the sensitivity required for the detection of early cancers.* Preoperative CEA levels have some bearing on prognosis because the level of elevation is correlated with body burden of tumor. In colon cancer, the levels correlate with the widely used Dukes grading system (Chapter 17). In patients with CEA-positive colon cancers, the presence of elevated CEA levels 6 weeks after therapy indicates residual disease. A rising CEA level indicates recurrence, with an increase in tumor marker level often preceding clinically detectable disease. Serum CEA is also useful in monitoring the treatment of metastatic breast cancer.

AFP is another well-established tumor marker (see Chapters 18 and 21). This glycoprotein is synthesized normally early in fetal life by the yolk sac, fetal liver, and fetal gastrointestinal tract. Abnormal plasma elevations are encountered in adults with cancer arising principally in the liver and germ cells of the testis. Elevated plasma AFP is also found less regularly in carcinomas of the colon, lung, and pancreas. Similar to CEA, non-neoplastic conditions, including cirrhosis, toxic liver injury, hepatitis, and pregnancy (especially with fetal distress or death), also may cause minimal to moderate plasma elevations of AFP. Although there is then some problem with specificity, marked elevations of the plasma AFP level have proved to be a useful indicator of hepatocellular carcinomas and germ cell tumors of the testis. AFP levels decline rapidly after surgical resection of liver cell cancer or treatment of germ cell tumors. Serial post-therapy measurements of AFP (and human chorionic gonadotropin) levels in patients with germ cell tumors of the testis provide a sensitive index of response to therapy and recurrence.

Other widely used markers include PSA and PSMA (prostate-specific antigen and prostate-specific membrane antigen) for prostate cancers, human chorionic gonadotropin for testicular tumors, and CA125 for ovarian tumors. The

TABLE 7–13 Selected Tumor Markers

Markers	Associated Cancers
Hormones	
Human chorionic gonadotropin	Trophoblastic tumors, nonseminomatous testicular tumors
Calcitonin	Medullary carcinoma of thyroid
Catecholamine and metabolites	Pheochromocytoma and related tumors
Ectopic hormones	See Paraneoplastic Syndromes in Table 7–12
Oncofetal Antigens	
α-Fetoprotein	Liver cell cancer, nonseminomatous germ cell tumors of testis
Carcinoembryonic antigen	Carcinomas of the colon, pancreas, lung, stomach, and heart
Isoenzymes	
Prostatic acid phosphatase	Prostate cancer
Neuron-specific enolase	Small cell cancer of lung, neuroblastoma
Specific Proteins	
Immunoglobulins	Multiple myeloma and other gammopathies
Prostate-specific antigen and prostate-specific membrane antigen	Prostate cancer
Mucins and Other Glycoproteins	
CA-125	Ovarian cancer
CA-19-9	Colon cancer, pancreatic cancer
CA-15-3	Breast cancer
New Molecular Markers	
p53, APC, RAS mutations in stool and serum	Colon cancer
p53 and *RAS* mutations in stool and serum	Pancreatic cancer
p53 and *RAS* mutations in sputum and serum	Lung cancer
p53 mutations in urine	Bladder cancer

development of tests to detect cancer markers in blood and body fluids is an active area of research. Some of the markers being evaluated include the detection of mutated *APC, p53,* and *RAS* in the stool of patients with colorectal carcinomas; the presence of mutated *p53* and of hypermethylated genes in the sputum of patients with lung cancer and in the saliva of patients with head and neck cancers; and the detection of mutated *p53* in the urine of patients with bladder cancer.[207]

REFERENCES

1. Parkin DM: Global cancer statistics in the year 2000. Lancet Oncol 2:533, 2001.
2. Pisani P, Bray F, Parkin DM: Estimates of the world-wide prevalence of cancer for 25 sites in the adult population. Int J Cancer 97:72, 2002.
3. Jemal A, et al: Cancer statistics, 2003. CA Cancer J Clin 53:5, 2003.
4. Simmonds MA: Cancer statistics, 2003: further decrease in mortality rate, increase in persons living with cancer. CA Cancer J Clin 53:4, 2003.
5. Willis RA: The Spread of Tumors in the Human Body. London, Butterworth & Co, 1952.
6. Dick JE: Stem cells: self-renewal writ in blood. Nature 423:231, 2003.
7. Al-Hajj M, et al: Prospective identification of tumorigenic breast cancer cells. Proc Natl Acad Sci U S A 100:3983, 2003.
8. Lessard J, Sauvageau G: BMI-1 determines the proliferative capacity of normal and leukaemic stem cells. Nature 423:255, 2003.
9. Dick JE: Breast cancer stem cells revealed. Proc Natl Acad Sci U S A 100:3547, 2003.
10. Park IK, et al: BMI-1 is required for maintenance of adult self-renewing haematopoietic stem cells. Nature 423:302, 2003.
11. Padera TP, et al: Lymphatic metastasis in the absence of functional intratumor lymphatics. Science 296:1883, 2002.
12. Couch FJ, Weber BL: Breast cancer. In Vogelstein B, Kinzler KW (eds): The Genetic Basis of Human Cancer, 2nd ed. New York, McGraw-Hill, 2002, p 549–581.
13. Choi SH, Barsky SH, Chang HR: Clinicopathologic analysis of sentinel lymph node mapping in early breast cancer. Breast J 9:153, 2003.
14. Covens A: Sentinel lymph nodes. Cancer 97:2945, 2003.
15. Weir HK, et al: Annual report to the nation on the status of cancer, 1975–2000, featuring the uses of surveillance data for cancer prevention and control. J Natl Cancer Inst 95:1276, 2003.
16. El-Serag HB: Hepatocellular carcinoma: an epidemiologic view. J Clin Gastroenterol 35:S72, 2002.
17. Ghafoor A, et al: Cancer statistics for African Americans. CA Cancer J Clin 52:326, 2002.
18. Brawley OW: Some perspective on black-white cancer statistics. CA Cancer J Clin 52:322, 2002.
19. O'Brien K, et al: Cancer statistics for Hispanics, 2003. CA Cancer J Clin 53:208, 2003.
20. Calle EE, et al: Overweight, obesity, and mortality from cancer in a prospectively studied cohort of U.S. adults. N Engl J Med 348:1625, 2003.
21. Knudson AG: Cancer genetics. Am J Med Genet 111:96, 2002.
22. Narod SA: Modifiers of risk of hereditary breast and ovarian cancer. Nat Rev Cancer 2:113, 2002.
23. Marsh D, Zori R: Genetic insights into familial cancers—update and recent discoveries. Cancer Lett 181:125, 2002.
24. Muller A, Fishel R: Mismatch repair and the hereditary non-polyposis colorectal cancer syndrome (HNPCC). Cancer Invest 20:102, 2002.
25. Wooster R, Weber BL: Breast and ovarian cancer. N Engl J Med 348:2339, 2003.

26. Houghton AN, Polsky D: Focus on melanoma. Cancer Cell 2:275, 2002.
27. King M-C et al: Breast and ovarian cancer risks due to inherited mutations in BRCA1 and BRCA2. Science 302:643, 2003.
28. Levy-Lahad E, Plon SE: A risky business—Assessing breast cancer risk. Science 302:574, 2003.
29. Coussens LM, Werb Z: Inflammation and cancer. Nature 420:860, 2002.
30. Balkwill F, Mantovani A: Inflammation and cancer: back to Virchow? Lancet 357:539, 2001.
31. DuBois RN: Cyclooxygenase-2 and colorectal cancer. Prog Exp Tumor Res 37:124, 2003.
32. Howe LR, Dannenberg AJ: A role for cyclooxygenase-2 inhibitors in the prevention and treatment of cancer. Semin Oncol 29:111, 2002.
33. Gale RE: Evaluation of clonality in myeloid stem-cell disorders. Semin Hematol 36:361, 1999.
34. Philipp-Staheli J, Payne SR, Kemp CJ: p27(Kip1): regulation and function of a haploinsufficient tumor suppressor and its misregulation in cancer. Exp Cell Res 264:148, 2001.
35. Loeb LA, Loeb KR, Anderson JP: Multiple mutations and cancer. Proc Natl Acad Sci U S A 100:776, 2003.
36. Hanahan D, Weinberg RA: The hallmarks of cancer. Cell 100:57, 2000.
37. Ekholm SV, Reed SI: Regulation of G(1) cyclin-dependent kinases in the mammalian cell cycle. Curr Opin Cell Biol 12:676, 2000.
38. Sherr CJ, McCormick F: The RB and p53 pathways in cancer. Cancer Cell 2:103, 2002.
39. Sherr CJ: The INK4a/ARF network in tumour suppression. Nat Rev Mol Cell Biol 2:731, 2001.
40. Lowe SW, Sherr CJ: Tumor suppression by Ink4a-Arf: progress and puzzles. Curr Opin Genet Dev 13:77, 2003.
41. Roberts JM, Sherr CJ: Bared essentials of CDK2 and cyclin E. Nat Genet 35:9, 2003.
42. Quelle DE, et al: Alternative reading frames of the INK4a tumor suppressor gene encode two unrelated proteins capable of inducing cell cycle arrest. Cell 83:993, 1995.
43. Walworth NC: Cell-cycle checkpoint kinases: checking in on the cell cycle. Curr Opin Cell Biol 12:697, 2000.
44. Bartek J, Lukas J: Mammalian G_1- and S-phase checkpoints in response to DNA damage. Curr Opin Cell Biol 13:738, 2001.
45. Kern SE: Progressive genetic abnormalities in human neoplasia. In Mendelsohn J, Howley PM, Israel MA, et al (eds): The Molecular Basis of Cancer, 2nd ed. Philadelphia, WB Saunders, 2001, p 41–69.
46. Ponder BA: Multiple endocrine neoplasia type 2. In Vogelstein B, Kinzler KW (eds): The Genetic Basis of Human Cancer, 2nd ed. New York, McGraw-Hill, 2002, p 501–513.
47. Cote GJ, Gagel RF: Lessons learned from the management of a rare genetic cancer. N Engl J Med 349:1566, 2003.
48. Ruco LP, et al: Met protein and hepatocyte growth factor (HGF) in papillary carcinoma of the thyroid: evidence for a pathogenetic role in tumourigenesis. J Pathol 194:4, 2001.
49. Ritter CA, Arteaga CL: The epidermal growth factor receptor-tyrosine kinase: a promising therapeutic target in solid tumors. Semin Oncol 30:3, 2003.
50. Maher EA, et al: Malignant glioma: genetics and biology of a grave matter. Genes Dev 15:1311, 2001.
51. Hayes DF, Thor AD: c-*erbB-2* in breast cancer: development of a clinically useful marker. Semin Oncol 29:231, 2002.
52. Goldman JM, Melo JV: Chronic myeloid leukemia—advances in biology and new approaches to treatment. N Engl J Med 349:1451, 2003.
53. George S, Desai J: Management of gastrointestinal stromal tumors in the era of tyrosine kinase inhibitors. Curr Treat Options Oncol 3:489, 2002.
54. Malumbres M, Barbacid M: *RAS* oncogenes: the first 30 years. Nat Rev Cancer 3:459, 2003.
55. Minna JD, Roth JA, Gazdar AF: Focus on lung cancer. Cancer Cell 1:49, 2002.
56. Markowitz SD, et al: Focus on colon cancer. Cancer Cell 1:233, 2002.
57. Jaffee EM, et al: Focus on pancreas cancer. Cancer Cell 2:25, 2002.
58. Hingorani SR, Tuveson DA: *Ras* redux: rethinking how and where *Ras* acts. Curr Opin Genet Dev 13:6, 2003.
59. Davies H, et al: Mutations of the *BRAF* gene in human cancer. Nature 417:949, 2002.
60. Pollock PM, et al: High frequency of *BRAF* mutations in nevi. Nat Genet 33:19, 2003.
61. Cox AD, Der CJ: *Ras* family signaling: therapeutic targeting. Cancer Biol Ther 1:599, 2002.
62. Kurzrock R, et al: Philadelphia chromosome-positive leukemias: from basic mechanisms to molecular therapeutics. Ann Intern Med 138:819, 2003.
63. Sattler M, Griffin JD: Molecular mechanisms of transformation by the *BCR-ABL* oncogene. Semin Hematol 40:4, 2003.
64. Eisenman RN: Deconstructing *myc.* Genes Dev 15:2023, 2001.
65. Grandori C, et al: The *Myc/Max/Mad* network and the transcriptional control of cell behavior. Annu Rev Cell Dev Biol 16:653, 2000.
66. Shiio Y, et al: Quantitative proteomic analysis of Myc oncoprotein function. EMBO J 21:5088, 2002.
67. Keyomarsi K, et al: Cyclin E and survival in patients with breast cancer. N Engl J Med 347:1566, 2002.
68. Murphy M, Levine AJ: Tumor suppressor genes. In Mendelsohn J, et al (eds): The Molecular Basis of Cancer, 2nd ed. Philadelphia, WB Saunders, 2001, p 95–114.
69. Knudson AG, Jr.: Retinoblastoma: a prototypic hereditary neoplasm. Semin Oncol 5:57, 1978.
70. Kim W, Kaelin WG: The von Hippel-Lindau tumor suppressor protein: new insights into oxygen sensing and cancer. Curr Opin Genet Dev 13:55, 2003.
71. Liu MC, Gelmann EP: *P53* gene mutations: case study of a clinical marker for solid tumors. Semin Oncol 29:246, 2002.
72. Baselga J, Norton L: Focus on breast cancer. Cancer Cell 1:319, 2002.
73. Frebourg T, et al: Germ-line *p53* mutations in 15 families with Li-Fraumeni syndrome. Am J Hum Genet 56:608, 1995.
74. Nichols KE, et al: Germ-line *p53* mutations predispose to a wide spectrum of early-onset cancers. Cancer Epidemiol Biomarkers Prev 10:83, 2001.
75. Onel K, Corden-Cardoc C: MDM2 and prognosis. Mol Cancer Res 2:1, 2004.
76. Shumeli A, Oren M: Regulation of p53 by MDM2: fate is in the numbers. Mol Cell 13(1):4–5.
77. Chresta CM, Hickman JA: Oddball p53 in testicular tumors. Nat Med 2:745, 1996.
78. Biederer C, et al: Replication-selective viruses for cancer therapy. J Mol Med 80:163, 2002.
79. Benard J, Douc-Rasy S, Ahomadegbe JC: *TP53* family members and human cancers. Hum Mutat 21:182, 2003.
80. Soussi T: *p53* mutations and resistance to chemotherapy: a stab in the back for *p73*. Bull Cancer 90:383, 2003.
81. Shibata H, et al: Rapid colorectal adenoma formation initiated by conditional targeting of the *Apc* gene. Science 278:120, 1997.
82. Reya T, et al: A role for *Wnt* signalling in self-renewal of haematopoietic stem cells. Nature 423:409, 2003.
83. van Es JH, Barker N, Clevers H: You wnt some, you lose some: oncogenes in the *Wnt* signaling pathway. Curr Opin Genet Dev 13:28, 2003.
84. Polakis P: The oncogenic activation of beta-catenin. Curr Opin Genet Dev 9:15, 1999.
85. Wei Y, et al: Activation of β-catenin in epithelial and mesenchymal hepatoblastomas. Oncogene 19:498, 2000.
86. Mendelsohn J, et al: Growth factors and their receptors in epithelial malignancies. In Mendelsohn J, et al (eds): The Molecular Basis of Cancer, 2nd ed. Philadelphia, WB Saunders, 2001, p 137–161.
87. Miyaki M, Kuroki T: Role of *Smad4 (DPC4)* inactivation in human cancer. Biochem Biophys Res Commun 306:799, 2003.
88. Gutmann DH, Collins FS: Neurofibromatosis 1. In Vogelstein B, Kinzler KW (eds): The Genetic Basis of Human Cancer, 2nd ed. New York, McGraw-Hill, 2002, p 417–437.
89. MacCollin M, Gusella J: Neurofibromatosis 2. In Vogelstein B, Kinzler W (eds): The Genetic Basis of Human Cancer, 2nd ed. New York, McGraw Hill, 2002, p 439–448.
90. Leslie NR, Downes CP: *PTEN*: the down side of PI 3-kinase signalling. Cell Signal 14:285, 2002.
91. Trotman LC, Pandolfi PP: *PTEN* and *p53:* who will get the upper hand? Cancer Cell 3:97, 2003.
92. Haber DA: Wilms tumor. In Vogelstein B, Kinzler W (eds): The Genetic Basis of Human Cancer, 2nd ed. New York, McGraw-Hill, 2002, p 403–415.

93. Hirohashi S, Kanai Y: Cell adhesion system and human cancer morphogenesis. Cancer Sci 94:575, 2003.
94. Narla G, et al: *KLF6*, a candidate tumor suppressor gene mutated in prostate cancer. Science 294:2563, 2001.
95. Dicker T, Siller G, Saunders N: Molecular and cellular biology of basal cell carcinoma. Australas J Dermatol 43:241, 2002.
96. Evan GI, Vousden KH: Proliferation, cell cycle and apoptosis in cancer. Nature 411:342, 2001.
97. Korsmeyer SJ: Programmed cell death and the regulation of homeostasis. Harvey Lect 95:21, 1999.
98. Igney FH, Krammer PH: Death and anti-death: tumour resistance to apoptosis. Nat Rev Cancer 2:277, 2002.
99. Zamzami N, Kroemer G: Apoptosis: mitochondrial membrane permeabilization—the (w)hole story? Curr Biol 13:R71, 2003.
100. Scorrano L, Korsmeyer SJ: Mechanisms of cytochrome *c* release by proapoptotic *BCL-2* family members. Biochem Biophys Res Commun 304:437, 2003.
101. Sax JK, et al: BID regulation by *p53* contributes to chemosensitivity. Nat Cell Biol 4:842, 2002.
102. Lawlor MA, Alessi DR: *PKB/Akt:* a key mediator of cell proliferation, survival and insulin responses? J Cell Sci 114:2903, 2001.
103. Hoeijmakers JH: Genome maintenance mechanisms for preventing cancer. Nature 411:366, 2001.
104. Lynch HT, de la Chapelle A: Hereditary colorectal cancer. N Engl J Med 348:919, 2003.
105. Ohmiya N, et al: Germline and somatic mutations in *hMSH6* and *hMSH3* in gastrointestinal cancers of the microsatellite mutator phenotype. Gene 272:301, 2001.
106. Jiricny J, Marra G: DNA repair defects in colon cancer. Curr Opin Genet Dev 13:61, 2003.
107. Friedberg EC: How nucleotide excision repair protects against cancer. Nat Rev Cancer 1:22, 2001.
108. Levitt NC, Hickson ID: Caretaker tumour suppressor genes that defend genome integrity. Trends Mol Med 8:179, 2002.
109. Hickson ID, et al: Role of the Bloom's syndrome helicase in maintenance of genome stability. Biochem Soc Trans 29:201, 2001.
109a. Livingston DM: EMSY, a BRCA-2 partner in crime. Nature Med 10:127, 2004.
110. Shiloh Y: ATM and related protein kinases: safeguarding genome integrity. Nat Rev Cancer 3:155, 2003.
111. D'Andrea AD: The Fanconi road to cancer. Genes & Dev 17:1933, 2003.
112. Venkitaraman AR: A growing network of cancer-susceptibility genes. N Engl J Med 348:1917, 2003.
113. El-Deiry WS: Transactivation of repair genes by *BRCA1*. Cancer Biol Ther 1:490, 2002.
114. Howlett NG, et al: Biallelic inactivation of *BRCA2* in Fanconi anemia. Science 297:606, 2002.
115. Thorstenson YR, et al: Contributions of *ATM* mutations to familial breast and ovarian cancer. Cancer Res 63:3325, 2003.
116. Blackburn EH: Switching and signaling at the telomere. Cell 106:661, 2001.
117. Samper E, Flores JM, Blasco MA: Restoration of telomerase activity rescues chromosomal instability and premature aging in *Terc-/-* mice with short telomeres. EMBO Rep 2:800, 2001.
118. Hiyama E, Hiyama K: Telomerase as tumor marker. Cancer Lett 194:221, 2003.
119. Blasco MA: Telomeres and cancer: a tale with many endings. Curr Opin Genet Dev 13:70, 2003.
120. Folkman J: Role of angiogenesis in tumor growth and metastasis. Semin Oncol 29:15, 2002.
121. Carmeliet P: Angiogenesis in health and disease. Nat Med 9:653, 2003.
122. Jain RK: Molecular regulation of vessel maturation. Nat Med 9:685, 2003.
123. Hendrix MJ, et al: Angiogenesis: vasculogenic mimicry and tumour-cell plasticity: lessons from melanoma. Nat Rev Cancer 3:411, 2003.
124. Ferrara N, Gerber HP, LeCouter J: The biology of VEGF and its receptors. Nat Med 9:669, 2003.
125. Bergers G, Benjamin LE: Angiogenesis: tumorigenesis and the angiogenic switch. Nat Rev Cancer 3:401, 2003.
126. Kalluri R: Basement membranes: structure, assembly and role in tumour angiogenesis. Nat Rev Cancer 3:422, 2003.
127. Fidler IJ: The pathogenesis of cancer metastasis: the "seed and soil" hypothesis revisited. Nat Rev Cancer 3:453, 2003.
128. Hynes RO: Metastatic potential: generic predisposition of the primary tumor or rare, metastatic variants—or both? Cell 113:821, 2003.
129. Ramaswamy S, et al: A molecular signature of metastasis in primary solid tumors. Nat Genet 33:49, 2003.
130. Radisky D, Muschler J, Bissell MJ: Order and disorder: the role of extracellular matrix in epithelial cancer. Cancer Invest 20:139, 2002.
131. Bissell MJ, Radisky D: Putting tumours in context. Nat Rev Cancer 1:46, 2001.
132. Lynch CC, Matrisian LM: Matrix metalloproteinases in tumor–host cell communication. Differentiation 70:561, 2002.
133. Ruoslahti E: Specialization of tumour vasculature. Nat Rev Cancer 2:83, 2002.
134. Muller A, et al: Involvement of chemokine receptors in breast cancer metastasis. Nature 410:50, 2001.
135. Yu Y, et al: Expression profiling identifies the cytoskeletal organizer ezrin and the developmental homeoprotein six-1 as key metastatic regulators. Nature Med 10:175, 2004.
136. Steeg PS, et al: Metastasis suppressor genes: basic biology and potential clinical use. Clin Breast Cancer 4:51, 2003.
136a. Cunha GR, et al: Role of stromal microenvironment in carcinogenesis of prostate. Int J Cancer 107:1, 2003.
137. Hogarty MD, Brodeur GM: Gene amplification in human cancers: biological and clinical significance. In Vogelstein B, Kinzler KW (eds): The Genetic Basis of Human Cancer, 2nd ed. New York, McGraw-Hill, 2002, p 115–128.
138. Esteller M: Relevance of DNA methylation in the management of cancer. Lancet Oncol 4:351, 2003.
139. Herman JG, Baylin S: Gene silencing in cancer in association with promoter hypermethylation. N Engl J Med 349:2042, 2003.
140. Gaudet F, et al: Induction of tumors in mice by genomic hypomethylation. Science 300:489, 2003.
141. Feinberg AP: Genomic imprinting and cancer. In Vogelstein B, Kinzler KW (eds): The Genetic Basis of Human Cancer, 2nd ed. New York, McGraw-Hill, 2002, p 43–55.
142. Sorlie T, et al: Repeated observation of breast tumor subtypes in independent gene expression data sets. Proc Natl Acad Sci U S A 100:8418, 2003.
143. Ross ME, et al: Classification of pediatric acute lymphoblastic leukemia by gene expression profiling. Blood, 2003.
144. Hahn WC, Weinberg RA: Rules for making human tumor cells. N Engl J Med 347:1593, 2002.
145. Kinzler KW, Vogelstein B: Colorectal tumors. In Vogelstein B, Kinzler KW (eds): The Genetic Basis of Human Cancer, 2nd ed. New York, McGraw-Hill, 2002, p 583.
146. Kunkel TA: Considering the cancer consequences of altered DNA polymerase function. Cancer Cell 3:105, 2003.
147. Fidler IJ: Critical determinants of metastasis. Semin Cancer Biol 12:89, 2002.
148. Tennant R: Chemical carcinogenesis. In Franks LM, Teich NM (eds): An Introduction to the Cellular and Molecular Biology of Cancer, 3rd ed. Oxford, Oxford University Press, 1997, p 106–125.
149. Perera FP: Environment and cancer: who are susceptible? Science 278:1068, 1997.
150. Vineis P, et al: *CYP1A1 T3801 C* polymorphism and lung cancer: a pooled analysis of 2451 cases and 3358 controls. Int J Cancer 104:650, 2003.
151. Palli D, et al: Biomarkers of dietary intake of micronutrients modulate DNA adduct levels in healthy adults. Carcinogenesis 24:739, 2003.
152. Mortelmans K, Zeiger E: The Ames *Salmonella*/microsome mutagenicity assay. Mutat Res 455:29, 2000.
153. Staib F, et al: *TP53* and liver carcinogenesis. Hum Mutat 21:201, 2003.
154. Mansbach JM, et al: Phenobarbital selectively promotes initiated cells with reduced TGF-β receptor levels. Carcinogenesis 17:171, 1996.
155. Montesano R, Hall J: Environmental causes of human cancers. Eur J Cancer 37 (Suppl 8):S67, 2001.
156. Hecht SS: Cigarette smoking and lung cancer: chemical mechanisms and approaches to prevention. Lancet Oncol 3:461, 2002.
157. Talaska G: Aromatic amines and human urinary bladder cancer: exposure sources and epidemiology. J Environ Sci Health Part C 21:29, 2003.
158. Preston DL, et al: Radiation effects on breast cancer risk: a pooled analysis of eight cohorts. Radiat Res 158:220, 2002.

159. Cleaver JE, Crowley E: UV damage, DNA repair and skin carcinogenesis. Front Biosci 7:1024, 2002.
160. Friedberg RC: Biological responses to DNA damage: a perspective in the new millennium. Cold Spring Harb Symp Quant Biol 65:593, 2000.
161. Williams D: Chernobyl, 15 years later, correlation of clinical, epidemiological and molecular outcomes. Ann Endocrinol 64:72, 2003.
162. Neronova E, Slozina N, Nikiforov A: Chromosome alterations in cleanup workers sampled years after the Chernobyl accident. Radiat Res 160:46, 2003.
163. zur Hausen H: Oncogenic DNA viruses. Oncogene 20:7820, 2001.
164. zur Hausen H: Papillomaviruses and cancer: from basic studies to clinical application. Nat Rev Cancer 2:342, 2002.
165. Munger K: Disruption of oncogene/tumor suppressor networks during human carcinogenesis. Cancer Invest 20:71, 2002.
166. Helt AM, Galloway DA: Mechanisms by which DNA tumor virus oncoproteins target the Rb family of pocket proteins. Carcinogenesis 24:159, 2003.
167. Munger K, Howley PM: Human papillomavirus immortalization and transformation functions. Virus Res 89:213, 2002.
168. zur Hausen H: Cervical cancer: papillomavirus and *p53*. Nature 393:217, 1998.
169. Dolcetti R, Masucci MG: Epstein-Barr virus: induction and control of cell transformation. J Cell Physiol 196:207, 2003.
170. Bornkamm GW, Hammerschimdt W: Molecular virology of Epstein-Barr virus. Philos Trans R Soc Lond B Biol Sci 356:437, 2001.
171. Lam N, Sugden B: CD40 and its viral mimic, LMP1: similar means to different ends. Cell Signal 15:9, 2003.
172. Thorley-Lawson DA: Epstein-Barr virus: exploiting the immune system. Nat Rev Immunol 1:75, 2001.
173. Tsao SW, et al: The significance of *LMP1* expression in nasopharyngeal carcinoma. Semin Cancer Biol 12:473, 2002.
174. Brennan P: Signalling events regulating lymphoid growth and survival. Semin Cancer Biol 11:415, 2001.
175. Thorley-Lawson DA, Gross A: Mechanism of disease: persistence of Epstein-Barr virus and the origins of associated lymphomas. N Engl J Med 350:1328, 2004.
176. Lindstrom MS, Wiman KG: Role of genetic and epigenetic changes in Burkitt lymphoma. Semin Cancer Biol 12:381, 2002.
177. Raab-Traub N: Epstein-Barr virus in the pathogenesis of NPC. Semin Cancer Biol 12:431, 2002.
178. Chen CJ, Chen DS: Interaction of hepatitis B virus, chemical carcinogen, and genetic susceptibility: multistage hepatocarcinogenesis with multifactorial etiology. Hepatology 36:1046, 2002.
179. Wang XW, et al: Molecular pathogenesis of human hepatocellular carcinoma. Toxicology 181:43, 2002.
180. Barmak K, et al: Human T cell leukemia virus type I-induced disease: pathways to cancer and neurodegeneration. Virology 308:1, 2003.
181. Mortreux F, Gabet AS, Wattel E: Molecular and cellular aspects of HTLV-1 associated leukemogenesis in vivo. Leukemia 17:26, 2003.
182. Haoudi A, Semmes OJ: The HTLV-1 *tax* oncoprotein attenuates DNA damage induced G_1 arrest and enhances apoptosis in *p53* null cells. Virology 305:229, 2003.
183. Covacci A, Rappuoli R: *Helicobacter pylori:* after the genomes, back to biology. J Exp Med 197:807, 2003.
184. Du MQ, Isaccson PG: Gastric MALT lymphoma: from aetiology to treatment. Lancet Oncol 3:97, 2002.
185. Burnet FM: The concept of immunological surveillance. Prog Exper Tumor Res 13:1, 1970.
186. Dunn GP, et al: Cancer immunoediting: from immunosurveillance to tumor escape. Nat Immunol 3:991, 2002.
187. Garcia-Lora A, Algarra I, Garrido F: MHC class I antigens, immune surveillance, and tumor immune escape. J Cell Physiol 195:346, 2003.
188. Dunn GP, Old LJ, Schreiber RD: The three Es of cancer immunoediting. Annu Rev Immunol 22, 2004.
189. Coulie PG, Hanagiri T, Takenoyama M: From tumor antigens to immunotherapy. Int J Clin Oncol 6:163, 2001.
190. Pardoll D: Does the immune system see tumors as foreign or self? Annu Rev Immunol 21:807, 2003.
191. Boon T, Van den Eynde B: Tumour immunology. Curr Opin Immunol 15:129, 2003.
192. Castelli C, et al: T-cell recognition of melanoma-associated antigens. J Cell Physiol 182:323, 2000.
193. Barker PA, Salehi A: The MAGE proteins: emerging roles in cell cycle progression, apoptosis, and neurogenetic disease. J Neurosci Res 67:705, 2002.
194. Cerwenka A, Lanier LL: Natural killer cells, viruses and cancer. Nat Rev Immunol 1:41, 2001.
195. Latour S, Veillette A: Molecular and immunological basis of X-linked lymphoproliferative disease. Immunol Rev 192:212, 2003.
196. Strand S, Galle PR: Immune evasion by tumours: involvement of the CD95 (APO-1/Fas) system and its clinical implications. Mol Med Today 4:63, 1998.
197. Hanahan D, Lanzavecchia A, Mihich E: The novel dichotomy of immune interactions with tumors. Cancer Res 63:3005, 2003.
198. Argiles JM, et al: Cancer cachexia: the molecular mechanisms. Int J Biochem Cell Biol 35:405, 2003.
199. Darnell RB, Posner JB: Paraneoplastic syndromes involving the nervous system. N Engl J Med 349:1543, 2003.
200. Mazzone PJ, Arroliga AC: Endocrine paraneoplastic syndromes in lung cancer. Curr Opin Pulm Med 9:313, 2003.
201. Hoey RP, et al: The parathyroid hormone-related protein receptor is expressed in breast cancer bone metastases and promotes autocrine proliferation in breast carcinoma cells. Br J Cancer 88:567, 2003.
202. Swansbury J: Some difficult choices in cytogenetics. Methods Mol Biol 220:245, 2003.
203. Rowland JM: Molecular genetic diagnosis of pediatric cancer: current and emerging methods. Pediatr Clin North Am 49:1415, 2002.
204. Bayani J, Squire JA: Advances in the detection of chromosomal aberrations using spectral karyotyping. Clin Genet 59:65, 2001.
205. Weiss MM, et al: Comparative genomic hybridisation as a supportive tool in diagnostic pathology. J Clin Pathol 56:522, 2003.
206. Louis DN, Pomeroy SL, Cairncross JG: Focus on central nervous system neoplasia. Cancer Cell 1:125, 2002.
207. Sidransky D: Emerging molecular markers of cancer. Nat Rev Cancer 2:210, 2002.
208. Lakhani SR, Ashworth A: Microarray and histopathological analysis of tumours: the future and the past? Nat Rev Cancer 1:151, 2001.
209. Riggins GJ, Morin PJ: Gene expression profiling in cancer. In Vogelstein B, Kinzler KW (eds): The Genetic Basis of Human Cancers, 2nd ed. New York, McGraw-Hill, 2002, p 131–141.
210. Benes V, Muckenthaler M: Standardization of protocols in cDNA microarray analysis. Trends Biochem Sci 28:244, 2003.
211. Ferrando AA, et al: Gene expression signatures define novel oncogenic pathways in T cell acute lymphoblastic leukemia. Cancer Cell 1:75, 2002.
212. Nutt CL, et al: Gene expression-based classification of malignant gliomas correlates better with survival than histological classification. Cancer Res 63:1602, 2003.
213. Ramaswamy S, et al: Multiclass cancer diagnosis using tumor gene expression signatures. Proc Natl Acad Sci U S A 98:15149, 2001.
214. van de Vijver MJ, et al: A gene-expression signature as a predictor of survival in breast cancer. N Engl J Med 347:1999, 2002.
215. Wulfkuhle JD, et al: Proteomic approaches to the diagnosis, treatment, and monitoring of cancer. Adv Exp Med Biol 532:59, 2003.

CHAPTER 8

Infectious Diseases

Alexander J. McAdam, MD, PhD • Arlene H. Sharpe, MD, PhD*

GENERAL PRINCIPLES OF MICROBIAL PATHOGENESIS

History

New and Emerging Infectious Diseases

Agents of Bioterrorism

Categories of Infectious Agents

Prions

Viruses

Bacteriophages, Plasmids, Transposons

Bacteria

Chlamydiae, Rickettsiae, Mycoplasmas

Fungi

Protozoa

Helminths

Ectoparasites

Transmission and Dissemination of Microbes

Host Barriers to Infection

Spread and Dissemination of Microbes

Release of Microbes from the Body

Sexually Transmitted Infections

How Microorganisms Cause Disease

Mechanisms of Viral Injury

Mechanisms of Bacterial Injury

Injurious Effects of Host Immunity

Immune Evasion by Microbes

Infections in Immunosuppressed Hosts

Special Techniques for Diagnosing Infectious Agents

Spectrum of Inflammatory Responses to Infection

Suppurative (Polymorphonuclear) Inflammation

Mononuclear and Granulomatous Inflammation

Cytopathic-Cytoproliferative Inflammation

Necrotizing Inflammation

Chronic Inflammation and Scarring

VIRAL INFECTIONS

Transient Infections

Measles

Mumps

Poliovirus Infection

West Nile Virus

Viral Hemorrhagic Fevers

Chronic Latent Infections (Herpesvirus Infections)

Herpes Simplex Virus

Cytomegalovirus

Varicella Zoster Virus

Chronic Productive Infections

Hepatitis B Virus

Transforming Infections

Epstein-Barr Virus

Human Papillomaviruses

BACTERIAL INFECTIONS

Gram-Positive Bacterial Infections

Staphylococcal Infections

Streptococcal Infections

Diphtheria

Listeriosis

Anthrax

Nocardia

Gram-Negative Bacterial Infections

Neisserial Infections

Whooping Cough

*The contributions of Dr. John Samuelson and Dr. Franz von Lichtenberg to the previous editions are gratefully acknowledged.

Pseudomonas Infection
Plague
Chancroid (Soft Chancre)
Granuloma Inguinale
Mycobacteria
Tuberculosis
Mycobacterium Avium-Intracellulare Complex
Leprosy
Spirochetes
Syphilis
Relapsing Fever
Lyme Disease
Anaerobic Bacteria
Abscesses
Clostridial Infections
Obligate Intracellular Bacteria
Chlamydial Infections
Rickettsial Infections
FUNGAL INFECTIONS
Yeasts
Candidiasis
Cryptococcosis
Molds
Aspergillosis
Zygomycosis (Mucormycosis)
PARASITIC INFECTIONS
Protozoa
Malaria
Babesiosis
Leishmaniasis
African Trypanosomiasis
Chagas Disease
Metazoa
Strongyloidiasis
Tapeworms (Cestodes): Cysticercosis and Hydatid Disease
Trichinosis
Schistosomiasis
Lymphatic Filariasis
Onchocerciasis

General Principles of Microbial Pathogenesis

Despite the availability and use of effective vaccines and antibiotics, infectious diseases remain an important cause of death in the United States and worldwide. In the United States, two of the top 10 leading causes of death are infectious diseases (pneumonia and influenza, and septicemia).[1] Infectious diseases are particularly important causes of death among the elderly and people with acquired immunodeficiency syndrome (AIDS), those with chronic diseases, and those receiving immunosuppressive drugs. In developing countries, unsanitary living conditions and malnutrition contribute to a massive burden of infectious diseases that kills more than 10 million people each year. Most of these deaths are among children, especially from respiratory and diarrheal infections.[2]

HISTORY

The history of infectious disease pathology is intertwined with that of microbiology. Some of the major historical events in these fields are briefly described here to provide a perspective for the concepts of pathogenesis to be discussed later. Some important experiments that were performed in the past would not be ethically acceptable today.

Louis Pasteur and Robert Koch were pioneers in establishing the microbiologic etiology of infectious diseases. Pasteur is credited with proving that microorganisms can cause disease (the germ theory of disease). Pasteur also created the first attenuated vaccines, including a rabies vaccine for humans in 1885. In 1882, Koch championed criteria for linking a specific microorganism to a disease. Koch's postulates require that (1) the organism is found in the lesions of the disease, (2) the organism can be isolated as single colonies on solid media, (3) inoculation of the organism causes lesions in experimental animals, and (4) the organism can be recovered from the experimental animal. Koch also isolated the bacteria that cause tuberculosis *(Mycobacterium tuberculosis)* and anthrax *(Bacillus anthracis)*.

Ronald Ross, an English military physician posted in India, demonstrated in 1897 that mosquitoes carry malaria. At the time, it was believed that malaria was caused by breathing the air near swamps ("malaria" comes from the Italian for "bad air"). Ross's demonstration that *Anopheles* mosquitoes transmit malaria led to public health efforts to reduce malaria through control of mosquitoes. This was successful in the United States, but malaria continues to be a major health problem in many parts of the world.

Walter Reed, an American military physician, led a team of investigators in Cuba in 1900 who demonstrated that yellow fever, like malaria, is transmitted by the bite of mosquitoes. Military volunteers allowed themselves to be bitten by mosquitoes that had previously bitten people sick with yellow fever. Following Reed's result, Dr. James Carroll showed in 1901 that yellow fever was caused by a virus. This was the first demonstration that a virus causes disease in humans.

F. Peyton Rous found the first evidence for an infectious cause of cancer in 1909. In 1911, Rous demonstrated that a virus causes sarcoma in chickens. Although a viral cause has not been found for most human cancers, we now know that viruses can contribute to the development of some; such associations include human papillomaviruses and cervical cancer.

The dawn of modern microbiology, which is based on molecular genetics, came in 1944, when Oswald Avery demonstrated that transfer of DNA from virulent to avirulent *Streptococcus pneumoniae* transformed the latter into a virulent phenotype. This showed that DNA is the genetic material, leading to an explosion of research in molecular genetics. Today, the entire genomic sequences of many species, including microbes and humans, are known, and this holds great promise for future research into the pathogenesis, diagnosis, and treatment of infectious diseases. Knowledge of the genomes of the host and pathogens promise to produce a much richer description of the host response to infectious agents than the morphologic descriptions of antimicrobial responses in this chapter.

NEW AND EMERGING INFECTIOUS DISEASES

Although infectious diseases such as leprosy have been known since biblical times and parasitic schistosomes and mycobacteria have been demonstrated in Egyptian mummies, a surprising number of new infectious agents continue to be discovered (Table 8–1). The infectious causes of some diseases with significant morbidity and mortality (e.g., *Helicobacter pylori* gastritis, hepatitis B and hepatitis C, human metapneumovirus respiratory disease, and Legionnaire's pneumonia) were previously unrecognized because the infectious agents are difficult to culture. Some infectious agents are genuinely new to humans, e.g., human immunodeficiency virus (HIV), which causes the acquired immunodeficiency syndrome (AIDS); *Borrelia burgdorferi*, which causes Lyme disease; and the coronavirus that may cause severe acute respiratory syndrome (SARS) (Chapter 15). Other infections are much more commonly seen because of immunosuppression caused by AIDS (e.g., cytomegalovirus [CMV], Kaposi sarcoma herpesvirus, *Mycobacterium avium-intracellulare, Pneumocystis jiroveci* (*carinii*), and *Cryptosporidium parvum*).[3,4] Finally, infectious diseases that are common in one area may be introduced into a new area. West Nile virus was common in Europe, Asia, and Africa when it was first described in the United States in 1999.

TABLE 8–1 Some Recently Recognized Infectious Agents and Manifestations

1977	Ebola virus	Epidemic hemorrhagic fever
	Hantaan virus	Hemorrhagic fever with renal disease
	Legionella pneumophila	Legionnaire's disease
	Campylobacter jejuni	Enteritis
1980	HTLV-I	T-cell lymphoma or leukemia
1981	*Staphylococcus aureus*	Toxic shock syndrome
1982	HTLV-II	Hairy cell leukemia
	Escherichia coli O157:H7	Hemolytic-uremic syndrome
	Borrelia burgdorferi	Lyme disease
1983	HIV	AIDS
	Helicobacter pylori	Gastric ulcers
1985	*Enterocytozoon bieneusi*	Chronic diarrhea
1988	HHV-6	Roseola subitum
	Hepatitis E	Enterically transmitted hepatitis
1989	Hepatitis C	Hepatitis C
	Ehrlichia chaffeensis	Human monocytic ehrlichiosis
1992	*Vibrio cholerae* O139	New epidemic cholera strain
	Bartonella henselae	Cat-scratch disease
1993	*Encephalitozoon cuniculi*	Opportunistic infections
1994	*Anaplasma phagocytophilium*	Human granulocytic ehrlichiosis (anaplasmosis)
1995	KSHV (HHV-8)	Kaposi sarcoma in AIDS
2001	Human metapneumovirus	Respiratory infections
2002	West Nile virus	Acute flaccid paralysis
2003	SARS coronavirus	Severe acute respiratory syndrome

Adapted from Lederberg J: Infectious disease as an evolutionary paradigm. Emerg Infect Dis 3:417, 1997.

Human demographics and behavior are among the many factors that contribute to the emergence of infectious diseases. AIDS has been predominantly (but not exclusively) a disease of homosexuals and drug abusers in the United States and Western countries, while in Africa, AIDS is predominantly a heterosexual disease that is much more frequent in areas where men remain uncircumcised.[5] Changes in the environment occasionally drive rates of infectious diseases. Reforestation of the eastern United States has led to massive increases in the populations of deer and mice, which carry the ticks that transmit Lyme disease, babesiosis, and ehrlichiosis.[6] Failure of DDT to control the mosquitoes that transmit malaria and the development of drug-resistant parasites have dramatically increased the morbidity and mortality of *Plasmodium falciparum* in Asia, Africa, and Latin America. Microbial adaptation to widespread antibiotic use contributed to the development of new drug-resistant strains of *Mycobacterium tuberculosis, Neisseria gonorrhoeae, Staphylococcus aureus*, and *Enterococcus faecium*.

AGENTS OF BIOTERRORISM

Sadly, the anthrax attacks in the United States in 2001 transformed the theoretical threat of bioterrorism into reality. The Centers for Disease Control and Prevention (CDC) have evaluated the microorganisms that pose the greatest danger as weapons on the basis of how efficiently disease can be transmitted, how hard the microorganisms are to produce and distribute, how well they can be defended against, and how likely they are to alarm the public and produce widespread fear. The CDC has ranked bioweapons into three categories, A, B, and C, based on these criteria. These agents are listed in Table 8–2.[7]

Category A agents are the highest-risk agents and can be readily disseminated or transmitted from person to person, can cause high mortality with potential for major public health impact, might cause public panic and social disruption, and require special action for public health preparedness. For example, smallpox is a category A agent owing to its high transmissibility in any climate or season, case mortality rate of 30% or greater, and lack of effective antiviral therapy. This agent can be easily disseminated because of the stability of the virus in aerosol form and the very small dose needed for infection. Smallpox naturally spreads from person to person mainly by respiratory aerosol or by direct contact with virus in skin lesions or contaminated clothing or bedding. Symptoms appear after 7 to 17 days. Initially, there is high fever, headache, and backache, followed by the appearance of the rash, which first appears on the mucosa of the mouth and pharynx, face, and forearms and later spreads to the trunk and legs and becomes vesicular and later pustular. Because people are infectious during the incubation period, this virus has the potential to continue to spread throughout an unprotected population. Since vaccination ended in the United States in 1972 and vaccination immunity has waned, the population is

TABLE 8–2 Potential Agents of Bioterrorism*

Category A Diseases/Agents	Category B Diseases/Agents	Category C Diseases/Agents
• Anthrax *(Bacillus anthracis)* • Botulism *(Clostridium botulinum* toxin*)* • Plague *(Yersinia pestis)* • Smallpox *(Variola major virus)* • Tularemia *(Francisella tularensis)* • Viral hemorrhagic fevers (filoviruses [e.g., Ebola, Marburg], arenaviruses [Lassa fever virus and New World arenaviruses], bunyaviruses [e.g. Crimean-Congo hemorrhagic fever and Rift Valley Fever viruses]	• Brucellosis (*Brucella* species) • Epsilon toxin of *Clostridium perfringens* • Food safety threats (e.g., *Salmonella* species, *Escherichia coli* 0157:H7, *Shigella*) • Glanders *(Burkholderia mallei)* • Melioidosis *(Burkholderia pseudomallei)* • Psittacosis *(Chlamydia psittaci)* • Q fever *(Coxiella burnetti)* • Ricin toxin from *Ricinus communis* (castor beans) • Staphylococcal enterotoxin B • Typhus fever *(Rickettsia prowazekii)* • Viral encephalitis (alphaviruses [e.g., Venezuelan equine encephalitis, eastern equine encephalitis, western equine encephalitis]) • Water safety threats (e.g., *Vibrio cholerae, Cryptosporidium parvum*)	• Emerging infectious disease threats such as Nipah virus and Hantavirus

*Adapted from Centers for Disease Control Information.

highly susceptible to smallpox. Recent concern that smallpox could be used for bioterrorism has led to a return of vaccination for selected groups in the U.S. and Israel.

Category B agents are moderately easy to disseminate, produce moderate morbidity but low mortality, and require specific diagnostic and disease surveillance. Many of these agents are foodborne or waterborne. Category C agents include emerging pathogens that could be engineered for mass dissemination because of availability, ease of production and dissemination, potential for high morbidity and mortality, and great impact on health.

CATEGORIES OF INFECTIOUS AGENTS

Infectious agents belong to a wide range of classes and vary in size from the ~27-kD nucleic acid–free prion to 20-nm poliovirus to 10-m tapeworms (Table 8–3).

Prions

Prions are apparently composed of abnormal forms of a host protein, termed prion protein (PrP).[8] These agents cause transmissible spongiform encephalopathies, including kuru (associated with human cannibalism), Creutzfeldt-Jakob disease (CJD; associated with corneal transplants), bovine spongiform encephalopathy (BSE; better known as mad cow disease), and variant Creutzfeldt-Jakob disease (vCJD; likely transmitted to humans from BSE-infected cattle).[9] PrP is normally found in neurons. Diseases occur when the prion protein undergoes a conformational change that confers resistance to proteases. The protease-resistant PrP promotes conversion of the normal protease-sensitive PrP to the abnormal form, explaining the infectious nature of these diseases. Accumulation of abnormal PrP leads to neuronal damage and distinctive spongiform pathologic changes in the brain.

TABLE 8–3 Classes of Human Pathogens and Their Habitats

Taxonomic	Size	Site of Propagation	Sample Species	Disease
Viruses	20–300 nm	Obligate intracellular	Poliovirus	Poliomyelitis
Chlamydiae	200–1000 nm	Obligate intracellular	*Chlamydia trachomatis*	Trachoma, urethritis
Rickettsiae	300–1200 nm	Obligate intracellular	*Rickettsia prowazekii*	Typhus fever
Mycoplasmas	125–350 nm	Extracellular	*Mycoplasma pneumoniae*	Atypical pneumonia
Bacteria	0.8–15 μm	Cutaneous Mucosal Extracellular Facultative intracellular	*Staphylococcus aureus* *Vibrio cholerae* *Streptococcus pneumoniae* *Mycobacterium tuberculosis*	Wound Cholera Pneumonia Tuberculosis
Fungi	2–200 μm	Cutaneous Mucosal Extracellular Facultative intracellular	*Trichophyton* sp. *Candida albicans* *Sporothrix schenckii* *Histoplasma capsulatum*	Tinea pedis (athlete's foot) Thrush Sporotrichosis Histoplasmosis
Protozoa	1–50 μm	Mucosal Extracellular Facultative intracellular Obligate intracellular	*Giardia lamblia* *Trypanosoma gambiense* *Trypanosoma cruzi* *Leishmania donovani*	Giardiasis Sleeping sickness Chagas disease Kala-azar
Helminths	3 mm–10 m	Mucosal Extracellular Intracellular	*Enterobius vermicularis* *Wuchereria bancrofti* *Trichinella spiralis*	Enterobiasis Filariasis Trichinosis

Spontaneous or inherited mutations in PrP, which make PrP protease resistant, have been observed in the sporadic and familial forms of CJD, respectively. These diseases are discussed in detail in Chapter 28.

Viruses

Viruses are obligate intracellular parasites that depend on the host cell's metabolic machinery for their replication. They consist of a nucleic acid genome surrounded by a protein coat (called a capsid) that is sometimes encased in a lipid membrane. Viruses are classified by their nucleic acid genome (DNA or RNA but not both), the shape of the capsid (icosahedral or helical), the presence or absence of a lipid envelope, their mode of replication, the preferred cell type for replication (called tropism), or the type of pathology (Table 8–4). Because viruses are only 20 to 300 nm in size, they are best visualized with the electron microscope (Fig. 8–1). However, some viral particles aggregate within the cells they infect and form characteristic inclusion bodies, which may be seen with the light microscope and are useful for diagnosis. For example, cytomegalovirus (CMV)-infected cells are enlarged and show a large eosinophilic nuclear inclusion and smaller basophilic cytoplasmic inclusions; herpesviruses form a large nuclear inclusion surrounded by a clear halo; and both smallpox and rabies viruses form characteristic cytoplasmic inclusions. Many viruses do not give rise to inclusions (e.g., Epstein Barr virus [EBV]).

TABLE 8–4 Selected Human Viral Diseases and Their Pathogens

Viral Pathogen	Virus Family	Genomic Type	Disease Expression
Respiratory			
Adenovirus	Adenoviridae	DS DNA	Upper and lower respiratory tract infections, conjunctivitis, diarrhea
Rhinovirus	Picornaviridae	SS RNA	Upper respiratory tract infection
Coxsackievirus	Picornaviridae	SS RNA	Pleurodynia, herpangina, hand-foot-and-mouth disease, SARS
Coronavirus	Coronaviridae	SS RNA	Upper respiratory tract infection
Influenza viruses A, B	Orthomyxoviridae	SS RNA	Influenza
Respiratory syncytial virus	Paramyxoviridae	SS RNA	Bronchiolitis, pneumonia
Digestive			
Mumps virus	Paramyxoviridae	SS RNA	Mumps, pancreatitis, orchitis
Rotavirus	Reoviridae	DS RNA	Childhood diarrhea
Norwalk agent	Caliciviridae	SS RNA	Gastroenteritis
Hepatitis A virus	Picornaviridae	SS RNA	Acute viral hepatitis
Hepatitis B virus	Hepadnaviridae	DS DNA	Acute or chronic hepatitis
Hepatitis D virus	Viroid-like	SS RNA	With HBV, acute or chronic hepatitis
Hepatitis C virus	Flaviviridae	SS RNA	Acute or chronic hepatitis
Hepatitis E virus	Norwalk-like	SS RNA	Enterically transmitted hepatitis
Systemic with Skin Eruptions			
Measles virus	Paramyxoviridae	SS RNA	Measles (rubeola)
Rubella virus	Togaviridae	SS RNA	German measles (rubella)
Parvovirus	Parvoviridae	SS DNA	Erythema infectiosum, aplastic anemia
Vaccinia virus	Poxviridae	DS DNA	Smallpox vaccine
Varicella-zoster virus	Herpesviridae	DS DNA	Chickenpox, shingles
Herpes simplex virus 1	Herpesviridae	DS DNA	"Cold sore"
Herpes simplex virus 2	Herpesviridae	DS DNA	Genital herpes
Systemic with Hematopoietic Disorders			
Cytomegalovirus	Herpesviridae	DS DNA	Cytomegalic inclusion disease
Epstein-Barr virus	Herpesviridae	DS DNA	Infectious mononucleosis
HTLV-I	Retroviridae	SS RNA	Adult T-cell leukemia; tropical spastic paraparesis
HIV-1 and HIV-2	Retroviridae	SS RNA	AIDS
Arboviral and Hemorrhagic Fevers			
Dengue virus 1–4	Togaviridae	SS RNA	Dengue, hemorrhagic fever
Yellow fever virus	Togaviridae	SS RNA	Yellow fever
Regional hemorrhagic fever viruses	Filoviridae	SS RNA	Ebola, Marburg disease
	Hantavirus	SS RNA	Korean, U.S. pneumonia
Warty Growths			
Papillomavirus	Papovaviridae	DS DNA	Condyloma; cervical carcinoma
Central Nervous System			
Poliovirus	Picornaviridae	SS RNA	Poliomyelitis
JC virus	Papovaviridae	DS DNA	Progressive multifocal leukoencephalopathy (opportunistic)
Arboviral encephalitis viruses	Togaviridae	SS RNA	Eastern, Western, Venezuelan, St. Louis,

DS, double-stranded; SS, single-stranded.

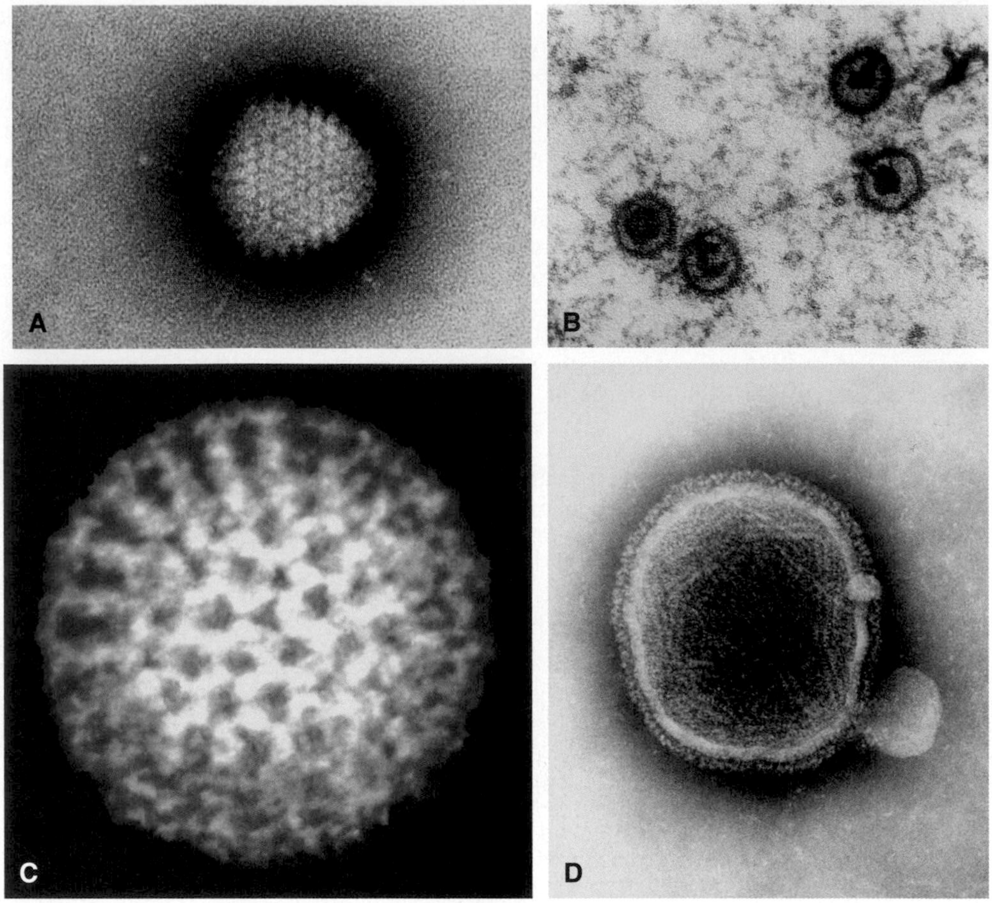

FIGURE 8–1 The variety of viral structures, as seen by electron microscopy. A, Adenovirus, an icosahedral nonenveloped DNA virus with fibers. B, Epstein Barr virus, an icosahedral enveloped DNA virus. C, Rotavirus, a nonenveloped, wheel-like, RNA virus. D, Paramyxovirus, a spherical enveloped RNA virus. RNA is seen spilling out of the disrupted virus. (Photos courtesy of Science Source; © Photo Researchers, Inc., New York, New York.)

Viruses account for a large share of human infections. Many viruses cause transient illnesses (e.g., colds, influenza). Other viruses are not eliminated from the body and persist within cells of the host for years, either continuing to multiply (e.g., chronic infection with hepatitis B virus) or surviving in some nonreplicating form (termed latent infection) with the potential to be reactivated later. For example, herpes zoster virus, the cause of chickenpox, can enter dorsal root ganglia and establish latency there and later be periodically activated to cause shingles, a painful skin condition. Some viruses can transform a host cell into a tumor or cancer cell (e.g., human papillomaviruses cause benign warts and have been implicated in cervical carcinoma). Different species of viruses can produce the same clinical picture (e.g., upper respiratory infection); conversely, a single virus can cause different clinical manifestations depending on host age or immune status (e.g., CMV).

Bacteriophages, Plasmids, Transposons

These are mobile genetic elements that infect bacteria and can indirectly cause human diseases by encoding bacterial virulence factors (e.g., adhesins, toxins, or enzymes that confer antibiotic resistance). Exchange of these elements between bacteria often endows the recipient with a survival advantage, with the capacity to cause disease, or both. Bacteriophages or plasmids can convert otherwise nonpathogenic bacteria into virulent ones. Plasmids or transposons encoding antibiotic resistance can convert an antibiotic-susceptible bacterium into a resistant one, making therapy difficult (e.g., vancomycin-resistant enterococci and methicillin-resistant staphylococci are endemic in many hospitals).

Bacteria

Bacterial cells are prokaryotes, meaning that they have a cell membrane but lack membrane-bound nuclei and other membrane-enclosed organelles (Table 8–5). Bacteria are bound by a cell wall usually consisting of peptidoglycan, a polymer of mixed sugars and amino acids. There are two forms of cell wall structures: a thick wall surrounding the cell membrane that retains crystal-violet stain (Gram-positive bacteria) or a thin cell wall sandwiched between two phospholipid bilayer membranes (Gram-negative bacteria) (Fig. 8–2). Bacteria are classified by Gram staining (positive or negative), shape (e.g., spherical ones are cocci; rod-shaped ones are bacilli), and form of respiration (aerobic or anaerobic) (Fig. 8–3). Many bacteria have flagella, long helical filaments extending from the cell surface, which enable bacteria to move in their environment. Some bacteria possess pili, another kind of surface projection, which can attach bacteria to host cells. Most bacteria synthesize their own DNA, RNA, and proteins, but they depend on the host for favorable growth conditions.

Normal healthy people can be colonized by as many as 10^{12} bacteria on the skin, 10^{10} bacteria in the mouth, and 10^{14} bacteria in the gastrointestinal tract. Bacteria colonizing the skin

TABLE 8–5 Examples of Bacterial, Spirochetal, and Mycobacterial Diseases

Clinical or Microbiologic Category	Species	Frequent Disease Presentations
Infections by pyogenic cocci	*Staphylococcus aureus, S. epidermidis*	Abscess, cellulitis, pneumonia, septicemia
	Streptococcus pyogenes, β-hemolytic	Upper respiratory tract infection, erysipelas, scarlet fever, septicemia
	Streptococcus pneumoniae (pneumoccoccus)	Lobar pneumonia, meningitis
	Neisseria meningitidis (meningococcus)	Cerebrospinal meningitis
	Neisseria gonorrhoeae (gonococcus)	Gonorrhea
Gram-negative infections, common	**Escherichia coli*	Urinary tract infection, wound infection, abscess, pneumonia, septicemia, endotoxemia, endocarditis
	**Klebsiella pneumoniae*	
	**Enterobacter (Aerobacter) aerogenes*	
	**Proteus* spp. *(P. mirabilis, P. morgagni)*	
	**Serratia marcescens*	
	**Pseudomonas* spp. *(P. aeruginosa)*	
	Bacteroides spp. *(B. fragilis)*	Anaerobic infection
	Legionella spp. *(L. pneumophila)*	Legionnaires disease
Contagious childhood bacterial diseases	*Haemophilus influenzae*	Meningitis, upper and lower respiratory tract infections
	Bordetella pertussis	Whooping cough
	Corynebacterium diphtheriae	Diphtheria
Enteropathic infections	Enteropathogenic *E. coli*	Invasive or noninvasive gastroenterocolitis, some with septicemia
	Shigella spp.	
	Vibrio cholerae	
	Campylobacter fetus, C. jejuni	
	Yersinia enterocolitica	
	Salmonella spp. (1000 strains)	
	Salmonella typhi	Typhoid fever
Clostridial infections	*Clostridium tetani*	Tetanus (lockjaw)
	Clostridium botulinum	Botulism (paralytic food poisoning)
	Clostridium perfringens, C. septicum	Gas gangrene, necrotizing cellulitis
	**Clostridium difficile*	Pseudomembranous colitis
Zoonotic bacterial infections	*Bacillus anthracis*	Anthrax (malignant pustule)
	**Listeria monocytogenes*	*Listeria* meningitis, listeriosis
	Yersinia pestis	Bubonic plague
	Francisella tularensis	Tularemia
	Brucella melitensis, B. suis, B. abortus	Brucellosis (undulant fever)
	Burkholderia mallei, B. pseudomallei	Glanders, melioidosis
	Leptospira spp. (many groups)	Leptospirosis, Weil disease
	Borrelia recurrentis	Relapsing fever
	Borrelia burgdorferi	Lyme borreliosis
	Bartonella henselae	Cat-scratch disease; bacillary angiomatosis
	Spirillum minus, Streptobacillus moniliformis	Rat-bite fever
Human treponemal infections	*Treponema pallidum*	Venereal, endemic syphilis (bejel)
	Treponema pertenue	Yaws (frambesia)
	Treponema carateum (T. herrejoni)	Pinta (carate, mal del pinto)
Mycobacterial infections	**Mycobacterium tuberculosis, M. bovis* (Koch bacillus)	Tuberculosis
	M. leprae (Hansen bacillus)	Leprosy
	**M. kansasii, M. avium, M. intracellulare*	Atypical mycobacterial infections
	M. ulcerans	Buruli ulcer
Actinomycetaceae	**Nocardia asteroides*	Nocardiosis
	Actinomyces israelii	Actinomycosis

*Important opportunistic infections.

include *Staphylococcus epidermidis* and *Propionibacterium acnes*, the cause of acne. Aerobic and anaerobic bacteria in the mouth, particularly *Streptococcus mutans*, contribute to dental plaque, a major cause of tooth decay. In the colon, 99.9% of bacteria are anaerobic, including *Bacteroides* species. Many bacteria remain extracellular when they invade the body, while others can survive and replicate either outside or inside of host cells (*facultative intracellular* bacteria) and some grow only inside host cells (*obligate intracellular* bacteria).

Chlamydiae, Rickettsiae, Mycoplasmas

These microbes are grouped together because, like other bacteria, they divide by binary fission and are sensitive to antibiotics, but they lack certain structures (e.g., *Mycoplasma* lack a cell wall) or metabolic capabilities (e.g., *Chlamydia* cannot synthesize adenosine triphosphate [ATP]). *Chlamydia* and *Rickettsiae* are obligate intracellular organisms that replicate in membrane-bound vacuoles in epithelial cells and the

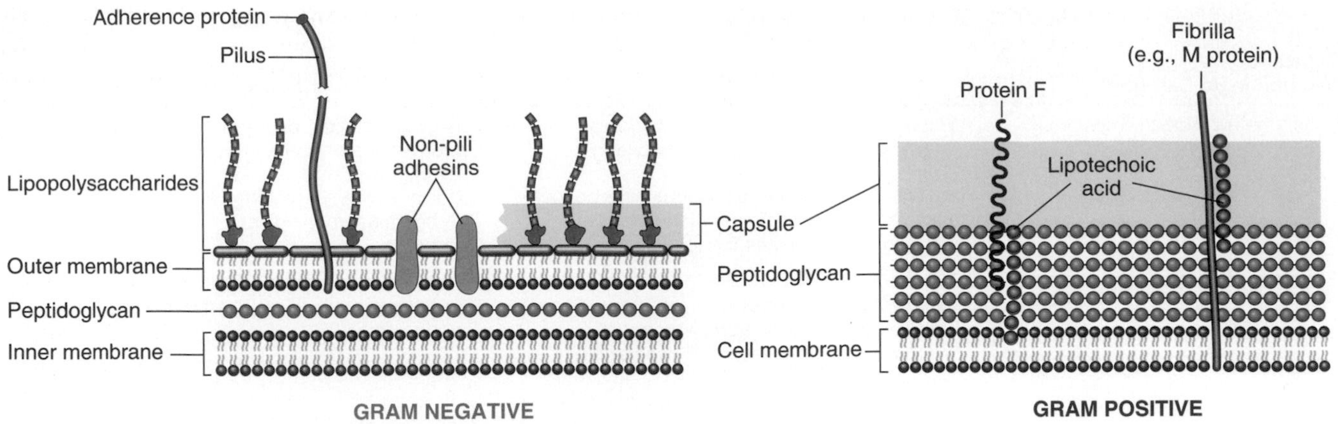

FIGURE 8–2 Molecules on the surface of Gram-negative and Gram-positive bacteria involved in pathogenesis. Not shown is the type 3 secretory apparatus of Gram-negative bacteria (see text).

cytoplasm of endothelial cells, respectively. *Chlamydia trachomatis* is the most frequent infectious cause of female sterility (by scarring and narrowing of the fallopian tubes) and blindness (by chronic inflammation of the conjuctiva that eventually scars and opacifies the cornea).

By injuring endothelial cells, rickettsiae cause a hemorrhagic vasculitis, often visible as a rash, but may also cause a transient pneumonia or hepatitis (Q fever) or injure the central nervous system (CNS) and cause death (Rocky Mountain spotted fever [RMSF] and epidemic typhus). *Rickettsiae* are transmitted by arthropod vectors, including lice (epidemic typhus), ticks (RMSF and ehrlichiosis), and mites (scrub typhus).[10]

Mycoplasma and the closely related genus *Ureaplasma* are the tiniest free-living organisms known (125 to 300 nm). *Mycoplasma pneumoniae* spreads from person to person by

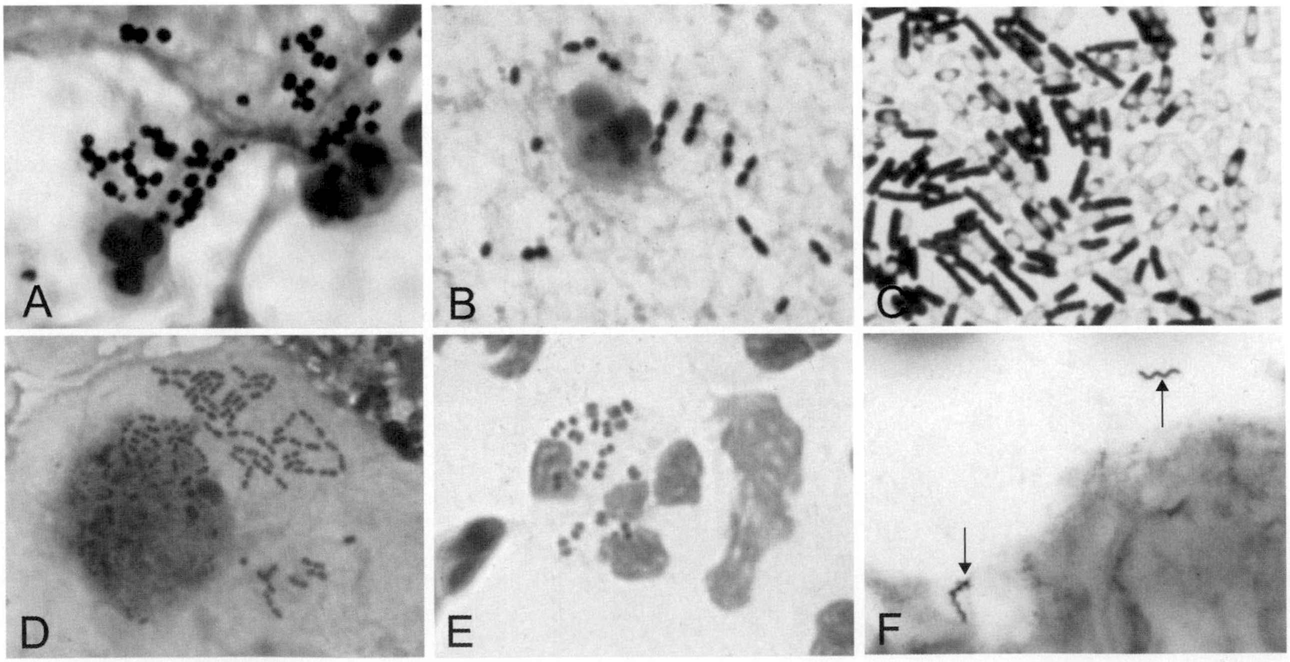

FIGURE 8–3 The variety of bacterial morphology. *A,* Gram stain of sputum from patient with pneumonia. There are Gram-positive cocci in clusters *(Staphylococcus aureus)* with degenerating neutrophils. *B,* Gram stain of sputum from a patient with pneumonia. Gram-positive, elongated cocci in pairs and short chains *(Streptococcus pneumoniae)* and a neutrophil is seen. *C,* Gram stain of *Clostridium sordellii* grown in culture. A mixture of Gram-positive and Gram-negative rods, many of which have subterminal spores (clear areas), are present. *Clostridia* species often stain as both Gram-positive and negative, although they are true Gram-positive bacteria. *D,* Gram stain of a bronchoalveolar lavage specimen showing Gram-negative intracellular rods typical of Enterobacteriaceae such as *Klebsiella pneumoniae* or *Escherichia coli*. *E,* Gram stain of urethral discharge from a patient with gonorrhea. Many Gram-negative diplococci *(Neisseria gonorrhoeae)* are present within a neutrophil. *F,* Silver stain of brain tissue from a patient with Lyme disease meningoencephalitis. Two helical spirochetes *(Borrelia burgdorferi)* are indicated by arrows. The panels are at different magnifications. (*D,* Courtesy of Dr. Karen Krisher, Clinical Microbiology Institute, Wilsonville, OR. All other panels courtesy of Dr. Kenneth Van Horn.)

aerosols, binds to the surface of epithelial cells in the airways, and causes an atypical pneumonia characterized by peribronchiolar infiltrates of lymphocytes and plasma cells (Chapter 15). Ureaplasma infections are transmitted venereally and may cause nongonococcal urethritis (NGU) (Chapter 21).

Fungi

Fungi are eukaryotes that possess thick chitin-containing cell walls and ergosterol-containing cell membranes. Fungi can grow either as budding yeast cells or as slender filamentous hyphae. Hyphae may be septate (with cell walls separating individual cells) or aseptate, which is an important distinguishing characteristic in clinical material. Some of the most important pathogenic fungi exhibit thermal dimorphism; that is, they grow as hyphal forms at room temperature but as yeast forms at body temperature. Fungi may produce sexual spores or, more commonly, asexual spores referred to as *conidia*. The latter are produced on specialized structures or fruiting bodies arising along the hyphal filament. Fungi may cause superficial or deep infections. Superficial infections involve the skin, hair, and nails. Fungal species that are confined to superficial layers of the human skin are known as dermatophytes. These infections are commonly referred to by the term "tinea" followed by the area of the body affected (e.g., tinea pedis: "athlete's foot," tinea capitis: "ringworm of the scalp"). Certain fungal species invade the subcutaneous tissue, causing abscesses or granulomas, (e.g., sporotrichosis and tropical mycoses).

Deep fungal infections can spread systemically and invade tissues, destroying vital organs in immunocompromised hosts, but usually heal or remain latent in otherwise normal hosts. Some deep fungal species are limited to a particular geographic region (e.g., *Coccidioides* in the southwestern United States and *Histoplasma* in the Ohio River Valley). Opportunistic fungi (e.g., *Candida, Aspergillus, Mucor*, and *Cryptococcus*), by contrast, are ubiquitous organisms that colonize normal human skin or gut without causing illness. Only in immunosuppressed individuals do opportunistic fungi give rise to life-threatening infections characterized by tissue necrosis, hemorrhage, and vascular occlusion, with minimal to no inflammatory response. In addition, AIDS patients are victims of the opportunistic fungus *Pneumocystis jiroveci (carinii)*.

Protozoa

Parasitic protozoa are single-celled eukaryotes that are major causes of disease and death in developing countries (Table 8–6). Protozoa can replicate intracellularly within a variety of cells (e.g., *Plasmodium* in red blood cells, *Leishmania* in macrophages) or extracellularly in the urogenital system, intestine, or blood. *Trichomonas vaginalis* are flagellated protozoal parasites that are sexually transmitted and can colonize the vagina and male urethra. The most prevalent intestinal protozoans, *Entamoeba histolytica* and *Giardia lamblia*, have two forms: (1) motile trophozoites that attach to the intestinal epithelial wall and may invade and (2) immobile cysts that are resistant to stomach acids and are infectious when ingested. Blood-borne protozoa (e.g., *Plasmodium, Trypanosoma*, and *Leishmania*) are transmitted by insect vectors, in which they replicate before being passed to new human hosts. *Toxoplasma gondii* is acquired either by contact with oocyst-shedding kittens or by eating cyst-ridden, undercooked meat.

Helminths

Parasitic worms are highly differentiated multicellular organisms. Their life cycles are complex; most alternate between sexual reproduction in the definitive host and asexual multiplication in an intermediary host or vector. Thus, depending on parasite species, humans may harbor either adult worms (e.g., *Ascarus lumbricoides*) or immature stages (e.g., *Toxocara canis*) or asexual larval forms (e.g., *Echinococcus* species). Once adult worms take up residence in humans,

TABLE 8–6 Protozoa Pathogenic for Humans

Species	Order	Form, Size	Disease
Luminal or Epithelial			
Entamoeba histolytica	Amebae	Trophozoite 15–20 μm	Amebic dysentery; liver abscess
Balantidium coli	Ciliates	Trophozoite 50–100 μm	Colitis
Naegleria fowleri	Ameboflagellates	Trophozoite 10–20 μm	Meningoencephalitis
Acanthamoeba sp.	Ameboflagellates	Trophozoite 15–30 μm	Meningoencephalitis or ophthalmitis
Giardia lamblia	Mastigophora	Trophozoite 11–18 μm	Diarrheal disease, malabsorption
Isospora belli	Coccidia	Oocyst 10–20 μm	Chronic enterocolitis or malabsorption or both
Cryptosporidium sp.	Coccidia	Oocyst 5–6 μm	
Trichomonas vaginalis	Mastigophora	Trophozoite 10–30 μm	Urethritis, vaginitis
Bloodstream			
Plasmodium species	Hemosporidia	Trophozoites, schizonts, gametes (all small and inside red cells)	Malaria
Babesia microti, B. bovis	Hemosporidia	Trophozoites inside red cells	Babesiosis
Trypanosoma species	Hemoflagellates	Trypomastigote 14–33 μm	African sleeping sickness
Intracellular			
Trypanosoma cruzi	Hemoflagellates	Trypomastigote 20 μm	Chagas disease
Leishmania donovani	Hemoflagellates	Amastigote 2 μm	Kala-azar
Leishmania species	Hemoflagellates	Amastigote 2 μm	Cutaneous and mucocutaneous leishmaniasis
Toxoplasma gondii	Coccidia	Tachyzoite 4–6 μm (cyst larger)	Toxoplasmosis

they do not multiply but generate eggs or larvae destined for the next phase of the cycle. An exception is *Strongyloides stercoralis*, the larvae of which can become infectious in the gut and cause overwhelming autoinfection in immunosuppressed persons. There are two important consequences of the lack of replication of adult worms: (1) Disease is often caused by inflammatory responses to the eggs or larvae rather than to the adults (e.g., schistosomiasis), and (2) disease is in proportion to the number of organisms that have infected the individual (e.g., 10 hookworms cause little disease, whereas 1000 hookworms cause severe anemia by consuming 100 mL of blood per day).

Ectoparasites

Ectoparasites are insects (lice, bedbugs, fleas) or arachnids (mites, ticks, spiders) that attach to and live on or in the skin. Arthropods may produce disease directly by damaging the human host or indirectly by serving as the vectors for transmission of an infectious agent into a human host. Some arthropods may cause itching and excoriations (e.g., pediculosis caused by lice attached to hair shafts, or scabies caused by mites burrowing into the stratum corneum). At the site of the bite, mouthparts may be found associated with a mixed infiltrate of lymphocytes, macrophages, and eosinophils. In addition, attached arthropods can be vectors for other pathogens. For example, deer ticks transmit the Lyme disease spirochete *Borrelia burgdorferi.*

TRANSMISSION AND DISSEMINATION OF MICROBES

Host Barriers to Infection

The outcome of infection is determined by the ability of the microbe to infect, colonize, and damage host tissues and the ability of host defense mechanisms to eradicate the infection. *Host barriers to infection prevent microbes from entering the body and consist of innate and adaptive immune defenses*[11] (see Fig. 6–1, Chapter 6). Innate immune defense mechanisms exist before infection and respond rapidly to microbes. These mechanisms include physical barriers to infection, phagocytic cells and natural killer cells, and plasma proteins, including the complement system proteins and other mediators of inflammatory responses (cytokines, collectins, acute phase reactants). Adaptive immune responses are stimulated by exposure to microbes and increase in magnitude, speed, and effectiveness with successive exposures to microbes. Adaptive immunity is mediated by T and B lymphocytes and their products (Chapter 6).

Microbes can enter the host by inhalation, ingestion, sexual transmission, insect or animal bites, or injection. The first barriers to infection are intact host skin and mucosal surfaces and their secretory products. In general, respiratory, gastrointestinal, or genitourinary tract infections occur in healthy persons and are caused by relatively virulent microorganisms that are capable of damaging or penetrating intact epithelial barriers. In contrast, most skin infections in healthy persons are caused by less virulent organisms entering the skin through damaged sites (cuts and burns).

Skin. The dense, keratinized outer layer of skin is a natural barrier to infection, and the low pH of the skin (about 5.5) and the presence of fatty acids inhibit growth of microorganisms other than residents of the normal flora. Human skin is normally inhabited by a variety of bacterial and fungal species, including some potential opportunists, such as *Staphyloccus epidermidis* and *Candida albicans.* Although skin is usually an effective barrier, certain types of fungi (dermatophytes) can infect the stratum corneum, hair, and nails, and a few microorganisms are able to traverse the unbroken skin. For example, *Schistosoma* larvae released from freshwater snails penetrate swimmers' skin by releasing collagenase, elastase, and other enzymes that dissolve the extracellular matrix. Most microorganisms, however, penetrate through breaks in the skin, including superficial pricks (fungal infections), wounds (staphylococci), burns *(Pseudomonas aeruginosa)*, and diabetic and pressure-related foot sores (multibacterial infections). Intravenous catheters in hospitalized patients can produce local or systemic infection (bacteremia). Needle sticks can expose the recipient to potentially infected blood and may transmit HBV, HCV, or HIV. Some pathogens penetrate the skin via an insect or animal bite. For instance, bites by fleas, ticks, mosquitoes, mites, and lice break the skin and transmit arboviruses (causes of yellow fever and encephalitis), rickettsiae (Rocky Mountain spotted fever), bacteria (plague, Lyme disease), protozoa (malaria, leishmaniasis), and helminths (filariasis). Animal bites can lead to infections with bacteria or with rabies virus.

Gastrointestinal Tract. Most gastrointestinal pathogens are transmitted by food or drink contaminated with fecal material. Where hygiene fails, diarrheal disease becomes rampant.

Acidic gastric secretions are important defenses within the gastrointestinal tract and are lethal for many gastrointestinal pathogens.[11] Healthy volunteers do not become infected by *Vibrio cholerae* unless they are fed 10^{11} organisms, whereas volunteers given *Vibrio cholerae* and sodium bicarbonate have a 10,000-fold increase in susceptibility to cholera. In contrast, some ingested agents, such as *Shigella* and *Giardia* cysts, are relatively resistant to gastric acid; hence, as few as 100 organisms of each are sufficient to cause illness.

Other normal defenses within the gastrointestinal tract include (1) the viscous mucous layer covering the gut, (2) lytic pancreatic enzymes and bile detergents, (3) mucosal antimicrobial peptides called defensins, (4) normal flora, and (5) secreted IgA antibodies. IgA antibodies are made by B cells located in mucosa-associated lymphoid tissues (MALT). These lymphoid aggregates are covered by a single layer of specialized epithelial cells called M cells. M cells are important for transport of antigens to MALT and for binding and uptake of numerous gut pathogens, including poliovirus, enteropathic *Escherichia coli, Vibrio cholerae, Salmonella typhi,* and *Shigella flexneri.*[12]

Infections via the gastrointestinal tract occur when local defenses are weakened or the organisms develop strategies to overcome these defenses. Host defenses are weakened by low gastric acidity, by antibiotics that unbalance the normal bacterial flora (e.g., in pseudomembranous colitis), or when there is stalled peristalsis or mechanical obstruction (e.g., in blind loop syndrome). Most enveloped viruses are killed by the bile and digestive enzymes, but nonenveloped viruses may be resistant (e.g., the hepatitis A virus, rotaviruses, reoviruses, and Norwalk agents).

Enteropathogenic bacteria elicit gastrointestinal disease by a variety of mechanisms:

- While growing on contaminated food, certain staphylococcal strains release powerful enterotoxins that cause food poisoning symptoms without any bacterial multiplication in the gut.
- *V. cholerae* and toxigenic *E. coli* multiply inside the mucous layer overlying the gut epithelium and release exotoxins that cause the gut epithelium to secrete high volumes of watery diarrhea.
- *Shigella, Salmonella,* and *Campylobacter* invade and damage the intestinal mucosa and lamina propria and so cause ulceration, inflammation, and hemorrhage, clinically manifested as dysentery.[13]
- *S. typhi* passes from the damaged mucosa through Peyer patches and mesenteric lymph nodes and into the bloodstream, resulting in a systemic infection.

Fungal infection of the gastrointestinal tract occurs mainly in immunologically compromised patients. *Candida*, part of the normal gastrointestinal flora, shows a predilection for stratified squamous epithelium, causing oral thrush or membranous esophagitis, but may also disseminate to the stomach, lower gastrointestinal tract, and systemic organs.

The cyst forms of intestinal protozoa are essential for their transmission because cysts resist stomach acid. In the gut, cysts convert to motile trophozoites and attach to sugars on the intestinal epithelia through surface lectins. Thereafter, there is wide species variation. *Giardia lamblia* attaches to the epithelial brush border, whereas cryptosporidia are taken up by enterocytes, in which they form gametes and spores. *Entamoeba histolytica* causes contact-mediated cytolysis through a channel-forming pore protein and thereby ulcerates and invades the colonic mucosa. Intestinal helminths, as a rule, cause disease only when they are present in large numbers or in ectopic sites, for example, by obstructing the gut or invading and damaging the bile ducts *(Ascaris lumbricoides)*. Hookworms may cause iron deficiency anemia by chronic loss of blood sucked from intestinal villi; the fish tapeworm *Diphyllobothrium latum* can deplete its host of vitamin B_{12}, giving rise to an illness resembling pernicious anemia. Finally, the larvae of several helminth parasites pass through the gut briefly on their way toward another organ habitat; for example, *Trichinella spiralis* larvae preferentially encyst in muscle, *Echinococcus* species larvae in the liver or lung.

Respiratory Tract. *Some 10,000 microorganisms, including viruses, bacteria, and fungi, are inhaled daily by every city inhabitant.* The distance these microorganisms travel into the respiratory system is inversely proportional to their size.[11] Large microbes are trapped in the mucociliary blanket that lines the nose and the upper respiratory tract. Microorganisms are trapped in the mucus secreted by goblet cells and are then transported by ciliary action to the back of the throat, where they are swallowed and cleared. Organisms smaller than 5 μm travel directly to the alveoli, where they are phagocytosed by alveolar macrophages or by neutrophils recruited to the lung by cytokines.

Damage to the mucociliary defense results from repeated insults in smokers and patients with cystic fibrosis, while acute injury occurs in intubated patients and in those who aspirate gastric acid. Successful respiratory microbes evade the mucociliary defenses in part by attaching to epithelial cells in the lower respiratory tract and pharynx. For example, influenza viruses possess hemagglutinin proteins that project from the surface of the virus and bind to sialic acid on the surface of epithelial cells. This attachment induces the host cell to engulf the virus, leading to viral entry and replication within the host cell. However, sialic acid binding prevents newly synthesized viruses from leaving the host cell. Influenza viruses have another cell surface protein, neuraminidase, which cleaves sialic acid and allows virus to release from the host cell. Neuraminidase also lowers the viscosity of mucus and facilitates viral transit within the respiratory tract. Interestingly, some anti-influenza drugs are sialic acid analogs that inhibit neuraminidase and prevent viral release from host cells.

Certain respiratory bacterial pathogens can impair ciliary activity. For instance, *Haemophilus influenzae* and *Bordetella pertussis* elaborate toxins that paralyze mucosal cilia; *Pseudomonas aeruginosa*, a cause of severe respiratory infection in persons with cystic fibrosis, and *Mycoplasma pneumoniae* produce ciliostatic substances. Some bacteria such as *Streptococcus pneumoniae* or *Staphylococcus* species lack specific adherence factors and often gain access after viral infection causes loss of ciliated epithelium, making individuals who have had viral respiratory infection more susceptible to secondary bacterial respiratory infection. *Mycobacterium tuberculosis*, in contrast, gains its foothold in normal alveoli because it is able to escape phagocytic killing by macrophages. Growth requirements for microorganisms can determine their site of infection in the respiratory tract. For example, rhinoviruses, which cause the common cold, grow optimally at 33°C, the temperature of the nasal mucosa, but grow poorly at 37°C, the temperature of the lower respiratory tract. Finally, opportunistic fungi infect the lungs when cellular immunity is depressed or when leukocytes are reduced in number (e.g., *P. jiroveci* [*carinii*] in AIDS patients and *Aspergillus* species in chemotherapy patients).

Urogenital Tract. The urinary tract is almost always invaded from the exterior via the urethra.[11] The regular flushing of the urinary tract with urine serves as a defense against invading microorganisms. Urine in the bladder is normally sterile, and successful pathogens (e.g., gonococci, *E. coli*) adhere to the urinary epithelium. Anatomy is an important factor for infection. Women have more than 10 times as many urinary tract infections (UTIs) as men, because the distance between the urinary bladder and skin (i.e., the length of the urethra) is 5 cm, in contrast to 20 cm in men. Obstruction of urinary flow and/or reflux can compromise normal defenses and increase susceptibility to UTIs. UTIs can spread retrogradely from the bladder to the kidney and cause acute and chronic pyelonephritis, which is the major preventable cause of renal failure.

From puberty until menopause, the vagina is protected from pathogens by a low pH resulting from catabolism of glycogen in the normal epithelium by lactobacilli. Antibiotics can kill the lactobacilli and make the vagina susceptible to infection. To be successful as pathogens, microorganisms have developed specific mechanisms for attaching to vaginal or cervical mucosa or enter via local breaks in the mucosa during sex (genital warts, syphilis).

Spread and Dissemination of Microbes

Some microorganisms proliferate locally, at the site of infection, whereas others penetrate the epithelial barrier and spread to other sites via the lymphatics, the blood, or nerves[11] (Fig. 8–4). Some of the superficial pathogens stay confined to the lumen of hollow viscera (e.g., cholera); others adhere to or proliferate exclusively in or on epithelial cells (e.g., papillomaviruses, dermatophytes). A variety of pathogenic bacteria, fungi, and helminths are invasive by virtue of their motility or ability to secrete lytic enzymes (e.g., streptococci and staphylococci secrete hyaluronidase, which degrades the extracellular matrix between host cells). Microbial spread initially follows tissue planes of least resistance and regional lymphatic and vascular anatomy. For example, staphylococcal infections may progress from a localized abscess or furuncle to regional lymphadenitis that sometimes leads to bacteremia and colonization of distant organs (heart, liver, brain, kidney, bone). Within the blood, microorganisms may be transported free or within host cells. Some viruses (e.g., poliovirus and HBV), most bacteria and fungi, some protozoa (e.g., African trypanosomes), and all helminths are transported free in the plasma. Leukocytes can carry herpesviruses, HIV, mycobacteria, and *Leishmania* and *Toxoplasma* organisms. Certain viruses (e.g., Colorado tick fever virus) and parasites (*Plasmodium* and *Babesia*) are carried by red blood cells. Viruses also may propagate from cell to cell by fusion or transport within nerves (e.g., rabies virus). Infectious foci disseminated by blood are called secondary foci. They can be single and large (a solitary abscess or tuberculoma) or multiple and tiny, the size of millet seeds (e.g., miliary tuberculosis or *Candida* microabscesses in many tissues). Bloodstream invasion by sporadic low-virulence or nonvirulent microbes is a common event but is quickly suppressed by the normal host defenses. By contrast, sustained bloodstream invasion with dissemination of pathogens, that is, viremia, bacteremia, fungemia, or parasitemia, is a serious insult and manifests itself by fever, low blood pressure, and multiple other systemic signs and symptoms of sepsis. Massive bloodstream invasion by bacteria or their endotoxins can rapidly become fatal, even for previously healthy individuals.

The major manifestations of infectious disease may arise at sites distant from those of microbe entry. For example, chickenpox and measles viruses enter through the airways but cause rashes in the skin; poliovirus enters through the intestine but kills motor neurons. *Schistosoma mansoni* parasites penetrate the skin but eventually localize in blood vessels of the portal system and mesentery, damaging the liver and intestine. The rabies virus travels to the brain in a retrograde fashion within nerves, while the varicella zoster virus hides in dorsal root ganglia, and on reactivation, travels along nerves to cause shingles.

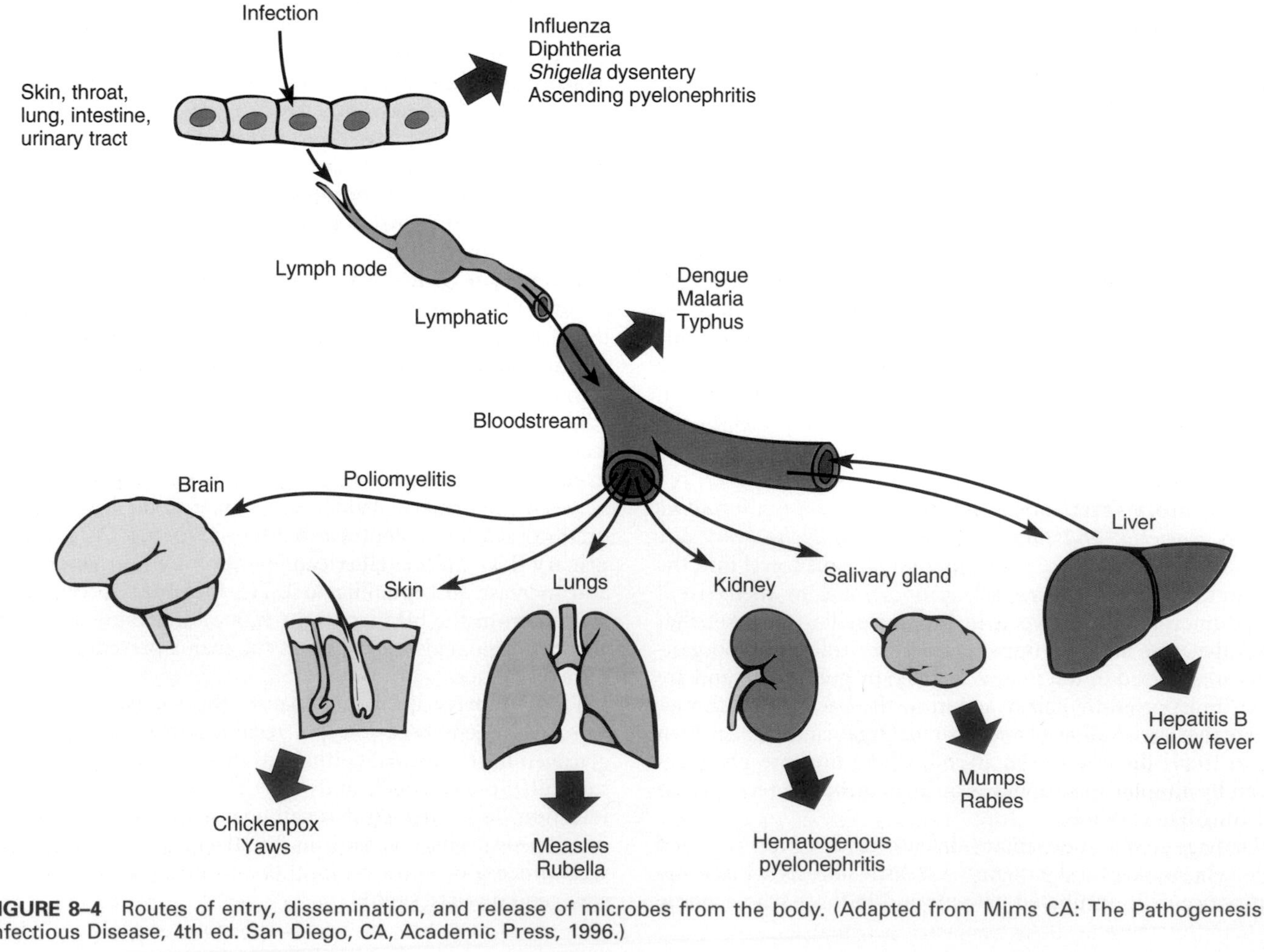

FIGURE 8–4 Routes of entry, dissemination, and release of microbes from the body. (Adapted from Mims CA: The Pathogenesis of Infectious Disease, 4th ed. San Diego, CA, Academic Press, 1996.)

The placental-fetal route is an important mode of transmission (Chapter 10). When infectious organisms reach the pregnant uterus through the cervical orifice or the bloodstream and are able to traverse the placenta, severe damage to the fetus can result. Bacterial or mycoplasmal placentitis can cause premature delivery or stillbirth. Viral infections can cause maldevelopment of the fetus, with infection early in pregnancy resulting in the most severe disease. Rubella infection during the first trimester can cause congenital heart disease, mental retardation, cataracts, or deafness in the infant, while little damage is caused by rubella infection during the third trimester. Transmission of treponemes leads to congenital syphilis only when *Treponema pallidum* infects the mother late in the second trimester but then causes severe fetal osteochondritis and periostitis that leads to multiple bony lesions. Infection also can occur during passage through the birth canal (e.g., gonoccocal or chlamydial conjunctivitis) or through maternal milk (e.g., CMV, hepatitis B, HTLV-1). Maternal transmission of HIV results in opportunistic infections in 50% of untreated children during the first year of life. Maternal transmission of HBV can subsequently cause chronic hepatitis or liver cancer.

Release of Microbes from the Body

For transmission of disease to occur, exit of a microorganism from the host's body is as important as entry into it. Depending on the location of infection, release may be accomplished by skin shedding, coughing, sneezing, or voiding of urine or feces, or through insect vectors.[11] Some microbes are hardy and can survive for extended periods in dust, food, or water. Bacterial spores, protozoan cysts, and thick-shelled helminth eggs can survive in a cool and dry environment. Some enteric pathogens are shed for long periods by asymptomatic carrier hosts (e.g., *Salmonella typhi*). Transmission from person to person can occur by respiratory, fecal-oral, or sexual routes (discussed below). Less hardy microorganisms must be quickly passed from person to person, often by direct contact. Viruses infecting the salivary glands (e.g., EBV, CMV, mumps viruses) are transmitted principally by kissing or talking. Other pathogens are spread mainly by prolonged intimate or mucosal contact, as occurs during sexual transmission, including viruses (HPV, herpesviruses, HBV, HIV), bacteria *(T. pallidum, N. gonorrhoeae, Chlamydiae trachomatis)*, fungi (*Candida* species), protozoa (*Trichomonas* species), and arthropods (*Phthirus pubis*, or crab lice). Bacteria and fungi transmitted by the respiratory route (e.g., *Mycobacterium tuberculosis*) are infective only when lesions are open to the airways. Many pathogens, ranging from viruses to helminths, can be transmitted by the fecal-oral route, that is, by ingestion of stool-contaminated food or water. Waterborne viruses involved in epidemic outbreaks include hepatitis A and E viruses, poliovirus, and rotavirus.[14] Some parasitic helminths (e.g., hookworms, schistosomes) shed eggs in stool that gain access to new hosts by larval penetration of the skin rather than by oral intake. Protozoa and helminths have evolved complex transmission cycles involving a chain of intermediate and vector hosts bearing successive developmental stages of the parasites. Transmission of HBV, HCV, and HIV infections through blood and blood products may be caused by human agency, that is, needle sharing by drug abusers, cuts, needle sticks, and other accidents.

Microorganisms also can be transmitted from animals to humans, either by invertebrate vectors or by vertebrates. Invertebrate vectors (insects, ticks, mites) can spread infection passively in some cases or serve as necessary hosts for replication and development of the pathogen. Transmission can occur from animal to human (termed *zoonotic infections*), either by direct contact or eating the animal or indirectly via an invertebrate vector (e.g., field mice are the reservoir hosts for Lyme disease).

Sexually Transmitted Infections

A number of organisms can be transmitted through sexual contact (Table 8–7). Some, such as *Chlamydia trachomatis* and *Neisseria gonorrhoeae*, are usually spread by sexual intercourse, while others, such as *Shigella* species and *Entamoeba histolytica*, are typically spread by other means but are also occasionally spread by sex. Groups that are at greater risk for some sexually transmitted infections (STIs) include adolescents, men who have sex with men, and people who use illegal drugs. While the increased risk among these groups is partially due to unsafe sexual practices, it is also due to limited access to health care. The presence of an STI in young children, unless acquired during birth, strongly suggests sexual abuse.

The initial site of infection with an STI may be the urethra, vagina, cervix, rectum, or oral pharynx. The organisms that cause these infections tend to be short-lived outside of the host, so they usually depend on direct person-to-person spread. Most of these agents can be infectious in the absence of symptoms, so transmission often occurs from people who do not realize that they have an infection. To reduce the spread of STIs, these infections are often reported to public health authorities so that people who have had intimate contact with the patient may be tested and treated.

Although the various pathogens that cause STIs differ in many ways, some general features should be noted.

- *Infection with one STI increases the risk for additional STIs.* This is mainly because the risk factors are the same for all STIs. This probably explains the association between two common STIs in the United States: chlamydia and gonorrhea. Coinfection with these two bacteria is so common that the diagnosis of either of them should lead to the treatment of both. In addition, biologic interactions between the organisms that cause STIs can increase the spread of infections. For example, the cervicitis caused by gonorrhea or chlamydia can increase the chance that a woman who is exposed to HIV will become infected with the virus. This appears to be because the local tissue damage associated with the cervicitis allows infection with HIV.
- *The microbes that cause STIs can be spread from a pregnant woman to the fetus and cause severe damage to the fetus or child.* Perinatally acquired *C. trachomatis* causes conjunctivitis, and neonatal herpes simplex virus infection is much more likely to cause visceral and CNS disease than is infection acquired later in life. Syphilis frequently causes miscarriage. HIV infection is always, eventually, fatal to children infected with the virus. Diagnosis of STIs in pregnant women is critical because intrauterine or neonatal STI transmission can often be prevented by treatment of the mother or newborn. Bacterial infections such as gonorrhea,

TABLE 8–7 Classification of Important Sexually Transmitted Diseases

	Disease or Syndrome and Population Principally Affected		
Pathogens	*Males*	*Both*	*Females*
Viruses			
Herpes simplex virus		Primary and recurrent herpes, neonatal herpes	
Hepatitis B virus		Hepatitis	
Human papillomavirus	Cancer of penis (some cases)	Condyloma acuminatum	Cervical dysplasia and cancer, vulvar cancer
Human immunodeficiency virus		Acquired immunodeficiency syndrome	
Chlamydiae			
Chlamydia trachomatis	Urethritis, epididymitis, proctitis	Lymphogranuloma venereum	Urethral syndrome, cervicitis, bartholinitis, salpingitis and sequelae
Mycoplasmas			
Ureaplasma urealyticum	Urethritis		
Bacteria			
Neisseria gonorrhoeae	Epididymitis, prostatitis, urethral stricture	Urethritis, proctitis, pharyngitis, disseminated gonococcal infection	Cervicitis, endometritis, bartholinitis, salpingitis, and sequelae (infertility, ectopic pregnancy, recurrent salpingitis)
Treponema pallidum		Syphilis	
Haemophilus ducreyi		Chancroid	
Calymmatobacterium granulomatis		Granuloma inguinale (donovanosis)	
Shigella	*Enterocolitis		
Campylobacter	*Enterocolitis		
Protozoa			
Trichomonas vaginalis	Urethritis, balanitis		Vaginitis
Entamoeba histolytica	*Amebiasis		
Giardia lamba	*Giardiasis		

*Most important in homosexual populations.
Modified and updated from Krieger JN: Biology of sexually transmitted diseases. Urol Clin North Am 11:15, 1984.

syphilis, and chlamydia can be easily cured with antibiotics. Antiretroviral treatment of pregnant women with HIV infection and treatment of the newborn can reduce transmission of HIV to children from 25% to less than 2%.

Syphilis is discussed later in this chapter, and other STIs are described in Chapters 21 and 22.

HOW MICROORGANISMS CAUSE DISEASE

Infectious agents establish infection and damage tissues in three ways:

- They can contact or enter host cells and directly cause cell death.
- They may release toxins that kill cells at a distance, release enzymes that degrade tissue components, or damage blood vessels and cause ischemic necrosis.
- They can induce host cellular responses that, although directed against the invader, cause additional tissue damage, usually by immune-mediated mechanisms. Thus, as we discussed in Chapters 2 and 6, the defensive responses of the host are a two-edged sword: They are necessary to overcome the infection but at the same time may directly contribute to tissue damage.

Here we describe some of the mechanisms whereby viruses and bacteria damage host tissues.

Mechanisms of Viral Injury

Viruses can directly damage host cells by entering them and replicating at the host's expense. The predilection for viruses to infect certain cells and not others is called tissue tropism and is determined by several factors, including (1) host cell receptors for the virus, (2) cellular transcription factors that recognize viral enhancer and promoter sequences, (3) anatomic barriers, and (4) local temperature, pH, and host defenses.[15] Each of these is described briefly.

A major determinant of tissue tropism is the presence of viral receptors on host cells. Viruses possess specific cell-surface proteins that bind to particular host cell-surface proteins. Many viruses use normal cellular receptors of the host to enter cells. For example, HIV gp120 binds to CD4 on T cells and to the chemokine receptors CXCR4 (mainly on T cells) and CCR5 (mainly on macrophages). Rhinoviruses bind to the same site on ICAM-1 as LFA-1, an integrin on the surface of lymphocytes that is an important adhesion molecule for lymphocyte activation and migration.[16] In some cases, host proteases are needed to enable binding of virus to host cells; for instance, a host protease cleaves and activates the influenza virus hemagglutinin. Another determinant of viral tropism is the ability of the virus to replicate inside some cells but not in others, and this is related to the presence of cell-type–specific transcription factors. For example, the JC virus, which causes leukoencephalopathy (Chapter 28), is restricted to oligodendroglia in the central nervous system because the promoter and enhancer DNA sequences upstream from the viral genes are active in glial cells but not in neurons or endothelial cells. Physical barriers also can contribute to tissue tropism. For example, enteroviruses replicate in the intestine in part because they can resist inactivation by acids, bile, and digestive enzymes. Rhinoviruses replicate only within the upper respiratory tract because they survive optimally at the lower temperature of the upper respiratory tract.

Once viruses are inside host cells, they can kill the cells and/or cause tissue damage in a number of ways (Fig. 8–5):

- Viruses may inhibit host cell DNA, RNA, or protein synthesis. For example, poliovirus inactivates cap-binding protein, which is essential for translation of host cell mRNAs, but leaves translation of poliovirus mRNAs unaffected.
- Viral proteins may insert into the host cell's plasma membrane and directly damage its integrity or promote cell fusion (HIV, measles virus, and herpesviruses).
- Viruses may lyse host cells. For example, respiratory epithelial cells are killed by influenza virus replication, liver cells by yellow fever virus, and neurons by poliovirus and rabies virus.
- Viruses may manipulate programmed cell death (apoptosis). Some virus-encoded proteins (including TAT and gp120 of HIV, adenovirus E1A) can induce cell death. In contrast, some viruses encode one or more genes that inhibit apoptosis (e.g., homologues of the cellular *bcl-2* gene), suggesting that apoptotic cell death may be a protective host response to eliminate virus-infected cells. It has been hypothesized that viral antiapoptotic strategies may enhance viral replication, promote persistent viral infections, or promote virus-induced cancers.[17]
- Viral proteins on the surface of the host cells may be recognized by the immune system, and the host lymphocytes may attack the virus-infected cells. Acute liver failure during hepatitis B infection may be accelerated by cytotoxic T lymphocyte (CTL)-mediated destruction of infected hepatocytes (a normal response to clear the infection). FAS ligand on CTLs, which bind to FAS receptors on the surface of hepatocytes, also can induce apoptosis in target cells.[18]
- Viruses may damage cells involved in host antimicrobial defense, leading to secondary infections. For example, viral damage to respiratory epithelium predisposes to the subsequent development of pneumonia by *Streptococcus pneumoniae* and *Haemophilus influenzae.* HIV depletes CD4+ helper lymphocytes and thereby causes opportunistic infections.
- Viral killing of one cell type may cause the death of other cells that depend on them. For example, denervation by the attack of poliovirus on motor neurons causes atrophy and sometimes death of distal skeletal muscle supplied by such neurons.
- Some viruses can cause *cell proliferation and transformation* (e.g., EBV, HBV, human papillomavirus, or HTLV-1), resulting in cancer. The mechanisms of viral transformation are numerous and are discussed in Chapter 7.

Mechanisms of Bacterial Injury

Bacterial Virulence. *Bacterial damage to host tissues depends on the ability of the bacteria to adhere to host cells, invade cells and tissues, or deliver toxins.* Pathogenic bacteria have virulence genes that encode proteins that confer these

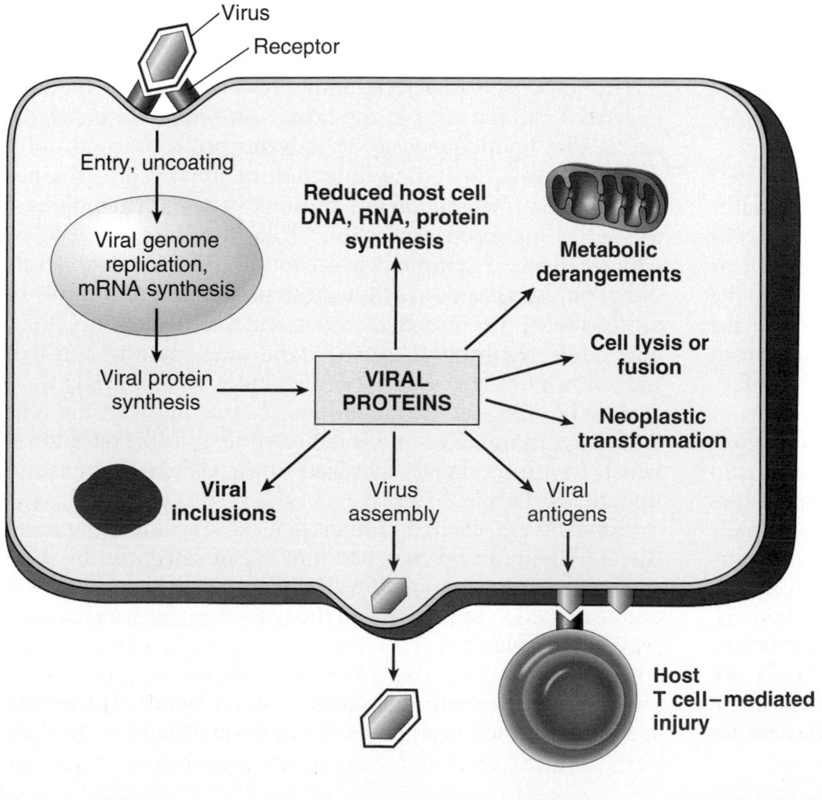

FIGURE 8–5 Mechanisms by which viruses cause injury to cells.

properties. Virulence genes are frequently found grouped together in clusters called *pathogenicity islands*. All of the *Salmonella* strains that infect humans are closely related enough to form a single species, meaning that they share many "housekeeping" genes.[19] Differences in a relatively small number of pathogenicity genes determine whether an isolate of *Salmonella* can cause the life-threatening infection, typhoid fever, or whether it is relatively avirulent.

Many bacteria induce expression of virulence factors as their concentration in the tissues increases. This may allow bacteria growing in discrete host sites, such as an abscess or consolidated pneumonia, to increase production of virulence factors, thereby overcoming host defenses. For example, Gram-positive organisms, such as *S. aureus*, coordinately regulate virulence factors by secreting *autoinducer* peptides.[20] As the bacteria grow to increasing concentrations, the level of the autoinducer peptide increases, inducing toxin expression.

Bacterial Adherence to Host Cells. *Adhesins* are bacterial surface molecules that bind to host cells. Bacterial adhesins that bind bacteria to host cells are limited in structural type but have a broad range of host cell specificity. The *fibrillae* covering the surface of the Gram-positive organism *Streptococcus pyogenes* are composed of lipoteichoic acids and M protein (Fig. 8–2). *Lipoteichoic acids* are hydrophobic and bind to fibronectin and to the surface of buccal epithelial cells. M protein, the second component of *S. pyogenes* fibrillae, prevents phagocytosis by host macrophages. *S. pyogenes* also expresses a nonfibrillar adhesin, *protein F*, which binds to fibronectin. Protein F may also help *S. pyogenes* to evade the immune response by entering epithelial cells.

Fimbriae or *pili* are filamentous proteins on the surface of Gram-negative bacteria. The stalks of pili are composed of conserved repeating subunits, while the variable amino acids on the tips of the pili determine the binding specificity of the bacteria. Strains of *Escherichia coli* that cause urinary tract infections uniquely express a specific P pilus, which binds to a gal(α1–4)gal moiety expressed on uroepithelial cells.[21] Pili on *Neisseria gonorrhoeae* mediate adherence of bacteria to host cells and can also act as targets of the antibody response against *N. gonorrhoeae*. Variation in the type of pili expressed is an important mechanism by which *N. gonorrhoeae* escapes the immune response.[22]

Virulence of Intracellular Bacteria. Unlike viruses, which infect a broad range of host cells, facultative intracellular bacteria infect either epithelial cells (*Shigella* and enteroinvasive *E. coli*), macrophages (*M. tuberculosis, M. leprae*), or both (*S. typhi*). The growth of bacteria in cells may allow the bacteria to escape from certain effector mechanisms of the immune response (e.g., antibodies), or it may facilitate spread of the bacteria, as migration of macrophages carries *M. tuberculosis* from the lung to other sites.

Bacteria have a number of mechanisms for entering host cells. Some bacteria use the host immune response to gain entry into macrophages. Coating of bacteria with antibodies or the complement protein C3b (opsonization) normally results in phagocytosis of bacteria by macrophages. Like many bacteria, *M. tuberculosis* activates the alternative complement pathway, resulting in opsonization with C3b. In addition, *M. tuberculosis* recruits a C2a fragment to form C3 convertase, generating additional C3b.[23] Once coated with C3b, *M. tuberculosis* binds to the CR3 complement receptor on macrophages and is endocytosed into the cell. Gram-negative bacteria use a complex secretion system delivered by projections from the bacterial surface to enter epithelial cells.[24] These projections bind to host cells, form pores in the host cell membrane, and then inject proteins that mediate rearrangement of the cell cytoskeleton, facilitating bacterial entry. Bacteria such as *L. monocytogenes* can manipulate the cell cytoskeleton to spread directly from cell to cell, perhaps allowing the bacteria to evade immune effector mechanisms.[25]

Once in the cytoplasm, bacteria have different strategies for interacting with the host cell. *Shigella* and *Escherichia coli* inhibit host protein synthesis, replicate rapidly, and lyse the host cell within 6 hours. Once within macrophages, most bacteria are killed when the phagosome fuses with an acidic lysosome to form a phagolysosome. Bacteria that grow inside macrophages must escape this destruction. To avoid being killed within the macrophage, *M. tuberculosis* blocks fusion of the lysosome with the phagosome.[26] This allows the *M. tuberculosis* to proliferate unchecked within the macrophage. Other bacteria avoid destruction in macrophages by escaping from the phagosome to proliferate in the cell cytoplasm. *L. monocytogenes* produces a pore-forming protein called listeriolysin O and two phospholipases to degrade the phagosome membrane, allowing the bacteria to escape into the cytoplasm.[25]

Bacterial Toxins. Any bacterial substance that contributes to illness can be considered a toxin. Toxins are classified as endotoxins, which are components of the bacterial cell, and exotoxins, which are proteins that are secreted by the bacterium. Historically, exotoxins were considered to be associated with Gram-positive bacteria, but it is now clear that both Gram-positive and Gram-negative bacteria produce exotoxins.

Bacterial endotoxin is a lipopolysaccharide (LPS) that is a large component of the outer cell wall of Gram-negative bacteria. Lipopolysaccharide is composed of a long-chain fatty acid anchor (lipid A) connected to a core sugar chain, both of which are very similar in all Gram-negative bacteria. Attached to the core sugar is a variable carbohydrate chain (O antigen), which is used to serotype and discriminate between different strains of bacteria.

The response to bacterial lipopolysaccharide can be both beneficial and harmful to the host.[27] The response is beneficial in that lipopolysaccharide activates protective immunity in several ways, including induction of important cytokines and chemoattractants of the immune systems (chemokines) as well as increased expression of costimulatory molecules, which enhance T-lymphocyte activation. However, high levels of lipopolysaccharide are thought to play an important role in septic shock, disseminated intravascular coagulation (DIC), and adult respiratory distress syndrome, mainly through induction of excessive levels of cytokines such as TNF, IL-1, and IL-12 (Chapter 4). Lipopolysaccharide binds to the cell-surface receptor CD14 and is delivered to Toll-like receptor 4, which transmits signals that lead to the cellular response to lipopolysaccharide.[28]

Exotoxins are secreted proteins that cause cellular injury and disease. They can be classified into broad categories by their site and mechanism of action. These are briefly described next and discussed in more detail in the specific sections about each type of bacteria.

- Bacteria secrete a variety of enzymes (proteases, hyaluronidases, coagulases, fibrinolysins) that act on their respective substrates in vitro, but the role of many of these enzymes in disease remains unclear. Proteases produced by *S. aureus* have a clearly defined role in splitting the epidermis from the deeper skin by cleaving proteins that link epidermal cells to one another.[29]

- Toxins that alter intracellular signaling or regulatory pathways work by affecting many pathways. Most of these toxins have an active (A) subunit with enzymatic activity and a binding (B) subunit that binds receptors on the cell surface and delivers the A subunit into the cell cytoplasm. The effect of these toxins depends on the binding specificity of the B domain and the cellular pathways affected by the A domain. A-B toxins are made by many bacteria including *Bacillus anthracis, Vibrio cholerae,* and some strains of *Escherichia coli.*
- Neurotoxins produced by *Clostridium botulinum* and *Clostridium tetani* inhibit release of neurotransmitters, resulting in paralysis.[30] These toxins do not kill neurons; instead, the A domains interact specifically with proteins involved in secretion of neurotransmitters at the synaptic junction. Both tetanus and botulism can result in death from respiratory failure due to paralysis of the chest and diaphragm muscles.
- Superantigens are bacterial toxins that stimulate very large number of T lymphocytes by binding to conserved portions of the T-cell receptor, leading to massive T-lymphocyte proliferation and cytokine release. The high levels of cytokines can lead to capillary leak and shock.[31] Superantigens made by *Staphlococcus aureus* and *Streptococcus pyogenes* cause toxic shock syndrome.

Injurious Effects of Host Immunity

As was mentioned earlier, the host immune response to microbes can sometimes be the cause of tissue injury. This is best exemplified by the immune response to mycobacteria. The granulomatous inflammatory reaction to *Mycobacterium tuberculosis* is a delayed hypersensitivity response that sequesters the bacilli and prevents spread, but also can produce tissue damage and fibrosis. Similarly, the liver damage following hepatitis B virus infection of hepatocytes is mainly due to the immune response to the infected liver cells and not to cytopathic effects of the virus. The humoral immune response to microbes also can have pathologic consequences. For example, following infection with β-hemolytic streptococci, antibodies produced to the streptococcal M protein can cross-react with cardiac proteins and become deposited in the heart, and lead to rheumatic fever. Poststreptococcal glomerulonephritis, which also can develop following infection with β-hemolytic streptococci, is caused by antistreptococcal antibodies that form complexes with streptococcal antigens and deposit in renal glomeruli and produce nephritis. Thus, antimicrobial immune responses can have beneficial and pathologic consequences.

IMMUNE EVASION BY MICROBES

Humoral and cellular immune responses that protect the host from most infections were discussed in Chapter 6. Throughout evolution, microbes have been engaged in a struggle for survival with their hosts. Not surprisingly, microorganisms have developed many means to resist and evade the immune system.[15] These mechanisms are important determinants of microbial virulence and pathogenicity. They include (1) remaining inaccessible to the host immune system, (2) varying or shedding antigens, (3) resisting innate immune defenses, and (4) preventing T-cell activation or impairing effective T-cell antimicrobial responses by specific or nonspecific immunosuppression.

Some microorganisms replicate in sites that are inaccessible to the host immune response. Microbes that propagate in the lumen of the intestine (e.g., toxin-producing *Clostridium difficile*) or gallbladder (e.g., *Salmonella typhi*) are concealed from many host immune defenses. Viruses that are shed from the luminal surface of epithelial cells (e.g., CMV in urine or milk and poliovirus in stool) or those that infect the keratinized epithelium (poxviruses, which cause molluscum contagiosum) are inaccessible to the host humoral immune system. Some organisms establish infections by rapidly invading host cells before the host humoral response becomes effective (e.g., malaria sporozoites entering liver cells, *Trichinella* and *Trypanosoma cruzi* entering skeletal or cardiac muscles). Some larger parasites (e.g., the larvae of tapeworms) form cysts in host tissues that are covered by a dense fibrous capsule and are thus inaccessible to host immune cells and antibodies. Viral latency is the ultimate strategy for hiding antigens from the immune system. During the latent state, many viral genes are not expressed.

Microbes can evade immune responses either by varying antigens or by shedding antigens. Neutralizing antibodies block the ability of microbes to infect cells. This highly specific immunity is the basis of vaccination, but it cannot protect against microbes with many variants of the antigens recognized by these antibodies. The low fidelity of viral RNA polymerases (HIV and many respiratory viruses) and reassortment of viral genomes (influenza viruses) lead to viral antigenic variation (Table 8–8). Other microbes also exhibit antigenic variation. There are at least 80 different serotypes of *S. pneumoniae*, each with different capsular polysaccharides. The spirochete *Borrelia recurrentis* repeatedly switches its surface antigens, and the Lyme disease *Borreliae* use similar mechanisms to vary their outer membrane proteins.[32] Cercariae of *Schistosoma mansoni* shed their antigens within minutes of penetrating the skin, preventing recognition by host antibodies.

Some microbes have devised methods for evading innate immune defenses, such as escaping killing by phagocytic cells and complement.[33,34] Cationic antimicrobial peptides (CAMPs), including defensins, cathelicidins, and thrombocidins, provide important initial defense against invading microbes. CAMP resistance is key to the virulence of a number of bacterial pathogens, enabling them to avoid killing by

TABLE 8–8 Pathogens with Significant Antigenic Variation

Rhinoviruses	Colds
Influenza virus	Influenza
Neisseria gonorrhoeae	Gonorrhea
Borrelia hermsii	Relapsing fever
Borrelia burgdorferi	Lyme disease
Trypanosoma brucei	African sleeping sickness
Giardia lamblia	Giardiasis
Plasmodium falciparum	Severe malaria

neutrophils and macrophages.[33] The carbohydrate capsule on the surface of all the major bacteria that cause pneumonia or meningitis (pneumococcus, meningococcus, *Haemophilus influenzae*) makes them more virulent by shielding bacterial antigens and by preventing phagocytosis of the organisms by neutrophils. For example, *E. coli* with the sialic acid-containing K1 capsule causes meningitis in newborns. Sialic acid will not bind C3b, which is critical for activation of the alternative complement pathway, so the bacteria escape from complement-mediated lysis and opsonization-directed phagocytosis. Many bacteria make toxic proteins that kill phagocytes, prevent their migration, or diminish their oxidative burst. Bacteria also can circumvent immune defenses by covering themselves with host proteins. *S. aureus* are covered by protein A molecules that bind the Fc portion of antibodies and so inhibit phagocytosis. *Neisseria, Haemophilus*, and *Streptococcus* all secrete proteases that degrade antibodies. Another successful strategy for circumventing phagocytic defense mechanisms is to replicate within phagocytic cells. A number of viruses, rickettsias, some intracellular bacteria (including mycobacteria, Listeria, and Legionella), fungi (e.g., *Cryptococcus neoformans*), and protozoa (e.g., leishmania, trypanosomes, toxoplasmas) can multiply within phagocytes.

Viruses can produce molecules that inhibit innate immunity.[15,35,36] Some viruses (e.g., herpesviruses and poxviruses) produce proteins that block complement activation. Viruses have developed a large number of strategies to combat interferons (IFN), an early host defense against viruses. Some viruses produce soluble homologues of IFN-α/β or IFN-γ receptors that inhibit actions of extracellular IFNs, or produce proteins that inhibit intracellular JAK/STAT signaling downstream of IFN receptors or inactivate or inhibit dsRNA-dependent protein kinase (PKR), a key mediator of the antiviral effects of IFN. Viruses also can produce homologues of chemokines or chemokine receptors, and these can function as antagonists and inhibit recruitment of inflammatory cells to favor survival of viruses. Viruses also can produce soluble cytokine mimics (e.g., EBV produces a homologue of the immunosuppressive cytokine IL-10) or soluble cytokine receptor homologues.

Some microbes can decrease recognition of infected cells by CD4+ helper T cells and CD8+ cytotoxic T cells. For example, several DNA viruses (e.g., herpesviruses, including HSV, HCMV, and EBV) can bind to or alter localization of MHC class I proteins, impairing peptide presentation to CD8+ T cells[36,37] (Fig. 8–6). Downregulation of MHC class I molecules might make it likely that virus-infected cells would be targets for NK cells. However, herpesviruses also express MHC class I homologues that act as effective inhibitors of NK cells by engaging killer inhibitory receptors (Chapter 6). Similarly, herpesviruses can target MHC class II molecules for degradation, impairing antigen presentation to CD4+ T helper cells. Viruses also can infect lymphocytes and directly compromise their function. HIV infects CD4+ T cells, macrophages, and dendritic cells, and EBV infects B lymphocytes.

INFECTIONS IN IMMUNOSUPPRESSED HOSTS

Different types of immunosuppression affect different cells of the immune system. The opportunistic infections that an immunosuppressed person contracts depend on the types of immune effector mechanisms that are not working correctly. Immunodeficiencies may be genetic (primary) or acquired (secondary) (Chapter 6).

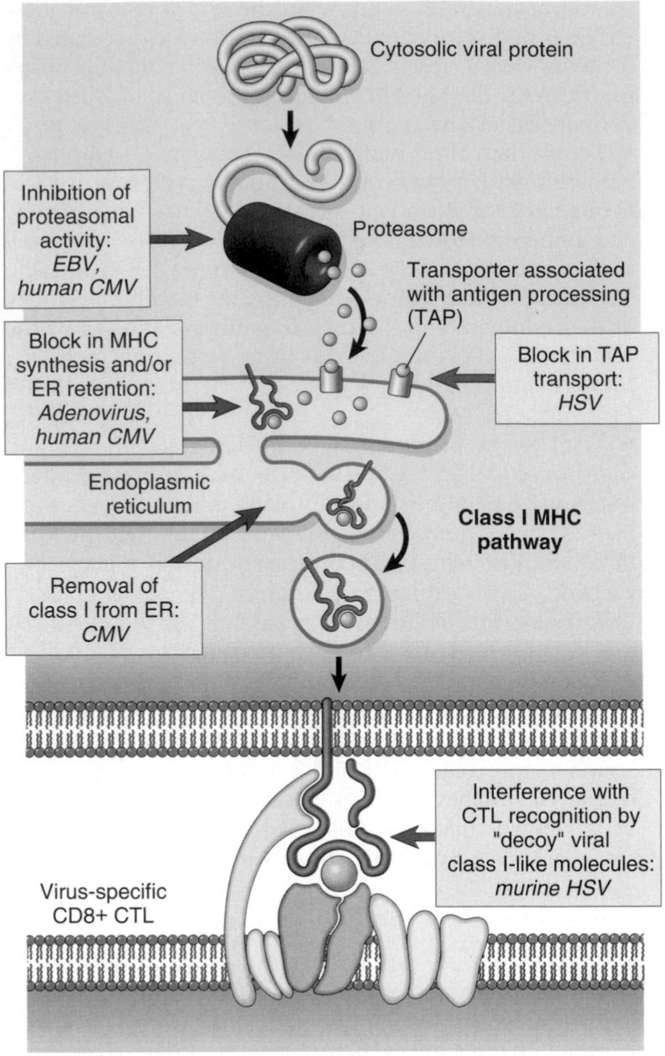

FIGURE 8–6 Inhibition of MHC expression by viruses. The steps at which different viruses inhibit the class I MHC antigen presentation pathway are shown. (Modified with permission from Abbas AK, Lichtman AH: Cellular and Molecular Immunology, 5th ed., Philadelphia, Saunders, 2003.)

Patients with antibody deficiency, as in X-linked agammaglobulinemia, contract severe bacterial infections, including *S. pneumoniae, H. influenzae*, and *S. aureus*, as well as a few viral infections (rotavirus and enteroviruses). Patients with deficiencies in complement proteins are particularly susceptible to bacterial infections such as *S. pneumoniae, H. influenzae*, and *N. meningitidis*. As discussed in Chapter 2, some children have deficiencies in neutrophil function, leading to increased infections with *S. aureus* as well as some Gram-negative bacteria and fungi.

Diseases of organ systems other than the immune system can also make patients susceptible to specific microorganisms. People with cystic fibrosis commonly get respiratory infections with *Pseudomonas aeruginosa, S. aureus*, and *Burkholdaria cepacia*.[38] The lack of splenic function in individuals with sickle-cell disease makes them susceptible to infection with encapsulated bacteria such as *S. pneumoniae*, which are normally opsonized and phagocytosed by splenic macrophages.

Acquired immunodeficiencies have a variety of causes, the most important being infection with the human immunodeficiency virus (HIV), which causes AIDS. HIV infects and eventually kills CD4+ helper T lymphocytes. As discussed in Chapter 6, this leads to profound immunosuppression and a multitude of infections. While most organisms that infect people with AIDS were common pathogens before the era of HIV, some were uncommon infections before HIV (cryptococcus, pneumocystis), and one, Kaposi sarcoma herpesvirus (KSHV), also called human herpesvirus-8 (HHV-8), was discovered as a result of research in HIV patients.[39]

Diseases that impair production of leukocytes, such as leukemia, which fills the bone marrow with cancerous cells, make patients vulnerable to opportunistic infections. Burns destroy skin, removing this barrier to microbes, allowing infection with pathogens such as *P. aeruginosa*. Iatrogenic causes of immunosuppression include immunosuppressive drugs used to treat patients with autoimmune diseases and organ transplant recipients as well as drugs used to treat cancer. Finally, malnutrition may impair the immune response.

Therapy to prevent organ transplant rejection leads to severe immunosuppression, making transplant recipients very susceptible to infectious diseases. Patients receiving bone marrow transplants are profoundly immunosuppressed during the time that the donated bone marrow is engrafting, and became susceptible to infection with almost any organism, including environmental organisms that seldom cause disease in healthy people (e.g., *Aspergillus* species and *Pseudomonas* species that are common in water).

SPECIAL TECHNIQUES FOR DIAGNOSING INFECTIOUS AGENTS

Some infectious agents or their products can be directly observed in hematoxylin- and eosin-stained sections (e.g., the inclusion bodies formed by CMV and herpesvirus; bacterial clumps, which usually stain blue; *Candida* and *Mucor* among the fungi; most protozoans; and all helminths). Many infectious agents, however, are best visualized by special stains that identify organisms on the basis of particular characteristics of their cell walls or coat—Gram, acid-fast, silver, mucicarmine, and Giemsa stains—or after labeling with specific antibody probes (Table 8–9). Regardless of the staining technique, organisms are usually best visualized at the advancing edge of a lesion rather than at its center, particularly if there is necrosis.

TABLE 8–9 Special Techniques for Diagnosing Infectious Agents

Gram stain	Most bacteria
Acid-fast stain	Mycobacteria, nocardiae (modified)
Silver stains	Fungi, legionellae, pneumocystis
Periodic acid–Schiff	Fungi, amebae
Mucicarmine	Cryptococci
Giemsa	Campylobacteria, leishmaniae, malaria parasites
Antibody probes	Viruses, rickettsiae
Culture	All classes
DNA probes	Viruses, bacteria, protozoa

Nucleic acid–based tests have become routine methods for detecting or quantifying several pathogens. Molecular diagnostics have become particularly important in the care of people infected with HIV.[40] Quantification of the viral RNA is an important guide to antiretroviral therapy. The management of hepatitis B and C infections is similarly guided by nucleic acid–based viral quantification or typing to predict resistance to antiviral drugs.

Nucleic acid amplification tests (NAATs), such as polymerase chain reaction (PCR) and transcription-mediated amplification, have become routine for diagnosis of gonorrhea, chlamydia, tuberculosis, and herpes encephalitis. In some cases, molecular assays are much more sensitive than conventional testing.[41,42] PCR testing of cerebrospinal fluid (CSF) for herpes simplex virus encephalitis has a sensitivity of about 80%, while viral culture of CSF has a sensitivity of less than 10%. Similarly, NAATs for genital chlamydia detect 10% to 30% more infections than does conventional chlamydia culture. In other cases, such as gonorrhea, the sensitivity of NAAT testing is similar to that of culture.

SPECTRUM OF INFLAMMATORY RESPONSES TO INFECTION

In contrast to the vast molecular diversity of microbes, the morphologic patterns of tissue responses to microbes are limited, as are the mechanisms directing these responses. At the microscopic level, therefore, many pathogens produce identical reaction patterns, and few features are unique or pathognomonic for a particular microorganism. Moreover, it is the interaction between the microorganism and the host that determines the histologic features of the inflammatory response. Thus, pyogenic bacteria, which normally evoke vigorous leukocyte responses, may cause rapid tissue necrosis with little leukocyte exudation in a profoundly neutropenic host. Similarly, in a normal patient, *M. tuberculosis* causes well-formed granulomas with few mycobacteria present, whereas in an AIDS patient, the same mycobacteria multiply profusely in macrophages, which fail to coalesce into granulomas.

There are five major histologic patterns of tissue reaction in infections.

Suppurative (Polymorphonuclear) Inflammation

This pattern is the reaction to acute tissue damage, described in Chapter 2, characterized by increased vascular permeability and leukocytic infiltration, predominantly of neutrophils (Fig. 8–7). The neutrophils are attracted to the site of infection by release of chemoattractants from the "pyogenic" bacteria that evoke this response, mostly extracellular Gram-positive cocci and Gram-negative rods. Massing of neutrophils forms pus. The sizes of exudative lesions vary from tiny microabscesses formed in multiple organs during bacterial sepsis secondary to a colonized heart valve to diffuse involvement of entire lobes of the lung during pneumonia. How destructive the lesions are depends on their location and the organism involved. For example, pneumococci usually spare alveolar walls and cause lobar pneumonia that resolves

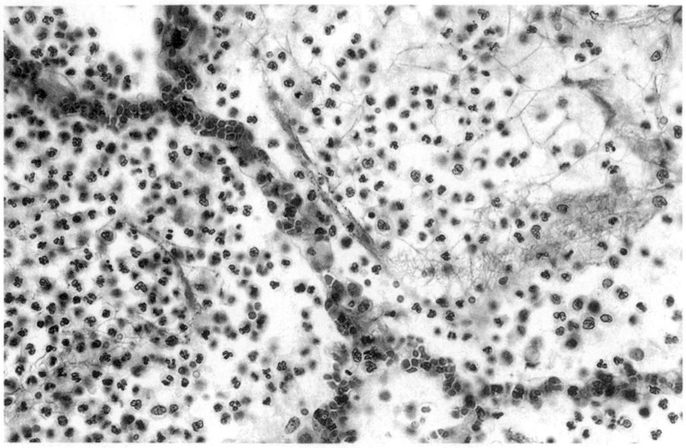

FIGURE 8–7 Pneumococcal pneumonia. Note the intra-alveolar polymorphonuclear exudate and intact alveolar septa.

completely, whereas staphylococci and *Klebsiella* species destroy alveolar walls and form abscesses that heal with scar formation. Bacterial pharyngitis resolves without sequelae, whereas untreated acute bacterial inflammation of a joint can destroy it in a few days.

Mononuclear and Granulomatous Inflammation

Diffuse, predominantly mononuclear, interstitial infiltrates are a common feature of all chronic inflammatory processes, but when they develop acutely, they often are a response to viruses, intracellular bacteria, or intracellular parasites. In addition, spirochetes and helminths provoke chronic inflammatory responses. Which mononuclear cell predominates within the inflammatory lesion depends on the host immune response to the organism. For example, mostly plasma cells are seen in the primary and secondary lesions of syphilis, whereas lymphocytes predominate in HBV infection or viral infections of the brain (Fig. 8–8). The presence of these lymphocytes reflects cell-mediated immune responses against the pathogen or pathogen-infected cells. At the other extreme, macrophages may become filled with organisms, as occurs in *Mycobacterium avium-intracellulare* infections in AIDS patients, who cannot mount an effective immune response to the organisms. *Granulomatous inflammation* is a distinctive form of mononuclear inflammation usually evoked by infectious agents that resist eradication (e.g., *M. tuberculosis, Histoplasma capsulatum*, schistosome eggs) and are capable of stimulating strong T cell–mediated immunity. Granulomatous inflammation is characterized by accumulation of activated macrophages called "epithelioid" cells, which may fuse to form giant cells. In some cases, there is a central area of caseous necrosis (see tuberculosis section in this chapter and Chapter 2).

Cytopathic-Cytoproliferative Inflammation

These reactions are usually produced by viruses. The lesions are characterized by cell necrosis or cellular proliferation, usually with sparse inflammatory cells. Some viruses replicate within cells and make viral aggregates that are visible as inclusion bodies (e.g., herpesviruses or adenovirus) or induce cells to fuse and form multinucleated cells called polykaryons (e.g., measles virus or herpesviruses). Focal cell damage in the skin may cause epithelial cells to become detached, forming blisters (Fig. 8–9). Some viruses can cause epithelial cells to proliferate (e.g., venereal warts caused by human papillomavirus or the umbilicated papules of molluscum contagiosum caused by poxviruses). Finally, viruses can cause dysplastic changes and contribute to the development of malignant neoplasms (Chapter 7).

Necrotizing Inflammation

Clostridium perfringens and other organisms that secrete powerful toxins can cause such rapid and severe necrosis (gangrenous necrosis) that tissue damage is the dominant feature. Because few inflammatory cells are present, these lesions resemble infarcts with disruption or loss of basophilic nuclear staining and preservation of cellular outlines. Clostridia are often opportunistic pathogens that are introduced into muscle tissue by penetrating trauma or infection of the bowel in a neutropenic host. Similarly, the parasite *Entamoeba histolytica* causes colonic ulcers and liver abscesses characterized by extensive tissue destruction with liquefactive necrosis and without a prominent inflammatory infiltrate. By entirely

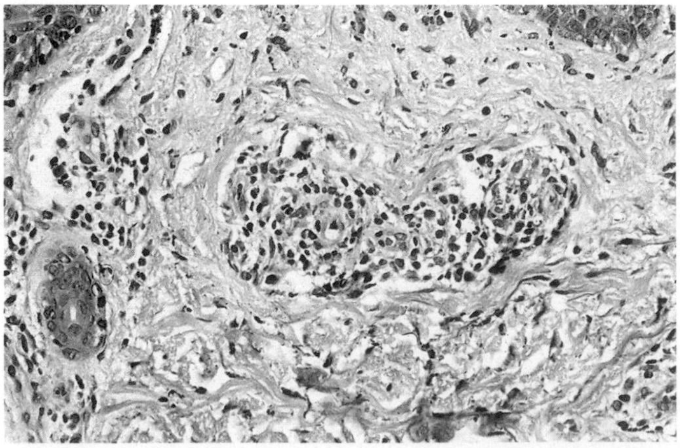

FIGURE 8–8 Secondary syphilis in the dermis with perivascular lymphoplasmacytic infiltrate and endothelial proliferation.

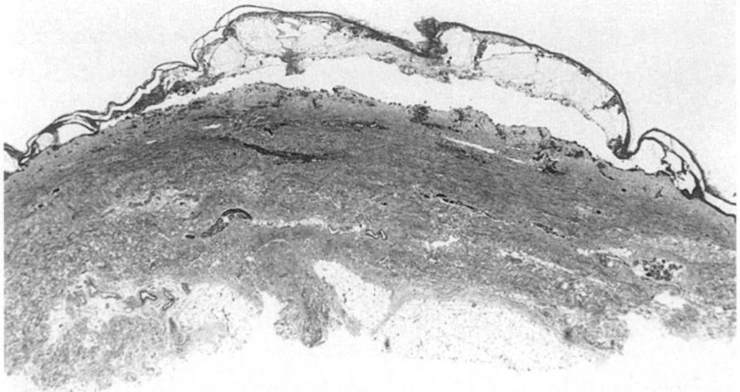

FIGURE 8–9 Herpesvirus blister in mucosa. See Figure 8–13 for viral inclusions.

different mechanisms, viruses can cause widespread and severe necrosis of host cells, with inflammation, as exemplified by total destruction of the temporal lobes of the brain by herpesvirus or the liver by HBV.

Chronic Inflammation and Scarring

The final common pathway of many infections is chronic inflammation, which can lead either to complete healing or to extensive scarring. For example, chronic HBV infection may cause cirrhosis of the liver, in which dense fibrous septae surround nodules of regenerating hepatocytes. Sometimes the exuberant scarring response is the major cause of dysfunction (e.g., the "pipe-stem" fibrosis of the liver or fibrosis of the bladder wall caused by schistosomal eggs or the constrictive fibrous pericarditis in tuberculosis) (Fig. 8–10).

These patterns of tissue reaction are useful guidelines for analyzing microscopic features of infectious processes, but they rarely appear in pure form because different types of host reactions often occur at the same time. For example, the lung of an AIDS patient may be infected with CMV, which causes cytolytic changes, and at the same time by *Pneumocystis*, which causes interstitial inflammation. Similar patterns of inflammation also can be seen in tissue responses to physical or chemical agents and in inflammatory diseases of unknown cause (Chapter 2).

This concludes our discussion of the general principles of the pathogenesis and pathology of infectious disease. We now turn to descriptions of specific infections caused by viruses, bacteria, fungi, and parasites. In this discussion, we emphasize *pathogenic mechanisms* and *pathologic changes*, rather than details of clinical features, which are available in clinical textbooks. Several infections that typically involve a specific organ are in the appropriate chapter.

Viral Infections

TRANSIENT INFECTIONS

The viruses that cause transient infections are structurally heterogeneous, but each elicits an effective immune response that eliminates the virus and may or may not confer lifelong protection. The mumps virus, for example, has only one serotype and infects people only once, whereas other transient viruses, such as influenza viruses, can repeatedly infect the same individual owing to antigenic variation. The immune response to some transient viruses wanes with time, allowing even the same serotype of virus to infect repeatedly (e.g., respiratory syncytial virus).

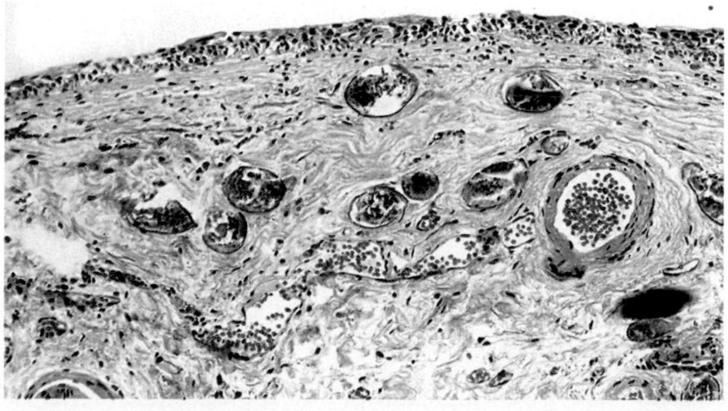

FIGURE 8–10 *Schistosoma haematobium* infection of the bladder with numerous calcified eggs and extensive scarring.

Measles

Measles (rubeola) virus is a leading cause of vaccine-preventable death and illness worldwide. In 2001, there were an estimated 30 million cases of measles, including 777,000 deaths, most of which occurred in developing countries. Because of poor nutrition, children in developing countries are 10 to 1000 times more likely to die of measles pneumonia than are Western children.[43] Epidemics of measles occur among unvaccinated individuals. Measles can produce severe disease in people with defects in cellular immunity (such as HIV-infected patients or patients with hematologic malignancy).[44] In the United States, the incidence of measles has decreased dramatically since 1963, when a measles vaccine was licensed.[45]

Pathogenesis Measles virus is a single-stranded RNA virus of the paramyxovirus family that includes mumps, respiratory syncytial virus (the major cause of lower respiratory infections in infants), parainfluenza virus (a cause of croup), and human metapneumovirus. There is only one strain of measles virus. Two cell-surface receptors have been identified for measles virus: CD46, a complement regulatory protein that inactivates C3 convertases, and signaling lymphocytic activation molecule (SLAM), a molecule involved in T-cell activation.[46,47] CD46 is expressed on all nucleated cells, while SLAM is expressed on cells of the immune system. Both these receptors bind the viral hemagglutinin protein. Measles virus is spread by respiratory droplets, initially multiplies within upper respiratory epithelial cells, and then spreads to lymphoid tissues, where it can replicate in mononuclear cells, including T lymphocytes, macrophages, and dendritic cells. Virus then spreads by the blood throughout the body. Most children develop T cell–mediated immunity to measles virus that controls the viral infection and produces the measles rash, a hypersensitivity reaction to viral antigens in the skin. Measles may cause croup, pneumonia, diarrhea with protein-losing enteropathy, keratitis with scarring and blindness, encephalitis, and hemorrhagic rashes ("black measles") in malnourished children with poor medical care. The rash does not occur in patients with deficiencies in cell-mediated immunity but does occur in agammaglobulinemic patients. Antibody-mediated immunity to measles virus protects against reinfection. Measles also can cause immunosuppression, and measles virus interactions with SLAM on T cells or dendritic cells may explain some of these immunosuppressive effects.[48,49] Subacute sclerosing panencephalitis (SSPE, described in Chapter 28) and measles inclusion body encephalitis (in immunocompromised individuals) are rare late complications of measles. The pathogenesis of SSPE is not well understood, but a replication-defective variant of measles may be involved in this persistent viral infection.[50]

Morphology. The blotchy, reddish brown rash of measles virus infection on the face, trunk, and proximal extremities is produced by dilated skin vessels, edema, and a moderate, nonspecific, mononuclear perivascular infiltrate. Ulcerated mucosal lesions in the oral cavity near the opening of Stensen ducts (the pathognomonic Koplik spots) are marked by necrosis, neutrophilic exudate, and neovascularization. The lymphoid organs typically have marked follicular hyperplasia, large germinal centers, and randomly distributed multinucleate giant cells, called Warthin-Finkeldey cells, which have eosinophilic nuclear and cytoplasmic inclusion bodies. These are pathognomonic of measles and are also found in the lung and sputum (Fig. 8–11). The milder forms of measles pneumonia show the same peribronchial and interstitial mononuclear cell infiltration that is seen in other nonlethal viral infections. In severe or neglected cases, bacterial superinfection may be a cause of death.

Mumps

Like measles virus, mumps virus is a member of the paramyxovirus family. Mumps virus has two types of surface glycoproteins, one with hemagglutinin and neuraminidase activities and the other with cell fusion and hemolytic activities. Mumps viruses enter the upper respiratory tract through inhalation of respiratory droplets, spread to draining lymph nodes where they replicate in lymphocytes (preferentially in activated T cells), and then spread through the blood to the salivary and other glands. Mumps virus infects salivary gland ductal epithelial cells, resulting in desquamation of involved cells, edema, and inflammation that leads to the classic signs of mumps: salivary gland pain and swelling. Mumps virus also can spread to other sites, including the central nervous system, testis and ovary, and pancreas. Aseptic meningitis is the most common extrasalivary gland complication of mumps infection, occurring in about 10% of cases. The mumps vaccine has reduced the incidence of mumps by 99% in the United States.[51]

Morphology. In **mumps parotitis**, which is bilateral in 70% of cases, affected glands are enlarged, have a doughy consistency, and are moist, glistening, and reddish brown on cross-section. On microscopic examination, the gland interstitium is edematous and diffusely infiltrated by macrophages, lymphocytes, and plasma cells, which compress acini and ducts. Neutrophils and necrotic debris may fill the ductal lumen and cause focal damage to the ductal epithelium.

In **mumps orchitis**, testicular swelling may be marked, caused by edema, mononuclear cell infiltration, and focal hemorrhages. Because the testis is tightly contained within the tunica albuginea, parenchymal swelling may compromise the blood supply and cause areas of infarction. Sterility, when it occurs, is caused by scars and atrophy of the testis after resolution of viral infection.

In the enzyme-rich **pancreas**, lesions may be destructive, causing parenchymal and fat necrosis and neutrophil-rich inflammation. **Mumps encephalitis** causes perivenous demyelination and perivascular mononuclear cuffing.

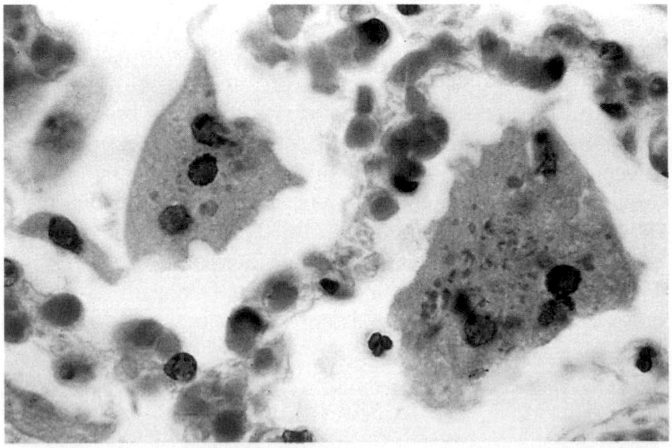

FIGURE 8–11 Measles giant cells in the lung. Note the glassy eosinophilic intranuclear inclusions.

Poliovirus Infection

Poliovirus is a spherical, unencapsulated RNA virus of the enterovirus genus. Other enteroviruses cause childhood diarrhea as well as rashes (coxsackievirus A), conjunctivitis (enterovirus 70), viral meningitis (coxsackieviruses and echovirus), myopericarditis (coxsackievirus B), and jaundice (hepatitis A virus). There are three major strains of poliovirus, each of which is included in the Salk formalin-fixed (killed) vaccine and the Sabin oral, attenuated (live) vaccine.[52] These vaccines, which have nearly eliminated poliovirus from the Western hemisphere, may get rid of polio from the earth, because the poliovirus, like smallpox virus, infects people but not other animals, is only briefly shed, does not undergo antigenic variation, and is effectively prevented by immunization.[53] Poliovirus is still present in India and Africa.

Poliovirus, like other enteroviruses, is transmitted by the fecal-oral route. It first infects tissues in the oropharynx, is secreted into the saliva and swallowed, and then multiplies in the intestinal mucosa and lymph nodes, causing a transient viremia and fever. The species specificity of poliovirus for humans is determined by particular amino acid residues that are present in the human receptor, CD155, which is an immunoglobulin superfamily member.[54] Although most polio infections are asymptomatic, in about 1 of 100 infected persons, poliovirus invades the central nervous system and replicates in motor neurons of the spinal cord (spinal poliomyelitis) or brain stem (bulbar poliomyelitis). Antiviral antibodies control the disease in most cases, and it is not known why they fail to contain the virus in some individuals. Virus spread to the nervous system may be secondary to viremia or by retrograde transport of the virus along axons of motor neurons.[55] Rare cases of poliomyelitis that occur after vaccination are caused by mutations of the attenuated viruses to wild type forms. The neurologic features and neuropathology of poliovirus infection are described in Chapter 28.

West Nile Virus

West Nile virus is an arthropod-borne virus (arbovirus) of the flavivirus group, which also includes viruses that cause dengue fever, Eastern encephalitis, and yellow fever. West Nile virus has a broad geographic distribution in the Old World, with outbreaks in Africa, the Middle East, Europe, Southeast Asia, and Australia. This virus was first detected in the United States in 1999 during an outbreak in New York City in which there were 62 cases of encephalitis and seven deaths.[56,57] West Nile virus is transmitted by mosquitoes to birds and to mammals. Wild birds develop prolonged viremia and are the major reservoir for the virus. Humans are usually incidental hosts. Virus has also been transmitted by transplanted organs.[58]

West Nile virus infection is usually asymptomatic, but in 20% of infected individuals, it gives rise to a mild, short-lived febrile illness associated with headache and myalgia. A maculopapular rash is seen in approximately half the cases.[58] CNS complications (meningitis, encephalitis, meningoencephalitis) are not frequent, occurring in about one in 150 clinically apparent infections. They manifest as acute flaccid paralysis, clinically indistinguishable from polio. There is a mortality of about 10% in patients with meningoencephalitis and long-term cognitive and neurologic impairment in many survivors. Perivascular and leptomeningeal chronic inflammation, microglial nodules, and neuronophagia predominantly involving the temporal lobes and brain stem have been observed in the brains of patients who died of West Nile virus infection. Immunosuppressed persons and the elderly appear to be at the greatest risk for severe disease. Rare complications include hepatitis, myocarditis, and pancreatitis.

The pathogenesis of severe CNS disease is not yet clear. Limited studies in animal models suggest that West Nile virus envelope proteins may be important for CNS tropism and that macrophage depletion may predispose to CNS disease.[59]

Viral Hemorrhagic Fevers

Viral hemorrhagic fevers (VHFs) are systemic infections characterized by fever and hemorrhage. They are caused by enveloped RNA viruses in four different families: arenaviruses, filoviruses, bunyaviruses, and flaviviruses. Although structurally distinct, these viruses all depend on an animal or insect host for survival and transmission. VHF viruses are restricted geographically to areas in which their hosts reside. Humans are infected when they come into contact with infected hosts or insect vectors, but humans are not the natural reservoir for any of these viruses. Although uncommon, human-to-human transmission can occur. The infectious dose for VHF viruses appears to be low. Hemorrhagic fever viruses produce a spectrum of illnesses, ranging from relatively mild acute disease characterized by fever, headache, myalgia, rash, neutropenia, and thrombocytopenia to severe, life-threatening disease in which there is sudden hemodynamic deterioration and shock. Human cases or outbreaks of hemorrhagic fevers are sporadic and unpredictable. There are no cures or effective drug therapy for viral hemorrhagic fevers. VHF viruses are potential biologic weapons owing to their infectious properties, morbidity and mortality, and the absence of therapy and vaccines.

The pathogenesis of hemorrhagic fever viruses is not well understood. These viruses enter the bloodstream by a number of routes, including the bite of an insect, and following inhalation or mucous membrane exposure. All (except for hantaviruses) cause disease during the period of viremia. Endothelial cell infection occurs with the majority of VHF viruses. The hemorrhagic manifestations are due to thrombocytopenia or severe platelet or endothelial dysfunction. Typically, there is increased vascular permeability. There may be necrosis and hemorrhage in many organs, and often there is widespread hepatocellular necrosis. Infection with many VHF viruses stimulates cytokine production, which may contribute to severe cytopathic effects or disseminated intravascular coagulation (DIC).

CHRONIC LATENT INFECTIONS (HERPESVIRUS INFECTIONS)

Herpesviruses are large encapsulated viruses that have a double-stranded DNA genome that encodes approximately 70 proteins. Herpesviruses cause acute infection followed by latent infection in which the viruses persist in a noninfectious form with periodic reactivation and shedding of infectious virus. Latency is operationally defined as the inability to recover infectious particles from cells that harbor the virus. There are nine types of human herpesviruses, belonging to three subgroups defined by the type of cell most frequently infected and the site of latency: *α-group viruses*, including herpes simplex virus-1 (HSV-1), HSV-2, and varicella zoster virus (VZV), which infect epithelial cells and produce latent infection in neurons; *lymphotropic β-group viruses*, including CMV, human herpesvirus 6 (which causes exanthem subitum, also known as roseola infantum and sixth disease, a benign rash of infants), and human herpesvirus 7 (which is not yet associated with a specific disease), which infect and produce latent infection in a variety of cell types; and the *γ-group viruses*: EBV and KSHV/HHV-8, the cause of Kaposi sarcoma,[60] which produce latent infection mainly in lymphoid cells. In addition, herpesvirus simiae is an Old World monkey virus that resembles HSV-1 and can cause fatal neurologic disease in animal handlers, usually resulting from an animal bite.

Herpes Simplex Virus

HSV-1 and HSV-2 differ serologically but are genetically similar and cause a similar set of primary and recurrent infections.[61] These viruses produce acute and latent infections. Both viruses replicate in the skin and the mucous membranes at the site of entrance of the virus (usually oropharynx or genitals), where they produce infectious virions and cause vesicular lesions of the epidermis. The viruses spread to sensory neurons that innervate these primary sites of replication. Viral nucleocapsids are transported along axons to the neuronal cell bodies, where the viruses establish latent infection. During latency, the viral DNA remains within the nucleus of the neuron, and only latency-associated viral mRNAs (called LATs or latency-associated transcripts) are synthesized.[62,63] In this state, no viral proteins appear to be produced, thus allowing the virus to evade immune recognition. In immunocompetent hosts, primary HSV infection resolves in a few weeks, although the virus remains latent in nerve cells. Reactivation of HSV-1 and HSV-2 may occur repeatedly with or without symptoms, and results in the spread of virus from the neurons to the skin or to mucous membranes. Reactivation from latency occurs in the presence of host immunity, and herpesviruses have developed ways to avoid immune recognition. Herpes simplex viruses can evade antiviral CTL by inhibiting the MHC class I recognition pathway, and elude humoral immune defenses by producing receptors for the Fc domain of immunoglobulin and inhibitors of complement.[15, 36, 37]

In addition to causing cutaneous lesions, HSV-1 is the major infectious cause of corneal blindness in the United States; corneal epithelial disease is thought to be due to direct viral damage, while corneal stromal disease appears to be immune mediated.[64] HSV-1 is also the major cause of fatal sporadic encephalitis in the United States, when the virus spreads to the brain, particularly the temporal lobes and orbital gyri of the frontal lobes. In addition, neonates and individuals with compromised cellular immunity (e.g., secondary to HIV infection or chemotherapy) may suffer disseminated herpesvirus infections.

Morphology. All HSV lesions are marked by formation of large, pink to purple intranuclear inclusions (Cowdry type A) that contain intact and disrupted virions and push darkly stained host cell chromatin to the edges of the nucleus (Fig. 8–12). Although cell and nuclear size increase only slightly, herpesvirus produces inclusion-bearing multinucleated syncytia.

HSV-1 and HSV-2 cause lesions ranging from self-limited cold sores and gingivostomatitis to life-threatening disseminated visceral infections and encephalitis. **Fever blisters or cold sores** favor the facial skin around mucosal orifices (lips, nose), where their distribution is frequently bilateral and independent of skin dermatomes. Intraepithelial vesicles (blisters), which are formed by intracellular edema and ballooning degeneration of epidermal cells, frequently burst and crust over, but some may result in superficial ulcerations.

Gingivostomatitis, which is usually encountered in children, is caused by HSV-1. It is a vesicular eruption extending from the tongue to the retropharynx and causing cervical lymphadenopathy. Swollen, erythematous HSV lesions of the fingers or palm (herpetic whitlow) occur in infants and, occasionally, in health care workers.

Genital herpes is usually caused by HSV-2, but HSV-1 can also cause genital lesions. Genital herpes is characterized by vesicles on the genital mucous membranes as well as on the external genitalia that are rapidly converted into superficial ulcerations, rimmed by an inflammatory infiltrate (Chapter 22). Herpesvirus (usually HSV-2) can be transmitted to neonates during passage through the birth canal of infected mothers. Although HSV-2 disease in the neonate may be mild, more often it is fulminating with generalized lymphadenopathy, splenomegaly, and necrotic foci throughout the lungs, liver, adrenals, and central nervous system.

Two forms of **corneal lesions** are caused by HSV (Chapter 29). **Herpes epithelial keratitis** shows typical virus-induced cytolysis of the superficial epithelium and is sensitive to antiviral drugs. In contrast, **herpes stromal keratitis** shows infiltrates of mononuclear cells around keratinocytes and endothelial cells, leading to neovascularization, scarring, opacification of the cornea, and eventual blindness. This is an immunologic reaction to the HSV infection and responds to corticosteroid therapy.

Herpes simplex encephalitis is described in Chapter 28.

Disseminated skin and visceral herpes infections are usually encountered in hospitalized patients with some form of underlying cancer or immunosuppression. **Kaposi varicelliform eruption** is a generalized vesiculating involvement of the skin, whereas **eczema herpeticum** is characterized by confluent, pustular, or hemorrhagic blisters, often with bacterial superinfection and viral dissemination to internal viscera. **Herpes esophagitis** is frequently complicated by superinfection with bacteria or fungi. **Herpes bronchopneumonia**, which may be introduced with an airway inserted through oral herpes lesions, is often necrotizing, and **herpes hepatitis** may cause liver failure.

As described in Chapter 6, KSHV/HHV8 is implicated in the pathogenesis of **Kaposi sarcoma**. KSHV encodes proteins that can evade host immune defenses, disrupt cell cycle regulation, inhibit apoptosis, and affect intracellular signal transduction.

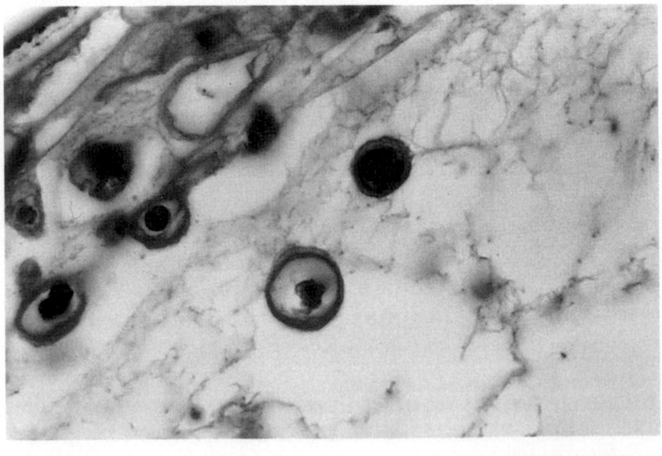

FIGURE 8–12 High-power view of cells from the blister in Figure 8–9 showing glassy intranuclear herpes simplex inclusion bodies.

Cytomegalovirus

Cytomegalovirus (CMV), a β-group herpesvirus, can produce a variety of disease manifestations, depending on the age of the host, and, more important, on the host's immune status. The major envelope glycoprotein of CMV binds to epidermal growth factor receptor;[60] it is not known if the virus uses this and other receptors to gain entry into different cell types in natural infections. CMV infects and remains latent in white blood cells and can be reactivated when cellular immunity is depressed. CMV causes an asymptomatic or mononucleosis-like infection in healthy individuals but devastating systemic infections in neonates and in immunocompromised patients. As its name implies, cytomegalovirus produces enlargement of infected cells. Infected cells exhibit gigantism of both the entire cell and its nucleus. Within the nucleus is a large inclusion surrounded by a clear halo (owl's eye).

Transmission of CMV can occur by several mechanisms, depending on the age group affected.[65,66] These include the following:

- Transplacental transmission from a newly acquired or primary infection in a mother who does not have protective antibodies ("congenital CMV").

- Transmission of the virus through cervical or vaginal secretions at birth or, later, through breast milk from a mother who has active infection ("perinatal CMV").
- Transmission through saliva during preschool years, especially in day care centers. Toddlers so infected readily transmit the virus to their parents.
- Transmission by the venereal route is the dominant mode after about 15 years of age, but spread may also occur via respiratory secretions and the fecal-oral route.
- Iatrogenic transmission can occur at any age through organ transplants or by blood transfusions.

CMV can induce transient but severe immunosuppression. Mouse CMV can infect dendritic cells and impair their function and maturation and their ability to stimulate T-cell responses, and it appears that human CMV also can infect dendritic cells and alter their function.[65,67] Similar to other herpesviruses, CMV can elude immune responses by down-modulating MHC class I and II molecules and producing homologues of TNF receptor, IL-10, and MHC class I receptors.[15,36,37,68] Interestingly, CMV can both activate and evade natural killer cells by inducing ligands for activating receptors and class I–like proteins that engage inhibitory receptors. Thus, CMV can both hide from immune defenses and actively suppress immune responses.

Morphology. The characteristic enlargement of infected cells can be appreciated histologically. Prominent intranuclear basophilic inclusions spanning half the nuclear diameter are usually set off from the nuclear membrane by a clear halo (Fig. 8–13). Within the cytoplasm of these cells, smaller basophilic inclusions can also be seen. In the glandular organs, the parenchymal epithelial cells are affected; in the brain, the neurons; in the lungs, the alveolar macrophages and epithelial and endothelial cells; and in the kidneys, the tubular epithelial and glomerular endothelial cells. Affected cells are strikingly enlarged, often to a diameter of 40 μm, and they show cellular and nuclear polymorphism. Disseminated CMV causes focal necrosis with minimal inflammation in virtually any organ.

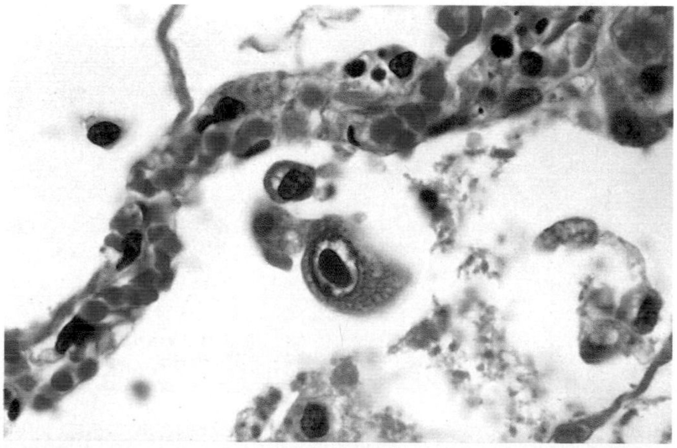

FIGURE 8–13 Cytomegalovirus: distinct nuclear and ill-defined cytoplasmic inclusions in the lung.

Congenital Infections. Infection acquired in utero may take many forms. In approximately 95% of cases, it is asymptomatic. However, sometimes when the virus is acquired from a mother with primary infection (who does not have protective immunoglobulins), classic *cytomegalic inclusion disease (CID)* develops. CID resembles erythroblastosis fetalis. Affected infants may suffer intrauterine growth retardation, be profoundly ill, and manifest jaundice, hepatosplenomegaly, anemia, bleeding due to thrombocytopenia, and encephalitis. In fatal cases, the brain is often smaller than normal (microcephaly) and may show foci of calcification.

The infants who survive usually bear permanent effects, including mental retardation, hearing loss, and other neurologic impairments. The congenital infection is not always devastating, however, and may take the form of interstitial pneumonitis, hepatitis, or a hematologic disorder. Most infants with this milder form of CID recover, although a few develop mental retardation later. Uncommonly, a totally asymptomatic infection may be followed months to years later by neurologic sequelae, including delayed-onset mental retardation and hearing deficits.

Perinatal Infections. Infection acquired during passage through the birth canal or from breast milk is asymptomatic in the vast majority of cases, although, uncommonly, infants may develop an interstitial pneumonitis, failure to thrive, skin rash, or hepatitis. These children have acquired maternal antibodies against CMV, which reduce the severity of disease. Despite the lack of symptoms, many of these patients continue to excrete CMV in their urine or saliva for months to years. Subtle effects on hearing and intelligence later in life have been reported in some studies.

Cytomegalovirus Mononucleosis. In healthy young children and adults, the disease is nearly always asymptomatic. In surveys around the world, 50% to 100% of adults demonstrate anti-CMV antibodies in the serum, indicating previous exposure. *The most common clinical manifestation of CMV infection in immunocompetent hosts beyond the neonatal period is an infectious mononucleosis-like illness, with fever, atypical lymphocytosis, lymphadenopathy, and hepatomegaly accompanied by abnormal liver function test results, suggesting mild hepatitis.* Most patients recover without any sequelae, although excretion of the virus may occur in body fluids for months to years.

Irrespective of the presence or absence of symptoms following infection, a person once infected becomes seropositive for life. The virus remains latent within leukocytes, which are the major reservoirs.

CMV in Immunosuppressed Individuals. This occurs most commonly in three groups of patients:

- *Recipients of solid organ transplants* (heart, liver, kidney) from seropositive donors. These patients typically receive immunosuppressive therapy, and the CMV is usually derived from the donor organ, but reactivation of latent CMV infection in the host may also occur.
- *Recipients of allogeneic bone marrow transplants.* These patients are immunosuppressed not only because of immunosuppressive therapy but also because of poor marrow function until it is engrafted. In this setting, there is usually reactivation of latent CMV in the recipient.
- *Patients with AIDS.* These immunosuppressed individuals have reactivation of latent infection and are also infected

by their sexual partners. *CMV is the most common opportunistic viral pathogen in AIDS.*

In all these settings, serious, life-threatening disseminated CMV infections primarily affect the lungs (pneumonitis), gastrointestinal tract (colitis), and retina (retinitis); the central nervous system is usually spared. In the pulmonary infection, an interstitial mononuclear infiltrate with foci of necrosis develops, accompanied by the typical enlarged cells with inclusions. The pneumonitis can progress to full-blown acute respiratory distress syndrome. Intestinal necrosis and ulceration can develop and be extensive, leading to the formation of pseudomembranes and debilitating diarrhea. CMV retinitis, by far the most common form of opportunistic CMV disease, can occur either alone or in combination with involvement of the lungs and intestinal tract. Diagnosis of CMV infections is made by demonstration of characteristic morphologic alterations in tissue sections, viral culture, rising antiviral antibody titer, detection of CMV antigens, and qualitative or quantitative PCR-based detection of CMV DNA. The PCR-based methods have revolutionized the approach to monitoring patients after transplantation.

Varicella-Zoster Virus

Two conditions—chickenpox and shingles—are caused by varicella zoster virus (VZV). Acute infection with VZV causes chickenpox; reactivation of latent VZV causes shingles (also called herpes zoster). Chickenpox is mild in children but more severe in adults and in immunocompromised patients. Shingles is a source of morbidity in elderly and immunosuppressed persons.[69] Like HSV, VZV infects mucous membranes, skin, and neurons and causes a self-limited primary infection in immunocompetent individuals. Also like HSV, VZV evades immune responses and establishes a latent infection in sensory ganglia.[62] In contrast to HSV, VZV is transmitted in epidemic fashion by aerosols, disseminates hematogenously, and causes widespread vesicular skin lesions. VZV infects neurons and/or satellite cells around neurons in the dorsal root ganglia and may recur many years after the primary infection, causing shingles. Localized recurrence of VZV is most frequent and painful in dermatomes innervated by the trigeminal ganglia, where VZV is most likely to exist in a state of latency. In contrast to numerous recurrences of HSV, VZV usually recurs only once, most frequently in immunosuppressed or elderly persons.

Morphology. The **chickenpox** rash occurs approximately 2 weeks after respiratory infection and travels in multiple waves centrifugally from the torso to the head and extremities. Each lesion progresses rapidly from a macule to a vesicle, which resembles a dewdrop on a rose petal. On histologic examination, chickenpox vesicles contain intranuclear inclusions in the epithelial cells like those of HSV-1 (Fig. 8–14). After a few days, most chickenpox vesicles rupture, crust over, and heal by regeneration, leaving no scars. Traumatic rupture of some vesicles with bacterial superinfection may lead to destruction of the basal epidermal layer and residual scarring.

Shingles occurs when VZVs that have long remained latent in the dorsal root ganglia after a previous chickenpox infection are reactivated and infect sensory nerves that carry viruses to one or more dermatomes. There, VZVs cause vesicular lesions, which are differentiated from chickenpox by the often intense itching, burning, or sharp pain because of the simultaneous radiculoneuritis. This pain is especially strong when the trigeminal nerves are involved; rarely, the geniculate nucleus is involved, causing facial paralysis (Ramsay Hunt syndrome). In the sensory ganglia, there is a dense, predominantly mononuclear infiltrate, with herpetic intranuclear inclusions within neurons and their supporting cells (Fig. 8–15). VZV also causes interstitial pneumonia, encephalitis, transverse myelitis, and necrotizing visceral lesions, particularly in immunosuppressed patients.

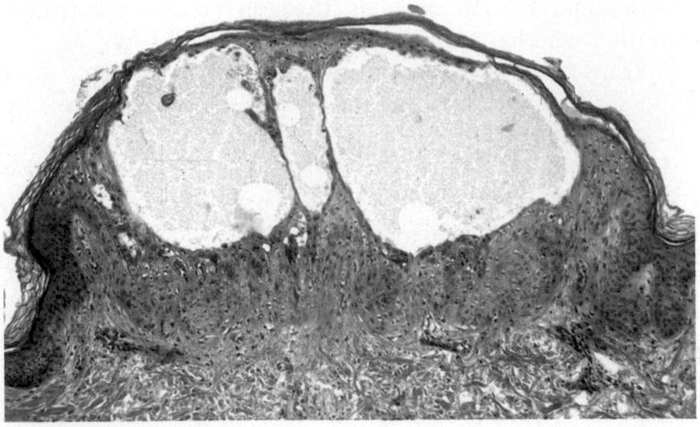

FIGURE 8–14 Skin lesion of chickenpox (varicella zoster virus) with intraepithelial vesicle.

CHRONIC PRODUCTIVE INFECTIONS

In some infections, the immune system is unable to eliminate the virus, and viral replication leads to persistent viremia.

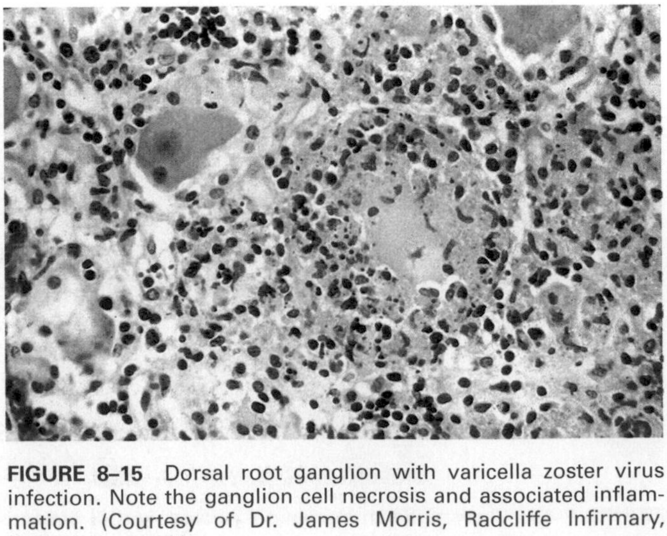

FIGURE 8–15 Dorsal root ganglion with varicella zoster virus infection. Note the ganglion cell necrosis and associated inflammation. (Courtesy of Dr. James Morris, Radcliffe Infirmary, Oxford, England.)

The high mutation rate of viruses such as HIV and hepatitis B may allow them to escape control by the immune system.

Hepatitis B Virus

Hepatitis B virus (HBV), the etiologic agent of "serum hepatitis," is a significant cause of acute and chronic liver disease worldwide.[70] Here we will briefly discuss HBV as an example of a chronic productive viral infection; viral hepatitis is discussed in detail in Chapter 18. HBV, a member of the hepadnavirus family, is a DNA virus that can be transmitted percutaneously (e.g., intravenous drug use or blood transfusion), perinatally, and sexually. HBV has a unique replicative cycle. It synthesizes its DNA genome by reverse transcription of an RNA template. The lack of proofreading function of the reverse transcriptase results in a high mutation rate for HBV and creates an opportunity for selection of mutants that have an advantage for growth or avoidance of immune recognition. Progeny viral DNA can integrate into the host genome, and this is associated with rearrangement of viral and host flanking sequences that can affect viral and host gene expression. HBV infects hepatocytes, and cellular injury occurs mainly due to the immune response to infected liver cells and not to cytopathic effects of the virus. HBV may evade immune defenses by inhibiting IFN-β production and by downregulating viral gene expression.[71] The effectiveness of the CTL response is a major determinant of whether a person clears the virus or becomes a chronic carrier. When infected hepatocytes are destroyed by CTLs, replicating virus is also eliminated and the infection is cleared. However, if the rate of infection of hepatocytes outpaces the ability of CTLs to eliminate infected cells, a chronic infection is established. This may happen in 5% to 10% of adults and up to 90% of children infected perinatally. In this setting, the liver develops a chronic hepatitis, with lymphocytic inflammation, apoptotic hepatocytes resulting from CTL-mediated killing, and progressive destruction of the liver parenchyma. Viral mutants arise during chronic infection, and it has been hypothesized that these might modulate the severity of disease by changing the expression of certain immunogenic epitopes or altering viral replication levels. Long-term viral replication can lead to cirrhosis of the liver and an increased risk for hepatocellular carcinoma. The morphology and pathogenesis of hepatocellular carcinoma and the role of HBV are discussed in Chapter 18. In some infected individuals, hepatocytes are infected but the CTL response is dormant, resulting in the establishment of a "carrier" state, without progressive liver damage.

TRANSFORMING INFECTIONS

This group includes viruses that have been implicated in the causation of human cancer: Epstein-Barr virus (EBV), human papilloma virus (HPV), HBV, and human T-cell leukemia virus-1 (HTLV-1). EBV and HPV are discussed here.

Epstein-Barr Virus (EBV)

EBV causes *infectious mononucleosis*, a benign, self-limited lymphoproliferative disorder, and is associated with the development of hairy leukoplakia and a number of neoplasms, most notably certain lymphomas and nasopharyngeal carcinoma. Infectious mononucleosis is characterized by fever, generalized lymphadenopathy, splenomegaly, sore throat, and the appearance in the blood of atypical activated T lymphocytes (mononucleosis cells). Some patients develop hepatitis, meningoencephalitis, and pneumonitis. Infectious mononucleosis occurs principally in late adolescents or young adults among upper socioeconomic classes in developed nations. In the rest of the world, primary infection with EBV occurs in childhood and is usually asymptomatic.

Pathogenesis. EBV is transmitted by close human contact, frequently with the saliva during kissing. An EBV envelope glycoprotein binds to CD21 (CR2), the receptor for the C3d component of complement (Chapter 2), present on B cells.[72] The viral infection begins in nasopharyngeal and oropharyngeal lymphoid tissues, particularly the tonsils (Fig. 8–16). Although EBV has the capacity to infect epithelial cells (mainly through binding to the integrin α_5/β_1), the role of epithelial infection in acute mononucleosis (and long-term viral shedding) remains uncertain. Either through transient

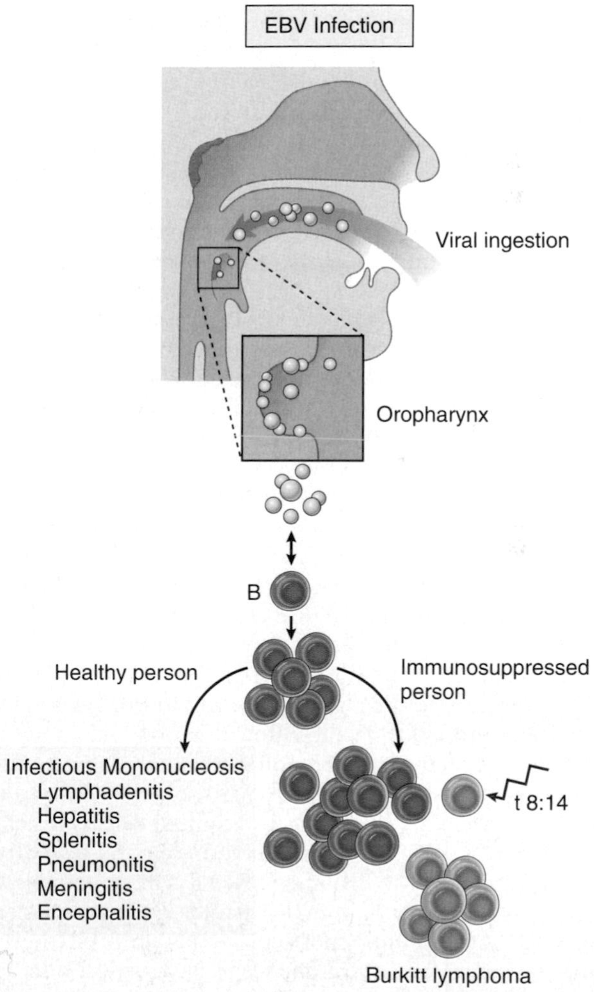

FIGURE 8–16 Pathways of transmission of the Epstein-Barr virus. In an individual with normal immune function, infection leads to mononucleosis. In the setting of cellular immunodeficiency, proliferation of infected B cells is uncontrolled and may cause B-cell neoplasms. One secondary genetic event that collaborates with Epstein-Barr virus (EBV) to cause B-cell transformation is a balanced 8;14 chromosomal translocation, which is seen in Burkitt lymphoma. EBV has also been implicated in the pathogenesis of nasopharyngeal carcinoma, Hodgkin disease, and certain other rare non-Hodgkin lymphomas.

infection of epithelium or transcytosis into the submucosa, EBV gains access to sub-mucosal lymphoid tissues. Here, infection of B cells may take one of two forms. In a minority of B cells, there is productive infection with lysis of infected cells and release of virions, which may infect other B cells. In most B cells, EBV establishes latent infection. Of note, patients with X-linked agammaglobulinemia, who lack B cells, do not become latently infected with EBV or shed virus, suggesting B cells are the main reservoir of latent infection. At least 11 EBV genes are involved in the establishment of latency, including EBNA1, which plays a role in EBV DNA replication, and EBNA2 and latent membrane protein-1 (LMP-1), which drive B cell activation and proliferation.[72] LMP-1 appears to act by binding to TNF receptor–associated factors (TRAFs), and activates signaling pathways that mimic B-cell activation by the TNF receptor homologue, CD40, which is involved in normal B-cell responses (Chapter 6). EBNA-2 stimulates transcription of many host cell genes, including cyclin D, which regulates cell cycle progression. The activated B cells then disseminate in the circulation and secrete antibodies with several specificities, including the heterophile anti–sheep red blood cell antibodies used for the diagnosis of infectious mononucleosis. Heterophile antibodies bind to antigens thought to differ from the antigens that induced them. People with mononucleosis make antibodies that agglutinate sheep or horse red blood cells in the laboratory, but these antibodies do not react with EBV.

The symptoms of infectious mononcleosis appear upon initiation of the host immune response. Cellular immunity mediated by cytotoxic CD8+ T cells and natural killer cells is the most important component of this response. The *atypical lymphocytes* seen in the blood, so characteristic of this disease, are mainly CD8+ cytotoxic T cells, but also include CD16+ NK cells. The reactive proliferation of T cells is largely centered in lymphoid tissues, which accounts for the lymphadenopathy and splenomegaly. Early in the course of the infection, IgM antibodies are formed against viral capsid antigens; later, IgG antibodies are formed that persist for life. In otherwise healthy persons, the fully developed humoral and cellular responses to EBV act as brakes on viral shedding, resulting in the elimination of B cells expressing the full complement of EBV latency-associated genes. However, EBV persists throughout life in a small population of resting B cells in which expression of EBV genes is limited to EBNA1 and latent membrane protein 2. Cells within this pool are thought to occasionally reactivate expression of the other latency-associated genes, such as EBNA2 and LMP1, causing them to proliferate. Particularly in hosts with acquired defects in cellular immunity (e.g., AIDS), this proliferation can progress through a multi-step process to EBV-associated B cell lymphomas. One example is Burkitt lymphoma (Chapter 7), in which a chromosomal translocation (most commonly an 8:14 translocation) involving the *c-myc* oncogene is a critical additional oncogenic event (Fig. 8–16).

Morphology. The major alterations involve the blood, lymph nodes, spleen, liver, central nervous system, and, occasionally, other organs. The **peripheral blood** shows absolute lymphocytosis with a total white cell count between 12,000 and 18,000 cells/μl, more than 60% of which are lymphocytes. Many of these are large, **atypical lymphocytes**, 12 to 16 μm in diameter, characterized by an abundant cytoplasm containing multiple clear vacuolations, an oval, indented, or folded nucleus, and scattered cytoplasmic azurophilic granules (Fig. 8–17). These atypical lymphocytes, most of which express CD8, are usually sufficiently distinctive to permit the diagnosis from examination of a peripheral blood smear.

The **lymph nodes** are typically discrete and enlarged throughout the body, principally in the posterior cervical, axillary, and groin regions. On histologic examination, the most striking feature is the expansion of paracortical areas by activated T cells (immunoblasts). A minor population of EBV-infected B cells expressing EBNA2, LMP-1, and other latency-specific genes can also be detected in the paracortex using specific antibodies. Occasionally, EBV-infected B cells resembling Reed-Sternberg cells may be found. B cell areas (follicles) may also be hyperplastic, but this is usually mild in degree. The T cell proliferation is sometimes so exuberant that it is difficult to distinguish the nodal morphology from that seen in malignant lymphomas. Similar changes commonly occur in the tonsils and lymphoid tissue of the oropharynx.

The **spleen** is enlarged in most cases, weighing between 300 and 500 gm. It is usually soft and fleshy, with a hyperemic cut surface. The histologic changes are analogous to those of the lymph nodes, showing an expansion of white pulp follicles and red pulp sinusoids due to the presence of numerous activated T cells. These spleens are especially vulnerable to rupture, possibly in part because the rapid increase in size produces a tense, fragile splenic capsule.

Liver function is almost always transiently impaired to some degree, although hepatomegaly is at most moderate. On histologic examination, atypical lymphocytes are seen in the portal areas and sinusoids, and scattered, isolated cells or foci of parenchymal necrosis filled with lymphocytes may be present. This histologic picture may be difficult to distinguish from that of other forms of viral hepatitis.

The **central nervous system** may show congestion, edema, and perivascular mononuclear infiltrates in the leptomeninges. Myelin degeneration and destruction of axis cylinders have been described in the peripheral nerves.

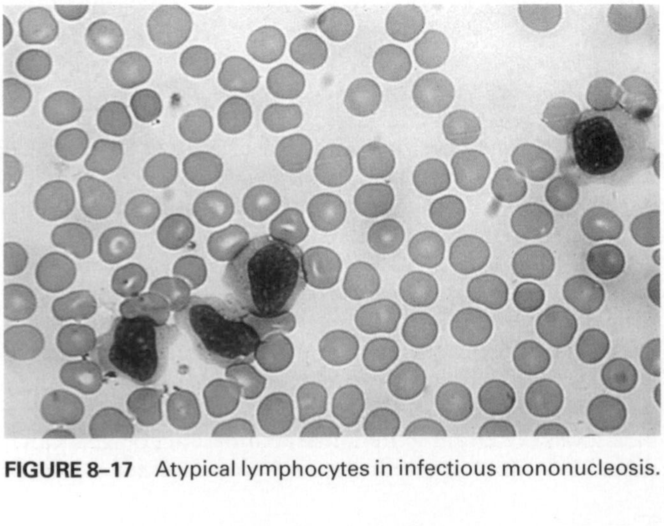

FIGURE 8–17 Atypical lymphocytes in infectious mononucleosis.

Although infectious mononucleosis classically presents with fever, sore throat, lymphadenitis, and the other features mentioned earlier, often its behavior is atypical. It may present with little or no fever and only malaise, fatigue, and lymphadenopathy, raising the specter of leukemia or lymphoma; as a fever of unknown origin without significant lymphadenopathy or other localized findings; as hepatitis that is difficult to differentiate from one of the hepatotropic viral syndromes; or as a febrile rash resembling rubella. *Ultimately, the diagnosis depends on the following findings (in increasing order of specificity): (1) lymphocytosis with the characteristic atypical lymphocytes in the peripheral blood, (2) a positive heterophile antibody reaction (monospot test), and (3) specific antibodies for EBV antigens (viral capsid antigens, early antigens, or Epstein-Barr nuclear antigen).* In most patients, infectious mononucleosis resolves within 4 to 6 weeks, but sometimes the fatigue lasts longer. One or more complications occasionally supervene. They may involve virtually any organ or system in the body. Perhaps most common is marked hepatic dysfunction with jaundice, elevated hepatic enzyme levels, disturbed appetite, and rarely even liver failure. Other complications involve the nervous system, kidneys, bone marrow, lungs, eyes, heart, and spleen (splenic rupture has been fatal). A more serious complication in those suffering from some form of immunodeficiency, such as AIDS, or receiving therapy that leads to defects of cellular immunity (e.g., bone marrow or solid organ transplant recipients) is that the B-cell proliferation may run amok, leading to death. In AIDS, this usually takes the form of monoclonal B-cell lymphomas, whereas in the setting of acute severe immunosuppression (e.g., bone marrow transplantation), even polyclonal proliferations may prove fatal.

These unfortunate consequences also occur in individuals suffering from the X-linked lymphoproliferation syndrome (XLP, also known as Duncan disease), a disorder caused by a defect in a gene, *SH2D1A*, that is expressed primarily in cytotoxic T cells and NK cells.[73] SH2D1A (also called SAP) participates in a signaling pathway critical for an effective cellular response to EBV-infected B cells. Patients are often normal until they are acutely infected with EBV, often during adolescence. The failure to control EBV infection variously leads to chronic infectious mononucleosis, agammaglobulinemia, and B cell lymphoma, each of which proves fatal in about a third of patients.

Human Papillomaviruses

Human papillomaviruses (HPVs) are nonenveloped DNA viruses that are members of the papovavirus family (which also includes polyomavirus, JC virus and SV-40). Based on DNA sequence, papillomaviruses are classified into over 100 types. Some HPVs cause papillomas (warts), benign tumors of squamous cells on the skin, and these are discussed in Chapter 25. Other HPVs are associated with warts that can progress to malignancy, particularly squamous cell carcinoma of the cervix (discussed in Chapter 22) and the anogenital area (discussed in Chapter 21). Papillomaviruses are mainly transmitted by skin or genital contact. HPVs infect squamous epithelial cells, but their life cycle is not well understood since these viruses cannot be cultured in vitro. The expression of viral genes depends on the differentiation state of the epithelial cells.[71] Papilloma viruses initially infect basal cells in the epithelium, but there is limited expression of viral genes in these cells. As the epithelial cells differentiate, additional HPV genes are expressed. Mature virions are produced in the cells within the granular layer and shed from the stratum corneum. In the upper spinous layers of the epithelium, HPV leads to a characteristic perinuclear vacuolization in the epithelial cells (koilocytosis). HPV DNA is maintained as an episomal plasmid, and virus-encoded proteins promote cell growth and malignancy. HPV E6 stimulates ubiquitination and degradation of p53, and HPV E7 binds to Rb, releasing the E2F transcription factor. Both these actions dysregulate the cell cycle and may promote cellular transformation and malignancy (Chapter 7).

Bacterial Infections

GRAM-POSITIVE BACTERIAL INFECTIONS

Common Gram-positive pathogens include *Staphylococcus* and *Streptococcus*, each of which causes many types of infections. Three less common diseases caused by Gram-positive rod-shaped organisms are also discussed here: diphtheria, listeriosis, and anthrax. *Nocardia* are environmental Gram-positive bacteria that cause infections mainly in immunocompromised people. *Clostridia*, which are Gram-positive, are discussed with the anaerobes.

Staphylococcal Infections

Staphylococcus aureus organisms are pyogenic, nonmotile, Gram-positive cocci that form grapelike clusters. *These bacteria cause a myriad of skin lesions (boils, carbuncles, impetigo, and scalded skin) and also cause osteomyelitis, pneumonia, endocarditis, food poisoning, and toxic shock syndrome* (Fig. 8–18). Here we review the general characteristics of *S. aureus* infection. Specific organ infections are described in other chapters. *Staphylococcus epidermidis*, a species that is related to *S. aureus*, causes opportunistic infections in catheterized patients, patients with prosthetic cardiac valves, and drug addicts. *Staphylococcus saprophyticus* is a common cause of urinary tract infections in young women.

Pathogenesis. *S. aureus* and other virulent staphylococci possess a multitude of virulence factors, which include surface proteins involved in adherence, secreted enzymes that degrade proteins, and secreted toxins that damage host cells. Staphylococci are distinguished by their large number of plasmids, which encode proteins involved in antibiotic resistance and other virulence factors.

S. aureus expresses surface receptors for fibrinogen (called clumping factor), fibronectin, and vitronectin, and uses these molecules as a bridge to bind to host endothelial cells.[75] Staphylococci infecting prosthetic valves and catheters have a polysaccharide capsule that allows them to attach to the artificial materials and to resist host cell phagocytosis. The lipase of *S. aureus* degrades lipids on the skin surface, and its expression is correlated with the ability of the bacteria to produce skin abscesses. Staphylococci also have protein A on their surface, which binds the Fc portion of immunoglobulins.

S. aureus produces multiple membrane-damaging (hemolytic) toxins, including α-toxin, which is a pore-forming protein that intercalates into the plasma membrane

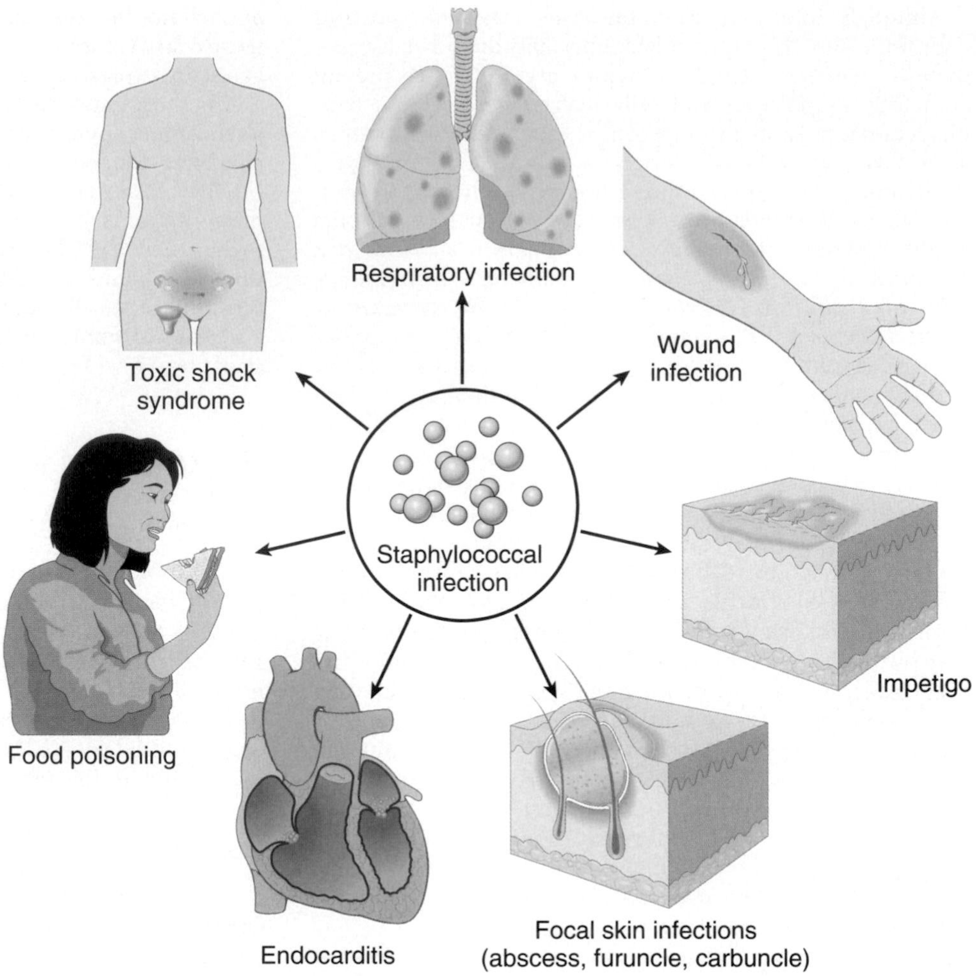

FIGURE 8–18 The many consequences of staphylococcal infection.

of host cells and depolarizes them;[76] β-toxin, a sphingomyelinase; and δ-toxin, which is a detergent-like peptide. Staphylococcal γ-toxin and leukocidin lyse erythrocytes and phagocytic cells, respectively.

The exfoliative toxins produced by *S. aureus* are serine proteases that split the skin by cleaving the protein desmoglein 1, which is part of the desmosomes that hold epidermal cells tightly together.[29] This can cause the superficial epidermis to split away from the deeper skin, making the patient vulnerable to secondary infections. Exfoliation can occur at the site of staphylococcal skin infection (bullous impetigo) or can be widespread, when secreted toxin from a localized infection causes disseminated loss of the superficial epidermis (staphylococcal scalded-skin syndrome).

Superantigens produced by *S. aureus* cause food poisoning and, of more concern, toxic shock syndrome (TSS). TSS came to public attention because of its association with the use of hyperabsorbent tampons, which became colonized with *S. aureus* during use. It is now clear that TSS can be caused by growth of *S. aureus* at many sites, most commonly the vagina and infected surgical sites. TSS is characterized by hypotension (shock), renal failure, coagulopathy, liver disease, respiratory distress, a generalized erythematous rash, and soft tissue necrosis at the site of infection. If not promptly treated, TSS can be fatal. TSS can also be caused by *Streptococcus pyogenes.*

As mentioned earlier, superantigens bind to conserved portions of MHC molecules and to relatively conserved portions of TCR β chains. In this manner, superantigens may stimulate up to 20% of T lymphocytes. The stimulation of so many T lymphocytes leads to massive T-lymphocyte proliferation and cytokine release. The high levels of cytokines can lead to capillary leak and shock and may cause vomiting by affecting the nervous system in the gut or the central nervous system.[77]

Morphology. Whether the lesion is located in the skin, lungs, bones, or heart valves, *S. aureus* causes pyogenic inflammation that is distinctive for its local destructiveness.

Excluding impetigo, which is a staphylococcal or streptococcal infection restricted to the superficial epidermis, staphylococcal skin infections are centered around the hair follicles. A **furuncle**, or **boil**, is a focal suppurative inflammation of the skin and subcutaneous tissue, either solitary or multiple or recurrent in successive crops. Furuncles are most frequent in moist, hairy areas, such as the face, axillae, groin, legs, and submammary folds. Beginning in a single hair follicle, a boil develops into a growing and deepening abscess that eventually "comes to a head" by thinning and rupturing the overlying skin. A **carbuncle** is associated with deeper suppuration that spreads laterally beneath the deep subcutaneous fascia and then burrows superficially to erupt in multiple adjacent skin sinuses. Carbuncles typically appear beneath the skin of the upper back and posterior neck, where fascial planes favor their spread. Chronic abscess formation of apocrine gland regions, most frequently of the axilla, is known as **hidradenitis suppurativa.** Those of the nail bed **(paronychia)** or on the palmar side of the fingertips **(felons)** are exquisitely painful. They may follow trauma or embedded splinters and, if deep enough, destroy the bone of the terminal phalanx or detach the fingernail.

Staphylococcal lung infections (Fig. 8–19) have a polymorphonuclear infiltrate similar to that of pneumococcus (see Fig. 8–7) but are much more destructive of lung tissues. *S. aureus* lung infections usually occur in patients with predisposing conditions such as influenza or hematogenous spread of infected thrombi.

Staphylococcal scalded skin syndrome, also called **Ritter disease,** is caused by the exfoliative A and B toxins. It is an exfoliative dermatitis that most frequently occurs in children with staphylococcal infections of the nasopharynx or skin. In staphylococcal scalded skin syndrome, there is a sunburnlike rash that spreads over the entire body and forms fragile bullae that lead to partial or total skin loss. The intraepithelial split in staphylococcal scalded skin syndrome is in the granulosa layer, distinguishing it from toxic epidermal necrolysis, or Lyell's disease, which is secondary to drug hypersensitivity and causes splitting at the epidermal-dermal junction (Chapter 25).

Streptococcal Infections

Streptococci are facultative or obligate anaerobic Gram-positive cocci that grow in pairs or chains and cause a myriad of suppurative infections of the skin, oropharynx, lungs, and heart valves and also cause poststreptococcal syndromes, including rheumatic fever (Chapter 12), immune complex glomerulonephritis (Chapter 20), and erythema nodosum (Chapter 25). β-hemolytic streptococci are typed according to their surface carbohydrate (Lancefield) antigens. *Streptococcus pyogenes* (group A) causes pharyngitis, scarlet fever, erysipelas, impetigo, rheumatic fever, toxic shock syndrome, and glomerulonephritis. *Streptococcus agalactiae* (group B) colonizes the female genital tract and causes sepsis and meningitis in neonates and chorioamnionitis in pregnancy. *Enterococcus faecalis* and *Enterococcus faecium* were, until recently, included in the *Streptococcus* genus but are now a separate genus. Enterococci cause endocarditis and urinary tract infections. *Streptococcus pneumoniae* is the most important α-hemolytic streptococcus. *S. pneumoniae* is a common cause of community-acquired pneumonia and meningitis in adults. The viridans group streptococci include several species of α-hemolytic streptococci that are part of the normal oral flora but are also a common cause of endocarditis. Finally, *Streptococcus mutans* is the major cause of dental caries.

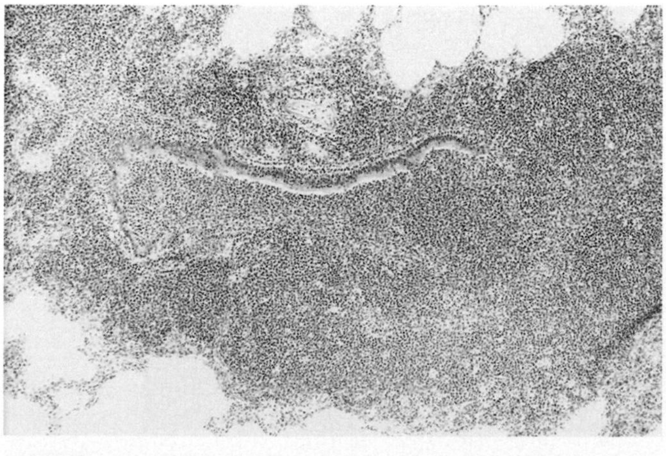

FIGURE 8–19 Staphylococcal abscess of the lung with extensive neutrophilic infiltrate and destruction of the alveoli (contrast with Figure 8–8).

Pathogenesis. The different species of streptococci produce many virulence factors and toxins. Many streptococci, including *S. pyogenes* and *S. pneumoniae*, have capsules that resist phagocytosis. *S. pyogenes* also expresses M protein, a surface protein that prevents bacteria from being phagocytosed, and a complement C5a peptidase, which degrades this chemotactic peptide.[78] Poststreptococcal acute rheumatic fever is probably an autoimmune disease caused by antistreptococcal M protein antibodies that cross-react with cardiac myosin.[79] Virulent *S. pyogenes* have been referred to as flesh-eating bacteria because they cause a rapidly progressive necrotizing fasciitis.[80] Pneumolysin is a cytosolic bacterial protein released on disruption of *S. pneumoniae.*[81] Pneumolysin inserts into target cell membranes and lyses them, greatly increasing tissue damage. This toxin also activates the classical pathway of complement, reducing complement available for opsonization of bacteria. Streptococci secrete a phage-encoded pyrogenic exotoxin that causes fever and rash in scarlet fever. *S. mutans* produces caries by metabolizing sucrose to lactic acid (which causes demineralization of tooth enamel) and by secreting high-molecular-weight glucans that promote aggregation of bacteria and plaque formation.[82]

Morphology. Streptococcal infections are characterized by diffuse interstitial neutrophilic infiltrates with minimal destruction of host tissues. The skin lesions caused by streptococci (furuncles, carbuncles, and impetigo) resemble those of staphylococci, although with streptococci there is less of a tendency to form discrete abscesses.

Erysipelas is most common among middle-aged persons in warm climates and is caused by exotoxins from superficial infection with *S. pyogenes.* It is characterized by rapidly spreading erythematous cutaneous swelling that may begin on the face or, less frequently, on the body or an extremity. The rash has a sharp, well-demarcated, serpiginous border and may form a "butterfly" distribution on the face (Fig. 8–20). On histologic examination, there is a diffuse, acute edematous, neutrophilic inflammatory reaction in the dermis and epidermis extending into the subcutaneous tissues. The leukocytic infiltration is more intense around vessels and the skin adnexa. Microabscesses may be formed, but tissue necrosis is usually minor.

Streptococcal pharyngitis, which is the major antecedent of poststreptococcal glomerulonephritis (Chapter 20), is marked by edema, epiglottic swelling, and punctate abscesses of the tonsillar crypts, sometimes accompanied by cervical lymphadenopathy. With extension of the pharyngeal infection, there may be encroachment on the airways, especially if there is

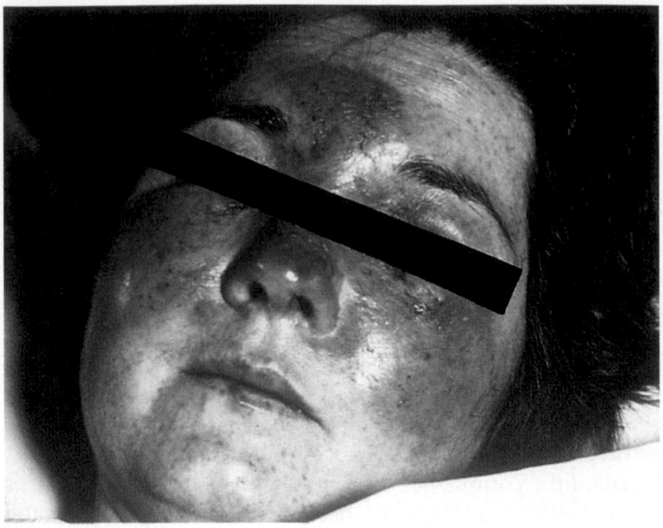

FIGURE 8–20 Streptococcal erysipelas.

peritonsillar or retropharyngeal abscess formation **(quinsy sore throat)**. On microscopic examination, these lesions show vasodilation, spreading edema, and intense, diffuse neutrophilic exudation, often with a liberal admixture of mononuclear phagocytes.

Scarlet fever, associated with tonsillitis caused by *S. pyogenes*, is most common between the ages of 3 and 15 years. It is manifested by a punctate erythematous rash that is most abundant over the trunk and inner aspects of the arms and legs. The face is also involved, but usually a small area about the mouth remains relatively unaffected to produce a circumoral pallor. On microscopic examination, there is a characteristic acute, edematous, neutrophilic inflammatory reaction within the affected tissues (i.e., the oropharynx, skin, and lymph nodes). The inflammatory involvement of the epidermis is usually followed by hyperkeratosis of the skin, which accounts for the scaling during defervescence.

Streptococcus pneumoniae is an important cause of lobar pneumonia (described in Chapter 15 and pictured in Fig. 8–7).

Diphtheria

Diphtheria is caused by a slender Gram-positive rod with clubbed ends, *Corynebacterium diphtheriae*, which is passed from person to person through aerosols or skin shedding. *C. diphtheriae* causes a range of illnesses: asymptomatic carriage; skin lesions in neglected wounds of combat troops in the tropics; and a life-threatening syndrome that includes formation of a tough pharyngeal membrane and toxin-mediated damage to the heart, nerves, and other organs. *C. diphtheriae* has only one toxin, which is a phage-encoded A-B toxin that blocks host cell protein synthesis.[83] In the cytosol of the cell, the A fragment catalyzes the covalent transfer of adenosine diphosphate (ADP)-ribose to elongation factor-2 (EF-2) which is involved in protein synthesis. A single molecule of diphtheria toxin can kill a cell by ADP-ribosylating, and thus inactivating, more than a million EF-2 molecules. Immunization with diphtheria toxoid (formalin-fixed toxin) does not prevent colonization with *C. diphtheriae* but protects immunized people from the lethal effects of the toxin. Recent large outbreaks of diphtheria in the former Soviet Union resulted from decreased vaccination rates, socioeconomic instability, and a deteriorating health infrastructure.[83]

Morphology. Inhaled *C. diphtheriae* proliferate at the site of attachment on the mucosa of the nasopharynx, oropharynx, larynx, or trachea but also form satellite lesions in the esophagus or lower airways. Release of exotoxin causes necrosis of the epithelium, accompanied by an outpouring of a dense fibrinosuppurative exudate. The coagulation of this exudate on the ulcerated necrotic surface creates a tough, dirty gray to black, superficial membrane (Fig. 8–21). Neutrophilic infiltration in the underlying tissues is intense and is accompanied by marked vascular congestion, interstitial edema, and fibrin exudation. When the membrane sloughs off its inflamed and vascularized bed, bleeding and asphyxiation may occur. With control of the infection, the membrane is coughed up or removed by enzymatic digestion, and the inflammatory reaction subsides.

Although the bacterial invasion remains localized, generalized hyperplasia of the spleen and lymph

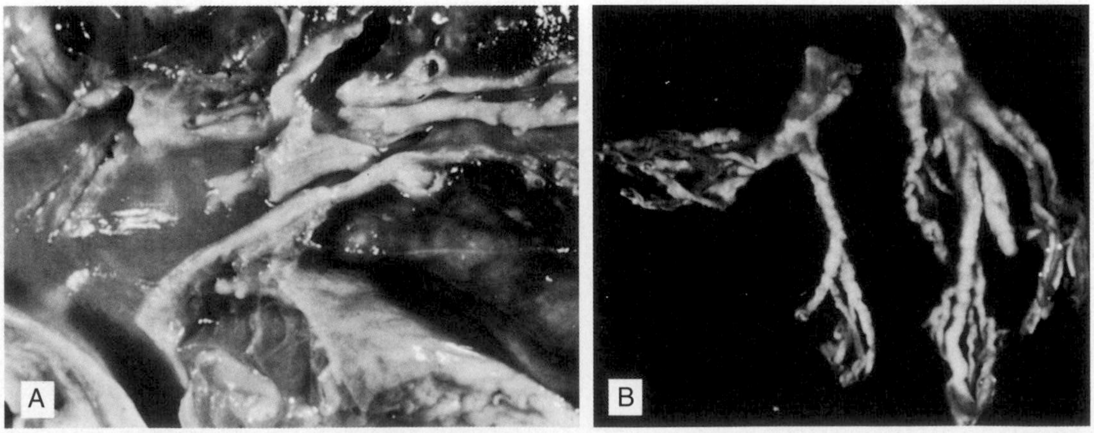

FIGURE 8–21 Membrane of diphtheria lying within a transverse bronchus (*A*) and forming a perfect cast (removed from the lung) of the branching respiratory tree (*B*).

nodes ensues owing to the absorption of soluble exotoxin into the blood. The exotoxin may cause fatty myocardial change with isolated myofiber necrosis, polyneuritis with degeneration of the myelin sheaths and axis cylinders, and (less commonly) fatty change and focal necroses of parenchymal cells in the liver, kidneys, and adrenals.

Listeriosis

Listeria monocytogenes is a Gram-positive, motile facultative intracellular bacterium that causes severe food-borne infections. Miniepidemics of *L. monocytogenes* have been linked to dairy products, chicken, and hot dogs. Pregnant women, their neonates, the elderly, and immunosuppressed persons (e.g., transplant recipients or AIDS patients) are particularly susceptible to severe *L. monocytogenes* infection. In pregnant women (and pregnant sheep and cattle), *L. monocytogenes* causes an amnionitis that may result in abortion, stillbirth, or neonatal sepsis. In neonates, *L. monocytogenes* may cause disseminated disease (granulomatosis infantiseptica) and an exudative meningitis, both of which are also seen in immunosuppressed adults.

L. monocytogenes has leucine-rich proteins on its surface called *internalins*, which bind to E-cadherin on host epithelial cells and induce internalization of the bacterium.[84] Inside the cell, the bacteria escape from the membrane-bound phagolysosome by the action of a pore-forming protein, listeriolysin O, and two phospholipases.[25] In the host cell cytoplasm, ACTA, a bacterial surface protein, binds to host cell cytoskeletal proteins and induces actin polymerization, which propels the bacteria into adjacent, uninfected host cells. Resting macrophages, which internalize *L. monocytogenes* through C3 activated on the bacterial surface, fail to kill the bacteria. In contrast, macrophages that are activated by IFN-γ phagocytose and kill the bacteria. Hence, unlike most other Gram-positive bacteria, protection against *L. monocytogenes* is mediated largely by IFN-γ produced by NK cells and T cells.

Morphology. In acute human infections, *L. monocytogenes* evokes an exudative pattern of inflammation with numerous neutrophils. The **meningitis** it causes is macroscopically and microscopically indistinguishable from that caused by other pyogenic bacteria (Chapter 28). The finding of Gram-positive, mostly intracellular, bacilli in the CSF is virtually diagnostic. More varied lesions may be encountered in neonates and immunosuppressed adults. Focal abscesses alternate with grayish or yellow nodules representing necrotic amorphous basophilic tissue debris. These can occur in any organ, including the lung, liver, spleen, and lymph nodes. In infections of longer duration, macrophages appear in large numbers, eventually to dispose of the necrotic remnants, but true epithelioid cell granulomas are rare. Infants born live with *L. monocytogenes* sepsis often have a papular red rash over the extremities, and listerial abscesses can be seen in the placenta. A smear of the meconium will disclose the Gram-positive organisms.

Anthrax

Bacillus anthracis is a large, spore-forming Gram-positive rod-shaped bacterium. These bacteria are common pathogens in farm and wild animals that have contact with soil contaminated with *B. anthracis* spores. Anthrax spores can be ground to a fine powder, making a potent biologic weapon. There are between 20,000 and 100,000 cases of anthrax each year, but recent use of the microbe as an agent of bioterrorism has heightened concern about in this organism. In 1979, accidental release of *B. anthracis* spores at a military research institute in Russia killed 66 people. In 2001, 22 people in the United States acquired *B. anthracis*; most cases were traced to powder (spores) delivered in the mail.

B. anthracis is typically acquired through exposure to animals or animal products such as wool or hides.[85] There are three major anthrax syndromes: cutaneous, inhalational, and gastrointestinal anthrax. *Cutaneous anthrax*, which makes up 95% of naturally occurring infections, begins as a painless, pruritic papule that develops into a vesicle within 2 days. As the vesicle enlarges, striking edema may form around it, and there is regional lymphadenopathy. After the vesicle ruptures, the remaining ulcer becomes covered with a characteristic black eschar, which dries and falls off as the patient recovers. Bacteremia is rare with cutaneous anthrax.

Inhalational anthrax occurs when spores are inhaled. The organism grows and is carried to lymph nodes by phagocytes where the spores germinate, and the release of toxins causes hemorrhagic mediastinitis. After a prodromal illness of 1 to 6 days characterized by fever, cough, and chest or abdominal pain, there is abrupt onset of increased fever, hypoxia, and sweating. Frequently, anthrax meningitis develops due to bacteremia. Inhalational anthrax rapidly leads to shock and frequently death within 1 to 2 days.

Gastrointestinal anthrax is an uncommon form of this infection that is usually contracted by eating undercooked meat contaminated with *B. anthracis*. Initially, the patient has nausea, abdominal pain, and vomiting. Severe, bloody diarrhea rapidly develops, and mortality is over 50%.

Pathogenesis. *B. anthracis* produces potent toxins and a polyglutamyl capsule that is antiphagocytic. The anthrax toxin, produced by *B. anthracis*, is well understood[86] (Fig. 8–22). The B subunit is referred to as the *protective antigen* because antibodies against this protein protect animals against the toxin. The protective antigen binds to a cell surface protein, and then a host protease clips off a 20-kDa fragment of the B subunit. The remaining 63-kDa fragments associate to form a heptamer. Anthrax toxin has two alternate A subunits: edema factor (EF) and lethal factor (LF), each named for the effect of the toxin in experimental animals. Three A subunits bind to the B heptamer, and this complex is endocytosed into the host cell. The low pH of the endosome causes a conformational change in the protective antigen heptamer, which then forms a selective channel in the endosome membrane through which EF and LF move into the cytoplasm. In the cytoplasm, EF binds to calcium and calmodulin to form an adenylate cyclase. The active EF converts adenosine triphosphate to cyclic adenosine monophosphate (cAMP). cAMP is an important signaling molecule in cells, and elevated cAMP leads to efflux of water from the cell to form edema. LF has a different mechanism of action. LF is a protease that destroys mitogen-activated protein kinase kinases (MAPKKs). MAPKKs regulate the activity of

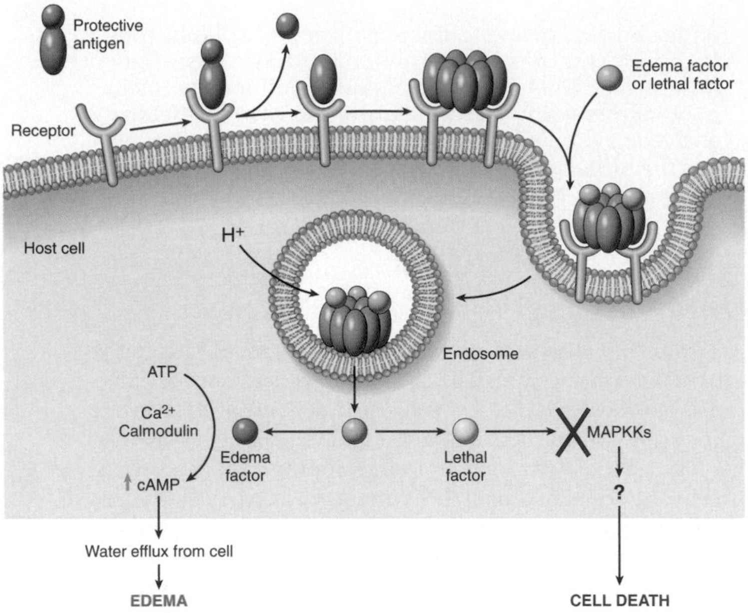

FIGURE 8–22 Mechanism of action of anthrax toxins. (Adapted from Mourez et al: 2001: a year of major advances in anthrax toxin research. Trends Microbiol 10(6):287, 2002.)

mitogen-activated protein kinases, which are important regulators of cell growth and differentiation (Chapter 3). The mechanism of cell death due to deregulation of mitogen-activated protein kinases is not understood.

Morphology. Anthrax lesions at any site are typified by necrosis and exudative inflammation with infiltration of neutrophils and macrophages. The presence of large, boxcar-shaped Gram-positive extracellular bacteria in chains, seen histopathologically or recovered in culture, should suggest the diagnosis.

Inhalational anthrax causes numerous foci of hemorrhage in the mediastinum with hemorrhagic, enlarged hilar and peribronchial lymph nodes.[87] Microscopic examination of the lungs typically shows perihilar interstitial pneumonia with infiltration of macrophages and neutrophils and pulmonary vasculitis. Hemorrhagic lesions associated with vasculitis are also present in about half of cases. Mediastinal lymph nodes show lymphocytosis, with phagocytosis of apoptotic lymphocytes by macrophages and a fibrin-rich edema (Fig. 8–23). *B. anthracis* is present predominantly in the alveolar capillaries and venules and, to a lesser degree, within the alveolar space. In fatal cases, *B. anthracis* is evident in multiple organs (spleen, liver, intestines, kidneys, adrenal glands, and meninges).

Nocardia

Nocardia are aerobic Gram-positive bacteria that grow in distinctive branched chains. In culture, *Nocardia* form aerial structures with terminal spores, resembling hyphae. Despite this morphological similarity to molds, *Nocardia* are true bacteria.

Nocardia are found in soil and cause opportunistic infections in immunocompromised people.[88] *Nocardia asteroides* causes respiratory infections while other species, mainly *Nocardia brasiliensis*, infect the skin. A fifth of *N. asteroides* infections involve the CNS, presumably after dissemination from the lungs. Most patients with *N. asteroides* have defects in T cell–mediated immunity, often due to prolonged steroid use, HIV infection, or diabetes mellitus. Respiratory infection with *N. asteroides* causes an indolent illness with fever, weight loss, and cough, which may be mistaken for tuberculosis or malignancy. CNS infections with *N. asteroides* are also indolent and cause neurologic deficits depending on the site of the infection. Skin infections have a range of manifestations, from rapidly progressive infections resembling those of *Staphylococcus* or *Streptococcus* to slowly progressive mycetoma.

Morphology. The diagnosis of nocardiosis depends on identification of slender Gram-positive organisms arranged in branching filaments (Fig. 8–24). Irregular staining gives the filaments a beaded appearance. *Nocardia* stain with modified acid fast stains (Fite-Faraco stain), unlike *Actinomyces*, which may appear similar on Gram stain of tissue. At any site of infection, *Nocardia* elicit a suppurative response with central liquefaction and surrounding granulation and fibrosis. Granulomas do not form.

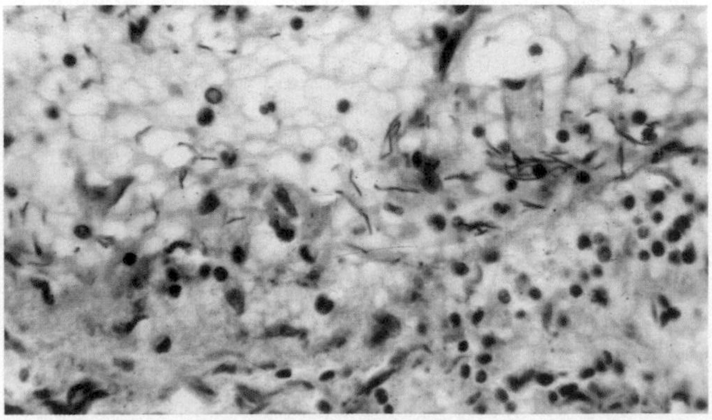

FIGURE 8–23 *B. anthracis* in the subcapsular sinus of a hilar lymph node of a patient who died of inhalational anthrax. (Courtesy of Dr. Lev Grinberg, Department of Pathology, Hospital 40, Ekaterinburg, Russia and Dr. David Walker, UTMB Center for Biodefense and Emerging Infectious Diseases, Galveston, TX.)

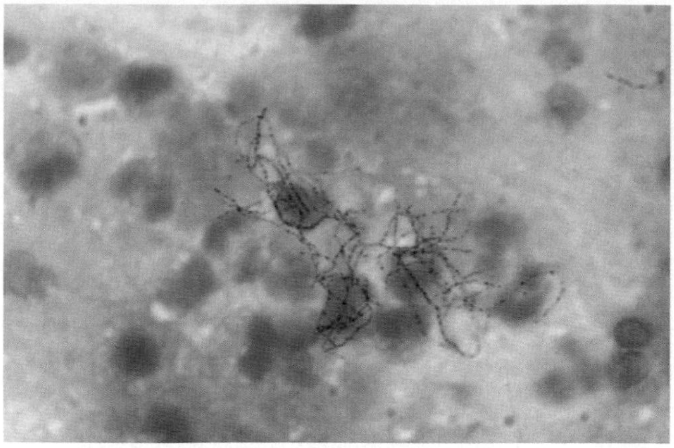

FIGURE 8–24 *Nocardia asteroides* in a Gram-stained sputum sample. Note the beaded, branched Gram-positive organisms and leukocytes. (Courtesy of Dr. Ellen Jo Baron, Stanford University Medical Center, Stanford, CA.)

GRAM-NEGATIVE BACTERIAL INFECTIONS

Only a few Gram-negative bacteria are considered in this section. A number of important Gram-negative pathogens are discussed in the appropriate chapters of organ systems, including bacterial causes of gastrointestinal infections and urinary tract infections. Anaerobic Gram-negative organisms are considered later in this chapter.

Neisserial Infections

Neisseria are Gram-negative diplococci that are flattened on the adjoining sides, giving the pair the shape of a coffee bean (Fig. 8–3*E*). These aerobic bacteria have stringent nutritional requirements and grow best on enriched media such as lysed sheep's blood agar ("chocolate" agar). The two clinically significant Neisseria are *Neisseria meningitidis* and *Neisseria gonorrhoeae*.

N. meningitidis is a significant cause of bacterial meningitis, particularly among people between 5 and 19 years old. The organism is a common colonizer of the oropharynx and is spread by the respiratory route. Approximately 10% of the population is colonized at any one time, and each episode of colonization lasts, on average, for several months. An immune response leads to clearance of colonization in most people, and this response is protective against subsequent disease with the same strain of bacteria. There are at least 13 serotypes of *N. meningitidis*. Invasive disease mainly occurs when people living in crowded quarters, such as military barracks or college dormitories, encounter new strains to which they have not previously made an immune response. An outbreak of 61 cases of serogroup C *N. meningitidis* occurred in Edmonton, Canada, in 1999–2001.[89] This serotype had not been previously identified in Edmonton, which presumably contributed to the high rate of disease. A vaccination campaign appears to have reduced the spread of disease.

Even in the absence of an immune response, only a small fraction of those infected with *N. meningitidis* get meningitis. The bacteria must invade respiratory epithelial cells and travel to the basolateral side of the cells to enter the blood.[90] Once in the blood, the capsule of the bacteria reduces opsonization and destruction of the bacteria by complement proteins. Despite this, the efficacy of complement against *N. meningitidis* is shown by the high rates of disease among people who are deficient in the complement proteins that form the membrane attack complex (C5 to C9). If *N. meningitidis* escapes the host response, the consequences can be severe. Although antibiotic treatment of meningitis has greatly reduced mortality of *N. meningitidis* infection, the death rate is still about 10%. The pathology of meningitis and other pyogenic meningitides is discussed in Chapter 28.

N. gonorrhoeae is an important cause of sexually transmitted disease, infecting about 600,000 people each year in the United States. It is second only to *Chlamydia trachomatis* as a causative agent of STI. Infection in men causes urethritis. In women, *N. gonorrhoeae* infection is often asymptomatic and so might go untreated. Untreated infection can lead to pelvic inflammatory disease, which can cause infertility or ectopic pregnancy (Chapter 22).

Although *N. gonorrhoeae* usually manifests as a local infection in the genital or cervical mucosa, pharynx, or anorectum, disseminated infections may occur. Like *N. meningitidis*, *N. gonorrhoeae* is much more likely to become disseminated in people who lack the complement proteins that form the membrane attack complex. Disseminated infection of adults and adolescents usually causes septic arthritis accompanied by a rash of hemorrhagic papules and pustules. Neonatal *N. gonorrhoeae* infection causes blindness and, rarely, sepsis. The eye infection, which is preventable by instillation of silver nitrate or antibiotics in the newborn's eyes, remains an important cause of blindness in some developing nations.

Pathogenesis. Both significant species of Neisseria use antigenic variation to escape the immune response. The existence of multiple serotypes of *N. meningitidis* results in meningitis in some people on exposure to a new strain, as discussed above. *Neisseria* species have additional mechanisms of antigenic variation such that a single clone of bacteria gives rise to multiple antigenic types,[91] allowing newly arisen antigenic variants to escape the immune response. Neisseria adhere to and invade non-ciliated epithelial cells at the site of entry (nasopharynx, urethra, or cervix). Bacterial persistence or invasion depends on escape from immune defenses. Two surface proteins of *Neisseria*, both of which adhere the bacteria to host cells, undergo antigenic variation through different mechanisms. Although both *N. meningitidis* and *N. gonorrhoeae* use these mechanisms, they appear to be more important in *N. gonorrhoeae*.

- There is a single complete gene for *pili* in the bacterial chromosome. Adherence of *N. gonorrhoeae* to epithelial cells is initially mediated by long pili, which bind to CD46, a complement-regulatory protein expressed by all human nucleated cells (Fig. 8–25). The expression pili loci include the regulatory elements for gene expression, as well as the entire protein-coding region. There are also 10 to 15 silent pili genes in the chromosome; these encode antigenically variant pili proteins, but they lack the regulatory elements (promoter) as well as the DNA encoding the N-terminal domain of the protein. Homologous recombination between the silent loci and the expression loci for pili shuttles variant genes into the complete loci, resulting in expression of new pili proteins. Because part or all of the coding

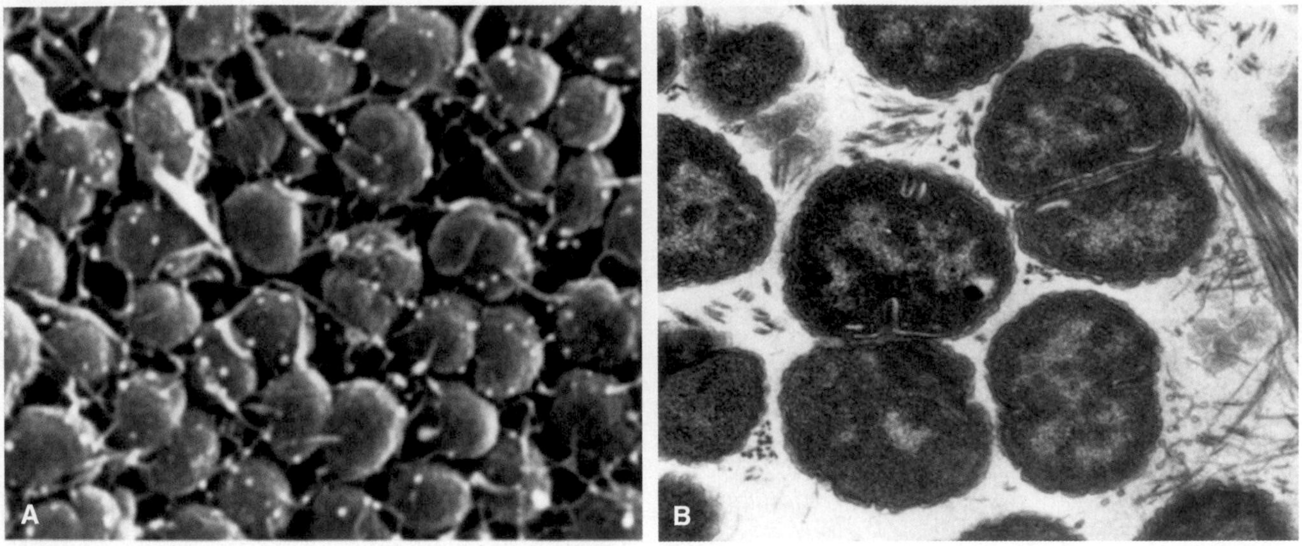

FIGURE 8–25 Gonococcal culture showing pili, as seen by scanning microscopy (*A*), and in clusters, as seen by transmission electron microscopy (*B*). (Courtesy of Dr. John Swanson, Rocky Mountain Laboratories, Hamilton, MT.)

region of a silent locus may recombine with the expression locus, variation can also be generated by the mixing of two or more coding regions.

- *N. gonorrhoeae* has three or four genes for OPA proteins, and *N. meningitidis* has up to 12. OPA proteins (so named because they make bacterial colonies opaque) are located in the outer membrane of the bacteria. They increase binding of Neisseria to epithelial cells and promote entry of bacteria into cells. Each *OPA* gene has several repeats of a 5-nucleotide sequence, which are frequently deleted or duplicated. These changes shift the reading frame of the gene so that it encodes new sequences. Stop codons are also introduced by the additions and deletions, which determine whether each *OPA* gene is expressed or silent. Thus, a single clone of *N. gonorrhoeae* can express none, one, or several *OPA* genes at a time but only a single gene for pili protein.

Whooping Cough

Whooping cough, caused by the Gram-negative coccobacillus *Bordetella pertussis*, is an acute, highly communicable illness characterized by paroxysms of violent coughing followed by a loud inspiratory "whoop." *B. pertussis* vaccination, whether with killed bacteria or the newer acellular vaccine, has been effective in preventing whooping cough. Since the 1980s, however, rates of pertussis have been increasing in areas such as the United States and the Netherlands, despite continued high rates of vaccination.[92,93] The cause of this increase is not known, but antigenic divergence of clinical strains from vaccine strains and waning immunity in young adults may play a role. In parts of the developing world, where vaccination is not widely practiced, pertussis kills hundreds of thousands of children each year.

Pathogenesis *B. pertussis* colonizes the brush border of the bronchial epithelium and also invades macrophages. Coordinated expression of virulence factors is regulated by the *Bordetella* virulence gene locus *(bvg)*.[94] BVGS is a transmembrane protein that "senses" signals that induce expression of virulence factors. On activation, BVGS phosphorylates the protein BVGA, which regulates transcription of mRNA for adhesins and toxins. The filamentous hemagglutinin adhesin binds to carbohydrates on the surface of respiratory epithelial cells, as well as to CR3 (Mac-1) integrins on macrophages. Pertussis toxin is an exotoxin composed of five distinct peptides, including a catalytic peptide S1 that shows homology with the catalytic peptides of cholera toxin and *E. coli* heat-labile toxin.[95] Like cholera toxin, pertussis toxin ADP-ribosylates and inactivates guanine nucleotide–binding proteins, so these G-proteins no longer transduce signals from host plasma membrane receptors. Indeed, inhibition of signals by pertussis toxin is considered a signature of seven-transmembrane G-protein–coupled receptors. The toxins produced by *B. pertussis* paralyze the cilia, thus impairing an important pulmonary defense.

Morphology. *Bordetella* bacteria cause a laryngotracheobronchitis that in severe cases features bronchial mucosal erosion, hyperemia, and copious mucopurulent exudate (Fig. 8–26). Unless superinfected, the lung alveoli remain open and intact. In parallel with a striking peripheral lymphocytosis (up to 90%), there is hypercellularity and enlargement of the mucosal lymph follicles and peribronchial lymph nodes.

Pseudomonas Infection

Pseudomonas aeruginosa is an opportunistic aerobic Gram-negative bacillus that is a frequent, deadly pathogen of

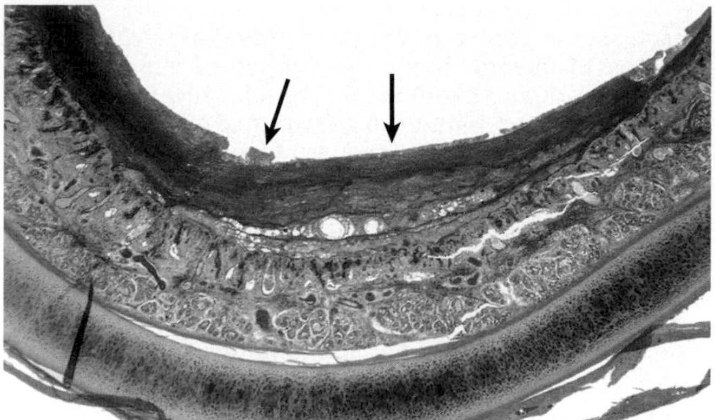

FIGURE 8–26 Whooping cough showing a haze of bacilli *(arrows)* etangled with the cilia of bronchial epithelial cells.

patients with cystic fibrosis, severe burns, or neutropenia.[96] Most patients with cystic fibrosis die of pulmonary failure secondary to chronic infection with *P. aeruginosa.* In addition, species in the *Burkholderia cepacia* complex, which are transmitted between cystic fibrosis patients, opportunistically infect people with cystic fibrosis and often cause fatal infections. Both *P. aeruginosa* and *B. cepacia* complex bacteria can be very resistant to antibiotics, making these infections difficult to treat. Although Gram-positive cocci are most frequently present soon after extensive skin burns, *P. aeruginosa* eventually predominates, spreads locally, and causes sepsis. *P. aeruginosa* is a common cause of hospital-acquired infections; it has been cultured from washbasins, respirator tubing, nursery cribs, and even antiseptic-containing bottles.

P. aeruginosa also causes corneal keratitis in wearers of contact lenses, endocarditis and osteomyelitis in intravenous drug abusers, external otitis (swimmer's ear) in healthy individuals, and severe external otitis in diabetics.

Pathogenesis. *P. aeruginosa* has pili and adherence proteins that bind to epithelial cells and lung mucin, as well as an endotoxin that causes the symptoms and signs of Gram-negative sepsis. *Pseudomonas* also has a number of virulence factors that are distinctive. In the lungs of patients with cystic fibrosis, these bacteria secrete a mucoid exopolysaccharide called *alginate*, forming a slimy biofilm in which bacteria are protected from antibodies, complement, phagocytes, and antibiotics. The organisms also secrete an exotoxin and several other virulence factors. Exotoxin A is similar in structure to diphtheria toxin and, like diphtheria toxin, it inhibits protein synthesis by ADP-ribosylating EF-2, a ribosomal guanine nucleotide–binding protein (G-protein).[97] *P. aeruginosa* also releases exoenzyme S, which ADP-ribosylates G-proteins, including p21 RAS, and so may interfere with host cell growth. The organisms also secrete a phospholipase C that lyses red blood cells and degrades pulmonary surfactant, and an elastase that degrades IgGs and extracellular matrix proteins. These enzymes may be important in tissue invasion and destruction of the cornea in keratitis.[5] Finally, *P. aeruginosa* produces iron-containing compounds that are extremely toxic to endothelial cells and so may cause the vascular lesions that are characteristic of this infection.[98]

Morphology. *Pseudomonas* pneumonia, particularly in the altered host, is the prototype of **necrotizing inflammation**, distributing through the terminal airways in a fleur-de-lis pattern, with striking whitish necrotic centers and red, hemorrhagic peripheral areas. On microscopic examination, masses of organisms cloud the tissue with a bluish haze, concentrating in the wall of blood vessels, where host cells undergo coagulation necrosis and nuclei fade away (Fig. 8–27). This picture of Gram-negative vasculitis accompanied by thrombosis and hemorrhage, although not pathognomonic, is highly suggestive of *P. aeruginosa* infection.

Bronchial obstruction caused by mucous plugging and subsequent *P. aeruginosa* infection are frequent complications of cystic fibrosis. Despite antibiotic treatment and the host immune response against the bacteria, chronic *P. aeruginosa* infection may result in bronchiectasis and pulmonary fibrosis (Chapter 15).

In skin burns, *P. aeruginosa* proliferates widely, penetrating deeply into the veins and spreading to cause massive bacteremias. Well-demarcated necrotic and hemorrhagic skin lesions of oval shape often arise during these bacteremias, called **ecthyma gangrenosum.** Disseminated intravascular coagulation (DIC) is a frequent complication of bacteremia.

Plague

Yersinia pestis is a Gram-negative facultative intracellular bacterium that is transmitted by fleabites or aerosols and causes a highly invasive, frequently fatal systemic infection called *plague.* Plague, also named Black Death, caused three great pandemics that killed an estimated 100 million people in Egypt and Byzantium in the sixth century; one quarter of Europe's population in the fourteenth and fifteenth centuries; and tens of millions in India, Myanmar, and China at the beginning of the twentieth century.[99] After 60 years of quiescence, plague epidemics occurred annually in Madagascar between 1995 and 1998, killing at least 40 people.[100] Currently, wild rodents in the western United States are infected with *Y. pestis*, although human infections are rare. *Y. enterocolitica* and

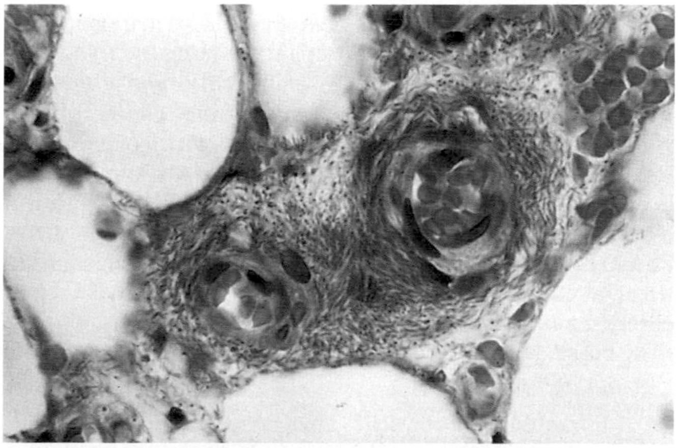

FIGURE 8–27 *Pseudomonas* vasculitis in which masses of organisms form a perivascular blue haze.

Y. pseudotuberculosis are genetically similar to *Y. pestis*; these bacteria cause fecal-orally transmitted ileitis and mesenteric lymphadenitis.

The pathogenic *Yersinia* proliferate within lymphoid tissue. These organisms have a complex of genes, called the Yop virulon, which enable the bacteria to kill host phagocytes, weakening the immune system.[101] The Yop virulon includes a type III secretion system, which is a hollow syringelike structure that projects from the bacterial surface, binds to host cells and injects bacterial toxins, called Yops, into the cell. YopE, YopH, and YopT block phagocytosis by inactivating molecules that regulate actin polymerization. YopPJ inhibits the signaling pathways that are activated by LPS, blocking the production of inflammatory cytokines. *Y. pestis* ensures that fleas will spread the bacteria by blocking the gut of the flea. The flea must regurgitate before it feeds, and in doing so, the flea infects the rodent or human that it is biting.

Morphology. *Y. pestis* causes lymph node enlargement (buboes), pneumonia, or sepsis, all with a striking neutrophilia. The distinctive histologic features of plague include (1) massive proliferation of the organisms, (2) early appearance of protein-rich and polysaccharide-rich effusions with few inflammatory cells but with marked tissue swelling, (3) necrosis of tissues and blood vessels with hemorrhage and thrombosis, and (4) neutrophilic infiltrates that accumulate adjacent to necrotic areas as healing begins.

In **bubonic plague**, the infected fleabite is usually on the legs and is marked by a small pustule or ulceration. The draining lymph nodes enlarge dramatically within a few days and become soft, pulpy, and plum colored and may infarct or rupture through the skin. In **pneumonic plague**, there is a severe, confluent, hemorrhagic, and necrotizing bronchopneumonia, often with fibrinous pleuritis. In **septicemic plague**, lymph nodes throughout the body as well as organs rich in mononuclear phagocytes develop foci of necrosis. Fulminant bacteremias also induce DIC with widespread hemorrhages and thrombi.

Chancroid (Soft Chancre)

Chancroid is an acute, sexually transmitted, ulcerative infection caused by *Hemophilus ducreyi*.[102] The disease is most common in tropical and subtropical areas and is more prevalent in lower socioeconomic groups and among men who have regular contact with prostitutes. *Chancroid is one of the most common causes of genital ulcers in Africa and Southeast Asia*, where it probably serves as an important cofactor in the transmission of HIV-1 infection. The incidence of chancroid has been increasing in the United States since the 1980s, mainly in discrete outbreaks, although it is endemic in some areas. Recent data suggest that chancroid may be underdiagnosed in the United States, since most sexually transmitted disease clinics do not have facilities for isolating *H. ducreyi*, and the PCR-based tests are not widely available.

Morphology. Four to 7 days after inoculation, the patient develops a tender, erythematous papule involving the external genitalia. In males, the primary lesion is usually on the penis; in females, most lesions occur in the vagina or the periurethral area. Over the course of several days, the surface of the primary lesion erodes to produce an irregular ulcer, which is more apt to be painful in males than in females. In contrast to the primary chancre of syphilis, the ulcer of chancroid is not indurated, and multiple lesions may be present. The base of the ulcer is covered by shaggy, yellow-gray exudate. The regional lymph nodes, particularly in the inguinal region, become enlarged and tender in about 50% of cases within 1 to 2 weeks of the primary inoculation. In untreated cases, the inflamed and enlarged nodes (buboes) may erode the overlying skin to produce chronic, draining ulcers.

Microscopically, the ulcer of chancroid contains a superficial zone of neutrophilic debris and fibrin, with an underlying zone of granulation tissue containing areas of necrosis and thrombosed vessels. A dense, lymphoplasmacytic inflammatory infiltrate is present beneath the layer of granulation tissue. Coccobacillary organisms are sometimes demonstrable in Gram or silver stains, but they are often obscured by the mixed bacterial growth that is frequently present at the ulcer base. In the majority of cases, *H. ducreyi* can be cultured from the ulcer when appropriate media are used.

Granuloma Inguinale

Granuloma inguinale, or donovanosis, is a chronic inflammatory disease caused by *Calymmatobacterium donovani*, a minute, encapsulated, coccobacillus that is closely related to the *Klebsiella* genus. The organism is sexually transmitted. Granuloma inguinale is uncommon in the United States and western Europe but is endemic in rural areas in certain tropical and subtropical regions.[103] Untreated cases are characterized by the development of extensive scarring, often associated with lymphatic obstruction and lymphedema (elephantiasis) of the external genitalia. Culture of the organism is difficult, and PCR assays are still in development, so the diagnosis is made by morphologic examination of smears or biopsies of the ulcer.[103]

Morphology. Granuloma inguinale begins as a raised, papular lesion involving the moist, stratified squamous epithelium of the genitalia or, rarely, extragenital sites including the oral mucosa or pharynx. The lesion eventually undergoes ulceration, accompanied by the development of abundant granulation tissue, which is manifested grossly as a protuberant, soft, painless mass. As the lesion enlarges, its borders become raised and indurated. Disfiguring scars may develop in untreated cases and are sometimes associated with urethral, vulvar, or anal strictures. Regional lymph nodes typically are spared or show only nonspecific reactive changes, in contrast to chancroid.

Microscopic examination of active lesions reveals marked epithelial hyperplasia at the borders of the ulcer, sometimes mimicking carcinoma **(pseudoepitheliomatous hyperplasia)**. A mixture of neutrophils and mononuclear inflammatory cells is present at the base of the ulcer and beneath the surrounding epithelium. The organisms are demonstrable in Giemsa-stained smears of the exudate as minute, encapsulated coccobacilli (Donovan bodies) in macrophages. Silver stains (e.g., the Warthin-Starry stain) may also be used to demonstrate the organism.

MYCOBACTERIA

Bacteria in the genus *Mycobacterium* are slender, aerobic rods that grow in straight or branching chains. *Mycobacterium* have a waxy cell wall composed of mycolic acid, which makes them *acid fast*, meaning they will retain stains even on treatment with a mixture of acid and alcohol. Mycobacteria stain weakly positive with Gram stain.

Tuberculosis

M. tuberculosis is responsible for most cases of tuberculosis; the reservoir of infection is humans with active tuberculosis. Oropharyngeal and intestinal tuberculosis contracted by drinking milk contaminated with *M. bovis* is rare in developed nations, but it is still seen in countries that have tuberculous dairy cows and unpasteurized milk.

Epidemiology. Tuberculosis is estimated to affect 1.7 billion individuals worldwide, with 8 to 10 million new cases and 1.7 million deaths each year. After HIV, tuberculosis is the leading infectious cause of death in the world. Infection with HIV makes people susceptible to rapidly progressive tuberculosis; over 50 million people are infected with both HIV and *M. tuberculosis*. From 1985 to 1992, the number of tuberculosis cases in the United States increased by 20% because of increase in disease among people with HIV, among immigrants, and among those in jail or homeless shelters. Because of increased public health efforts, the number of cases of tuberculosis has declined since 1993. Currently, there are about 16,000 new cases of active tuberculosis in the United States annually, and about 45% of these are in immigrants.

Tuberculosis flourishes wherever there is poverty, crowding, and chronic debilitating illness. In the United States, tuberculosis is mainly a disease of the elderly, the urban poor, and people with AIDS. *Certain disease states also increase the risk*: diabetes mellitus, Hodgkin's lymphoma, chronic lung disease (particularly silicosis), chronic renal failure, malnutrition, alcoholism, and immunosuppression.

It is important that *infection* with *M. tuberculosis* be differentiated from *disease*. Infection is the presence of organisms, which may or may not cause clinically significant disease. Most infections are acquired by person-to-person transmission of airborne droplets of organisms from an active case to a susceptible host. In most people, primary tuberculosis is asymptomatic, although it may cause fever and pleural effusion. Generally, the only evidence of infection, if any remains, is a tiny, fibrocalcific nodule at the site of the infection. Viable organisms may remain dormant in such lesions for decades. When the person's immune defenses are lowered, the infection may reactivate to produce communicable and potentially life-threatening disease.

Infection with *M. tuberculosis* typically leads to the development of delayed hypersensitivity to *M. tuberculosis* antigens, which can be detected by the tuberculin (Mantoux) test. About 2 to 4 weeks after infection, intracutaneous injection of purified protein derivative of *M. tuberculosis* (PPD) induces a visible and palpable induration that peaks in 48 to 72 hours. *A positive tuberculin test result* signifies cell-mediated hypersensitivity to tubercular antigens. It does not differentiate between infection and disease. False-negative reactions may be produced by certain viral infections, sarcoidosis, malnutrition, Hodgkin disease, immunosuppression, and (notably) overwhelming active tuberculous disease. False-positive reactions may also result from infection by atypical mycobacteria.

Pathogenesis. The pathogenesis of tuberculosis in a previously unexposed, immunocompetent person depends on the development of anti-mycobacterial cell-mediated immunity, which confers resistance to the bacteria and results in development of hypersensitivity to tubercular antigens. The pathological manifestations of tuberculosis, such as caseating granulomas and cavitation, are the result of the hypersensitivity that is part and parcel of the host immune response. Because the effector cells that mediate immunity also mediate hypersensitivity and tissue destruction, the appearance of hypersensitivity also signals the acquisition of immunity to the organism. A summary of the pathogenesis of tuberculosis is shown in Figure 8–28.

Macrophages are the primary cells infected by *M. tuberculosis*. Early in infection, tuberculosis bacilli replicate essentially unchecked, while later in infection, the T-helper response stimulates macrophages to contain the proliferation of the bacteria.

- *M. tuberculosis* enters macrophages by endocytosis mediated by several macrophage receptors: mannose receptors bind lipoarabinomannan, a glycolipid in the bacterial cell wall, and complement receptors (already discussed) bind opsonized mycobacteria.[26]
- Once inside the macrophage, *M. tuberculosis* replicates within the phagosome by blocking fusion of the phagosome and lysosome.[104,105] This is an active process as live, but not dead, mycobacteria block phagolysosome formation. *M. tuberculosis* has several mechanisms for blocking phagolysosome formation, including inhibition of Ca^{2+} signals and blocking recruitment and assembly of the proteins which mediate phagosome-lysosome fusion. Thus the earliest stage of primary tuberculosis (<3 weeks) in the nonsensitized individual is characterized by proliferation of bacteria in the pulmonary alveolar macrophages and airspaces, with resulting bacteremia and seeding of multiple sites. *Despite the bacteremia, most patients at this stage are asymptomatic or have a mild flulike illness.*
- The genetic make-up of the host may influence the course of the disease. In some people with polymorphisms in the *NRAMP1* gene, the disease may progress from this point without development of an effective immune response. NRAMP1 protein is a transmembrane protein found in endosomes and lysosomes that pumps divalent cations into the lysosome. This may have role in generation of anti-microbial oxygen radicals.[106]
- About 3 weeks after infection, a T_H1 response against *M. tuberculosis* is mounted that activates macrophages to become bactericidal.[107,108] T_H1 cells are stimulated by mycobacterial antigens drained to the lymph node, which are presented with class II major histocompatibility proteins by antigen presenting cells. Differentiation of T_H1 cells depends on the presence of IL-12, which is produced by

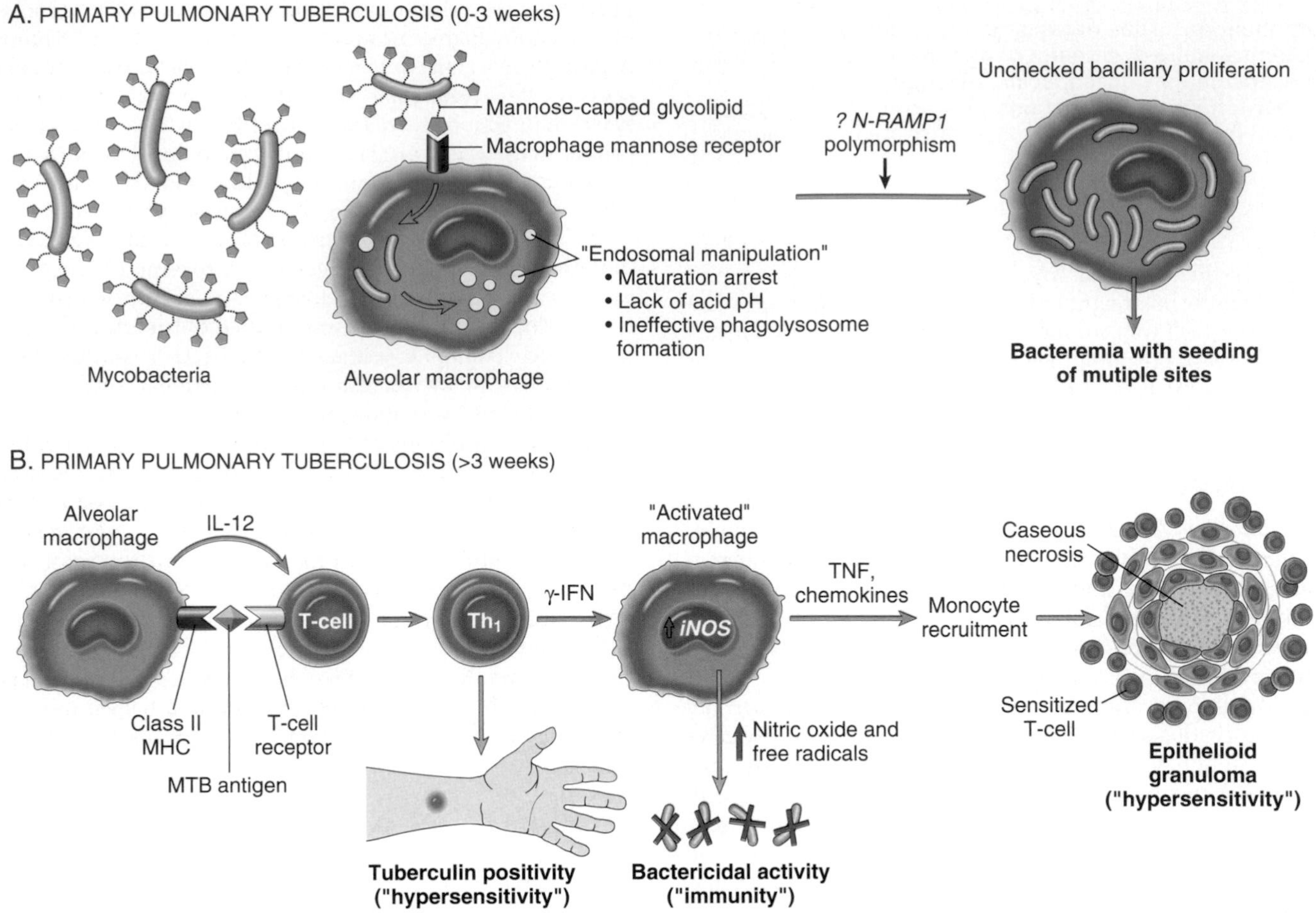

FIGURE 8–28 The sequence of events in primary pulmonary tuberculosis, commencing with inhalation of virulent *M. tuberculosis* and culminating with the development of cell-mediated immunity to the organism. *A*, Events occurring in the first 3 weeks after exposure. *B*, events thereafter. The development of resistance to the organism is accompanied by the appearance of a positive tuberculin test. Cells and bacteria are not drawn to scale. iNOS, inducible nitric oxide synthase; MHC, major histocompatibility complex; MTB, *M. tuberculosis*; NRAMP1, natural resistance-associated macrophage protein.

antigen presenting cells that have encountered the mycobacteria.

- Mature T_H1 cells, both in lymph nodes and in the lung, produce IFN-γ. *IFN-γ is the critical mediator which drives macrophages to become competent to contain the M. tuberculosis infection.* IFN-γ stimulates formation of the phagolysosome in infected macrophages, exposing the bacteria to an inhospitable acidic environment. IFN-γ also stimulates expression of inducible nitric oxide synthase (iNOS), which produces nitric oxide (NO). NO generates reactive nitrogen intermediates and other free radicals capable of oxidative destruction of several mycobacterial constituents, from cell wall to DNA.
- *In addition to stimulating macrophages to kill mycobacteria, the T_H1 response orchestrates the formation of granulomas and caseous necrosis.* Activated macrophages, stimulated by IFN-γ, produce TNF, which recruits monocytes. These monocytes differentiate into the "epithelioid histiocytes" that characterize the granulomatous response. In many people, this response contains the bacteria and doesn't cause significant tissue destruction or illness. In other people, the infection progresses due to age or immunosuppression, and the ongoing immune response results in tissue destruction due to caseation and cavitation. The importance of TNF in this response is underscored by the fact that patients with rheumatoid arthritis who are treated with a TNF antagonist have an increased risk of tuberculosis reactivation.
- In addition to the T_H1 response, unusual T cells which recognize mycobacterial lipid antigens bound to CD1 on antigen presenting cells, or which express a γδ T cell receptor, also make IFN-γ. However, it is clear that T_H1 cells have a central role in this process as *defects in any of the steps in generating a T_H1 response results in absence of resistance and disease progression.*

In summary, immunity to *M. tuberculosis* is primarily mediated by T_H1 cells, which stimulate macrophages to kill the bacteria. This immune response, while largely effective, comes at the cost of hypersensitivity and the accompanying tissue destruction. Reactivation of the infection or re-exposure to the bacilli in a previously sensitized host results in rapid mobilization of a defensive reaction but also increased tissue necrosis. Just as hypersensitivity and resistance appear in parallel, so, too, the loss of hypersensitivity (indicated by tuberculin negativity in a previously tuberculin-positive individual) may be an ominous sign that resistance to the organism has faded.

Clinical Features of Tuberculosis. The many clinical-pathologic patterns of tuberculosis are shown in Figure 8–29. *Primary tuberculosis is the form of disease that develops in a previously unexposed, and therefore unsensitized, person.* About 5% of newly infected people develop clinically significant disease. The elderly and profoundly immunosuppressed persons may lose their immunity to the tubercle bacillus and so may develop primary tuberculosis more than once. With primary tuberculosis, the source of the organism is exogenous.

While most patients with primary tuberculosis go on to have latent disease, progressive infection, with continued lung pathology, occurs in some. The diagnosis of progressive primary tuberculosis in adults can be difficult. Contrary to the usual picture of "adult type" (or reactivation) tuberculosis (apical disease with cavitation; see below), progressive primary tuberculosis more often resembles an acute bacterial pneumonia, with lower and middle lobe consolidation, hilar adenopathy, and pleural effusion; cavitation is rare, especially in patients with severe immunosuppression. Lymphohematogenous dissemination is a dreaded complication and may result in the development of *tuberculous meningitis* and *miliary tuberculosis.* Since similar lesions also occur following progression of secondary tuberculosis, these will be discussed with the latter.

Secondary tuberculosis is the pattern of disease that arises in a previously sensitized host. It may follow shortly after primary tuberculosis, but more commonly, it arises from reactivation of dormant primary lesions many decades after initial infection, particularly when host resistance is weakened. It may also result from exogenous reinfection because of waning of the protection afforded by the primary disease or because of a large inoculum of virulent bacilli. Reactivation of tuberculosis is more common in low-prevalence areas, while reinfection plays an important role in regions of high contagion.

Secondary pulmonary tuberculosis is classically localized to the apex of the upper lobes of one or both lungs. This may be because the high oxygen tension in the apices promotes growth of the bacteria. Because of the preexistence of hypersensitivity, the bacilli elicit a prompt and marked tissue response that tends to wall off the focus of infection. As a result of this localization, the regional lymph nodes are less prominently involved early in the secondary disease than they are in primary tuberculosis. On the other hand, cavitation occurs readily in the secondary form, resulting in dissemination of mycobacteria along the airways. Indeed, cavitation is almost inevitable in neglected secondary tuberculosis, and erosion into an airway becomes an important source of infection because the patient now coughs sputum that contains bacilli.

Localized secondary tuberculosis may be asymptomatic. When manifestations appear, they are usually *insidious* in onset. Systemic symptoms, probably related to cytokines

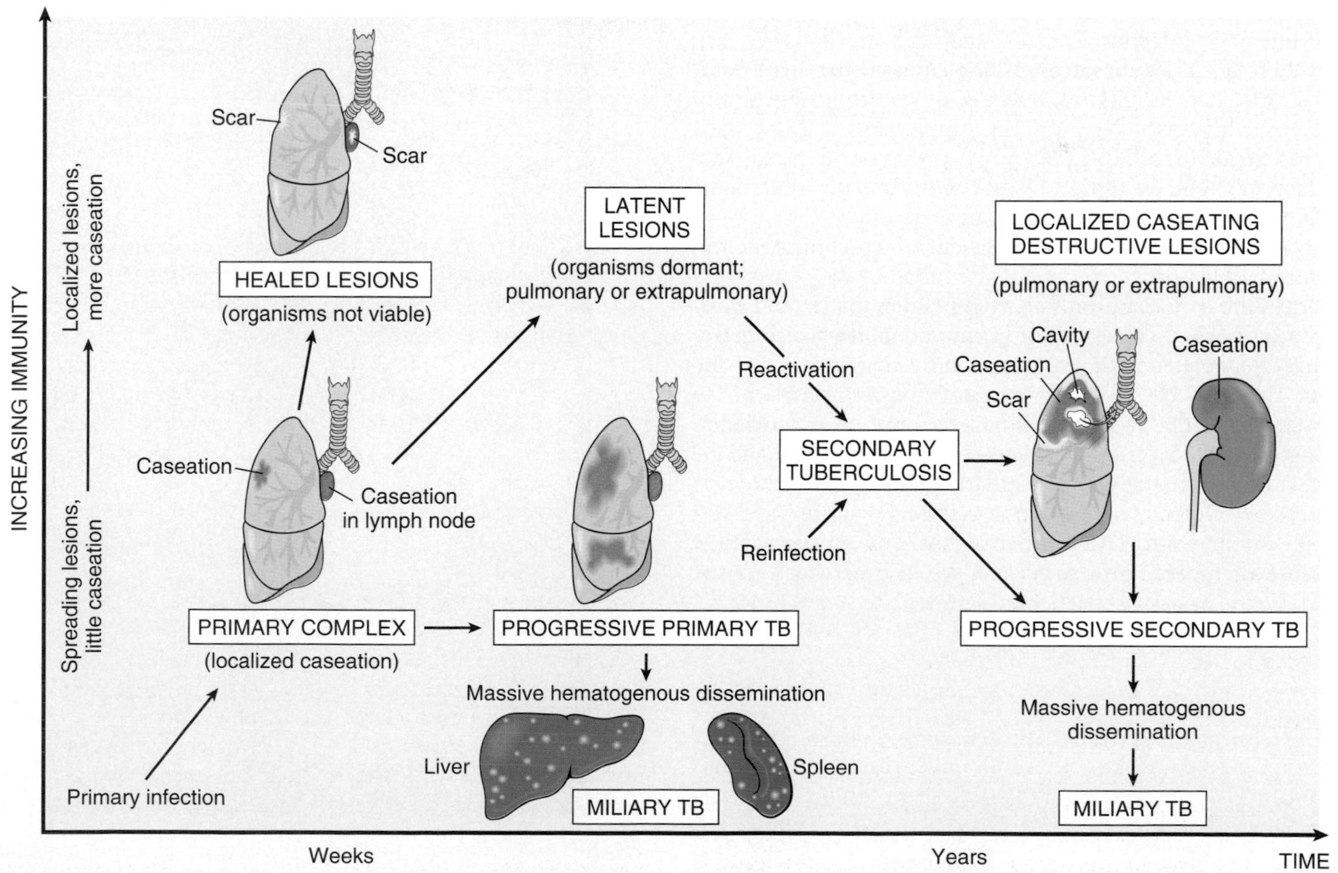

FIGURE 8–29 The natural history and spectrum of tuberculosis. (Adapted from a sketch provided by Dr. R. K. Kumar, The University of New South Wales, School of Pathology, Sydney, Australia.)

released by activated macrophages (e.g., TNF and IL-1), often appear early in the course and include malaise, anorexia, weight loss, and fever. Commonly, the *fever is low grade* and remittent (appearing late each afternoon and then subsiding), and *night sweats* occur. With progressive pulmonary involvement, increasing amounts of sputum, at first mucoid and later purulent, appear. Some degree of *hemoptysis* is present in about half of all cases of pulmonary tuberculosis. *Pleuritic pain* may result from extension of the infection to the pleural surfaces. Extrapulmonary manifestations of tuberculosis are legion and depend on the organ system involved.

The diagnosis of pulmonary disease is based in part on the history and on physical and radiographic findings of consolidation or cavitation in the apices of *the lungs*. Ultimately, however, *tubercle bacilli must be identified.* Acid-fast smears and cultures of the sputum of patients suspected of having tuberculosis should be performed. Conventional cultures required up to 10 weeks, but liquid media–based culture can provide an answer within 2 weeks. PCR amplification of *M. tuberculosis* DNA allows for even more rapid diagnosis. PCR assays can detect as few as 10 organisms in clinical specimens, compared to more than 10,000 organisms required for smear-positivity. However, culture remains the gold standard because it also allows testing of drug susceptibility. Multidrug resistance is now seen more commonly than it was in past years; hence, currently, all newly diagnosed cases in the United States are treated with multiple drugs. The prognosis is generally good if infections are localized to the lungs, except when they are caused by drug-resistant strains or occur in aged, debilitated, or immunosuppressed individuals, who are at high risk for developing miliary tuberculosis (see below).

While HIV infection is associated with an increased risk of tuberculosis at all stages of the disease, the manifestations differ depending on the degree of immunosuppression. Patients with less severe immunosuppression (CD4+ T-cell counts greater than 300 cells/mm^3) present with usual secondary tuberculosis (apical disease with cavitation). Patients with more advanced immunosuppression (CD4+ T-cell counts less than 200 cells/mm^3) present with a clinical picture that resembles progressive primary tuberculosis (lower and middle lobe consolidation, hilar lymphadenopathy, and non-cavitary disease). The extent of immunodeficiency also determines the frequency of extrapulmonary involvement, rising from 10% to 15% in mildly immunosuppressed patients to greater than 50% in those with severe immune deficiency. Other atypical features in HIV-positive patients that make the diagnosis of tuberculosis particularly challenging include an increased frequency of sputum-smear negativity for acid-fast bacilli compared to HIV-negative controls, false-negative PPD because of tuberculin anergy, and the lack of characteristic granulomas in tissues, particularly in the late stages of HIV.

Morphology

Primary Tuberculosis. In countries where bovine tuberculosis and infected milk have been eliminated, primary tuberculosis almost always begins in the lungs. Typically, the inhaled bacilli implant in the distal airspaces of the lower part of the upper lobe or the upper part of the lower lobe, usually close to the pleura. As sensitization develops, a 1- to 1.5-cm area of gray-white inflammatory consolidation emerges, known as the Ghon focus. In most cases, the center of this focus undergoes caseous necrosis. Tubercle bacilli, either free or within phagocytes, drain to the regional nodes, which also often caseate. This combination of parenchymal lung lesion and nodal involvement is referred to as the Ghon complex (Fig. 8–30). During the first few weeks, there is also lymphatic and hematogenous dissemination to other parts of the body. In approximately 95% of cases, development of cell-mediated immunity controls the infection. Hence, the Ghon complex undergoes progressive fibrosis, often followed by radiologically detectable calcification (Ranke complex), and despite seeding of other organs, no lesions develop.

Histologically, sites of active involvement are marked by a characteristic granulomatous inflammatory reaction that forms both caseating and noncaseating tubercles (Figs. 8–31*A* to *C*). Individual tubercles are microscopic; it is only when multiple granulomas coalesce that they become macroscopically visible. The granulomas are usually enclosed within a fibroblastic rim punctuated by lymphocytes. Multinucleate giant cells are present in the granulomas. Immunocompromised people do not form the characteristic granulomas (Fig. 8–31*D*).

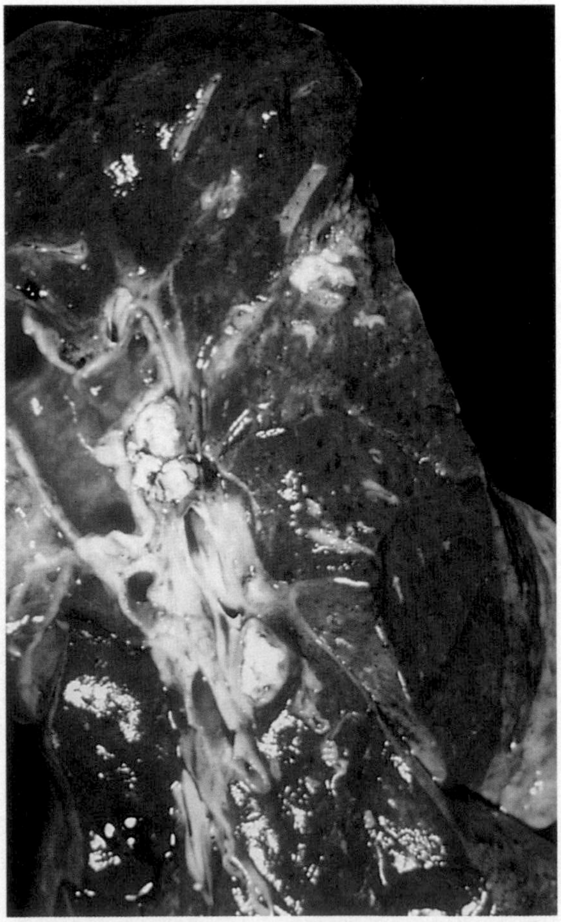

FIGURE 8–30 Primary pulmonary tuberculosis, Ghon complex. The gray-white parenchymal focus is under the pleura in the lower part of the upper lobe. Hilar lymph nodes with caseation are seen on the left.

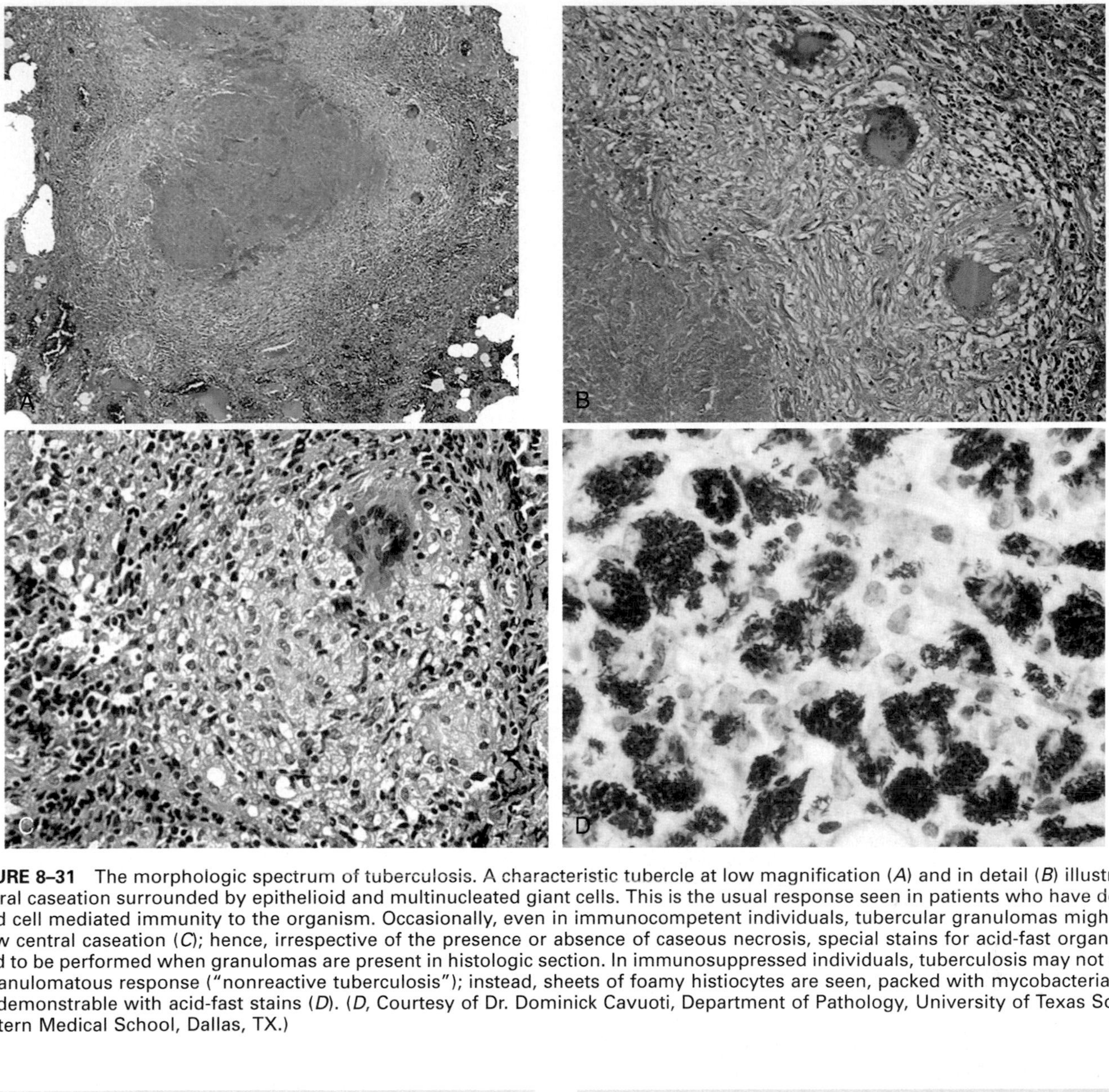

FIGURE 8–31 The morphologic spectrum of tuberculosis. A characteristic tubercle at low magnification (*A*) and in detail (*B*) illustrates central caseation surrounded by epithelioid and multinucleated giant cells. This is the usual response seen in patients who have developed cell mediated immunity to the organism. Occasionally, even in immunocompetent individuals, tubercular granulomas might not show central caseation (*C*); hence, irrespective of the presence or absence of caseous necrosis, special stains for acid-fast organisms need to be performed when granulomas are present in histologic section. In immunosuppressed individuals, tuberculosis may not elicit a granulomatous response ("nonreactive tuberculosis"); instead, sheets of foamy histiocytes are seen, packed with mycobacteria that are demonstrable with acid-fast stains (*D*). (*D*, Courtesy of Dr. Dominick Cavuoti, Department of Pathology, University of Texas Southwestern Medical School, Dallas, TX.)

Secondary Tuberculosis. **The initial lesion is usually a small focus of consolidation, less than 2 cm in diameter, within 1 to 2 cm of the apical pleura.** Such foci are sharply circumscribed, firm, gray-white to yellow areas that have a variable amount of central caseation and peripheral fibrosis (Fig. 8–32). In favorable cases, the initial parenchymal focus undergoes progressive fibrous encapsulation, leaving only fibrocalcific scars. Histologically, the active lesions show characteristic coalescent tubercles with central caseation. Although tubercle bacilli can be demonstrated by appropriate methods in early exudative and caseous phases of granuloma formation, it is usually impossible to find them in the late, fibrocalcific stages. Localized, apical, secondary pulmonary tuberculosis may heal with fibrosis either spontaneously or after therapy, or the disease may progress and extend along several different pathways.

Progressive pulmonary tuberculosis may ensue in the elderly and immunosuppressed. The apical lesion enlarges with expansion of the area of caseation. Erosion into a bronchus evacuates the caseous center, creating a ragged, irregular cavity lined by caseous material that is poorly walled off by fibrous tissue. Erosion of blood vessels results in hemoptysis. With adequate treatment, the process may be arrested, although healing by fibrosis often distorts the pulmonary architecture. Irregular cavities, now free of caseation necrosis, may remain or collapse in the surrounding fibrosis. If the treatment is inadequate or if host defenses are impaired, the infection may spread by direct expansion via dissemination through airways, lymphatic channels, or the vascular system. **Miliary pulmonary disease** occurs when organisms drain through lymphatics into the lymphatic ducts, which empty into the venous return to the right side of the heart and thence into the pulmonary arteries. Individual lesions are either microscopic or small, visible (2-mm) foci of yellow-white consolidation scattered through the lung parenchyma (the word

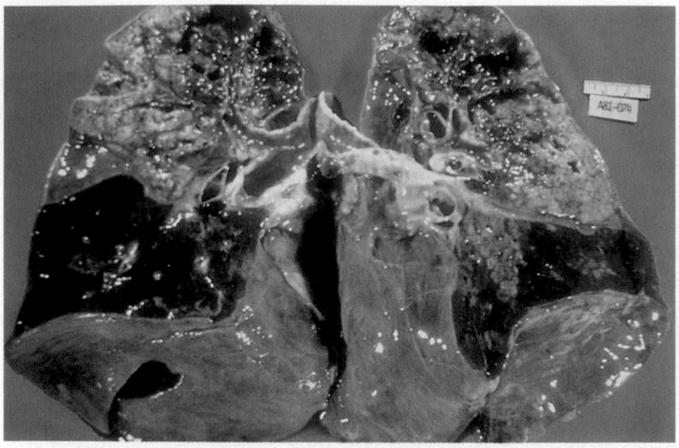

FIGURE 8–32 Secondary pulmonary tuberculosis. The upper parts of both lungs are riddled with gray-white areas of caseation and multiple areas of softening and cavitation.

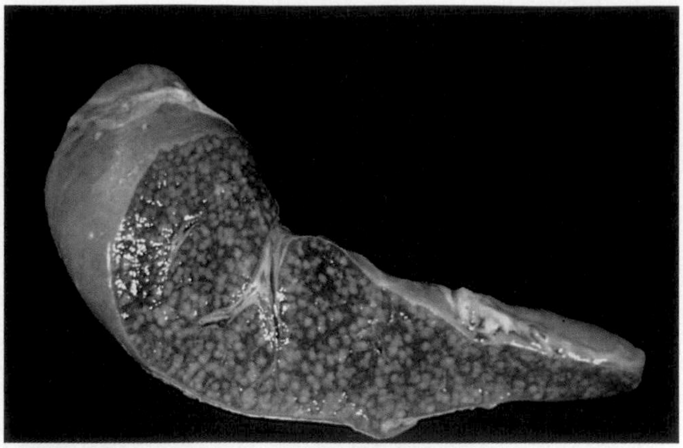

FIGURE 8–33 Miliary tuberculosis of the spleen. The cut surface shows numerous gray-white granulomas.

"miliary" is derived from the resemblance of these foci to millet seeds). Miliary lesions may expand and coalesce to yield almost total consolidation of large regions or even whole lobes of the lung. With progressive pulmonary tuberculosis, the pleural cavity is invariably involved, and serous **pleural effusions, tuberculous empyema**, or **obliterative fibrous pleuritis** may develop.

Endobronchial, endotracheal, and laryngeal tuberculosis may develop when infective material is spread either through lymphatic channels or from expectorated infectious material. The mucosal lining may be studded with minute granulomatous lesions, sometimes apparent only on microscopic examination.

Systemic miliary tuberculosis ensues when infective foci in the lungs seed the pulmonary venous return to the heart; the organisms subsequently disseminate through the systemic arterial system. Almost every organ in the body can be seeded. Lesions resemble those in the lung. Miliary tuberculosis is most prominent in the liver, bone marrow, spleen, adrenals, meninges, kidneys, fallopian tubes, and epididymis (Fig. 8–33).

Isolated-organ tuberculosis may appear in any of the organs or tissues seeded hematogenously and may be the presenting manifestation of tuberculosis. Organs that are typically involved include the meninges (tuberculous meningitis), kidneys (renal tuberculosis), adrenals (formerly an important cause of Addison disease), bones (osteomyelitis), and fallopian tubes (salpingitis). When the vertebrae are affected, the disease is referred to as Pott's disease. Paraspinal "cold" abscesses in these patients may track along the tissue planes to present as an abdominal or pelvic mass.

Lymphadenitis is the most frequent form of extrapulmonary tuberculosis, usually occurring in the cervical region ("scrofula"). In HIV-negative individuals, lymphadenopathy tends to be unifocal, and most patients do not have evidence of ongoing extranodal disease. HIV-positive patients, on the other hand, almost always demonstrate multifocal disease, systemic symptoms, and either pulmonary or other organ involvement by active tuberculosis.

In years past, **intestinal tuberculosis** contracted by the drinking of contaminated milk was fairly common as a primary focus of tuberculosis. In developed countries today, intestinal tuberculosis is more often a complication of protracted advanced secondary tuberculosis, secondary to the swallowing of coughed-up infective material. Typically, the organisms are trapped in mucosal lymphoid aggregations of the small and large bowel, which then undergo inflammatory enlargement with ulceration of the overlying mucosa, particularly in the ileum.

Mycobacterium Avium-Intracellulare Complex

Mycobacterium avium (which includes three subspecies) and *Mycobacterium intracellulare* are separate species, but the infections they cause are so similar that they are simply referred to as *Mycobacterium avium-intracellulare* complex, or MAC. MAC is common in soil, water, dust, and domestic animals. Clinically significant infection with MAC is uncommon except among people with AIDS and low levels of CD4+ lymphocytes (<60 cells/mm^3).

In AIDS patients, MAC causes widely disseminated infections, and organisms proliferate abundantly in many organs, commonly including the lungs and gastrointestinal system. Unchecked by the immune response, the organisms reach very high levels: up to 10^4 organisms/mL of blood and 10^6 organisms/gm in tissue. Patients are feverish, with drenching night sweats and weight loss. In the rare case of MAC in a patient without HIV, the organisms primarily infect the lung, causing a productive cough and sometimes fever and weight loss.

Morphology. The hallmark of MAC infections in patients with HIV is abundant acid-fast bacilli within macrophages (Fig. 8–34). MAC infections are usually widely disseminated throughout the mononuclear systems, causing enlargement of involved lymph nodes, liver, and spleen. There may be a yellowish pigmentation to these organs secondary to the large number of organisms present in swollen macrophages. Granulomas, lymphocytes, and tissue destruction are rare.

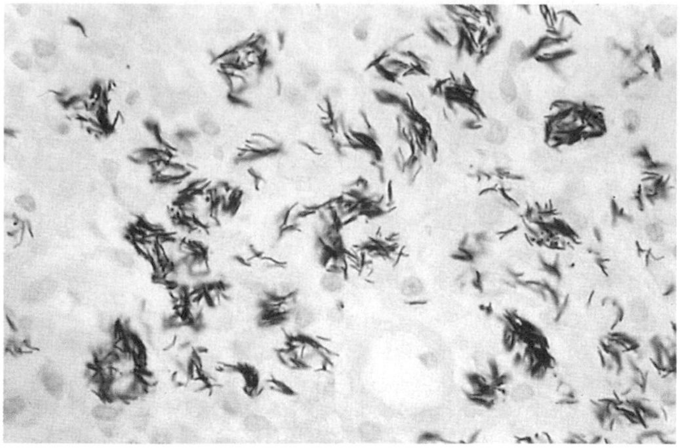

FIGURE 8–34 *Mycobacterium avium* infection in a patient with AIDS, showing massive infection with acid-fast organisms.

Leprosy

Leprosy, or Hansen disease, is a slowly progressive infection caused by *Mycobacterium leprae*, affecting the skin and peripheral nerves and resulting in disabling deformities. *M. leprae* is, for the most part, contained within the skin, but leprosy is likely to be transmitted from person to person through aerosols from lesions in the upper respiratory tract. Inhaled *M. leprae*, like *M. tuberculosis*, is taken up by alveolar macrophages and disseminates through the blood, but grows only in relatively cool tissues of the skin and extremities. Despite its low communicability, leprosy remains endemic among an estimated 10 to 15 million people living in poor tropical countries.

Pathogenesis. *M. leprae* is an acid-fast obligate intracellular organism that grows very poorly in culture but can be grown in the armadillo. It grows more slowly than other mycobacteria and grows best at 32° to 34°C, the temperature of the human skin and the core temperature of armadillos. Like *M. tuberculosis*, *M. leprae* secretes no toxins, and its virulence is based on properties of its cell wall. The cell wall is similar enough to that of *M. tuberculosis* that immunization with bacille Calmette-Guérin confers some protection against *M. leprae* infection. Cell-mediated immunity is reflected by delayed type hypersensitivity reactions to dermal injections of a bacterial extract called *lepromin*.

Leprosy has two strikingly different patterns of disease. Patients with the less severe form, *tuberculoid leprosy*, have dry, scaly skin lesions that lack sensation. They often have large, asymmetric peripheral nerve involvement. The more severe form of leprosy, *lepromatous leprosy*, includes symmetric skin thickening and nodules. This is also called *anergic leprosy*, because of the unresponsiveness (anergy) of the host immune system. Cooler areas of skin, including the earlobes and feet, are more severely affected than warmer areas, such as the axilla and groin. In lepromatous leprosy, damage to the nervous system comes from widespread invasion of the mycobacteria into Schwann cells and into endoneural and perineural macrophages. In advanced cases of lepromatous leprosy, *M. leprae* is present in sputum and blood. People can also have intermediate forms of disease, called *borderline leprosy*.

The T-helper lymphocyte response to *M. leprae* determines whether an individual has tuberculoid or lepromatous leprosy.[109] Patients with tuberculoid leprosy have a T_H1 response, with production of IL-2 and IFN-γ. As with *M. tuberculosis*, IFN-γ is critical to mobilizing an effective host macrophage response. IL-12, which is produced by antigen presenting cells, is important to the generation of T_H1 cells (Chapter 6). Low levels of IL-12 or unresponsiveness of T cells to this cytokine may reduce the T_H1 response, leading to lepromatous leprosy. In addition to T_H1 cells, lymphocytes bearing the γ/δ T-cell receptor infiltrate the lesions of leprosy and produce IFN-γ in patients with tuberculoid leprosy. Patients with lepromatous leprosy have a defective T_H1 response or a dominant T_H2 response, with production of IL-4, IL-5, and IL-10, which may suppress macrophage activation in response to *M. leprae*. In some cases, antibodies are produced against *M. leprae* antigens. Paradoxically, these antibodies are usually not protective, but they may form immune complexes with free antigens that can lead to erythema nodosum, vasculitis and glomerulonephritis.

Morphology. Tuberculoid leprosy begins with localized skin lesions that are at first flat and red but enlarge and develop irregular shapes with indurated, elevated, hyperpigmented margins and depressed pale centers (central healing). Neuronal involvement dominates tuberculoid leprosy. Nerves become enclosed within granulomatous inflammatory reactions and, if small enough (e.g., the peripheral twigs), are destroyed (Fig. 8–35). Nerve degeneration causes skin anesthesias and skin and muscle atrophy that render the patient liable to trauma of the affected parts, with the development of indolent skin ulcers. Contractures, paralyses, and autoamputation of fingers or toes may ensue. Facial nerve involvement can lead to paralysis of the eyelids, with keratitis and corneal ulcerations. On microscopic examination, all sites of involvement disclose granulomatous lesions closely resembling those found in tuberculosis, and bacilli are almost never found. The presence of granulomas and absence of bacteria reflect strong T-cell immunity. Because leprosy pursues an extremely slow course, spanning decades, most patients die with leprosy rather than of it.

Lepromatous leprosy involves the skin, peripheral nerves, anterior chamber of the eye, upper airways (down to the larynx), testes, hands, and feet. The vital organs and central nervous system are rarely affected, presumably because the core temperature is too high for growth of *M. leprae*. Lepromatous lesions contain large aggregates of lipid-laden macrophages (lepra cells), often filled with masses of acid-fast bacilli (globi; Fig. 8–36). The failure to contain the infection and to form granulomas reflects failure of the T_H1 response. Macular, papular, or nodular lesions form on the face, ears, wrists, elbows, and knees. With progression, the nodular lesions coalesce to yield a distinctive leonine facies. Most skin lesions are hypoesthetic or anesthetic. Lesions in the nose may cause persistent inflammation and bacilli-laden discharge. The peripheral nerves, particularly the ulnar and peroneal nerves where they approach the skin surface, are symmetrically invaded with mycobacteria, with minimal inflammation. Loss of sensation and trophic changes in the hands and feet follow the nerve lesions. Lymph nodes show aggregation of foamy

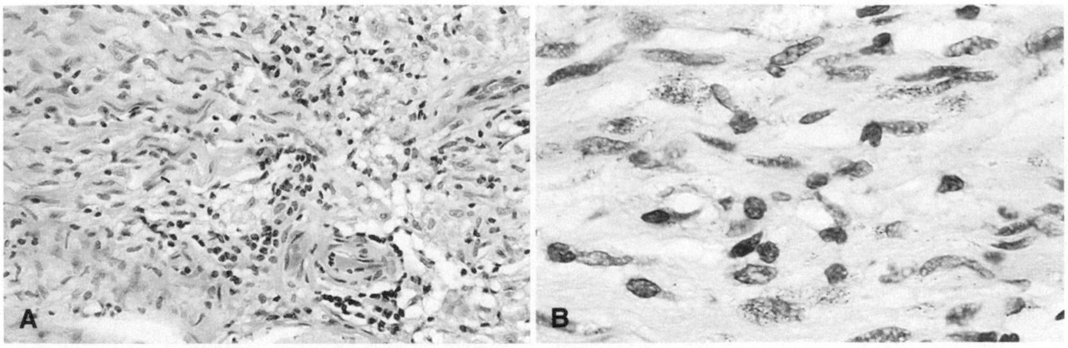

FIGURE 8–35 Leprosy. *A,* Peripheral nerve. Note the inflammatory cell infiltrates in the endoneural and epineural compartments. *B,* Cells within the endoneurium contain acid-fast positive lepra bacilli. (Courtesy of E.P. Richardson, Jr. and U. De Girolami, Harvard Medical School.)

macrophages in the paracortical (T-cell) areas, with enlargement of germinal centers. In advanced disease, aggregates of macrophages are also present in the splenic red pulp and the liver. The testes are usually extensively involved, with destruction of the seminiferous tubules and consequent sterility.

SPIROCHETES

Spirochetes are Gram-negative, slender corkscrew-shaped bacteria with axial periplasmic flagella wound around a helical protoplasm. The bacteria are covered in a membrane called an outer sheath, which may mask bacterial antigens from the host immune response.

Syphilis

Treponema pallidum subspecies pallidum is the microaerophilic spirochete that causes syphilis, a chronic venereal disease with multiple clinical presentations. Other closely related treponemes cause yaws *(Treponema pallidum subspecies pertenue)* and pinta *(Treponema pallidum subspecies carateum). T. pallidum subspecies pallidum,* hereafter referred to simply as *T. pallidum,* is too slender to be seen in conventional stains such as Gram stain, but it can be visualized by silver stains, dark-field examination, and immunofluorescence techniques (Fig. 8–37). Sexual intercourse is the usual mode of spread. Transplacental transmission of *T. pallidum* occurs readily, and active disease during pregnancy results in congenital syphilis.

Public health programs and penicillin treatment reduced the number of cases of syphilis in the United States from the late 1940s until the 1970s. Cases of syphilis surged upward in the mid-1980s, reaching a total of 50,223 cases in 1990. Renewed public health efforts led to a sharp drop in the incidence of syphilis over the next 10 years, with 5979 cases reported in 2000. In 2001, there was a small but concerning increase to 6103 cases. Syphilis is 16 times more common among black people than among white people; however, this disparity is shrinking owing to falling rates in blacks and rising rates in whites. The disease is more common in the southern United States, but the rate is dropping in the South and rising in the Northeast and West. In 1999, the Centers for Disease Control announced a National Syphilis Elimination Plan, with the goal of reducing the number of new syphilis cases in the United States to fewer than 1000 each year.

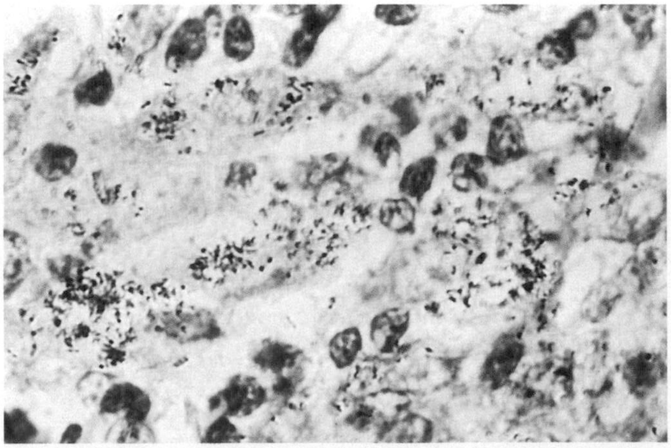

FIGURE 8–36 Lepromatous leprosy. Acid-fast bacilli ("red snappers") within macrophages.

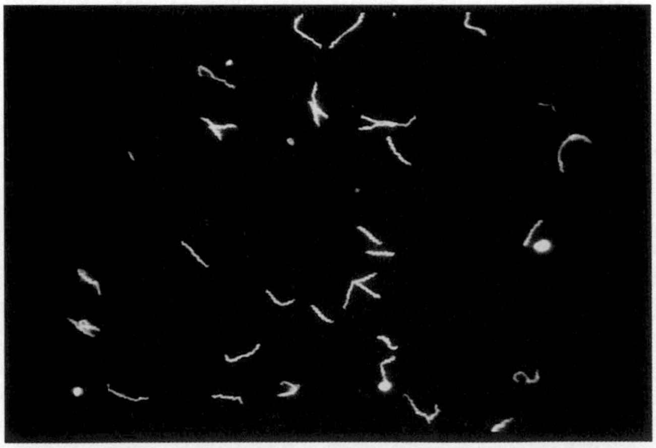

FIGURE 8–37 *Treponema pallidum* (dark-field microscopy) showing several spirochetes in scrapings from the base of a chancre. (Courtesy of Dr. Paul Southern, Department of Pathology, University of Texas Southwestern Medical School, Dallas, TX.)

Syphilis is divided into three stages, which have distinct clinical and pathologic manifestations (Fig. 8–38).

Primary Syphilis. The *primary stage* of syphilis, occurring approximately 3 weeks after contact with an infected individual, features a single firm, nontender, raised, red lesion (chancre) located at the site of treponemal invasion on the penis, cervix, vaginal wall, or anus. The chancre heals in 3 to 6 weeks with or without therapy. *Spirochetes are plentiful within the chancre and can be seen by dark-field microscopy or immunofluorescent stains of serous exudate.* Treponemes spread throughout the body by hematologic and lymphatic dissemination even before the appearance of the chancre.

Secondary Syphilis. The *secondary stage* of syphilis usually occurs 2 to 10 weeks after the primary chancre and is due to spread and proliferation of the spirochetes within the skin and mucocutaneous tissues. Secondary syphilis occurs in approximately 75% of untreated patients. *The skin lesions, which frequently occur on the palms or soles of the feet, may be maculopapular, scaly, or pustular.* Moist areas of the skin, such as the anogenital region, inner thighs, and axillae, may have *condylomata lata*, which are broad-based, elevated plaques. Silvery-gray superficial erosions may form on any of the mucous membranes but are particularly common in the mouth, pharynx, and external genitalia. All these painless superficial lesions contain spirochetes and so are infectious. Lymphadenopathy, mild fever, malaise, and weight loss are also common in secondary syphilis. The symptoms of secondary syphilis last several weeks, after which the patient enters the latent phase of the disease. Superficial lesions may recur during the early latent phase, although they are milder.

Tertiary Syphilis. The *tertiary stage* of syphilis is rare where adequate medical is available, but it occurs in approximately one-third of untreated patients, usually after a latent period of 5 years or more. Tertiary syphilis has three main manifestations: cardiovascular syphilis, neurosyphilis and so-called benign tertiary syphilis. These may occur alone or in combination.

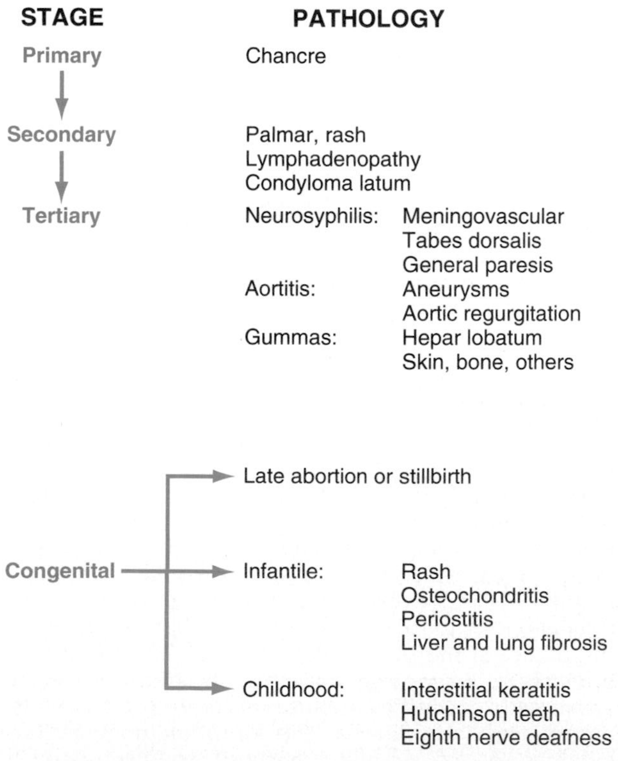

FIGURE 8–38 Protean manifestations of syphilis.

Cardiovascular syphilis, in the form of syphilitic aortitis, accounts for more than 80% of cases of tertiary disease. The aortitis leads to slowly progressive dilation of the aortic root and arch, which causes aortic valve insufficiency and aneurysms of the proximal aorta (see Chapter 11).

Neurosyphilis may be symptomatic or asymptomatic. Symptomatic disease manifests in several ways, including chronic meningovascular disease, tabes dorsalis, and a generalized brain parenchymal disease called *general paresis*. These are discussed in Chapter 28. Asymptomatic neurosyphilis, which accounts for about one third of neurosyphilis, is detected when a patient's CSF exhibits abnormalities such as pleocytosis, elevated protein levels, or decreased glucose. Antibodies stimulated by the spirochetes, discussed below, can also be detected in CSF, and this is the most specific test for neurosyphilis. Asymptomatic people are tested for neurosyphilis because antibiotics are given for a longer time if the spirochetes have spread to the central nervous system.

So-called benign tertiary syphilis is characterized by the formation of gummas in various sites. These are nodular lesions probably related to the development of delayed hypersensitivity to the bacteria. Gummas occur most commonly in bone, skin, and the mucous membranes of the upper airway and mouth, although any organ may be affected. Skeletal involvement characteristically causes local pain, tenderness, swelling, and sometimes pathologic fractures. Involvement of skin and mucous membranes may produce nodular lesions or, rarely, destructive, ulcerative lesions that mimic malignant neoplasms. Gummas, once common, are now very rare because of the use of effective antibiotics.

Congenital Syphilis. Congenital syphilis occurs when *T. pallidum* crosses the placenta from an infected mother to the fetus. Maternal transmission happens most frequently during primary or secondary syphilis, when the spirochetes are most numerous. Congenital syphilis is rare if maternal syphilis has been present for more than 5 years. Because the manifestations of maternal syphilis may be subtle, routine serologic testing for syphilis is mandatory in all pregnancies. Intrauterine death and perinatal death each occurs in approximately 25% of cases of untreated congenital syphilis.

Manifestations of congenital disease are divided into early (infantile) and late (tardive) syphilis, depending on whether they usually occur in the first 2 years of life or later. Early congenital syphilis is often manifested by nasal discharge and congestion (snuffles) in the first few months of life. A desquamating or bullous rash can lead to sloughing of the skin, particularly of the hands and feet and around the mouth and anus. Hepatomegaly and skeletal abnormalities are also common.

Nearly half of untreated children with neonatal syphilis will develop late manifestations. Classic manifestations include the Hutchinson triad: notched central incisors, interstitial keratitis with blindness, and deafness from eighth cranial nerve injury. Skeletal, neurologic, and facial abnormalities may also occur and are discussed below.

Serologic Tests for Syphilis. Although PCR tests for syphilis have been developed, serology remains the mainstay of diagnosis. Serologic tests for syphilis include nontreponemal antibody tests and antitreponemal antibody tests. Nontreponemal tests measure antibody to cardiolipin, a phospholipid that is present in both host tissues and the *T. pallidum.* These antibodies are detected in the rapid plasma reagin (RPR) and Venereal Disease Research Laboratory (VDRL) tests. Nontreponeal tests typically become positive 4 to 6 weeks after infection and are nearly always positive in secondary syphilis. They may become negative in late or tertiary syphilis, despite the presence of low levels of spirochetes. The VDRL and RPR are used as screening tests for syphilis and to monitor response to therapy as these tests become negative after successful treatment of infection. Two additional points about nontreponemal tests deserve emphasis:

- *Nontreponemal antibody tests are often negative during the early stages of disease*, even in the presence of a primary chancre. Dark-field microscopy should always be performed in the evaluation of a suspected chancre, even if serologic tests for syphilis are negative.
- Up to 15% of positive VDRL tests represent *biologic false-positive* results. These false-positive tests, which may be transient or persistent, increase in frequency with age. Conditions associated with false-positive VDRL results include certain acute infections, collagen vascular diseases (e.g., systemic lupus erythematosus), drug addiction, pregnancy, hypergammaglobulinemia of any cause, and lepromatous leprosy.

Treponemal antibody tests measure antibodies reactive with *T. pallidum* after absorption of the serum with nonpathogenic treponemal antigens. These include the fluorescent treponemal antibody absorption test (FTA-Abs) and the microhemaggluination assay for *T. pallidum* antibodies (MHATP). These tests also become positive 4 to 6 weeks after infection, but unlike nontreponemal antibody tests, they remain positive indefinitely, even after successful treatment. They are not recommended as primary screening tests because they are significantly more expensive than nontreponemal tests. While they are more specific than the nontreponemal tests, false-positive treponemal antibody tests occur in up to 2% of the general population.

Serologic response may be delayed, exaggerated (false-positive results), or even absent in some patients with syphilis and HIV infection. However, in most cases, these tests remain extremely useful in the diagnosis and management of syphilis in patients with acquired immunodeficiency syndrome.

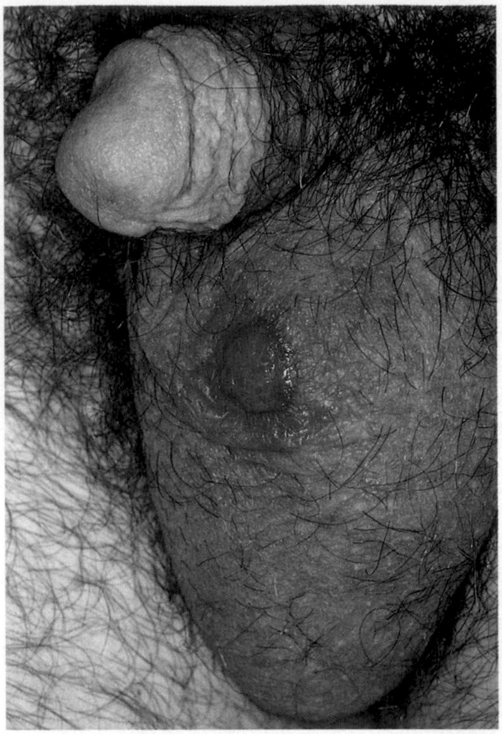

FIGURE 8–39 Syphilitic chancre in the scrotum (see Figure 8–8 for the histopathology of syphilis). (Courtesy of Dr. Richard Johnson, Beth Israel-Deaconess Hospital, Boston, MA.)

Morphology. In **primary syphilis**, a chancre occurs on the penis or scrotum of 70% of men and on the vulva or cervix of 50% of women. The chancre is a slightly elevated, firm, reddened papule, up to several centimeters in diameter, that erodes to create a clean-based shallow ulcer. The contiguous induration creates a buttonlike mass directly adjacent to the eroded skin, providing the basis of the designation hard chancre (Fig. 8–39). On histologic examination, treponemes are visible at the surface of the ulcer with silver stains (e.g., Warthin-Starry stain) or immunofluorescence techniques. The chancre contains an intense infiltrate of plasma cells, with scattered macrophages and lymphocytes and a proliferative endarteritis (Fig. 8–8). The endarteritis, which is seen in all stages of syphilis, starts with endothelial hypertrophy and proliferation followed by intimal fibrosis. The regional nodes are usually enlarged and may show nonspecific acute or chronic lymphadenitis, plasma cell–rich infiltrates, or focal epithelioid granulomas.

In **secondary syphilis**, widespread mucocutaneous lesions involve the oral cavity, palms of the hands, and soles of the feet. The rash is frequently macular, with discrete red-brown spots less than 5 mm in diameter, but it may be follicular, pustular, annular, or scaling. Reddened mucous patches in the mouth or vagina contain the most organisms and are the most infectious. Histologically, the mucocutaneous lesions of secondary syphilis show the same plasma cell infiltrate and obliterative endarteritis as the primary chancre, although the inflammation is often less intense.

Tertiary syphilis occurs years after the initial infection and most frequently involves the aorta (80% to 85%); the central nervous system (5% to 10%); and the liver, bones, and testes. The aortitis is caused by endarteritis of the vasa vasorum of the proximal aorta. Occlusion of the vasa vasorum results in scarring of the media of the proximal aortic wall, causing a loss of elasticity. There may be narrowing of the coronary artery ostia caused by subintimal scarring with resulting myocardial ischemia. The morphologic and clinical features of syphilitic aortitis are discussed in greater detail with diseases of the blood vessels

(Chapter 11). **Neurosyphilis** takes one of several forms, designated meningovascular syphilis, tabes dorsalis, and general paresis (Chapter 28). **Syphilitic gummas** are white-gray and rubbery, occur singly or multiply, and vary in size from microscopic defects resembling tubercles to large tumorlike masses. They occur in most organs but particularly in skin, subcutaneous tissue, bone, and joints. In the liver, scarring as a result of gummas may cause a distinctive hepatic lesion known as hepar lobatum (Fig. 8–40). On histologic examination, the gummas contain a center of coagulated, necrotic material and margins composed of plump or palisaded macrophages and fibroblasts surrounded by large numbers of mononuclear leukocytes, chiefly plasma cells. Treponemes are scant in these gummas and are difficult to demonstrate.

The rash of **congenital syphilis** is more severe than that of adult secondary syphilis, with bullous eruption of the palms and soles of the feet and epidermal sloughing. **Syphilitic osteochondritis and periostitis** affect all bones, although lesions of the nose and lower legs are most distinctive. Destruction of the vomer causes collapse of the bridge of the nose and, later on, the characteristic saddle nose deformity. Periostitis of the tibia leads to excessive new bone growth on the anterior surfaces and anterior bowing, or saber shin. There is also widespread disturbance in endochondral bone formation. The epiphyses become widened as the cartilage overgrows, and cartilage is found as displaced islands within the metaphysis.

The **liver** is often severely affected in congenital syphilis. Diffuse fibrosis permeates lobules to isolate hepatic cells into small nests, accompanied by the characteristic white cell infiltrate and vascular changes. Gummas are occasionally found in the liver, even in early cases. The **lungs** may be affected by a diffuse interstitial fibrosis. In the syphilitic stillborn, the lungs appear as pale, airless organs (pneumonia alba). The generalized spirochetemia may lead to diffuse interstitial inflammatory reactions in virtually any other organ of the body (e.g., the pancreas, kidneys, heart, spleen, thymus, endocrine organs, and central nervous system).

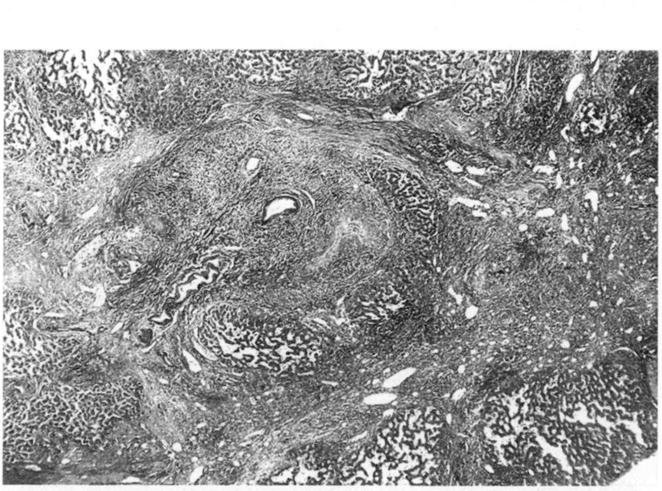

FIGURE 8–40 Trichrome stain of liver shows liver gumma (scar), stained blue, which is caused by tertiary syphilis (also known as hepar lobatum). Compare with nodules of alcoholic cirrhosis (Chapter 18).

The late-occurring form of congenital syphilis is distinctive for the **triad of interstitial keratitis, Hutchinson teeth, and eighth nerve deafness**. Eye changes consist of interstitial keratitis and choroiditis with abnormal pigment production causing a spotted retina. The dental changes involve the incisor teeth, which are small and shaped like a screwdriver or a peg, often with notches in the enamel (Hutchinson teeth). Eighth nerve deafness and optic nerve atrophy develop secondary to meningovascular syphilis.

Pathogenesis. There are no good animals models of syphilis available, and *T. pallidum* has never been grown in culture (it lacks genes for making nucleotides, fatty acids, and most amino acids). As a result, our scant knowledge of *T. pallidum* pathogenesis comes mainly from observations of the disease in humans.

The immune response to *T. pallidum* reduces the burden of bacteria, but it may also have a central role in the pathogenesis of the disease. The T-helper cells that infiltrate the chancre are T_H1 cells, suggesting that activation of macrophages to kill bacteria may cause resolution of the local infection.[110] Although there are many plasma cells in the syphilitic lesions and treponeme-specific antibodies are readily detectable, the antibody response does not eliminate the infection. The outer membrane of *T. pallidum* appears to protect the bacteria from antibody binding. The mechanism of this is not well understood, but either the paucity of bacterial proteins in the membrane or absorption (coating) of the membrane by host proteins may play a role.[111] The immune response is ultimately inadequate, as the spirochetes disseminate, persist, and cause secondary and tertiary syphilis.

Proliferative endarteritis occurs in all stages of syphilis. The pathophysiology of the endarteritis is not known, although the scarcity of treponemes and the intense inflammatory infiltrate suggest that the immune response plays a role in the development of these lesions. Regardless of the mechanism by which the endarteritis forms, much of the pathology of the disease, such as syphilitic aortitis, can be ascribed to the vascular abnormalities.

Relapsing Fever

Relapsing fever is an insect-transmitted disease characterized by recurrent fevers with spirochetemia. *Epidemic relapsing fever* is caused by body louse–transmitted *Borrelia recurrentis*, which infects only humans. *B. recurrentis*, which is associated with overcrowding due to poverty or war, caused multiple large epidemics in Africa, Eastern Europe, and Russia in the first half of the twentieth century, infecting 15 million people and killing 5 million, and is still a problem in some developing countries. *Endemic relapsing fever* is caused by several *Borrelia* species, which are transmitted from small animals to humans by *Ornithodorus* (soft-bodied) ticks.

In both louse- and tick-transmitted borreliosis, there is a 1- to 2-week incubation period after the bite as the spirochetes multiply in the blood. Clinical infection is heralded by shaking chills, fever, headache, and fatigue, followed by disseminated intravascular coagulation and multiorgan failure. Spirochetes are temporarily cleared from the blood by anti-*Borrelia* antibodies, which target a single major surface protein called the variable major protein.[112] After a few days, bacteria bearing a different surface antigen emerge and reach high densities in the blood, and symptoms return until a second set of host antibodies clears these organisms. The lessening severity of successive attacks of relapsing fever and its spontaneous cure in many untreated patients have been attributed to the limited genetic repertoire of *Borrelia*, enabling the host to build up cross-reactive as well as clone-specific antibodies. Antibiotic treatment of *Borrelia* infections may cause a massive release of endotoxin, resulting in the production of cytokines that cause fever with rigors, fall in blood pressure, and leukopenia (the Jarisch-Herxheimer reaction).[113]

Morphology. Diagnosis of relapsing fever can be made by identification of spirochetes in blood smears obtained during febrile periods. In fatal louse-borne disease, the spleen is moderately enlarged (300 to 400 gm) and contains focal necroses and miliary collections of leukocytes, including neutrophils, and numerous borreliae. There is congestion and hypercellularity of the red pulp with erythrophagocytosis. The liver may also be enlarged and congested with prominent Kupffer cells and septic foci. Scattered hemorrhages resulting from DIC may be found in serosal and mucosal surfaces, skin, and viscera. Pulmonary bacterial superinfection is a frequent complication.

Lyme Disease

Lyme disease, named for the Connecticut town where, in the mid-1970s, there was an epidemic of arthritis associated with skin erythema, is caused by several subspecies of the spirochete *Borrelia burgdorferi*.[114,115] The disease, transmitted from rodents to people by *Ixodes* deer ticks (Fig. 8–41), is a common arthropod-borne disease in the United States, Europe, and Japan. In the United States, the incidence of Lyme disease has risen steadily, with approximately 17,000 cases in 2000, almost as many as new cases of tuberculosis. Most cases occur in the Northeastern states and in some parts of Midwestern states. In endemic areas, as many as 50% of ticks are infected with *B. burgdorferi*, and ticks may also be infected with *Ehrlichia* and *Babesia* (discussed later).

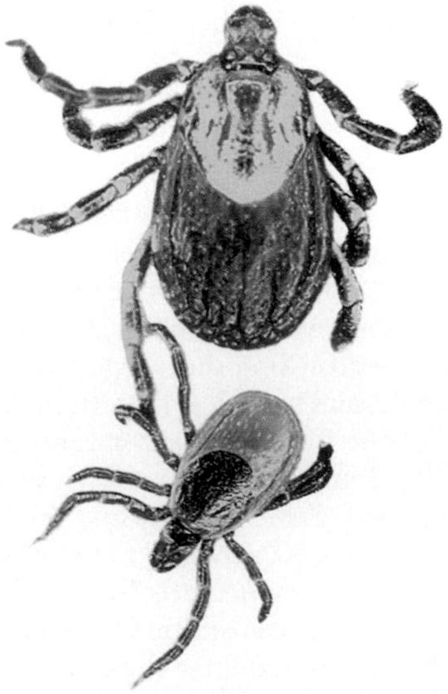

FIGURE 8–41 Tiny deer tick *(bottom)*, which transmits Lyme disease and Babesia and Ehrlichia organisms, contrasted with a larger dog tick *(top)*, which is not thought to transmit human infections. (Courtesy of Dr. F.R. Matuschka, Free University of Berlin, Germany.)

Lyme disease involves multiple organ systems and is divided into three stages. In *stage 1* (Fig. 8–42) spirochetes multiply and spread in the dermis at the site of a tick bite, causing an expanding area of redness, often with a pale center. This skin lesion, called *erythema chronicum migrans*, may be accompanied by fever and lymphadenopathy but usually disappears in 4 to 12 weeks. In *stage 2, the early disseminated stage*, spirochetes spread hematogenously throughout the body and cause secondary skin lesions, lymphadenopathy, migratory joint and muscle pain, cardiac arrhythmias, and meningitis often with cranial nerve involvement. In *stage 3, the late disseminated stage*, 2 or 3 years after the initial bite, Lyme borreliae cause a chronic arthritis sometimes with severe damage to large joints and an encephalitis that varies from mild to debilitating.

Pathogenesis. *B. burgdorferi* does not produce lipopolysaccharide (LPS), and the initial immune response is instead stimulated by binding of bacterial lipoproteins to toll-like receptor 2 expressed by macrophages. In response, these cells release proinflammatory cytokines (IL-6 and TNF) and generate bactericidal nitric oxide, reducing but usually not eliminating the infection.

The adaptive immune response to Lyme disease is mediated by CD4+ T-helper cells and B-cells. Borrelia-specific antibodies, made 2–4 weeks after infection, drive complement-mediated killing of the bacteria, however *B. burgdorferi* escapes the antibody response through antigenic variation. Similar to *Borrelia hermsii*, a cause of relapsing fever, *B. burgdorferi* has a plasmid with a single complete expression site for a gene encoding an antigenic surface protein, VlsE, and several variant coding sequences for VlsE that can shuttle into the expression site. Thus, as the antibody response to one VlsE protein is mounted, bacteria expressing an alternate VlsE protein can escape immune recognition. Chronic manifestations of Lyme disease, such as the late arthritis, are probably

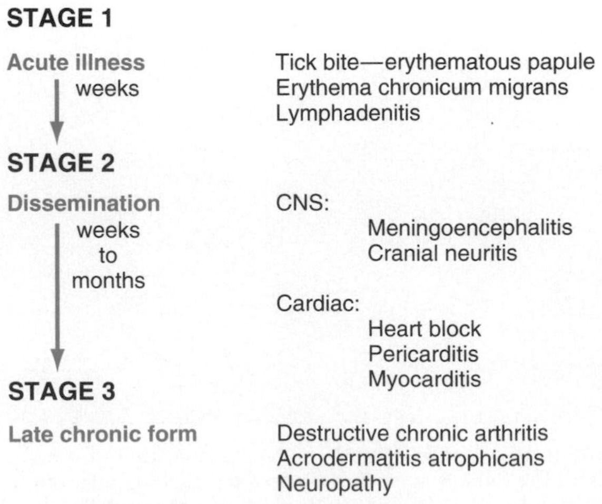

FIGURE 8–42 Clinical stages of Lyme disease.

caused by persistence of bacteria, although an autoimmune response stimulated by the bacteria has also been suggested to have a role.[115]

Morphology. Skin lesions caused by *B. burgdorferi* are characterized by edema and a lymphocytic–plasma cell infiltrate. In early Lyme arthritis, the synovium resembles that of early rheumatoid arthritis, with villous hypertrophy, lining cell hyperplasia, and abundant lymphocytes and plasma cells in the subsynovium. A distinctive feature of Lyme arthritis is an arteritis, with onionskin-like lesions resembling those seen in lupus (Chapter 6). In late Lyme disease, there may be extensive erosion of the cartilage in large joints. In Lyme meningitis, the CSF is hypercellular, shows a marked lymphoplasmacytic infiltrate, and contains anti-spirochete IgGs.

ANAEROBIC BACTERIA

Many anaerobic bacteria are normal flora in sites of the body that have low oxygen levels. The anaerobic flora cause disease (abscesses or peritonitis) when they are introduced into sterile sites or when the balance of organisms is upset and pathogenic anaerobes predominate (*Clostridium difficile* colitis with antibiotic treatment). Environmental anaerobes also cause disease (tetanus, botulism, and gas gangrene).

Abscesses

Abscesses are usually caused by mixed anaerobic and facultative (able to grow with or without oxygen) bacteria. On average, abscesses have 2.5 species of bacteria, 1.6 of which are anaerobes and 0.9 of which are aerobic or facultative bacteria.[116] *Commensal bacteria from adjacent sites (oropharynx, intestine, and female genital tract) are the usual cause of abscesses, so the species found in the abscess reflect the species found in the normal flora.* Since most anaerobes that cause abscesses are part of the normal flora, it is not surprising that these organisms do not produce significant toxins.

The bacteria found in head and neck abscesses reflect the oral and pharyngeal flora. Common anaerobes at this site include the Gram-negative bacilli *Prevotella* and *Porphyromonas* species, often mixed with the facultative *S. aureus* and *S. pyogenes*. *Fusobacterium necrophorum*, an oral commensal, causes Lemierre syndrome, characterized by infection of the lateral pharyngeal space and septic jugular vein thrombosis. Abdominal abscesses are caused by the anaerobes of the gastrointestinal tract, including Gram-positive *Peptostreptococcus* and *Clostridium* species, as well as the Gram-negative *Bacteriodes fragilis* and *Escherichia coli*. Genital tract infections in women are caused by anaerobic Gram-negative bacilli, including *Prevotella* species that are found in Bartholin cyst abscesses and tubo-ovarian abscesses, often mixed with *E. coli* or *Streptococcus agalactiae*.

Morphology. The pus of abscesses is discolored and foul smelling owing to the presence of anaerobes, especially in lung abscesses, and the suppuration is often poorly walled off. Otherwise, these lesions pathologically resemble those of the common pyogenic infections. Gram stain will reflect the mixed infection including Gram-positive and Gram-negative rods and Gram-positive cocci mixed with neutrophils.

Clostridial Infections

Clostridium species are Gram-positive bacilli that grow under anaerobic conditions and produce spores that are frequently present in the soil. Four types of disease are caused by *Clostridium*:

- *Clostridium perfringens, Clostridium septicum*, and other species cause cellulitis and myonecrosis of traumatic and surgical wounds *(gas gangrene)*, uterine myonecrosis often associated with illegal abortions, mild food poisoning, and infection of the small bowel of ischemic or neutropenic patients often leading to severe sepsis.
- *Clostridium tetani* proliferates in puncture wounds and in the umbilical stump of newborn infants in developing countries and releases a potent neurotoxin, called tetanospasmin, that causes convulsive contractions of skeletal muscles (lockjaw). Tetanus toxoid (formalin-fixed neurotoxin) is part of the DPT (diphtheria, pertussis, and tetanus) immunizations given to children, and this has greatly decreased the incidence of tetanus in the United States and in developing countries.
- *Clostridium botulinum* grows in inadequately sterilized canned foods and releases a potent neurotoxin that blocks synaptic release of acetylcholine and causes a severe paralysis of respiratory and skeletal muscles (botulism).
- *Clostridium difficile* overgrows other intestinal flora in antibiotic-treated patients, releases toxins, and causes pseudomembranous colitis (Chapter 17).

Pathogenesis. *C. perfringens* will not grow in the presence of oxygen, so tissue death allows the bacteria to proliferate within the host. These bacteria release collagenase and hyaluronidase that degrade extracellular matrix proteins and contribute to bacterial invasiveness, but their most powerful virulence factors are the many toxins they produce. *C. perfringens* secretes 14 toxins, the most important of which is *α-toxin.*[117] This toxin has multiple actions. It is a phospholipase C that degrades lecithin, a major component of cell membranes, and so destroys red blood cells, platelets, and muscle cells, causing myonecrosis; it also has a sphingomyelinase activity that contributes to nerve sheath damage; α-toxin releases phospholipid derivatives such as inositol triphosphate, prostaglandins, and thromboxanes, and these may dysregulate cellular metabolism, increasing cell death.

Ingestion of food contaminated with *C. perfringens* causes a brief diarrhea. Spores, usually in contaminated meat, survive cooking, and the organism proliferates in cooling food. *C. perfringens* enterotoxin forms pores in the epithelial cell membranes, lysing the cells and disrupting tight junctions between epithelial cells.[118]

The neurotoxins produced by *C. botulinum* and *C. tetani* both inhibit release of neurotransmitters, resulting in paralysis.[30] Botulism toxin, eaten in contaminated foods or absorbed from wounds infected with *C. botulinum*, binds gangliosides on motor neurons and is transported into the cell. In the cytoplasm, the A fragment of botulism toxin cleaves a protein, called synaptobrevin, which mediates fusion of neurotransmitter-containing vesicles with the neuron membrane. By blocking vesicle fusion, botulism toxin blocks release of acetylcholine at the neuromuscular junction, resulting in flaccid paralysis. If the respiratory muscles are affected, botulism can lead to death. Indeed, the widespread use of botulism toxin (Botox) in cosmetic surgery is based on its ability to cause paralysis of strategically placed muscles on the face. The mechanism of tetanus toxin is similar to that of botulism toxin, but tetanus toxin causes a violent spastic paralysis by blocking release of the neurotransmitter γ-aminobutyric acid from motor neurons.

C. difficile produces toxin A, an enterotoxin that stimulates chemokine production and thus attracts leukocytes, and toxin B, a cytotoxin, which causes distinctive cytopathic effects in cultured cells and is used in the diagnosis of *C. difficile* infections. Both toxins are glucosyl transferases and are part of a pathogenicity island, which is absent from the chromosomes of nonpathogenic strains of *C. difficile*.[119]

Morphology. Clostridial cellulitis, which originates in wounds, can be differentiated from infection caused by pyogenic cocci by its foul odor, its thin, discolored exudate, and the relatively quick and wide tissue destruction. On microscopic examination, the amount of tissue necrosis is disproportionate to the number of neutrophils and Gram-positive bacteria present (Fig. 8–43). Clostridial cellulitis, which often has granulation tissue at its borders, is treatable by debridement and antibiotics.

In contrast, **clostridial gas gangrene** is life threatening and is characterized by marked edema and enzymatic necrosis of involved muscle cells 1 to 3 days after injury. An extensive fluid exudate, which is lacking in inflammatory cells, causes swelling of the affected region and the overlying skin, forming large, bullous vesicles that rupture. Gas bubbles caused by bacterial fermentation appear within the gangrenous tissues. As the infection progresses, the inflamed muscles become soft, blue-black, friable, and semifluid as a result of the massive proteolytic action of the released bacterial enzymes. On microscopic examination, there is severe **myonecrosis**, extensive hemolysis, and marked vascular injury, with thrombosis. *C. perfringens* is also associated with dusk-colored, wedge-shaped infarcts in the small bowel, particularly in neutropenic patients. Regardless of the site of entry, when *C. perfringens* disseminates hematogenously, there is widespread formation of gas bubbles.

Despite the severe neurologic damage caused by botulinum and tetanus toxins, the neuropathologic changes are subtle and nonspecific.

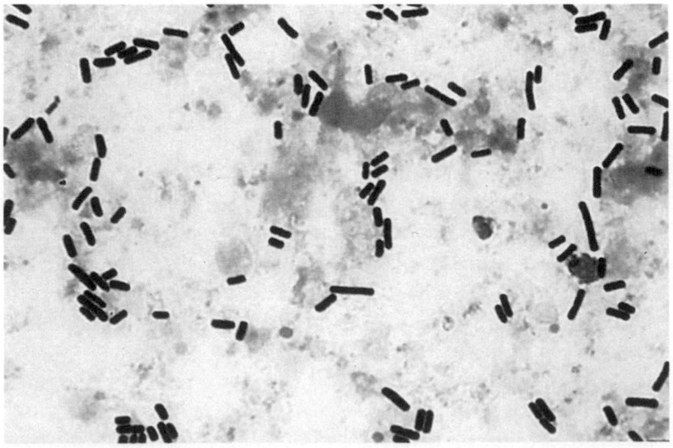

FIGURE 8–43 Boxcar-shaped Gram-positive *Clostridium perfringens* in gangrenous tissue.

OBLIGATE INTRACELLULAR BACTERIA

Obligate intracellular bacteria proliferate only within host cells, although some may survive outside of cells. These organisms are well adapted to the intracellular environment, with pumps to capture amino acids and adenosine triphosphate (ATP) for energy in their membranes. Some are unable to synthesize ATP at all (e.g., *Chlamydia*), while others synthesize at least some of their own ATP (e.g., the *Rickettsiae*).

Chlamydial Infections

Chlamydia trachomatis is a small Gram-negative bacterium that is an obligate intracellular parasite. The various diseases caused by *C. trachomatis* infection are associated with different serotypes of the bacteria: urogenital infections and inclusion conjunctivitis (serotypes D through K), lymphogranuloma venereum (serotypes L1, L2, and L3), and an ocular infection of children, trachoma (serotypes A, B, and C). The venereal infections caused by *C. trachomatis* will be discussed here.

C. trachomatis exists in two forms during its unique life cycle. The infectious form, the elementary body (EB), is a metabolically inactive, sporelike structure. The EB is taken up by host cells, primarily by receptor-mediated endocytosis. The bacteria prevent fusion of the endosome and lysosome, but the mechanism of this is not known. Inside the endosome, the EB differentiates into a metabolically active form, called the reticulate body (RB). Using energy sources and amino acids from the host cell, the RB replicates and ultimately forms new EBs that are capable of infecting additional cells.

Genital infection by *C. trachomatis (serotypes D through K) is the most common bacterial sexually transmitted disease in the world*.[120] In 2001, approximately 780,000 cases of genital chlamydia were reported to the Centers for Disease Control; this is about twice the number of cases of gonorrhea. Before the identification of *C. trachomatis*, patients infected with this organism were diagnosed with *nongonococcal urethritis* (NGU). Indeed, *C. trachomatis* is the cause of about half the cases of NGU. Other organisms that cause NGU include *Ureaplasma urealyticum, Mycoplasma hominis, Mycoplasma genitalium*, and *Trichomonas vaginalis*.[121] In the past, it was recommended that patients with urethritis who did not respond to treatment for *N. gonorrhoeae* be tested or treated for *C. trachomatis*. Since the current CDC recommendations call for treatment of both bacteria in patients who are diagnosed with either infection, such "relapses" should no longer occur.

Genital *C. trachomatis* infections (other than lymphogranuloma venereum, discussed below) are associated with clinical features that are similar to those caused by *N. gonorrhoeae.* Patients may develop epididymitis, prostatitis, pelvic inflammatory disease, pharyngitis, conjunctivitis, perihepatic inflammation, and, among people engaging in anal intercourse, proctitis. Unlike *N. gonorrhoeae* urethritis, *C. trachomatis* urethritis in men may be asymptomatic, so infected men might not seek treatment. Both *N. gonorrhoeae* and *C. trachomatis* frequently cause asymptomatic infections in women. *C. trachomatis* urethritis can be diagnosed by culture of the bacteria in human cell lines, but amplified nucleic acid tests performed on genital swabs or urine specimens are more sensitive and have supplanted cultures.

Genital infection with the L serotypes of *C. trachomatis* causes *lymphogranuloma venereum,* a chronic, ulcerative disease.[122] Lymphogranuloma venereum is a sporadic disease in the United States and Western Europe, but it is endemic in parts of Asia, Africa, the Caribbean region, and South America. The infection is initially manifested by a small, often unnoticed, papule on the genital mucosa or nearby skin. Two to 6 weeks later, growth of the organism and the host response in draining lymph nodes produce swollen, tender lymph nodes, which may coalesce and rupture. If not treated, the infection can subsequently cause fibrosis and strictures in the anogenital tract. Rectal strictures are particularly common in women.

Morphology. The morphologic features of *C. trachomatis* **urethritis** are virtually identical to those of gonorrhea. The primary infection is characterized by a mucopurulent discharge containing a predominance of neutrophils. Organisms are not visible in Gram-stained smears or sections.

The lesions of **lymphogranuloma venereum** contain a mixed granulomatous and neutrophilic inflammatory response, with a variable number of chlamydial inclusions in the cytoplasm of epithelial cells or inflammatory cells. Regional lymphadenopathy is common, usually occurring within 30 days of the time of infection. Lymph node involvement is characterized by a granulomatous inflammatory reaction associated with irregularly shaped foci of necrosis and neutrophilic infiltration (stellate abscesses). With time, the inflammatory reaction is dominated by nonspecific chronic inflammatory infiltrates and extensive fibrosis. The latter, in turn, may cause local lymphatic obstruction with lymphedema and strictures. In active lesions, the diagnosis of lymphogranuloma venereum may be made by demonstration of the organism in biopsy sections or smears of exudate. In more chronic cases, the diagnosis rests with the demonstration of antibodies to the appropriate chlamydial serotypes in the patient's serum.

Rickettsial Infections

Members of the order *Rickettsiales* are vector-borne obligate intracellular bacteria that cause epidemic typhus *(Rickettsia prowazekii),* scrub typhus *(Orienta tsutsugamushi),* and spotted fevers (*Rickettsia rickettsii* and others) (Table 8–10).[123] These organisms have the structure of Gram-negative, rod-shaped bacteria, although they stain poorly with Gram stain. Epidemic typhus, which is transmitted from person to person by body lice, is associated with wars and human suffering, when individuals are forced to live in close contact without changing clothes (e.g., a 1996 outbreak in a Burundi prison).[124] Scrub typhus, transmitted by chiggers, was a major problem for U.S. soldiers in the Pacific in World War II and in Vietnam. Rocky Mountain spotted fever (RMSF), transmitted to humans by dog ticks, is most frequent in the southeastern and south-central United States. Rickettsiae of Rocky Mountain spotted fever are transmitted after several hours of the tick feeding or, less commonly, when the tick is crushed during removal from the skin.

Ehrlichiosis is a recently discovered, tick-transmitted disease caused by *Rickettsiales.* The bacteria predominantly infect neutrophils *(Anaplasma phagocytophilum* and *Ehrlichia ewingii)* or macrophages *(Ehrlichia chaffeensis).* Characteristic cytoplasmic inclusions (morulae), occasionally shaped like mulberries and composed of masses of bacteria, can be seen in the appropriate leukocytes in ehrlichiosis (Fig. 8–44). Ehrlichiosis is characterized by abrupt onset of fever, headache, and malaise, which may progress to respiratory insufficiency, renal failure, and shock. Rash occurs in approximately 40% of patients with *E. chaffeensis* infections.

Pathogenesis. Rickettsiae do not produce significant toxins, and their LPS is not toxic. The rickettsiae that cause typhus and spotted fevers predominantly infect vascular endothelial cells, especially those in the lungs and brain. The bacteria enter the endothelial cells by endocytosis, but they escape from the endosome into the cytoplasm before formation of the acidic phagolysosome. The organisms proliferate in the endothelial cell cytoplasm and then either burst the cell (typhus group) or spread from cell to cell through actin-mobilized motion (spotted fever group). *The severe manifestations of rickettsial infection are primarily due to vascular leakage secondary to endothelial cell damage.*[125] This causes hypovolemic shock with peripheral edema, as well as pulmonary edema, renal failure, and a variety of CNS manifestations that can include coma.

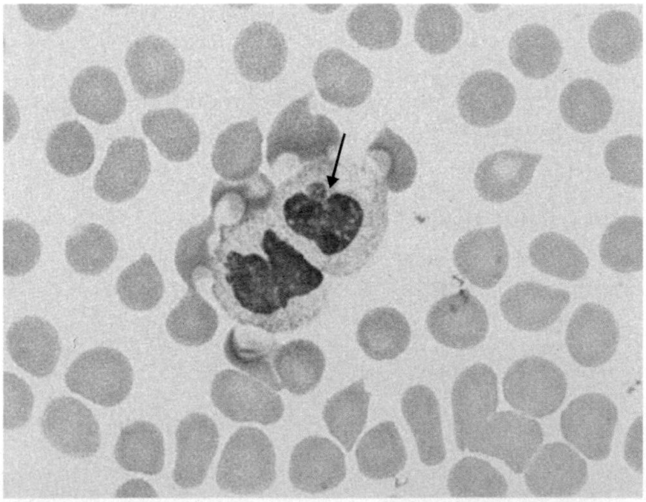

FIGURE 8–44 Peripheral blood granulocyte (band neutrophil) containing an Ehrlichia inclusion (*arrow*). (Courtesy of Dr. Stephen Dumler, Johns Hopkins Medical Institutions, Baltimore, MD.)

TABLE 8–10 Rickettsial Diseases and Pathogens

Organism	Disease	Geography	Transmission	Distinctive Features
Typhus Group (No Eschar)				
R. prowazekii	Epidemic typhus Brill-Zinsser disease	Worldwide (war, famine)	Louse feces	Endothelial infection; centrifugal rash; reactivation with mild disease
R. typhi	Murine typhus	Worldwide (rat related)	Rat flea feces	Similar to epidemic typhus, but mortality is lower
Spotted Fever Group				
R. rickettsii	Rocky Mountain spotted fever	North and South America	Tick bite	Endothelia and vascular smooth muscle infected; centripetal rash, eschar rare
R. conorii	Boutonneuse fever	Africa, Southern Europe, India	Tick bite	Prominent eschar, tache noire
R. africae	African tick fever	Africa, Caribbean	Tick bite	Multiple eschars
R. sibirica	North Asia tick typhus	Eurasia	Tick bite	Typical spotted fever with eschar
R. japonica	Japanese spotted fever	Japan	Tick bite	Typical spotted fever with eschar
R. australis	Queensland tick typhus	Eastern Australia	Tick bite	Typical spotted fever with eschar
R. akari	Rickettsialpox	United States, Ukraine, Korea, Croatia	Mite bite	Mild spotted fever with eschar
R. felis	Similar to murine typhus	United States	Opossum flea	Similar to murine typhus
Orientia tsutsugamushi	Scrub typhus	Eastern Asia and Western Pacific region	Chigger bite	Eschar common, insects present in scrub vegetation
Ehrlichiosis Group				
Ehrlichia chaffeensis	Monocytic ehrlichiosis	United States, Europe	Tick bite	Fever, lymphadenopathy, no eschar, rash in 40%
Anaplasma phagocytophilum and *E. ewingii*	Granulocytic ehrlichiosis	United States, Europe	Tick bite	Fever, lymphadenopathy, no eschar or rash

The innate immune response to rickettsial infection is mounted by natural killer cells, which produce γ-interferon, reducing bacterial proliferation. Cytotoxic T-lymphocyte responses are critical for elimination of rickettsial infections. IFN-γ and TNF, from activated natural killer cells, CD4+, and CD8+ T lymphocytes, stimulate the production of bactericidal nitric oxide. Cytotoxic T lymphocytes lyse infected cells, reducing bacterial proliferation. Rickettsial infections are diagnosed by immunostaining of organisms or by detection of antirickettsial antibodies in the serum.

Morphology

Typhus Fever. In mild cases, the gross changes are limited to a rash and small hemorrhages due to the vascular lesions. In more severe cases, there may be areas of necrosis of the skin with gangrene of the tips of the fingers, nose, earlobes, scrotum, penis, and vulva. In such cases, irregular ecchymotic hemorrhages may be found internally, principally in the brain, heart muscle, testes, serosal membrane, lungs, and kidneys.

The most prominent microscopic changes are the small-vessel lesions that underlie the rash and the focal areas of hemorrhage and inflammation in the various organs and tissues affected. Endothelial swelling in the capillaries, arterioles, and venules may narrow the lumina of these vessels. A cuff of mononuclear inflammatory cells usually surrounds the affected vessel. The vascular lumina are sometimes thrombosed, but necrosis of the vessel wall is unusual in typhus compared with RMSF. Vascular thromboses lead to the gangrenous necroses of the skin and other structures in a minority of cases. In the brain, characteristic typhus nodules are composed of focal microglial proliferations with an infiltrate of mixed T lymphocytes and macrophages (Fig. 8–45).

Scrub typhus, or mite-borne infection, is usually a milder version of typhus fever. The rash is usually transitory or might not appear. Vascular necrosis or thrombosis is rare, but there may be a prominent inflammatory lymphadenopathy.

Rocky Mountain spotted fever. A hemorrhagic rash that extends over the entire body, including the palms of the hands and soles of the feet, is the hall-

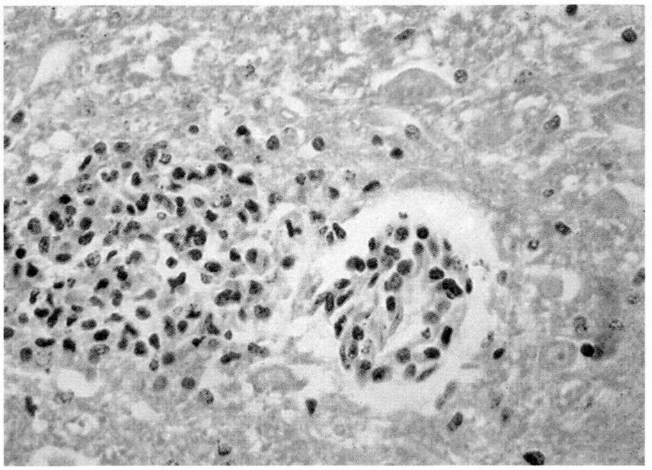

FIGURE 8–45 Typhus nodule in the brain.

mark of RMSF. An eschar at the site of the tick bite is uncommon with RMSF but is common with *R. akari*, *R. africae*, and *R. conorii* infection. The vascular lesions that underlie the rash often lead to acute necrosis, fibrin extravasation, and occasionally thrombosis of the small blood vessels, including arterioles (Fig. 8–46). In severe RMSF, foci of necrotic skin are thus induced, particularly on the fingers, toes, elbows, ears, and scrotum. The perivascular inflammatory response is similar to that of typhus, particularly in the brain, skeletal muscle, lungs, kidneys, testes, and heart muscle. The vascular necroses in the brain may involve larger vessels and produce microinfarcts. A noncardiogenic pulmonary edema causing adult respiratory distress syndrome is the major cause of death with RMSF.

Fungal Infections

Fungal infections are called *mycoses*. Fungi are eukaryotes that grow predominantly by budding (yeasts) or by filamentous extensions called hyphae (molds). The distinction between yeasts and molds is not absolute and is based on the usual morphology of the organism. Some fungi, such as *Candida albicans*, tend to grow predominantly as yeast but may also form hyphae. Dimorphic fungi have both a yeast form (at human body temperature) and a mold form (at room temperature).[126] Some of the fungi that can cause disseminated disease are discussed below. Others are discussed in other chapters, depending on the primary organ involved.

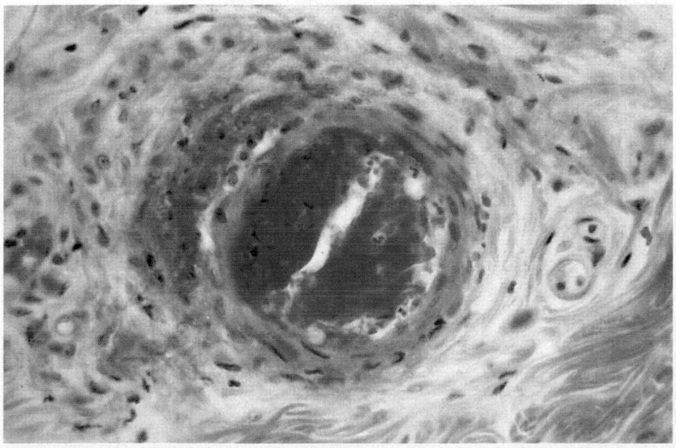

FIGURE 8–46 Rocky Mountain spotted fever with a thrombosed vessel and vasculitis.

YEASTS

Candidiasis

Residing normally in the skin, mouth, gastrointestinal tract, and vagina, *Candida* species are versatile microorganisms. In healthy people, *Candida* species usually live as benign commensals and produce no disease. However, *Candida* species, most often *C. albicans*, are the most frequent cause of human fungal infections. These infections range from superficial lesions in healthy persons to disseminated infections in immunocompromised patients.[126] *C. albicans* grows best on warm, moist surfaces and so frequently causes oral thrush, vaginitis, and diaper rash. Diabetics and burn patients are particularly susceptible to superficial candidiasis. *Candida* can be directly introduced into the blood by intravenous lines, catheters, peritoneal dialysis, cardiac surgery, or intravenous drug abuse. Severe disseminated candidiasis is associated with neutropenia secondary to leukemia or anticancer therapy, immunosuppression after transplantation, and neutrophil disorders such as chronic granulomatous disease. Although the course of candidal sepsis is less rampant than that of bacterial sepsis, disseminated *Candida* eventually may cause shock and DIC.

Pathogenesis. A single strain of *Candida* can be successful as a commensal or a pathogen. *Candida* species have highly developed mechanisms to adapt rapidly to changes in the host environment (produced by antibiotic therapy, the immune response, or altered host physiology). *Candida* can shift between different phenotypes in a reversible and apparently random fashion. Phenotypic switching involves coordinated regulation of phase-specific genes and provides a way for *Candida* to adapt to changes in the host environment. *C. albicans* produces genetically altered variants at a high rate. These variants can exhibit altered colony morphology, cell shape, antigenicity, and virulence.[127]

Candida produce a large number of functionally distinct adhesins that mediate adherence to host cells, and some of them also function in *Candida* morphogenesis or signaling.[128,129] These adhesins include (1) an integrin-like protein, which binds arginine-glycine-aspartic acid (RGD) groups on fibrinogen, fibronectin, and laminin; (2) a protein that resembles transglutaminase substrates and binds to epithelial cells; and (3) several agglutinins that bind to endothelial cells or fibronectin. Adhesion is an important determinant of virulence, since strains with reduced adherence to cells in vitro are avirulent in experimental models in vivo. Differential expression of adhesins by yeast and hyphae leads to recognition of distinct receptors on host cells. *Candida* yeast mainly bind mannose receptors, while *Candida* hyphae primarily bind complement receptor 3 (CR3) and Fcγ receptor.

The immune response to *Candida* is complex. Innate immunity and T-cell responses are important for protection against mucosal and cutaneous *Candida* infection, while neutrophils and mononuclear phagocytes appear to be more important for resistance to systemic *Candida* infections. Dendritic cells phagocytose yeast and hyphal forms in different ways. Hyphae, but not yeast, can escape from phagosomes and enter the cytoplasm. The differential interactions of yeast and hyphae with dendritic cells lead to the production of distinct cytokines and activation of distinct subsets of T cells. T_H1 responses are needed for protective antifungal immunity. It has been speculated that the interaction of *Candida* adhesins with distinct recognition receptors on dendritic cells may determine commensalism of *Candida* on mucosal surfaces.[128, 129]

Candida produce a number of enzymes that contribute to invasiveness, including at least nine secreted aspartyl proteinases, which may be involved in tissue invasion by degrading extracellular matrix proteins, and catalases, which may aid intracellular survival and resist oxidative killing by phagocytic cells.[128,130] *Candida* also secrete adenosine, which blocks neutrophil oxygen radical production and degranulation.

Morphology. In tissue sections, *C. albicans* can appear as yeastlike forms (blastoconidia), pseudohyphae, and, less commonly, true hyphae, defined by the presence of septae (Fig. 8–47). Pseudohyphae are an important diagnostic clue for *C. albicans* and represent budding yeast cells joined end to end at constrictions, thus simulating true fungal hyphae. All forms may be present together in the same tissue. The organisms may be visible with routine hematoxylin and eosin stains, but a variety of special "fungal" stains (Gomori methenamine-silver, periodic acid-Schiff) are commonly used to better visualize them.

Most commonly candidiasis takes the form of a superficial infection on mucosal surfaces of the oral cavity **(thrush)**. Florid proliferation of the fungi creates gray-white, dirty-looking pseudomembranes composed of matted organisms and inflammatory debris. Deep to the surface, there is mucosal hyperemia and inflammation. This form of candidiasis is seen in newborns, debilitated patients, and children receiving oral steroids for asthma and following a course of broad-spectrum antibiotics that destroy competing normal bacterial flora. The other major risk group includes HIV-positive patients; patients with oral thrush for no obvious reason should be evaluated for HIV infection.

Candida esophagitis is commonly seen in AIDS patients and in those with hematolymphoid malignancies. These patients present with dysphagia (painful swallowing) and retrosternal pain; endoscopy demonstrates white plaques and pseudomembranes resembling oral thrush on the esophageal mucosa (Fig. 8–47).

Candida vaginitis is a common form of vaginal infection in women, especially those who are diabetic or pregnant or on oral contraceptive pills. It is usually associated with intense itching and a thick, curdlike discharge.

Cutaneous candidiasis can present in many different forms, including infection of the nail proper ("onychomycosis"), nail folds ("paronychia"), hair follicles ("folliculitis"), moist, intertriginous skin such as armpits or webs of the fingers and toes ("intertrigo"), and penile skin ("balanitis"). "Diaper rash" is a cutaneous candidial infection seen in the perineum of infants, in the region of contact of wet diapers.

Chronic mucocutaneous candidiasis is a chronic refractory disease afflicting the mucous membranes, skin, hair, and nails; it is associated with underlying T-cell defects. Predisposing conditions include

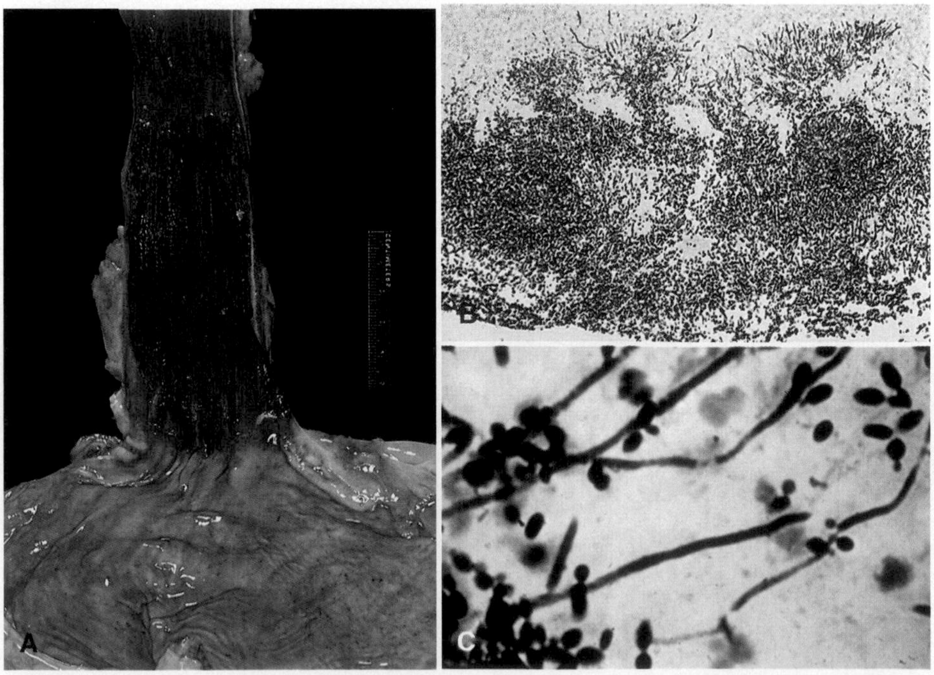

FIGURE 8–47 The morphology of *Candida* infections. *A*, Severe candidiasis of the distal esophagus. *B*, Silver stain of esophageal candidiasis reveals the dense mat of *Candida*. *C*, Characteristic pseudohyphae and blastoconidia (budding yeast) of *Candida*. (*C*, Courtesy of Dr. Dominick Cuvuoti, Department of Pathology, University of Texas Southwestern Medical School, Dallas, TX.)

endocrinopathies (most commonly hypoparathyroidism and Addison's disease). Disseminated candidiasis is rare in this disease.

Invasive candidiasis is caused by blood-borne dissemination of organisms to various tissues or organs. Common patterns include (1) renal abscesses, (2) myocardial abscesses and endocarditis, (3) brain involvement (most commonly meningitis, but parenchymal microabscesses occur), (4) endophthalmitis (virtually any eye structure can be involved), (5) hepatic abscesses, and (6) *Candida* pneumonia, usually presenting as bilateral nodular infiltrates, resembling *Pneumocystis* pneumonia. In any of these locations, the fungus may evoke little or no inflammatory reaction, cause the usual suppurative response, or occasionally produce granulomas. Patients with acute leukemias who are profoundly neutropenic post-chemotherapy are particularly prone to developing systemic disease. *Candida* endocarditis is the most common fungal endocarditis, usually occurring in the setting of prosthetic heart valves or in intravenous drug abusers.

Cryptococcosis

Cryptococcus neoformans is an encapsulated yeast that causes meningoencephalitis in normal individuals but more frequently presents as an opportunistic infection in patients with AIDS, leukemia, lymphoma, systemic lupus erythematosus, Hodgkin lymphoma, or sarcoidosis and in transplant recipients. Many of these patients receive high-dose corticosteroids, a major risk factor for *Cryptococcus* infection.

Pathogenesis. *C. neoformans* is present in the soil and in bird (particularly pigeon) droppings and infects patients when it is inhaled. Several virulence factors enable it to evade host defenses. The virulence factors include (1) a polysaccharide capsule, (2) melanin production, and (3) enzymes.[131] These mechanisms are not very effective when *C. neoformans* infects hosts with intact immune defenses, but they can lead to disseminated disease in immunosuppressed individuals.

The polysaccharide capsule of *C. neoformans* is a major virulence factor, preventing phagocytosis of cryptococci by alveolar macrophages. Capsular polysaccharide inhibits phagocytosis, leukocyte migration, and recruitment of inflammatory cells. Acapsular strains are less virulent in animal models. *C. neoformans* can undergo phenotypic switching, which leads to changes in the structure and size of the capsule polysaccharide, providing a means to evade immune responses.[132]

C. neoformans makes laccase, which catalyzes the formation of a melaninlike pigment.[133] Laccase mutants of *C. neoformans* have reduced virulence in animal models.[131] The role of melanin in cryptococcal pathogenesis may be related to the antioxidant properties of melanin. The melanin synthetic pathway consumes host epinephrine in the synthesis of fungal melanin, protecting the fungi from the epinephrine oxidative system present in the host nervous system. This suggests a potential mechanism for the neurotropism of *C. neoformans.* These fungi make a number of other enzymes, including a serine proteinase that cleaves fibronectin and other basement membrane proteins, which may aid tissue invasion.[134] *C. neoformans* can establish latent infections accompanied by granuloma formation but can reactivate in immunosuppressed hosts. Studies in rat models indicate that yeast cells can persist in macrophages within granulomas.[131]

Morphology. In contrast to *Candida*, cryptococcus has yeast but not pseudohyphal or hyphal forms. The 5- to 10-μm cryptococcal yeast has a thick gelatinous capsule that is valuable for diagnosis. Capsular polysaccharide stains intense red with periodic acid-Schiff and mucicarmine in tissues and can be detected with antibody-coated beads in an agglutination assay. India ink preparations create a negative image, visualizing the thick capsule as a clear halo within a dark background, but do not stain the yeast. Although the lung is the primary site of localization, pulmonary infection with *C. neoformans* is usually mild and asymptomatic, even while the fungus is spreading to the central nervous system. *C. neoformans*, however, may form a solitary pulmonary granuloma similar to the circumscribed (coin) lesions caused by *Histoplasma.* The major lesions caused by *C. neoformans* are in the central nervous system, involving the meninges, cortical gray matter, and basal nuclei. The tissue response to cryptococci is extremely variable. In immunosuppressed patients, organisms may evoke virtually no inflammatory reaction, so gelatinous masses of fungi grow in the meninges or expand the perivascular Virchow-Robin spaces within the gray matter, producing the so-called soap-bubble lesions (Fig. 8–48). In nonimmunosuppressed patients or in those with protracted disease, the fungi induce a chronic granulomatous reaction composed of macrophages, lymphocytes, and foreign body type giant cells. Neutrophils and suppuration also may occur, as well as a rare granulomatous arteritis of the circle of Willis. In severely immunosuppressed persons, *C. neoformans* may disseminate widely to the skin, liver, spleen, adrenals, and bones.

MOLDS

Aspergillosis

Aspergillus is a ubiquitous mold that causes allergies (brewer's lung) in otherwise healthy people and serious *sinusi-*

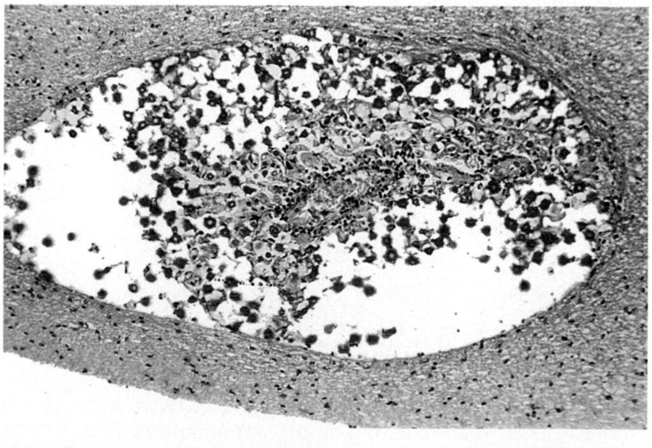

FIGURE 8–48 Mucicarmine stain of cryptococci (staining red) in a Virchow-Robin perivascular space of the brain (soap-bubble lesion).

tis, pneumonia, and *fungemia* in immunocompromised individuals. The major factors that predispose to *Aspergillus* infection are neutropenia and corticosteroids. This saprophytic fungus sporulates and produces abundant conidia (asexual spores) that are readily aerosolized. Molecular epidemiologic studies of *Aspergillus* isolated from opportunistic infections show many different strains of *Aspergillus*, suggesting that the immune status of the host is more important than fungal pathogenicity.[135] *Aspergillus fumigatus* is the most common species to cause disease, and it produces severe invasive infections in immunocompromised individuals.[126,136]

Pathogenesis. *Aspergillus* species are transmitted by airborne conidia, and the lung is the major portal of entry. The small size of *Aspergillus fumigatus* spores, approximately 2 to 3 μm, enables them to reach alveoli. In the lung, *Aspergillus* conidia are encountered initially by alveolar macrophages, which can engulf and kill the germinating conidia and secrete cytokines and chemokines to elicit adaptive immune responses. Germinating conidia and hyphae that evade unactivated alveolar macrophages are killed mainly by activated macrophages. T lymphocytes confer protective immunity, but little is known about the effector cells and defense mechanisms.

Aspergillus produces several virulence factors, including adhesins, antioxidants, enzymes, and toxins.[136] Conidia can bind to fibrinogen, laminin, complement, fibronectin, collagen, albumin, and surfactant proteins,[136] but receptor-ligand interactions are not well defined. *Aspergillus* produces several antioxidant defenses, including melanin pigment, mannitol, catalases, and superoxide dismutases. This fungus also produces phospholipases, proteases, and toxins, but their roles in pathogenicity are not yet clear. *Restrictocin* and *mitogillin* are ribotoxins that inhibit host-cell protein synthesis by degrading mRNAs.[136] The carcinogen *aflatoxin* is made by *Aspergillus* species growing on the surface of peanuts and may be a major cause of liver cancer in Africa.[137] Sensitization to *Aspergillus* spores produces an allergic alveolitis by T_H2 reactions[138] (Chapter 15). *Allergic bronchopulmonary aspergillosis,* which is associated with hypersensitivity arising from superficial colonization of the bronchial mucosa and often occurs in asthmatic patients, may eventually result in chronic obstructive lung disease.

Morphology. Colonizing aspergillosis (aspergilloma) usually implies growth of the fungus in pulmonary cavities with minimal or no invasion of the tissues (the nose also is often colonized). The cavities usually result from preexisting tuberculosis, bronchiectasis, old infarcts, or abscesses. Proliferating masses of fungal hyphae called fungus balls form brownish masses lying free within the cavities. The surrounding inflammatory reaction may be sparse, or there may be chronic inflammation and fibrosis. Patients with aspergillomas usually have recurrent hemoptysis.

Invasive aspergillosis is an opportunistic infection that is confined to immunosuppressed and debilitated hosts. The primary lesions are usually in the lung, but widespread hematogenous dissemination with involvement of the heart valves, brain, and kidneys is common. The pulmonary lesions take the form of necrotizing pneumonia with sharply delineated, rounded, gray foci with hemorrhagic borders, often referred to as **target lesions** (Fig. 8–49*A*). Aspergillus forms fruiting bodies (particularly in cavities) and septate filaments, 5 to 10 μm thick, branching at acute angles (40 degrees) (Fig. 8–49*B*). *Aspergillus* has a tendency to invade blood vessels; therefore, areas of hemorrhage and infarction are usually superimposed on the necrotizing, inflammatory tissue reactions. Rhinocerebral *Aspergillus* infection in immunosuppressed individuals resembles that caused by Zygomycetes (e.g., mucormycosis).

Zygomycosis (Mucormycosis)

Zygomycosis (mucormycosis, phycomycosis) is an opportunistic infection caused by "bread mold fungi," including *Rhizopus, Absidia, Cunninghamella,* and *Mucor*, which belong to the class Zygomycetes.[139] These fungi are widely distributed

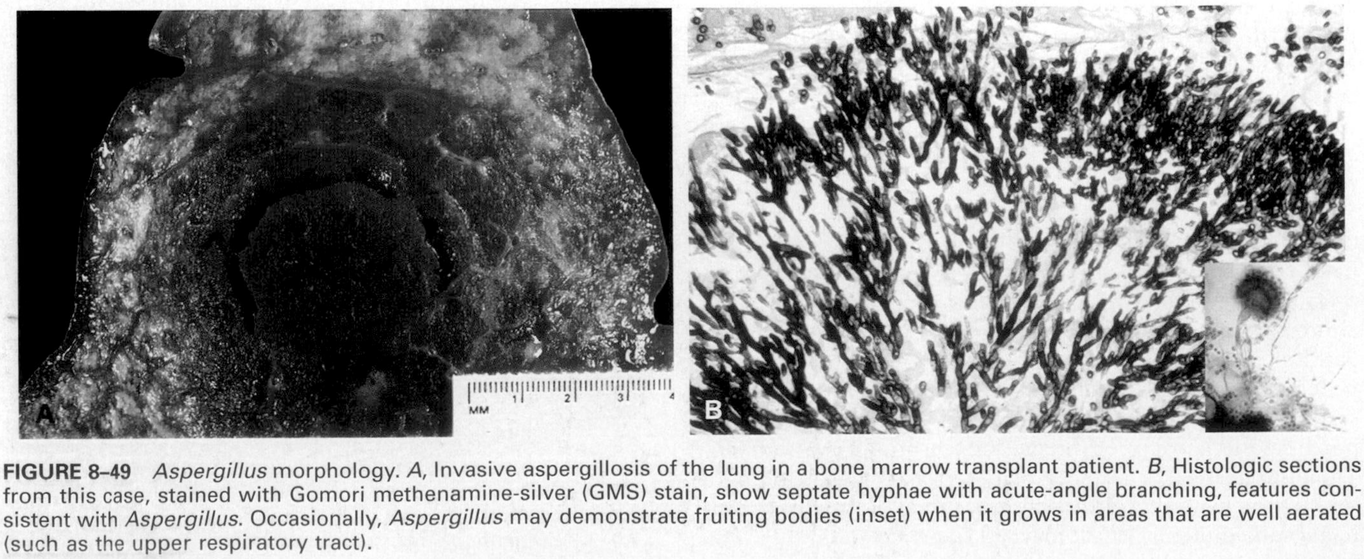

FIGURE 8–49 *Aspergillus* morphology. *A*, Invasive aspergillosis of the lung in a bone marrow transplant patient. *B*, Histologic sections from this case, stained with Gomori methenamine-silver (GMS) stain, show septate hyphae with acute-angle branching, features consistent with *Aspergillus*. Occasionally, *Aspergillus* may demonstrate fruiting bodies (inset) when it grows in areas that are well aerated (such as the upper respiratory tract).

in nature and cause no harm to immunocompetent individuals, but they infect immunosuppressed patients, albeit somewhat less frequently than do *Candida* and *Aspergillus.* The major predisposing factors are neutropenia, corticosteroid use, diabetes mellitus and breakdown of the cutaneous barrier (e.g., as a result of burns, surgical wounds, trauma).

Pathogenesis. Similar to *Aspergillus*, zygomycetes are transmitted by airborne asexual spores. Most commonly, inhaled spores produce infection in the sinuses and the lungs, but spores can also lead to infection following percutaneous exposure or ingestion. Macrophages provide the initial defenses by phagocytosis and oxidative killing of germinating spores.[139] Neutrophils have a key role in killing fungi during established infection. Proteolytic and lipolytic enzymes and mycotoxins have been identified for some of the zygomycetes, but whether these contribute to disease is not yet known. The thermotolerance of the spores of some species of zygomycetes might contribute to their spread.

Morphology. Zygomycetes form nonseptate, irregularly wide (6 to 50 μm) fungal hyphae with frequent right-angle branching, which are readily demonstrated in the necrotic tissues by hematoxylin and eosin or special fungal stains (Fig. 8–50). The three primary sites of invasion are the nasal sinuses, lungs, and gastrointestinal tract, depending on whether the spores (which are widespread in dust and air) are inhaled or ingested. Most commonly in diabetics, the fungus may spread from nasal sinuses to the orbit and brain, giving rise to **rhinocerebral mucormycosis.** The zygomycetes cause local tissue necrosis, invade arterial walls, and penetrate the periorbital tissues and cranial vault. Meningoencephalitis follows, sometimes complicated by cerebral infarctions when fungi invade arteries and induce thrombosis.

Lung involvement with zygomycetes may be secondary to rhinocerebral disease, or it may be primary in patients with hematologic neoplasms. The lung lesions combine areas of hemorrhagic pneumonia with vascular thrombi and distal infarctions.

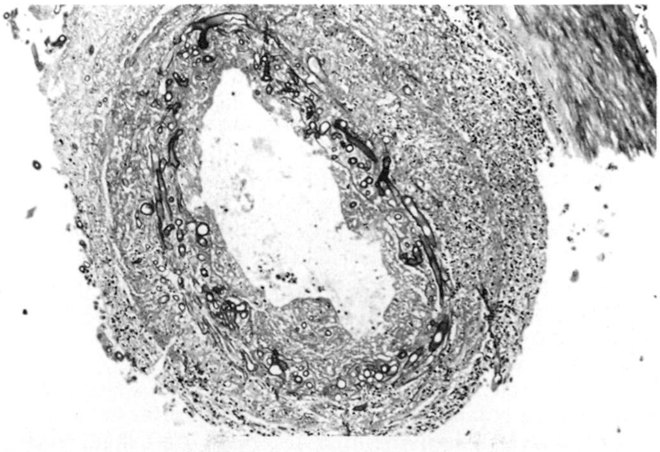

FIGURE 8–50 PAS stain of mucormycosis showing hyphae, which have an irregular width and right-angle branching, invading an artery wall.

Parasitic Infections

PROTOZOA

Protozoa are unicellular, eukaryotic organisms. The parasitic protozoa are transmitted by insects or by the fecal-oral route and, in humans, mainly occupy the blood or intestine.

Malaria

Malaria, caused by the intracellular parasite *Plasmodium*, is a worldwide infection that affects 300 million and kills 1 million people each year. According to the World Health Organization, 90% of deaths from malaria occur in sub-Saharan Africa, where malaria is the leading cause of death in children younger than 5 years old. *Plasmodium falciparum*, which causes severe malaria, and the three other malaria parasites that infect humans (*P. vivax*, *P. ovale*, and *P. malariae*) are transmitted by female *Anopheles* mosquitoes that are widely distributed throughout Africa, Asia, and Latin America. Nearly all of the approximately 1500 new cases of malaria each year in the United States occur in travelers or immigrants, although rare cases transmitted by *Anopheles* mosquitoes or blood transfusion do occur. Worldwide public health efforts to control malaria in the 1950s through 1980s failed, leaving mosquitoes resistant to DDT and malathion and *Plasmodium* resistant to chloroquine and pyrimethamine.

Life Cycle and Pathogenesis. *P. vivax*, *P. ovale*, and *P. malariae* cause low parasitemia, mild anemia, and, in rare instances, splenic rupture and nephrotic syndrome. *P. falciparum* causes high levels of parasitemia, severe anemia, cerebral symptoms, renal failure, pulmonary edema, and death. The life cycles of the *Plasmodium* species are similar, although *P. falciparum* differs in ways that contribute to its greater virulence.

The infectious stage of malaria, the *sporozoites*, is found in the salivary glands of female mosquitoes. When the mosquito takes a blood meal, sporozoites are released into the human's blood and within minutes attach to and invade liver cells by binding to the hepatocyte receptor for the serum proteins thrombospondin and properdin[140] (Fig. 8–51). Within liver cells, malaria parasites multiply rapidly, so as many as 30,000 *merozoites* (asexual, haploid forms) are released when each infected hepatocyte ruptures. *P. vivax* and *P. ovale* form latent *hypnozoites* in hepatocytes, which cause relapses of malaria long after initial infection.

Once released from the liver, *Plasmodium* merozoites bind by a parasite lectinlike molecule to sialic residues on glycophorin molecules on the surface of red blood cells. Within the red blood cells, the parasites grow in a membrane-bound digestive vacuole, hydrolyzing hemoglobin through secreted enzymes. The *trophozoite* is the first stage of the parasite in the red blood cell and is defined by the presence of a single chromatin mass. The next stage, the *schizont*, has multiple chromatin masses, each of which develops into a merozoite. On lysis of the red blood cell, the new merozoites infect additional red blood cells. Although most malaria parasites within the red blood cells develop into merozoites, some parasites develop into sexual forms called *gametocytes* that infect the mosquito when it takes its blood meal.

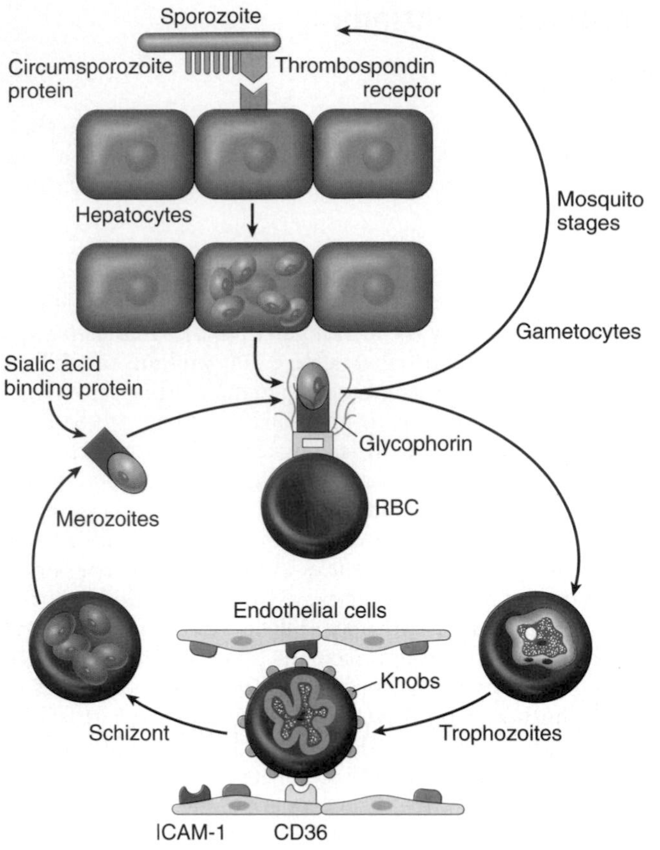

FIGURE 8–51 Life cycle of *Plasmodium falciparum.* (Drawn by Dr. Jeffrey Joseph, Beth Israel-Deaconess Hospital, Boston, MA.)

P. falciparum causes more severe disease than the other *Plasmodium* species do. Several features of *P. falciparum* account for its greater pathogenicity:

- *P. falciparum* is able to infect red blood cells of any age, leading to high parasite burdens and profound anemia. The other species infect only new or old red blood cells, which are a smaller fraction of the red blood cell pool.
- *P. falciparum* causes infected red blood cells to clump together (rosetting) and to stick to endothelial cells lining small blood vessels (sequestration), which blocks blood flow. Several proteins, including *P. falciparum* erythrocyte membrane protein 1 (PfEMP1), form knobs on the surface of red blood cells.[141] PfEMP1 binds to ligands on endothelial cells, including CD36, thrombospondin, VCAM-1, ICAM-1, and E-selectin. *Ischemia due to poor perfusion causes the manifestations of cerebral malaria, which is the main cause of death due to malaria in children.*
- *P. falciparum* stimulates production of high levels of cytokines, including TNF, IFN-γ, and IL-1.[141] GPI-linked proteins, including merozoite surface antigens, are released from infected red blood cells and induce cytokine production by host cells by a mechanism that is not yet understood. These cytokines suppress production of red blood cells, increase fever, induce nitric oxide production, leading to tissue damage, and induce expression of endothelial receptors for PfEMP1, increasing sequestration.

Host Resistance to Plasmodium. There are two general mechanisms of host resistance to *Plasmodium*. First, inherited alterations in red blood cells make people resistant to *Plasmodium*. Second, repeated or prolonged exposure to *Plasmodium* species stimulates an immune response that reduces the severity of the illness caused by malaria.

Several common mutations in hemoglobin genes confer resistance to malaria. People who are heterozygous for the sickle cell trait (HbS) become infected with *P. falciparum*, but they are less likely to die from infection. The HbS trait causes the parasites to grow poorly or die at low oxygen concentrations, perhaps because of low potassium levels caused by potassium efflux from red blood cells on hemoglobin sickling. The geographic distribution of the HbS trait is similar to that of *P. falciparum*, suggesting evolutionary selection of the HbS trait in people by the parasite. HbC, another common hemoglobin mutation, also protects against severe malaria by reducing parasite proliferation. People can also be resistant to malaria due to the absence of proteins to which the parasites bind. *P. vivax* enters red blood cells by binding to the Duffy blood group antigen. Many Africans, including most Gambians, are not susceptible to infection by *P. vivax* because they do not have the Duffy antigen.

Individuals living where *Plasmodium* is endemic often gain partial immune-mediated resistance to malaria, evidenced by reduced illness despite infection. Antibodies and T lymphocytes specific for *Plasmodium* reduce disease manifestations, although the parasite has developed strategies to evade the host immune response. *P. falciparum* uses antigenic variation to escape from antibody responses to PfEMP1.[141] Each haploid *P. falciparum* genome has about 50 *var* genes, each encoding a different form of PfEMP1. The mechanism of *var* regulation is not known, but at least 2% of the parasites switch PfEMP1 genes each generation. Cytotoxic T lymphocytes may also be important in resistance to *P. falciparum*. Individuals with the HLA allele B53 are resistant to *P. falciparum*, perhaps because HLA-B53 presents liver stage-specific malaria antigens to cytotoxic T lymphocytes, which then kill malaria-infected hepatocytes.[142] The parasite has also evolved to evade this mechanism of the immune response: *Plasmodia*-infected red blood cells inhibit cytotoxic T-lymphocyte development by blocking maturation and antigen presentation by dendritic cells.[143] Despite enormous efforts, there has been little success in developing a vaccine for malaria.

Morphology. *P. falciparum* infection initially causes congestion and enlargement of the spleen, which may eventually exceed 1000 gm in weight. Parasites are present within red blood cells, and there is increased phagocytic activity of the macrophages in the spleen. In chronic malaria infection, the spleen becomes increasingly fibrotic and brittle, with a thick capsule and fibrous trabeculae. The parenchyma is gray or black because of phagocytic cells containing granular, brown-black, faintly birefringent hemozoin pigment. In addition, macrophages with engulfed parasites, red blood cells, and debris are numerous.

With progression of malaria, the liver becomes progressively enlarged and pigmented. Kupffer cells are heavily laden with malarial pigment, parasites, and cellular debris, while some pigment is also present in the parenchymal cells. Pigmented phagocytic cells may be found dispersed throughout the bone marrow, lymph nodes, subcutaneous tissues, and lungs. The kidneys are often enlarged and congested with a dusting of pigment in the glomeruli and hemoglobin casts in the tubules.

In **malignant cerebral malaria** caused by *P. falciparum*, brain vessels are plugged with parasitized red cells, each cell containing dots of hemozoin pigment (Fig. 8–52). About the vessels, there are ring hemorrhages that are probably related to local hypoxia incident to the vascular stasis and small focal inflammatory reactions (called *malarial* or *Dürck granulomas*). With more severe hypoxia, there is degeneration of neurons, focal ischemic softening, and occasionally scant inflammatory infiltrates in the meninges.

Nonspecific focal hypoxic lesions in the heart may be induced by the progressive anemia and circulatory stasis in chronically infected patients. In some, the myocardium shows focal interstitial infiltrates. Finally, in the nonimmune patient, pulmonary edema or shock with DIC may cause death, sometimes in the absence of other characteristic lesions.

Babesiosis

Babesia microti is a malaria-like protozoan transmitted by the same deer ticks that carry Lyme disease and granulocytic ehrlichiosis.[144] The white-footed mouse is the reservoir for *B. microti*, and in some areas, nearly all mice have a persistent low-level parasitemia. *B. microti* survives well in refrigerated blood, and several cases of transfusion-acquired Babesiosis have been reported. Babesiae parasitize red blood cells and cause fever and hemolytic anemia. The symptoms are mild except in debilitated or splenectomized individuals, who develop severe and fatal parasitemias.

Morphology. In blood smears, *Babesia* resemble *P. falciparum* ring stages, although they lack hemozoin pigment and are more pleomorphic. They form characteristic tetrads (Maltese cross), which are diagnostic if found (Fig. 8–53). The level of *B. microti* parasitemia is a good indication of the severity of infection: 1% in mild cases and up to 30% in splenectomized persons, who also show marked erythrophagocytosis associated with the red blood cell destruction. In fatal cases, the anatomic findings are related to shock and hypoxia and include jaundice, hepatic necrosis, acute renal tubular necrosis, adult respiratory distress syndrome, hemolysis, and visceral hemorrhages.

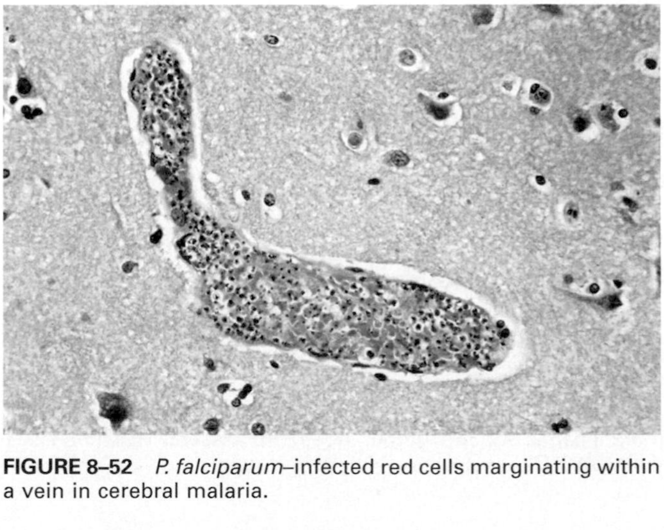

FIGURE 8–52 *P. falciparum*–infected red cells marginating within a vein in cerebral malaria.

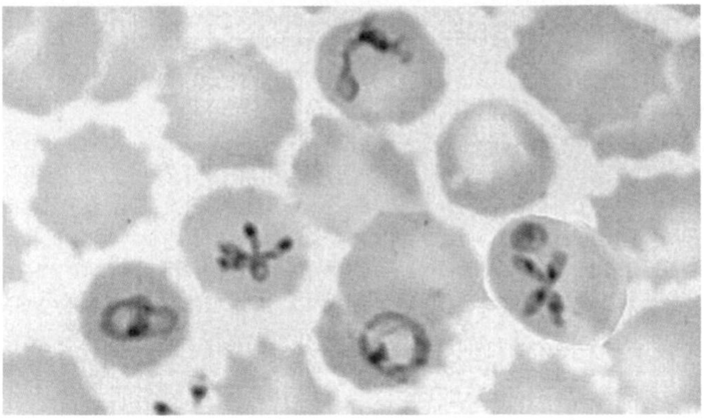

FIGURE 8–53 Erythrocytes with *Babesia*, including the distinctive Maltese cross form. (Courtesy of Lynne Garcia, LSG and Associates, Santa Monica, CA.)

Leishmaniasis

Leishmaniasis is a chronic inflammatory disease of the skin, mucous membranes, or viscera caused by obligate intracellular, kinetoplastid protozoan parasites transmitted through the bite of infected sandflies. Leishmaniasis is endemic throughout the Middle East, South Asia, Africa, and Latin America. Numerous U.S. soldiers were infected with *Leishmania* in the Persian Gulf during Operation Desert Storm.[145] Leishmaniasis may also be epidemic, as is tragically the case in Sudan, India, Bangladesh, and Brazil, where tens of thousands of people have died of visceral leishmaniasis. Finally, leishmanial infection, like other intracellular organisms (mycobacteria, *Histoplasma*, *Toxoplasma*, and trypanosomes), is exacerbated by AIDS.

Pathogenesis. The life cycle of *Leishmania* involves two forms: the promastigote, which develops and lives extracellularly in the sandfly vector, and the amastigote, which multiplies intracellularly in host macrophages. Mammals, including rodents, dogs, and foxes, are reservoirs of *Leishmania*. When sandflies bite infected humans or animals, macrophages harboring amastigotes are ingested. The amastigotes differentiate into promastigotes and multiply within the digestive tract of the sandfly and migrate to the pharynx, where they are poised for transmission by a sandfly bite. When the infected sandfly bites a person, the infectious slender, flagellated promastigotes are released into the host dermis along with the sandfly saliva, which potentiates parasite infectivity.[146] The promastigotes are phagocytosed by macrophages, and the acidity within the phagolysosome induces them to transform into round amastigotes that lack flagella but contain a single DNA-containing specialized mitochondrion called the kinetoplast.[147] Amastigotes proliferate within macrophages, and dying macrophages release progeny amastigotes which can infect additional macrophages.

How far the amastigotes spread throughout the body depends on the *Leishmania* species. Cutaneous disease is caused primarily by *Leishmania major* and *Leishmania aethiopica* in the Old World and *Leishmania mexicana* and *Leishmania braziliensis* in the New World; mucocutaneous disease (also called espundia) is caused by *L. braziliensis*; and visceral disease involving the liver and spleen is caused by *Leishmania donovani* in the Old World and *Leishmania chagasi* in the New World. Tropism of *Leishmania* species appears to be linked to the optimal temperature for their growth. Parasites that cause visceral disease grow at 37°C in vitro, whereas parasites that cause mucocutaneous disease grow only at lower temperatures.

Leishmania manipulate innate host defenses to facilitate their entry and survival in host macrophages.[148] Promastigotes produce two abundant surface glycoconjugates, which appear to be important for their virulence.[149] The first, *lipophosphoglycan*, forms a dense glycocalyx that both activates complement (leading to C3b deposition on the parasite surface) and inhibits complement action (by preventing membrane attack complex insertion into the parasite membrane). Thus, the parasite becomes coated with C3 but avoids destruction by the membrane attack complex. The C3b on the surface of the parasite binds to Mac-1 and CR1 on macrophages, targeting the promastigote for phagocytosis by the macrophage. Once inside the cell, lipophosphoglycan protects the parasites within the phagolysosomes by scavenging oxygen radicals and by inhibiting lysosomal enzymes. The second surface glycoprotein, *gp63*, is a zinc-dependent proteinase that cleaves complement and some lysosomal antimicrobial enzymes. Gp63 also binds to fibronectin receptors on macrophages and promotes promastigote adhesion to macrophages. *Leishmania* amastigotes also produce molecules that facilitate their survival and replication within macrophages. Amastigotes reproduce in macrophage phagolysosomes, which have a pH of 4.5. However, the amastigotes are protected from this hostile environment by a proton-transporting ATPase, which maintains the intracellular parasite pH at 6.5.

Much of our knowledge of mechanisms of resistance and susceptibility to *Leishmania* comes from experimental mouse models.[150] Parasite-specific CD4+ helper T lymphocytes of the T_H1 subset are needed to control *Leishmania* in mice and humans. *Leishmania* evade host immunity by altering macrophage gene expression and impairing the development of the T_H1 response. In animal models, mice that are resistant to *Leishmania* infection produce high levels of T_H1-derived IFN-γ, which activates macrophages to kill the parasites through toxic metabolites of oxygen and nitric oxide. In contrast, in mouse strains that are susceptible to leishmaniasis, there is a dominant T_H2 response, and T_H2 cytokines such as IL-4, IL-13, and IL-10 prevent effective killing of *Leishmania* by inhibiting activation of macrophages.

Morphology. *Leishmania* species produce four different lesions in humans: visceral, cutaneous, mucocutaneous, and diffuse cutaneous. In **visceral leishmaniasis**, *L. donovani* or *L. chagasi* parasites invade macrophages throughout the mononuclear phagocyte system and cause severe systemic disease marked by hepatosplenomegaly, lymphadenopathy, pancytopenia, fever, and weight loss. The spleen may weigh as much as 3 kg, and the lymph nodes may measure 5 cm in diameter. Phagocytic cells are enlarged and filled with *Leishmania*, many plasma cells are present, and the normal architecture of the spleen is obscured (Fig. 8–54). In the late stages, the liver becomes increasingly fibrotic. Phagocytic cells crowd the bone marrow and also may be found in the lungs, gastrointestinal tract, kidneys, pancreas, and testes. Often there is hyperpigmentation of the skin in the extremities, which is why the disease is called kala-azar or "black fever" in Hindi. In the kidneys, there may be an immune complex–mediated mesangioproliferative glomerulonephritis, and in advanced cases, there may be amyloid deposition. The overloading of phagocytic cells with parasites predisposes the patients to bacterial infections, the usual cause of death. Hemorrhages related to thrombocytopenia may also be fatal.

Cutaneous leishmaniasis, caused by *L. major, L. mexicana*, and *L. braziliensis*, is a relatively mild, localized disease consisting of a single ulcer on exposed skin. The lesion (often called **tropical sore**) begins as an itching papule surrounded by induration, changes into a shallow and slowly expanding ulcer with irregular borders, and usually heals by involution within 6 months without treatment. On microscopic examination, the lesion is granulomatous, usually with many giant cells and few parasites.

Mucocutaneous leishmaniasis, caused by *L. braziliensis*, is found only in the New World. Moist, ulcerating or nonulcerating lesions, which may be disfiguring, develop in the larynx and at the mucocutaneous junctions of the nasal septum, anus, or vulva. On microscopic examination, there is a mixed inflammatory infiltrate with parasite-containing histiocytes in association with lymphocytes and plasma cells. Later, the tissue reaction becomes granulomatous, and the number of parasites declines. Eventually, the lesions remit and scar, although reactivation may occur after long intervals by mechanisms that are not currently understood.

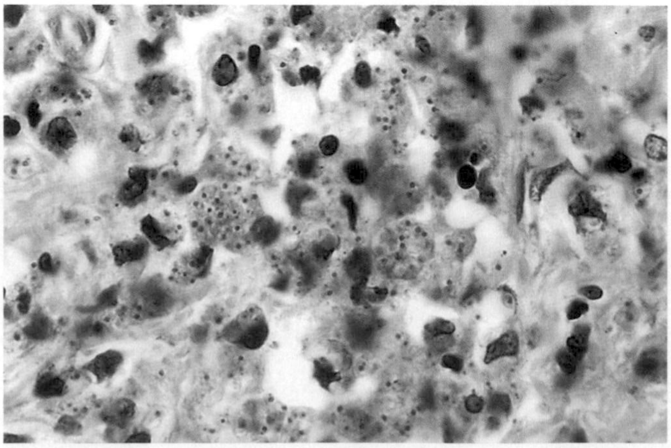

FIGURE 8–54 *Leishmania donovani* parasites within the macrophages of a lymph node in visceral leishmaniasis (kala-azar).

Diffuse cutaneous leishmaniasis is a rare form of dermal infection, thus far found in Ethiopia and adjacent East Africa and in Central and South America. Diffuse cutaneous leishmaniasis begins as a single skin nodule, which continues spreading until the entire body is covered by bizarre nodular lesions. These lesions, which resemble keloids or large verrucae, are frequently confused with the nodules of lepromatous leprosy. The lesions do not ulcerate but contain vast aggregates of foamy macrophages stuffed with leishmania. Patients are usually immunologically unresponsive not only to leishmanin but also to other skin antigens, and the lesions often respond poorly to treatment.

African Trypanosomiasis

African trypanosomes are kinetoplastid parasites that proliferate as extracellular forms in the blood and cause sustained or intermittent fevers, lymphadenopathy, splenomegaly, progressive brain dysfunction (sleeping sickness), cachexia, and death (Fig. 8–55). *Trypanosoma brucei rhodesiense* infections, which occur in East Africa, are often acute and virulent. *Trypanosoma brucei gambiense* infection tends to be chronic and occurs most frequently in the West African bush. Tsetse flies (genus *Glossina*) transmit African *Trypanosoma* to humans either from the reservoir of parasites found in wild and domestic animals *(T. brucei rhodesiense)* or from other humans *(T. brucei gambiense)*. Within the fly, the parasites multiply in the stomach and then in the salivary glands before developing into nondividing trypomastigotes, which are transmitted to humans and animals.

Pathogenesis. African trypanosomes are covered by a single, abundant, glycolipid-anchored protein called the *variant surface glycoprotein (VSG)*.[151] As parasites proliferate in the bloodstream, the host produces antibodies to the VSG, which, in association with phagocytes, kill most of the organisms, causing a spike of fever. A small number of parasites, however, undergo a genetic rearrangement and produce a different VSG on their surface and so escape the host immune response. These successor trypanosomes multiply until the host mounts an antibody response against their VSG and kills them, allowing another clone with a new VSG to take over. In this way, African trypanosomes escape the immune response to cause waves of fever before they finally invade the central nervous system.

Trypanosomes have about 1000 VSG genes, only one of which is expressed at a time. The parasite uses an elegant mechanism to turn VSG genes on and off.[151] Although VSG genes are scattered throughout the trypanosome genome, only VSG genes found within chromosomal regions called *bloodstream expression sites*, located in telomeres (the ends of chromosomes), can be expressed. New VSG genes are moved into the bloodstream expression sites mainly by homologous recombination.[152] A poorly understood transcription apparatus, which includes the RNA polymerase that transcribes VSG genes, associates with a single bloodstream expression site to limit expression to a single VSG gene.

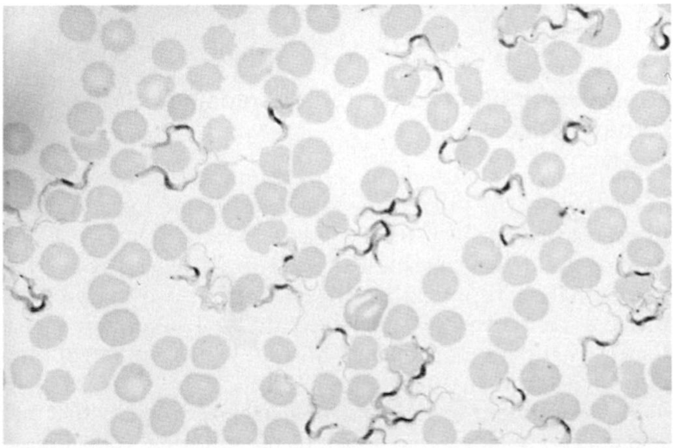

FIGURE 8–55 Slender bloodstream parasites of African trypanosomiasis.

Morphology. A large, red, rubbery chancre forms at the site of the insect bite, where large numbers of parasites are surrounded by a dense, largely mononuclear, inflammatory infiltrate. With chronicity, the lymph nodes and spleen enlarge owing to hyperplasia and infiltration by lymphocytes, plasma cells, and macrophages, which are filled with dead parasites. Trypanosomes, which are small and difficult to visualize, concentrate in capillary loops, such as the choroid plexus and glomeruli. When parasites breach the blood-brain barrier and invade the central nervous system, a leptomeningitis extends into the perivascular Virchow-Robin spaces, and eventually a demyelinating panencephalitis occurs. Plasma cells containing glycoprotein globules are frequent and are referred to as **flame cells** or **Mott cells**. Chronic disease leads to progressive cachexia, and patients, devoid of energy and normal mentation, waste away.

Chagas Disease

Trypanosoma cruzi is a kinetoplastid, intracellular protozoan parasite that causes American trypanosomiasis, or Chagas disease. Chagas disease occurs rarely in the United States and Mexico but is more common in South America, particularly Brazil. *T. cruzi* parasites infect many animals, including cats, dogs, and rodents. *T. cruzi* parasites are transmitted between animals and to humans by "kissing bugs" (triatomids), which hide in the cracks of loosely constructed houses, feed on the sleeping inhabitants, and pass infectious parasites in the feces; the infectious parasites enter the host through damaged skin or through mucous membranes. At the site of skin entry, there may be a transient, erythematous nodule called a *chagoma*.

Pathogenesis. *T. cruzi* has on its surface a homologue of the human complement regulatory protein decay-accelerating factor (DAF).[153] Like human DAF, the parasite homologue is anchored by means of a glycosyl phosphatidylinositol linkage, binds C3b, and inhibits C3 convertase formation and alternative pathway complement activation.

While most intracellular pathogens avoid the toxic contents of lysosomes, *T. cruzi* actually requires brief exposure to the acidic phagolysosome to stimulate development of amastigotes, the intracellular stage of the parasite.[154] To gain exposure to lysosomes, *T. cruzi* trypomastigotes stimulate an increase in the concentration of cytoplasmic calcium in host cells, which promotes fusion of the phagosome and lysosome. In addition to stimulating amastigote development, the low pH of the lysosome activates hemolysins that disrupt the lysosomal membrane, releasing the parasite into the cell cytoplasm. Parasites reproduce as rounded amastigotes in the cytoplasm of host cells and then develop flagella, burst host cells, enter the bloodstream, and penetrate smooth, skeletal, and heart muscles or infect kissing bugs when the insects take a blood meal.

In *acute Chagas disease*, which is mild in most individuals, cardiac damage results from direct invasion of myocardial cells by the organisms and from the consequent inflammatory changes. Rarely, acute Chagas disease patients present with high parasitemia, fever, or progressive cardiac dilation and failure, often with generalized lymphadenopathy or splenomegaly. In *chronic Chagas disease*, which occurs in 20% of infected patients 5 to 15 years after initial infection, the mechanism of cardiac and digestive tract damage is controversial; it likely results from an immune response induced by *T. cruzi* parasites, which are still present in small numbers. The striking inflammatory infiltration of the myocardium may be induced by the scant organisms.[155] Alternatively, parasites may induce an autoimmune response, such that antibodies and T cells that react with parasite proteins cross-react with host myocardial and nerve cells and extracellular proteins such as laminin. Damage to myocardial cells and to conductance pathways causes a dilated cardiomyopathy and cardiac arrhythmias, whereas damage to the myenteric plexus causes dilated colon (megacolon) and esophagus.

Morphology. In lethal **acute myocarditis**, the changes are diffusely distributed throughout the heart. Clusters of amastigotes cause swelling of individual myocardial fibers and create intracellular pseudocysts. There is focal myocardial cell necrosis accompanied by extensive, dense, acute interstitial inflammatory infiltration throughout the myocardium, and there is often four-chamber cardiac dilation (Chapter 12).

In **chronic Chagas disease,** the heart is typically dilated, rounded, and increased in size and weight. Often, there are mural thrombi that, in about half of autopsy cases, have given rise to pulmonary or systemic emboli or infarctions. On histologic examination, interstitial and perivascular inflammatory infiltration is composed of lymphocytes, plasma cells, and monocytes and is heaviest in the right bundle branch of the cardiac conduction system. There are scattered foci of myocardial cell necrosis and interstitial fibrosis, especially toward the apex of the left ventricle, which may undergo aneurysmal dilation and thinning. In the Brazilian endemic foci, as many as half of the patients with lethal carditis also have dilation of the esophagus or colon, apparently related to damage to the intrinsic innervation of these organs. At the late stages, however, when such changes appear, parasites cannot be found within these ganglia. Chronic Chagas cardiomyopathy is often treated by cardiac transplantation.

METAZOA

Metazoa are multicellular, eukaryotic organisms. The parasitic metazoa are contracted by eating the parasite, often in undercooked meat, and by direct invasion of the host through the skin and through insect bites. They dwell in many sites of the body, including the intestine, skin, lung, liver, muscle, blood vessels, and lymphatics.

Strongyloidiasis

Strongyloides stercoralis infects 30 to 100 million people worldwide. It is endemic in the southeastern United States, South America, sub-Saharan Africa, and Southeast Asia.[156] The worms live in the soil and infect humans when larvae penetrate the skin, travel in the circulation to the lungs, and then travel up the trachea to be swallowed. Female worms reside in the mucosa of the small intestine, where they produce eggs by asexual reproduction (parthenogenesis). Most of the larvae are passed in the stool and then may contaminate soil to continue the cycle of infection.

In immunocompetent hosts, *S. stercoralis* may cause diarrhea, bloating, and occasionally malabsorption. Unlike other parasitic worms, *S. stercoralis* larvae hatched in the gut can invade the colon mucosa and reinitiate infection (autoinfection). *Immunocompromised hosts, particularly people on prolonged corticosteroid therapy, can have very high levels of disseminated worms due to uncontrolled autoinfection.* This hyperinfection can be complicated by sepsis caused by bacteria from the intestine, which are carried into the host's blood by the invading larvae.

Morphology. In mild strongyloidiasis, worms, mainly larvae, are present in the duodenal crypts but are not seen in the underlying tissue. There is an eosinophil-rich infiltrate in the lamina propria with mucosal edema. Hyperinfection with *S. stercoralis* results in invasion of larvae into the colonic submucosa, lymphatics, and blood vessels, with an associated mononuclear infiltrate. There are many adult worms, larvae, and eggs in the crypts of the duodenum and ileum (Fig. 8–56). Worms of all stages may be found in other organs, including skin and lungs, and may even be found in large numbers in sputum.

Tapeworms (Cestodes): Cysticercosis and Hydatid Disease

Taenia solium and *Echinococcus granulosus* are cestode parasites (tapeworms) that cause cysticercosis and hydatid infections, respectively.[157,158] Both diseases are caused by larvae that develop following ingestion of tapeworm eggs. These tapeworms have a complex life cycle requiring two mammalian hosts: a definitive host, in which the worm reaches sexual maturity, and an intermediate host, in which the worm does not reach sexual maturity.

T. solium tapeworms consist of a head (scolex) that has suckers and hooklets that attach to the intestinal wall, a neck, and many flat segments called proglottids that contain male and female reproductive organs. New proglottids develop behind the scolex. The most distal proglottids are mature and

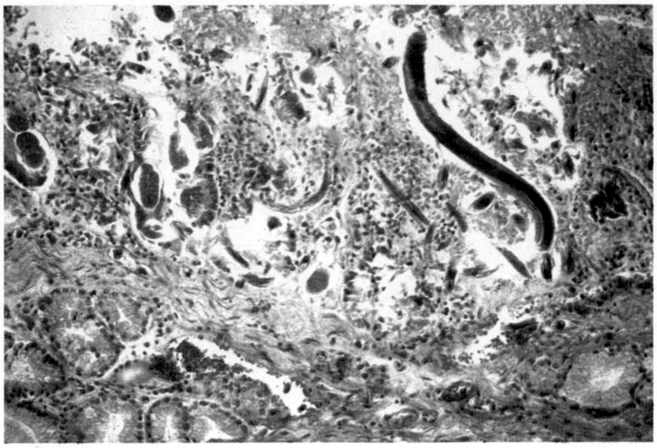

FIGURE 8–56 Strongyloides hyperinfection in a patient treated with high-dose cortisone. A female, her eggs and rhabditoid larvae are in the duodenal crypts; filariform larvae are entering the blood vessels and muscularis mucosa. (Courtesy of Dr. Franz C. Von Lichtenberg, Brigham and Women's Hospital, Boston, MA.)

contain many eggs, and they can detach and be shed in the feces. *T. solium* can be transmitted to humans in two ways, with distinct outcomes. (1) Ingestion of undercooked pork containing larval cysts, called cysticerci, leads to development of adult tapeworms in the intestine. Ingested cysticerci attach to the intestinal wall and develop into mature adult tapeworms, which can grow to many meters in length and can produce mild abdominal symptoms. (2) When intermediate hosts (pigs or humans) ingest eggs in food or water contaminated with human feces, the larvae hatch, penetrate the gut wall, disseminate hematogenously, and encyst in many organs. Convulsions, increased intracranial pressure, and neurologic disturbances are caused by *T. solium* cysts in brain tissue.[159] Adult tapeworms are not produced with this mode of infection. Viable *T. solium* cysts do not produce symptoms and can evade host immune defenses by producing taeniaestatin, a serine proteinase inhibitor that inhibits complement activation, and paramyosin, which appears to inhibit the classical pathway of complement activation.[160] When the cysticerci degenerate, an inflammatory response develops. *Taenia saginata*, the beef tapeworm, and *Diphyllobothrium latum*, the fish tapeworm, are acquired by eating undercooked meat or fish. In humans, these parasites live only in the gut, and they do not form cysticerci.

Hydatid disease is caused by ingestion of eggs of echinoccal species.[158,161] For *Echinococcus granulosus*, the definitive hosts are dogs, and sheep are the usual intermediate hosts. For *Echinoccus multilocularis*, foxes are the most important definitive host, and rodents are intermediate hosts. Humans are accidental intermediate hosts, infected by ingestion of food contaminated with eggs shed by dogs or foxes. Eggs hatch in the duodenum and invade the liver, lungs, or bones. Unilocular cysts caused by *E. granulosus* are most common. Multilocular cysts are caused by *E. multilocularis*.

Morphology. Cysticerci may be found in any organ, but the more common locations include the brain, muscles, skin, and heart. Cerebral symptoms depend on the precise location of the cysts, which includes the meninges, gray and white matter, sylvian aqueduct, and ventricular foramina. The cysts are ovoid and white to opalescent, rarely exceeding 1.5 cm, and contain an invaginated scolex with hooklets that are bathed in clear cyst fluid (Fig. 8–57). The cyst wall is more than 100 µm thick, is rich in glycoproteins, and evokes little host reaction when it is intact. When cysts degenerate, however, there is inflammation, followed by focal scarring, and calcifications, which may be visible by radiography.

About two-thirds of human *E. granulosus* cysts are found in the liver, 5% to 15% in the lung, and the rest in bones and brain or other organs. In the various organs, the larvae lodge within the capillaries and first incite an inflammatory reaction composed principally of mononuclear leukocytes and eosinophils. Many such larvae are destroyed, but others encyst. The cysts begin at microscopic levels and progressively increase in size, so that in 5 years or more, they may have achieved dimensions of more than 10 cm in diameter. Enclosing an opalescent fluid is an inner, nucleated, germinative layer and an outer, opaque, nonnucleated layer. The outer nonnucleated layer is distinctive and has innumerable delicate laminations as though made up of many layers of gelatin. Outside this opaque layer, there is a host inflammatory reaction that produces a zone of fibroblasts, giant cells, and mononuclear and eosinophilic cells. In time, a dense fibrous capsule forms. When these cysts have been present for about 6 months, daughter cysts develop within them. These appear first as minute projections of the germinative layer that develop central vesicles and thus form tiny brood capsules. Scolices of the worm develop on the inner aspects of these brood capsules and separate from the germinative layer to produce a fine, sandlike sediment within the hydatid fluid.

Trichinosis

Trichinella spiralis is a nematode parasite that is acquired by ingestion of larvae in undercooked meat from pigs that have themselves been infected by eating *T. spiralis*-infected

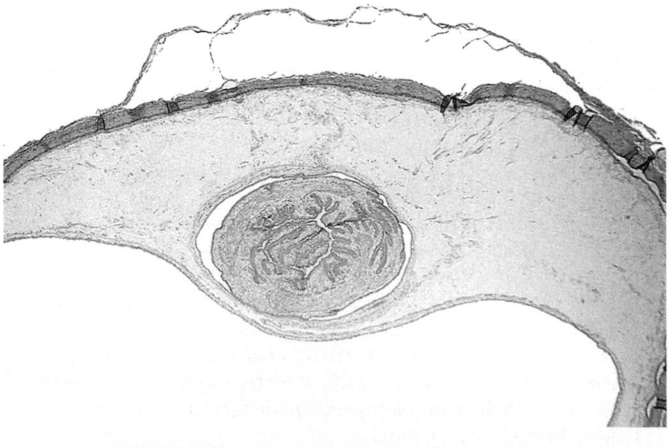

FIGURE 8–57 Portion of a cysticercus cyst.

rats or pork. In the United States, the number of *T. spiralis*-infected pigs has been greatly reduced by laws requiring cooking of hog food, and this has reduced the number of reported human infections in the United States to about 100 each year. Still, trichinosis is widespread where undercooked pork is eaten.

In the human gut, *T. spiralis* larvae develop into adults that mate and release new larvae, which penetrate into the tissues. Larvae disseminate hematogenously and penetrate muscle cells, causing fever, myalgias, marked eosinophilia, and periorbital edema. Much less commonly, patients develop dyspnea (because of invasion of the diaphragm), encephalitis, and cardiac failure. In striated skeletal muscle, *T. spiralis* larvae become intracellular parasites, increase dramatically in size, and modify the host muscle cell (referred to as the nurse cell) so that it loses its striations, gains a collagenous capsule, and develops a plexus of new blood vessels around itself.[162] The nurse cell–parasite complex is largely asymptomatic, and the worm may persist for years before it dies and calcifies. Antibodies to larval antigens, which include an immunodominant carbohydrate epitope called *tyvelose*, may reduce reinfection and are useful for serodiagnosis of the disease.[163]

T. spiralis and other invasive nematodes stimulate a T_H2 response, with production of IL-4, IL-5, IL-10, and IL-13. The cytokines produced by T_H2 cells activate eosinophils and mast cells, both of which are associated with the inflammatory response to these parasites. In animal models of *T. spiralis* infection, the T_H2 response is associated with increased contractility of the intestine, which expels adult worms from the gut and subsequently reduces the number of larvae in the muscles.[164] The mechanism by which the T_H2 response increases intestinal motility is unclear, although IL-4, IL-13, and mast cell degranulation have each been implicated.[165] While the T_H2 response indirectly reduces the number of larvae in muscle by eliminating adults from the intestine, it is not clear whether the intramuscular inflammatory response, which is composed of mononuclear cells and eosinophils, is effective against the larvae.

Morphology. During the invasive phase of trichinosis, cell destruction can be widespread but is rarely lethal. In the heart, there is a patchy interstitial myocarditis characterized by many eosinophils and scattered giant cells. The myocarditis can lead to scarring. Larvae in the heart do not encyst and are difficult to identify, because they die and disappear. In the lungs, trapped larvae cause focal edema and hemorrhages, sometimes with an allergic eosinophilic infiltrate. In the CNS, larvae cause a diffuse lymphocytic and eosinophilic infiltrate, with focal gliosis in and about small capillaries of the brain.

T. spiralis preferentially encysts in striated skeletal muscles with the richest blood supply, including the diaphragm; the extraocular; and the laryngeal, deltoid, gastrocnemius, and intercostal muscles (Fig. 8–58). Coiled larvae are approximately 1 mm long and are surrounded by membrane-bound vacuoles within nurse cells, which in turn are surrounded by new blood vessels and an eosinophil-rich mononuclear cell infiltrate. This infiltrate is greatest around dying parasites, which eventually calcify and leave behind characteristic scars, which are useful for retrospective diagnosis of trichinosis.

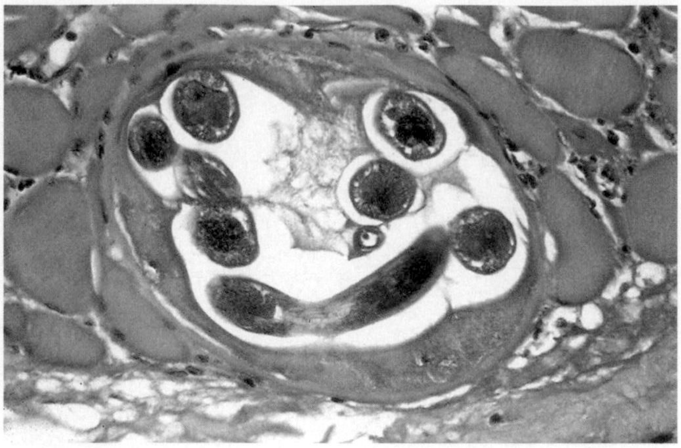

FIGURE 8–58 Coiled *Trichinella spiralis* larva within a skeletal muscle cell.

Schistosomiasis

Schistosomiasis infects approximately 200 million persons and kills approximately 280,000 annually. Most of the mortality comes from hepatic granulomas and fibrosis, caused by *Schistosoma mansoni* in Latin America, Africa, and the Middle East and *Schistosoma japonicum* and *Schistosoma mekongi* in East Asia.[166] In addition, *Schistosoma haematobium*, found in Africa, causes hematuria and granulomatous disease of the bladder, resulting in chronic obstructive uropathy.

Pathogenesis. Schistosomiasis is transmitted by freshwater snails that live in the slow-moving water of tropical rivers, lakes, and irrigation ditches, ironically linking agricultural development with spread of the disease (Fig. 8–59). Infectious schistosome larvae (cercariae) swim through fresh water and penetrate human skin with the aid of powerful proteolytic enzymes that degrade the keratinized layer. Within the skin, schistosome larvae shed a surface glycocalyx that protects the organisms from osmotic shock; this glycocalyx, however, activates complement by the alternative pathway and is recognized by many human antischistosome antibodies. Schistosomes migrate into the peripheral vasculature, traverse to the lung, and settle in the portal or pelvic venous system, where

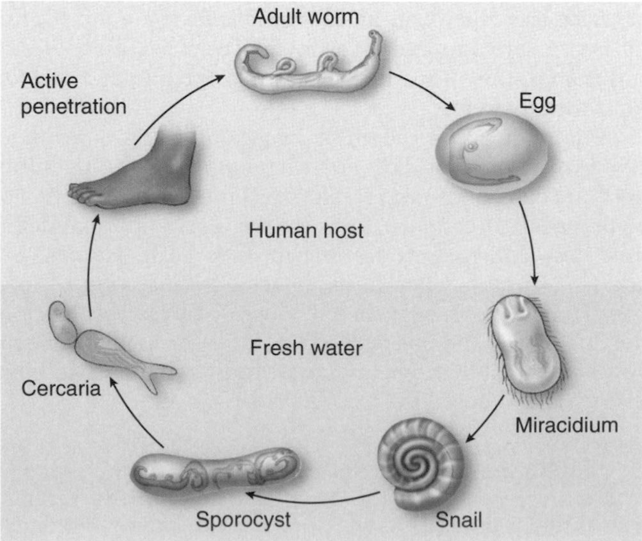

FIGURE 8–59 Schistosome life cycle.

they develop into adult male and female schistosomes. Females produce hundreds of eggs per day, around which granulomas and fibrosis form. Some schistosome eggs are passed from the portal veins through the intestinal wall into the colonic lumen, are shed with the feces, and release into freshwater miracidia that infect the snails to complete the life cycle.

The immune response to *S. mansoni* and *S. japonicum* eggs in the liver causes the severe pathology of schistosomiasis.[167] While the immune response does provide some protection in animal models, the price of this response is granuloma formation and hepatic fibrosis. Acute schistosomiasis in humans can be a severe febrile illness that peaks about 2 months after infection. The T-helper response in this early stage is dominated by T_H1 cells, and the IFN-γ produced by T cells may stimulate macrophages to produce high levels of the pyrogens TNF, IL-1, and IL-6. Chronic schistosomiasis is associated with a dominant T_H2 response, although T_H1 cells persist. Stimulation of T_H2 cells may be due to proteins in the parasite egg that cause mast cells to produce IL-4, which induces further T_H2 differentiation and amplifies the response. Both types of T-helper cells appear to stimulate formation of granulomas in the liver. Eggs become surrounded by granulomatous lesions composed of macrophages, lymphocytes, eosinophils, and connective tissue. Severe hepatic fibrosis is a serious manifestation of chronic schistosomiasis. In animal models, IL-13, produced by T_H2 cells, increases fibrosis by increasing synthesis of proline, an important amino acid in collagen.

Morphology. In mild *S. mansoni* or *S. japonicum* infections, white, pinhead-sized granulomas are scattered throughout the gut and liver. At the center of the granuloma is the schistosome egg, which contains a miracidium; this degenerates over time and calcifies. The granulomas are composed of macrophages, lymphocytes, neutrophils, and eosinophils; the last-mentioned are distinctive for helminth infections (Fig. 8–60). The liver is darkened by regurgitated heme-derived pigments from the schistosome gut, which, like malaria pigments, are iron-negative and accumulate in Kupffer cells and splenic macrophages.

In severe *S. mansoni* or *S. japonicum* infections, inflammatory patches or pseudopolyps may form in the colon. The surface of the liver is bumpy, whereas cut surfaces reveal granulomas and a widespread fibrous portal enlargement without distortion of the intervening parenchyma by regenerative nodules. Because these fibrous triads resemble the stem of a clay pipe, the lesion is named **pipe-stem fibrosis** (Fig. 8–61). Many of these portal triads lack a vein lumen, causing presinusoidal portal hypertension and severe congestive splenomegaly, esophageal varices, and ascites. Schistosome eggs, diverted to the lung through portal collaterals, may produce granulomatous pulmonary arteritis with intimal hyperplasia, progressive arterial obstruction, and ultimately heart failure (cor pulmonale). On histologic examination, arteries in the lungs show disruption of the elastica layer by granulomas and scars, luminal organizing thrombi, and angiomatoid lesions similar to those of idiopathic pulmonary hypertension (Chapter 15). Patients with hepatosplenic schistosomiasis also have an increased frequency of mesangioproliferative or membranous glomerulopathy (Chapter 20), in which glomeruli contain deposits of immunoglobulin and complement but rarely schistosome antigen.

In *S. haematobium* infection, bladder inflammatory patches due to massive egg deposition and granulomas appear early, and when they erode, they cause hematuria (Fig. 8–10). Later, the granulomas calcify and develop a "sandy" appearance, which, if severe, may line the wall of the bladder and cause a dense concentric rim (calcified bladder) on radiographic films. The most frequent complication of *S. haematobium* infection is inflammation and fibrosis of the ureteral walls, leading to obstruction, hydronephrosis, and chronic pyelonephritis. There is also an association between urinary schistosomiasis and squamous cell carcinoma of the bladder (Chapter 21).

Lymphatic Filariasis

Lymphatic filariasis is transmitted by mosquitoes and is caused by two closely related nematodes, *Wuchereria bancrofti*

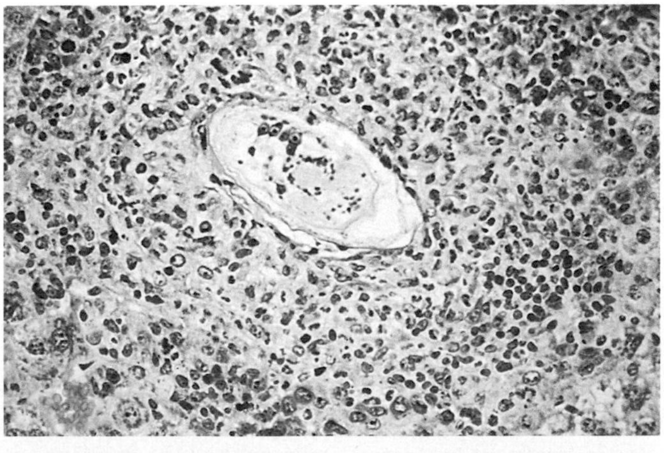

FIGURE 8–60 *Schistosoma mansoni* granuloma with a miracidium-containing egg *(center)* and numerous, adjacent, scattered eosinophils.

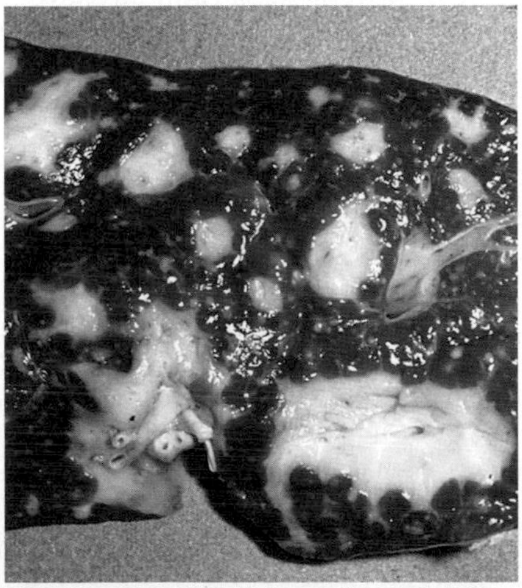

FIGURE 8–61 Pipe-stem fibrosis of the liver due to chronic *Schistosoma japonicum* infection.

and *Brugia malayi*, which are responsible for 90% and 10%, respectively, of the 90 million infections worldwide. In endemic areas, which include parts of Latin America, sub-Saharan Africa, and Southeast Asia, filariasis causes a spectrum of diseases, including (1) asymptomatic microfilaremia, (2) chronic lymphadenitis with swelling of the dependent limb or scrotum (elephantiasis), and (3) tropical pulmonary eosinophilia. As is the case with leprosy and leishmanial infections, some of the different disease manifestations caused by lymphatic filariae may be understood in the context of varying patterns of host T-cell responses to the parasites.[168,169]

Pathogenesis. Infective larvae released by mosquitoes into the tissues during the blood meal develop within lymphatic channels into adult males and females, which mate and release microfilariae that enter into the bloodstream. When mosquitoes bite infected individuals, they can take up the microfilariae and transmit the disease. Experiments in athymic (nude) mice suggest that adult filariae secrete factors that, by themselves, are capable of causing lymphatic dilation, lymphedema, and elephantiasis. In contrast, microfilariae, even in massive numbers in microfilaremic hosts, are not directly toxic to the host. The filarial genome project has led to the identification of a number of filarial molecules that can evade or inhibit immune defenses. *Brugia malayi* produces (1) several surface glycoproteins with antioxidant function, which may protect from superoxide and free oxygen radicals; (2) homologues of cystatins, cysteine protease inhibitors, which can impair the MHC class II antigen-processing pathway; (3) serpins, serine protease inhibitors, which can inhibit neutrophil proteases, critical inflammatory mediators; and (4) homologues of TGF-β, which can bind to mammalian TGF-β receptors and may downregulate inflammatory responses.[170–172] Recent studies have revealed that endosymbiotic rickettsia-like *Wolbachia* bacteria infect filarial nematodes and might contribute to pathogenesis of disease.[173] *Wolbachia* appear to be needed for nematode development and reproduction, since antibiotics that eradicate *Wolbachia* impair nematode survival and fertility. It has been hypothesized that LPS from *Wolbachia* may stimulate inflammatory responses.

In chronic lymphatic filariasis, damage to the lymphatics is caused directly by the adult parasites and by a T_H1–mediated immune response, which stimulates the formation of granulomas around the adult parasites. Microfilariae are absent from the bloodstream, because the immune response damages the adults such that they do not breed successfully. In contrast, there is an *inadequate response* to circulating parasites in microfilaremic individuals.[168,169] Because most microfilaremic individuals come from areas where filariasis is endemic, there is speculation that the inadequate response is caused by prenatal exposure to parasite antigens that may induce immunologic tolerance in the host.

Finally, there is an *IgE-mediated hypersensitivity* to microfilariae in *tropical pulmonary eosinophilia.* IgE and eosinophils may be stimulated by IL-4 and IL-5, respectively, secreted by filaria-specific T_H2 helper T cells. Tropical pulmonary eosinophilia results in restrictive lung disease, discussed in Chapter 15.

Morphology. Chronic filariasis is characterized by persistent lymphedema of the scrotum, penis, vulva, leg, or arm (Fig. 8–62). Frequently, there is hydrocele and lymph node enlargement. In severe and long-lasting infections, chylous weeping of the enlarged scrotum may ensue, or a chronically swollen leg may develop tough subcutaneous fibrosis and epithelial hyperkeratosis, termed **elephantiasis**. Elephantoid skin shows dilation of the dermal lymphatics with widespread lymphocytic infiltrates and focal cholesterol deposits; the epidermis is thickened and hyperkeratotic. Adult filarial worms—live, dead, or calcified—are present in the scrotal draining lymphatics or nodes, surrounded by (1) mild or no inflammation, (2) an intense eosinophilia with hemorrhage and fibrin (recurrent filarial funiculoepididymitis), or (3) granulomas not dissimilar to those found in mycobacterial infections. Organization of the endolymphatic exudate results in polypoid infoldings of the vessels with persisting eosinophilic and lymphocytic infiltrates. In time, hydrocele fluid, which often contains cholesterol crystals, red cells, and hemosiderin, induces thickening and calcification of the tunica vaginalis.

Lung involvement by microfilariae is marked by eosinophilia caused by T_H2 responses and cytokine production (tropical eosinophilia) or by dead microfilariae surrounded by stellate, hyaline, eosinophilic precipitates embedded in small epithelioid granulomas (Meyers-Kouvenaar bodies). Typically, these patients lack any other manifestations of filarial disease.

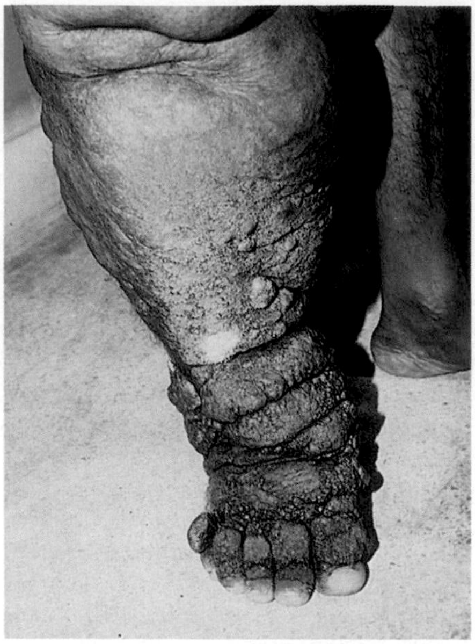

FIGURE 8–62 Massive edema and elephantiasis caused by filariasis of the leg. (Courtesy of Dr. Willy Piessens, Harvard School of Public Health, Boston, MA.)

Onchocerciasis

Onchocerca volvulus, a filarial nematode transmitted by black flies, affects more than 17 million people in Africa, South America, and Yemen.[174] An aggressive campaign of ivermectin treatment has dramatically reduced the incidence of *Onchocerca* infection in West Africa; however, *O. volvulus* remains the second most common preventable cause of blindness in sub-Saharan Africa.

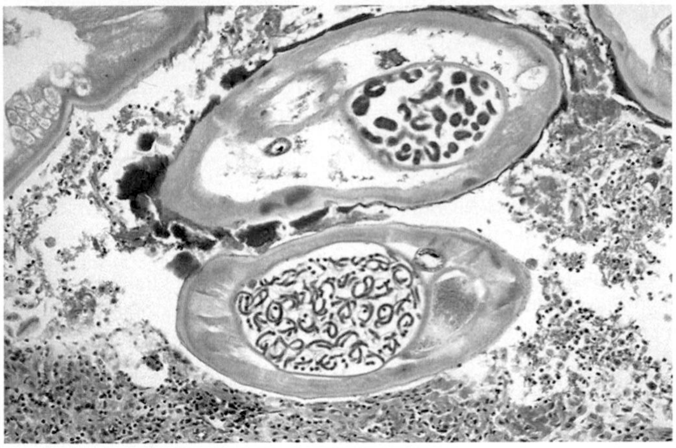

FIGURE 8–63 Microfilaria-laden gravid female of *Onchocerca volvulus* in a subcutaneous fibrous nodule.

Adult *O. volvulus* parasites mate in the dermis, where they are surrounded by a mixed infiltrate of host cells that produces a characteristic subcutaneous nodule *(onchocercoma)*. The major pathologic process, which includes blindness and chronic pruritic dermatitis, is caused by large numbers of microfilariae, released by females, that accumulate in the skin and in the eye chambers. *Punctate keratitis* is caused by inflammation around a degenerating microfilaria. It is sometimes accentuated by treatment with antifilarial drugs (Mazzotti reaction), resulting in blindness. Ivermectin kills only immature worms, not adult worms, so parasites repopulate the host a few months after treatment. Recently, doxycycline treatment has been shown to block reproduction of *O. volvus* for up to 24 months.[175] Doxycycline kills *Wolbachia*, which are symbiotic bacteria that live inside adult *O. volvulus* and are required for worm fertility, similar to filarial nematodes.

Morphology. *O. volvulus* causes chronic, itchy dermatitis with focal darkening or loss of pigment and scaling, referred to as leopard, lizard, or elephant skin. Foci of epidermal atrophy and elastic fiber breakdown may alternate with areas of hyperkeratosis, hyperpigmentation with pigment incontinence, dermal atrophy, and fibrosis. The subcutaneous onchocercoma is composed of a fibrous capsule surrounding adult worms and a mixed chronic inflammatory infiltrate that includes fibrin, neutrophils, eosinophils, lymphocytes, and giant cells (Fig. 8–63). The progressive eye lesions begin with punctate keratitis along with small, fluffy opacities of the cornea caused by degenerating microfilariae, which evoke an eosinophilic infiltrate. This is followed by a sclerosing keratitis that opacifies the cornea, beginning at the scleral limbus. Microfilariae in the anterior chamber cause iridocyclitis and glaucoma, whereas involvement of the choroid and retina results in atrophy and loss of vision.

REFERENCES

1. Arias E, Smith BL: Deaths: preliminary data for 2001. Natl Vital Stat Rep 51:1, 2003.
2. Murray CJ, Lopez AD: Global mortality, disability, and the contribution of risk factors: Global Burden of Disease Study. Lancet 349:1436, 1997.
3. Ksiazek TG, Erdman D, Goldsmith CS, et al: A novel coronavirus associated with severe acute respiratory syndrome. N Engl J Med 348:1953, 2003.
4. Drosten C, Gunther S, Preiser W, et al: Identification of a novel coronavirus in patients with severe acute respiratory syndrome. N Engl J Med 348:1967, 2003.
5. Weiss HA, Quigley MA, Hayes RJ: Male circumcision and risk of HIV infection in sub-Saharan Africa: a systematic review and meta-analysis. AIDS 14:2361, 2000.
6. Barbour AG, Fish D: The biological and social phenomenon of Lyme disease. Science 260:1610, 1993.
7. Centers for Disease Control and Prevention: Biological and chemical terrorism: strategic plan for preparedness and response. Recommendations of the CDC Strategic Planning Workgroup. MMWR 49:5, 2000.
8. Uptain SM, Lindquist S: Prions as protein-based genetic elements. Annu Rev Microbiol 56:703, 2002.
9. Prusiner SB: Shattuck lecture: neurodegenerative diseases and prions. N Engl J Med 344:1516, 2001.
10. Walker D, Tumler JS: Emergence of the ehrlichioses as human health problems. Emerg Infect Dis 2:18, 1996.
11. Mims C: The Pathogenesis of Infectious Disease, 5th ed. San Diego, CA, Academic Press, 2001.
12. Neutra MR, Pringault E, Kraehenbuhl JP: Antigen sampling across epithelial barriers and induction of mucosal immune responses. Annu Rev Immunol 14:275, 1996.
13. Berg RD: Bacterial translocation from the gastrointestinal tract. Trends Microbiol 3:149, 1995.
14. Metcalf TG, Melnick JL, Estes MK: Environmental virology: from detection of virus in sewage and water by isolation to identification by molecular biology—a trip of over 50 years. Annu Rev Microbiol 49:461, 1995.
15. Kaufmann SHE, Sher A, Ahmed R: Immunology of Infectious Diseases. Washington, DC, ASM Press, 2002.
16. Rossmann MG, et al: Cell recognition and entry by rhino- and enteroviruses. Virology 269:239, 2000.
17. Derfuss T, Meinl E: Herpesviral proteins regulating apoptosis. Curr Top Microbiol Immunol 269:257, 2002.
18. Kondo T, Suda T, Fukuyama H, Adachi M, Nagata S: Essential roles of the Fas ligand in the development of hepatitis. Nat Med 3:409, 1997.
19. Edwards RA, Olsen GJ, Maloy SR: Comparative genomics of closely related salmonellae. Trends Microbiol 10:94, 2002.
20. Novick RP, Muir TW: Virulence gene regulation by peptides in staphylococci and other Gram-positive bacteria. Curr Opin Microbiol 2:40, 1999.
21. Mulvey MA: Adhesion and entry of uropathogenic *Escherichia coli*. Cell Microbiol 4:257, 2002.
22. Seifert HS: Questions about gonococcal pilus phase- and antigenic variation. Mol Microbiol 21:433, 1996.
23. Ernst JD: Macrophage receptors for Mycobacterium tuberculosis. Infect Immun 66:1277, 1998.
24. Anderson DM, Schneewind O: Type III machines of Gram-negative pathogens: injecting virulence factors into host cells and more. Curr Opin Microbiol 2:18, 1999.
25. Portnoy DA, Auerbuch V, Glomski IJ: The cell biology of Listeria monocytogenes infection: the intersection of bacterial pathogenesis and cell-mediated immunity. J Cell Biol 158:409, 2002.
26. Pieters J, Gatfield J: Hijacking the host: survival of pathogenic mycobacteria inside macrophages. Trends Microbiol 10:142, 2002.
27. Triantafilou M, Triantafilou K: Lipopolysaccharide recognition: CD14, TLRs and the LPS-activation cluster. Trends Immunol 23:301, 2002.
28. Dobrovolskaia MA, Vogel SN: Toll receptors, CD14, and macrophage activation and deactivation by LPS. Microbes Infect 4:903, 2002.
29. Amagai M, Matsuyoshi N, Wang ZH, Andl C, Stanley JR: Toxin in bullous impetigo and staphylococcal scalded-skin syndrome targets desmoglein 1. Nat Med 6:1275, 2000.
30. Turton K, Chaddock JA, Acharya KR: Botulinum and tetanus neurotoxins: structure, function and therapeutic utility. Trends Biochem Sci 27:552, 2002.
31. Papageorgiou AC, Acharya KR: Microbial superantigens: from structure to function. Trends Microbiol 8:369, 2000.
32. Zhang JR, Hardham JM, Barbour AG, Norris SJ: Antigenic variation in Lyme disease borreliae by promiscuous recombination of VMP-like sequence cassettes. Cell 89:275, 1997.
33. Peschel A: How do bacteria resist human antimicrobial peptides? Trends Microbiol 10:179, 2002.

34. Hornef MW, Wick MJ, Rhen M, Normark S: Bacterial strategies for overcoming host innate and adaptive immune responses. Nat Immunol 3:1033, 2002.
35. Orange JS, Fassett MS, Koopman LA, Boyson JE, Strominger JL: Viral evasion of natural killer cells. Nat Immunol 3:1006, 2002.
36. Yewdell JW, Hill AB: Viral interference with antigen presentation. Nat Immunol 3:1019, 2002.
37. Furman MH, Ploegh HL: Lessons from viral manipulation of protein disposal pathways. J Clin Invest 110:875, 2002.
38. Lyczak JB, Cannon CL, Pier GB: Lung infections associated with cystic fibrosis. Clin Microbiol Rev 15:194, 2002.
39. Schalling M, Ekman M, Kaaya EE, Linde A, Biberfeld P: A role for a new herpes virus (KSHV) in different forms of Kaposi's sarcoma. Nat Med 1:707, 1995.
40. Clarke JR: Molecular diagnosis of HIV. Expert Rev Mol Diagn 2:233, 2002.
41. Cinque P, Bossolasco S, Lundkvist A: Molecular analysis of cerebrospinal fluid in viral diseases of the central nervous system. J Clin Virol 26:1, 2003.
42. Watson EJ, Templeton A, Russell I, et al: The accuracy and efficacy of screening tests for Chlamydia trachomatis: a systematic review. J Med Microbiol 51:1021, 2002.
43. Weiss R: Measles battle loses potent weapon. Science 258:546, 1992.
44. Moss WJ, Cutts F, Griffin DE: Implications of the HIV epidemic for control and eradication of measles. Clin Infect Dis 29:106, 1999.
45. Hutchins S, Markowitz L, Atkinson W, Swint E, Hadler S: Measles outbreaks in the United States, 1987 through 1990. Pediatr Infect Dis J 15:31, 1996.
46. Hsu EC, Dorig RE, Sarangi F, Marcil A, Iorio C, Richardson CD: Artificial mutations and natural variations in the CD46 molecules from human and monkey cells define regions important for measles virus binding. J Virol 71:6144, 1997.
47. Tatsuo H, Ono N, Tanaka K, Yanagi Y: SLAM (CDw150) is a cellular receptor for measles virus. Nature 406:893, 2000.
48. Hahm B, Arbour N, Naniche D, Homann D, Manchester M, Oldstone MB: Measles virus infects and suppresses proliferation of T lymphocytes from transgenic mice bearing human signaling lymphocytic activation molecule. J Virol 77:3505, 2003.
49. Sidorenko SP, Clark EA: The dual-function CD150 receptor subfamily: the viral attraction. Nat Immunol 4:19, 2003.
50. Norrby E, Kristensson K: Measles virus in the brain. Brain Res Bull 44:213, 1997.
51. van Loon FP, et al: Mumps surveillance: United States, 1988–1993. MMWR CDC Surveill Summ 44:1, 1995.
52. Minor PD: The molecular biology of polioviruses vaccines. J Gen Virol 73:3065, 1992.
53. Dowdle WR, Birmingham ME: The biologic principles of poliovirus eradication. J Infect Dis 175 (Suppl 1):S286, 1997.
54. Hogle JM: Poliovirus cell entry: common structural themes in viral cell entry pathways. Annu Rev Microbiol 56:677, 2002.
55. Racaniello VR, Ren R: Poliovirus biology and pathogenesis. Curr Top Microbiol Immunol 206:305, 1996.
56. Nash D, Mostashari F, Fine A, et al: The outbreak of West Nile virus infection in the New York City area in 1999. N Engl J Med 344:1807, 2001.
57. Petersen LR, Roehrig JT: West Nile virus: a reemerging global pathogen. Emerg Infect Dis 7:611, 2001.
58. Petersen LR, Marfin AA: West Nile virus: a primer for the clinician. Ann Intern Med 137:173, 2002.
59. Chambers TJ, Halevy M, Nestorowicz A, Rice CM, Lustig S: West Nile virus envelope proteins: nucleotide sequence analysis of strains differing in mouse neuroinvasiveness. J Gen Virol 79 (Pt 10):2375, 1998.
60. Wang X, et al: Epidermal growth factor receptor is a cellular receptor for human cytomegalovirus. Nature 424:456, 2003.
61. Stanbury L: Pathogenesis of herpes simplex virus infection and animal models for its study. Curr Top Microbiol Immunol 179:15, 1992.
62. Jones C: Herpes simplex virus-1 and bovine herpesvirus-1 latency. Clin Microbiol Rev 16:79, 2003.
63. Steiner I: Human herpes viruses latent infection in the nervous system. Immunol Rev 152:157, 1996.
64. Keadle TL, Morris JL, Pepose JS, Stuart PM: CD4+(+) and CD8(+) cells are key participants in the development of recurrent herpetic stromal keratitis in mice. Microb Pathog 32:255, 2002.
65. Lehner PJ, Wilkinson GW: Cytomegalovirus: from evasion to suppression? Nat Immunol 2:993, 2001.
66. Sinzger C, Jahn G: Human cytomegalovirus cell tropism and pathogenesis. Intervirology 39:302, 1996.
67. Andrews DM, Andoniou CE, Granucci F, Ricciardi-Castagnoli P, Degli-Esposti MA: Infection of dendritic cells by murine cytomegalovirus induces functional paralysis. Nat Immunol 2:1077, 2001.
68. Benedict C, Norris P, Ware C: To kill or be killed:viral evasion of apoptosis. Nat Immunol 11:1013, 2002.
69. White CJ: Varicella-zoster virus vaccine. Clin Infect Dis 24:753, 1997.
70. Chisari F: Viruses, immunity and cancer: lessons from hepatitis B. Am J Path 156:1117, 2000.
71. Nathanson N, Ahmed R, Gonzalez-Scarano F, et al: Viral Pathogenesis. Philadelphia, Lippincott-Raven, 1997.
72. Thorley-Lawson DA: Epstein-Barr virus: exploiting the immune system. Nat Rev Immunol 1:75, 2001.
73. Morra M, et al: X-linked lymphoproliferative syndrome: a progressive immunodeficiency. Annu Rev Immunol 19:657, 2001.
74. Sixbey JW, Yao QY: Immunoglobulin A-induced shift of Epstein-Barr virus tissue tropism. Science 255:1578, 1992.
75. Foster TJ, McDevitt D: Surface-associated proteins of Staphylococcus aureus: their possible roles in virulence. FEMS Microbiol Lett 118:199, 1994.
76. Kaneko J, Ozawa T, Tomita T, Kamio Y: Sequential binding of Staphylococcal gamma-hemolysin to human erythrocytes and complex formation of the hemolysin on the cell surface. Biosci Biotechnol Biochem 61:846, 1997.
77. Proft T, Fraser JD: Bacterial superantigens. Clin Exp Immunol 133:299, 2003.
78. Bisno AL, Brito MO, Collins CM: Molecular basis of group A streptococcal virulence. Lancet Infect Dis 3:191, 2003.
79. Gibofsky A, Kerwar S, Zabriskie JB: Rheumatic fever. The relationships between host, microbe, and genetics. Rheum Dis Clin North Am 24:237, 1998.
80. Stevens DL: The toxins of group A streptococcus, the flesh eating bacteria. Immunol Invest 26:129, 1997.
81. Paton JC: The contribution of pneumolysin to the pathogenicity of Streptococcus pneumoniae. Trends Microbiol 4:103, 1996.
82. Loeche WJ: Role of Streptococcus mutans in human dental decay. Microbiol Rev 50:353, 1986.
83. Hadfield TL, McEvoy P, Polotsky Y, Tzinserling VA, Yakovlev AA: The pathology of diphtheria. J Infect Dis 181 (Suppl 1):S116, 2000.
84. Mengaud J, Ohayon H, Gounon P, Mege RM, Cossart P: E-cadherin is the receptor for internalin, a surface protein required for entry of *L. monocytogenes* into epithelial cells. Cell 84:923, 1996.
85. Swartz MN: Recognition and management of anthrax: an update. N Engl J Med 345:1621, 2001.
86. Mourez M, Lacy DB, Cunningham K, et al: 2001: a year of major advances in anthrax toxin research. Trends Microbiol 10:287, 2002.
87. Grinberg LM, Abramova FA, Yampolskaya OV, Walker DH, Smith JH: Quantitative pathology of inhalational anthrax I: quantitative microscopic findings. Mod Pathol 14:482, 2001.
88. Torres HA, Reddy BT, Raad, II, et al: Nocardiosis in cancer patients. Medicine (Baltimore) 81:388, 2002.
89. Tyrrell GJ, Chui L, Johnson M, Chang N, Rennie RP, Talbot JA: Outbreak of Neisseria meningitidis, Edmonton, Alberta, Canada. Emerg Infect Dis 8:519, 2002.
90. Pathan N, Faust SN, Levin M: Pathophysiology of meningococcal meningitis and septicaemia. Arch Dis Child 88:601, 2003.
91. Serkin CD, Seifert HS: Frequency of pilin antigenic variation in *Neisseria gonorrhoeae.* J Bacteriol 180:1955, 1998.
92. Mooi FR, van Loo IH, King AJ: Adaptation of Bordetella pertussis to vaccination: a cause for its reemergence? Emerg Infect Dis 7:526, 2001.
93. Hardwick TH, Cassiday P, Weyant RS, Bisgard KM, Sanden GN: Changes in predominance and diversity of genomic subtypes of Bordetella pertussis isolated in the United States, 1935 to 1999. Emerg Infect Dis 8:44, 2002.
94. Locht C, Antoine R, Jacob-Dubuisson F: Bordetella pertussis, molecular pathogenesis under multiple aspects. Curr Opin Microbiol 4:82, 2001.
95. Gierschik P: ADP-ribosylation of signal-transducing guanine nucleotide-binding proteins by pertussis toxin. Curr Top Microbiol Immunol 175:69, 1992.
96. Govan JR, Deretic V: Microbial pathogenesis in cystic fibrosis: mucoid Pseudomonas aeruginosa and Burkholderia cepacia. Microbiol Rev 60:539, 1996.

97. Kreitman RJ, Pastan I: Targeting Pseudomonas exotoxin to hematologic malignancies. Semin Cancer Biol 6:297, 1995.
98. Britigan BE, Roeder TL, Rasmussen GT, Shasby DM, McCormick ML, Cox CD: Interaction of the Pseudomonas aeruginosa secretory products pyocyanin and pyochelin generates hydroxyl radical and causes synergistic damage to endothelial cells: implications for Pseudomonas-associated tissue injury. J Clin Invest 90:2187, 1992.
99. Cravens G, J.S. Marr: The Black Death. New York, Ballantine Books, 1977.
100. Boisier P, Rahalison L, Rasolomaharo M, et al: Epidemiologic features of four successive annual outbreaks of bubonic plague in Mahajanga, Madagascar. Emerg Infect Dis 8:311, 2002.
101. Cornelis GR: Molecular and cell biology aspects of plague. Proc Natl Acad Sci U S A 97:8778, 2000.
102. Lewis DA: Chancroid: clinical manifestations, diagnosis, and management. Sex Transm Infect 79:68, 2003.
103. O'Farrell N: Donovanosis. Sex Transm Infect 78:452, 2002.
104. Glickman MS, Jacobs WR: Microbial pathogenesis of Mycobacterium tuberculosis: dawn of a discipline. Cell 104:477, 2003.
105. Fratti RA, Backer JM, Gruenberg J, Corvera S, Deretic V: Role of phosphatidylinositol 3-kinase and Rab5 effectors in phagosomal biogenesis and mycobacterial phagosome maturation arrest. J Cell Biol 154:631, 2001.
106. Bellamy R, Ruwende C, Corrah T, McAdam KP, Whittle HC, Hill AV: Variations in the NRAMP1 gene and susceptibility to tuberculosis in West Africans. N Engl J Med 338:640, 1998.
107. Young D, Hussell T, Dougan G: Chronic bacterial infections: living with unwanted guests. Nat Immunol 3:1026, 2002.
108. Flynn J, Chan J: Immunology of tuberculosis. Annu Rev Immunol 19:93, 2001.
109. Yamamura M, Uyemura K, Deans RJ, et al: Defining protective responses to pathogens: cytokine profiles in leprosy lesions. Science 254:277, 1991.
110. Van Voorhis WC, Barrett LK, Koelle DM, Nasio JM, Plummer FA, Lukehart SA: Primary and secondary syphilis lesions contain mRNA for Th1 cytokines. J Infect Dis 173:491, 1996.
111. Blanco DR, Miller JN, Lovett MA: Surface antigens of the syphilis spirochete and their potential as virulence determinants. Emerg Infect Dis 3:11, 1997.
112. Barbour AG, Burman N, Carter CJ, Kitten T, Bergstrom S: Variable antigen genes of the relapsing fever agent Borrelia hermsii are activated by promoter addition. Mol Microbiol 5:489, 1991.
113. Fekade D, Knox K, Hussein K, et al: Prevention of Jarisch-Herxheimer reactions by treatment with antibodies against tumor necrosis factor alpha. N Engl J Med 335:311, 1996.
114. Hengge UR, et al: Lyme borreliosis. Lancet Infect Dis 3:489, 2000.
115. Steere AC: Lyme disease. N Engl J Med 345:115, 2001.
116. Brook I: Microbiology of polymicrobial abscesses and implications for therapy. J Antimicrob Chemother 50:805, 2002.
117. Songer JG: Bacterial phospholipases and their role in virulence. Trends Microbiol 5:156, 1997.
118. McClane BA: Clostridium perfringens enterotoxin and intestinal tight junctions. Trends Microbiol 8:145, 2000.
119. Hammond GA, Lyerly DM, Johnson JL: Transcriptional analysis of the toxigenic element of Clostridium difficile. Microb Pathog 22:143, 1997.
120. Coonrod DV: Chlamydial infections. Curr Womens Health Rep 2:266, 2002.
121. Burstein GR, Zenilman JM: Nongonococcal urethritis: a new paradigm. Clin Infect Dis 28 (Suppl 1):S66, 1999.
122. Mabey D, Peeling RW: Lymphogranuloma venereum. Sex Transm Infect 78:90, 2002.
123. Azad AF, Beard CB: Rickettsial pathogens and their arthropod vectors. Emerg Infect Dis 4:179, 1998.
124. Bise G, Coninx R: Epidemic typhus in a prison in Burundi. Trans R Soc Trop Med Hyg 91:133, 1997.
125. Valbuena G, Feng HM, Walker DH: Mechanisms of immunity against rickettsiae: new perspectives and opportunities offered by unusual intracellular parasites. Microbes Infect 4:625, 2002.
126. Latge JP, Calderone R: Host-microbe interactions: fungi invasive human fungal opportunistic infections. Curr Opin Microbiol 5:355, 2002.
127. Soll DR: Candida commensalism and virulence: the evolution of phenotypic plasticity. Acta Trop 81:101, 2002.
128. Calderone RA, Fonzi WA: Virulence factors of Candida albicans. Trends Microbiol 9:327, 2001.
129. Romani L, Bistoni F, Puccetti P: Fungi, dendritic cells and receptors: a host perspective of fungal virulence. Trends Microbiol 10:508, 2002.
130. Sanglard D, Hube B, Monod M, Odds FC, Gow NA: A triple deletion of the secreted aspartyl proteinase genes SAP4, SAP5, and SAP6 of Candida albicans causes attenuated virulence. Infect Immun 65:3539, 1997.
131. Rodrigues ML, Alviano CS, Travassos LR: Pathogenicity of Cryptococcus neoformans: virulence factors and immunological mechanisms. Microbes Infect 1:293, 1999.
132. Fries BC, Goldman DL, Casadevall A: Phenotypic switching in Cryptococcus neoformans. Microbes Infect 4:1345, 2002.
133. Williamson PR: Laccase and melanin in the pathogenesis of Cryptococcus neoformans. Front Biosci 2:99, 1997.
134. Rodrigues ML, dos Reis FC, Puccia R, Travassos LR, Alviano CS: Cleavage of human fibronectin and other basement membrane-associated proteins by a Cryptococcus neoformans serine proteinase. Microb Pathog 34:65, 2003.
135. Debeaupuis JP, Sarfati J, Chazalet V, Latge JP: Genetic diversity among clinical and environmental isolates of Aspergillus fumigatus. Infect Immun 65:3080, 1997.
136. Latge JP: Aspergillus fumigatus and aspergillosis. Clin Microbiol Rev 12:310, 1999.
137. Prieto R, Yousibova GL, Woloshuk CP: Identification of aflatoxin biosynthesis genes by genetic complementation in an Aspergillus flavus mutant lacking the aflatoxin gene cluster. Appl Environ Microbiol 62:3567, 1996.
138. Arruda LK, Platts-Mills TA, Fox JW, Chapman MD: Aspergillus fumigatus allergen I, a major IgE-binding protein, is a member of the mitogillin family of cytotoxins. J Exp Med 172:1529, 1990.
139. Ribes J, Vanover-Sams C, Baker D: Zygomycetes in human disease. Clinical Microbiology Reviews 13:236, 2000.
140. Cerami C, Frevert U, Sinnis P, et al: The basolateral domain of the hepatocyte plasma membrane bears receptors for the circumsporozoite protein of Plasmodium falciparum sporozoites. Cell 70:1021, 1992.
141. Chen Q, Schlichtherle M, Wahlgren M: Molecular aspects of severe malaria. Clin Microbiol Rev 13:439, 2000.
142. Hill AV, Elvin J, Willis AC, et al: Molecular analysis of the association of HLA-B53 and resistance to severe malaria. Nature 360:434, 1992.
143. Ocana-Morgner C, Mota MM, Rodriguez A: Malaria blood stage suppression of liver stage immunity by dendritic cells. J Exp Med 197:143, 2003.
144. Boustani MR, Gelfand JA: Babesiosis. Clin Infect Dis 22:611, 1996.
145. Magill AJ: Epidemiology of the leishmaniases. Dermatol Clin 13:505, 1995.
146. Titus RG, Ribeiro JM.: Salivary gland lysates from the sand fly Lutzomyia longipalpis enhance Leishmania infectivity. Science 239:1306. 1988.
147. Zilberstein D, Shapira M: The role of pH and temperature in the development of Leishmania parasites. Annu Rev Microbiol 48:449, 1994.
148. Sacks D, Sher A: Evasion of innate immunity by parasitic protozoa. Nat Immunol 3:1041, 2002.
149. Beverley SM, Turco SJ: Identification of genes mediating lipophosphoglycan biosynthesis by functional complementation of Leishmania donovani mutants. Ann Trop Med Parasitol 89 (Suppl 1):11, 1995.
150. Sacks D, Noben-Trauth N: The immunology of susceptibility and resistance to Leishmania major in mice. Nat Rev Immunol 2:845, 2002.
151. Navarro M, Gull K: A pol I transcriptional body associated with VSG mono-allelic expression in Trypanosoma brucei. Nature 414:759, 2001.
152. Robinson NP, Burman N, Melville SE, Barry JD: Predominance of duplicative VSG gene conversion in antigenic variation in African trypanosomes. Mol Cell Biol 19:5839, 1999.
153. Norris KA, Bradt B, Cooper NR, So M: Characterization of a Trypanosoma cruzi C3 binding protein with functional and genetic similarities to the human complement regulatory protein, decay-accelerating factor. J Immunol 147:2240, 1991.
154. Andrews NW: Lysosomes and the plasma membrane: trypanosomes reveal a secret relationship. J Cell Biol 158:389, 2002.
155. Tarleton RL, Zhang L, Downs MO: "Autoimmune rejection" of neonatal heart transplants in experimental Chagas disease is a parasite-

specific response to infected host tissue. Proc Natl Acad Sci U S A 94:3932, 1997.
156. Siddiqui AA, Berk SL: Diagnosis of Strongyloides stercoralis infection. Clin Infect Dis 33:1040, 2001.
157. Hoberg EP: Taenia tapeworms: their biology, evolution and socioeconomic significance. Microbes Infect 4:859, 2002.
158. Zhang W, Li J, McManus DP: Concepts in immunology and diagnosis of hydatid disease. Clin Microbiol Rev 16:18, 2003.
159. Kristensson K, Mhlanga JD, Bentivoglio M: Parasites and the brain: neuroinvasion, immunopathogenesis and neuronal dysfunctions. Curr Top Microbiol Immunol 265:227, 2002.
160. White AJ: Neurocysticercosis: updates on epidemiology, pathogenesis, diagnosis, and management. Annu Rev Med 51:187, 2000.
161. McManus DP: The molecular epidemiology of Echinococcus granulosus and cystic hydatid disease. Trans R Soc Trop Med Hyg 96 (Suppl 1):S151, 2002.
162. Polvere RI, Kabbash CA, Capo VA, Kadan I, Despommier DD: Trichinella spiralis: synthesis of type IV and type VI collagen during nurse cell formation. Exp Parasitol 86:191, 1997.
163. Ortega-Pierres MG, Yepez-Mulia L, Homan W, et al: Workshop on a detailed characterization of Trichinella spiralis antigens: a platform for future studies on antigens and antibodies to this parasite. Parasite Immunol 18:273, 1996.
164. Urban JF, Jr, Noben-Trauth N, Schopf L, Madden KB, Finkelman FD: Cutting edge: IL-4 receptor expression by non-bone marrow-derived cells is required to expel gastrointestinal nematode parasites. J Immunol 167:6078, 2001.
165. Akiho H, Blennerhassett P, Deng Y, Collins SM: Role of IL-4, IL-13, and STAT6 in inflammation-induced hypercontractility of murine smooth muscle cells. Am J Physiol Gastrointest Liver Physiol 282:G226, 2002.
166. Ross AG, Bartley PB, Sleigh AC, et al: Schistosomiasis. N Engl J Med 346:1212, 2002.
167. Pearce EJ, MacDonald AS: The immunobiology of schistosomiasis. Nat Rev Immunol 2:499, 2002.
168. Allen JE, Loke P: Divergent roles for macrophages in lymphatic filariasis. Parasite Immunol 23:345, 2001.
169. King CL: Transmission intensity and human immune responses to lymphatic filariasis. Parasite Immunol 23:363, 2001.
170. Maizels RM, Blaxter ML, Scott AL: Immunological genomics of Brugia malayi: filarial genes implicated in immune evasion and protective immunity. Parasite Immunol 23:327, 2001.
171. Lawrence RA, Devaney E: Lymphatic filariasis: parallels between the immunology of infection in humans and mice. Parasite Immunol 23:353, 2001.
172. Maizels RM, Gomez-Escobar N, Gregory WF, Murray J, Zang X: Immune evasion genes from filarial nematodes. Int J Parasitol 31:889, 2001.
173. Taylor MJ, Cross HF, Ford L, Makunde WH, Prasad GB, Bilo K: Wolbachia bacteria in filarial immunity and disease. Parasite Immunol 23:401, 2001.
174. Hoerauf A, Buttner DW, Adjei O, Pearlman E: Onchocerciasis. BMJ 326:207, 2003.
175. Hoerauf A, Mand S, Adjei O, Fleischer B, Buttner DW: Depletion of wolbachia endobacteria in Onchocerca volvulus by doxycycline and microfilaridermia after ivermectin treatment. Lancet 357:1415, 2001.

CHAPTER 9

Environmental and Nutritional Pathology

Agnes B. Kane, MD, PhD • Vinay Kumar, MD

ENVIRONMENT AND DISEASE

Recognition of Occupational and Environmental Diseases

Mechanisms of Toxicity

COMMON ENVIRONMENTAL AND OCCUPATIONAL EXPOSURES

Personal Exposures

Tobacco Use

Alcohol Abuse

Drug Abuse

Therapeutic Drugs

Oral Contraceptives and Hormone Replacement Therapy

Acetaminophen

Aspirin (Acetylsalicylic Acid)

Outdoor Air Pollution

Indoor Air Pollution

Industrial Exposures

Volatile Organic Compounds

Polycyclic Aromatic Hydrocarbons

Plastics, Rubber, and Polymers

Metals

Agricultural Hazards

Natural Toxins

Radiation Injury

Ionizing Radiation

Ultraviolet Radiation

Electromagnetic Fields

Physical Environment

Mechanical Force

Thermal Injuries

Electrical Injuries

Injuries Related to Changes in Atmospheric Pressure

NUTRITION AND DISEASE

Food Safety: Additives and Contaminants

Nutritional Deficiencies

Protein–Energy Malnutrition

Anorexia Nervosa and Bulimia

Vitamin Deficiencies

Mineral Deficiencies

Obesity

Diet and Systemic Diseases

Chemoprevention of Cancer

Environment and Disease

Environmental and occupational health encompasses the diagnosis, treatment, and prevention of injuries and illnesses resulting from exposure to exogenous chemical or physical agents. Such exposure may occur in the workplace, or people may voluntarily expose themselves to these hazards, for example, by abusing drugs or ethanol and smoking cigarettes. These personal habits may lead to involuntary exposure of fetuses and infants to drugs, ethanol, or environmental tobacco smoke.

People are often confused about the magnitude of the adverse health effects of exogenous physical and chemical agents. There is widespread concern about the potential chronic or delayed effects of exposure to low levels of contaminants in air, water, and food, and hence patients frequently seek advice and information from their health care professionals about the risk of disease associated with specific environmental and occupational exposures. This chapter provides a basic foundation in the most important diseases associated with environmental and occupational exposures, emphasizing the mechanisms leading to these diseases. This framework will help physicians to recognize and treat injuries and illness resulting from environmental and occupational exposures and to educate their patients about the risks of these exposures.[1]

RECOGNITION OF OCCUPATIONAL AND ENVIRONMENTAL DISEASES

Accidents, illness, and premature deaths threaten the health of 130 million workers in the United States. Occupational health risks are even greater in developing countries, where children and women constitute a larger proportion of the work force. In the United States, the annual rate of occupational injuries is 7400 per 100,000 workers. The overall fatality rate is 4.8 per 100,000 workers; the highest rates occur in the mining, agricultural, construction, transportation, and public utility industries. In addition to physical injury, occupational exposures contribute to a wide range of illnesses that may lead to premature death (Table 9–1). The magnitude of occupational diseases is most likely underestimated because workers and their employers fear economic or legal pressures, physicians may not recognize that an illness is work related, and there may be a long latent period between exposure and the development of clinical illness. Nevertheless, occupational diseases are preventable if there is adequate surveillance by state and federal governments, responsible leadership in industry, and access to health professionals trained in occupational safety and health.[1]

The magnitude and extent of illness related to environmental exposures are difficult to ascertain. The Environmental Protection Agency estimates that more than 80,000 chemicals are currently used in the United States; approximately 1500 are pesticides and 5500 are food additives that affect our water and food supplies. Although only 600 of these chemicals have been tested, 10% have produced cancer in at least one rodent species.[2] Industrial chemicals, production byproducts, and metals are commonly detected at hazardous waste sites (Table 9–2). There are currently 11,300 Superfund-designated waste sites in the United States. The potential human health hazards associated with exposure to chemical mixtures is a major concern.[2]

There is considerable difference in the magnitudes of exposure in the occupational and environmental settings. Occupational exposures affect a defined cohort of workers who are exposed to chemicals in the range of parts per million (ppm); by contrast, environmental exposures to these same chemicals in the air, water, or hazardous waste sites may be in the parts per billion (ppb) or parts per trillion (ppt) range. The health effects of such chronic, low-level exposures are unknown.

In the United States, four regulatory agencies determine exposure limits for environmental and occupational hazards: the Environmental Protection Agency, the Food and Drug Administration (FDA), the Occupational Safety and Health Administration, and the Consumer Products Safety Commission. The Environmental Protection Agency regulates exposure to pesticides, toxic chemicals, water and air pollutants, and hazardous wastes. The FDA regulates drugs, medical devices, food additives, and cosmetics. The Occupational Safety and Health Administration mandates that employers (including hospitals and physicians) provide safe working conditions for employees. All other products sold for use in homes, schools, or recreation are regulated by the Consumer Products Safety Commission.

Physicians should be familiar with current approaches used by regulatory agencies in the United States and be prepared to explain the strengths and limitations of the scientific evidence in nontechnical terms. Health care providers must be prepared to counsel patients about the primary prevention of disease related to occupational and environmental exposures, taking into account potential synergistic effects of mixed exposures and individual genetic susceptibility. Prevention of tobacco smoking would prevent 80% to 90% of lung cancers; however, this objective has been difficult to achieve, especially in teenagers. Strategies for secondary prevention of lung cancer in former or current smokers (e.g., chemoprevention) have been disappointing so far.[3] Prevention of occupationally

TABLE 9–1 Reported Occupational Diseases in the United States in 1997

Disease	Number of Workers	Percentage
Repeated trauma	276,600	64
Skin disorders	57,900	13
Lung conditions due to toxic exposures	20,300	5
Physical injury	16,600	4
Poisoning	5100	1
Lung disease due to dusts	2900	1
All other illnesses	50,600	12
Total	430,000	100

Data from Levy BS, Wegman DH: Occupational health – an overview. In Levy BS, et al. (eds): Occupational Health. Recognizing and Preventing Work-Related Disease and Injury, fourth ed. Philadelphia, Lippincott Williams & Wilkins, 2000, p. 3; and Bureau of Labor Statistics, U.S. Department of Labor, www.hls.gov.

TABLE 9–2 Common Chemicals at Hazardous Waste Sites

Acetone	DDT, DDE, DDD
Aldrin/Dieldrin	1,1 and 1,2-Dichloroethane
Arsenic	Lead
Barium	Mercury
Benzene	Methylene chloride
2-Butanone	Nickel
Cadmium	Pentachlorophenol
Carbon tetrachloride	Polychlorinated biphenyls
Chlordane	Tri- and Tetrachloroethylene
Chloroform	Toluene
Chromium	Vinyl Chloride
Cyanide	Zinc

Data from U.S. Environmental Protection Agency, www.epa.gov/superfund/resources/chemicals.htm.

related diseases rests on defining and enforcing safe exposure levels, developing new technologies to reduce industrial exposures, and identifying less toxic substitutes for industrial and chemical agents. These strategies require a basic understanding of biochemical and molecular mechanisms of toxicity.

MECHANISMS OF TOXICITY

Toxicology is the scientific discipline that studies the detection, effects, and mechanisms of action of poisons and toxic chemicals. *Toxicity* is a relative phenomenon that depends on the inherent structure and properties of a chemical and on its dose. Dose–response curves are typically generated in laboratory animals exposed to various amounts of a chemical. A typical dose–response curve for acute toxicity is illustrated in Figure 9–1. In this example, a measurable response occurs at a dose of 0.1 mg/kg; this is defined as the *threshold dose.* To the left of this dose, at subthreshold levels, there is no measurable response. For this chemical, this is the *no observed effect level* and can be considered a safe dose. This information is used to establish a daily or annual *threshhold limit value* or *permissible exposure level* for occupational exposures. Frequently, a plateau is reached at higher doses; this is defined as the *ceiling effect.* It is uncertain whether carcinogens show a threshold effect or whether the dose–response curve should be extrapolated linearly to zero.[4]

Despite the inherent limitations of toxicity testing in animals, several important toxicologic principles have been established by this experimental approach. Exogenous chemicals are absorbed after ingestion, inhalation, or skin contact, and then distributed to various organs (Fig. 9–2). Chemicals are frequently metabolized, often by multiple enzymatic pathways, to products that may be more toxic or less toxic than the parent chemical. One or more of these products then interacts with the target macromolecule, resulting in a toxic effect.[5] The site of toxicity is frequently the site where metabolism or excretion of toxic metabolites occurs. The dose administered (external dose) may not be the same as the *biologic effective dose* delivered to the target organ and target macromolecule.

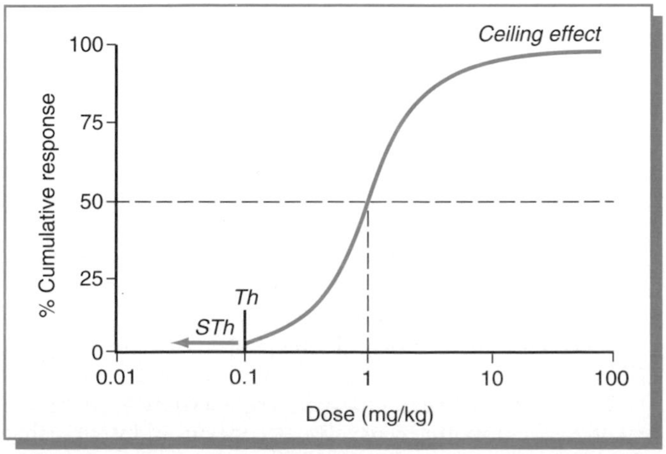

FIGURE 9–1 The dose-response curve for acute chemical toxicity. Th, threshold dose; STh, subthreshold levels. (Data from Hughes WW: Essentials of Environmental Toxicology: The Effects of Environmentally Hazardous Substances on Human Health. Washington, DC, Taylor & Francis, 1996, p. 33.)

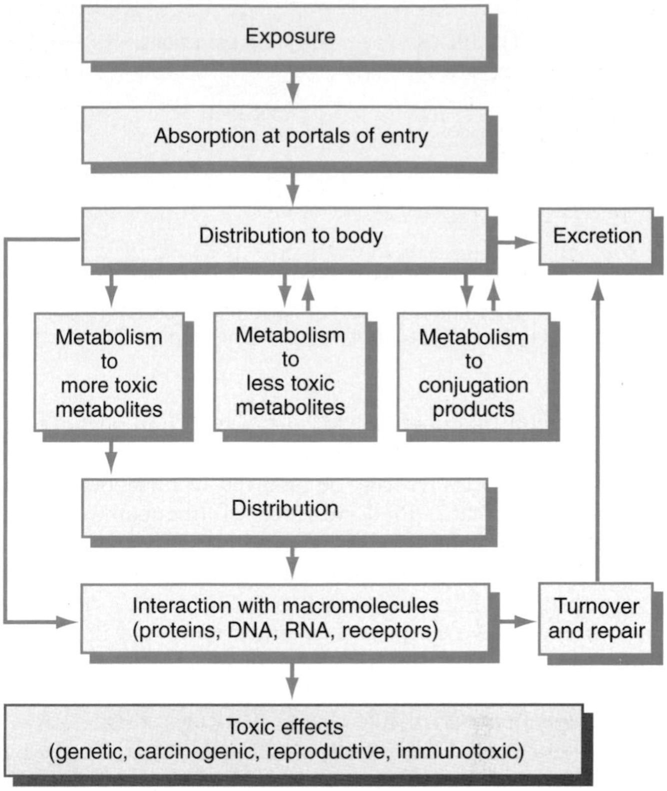

FIGURE 9–2 Absorption and distribution of toxicants. (From Hodgson E, Levi PE: Absorption and distribution of toxicants. In Hodgson E, Levi PE [eds]: A Textbook of Modern Toxicology. Stamford, CT, Appleton & Lange, 1997, p. 52.)

The basic principles of xenobiotic metabolism with some specific examples are discussed next.

- *Most xenobiotics are lipophilic*; this property facilitates their transport in the bloodstream by lipoproteins and penetration through lipid membranes.
- Lipophilic toxicants are metabolized to hydrophilic metabolites in two steps (Fig. 9–3). In *phase I reactions,* a polar functional group is added to the parent compound. These are frequently oxidation reactions that produce reactive, electrophilic intermediates as a primary metabolite. This metabolite may be eliminated, or it may participate in *phase II reactions.* These reactions produce conjugation products with endogenous substrates that are more water soluble and more readily excreted than the original compound.
- *There are genetic variations in the level of activity of these xenobiotic-metabolizing enzymes.* For example, the mixed-function oxidase system, or cytochrome P-450–dependent monooxygenase system (P-450), has multiple isozymes. Cytochrome P-450 enzymes are involved in the detoxification of endogenous hormones and natural products as well as in the activation of xenobiotics to reactive intermediates or ultimate carcinogens. The cytochrome P-450 gene, *CYP1A1*, is induced by polycyclic aromatic hydrocarbons present in tobacco smoke.[6] Smokers who have inherited alleles of the *CYP1A1* gene that confer higher activity and increased inducibility of this enzyme may be at higher risk of developing lung cancer (Chapter 7).[7] Glutathione-*S*-transferases are enzymes involved in detoxification of xenobiotic metabolites by conjugation to glutathione (GSH).

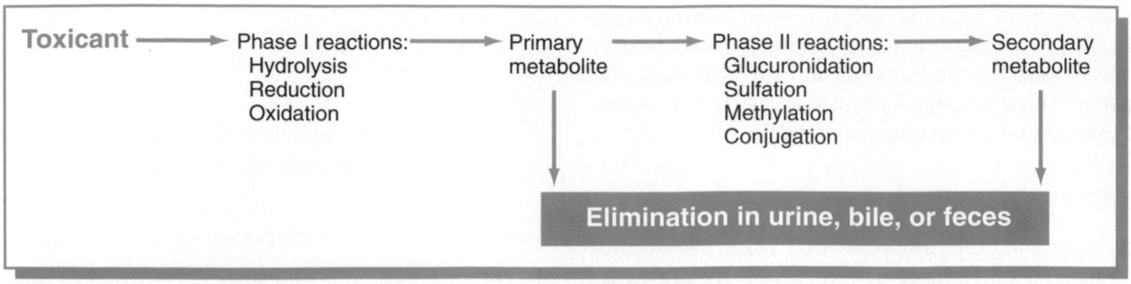

FIGURE 9–3 Biotransformation of lipophilic toxicants to hydrophilic metabolites. (Adapted from Hodgson E: Metabolism of toxicants. In Hodgson E, Levi PE [eds]: A Textbook of Modern Toxicology. Stamford, CT, Appleton & Lange, 1997, p. 57.)

People with inherited GSTM1 deficiency (null phenotype) may be at increased risk for lung, bladder, and colon cancers.[7]

- Multiple pathways may be involved in metabolism of a chemical toxicant. Predominance of one pathway over another may account for variations in toxicity and carcinogenicity assays between different species, sexes, and age groups.
- Endogenous factors such as nutritional and hormonal status alter enzyme activities involved in xenobiotic metabolism.
- Exogenous factors (e.g., chemicals, drugs, ethanol, stress) can induce or inhibit activities of xenobiotic-metabolizing enzymes.
- Other repair pathways may modify the interaction between the ultimate metabolite and target macromolecule, resulting in increased or decreased sensitivity to the toxic and carcinogenic effects of xenobiotics.

With this background of the principles of xenobiotic metabolism, we now examine some biochemical pathways that are involved in the processing of toxic chemicals using specific examples that are relevant to human disease. Each of the two phases of xenobiotic metabolism is discussed separately. The most important phase I reactions are the following:

1. *Cytochrome P-450–dependent monooxygenase system.* This system, located in the smooth endoplasmic reticulum, is composed of a heme protein (cytochrome P-450); NADPH P-450 reductase, which transfers electrons from the reduced form of nicotinamide adenine dinucleotide phosphate (NADPH) to cytochrome P-450; and phosphatidylcholine. The activity of this system is highest in the liver, followed by the skin, lung, and gastrointestinal mucosa. Different P-450 isozymes have different tissue distributions; these isozymes show preferential activity toward different substrates. An example of activation of a xenobiotic by cytochrome P-450 is metabolism of benzo[a]pyrene to a secondary metabolite that binds covalently to DNA and causes lung and skin tumors (Fig. 9–4*A*). Benzo[a]pyrene is one of several chemical carcinogens present in cigarette smoke.
2. *Flavin-containing monooxygenase system.* This is located in the smooth endoplasmic reticulum in the liver. As shown in Figure 9–4*A*, it oxidizes nicotine in cigarette smoke as well as other amines.
3. *Peroxidase-dependent cooxidation.* This reaction is catalyzed by prostaglandin-H synthase, an enzyme involved in arachidonic acid metabolism. It is also located in the smooth endoplasmic reticulum with high activity in seminal vesicles, kidneys, and the urinary bladder. It is involved in the metabolism of 2-naphthylamine, a chemical found in synthetic dyes that is associated with an increased risk of bladder cancer (see Fig. 9–4*B*).

All of these oxidative reactions may generate oxygen free radicals as byproducts. Some of the primary metabolites are also highly reactive radicals with unpaired electrons (e.g., nitrogen- and carbon-centered radicals derived from 2-naphthylamine; see Fig. 9–4). As discussed in Chapter 1, our cells have multiple defense mechanisms against free radicals, including enzymes such as superoxide dismutases, catalase, and glutathione peroxidase. Vitamins C and E, as well as beta-carotene, also serve as endogenous antioxidants. Reduced GSH and the mammalian thioredoxin system are major antioxidant defense mechanisms. GSH also detoxifies xenobiotic metabolites catalyzed by glutathione S-transferases.[8] Xenobiotic metabolism may lead to depletion of cellular GSH due to excessive redox cycling of chemicals such as the herbicide paraquat (see Fig. 9–4*A*). This compound undergoes cyclic oxidation and reduction in the lungs, resulting in generation of excess reactive oxygen species that cause acute lung injury and pulmonary edema. Oxidant stress occurs when endogenous free radical defense mechanisms are overwhelmed.

As mentioned earlier, the products of phase I reactions are often conjugated with endogenous substrates to yield water-soluble end products that can be excreted from the body. Examples of such phase II reactions are as follows:

1. *Glucuronidation.* An alternative pathway for metabolism of naphthylamine is oxidation by cytochrome P-450 followed by glucuronidation in the liver. The secondary glucuronide metabolite is excreted in the urine and under the acidic conditions in the urine, gives rise to the ultimate carcinogen, *N*-hydroxy-2-naphthylamine (see Fig. 9–4*B*). This sequence of metabolic reactions ultimately leads to an increased incidence in cancer of the urinary bladder in workers exposed to synthetic dyes.
2. *Biomethylation.* Inorganic mercury, usually in the form of $HgCl_2$, causes necrosis of the proximal convoluted tubules of the kidneys. Occupational exposure to inorganic mercury compounds usually occurs in industries that manufacture germicides, fungicides, electronics, and plastics. Mercury can be methylated by aquatic microorganisms that are subsequently ingested by herbivorous fish (see Fig. 9–4*B*). These fish are ingested by carnivorous fish, which may be eaten by humans. This is an example of

bioaccumulation of a toxic chemical in the environment. The tragic consequences of human exposure to methylmercury were realized in the 1950s and 1960s after an epidemic of poisoning in Minamata, Japan. Industrial discharge of mercury into a bay resulted in bioaccumulation of this toxicant a million-fold in fish, reaching concentrations greater than 10 ppm. People who ingested these fish developed delayed paralysis and death. Methylmercury is more easily absorbed from the gastrointestinal tract than is inorganic mercury and readily crosses the blood-brain barrier and the placenta. The fetus is especially susceptible to methylmercury; the consequences of maternal exposure are fetal brain damage, mental retardation, and death. In view of this, the FDA has recently recommended that pregnant women should avoid eating certain types of fish (e.g., swordfish, tilefish, shark, and king mackerel) that contain mercury at levels as low as 1 ppm.[9] A mercury preservative, thimerosal or ethyl mercury, has been widely used in vaccines; it was eliminated from all vaccines used in the United States in 2000 due to concerns about the health effects of ethyl mercury in infants.[10]

3. *Glutathione conjugation.* A common pathway for detoxification of primary metabolites is conjugation to reduced glutathione; these water-soluble secondary metabolites are readily excreted in the bile and urine. Vinyl chloride monomer is widely used in the manufacture of plastics, and it can cause angiosarcoma of the liver in exposed workers. Vinyl chloride is activated to a reactive intermediate by cytochrome P-450 in the liver. This intermediate can bind covalently to cellular macromolecules or be metabolized to chloroacetaldehyde and conjugated to reduced glutathione and excreted (Fig. 9–4*B*).

TABLE 9–3 Organ-Specific Carcinogens in Tobacco Smoke

Organ	Carcinogen
Lung, larynx	Polycyclic aromatic hydrocarbons 4-(Methylnitrosoamino)-1-(3-pyridyl)-1-butanone (NNK) Polonium 210
Esophagus	*N*′-Nitrosonornicotine (NNN)
Pancreas	NNK (?)
Bladder	4-Aminobiphenyl, 2-naphthylamine
Oral cavity (smoking)	Polycyclic aromatic hydrocarbons, NNK, NNN
Oral cavity (snuff)	NNK, NNN, polonium 210

Data from Szczesny LB, Holbrook JH: Cigarette smoking. In Rom WH (ed): Environmental and Occupational Medicine, 2nd ed. Boston, Little, Brown, 1992, p. 1211.

Common Environmental and Occupational Exposures

PERSONAL EXPOSURES

Tobacco Use

Use of tobacco products, including cigarettes, cigars, pipes, and snuff, is associated with more mortality and morbidity than any other personal, environmental, or occupational exposure. Cigarette smoking contributes to 440,000 premature deaths per year in the United States, resulting in an annual economic loss of $157 billion from health-related costs. Lung cancer, cardiovascular disease, and chronic respiratory disease account for most of the deaths related to smoking.[11]

Beginning in World War I, annual cigarette consumption increased in men, followed by women, reaching a peak of 4336 cigarettes per capita in 1963. After the Surgeon General's Advisory Committee report, released in 1964, concluded that cigarette smoking is one of the most important risk factors for lung cancer, per capita consumption of cigarettes declined to less than 3000 in 1995. Among children and adolescents, smoking continues to be a major public health problem; early exposure to carcinogens in tobacco smoke may increase the risk of developing lung cancer.[12] Smoking also interacts with other environmental and occupational exposures in an additive or synergistic fashion. The most important example of such synergism is the increase in risk of lung cancer in cigarette smokers exposed to asbestos.[13]

Mainstream cigarette smoke inhaled by the smoker is composed of a particulate phase and a gas phase; tar is the total particulate phase without water or nicotine. There are 0.3 to 3.3 billion particles per milliliter of mainstream smoke and more than 4000 constituents, including 43 known carcinogens. Examples of the organ-specific carcinogens found in tobacco smoke and snuff are listed in Table 9–3. In addition to these chemical carcinogens, cigarette smoke contains carcinogenic metals such as arsenic, nickel, cadmium, and chromium; potential promoters such as acetaldehyde and phenol; irritants such as nitrogen dioxide and formaldehyde; cilia toxins such as hydrogen cyanide; and carbon monoxide. Carbon monoxide is a colorless, odorless gas produced during incomplete combustion of fossil fuels or tobacco. It has 200 times higher affinity for hemoglobin than oxygen does and it impairs release of oxygen from hemoglobin. Thus, carbon monoxide exposure decreases the delivery of oxygen to peripheral tissues. Carbon monoxide also binds to other heme-containing proteins such as myoglobin and cytochrome oxidase. Nicotine is an important constituent of cigarette smoke. It is an alkaloid that readily crosses the blood-brain barrier and stimulates nicotine receptors in the brain. It is also responsible for the acute pharmacologic effects associated with tobacco use that are most likely mediated by catecholamines: increased heart rate and blood pressure, increased coronary artery blood flow, increased contractility and cardiac output, and mobilization of free fatty acids. Nicotine is responsible for tobacco addiction.

The inhaled agents in cigarette smoke may act directly on the mucous membranes, may be swallowed in saliva, or may be absorbed into the bloodstream from the abundant alveolar capillary bed. By various routes of delivery, the constituents of cigarette smoke act on distant target organs and cause a variety of systemic diseases, listed in Table 9–4. The greatest numbers of deaths attributable to cigarette smoking are due to lung cancer, ischemic heart disease, and chronic obstructive lung disease. Lung cancer is caused by multiple carcinogens and promoters in cigarette smoke. As described in Chapter 15, specific preneoplastic changes are found in the tracheobronchial lining of cigarette smokers. These cellular changes

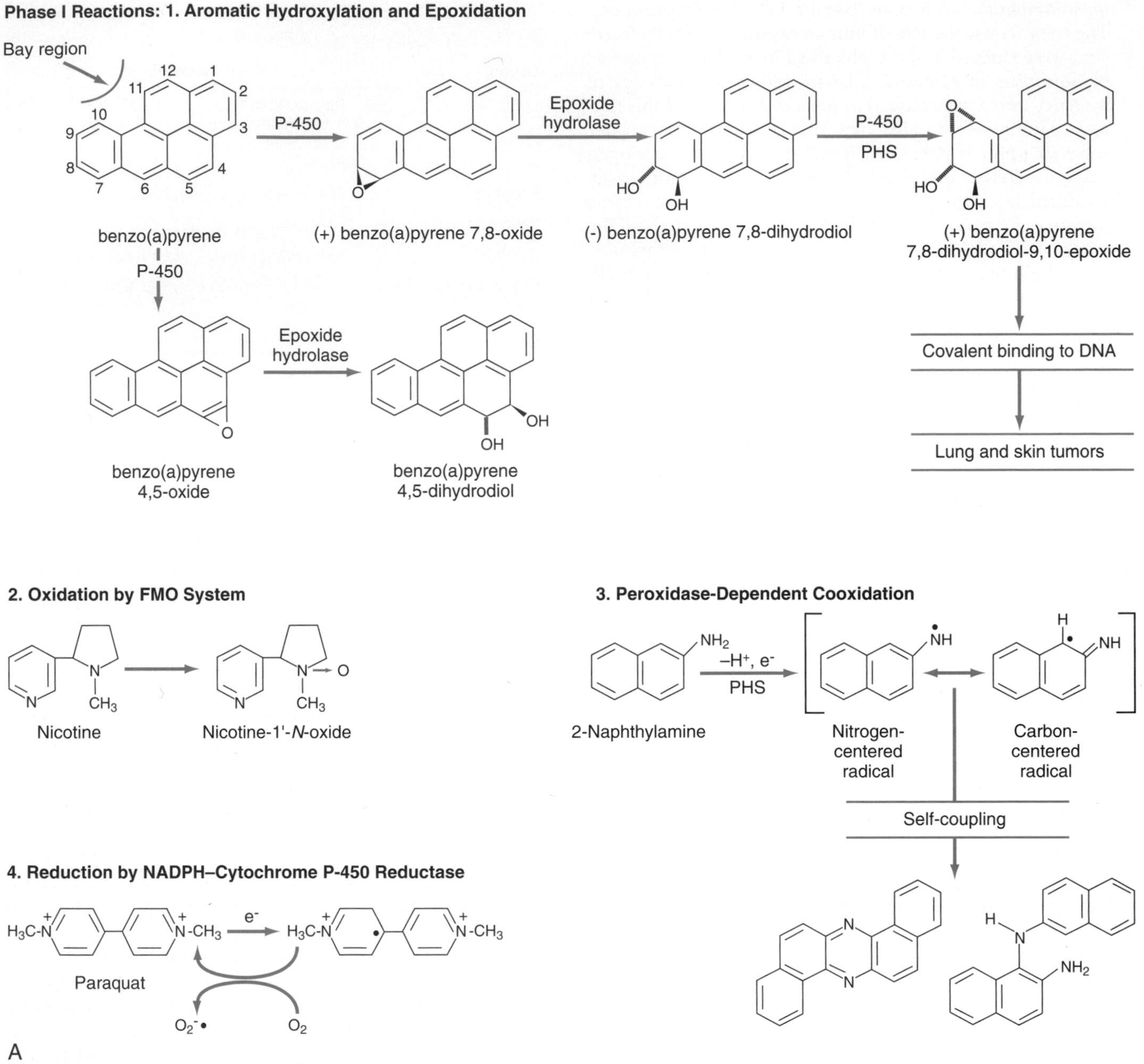

FIGURE 9–4 *A,* Xenobiotic metabolism: phase I reactions. FMO, flavin-containing monooxygenase; PHS, prostaglandin-H synthases. *Illustration continued on following page*

are dose related, and the incidence of lung cancer is directly related to the number of cigarettes smoked. Cessation of smoking reduces but does not completely eliminate the risks of lung cancer and coronary artery disease. It is estimated that 30% of all cancer deaths and up to 90% of all lung cancer deaths are attributable to cigarette smoking. Cigarette smoking is a multiplicative risk factor with hypertension and hypercholesterolemia for development of coronary artery disease and arteriosclerosis. It is also a multiplicative risk factor for acute myocardial infarction and stroke in women who take oral contraceptives. Smoking may contribute to cardiac arrest by increasing platelet adhesion and aggregation, triggering arrhythmia, and by causing an imbalance between the demand for oxygen and supply to the myocardium. Smokers also suffer from increased morbidity due to acute respiratory tract infections, including influenza, and acute and chronic sinusitis. Ciliatoxins in cigarette smoke impair tracheobronchial clearance, and many of the gas phase constituents of smoke are direct irritants of the respiratory epithelium. The pathogenesis of chronic obstructive lung disease associated with cigarette smoking is discussed in Chapter 15.

The fetus is especially vulnerable to the consequences of maternal smoking. Even 10 cigarettes per day can cause fetal hypoxia; fetal carboxyhemoglobin levels are higher than maternal levels. The consequences of fetal hypoxia are low birth weight, prematurity, and increased incidence of spontaneous abortion; serious complications at the time of delivery

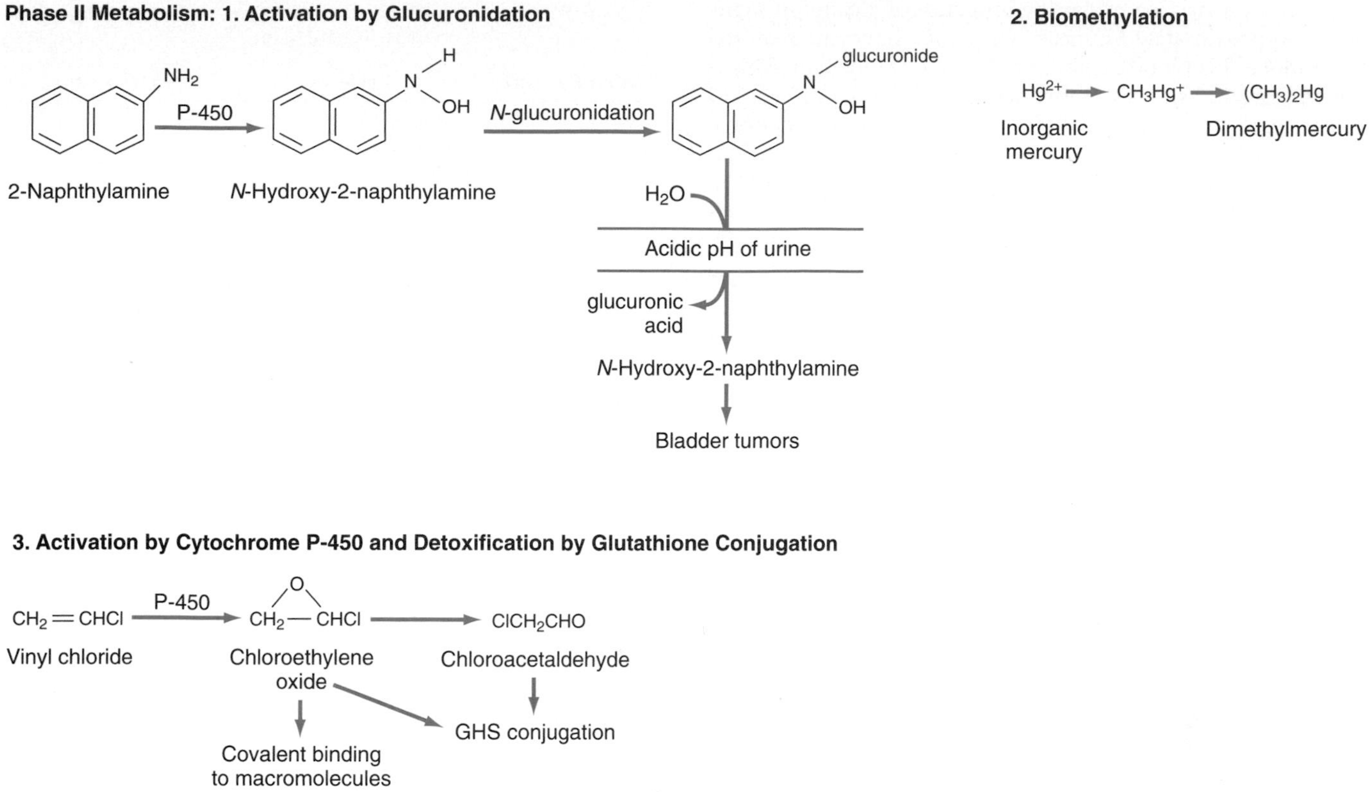

B

FIGURE 9–4 *con't—B,* Xenobiotic metabolism: phase II reactions (see text for details). (Adapted from Parkinson A: Biotransformation of xenobiotics. In Klaasen CD [ed]: Casarett and Doull's Toxicology: The Basic Science of Poisons, 5th ed. New York, McGraw-Hill, 1996, pp. 113–186; and Hodgson E, Levi PE [(eds]: A Textbook of Modern Toxicology. Stamford, CT, Appleton & Lange, 1997, pp. 57, 95.)

include premature rupture of the membranes, placenta previa, and abruptio placentae, as described in Chapter10.

Cigarette smoking is especially hazardous in the workplace. Smokers have higher rates of accidental injuries, and cigarette smoke may act as a vector to transport other hazardous agents into the lungs, such as radon gas in miners. Similar to asbestos exposure, cigarette smoke is synergistic with radon decay products in causing lung cancer. Cigarette smoke exacerbates bronchitis, asthma, and pneumoconiosis associated with exposure to silica, coal dust, grain dust, cotton dust, and welding fumes.

Tobacco use also increases the prevalence of peptic ulcers; smoking impairs healing of ulcers and increases the likelihood of recurrence. Smoking may also increase pyloric reflux and decrease bicarbonate secretion from the pancreas.

In addition to the health hazards of mainstream tobacco smoke, there are risks associated with exposure to sidestream smoke, also called passive smoking or environmental tobacco smoke (ETS). In 1986, two reports issued by the National Research Council and the Surgeon General concluded that ETS increases the risk of lung cancer, ischemic heart disease, and acute myocardial infarction.[14] The Environmental Protection Agency classified ETS as a known human carcinogen in 1992. ETS is especially hazardous for infants and young children. Maternal smoking increases the incidence of sudden infant death syndrome. Young children in households of cigarette smokers suffer from an increased incidence of respiratory and ear infections and exacerbation of asthma.

TABLE 9–4 Deaths per Year Attributable to Cigarette Smoking in the United States

	Number of Deaths	
Cause of Death	*Men*	*Women*
Cancer	102,812	54,664
Cardiovascular disease	90,906	57,699
Respiratory disease	53,713	44,429
Residential fires	589	377
Perinatal deaths	598	407
Lung cancer and heart disease attributable to passive smoking	15,517	22,536
Total	264,135	80,112

Data from CDC. Annual smoking-attributable mortality, years of potential life lost, and economic costs—United States, 1995–1999. MMWR 51:300, 2002.

Alcohol Abuse

Ethanol is the most widely used and abused agent throughout the world. There are 15 to 20 million alcoholics in the United States; approximately 100,000 deaths in the United States are attributed to alcohol abuse per year, with an economic cost of $100 to $130 billion.[15] Ethanol is ingested in alcoholic beverages such as beer, wine, and distilled spirits. A blood alcohol concentration of 80 to 100 mg/dL is the legal definition for driving under the influence of alcohol in many states. Approximately 3 ounces (44 ml) of ethanol are required to produce this blood alcohol level in a 70-kg person. This is equivalent to 12 ounces of fortified wine, 8 bottles of beer (12 ounces each), or 6 ounces of 100-proof whiskey. In occasional drinkers, a blood alcohol level of 200 mg/dL produces inebriation, with coma, death, and respiratory arrest at 300 to 400 mg/dL. Habitual drinkers can tolerate blood alcohol levels up to 700 mg/dL. This metabolic tolerance is partially explained by a fivefold to tenfold induction of the cytochrome P-450 xenobiotic-metabolizing enzyme CYP2E1. Such induction increases the metabolism of ethanol as well as that of other drugs and chemicals, including cocaine and acetaminophen. Although no specific receptor for ethanol has been identified, chronic use results in psychologic and physical dependence. The biologic basis for ethanol addiction is unknown, although genetic factors may be involved.

Ethanol is metabolized to acetaldehyde by alcohol dehydrogenase in the gastric mucosa and liver, and by cytochrome P-450 (CYP2E1) and catalase in the liver (Fig. 9–5). Acetaldehyde is converted to acetic acid by aldehyde dehydrogenase. There are genetic polymorphisms in aldehyde dehydrogenase that affect ethanol metabolism; approximately 50% of Chinese, Vietnamese, and Japanese people have reduced activity of this enzyme due to a point mutation that converts glutamine to lysine at amino acid 487. These ethnic groups also rapidly convert ethanol to acetaldehyde, which builds up and triggers a facial flushing syndrome. Women have lower levels of gastric alcohol dehydrogenase activity than men do; therefore, they may develop higher blood alcohol levels than men after drinking the same quantity of ethanol.[15]

The metabolism of ethanol is directly responsible for most of its toxic effects. In addition to its acute action as a central nervous system depressant, chronic ethanol use can cause a wide range of systemic effects (Table 9–5). Some of these chronic effects can be attributed to specific vitamin deficiencies; for example, damage to the peripheral and central nervous systems is related to thiamine deficiency, whereas

TABLE 9–5 Mechanisms of Disease Caused by Ethanol Abuse

Organ System	Lesion	Mechanism
Liver	Fatty change Acute hepatitis Alcoholic cirrhosis	Toxicity
Nervous system	Wernicke syndrome Korsakoff syndrome Cerebellar degeneration Peripheral neuropathy	Thiamine deficiency Toxicity and thiamine deficiency Nutritional deficiency Thiamine deficiency
Cardiovascular system	Cardiomyopathy Hypertension	Toxicity Vasopressor
Gastrointestinal tract	Gastritis Pancreatitis	Toxicity Toxicity
Skeletal muscle	Rhabdomyolysis	Toxicity
Reproductive system	Testicular atrophy Spontaneous abortion	? ?
Fetal alcohol syndrome	Growth retardation Mental retardation Birth defects	Toxicity

Data from Rubin E: Alcohol abuse. In Craighead JE (ed): Pathology of Environmental and Occupational Disease. St. Louis, Mosby–Year Book, 1996, p. 249; and Lewis DD, Woods SE: Fetal alcohol syndrome. Am Fam Physician 50:1025, 1994.

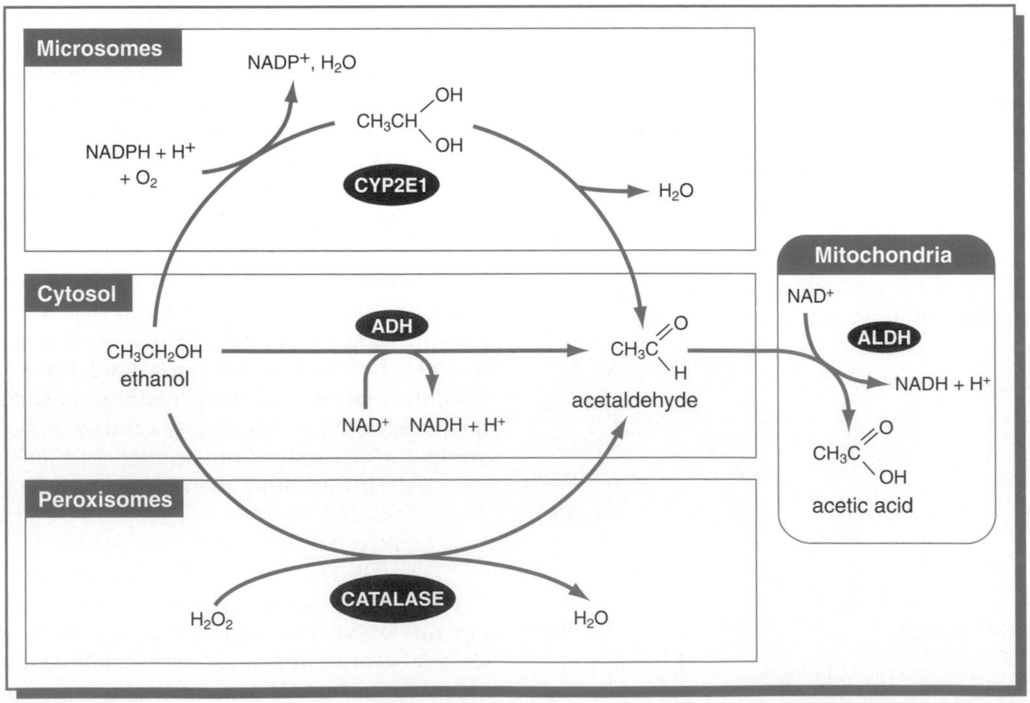

FIGURE 9–5 Metabolism of ethanol. ADH, alcohol dehydrogenase; ALDH, aldehyde dehydrogenase. (From Parkinson A: Biotransformation of xenobiotics. In Klassen CD [ed]: Casarett and Doull's Toxicology: The Basic Science of Poisons, 5th ed. New York, McGraw-Hill, 1996, p. 128.)

other systemic effects result from direct toxicity. The effects of ethanol on various organ systems are discussed next.

Liver. Ethanol can cause fatty change, acute alcoholic hepatitis, and cirrhosis. *Fatty change* is an acute, reversible manifestation of ethanol ingestion. In chronic alcoholism, fat accumulation can cause massive enlargement of the liver. The biochemical mechanisms responsible for fat accumulation in hepatocytes are the following:

- Catabolism of fat by peripheral tissues is increased, and there is increased delivery of free fatty acids to the liver.
- Metabolism of ethanol in the cytosol and of its derivative, acetaldehyde, in the mitochondria converts the oxidized form of nicotinamide adenine dinucleotide (NAD^+) to the reduced form (NADH); an excess of NADH over NAD stimulates lipid biosynthesis.
- Oxidation of fatty acids by mitochondria is decreased.
- Acetaldehyde forms adducts with tubulin and impairs function of microtubules, resulting in decreased transport of lipoproteins from the liver.

Acute alcoholic hepatitis is another potentially reversible form of liver injury (Chapter 18). Although fatty change is asymptomatic except for liver enlargement, alcoholic hepatitis can produce fever, liver tenderness, and jaundice. On histologic examination, there are focal areas of hepatocyte necrosis and cell injury manifest by fat accumulation and alcoholic hyalin, or Mallory bodies. Neutrophils accumulate around foci of necrosis (Fig. 9–6). Ethanol and its metabolites are directly toxic to hepatocytes; this toxicity is believed to be mediated by glutathione depletion, mitochondrial injury, altered metabolism of methionine, and cytokine release from Kupffer cells.[16] Hepatocellular necrosis, as well as fibrosis, begins around the central vein, suggesting that hypoxia may contribute to this injury. With chronic ethanol use, 10% to 15% of alcoholics develop irreversible liver damage, or *alcoholic cirrhosis*. This is characterized by a hard, shrunken liver with formation of micronodules of regenerating hepatocytes surrounded by dense bands of collagen (Fig. 9–7). Alcoholic cirrhosis is a serious, potentially fatal disease accompanied by weakness, muscle wasting, ascites, gastrointestinal hemorrhage, and coma. Perisinusoidal fibrosis occurs initially, with

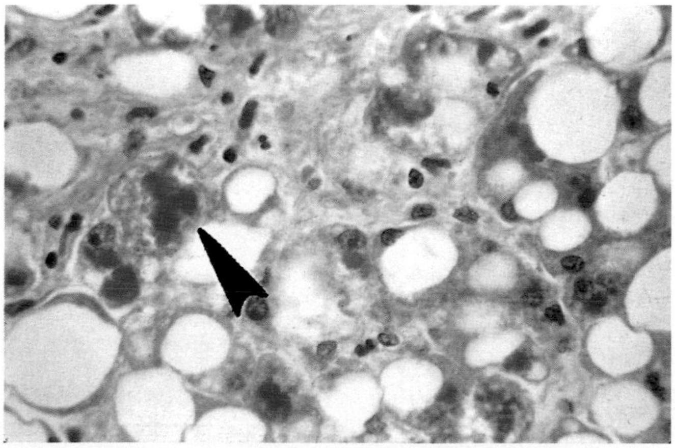

FIGURE 9–6 Acute alcoholic hepatitis. The liver cells show cytoplasmic accumulation of fat and hyalin *(arrow)*. A scattered inflammatory infiltrate is present. (MEDCOM © 1976.)

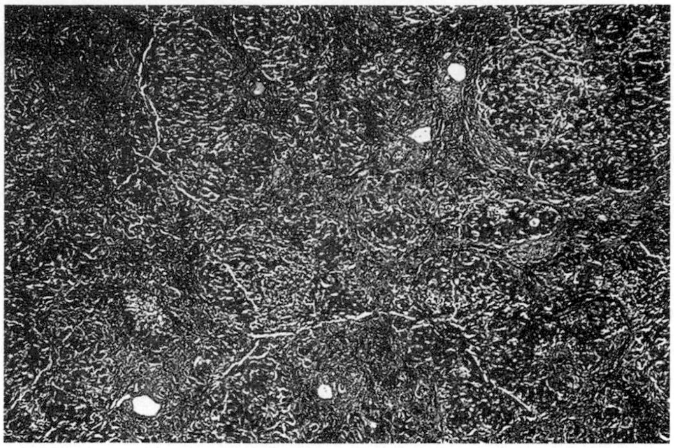

FIGURE 9–7 Micronodular cirrhosis is a late complication of chronic alcoholism. The liver architecture is distorted by regenerating nodules of hepatocytes surrounded by dense bands of fibrous tissue that stain blue (Masson trichrome stain). (Courtesy of Dr. Steve Kroft, Department of Pathology, Southwestern Medical School, Dallas, TX.)

deposition of collagen by perisinusoidal stellate cells (Ito cells) in the spaces of Disse. Stimulation of collagen synthesis by Ito cells may be caused by direct toxic effect of ethanol or its metabolites, or it may be mediated by cytokines. Patients with cirrhosis have depleted liver stores of α-tocopherol, which increases their vulnerability to oxidative injury.

Nervous System. The acute depressive effects and addiction produced by ethanol are hypothesized to be related to fluidization of membrane phospholipids and altered signal transduction. A deficiency of thiamine is common in chronic alcoholics. Chronic thiamine deficiency contributes to degeneration of nerve cells, reactive gliosis, and atrophy of the cerebellum and peripheral nerves. It produces the ataxia, disturbed cognition, ophthalmoplegia, and nystagmus characteristic of *Wernicke syndrome.* Some alcoholics with poor nutrition develop the severe memory loss characteristic of *Korsakoff syndrome*; this is believed to result from a combination of toxicity and thiamine deficiency. These effects are discussed further under thiamine deficiency, later in this chapter and in Chapter 28.

Cardiovascular System. Chronic ethanol abuse can cause cardiomyopathy, a degenerative disease of the heart muscle, resulting in dilation of the heart (Chapter 12). The exact mechanism responsible for myocardial injury and altered contractility is unknown, although it is most likely due to direct toxicity rather than thiamine deficiency. Hypertension is also more common in chronic alcoholics, secondary to the vasopressor effects of ethanol triggered by increased release of catecholamines. Paradoxically, moderate consumers (one to two drinks per day) show a protective effect of ethanol on the cardiovascular system. At this level of consumption, drinkers show increased levels of high-density lipoprotein and decreased platelet aggregation.

Gastrointestinal Tract. Acute gastritis is a direct toxic effect of ethanol use (Chapter 17). Chronic users are vulnerable to acute and chronic pancreatitis, which may lead to destruction of pancreatic acini and islets. Pancreatic acinar destruction leads to impaired intestinal absorption of nutrients and contributes to vitamin deficiencies.

Skeletal Muscle. Direct ethanol toxicity can also injure skeletal muscles, leading to muscle weakness, pain, and breakdown of myoglobin.

Reproductive System. Chronic ethanol use leads to testicular atrophy and decreased fertility in both men and women. Women who drink alcohol also have an increased risk of spontaneous abortion. The mechanisms responsible for these adverse reproductive effects are unknown.

Fetal Alcohol Syndrome. A tragic consequence of maternal ethanol consumption at levels of only one drink per day is the *fetal alcohol syndrome*, first recognized in 1968. This syndrome is characterized by growth and developmental defects, including microcephaly; facial dysmorphology; and malformations of the brain, cardiovascular system, and genitourinary system (Chapter 10). Affected infants show growth retardation, microcephaly, atrial septal defect, short palpebral fissures, maxillary hypoplasia, and several other minor anomalies. This is the most common type of preventable mental retardation in the United States, and it affects at least 1200 children per year.[17] The pathogenesis of fetal alcohol syndrome is not entirely clear. It is hypothesized that acetaldehyde, a metabolite of ethanol (see Fig. 9–5), crosses the placenta and damages the fetal brain.

Ethanol and Cancer. Use of alcoholic beverages is associated with an increased incidence of cancer of the oral cavity, pharynx, esophagus, liver, and possibly the breast. Although ethanol is not a direct-acting carcinogen, one of its metabolites, acetaldehyde, may act as a tumor promoter.[18] Ethanol inhibits the detoxification of chemical carcinogens such as nitrosamines, which have been associated with tumors of the upper gastrointestinal tract. Heavy alcohol use synergizes with chronic hepatitis B or C infection in predisposing to the development of hepatocellular carcinoma.[18]

Two other chemicals, *methanol* and *ethylene glycol*, may be ingested accidentally or used as inexpensive substitutes for ethanol. They are metabolized by alcohol dehydrogenase, but more slowly than ethanol, resulting in initial symptoms of intoxication, followed by toxic effects after several hours or days. *Methanol* is metabolized to formaldehyde and formic acid, resulting in metabolic acidosis, dizziness, vomiting, blurred vision or blindness, and respiratory depression. Methanol has been proposed as a gasoline additive or substitute, but there is concern that chronic inhalation of methanol-containing fumes may cause central nervous system depression. The lethal dose of *ethylene glycol* is only 1.4 mL/kg; it is metabolized by alcohol dehydrogenase to aldehydes, glycolate, oxalate, and lactate. If a person survives the initial toxicity, acute renal failure may occur several days later because of obstruction of the kidney tubules by calcium oxalate crystals. Acute methanol or ethylene glycol poisoning is treated by administration of ethanol, which slows the production of toxic metabolites.

Drug Abuse

Drug abuse, addiction, and overdose are serious public health problems. In a recent survey, 8% to 23% of teenagers reported marijuana use, and 2% reported cocaine use during the previous month. A National Comorbidity Survey conducted in 1995 discovered that 7.5% of US residents 15 to 54 years old had a history of drug dependence. Risk factors for drug use include family history, male sex, psychiatric disorders, ethanol abuse, easy access to drugs, and peer pressure.[21] The molecular targets of many commonly abused drugs have recently been identified, as summarized in Table 9–6. Identification of specific neurotransmitter pathways that may activate reward circuits in the brain, as diagrammed in Figure 9–8, may lead to more effective therapies for drug abuse and addiction.[19]

Sedative-Hypnotics. Ethanol is the most widely abused central nervous system depressant, as discussed before. Barbiturates are circulated illegally and are known as downers. They

TABLE 9–6 Common Drugs of Abuse

Class	Molecular Target	Example
Opioid narcotics	Mu opioid receptor (agonist)	Heroin, hydromorphone (Dilaudid) Oxycodone (Percodan, Percocet, Oxycontin) Methadone (Dolophine) Meperidine (Demerol)
Sedative-hypnotics	$GABA_A$ receptor (agonist)	Barbiturates Ethanol Methaqualone (Quaalude) Glutethimide (Doriden) Ethchlorvynol (Placidyl)
Psychomotor stimulants	Dopamine transporter (antagonist) Serotonin receptors (toxicity)	Cocaine Amphetamine 3,4-methylenedioxymethamphetamine (MDMA, ecstasy)
Phencyclidine-like drugs	NMDA glutamate receptor channel (antagonist)	Phencyclidine (PCP, angel dust) Ketamine
Cannabinoids	CBI cannabinoid receptors (agonist)	Marijuana Hashish
Nicotine	Nicotine acetylcholine receptor (agonist)	Tobacco products
Hallucinogens	Serotonin 5-HT_2 receptors (agonist)	Lysergic acid diethylamide (LSD) Mescaline Psilocybin

Data from Hyman SE: A 28-year-old man addicted to cocaine. JAMA 286:2586, 2001.

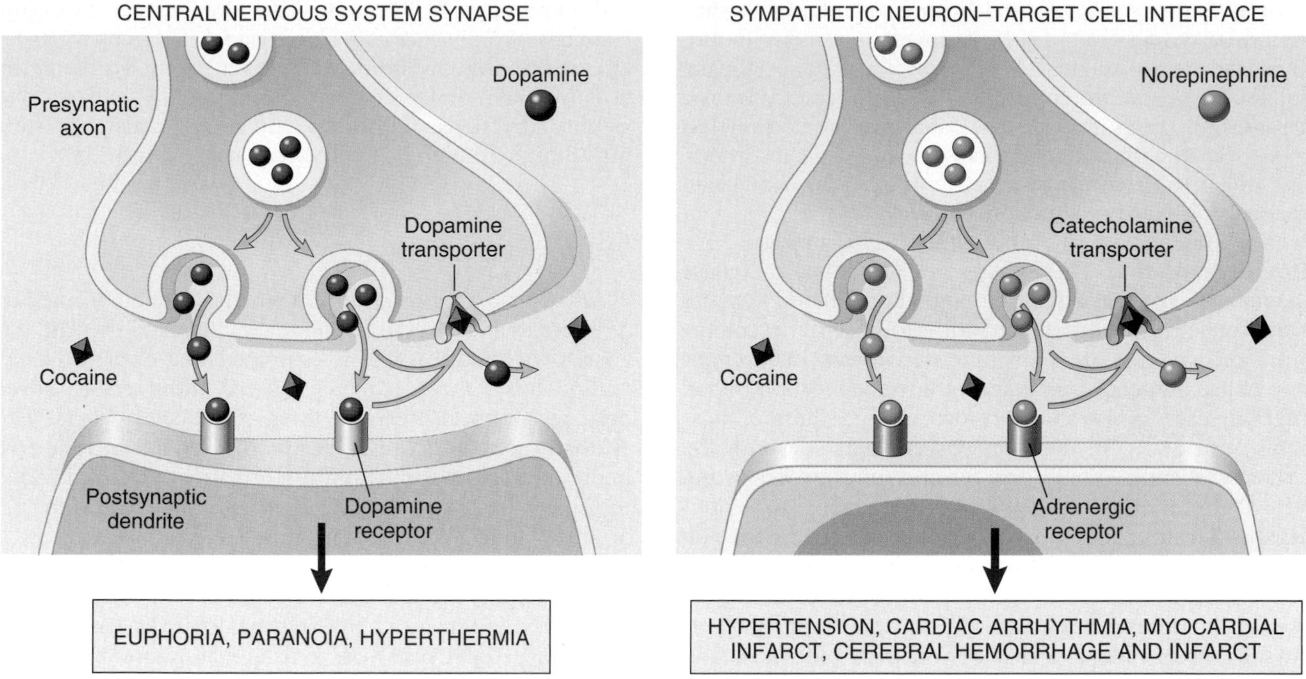

FIGURE 9–8 Effects of cocaine on neurotransmitters. Cocaine inhibits the reuptake of the neurotransmitters dopamine and norepinephrine in the central and peripheral nervous systems.

induce sedation and decrease anxiety. Tolerance develops rapidly, causing drug users to increase the dose. Simultaneous use of barbiturates and ethanol is potentially lethal, causing coma and cardiopulmonary arrest. Chronic use of barbiturates induces cytochrome P-450 activity, increasing the metabolism of drugs such as dicumarol, tetracycline, digoxin, and oral contraceptives. Barbiturates have been replaced by safer sedatives such as diazepam (Valium), a member of the benzodiazepines. These drugs have a wider margin of safety and infrequently produce addiction or tolerance. At high doses, these sedatives can cause drowsiness, dizziness, and coma, but they do not induce cytochrome P-450 activity.

Psychomotor Stimulants. Cocaine is an alkaloid extracted from the leaves of *Erythroxylon coca.* The leaves have been chewed by South American Indians for two centuries to relieve fatigue and hunger. Cocaine abuse is a serious public health problem. Beginning in the 1960s, cocaine sniffing and smoking of freebase cocaine (also called "crack" because of the sound it produces when heated) have escalated in the United States. Cocaine produces a rapid "high" of short duration characterized by euphoria, increased energy, and stimulation. Chronic abuse can also cause insomnia, increased anxiety, paranoia, and hallucinations. *Acute overdose produces seizures, cardiac arrhythmias, and respiratory arrest;* these usually occur after intravenous injection or smoking of crack. The fundamental mechanism of cocaine action is to block the reuptake of dopamine, serotonin, and catecholamines (epinephrine, nor-epinephrine) in the presynaptic terminals where these transmitters are released. In the central nervous system, after the release of dopamine by the presynaptic axon, a membrane bound dopamine transporter binds to the free dopamine in the extracellular space and carries it back to the presynaptic neuron. Cocaine inhibits this process by binding strongly to this reuptake transporter. Thus cocaine prolongs the dopaminergic effects in the brain's pleasure centers (limbic system) producing intense euphoria. In the periphery, cocaine blocks reuptake of epinephrine and norepinephrine, resulting in excess catecholamine stimulation (Fig. 9–8)[20,21] inducing systemic vasoconstriction.

The cardiovascular effects of cocaine are clinically important and potentially fatal. Acutely, accumulation of catecholamines causes potent stimulation of α- and β-adrenergic receptors. This results in increased blood pressure and heart rate, along with coronary spasms. Together these effect increase myocardial oxygen demand, and decrease oxygen supply and can lead to cardiac arrhythmias and ischemia that may be sufficiently severe to cause infarction. The typical patient who presents with cocaine-induced myocardial infarction is a man in his early 30's; cigarette smoking compounds the risk. Chronically, cocaine use accelerates atherosclerosis by enhancing platelet activation and aggregation, and increasing the concentration of plasminogen-activator inhibitor, and increasing endothelial permeability. Other chronic effects in the heart with uncertain pathogenesis are cardiomyopathy and myocarditis. These entities are discussed more fully in Chapter 11.

The fetus is particularly at risk: decreased blood flow to the placenta causes fetal hypoxia resulting in increased spontaneous abortion, abruption placentae, and hemorrhages in newborn infants. Metabolites of cocaine can be detected in at least 6% of newborn infants; these babies show evidence of neurologic impairment and a diminished response to external stimuli. Cocaine addiction is a complex problem with economic, social, and health implications. As with all drug and ethanol addictions, treatment requires behavioral and pharmacologic approaches. Interestingly, in the case of cocaine vaccination to produce cocaine specific antibodies are currently in clinical trials.[22]

Amphetamines are also potent central nervous system stimulants. Overdose causes sweating, tremors, restlessness, and confusion that may progress to delirium, convulsions, cardiac arrhythmias, coma, and death. Amphetamines can induce fetal malformations and withdrawal symptoms in the neonate. A popular amphetamine congener, MDMA, or ecstasy, is toxic to serotonin neurons in the brain. Imbalance in serotonin has been associated with anxiety, depression, and panic disorder.[23] These addictive drugs cause short-term adaptive changes in intracellular signal transduction pathways in the brain that may contribute to tolerance and withdrawal symptoms.[21]

Opioid Narcotics. These drugs are prescribed to relieve pain, but they also cause sedation and altered mood. Opiates can be isolated from opium or synthesized from morphine. Heroin and codeine are morphine derivatives. Intravenous heroin abuse induces suppression of anxiety, sedation, mood changes, nausea, and respiratory depression. Chronic abuse induces tolerance as well as psychologic dependence. Overdose can cause convulsions, cardiorespiratory arrest, and death. All intravenous drug users are susceptible to serious infections. The four sites most commonly affected are the skin and subcutaneous tissue, heart valves, liver, and lungs. In a series of addicts admitted to the hospital, more than 10% had endocarditis, which often takes a distinctive form involving right-sided heart valves, particularly the tricuspid. Most cases are caused by *Staphylococcus aureus*, but fungi and a multitude of other organisms have also been implicated. Viral hepatitis is the most common infection among addicts and is acquired by the casual sharing of dirty needles. In the United States, this practice has also led to a high incidence of AIDS in drug addicts.

Cannabinoids and Hallucinogens. Both natural and chemical substances have hallucinogenic or psychedelic properties. Among the natural hallucinogens are the alkaloid mescaline, isolated from the peyote cactus, which is chewed; psilocybin, isolated from seeds of the morning glory flower or sacred teonanacatl mushrooms; and marijuana, isolated from the hemp plant, *Cannabis sativa.* The active ingredient in marijuana, isolated from the leaves and flowers, or in hashish, the resin isolated from the plants, is Δ^9-tetrahydrocannabinol (THC). Smoking rapidly delivers THC to the brain, producing a state of relaxation and heightened sensation. Intoxication impairs cognitive and motor functions. Chronic marijuana smoking may induce lung damage similar to that caused by tobacco smoke; however, it is not carcinogenic.

Phencyclidine (PCP) was formerly used as an anesthetic; it is now available as a street drug and is ingested, smoked, or snorted. Drug users experience inebriation, disorientation, and numbness. PCP characteristically induces nystagmus. High doses can induce coma lasting a few hours up to 10 days. Lysergic acid diethylamide (LSD) is a potent synthetic drug usually taken orally. It is absorbed rapidly and produces psychic effects, visual illusions, and altered perception for up to 12 hours. In high doses, LSD can cause death.

THERAPEUTIC DRUGS

An adverse drug reaction is defined as a toxic or undesired response to a drug used at therapeutic doses to prevent, diagnose, or treat disease. It is estimated that approximately 2 million hospitalized patients suffered from serious adverse drug reactions in 1994, resulting in 106,000 deaths. These estimates are conservative because they do not include errors in drug dosage or administration or patient noncompliance.[24] In Table 9–7, adverse drug reactions are classified on the basis of their underlying mechanisms. Predictable reactions are based on the known toxicity or mechanism of action of a drug; these reactions are usually related to dose. Individual variations or polymorphisms in drug-metabolizing enzymes contribute to variable responses to drug therapy and an increased incidence of side effects. At least 5% of commonly prescribed drugs are metabolized by the cytochrome P-450 CYP1A2 pathway; approximately 12% of Caucasians carry variant alleles that reduce drug metabolism by this pathway.[25] *Pharmacogenomics* is a new field that uses genotyping to predict and prevent adverse drug reactions; for example, children with leukemia are screened for thiopurine methyltransferase variants to determine the optimal dose of azathiopurine,[26] and genotyping for the cytochrome P-450 CYP2D6 enzyme will help individualize doses of antipsychotic drugs to reduce side effects.[27] In contrast to these predictable types of adverse drug reactions, idiopathic or idiosyncratic reactions are rare and unpredictable, although the consequences may be severe or even fatal.

Herbal medicines are widely used in the United States and throughout the world; although many of these preparations have been shown to be effective in short-term trials, there is lack of quality control in this industry and few long-term studies of effectiveness and safety. As summarized in Table 9–8, the most commonly used herbal medicines in the United States can produce adverse effects, including allergic or hypersensitivity reactions, and potentially serious interactions with prescription drugs.[28]

TABLE 9–7 Mechanisms of Adverse Drug Reactions

Mechanism	Example	Adverse Effect
Toxicity due to overdose	Acetaminophen	Liver necrosis and failure
Predictable reaction based on pharmacologic mechanism	Nonselective, nonsteroidal anti-inflammatory drugs	Peptic ulcer
Altered drug metabolism related to:		
Thiopurine S-methyltransferase deficiency	Azathioprine	Bone marrow failure
Cytochrome P-450 CYP2C9 variants	Oral anticoagulants	Bleeding
Cytochrome P-450 CYP2D6 variants	Some antipsychotic drugs	Excessive sedation; parkinsonism
N-acetyltransferase, slow acetylator phenotype	Hydralazine	Lupus
Idiopathic	Chloramphenicol	Aplastic anemia

Oral Contraceptives and Hormone Replacement Therapy

Estrogens, alone or in combination with progestin, have been widely used for over 35 years as oral contraceptives or as hormone replacement therapy by perimenopausal and postmenopausal women. Most oral contraceptives combine synthetic ethinyl estradiol or mestranol with a progestin or use progestin alone; hormone replacement therapy uses natural estrogens alone or in combination with progesterone. Recent epidemiologic evidence has clarified the potential benefits and risks of these widely used drugs.

Oral Contraceptives. There has been considerable concern and controversy about the safety of oral contraceptives, especially in relation to breast cancer. Two population-based, case-control studies, the Cancer and Steroid Hormone Study published in 1986 and the Women's Contraceptive and Reproductive Experiences Study published in 2002, explored the association between past or current use of oral contraceptives and breast cancer.[29] The most recent study included women between ages 35 and 64 diagnosed with breast cancer between 1994 and 1998. Potential effects of duration, formulations containing a high dose of estrogen, and family history of breast cancer were compared in women diagnosed with breast cancer or in control women without cancer. Past or current use of oral contraceptives was not found to be associated with an increased risk of breast cancer in white or black women in the United States.[30] Previous studies of other hormone-responsive cancers have also shown no increased risk of cancer; in fact, oral contraceptive use was found to decrease the risk of endometrial and ovarian cancers. In contrast, women infected with human papillomavirus have an increased risk of developing cervical cancer if they use oral contraceptives, although this risk may be related to other lifestyle factors (Chapter 22).

Uncommon adverse effects of oral contraceptives include:

- *Venous thrombosis and pulmonary embolism.* Oral contraceptives increase the risk of thrombosis; this risk is higher in carriers of mutations in factor V or prothrombin,[26] as described in Chapter 4. The older, high-dose preparations incurred a greater risk, but a smaller risk persists even with the low-estrogen–containing oral contraceptives. The newer, third-generation oral contraceptives that combine low-dose estrogen with synthetic progestins confer an even higher risk.
- *Cardiovascular disease.* Estrogens and progestins have opposing effects on high-density lipoprotein (HDL) and low-density lipoprotein (LDL) levels. The overall effect on lipoproteins depends on the preparations used, especially the dose of progestin in the formulation. Recent epidemiologic evidence suggests that nonsmoking healthy women younger than age 45 who use the newer low-estrogen formulations do not have an increased risk of atherosclerosis or myocardial infarction. However, the risk of myocardial infarction is increased in women older than age 35 who smoke. The risk of ischemic stroke is also increased, regardless of age or smoking history.
- *Liver tumors.* Benign hepatic adenomas may occur, especially in older women who have used oral contraceptives for prolonged periods. These tumors may rupture and cause intra-abdominal bleeding.

Hormone Replacement Therapy. In the United States, approximately one third of perimenopausal and postmenopausal women use hormone replacement therapy (HRT), either estrogen in combination with a progestin or a natural estrogen alone. There has been recent controversy about the risks and benefits of HRT. Short-term benefits include reduction in symptoms that accompany menopause, including hot flashes, vaginal dryness, and sleep disturbances. Long-term benefits include maintenance of bone mineral density and prevention of osteoporotic fractures. The major controversies surrounding HRT are the potential increased risk of cancer versus the potential benefits associated with prevention of ischemic heart disease and dementia. Recent results from the Women's Health Initiative and the Heart and Estrogen/Progestin Replacement Study have provided new information about the risks and benefits of HRT:[31]

- *Cancer.* Unopposed estrogen therapy greatly increases the risk of endometrial hyperplasia and cancer; therefore, most postmenopausal women now use estrogen in combination with a progestin. This combination drastically reduces or eliminates the risk of endometrial cancer. The risk of colon cancer was reduced in women who used HRT in some studies, but not in the Heart and Estrogen/Progestin Replacement Study. Recent results from the Women's Health Initiative indicate an increased risk of breast cancer in women who used HRT combined therapy for 5 years.
- *Venous thrombosis and pulmonary embolism.* The risk of thromboembolic events, including deep vein thrombosis,

TABLE 9–8 Adverse Effects of Herbal Medicines

Example	Adverse Effects	Drug Interactions
Echinacea	Allergic reactions	None described
Ginkgo	Headache, nausea	Potentiates anticoagulants
Ginseng	Headache, insomnia, euphoria, diarrhea	Interacts with monamine oxidase inhibitors, hypoglycemic drugs, anticoagulants
Saw palmetto	Constipation, decreased libido, urine retention	None described
St. John's wort	Allergic reactions, nausea, photosensitivity	Accelerated drug metabolism (oral contraceptives, anticoagulants)

Data from Ernst E: The risk-benefit profile of commonly used herbal therapies: ginkgo, St. John's wort, ginseng, echinacea, saw palmetto, and kava. Ann Intern Med 136:42, 2002.

pulmonary embolism, stroke, and retinal thrombosis, is elevated approximated twofold in HRT users, especially within the first 2 years.

- *Cardiovascular disease.* The recent Women's Health Initiative reported an approximate 29% increased risk of myocardial infarction, especially during the first year of combined HRT use. This is in contrast to earlier studies in which either no effect or slight protection against cardiovascular diseases was reported. Methodologic differences probably underlie these divergent results.[32]
- *Cholecystitis.* There is an increased risk of gallbladder disease in HRT users that increases with time.
- *Dementia.* The current studies are not adequate to evaluate whether HRT use prevents dementia.

Overall, the risks and benefits associated with the use of oral contraceptives and HRT must be evaluated for each individual patient in the context of her overall health, individual risk factors, and family history.

Acetaminophen

When taken in large doses, this widely used nonprescription analgesic and antipyretic causes *hepatic necrosis.* The window between the usual therapeutic dose (0.5 gm) and the toxic dose (15 to 25 gm) is large, however, and the drug is ordinarily safe in adults. Doses should be reduced for infants and children, especially in the setting of fever, reduced food intake, or dehydration, since these conditions may predispose to liver injury.[33] Toxicity begins with nausea, vomiting, diarrhea, and sometimes shock, followed in a few days by evidence of jaundice; with serious overdosage, liver failure ensues, with centrilobular necrosis that may extend to the entire lobule. Some patients show evidence of concurrent renal and myocardial damage.

Aspirin (Acetylsalicylic Acid)

Overdose may result from accidental ingestion by young children; in adults, overdose is frequently suicidal. The major untoward consequences are metabolic with few morphologic changes. At first respiratory alkalosis develops, followed by metabolic acidosis that often proves fatal before anatomic changes can appear. Ingestion of as little as 2 to 4 gm by children or 10 to 30 gm by adults may be fatal, but survival has been reported after doses five times larger.

Chronic aspirin toxicity (salicylism) may develop in persons who take 3 gm or more daily, the dose required to treat chronic inflammatory conditions. Chronic salicylism is manifested by headache, dizziness, ringing in the ears (tinnitus), difficulty in hearing, mental confusion, drowsiness, nausea, vomiting, and diarrhea. The central nervous system changes may progress to convulsions and coma. The morphologic consequences of chronic salicylism are varied. Most often there is an acute erosive gastritis (Chapter 17), which may produce overt or covert gastrointestinal bleeding and lead to gastric ulceration. A bleeding tendency may appear concurrently with chronic toxicity, because aspirin acetylates platelet cyclooxygenase and blocks the ability to make thromboxane A_2, an activator of platelet aggregation. Petechial hemorrhages may appear in the skin and internal viscera, and bleeding from gastric ulcerations may be exaggerated.

Proprietary analgesic mixtures of aspirin and phenacetin or its active metabolite, acetaminophen, when taken for a span of years, have caused renal papillary necrosis, referred to as *analgesic nephropathy* (Chapter 20).

OUTDOOR AIR POLLUTION

Air pollution is a serious problem in the United States and many other industrialized countries. In the United States, the Environmental Protection Agency is charged with identification and regulation of pollutants in the ambient air that may cause adverse health effects. The current National Ambient Air Quality Standards for the six major pollutants are listed in Table 9–9. Despite federal and state regulations, many cities and regions in the United States currently do not meet these primary standards. Epidemiologic research, human clinical studies, and animal toxicologic studies continue to provide evidence for adverse health effects of ambient air pollutants, even at exposure levels below the current standards. The major sources of ambient air pollutants are:

- *Combustion of fossil fuels.* These are divided into mobile sources such as motor vehicles, stationary sources such as power plants and factories, and other sources such as barbecues and fireplaces. Tailpipe emissions from motor vehicles are a complex mixture of carbon monoxide, oxides of nitrogen, hydrocarbons, diesel exhaust particles, and other particulates including lead oxide from tetraethyl lead contained in leaded gasoline.

TABLE 9–9 National Ambient Air Quality Standards: Sources and Number of People at Risk

Pollutant	Primary Standard	Tons Emitted (Millions)	People at Risk (Millions)
Ozone	0.08 ppm 8 hr average	Not applicable	143
Nitrogen oxides	0.053 ppm annual arithmetic mean	25	Not available
Sulfur dioxide	0.03 ppm annual arithmetic mean	19	0.3
Particulates (PM_{10})	50 μg/μL annual arithmetic mean	24	8.7
Carbon monoxide	9 ppm 8 hr average	97	31
Lead	1.5 μg/μL quarterly average	30	2.5

Data from U.S. Environmental Protection Agency: epa.gov/oar/oaqps, www.scorecard.org/env-releases, the American Lung Association: www.lungusa.org/air, and Goldman LR: Environmental health and its relationship to occupational health. In Levy BS, et al. (eds): Occupational Health. Recognizing and Preventing Work-Related Disease and Injury, fourth ed. Philadelphia, Lippincott Williams & Wilkins, 2000, p. 51.

- *Photochemical reactions.* Oxides of nitrogen and volatile hydrocarbons interact in the atmosphere to produce ozone (O_3) as a secondary pollutant.
- *Power plants.* These release sulfur dioxide (SO_2) and particulates into the atmosphere. Coal and oil contain sulfur, leading to atmospheric formation of sulfates. Automobiles release oxides of nitrogen, leading to atmospheric formation of nitrates. Aerosolized acid sulfates contribute to acid rain.
- *Waste incinerators, industry, smelters.* These point sources release acid aerosols, metals, mercury vapor, and organic compounds that may be hazardous for human health. One example of the numerous hazardous chemicals emitted by these sources is methyl isocyanate that was accidentally released at Bhopal in India in 1984, resulting in 3000 deaths due to pulmonary edema. Some of the air toxins, such as polycyclic aromatic hydrocarbons, are known carcinogens.[34]

Lungs are the major target of common outdoor air pollutants; especially vulnerable are children, asthmatics, and people with chronic lung or heart disease, as summarized in Table 9–10. The serious toxicity associated with lead exposure is discussed subsequently under Industrial Exposures. The major air pollutants and the mechanisms responsible for their adverse health effects are summarized briefly.[34]

Ozone. Ozone is a major component of smog that accompanies summer heat waves over much of the United States. Exposure of exercising children and adults to as little as 0.08 ppm produces cough, chest discomfort, and inflammation in the lungs. Asthmatics are especially sensitive and require more frequent visits to emergency rooms and more hospitalizations during smog episodes. It is not known whether these acute changes lead to chronic, irreversible lung injury. Ozone is highly reactive and oxidizes polyunsaturated lipids to hydrogen peroxide and lipid aldehydes. These products act as irritants and induce release of inflammatory mediators, cause increased epithelial permeability and reactivity of the airways, and decrease ciliary clearance. The highest inhaled dose is delivered at the bronchoalveolar junction; however, ozone also causes inflammation of the upper respiratory tract.

Nitrogen Dioxide. Oxides of nitrogen include NO and NO_2. These have lower reactivity than ozone. Nitrogen dioxide dissolves in water in the airways to form nitric and nitrous acids, which damage the airway epithelial lining. Children and patients with asthma have increased susceptibility to nitrogen dioxide; there is a wide variation in individual responses to this pollutant.

Sulfur Dioxide. This pollutant is highly soluble in water; it is absorbed in the upper and lower airways, where it releases H^+, HSO_3^- (bisulfite), and SO_3^- (sulfite), which cause local irritation.

Acid Aerosols. Primary combustion products of fossil fuels are emitted by tall smoke stacks at high altitudes and are transported by air. In the atmosphere, sulfur and nitrogen dioxide are oxidized to sulfuric acid and nitric acid, respectively, which are dissolved in water droplets or adsorbed to particulates. These acid aerosols are irritants to the airway epithelium and alter mucociliary clearance. Asthmatics have decreased lung function and increased hospitalizations when exposed to acid aerosols, although there is a wide variation in airway responses.

Particulates. As discussed in Chapter 15, the deposition and clearance of particulates inhaled into the lungs depend on their size. Ambient particulates are highly heterogeneous in size and in chemical composition. It is uncertain which characteristics of ambient particulates contribute to their adverse health effects. Recent epidemiologic and toxicologic studies suggest that ultrafine particles (less than 0.1 μm in aerodynamic diameter) are more hazardous. They contribute to increased morbidity and mortality, especially among infants, the elderly, and people with chronic cardiopulmonary disease. The mechanisms responsible for these adverse health effects are suspected to involve: (1) systemic cytokine release

TABLE 9–10 Health Effects of Outdoor Air Pollutants

Pollutant	Populations at Risk	Effects
Ozone	Healthy adults and children	Decreased lung function Increased airway reactivity Lung inflammation
	Athletes, outdoor workers Asthmatics	Decreased exercise capacity Increased hospitalizations
Nitrogen dioxide	Healthy adults Asthmatics Children	Increased airway reactivity Decreased lung function Increased respiratory infections
Sulfur dioxide	Healthy adults Patients with chronic lung disease	Increased respiratory symptoms Increased mortality Increased hospitalization
	Asthmatics	Decreased lung function
Acid aerosols	Healthy adults Children Asthmatics	Altered mucociliary clearance Increased respiratory infections Decreased lung function Increased hospitalizations
Particulates	Children	Increased respiratory infections Decreased lung function
	Patients with chronic lung or heart disease Asthmatics	Excess mortality Increased attacks

Data from Bascom R, et al: Health effects of outdoor air pollution, Am J Respir Crit Care Med 153:3, 477, 1996.

associated with pulmonary inflammation; (2) increased blood viscosity; and (3) autonomic changes associated with variable heart rates and arrhythmias.[35]

INDOOR AIR POLLUTION

Rising energy costs during the past 30 years have led to increased insulation and decreased ventilation of homes, which elevates the level of indoor air pollutants. The health hazards of environmental tobacco smoke have already been discussed. Other sources of indoor air pollutants are gas cooking stoves and furnaces, wood stoves, construction materials, furniture, radon, allergens associated with pets, dust mites, and fungal spores and bacteria. The major categories of indoor air pollutants and their health effects are summarized in Table 9–11 and discussed briefly next.[36]

Carbon Monoxide. This odorless, colorless gas is a byproduct of combustion produced from burning gasoline, oil, coal, wood, and natural gas. It is also a major pollutant in tobacco smoke, and its untoward effects were discussed earlier along with cigarette smoking. Here we should note that carbon monoxide levels in ambient air should not exceed 9 ppm; however, indoor levels of 2 to 4 ppm have been measured in homes during the winter. Such carbon monoxide pollution of indoor air can reduce exercise capacity and aggravate myocardial ischemia. Higher levels can cause poisoning manifested as headaches, dizziness, loss of motor control, and coma. Approximately 900 accidental deaths due to asphyxia are caused by indoor carbon monoxide pollution each year in the United States.

Nitrogen Dioxide. Gas stoves and kerosene space heaters can raise indoor levels of nitrogen dioxide to 20 to 40 ppm in homes; this is several orders of magnitude higher than outdoor air levels. Children are more susceptible to the untoward effects of nitrogen dioxide. It impairs lung defenses and is hence associated with increased respiratory infections.

Wood Smoke. This is a complex mixture of nitrogen oxides, particulates, and polycyclic aromatic hydrocarbons. High concentrations of wood smoke in poorly ventilated homes can increase the incidence of respiratory infections in children.

Formaldehyde. This highly soluble, volatile chemical has been used in the manufacture of many consumer products, including textiles, pressed wood, furniture, and urea formaldehyde foam insulation. Although indoor levels are usually less than 1 ppm, it can cause acute irritation of the eyes and upper respiratory tract and exacerbation of asthma. Formaldehyde is frequently emitted with acrolein and acetaldehyde, which may have additive or synergistic irritant effects. Additional volatile organic compounds that may be present at low levels in indoor air include benzene, tetrachloroethylene, polycyclic aromatic hydrocarbons, and chloroform. The potential for toxicity or carcinogenicity at these exposure levels is low, although occupational exposure to these volatile compounds can be hazardous. Formaldehyde at high doses (6 to 14 ppm) has produced nasal tumors in rats.[37]

Radon. Radon, a radioactive gas, is a decay product of uranium widely distributed in the soil. Radon gas emanating from the earth is prevalent in homes. Indoor levels of radon average around 1.5 pCi/L; approximately 4% of homes have an annual average level greater than 4 pCi/L. Radon gas is inhaled into the lungs; its decay products emit alpha radiation, which has been associated with lung cancer in miners. According to some estimates, the low levels found in indoor air account for 10,000 lung cancers per year in the United States.[38]

Asbestos Fibers. Homes and public buildings built before the 1970s in the United States contain asbestos insulation, pipe covers, ceiling tiles, and flooring. If these materials are nonfriable and undisturbed, low levels of fibers can be measured in indoor air. Maintenance and abatement workers who repair or remove asbestos-containing materials are at risk for lung cancer and mesothelioma if they do not use respirators.[39,40]

Manufactured Mineral Fibers. Fiberglass has been widely used as an asbestos substitute for home insulation. Low levels of these fibers can be measured in indoor air. Maintenance and construction workers can develop skin and lung irritation when using these materials.[41]

Bioaerosols. Aerosolization of bacteria responsible for *Legionella* pneumonia has been associated with contaminated heating and cooling systems in public buildings (Chapter 8). More common hazards in indoor air are allergens associated with pets, dust mites, cockroaches, fungi, and molds. These allergens cause allergic rhinitis and exacerbate asthma.[41]

The etiology of the so-called *sick building syndrome*, or *multiple chemical sensitivity syndrome*, is less clear. In some cases, high levels of one or more of these indoor air pollutants may be responsible. In most cases, poor ventilation is at fault.[41]

TABLE 9–11 Health Effects of Indoor Air Pollutants

Pollutant	Populations at Risk	Effects
Carbon monoxide	Adults and children	Acute poisoning
Nitrogen dioxide	Children	Increased respiratory infections
Wood smoke	Children	Increased respiratory infections
Formaldehyde	Adults and children	Eye and nose irritation, asthma
Radon	Adults and children	Lung cancer
Asbestos fibers	Maintenance and abatement workers	Lung cancer, mesothelioma
Manufactured mineral fibers	Maintenance and construction workers	Skin and airway irritation
Bioaerosols	Adults and children	Allergic rhinitis, asthma

Data from Lambert WE, Samet JM: Indoor air pollution. In Harber P, et al (eds): Occupational and Environmental Respiratory Disease. St. Louis, Mosby–Year Book, 1996, p. 784; and Menzies D, Bourbeau J: Building-related illnesses. N Engl J Med 337:1524, 1997.

INDUSTRIAL EXPOSURES

For centuries, physicians have recognized that occupational exposures contribute to human disease. The spectrum of human diseases associated with occupational exposures is summarized in Table 9–12. Almost all organ systems can be affected, resulting in acute toxicity or irritation, hypersensitivity reactions, chronic toxicity, fibrosis, and cancer. The chronic effects of occupational exposures are complex; they include degenerative changes in the nervous system, reproductive dysfunction, lung fibrosis, and cancer. The mechanisms responsible for these effects are not well understood. Some examples of acute and chronic diseases resulting from occupational exposures and potential hazards of environmental exposures are discussed in the following sections.

Volatile Organic Compounds

Large volumes of organic solvents and vapors are used in industry and in homes. These chemicals are known as volatile organic compounds (VOCs). They are used in manufacturing, degreasing, and dry cleaning and as components of paint removers and aerosol sprays. VOCs and petroleum products such as kerosene, mineral oil, and turpentine are stored in underground tanks. Surface spills and leakage from storage tanks can cause contamination of underground water supplies. In general, high levels of exposure encountered in industry cause headache, dizziness, and liver or kidney toxicity. At lower levels of exposure, there is concern about potential carcinogenicity and adverse reproductive effects. Some VOCs and their adverse effects are described next.

Aliphatic Hydrocarbons. These compounds are the most widely used industrial solvents and dry-cleaning agents. All of these chemicals are readily absorbed through the lungs, skin, and gastrointestinal tract. In addition to acute central nervous system depression, they can cause liver and kidney toxicity. Common examples of these chemicals are chloroform and carbon tetrachloride; both are carcinogenic in rodents. Methylene chloride, another such chemical, is used in paint removers and aerosols. In enclosed areas, high concentrations of methylene chloride can be reached because it is highly volatile. Methylene chloride is metabolized by cytochrome P-450 to carbon dioxide and carbon monoxide. Carbon monoxide can form carboxyhemoglobin, causing respiratory depression and death. Perchloroethylene and related compounds are widely used in the dry-cleaning industry. Acute exposure causes central nervous system depression, confusion, dizziness, impaired gait, and nausea. Repeated exposures may cause dermatitis. Perchloroethylene is a potential human carcinogen.

Petroleum Products. Gasoline, kerosene, mineral oil, and turpentine are highly volatile and are a common cause of poisoning in children. Inhalation of these vapors causes dizziness, incoordination, and central nervous system depression.

Aromatic Hydrocarbons. Benzene, toluene, and xylene are widely used solvents in the rubber and shoe industries and in printing and paper-coating. Although toluene and xylene are not carcinogenic, inhalation of benzene is hazardous because it can cause bone marrow toxicity, aplastic anemia, and acute leukemia. Benzene is metabolized by the cytochrome P-450 system in liver, producing benzoquinone and muconaldehyde. These metabolic products are believed to cause bone marrow toxicity.

Polycyclic Aromatic Hydrocarbons

Polycyclic aromatic hydrocarbons are among the most potent chemical carcinogens (Chapter 7). The carcinogenicity of these compounds was recognized in 1775, with the description of scrotal cancer in English chimney sweeps exposed to soot. A variety of polycyclic aromatic hydrocarbons charac-

TABLE 9–12 Human Diseases Associated with Occupational Exposures

Organ	Effect	Toxicant
Cardiovascular system	Heart disease	Carbon monoxide, lead, solvents, cobalt, cadmium
Respiratory system	Nasal cancer	Isopropyl alcohol, wood dust
	Lung cancer	Radon, asbestos, silica, bis(chloromethyl)ether, nickel, arsenic, chromium, mustard gas
	Chronic obstructive lung disease	Grain dust, coal dust, cadmium
	Hypersensitivity	Beryllium, isocyanates
	Irritation	Ammonia, sulfur oxides, formaldehyde
	Fibrosis	Silica, asbestos, cobalt
Nervous system	Peripheral neuropathies	Solvents, acrylamide, methyl chloride, mercury, lead, arsenic, DDT
	Ataxic gait	Chlordane, toluene, acrylamide, mercury
	Central nervous system depression	Alcohols, ketones, aldehydes, solvents
	Cataracts	Ultraviolet radiation
Urinary system	Toxicity	Mercury, lead, glycol ethers, solvents
	Bladder cancer	Naphthylamines, 4-aminobiphenyl, benzidine, rubber products
Reproductive system	Male infertility	Lead, phthalate plasticizers
	Female infertility	Cadmium, lead
	Teratogenesis	Mercury, polychlorinated biphenyls
Hematopoietic system	Leukemia	Benzene, radon, uranium
Skin	Folliculitis and acneiform dermatosis	Polychlorinated biphenyls, dioxins, herbicides
	Cancer	Ultraviolet radiation
Gastrointestinal tract	Liver angiosarcoma	Vinyl chloride

Data from Leigh JP, et al: Occupational injury and illness in the United States. Estimates of costs, morbidity, and mortality. Arch Intern Med 157:1557, 1997; Mitchell FL: Hazardous waste. In Rom WN (ed): Environmental and Occupational Medicine, 2nd ed. Boston, Little, Brown, 1992, p. 1275; and Levi PE: Classes of toxic chemicals. In Hodgson E, Levi PE (eds): A Textbook of Modern Toxicology, Stamford, CT, Appleton & Lange, 1997, p. 229.

terized by three or more fused benzene rings are produced by combustion of fossil fuels; high-temperature processing of coke, coal, and crude oil; and iron and steel foundries. Benzo[a]pyrene is the prototype of polycyclic aromatic hydrocarbons. As described earlier (see Fig. 9–4*A*), it is metabolized by cytochrome P-450, prostaglandin H synthetase, and epoxide hydrolase, an inducible microsomal enzyme in the liver. Activated epoxide intermediates bind to DNA; these adducts have been used as markers of polycyclic aromatic hydrocarbon exposure. Occupational exposure to polycyclic aromatic hydrocarbons is associated with an increased risk of lung and bladder cancers.[42] Cigarette smoking is another important source of benzo[a]pyrene. Mutations in the *p53* tumor-suppressor gene found in lung cancers associated with cigarette smoking are most commonly G:C→T:A transversions. This mutational spectrum is consistent with metabolism of benzo[a]pyrene to reactive intermediates that attack deoxyguanines on the nontranscribed DNA strand.[7]

Plastics, Rubber, and Polymers

Millions of tons of synthetic plastics, rubber, and polymers are produced throughout the world. These products are then fabricated into latex fabrics, pipe, cables, flooring, home and recreational products, medical products, and containers. In 1974, occupational exposure to vinyl chloride monomers used to produce polyvinyl chloride resins was found to be associated with angiosarcoma of the liver. Vinyl chloride is a colorless gas that is flammable and explosive. Before the polymerization step in the manufacturing of polyvinyl chloride, it can be absorbed through the skin or lungs. Vinyl chloride is metabolized by the cytochrome P-450 system in the liver to chloroacetaldehyde. This metabolite covalently binds to DNA and is mutagenic. Exposure of rubber workers to 1,3-butadiene has been shown to be associated with an increased risk of leukemia. Plastics are widely used in consumer products, including food and beverage containers. Public exposure to plasticizers, such as phthalate esters, and to additives such as bisphenol-A raises concern about potential adverse reproductive effects of these synthetic chemicals. Phthalate esters have been shown to induce testicular injury in rats, and bisphenol-A mimics the proliferative effects of estrogen.

Metals

Occupational exposure to metals in mining and manufacturing is associated with acute and chronic toxicity, as well as carcinogenicity, as summarized in Table 9–13.[43] Occupational as well as environmental exposure to lead continues to be a serious public health problem. Agricultural exposure to arsenic-containing pesticides is discussed subsequently. The pulmonary effects of beryllium are described in Chapter 15. The health effects of inorganic and organic mercury were discussed earlier in this chapter under "Mechanisms of Toxicity." The untoward effects of some of the remaining metals listed in Table 9–13 are described here.

Lead. More than 4 million tons of lead are produced each year for use in batteries, alloys, exterior red lead paint, and ammunition. Workers employed in these industries as well as in mining, smelting, spray painting, recycling, and radiator repair are exposed to lead. In some countries, tetraethyl lead is still used as a gasoline additive, thus polluting the air. *Inhalation is the most important route of occupational exposure.* Environmental sources of lead are urban air due to use of leaded gasoline, soil contaminated with exterior lead paint, the water supply due to lead plumbing, and house dust in homes with interior lead paint. Consumers may be exposed to lead-glazed ceramics, lead solder in food and soft drink cans, and illegally

TABLE 9–13 Toxic and Carcinogenic Metals

Metal	Disease	Occupation
Lead	Renal toxicity Anemia, colic Peripheral neuropathy Insomnia, fatigue Cognitive deficits	Battery and ammunition workers, foundry workers, spray painting, radiator repair
Mercury	Renal toxicity Muscle tremors, dementia Cerebral palsy Mental retardation	Chlorine-alkali industry
Arsenic	Cancer of skin, lung, liver	Miners, smelters, oil refinery workers, farm workers
Beryllium	Acute lung irritant Chronic lung hypersensitivity ? Lung cancer	Beryllium refining, aerospace manufacturing, ceramics
Cobalt and tungsten carbide	Lung fibrosis Asthma	Toolmakers, grinders, diamond polishers
Cadmium	Renal toxicity ? Prostate cancer	Battery workers, smelters, welders, soldering
Chromium	Cancer of lung and nasal cavity	Pigment workers, smelters, steel workers
Nickel	Cancer of lung and nasal sinuses	Smelters, steel workers, electroplating

Data from Levi PE: Classes of toxic chemicals. In Hodgson E, Levi PE (eds): A Textbook of Modern Toxicology. Stamford, CT, Appleton & Lange, 1997, p. 229; and Sprince NL: Hard metal disease. In Rom WN (eds): Environmental and Occupational Medicine, 2nd ed. Boston, Little, Brown, 1992, p. 791.

produced alcoholic beverages (moonshine). Lead ingested in this manner is absorbed through the gastrointestinal tract. Intestinal absorption of lead is enhanced by calcium, iron, or zinc deficiency; compared with adults, the absorption is greater in children and infants and hence they are particularly vulnerable to lead toxicity. Absorbed lead is mainly (80% to 85%) taken up by bone and developing teeth in children; the blood accumulates 5% to 10%, and the remainder is distributed throughout the soft tissues. Lead clears rapidly from blood, but that deposited in bones has a half-life of 30 years. Thus, the presence of lead in blood indicates recent exposure, and it does not allow the determination of total body burden. The toxicity of lead is related to its multiple biochemical effects:

- *High affinity for sulfhydryl groups.* The most important enzymes inhibited by lead due to this mechanism are involved in heme biosynthesis: δ-aminolevulinic acid dehydratase and ferroketolase. These enzymes catalyze the incorporation of iron into the heme molecule, and hence patients develop hypochromic anemia.
- *Competition with calcium ions.* As a divalent cation, lead competes with calcium and is stored in bone. It also interferes with nerve transmission and brain development.
- *Inhibition of membrane-associated enzymes.* Lead inhibits 5′-nucleotidase activity and sodium-potassium ion pumps, leading to decreased survival of red blood cells (hemolysis), renal damage, and hypertension.
- *Impaired production* of 1,25-dihydroxyvitamin D, the active metabolite of vitamin D.

Lead contributes to multiple chronic health effects, illustrated in Figure 9–9. *Injury to the central and peripheral nervous systems* causes headache, dizziness, memory deficits, and decreased nerve conduction velocity. *Blood changes* occur early and are characteristic. Because lead interferes with heme biosynthesis, it causes a microcytic hypochromic anemia; punctate basophilic stippling of erythrocytes is characteristic. There is also an element of hemolysis because lead inhibits membrane-associated red cell enzymes. Because lead inhibits incorporation of iron into heme, the iron is displaced, and zinc protoporphyrin is formed. Thus, an elevated blood level of zinc protoporphyrin or its product, free erythrocyte protoporphyrin, is an important indicator of lead poisoning. *Gastrointestinal symptoms* include colic and anorexia. The kidneys are a major route of excretion of lead. Acutely, there is *damage to the proximal tubules*, with intranuclear lead inclusions and clinical evidence of renal tubule dysfunction. Chronically, lead can cause diffuse interstitial fibrosis, gout, and renal failure. Even in the absence of overt clinical symptoms of kidney damage, lead causes hypertension. Lead can cause infertility in men due to testicular injury; failure of implantation of the fertilized ovum can occur in women.[44]

Infants and children are especially vulnerable to lead toxicity. It is estimated by the CDC that in the year 2000 approximately 454,000 children in the United States had blood lead levels greater than 10 μg/dL. A recent study indicates that even below this level there is an inverse correlation between blood lead concentration and IQ scores. Very slightly elevated blood levels (~3 μg/dL) in young females have also been reported to delay puberty.[45] Thus, lead toxicity continues to be a matter of concern. Lead may be mobilized from the maternal skeleton during pregnancy and it readily crosses the placental barrier.

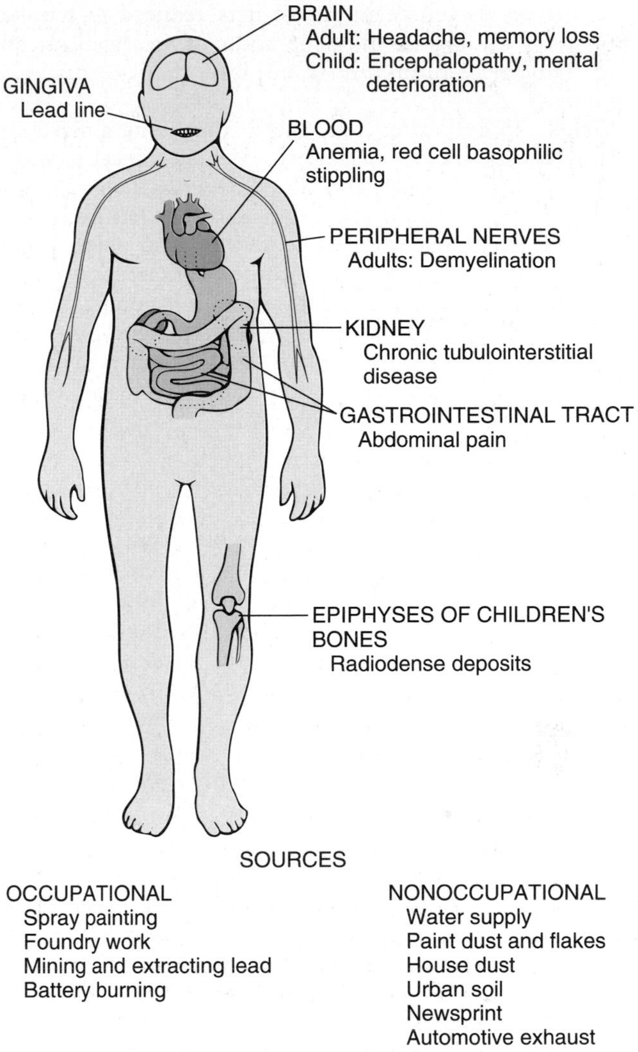

FIGURE 9–9 Consequences of lead exposure.

Hence lead exposure can begin in utero. Similar to neurotoxicity caused by methylmercury, the developing nervous system of the fetus and infants is extremely susceptible to lead toxicity.[46]

Cobalt and Tungsten Carbide. Cutting tools, metal grinders, polishers, and drilling equipment are fabricated from tungsten carbide with cobalt as a binder. Workers who use these tools or work in related industries can develop asthma and interstitial lung fibrosis (called *hard metal disease*). Asthma and lung injury appear to be caused by cobalt, although lung damage may be exacerbated by metal mixtures.

Cadmium. Occupational exposure to cadmium occurs near mines and smelters; this metal is also used in paint pigments, alloys, solder, electroplating, and batteries. Acute effects are lung edema and irritation. Chronic toxicity affects the kidney. Cadmium induces the synthesis of metallothionein, a metal-binding protein, in the liver and kidney. When this defense mechanism is overwhelmed, cadmium damages the proximal convoluted tubules, causing proteinuria.

Chromium. Occupational exposure to chromium occurs in mining and smelting. Chromium is also used in stainless steel, pigments, and alloys. Hexavalent chromium is readily absorbed across cell membranes; it is reduced to trivalent chromium, leading to the generation of free radicals and DNA damage. Chromium is an important occupational carcinogen.

Nickel. Topical exposure to metals that contain nickel frequently causes contact dermatitis. Metallic nickel is widely used in industry in steels and alloys, batteries, fuel cells, electroplating, and ceramics. Nickel is also recycled from scrap metal and is emitted from waste incinerators, power plants, and cigarette smoke. The major route of occupational exposure is by inhalation. Particulate nickel compounds are carcinogenic; they enter target cells after phagocytosis, with release of nickel ions intracellularly. Nickel appears to damage heterochromatin selectively and can inactivate tumor-suppressor genes by hypermethylation.[47]

AGRICULTURAL HAZARDS

Although agricultural productivity has been improved by the use of fertilizers and pesticides, these chemicals are not an unalloyed blessing. They cause disease in those exposed to them, particularly farmers. However, the potential health hazards of pesticides extend beyond the farming community because pesticide residues are found on foods and contaminate soil and water supplies. Environmental contamination is a threat to wildlife; some pesticides undergo bioaccumulation and persist in wildlife and humans for decades. Bioaccumulation and biopersistence are characteristic of organochlorines, such as DDT (dichlorodiphenyltrichloroethane), and dioxins, such as TCDD (2,3,7,8-tetrachlorodibenzo-*p*-dioxin). There is considerable controversy about the adverse health effects of these persistent pesticides and their metabolites, especially concerning their relationship to breast cancer,[48] reproductive abnormalities,[49] and cognitive deficits.[50]

Agricultural pesticides are divided into five categories, depending on the target pest: insecticides, herbicides, fungicides, rodenticides, and fumigants (Table 9–14). All pesticides are toxic to some plant or rodent species; at higher doses, they can also be toxic to farm animals, pets, and humans. In general, herbicides used to control weeds have low acute toxicity for mammals; fungicides are characterized as moderately toxic. Acute toxicity of insecticides for mammals ranges from low to high. For example, DDT was widely used as an insecticide in the 1940s and 1950s because it has low acute toxicity for humans. However, DDT persists in the environment and accumulates in the food chain. Birds that ingested DDT-contaminated insects and fish suffered reproductive defects. DDT and its major metabolite, DDE

TABLE 9–14 Health Effects of Agricultural Pesticides

Category	Example	Effects and Disease Associations
Insecticides	Organochlorines	Neurotoxicity; hepatotoxicity
	DDT	
	Chlordane	
	Lindane	
	Methoxychlor	
	Organophosphates	Neurotoxicity; delayed neuropathy
	Parathion	
	Diazinon	
	Malathion	
	Carbamates	Neurotoxicity (reversible)
	Aldicarb	
	Carbaryl	
	Botanical agents	Paresthesia; lung irritant; allergic dermatitis
	Nicotine	
	Pyrethrins	
	Rotenone	
Herbicides	Arsenic compounds	Hyperpigmentation; gangrene; anemia; sensory neuropathy; cancer
	Dinitrophenols	Hyperthermia; sweating
	Chlorophenoxy herbicides	
	2,4-D and 2,4,5-T	? Lymphoma; sarcoma
	TCDD	Fetotoxicity; immunotoxicity; cancer
	Paraquat	Acute lung injury
	Atrazine	? Cancer
	Alachlor	? Cancer
Fungicides	Captan	? Reproductive toxicity
	Maneb	
	Benomyl	
Rodenticides	Fluoroacetate	Cardiac and respiratory failure
	Warfarin	Hemorrhage
	Strychnine	Respiratory failure
Fumigants	Carbon disulfide	Cardiac toxicity
	Ethylene dibromide	Neurotoxicity
	Phosphine	Lung edema; brain damage
	Chloropicrin	Eye irritation; lung edema; arrhythmias

Data from Hodgson E: Introduction to toxicology. In Hodgson E, Levi PE (eds): A Textbook of Modern Toxicology. Stamford, CT, Appleton & Lange, 1997, p. 1; and Levi PE: Classes of toxic chemicals. In Hodgson E, Levi PE (eds): A Textbook of Modern Toxicology. Stamford, CT, Appleton & Lange, 1997, p. 229.

(1,1-dichloro-2,2-bis(*p*-chlorophenyl) ethylene), accumulate in fat tissue and have been detected in human milk. Organochlorines, as well as industrial chemicals such as polychlorinated biphenyls (PCBs), are weakly estrogenic. Some of these chemicals are carcinogenic in rodents and cause reproductive dysfunction in amphibians, birds, and fish.[48] Although several epidemiologic studies have not found increased levels of DDE or PCBs in women with breast cancer compared with matched control subjects, there is still concern that these persistent organochlorines, other potentially estrogenic pesticides, and natural phytoestrogens in plants such as soybeans may have adverse reproductive effects in humans. The mechanisms of action of these xenoestrogens, alone or in combination, in the development of cancer and in reproductive dysfunction are unknown.[48,49]

The major health effects of the most common agricultural pesticides are summarized in Table 9–14. Selected examples are discussed here.

- *Organochlorines,* such as DDT, have low acute toxicity for humans; however, they bioaccumulate and persist in the environment and in fat tissue. These chemicals are absorbed through the skin, gastrointestinal tract, and lungs. As alluded to earlier, the role of DDT and its metabolites as an endocrine-disrupting agent is controversial. *Chlordane* is representative of cyclodienes that are used to control termites and other soil insects. Acute toxicity causes hypothermia, tremor, and convulsions. Chlordane also causes immune dysfunction and may act as a nongenotoxic carcinogen. These effects may contribute to the increased incidence of lymphoma observed in some farm workers. *Lindane* is an isomer of benzene hexachloride that is used to control lice and scabies, as a wood preservative, and as a household fumigant. It has been reported to cause immune dysfunction and reproductive problems in women.
- *Organophosphates* are irreversible inhibitors of cholinesterases resulting in abnormal transmission at peripheral and central nerve endings. These chemicals are absorbed through the skin, gastrointestinal tract, and lungs. Up to 40% of farm workers in the United States show measurable inhibition of red blood cell or plasma cholinesterase activity; fatalities have been reported from organophosphate exposure. *Carbamates* are reversible inhibitors of cholinesterase that produce acute neurotoxic effects similar to those of organophosphate insecticides. Carbaryl (Sevin) is potentially mutagenic and teratogenic because it poisons the mitotic spindle.
- *Herbicides* like the dioxin TCDD has received much attention. During the Vietnam War, the defoliant Agent Orange was contaminated with TCDD. A chemical factory explosion in Seveso, Italy, in 1976 caused local environmental contamination and human exposure to TCDD, resulting in chloracne and an increased incidence of leukemia, lymphoma, and sarcomas. TCDD and structurally similar dioxins are also produced in the paper pulp industry using chlorine bleach and by waste incinerators. Low doses of dioxin are present in our food, soil, and water. In some laboratory animals, TCDD is highly toxic, immunosuppressive, teratogenic, and carcinogenic. The sensitivity of some strains of laboratory mice to dioxin is linked to the aryl hydrocarbon hydroxylase receptor. TCDD can induce liver cytochrome P-450 enzyme activity, increase estrogen metabolism, and interfere with development of the male reproductive tract. TCDD also decreases thyroxine levels in adult rats. Extrapolation of these multiple adverse effects observed in laboratory animals to low-dose exposure of humans is difficult.[51]
- *Rodenticides* are highly toxic chemicals with restricted use. The major health threat is death from suicidal or accidental ingestion.

NATURAL TOXINS

In addition to manufactured pesticides, potent toxins and carcinogens are present in the natural environment, as summarized in Table 9–15. These mycotoxins and phytotoxins may contaminate foods. For example, cycad flour is used in arid climates. This plant contains the toxin cycasin (methylazoxymethanol β-glucoside). If the plant and seeds are cut into small pieces, soaked in water, and dried, the toxin is leached. However, if these precautions are not followed, a degenerative neurologic disorder (amyotrophic lateral sclerosis) is produced by ingestion of cycasin. Animal toxins can be ingested by eating fish, snails, or mollusks. The most common poisoning results from eating tropical fish and snails that have ingested dinoflagellates containing ciguatoxin. Ciguatera

TABLE 9–15 Natural Toxins

Category	Example	Source	Effects and Associated Diseases
Mycotoxins	Ergot alkaloids	*Claviceps* fungi	Gangrene, convulsions, abortion
	Aflatoxins	*Aspergillus flavus*	Liver cancer
	Tricothecenes	*Fusarium, Trichoderma*	Diarrhea, ataxia
Phytotoxins	Cycasin	Cycad flour	Amyotrophic lateral sclerosis
	Monocrotaline	*Senecio* plants	Hepatitis
	Safrole	Black pepper; oil of Sassafras	Cancer
	Solanine	Solanaceae plants (potato)	Neurotoxin
Animal toxins	Venoms	Snakes	Cardiotoxin, neurotoxin
		Bees	Direct toxicity, cardiotoxin
	Saxitoxin	Dinoflagellates	Neurotoxin, paralysis
	Ciguatoxin	Dinoflagellates	Paresthesia, paresis, vomiting, diarrhea
	Tetrodotoxin	Puffer fish	Neurotoxin, shock

Data from Hodgson E: Introduction to toxicology. In Hodgson E, Levi PE (eds): A Textbook of Modern Toxicology. Stamford, CT, Appleton & Lange, 1997, p. 1.

poisoning can be severe and occurs in the South Pacific and the Caribbean. Paralytic shellfish poisoning occurs in North America after eating mollusks that have ingested dinoflagellates that contain saxitoxin. Aflatoxin B_1 is produced by fungi that contaminate peanuts, corn, and cottonseed. It is a potent carcinogen that contributes to the high incidence of liver cancer in some regions of Africa and the Far East (Chapters 7 and 18).

RADIATION INJURY

Radiation is energy distributed across the electromagnetic spectrum as waves (long wavelengths, low frequency) or particles (short wavelengths, high frequency). The types, frequencies, and biologic effects of electromagnetic radiation are summarized in Table 9–16. Approximately 80% of radiation is derived from natural sources, including cosmic radiation, ultraviolet light, and natural radioisotopes, especially radon gas. The remaining 20% is derived from manufactured sources that include instruments used in medicine and dentistry, consumer products that emit radio waves or microwaves, and nuclear power plants. The potentially catastrophic effects of radiation are most vividly illustrated by the effects of nuclear explosions. The atomic bombs dropped on Hiroshima and Nagasaki in 1945 not only caused acute injury and death but also increased incidence of various cancers among the survivors. Numerous historical incidents document the deleterious effects of therapeutic radiation. For example, early in the 20th century, American radiologists experienced an increased incidence of aplastic anemia and neoplasms of the skin, brain, and hematopoietic system. Children who were treated with radiation for an enlarged thymus or benign skin lesions between 1910 and 1959 suffered from an increased incidence of thyroid abnormalities, thyroid tumors, and leukemias and lymphomas. Exposure of the fetus to radiation can produce mental retardation, congenital anomalies, leukemia, and solid tumors. Investigation of these deliberate or accidental exposures to radiation led to an understanding of the relationship between the dose and timing of radiation and the acute and chronic health effects. However, in general, these historical exposures were higher than radiation currently received by the general population from natural and manufactured sources, by patients undergoing diagnostic procedures such as mammography or chest radiography, and by nuclear power plant workers. Unfortunately, fear of widespread radiation exposure following a terrorist attack reinforces the importance of understanding the mechanisms and clinical manifestations of radiation injury.[52] Despite our understanding of the health effects of high doses of radiation, the potential adverse effects of low doses are controversial. Furthermore, accidents at nuclear power plants in Windscale, England, in 1957, at Three Mile Island in Pennsylvania in 1979, and at Chernobyl in the former Soviet Union in 1986 perpetuate public anxiety about excess cancers associated with the medical, commercial, and military uses of radioactivity.[53]

TABLE 9–16 Ionizing and Nonionizing Electromagnetic Radiation

Frequency (Hz)	Radiation	Biologic Effects
1–50	Electric power	?
10^6–10^{11}	Radio waves and radar	Thermal effects, cataracts
10^9–10^{10}	Microwaves	Lens opacities
10^{11}–10^{14}	Infrared	Cataracts
10^{15}	Visible light	Retinal burns (lasers)
10^{15}–10^{18}	Ultraviolet light	Skin burns, cancer
10^{18}–10^{20}	X-rays and gamma rays	Acute and delayed injury; cancer
10^{27}	Cosmic radiation	?

Electromagnetic radiation characterized by long wavelengths and low frequencies is described as *nonionizing radiation.* Electric power, radio waves and microwaves, infrared, and ultraviolet light are examples of nonionizing radiation. They produce vibration and rotation of atoms in biologic molecules. Radiation energy of short wavelengths and high frequency can ionize biologic target molecules and eject electrons. X-rays, gamma rays, and cosmic rays are forms of *ionizing radiation.* Ionizing radiation can be in the form of electromagnetic waves, such as x-rays produced by a roentgen tube or gamma rays emitted from natural sources, or particles that are released by natural decay of radioisotopes or by artificial acceleration of subatomic particles. *Particulate radiation* is classified by the type of particles emitted: alpha particles, beta particles or electrons, protons, neutrons, mesons, or deuterons. The energy of these particles is measured in million electron volts (MeV). Radioisotopes decay by emission of alpha or beta particles or by capture of electrons. In the case of radon gas, unstable daughter nuclei are produced that subsequently disintegrate, releasing alpha particles. *Alpha particles* consist of two neutrons and two protons; they have strong ionizing power but low penetration because of their large size. In contrast, *beta particles* are electrons emitted from the nucleus of an atom; these have weaker ionizing power but higher penetration than alpha particles. The decay of radioisotopes is expressed by the *curie* (Ci), 3.7×10^{10} disintegrations per second, or the *becquerel* (Bq), 1 disintegration per second. The rate of decay of radioisotopes is usually expressed as the half-life ($t_{1/2}$) and ranges from a few seconds to centuries. Internal deposition of radioisotopes with long half-lives is especially dangerous because it results in continuous release of radioactive particles and gamma rays. For example, radium was used to paint watch dials and treat cancer in the first half of the 20th century; its long half-life of 1638 years and ability to be concentrated in the skeleton result in delayed appearance of bone tumors.

Ionizing Radiation

The dose of ionizing radiation is measured in several units:

- *roentgen:* unit of charge produced by x-rays or gamma rays that ionize a specific volume of air
- *rad:* the dose of radiation that will produce absorption of 100 ergs of energy per gram of tissue; 1 gm of tissue exposed to 1 roentgen of gamma rays is equal to 93 ergs
- *gray* (Gy): the dose of radiation that will produce absorption of 1 joule of energy per kilogram of tissue; 1 Gy corresponds to 100 rad

- *rem:* the dose of radiation that causes a biologic effect equivalent to 1 rad of x-rays or gamma rays
- *sievert* (Sv): the dose of radiation that causes a biologic effect equivalent to 1 Gy of x-rays or gamma rays; 1 Sv corresponds to 100 rem.[53]

These measurements do not directly quantify energy transferred per unit of tissue and therefore do not predict the biologic effects of radiation. The following terms provide a better approximation of such information.

- *Linear energy transfer* (LET) expresses energy loss per unit of distance traveled as electron volts per micrometer. This value depends on the type of ionizing radiation. LET is high for alpha particles, less so for beta particles, and even less for gamma rays and x-rays. Thus, alpha and beta particles penetrate short distances and interact with many molecules within that short distance. Gamma rays and x-rays penetrate deeply but interact with relatively few molecules per unit distance. It should be evident that if equivalent amounts of energy entered the body in the form of alpha and gamma radiation, the alpha particles would induce heavy damage in a restricted area, whereas gamma rays would dissipate energy over a longer course and produce considerably less damage per unit of tissue.
- *Relative biologic effectiveness* (RBE) is simply a ratio that represents the relationship of the LETs of various forms of irradiation to cobalt gamma rays and megavolt x-rays, both of which have an RBE of unity (1).

In addition to the physical properties of the radioactive material and the dose, the biologic effects of ionizing radiation depend on several factors:

- Dose rate: a single dose can cause greater injury than divided or fractionated doses that allow time for cellular repair.
- Since DNA is the most important subcellular target of ionizing radiation, rapidly dividing cells are more radiosensitive than are quiescent cells. Hematopoietic cells, germ cells, gastrointestinal epithelium, squamous epithelium, endothelial cells, and lymphocytes are highly susceptible to radiation injury; bone, cartilage, muscle, and peripheral nerves are more resistant.
- A single dose of external radiation administered to the whole body is more lethal than regional doses with shielding. For example, the median lethal dose (LD_{50}) of ionizing radiation is 2.5 to 4.0 Gy (250 to 400 rad), whereas doses of 40 to 70 Gy (4000 to 7000 rad) can be delivered in a fractionated manner during several weeks for cancer therapy.
- Cells in the G_2 and mitotic phases of the cell cycle are most sensitive to ionizing radiation.
- Different cell types differ in the extent of their adaptive and reparative responses.
- Since ionizing radiation produces oxygen-derived radicals from the radiolytic cleavage of water (Chapter 1), cell injury induced by x-rays and gamma rays is enhanced by hyperbaric oxygen. Halogenated pyrimidines can also increase radiosensitivity to tumor cells. Conversely, free radical scavengers and antioxidants protect against radiation injury.

Cellular Mechanisms of Radiation Injury. The acute effects of ionizing radiation range from overt necrosis at high doses (>10 Gy), killing of proliferating cells at intermediate doses (1 to 2 Gy), and no histopathologic effect at doses less than 0.5 Gy. Subcellular damage does occur at these lower doses, primarily targeting DNA; however, most cells show adaptive and reparative responses to low doses of ionizing radiation. If cells undergo extensive DNA damage or if they are unable to repair this damage, they undergo apoptosis (Chapter 7). Surviving cells may show delayed effects of radiation injury: mutations, chromosome aberrations, and genetic instability. These genetically damaged cells may become malignant; tissues with rapidly proliferating cell populations are especially susceptible to the carcinogenic effects of ionizing radiation. Most cancers induced by ionizing radiation have occurred after doses greater than 0.5 Gy. Acute cell death, especially of vascular endothelial cells, can cause delayed organ dysfunction several months or years after radiation exposure. In general, this delayed injury is caused by a combination of atrophy of parenchymal cells, ischemia due to vascular damage, and fibrosis.[53] Acute and delayed effects of ionizing radiation are listed in Table 9–17, and their mechanisms are described next.

Acute Effects. Ionizing radiation can produce a variety of lesions in DNA, including DNA–protein cross-links, cross-linking of DNA strands, oxidation and degradation of bases, cleavage of sugar–phosphate bonds, and single-stranded or double-stranded DNA breaks. This damage may be produced directly by particulate radiation, x-rays, or gamma rays or indirectly by oxygen-derived free radicals or soluble products derived from peroxidized lipids.[54] Even relatively low doses of ionizing radiation (less than 0.5 Gy) induce alterations in gene expression in some target cell populations. Free radicals generated directly or indirectly by exposure to ionizing radiation may produce oxidant stress that activates transcription factors (such as NF-κB) that increase gene expression.[55] DNA damage itself stimulates the expression of several genes involved in DNA repair, cell-cycle arrest, and apoptosis. As discussed in Chapter 7, the tumor-suppressor gene *p53* is activated after many different forms of DNA damage. The end-points resulting from activation of this p53-mediated DNA damage response are discussed in Chapter 7. Briefly, activation of p53 induces cell-cycle arrest, DNA repair and, in some cases, apoptosis. Apoptosis of microvascular endothelial cells may be the primary target of acute radiation in the GI tract, resulting in secondary damage to intestinal crypt stem cells[56] and the GI syndrome (see Table 9–18).

Fibrosis. An important delayed complication of ionizing radiation, usually at doses used for cancer therapy, is replacement of normal parenchymal tissue by fibrosis, resulting in scarring and loss of function. These fibrotic changes may be secondary to ischemic injury caused by vascular damage, death of parenchymal cells, or deletion of stem cells.[57] The mechanisms responsible for fibrosis have been explored in a murine model of radiation-induced pulmonary fibrosis using microarray analysis of gene expression. Up-regulation of chemokines that recruit inflammatory cells to the lungs as well as cytokines and growth factors involved in fibroblast activation and collagen deposition are central components of radiation-induced fibrosis.[58] As described in Chapter 3, these chemokines, cytokines, and growth factors also play important roles in wound healing.

TABLE 9–17 Acute Injury and Delayed Complications Caused by Ionizing Radiation

Organ	Acute Injury	Delayed Complications
Bone marrow	Atrophy	Hypoplasia, leukemia
Skin	Erythema	Atrophy of epidermis and fibrosis of dermis; cancer
Heart	—	Interstitial fibrosis
Lung	Edema, endothelial and epithelial cell death	Interstitial and intra-alveolar fibrosis; cancer
Gastrointestinal tract	Edema, mucosal ulcers	Ulcers; fibrosis; strictures; adhesions; cancer
Liver	Veno-occlusive disease	Cirrhosis; liver tumors
Kidney	Vasodilation	Cortical atrophy, interstitial fibrosis
Urinary bladder	Mucosal erosion	Submucosal fibrosis; cancer
Brain	Edema, necrosis	Necrosis of white matter, gliosis; brain cancer
Testis	Necrosis	Tubular atrophy
Ovary	Atresia of follicles	Stromal fibrosis
Thyroid	—	Hypothyroidism; cancer
Breast	—	Fibrosis; cancer
Thymus, lymph nodes	Atrophy	Lymphoma

Carcinogenesis. Occupational or accidental exposures to ionizing radiation produce an increased incidence of various types of cancer, including skin cancers, leukemia, osteogenic sarcomas, and lung cancer. There is usually a latent period of 10 to 20 years before appearance of these cancers. In survivors of the atomic blasts at Hiroshima and Nagasaki, all types of leukemias were especially common, with the exception of chronic lymphocytic leukemia. Exposure of children to irradiation causes an increased incidence of breast and thyroid cancers as well as gastrointestinal and urinary tract tumors. The nuclear power accident at Chernobyl in 1986 caused more than 50 deaths, with estimated exposures of 50 to 300 rad. More than 20,000 people were exposed to up to 40 rem. As early as 1990, an increased incidence of thyroid cancer was seen in exposed children. Approximately 2 million people living near Three Mile Island were exposed to low doses of 100 mrem in 1979; no adverse effects have yet been reported. Workers in the nuclear energy industry and in health care and research are exposed annually to doses ranging from 1 to 9 mSv. The annual maximal permissible exposure level for these workers is 50 mSv or 1 rem. There is uncertainty about the potential carcinogenic risk at these low exposures because the shape of the dose–response curve is unknown.

The mechanisms responsible for the delayed carcinogenic effects of ionizing radiation are not completely understood. The latent period between acute exposure to ionizing radiation and the delayed appearance of cancer may be due to a phenomenon called *induced genetic instability.* Quantitative analysis of mutation rates in irradiated cells in culture shows that mutations continue to be expressed in surviving cells after several generations. Accumulation of these delayed mutations may be the result of persistent DNA lesions that are not repaired or due to an epigenetic mechanism, such as altered methylation at CpG sites or shortening of telomeres. Delayed chromosome aberrations are also observed after exposure to ionizing radiation, especially in human lymphocytes.[59] These mechanisms may be responsible for induction of secondary cancers, especially leukemias, in cancer patients treated with radiation therapy.

TABLE 9–18 Clinical Features of the Acute Radiation Syndrome

Category	Whole-Body Dose (rem)	Symptoms	Prognosis
Subclinical	<200	Mild nausea and vomiting Lymphocytes <1500/μL	100% survival
Hematopoietic	200–600	Intermittent nausea and vomiting Petechiae, hemorrhage Maximum neutrophil and platelet depression in 2 wk Lymphocytes <1000/μL	Infections May require bone marrow transplant
Gastrointestinal	600–1000	Nausea, vomiting, diarrhea Hemorrhage and infection in 1–3 wk Severe neutrophil and platelet depression Lymphocytes <500/μL	Shock and death in 10–14 days even with replacement therapy
Central nervous system	>1000	Intractable nausea and vomiting Confusion, somnolence, convulsions Coma in 15 min–3 hr Lymphocytes absent	Death in 14–36 hr

Clinical Manifestations of Exposure to Ionizing Radiation

The clinical effects of ionizing radiation depend on the dose, duration, and mode of exposure. These are described next.

Acute, Whole-Body Exposure. Whole-body irradiation is potentially lethal; the clinical manifestations are dose dependent and described as the *acute radiation syndrome* or *radiation sickness.* On the basis of calculated doses delivered in nuclear reactor accidents or the atomic bombing of Japan, the LD_{50} at 60 days for humans exposed to a single dose of x-rays or gamma radiation is 2.5 to 4.0 Gy (250 to 400 rad). Depending on the dose, four clinical syndromes are produced: a subclinical or prodromal syndrome, hematopoietic syndrome, gastrointestinal syndrome, or central nervous system syndrome. These are summarized in Table 9–18. The acute symptoms are manifestations of the high sensitivity of rapidly proliferating tissues, such as the lymphohematopoietic cells and gastrointestinal epithelium, to acute radiation-induced necrosis or apoptosis (Fig. 9–10). If the patient survives the acute radiation syndrome, sublethally injured cells may repair the radiation damage, and the necrotic or apoptotic cells may be replaced by the progeny of more radioresistant stem cells.

Effects of Radiation Therapy. External radiation is delivered to malignant neoplasms at fractionated doses up to 40 to 70 Gy (4000 to 7000 rad), with shielding of adjacent normal tissues. Radiation therapy, especially when it is delivered to the chest or abdomen, can cause acute radiation sickness and neutrophil and platelet depression. These patients may experience transient fatigue, vomiting, and anorexia that may require reduction of the dose. Acutely, radiation therapy may shrink the tumor mass and relieve pain or compression of adjacent tissues. Unfortunately, cancer patients treated with radiation therapy may develop sterility, a secondary malignant neoplasm, or delayed radiation injury (described later).[53]

Effects on Growth and Development. The developing fetus and young children are highly sensitive to growth and developmental abnormalities induced by ionizing radiation. Four susceptible phases can be defined:

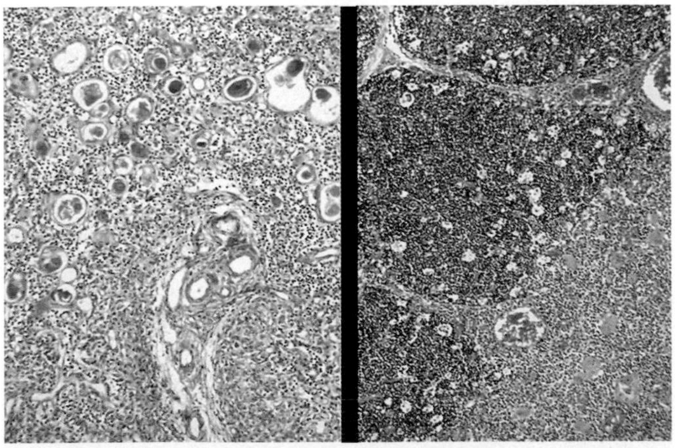

FIGURE 9–10 Atrophy of the thymus gland after exposure to ionizing radiation. The right panel shows a normal thymus with deeply staining cortex and pale staining medulla; the left panel shows depletion of lymphocytes with preservation of (pink, concentric) Hassall corpuscles. (American Registry of Pathology © 1990.)

- Preimplantation embryo. Before implantation, irradiation of the mother can be lethal to the embryo.
- Critical stages of organogenesis. From the time of implantation until 9 weeks of gestation, exposure of the mother even to diagnostic radiation can produce a wide range of congenital malformations. This is the period of maximal growth and differentiation in the developing fetus, when it is most susceptible to a wide range of teratogenic agents, as discussed in Chapter 10.
- Fetal period. From 9 weeks of gestation until birth, functional abnormalities of the central nervous system and reproductive system may be produced by maternal irradiation. The reproductive organs may be underdeveloped. Mental retardation affected offspring of Japanese mothers who were exposed to the atomic bomb in the first trimester of pregnancy. Newborns exposed to irradiation in utero have an increased incidence of childhood leukemia and brain tumors.
- Postnatal period. In infants and young children exposed to radiation, bone growth and maturation may be retarded. Development of the central nervous system, eyes, and teeth may also be perturbed. Although external radiation has been shown to shorten the life span of rodents, it is controversial whether ionizing radiation accelerates the process of aging in humans.

Induction of Mutations. *Drosophila* and laboratory mice show heritable mutations and chromosome abnormalities when exposed to ionizing radiation. Although chromosome aberrations have been demonstrated in the peripheral blood lymphocytes of atomic bomb survivors and radiation workers, there is no evidence so far that radiation-induced mutations have been transmitted to future generations. Geneticists are concerned, however, that recessive mutations induced by radiation may be accumulating in the human population. In addition, there are no dose–response data for the frequency of mutations induced by ionizing radiation in human germ cells.[53]

Delayed Radiation Injury. Months or years after irradiation, delayed complications, other than carcinogenesis, may occur. Radiation damage to the heart, lungs, central nervous system, or kidneys can be life threatening. Infertility can occur in men or women. Cataracts can impair vision, and excess connective tissue can cause intestinal obstruction. Fibrous strictures and chronic ulcers may affect the skin, gastrointestinal tract, urinary bladder, and vagina. Chronic vascular insufficiency and excess connective tissue also complicate subsequent surgical procedures. Wound healing is impaired, and infections are more common. Unfortunately, cancer patients who have received fractionated doses of radiation may also suffer from these delayed complications. The following tissues are the most vulnerable sites of delayed radiation injury:

- **Blood vessels.** After an initial inflammatory reaction that may be accompanied by death of endothelial cells (Fig. 9–11), blood vessels in the field of irradiation show subintimal fibrosis, fibrosis of the muscle wall, degeneration of the internal elastic lamina, and severe narrowing of the lumen (Fig. 9–12). Capillaries may become thrombosed and obliterated or ectatic. The organs supplied by these

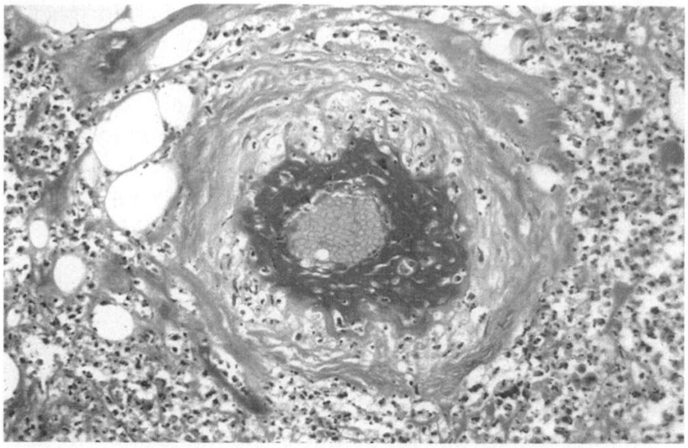

FIGURE 9–11 Acute vascular injury with fibrinoid necrosis and edema after exposure to ionizing radiation. (American Registry of Pathology © 1990.)

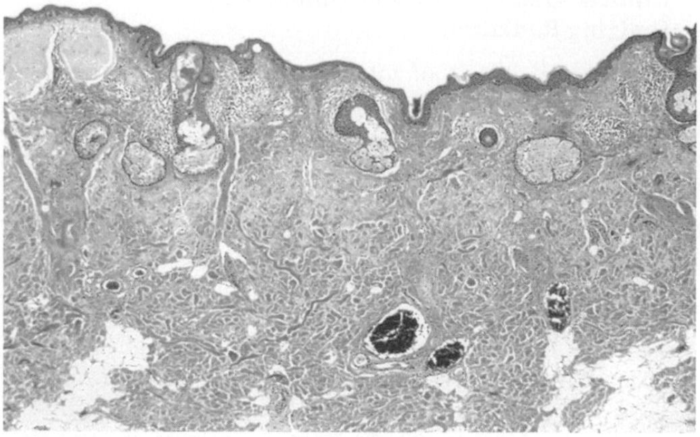

FIGURE 9–13 Chronic radiation dermatitis with atrophy of the epidermis, dermal fibrosis, and telangiectasia of the subcutaneous blood vessels. (American Registry of Pathology © 1990.)

damaged vessels will show ischemic changes, atrophy, and fibrosis.

- **Skin**. Hair follicles and the epidermis are sensitive to acute radiation-induced injury. Desquamation can occur, resulting in replacement of the normal epidermis by atrophic epidermis characterized by hyperkeratosis, hyperpigmentation, and hypopigmentation. The subcutaneous vessels may be weakened and dilated; they are surrounded by dense bands of collagen in the dermis (Fig. 9–13). Impaired healing, increased susceptibility to infection, and ulceration may occur. These changes are called *radiation dermatitis.* As described earlier, skin cancer, especially basal cell and squamous cell carcinomas, may occur as long as 20 years after exposure.
- **Heart**. Radiotherapy delivered to the chest for malignant lymphoma, lung cancer, or breast cancer may damage the heart and pericardium. Fibrosis of the pericardium can cause constrictive pericarditis (Fig. 9–14). Less commonly, radiation-induced injury of capillaries and the coronary arteries can cause myocardial ischemia and fibrosis.
- **Lungs**. The lungs are highly susceptible to radiation-induced injury, leading to acute lung injury and delayed radiation pneumonitis. Delayed injury causes dyspnea, chronic cough, and diminished lung function. This is caused by intra-alveolar and interstitial fibrosis. Both internal and external irradiation increase the incidence of lung cancer; this effect is synergistic with cigarette smoking. In addition to carcinogenic chemicals, cigarette smoke contains two radionuclides: lead 210 and polonium 210. Underground miners are exposed to radon 222, which increases their risk of developing lung cancer. Lung cancers that develop in underground miners have a characteristic mutation (G → T) at codon 249 of the *p53* tumor-suppressor gene.[60]
- **Kidneys and urinary bladder**. The kidneys are moderately susceptible to radiation-induced injury. Delayed peritubular fibrosis, vascular damage, and hyalinization of glomeruli develop gradually, leading to hypertension and atrophy. The urinary bladder is sensitive to radiation injury, with

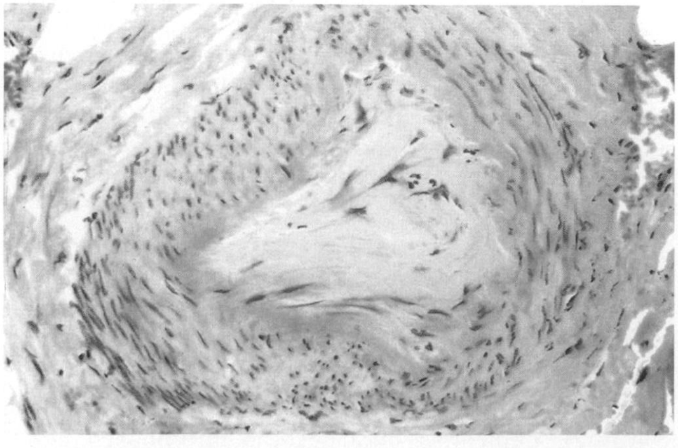

FIGURE 9–12 Chronic vascular injury with subintimal fibrosis occluding the lumen. (American Registry of Pathology © 1990.)

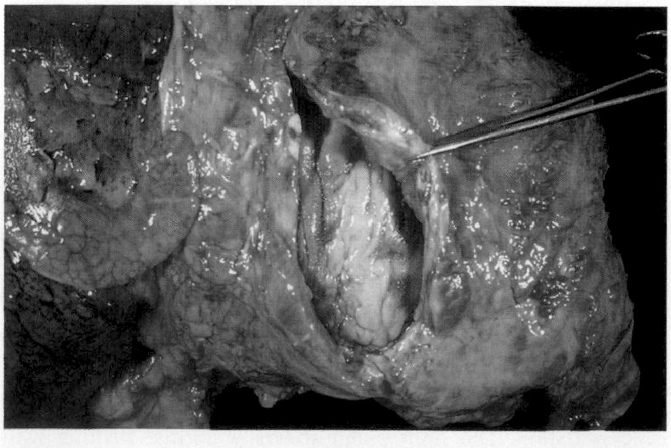

FIGURE 9–14 Extensive mediastinal fibrosis after radiotherapy for carcinoma of the lung. Note the markedly thickened pericardium. (From the teaching collection of the Department of Pathology, Southwestern Medical School, Dallas, TX.)

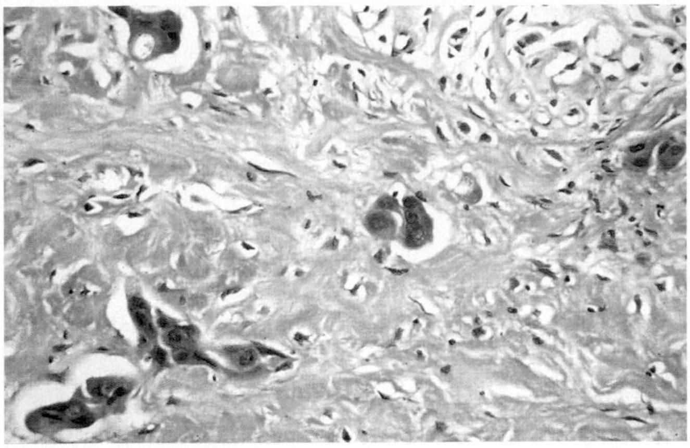

FIGURE 9–15 Radiation fibrosis of the breast stroma after radiotherapy for infiltrating ductal carcinoma. The nests of remaining tumor cells are pleomorphic and multinucleated. (American Registry of Pathology © 1990.)

acute necrosis of the epithelium followed by submucosal fibrosis, contracture, bleeding, and ulceration. Tumors of the bladder and kidney have been reported in Japanese atomic bomb survivors and in women irradiated for treatment of cervical carcinoma.

- **Gastrointestinal tract.** Esophagitis, gastritis, enteritis, colitis, and proctitis can result from irradiation. These are associated with exfoliation of the epithelial mucosa, susceptibility to infection, and loss of electrolytes and fluid. Delayed injury to small blood vessels causes chronic ischemia, ulceration and atrophy of the mucosa, and fibrosis that can cause strictures and obstruction.
- **Breast.** Diagnostic doses of ionizing radiation administered during adolescence increase the incidence of breast cancer after 15 to 20 years. Radiotherapy for breast cancer causes a dense, fibrotic reaction with extreme pleomorphism of epithelial cells (Fig. 9–15).
- **Ovary and testis.** The spermatogonia are extremely sensitive to irradiation; even low doses may cause suppression of meiosis and infertility. Blood vessels may be obliterated and the seminiferous tubules become fibrotic, leaving the Sertoli cells and interstitial Leydig cells intact. Ovarian follicles degenerate acutely after irradiation; usually a few primordial oocytes and their follicular epithelium remain scattered in a fibrous stroma.
- **Eyes and central nervous system.** The lens is sensitive to ionizing radiation, and hence radiation gives rise to cataracts; the retinal and ciliary arteries may also be damaged. The brain may show focal necrosis and demyelination of the white matter. Irradiation of the spinal cord can damage small blood vessels, leading to necrosis, demyelination, and paraplegia. This is called *transverse myelitis.*

Ultraviolet Radiation

Solar radiation spans the spectrum of wavelengths between 200 and 4000 nm, including ultraviolet, visible, and infrared radiation. Ultraviolet radiation is divided into ultraviolet A (UVA), ultraviolet B (UVB), and ultraviolet C (UVC); 3% to 5% of the total solar radiation that penetrates the earth's surface is ultraviolet radiation. Ozone in the atmosphere is an important protective agent against ultraviolet radiation because it completely absorbs all UVC and partially absorbs UVB. Chlorofluorocarbons, used commercially as propellants, as solvents, and in refrigerators and air conditioners, interact with and deplete ozone. Such depletion is predicted to contribute to an increase in UVB and possibly UVC exposure, thus triggering a 2% to 4% increase in the incidence of skin cancers. Some protection from the effects of UV light is afforded by window glasses: they absorb UVB radiation, but they transmit UVA radiation. Sunblocks and sunscreens offer greater protection because they absorb or block UVB and UVA to variable degrees. There are two major health effects of ultraviolet radiation: premature aging of the skin and skin cancer (Table 9–19). The carcinogenic effects of ultraviolet light are discussed in Chapter 7. Here we focus on other effects of ultraviolet radiation.

The acute effects of UVA and UVB are short-lived and reversible. They include erythema, pigmentation, and injury to Langerhans cells and keratinocytes in the epidermis. The kinetics and chemical mediators of these reactions differ in response to UVA and UVB. Depending on the intensity and length of exposure, erythema, edema, and acute inflammation are mediated by release of histamine from mast cells in the dermis, synthesis of arachidonic acid metabolites, and the production of pro-inflammatory cytokines like IL-1. UVA produces oxidation of melanin with transient, immediate

TABLE 9–19 Acute and Delayed Effects of Ultraviolet Radiation

Radiation	Wavelength (nm)	Acute Effects	Delayed Effects
UVA	320–400	Erythema 8–48 hr Depletion of Langerhans cells Pigment darkening Dermal inflammation	Tanning ? Skin cancer
UVB	290–320	Erythema 3–24 hr Apoptosis of keratinocytes Depletion of Langerhans cells	Tanning Solar elastosis Premature aging Actinic keratosis Skin cancer
UVC	200–290		? Skin cancer

Data from Rosen CF: Ultraviolet radiation. In Craighead JE (ed): Pathology of Environmental and Occupational Disease. St. Louis, Mosby–Year Book, 1996, p. 193.

darkening, especially in individuals with darker skin. Tanning induced by UVA and UVB is due to a delayed increase in the number of melanocytes, elongation and extension of dendritic processes, and transfer of melanin to keratinocytes. Tanning induced by UVB is protective against subsequent exposures; tanning induced by UVA provides limited protection. Both UVA and UVB deplete Langerhans cells and thus reduce the processing of antigens introduced through the epidermis. UVB causes apoptosis of keratinocytes in the epidermis, resulting in dyskeratotic, sunburn cells.

Repeated exposures to ultraviolet radiation give rise to changes in the skin that are characteristic of premature aging (e.g., wrinkling, solar elastosis, and irregularities in pigmentation). In contrast to ionizing radiation that increases deposition of collagen in the dermis, ultraviolet radiation causes degenerative changes in elastin and collagen, leading to wrinkling, increased laxity, and a leathery appearance. These connective tissue alterations accumulate over time and are largely irreversible. They are caused by increased expression of the elastin gene, increased expression of matrix metalloproteinases that degrade collagen, and induction of a tissue inhibitor of matrix metalloproteinase. The end result of these changes in connective tissue enzymes is degradation of type I collagen fibrils and disorganization and degeneration of the dermal connective tissue[61] (Fig. 9–16).

Skin damage induced by UVB is believed to be caused by the generation of reactive oxygen species and by damage to endogenous chromophores such as melanin. Ultraviolet radiation also damages DNA, resulting in the formation of pyrimidine dimers between adjacent pyrimidines on the same DNA strand. Other forms of DNA damage, for example, formation of pyrimidine–pyrimidone (6-4) photoproducts, single-stranded breaks, and DNA–protein cross-links, are also noted.[61] A unique spectrum of mutations has been identified in premalignant and malignant skin lesions in humans, involving adjacent pyrimidine bases in *p53*: C→T or CC→TT double-base substitutions. This observation provides strong evidence for an etiologic role of ultraviolet light in induction of skin cancer.

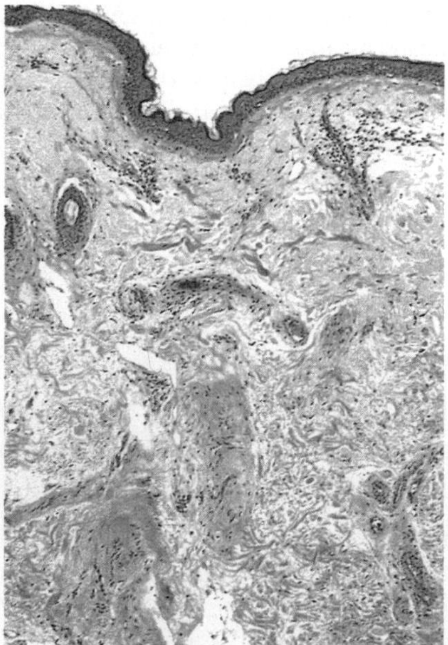

FIGURE 9–16 Solar elastosis with basophilic degeneration of the connective tissue in the upper layer of the dermis. (American Registry of Pathology © 1990.)

Exposure to UV radiation induces a series of molecular changes collectively referred to as the *ultraviolet response pathway*. The triggering of this pathway involves activation of *RAS* signalling with activation of mitogenactivated protein kinases and induction of cellular protooncogenes and other genes involved in cell proliferation. This effect is believed to be independent of DNA damage. Subsequently, thymidine dinucleotides produced by ultraviolet radiation activate the *p53* pathway in a manner analogous to DNA breaks produced by ionizing radiation. Thus, exposure to ultraviolet radiation can induce a protective cellular response leading to DNA repair, cell-cycle arrest, or apoptosis, depending on the intensity of exposure and the sensitivity of the target cell. The importance of DNA repair as a defense mechanism against skin cancer is illustrated by increased susceptibility of patients with xeroderma pigmentosum to ultraviolet light–induced skin cancers (Chapter 7).

Electromagnetic Fields

Nonionizing electromagnetic fields range from less than 1 cycle/second (Hertz, or Hz) for DC power lines up to 100 GHz for long-distance microwaves and radar.[63] There is public concern that residential exposure to ambient 50- to 60-Hz magnetic fields is a health threat that may contribute to an increased incidence of leukemia in children. However, epidemiologic studies have failed to establish a significant relationship between residential electromagnetic fields and an increased incidence of childhood leukemia except perhaps at very high exposures. Occupational exposures at higher levels have also not consistently been associated with an increased risk of leukemia, brain cancer, breast cancer, or neurodegenerative disease.[64] Animal studies have not provided any evidence for a causal relationship between exposure to electromagnetic fields and brain cancer.[65] Thus, cell phone users can be assured that going wireless is unlikely to predispose them to the development of brain tumors.

PHYSICAL ENVIRONMENT

Trauma, with its associated death and disability, remain a major public health problem in modern industrialized societies. Unintentional injuries, including motor vehicle accidents, homicide, and suicide, are the leading causes of death for adolescents and adults up to age 44 in the United States (Table 9–20). Identification of risk factors and the factors responsible for the racial and ethnic differences shown in the table are important for the prevention of these premature, tragic deaths. Physicians and health care personnel play an important role in educating their patients about potential risk factors and in encouraging active preventive strategies. For example, motor vehicles are a major cause of injury: approximately 40% of deaths resulting from motor vehicle accidents involve ethanol. Physicians can discourage their patients from drinking and driving, encourage the use of seat belts, air bags, and safety seats for infants and children, and discourage the use of cell phones while driving. Violence, in association with use of firearms, drug and alcohol use, and physical and mental

TABLE 9–20 Adult Mortality Rates in the United States, Ages 25–44, in 1998

	Rate per 100,000 population		
Cause	*Hispanic*	*Black*	*White*
Unintentional injuries	33.4	40.1	31.6
Cancer	16.8	38.0	25.3
Homicide	13.1	36.2	4.7
Human immunodeficiency virus	12.1	43.3	4.8
Heart disease	10.3	43.5	18.3
Suicide	7.8	—	17.0
Total	130.2	303.7	139.4

Data from CDC Fact Book, 2000/2001, Department of Health and Human Services, Centers for Disease Control and Prevention.

abuse, is a major concern in the United States. Hence, firearm safety and access are important matters of public health.[66]

Injuries caused by the physical environment, resulting from human activities as well as from external forces, can be divided into four categories: mechanical force, heat and cold, electrical injuries, and high altitudes.

Mechanical Force

Mechanical force may inflict soft-tissue injuries, bone injuries, and head injuries. Injuries of the bones and of the head are considered in Chapter 28. Soft-tissue injuries can be superficial, involving mainly the skin, or deep, associated with visceral damage. The skin injuries can be further described as follows.

Abrasion. This type of skin injury represents basically a scrape, in which the superficial epidermis is torn off by friction or force (Fig. 9–17). Regeneration without scarring usually occurs promptly unless infection complicates the process.

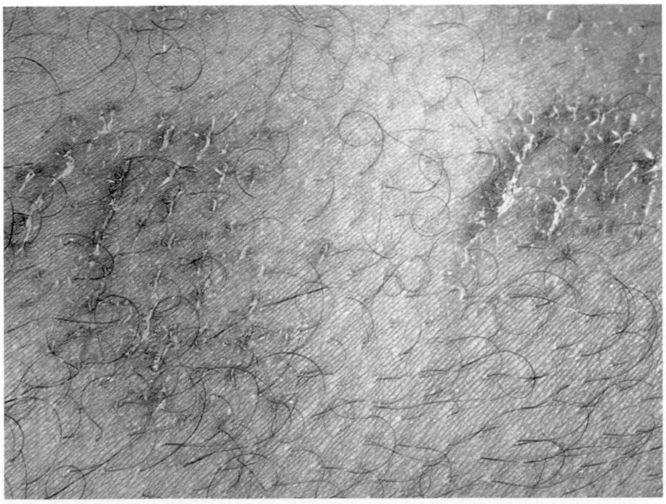

FIGURE 9–17 Abrasion. Note the superficial tears in the epidermis. There is bleeding under the skin as well. (From the teaching collection of the Department of Pathology, Southwestern Medical School, Dallas, TX.)

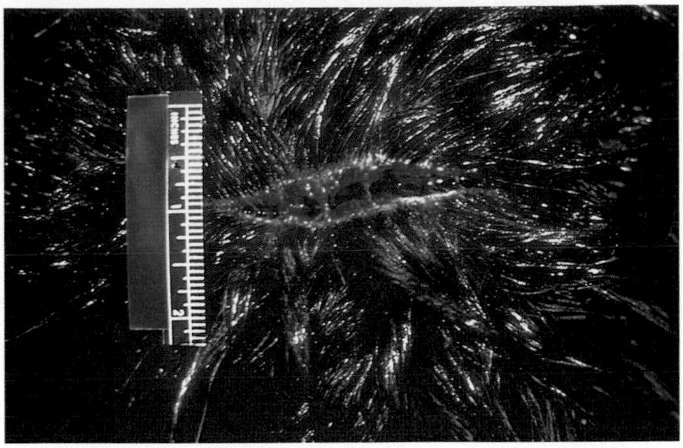

FIGURE 9–18 Laceration of the scalp. The bridging strands of the fibrous tissue are evident. (From the teaching collection of the Department of Pathology, Southwestern Medical School, Dallas, TX.)

Laceration Versus Incision. A laceration is an irregular tear in the skin produced by overstretching. It may be linear or stellate, depending on the tearing force. Typical of a laceration are the bridging strands of fibrous tissue or blood vessels across the wound, not seen in an incision (Fig. 9–18). The immediate margins of the laceration are frequently hemorrhagic and traumatized. In contrast, an incision is made by a sharp cutting object, such as a knife (scalpel) or a piece of glass. The margins of the incision are usually relatively clean, and there are no bridging strands of tissue. The incision, in contrast with the laceration, can usually be neatly approximated by sutures, leaving little or no scar. Deep tissues and organs may sustain lacerations from an external blow with or without apparent superficial injury. For example, when the unrestrained body impacts on the steering wheel in a head-on collision, the liver or spleen may sustain fatal lacerations.

Contusion. This is an injury caused by a blunt force that damages small blood vessels and causes interstitial bleeding, usually without disruption of the continuity of the tissue (Fig. 9–19). With superficial contusions, the bleeding is usually

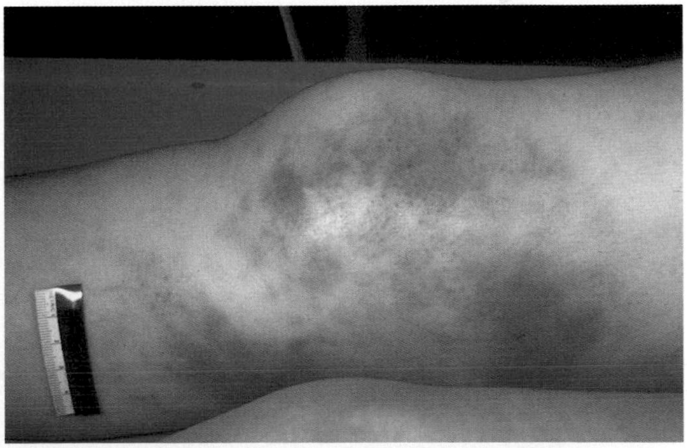

FIGURE 9–19 Contusion resulting from blunt trauma. The skin is intact, but there is hemorrhage in subcutaneous vessels, producing extensive discoloration. (From the teaching collection of the Department of Pathology, Southwestern Medical School, Dallas, TX.)

evident almost at once, but with deeper contusions, of skeletal muscle, for example, the bleeding may not be evident for many hours and may leave only swelling and tenderness at the site. Older individuals with small-vessel fragility may sustain extensive hematomas at contused sites.

Gunshot Wounds. Injuries of this nature fall largely into the domain of forensic pathology, a specialty dealing with trauma and medicolegal issues. The character of a gunshot wound at entry and exit and the extent of injury depend on the type of gun used (handgun or rifle) and on a large number of variables, including the caliber of the bullet, the type of ammunition, the distance of the firearm from the body, the locus of the injury, the trajectory of the missile (at right angles to the skin or oblique), and the gyroscopic stability of the bullet (the presence or absence of wobbling or tumbling).

With handguns held at close range (within a foot of the skin surface), there is a gray-black discoloration about the wound of entrance (fouling) produced by the heat, smoke, and burned powder deposits exiting with the bullet from the muzzle. In addition, there may be discrete, larger particles of unburned powder producing a halo of stippling about the entrance wound, the diameter of which depends on the distance of the gun from the body. When firearms are held more than a foot away, but within 3 feet, there may be only stippling without fouling. At greater distances, neither is present (Fig. 9–20). In general, the perforating cutaneous wound is slightly smaller than the diameter of the bullet and has a narrow enclosing rim of abrasion. When the trajectory of the bullet is angled into the skin, the abrasion is asymmetric, having its greatest width at the margin closest to the origin of the bullet. Depending on the size and velocity of the bullet and the distance between the target and the muzzle to the firearm, when the skin is closely applied to underlying bone as in the scalp, entering gas may elevate the overlying skin and, in some instances, produce stellate lacerations about the perforating wound. Similarly, large-caliber, high-velocity missiles, after penetrating the skin and subcutaneous tissues, may traverse internal organs and, by their mass and velocity, cause extending massive lacerations through the liver or other viscera. In contrast, smaller, low-velocity bullets, even though they penetrate the organ, may produce only fairly restricted burrowing or through-and-through tracts with limited surrounding injury.

Cutaneous exit wounds are generally more irregular than are wounds of entrance, because in passing through the tissues, the bullet almost inevitably develops a wobbling trajectory. In fact, with high-velocity rifle bullets, the exit wound may be considerably larger than the entrance wound. The margins of the wound may be everted, and there is no fouling or stippling and often little surrounding abrasion. To the experienced eye, it is evident that gunshot wounds tell a story.

Thermal Injuries

Both excess heat and excess cold are important causes of injury. Burns are all too common and are discussed first; a brief discussion of hyperthermia and hypothermia follows.

Thermal Burns. In the United States, burns cause 5000 deaths per year and result in the hospitalization of more than ten times that many persons. Many victims are children, who are often scalded by hot liquids. Fortunately, marked decreases have been seen in both mortality rates and length of hospitalizations since the 1970s. This improved prognosis results from a better understanding of the systemic effects of massive burns and discoveries of better ways to prevent wound infection and facilitate healing of skin surfaces.

The clinical significance of burns depends on the following important factors:

- Depth of the burn
- Percentage of body surface involved
- Possible presence of internal injuries from inhalation of hot and toxic fumes
- Promptness and efficacy of therapy, especially fluid and electrolyte management and prevention or control of wound infections.

A *full-thickness burn* involves total destruction of the epidermis and dermis, with loss of the dermal appendages that would have provided cells for epithelial regeneration. Both *third-* and *fourth-degree burns* are in this category. In *partial-*

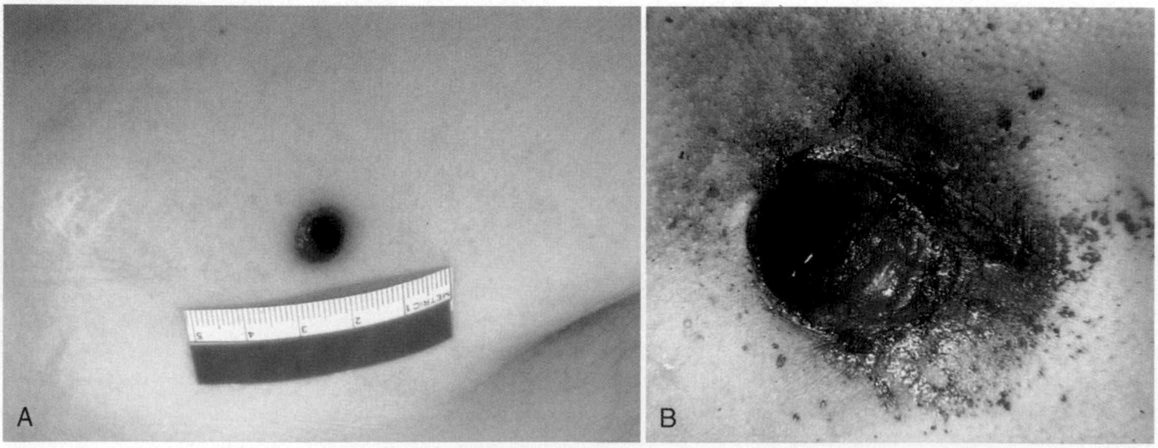

FIGURE 9–20 *A,* Gunshot wound of entry from a long distance. (From the teaching collection of the Department of Pathology, Southwestern Medical School, Dallas, TX.) *B,* An entry gunshot wound at close range revealing the prominent black discoloration produced by unburned powder, heat, and smoke as well as the more peripheral stippling resulting from larger particles of unburned powder. (Courtesy of George Katsas, MD, Forensic Pathologist, Boston, MA.)

thickness burns, at least the deeper portions of the dermal appendages are spared. Partial-thickness burns include *first-degree burns* (epithelial involvement only) and *second-degree burns* (both epidermis and superficial dermis).

Morphology. On gross inspection, full-thickness burns are white or charred, dry, and anesthetic (because of nerve ending destruction); depending on the depth, partial-thickness burns are pink or mottled with blisters and are painful. On histologic examination, devitalized tissue demonstrates coagulative necrosis; adjacent vital tissue quickly develops inflammatory changes with an accumulation of inflammatory cells and marked exudation.

Despite continuous improvement in therapy, any burn exceeding 50% of the total body surface, whether superficial or deep, is grave and potentially fatal. With burns of more than 20% of the body surface, there is a rapid shift of body fluids into the interstitial compartments, both at the burn site and systemically, which can result in hypovolemic shock (Chapter 4). The mechanisms include an increase in local interstitial osmotic pressure (from release of osmotically active constituents of dying cells) and both neurogenic and mediator-induced increases in vascular permeability. Because protein from the blood is lost into interstitial tissue, generalized edema, including pulmonary edema, may become severe if fluids used for volume replacement are not osmotically active.

Another important consideration in patients with burns is the degree of *injury to the airways and lungs.* Inhalation injury is frequent in persons trapped in burning buildings and may result from the direct effect of heat on the mouth, nose, and upper airways or from the inhalation of toxic components in smoke. Water-soluble gases such as chlorine, sulfur oxides, and ammonia may react with water to form acids or alkalis, particularly in the upper airways, to produce inflammation and swelling, which may lead to partial or complete airway obstruction. Lipid-soluble gases such as nitrous oxide and products of burning plastics are more likely to reach deeper airways, producing pneumonitis. Unlike shock, which develops within hours, pulmonary manifestations may not develop for 24 to 48 hours. Thus, the initial absence of respiratory symptoms does not necessarily imply that there has been no respiratory injury.

Secondary *infection* is an important complication in all burn patients who have lost epidermis. Organ system failure resulting from sepsis continues to be the leading cause of death in burn patients. The burn site is ideal for growth of microorganisms: serum and debris provide nutrients, and the burn injury compromises blood flow, blocking effective inflammatory responses. Furthermore, cellular and humoral defenses against infections are compromised, and both lymphocyte and phagocyte functions are impaired. The most common offender is the opportunist *Pseudomonas aeruginosa*, but antibiotic-resistant strains of other common hospital-acquired bacteria, such as *S. aureus*, and fungi, particularly *Candida* species, may also be involved. Direct bacteremic spread and release of toxic substances such as endotoxin from the local site exert dire consequences. Pneumonia or septic shock with renal failure and the acute respiratory distress syndrome (Chapter 15) are the most common serious sequelae. Aggressive, early debridement of burn wounds is designed not only to provide a clean, vascular surface on which wound repair can proceed, but also to provide phagocytes ready access to infecting microorganisms. Topical antibiotics may help, but burn infection continues to be an important problem.

Another important pathophysiologic effect of burns is the *development of a hypermetabolic state* with excess heat loss and an increased need for nutritional support. It is estimated that when more than 40% of the body surface is burned, the resting metabolic rate may approach twice normal. The consequence is breakdown of tissue, which may result in loss of essential protein stores, reaching lethal proportions comparable to starvation within several weeks. Thus, it is essential to keep the patient's room temperature elevated to reduce body heat loss and to implement appropriate nutritional supplementation.

Hyperthermia. Prolonged exposure to elevated ambient temperatures can result in heat cramps, heat exhaustion, and heat stroke.

- *Heat cramps* result from loss of electrolytes through sweating. Cramping of voluntary muscles, usually in association with vigorous exercise, is the hallmark. Heat-dissipating mechanisms are able to maintain normal core body temperature.
- *Heat exhaustion* is probably the most common heat syndrome. Its onset is sudden, with prostration and collapse, and it results from a failure of the cardiovascular system to compensate for hypovolemia, secondary to water depletion. After a period of collapse, which is usually brief, equilibrium is spontaneously re-established.
- *Heat stroke* is associated with high ambient temperatures and high humidity. Thermoregulatory mechanisms fail, sweating ceases, and core body temperature rises. Body temperatures of 112° to 113°F have been recorded in some terminal cases. Clinically, a rectal temperature of 106°F or higher is considered a grave prognostic sign, and the mortality rate for such patients exceeds 50%. The underlying mechanism is marked generalized peripheral vasodilation with peripheral pooling of blood and a decreased effective circulating blood volume. Necrosis of the muscles and myocardium may occur. Arrhythmias, disseminated intravascular coagulation, and other systemic effects are common. Elderly persons, individuals undergoing intense physical stress (including young athletes and military recruits), and persons with cardiovascular disease are prime candidates for heat stroke.

Hypothermia. Prolonged exposure to low ambient temperature leads to hypothermia, a condition seen all too frequently in homeless persons. Lowering of body temperature is hastened by high humidity in cold, wet clothing and dilation of superficial blood vessels as a result of the ingestion of alcohol. At about 90°F, loss of consciousness occurs, followed by bradycardia and atrial fibrillation at lower core temperatures.

Local Reactions. Chilling or freezing of cells and tissues causes injury in two ways:

1. Direct effects are probably mediated by physical disruption of organelles within cells and high salt concentrations incident to the crystallization of the intracellular and extracellular water.

2. Indirect effects are exerted by circulatory changes. Depending on the rate at which the temperature drops and the duration of the drop, slowly developing chilling may induce vasoconstriction and increased permeability, leading to edematous changes. Such changes are typical of "trench foot." Atrophy and fibrosis may follow. Alternatively, with sudden sharp drops in temperature that are persistent, the vasoconstriction and increased viscosity of the blood in the local area may cause ischemic injury and degenerative changes in peripheral nerves. In this situation, only after the temperature begins to return toward normal do the vascular injury and increased permeability with exudation become evident. However, during the period of ischemia, hypoxic changes and infarction of the affected tissues may develop (e.g., gangrene of toes or feet).

Electrical Injuries

The passage of an electric current through the body may be without effect; may cause sudden death by disruption of neural regulatory impulses, producing, for example, cardiac arrest; or may cause thermal injury to organs interposed in the pathway of the current. Many variables are involved, but most important are the resistance of the tissues to the conductance of the electric current and the intensity of the current. The greater the resistance of tissues, the greater the heat generated. Although all tissues of the body are conductors of electricity, their resistance to flow varies inversely with their water content. Dry skin is particularly resistant, but when skin is wet or immersed in water, its resistance is greatly decreased. Thus, an electric current may cause only a surface burn of dry skin but may cause death by disruption of regulatory pathways when it is transmitted through wet skin, producing, for example, ventricular fibrillation or respiratory paralysis without injury to the skin.

The thermal effects of the passage of the electric current depend on its intensity. High-intensity current, such as lightning coursing along the skin, produces linear arborizing burns known as *lightning marks.* Sometimes intense current is conducted around the victim (so-called *flashover*), blasting and disrupting the clothing but doing little injury. When lightning is transmitted internally, it may produce sufficient heat and steam to explode solid organs, fracture bones, or char areas of organs. Focal hemorrhages from rupture of small vessels may be seen in the brain. Sometimes, death is preceded by violent convulsions related to brain damage. Less intense voltage may heat, coagulate, or rupture vessels and cause hemorrhages or, in solid organs such as the spleen and kidneys, cause infarctions or ruptures.

Injuries Related to Changes in Atmospheric Pressure

Depending on the direction of change (increase or decrease) in atmospheric pressure, its rate of development, and the magnitude of change, four syndromes can be produced:

- High-altitude illness
- Blast injury
- Decompression disease—also known as *caisson disease*—which is sometimes referred to as barotrauma.

High-Altitude Illness. As is well known, this is encountered in mountain climbers in the rarefied atmosphere of altitudes above 4000 m. The lowered oxygen tension produces progressive mental obtundation and may be accompanied by poorly understood increased capillary permeability with systemic and, in particular, pulmonary edema.

Blast Injury. This form of injury obviously implies a violent increase in pressure either in the atmosphere (air blast) or in water (immersion blast). With *air blast,* the compression wave impinges on the side toward the explosion and so may collapse the thorax or violently compress the abdomen, with rupture of internal organs. The pressure wave may enter the airways and damage the alveoli. The following wave of decreased pressure, with its sudden expansion of the abdomen and thorax, may rupture the intestines or lungs. In *immersion blast,* the pressure is supplied to the body from all sides, inducing injuries similar to those of air blast.

Decompression (Caisson) Disease. As the name implies, this disorder is encountered in deep-sea divers and underwater workers who spend long periods in caissons or tunnels, under increased atmospheric pressure. The injury, encountered with too rapid decompression, is a function of Henry's law, which in essence states that the solubility of a gas in a liquid (e.g., blood) is proportional to the partial pressure of that gas in the environment. As the underwater depth and consequent atmospheric pressure increase, increasing amounts of oxygen and accompanying gases (nitrogen or helium) dissolve in the blood and tissue fluids. Once ascent begins (decompression), the dissolved gases come out of solution and form minute bubbles in the bloodstream and tissues. Coalescence of these bubbles produces even larger masses capable of becoming significant emboli in the bloodstream. The oxygen bubbles are soluble in blood and tissues and so redissolve. The nitrogen and helium dissolve only slowly. Periarticular bubbles produce the *bends.* Bubbles formed within the lung or gaseous emboli give rise to respiratory difficulties, with severe substernal pain referred to as the *chokes.* Various central nervous system manifestations may appear, ranging from headache and visual disturbances to behavioral disorientation. Involvement of the inner ear may produce vertigo and the *staggers.* All these manifestations may appear within hours of the too rapid ascent, but skeletal manifestations—*caisson disease of bone*—may sometimes appear days later. These take the form of foci of aseptic necrosis, typically of femoral and humeral heads, and medullary foci, particularly in the lower femur and upper tibia, attributed to embolic occlusion of the vascular supply.

Nutrition and Disease

FOOD SAFETY: ADDITIVES AND CONTAMINANTS

Food is essential for life, yet it contains numerous natural constituents and additives that may threaten human health. This mixture of natural compounds and chemical additives is the most complex and variable environmental exposure that humans experience. A wide range of chemicals are natural constituents of foods, including carcinogens such as safrole in nutmeg and parsley and estragole in basil and fennel. Coffee contains more than 200 compounds, including tannins that may be carcinogenic. Natural pesticides are also found in plants, for example, 5- and 8-methoxypsoralen in celery, parsnips, and parsley.[67] Some scientists contend that natural plant pesticides and carcinogens are a greater threat to humans than are agricultural pesticide residues or industrial toxicants. Food may be contaminated by natural toxicants or microorganisms, for example, the liver carcinogen aflatoxin B_1 or the deadly botulinum toxin. Contamination with pathogenic viruses and bacteria continues to threaten public health. Hepatitis A virus, *Salmonella enteritidis, Escherichia coli, Listeria monocytogenes, Campylobacter,* and *Cryptosporidium* are common examples of food-borne infections. Additional toxicants can be generated in foods during preservation or preparation. Broiling meat produces oxidized fats, pyrolysis products of amino acids, and carcinogenic polycyclic aromatic hydrocarbons. Foods preserved by smoking or by nitrate and nitrite additives may contain precursors of *N*-nitrosamines. These chemicals are potent carcinogens in many animal species, producing cancers of the mouth, esophagus, larynx, liver, and kidney.[67]

Additional chemicals are added to foods either directly (chemical sweeteners, preservatives, food colors) or indirectly. Indirect additives include residues of drugs or hormones fed to animals, agricultural pesticides, industrial contaminants, and residues from food packaging. Low levels of metals such as mercury and lead, PCBs, and chlorinated hydrocarbons are present in our food supply. Other metals, such as arsenic and cadmium, may be natural contaminants of water and soil in some geographic locations. The Food and Drug Administration monitors the levels of pesticides, metals, and industrial contaminants in food samples in the United States. The level of some contaminants, such as dieldrin, approaches the acceptable daily intake that has been established as a safe threshold dose. Despite the considerable concern about additives and contaminants, regulation of their content in food is complicated by the detection limit of potential carcinogens, reliance on toxicologic assays using high doses of chemicals in rodents, and uncertainties in extrapolation of risk for humans under lifetime exposures at low doses.[67]

NUTRITIONAL DEFICIENCIES

Although the potential health hazards associated with food additives and contaminants are of concern, much more significant are the global health problems associated with inadequate nutrition. In third world countries, undernutrition or protein–energy malnutrition (PEM) continues to be common; in industrialized societies, the most frequent diseases (atherosclerosis, cancer, diabetes, and hypertension) have all been linked to some form of dietary impropriety.

An adequate diet should provide: (1) energy, in the form of carbohydrates, fats, and proteins; (2) essential (as well as nonessential) amino acids and fatty acids to be used as building blocks for synthesis of structural and functional proteins and lipids; and (3) vitamins and minerals, which function as coenzymes or hormones in vital metabolic pathways or, as in the case of calcium and phosphate, as important structural components.

In *primary malnutrition*, one or all of these components are missing from the diet. By contrast, in *secondary* or *conditional malnutrition*, the supply of nutrients is adequate, but malnutrition may result from nutrient malabsorption, impaired nutrient use or storage, excess nutrient losses, or increased need for nutrients.

In developing nations, the incidence of overt hunger is high, and the incidence of more subtle forms of undernutrition is even higher. Vitamin A deficiencies are rampant in certain parts of Africa, iodine deficiencies occur in regions where iodized salt is not available, and iron deficiency is often seen in infants fed exclusively milk diets. Thus, ignorance about the nutritional value of foods also plays an important role in malnutrition. In the United States, the National Research Council recommends daily allowances for protein, vitamins, and minerals for healthy adults, specifying ranges for both men and women. These standards represent the scientifically based general consensus of the safe (not minimal) amounts of each nutrient necessary to maintain good health. Debates continue as to optimal levels of fat and fiber to prevent cardiovascular disease and cancer, and this subject is briefly discussed later.

Affluent societies are not immune to a significant incidence of undernutrition. The following listing of common causes in the United States highlights this point:

- *Ignorance and poverty.* Homeless persons, aged individuals, and children of the poor demonstrate effects of PEM as well as trace nutrient deficiencies. Even the affluent may fail to recognize that infants, adolescents, and pregnant women have increased nutritional needs.
- *Chronic alcoholism.* Alcoholics may sometimes suffer PEM but are more frequently deficient in several vitamins, especially thiamine, pyridoxine, folate, and vitamin A, owing to a combination of dietary deficiency, defective gastrointestinal absorption, abnormal nutrient use and storage, increased metabolic needs, and an increased rate of loss. A failure to recognize the likelihood of thiamine deficiency in chronic alcoholics may result in irreversible brain damage (e.g., Korsakoff psychosis, discussed later).
- *Acute and chronic illnesses.* The basal metabolic rate becomes accelerated in many illnesses (in patients with extensive burns, it may double), resulting in an increased daily requirement for all nutrients. Failure to appreciate this fact can compromise recovery.
- *Self-imposed dietary restriction.* Anorexia nervosa, bulimia nervosa, and less overt eating disorders affect a large population of individuals who are concerned about body image or suffer from an unreasonable fear of cardiovascular disease.

Other, less common causes of malnutrition include the malabsorption syndromes, genetic diseases, specific drug therapies (which block uptake or use of particular nutrients), and total parenteral nutrition.

In the sections that follow, we barely skim the surface of nutritional disorders. Included in the discussion are PEM, deficiencies of most of the vitamins and trace minerals, obesity, and a brief overview of the relationships of diet to atherosclerosis and cancer. Several other nutrients and nutritional issues are discussed in the context of specific disorders throughout the text.

Protein–Energy Malnutrition

Severe PEM is a disastrous disease. It is far too common in third world countries, where up to 25% of children may be affected; in these countries, it is a major factor in the high death rates among children younger than age 5 years.

PEM refers to a *range of clinical syndromes* characterized by an inadequate dietary intake of protein and calories to meet the body's needs. From a functional standpoint, there are two protein compartments in the body: the *somatic protein compartment*, represented by the skeletal muscles; and the *visceral protein compartment*, represented by protein stores in the visceral organs, primarily the liver. These two compartments are regulated differently, and as we shall see, the somatic compartment is affected more severely in marasmus (calorie deficiency), while the visceral compartment is depleted more severely in kwashiorkor (protein deficiency). Before the clinical presentations of the two polar forms of severe malnutrition (marasmus and kwashiorkor) are discussed, some comments are made on the clinical assessment of undernutrition and some of its general metabolic characteristics.

The diagnosis of PEM is obvious in its most severe forms. In mild to moderate forms, the usual approach is to compare the body weight for a given height with standard tables; other parameters are also helpful, including evaluation of fat stores, muscle mass, and serum proteins. With a loss of fat, the major storage form of energy, the thickness of skin folds (which includes skin and subcutaneous tissue) is reduced. If the somatic protein compartment is catabolized, the resultant reduction in muscle mass is reflected by reduced circumference of the midarm. Measurement of serum proteins (albumin, transferrin, and others) provides a measure of the adequacy of the visceral protein compartment. The most common victims of PEM worldwide are children. A child whose weight falls to less than 80% of normal is considered malnourished.

Malnutrition can present in many forms. Marasmus and kwashiorkor are two ends of a specimen and considerable overlap exists. *Marasmus* refers to malnutrition caused primarily by severe reduction in caloric intake. It results in greater than 60% reduction in body weight adjusted for height and sex. A child with marasmus suffers growth retardation and loss of muscle. The loss of muscle mass results from catabolism and depletion of the somatic protein compartment. This seems to be an adaptational response that serves to provide the body with amino acids as a source of energy. Interestingly, the visceral protein compartment, which is presumably more precious and critical for survival, is depleted only marginally, and hence *serum albumin levels are either normal or only slightly reduced.* In addition to muscle proteins, subcutaneous fat is also mobilized and used as a fuel. With such losses of muscle and subcutaneous fat, the *extremities are emaciated*; by comparison, the head appears too large for the body. Anemia and manifestations of multivitamin deficiencies are present, and there is evidence of *immune deficiency*, particularly of T cell–mediated immunity. Hence, concurrent infections are usually present, and they impose an additional stress on an already weakened body.

Kwashiorkor, in contast to marasmus, occurs when protein deprivation is relatively greater than the reduction in total calories. This is the most common form seen in African children who have been weaned (often too early, owing to the arrival of another child) and are subsequently fed an exclusively carbohydrate diet. The prevalence of kwashiorkor is also high in impoverished countries of Southeast Asia. Less severe forms may occur worldwide in persons with chronic diarrheal states in which protein is not absorbed or in those with conditions in which chronic protein loss occurs (e.g., protein-losing enteropathies, the nephrotic syndrome, or after extensive burns).

Kwashiorkor is a more severe form of malnutrition than marasmus. Unlike marasmus, marked protein deprivation is associated with severe loss of the visceral protein compartment, and the resultant hypoalbuminemia gives rise to generalized, or dependent, edema (Fig. 9–21). The weight of children with severe kwashiorkor is typically 60% to 80% of normal. However, the true loss of weight is masked by the increased fluid retention (edema). In further contrast to marasmus, there is relative sparing of subcutaneous fat and muscle mass. The modest loss of these compartments may also be masked by edema. Children with kwashiorkor have characteristic skin lesions, with alternating zones of hyperpigmentation, areas of desquamation, and hypopigmentation, giving a "flaky paint" appearance. Hair changes include overall loss of color or alternating bands of pale and darker hair, straightening, line texture, and loss of firm attachment to the scalp. Other features that differentiate kwashiorkor from marasmus include an enlarged, *fatty liver* (resulting from reduced synthesis of carrier proteins) and a tendency to develop early apathy, listlessness, and loss of appetite. As in marasmus, other vitamin deficiencies are likely to be present, as are *defects in immunity* and *secondary infections.* The latter add to the catabolic state, thus setting up a vicious circle.

Secondary PEM is not uncommon in chronically ill or hospitalized patients within the United States. Both marasmus-like and kwashiorkor-like syndromes (with intermediate forms) may develop. Table 9–21 summarizes the secondary forms of these two syndromes.

Secondary PEM is a common complication in advanced cancer patients and in patients with AIDS. The malnutrition in these settings is sometimes called *cachexia*. Individuals with chronic gastrointestinal disease and elderly patients who are

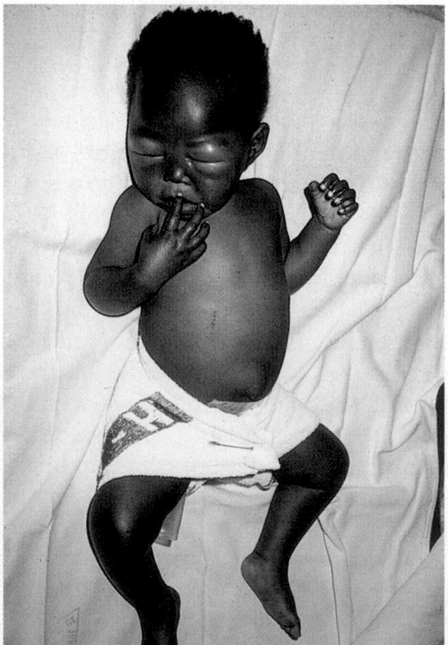

FIGURE 9–21 Kwashiorkor. The infant shows generalized edema, seen in the form of puffiness of the face, arms, and legs.

TABLE 9–21 Comparison of Severe Marasmus-Like and Kwashiorkor-Like Secondary Protein–Energy Malnutrition

Syndrome	Clinical Setting	Time Course	Clinical Features	Laboratory Findings	Prognosis
Marasmus-like protein–energy malnutrition	Chronic illness (e.g., chronic lung disease, cancer)	Months	History of weight loss Muscle wasting Absent subcutaneous fat	Normal or mildly reduced serum proteins	Variable; depends on underlying disease
Kwashiorkor-like protein–energy malnutrition	Acute, catabolic illness (e.g., severe trauma, burns, sepsis)	Weeks	Normal fat and muscle Edema Easily pluckable hair	Serum albumin <2.8 gm/dL	Poor

Data from Bennett JC, Plum F (eds): Cecil Textbook of Medicine, 20th ed. Philadelphia, WB Saunders, 1996, p. 1156.

weak and bedridden may show physical signs of protein and energy malnutrition: (1) depletion of subcutaneous fat in the arms, chest wall, shoulders, or metacarpal regions; (2) wasting of the quadriceps femoris and deltoid muscles; and (3) ankle or sacral edema.

Bedridden or hospitalized malnourished patients have an increased risk of infection, sepsis, impaired wound healing, and death after surgery.[68] The biochemical mechanisms responsible for secondary PEM in patients with cachexia are complex. In contrast to patients with anorexia nervosa, described next, patients with cachexia show loss of fat as well as muscle mass, which may occur before a decrease in appetite. Cachectic patients show increased expenditure of resting energy; in contrast, in chronic starvation, the basal metabolic rate is decreased. Cytokines produced by the host during sepsis, for example, or by tumors have been postulated to be involved in cachexia: tumor necrosis factor, interleukin-1, interleukin-6, and interferon-γ. In addition, as discussed in Chapter 7, lipid- and protein-mobilizing factors have been isolated from animals and people with cancer cachexia.[69]

Morphology. The central anatomic changes in PEM are (1) growth failure; (2) peripheral edema in kwashiorkor; and (3) loss of body fat and atrophy of muscle, more marked in marasmus.

The **liver** in kwashiorkor, but not in marasmus, is enlarged and fatty; superimposed cirrhosis is rare.

In kwashiorkor (rarely in marasmus), the **small bowel** shows a decrease in the mitotic index in the crypts of the glands, associated with mucosal atrophy and loss of villi and microvilli. In such cases, concurrent loss of small intestinal enzymes occurs, most often manifested as disaccharidase deficiency. Hence, infants with kwashiorkor initially may not respond well to a full-strength, milk-based diet. With treatment, the mucosal changes are reversible.

The **bone marrow** in both kwashiorkor and marasmus may be hypoplastic, mainly because of decreased numbers of red cell precursors. How much of this derangement is due to a deficiency of protein and folates or to reduced synthesis of transferrin and ceruloplasmin is uncertain. Thus, anemia is usually present, most often hypochromic microcytic anemia, but a concurrent deficiency of folates may lead to a mixed microcytic–macrocytic anemia.

The **brain** in infants who are born to malnourished mothers and who suffer PEM during the first 1 or 2 years of life has been reported by some observers to show cerebral atrophy, a reduced number of neurons, and impaired myelinization of the white matter, but there is no universal agreement on the validity of these findings.

Many **other changes** may be present, including (1) thymic and lymphoid atrophy (more marked in kwashiorkor than in marasmus); (2) anatomic alterations induced by intercurrent infections, particularly with all manner of endemic worms and other parasites; and (3) deficiencies of other required nutrients, such as iodine and vitamins.

Anorexia Nervosa and Bulimia

Anorexia nervosa is self-induced starvation, resulting in marked weight loss; bulimia is a condition in which the patient binges on food and then induces vomiting. These eating disorders occur primarily in previously healthy young women who have developed an obsession with attaining thinness.

The clinical findings in anorexia nervosa are generally similar to those in severe PEM. In addition, effects on the endocrine system are prominent. *Amenorrhea*, resulting from decreased secretion of gonadotropin-releasing hormone (and subsequent decreased secretion of luteinizing hormone and follicle-stimulating hormone), is so common that its presence is a diagnostic feature for the disorder. Other common findings, related to decreased thyroid hormone release, include cold intolerance, bradycardia, constipation, and changes in the skin and hair. The skin becomes dry and scaly and may be yellow because of excess carotene in the blood. Body hair may be increased but is usually fine and pale (lanugo). Bone density is decreased, most likely owing to low estrogen levels, which mimic the postmenopausal acceleration of osteoporosis. As expected with severe PEM, anemia, lymphopenia, and hypoalbuminemia may be present. A major complication of anorexia nervosa is an increased susceptibility to cardiac arrhythmia and sudden death, resulting in all likelihood from hypokalemia.

In bulimia, binge eating is the norm. Huge amounts of food, principally carbohydrates, are ingested, only to be followed by induced vomiting. Although menstrual irregularities are common, amenorrhea occurs in less than 50% of bulimia patients, probably because weight and gonadotropin levels are maintained near normal. The major medical complications relate to continual induced vomiting and include (1) electrolyte imbalances (hypokalemia), which predispose the patient to cardiac arrhythmias; (2) pulmonary aspiration of gastric contents; and (3) esophageal and cardiac rupture.

Vitamin Deficiencies

Thirteen vitamins are necessary for health; four—A, D, E, and K—are fat-soluble, and the remainder are water-soluble. The distinction between fat- and water-soluble vitamins is important, because although fat-soluble vitamins are more readily stored in the body, they are likely to be poorly absorbed in gastrointestinal disorders of fat malabsorption (Chapter 17). Small amounts of some vitamins can be synthesized endogenously—vitamin D from precursor steroids; vitamin K and biotin by the intestinal microflora; and niacin from tryptophan, an essential amino acid—but the rest must be supplied in the diet. A deficiency of vitamins may be primary (dietary in origin) or secondary (because of disturbances in intestinal absorption, transport in the blood, tissue storage, or metabolic conversion). In the following sections, the major vitamins, together with their well-defined deficiency states, are discussed individually (with the exception of vitamin B_{12} and folate, which are discussed in Chapter 13) beginning with the fat-soluble vitamins. However, deficiencies of a single vitamin are uncommon, and the expression of a deficiency of a combination of vitamins may be submerged in concurrent PEM. A summary of all the essential vitamins, along with their functions and deficiency syndromes, is presented in Table 9–22.

Vitamin A. Vitamin A is actually a group of related natural and synthetic chemicals that exert a hormone-like activity or function. The relationship of some important members of this group is presented in Figure 9–22. *Retinol*, perhaps the most important form of vitamin A, is the transport form and, as the retinol ester, also the storage form. It is oxidized in vivo to the aldehyde *retinal* (the form used in visual pigment) and the acid *retinoic acid.* Important dietary sources of vitamin A are animal derived (e.g., liver, fish, eggs, milk, butter). Yellow and leafy green vegetables such as carrots, squash, and spinach supply large amounts of carotenoids, many of which are provitamins that can be metabolized to active vitamin A in vivo; the most important of these is beta-carotene. A widely used term, *retinoids*, refers to both natural and synthetic chemicals that are structurally related to vitamin A but do not necessarily have vitamin A activity.

As with all fats, the digestion and absorption of carotenes and retinoids require bile, pancreatic enzymes, and some level of antioxidant activity in the food. *Retinol*, whether derived from ingested esters or from beta-carotene (through an intermediate oxidation step involving retinal), is transported in chylomicrons to the liver for esterification and storage. More than 90% of the body's vitamin A reserves are stored in the liver, predominantly in the perisinusoidal stellate (Ito) cells. In normal persons who consume an adequate diet, these reserves are sufficient for at least 6 months' deprivation. *Retinoic acid*, on the other hand, can be absorbed unchanged; it represents a small fraction of vitamin A in the blood and is active in epithelial differentiation and growth but not in the maintenance of vision.

TABLE 9-22 Vitamins: Major Functions and Deficiency Syndromes

Vitamin	Functions	Deficiency Syndromes
Fat-Soluble		
Vitamin A	A component of visual pigment Maintenance of specialized epithelia Maintenance of resistance to infection	Night blindness, xerophthalmia, blindness Squamous metaplasia Vulnerability to infection, particularly measles
Vitamin D	Facilitates intestinal absorption of calcium and phosphorus and mineralization of bone	Rickets in children Osteomalacia in adults
Vitamin E	Major antioxidant; scavenges free radicals	Spinocerebellar degeneration
Vitamin K	Cofactor in hepatic carboxylation of procoagulants—factors II (prothrombin), VII, IX, and X; and protein C and protein S	Bleeding diathesis
Water-Soluble		
Vitamin B_1 (thiamine)	As pyrophosphate, is coenzyme in decarboxylation reactions	Dry and wet beriberi, Wernicke syndrome, ?Korsakoff syndrome
Vitamin B_2 (riboflavin)	Converted to coenzymes flavin mononucleotide and flavin adenine dinucleotide, cofactors for many enzymes in intermediary metabolism	Ariboflavinosis, cheilosis, stomatitis, glossitis, dermatitis, corneal vascularization
Niacin	Incorporated into nicotinamide adenine dinucleotide (NAD) and NAD phosphate, involved in a variety of redox reactions	Pellagra—three "D's": dementia, dermatitis, diarrhea
Vitamin B_6 (pyridoxine)	Derivatives serve as coenzymes in many intermediary reactions	Cheilosis, glossitis, dermatitis, peripheral neuropathy
Vitamin B_{12}	Required for normal folate metabolism and DNA synthesis Maintenance of myelinization of spinal cord tracts	Combined system disease (megaloblastic pernicious anemia and degeneration of posterolateral spinal cord tracts)
Vitamin C	Serves in many oxidation-reduction (redox) reactions and hydroxylation of collagen	Scurvy
Folate	Essential for transfer and use of 1-carbon units in DNA synthesis	Megaloblastic anemia, neural tube defects
Pantothenic acid	Incorporated in coenzyme A	No nonexperimental syndrome recognized
Biotin	Cofactor in carboxylation reactions	No clearly defined clinical syndrome

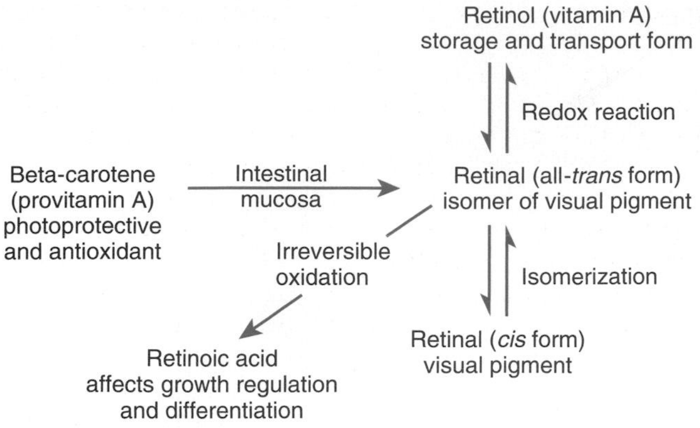

FIGURE 9–22 Interrelationships of retinoids and their major functions.

When dietary intake of vitamin A is inadequate, the retinol esters in the liver are mobilized, and released retinol is then bound to a specific retinol-binding protein, synthesized in liver. The uptake of retinol by the various cells of the body is dependent on surface receptors specific for retinol-binding protein, rather than receptors specific for the retinol. Retinol is transported across the cell membrane, where it binds to a cellular retinol-binding protein, and the retinol-binding protein is released back into the blood.

Function. In humans, the best-defined functions of vitamin A are as follows:

- Maintaining normal vision in reduced light
- Potentiating the differentiation of specialized epithelial cells, mainly mucus-secreting cells
- Enhancing immunity to infections, particularly in children.

In addition, the retinoids, beta-carotene, and some related carotenoids have been shown to function as photoprotective and antioxidant agents.

The *visual process* involves four forms of vitamin A–containing pigments: rhodopsin in the rods, the most light-sensitive pigment and therefore important in reduced light, and three iodopsins in cone cells, each responsive to specific colors in bright light. The synthesis of rhodopsin from retinol involves (1) oxidation to all-*trans*-retinal; (2) isomerization to 11-*cis*-retinal; and (3) interaction with the rod protein opsin to form rhodopsin.

When a photon of light impinges on the dark-adapted retina, rhodopsin undergoes a sequence of configurational changes to ultimately yield all-*trans*-retinal and opsin. In the process, a nerve impulse is generated (by changes in membrane potential) that is transmitted by neurons from the retina to the brain. During dark adaptation, some of the all-*trans*-retinal is reconverted to 11-*cis*-retinal, but most is reduced to retinol and lost to the retina, dictating the need for continuous input of retinol.

Vitamin A plays an important role in the orderly *differentiation of mucus-secreting epithelium*; when a deficiency state exists, the epithelium undergoes squamous metaplasia and differentiation to a keratinizing epithelium. The mechanism is not precisely understood; but in cell culture systems, retinoic acid (retinol is much less potent) regulates the expression of genes encoding a number of cell receptors and secreted proteins, including receptors for growth factors.

Vitamin A plays a role in *host resistance to infections.*[70] This beneficial effect of vitamin A seems to derive in part from its ability to stimulate the immune system, possibly through the formation of a metabolite called *14-hydroxyretinol.* In addition, it appears that during infections, the bioavailability of vitamin A is reduced. The acute-phase response that accompanies many infections reduces the formation of retinol-binding protein in the liver, resulting in depression of circulating retinol levels, which in turn leads to reduced tissue availability of vitamin A. In keeping with this, supplements of the vitamin during the course of infections such as measles dramatically improve the clinical outcome.

Deficiency State. Vitamin A deficiency occurs worldwide either on the basis of general undernutrition or as a conditioned deficiency among individuals having some cause for malabsorption of fats. It is rarely seen in the United States and other industrialized countries, but it is not uncommon in the underprivileged populations of the world. One of the earliest manifestations of vitamin A deficiency is impaired vision, particularly in reduced light (night blindness). Because vitamin A and retinoids are involved in maintaining the differentiation of epithelial cells, persistent deficiency gives rise to a series of changes, the most devastating of which occur in the eyes. Collectively, the ocular changes are referred to as *xerophthalmia* (dry eye). First, there is dryness of the conjunctivae (xerosis) as the normal lacrimal and mucus-secreting epithelium is replaced by keratinized epithelium. This is followed by the build-up of keratin debris in small opaque plaques (*Bitot spots*) and, eventually, erosion of the roughened corneal surface with softening and destruction of the cornea (*keratomalacia*) and total blindness.

In addition to the ocular epithelium, the epithelium lining the upper respiratory passages and urinary tract is replaced by keratinizing squamous cells (*squamous metaplasia*). Loss of the mucociliary epithelium of the airways predisposes to secondary pulmonary infections, and desquamation of keratin debris in the urinary tract predisposes to renal and urinary bladder stones. Hyperplasia and hyperkeratinization of the epidermis with plugging of the ducts of the adnexal glands may produce follicular or papular dermatosis. The pathologic effects of vitamin A deficiency are summarized in Figure 9–23.

Another serious consequence of avitaminosis A is *immune deficiency*. This impairment of immunity leads to higher mortality rates from common infections such as measles, pneumonia, and infectious diarrhea. In parts of the world where vitamin A deficiency is endemic, dietary supplements reduce mortality by 20% to 30%.

Vitamin A Toxicity. Both short- and long-term excess of vitamin A may produce toxic manifestations, a point of some concern because of the megadoses being popularized by certain health food stores. The clinical consequences of acute hypervitaminosis A include headache, vomiting, stupor, and papilledema, symptoms also suggestive of brain tumor. Chronic toxicity is associated with weight loss, nausea, and vomiting; dryness of the mucosa of the lips; bone and joint pain; hyperostosis; and hepatomegaly with parenchymal damage and fibrosis. Although synthetic retinoids used for the treatment of acne are not associated with the complications listed, their use in pregnancy should be avoided owing to a well-established increase in the incidence of congenital malformations (Chapter 10). Recent studies indicate other

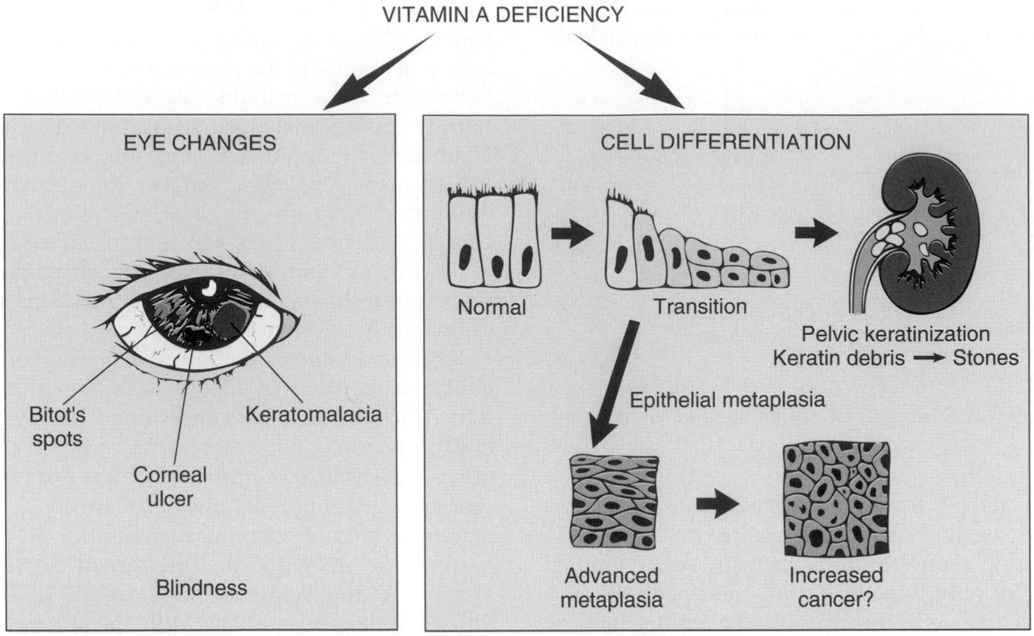

FIGURE 9–23 Vitamin A deficiency: its major consequences in the eye and in the production of keratinizing metaplasia of specialized epithelial surfaces, and its possible role in potentiating neoplasia.

untoward effects of chronic hypervitaminosis A. Vitamin A stimulates osteoclast formation, thus leading to increased bone resorption and osteoporosis and predisposition to fractures. This is particularly true in older individuals, who are prone to osteoporosis[71] (Chapter 26).

Vitamin D. The major function of vitamin D is the *maintenance of normal plasma levels of calcium and phosphorus.* In this capacity, it is required for the prevention of bone diseases (rickets in growing children whose epiphyses have not already closed and osteomalacia in adults) and of hypocalcemic tetany. With respect to tetany, vitamin D maintains the correct concentration of ionized calcium in the extracellular fluid compartment required for normal neural excitation and relaxation of muscle. Insufficient ionized calcium in the extracellular fluid results in continuous excitation of muscle, leading to the convulsive state, hypocalcemic tetany. Our attention here is focused on the function of vitamin D in the regulation of serum calcium levels.

Metabolism of Vitamin D. Humans have two possible sources of vitamin D: endogenous synthesis in the skin and diet.[72] There are large amounts of the precursor 7-dehydrocholesterol in the skin; ultraviolet light in sunlight converts it to vitamin D_3. Depending on the skin's level of melanin pigmentation, which absorbs ultraviolet light, and the amount of exposure to sunlight, about 80% of the vitamin D needed can be endogenously derived. The remainder must be obtained from dietary sources such as deep-sea fish, plants, and grains. In plant sources, vitamin D is present in its precursor form (ergosterol), which is converted to vitamin D_2 in the body. In many countries, various foods are fortified with vitamin D_2. Since D_3 and D_2 undergo identical metabolic transformations and have identical functions, both are hereafter referred to as vitamin D.

The metabolism of vitamin D can be outlined as follows:

1. Absorption of vitamin D in the gut or synthesis from precursors in the skin
2. Binding to a plasma α_1-globulin (D-binding protein) and transport to liver
3. Conversion to 25-hydroxyvitamin D, 25(OH)D by 25-hydroxylase in the liver
4. Conversion of 25(OH)D to 1,25$(OH)_2$D by α_1-hydroxylase in the kidney; *biologically this is the most active form of vitamin D.*

The production of 1,25$(OH)_2$D by the kidney is regulated by three mechanisms:

1. In a feedback loop, increased levels of 1,25$(OH)_2$D down-regulate synthesis of this metabolite by inhibiting the action of α_1-hydroxylase, and decreased levels have the opposite effect.
2. Hypocalcemia stimulates secretion of parathyroid hormone (PTH), which in turn augments the conversion of 25(OH)D to 1,25$(OH)_2$D by activating α_1-hydroxylase.
3. Hypophosphatemia directly activates α_1-hydroxylase and thus increases formation of 1,25$(OH)_2$D.

Functions of Vitamin D. 1,25$(OH)_2$D, the biologically active form of vitamin D, is best regarded as a steroid hormone. Like other steroid hormones, it acts by binding to a high-affinity receptor that is widely distributed. However, the essential function of vitamin D—the maintenance of normal plasma levels of calcium and phosphorus—involves actions on the intestines, bones, and kidneys. The active form of vitamin D has several important actions:

- Stimulates intestinal absorption of calcium and phosphorus
- Collaborates with PTH in the mobilization of calcium from bone

- Stimulates the PTH-dependent reabsorption of calcium in the distal renal tubules.

How $1,25(OH)_2D$ stimulates intestinal absorption of calcium and phosphorus is still somewhat unclear. The weight of evidence favors the view that it binds to epithelial receptors, activating the synthesis of calcium transport proteins. The increased absorption of phosphorus is independent of the effects on calcium transport.

The effects of vitamin D on bone depend on the plasma levels of calcium. On the one hand, with hypocalcemia, $1,25(OH)_2D$ collaborates with PTH in the resorption of calcium and phosphorus from bone to support blood levels. On the other hand, vitamin D is required for normal mineralization of epiphyseal cartilage and osteoid matrix. It is still not clear how the resorptive function is mediated, but direct activation of osteoclasts is ruled out. It is more likely that vitamin D favors differentiation of osteoclasts from their precursors (monocytes). The precise details of mineralization of bone when vitamin D levels are adequate are also uncertain. It is widely believed that the main function of vitamin D is to maintain calcium and phosphorus at supersaturated levels in the plasma. However, vitamin D–mediated increases in the synthesis of the calcium-binding proteins osteocalcin and osteonectin in the osteoid matrix may also play a role.

Equally unclear is the role of vitamin D in renal reabsorption of calcium. PTH is clearly necessary, but it is believed that vitamin D is also. There is no convincing evidence that vitamin D participates in renal reabsorption of phosphorus. An overview of the normal metabolism of vitamin D and the consequences of a deficiency are depicted in Figure 9–24.

Deficiency States. Rickets in growing children and osteomalacia in adults are worldwide skeletal diseases; but in developed countries, they rarely occur as a result of dietary deficiencies. Recent studies suggest, however, that deficiency of vitamin D is far more common than was suspected earlier. It is especially prevalent in the elderly because of inadequate sun exposure and inadequate intake. Even healthy young adults living in northern climates develop vitamin D deficiencies in winter.[73] Both rickets and osteomalacia may result from deranged vitamin D absorption or metabolism or, less commonly, from disorders that affect the function of vitamin D or disturb calcium or phosphorus homeostasis. A summary of the causes of rickets and osteomalacia is given in Table 9–23.

Whatever the basis, a deficiency of vitamin D tends to cause hypocalcemia. When hypocalcemia occurs, PTH production is increased, which (1) activates renal α_1-hydroxylase, thus increasing the amount of active vitamin D and calcium absorption; (2) mobilizes calcium from bone; (3) decreases renal calcium excretion; and (4) increases renal excretion of phosphate.

Thus, the serum level of calcium is restored to nearly normal, but hypophosphatemia persists, and so mineralization of bone is impaired.

An understanding of the morphologic changes in rickets and osteomalacia is facilitated by a brief summary of normal bone development and maintenance. The development of flat bones in the skeleton involves intramembranous ossification, while the formation of long tubular bones reflects endochondral ossification. With intramembranous bone formation, mesenchymal cells differentiate directly into osteoblasts, which synthesize the collagenous osteoid matrix on which calcium is deposited. In contrast, with endochondral ossification, growing cartilage at the epiphyseal plates is provisionally mineralized and then progressively resorbed and replaced by osteoid matrix, which undergoes mineralization to create bone (Fig. 9–25*B*).

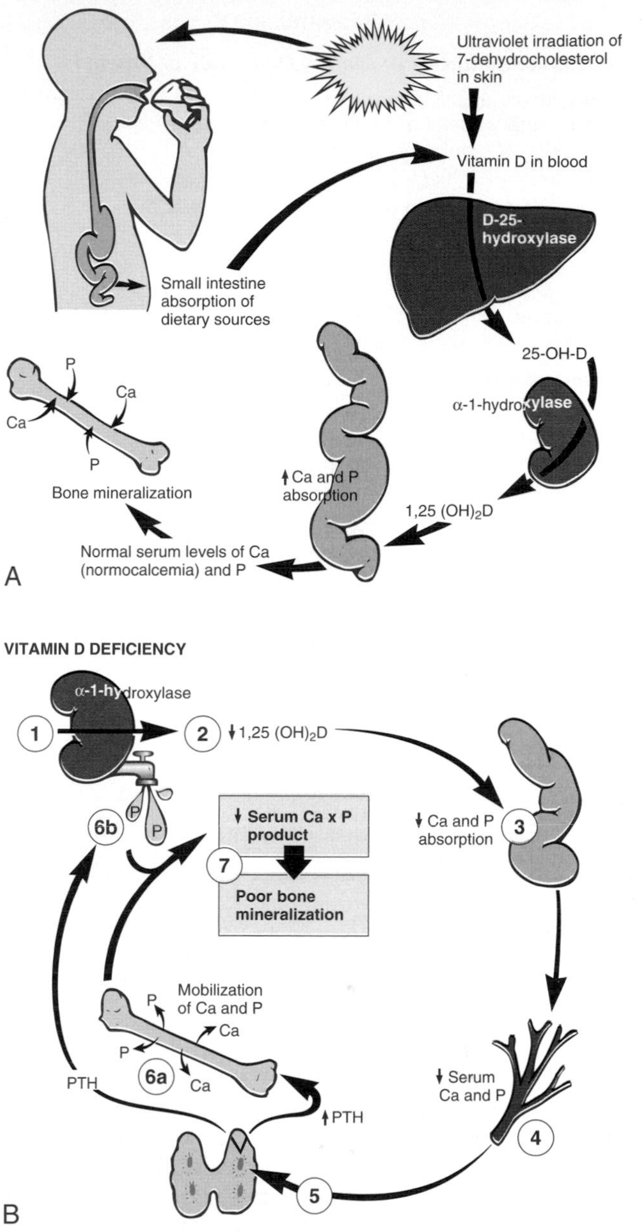

FIGURE 9–24 *A,* Schema of normal vitamin D metabolism. *B,* Vitamin D deficiency. There is inadequate substrate for the renal hydroxylase (1), yielding a deficiency of $1,25(OH)_2D$ (2), and deficient absorption of calcium and phosphorus from the gut (3), with consequent depressed serum levels of both (4). The hypocalcemia activates the parathyroid glands (5), causing mobilization of calcium and phosphorus from bone (6a). Simultaneously, the parathyroid hormone (PTH) induces wasting of phosphate in the urine (6b) and calcium retention. Consequently, the serum levels of calcium are normal or nearly normal, but the phosphate is low; hence, mineralization is impaired (7).

TABLE 9–23 Predisposing Conditions for Rickets or Osteomalacia

Inadequate Synthesis or Dietary Deficiency of Vitamin D

Inadequate exposure to sunlight
Limited dietary intake of fortified foods
Poor maternal nutrition
Dark skin pigmentation

Decreased Absorption of Fat-Soluble Vitamin D

Cholestatic liver disease
Pancreatic insufficiency
Biliary tract obstruction
Celiac sprue
Extensive small-bowel disease

Derangements in Vitamin D Metabolism

Increased degradation of vitamin D and 25(OH)D
  Induction of cytochrome P-450 enzymes (phenytoin, phenobarbital, rifampin)
Impaired synthesis of 25(OH)D
  Diffuse liver disease
Decreased synthesis of $1,25(OH)_2D$
  Advanced renal disease
  Inherited deficiency of renal α_1-hydroxylase (vitamin D–dependent rickets type I)

End-Organ Resistance to $1,25(OH)_2D$

Inherited absence of or defective receptors for acute metabolite of vitamin D (vitamin D–dependent rickets type II)

Phosphate Depletion

Poor absorption of phosphate due to chronic use of antacids—binding by aluminum hydroxide
Excess renal tubule excretion of phosphate (X-linked hypophosphatemic rickets)

Morphology. The basic derangement in both rickets and osteomalacia is an excess of unmineralized matrix. The changes that occur in the growing bones of children with rickets, however, are complicated by inadequate provisional calcification of epiphyseal cartilage deranging endochondral bone growth. The following sequence ensues in rickets:

- Overgrowth of epiphyseal cartilage due to inadequate provisional calcification and failure of the cartilage cells to mature and disintegrate
- Persistence of distorted, irregular masses of cartilage, many of which project into the marrow cavity (Fig. 9–25*A*)
- Deposition of osteoid matrix on inadequately mineralized cartilaginous remnants
- Disruption of the orderly replacement of cartilage by osteoid matrix, with enlargement and lateral expansion of the osteochondral junction
- Abnormal overgrowth of capillaries and fibroblasts in the disorganized zone because of microfractures and stresses on the inadequately mineralized, weak, poorly formed bone
- Deformation of the skeleton due to the loss of structural rigidity of the developing bones.

The conformation of the gross skeletal changes depends on the severity of the rachitic process, its duration, and in particular the stresses to which individual bones are subjected. During the nonambulatory stage of infancy, the head and chest sustain the greatest stresses. The softened occipital bones may become flattened, and the parietal bones can be buckled inward by pressure; with the release of the

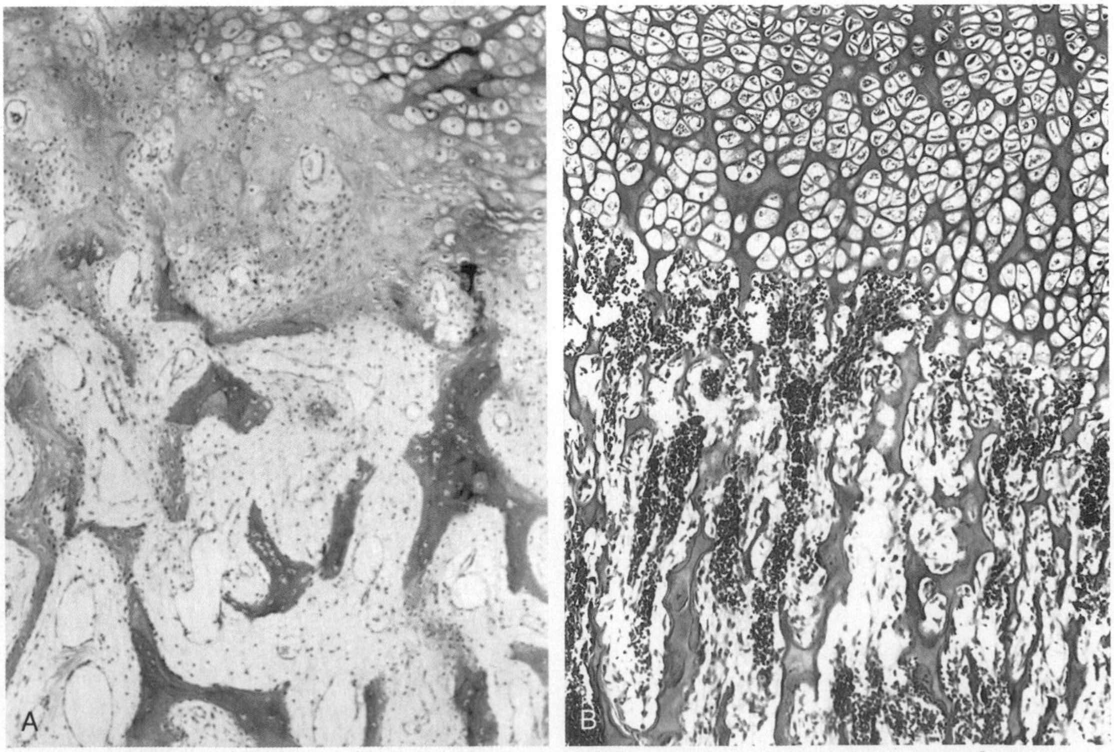

FIGURE 9–25 *A,* Detail of a rachitic costochondral junction. The palisade of cartilage is lost. Some of the trabeculae are old, well-formed bone, but the paler ones consist of uncalcified osteoid. *B,* For comparison, normal costochondral function from a young child demonstrates the orderly transition from cartilage to new bone formation.

pressure, elastic recoil snaps the bones back into their original positions **(craniotabes)**. An excess of osteoid produces **frontal bossing** and a **squared appearance to the head.** Deformation of the chest results from overgrowth of cartilage or osteoid tissue at the costochondral junction, producing the **"rachitic rosary."** The weakened metaphyseal areas of the ribs are subject to the pull of the respiratory muscles and thus bend inward, creating anterior protrusion of the sternum **(pigeon breast deformity)**. The inward pull at the margin of the diaphragm creates **Harrison's** groove, girdling the thoracic cavity at the lower margin of the rib cage. The pelvis may become deformed. When an ambulating child develops rickets, deformities are likely to affect the spine, pelvis, and long bones (e.g., tibia), causing, most notably, **lumbar lordosis** and **bowing of the legs** (Fig. 9–26).

In adults, the lack of vitamin D deranges the normal bone remodeling that occurs throughout life. The newly formed osteoid matrix laid down by osteoblasts is inadequately mineralized, thus producing the excess of persistent osteoid characteristic of **osteomalacia.** Although the contours of the bone are not affected, the bone is weak and vulnerable to gross fractures or microfractures, which are most likely to affect vertebral bodies and femoral necks.

On histologic examination, the unmineralized osteoid can be visualized as a thickened layer of matrix (which stains pink in hematoxylin and eosin preparations) arranged about the more basophilic, normally mineralized trabeculae.

Persistent failure of mineralization in adults leads eventually to loss of skeletal mass, referred to as *osteopenia.* It is then difficult to differentiate osteomalacia from other osteopenias

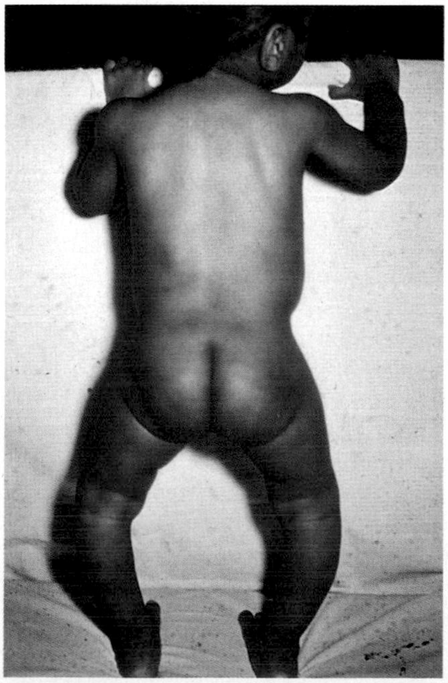

FIGURE 9–26 Rickets. The bowing of legs in a toddler due to the formation of poorly mineralized bones is evident.

such as osteoporosis (Chapter 26). Osteoporosis, unlike osteomalacia, results from reduced production of osteoid, the protein matrix of the bone. Studies suggest that vitamin D may also be essential for preventing demineralization of bones. In certain familial forms of osteoporosis, the defect has been localized to the vitamin D receptor. It appears that certain genetically determined variants of the vitamin D receptor are associated with an accelerated loss of bone minerals with aging.

Vitamin E. A group of eight closely related fat-soluble compounds—four tocopherols and four tocotrienols—all exhibit vitamin E biologic activity, but α-tocopherol is the most active and the most widely available. Vitamin E is abundant in so many foods—vegetables, grains, nuts and their oils, dairy products, fish, and meat—that a diet sufficient to sustain life is unlikely to be insufficient in vitamin E. The absorption of tocopherols, as of all fat-soluble vitamins, requires normal biliary tract and pancreatic function. After absorption, vitamin E is transported in the blood in the form of chylomicrons, which rapidly equilibrate with the plasma lipoproteins, mainly LDLs. Unlike vitamin A, which is stored predominantly in the liver, vitamin E accumulates throughout the body, mostly in fat depots but also in liver and muscle.

Vitamin E is one of a group of *antioxidants that serve to scavenge free radicals formed in redox reactions throughout the body* (Chapter 1). It plays a role in termination of free radical–generated lipid peroxidation chain reactions, particularly in cellular and subcellular membranes that are rich in polyunsaturated lipids. These chain-terminating nutrients are complemented by selenium, which is converted to selenocysteine and is essential for the activities of glutathione peroxidase and thioredoxin reductase. These antioxidants metabolize peroxides before they can initiate membrane damage, thus maintaining intracellular redox status.[8] For reasons that are not clear, the nervous system is a particular target of vitamin E deficiency. Although the basis for this affinity is not entirely clear, it is speculated that neurons with long axons are particularly vulnerable because of their large membrane surface area. Mature red cells may also be vulnerable to vitamin E deficiency because they are at risk for oxidative injury imposed by the generation of superoxide radicals during oxygenation of hemoglobin.

Hypovitaminosis E resulting from a deficient diet is uncommon in the Western world and occurs almost exclusively in association with (1) fat malabsorption that accompanies cholestasis, cystic fibrosis, and primary small intestinal disease; (2) infant low birth weight with immature liver and gastrointestinal tract; (3) abetalipoproteinemia, a rare autosomal recessive disorder in which transport of vitamin E is abnormal because the apoprotein B component of chylomicrons, LDLs, and very-low-density lipoproteins (VLDLs) is not synthesized; and (4) rare autosomal recessive syndrome of impaired vitamin E metabolism.

Morphology. The anatomic changes found in the nervous system depend on the duration and severity of the deficiency state. Most consistent is **degeneration of the axons in the posterior columns of the spinal cord, with focal accumulation of lipopigment and loss of nerve cells in the dorsal root ganglia, attributed to a dying-back type of axonopathy.** Myelin degeneration in sensory axons of peripheral nerves may also be present, and in more marked cases, degenerative changes in the spinocerebellar tracts may occur as well. In occasional cases, features of both primary and denervation muscle disease have been observed in skeletal muscle.

Vitamin E–deficient erythrocytes are more susceptible to oxidative stress and have a shorter half-life in the circulating blood.

The neurologic manifestations of vitamin E deficiency are depressed or, more often, absent tendon reflexes; ataxia; dysarthria; loss of position and vibration sense; and loss of pain sensation. Muscle weakness is also common. In addition, there may be impaired vision and disorders of eye movement, sometimes progressing to total ophthalmoplegia. Anemia is not a feature of the deficiency state in adults but is often found in premature infants and is probably multifactorial in origin.

In closing, attention should be drawn to the ongoing interest in the possible protective effects of vitamin E and other antioxidants against atherosclerosis and cancer, the two most common causes of death in the United States. In the case of atherosclerosis, it is suggested that vitamin E may inhibit atheroma formation by reducing the oxidation of LDL (Chapter 11). However, there is no conclusive evidence to support an atheroprotective effect of supplemental vitamin E. In the context of cancer, antioxidants are postulated to scavenge free radicals, thereby preventing DNA damage and mutagenesis. There is limited epidemiologic evidence supporting a protective effect of supplemental vitamin E and lycopene-rich foods against prostate cancer.[74]

Vitamin K. Vitamin K is a required cofactor for a liver microsomal carboxylase that is necessary to convert glutamyl residues in certain protein precursors to γ-carboxyglutamates. *Clotting factors VII, IX, and X and prothrombin all require carboxylation of glutamate residues for functional activity.* Carboxylation provides calcium-binding sites and thus allows calcium-dependent interaction of these clotting factors with a phospholipid surface involved in the generation of thrombin (Chapter 4). In addition, activation of anticoagulant proteins C and S also requires glutamate carboxylation. In recent years, a diverse group of proteins with no connection to coagulation have also been found to be vitamin K-dependent. Such proteins have been found in a wide variety of tissues, including kidney, bone, placenta, and lung. As with the proteins involved in coagulation, vitamin K serves to facilitate carboxylation of glutamyl residues in these other proteins as well. Of particular interest is osteocalcin, a noncollagenous protein secreted by osteoblasts; as with the coagulation proteins, γ-carboxylation of osteocalcin facilitates binding to calcium. Thus, *it appears that vitamin K may favor calcification of bone proteins.* Studies also reveal that vitamin K can inhibit bone resorption by reducing the expression of the osteoclast differentiation factor, RANK-ligand (Chapter 26).[75] On the basis of these results, there are ongoing trials of vitamin K supplementation in osteoporosis, and some studies suggest that it is beneficial, especially in combination with vitamin D.

In the course of the reaction of vitamin K with its substrate proteins, its active (reduced) form is oxidized to an epoxide but then is promptly reduced back by a liver epoxide reductase. Thus, in a healthy liver, vitamin K is efficiently recycled, and the daily dietary requirement is low. Furthermore, endogenous intestinal bacterial flora readily synthesize the vitamin. Nevertheless, there is a small but definite need for exogenous vitamin, which fortunately is widely available in the usual Western diet. Deficiency usually occurs (1) in fat malabsorption syndromes, particularly with biliary tract disease, as with the other fat-soluble vitamins; (2) after destruction of the endogenous vitamin K–synthesizing flora, particularly with ingestion of broad-spectrum antibiotics; (3) in the neonatal period, when liver reserves are small, the bacterial flora is not yet developed, and the level of vitamin K in breast milk is low; and (4) in diffuse liver disease, even in the presence of normal vitamin K stores, because hepatocyte dysfunction interferes with synthesis of the vitamin K–dependent coagulation factors.

In patients with thromboembolic disease, therapeutically desirable vitamin K deficiency is induced by coumarin anticoagulants (e.g., warfarin). These agents block the activity of liver epoxide reductase and thereby prevent regeneration of reduced vitamin K.

The major consequence of vitamin K deficiency (or of inefficient use of vitamin K by the liver) is the development of a *bleeding diathesis.* In neonates, it causes hemorrhagic disease of the newborn. Its most serious manifestation is intracranial hemorrhage, but bleeding may occur at any site, including skin, umbilicus, and viscera. The estimated 3% prevalence of vitamin K–dependent bleeding diathesis among neonates warrants routine prophylactic vitamin K therapy for all newborns. However, in normal full-term infants, by 1 week of age, endogenous flora provide sufficient vitamin K to correct any lingering deficit. In adults suffering from vitamin K deficiency or decreased synthesis of vitamin K–dependent factors, a bleeding diathesis may occur, characterized by *hematomas, hematuria, melena, ecchymoses,* and *bleeding from the gums.*

Thiamine. Thiamine is widely available in the diet, although refined foods such as polished rice, white flour, and white sugar contain little. During absorption from the gut, thiamine undergoes phosphorylation to produce thiamine pyrophosphate, the functionally active coenzyme form of the vitamin. Thiamine pyrophosphate has three major functions: (1) it regulates oxidative decarboxylation of α-keto acids, leading to the synthesis of adenosine triphosphate; (2) it acts as a cofactor for transketolase in the pentose phosphate pathway; and (3) in a little-understood manner, it maintains neural membranes and normal nerve conduction (chiefly of peripheral nerves).

In underdeveloped countries where a large part of the scant diet consists of polished rice, as occurs in many areas of Southeast Asia, thiamine deficiency sometimes develops. In developed countries, clinically evident thiamine deficiency, although uncommon on a strictly dietary basis, *affects as many as one fourth of chronic alcoholics admitted to general hospitals.* A thiamine deficiency state may also result from the pernicious vomiting of pregnancy or from debilitating illnesses that impair the appetite, predispose to vomiting, or cause protracted diarrhea. Because a subclinical deficiency state may be converted to overt disease by extended intravenous glucose therapy or refeeding of chronically malnourished persons (particularly alcoholics), care must be taken that adequate amounts of thiamine are administered concurrently.

The major targets of thiamine deficiency are the peripheral nerves, the heart, and the brain, so persistent thiamine deficiency gives rise to three distinctive syndromes:

- A polyneuropathy (dry beriberi)
- A cardiovascular syndrome (wet beriberi)
- Wernicke-Korsakoff syndrome.

Typically, these three syndromes appear in this sequence, but on occasion the deficiency manifests as only one of them. The *polyneuropathy is usually symmetric and takes the form of a nonspecific peripheral neuropathy with myelin degeneration* and disruption of axons involving motor, sensory, and reflex arcs. It usually first appears in the legs, but it may also extend to the arms, so classically these patients present with toe drop, foot drop, and wrist drop. The progressive sensory loss is accompanied by muscle weakness and hyporeflexia or areflexia.

Beriberi heart disease (wet beriberi) is associated with peripheral vasodilation, leading to more rapid arteriovenous shunting of blood, high-output cardiac failure, and eventually peripheral edema. The heart may be normal, have subtle changes, or be markedly enlarged and globular (owing to four-chamber dilation), with pale, flabby myocardium. The dilation thins the ventricular walls. Mural thrombi are often present, particularly in the dilated atria.

In protracted severe deficiency states, most often encountered in chronic alcoholics in the Western world, Wernicke-Korsakoff syndrome may appear. It usually develops against a background of peripheral neuropathy and cardiac insufficiency, but in some instances it is the only manifestation of thiamine deficiency. The details of this syndrome are presented in Chapter 28. Briefly, Wernicke encephalopathy is marked by ophthalmoplegia; nystagmus; ataxia of gait and stance; and derangement of mental function, characterized by global confusion, apathy, listlessness, and disorientation. Korsakoff psychosis takes the form of serious impairment of remote recall (retrograde amnesia), inability to acquire new information, and confabulation. Wernicke encephalopathy and Korsakoff psychosis are not distinct syndromes but rather are successive stages of a single central nervous system disease that have the same pathophysiologic substrate.

The central nervous system lesions affect *the mamillary bodies, the periventricular regions of the thalamus, the floor of the fourth ventricle, and the anterior region of the cerebellum.* There are hemorrhages and degenerative changes in the neurons (Chapter 28). The three major syndromes of thiamine deficiency are summarized in Figure 9–27.

Riboflavin. Riboflavin is a critical component of the coenzymes flavin mononucleotide and flavin adenine dinucleotide, which participate in a wide range of oxidation-reduction reactions. In addition, flavin in covalent linkage is incorporated into succinic dehydrogenase and monoamine oxidase as well as into other mitochondrial enzymes. It is widely distributed in meat, dairy products, and vegetables as free riboflavin or riboflavin phosphate and is absorbed in the upper gastrointestinal tract.

Ariboflavinosis still occurs as a primary deficiency state among persons in economically deprived and developing countries. Under such circumstances, it is frequently accompanied by deficiencies of other vitamins and proteins. In industrialized nations, a deficiency is most likely to be encountered in alcoholics and in persons who have chronic infections, advanced cancer, or other debilitating diseases. It is also seen in individuals with eating disorders such as anorexia nervosa and in individuals who avoid dairy products, since milk is a good source of riboflavin.

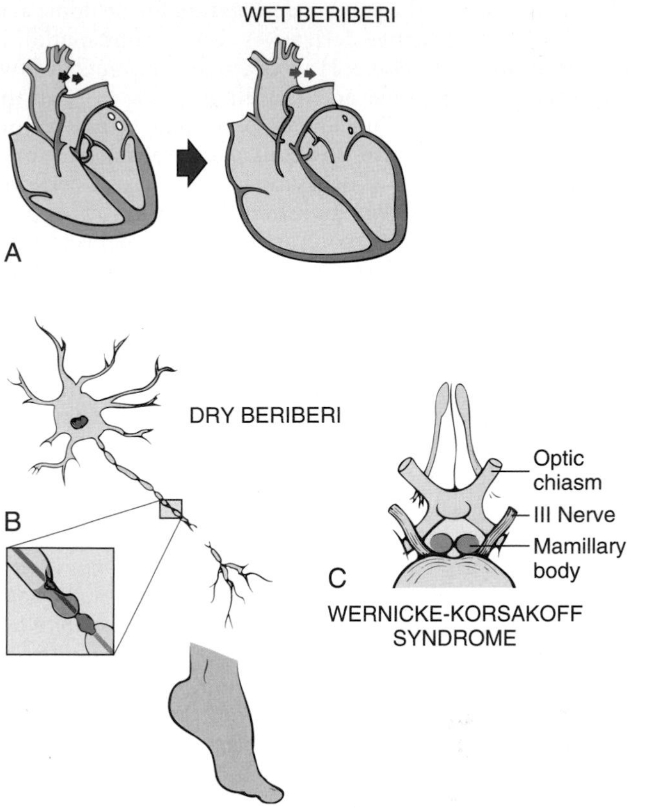

FIGURE 9–27 *A,* The flabby, four-chambered, dilated heart of wet beriberi. *B,* The peripheral neuropathy with myelin degeneration leading to footdrop, wristdrop, and sensory changes in dry beriberi. *C,* Hemorrhages into the mamillary bodies in the Wernicke-Korsakoff syndrome.

Morphology. Ariboflavinosis is associated with changes at the angles of the mouth (known as cheilosis or cheilitis), glossitis, and ocular and skin changes.

Cheilosis is usually the first and most characteristic sign of this deficiency state. It begins as areas of pallor at the angles of the mouth. Later, cracks or fissures may appear, radiating from the corners of the mouth, which tend to become secondarily infected.

With **glossitis**, the tongue becomes atrophic, taking on a magenta hue strongly resembling the red-blue coloration of cyanosis.

The **eye change** is a superficial interstitial keratitis. In the earlier stages, the superficial layers of the cornea are invaded by capillaries. Interstitial inflammatory infiltration and exudation follow, producing opacities and sometimes ulcerations of the corneal surface.

A greasy, scaling **dermatitis** over the nasolabial folds may extend into a butterfly distribution to involve the cheeks and skin about the ears. Scrotal and vulvar lesions are common. In well-defined cases, atrophy of the skin may also develop. Erythroid hypoplasia in the **bone marrow** is typically present but is usually not marked.

Niacin. Niacin is the generic designation for nicotinic acid and its functionally active derivatives (e.g., nicotinamide). In the form of nicotinamide, it is an essential component of two coenzymes, nicotinamide adenine dinucleotide (NAD) and nicotinamide adenine dinucleotide phosphate (NADP), both of which play central roles in cellular intermediary metabolism. NAD functions as a coenzyme for a variety of dehydrogenases involved in the metabolism of fat, carbohydrates, and amino acids. NADP participates in a variety of dehydrogenation reactions, particularly in the hexose–monophosphate shunt of glucose metabolism.

Niacin can be derived from the diet or may be synthesized endogenously. It is widely available in grains, legumes, and seed oils and in much smaller quantities in meats. In some grains, it is present in bound form and therefore not absorbable; the niacin in maize (corn), in particular, is bound, so the niacin deficiency syndrome *pellagra* has appeared with unexpected frequency among native populations that subsist largely on maize. Niacin can also be synthesized endogenously from tryptophan. Thus, pellagra may result from either a niacin or a tryptophan deficiency. *In industrialized countries, pellagra is encountered sporadically (usually in combination with other vitamin deficiencies), principally among alcoholics and persons suffering from chronic debilitating illnesses, including HIV infection.* It may also occur with protracted diarrheal states, with diets that are grossly deficient in protein, and with long-term administration of drugs such as isoniazid and 6-mercaptopurine.

In pharmacologic doses, nicotinic acid lowers plasma LDL levels by reducing hepatic synthesis of VLDL, and hence it is used in the treatment of hypercholesterolemia.

Morphology. The term **pellagra**, strictly speaking, refers to rough skin. The clinical syndrome, however, is classically identified by most clinicians by the "three Ds": dermatitis, diarrhea, and dementia.

Dermatitis is usually bilaterally symmetric and is found mainly on exposed areas of the body. The changes at first comprise redness, thickening, and roughening of the skin, which may be followed by extensive scaling and desquamation, producing fissures and chronic inflammation (Fig. 9–28). Similar lesions may occur in the mucous membranes of the mouth and vagina.

Diarrhea is caused by atrophy of the columnar epithelium of the gastrointestinal tract mucosa, followed by submucosal inflammation. Atrophy may be followed by ulceration.

Dementia results from degeneration of the neurons in the brain, accompanied by degeneration of the corresponding tracts in the spinal cord. The spinal cord lesions bear a close resemblance to the posterior column alterations observed in pernicious anemia.

Pyridoxine (Vitamin B_6). A primary, clinically overt deficiency of vitamin B_6 is rare in humans, but subclinical conditioned deficiency states, paradoxically, are thought to be common. Three naturally occurring substances—pyridoxine, pyridoxal, and pyridoxamine—together with the phosphate forms of each possess vitamin B_6 activity and are generically referred to as *pyridoxine.* All are equally active metabolically, and all are converted in the tissues to the coenzyme form, pyridoxal 5-phosphate. This coenzyme participates as a cofactor for a large number of enzymes involved in transaminations, carboxylations, and deaminations in the metabolism of lipids and amino acids.

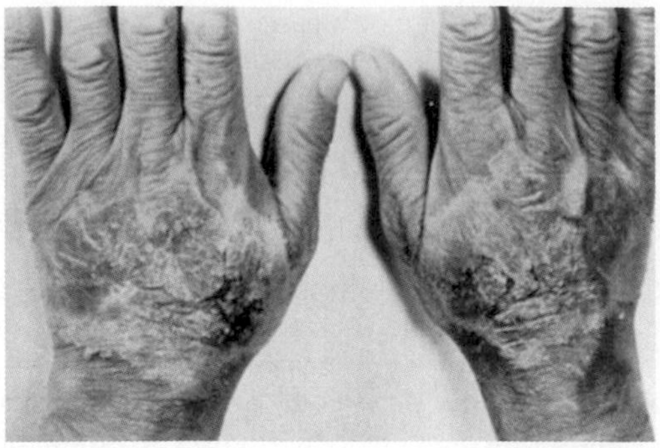

FIGURE 9–28 The sharply demarcated, characteristic scaling dermatitis of pellagra.

Vitamin B_6 is present in virtually all foods; however, food processing may destroy pyridoxine and in the past was responsible for severe deficiency in infants fed poorly controlled dried milk preparations. Secondary hypovitaminosis B_6 is produced most often by long-term use of any of a variety of drugs that act as pyridoxine antagonists. These include isoniazid (used to treat tuberculosis), estrogens, and penicillamine. Alcoholics are also prone to develop vitamin B_6 deficiency because acetaldehyde, an alcohol metabolite, enhances pyridoxine degradation. Pregnancy is associated with increased demand. Thus, pyridoxine supplementation is required in these conditions. A deficiency of vitamin B_6 is associated with high levels of plasma homocysteine. The latter is a risk factor for atherosclerosis, but currently there is no evidence that vitamin B_6 supplements reduce the risk of cardiovascular disease.

Clinical findings in vitamin B_6–deficient patients resemble those seen in patients with riboflavin and niacin deficiency. Patients may have seborrheic dermatitis, cheilosis, glossitis, peripheral neuropathy, and sometimes convulsions.

Vitamin C (Ascorbic Acid). A deficiency of vitamin C leads to the development of scurvy, characterized principally by bone disease in growing children and hemorrhages and healing defects in both children and adults. Unlike some other vitamins, ascorbic acid cannot be synthesized endogenously, and therefore humans are dependent on intake with food. Ascorbic acid is present in milk and some animal products (liver, fish) and is abundant in a variety of fruits and vegetables. All but the most restricted diets provide adequate amounts of vitamin C.

With the abundance of ascorbic acid in many foods, scurvy has ceased to be a global problem, although it is sometimes encountered even in affluent populations as a conditioned deficiency, particularly among elderly individuals, persons who live alone, and alcoholics—all groups that often have erratic and inadequate eating patterns. Scurvy occasionally appears in patients undergoing peritoneal dialysis and hemodialysis and among food faddists. Tragically, the condition sometimes appears in infants who are maintained on formulas of processed milk without supplementation.

Ascorbic acid functions in a variety of biosynthetic pathways by accelerating hydroxylation and amidation reactions. The most clearly established *function of vitamin C is the acti-*

vation of prolyl and lysyl hydroxylases from inactive precursors, providing for hydroxylation of procollagen. Inadequately hydroxylated precursors cannot acquire a stable helical configuration and cannot be adequately cross-linked, so they are poorly secreted from the fibroblast. Those that are secreted lack tensile strength, are more soluble, and are more vulnerable to enzymatic degradation. Collagen, which normally has the highest content of hydroxyproline, is most affected, particularly in blood vessels, accounting for the predisposition to hemorrhages in scurvy. In addition, it appears that a deficiency of vitamin C leads to *suppression of the rate of synthesis of pro-collagen peptides*, independent of an effect on proline hydroxylation.

While the role of vitamin C in collagen synthesis has been known for many decades, it is only in relatively recent years that its antioxidant properties have been recognized. Vitamin C can scavenge free radicals directly in aqueous phases of the cell and can act indirectly by regenerating the antioxidant form of vitamin E. Thus, vitamins E and C act in concert. It is because of these synergistic actions that both of these vitamins have attracted interest as agents that may retard atherosclerosis by reducing the oxidation of LDL (Chapter 11). However, at present, there is no conclusive evidence that vitamin C supplementation is useful in primary or secondary prevention of coronary artery disease. Similarly, despite much attention in the lay press, there is no evidence that vitamin C supplements prevent the common cold; high doses may reduce the duration of symptoms.

Morphology. Scurvy in a growing child is far more dramatic than in an adult. **Hemorrhages** constitute one of the most striking features. Because the defect in collagen synthesis results in inadequate support of the walls of capillaries and venules, purpura and ecchymoses often appear in the skin and in the gingival mucosa. Furthermore, the loose attachment of the periosteum to bone, together with the vascular wall defects, leads to extensive **subperiosteal hematomas** and **bleeding into joint spaces** after minimal trauma. Retrobulbar, subarachnoid, and intracerebral hemorrhages may prove fatal.

Skeletal changes may also develop in infants and children. The primary disturbance is in the formation of osteoid matrix, rather than in mineralization or calcification, such as occurs in rickets. In scurvy, the palisade of cartilage cells is formed as usual and is provisionally calcified. However, there is insufficient production of osteoid matrix by osteoblasts. Resorption of the cartilaginous matrix then fails or slows; as a consequence, there is cartilaginous overgrowth, with long spicules and plates projecting into the metaphyseal region of the marrow cavity, and sometimes widening of the epiphysis (Fig. 9–29). The scorbutic bone yields to the stresses of weight bearing and muscle tension, with bowing of the long bones of the lower legs and abnormal depression of the sternum with outward projection of the ends of the ribs. The bone changes in adults are similar to those in children, with decreased formation of osteoid matrix, but deformation does not occur.

In severely scorbutic children and adults, **gingival swelling, hemorrhages, and secondary bacterial periodontal infection** are common. A distinctive **perifollicular, hyperkeratotic, papular rash** that may be ringed by hemorrhage often appears. **Wound healing and localization of focal infections are impaired** because of the derangement in collagen synthesis. Anemia is common, resulting from bleeding and from a secondary decrease in iron absorption (Chapter 13). The major features of scurvy are summarized in Figure 9–30.

Folate. Marginal body stores and inadequate dietary intake contribute to folate deficiency throughout the world. Folates are essential cofactors in nucleic acid synthesis; the conversion of 5-methyltetrahydrofolate to tetrahydrofolate requires vitamin B_{12}. Therefore, deficiency of either folate or vitamin B_{12} results in megaloblastic anemia. Rapidly dividing cells in the fetus are especially vulnerable to folate deficiency. The requirement for folate, similar to that of pyridoxine, is increased in pregnancy. Poor diet during the first trimester of pregnancy has been shown to be associated with an increased incidence of neural tube defects in the fetus. Folate supplements have been shown to decrease the risk of neural tube defects.[76] Since neural tube defects occur within the first few weeks post-conception, folic acid must be taken by all women who expect to be pregnant.[77] As with vitamins B_6 and B_{12}, low plasma folate is associated with high levels of plasma homocysteine. Although elevations in homocysteine predispose to atherosclerosis, as with other vitamins that affect homocysteine levels, there is no clear evidence that folate supplements reduce atherosclerotic disease.

Folate is found in whole-wheat flour, beans, nuts, liver, and green leafy vegetables. It is heat labile and depleted in cooked and processed foods. In the United States, it is estimated that 15% to 20% of adults have low serum folate. In developing countries that rely on diets based on corn with few fresh vegetables, folate deficiency is more common. Even in those people with adequate diets, oral contraceptives, anticonvulsants, ethanol, and cigarette smoking interfere with folate absorption and metabolism. Chronic diseases such as intestinal malabsorption and metastatic cancer are also associated with folate deficiency.[76]

Combined folate and vitamin B_{12} deficiency has been postulated to contribute to the development of colon cancer. The following mechanisms have been proposed: (1) altered DNA methylation; (2) accumulation of cells in S phase with increased susceptibility in induction of DNA damage; and (3) perturbations of nucleotide pools that impair DNA synthesis and repair.[76]

The consequences of vitamin B_{12} deficiency and pernicious anemia are described in Chapter 13. In contrast to folate deficiency, vitamin B_{12} deficiency is associated with myelin degeneration in both sensory and motor pathways of the spinal cord as described in Chapter 28.

Mineral Deficiencies

A number of minerals are essential for health. Calcium and phosphorus are required in large amounts and are considered in the discussion of vitamin D. Trace elements are metals that occur at concentrations smaller than 1 μg per gram of wet tissue. *Of the various trace elements found in the body, only five—iron, zinc, copper, selenium, and iodine—have been*

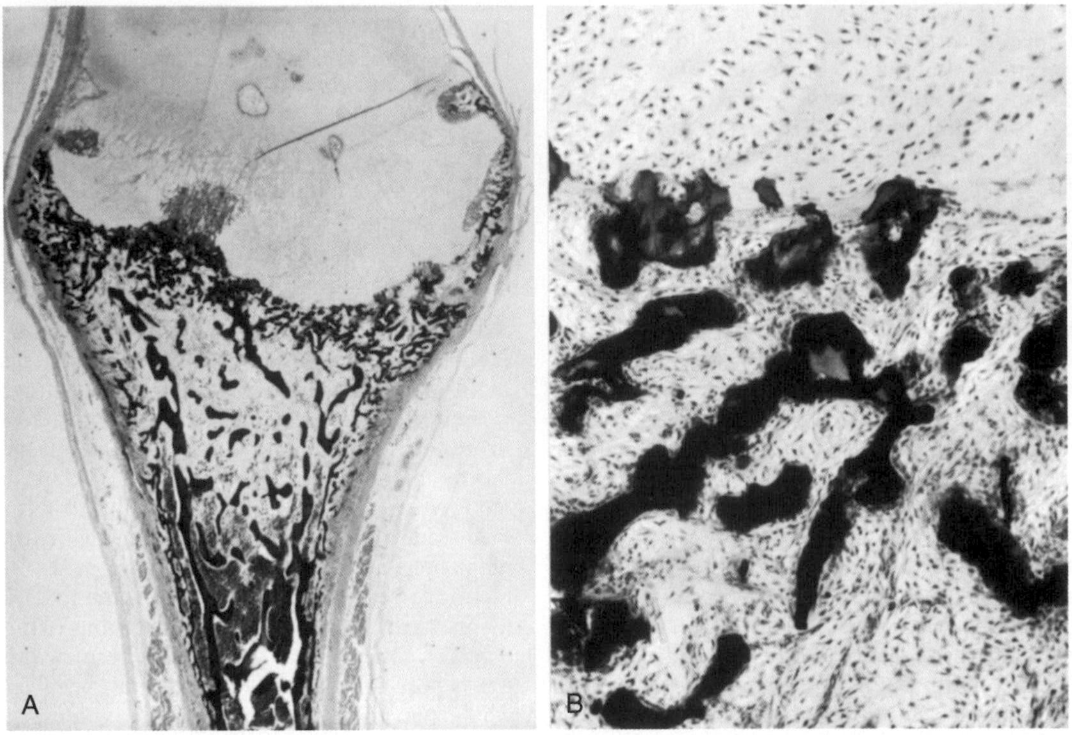

FIGURE 9–29 *A,* Longitudinal section of a scorbutic costochondral junction with widening of the epiphyseal cartilage and projection of masses of cartilage into the adjacent bone. *B,* Detail of a scorbutic costochondral junction. The orderly palisade is totally destroyed. There is dense mineralization of the spicules but no evidence of newly formed osteoid.

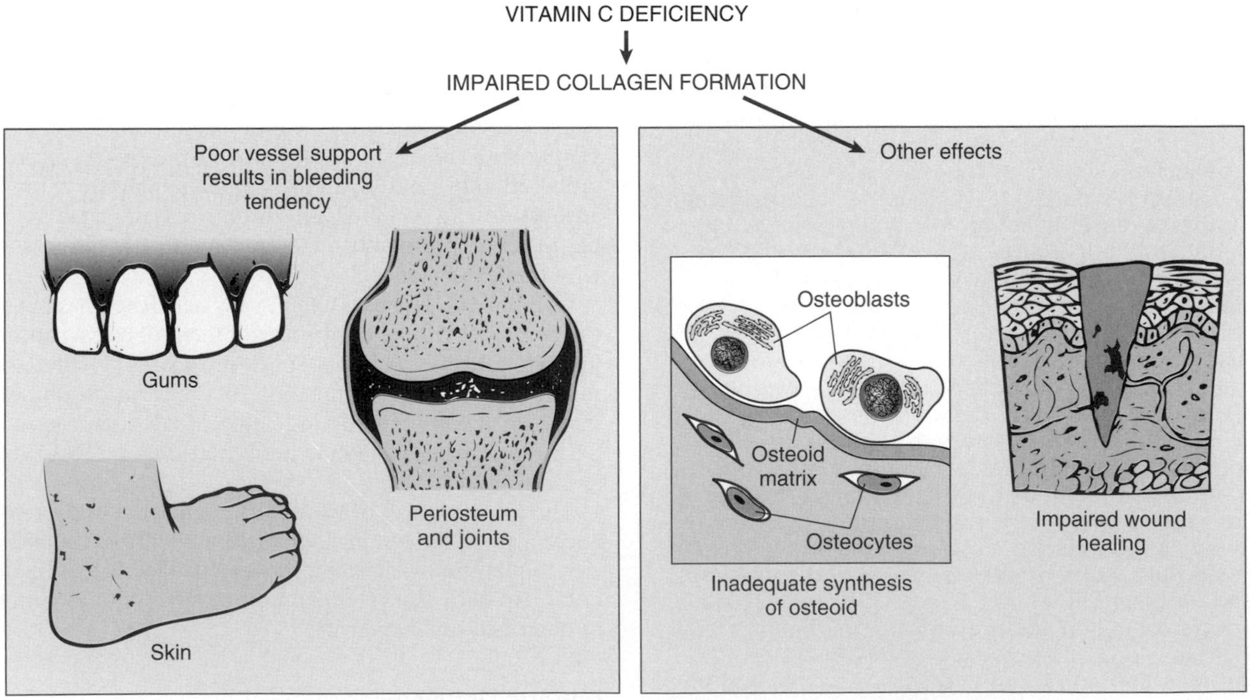

FIGURE 9–30 The major consequences of vitamin C deficiency.

associated with well-characterized deficiency states. In theory, a deficiency of a trace element might occur for many of the same reasons as a vitamin deficiency does, but three influences are particularly relevant: (1) inadequate supplementation in preparations used for total parenteral nutrition; (2) interference with absorption by dietary constituents; and (3) inborn errors of metabolism leading to abnormalities of trace metal absorption.

Dietary interference as a mechanism was first noted among inhabitants of Egypt and Iran who subsisted largely on unrefined cereals; sufficient phytic acid and fiber were present in the diet to bind zinc and block its absorption. Genetic malabsorption syndromes involving a trace element are rare. In one, failure to synthesize metallothionein (a metal-binding protein) in intestinal mucosal cells blocks absorption of both copper and zinc.

Table 9–24 provides brief comments on the role of several trace elements in health and disease. Additional comments are offered only for zinc and selenium deficiency.

Zinc Deficiency. A lack of zinc is unusual because it is reasonably abundant in meats, fish, shellfish, whole-grain cereals, and legumes. Most cases of zinc deficiency have been related to either total parenteral nutrition unsupplemented by zinc or the aforementioned rare genetic syndrome that interferes with absorption.

The essential features of zinc deficiency are (1) a distinctive rash, most often around the eyes, nose, mouth, anus, and distal parts, called *acrodermatitis enteropathica* (Fig. 9–31); (2) anorexia, often accompanied by diarrhea; (3)growth retardation in children; (4) impaired wound healing; (5) hypogonadism with diminished reproductive capacity; (6) altered immune function; (7) impaired night vision related to altered vitamin A metabolism; (8) depressed mental function; and (9) an increased incidence of congenital malformations in infants of zinc-deficient mothers.

Zinc deficiency should be suspected in any case of obscure growth retardation or infertility associated with a distinctive rash (acrodermatitis enteropathica). Oral zinc supplementation is promptly curative.

Selenium Deficiency. Selenium, like vitamin E, protects against oxidative damage of membrane lipids. The deficiency of this element is well known in China as *Keshan disease,* which presents as a congestive cardiomyopathy, mainly in children and young women. It results from a markedly low level of the metal in soil, water, and food.

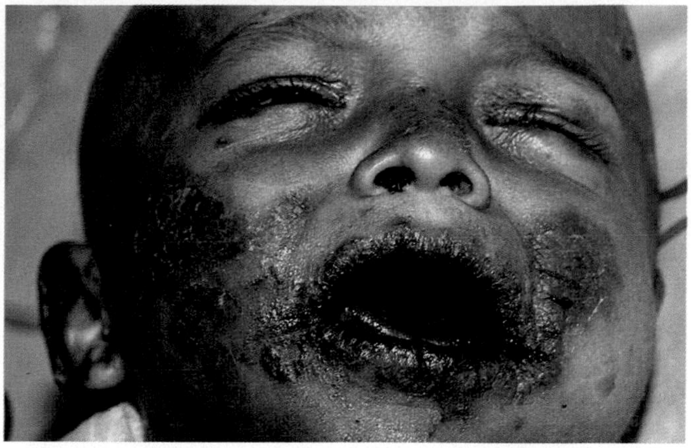

FIGURE 9–31 Zinc deficiency with hemorrhagic dermatitis around the mouth and eyes.

OBESITY

Obesity is a global epidemic resulting from sedentary lifestyles, improved socioeconomic conditions, and availability of processed, high calorie foods and soft drinks in industrialized societies. Approximately 35% of the US adult population is overweight, and an additional 30% of adults are obese; the prevalence of obesity in children and adolescents is also increasing; indeed, reaching epidemic proportions.[78] Because obesity is correlated with increased morbidity and mortality, it is important to define and recognize it, to understand its causes, and to be able to initiate appropriate measures to prevent or manage it. Behavioral and dietary changes are the initial therapeutic strategies; weight-loss drugs should be used with caution, especially herbal preparations that combine ephedra alkaloids and caffeine, because there are serious potential adverse reactions.

How does one measure fat accumulation? There are several highly technical ways to approximate the measurement, but for practical considerations, the following ones are commonly used:

- Some expression of weight in relation to height, especially the measurement referred to as the *body mass index* (BMI)
- Skin fold measurements

TABLE 9–24 Functions of Trace Metals and Deficiency Syndromes

Nutrient	Functions	Deficiency Syndromes
Iron	Essential component of hemoglobin as well as a number of iron-containing metalloenzymes	Hypochromic microcytic anemia
Zinc	Component of enzymes, principally oxidases	Acrodermatitis enteropathica, growth retardation, infertility
Iodine	Component of thyroid hormone	Goiter and hypothyroidism
Selenium	Component of glutathione peroxidase	Myopathy, rarely cardiomyopathy
Copper	Component of cytochrome *c* oxidase, dopamine β-hydroxylase, tyrosinase, lysyl oxidase, and unknown enzyme involved in cross-linking keratin	Muscle weakness, neurologic defects, hypopigmentation, abnormal collagen cross-linking
Manganese	Component of metalloenzymes, including oxidoreductases, hydrolases, and lipases	No well-defined deficiency syndrome
Fluoride	Mechanism unknown	Dental caries

- Various body circumferences, particularly the ratio of the waist to hip circumference.

The BMI, expressed in kilograms per square meter, is closely correlated with body fat. A BMI of approximately 25 kg/m^2 is considered normal. Individuals with BMI ≥30 kg/m^2 are considered obese, and those whose BMI falls between 25.0 to 29.9 kg/m^2 are considered overweight[79] (Table 9–25). As noted, the prevalence of obesity-related diseases, such as diabetes, hypertension, and coronary artery disease, begins to increase at BMI values >25.0 kg/m^2 and then continues the ascent at higher values.

The untoward effects of obesity are related not only to the total body weight, but also to the distribution of the stored fat. *Central or visceral obesity,* in which fat accumulates in the trunk and in the abdominal cavity (in the mesentery and around viscera), is associated with a much higher risk for several diseases than is excess accumulation of fat diffusely in subcutaneous tissue.

The etiology of obesity is complex and incompletely understood. Involved are genetic, environmental, and psychological factors. However, simply put, *obesity is a disorder of energy balance. When food-derived energy chronically exceeds energy expenditure, the excess calories are stored as triglycerides in adipose tissue.* The two sides of the energy equation, intake and expenditure, are finely regulated by neural and hormonal mechanisms (Fig. 9–32). In most individuals, when food intake increases, so does the consumption of calories, and vice versa. Hence, body weight is maintained within a narrow range for many years. Apparently, this fine balance is maintained by an internal set point, or "lipostat," that can sense the quantity of the energy stores (adipose tissue) and appropriately regulate the food intake as well as the energy expenditure. The molecular nature of the lipostat remained obscure for many years, but with the identification of leptin in 1994, a series of breathtaking discoveries changed the picture.

A simplified scheme of the current understanding of the neurohumoral mechanisms that regulate the energy equation and therefore influence body weight is shown in Figure 9–32. Broadly speaking, there are three components of this system:

1. The afferent system, which generates humoral signals from the adipose tissue (leptin), pancreas (insulin), and stomach (ghrelin)
2. The central processing unit, located primarily in the hypothalamus, which integrates the afferent signals
3. The effector system, which carries out "orders" from the hypothalamic nuclei in the form of feeding behavior and energy expenditure.

TABLE 9–25 Body Mass Index Associated Disease Risk

Obesity Class		BMI (kg/m^2)	Risk
Underweight		<18.5	Increased
Normal		18.5–24.9	Normal
Overweight		25.0–29.9	Increased
Obesity	I	30.0–34.9	High
	II	35.0–39.9	Very high
Extreme Obesity	III	≥40.0	Extremely high

Data from National Institutes of Health, National Heart, Lung, and Blood Institute. Clinical guidelines on the identification, evaluation, and treatment of overweight and obesity in adults—The evidence report. Obes Res 6 (suppl 2):515, 1998.

These three components are described next.[80] Not shown in Figure 9–32 is that energy expenditure occurs through a variety of hormonal (e.g., thyrotropin-releasing hormone) and autonomic intermediaries.

Among the afferent signals, insulin and leptin exert long-term control over the energy cycle by activating catabolic circuits and inhibiting anabolic pathways, as discussed in greater detail below. By contrast, ghrelin is predominately a short-term mediator. Produced in the stomach, ghrelin levels rise sharply before every meal and fall promptly when the stomach is "filled." In fact, it is thought that the success of gastric bypass surgery in massively obese individuals may relate more to the associated suppression of ghrelin levels than to an anatomic reduction in stomach capacity.

Whereas both insulin and leptin influence the energy cycle, available data suggest that leptin has a more important role than insulin in the central nervous system control of energy homeostasis.[81,81a] Hence, our discussion will be focused on leptin, recognizing that leptin and insulin share some of their actions.

It is now established that adipocytes communicate with the hypothalamic centers that control appetite and energy expenditure by secreting leptin, a member of the cytokine family. When there is an abundance of stored energy in the form of adipose tissue, the resultant high levels of leptin cross the blood-brain barrier, binding to leptin receptors. Leptin receptor signaling has two effects: it inhibits anabolic circuits that normally promote food intake and inhibit energy expenditure, and, through a distinct set of neurons, leptin triggers catabolic circuits (Fig. 9–32). *The net effect of leptin, therefore, is to reduce food intake and promote energy expenditure.* Hence, over a period of time, energy stores (adipocytes) are reduced, and weight is lost. This in turn reduces the circulating levels of leptin, and a new equilibrium is reached. This cycle is reversed when adipose tissue is lost and leptin levels are reduced below a threshold. Equilibrium is again reached, since with low leptin levels, the anabolic circuits are relieved of inhibition and catabolic circuits are not activated, resulting in net gain of weight.

The molecular basis of leptin action is extremely complex and not yet fully unraveled. For the most part, leptin exerts its function through a series of integrated neural pathways referred to as the *leptin–melanocortin circuit,* described in Box 9–1 and illustrated in Figure 9–33. The understanding of this circuitry is important since obesity is a serious public health problem, and development of antiobesity drugs will depend on a full understanding of these pathways.

Obesity, particularly *central obesity, increases the risk for a number of conditions,*[79] including diabetes, hypertension, osteoarthritis, pancreatitis, and many others, listed in Table 9–26. Only some of these complications are discussed here. The mechanisms underlying these associations are complex and likely to be interrelated. Obesity, for instance, is associated with *insulin resistance* and hyperinsulinemia, important features of non–insulin-dependent, or type II, diabetes, and weight loss is associated with improvement. It has been speculated that excess insulin, in turn, may play a role in the retention of sodium, expansion of blood volume, production of

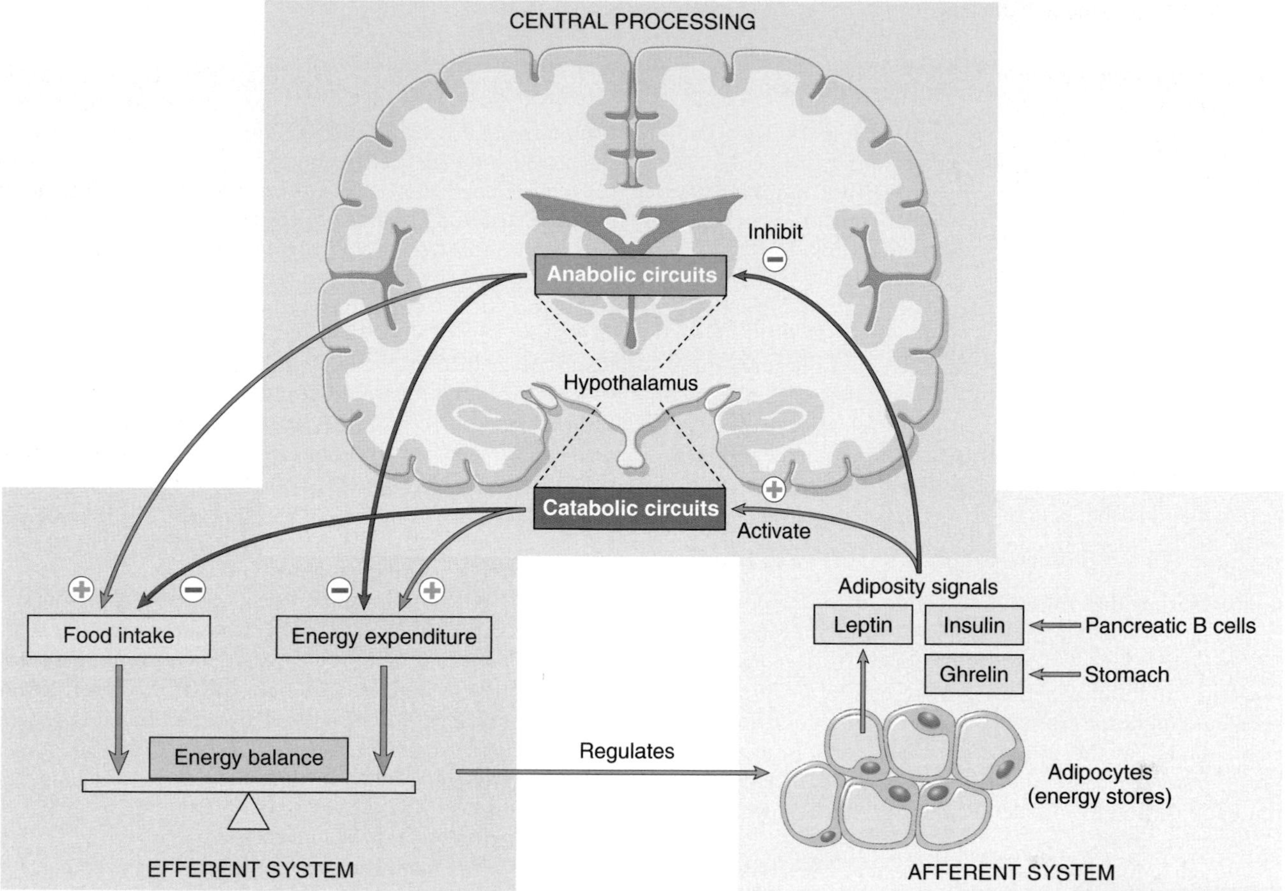

FIGURE 9–32 A simplified schema of the circuitry that regulates energy balance. When sufficient energy is stored in adipose tissue and the individual is well fed, afferent adiposity signals (insulin, leptin, ghrelin) are delivered to the central neuronal processing units, in the hypothalamus. Here the adiposity signals inhibit anabolic circuits and activate catabolic circuits. The effector arms of these central circuits then impact on energy balance by inhibiting food intake and promoting energy expenditure. This in turn reduces the energy stores and the adiposity signals are obtunded. Conversely, when energy stores are low, the available anabolic circuits take over at the expense of catabolic circuits to generate energy stores in the form of adipose tissue, thus generating an equilibrium.

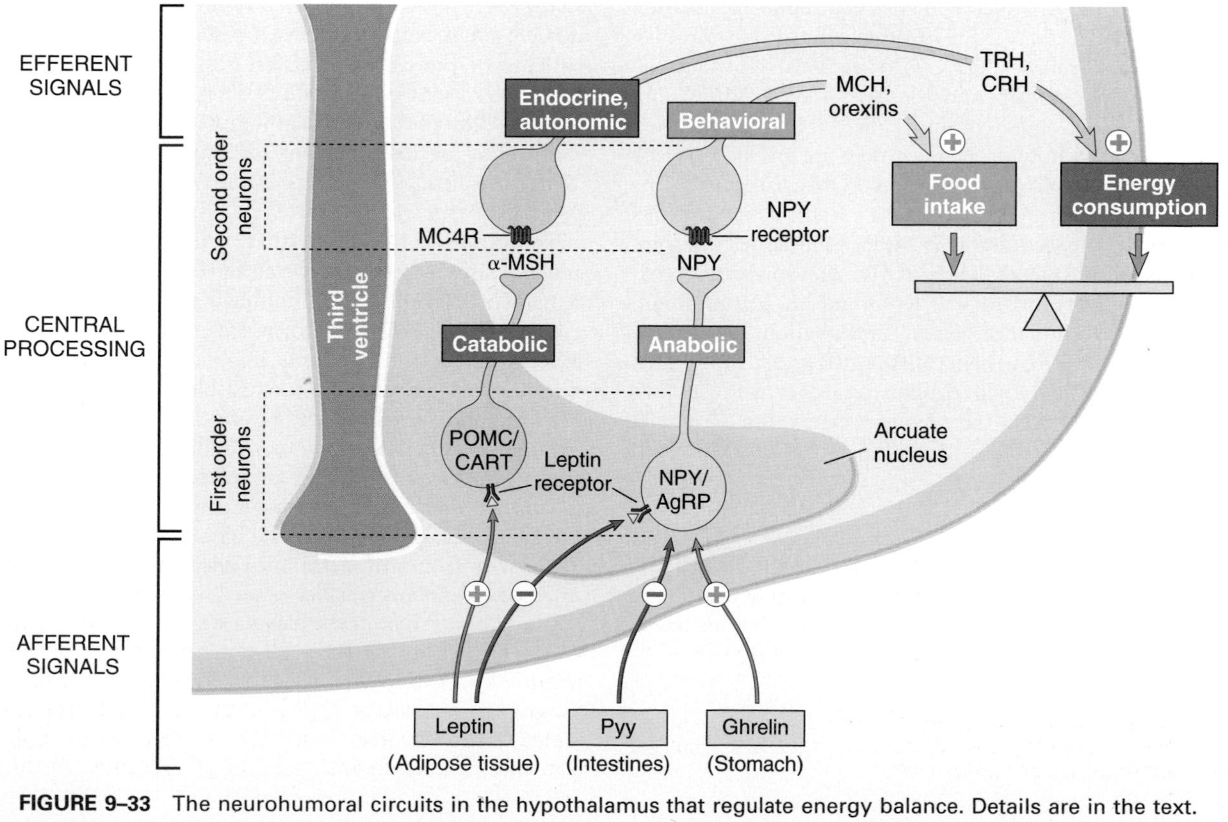

FIGURE 9–33 The neurohumoral circuits in the hypothalamus that regulate energy balance. Details are in the text.

Box 9–1 Genetics of Obesity

Obesity is a disorder with a multifactorial etiology. Only rarely does it result from single gene disorders. Evidence supporting an important role for genes in weight control includes familial clustering of obesity and higher concordance of body mass index (BMI) among monozygotic twins (74%) versus dizygotic twins (32%) living in the same environment. Although monogenic forms of obesity in humans are rare, studies of these genetic forms of obesity and their murine counterparts have significantly advanced our understanding of the molecular basis of obesity. Some of these are discussed below.

In recent years many "obesity" genes have been identified. As might be expected, they encode the molecular components of the neuroendocrine system that regulates energy balance. Leptin, the key player in energy homeostasis, is the product of the *OB* gene. Its role as an antiobesity factor is buttressed by the observation that mice homozygous for mutations in the leptin gene (*OB/OB*) do not secrete leptin, are massively obese, and are "cured" by the administration of exogenous leptin. Mice with mutations in the leptin receptor (*db/db*) are also obese, but, unlike the case with *ob/ob* mice, their obesity cannot be ameliorated by the administration of leptin. In these mice, obesity occurs because the leptin-mediated afferent signals impinging on the hypothalamus fail to regulate appetite and energy expenditure.

Although leptin receptors are expressed at several sites in the brain, those most critical for regulation of the leptin–melanocortin circuit are expressed in the arcuate nucleus of the hypothalamus. There are two major types of neurons in this locale that bear leptin receptors: one set (*oraxogenic*) produces appetite-stimulating neurotransmitters called neuropeptide Y (NPY) and agouti-related peptide (AgRP). These are appropriately called NPY/AgRP neurons (see Fig. 9–33). As can be surmised from the discussion in the text, leptin reduces the expression of NPY and AgRP. The other set of leptin-sensitive neurons, the so-called POMC/CART neurons, transcribe two *anorexigenic* neuropeptides—α-melanocyte-stimulating hormone (α-MSH) and cocaine and amphetamine-related transcript (CART). Both of these peptides are products of pro-opiomelanocortin (POMC). When the POMC/CART neurons are activated by leptin signals, they exert catabolic effects mainly through the secretion of α-MSH. As indicated in Figure 9–33, the NPY/AgRP and POMC/CART neurons are referred to as first-order neurons of the leptin–melanocortin circuit, since they are the initial targets of leptin action. The neurotransmitters produced by them (NPY, AgRP, and α-MSH) then interact through their own specific receptors with second-order neurons that trigger the efferent systems with peripheral actions. The effects of these neurotransmitters are described next.

In the anabolic pathway, the first-order NPY/AgRP neurons make monosynaptic connections to second-order neurons, which express oraxogenic peptides melanin-concentrating hormone (MCH) and oraxins A and B. As illustrated in Figure 9–33, NPY released from first-order neurons binds to its receptor on second-order neurons and thus transmits feeding signals. Such signals are attenuated when leptin is in excess and are activated by low levels of leptin. AgRP, like NPY, exerts anabolic effects but by a somewhat distinct mechanism.

α-MSH produced by the POMC/CART neurons exerts its catabolic effects by binding to a set of second-order neurons (in the paraventricular nucleus) that express the melanocortin 4 receptor (MC4R). Catabolic output from the MC4R neurons is relayed to the periphery via the endocrine and autonomic systems. This reduces feeding and increases energy expenditure. The energy-consuming actions of MC4R neurons are mediated in part by the release of thyrotropin-releasing hormone (TRH), which activates the thyroxine axis through the anterior pituitary; TRH not only increases thermogenesis via secretion of thyroxine, but it is also an appetite suppressant. Corticotropin-releasing hormone (CRH) is another product of MC4R neurons. It induces anorexia and also activates the sympathetic nervous system. A subset of MC4R neurons projects to sympathetic motor output areas. Fibers from these areas innervate brown adipose tissue, rich in β_3-adrenergic receptors. When these receptors are stimulated, they cause fatty acid hydrolysis and also uncouple energy production from storage. Thus, the fats are literally burned, and energy so produced is dissipated as heat.

It is noteworthy that each of the six single gene defects that give rise to human obesity involves proteins in the leptin–melanocortin pathway. Four of these are autosomal recessive and affect the leptin receptor, POMC, and PC1. (The last mentioned is a prohormone convertase that cleaves POMC). In all these cases, there is profound hyperphagia and childhood-onset massive obesity. While these four forms of genetic obesity are quite rare, those caused by mutations in the melanocortin receptor, MC4R, are by comparison quite common. In a recent study, 5% to 8% of a cohort of 500 obese individuals had functionally important mutations in the MC4R gene.[83] In these patients, despite abundant fat stores and leptin, energy consumption cannot be stimulated. The sixth monogenic form of human obesity results from mutation in a transcription factor (SIM1) that is essential for the formation of second-order leptin neurons.

Despite the remarkable advances in our understanding of genetic control of pathways that regulate energy balance, the genetic basis of the most common forms of human obesity remains mysterious. As a multifactorial disorder, one might expect mutations or polymorphisms in several genes of small effect that give rise to obesity in concert with environmental factors. It is interesting to note that blood leptin levels are elevated in most humans with obesity. Clearly, the high levels of leptin are unable to down-regulate the anabolic pathways or activate the catabolic pathways. The basis of such leptin resistance is unclear but it may be contributed to by a decrease in the ability of leptin to cross the blood-brain barrier, possibly due to defective transport across endothelial cells. The fact that in some obese individuals leptin levels in the cerebrospinal fluid are lower than in the plasma supports this hypothesis.

TABLE 9–26 Medical Complications Associated with Obesity

Gastrointestinal	Gallstones, pancreatitis, abdominal hernia, NAFLD (steatosis, steatohepatitis, and cirrhosis), and possibly GERD
Endocrine/metabolic	Metabolic syndrome, insulin resistance, impaired glucose tolerance, type II diabetes mellitus, dyslipidemia, polycystic ovary syndrome
Cardiovascular	Hypertension, coronary artery disease, congestive heart failure, arrhythmias, pulmonary hypertension, ischemic stroke, venous stasis, deep vein thrombosis, pulmonary embolus
Respiratory	Abnormal pulmonary function, obstructive sleep apnea, obesity hypoventilation syndrome
Musculoskeletal	Osteoarthritis, gout, low back pain
Gynecologic	Abnormal menses, infertility
Genitourinary	Urinary stress incontinence
Ophthalmologic	Cataracts
Neurologic	Idiopathic intracranial hypertension (pseudotumor cerebri)
Cancer	Esophagus, colon, gallbladder, prostate, breast, uterus, cervix, kidney
Postoperative events	Atelectasis, pneumonia, deep vein thrombosis, pulmonary embolus

Data from Klein S, Wadden T, Sugerman HJ: AGA technical review on obesity. Gastroenterol 123:882, 2002. NAFLD, non-alcoholic fatty liver disease; GERD, gastroesophageal reflux disease.

excess norepinephrine, and smooth muscle proliferation that are the hallmarks of hypertension. Regardless of whether these pathogenic mechanisms are actually operative, *the risk of developing hypertension among previously normotensive persons increases proportionately with weight.* Obesity is also associated with a somewhat distinctive metabolic syndrome, the so-called *syndrome X*, which is characterized by abdominal obesity, insulin resistance, hypertriglyceridemia, low serum HDL, hypertension, and increased risk for coronary artery disease.[82]

Obese persons are likely to have hypertriglyceridemia and a low HDL cholesterol value, and these factors may increase the risk of *coronary artery disease*. The association between obesity and heart disease is not straightforward, and the linkage may be related to the associated diabetes and hypertension rather than to weight. Nevertheless, the American Heart Association has recently added obesity to its list of major risk factors.[79]

Nonalcoholic steatohepatitis occurs in adolescents and adults who are obese and have type II diabetes. Fatty change accompanied by liver cell injury and inflammation may progress to fibrosis or regress following weight loss.

Cholelithiasis (gallstones) is six times more common in obese than in lean subjects. The mechanism is mainly an increase in total body cholesterol, increased cholesterol turnover, and augmented biliary excretion of cholesterol in the bile, which in turn predisposes to the formation of cholesterol-rich gallstones (Chapter 18).

Hypoventilation syndrome is a constellation of respiratory abnormalities in very obese persons. It has been called the *pickwickian syndrome,* after the fat lad who was constantly falling asleep in Charles Dickens' *Pickwick Papers.* Hypersomnolence, both at night and during the day, is characteristic and is often associated with apneic pauses during sleep, polycythemia, and eventual right-sided heart failure.

Marked adiposity predisposes to the development of degenerative joint disease (*osteoarthritis*). This form of arthritis, which typically appears in older persons, is attributed in large part to the cumulative effects of wear and tear on joints. It is reasonable to assume that the greater the body burden of fat, the greater the trauma to joints with passage of time.

Obesity increases the risk of *ischemic stroke* in both men and women. Abdominal obesity is associated with increased risk of *venous thrombosis*.

Somewhat controversial is the association between obesity and cancer. A recent large prospective study has revealed an association between increasing BMI and mortality from many forms of cancer, including cancers of the esophagus, colon, rectum, liver, and non-Hodgkin lymphoma.[84] The basis of this association is difficult to discern. With hormone-dependent cancers, such as those arising in the endometrium, the blame can be placed on hormonal imbalance since obesity is known to raise estrogen levels, but for others we remain in the dark.

DIET AND SYSTEMIC DISEASES

The problems of undernutrition and overnutrition, as well as specific nutrient deficiencies, have been discussed; however, the composition of the diet, even in the absence of any of these problems, may make a significant contribution to the causation and progression of a number of diseases. A few examples suffice here.

Currently one of the most important and controversial issues is the contribution of diet to atherogenesis. The central question is, Can dietary modification prevent or retard the development of atherosclerosis (most importantly, coronary artery disease)? The average adult in the United States consumes an inordinate amount of fat and cholesterol daily, with a ratio of saturated fatty acids to polyunsaturated fatty acids of about 3:1. Vegetable oils (e.g., corn and safflower oils) and fish oils contain polyunsaturated fatty acids and are good sources of cholesterol-lowering lipids. Fish oil fatty acids belonging to the omega-3, or n-3, family have more double bonds than do the omega-6, or n-6, fatty acids found in vegetable oils. A recent meta-analysis of 11 studies with over 16,000 patients revealed that a diet enriched in omega-3 fatty acids (vs. placebo) significantly reduced the incidence of fatal myocardial infarction and sudden cardiac death.[85]

There are other examples of the effect of diet on disease:

- Hypertension is beneficially affected by restricting sodium intake.
- Dietary fiber, or roughage, resulting in increased fecal bulk, has a preventive effect against diverticulosis of the colon.
- People who consume diets that contain abundant fresh fruits and vegetables with limited intake of meats and processed foods have a lower risk of myocardial infarction. One mechanism that may explain these epidemiologic observations is the association of hyperhomocysteinemia with increased intake of meats and decreased intake of vitamin B_6, vitamin B_{12}, and folate. Excess levels of homocysteine are hypothesized to contribute to atherosclerosis (Chapter 11).
- Calorie restriction has been convincingly demonstrated to increase life span in experimental animals. The basis of this striking observation is not entirely clear (Chapter 1).
- Even lowly garlic has been touted to protect against heart disease (and also, alas, kisses), although research has yet to prove the effect on heart disease unequivocally.

CHEMOPREVENTION OF CANCER

Epidemiologic studies have provided evidence that populations who consume large quantities of fruits and vegetables in their diets have a lower risk of cancer. It is hypothesized that carotenoids that are converted to vitamin A in the liver and intestine may be important in the primary chemoprevention of cancer.[86] The following mechanisms are proposed for the anticarcinogenic effects of carotenoids and retinoids:

- Retinoic acid promotes differentiation of mucus-secreting epithelial tissues. Supplementation of the diet with beta-carotene and retinol is hypothesized to reverse squamous metaplasia and preneoplastic lesions in the respiratory tract of cigarette smokers and workers exposed to asbestos.
- Fruits and vegetables provide antioxidants such as beta-carotene, vitamins C and E, and selenium that prevent oxidative damage to DNA.
- Vitamin A can enhance immune responses; other retinoids may modulate inflammatory reactions that are potential sources of reactive oxygen and nitrogen intermediates.

Notwithstanding such theoretical considerations, clinical studies on the role of vitamin A supplementation and cancer risk have failed to provide clear answers. Clinical trials using beta-carotene and retinyl palmitate as primary preventive agents against lung cancer were terminated because the participants showed an excess of lung cancers and increased mortality. On the other hand, 13-*cis*-retinoic acid was effective in prevention of secondary squamous cell carcinomas of the head and neck region. These apparently conflicting results are not easily explained; however, there are multiple chemical forms of retinoids that alter gene expression, cell proliferation, differentiation, and apoptosis by binding to six different nuclear receptors. Some retinoids are associated with significant toxicity, including dry skin, conjunctivitis, and hypertriglyceridemia. Until the biochemical and molecular mechanisms of action of individual retinoids and other antioxidants are understood, it is unwise to recommend dietary supplements for the primary chemoprevention of cancer. However, a diet rich in fruits, vegetables, and unprocessed grains that is low in fat and animal protein has been associated with a decreased risk of cardiovascular disease and some types of cancer.[84]

High animal fat intake combined with low fiber intake has been implicated in the causation of colon cancer. The most convincing explanation for these associations is as follows: high fat intake increases the level of bile acids in the gut, which in turn modifies intestinal flora, favoring the growth of microaerophilic bacteria. The bile acids or bile acid metabolites produced by these bacteria might serve as carcinogens or promoters. The protective effect of a high-fiber diet might relate to (1) increased stool bulk and decreased transit time, which decrease the exposure of mucosa to putative offenders, and (2) the capacity of certain fibers to bind carcinogens and thereby protect the mucosa.

Attempts to document these theories in clinical and experimental studies have, on the whole, led to contradictory results.

Thus, we must conclude that, despite many tantalizing trends and proclamations by "diet gurus," to date there is no definite proof that diet can cause or protect against cancer. Nonetheless, concern persists that carcinogens lurk in things as pleasurable as a juicy steak and rich ice cream.

REFERENCES

1. Levy BS, Wegman DH: Occupational health—an overview. In Levy BS, et al. (eds): Occupational Health. Recognizing and Preventing Work-Related Disease and Injury, 4th ed. Philadelphia, Lippincott Williams & Wilkins, 2000, pp 3–13.
2. Carpenter DO, et al: Understanding the human health effects of chemical mixtures. Environ Health Perspect 110 (suppl A):25, 2002.
3. Minna JD, et al: Focus on lung cancer. Cancer Cell 1:49, 2002.
4. Hodgson E: Introduction to toxicology. In Hodgson E, Levi PE (eds): Textbook of Modern Toxicology. Stamford, CT, Appleton & Lange, 1997, pp 1–25.
5. Hodgson E, Levi PE: Absorption and distribution of toxicants. In Hodgson E, Levi PE (eds): A Textbook of Modern Toxicology. Stamford, CT, Appleton & Lange, 1997, pp 27–56.
6. Nebert DW, Russell DW: Clinical importance of the cytochromes P450. Lancet 360:1155, 2002.
7. Perera FP: Environment and cancer: who are susceptible? Science 278:1068, 1997.
8. Nordberg J, Arnér ESJ: Reactive oxygen species, antioxidants, and the mammalian thioredoxin system. Free Radical Biol Med 31:1287, 2001.
9. Bolger PM, Schwetz, BA: Mercury and Health. N Engl J Med 347:1735, 2002.
10. Clarkson TW: The three modern faces of mercury. Environ Health Perspect 110 (suppl 1):11, 2002.
11. Fellows JL, et al: Annual smoking-attributable mortality, years of potential life lost, and economic costs—United States, 1995–1999. MMWR 51:300, 2002.
12. Wiencke JK, Kelsey KT: Teen smoking, field cancerization, and a "critical period" hypothesis for lung cancer susceptibility. Environ Health Perspect 110:555, 2002.
13. Pinkerton KE, et al: Interaction of tobacco smoking with occupational and environmental factors. In Harber PH, et al (eds.): Occupational and Environmental Respiratory Disease. St. Louis, Mosby, 1996, pp 827–835.
14. Hanrahan JP, Weiss ST: Environmental tobacco smoke. In Harber PH, et al (eds): Occupational and Environmental Respiratory Disease. St. Louis, Mosby, 1996, pp 767–783.
15. Lieber CS: Medical disorders of alcoholism. N Engl J Med 333:1058, 1995.
16. Tsukamoto H, Lu SC: Current concepts in the pathogenesis of alcoholic liver injury. FASEB J 15:1335, 2001.

17. Thackray H, Tifft C: Fetal alcohol syndrome. Pediatr Rev 22(2):47, 2001.
18. Montesano R, Hill J: Environmental causes of human cancers. Eur J Cancer 37:S67, 2001.
19. Cami J, et al.: Drug addiction. N Engl J Med 349:975, 2003.
20. Hyman SE: A 28-year-old man addicted to cocaine. JAMA 286:2586, 2001.
21. Lange RA, Hillis LD: Cardiovascular complications of cocaine. N Engl J Med 345:351, 2001.
22. Kantak KM: Vaccines against drugs of abuse: a viable treatment option? Drugs 63:341, 2003.
23. Reneman L, et al: Effects of dose, sex, and long-term abstention from use on toxic effects of MDMA (ecstasy) on brain serotonin neurons. Lancet 358:1864, 2001.
24. Lazarou J, et al: Incidence of adverse drug reactions in hospitalized patients: A meta-analysis of prospective studies JAMA 279:1200, 1998.
25. Philips KA, et al: Potential role of pharmacogenomics in reducing adverse drug reactions: a systematic review. JAMA 286:2270, 2001.
26. Evans WE, Johnson JA: Pharmacogenomics: the inherited basis for interindividual differences in drug response. Annu Rev Genomics Hum Genet 2:9, 2001.
27. Dahl M-L: Cytochrome P450 phenotyping/genotyping in patients receiving antipsychotics: useful aid to prescribing? Clin Pharmacokinet 41:453, 2002.
28. Ernst E: The risk–benefit profile of commonly used herbal therapies: ginkgo, St. John's wort, ginseng, echinacea, saw palmetto, and kava. Ann Intern Med 136:42, 2002.
29. Davidson NE, Helzlsouer KJ: Good news about oral contraceptives. N Engl J Med 346:2078, 2002.
30. Marchbanks PA, et al: Oral contraceptives and the risk of breast cancer. N Engl J Med 346:2025, 2002.
31. Nelson HID, et al: Postmenopausal hormone replacement therapy: scientific review. JAMA 288:872, 2002.
32. Grodstein F, Clarkson TB, Manson JE: Understanding divergent data on postmenopausal hormone therapy. N Engl J Med. 348:645, 2003.
33. Berde CB, Sethna NF: Analgesics for the treatment of pain in children. N Engl J Med 347:1094, 2002.
34. Bascom R, et al: Health effects of outdoor air pollution. Am J Respir Crit Care Med 153:3, 477, 1996.
35. Pope CA: Epidemiology of fine particulate air pollution and human health: biologic mechanisms and who's at risk? Environ Health Perspect 108 (suppl 4):713, 2000.
36. Lambert WE, Samet JM: Indoor air pollution. In Harber P, et al (eds): Occupational and Environmental Respiratory Disease. St. Louis, Mosby, 1996, pp 784–807.
37. Morgan KT: A brief review of formaldehyde carcinogenesis in relation to rat nasal pathology and human health risk assessment. Toxicol Pathol 25:291, 1997.
38. Samet JM, Eradze GR: Radon and lung cancer risk: taking stock at the millennium. Environ Health Perspect 108 (suppl 4):635, 2000.
39. Billings CH, Howard P: Asbestos exposure, lung cancer and asbestosis. Moraldi Arch Dis 55:151, 2000.
40. Manning CB, Vallyathan V, Mossman BT: Diseases caused by asbestos: mechanisms of injury and disease development. Intl Immunopharmacol 2:191, 2002.
41. Menzies D, Bourbeau J: Building-related illnesses. N Engl J Med 337:1524, 1997.
42. Mastrangelo G, et al: Polycyclic aromatic hydrocarbons and cancer in man. Environ Health Perspect 104:1166, 1996.
43. Kelleher P, et al: Inorganic dust pneumonias: the metal-related parenchymal disorders. Environ Health Perspect 108 (suppl 4):685, 2000.
44. Fischbein A: Occupational and environmental lead exposure. In Rom WN (ed.): Environmental and Occupational Medicine, 2nd ed. Boston, Little, Brown, 1992, pp 735–758.
45. Rogan WJ, Ware JH: Exposure to lead in children—how low is low enough? N Engl J Med 348:1515, 2003.
46. Goyer RA: Results of lead research: prenatal exposure and neurological consequences. Environ Health Perspect 104:1050, 1996.
47. Costa M, et al: Molecular mechanisms of nickel carcinogenesis. Environ Health Perspect 102 (Suppl 3):127, 1994.
48. Goldman LR: Environmental health and its relationship to occupational health. In Levy BS, et al. (eds): Occupational Health. Recognizing and Preventing Work-Related Disease and Injury, 4th ed. Philadelphia, Lippincott Williams & Wilkins, 2000, pp 51–96.
49. Moline JM, et al: Exposure to hazardous substances and male reproductive health: a research framework. Environ Health Perspect 108:803, 2000.
50. Schantz SL, Widholm JJ: Cognitive effects of endocrine-disrupting chemicals in animals. Environ Health Perspect 109:1197, 2001.
51. Huff J, et al: Carcinogenicity of TCDD: experimental, mechanistic, and epidemiologic evidence. Annu Rev Pharmacol Toxicol 34:343, 1994.
52. Mettler FA, Voelz GL: Major radiation exposure—what to expect and how to respond. N Engl J Med 346:1554, 2002.
53. Upton AC: Ionizing radiation. In Craighead JE (ed): Pathology of Environmental and Occupational Disease. St. Louis, Mosby, 1996, pp 205–214.
54. Karanjawla ZE et al.: Supplementary oxygen metabolism causes chromosome breaks and is associated with neuronal apoptosis observed in double stranded DNA strand repair mutants. Curr Biol 12:397, 2002.
55. Smith ML, Fornace AJ Jr: Mammalian DNA damage-inducible genes associated with growth arrest and apoptosis. Mutat Res 340:109, 1996.
56. Paris F, et al: Endothelial apoptosis as the primary lesion initiating intestinal radiation damage in mice. Science 293:293, 2001.
57. Belka C, et al: Radiation induced CNS toxicity—molecular and cellular mechanisms. Brit J Cancer 85:1233, 2001.
58. Johnston CJ, et al: Radiation-induced pulmonary fibrosis: examination of chemokine and chemokine receptor families. Radiation Res 157:256, 2002.
59. Murnane JP: Role of induced genetic instability in the mutagenic effects of chemicals and radiation. Mutat Res 367:11, 1996.
60. Greenblatt MS, et al: Mutations in the *p53* tumor suppressor gene: clues to cancer etiology and molecular pathogenesis. Cancer Res 54:4855, 1994.
61. Rittie L, Fisher GJ: UV light-induced signal cascades and skin aging. Aging Res Rev 1:705, 2002.
62. Cleaver JE, Crowley E: UV damage, DNA repair and skin carcinogens. Front Biosci 7:1024, 2002.
63. Cleary SF: Electromagnetic energy. In Craighead JE (ed): Pathology of Environmental and Occupational Disease. St. Louis, Mosby, 1996, pp 215–228.
64. Ahlbom A, et al: Review of the epidemiologic literature on EMF and health. Environ Health Perspect 109 (Suppl 6):911, 2001.
65. Adey WR, et al: Spontaneous and nitrosourea-induced primary tumors of the central nervous system in Fischer 344 rats exposed to frequency-modulated microwave fields. Cancer Res 60:1857, 2000.
66. Rivara FP, et al: Injury prevention. N Engl J Med 337:543, 613, 1997.
67. Rodricks JV, Jackson BA: Food constituents and contaminants. In Lippmann M (ed): Environmental Toxicants: Human Exposures and Their Health Effects. New York, Van Nostrand Reinhold, 1992, pp 266–298.
68. Detsky AL, et al: Is this patient malnourished? JAMA 271:54, 1994.
69. Tisdale MJ: Biology of cachexia. J Natl Cancer Inst 89:1763, 1997.
70. Stephensen CB: Vitamin A, infection and immune function. Ann Rev Nutr 21:167, 2001.
71. Lips P: Hypervitaminosis A and fractures. N Engl J Med. 348:347, 2003.
72. Willett WC, Stampfer MJ: What vitamins should I be taking, Doctor? N Engl J Med 345:1819, 2001.
73. Tangpricha V, et al: Vitamin D insufficiency among free living healthy young adults. Am J Med 112:659, 2002.
74. Fairfield KM, Fletcher RH: Vitamins for chronic disease prevention in adults: scientific review. JAMA 287:3116, 2002.
75. Koshihara Y, et al: Vitamin K stimulates osteoblastogenesis and inhibits osteoclastogenesis in human bone marrow culture. J Endocrinol 176:339, 2003.
76. Branda RF: Folic acid deficiency. In Craighead JM (ed): Pathology of Environmental and Occupational Disease. St. Louis, Mosby, 1996, pp 170–174.
77. Lumley J, et al: Periconceptional supplementation with folate and/or multivitamins for preventing neural tube defects. Cochrane Database of Systematic Reviews, June 1, 2002.
78. Marx J: Cellular warriors at the battle of the bulge. Science 299:846, 2003.
79. Klein S, Wadden T, Sugerman HJ: AGA technical review on obesity. Gastroenterol 123:882, 2002.
80. Lustig RH: The neuroendocrinology of obesity. Endocrinol Metab Clin North Am 30(3):765, 2001.
81. Cummings DE, Schwartz MW: Genetics and pathophysiology of human obesity: Annu Rev Med 54:453, 2003.
81a. Elmquist JK, Flier JS: The fat-brain axis enters a new dimension. Science 304:63, 2004.

82. Lakka HM, et al: The metabolic syndrome and total and cardiovascular disease mortality in middle-aged men. JAMA 288:2709, 2002.
83. List JF, Havener JF: Defective melanocortin 4 receptors in hyperphagia and morbid obesity. N Engl J Med 384:1160, 2003.
84. Calle EE, et al: Overweight, obesity, and mortality from cancer in a prospectively studied cohort of US adults. N Engl J Med 348:1625, 2003.
85. Bucher HC, et al: N-3 polyunsaturated fatty acids in coronary heart disease: a meta-analysis of randomized controlled trials. Am J Med 112:298, 2002.
86. Hong WK, Sporn MB: Recent advances in chemoprevention of cancer. Science 278:1073, 1997.

CHAPTER 10

Diseases of Infancy and Childhood

Anirban Maitra, MBBS • Vinay Kumar, MD

CONGENITAL ANOMALIES

Definitions

Causes of Anomalies

Genetic Causes

Environmental Causes

Multifactorial Causes

Pathogenesis of Congenital Anomalies

BIRTH WEIGHT AND GESTATIONAL AGE

Prematurity and Fetal Growth Restriction

Immaturity of Organ Systems

Lungs

Kidneys

Brain

Liver

Apgar Score

BIRTH INJURIES

PERINATAL INFECTIONS

Transcervical (Ascending) Infections

Transplacental (Hematologic) Infections

Onset of Sepsis

NEONATAL RESPIRATORY DISTRESS SYNDROME

NECROTIZING ENTEROCOLITIS

GERMINAL MATRIX—INTRAVENTRICULAR HEMORRHAGE

FETAL HYDROPS

Immune Hydrops

Nonimmune Hydrops

INBORN ERRORS OF METABOLISM AND OTHER GENETIC DISORDERS

Phenylketonuria

Galactosemia

Cystic Fibrosis (Mucoviscidosis)

SUDDEN INFANT DEATH SYNDROME (SIDS)

TUMORS AND TUMOR-LIKE LESIONS OF INFANCY AND CHILDHOOD

Benign Tumors and Tumor-Like Lesions

Malignant Tumors

Incidence and Types

Neuroblastic Tumors

Wilms Tumor

Children are not merely little adults, and the diseases they get are not merely variants of adult diseases. Many childhood conditions are unique to, or at least take distinctive forms in, this stage of life and so are discussed separately in this chapter. Diseases originating in the perinatal period are important in that they account for significant morbidity and mortality. As would be expected, the chances for survival of live-born infants improve with each passing week. This differential represents, at least in part, a triumph of improved medical care. Better prenatal care, more effective methods of monitoring the condition of the fetus, and judicious resort to cesarean section before term when there is evidence of fetal distress all contribute to bringing into this "mortal coil" live-born infants who in past years might have been stillborn. These infants represent an increased number of *high-risk* infants. Nonetheless, the infant mortality rate in the United States has shown a decline from a level of 20.0 deaths per 1000 live births in 1970 to about 6.9 deaths in 2000.[1] Although the death rate has con-

The contributions of Dr. Deborah Scofield to this chapter in earlier editions are gratefully acknowledged.

tinued to decline for all infants, American blacks continue to have an infant mortality rate more than twice (13.9 deaths per 1000 live births) that of American whites (6.0 deaths). Worldwide, the infant mortality rates vary widely, from as low as 3 deaths per 1,000 live births in Sweden, to as high as 82 deaths in the Indian subcontinent.

Each stage of development of the infant and child is prey to a somewhat different group of disorders. The data available permit a survey of four time spans: (1) the neonatal period (the first 4 weeks of life), (2) infancy (the first year of life), (3) age 1 to 4 years, and (4) age 5 to 14 years.

The major causes of death in infancy and childhood are cited in Table 10–1. Congenital anomalies, disorders relating to short gestation (prematurity) and low birth weight, and sudden infant death syndrome (SIDS) represent the leading causes of death in the first 12 months of life. Once the infant survives the first year of life, the outlook brightens measurably. In the next two age groups—1 to 4 years and 5 to 14 years—injuries resulting from accidents have become the leading cause of death (see Table 10–1). Among the natural diseases, in order of importance, congenital anomalies and malignant neoplasms assume major significance. It would appear then that, in a sense, life is an obstacle course. For the great majority, the obstacles are surmounted or, even better, bypassed. We now take a closer look at the specific conditions encountered during the various stages of infant and child development.

TABLE 10–1 Cause of Death Related with Age

Causes*	Rate†
Under 1 Year: All Causes	**727.4**
Congenital malformations, deformations, and chromosomal anomalies	
Disorders related to short gestation and low birth weight	
Sudden infant death syndrome (SIDS)	
Newborn affected by maternal complications of pregnancy	
Newborn affected by complications of placenta, cord, and membranes	
Respiratory distress of newborn	
Accidents (unintentional injuries)	
Bacterial sepsis of newborn	
Intrauterine hypoxia and birth asphyxia	
Diseases of the circulatory system	
1–4 Years: All Causes	**32.6**
Accidents and adverse effects	
Congenital malformations, deformations, and chromosomal abnormalities	
Malignant neoplasms	
Homicide and legal intervention	
Diseases of the heart‡	
Influenza and pneumonia	
5–14 Years: All Causes	**18.5**
Accidents and adverse effects	
Malignant neoplasms	
Homicide and legal intervention	
Congenital malformations, deformations, and chromosomal abnormalities	
Suicide	
Diseases of the heart	
15–24 Years: All Causes	**80.7**
Accidents and adverse effects	
Homicide	
Suicide	
Malignant neoplasms	
Diseases of the heart	

*Causes are listed in decreasing order of frequency. All causes and rates are preliminary 2000 statistics. (Minino AM, Smith BL. Deaths: Preliminary data for 2000. National Vital Statistics Report, 49:12, 2001).

†Rates are expressed per 100,000 population.

‡Excludes congenital heart disease.

Congenital Anomalies

Congenital anomalies are morphologic defects that are present at birth, but some, such as cardiac defects and renal anomalies, may not become clinically apparent until years later. The term *congenital* does not imply or exclude a genetic basis for the birth defect. It is estimated that about 3% of newborns have a *major anomaly*, defined as an anomaly having either cosmetic or functional significance. As indicated in Table 10–1, they are the most common cause of mortality in the first year of life and contribute significantly to morbidity and mortality throughout the early years of life. In a real sense, anomalies found in live-born infants represent the less serious developmental failures in embryogenesis that are compatible with live birth. Perhaps 20% of fertilized ova are so anomalous that they are blighted from the outset. Others may be compatible with early fetal development, only to lead to spontaneous abortion. Less severe anomalies allow more prolonged intrauterine survival, with some disorders terminating in stillbirth and those still less significant permitting live birth despite the handicaps imposed.

DEFINITIONS

Before proceeding, we define some of the terms used for various kinds of errors in morphogenesis—*malformations, disruptions, deformations, sequences*, and *syndromes.*

- *Malformations* represent primary errors of morphogenesis, in other words there is an *intrinsically abnormal developmental process* (Fig. 10–1). They are usually multifactorial rather than the result of a single gene or chromosomal defect. Malformations may present in several patterns. Some, such as congenital heart defects and anencephaly (absence of brain), involve single body systems, whereas in other cases multiple malformations involving many organs may coexist.
- *Disruptions* result from secondary destruction of an organ or body region that was previously normal in development; thus, in contrast to malformations, disruptions arise from an *extrinsic disturbance in morphogenesis. Amni-*

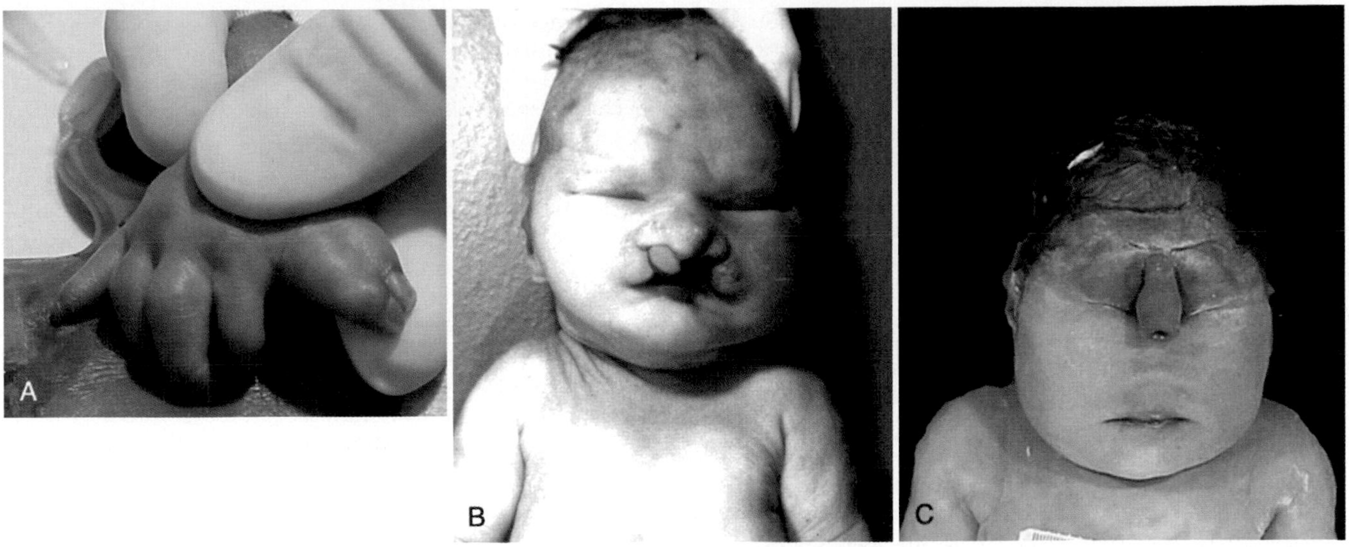

FIGURE 10–1 Malformations. Human malformations can range in severity from the incidental to the lethal. *Polydactyly* (one or more extra digits) and *syndactyly* (fusion of digits), both of which are illustrated in *A*, have little functional consequence when they occur in isolation. Similarly, *cleft lip (B)*, with or without associated *cleft palate*, is compatible with life when it occurs as an isolated anomaly; in the present case, however, this child had an underlying *malformation syndrome* (trisomy 13) and expired because of severe cardiac defects. The stillbirth illustrated in *C* represents a severe and essentially lethal malformation, where the midface structures are fused or ill-formed; in almost all cases, this degree of external dysmorphogenesis is associated with severe internal anomalies such as maldevelopment of the brain and cardiac defects. (Pictures *A* and *C* courtesy of Dr. Reade Quinton, and *B* courtesy of Dr. Beverly Rogers, Department of Pathology, University of Texas Southwestern Medical Center, Dallas, TX.)

otic bands, denoting rupture of amnion with resultant formation of "bands" that encircle, compress, or attach to parts of the developing fetus, are the classic example of a disruption (Fig. 10–2). A variety of environmental agents may cause disruptions (see below). Understandably, disruptions are not heritable and hence are not associated with risk of recurrence in subsequent pregnancies.

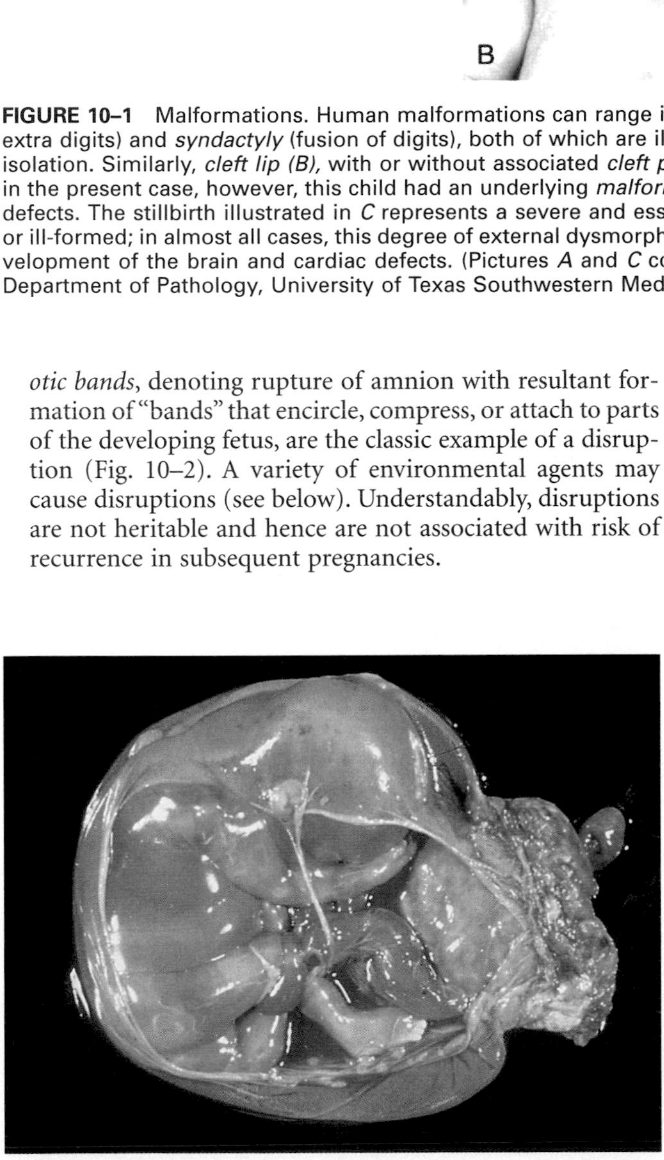

FIGURE 10–2 Disruption. Disruptions occur in a normally developing organ because of an extrinsic abnormality that interferes with normal morphogenesis. *Amniotic bands* are a frequent cause of disruptions. In the illustrated example, note the placenta at the right of the diagram and the band of amnion extending from the top portion of the amniotic sac to encircle the leg of the fetus. (Courtesy of Dr. Theonia Boyd, Children's Hospital of Boston, MA.)

- *Deformations*, like disruptions, also represent an *extrinsic disturbance of development* rather than an intrinsic error of morphogenesis. Deformations are common problems, affecting approximately 2% of newborn infants to varying degrees. Fundamental to the pathogenesis of deformations is localized or generalized compression of the growing fetus by *abnormal biomechanical forces*, leading eventually to a variety of structural abnormalities. The most common underlying factor responsible for deformations is *uterine constraint.* Between the 35th and 38th weeks of gestation, rapid increase in the size of the fetus outpaces the growth of the uterus, and the relative amount of amniotic fluid (which normally acts as a cushion) also decreases. Thus, even the normal fetus is subjected to some form of uterine constraint. Several factors increase the likelihood of excessive compression of the fetus resulting in deformations. *Maternal factors* include first pregnancy, small uterus, malformed (bicornuate) uterus, and leiomyomas. *Fetal or placental factors* include oligohydramnios, multiple fetuses, and abnormal fetal presentation. An example of a deformation is clubfeet, often a component of Potter sequence, described later.
- A *sequence* is a pattern of cascade anomalies. Approximately half the time, congenital anomalies occur singly; in the remaining cases, multiple congenital anomalies are recognized. In some instances, the constellation of anomalies may be explained by a single, localized aberration in organogenesis (malformation, disruption, or deformation) leading to secondary effects in other organs. A good example of a sequence is the *oligohydramnios* (or *Potter*) *sequence* (Fig. 10–3). Oligohydramnios (decreased amniotic fluid) may be caused by a variety of unrelated maternal, placental, or fetal abnormalities. Chronic leakage of amniotic fluid because of rupture of the amnion, uteroplacental

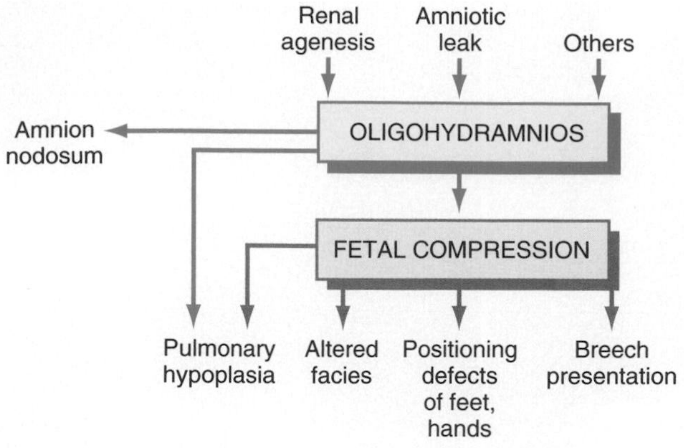

FIGURE 10–3 Schematic diagram of the pathogenesis of the oligohydramnios sequence.

insufficiency resulting from maternal hypertension or severe toxemia, and renal agenesis in the fetus (as fetal urine is a major constituent of amniotic fluid) are all causes of oligohydramnios. The fetal compression associated with significant oligohydramnios, in turn, results in a classic phenotype in the newborn infant, including flattened facies and positional abnormalities of the hands and feet (Fig. 10–4). The hips may be dislocated. Growth of the chest wall and the contained lungs is also compromised so that the lungs are frequently hypoplastic, occasionally to the degree that they are the cause of fetal demise. Nodules in the amnion *(amnion nodosum)* are frequently present.

- A *syndrome* is a constellation of congenital anomalies, believed to be pathologically related, that, in contrast to a sequence, *cannot* be explained on the basis of a single, localized, initiating defect. Syndromes are most often caused by a single etiologic agent, such as a viral infection or specific chromosomal abnormality, which simultaneously affects several tissues.

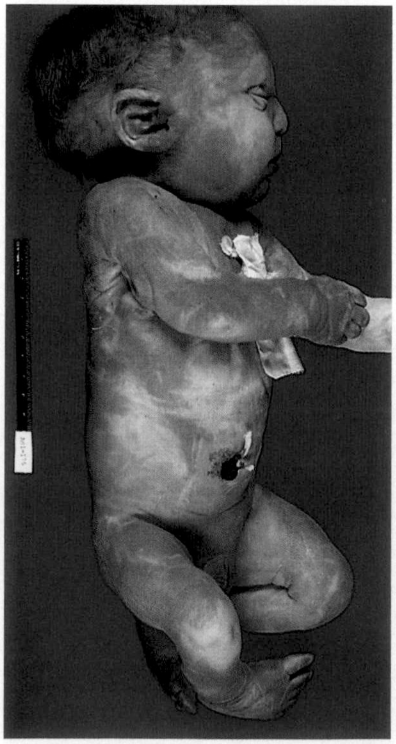

FIGURE 10–4 Infant with oligohydramnios sequence. Note the flattened facial features and deformed right foot (talipes equinovarus).

In addition to the aforementioned global definitions, a few organ-specific terms should be defined. *Agenesis* refers to the complete absence of an organ and its associated primordium. A closely related term, *aplasia*, refers also to the absence of an organ but one owing to failure of development of the primordium. *Atresia* describes the absence of an opening, usually of a hollow visceral organ, such as the trachea and intestine. *Hypoplasia* refers to incomplete development or underdevelopment of an organ with decreased numbers of cells, whereas *hyperplasia* refers to the converse, that is, overdevelopment of an organ associated with increased numbers of cells. An abnormality in an organ or a tissue as a result of an increase or a decrease in the size (rather than the number) of individual cells defines *hypertrophy* or *hypotrophy.* Finally, *dysplasia*, in the context of malformations (*versus* neoplasia) describes an abnormal organization of cells.

CAUSES OF ANOMALIES

At one time, it was believed that the presence of a visible, external anomaly was divine punishment for wickedness, a belief that occasionally jeopardized the mother's life. Although we are learning a great deal about some of the molecular bases of malformations, *the exact cause remains unknown in at least half the cases.* The common known causes of congenital anomalies can be grouped into three major categories: genetic, environmental, and multifactorial (Table 10–2).

Genetic Causes

Anomalies that are known to be genetic in origin can be divided into two groups:

- Those associated with karyotypic aberrations
- Those arising from single gene mutations.

A third group is suspected of resulting from *multifactorial inheritance*, a term that implies the interaction of two or more genes of small effect with environmental factors, and is discussed separately.

Virtually all the *chromosomal syndromes* (Chapter 5) are characterized by congenital anomalies. Karyotypic abnormalities are present in approximately 10% to 15% of live-born infants with congenital anomalies, but only one approaches a birth frequency of 1 in 1000 total births—trisomy 21 (Down syndrome). Next in order of frequency are Klinefelter syndrome, Turner syndrome, and trisomy 13 (Patau syndrome). The remaining chromosomal syndromes associated with malformations are far more rare. *The great preponderance of these cytogenetic aberrations arises as defects in gametogenesis and so are not familial.* There are, however, several transmissible chromosomal abnormalities, for example, the form of Down syndrome associated with a Robertsonian translocation in the parent, which is passed from one generation to the next, thus constituting a familial pattern of structural abnormalities. It should come as a sobering thought that *80% to 90% of fetuses with aneuploidy and other abnormalities of chromosome number die in utero, the majority in the earliest stages of gestation.*

TABLE 10–2 Causes of Congenital Anomalies in Humans

Cause	Frequency (%)
Genetic	
Chromosomal aberrations	10–15
Mendelian inheritance	2–10
Environmental	
Maternal/placental infections	2–3
Rubella	
Toxoplasmosis	
Syphilis	
Cytomegalovirus	
Human immunodeficiency virus (HIV)	
Maternal disease states	6–8
Diabetes	
Phenylketonuria	
Endocrinopathies	
Drugs and chemicals	1
Alcohol	
Folic acid antagonists	
Androgens	
Phenytoin	
Thalidomide	
Warfarin	
13-*cis*-retinoic acid	
Others	
Irradiations	1
Multifactorial (Multiple Genes ? Environment)	**20–25**
Unknown	**40–60**

Adapted from Stevenson RE, et al (eds): Human Malformations and Related Anomalies. New York, Oxford University Press, 1993, p. 115.

Single gene mutations of large effect may underlie major congenital anomalies, which, as expected, follow mendelian patterns of inheritance.[2] Of these, approximately 90% are inherited in an autosomal dominant or recessive pattern, while the remainder segregates in an X-linked pattern. Not surprisingly, many of the mutations that give rise to birth defects involve abrogation of function of genes involved in normal organogenesis and development. For example, holoprosencephaly is the most common developmental defect of the forebrain and midface in humans (see Chapter 28); mutations of *sonic hedgehog*, a gene involved in developmental patterning (see below), have been reported in a subset of patients with holoprosencephaly.[3] Similarly, mutations of a downstream target of sonic hedgehog signaling, *GLI3*, have been reported in patients with anomalies of digits, either conjoined digits *(syndactyly)* or supernumerary digits *(polydactyly)*.

Environmental Causes

Environmental influences, such as viral infections, drugs, and irradiation, to which the mother was exposed during pregnancy may cause fetal malformations (the appellation of "malformation" is loosely used in this context, since technically, these anomalies represent *disruptions*).

Viruses. Many viruses have been implicated in causing malformations, including the agents responsible for rubella, cytomegalic inclusion disease, herpes simplex, varicella-zoster infection, influenza, mumps, human immunodeficiency virus (HIV), and enterovirus infections. Among these, the rubella virus and cytomegalovirus are the most extensively investigated. With all viruses, the gestational age at which the infection occurs in the mother is critically important. *The at-risk period for rubella infection extends from shortly before conception to the 16th week of gestation,* the hazard being greater in the first 8 weeks than in the second 8 weeks.[4] The incidence of malformations is reduced from 50% to 20% to 7% if infection occurs in the first, second, or third month of gestation. The fetal defects are varied, but the major tetrad comprises cataracts, heart defects (persistent ductus arteriosus, pulmonary artery hypoplasia or stenosis, ventricular septal defect, tetralogy of Fallot), deafness, and mental retardation, referred to as *rubella embryopathy.*

Intrauterine infection with cytomegalovirus, mostly asymptomatic, is the most common fetal viral infection. This viral disease is considered in detail in Chapter 8; *the highest at-risk period is the second trimester of pregnancy.* Because organogenesis is largely completed by the end of the first trimester, congenital malformations occur less frequently than in rubella; nevertheless, the effects of virus-induced injury on the formed organs are often severe. Involvement of the central nervous system is a major feature, and the most prominent clinical changes are mental retardation, microcephaly, deafness, and hepatosplenomegaly.

Drugs and Other Chemicals. A variety of drugs and chemicals have been suspected to be teratogenic, but perhaps less than 1% of congenital malformations are caused by these agents. The list includes thalidomide, folate antagonists, androgenic hormones, alcohol, anticonvulsants, warfarin (oral anticoagulant), and 13-*cis*-retinoic acid used in the treatment of severe acne.[5] For example, *thalidomide,* once used as a tranquilizer in Europe, caused an extremely high frequency (50% to 80%) of limb abnormalities in exposed fetuses.[6] *Alcohol,* perhaps the most widely used agent today, is a teratogen. Affected infants show growth retardation, microcephaly, atrial septal defect, short palpebral fissures, maxillary hypoplasia, and several other minor anomalies. These together are labeled the *fetal alcohol syndrome.*[7] While cigarette smoke–derived nicotine has not been convincingly demonstrated to be a teratogen, there is a high incidence of spontaneous abortions, premature labor, and placental abnormalities in pregnant smokers; babies born to smoking mothers often have a low birth weight and may be prone to sudden infant death syndrome (see later). *In light of these findings, it is best to avoid nicotine exposure altogether during pregnancy.*

Radiation. In addition to being mutagenic and carcinogenic, radiation is teratogenic. Exposure to heavy doses of radiation during the period of organogenesis leads to malformations, such as microcephaly, blindness, skull defects, spina bifida, and other deformities. Such exposure occurred in the past when radiation was used to treat cervical cancer.

Maternal Diabetes. Among maternal conditions listed in Table 10–2, diabetes mellitus is a common entity, and despite advances in antenatal obstetric monitoring and glucose control, the incidence of major malformations in infants of diabetic mothers stands between 6% and 10% in most series. Maternal hyperglycemia-induced fetal hyperinsulinemia results in increased body fat, muscle mass, and organomegaly *(fetal macrosomia)*; cardiac anomalies, neural tube defects, and other central nervous system malformations are some of the major anomalies seen in *diabetic embryopathy.*[8]

Multifactorial Causes

The genetic and environmental factors just discussed account for no more than half of human congenital anomalies. The causes of the vast majority of birth defects, including some relatively common disorders such as cleft lip and cleft palate, remain unknown. In these anomalies, it would appear that inheritance of a certain number of mutant genes and their interaction with the environment is required before the disorder is expressed. In the case of congenital dislocation of the hip, for example, depth of the acetabular socket and laxity of the ligaments are believed to be genetically determined, whereas a significant environmental factor is believed to be frank breech position in utero, with hips flexed and knees extended. The importance of environmental contribution to multifactorial inheritance is underscored by a dramatic reduction in the incidence of neural tube defects by periconceptional intake of folic acid in the diet.[9,10] The approximate frequency of some common congenital anomalies in the United States is presented in Table 10–3. Both temporal and regional variability are common in the reporting of many malformations. For example, between 1979 and 1989, there was a mean annual percent decrease in the incidence of anencephaly of 6.4 and a mean annual increase in the incidence of atrial septal defect of 22.0.[11]

PATHOGENESIS OF CONGENITAL ANOMALIES

The pathogenesis of congenital anomalies is complex and still poorly understood, but certain general principles of developmental pathology are relevant regardless of the etiologic agent.

The timing of the prenatal teratogenic insult has an important impact on the occurrence and the type of anomaly produced (Fig. 10–5). The intrauterine development of humans can be divided into two phases: (1) the embryonic period occupying the first 9 weeks of pregnancy and (2) the fetal period terminating at birth.

In the *early embryonic period* (first 3 weeks after fertilization), an injurious agent damages either enough cells to cause death and abortion or only a few cells, presumably allowing the embryo to recover without developing defects. *Between the third and the ninth weeks, the embryo is extremely susceptible to teratogenesis,* and the peak sensitivity during this period occurs between the fourth and the fifth weeks. During this period, organs are being crafted out of the germ cell layers. The *fetal period* that follows organogenesis is marked chiefly by the further growth and maturation of the organs, with greatly reduced susceptibility to teratogenic agents. Instead the fetus is susceptible to growth retardation or injury to already formed organs. It is therefore possible for a given agent to produce different anomalies if exposure occurs at different times of gestation.

Teratogens and genetic defects may act at several steps involved in normal morphogenesis. These include the following:[12]

- Proper *cell migration* to predetermined locations that influence the development of other structures
- *Cell proliferation,* which determines the size and form of embryonic organs
- *Cellular interactions* among tissues derived from different structures (e.g., ectoderm, mesoderm), which affect the differentiation of one or both of these tissues
- *Cell–matrix associations,* which affect growth and differentiation
- *Programmed cell death (apoptosis),* which, as we have seen, allows orderly organization of tissues and organs during embryogenesis (Chapter 1)
- *Hormonal influences* and *mechanical forces,* which affect morphogenesis at many levels.

The complex interplay between environmental teratogens and intrinsic genetic defects is underscored by the fact that features of dysmorphogenesis caused by environmental insults can be recapitulated by certain genetic defects. This is exemplified in the relationship between the teratogen, retinoic acid (see below and Fig. 10–6), and two growth factors—transforming growth factor (TGF) and fibroblast growth factor (FGF)—both involved in morphogenesis. As discussed later, retinoic acid can induce defects in palatal development *(cleft lip and cleft palate),* possibly by impacting on multiple targets associated with secondary palatal development. In experimental models of retinoic acid teratogenesis, abnormal expression of TGF and FGF has been reported in the developing palate.[13,14] Not unexpectedly, therefore, rare single gene mutations in one or more of these growth factors or their receptors may also cause palatal abnormalities. There is an association, for example, between rare mutations of the *TGF-α* gene and nonsyndromic cleft lip or cleft palate in humans;[15] in addition, loss of function of the epidermal growth factor receptor, which acts as a receptor for TGF-α, can result in abnormal palatogenesis.[16] Disruption of TGF-β3 in mice also results in cleft palate.[17]

TABLE 10–3 Approximate Frequency of the More Common Congenital Malformations in the United States

Malformation	Frequency per 10,000 Total Births
Clubfoot without central nervous system anomalies	25.7
Patent ductus arteriosus	16.9
Ventricular septal defect	10.9
Cleft lip with or without cleft palate	9.1
Spina bifida without anencephalus	5.5
Congenital hydrocephalus without anencephalus	4.8
Anencephalus	3.9
Reduction deformity (musculoskeletal)	3.5
Rectal and intestinal atresia	3.4

Adapted from James LM: Maps of birth defects occurrence in the U.S., birth defects monitoring program (BDMP)/CPHA, 1970–1987. Teratology 48:551, 1993.

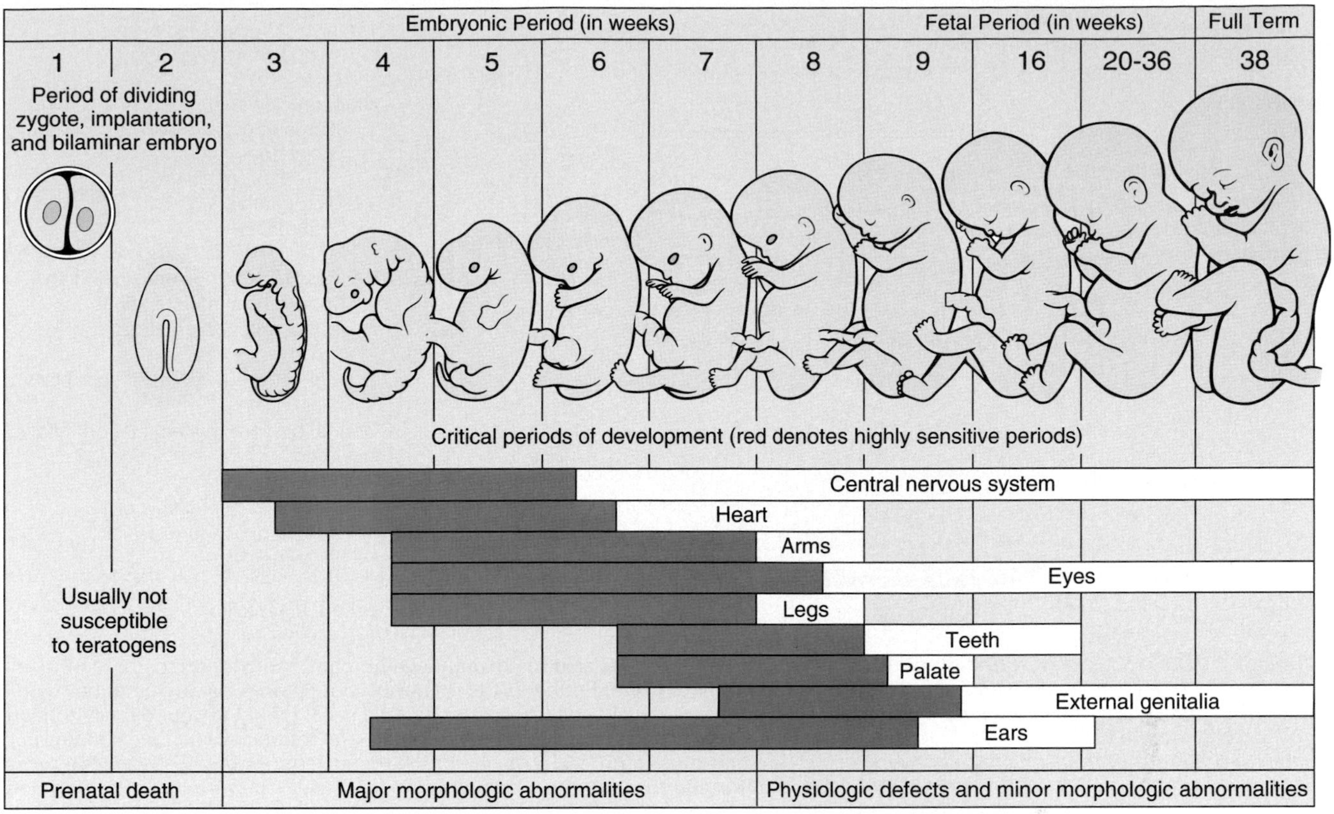

FIGURE 10–5 Critical periods of development for various organ systems and the resultant malformations. (Modified and redrawn from Moore KL: The Developing Human, 5th ed. Philadelphia, WB Saunders, 1993, p. 156.)

Since many congenital malformations reflect failure of normal *morphogenesis* during development, it is reasonable to expect that alterations of genes that control these events might cause birth defects. Two such classes of genes deserve special mention.

Homeobox Genes. Classes of genes known to be important in embryonic patterning include those that contain conserved regions involved in transcriptional regulation. One such class, *the HOX genes*, were first identified from study of the *Drosophila* mutant, *antennapedia*, in which legs appear in the position normally occupied by the antennae.[18] *HOX* genes have a 180-nucleotide motif, dubbed the *homeobox*, which has DNA-binding properties and is conserved between species as divergent as insects and humans. In vertebrates, *these genes have been implicated in the patterning of limbs, vertebrae, and craniofacial structures.* Introduction of altered *Hox* genes in transgenic mice, embryonic exposure to chemical agents known to increase or decrease expression of *Hox* genes, mutations, and experimental deletion of those genes *(knockouts)* produce malformations concordant with their presumed role in embryonic patterning. In humans, mutations of *HOXD13* cause *synpolydactyly* (extra digits) in heterozygous individuals, and mutations of *HOXA13* cause *hand-foot-genital syndrome*, characterized by distal limb and distal urinary tract malformations.[19]

Homeobox genes themselves are regulated by upstream genes and interact with downstream target genes. Upstream regulators of *HOX* genes are also implicated in teratogenesis. For example, the vitamin A (retinol) derivative, *all-trans-retinoic acid*, is essential for normal development, and its *absence* during embryogenesis results in a constellation of malformations affecting multiple organ systems, including the eyes, genitourinary system, cardiovascular system, diaphragm, and lungs (Fig. 10–6, *left*).[20] Conversely, *retinoic acid itself is a known human teratogen.* Infants born to mothers treated with retinoic acid for severe acne have a predictable phenotype *(retinoic acid embryopathy)*, including central nervous system, cardiac, and craniofacial defects (Fig. 10–6, *right*).[21] In animals, retinoic acid exposure produces reproducible changes in *Hox* gene expression and causes a wide range of structural congenital malformations, the nature of which is determined by the dosage and timing of exposure.[22] The precise mechanisms by which retinoic acid interacts with these genes in a normal embryo and the manner by which *malformations* are caused are still being determined. One scenario (Fig. 10–6, *center*) is that the malformations are caused by differential temporal and spatial expression of nuclear retinoic acid receptors (RAR; RXR) and cellular retinoic acid–binding proteins (CRABP), which determine the activity of retinoic acid receptor complexes as transcriptional regulators of *HOX* genes.[23,24] Recent evidence also suggests that *HOX* genes possess retinoic acid response elements *(RAREs)*, and that the latter are required for mediating both physiologic and pathologic effects of retinoids during development.[25] Finally, *HOX* gene expression may be modulated through families of intermediary proteins, which are themselves transcription factors, but are in turn regulated by retinoic acid.[26] Not surprisingly, a variety of other teratogens (e.g., the anticonvulsant sodium valproate) may also mediate their effects through disruption of *HOX* gene expression.[27] Once again, these examples illustrate the principle that interactions between patterning genes and environmental teratogens are important in the genesis of congenital anomalies.

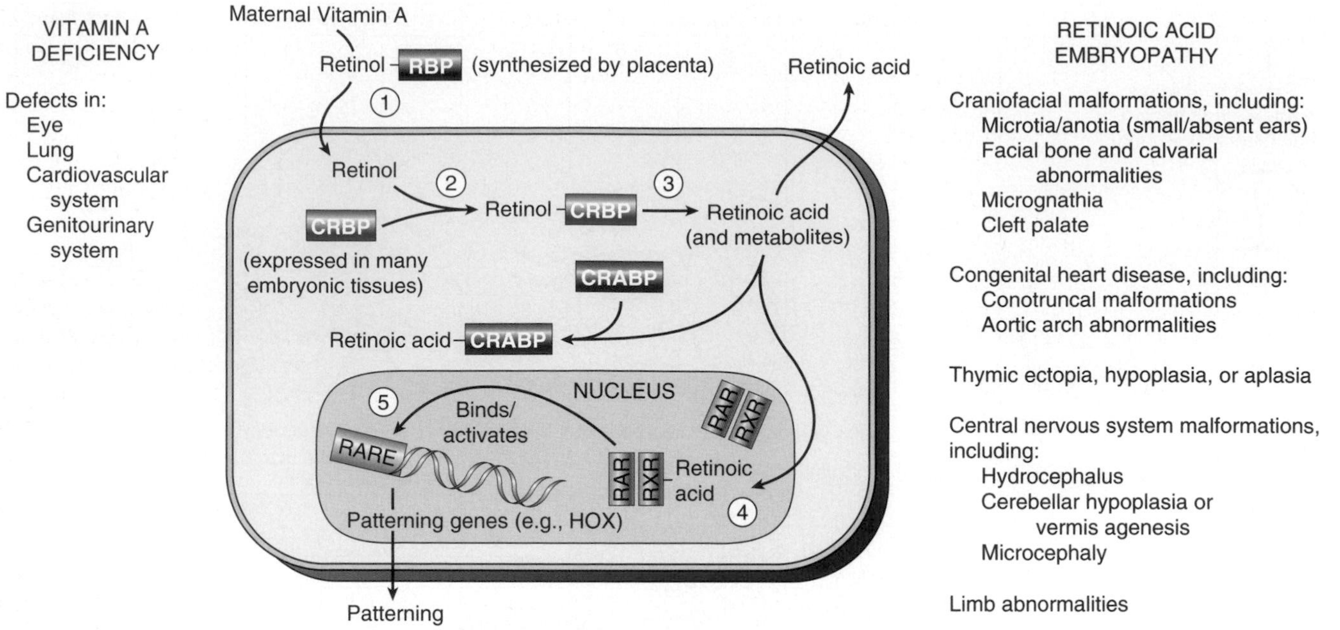

FIGURE 10–6 Schematic representation of the postulated role of retinoic acid in normal development, the general features of its deficiency (vitamin A deficiency) *(left)* and retinoic acid embryopathy *(right)*. *1,* Retinol in the maternal circulation is bound by retinol-binding protein (RBP), which is synthesized by the placenta and enters the fetal circulation. *2,* Once in fetal cells, retinol is bound by cytoplasmic retinol-binding protein (CRBP), which *(3)* regulates the conversion to retinoic acid and metabolites. The retinoic acid either remains in the cytoplasm (bound to cytoplasmic/cellular retinoic acid–binding protein *[CRABP]*) or *(4)* enters the nucleus, where it is bound to nuclear retinoic acid receptors *(RAR, RXR)*. The retinoic acid–receptor complex acts as a transcriptional regulator of various patterning genes (e.g., *HOX*) that have the appropriate retinoic acid response element *(RARE)*. Expression of the binding proteins and receptors in various tissues and at various times during embryogenesis may be a mechanism of selectively modulating the action of retinoic acid. This differential expression may also explain the pattern of abnormalities seen in vitamin A deficiency and retinoic acid embryopathy.

PAX Genes. Another family of developmental genes is the *PAX* genes, which are characterized by a 384 base pair sequence—the *paired box.* Similar to the *HOX* genes, the *PAX* genes are highly conserved throughout evolution; they code for DNA-binding proteins that are believed to function as transcription factors. In contrast to *HOX* genes, however, their expression patterns suggest that they act singly, rather than in a temporal or spatial combination. Mutations in several of the *PAX* genes cause human malformations. *PAX3* is mutated in Waardenburg syndrome, characterized by congenital pigment abnormalities and deafness; *PAX6* mutations cause congenital absence of the iris—aniridia; and *PAX2* mutations cause the "renal-coloboma" syndrome, characterized by developmental defects of the kidneys, eyes, ears, and brain.[28] Parenthetically, *PAX* genes may function also as proto-oncogenes, in that their overexpression is associated with tumorigenesis. Translocations involving *PAX3* and *PAX7* have been identified in the majority of alveolar rhabdomyosarcomas,[29] and translocations involving *PAX5* and *PAX8* are observed in subsets of lymphomas[30] and thyroid cancers,[31] respectively.

Birth Weight and Gestational Age

Infants born before completion of the normal gestation period or who have failed to grow normally during gestation have higher morbidity and mortality rates than full-term infants. For example, an infant weighing 2300 gm and born at 34 weeks of gestation is likely to be physiologically immature and therefore at greater risk for suffering the consequences of organ system immaturity (e.g., respiratory distress syndrome [RDS] or transient hyperbilirubinemia) than a full-term infant also weighing 2300 gm but with corresponding functional maturity of most organ systems. Therefore, a system of classification that takes into account *both birth weight and gestational age* has been adopted. Based on birth weight, infants are classified as being

- *Appropriate for gestational age (AGA)*
- *Small for gestational age (SGA)*
- *Large for gestational age (LGA)*

Infants whose birth weight falls between the 10th and the 90th percentiles for a given gestational age are considered AGA, whereas those who fall above or below these norms are classified as LGA or SGA, respectively. With respect to gestational age, infants born before 37 weeks are considered *preterm,* whereas those delivered after the 42nd week are considered *post-term.* Such a classification is useful in risk stratification. For example, an AGA 1500-gm infant born at 32 weeks' gestation has a much lower mortality risk than an SGA, 700-gm infant born at a similar gestational age. We briefly discuss the subgroups of infants that are SGA and/or preterm, since they account for a significant proportion of perinatal mortality.

PREMATURITY AND FETAL GROWTH RESTRICTION

Prematurity is the second most common cause of neonatal mortality (second only to congenital anomalies), and it is defined by a gestational age less than 37 weeks. As might be expected, those born before completion of gestation also weigh less than 2500 gm. The major risk factors for prematurity include:

- *Preterm premature rupture of placental membranes* (PPROM): PPROM accounts for 30% to 40% of preterm deliveries and is the single most common identifiable cause of prematurity.[32] Rupture of membranes (ROM) before the onset of labor can be spontaneous or induced. PPROM refers to spontaneous ROM occurring *prior* to 37 weeks' gestation (hence the annotation "preterm"). In contrast, PROM refers to spontaneous ROM occurring *after* 37 weeks' gestation. This distinction is important because after 37 weeks the associated risk to the fetus is considerably decreased. The three most common risk factors for PPROM are maternal smoking, a prior history of preterm delivery, and vaginal bleeding at any time during the index pregnancy.[33] The fetal and maternal outcome after PPROM depends on the gestation age of the fetus (second-trimester PPROM has a dismal prognosis), and the effective prophylaxis of infections in the exposed amniotic cavity.
- *Intrauterine infection:* This is a major cause of premature labor with and without intact membranes. Intrauterine infection is present in approximately 25% of all preterm births and the earlier the gestational age at delivery, the higher the frequency of intra-amniotic infection. The histologic correlates of intrauterine infection are inflammation of the placental membranes *(chorioamnionitis)* and inflammation of the fetal umbilical cord *(funisitis)*. The most common microorganisms implicated in intrauterine infections are *Ureaplasma urealyticum, Mycoplasma hominis, Gardnerella vaginalis, Trichomonas, gonorrhea,* and *Chlamydia.*[34] Intrauterine infections can be clinically silent or culture-negative; in these instances, elevated intra-amniotic levels of cytokines (e.g., IL-6)[35] or maternal granulocyte colony stimulating factor are usually demonstrable.[36] Inflammatory cells recruited to the site of infection initiate the onset of preterm labor by (1) the release of collagenases and elastases, with consequent ROM, or (2) release of prostaglandins that induce uterine smooth muscle contractions.
- *Uterine, cervical, and placental structural abnormalities:* uterine distortion (e.g., uterine fibroids), compromised structural support of the cervix ("cervical incompetence"), *placenta previa,* and *abruptio placentae* (Chapter 22) are associated with an increased risk of prematurity.
- *Multiple gestation* (twin pregnancy).

Many of the causes of preterm labor and prematurity described above can also result in fetal growth restriction, making them especially vulnerable to several complications, including

- Hyaline membrane disease (respiratory distress syndrome)
- Necrotizing enterocolitis
- Sepsis
- Intraventricular hemorrhage
- Long-term complications, including developmental delay.

Although preterm infants have low birth weights, it is often appropriate once adjusted for their gestational age. In contrast, *at least one third of infants who weigh less than 2500 gm are born at term and therefore are undergrown rather than immature. Hence, fetal growth restriction (FGR) commonly underlies SGA.* FGR has also been called intrauterine growth retardation (IUGR); however, the usage of the term FGR probably better reflects the pathophysiology of this disorder. FGR can be detected before delivery by ultrasonographic measurement of various fetal dimensions, such as biparietal diameter, head circumference, abdominal circumference, femur length (as an indicator of fetal length), head-to-abdominal circumference ratio, femur length-to-abdominal circumference ratio, and total intrauterine volume.[37] Factors known to result in FGR can be divided into three main groups: fetal, placental, and maternal.

Fetal. Fetal factors are those that intrinsically reduce growth potential of the fetus despite an adequate supply of nutrients from the mother. Prominent among such fetal conditions are *chromosomal disorders, congenital anomalies, and congenital infections.* Chromosomal abnormalities may be detected in up to 17% of fetuses sampled for FGR and in up to 66% of fetuses with documented ultrasonographic malformations. Among the first group, the abnormalities include triploidy (7%), trisomy 18 (6%), trisomy 21 (1%), trisomy 13 (1%), and a variety of deletions and translocations (2%). *Fetal infection* should be considered in all infants with FGR. Those most commonly responsible for FGR are the TORCH group of infections (*T*oxoplasmosis, *R*ubella, *C*ytomegalovirus, *He*rpesvirus, and *O*ther viruses and bacteria, such as syphilis). Infants who are SGA because of fetal factors are usually characterized by symmetric growth restriction (also referred to as *proportionate FGR*), meaning that all organ systems are similarly affected.

Placental. During the third trimester of pregnancy, vigorous fetal growth places particularly heavy demands on the uteroplacental supply line. Therefore, the adequacy of placental growth in the preceding midtrimester is extremely important, and *uteroplacental insufficiency is an important cause of growth restriction.* This insufficiency may result from *umbilical–placental vascular anomalies* (such as single umbilical artery, abnormal cord insertion, placental hemangioma), *placenta abruptio, placenta previa, placental thrombosis and infarction, placental infection,* or *multiple gestations* (Chapter 22). In some cases, the placenta may be small without any detectable underlying cause. Placental causes of FGR tend to result in *asymmetric* (or disproportionate) growth retardation of the fetus with relative sparing of the brain. Physiologically, this general type of FGR is viewed as a down-regulation of growth in the latter half of gestation because of limited availability of nutrients or oxygen.

Confined placental mosaicism is a more recently discovered cause of FGR and has been documented in up to 2% of viable pregnancies studied by chorionic villus sampling at 9 to 11 weeks' gestation. Chromosomal mosaicism, in general, results from viable genetic mutations occurring after zygote formation. Depending on the developmental timing and cell of origin of the mutation, variable forms of chromosomal mosaicism result. For example, genetic mutations occurring at the time of the first or second postzygotic division result in generalized constitutional mosaicism of the fetus and placenta. Conversely, if the mutation occurs later and within dividing trophoblast or extraembryonic progenitor cells of the inner cell mass (approximately 90% of the time), a genetic abnormality limited to the placenta results—confined placental mosaicism (Fig. 10–7).[38] The phenotypic consequences of such placental mosaicism depend on both the specific cytogenetic abnormality and the percentage of cells involved. Chromosomal trisomies, in particular trisomy 7, are the most frequent abnormality documented.

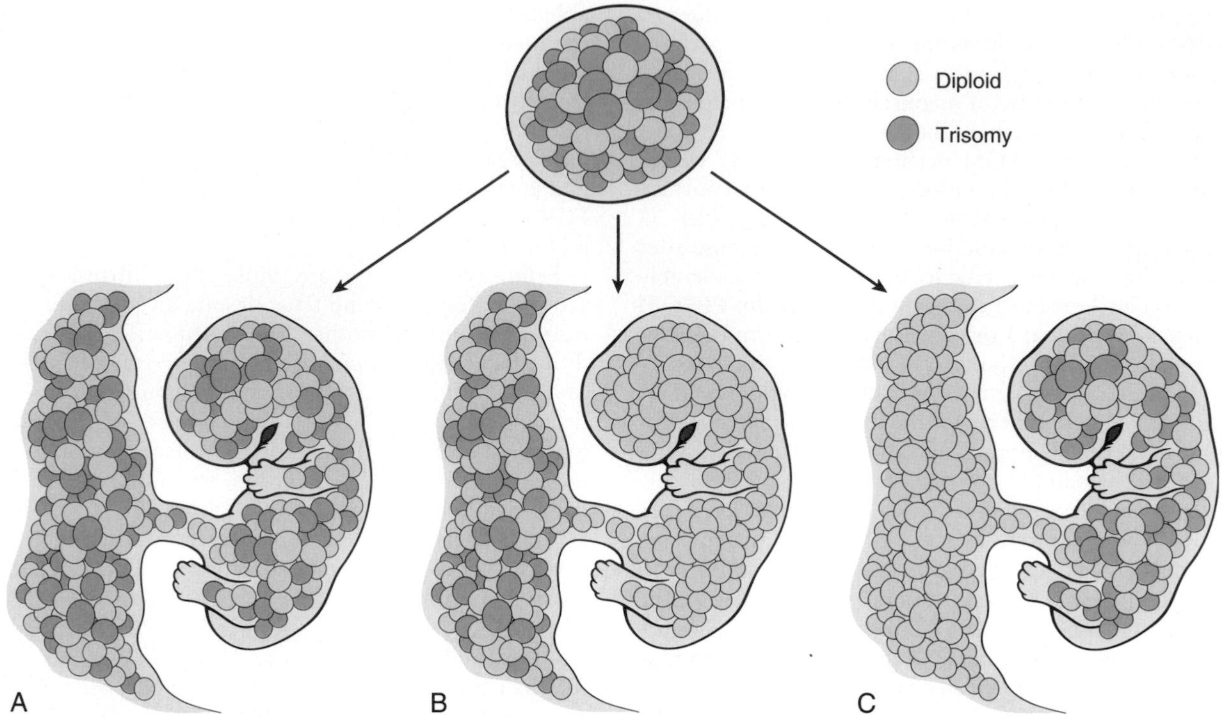

FIGURE 10–7 Diagrammatic representation of constitutional chromosomal mosaicism. *A*, Generalized. *B*, Confined to the placenta. *C*, Confined to the embryo. (Modified and redrawn from Kalousek DK: Confined placental mosaicism and intrauterine development. Pediatr Pathol 10:69, 1990.)

Maternal. By far the most common factors associated with SGA infants are maternal because many conditions affecting the mother's health result in decreased placental blood flow. Vascular diseases, such as *preeclampsia (toxemia of pregnancy)* and *chronic hypertension*, are often the underlying cause. The list of other maternal conditions associated with SGA infants is long, but some of the avoidable factors worth mentioning are maternal *narcotic abuse, alcohol intake*, and *heavy cigarette smoking. Drugs* causing FGR include both classic teratogens, such as antimetabolites, and some commonly administered therapeutic agents, such as phenytoin (Dilantin). *Maternal malnutrition* (in particular, prolonged hypoglycemia) may also affect fetal growth, but the association between SGA infants and the nutritional status of the mother is complex.

The SGA infant faces a difficult course, not only in the perinatal period, when struggle for survival is the main objective, but also in childhood and adult life. Depending on the underlying cause of FGR and, to a lesser extent, the degree of prematurity, there is a significant risk of morbidity in the form of a major handicap, cerebral dysfunction, learning disability, or hearing and visual impairment.

IMMATURITY OF ORGAN SYSTEMS

A major problem confronting the preterm infant regardless of birth weight is the functional, and sometimes structural, immaturity of various organs. Those who are also SGA are the most seriously handicapped. Because immaturity may be the direct cause of death in early preterm infants and significantly biases the probable outcome in others, it is appropriate to consider the features of immaturity of the more vital organs.

Lungs. During the first half of fetal life, the development of the lungs consists essentially of the formation of a system of branching tubes from the foregut that eventually give rise to the trachea, bronchi, and bronchioles. The alveoli begin to differentiate only at approximately the seventh month of gestation. They are at first imperfectly formed, with thick walls, large amounts of interlobular and intralobular connective tissue, and a cuboidal epithelium ("glandular stage"). The vascularization is buried within this connective tissue and is not in immediate contact with the alveolar spaces (Fig. 10–8). Between the 26th and 32nd weeks of gestation, the cuboidal epithelium shows transition to the flat, type I alveolar epithelial cells as well as type II cells that contain lamellar bodies ("saccular stage") (Chapter 15). Further maturation of the lungs ("alveolar stage") leads to reduction in the interstitial tissues and increasing numbers of capillaries. Even at full term, however, the alveoli are small and the septa are considerably thicker than in the adult. Development of alveoli continues after birth, and the full adult complement of alveoli is reached at about age 8. The immature lungs are grossly unexpanded, red, and meaty. The alveolar spaces are incompletely expanded and often lined by cuboidal epithelium and usually contain pink proteinaceous precipitate and occasional squamous epithelial cells.

Kidneys. In the preterm infant, the formation of glomeruli is incomplete. Primitive glomeruli can be seen in the subcapsular zone. These structures have an organoid, glandular

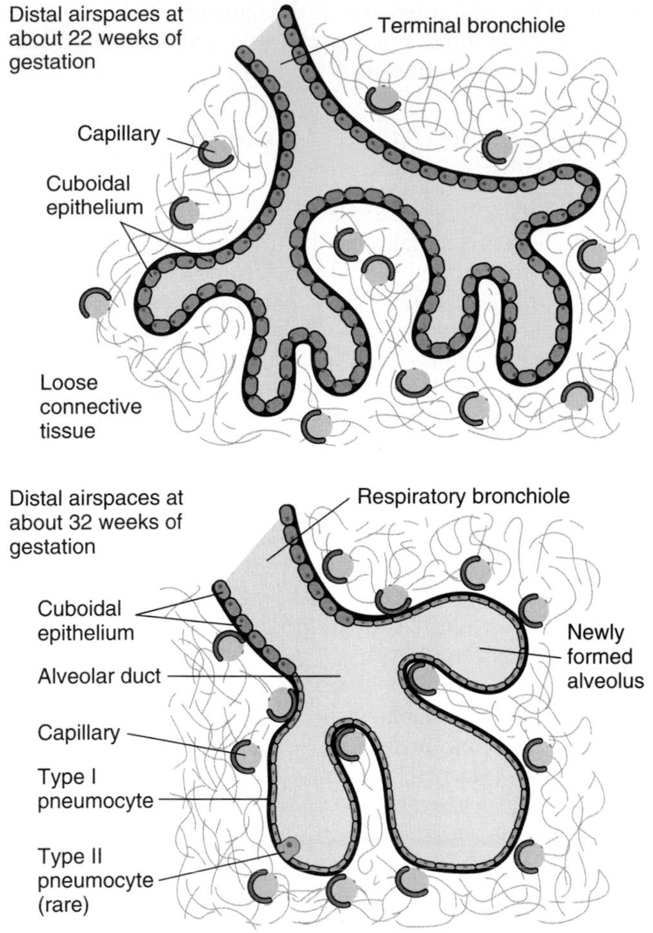

FIGURE 10–8 Schematic diagrams of fetal lung maturation.

appearance imparted by the presence of cuboidal cells in the parietal and visceral layers of Bowman capsule. The deeper glomeruli are well formed, however, and renal function is adequate to permit survival.

Brain. The brain is also incompletely developed in the preterm infant. The surface is relatively smooth and devoid of the typical convolutions found in the cerebral hemispheres of the adult. The brain substance is soft, gelatinous, and easily torn. There is poorly developed myelination of the nerve fibers. Despite this underdevelopment, the vital brain centers are sufficiently developed, even in the very immature infant, to sustain normal central nervous system function. Homeostasis is not perfect, however, and the preterm infant has difficulty in maintaining a constant normal level of temperature and has poor vasomotor control, irregular respirations, muscular inertia, and feeble sweating.

Liver. The liver, although large relative to the size of the preterm infant, suffers from lack of physiologic maturity. Many or most of the functions of the liver are marginally adequate to carry out the demands placed on them. Almost all newborns and particularly those of low birth weight have a transient period of *physiologic jaundice* within the first postnatal week. This jaundice stems from both breakdown of fetal red cells and inadequacy of the biliary excretory function of liver cells.

APGAR SCORE

The Apgar score, devised by Virginia Apgar, represents a clinically useful method of evaluating the physiologic condition and responsiveness of newborn infants and hence their chances of survival.[39] Table 10–4 indicates the five parameters to be scored and how they are quantitated. The newborn infant may be evaluated at 1 minute and at 5 minutes. A total score of 10 indicates an infant in the best possible condition. The correlation between the Apgar score and the mortality during the first 28 days of life is impressive. Infants with a 5-minute Apgar score of 0 to 1 have 50% mortality within the first month of life. This drops to 20% with a score of 4 and to almost 0% when the score is 7 or better. Despite the established value of the Apgar score in predicting perinatal morbidity, particularly in normal-birthweight infants, it is not a reliable indicator of long-term neurologic morbidity.

Birth Injuries

Birth injuries constitute important causes of illness or death in infants as well as in children during the first years of life. No infant is immune to birth injury, although the risk and type of injury vary from the LGA infant to the preterm AGA or SGA infant. These injuries most commonly involve the head, skeletal system, liver, adrenals, and peripheral nerves. Considering the violent expulsive forces to which the fragile fetus is exposed, it is quite surprising that birth injuries are so relatively uncommon.

Morbidity associated with birth injury may be acute (e.g., that due to fractures) or the result of later-appearing sequelae (e.g., after damage to nerves or the brain). The distribution of injuries in a large municipal hospital, in descending order of frequency, is as follows: clavicular fracture, facial nerve injury, brachial plexus injury, intracranial injury, humeral fracture, and lacerations. Not surprisingly, LGA infants are at greater

TABLE 10–4 Evaluation of the Newborn Infant*

Sign	0	1	2
Heart rate	Absent	Below 100	Over 100
Respiratory effort	Absent	Slow, irregular	Good, crying
Muscle tone	Limp	Some flexion of extremities	Active motion
Response to catheter in nostril (tested after oropharynx is clear)	No response	Grimace	Cough or sneeze
Color	Blue, pale	Body pink, extremities blue	Completely pink

*Sixty seconds after the complete birth of the infant (disregarding removal of the cord and placenta), the five objective signs are evaluated and each is given a score of 0, 1, or 2. A total score of 10 indicates an infant in the best possible condition.

Data from Apgar V: A proposal for a new method of evaluation of the newborn infant. Anesth Analg 32:260, 1953.

risk for birth injury, in particular those involving the skeletal system and peripheral nerves. We briefly discuss only injuries involving the head because they are the most ominous.

Intracranial hemorrhages are the most common important birth injury. These hemorrhages are generally related to excessive molding of the head or sudden pressure changes in its shape as it is subjected to the pressure of forceps or sudden precipitate expulsion. Prolonged labor, hypoxia, hemorrhagic disorders, or intracranial vascular anomalies are important predispositions. The hemorrhage may arise from tears in the dura or from rupture of vessels that traverse the brain. The substance of the brain may be torn or bruised, leading to intraventricular hemorrhages or bleeding into the brain substance. The consequences of intracranial hemorrhages are mentioned later under germinal matrix hemorrhage.

Caput succedaneum and *cephalhematoma* are so common, even in normal uncomplicated births, that they hardly merit the designation *birth injury.* The first refers to progressive accumulation of interstitial fluid in the soft tissues of the scalp, giving rise to a usually circular area of edema, congestion, and swelling at the site where the head begins to enter the lower uterine canal. Hemorrhage may occur into the scalp, producing a cephalhematoma. Both forms of injury are of little clinical significance and are important only insofar as they must be differentiated from skull fractures with attendant hemorrhage and edema. In approximately 25% of cephalhematomas, there is an underlying skull fracture. Such skull fractures may occur in cases of precipitate delivery, inappropriate use of forceps, or prolonged labor with disproportion between the size of the fetal head and birth canal.

Perinatal Infections

Infections of the embryo, fetus, and neonate are manifested in a variety of ways and are mentioned as etiologic factors in numerous other sections within this chapter. Here we discuss only the general routes and timing of infections. In general, fetal and perinatal infections are acquired via one of two primary routes—*transcervically* (also referred to as *ascending*) or *transplacentally (hematologic).* Occasionally, infections occur by a combination of the two routes in that an ascending microorganism infects the endometrium and then the fetal bloodstream via the chorionic villi.

TRANSCERVICAL (ASCENDING) INFECTIONS

Most bacterial and a few viral (e.g., herpes simplex II) infections are acquired by the cervicovaginal route. Such infections may be acquired in utero or around the time of birth. In general, the fetus acquires the infection either by inhaling infected amniotic fluid into the lungs shortly before birth or by passing through an infected birth canal during delivery. As previously stated, preterm birth is often an unfortunate consequence and may be related either to damage and rupture of the amniotic sac as a direct consequence of the inflammation or to the induction of labor associated with a release of prostaglandins by the infiltrating neutrophils. Chorioamnionitis of the placental membranes and funisitis are usually demonstrable, although the presence or absence and severity of chorioamnionitis do not necessarily correlate with the severity of the fetal infection. In the fetus infected via inhalation of amniotic fluid, pneumonia, sepsis, and meningitis are the most common sequelae.

TRANSPLACENTAL (HEMATOLOGIC) INFECTIONS

Most parasitic (e.g., toxoplasma, malaria) and viral infections and a few bacterial infections (i.e., *Listeria, Treponema*) gain access to the fetal bloodstream transplacentally via the chorionic villi. This hematogenous transmission may occur at any time during gestation or occasionally, as may be the case with hepatitis B and HIV, at the time of delivery via maternal-to-fetal transfusion. The clinical manifestations of these infections are highly variable, depending largely on the gestational timing and microorganism involved.

Some infections, such as those with *parvovirus B19* (which causes *fifth disease* in the mother), may induce spontaneous abortion, stillbirth, hydrops fetalis, and congenital anemia.[40] While the virus can bind to different cell types, replication occurs only in erythroid cells, and diagnostic viral cytopathic effect can be recognized in late erythroid progenitor cells of infected infants (Fig. 10–9).

The *TORCH group of infections* (see above) are grouped together because they may evoke similar clinical and pathologic manifestations, including *fever, encephalitis, chorioretinitis, hepatosplenomegaly, pneumonitis, myocarditis, hemolytic anemia, and vesicular or hemorrhagic skin lesions.* Such infections occurring early in gestation may also cause chronic sequelae in the child, including growth and mental retardation, cataracts, congenital cardiac anomalies, and bone defects.

ONSET OF SEPSIS

Perinatal infections can also be grouped clinically by whether they tend to result in *early-onset* (within the first 7 days of life) versus *late-onset* sepsis (from 7 days to 3 months). Most cases of early-onset sepsis are acquired at or shortly before birth and tend to result in clinical signs and symptoms of pneumonia, sepsis, and occasionally meningitis within 4 or 5 days of life. Group B streptococcus is the most common

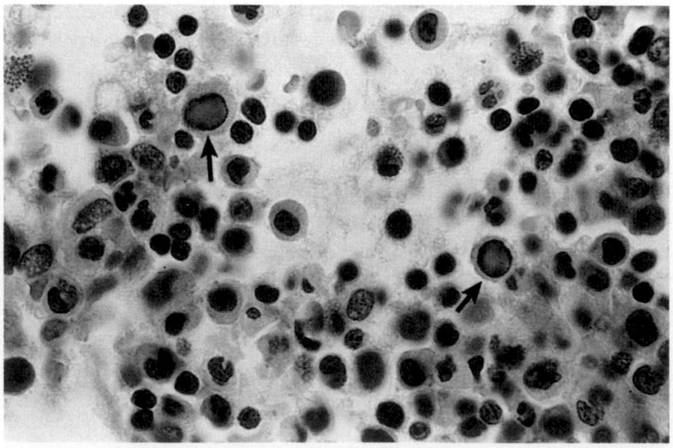

FIGURE 10–9 Bone marrow from an infant infected with parvovirus B19. The arrows point to two erythroid precursors with large homogeneous intranuclear inclusions and a surrounding peripheral rim of residual chromatin.

organism isolated in early-onset sepsis and is also the most common cause of bacterial meningitis. Infections with *Listeria* and *Candida* require a latent period between the time of microorganism inoculation and the appearance of clinical symptoms and present as late-onset sepsis.

Neonatal Respiratory Distress Syndrome (RDS)

There are many causes of respiratory distress in the newborn, including excessive sedation of the mother, fetal head injury during delivery, aspiration of blood or amniotic fluid, and intrauterine hypoxia brought about by coiling of the umbilical cord about the neck. The most common cause, however, is RDS, also known as *hyaline membrane disease* because of the formation of *membranes* in the peripheral airspaces of infants who succumb to this condition. Approximately 60,000 cases of RDS are reported each year in the United States, with annual deaths totaling 5000.

In untreated infants (not receiving surfactant), RDS presents in a stereotyped fashion, characterized by the following characteristic clinical setting. The infant is almost always *preterm* and AGA, and there are strong, but not invariable, associations with *male gender, maternal diabetes*, and delivery by *cesarean section*. Resuscitation may be necessary at birth, but usually within a few minutes rhythmic breathing and normal color are reestablished. Soon afterward, often within 30 minutes, breathing becomes more difficult, and within a few hours cyanosis becomes evident. Fine rales can now be heard over both lung fields. A chest x-ray film at this time usually reveals uniform minute reticulogranular densities, producing a so-called *ground-glass picture*. In the full-blown condition the respiratory distress persists, cyanosis increases, and even the administration of 80% oxygen by a variety of ventilatory methods fails to improve the situation. If therapy staves off death for the first 3 or 4 days, however, the infant has an excellent chance of recovery.[41]

Etiology and Pathogenesis. Immaturity of the lungs is the most important subsoil on which this condition develops. It may be encountered in full-term infants but is much less frequent than in those "born before their time into this breathing world."[42] The incidence of RDS is inversely proportional to gestational age. It occurs in about 60% of infants born at less than 28 weeks of gestation, 15% to 20% of those born between 32 and 36 weeks' gestation, and less than 5% of those born after 37 weeks' gestation.

The *fundamental defect in RDS is a deficiency of pulmonary surfactant*. As described in Chapter 15, surfactant consists predominantly of dipalmitoyl phosphatidylcholine (lecithin), smaller amounts of phosphatidylglycerol, and two groups of surfactant-associated proteins. The first group is comprised of hydrophilic glycoproteins SP-A and SP-D, which play a role in pulmonary host defense (innate immunity). The second group consists of hydrophobic surfactant proteins SP-B and SP-C, which, in concert with the surfactant lipids, are involved in the reduction of surface tension at the air-liquid barrier in the alveoli of the lung.[43] With reduced surface tension in the alveoli, less pressure is required to keep them patent and hence aerated. The importance of surfactant proteins in normal lung function can be gauged by the occurrence of severe respiratory failure in neonates with congenital SP-B deficiency caused by mutations in the *SP-B* gene.[44]

Surfactant is synthesized by type II alveolar cells, most abundantly after the 35th week of gestation in the fetus. At birth, the first breath of life requires high inspiratory pressures to expand the lungs. With normal levels of surfactant, the lungs retain up to 40% of the residual air volume after the first breath; thus, subsequent breaths require far lower inspiratory pressures. With a deficiency of surfactant, the lungs collapse with each successive breath, and so infants must work as hard with each successive breath as they did with the first. The problem of *stiff* atelectatic lungs is compounded by the *soft* thoracic wall that is pulled in as the diaphragm descends. Progressive atelectasis and reduced lung compliance then lead to a train of events as depicted in Figure 10–10, resulting in a protein-rich, fibrin-rich exudation into the alveolar spaces with the formation of hyaline membranes. The fibrin–hyaline membranes constitute barriers to gas exchange, leading to carbon dioxide retention and hypoxemia. The hypoxemia itself further impairs surfactant synthesis, and a vicious cycle ensues.

Surfactant synthesis is modulated by a variety of hormones and growth factors, including cortisol, insulin, prolactin, thyroxine, and TGF-β.[45] *The role of glucocorticoids is particularly important.* Corticosteroids induce the formation of surfactant lipids and surfactant-associated proteins in fetal lung; thyrox-

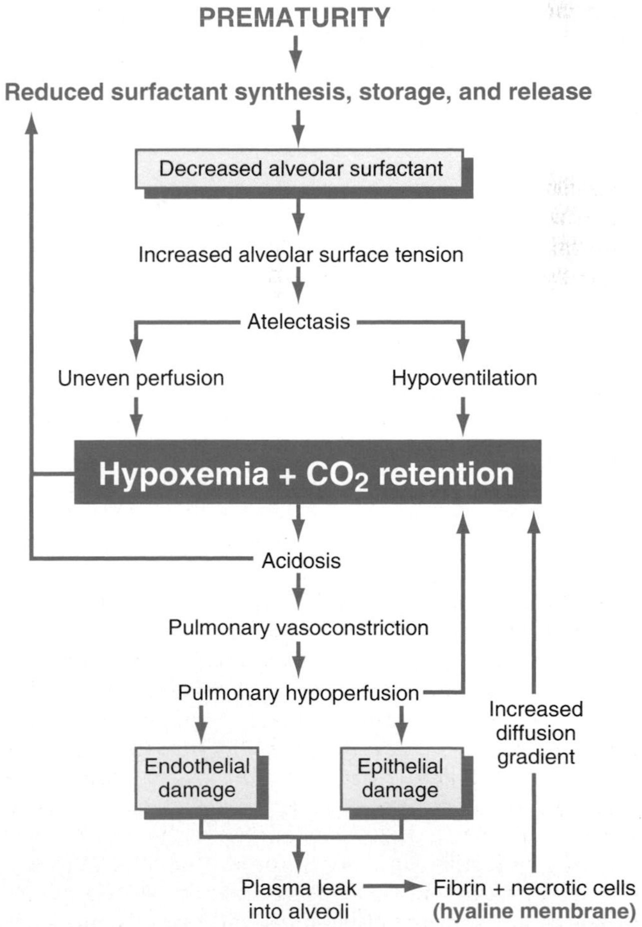

FIGURE 10–10 Schematic outline of the pathophysiology of the respiratory distress syndrome (see text).

ine acts synergistically with corticosteroids in this regard.[46] Conditions associated with intrauterine stress and FGR that increase corticosteroid release lower the risk of developing RDS. Surfactant synthesis can be suppressed by the compensatory high blood levels of insulin in infants of diabetic mothers, which counteracts the effects of steroids. This may explain, in part, why infants of diabetic mothers have a higher risk of developing RDS. Labor is known to increase surfactant synthesis; hence, cesarean section before the onset of labor may increase the risk of RDS. Recently, certain genetic polymorphisms in both *SP-A* and *SP-B* genes have been reported as being synergistic determinants of increased RDS risk in preterm infants.[47]

Morphology. The lungs are distinctive on gross examination. Although of normal size, they are solid, airless, and reddish purple, similar to the color of the liver, and they usually sink in water. Microscopically, alveoli are poorly developed, and those that are present are collapsed (Fig. 10–11). When the infant dies early in the course of the disease, necrotic cellular debris is present in the terminal bronchioles and alveolar ducts. The necrotic material becomes incorporated within eosinophilic hyaline membranes lining the respiratory bronchioles, alveolar ducts, and random alveoli. The membranes are largely made up of fibrinogen and fibrin admixed with cell debris derived chiefly from necrotic type II pneumocytes. The sequence of events that leads to the formation of hyaline membranes is depicted in Figure 10–10. There is a remarkable paucity of neutrophilic inflammatory reaction associated with these membranes. The lesions of hyaline membrane disease are never seen in stillborn infants.

In infants who survive more than 48 hours, reparative changes occur in the lungs. The alveolar epithelium proliferates under the surface of the membrane, which may be desquamated into the airspace, where it may undergo partial digestion or phagocytosis by macrophages.

Clinical Course. Although a classic clinical presentation before the era of treatment with exogenous surfactant was described earlier, the actual clinical course and prognosis for neonatal RDS vary, dependent on the maturity and birth weight of the infant and the promptness of institution of therapy. A major thrust in the control of RDS focuses on prevention, either by delaying labor until the fetal lung reaches maturity or by inducing maturation of the lung in the fetus at risk. Critical to these objectives is the ability to assess fetal lung maturity accurately. Because pulmonary secretions are discharged into the amniotic fluid, analysis of amniotic fluid phospholipids provides a good estimate of the level of surfactant in the alveolar lining. Prophylactic administration of exogenous surfactant at birth to extremely premature infants (gestational age <26 to 28 weeks) and administration of surfactant to older premature infants who are symptomatic have been shown to be extremely beneficial, such that it is now uncommon for infants to die of acute RDS.[48] In addition, antenatal corticosteroids decrease neonatal morbidity and mortality when administered to mothers with threatened premature delivery at 24 to 34 weeks' gestation.[49] Once the infant is born, the cornerstone of treatment is the delivery of surfactant replacement therapy and oxygen, usually accomplished by a variety of ventilatory assistance methods, including high-frequency ventilation.

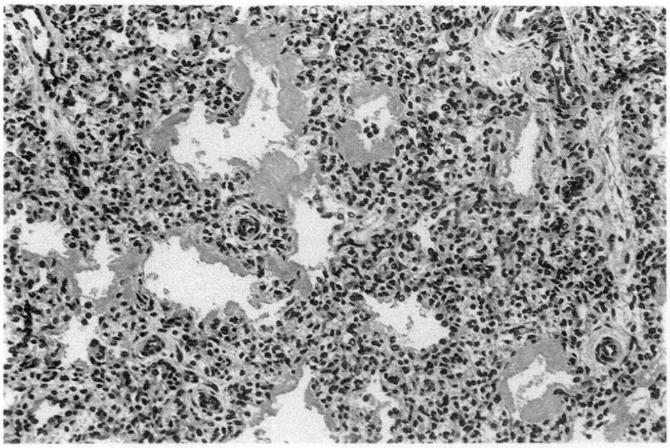

FIGURE 10–11 Hyaline membrane disease. There is alternating atelectasis and dilation of the alveoli. Note the eosinophilic thick hyaline membranes lining the dilated alveoli.

In uncomplicated cases, recovery begins to occur within 3 or 4 days. Therapy, however, carries with it the now well-recognized hazard of *oxygen toxicity*, caused by oxygen-derived free radicals. High concentrations of oxygen administered for prolonged periods cause two well-known complications: *retrolental fibroplasia* (also called *retinopathy of prematurity*) *in the eyes* (Chapter 29) and *bronchopulmonary dysplasia.* The retinopathy has been ascribed to changes in expression of vascular endothelial growth factor (VEGF), which is strongly induced by hypoxia, and also serves as a survival factor for endothelial cells and causes angiogenesis (Chapter 3).[50] During the initial *hyperoxic* phase of RDS therapy (phase I), VEGF is markedly decreased, causing endothelial cell apoptosis; VEGF increases after return to relatively hypoxic room air ventilation, inducing the retinal vessel proliferation *(neovascularization)* characteristic of the lesions in the retina. The occurrence of retinopathy of prematurity even with careful use of oxygen supplementation suggests that factors besides VEGF may also be involved. It is thought that *insulin-like growth factor-1* (IGF-1), a key upstream regulatory element for VEGF-induced neovascularization in the retina, may also play a role. Low IGF-1 suppresses VEGF signaling in retinal endothelial cells.[51]

Bronchopulmonary dysplasia (BPD), originally described in 1967, is now infrequent in infants of more than 1200 gm birth weight or with gestations exceeding 30 weeks. Gentler ventilation techniques, antenatal glucocorticoid therapy, and surfactant treatments have minimized severe lung injury in larger and more mature infants. Clinically, BPD is diagnosed in a neonate under 32 weeks' gestational age who requires at least 28 days of oxygen therapy; the degree of BPD is classified as *mild, moderate, or severe* depending on the need for supplemental oxygen and positive-pressure ventilation.[52] The original histopathologic descriptions of BPD reported airway epithelial hyperplasia and squamous metaplasia, alveolar wall thickening, and peribronchial as well as interstitial fibrosis.[53] In recent years, the histologic changes seen in infants who have died with BPD differ. *The major abnormality in "new" BPD is a decrease in alveolar number, referred to as alveolar hypoplasia.*[54] Thus, the current view is that BPD is caused by an arrested development of alveolar septation at the saccular stage (see above for stages of lung development).

Multiple factors contribute to BPD and probably act additively or synergistically to promote injury. Oxygen alone can arrest septation of lungs that are in the saccular stage of development, with infants receiving higher levels of supplemental oxygen having more persistent lung disease.[55] Mechanical ventilation of preterm animals without simultaneous exposure to high levels of supplemental oxygen also results in the pathologic lesion of BPD. The levels of a variety of pro-inflammatory cytokines (tumor necrosis factor, macrophage inflammatory protein-1, and interleukin-8 [IL-8]) are increased in the alveoli of infants who develop BPD, suggesting a role for these cytokines in arresting pulmonary development.[56,57] If oxygen toxicity is avoided, as is usually the case in current clinical settings, and the infant can be kept alive for about 3 or 4 days, recovery of infants of 31 weeks' gestation or more can be anticipated without permanent sequelae.

Infants who recover from RDS are at increased risk for developing a variety of other complications associated with preterm birth; most important among these are *patent ductus arteriosus, intraventricular hemorrhage*, and *necrotizing enterocolitis.* Thus, although current high technology saves many infants with RDS, it also brings to the surface the exquisite fragility of the immature neonate.

Necrotizing Enterocolitis

Necrotizing enterocolitis (NEC) most commonly occurs in premature infants, with the incidence of the disease being inversely proportional to the gestational age. It occurs in approximately 1 out of 10 very low birthweight infants (<1500 gm). Approximately 2500 cases occur annually in the United States.

The etiology of NEC is controversial, but is in all likelihood multifactorial. In most preterm infants, the symptoms of NEC do not appear until after oral feeding is instituted, suggesting that some postnatal insult (such as introduction of bacteria) sets in motion the cascade culminating in tissue destruction. *Intestinal ischemia* appears to be a prerequisite and may result from either generalized hypoperfusion or from selective reduction of blood flow to the intestines in order to divert oxygen to vital organs such as the brain.[58] Inflammatory mediators, particularly *platelet-activating factor*, have been implicated in increasing mucosal permeability, thus adding "fuel to the fire."[59] Ultimately, breakdown of mucosal barrier functions permits transluminal migration of gut bacteria, leading to a vicious cycle of inflammation, mucosal necrosis, and further bacterial entry, eventually culminating in sepsis and shock (Chapter 4).

The clinical course is fairly typical, with the onset of bloody stools, abdominal distention, and development of circulatory collapse. Abdominal radiographs often demonstrate gas within the intestinal wall *(pneumatosis intestinalis)*. NEC typically involves the terminal ileum, cecum, and right colon, although any part of the small or large intestines may be involved. The involved segment is distended, friable, and congested, or it can be frankly gangrenous; intestinal perforation with accompanying peritonitis may be seen. Microscopically, mucosal or transmural coagulative necrosis, ulceration, bacterial colonization, and submucosal gas bubbles may be seen (Fig. 10–12). Reparative changes, such as the formation of granulation tissue and fibrosis, may begin shortly after the acute episode. When detected early on, NEC can be often managed conservatively, but many cases (20% to 60%) require resection of the necrotic segments of bowel. NEC is associated with high perinatal mortality; those who survive often develop *post-NEC strictures* from fibrosis caused by the healing process.

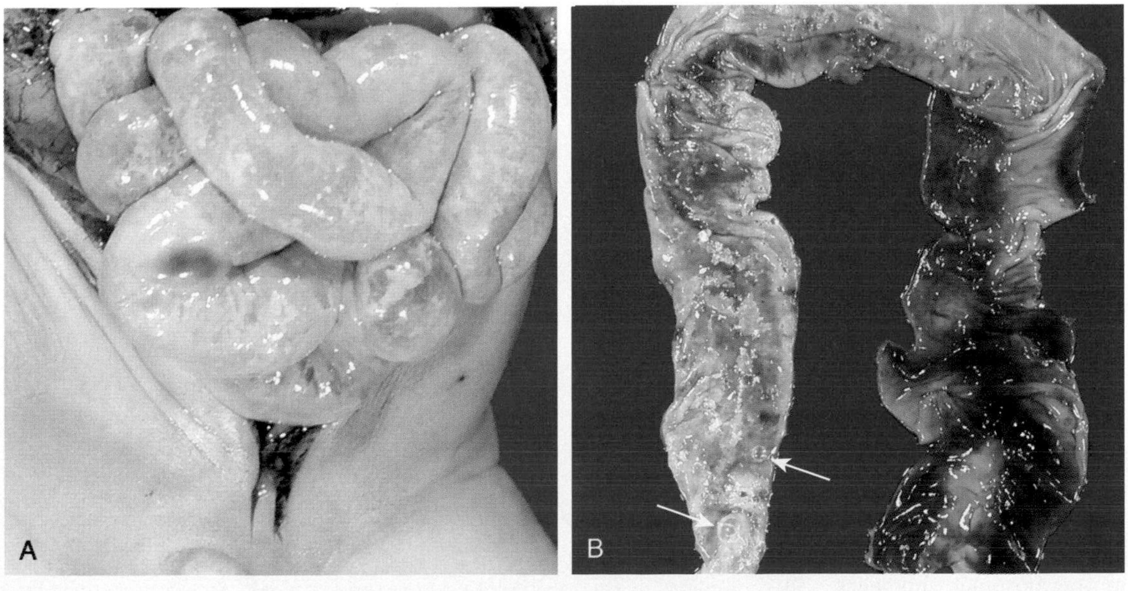

FIGURE 10–12 Necrotizing enterocolitis. *A,* Postmortem examination in a severe case of NEC shows the entire small bowel is markedly distended with a perilously thin wall (usually this implies impending perforation). *B,* The congested portion of the ileum corresponds to areas of hemorrhagic infarction and transmural necrosis microscopically. Submucosal gas bubbles *(pneumatosis intestinalis)* can be seen in several areas *(arrows).*

Germinal Matrix—Intraventricular Hemorrhage

Subependymal (germinal matrix) hemorrhage, with secondary bleeding into the ventricles, is particularly prone to occur in preterm infants. This condition can occur in as many as 40% to 50% of infants weighing less than 1500 gm who are admitted to neonatal intensive care units. The microcirculation within the germinal matrix is particularly susceptible to damage from hypoxia and changes in perfusion pressure, both relatively common occurrences in apneic preterm babies. Whatever their origin, intracranial hemorrhages are of great importance because they cause sudden increases in intracranial pressure, damage to the brain substance, herniation of the medulla or base of the brain into the foramen magnum, and serious, frequently fatal depression of function of the vital medullary centers.

Fetal Hydrops

Fetal hydrops refers to the accumulation of edema fluid in the fetus during intrauterine growth. The causes of fetal hydrops are manifold; the most important are listed in Table 10–5. Until recently, hemolytic anemia caused by Rh blood group incompatibility between mother and fetus *(immune hydrops)* was the most common cause, but with the successful prophylaxis of this disorder during pregnancy, causes of *nonimmune hydrops* have emerged as the principal culprits. Notably, the intrauterine fluid accumulation can be quite variable, from progressive, generalized edema of the fetus *(hydrops fetalis),* a usually lethal condition (Fig. 10–13), to more localized degrees of edema, such as isolated pleural and peritoneal effusions, or postnuchal fluid accumulation (*cystic hygroma,* see later) that are compatible with life.

TABLE 10–5 Selected Causes of Hydrops Fetalis (in decreasing order of frequency)

Cardiovascular
Malformations
Tachyarrhythmia
High-output failure
Chromosomal
Turner syndrome
Trisomy 21, trisomy 18
Thoracic Causes
Cystic adenomatoid malformation
Diaphragmatic hernia
Fetal Anemia
Homozygous alpha-thalassemia
Parvovirus B19
Immune hydrops (Rh and ABO)
Twin Gestation
Twin-to-twin transfusion
Infection (excluding parvovirus)
Cytomegalovirus
Syphilis
Toxoplasmosis
Major Malformations
Tumors
Metabolic disorders

Note: The cause of fetal hydrops may be undetermined ("idiopathic") in up to 20% of cases. Data from Machin GA: Hydrops, cystic hygroma, hydrothorax, pericardial effusions, and fetal ascites, In Gilbert-Barness E (ed): Potter's Pathology of Fetus and Infant. St. Louis, Mosby-Year Book, 1997.

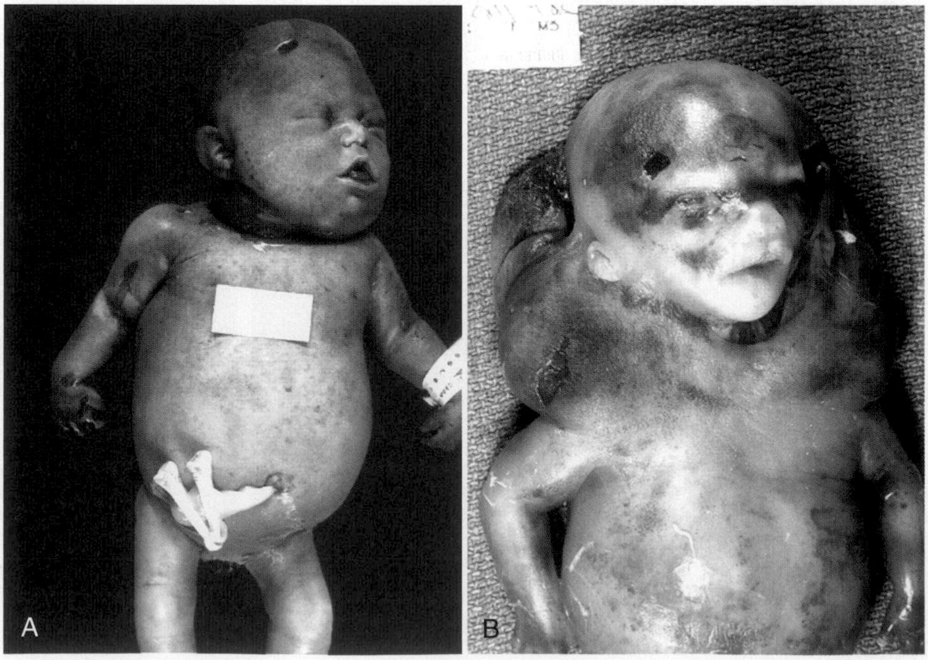

FIGURE 10–13 Hydrops fetalis. There is generalized accumulation of fluid in the fetus. In *B,* fluid accumulation is particularly prominent in the soft tissues of the neck, and this condition has been termed *cystic hygroma.* Cystic hygromas are characteristically seen, but not limited to, constitutional chromosomal anomalies such as 45,X0 karyotypes. (Courtesy of Dr. Beverly Rogers, Department of Pathology, University of Texas Southwestern Medical Center, Dallas, TX.)

IMMUNE HYDROPS

Immune hydrops is defined as a hemolytic disease in the newborn caused by blood-group incompatibility between mother and child. When the fetus inherits red cell antigenic determinants from the father that are foreign to the mother, a maternal immune reaction may occur, leading to hemolytic disease in the infant. Any of the numerous red cell antigenic systems may theoretically be involved, but the major antigens known to induce clinically significant immunologic disease are the ABO and certain of the Rh antigens. The incidence of immune hydrops in urban populations has declined remarkably, owing largely to the current methods of preventing Rh immunization in at-risk mothers. Successful prophylaxis of this disorder has resulted directly from an understanding of its pathogenesis.

Etiology and Pathogenesis. The underlying basis of immune hydrops is the immunization of the mother by blood group antigens on fetal red cells and the free passage of antibodies from the mother through the placenta to the fetus (Fig. 10–14). Fetal red cells may reach the maternal circulation during the last trimester of pregnancy, when the cytotrophoblast is no longer present as a barrier, or during childbirth itself. The mother thus becomes sensitized to the foreign antigen.

Of the numerous antigens included in the Rh system, only the D antigen is the major cause of Rh incompatibility. Several factors influence the immune response to Rh-positive fetal red cells that reach the maternal circulation.

- Concurrent ABO incompatibility protects the mother against Rh immunization because the fetal red cells are promptly coated by isohemagglutinins (anti-A or anti-B) and removed from the maternal circulation.
- The antibody response depends on the dose of immunizing antigen; hence, hemolytic disease develops only when the mother has experienced a significant transplacental bleed (more than 1 mL of Rh-positive red cells).
- The isotype of the antibody is important because immunoglobulin G (IgG) (but not immunoglobulin M [IgM]) antibodies can cross the placenta. The initial exposure to Rh antigen evokes the formation of IgM antibodies, so Rh disease is uncommon with the first pregnancy. Exposure during a subsequent pregnancy generally leads to a brisk IgG antibody response.

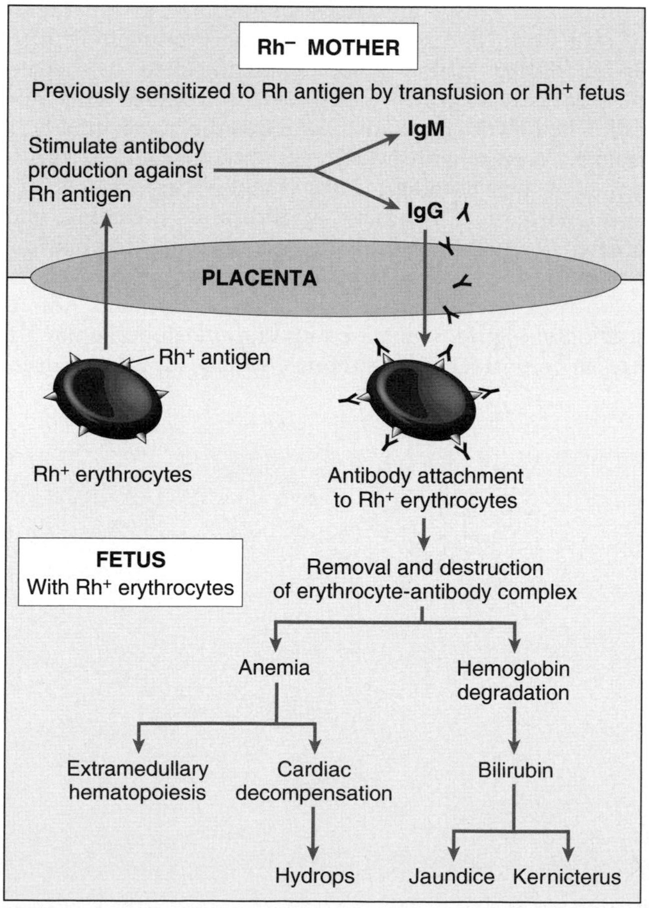

FIGURE 10–14 Pathogenesis of immune hydrops fetalis (see text).

The incidence of maternal Rh isoimmunization has significantly decreased since the use of Rhesus immune globulin (RhIg) containing anti-D antibodies. Administration of RhIg at 28 weeks and within 72 hours of delivery to Rh-negative mothers significantly decreases the risk for hemolytic disease in Rh-positive neonates and in subsequent pregnancies. Moreover, antenatal identification and management of the at-risk fetus have been greatly facilitated by amniocentesis and the advent of chorionic villus and fetal blood sampling. In addition, cloning of the *RhD* gene has resulted in efforts to determine fetal Rh status using maternal blood. When identified, cases of severe intrauterine hemolysis may be treated by fetal intravascular transfusions via the umbilical cord and early delivery.

The pathogenesis of fetal hemolysis caused by maternal/fetal ABO incompatibility is slightly different than that caused by differences in the Rh antigens. ABO incompatibility occurs in approximately 20% to 25% of pregnancies, but laboratory evidence of hemolytic disease occurs only in 1 in 10 of such infants, and the hemolytic disease is severe enough to require treatment in only 1 in 200 cases. Several factors account for this. First, most anti-A and anti-B antibodies are of the IgM type and hence do not cross the placenta. Second, neonatal red cells express blood group antigens A and B poorly. Third, many cells other than red cells express A and B antigens and thus sop up some of the transferred antibody. ABO hemolytic disease occurs almost exclusively in infants of group A or B who are born of group O mothers. The normal anti-A and anti-B isohemagglutinins in group O mothers are usually of the IgM type and so do not cross the placenta. However, for reasons not well understood, certain group O women possess IgG antibodies directed against group A or B antigens (or both) even without prior sensitization. Therefore, the firstborn may be affected. Fortunately, even with transplacentally acquired antibodies, lysis of the infant's red cells is minimal. There is no effective protection against ABO reactions.

There are two consequences of excessive destruction of red blood cells in the neonate (see Fig. 10–14). One is *anemia*, and the other is the accumulation of bilirubin *(jaundice)*. The severity of these changes varies considerably, however, depending on the degree of hemolysis and the maturity of the infant organ systems. Extramedullary hematopoiesis in the liver and spleen may suffice to maintain normal red cell levels if the hemolysis is mild. If the hemolytic reaction is marked, anemia associated with jaundice and the presence of unconjugated bilirubin occurs. Because unconjugated bilirubin is water insoluble and has an affinity for lipids, it binds to lipids in the brain owing to the poorly developed blood-brain barrier in the infant, resulting in serious damage to the central nervous system, termed *kernicterus*. In addition, the anemia may be associated with hypoxic injury to the heart and liver, resulting in circulatory and hepatic failure and edema (see below). If severe, plasma protein levels may drop to as low as 2.0 to 2.5 gm/dL because of reduced hepatic synthesis. *This decrease in oncotic pressure within the circulation, combined with a secondary increase in venous capillary pressure owing to cardiac failure, results in generalized edema and ascites* (anasarca). As alluded to previously, this latter condition is referred to as *hydrops fetalis*.

NONIMMUNE HYDROPS

The three major causes of nonimmune hydrops include *cardiovascular defects, chromosomal anomalies*, and *fetal anemia* (see Table 10–5).[60] Both structural and functional cardiovascular defects, such as congenital cardiac defects and arrhythmias, may result in intrauterine cardiac failure and hydrops. Among the chromosomal anomalies, 45,X karyotype (Turner syndrome) and the trisomies 21 and 18 are associated with fetal hydrops. Most often, underlying structural cardiac anomalies associated with the chromosomal aberrations form the basis of fetal hydrops. In the Turner phenotype, however, abnormalities of lymphatic drainage from the neck may lead to postnuchal fluid accumulation *(cystic hygromas)*. Fetal anemia, not caused by Rh- or ABO-associated antibodies, also results in hydrops. In fact, in some parts of the world (e.g., Southeast Asia), severe fetal anemia due to homozygous α-thalassemia is probably the most common cause of nonimmune hydrops.[61] Transplacental infection by parvovirus B19 is rapidly emerging as an important cause of hydrops. The virus gains entry into erythroid precursors (normoblasts), where it replicates, leading to erythrocyte maturation arrest and aplastic anemia. Parvoviral intranuclear inclusions can be seen within circulating and marrow erythroid precursors (see Fig. 10–9). The basis for hydrops in fetal anemia of both immune and nonimmune etiology is tissue ischemia with secondary myocardial dysfunction and circulatory failure. Additionally, secondary liver failure may ensue, with loss of synthetic function contributing to hypoalbuminemia, reduced oncotic pressure, and edema. Approximately 10% of cases of nonimmune hydrops are related to monozygous twin pregnancies and twin-to-twin transfusion occurring through anastomoses between the two circulations.

Morphology of Hydrops Fetalis. The anatomic findings in fetuses with intrauterine fluid accumulation vary with both the severity of the disease and the underlying etiology. As previously noted, hydrops fetalis represents the most severe and generalized manifestation, and lesser degrees of edema such as isolated pleural, peritoneal, or postnuchal fluid collections can occur. Accordingly, infants may be stillborn, die within the first few days, or recover completely. The presence of dysmorphic features suggests the presence of a constitutional chromosomal abnormality; postmortem examination may reveal an underlying cardiac anomaly. In hydrops associated with fetal anemia, both fetus and placenta are characteristically pale; in most cases the liver and spleen are enlarged from cardiac failure and congestion. Additionally, the bone marrow demonstrates compensatory hyperplasia of erythroid precursors (parvovirus-associated aplastic anemia being a notable exception), and extramedullary hematopoiesis is present in the liver, spleen, and possibly other tissues such as the kidneys, lungs, and even the heart. The increased hematopoietic activity accounts for the presence in the peripheral circulation of large numbers of immature red cells, including reticulocytes, normoblasts, and erythroblasts **(erythroblastosis fetalis)** (Fig. 10–15).

The most serious threat in fetal hydrops is central nervous system damage known as **kernicterus** (Fig. 10–16). The affected brain is enlarged and edematous and, when sectioned, is found to have a bright yellow pigmentation (kernicterus), particularly in the basal ganglia, thalamus, cerebellum, cerebral gray matter, and spinal cord. The precise level of bilirubin that induces kernicterus is unpredictable, but neural damage usually requires a blood bilirubin level greater than 20 mg/dL in term infants; in premature infants this threshold may be considerably lower.

Clinical Features. The clinical manifestations of fetal hydrops vary with the severity of the disease and can be inferred from the preceding discussion. Minimally affected infants display pallor, possibly accompanied by hepatosplenomegaly (to which may be added jaundice with more severe hemolytic reactions), whereas the most gravely ill neonates present with intense jaundice, generalized edema, and signs of neurologic involvement. These infants may be supported by a variety of measures, including phototherapy (visual light oxidizes toxic unconjugated bilirubin to harmless, readily excreted, water-soluble dipyrroles) and, in severe cases, total exchange transfusion of the infant. Administration of high-dose intravenous immunoglobulin may also play an important role, although specific details regarding

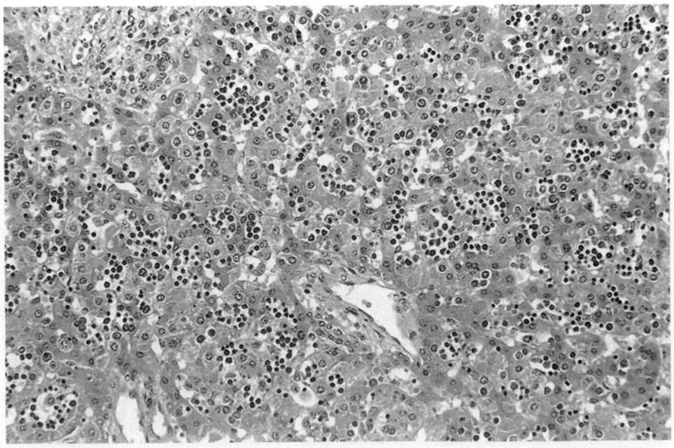

FIGURE 10–15 Numerous islands of extramedullary hematopoiesis (small blue cells) are scattered among mature hepatocytes in this infant with nonimmune hydrops fetalis.

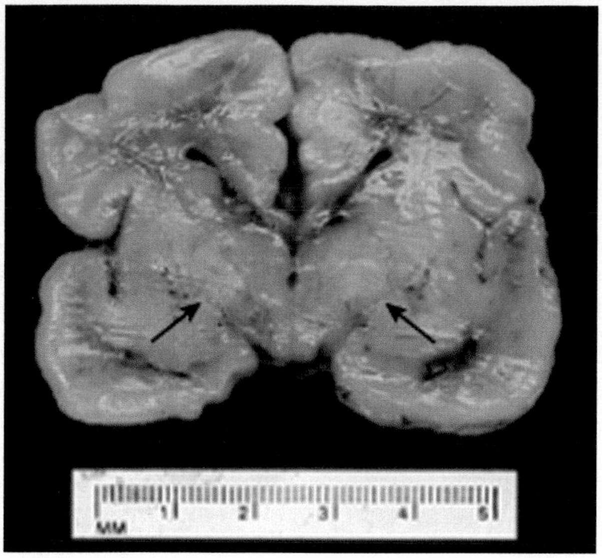

FIGURE 10–16 Kernicterus. Severe hyperbilirubinemia in the neonatal period, for example, secondary to immune hemolysis, results in deposition of bilirubin pigment in the brain parenchyma. This occurs because the blood-brain barrier is less well developed in the neonatal period than it is in adulthood. Infants who survive develop long-term neurologic sequelae.

optimal dosage and timing of this therapy still need to be determined.

Inborn Errors of Metabolism and Other Genetic Disorders

Sir Archibald Garrod coined the term "inborn errors of metabolism" in 1908; since that time the number of well-characterized genetic disorders giving rise to inborn errors of metabolism has increased exponentially and is beyond the scope of this chapter. *Most inborn errors of metabolism are rare, and some were discussed in Chapter 5. They are inherited, most commonly, as autosomal recessive or X-linked diseases*; a few are inherited as dominant traits. Mitochondrial disorders (Chapter 5) form a distinct entity by themselves. Some of the clinical features that suggest an underlying metabolic disorder in a neonate are tabulated in Table 10–6. Three metabolic genetic defects, phenylketonuria (PKU), galactosemia, and cystic fibrosis, are selected for discussion here. PKU and galactosemia are reviewed because their early diagnosis (via neonatal screening programs) is particularly important, since appropriate dietary regimen can prevent early death or mental retardation. Cystic fibrosis is included because it is one of the most common, potentially lethal diseases occurring in individuals of Caucasian descent. Neonatal screening for cystic fibrosis remains a controversial topic, with the benefits and risks much less clear than in the other two diseases.

PHENYLKETONURIA (PKU)

There are several variants of PKU. The most common form, referred to as *classic PKU* (or Type 1 PKU), is quite common in persons of Scandinavian descent and is distinctly uncommon in individuals of African-American and Jewish descent.

TABLE 10–6 Abnormalities Suggesting Inborn Errors of Metabolism

General
Dysmorphic features
Deafness
Self-mutilation
Abnormal hair
Abnormal body or urine odor ("sweaty feet"; "mousy or musty"; "maple syrup")
Hepatosplenomegaly; cardiomegaly
Hydrops
Neurologic
Hypotonia or hypertonia
Coma
Persistent lethargy
Seizures
Gastrointestinal
Poor feeding
Recurrent vomiting
Jaundice
Eyes
Cataract
Cherry red macula
Dislocated lens
Glaucoma
Muscle, Joints
Myopathy
Abnormal mobility

Adapted from Barness LA and Gilbert-Barness E: Metabolic diseases, In Gilbert-Barness E (ed): Potter's Pathology of Fetus and Infant. St. Louis, Mosby-Year Book, 1997.

Homozygotes with this autosomal recessive disorder classically have a severe deficiency of phenylalanine hydroxylase, leading to hyperphenylalaninemia and its pathologic consequences. Affected infants are normal at birth but within a few weeks develop a rising plasma phenylalanine level, which in some way impairs brain development. Usually by 6 months of life *severe mental retardation* becomes evident; fewer than 4% of untreated PKU children have intelligence quotient values greater than 50 or 60. About one third of these children are never able to walk, and two thirds cannot talk. *Seizures*, other neurologic abnormalities, *decreased pigmentation of hair* and skin, and eczema often accompany the mental retardation in untreated children. Hyperphenylalaninemia and the resultant mental retardation can be avoided by restriction of phenylalanine intake early in life. Hence, a number of screening procedures are routinely used for detection of PKU in the immediate postnatal period.

Many clinically normal female PKU patients who are treated with dietary control early in life reach childbearing age. Most of them discontinue dietary treatment and have marked hyperphenylalaninemia. Between 75% and 90% of children born to such women are mentally retarded and microcephalic, and 15% have congenital heart disease, even though the infants themselves are heterozygotes. This syndrome, termed *maternal PKU*, results from the teratogenic effects of phenylalanine or its metabolites that cross the placenta and affect specific fetal organs during development.[62] The presence and severity of the fetal anomalies directly correlate with the maternal phenylalanine level, so *it is imperative that maternal dietary restriction of phenylalanine is initiated before conception and continues throughout the pregnancy.*

The biochemical abnormality in PKU is an inability to convert phenylalanine into tyrosine. In normal children, less than 50% of the dietary intake of phenylalanine is necessary for protein synthesis. The rest is irreversibly converted to tyrosine by a complex *hepatic phenylalanine hydroxylase system* (Fig. 10–17), which, in addition to the enzyme *phenylalanine hydroxylase,* has two other components: the cofactor *tetrahydrobiopterin (BH_4)* and the enzyme *dihydropteridine reductase,* which regenerates BH_4. Although neonatal hyperphenylalaninemia can be caused by deficiencies in any of these components, 98% to 99% of cases are attributable to abnormalities in phenylalanine hydroxylase. With a block in phenylalanine metabolism owing to lack of phenylalanine hydroxylase, minor shunt pathways come into play, yielding phenylpyruvic acid, phenyllactic acid, phenylacetic acid, and *o*-hydroxyphenylacetic acid, which are excreted in large amounts in the urine in PKU. Some of these abnormal metabolites are excreted in the sweat, and phenylacetic acid in particular imparts a strong *musty* or *mousy odor* to affected infants. It is believed that excess phenylalanine or its metabolites contribute to the brain damage in PKU.

At the molecular level, several mutant alleles of the phenylalanine hydroxylase gene have been identified. Each mutation induces a particular alteration in the enzyme resulting in a corresponding quantitative effect on residual enzyme activity ranging from complete absence to 50% of normal values. The degree of hyperphenylalaninemia and clinical phenotype is inversely related to the amount of residual enzyme activity. Infants with mutations resulting in a lack of phenylalanine hydroxylase activity present with the classic features of PKU, while those with up to 6% residual activity present with milder disease. Moreover, some mutations result in only modest elevations of phenylalanine levels, and the affected children have no neurologic damage. This latter condition, referred to as *benign hyperphenylalaninemia*, or *mild PKU*, is important to recognize because the individuals may well test *positive* in screening tests but do not develop the stigmata of classic PKU.[63] Measurement of serum phenylalanine levels differentiates benign hyperphenylalaninemia and classic PKU.

Although dietary restriction of phenylalanine is relatively successful in reducing or preventing the mental retardation associated with PKU, there are problems with long-term compliance (resulting in a decline in mental or behavioral status) and nutritional imbalances involving trace minerals, fatty acids, and lipids. There is great interest in somatic gene therapy as alternative treatment for these patients, since adenovirus-mediated transfer and transient expression of a functional recombinant phenylalanine hydroxylase gene have been accomplished in animal systems.[64] As alluded to earlier, a number of variant forms of PKU have been identified, resulting from deficiencies of enzymes other than phenylalanine hydroxylase. For example, some patients lack the enzyme responsible for BH_4 regeneration, *dihydropteridine reductase* (Type 2 PKU) (see Fig. 10–17), while others lack the biopterin synthetic enzyme, *dihydrobiopterin synthetase* (Type 3 PKU). BH_4 is not only an essential cofactor for phenylalanine hydroxylase, but is also required for tyrosine and tryptophan metabolism. The concomitant impairment of tyrosine and tryptophan hydroxylation leads to disturbance in the synthesis of neurotransmitters, and neurologic damage is not arrested despite normalization of phenylalanine levels. Although they account for a small minority of patients with hyperphenylalaninemia, *it is important to recognize these PKU variants because the ongoing neurologic disturbances cannot be treated by dietary control of phenylalanine levels alone.*

GALACTOSEMIA

Galactosemia is an autosomal recessive disorder of galactose metabolism. Normally, lactose, the major carbohydrate of mammalian milk, is split into glucose and galactose in the intestinal microvilli by lactase. Galactose is then converted to glucose in three steps (Fig. 10–18). *Two variants of galactosemia have been identified. In the more common variant, there is a total lack of galactose-1-phosphate uridyl transferase involved in reaction 2. The rare variant arises from a deficiency of galactokinase, involved in reaction 1.* Because galactokinase deficiency leads to a milder form of the disease not associated with mental retardation, it is not considered in this discussion. As a result of the transferase lack, *galactose-1-phosphate* accumulates in many locations, including the liver, spleen, lens of the eye, kidneys, heart muscle, cerebral cortex, and erythrocytes. Alternative metabolic pathways are activated, leading to the production of *galactitol,* which also accumulates in the tissues. Heterozygotes may have a mild deficiency but are spared the clinical and pathologic consequences of the homozygous state.

The clinical picture is variable, probably reflecting the heterogeneity of mutations in the *galactose-1-phosphate uridyl transferase* gene (also known as *GALT*) leading to galactosemia. The liver, eyes, and brain bear the brunt of the damage. The early-to-develop *hepatomegaly* is due largely to fatty change, but in time widespread scarring that closely resembles the cirrhosis of alcohol abuse may supervene (Fig. 10–19). *Opacification of the lens (cataracts)* develops,

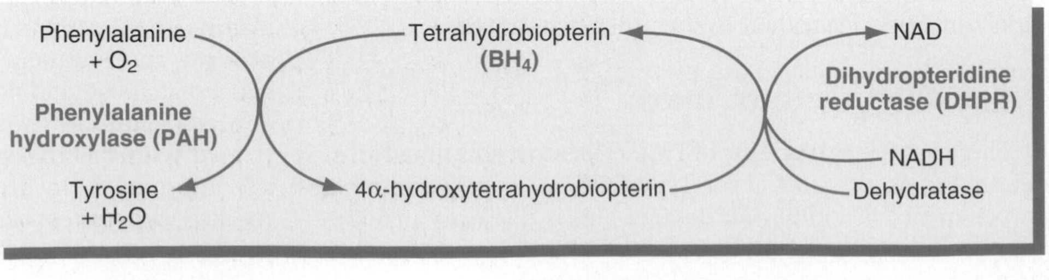

FIGURE 10–17 The phenylalanine hydroxylase system.

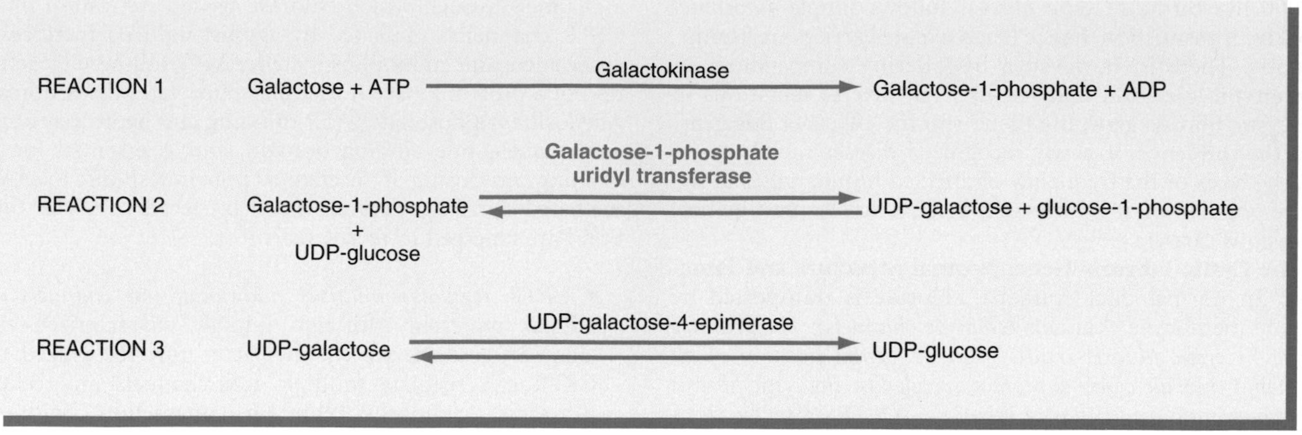

FIGURE 10–18 Pathways of galactose metabolism.

probably because the lens absorbs water and swells as galactitol, produced by alternative metabolic pathways, accumulates and increases its tonicity. *Nonspecific alterations appear in the central nervous system*, including loss of nerve cells, gliosis, and edema, particularly in the dentate nuclei of the cerebellum and the olivary nuclei of the medulla. Similar changes may occur in the cerebral cortex and white matter.

There is still no clear understanding of the mechanism of injury to the liver and brain. Long-term toxicity has been variously imputed to several metabolic intermediates, including *galactose-1-phosphate, galactitol* (a polyol metabolite of galactose), and *UDP-galactose.*[65,66]

Almost from birth these infants *fail to thrive. Vomiting* and *diarrhea* appear within a few days of milk ingestion. *Jaundice* and *hepatomegaly* usually become evident during the first week of life and may seem to be a continuation of the physiologic jaundice of the newborn. The *cataracts* develop within a few weeks, and within the first 6 to 12 months of life mental retardation may be detected. Even in untreated infants, the mental deficit is usually not as severe as that with PKU. Accumulation of galactose and galactose-1-phosphate in the kidney impairs amino acid transport, resulting in *aminoaciduria.* There is an increased frequency of fulminant

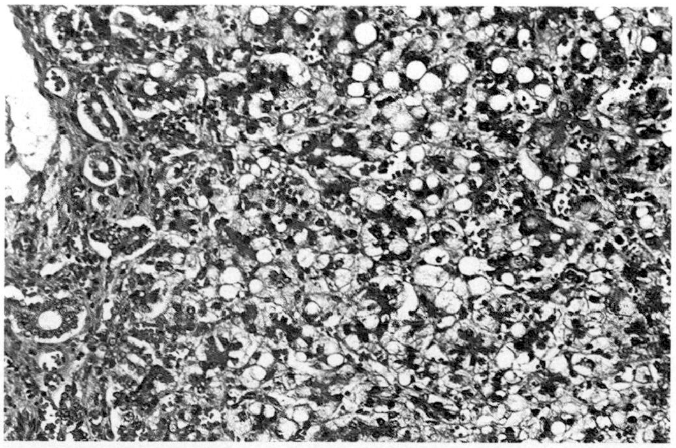

FIGURE 10–19 Galactosemia. The liver shows extensive fatty change and a delicate fibrosis. (Courtesy of Dr. Wesley Tyson, The Children's Hospital, Denver, CO.)

Escherichia coli septicemia, possibly arising from depressed neutrophil bactericidal activity.[67] *Hemolysis* and *coagulopathy* in the newborn period can occur as well.

The diagnosis of galactosemia can be suspected by the demonstration in the urine of a reducing sugar other than glucose, but tests that directly identify the deficiency of the transferase in leukocytes and erythrocytes are more reliable. Antenatal diagnosis is possible by the assay of GALT activity in cultured amniotic fluid cells or determination of galactitol level in amniotic fluid supernatant. Over 140 mutations have been documented in *GALT*; among these, a glutamine to arginine substitution at codon 188 *(Gln188Arg)* is the most prevalent mutation in non-Hispanic whites, while a serine-to-leucine substitution at codon 135 *(Ser135Leu)* is the most common mutation in African Americans.[68]

Many of the clinical and morphologic changes of galactosemia can be prevented or ameliorated by early removal of galactose from the diet for at least the first 2 years of life. Control instituted soon after birth prevents the cataracts and liver damage and permits almost normal development. Even with dietary restrictions, however, it is now well established that older patients are frequently affected by a speech disorder and gonadal failure (especially premature ovarian failure) and, less commonly, by an ataxic condition.[69,70]

CYSTIC FIBROSIS (MUCOVISCIDOSIS)

Cystic fibrosis is fundamentally a *widespread disorder in epithelial transport affecting fluid secretion in exocrine glands and the epithelial lining of the respiratory, gastrointestinal, and reproductive tracts.* In many infants, this disorder leads to abnormally viscid mucous secretions, which obstruct organ passages, resulting in most of the clinical features of this disorder, such as recurrent pulmonary infections leading to *chronic lung disease, pancreatic insufficiency, steatorrhea, malnutrition, hepatic cirrhosis, intestinal obstruction, and male infertility.* These manifestations may appear at any point in life from before birth to much later in childhood or even in adolescence.

With an incidence of 1 in 3200 live births in the United States, *cystic fibrosis is the most common lethal genetic disease that affects Caucasian populations.* It is uncommon among Asians (1 in 31,000 live births) and African Americans (1 in

15,000 live births). Cystic fibrosis follows simple *autosomal recessive* transmission, hence heterozygote carriers are asymptomatic. There is, however, a bewildering compendium of phenotypic variation that results from diverse mutations in the cystic fibrosis gene, the tissue-specific effects of this gene, and the influence of newly recognized disease modifiers.[71,72] On the basis of the frequency of affected homozygotes in the white population, it is estimated that 2% to 4% must be heterozygous carriers.

The Cystic Fibrosis Gene: Normal Structure and Function. In normal duct epithelia, chloride is transported by plasma membrane channels *(chloride channels). The primary defect in cystic fibrosis results from abnormal function of an epithelial chloride channel protein encoded by the cystic fibrosis transmembrane conductance regulator (CFTR) gene on chromosome band 7q31.2.* The protein encoded by *CFTR* has two transmembrane domains, two cytoplasmic nucleotide-binding domains (NBD), and a regulatory domain (R domain) that contains protein kinase A and C phosphorylation sites (Fig. 10–20). The two transmembrane domains form

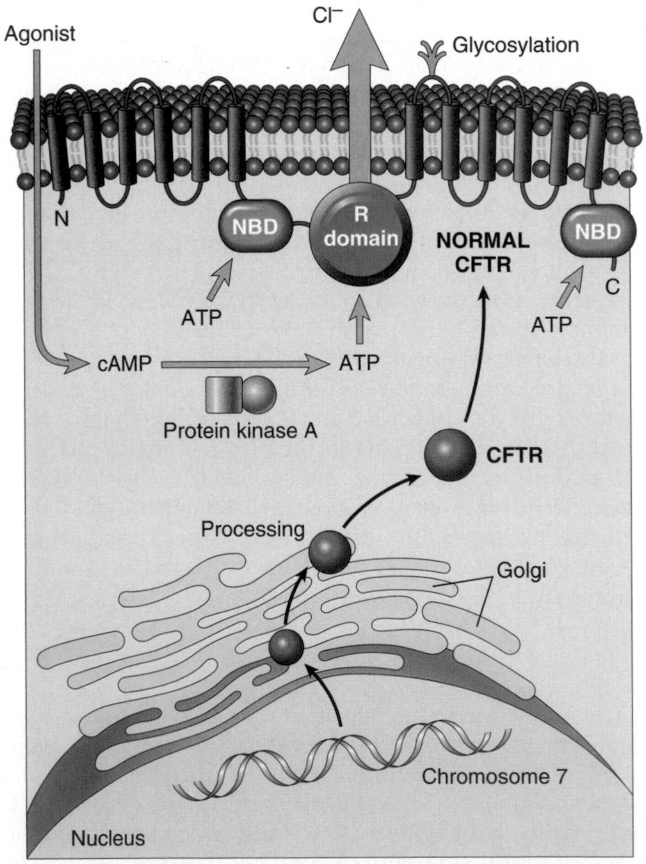

FIGURE 10–20 *Top,* Normal cystic fibrosis transmembrane conductance regulator (CFTR) structure and activation. CFTR consists of two transmembrane domains, two nucleotide-binding domains (NBD), and a regulatory R domain. Agonists (e.g., acetylcholine) bind to epithelial cells and increase cAMP, which activates protein kinase A, the latter phosphorylating the CFTR at the R domain, resulting in opening of the chloride channel. *Bottom,* CFTR from gene to protein. The most common mutation in the *CFTR* gene results in defective protein folding in the Golgi/ER and degradation of CFTR before it reaches the cell surface. Other mutations affect synthesis of CFTR, nucleotide-binding and R domains, and membrane-spanning domains.

a channel through which chloride passes. Activation of the CFTR channel is mediated by agonist-induced increases in cyclic adenosine monophosphate (cAMP), followed by activation of a protein kinase A that phosphorylates the R domain. Adenosine triphosphate (ATP) binding and hydrolysis occurs at the nucleotide-binding domain, and is essential for the opening and closing of the channel pore in response to cAMP-mediated signaling. Several important facets of CFTR function have emerged in recent years:

- *CFTR regulates multiple additional ion channels and cellular processes.* Although initially characterized as a chloride-conductance channel, it is now recognized that CFTR can regulate multiple ion channels and cellular processes, primarily through interaction with its nucleotide-binding domain.[73–75] These include so-called outwardly rectified chloride channels, inwardly rectified potassium channels (Kir6.1), the epithelial sodium channel (ENaC), gap junction channels, and cellular processes involved in ATP transport and mucus secretion. Of these, the interaction of CFTR with the ENaC has possibly the most pathophysiologic relevance in cystic fibrosis. The ENaC is situated on the apical surface of exocrine epithelial cells, and is responsible for intracytoplasmic sodium transport from the luminal fluid, rendering it (the luminal fluid) hypotonic. The ENaC is *inhibited* by normally functioning CFTR; hence, *in cystic fibrosis, ENaC activity increases, markedly augmenting sodium transport across the apical membrane.*[76] The importance of this phenomenon is discussed below in the context of pulmonary and gastrointestinal pathology in cystic fibrosis. The one exception to this rule happens to be the human sweat ducts, where ENaC activity *decreases* as a result of *CFTR* mutations; therefore, a hypertonic luminal fluid containing both high sweat chloride (the *sine qua non* of classic cystic fibrosis) and high sodium content is formed.[77] This is the basis for the "salty" sweat that mothers can often detect in their affected infants.
- *The functions of* CFTR *are tissue-specific; therefore, impact of a mutation in* CFTR *is also tissue-specific.* The major function of CFTR in the *sweat gland ducts* is to reabsorb luminal chloride ions and augment sodium reabsorption via the ENaC (see above). Therefore, in the sweat ducts, loss of CFTR function leads to decreased reabsorption of sodium chloride and production of hypertonic sweat (Fig. 10–21). The CFTR channel is, however, not only responsible for chloride absorption, but also, in the *respiratory and intestinal epithelium*, forms one of the most important avenues for *active luminal secretion of chloride.* At these sites, *CFTR* mutations result in loss or reduction of chloride secretion into the lumen (see Fig. 10–21). Active luminal sodium absorption is also increased (due to loss of inhibition of ENaC activity), and both of these ion changes increase passive water reabsorption from the lumen, *lowering the water content of the surface fluid layer coating mucosal cells.*[78] Thus, unlike the sweat ducts, there is no difference in the salt concentration of the surface fluid layer coating the respiratory and intestinal mucosal cells in normal individuals versus those with cystic fibrosis. Instead, *the pathogenesis of respiratory and intestinal complications in cystic fibrosis appears to stem from an isotonic but low-volume surface fluid layer.* In the lungs, this dehydration leads to defective mucociliary action and the accumulation of hyperconcen-

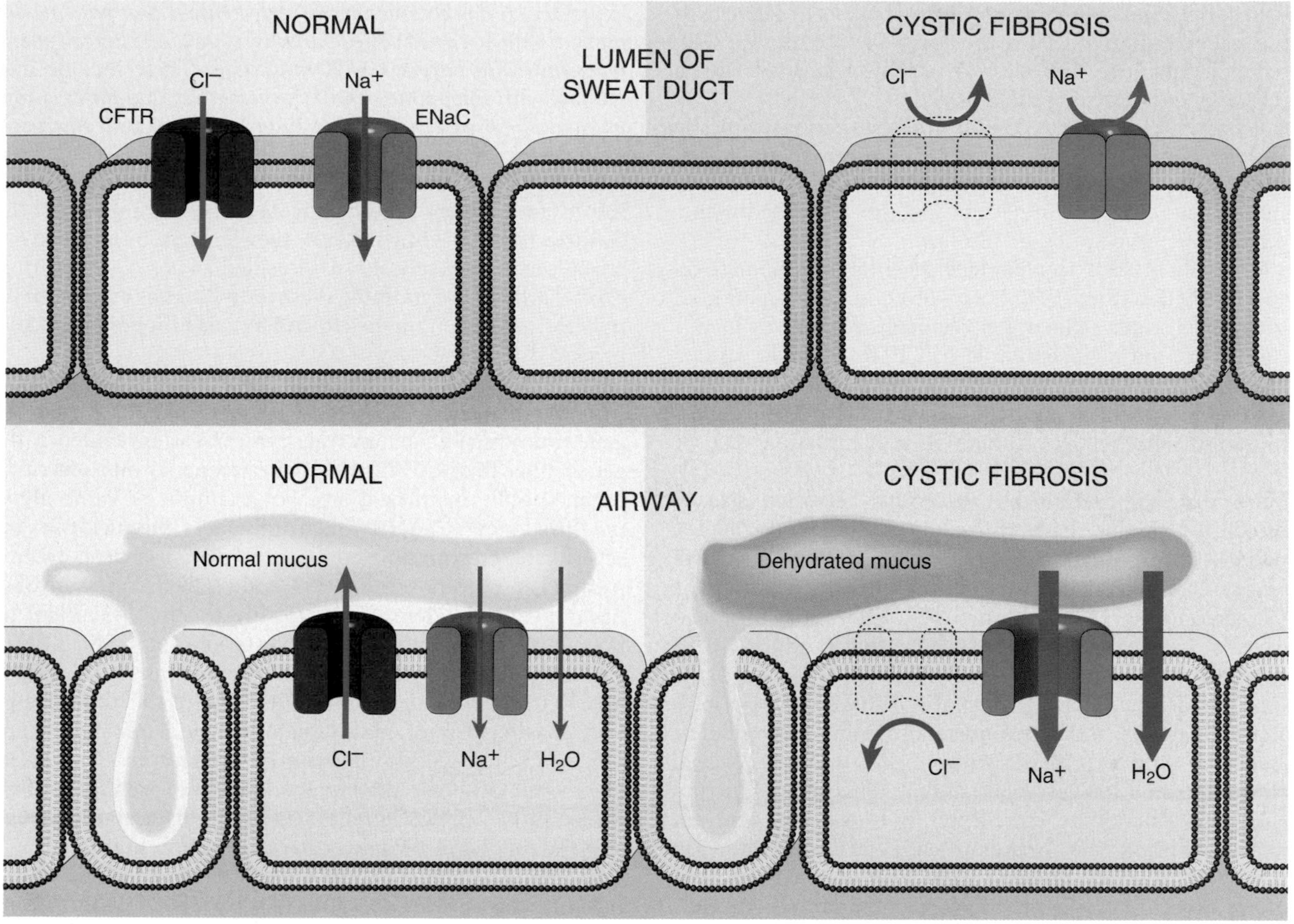

FIGURE 10–21 Chloride channel defect in the sweat duct *(top)* causes increased chloride and sodium concentration in sweat. In the airway *(bottom)*, cystic fibrosis patients have decreased chloride secretion and increased sodium and water reabsorption leading to dehydration of the mucus layer coating epithelial cells, defective mucociliary action, and mucus plugging of airways. CFTR, Cystic fibrosis transmembrane conductance regulator; EnaC, Epithelial sodium channel.

trated, viscid secretions that obstruct the air passages and predispose to recurrent pulmonary infections.

- CFTR *mediates transport of bicarbonate ions.* It has recently been demonstrated that CFTR can also transport bicarbonate ions, and in some *CFTR* mutant variants, chloride transport is completely or substantially preserved, while *bicarbonate transport is markedly abnormal.*[79] Alkaline fluids are secreted by normal tissues, while acidic fluids (due to absence of bicarbonate ions) are secreted by epithelia harboring these mutant *CFTR*. The decreased luminal pH can lead to a variety of adverse effects such as increased mucin precipitation and plugging of ducts, and increased binding of bacteria to plugged mucins. Pancreatic insufficiency, a feature of classic cystic fibrosis, is virtually always present when there are *CFTR* mutations with abnormal bicarbonate conductance.

The Cystic Fibrosis Gene: Mutational Spectra and Genotype–Phenotype Correlation. Since the *CFTR* gene was cloned in 1989, more than 800 disease-causing mutations have been identified. Various mutations can be grouped into six "classes" based on their effect on the CFTR protein:[80]

- Class I: *Defective protein synthesis.* These mutations are associated with complete lack of CFTR protein at the apical surface of epithelial cells.
- Class II: *Abnormal protein folding, processing, and trafficking.* These mutations result in defective processing of the protein from the endoplasmic reticulum to the Golgi apparatus; the protein does not become fully folded and glycosylated and is instead degraded before it reaches the cell surface. The most common cystic fibrosis gene abnormality in patients with this disease is a Class II mutation that leads to a deletion of three nucleotides coding for phenylalanine at amino acid position 508 (ΔF508). Worldwide, this mutation can be found in approximately 70% of cystic fibrosis patients. Class II mutations are also associated with complete lack of CFTR protein at the apical surface of epithelial cells.
- Class III: *Defective regulation.* Mutations in this class prevent activation of CFTR by preventing ATP binding and hydrolysis, an essential prerequisite for ionic passage (see above). Thus, there is a normal amount of CFTR on the apical surface, but it is nonfunctional.
- Class IV: *Decreased conductance.* These mutations typically occur in the transmembrane domain of *CFTR*, which

forms the ionic pore for chloride transport. There is a normal amount of CFTR at the apical membrane, but with reduced function. This class is usually associated with a milder phenotype of cystic fibrosis.

- Class V: *Reduced abundance.* These mutations typically affect intronic splice sites or the *CFTR* promoter, such that there is a reduced amount of normal protein. As discussed subsequently, Class V mutations are also associated with a milder phenotype of cystic fibrosis.
- Class VI: *Altered regulation of separate ion channels.* As previously described, CFTR is involved in the regulation of multiple distinct cellular ion channels. Mutations in this class affect the regulatory role of CFTR. In some cases, a given mutation affects the conductance by CFTR as well as regulation of other ion channels. For example, the ΔF508 mutation is both a Class II and Class VI mutation.

Since cystic fibrosis is an autosomal recessive disease, affected individuals harbor mutations on both alleles. However, the combination of mutations on the two alleles can have a remarkable effect on the overall phenotype, as well as on organ-specific manifestations (Fig. 10–22). Thus, two "severe" (Class I, II, and III) mutations that produce virtual absence of membrane CFTR are associated with the *classic* cystic fibrosis phenotype (pancreatic insufficiency, sinopulmonary infections, and gastrointestinal symptoms), while the presence of a "mild" (Class IV or V) mutation on *one or both* alleles results in a less severe phenotype. This general dictum of genotype-phenotype correlation is most consistent for pancreatic disease, wherein the presence of a "mild" mutation in one allele can revert the pancreatic insufficiency phenotype conferred by homozygosity for "severe" mutations. By contrast, genotype-phenotype correlations are far less consistent in pulmonary disease, reflecting an effect of secondary modifiers (see below). As genetic testing for *CFTR* mutations has expanded, *it has become increasingly evident that patients who present with a variety of apparently unrelated clinical phenotypes may also harbor* CFTR *mutations.* These include individuals with *idiopathic chronic pancreatitis, late-onset chronic pulmonary disease, idiopathic bronchiectasis,* and *obstructive azoospermia* caused by bilateral absence of the vas deferens (see detailed discussion of individual phenotypes later).[81] Importantly, most of these patients do not demonstrate other features of cystic fibrosis, yet they harbor bi-allelic *CFTR* mutations. These subsets are classified as *nonclassic* or *atypical cystic fibrosis.* Identifying these individuals is important not only for subsequent management, but also for the purposes of genetic counseling.

Genetic and Environmental Modifiers. Although cystic fibrosis remains one of the best-known examples of the "one gene, one disease" axiom, there is increasing evidence that genes other than *CFTR* modify the frequency and severity of organ-specific manifestations. For example, a *"cystic fibrosis modifier locus" (CFM1)*, which influences the incidence and severity of meconium ileus (see below), has been recently mapped to chromosome 19q13, although the gene involved has not yet been identified.[82] Notably, this modifier locus has no effects on pulmonary manifestations of cystic fibrosis. Another candidate genetic modifier is *mannose-binding lectin*, a key effector of innate immunity involved in opsonization and phagocytosis of microorganisms. Functional polymorphisms in one or both mannose-binding lectin alleles associated with lower circulating levels of the protein confer a threefold higher risk of end-stage lung disease and reduced survival following chronic bacterial infection in the setting of cystic fibrosis.[83] Similarly, in a recent study of cystic fibrosis patients who were homozygous for the ΔF508 mutation, functional polymorphisms in mannose-binding lectin independently influenced the severity of liver disease and the onset of cirrhosis.[84]

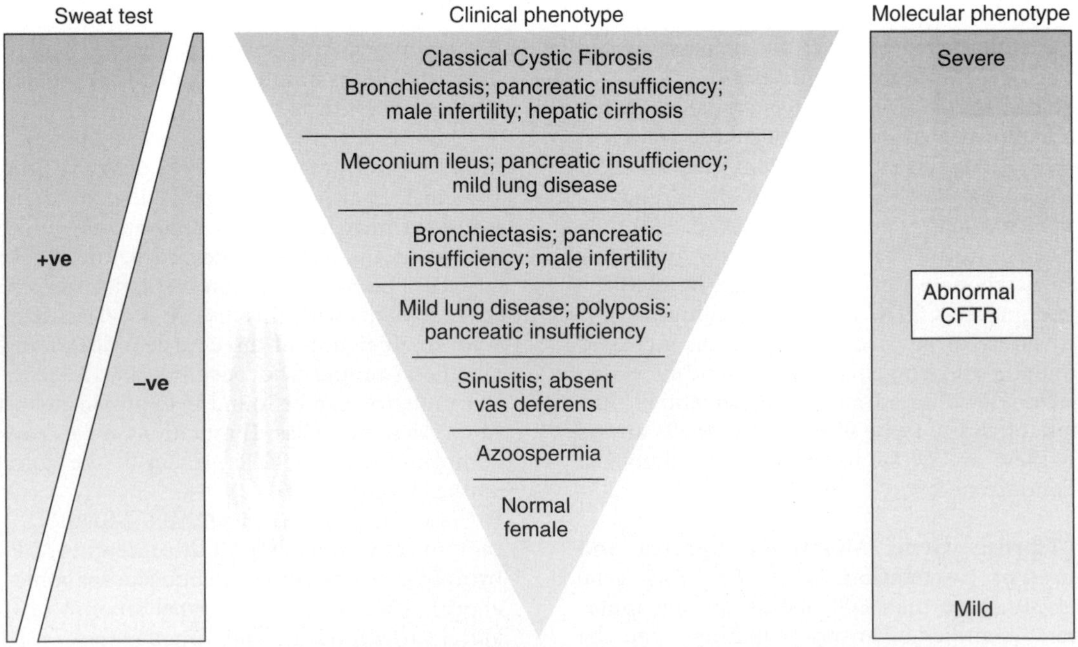

FIGURE 10–22 The many clinical manifestations of mutations in the cystic fibrosis gene, from most severe to asymptomatic. (Redrawn from Wallis C: Diagnosing cystic fibrosis: blood, sweat, and tears. Arch Dis Child 76:85, 1997.)

Environmental modifiers may also cause significant phenotypic differences between individuals who share the same *CFTR* genotype. This is best exemplified in pulmonary disease, where *CFTR* genotype and phenotype correlations can be perplexing. As previously stated, defective mucociliary action because of deficient hydration of the mucus results in inability of the airways to clear bacteria. *Pseudomonas aeruginosa* species, in particular, colonize the lower respiratory tract, first intermittently and then chronically. Concurrent viral infections predispose to such colonization. The static mucus creates a hypoxic microenvironment in the airway surface fluid, which in turn favors the production of *alginate,* a mucoid polysaccharide capsule. Alginate production permits the formation of a protective biofilm that protects the bacteria from antibodies or antibiotics, allows them to evade host defenses, and produce a chronic destructive lung disease. At this stage, antibody and cell-mediated reactions induced by the organisms result in further pulmonary destruction while sparing the organism. It is evident, therefore, that in addition to genetic factors (e.g., class of mutation), a plethora of environmental modifiers (e.g., virulence of organisms, efficacy of therapy, intercurrent and concurrent infections by other organisms, exposure to smoking and allergens) can influence the severity and progression of lung disease in cystic fibrosis.

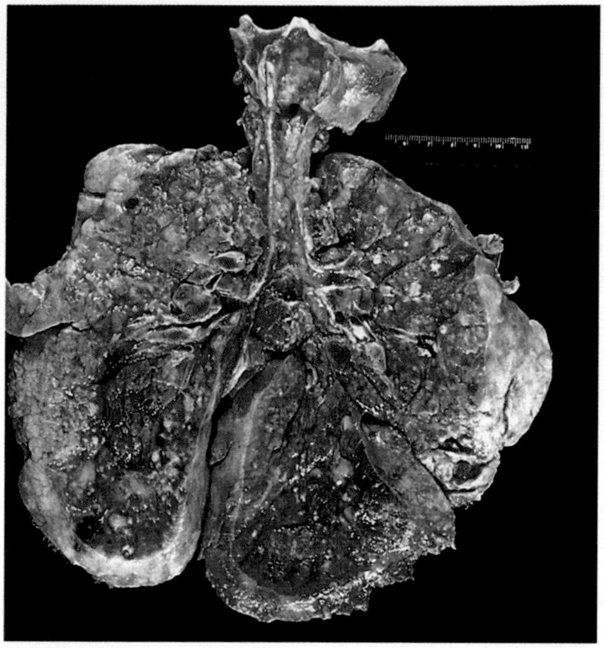

FIGURE 10–23 Lungs of a patient dying of cystic fibrosis. There is extensive mucus plugging and dilation of the tracheobronchial tree. The pulmonary parenchyma is consolidated by a combination of both secretions and pneumonia—the green color associated with *Pseudomonas* infections. (Courtesy of Dr. Eduardo Yunis, Children's Hospital of Pittsburgh, Pittsburgh, PA.)

Morphology. The anatomic changes are highly variable and depend on which glands are affected and on the severity of this involvement. In individuals with nonclassic cystic fibrosis, the disease is quite mild and does not seriously disturb their growth and development, and they readily survive into adolescence or adulthood. In others, the pancreatic involvement is severe and impairs intestinal absorption because of the pancreatic achylia, and so malabsorption, inanition, and stunted development not only seriously hamper life but also shorten survival. In others, the mucus secretion defect leads to defective mucociliary action, obstruction of bronchi and bronchioles, and crippling fatal pulmonary infections (Fig. 10–23). Thus, cystic fibrosis may be compatible with long life or may cause death in infancy. Significantly, the sweat glands, producing a hypertonic but watery secretion, are morphologically unaffected.

Pancreatic abnormalities are present in approximately 85% to 90% of patients with cystic fibrosis. In the milder cases, there may be only accumulations of mucus in the small ducts with some dilation of the exocrine glands. In more advanced cases, usually seen in older children or adolescents, the ducts are totally plugged, causing atrophy of the exocrine glands and progressive fibrosis (Fig. 10–24). Total atrophy of the exocrine portion of the pancreas may occur, leaving only the islets within a fibrofatty stroma. The total loss of pancreatic exocrine secretion impairs fat absorption, and so avitaminosis A may contribute to squamous metaplasia of the lining epithelium of the ducts in the pancreas, which are already injured by the inspissated mucus secretions. Thick viscid plugs of mucus may also be found in the small intestine of infants. Sometimes these cause small-bowel obstruction, known as **meconium ileus.**

The **liver involvement** follows the same basic pattern. Bile canaliculi are plugged by mucinous material, accompanied by ductular proliferation and portal inflammation. Hepatic **steatosis** is not an uncommon finding in liver biopsies. Over time, **focal biliary cirrhosis** develops (Chapter 18), which eventually involves the entire liver, resulting in diffuse hepatic nodularity. Such severe hepatic involvement is encountered in only approximately 5% of patients.

The **salivary glands** are frequently involved, with histologic changes similar to those described in the pancreas: progressive dilation of ducts, squamous metaplasia of the lining epithelium, and glandular atrophy followed by fibrosis.

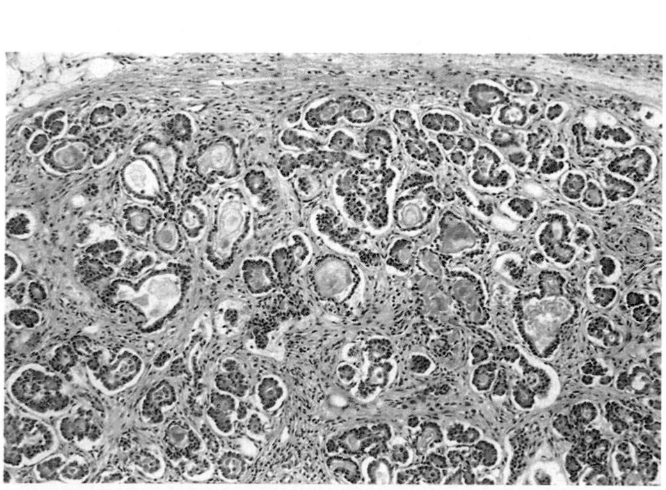

FIGURE 10–24 Mild to moderate cystic fibrosis changes in the pancreas. The ducts are dilated and plugged with eosinophilic mucin, and the parenchymal glands are atrophic and replaced by fibrous tissue.

The **pulmonary changes** are the most serious complications of this disease. These stem from the viscous mucus secretions of the submucosal glands of the respiratory tree with secondary obstruction and infection of the air passages. The bronchioles are often distended with thick mucus associated with marked hyperplasia and hypertrophy of the mucus-secreting cells. Superimposed infections give rise to severe chronic bronchitis and bronchiectasis (Chapter 15). In many instances, lung abscesses develop. *Staphylococcus aureus, Hemophilus influenzae,* and *Pseudomonas aeruginosa* are the three most common organisms responsible for lung infections. As mentioned previously, a mucoid form of *P. aeruginosa* (alginate-producing) is particularly frequent and causes chronic inflammation. Even more sinister is the increasing frequency of infection with another pseudomonad, *Burkholderia cepacia.* This opportunistic bacterium is particularly hardy, and infection with this organism has been associated with fulminant illness. Other emerging opportunistic bacterial pathogens include *Stenotrophomonas maltophila* and *nontuberculous mycobacteria,* while *allergic bronchopulmonary aspergillosis* also occurs with increased frequency in cystic fibrosis.

Azoospermia and infertility are found in 95% of the males who survive to adulthood; **congenital bilateral absence of the vas deferens** (CBAVD) is a frequent finding in these patients. In some males, CBAVD may be the only feature suggesting an underlying *CFTR* mutation.

Clinical Course. Few childhood diseases are as protean as cystic fibrosis in clinical manifestations (Table 10–7). The symptoms are extremely varied and range from mild to severe, from onset at birth to onset years later, and from involvement of one organ system to involvement of many. Approximately 5% to 10% of the cases come to clinical attention at birth or soon after because of an attack of *meconium ileus.* Distal intestinal obstruction can also occur in older individuals, manifesting as recurrent episodes of right lower quadrant pain sometimes associated with a palpable mass in the right iliac fossa.

Exocrine pancreatic insufficiency occurs in the majority (85–90%) of patients with cystic fibrosis and is associated with "severe" *CFTR* mutations on *both* alleles (e.g., *ΔF508/ΔF508*), whereas 10% to 15% of patients with one "severe" and one "mild" *CFTR* mutation *(ΔF508/R117H)* or two "mild" *CFTR* mutations retain enough pancreatic exocrine function so as not to require enzyme supplementation (*pancreas sufficient* phenotype).[80] Pancreatic insufficiency is associated with protein and fat malabsorption and increased fecal loss. Manifestations of malabsorption (e.g., large, foul stools, abdominal distention, and poor weight gain) appear during the first year of life. The faulty fat absorption may induce deficiency of the fat-soluble vitamins, resulting in manifestations of avitaminosis A, D, or K. Hypoproteinemia may be severe enough to cause generalized edema. Persistent diarrhea may result in rectal prolapse in up to 10% of children with cystic fibrosis. The *pancreas sufficient* phenotype is usually not associated with other gastrointestinal complications, and in general, these individuals demonstrate excellent growth and development. The diagnosis of an underlying *CFTR* mutation in individuals with pancreas sufficient cystic fibrosis is suspected because of abnormal or borderline sweat chloride levels, a positive family history, or because of concomitant infertility in a male patient. *"Idiopathic" chronic pancreatitis* occurs in a subset of patients with pancreas sufficient cystic fibrosis and is associated with recurrent abdominal pain with

TABLE 10–7 Clinical Features and Diagnostic Criteria for Cystic Fibrosis

1. *Chronic sinopulmonary disease manifested by*
   a. Persistent colonization/infection with typical cystic fibrosis pathogens, including *Staphylococcus aureus*, nontypeable *Hemophilus influenzae*, mucoid and nonmucoid *Pseudomonas aeruginosa, Burkholderia cepacia*
   b. Chronic cough and sputum production
   c. Persistent chest radiograph abnormalities (e.g., bronchiectasis, atelectasis, infiltrates, hyperinflation)
   d. Airway obstruction manifested by wheezing and air trapping
   e. Nasal polyps; radiographic or computed tomographic abnormalities of paranasal sinuses
   f. Digital clubbing
2. *Gastrointestinal and nutritional abnormalities, including*
   a. Intestinal: meconium ileus, distal intestinal obstruction syndrome, rectal prolapse
   b. Pancreatic: pancreatic insufficiency, recurrent pancreatitis
   c. Hepatic: chronic hepatic disease manifested by clinical or histologic evidence of focal biliary cirrhosis, or multilobular cirrhosis
   d. Nutritional: failure to thrive (protein–calorie malnutrition), hypoproteinemia, edema, complications secondary to fat-soluble vitamin deficiency
3. *Salt-loss syndromes: acute salt depletion, chronic metabolic acidosis*
4. *Male urogenital abnormalities resulting in obstructive azoospermia (congenital bilateral absence of vas deferens)*

Criteria for Diagnosis of Cystic Fibrosis

One or more characteristic phenotypic features,
OR a history of cystic fibrosis in a sibling,
OR a positive newborn screening test result

AND

An increased sweat chloride concentration on two or more occasions
OR identification of two cystic fibrosis mutations,
OR demonstration of abnormal epithelial nasal ion transport

Adapted with permission from Rosenstein BJ, Cutting GR: The diagnosis of cystic fibrosis: a consensus statement. J Pediatrics 132:589;1998.

life-threatening complications.[85] These patients have other features of cystic fibrosis, such as pulmonary disease. By contrast, "idiopathic" chronic pancreatitis can also occur as an isolated late-onset finding in the absence of other stigmata of cystic fibrosis (Chapter 19); bi-allelic *CFTR* mutations (usually one "mild", one "severe") are demonstrable in the majority of these individuals, qualifying their inclusion as *nonclassic or atypical cystic fibrosis. Endocrine pancreatic insufficiency* (i.e., diabetes) is uncommon in cystic fibrosis, and usually accompanied by substantial destruction of pancreatic parenchyma.

Cardiorespiratory complications, such as persistent lung infections, obstructive pulmonary disease, and *cor pulmonale*, are the single most common cause of death (~80%) in patients in the United States. By age 18, 80% of patients with classic cystic fibrosis harbor *P. aeruginosa*, and 3.5% harbor *Burkholderia cepacia*.[86] With the indiscriminate use of antibiotic prophylaxis against *Staphylococcus*, there has been an unfortunate resurgence of resistant strains of *Pseudomonas* in many patients. Individuals who carry a "severe" *CFTR* mutation on one allele and a "mild" *CFTR* mutation on the other allele may exhibit late-onset mild pulmonary disease, another example of nonclassic or atypical cystic fibrosis.[81] Patients with mild pulmonary disease usually have mild or no pancreatic disease. *Idiopathic bronchiectasis*, a poorly defined entity in adults where no discernible cause for the bronchiectasis can be found, has been linked to *CFTR* mutations in a subset of cases. *Recurrent sinonasal polyps* can occur in up to 25% of patients with cystic fibrosis; hence, children who present with this finding should be tested for abnormalities of sweat chloride.

Significant *liver disease* occurs late in the natural history of cystic fibrosis and used to be foreshadowed by pulmonary and pancreatic involvement; however, with increasing life expectancies, liver disease has also received increasing attention. In fact, after cardiopulmonary and transplantation-related complications, liver disease is the most common cause of death in cystic fibrosis. Most studies suggest that symptomatic or biochemical liver disease in cystic fibrosis has its onset at or around puberty, with a prevalence of approximately 13% to 17%.[87] However, *asymptomatic hepatomegaly* may be present in up to a third of the individuals. Obstruction of the common bile duct may occur due to stones or sludge; it presents with abdominal pain and the acute onset of jaundice. As previously noted, *diffuse biliary cirrhosis* may develop in up to 5% of individuals with cystic fibrosis.

Approximately 95% of males with cystic fibrosis are *infertile*, as a result of obstructive azoospermia. As mentioned earlier, this is most commonly due to bilateral absence of vas deferens (also called CBAVD). CBAVD can occur as a consequence of several conditions, but bi-allelic *CFTR* mutations are the most common cause (present in 50% to 75% of cases).[88,89]

In most cases, the diagnosis of cystic fibrosis is based on persistently elevated sweat electrolyte concentrations (often the mother makes the diagnosis because her infant tastes salty), characteristic clinical findings (sinopulmonary disease and gastrointestinal manifestations), or a family history. A minority of patients with cystic fibrosis, especially those with at least one "mild" *CFTR* mutation, may have a normal or near-normal sweat test (<60 mM/L). Measurement of nasal transepithelial potential difference in vivo can be a useful adjunct under these circumstances; individuals with cystic fibrosis demonstrate a significantly more negative baseline nasal potential difference than controls. Sequencing the *CFTR* gene is, of course, the "gold standard" for diagnosis of cystic fibrosis. Therefore, in patients with suggestive clinical findings or family history (or both), genetic analysis may be warranted. It is important to inform the molecular laboratory whether the individual has classic cystic fibrosis or conforms to one of the nonclassic or atypical variants (CBAVD, late-onset pulmonary disease, or idiopathic chronic pancreatitis), so the appropriate "mild" *CFTR* mutations are also analyzed. A recent study has demonstrated that a subset of patients with nonclassic or atypical cystic fibrosis may not reveal *CFTR* mutations in one or both alleles.[90] This indicates that other genetic loci (perhaps those that encode proteins interacting with CFTR) may also produce a partial phenotype resembling cystic fibrosis.

Advances in management of cystic fibrosis include both improved control of infections and bilateral lung (or lobar), heart-lung, liver, pancreas, or liver-pancreas transplantation. Children and adolescents undergoing bilateral lung transplantation have overall survival rates around 70%. These improvements in management mean that more patients are now surviving to adulthood; the median life expectancy is close to 30 years and continues to increase. In principle, cystic fibrosis, like other single gene disorders, should be amenable to gene therapy. In vitro, it has been possible to correct the chloride defect in epithelial cells of cystic fibrosis patients by both viral and nonviral vector-based transfer of the *CFTR* gene; even a single copy of the wild-type *CFTR* gene is able to revert the cystic fibrosis phenotype. Clinical trials with gene therapy in humans are still in their early stages but provide a source of hope for millions of cystic fibrosis patients worldwide.

Sudden Infant Death Syndrome (SIDS)

SIDS is a disease of unknown cause. The National Institute of Child Health and Human Development defines SIDS as "the sudden death of an infant under 1 year of age which remains unexplained after a thorough case investigation, *including performance of a complete autopsy, examination of the death scene, and review of the clinical history*."[91] An aspect of SIDS that is not stressed in the definition is that the infant usually dies while asleep, hence the pseudonyms of *crib death* or *cot death*.

Epidemiology. As infantile deaths owing to nutritional problems and microbiologic infections have come under control in countries with higher standards of living, SIDS has assumed greater importance in many countries, including the United States. SIDS is the leading cause of death between age 1 month and 1 year in this country and the third leading cause of death overall in infancy, after congenital anomalies and diseases of prematurity and low birth weight. Due largely to nationwide SIDS awareness campaigns by organizations such as the American Academy of Pediatrics, there has been a significant drop in SIDS-related mortality in the past decade, from over 5000 annual deaths in 1990 to approximately 2600 deaths in 1999. Worldwide, in countries where unexpected infant deaths are diagnosed as SIDS only after postmortem examination, the death rates from SIDS (20 to 100/100,000 live births) are comparable to death rates in the United States (77/100,000 live births).

Approximately 90% of all SIDS deaths occur during the first 6 months of life, most between ages 2 and 4 months. This narrow window of peak susceptibility is a unique characteristic that is independent of other risk factors (to be described) and the geographic locale. Most infants who die of SIDS, die at home, usually during the night after a period of sleep. Only rarely is the catastrophic event observed, but even when seen, it is reported that the apparently healthy infant suddenly turns blue, stops breathing, and becomes limp without emitting a cry or struggling. Most infants have had minor manifestations of an upper respiratory infection preceding the fatal event. The term *apparent life-threatening event (ALTE)* has been applied to those infants who could be resuscitated after such an episode.[92] Infants with ALTE are often siblings of SIDS victims and harbor a range of physiologic abnormalities such as frequent or prolonged apnea, diminished chemoreceptor sensitivity to hypercarbia and hypoxia, and impaired control of heart, respiratory rate, and vagal tone.[92] Some of these infants later succumb to SIDS.

Morphology. At autopsy, a variety of findings have been reported. They are usually subtle and of uncertain significance and are not present in all cases. **Multiple petechiae** are the most common finding in the typical SIDS autopsy (~80% of cases); these are usually present on the thymus, visceral and parietal pleura, and epicardium. Grossly, the lungs are usually congested, and **vascular engorgement** with or without **pulmonary edema** is demonstrable microscopically in the majority of cases. These changes possibly represent agonal events, since they are found with comparable frequencies in *explained* sudden deaths in infancy. Within the upper respiratory system (larynx and trachea), there may be some histologic evidence of recent infection (correlating with the clinical symptoms), although the changes are not sufficiently severe to account for death and should not detract from the diagnosis of SIDS. The central nervous system demonstrates **astrogliosis** of the brain stem and cerebellum. Sophisticated morphometric studies have revealed quantitative brainstem abnormalities such as **hypoplasia of the arcuate nucleus** or a subtle decrease in brain stem neuronal populations in several cases;[93,94] these observations are not uniform, however, and not amenable to most "routine" autopsy procedures. Nonspecific findings include frequent persistence of hepatic **extramedullary hematopoiesis** and **periadrenal brown fat**; it is tempting to speculate that these latter findings relate to chronic hypoxemia, retardation of normal development, and chronic stress. Thus, autopsy usually fails to provide a clear cause of death, and this may well be related to the etiologic heterogeneity of SIDS. The importance of a postmortem examination rests in identifying other causes of sudden unexpected death in infancy, such as unsuspected infection, congenital anomaly, or a genetic disorder (Table 10–8), the presence of any of which would *exclude* a diagnosis of SIDS, and in ruling out the unfortunate possibility of traumatic child abuse.

Pathogenesis. The circumstances surrounding SIDS have been explored in great detail, and it is generally accepted that

TABLE 10–8 Risk Factors and Postmortem Findings Associated with Sudden Infant Death Syndrome

Parental
Young maternal age (age <20 years)
Maternal smoking during pregnancy
Drug abuse in *either* parent, specifically paternal marijuana and maternal opiate, cocaine use
Short intergestational intervals
Late or no prenatal care
Low socioeconomic group
African American and American Indian ethnicity (? socioeconomic factors)
Infant
Brain stem abnormalities, associated defective arousal, and cardiorespiratory control
Prematurity and/or low birth weight
Male sex
Product of a multiple birth
SIDS in a prior sibling
Antecedent respiratory infections
? Gastroesophageal reflux
Environment
Prone sleep position
Sleeping on a soft surface
Hyperthermia
Postnatal passive smoking
Postmortem Abnormalities Detected in Cases of Sudden Unexpected Infant Death*
Infections
• Viral myocarditis
• Bronchopneumonia
Unsuspected congenital anomaly
• Congenital aortic stenosis
• Anomalous origin of the left coronary artery from the pulmonary artery (ALCAPA)
Traumatic child abuse
• Intentional suffocation (filicide)
Genetic and metabolic defects
• Long QT syndrome (*SCN5A* and *KCNQ1* mutations)
• Fatty acid oxidation disorders (*MCAD, LCHAD, SCHAD* mutations)
• Histiocytoid cardiomyopathy (*MTCYB* mutations)
• Abnormal inflammatory responsiveness (partial deletions in *C4a* and *C4b*)

*SIDS is not the only cause of sudden unexpected death in infancy but rather is *a diagnosis of exclusion*. Therefore, performance of an autopsy may often reveal findings that would explain the cause of sudden unexpected death. These cases should *not*, strictly speaking, be labeled as "SIDS." SCN5A, sodium channel, voltage-gated, type V, alpha polypeptide; KCNQ1, potassium voltage-gated channel, KQT-like subfamily, member 1; MCAD, medium-chain acyl coenzyme A dehydrogenase; LCHAD, long-chain 3-hydroxyacyl coenzyme A dehydrogenase; SCHAD, short-chain 3-hydroxyacyl coenzyme A dehydrogenase; MTCYB, mitochondrial cytochrome b; C4, complement component 4.

it is a *multifactorial condition,* with a variable mixture of contributing factors. A "triple risk" model of SIDS has been proposed, which postulates the intersection of three overlapping factors: (1) *a vulnerable infant,* (2) *a critical developmental period in homeostatic control,* and (3) *an exogenous stressor(s).*[95] According to this model, several factors make the infant vulnerable to sudden death during the critical developmental period (i.e., age 1 month to 1 year). These vulnerability factors may be attributable to the parents or the infant, while the exogenous stressor(s) is attributable to the environment (Table 10–8).

While numerous factors have been proposed to account for a vulnerable infant, *the most compelling hypothesis is that SIDS reflects a delayed development of arousal and cardiorespiratory control.*[96] Regions of the brain stem, particularly the *arcuate nucleus,* located in the ventral medullary surface, play a critical role in the body's "arousal" response to noxious stimuli such as hypercarbia, hypoxia, and thermal stress encountered during sleep. In addition, these areas regulate breathing, heart rate, and body temperature. In certain infants, for yet unexplained reasons, there may be a maldevelopment or delay in maturation of this region, compromising the arousal response to noxious stimuli. This physiologic impairment is compounded by other factors, such as sleeping position or infection (see below). Support of this hypothesis comes from postmortem studies in SIDS victims demonstrating both *quantitative* abnormalities (e.g., arcuate hypoplasia and decrease in neuronal density) as well as *qualitative* abnormalities (e.g., reduced serotonergic and muscarinic receptor binding) in the brain stem.[93,97,98] Whether these changes are primary or merely the manifestation of a more "upstream" deficit remains to be elucidated. Recently, some candidate genes have been identified from experimental animal models, which may provide a genetic basis to abnormal neural regulation in the brainstem. For example, *Krox20,* a homeobox gene, appears to be required for hindbrain segmentation and myelination. Mouse models lacking *Krox20* function exhibit abnormally slow respiratory rhythm and prolonged apnea.[99] Similarly, brain-derived neurotrophic factor (BDNF) is required for normal development of the central respiratory rhythm, including the stabilization of central respiratory output that occurs after birth. Loss of one or both *BDNF* alleles results in an approximately 50% depression of central respiratory frequency compared with wild-type controls, while hypoxic ventilatory drive is deficient or absent.[100] Whether knowledge gleamed from these animal models of central respiratory dysfunction will be applicable to humans remains to be seen.

Epidemiologic studies of infant deaths have found additional risk factors for SIDS (Table 10–8). Infants who are born before term or who are low birth weight are at increased risk, and risk increases with decreasing gestational age or birth weight. Male sex is associated with a slightly greater incidence of SIDS. SIDS in a prior sibling is associated with a fivefold relative risk of recurrence, underscoring the importance of a genetic and/or shared environmental predisposition; *traumatic child abuse needs to be carefully excluded under these circumstances.* Most SIDS babies have an immediate prior history of a mild respiratory tract infection, but no single causative organism has been isolated. These infections may predispose an already vulnerable infant to even greater impairment of cardiorespiratory control and delayed arousal. In this context, laryngeal chemoreceptors have emerged as a putative "missing link" between upper respiratory tract infections, the prone position (see below), and SIDS. When stimulated, these laryngeal chemoreceptors elicit an apneic and bradycardic reflex.[101] Stimulation of the chemoreceptors is augmented by respiratory tract infections, which increase the volume of secretions, and by the prone position, which impairs swallowing and clearing of the airways even in healthy infants. In a previously vulnerable infant with impaired arousal, the apneic and bradycardic reflex may prove fatal.

Maternal smoking during pregnancy has consistently emerged as a risk factor in epidemiologic studies of SIDS, with children exposed to in utero nicotine having more than double the risk of SIDS compared to children born to nonsmokers.[102] Young maternal age, frequent childbirths, and inadequate prenatal care are all risk factors associated with increased incidence of SIDS in the offspring. African Americans and American Indians have significantly higher rates of SIDS deaths than Caucasians. It is not obvious whether these ethnic trends represent the effects of genetic make up or the effects of lower socioeconomic status, which by itself is a risk factor for SIDS.

Among the potential environmental factors, prone sleeping position, sleeping on soft surfaces, and thermal stress are possibly the most important modifiable risk factors for SIDS.[103] The prone position predisposes an infant to one or more recognized noxious stimuli (hypoxia, hypercarbia, and thermal stress) during sleep. In addition, the prone position is also associated with decreased arousal responsiveness compared to the supine position. Results of studies from Europe, Australia, New Zealand, and the United States showed clearly increased risk for SIDS in infants who sleep in a prone position, prompting the American Academy of Pediatrics to recommend placing *healthy infants on their back* when laying them down to sleep. This "Back To Sleep" campaign has resulted in substantial decreases in SIDS-related deaths since its inception in 1994.[104]

It should be noted that SIDS is not the only cause of sudden unexpected deaths in infancy. In fact, SIDS is a diagnosis of exclusion, requiring careful examination of the death scene and a complete postmortem examination. The latter can reveal an unsuspected cause of sudden death in up to 20% or more of "SIDS" babies (Table 10–8). Infections (e.g., viral myocarditis or bronchopneumonia) are the most common causes of sudden "unexpected" death, followed by an unsuspected congenital anomaly. In part due to advancements in molecular diagnostics and knowledge of the human genome, several genetic causes of sudden "unexpected" infant death have emerged. For example, fatty acid oxidation disorders, characterized by defects in mitochondrial fatty acid oxidative enzymes, may be responsible for up to 5% of sudden death in infancy; of these, a *deficiency in medium-chain acyl-coenzyme A dehydrogenase* is the most common.[105] Retrospective analyses of SIDS cases have also revealed mutations of cardiac sodium and potassium channels, which result in a form of cardiac arrhythmia characterized by prolonged QT intervals; these account for no more than 1% of SIDS deaths.[106] Other newly emerging genetic causes of *explained* sudden death are listed in Table 10–8.

Tumors and Tumor-Like Lesions of Infancy and Childhood

Only 2% of all malignant tumors occur in infancy and childhood; nonetheless, cancer (including leukemia) is a leading cause of death from disease in the United States in children over age 4 and up to age 14. Neoplastic disease accounts for approximately 9% of all deaths in this cohort; only accidents cause significantly more deaths. Benign tumors are even more common than cancers. Most benign tumors are of little concern, but on occasion they cause serious disease by virtue of their location or rapid increase in size.

It is sometimes difficult to segregate, on morphologic grounds, true tumors or neoplasms from tumor-like lesions in the infant and child. In this context, two special categories of tumor-like lesions should be distinguished from true tumors.

The term *heterotopia* (or *choristoma*) is applied to microscopically normal cells or tissues that are present in abnormal locations. Examples of heterotopias include a rest of pancreatic tissue found in the wall of the stomach or small intestine or a small mass of adrenal cells found in the kidney, lungs, ovaries, or elsewhere. The heterotopic rests are usually of little significance, but they can be confused clinically with neoplasms. Rarely, they are sites of origin of true neoplasms, producing the paradox of an adrenal carcinoma arising in the ovary.

The term *hamartoma* refers to an excessive but focal overgrowth of cells and tissues native to the organ in which it occurs. Although the cellular elements are mature and identical to those found in the remainder of the organ, they do not reproduce the normal architecture of the surrounding tissue. Hamartomas can be thought of as the linkage between malformations and neoplasms—the line of demarcation between a hamartoma and a benign neoplasm is frequently tenuous and is variously interpreted. Hemangiomas, lymphangiomas, rhabdomyomas of the heart, adenomas of the liver, and developmental cysts within the kidneys, lungs, or pancreas are interpreted by some as hamartomas and by others as true neoplasms. The frequency of these lesions in infancy and childhood and their clinical behavior give credence to the belief that many are developmental aberrations. Their unequivocally benign histology, however, does not preclude bothersome and rarely life-threatening clinical problems in some cases.

BENIGN TUMORS AND TUMOR-LIKE LESIONS

Virtually any tumor may be encountered in children, but within this wide array hemangiomas, lymphangiomas, fibrous lesions, and teratomas deserve special mention. You will notice that most common neoplasms of childhood are so-called soft tissue tumors, with a mesenchymal derivation. This contrasts with adults, where the most common tumors, benign or malignant, have an epithelial origin. Benign tumors of various tissues are described in greater detail in appropriate chapters, but here a few comments are made about their special features in childhood.

Hemangioma. Hemangiomas (Chapter 11) are the most common tumors of infancy. Architecturally, they do not differ from those encountered in adults. Both cavernous and capillary hemangiomas may be encountered, although the latter are often more cellular than in adults, a feature that is deceptively worrisome. In children, most are located in the skin, particularly on the face and scalp, where they produce flat-to-elevated, irregular, red-blue masses; some of the flat, larger lesions (considered by some to represent vascular ectasias) are referred to as *port-wine stains.* Hemangiomas may enlarge along with the growth of the child, but in many instances they spontaneously regress (Fig. 10–25). In addition to their cosmetic significance, they can represent one facet of the hereditary disorder von Hippel-Lindau disease (Chapter 20). Rarely, vascular tumors, particularly those in the liver and soft tissues, become malignant.

Lymphatic Tumors. A wide variety of lesions are of lymphatic origin. Some of them—*lymphangiomas*—are hamartomatous or neoplastic in origin, whereas others appear to represent abnormal dilations of preexisting lymph channels known as *lymphangiectasis.* The *lymphangiomas* are usually characterized by cystic and cavernous spaces. Lesions of this nature may occur on the skin but, more important, are encountered in the deeper regions of the neck, axilla, medi-

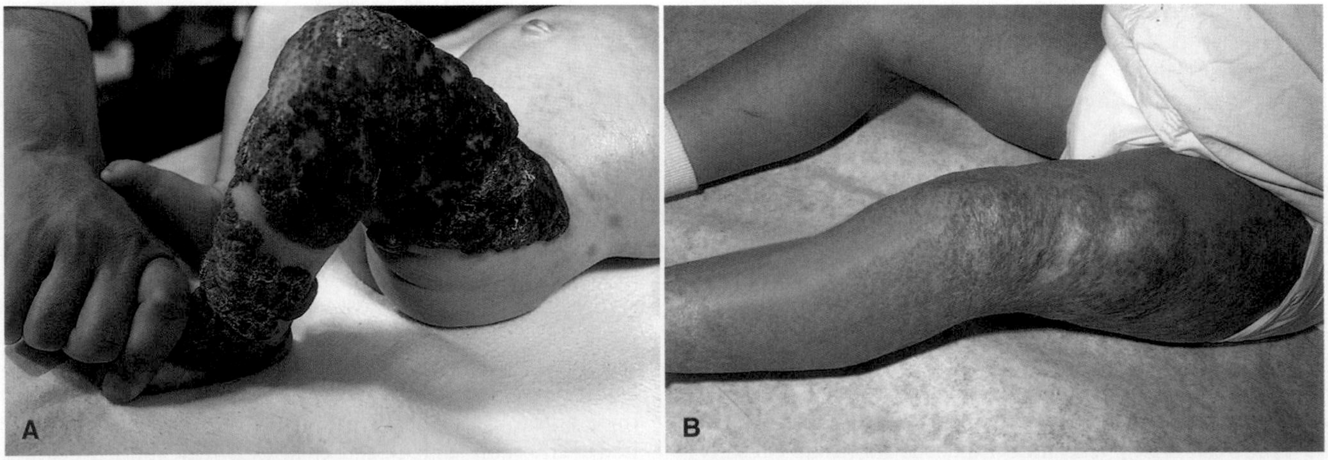

FIGURE 10–25 Congenital capillary hemangioma at birth (*A*) and at age 2 years (*B*) after spontaneous regression. (Courtesy of Dr. Eduardo Yunis, Children's Hospital of Pittsburgh, Pittsburgh, PA.)

astinum, retroperitoneal tissue, and elsewhere. Although histologically benign, they tend to increase in size after birth, both by the collection of fluid and by the budding of preexisting spaces. In this manner, they may encroach on vital structures, such as those in the mediastinum or nerve trunks in the axilla, and give rise to clinical problems. *Lymphangiectasis*, in contrast, usually presents as a diffuse swelling of part or all of an extremity; considerable distortion and deformation may result as a consequence of the spongy, dilated subcutaneous and deeper lymphatics. The lesion is not progressive, however, and does not extend beyond its original location. Nonetheless, it creates difficult corrective cosmetic problems.

Fibrous Tumors. Fibrous tumors occurring in infants and children range from sparsely cellular proliferations of spindle-shaped cells (designated as *fibromatosis*) to richly cellular lesions indistinguishable from fibrosarcomas occurring in adults (designated as *congenital-infantile fibrosarcomas*). Biologic behavior cannot be predicted based on histology alone, however, despite their histologic similarities with adult fibrosarcomas, the congenital-infantile variants have an excellent prognosis. Recently, a characteristic chromosomal translocation—t(12;15)(p13;q25)—has been described in congenital-infantile fibrosarcomas and aids in its distinction from other fibrous soft-tissue lesions of childhood.[107] In some soft-tissue fibrous lesions, a variable proportion of the cells acquire a moderate amount of pink cytoplasm and express muscle-specific actin. These *myofibromatoses* present in infants and younger children, and although usually solitary, they may be multifocal, involving any organ. Solitary lesions are benign, but multifocal lesions may result in significant morbidity and mortality when they involve vital organs.

Teratomas. Teratomas illustrate the relationship of histologic maturity to biologic behavior. They may occur as benign, well-differentiated cystic lesions (mature teratomas), as lesions of indeterminate potential (immature teratomas), or as unequivocally malignant teratomas (usually admixed with another germ cell tumor component such as endodermal sinus tumor) (Chapter 21). They exhibit two peaks in incidence: the first at approximately 2 years of age and the second in late adolescence or early adulthood. The first peak represents congenital neoplasms; the later-occurring lesions may also be of prenatal origin but are more slowly growing. *Sacrococcygeal teratomas* are the most common teratomas of childhood, accounting for 40% or more of cases (Fig. 10–26). They occur with a frequency of 1 in 20,000 to 40,000 live births, four times more commonly in girls than in boys. In view of the overlap in the mechanisms underlying teratogenesis and oncogenesis, it is interesting that approximately 10% of sacrococcygeal teratomas are associated with congenital anomalies, primarily defects of the hindgut and cloacal region and other midline defects (e.g., meningocele, spina bifida) not believed to result from local effects of the tumor. Approximately 75% of these tumors are mature teratomas, and about 12% are unequivocally malignant and lethal. The remainder are immature teratomas, and their malignant potential correlates with the amount of immature tissue, usually immature neuroepithelial elements, present. Most of the benign teratomas are encountered in younger infants (<4 months), whereas children with malignant lesions tend to be somewhat older. Other sites for teratomas in childhood include the testis (Chapter 21), ovaries (Chapter 22), and various midline locations, such as the mediastinum, retroperitoneum, and head and neck.

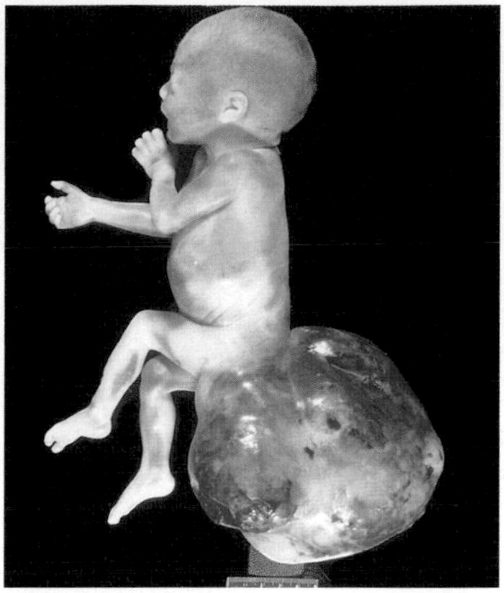

FIGURE 10–26 Sacrococcygeal teratoma. Note the size of the lesion compared with that of the infant.

MALIGNANT TUMORS

Cancers of infancy and childhood differ biologically and histologically from their counterparts occurring later in life. The main differences, some of which have already been alluded to, include the following:

- Incidence and type of tumor.
- Relatively frequent demonstration of a close relationship between abnormal development (teratogenesis) and tumor induction (oncogenesis)
- Prevalence of underlying familial or genetic aberrations
- Tendency of fetal and neonatal malignancies to regress spontaneously or cytodifferentiate
- Improved survival or cure of many childhood tumors, so that more attention is now being paid to minimizing the adverse delayed effects of chemotherapy and radiotherapy in survivors, including the development of second malignancies.

Incidence and Types

The most frequent childhood cancers arise in the hematopoietic system, nervous tissue (including the central and sympathetic nervous system, adrenal medulla, and retina), soft tissues, bone, and kidney. This is in sharp contrast to adults, in whom the skin, lung, breast, prostate, and colon are the most common sites of tumors.

Neoplasms that exhibit sharp peaks in incidence in children younger than age 10 years include (1) leukemia (principally acute lymphoblastic leukemia), (2) neuroblastoma, (3) Wilms tumor, (4) hepatoblastoma, (5) retinoblastoma, (6) rhabdomyosarcoma, (7) teratoma, (8) Ewing sarcoma and, finally, posterior fossa neoplasms—principally (9) juvenile astrocytoma, (10) medulloblastoma, and (11) ependymoma. Other forms of cancer are also common in childhood but do not have the same striking early peak. The age distribution of these cancers is approximately indicated in Table 10–9. Within this large array, leukemia alone accounts for more deaths in children younger than age 15 years than all of the other tumors combined.

TABLE 10–9 Common Malignant Neoplasms of Infancy and Childhood

0 to 4 Years	5 to 9 Years	10 to 14 Years
Leukemia	Leukemia	
Retinoblastoma	Retinoblastoma	
Neuroblastoma	Neuroblastoma	
Wilms tumor		
Hepatoblastoma	Hepatocarcinoma	Hepatocarcinoma
Soft tissue sarcoma (especially rhabdomyosarcoma)	Soft tissue sarcoma	Soft tissue sarcoma
Teratomas		
Central nervous system tumors	Central nervous system tumors	
	Ewing sarcoma	
	Lymphoma	Osteogenic sarcoma
		Thyroid carcinoma
		Hodgkin disease

Histologically, many of the malignant pediatric neoplasms are unique. In general, they tend to have a more primitive *(embryonal)* rather than pleomorphic–anaplastic microscopic appearance, are often characterized by sheets of cells with small, round nuclei, and frequently exhibit features of organogenesis specific to the site of tumor origin. Because of this latter characteristic, these tumors are frequently designated by the suffix *-blastoma*, for example, nephroblastoma (Wilms tumor), hepatoblastoma, and neuroblastoma. Owing to their primitive histologic appearance, many childhood tumors have been collectively referred to as *small round blue cell tumors.* The differential diagnosis of such tumors includes neuroblastoma, Wilms tumor, lymphoma, rhabdomyosarcoma, and Ewing sarcoma/primitive neuroectodermal tumor. Rendering a definitive diagnosis is usually possible on histologic examination alone, or in combination with chromosome analysis, immunoperoxidase stains, and electron microscopy. The diagnostic features associated with the more common childhood neoplasms are summarized in Table 10–10. Two of these tumors are particularly illustrative and are discussed here: the neuroblastic tumors, specifically neuroblastoma, and Wilms tumor. The remaining tumors are discussed in their respective organ-specific chapters.

The Neuroblastic Tumors

The term "neuroblastic tumor" includes tumors of the sympathetic ganglia and adrenal medulla that are derived from primordial neural crest cells populating these sites. As a family, neuroblastic tumors demonstrate certain characteristic features such as *spontaneous or therapy-induced differentiation of primitive neuroblasts into mature elements, spontaneous tumor regression*, and a *wide range of clinical behavior and prognosis*, which often mirror the extent of histologic differentiation. Neuroblastoma is the most important member of this family. It is the second most common solid malignancy of childhood

TABLE 10–10 Genetic and Other Useful Markers of Small Round Cell Tumors of Childhood

Tumor Type	Genetic Markers	Other Diagnostically Useful Features
Neuroblastoma	17q gain,* 1p deletion* N-*myc* amplification* DNA hyperdiploidy, near triploidy†	Clinical elevation in level of urinary catecholamines Neurosecretory granules by electron microscopy Neuron-specific enolase expression
Ewing sarcoma/PNET	t(11;22),‡ t(21;22), t(7;22) *EWS-FLI1* or *EWS-ERG* fusion transcript	*MIC2* (CD99) gene expression
Rhabdomyosarcoma	t(2;13),‡* t(1;13)—alveolar rhabdomyosarcoma (ARMS) 11p15.5 deletion—embryonal rhabdomyosarcoma (ERMS) *PAX3-FKHR* and *PAX7-FKHR* fusion transcript (ARMS)	Myogenin and Myo D1 expression (all subtypes) Alternating thick and thin filaments by electron microscopy
Burkitt lymphoma	t(8;14),‡ t(2;8), t (8;22)	B-cell phenotype expressing CD19, CD20, CD10, IgM Epstein-Barr virus latent infection (endemic cases)
Lymphoblastic lymphoma/acute lymphoblastic leukemia	Hyperdiploidy (>50),† Hypodiploidy (<46)* B-lineage: various translocations, including t(12;21) (*TEL-AML1*),‡,† t(9;22) (*BCR-ABL*, Philadelphia chromosome),* t(4;11) (AF4-MLL)*, t(1;19) (*PBX-E2A*) T-lineage: 1p32 abnormalities (*TAL1* gene)	Terminal deoxynucleotidyl transferase (TdT)+ Various B- and T-lineage antigens
Wilms tumor	11p13 (*WT1*) deletion/mutation 11p15.5 abnormalities of imprinting (e.g., *IGF2, H19,* $p57^{KIP2}$) 16q,* 1p,* 7p deletion	
Retinoblastoma	13q14 (*RB*) deletion/mutation	Retinal S antigen expression
Medulloblastoma	17p deletion Isochromosome 17q	Evidence of neuronal differentiation (synaptophysin expression) or glial differentiation (glial fibrillary acid protein [GFAP] expression)

*Generally associated with a poorer prognosis.
†Generally associated with a better prognosis.
‡Most common translocation.
PNET, peripheral neuroectodermal tumor.

after brain tumors, accounting for 7% to 10% of all pediatric neoplasms, and as many as 50% of malignancies diagnosed in infancy.[108] Approximately 650 new cases are diagnosed in the United States each year, accounting for an incidence of approximately 9.5 cases per million children. The median age at diagnosis is 22 months; a little more than a third of the cases are diagnosed in infancy. There is a higher incidence of neuroblastoma in Caucasian as compared to African American populations, and males are at a marginally greater risk than females. Alone, it accounts for at least 15% of all childhood cancer deaths, although the 5-year survival rate has improved from 25% in the early 1960s to almost 55% in the mid-1990s. As will be evident later, age and stage have a remarkable effect on prognosis, and, in general, infants tend to have a significantly better prognosis than older individuals. Most occur sporadically, but a few are familial with autosomal dominant transmission, and in such cases the neoplasms may involve both of the adrenals or multiple primary autonomic sites.

Morophology. In childhood, about 40% of neuroblastomas arise in the adrenal medulla. The remainder occur anywhere along the sympathetic chain, with the most common locations being the paravertebral region of the abdomen (25%) and posterior mediastinum (15%). Tumors may arise in numerous other sites, including the pelvis and neck and within the brain (cerebral neuroblastomas).

Macroscopically, neuroblastomas range in size from minute nodules (the **in situ lesions**) to large masses more than 1 kg in weight (Fig. 10–27). In situ neuroblastomas are reported to be 40 times more frequent than overt tumors. The great majority of these silent lesions spontaneously regress, leaving only a focus of fibrosis or calcification in the adult. Some neuroblastomas are often sharply demarcated with a fibrous pseudocapsule, but others are far more infiltrative and invade surrounding structures, including the kidneys, renal vein, and vena cava, and envelop the aorta. On transection, they are composed of soft, gray-tan, brainlike tissue. Larger tumors have areas of necrosis, cystic softening, and hemorrhage. Occasionally, foci of punctate calcification can be palpated.

Histologically, classic neuroblastomas are composed of small, primitive-appearing cells with dark nuclei, scant cytoplasm, and poorly defined cell borders growing in solid sheets.[109] Such tumors may be difficult to differentiate microscopically from other **small, blue, round cell tumors**. Mitotic activity, nuclear breakdown ("karyorrhexis"), and pleomorphism may be prominent. The background often demonstrates a faintly eosinophilic fibrillary material **(neuropil)** that corresponds to neuritic processes of the primitive neuroblasts. Typically, rosettes **(Homer-Wright pseudorosettes)** can be found in which the tumor cells are concentrically arranged about a central space filled with neuropil (Fig. 10–28). Other helpful features include immunochemical reactions for neuron-specific enolase and ultrastructural demonstration of small, membrane-bound, cytoplasmic catecholamine-containing secretory granules; the latter contain characteristic central dense cores surrounded by a peripheral halo (dense core granules). Some neoplasms show signs of maturation that can be spontaneous or therapy-induced. Larger cells having more abundant cytoplasm with large vesicular nuclei and a prominent nucleolus, representing *ganglion cells* in various stages of maturation, may be found in tumors admixed with primitive neuroblasts **(ganglioneuroblastoma)**. Even better-differentiated lesions contain many more large cells resembling mature ganglion cells with no or minimal residual neuroblasts; such neoplasms merit the designation **ganglioneuroma** (Fig. 10–29). Maturation of neuroblasts into ganglion cells is usually accompanied by the appearance of **Schwann cells.** In fact, the presence of a so-called "schwannian stroma" comprised of organized fascicles of neuritic processes, mature Schwann cells, and fibroblasts is a histologic prerequisite for the designation of ganglioneuroblastoma and ganglioneuroma; ganglion cells in and of themselves do not fulfill

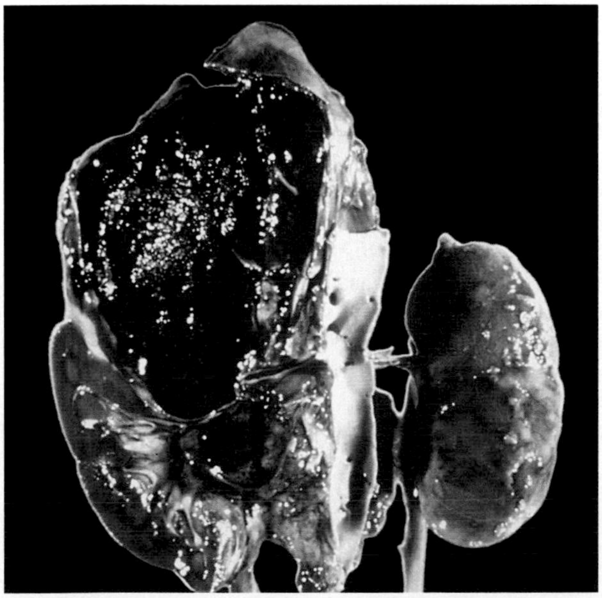

FIGURE 10–27 Adrenal neuroblastoma in a 6-month-old child. The hemorrhagic, partially encapsulated tumor has displaced the opened left kidney and is impinging on the aorta and left renal artery. (Courtesy of Dr. Arthur Weinberg, University of Texas Southwestern Medical School, Dallas, TX.)

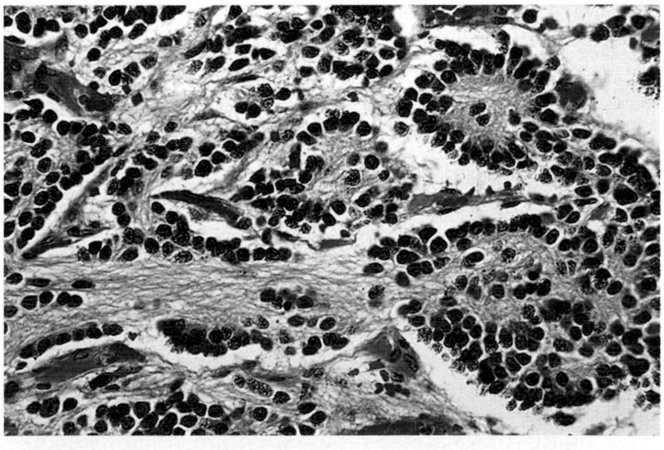

FIGURE 10–28 Adrenal neuroblastoma. This tumor is composed of small cells embedded in a finely fibrillar matrix.

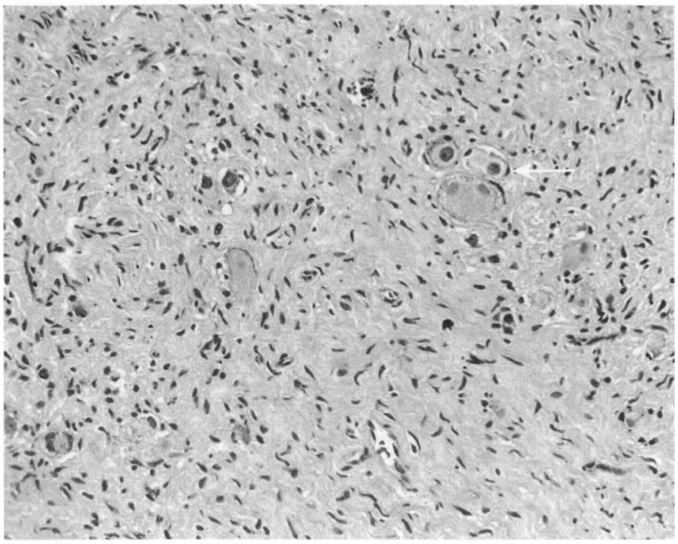

FIGURE 10–29 Ganglioneuromas, arising from spontaneous or therapy-induced maturation of neuroblastomas, are characterized by clusters of large cells with vesicular nuclei and abundant eosinophilic cytoplasm, representing neoplastic ganglion cells *(arrow)*. Spindle-shaped Schwann cells are present in the background stroma.

the criteria for maturation.[109] The origin of Schwann cells in neuroblastoma remains an issue of contention; some investigators believe they represent a reactive population recruited by the tumor cells.[110] Others, however, have demonstrated that Schwann cells carry the same genetic changes as the neuroblasts and therefore are an integral component of the tumor.[111] Irrespective of histogenesis, documenting the presence of schwannian stroma is essential, since its presence is associated with a **favorable histology** (Table 10–11).[112]

Metastases, when they develop, appear early and widely. In addition to local infiltration and lymph node spread, there is a pronounced tendency to spread through the bloodstream to involve the liver, lungs, bone marrow, and bones. Several staging systems have been proposed for neuroblastomas; the International Neuroblastoma Staging System is detailed below:[113]

Stage 1: Localized tumor with complete gross excision, with or without microscopic residual disease. Representative ipsilateral nonadherent lymph nodes negative for tumor (nodes adherent to the primary tumor may be positive for tumor).

Stage 2A: Localized tumor with incomplete gross resection. Representative ipsilateral nonadherent lymph nodes negative for tumor microscopically.

Stage 2B: Localized tumor with or without complete gross excision, ipsilateral nonadherent lymph nodes positive for tumor. Enlarged contralateral lymph nodes, which are negative for tumor microscopically.

Stage 3: Unresectable unilateral tumor infiltrating across the midline with or without regional lymph node involvement; or localized unilateral tumor with contralateral regional lymph node involvement.

Stage 4: Any primary tumor with dissemination to distant lymph nodes, bone, bone marrow, liver, skin, and/or other organs *(except as defined for stage 4S)*.

Stage 4S ("S" = special): Localized primary tumor (as defined for Stages 1, 2A, or 2B) with dissemination limited to skin, liver, and/or bone marrow; *Stage 4S is limited to infants <1 yr.*

Unfortunately, most (60% to 80%) children present with Stage 3 or 4 tumors, and only 20% to 40% present with Stage 1, 2A, 2B, or 4S neuroblastomas. The staging system is of paramount importance in determining prognosis.

Clinical Course and Prognostic Features. In young children, under age 2 years, neuroblastomas generally present with large abdominal masses, fever, and possibly weight loss. In older children, they may not come to attention until metastases produce manifestations, such as bone pain, respiratory symptoms, or gastrointestinal complaints. Neuroblastomas may metastasize widely through the hematogenous and lymphatic systems, particularly to liver, lungs, and bones, in addition to the bone marrow. Proptosis and ecchymosis may also be present because the periorbital region is a common metastatic site. Bladder and bowel dysfunction may be caused by paraspinal neuroblastomas that impinge on nerves. In neonates, disseminated neuroblastomas may present with multiple cutaneous metastases with deep blue discoloration to the skin (earning the rather unfortunate designation of "*blueberry muffin baby*"). *About 90% of neuroblastomas, regardless of location, produce catecholamines* (similar to the catecholamines associated with pheochromocytomas), which are an important diagnostic feature (i.e., elevated blood levels of catecholamines and elevated urine levels of metabolites, vanillylmandelic acid [VMA], and homovanillic acid [HVA]). Despite the elaboration of catecholamines, hypertension is much less frequent with these neoplasms than with pheochromocytomas (Chapter 24). Ganglioneuromas, unlike their malignant counterparts, tend to produce either asymptomatic mass lesions or symptoms related to compression.

The course of neuroblastomas is extremely variable. Several clinical, histopathologic, molecular, and biochemical factors have been identified in neuroblastomas that have a bearing on prognosis (see Table 10–11):

Age and stage are the most important determinants of outcome. Infants younger than age 1 year have an excellent prognosis regardless of the stage of the neoplasm. Most often in this age group, the neoplasms are Stage 1, 2A, or 2B, and therapy yields a greater than 90% 5-year survival.[114] At this early age, even when metastases are present, in about half the spread is limited to the liver, bone marrow, and skin (stage 4S), and such infants have at least an 80% 5-year survival with only minimal therapy. In fact, with Stage 4S disease, it is not uncommon for the primary or metastatic tumors to undergo spontaneous regression.[115] The biologic basis of this welcome behavior is not clear. Even when the dissemination is more widespread in the first year of life or the tumor is accompanied by unfavorable biologic characteristics such as N-*myc* amplification (see below), the survival is greater than 50%. Children between ages 1 and 5 years have an intermediate prognosis for low-stage tumors that have otherwise favorable

TABLE 10–11 Prognostic Factors in Neuroblastomas

Variable	Favorable	Unfavorable
Stage*	Stage 1, 2A, 2B, 4S	Stage 3, 4
Age*	≤ 1 year	>1 year
Histology*		
Evidence of schwannian stroma and gangliocytic differentiation[a]	Present	Absent
Mitotic rate[b]	Low	High
Mitosis–karyorrhexis index[c]	≤200/5000 cells	>200/5000 cells
Intratumoral calcification	Present	Absent
DNA ploidy*	Hyperdiploid or near-triploid	Diploid, near-diploid, or near-tetraploid
N-myc*	Not amplified	Amplified
Chromosome 17q Gain	Absent	Present
Chromosome 1p Loss	Absent	Present
Trk-A Expression	Present	Absent
Telomerase Expression	Low or absent	Highly expressed
MRP Expression	Absent	Present
CD44 Expression	Present	Absent
Serum Biochemical Markers		
Ferritin	Normal	Elevated
Lactate Dehydrogenase	≤1500 U/mL	>1500 U/mL

*Corresponds to the most commonly used parameters in clinical practice for assessment of prognosis and risk stratification.
[a]It is not only the presence but also the *amount* of schwannian stroma that confers the designation of a favorable histology. At least *50% or more schwannian stroma* is required before a neoplasm can be classified as ganglioneuroblastoma or ganglioneuroma.
[b]Mitotic rate is classified as *low* (≤10 mitoses/10 high power fields) or *high* (>10 mitoses/10 high power fields).
[c]Mitotic karyorrhexis index (MKI) is defined as the number of mitotic or karyorrhectic cells per 5000 tumor cells in random foci.
Trk-A, tyrosine kinase receptor A; *MRP*, multidrug resistance–associated protein.

biologic characteristics (see below), while those with advanced stage disease have <20% 5-year survival, irrespective of other prognostic variables. In contrast, children older than age 5 years usually have extremely poor outcomes irrespective of stage.

Morphology is an independent prognostic variable in neuroblastic tumors.[112] An age-linked morphologic classification of neuroblastic tumors has recently been proposed that divides them into *favorable* and *unfavorable* histologic subtypes. The specific morphologic features that bear in prognosis are listed in Table 10–11.

Ploidy of the tumor cells correlates with outcome. In general, *hyperdiploidy* and *near-triploidy* have a correlation with young age, low stage, and a good prognosis, whereas *diploidy*, *near-diploidy*, and *near-tetraploidy* are associated with an unfavorable outcome irrespective of age. For example, in infants and children younger than age 2 years who have advanced disease, the presence of hyperdiploidy or near-triploidy correlates with response to chemotherapy and long-term disease-free survival, while corresponding diploid tumors have a significantly worse prognosis (the beneficial prognostic effects of ploidy tend to be negated in older children with advanced disease).

Amplification of the N-myc oncogene in neuroblastomas is a molecular event that has possibly the most profound impact on prognosis.[116] N-*myc* is located on the distal short arm of chromosome 2 (2p23-24). Amplification of N-*myc* does not karyotypically manifest at the resident 2p23-24 site, but rather as extrachromosomal *double minute chromatin bodies* or *homogeneously staining regions* on other chromosomes (Fig. 10–30). N-*myc* amplification is present in about 25% to 30% of primary tumors, most in advanced-stage disease. Up to 300 copies of N-*myc* have been observed in some tumors; the greater the number of copies, the worse the prognosis. N-*myc* amplification is currently the most important genetic abnormality used in risk stratification of neuroblastic tumors (see below).

Partial gain of the distal long arm of chromosome 17 is the most common karyotypic abnormality in neuroblastomas, present in up to 50% of tumors.[117] The mechanism of 17q gain is via an *unbalanced translocation*, where a portion of 17q is translocated to a partner chromosome (most commonly the distal short arm of chromosome 1, or the distal long arm of chromosome 11). Partial gain of 17q demonstrates significant association with adverse outcome in neuroblastomas, independent of other prognostic variables.

Deletion of the distal short arm of chromosome 1 in the region of band p36 has been demonstrated in 25% to 35% of primary tumors.[118] In addition, constitutional deletions of 1p36 have been demonstrated in a subset of patients with neuroblastomas. The loss of genetic material implies that one or more putative tumor suppressor genes in this region may be important in the pathogenesis of neuroblastomas, but their identity remains elusive. At least two distinct loci of deletions on 1p36 have been identified. The first, more distal region appears to demonstrate preferential loss of the maternal allele in tumors,

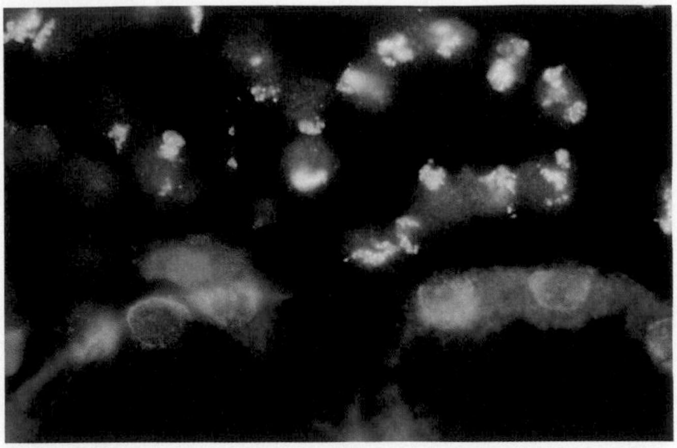

FIGURE 10–30 Fluorescence in situ hybridization using a fluorescein-labeled cosmid probe for N-*myc* on a tissue section. Note the neuroblastoma cells on the upper half of the photo with large areas of staining *(yellow-green)*; this corresponds to amplified N-*myc* in the form of homogeneously staining regions. Renal tubular epithelial cells in the lower half of the photograph show no nuclear staining and background *(green)* cytoplasmic staining. (Courtesy of Dr. Timothy Triche, Children's Hospital, Los Angeles, CA.)

suggesting the possibility of *genomic imprinting* (Chapter 5); deletions in this region do not correlate with N-*myc* amplification. The second, more proximal region does not demonstrate a parent-of-origin specific allele loss, but correlates with concurrent N-*myc* amplification.[119]

The expression of specific proteins is also a prognostic marker for neuroblastoma. *TRK-A* (tyrosine kinase receptor A) is the high-affinity receptor for nerve growth factor, which induces terminal neuronal differentiation in developing sympathetic neuroblasts. High levels of expression of the *TRK-A* gene are associated with a favorable outcome and almost always occur in tumors lacking N-*myc* amplification. Tumors with high *TRK-A* expression are more likely to regress spontaneously or respond to therapy.[120] The immortality enzyme *telomerase* (Chapter 1) is overexpressed in neuroblastomas associated with unfavorable clinical and genetic features, and with reduced survival probability.[121] Low or absent telomerase expression is postulated to be one of the mechanisms for spontaneous regression of neuroblastomas. Overexpression of the *multidrug resistance associated protein (MRP)* may confer resistance to a variety of chemotherapeutic agents; high *MRP* expression in neuroblastomas tends to closely correlate with N-*myc* amplification. Finally, *CD44* is a cell adhesion molecule whose expression is lost in high-stage tumors. *CD44* appears to be an independent predictor of survival in some series.

In general, based on many of the aforementioned factors, neuroblastomas can be classified into *three risk groups.* The first, *low-risk* group occurs in infants with low stage (1, 2A, 2B), or if disseminated, with 4S disease, and is characterized by hyperdiploid or near-triploid content of DNA and high levels of *TRK-A* expression in the *absence* of N-*myc* amplification, chromosome 17q gain, or chromosome 1p deletions. These low-risk tumors have a cure rate greater than 90%. The second, *intermediate-risk* group consists of more advanced stage (3 or 4) occurring in either infants or older patients, with favorable histologic features, and absence of N-*myc* amplification; these tumors usually exhibit low levels of *TRK-A* expression, and are slowly progressive with a cure rate of 25% to 50%. The third and final, *high-risk* group of neuroblastomas has multiple unfavorable features and is associated with the worst prognosis and a cure rate of less than 20%. These neuroblastomas tend to occur in children older than age 1 year with advanced-stage disease and are characterized by unfavorable histology, N-*myc* amplification, chromosome 17q and 1p abnormalities, near-diploid or tetraploid DNA content, and minimal *TRK-A* expression.

Since the vast majority of neuroblastomas release catecholamines into the circulation, detection of catecholamine metabolites (VMA/HVA) in urine could, in principle, form the basis for screening for this tumor.[122,123] However, benefits of such screening have not yet been established. Currently, therefore, community-based screening programs for neuroblastomas are not advocated.

Wilms Tumor

Wilms tumor is the most common primary renal tumor of childhood and the fourth most common pediatric malignancy in the United States. It arises in approximately 10 children per million under age 15 years and is usually diagnosed between ages 2 and 5 years. Approximately 5% to 10% of Wilms tumors involve both kidneys, either simultaneously *(synchronous)* or one after the other *(metachronous).* Bilateral Wilms tumors have a median age of onset approximately 10 months earlier than tumors restricted to one kidney.[124] The biology of this tumor illustrates several important aspects of childhood neoplasms, such as the relationship between *malformations* and *neoplasia*, the histologic similarities between *organogenesis* and *oncogenesis*, the *two-hit theory* of recessive tumor suppressor genes (Chapter 7), the role of *premalignant lesions*, and perhaps most importantly, the potential for *judicious treatment modalities* to dramatically affect prognosis and outcome.

Pathogenesis and Genetics. The risk of Wilms tumor is increased in association with at least three recognizable groups of congenital malformations associated with distinct chromosomal loci. Although Wilms tumors arising in this setting account for no more than 10% of cases, these syndromic tumors have provided important insight into the biology of this neoplasm.

The first group of patients has the *WAGR syndrome*, characterized by *a*niridia, *g*enital anomalies, and mental *r*etardation and a 33% chance of developing *W*ilms tumor. Patients with WAGR syndrome carry constitutional (germline) deletions of 11p13. Studies on these patients led to the identification of the first Wilms tumor–associated gene, *WT1,* and a contiguously deleted autosomal dominant gene for aniridia, *PAX6*, both located at chromosome 11p13.[125] Patients with deletions restricted to *PAX6*, with normal *WT1* function, develop sporadic aniridia, but they are *not* at an increased risk for development of Wilms tumors. The presence of germline *WT1* deletions in WAGR syndrome represents the "first hit"; the development of Wilms tumor in these patients frequently correlates with the occurrence of a nonsense or frameshift mutation in the second *WT1* allele ("second hit").

A second group of patients at a much higher risk for Wilms tumor (~90%) have the *Denys-Drash syndrome*, which is characterized by *gonadal dysgenesis* (male pseudohermaphroditism) and *early-onset nephropathy* leading to renal failure. The characteristic glomerular lesion in these patients is a *diffuse mesangial sclerosis* (Chapter 20). As in patients with

WAGR, these patients also demonstrate germline abnormalities in *WT1*. In patients with the Denys-Drash syndrome, however, the genetic abnormality is a *dominant negative missense mutation* in the zinc-finger region of *WT1* gene that affects its DNA-binding properties.[126] This mutation interferes with the function of the remaining wild-type allele, yet strangely, it is sufficient only in causing genitourinary abnormalities, but not tumorigenesis—Wilms tumors arising in Denys-Drash syndrome demonstrate bi-allelic inactivation of *WT1*. In addition to Wilms tumors, these individuals are also at increased risk for developing germ-cell tumors called *gonadoblastomas* (Chapter 21), almost certainly a consequence of disruption in normal gonadal development.

WT1 encodes a transcription factor that is expressed within the kidney and gonads of the developing human fetus.[127] This gene can function as both a transcriptional activator and repressor, depending on the cellular context. For example, the cell-cycle inhibitor *p21* can be induced by *WT1*, thus mediating growth arrest.[128] Other transcriptional targets of *WT1* include *amphiregulin*, a member of the epidermal growth factor family expressed in developing kidneys, the antiapoptotic gene, *BCL2*, *connective tissue growth factor, the vitamin D receptor*, and additional genes implicated in cellular differentiation pathways.[129] The *WT1* gene is critical to normal renal and gonadal development, and transgenic mice lacking functional *Wt1* have agenesis of both organs. It is not surprising therefore that constitutional inactivation of one copy of this gene results in genitourinary abnormalities in humans. Despite the importance of *WT1* in nephrogenesis and its unequivocal role as a tumor suppressor gene, only about 15% of patients with *sporadic* (nonsyndromic) Wilms tumors demonstrate *WT1* mutations, suggesting that the majority of Wilms tumors arise by genetically distinct pathways.

Clinically distinct from these previous two groups of patients but also having an increased risk of developing Wilms tumor are children with *Beckwith-Wiedemann syndrome,* characterized by enlargement of body organs (organomegaly), macroglossia, hemihypertrophy, omphalocele, and abnormal large cells in adrenal cortex (adrenal cytomegaly). The genetic locus that is involved in these patients is in band p15.5 of chromosome 11 distal to the *WT1* locus. Although this locus is called "*WT2*" for the second Wilms tumor locus, the gene involved has not been identified.

The "*WT2*" locus has served as a model for another mechanism of tumorigenesis in humans—*genomic imprinting* (Chapter 5).[130] This region contains at least 10 genes that are normally expressed from only *one* of the two parental alleles, with transcriptional silencing of the other parental homologue by methylation of the promoter region. One of the candidate genes in this region—insulin-like growth factor-2 (*IGF2*)—is normally expressed solely from the *paternal allele*, while the maternal allele is imprinted (i.e., silenced) by methylation. In some Wilms tumors, *loss of imprinting* (i.e., re-expression of *IGF2* by the maternal allele) can be demonstrated, leading to overexpression of the *IGF-2* protein.[131] In other instances, there is a selective deletion of the imprinted maternal allele, combined with duplication of the transcriptionally active paternal allele in the tumor *(uniparental paternal disomy)*, which has an identical functional effect in terms of overexpression of *IGF-2*. Since the *IGF-2* protein is an embryonal growth factor, it could conceivably explain the features of overgrowth associated with Beckwith-Wiedemann syndrome, as well as the increased risk for Wilms tumors in these patients. In addition to Wilms tumors, patients with Beckwith-Wiedemann syndrome are also at increased risk for developing hepatoblastoma, adrenocortical tumors, rhabdomyosarcomas, and pancreatic tumors.

Familial predisposition to Wilms tumors is rare,[132,133] and most patients with the syndromes described above are likely to represent de novo mutations.

In addition to the loci affected in syndromic Wilms tumors, recent studies indicate the involvement of β-catenin. It will be recalled (Chapter 7) that β-catenin belongs to the developmentally important *wnt (wingless)* signaling pathway. β-catenin mutations have been demonstrated in 15% of Wilms tumors; there is a significant correlation between the presence of *WT1* and β-catenin mutations, suggesting a synergistic role for these events in the genesis of Wilms tumors.[135]

Nephrogenic Rests

Nephrogenic rests are putative precursor lesions of Wilms tumors and are seen in the renal parenchyma adjacent to approximately 40% of unilateral tumors; this frequency rises to nearly 100% in cases of bilateral Wilms tumors.[136] The appearance of nephrogenic rests varies from expansile masses that resemble Wilms tumors (hyperplastic rests) to sclerotic rests consisting predominantly of fibrous tissue and occasional admixed immature tubules or glomeruli. It is important to document the presence of nephrogenic rests in the resected specimen, since these patients are at an increased risk of developing Wilms tumors in the *contralateral* kidney and require frequent and regular surveillance for many years.

Morphology. Grossly, Wilms tumor tends to present as a large, solitary, well-circumscribed mass, although 10% are either bilateral or multicentric at the time of diagnosis. On cut section, the tumor is soft, homogeneous, and tan to gray with occasional foci of hemorrhage, cyst formation, and necrosis (Fig. 10–31).

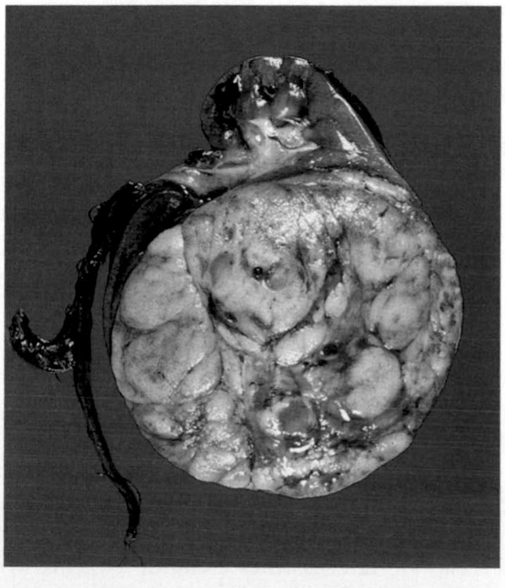

FIGURE 10–31 Wilms tumor in the lower pole of the kidney with the characteristic tan-to-gray color and well-circumscribed margins.

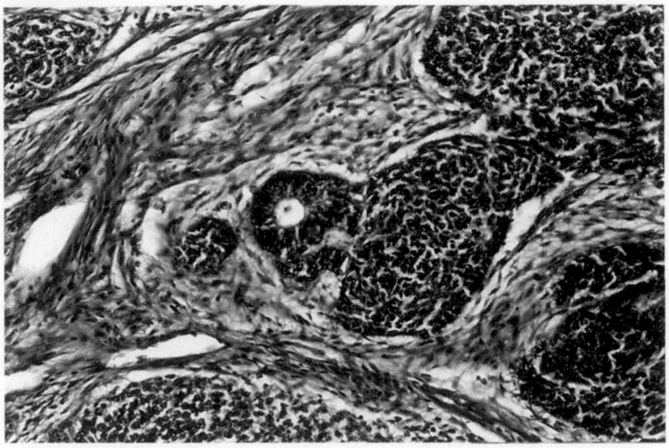

FIGURE 10–32 Triphasic histology of Wilms' tumor: the stromal component is comprised of spindle-shaped cells in the less cellular area on the left; the immature tubule in the center is an example of the epithelial component and the tightly packed blue cells, of the blastemal elements. (Courtesy of Dr. Charles Timmons, Department of Pathology, University of Texas Southwestern Medical School, Dallas, TX.) Anaplasia in Wilms' tumor is characterized by cells with large, hyperchromatic, pleomorphic nuclei and abnormal mitoses *(inset).*

Microscopically, Wilms tumors are characterized by recognizable attempts to recapitulate different stages of nephrogenesis. The classic triphasic combination of blastemal, stromal, and epithelial cell types is observed in the vast majority of lesions, although the percentage of each component is variable (Fig. 10–32). Sheets of small blue cells, with little distinctive features, characterize the blastemal component. Epithelial differentiation is usually in the form of abortive tubules or glomeruli. Stromal cells are usually fibrocytic or myxoid in nature, although skeletal muscle differentiation is not uncommon. Rarely, other heterologous elements are identified, including squamous or mucinous epithelium, smooth muscle, adipose tissue, cartilage, and osteoid and neurogenic tissue. Approximately 5% of tumors reveal **anaplasia**, defined as the presence of cells with large, hyperchromatic, pleomorphic nuclei and abnormal mitoses.[137] The presence of anaplasia correlates with underlying *p53* mutations[138] and the emergence of resistance to chemotherapy.

Clinical Features. Most children with Wilms tumors present with a large abdominal mass that may be unilateral or, when very large, may extend across the midline and down into the pelvis. Hematuria, pain in the abdomen after some traumatic incident, intestinal obstruction, and appearance of hypertension are other patterns of presentation. In a considerable number of these patients, pulmonary metastases are present at the time of primary diagnosis.

The prognosis for Wilms tumor is currently very good, and excellent results are obtained with a combination of nephrectomy and chemotherapy in most cases. Two-year survival rates are as high as 90%, even for tumors that have spread beyond the kidney, and survival for 2 years usually implies a cure. Even recurrences can be successfully treated. Tumors with *diffuse anaplasia*, especially those with extrarenal spread, have the least favorable outcome, underscoring the need for correctly identifying this histologic pattern.

Along with the increased survival of patients with Wilms tumor have come reports of an increased relative risk of developing second primary tumors.[139] Although many of these tumors can be attributed to therapy, studies of families of these patients suggest a possible association of Wilms tumor with bone and soft-tissue sarcomas, leukemia and lymphomas, brain tumors, and genitourinary tumors.

REFERENCES

1. Minino AM, Smith BL: Deaths: preliminary data for 2000. Natl Vital Stat Rep 49(12):1, 2001.
2. Opitz JM, Wilson GN: Causes and pathogenesis of birth defects. In Gilbert-Barness E (ed): Pathology of the Fetus and Infant, Vol. 1. St. Louis, Mosby-Year Book, 1997, p 44–64.
3. Villavicencio EH, Walterhouse DO, Iannaccone PM: The sonic hedgehog-patched-gli pathway in human development and disease. Am J Hum Genet 67:1047, 2000.
4. Miller E, Cradock-Watson JE, Pollock TM: Consequences of confirmed maternal rubella at successive stages of pregnancy. Lancet 2:781, 1982.
5. Cohen MM, Jr: Syndromology: an updated conceptual overview. VII. Aspects of teratogenesis. Int J Oral Maxillofac Surg 19:26, 1990.
6. Finnell RH, et al: Molecular basis of environmentally induced birth defects. Ann Rev Pharmacol Toxicol 42:181, 2002.
7. Thackray H, Tifft C: Fetal alcohol syndrome. Pediatr Rev 22:47, 2001.
8. Kousseff BG: Diabetic embryopathy. Curr Opin Pediatr 11:348, 1999.
9. Olney RS, Mulinare J: Trends in neural tube defect prevalence, folic acid fortification, and vitamin supplement use. Semin Perinatol 26:277, 2002.
10. Williams LJ, et al: Prevalence of spina bifida and anencephaly during the transition to mandatory folic acid fortification in the United States. Teratology 66:33, 2002.
11. Edmonds LD, James LM: Temporal trends in the birth prevalence of selected congenital malformations in the Birth Defects Monitoring Program/Commission on Professional and Hospital Activities, 1979–1989. Teratology 48:647, 1993.
12. Stevenson RE: The environmental basis of human anomalies. In Stevenson RE, et al (eds): Human Malformations and Related Anomalies, Vol. 1. New York, Oxford University Press, 1993.
13. Abbott BD, Birnbaum LS: Retinoic acid–induced alterations in the expression of growth factors in embryonic mouse palatal shelves. Teratology 42:597, 1990.
14. Nugent P, Greene RM: Interactions between the transforming growth factor beta (TGF-β) and retinoic acid signal transduction pathways in murine embryonic palatal cells. Differentiation 58:149, 1994.
15. Machida J, et al: Transforming growth factor-alpha (TGFα): genomic structure, boundary sequences, and mutation analysis in nonsyndromic cleft lip/palate and cleft palate only. Genomics 61:237, 1999.
16. Miettinen PJ, et al: Epidermal growth factor receptor function is necessary for normal craniofacial development and palate closure. Nat Genet 22:69, 1999.
17. Proetzel G, et al: Transforming growth factor-beta 3 is required for secondary palate fusion. Nat Genet 11:409, 1995.
18. Qian YQ, et al: The structure of the *Antennapedia* homeodomain determined by NMR spectroscopy in solution: comparison with prokaryotic repressors. Cell 59:573, 1989.
19. D'Elia AV, et al: Missense mutations of human homeoboxes: a review. Hum Mutat 18:361, 2001.
20. Ross SA, et al: Retinoids in embryonal development. Physiol Rev 80:1021, 2000.
21. Zile MH: Vitamin A and embryonic development—an overview. J Nutr 128 (suppl 2):455S, 1998.
22. Lufkin T: Transcriptional regulation of vertebrate *Hox* genes during embryogenesis. Crit Rev Eukaryot Gene Expr 7:195, 1997.
23. Clagett-Dame M, Plum LA: Retinoid-regulated gene expression in neural development. Crit Rev Eukaryot Gene Expr 7:299, 1997.
24. Leonard L, et al: Anteriorization of CRABP-I expression by retinoic acid in the developing mouse central nervous system and its relationship to teratogenesis. Dev Biol 168:514, 1995.
25. Marshall H, et al: Retinoids and *Hox* genes. Faseb J 10:969, 1996.
26. Houle M, et al: Retinoic acid regulation of *Cdx1:* an indirect mechanism for retinoids and vertebral specification. Mol Cell Biol 20:6579, 2000.

27. Faiella A, et al: A mouse model for valproate teratogenicity: parental effects, homeotic transformations, and altered *HOX* expression. Hum Mol Genet 9:227, 2000.
28. Dahl E, Koseki H, Balling R: *Pax* genes and organogenesis. Bioessays 19:755, 1997.
29. Mansouri A: The role of *Pax3* and *Pax7* in development and cancer. Crit Rev Oncog 9:141, 1998.
30. Ohno H, Ueda C, Akasaka T: The t(9;14)(p13;q32) translocation in B-cell non-Hodgkin's lymphoma. Leuk Lymphoma 36:435, 2000.
31. Fuhrer D: A nuclear receptor in thyroid malignancy: is *PAX8/PPARγ* the Holy Grail of follicular thyroid cancer? Eur J Endocrinol 144:453, 2001.
32. Ernest JM: Neonatal consequences of preterm PROM. Clin Obstet Gynecol 41:827, 1998.
33. Lee T, Silver H: Etiology and epidemiology of preterm premature rupture of the membranes. Clin Perinatol 28:721, 2001.
34. Goldenberg RL, Hauth JC, Andrews WW: Intrauterine infection and preterm delivery. N Engl J Med 342:1500, 2000.
35. Greig PC, et al: Amniotic fluid interleukin-6 levels correlate with histologic chorioamnionitis and amniotic fluid cultures in patients in premature labor with intact membranes. Am J Obstet Gynecol 169:1035, 1993.
36. Goldenberg RL, et al: The preterm prediction study: granulocyte colony-stimulating factor and spontaneous preterm birth. National Institute of Child Health and Human Development Maternal-Fetal Medicine Units Network. Am J Obstet Gynecol 182:625, 2000.
37. Resnik R: Intrauterine growth restriction. Obstet Gynecol 99:490, 2002.
38. Kalousek DK: Current topic: confined placental mosaicism and intrauterine fetal development. Placenta 15:219, 1994.
39. Apgar V: A proposal for a new method of evaluation of the newborn infant. Anesth Analg 32:260, 1953.
40. Rogers BB, Over CE: Parvovirus B19 in fetal hydrops. Hum Pathol 30:247, 1999.
41. Stark AR, Frantz ID, III: Respiratory distress syndrome. Pediatr Clin North Am 33:533, 1986.
42. Editorial. Born before their time into this breathing world. BMJ 2:1403, 1976.
43. Goerke J: Pulmonary surfactant: functions and molecular composition. Biochim Biophys Acta 1408:79, 1998.
44. Nogee LM, et al: A mutation in the surfactant protein B gene responsible for fatal neonatal respiratory disease in multiple kindreds. J Clin Invest 93:1860, 1994.
45. Li C, et al: TGF-β inhibits pulmonary surfactant protein-B gene transcription through *SMAD3* interactions with *NKX2.1* and HNF-3 transcription factors. J Biol Chem, 2002.
46. Gonzales LW, et al: Glucocorticoids and thyroid hormones stimulate biochemical and morphological differentiation of human fetal lung in organ culture. J Clin Endocrinol Metab 62:678, 1986.
47. Haataja R, et al: Surfactant proteins A and B as interactive genetic determinants of neonatal respiratory distress syndrome. Hum Mol Genet 9:2751, 2000.
48. Ishisaka DY: Exogenous surfactant use in neonates. Ann Pharmacother 30:389, 1996.
49. Effect of corticosteroids for fetal maturation on perinatal outcomes. NIH Consensus Development Panel on the Effect of Corticosteroids for Fetal Maturation on Perinatal Outcomes. JAMA 273:413, 1995.
50. Aiello LP: Clinical implications of vascular growth factors in proliferative retinopathies. Curr Opin Ophthalmol 8:19, 1997.
51. Hellstrom A, et al: Low IGF-I suppresses VEGF-survival signaling in retinal endothelial cells: direct correlation with clinical retinopathy of prematurity. Proc Natl Acad Sci USA 98:5804, 2001.
52. Jobe AH, Bancalari E: Bronchopulmonary dysplasia. Am J Respir Crit Care Med 163:1723, 2001.
53. Northway WH, Jr., Rosan RC, Porter DY: Pulmonary disease following respirator therapy of hyaline-membrane disease. Bronchopulmonary dysplasia. N Engl J Med 276:357, 1967.
54. Husain AN, Siddiqui NH, Stocker JT: Pathology of arrested acinar development in postsurfactant bronchopulmonary dysplasia. Hum Pathol 29:710, 1998.
55. Supplemental Therapeutic Oxygen for Prethreshold Retinopathy Of Prematurity (STOP-ROP), a randomized, controlled trial. I: primary outcomes. Pediatrics 105:295, 2000.
56. Baier RJ, Loggins J, Kruger TE: Monocyte chemoattractant protein-1 and interleukin-8 are increased in bronchopulmonary dysplasia: relation to isolation of *Ureaplasma urealyticum.* J Investig Med 49:362, 2001.
57. Groneck P, Speer CP: Inflammatory mediators and bronchopulmonary dysplasia. Arch Dis Child Fetal Neonatal Ed 73:F1, 1995.
58. Hsueh W, et al: Necrotizing enterocolitis of the newborn: pathogenetic concepts in perspective. Pediatr Dev Pathol 1:2, 1998.
59. Gonzalez-Crussi F, Hsueh W: Experimental model of ischemic bowel necrosis. The role of platelet-activating factor and endotoxin. Am J Pathol 112:127, 1983.
60. Lallemand AV, Doco-Fenzy M, Gaillard DA: Investigation of nonimmune hydrops fetalis: multidisciplinary studies are necessary for diagnosis—review of 94 cases. Pediatr Dev Pathol 2:432, 1999.
61. Hsieh FJ, Ko TM, Chen HY: Hydrops fetalis caused by severe alpha-thalassemia. Early Hum Dev 29:233, 1992.
62. Levy HL: Maternal phenylketonuria. Review with emphasis on pathogenesis. Enzyme 38:312, 1987.
63. Svensson E, et al: Two missense mutations causing mild hyperphenylalaninemia associated with DNA haplotype 12. Hum Mutat 1:129, 1992.
64. Nagasaki Y, et al: Reversal of hypopigmentation in phenylketonuria mice by adenovirus-mediated gene transfer. Pediatr Res 45 (4 Pt 1): 465, 1999.
65. Liu G, Hale GE, Hughes CL: Galactose metabolism and ovarian toxicity. Reprod Toxicol 14:377, 2000.
66. Ning C, et al: Galactose metabolism in mice with galactose-1-phosphate uridyltransferase deficiency: sucklings and 7-week-old animals fed a high-galactose diet. Mol Genet Metab 72:306, 2001.
67. Litchfield WJ, Wells WW: Effect of galactose on free radical reactions of polymorphonuclear leukocytes. Arch Biochem Biophys 188:26, 1978.
68. Elsas LJ 2nd, Lai K: The molecular biology of galactosemia. Genet Med 1:40, 1998.
69. Kaufman F, et al: Ovarian failure in galactosaemia. Lancet 2:737, 1979.
70. Schweitzer S, et al: Long-term outcome in 134 patients with galactosaemia. Eur J Pediatr 152:36, 1993.
71. Acton JD, Wilmott RW: Phenotype of CF and the effects of possible modifier genes. Paediatr Respir Rev 2:332, 2001.
72. Mickle JE, Cutting GR: Genotype–phenotype relationships in cystic fibrosis. Med Clin North Am 84:597, 2000.
73. Greger R: Role of CFTR in the colon. Annu Rev Physiol 62:467, 2000.
74. Schwiebert EM, et al: Both CFTR and outwardly rectifying chloride channels contribute to cAMP-stimulated whole cell chloride currents. Am J Physiol 266 (5 Pt 1):C1464, 1994.
75. Stutts MJ, et al: CFTR as a cAMP-dependent regulator of sodium channels. Science 269:847, 1995.
76. Stutts MJ, Rossier BC, Boucher RC: Cystic fibrosis transmembrane conductance regulator inverts protein kinase A–mediated regulation of epithelial sodium channel single channel kinetics. J Biol Chem 272:14037, 1997.
77. Reddy MM, Light MJ, Quinton PM: Activation of the epithelial Na^+ channel (ENaC) requires CFTR Cl^- channel function. Nature 402:301, 1999.
78. Knowles MR, Boucher RC: Mucus clearance as a primary innate defense mechanism for mammalian airways. J Clin Invest 109:571, 2002.
79. Choi JY, et al: Aberrant CFTR-dependent $HCO3^-$ transport in mutations associated with cystic fibrosis. Nature 410:94, 2001.
80. Zielenski J: Genotype and phenotype in cystic fibrosis. Respiration 67:117, 2000.
81. Noone PG, Knowles MR: "CFTR-opathies": disease phenotypes associated with cystic fibrosis transmembrane regulator gene mutations. Respir Res 2:328, 2001.
82. Larriba S, et al: ATB(O)SLC1A5 gene. Fine localization and exclusion of association with the intestinal phenotype of cystic fibrosis. Eur J Human Genet 11:860, 2001.
83. Garred P, et al: Association of mannose-binding lectin gene heterogeneity with severity of lung disease and survival in cystic fibrosis. J Clin Invest 104:431, 1999.
84. Gabolde M, et al: The mannose-binding lectin gene influences the severity of chronic liver disease in cystic fibrosis. J Med Genet 38:310, 2001.
85. Noone PG, et al: Cystic fibrosis gene mutations and pancreatitis risk: relation to epithelial ion transport and trypsin inhibitor gene mutations. Gastroenterology 121:1310, 2001.
86. Rajan S, Saiman L: Pulmonary infections in patients with cystic fibrosis. Semin Respir Infect 17:47, 2002.

87. Diwakar V, Pearson L, Beath S: Liver disease in children with cystic fibrosis. Paediatr Respir Rev 2:340, 2001.
88. Chillon M, et al: Mutations in the cystic fibrosis gene in patients with congenital absence of the vas deferens. N Engl J Med 332:1475, 1995.
89. Mak V, et al: Proportion of cystic fibrosis gene mutations not detected by routine testing in men with obstructive azoospermia. JAMA 281: 2217, 1999.
90. Groman JD, et al: Variant cystic fibrosis phenotypes in the absence of *CFTR* mutations. N Engl J Med 347:401, 2002.
91. Willinger M, James LS, Catz C: Defining the sudden infant death syndrome (SIDS): deliberations of an expert panel convened by the National Institute of Child Health and Human Development. Pediatr Pathol 11:677, 1991.
92. Hunt CE: Sudden infant death syndrome and other causes of infant mortality: diagnosis, mechanisms, and risk for recurrence in siblings. Am J Respir Crit Care Med 164:346, 2001.
93. Filiano JJ, Kinney HC: Arcuate nucleus hypoplasia in the sudden infant death syndrome. J Neuropathol Exp Neurol 51:394, 1992.
94. Kinney HC, et al: Subtle developmental abnormalities in the inferior olive: an indicator of prenatal brainstem injury in the sudden infant death syndrome. J Neuropathol Exp Neurol 61:427, 2002.
95. Filiano JJ, Kinney HC: A perspective on neuropathologic findings in victims of the sudden infant death syndrome: the triple-risk model. Biol Neonate 65:194, 1994.
96. Harper RM, et al: Sleep influences on homeostatic functions: implications for sudden infant death syndrome. Respir Physiol 119:123, 2000.
97. Kinney HC, et al: Decreased muscarinic receptor binding in the arcuate nucleus in sudden infant death syndrome. Science 269:1446, 1995.
98. Panigrahy A, et al: Decreased kainate receptor binding in the arcuate nucleus of the sudden infant death syndrome. J Neuropathol Exp Neurol 56:1253, 1997.
99. Jacquin TD, et al: Reorganization of pontine rhythmogenic neuronal networks in *Krox-20* knockout mice. Neuron 17:747, 1996.
100. Balkowiec A, Katz DM: Brain-derived neurotrophic factor is required for normal development of the central respiratory rhythm in mice. J Physiol 510 (Pt 2):527, 1998.
101. Lindgren C: Respiratory control during upper airway infection mechanism for prolonged reflex apnoea and sudden infant death with special reference to infant sleep position. FEMS Immunol Med Microbiol 25:97, 1999.
102. Nagler J: Sudden infant death syndrome. Curr Opin Pediatr 14:247, 2002.
103. Changing concepts of sudden infant death syndrome: implications for infant sleeping environment and sleep position. American Academy of Pediatrics. Task Force on Infant Sleep Position and Sudden Infant Death Syndrome. Pediatrics 105 (3 Pt 1):650, 2000.
104. Moon RY, Biliter WM: Infant sleep position policies in licensed child care centers after back to sleep campaign. Pediatrics 106:576, 2000.
105. Treem WR: New developments in the pathophysiology, clinical spectrum, and diagnosis of disorders of fatty acid oxidation. Curr Opin Pediatr 12:463, 2000.
106. Valdes-Dapena M, Gilbert-Barness E: Cardiovascular causes for sudden infant death. Pediatr Pathol Mol Med 21:195, 2002.
107. Bourgeois JM, et al: Molecular detection of the *ETV6-NTRK3* gene fusion differentiates congenital fibrosarcoma from other childhood spindle cell tumors. Am J Surg Pathol 24:937, 2000.
108. Kelly DR, Joshi VV: Neuroblastoma and related tumors. In Parham D (ed): Pediatric Neoplasia Morphology and Biology. Philadelphia, Lippincott-Raven, 1996, pp. 105–152.
109. Shimada H, et al: Terminology and morphologic criteria of neuroblastic tumors: recommendations by the International Neuroblastoma Pathology Committee. Cancer 86:349, 1999.
110. Ambros IM, et al: Role of ploidy, chromosome 1p, and Schwann cells in the maturation of neuroblastoma. N Engl J Med 334:1505, 1996.
111. Mora J, et al: Neuroblastic and Schwannian stromal cells of neuroblastoma are derived from a tumoral progenitor cell. Cancer Res 61:6892, 2001.
112. Shimada H, et al: The International Neuroblastoma Pathology Classification (the Shimada system). Cancer 86:364, 1999.
113. Smith EI, et al: A surgical perspective on the current staging in neuroblastoma—the International Neuroblastoma Staging System proposal. J Pediatr Surg 24:386, 1989.
114. Brodeur GM, Castleberry RP: Neuroblastoma. In Pizzo PA, Poplack DG (eds): Principles and Practice of Pediatric Oncology. Philadelphia, JB Lippincott, 1993, pp. 739–767.
115. Evans AE, Gerson J, Schnaufer L: Spontaneous regression of neuroblastoma. Natl Cancer Inst Monogr 44:49, 1976.
116. Schwab M: Human neuroblastoma: from basic science to clinical debut of cellular oncogenes. Naturwissenschaften 86:71, 1999.
117. Lastowska M, et al: Breakpoint position on 17q identifies the most aggressive neuroblastoma tumors. Genes Chromosomes Cancer 34:428, 2002.
118. Bown N: Neuroblastoma tumour genetics: clinical and biological aspects. J Clin Pathol 54:897, 2001.
119. Caron H, et al: Evidence for two tumour suppressor loci on chromosomal bands 1p35-36 involved in neuroblastoma: one probably imprinted, another associated with N-*myc* amplification. Hum Mol Genet 4:535, 1995.
120. Nakagawara A, et al: Association between high levels of expression of the *TRK* gene and favorable outcome in human neuroblastoma. N Engl J Med 328:847, 1993.
121. Hiyama E, et al: Correlating telomerase activity levels with human neuroblastoma outcomes. Nat Med 1:249, 1995.
122. Schilling FH, et al: Neuroblastoma screening at one year of age. N Engl J Med 346:1047, 2002.
123. Woods WG, et al: Screening of infants and mortality due to neuroblastoma. N Engl J Med 346:1041, 2002.
124. Blute ML, et al: Bilateral Wilms tumor. J Urol 138 (4 Pt 2):968, 1987.
125. Grundy P, Coppes MJ, Haber D: Molecular genetics of Wilms tumor. Hematol Oncol Clin North Am 9:1201, 1995.
126. Mueller RF: The Denys-Drash syndrome. J Med Genet 31:471, 1994.
127. Scharnhorst V, van der Eb AJ, Jochemsen AG: WT1 proteins: functions in growth and differentiation. Gene 273:141, 2001.
128. Englert C, et al: Induction of *p21* by the Wilms tumor suppressor gene *WT1*. Cancer Res 57:1429, 1997.
129. Dome JS, Coppes MJ: Recent advances in Wilms tumor genetics. Curr Opin Pediatr 14:5, 2002.
130. Feinberg AP: Imprinting of a genomic domain of 11p15 and loss of imprinting in cancer: an introduction. Cancer Res 59 (7 Suppl):1743s, 1999.
131. Steenman MJ, et al: Loss of imprinting of *IGF2* is linked to reduced expression and abnormal methylation of H19 in Wilms tumour. Nat Genet 7:433, 1994.
132. Breslow NE, et al: Familial Wilms tumor: a descriptive study. Med Pediatr Oncol 27:398, 1996.
133. Rahman N, et al: Confirmation of *FWT1* as a Wilms tumour susceptibility gene and phenotypic characteristics of Wilms tumour attributable to *FWT1*. Hum Genet 103:547, 1998.
134. McDonald JM, et al: Linkage of familial Wilms tumor predisposition to chromosome 19 and a two-locus model for the etiology of familial tumors. Cancer Res 58:1387, 1998.
135. Maiti S, et al: Frequent association of β-catenin and *WT1* mutations in Wilms tumors. Cancer Res 60:6288, 2000.
136. Hennigar RA, O'Shea PA, Grattan-Smith JD: Clinicopathologic features of nephrogenic rests and nephroblastomatosis. Adv Anat Pathol 8:276, 2001.
137. Faria P, et al: Focal versus diffuse anaplasia in Wilms tumor—new definitions with prognostic significance: a report from the National Wilms Tumor Study Group. Am J Surg Pathol 20:909, 1996.
138. Bardeesy N, Beckwith JB, Pelletier J: Clonal expansion and attenuated apoptosis in Wilms tumors are associated with *p53* gene mutations. Cancer Res 55:215, 1995.
139. Shearer P, et al: Secondary acute myelogenous leukemia in patients previously treated for childhood renal tumors: a report from the National Wilms Tumor Study Group. J Pediatr Hematol Oncol 23:109, 2001.

UNIT II

Diseases of Organ Systems

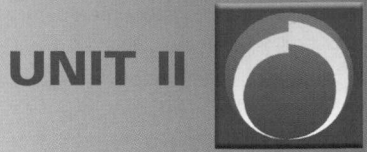

CHAPTER 11

Blood Vessels

Frederick J. Schoen, MD, PhD

VASCULAR WALL CELLS AND THEIR RESPONSE TO INJURY
Endothelial Cells
Vascular Smooth Muscle Cells
Vessel Development, Growth, and Remodeling
Intimal Thickening—A Response to Vascular Intimal Injury
CONGENITAL ANOMALIES
ARTERIOSCLEROSIS
ATHEROSCLEROSIS
Natural History and Main Consequence
Epidemiology and Risk Factors
Pathogenesis
Other Factors in Atherogenesis
Clinicopathologic Effects of Atherosclerotic Coronary Artery Disease
Prevention
HYPERTENSIVE VASCULAR DISEASE
Hypertension
ANEURYSMS AND DISSECTIONS
Abdominal Aortic Aneurysms
Syphilitic (Luetic) Aneurysms
Aortic Dissection (Dissecting Hematoma)
INFLAMMATORY DISEASE—THE VASCULITIDES
Giant Cell (Temporal) Arteritis
Takayasu Arteritis
Polyarteritis Nodosa (PAN)
Kawasaki Disease (Mucocutaneous Lymph Node Syndrome)
Microscopic Polyangiitis (Microscopic Polyarteritis, Hypersensitivity or Leukocytoclastic Vasculitis)
Wegener Granulomatosis
Thromboangiitis Obliterans (Buerger Disease)
Vasculitis Associated with Other Disorders
Infectious Arteritis
RAYNAUD PHENOMENON
VEINS AND LYMPHATICS
Varicose Veins
Thrombophlebitis and Phlebothrombosis
Superior and Inferior Vena Caval Syndromes
Lymphangitis and Lymphedema
TUMORS
Benign Tumors and Tumor-Like Conditions
Hemangioma
Lymphangomas
Glomus Tumor (Glomangioma)
Vascular Ectasias
Bacillary Angiomatosis
Intermediate-Grade (Borderline, Low-Grade Malignant) Tumors
Kaposi Sarcoma
Hemangioendothelioma

Malignant Tumors
Angiosarcoma
Hemangiopericytoma
PATHOLOGY OF VASCULAR INTERVENTIONS
Balloon Angioplasty and Endovascular Stents
Vascular Replacement
Coronary Artery Bypass Graft Surgery

Diseases of arteries are responsible for more morbidity and mortality than any other type of human disease. Disorders of veins less commonly cause clinically significant problems. Vascular abnormalities cause clinical disease by two principal mechanisms:

- *Narrowing* or *completely obstructing* the lumens, either progressively (e.g., by atherosclerosis) or precipitously (e.g., by thrombosis or embolism).
- *Weakening* of the walls, leading to dilation or rupture.

To understand the diseases that affect blood vessels, we first consider some of the anatomic and functional characteristics of these highly specialized and dynamic tissues.

Normal

The general architecture and cellular composition of blood vessels are the same throughout the cardiovascular system. However, certain features of the vasculature vary with and reflect distinct functional requirements at different locations (see below). To withstand the pulsatile flow and higher blood pressures in arteries, arterial walls are generally thicker than the walls of veins. Arterial wall thickness gradually diminishes as the vessels become smaller, but the ratio of wall thickness to lumen diameter becomes greater.

The basic constituents of the walls of blood vessels are endothelial cells and smooth muscle cells, and extracellular matrix (ECM), including elastin, collagen, and glycosoaminoglycans. The three concentric layers—*intima, media,* and *adventitia*—are most clearly defined in the larger vessels, particularly arteries (Fig. 11–1). In normal arteries, the intima consists of a single layer of endothelial cells with minimal underlying subendothelial connective tissue. It is separated from the media by a dense elastic membrane called the *internal elastic lamina.* The smooth muscle cell layers of the media near the vessel lumen receive oxygen and nutrients by direct diffusion from the vessel lumen, facilitated by holes in the internal elastic membrane. However, diffusion from the lumen is inadequate for the outer portions of the media in large and medium-sized vessels, therefore these areas are nourished by small arterioles arising from outside the vessel (called *vasa vasorum*, literally "vessels of the vessels") coursing into the outer one half to two thirds of the media. The outer limit of the media of most arteries is a well-defined *external elastic lamina.* External to the media is the adventitia, consisting of connective tissue with nerve fibers and the vasa vasorum.

Based on their size and structural features, *arteries* are divided into three types: (1) large or *elastic arteries*, including the aorta, its large branches (particularly the innominate, subclavian, common carotid, and iliac), and pulmonary arteries; (2) medium-sized or *muscular arteries*, comprising other branches of the aorta (e.g., coronary and renal arteries); and (3) small arteries (less than approximately 2 mm in diameter) and *arterioles* (20 to 100 micrometers in diameter), within the substance of tissues and organs.

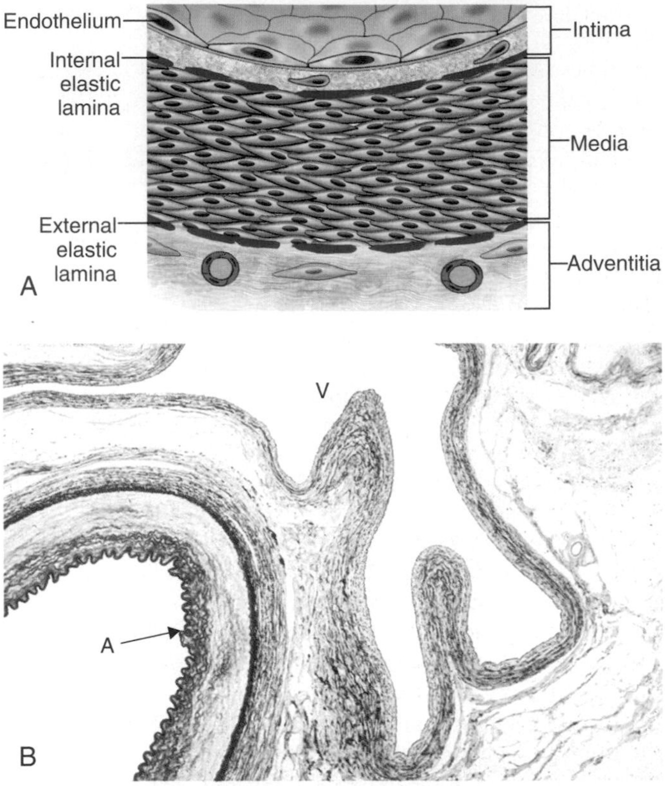

FIGURE 11–1 The vascular wall. *A,* Graphic representation of the cross section of a small muscular artery (e.g., renal or coronary artery). *B,* Photomicrograph of histologic section containing a portion of an artery (A) and adjacent vein (V). Elastic membranes are stained black (internal elastic membrane of artery highlighted by *arrow*). Because it is exposed to higher pressures, the artery has a thicker wall that maintains an open, round lumen, even when blood is absent. Moreover, the elastin of the artery is more organized than in the corresponding vein. In contrast, the vein has a larger, but collapsed, lumen, and the elastin in its wall is diffusely distributed. (*B,* Courtesy of Mark Flomenbaum, M.D., Ph.D., Office of the Chief Medical Examiner, New York City.)

The relative amount and configuration of the basic constituents vary along the arterial system owing to local adaptations to mechanical or metabolic needs. These structural changes, from location to location, are principally in the media and in the ECM. In the elastic arteries the media is rich in elastic fibers, which are arranged in fairly compact layers separated by and alternating with layers of smooth muscle cells. The elastic components of the aorta allow it to expand during systole, thereby storing some of the energy of each heartbeat. In between cardiac contractions during the diastolic phase of the cardiac cycle, elastic recoil of the vascular wall propels blood through the peripheral vascular system. With aging, the aorta loses elasticity, and large vessels expand less readily, particularly when blood pressure is increased. Thus the arteries of older individuals often become progressively tortuous and dilated *(ectatic)*. In *muscular arteries* the media is composed predominantly of circularly or spirally arranged smooth muscle cells. Elastin is limited to the internal and external membranes. In the muscular arteries and arterioles (see below), regional blood flow and blood pressure are regulated by changes in lumen size through smooth muscle cell contraction *(vasoconstriction)* or relaxation *(vasodilation)*, controlled in part by the autonomic nervous system and in part by local metabolic factors and cellular interactions.

In arterioles, medial smooth muscle cell contraction causes dramatic adjustments in lumen diameter that regulate systemic arterial blood pressure and significantly influence blood flow distribution among various capillary beds. Since the resistance of a tube to fluid flow is inversely proportional to the fourth power of the diameter (i.e., halving the diameter increases resistance 16-fold), small changes in the lumen size of small arteries caused by structural change or vasoconstriction can have a profound effect. Thus *arterioles are the principal points of physiologic resistance to blood flow.*

Capillaries, approximately the diameter of a red blood cell (7 to 8 μm), have an endothelial cell lining but no media. Collectively, capillaries have a very large total cross-sectional area; within the capillaries, the flow rate slows dramatically. With thin walls only one cell thick and slow flow, capillaries are ideally suited to the rapid exchange of diffusible substances between blood and tissues. As normal tissue function depends on an adequate supply of oxygen through blood vessels, and since diffusion of oxygen in even minimally demanding solid tissues is inefficient over distances of greater than approximately 100 μm,[1] the capillary network of most tissues is very rich. Metabolically highly active tissues, such as the myocardium, have the highest density of capillaries.

Blood from capillary beds flows initially into the *postcapillary venules* and then sequentially through collecting venules and small, medium, and large veins. *In many types of inflammation, vascular leakage and leukocyte exudation occur preferentially in postcapillary venules* (see Chapter 2).

Relative to arteries, veins have larger diameters, larger lumens, and thinner and less well organized walls (see Fig. 11–1*B*). Thus, because of their poor support, *veins are predisposed to irregular dilation, compression, degeneration, and easy penetration by tumors and inflammatory processes.* The venous system collectively has a large capacity; approximately two thirds of all the blood is in veins. Reverse flow is prevented by venous valves in the extremities, where blood flows against gravity.

Lymphatics are thin-walled, endothelium-lined channels that serve as a drainage system for returning interstitial tissue fluid and inflammatory cells to the blood. *Lymphatics constitute an important pathway for disease dissemination through transport of bacteria and tumor cells to distant sites.*

Some pathologic lesions involve vessels of a characteristic size, range, and/or type. As will been seen later, atherosclerosis affects elastic and muscular arteries, hypertension affects small muscular arteries and arterioles, and specific types of vasculitis involve characteristic vascular segments.

Pathology

Vascular Wall Cells and Their Response to Injury

As the main cellular components of the blood vessels, *endothelial cells (ECs)* and *smooth muscle cells (SMCs)* play an important role in vascular biology and pathology. The integrated function of these cells is critical to the mechanisms by which the vasculature develops and responds to hemodynamic and biochemical stimuli. Knowing how blood vessels function, adapt to unusual need, and respond to injury helps our understanding of specific pathologic conditions, their mechanisms, and their complications. Furthermore, unraveling these mechanisms may foster new therapeutic options for treating or preventing diseases that are important causes of mortality and morbidity.

ENDOTHELIAL CELLS

ECs comprise the single cell–thick, continuous lining of the entire cardiovascular system, collectively called the *endothelium.* Endothelial structural and functional integrity is fundamental to the maintenance of vessel wall homeostasis and normal circulatory function. ECs uniquely contain *Weibel-Palade bodies*, 0.1 μm-wide, 3 μm-long membrane-bound storage organelles that contain von Willebrand factor (vWF). ECs can be identified immunohistochemically with antibodies to PECAM-1 (CD31, a protein localized to interendothelial junctions), CD34, and vWF.

Vascular endothelium is a versatile, multifunctional tissue having many synthetic and metabolic properties (listed in Table 11–1), and it is an active participant in blood–tissue interactions. As a semipermeable membrane, endothelium controls the transfer of small and large molecules across the vascular wall. In most regions the intercellular junctions are normally impermeable to large molecules such as plasma proteins; however, the relatively labile junctions between ECs may widen under the influence of hemodynamic factors (e.g., high blood pressure) and vasoactive agents (e.g., histamine in inflammation) (Chapter 2). Moreover, ECs play a role in the maintenance of a nonthrombogenic blood–tissue interface (Chapter 4), the modulation of blood flow and vascular resistance, the metabolism of hormones, the regulation of immune and inflammatory reactions, and the growth regulation of other cell types, particularly SMCs. Frank loss (denudation) of EC stimulates thrombosis (see Chapter 4) and SMC proliferation (see below).

The vascular endothelium has substantial phenotypic variability based on anatomic site and dynamic adaptation to local environmental cues. For example, EC populations that develop embryologically from different sites (large vessels vs. capillaries, arterial vs. venous) may have different characteristics.[2] Lymphatic endothelium is of particular interest owing to the role of lymphatics in tumor metastasis.[3]

TABLE 11–1 Endothelial Cell Properties and Functions

Maintenance of Permeability Barrier
Elaboration of Anticoagulant, Antithrombotic, Fibrinolytic Regulators
Prostacyclin Thrombomodulin Heparin-like molecules Plasminogen activator
Elaboration of Prothrombotic Molecules
Von Willebrand factor Tissue factor Plasminogen activator inhibitor
Extracellular Matrix Production (collagen, proteoglycans)
Modulation of Blood Flow and Vascular Reactivity
Vasconstrictors: endothelin, ACE Vasodilators: NO, prostacyclin
Regulation of Inflammation and Immunity
IL-1, IL-6, chemokines Adhesion molecules: VCAM-1, ICAM, E-selectin P-selectin Histocompatibility antigens
Regulation of Cell Growth
Growth stimulators: PDGF, CSF, FGF Growth inhibitors: heparin, TGF-β
Oxidation of LDL

ACE, angiotensin converting enzyme; NO, nitric oxide; IL, interleukin; PDGF, platelet-derived growth factor; CSF, colony-stimulating factor; FGF, fibroblast growth factor; TGF-β, transforming growth factor-beta; LDL, low-density lipoprotein.

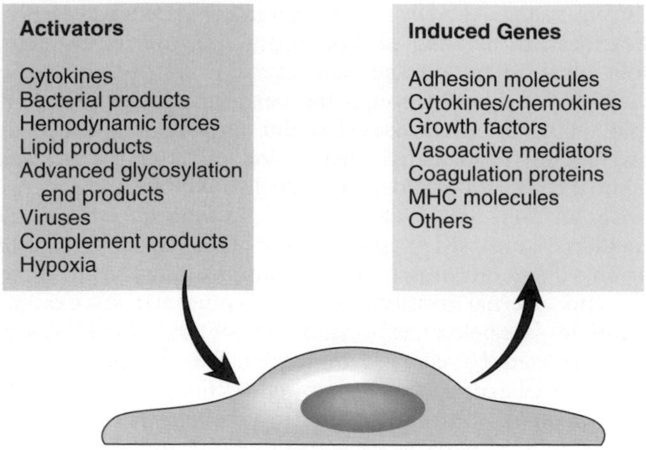

FIGURE 11–2 Endothelial cell response to environmental stimuli: causes (activators) and consequences (induced genes).

Structurally intact ECs can respond to various pathophysiologic stimuli by adjusting their usual (constitutive) functions and by expressing newly acquired (inducible) properties—a process termed *endothelial activation* (Fig. 11–2).[4,5] Inducers of endothelial activation include cytokines and bacterial products, which cause inflammation and septic shock (Chapter 2); hemodynamic stresses and lipid products, critical to the pathogenesis of atherosclerosis (see later); advanced glycosylation end products (important in diabetes, Chapter 24), as well as viruses, complement components, and hypoxia. Activated ECs, in turn, express adhesion molecules (Chapter 2), and produce other cytokines and chemokines, growth factors, vasoactive molecules that result either in vasoconstriction or in vasodilation, major histocompatibility complex molecules, procoagulant and anticoagulant moieties, and a variety of other biologically active products. ECs influence the vasoreactivity of the underlying smooth muscle cells through the production of both relaxing factors (e.g., nitric oxide [NO]) and contracting factors (e.g., endothelin). Normal endothelial function is characterized by a balance of these factors and the ability of the vessel to respond appropriately to various pharmacologic stimuli (e.g., vasorelaxation in response to acetylcholine).

Endothelial dysfunction, as defined by an altered phenotype that impairs vasoreactivity or induces a surface that is thrombogenic or abnormally adhesive to inflammatory cells, is responsible, at least in part, for the initiation of thrombus formation, atherosclerosis, and the vascular lesions of hypertension and other disorders. Certain forms of EC dysfunction are rapid in onset (within minutes), reversible, and independent of new protein synthesis (e.g., EC contraction induced by histamine and other vasoactive mediators that cause gaps in venular endothelium Chapter 2). Other changes involve alterations in gene expression and protein synthesis and may require hours or even days to develop.

VASCULAR SMOOTH MUSCLE CELLS

As the predominant cellular element of the vascular media, SMCs are responsible for vasoconstriction and dilation in response to normal or pharmacologic stimuli. They also synthesize collagen, elastin, and proteoglycans; and elaborate growth factors and cytokines. They migrate to the intima and proliferate following vascular injury. Thus, SMCs are important elements of both normal vascular repair and pathologic processes such as atherosclerosis.

The migratory and proliferative activities of SMCs are regulated by growth promoters and inhibitors. Promoters include platelet-derived growth factor (PDGF), as well as endothelin-1, thrombin, fibroblast growth factor (FGF), interferon-gamma (IFN-γ), and interleukin-1 (IL-1). Inhibitors include heparan sulfates, NO and transforming growth factor-beta (TGF-β). Other regulators include the renin-angiotensin system (e.g., angiotensin II), catecholamines, the estrogen receptor, and osteopontin, a component of the extracellular matrix.[6]

VESSEL DEVELOPMENT, GROWTH, AND REMODELING

Much has been learned over the past decade about how new blood vessels form and change over time.[7,8] Study of the zebra fish, aided by the translucency and rapidly understood genetics of this small organism, has facilitated extraordinary insights into cardiovascular development, including blood vessel formation in the embryo *(vasculogenesis)* (see also Chapter 12).[9]

Vessel formation is a complex process involving highly directed and specific cellular interactions with regulatory factors and adhesive substrates. As was discussed earlier in Chapter 3, angiogenesis involves differentiation, proliferation, and interaction of endothelial and smooth muscle cells to create mature new blood vessels. The formation of a muscular coat endows blood vessels with vascoelastic and vasomotor properties, which accommodate the changing needs of tissue perfusion. Stimulation of angiogenesis to enhance tissue perfusion in ischemic disease is a therapeutic goal. In contrast, angiogenesis contributes to the pathogenesis of tumor growth, arthritis, diabetic retinopathy, and other diseases.[1,10] Therefore, an understanding of the basic cellular and molecular mechanisms of angiogenesis should lead to future therapies to stimulate or inhibit angiogenesis.[11]

INTIMAL THICKENING—A RESPONSE TO VASCULAR INTIMAL INJURY

Vascular injury (acute EC loss or chronic endothelial injury/dysfunction) stimulates SMC growth. Reconstitution of the damaged vascular wall is a physiologic healing response that includes the formation of a *neointima,* in which SMCs (1) migrate from the media to the intima, (2) multiply as intimal SMCs, and (3) synthesize and deposit ECM (Fig. 11–3).

During the healing response, SMCs undergo changes that resemble dedifferentiation. In the intima they lose the capacity to contract and gain the capacity to divide. Concurrently, there is a decrease in contractile filaments and an increase in organelles involved in protein synthesis, such as rough endoplasmic reticulum and Golgi apparatus. Intimal SMCs may return to a nonproliferative state when either the overlying endothelial layer is re-established following acute injury or the chronic stimulation ceases. However, an exaggerated healing response leads to *intimal thickening* or *intimal hyperplasia,* which, when excessive, can cause stenosis or occlusion of small and medium-sized blood vessels. It is important to note that intimal thickening occurs in otherwise normal arteries as a result of maturation and aging. In many adults, the intima and the media of otherwise normal arteries, such as the coronary arteries, are of approximately equal thickness. The lack of harmful consequences of this type of intimal thickness suggests that it is not an early lesion of atherosclerosis, nor is it necessarily a harbinger of other disease.

Congenital Anomalies

Aberrations of the usual anatomic pattern of branching and anastomosing are important in surgery, during which an unexpected vessel can be injured. They are rarely symptomatic, except in the coronary arterial tree.[12] Among other diverse congenital vascular anomalies, several have importance: *developmental or berry aneurysms,* and *arteriovenous fistulas* or *aneurysms.* Berry aneurysms involve cerebral vessels and are discussed in Chapter 28.

Arteriovenous Fistulas. These are rare, usually small, abnormal communications between arteries and veins. They arise as developmental defects, but can also be produced from rupture of an arterial aneurysm into the adjacent vein, from penetrating injuries that pierce the walls of artery and vein, or from inflammatory necrosis of adjacent vessels. Arteriovenous fistulas may be of clinical significance because they short-circuit blood from the arterial to the venous side, thereby causing the heart to pump additional volume; sometimes high-output cardiac failure ensues. Moreover, they can rupture and cause hemorrhage, especially in the brain.[13] In contrast, intentionally created arteriovenous fistulas are used to provide vascular access for chronic hemodialysis.

Arteriosclerosis

Arteriosclerosis (literally, "hardening of the arteries") is a generic term for thickening and loss of elasticity of arterial walls. Three patterns of arteriosclerosis are recognized; they vary in pathophysiology and clinical and pathological consequences.

- *Atherosclerosis,* the most frequent and important pattern, will be discussed first and in detail below.
- *Mönckeberg medial calcific sclerosis* is characterized by calcific deposits in muscular arteries in persons older than

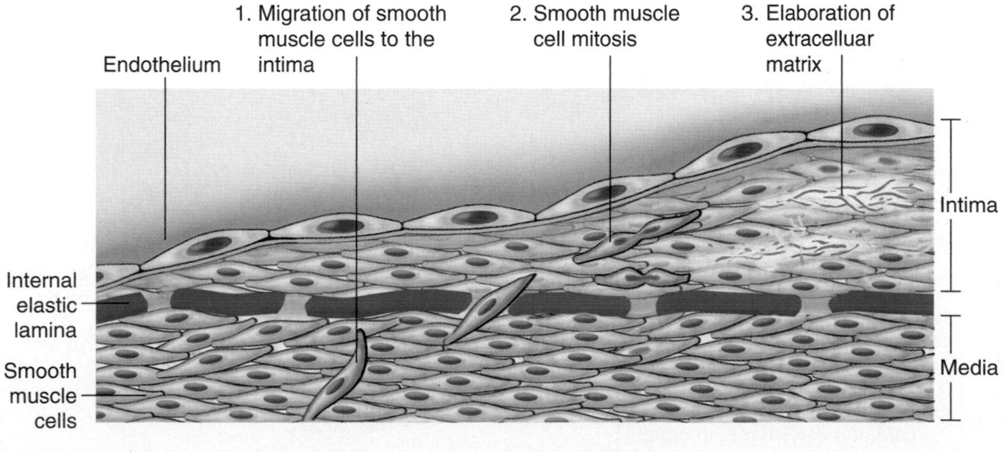

FIGURE 11–3 Schematic diagram of the mechanism of intimal thickening, emphasizing smooth muscle cell migration to, and proliferation and extracellular matrix elaboration in, the intima. (Modified and redrawn from Schoen FJ: Interventional and Surgical Cardiovascular Pathology: Clinical Correlations and Basic Principles. Philadelphia, W.B. Saunders Co., 1989, p. 254.)

age 50. The radiographically visible, often palpable calcifications, do not encroach on the vessel lumen.

- *Arteriolosclerosis* affects small arteries and arterioles. There are two anatomic variants, hyaline and hyperplastic, both associated with thickening of vessel walls with luminal narrowing that may cause downstream ischemic injury. Most often associated with hypertension and diabetes mellitus, arteriolosclerosis will be described later in this chapter in the section on hypertension.

Atherosclerosis

Atherosclerosis is characterized by intimal lesions called *atheromas*, or *atheromatous or fibrofatty plaques*, which protrude into and obstruct vascular lumens and weaken the underlying media. They may lead to serious complications. Global in distribution, atherosclerosis overwhelmingly contributes to more mortality—approximately half of all deaths—and serious morbidity in the Western world than any other disorder. Epidemiologic data on atherosclerosis are usually presented in terms of frequency of the number of deaths caused by ischemic heart disease (IHD) (see Chapter 12). Myocardial infarction alone is responsible for 20% to 25% of all deaths in the United States.

NATURAL HISTORY AND MAIN CONSEQUENCES

The American Heart Association classification divides atherosclerotic lesions into six types, beginning with isolated foam cells ("fatty dots"), through stages of fatty streaks, atheromas, and fibroatheromas, to the complicated lesions (Fig. 11–4). The natural history, morphologic features, and main pathogenetic events of atherosclerosis are summarized in Figure 11–5, which serves as a road map for the discussion that follows.

Fatty streaks are the earliest lesion of atherosclerosis. They are composed of lipid-filled foam cells (Fig. 11–6). They are not significantly raised and thus do not cause any disturbance in blood flow. Fatty streaks begin as multiple yellow, flat spots less than 1 mm in diameter that coalesce into elongated streaks, 1 cm long or longer. They contain T lymphocytes and extracellular lipid in smaller amounts than in plaques.

Fatty streaks appear in the aortas of some children younger than age 1 year and all children older than age 10 years, regardless of geography, race, sex, or enviroment. Coronary fatty streaks begin to form in adolescence and at anatomic sites that may be prone to develop plaques. The relationship of fatty streaks to atherosclerotic plaques is complex. Fatty streaks are related to the known risk factors of atherosclerosis in adults (especially serum lipoprotein cholesterol concentrations and smoking), and some experimental evidence supports the concept of the evolution of fatty streaks into plaques. Fatty streaks, however, often occur in areas of the vasculature that are not particularly susceptible to developing atheromas later in life. Moreover, they frequently affect individuals in geographic locales and populations in which atherosclerotic plaque is uncommon. Thus, although fatty streaks may be precursors of plaques, not all fatty streaks are destined to become fibrous plaques or more advanced lesions.

Atherosclerotic plaques develop primarily in elastic arteries (e.g., aorta, carotid, and iliac arteries) and large and medium-sized muscular arteries (e.g., coronary and popliteal arteries). *Symptomatic atherosclerotic disease most often involves the arteries supplying the heart, brain, kidneys, and lower extremities. Myocardial infarction (heart attack), cerebral infarction (stroke), aortic aneurysms, and peripheral vascular disease (gangrene of the legs) are the major consequences of atherosclerosis.* Atherosclerosis also takes a toll through other consequences

Nomenclature and main histology	Sequences in progression	Main growth mechanism	Earliest onset	Clinical correlation
Type I (initial) lesion Isolated macrophage foam cells	I ↓	Growth mainly by lipid accumulation	From first decade	Clinically silent
Type II (fatty streak) lesion Mainly intracellular lipid accumulation	II ↓			
Type III (intermediate) lesion Type II changes and small extracellular lipid pools	III ↓		From third decade	
Type IV (atheroma) lesion Type II changes and core of extracellular lipid	IV ↓ (→ VI)			Clinically silent or overt
Type V (fibroatheroma) lesion Lipid core and fibrotic layer, or multiple lipid cores and fibrotic layers, or mainly calcific, or mainly fibrotic	V ↓	Accelerated smooth muscle and collagen increase	From fourth decade	
Type VI (complicated) lesion Surface defect, hematoma-hemorrhage, thrombus	VI	Thrombosis, hematoma		

FIGURE 11–4 American Heart Association classification of human atherosclerotic lesions from the fatty dot (type I) to the complicated type VI lesion. The diagram also includes growth mechanisms and clinical correlations. (Modified from Stary HC, et al: A definition of advanced types of atherosclerotic lesions and a histological classification of atherosclerosis. Circulation 92:1355, 1995.)

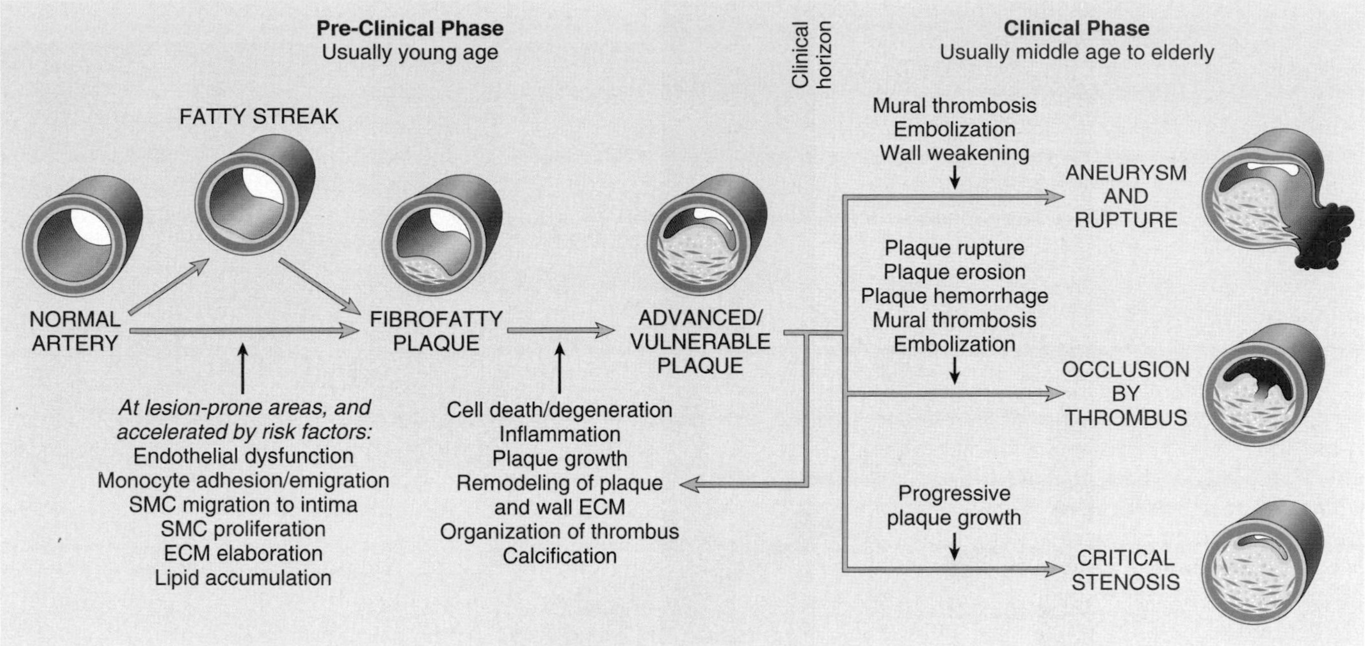

FIGURE 11–5 Schematic summary of the natural history, morphologic features, main pathogenetic events, and clinical complications of atherosclerosis in the coronary arteries.

of acutely or chronically diminished arterial perfusion, *such as mesenteric occlusion, sudden cardiac death, chronic ischemic heart disease, and ischemic encephalopathy.*

In small arteries, atheromas can occlude lumens, compromise blood flow to distal organs, and cause ischemic injury. Plaques can undergo disruption and precipitate thrombi that further obstruct blood flow. In large arteries, plaques encroach on the subjacent media and weaken the affected vessel wall, causing aneurysms that may rupture. Moreover, extensive atheromas can be friable, and shed emboli into the distal circulation.

Morphology. The key processes in atherosclerosis are intimal thickening and lipid accumulation. An atheroma (derived from the Greek word for gruel) or atheromatous plaque consists of a raised focal lesion initiating within the intima, having a soft, yellow, grumous core of lipid (mainly cholesterol and cholesterol esters), covered by a firm, white fibrous cap (Fig. 11–7). Also called fibrous, fibrofatty, lipid, or fibrolipid plaques, atheromatous plaques appear white to whitish yellow and impinge on the lumen of the artery. They vary in size from approximately 0.3 to 1.5 cm in diameter but sometimes coalesce to form larger masses. Atherosclerotic lesions usually involve only a partial circumference of the arterial wall ("eccentric" lesions) and are patchy and variable along the vessel length. Focal and sparsely distributed at first, atherosclerosis lesions become increasingly numerous and diffuse as the disease progresses.

In the characteristic distribution of atherosclerotic plaques in humans the abdominal aorta (Fig. 11–8) is usually much more involved than the thoracic aorta, and lesions tend to be much more prominent around the origins (ostia) of major branches. In descending order (after the lower abdominal aorta), the most heavily involved vessels are the coronary arteries, the popliteal arteries, the internal carotid arteries, and the vessels of the circle of Willis. Vessels of the upper extremities are usually spared, as are the mesenteric and renal arteries, except at their ostia. Nevertheless, in an individual case, the severity of atherosclerosis in one artery does not predict the severity in another. In an individual, and indeed within a particular artery, lesions at various stages often coexist.

Atherosclerotic plaques have three principal components: (1) cells, including SMCs, macrophages, and other leukocytes; (2) ECM, including collagen, elastic fibers, and proteoglycans; and (3) intracellular and extracellular lipid (Fig. 11–9). These components occur in varying proportions and configurations in different lesions. Typically, the superficial fibrous cap is composed of SMCs and relatively dense ECM. Beneath and to the side of the cap (the "shoulder") is a cellular area consisting of macrophages, SMCs, and T lymphocytes. Deep to the fibrous cap is a necrotic core, containing a disorganized mass of lipid (primarily cholesterol and cholesterol esters), cholesterol clefts, debris from dead cells, foam cells, fibrin, variably organized thrombus, and other plasma proteins. Foam cells are large, lipid-laden cells that derive predominantly from blood monocytes (tissue macrophages), but SMCs can also imbibe lipid to become foam cells. Finally, particularly around the periphery of the lesions, there is usually evidence of neovascularization (proliferating small blood vessels). Typical atheromas contain relatively abundant lipid.

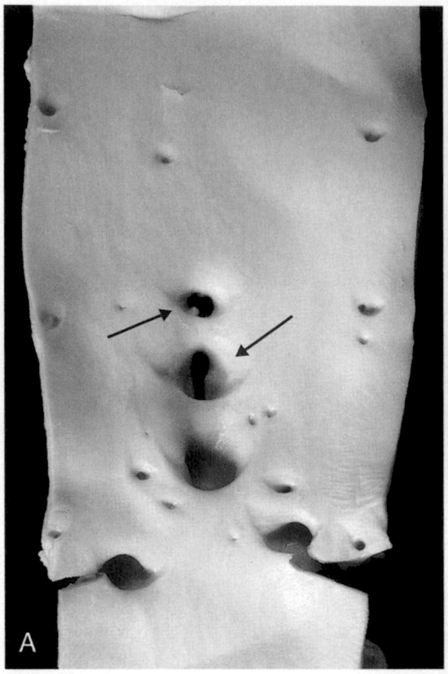

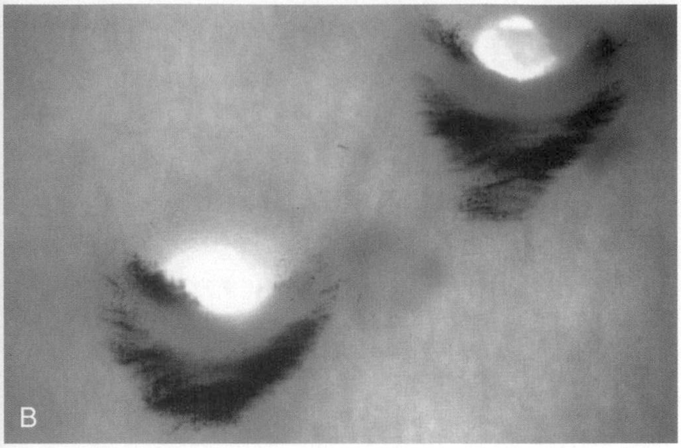

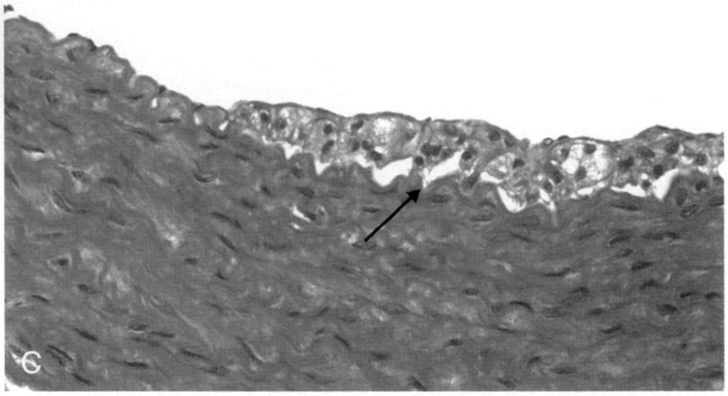

FIGURE 11–6 Fatty streak—a collection of foam cells in the intima. *A,* Aorta with fatty streaks (arrows), associated largely with the ostia of branch vessels. *B,* Close-up photograph of fatty streaks from aorta of experimental hypercholesterolemic rabbit shown following staining with Sudan red, a lipid-soluble dye, again illustrating the relationship of lesions to branch vessel ostia. *C,* Photomicrograph of fatty streak in experimental hypercholesterolemic rabbit, demonstrating intimal, macrophage-derived foam cells *(arrow).* (*B* and *C,* Courtesy of Myron I. Cybulsky, M.D., University of Toronto, Canada).

Nevertheless, many so-called fibrous plaques are composed mostly of SMCs and fibrous tissue.

Plaques generally continue to change and progressively enlarge through cell death and degeneration, synthesis and degradation (remodeling) of ECM, and organization of thrombus. Moreover, atheromas often undergo **calcification** (Fig. 11–9*C*). Patients with advanced coronary calcification appear to be at increased risk for coronary events.

The **advanced lesion** of atherosclerosis is at risk for the following pathological changes that have clinical significance:

- Focal **rupture, ulceration,** or **erosion** of the luminal surface of atheromatous plaques may result in exposure of highly thrombogenic substances that induce thrombus formation (Fig. 11–8*B*) or discharge of debris into the bloodstream, producing

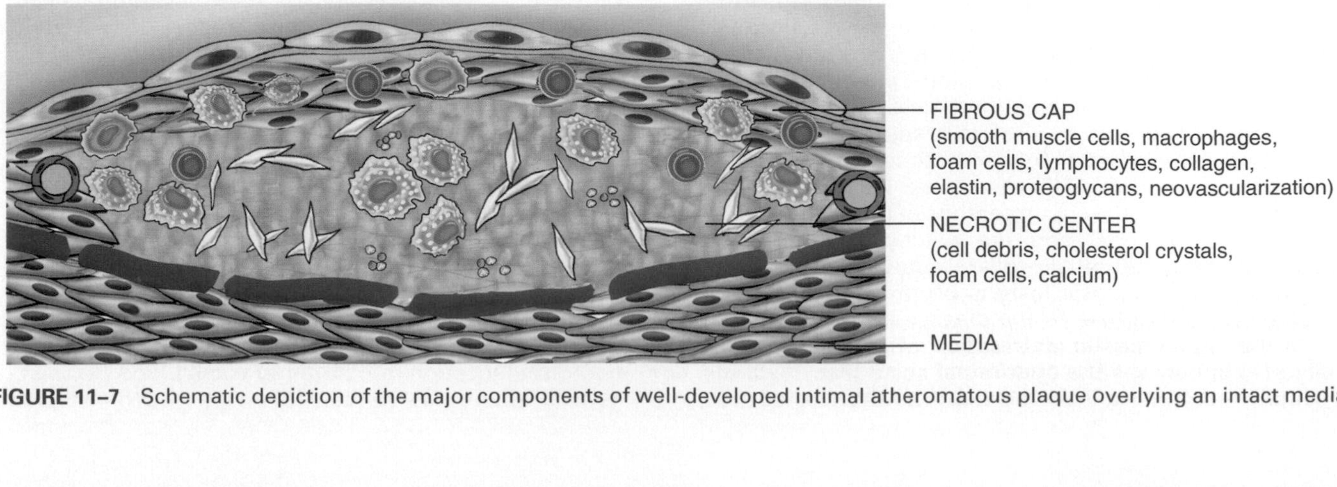

FIGURE 11–7 Schematic depiction of the major components of well-developed intimal atheromatous plaque overlying an intact media.

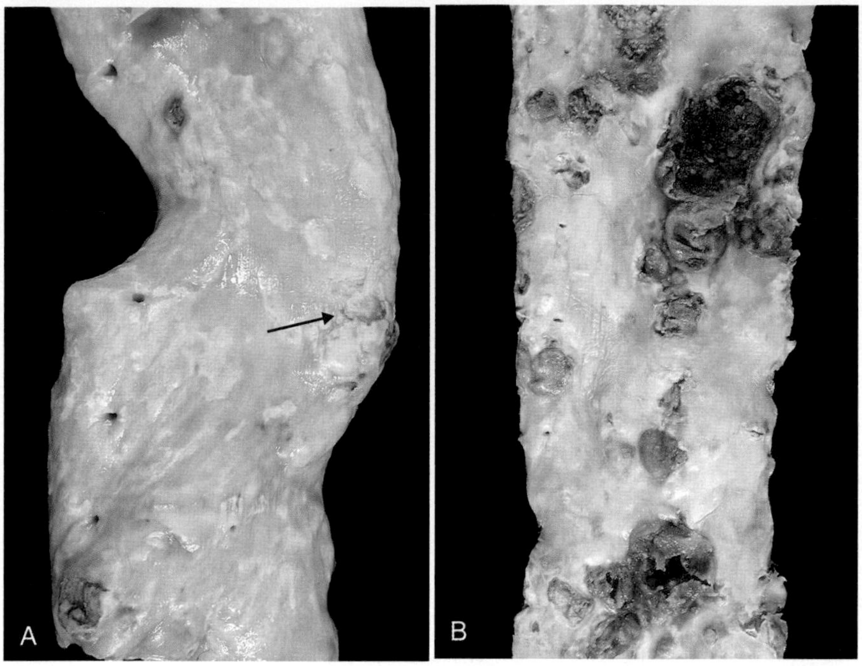

FIGURE 11–8 Gross views of atherosclerosis in the aorta. *A,* Mild atherosclerosis composed of fibrous plaques, one of which is denoted by the *arrow. B,* Severe disease with diffuse and complicated lesions.

microemboli composed of lesion contents **(cholesterol emboli or atheroemboli)**.

- **Hemorrhage** into a plaque, especially in the coronary arteries, may be initiated by rupture of either the overlying fibrous cap or the thin-walled capillaries that vascularize the plaque. A contained hematoma may expand the plaque or induce plaque rupture.
- Superimposed **thrombosis**, the most feared complication, usually occurs on disrupted lesions (those with rupture, ulceration, erosion, or hemorrhage) and may partially or completely occlude the lumen. Thrombi may heal and become incorporated into and thereby enlarge the intimal plaque.
- **Aneurysmal dilation** may result from ATH-induced atrophy of the underlying media, with loss of elastic tissue, causing weakness and potential rupture, discussed later.

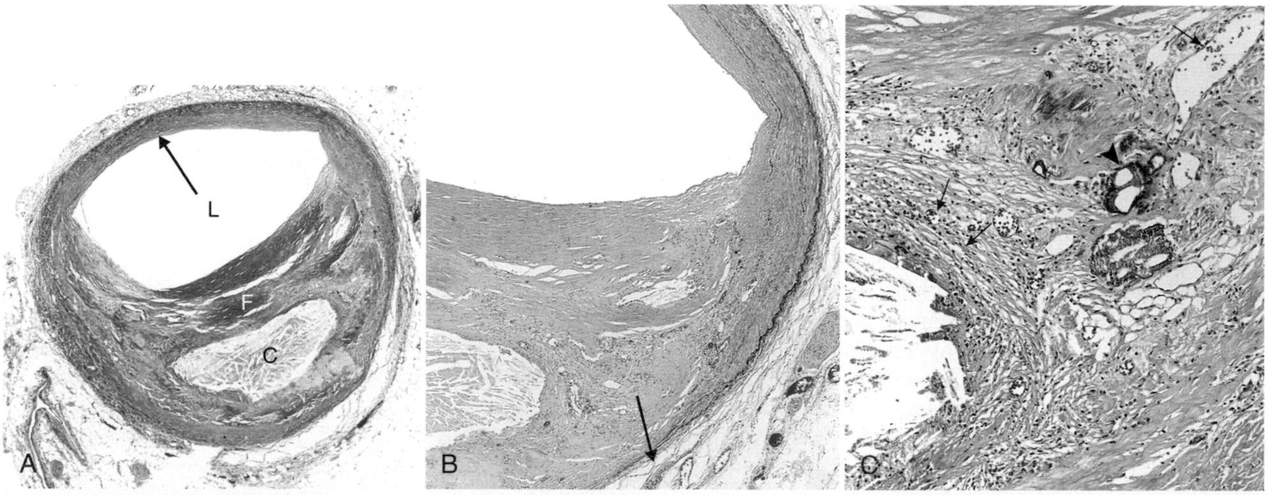

FIGURE 11–9 Histologic features of atheromatous plaque in the coronary artery. *A,* Overall architecture demonstrating fibrous cap (F) and a central necrotic (largely lipid) core (C). The lumen (L) has been moderately narrowed. Note that a segment of the wall is plaque free *(arrow).* In this section, collagen has been stained blue (Masson's trichrome stain). *B,* Higher-power photograph of a section of the plaque shown in *A,* stained for elastin (black), demonstrating that the internal and external elastic membranes are destroyed and the media of the artery is thinned under the most advanced plaque *(arrow). C,* Higher-magnification photomicrograph at the junction of the fibrous cap and core, showing scattered inflammatory cells, calcification *(broad arrow),* and neovascularization *(small arrows).*

EPIDEMIOLOGY AND RISK FACTORS

Virtually ubiquitous among most developed nations, atherosclerosis is much less prevalent in Central and South America, Africa, and Asia. The mortality rate for ischemic heart disease (IHD) in the United States is among the highest in the world and is approximately five times higher than that in Japan. Nevertheless, IHD has been increasing in Japan and is now that country's second leading cause of death.[15] Moreover, Japanese who immigrate to the United States and adopt the lifestyles and dietary customs of their new home acquire the predisposition to atherosclerosis typical of the American population.

Considerable progress on the health impact of atherosclerosis-related disease has been made over recent decades in the United States and elsewhere. Between 1963 (the peak year) and 2000 there was an approximately 50% decrease in the death rate from IHD and a 70% decrease in death from strokes, a reduction in mortality that increased the average life expectancy in the United States by approximately 3 years. Three factors contribute to this impressive improvement: (1) prevention of atherosclerosis through changes in lifestyle, including reduced cigarette smoking, altered dietary habits with reduced consumption of cholesterol and saturated animal fats, and control of hypertension; (2) improved methods of treatment of myocardial infarction and other complications of IHD; and (3) prevention of recurrences in patients who have previously suffered serious atherosclerosis-related clinical events.

The prevalence and severity of the disease among individuals and groups—and therefore the age when it is likely to cause tissue or organ injury—are related to a number of factors, some constitutional but others acquired and potentially controllable. The risk factors that predispose to ATH and resultant IHD have been identified by means of a number of prospective studies in well-defined population groups, most notably the Framingham (Massachusetts) Study and the Multiple Risk Factor Intervention Trial[16,17] (Table 11–2 and Fig. 11–10). The constitutional factors include age, sex, and genetics.

Age. Age is a dominant influence. Death rates from IHD rise with each decade even into advanced age. atherosclerosis is not usually clinically evident until middle age or later, when the arterial lesions precipitate organ injury. Between ages 40 and 60 the incidence of myocardial infarction increases fivefold.

Sex. Other factors being equal, males are much more prone to atherosclerosis and its consequences than are females. Myocardial infarction and other complications of atherosclerosis are uncommon in premenopausal women unless they are predisposed by diabetes, hyperlipidemia, or severe hypertension. After menopause, however, the incidence of atherosclerosis-related diseases increases, probably owing to a decrease in natural estrogen levels. Indeed, the frequency of myocardial infarction equalizes by the seventh to eighth decade of life.

Genetics. The well-established familial predisposition to atherosclerosis and IHD is most likely polygenic. Most commonly, the genetic propensity relates to familial clustering of other risk factors, such as hypertension or diabetes, while less commonly it involves well-defined hereditary genetic derangements in lipoprotein metabolism that result in excessively high blood lipid levels, such as familial hypercholesterolemia, which was discussed in Chapter 5.

TABLE 11–2 Risk Factors for Atherosclerosis

Major	Lesser, Uncertain, or Nonquantitated
Nonmodifiable	
Increasing age	Obesity
Male gender	Physical inactivity
Family history	Stress ("type A" personality)
Genetic abnormalities	Postmenopausal estrogen deficiency
	High carbohydrate intake
Potentially Controllable	
Hyperlipidemia	Alcohol
Hypertension	Lipoprotein Lp(a)
Cigarette smoking	Hardened (trans)unsaturated fat intake
Diabetes	*Chlamydia pneumoniae*

Other, nongenetic *risk factors, particularly diet, lifestyle, and personal habits, are to a large extent potentially reversible.* The four major risk factors potentially responsive to change are hyperlipidemia, hypertension, cigarette smoking, and diabetes.

Hyperlipidemia. Hyperlipidemia is a major risk factor for atherosclerosis. Most of the evidence specifically implicates *hypercholesterolemia.* Elevated levels of serum cholesterol are sufficient to stimulate lesion development, even if other risk

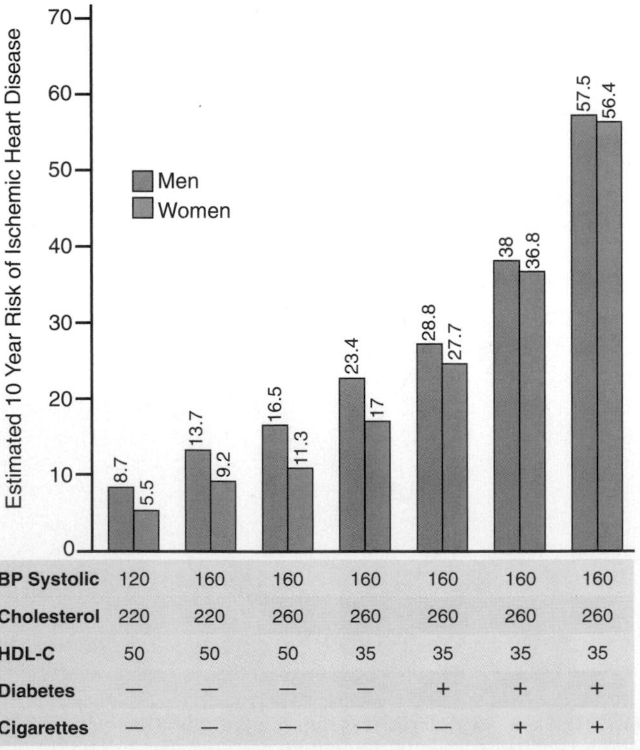

BP Systolic	120	160	160	160	160	160	160
Cholesterol	220	220	260	260	260	260	260
HDL-C	50	50	50	35	35	35	35
Diabetes	—	—	—	—	+	+	+
Cigarettes	—	—	—	—	—	+	+

FIGURE 11–10 Estimated 10-year risk of coronary artery disease according to various combinations of risk factor levels, expressed as the probability of an event in 10 years. HDL-C, high density lipoprotein cholesterol (From Kannel WB, et al: An update on coronary risk factors. Med Clin North Am 79:951, 1995.)

factors are absent.[18] The major component of total serum cholesterol associated with increased risk is low-density lipoprotein (LDL) cholesterol, which has an essential physiologic role as a vehicle for the delivery of cholesterol to peripheral tissues. In contrast, high-density lipoprotein (HDL) is believed to mobilize cholesterol from developing and existing atheromas and transport it to the liver for excretion in the bile, hence its designation as the "good cholesterol." Therefore, the higher the level of HDL, the lower is the risk. Understandably, there is thus great interest in dietary, pharmacologic, and behavioral methods of lowering serum LDL and raising serum HDL. Exercise and moderate consumption of ethanol both raise the HDL level, whereas obesity and smoking lower it.

High dietary intake of cholesterol and saturated fats, such as those present in egg yolk, animal fats, and butter, raises the plasma cholesterol level. Conversely, a diet low in cholesterol and low in the ratio of saturated-to-polyunsaturated fats lowers plasma cholesterol levels. Moreover, omega-3 fatty acids, abundant in fish oils, are likely beneficial, whereas hardened (trans)unsaturated fats produced by artificial hydrogenation of polyunsaturated vegetable fats and used in baked goods and margarine may adversely affect cholesterol profiles and contribute to atherosclerosis. The drugs called *statins* lower circulating cholesterol indirectly by inhibiting HMG CoA reductase, a key enzyme required for cholesterol biosynthesis in the liver (see Chapter 5).

Hypertension. Hypertension (see later) is a major risk factor for atherosclerosis at all ages. Men between ages 45 and 62 whose blood pressure exceeds 169/95 mm Hg have a more than fivefold greater risk of IHD than those with blood pressures of 140/90 mm Hg or lower. Both systolic and diastolic levels are important in increasing risk. Antihypertensive therapy reduces the incidence of atherosclerosis-related diseases, particularly strokes and IHD.

Cigarette Smoking. Cigarette smoking is a well-established risk factor in men and is thought to account for the relatively recent increase in the incidence and severity of atherosclerosis in women. Smoking one or more packs of cigarettes per day for several years increases the death rate from IHD by up to 200%. Cessation of smoking reduces the increased risk substantially.

Diabetes Mellitus. Diabetes mellitus induces hypercholesterolemia and a markedly increased predisposition to atherosclerosis. Other factors being equal, the incidence of myocardial infarction is twice as high in diabetics as in nondiabetics. There is also an increased risk of strokes and, even more striking, perhaps a 100-fold increased risk of atherosclerosis-induced gangrene of the lower extremities. The complex mechanisms of increased atherosoclrosis in diabetes are discussed in Chapter 24.

Other Factors. Patients with homocystinuria, a rare inborn error of metabolism resulting in high levels of circulating homocysteine (>100 μmol/L) and urinary homocysteine, have premature vascular disease. Beyond these individuals, clinical and epidemiologic studies have shown a more general relationship between total serum homocysteine levels and coronary artery disease, peripheral vascular disease, stroke, and venous thrombosis. Hyperhomocystinemia can potentially be caused by low folate and vitamin B intake, and recent evidence (obtained in women) suggests that folate and vitamin B_6 ingestion beyond conventional dietary recommendations may reduce the incidence of cardiovascular disease. However, this remains to be firmly establised.

Epidemiologic evidence also indicates that several markers of hemostatic and thrombotic function and inflammation are potent predictors of risk for major atherosclerotic events, including myocardial infarction and stroke. Such markers include those related to fibrinolysis (e.g., elevated plasminogen activator inhibitor-1) and inflammation (e.g., C-reactive protein; see below).

Lipoprotein Lp(a) is an altered form of LDL that contains the apolipoprotein B-100 portion of the LDL linked to apolipoprotein A. Epidemiologic studies suggest a correlation between increased blood levels of Lp(a) and coronary and cerebrovascular disease, independent of the level of total cholesterol or LDL.

Factors associated with a less pronounced and/or difficult-to-quantitate risk include lack of exercise; competitive, stressful life style with "type A" personality behavior; and unrestrained weight gain (largely because obesity induces hypertension, diabetes, hypertriglyceridemia, and decreased HDL). Epidemiologic data also indicate a protective role for moderate intake of alcohol.

Multiple risk factors may have a multiplicative effect; two major risk factors increase the risk approximately fourfold. When three risk factors are present (e.g., hyperlipidemia, hypertension, and smoking), the rate of myocardial infarction is increased seven times. However, atherosclerosis and its consequences may develop in the absence of any apparent risk factors, so that even those who live "the prudent life" and have no apparent genetic predispositions are not immune to this killer disease.

PATHOGENESIS

Understandably, the overwhelming importance of atherosclerosis has stimulated enormous efforts to discover its cause. Historically, two hypotheses for atherogenesis were dominant: One emphasized cellular proliferation in the intima, whereas the other emphasized organization and repetitive growth of thrombi. The contemporary view of the pathogenesis of atherosclerosis incorporates elements of both older theories and accommodates the risk factors previously discussed.[19,20] This concept, called *the response to injury hypothesis, considers atherosclerosis to be a chronic inflammatory response of the arterial wall initiated by injury to the endothelium. Moreover, lesion progression is sustained by interaction between modified lipoproteins, monocyte-derived macrophages, T lymphocytes, and the normal cellular constituents of the arterial wall* (Fig. 11–11). Central to this thesis are the following:

- *Chronic endothelial injury*, usually subtle, with resultant endothelial dysfunction, yielding increased permeability, leukocyte adhesion, and thrombotic potential
- Accumulation of *lipoproteins*, mainly LDL, with its high cholesterol content, in the vessel wall
- Modification of lesional lipoproteins by *oxidation*
- Adhesion of *blood monocytes* (and other leukocytes) to the endothelium, followed by their migration into the intima and their transformation into *macrophages* and *foam cells*
- Adhesion of *platelets*
- Release of factors from activated platelets, macrophages, or vascular cells that cause *migration of SMCs* from media into the intima

- Proliferation of smooth muscle cells in the intima, and elaboration of extracellular matrix, leading to the accumulation of collagen and proteoglycans
- *Enhanced accumulation of lipids* both within cells (macrophages and SMCs) and extracellularly.

Several aspects of the atherogenic process will now be considered in detail.

The Role of Endothelial Injury. Chronic or repetitive endothelial injury is the cornerstone of the response-to-injury hypothesis. Endothelial injury induced in experimental animals by mechanical denudation, hemodynamic forces, immune complex deposition, irradiation, and chemicals causes intimal thickening and, in the presence of high-lipid diets, typical atheromas. However, *early human lesions begin at sites of morphologically intact endothelium.* Thus, in the human disease, the initiating abnormality may be nondenuding endothelial dysfunction causing increased endothelial permeability, enhanced leukocyte adhesion, and alterations in expression of endothelial cell gene products.

The specific cause of endothelial dysfunction in early atherosclerosis is unknown: potential culprits include circulating derivatives of cigarette smoke, homocysteine, and possibly viruses and other infectious agents. Inflammatory cytokines, such as tumor necrosis factor (TNF), stimulate expression of endothelial genes that may promote atherosclerosis. However, the two most important determinants of endothelial alterations, perhaps acting in concert, are thought to be hemodynamic disturbances that accompany normal circulatory function and adverse effects of hypercholesterolemia.

In support of a hemodynamic effect is the well-defined tendency for plaques to occur at ostia of the vessels arising from the aorta, branch points, and along the posterior wall of the abdominal aorta where there are disturbed flow patterns. Areas of disturbed, turbulent flow and low shear stress are prone to atherosclerosis while those with smooth, laminar flow seem protected. The normal laminar flow typically encountered in *lesion-protected areas* of the arterial vasculature blocks inflammatory mechanisms that mediate endothelial dysfunction and apoptosis of endothelial cells believed to be important in plaque erosion (see Chapter 12). It also induces endothelial genes whose products (such as the antioxidant superoxide dismutase) *protect* against the development of lesions.[21,22] Thus, steady laminar flow protects against atherosclerosis, and induction of so-called atheroprotective genes in areas of laminar flow could in large part explain the nonrandom localization of early atherosclerotic lesions.

The Role of Inflammation. Inflammatory mechanisms mediate initiation, progression, and (as we will see in Chapter 12) the complications of atherosclerotic lesions.[23,24] The normal endothelium does not support binding of white blood

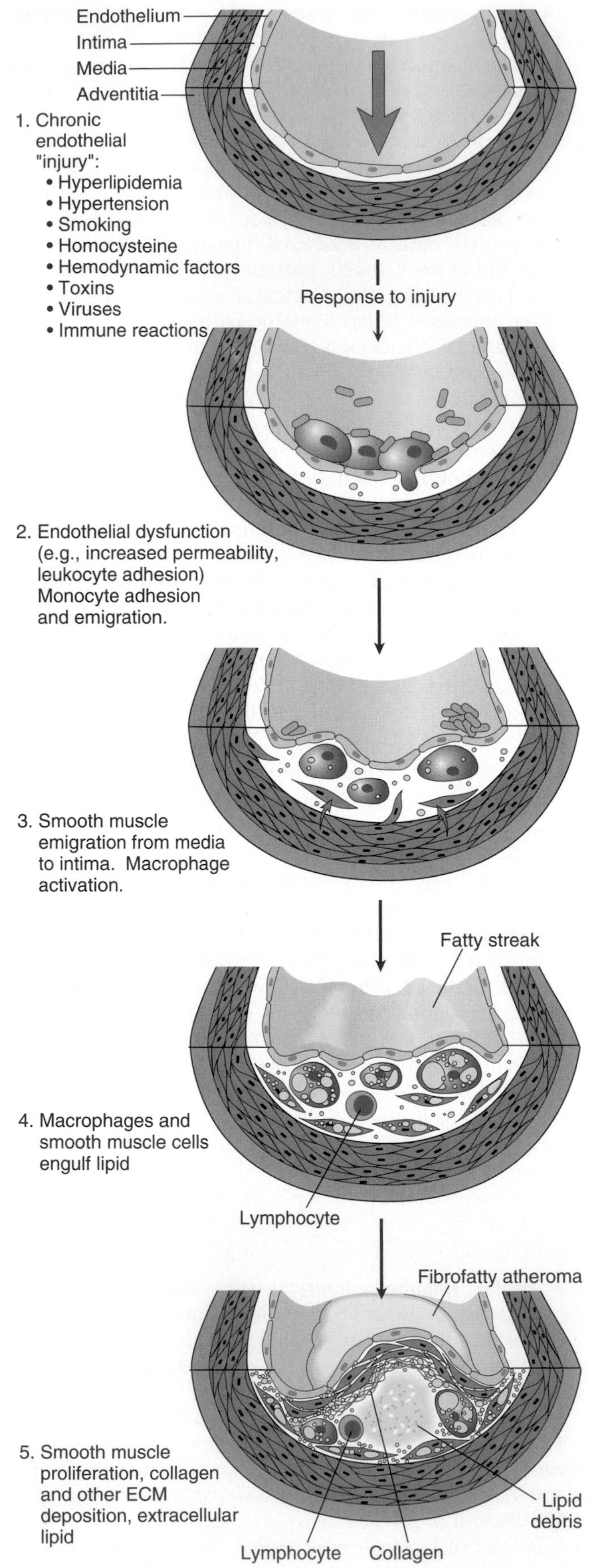

FIGURE 11–11 Evolution of arterial wall changes in the response to injury hypothesis. *1,* Normal. *2,* Endothelial injury with adhesion of monocytes and platelets (the latter to denuded endothelium). *3,* Migration of monocytes (from the lumen) and smooth muscle cells (from the media) into the intima. *4,* Smooth muscle cell proliferation in the intima. *5,* Well-developed plaque (see Fig. 11–7 for details of mature plaque structure).

cells. However, early in atherogenesis arterial endothelial cells begin to express on their surface selective adhesion molecules that bind various classes of leukocytes. Vascular cell adhesion molecule-1 (VCAM-1) binds precisely the types of leukocytes found in early human and experimental atheroma, the monocyte and T lymphocyte. After monocytes adhere to the endothelium, they (1) migrate between ECs to localize in the intima, largely stimulated by chemokines; and (2) transform into macrophages and avidly engulf lipoproteins, largely oxidized LDL.

Although recruitment of monocytes and their subsequent differentiation into macrophages and ultimately into foam cells is initially protective as they remove potentially harmful lipid particles, progressive accumulation ultimately results in lesion progression. Macrophages produce IL-1 and TNF, which increase adhesion of leukocytes. Several chemokines generated by macrophages, including monocyte chemotactic protein-1 (MCP-1), may recruit more leukocytes into the plaque. Macrophages produce toxic oxygen species that also cause oxidation of the LDL in the lesions, and they elaborate growth factors that may contribute to SMC proliferation.

T lymphocytes (both CD4+ and CD8+) are also recruited to the intima by chemoattractants. Cross-talk between macrophages and T cells results in cellular and humoral immune activation characteristic of a chronic inflammatory state. For example, T cells encounter signals that cause them to elaborate inflammatory cytokines, such as IFN-γ and lymphotoxin, which in turn can stimulate macrophages as well as vascular endothelial cells and SMCs. The identity of the antigens responsible for this immune activation is undetermined, but bacterial and viral antigens or heat-shock proteins (see later), and new antigens induced by modified arterial wall constituents or lipoproteins, are possibilities. The activated leukocytes and intrinsic arterial cells can release fibrogenic mediators, including a variety of peptide growth factors that can promote replication of SMCs and contribute to elaboration by these cells of a dense extracellular matrix characteristic of the more advanced atherosclerotic lesion.

The Role of Lipids. Recall from an earlier discussion (Chapter 5) that the various classes of blood lipids are transported as lipoproteins complexed to specific apoproteins. Dyslipoproteinemias result from either mutations that yield defective apolipoproteins or some other underlying disorder, such as the nephrotic syndrome, alcoholism, hypothyroidism, or diabetes mellitus. Examples of lipoprotein abnormalities frequently found in the population (and, indeed, present in many myocardial infarction survivors) are: (1) increased LDL cholesterol levels, (2) decreased HDL cholesterol levels, and (3) increased levels of the abnormal lipoprotein Lp(a) (see earlier).

The evidence implicating hypercholesterolemia in the genesis of atherosclerosis includes the following:

- The major lipids in atheromatous plaques are plasma-derived cholesterol and cholesterol esters.
- *Oxidized LDL* is observed in macrophages in arteries at sites of fatty streaks. Antioxidant treatment protects against the development of atherosclerosis in hypercholesterolemic experimental animals.
- *Genetic defects* in lipoprotein metabolism causing hyperlipoproteinemia are associated with accelerated atherosclerosis.[25] For example, homozygous familial hypercholesterolemia, which often results in myocardial infarction before age 20 years, is caused by defects in the LDL receptor, leading to inadequate hepatic uptake of LDL and markedly increased circulating LDL (see Chapter 5). This is also seen experimentally when atherosclerosis is induced in animals genetically modified to have abnormal lipid metabolism (such as apolipoprotein-deficient and LDL receptor-deficient mice).[26]
- Other genetic or acquired disorders (e.g., diabetes mellitus, hypothyroidism) that cause hypercholesterolemia lead to premature and severe atherosclerosis.
- Experimental animals fed high-cholesterol diets develop atherosclerosis-like vascular lesions.
- Epidemiologic analyses demonstrate a significant correlation between the severity of atherosclerosis and the levels of total plasma cholesterol or LDL cholesterol.
- Lowering levels of serum cholesterol by diet or drugs slows the rate of progression of atherosclerosis, causes regression of some plaques, and reduces the risk of cardiovascular events. Indeed, lowering cholesterol increases overall survival and reduces risk of atherosclerosis-related events in patients with established coronary heart disease who have elevated or average cholesterol levels, as well as in patients with hypercholesterolemia, but without overt atherosclerosis-related disease.

The mechanisms by which hyperlipidemia contributes to atherogenesis include the following:

- Chronic hyperlipidemia, particularly hypercholesterolemia, may directly impair EC function through increased production of oxygen free radicals that deactivate NO, the major endothelial-relaxing factor.
- With chronic hyperlipidemia, lipoproteins accumulate within the intima at sites of increased endothelial permeability.
- Chemical change of lipid induced by free radicals generated in macrophages or ECs in the arterial wall yields *oxidized (modified) LDL*. Oxidized LDL (1) is ingested by macrophages through the *scavenger receptor*, distinct from the LDL receptor (Chapter 5), thus forming foam cells; (2) increases monocyte accumulation in lesions; (3) stimulates release of growth factors and cytokines; and (4) is cytotoxic to ECs and SMCs.

The Role of Smooth Muscle Cells. *SMCs migrate from the media to the intima, where they proliferate and deposit ECM components, converting a fatty streak into a mature fibrofatty atheroma, and contribute to the progressive growth of atherosclerotic lesions.* Several growth factors have been implicated in the proliferation of SMCs, including PDGF (released by platelets adherent to a focus of endothelial injury, and by macrophages, ECs, and SMCs), FGF, and TGF-α. SMCs may also take up modified lipids, contributing to foam cell formation.

Vascular SMCs synthesize extracellular matrix molecules (notably collagen) that stabilize atherosclerotic plaques. However, activated inflammatory and immune cells in the plaque can lead to the death of intimal SMCs by apoptosis.[27]

The above discussion emphasizes that the evolving atheroma consists of a chronic inflammatory reaction, with macrophages, lymphocytes, ECs, and SMCs all expressing or contributing a variety of factors that influence cell function. At an early stage, the intimal plaque is an aggregation of foam cells of macrophage and SMC origin, some of which have died and released lipid and debris. With progression, the atheroma is modified by SMC-synthesized collagen and proteoglycans. Connective tissue is particularly prominent on the intimal aspect, producing the fibrous cap, but many lesions retain a central core of lipid-laden cells and fatty debris. Disruption of the fibrous cap with superimposed thrombus is often associated with catastrophic clinical events (Fig. 11–5 and below). Moreover, and as we will see in Chapter 12, inflammatory processes make a significant contribution to the precipitation of the acute complications of atherosclerosis.

OTHER FACTORS IN ATHEROGENESIS

Oligoclonality of Lesions. The monoclonal hypothesis of atherogenesis, put forth in 1977, was based on the observation that some human plaques are monoclonal or at most oligoclonal.[28] One interpretation of oligoclonality is that plaques may be equivalent to benign neoplastic growths, perhaps induced by an exogenous chemical (e.g., cholesterol or some of its oxidized products) or an oncogenic virus. A recent study showed, however, that clonal patches exist and are often greater than 4 mm in size in not only atherosclerotic but also normal arteries, consistent with the possibility that atherosclerotic plaques could arise in a pre-existing clonal patch.[29]

Infection. There is considerable interest in the possibility that infections may contribute to atherosclerosis; bacteria and viruses have been implicated, notably *Chlamydia pneumoniae* and *cytomegalovirus*, respectively.[30] Both organisms are widely distributed, can infect cells of the blood vessel wall, and exhibit persistence, latency, and recurrence of infection.

Evidence for participation of *C. pneumoniae* is strongest, and studies suggest that antibiotic therapy appropriate for this organism reduces recurrent clinical events in patients with IHD. Lines of evidence associating *C. pneumoniae* with atherosclerotic cardiovascular disease include seroepidemiologic studies, direct detection of bacterial components in atherosclerotic lesions, occasional isolation of viable organisms from coronary and carotid atheromatous tissue, and in vitro and animal experiments. The strongest evidence has been detection of bacterial components in atherosclerotic lesions.

However, proof of specific mechanisms by which bacteria or viruses can cause atherosclerosis remains elusive. Secondary infection of the lesions might potentiate the local effects of known risk factors, such as hypercholesterolemia, by accelerating the chronic inflammatory pathways that are associated with atherosclerotic lesions or by altering the response of vascular wall cells to injury.[31] Moreover, extravascular infection might influence the development of atheromatous lesions and their complications by altering systemic lipid metabolism or through circulating inflammatory mediators. For example, endotoxin or pro-inflammatory cytokines (such as IL-6) produced in response to a remote infection could promote the activation of vascular wall cells and leukocytes in pre-existing lesions.

In addition, infectious organisms might potentiate the complications of existing lesions. For example, *C. pneumoniae* heat-shock protein can activate macrophages to produce matrix-degrading proteinases that may weaken atherosclerotic plaques, rendering them susceptible to rupture and hence to thrombosis. Moreover, hepatic synthesis of acute-phase reactants at a nonvascular site of infection might promote thrombotic complications of atherosclerosis by altering the balance between coagulation and fibrinolysis.

Figure 11–12 summarizes the major proposed cellular mechanisms of atherogenesis, emphasizing the multifactorial pathogenesis of this disease. This schema considers atherosclerosis as a chronic inflammatory response of the vascular wall to a variety of events that are initiated early in life. Multiple mechanisms contribute to plaque formation and progression, including endothelial dysfunction, monocyte adhesion and infiltration, lipid accumulation and oxidation, smooth muscle proliferation, extracellular matrix deposition, and thrombosis.

CLINICOPATHOLOGIC EFFECTS OF ATHEROSCLEROTIC CORONARY ARTERY DISEASE

The complications of atherosclerotic coronary artery disease occur through impaired coronary perfusion relative to myocardial demand (myocardial ischemia). The vascular changes that may cause ischemia in the heart and other organs involve a complex dynamic interaction among fixed atherosclerotic narrowing of the epicardial coronary arteries, intraluminal thrombosis overlying a disrupted atherosclerotic plaque, platelet aggregation, and vasospasm. These factors and critical events in the clinical manifestations of coronary arterial atherosclerotic disease and its downstream consequences in the myocardium are summarized in Figure 11–5 and discussed in depth in Chapter 12.

PREVENTION

Efforts to reduce the consequences and impact of atherosclerosis include: *primary prevention* programs, aimed at either delaying atheroma formation or causing regression of established lesions in persons who have never suffered a serious complication of atherosclerotic coronary artery disease, and *secondary prevention* programs, intended to prevent recurrence of events such as myocardial infarction in patients with symptomatic disease.

As detailed above, there is ample justification for the following recommendations for primary prevention of atherosclerosis-related complications in adults, based on risk factor modification: abstention from or cessation of cigarette smoking, control of hypertension, weight reduction and increased exercise, moderation of alcohol consumption, and, most importantly, lowering total and LDL blood cholesterol levels while increasing HDL.

Moreover, several lines of evidence suggest that risk-factor evaluation and prevention directed at modification should begin in childhood:

- Pathology studies have established that atherosclerotic coronary artery disease begins in childhood.
- Cardiovascular risk factors in children predict the adult profile and have distinct ethnic and sex differences that relate to adult heart disease.
- Serum cholesterol concentrations and smoking are important determinants of the early stages of atherosclerosis noted at autopsy in adolescents and young adults.

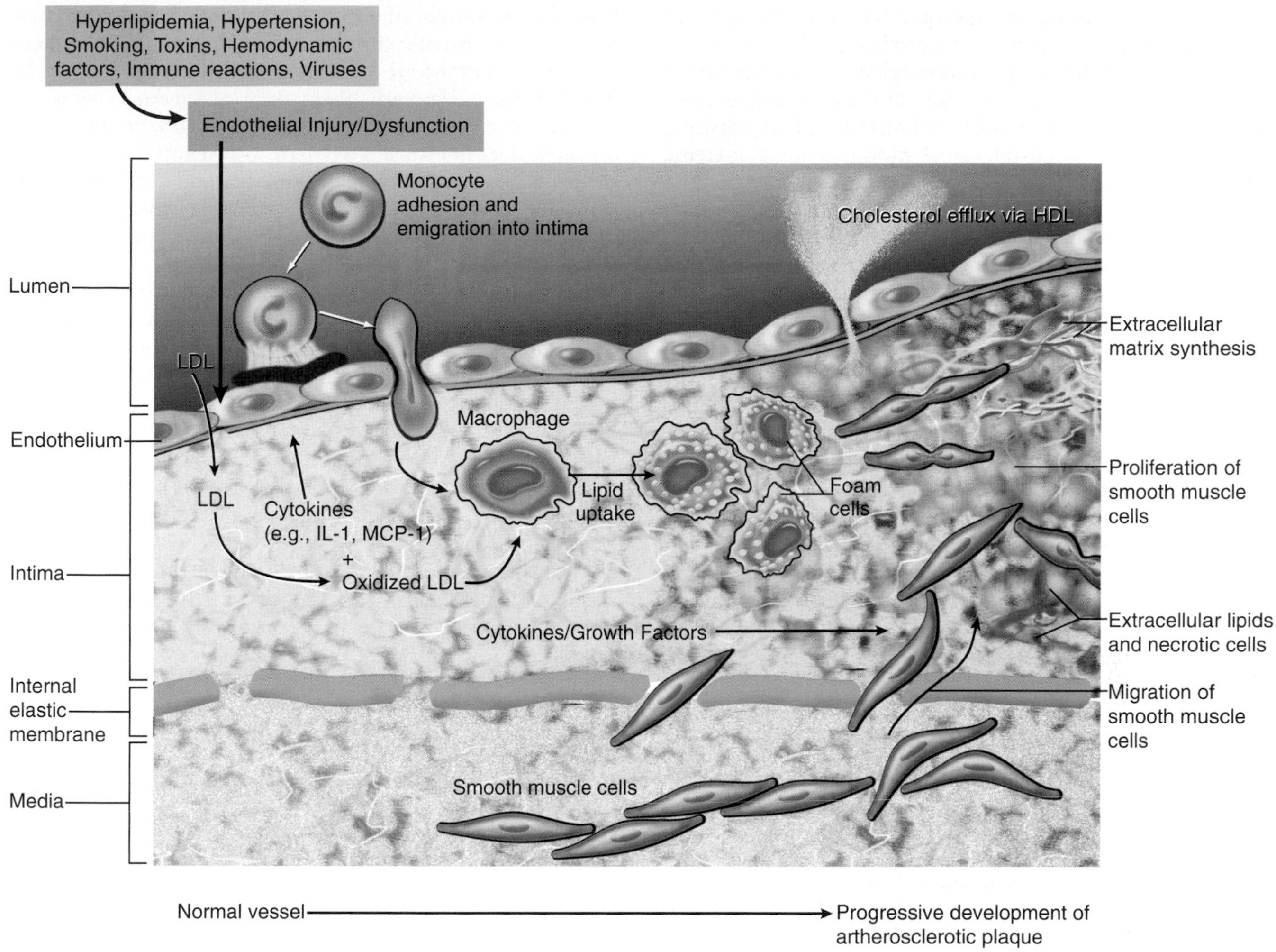

FIGURE 11–12 Schematic diagram of hypothetical sequence of cellular interactions in atherosclerosis. Hyperlipidemia and other risk factors are thought to cause endothelial injury, resulting in adhesion of platelets and monocytes and release of growth factors, including platelet-derived growth factor (PDGF), which lead to smooth muscle cell migration and proliferation. Foam cells of atheromatous plaques are derived from both macrophages and smooth muscle cells—from macrophages via the very-low-density lipoprotein (VLDL) receptor and low-density lipoprotein (LDL) modifications recognized by scavenger receptors (e.g., oxidized LDL), and from smooth muscle cells by less certain mechanisms. Extracellular lipid is derived from insudation from the vessel lumen, particularly in the presence of hypercholesterolemia, and also from degenerating foam cells. Cholesterol accumulation in the plaque reflects an imbalance between influx and efflux, and high-density lipoprotein (HDL) likely helps clear cholesterol from these accumulations. Smooth muscle cells migrate to the intima, proliferate, and produce extracellular matrix, including collagen and proteoglycans.

Hypertensive Vascular Disease

Systemic and local blood pressure must be tightly regulated. Low pressure causes inadequate organ perfusion, leading to dysfunction and ultimately death of underperfused tissues. In contrast, higher pressures that drive blood flow in excess of metabolic demand provide no benefit but may induce blood vessel and organ dysfunction and damage. Elevated blood pressure is called *hypertension.* As discussed above, hypertension is a risk factor for atherosclerosis. In this section, we shall discuss first the mechanisms of normal blood pressure control, next the possible mechanisms of hypertension, and finally the pathologic changes in the small blood vessels associated with the disorder.

HYPERTENSION

Hypertension is a common health problem with sometimes devastating consequences, and often remains asymptomatic until late in its course. Hypertension is one of the most important risk factors for both coronary artery disease and cerebrovascular accidents; hypertension can lead to cardiac hypertrophy and, potentially, heart failure *(hypertensive heart disease*; Chapter 12*)*, aortic dissection, and renal failure.

It is widely acknowledged that hypertension is a complex, multifactorial disease that has both genetic and environmental determinants. Molecular pathways underlying blood pressure variation have been recently elucidated,[32,33] creating possible targets for therapeutic intervention. Nevertheless, the pathogenic mechanisms of hypertension in the majority of affected individuals remain largely unknown.

Blood pressure (like height and weight) is considered to be a continuously distributed variable, and essential hypertension is one extreme of this distribution rather than a distinct disease. The detrimental effects of blood pressure increase continuously as the pressure rises, and no rigidly defined threshold level of blood pressure distinguishes risk from safety. Regardless, a sustained diastolic pressure greater than 90 mm Hg or a sustained systolic pressure in excess of 140 mm Hg is considered to constitute hypertension. By these criteria, screening programs reveal that 25% of persons in the general population are hypertensive. Hypertension affects more than 800 million individuals worldwide. The prevalence and vulnerability to complications increase with age and, for unknown reasons, are high in African Americans. Epidemiologic data indicate that systolic blood pressure is more important than diastolic blood pressure as a determinant of cardiovascular risk, except in young individuals.[34]

Reduction of blood pressure dramatically reduces the incidence and death rates from IHD, heart failure, and stroke. However, more than one fourth of those with hypertension are not aware that they have the disorder and, in as many as three fourths of those with known hypertension, the condition may be poorly controlled.[35]

Table 11–3 lists the major causes of hypertension. A small number of patients (approximately 5%) have underlying renal or adrenal disease (such as primary aldosteronism, Cushing syndrome, pheochromocytoma), narrowing of the renal artery, usually by an atheromatous plaque (renovascular hypertension) or other identifiable cause (secondary hypertension). *However, about 95% of hypertension is idiopathic (called essential hypertension). This form of hypertension generally does not cause short-term problems;* especially when controlled, is compatible with long life and is asymptomatic, unless a myocardial infarction, cerebrovascular accident, or other complication supervenes. Thus, this subgroup is often called *benign hypertension.*

A small percentage, perhaps 5%, of hypertensive persons show a rapidly rising blood pressure that if untreated, leads to death within a year or two. Called *accelerated* or *malignant hypertension*, the clinical syndrome is characterized by severe hypertension (i.e., systolic pressure over 200 mm Hg, diastolic pressure over 120 mm Hg), renal failure, and retinal hemorrhages and exudates, with or without papilledema. It may develop in previously normotensive persons but more often is superimposed on pre-existing benign hypertension, either essential or secondary.

TABLE 11–3 Types and Causes of Hypertension

Essential Hypertension
Secondary Hypertension
Renal
Acute glomerulonephritis
Chronic renal disease
Polycystic disease
Renal artery stenosis
Renal artery fibromuscular dysplasia
Renal vasculitis
Renin-producing tumors
Endocrine
Adrenocortical hyperfunction (Cushing syndrome, primary aldosteronism, congenital adrenal hyperplasia, licorice ingestion)
Exogenous hormones (glucocorticoids, estrogen [including pregnancy-induced and oral contraceptives], sympathomimetics and tyramine-containing foods, monoamine oxidase inhibitors)
Pheochromocytoma
Acromegaly
Hypothyroidism (myxedema)
Hyperthyroidism (thyrotoxicosis)
Pregnancy-induced
Cardiovascular
Coarctation of aorta
Polyarteritis nodosa (or other vasculitis)
Increased intravascular volume
Increased cardiac output
Rigidity of the aorta
Neurologic
Psychogenic
Increased intracranial pressure
Sleep apnea
Acute stress, including surgery

Pathogenesis of Hypertension. The multiple mechanisms of hypertension constitute aberrations of the normal physiologic regulation of blood pressure.[36] *Arterial hypertension occurs when the relationship between cardiac output and total peripheral resistance is altered.* For many of the secondary forms of hypertension, these factors are reasonably well understood. For example, in *renovascular hypertension*, renal artery stenosis causes decreased glomerular flow and pressure in the afferent arteriole of the glomerulus. This (1) induces renin secretion, initiating angiotensin II–mediated vasoconstriction and increased peripheral resistance, and (2) increases sodium reabsorption and therefore blood volume through the aldosterone mechanism. In pheochromocytoma, a tumor of the adrenal medulla (see Chapter 24), catecholamines produced by tumor cells cause episodic vasoconstriction and thus induce hypertension.

Regulation of Normal Blood Pressure. *Blood pressure is proportional to cardiac output and peripheral vascular resistance* (Fig. 11–13). *Indeed, the blood pressure level is a complex trait that is determined by the interaction of multiple genetic, environmental, and demographic factors that influence cardiac output and vascular resistance.* The major factors that determine blood pressure variation within and between populations include age, gender, body mass index, and diet, principally sodium intake.

Cardiac output is highly dependent on blood volume, itself greatly influenced by the whole body sodium homeostasis. Peripheral vascular resistance is determined mainly at the level of the arterioles and is affected by neural and hormonal factors. Normal vascular tone reflects the balance between humoral vasoconstricting influences (including angiotensin II, catecholamines, and endothelin) and vasodilators (including kinins, prostaglandins, and NO). Resistance vessels also exhibit *autoregulation*, whereby increased blood flow induces vasoconstriction to protect against tissue hyperperfusion. Other local factors such as pH and hypoxia, and the α- and β-adrenergic systems, which influence heart rate, cardiac contraction, and vascular tone, may be important. The integrated function of these systems ensures adequate perfusion of all tissues, despite regional differences in demand.

The kidneys play an important role in blood pressure regulation as follows:

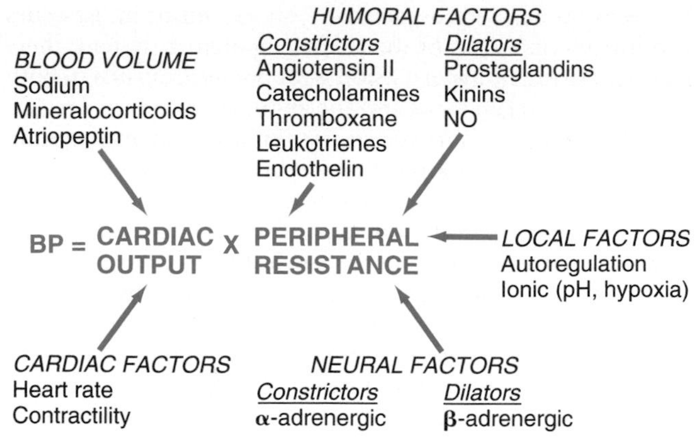

FIGURE 11–13 The critical roles of cardiac output and peripheral resistance in blood pressure regulation. NO, nitric oxide.

■ Through the renin-angiotensin system, the kidney influences both peripheral resistance and sodium homeostasis. Renin elaborated by the juxtaglomerular cells of the kidney converts *plasma angiotensinogen* to *angiotensin I*, which is then converted to *angiotensin II* by angiotensin-converting enzyme (Fig. 11–14). Angiotensin II raises blood pressure by increasing both peripheral resistance (direct action on vascular SMCs) and blood volume (stimulation of aldosterone secretion, increase in distal tubular reabsorption of sodium).

■ The kidney also produces a variety of vascular relaxing, or antihypertensive, substances (including prostaglandins and NO), which presumably counterbalance the vasopressor effects of angiotensin.

■ When blood volume is reduced, the *glomerular filtration rate* falls, leading to increased reabsorption of sodium by proximal tubules and thereby conserving sodium and expanding blood volume.

■ *Natriuretic factors*, including the natriuretic peptides secreted by atrial and ventricular myocardium in response to volume expansion, inhibit sodium reabsorption in distal tubules and thereby cause sodium excretion and diuresis. Natriuretic peptides also induce vasodilation and may be considered to represent endogenous inhibitors of the renin-angiotensin system.[37]

■ When renal excretory function is impaired, increased arterial pressure is a compensatory mechanism that helps restore fluid and electrolyte balance.

Mechanisms of Essential Hypertension. It is now thought that essential hypertension results from an interaction of

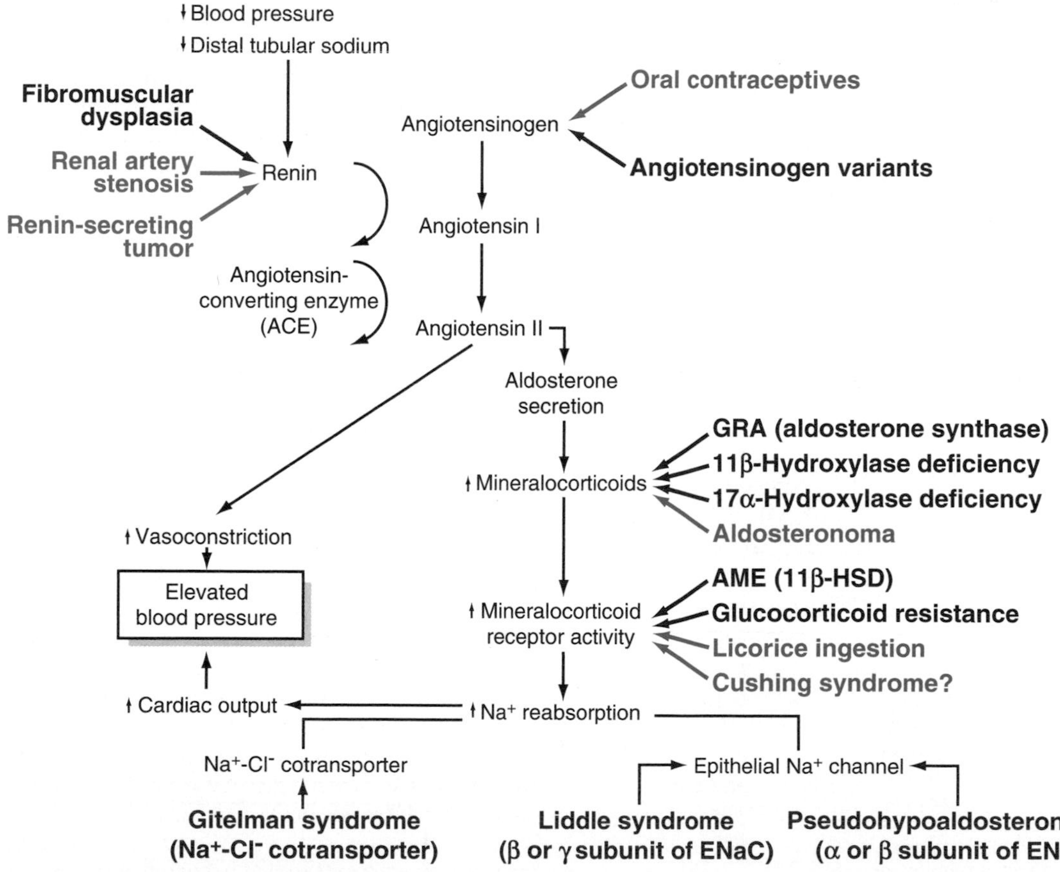

FIGURE 11–14 Blood pressure regulation by the renin-angiotensin system and the central roles of sodium metabolism in specific causes of inherited and acquired forms of hypertension. Components of the systemic renin-angiotensin system are shown in black. Genetic disorders that affect blood pressure by altering activity of this pathway are indicated in red; *arrows* indicate sites in the pathway altered by mutation. Genes that are mutated in these disorders are indicated in parentheses. Acquired disorders that alter blood pressure through effects on this pathway are indicated in blue. (From Lifton RP, et al: Molecular genetics of human blood pressure variation. Science 272:676, 1996.)

genetic and environmental factors that affect cardiac output, peripheral resistance, or both (Fig. 11–15).

Genetic factors clearly play a role in determining blood pressure levels, as shown by studies comparing blood pressure in monozygotic and dizygotic twins, studies of familial aggregation of hypertension comparing the blood pressure of biologic and adoptive siblings, and adoption studies. Moreover, several single-gene disorders cause relatively rare forms of hypertension (and hypotension) (see Fig. 11–16) by altering net sodium reabsorption in the kidney. The strong effect of sodium balance is emphasized by considering that the kidneys filter 170 liters of plasma containing 23 moles of salt daily; on a typical 100-mEq sodium diet, this means that 99.5% of the filtered salt must be reabsorbed. This is accomplished by an integrated system of ion channels, exchangers, and transporters. Absorption of the last 2% of sodium occurs via the epithelial Na^+ channel (ENaC), highly regulated by the renin-angiotensin system in the cortical collecting tubule; this site determines net sodium balance (see below).

Single-gene disorders cause relatively rare and severe forms of hypertension through several mechanisms (see Figs. 11–14 and 11–16). These include:

- Gene defects in enzymes involved in aldosterone metabolism (e.g., aldosterone synthase, 11β-hydroxylase, 17α-hydroxylase). These lead to an adaptive increase in secretion of aldosterone, increased salt and water resorption, plasma volume expansion and, ultimately, hypertension.
- Mutations in proteins that affect sodium reabsorption. For example, the moderately severe form of salt-sensitive hypertension, called *Liddle syndrome*, is caused by mutations in an ENaC protein that lead to increased distal tubular reabsorption of sodium induced by aldosterone.

Inherited variations in blood pressure may also depend on the cumulative effects of allelic forms of several genes that affect blood pressure. For example, predisposition to essential hypertension has been associated with variations in the genes encoding components of the renin-angiotensin system: there is an association of hypertension with polymorphisms in both the angiotensinogen locus and the angiotensin II type I receptor locus.[38] Genetic variants in the renin-angiotensin system may contribute to the known racial differences in blood pressure regulation.

Reduced renal sodium excretion in the presence of normal arterial pressure may well be the key initiating event in essential hypertension and, indeed, a final common pathway for the pathogenesis of hypertension (see bottom of Fig. 11–14). Decreased sodium excretion might lead sequentially to an increase in fluid volume, increased cardiac output, and peripheral vasoconstriction, thereby elevating blood pressure (Fig. 11–15). At the higher setting of blood pressure, enough additional sodium could be excreted by the kidneys to equal intake and prevent fluid retention. Thus, an altered but steady state of sodium excretion would be achieved ("resetting of pressure natriuresis"), but at the expense of stable increases in blood pressure.

An alternative hypothesis implicates *vasoconstrictive influences* (either factors that induce functional vasoconstriction or stimuli that induce direct structural changes in the vessel wall, causing increased peripheral resistance) as the primary cause of hypertension. Moreover, chronic or repeated vasoconstrictive influences could cause structural thickening of the resistant vessels. In this model, the structural changes in the vessel wall may occur early in hypertension, preceding rather than being strictly secondary to the vasoconstriction.

Environmental factors could modify expression of the genetic determinants of increased pressure. Stress, obesity, smoking, physical inactivity, and heavy consumption of salt have all been implicated as exogenous factors in hypertension. Indeed, evidence linking the level of dietary sodium intake with the prevalence of hypertension in different population groups is particularly impressive. Moreover, in both essential

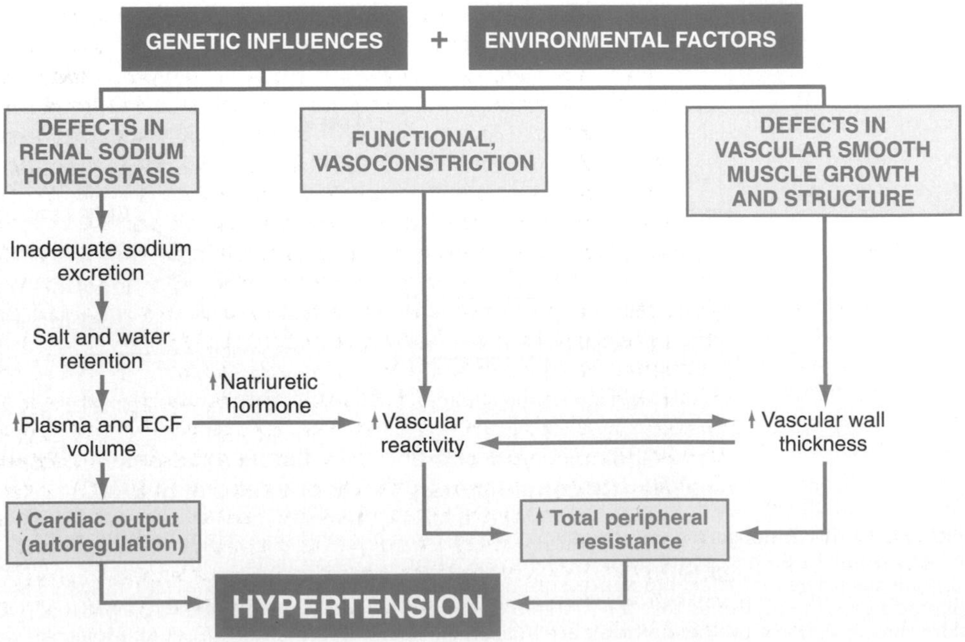

FIGURE 11–15 Hypothetical scheme for the pathogenesis of essential hypertension, implicating genetic defects in renal excretion of sodium, functional regulation of vascular tone, and structural regulation of vascular caliber. Environmental factors, especially increased salt intake, may potentiate the effects of genetic factors. The resultant increases in cardiac output and peripheral resistance contribute to hypertension. ECF, extracellular fluid.

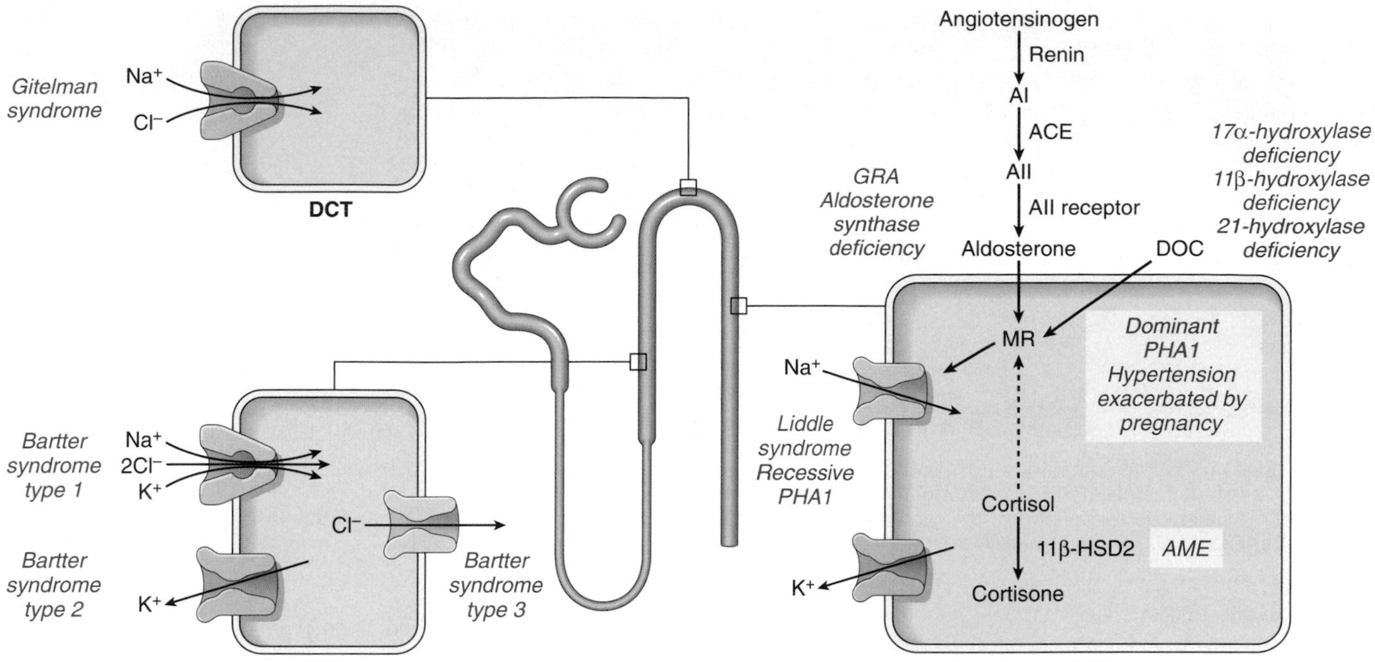

FIGURE 11–16 Mutations altering blood pressure in humans. A diagram of a nephron, the filtering unit of the kidney, is shown. The molecular pathways mediating NaCl reabsorption in individual renal cells in the thick ascending limb of the loop of Henle (TAL), distal convoluted tubule (DCT), and the cortical collecting tubule (CCT) are indicated, along with the pathway of the renin-angiotensin system, the major regulator of renal salt reabsorption. Single gene defects that manifest as inherited diseases affecting these pathways are indicated, with hypertensive disorders in red and hypotensive disorders in blue. Abbreviations: AI, angiotensin I; ACE, angiotensin converting enzyme; AII, angiotensin II; MR, mineralocorticoid receptor; GRA, glucocorticoid-remediable aldosteronism; PHA1, pseudo-hypoaldosteronism, type 1; AME, apparent mineralocorticoid excess; 11β–HSD2, 11β-hydroxysteroid dehydrogenase-2; and DOC, deoxycorticosterone. (From Lifton RP, et al: Molecular mechanisms of human hypertension. Cell 104:545, 2001.)

and secondary hypertension, heavy sodium intake augments the condition.

To summarize, essential hypertension is a complex, multifactorial disorder. Although single gene disorders can be responsible for hypertension in unusual cases, it is unlikely that a mutation at a single gene locus is a major cause of essential hypertension in the larger population. It is more likely that essential hypertension results from the combined effect of mutations or polymorphisms at several gene loci that influence blood pressure, interacting with a variety of environmental factors. Thus, environmental factors (e.g., stress, salt intake) affect the variables that control blood pressure in the genetically predisposed individual. Mendelian forms of hypertension and hypotension are rare but yield insights into pathways and mechanisms of blood pressure regulation, and they may help define rational targets for therapeutic intervention. Sustained hypertension requires participation of the kidney, since the kidney normally responds to hypertension by eliminating salt and water. Susceptibility genes for essential hypertension in the larger population are currently unknown but may well include genes that govern responses to an increased renal sodium load, levels of pressor substances, reactivity of vascular SMCs to pressor agents, or SMC growth. In established hypertension, both increased blood volume and increased peripheral resistance contribute to the increased pressure.

Vascular Pathology in Hypertension. Hypertension not only accelerates atherogenesis but also causes degenerative changes in the walls of large and medium arteries that potentiate both aortic dissection and cerebrovascular hemorrhage. Hypertension is also associated with two forms of small blood vessel disease: hyaline arteriolosclerosis and hyperplastic arteriolosclerosis (Fig. 11–17).

Morphology

Hyaline Arteriolosclerosis. This vascular lesion consists of a homogeneous, pink, hyaline thickening of the walls of arterioles with loss of underlying structural detail, and with narrowing of the lumen (Fig. 11–17*A*). Encountered frequently in elderly patients, whether normotensive or hypertensive, hyaline arteriolosclerosis is more generalized and more severe in patients with hypertension. It is also common in diabetes as part of the characteristic microangiography (Chapter 24).

The lesions reflect leakage of plasma components across vascular endothelium and excessive extracellular matrix production by SMCs secondary to the chronic hemodynamic stress of hypertension or a metabolic stress in diabetes that accentuates EC injury. **Hyaline arteriolosclerosis is a major morphologic characteristic of benign nephrosclerosis,** in which the arteriolar narrowing causes diffuse impairment of renal blood supply, loss of nephrons, and symmetric contraction of the kidneys (Chapter 20).

Hyperplastic Arteriolosclerosis. Related to more acute or severe elevations of blood pressure, hyper-

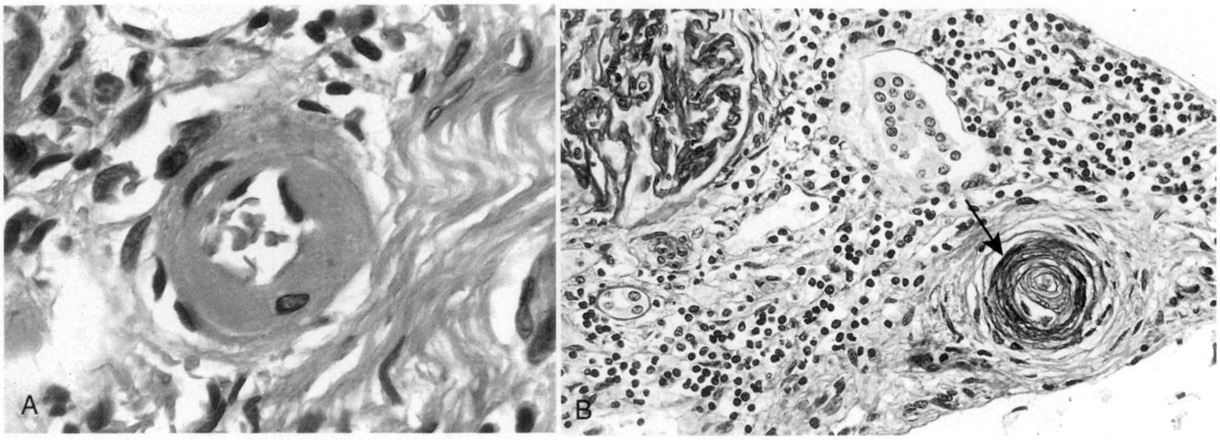

FIGURE 11–17 Vascular pathology in hypertension. *A,* Hyaline arteriolosclerosis. The arteriolar wall is hyalinized, and the lumen is markedly narrowed. *B,* Hyperplastic arteriolosclerosis (onionskinning) causing luminal obliteration *(arrow),* with secondary ischemic changes, manifested by wrinkling of the glomerular capillary vessels at the upper left (periodic acid-Schiff [PAS] stain). (Courtesy of Helmut Rennke, M.D., Brigham and Women's Hospital, Boston, MA.)

plastic arteriolosclerosis is characteristic of but not limited to malignant hypertension (diastolic pressures usually over 120 mm Hg). Hyperplastic arteriolosclerosis has onionskin, concentric, laminated thickening of the walls of arterioles with progressive narrowing of the lumina (see Fig. 11–17*B*). With the electron microscope, the laminations are seen to consist of SMCs and thickened and reduplicated basement membrane. In malignant hypertension, these hyperplastic changes are accompanied by deposits of fibrinoid and acute necrosis of the vessel walls, referred to as **necrotizing arteriolitis**, particularly in the kidney (see Chapter 20).

Aneurysms and Dissections

An *aneurysm* is a *localized abnormal dilation of a blood vessel or the wall of the heart* (Fig. 11–18). When an *aneurysm* is bounded by arterial wall components or the attenuated wall of the heart, it is called a *true aneurysm*. Atherosclerotic, syphilitic, and congenital vascular aneurysms and the left ventricular aneurysm that can follow a myocardial infarction are of this type. In contrast, a *false aneurysm* (also called *pseudoaneurysm*) is a breach in the vascular wall leading to an extravascular hematoma that freely communicates with the intravascular space ("pulsating hematoma"). The most common false aneurysm is a post-myocardial infarction rupture that has been contained by a pericardial adhesion, or a leak at the junction *(anastomosis)* of a vascular graft with a natural artery. An arterial *dissection* arises when blood enters the wall of the artery, as a hematoma dissecting between its layers (see Fig. 11–20). Dissections may, but do not always, arise in aneurysmal arteries. Aneurysms and dissections are most important when they involve the aorta.[39] Both true and false aneurysms, as well as dissections, can rupture.

The two most important causes of aortic aneurysms are atherosclerosis and cystic medial degeneration of the arterial media. However, any vessel may be affected by a wide variety of disorders that weaken the wall, including trauma (traumatic aneurysms or arteriovenous aneurysms), congenital defects

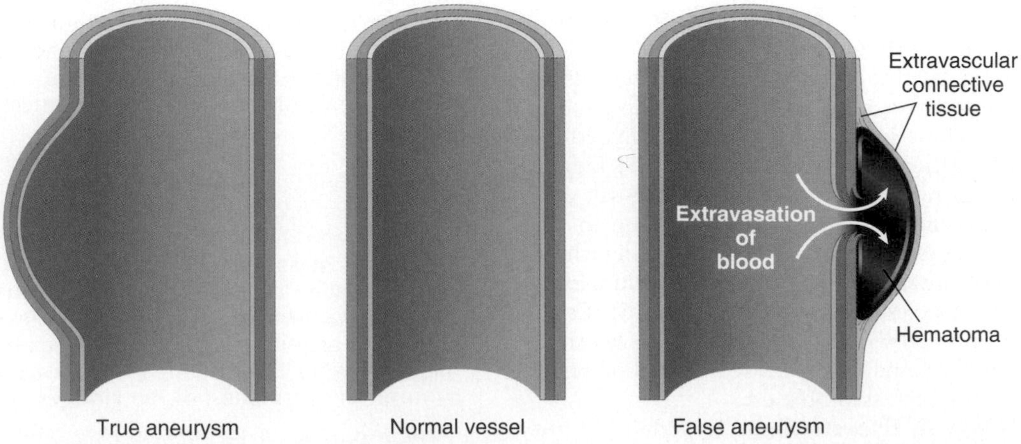

FIGURE 11–18 True and false aneurysms. *Center,* Normal vessel. *Left,* True aneurysm. The wall bulges outward and may be attenuated but is intact. *Right,* False aneurysm. The wall is ruptured, and there is a collection of blood (hematoma) that is bounded externally by adherent extravascular tissues.

such as those potentiating *berry* aneurysms, which are small, spherical dilatations, most frequently in the brain (see Chapter 28); infections (mycotic aneurysms, see below); syphilis; or trauma. Arterial aneurysms can also be caused by systemic diseases, as in some vasculitides (see later).

Infection of a major artery that weakens its wall gives rise to *mycotic aneurysm.* Thrombosis and rupture are possible complications. Mycotic aneurysms may originate either (1) from embolization and arrest of a septic embolus at some point within a vessel, usually as a complication of infective endocarditis; (2) as an extension of an adjacent suppurative process; or (3) by circulating organisms directly infecting the arterial wall.

For descriptive purposes, aneurysms can be classified by macroscopic shape and size. *Saccular* aneurysms are essentially spherical (involving only a portion of the vessel wall) and vary in size from 5 to 20 cm in diameter, often partially or completely filled by thrombus. Alternatively, aneurysms may be *fusiform* (involving a long segment). Fusiform aneurysms vary in diameter (up to 20 cm) and in length; many involve the entire ascending and transverse portions of the aortic arch, whereas others may involve large segments of the abdominal aorta or even the iliacs. However, these shapes are not specific for any disease or clinical manifestations.

ABDOMINAL AORTIC ANEURYSMS

Atherosclerosis, the most frequent etiology of aneurysms, causes arterial wall thinning through medial destruction secondary to plaque that originates in the intima. *Atherosclerotic aneurysms occur most frequently in the abdominal aorta (abdominal aortic aneurysm,* often abbreviated AAA),[40] but the common iliac arteries, the arch, and descending parts of the thoracic aorta can be involved.

Morphology. Usually positioned below the renal arteries and above the bifurcation of the aorta (Fig. 11–19), AAAs are saccular or fusiform, sometimes up to 15 cm in greatest diameter and of variable length (up to 25 cm). In areas of severe complicated atherosclerosis, destruction and thinning of the underlying aortic media can weaken the wall. The aneurysm and the nearby aorta often contain atheromatous ulcers covered by granular mural thrombi, prime sites for the formation of atheroemboli that may lodge in the vessels of the kidneys or lower extremities. Additionally, a thrombus frequently fills at least part of the dilated segment. Occasionally the aneurysm may affect the origins of the renal and superior or inferior mesenteric arteries, either by producing direct pressure on these vessels or by narrowing or occluding their ostia with mural thrombi. Not infrequently, AAAs are accompanied by smaller fusiform or saccular dilations of the iliac arteries.

Two variants of AAAs merit special mention. **Inflammatory abdominal aortic aneurysms** are characterized by dense periaortic fibrosis containing an abundant, inflammatory reaction rich in lymphocytes and plasma cells with many macrophages and often giant cells. Their cause is uncertain. **Mycotic abdominal aortic aneurysms** are atherosclerotic AAAs that have become infected by lodgment of circulating organisms in the wall, particularly in bacteremia from a primary *Salmonella* gastroenteritis. In such cases, suppuration can further destroy the media, potentiating rapid dilation and rupture.

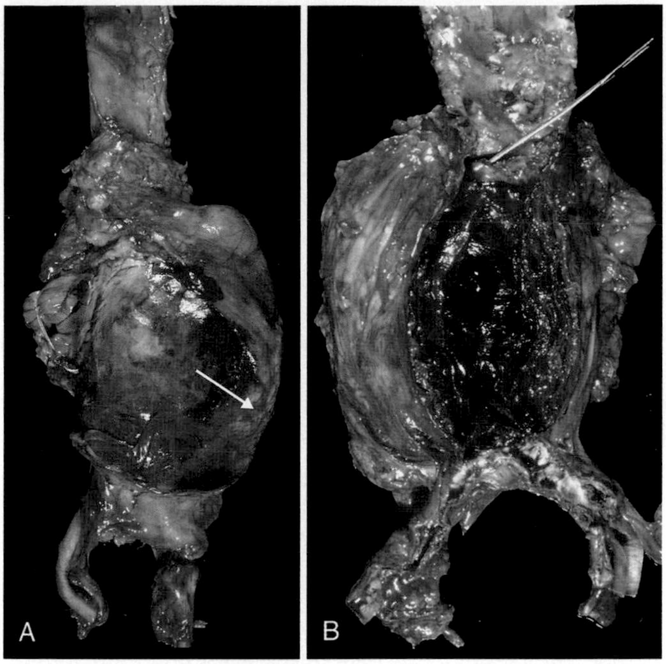

FIGURE 11–19 Abdominal aortic aneurysm. *A,* External view, gross photograph of a large aortic aneurysm that ruptured; the rupture site is indicated by the *arrow. B,* Opened view, with the location of the rupture tract indicated by a probe. The wall of the aneurysm is exceedingly thin, and the lumen is filled by a large quantity of layered but largely unorganized thrombus.

Pathogenesis. Atherosclerosis is a major cause of AAAs, but other factors may contribute. AAAs rarely develop before age 50 and are more common in men. There is a genetic susceptibility to AAA beyond the genetic predisposition to atherosclerosis or hypertension. For example, as discussed subsequently in the section on Marfan syndrome and aortic dissection, genetic defects in a connective tissue component responsible for the strength of the aorta can themselves produce aneurysms and dissections. Recent attention has focused on an altered balance of collagen degradation and synthesis mediated by local inflammatory infiltrates and the destructive proteolytic enzymes they produce and regulate. The genetic predisposition may be related to the quality of the aortic connective tissue. Thus, abnormal collagen or its remodeling could provide a susceptible substrate on which atherosclerosis or hypertension, or both, could act to weaken the aortic wall. In this regard, the matrix metalloproteinases (MMPs) have been implicated in the development of aortic aneurysms through increased proteolysis of extracellular matrix proteins. MMPs are expressed in aortic aneurysms at elevated levels compared with normal vessel wall, particularly in macrophages. These enzymes have the capacity to degrade virtually all components of the extracellular matrix in the arterial wall (collagens, elastin, proteoglycans, laminin, fibronectin). A decreased level of tissue inhibitor of metalloproteinases (TIMP) has been reported in aortic aneurysms.

Moreover, in experimental models, inhibitors of MMPs, MMP gene disruption, or the overexpression of TIMP-1 may block aneurysm development.[41–44]

Clinical Course. The clinical consequences of AAAs include:

- Rupture into the peritoneal cavity or retroperitoneal tissues with massive, potentially fatal, hemorrhage
- Obstruction of a vessel, particularly of the iliac, renal, mesenteric, or vertebral branches that supply the spinal cord leading to ischemic tissue injury
- Embolism from atheroma or mural thrombus
- Impingement on an adjacent structure, such as compression of a ureter or erosion of vertebrae
- Presentation as an abdominal mass (often palpably pulsating) that simulates a tumor.

The risk of rupture is directly related to the size of the aneurysm.[45] Risk varies from zero for a small AAA (less than approximately 4 cm in diameter), to 1% per year for aneurysms measuring 4.0 to 4.9 cm indiameter, 11% per year for aneurysms between 5.0 and 5.9 cm in diameter, and 25% per year for those larger than 6.0 cm. Most aneurysms expand at a rate of 0.2 to 0.3 cm/year, but 20% expand more rapidly. The most important clinical factor affecting aneurysm growth is blood pressure, based on La Place's law describing the wall tension as proportional to both diameter and internal pressure in the lumen. Large aneurysms are managed aggressively; operative mortality for unruptured aneurysms is approximately 5%, whereas emergency surgery after rupture carries a mortality rate of more than 50%. As a reflection of the systemic nature of ATH and its complications, patients with AAAs are also at significantly increased risk for myocardial infarction and stroke.

The treatment of abdominal and thoracic aortic aneurysms is evolving toward endoluminal approaches using stent grafts (expandable wire frames covered by a cloth sleeve) rather than surgery for some patients.[46,47]

SYPHILITIC (LUETIC) ANEURYSMS

The obliterative endarteritis characteristic of the tertiary stage of syphilis (lues) shows a predilection for small vessels, with complications especially in the aorta and nervous system (Chapter 8). Syphilitic involvement of the vasa vasorum of the thoracic aorta can lead to aneurysmal dilation that can include the aortic annulus. Fortunately, better control and treatment of syphilis in its early stages have decreased the frequency of these complications.

Morphology. Inflammatory involvement begins in the aortic adventitia, particularly involving the vasa vasorum, inducing obliterative endarteritis rimmed by an infiltrate of lymphocytes and plasma cells **(syphilitic aortitis)**. The narrowing of the lumina of the vasa causes ischemic injury of the aortic media, with patchy loss of the medial elastic fibers and muscle cells followed by inflammation and scarring. With destruction of the media, the aorta loses its elastic recoil and may become dilated, producing a syphilitic aneurysm. Contraction of fibrous scars may lead to wrinkling of intervening segments of aortic intima, noted grossly as "tree-barking." Luetic involvement of the aorta favors the development of superimposed atheromatosis of the aortic root (an unusual location for typical atherosclerosis), which can envelop and occlude the coronary ostia.

Luetic aortitis may also cause aortic valve ring dilation, resulting in valvular insufficiency through circumferential stretching of the valve cusps, widening of the commissures between the cusps, and turbulence-induced thickening and rolling of the free margins. Owing to aortic insufficiency, the left ventricular wall can undergo massive volume overload hypertrophy, sometimes to 1000 gm (about three times normal weight), descriptively referred to as "cor bovinum" (cow's heart).

Thoracic aortic aneurysms (regardless of etiology) can give rise to signs and symptoms referable to (1) encroachment on mediastinal structures, (2) respiratory difficulties due to encroachment on the lungs and airways, (3) difficulty in swallowing due to compression of the esophagus, (4) persistent cough due to irritation of or pressure on the recurrent laryngeal nerves, (5) pain caused by erosion of bone (i.e., ribs and vertebral bodies), (6) cardiac disease as the aortic aneurysm leads to aortic valve dilation with valvular insufficiency or narrowing of the coronary ostia causing myocardial ischemia, and (7) rupture. Most patients with syphilitic aneurysms die of heart failure induced by aortic valvular incompetence.

AORTIC DISSECTION (DISSECTING HEMATOMA)

Aortic dissection is a catastrophic illness characterized by dissection of blood between and along the laminar planes of the media, with the formation of a blood-filled channel within the aortic wall (Fig. 11–20), which often ruptures outward, causing massive hemorrhage.[48] In contrast to atherosclerotic and syphilitic aneurysms, aortic dissection may or may not be associated with marked dilatation of the aorta. For this reason, the older term "dissecting aneurysm" is discouraged.

Aortic dissection occurs principally in two groups of patients: More than 90% of dissections occur in men between the ages of 40 and 60 with antecedent hypertension. The second major group of patients, usually younger, has a systemic or localized abnormality of connective tissue that affects the aorta (e.g., Marfan syndrome, discussed in Chapter 5). Dissection can also be iatrogenic, as a complication of arterial cannulation (e.g., during diagnostic catheterization or cardiopulmonary bypass). Rarely, for unknown reasons, dissection of the aorta or its branches, including the coronary arteries, occurs during or following pregnancy. Dissection is unusual in the face of substantial atherosclerosis or other cause of medial scarring such as syphilis.

Morphology. In spontaneous dissection, an intimal tear that is presumably the origin extends into but not through the media of the ascending aorta, usually within 10 cm of the aortic valve (Fig. 11–20*A*). Such tears are typically transverse or oblique, 1 to 5 cm in length, with sharp but jagged edges. The dissection can extend along the aorta proximally toward the

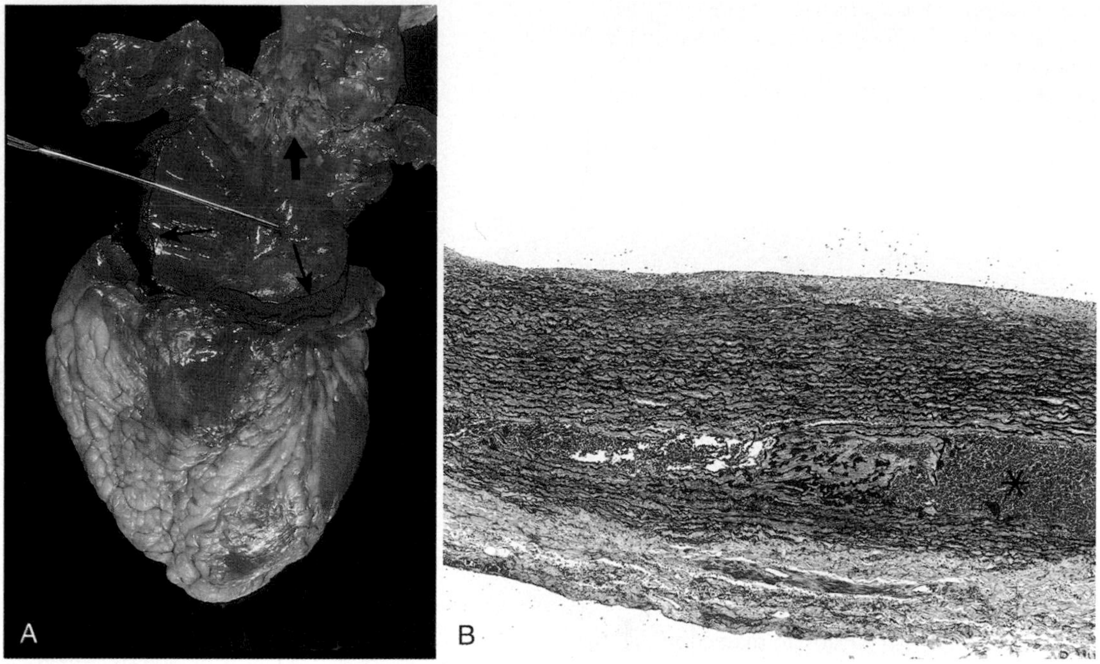

FIGURE 11–20 Aortic dissection. *A,* Gross photograph of opened aorta with proximal dissection, demonstrating a small, oblique intimal tear (demarcated by probe), allowing blood to enter the media, creating an intramural hematoma *(thin arrows).* Note that the intimal tear has occurred in a region largely free from atherosclerotic plaque, and that propagation of the intramural hematoma was arrested at a site more distally, where atherosclerosis begins *(broad arrow). B,* Histologic view of the dissection demonstrating an aortic intramural hematoma *(asterisk).* Aortic elastic layers are black, and blood is red in this section, stained with the Movat stain.

heart as well as distally, sometimes all the way into the iliac and femoral arteries. The dissecting hematoma spreads characteristically along the laminar planes of the aorta, usually between the middle and outer thirds (Fig. 11–20*B*). It often ruptures out, causing massive hemorrhage. In some instances, the blood reruptures into the lumen of the aorta, producing a second or distal intimal tear and a new vascular channel within the media of the aortic wall (to produce a "double-barreled aorta" with a "false channel"). In the course of time, false channels may become endothelialized ("chronic dissection").

Morphologically detectable aortic wall pathology is not always present in dissection. The most frequent preexisting histologically detectable lesion is **medial degeneration**, often called cystic medial degeneration. Medial degeneration is characterized by elastic tissue fragmentation and separation of the elastic and fibromuscular elements of the tunica media by small cleftlike spaces where the normal elastic tissue is lost; these areas are filled with the amorphous extracellular matrix of connective tissue and resemble but are not truly "cysts." Ultimately there may be large-scale loss of elastic laminae (Fig. 11–21). Thus, the terminology "cystic medial necrosis," as medial degeneration is often called, is inaccurate because neither necrosis nor cysts are present. Inflammation is absent. Medial degeneration of the aorta frequently accompanies Marfan syndrome.

Patients with dissection due to hypertension have variable non-specific changes in aortic wall histology, ranging from mild fragmentation of elastic tissue (most commonly) to overt medial degeneration.

Pathogenesis. Hypertension is clearly the major risk factor in dissection overall, but its contribution to aortic medial damage is uncertain. Severe degenerative changes may be found incidentally at autopsy of patients who are free from dissection. Thus, medial structural lesions do not always lead to dissection, and abnormal medial histology is not prerequisite to dissection. Some dissections are related to the inherited connective tissue disorders that cause abnormal vascular structure, most prominently Marfan syndrome, an autosomal dominant disease of connective tissue fibrillin characterized by skeletal, cardiovascular, and ocular manifestations (see Chapter 5). The cause of spontaneous dissections not associated with hypertension or genetic disorders is unknown.

Regardless of the underlying etiology, the trigger for the intimal tear and intramural aortic hemorrhage is unknown in most cases. Nevertheless, once the tear has occurred, increased systemic blood pressure fosters progression of the medial hematoma. Aggressive antihypertensive therapy is often effective in limiting an evolving dissection.

Clinical Course. The risk and nature of serious complications of dissection depend strongly on the level of the aorta affected, with the most serious complications occurring from the aortic valve to the arch. Thus, aortic dissections are generally classified into two types (Fig. 11–22):

- The more common (and serious or potentially damaging) *proximal* lesions, involving either the ascending portion only or both the ascending and the descending aorta (collectively called type A)
- *Distal lesions not involving the ascending part* and usually beginning distal to the subclavian artery (called type B).

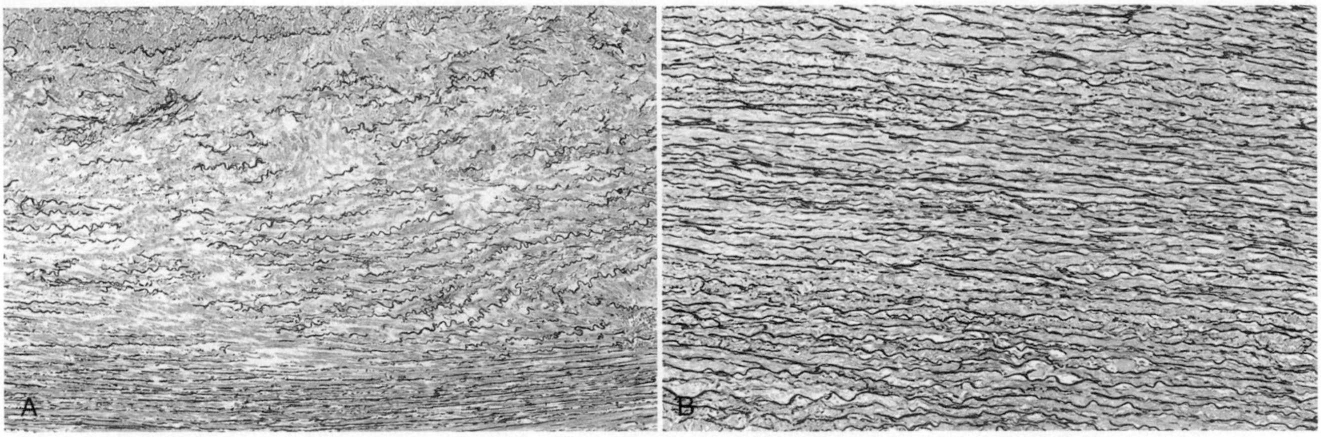

FIGURE 11–21 Medial degeneration. *A,* Cross-section of aortic media with marked elastin fragmentation and formation of areas devoid of elastin that resemble cystic spaces, from a patient with Marfan syndrome. *B,* Normal media for comparison, showing the regular layered pattern of elastic tissue. In both *A* and *B,* the tissue section is stained to highlight elastin as black.

The classic clinical symptoms of aortic dissection are the sudden onset of excruciating pain, usually beginning in the anterior chest, radiating to the back, and moving downward as the dissection progresses. This intense pain can be readily confused with that of acute myocardial infarction.

The most common cause of death is rupture of the dissection outward into any of the three body cavities (i.e., pericardial, pleural, or peritoneal). Retrograde dissection into the aortic root can cause disruption of the aortic valvular apparatus. Thus, common clinical manifestations include cardiac tamponade, aortic insufficiency, and myocardial infarction or extension of the dissection into the great arteries of the neck or into the coronary, renal, mesenteric, or iliac arteries, causing critical vascular obstruction; compression of spinal arteries may cause transverse myelitis.

At one time, aortic dissection was usually fatal, but the prognosis has improved markedly. The development of techniques for surgical repair of the aortic wall and the early institution of intensive antihypertensive therapy permit salvage of 65% to 75% of patients with dissections.

Inflammatory Disease—The Vasculitides

Inflammation of the walls of vessels, called *vasculitis,* is encountered in diverse clinical settings. Vessels of any type in virtually any organ can be affected. Clinical manifestations often include constitutional signs and symptoms such as fever, myalgias, arthralgias, and malaise, or local manifestations of downstream tissue ischemia. Of these so-called *systemic necrotizing vasculitides*, several types affect the aorta and medium-sized vessels, but most affect small vessels, such as arterioles, venules, and capillaries (designated *small vessel vasculitis*).[49] Some entities involve vessels of several types and/or sizes. Moreover, some patients have disorders that do not fit neatly into a single, well-defined category and have features of several of the entities; thus, they are considered "overlap" syndromes.

The two most common mechanisms of vasculitis are the direct invasion of vascular walls by infectious pathogens and immune-mediated mechanisms (Table 11–4). Nevertheless, it is important to recognize that infections can indirectly induce a noninfectious, systemic immune-mediated vasculitis, for example, by generating immune complexes or triggering cross-reactivity. In a particular patient, it is critical to distinguish between infectious and immunologic mechanisms, since anti-inflammatory/immunosuppressive therapy is appropriate for immune-mediated vasculitis but would be potentially harmful for infectious vasculitis. Physical and

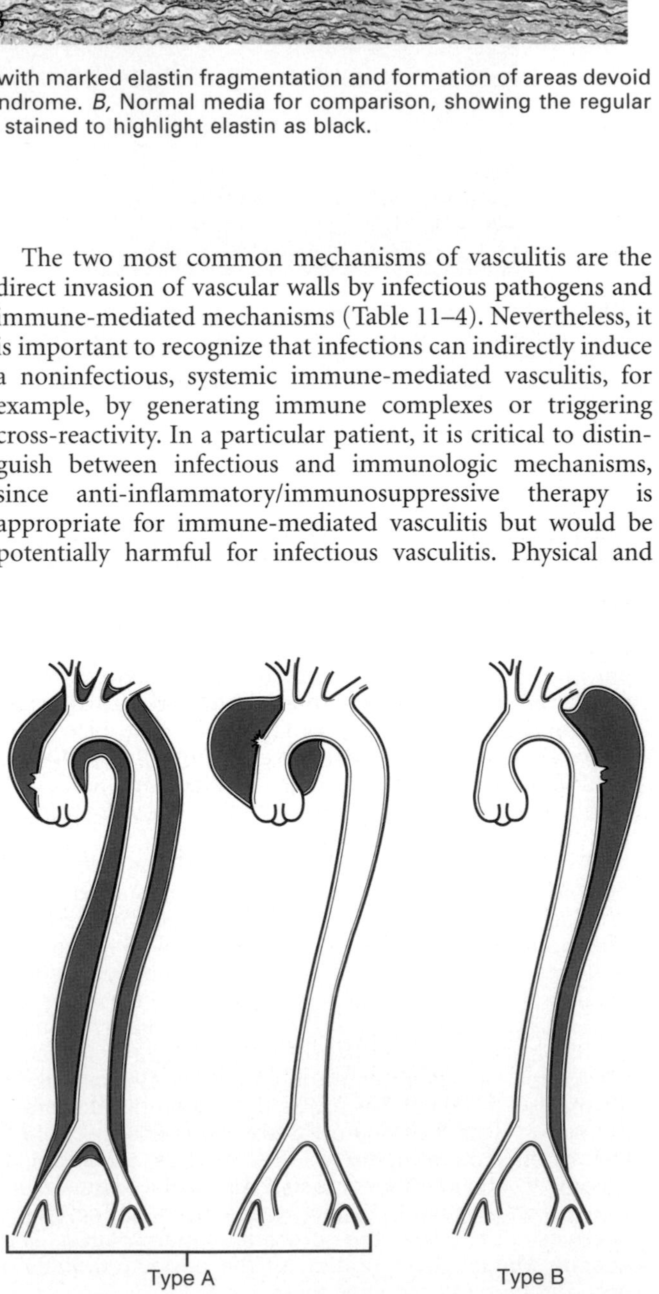

FIGURE 11–22 Classification of dissection into types A and B. Type A (proximal) involves the ascending aorta, whereas type B (distal) does not. The serious complications predominantly occur in the region from the aortic valve through the arch.

TABLE 11–4 Classification of Vasculitis Based on Pathogenesis

Direct Infection
Bacterial (e.g., *Neisseria*)
Rickettsial (e.g., Rocky Mountain spotted fever)
Spirochetal (e.g., syphilis)
Fungal (e.g., aspergillosis, mucormycosis)
Viral (e.g., herpes zoster-varicella)
Immunologic
Immune complex–mediated
Infection-induced (e.g., hepatitis B and C virus)
Henoch-Schönlein purpura
SLE and rheumatoid arthritis
Drug-induced
Cryoglobulinemia
Serum sickness
Antineutrophil cytoplasmic antibody (ANCA)–mediated
Wegener granulomatosis
Microscopic polyangiitis (microscopic polyarteritis)
Churg-Strauss syndrome
Direct antibody mediated
Goodpasture syndrome (anti-GBM antibodies)
Kawasaki disease (anti-endothelial antibodies)
Cell-mediated
Organ allograft rejection
Inflammatory bowel disease
Paraneoplastic vasculitis
Unknown
Giant cell (temporal) arteritis
Takayasu arteritis
Polyarteritis nodosa (classic polyarteritis nodosa)

GBM, glomerular basement membrane; SLE, systemic lupus erythematosus.

Data from Jennette JC, Falk RJ: Update on the pathobiology of vasculitis. In Schoen FJ, Gimbrone MA (eds); Cardiovascular Pathology: Clinicopathologic Correlations and Pathogenetic Mechanisms. Baltimore, Williams & Wilkins, 1995, p 156.

chemical injury, such as irradiation, mechanical trauma, and toxins can also cause vascular damage.

Pathogenesis of Noninfectious Vasculitis. The main immunologic mechanisms that initiate noninfectious vasculitis are: (1) immune complex deposition, (2) antineutrophil cytoplasmic antibodies, and (3) anti-endothelial cell antibodies.

Immune Complexes. The evidence for involvement of immune complexes in vasculitides can be summarized as follows:

- The vascular lesions resemble those found in experimental immune complex–mediated conditions, such as the local Arthus phenomenon and serum sickness (Chapter 6). Immune reactants and complement can be detected in the serum or vessels of patients with vasculitis (e.g., DNA–anti-DNA complexes are present in the vascular lesions of systemic lupus erythematosus–associated vasculitis and IgG, IgM, and complement in cryoglobulinemic vasculitis).
- Hypersensitivity to drugs causes approximately 10% of vasculitic skin lesions, largely through vascular deposits of immune complexes. Some, such as penicillin, conjugate serum proteins; others, like streptokinase, are themselves foreign proteins. The manifestations vary and range from small-vessel hypersensitivity and leukocytoclastic vasculitis to polyarteritis nodosa, Wegener granulomatosis, and Churg-Strauss syndrome (see later for descriptions of these entities), and from mild and self-limiting to severe and even fatal. Identification of the disorder as a drug reaction is particularly important, as discontinuation of the offending agent is often followed by rapid improvement.[50]
- In vasculitis associated with viral infections, immune complexes can be found in the serum and in the vascular lesions of some patients, particularly in cases of polyarteritis nodosa (for example, HBsAg–anti-HbsAg in hepatitis-induced vasculitis).

Whether immune complexes deposit in vessel walls from the circulation, or are formed in situ, or both, is not known (see Chapter 6). However, many small vessel vasculitides show a paucity of vascular immune deposits and therefore other mechanisms have been sought for these so-called pauci-immune vasculitides.

Antineutrophil Cytoplasmic Antibodies. Serum from many patients with vasculitis reacts with cytoplasmic antigens in neutrophils, indicating the presence of *antineutrophil cytoplasmic antibodies (ANCAs)*.[51] ANCAs are a heterogeneous group of autoantibodies directed against enzymes mainly found within the azurophil or primary granules in neutrophils, in the lysosomes of monocytes, and in ECs. The description of these autoantibodies is based on the immunofluorescent patterns of staining of ethanol-fixed neutrophils. Two main patterns are recognized: one shows cytoplasmic localization of the staining (c-ANCA), and the most common target antigen is proteinase-3 (PR3), a neutrophil granule constituent. The second shows perinuclear staining (p-ANCA) and is usually specific for myeloperoxidase (MPO). Either ANCA specificity may occur in a patient with ANCA-associated small-vessel vasculitis but c-ANCA is typically found in Wegener granulomatosis and p-ANCA is found in most cases of microscopic polyangiitis and Churg-Strauss syndrome. The disorders characterized by circulating ANCAs are called the *ANCA-associated vasculitides*.

ANCAs serve as useful quantitative diagnostic markers for these conditions, and their levels may reflect the degree of inflammatory activity.[52] ANCAs rise in episodes of recurrence, and thus are useful in management. In addition, the close association between ANCA titers and disease activity, particularly c-ANCA in Wegener granulomatosis, suggests that they may be important in the pathogenesis of this disease. Experimental data are consistent with a pathophysiologic mechanism for ANCA and/or ANCA antigen autoimmune responses in these diseases, but the precise mechanisms are unknown. However, there is yet no definitive proof that ANCAs play a causative role in the development of systemic vasculitis.

One plausible hypothesis for a causative role of ANCAs in vasculitis is summarized briefly as follows:[53] (1) An underlying disorder (e.g., an infection) elicits pro-inflammatory cytokines such as TNF, and granulocyte-macrophage colony-stimulating factor, and microbial products such as endotoxin, which together cause neutrophils and other inflammatory cells to express PR3 and MPO on their surfaces. (2) These stimulate the formation of ANCAs. (3) ANCAs react with circulating cytokine-primed neutrophils and cause them to degranulate (4) PMNs activated by ANCA cause endothelial cell toxicity and other direct tissue injury. Interestingly, ANCAs directed against neutrophil constituents other than PR3 and MPO are also found in some patients with a wide range of inflammatory but nonvasculitic disorders such as inflammatory bowel disease, autoimmune liver disease, primary sclerosing cholangitis, and rheumatoid arthritis, and in some patients with malignancies and infections.

Anti-endothelial Cell Antibodies. Antibodies to ECs, perhaps induced by defects in immune regulation, may predispose to certain vasculitides, such as those associated with SLE and Kawasaki disease.

Classification. The systemic vasculitides are classified on the basis of the size and anatomic site of the involved blood vessels (Fig. 11–23), histologic characteristics of the lesion, and clinical manifestations. There is considerable clinical and pathologic overlap among these disorders summarized in Table 11–5 and discussed below.

GIANT CELL (TEMPORAL) ARTERITIS

Giant cell (temporal) arteritis, the most common form of systemic vasculitis in adults, is an acute and chronic, often granulomatous, inflammation of arteries of large to small size.[54] It affects principally the arteries in the head—especially the temporal arteries—but also the vertebral and ophthalmic arteries and the aorta, where it may cause thoracic aortic aneurysm. Ophthalmic arterial involvement may lead to permanent blindness. Therefore, visual loss caused by giant cell arteritis is a medical emergency that requires prompt recognition and treatment. Lesions can be found in other arteries throughout the body, including the aorta *(giant cell aortitis).*

Morphology. Characteristically, segments of affected arteries develop **nodular thickenings with reduction of the lumen** and may become thrombosed. In the more common variant there is **granulomatous inflammation** of the inner half of the media centered on the internal elastic membrane marked by a mononuclear infiltrate, **multinucleate giant cells** of both foreign body and Langhans type (present in two thirds of cases), and **fragmentation of the internal elastic lamina** (Fig. 11–24). In the less common pattern, granulomas and giant cells are rare or absent, and there is a nonspecific panarteritis with a mixed inflammatory infiltrate composed largely of lymphocytes and macrophages admixed with neutrophils and eosinophils. The healed stage of both of these patterns reveals collagenous thickening of the vessel wall; organization of the luminal thrombus sometimes transforms the artery into a fibrous cord. However, the scarring may be difficult to distinguish from aging-related changes.

Pathogenesis. The morphologic alterations suggest an immunologic reaction against a component of the arterial wall, such as elastin, but an understanding of the pathogenesis remains elusive. The granulomatous nature of the inflammation, association with certain human leukocyte

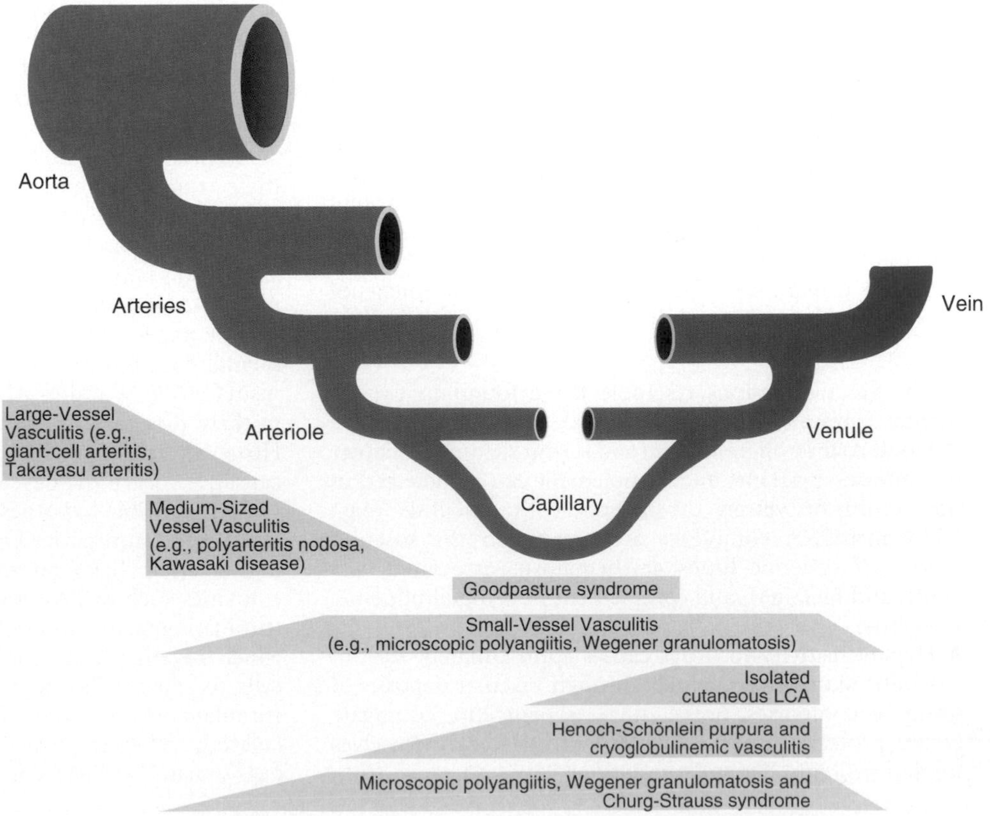

FIGURE 11–23 Diagrammatic representation of the sites of the vasculature involved by the major forms of vasculitis. The widths of the trapezoids indicate the frequencies of involvement of various portions. LCA, leukocytoclastic angiitis. (Reproduced from Jennette JC, and Falk RJ: Small-vessel vasculitis. New Engl J Med 337:1512, 1997.)

TABLE 11–5 Classification and Characteristics of Selected Vasculitis

Large Vessel Vasculitis*[*,†]	
Giant cell (temporal) arteritis	Granulomatous arteritis of the aorta and its major branches, with a predilection for the extracranial branches of the carotid artery. Often involves the temporal artery. Usually occurs in patients older than age 50 and often is associated with polymyalgia rheumatica.
Takayasu arteritis	Granulomatous inflammation of the aorta and its major branches. Usually occurs in patients younger than age 50.
***Medium-Sized Vessel Vasculitis*[‡]**	
Polyarteritis nodosa (classic polyarteritis nodosa)	Necrotizing inflammation of medium-sized or small arteries without glomerulonephritis or vasculitis in arterioles, capillaries, or venules
Kawasaki disease	Arteritis involving large, medium-sized, or small arteries and associated with mucocutaneous lymph node syndrome. Coronary arteries are often involved. Aorta and veins may be involved. Usually occurs in children.
***Small Vessel Vasculitis*[§]**	
Wegener granulomatosis[∞]	Granulomatous inflammation involving the respiratory tract and necrotizing vasculitis affecting small to medium-sized vessels (e.g., capillaries, venules, arterioles, and arteries). Necrotizing glomerulonephritis is common.
Churg-Strauss syndrome[∞]	Eosinophil-rich and granulomatous inflammation involving the respiratory tract and necrotizing vasculitis affecting small to medium-sized vessels associated with asthma and blood eosinophilia.
Microscopic polyangiitis (microscopic polyarteritis)[∞]	Necrotizing vasculitis with few or no immune deposits affecting small vessels (i.e., capillaries, venules, or arterioles). Necrotizing arteritis involving small and medium-sized arteries may be present. Necrotizing glomerulonephritis is common. Pulmonary capillaritis often occurs.

*Note that some small and large vessel vasculitides may involve medium-sized arteries, but large and medium-sized vessel vasculitides do not involve vessels smaller than arteries.

†Aorta and its largest branches to extremities and head and neck.

‡Main visceral arteries and their branches.

§Arterioles, venules, capillaries (occasionally small arteries).

∞Strongly associated with antineutrophil cytoplasmic autoantibodies (ANCA), predominantly cytoplasmic (antiproteinase 3), c-ANCA in Wegener granulomatosis, and perinuclear (antimyeloperoxidase) p-ANCA in microscopic polyangiitis and Churg-Strauss syndrome.

Modified from Jennette JC, et al: Nomenclature of systemic vasculitides: the proposal of an international consensus conference. Arthritis Rheum 37:187, 1994.

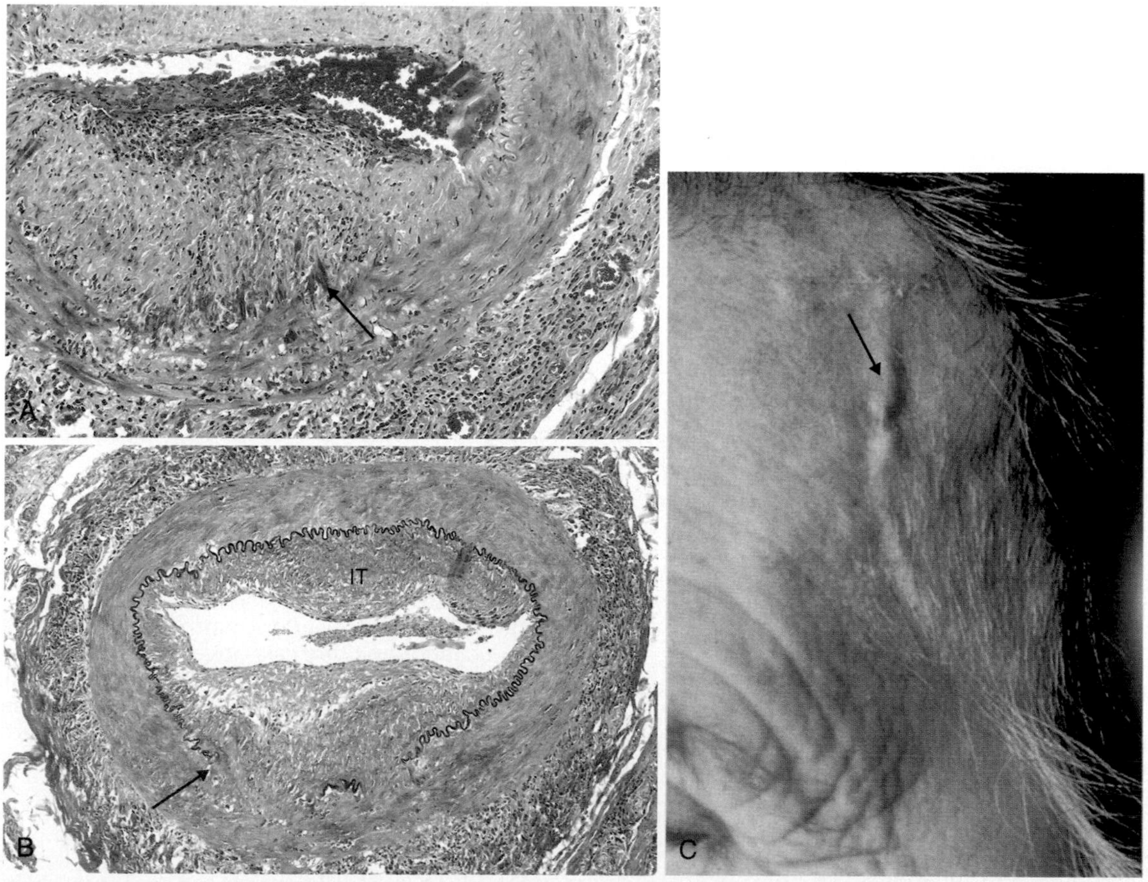

FIGURE 11–24 Temporal (giant cell) arteritis. *A,* H&E stain of section of temporal artery showing giant cells at the degenerated internal elastic membrane in active arteritis (*arrow*). *B,* Elastic tissue stain demonstrating focal destruction of internal elastic membrane (*arrow*) and intimal thickening (IT) characteristic of long-standing or healed arteritis. *C,* Examination of the temporal artery of a patient with giant-cell arteritis shows a thickened, nodular, and tender segment of a vessel on the surface of head (*arrow*). (*C* Reproduced from Salvarani C, et al. Polymyalgia rheumatica and giant-cell arteritis. N Engl J Med 347:261, 2002.)

DR antigens (HLA-DR), and the response to corticosteroid therapy, are consistent with T cell–mediated and antigen-driven injury. Clinical subsets appear to result from variable cytokine expression. Striking features of the disorder are the rarity of the disease in persons younger than age 50, the predilection for the superficial temporal arteries, and the high incidence in populations of Nordic origins.[55] The extraordinary trophism for a single arterial site remains unexplained.

Clinical Features. Temporal arteritis is most common in older individuals and rare before age 50. Symptoms are either only vague and constitutional—fever, fatigue, weight loss—without localizing signs or symptoms, or facial pain or headache, often most intense along the course of the superficial temporal artery, which may be painful to palpation. More serious are ocular symptoms (associated with involvement of the ophthalmic artery), which appear quite abruptly in about half of patients and range from diplopia to transient or complete vision loss. The diagnosis depends on biopsy and histologic confirmation, but because of the segmental nature of the involvement, adequate biopsy requires at least a 2- to 3-cm length of artery, and negative or atypical findings on biopsy do not rule out the condition. Treatment with anti-inflammatory agents is generally very effective.

TAKAYASU ARTERITIS

This granulomatous vasculitis of medium and larger arteries, described in 1908 by Takayasu, is *characterized principally by ocular disturbances and marked weakening of the pulses in the upper extremities (pulseless disease). The pathologic findings that account for the clinical picture are vasculitis and subsequent fibrous thickening of the aorta, particularly the aortic arch and its branches, with narrowing or virtual obliteration of the origins or more distal portions* (Fig. 11–25).[56] The illness is seen predominantly in females younger than age 40. The cause and pathogenesis are unknown, although autoimmune mechanisms are suspected. A high frequency of the HLA haplotype A24-B52-DR2 has been found in Japanese patients but not in other populations.

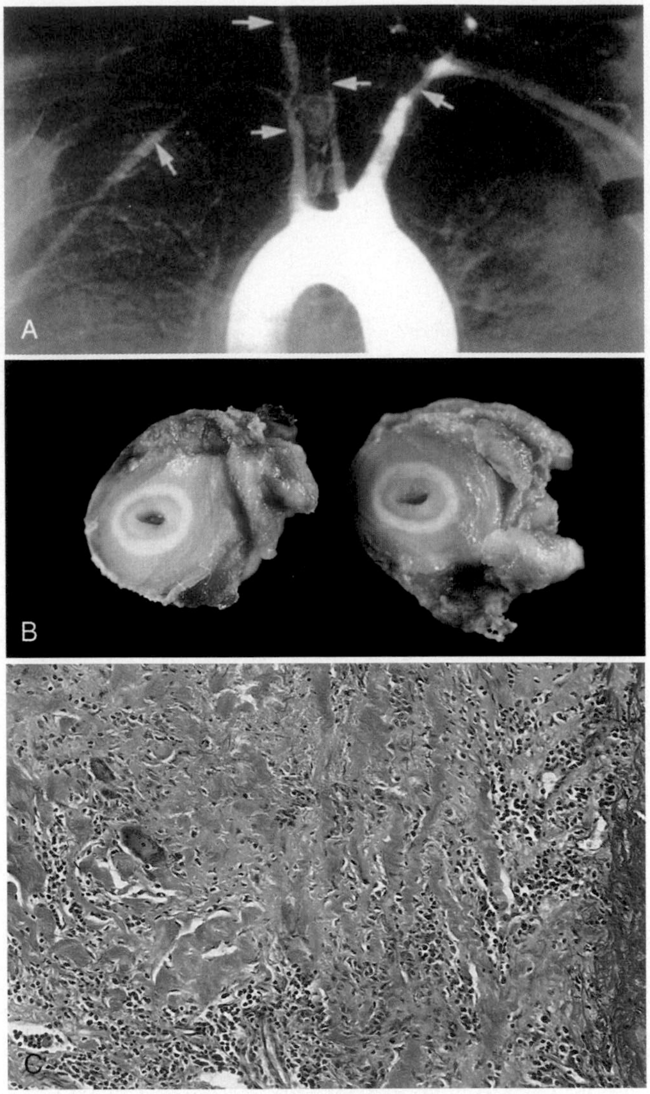

FIGURE 11–25 Takayasu arteritis. *A,* Aortic arch angiogram showing narrowing of brachiocephalic, carotid, and subclavian arteries *(arrows). B,* Gross photograph of two cross-sections of the right carotid artery taken at autopsy of the patient shown in *A,* demonstrating marked intimal thickening with minimal residual lumen. *C,* Histologic view of active Takayasu aortitis, illustrating destruction of the arterial media by mononuclear inflammation with giant cells.

Morphology. Takayasu arteritis classically involves the aortic arch, but in one third of cases it also affects the remainder of the aorta and its branches, often for some distance; in half the cases, it affects the pulmonary arteries. The gross morphologic changes include, in most cases, irregular thickening of the aortic or branch vessel wall with intimal wrinkling (Fig. 11–25*A*). When the aortic arch is involved, the orifices of the major arteries to the upper portion of the body may be markedly narrowed or even obliterated by intimal thickening (Fig. 11–25*B*). The coronary and renal arteries may be similarly affected. Histologically, the changes range from an adventitial mononuclear infiltrate with perivascular cuffing of the vasa vasorum to intense mononuclear inflammation in the media. Granulomatous inflammation, replete with giant cells and patchy necrosis of the media in some cases (see Fig. 11–25*C*) may be indistinguishable from those in giant cell (temporal) arteritis. **Thus, distinctions among active giant cell lesions of the aorta are based largely on the age of the patient, and most giant cell lesions of the aorta in young patients are designated Takayasu arteritis.** Later, as the disease runs its course, or after treatment with steroids, there is collagenous fibrosis involving all layers of the vessel wall but particularly the intima, accompanied by lymphocytic infiltration. Involvement of the root of the aorta may cause dilation, producing aortic valve insufficiency. Narrowing of the coronary ostia may lead to myocardial infarction.

Clinical Features. The salient clinical features include markedly lower blood pressure and weaker pulses in the upper extremities (than in the lower) with coldness or numbness of the fingers; ocular disturbances, including visual defects, retinal hemorrhages, and total blindness; hypertension; and neurologic deficits. Involvement of the more distal aorta may lead to claudication of the legs; that of the pulmonary arteries may lead to pulmonary hypertension. The course of the disease is variable. In some persons there is rapid progression, but in others a quiescent stage is reached in 1 or 2 years, permitting long-term survival, albeit sometimes with visual or neurologic deficits.

POLYARTERITIS NODOSA (PAN)

PAN is a systemic vasculitis of small or medium-sized muscular arteries (but not arterioles, capillaries, or venules), typically involving renal and visceral vessels but sparing the pulmonary circulation.[57] Clinical manifestations result from ischemia and infarction of affected tissues and organs.

Morphology. Classic PAN occurs as segmental transmural necrotizing inflammation of **arteries of medium to small size, in any organ** with the possible exception of the lung, and most frequently kidneys, heart, liver, and gastrointestinal tract. Individual lesions may involve only a portion of the vessel circumference and have a predilection for branching points and bifurcations. Segmental erosion with weakening of the arterial wall due to the inflammatory process may cause aneurysmal dilation or localized rupture. Impairment of perfusion, causing ulcerations, infarcts, ischemic atrophy, or hemorrhages in the area supplied by these vessels, may provide the first clue to the existence of the underlying disorder.

The histologic picture during the acute phase is characterized by **transmural inflammation of the arterial wall** with neutrophils, eosinophils, and mononuclear cells, frequently accompanied by **fibrinoid necrosis** (Fig. 11–26*A*). The lumen may become thrombosed. Later, the acute inflammatory infiltrate disappears and is replaced by **fibrous thickening of the vessel wall** that may extend into the adventitia. Firm nodularity sometimes marks the lesions. **Particularly characteristic of PAN is that all stages of activity may coexist in different vessels or even within the same vessel.**

Clinical Course. Although a disease of young adults, classic PAN may occur in children and older individuals. The course may be acute, subacute, or chronic and is frequently remittent and episodic, with long symptom-free intervals. Because the vascular involvement is widely scattered, the clinical signs and symptoms of PAN may be varied and puzzling. The most common manifestations are malaise, fever of unknown cause, and weight loss; hypertension, usually developing rapidly; abdominal pain and melena (bloody stool) due to vascular lesions in the gastrointestinal tract; diffuse muscular aches and pains; and peripheral neuritis, which is predominantly motor. Renal arterial involvement is often prominent and is a major cause of death. However, small-vessel involvement is absent, and there is no glomerulonephritis. About 30% of patients with PAN have hepatitis B antigen in their serum. There is no association with ANCA. Untreated, the disease is fatal in most cases, either during an acute fulminant attack or following a protracted course, but therapy with corticosteroids and cyclophosphamide results in remissions or cures in 90% of cases.

KAWASAKI DISEASE (MUCOCUTANEOUS LYMPH NODE SYNDROME)

Kawasaki disease is an arteritis that often involves the coronary arteries, usually in young children and infants (80% of cases are <4 years old), and is the leading cause of acquired heart disease in children in North America and Japan. It is associated with the *mucocutaneous lymph node syndrome,* an acute but usually self-limited illness manifested by fever, conjunctival and oral erythema and erosion, edema of the hands and feet, erythema of the palms and soles, a skin rash often with desquamation, and enlargement of cervical lymph nodes. Epidemic in Japan, the disease has also been reported in Hawaii and increasingly in the continental United States. Approximately 20% of patients develop cardiovascular sequelae, ranging in severity from asymptomatic vasculitis of the coronary arteries, coronary artery ectasia, or aneurysm formation to giant coronary artery aneurysms (7 to 8 mm) with rupture or thrombosis, myocardial infarction, or sudden death. Acute fatalities occur in approximately 1% of patients. Pathologic changes outside the cardiovascular system are rarely significant. The use of aspirin and intravenous gammaglobulin has had a significant effect on lowering the rate of coronary artery aneurysms and death from the disease.[58]

Morphology. The vasculitis is PAN-like, with necrosis and pronounced inflammation affecting the entire thickness of the vessel wall, but fibrinoid necrosis is usually less prominent in Kawasaki disease. Although the acute vasculitis subsides spontaneously or in response to treatment, it can be complicated by aneurysm formation, thrombosis, and/or myocardial infarction. As with other causes of arteritis, healed lesions may cause obstructive intimal thickening.

The cause of the condition is uncertain, but there is evidence that the vasculitis results from an immune reaction characterized by T-cell and macrophage activation to an unknown antigen, secretion of cytokines, polyclonal B-cell hyperactivity, and the formation of autoantibodies to endothelial cells and smooth muscle cells, leading to acute vasculitis. It is currently speculated that in genetically susceptible persons, a variety of common infectious agents (most likely viral) may trigger the disease.[59]

MICROSCOPIC POLYANGIITIS (MICROSCOPIC POLYARTERITIS, HYPERSENSITIVITY, OR LEUKOCYTOCLASTIC VASCULITIS)

This type of necrotizing vasculitis generally affects arterioles, capillaries, and venules—vessels smaller than those involved in PAN.[60] *In unusual cases larger arteries may be involved. In contrast to PAN, all lesions tend to be of the same age.* It typically presents as "palpable purpura" involving the skin, or involvement of the mucous membranes, lungs, brain, heart, gastrointestinal tract, kidneys, and muscle. Skin biopsy is often diagnostic. In contrast to PAN, necrotizing glomerulonephritis (90% of patients) and pulmonary capillaritis are particularly common. The major clinical features are hemoptysis, arthralgia, abdominal pain, hematuria, proteinuria, hemorrhage, and muscle pain or weakness. In many cases, an immunologic reaction to an antigen such as drugs (e.g., penicillin), microorganisms

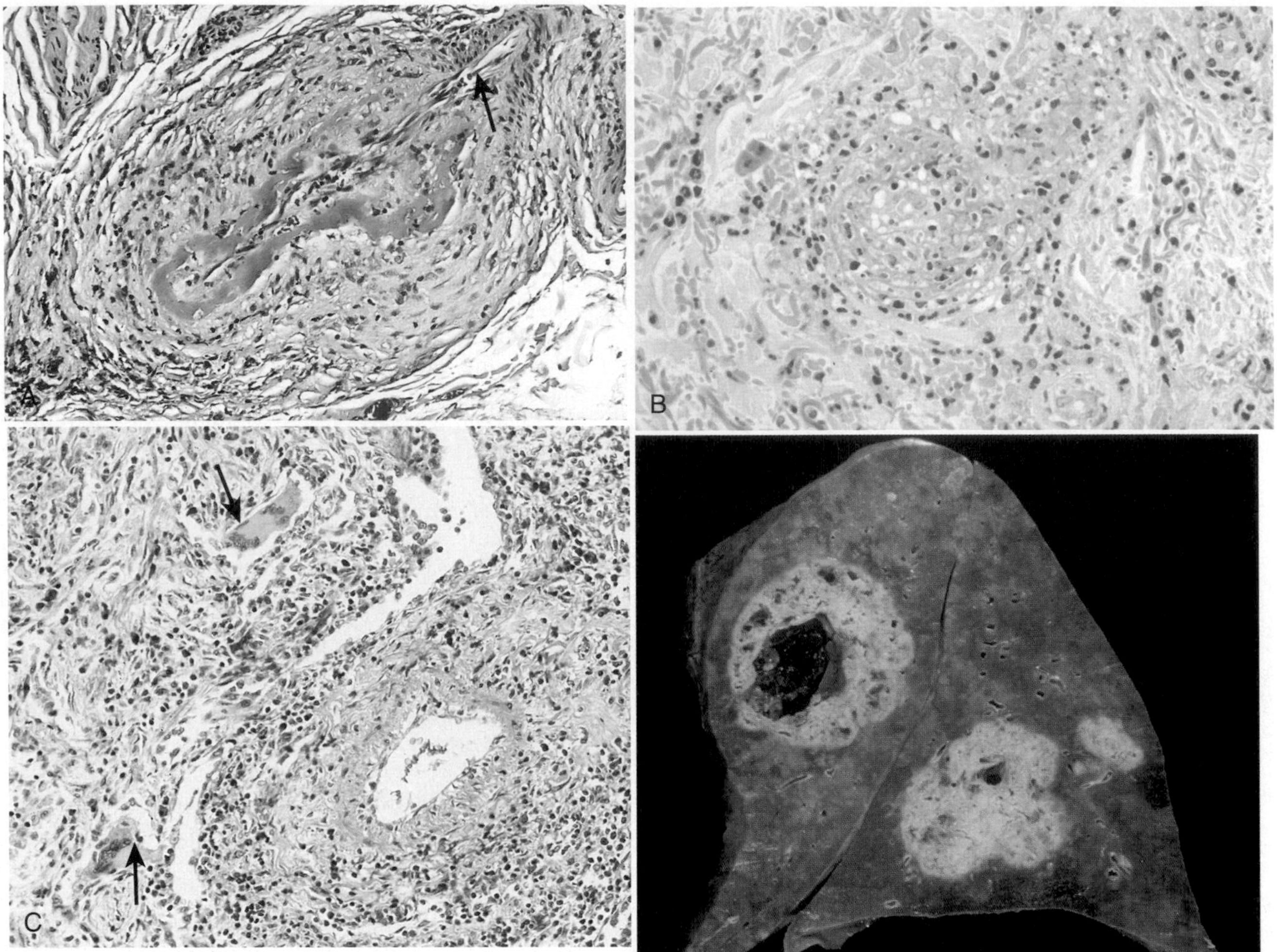

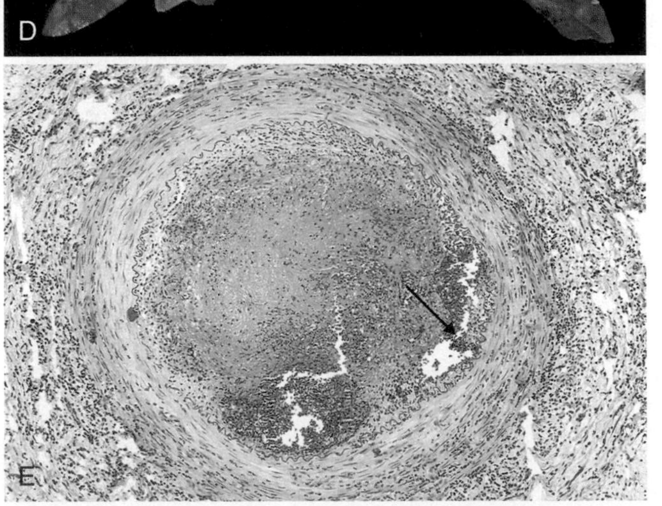

FIGURE 11–26 Representative forms of systemic medium-sized to small vessel vasculitis. *A,* Polyarteritis nodosa. *B,* Leukocytoclastic vasculitis. *C* and *D,* Wegener granulomatosis. *E,* Thromboangiitis obliterans (Buerger disease). In polyarteritis nodosa (*A*), there is segmental fibrinoid necrosis and thrombotic occlusion of the lumen of this small artery. Note that part of the vessel wall at the upper right *(arrow)* is uninvolved. In leukocytoclastic vasculitis (*B*), shown here from a skin biopsy, there is fragmentation of neutrophils in and around blood vessel walls. In Wegener granulomatosis (*C*), there is inflammation (vasculitis) of a small artery along with adjacent granulomatous inflammation, in which epithelioid cells and giant cells *(arrows)* are seen. *D,* Gross photo from the lung of a patient with fatal Wegener granulomatosis, demonstrating large nodular lesions. In a typical case of Buerger disease (*E*), the lumen is occluded by a thrombus containing two abscesses *(arrow).* The vessel wall is infiltrated with leukocytes. (*A,* and *D,* courtesy of Sidney Murphree, MD, Department of Pathology, University of Texas Southwestern Medical School, Dallas, TX; *B,* courtesy of Scott Granter, M.D., Brigham and Women's Hospital, Boston.)

(e.g., streptococci), heterologous proteins, and tumor antigens are the precipitating cause. In 70% of patients, p-ANCAs are present.

Morphology. The lesions of microscopic polyangiitis are often histologically similar to those of PAN. In contrast to PAN, muscular and large arteries are usually spared; thus, macroscopic infarcts similar to those seen in PAN are uncommon. Although microscopic polyangiitis has the same spectrum of manifestations as Wegener granulomatosis, granulomatous inflammation is absent. Histologically, segmental fibrinoid necrosis of the media may be present, but in some lesions the change is limited to infiltration with neutrophils, which become fragmented as they follow the vessel wall (leukocytoclasia). The term leukocytoclastic angiitis (LCA) is given to such lesions, most commonly found in postcapillary venules (Fig. 11–26*B*). Immunoglobulins and complement components are often present in the vascular lesions of the skin, especially if these are examined within 24 hours of development, but in general, there is a paucity of immunoglobulin demonstrable by immunofluorescence microscopy ("pauci-immune injury").

With the exception of those who develop widespread renal or brain involvement, most patients respond well simply to removal of the offending agent. Disseminated vascular lesions of hypersensitivity angiitis may also appear in Henoch-Schönlein purpura, essential mixed cryoglobulinemia, vasculitis associated with some of the connective tissue disorders, and vasculitis associated with malignancy.

In *allergic granulomatosis and angiitis* (Churg-Strauss syndrome), vascular lesions may be histologically similar to those of classic PAN or microscopic polyangiitis, but they characteristically have necrotizing vasculitis accompanied by granulomas with eosinophilic necrosis.[61] p-ANCAs are present in approximately 50% of patients. There is a strong association with allergic rhinitis, bronchial asthma, and eosinophilia. Vessels in the lung, heart, spleen, peripheral nerves, and skin are frequently involved by intravascular and extravascular granulomas, and infiltration of vessels and perivascular tissues by eosinophils is striking. However, an early, prevasculitic phase marked by tissue infiltration by eosinophils without overt vasculitis may be present in some cases.[62] Severe renal disease is infrequent. Coronary arteritis and myocarditis are the principal causes of morbidity and mortality. The disorder is thought to result from hyperresponsiveness to an allergic stimulus; in asthmatics, cysteinyl leukotriene receptor type 1 antagonists are reported to trigger it.

WEGENER GRANULOMATOSIS

Wegener granulomatosis is a necrotizing vasculitis characterized by the triad of (1) *acute necrotizing granulomas* of the upper respiratory tract (ear, nose, sinuses, throat), the lower respiratory tract (lung), or both; (2) *necrotizing or granulomatous vasculitis* affecting small to medium-sized vessels (e.g., capillaries, venules, arterioles, and arteries), most prominent in the lungs and upper airways but affecting other sites as well; and (3) renal disease in the form of *focal necrotizing, often crescentic, glomerulitis*. Some patients who do not manifest the full triad are said to have "limited" Wegener granulomatosis, in which the involvement is restricted to the respiratory tract. Conversely, widespread Wegener granulomatosis affects the eye, skin, and (rarely) other organs, notably the heart, and the clinical syndromes may be very similar to PAN with the addition of respiratory involvement.

Morphology. The upper respiratory tract lesions range from inflammatory sinusitis resulting from **mucosal granulomas** to **ulcerative lesions of the nose, palate**, or **pharynx, rimmed by necrotizing granulomas and accompanying vasculitis**. Microscopically, the granulomas reveal a geographic pattern of necrosis surrounded by lymphocytes, plasma cells, macrophages, and variable numbers of giant cells. In association with such lesions there is a **necrotizing or granulomatous vasculitis** of small and sometimes larger arteries and veins (Fig. 11–26*C*). These areas are generally surrounded by a zone of fibroblastic proliferation with giant cells and a leukocytic infiltrate in the lungs; dispersed focal necrotizing granulomas may coalesce to produce radiographically visible nodules that may undergo cavitation. The late stage of the disease may show striking pulmonary involvement by necrotizing granulomas (Fig. 11–26*D*). Since smaller lesions show radiographic resemblance to a tubercle, a mycobacterial or fungal infection must be considered. Lesions may ultimately undergo progressive fibrosis and organization. Alveolar hemorrhage may be prominent in lung lesions.

The **renal lesions** are of two types (see Chapter 20). In milder or early forms, there is acute focal proliferation and necrosis in the glomeruli, with thrombosis of isolated glomerular capillary loops (focal necrotizing glomerulonephritis). More advanced glomerular lesions are characterized by diffuse necrosis, proliferation, and crescent formation (**crescentic glomerulonephritis**). Patients with focal lesions may have only hematuria and proteinuria responsive to therapy, whereas those with diffuse disease can develop rapidly progressive renal failure.

Pathogenesis. The resemblance to PAN and serum sickness suggests that Wegener granulomatosis may represent some form of hypersensitivity, possibly to an inhaled infectious or other environmental agent, but this is unproved. Immune complexes have been seen in the glomeruli and vessel walls in occasional patients. The presence of granulomas and dramatic response to immunosuppressive therapy also strongly support an immunologic mechanism, perhaps of the cell-mediated type.

Clinical Features. Males are affected more often than females, at an average age of about 40 years, with peak incidence in the fifth decade. Typical clinical features include persistent pneumonitis with bilateral nodular and cavitary infiltrates (95%), chronic sinusitis (90%), mucosal ulcerations of the nasopharynx (75%), and evidence of renal disease (80%). Other features include skin rashes, muscle pains, articular involvement, mononeuritis or polyneuritis, and fever. Untreated, the course of the disease is malignant; 80% of patients die within 1 year. c-ANCAs are present in the serum in up to 95% of patients with active generalized disease, and this appears to be a good marker for disease activity. During treatment, a rising titer of c-ANCA suggests a relapse; most patients in remission have a negative test or the titer falls significantly.

Lymphomatoid granulomatosis, characterized by pulmonary nodules of lymphoid and plasmacytoid cells, often with cellular atypia, is a condition that is sometimes difficult to differentiate from Wegener granulomatosis. These infiltrates invade vessels, giving the histologic appearance of a vasculitis. About one third of patients have similar lesions in other organs. Lymphomatoid granulomatosis probably represents an evolving lymphoproliferative disorder, because up to 50% of patients develop a lymphoid malignancy, most commonly non-Hodgkin lymphoma.

THROMBOANGIITIS OBLITERANS (BUERGER DISEASE)

Thromboangiitis obliterans (Buerger disease), a distinctive disease that often leads to vascular insufficiency, is characterized by segmental, thrombosing, acute and chronic inflammation of medium-sized and small arteries, principally the tibial and radial arteries and sometimes secondarily extending to veins and nerves of the extremities.[62a] Previously a condition that occurred almost exclusively among heavy cigarette-smoking men, Buerger disease has been increasingly reported in women, probably reflecting smoking increases. The disease begins before age 35 in most cases.

The relationship to cigarette smoking is one of the most consistent aspects of this disorder; most patients have hypersensitivity to intradermally injected tobacco extracts. Several possibilities have been proposed for this association, including direct endothelial cell toxicity by some tobacco products or hypersensitivity to them. There is an increased prevalence of HLA-A9 and HLA-B5 in these patients, and the condition is far more common in Israel, Japan, and India than in the United States and Europe, all of which hints at genetic influences.

Morphology. Thromboangiitis obliterans is characterized by **sharply segmental acute and chronic vasculitis of medium-sized and small arteries**, mostly of the upper and lower extremities. Microscopically, acute and chronic inflammation permeates the arterial walls, accompanied by thrombosis of the lumen, which may undergo organization and recanalization. Typically, the thrombus contains small **microabscesses** with a central focus of neutrophils surrounded by granulomatous inflammation (Fig. 11–26*E*). The inflammatory process extends into contiguous veins and nerves (rare with other forms of vasculitis), and in time all three structures become encased in fibrous tissue.

Later complications are chronic ulcerations of the toes, feet, or fingers and frank gangrene in some patients. In contrast to atherosclerosis, Buerger disease involves smaller arteries and is accompanied by severe pain, even at rest, related undoubtedly to the neural involvement. Abstinence from cigarette smoking in the early stages of the disease often prevents further attacks.

VASCULITIS ASSOCIATED WITH OTHER DISORDERS

Vasculitis resembling hypersensitivity angiitis or classic PAN may sometimes be associated with an underlying disorder, such as rheumatoid arthritis, SLE, malignancy, or systemic illnesses such as mixed cryoglobulinemia and Henoch-Schönlein purpura. Distinguishing between *lupus vasculitis* (Fig. 11–27) and the antiphospholipid antibody syndrome is clinically important, as aggressive anti-inflammatory therapy is required in the former and aggressive antithrombotic/anticoagulant therapy in the latter.[63] *Rheumatoid vasculitis* occurs predominantly after long-standing, severe rheumatoid arthritis and usually affects small and medium-sized arteries leading to visceral infarction, but it may cause a clinically significant aortitis.

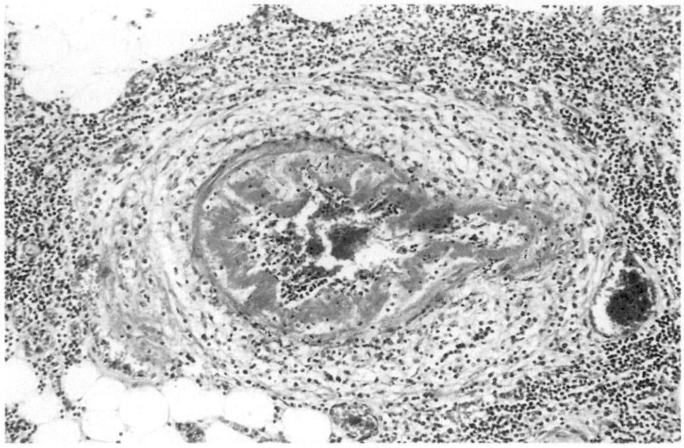

FIGURE 11–27 Vasculitis with fibrinoid necrosis in a patient with active systemic lupus erythematosus.

INFECTIOUS ARTERITIS

Localized arteritis may be caused by the direct invasion of infectious agents, usually bacteria or fungi, particularly *Aspergillus* and mucormycosis. Vascular lesions frequently accompany bacterial pneumonia or occur adjacent to caseous tuberculous abscesses or in the superficial cerebral vessels in cases of meningitis. Much less commonly, they arise from the hematogenous spread of bacteria, in cases of septicemia or embolization from infective endocarditis.

Vascular infections may weaken the arterial wall to result in a *mycotic aneurysm* (see earlier) or induce thrombosis and infarction. For example, inflammation of the superficial vessels of the brain in bacterial meningitis may predispose to thrombosis, with subsequent brain infarction and extension of the subarachnoid infection into brain parenchyma.

Raynaud Phenomenon

Raynaud phenomenon refers to paroxysmal pallor or cyanosis of the digits of the hands or feet and, infrequently, the tips of the nose or ears (acral parts) owing to cold-induced vasoconstriction of the digital arteries, precapillary arterioles, and cutaneous arteriovenous shunts.[64] Characteristically, the fingers change color in the sequence white—blue—red (Fig. 11–28). *Structural changes in the arterial walls are absent except late in the course, when intimal thickening can appear.* Raynaud phenomenon reflects an exaggeration of normal central and local vasomotor responses to cold or emotion. The prevalence in the overall population is approximately 3% to 5%; the median age of those affected is 14 years. One quarter of patients have a family history of Raynaud phenomenon in a first-degree relative. The course of Raynaud phenomenon is usually benign, but long-standing cases can have atrophy of the skin, subcutaneous tissues, and muscles. Ulceration and ischemic gangrene are rare.

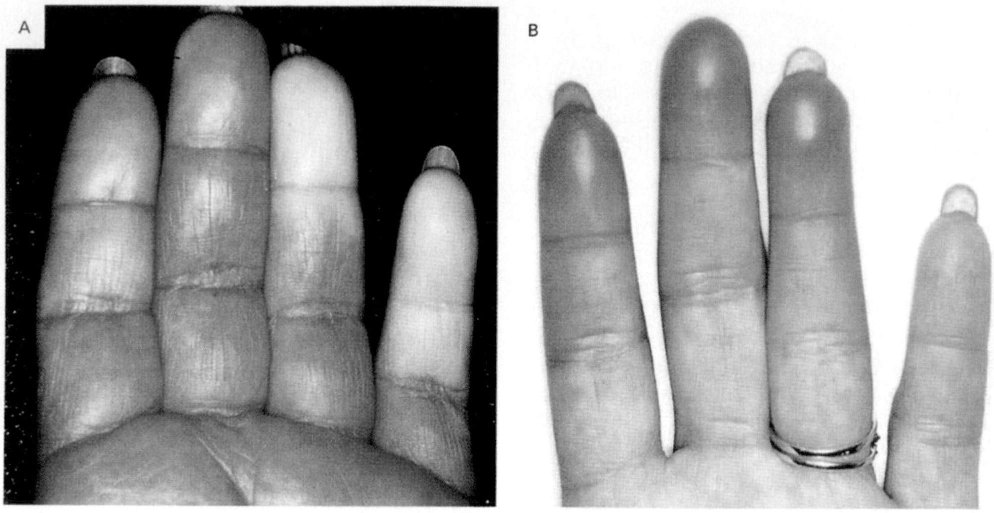

FIGURE 11–28 Raynaud phenomenon. *A,* Sharply demarcated pallor of the distal fingers resulting from the closure of digital arteries. *B,* Cyanosis of the fingertips. (Reproduced from Salvarani C, et al.: Polymyalgia rheumatica and giant-cell arteritis. N Engl J Med 347:261, 2002.)

In contrast to uncomplicated, or primary, Raynaud phenomenon, *secondary Raynaud phenomenon* refers to arterial insufficiency of the extremities *caused by various conditions, including SLE, systemic sclerosis (scleroderma), atherosclerosis, or Buerger disease* (see above). Indeed, since Raynaud phenomenon may be the first manifestation of such conditions, all patients who manifest the condition should undergo evaluation to rule out an underlying cause, which will be apparent at presentation or will develop later in approximately 10% of patients. Features suggestive of secondary Raynaud phenomenon include age of onset >30 years, more severe episodes, associated skin lesions, and clinical features of connective tissue disease.

Veins and Lymphatics

Varicose veins and phlebothrombosis/thrombophlebitis together account for at least 90% of clinical venous disease and are discussed below.

VARICOSE VEINS

Varicose veins are abnormally dilated, tortuous veins produced by prolonged, increased intraluminal pressure and loss of vessel wall support. The *superficial veins* of the upper and lower leg are the main sites of involvement (Fig. 11–29). When the legs are dependent for long periods of time, venous pressures in these sites are markedly elevated (up to ten times normal). Therefore, occupations that require long periods of standing and long automobile or airplane rides frequently lead to marked venous stasis and pedal edema, even in individuals with essentially normal veins *(simple orthostatic edema).* This also contributes to varicosities. In the long term, persons >50 years old, obese individuals, and women (owing to elevated venous pressure in the lower legs caused by pregnancy) are also at risk. A *familial tendency* toward premature varicosities is thought to be due to defective venous wall development. It is estimated that 15% to 20% of the general population eventually develop varicose veins in the lower legs.

Morphology. Veins with varicosities are dilated, tortuous, elongated, and scarred, with thinning at the points of maximal dilation. Intraluminal thrombosis and valvular deformities (thickening, rolling, and shortening of the cusps) are frequently discovered when these vessels are opened. Microscopically, the

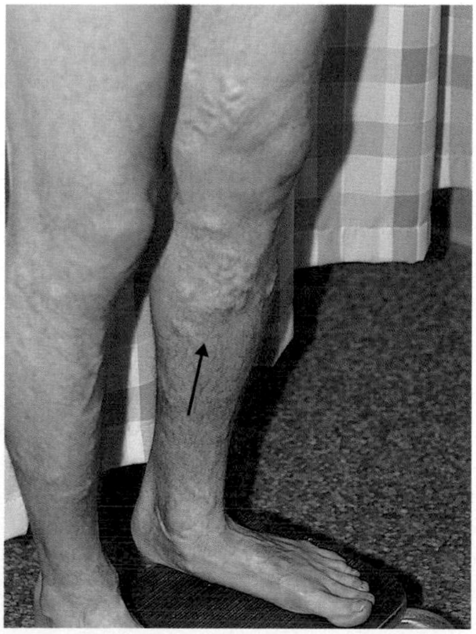

FIGURE 11–29 Varicose veins of the leg, highlighted by *arrow* (Courtesy of Magruder C. Donaldson, M.D., Brigham and Women's Hospital, Boston, MA.)

changes consist of variations in the thickness of the vein wall caused by dilation in some areas and by compensatory hypertrophy of the smooth muscle and subintimal fibrosis in others. Frequently there is elastic tissue degeneration and spotty calcifications within the media **(phlebosclerosis)**.

Clinical Course. Varicose dilation of veins renders the valves incompetent and leads to venous stasis, congestion, edema, pain, and thrombosis. The most disabling sequelae include persistent edema in the extremity and trophic changes in the skin that lead to stasis dermatitis, ulcerations, vulnerability to injury, and poorly healing wounds and infections that may become chronic *varicose ulcers. However, embolism or other serious complication is very rare. This is in sharp contrast to the relatively frequent thromboembolism that arises from thrombosed deep veins* (see below).

Varicosities also occur in two other sites that deserve mention. *Esophageal varices* form in patients who have cirrhosis of the liver and its attendant portal hypertension (Chapter 18); rupture of esophageal varices can lead to massive upper gastrointestinal hemorrhage. *Hemorrhoids* result from varicose dilation of the hemorrhoidal plexus of veins at the anorectal junction. Presumed to be caused by prolonged pelvic congestion resulting from repeated pregnancies or straining at stools, hemorrhoids are uncomfortable and may be a source of bleeding. They sometimes thrombose; in this distended state, they are prone to painful ulceration.

THROMBOPHLEBITIS AND PHLEBOTHROMBOSIS

The deep leg veins account for more than 90% of cases of thrombophlebitis and phlebothrombosis, two designations for inflammation and venous thrombosis. *Cardiac failure, neoplasia, pregnancy, obesity, the postoperative state, and prolonged bed rest or immobilization are the most important clinical predispositions.* Genetic hypercoagulability syndromes can also be associated with venous thrombosis.

In patients with cancer, particularly adenocarcinomas of the pancreas, colon, or lung, hypercoagulability occurs as a paraneoplastic syndrome (see Chapter 7). The resultant venous thromboses have a tendency to appear in one site, only to disappear and be followed by thromboses in other veins, giving rise to so-called *migratory thrombophlebitis (Trousseau sign)*. The periprostatic venous plexus in the male and the pelvic veins in the female are additional sites, as are the large veins in the skull and the dural sinuses when these channels become inflamed by bacterial infections of the meninges, middle ears, or mastoids. Similarly, infections in the abdominal cavity, such as peritonitis, acute appendicitis, acute salpingitis, and pelvic abscesses, may lead to inflammation and thrombosis of the portal vein.

Thrombi in the legs tend to produce few, if any, signs or symptoms in the early stages. Indeed, local manifestations, including edema distal to the occluded vein, dusky cyanosis, dilatation of superficial veins, heat, tenderness, redness, swelling, and pain may be absent in a bedridden patient. In some cases, however, pain can be elicited by pressure over affected veins, squeezing the calf muscles or forced dorsiflexion of the foot (Homan sign).

Pulmonary embolism is a common and serious clinical sequel to deep leg vein thrombosis. The contraction of surrounding muscles tends to "milk" the contents loose from their attachments to the vein walls. *Not infrequently, the first manifestation of thrombophlebitis is the development of an embolic episode*; in a very ill patient pulmonary embolization often constitutes the final blow.

A special variant of primary phlebothrombosis is *plegmasia alba dolens* (painful white leg), referring to iliofemoral venous thrombosis occurring in pregnant women prior to or following delivery (aptly also called "milk leg"). It is postulated that the thrombus (predisposed by stasis caused by the pressure of the gravid uterus and to a hypercoagulable state during pregnancy) initiates phlebitis, and the perivenous inflammatory response induces lymphatic blockage with painful swelling.

SUPERIOR AND INFERIOR VENA CAVAL SYNDROMES

The superior vena caval syndrome is usually caused by neoplasms that compress or invade the superior vena cava, most commonly a primary bronchogenic carcinoma or mediastinal lymphoma. The consequent obstruction produces a distinctive clinical complex manifested by dusky cyanosis and marked dilation of the veins of the head, neck, and arms. Commonly the pulmonary vessels are also compressed, inducing respiratory distress.

The inferior vena caval syndrome may be caused by neoplasms that either compress or penetrate the walls of the inferior vena cava or a thrombus from the femoral or iliac vein that propagates upward. Moreover, certain neoplasms, particularly hepatocellular carcinoma and renal cell carcinoma, show a striking tendency to grow within veins, with ultimate extension into the inferior vena cava, and, occasionally, into the right atrium. Obstruction of the inferior vena cava causes marked edema of the legs, distention of the superficial collateral veins of the lower abdomen, and, when the renal veins are involved, massive proteinuria.

LYMPHANGITIS AND LYMPHEDEMA

Primary disorders of the lymphatic vessels are extremely uncommon; secondary processes develop in association with inflammation or cancer.

Bacterial infections may spread into and through the lymphatics to create acute inflammatory involvement in these channels *(lymphangitis)*. The most common etiologic agents are the group A beta-hemolytic streptococci, although any virulent pathogen may cause acute lymphangitis. Anatomically, the affected lymphatics are dilated and filled with an exudate, chiefly of neutrophils and histiocytes, which usually extends through the wall into the perilymphatic tissues and in severe cases produces cellulitis or focal abscesses. Clinically, lymphangitis is recognized by painful subcutaneous red streaks that extend along the course of lymphatics, with painful enlargement of the regional lymph nodes *(acute lymphadenitis)*. If the lymph nodes fail to block the spread of bacteria, spillage into the venous system can initiate a bacteremia or septicemia.

Occlusion of lymphatic drainage is followed by the abnormal accumulation of interstitial fluid in the affected part, called *obstructive lymphedema*. Lymphatic blockage is most commonly secondary to (1) spread of malignant tumors obstructing either the lymphatic channels or the regional lymph nodes, (2) radical surgical procedures with removal of regional groups of lymph nodes (e.g., the axillary dissection of radical mastectomy), (3) postirradiation fibrosis, (4) filariasis, and (5) postinflammatory thrombosis and scarring. *Chylous ascites, chylothorax,* and *chylopericardium* are caused by rupture of obstructed, dilated lymphatics into the peritoneum, pleural cavity, or pericardium, usually due to obstruction of lymphatics by an infiltrating tumor mass.

In contrast, *primary lymphedema* may occur as an isolated congenital defect (simple congenital lymphedema) or as the familial *Milroy disease (heredofamilial congenital lymphedema)*. A third form of primary lymphedema, known as *lymphedema praecox*, appears between ages 10 and 25 years, usually in females. Of unknown cause, the edema begins in the feet and slowly accumulates throughout life. The involved extremity may swell to many times its normal size, and the process may extend upward to affect the trunk. Potential consequences are disability owing to the size of the limb, superimposed infection, or chronic ulcerations.

Lymphedema causes dilation of lymphatics up to the points of obstruction, accompanied by increases of interstitial fluid. Persistence of the edema leads to increased subcutaneous interstitial fibrous tissue, with consequent enlargement of the affected part, brawny induration, "peau d'orange" appearance of the skin, and skin ulcers.

TABLE 11–6 Classification of Vascular Tumors and Tumor-Like Conditions

Benign Neoplasms, Developmental and Acquired Conditions
Hemangioma
Capillary hemangioma
Cavernous hemangioma
Pyogenic granuloma (lobular capillary hemangioma)
Lymphangioma
Simple (capillary) lymphangioma
Cavernous lymphangioma (cystic lymphangioma)
Glomus tumor
Vascular ectasias
Nevus flammeus
Spider telangiectasia (arterial spider)
Hereditary hemorrhagic telangiectasis (Osler-Weber-Rendu disease)
Reactive vascular proliferations
Bacillary angiomatosis
Intermediate-Grade Neoplasms
Kaposi sarcoma
Hemangioendothelioma
Malignant Neoplasms
Angiosarcoma
Hemangiopericytoma

Tumors

Tumors of the blood and lymphatic vessels include a spectrum from the benign hemangiomas (some of which are regarded as hamartomas), to intermediate lesions that are locally aggressive but infrequently metastasize, to relatively rare, highly malignant angiosarcomas (Table 11–6). In addition, congenital or developmental malformations may present as tumor-like lesions, as do some non-neoplastic reactive vascular proliferations, such as *bacillary angiomatosis.* For these reasons, vascular neoplasms are difficult to categorize clinically and histologically. Neoplasms of this group display endothelial cell differentiation (e.g., hemangioma, lymphangioma, angiosarcoma) or appear to be derived from cells that support and/or surround blood vessels (e.g., glomus tumor, hemangiopericytoma). Most such lesions occur in soft tissues and viscera. Primary tumors of the large vessels, such as the aorta, pulmonary artery, and vena cava, are extremely rare, most being connective tissue sarcomas.

Although in most cases a well-differentiated benign hemangioma can be readily distinguished from an anaplastic, high-grade angiosarcoma, the line dividing benign from malignant is poorly defined in some cases. However, the following criteria are helpful:

- Benign tumors produce readily recognized vascular channels filled with blood cells or lymphatics with transudate; these channels are lined by a layer of normal endothelial cells, without atypia.
- Malignant tumors are more solidly cellular, with cytologic anaplasia, including mitotic figures, and usually do not form well-organized vessels.

The endothelial derivation of neoplastic proliferations that do not form distinct vascular lumina can usually be confirmed by immunohistochemical demonstration of endothelium-specific markers such as CD31, CD34, or vWF. Because these lesions constitute abnormalities of unregulated vascular proliferation, the possibility of controlling such growth by agents that inhibit blood vessel formation (anti-angiogenic factors) is particularly exciting.

BENIGN TUMORS AND TUMOR-LIKE CONDITIONS

Hemangioma

Difficult to distinguish with certainty from malformations or hamartomas, *hemangiomas (angiomas)* are most commonly localized; however, some involve large segments of the body such as an entire extremity (called *angiomatosis*). The majority are superficial lesions, often of the head or neck, but they may occur internally, with nearly one third in the liver. Malignant transformation occurs rarely if at all (Fig. 11–30).

Hemangiomas constitute 7% of all benign tumors in infancy and childhood (Chapter 10). Most are present from birth and expand along with the growth of the child. Nevertheless, many of the capillary lesions regress spontaneously at or before puberty. There are several histologic and clinical variants.

Capillary Hemangioma. *Capillary hemangiomas,* the largest single type of vascular tumor, are most common in the skin, subcutaneous tissues, and mucous membranes of the oral cavities and lips, but they may also occur in the liver, spleen, and kidneys. The "strawberry type" of capillary hemangioma *(juvenile hemangioma)* of the skin of newborns is extremely common (1 in 200 births), may be multiple, grows rapidly in the first few months, begins to fade when the

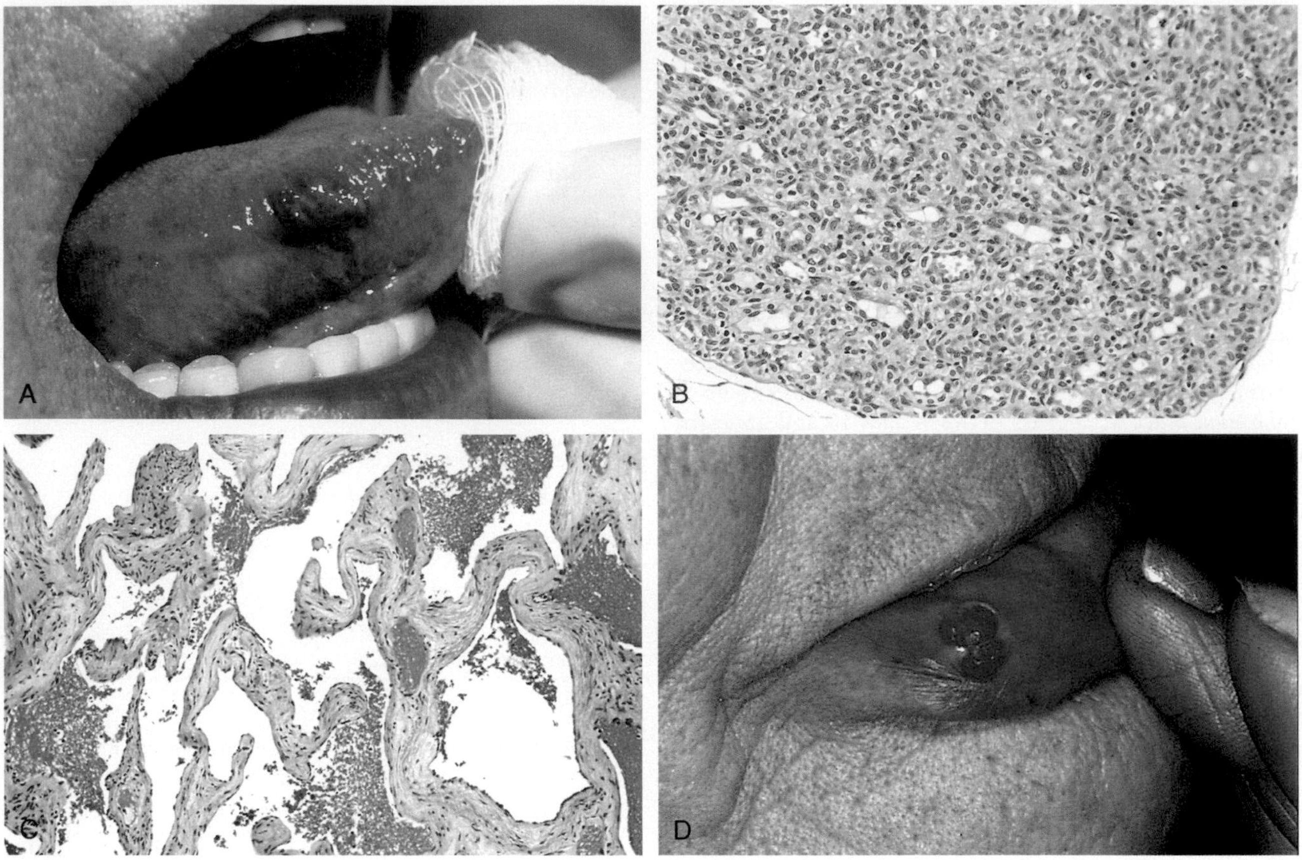

FIGURE 11–30 Hemangiomas. *A,* Hemangioma of the tongue. *B,* Histology of juvenile capillary hemangioma. *C,* Histology of cavernous hemangioma. *D,* Pyogenic granuloma of the lip. (*A* and *D,* courtesy of John Sexton, M.D., Beth Israel Hospital, Boston; *B,* courtesy of Christopher D.M. Fletcher, M.D., Brigham and Women's Hospital, Boston; and *C,* courtesy of Thomas Rogers, M.D., University of Texas Southwestern Medical School, Dallas, TX.)

child is between ages 1 and 3 years, and regresses by age 7 in 75% to 90% of cases.

Morphology. Varying in size from a few millimeters to several centimeters in diameter, hemangiomas are bright red to blue and are level with the surface of the skin or slightly elevated, with intact covering epithelium (Fig. 11–30*A*). Occasionally, they are pedunculated. Histologically, capillary hemangiomas are usually lobulated but unencapsulated aggregates of **closely packed, thin-walled capillaries**, usually blood-filled and lined by a flattened endothelium, separated by scant connective tissue stroma (Fig. 11–30*B*). The lumina may be partially or completely thrombosed and organized. Rupture of vessels causes scarring and accounts for the hemosiderin pigment occasionally found.

Cavernous Hemangioma. Less common than the capillary variety, *cavernous hemangiomas* share age and anatomic distribution, but they are usually larger, less well circumscribed, and more frequently involve deep structures than do capillary hemangiomas. As they may be locally destructive and show no tendency to regress, many require surgery.

Morphology. Grossly, the usual cavernous hemangioma is a red-blue, soft, spongy mass 1 to 2 cm in diameter. Rarely, giant forms occur that affect large subcutaneous areas of the face, extremities, or other regions of the body. Histologically, the mass is sharply defined, but not encapsulated, and is made up of **large, cavernous vascular spaces**, partly or completely filled with blood separated by a scant connective tissue stroma (Fig. 11–30*C*). Intravascular thrombosis with associated dystrophic calcification is common.

In most situations, the tumors are of little clinical significance; however, they can be a cosmetic disturbance and are vulnerable to traumatic ulceration and bleeding. Moreover, when picked up in internal organs by computed tomography or magnetic resonance imaging scans, they must be distinguished from more ominous lesions. Those in the brain are most threatening, since they may cause pressure symptoms or rupture. In one rare systemic entity, *von Hippel-Lindau disease* (discussed in Chapters 20 and 28), cavernous hemangiomas occur within the cerebellum, brain stem, and eye, along with similar angiomatous lesions or cystic neoplasms in the pancreas and liver and other visceral neoplasms.

Pyogenic Granuloma (Lobular Capillary Hemangioma). This polypoid form of capillary hemangioma occurs as a rapidly growing exophytic red nodule attached by a stalk to the skin and gingival or oral mucosa. The lesion bleeds easily and is often ulcerated (Fig. 11–30*D*). Approximately one third of lesions develop after trauma, growing rapidly to reach a maximum size of 1 to 2 cm within a few weeks. The proliferating capillaries are often accompanied by extensive edema and an acute and chronic inflammatory infiltrate, especially when ulcerated. On histologic examination they have a striking resemblance to exuberant granulation tissue, sometimes suggesting an infectious etiology. Recurrence occurs infrequently as a solitary nodule or as satellite nodules. *Granuloma gravidarum* is a pyogenic granuloma that occurs in the gingiva of 1% of pregnant women and regresses after delivery. These lesions, like the spider telangiectasias discussed below, highlight the role of estrogen in vascular growth and proliferation.

Lymphangomas

Lymphangiomas are the benign lymphatic analog of the hemangiomas of blood vessels.

Lymphangioma Circumscriptum (Capillary Lymphangioma). These lesions are composed of small lymphatic channels and tend to occur subcutaneously in the head and neck region and in the axilla. They are slightly elevated or sometimes pedunculated lesions, 1 to 2 cm in diameter, blister-like blebs that are filled with exudate. Histologically, they are composed of a network of endothelium-lined lymph spaces beneath the epidermis and can be *distinguished from capillary channels only by the absence of blood cells.*

Analogous to the cavernous hemangioma, *cavernous lymphangioma (cystic hygroma)* occurs in children in the neck or axilla, and only rarely, retroperitoneally. They occasionally achieve considerable size, up to 15 cm in diameter, and may fill the axilla or produce gross deformities in and about the neck. The tumors are made up of massively dilated, cystic lymphatic spaces lined by endothelial cells and separated by a scant intervening connective tissue stroma that often contains lymphoid aggregates. Because the margins of the tumor are not discrete and these lesions are not encapsulated, removal can be difficult. Cystic hygromas of the neck occur in Turner syndrome (Chapter 5).

Glomus Tumor (Glomangioma)

A *glomus tumor* is a biologically benign but often exquisitely painful tumor that arises from the modified smooth muscle cells of the glomus body, a specialized arteriovenous anastomosis that is involved in thermoregulation. Glomus tumors *are most commonly found in the distal portion of the digits*, especially under the fingernails. Excision is curative.

Morphology. Grossly, the lesions are usually small (under 1 cm in diameter), slightly elevated, rounded, red-blue, and firm nodules, which may appear as minute foci of fresh hemorrhage under the nail. Histologically, there are branching vascular channels separated by a connective tissue stroma that contains **aggregates, nests, and masses of the specialized glomus cells that typically are arranged around vessels.** Individual cells are usually small, regular in size, and round or cuboidal, with scant cytoplasm and features very similar to smooth muscle cells on electron microscopy. Although they resemble cavernous hemangiomas, glomangiomas constitute a distinct subgroup.

Vascular Ectasias

Not true neoplasms, *vascular ectasias* include a common group of lesions characterized by localized dilation of preexisting vessels. The term *telangiectasis* designates a congenital anomaly or an acquired exaggeration of preformed vessels, composed of prominent capillaries, venules, and arterioles that creates a small focal red lesion, usually in the skin or mucous membranes.

Nevus Flammeus. As the ordinary birthmark, this most common form of ectasia characteristically forms on the head and neck, is flat, and ranges in color from light pink to deep purple. Histologically, such lesions show only dilation of vessels in the dermis. The vast majority ultimately fade and regress.

A special form of nevus flammeus, the so-called *port-wine stain,* may grow proportionately with a child, thicken the skin surface, become unsightly, and demonstrate no tendency to fade. Port-wine stains in the distribution of the trigeminal nerve may be associated with the *Sturge-Weber syndrome* (also called *encephalotrigeminal angiomatosis*), an extremely uncommon congenital disorder attributed to the faulty development of certain mesodermal and ectodermal elements. Sturge-Weber syndrome is characterized by venous angiomatous masses in the leptomeninges over the cortex and by ipsilateral port-wine nevi of the face. It is often associated with mental retardation, seizures, hemiplegia, and radiopacities in the skull. Thus, a large vascular malformation in the face may indicate the presence of more extensive vascular malformation in a child who exhibits some evidence of mental deficiency.

Spider Telangiectasia (Arterial Spider). Another clearly non-neoplastic vascular lesion is the *spider telangiectasia*, a more or less radial and often pulsatile array of dilated subcutaneous arteries or arterioles about a central core that blanches when pressure is applied to its center. These lesions tend to be on the face, neck, or upper chest and are most frequent in pregnant women and in patients with cirrhosis. The hyperestrinism found in these two settings is believed in some way to play a role in the development of these telangiectases.

Hereditary Hemorrhagic Telangiectasia (Osler-Weber-Rendu Disease). In the autosomal dominant *Osler-Weber-Rendu disease*, telangiectases are genetic malformations consisting of dilated capillaries and veins. They are present from birth and distributed widely over the skin and mucous membranes of the oral cavity, lips, and respiratory, gastrointestinal, and urinary tracts. Rupture may occur, causing (rarely) serious nosebleeds, bleeding into the gut, or hematuria.

Bacillary Angiomatosis

First described in patients with the acquired immunodeficiency syndrome (AIDS), *bacillary angiomatosis* is an opportunistic infection of immunocompromised persons manifest as vascular proliferations that clinically resemble tumors and involve skin, bone, brain, and other organs. Along with the closely related vascular lesion of the liver and spleen called *bacillary peliosis*, bacillary angiomatosis is caused by infection with gram-negative bacilli of the *Bartonella* family, particularly *Bartonella henselae*, the organism that causes cat-scratch disease in immunocompetent persons, and *B. quintana*, the cause of trench fever affecting soldiers during World War I. Difficult to cultivate in the laboratory, these organisms can be demonstrated using molecular methods (polymerase chain reaction with species-specific primers). How these organisms cause the exuberant vessel lesions is unclear.

Morphology. Grossly, cutaneous bacillary angiomatosis is marked by one to numerous red papules and nodules or rounded subcutaneous masses (Fig. 11–31). Histologically, there is a tumor-like growth pattern involving the proliferation of capillaries that exhibit protuberant epithelioid endothelial cells with nuclear atypia and mitoses. Numerous stromal neutrophils, nuclear dust, and purplish granular material consisting of the causative bacteria distinguish this from pyogenic granuloma, Kaposi sarcoma, or angiosarcoma, which it resembles (see later).

The domestic cat is the principal reservoir of *B. henselae* and the cat flea its vector, while the human body louse plays an important role in infection due to *B. quintana*. These infections are cured by macrolide antibiotics (including erythromycin).

INTERMEDIATE-GRADE (BORDERLINE, LOW-GRADE MALIGNANT) TUMORS

Kaposi Sarcoma

Kaposi sarcoma (KS) has come to the forefront because of its frequent occurrence in patients with AIDS. Four forms of the disease are recognized (but as we will see later, these variants likely share a common pathogenesis):[65]

- *Chronic*, also called *classic or European KS*, first described by Kaposi in 1872, occurs primarily (90%) in older men of Eastern European (especially Ashkenazi Jews) or Mediterranean descent but is uncommon in the United States. This form is not associated with human immunodeficiency virus (HIV), but homosexual men may be at increased risk. Clinically, chronic KS commences with multiple red to purple skin plaques or nodules, primarily on the arms or legs, slowly increasing in size and number, spreading to more proximal sites and often becoming confluent. The tumors frequently remain asymptomatic and localized to the skin and subcutaneous tissue but are locally persistent, with an erratic course of lapses and remissions. The viscera or mucosa becomes involved in approximately 10% of patients.
- *Lymphadenopathic*, also called *African* or *endemic KS*, is common in portions of Africa and particularly prevalent among young Bantu children of South Africa (same geographic distribution as Burkitt lymphoma), who present with localized or generalized lymphadenopathy, and in whom the disease is extremely aggressive. Skin lesions are sparse. With the high prevalence of HIV-associated disease in Africa and the association of AIDS with KS (see below), KS in HIV-negative and HIV-positive patients is now the most frequently occurring tumor in Central Africa (50% of all tumors in men in some countries).
- *Transplant-associated* (or *immunosuppression-associated*) *KS* occurs typically several months to a few years postoperatively in organ transplant recipients who receive high doses of immunosuppressive therapy. This type of KS tends to be

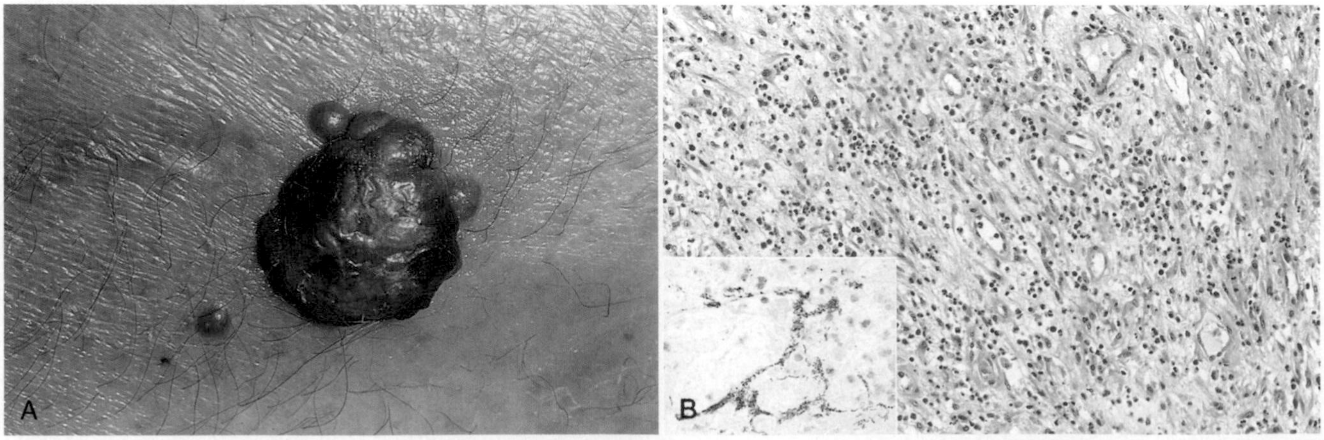

FIGURE 11–31 Bacillary angiomatosis. *A,* Photograph of a moist, erosive cutaneous lesion. *B,* Histologic appearance with acute neutrophilic inflammation and vascular (capillary) proliferation. *Inset,* demonstration by modified silver (Warthin-Starry) stain of clusters of tangled bacilli (black). (*A,* courtesy of Richard Johnson, M.D., Beth Israel Deaconess Medical Center, Boston, MA; *B* and *inset,* courtesy of Scott Granter, M.D., Brigham and Women's Hospital, Boston, MA.)

aggressive, involving lymph nodes, mucosa, and visceral organs in half of patients, and skin lesions may be absent. Lesions sometimes regress when immunosuppressive therapy is markedly reduced, but organ or internal involvement is usually fatal.

- *KS is the most common AIDS-associated cancer in the United States and* was originally present in approximately one third of AIDS patients, particularly male homosexuals. With the use of HAART (discussed in Chapter 6) KS incidence has declined to less than 1%. Diagnosis of the tumor may precede the clinical recognition of the syndrome. AIDS-associated KS lesions have no site of predilection, but involvement of lymph nodes and the gut and wide dissemination tend to occur early in the course. Most patients eventually succumb to the opportunistic infectious complications of AIDS rather than directly to the consequences of KS.

Morphology. The morphology of KS is illustrated in Figure 11–32. In the relatively indolent, classic disease of older men and sometimes in the other variants, three stages can be identified: patch, plaque, and nodule. The **patches** are pink to red to purple solitary or multiple macules that in the classic disease are usually confined to the distal lower extremities or feet. Microscopic examination discloses only dilated, perhaps irregular, and angulated blood vessels lined by endothelial cells with an interspersed infiltrate of lymphocytes, plasma cells, and macrophages (sometimes containing hemosiderin), lesions difficult to distinguish from granulation tissue. Over time, lesions in the classic disease spread proximally and usually convert into larger, violaceous, **raised plaques** that reveal dermal, dilated, jagged vascular channels lined by somewhat plump spindle cells accompanied by perivascular aggregates of similar spindled cells (Fig. 11–32*B*). Scattered between the vascular channels are red cells, hemosiderin-laden macrophages, lymphocytes, and plasma cells. Pink, hyalin, globules of uncertain nature may be found in the spindled cells and macrophages. Occasional mitotic figures may be present.

At a still later stage, the lesions may become **nodular** and more distinctly neoplastic and may be composed of sheets of plump, proliferating spindle cells, mostly in the dermis or subcutaneous tissues. Particularly characteristic in this cellular background are scattered small vessels and slit-like spaces that often contain rows of red cells and hyalin droplets. Marked hemorrhage, hemosiderin pigment, lymphocytes, and occasional macrophages may be admixed with this cellular background. Mitotic figures are common, as are the round, pink, cytoplasmic globules. The nodular stage is often accompanied by involvement of lymph nodes and of viscera, particularly in the African and AIDS-associated diseases.

Pathogenesis. The epidemiologic features of KS have long suggested an infectious cause with the possibility of sexual transmission. In 1994, DNA fragments of a previously unrecognized herpesvirus (called *human herpesvirus 8 [HHV-8]*, also known as KS-associated herpesvirus [KSHV]), were isolated from a skin lesion of a patient with AIDS.[66] Subsequent studies have shown that, regardless of clinical subtype, 95% of KS lesions are infected with KSHV, and this agent is both necessary and sufficient for KS development. However, in many patients, immunosuppression appears to be an important cofactor in the pathogenesis and clinical expression of this disease. KSHV (like Epstein-Barr virus) is a member of the gamma-herpesvirus subfamily, notable for causing lymphomas, lymphoproliferative disorders, and other tumors. Rates of infection with KSHV parallel the incidence of KS, being low in the United States and Europe, intermediate in Mediterranean countries, and high in Africa. KSHV is transmitted sexually and by poorly understood nonsexual routes.

Like other herpesviruses, KSHV establishes a latent form of infection. In the early stages, KS appears to be a reactive, polyclonal lesion associated with immune dysregulation. KSHV proteins may disrupt the control of cellular proliferation and prevent apoptosis of endothelial cells, through the production of p53 inhibitors and a viral homologue of cyclin D[67] (Chapter 6). Only a few cells are infected in early lesions. The number

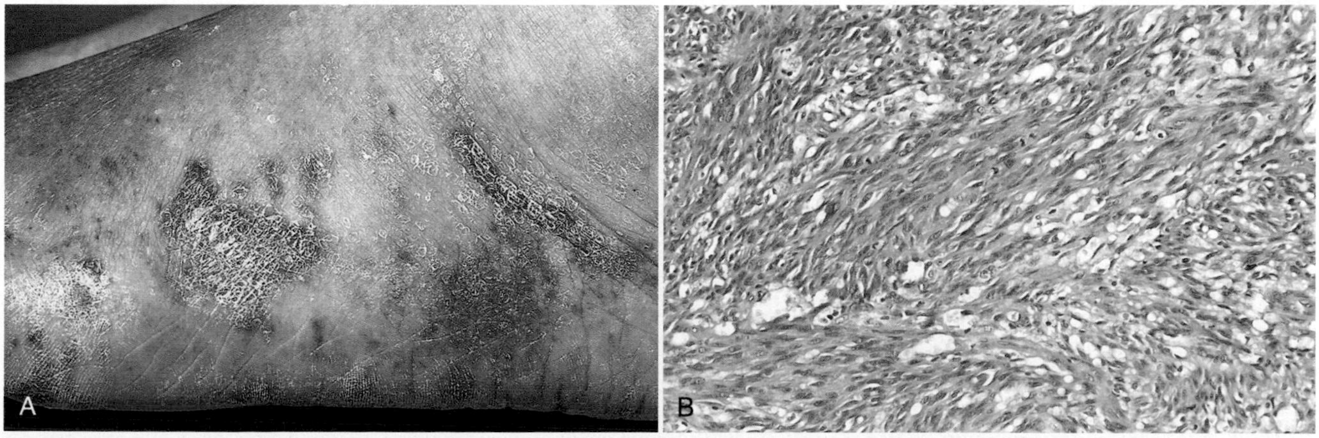

FIGURE 11–32 Kaposi sarcoma. *A,* Gross photograph, illustrating coalescent red-purple macules and plaques of the skin. *B,* Histology of nodular form, demonstrating sheets of plump, proliferating spindle cells. (*B,* courtesy of Christopher D.M. Fletcher, M.D., Brigham and Women's Hospital, Boston, MA.)

of cells infected increases with lesion stage, ultimately involving nearly all spindle cells of late-stage lesions. AIDS is thought to be a cofactor, but the specific mechanisms are yet uncertain.[68]

Clinical Course. The presentation and natural course of KS vary widely and are significantly affected by the clinical setting. Most primary KSHV infections are asymptomatic. The classic form of KS is, at the outset, largely restricted to the surface of the body, and resection of primary lesions and recurrences is usually adequate treatment, yielding an excellent prognosis. Radiation is used for multiple lesions in a restricted area; chemotherapy is used for extensive or disseminated disease. Endemic KS is also treated with chemotherapy or radiotherapy with good results. In immunosuppression-associated KS, withdrawal or reduction of immunosuppression, possibly supplemented with chemotherapy or radiotherapy is often effective. In persons who have AIDS, antiretroviral therapy for HIV is usually done, with or without chemotherapy or radiotherapy for the KS lesions. Interferon alpha may be used, and angiogenesis inhibitors have also proved effective in limited cases.

Hemangioendothelioma

The term *hemangioendothelioma* is used to denote a wide spectrum of vascular neoplasms showing histologic features and clinical behavior *intermediate between the benign, well-differentiated hemangiomas and the frankly malignant angiosarcomas* (see later).

Representative of this group is the *epithelioid hemangioendothelioma*, a unique vascular tumor occurring around medium-sized and large veins in the soft tissue of adults. In such tumors, well-defined vascular channels are inconspicuous, and the tumor cells are plump and often cuboidal, thus resembling epithelial cells. The differential diagnosis includes metastatic carcinoma, melanoma, and those sarcomas that can assume an epithelioid appearance. Clinical behavior of epithelioid hemangioendothelioma is variable; most are cured by excision, but up to 40% recur, 20% to 30% eventually metastasize, and perhaps 15% of patients die of the tumors.

MALIGNANT TUMORS

Angiosarcoma

Angiosarcomas are malignant endothelial neoplasms (Fig. 11–33) with structure varying from highly differentiated tumors that resemble hemangiomas *(hemangiosarcoma)* to those whose anaplasia makes them difficult to distinguish from malignant epithelial neoplasms such as carcinoma or melanoma. They occur in both sexes, more often in older adults, anywhere in the body but most commonly in the skin, soft tissue, breast, and liver.

The rare *hepatic angiosarcomas* are associated with distinct carcinogens, including arsenic (exposure to arsenical pesticides), Thorotrast (a radioactive contrast medium formerly widely used in radiology), and polyvinyl chloride (PVC) (a widely used plastic). The increased frequency of angiosarcomas among workers in the PVC industry is one of the well-documented instances of chemical carcinogenesis in humans (Chapter 9). With all three agents, there is a very long latent period of many years between exposure and the development of tumors.

Angiosarcomas may also arise in the setting of lymphedema, most typically approximately 10 years following radical mastectomy for breast cancer. In such cases, the tumor presumably arises from dilated lymphatic vessels *(lymphangiosarcoma)*. Angiosarcomas can be induced by radiation and

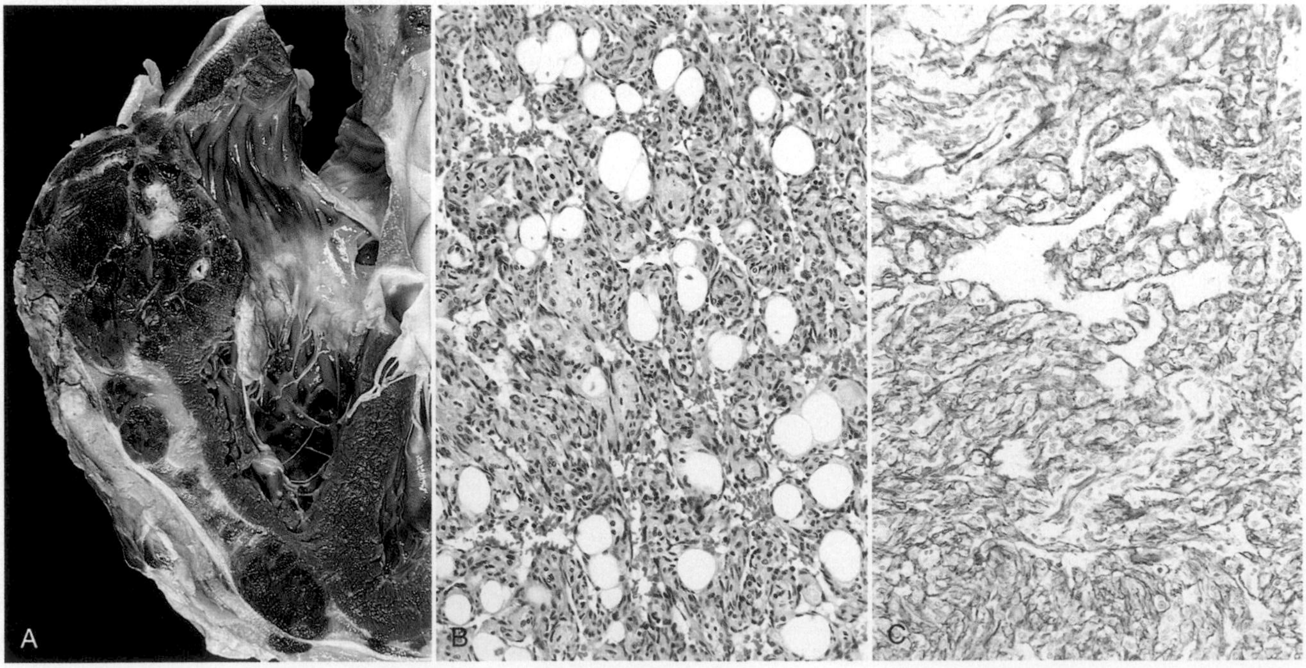

FIGURE 11–33 Angiosarcoma. *A,* Gross photograph of angiosarcoma of the heart (right ventricle). *B,* Photomicrograph of moderately well-differentiated angiosarcoma with dense clumps of irregular, moderate anaplastic cells and distinct vascular lumens. *C,* Positive immunohistochemical staining of angiosarcoma for the endothelial cell marker CD31, proving the endothelial nature of the tumor cells.

may be associated with foreign material introduced into the body, either iatrogenically or accidentally.

Morphology. Grossly, cutaneous angiosarcoma may begin as deceptively small, sharply demarcated, asymptomatic, often multiple red nodules, but eventually most such tumors become large, fleshy masses of pale, gray-white, soft tissue (Fig. 11–33*A*). The margins blend imperceptibly with surrounding structures. Central softening and areas of necrosis and hemorrhage are frequent.

Microscopically, **all degrees of differentiation of these tumors may be found,** from those that are largely vascular with plump, anaplastic but recognizable endothelial cells producing vascular channels (Fig. 11–33*B*) to tumors that are quite undifferentiated, produce no definite blood vessels, are markedly atypical, and have a solid spindle cell appearance. EC derivation is demonstrated by staining for CD31, CD34, or vWF (Fig. 11–33*C*).

Clinically, angiosarcomas show local invasion and distal metastatic spread. The majority of patients have a poor outcome with very few surviving 5 years.

Hemangiopericytoma

Hemangiopericytoma is a term that has been loosely used to describe a heterogeneous group of neoplasms with a grossly fleshy or spongy consistency and a thin-walled branching ("staghorn") vascular pattern microscopically. They are believed (though not proven) to be derived from pericytes, the cells normally arranged along capillaries and venules. Tumors classified as hemangiopericytoma most commonly arise as slowly growing masses in the pelvic retroperitoneum or the lower extremities (especially the thigh) of middle aged women, reaching 5 to 15 cm in maximum diameter. Approximately two-thirds of these tumors have a benign course, but one-third are malignant; the presence of necrosis, a high mitotic rate, and nuclear pleomorphism, especially in a large tumor, is associated with aggressive behavior. Several types of neoplasms, most notably solitary fibrous tumor, were previously classified as hemangiopericytoma.

Pathology of Vascular Interventions

Characteristic morphologic changes are introduced by current modes of therapy of vascular disease, such as balloon angioplasty and vascular replacement. Some key morphologic considerations of each of these and related interventions are discussed briefly.

BALLOON ANGIOPLASTY AND ENDOVASCULAR STENTS

Balloon angioplasty (dilation of a stenosis of an artery by a percutaneously inserted balloon catheter) is used extensively, especially for coronary arterial dilation *(percutaneous transluminal coronary angioplasty [PTCA])*. The morphologic effects of angioplasty and the frequently used *endovascular stents* are demonstrated in Figure 11–34.

The process of balloon dilation of an atherosclerotic vessel characteristically causes plaque fracture, often with accompanying localized hemorrhagic dissection of the adjacent arterial wall (Fig. 11–34*A*). *The key elements of luminal expansion in angioplasty are plaque rupture, medial dissection, and stretching of the media of the dissected segment.*

Most patients improve symptomatically following angioplasty, at least in the short-term. *Abrupt reclosure* may occur as a result of compression of the lumen by an extensive circumferential or longitudinal dissection or by thrombosis. The long-term success of angioplasty is limited by the development of *proliferative restenosis*, which results from intimal thickening and occurs in approximately 30% to 50% of patients within the first 4 to 6 months following angioplasty (Fig. 11–34*B*). The factors causing restenosis are complex but probably relate primarily to endothelial cell and smooth muscle cell injury, elaboration of cytokines and growth factors from the inflammatory cells in the plaque, local thrombosis, and elastic recoil of the dilated segment. The end result is an occlusive, rapidly progressive fibrous lesion that contains abundant smooth muscle cells and extracellular matrix.

Coronary stents are expandable tubes of metallic mesh that are inserted percutaneously to preserve luminal patency, particularly at sites of balloon angioplasty. They are now used in 70% of angioplasty procedures. Stents may reverse the untoward effects of PTCA by providing a larger and more regular lumen, initially acting as a scaffold to support the intimal flaps and dissections that occur in PTCA, limit elastic recoil, mechanically prevent vascular spasm, and increase blood flow, all of which could minimize thrombus formation and reduce the impact of postangioplasty restenosis.[69]

Nevertheless, both early thrombosis and late intimal thickening may occur and lead to in-stent restenosis (Fig. 11–34*C*). Stent implantation is accompanied by damage to the endothelial lining and stretching of the vessel wall, stimulating early adherence and accumulation of platelets and leukocytes. Stent wires are covered initially by a variable platelet–fibrin coating and later by an endothelium-lined neointima, with the wires embedded in a layer of intimal thickening consisting of α-actin–positive smooth muscle cells in a collagenous matrix. This layer of connective tissue may thicken, and proliferative restenosis is not necessarily prevented by stenting. Indeed, in-stent restenosis is the major limitation of coronary stenting. Approaches to inhibiting in-stent restenosis have included local administration of either irradiation or antiproliferative drugs at the precise site and time of vessel injury; the latter has shown excellent promise.[70]

VASCULAR REPLACEMENT

Many patients now receive synthetic or autologous grafts that replace a segment of vessel or bypass diseased arteries. The clinical performance of a vascular graft depends primarily on its type and location. Large-diameter (12- to 18-mm) Dacron grafts in current use function well in high-flow locations such as the aorta. In contrast, small-diameter fabric vascular grafts (up to 6 to 8 mm in diameter) used in the periphery or as coronary artery bypass perform less well.[71]

The most widely used small vessel replacements are *autologous saphenous vein* (the patient's own vein) and *expanded-polytetrafluoroethylene* (a spongy Teflon fabric). Failure of small-diameter vascular prostheses (6-mm-diameter) is most

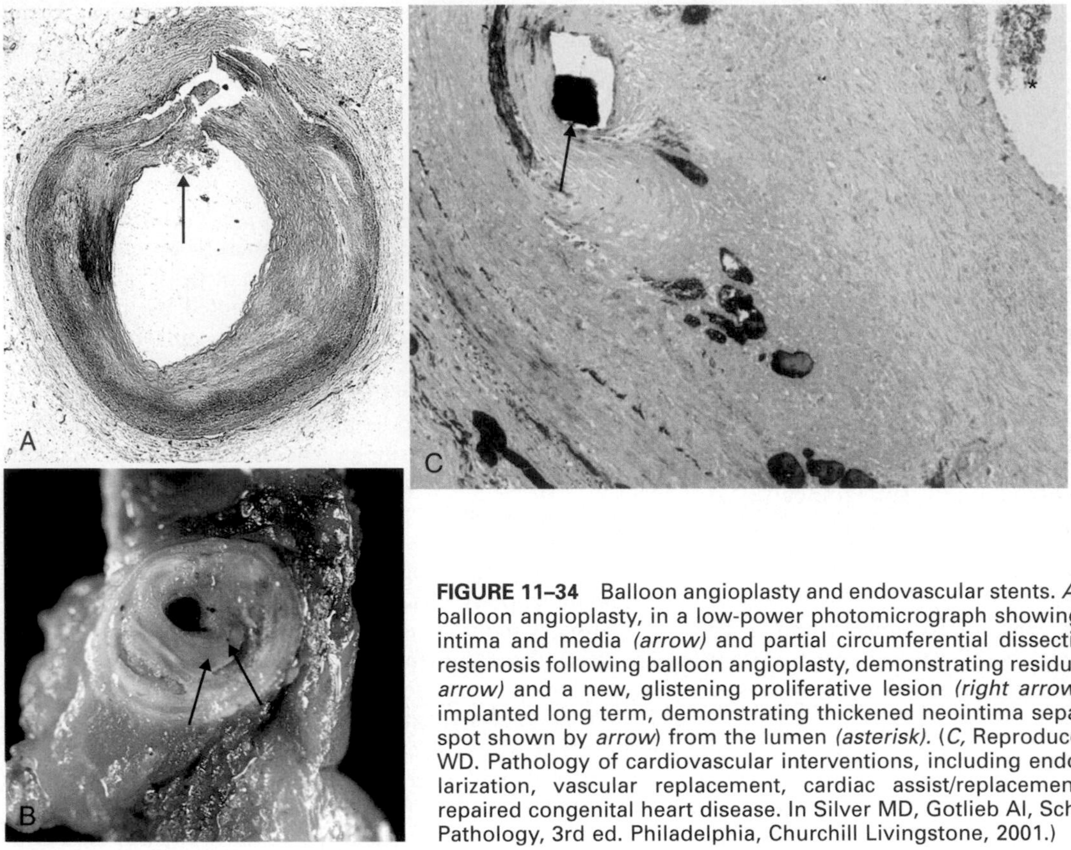

FIGURE 11–34 Balloon angioplasty and endovascular stents. *A,* Coronary artery with recent balloon angioplasty, in a low-power photomicrograph showing the split encompassing the intima and media *(arrow)* and partial circumferential dissection. *B,* Gross photograph of restenosis following balloon angioplasty, demonstrating residual atherosclerotic plaque *(left arrow)* and a new, glistening proliferative lesion *(right arrow). C,* Coronary arterial stent implanted long term, demonstrating thickened neointima separating the stent wires (black spot shown by *arrow*) from the lumen *(asterisk).* (*C,* Reproduced from Schoen FJ, Edwards WD. Pathology of cardiovascular interventions, including endovascular therapies, revascularization, vascular replacement, cardiac assist/replacement, arrhythmia control, and repaired congenital heart disease. In Silver MD, Gotlieb AI, Schoen FJ (eds): Cardiovascular Pathology, 3rd ed. Philadelphia, Churchill Livingstone, 2001.)

frequently due to thrombotic occlusion, intimal fibrous hyperplasia, either generalized (in vein grafts) or primarily at the junction of the graft with the native vasculature (in synthetic grafts) (Fig. 11–35) or, occasionally, atherosclerosis.

Healing of a vascular graft depends on the migration and proliferation of endothelial cells and smooth muscle cells, (derived from the adjacent artery) at the junction of the graft with the native vessel *(anastomosis).* The ability to endothelialize cardiovascular prostheses is limited in humans, and full endothelialization of clinical grafts is unusual. Luminal covering develops relatively slowly and incompletely; formation of *neointima* (a surface covered by endothelial cells) is gener-

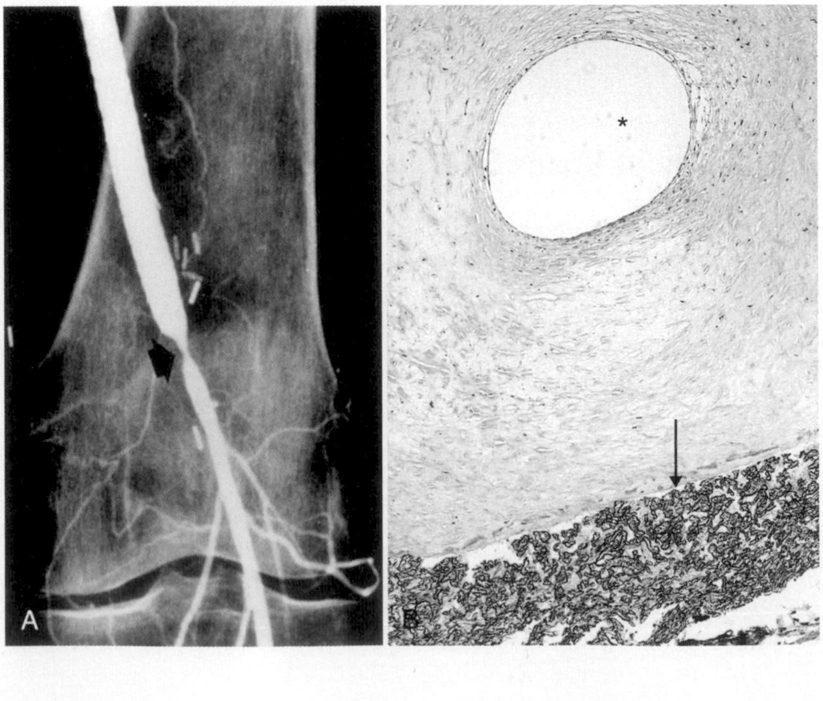

FIGURE 11–35 Anastomotic hyperplasia at the distal anastomosis of synthetic femoropopliteal graft. *A,* Angiogram demonstrating constriction *(arrow). B,* Photomicrograph demonstrating Gore-Tex graft *(arrow)* with prominent intimal proliferation and very small residual lumen (asterisk). (*A,* courtesy of Anthony D. Whittemore, M.D., Brigham and Women's Hospital, Boston, MA.)

ally restricted to a 12- to 15-mm zone near the anastomosis, and the remainder of the graft surface constitutes a *pseudointima* (thrombus or cells other than endothelial cells).

Coronary Aftery Bypass Graft Surgery

Coronary artery bypass graft surgery (aortocoronary bypass) is one of the most frequently performed major surgical procedures in the United States (more than 400,000 per year). Bypasses are done using grafts of either reversed autologous saphenous vein (taken from the patient's own leg) or internal mammary artery (usually the left internal mammary artery, owing to proximity to the heart). The long-term patency of saphenous vein grafts is 50% at 10 years, owing to pathologic changes, including thrombosis (usually early), intimal thickening (usually several months to several years postoperatively), and atherosclerosis in the graft, sometimes with superimposed plaque rupture, thrombi, or aneurysms (usually more than 2 to 3 years).[72] In contrast, internal mammary artery grafts have a greater than 90% patency at 10 years.

REFERENCES

1. Carmeliet P, Jain RK: Angiogenesis in cancer and other diseases. Nature 407:249, 2000.
2. Shin D, et al: Expression of ephrin-B2 identifies a stable genetic difference between arterial and venous vascular smooth muscle as well as endothelial cells, and marks subsets of microvessels at sites of adult neovascularization. Dev Biol 230:139, 2001.
3. Karkkainen MJ, et al: Lymphatic endothelium: a new frontier of metastasis research. Nat Cell Biol 4:E2, 2002.
4. Garcia-Cardena G, et al: Biomechanical activation of vascular endothelium as a determinant of its functional phenotype. Proc Nat Acad Sci USA 98:4478, 2001.
5. Stevens T, et al: NHLBI workshop report: endothelial cell phenotypes in heart, lung and blood diseases. Am J Physiol Cell Physiol 281:C1422, 2001.
6. Berk BC: Vascular smooth muscle growth: autocrine growth mechanisms. Physiol Rev 81:999, 2001.
7. Carmeliet P: Mechanisms of angiogenesis and arteriogenesis. Nat Med 6:389, 2000.
8. Yancopoulos GD, et al: Vascular-specific growth factors and blood vessel formation. Nature 407:242, 2000.
9. Shin JT, Fishman MC: From zebrafish to humans: modular medical models. Annu Rev Genomics Hum Genet 3:311, 2002.
10. Folkman J: Angiogenesis-dependent diseases. Semin Oncol 28:536, 2001.
11. Folkman J, et al: Angiogenesis research: guidelines for translation to clinical application. Thromb Haemost 86:23, 2001.
12. Angelini P, et al: Coronary anomalies: incidence, pathophysiology, and clinical relevance. Circulation 105:2449, 2002.
13. Fleetwood IG, Steinberg GK: Arteriovenous malformations. Lancet 359:863, 2002.
14. Stary HC, et al: A definition of advanced types of atherosclerotic lesions and a histological classification of atherosclerosis. Circulation 92:1355, 1995.
15. Komatsu A, Sakurai I: A study of the development of atherosclerosis in childhood and young adults: risk factors and the prevention of progression in Japan and the USA. The Pathological Determinants of Atherosclerosis in Youth (PDAY) Research Group. Pathol Intern 46:541, 1996.
16. Kannel WB, Wilson PWF: An update on coronary risk factors. Med Clin North Am 79:951, 1995.
17. Ridker PM, et al: Risk factors for atherosclerotic disease. In Braunwald E, Zipes DP, Libby P (eds): Heart Disease, 6th ed. Philadelphia, WB Saunders Co., 2001, p. 1010–1039.
18. Glass CK, Witzum JL: Atherosclerosis: the road ahead. Cell 104:503, 2001.
19. Libby P: The vascular biology of atherosclerosis. In Braunwald E, Zipes DP, Libby P (eds): Heart Disease, 6th ed. Philadelphia, WB Saunders Co., 2001, p. 995–1009.
20. Lusis AJ: Atherosclerosis. Nature 407:233, 2000.
21. Gimbrone MA Jr, et al: Endothelial dysfunction, hemodynamic forces, and atherogenesis. Ann NY Acad Sci 902:239, 2000.
22. Berk BC, et al: Endothelial atheroprotective and anti-inflammatory mechanisms. Ann NY Acad Sci 947:93, 2001.
23. Ross R: Atherosclerosis—an inflammatory disease N Engl J Med 340:115, 1999.
24. Libby P, et al: Inflammation and atherosclerosis. Circulation 105:1135, 2002.
25. Breslow JL: Genetics of lipoprotein abnormalities associated with coronary artery disease susceptibility. Annu Rev Genet 34:233, 2000.
26. Reardon CA, Getz GS: Mouse models of atherosclerosis. Curr Opin Lipidol 12:167, 2001.
27. Geng Y-J, Libby P: Progression of atheroma: a struggle between death and procreation. Arterioscler Thromb Vasc Biol 22:1370, 2002.
28. Benditt EP: Implications of the monoclonal character of human atherosclerotic plaques. Am J Path 86:693, 1977.
29. Chung IM, et al: Clonal architecture of normal and atherosclerotic aorta: implications for atherogenesis and vascular development. Am J Pathol 152:913, 1998.
30. O'Connor S, et al: Potential infectious etiologies of atherosclerosis: a multifactorial perspective. Emerg Infect Dis 7:780, 2001.
31. Streblow DN, et al: Do pathogens accelerate atherosclerosis? J Nutr 131:2798S, 2001.
32. Lifton RP, et al: Molecular mechanisms of human hypertension. Cell 104:545, 2001.
33. Hingorani AD, Brown MJ: Identifying the genes for human hypertension. Nephrol Dial Transplant 11:575, 1996.
34. Kannel WB: Elevated systolic blood pressure as a cardiovascular risk factor. Am J Cardiol 85:251, 2000.
35. Hyman DJ, Pavlik VN: Characteristics of patients with uncontrolled hypertension in the United States. N Engl J Med 345:479, 2002.
36. Kaplan NM: Systemic hypertension: mechanisms and diagnosis. In Braunwald E, Zipes DP, Libby P (eds): Heart Disease, 6th ed. Philadelphia, WB Saunders Co., 2001, p. 941–971.
37. Corti R, et al: Vasopeptidase inhibitors: a new therapeutic concept in cardiovascular disease? Circulation 104:1856, 2001.
38. Thibonnier M, Schork NJ: The genetics of hypertension. Curr Opin Genet Develop 5:362, 1995.
39. Beckman JA, O'Gara PT: Diseases of the aorta. Adv Int Med 44:267, 1999.
40. Ernst CB: Abdominal aortic aneurysm. N Engl J Med 328:1167, 1993.
41. Curci JA, et al: Expression and localization of macrophage elastase (matrix metalloproteinase-12) in abdominal aortic aneurysms. J Clin Invest 102:1900, 1998.
42. Yoon S, et al: Genetic analysis of MMP3, MMP9, and PAI-1 in Finnish patients with abdominal aortic or intracranial aneurysms. Biochem Biophys Res Commun 265:563, 1999.
43. Carrell TWG, et al: Stromelysin-1 (matrix metalloproteinase-3) and tissue inhibitor of metalloproteinase-3 are overexpressed in the wall of abdominal aortic aneurysms. Circulation 105:477, 2001.
44. Knox J, et al: Evidence for altered balance between matrix metalloproteinases and their inhibitors in human aortic diseases. Circulation 95:205, 1997.
45. Hallett JW Jr: Management of abdominal aortic aneurysms. Mayo Clin Proc 75:395, 2000.
46. Arko FR, et al: Endovascular stent-grafts for the repair of infrarenal abdominal aortic aneurysms: a brief review. J Interv Cardiol 14:475, 2001.
47. Najibi S, et al: Endovascular aortic aneurysm operations. Arch Surg 137:211, 2002.
48. Khan IA, Nair CK: Clinical, diagnostic, and management perspectives of aortic dissection. Chest 122:311, 2002.
49. Jennette JC, Falk RJ: Small-vessel vasculitis. N Engl J Med 337:1512, 1997.
50. Cuellar ML: Drug-induced vasculitis. Curr Rheumatol Rep 4:55, 2002.
51. Frannsen CFM, et al: Antiproteinase 3 and antimyeloperoxidase associated vasculitis. Kidney Internat 57:2195, 2000.
52. Savige J, et al: Antineutrophil cytoplasmic antibodies and associated diseases: a review of the clinical and laboratory features. Kidney Internat 57:846, 2000.
53. Harper L, Savage COS: Leukocyte–endothelial interactions in antineutrophil cytoplasmic antibody-associated systemic vasculitis. Rheum Dis Clin North Am 27:887, 2001.

54. Salvarani C, et al: Polymyalgia rheumatica and giant-cell arteritis N Engl J Med 347:261, 2002.
55. Gran JT: Some thoughts about the etiopathogenesis of temporal arteritis—a review. Scand J Rheumatol 31:1, 2002.
56. Fraga A, Medina F: Takasayu's arteritis. Curr Rheumatol Rep 4:30, 2002.
57. Hughes LB, Bridges SL Jr: Polyarteritis nodosa and microscopic polyangiitis: etiologic and diagnostic considerations. Curr Rheumatol Rep 4:75, 2002.
58. Gedalia A: Kawasaki disease: an update. Curr Rheumatol Rep 4:25, 2002.
59. Freeman AF, Shulman ST: Recent developments in Kawasaki disease. Curr Opin Infect Dis 14:357, 2001.
60. Koutkia P, et al: Leucocytoclastic vasculitis: an update for the clinician. Scand J Rheumatol 30:315, 2001.
61. Gross W: Churg-Strauss syndrome: update on recent developments. Curr Opin Rheumatol 14:11, 2002.
62. Churg A: Recent advances in the Churg-Strauss syndrome. Mod Pathol 14:1284, 2001.
62a. Olin JW: Thromboanglitis obliterans. N Engl J Med 343:864, 2004.
63. Golan TD: Lupus vasculitis: differential diagnosis with antiphospholipid syndrome. Curr Rheumatol Rep 4:18, 2002.
64. Wigley FM: Raynaud's phenomenon. N Engl J Med 347:1001, 2002.
65. Antman K, Chang Y: Kaposi's sarcoma. N Engl J Med 342:1027, 2000.
66. Chang Y, et al: Identification of herpesvirus-like DNA sequences in AIDS-associated Kaposi's sarcoma. Science 266:1865, 1994.
67. Ensoli B, et al: Reactivation and role of HHV-8 in Kaposi sarcoma initiation. Adv Cancer Res 81:161, 2001.
68. Boshoff C, Weiss R: AIDS-related malignancies. Nature Rev Cancer 2:373, 2002.
69. Regar E, et al: Stent development and local drug delivery. Br Med Bull 59:227, 2001.
70. Lowe HC, et al: Coronary in-stent restenosis: current status and future strategies. J Am Coll Cardiol 39:183, 2002.
71. Schoen FJ, Edwards WD: Pathology of cardiovascular interventions, including endovascular therapies, revascularization, vascular replacement, cardiac assist/replacement, arrhythmia control and repaired congenital heart disease. In Silver MD, Gotlieb AI, Schoen FJ (eds): Cardiovascular Pathology. Philadelphia, Churchill Livingstone, 2001, p. 678.
72. Safian RD: Accelerated atherosclerosis in saphenous vein bypass grafts: a spectrum of diffuse plaque instability. Prog Cardiovasc Dis 44:437, 2002.

CHAPTER 12

The Heart

Frederick J. Schoen, MD, PhD

MYOCARDIUM

BLOOD SUPPLY

VALVES

EFFECTS OF AGING ON THE HEART

HEART FAILURE

Cardiac Hypertrophy: Pathophysiology and Progression to Failure

Left-Sided Heart Failure

Right-Sided Heart Failure

HEART DISEASE

CONGENITAL HEART DISEASE

Left-to-Right Shunts

Atrial Septal Defect

Ventricular Septal Defect

Patent Ductus Arteriosus

Atrioventricular Septal Defect (AVSD)

Right-to-Left Shunts

Tetralogy of Fallot

Transposition of the Great Arteries (TGA)

Truncus Arteriosus

Tricuspid Atresia

Total Anomalous Pulmonary Venous Connection (TAPVC)

Obstructive Congenital Anomalies

Coarctation of Aorta

Pulmonary Stenosis and Atresia

Aortic Stenosis and Atresia

ISCHEMIC HEART DISEASE

Angina Pectoris

Myocardial Infarction (MI)

Infarct Modification by Reperfusion

Chronic Ischemic Heart Disease

Sudden Cardiac Death

HYPERTENSIVE HEART DISEASE

Systemic (Left-Sided) Hypertensive Heart Disease

Pulmonary (Right-Sided) Hypertensive Heart Disease (Cor Pulmonale)

VALVULAR HEART DISEASE

Valvular Degeneration Caused by Calcification

Calcific Aortic Stenosis

Calcific Stenosis of Congenitally Bicuspid Aortic Valve

Mitral Annular Calcification

Myxomatous Degeneration of the Mitral Valve (Mitral Valve Prolapse)

Rheumatic Fever and Rheumatic Heart Disease

Infective Endocarditis (IE)

Noninfected Vegetations

Nonbacterial Thrombotic Endocarditis (NBTE)

Endocarditis of Systemic Lupus Erythematosus (Libman-Sacks Disease)

Carcinoid Heart Disease

Complications of Artificial Valves

CARDIOMYOPATHIES

Dilated Cardiomyopathy

Arrhythmogenic Right Ventricular Cardiomyopathy (Arrhythmogenic Right Ventricular Dysplasia)

Hypertrophic Cardiomyopathy

Restrictive Cardiomyopathy

Myocarditis

Other Specific Causes of Myocardial Disease

PERICARDIAL DISEASE
Pericardial Effusion and Hemopericardium
Pericarditis
Acute Pericarditis
Chronic or Healed Pericarditis
Rheumatoid Heart Disease
TUMORS OF THE HEART
Primary Cardiac Tumors
Myxoma
Lipoma
Papillary Fibroelastoma
Rhabdomyoma
Sarcoma
Cardiac Effects of Noncardiac Neoplasms
CARDIAC TRANSPLANTATION

The human heart is a remarkably efficient, durable, and reliable pump that propels over 6000 liters of blood through the body daily and beats more than 40 million times a year during an individual's lifetime, thereby providing the tissues with a steady supply of vital nutrients and facilitating the excretion of waste products. As might be anticipated, cardiac dysfunction can be associated with devastating physiologic consequences. Heart disease is the predominant cause of disability and death in industrialized nations. In the United States, it accounts for about 40% of all postnatal deaths, totaling about 750,000 individuals annually and nearly twice the number of deaths caused by all forms of cancer combined. The yearly economic burden of ischemic heart disease, the most prevalent subgroup, is estimated to be in excess of $100 billion. The major categories of cardiac diseases considered in this chapter include congenital heart abnormalities, ischemic heart disease, heart disease caused by systemic hypertension, heart disease caused by pulmonary diseases (cor pulmonale), diseases of the cardiac valves, and primary myocardial diseases. A few comments about pericardial diseases and cardiac neoplasms as well as cardiac transplantation are also offered. Before considering details of specific conditions, we will review salient features of normal anatomy and function as well as the principles of cardiac hypertrophy and failure, the common end points of many different types of heart disease.

Normal

The normal heart weight varies with body height and weight; it averages approximately 250 to 300 g in females and 300 to 350 g in males. The usual thickness of the free wall of the right ventricle is 0.3 to 0.5 cm and that of the left ventricle 1.3 to 1.5 cm. As will be seen, increases in cardiac size and weight accompany many forms of heart disease. Greater heart weight or ventricular thickness indicates *hypertrophy,* and an enlarged chamber size implies *dilation.* An increase in cardiac weight or size (owing to hypertrophy and/or dilation) is termed *cardiomegaly.*

Myocardium

Basic to the heart's function is the near-inexhaustible cardiac muscle, the *myocardium*, composed primarily of a collection of specialized muscle cells called *cardiac myocytes* (Fig. 12–1). They are arranged largely in a circumferential and

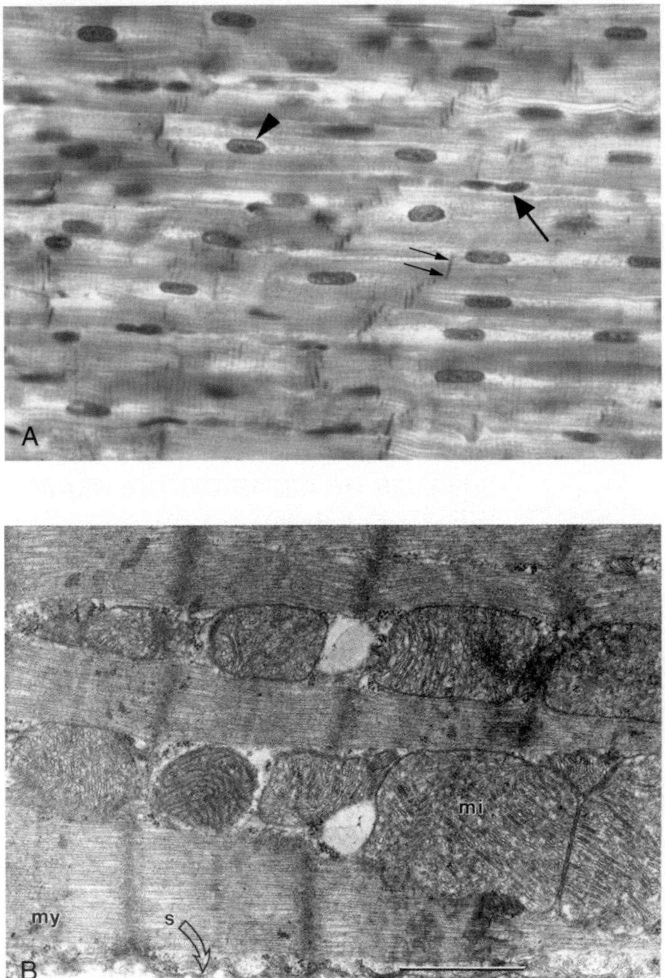

FIGURE 12–1 Myocardium (cardiac muscle). *A* The histology of myocardium is shown, emphasizing the centrally-placed nuclei of the cardiac myocytes (arrowhead), intercalated discs (representing specialized end-to-end junctions of adjoining cells; highlighted by a double arrow) and the sarcomeric structure visible as cross-striations within myocytes. A capillary endothelial cell is indicated by an arrow. (Photomicrograph courtesy of Mark Flomenbaum, M.D., Ph.D., Office of the Chief Medical Examiner, New York City, NY.) *B* Electron microscopy of myocardium, showing myofibrillar (my) and mitochondrial (mi) architecture and the sarcolemmal membrane (s). Z bands are indicated by arrows. Bar = 1 μm. (Reproduced by permission from Vivaldi MT, et al. Triphenyltetrazolium staining of irreversible injury following coronary artery occlusion in rats. Am J Pathol 121:522, 1985. Copyright J.B. Lippincott, 1985.)

spiral orientation around the left ventricle, the chamber that pumps blood to the systemic circulation. Cardiac myocytes have five major components: (1) cell membrane (sarcolemma) and T-tubules, for impulse conduction; (2) sarcoplasmic reticulum, a calcium reservoir needed for contraction; (3) contractile elements; (4) mitochondria; and (5) nucleus. Cardiac muscle cells contain many more mitochondria between myofibrils than do skeletal muscle cells (approximately 23% of cell volume vs. 2%), reflecting the almost complete dependence of cardiac muscle on aerobic metabolism. Cardiac muscle cells each usually contain one spindle-shaped nucleus. Ventricular muscle contracts during *systole* and relaxes during *diastole.*

The functional intracellular contractile unit of cardiac muscle (like skeletal muscle) is the *sarcomere,* an orderly arrangement of thick filaments composed principally of *myosin,* and thin filaments containing *actin.* Sarcomeres also contain the regulatory proteins troponin and tropomyosin. Cardiac muscle cells are composed of many parallel myofilaments (arrays of sarcomeres in series), which are responsible for the striated appearance of these cells. Contraction of cardiac muscle occurs by the cumulative effort of sliding of the actin filaments between the myosin filaments toward the center of each sarcomere. The lengths of sarcomeres range from 1.6 to 2.2 μm, depending on the state of contraction. Shorter sarcomeres have considerable overlap of actin and myosin filaments, with consequent reduction in contractile force, whereas longer lengths enhance contractility (Frank-Starling mechanism). Thus, moderate ventricular dilation during diastole increases the subsequent force of contraction during systole. With progressive dilation, however, there is a point at which effective overlap of the actin and myosin filaments is reduced, and the force of contraction turns sharply downward, as occurs in heart failure.

The myocytes comprise only approximately 25% of the total number of cells in the heart. However, because cardiac myocytes are so much larger than the intervening cells, they account for more than 90% of the volume of the myocardium. The remainder are endothelial cells, mostly associated with the rich myocardial capillary network, and fibroblasts. Inflammatory cells are rare and collagen is sparse in normal myocardium.

Reflecting their different functional requirements, atrial myocytes are generally smaller in diameter and less structured than their ventricular counterparts. Some atrial cells also differ from ventricular cells in having distinctive electron-dense granules in the cytoplasm called *specific atrial granules.* They are the sites of storage of *atrial natriuretic peptide (ANP, or A-type natriuretic peptide),* a polypeptide secreted into the blood under conditions of atrial distention. ANP can produce a variety of physiologic effects, including vasodilation, natriuresis, and diuresis, actions beneficial in pathologic states such as hypertension and congestive heart failure.[1] Other natriuretic peptides are produced by the ventricles in response to elevations of ventricular pressure and volume (B-type, initially called *brain natriuretic peptide*) and by the vascular endothelium (C-type) in response to elevated shear stress.[2]

Functional integration of myocytes is mediated by structures unique to cardiac muscle called *intercalated disks,* which join individual cells and within which specialized intercellular junctions permit both mechanical and electrical (ionic) coupling. One of the components of intercalated disks are *gap junctions,* which facilitate synchronous myocyte contraction by providing electrical coupling with relatively unrestricted passage of ions across the membranes of adjoining cells. Gap junctions consist of clusters of plasma membrane channels that directly link the cytoplasmic compartments of neighboring cells. Abnormalities in the spatial distribution of gap junctions and their respective proteins in ischemic and myocardial heart disease may contribute to electromechanical dysfunction (arrhythmias).[3]

In addition, specialized excitatory and conducting myocytes within the cardiac conduction system are involved in regulating the rate and rhythm of the heart. Components include (1) the sinoatrial (SA) pacemaker of the heart, the *SA node,* located near the junction of the right atrial appendage with the superior vena cava; (2) the *atrioventricular (AV) node,* located in the right atrium along the atrial septum; (3) the *bundle of His,* which courses from the right atrium to the summit of the ventricular septum; and its division into (4) right and left bundle branches that further arborize in the respective ventricles.

Blood Supply

Generating energy almost exclusively by the oxidation of substrates, the heart relies heavily on an adequate flow of oxygenated blood through the coronary arteries. With origins from the aorta immediately distal to the aortic valve in the sinuses of Valsalva, the coronary arteries consist of 5- to 10-cm long, 2- to 4-mm diameter conduits that run along the external surface of the heart *(epicardial coronary arteries)* and smaller vessels that penetrate the myocardium *(intramural arteries).* These small arteries yield arterioles and, ultimately, a rich network of capillaries in which there is nearly one vessel adjacent to each cardiac muscle cell.

The three major epicardial coronary arteries are (1) the left anterior descending (LAD) and (2) the left circumflex (LCX) arteries, both arising from bifurcation branches of the left (main) coronary artery, and (3) the right coronary artery (RCA). Branches of the LAD are called diagonal and septal perforators, and those of the LCX are obtuse marginals. Most coronary arterial blood flow to the myocardium occurs during ventricular diastole, when the microcirculation is not compressed by the cardiac contraction.

Knowledge of the areas of supply *(perfusion)* of the three major coronary arteries helps correlate sites of vascular obstruction with regions of myocardial infarction (MI). Typically, the LAD supplies most of the apex of the heart (the rounded point at the distal parts of the ventricles as contrasted with the wide proximal part, the base), the anterior wall of the left ventricle, and the anterior two-thirds of the ventricular septum. By convention, the coronary artery (either RCA or LCX) that gives rise to the posterior descending branch and thereby perfuses the posterior third of the septum is called "dominant" (despite the fact that the LAD and LCX collectively perfuse the majority of the left ventricular myocardium—the LAD itself about 50%). In a *right dominant circulation,* present in approximately four-fifths of individuals, the circumflex branch of the left coronary artery generally perfuses only the lateral wall of the left ventricle, and the RCA supplies the entire right ventricular free wall and the posterobasal wall of the left ventricle and the posterior third of the ventricular septum. *Thus, occlusions of the right as well as the left coronary artery can cause left ventricular damage.*

The right and left coronary arteries function as end arteries, although anatomically most hearts have numerous intercoronary anastomoses (called the *collateral circulation*). Little blood courses through these channels in the normal heart. However, when one artery is severely narrowed, blood flows via collaterals from the high to the low pressure system, and causes the channels to enlarge. Progressive dilation of collaterals, stimulated by ischemia, may play a role in providing blood flow to areas of the myocardium otherwise deprived of adequate perfusion. However, when the principal blood flow is compromised and collateral blood flow is inadequate, the subendocardium (myocardium adjacent to the ventricular cavities) is the area most susceptible to ischemic damage.

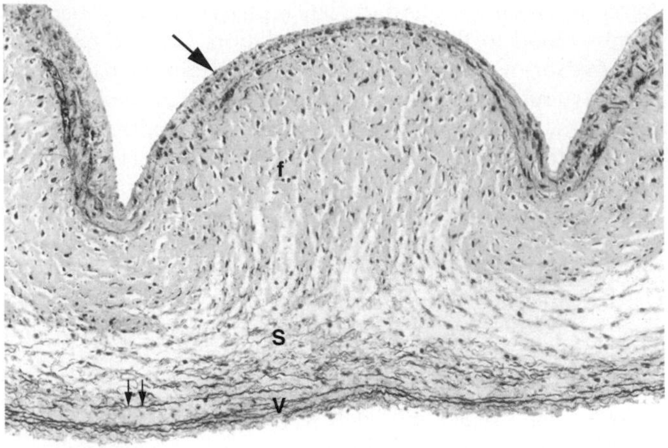

FIGURE 12–2 Aortic valve histology, shown as a low-magnification photomicrograph of cuspal cross-section in the systolic (nondistended) state, emphasizing three major layers (ventricularis [v], spongiosa [s], and fibrosa [f]). Superficial endothelial cells *(arrow)* and diffusely distributed deep interstitial cells are noted. The strength of the valve is predominantly derived from the fibrosa, with its dense collagen *(yellow).* This section highlights the dense, laminated elastic tissue in the ventricularis *(double arrow).* The outflow surface is at top. (Reproduced by permission from Schoen FJ: Aortic valve structure–function correlations: Role of elastic fibers no longer a stretch of the imagination. J Heart Valve Dis 6:1, 1997.)

Valves

The four cardiac valves (tricuspid, pulmonary, mitral, and aortic) maintain unidirectional blood flow. The ability of the valves to permit unobstructed forward flow depends on the mobility and pliability of their leaflets, which appear thin and translucent on gross inspection. The competency (ability to prevent reverse flow) of the *semilunar* valves (aortic and pulmonary) depends on the stretching and molding of their three leaflets (often called cusps) to fill the orifice in diastole (the closed phase), when there is backpressure from the blood in the aorta or pulmonary artery. This requires the cusps to stretch to 40% to 50% larger than their area during systole (open phase), when they are relaxed. During the closed phase, the cusps overlap along an area (the lunula) beneath the free edge. Only the portion of the cusps below the closing edge separates aortic from left ventricular cavity blood; thus, defects or fenestrations of the cusp in the lunula usually do not compromise valve competence, but those below it will induce regurgitation. The function of the semilunar valves also depends on the integrity and coordinated movements of the cuspal attachments. Thus, dilation of the aortic root can hinder coaptation of the aortic valve cusps during closure, yielding regurgitation. Each aortic cusp has a small nodule *(nodule of Arantius)* in the center of the free edge, which facilitates closure. The pulmonary valve has structure and function analogous to the aortic.

The atrioventricular (AV) valves (mitral and tricuspid) have a different method of maintaining closure. Their free margins are tethered to the ventricular wall by many delicate tendinous cords *(chordae tendineae)*, attached to papillary muscles that are contiguous with the underlying ventricular walls. Left ventricular papillary muscles are positioned beneath the commissures and thereby receive cords from two adjacent leaflets. Thus, normal mitral valve competency depends on the coordinated actions of annulus (the outer edge of the value orifice, where the leaflets attach), leaflets, cords, papillary muscles, and associated left ventricular wall (collectively the *mitral apparatus*) acting to maintain leaflet coaptation in the annulus. Left ventricular dilation or a ruptured cord or papillary muscle can interfere with mitral closure, resulting in regurgitant flow. Tricuspid valve function depends on analogous structures.

The microstructure of the cardiac valves reflects their function (Fig. 12–2). The cardiac valves are lined with endothelium; all have a similar, layered architecture consisting predominantly of a dense collagenous core *(fibrosa)* close to the outflow surface and continuous with valvular supporting structures, a central core of loose connective tissue *(spongiosa),* and a layer rich in elastin *(ventricularis)* below the inflow surface.[4] The collagen of the fibrosa is responsible for the mechanical integrity of a valve, and the spongiosa functions as a shock absorber. In systole, the elastin of the ventricularis contracts the cusps that were enlarged during diastole. The valve is populated throughout by interstitial cells, which produce and repair the extracellular matrix (especially collagen) of the valve. In general, normal leaflets and cusps have scant blood vessels limited to the proximal portion because they are thin enough to be nourished by diffusion from the heart's blood. Pathological changes of valves are largely of three types: damage to the collagen with weakness of the leaflets in myxomatous mitral valve disease, nodular calcification beginning in interstitial cells in calcific aortic stenosis, and fibrotic thickening in rheumatic heart disease (see later).

Effects of Aging on the Heart

With an increasing number of persons surviving into their eighth decade and beyond, knowledge of changes in the cardiovascular system that are expected to occur with aging is important. Indeed, the number of individuals aged 65 years and older will approximately double from 2000 to 2050 (from 35 million to 79 million in the United States). Changes associated with aging occur in the pericardium, cardiac chambers, valves, epicardial coronary arteries, conduction system, myocardium, and aorta (Table 12–1).[5]

TABLE 12–1 Changes in the Aging Heart

Chambers
Increased left atrial cavity size
Decreased left ventricular cavity size
Sigmoid-shaped ventricular septum
Valves
Aortic valve calcific deposits
Mitral valve annular calcific deposits
Fibrous thickening of leaflets
Buckling of mitral leaflets toward the left atrium
Lambl excrescences
Epicardial Coronary Arteries
Tortuosity
Increased cross-sectional luminal area
Calcific deposits
Atherosclerotic plaque
Myocardium
Increased mass
Increased subepicardial fat
Brown atrophy
Lipofuscin deposition
Basophilic degeneration
Amyloid deposits
Aorta
Dilated ascending aorta with rightward shift
Elongated (tortuous) thoracic aorta
Sinotubular junction calcific deposits
Elastic fragmentation and collagen accumulation
Atherosclerotic plaque

With advancing age, the amount of epicardial fat increases, particularly over the anterior surface of the right ventricle and in the atrial septum. A reduction in the size of the left ventricular cavity, particularly in the base-to-apex dimension, is associated with increasing age and accentuated by systemic hypertension. Accompanied by a rightward shift and tortuosity of a dilated ascending aorta, this chamber alteration causes the basal ventricular septum to bend leftward, bulging into the left ventricular outflow tract (termed *sigmoid septum*). Such reduction in the size of the left ventricular cavity can simulate the obstruction to blood leaving the left ventricle that often occurs with hypertrophic cardiomyopathy, discussed later in this chapter.

Several changes of the valves are noted with aging, including calcification of the mitral annulus and aortic valve, the latter frequently leading to aortic stenosis. In addition, the valves can develop fibrous thickening, and the mitral leaflets tend to buckle back toward the left atrium during ventricular systole, simulating a prolapsing (myxomatous) mitral valve (see later). Moreover, many older persons develop small filiform processes *(Lambl excrescences)* on the closure lines of aortic and mitral valves, probably arising from the organization of small thrombi on the valve contact margins.

Compared with younger myocardium, "elderly" myocardium also has fewer myocytes, increased collagenized connective tissue and, in some individuals, deposition of amyloid. In the muscle cells, lipofuscin deposits (Chapter 1), and *basophilic degeneration*, an accumulation within cardiac myocytes of a gray-blue byproduct of glycogen metabolism, may be present. Extensive lipofuscin deposition in a small, atrophied heart is called *brown atrophy*; this change often accompanies cachectic weight loss, as seen in terminal cancer.

Although the morphologic changes described are common in elderly patients at necropsy, and they may mimic disease, in only a minority are they associated with clinical cardiac dysfunction.

Pathology

Although many diseases can involve the heart and blood vessels,[6,7] cardiovascular dysfunction results from one or more of five principal mechanisms:

- *Failure of the pump.* In the most common circumstance, the cardiac muscle contracts weakly or inadequately, and the chambers cannot empty properly. In some conditions, however, the muscle cannot relax sufficiently to permit ventricular filling.
- *An obstruction to flow,* owing to a lesion preventing valve opening or otherwise causing increased ventricular chamber pressure (e.g., aortic valvular stenosis, systemic hypertension, or aortic coarctation). The increased pressure overworks the chamber that pumps against the obstruction.
- *Regurgitant flow* causes some of the output from each contraction to flow backward, adding a volume workload to each of the chambers, which must pump the extra blood (e.g., left ventricle in aortic regurgitation; left atrium and left ventricle in mitral regurgitation).
- *Disorders of cardiac conduction.* Heart block or arrhythmias owing to uncoordinated generation of impulses (e.g., atrial or ventricular fibrillation) lead to nonuniform and inefficient contractions of the muscular walls.
- *Disruption of the continuity of the circulatory system* that permits blood to escape (e.g., gunshot wound through the thoracic aorta).

Most cardiovascular disease arises from the interaction of environmental factors and genetic susceptibility. *The contemporary view holds that most clinical cardiovascular diseases result from a complex interplay of genetics and environmental factors that disrupt networks controlling morphogenesis, myocyte survival, biomechanical stress responses, contractility, and electrical conduction.*[8] For example, there is growing recognition that pathogenesis of congenital heart defects, in many cases, involves an underlying genetic abnormality whose expression is strongly modified by external (environmental or maternal) factors. Moreover, since a diverse group of cytoskeletal protein mutations have been linked with cardiac muscle cell dysfunction in the cardiomyopathies, perhaps subtle mutations or polymorphisms in these genes could confer an increased risk or more rapid onset of heart failure in response to acquired cardiac injury. In these and other examples, the clinical expression of cardiac disease represents the end result of multiple internal and external cues for growth, death, and survival of cardiac myocytes. These factors and pathways are shared with other normal tissues and pathological processes.[9]

Heart Failure

The abnormalities described above often culminate in heart failure, an extremely common result of many forms of heart disease. In heart failure, often called *congestive heart failure (CHF)*, the heart is unable to pump blood at a rate commensurate with the requirements of the metabolizing tissues or can do so only at an elevated filling pressure. Although usually caused by a slowly developing intrinsic deficit in myocardial contraction, a similar clinical syndrome is present in some patients with heart failure caused by conditions in which the normal heart is suddenly presented with a load that exceeds its capacity (e.g., fluid overload, acute myocardial infarction, acute valvular dysfunction) or in which ventricular filling is impaired (see below). CHF is a common and often recurrent condition with a poor prognosis. The magnitude of the problem is exemplified by the impact of CHF in the United States, where each year it affects nearly 5 million individuals, is the underlying or contributing cause of death of an estimated 300,000, and necessitates over 1 million hospitalizations.[10] Moreover, CHF is the leading discharge diagnosis in hospitalized patients over age 65 and has an associated annual cost of $18 billion. In many pathologic states, the onset of heart failure is preceded by *cardiac hypertrophy*, the compensatory response of the myocardium to increased mechanical work (see below).

The cardiovascular system maintains arterial pressure and perfusion of vital organs in the presence of excessive hemodynamic burden or disturbance in myocardial contractility by a number of mechanisms.[11] The most important are:

- *The Frank-Starling mechanism*, in which the increased preload of dilation (thereby increasing cross-bridges within the sarcomeres) helps to sustain cardiac performance by enhancing contractility
- *Myocardial structural changes, including augmented muscle mass (hypertrophy) with or without cardiac chamber dilation*, in which the mass of contractile tissue is augmented
- *Activation of neurohumoral systems*, especially (1) release of the neurotransmitter norepinephrine by adrenergic cardiac nerves (which increases heart rate and augments myocardial contractility and vascular resistance), (2) activation of the renin-angiotensin-aldosterone system, and (3) release of atrial natriuretic peptide.

These adaptive mechanisms may be adequate to maintain the overall pumping performance of the heart at relatively normal levels, but their capacity to sustain cardiac performance may ultimately be exceeded. Moreover, pathologic changes, such as apoptosis, cytoskeletal alterations, and extracellular matrix (particularly collagen) synthesis and remodeling, may also occur, causing structural and functional disturbances. Most instances of heart failure are the consequence of progressive deterioration of myocardial contractile function *(systolic dysfunction)*, as often occurs with ischemic injury, pressure or volume overload, or dilated cardiomyopathy. The most frequent specific causes are ischemic heart disease and hypertension. Sometimes, however, failure results from an inability of the heart chamber to relax, expand, and fill sufficiently during diastole to accommodate an adequate ventricular blood volume *(diastolic dysfunction)*, as can occur with massive left ventricular hypertrophy, myocardial fibrosis, deposition of amyloid, or constrictive pericarditis.[12] *Whatever its basis, CHF is characterized by diminished cardiac output (sometimes called forward failure) or damming back of blood in the venous system (so-called backward failure), or both.*

The molecular, cellular, and structural changes in the heart that occur as a response to injury, and cause changes in size, shape, and function, are often called *left ventricular remodeling*. Our discussion focuses on structural changes and considers heart failure to be a progressive disorder, which can culminate in a clinical syndrome characterized by impaired cardiac function and circulatory congestion. Nevertheless, we recognize that the modern treatment of chronic heart failure emphasizes the neurohumoral hypothesis, in which neuroendocrine activation is important in the progression of heart failure. Thus, inhibition of neurohormones may have long-term beneficial effects on morbidity and mortality.[13] In the future, patients with CHF may be helped by implanted mechanical cardiac assist devices, an area in which considerable progress has recently been made.[14]

CARDIAC HYPERTROPHY: PATHOPHYSIOLOGY AND PROGRESSION TO FAILURE

The cardiac myocyte is generally considered a terminally differentiated cell that has lost its ability to divide. Under normal circumstances, functionally useful augmentation of myocyte number *(hyperplasia)* cannot occur. Increased mechanical load causes an increase in the content of subcellular components and a consequent increase in cell size *(hypertrophy)*. Increased mechanical work owing to pressure or volume overload or trophic signals (e.g., hyperthyroidism through stimulation of beta-adrenergic receptors) increases the rate of protein synthesis, the amount of protein in each cell, the number of sarcomeres and mitochondria, the dimension and mass of myocytes and, consequently, the size of the heart. Nevertheless, the extent to which adult cardiac myocytes have some capacity to synthesize DNA and whether this leads to some degree of cell division is an area of considerable recent attention and debate.[15]

The extent of hypertrophy varies for different underlying causes. Heart weight usually ranges from 350 to 600 gm (up to approximately two times normal) in pulmonary hypertension and ischemic heart disease; from 400 to 800 gm (up to two to three times normal) in systemic hypertension, aortic stenosis, mitral regurgitation, or dilated cardiomyopathy; from 600 to 1000 gm (three or more times normal) in aortic regurgitation or hypertrophic cardiomyopathy. Hearts weighing more than 1000 gm are rare.

The pattern of hypertrophy reflects the nature of the stimulus (Fig. 12–3). Pressure-overloaded ventricles (e.g., in hypertension or aortic stenosis) develop *pressure-overload* (also called *concentric*) *hypertrophy* of the left ventricle, with an increased wall thickness. In the left ventricle the augmented muscle may reduce the cavity diameter. In pressure overload, the predominant deposition of sarcomeres is parallel to the long axes of cells; cross-sectional area of myocytes is expanded (but cell length is not). In contrast, volume overload stimulates deposition of new sarcomeres and cell length (as well as width) is increased. Thus, *volume-overload hypertrophy* is characterized by dilation with increased ventricular diameter. In volume overload, muscle mass and wall thickness are increased approximately in proportion to chamber diameter. However, owing to dilation, wall thickness of a heart in which both hypertrophy and dilation have occurred is not necessarily increased, and it may be normal or less than normal. Thus, wall thickness is by itself not an adequate measure of volume-overload hypertrophy.

Cardiac hypertrophy is also accompanied by numerous transcriptional and morphologic changes. With prolonged hemodynamic overload, gene expression is altered, leading to re-expression of a pattern of protein synthesis analogous to that seen in fetal cardiac development; other changes are analogous to events that occur during mitosis of normally proliferating cells (Chapter 1). Early mediators of hypertrophy include the immediate-early genes (e.g., *c-fos, c-myc, c-jun* and *EGR1*). Selective up-regulation or re-expression of embryonic/fetal forms of contractile and other proteins also occurs, including β-myosin heavy chain, ANP, and collagen (see Chapter 1). The increased myocyte size that occurs in cardiac hypertrophy is usually accompanied by decreased capillary density, increased intercapillary distance, and deposition of fibrous tissue. Nevertheless, the enlarged muscle mass has increased metabolic requirements and increased wall tension, both major determinants of the oxygen consumption of the heart. The other major factors in oxygen consumption are heart rate and contractility (inotropic state, or force of contraction), both of which are often increased in hypertrophic states.

Thus, the geometry, structure, and composition (cells and extracellular matrix) of the hypertrophied heart are not normal. Cardiac hypertrophy constitutes a tenuous balance between adaptive characteristics (including new sarcomeres) and potentially deleterious structural and biochemical/molecular alterations (including decreased capillary-to-myocyte ratio, increased fibrous tissue, and synthesis of abnormal proteins). Thus, sustained cardiac hypertrophy often evolves to cardiac failure. Ultimately, the primary cardiac disease and the superimposed compensatory burdens further encroach on the myocardial reserve. Then begins the downward slide of stroke volume and cardiac output that often ends in death. The proposed sequence of initially beneficial and later harmful events in the response to increased cardiac work is summarized in Figure 12–4.

The structural, biochemical, and molecular basis for myocardial contractile failure is obscure in many cases. Nevertheless, in some instances (e.g., myocardial infarction), there is obvious death of myocytes and loss of vital elements of the "pump"; consequently, noninfarcted regions of cardiac muscle are overworked. In contrast, in valvular heart disease, increased pressure or volume work affects the myocardium globally. *The molecular and cellular changes in hypertrophied hearts that initially mediate enhanced function may contribute to the development of heart failure.*[16–18] Proteins related to contractile elements, excitation–contraction coupling, and energy utilization may be significantly altered through production of different isoforms that either may be less functional than normal or may be reduced or increased in amount. Alterations of intracellular handling of calcium ions may also contribute to impaired contraction and relaxation.[19] Loss of myocytes due to apoptosis may contribute to progressive myocardial dysfunction in cardiac disease with hypertrophy.[20]

Increased heart mass predicts excess cardiac mortality and morbidity. Indeed, besides predisposing to CHF, left ventricular hypertrophy is an independent risk factor for sudden death.[21] Interestingly, and in contrast to the *pathologic hypertrophy* just discussed, hypertrophy that is induced by regular strenuous exercise *(physiologic hypertrophy)* seems to be an extension of normal growth and has minimal or no deleterious effect. A suitable explanation for this discrepancy is yet lacking.

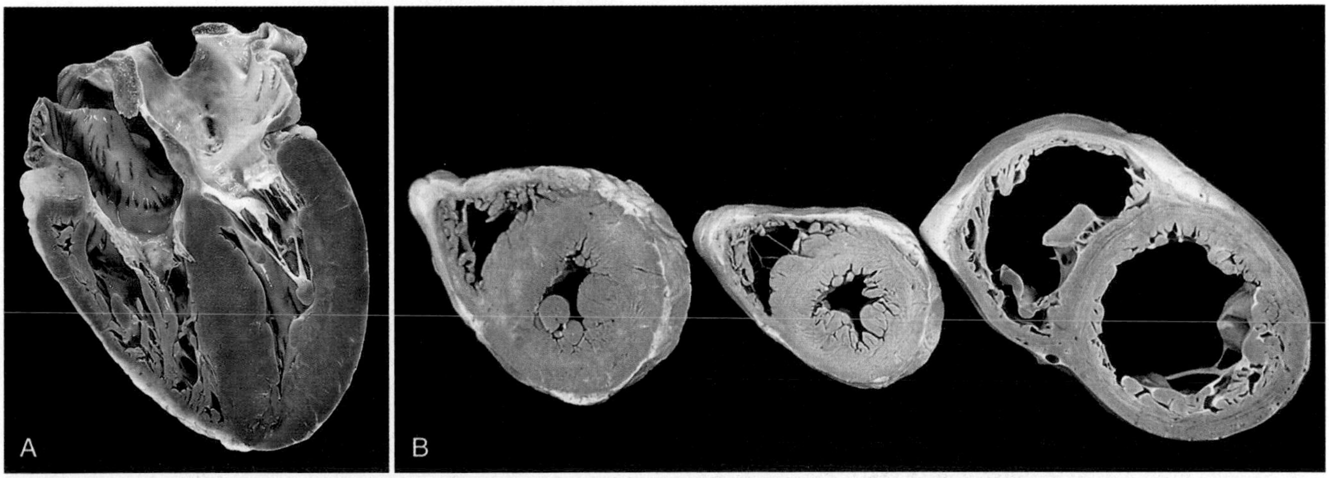

FIGURE 12–3 Left ventricular hypertrophy. *A,* Pressure hypertrophy due to left ventricular outflow obstruction. The left ventricle is on the lower right in this apical four-chamber view of the heart. *B,* Altered cardiac configuration in left ventricular hypertrophy without and with dilation, viewed in transverse heart sections. Compared with a normal heart (*center*), the pressure-hypertrophied hearts (*left* and in *A*) have increased mass and a thick left ventricular wall, but the hypertrophied and dilated heart *(right)* has increased mass but a normal wall thickness. (Reproduced by permission from Edwards WD: Cardiac anatomy and examination of cardiac specimens. In Emmanouilides GC, Riemenschneider TA, Allen HD, Gutgesell HP (eds): Moss and Adams Heart Disease in Infants, Children, and Adolescents: Including the Fetus and Young Adults, 5th ed. Philadelphia, Williams and Wilkins, 1995, p. 86.)

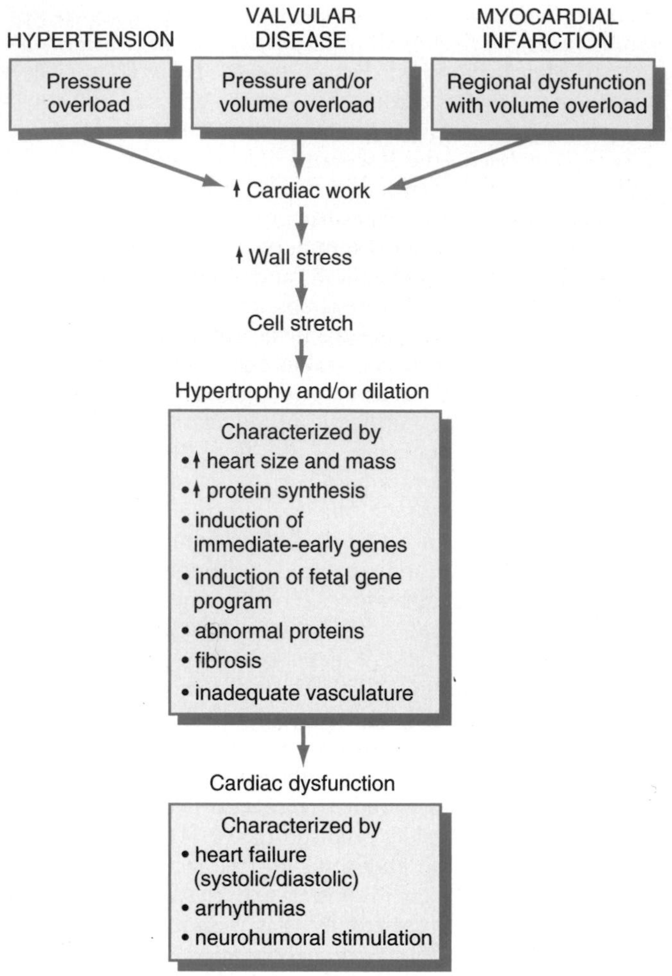

FIGURE 12–4 Schematic representation of the sequence of events in cardiac hypertrophy and its progression to heart failure, emphasizing cellular and extracellular changes.

The degree of structural abnormality of the heart in CHF does not always reflect the level of dysfunction and, indeed, it may be impossible from morphologic examination of the heart to distinguish a damaged but compensated heart from one that has decompensated. At autopsy, the heart of patients having CHF is generally characterized by increased weight, chamber dilation, thin walls, and microscopic changes of hypertrophy, but the extent of these changes varies from one patient to the next. *Moreover, many of the significant adaptations and morphologic changes noted in CHF are distant from the heart and are produced by the hypoxic and congestive effects of the failing circulation on other organs and tissues.* Thus CHF represents a clinical syndrome characterized primarily by findings outside the cardiovascular system—in both "forward" (e.g., poor organ perfusion) and "backward" (dyspnea and peripheral edema) directions.

To some extent, the right and left sides of the heart act as two distinct anatomic and functional units. Thus left-sided and right-sided failure can occur independently. Nevertheless, because the cardiovascular system is a closed circuit, failure of one side (particularly the left side) often produces excessive strain on the other, terminating in global heart failure. Despite this interdependency, the clearest understanding of the pathologic physiology and anatomy of heart failure is derived from a consideration of each side separately.

LEFT-SIDED HEART FAILURE

As discussed, left-sided heart failure is most often caused by (1) ischemic heart disease, (2) hypertension, (3) aortic and mitral valvular diseases, and (4) nonischemic myocardial diseases. The morphologic and clinical effects of left-sided CHF primarily result from progressive damming of blood within the pulmonary circulation and the consequences of diminished peripheral blood pressure and flow.

Morphology. The findings in the **heart** vary depending on the cause of the disease process; abnormalities such as myocardial infarction or a valvular deformity may be present. Except with obstruction at the mitral valve or other processes that restrict the size of the left ventricle, this chamber is usually hypertrophied and often dilated, sometimes quite massively. There are usually nonspecific changes of hypertrophy and fibrosis in the myocardium. Secondary enlargement of the left atrium with resultant atrial fibrillation (i.e., uncoordinated, chaotic contraction of the atrium) may either compromise stroke volume or cause blood stasis and possible thrombus formation (particularly in the atrial appendage). A fibrillating left atrium carries a substantially increased risk of embolic stroke.[22] The extracardiac effects of left-sided heart failure are manifested most prominently in the lungs, although the kidneys and brain may also be affected.

Lungs. Pressure in the pulmonary veins mounts and is ultimately transmitted retrograde to the capillaries and arteries. The result is pulmonary congestion and edema, with heavy, wet lungs as described in detail in Chapters 4 and 15. It is sufficient to note here that the pulmonary changes include, in sequence, (1) a perivascular and interstitial transudate, particularly in the interlobular septa, responsible for Kerley's B lines on x-ray; (2) progressive edematous widening of alveolar septa; and (3) accumulation of edema fluid in the alveolar spaces. Moreover, iron-containing proteins in edema fluid and hemoglobin from erythrocytes, which leak from congested capillaries, are phagocytosed by macrophages and converted to hemosiderin. Hemosiderin-containing macrophages in the alveoli (called **siderophages**, or **heart failure cells**) denote previous episodes of pulmonary edema.

These anatomic changes are associated with striking clinical manifestations. **Dyspnea** (breathlessness), usually the earliest and the cardinal complaint of patients in left-sided heart failure, is an exaggeration of the normal breathlessness that follows exertion. With further impairment, there is **orthopnea**, which is dyspnea on lying down that is relieved by sitting or standing. Thus the orthopneic patient must sleep while sitting upright. **Paroxysmal nocturnal dyspnea** is an extension of orthopnea that consists of attacks of extreme dyspnea bordering on suffocation, usually occurring at night. Cough is a common accompaniment of left-sided failure.

Kidneys. Decreased cardiac output causes a reduction in renal perfusion, which activates the renin-angiotensin-aldosterone system, inducing retention of salt and water with consequent expansion of the interstitial fluid and blood volumes. This compensatory reaction can contribute to the pulmonary edema in left-sided heart failure and is counteracted by the release of ANP through atrial dilation, which acts to decrease excessive blood volume. If the perfusion deficit of the kidney becomes sufficiently severe, impaired excretion of nitrogenous products may cause azotemia, in this instance **prerenal azotemia** (Chapter 20).

Brain. In far-advanced CHF, cerebral hypoxia may give rise to **hypoxic encephalopathy** (see Chapter 28), with irritability, loss of attention span, and restlessness, which may even progress to stupor and coma.

RIGHT-SIDED HEART FAILURE

Isolated right-sided heart failure occurs in only a few diseases. Usually it is a secondary consequence of left-sided heart failure because any increase in pressure in the pulmonary circulation incidental to left-sided heart failure inevitably produces an increased burden on the right side of the heart. The causes of right-sided heart failure must then include all those that induce left-sided heart failure.

Pure right-sided heart failure most often occurs with chronic severe pulmonary hypertension and thus is called *cor pulmonale.* In this condition, the right ventricle is burdened by a pressure workload due to increased resistance within the pulmonary circulation. Hypertrophy and dilation are generally confined to the right ventricle and atrium, although bulging of the ventricular septum to the left can cause dysfunction of the left ventricle.

The major morphologic and clinical effects of pure right-sided heart failure differ from those of left-sided heart failure in that pulmonary congestion is minimal, whereas engorgement of the systemic and portal venous systems may be pronounced.

Morphology.

Liver and Portal System. The liver is usually increased in size and weight **(congestive hepatomegaly)**, and a cut section displays prominent **passive congestion** (see Chapter 18). Congested red centers of the liver lobules are surrounded by paler, sometimes fatty, peripheral regions. In some instances, especially when left-sided heart failure is also present, the severe central hypoxia produces **centrilobular necrosis** along with the sinusoidal congestion. With long-standing severe right-sided heart failure, the central areas can become fibrotic, creating so-called **cardiac sclerosis** or **cardiac cirrhosis** (Chapter 18).

Right-sided heart failure also leads to elevated pressure in the portal vein and its tributaries. Congestion produces a tense, enlarged spleen **(congestive splenomegaly)**. Microscopically there may be marked sinusoidal dilation. With long-standing congestion, the enlarged spleen may achieve a weight of 300 to 500 gm (normal, approximately 150 gm). Chronic edema of the bowel wall can also occur and in some patients may interfere with absorption of nutrients. In addition, accumulations of transudate in the peritoneal cavity may give rise to **ascites.**

Kidneys. Congestion of the kidneys is more marked with right-sided heart failure than with left-sided heart failure, leading to greater fluid retention, peripheral edema, and more pronounced azotemia.

Brain. Symptoms essentially identical to those described in left-sided heart failure may occur, representing venous congestion and hypoxia of the central nervous system.

Pleural and Pericardial Spaces. Accumulation of fluid in the pleural space (particularly right) and pericardial space (effusions) may appear. Thus, while pulmonary edema indicates left-sided heart failure, pleural effusions accompany right-sided heart failure. Pleural effusions can range from 100 ml to well over 1 liter and can cause partial atelectasis of the corresponding lung.

Subcutaneous Tissues. Peripheral edema of dependent portions of the body, especially ankle (pedal) and pretibial edema, is a hallmark of right-sided heart failure. In chronically bedridden patients, the edema may be primarily presacral. Generalized massive edema is called **anasarca.**

The symptoms of pure left-sided heart failure are largely due to pulmonary congestion and edema. In contrast, in right-sided heart failure, respiratory symptoms may be absent or quite insignificant, and there is a systemic (and portal) venous congestive syndrome, with hepatic and splenic enlargement, peripheral edema, pleural effusion, and ascites. *In many cases of chronic cardiac decompensation, however, the patient presents with the picture of biventricular CHF, encompassing the clinical syndromes of both right-sided and left-sided heart failure.*

Heart Disease

With the introduction to general principles of cardiac functional anatomy and heart failure, we now turn to a discussion of the major forms of heart disease. Five categories of disease account for nearly all cardiac mortality:

- Congenital heart disease
- Ischemic heart disease
- Hypertensive heart disease (systemic and pulmonary)
- Valvular heart disease
- Nonischemic (primary) myocardial disease.

Although congenital heart disease is discussed first, it is important to keep in mind that ischemic heart disease is responsible for 80% to 90% of cardiovascular deaths and is the leading cause of all mortality in the developed world.

Congenital Heart Disease

Congenital heart disease is a general term used to describe abnormalities of the heart or great vessels that are present from birth. Most such disorders arise from faulty embryogenesis during gestational weeks 3 through 8, when major cardiovascular structures develop. The most severe anomalies may be incompatible with intrauterine survival. Congenital heart defects compatible with embryologic maturation and birth are generally morphogenetic defects of individual chambers or regions of the heart, with the remainder of the heart developing relatively normally. Examples are infants born with a defect in septation ("hole in the heart"), such as an atrial septal defect (ASD) or a ventricular septal defect (VSD), or a hypoplastic right or left ventricle, in which the unaffected ventricle is morphologically, electrically, and physiologically normal. Alternatively, the development of the muscular component of the heart may proceed normally, but vessels that arise from the heart may not have the appropriate connections with specific cardiac chambers. Some forms of congenital heart disease produce manifestations soon after birth, frequently accompanying the change from fetal to postnatal circulatory patterns (with reliance on the lungs, rather than placenta, for oxygenation). Others, however, do not necessarily become evident until adulthood (e.g., aortic coarctation or ASD).

Owing largely to surgical advances in the correction of simple and complex structural heart defects, the number of adults who have survived with congenital heart disease is increasing rapidly. It is estimated that by 2020 there will be at least 750,000 adults with congenital heart disease who require a very specialized form of care with novel medical, psychologic, and social dimensions.[23] They include those who have never had cardiac surgery, those who have had reparative cardiac surgery and require no further intervention, and those who have had incomplete or palliative surgery.[24]

Although surgery may fully correct the hemodynamic abnormalities of congenital heart disease, the heart following repair of a congenital defect may not be fully normal. Myocardial hypertrophy and other changes of cardiac remodeling brought about by the congenital defect may be irreversible or even necessary for survival and growth. Although adaptive initially, such changes can elicit late-onset arrhythmias, ischemia, and myocardial dysfunction, sometimes after many uneventful years subsequent to the surgery. Associated prosthetic materials and devices, such as substitute valves or myocardial patches, yield an additional risk of complications, most prominently thromboembolism, infection, or dysfunction of the material or device. Moreover, there may be specific difficulties resulting from hyperviscosity of the blood owing to increased hematocrit, and maternal risks associated with childbearing in those with cyanotic congenital disease.

Incidence. Congenital heart disease is the most common type of heart disease among children. Although figures vary, a generally accepted incidence is approximately 1% of live births. The incidence is higher in premature infants and in stillborns. Twelve disorders account for about 85% of cases; their frequencies are presented in Table 12–2.

TABLE 12–2 Frequencies of Congenital Cardiac Malformations*

Malformation	Incidence per Million Live Births	%
Ventricular septal defect	4482	42
Atrial septal defect	1043	10
Pulmonary stenosis	836	8
Patent ductus arteriosus	781	7
Tetralogy of Fallot	577	5
Coarctation of aorta	492	5
Atrioventricular septal defect	396	4
Aortic stenosis	388	4
Transposition of great arteries	388	4
Truncus arteriosus	136	1
Total anomalous pulmonary venous connection	120	1
Tricuspid atresia	118	1
TOTAL	9757	

*Presented as upper quartile of 44 published studies. Percentages do not add to 100% owing to rounding.

Source: Hoffman JIE, Kaplan S: The incidence of congenital heart disease. J Am Coll Cardiol 39:1890, 2002.

In the past few decades, the reported incidence of structural heart defects in newborns has increased owing to increased diagnostic sensitivity (especially cross-sectional and Doppler echocardiography and magnetic resonance imaging). The enhanced resolving power of noninvasive methods should prove particularly useful in the study of familial structural defects, because apparently unaffected relatives can be evaluated for subclinical evidence of anomalies.

Etiology and Pathogenesis. The etiology of congenital malformations in general was discussed in Chapter 10. We therefore confine our remarks to factors of particular relevance to congenital cardiac malformations.

Congenital heart defects are caused by developmental abnormalities. However, the genes that may be involved in these defects have been identified in only a minority of conditions. In fact, well-defined genetic or environmental influences are identifiable in only about 10% of cases of congenital heart disease, but the understanding of probable genetic links is increasing. The obvious role of genetic factors in some cases is demonstrated by the occurrence of familial forms of congenital heart disease and by an association of congenital cardiac malformations with certain chromosomal abnormalities (e.g., trisomies 13, 15, 18, and 21, and the Turner syndrome). Indeed, a congenital heart defect in a parent or preceding sibling is the greatest risk factor for developing a cardiac malformation. Trisomy 21 (associated with Down syndrome) is the most common known genetic cause of congenital heart disease. *Environmental factors*, such as congenital rubella infection or teratogens, are responsible for some additional cases. Multifactorial genetic, environmental, and maternal factors probably account for the remaining majority of cases in which a cause is not apparent.

The growing understanding of the genetics of congenital heart disease has also led to the recognition that powerful disease modifiers must exist. There is wide variation in the nature and severity of lesions in patients with identical genetic abnormalities. This suggests that altering key environmental or maternal factors could modify disease in high-risk individuals, whether or not the disease is caused by a distinct genetic abnormality. For instance, this type of strategy has resulted in marked reduction in neural tube defects by increasing maternal dietary folate.[25]

Genetics of Cardiac Development and Congenital Heart Disease. Composed of diverse cell lineages, the heart is among the first organs to form and function in vertebrate embryos. Cardiac morphogenesis involves a myriad of genes and is tightly regulated to ensure an effective embryonic circulation. Key steps involve specification of cardiac cell fate, morphogenesis and looping of the heart tube, segmentation and growth of the cardiac chambers, cardiac valve formation, and connection of the great vessels to the heart.[26] The genetic regulation of heart formation has been widely studied in model organisms, including chick, frog, mouse, and zebrafish. In recent years, the zebrafish, an organism that is transparent and has external fertilization, a brief generation time, and no requirement of a functional cardiovascular system for survival during embryogenesis, has permitted detailed genetic analysis of both normal development and cardiac defects.[27,28] The molecular pathways controlling cardiac development provide a foundation for understanding the basis of some congenital heart defects and can be used to reveal pathways and interactions important in human disease.[29]

Several congenital heart diseases are associated with mutations in transcription factors. For example, mutation of the gene that encodes the transcription factor, TBX5, has been shown to cause the ASD and VSD observed in the Holt-Oram syndrome, a rare hereditary condition associated with heart, arm, and hand defects.[30] Another gene, encoding the transcription factor NKX2.5, causes nonsyndromic (isolated) ASD in humans when one copy is missing. This gene is the human counterpart of the *tinman* gene of the fruit fly (so named because, like the Tin Man in *The Wizard of Oz*, fruit fly embryos lacking both copies of *tinman* have no hearts). Nevertheless, most ASDs do not have an identifiable genetic etiology, and the mechanisms by which mutated transcription factors cause clinically important heart defects are just beginning to be understood.[31]

Until recently, in most studies, defects were classified by their pathology; for example, all VSDs were considered as one group. A major advance has been to examine familial aggregation of defects based on presumed pathogenesis. Since some cardiac structures share developmental pathways, anatomically and clinically distinct lesions may be related by a common genetic defect. Thus, the occurrence of distinct defects in the same family remains consistent with a genetic model. Defects unrelated by pathogenesis would require a different interpretation.

Developmental errors in mesenchymal tissue migration exemplify the concept that distinct syndromes share a common pathogenesis. Included in this category is a wide range of anomalies of the outflow tract, some due to failure of fusion and others due to failure of septation. These lesions include isolated interruption of the aortic arch, persistent truncus arteriosus (failure of separation of aorta and pulmonary arteries), and tetralogy of Fallot (malalignment of aorta and pulmonary artery with the ventricles). Comprising 15% of congenital heart defects, outflow tract defects may be caused by the abnormal development of neural crest–derived cells, whose migration into the embryonic heart is required for formation of the outflow tracts of the heart (Fig. 12–5). Considerable progress has been made during the past few years in identifying a region of chromosome 22 that has a major role in development of the conotruncus, the branchial arches, and the face. Chromosome 22q11.2 deletions are seen in 15% to 50% of these disorders, rendering this abnormality a common genetic cause of congenital heart defects (see also Chapter 5). This condition includes developmental anomalies of the fourth branchial arch and derivatives of the third and fourth pharyngeal pouches. Hypoplasia of the thymus and parathyroids causes immune deficiency (Di George syndrome, Chapter 5) and hypocalcemia.

Other common mechanisms of congenital heart disease include extracellular matrix abnormalities and situs and looping defects. The endocardial cushions have received the most attention as an area where defects in cell–cell and cell–extracellular matrix interactions might produce malformations, as evidenced by a high frequency of endocardial cushion defects and atrioventricular septal defects in Down syndrome. Situs and looping defects may arise from single genes that have a major effect on determining laterality.

Clinical Features. The varied structural anomalies in congenital heart disease fall primarily into three major categories:

- Malformations causing a *left-to-right shunt*
- Malformations causing a *right-to-left shunt*
- Malformations causing an *obstruction.*

A *shunt* is an abnormal communication between chambers or blood vessels. Abnormal channels permit the flow of blood from left to right or the reverse, depending on pressure relationships. When blood from the right side of the heart enters the left side *(right-to-left shunt)*, a dusky blueness of the skin and mucous membranes *(cyanosis)* results because there is diminished pulmonary blood flow, and poorly oxygenated blood enters the systemic circulation (called *cyanotic congenital heart disease*). The most important examples of right-to-left shunts are tetralogy of Fallot, transposition of the great arteries, persistent truncus arteriosus, tricuspid atresia, and total anomalous pulmonary venous connection. Moreover, with right-to-left shunts, bland or septic emboli arising in peripheral veins can bypass the normal filtration action of the lungs and thus directly enter the systemic circulation *(paradoxical embolism)*; brain infarction and abscess are potential consequences. Clinical findings frequently associated with severe, long-standing cyanosis include *clubbing of the tips of the fingers and toes* (hypertrophic osteoarthropathy) and polycythemia.

In contrast, *left-to-right shunts* (such as ASD, VSD, and patent ductus arteriosus [PDA]) increase pulmonary blood flow and are not initially associated with cyanosis. However, they expose the postnatal, low-pressure, low-resistance pulmonary circulation to increased pressure and/or volume, which can result in right ventricular hypertrophy and, potentially, failure. Shunts associated with increased pulmonary blood flow include ASDs; shunts associated with both increased pulmonary blood flow and pressure include VSDs and PDA. The muscular pulmonary arteries ($<$1 mm diameter) first respond to increased pressure by medial hypertrophy

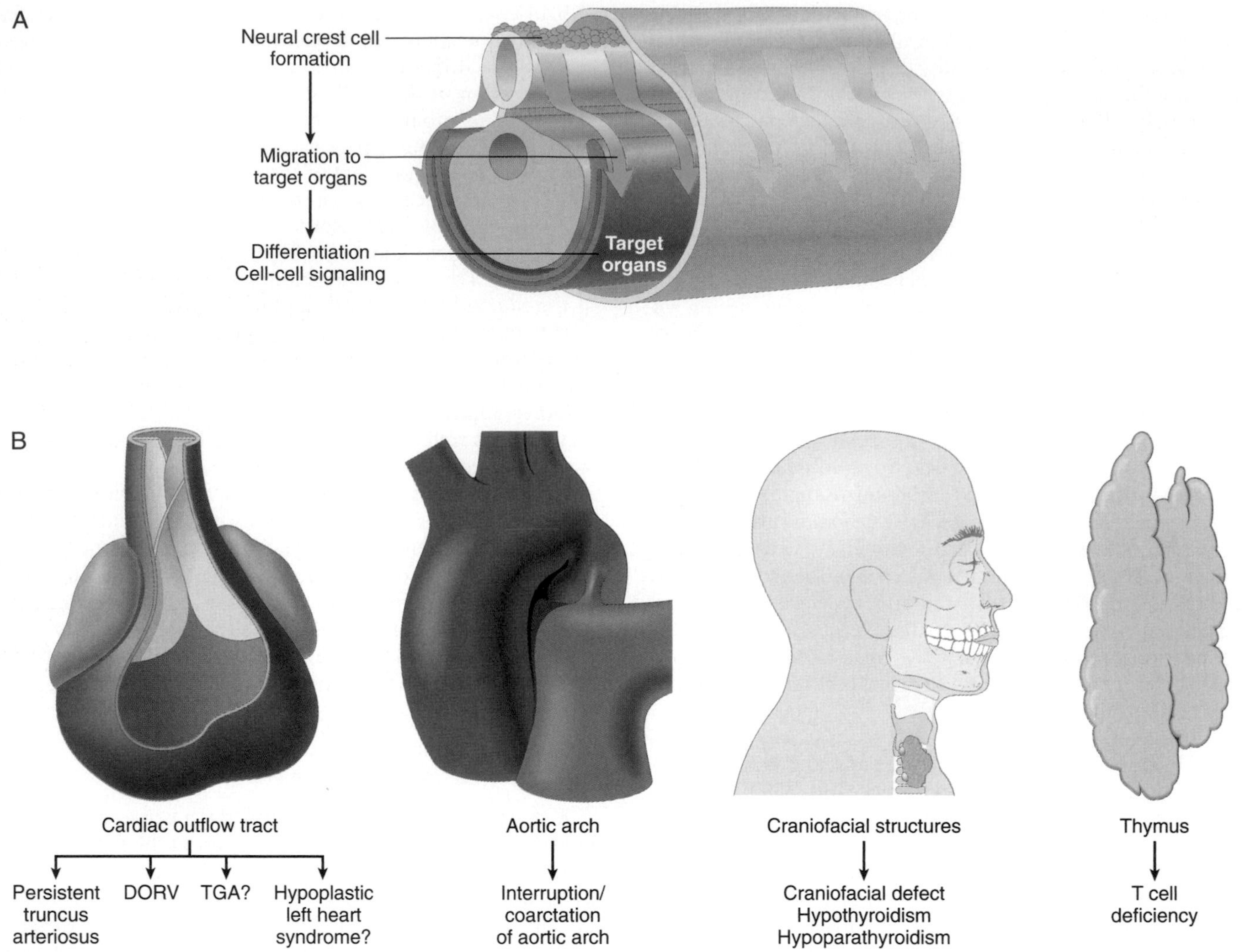

FIGURE 12–5 Cardiac defects related to neural crest abnormalities. *A,* Biologic pathways for cardiac neural crest-related defects. *B,* Disease phenotypes. DORV, double-outlet right ventricle; TGA, transposition of the great arteries. (Reproduced by permission from Chien KR: Genomic circuits and the integrative biology of cardiac diseases. Nature 407:227, 2000.)

and vasoconstriction, which maintains relatively normal distal pulmonary capillary and venous pressures, helping to prevent pulmonary edema. Prolonged pulmonary arterial vasoconstriction, however, stimulates the development of irreversible obstructive intimal lesions. Eventually pulmonary vascular resistance increases toward systemic levels, thereby reversing the shunt to right-to-left with unoxygenated blood in the systemic circulation *(late cyanotic congenital heart disease, or Eisenmenger syndrome).*

Once significant irreversible pulmonary hypertension develops, the structural defects of congenital heart disease are considered irreparable. The secondary pulmonary vascular changes can eventually lead to the patient's death. This is the rationale for early intervention, either surgical or nonsurgical.

Some developmental anomalies of the heart (e.g., coarctation of the aorta, aortic valvular stenosis, and pulmonary valvular stenosis) produce obstructions to flow because of abnormal narrowing of chambers, valves, or blood vessels and therefore are called *obstructive congenital heart disease.* A complete obstruction is called an *atresia.* In some disorders (e.g., tetralogy of Fallot), an obstruction (pulmonary stenosis) is associated with a shunt (right-to-left through a VSD).

In congenital heart disease, altered hemodynamics usually cause cardiac dilation or hypertrophy (or both). A decrease in the volume and muscle mass of a cardiac chamber is called *hypoplasia* if it occurs before birth and *atrophy* if it develops after birth.

LEFT-TO-RIGHT SHUNTS

The diseases in this group cause cyanosis several months or years after birth. The most commonly encountered left-to-right shunts include atrial septal defects, ventricular septal defects, patent (or persistent) ductus arteriosus, and AV septal defects, and are shown in Figure 12–6. (For ease of recall, note that each is designated by an abbreviation containing the letter "D" as in ASD, VSD, PDA, and AVSD).

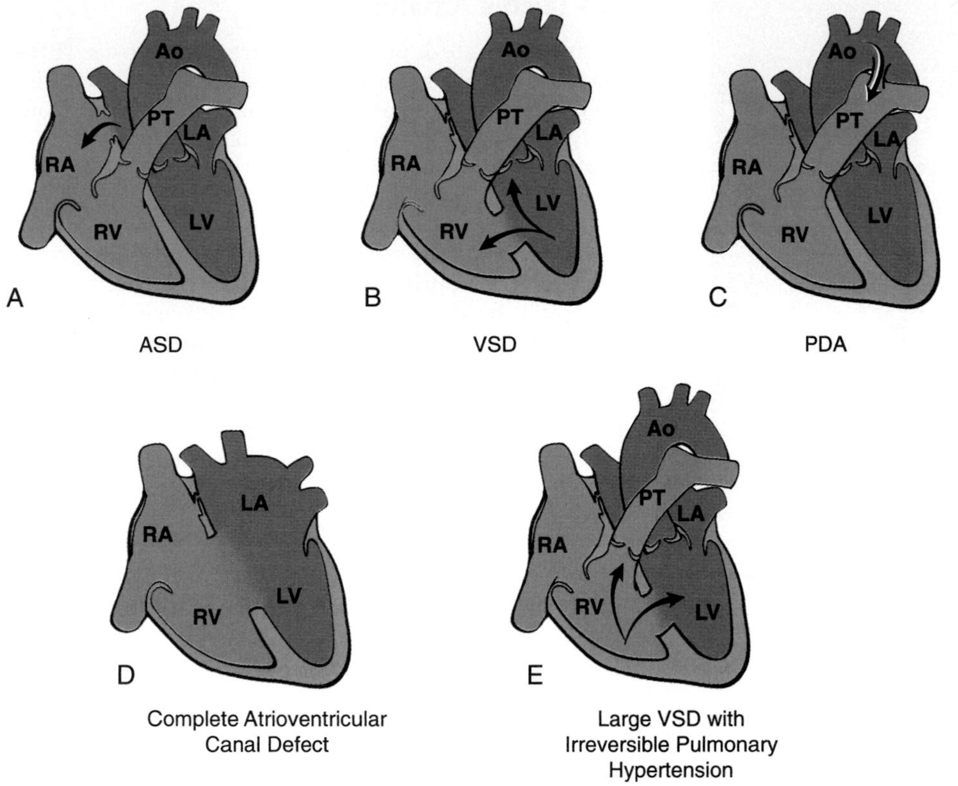

FIGURE 12–6 Schematic diagram of congenital left-to-right shunts. *A,* Atrial septal defect (ASD). *B,* Ventricular septal defect (VSD). With VSD the shunt is left-to-right, and the pressures are the same in both ventricles. Pressure hypertrophy of the right ventricle and volume hypertrophy of the left ventricle are generally present. *C,* Patent ductus arteriosus (PDA). *D,* Atrioventricular septal defect (AVSD). *E,* Large VSD with irreversible pulmonary hypertension. The shunt is right-to-left (shunt reversal). Volume hypertrophy and pressure hypertrophy of the right ventricle are present. Arrow indicates the direction of blood flow. The right ventricular pressure is now sufficient to yield a right-to-left shunt (Ao, aorta; LA, left atrium; LV, left ventricle; PT, pulmonary trunk; RA, right atrium; RV, right ventricle.)

Atrial Septal Defect

An ASD is an abnormal opening in the atrial septum that allows communication of blood between the left and right atria (not to be confused with a *patent foramen ovale,* present in up to one-third of normal individuals). ASD is the most common congenital cardiac anomaly *seen in adults.* Indeed, it is usually asymptomatic until adulthood (see Fig. 12–6*A*).

Morphology. The three major types of ASDs, classified according to their location in the septum, are secundum, primum, and sinus venosus. The **secundum ASD,** accounting for approximately 90% of all ASDs, is a defect located at and resulting from a deficient or fenestrated oval fossa. ASDs are usually isolated (i.e., not associated with other anomalies). When associated with another defect, such as tetralogy of Fallot, the other defect is usually hemodynamically dominant. The atrial aperture may be of any size and may be single, multiple, or fenestrated. **Primum** anomalies (5% of ASDs) occur adjacent to the AV valves and are usually associated with a cleft anterior mitral leaflet. This combination is known as a partial AV septal defect (see later). **Sinus venosus** defects (5%) are located near the entrance of the superior vena cava. They are commonly accompanied by anomalous connections of right pulmonary veins to the superior vena cava or right atrium.

ASDs result in a left-to-right shunt, largely because pulmonary vascular resistance is considerably less than systemic vascular resistance and because the compliance (distensibility) of the right ventricle is much greater than that of the left. Pulmonary blood flow may be 2 to 4 times normal. Although some neonates may be in profound CHF, most isolated ASDs are well tolerated and usually do not become symptomatic before age 30. A murmur is often present as a result of excessive flow through the pulmonary valve. Eventually, volume hypertrophy of the right atrium and right ventricle develops.

Irreversible pulmonary hypertension develops in fewer than 10% of subjects with an isolated uncorrected ASD. The objectives of surgical closure of an ASD are the reversal of the hemodynamic abnormalities and the prevention of complications, including heart failure, paradoxical embolization, and irreversible pulmonary vascular disease. Mortality is low, and postoperative survival is comparable to that of a normal population.

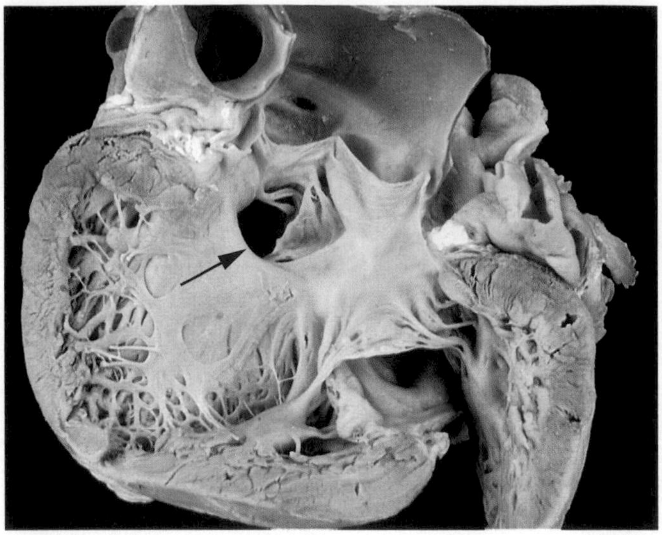

FIGURE 12–7 Gross photograph of a ventricular septal defect (membranous type); defect denoted by arrow. (Courtesy of William D. Edwards, M.D., Mayo Clinic, Rochester, MN.)

Ventricular Septal Defect

Incomplete closure of the ventricular septum, allowing free communication and thus a shunt from left to right ventricles, is the most common congenital cardiac anomaly overall (see Fig. 12–6*B*). Frequently, VSD is associated with other structural defects, such as tetralogy of Fallot. About 30% occur as isolated anomalies. Depending on the size of the defect, it may produce difficulties virtually from birth or, with smaller lesions, may not be recognized until later or may even spontaneously close.

Morphology. VSDs are classified according to size and location. Most are about the size of the aortic valve orifice. About 90% involve the region of the membranous septum (membranous VSD) (Fig. 12–7). The remainder lie below the pulmonary valve (infundibular VSD) or within the muscular septum. Although most often single, VSDs in the muscular septum may be multiple (so-called Swiss-cheese septum).

The functional significance of a VSD depends on the size of the defect and the presence of other anomalies. About 50% of small muscular VSDs close spontaneously, and the remainder are generally well tolerated for years. Large defects are usually membranous or infundibular, and they generally remain patent and permit a significant left-to-right flow. Right ventricular hypertrophy and pulmonary hypertension are present from birth. Over time, irreversible pulmonary vascular disease develops in virtually all patients with large unoperated VSDs, leading to shunt reversal, cyanosis, and death.

Large defects may become manifest virtually at birth with signs of cardiac failure accompanying the murmur. Surgical closure of asymptomatic VSDs is generally not attempted during infancy, in hope of spontaneous closure. Correction, however, is indicated at age 1 year with large defects, before obstructive pulmonary vascular disease becomes irreversible.

Patent Ductus Arteriosus

Patent (also called persistent) ductus arteriosus (PDA) results when the ductus arteriosus remains open after birth (see Fig 12–6*C*). About 90% of PDAs occur as an isolated anomaly. The remainder are most often associated with VSD, coarctation of the aorta, or pulmonary or aortic stenosis. The length and diameter of the ductus vary widely.

Most often PDA does not produce functional difficulties at birth. Indeed, a narrow ductus may have no effect on growth and development during childhood. Its existence, however, can generally be detected by a continuous harsh murmur, described as "machinery-like." Because the shunt is at first left-to-right, there is no cyanosis. Obstructive pulmonary vascular disease eventually ensues, however, with ultimate reversal of flow and its associated consequences.

There is general agreement that an isolated PDA should be closed as early in life as is feasible. Conversely, preservation of ductal patency (by administering prostaglandin E) assumes great importance in the survival of infants with various forms of congenital heart disease with obstructed pulmonary or systemic blood flow, such as aortic valve atresia. Ironically, therefore, the ductus may be either life-threatening or life-saving.

Atrioventricular Septal Defect (AVSD)

AVSD (also called complete atrioventricular canal defect) results from abnormal development of the embryologic AV canal, in which the superior and inferior endocardial cushions fail to fuse adequately, resulting in incomplete closure of the AV septum and inadequate formation of the tricuspid and mitral valves (see Fig. 12–6*D*). The two most common forms are *partial* AVSD (consisting of a primum ASD and a cleft anterior mitral leaflet, causing mitral insufficiency) and *complete* AVSD (consisting of a large combined AV septal defect and a large common AV valve—essentially a hole in the center of the heart). In the complete form, all four cardiac chambers freely communicate, inducing volume hypertrophy of each. More than one-third of all patients with the complete AVSD have Down syndrome. Surgical repair is possible.

RIGHT-TO-LEFT SHUNTS

The diseases in this group cause cyanosis early in postnatal life. Although a VSD is the most common congenital cardiac malformation, tetralogy of Fallot constitutes the most common form of *cyanotic* congenital heart disease. Other relatively frequently encountered anomalies in this category include transposition of the great arteries, tricuspid atresia, total anomalous pulmonary venous connection, and truncus arteriosus (note that each entity begins with the letter "T"). Tetralogy of Fallot and transposition of the great arteries are illustrated schematically in Figure 12–8.

Tetralogy of Fallot

The four features of the tetralogy of Fallot are (1) VSD, (2) obstruction to the right ventricular outflow tract (subpulmonary stenosis), (3) an aorta that overrides the VSD, and (4) right ven-

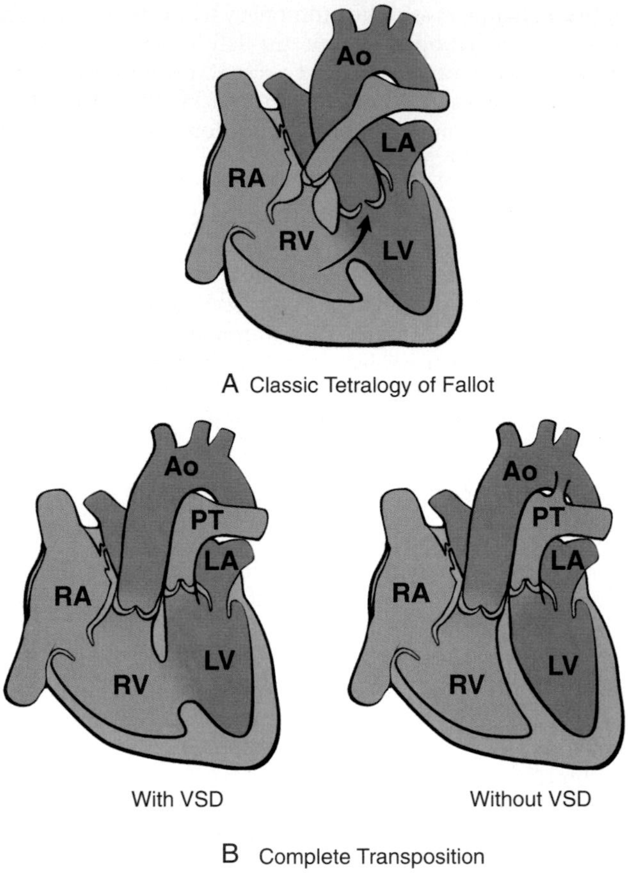

FIGURE 12–8 Schematic diagram of the most important right-to-left shunts *(cyanotic congenital heart disease). A,* Tetralogy of Fallot. Diagrammatic representation of anatomic variants, indicating that the direction of shunting across the VSD depends on the severity of the subpulmonary stenosis. Arrows indicate the direction of the blood flow. *B,* Transposition of the great vessels with and without VSD. (Ao, aorta; LA, left atrium; LV, left ventricle; PT, pulmonary trunk; RA, right atrium; RV, right ventricle.) (Courtesy of William D. Edwards, M.D., Mayo Clinic, Rochester, MN.)

tricular hypertrophy (see Fig. 12–8*A*). All of the features result embryologically from anterosuperior displacement of the infundibular septum. Even untreated, some patients with tetralogy of Fallot often survive into adult life (in a large series of untreated patients with this condition, 10% were alive at 20 years and 3% at 40 years). The clinical consequences of tetralogy of Fallot depend primarily on the severity of subpulmonary stenosis.

Morphology. The heart is often enlarged and may be "boot-shaped" owing to marked right ventricular hypertrophy, particularly of the apical region. The VSD is usually large and approximates the diameter of the aortic orifice. The aortic valve forms the superior border of the VSD, thereby overriding the defect and both ventricular chambers. The obstruction to right ventricular outflow is most often due to narrowing of the infundibulum (subpulmonic stenosis) but is often accompanied by pulmonary valvular stenosis. Sometimes there is complete atresia of the pulmonary valve and variable portions of the pulmonary arteries, such that blood flow through a patent ductus or dilated bronchial arteries, or through both, is necessary for survival. Aortic valve insufficiency or ASD may also be present, and a right aortic arch is present in about 25% of cases.

The severity of obstruction to right ventricular outflow determines the direction of blood flow. If the subpulmonary stenosis is mild, the abnormality resembles an isolated VSD, and the shunt may be left-to-right, without cyanosis (so-called pink tetralogy). *As the obstruction increases in severity, there is commensurately greater resistance to right ventricular outflow. As it approaches the level of systemic vascular resistance, right-to-left shunting predominates and, along with it, cyanosis (classic tetralogy of Fallot).* With increasing severity of subpulmonic stenosis, the pulmonary arteries are progressively smaller and thinner walled (hypoplastic), and the aorta is progressively larger in diameter. As the child grows and the heart increases in size, the pulmonic orifice does not expand proportionally, making the obstruction progressively worse. Thus most infants with tetralogy are cyanotic from birth or soon thereafter. The subpulmonary stenosis, however, protects the pulmonary vasculature from pressure overload, and right ventricular failure is rare because the right ventricle is decompressed into the left ventricle and aorta. Complete surgical repair is possible for classic tetralogy of Fallot but is more complicated for patients with pulmonary atresia and dilated bronchial arteries.

Transposition of the Great Arteries (TGA)

Transposition of the great arteries implies ventriculoarterial discordance, such that the aorta arises from the right ventricle and the pulmonary artery emanates from the left ventricle (see Fig. 12–8*B*). The AV connections are normal (concordant), with right atrium joining right ventricle and left atrium emptying into left ventricle.

The essential embryologic defect in complete TGA is abnormal formation of the truncal and aortopulmonary septa. *The aorta arises from the right ventricle and lies anterior and to the right of the pulmonary artery* (Fig. 12–9); *in contrast, in the normal heart, the aorta is posterior and to the left.* The result is separation of the systemic and pulmonary circulations, a condition incompatible with postnatal life unless a shunt exists for adequate mixing of blood. Patients with TGA and a VSD (about 35%) have a stable shunt. Those with only a patent foramen ovale or PDA (about 65%), however, have unstable shunts that tend to close and therefore require immediate intervention to create a shunt (such as balloon atrial septostomy) within the first few days of life. Right ventricular hypertrophy becomes prominent because this chamber functions as the systemic ventricle. Concurrently the left ventricle becomes thin-walled (atrophic) as it supports the low-resistance pulmonary circulation.

The outlook for infants with TGA depends on the degree of "mixing" of the blood, the magnitude of the tissue hypoxia, and the ability of the right ventricle to maintain the systemic circulation. Without surgery, most patients die within the first months of life. Currently, most patients undergo a reparative operation (usually entailing transection and "switching" of the great arteries as well as of the coronary arteries) during the first several weeks of life.

Truncus Arteriosus

The persistent truncus arteriosus anomaly arises from a developmental failure of separation of the embryologic

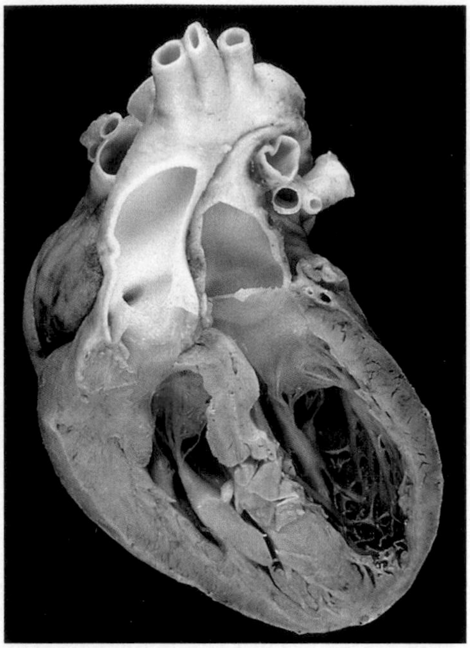

FIGURE 12–9 Transposition of the great arteries. (Courtesy of William D. Edwards, M.D., Mayo Clinic, Rochester, MN.)

truncus arteriosus into the aorta and pulmonary artery. This results in a single great artery that receives blood from both ventricles, accompanied by an underlying VSD, and that gives rise to the systemic, pulmonary, and coronary circulations. Because blood from the right and left ventricles mixes, there is early systemic cyanosis as well as increased pulmonary blood flow, with the danger of irreversible pulmonary hypertension.

Tricuspid Atresia

Complete occlusion of the tricuspid valve orifice is known as *tricuspid atresia.* It results embryologically from unequal division of the AV canal, and thus the mitral valve is larger than normal. This lesion is almost always associated with underdevelopment (hypoplasia) of the right ventricle. The circulation is maintained by a right-to-left shunt through an interatrial communication (ASD or patent foramen ovale). A VSD is also present and affords communication between the left ventricle and the great artery that arises from the hypoplastic right ventricle. Cyanosis is present virtually from birth, and there is a high mortality in the first weeks or months of life.

Total Anomalous Pulmonary Venous Connection (TAPVC)

TAPVC, in which no pulmonary veins directly join the left atrium, results embryologically when the common pulmonary vein fails to develop or becomes atretic, causing primitive systemic venous channels from the lungs to remain patent. TAPVC usually drains into the left innominate vein or to the coronary sinus. Either a patent foramen ovale or an ASD is always present, allowing pulmonary venous blood to enter the left atrium. Consequences of TAPVC include volume and pressure hypertrophy of the right atrium and right ventricle, and these chambers and the pulmonary trunk are dilated. The left atrium is hypoplastic, but the left ventricle is usually normal in size. Cyanosis may be present, owing to mixing of well-oxygenated and poorly oxygenated blood at the site of anomalous pulmonary venous connection and a large right-to-left shunt at the ASD.

OBSTRUCTIVE CONGENITAL ANOMALIES

Congenital obstruction to blood flow may occur at the level of the heart valves or within a great vessel. Relatively common examples include stenosis of the pulmonary valve, stenosis or atresia of the aortic valve, and coarctation of the aorta. Obstruction can also occur within a chamber, as with subpulmonary stenosis in tetralogy of Fallot.

Coarctation of the Aorta

Coarctation (narrowing, constriction) of the aorta ranks high in frequency among the common structural anomalies. Males are affected twice as often as females, although females with Turner syndrome frequently have a coarctation (see Chapter 5). Two classic forms have been described: (1) an "infantile" form with tubular hypoplasia of the aortic arch proximal to a PDA that is often symptomatic in early childhood and (2) an "adult" form in which there is a discrete ridgelike infolding of the aorta, just opposite the closed ductus arteriosus (ligamentum arteriosum) distal to the arch vessels (Fig. 12–10). Encroachment on the aortic lumen is of variable severity, sometimes leaving only a small channel and at other times producing only minimal narrowing. Clinical manifestations depend almost entirely on the severity of the narrowing and the patency of the ductus arteriosus. Although coarctation of the aorta may occur as a solitary defect, it is accompanied by a bicuspid aortic valve in 50% of cases and may also be associated with congenital aortic stenosis, ASD, VSD, mitral regurgitation, and berry aneurysms of the circle of Willis.

Coarctation of the aorta with a PDA usually leads to manifestations early in life; indeed, it may cause signs and symp-

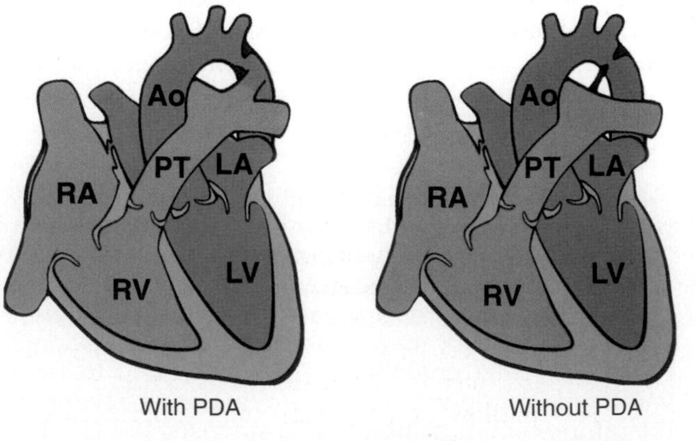

FIGURE 12–10 Diagram showing coarctation of the aorta with and without PDA. (Ao, aorta; LA, left atrium; LV, left ventricle; PT, pulmonary trunk; RA, right atrium; RV, right ventricle; PDA, persistent ductus arteriosus.) (Courtesy of William D. Edwards, M.D., Mayo Clinic, Rochester, MN.)

toms immediately after birth. Many infants with this anomaly do not survive the neonatal period without surgical or catheter-based intervention. In such cases, the delivery of unsaturated blood through the ductus arteriosus produces cyanosis localized to the lower half of the body.

The outlook is different with *coarctation of the aorta without a PDA,* unless it is very severe. Most of the children are asymptomatic, and the disease may go unrecognized until well into adult life. Typically there is hypertension in the upper extremities, but there are weak pulses and a lower blood pressure in the lower extremities, associated with manifestations of arterial insufficiency (i.e., claudication and coldness). Particularly characteristic in adults is the development of collateral circulation between the precoarctation arterial branches and the postcoarctation arteries through enlarged intercostal and internal mammary arteries and the radiographically visible erosions ("notching") of the undersurfaces of the ribs.

With all significant coarctations, murmurs are often present throughout systole. Sometimes a thrill may be present, and there is cardiomegaly owing to left ventricular hypertrophy. With uncomplicated coarctation of the aorta, surgical resection and end-to-end anastomosis or replacement of the affected aortic segment by a prosthetic graft yields excellent results.

Pulmonary Stenosis and Atresia

This relatively frequent malformation constitutes an obstruction at the pulmonary valve, which may be mild to severe. It may occur as an isolated defect, or as part of a more complex anomaly—either tetralogy of Fallot or TGA. Right ventricular hypertrophy often develops, and there is sometimes poststenotic dilation of the pulmonary artery owing to jetstream injury to the wall. With coexistent subpulmonary stenosis (as in tetralogy of Fallot), the high ventricular pressure is not transmitted to the valve, and the pulmonary trunk is not dilated and may in fact be hypoplastic. When the valve is entirely atretic, there is no communication between the right ventricle and lungs, and so the anomaly is commonly associated with a hypoplastic right ventricle and an ASD; flow enters the lungs through a PDA. Mild stenosis may be asymptomatic and compatible with long life. The smaller the valvular orifice, the more severe is the cyanosis and the earlier its appearance.

Aortic Stenosis and Atresia

Here we are concerned with the narrowings and obstructions of the aortic valve present from birth. There are three major types of stenosis: valvular, subvalvular, and supravalvular. With *valvular aortic stenosis,* the cusps may be hypoplastic (small), dysplastic (thickened, nodular), or abnormal in number (usually acommissural or unicommissural). In severe congenital aortic stenosis or atresia, obstruction of the left ventricular outflow tract leads to underdevelopment (hypoplasia) of the left ventricle and ascending aorta. There may be dense, porcelain-like left ventricular endocardial fibroelastosis (see section on restrictive cardiomyopathy, later in this chapter). The ductus must be open to allow blood flow to the aorta and coronary arteries. This constellation of findings, called the *hypoplastic left heart syndrome,* is nearly always fatal in the first week of life, when the ductus closes. Less severe degrees of congenital aortic stenosis may be compatible with long survival. Cogenital aortic stenosis is an isolated lesion in 80% of cases.

Subaortic stenosis represents either a thickened ring (discrete type) or collar (tunnel type) of dense endocardial fibrous tissue below the level of the cusps. *Supravalvular aortic stenosis* represents an inherited form of aortic dysplasia in which the ascending aortic wall is greatly thickened, causing luminal constriction. It may be related to a developmental disorder affecting multiple organ systems, including the vascular system, which includes hypercalcemia of infancy (Williams syndrome). Mutations in the elastin gene cause supravalvular aortic stenosis, probably via disruption of an important elastin-smooth muscle cell interactions in arterial morphogenesis.[32]

A prominent systolic murmur is usually detectable and sometimes a thrill, which does not distinguish the site of stenosis. Pressure hypertrophy of the left ventricle develops as a consequence of the obstruction to blood flow. In general, congenital stenoses are well tolerated unless very severe. Mild stenoses can be managed conservatively with antibiotic prophylaxis and avoidance of strenuous activity, but the threat of sudden death with exertion always looms.

Ischemic Heart Disease

Ischemic heart disease (IHD) is the generic designation for a group of closely related syndromes resulting from myocardial *ischemia*—an imbalance between the supply (perfusion) and demand of the heart for oxygenated blood. Ischemia comprises not only insufficiency of oxygen, but also reduced availability of nutrient substrates and inadequate removal of metabolites (see Chapter 1). Isolated hypoxemia (i.e., diminished transport of oxygen by the blood) induced by cyanotic congenital heart disease, severe anemia, or advanced lung disease is less deleterious than ischemia because perfusion (including metabolic substrate delivery and waste removal) is maintained.

In more than 90% of cases, the cause of myocardial ischemia is reduction in coronary blood flow due to atherosclerotic coronary arterial obstruction. Thus, IHD is often termed *coronary artery disease (CAD) or coronary heart disease.* In most cases, there is a long period (decades) of silent, slowly progressive, coronary atherosclerosis before these disorders become manifest. Thus, *the syndromes of IHD are only the late manifestations of coronary atherosclerosis that probably began during childhood or adolescence* (see Chapter 11).

The clinical manifestations of IHD can be divided into four syndromes:

- *Myocardial infarction (MI),* the most important form of IHD, in which the duration and severity of ischemia is sufficient to cause death of heart muscle.
- *Angina pectoris, in which the ischemia is less severe and does not cause death of cardiac muscle.* Of the three variants—stable angina, Prinzmetal angina, and unstable angina—the latter is the most threatening as a frequent harbinger of MI.
- *Chronic IHD* with heart failure.
- *Sudden cardiac death.*

As will be discussed in more detail later, acute myocardial infarction, unstable angina, and sudden cardiac death are sometimes referred to as *acute coronary syndromes.*

Certain conditions aggravate ischemia through either an increase in cardiac energy demand (e.g., hypertrophy) or by diminished availability of blood or oxygen due to lowered systemic blood pressure (e.g., shock) or hypoxemia as discussed above. Moreover, increased heart rate not only increases demand through more contractions per unit time but also decreases supply (by decreasing the relative time spent in diastole—when coronary perfusion occurs).

The risk of an individual developing detectable IHD depends in part on the number, distribution, and structure of atheromatous plaques, and the degree of narrowing they cause. However, the clinical manifestations of IHD are not entirely predicted by these anatomic observations of disease burden. Moreover, there is an extraordinarily broad spectrum of the expression of disease from elderly individuals with extensive coronary atherosclerosis who have never had a symptom, to the previously asymptomatic young adult in whom modestly obstructive disease comes unexpectedly to medical attention as a result of acute MI or sudden cardiac death. The reasons for clinical heterogeneity of the disease are complex, but the often precipitous and variable onset and natural history largely depend on the pathologic basis of the so-called acute coronary syndromes of IHD (comprising unstable angina, acute MI, and sudden death). *The acute coronary syndromes are frequently initiated by an unpredictable and abrupt conversion of a stable atherosclerotic plaque to an unstable and potentially life-threatening atherothrombotic lesion through superficial erosion, ulceration, fissuring, rupture, or deep hemorrhage, usually with superimposed thrombosis.* For purposes of simplicity, this spectrum of alteration in atherosclerotic lesions will be termed either *plaque disruption* or *acute plaque change.*

Epidemiology. IHD in its various forms is the leading cause of death for both males and females in the United States and other industrialized nations. Each year, nearly 500,000 Americans die of IHD. Awesome as these numbers may be, they represent an improvement over those that prevailed several decades ago. Since its peak in 1963, the overall death rate from IHD has fallen in the United States by approximately 50%. This decline is a spectacular achievement that has resulted primarily from (1) *prevention* achieved by modification of determinants of risk, such as smoking, elevated blood cholesterol, hypertension, and a sedentary lifestyle,[33,34] and (2) *diagnostic and therapeutic advances*, allowing earlier, more effective, and safer treatments, including new medications, coronary care units, thrombolysis for MI, percutaneous transluminal coronary angioplasty (PTCA), endovascular stents, coronary artery bypass graft (CABG) surgery, and improved control of arrhythmias.[35,36] Additional risk reduction may potentially be associated with maintenance of normal blood glucose levels in diabetic patients, control of obesity, and aspirin prophylaxis in middle-aged men.[37] Nevertheless, continuing this progress in the 21st century will be particularly challenging, in view of a predicted increased longevity of "baby boomers" and others. The anticipated doubling of the population of individuals over age 65 by 2050 is expected to contribute to a dramatic increase in IHD and associated deaths.

Pathogenesis. *The dominant influence in the causation of the IHD syndromes is diminished coronary perfusion relative to myocardial demand, owing largely to a complex and dynamic interaction among fixed atherosclerotic narrowing of the epicardial coronary arteries, intraluminal thrombosis overlying a disrupted atherosclerotic plaque, platelet aggregation, and vasospasm.* The individual elements and their interactions are discussed below.

More than 90% of patients with IHD have atherosclerosis of one or more of the coronary arteries. The clinical manifestations of coronary atherosclerosis are generally due to progressive encroachment of the lumen leading to stenosis (chronic, "fixed" obstructions) or to acute plaque disruption with thrombosis (generally both sudden and dynamic), which compromises blood flow. A fixed obstructive lesion of 75% or greater (i.e., only 25% or less lumen remaining) generally causes symptomatic ischemia induced by exercise; with this degree of obstruction, the augmented coronary flow provided by compensatory vasodilation is no longer sufficient to meet even moderate increases in myocardial demand. A 90% stenosis can lead to inadequate coronary blood flow even at rest. Slowly developing occlusions may stimulate collateral vessels over time, which protect against distal myocardial ischemia and infarction even with an eventual high-grade stenosis.

Although only a single major coronary epicardial trunk may be affected, two or all three—lateral anterior descending (LAD), left circumflex (LCX), and right coronary artery (RCA)—are often involved. Clinically significant stenosing plaques may be located anywhere within these vessels but tend to predominate within the first several centimeters of the LAD and LCX and along the entire length of the RCA. Sometimes the major secondary epicardial branches are also involved (i.e., diagonal branches of the LAD, obtuse marginal branches of the LCX, or posterior descending branch of the RCA), but atherosclerosis of the intramural branches is rare. However, as mentioned above, the onset of symptoms and prognosis of IHD depend not only on the extent and severity of fixed, chronic anatomic disease, but also critically on dynamic changes in coronary plaque morphology (discussed below).

Role of Acute Plaque Change. *In most patients the myocardial ischemia underlying unstable angina, acute MI, and (in many cases) sudden cardiac death is precipitated by abrupt plaque change followed by thrombosis* (Fig. 12–11 and Fig. 12–12).[38–40] Thus, these important manifestations are termed the acute coronary syndromes. Most often, the initiating event is disruption of previously only partially stenosing plaques with any of the following:

- *Rupture/fissuring*, exposing the highly thrombogenic plaque constituents
- *Erosion/ulceration*, exposing the thrombogenic subendothelial basement membrane to blood
- *Hemorrhage into the atheroma*, expanding its volume.

The events that trigger abrupt changes in plaque configuration and superimposed thrombosis are complex and poorly understood. Influences, both intrinsic (e.g., plaque structure and composition) and extrinsic (e.g., blood pressure, platelet reactivity) are important.[41,42] Acute alterations in plaque imply the inability of a plaque to withstand mechanical stresses.

The structure and composition of a plaque are dynamic and contribute to a propensity to disruption. Plaques that contain large areas of foam cells and extracellular lipid, and those in which the fibrous caps are thin or contain few smooth muscle cells or have clusters of inflammatory cells, are more likely to rupture, and are therefore called "vulnerable plaques." Fissures frequently occur at the junction of the fibrous cap and the adjacent normal plaque-free arterial segment, a location at which the blood flow–inducing mechanical stresses within the plaque are highest and the fibrous cap is thinnest. It is now recognized that the fibrous cap can undergo continuous remodeling. The balance of synthetic and degradative activity of collagen, the major structural component of the fibrous cap, accounts for its mechanical strength and determines plaque stability and prognosis. Collagen is produced by smooth muscle cells and degraded by the action of metalloproteinases, enzymes elaborated by macrophages in atheroma. Thus, there is considerable evidence that inflammation destabilizes the mechanical integrity of plaques (see below). Moreover, drugs such as statins (inhibitors of HMG Co-A reductase, a key enzyme in the synthesis of cholesterol) that reduce clinical events associated with IHD, are thought to stabilize plaques by their lipid-lowering effect, as well as by reducing plaque inflammation.[43]

Influences extrinsic to plaque are also important. Adrenergic stimulation can elevate physical stresses on the plaque through systemic hypertension or local vasospasm. Indeed, the adrenergic stimulation associated with awakening and arising induces a pronounced circadian periodicity for the time of onset of acute MI, with a peak incidence between 6 a.m. and 12 noon, concurrent with a surge in blood pressure and immediately following heightened platelet reactivity. Intense emotional stress can also contribute to plaque disruption; this is most dramatically illustrated by the marked increase in the incidence of sudden death that is associated with natural or other disasters such as earthquakes and the September 11, 2001 attacks in New York and Washington, DC.[44]

It is now recognized that the preexisting culprit lesion in patients who develop myocardial infarction and other acute coronary syndromes is not necessarily a severely stenotic and hemodynamically significant lesion prior to its acute change. Pathologic and clinical studies show that plaques that undergo abrupt disruption leading to coronary occlusion often are those that previously produced only mild to moderate luminal stenosis. Approximately two thirds of plaques that rupture with subsequent occlusive thrombosis caused occlusion of only 50% or less before plaque rupture, and 85% had initial stenosis less than 70%.[45] Thus, the worrisome conclusion is that a rather large number of now asymptomatic adults in the industrial world have a real but unpredictable risk of a catastrophic coronary event. Regrettably, it is presently impossible to reliably predict plaque disruption or subsequent thrombosis in an individual patient.

Accumulating evidence indicates that plaque disruption and the ensuing platelet aggregation and intraluminal thrombosis are common, repetitive, and often clinically silent complications of atheroma. Moreover, healing of subclinical plaque disruption and overlying thrombosis is an important mechanism of growth of atherosclerotic lesions.

Role of Inflammation. Inflammatory processes play important roles at all stages of atherosclerosis, from its inception to the development of complications.[46,47] The establishment of the initial lesion requires the interaction between endothelial cells and circulating leukocytes, leading to the accumulation of T cells and macrophages in the arterial wall. Entry of leukocytes into the wall is a consequence of the release of chemokines by endothelial cells, and the increased expression of adhesion proteins (ICAM-1, VCAM-1, E-selectin and P-selectin) in these cells. T cells located in the arterial wall produce cytokines such as TNF, IL-6 and IFN-γ that stimulate endothelial cells and activate macrophages, which become loaded with oxidized LDL. At later stages of atherosclerosis, destabilization and rupture of the plaque may involve the secretion of metalloproteinases by macrophages.[48] These enzymes weaken the plaque by digesting collagen at the fibrous cap or the shoulder of the lesion.

Because of the important role of inflammation in the pathogenesis of atherosclerosis, several proteins involved in inflammation may serve as potential markers of atherosclerosis. C-reactive protein (CRP), an acute phase reactant made in the liver, has been suggested as a predictor of risk of coronary heart disease.[49,50] In some, but not all, studies CRP predicts risk independently from risk estimates provided by serum lipid levels.[51,52,52a] It could be used to estimate the risk of myocardium infarct in patients with angina, and the risk of new infarcts in patients who are infarct survivors.

Role of Coronary Thrombus. As mentioned above, partial or total thrombosis associated with a disrupted plaque is crit-

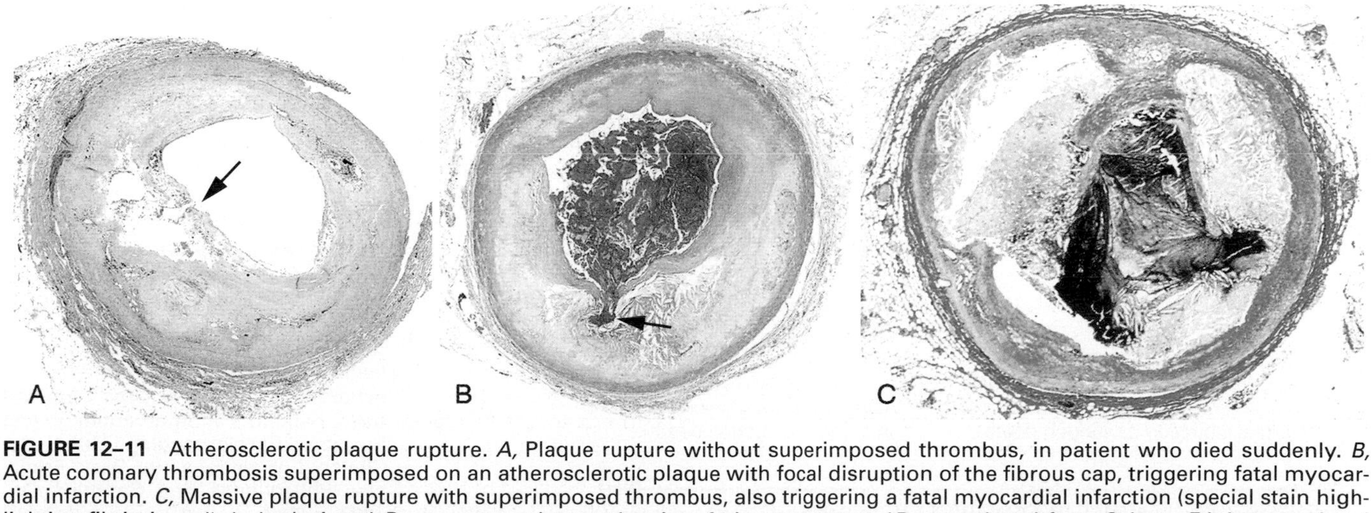

FIGURE 12–11 Atherosclerotic plaque rupture. *A,* Plaque rupture without superimposed thrombus, in patient who died suddenly. *B,* Acute coronary thrombosis superimposed on an atherosclerotic plaque with focal disruption of the fibrous cap, triggering fatal myocardial infarction. *C,* Massive plaque rupture with superimposed thrombus, also triggering a fatal myocardial infarction (special stain highlighting fibrin in red). In both *A* and *B*, an arrow points to the site of plaque rupture. (*B,* reproduced from Schoen FJ: Interventional and Surgical Cardiovascular Pathology: Clinical Correlations and Basic Principles. Philadelphia, W.B. Saunders, 1989, p. 61.)

ical to the pathogenesis of the acute coronary syndromes. In the most serious form, acute transmural MI (see later for distinction of transmural vs. subendocardial infarcts), thrombus superimposed on a disrupted but previously only partially stenotic plaque converts it to a total occlusion. In contrast, with unstable angina, acute subendocardial infarction, or sudden cardiac death, the extent of luminal obstruction by thrombosis is usually incomplete (mural thrombus), and it may wax and wane with time.

Mural thrombus in a coronary artery can also embolize. Indeed, small fragments of thrombotic material in the distal intramyocardial circulation or microinfarcts may be found at autopsy of patients who have had unstable angina or sudden death. Finally, thrombus is a potent activator of multiple growth-related signals in smooth muscle cells, which can contribute to the growth of atherosclerotic lesions (see Chapter 11).

Role of Vasoconstriction. Vasoconstriction compromises lumen size, and, by increasing the local mechanical forces, can potentiate plaque disruption. Vasoconstriction at sites of atheroma is stimulated by: (1) circulating adrenergic agonists, (2) locally released platelet contents, (3) impaired secretion of endothelial cell relaxing factors relative to contracting factors (e.g., endothelin) due to atheroma-associated endothelial dysfunction (see Chapter 11), and possibly (4) mediators released from perivascular inflammatory cells.

To summarize (Fig. 12–12 and Table 12–3), *the acute coronary syndromes—angina, acute MI, and sudden death—share a common pathophysiologic basis in coronary atherosclerotic plaque disruption and associated intraluminal platelet–fibrin thrombus formation.* The critical consequence is downstream myocardial ischemia. *Stable angina* results from increases in myocardial oxygen demand that outstrip the ability of markedly stenosed coronary arteries to increase oxygen delivery but is not usually associated with plaque disruption. *Unstable angina* derives from a sudden change in plaque morphology, which induces partially occlusive platelet aggregation or mural thrombus, and vasoconstriction leading to severe but transient reductions in coronary blood flow. In some cases, distal microinfarcts occur secondary to thromboemboli. In *MI*, acute plaque change induces total thrombotic occlusion. Finally, *sudden cardiac death* frequently involves a coronary lesion in which disrupted plaque and often partial thrombus and possibly embolus have led to regional myocardial ischemia that induces a fatal ventricular arrhythmia. Each of these important syndromes is discussed in detail first. Then we turn to the important consequences in the myocardium.

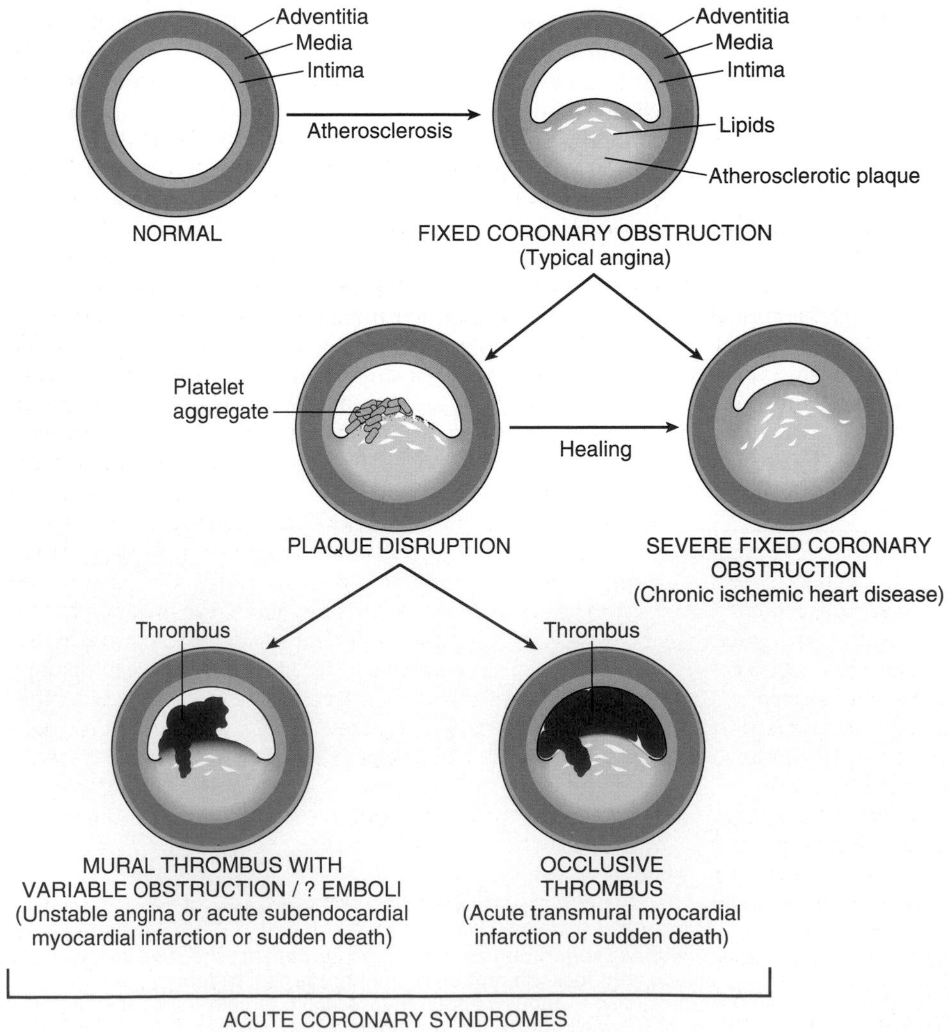

FIGURE 12–12 Schematic representation of sequential progression of coronary artery lesion morphology, beginning with stable chronic plaque responsible for typical angina and leading to the various acute coronary syndromes. (Modified and redrawn from Schoen FJ: Interventional and Surgical Cardiovascular Pathology: Clinical Correlations and Basic Principles. Philadelphia, W.B. Saunders Co., 1989, p. 63.)

TABLE 12–3 Coronary Artery Pathology in Ischemic Heart Disease

Syndrome	Stenoses	Plaque Disruption	Plaque-Associated Thrombus
Stable angina	>75%	No	No
Unstable angina	Variable	Frequent	Nonocclusive, often with thromboemboli
Transmural myocardial infarction	Variable	Frequent	Occlusive
Subendocardial myocardial infarction	Variable	Variable	Widely variable, may be absent, partial/complete, or lysed
Sudden death	Usually severe	Frequent	Often small platelet aggregates or thrombi and/or thromboemboli

ANGINA PECTORIS

Angina pectoris is a symptom complex of IHD characterized by paroxysmal and usually recurrent attacks of substernal or precordial chest discomfort (variously described as constricting, squeezing, choking, or knifelike) caused by transient (15 seconds to 15 minutes) myocardial ischemia that falls short of inducing the cellular necrosis that defines infarction. There are three overlapping patterns of angina pectoris: (1) stable or typical angina, (2) Prinzmetal or variant angina, and (3) unstable or crescendo angina. They are caused by varying combinations of increased myocardial demand and decreased myocardial perfusion, owing to fixed stenosing plaques, disrupted plaques, vasospasm, thrombosis, platelet aggregation, and embolization. Moreover, it is being increasingly recognized that not all ischemic events are perceived by patients, even though such events may have adverse prognostic implications *(silent ischemia).*

Stable angina, the most common form and therefore called *typical angina pectoris, appears to be caused by the reduction of coronary perfusion to a critical level by chronic stenosing coronary atherosclerosis;* this renders the heart vulnerable to further ischemia whenever there is increased demand, such as that produced by physical activity, emotional excitement, or any other cause of increased cardiac workload. Typical angina pectoris is usually relieved by rest (thereby decreasing demand) or nitroglycerin, a strong vasodilator. Although the coronary arteries are usually maximally dilated by intrinsic regulatory influences, nitroglycerin also decreases cardiac work by dilating the peripheral vasculature. In particular instances, local vasospasm may contribute to the imbalance between supply and demand.

Prinzmetal variant angina is an uncommon pattern of episodic angina that occurs at rest and is due to coronary artery spasm. Usually there is an elevated ST segment on the electrocardiogram (ECG), indicative of transmural ischemia. Although individuals with this form of angina may well have significant coronary atherosclerosis, the anginal attacks are unrelated to physical activity, heart rate, or blood pressure. Prinzmetal angina generally responds promptly to vasodilators, such as nitroglycerin and calcium channel blockers.

Unstable or *crescendo angina* refers to a pattern of pain that occurs with progressively increasing frequency, is precipitated with progressively less effort, often occurs at rest, and tends to be of more prolonged duration. *As discussed above, in most patients, unstable angina is induced by disruption of an atherosclerotic plaque with superimposed partial (mural) thrombosis and possibly embolization or vasospasm (or both).* Although the ischemia that occurs in unstable angina falls precariously close to inducing clinically detectable infarction, unstable angina is often the prodrome of subsequent acute MI. Thus this syndrome is sometimes referred to as *preinfarction angina*, and in the spectrum of IHD, unstable angina lies intermediate between stable angina on the one hand and MI on the other.

MYOCARDIAL INFARCTION (MI)

MI, also known as "heart attack," is the death of cardiac muscle resulting from ischemia. It is by far the most important form of IHD and alone is the leading cause of death in the United States and industrialized nations. About 1.5 million individuals in the United States suffer an acute MI annually and approximately one third of them die. At least 250,000 people a year die of a heart attack before they reach the hospital.

Transmural versus Subendocardial Infarction. Most myocardial infarcts are *transmural*, in which the ischemic necrosis involves the full or nearly full thickness of the ventricular wall in the distribution of a single coronary artery. This pattern of infarction is usually associated with coronary atherosclerosis, acute plaque change, and superimposed thrombosis (as discussed previously). In contrast, a *subendocardial (nontransmural) infarct* constitutes an area of ischemic necrosis limited to the inner one third or at most one half of the ventricular wall; under some circumstances, it may extend laterally beyond the perfusion territory of a single coronary artery. As previously pointed out, the subendocardial zone is normally the least well-perfused region of myocardium and therefore is most vulnerable to any reduction in coronary flow. A subendocardial infarct can occur as a result of a plaque disruption followed by coronary thrombus that becomes lysed before myocardial necrosis extends across the major thickness of the wall; in this case the infarct will be limited to the distribution of one coronary artery with plaque change. However, subendocardial infarcts can also result from sufficiently prolonged and severe reduction in systemic blood pressure, as in shock, often superimposed on chronic, otherwise noncritical, coronary stenoses. In cases of global hypotension, resulting subendocardial infarcts are usually circumferential or nearly so, rather than limited to the distribution of a single major coronary artery.

Incidence and Risk Factors. The risk factors for atherosclerosis, the major underlying cause of IHD in general, are discussed in Chapter 11 and are not reiterated here. Suffice it to say that *MI may occur at virtually any age, but the frequency rises progressively with increasing age and when predispositions* *to atherosclerosis are present,* such as hypertension, cigarette smoking, diabetes mellitus, genetic hypercholesterolemia, and other causes of hyperlipoproteinemia. Nearly 10% of myocardial infarcts occur in people under age 40, and 45% occur in people under age 65. Blacks and whites are equally affected. Throughout life, men are at significantly greater risk of MI than women; the differential progressively declines with advancing age. *Except for those having some predisposing atherogenic condition, women are remarkably protected against MI during the reproductive years.* Nevertheless, the decrease of estrogen following menopause can permit rapid development of coronary artery disease (CAD), and IHD is the overwhelming cause of death in elderly women. Moreover, recent epidemiologic evidence suggests that postmenopausal hormone replacement therapy does not protect women against MI.[53]

Pathogenesis. We now consider the basis for and subsequent consequences of myocardial ischemia, particularly as they relate to the typical transmural myocardial infarct.

Coronary Arterial Occlusion. As discussed above, transmural acute MI results from a dynamic interaction among several or all of the following—coronary atherosclerosis, acute atheromatous plaque change (such as rupture), superimposed platelet activation, thrombosis, and vasospasm—resulting in an occlusive intracoronary thrombus overlying a disrupted plaque. In addition, either increased myocardial demand (as with hypertrophy or tachycardia) or hemodynamic compromise (as with a drop in blood pressure) can worsen the situation. Recall also that collateral circulation may provide perfusion to ischemic zones from a relatively unobstructed branch of the coronary tree, bypassing the point of obstruction and protecting against the effects of an acute coronary occlusion.

In the typical case of MI, the following sequence of events can be proposed:

- *The initial event is a sudden change in the morphology of an atheromatous plaque,* that is, disruption—manifest as intraplaque hemorrhage, erosion or ulceration, or rupture or fissuring.
- Exposed to subendothelial collagen and necrotic plaque contents, *platelets undergo adhesion, aggregation, activation, and release of potent aggregators* including thromboxane A_2, serotonin, and platelet factors 3 and 4.
- Vasospasm is stimulated by platelet aggregation and the release of mediators.
- Other mediators activate the extrinsic pathway of coagulation, adding to the bulk of the thrombus.
- *Frequently within minutes, the thrombus evolves to completely occlude the lumen of the coronary vessel.*

The evidence for this sequence is compelling and derives from (1) autopsy studies of patients dying with acute MI, (2) angiographic studies demonstrating a high frequency of thrombotic occlusion early after MI, (3) the high success rate of therapeutic thrombolysis and primary angioplasty, and (4) the demonstration of residual disrupted atherosclerotic lesions by angiography after thrombolysis. Although coronary angiography performed within 4 hours of the onset of apparent MI shows a thrombosed coronary artery in almost 90% of cases, the observation of occlusion is seen in only about 60% when angiography is delayed until 12 to 24 hours after onset.[54] Thus with the passage of time, at least some occlusions appear to clear spontaneously owing to lysis of the thrombus or relaxation of spasm or both.

In approximately 10% of cases, transmural acute MI is not associated with atherosclerotic plaque thrombosis stimulated by disruption. In such situations, other mechanisms may be involved:

- *Vasospasm*: isolated, intense, and relatively prolonged, with or without coronary atherosclerosis, perhaps in association with platelet aggregation (sometimes related to cocaine abuse).
- *Emboli*: from the left atrium in association with atrial fibrillation, a left-sided mural thrombus or vegetative endocarditis; or *paradoxical emboli* from the right side of the heart or the peripheral veins which cross to the systemic circulation, through a patent foramen ovale, causing coronary occlusion.
- *Unexplained*: cases without detectable coronary atherosclerosis and thrombosis may be caused by diseases of small intramural coronary vessels such as vasculitis, hematologic abnormalities such as hemoglobinopathies, amyloid deposition in vascular walls, or other unusual disorders, such as vascular dissection and inadequate protection during cardiac surgery.

Myocardial Response. *The consequence of coronary arterial obstruction is the loss of critical blood supply to the myocardium* (Fig. 12–13), *which induces profound functional, biochemical, and morphologic consequences.* Occlusion of a major coronary artery results in ischemia and, potentially, cell death through-

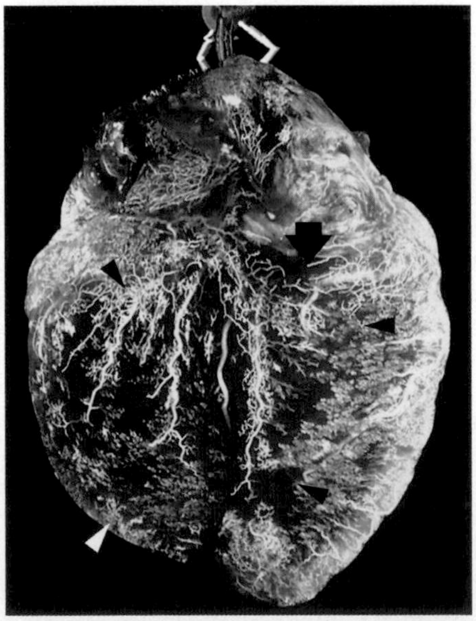

FIGURE 12–13 Postmortem angiogram showing the posterior aspect of the heart of a patient who died during the evolution of acute myocardial infarction, demonstrating total occlusion of the distal right coronary artery by an acute thrombus *(arrow)* and a large zone of myocardial hypoperfusion involving the posterior left and right ventricles, as indicated by arrowheads, and having almost absent filling of capillaries, that is, less white. The heart has been fixed by coronary arterial perfusion with glutaraldehyde and cleared with methyl salicylate, followed by intracoronary injection of silicone polymer. Photograph courtesy of Lewis L. Lainey. (Reproduced by permission from Schoen FJ: Interventional and Surgical Cardiovascular Pathology: Clinical Correlations and Basic Principles. Philadelphia, WB Saunders, 1989, p. 60.)

out the anatomic region supplied by that artery (called the area at risk), most pronounced in the subendocardium. The outcome depends largely on the severity and duration of flow deprivation.

The principal early biochemical consequence of myocardial ischemia is the cessation of aerobic glycolysis (and therefore initiating anaerobic glycolysis) within seconds, leading to inadequate production of high-energy phosphates (e.g., creatine phosphate and adenosine triphosphate) and accumulation of potentially noxious breakdown products (such as lactic acid). Myocardial function is exceedingly sensitive to severe ischemia; striking loss of contractility occurs within 60 seconds of onset of ischemia. This can precipitate acute heart failure long before myocardial cell death. As detailed in Chapter 1, ultrastructural changes (including myofibrillar relaxation, glycogen depletion, cell and mitochondrial swelling) also develop within a few minutes after onset of ischemia. Nevertheless, these early changes are potentially *reversible*, and cell death is not immediate. As demonstrated experimentally, only severe ischemia lasting at least 20 to 40 minutes or longer leads to irreversible damage (necrosis) of some cardiac myocytes. Ultrastructural evidence of *irreversible* myocyte injury (primary structural defects in the sarcolemmal membrane) develops only after 20 to 40 minutes in severely ischemic myocardium (with blood flow of 10% or less of normal).[56] With prolonged ischemia, injury to the microvasculature then follows. This time frame is summarized in Table 12–4.

Thus, myocardial necrosis begins at approximately 30 minutes after coronary occlusion. Classic acute MI with extensive damage occurs when the perfusion of the myocardium is reduced severely below its needs for an extended interval (usually at least 2 to 4 hours), causing profound, prolonged ischemia and resulting in permanent loss of function of large regions in which cell death has occurred. The predominant mechanism of cell death is coagulation necrosis; apoptosis may also be important, but this is as yet uncertain. In contrast, if restoration of myocardial blood flow (known as reperfusion) follows briefer periods of flow deprivation (less than 20 minutes in the most severely ischemic myocardium), loss of cell viability can be prevented. This provides the rationale for the very early clinical detection of acute MI—to permit early therapy such as thrombolysis, establish reperfusion of the area at risk, salvage as much ischemic but not yet dead myocardium as possible, and consequently minimize infarct size.

Myocardial ischemia contributes to arrhythmias through complex and poorly understood mechanisms, probably involving electrical instability (irritability).[56] Sudden death, a leading cause of mortality in IHD patients, can be caused by massive cell injury with mechanical failure but is most often due to ventricular fibrillation caused by myocardial irritability induced by ischemia or infarction. Interestingly, studies of resuscitated survivors of "sudden death" show that the majority do not develop acute MI; in such cases, myocardial irritability induced by ischemia presumably led directly to the serious arrhythmia.

TABLE 12–4 Approximate Time of Onset of Key Events in Ischemic Cardiac Myocytes

Feature	Time
Onset of ATP depletion	Seconds
Loss of contractility	<2 min
ATP reduced to 50% of normal to 10% of normal	 10 min 40 min
Irreversible cell injury	20–40 min
Microvascular injury	>1 hr

ATP, adenosine triphosphate.

The progression of ischemic necrosis in the myocardium is summarized in Figure 12–14. Irreversible injury of ischemic myocytes occurs first in the subendocardial zone. With more extended ischemia, a *wavefront* of cell death moves through the myocardium to involve progressively more of the transmural thickness of the ischemic zone. The precise location, size, and specific morphologic features of an acute myocardial infarct depend on:

- The location, severity, and rate of development of coronary atherosclerotic obstructions
- The size of the vascular bed perfused by the obstructed vessels
- The duration of the occlusion
- The metabolic/oxygen needs of the myocardium at risk
- The extent of collateral blood vessels
- The presence, site, and severity of coronary arterial spasm
- Other factors, such as alterations in blood pressure, heart rate, and cardiac rhythm.

The necrosis is largely complete within 6 hours in experimental models and humans, involving nearly all of the ischemic myocardial bed at risk supplied by the occluded coronary artery. Progression of necrosis, however, may follow a more protracted course in some patients (possibly over 6 to 12 hours or longer) in whom the coronary arterial collateral system, stimulated by chronic ischemia, is better developed and thereby more effective.

Morphology. The evolution of the morphologic changes in acute MI and its healing are summarized in Table 12–5.

Nearly all transmural infarcts involve at least a portion of the left ventricle (including the ventricular septum). About 15% to 30% of those that affect the posterior free wall and posterior portion of the septum transmurally extend into the adjacent right ventricular wall. Isolated infarction of the right ventricle, however, occurs in only 1% to 3% of cases. Associated infarction of atrial tissue accompanies a large posterior left ventricular infarct in some cases. Transmural infarcts usually encompass nearly the entire perfusion zone of the occluded coronary artery. Almost always there is a narrow rim (approximately 0.1 mm) of preserved subendocardial myocardium sustained by diffusion of oxygen and nutrients from the lumen.

The frequencies of critical narrowing (and thrombosis) of each of the three main arterial trunks and the corresponding sites of myocardial lesions resulting in infarction (in the typical right dominant heart) are as follows:

- Left anterior descending coronary artery (40% to 50%): infarct involves anterior wall of left ventri-

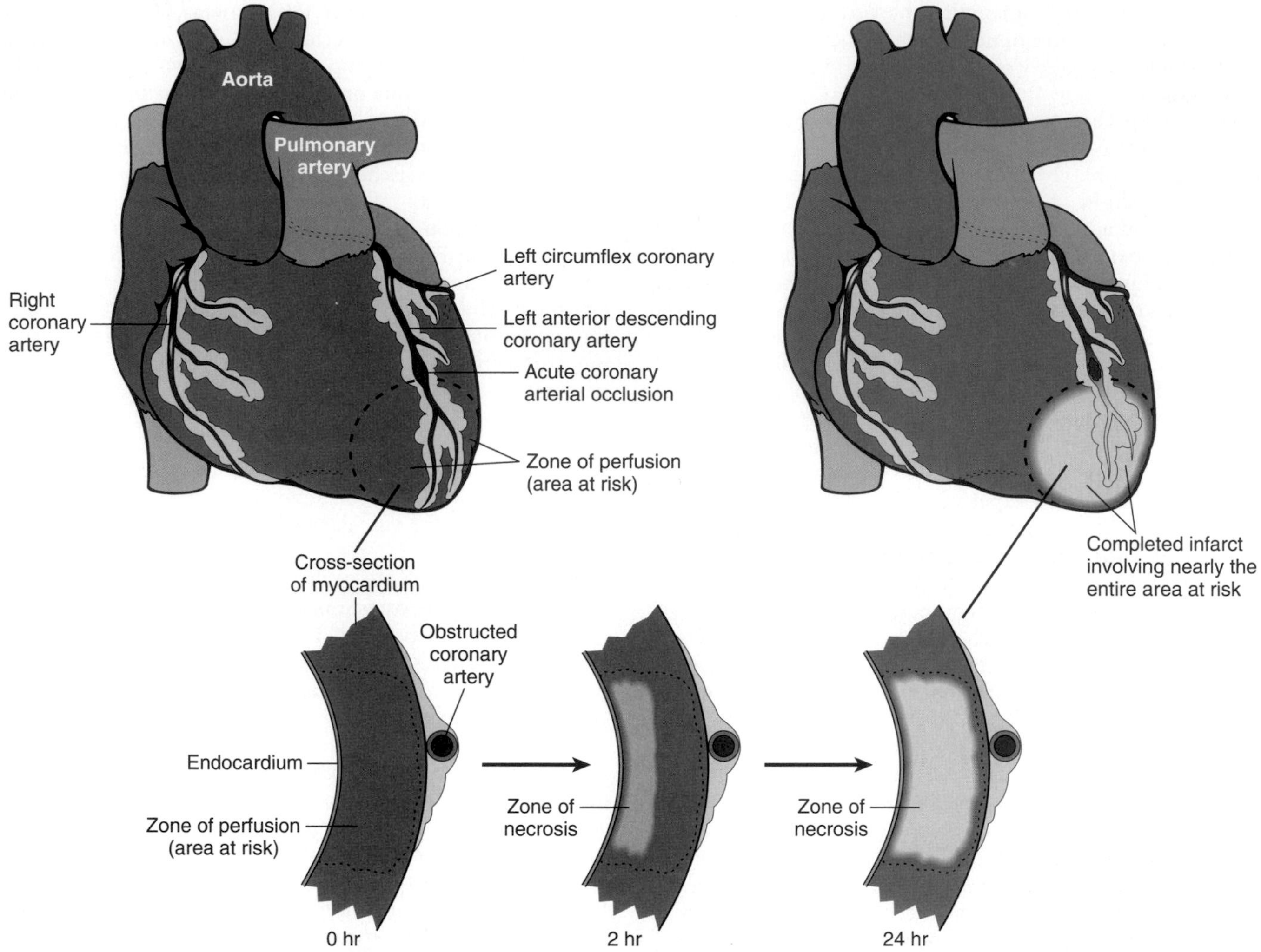

FIGURE 12–14 Schematic representation of the progression of myocardial necrosis after coronary artery occlusion. Necrosis begins in a small zone of the myocardium beneath the endocardial surface in the center of the ischemic zone. This entire region of myocardium *(shaded)* depends on the occluded vessel for perfusion and is the area at risk. Note that a very narrow zone of myocardium immediately beneath the endocardium is spared from necrosis because it can be oxygenated by diffusion from the ventricle. The end result of the obstruction to blood flow is necrosis of the muscle that was dependent on perfusion from the coronary artery obstructed. Nearly the entire area at risk loses viability. The process is called *myocardial infarction,* and the region of necrotic muscle is a *myocardial infarct.*

cle near apex; anterior portion of ventricular septum; apex circumferentially

- Right coronary artery (30% to 40%): infarct involves inferior/posterior wall of left ventricle; posterior portion of ventricular septum; inferior/posterior right ventricular free wall in some cases
- Left circumflex coronary artery (15% to 20%): infarct involves lateral wall of left ventricle except at apex

Other locations of critical coronary arterial lesions causing infarcts are sometimes encountered, such as the left main coronary artery or the secondary branches (e.g., diagonal branches of the LAD artery or marginal branches of the LCX artery). In contrast, stenosing atherosclerosis or thrombosis of a penetrating intramyocardial branch of the coronary arteries is almost never encountered. Occasionally the observation of multiple severe stenoses or thromboses in the absence of myocardial damage suggests that formation of collateral connections between coronary arteries was protective.

The gross and microscopic appearance of an infarct at autopsy depends on the duration of survival of the patient following the MI. Areas of damage undergo a progressive sequence of morphologic changes that consist of typical ischemic coagulative necrosis, followed by inflammation and repair that closely parallels that occurring after injury at other, noncardiac sites.

Early recognition of acute myocardial infarcts by pathologists can be difficult, particularly when death has occurred within a few hours after the onset of symptoms.[57] Myocardial infarcts less than 12 hours old are usually not apparent on gross examination. It is often possible, however, to highlight the area of necrosis that first becomes apparent after 2 to 3 hours after the infarct, by immersion of tissue slices in a

TABLE 12–5 Evolution of Morphologic Changes in Myocardial Infarction

Time	Gross Features	Light Microscope	Electron Microscope
Reversible Injury			
0–½ hr	None	None	Relaxation of myofibrils; glycogen loss; mitochondrial swelling
Irreversible Injury			
½–4 hr	None	Usually none; variable waviness of fibers at border	Sarcolemmal disruption; mitochondrial amorphous densities
4–12 hr	Occasionally dark mottling	Beginning coagulation necrosis; edema; hemorrhage	
12–24 hr	Dark mottling	Ongoing coagulation necrosis; pyknosis of nuclei; myocyte hypereosinophilia; marginal contraction band necrosis; beginning neutrophilic infiltrate	
1–3 days	Mottling with yellow-tan infarct center	Coagulation necrosis, with loss of nuclei and striations; interstitial infiltrate of neutrophils	
3–7 days	Hyperemic border; central yellow-tan softening	Beginning disintegration of dead myofibers, with dying neutrophils; early phagocytosis of dead cells by macrophages at infarct border	
7–10 days	Maximally yellow-tan and soft, with depressed red-tan margins	Well-developed phagocytosis of dead cells; early formation of fibrovascular granulation tissue at margins	
10–14 days	Red-gray depressed infarct borders	Well-established granulation tissue with new blood vessels and collagen deposition	
2–8 wk	Gray-white scar, progressive from border toward core of infarct	Increased collagen deposition, with decreased cellularity	
>2 mo	Scarring complete	Dense collagenous scar	

solution of *triphenyltetrazolium chloride* (TTC). This histochemical stain imparts a brick-red color to intact, noninfarcted myocardium where the dehydrogenase enzymes are preserved. Because dehydrogenases are depleted in the area of ischemic necrosis (they leak out through the damaged cell membranes), an infarcted area is revealed as an unstained pale zone (while old scarred infarcts appear white and glistening) (Fig. 12–15). Subsequently, by 12 to 24 hours, an infarct can be identified in routinely fixed gross slices owing to a red-blue hue caused by stagnated, trapped blood. Progressively thereafter, the infarct becomes a more sharply defined, yellow-tan, somewhat softened area that by 10 days to 2 weeks is rimmed by a hyperemic zone of highly vascularized granulation tissue. Over the succeeding weeks, the injured region evolves to a fibrous scar.

The histopathologic changes also have a fairly predictable sequence (summarized in Table 12–5 and Figure 12–16). Using light microscopic examination of routinely stained tissue sections, the typical changes of coagulative necrosis become detectable variably in the first 4 to 12 hours. "Wavy fibers" may be present at the periphery of the infarct; these changes probably result from the forceful systolic tugs by the viable fibers immediately adjacent to the noncontractile dead fibers, thereby stretching and buckling them. An additional but sublethal ischemic change may be seen in the margins of infarcts: so-called vacuolar degeneration or **myocytolysis**, involving large vacuolar spaces within cells, probably containing water. This potentially reversible alteration is particularly frequent in the thin zone of viable subendocardial cells.

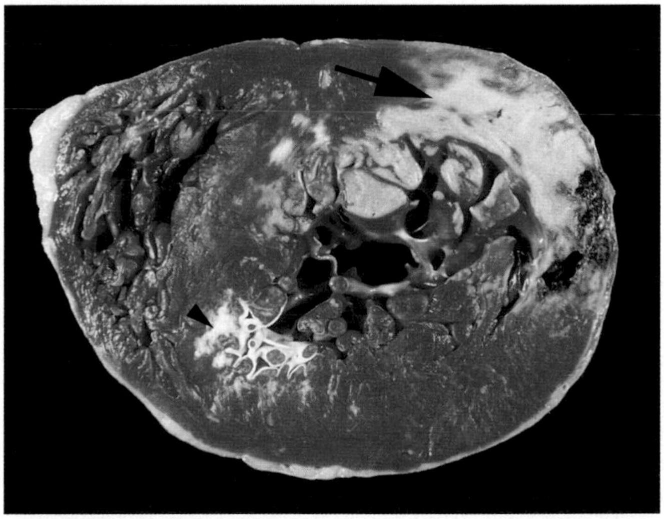

FIGURE 12–15 Acute myocardial infarct, predominantly of the posterolateral left ventricle, demonstrated histochemically by a lack of staining by the triphenyltetrazolium chloride (TTC) stain in areas of necrosis *(arrow)*. The staining defect is due to the enzyme leakage that follows cell death. Note the myocardial hemorrhage at one edge of the infarct that was associated with cardiac rupture, and the anterior scar *(arrowhead)*, indicative of old infarct. (Specimen the oriented with the posterior wall at the top.)

Subendocardial myocyte vacuolization in other contexts may signify severe chronic ischemia.

The necrotic muscle elicits acute inflammation (typically most prominent at 2 to 3 days). Thereafter macrophages remove the necrotic myocytes (most

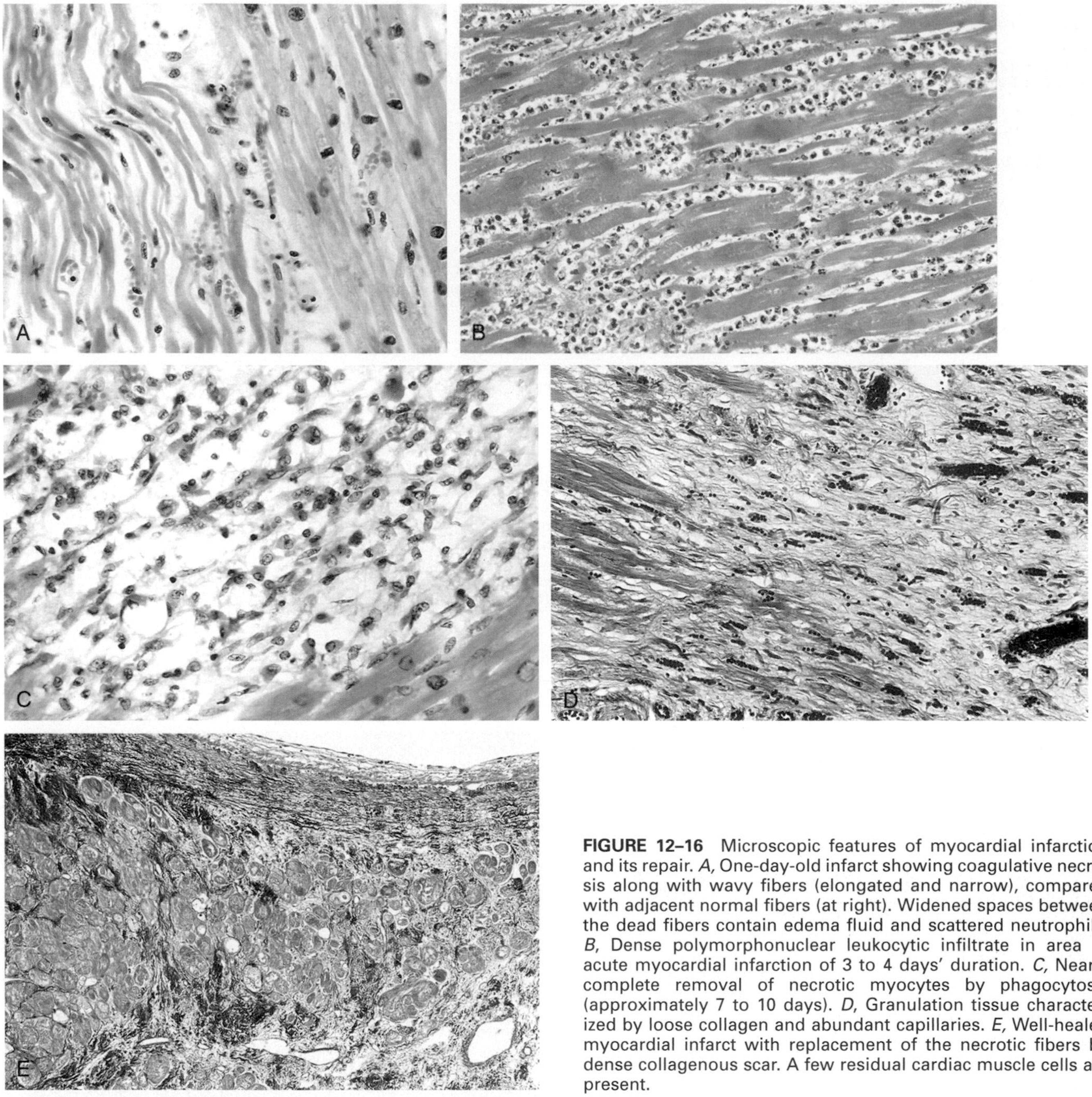

FIGURE 12–16 Microscopic features of myocardial infarction and its repair. *A,* One-day-old infarct showing coagulative necrosis along with wavy fibers (elongated and narrow), compared with adjacent normal fibers (at right). Widened spaces between the dead fibers contain edema fluid and scattered neutrophils. *B,* Dense polymorphonuclear leukocytic infiltrate in area of acute myocardial infarction of 3 to 4 days' duration. *C,* Nearly complete removal of necrotic myocytes by phagocytosis (approximately 7 to 10 days). *D,* Granulation tissue characterized by loose collagen and abundant capillaries. *E,* Well-healed myocardial infarct with replacement of the necrotic fibers by dense collagenous scar. A few residual cardiac muscle cells are present.

pronounced at 5 to 10 days), and the damaged zone is progressively replaced by the ingrowth of highly vascularized granulation tissue (most prominent at 2 to 4 weeks), which progressively becomes less vascularized and more fibrous. In most instances, scarring is well advanced by the end of the sixth week, but the efficiency of repair depends on the size of the original lesion. As healing requires the participation of inflammatory cells that migrate to the region of damage through intact blood vessels, which often survive only at the infarct margins, the infarct heals from its borders toward the center. Thus, a large infarct may not heal as readily nor as completely as a small one. A healing infarct may appear nonuniform, with the most advanced healing at the periphery. Once a lesion is completely healed, it is impossible to distinguish its age (i.e., the dense fibrous tissue scar of an 8-week-old and a 10-year-old lesion may look similar).

Several infarcts of varying age are frequently found in the same heart. Repetitive necrosis of adjacent regions yields progressive **extension** of an individual infarct over a period of days to weeks. Examination of the heart in such cases often reveals a central zone of repairing infarct that is days to weeks older and whose healing is more advanced than that of a peripheral margin of more recent ischemic necrosis. This contrasts with the appearance of a single-event infarct described above, in which the most advanced repair was peripheral. An initial infarct may extend because of retrograde propagation of a thrombus, proximal vasospasm, progressively impaired cardiac contractility that renders flow through moderate stenoses critically insufficient, the development of platelet-fibrin microemboli, the appearance of an arrhythmia that impairs cardiac function, or poor perfusion owing to progressively impaired myocardial function. In general, the sequential morphology of evolving subendocardial and transmural infarcts is qualitatively similar, but subendocardial infarcts tend to be smaller.

The temporal sequence of morphologic events in MI is summarized in Figure 12–17, emphasizing the possibility of interventions that might limit infarct size, since myocardium that is not yet necrotic is potentially salvageable.

Infarct Modification by Reperfusion. The most effective way to salvage ischemic myocardium threatened by infarction is to restore tissue perfusion as rapidly as possible. This is best accomplished by restoration of coronary flow *(reperfusion)* by thrombolysis, balloon angioplasty (also known as percutaneous transluminal coronary angioplasty, or PTCA), or coronary arterial bypass graft (CABG). Reperfusion-associated pathologies, including reperfusion-induced arrhythmias, myocardial hemorrhage with contraction bands, irreversible cell damage distinct from and additional to the injury associated with the original ischemic event *(reperfusion injury)*, microvascular injury, and prolonged ischemic dysfunction *(myocardial stunning)*, are discussed below and summarized in Figure 12–18. Thrombolytic therapy (dissolution of the offending thrombus by streptokinase or tissue-type plasminogen activator [t-PA] through activation of the fibrinolytic system) or PTCA is often used in an attempt to dissolve or mechanically disrupt the thrombus that initiated acute MI. The

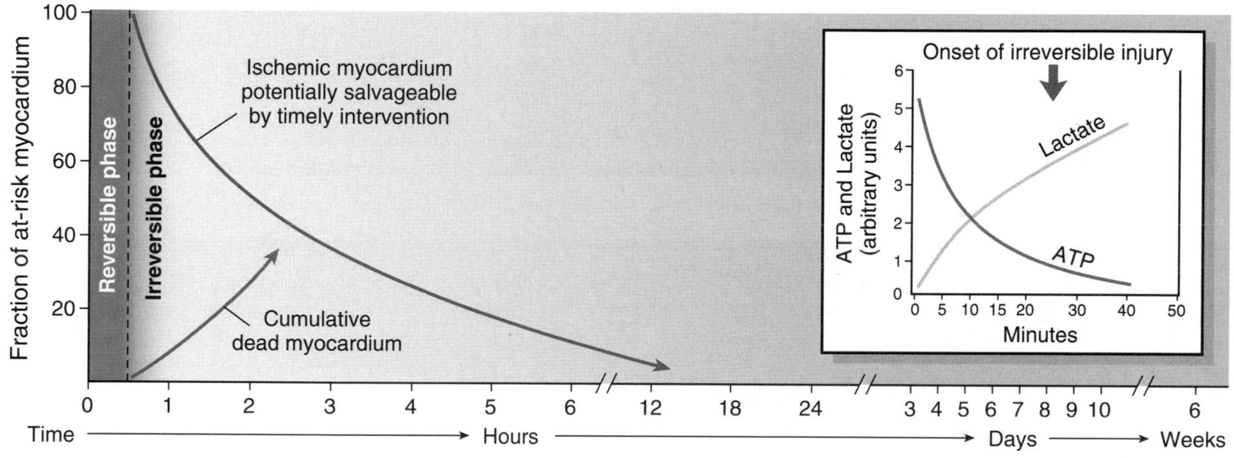

Electron microscopy	**Reversible phase:** Glycogen depletion; mitochondrial swelling and relaxation of myofibrils **Irreversible phase:** Sarcolemmal disruption; mitochondrial amorphous densities						
Histochemistry	TTC staining defect →						
Light microscopy	Waviness of fibers at border	Beginning coagulation necrosis; edema; focal hemorrhage; beginning neutrophilic infiltrate	Continuing coagulation necrosis; pallor (shrunken nuclei and eosinophilic cytoplasm); myocyte contraction bands	Coagulation necrosis with loss of nuclei and striations; neutrophilic infiltrate	Disintegration of myofibers and phagocytosis by macrophages	Completion of phagocytosis; prominent granulation tissue with neovascularization and fibrovascular reaction	Mature fibrous scar
Gross changes			Pallor	Pallor, sometimes hyperemia; yellowing at periphery	Hyperemic border; central yellow-brown softening	Maximally yellow and soft vascularized edges; red-brown and depressed	

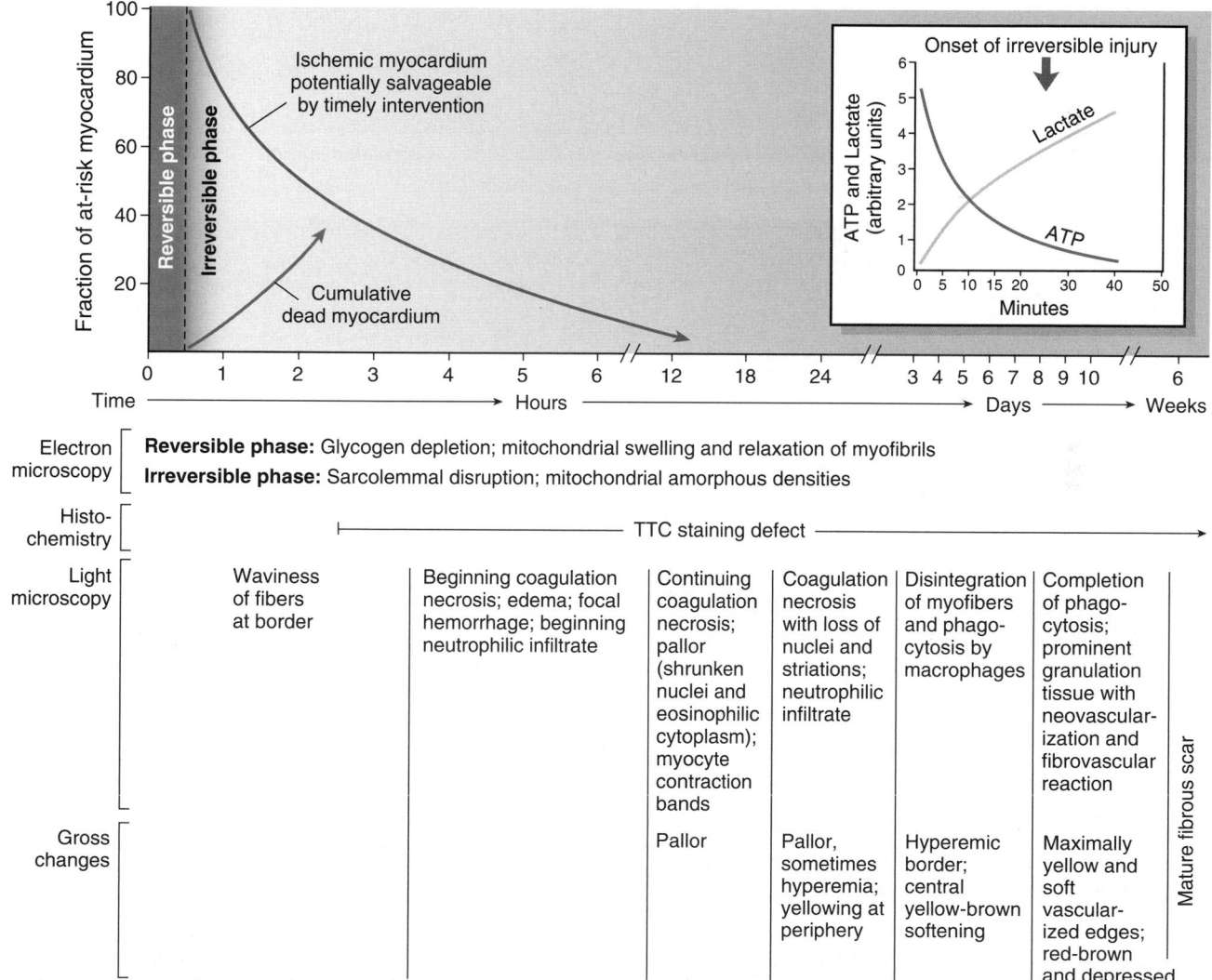

FIGURE 12–17 Temporal sequence of early biochemical, ultrastructural, histochemical, and histologic findings after onset of severe myocardial ischemia. For approximately 30 minutes after the onset of even the most severe ischemia, myocardial injury is potentially reversible. Thereafter, progressive loss of viability occurs that is complete by 6 to 12 hours. The benefits of reperfusion are greatest when it is achieved early, with progressively smaller benefit occurring as reperfusion is delayed. (Modified with permission from Antman E: Acute myocardial infarction. In Braunwald E, Zipes DP, Libby P (eds): Heart Disease: A Textbook of Cardiovascular Medicine, 6th ed. Philadelphia, WB Saunders, 2001, pp. 1114–1231.)

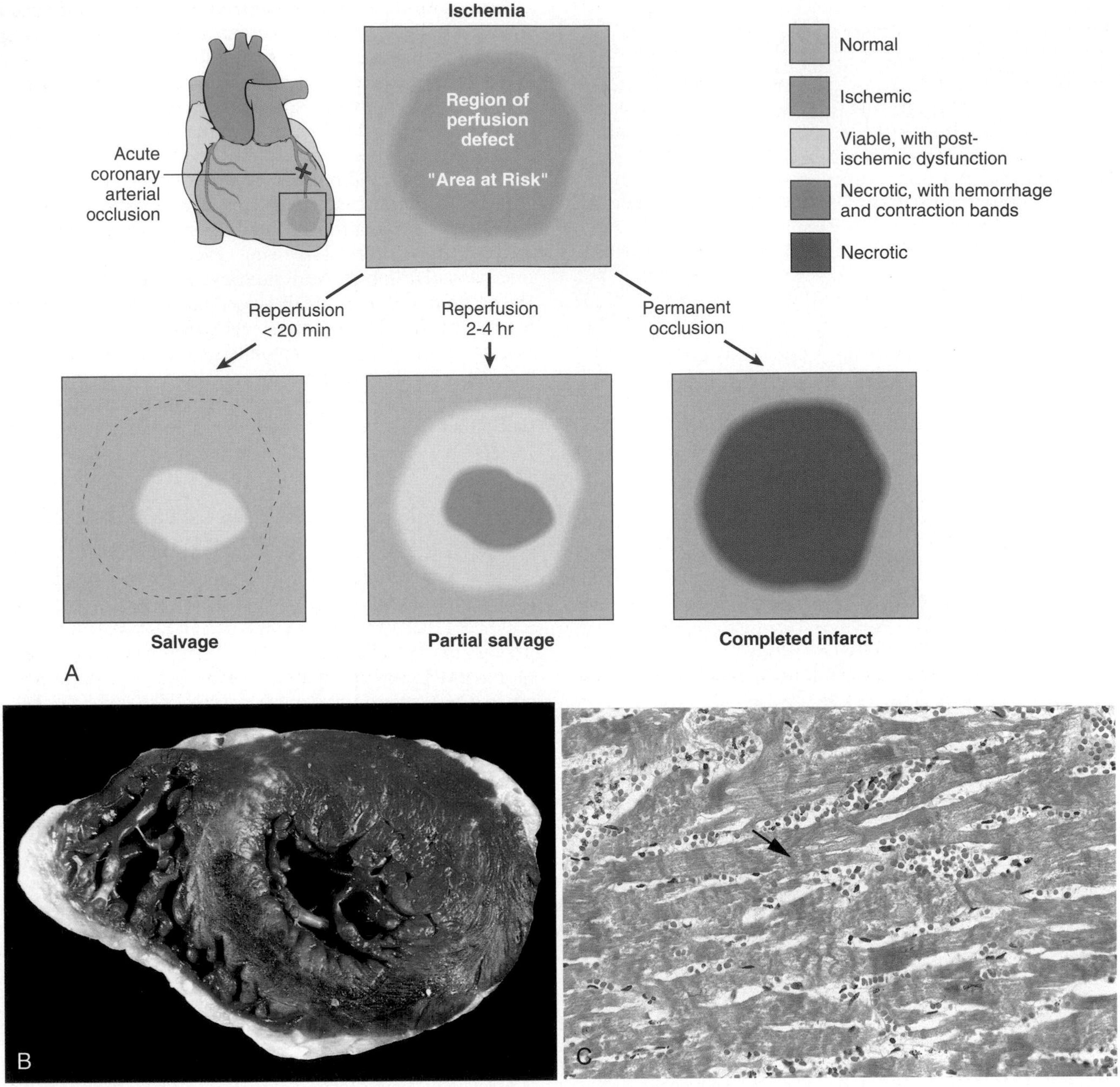

FIGURE 12–18 Consequences of myocardial ischemia followed by reperfusion. *A,* Schematic illustration of the progression of myocardial ischemic injury and its modification by restoration of flow (reperfusion). Hearts suffering brief periods of ischemia of <20 minutes followed by reperfusion do not develop necrosis (reversible injury). Brief ischemia followed by reperfusion results in stunning. If coronary occlusion is extended beyond 20 minutes' duration, a wavefront of necrosis progresses from subendocardium to subepicardium over time. Reperfusion before 3 to 6 hours of ischemia salvages ischemic but viable tissue. (This salvaged tissue may demonstrate stunning.) Reperfusion beyond 6 hours does not appreciably reduce myocardial infarct size. Late reperfusion may still have a beneficial effect on reducing or preventing myocardial infarct expansion and left ventricular remodeling. *B,* Gross and *C,* microscopic appearance of myocardium modified by reperfusion. *B,* Large, densely hemorrhagic, anterior wall acute myocardial infarction from patient with left anterior descending artery thrombus treated with streptokinase intracoronary thrombolysis (triphenyl tetrazolium chloride–stained heart slice). (Specimen oriented with posterior wall at top.) *C,* Myocardial necrosis with hemorrhage and contraction bands, visible as dark bands spanning some myofibers *(arrow).* This is the characteristic appearance of markedly ischemic myocardium that has been reperfused.

purpose of these treatments is to restore blood flow to the area at risk for infarction and possibly rescue the ischemic (but not yet necrotic) heart muscle. Removal of thrombus re-establishes flow through the occluded coronary artery in most cases; early reperfusion can salvage myocardium and thereby limit infarct size, with consequent improvement in both short- and long-term function and survival.[58] As discussed above, loss of myocardial viability in infarction is progressive, occurring over a period of at least several hours. Thus, reperfusion of at risk myocardium offers an effective approach for restoring the balance between myocardial perfusion and need. The potential benefit is clearly related to the rapidity with which the coronary occlusion is alleviated; the first 3 to 4 hours following onset of symptoms are critical. Moreover, thrombolysis can at best remove a thrombus occluding a coronary artery; it does not significantly alter the underlying disrupted atherosclerotic plaque that initiated it. In contrast, PTCA not only eliminates a thrombotic occlusion, but also can relieve some of the original obstruction caused by the underlying plaque.[59] CABG provides flow around it.

Recall that severe ischemia does not cause immediate cell death even in the most severely affected regions of myocardium, and not all regions of myocardium are equally ischemic. Therefore, the outcome distal to the occlusion following restoration of flow to previously ischemic myocardium may vary from region to region. As indicated in Figure 12–18*A*, reperfusion of myocardium sufficiently early (within 15 to 20 minutes) after onset of ischemia may prevent all necrosis. Reperfusion after a longer interval may not prevent all necrosis but can salvage (i.e., prevent necrosis of) at least some myocytes that would have died with more prolonged or permanent ischemia.

The typical appearance of ischemic then reperfused myocardium is illustrated in Figure 12–18*B* and *C*. A partially completed then reperfused infarct usually has hemorrhage because the vasculature injured during the period of ischemia becomes leaky on restoration of flow. Moreover, disintegration of myocytes that were lethally damaged by the preceding ischemia may be accentuated or accelerated by reperfusion. Microscopic examination reveals that myocytes already irreversibly injured at the time of reflow often have *necrosis with contraction bands.* Contraction bands are intensely eosinophilic transverse bands composed of closely packed hypercontracted sarcomeres. They are most likely produced by exaggerated contraction of myofibrils at the instant perfusion is reestablished, at which time the internal portions of an already dead cell whose membranes have been damaged by ischemia are exposed to a high concentration of calcium ions from the plasma. Thus *reperfusion not only salvages reversibly injured cells but also alters the morphology of cells already lethally injured at the time of reflow.*

However, despite the potential for myocardial salvage by reperfusion of ischemic myocardium, some small amount of *new* cellular damage may occur that blunts the beneficial effect of reperfusion itself *(reperfusion injury)*.[60,61] The clinical significance of myocardial reperfusion injury is uncertain. As discussed in Chapter 1, reperfusion injury is mediated, at least in part, by the generation of oxygen free radicals from infiltrating leukocytes during reperfusion. Recent advances in the understanding of cell death in ischemia and reperfusion suggest that apoptosis may be prominent at reperfusion; thus, prevention of apoptosis may be a potential therapeutic target to limit reperfusion injury.[62] Reperfusion-induced microvascular injury causes not only hemorrhage, but also endothelial swelling that occludes capillaries and may prevent local reperfusion to areas of critically injured myocardium (called *no-reflow*).

Ischemic myocardium may have profound functional changes despite complete salvage of viability.[63] Although most of the viable myocardium existing at the time of reflow ultimately recovers after alleviation of ischemia, critical abnormalities in cellular biochemistry and function of myocytes salvaged by reperfusion may persist for as long as several days *(prolonged postischemic ventricular dysfunction,* or *stunned myocardium).* Stunning may induce a state of reversible cardiac failure that may benefit from temporary cardiac assist. Paradoxically, short-lived transient severe ischemia, as might occur in repetitive angina pectoris or silent ischemia, may protect the myocardium against a greater subsequent ischemic insult (a phenomenon known as *preconditioning*) by mechanisms that are not well known. Myocardium that is subjected to persistently low flow has chronically depressed function and is said to be *hibernating.*[64] This portion of the myocardium may undergo profound restoration of function following revascularization by CABG surgery or balloon angioplasty.

Clinical Features. MI is diagnosed classically by typical symptoms, biochemical evidence, and by the ECG pattern. Patients with MI have rapid, weak pulse and are often sweating profusely (diaphoretic). Dyspnea due to impaired contractility of the ischemic myocardium and the resultant pulmonary congestion and edema is common. In about 10% to 15% of MI patients, the onset is entirely asymptomatic and the disease is discovered only later by ECG changes, usually consisting of new Q waves. Such "silent" MIs are particularly common in patients with diabetes mellitus and in elderly patients.

Laboratory evaluation is based on measuring the blood levels of intracellular macromolecules that leak out of fatally injured myocardial cells through damaged cell membranes; these molecules include myoglobin, cardiac troponins T and I (TnT, TnI), creatine kinase (CK), lactate dehydrogenase, and many others. Although these markers have become increasingly sensitive indicators of myocardial damage, they do not reflect its mechanism.[65] From a biochemical perspective, the diagnosis of myocardial injury is established when blood levels of sensitive and specific biomarkers, such as cardiac troponin and the MB fraction of creatine kinase (CK-MB), are increased in the clinical setting of acute ischemia. *The preferred biomarkers for myocardial damage are cardiac-specific proteins, particularly Troponin-I (TnI) and Troponin-T.* Troponins are proteins that regulate calcium-mediated contraction of cardiac and skeletal muscle. These markers have nearly complete tissue specificity and high sensitivity. TnI and TnT are not normally detectable in the circulation, but after acute MI, levels of both cardiac troponins rise at 2 to 4 hours and peak at 48 hours. Troponin levels remain elevated for 7 to 10 days after the acute event.

Formerly the "gold standard," cardiac creatine kinase (CK-MB) remains the best alternative to troponin measurement. *Creatine kinase* is an enzyme that is highly concentrated in brain, myocardium, and skeletal muscle and is composed of two dimers, designated "M" and "B." The isoenzyme CK-MM is derived predominantly from skeletal muscle and heart; CK-BB from brain, lung, and many other tissues; and CK-MB principally from myocardium, although variable amounts of the MB form are also present in skeletal muscle. Total CK activity is sensitive but not specific, as CK is elevated in other conditions such as skeletal muscle injury. CK-MB activity begins to rise within 2 to 4 hours of onset of MI, peaks at about 24 hours, and returns to normal within approximately 72 hours. Although the diagnostic sensitivities of cardiac troponin and CK-MB measurements are similar in the early stages of MI, persistence of elevated troponin levels for approximately 10 days allows the diagnosis of acute MI long after CK-MB levels have returned to normal. The peak of either troponin or CK-MB is accelerated in patients who have had reperfusion, owing to washing out of the enzyme from the necrotic tissue. *An absence of a change in the levels of CK and CK-MB during the first 2 days of chest pain and of troponin in the days following essentially excludes the diagnosis of MI.*

As discussed, C-reactive protein (CRP) may serve as a marker to predict the risk of myocardial infarct in patients with angina, and the risk of new infarcts in patients who recover from infarcts.[49,50] Using highly sensitive methods, serum CRP, levels of more than 3 mg/L are associated with the highest risk of cardiovascular disease, while levels of 1 to 3 mg/L are associated with moderate risk.[51,52]

Other diagnostic modalities such as echocardiography (for visualization of abnormalities of regional wall motion), radioisotope studies such as radionuclide angiography (for chamber configuration), perfusion scintigraphy (for regional perfusion), and magnetic resonance imaging (for structural characterization) sometimes provide additional anatomic, biochemical, and functional data.

Consequences and Complications of Myocardial Infarction. Extraordinary progress has been made in improving the outcome of patients with acute MI. Concurrent with the marked decrease in the overall mortality of IHD since the 1960s, the in-hospital death rate has declined from approximately 30% to an overall rate of between 10% and 13% today (and to approximately 7% for patients receiving aggressive reperfusion therapy). Nevertheless, half of the deaths associated with acute MI occur within 1 hour of onset; these individuals never reach the hospital. In general, factors associated with a poor prognosis include advanced age, female gender, diabetes mellitus and, owing to a loss of functional myocardium, previous MI.

Nearly three-fourths of patients have one or more complications following acute MI, which include the following (some of which are illustrated in Fig. 12–19):

- *Contractile dysfunction. Myocardial infarcts produce abnormalities in left ventricular function approximately proportional to their size.* Most often, there is some degree of left ventricular failure with hypotension, pulmonary vascular congestion, and transudation into the interstitial pulmonary spaces, which may progress to pulmonary edema with respiratory impairment. Severe "pump failure" *(cardiogenic shock)* occurs in 10% to 15% of patients following acute MI, generally with a large infarct (often greater than 40% of the left ventricle). Cardiogenic shock has a nearly 70% mortality rate and accounts for two thirds of in-hospital deaths.
- *Arrhythmias.* Many patients have *conduction disturbances and myocardial irritability* following MI, which undoubtedly are responsible for many of the sudden deaths. MI-associated arrhythmias include sinus bradycardia, heart block (asystole), tachycardia, ventricular premature contractions or ventricular tachycardia, and ventricular fibrillation. Owing to the location of portions of the atrioventricular conduction system (bundle of His) in the inferoseptal myocardium, infarcts of this region may also be associated with heart block. Prompt intervention by mobile and hospital coronary care units can control potentially lethal arrhythmias in many patients.
- *Myocardial rupture.* The *cardiac rupture syndromes* result from the mechanical weakening that occurs in necrotic and subsequently inflamed myocardium and include (1) rupture of the ventricular free wall (most commonly), with hemopericardium and cardiac tamponade, usually fatal (see Fig. 12–19*A*); (2) rupture of the ventricular septum (less commonly), leading to a left-to-right shunt (see Fig. 12–19*B*); and (3) papillary muscle rupture (least commonly), resulting in the acute onset of severe mitral regurgitation (see Fig. 12–19*C*). Free-wall rupture may occur at almost any time after MI but is most frequent 3 to 7 days after onset, when coagulative necrosis, neutrophilic infiltration, and lysis of the myocardial connective tissue have appreciably weakened the infarcted myocardium (mean, 4 to 5 days; range, 1 to 10 days). However, as many as one quarter of cardiac ruptures occur within 24 hours. The lateral wall at the midventricular level is the most common site for postinfarction free-wall rupture. Risk factors for free-wall rupture include age older than 60, female gender, pre-existing hypertension, and lack of left ventricular hypertrophy. Moreover, this complication occurs more readily in patients without prior MI owing to an absence of fibrosis, which tends to block myocardial tearing. Acute free-wall ruptures are usually rapidly fatal. However, a strategically located pericardial adhesion that aborts a rupture may result in the formation of a *false aneurysm* (that is, a contained rupture that results in a hematoma communicating with the ventricular cavity). The wall of a false aneurysm consists only of epicardium and adherent parietal pericardium. Many false aneurysms are filled with mural thrombus, and half ultimately rupture. Postinfarction rupture of septal myocardium causing an *(acute) ventricular septal defect* complicates 1% to 2% of infarcts.[66]
- *Pericarditis.* A fibrinous or fibrohemorrhagic pericarditis usually develops about the second or third day following a transmural infarct and usually resolves over time (see Fig. 12–19*D*). Pericarditis is the epicardial manifestation of the underlying myocardial inflammation.
- *Right ventricular infarction.* Although isolated infarction of the right ventricle is unusual, infarction of the right ventricular myocardium often accompanies ischemic injury of the adjacent posterior left ventricle and ventricular septum. A right ventricular infarct of either type can yield serious functional impairment.
- Infarct *extension.* New necrosis may occur adjacent to an existing infarct.
- Infarct *expansion.* Owing to the weakening of necrotic muscle, there may be disproportionate stretching, thinning, and dilation of the infarct region (especially with anteroseptal infarcts), which is often associated with mural thrombus (see Fig. 12–19*E*).
- *Mural thrombus.* With any infarct, the combination of a local myocardial abnormality in contractility (causing stasis) with endocardial damage (causing a thrombogenic surface) can foster *mural thrombosis* (Chapter 4) and, potentially, *thromboembolism.*
- *Ventricular aneurysm.* In contrast to *false aneurysms* mentioned above, *true* aneurysms of the ventricular wall are bounded by myocardium that has become scarred. A late complication, aneurysms of the ventricular wall most commonly result from a large transmural anteroseptal infarct (often one that has undergone expansion) that heals

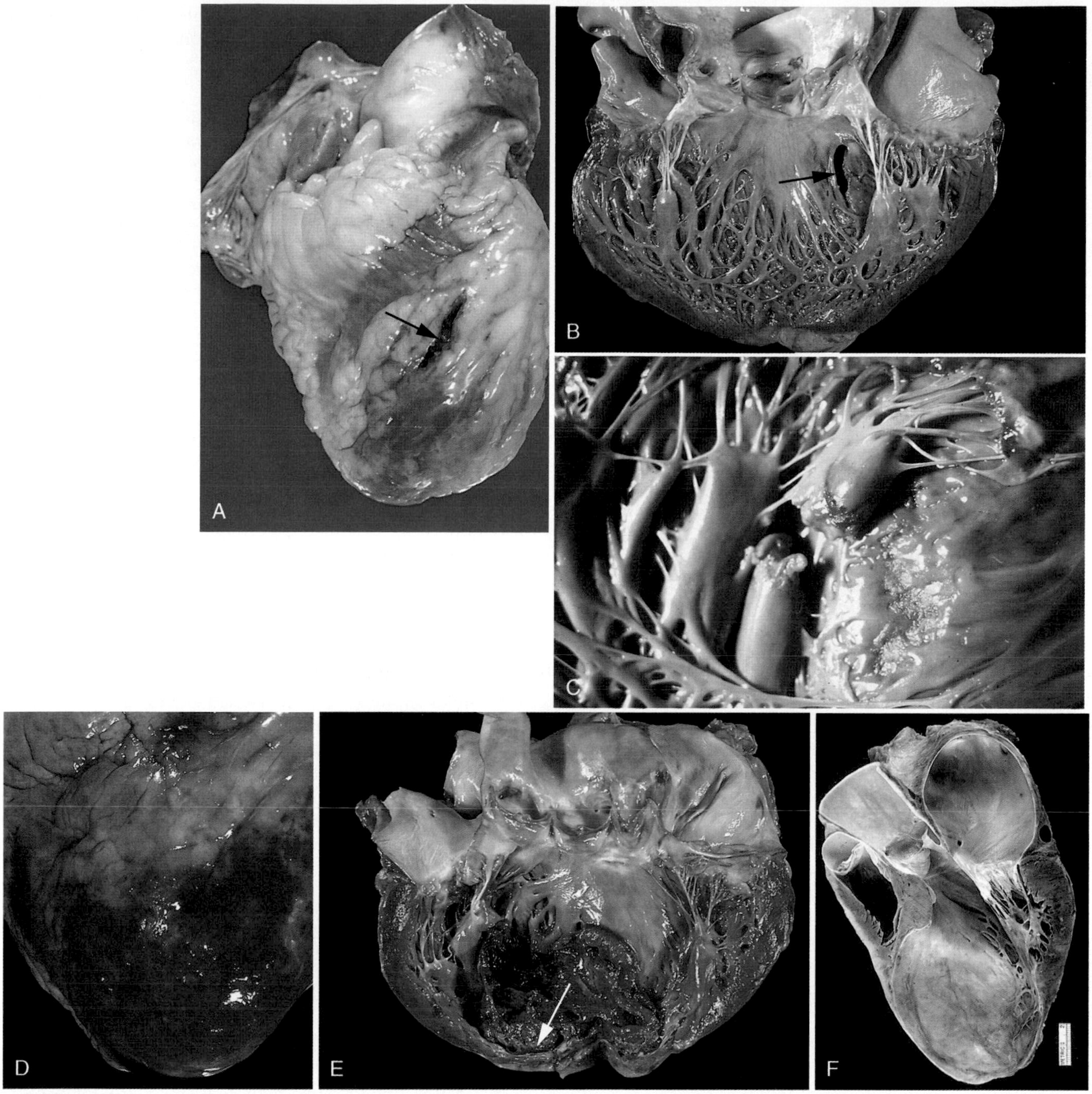

FIGURE 12–19 Complications of myocardial infarction. Cardiac rupture syndromes *(A, B,* and *C). A,* Anterior myocardial rupture in an acute infarct *(arrow). B,* Rupture of the ventricular septum *(arrow). C,* Complete rupture of a necrotic papillary muscle. *D,* Fibrinous pericarditis, showing a dark, roughened epicardial surface overlying an acute infarct. *E,* Early expansion of anteroapical infarct with wall thinning *(arrow)* and mural thrombus. *F,* Large apical left ventricular aneurysm. The left ventricle is on the right in this apical four-chamber view of the heart. (*A–E,* Reproduced by permission from Schoen FJ: Interventional and Surgical Cardiovascular Pathology: Clinical Correlations and Basic Principles, Philadelphia, WB Saunders, 1989.) (*F,* Courtesy of William D. Edwards, M.D., Mayo Clinic, Rochester, MN.)

into a large region of thin scar tissue, which paradoxically bulges during systole (see Fig. 12–19*F*). Complications of ventricular aneurysms include mural thrombus, arrhythmias and heart failure, but rupture of the fibrotic wall does not occur.

■ *Papillary muscle dysfunction.* As mentioned above, rarely, early dysfunction of a papillary muscle following MI occurs due to its rupture. More frequently, postinfarct mitral regurgitation results from early ischemic dysfunction of a papillary muscle and underlying myocardium and later from papillary muscle fibrosis and shortening or ventricular dilation (see below).

- *Progressive late heart failure* is discussed as chronic IHD below.

The propensity toward specific complications and the prognosis after MI depend primarily on infarct size, site, and fractional thickness of the myocardial wall that is damaged (subendocardial or transmural infarct). Large transmural infarcts yield a higher probability of cardiogenic shock, arrhythmias, and late CHF. Patients with anterior transmural infarcts are at greatest risk for free-wall rupture, expansion, mural thrombi, and aneurysm. In contrast, posterior transmural infarcts are more likely to be complicated by serious conduction blocks, right ventricular involvement, or both, and when acute ventricular septal defects occur in this area, they are more difficult to manage. Overall, however, patients with anterior infarcts have a substantially worse clinical course than those with inferior (posterior) infarcts. With subendocardial infarcts, thrombi may form on the endocardial surface, but pericarditis, rupture, and aneurysms rarely occur.

Multiple dynamic structural changes maintain cardiac output after acute MI. Both the necrotic zone and the noninfarcted segments of the ventricle undergo progressive changes in size, shape and thickness comprising early wall thinning, healing, hypertrophy and dilation, and late aneurysm formation, collectively termed *ventricular remodeling.*[67–69] Clearly, the initial compensatory hypertrophy of noninfarcted myocardium is hemodynamically beneficial. However, the adaptive effect of remodeling may be overwhelmed by expansion and ventricular aneurysm or late depression of regional and global contractile function owing to degenerative changes in viable myocardium. This may lead to late impairment of ventricular performance.

Long-term prognosis after MI depends on many factors, the most important of which are the quality of left ventricular function and the extent of vascular obstructions in vessels that perfuse viable myocardium. The overall total mortality within the first year is about 30%, including those victims who die before reaching the hospital. Thereafter there is a 3% to 4% mortality among survivors with each passing year. Infarct prevention through control of risk factors in individuals who have never experienced MI *(primary prevention)* and *prevention of reinfarction* in those who have recovered from an acute MI *(secondary prevention)* are important strategies that have received much attention and have achieved considerable success.

CHRONIC ISCHEMIC HEART DISEASE

The designation chronic ischemic heart disease (CIHD) is used here to describe the cardiac findings in patients, often but not exclusively elderly, who develop progressive heart failure as a consequence of ischemic myocardial damage. The term *ischemic cardiomyopathy* is often used by clinicians to describe CIHD. In most instances, there has been prior MI and sometimes previous coronary arterial bypass graft surgery or other interventions. CIHD usually constitutes postinfarction cardiac decompensation owing to exhaustion of the compensatory hypertrophy of noninfarcted viable myocardium that is itself in jeopardy of ischemic injury (see earlier discussion of cardiac hypertrophy). However, in other cases severe obstructive CAD may be present without acute or healed infarction but with diffuse myocardial dysfunction.

Morphology. Hearts from patients with CIHD are usually enlarged and heavy, secondary to left ventricular hypertrophy and dilation. Invariably there is moderate to severe stenosing atherosclerosis of the coronary arteries and sometimes total occlusion. Discrete, gray-white scars of healed infarcts are usually present. The mural endocardium is generally normal except for some superficial, patchy, fibrous thickenings, although mural thrombi may be present. The major microscopic findings include myocardial hypertrophy, diffuse subendocardial vacuolization, and scars of previously healed infarcts.

The clinical diagnosis is made largely by the insidious onset of CHF in patients who have had past episodes of MI or anginal attacks. In some individuals, however, progressive myocardial damage is entirely silent, and heart failure is the first indication of CIHD. The diagnosis rests largely on the exclusion of other forms of cardiac involvement. Such patients make up nearly half of cardiac transplant recipients.

SUDDEN CARDIAC DEATH

This catastrophe strikes down about 300,000 to 400,000 individuals annually in the United States. Sudden cardiac death (SCD) is most commonly defined as unexpected death from cardiac causes early after symptom onset (usually within 1 hour) or without the onset of symptoms. In many adults, SCD is a complication and often the first clinical manifestation of IHD. With decreasing age of the victim, the following nonatherosclerotic causes of SCD become increasingly probable:[70,71]

- Congenital structural or coronary arterial abnormalities
- Aortic valve stenosis
- Mitral valve prolapse
- Myocarditis
- Dilated or hypertrophic cardiomyopathy
- Pulmonary hypertension
- Hereditary or acquired abnormalities of the cardiac conduction system
- Isolated hypertrophy, hypertensive or unknown cause. Increased cardiac mass is an independent risk factor for cardiac death; thus, some young patients who die suddenly, including athletes, have hypertensive hypertrophy or unexplained increased cardiac mass as the only finding.

The ultimate mechanism of SCD is most often a lethal arrhythmia (e.g., asystole, ventricular fibrillation). Although ischemic injury can impinge on the conduction system and create electromechanical cardiac instability, in most cases the fatal arrhythmia is triggered by electrical irritability of myocardium that may be distant from the conduction system, induced by ischemia or other cellular abnormalities. The prognosis of patients vulnerable to SCD, especially those with chronic IHD, is markedly improved by implantation of an automatic cardioverter defibrillator, which senses and electrically counteracts an episode of ventricular fibrillation.[72]

Morphology. Marked coronary atherosclerosis with critical (>75%) stenosis involving one or more of the three major vessels is present in 80% to 90% of SCD victims; only 10% to 20% of cases are of nonatherosclerotic origin. Usually there are high-grade stenoses (>90%), and acute plaque disruption is common. A healed myocardial infarct is present in about 40%, but in those who were successfully resuscitated from sudden cardiac arrest, new MI is found in only 25% or less. Subendocardial myocyte vacuolization indicative of severe chronic ischemia is common.

Arrhythmias that occur in the absence of structural cardiac pathology can also precipitate sudden death. The most important cause is the autosomal dominant long QT syndrome (Romano-Ward syndrome), which causes heightened cardiac excitability and episodic ventricular arrhythmias. Mutations causing this disorder have been demonstrated in at least five different genes that encode components of cardiac ion channels including potassium and sodium channels.[73]

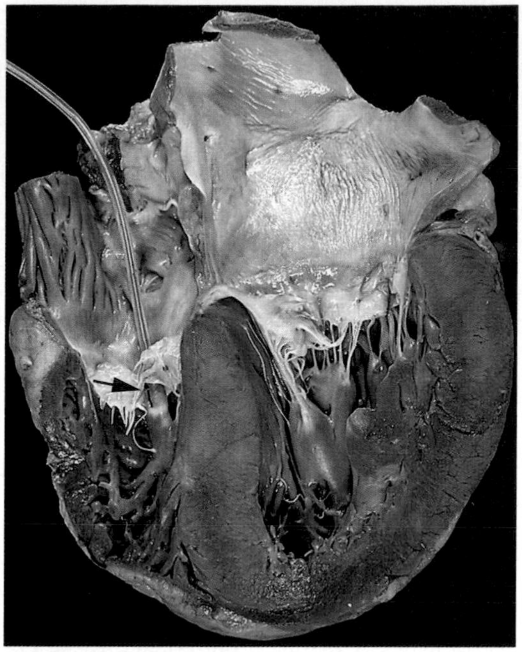

FIGURE 12–20 Hypertensive heart disease with marked concentric thickening of the left ventricular wall causing reduction in lumen size. The left ventricle is on the right in this apical four-chamber view of the heart. A pacemaker is incidentally present in the right ventricle *(arrow)*.

Hypertensive Heart Disease

Hypertensive heart disease (HHD) is the response of the heart to the increased demands induced by systemic hypertension.[74] Pulmonary hypertension also causes heart disease and is referred to as right-sided HHD, or cor pulmonale.

SYSTEMIC (LEFT-SIDED) HYPERTENSIVE HEART DISEASE

In hypertension, hypertrophy of the heart is an adaptive response to pressure overload that can lead to myocardial dysfunction, cardiac dilation, CHF, and sudden death (see section on cardiac hypertrophy, earlier in this chapter). *The minimal criteria for the diagnosis of systemic HHD are the following: (1) left ventricular hypertrophy (usually concentric) in the absence of other cardiovascular pathology that might have induced it and (2) a history or pathologic evidence of hypertension.* Notwithstanding, the Framingham Study established unequivocally that even mild hypertension (levels only slightly above 140/90 mm Hg), if sufficiently prolonged, induces left ventricular hypertrophy. Approximately 25% of the population of the United States suffers from hypertension of at least this degree. The pathogenesis of hypertension is discussed in Chapter 11.

Morphology. Hypertension induces left ventricular pressure overload hypertrophy without dilation of the left ventricle. The thickening of the left ventricular wall increases the ratio of its wall thickness to radius, and increases the weight of the heart disproportionately to the increase in overall cardiac size (Fig. 12–20). The left ventricular wall thickness may exceed 2.0 cm and the heart weight may exceed 500 gm. In time, the increased thickness of the left ventricular wall imparts a stiffness that impairs diastolic filling. This often induces left atrial enlargement.

Microscopically, the earliest change of systemic HHD is an increase in the transverse diameter of myocytes, which may be difficult to appreciate on routine microscopy. At a more advanced stage, the cellular and nuclear enlargement becomes somewhat more irregular, with variation in cell size among adjacent cells, and interstitial fibrosis. The biochemical, molecular, and morphologic changes that occur in hypertensive hypertrophy are similar to those noted in other conditions of myocardial overload (see section on cardiac hypertrophy, earlier in this chapter).

Compensated systemic HHD may be asymptomatic and suspected only in the appropriate clinical setting by ECG or echocardiographic indications of left ventricular enlargement. Other causes for such hypertrophy must be excluded. In many patients, systemic HHD comes to attention by the onset of atrial fibrillation (owing to left atrial enlargement) or CHF with cardiac dilation, or both. Depending on the severity, duration, and underlying basis of the hypertension, and on the adequacy of therapeutic control, the patient may (1) enjoy normal longevity and die of unrelated causes, (2) develop progressive IHD owing to the effects of hypertension in potentiating coronary atherosclerosis, (3) suffer progressive renal damage or cerebrovascular stroke, or (4) experience progressive heart failure. The risk of sudden cardiac death is also increased. Effective control of hypertension can prevent or lead to regression of cardiac hypertrophy and its associated risks.[75]

PULMONARY (RIGHT-SIDED) HYPERTENSIVE HEART DISEASE (COR PULMONALE)

Cor pulmonale, as pulmonary HHD is frequently called, consists of right ventricular hypertrophy, dilation, and potentially failure secondary to pulmonary hypertension caused by disorders of the lungs or pulmonary vasculature (Table 12–6). Pulmonary HHD is the right-sided counterpart of left-sided (systemic) HHD. Although right ventricular dilation and thickening caused either by diseases of the left side of the heart or congenital heart diseases are generally excluded by this definition of cor pulmonale, pulmonary venous hypertension that follows left-sided heart diseases of various etiologies is quite common.

Cor pulmonale may be acute or chronic, depending on the suddenness of development of the pulmonary hypertension. *Acute cor pulmonale* can follow massive pulmonary embolism. *Chronic cor pulmonale* usually implies right ventricular hypertrophy (and dilation) secondary to prolonged pressure overload caused by obstruction of the pulmonary arteries or arterioles or compression or obliteration of septal capillaries (e.g., owing to primary pulmonary hypertension or emphysema).

Morphology. In acute cor pulmonale, there is marked dilation of the right ventricle without hypertrophy. On cross-section, the normal crescent shape of the right ventricle is transformed to a dilated ovoid. In chronic cor pulmonale, the right ventricular wall thickens, sometimes up to 1.0 cm or more, and may even come to approximate that of the left ventricle (Fig. 12–21). More subtle stages of right ventricular hypertrophy may be observed as thickening of the muscle bundles in the outflow tract, immediately below the pulmonary valve, or of the moderator band, the muscle bundle that connects the ventricular septum to the anterior right ventricular papillary muscle. Sometimes there is secondary compression of the left ventricular chamber or tricuspid regurgitation with fibrous thickening of this valve.

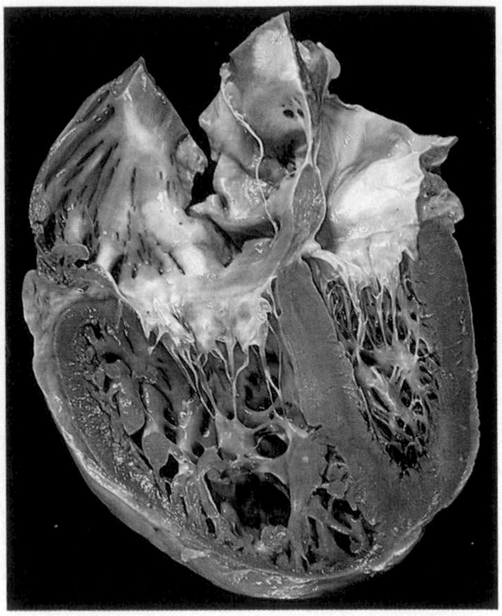

FIGURE 12–21 Chronic cor pulmonale, characterized by a markedly dilated and hypertrophied right ventricle, with thickened free wall and hypertrophied trabeculae (apical four-chamber view of heart, right ventricle on left). The shape of the left ventricle (to the right) has been distorted by the right ventricular enlargement. Compare with Figure 12–20.

TABLE 12–6 Disorders Predisposing to Cor Pulmonale

Diseases of the Pulmonary Parenchyma
Chronic obstructive pulmonary disease
Diffuse pulmonary interstitial fibrosis
Pneumoconioses
Cystic fibrosis
Bronchiectasis
Diseases of the Pulmonary Vessels
Recurrent pulmonary thromboembolism
Primary pulmonary hypertension
Extensive pulmonary arteritis (e.g., Wegener granulomatosis)
Drug-, toxin-, or radiation-induced vascular obstruction
Extensive pulmonary tumor microembolism
Disorders Affecting Chest Movement
Kyphoscoliosis
Marked obesity (pickwickian syndrome)
Neuromuscular diseases
Disorders Inducing Pulmonary Arterial Constriction
Metabolic acidosis
Hypoxemia
Chronic altitude sickness
Obstruction to major airways
Idiopathic alveolar hypoventilation

Valvular Heart Disease

Valvular involvement by disease causes stenosis, insufficiency (regurgitation or incompetence), or both. *Stenosis is the failure of a valve to open completely, thereby impeding forward flow. Insufficiency, in contrast, results from failure of a valve to close completely, thereby allowing reversed flow.* These abnormalities can be either *pure*, when only stenosis or regurgitation is present, or *mixed*, when both stenosis and regurgitation coexist in the same valve, but one of these defects usually predominates. *Isolated* disease refers to disease affecting one valve, and *combined* disease implies that more than one valve may be dysfunctional. *Functional regurgitation* results when a valve becomes incompetent owing to either (1) dilation of the ventricle, which causes the right or left ventricular papillary muscles to be pulled down and outward, thereby preventing coaptation of otherwise intact mitral or tricuspid leaflets during systole, or (2) dilation of the aortic or pulmonary artery, pulling the valve commissures apart and preventing full closure of the aortic or pulmonary valve cusps. Abnormalities of flow often produce abnormal heart sounds known as *murmurs.*

Valvular dysfunction can vary in degree from slight and physiologically unimportant to severe and rapidly fatal. The clinical consequences depend on the valve involved, the degree of impairment, the rate of its development, and the rate and quality of compensatory mechanisms. For example, sudden destruction of an aortic valve cusp by infection (as in infective endocarditis; see later) may cause rapidly fatal cardiac failure owing to massive regurgitation. In contrast, rheumatic mitral stenosis usually develops over years and its clinical effects are remarkably well tolerated. Depending on degree, duration, and etiology, valvular stenosis or insufficiency often produces secondary changes in the heart, blood vessels, and other organs, both proximal and distal to the valvular lesion. Most important are the myocardial hypertrophy and the pulmonary and systemic changes discussed earlier. Moreover, a patch of endocardial thickening often occurs at the point where a jet lesion impinges, such as the focal endocardial fibrosis in the left atrium secondary to a regurgitant jet of mitral insufficiency.

Valvular abnormalities may be caused by congenital disorders (discussed earlier) or by a variety of acquired diseases. *Most frequent are acquired stenoses of the aortic and mitral valves, which account for approximately two-thirds of all valve disease.* Valvular stenosis almost always is due to a primary cuspal abnormality and is virtually always a chronic process. In contrast, valvular insufficiency may result from either intrinsic disease of the valve cusps or damage to or distortion of the supporting structures (e.g., the aorta, mitral annulus, tendinous cords, papillary muscles, ventricular free wall) without primary changes in the cusps. It may appear acutely, as with rupture of cords, or chronically with leaflet scarring and retraction.

The most important causes of acquired heart valve diseases are summarized in Table 12–7 and are discussed in the following sections.[76] In contrast to the many potential causes of valvular insufficiency, only a relatively few mechanisms produce acquired valvular stenosis. The most frequent causes of the major functional valvular lesions are as follows:

- Aortic stenosis: calcification of anatomically normal and congenitally bicuspid aortic valves
- Aortic insufficiency: dilation of the ascending aorta, related to hypertension and aging.
- Mitral stenosis: rheumatic heart disease
- Mitral insufficiency: myxomatous degeneration (mitral valve prolapse)

VALVULAR DEGENERATION CAUSED BY CALCIFICATION

The heart valves are subjected to high repetitive mechanical stresses, particularly at the hinge points of the cusps and leaflets owing to (1) 40 million or more cardiac cycles per year, (2) substantial tissue deformations at each cycle, and (3) transvalvular pressure gradients in the closed phase of approximately 120 mm for the mitral and 80 mm for the aortic valve. It is therefore not surprising that these normally delicate structures suffer cumulative damage complicated by formation of calcific deposits (composed of calcium phosphate mineral), which may lead to clinically important disease (see Chapter 1). The most frequent calcific valvular diseases, illustrated in Figure 12–22, are calcific aortic stenosis, calcification of a congenitally bicuspid aortic valve, and mitral annular calcification. Each comprises primarily dystrophic calcification without significant lipid deposition or cellular proliferation, a process distinct from but with some features of atherosclerosis.

TABLE 12–7 Major Etiologies of Acquired Heart Valve Disease

Mitral Valve Disease	Aortic Valve Disease
Mitral Stenosis	*Aortic Stenosis*
Postinflammatory scarring (rheumatic heart disease)	Postinflammatory scarring (rheumatic heart disease) Senile calcific aortic stenosis Calcification of congenitally deformed valve
Mitral Regurgitation	*Aortic Regurgitation*
Abnormalities of Leaflets and Commissures	***Intrinsic Valvular Disease***
Postinflammatory scarring Infective endocarditis Mitral valve prolapse Fen-phen–induced valvular fibrosis	Postinflammatory scarring (rheumatic heart disease) Infective endocarditis
Abnormalities of Tensor Apparatus	***Aortic Disease***
Rupture of papillary muscle Papillary muscle dysfunction (fibrosis) Rupture of chordae tendineae	Degenerative aortic dilation Syphilitic aortitis Ankylosing spondylitis Rheumatoid arthritis Marfan syndrome
Abnormalities of Left Ventricular Cavity and/or Annulus	
LV enlargement (myocarditis, dilated cardiomyopathy) Calcification of mitral ring	

LV, Left ventricular.
Modified from Schoen, FJ: Surgical pathology of removed natural and prosthetic valves. Hum Pathol 18:558, 1987.

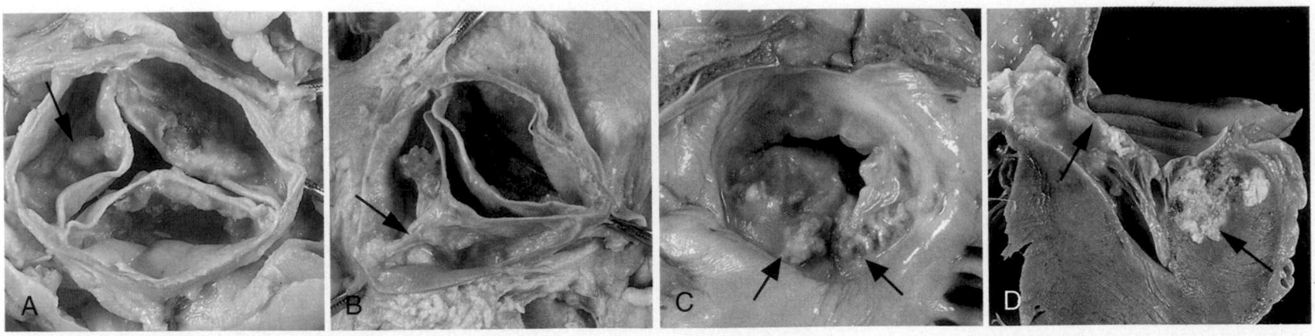

FIGURE 12–22 Calcific valvular degeneration. *A,* Calcific aortic stenosis of a previously normal valve having three cusps (viewed from aortic aspect). Nodular masses of calcium are heaped-up within the sinuses of Valsalva *(arrow).* Note that the commissures are not fused, as in postrheumatic aortic valve stenosis (see Fig. 12–24*E*). *B,* Calcific aortic stenosis occurring on a congenitally bicuspid valve. One cusp has a partial fusion at its center, called a *raphe* (arrow). *C and D,* Mitral annular calcification, with calcific nodules at the base (attachment margin) of the anterior mitral leaflet *(arrows). C,* Left atrial view. *D,* Cut section of myocardium.

Calcific Aortic Stenosis

Aortic stenosis is the most common of all valvular abnormalities. *Acquired aortic stenosis* is usually the consequence of calcification owing to progressive and advanced age-associated "wear and tear" of either previously anatomically normal aortic valves or congenitally bicuspid valves (with which approximately 1% of the population is born, see later). The incidence of aortic stenosis is increasing with the rising average age of the population. With the decline in the incidence of rheumatic fever in North America, rheumatic aortic stenosis now accounts for less than 10% of cases of acquired aortic stenosis. Aortic stenosis comes to clinical attention primarily in the sixth to seventh decades of life with congenitally bicuspid valves but not until the eighth and ninth decades with previously normal valves; hence the term *senile calcific aortic stenosis* is used to describe the latter condition.

Morphology. The morphologic hallmark of nonrheumatic, calcific aortic stenosis (with either tricuspid or bicuspid valves) is heaped-up calcified masses within the aortic cusps that ultimately protrude through the outflow surfaces into the sinuses of Valsalva, preventing the opening of the cusps. The calcific deposits distort the cuspal architecture, primarily at the bases; the free cuspal edges are usually not involved (see Fig. 12–22*A*). The calcific process begins in the valvular fibrosa, at the points of maximal cusp flexion (the margins of attachment), and the microscopic layered architecture is largely preserved. An earlier, hemodynamically inconsequential stage of the calcification process is called **aortic valve sclerosis.** In aortic stenosis, the functional valve area is decreased sufficiently to cause measurable obstruction to outflow; this subjects the left ventricular myocardium to progressively increasing pressure overload.

Notably, in contrast to rheumatic (and congenital) aortic stenosis (see Fig. 12–24*E*), commissural fusion is not a usual feature of degenerative aortic stenosis. By the time valves with aortic stenosis are seen at surgical resection or postmortem examination, however, the cusps may be secondarily fibrosed and thickened. The mitral valve is generally normal in patients with calcific aortic stenosis, although some patients may have direct extension of aortic valve calcific deposits onto the mitral anterior leaflet or independent calcification of the mitral annulus. In contrast, virtually all patients with rheumatic aortic stenosis have concomitant and characteristic structural abnormalities of the mitral valve (see later).

Clinical Features. In calcific aortic stenosis (superimposed on a previously normal or bicuspid aortic valve), the obstruction to left ventricular outflow leads to a gradually increasing pressure gradient across the calcified valve, which may reach 75 to 100 mm Hg in severe cases. These pressures imply severe aortic stenosis with a valve area of approximately 0.5 to 1 cm^2 (normal, approximately 4 cm^2). Left ventricular pressure must consequently rise to 200 mm Hg or more in such instances, and cardiac output is maintained by the development of concentric left ventricular (pressure overload) hypertrophy. The hypertrophied myocardium tends to be ischemic (owing to decreased coronary blood flow reserve and impaired microcirculatory perfusion even in the presence of unobstructed coronary arteries), and angina pectoris may appear. There may be impairment of both systolic and diastolic myocardial function, with symptoms of CHF. Eventually, cardiac decompensation may ensue. The onset of symptoms (angina, CHF, or syncope, for which the pathophysiologic basis is poorly understood) in aortic stenosis heralds the exhaustion of compensatory cardiac hyperfunction and carries a poor prognosis (approximately 50% with angina will die within 5 years and 50% with CHF will die within 2 years) if not treated by surgery.[77] Since medical therapy is ineffective in severe symptomatic aortic stenosis, such patients require prompt relief of the obstruction by surgical valve replacement. In contrast, most asymptomatic patients have an excellent prognosis. Thus, the presence or absence of symptoms is the crucial factor that determines management of aortic stenosis.

Calcific Stenosis of Congenitally Bicuspid Aortic Valve

Occurring with an estimated frequency of approximately 1.4% of live births,[78] bicuspid aortic valves are generally neither stenotic nor symptomatic at birth or throughout early life. However, they are predisposed to progressive degenerative calcification, similar to that occurring in aortic valves with initially normal anatomy (see Fig. 12–22*B*). In a congenitally bicuspid aortic valve, there are only two functional cusps. The two cusps are usually of unequal size, with the larger cusp having a midline *raphe*, resulting from incomplete separation during development; less frequently the cusps are of the same size and the raphe is absent.[79] The raphe that represents the incomplete commissure is frequently a major site of calcific deposits. Once stenosis is present, the clinical course is similar to that described above for calcific aortic stenosis. Valves that become bicuspid owing to an acquired deformity (e.g., postinflammatory commissural fusion in rheumatic valve disease) have a conjoined cusp containing the fused commissure that is generally twice the size of the nonconjoined cusp. The mitral valve is normal in patients with a congenitally bicuspid aortic valve. Bicuspid aortic valves may also become incompetent as a result of aortic dilation, cusp prolapse, or infective endocarditis.

Mitral Annular Calcification

Degenerative calcific deposits can develop in the fibrous ring *(annulus)* of the mitral valve, visualized on gross inspection as irregular, stony hard, and occasionally ulcerated nodules (2–5 mm in thickness) that lie behind the leaflets (see Fig. 12–22*C* and *D*). The process generally does not affect valvular function. In unusual cases, however, it may lead either to regurgitation by interfering with systolic contraction of the mitral valve ring, to stenosis by impairing opening of the mitral leaflets, or to arrhythmias and occasionally sudden death by the calcium deposits penetrating sufficiently deeply to impinge on the atrioventricular conduction system. Because calcific nodules may provide a site for thrombi that can embolize, some patients with mitral annular calcification have an increased risk of stroke. The calcific nodules can also be the nidus for infective endocarditis. Heavy calcific deposits are sometimes visualized on echocardiography or seen as a distinctive, ring-like opacity on chest radiographs. Mitral annular calcification is most common in women over age 60 and individuals with myxomatous mitral valve (see below) or elevated left ventricular pressure (as in systemic hypertension, aortic stenosis, or hypertrophic cardiomyopathy).

MYXOMATOUS DEGENERATION OF THE MITRAL VALVE (MITRAL VALVE PROLAPSE)

In this valvular abnormality, one or both mitral leaflets are "floppy" and *prolapse*, or balloon back into the left atrium during systole. *Mitral valve prolapse*, as it is known clinically, is estimated to affect 3% or more of adults in the United States, most often young women. *Myxomatous degeneration of the mitral valve*, as it is known pathologically, is one of the most common forms of valvular heart disease in the industrialized world. Usually an incidental finding on physical examination, mitral valve prolapse may lead to serious complications in a small minority of those who are affected.

Morphology. The characteristic anatomic change in myxomatous degeneration is intercordal ballooning (hooding) of the mitral leaflets or portions thereof (Fig. 12-23). The affected leaflets are often enlarged, redundant, thick, and rubbery. Frequently involved, the tendinous cords are elongated, thinned, and occasionally ruptured. Annular dilation is characteristic, a finding that is rare in other causes of mitral insufficiency. Concomitant involvement of the tricuspid valve is present in 20% to 40% of cases, and the aortic or pulmonic valve (or both) may also be affected. Commissural fusion that typifies rheumatic heart disease is absent. Histologically, the essential change is attenuation of the fibrosa layer of the valve, on which the structural integrity of the leaflet depends, accompanied by focally marked thickening of the spongiosa layer with deposition of mucoid (myxomatous) material. The collagenous structure of the cords is attenuated.

Secondary changes reflect the stresses and injury incident to the billowing leaflets: (1) fibrous thickening of the valve leaflets, particularly where they rub against each other; (2) linear fibrous thickening of the left ventricular endocardial surface where abnormally long cords snap against it; (3) thickening of the mural endocardium of the left ventricle or atrium as a consequence of friction-induced injury induced by the prolapsing leaflets; (4) thrombi on the atrial surfaces of the leaflets, particularly in the recesses behind the ballooned cusps, and on the atrial walls these thrombi contact; and (5) focal calcifications at the base of the posterior mitral leaflet.

Secondary changes of myxomatous degeneration can also occur in mitral valves having regurgitation of another etiology (e.g., ischemic dysfunction).

Pathogenesis. The basis for the changes within the valve leaflets and associated structures is unknown. Favored is the proposition that there is an underlying developmental defect of connective tissue, possibly systemic. In keeping with this, myxomatous is degeneration of the mitral valve is a common feature of Marfan syndrome (caused by mutations in the gene encoding fibrillin-1; Chapter 5), and occasionally occurs in other hereditary disorders of connective tissues. Even in the absence of these well-defined conditions, in some individuals with the floppy mitral valve syndrome, there are hints of systemic structural abnormalities in connective tissue, such as scoliosis, straight back, and high-arched palate. Subtle defects in structural proteins may predispose connective tissues rich in microfibrils and elastin (such as cardiac valves) to damage by long-standing hemodynamic stress. Alternatively, the prominent destruction and remodeling of the valvular connective tissue evident in this disorder may be induced by a primary hemodynamic, cellular, or metabolic abnormality.[80]

Clinical Features. Mitral valve prolapse is defined and revealed by echocardiography. Most patients with mitral valve prolapse are asymptomatic, and the condition is discovered only on routine examination by the presence of a midsystolic click as an incidental finding on physical examination. In those cases where mitral regurgitation occurs, there is a late systolic or sometimes holosystolic murmur. A minority of patients have chest pain mimicking angina, dyspnea, and

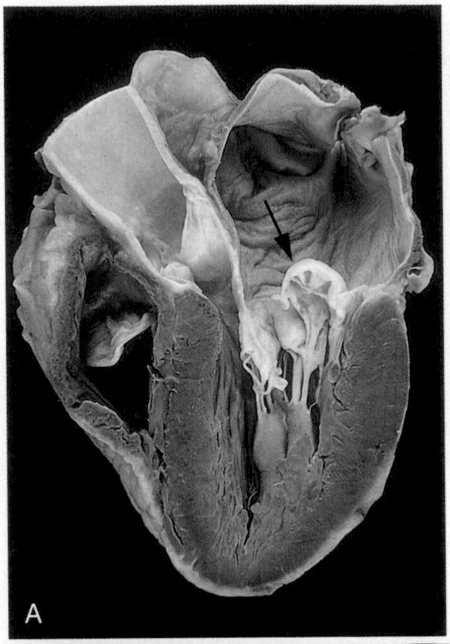

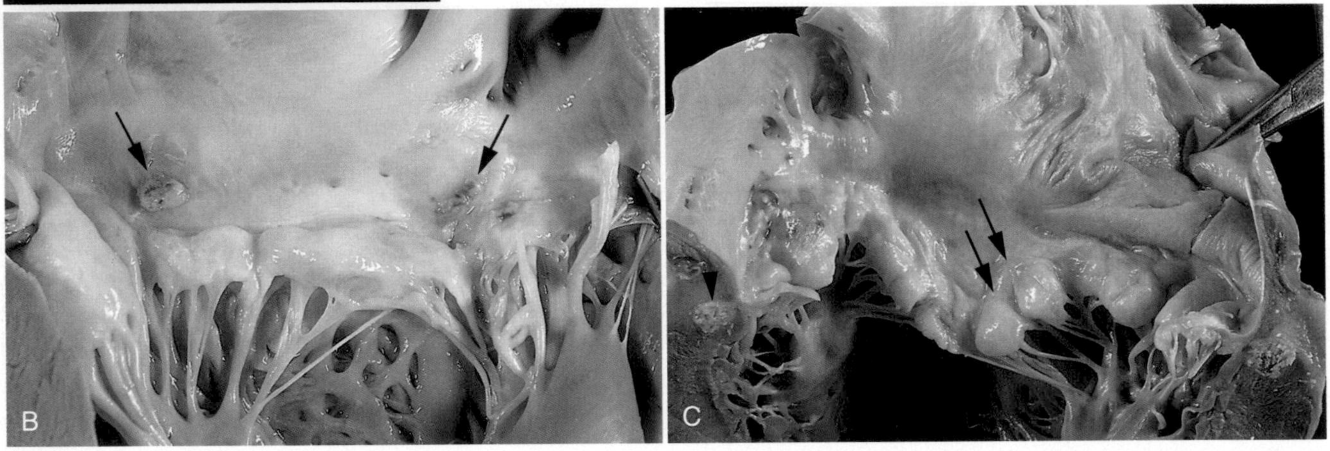

FIGURE 12–23 Myxomatous degeneration of the mitral valve. *A,* Long axis of left ventricle demonstrating hooding with prolapse of the posterior mitral leaflet into the left atrium *(arrow).* The left ventricle is on right in this apical four-chamber view. (Courtesy of William D. Edwards, M.D., Mayo Clinic, Rochester, MN.) *B,* Opened valve, showing pronounced hooding of the posterior mitral leaflet with thrombotic plaques at sites of leaflet–left atrium contact *(arrows). C,* Opened valve with pronounced hooding from patient who died suddenly *(double arrows).* Note also mitral annular calcification *(arrowhead).*

fatigue or, curiously, psychiatric manifestations, such as depression, anxiety reactions, and personality disorders. Although the great majority of patients with mitral valve prolapse have no untoward effects, approximately 3% develop one of four serious complications:

- *Infective endocarditis,* much more frequent in these patients than in the general population
- *Mitral insufficiency* requiring surgery, either slow onset attributed to leaflet deformity, dilation of the mitral annulus, or cordal lengthening, or sudden onset owing to cordal rupture
- *Stroke or other systemic infarct,* resulting from embolism of leaflet thrombi
- *Arrhythmias,* both ventricular and atrial. Sudden death occurs occasionally (see Fig. 12–23*C*). The mechanism of ventricular arrhythmia is unknown in most cases.

The risk of these complications is higher in men, older patients, and those with either arrhythmias or some mitral regurgitation, as evidenced by holosystolic murmurs and left-sided chamber enlargement.[81] For patients with symptoms or at high risk for serious complications, surgical valve repair is often done.

RHEUMATIC FEVER AND RHEUMATIC HEART DISEASE

Rheumatic fever (RF) is an acute, immunologically mediated, multisystem inflammatory disease that occurs a few weeks following an episode of group A streptococcal pharyngitis. Acute rheumatic carditis during the active phase of RF may progress to chronic rheumatic heart disease (RHD).

The most important consequence of RF are chronic valvular deformities, characterized principally by deforming fibrotic valvular disease (particularly mitral stenosis), which produces permanent dysfunction and severe, sometimes fatal, cardiac problems decades later. Rheumatic fever does not follow infections by streptococci at other sites, such as the skin. The incidence and mortality rate of RF have declined remarkably in many parts of the world over the past 30 years, owing to improved socioeconomic conditions, rapid diagnosis and treatment of streptococcal pharyngitis, and an unexplained decrease in the virulence of group A streptococci.[82] Nevertheless, in developing countries, and in many crowded, economically depressed urban areas in the Western world, RHD remains an important public health problem.

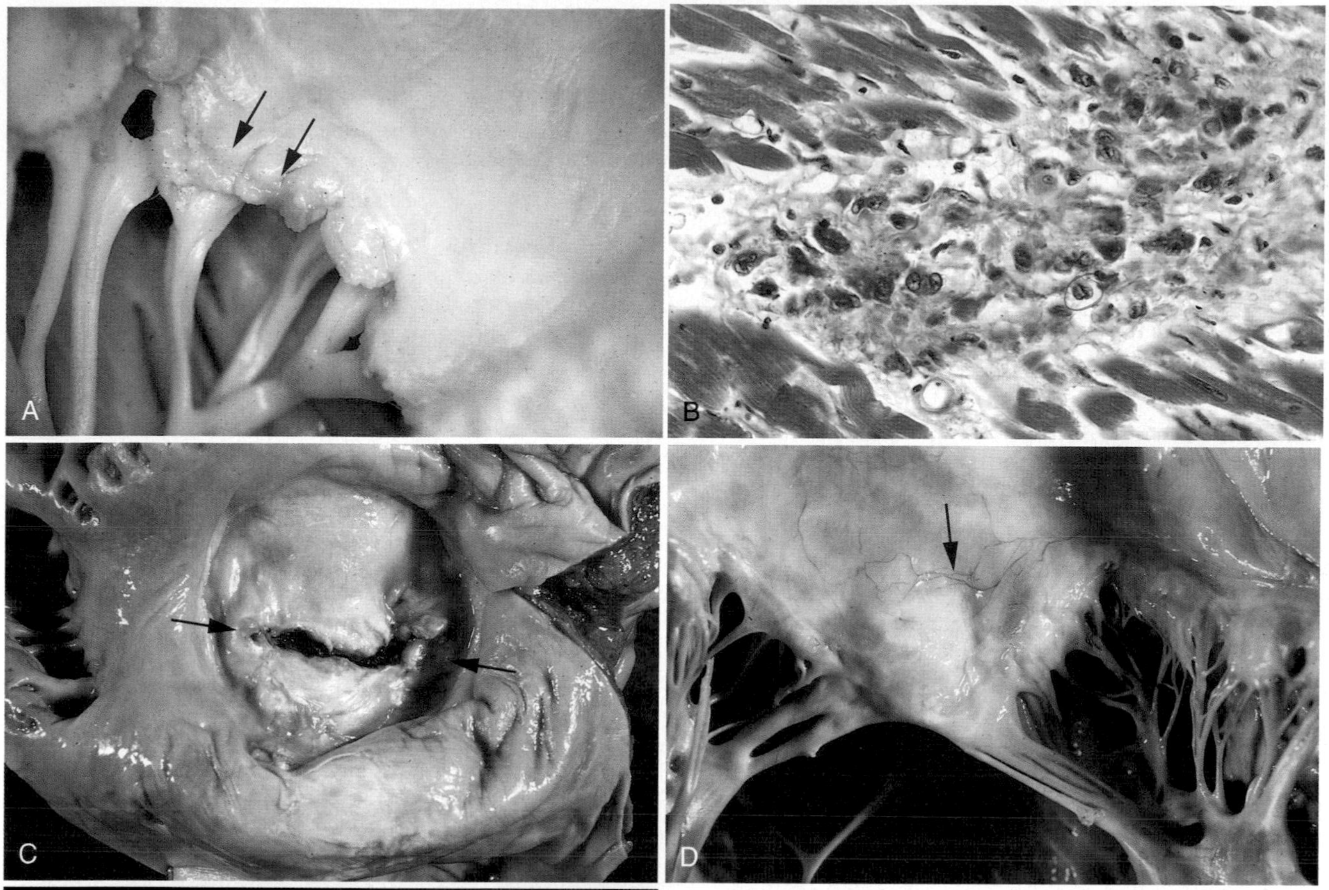

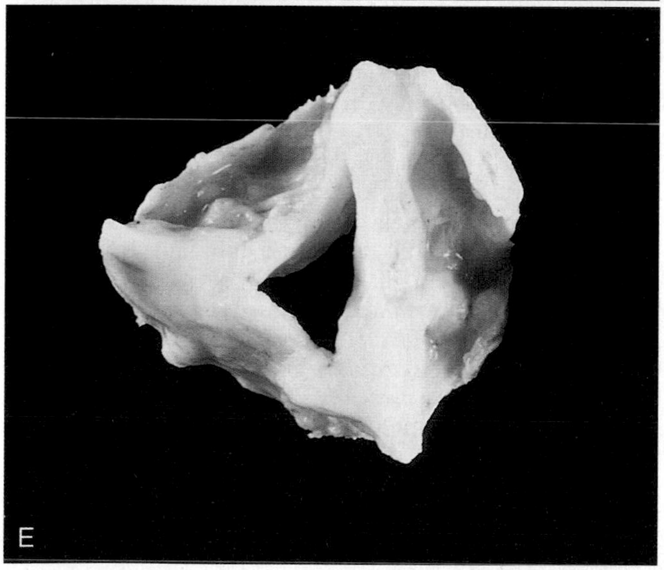

FIGURE 12–24 Acute and chronic rheumatic heart disease. *A,* Acute rheumatic mitral valvulitis superimposed on chronic rheumatic heart disease. Small vegetations (verrucae) are visible along the line of closure of the mitral valve leaflet *(arrows).* Previous episodes of rheumatic valvulitis have caused fibrous thickening and fusion of the chordae tendineae. *B,* Microscopic appearance of Aschoff body in a patient with acute rheumatic carditis. The myocardial interstitium has a circumscribed collection of mononuclear inflammatory cells, including some large histiocytes with prominent nucleoli and a prominent binuclear histiocyte, and central necrosis. *C and D,* Mitral stenosis with diffuse fibrous thickening and distortion of the valve leaflets, commissural fusion *(arrows),* and thickening and shortening of the chordae tendineae. Marked dilation of the left atrium is noted in the left atrial view *(C). D,* Opened valve. Note neovascularization of anterior mitral leaflet *(arrow). E,* Surgically removed specimen of rheumatic aortic stenosis, demonstrating thickening and distortion of the cusps with commissural fusion (*E,* reproduced from Schoen FJ, St. John-Sutton M: Contemporary issues in the pathology of valvular heart disease. Human Pathol 18:568, 1967.)

Morphology. Key pathologic features of acute RF and chronic RHD are shown in Figure 12–24. During acute RF, focal inflammatory lesions are found in various tissues. They are most distinctive within the heart, where they are called **Aschoff bodies**. They consist of foci of swollen eosinophilic collagen surrounded by lymphocytes (primarily T cells), occasional plasma cells, and plump macrophages called Anitschkow cells (pathognomonic for RF). These distinctive cells have abundant cytoplasm and central round-to-ovoid nuclei in which the chromatin is disposed in a central, slender, wavy ribbon (hence the designation "caterpillar cells"). Some of the larger macrophages become multinucleated to form Aschoff giant cells.

During acute RF, diffuse inflammation and Aschoff bodies may be found in any of the three layers of the heart—pericardium, myocardium, or endocardium—hence the lesion is called a **pancarditis**. In the pericardium, the inflammation is accompanied by a fibrinous or serofibrinous pericardial exudate, described as a "bread-and-butter" pericarditis, which generally resolves without sequelae. The myocardial involvement—myocarditis—takes the form of scattered Aschoff bodies within the interstitial connective tissue, often perivascular.

Concomitant involvement of the endocardium and the left-sided valves by inflammatory foci typically results in fibrinoid necrosis within the cusps or along the tendinous cords on which sit small (1- to 2-mm) vegetations—verrucae—along the lines of closure. These irregular, warty projections probably arise from the precipitation of fibrin at sites of erosion, related to underlying inflammation and collagen degeneration, and cause little disturbance in cardiac function. Subendocardial lesions, perhaps exacerbated by regurgitant jets, may induce irregular thickenings called **MacCallum plaques,** usually in the left atrium.

Chronic RHD is characterized by organization of the acute inflammation and subsequent fibrosis. In particular, the valvular leaflets become thickened and retracted, causing permanent deformity. The cardinal anatomic changes of the mitral (or tricuspid) valve are **leaflet thickening, commissural fusion and shortening, and thickening and fusion of the tendinous cords** (see Fig. 12–24). In chronic disease, the mitral valve is virtually always abnormal, but involvement of another valve, such as the aortic, may be the most clinically important in some cases. Microscopically there is diffuse fibrosis and often neovascularization that obliterate the originally layered and avascular leaflet architecture. Aschoff bodies are replaced by fibrous scar so that diagnostic forms of these lesions are rarely seen in surgical specimens or autopsy tissue from patients with chronic RHD. Fibrosis resulting from healed inflammation outside the valves is usually of no consequence.

RHD is overwhelmingly the most frequent cause of mitral stenosis (99% of cases). In patients with RHD, the mitral valve alone is involved in 65% to 70% of cases, and mitral and aortic in about 25%; similar but generally less severe fibrous thickenings and stenoses can occur in the tricuspid valve and rarely in the pulmonic. Fibrous bridging across the valvular commissures and calcification create "fish mouth" or "buttonhole" stenoses. With tight mitral stenosis, the left atrium progressively dilates and may harbor mural thrombus either in the appendage or along the wall. Long-standing congestive changes in the lungs may induce pulmonary vascular and parenchymal changes and in time lead to right ventricular hypertrophy. The left ventricle is generally normal with isolated pure mitral stenosis.

Pathogenesis. It is strongly suspected that *acute rheumatic fever is a hypersensitivity reaction induced by group A streptococci*, but the exact pathogenesis remains uncertain despite many years of investigation.[83] It is thought that antibodies directed against the M proteins of certain strains of streptococci cross-react with glycoprotein antigens in the heart, joints, and other tissues. The onset of symptoms 2 to 3 weeks after infection and the absence of streptococci from the lesions support the concept that RF results from an immune response against the offending bacteria. Because the nature of cross-reacting antigens has been difficult to define, it has also been suggested that the streptococcal infection evokes an autoimmune response against self-antigens. Only a minority of infected patients develop RF, suggesting that genetic susceptibility influences the hypersensitivity reaction. The proposed pathogenetic sequence and time course of the disease are summarized in Figure 12–25. The chronic sequelae result from progressive fibrosis due to both healing of the acute inflammatory lesions and the turbulence induced by ongoing valvular deformities.

Clinical Features. *RF is characterized by a constellation of findings that includes as major manifestations (1) migratory polyarthritis of the large joints, (2) carditis, (3) subcutaneous nodules, (4) erythema marginatum of the skin, and (5) Sydenham chorea, a neurologic disorder with involuntary purposeless, rapid movements.* The diagnosis is established by the so-called Jones criteria: evidence of a preceding group A streptococcal infection, with the presence of two of the major manifestations listed above or one major and two minor manifestations (nonspecific signs and symptoms that include fever, arthralgia, or elevated blood levels of acute phase reactants).

Acute rheumatic fever typically occurs 10 days to 6 weeks after an episode of pharyngitis caused by group A streptococci in about 3% of patients. Acute RF appears most often in children between ages 5 and 15, but about 20% of first attacks occur in middle to later life. Although pharyngeal cultures for streptococci are negative by the time the illness begins, antibodies to one or more streptococcal enzymes, such as streptolysin O and DNAse B, are present and can be detected in the sera of most patients. The predominant clinical manifestations are those of arthritis and carditis. *Arthritis* is far more common in adults than in children. It typically begins with migratory polyarthritis accompanied by fever in which one large joint after another becomes painful and swollen for a period of days and then subsides spontaneously, leaving no residual disability. Clinical features related to *acute carditis* include pericardial friction rubs, weak heart sounds, tachycardia, and arrhythmias. The myocarditis may cause cardiac dilation that may evolve to functional mitral valve insufficiency or even heart failure. Overall the prognosis for the primary attack is generally good, and only 1% of patients die from fulminant RF.

After an initial attack, there is increased vulnerability to reactivation of the disease with subsequent pharyngeal infections, and the same manifestations are likely to appear with each recurrent attack. Carditis is likely to worsen with each recurrence, and damage is cumulative. Other hazards include embolization from mural thrombi, primarily within the atria or their appendages, and infective endocarditis superimposed on deformed valves. *Chronic rheumatic carditis* usually does not cause clinical manifestations for years or even decades after the initial episode of RF. The signs and symptoms of valvular disease depend on which cardiac valve(s) are involved. In addition to various cardiac murmurs, cardiac hypertrophy and dilation, and heart failure, patients with chronic rheumatic heart disease may suffer from arrhythmias (particularly atrial fibrillation in the setting of mitral stenosis), thromboembolic complications, and infective endocarditis. The long-term prognosis is highly variable. In some cases, there is a relentless cycle of valvular deformity yielding hemodynamic abnormality, which begets further deforming fibrosis. Surgical repair of diseased valves by incising the fused mitral valve commissures and replacement with prosthetic devices has greatly improved the outlook for patients with RHD.

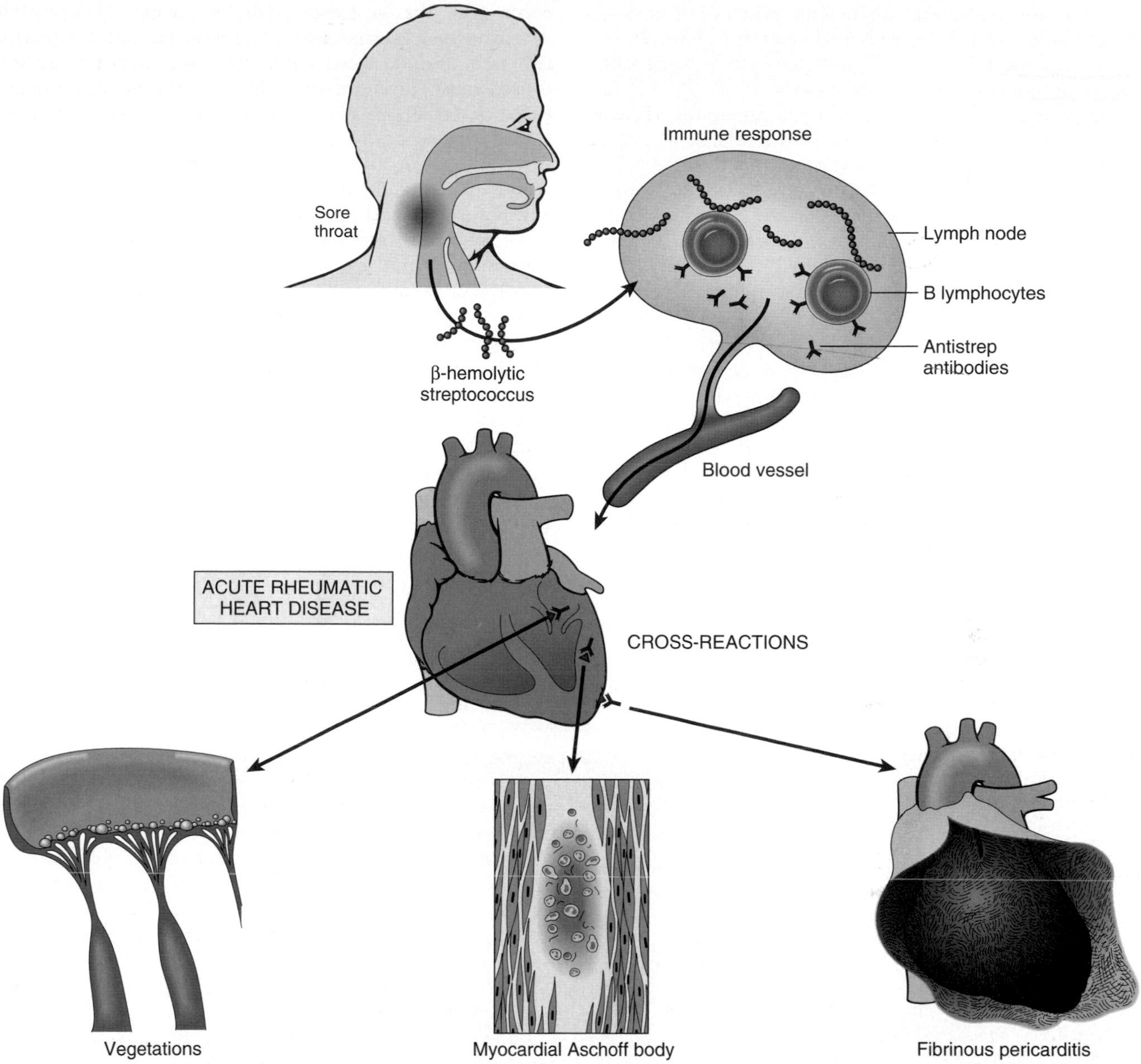

FIGURE 12–25 The pathogenetic sequence and key morphologic features of acute rheumatic heart disease.

INFECTIVE ENDOCARDITIS (IE)

Infective endocarditis, one of the most serious of all infections, is characterized by colonization or invasion of the heart valves or the mural endocardium by a microbe, leading to the formation of bulky, friable *vegetations* composed of thrombotic debris and organisms, often associated with destruction of the underlying cardiac tissues.[84] The aorta, aneurysmal sacs, other blood vessels, and prosthetic devices can also become infected. Although fungi, rickettsiae (Q fever), and chlamydiae have at one time or another been responsible for these infections, most cases are bacterial *(bacterial endocarditis).* Prompt diagnosis and effective treatment of IE can significantly alter the outlook for the patient.

Traditionally, IE has been classified on clinical grounds into acute and subacute forms. This subdivision expresses the range of severity of the disease and its tempo, determined in large part by the virulence of the infecting microorganism and whether underlying cardiac disease is present. *Acute endocarditis* describes a destructive, tumultuous infection, frequently of a previously normal heart valve, with a highly virulent organism, that leads to death within days to weeks of more than 50% of patients despite antibiotics and surgery. In contrast, organisms of low virulence can cause infection in a previously abnormal heart, particularly on deformed valves. In such cases, the disease may appear insidiously and, even untreated, pursue a protracted course of weeks to months *(subacute endocarditis).* Most patients with subacute IE recover after appropriate antibiotic therapy.

The highly virulent organisms of acute endocarditis tend to produce necrotizing, ulcerative, invasive valvular infections that are difficult to cure by antibiotics and usually require surgery. In contrast, the lower-virulence organisms of subacute disease are less destructive than those of acute endocarditis, and the vegetations often show evidence of healing. Both the clinical and the morphologic patterns, however, are points along a spectrum, and a clear delineation between acute and subacute disease does not always exist.

Etiology and Pathogenesis. As stated previously, IE may develop on previously normal valves, but a variety of cardiac and vascular abnormalities predispose to this form of infection. In years past, RHD was the major antecedent disorder, but more common now are myxomatous mitral valve, degenerative calcific valvular stenosis, bicuspid aortic valve (whether calcified or not), and artificial (prosthetic) valves. Host factors such as neutropenia, immunodeficiency, malignancy, therapeutic immunosuppression, diabetes mellitus, and alcohol or intravenous drug abuse are predisposing influences. Sterile platelet–fibrin deposits that accumulate at sites of impingement of jet streams caused by pre-existing cardiac disease or indwelling vascular catheters may also be important in the development of endocarditis.

The causative organisms differ somewhat in the major high-risk groups. Endocarditis of native but previously damaged or otherwise abnormal valves is caused most commonly (50% to 60% of cases) by *Streptococcus viridans*; this is *not* the organism responsible for rheumatic disease discussed earlier. In contrast, the more virulent *S. aureus* organisms commonly found on the skin can attack either healthy or deformed valves and are responsible for 10% to 20% of cases overall; *S. aureus* is the major offender in intravenous drug abusers. The roster of the remaining bacteria includes enterococci and the so-called HACEK group (*Haemophilus, Actinobacillus, Cardiobacterium, Eikenella,* and *Kingella*), all commensals in the oral cavity. Prosthetic valve endocarditis is caused most commonly by coagulase-negative staphylococci (e.g., *S. epidermidis*). Other agents causing endocarditis include gram-negative bacilli and fungi. In about 10% of all cases of endocarditis, no organism can be isolated from the blood ("culture-negative" endocarditis) because of prior antibiotic therapy, difficulties in isolating the offending agent, or because deeply embedded organisms within the enlarging vegetation are not released into the blood.

Foremost among the factors predisposing to the development of endocarditis is seeding of the blood with microbes. The portal of entry of the agent into the bloodstream may be an obvious infection elsewhere, a dental or surgical procedure that causes a transient bacteremia, injection of contaminated material directly into the bloodstream by intravenous drug users, or an occult source from the gut, oral cavity, or trivial injuries. Recognition of predisposing anatomic substrates and clinical conditions causing bacteremia facilitates prevention by appropriate antibiotic prophylaxis.[85]

Morphology. In both the subacute and acute forms of the disease, friable, bulky, and potentially destructive vegetations containing fibrin, inflammatory cells, and bacteria or other organisms are present on the heart valves (Fig. 12–26). The aortic and mitral valves

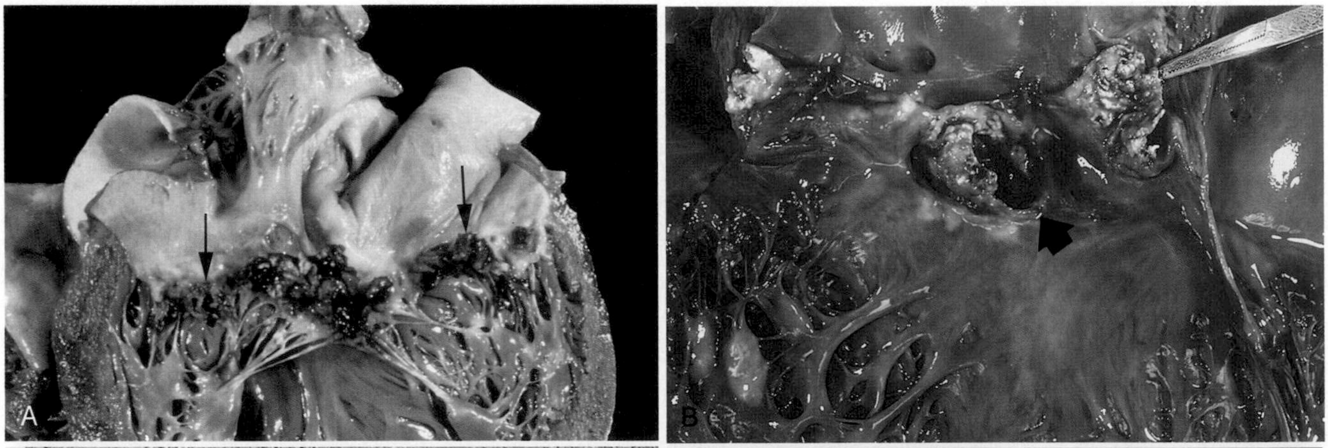

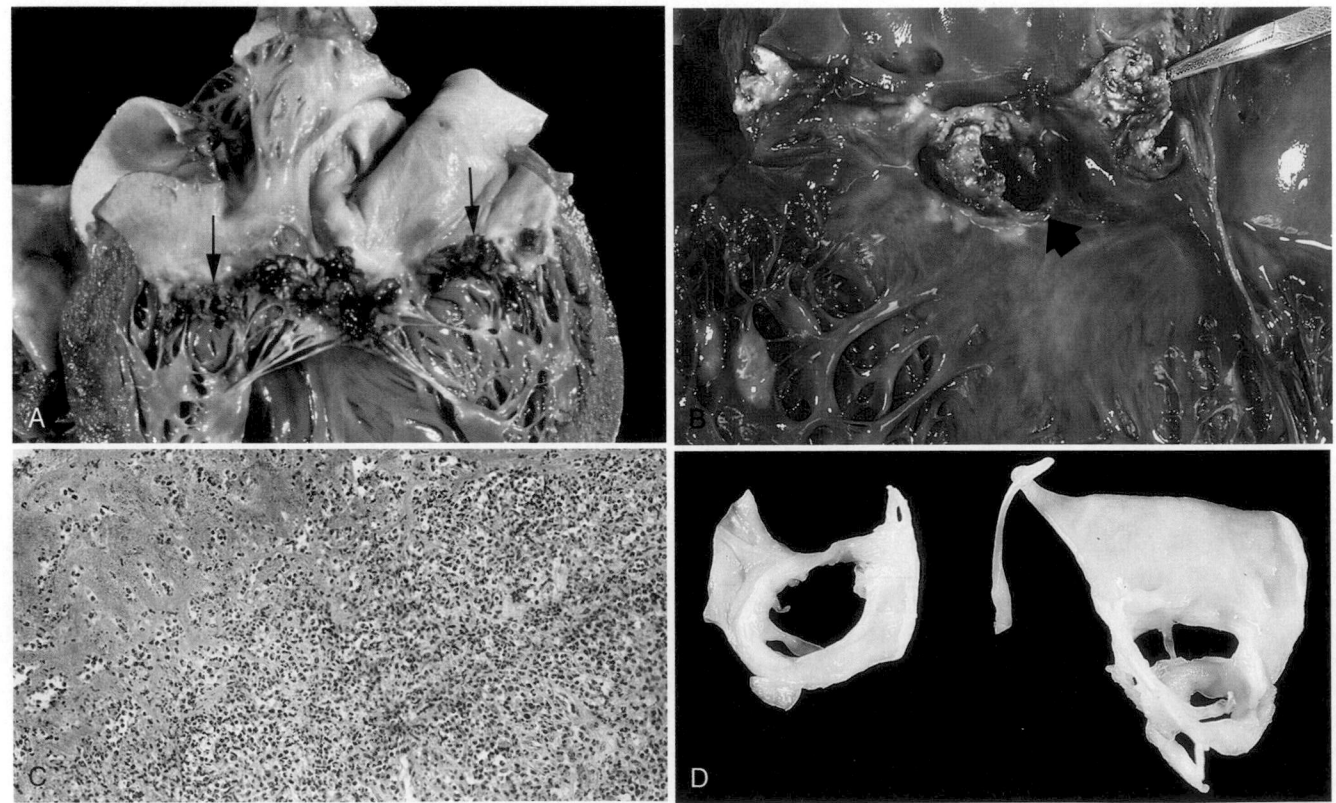

FIGURE 12–26 Infective (bacterial) endocarditis. *A,* Endocarditis of mitral valve (subacute, caused by *Strep. viridans*). The large, friable vegetations are denoted by arrows. *B,* Acute endocarditis of congenitally bicuspid aortic valve (caused by *Staph. aureus*) with extensive cuspal destruction and ring abscess *(arrow)*. *C,* Histologic appearance of vegetation of endocarditis with extensive acute inflammatory cells and fibrin. Bacterial organisms were demonstrated by tissue Gram stain. (*C,* reproduced from Schoen FJ: Surgical pathology of removed natural and prosthetic heart valves. Human Pathol 18:558, 1987.) *D,* Healed endocarditis, demonstrating mitral valvular destruction but no active vegetations.

are the most common sites of infection, although the valves of the right heart may also be involved, particularly in intravenous drug abusers. The vegetations may be single or multiple and may involve more than one valve. Vegetations sometimes erode into the underlying myocardium to produce an abscess cavity **(ring abscess)**, one of several important complications. The appearance of the vegetations is influenced by the type of organism responsible, the degree of host reaction to the infection, and previous antibiotic therapy. **Fungal endocarditis**, for example, tends to cause larger vegetations than does bacterial infection. **Systemic emboli** may occur at any time because of the friable nature of the vegetations, and they may cause infarcts in the brain, kidneys, myocardium, and other tissues. Because the embolic fragments contain large numbers of virulent organisms, abscesses often develop at the sites of such infarcts **(septic infarcts)**.

The vegetations of **subacute endocarditis** are associated with less valvular destruction than those of acute endocarditis, although the distinction between the two forms may be difficult. Microscopically, the vegetations of typical subacute IE often have granulation tissue at their bases (suggesting chronicity). With the passage of time, fibrosis, calcification, and a chronic inflammatory infiltrate may develop.

Figure 12–27 compares the gross appearance of the vegetations of infective endocarditis with those of the valve lesions characterized by noninfective thrombotic vegetations (NBTE), and with the endocarditis of systemic lupus erythematosus (SLE), called Libman-Sacks endocarditis (see later).

Clinical Features. Fever is the most consistent sign of IE. However, with subacute disease, particularly in the elderly, fever may be slight or absent, and the only manifestations are sometimes nonspecific fatigue, loss of weight, and a flulike syndrome. In contrast, acute endocarditis has a stormy onset with rapidly developing fever, chills, weakness, and lassitude. Complications generally begin within the first weeks of the onset of the disease. They may be immunologically mediated as exemplified by glomerulonephritis, owing to trapping of antigen-antibody complexes, which can cause hematuria, albuminuria, or renal failure (Chapter 20). Sometimes complications involving the heart or extracardiac sites call attention to endocarditis. Murmurs are present in 90% of patients with left-sided lesions but may merely relate to the pre-existing cardiac abnormality predisposing to IE. The so-called Duke criteria (Table 12–8) provide a standardized assessment of patients with suspected IE that integrates factors predisposing patients to the development of IE, blood-culture evidence of infection, echocardiographic findings, and clinical and laboratory information in assessing patients with potential IE.[86] Previously important clinical findings secondary to microemboli are now uncommon. They include petechiae, red, linear, or flame-shaped streaks in the nail bed of the digits (splinter or subungual hemorrhages), erythematous or hemorrhagic nontender lesions on the palms or soles (Janeway lesions), subcutaneous nodules in the pulp of the digits (Osler nodes). Also included are retinal hemorrhages (Roth spots) in the eyes owing to the shortened clinical course of the disease as a result of antibiotic therapy.

Prevention of IE is important and is done by the prophylactic use of antibiotics in the patient with some form of cardiac anomaly or artificial valve who is about to have a dental, surgical, or other invasive procedure.

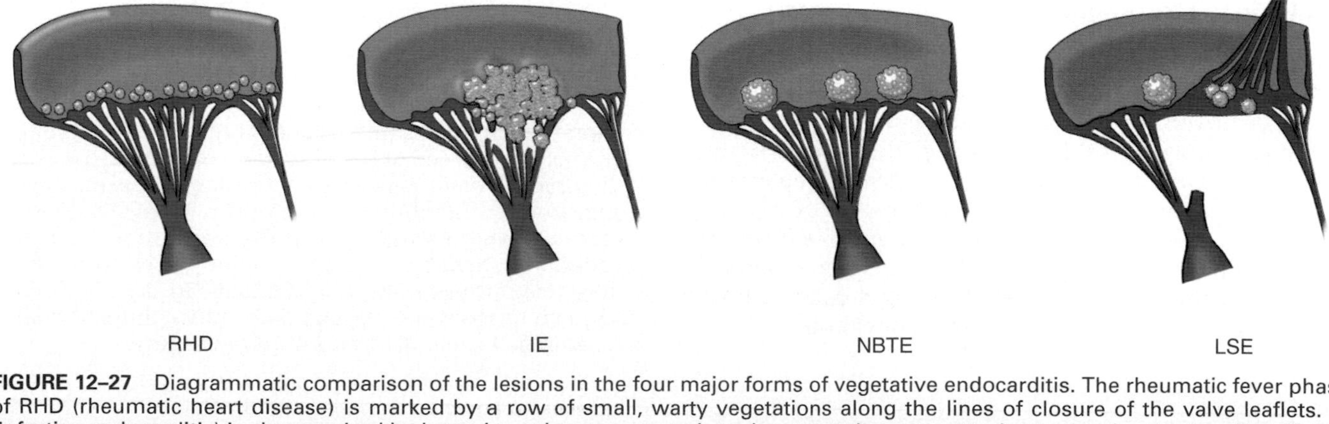

FIGURE 12–27 Diagrammatic comparison of the lesions in the four major forms of vegetative endocarditis. The rheumatic fever phase of RHD (rheumatic heart disease) is marked by a row of small, warty vegetations along the lines of closure of the valve leaflets. IE (infective endocarditis) is characterized by large, irregular masses on the valve cusps that can extend onto the chordae (see Fig. 12–26). NBTE (nonbacterial thrombotic endocarditis) typically exhibits small, bland vegetations, usually attached at the line of closure. One or many may be present (see Fig. 12–28). LSE (Libman-Sacks endocarditis) has small or medium-sized vegetations on either or both sides of the valve leaflets.

TABLE 12–8 Diagnostic Criteria for Infective Endocarditis*

Pathologic Criteria

Microorganisms, demonstrated by culture or histologic examination, in a vegetation, embolus from a vegetation, or intracardiac abscess
Histologic confirmation of active endocarditis in vegetation or intracardiac abscess

Clinical Criteria

Major

Positive blood culture(s) indicating characteristic organism or persistence of unusual organism
Echocardiographic findings, including valve-related or implant-related mass or abscess, or partial separation of artificial valve
New valvular regurgitation

Minor

Predisposing heart lesion or intravenous drug use
Fever
Vascular lesions, including arterial petechiae, subungual/splinter hemorrhages, emboli, septic infarcts, mycotic aneurysm, intracranial hemorrhage, Janeway lesions†
Immunologic phenomena, including glomerulonephritis, Osler nodes,‡ Roth spots,§ rheumatoid factor
Microbiologic evidence, including single culture showing uncharacteristic organism
Echocardiographic findings consistent with but not diagnostic of endocarditis, including new valvular regurgitation, pericarditis

*Diagnosis by these guidelines, often called the Duke Criteria, requires either pathologic or clinical criteria; if clinical criteria are used, 2 major, 1 major + 3 minor, or 5 minor criteria are required for diagnosis. Modified from Durack DT, et al: Am J Med, 96:200, 1994 and Karchmer AW, In Braunwald E, Zipes DP, Libby P (eds): Heart Disease. A Textbook of Cardiovascular Medicine, 6th ed. Philadelphia, WB Saunders Co., 2001, p. 1723.
†Janeway lesions are small erythematous or hemorrhagic, macular, nontender lesions on the palms and soles and are the consequence of septic embolic events.
‡Osler nodes are small, tender subcutaneous nodules that develop in the pulp of the digits or occasionally more proximally in the fingers and persist for hours to several days.
§Roth spots are oval retinal hemorrhages with pale centers.

NONINFECTED VEGETATIONS

Nonbacterial Thrombotic Endocarditis (NBTE)

NBTE is characterized by the deposition of small masses of fibrin, platelets, and other blood components on the leaflets of the cardiac valves. In contrast to the vegetations of IE, discussed previously, *the valvular lesions of NBTE are sterile and do not contain microorganisms.* NBTE is often encountered in debilitated patients, such as those with cancer or sepsis—hence the previously used term *marantic endocarditis.* Although the local effect on the valves is usually unimportant, NBTE may achieve clinical significance by producing emboli and resultant infarcts in the brain, heart, or elsewhere.

Morphology. In contrast to IE, the vegetations of NBTE are sterile, nondestructive, and small (1 to 5 mm), and occur singly or multiply along the line of closure of the leaflets or cusps (Fig. 12–28). Histologically, they are composed of bland thrombus without accompanying inflammatory reaction or induced valve damage. Should the patient survive the underlying disease, organization may occur, leaving delicate strands of fibrous tissue.

Pathogenesis. NBTE frequently occurs concomitantly with venous thromboses or pulmonary embolism, suggesting *a common origin in a hypercoagulable state with systemic activation of blood coagulation such as disseminated intravascular coagulation* (Chapter 4). *This may be related to some underlying disease, such as a cancer,* and, in particular, mucinous adenocarcinomas of the pancreas. The striking association with mucinous adenocarcinomas in general may relate to the procoagulant effect of circulating mucin, and thus NBTE can be a part of the Trousseau syndrome (Chapter 7). Lesions of NBTE, however, are also seen occasionally in association with nonmucin-producing malignancy, such as acute promyelocytic leukemia, and in other debilitating diseases or conditions (e.g., hyperestrogenic states, extensive burns, or sepsis) promoting hypercoagulability. Endocardial trauma, as from an indwelling catheter, is also a well-recognized predisposing condition, and one frequently notes right-sided valvular and endocardial thrombotic lesions along the track of a Swan-Ganz pulmonary artery catheter.

Endocarditis of Systemic Lupus Erythematosus (Libman-Sacks Disease)

In SLE, mitral and tricuspid valvulitis with small, sterile vegetations, called *Libman-Sacks endocarditis* is occasionally encountered.

Morphology. The lesions are small single or multiple, sterile, granular pink vegetations ranging from 1 to 4 mm in diameter. The lesions may be located on the undersurfaces of the atrioventricular valves, on the valvular endocardium, on the cords, or on the mural endocardium of atria or ventricles. Histologically the verrucae consist of a finely granular, fibrinous eosinophilic material that may contain hematoxylin bodies (the tissue equivalent of the lupus erythematosus cell of the blood and bone marrow, see Chapter 6). An intense valvulitis may be present, characterized by fibrinoid necrosis of the valve substance that is often contiguous with the vegetation. Leaflet vegetations can be difficult in some cases to distinguish from those of IE or NBTE (see Fig. 12–27). Subsequent fibrosis and serious deformity can result that resemble chronic RHD and require surgery.

Thrombotic heart valve lesions with sterile vegetations or rarely fibrous thickening commonly occur with the antiphos-

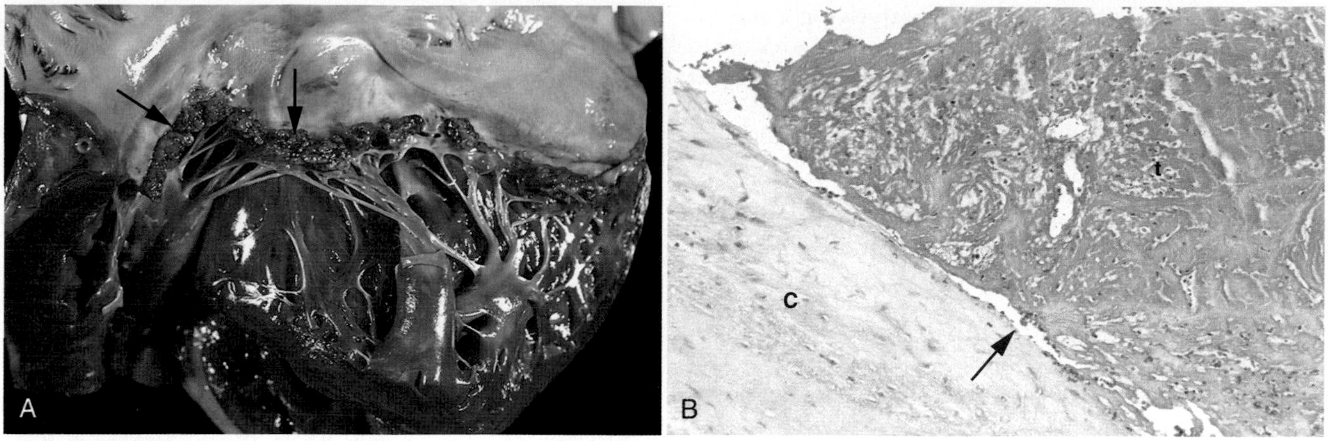

FIGURE 12–28 Nonbacterial thrombotic endocarditis (NBTE). *A,* Nearly complete row of thrombotic vegetations along the line of closure of the mitral valve leaflets *(arrows). B,* Photomicrograph of NBTE, showing bland thrombus, with virtually no inflammation in the valve cusp *(c)* or the thrombotic deposit *(t).* The thrombus is only loosely attached to the cusp *(arrow).*

pholipid syndrome[87,88] (discussed in Chapter 4). Circulating antiphospholipid antibodies are also commonly associated with venous or arterial thrombosis, recurrent pregnancy loss, or thrombocytopenia. The mitral valve is more frequently involved than the aortic; regurgitation is the usual functional abnormality.

CARCINOID HEART DISEASE

Carcinoid heart disease is the cardiac manifestation of the systemic syndrome caused by carcinoid tumors. It involves the endocardium and valves of the right heart. Cardiac lesions are present in one half of patients with the *carcinoid syndrome* which is characterized by *episodic flushing of the skin, cramps, nausea, vomiting, and diarrhea* (see Chapter 17).

Morphology. The cardiovascular lesions associated with the carcinoid syndrome are distinctive, consisting of fibrous intimal thickenings on the inside surfaces of the cardiac chambers and valvular leaflets. They are located mainly in the right ventricle, tricuspid and pulmonic valves, and occasionally in the major blood vessels (Fig. 12–29).[89] The endocardial plaquelike thickenings are composed predominantly of smooth muscle cells and sparse collagen fibers embedded in an acid mucopolysaccharide-rich matrix material. Elastic fibers are not present. Underlying structures are intact, including the valve layers and the subendocardial elastic tissue layer. Occasionally, left-sided lesions are also encountered.

The clinical and pathologic findings relate to the elaboration by carcinoid tumors of a variety of bioactive products, such as serotonin (5-hydroxytryptamine), kallikrein, bradykinin, histamine, prostaglandins, and tachykinins. Which of the secretory products induces the syndrome or the cardiac pathology is still not clear. Nevertheless, plasma levels of serotonin and urinary excretion of the serotonin metabolite 5-hydroxyindoleacetic acid correlate with the severity of the right heart lesions.[90]

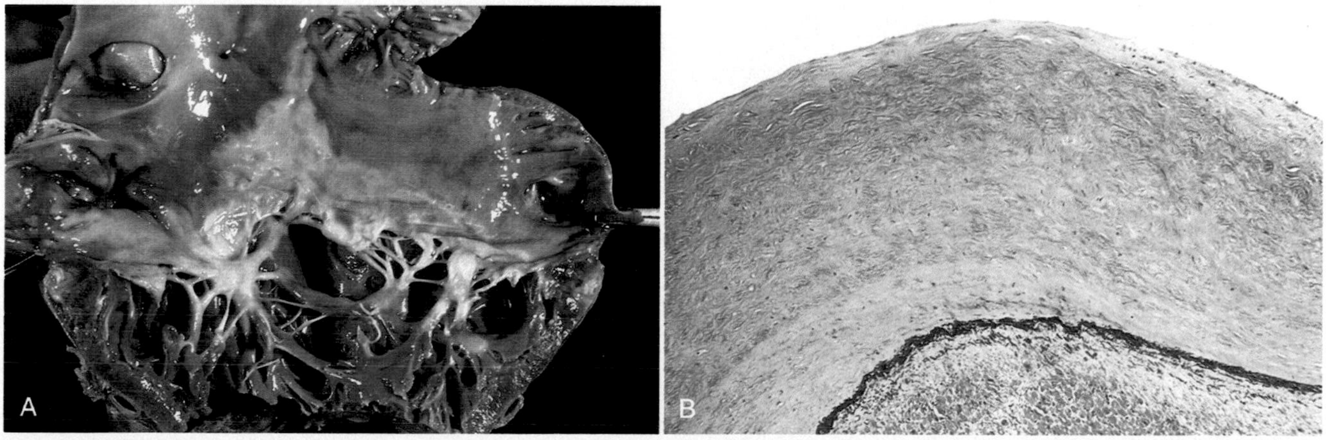

FIGURE 12–29 Carcinoid heart disease. *A,* Characteristic endocardial fibrotic lesion involving the right ventricle and tricuspid valve. *B,* Microscopic appearance of carcinoid heart disease with intimal thickening. Movat stain shows underlying myocardial elastic tissue black and acid mucopolysaccharides blue-green.

The fact that the cardiac changes are largely right-sided is explained by inactivation of both serotonin and bradykinin in the blood during passage through the lungs by the monoamine oxidase present in the pulmonary vascular endothelium. In the absence of hepatic metastases, gastrointestinal carcinoids (with venous drainage via the portal system) do not usually induce the carcinoid syndrome because there is rapid metabolism of serotonin during passage of blood through the liver. In contrast, primary carcinoid tumors in organs outside of the portal system of venous drainage (e.g., ovary and lung), may induce the syndrome without producing hepatic metastases. Left-sided lesions can occur when blood containing the responsible mediator enters the left heart owing to incomplete inactivation because of very high blood levels. Left side lesions may also be a consequence of a pulmonary carcinoid or patent foramen ovale with right to left flow.

Left-sided valve lesions with pathologic features similar to those seen in the carcinoid syndrome have been reported to complicate the use of fenfluramine and phentermine (fen-phen), appetite suppressants used for the treatment of obesity; these agents may affect systemic serotonin metabolism.[91] Occasionally, similar left-sided plaques are found in patients who receive methysergide or ergotamine therapy for migraine headaches; these serotonin analogs are metabolized to serotonin as they pass through the pulmonary vasculature.

COMPLICATIONS OF ARTIFICIAL VALVES

Replacement of damaged cardiac valves with prostheses has now become a common and often life-saving mode of therapy.[92,93] Artificial valves fall primarily into two categories: (1) *mechanical prostheses* using different types of rigid, mobile occluders composed of nonphysiologic biomaterials, such as caged balls, tilting disks, or hinged semicircular flaps, and (2) *tissue valves*, usually *bioprostheses* consisting of chemically treated animal tissue, especially porcine aortic valve tissue, which has been preserved in a dilute glutaraldehyde solution and subsequently mounted on a prosthetic frame. Tissue valves are flexible and function somewhat like natural semilunar valves.

Approximately 60% of substitute valve recipients develop a serious prosthesis-related problem within 10 years postoperatively.[94] Although the *frequency* of total prosthetic valve-related events is similar among valve types, the *nature* of these complications differs among types (Table 12–9 and Fig. 12–30).

- *Thromboembolic complications* constituting local obstruction of the prosthesis by thrombus or distant thromboemboli are the major problem with mechanical valves (Fig. 12–30*A*). This necessitates long-term anticoagulation in patients with these devices. However, hemor-

TABLE 12–9 Causes of Failure of Cardiac Valve Prostheses

Thrombosis/thromboembolism
Anticoagulant-related hemorrhage
Prosthetic valve endocarditis
Structural deterioration (intrinsic) Wear, fracture, poppet failure in ball valves, cuspal tear, calcification
Nonstructural dysfunction Granulation tissue, suture, tissue entrapment, paravalvular leak, disproportion, hemolytic anemia, noise

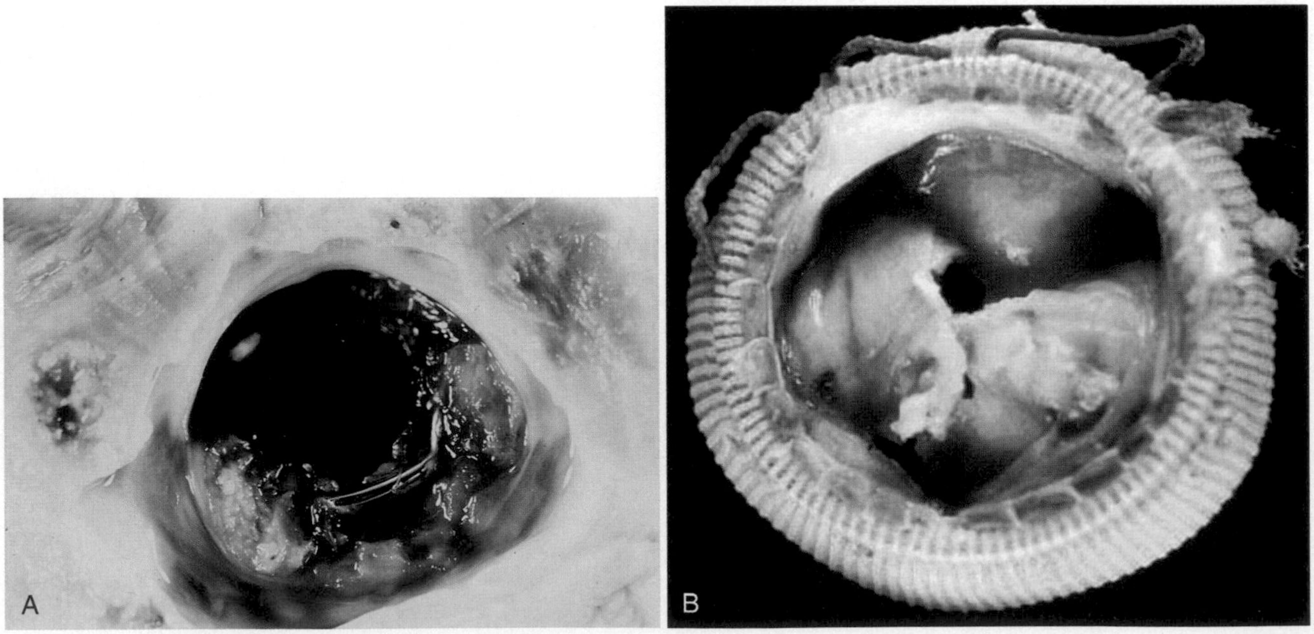

FIGURE 12–30 Complications of artificial heart valves. *A,* Thrombosis of a mechanical prosthetic valve. *B,* Calcification with secondary tearing of a porcine bioprosthetic heart valve, viewed from the inflow aspect.

rhagic complications such as stroke or gastrointestinal bleeding may arise secondarily in patients who receive long-term anticoagulation.

- *Infective endocarditis* is an infrequent but potentially serious complication. Endocarditis is located at the prosthesis-tissue interface, causing a ring abscess, which can eventually lead to a paravalvular regurgitant blood leak. In addition, vegetations may directly involve bioprosthetic valvular cusps. The major organisms causing such infections are staphylococcal skin contaminants (e.g., *S. aureus, S. epidermidis*), streptococci, and fungi.
- *Structural deterioration* uncommonly causes failure of contemporary mechanical valves. However, it is a major failure mode of bioprostheses, with calcification and/or tearing causing secondary regurgitation (see Fig. 12–30*B*).
- Other complications include hemolysis induced by high blood shear, mechanical obstruction to flow inherent in all artificial valves, and inadequate or exuberant healing, causing a paravalvular leak or overgrowth of fibrous tissue, respectively.

Cardiomyopathies

The previous sections emphasize that myocardial dysfunction occurs commonly but secondarily in a number of different conditions such as ischemic heart disease, hypertension, and valvular heart disease. Far less frequently observed is disease whose cause is intrinsic to the myocardium. Myocardial diseases are a diverse group that includes inflammatory disorders *(myocarditis)*, immunologic diseases, systemic metabolic disorders, muscular dystrophies, genetic abnormalities in cardiac muscle cells, and an additional group of diseases of unknown etiology.

The term *cardiomyopathy* (literally, heart muscle disease) is used to describe *heart disease resulting from a primary abnormality in the myocardium.*[95] Although chronic myocardial dysfunction due to ischemia should be excluded from the cardiomyopathy rubric, the term *ischemic cardiomyopathy* has gained some popularity among clinicians to describe CHF caused by CAD (as discussed in the section "Chronic Ischemic Heart Disease").

In many cases cardiomyopathies are *idiopathic* (i.e., of unknown cause). However, a major advance in our understanding of myocardial diseases, previously considered idiopathic, has been the demonstration that specific genetic abnormalities in cardiac energy metabolism or structural and contractile proteins underlie myocardial dysfunction in many patients.[96–98] Thus, etiologic distinctions have become somewhat blurred in recent years. Moreover, myocardial disease of diverse and even unknown etiologies may have a similar morphologic appearance. Therefore, our discussion avoids the controversies associated with classification schemes and emphasizes clinicopathologic, etiologic, and mechanistic concepts.

Without additional data, the clinician encountering a patient with myocardial disease is usually unaware of the etiology. Hence the clinical approach is largely determined by one of the following three clinical, functional, and pathologic patterns (Fig. 12–31 and Table 12–10):

- Dilated cardiomyopathy
- Hypertrophic cardiomyopathy
- Restrictive cardiomyopathy

Among these three categories, the dilated form is most common (90% of cases), and the restrictive is least prevalent. Within the hemodynamic patterns of myocardial dysfunction, there is a spectrum of clinical severity, and overlap of clinical features often occurs between groups. Moreover, each of these patterns can be either idiopathic or due to a specific identifiable cause (Table 12–11) or secondary to primary extramyocardial disease.

Endomyocardial biopsies are used in the diagnosis and management of patients with myocardial disease and in cardiac transplant recipients. Endomyocardial biopsy involves inserting a device (called a *bioptome*) transvenously into the right side of the heart and snipping a small piece of septal myocardium in its jaws, which is then analyzed by a pathologist.[99]

DILATED CARDIOMYOPATHY

The term *dilated cardiomyopathy* (DCM) is applied to a form of cardiomyopathy characterized by *progressive cardiac dilation and contractile (systolic) dysfunction*, usually with concomitant hypertrophy. It is sometimes called congestive car-

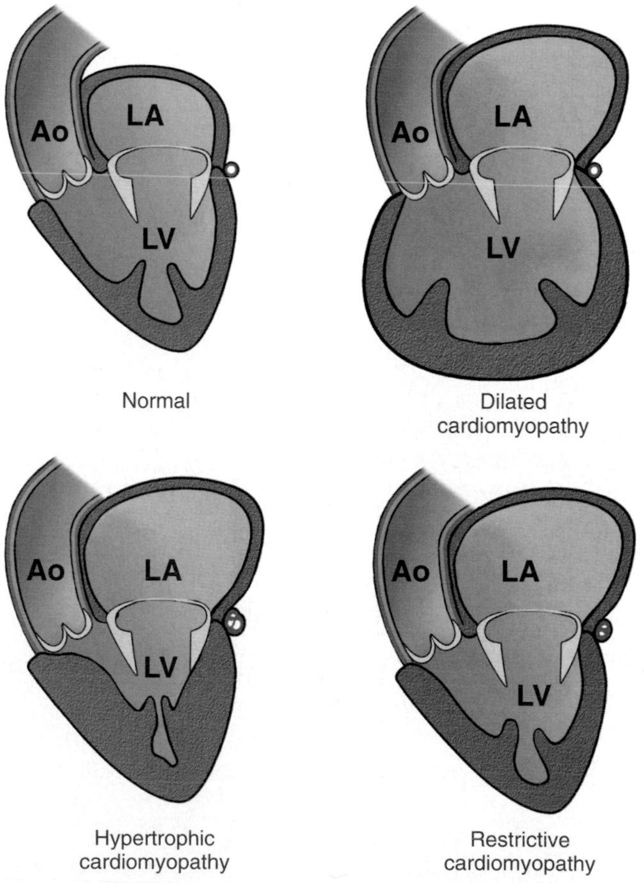

FIGURE 12–31 Graphic representation of the three distinctive and predominant clinical–pathologic–functional forms of myocardial disease.

TABLE 12–10 Cardiomyopathy and Indirect Myocardial Dysfunction: Functional Patterns and Causes

Functional Pattern	Left Ventricular Ejection Fraction*	Mechanisms of Heart Failure	Causes	Indirect Myocardial Dysfunction (Not Cardiomyopathy)
Dilated	<40%	Impairment of contractility (systolic dysfunction)	Idiopathic; alcohol; peripartum; genetic; myocarditis; hemochromatosis; chronic anemia; doxorubicin (Adriamycin); sarcoidosis	Ischemic heart disease; valvular heart disease; hypertensive heart disease; congenital heart disease
Hypertrophic	50–80%	Impairment of compliance (diastolic dysfunction)	Genetic; Friedreich ataxia; storage diseases; infants of diabetic mothers	Hypertensive heart disease; aortic stenosis
Restrictive	45–90%	Impairment of compliance (diastolic dysfunction)	Idiopathic; amyloidosis; radiation-induced fibrosis	Pericardial constriction

*Normal, approximately 50–65%.

TABLE 12–11 Conditions Associated with Heart Muscle Diseases

Cardiac Infections

Viruses
Chlamydia
Rickettsia
Bacteria
Fungi
Protozoa

Toxins

Alcohol
Cobalt
Catecholamines
Carbon monoxide
Lithium
Hydrocarbons
Arsenic
Cyclophosphamide
Doxorubicin (Adriamycin) and daunorubicin

Metabolic

Hyperthroidism
Hypothyroidism
Hyperkalemia
Hypokalemia
Nutritional deficiency (protein, thiamine, other avitaminoses)
Hemochromatosis

Neuromuscular Disease

Friedreich ataxia
Muscular dystrophy
Congenital atrophies

Storage Disorders and Other Depositions

Hunter-Hurler syndrome
Glycogen storage disease
Fabry disease
Amyloidosis

Infiltrative

Leukemia
Carcinomatosis
Sarcoidosis
Radiation-induced fibrosis

Immunologic

Myocarditis (several forms)
Post-transplant rejection

diomyopathy. Although it is recognized that approximately 25% to 35% of individuals with DCM have a familial (genetic) form, DCM can result from a number of acquired myocardial insults that ultimately yield a similar clinicopathologic pattern. These include toxicities (including chronic alcoholism, a history of which can be elicited in 10% to 20% of patients), myocarditis (an inflammatory disorder that precedes the development of cardiomyopathy in at least some cases, as documented by endomyocardial biopsy), and pregnancy-associated nutritional deficiency or immunologic reaction. In some patients, the cause of DCM is unknown; such cases are appropriately designated as *idiopathic dilated cardiomyopathy*.

Morphology. In DCM, the heart is usually heavy, often weighing two to three times normal, and large and flabby, with dilation of all chambers (Fig. 12–32). Nevertheless, because of the wall thinning that accompanies dilation, the ventricular thickness may be less than, equal to, or greater than normal. Mural thrombi are common and may be a source of thromboemboli. There are no primary valvular alterations, and mitral or tricuspid regurgitation, when present, results from left ventricular chamber dilation (functional regurgitation). The coronary arteries are usually free of significant narrowing, but any coronary artery obstructions present are insufficient to explain the degree of cardiac dysfunction.

The histologic abnormalities in idiopathic DCM also are nonspecific and usually do not reflect a specific etiologic agent. Moreover, their severity does not necessarily reflect the degree of dysfunction or the patient's prognosis. Most muscle cells are hypertrophied with enlarged nuclei, but many are attenuated, stretched, and irregular. Interstitial and endocardial fibrosis of variable degree is present, and small subendocardial scars may replace individual cells or groups of cells, probably reflecting healing of previous secondary myocyte ischemic necrosis caused by hypertrophy-induced imbalance between perfusion, supply and demand.

Pathogenesis. Historically, the etiologic associations in dilated cardiomyopathy have included myocardial inflamma-

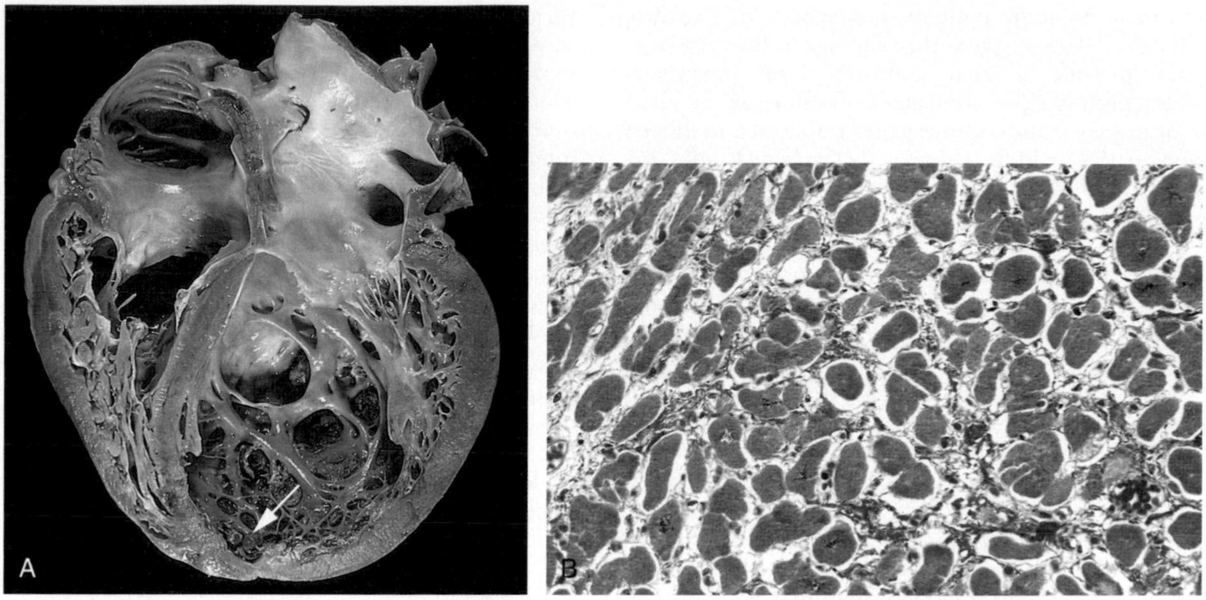

FIGURE 12–32 Dilated cardiomyopathy. *A*, Gross photograph. Four-chamber dilatation and hypertrophy are evident. There is granular mural thrombus at the apex of the left ventricle (on the right in this apical four-chamber view). The coronary arteries were unobstructed. *B*, Histology demonstrating variable myocyte hypertrophy and interstitial fibrosis (collagen is highlighted as blue in this Masson trichrome stain).

tory disease (myocarditis), toxicities (especially alcohol), and the peripartum state. More recently, the importance of genetic factors has been appreciated, and many cases that in past years would have been called "idiopathic" can now be demonstrated to result from specific molecular defects related to cardiac muscle functions. Each of these subgroups will be described below.

- *Myocarditis. Viral nucleic acids* from coxsackievirus B and other enteroviruses have been detected in the myocardium of some patients, and sequential endomyocardial biopsies have demonstrated progression from myocarditis to DCM in others, suggesting that, in at least some cases, DCM was a consequence of myocarditis. Myocarditis is discussed in more detail below.
- *Alcohol or other toxicity. Alcohol abuse* is also strongly associated with the development of dilated cardiomyopathy, raising the possibility that ethanol toxicity (Chapter 9) or a secondary nutritional disturbance may be the cause of the myocardial injury. Alcohol or its metabolites (especially acetaldehyde) have a direct toxic effect on the myocardium. Nevertheless, the cause-and-effect relationship with alcohol alone remains uncertain, and no morphologic features serve to distinguish *alcoholic cardiomyopathy* from DCM of other etiology. Moreover, chronic alcoholism may be associated with thiamine deficiency, introducing an element of beriberi heart disease (also indistinguishable from DCM) (see Chapter 9). In yet other cases, a nonalcoholic *toxic insult* is the cause of the myocardial failure. Particularly important in this last group is myocardial injury caused by certain chemotherapeutic agents, including doxorubicin (Adriamycin), discussed later. In the past, cobalt has also caused CHF.
- *Pregnancy-associated.* A special form of dilated cardiomyopathy, termed *peripartum cardiomyopathy*, occurs late in pregnancy or several weeks to months postpartum. The cause of peripartum cardiomyopathy is poorly understood but is probably multifactorial. Pregnancy-associated hypertension, volume overload, nutritional deficiency, other metabolic derangement, or an as yet poorly characterized immunologic reaction may be involved.
- *Genetic influences.* DCM has a familial occurrence in 25% to 35% of cases. In the genetic forms of DCM, autosomal dominant inheritance is the predominant pattern; X-linked, autosomal recessive, and mitochondrial inheritance are less common. The genetic abnormalities identified as causes of familial DCM in humans largely affect the cytoskeleton. In some families there are deletions in the mitochondrial genes resulting in abnormal oxidative phosphorylation, in others, there are mutations in genes encoding enzymes involved in beta-oxidation of fatty acids. The mitochendrial defects most frequently cause dilated cardiomyopathy in children. Although X-linked dilated cardiomyopathy is not the dominant form, it is the best understood. This disorder typically presents in the teenage years or in the early 20s and usually is rapidly progressive. X-linked cardiomyopathy has been linked to the gene for dystrophin, a cell membrane–based cytoskeletal protein that plays a critical role in linking the internal cytoskeleton with the external basement membrane. Recall that dystrophin is mutated in the most common skeletal myopathies (i.e., Duchenne and Becker muscular dystrophies, see Chapter 27). Interestingly, some patients and families with dystrophin gene mutations have DCM as the primary clinical feature. Myocarditis-associated enteroviral protease 2A has been shown to cleave dystrophin directly, suggesting a mechanism for the development of postmyocarditis DCM.[100] Moreover, disruption of dystrophin is a common finding in end-stage cardiomyopathy, dilated or ischemic. This disruption is reversible, correlating with

improvements in some patients, managed with a cardiac assist device.[101] This suggests that damage to the cytoskeleton may provide a final common (and potentially reversible) pathway for contractile dysfunction in heart failure of diverse causes. Other genes implicated in dilated cardiomyopathy include α-cardiac actin (which links the sarcomere with dystrophin), desmin, and the nuclear lamina proteins, lamin A and lamin C.

Clinical Features. DCM may occur at any age, including in childhood, but it most commonly affects individuals between the ages of 20 and 50. It presents with slowly progressive signs and symptoms of CHF such as shortness of breath, easy fatigability, and poor exertional capacity, but patients may slip precipitously from a compensated to a decompensated functional state. In the end stage, patients often have ejection fractions of less than 25% (normal, approximately 50% to 65%). Fifty percent of patients die within 2 years, and only 25% survive longer than 5 years, but some severely affected patients may unexpectedly improve on therapy. Secondary mitral regurgitation and abnormal cardiac rhythms are common. Death is usually attributable to progressive cardiac failure or arrhythmia and can occur suddenly. Embolism from dislodgment of an intracardiac thrombus may occur. Cardiac transplantation is frequently recommended.

Arrhythmogenic Right Ventricular Cardiomyopathy (Arrhythmogenic Right Ventricular Dysplasia)

Arrhythmogenic right ventricular cardiomyopathy, or *arrhythmogenic right ventricular dysplasia*, is a poorly understood condition with a distinct clinical presentation. It is most commonly associated with right-sided heart failure and various rhythm disturbances, particularly ventricular tachycardia. Left-sided involvement with left-sided heart failure may also occur. In some cases it gives rise to sudden death. Morphologically, the right ventricular wall is severely thinned due to loss of myocytes, with extensive fatty infiltration and interstitial fibrosis (Fig. 12–33). Most cases have no family history, but familial forms do occur. Although a gene defect was recently localized on chromosome 14, the pathogenesis remains obscure.[102,103] Pedigree analyses of large kindreds indicate autosomal dominant inheritance with variable penetrance.

Naxos syndrome appears to be a related disorder that has similar cardiac findings, in addition to hyperkeratosis of plantar palmar skin surfaces. The abnormal gene in Naxos disease codes for plakoglobin,[104] also known as γ-catenin, an intracellular protein that links transmembrane adhesion molecules in desmosomes to desmin, the principal intermediate filament protein in cardiac myocytes.

HYPERTROPHIC CARDIOMYOPATHY

Hypertrophic cardiomyopathy (HCM) is also known by such terms as *idiopathic hypertrophic subaortic stenosis* and *hypertrophic obstructive cardiomyopathy.* It is characterized by *myocardial hypertrophy, abnormal diastolic filling* and, in about one third of cases, *intermittent ventricular outflow obstruction.* The heart is thick-walled, heavy, and *hyper*contracting, in striking contrast to the flabby, *hypo*contracting heart of DCM. HCM causes primarily diastolic dysfunction; systolic function is usually preserved. The two most common diseases that must be distinguished clinically from HCM are amyloidosis and hypertensive heart disease coupled with age-related subaortic septal hypertrophy (see earlier section on hypertensive heart disease). Occasionally, valvular or congenital subvalvular aortic stenosis can also mimic HCM.

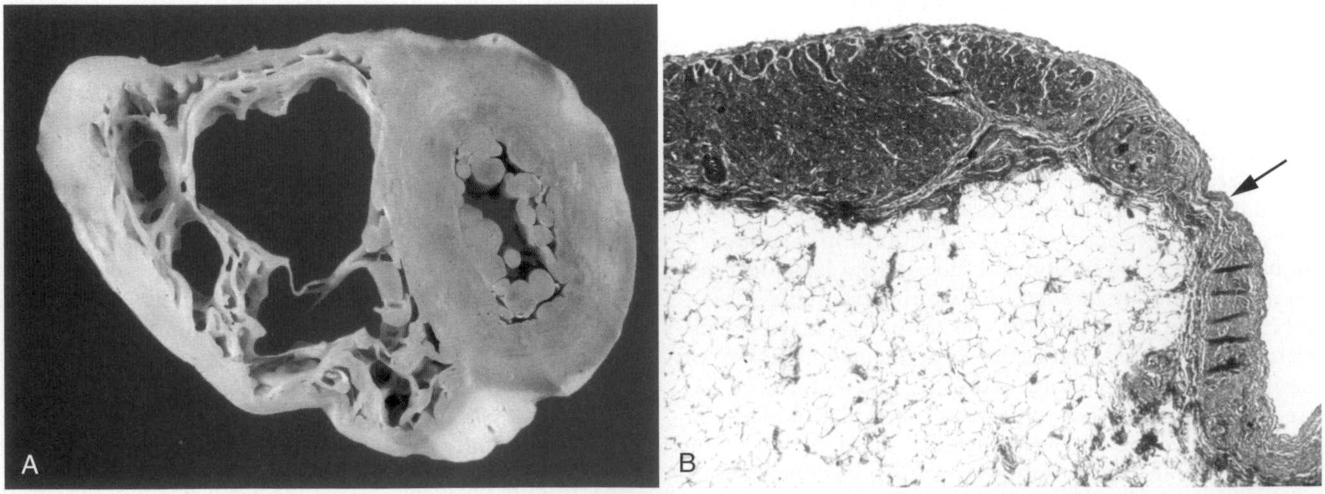

FIGURE 12–33 Arrythmogenic right ventricular cardiomyopathy. *A,* Gross photograph, showing dilation of the right ventricle and near transmural replacement of the right ventricular free-wall myocardium by fat and fibrosis. The left ventricle has a virtually normal configuration. *B,* Histologic section of the right ventricular free wall, demonstrating replacement of myocardium *(red)* by fibrosis *(blue, arrow)* and fat (collagen is blue in this Masson trichrome stain).

Morphology. The essential feature of HCM is massive myocardial hypertrophy without ventricular dilation (Fig. 12–34*A,B*). The classic pattern is disproportionate thickening of the ventricular septum as compared with the free wall of the left ventricle (with a ratio greater than 1:3), frequently termed asymmetrical septal hypertrophy. In about 10% of cases, however, the hypertrophy is symmetrical throughout the heart. On cross-section, the ventricular cavity loses its usual round-to-ovoid shape and may be compressed into a "banana-like" configuration by bulging of the ventricular septum into the lumen (see Fig. 12–34*A*). Although disproportionate hypertrophy can involve the entire septum, it is usually most prominent in the subaortic region. Often present are endocardial thickening or mural plaque formation in the

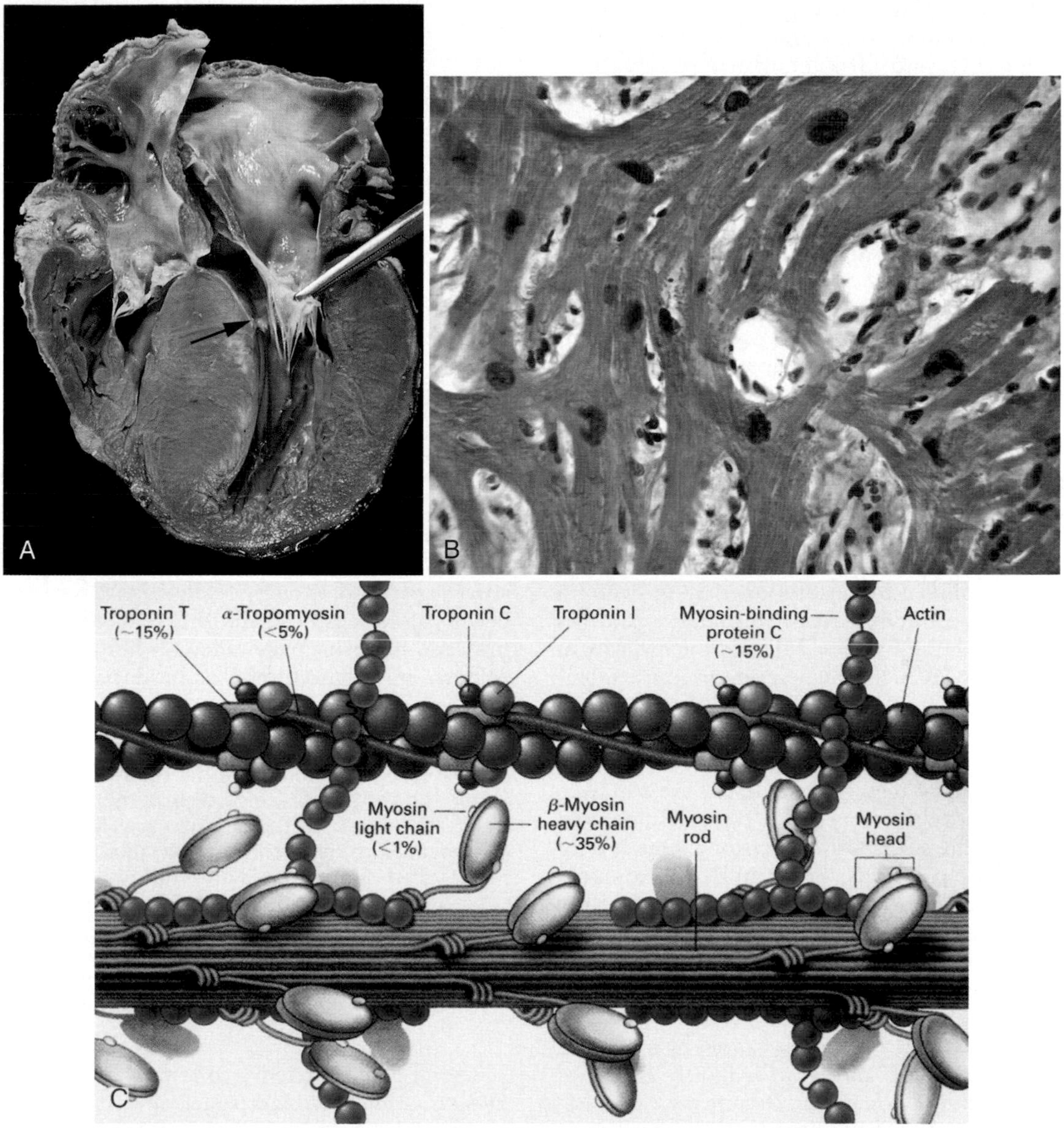

FIGURE 12–34 Hypertrophic cardiomyopathy with asymmetric septal hypertrophy. *A,* The septal muscle bulges into the left ventricular outflow tract, and the left atrium is enlarged. The anterior mitral leaflet has been moved away from the septum to reveal a fibrous endocardial plaque *(arrow)* (see text). *B,* Histologic appearance demonstrating disarray, extreme hypertrophy, and characteristic branching of myocytes as well as the interstitial fibrosis characteristic of hypertrophic cardiomyopathy (collagen is blue in this Masson trichrome stain). *C,* Schematic structure of the sarcomere of cardiac muscle, highlighting proteins in which mutations cause defective contraction, hypertrophy, and myocyte disarray in hypertrophic cardiomyopathy. The frequency of a particular gene mutation is indicated as a percentage of all cases of HCM; most common are mutations in β-myosin heavy chain. Normal contraction of the sarcomere involves myosin–actin interaction initiated by calcium binding to troponin C, I, and T and α-tropomyosin. Actin stimulates ATPase activity in the myosin head and produces force along the actin filaments. Myocyte-binding protein C modulates contraction. (*A,* reproduced by permission from Schoen FJ: Interventional and Surgical Cardiovascular Pathology: Clinical Correlations and Basic Principles. Philadelphia, W.B. Saunders, 1989. *C,* from Spirito P, et al: The management of hypertrophic cardiomyopathy. N Engl J Med 336:775, 1997.)

left ventricular outflow tract and thickening of the anterior mitral leaflet. Both findings are a result of contact of the anterior mitral leaflet with the septum during ventricular systole, and they correlate with echocardiographically demonstrated functional left ventricular outflow tract obstruction during midsystole present in some cases.

The most important histologic features of the myocardium in HCM are (1) extensive myocyte hypertrophy to a degree unusual in other conditions, with transverse myocyte diameters frequently greater than 40 μm (normal, approximately 15 μm); (2) haphazard disarray of bundles of myocytes, individual myocytes, and contractile elements in sarcomeres within cells (myofiber disarray); and (3) interstitial and replacement fibrosis (see Fig. 12–34*B*).

Pathogenesis. Hypertrophic cardiomyopathy is caused by a mutation in any one of several genes that encode proteins that are part of the sarcomere, the contractile unit of cardiac and skeletal muscle[105–107] (Fig. 12–34*C*). Thus, HCM is a genetic disease of force generation within the cardiac myocyte. Most cases are familial and the pattern of transmission is autosomal dominant with variable expression. Remaining cases appear to be sporadic. Mutations causing HCM have been found in at least 12 sarcomeric genes, including β-myosin heavy chain (β-MHC), cardiac troponinT, α-tropomyosin, and myosin-binding protein C (MYBP-C). Of these, mutations in the β-MHC (β-myosin heavy chain) gene are most common; MYBP-C and troponinT are next in frequency. Mutations in these three genes account for 70% to 80% of all cases of HCM. The amino acid substitution 403 Arg→Gln (in β-MHC) is the most commonly reported mutation and has been described in multiple families. This and the majority of the mutations causing HCM are single-point missense mutations. All told, more than 100 other mutations have been found in HCM, and hence the disease is genetically quite heterogeneous.

Although it is clear that these genetic defects are critical to the etiology of this entity, the sequence of events leading from mutations to disease are still poorly understood. One current hypothesis considers cardiac hypertrophy in HCM a compensatory phenomenon owing to impaired contraction of cardiac myocytes, which triggers the release of growth factors that result in intense compensatory hypertrophy (leading to myofiber disarray) and fibroblast proliferation (causing interstitial fibrosis).[108]

As discussed above, HCM is a disease caused by mutations in proteins of the sarcomere, and DCM is mostly associated with abnormalities of the cytoskeleton. Despite these etiologic differences, there are some common mechanistic and clinicopathologic threads between the genetic forms of dilated and hypertrophic cardiomyopathy, as summarized in Figure 12–35.

Clinical Features. The basic physiologic abnormality in HCM is reduced chamber size and poor compliance with reduced stroke volume that results from *impaired diastolic filling of the massively hypertrophied left ventricle.* In addition, approximately 25% of patients with HCM have dynamic obstruction to the left ventricular outflow. The limitation of cardiac output and a secondary increase in pulmonary venous pressure cause exertional dyspnea. Auscultation discloses a *harsh systolic ejection murmur*, caused by ventricular outflow obstruction as the anterior mitral leaflet moves toward the ventricular septum during systole. Owing to the massive hypertrophy, high left ventricular chamber pressure, and potentially abnormal intramural arteries, focal myocardial ischemia commonly results, even in the absence of concomitant CAD, and thus anginal pain is frequent. The major clinical problems in HCM are atrial fibrillation with mural thrombus formation and possibly embolization, infective endocarditis of the mitral valve, intractable cardiac failure, ventricular arrhythmias, and sudden death. Hypertrophic cardiomyopathy is one of the most common causes of sudden, otherwise unexplained, death in young athletes.

Given the heterogeneous genetic defects of HCM, it should not be surprising that the clinical and morphologic features are markedly heterogeneous among affected patients. Many patients are stable over the many years of observation, and some improve. Most patients can be significantly helped by medical therapy that enhances ventricular relaxation. Reduction of the mass of the septum by surgical excision of muscle is done in some cases to relieve outflow tract obstruction, if present. In a recently introduced nonsurgical myocardial reduction, alcohol is infused through a catheter to induce infarction of the myocardium.

RESTRICTIVE CARDIOMYOPATHY

Restrictive cardiomyopathy is a disorder characterized by a *primary decrease in ventricular compliance, resulting in impaired ventricular filling during diastole*; the contractile (systolic) function of the left ventricle is usually unaffected.[109] Thus, the functional state can be confused with that of constrictive pericarditis or HCM. Restrictive cardiomyopathy can be idiopathic or associated with distinct diseases that affect the myocardium, principally radiation fibrosis, amyloidosis, sarcoidosis, metastatic tumor, or products of inborn errors of metabolism.

Morphology. In idiopathic **restrictive cardiomyopathy,** the ventricles are of approximately normal size or slightly enlarged, the cavities are not dilated, and the myocardium is firm. Biatrial dilation is commonly observed. Microscopically, there is often only patchy or diffuse interstitial fibrosis, which can vary from minimal to extensive. Restrictive cardiomyopathy of disparate causes may have similar gross morphology. However, endomyocardial biopsy often reveals features that are disease-specific histologically.

Several other restrictive conditions require brief mention. *Endomyocardial fibrosis* is principally a disease of children and young adults in Africa and other tropical areas, characterized by fibrosis of the ventricular endocardium and subendocardium that extends from the apex toward, and often involves the tricuspid and mitral valves. The fibrous tissue markedly diminishes the volume and compliance of affected chambers and so induces a restrictive functional defect. Ventricular mural thrombi sometimes develop, and indeed there is a suggestion that the fibrous tissue results from the organization of mural thrombi. The etiology is unknown.

Loeffler endomyocarditis is also marked by endomyocardial fibrosis, typically with large mural thrombi similar to those

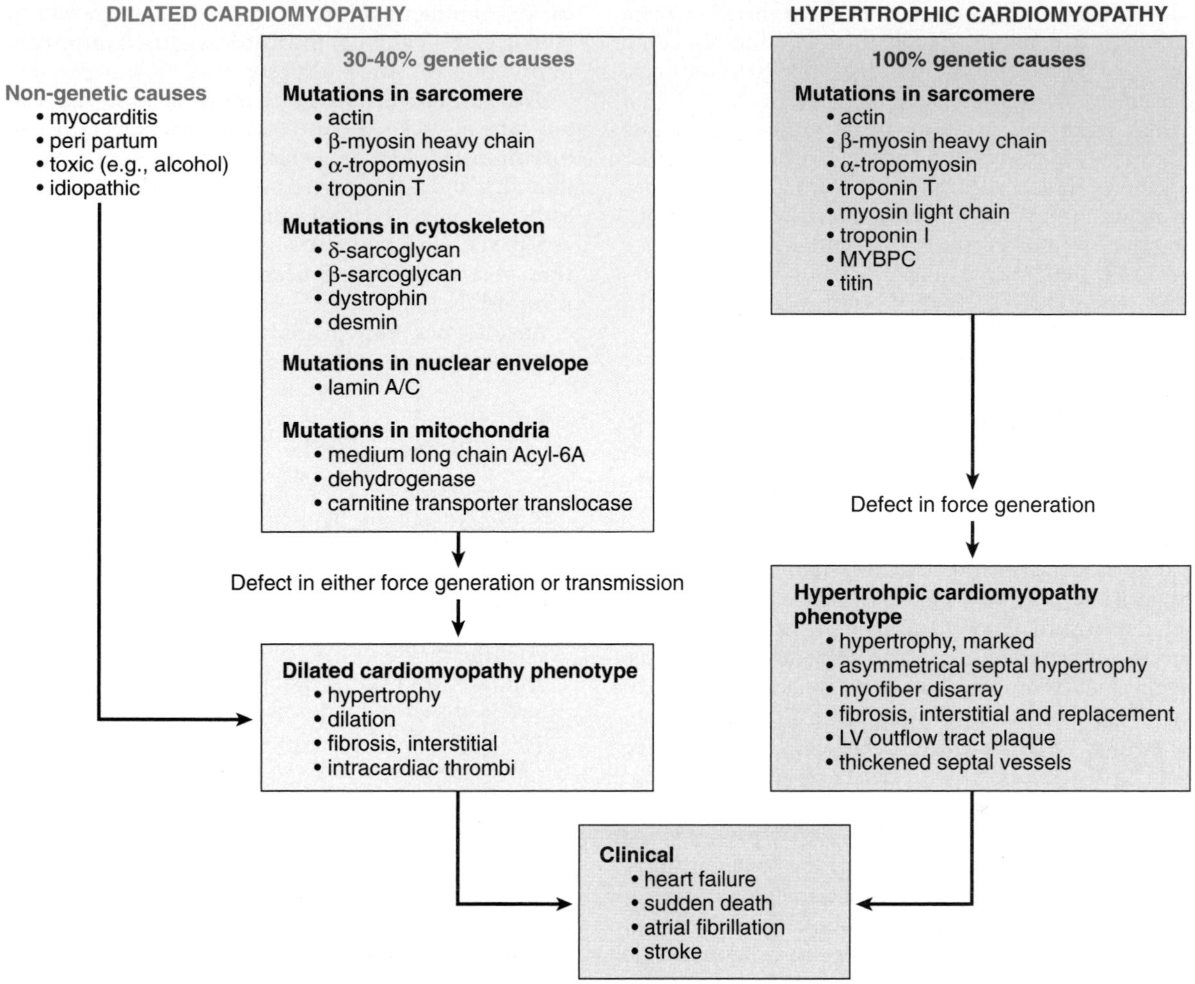

DILATED CARDIOMYOPATHY
Non-genetic causes
• myocarditis
• peri partum
• toxic (e.g., alcohol)
• idiopathic
30-40% genetic causes
Mutations in sarcomere
• actin
• β-myosin heavy chain
• α-tropomyosin
• troponin T
Mutations in cytoskeleton
• δ-sarcoglycan
• β-sarcoglycan
• dystrophin
• desmin
Mutations in nuclear envelope
• lamin A/C
Mutations in mitochondria
• medium long chain Acyl-6A
• dehydrogenase
• carnitine transporter translocase
Defect in either force generation or transmission
Dilated cardiomyopathy phenotype
• hypertrophy
• dilation
• fibrosis, interstitial
• intracardiac thrombi
HYPERTROPHIC CARDIOMYOPATHY
100% genetic causes
Mutations in sarcomere
• actin
• β-myosin heavy chain
• α-tropomyosin
• troponin T
• myosin light chain
• troponin I
• MYBPC
• titin
Defect in force generation
Hypertrohpic cardiomyopathy phenotype
• hypertrophy, marked
• asymmetrical septal hypertrophy
• myofiber disarray
• fibrosis, interstitial and replacement
• LV outflow tract plaque
• thickened septal vessels
Clinical
• heart failure
• sudden death
• atrial fibrillation
• stroke

FIGURE 12–35 Pathways of dilated and hypertrophic cardiomyopathy, emphasizing several important concepts. Some forms of dilated cardiomyopathy (others are caused by myocarditis, alcohol, and other toxic injury or the peripartum state) and virtually all forms of hypertrophic cardiomyopathy are genetic in origin. The genetic causes of dilated cardiomyopathy involve mutations in any of a wide variety of proteins, predominantly of the cytoskeleton, but also the sarcomere, mitochondria, and nuclear envelope. In contrast, the mutated genes that cause hypertrophic cardiomyopathy encode proteins of the sarcomere. Although these two forms of cardiomyopathy differ greatly in subcellular basis and morphologic phenotypes, they share a common pathway of clinical complications.

seen in the tropical disease, but cases are not restricted to a specific geographic area. In addition to the cardiac changes, there is often an eosinophilic leukemia, which can result in infiltration of other organs by eosinophils and a rapidly fatal downhill course. The circulating eosinophils are abnormal, and many are degranulated. The release of toxic products of eosinophils, especially major basic protein, is postulated to initiate endocardial damage, with subsequent foci of endomyocardial necrosis accompanied by an eosinophilic infiltrate. This is followed by scarring of the necrotic area, layering of the endocardium by thrombus, and finally organization of the thrombus. Eosinophilic endomyocardial disease has a poor prognosis, but benefits are reported from surgical removal of the fibrous/thrombotic layer of tissue (called endomyocardial stripping).

Endocardial fibroelastosis is an uncommon heart disease of obscure etiology characterized by focal or diffuse fibroelastic thickening usually involving the mural left ventricular endocardium. Most common in the first 2 years of life, it is often accompanied by some form of congenital cardiac anomaly, aortic valve obstruction in about one third of all cases. Focal disease may have no functional importance, but diffuse involvement may be responsible for rapid and progressive cardiac decompensation and death.

MYOCARDITIS

Under this category are grouped inflammatory processes of the myocardium that result in injury to cardiac myocytes.[110,111] However, the presence of inflammation alone is not diagnostic of myocarditis, because inflammatory infiltrates may also be seen as a secondary response in conditions such as ischemic injury. *In myocarditis, by contrast, the inflammatory process is the cause of rather than a response to myocardial injury.*

Etiology and Pathogenesis. In the United States, *infections* and particularly *viruses* are the most common cause of myocarditis. *Coxackieviruses A* and *B* and other enteroviruses probably account for most of the cases. Other less common etiologic agents include cytomegalovirus, human immunodeficiency virus (HIV), and a host of other agents listed in Table 12–12. Although it is often difficult to isolate the offending virus from the tissues after the onset of clinical symptoms, serologic studies and, more recently, the identification of viral DNA or RNA sequences in the myocardium by polymerase chain reaction may identify the culprit in some cases. Whether the viruses are the direct cause of the myocardial injury or they initiate an immune response that cross-reacts with myocardial cells is unclear in most cases.[112] As with hepatitis viruses (Chapter 18), T cells may damage virus-infected myocytes by reacting against viral antigens expressed on the cell membrane.

Nonviral biologic agents are an important cause of myocarditis, particularly direct cardiac infection caused by the protozoa *Trypanosoma cruzi*, the agent of Chagas disease. Although uncommon in the northern hemisphere, Chagas disease affects up to one half of the population in endemic areas of South America, and myocardial involvement is found in approximately 80% of infected individuals.[113] About 10% of patients die during an acute attack; others may enter a chronic immune-mediated phase and develop progressive signs of cardiac insufficiency 10 to 20 years later. Trichinosis is the most common helminthic disease with associated cardiac involvement. Parasitic diseases, including toxoplasmosis, and bacterial infections, including Lyme disease and diphtheria, can also cause myocarditis. In the case of diphtheritic myocarditis, toxins released by *Corynebacterium diphtheriae* appear to be responsible for the myocardial injury.

Myocarditis occurs in approximately 5% of patients with Lyme disease, a systemic illness caused by the bacterial spirochete *Borrelia burgdorferi*, which has dermatologic, neurologic, and rheumatologic manifestations. Lyme carditis (myocarditis) manifests primarily as self-limited conduction system disease.[114] Nevertheless, a temporary pacemaker is required for AV block in approximately 30% of patients.

Myocarditis occurs in many patients with acquired immunodeficiency syndrome (AIDS).[115,116] Two types have been identified: (1) inflammation and myocyte damage without a clear etiologic agent and (2) myocarditis caused directly by HIV or by an opportunistic pathogen.

There are also noninfectious causes of myocarditis. Myocarditis can be related to allergic reactions *(hypersensitivity myocarditis)*, often to a particular drug such as antibiotics, diuretics, and antihypertensive agents. Myocarditis can also be associated with systemic diseases of immune origin, such as RF, SLE, and polymyositis. Cardiac sarcoidosis and rejection of a transplanted heart are also considered forms of myocarditis.

Against this background we can turn to the anatomic changes seen in the major forms of myocarditis.

TABLE 12–12 Major Causes of Myocarditis

Infections
Viruses (e.g., coxsackievirus, ECHO, influenza, HIV, cytomegalovirus)
Chlamydiae (e.g., *C. psittaci*)
Rickettsiae (e.g., *R. typhi*, typhus fever)
Bacteria (e.g., *Corynebacterium diphtheriae, Neisseria meningococcus, Borrelia* (Lyme disease)
Fungi (e.g., *Candida*)
Protozoa (e.g., *Trypanosoma* Chagas disease, toxoplasmosis)
Helminths (e.g., trichinosis)
Immune-Mediated Reactions
Postviral
Poststreptococcal (rheumatic fever)
Systemic lupus erythematosus
Drug hypersensitivity (e.g., methyldopa, sulfonamides)
Transplant rejection
Unknown
Sarcoidosis
Giant cell myocarditis

HIV, human immunodeficiency virus.

Morphology. During the active phase of myocarditis, the heart may appear normal or dilated; some hypertrophy may be present. The lesions may be diffuse or patchy. The ventricular myocardium is typically flabby and often mottled by either pale foci or minute hemorrhagic lesions. Mural thrombi may be present in any chamber.

During active disease, myocarditis is most frequently characterized by an interstitial inflammatory infiltrate and focal necrosis of myocytes adjacent to the inflammatory cells (Fig. 12–36).[74] Myocarditis in which the infiltrate is mononuclear and predominantly lymphocytic is most common (see Fig. 12–36*A*). Although endomyocardial biopsies are diagnostic in some cases, they can be spuriously negative because inflammatory involvement may be focal or patchy. If the patient survives the acute phase of myocarditis, the inflammatory lesions either resolve, leaving no residual changes, or heal by progressive fibrosis, as mentioned earlier.

Hypersensitivity myocarditis has interstitial infiltrates, principally perivascular, composed of lymphocytes, macrophages, and a high proportion of eosinophils (see Fig. 12–36*B*).

A morphologically distinctive form of myocarditis of uncertain cause, called **giant cell myocarditis**, is characterized by a widespread inflammatory cellular infiltrate containing multinucleate giant cells interspersed with lymphocytes, eosinophils, plasma cells, and macrophages and having at least focal but frequently extensive necrosis (Fig.12–36*C*). The giant cells are of either macrophage or myocyte origin. This variant carries a poor prognosis.[117]

The myocarditis of **Chagas disease** is rendered distinctive by parasitization of scattered myofibers by trypanosomes accompanied by an inflammatory infiltrate of neutrophils, lymphocytes, macrophages, and occasional eosinophils (Fig. 12–36*D*).

Clinical Features. The clinical spectrum of myocarditis is broad; at one end the disease is entirely asymptomatic, and such patients recover completely without sequelae. At the other extreme is the precipitous onset of heart failure or arrhythmias, occasionally with sudden death. A systolic murmur may appear, indicating functional mitral regurgitation related to dilation of the left ventricle. Between these extremes are the many levels of involvement associated with such symptoms as fatigue, dyspnea, palpitations, precordial discomfort, and fever. The clinical features of myocarditis can

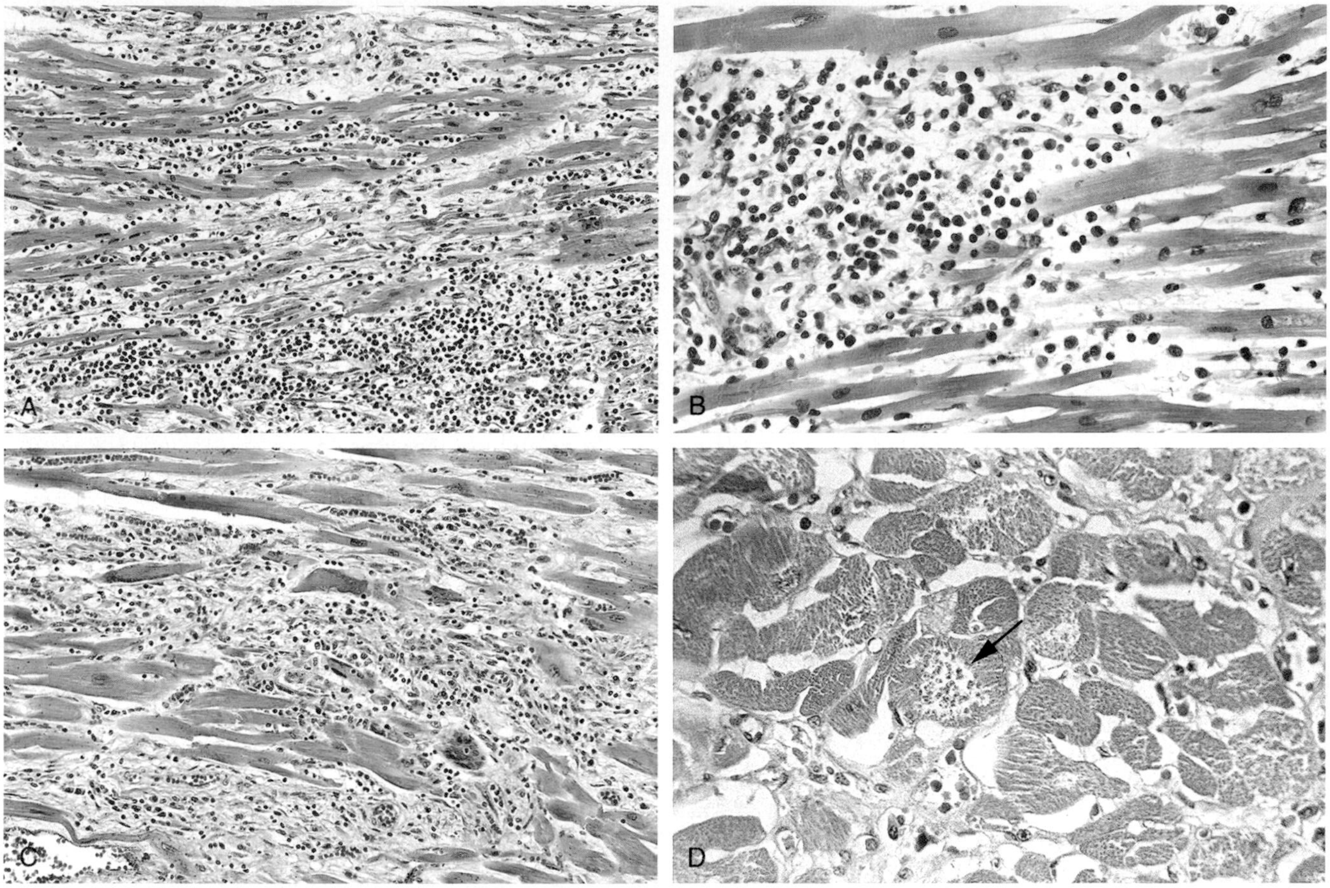

FIGURE 12–36 Myocarditis. *A,* Lymphocytic myocarditis, with mononuclear inflammatory cell infiltrate and associated myocyte injury. *B,* Hypersensitivity myocarditis, characterized by interstitial inflammatory infiltrate composed largely of eosinophils and mononuclear inflammatory cells, predominantly localized to perivascular and large interstitial spaces. This form of myocarditis is associated with drug hypersensitivity. *C,* Giant cell myocarditis, with mononuclear inflammatory infiltrate containing lymphocytes and macrophages, extensive loss of muscle, and multinucleated giant cells. *D,* The myocarditis of Chagas disease. A myofiber is distended with trypanosomes *(arrow).* There is a surrounding inflammatory reaction and individual myofiber necrosis.

mimic those of acute MI. Occasionally, years later, when an attack of myocarditis is forgotten, the patient may be diagnosed as having dilated cardiomyopathy. Indeed, many patients have been observed to progress clinically from unequivocal myocarditis to DCM; endomyocardial biopsy findings of evolving disease have been documented in some.

OTHER SPECIFIC CAUSES OF MYOCARDIAL DISEASE

Adriamycin and Other Drugs. The anthracycline chemotherapeutic agents doxorubicin (Adriamycin) and daunorubicin are well-recognized causes of toxic myocardial injury that can cause DCM.[118] The hazard is dose-dependent (cardiotoxicity becomes progressively more frequent above a total dose of 500 mg/m^2) and is attributed primarily to lipid peroxidation of myocyte membranes. Many other agents, such as lithium, phenothiazines, chloroquine, and cocaine have been implicated in myocardial injury and sometimes sudden death. Common morphologic threads running throughout the cardiotoxicity of many chemicals and drugs (including diphtheria exotoxin) are myofiber swelling and vacuolization, fatty change, individual cell lysis (myocytolysis), and sometimes patchy foci of necrosis. Electron microscopy usually reveals cytoplasmic vacuolization and lysis of myofibrils, typified by Adriamycin cardiotoxicity. With discontinuance of the toxic agent, these changes may resolve completely, leaving no apparent sequelae. Sometimes, however, nonspecific hypertrophy with interstitial fibrosis or small focal replacement scars remain, and both the physiologic and morphologic patterns can be indistinguishable from those of DCM.

Another chemotherapeutic agent with cardiac toxicity is cyclophosphamide (Cytoxan), which, like Adriamycin, has dose-dependent cardiotoxic effects, but severe cardiomyopathy may occur following single high-dose therapy. In contrast to the primary myocyte injury with Adriamycin, the principal insult with cyclophosphamide appears to be vascular, leading to myocardial hemorrhage.

Catecholamines. Foci of myocardial necrosis with contraction bands, often associated with a sparse mononuclear inflammatory infiltrate consisting mostly of macrophages, are frequently observed in patients who have a pheochromocytoma, with its elaboration of catecholamines (Chapter 24). This is considered to be a manifestation of the general problem of "catecholamine effect", which is also seen in association with the administration of large doses of vasopressor agents such as dopamine. Cocaine also causes catecholamine-induced cell damage.[119] The mechanism of catecholamine cardiotoxicity is uncertain, but it appears to relate either to direct toxicity of catecholamines to cardiac myocytes via calcium overload or to vasoconstriction in the myocardial circulation in the face of an increased heart rate. The mononuclear cell infiltrate is likely a secondary reaction to the foci of myocyte cell death. Similar morphology may be encountered in patients who have recovered from hypotensive episodes or have been resuscitated from a frank cardiac arrest; in such cases, the damage is a result of ischemia-reperfusion (see earlier) and inflammation follows. Curiously, some patients with intracranial lesions associated with elevated cerebrospinal fluid pressure and neurostimulation also develop focal myocardial necrosis with contraction bands.[120]

Amyloidosis. Cardiac amyloidosis may appear along with systemic amyloidosis (Chapter 6) or may be isolated to the heart, particularly in the aged.[121,122] Cardiac amyloid deposits may occur in the ventricles and atria (*senile cardiac amyloidosis [SCA]* or systemic senile amyloidosis with cardiac involvement) or be limited to the atria *(isolated atrial amyloidosis).* In SCA the protein deposits derive from transthyretin, a normal serum protein that transports both thyroxine and retinol-binding protein. The cardiac manifestations of isolated SCA may be histologically indistinguishable from those of primary amyloidosis (Chapter 6), but SCA can be identified by immunohistochemical staining of tissue with antisera to transthyretin.[123] SCA has a far better prognosis than systemic amyloidosis. Although SCA is exclusively a disease of elderly people, mutant forms of transthyretin can accelerate cardiac (and indeed systemic) amyloidosis. For example, the risk of isolated cardiac amyloidosis is four times greater in African Americans than in Caucasians after age 60; 4% of African Americans have a gene mutation in which isoleucine is substituted for valine at position 122 (Ile 122) that produces an amyloidogenic/fibrillogenic form of transthyretin (autosomal dominant familial transthyretin amyloidosis).[124] In isolated atrial amyloidosis, the deposits consist of atrial natriuretic peptide.

Cardiac amyloidosis most frequently produces restrictive hemodynamics, but it can be asymptomatic or can be manifested by dilation, arrhythmias, or features mimicking those of ischemic or valvular disease owing to deposits in the interstitium, conduction system, vasculature, and valves, respectively.

Morphology. Grossly, the heart in cardiac amyloidosis varies from normal to firm, rubbery, and noncompliant with thickened walls. Usually the chambers are of normal size, but in some cases they are dilated. Numerous small, semitranslucent nodules resembling drips of wax may be seen at the atrial endocardial surface, particularly on the left. Amyloid deposits occur outside of the myocytes in the myocardial interstitium, conduction tissue, valves, endocardium, pericardium, and small intramural coronary arteries, and they are highlighted by the classic apple-green birefringence demonstrated by polarization of tissue sections stained with Congo red or by the sulfated Alcian blue stain. In the interstitium, amyloid deposits often form rings around cardiac myocytes and capillaries. Intramural arteries and arterioles may have sufficient amyloid in their walls to compress and occlude their lumens, inducing myocardial ischemia ("small vessel disease").

Iron Overload. *Iron overload* can occur in either hereditary hemochromatosis (Chapter 18) or hemosiderosis owing to multiple blood transfusions. The heart in each is usually dilated and the morphology does not belie the cause. Iron deposition is more prominent in ventricles than atria and in the working myocardium than in the conduction system. It is thought that iron causes systolic dysfunction by interfering with metal-dependent enzyme systems.

Morphology. Grossly, the myocardium of the iron-overloaded heart is rust-brown in color but is usually otherwise indistinguishable from that of idiopathic DCM. Microscopically, there is marked accumulation of hemosiderin within cardiac myocytes (contrasted with the extracellular deposition of amyloid discussed previously), particularly in the perinuclear region, demonstrable with a Prussian blue stain. This is associated with varying degrees of cellular degeneration and fibrosis. Ultrastructurally, the cardiac myocytes contain abundant perinuclear siderosomes (iron-containing lysosomes).

Hyperthyroidism and Hypothyroidism. Cardiac manifestations are among the earliest, most consistent features of hyperthyroidism and hypothyroidism and reflect direct and indirect effects of thyroid hormones on the cells of the heart. In *hyperthyroidism* (Chapter 24), tachycardia, palpitations, and cardiomegaly are common; supraventricular arrhythmias occasionally appear. Cardiac failure occurs uncommonly, usually in the elderly superimposed on other cardiac diseases. In *hypothyroidism* (Chapter 24), cardiac output is decreased, with reduced stroke volume and heart rate. Increased peripheral vascular resistance and decreased blood volume result in narrowing of the pulse pressure, prolongation of circulation time, and decreased flow to peripheral tissues. Reduced circulation in the skin accounts for the characteristic cold sensitivity.

Morphology. In hyperthyroidism, the gross and histologic features are those of nonspecific hypertrophy. In well-advanced hypothyroidism (myxedema), the heart is flabby, enlarged, and dilated. Histologic features of hypothyroidism include myofiber swelling with loss of striations and basophilic degeneration, accompanied by interstitial mucopolysaccharide-rich edema fluid. A similar fluid sometimes accumulates within the pericardial sac. The term **myxedema heart** has been applied to these changes.

Pericardial Disease

Pericardial lesions are almost always associated with disease in other portions of the heart or surrounding structures, or are secondary to a systemic disorder; isolated pericardial disease is unusual.

PERICARDIAL EFFUSION AND HEMOPERICARDIUM

Normally, there is about 30 to 50 mL of thin, clear, straw-colored fluid in the pericardial sac. Under various circumstances, the parietal pericardium undergoes distention by fluid of variable composition *(pericardial effusion)*, blood (hemopericardium), or pus (purulent pericarditis). The consequences depend on the ability of the parietal pericardium to stretch, based on the speed of accumulation and the amount of fluid. Thus, with slowly accumulating effusions of less than 500 mL, the only clinical significance is a characteristic globular enlargement of the heart shadow noted on chest x-ray. In contrast, rapidly developing fluid collections of as little as 200 to 300 mL—for example, in the hemopericardium caused by ruptured MI, traumatic perforation, infective endocarditis, or ruptured aortic dissection—may produce compression of the thin-walled atria and venae cavae, or the ventricles themselves. As a consequence, cardiac filling is restricted, producing potentially fatal *cardiac tamponade.*

PERICARDITIS

Pericardial inflammation is usually secondary to a variety of cardiac diseases, thoracic or systemic disorders, metastases from neoplasms arising in remote sites, or a surgical procedure on the heart. Primary pericarditis is unusual and almost always of viral origin. The major causes of pericarditis are listed in Table 12–13. Most evoke an acute pericarditis, but a few, such as tuberculosis and fungi, produce chronic reactions. Since it is often impossible from pathologic examination to determine the etiologic basis for the reaction, a morphologic classification follows.

Acute Pericarditis

Serous Pericarditis. Serous inflammatory exudates are characteristically produced by noninfectious inflammations, such as RF, SLE, scleroderma, tumors, and uremia. An infection in the tissues contiguous to the pericardium, for example, a bacterial pleuritis, may cause sufficient irritation of the parietal pericardial serosa to cause a sterile serous effusion that may progress to serofibrinous pericarditis and ultimately to a frank suppurative reaction. In some instances, a well-defined viral infection elsewhere—upper respiratory tract infection, pneumonia, parotitis—antedates the pericarditis and serves as the primary focus of infection. Infrequently, usually in young adults, a viral pericarditis occurs as an apparent primary involvement that may accompany myocarditis *(myopericarditis).*

TABLE 12–13 Causes of Pericarditis

Infectious Agents
Viruses
Pyogenic bacteria
Tuberculosis
Fungi
Other parasites
Presumably Immunologically Mediated
Rheumatic fever
Systemic lupus erythematosus
Scleroderma
Postcardiotomy
Postmyocardial infarction (Dressler) syndrome
Drug hypersensitivity reaction
Miscellaneous
Myocardial infarction
Uremia
Following cardiac surgery
Neoplasia
Trauma
Radiation

Morphology. Whatever the cause, there is an inflammatory reaction in the epicardial and pericardial surfaces with scant numbers of polymorphonuclear leukocytes, lymphocytes, and macrophages. Usually the volume of fluid is not large (50 to 200 mL) and accumulates slowly. Dilation and increased permeability of the vessels due to inflammation produces a fluid of high specific gravity and rich protein content. A mild inflammatory infiltrate in the epipericardial fat consisting predominantly of lymphocytes is frequently termed chronic pericarditis. Organization into fibrous adhesions rarely occurs.

Fibrinous and Serofibrinous Pericarditis. These two anatomic forms are *the most frequent type of pericarditis* and are composed of serous fluid mixed with a fibrinous exudate. Common causes include acute MI (recall Fig. 12–19D), the postinfarction (Dressler) syndrome (likely an autoimmune condition appearing several weeks after a MI), uremia, chest radiation, RF, SLE, and trauma. A fibrinous reaction also follows routine cardiac surgery.

Morphology. In fibrinous pericarditis, the surface is dry, with a fine granular roughening. In serofibrinous pericarditis, an increased inflammatory process induces more and thicker fluid, which is yellow and cloudy owing to leukocytes and erythrocytes (which may be sufficient to give a visibly bloody appearance), and often fibrin. As with all inflammatory exudates, **fibrin may be digested with resolution of the exudate** or **it may become organized** (see Chapter 3).

From the clinical standpoint, *the development of a loud pericardial friction rub is the most striking characteristic of fibrinous pericarditis,* and pain, systemic febrile reactions, and signs suggestive of cardiac failure may be present. However, a collection of serous fluid may obliterate the rub by separating the two layers of the pericardium.

Purulent or Suppurative Pericarditis. This almost invariably denotes the invasion of the pericardial space by infective organisms, which may reach the pericardial cavity by several routes: (1) direct extension from neighboring inflammation, such as an empyema of the pleural cavity, lobar pneumonia, mediastinal infections, or extension of a ring abscess through the myocardium or aortic root in infective endocarditis; (2) seeding from the blood; (3) lymphatic extension; or (4) direct introduction during cardiotomy. Immunosuppression predisposes to infection by all of these pathways.

Morphology. The exudate ranges from a thin to a creamy pus of up to 400 to 500 mL in volume. The serosal surfaces are reddened, granular, and coated with the exudate (Fig. 12–37). Microscopically there is an acute inflammatory reaction. Sometimes the inflammatory process extends into surrounding structures to induce a so-called **mediastinopericarditis.** Organization is the usual outcome; resolution is infrequent. Because of the great intensity of the inflammatory response, the organization frequently produces **constrictive pericarditis**, a serious consequence (see later).

The clinical findings in the active phase are essentially the same as those present in fibrinous pericarditis, but signs of systemic infection are usually marked: for example, spiking temperatures, chills, and fever.

Hemorrhagic Pericarditis. An exudate composed of blood mixed with a fibrinous or suppurative effusion is most commonly caused by malignant neoplastic involvement of the pericardial space; in such cases, cytologic examination of fluid removed through a pericardial tap may yield neoplastic cells. Hemorrhagic pericarditis may also be found in bacterial infections, in patients with an underlying bleeding diathesis, and in tuberculosis. Hemorrhagic pericarditis often follows cardiac surgery and sometimes is responsible for significant blood loss or even tamponade, requiring a "second-look" operation. The clinical significance is similar to that of the spectrum of fibrinous or suppurative pericarditis.

Caseous Pericarditis. Caseation within the pericardial sac is, until proved otherwise, tuberculous in origin; infrequently, fungal infections evoke a similar reaction. Pericardial involvement occurs by direct spread from tuberculous foci within the tracheobronchial nodes. Caseous pericarditis is rare but is the most frequent antecedent of disabling, fibrocalcific, chronic constrictive pericarditis.

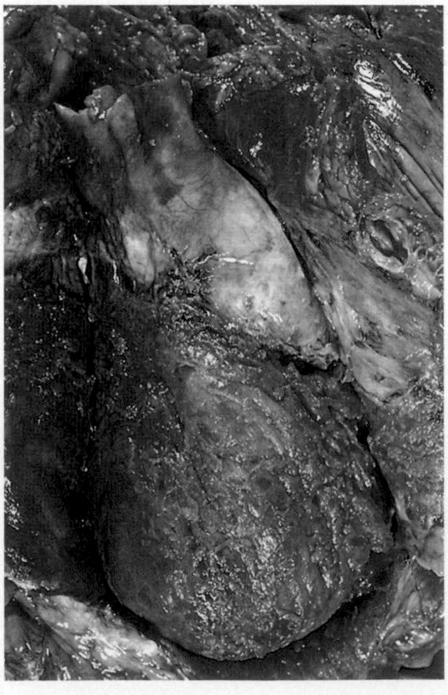

FIGURE 12–37 Acute suppurative pericarditis as an extension from a pneumonia. Extensive purulent exudate is evident in this in situ photograph.

Chronic or Healed Pericarditis

In some cases, organization merely produces plaque-like fibrous thickenings of the serosal membranes ("soldier's plaque") or thin, delicate adhesions of obscure origin that are observed fairly frequently at autopsy and rarely cause impairment of cardiac function. In other cases, organization results in complete obliteration of the pericardial sac. This fibrosis yields a delicate, stringy type of adhesion between parietal and visceral pericardium called *adhesive pericarditis,* which by itself rarely hampers or restricts cardiac action.

Adhesive Mediastinopericarditis. This form of pericardial fibrosis may follow a suppurative or caseous pericarditis, previous cardiac surgery, or irradiation to the mediastinum. The pericardial sac is obliterated, and adherence of the external aspect of the parietal layer to surrounding structures produces a great strain on cardiac function. With each systolic contraction, the heart is pulling not only against the parietal pericardium, but also against the attached surrounding structures. Systolic retraction of the rib cage and diaphragm, pulsus paradoxus, and a variety of other characteristic clinical findings may be observed. *The increased workload causes cardiac hypertrophy and dilation, which may be quite massive in more severe cases, mimicking DCM* (see earlier).

Constrictive Pericarditis. The heart may be encased in a dense, fibrous or fibrocalcific scar that limits diastolic expansion and seriously restricts cardiac output, resembling restrictive cardiomyopathy. A well-defined history of previous pericarditis may or may not be present. In constrictive pericarditis, the pericardial space is obliterated, and the heart is surrounded by a dense, adherent layer of scar with or without calcification, often 0.5 to 1.0 cm thick, that can resemble a plaster mold in extreme cases *(concretio cordis).*

Although the signs of cardiac failure may resemble those produced by adhesive mediastinopericarditis, cardiac hypertrophy and dilation cannot occur because of the dense enclosing scar, and the heart is consequently quiet with reduced output. The major therapy is surgical removal of the shell of constricting fibrous tissue (pericardiectomy).

RHEUMATOID HEART DISEASE

Rheumatoid arthritis is mainly a disorder of the joints, but it is also associated with many nonarticular involvements (e.g., subcutaneous rheumatoid nodules, acute vasculitis, and Felty syndrome; see Chapter 26). The heart is also involved in 20% to 40% of cases of severe prolonged rheumatoid arthritis. The most common finding is a *fibrinous pericarditis* that may progress to fibrous thickening of the visceral and parietal pericardium with dense fibrous adhesions. Rheumatoid inflammatory granulomatous nodules resembling those that occur subcutaneously may also be identifiable in the myocardium. Much less frequently, rheumatoid nodules involve endocardium, valves of the heart, and root of the aorta. *Rheumatoid valvulitis* can lead to marked fibrous thickening and secondary calcification of the aortic valve cusps, producing changes resembling those of chronic rheumatic valvular disease, but intercommissural adhesion is rarely present.

Tumors of the Heart

Primary tumors of the heart are rare; in contrast, metastatic tumors to the heart occur in about 5% of patients dying of cancer. The most common primary tumors, in descending order of frequency (overall, including adults and children), are myxomas, fibromas, lipomas, papillary fibroelastomas, rhabdomyomas, angiosarcomas, and other sarcomas. The five most common tumors are all benign and collectively account for 80% to 90% of primary tumors of the heart.[125]

PRIMARY CARDIAC TUMORS

Myxoma

Myxomas are the most common primary tumor of the heart in adults (Fig. 12–38).[126] Although they may arise in any of the four chambers or, rarely, on the heart valves, about 90% are located in the atria, with a left-to-right ratio of approximately 4:1 *(atrial myxomas).*

It has long been questioned whether cardiac myxomas are truly neoplastic lesions, hamartomas, or organized thrombi, but the weight of evidence is on the side of benign neoplasia. All the tumor cell types present are thought to derive from differentiation of primitive multipotential mesenchymal cells.

Morphology. The tumors are almost always single, but rarely several occur simultaneously. The region of the fossa ovalis in the atrial septum is the favored site of origin. Myxomas range from small (less than 1 cm) to large (up to 10 cm), sessile or pedunculated masses (Fig. 12–38*A*) that vary from globular hard masses mottled with hemorrhage to soft, translucent, papillary, or villous lesions having a gelatinous appearance. The pedunculated form is frequently sufficiently mobile to move into or sometimes through the AV valves during systole, causing intermittent and often position-dependent obstruction. Sometimes, such mobility exerts a "wrecking-ball" effect, causing damage to the valve leaflets.

Histologically, myxomas are composed of stellate or globular myxoma ("lepidic") cells, endothelial cells, smooth muscle cells, and undifferentiated cells embedded within an abundant acid mucopolysaccharide ground substance and covered on the surface by endothelium (Fig. 12–38*B*). Peculiar structures that variably resemble poorly formed glands or vessels are characteristic. Hemorrhage and mononuclear inflammation are usually present.

The major clinical manifestations are due to valvular "ball-valve" obstruction, embolization, or a syndrome of constitutional symptoms, such as fever and malaise. Sometimes fragmentation with systemic embolization calls attention to these lesions. Constitutional symptoms are likely due to the elaboration by some myxomas of the cytokine interleukin-6, a major mediator of the acute phase response. Echocardiography provides the opportunity to identify these masses noninvasively. Surgical removal is usually curative, although rarely, the neoplasm recurs months to years later.

Approximately 10% of patients with myxoma have a familial cardiac myxoma syndrome (known as *Carney syndrome*) characterized by autosomal dominant transmission, multiple cardiac and often extracardiac (e.g., skin) myxomas, spotty pigmentation, and endocrine overactivity. A careful history and physical examination in patients with cardiac myxoma is

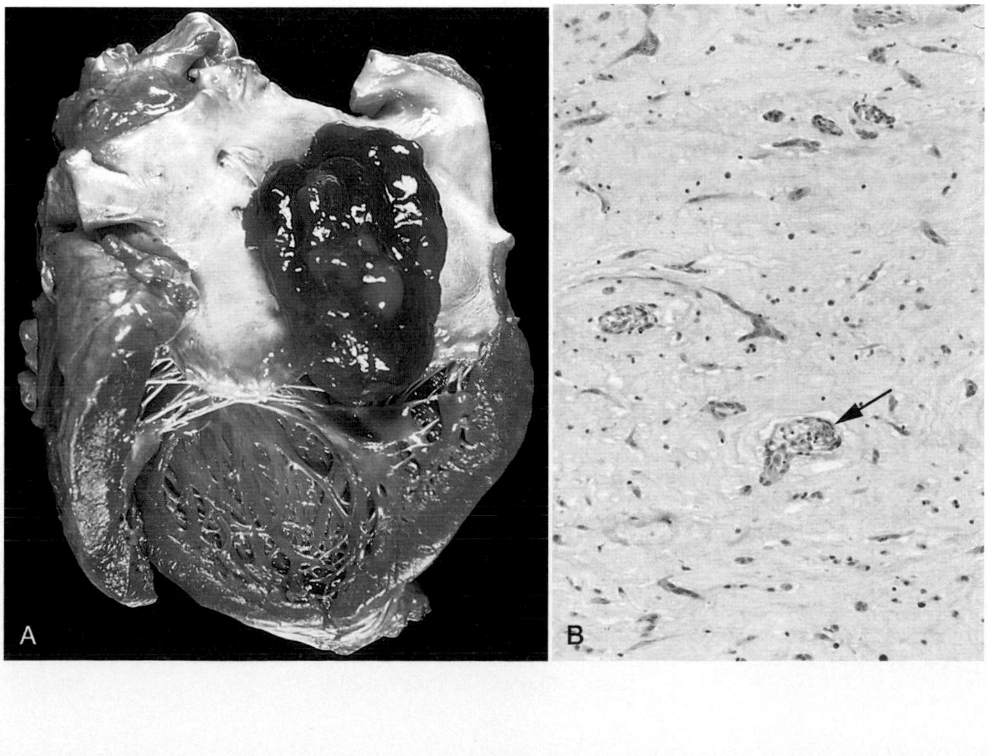

FIGURE 12–38 Left atrial myxoma. *A,* Gross photograph showing large pedunculated lesion arising from the region of the fossa ovalis and extending into the mitral valve orifice. *B,* Microscopic appearance, with abundant amorphous extracellular matrix in which are scattered collections of myxoma cells in various groupings, including abnormal vascular formations *(arrow).*

important to identify other signs of the Carney complex, as this diagnosis carries implications for family members of the patient. The gene *PRKAR1* on chromosome 17 (encoding a regulatory subunit of cAMP-dependent protein kinase A, possibly a tumor suppressor gene) is mutated in about half of known Carney complex kindreds, while most of the other kindreds have abnormalities in the locus 2p16.[127]

Lipoma

Lipomas (excessive fat accumulations) may occur in the subendocardium or in the subepicardium, or within the myocardium, as localized, poorly encapsulated masses, which may be asymptomatic, can create ball-valve obstructions as with myxomas, or may produce arrhythmias. Lipomas are most often located in the left ventricle, right atrium, or atrial septum and are not necessarily neoplastic. In the atrial septum, non-neoplastic depositions of fat are called "lipomatous hypertrophy."

Papillary Fibroelastoma

Papillary fibroelastomas are curious, usually incidental, lesions, most often identified at autopsy. They may embolize and become clinically important. Although these masses are called neoplasms, it is possible that at least some fibroelastomas represent organized thrombi. Fibroelastomas resemble the much smaller, usually trivial, *Lambl excrescences* that are frequently found on the aortic valves of older individuals.

Morphology. Papillary fibroelastomas are generally located on valves, particularly the ventricular surfaces of semilunar valves and the atrial surfaces of AV valves. They constitute a distinctive cluster of hair-like projections up to 1 cm in diameter, covering up to several centimeters in diameter of the endocardial surface. Histologically, they are covered by endothelium, deep to which is myxoid connective tissue containing abundant mucopolysaccharide matrix and elastic fibers.

Rhabdomyoma

Rhabdomyomas are the most frequent primary tumor of the heart in infants and children and are frequently discovered in the first years of life because of obstruction of a valvular orifice or cardiac chamber. That rhabdomyomas are hamartomas or malformations rather than true neoplasms is supported by a high frequency of tuberous sclerosis (see Chapter 28) in patients with cardiac rhabdomyomas. A recent study suggested that cardiac rhabdomyomas may be due to a defect in apoptosis during developmental cardiac remodeling.[128]

Morphology. Rhabdomyomas are generally small, gray-white myocardial masses up to several centimeters in diameter located on either the left or the right side of the heart and protruding into the ventricular chambers. Histologically they are composed of a mixed population of cells, the most characteristic of which are large, rounded, or polygonal cells containing numerous glycogen-laden vacuoles separated by strands of cytoplasm running from the plasma membrane to the more or less centrally located nucleus, the so-called **spider cells**. These cells can be shown to have myofibrils.

Sarcoma

Cardiac *angiosarcomas* and other sarcomas are not clinically or morphologically distinctive from their counterparts in other locations (Fig. 11–34 and Chapter 26) and so require no further comment here.

CARDIAC EFFECTS OF NONCARDIAC NEOPLASMS

With enhanced patient survival due to diagnostic and therapeutic advances, significant cardiovascular effects of noncardiac neoplasms and their therapy are now commonly encountered (Table 12–14). Pathology derives from infiltration of tumor tissue, circulating mediators, or tumor therapy.

The most frequent tumors involving the heart as metastases are carcinomas of the lung and breast, melanomas, leukemias, and lymphomas. Metastases can reach the heart and pericardium by retrograde lymphatic extension (most carcinomas), by hematogenous seeding (many tumors), by direct contiguous extension (primary carcinoma of the lung, breast, or esophagus), or by direct contiguous venous extension (tumors of the kidney or liver). Clinical symptoms are most often associated with pericardial spread, by either a pericardial effusion that causes tamponade or by tumor bulk that is sufficient to directly restrict cardiac filling. Myocardial metastases are usually clinically silent or have nonspecific features, such as a generalized defect in ventricular contractility or

TABLE 12–14 Cardiovascular Effects of Noncardiac Neoplasms

Direct Consequences of Tumor
Pericardial and myocardial metastases
Large vessel obstruction
Pulmonary tumor emboli
Indirect Consequences of Tumor (Complications of Circulating Mediators)
Nonbacterial thrombotic endocarditis (NBTE)
Carcinoid heart disease
Pheochromocytoma-associated heart disease
Myeloma-associated amyloidosis
Effects of Tumor Therapy
Chemotherapy
Radiation therapy

Modified from Schoen, FJ, et al: Cardiac effects of non-cardiac neoplasms. Cardiol Clin 2:657, 1984.

compliance. Bronchogenic carcinoma or malignant lymphoma may infiltrate the mediastinum extensively, causing encasement, compression, or invasion of the superior vena cava with resultant obstruction to blood coming from the head and upper extremities *(superior vena cava syndrome)*. Renal cell carcinoma, because of its high propensity to invade the renal vein, can grow in the lumen of the renal vein into and along the inferior vena cava and can, occasionally, extend into the right atrium, blocking venous return to the heart.

Noncardiac tumors cause indirect cardiac effects, sometimes via circulating tumor-derived substances (e.g., NBTE [see earlier], carcinoid heart disease, pheochromocytoma-associated myocardial damage, multiple myeloma–derived immunoglobulin-causing amyloidosis). Complications of chemotherapy were discussed earlier in this chapter. Radiation used to treat breast, lung, or mediastinal neoplasms can cause pericarditis, pericardial effusion, myocardial fibrosis, and chronic pericardial disorders. Other cardiac effects of radiotherapy include accelerated coronary artery disease and mural and valvular endocardial fibrosis.

Cardiac Transplantation

Transplantation of cardiac allografts is now frequently performed (approximately 3000 per year worldwide) for severe, intractable heart failure of diverse causes, the two most common of which are DCM and IHD. Three major factors contribute to the widespread success of cardiac transplantation since the first successful human to human transplant in 1967: (1) careful selection of candidates, (2) improved maintenance (including the use of cyclosporin A, along with steroids and other drugs), and (3) early histopathologic diagnosis of acute allograft rejection by sequential endomyocardial biopsy.[129]

Of the major complications (illustrated in Fig. 12–39), allograft rejection is the primary problem requiring surveillance; scheduled endomyocardial biopsy is the only reliable means of diagnosing acute cardiac rejection before substantial myocardial damage (and clinical recognition) has occurred and at a stage that is reversible in the majority of instances. Rejection is characterized by interstitial lymphocytic inflammation that, in its more advanced stages, damages adjacent myocytes (see Fig. 12-39*A*). When myocardial injury is not extensive, the "rejection episode" is usually either self-limited or successfully reversed by increased immunosuppressive therapy. Advanced rejection may be irreversible and fatal when not properly treated.

The major current limitation to the long-term success of cardiac transplantation is late, progressive, diffuse stenosing intimal proliferation of the coronary arteries *(graft arteriopathy)* (Fig. 12–39*B*). This is a particularly vexing problem because it may lead to silent MI (especially difficult to diagnose because these patients, with denervated hearts, do not experience chest pain); in this situation, CHF or sudden death is the usual outcome. The mechanism of formation of these diffuse arterial lesions is uncertain. However, it is clear that low-level, chronic immunologic responses induce inflammatory cells and vascular wall cells to secrete growth factors that promote intimal smooth muscle cell recruitment and proliferation, and synthesis of extracellular matrix, thereby expanding the intima.[130] Other postoperative problems include infection and development of malignancies, particularly lymphomas (generally related to Epstein-Barr virus in the presence of profound chronic therapeutic immunosuppression). Despite these problems, the outlook is good, with a 1-year survival of 70% to 80% and 5-year survival of more than 60%.

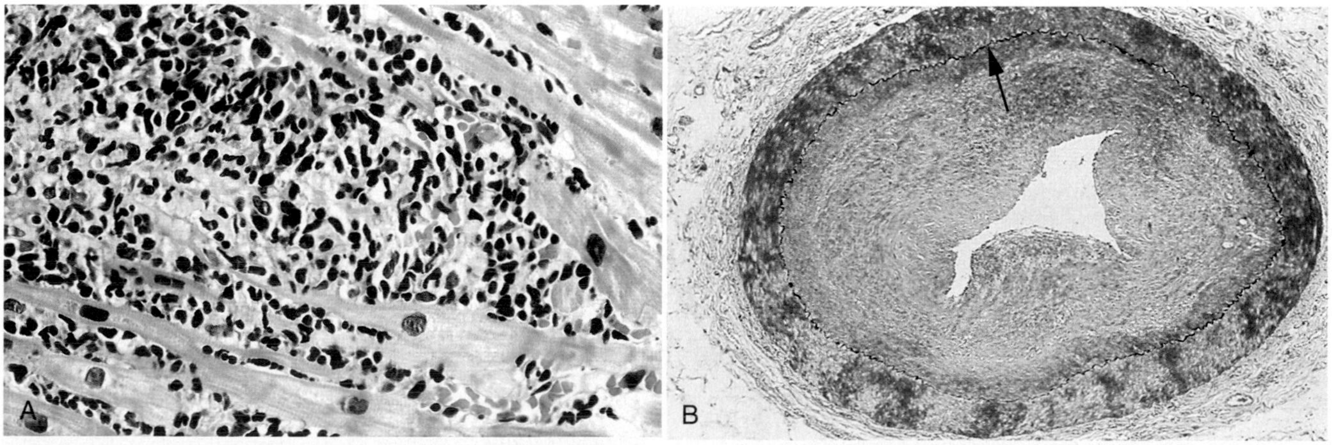

FIGURE 12–39 Complications of heart transplantation. *A,* Cardiac allograft rejection typified by lymphocytic infiltrate, with associated damage to cardiac myocytes. *B,* Graft coronary arteriosclerosis, demonstrating severe diffuse concentric intimal thickening producing critical stenosis. The internal elastic lamina *(arrow)* and media are intact (Movat pentachrome stain, elastin black). (*B,* reproduced by permission from Salomon RN, et al: Human coronary transplantation-associated arteriosclerosis. Evidence for chronic immune reaction to activated graft endothelial cells. Am J Pathol 138:791, 1991.)

REFERENCES

1. Sagnella GA: Practical implications of current natriuretic peptide research. J Renin Angioten Aldost Syst 1:304, 2000.
2. Maisel AS, et al: Rapid measurement of B-type natriuretic peptide in the emergency diagnosis of heart failure. N Engl J Med 347:161, 2002.
3. Lerner DL, et al: The role of altered intercellular coupling in arrhythmias induced by acute myocardial ischemia. Cardiovasc Res 50:263, 2001.
4. Schoen FJ: Aortic valve structure–function correlations: role of elastic fibers no longer a stretch of the imagination. J Heart Valve Dis 6:1, 1997.
5. Duncan AK, et al: Cardiovascular disease in elderly patients. Mayo Clin Proc 71:184, 1996.
6. Braunwald E, Zipes DP, Libby P (eds): Heart Disease. A Textbook of Cardiovascular Medicine, 6th ed. Philadelphia, WB Saunders Co., 2001.
7. Silver, MD, Gotlieb AI, Schoen FJ (eds): Cardiovascular Pathology, 3rd ed. New York, Churchill Livingstone, 2001.
8. Chien KR: Genomic circuits and the integrative biology of cardiac diseases. Nature 407:227, 2000.
9. Hoshijima M, Chien KR: Mixed signals in heart failure: cancer rules. J Clin Invest 109:849, 2002.
10. Cohn JN, et al: Report of the National Heart, Lung, and Blood Institute Special Emphasis Panel on Heart Research. Circulation 95:766, 1997.
11. Lorell BH, Carabello BA: Left ventricular hypertrophy: pathogenesis, detection, and prognosis. Circulation 102:470, 2000.
12. Zile MR, Brutsaert DL: New concepts in diastolic dysfunction and diastolic heart failure. Parts I and II. Circulation 105:1387, 1503, 2002.
13. Francis GS: Pathophysiology of chronic heart failure. Am J Med 110:37S, 2001.
14. Rose EA, et al: Long-term mechanical left ventricular assistance for end-stage heart failure. N Engl J Med 345:1435, 2001.
15. Pasumarthi KBS, Field LJ: Cardiomyocyte cell cycle regulation. Circ Res 90:1044, 2002.
16. Johnatty SE, et al: Identification of genes regulated during mechanical load–induced cardiac hypertrophy. J Mol Cell Cardiol 32:805, 2000.
17. Razeghi P, et al: Metabolic gene expression in fetal and failing human heart. Circulation 104:2923, 2001.
18. MacLellan WR: Advances in the molecular mechanisms of heart failure. Curr Opin Cardiol 15:128, 2000.
19. Frey N, et al: Decoding calcium signals involved in cardiac growth and function. Nature Med 6:1221, 2000.
20. Kang PM, Izumo S: Apoptosis and heart failure: a critical review of the literature. Circ Res 86:1107, 2000.
21. Levy D, et al: Prognostic implications of echocardiographically determined left ventricular mass in the Framingham Heart Study. N Engl J Med 322:1561, 1990.
22. Hart RG, Halperin JL: Atrial fibrillation and stroke: concepts and controversies. Stroke 32:803, 2001.
23. Webb CL, et al: Collaborative care for adults with congenital heart disease. Circulation 105:2318, 2002.
24. Schoen FJ, Edwards WD: Pathology of cardiovascular interventions, including endovascular therapies, revascularization, vascular replacement, cardiac assist/replacement, arrhythmia control and repaired congenital heart disease. In Silver MD, Gotlieb AI, Schoen FJ (eds): Cardiovascular Pathology. Philadelphia, Churchill Livingstone, 2001, p 678–721.
25. Fleming A, Copp AJ: Embryonic folate metabolism and mouse neural tube defects. Science 280:2107, 1998.
26. Olson EN, Schneider MD: Sizing up the heart: development REDUX in disease. Genes Dev 17: 1937, 2003.
27. Yelon D: Cardiac patterning and morphogenesis in zebrafish. Dev Dyn 222:552, 2001.
28. Chen J-N, Fishman MC: Genetics of heart development. Trends Genetics 16:383, 2000.
29. Srivastava D: Genetic assembly of the heart: implications for congenital heart disease. Ann Rev Physiol 63:452, 2001.
30. Vaughn CJ, Basson CT: Molecular determinants of atrial and ventricular septal defects and patent ductus arteriosus. Am J Med Genetics (Sem Med Genet) 97:304, 2001.
31. Cripps RM, Olson EN: Control of cardiac development by an evolutionarily conserved transcriptional network. Dev Biol 246:14, 2002.
32. Milewicz DM, Seidman CE: Genetics of cardiovascular disease. Circulation 102:IV–103, 2000.
33. Manson JE, et al: The primary prevention of myocardial infarction. N Engl J Med 326:1406, 1992.
34. Rich Edwards JW, et al: The primary prevention of coronary heart disease in women. N Engl J Med 332:1758, 1995.
35. Braunwald E: Cardiovascular medicine at the turn of the millennium: triumphs, concerns, and opportunities. N Engl J Med 337:1360, 1997.
36. Hunink MG, et al: The recent decline in mortality from coronary heart disease, 1980–1990. The effect of secular trends in risk factors and treatment. J Am Med Assoc 277:535, 1997.
37. Lauer MS: Aspirin for primary prevention of coronary events. New Engl J Med 346:1468, 2002.
38. Libby P: Current concepts of the pathogenesis of the acute coronary syndromes. Circulation 104:365, 2001.
39. Fuster V, et al: 27th Bethesda Conference: Matching the intensity of risk factor management with the hazard for coronary disease events. Task Force 1. Pathogenesis of coronary disease: the biologic role of risk factors. J Am Coll Cardiol 27:964, 1996.
40. Yeghiazarians Y, et al: Unstable angina pectoris. New Engl J Med 342:101, 2000.
41. Willich SN: Circadian variation and triggering of cardiovascular events. Vasc Med 4:41, 1999.
42. Muller JE: Circadian variation in cardiovascular events. Am J Hyperten 12:35S, 1999.
43. Ambrose JA, Martinez EE: A new paradigm for plaque stabilization. Circulation 105:2000, 2002.
44. Leor J, et al: Sudden cardiac death triggered by an earthquake. N Engl J Med 334:413, 1996.
45. Falk E, et al: Coronary plaque disruption. Circulation 92:657, 1995.
46. Ross R: Atherosclerosis: an inflammatory disease. N Engl J Med 340:115, 1999.
47. Libby P, Ridker PM, Maseri A: Inflammation and atherosclerosis. Circulation 105:1135, 2002.
48. Plutzky J: Inflammatory pathways in atherosclerosis and acute coronary syndromes. Am J Cardiol 88:10K, 2001.
49. Blake GJ, Ridker P: C-reactive protein: a surrogate risk marker or mediator of atherothrombosis? Am J Physiol Reg Integr Comp Physiol 285:R1252, 2003.
50. Ridker PM, Morrow DA: C-reactive protein, inflammation and coronary risk. Cardiol Clin 21:315, 2003.
51. Ridker PM, Rifai N, Rose L, Buring JE, Cook NR: Comparison of C-reactive protein and low-density lipoprotein cholesterol levels in the prediction of first cardiovascular events. N Engl J Med 348:1059, 2002.
52. Torres JL, Ridker PM: Clinical use of high sensitivity C-reactive protein for the prediction of adverse cardiovascular events. Curr Opin Cardiol 18:471, 2003.

52a. Tall AR: C-reactive protein reassessed. N Engl J Med 350:1450, 2004.

53. Manson JE, Martin KA: Postmenopausal hormone-replacement therapy. N Engl J Med 345:34, 2001.
54. DeWood MA, et al: Prevalence of total coronary occlusion during the early hours of transmural myocardial infarction. N Engl J Med 303:897, 1980.
55. Jennings RB, et al: Development of cell injury in sustained acute ischemia. Circulation 82:II–2, 1990.
56. Huikuri HV, et al: Sudden death due to cardiac arrhythmias. N Engl J Med 345:1473, 2001.
57. Vargas SO, et al: Pathologic detection of early myocardial infarction: a critical review of the evolution and usefulness of modern techniques. Mod Pathol 12:635, 1999.
58. Huber K, Maurer G: Thrombolytic therapy in acute myocardial infarction. Semin Thromb Hemost 22:15, 1996.
59. Bittl JA: Advances in coronary angioplasty. N Engl J Med 335:1290, 1996.
60. Hansen PR: Role of neutrophils in myocardial ischemia and reperfusion. Circulation 91:1872, 1995.
61. Verma S, et al: Fundamentals of reperfusion injury for the clinical cardiologist. Circulation 105:2332, 2002.
62. Yellon DM, Baxter GF: Protecting the ischemic and reperfused myocardium in acute myocardial infarction: distant dream or near reality? Heart 83:381, 2000.

63. Kloner RA, Jennings RB: Consequences of brief ischemia: stunning, preconditioning, and their clinical implications. Parts I and II. Circulation 104:2981, 3158, 2001.
64. Wijns W, et al: Hibernating myocardium. N Engl J Med 339:173, 1998.
65. Wagner GS, et al: Moving toward a new definition of acute myocardial infarction for the 21st century: status of the ESC/ACC consensus conference. European Society of Cardiology and American College of Cardiology. J Electrocardiol 33:57, 2000.
66. Birnbaum Y, et al: Ventricular septal rupture after acute myocardial infarction. N Engl J Med 347:1426, 2002.
67. St. John Sutton MG, Sharpe N: Left ventricular remodeling after myocardial infarction. Pathophysiology and therapy. Circulation 101:2981, 2000.
68. Cohn JN, et al: Cardiac remodeling—Concepts and clinical implications: a consensus paper from an international forum on cardiac remodeling. J Am Coll Cardiol 35:569, 2000.
69. Anversa P, Nadal-Ginard B: Myocyte renewal and ventricular remodelling. Nature 415:240, 2002.
70. Liberthson RR: Sudden death from cardiac causes in children and young adults. N Engl J Med 334:1039, 1996.
71. Futterman LG, Myerburg R: Sudden death in athletes: an update. Sports Med 26:335, 1998.
72. Bigger JT: Expanding indications for implantable cardiac defibrillators. N Engl J Med 346:931, 2002.
73 Roberts R, Brugada R: Genetic aspects of arrhythmias. Am J Med Gen 97:310, 2000.
74. Varagic J, Susic D, Frohlich E: Heart, aging, and hypertension. Curr Opin Cardiol 16:336, 2001.
75. Kannel WB: Blood pressure as a cardiovascular risk factor. Prevention and treatment. JAMA 275:1571, 1996.
76. Bonow RO, et al: ACC/AHA Guidelines for the Management of Patients with Valvular Heart Disease. Executive Summary. A report of the American College of Cardiology/American Heart Association Task Force on Practice Guidelines (Committee on Management of Patients with Valvular Disease). J Heart Valve Dis 7:672, 1998.
77. Carabello BA: Aortic stenosis. N Engl J Med 346:677, 2002.
78. Hoffman JIE, Kaplan S: The incidence of congenital heart disease. J Am Coll Cardiol 39:1890, 2002.
79. Sabet HY, et al: Congenitally bicuspid aortic valves: a surgical pathology study of 542 cases (1991 through 1996) and a literature review of 2,715 additional cases. Mayo Clin Proc 74:14, 1999.
80. Rabkin E, et al: Activated interstitial myofibroblasts express catabolic enzymes and mediate matrix remodeling in myxomatous heart valves. Circulation 104:2525, 2001.
81. Zuppiroli A, et al: Natural history of mitral valve prolapse. Am J Cardiol 75:1028, 1995.
82. Stollerman GH: Rheumatic fever in the 21st century. Clin Infect Dis 33:806, 2001.
83. Veasy LG, Hill HR: Immunologic and clinical correlations in rheumatic fever and rheumatic heart disease. Pediatr Infect Dis J 16:400, 1997.
84. Mylonakis E, Calderwood SB: Infective endocarditis in adults. N Engl J Med 345:1318, 2001.
85. Dajani AS, et al: Prevention of bacterial endocarditis. Recommendations by the American Heart Association. Circulation 96:358, 1997.
86. Durack DT, et al: New criteria for diagnosis of infective endocarditis: utilization of specific echocardiographic findings. Am J Med 96:200, 1994.
87. Hojnik M, et al: Heart valve involvement (Libman-Sacks endocarditis) in the antiphospholipid syndrome. Circulation 93:1579, 1996.
88. Levine JS, et al: The antiphospholipid syndrome. N Engl J Med 346:752, 2002.
89. Simula DV, et al: Surgical pathology of cardinoid heart disease: a study of 139 valves from 75 patients spanning 20 years. Mayo Clin Proc 77:139, 2002.
90. Robiolio PA, et al: Carcinoid heart disease: correlation of high serotonin levels with valvular abnormalities detected by cardiac catheterization and echocardiography. Circulation 92:790, 1995.
91. Connolly HM, et al: Fenfluramine–phentermine associated valvular heart disease: a new observation. N Engl J Med 337:581, 1997.
92. Vongpatanasin W, et al: Prosthetic heart valves. N Engl J Med 355:407, 1996.
93. Schoen FJ: Pathology of heart valve substitution with mechanical and tissue prostheses. In Silver MD, Gotlieb AI, Schoen FJ (eds), Cardiovascular Pathology, 3rd ed. Philadelphia, Churchill Livingstone, 2001, p 629–677.
94. Hammermeister K, et al: Outcomes 15 years after valve replacement with a mechanical versus a bioprosthetic valve: final report of the Veterans Affairs randomized trial. J Am Coll Cardiol 36:1152, 2000.
95. Richardson P, et al: Report of the 1995 World Health Organization/International Society and Federation of Cardiology Task Force on the definition and classification of cardiomyopathies. Circulation 93:841, 1996.
96. Roberts R, Schwartz K: Myocardial disease. Circulation 102:IV–34, 2000.
97. Franz WM, et al: Cardiomyopathies: from genetics to the prospect of treatment. Lancet 358:1627, 2001.
98. Towbin JA, Bowles NE: The failing heart. Nature 415:227, 2002.
99. Veinot JP: Diagnostic endomyocardial biopsy pathology—general biopsy considerations, and its use for myocarditis and cardiomyopathy: a review. Can J Cardiol 18:55, 2002.
100. Badorff C, et al: Enteroviral protease 2A cleaves dystrophin: evidence of cytoskeletal disruption in an acquired cardiomyopathy. Nature Med 5:320, 1999.
101. Vatta M, et al: Molecular remodelling of dystrophin in patients with end-stage cardiomyopathies and reversal on assistance-device therapy. Lancet 359:936, 2002.
102. Gemayel C, et al: Arrhythmogenic right ventricular cardiomyopathy. J Am Coll Cardiol 38:1773, 2001.
103. Thienne G, Basso C: Arrhythmogenic right ventricular cardiomyopathy: an update. Cardiovasc Pathol 10:109, 2001.
104. McKoy G, et al: Identification of a detection of phakaglobin in arrhythmic right ventricular cardiomyopathy with palm plantar keratoderma and wooly hair (Naxos disease). Lancet 355:2119, 2000.
105. Seidman JG, Seidman C: The genetic basis for cardiomyopathy: from mutation identification to mechanistic paradigms. Cell 104:557, 2001.
106. Roberts R, Sigwart U: New concepts in hypertrophic cardiomyopathies. Parts I and II. Circulation 104:2113, 2249, 2001.
107. Maron BJ: Hypertrophic cardiomyopathy. JAMA 287:1308, 2002.
108. Marian AJ: Pathogenesis of diverse clinical and pathological phenotypes in hypertrophic cardiomyopathy. Lancet 355:58, 2000.
109. Kushwaha SS, et al: Restrictive cardiomyopathy. N Engl J Med 335:267, 1997.
110. Feldman AM, McNamara D: Myocarditis. N Engl J Med 343:1388, 2000.
111. Winters GL, McManus BM: Myocarditis. In Silver MD, Gotlieb AI, Schoen FJ, (eds): Cardiovascular Pathology, 3rd ed. Philadelphia, Churchill Livingstone, 2001, p 256–284.
112. Huber SA: Autoimmunity in myocarditis: relevance of animal models. Clin Immunol Immunopathol 83:93, 1997.
113. Morris SA, et al: Pathophysiological insights into the cardiomyopathy of Chagas' disease. Circulation 82:1900, 1990.
114. Pinto DS: Cardiac manifestations of Lyme disease. Med Clin North Am 86:285, 2002.
115. Lewis W: Cardiomyopathy in AIDS: A pathophysiological perspective. Prog Cardiovasc Dis 43:151, 2000.
116. Rerkpattanapipat P, et al: Cardiac manifestations of acquired immunodeficiency syndrome. Arch Intern Med 160:602, 2000.
117. Cooper LT Jr, et al: Idiopathic giant cell myocarditis in natural history and treatment. Multicenter Giant Cell Myocarditis Study Group Investigators. N Engl J Med 336:1860, 1997.
118. Shan K, et al: Anthracycline-induced cardiotoxicity. Ann Intern Med 125:47, 1996.
119. Kloner RA, et al: The effects of acute and chronic cocaine use on the heart. Circulation 85:407, 1992.
120. Samuels MA: Neurally induced cardiac damage. Definition of the problem. Neurol Clin 11:273, 1993.
121. Falk RH, et al: The systemic amyloidoses. N Engl J Med 337:898, 1997.
122. McCarthy RE III, Kasper EK: A review of the amyloidoses that infiltrate the heart. Clin Cardiol 21:547, 1998.
123. Kyle RA, et al: The premortem recognition of systemic senile amyloidosis with cardiac involvement. Am J Med 171:395, 1996.
124. Jacobson DR, et al: Variant-sequence transthyretin (isoleucine 122) in late-onset cardiac amyloidosis in black Americans. N Engl J Med 336:466, 1997.
125. Tazelaar HD, et al: Pathology of surgically excised primary cardiac tumors. Mayo Clin Proc 67:957, 1992.

126. Reynen K: Cardiac myxomas. N Engl J Med 333:1610, 1995.
127. Vaughan CJ, et al: Tumors of the heart: molecular genetic advances. Curr Opin Cardiol 16:195, 2001.
128. Smith M, Sperling D: Novel 23-base-pair duplication mutation in TSCI exon 15 in an infant presenting with cardiac rhabdomyomas. Am J Med Gen 84:346, 1999.
129. Winters GL, Schoen FJ: Pathology of cardiac transplantation. In Silver MD, Gotlieb AI, Schoen FJ (eds): Cardiovascular Pathology. 3rd ed. Philadelphia, Churchill Livingstone, 2001, p 725–762.
130. Libby P, Pober JS: Chronic rejection. Immunity 14:387, 2001.

CHAPTER 13

Red Blood Cell and Bleeding Disorders

Jon C. Aster, MD, PhD

NORMAL DEVELOPMENT OF BLOOD CELLS

Origin and Differentiation of Hematopoietic Cells

ANEMIAS

Anemias of Blood Loss

Acute Blood Loss

Chronic Blood Loss

Hemolytic Anemias

Hereditary Spherocytosis (HS)

Hemolytic Disease Due to Red Cell Enzyme Defects: Glucose-6-Phosphate Dehydrogenase Deficiency

Sickle Cell Disease

Thalassemia Syndromes

Paroxysmal Nocturnal Hemoglobinuria

Immunohemolytic Anemia

Hemolytic Anemia Resulting from Trauma to Red Cells

Anemias of Diminished Erythropoiesis

Megaloblastic Anemias

Iron Deficiency Anemia

Anemia of Chronic Disease

Aplastic Anemia

Pure Red Cell Aplasia

Other Forms of Marrow Failure

POLYCYTHEMIA

BLEEDING DISORDERS: HEMORRHAGIC DIATHESES

Bleeding Disorders Caused by Vessel Wall Abnormalities

Bleeding Related to Reduced Platelet Number: Thrombocytopenia

Immune Thrombocytopenic Purpura (ITP)

Acute Immune Thrombocytopenic Purpura

Drug-Induced Thrombocytopenia: Heparin-Induced Thrombocytopenia

HIV-Associated Thrombocytopenia

Thrombotic Microangiopathies: Thrombotic Thrombocytopenic Purpura (TTP) and Hemolytic-Uremic Syndrome (HUS)

Bleeding Disorders Related to Defective Platelet Functions

Hemorrhagic Diatheses Related to Abnormalities in Clotting Factors

Deficiencies of Factor VIII–vWF Complex

Von Willebrand Disease

Hemophilia A (Factor VIII Deficiency)

Hemophilia B (Christmas Disease, Factor IX Deficiency)

Disseminated Intravascular Coagulation (DIC)

The organs and tissues involved in hematopoiesis have been traditionally divided into *myeloid tissue,* which includes the bone marrow and the cells derived from it (e.g., erythrocytes, platelets, granulocytes, and monocytes), and *lymphoid tissue,* consisting of thymus, lymph nodes, and spleen. This subdivision is artificial with respect to both the normal physiology of hematopoietic cells and the diseases affecting them. For example, although bone marrow is not where most mature lymphoid cells are found, it is the source of lymphoid stem cells. Similarly, myeloid leukemias, neoplastic disorders of myeloid stem cells, originate in the bone marrow but secondarily involve the spleen and (to a lesser degree) lymph nodes. Some red cell disorders (hemolytic anemias) result from the formation of autoantibodies, signifying a primary disorder of lymphocytes. Thus, it is not possible to draw neat lines between diseases involving the myeloid and lymphoid tissues. Recognizing this difficulty, we somewhat arbitrarily divide diseases of the hematopoietic tissues into two chapters. In the first, we consider diseases of red cells and those affecting hemostasis. In the second, we discuss white cell diseases and disorders affecting primarily the spleen and thymus.

NORMAL

A complete discussion of normal hematopoiesis is beyond our scope, but certain features are helpful to an understanding of the diseases of blood.

Normal Development of Blood Cells

Blood cells first appear during the third week of fetal embryonic development in the yolk sac, but these cells are generated from a primitive stem cell population restricted to the production of myeloid cells. The origin of definitive hematopoietic stem cells that give rise to lymphoid and myeloid cells is still unsettled. Most studies suggest they arise in the mesoderm of the intraembryonic aorta/gonad/mesonephros (AGM) region,[1] but evidence also exists for an origin within a small subset of yolk sac–derived cells. By the third month of embryogenesis, stem cells derived from the AGM and/or yolk sac migrate to the liver, which is the chief site of blood cell formation until shortly before birth. Beginning in the fourth month of development, stem cells migrate to the bone marrow to commence hematopoiesis at this site. By birth, marrow throughout the skeleton is hematopoietically active and virtually the sole source of blood cells. In full-term infants, hepatic hematopoiesis dwindles to a trickle, persisting only in widely scattered small foci that become inactive soon after birth. Up to the age of puberty, marrow throughout the skeleton remains red and hematopoietically active. By age 18 only the vertebrae, ribs, sternum, skull, pelvis, and proximal epiphyseal regions of the humerus and femur retain red marrow, the remaining marrow becoming yellow, fatty, and inactive. Thus, in adults, only about half of the marrow space is active in hematopoiesis.

Several features of this normal sequence should be emphasized. By birth, the bone marrow is virtually the sole source of all forms of blood cells, including lymphocyte precursors. In the premature infant, foci of hematopoiesis are frequently evident in the liver and, rarely, in the spleen, lymph nodes, or thymus. Significant postembryonic extramedullary hematopoiesis is abnormal in the full-term infant. With an increased demand for blood cells in the adult, the fatty marrow can transform to red, active marrow. For example, in the face of red cell deficiency (anemia), the marrow can increase red cell production (erythropoiesis) as much as eightfold. If the marrow stem cells and microenvironment are normal and the necessary nutrients are available (e.g., adequate amounts of iron, protein, requisite vitamins), premature loss of red cells (as occurs in hemolytic disorders) produces anemia only when marrow compensatory mechanisms are outstripped. Under these circumstances, extramedullary hematopoiesis can reappear within the spleen, liver, and even lymph nodes.

ORIGIN AND DIFFERENTIATION OF HEMATOPOIETIC CELLS

The formed elements of blood—red cells, granulocytes, monocytes, platelets, and lymphocytes—have a common origin from pluripotent hematopoietic stem cells sitting at the apex of a complex hierarchy of progenitors (Fig. 13–1). Most of the work supporting this scheme comes from studies conducted in mice, but it is believed hematopoiesis in man proceeds in a highly analogous fashion. The pluripotent stem cell gives rise to two types of multipotent progenitors, the common lymphoid and the common myeloid stem cell. The common lymphoid stem cell in turn gives rise to precursors of T cells (pro-T cells), B cells (pro-B cells), and natural killer cells.[2] The details of lymphoid differentiation are not discussed here, but it is worth pointing out that morphologic distinctions among lymphoid cells at various stages of differentiation are subtle at best. As a result, monoclonal antibodies recognizing differentiation-stage–specific antigens are used widely to define normal lymphocyte subsets (Chapter 14). From the common myeloid stem cell arise at least three types of *committed stem cells* capable of differentiating along the erythroid/megakaryocytic, eosinophilic, and granulocyte-macrophage pathways.[3] In functional assays the committed stem cells are called colony-forming units (CFU), because each can give rise to colonies of differentiated progeny in vitro (see Fig. 13–1). From the various committed stem cells are derived intermediate stages and ultimately the morphologically recognizable precursors of the differentiated cells, such as proerythroblasts, myeloblasts, megakaryoblasts, monoblasts, and eosinophiloblasts, which in turn give rise to mature progeny.

The specific characteristics of rare cells lying high up in the hierarchy shown in Figure 13–1 are still debated. What are agreed upon are certain overarching themes that apply to hematopoiesis. Since mature blood elements are terminally differentiated cells with finite life spans, their numbers must be replenished constantly. It follows that stem cells must not only differentiate, but also *self-renew, a critical property of stem cells.* Pluripotent stem cells have the greatest capacity for self-renewal, but normally most are not in cell cycle. As commitment to particular lines of differentiation proceeds, self-renewal becomes limited, but a greater fraction of committed cells divide actively. For example, few common myeloid stem cells are normally in cell cycle, but up to 50% of CFU-

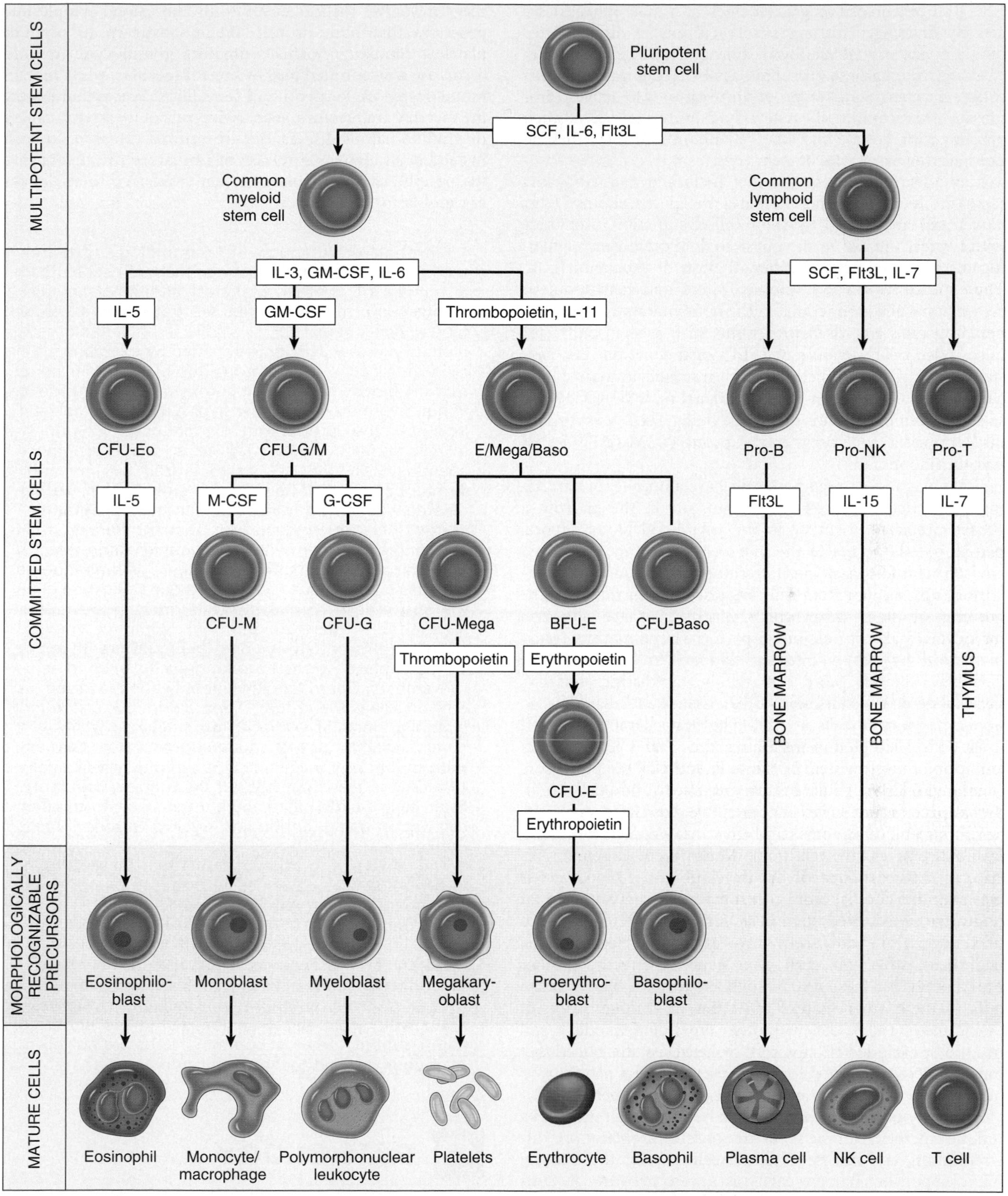

FIGURE 13–1 Differentiation of hematopoietic cells. SCF, stem cell factor; Flt3L, Flt3 ligand; GM-CSF, granulocyte-macrophage colony-stimulating factor; M-CSF, macrophage colony-stimulating factor; G-CSF, granulocyte colony-stimulating factor. (Modified from Wyngaarden JB, et al [eds]: Cecil Textbook of Medicine, 19th ed. Philadelphia, WB Saunders, 1992, p. 820.)

GM (the precursors of granulocytes and macrophages) are actively dividing. This suggests that pools of differentiated cells are replenished mainly by lineage-restricted stem cells. Although the earliest morphologically recognizable precursors (e.g., myeloblasts or proerythroblasts) also actively proliferate, they cannot self-renew, and eventually all of their progeny differentiate and "die." By definition, then, they do not have the properties of stem cells.

Many disorders of the marrow, including marrow failure (aplastic anemias) and hematopoietic neoplasms (e.g., leukemias) are caused by stem cell dysfunction, and there is thus great interest in the physiologic mechanisms regulating the proliferation and differentiation of progenitor cells. These processes involve soluble factors and hematopoietic cell–stromal cell interactions in the bone marrow. Among the hematopoietic growth factors, some, such as stem cell factor (also called c-KIT ligand) and FLT3-ligand, act on very early stem cells. Others, such as the granulocyte-macrophage colony-stimulating factor (GM-CSF), act on CFU-GM. Some recombinant factors are currently being used to stimulate hematopoiesis, including erythropoietin, GM-CSF, G-CSF, and thrombopoietin.

Bone marrow–derived stem cells have a number of surprising properties. Although residing mainly in the marrow, a subset circulates normally in the peripheral blood. Hence, hematopoiesis occurs in the marrow because its specialized environment fosters stem cell homing, survival, and differentiation, not because stem cells are restricted to this site. The homing of stem cells, which involves surface adhesion molecules, makes it possible to perform bone marrow transplantation by simply infusing donor stem cells into the peripheral blood. More remarkably, circulating marrow-derived stem cells can "seed" other tissues and develop into nonhematopoietic cells as well. The best characterized and most widely accepted of these alternative "fates" is the differentiation of marrow stem cells into endothelial cell precursors (hemangioblasts)[4], which in turn give rise to endothelial cells. This capacity is not surprising, given the close functional relationship of blood elements and the cardiovascular system. In fact, many genes involved in the development of hematopoietic cells also participate in the development of blood vessels and endothelial cells. More controversial studies suggest that bone marrow-derived stem cells can also differentiate into hepatocytes, bile duct cells, myocardium, skeletal muscle, endothelial cells, glia, and even neurons directly.[5,6] Other explanations for these results, such as fusion of marrow stem cells to these other mature cell types or contamination of hematopoietic stem cells with other types of stem cells,[4,7] still need to be excluded (Chapter 3). Nonetheless, it is hoped that marrow-derived stem cells will have sufficient plasticity to permit their use in a variety of stem cell-based therapies.

Anatomy of Bone Marrow. The bone marrow provides a unique microenvironment for the orderly proliferation, differentiation, and release of blood cells. Under the electron microscope, the marrow cavity is a vast network of thin-walled sinusoids lined by a single layer of endothelial cells underlaid by a discontinuous layer of basement membrane and adventitial cells. Within the interstitium lie clusters of hematopoietic cells and fat cells. Differentiated blood cells enter sinusoids by transcellular migration through the endothelial cells. The normal marrow is organized anatomically in subtle but important ways. For example, normal megakaryocytes lie next to sinusoids and extend cytoplasmic processes that bud off into the bloodstream to produce platelets. Similarly, normal immature granulocytic myeloid forms are concentrated next to bone trabeculae, while mature granulocytes are located more centrally. Diseases that distort the marrow architecture, such as deposits of metastatic cancer or granulomatous disease, disturb normal function. In such instances, an abnormal release of immature precursors into the peripheral blood can occur that is referred to as "leukoerythroblastosis."

Morphology. Although the morphology of hematopoietic cells within the bone marrow is best studied in smears of marrow aspirates, additional complementary information is obtained from bone marrow biopsy specimens. For example, a reasonable estimate of marrow activity is obtained by examining the ratio of fat cells to hematopoietic elements in bone marrow biopsy samples. In normal adults, this ratio is about 1:1, but with marrow hypoplasia (e.g., aplastic anemia), the proportion of fat cells is greatly increased; conversely, fat cells may disappear completely in diseases characterized by increased hematopoiesis (e.g., hemolytic anemias). Also, certain disorders (such as metastatic cancers and granulomatous diseases) induce local marrow fibrosis, rendering the lesional cells "inaspirable"; here too, a biopsy is the examination of choice. The limitation of biopsies is that tissue fixation and decalcification alter the appearance of marrow cells, making them less recognizable than in air-dried aspirate smears. However, it is not always possible to differentiate the various "blast" forms morphologically, even in aspirate smears. Often, tentative identification is based on "the company they keep." Thus, a primitive cell found within a focus of maturing granulocytes is likely a myeloblast. Pluripotent and multipotent stem cells are morphologically inconspicuous lymphocyte-like cells constituting less than 0.1% of the marrow cellularity. Stem cells are identified and purified away from other cell types using antibodies against discriminating markers (e.g., CD34).

The relative proportion of hematopoietic precursors is almost always deranged in diseases of the blood and bone marrow, which normally contains about 65% granulocytes and their precursors; 25% erythroid precursors; and 10% lymphocytes and monocytes and their precursors. Thus, the normal myeloid to erythroid ratio is 2 to 3:1. Prevalent cell types in the myeloid compartment include myelocytes, metamyelocytes, and granulocytes. In the erythroid compartment, the most common forms are polychromatophilic and orthochromic normoblasts.

PATHOLOGY

Anemias

The function of red cells is to transport oxygen to peripheral tissues. Reduced oxygen-carrying capacity of blood usually results from a deficiency of red cells, or *anemia,* defined as *a reduction below normal limits of the total circulat-*

ing red cell mass. Measurement of red cell mass is not easy, however, and in routine practice anemia is defined as a reduction below normal in the volume of packed red cells, as measured by the *hematocrit,* or a reduction in the *hemoglobin concentration* of the blood. On occasion, fluid retention can expand plasma volume and dehydration can contract plasma volume, creating spurious abnormalities in these values.

There are innumerable classifications of anemia. An acceptable one based on underlying mechanisms is presented in Table 13–1. A second useful approach classifies anemia according to alterations in red cell morphology, which often correlates with the cause of red cell deficiency. Morphologic characteristics providing etiologic clues include red cell size (normocytic, microcytic, or macrocytic); degree of hemoglobinization, reflected in the color of red cells (normochromic or hypochromic); and other special features, such as shape. These red cell indices are often judged qualitatively by physicians, but precise quantitation is done in clinical laboratories using special instrumentation. The most useful red cell indices are as follows:

- *Mean cell volume:* the average volume of a red blood cell, expressed in femtoliters (cubic micrometers)
- *Mean cell hemoglobin:* the average content (mass) of hemoglobin per red blood cell, expressed in picograms
- *Mean cell hemoglobin concentration:* the average concentration of hemoglobin in a given volume of packed red blood cells, expressed in grams per deciliter
- *Red blood cell distribution width:* the coefficient of variation of red blood cell volume

Adult reference ranges for red cell indices are shown in Table 13–2.

Whatever its cause, anemia leads to certain clinical features when sufficiently severe. Patients appear pale. Weakness, malaise, and easy fatigability are common complaints. The lowered oxygen content of the circulating blood leads to dyspnea on mild exertion. The nails can become brittle, lose their usual convexity, and assume a concave spoon shape (koilonychia). Anoxia can cause fatty change in the liver, myocardium, and kidney. If fatty changes in the myocardium are sufficiently severe, cardiac failure can develop and compound the respiratory difficulty caused by reduced oxygen transport. On occasion, the myocardial hypoxia manifests as angina pectoris, particularly when complicated by preexisting coronary artery disease. With acute blood loss and shock, oliguria and anuria can develop due to renal hypoperfusion. Central nervous system hypoxia can cause headache, dimness of vision, and faintness.

TABLE 13–1 Classification of Anemia According to Underlying Mechanism

Blood Loss

Acute: trauma
Chronic: lesions of gastrointestinal tract, gynecologic disturbances

Increased Rate of Destruction (Hemolytic Anemias)

Intrinsic (intracorpuscular) abnormalities of red cells
- *Hereditary*
  - Red cell membrane disorders
    - Disorders of membrane cytoskeleton: spherocytosis, elliptocytosis
    - Disorders of lipid synthesis: selective increase in membrane lecithin
  - Red cell enzyme deficiencies
    - Glycolytic enzymes: pyruvate kinase deficiency, hexokinase deficiency
    - Enzymes of hexose monophosphate shunt: G6PD, glutathione synthetase
  - Disorders of hemoglobin synthesis
    - Deficient globin synthesis: thalassemia syndromes
    - Structurally abnormal globin synthesis (hemoglobinopathies): sickle cell anemia, unstable hemoglobins
- *Acquired*
  - Membrane defect: paroxysmal nocturnal hemoglobinuria

Extrinsic (extracorpuscular) abnormalities
- Antibody mediated
  - Isohemagglutinins: transfusion reactions, erythroblastosis fetalis
  - Autoantibodies: idiopathic (primary), drug-associated, systemic lupus erythematosus, malignant neoplasms, mycoplasmal infection
- Mechanical trauma to red cells
  - Microangiopathic hemolytic anemias: thrombotic thrombocytopenic purpura, disseminated intravascular coagulation
  - Cardiac traumatic hemolytic anemia
- Infections: malaria, hookworm
- Chemical injury: lead poisoning
- Sequestration in mononuclear phagocyte system: hypersplenism

Impaired Red Cell Production

Disturbance of proliferation and differentiation of stem cells: aplastic anemia, pure red cell aplasia, anemia of renal failure, anemia of endocrine disorders
Disturbance of proliferation and maturation of erythroblasts
- Defective DNA synthesis: deficiency or impaired use of vitamin B_{12} and folic acid (megaloblastic anemias)
- Defective hemoglobin synthesis
  - Deficient heme synthesis: iron deficiency
  - Deficient globin synthesis: thalassemias
- Unknown or multiple mechanisms: sideroblastic anemia, anemia of chronic infections, myelophthisic anemias due to marrow infiltrations

ANEMIAS OF BLOOD LOSS

Acute Blood Loss

The clinical and morphologic reactions to blood loss depend on the rate of hemorrhage and whether the bleeding

TABLE 13–2 Adult Reference Ranges for Red Blood Cells*

Measurement (units)	Men	Women
Hemoglobin (gm/dL)	13.6–17.2	12.0–15.0
Hematocrit (%)	39–49	33–43
Red cell count ($10^6/\mu L$)	4.3–5.9	3.5–5.0
Reticulocyte count (%)	0.5–1.5	
Mean cell volume (μm^3)	82–96	
Mean corpuscular hemoglobin (pg)	27–33	
Mean corpuscular hemoglobin concentration (gm/dL)	33–37	
RBC distribution width	11.5–14.5	

*Reference ranges vary among laboratories. The reference ranges for the laboratory providing the result should always be used in interpreting the test result.
RBC, red blood cell.

is external or internal. The effects of acute blood loss are mainly due to the loss of intravascular volume, which can lead to cardiovascular collapse, shock, and death. If the patient survives, the blood volume is rapidly restored by shift of water from the interstitial fluid compartment. The resulting hemodilution lowers the hematocrit. Reduction in the oxygenation of renal juxtaglomerular cells triggers increased production of erythropoietin, which stimulates the proliferation of committed erythroid stem cells (CFU-E) in the marrow. It takes about 5 days for the progeny of these CFU-Es to fully differentiate, an event marked by the appearance of increased numbers of newly released red cells (reticulocytes) in the peripheral blood. The iron in hemoglobin is recaptured if red cells are lost internally, as into the peritoneal cavity, but external bleeding leads to iron loss and possible iron deficiency, which can hamper restoration of normal red cell counts.

The earliest change in the peripheral blood immediately after acute blood loss is *leukocytosis,* due to the mobilization of granulocytes from marginal pools. Initially, red cells appear normal in size and color (normocytic, normochromic). However, as marrow production increases, *there is a striking increase in the reticulocyte count, reaching 10% to 15% after 7 days.* Reticulocytes are recognizable as polychromatophilic macrocytes in the usual blood smear. Early recovery from blood loss is often accompanied by *thrombocytosis,* which is caused by increased platelet production.

Chronic Blood Loss

Chronic blood loss induces anemia only when the rate of loss exceeds the regenerative capacity of the marrow or when iron reserves are depleted. Iron deficiency anemia, which has identical features regardless of underlying cause (e.g., bleeding, malnutrition, malabsorption states), will be discussed later.

HEMOLYTIC ANEMIAS

Hemolytic anemias share the following features:

- *A shortened red cell life span (normal = 120 days); that is, premature destruction of red cells*
- *Elevated erythropoietin levels and increased erythropoiesis in the marrow and other sites,* to compensate for the loss of red cells
- *Accumulation of the products of hemoglobin catabolism, due to an increased rate of red cell destruction*

The physiologic destruction of senescent red cells takes place within the mononuclear phagocytic cells of the spleen. In the great majority of hemolytic anemias, the premature destruction of red cells also occurs within the mononuclear phagocyte system (extravascular hemolysis), which undergoes a form of work-related hyperplasia marked by splenomegaly. Much less commonly, lysis of red cells within the vascular compartment (intravascular hemolysis) predominates.

Intravascular hemolysis of red cells is caused by mechanical injury, complement fixation, infection by intracellular parasites such as falciparum malaria (Chapter 8), or exogenous toxic factors. Mechanical injury caused by defective cardiac valves, thrombi within the microcirculation, or repetitive physical trauma (marathon running, bongo drum beating) can physically lyse red cells. Complement fixation can occur on antibody-coated cells during transfusion of mismatched blood. Toxic injury is exemplified by clostridial sepsis, which releases toxins that attack the red cell membrane.

Whatever the mechanism, *intravascular hemolysis is manifested by (1) hemoglobinemia, (2) hemoglobinuria, (3) jaundice, and (4) hemosiderinuria.* Free hemoglobin in plasma is promptly bound by an α_2-globulin (haptoglobin), producing a complex that is rapidly cleared by the mononuclear phagocyte system, thus preventing excretion into the urine. *Decreased serum haptoglobin is characteristic of intravascular hemolysis.* When the haptoglobin is depleted, free hemoglobin is prone to oxidation to methemoglobin, which is brown in color. The renal proximal tubular cells reabsorb and catabolize much of the filtered hemoglobin and methemoglobin, but some passes out with the urine, imparting a red-brown color. Iron released from hemoglobin can accumulate within tubular cells, giving rise to renal hemosiderosis. Concomitantly, heme groups derived from the complexes are catabolized to bilirubin within the mononuclear phagocyte system, leading to jaundice. In hemolytic anemias, the serum bilirubin is unconjugated and the level of hyperbilirubinemia depends on the functional capacity of the liver and the rate of hemolysis. When the liver is normal, jaundice is rarely severe. Excessive bilirubin excreted by the liver into the gastrointestinal tract leads to increased formation and fecal excretion of urobilin (Chapter 18).

Extravascular hemolysis takes place whenever red cells are rendered "foreign" or become less deformable. Since extreme alterations in shape are required for red cells to navigate the splenic sinusoids successfully, reduced deformability makes the passage difficult and leads to sequestration within the cords, followed by phagocytosis (Fig. 13–2). This is an important pathogenetic mechanism of extravascular hemolysis in a variety of hemolytic anemias. With extravascular hemolysis,

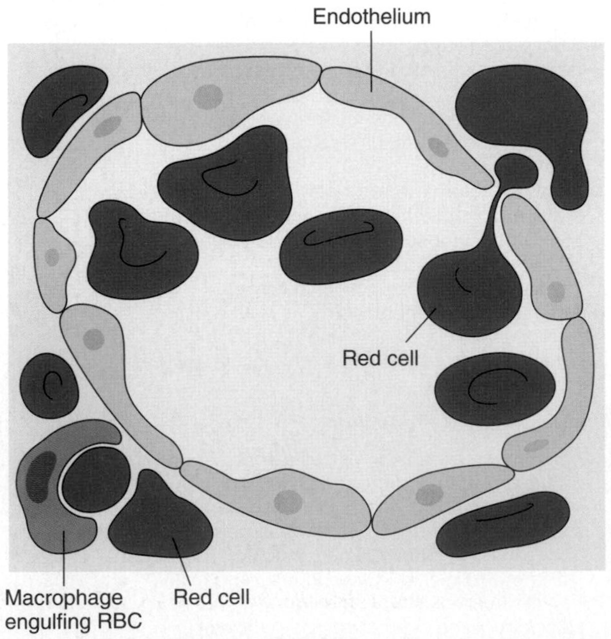

FIGURE 13–2 Schematic of splenic sinus (electron micrograph). A red cell is in the process of squeezing from the red pulp cords into the sinus lumen. Note the degree of deformability required for red cells to pass through the wall of the sinus.

hemoglobinemia and hemoglobinuria are not observed, and its principal features are anemia and jaundice. However, some hemoglobin inevitably escapes from phagocytes, leading to decreases in plasma haptoglobin. The morphologic changes are identical to those in intravascular hemolysis, except that "work" hyperplasia of the mononuclear phagocyte system often leads to splenomegaly.

Morphology. Certain morphologic changes are common in hemolytic anemias, regardless of cause or type. Anemia and lowered tissue oxygen tension stimulate increased production of erythropoietin, which leads to the appearance of **increased numbers of erythroid precursors (normoblasts) in the marrow** (Fig. 13–3). If the anemia is severe, extramedullary hematopoiesis can appear in the liver, spleen, and lymph nodes. The accelerated erythropoiesis leads to a **prominent reticulocytosis in the peripheral blood.** Elevated biliary excretion of bilirubin promotes the formation of pigment gallstones (cholelithiasis). If chronic, phagocytosis of red cells leads to hemosiderosis, usually confined to the mononuclear phagocyte system.

The hemolytic anemias are classified in a variety of ways. One has already been mentioned, namely, division into intravascular and extravascular hemolytic disorders. However, since disorders with predominantly intravascular hemolysis are quite uncommon, this classification is not entirely satisfactory. A second pathogenetic classification is based on whether the underlying cause of red cell destruction is extrinsic (extracorpuscular mechanism) or intrinsic to the red cell (intracorpuscular defect). These anemias can also be divided into hereditary and acquired disorders. *In general, hereditary disorders are due to intrinsic defects and the acquired disorders to extrinsic factors such as autoantibodies.* Each of the classifications has value. Here we follow the intrinsic-extrinsic outline given in Table 13–1, limiting our discussion to the more common entities.

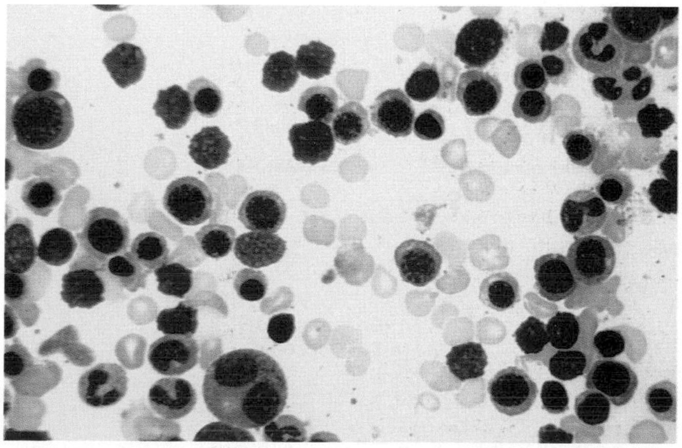

FIGURE 13–3 Marrow smear from a patient with hemolytic anemia. The marrow reveals greatly increased numbers of maturing erythroid progenitors (normoblasts). (Courtesy of Dr. Steven Kroft, Department of Pathology, University of Texas Southwestern Medical School, Dallas, TX.)

Hereditary Spherocytosis (HS)

This inherited disorder is caused by intrinsic defects in the red cell membrane that render red cells spheroid, less deformable, and vulnerable to splenic sequestration and destruction. The prevalence of HS is highest in northern Europe, where rates of 1 in 5000 are reported. An autosomal dominant inheritance pattern is seen in three fourths of cases. The remaining patients have a more severe autosomal recessive form of the disease.

Molecular Pathology. The remarkable elasticity and durability of the normal red cell are attributable to the physicochemical properties of its specialized membrane skeleton (Fig. 13–4), which lies closely apposed to the internal surface of the plasma membrane. Its chief protein component, spectrin, consists of two polypeptide chains, α and β, which form intertwined (helical) flexible heterodimers. The "head" regions of spectrin dimers self-associate to form tetramers, while the "tails" associate with actin oligomers. Each actin oligomer can bind multiple spectrin tetramers, thus creating a 2-dimensional spectrin–actin skeleton that is connected to the cell membrane by two distinct interactions. The first, involving the proteins ankyrin and band 4.2, binds spectrin to the transmembrane ion transporter, band 3. The second, involving protein 4.1, binds the "tail" of spectrin to another transmembrane protein, glycophorin A.

HS is caused by diverse mutations affecting ankyrin, band 3, spectrin, or band 4.2, the proteins involved in the first of these two tethering interactions,[8] presumably because this complex is particularly important in stabilizing the lipid bilayer. *The most common cause of autosomal dominant HS is mutation of red cell ankyrin.*[9] Another 20% of autosomal dominant HS cases are caused by mutations in band 3.[10] The remaining cases are associated mostly with mutations in α-spectrin, β-spectrin, or band 4.2. Regardless of the molecular defect, *reduced membrane stability leads to loss of membrane fragments during exposure to shear stresses in the circulation* (see Fig. 13–4). The loss of membrane relative to cytoplasm "forces" the cells to assume the smallest possible diameter for a given volume, namely, a sphere.

Although there is much to learn about the molecular defects in HS, the travails of the spherocytic red cells are fairly well defined (Fig. 13–5). In the life of the "portly," inflexible spherocyte, the spleen is the villain. Red cells must undergo extreme deformation to leave the cords of Billroth and enter the sinusoids. Because of their spheroidal shape and reduced membrane plasticity, spherocytes attempting to squeeze out of the cords are like an "obese man attempting to bend at the waist."[11] As spherocytes are trapped in the spleen, the already sluggish circulation of the cords stagnates further, producing a progressively more hostile environment. Lactic acid accumulates and the pH falls, inhibiting glycolysis. The inability to generate adenosine triphosphate impairs the ability of red cells to extrude sodium, adding an element of osmotic injury. Stagnation in the cords also promotes contact with plentiful macrophages, which phagocytose the hapless spherocytes. The cardinal role of the spleen in the premature demise of the spherocytes is proved by the invariably beneficial effect of splenectomy. The spherocytes persist, but the anemia is corrected.

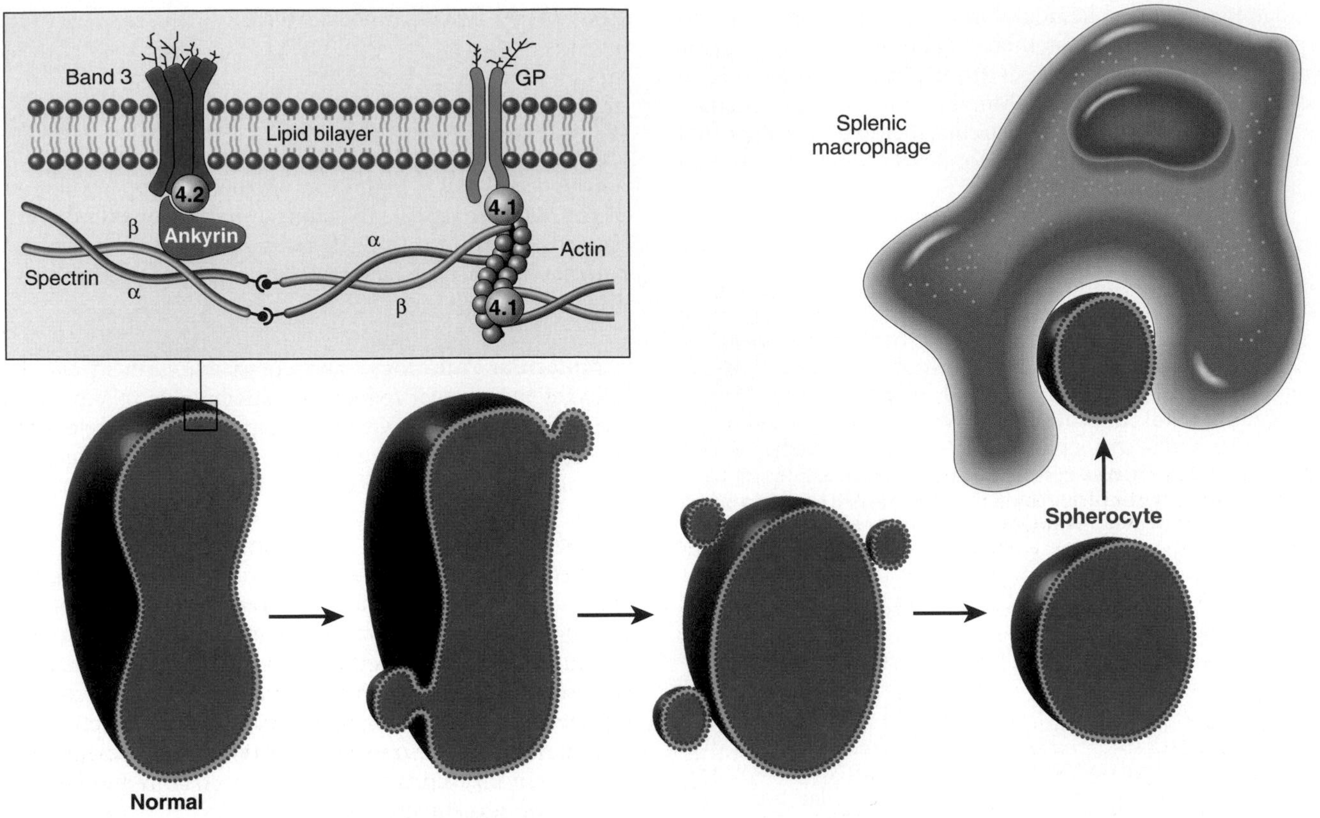

FIGURE 13–4 Schematic representation of the red cell membrane cytoskeleton and alterations leading to spherocytosis and hemolysis. Mutations weakening interactions involving α-spectrin, β-spectrin, ankyrin, band 4.2, or band 3 all cause the normal biconcave red cell to lose membrane fragments and adopt a spherical shape. Such spherocytic cells are less deformable than normal and therefore become trapped in the splenic cords, where they are phagocytosed by macrophages.

Morphology. The most outstanding morphologic finding in this disease are spherocytes, apparent on smears as abnormally small, dark-staining (hyperchromic) red cells lacking the normal central zone of pallor (Fig. 13–6). Spherocytosis, although distinctive, is not pathognomonic, as it is also seen in autoimmune hemolytic anemias. Present also are changes associated with all hemolytic anemias, including reticulocytosis, marrow hyperplasia due to increased erythropoiesis, hemosiderosis, and mild jaundice. Cholelithiasis (pigment stones) occurs in 40% to 50% of the affected adults. Other alterations are fairly distinctive. Moderate splenic enlargement is characteristic (500 to 1000 gm); in few other hemolytic anemias is the spleen enlarged as much or as often. It results from congestion of the cords of Billroth and "work hyperplasia" due to markedly increased erythrophagocytosis.

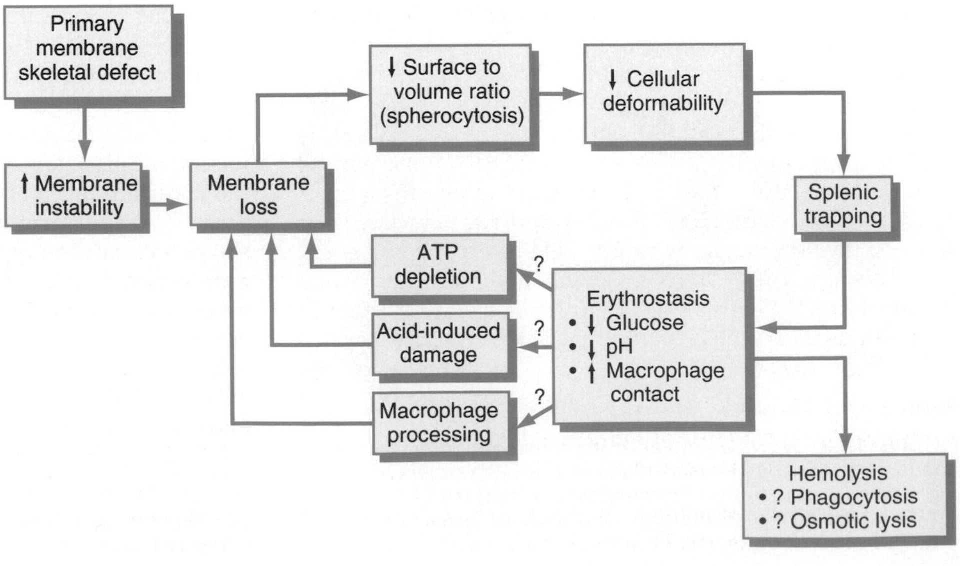

FIGURE 13–5 Model of the pathophysiology of hereditary spherocytosis. (Adapted from Wyngaarden JB, et al [eds]: Cecil Textbook of Medicine, 19th ed. Philadelphia, WB Saunders, 1992, p. 859.)

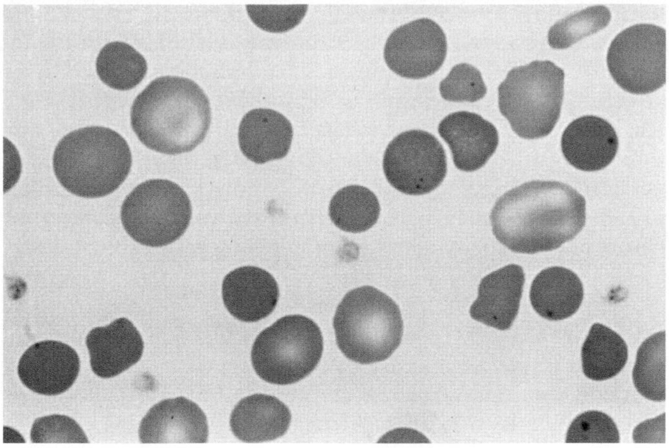

FIGURE 13–6 Hereditary spherocytosis (peripheral smear). Note the anisocytosis and several dark-appearing spherocytes with no central pallor. Howell-Jolly bodies (small dark nuclear remnants) are also present in red cells of this asplenic patient. (Courtesy of Dr. Robert W. McKenna, Department of Pathology, University of Texas Southwestern Medical School, Dallas, TX.)

Clinical Course. The characteristic clinical features are anemia, splenomegaly, and jaundice. The severity of the disease varies greatly from one patient to another. In a minority, HS presents at birth with marked jaundice, requiring exchange transfusion. In 20% to 30% of patients, the disease is virtually asymptomatic because the decreased red cell survival is readily compensated for by increased erythropoiesis. In most, however, the compensatory changes are outpaced, producing a chronic hemolytic anemia, usually of mild to moderate severity. The generally stable clinical course is sometimes punctuated by an *aplastic crisis,* usually triggered by an acute parvovirus infection. Parvovirus infects and kills red cell progenitors, causing red cell production to cease until an effective immune response commences, generally in 1 to 2 weeks. Because the lifespan of red cells in HS is shortened to 10 to 20 days, cessation of erythropoiesis for even short time periods leads to sudden worsening of the anemia accompanied by reticulocytopenia. Transfusions may be necessary to support the patient until the immune response clears the infection. *Hemolytic crises* are produced by intercurrent events leading to increased splenic destruction of red cells (e.g., infectious mononucleosis); these are clinically less significant than aplastic crises. Gallstones, found in many patients, can also produce symptoms. Diagnosis of HS is based on family history, hematologic findings, and several pieces of laboratory evidence. In two thirds of the patients, the red cells are abnormally sensitive to *osmotic lysis* when incubated in solutions of hypotonic salt, which induce the influx of water into spherocytes with little margin for expansion. Spherocytes retain most of the cytoplasm they were "born" with and lose sodium and water during conditioning in the circulation, leading to an *increased mean cell hemoglobin concentration* in most patients. As mentioned earlier, splenectomy is often beneficial.

Hemolytic Disease Due to Red Cell Enzyme Defects: Glucose-6-Phosphate Dehydrogenase Deficiency

The red cell is vulnerable to injury by exogenous and endogenous oxidants. *Abnormalities in the hexose monophosphate shunt or glutathione metabolism resulting from deficient or impaired enzyme function reduce the ability of red cells to protect themselves against oxidative injuries, leading to hemolytic disease.* The most important of these enzyme derangements is the hereditary deficiency of glucose-6-phosphate dehydrogenase (G6PD) activity. As noted in Figure 13–7, G6PD reduces NADP to NADPH while oxidizing glucose-6-phosphate. NADPH then provides reducing equivalents needed for conversion of oxidized glutathione to reduced glutathione, which protects against oxidant injury by catalyzing the breakdown of compounds such as H_2O_2.

Several hundred G6PD genetic variants are known, but most are harmless. Only two variants, designated G6PD A^- and G6PD Mediterranean, cause most clinically significant hemolytic anemias.[12] G6PD A^- is present in about 10% of American blacks; G6PD Mediterranean, as the name implies, is prevalent in the Middle East. The high frequency of these variants in each population is believed to stem from a protective effect against *Plasmodium falciparum* malaria.[13]

G6PD variants associated with hemolysis destabilize the enzyme. Compared to the most common normal variant, G6PD B, the half-life of G6PD A^- is moderately reduced, whereas that of G6PD Mediterranean is more markedly abnormal. Elucidation of the crystal structure of G6PD has revealed that both disease-associated mutations result in misfolding of the protein, making it more susceptible to proteolytic degradation.[14] Because mature red cells do not synthesize new proteins, G6PD A^- or G6PD Mediterranean enzyme activities fall quickly as red cells age to levels inadequate to protect against oxidant stress.

G6PD deficiency is a recessive X-linked trait, placing males at highest risk for symptomatic disease. G6PD deficiency manifests in several distinct clinical patterns. Most common

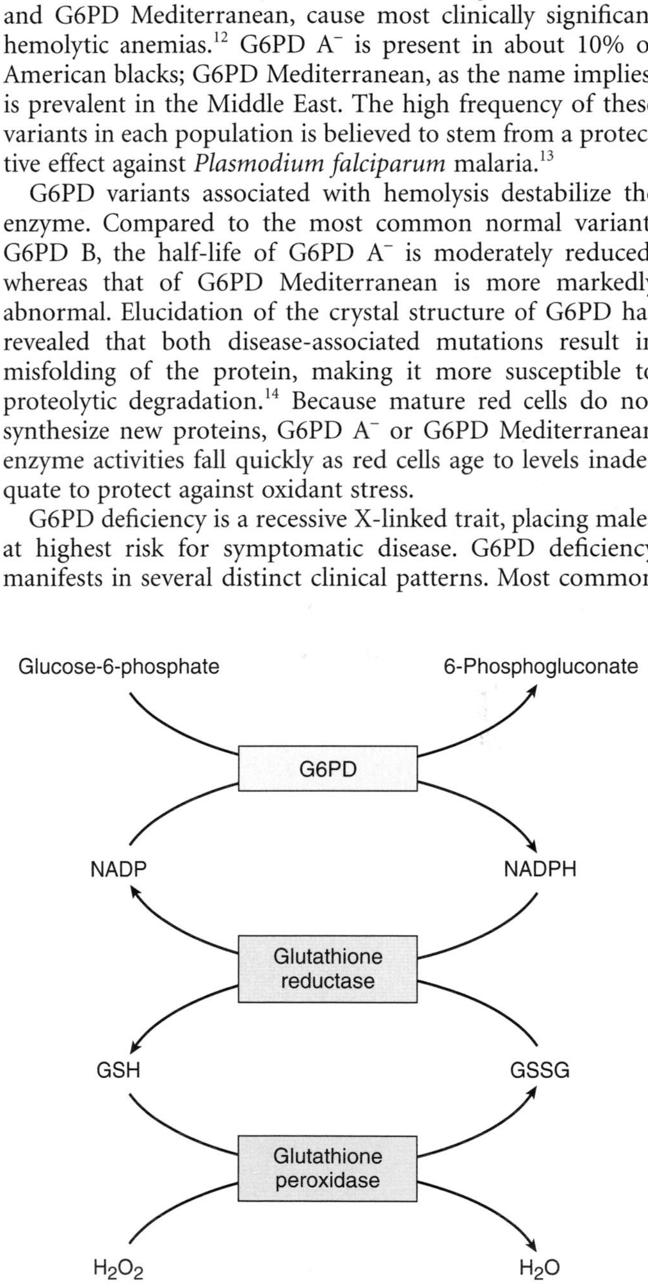

FIGURE 13–7 Role of glucose-6-phosphate dehydrogenase (G6PD) in defense against oxidant injury. The disposal of H_2O_2, a potential oxidant, is dependent on the adequacy of reduced glutathione (GSH), which is generated by the action of NADPH. The synthesis of NADPH is dependent on the activity of G6PD. GSSG, oxidized glutathione.

is hemolysis after exposure to oxidant stress. This can occur due to ingestion of certain *drugs* or foods, or (more commonly) exposure to oxidant free radicals generated by leukocytes in the course of *infections.* The oxidant drugs implicated are numerous, including antimalarials (e.g., primaquine and chloroquine), sulfonamides, nitrofurantoins, and others. Some drugs cause hemolysis only in those with the more severe Mediterranean variant. Many infections can trigger hemolysis; viral hepatitis, pneumonia, and typhoid fever are among those most likely to do so. Hemolysis can also occur after ingestion of fava beans *(favism),* which generate oxidants when metabolized. Favism is endemic in the Mediterranean, Middle East, and parts of Africa where consumption of fava beans is prevalent. Uncommonly, G6PD deficiency presents as neonatal jaundice or a chronic low-grade hemolytic anemia in the absence of infection or known environmental triggers.

G6PD deficiency causes episodic intravascular and extravascular hemolysis, which seems to involve the following sequence. When G6PD-deficient red cells are exposed to high levels of oxidants, there is oxidation of reactive sulfhydryl groups on globin chains, which become denatured and form membrane-bound precipitates known as *Heinz bodies.* These are seen within red cells stained with crystal violet as dark inclusions (Fig. 13–8). Heinz bodies can damage the membrane sufficiently to cause intravascular hemolysis. Less severe membrane damage results in decreased red cell deformability. As inclusion-bearing red cells pass through the splenic cords, macrophages pluck out the Heinz bodies. Due to membrane damage, some of these partially devoured cells retain an abnormal shape, appearing to have a bite of cytoplasm removed ("bite cells") (see Fig. 13–8). Other less severely damaged cells revert to a spherocytic shape due to loss of membrane surface area. Both bite cells and spherocytes are highly prone to trapping in splenic cords and rapid removal via erythrophagocytosis.

Acute intravascular hemolysis marked by anemia, hemoglobinemia, and hemoglobinuria usually begins 2 to 3 days following exposure of G6PD-deficient individuals to oxidants. The hemolysis tends to be greater in individuals with highly unstable G6PD Mediterranean. Since only older red cells are at risk for lysis, the episode is *self-limited,* as hemolysis stops when only the younger red cells remain (even if administration of an offending drug continues). The recovery phase is heralded by reticulocytosis. Since hemolytic episodes related to G6PD deficiency occur intermittently, most features of chronic hemolytic anemias (e.g., splenomegaly, cholelithiasis) are absent.

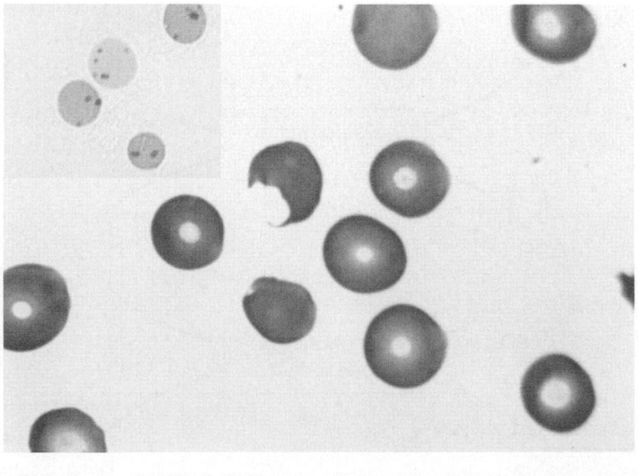

FIGURE 13–8 G6PD deficiency: effects of oxidant drug exposure (peripheral blood smear). *Inset,* Red cells with precipitates of denatured globin (Heinz bodies) revealed by supravital staining. As the splenic macrophages pluck out these inclusions, "bite cells" like the one in this smear are produced. (Courtesy of Dr. Robert W. McKenna, Department of Pathology, University of Texas Southwestern Medical School, Dallas, TX.)

Sickle Cell Disease

Sickle cell disease is an important *hereditary hemoglobinopathy, a type of disease characterized by production of defective hemoglobins.* Hemoglobin, as you recall, is a tetrameric protein composed of two like pairs of globin chains, each with its own heme group. Normal adult red cells contain mainly HbA ($\alpha_2\beta_2$) along with small amounts of HbA_2 ($\alpha_2\delta_2$) and fetal hemoglobin ($\alpha_2\gamma_2$). The clinically significant hemoglobinopathies result from mutations in the β-globin gene. Sickle cell anemia is caused by a point mutation at the sixth position of the β-globin chain leading to the substitution of a valine residue for a glutamic acid residue. The abnormal physiochemical properties of the resulting sickle hemoglobin (HbS) are responsible for sickle cell disease. Several hundred other abnormal hemoglobins have been identified containing point mutations or deletions in one of the globin chains.

About 8% of black Americans are heterozygous for HbS. If an individual is homozygous for the sickle mutation, almost all the hemoglobin in the red cell is HbS ($\alpha_2\beta^s{}_2$). In heterozygotes, only about 40% of the hemoglobin is HbS, the remainder being normal hemoglobins. Where malaria is endemic in Africa, as many as 30% of the native population are heterozygous. This high frequency is likely related to protection against falciparum malaria afforded by HbS, particularly in infants.[15]

Pathogenesis. *When deoxygenated, HbS molecules undergo aggregation and polymerization.* Initially, the red cell cytosol converts from a freely flowing liquid to a viscous gel as HbS aggregates form. With continued deoxygenation, aggregated HbS molecules assemble into long needle-like fibers within red cells, producing a distorted sickle or holly-leaf shape (Fig. 13–9).

Sickling of red cells is initially a reversible phenomenon; with oxygenation, HbS depolymerizes and the cell shape normalizes. However, with repeated episodes of sickling, membrane damage occurs and cells become irreversibly sickled, retaining their abnormal shape even when fully oxygenated. The precipitation of HbS fibers also *causes oxidant damage, not only in irreversibly sickled cells but also in normal-appearing cells.* With membrane injury, red cells become loaded with calcium, which is normally excluded rigorously. Calcium ions activate a potassium ion channel, leading to the efflux of potassium and water, intracellular dehydration, and an increase in the mean cell hemoglobin concentration.[16] In addition, lesions produced by repeated episodes of deoxygenation render sickle red cells abnormally sticky.[17] These membrane changes are important in the pathogenesis of microvascular occlusions, described later.

A number of factors affect the rate and degree of sickling.

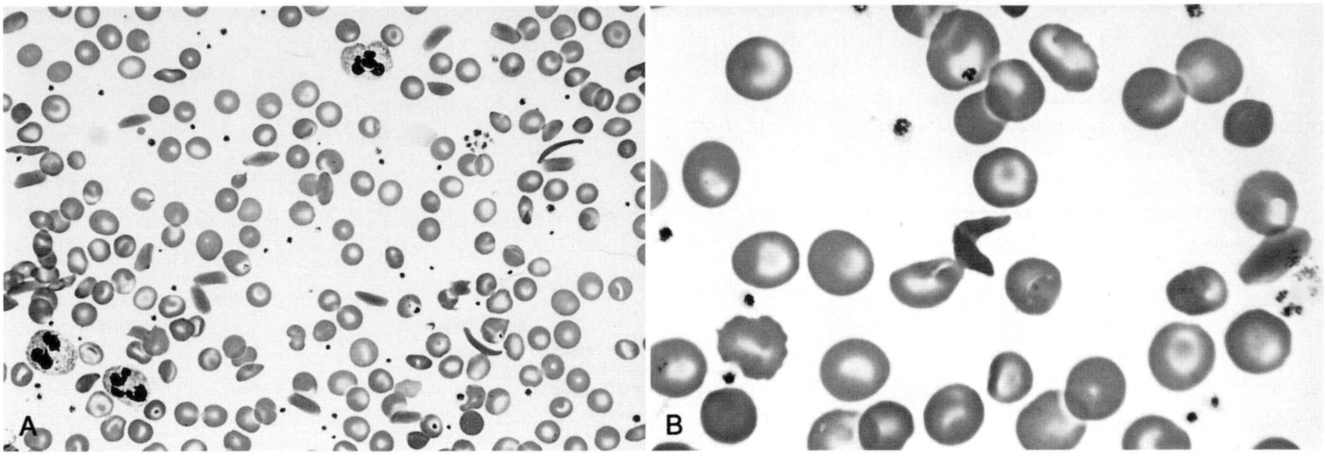

FIGURE 13–9 Sickle cell anemia (peripheral blood smear). *A*, Low magnification shows sickle cells, anisocytosis, and poikilocytosis. *B*, Higher magnification shows an irreversibly sickled cell in the center. (Courtesy of Dr. Robert W. McKenna, Department of Pathology, University of Texas Southwestern Medical School, Dallas, TX.)

- *Perhaps most important is the amount of HbS and its interaction with the other hemoglobin chains in the cell.* In heterozygotes, approximately 40% of the hemoglobin is HbS, the rest being HbA, which interacts only weakly with HbS when deoxygenated. Both the relatively low concentration of HbS and the presence of interfering HbA act to prevent efficient HbS aggregation and polymerization, and thus red cells in heterozygous individuals do not sickle except under conditions of severe hypoxia. Such individuals have *sickle cell trait,* an asymptomatic carrier state. In contrast, *homozygous HbS individuals have full-blown sickle cell anemia.* Hemoglobins other than the normal HbA also influence the aggregation and polymerization of HbS and thus the severity of sickle cell anemia profoundly. *Fetal hemoglobin (HbF) inhibits the polymerization of HbS,* and hence newborns do not manifest the disease until they are 5 to 6 months of age, when the amount of HbF in the cells falls close to adult levels. Another hemoglobin modifying the effect of HbS is HbC, which has a point mutation in the β-globin chain leading to substitution of lysine for glutamate at position 6. HbC has a greater tendency to form aggregates with deoxygenated HbS than HbA. As a result, individuals with HbS and HbC have a symptomatic sickling disorder (designated *HbSC disease*) that is generally milder than sickle cell anemia. About 2% to 3% of American blacks are asymptomatic HbC/HbA heterozygotes, and about 1 in 1250 has HbSC disease.
- *The rate of HbS polymerization is strongly dependent upon the hemoglobin concentration per cell,* that is, the mean corpuscular hemoglobin concentration (MCHC). Higher HbS concentrations increase the probability that aggregation and polymerization will occur during any given period of deoxygenation. Thus, *intracellular dehydration, which increases the MCHC, facilitates sickling and vascular occlusion* (see later). Conversely, conditions that decrease the MCHC reduce disease severity. This is most clearly illustrated when homozygous sickle cell anemia co-exists with α-thalassemia. These patients have milder disease because thalassemia reduces globin synthesis and limits the total hemoglobin concentration per cell.
- *A decrease in pH* reduces the oxygen affinity of hemoglobin, thereby increasing the fraction of deoxygenated HbS at any given oxygen tension and augmenting the tendency for sickling.
- *The length of time red cells are exposed to low oxygen tension is an important variable.* Normal transit times for red cells passing through capillaries are not sufficient for significant aggregation of deoxygenated HbS to occur. Hence, sickling of red cells is confined to microvascular beds where blood flow is sluggish. This is normally the case in the spleen and the bone marrow, which are prominently affected by sickle cell disease. Two factors play particularly important pathogenic roles in occlusive episodes involving other vascular beds: inflammation and increased red cell adhesion. As you will recall, the exodus of blood from inflamed tissues is slowed, due to the adhesion of leukocytes and red cells to activated endothelium and the transudation of fluid through leaky vessels. As a result, inflamed vascular beds have longer red cell transit times and are prone to induce clinically significant sickling. For reasons that are unclear, sickle red cells also express adhesion molecules at increased levels on their surfaces. In fact, adhesion of sickle red cells to cultured endothelial cells in vitro correlates with clinical severity, presumably because "stickiness" influences transit time in vivo.[17]

The clinical manifestations of sickle cell disease are dominated by chronic hemolysis and ischemic tissue damage resulting from occlusion of small blood vessels (Fig. 13–10).

Irreversibly sickled cells have rigid, nondeformable cell membranes that lead to difficulty in negotiating the splenic sinusoids, sequestration, and rapid phagocytosis. Some intravascular hemolysis can also occur because of the increased mechanical fragility of severely damaged cells. *The red cell survival correlates with the percentage of irreversibly sickled cells in the circulation,* supporting the concept that the hemolytic anemia results primarily from premature removal of irreversibly sickled cells.

The pathogenesis of microvascular occlusions, a clinically important component of sickle cell anemia, is less certain. There is no correlation between the number of irreversibly sickled cells and the frequency or severity of ischemic episodes, suggesting that reversibly sickled cells initiate microvascular occlusion. As mentioned above, reversibly sickled cells express higher than normal levels of adhesion

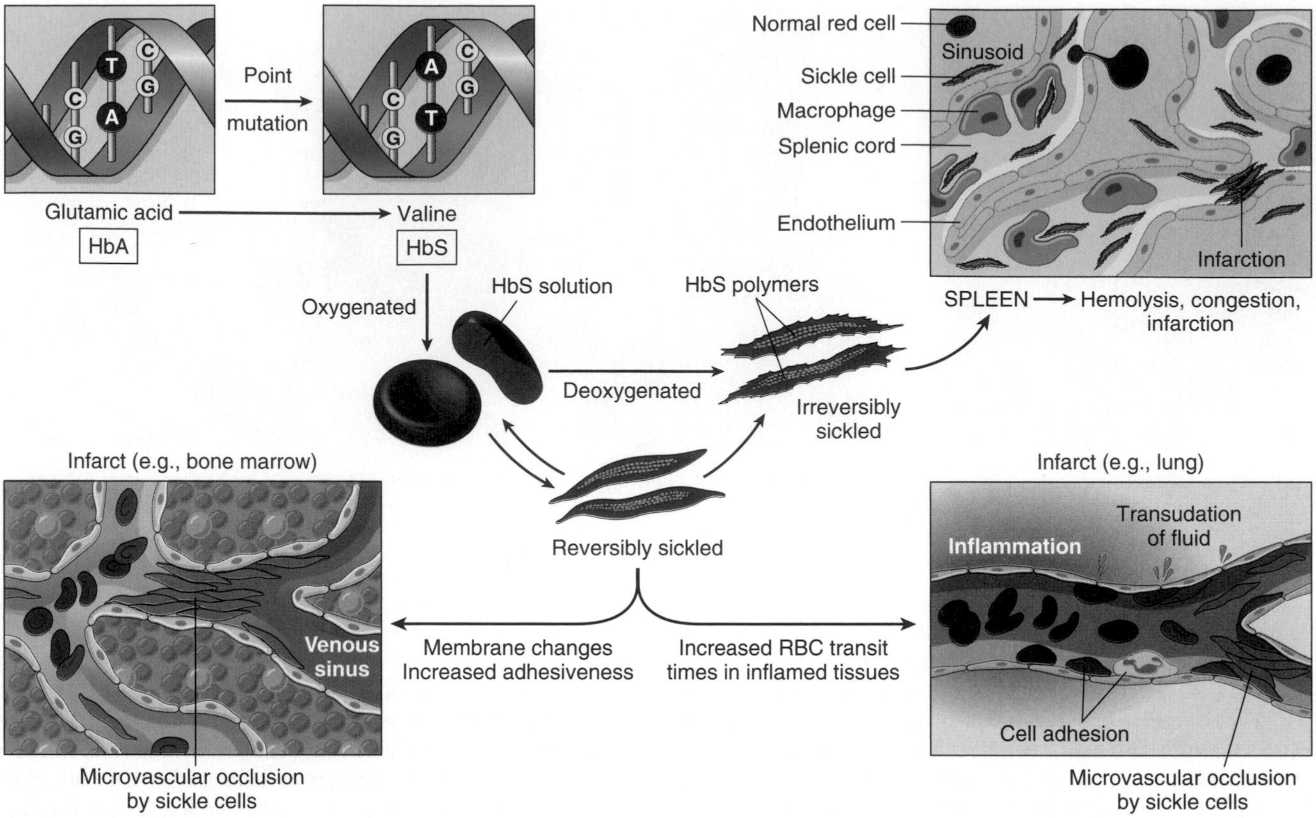

FIGURE 13–10 Pathophysiology of sickle cell anemia.

molecules and appear abnormally sticky in certain assays. In vivo, it is hypothesized that increased adhesiveness makes reversibly sickled red cells more likely to arrest during transit through the microvasculature, particularly in areas of sluggish flow. This tendency is likely enhanced by inflammation, which up-regulates the expression of adhesion molecules on endothelial cells (Chapter 2), making adherence of granulocytes, monocytes, and reversibly sickled cells more likely. An important role for pro-inflammatory granulocytes is supported by observations showing that leukocytosis correlates with disease severity.[18] The arrest of sickle red cells within hypoxic, inflamed vascular beds results in an extended exposure to a low oxygen tension, causing sickling and vascular obstruction. Indeed it appears that sickled cells, themselves, can induce adhesion molecules on the endothelium.[19] Once this process starts, it is easy to envision how a vicious cycle of sickling, obstruction, hypoxia, and more sickling ensues.[20] In recent years increasing attention is being focused on the role of nitric oxide (NO) in microvascular occlusions. It is thought that in patients with sickle cell anemia, plasma hemoglobin (released from lysed RBC) binds to and inactivates NO. Recall that NO is a potent vasodilator and inhibits platelet aggregation. Such reduction in bioavailable NO predisposes to increased vascular tone (narrowing) and platelet aggregation. These findings provide rationale for NO therapy in sickle cell disease.[21]

Morphology. The anatomic alterations are caused by chronic hemolysis, increased formation of bilirubin, and small vessel stasis and thrombosis. The consequences of the increased red cell destruction and anemia have been detailed in the general discussion of all hemolytic anemias. The bone marrow is hyperplastic because of a compensatory hyperplasia of erythroid progenitors. Expansion of the marrow leads to bone resorption and secondary new bone formation, resulting in prominent cheekbones and changes in the skull that resemble a crew-cut in roentgenograms. Extramedullary hematopoiesis can also appear.

In children, during the early phase of the disease, the spleen is commonly enlarged up to 500 gm. On histologic examination, there is marked congestion of the red pulp, due mainly to the trapping of sickled red cells in the splenic cords and sinuses (Fig. 13–11). This erythrostasis in the spleen leads to marked tissue hypoxia, thrombosis, infarction, and fibrosis. Continued scarring causes progressive shrinkage of the spleen so that by adolescence or early adulthood only a small nubbin of fibrous tissue is left; this process is called **autosplenectomy** (Fig. 13–12). Infarction secondary to vascular occlusions and anoxia can occur in many other tissues as well, including the bones, brain, kidney, liver, retina, and pulmonary vessels, the latter sometimes producing cor pulmonale. Vascular stagnation in subcutaneous tissues often leads to leg ulcers in adult patients; this complication is rare in children. As in other hemolytic anemias, increased breakdown of hemoglobin can cause pigment gallstones, and all patients develop hyperbilirubinemia during periods of active hemolysis.

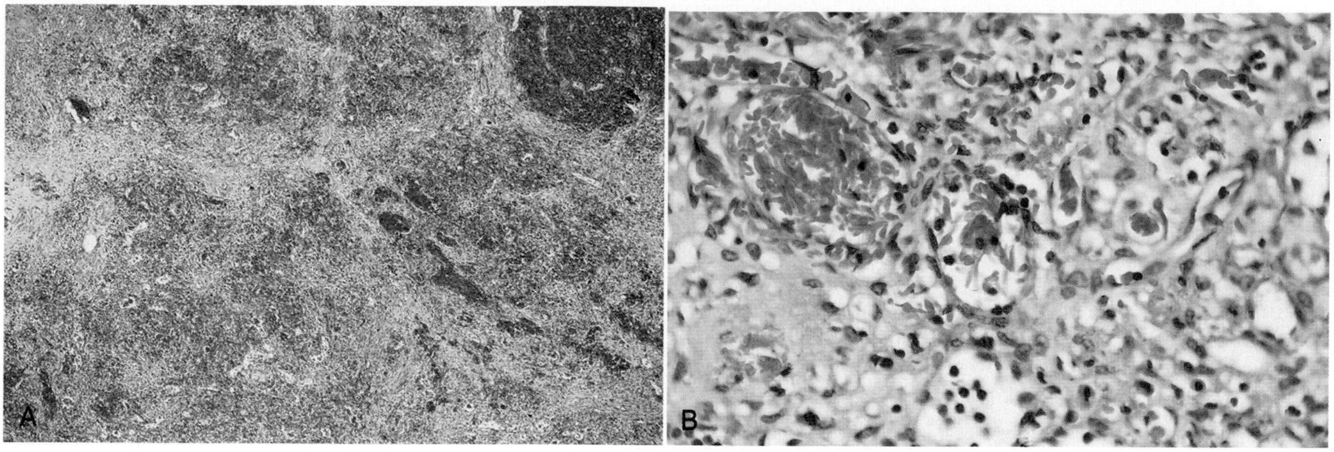

FIGURE 13–11 *A,* Spleen in sickle cell anemia (low power). Red pulp cords and sinusoids are markedly congested; between the congested areas, pale areas of fibrosis resulting from ischemic damage are evident. *B,* Under high power, splenic sinusoids are dilated and filled with sickled red cells. (Courtesy of Dr. Darren Wirthwein, Department of Pathology, University of Texas Southwestern Medical School, Dallas, TX.)

Clinical Course. *From the description of the disease to this point, it is evident that patients are beset with problems stemming from (1) severe anemia, (2) vaso-occlusive complications, and (3) chronic hyperbilirubinemia.*[22] Increased susceptibility to infection with encapsulated organisms, another threat, has at least two causes. First, splenic function is severely impaired, in children because of congestion and poor blood flow, and in adults because of infarction and autosplenectomy. Secondly, defects in the alternative complement pathway impair opsonization of encapsulated bacteria such as pneumococci and *Haemophilus influenzae.* Septicemia and meningitis caused by these two organisms are the most common causes of death in children with sickle cell anemia.

Chronic hemolysis induces moderately severe anemia (hematocrit values between 18% and 30%) associated with striking reticulocytosis and hyperbilirubinemia. Irreversibly sickled cells, ranging in frequency from 5% to 15%, are seen in peripheral smears.

The protracted course is frequently exacerbated by a variety of "crises." *Vaso-occlusive crises,* also called *pain crises,* represent episodes of hypoxic injury and infarction associated with severe pain in the affected region. Although infection, dehydration, and acidosis (all of which favor sickling) sometimes act as triggers, in most instances no predisposing causes are identified. The most commonly involved sites are the bones, lungs, liver, brain, spleen, and penis. *In children, painful bone crises are extremely common and often difficult to distinguish from acute osteomyelitis.* They frequently manifest as the hand-foot syndrome, a dactylitis of the bones of the hands or feet or both.[23] Particularly dangerous are vaso-occlusive crises involving the lungs, which typically present with fever, cough, chest pain, and a pulmonary infiltrate. Also known as *acute chest syndrome,* these are sometimes initiated by a simple lung infection.[24] Due to inflammation, blood flow becomes sluggish and "spleenlike," leading to sickling and vaso-occlusion within pulmonary vascular beds. This further compromises pulmonary function, creating a potentially fatal cycle of worsening pulmonary and systemic hypoxemia, sickling, and vaso-occlusion. Other organs affected by vaso-occlusive crises include the central nervous system, where hypoxia can provoke seizures or strokes, and the cutaneous tissues of the leg, leading to the appearance of ulcers.

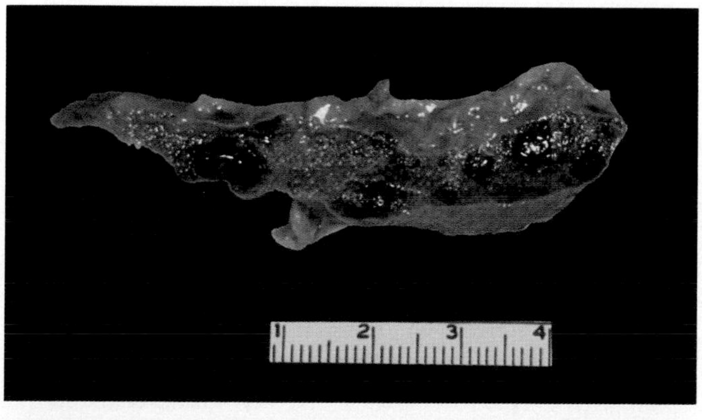

FIGURE 13–12 Splenic remnant in sickle cell anemia. (Courtesy of Drs. Dennis Burns and Darren Wirthwein, Department of Pathology, University of Texas Southwestern Medical School, Dallas, TX.)

Although pain crises are the most common cause of patient morbidity and mortality, several other acute events complicate the course of sickle cell disease. *Sequestration crises* occur in children with intact spleens. Massive sequestration of sickled red cells leads to rapid splenic enlargement, hypovolemia, and sometimes shock. Both sequestration crises and the acute chest syndrome may require treatment with exchange transfusions if the patient is to survive. In *aplastic crises,* there is a transient cessation of bone marrow erythropoiesis due to an acute infection of erythroid progenitor cells by parvovirus B19. Reticulocytes disappear from the peripheral blood, causing a sudden and rapid worsening of anemia.

In addition to these dramatic crises, chronic tissue hypoxia also takes a subtle yet important toll. Chronic hypoxia is responsible for a generalized impairment of growth and development as well as organ damage affecting spleen, heart, kidneys, and lungs. Damage to the renal medulla leads to hyposthenuria (inability to concentrate urine), which causes an increased propensity for dehydration and its attendant risks. It must be emphasized that there is great variation in the clinical manifestations of sickle cell anemia. Some individuals are crippled by repeated vaso-occlusive crises, whereas others have only mild symptoms. The basis for this wide range in disease expression is not understood, but variation in unidentified modifying genes seems likely.

The diagnosis is suggested by clinical findings and the presence of irreversibly sickled cells in peripheral blood smears and is confirmed by various tests for sickle hemoglobin. In general, these involve mixing a blood sample with an oxygen-consuming reagent, such as metabisulfite, which induces sickling of red cells if HbS is present. Hemoglobin electrophoresis is also used to demonstrate the presence of HbS and exclude other sickle syndromes, such as HbSC disease. Prenatal diagnosis is possible based on analysis of fetal DNA obtained by amniocentesis or chorionic biopsy. The outlook for patients with sickle cell anemia has improved considerably as a result of better supportive care. Approximately 90% of patients survive to age 20, and close to 50% survive beyond the fifth decade. A major recent advance in sickle cell anemia is treatment with the cancer therapeutic drug hydroxyurea, which has several beneficial effects.[25] Through uncertain mechanisms, hydroxyurea causes a significant increase in the concentration of HbF in red cells, which (as we have discussed) interferes with the polymerization of HbS. However, the therapeutic response to hydroxyurea often precedes the rise in HbF levels, implying that other mechanisms are also important, several of which have been proposed. Firstly, hydroxyurea acts as an anti-inflammatory agent by inhibiting the production of white cells, which may reduce inflammation-related red cell stasis and sickling. Secondly, hydroxyurea increases the mean red cell volume and thereby decreases the concentration of HbS. Thirdly, hydroxyurea can be oxidized by heme groups to produce NO. It is hypothesized all of these actions contribute to ability of hydroxyurea to reduce pain crises in children and adults.[26,27]

Thalassemia Syndromes

The thalassemia syndromes are a heterogeneous group of inherited disorders caused by genetic lesions leading to decreased synthesis of either the α- or β-globin chain of HbA ($\alpha_2\beta_2$). *β-Thalassemia is caused by deficient synthesis of the β chain, whereas α-thalassemia is caused by deficient synthesis of the α chain. The hematologic consequences of diminished synthesis of one globin chain stem not only from low intracellular hemoglobin (hypochromia), but also from a relative excess of the unimpaired chain.* For example, in β-thalassemia, excess free α chains aggregate into insoluble inclusions within red cells and their precursors, leading to premature destruction of maturing erythroblasts in the marrow *(ineffective erythropoiesis)* and lysis of mature red cells in the spleen *(hemolysis)*.

β-Thalassemias

The abnormality common to all β-thalassemias is diminished synthesis of structurally normal β-globin chains, coupled with unimpaired synthesis of α chains. The clinical severity of the anemia varies due to heterogeneity in the causative mutations. We begin our discussion with the molecular lesions in β-thalassemia, and then relate the clinical variants to specific underlying molecular defects.

Molecular Pathogenesis. Adult hemoglobin (HbA) is a tetramer composed of two α chains and two β chains encoded by a pair of functional α-globin genes on chromosome 16 and a single β-globin gene on chromosome 11. β-Thalassemia syndromes are classified into two categories: (1) *β^0-thalassemia*, associated with total absence of β-globin chains in the homozygous state, and (2) *β^+-thalassemia*, characterized by reduced (but detectable) β-globin synthesis in the homozygous state. Sequencing of β-thalassemia genes has revealed approximately 100 different causative mutations.[28] Most are point mutations; unlike α-thalassemia, gene deletions are uncommon in β-thalassemia. Details of these mutations and their effects on β-globin synthesis are found in specialized texts. A few illustrative examples are cited (Fig. 13–13).

- *Promoter region mutations.* Point mutations within promoter sequences prevent RNA polymerase from binding normally, reducing transcription by 75% to 80%. Some normal β-globin is synthesized, producing β^+-thalassemia.
- *Chain terminator mutations.* Two types of mutations cause premature termination of mRNA translation. One creates a new stop codon within an exon; the second consists of small insertions or deletions that shift the mRNA reading frames and introduce downstream stop codons that terminate protein synthesis (frameshift mutations; see Chapter 5). In both cases, synthesis of functional β-globin is prevented by premature chain termination, leading to β^0-thalassemia.
- *Splicing mutations. Mutations leading to aberrant splicing are the most common cause of β-thalassemia.* Most affect

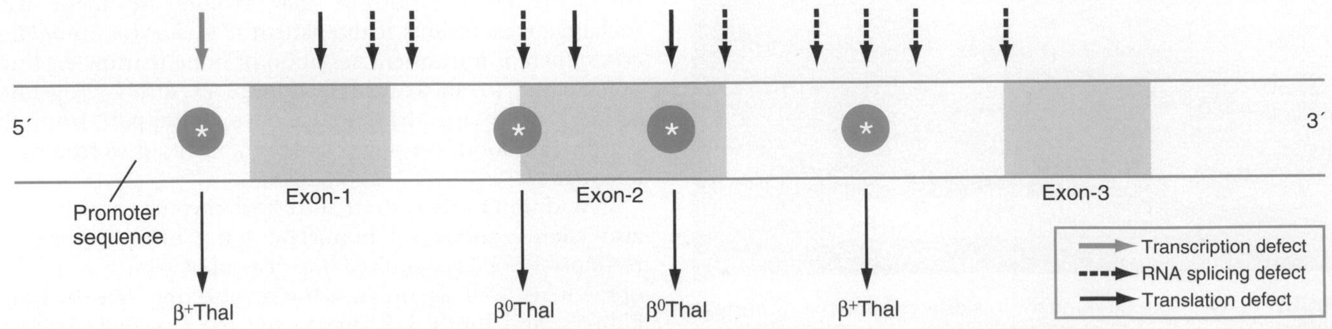

FIGURE 13–13 Diagrammatic representation of the β-globin gene. Arrows denote sites where point mutations giving rise to thalassemia have been identified.

introns; others are located within exons. Some of these mutations alter normal splice junctions, such that normal splicing does not occur at all. Unspliced mRNA is degraded within the nucleus, and β^0-thalassemia results. Other mutations occurring in introns create new "ectopic" splice sites at abnormal locations—within an intron, for example. Because normal splice sites remain, both normal and abnormal splicing occurs, giving rise to normal and abnormal β-globin mRNA. These mutations cause β^+-thalassemia.

Impaired β-globin synthesis results in anemia by two mechanisms (Fig. 13–14). The deficit in HbA synthesis produces "under-hemoglobinized," hypochromic, microcytic red cells with subnormal oxygen transport capacity. A more important factor is diminished survival of red cells and their precursors, resulting from the imbalance in α- and β-chain synthesis. Free α chains precipitate within the normoblasts, forming insoluble inclusions. These inclusions cause a variety of untoward effects, but *cell membrane damage is the proximal cause of most red cell pathology.* Many developing normoblasts in the marrow succumb to these membrane lesions, undergoing apoptosis. In severe β-thalassemia, it is estimated that 70% to 85% of normoblasts suffer this fate, leading to ineffective erythropoiesis.[28] The inclusion-bearing red cells derived from precursors escaping intramedullary death are prone to splenic sequestration and destruction due to cell membrane damage and decreased deformability.

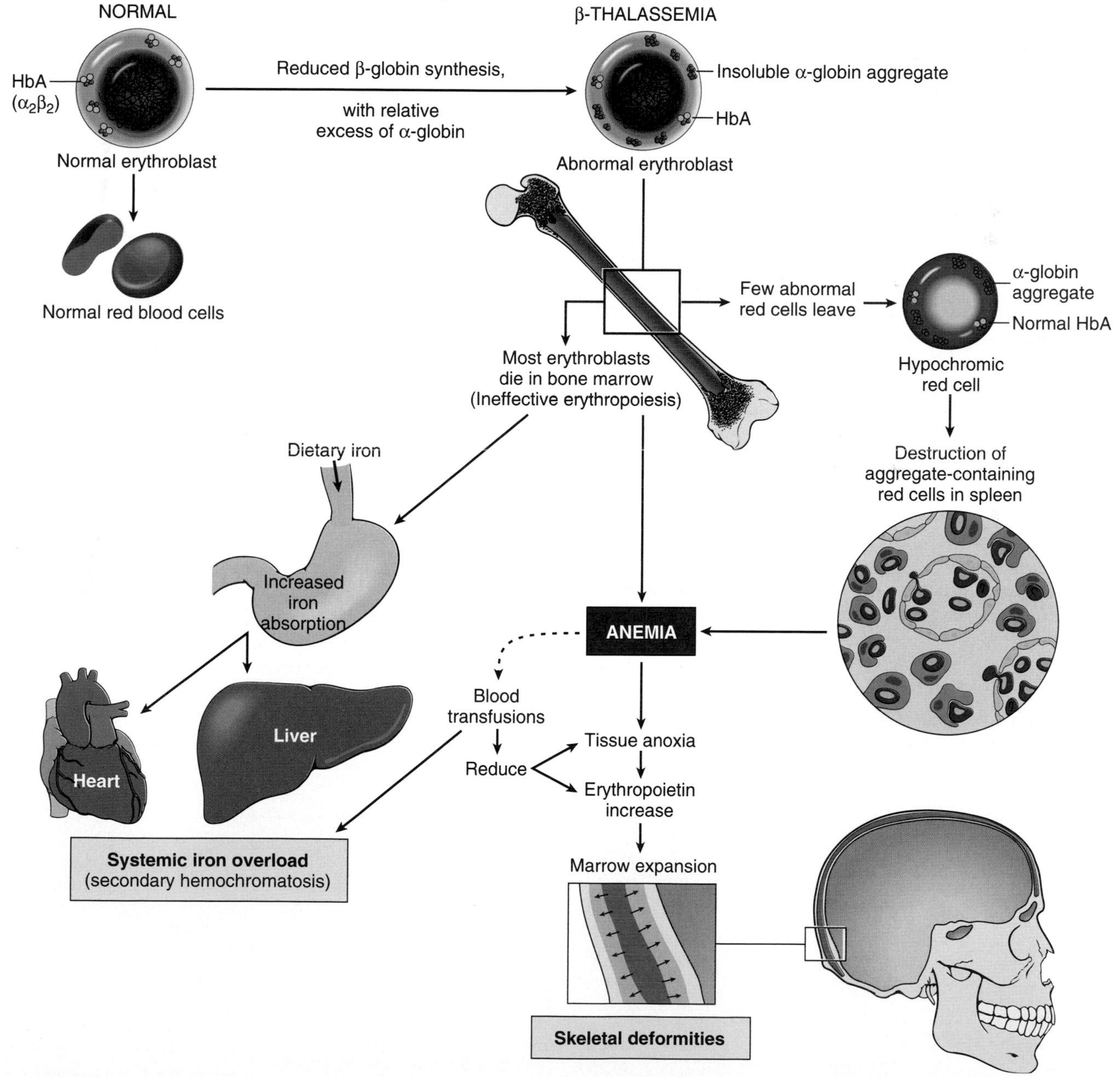

FIGURE 13–14 Pathogenesis of β-thalassemia major. Note that aggregates of unpaired α-globin chains are not visible in routinely stained blood smears. Blood transfusions are a double-edged sword, correcting the anemia and thereby reducing the stimulus for marrow expansion, but also adding to systemic iron overload.

In severe β-thalassemia, marked anemia produced by ineffective erythropoiesis and hemolysis leads to several additional problems. Erythropoietin secretion in the setting of severe uncompensated anemia leads to massive erythroid hyperplasia in the marrow and sites of extramedullary hematopoiesis. The expanding mass of erythropoietic marrow invades the bony cortex, impairs bone growth, and produces other skeletal abnormalities, described later. Extramedullary hematopoiesis involves the liver, spleen, and lymph nodes, and in extreme cases produces extraosseous masses in the thorax, abdomen, and pelvis. The metabolically active erythroid progenitors steal nutrients from other tissues that are already oxygen starved, causing severe cachexia in untreated patients. *Another disastrous complication seen in severe β-thalassemia (as well as in other causes of ineffective erythropoiesis) is excessive absorption of dietary iron.* This, coupled with the iron accumulation due to the repeated blood transfusions required by these patients, leads to a state of severe iron overload. Secondary injury to parenchymal organs, particularly the iron-laden liver, often follows and sometimes induces secondary hemochromatosis (Chapter 18).

Clinical Syndromes. Clinical classification of β-thalassemias is based on the severity of the anemia, which in turn depends on the type of genetic defect (β^+ or β^0) and the gene dosage (homozygous or heterozygous).[29] In general, individuals homozygous for β-thalassemia genes (β^+/β^+ or β^0/β^0) have a severe, transfusion-dependent anemia called *β-thalassemia major.* Heterozygotes with one β-thalassemia gene and one normal gene (β^+/β or β^0/β) usually have a mild microcytic anemia that causes no symptoms. This condition is referred to as *β-thalassemia minor* or *β-thalassemia trait.* A third clinical variant of intermediate severity is called *β-thalassemia intermedia.* β-thalassemia intermedia is genetically heterogeneous. This category includes milder variants of β^+/β^+ or β^+/β^0-thalassemia and unusually severe variants of heterozygous β-thalassemia (β^0/? or β^+/?). Ironically, the presence of an α-thalassemia gene defect often decreases the severity of β-thalassemia major, since the imbalance in α- and β-chain synthesis is lessened; this combination can also result in a clinical phenotype resembling β-thalassemia intermedia. The clinical and morphologic features of thalassemia intermedia are not described separately but can be surmised from the following discussions of thalassemia major and minor (Table 13–3).

Thalassemia Major. β-Thalassemia is most common in Mediterranean countries and parts of Africa and Southeast Asia. In the United States, the incidence is highest in immigrants from these areas. As indicated in Table 13–3, the genotype of affected patients can be β^+/β^+, β^0/β^0, or β^0/β^+. With all these genotypes, the anemia manifests 6 to 9 months after birth, as hemoglobin synthesis switches from HbF to HbA. In untransfused patients, hemoglobin levels range between 3 and 6 gm/dL. The peripheral blood smear shows severe red cell morphologic abnormalities, including marked anisocytosis and poikilocytosis (variation in size and shape, respectively), microcytosis (small size), and hypochromia (poor hemoglobinization). Target cells (so called because hemoglobin collects in the center of the cells), basophilic stippling, and fragmented red cells are also common. Inclusions of aggregated α chains are efficiently removed by the spleen and not easily found in peripheral blood smears. The reticulocyte count is elevated, but because of ineffective erythropoiesis is lower than expected for the severity of anemia. Variable numbers of poorly hemoglobinized normoblasts are seen in the peripheral blood due to "stress" erythropoiesis and abnormal release of progenitors from sites of extramedullary hematopoiesis. The red cells can completely lack HbA (β^0/β^0 genotype) or contain small amounts (β^+/β^+ or β^0/β^+ genotypes). HbF is markedly increased and indeed constitutes the major red cell hemoglobin. HbA_2 levels may be normal, low, or high.

Morphology. The major morphologic alterations, in addition to those found in all hemolytic anemias, involve the bone marrow and spleen. In the untransfused patient, there is striking expansion of hematopoietically active marrow, particularly in facial bones. This erodes existing cortical bone and induces new bone formation, giving rise to a "crew-cut" appearance on X-rays (Fig. 13–15). Both mononuclear phagocytic cell hyperplasia and extramedullary hematopoiesis contribute to enlargement of the spleen, which can weigh up to 1500 gm.

TABLE 13–3 Clinical and Genetic Classification of Thalassemias

Clinical Nomenclature	Genotype	Disease	Molecular Genetics
β-Thalassemias			
Thalassemia major	Homozygous β^0-thalassemia (β^0/β^0) Homozygous β^+-thalassemia (β^+/β^+)	Severe; requires blood transfusions	Rare gene deletions in β^0/β^0 Defects in transcription, processing, or translation of β-globin mRNA
Thalassemia intermedia	β^0/β β^+/β^+	Severe, but does not require regular blood transfusions	
Thalassemia minor	β^0/β β^+/β	Asymptomatic with mild or absent anemia; red cell abnormalities seen	
α-Thalassemias			
Hydrops fetails	–/– –/–	Lethal in utero without transfusions	Mainly gene deletions
HbH disease	–/– –/α	Severe; resembles β-thalassemia intermedia	
α-Thalassemia trait	–/– α/α (Asian) –/α –/α (black African)	Asymptomatic, like β-thalassemia minor	
Silent carrier	–/α α/α	Asymptomatic; no red cell abnormality	

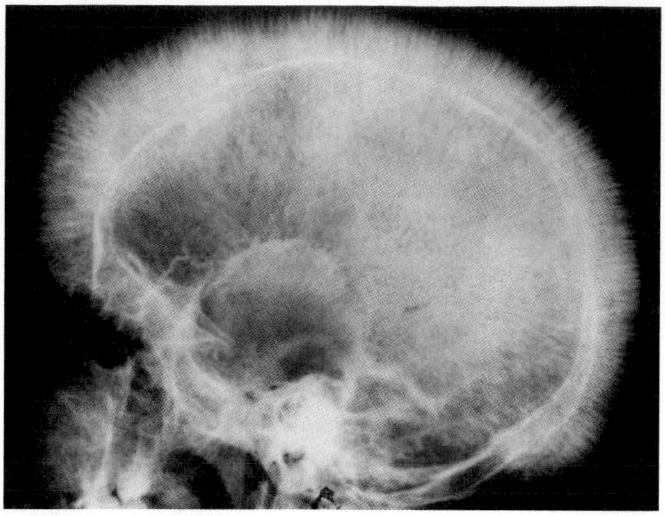

FIGURE 13–15 Thalassemia: x-ray film of the skull showing new bone formation on the outer table, producing perpendicular radiations resembling a crew-cut. (Courtesy of Dr. Jack Reynolds, Department of Radiology, University of Texas Southwestern Medical School, Dallas, TX.)

> Hemosiderosis and secondary hemochromatosis, the two manifestations of iron overload (Chapter 18), occur in almost all patients due to numerous blood transfusions and increased absorption of dietary iron. Iron deposition often causes damage to several organs, most notably the heart, liver, and pancreas (Chapter 18).

The clinical course of β-thalassemia major is brief unless blood transfusions are given. Untreated children suffer from growth retardation and die at an early age from the profound effects of anemia. Blood transfusions not only improve the anemia but also suppress secondary features related to excessive erythropoiesis. In those who survive long enough, the cheekbones and other bony prominences are enlarged and distorted. Hepatosplenomegaly due to extramedullary hematopoiesis is usually present. Cardiac disease resulting from progressive iron overload and secondary hemochromatosis (Chapter 18) is an important cause of death, particularly in heavily transfused patients. Administration of iron chelators can forestall or prevent this complication. With transfusions and iron chelation, survival into the third decade is possible, but the overall outlook remains guarded. Bone marrow transplantation from an HLA-identical sibling is currently the only therapy offering a cure. Prenatal diagnosis is possible by molecular analysis of DNA.

Thalassemia Minor. Thalassemia minor is much more common than thalassemia major and understandably affects the same ethnic groups. Most patients are heterozygous carriers of a β^+ or β^0 gene. Thalassemia trait may offer resistance against falciparum malaria, accounting for its prevalence in parts of the world where malaria is endemic. These patients are usually asymptomatic, and anemia is mild if present. The peripheral blood smear typically shows some red cell abnormalities, including hypochromia, microcytosis, basophilic stippling, and target cells. Mild erythroid hyperplasia is seen in the bone marrow. Hemoglobin electrophoresis characteristically reveals an increase in HbA_2 to 4% to 8% of the total hemoglobin (normal, 2.5% ± 0.3%). HbF levels can be normal or slightly increased. Recognition of β-thalassemia trait is important on two counts: (1) differentiation from the hypochromic microcytic anemia of iron deficiency and (2) genetic counseling. Iron deficiency can usually be excluded as the cause of a microcytic anemia through measurement of serum iron, total iron-binding capacity, and serum ferritin (see Iron Deficiency Anemia). Hemoglobin electrophoresis is a very helpful confirmatory test for β-thalassemia trait, particularly in individuals (such as women of childbearing age) at risk for both thalassemia trait and iron deficiency.

α-Thalassemias

The α-thalassemia disorders are characterized by reduced or absent synthesis of α-globin chains. There are normally four α-globin genes. The severity of α-thalassemia varies greatly depending on the number of α-globin genes affected. As in β-thalassemias, the anemia stems both from lack of adequate hemoglobin and the effects of excess unpaired non-α chains (β, γ, δ). However, the situation is complicated somewhat by synthesis of different non-α chains at varying times of development. Thus, in the newborn with α-thalassemia, excess unpaired γ-globin forms γ_4-tetramers known as hemoglobin Barts, whereas in adults excess β-globin chains form β_4 tetramers known as HbH. Since free β and γ chains are more soluble than free α chains and form fairly stable homotetramers, hemolysis and ineffective erythropoiesis are less severe than in β-thalassemias. A variety of molecular lesions result in α-thalassemia, but the most common cause of reduced α-chain synthesis is deletion of α-globin genes.[29]

Clinical Syndromes. Clinical syndromes are determined and classified by the number and position of deleted α-globin genes. Each of the four α-globin genes, which occur in two linked pairs on each copy of chromosome 16, normally contributes approximately 25% of the α-globin chains. α-Thalassemia syndromes stem from combinations of deletions that remove one to four α-globin gene copies. Not surprisingly, the severity of the clinical syndrome is proportional to the number of missing α-globin genes. Categories of α-thalassemias are given in Table 13–3, which lists clinical terms, along with their genetic equivalents and salient clinical features.

Silent Carrier State. This occurs if a single α-globin gene is deleted. It is associated with a barely detectable reduction in α-globin chain synthesis that is insufficient to result in anemia. These individuals are completely asymptomatic.

α-Thalassemia Trait. This is caused by deletion of two α-globin genes. The two involved genes can be from the same chromosome (α/α –/–), or one α-globin gene can be deleted from each of the two chromosomes (α/– α/–) (see Table 13–3). The former genotype is more common in Asian populations, the latter in regions of Africa. Both genotypes produce similar quantitative deficiencies of α-globin chains and are clinically identical, but only matings involving individuals with the α/α –/– genotype are at risk for producing offspring with severe α-thalassemia (HbH disease or hydrops fetalis). As is evident from Table 13–3, in black African populations, α-thalassemia trait is associated with an α/– α/– genotype, and mating of two such individuals cannot result in progeny with HbH disease or hydrops fetalis.

The clinical picture in α-thalassemia trait is identical to that described for β-thalassemia minor, that is, small red cells (microcytosis), minimal or no anemia, and no abnormal physical signs.

Hemoglobin H Disease. This is caused by deletion of three α-globin genes. As already discussed, HbH disease is seen most commonly in Asian populations and rarely in those of African origin. With only one normal α-globin gene, the synthesis of α chains is markedly reduced and tetramers of excess β-globin, called HbH, form. HbH has extremely high affinity for oxygen and therefore is not useful for oxygen exchange, leading to tissue hypoxia disproportionate to the level of hemoglobin. Additionally, HbH is prone to oxidation, leading to the formation of intracellular inclusions that can be demonstrated by staining with vital dyes. The instability of HbH is a major cause of anemia, as precipitates of oxidized HbH form in older red cells, which are then removed by splenic macrophages. This produces a moderately severe anemia resembling β-thalassemia intermedia.

Hydrops Fetalis. This most severe form of α-thalassemia is caused by deletion of all four α-globin genes. In the fetus, excess γ-globin chains form tetramers (hemoglobin Barts) with such a high affinity for oxygen that they deliver almost no oxygen to tissues. Survival in early development is due to the expression of ζ chains, an embryonic globin that pairs with γ chains to form a functional Hb tetramer ($\zeta_2\gamma_2$). Signs of fetal distress usually become evident by the third trimester of pregnancy. In the past, severe tissue anoxia invariably led to intrauterine fetal death; with intrauterine transfusion, many such infants can be saved. The fetus shows severe pallor, generalized edema, and massive hepatosplenomegaly similar to that seen in erythroblastosis fetalis (Chapter 10).

Paroxysmal Nocturnal Hemoglobinuria

Despite its rarity, paroxysmal nocturnal hemoglobinuria (PNH) has fascinated hematologists because it is the only hemolytic anemia caused by an acquired intrinsic defect in the cell membrane. Before we describe its molecular basis, it is instructive to recall that proteins are anchored into the lipid bilayer in two ways. Most have a hydrophobic sequence that spans the cell membrane (Fig. 13–16); these are called transmembrane proteins. The remainder are attached to the cell membrane by covalent linkage to a specialized phospholipid called glycosylphosphatidylinositol (GPI). *PNH results from acquired mutations in phosphatidylinositol glycan A (PIGA), which is essential for the synthesis of the GPI anchor.*[30] Because *PIGA* is X-linked and subject to lyonization (see Chapter 5), only the active *PIGA* gene needs to be mutated to produce a functional deficiency. The causative somatic mutations occur in pluripotent stem cells; hence, all its clonal progeny (red cells, white cells, and platelets) are deficient in proteins attached to the cell membrane via GPI. Several GPI-linked proteins inactivate complement. Their absence in PNH renders blood cells unusually sensitive to lysis by complement. Not all blood cells are affected in PNH patients, indicating that the mutant clone exists side by side with progeny of normal stem cells.

Three GPI-linked proteins that regulate complement activity—decay-accelerating factor, or CD55; membrane inhibitor of reactive lysis, or CD59; and a C8 binding protein—are deficient in PNH. Of these, CD59 is the most

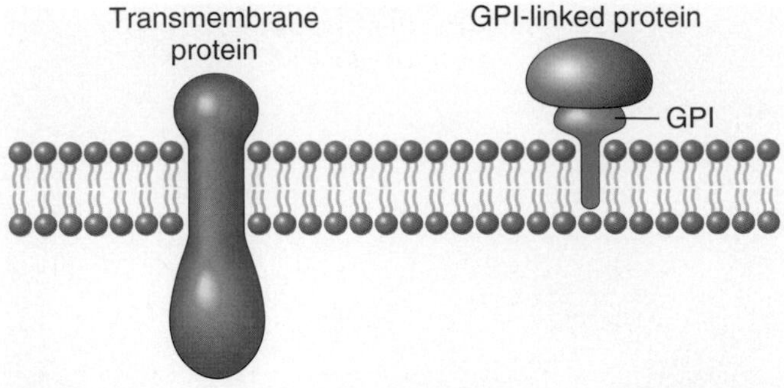

FIGURE 13–16 Two kinds of membrane proteins: transmembrane and glycosyl phosphatidyl inositol (GPI)-linked. The latter are anchored to cell membranes through a covalent attachment to a glycosyl phospatidyl inositol moiety. In PNH, GPI cannot be synthesized, leading to a global deficiency of GPI-linked membrane proteins.

important. It is a potent inhibitor of C3 convertase, and thereby prevents spontaneous activation of the alternative complement pathway in vivo. These defects are not limited to red blood cells, as deficient platelets and granulocytes are also more sensitive to lysis by complement.

The intravascular hemolysis is actually paroxysmal and nocturnal in only 25% of cases. Chronic hemolysis without dramatic hemoglobinuria is more common. During the disease course, hemosiderinuria eventually leads to iron deficiency. An inconstant but severe clinical manifestation is episodic venous thrombosis, often involving the hepatic, portal, or cerebral veins; this thrombosis is fatal in 50% of cases. Dysfunction of platelets due to the absence of certain GPI-linked proteins contributes to the prothrombotic state. PNH patients are also at increased risk for developing acute myelogenous leukemia. The basis for this association is unclear.

Remarkably, it is now appreciated that normal individuals harbor small numbers of bone marrow cells with *PIGA* mutations identical to those causing PNH.[30] It is assumed that these cells increase in numbers (thus producing clinically evident PNH) only in very rare instances where they have a selective advantage. Consistent with this view, PNH often arises in the setting of primary bone marrow failure (aplastic anemia), which can be caused by immune-mediated destruction or suppression of marrow stem cells. Based on this scenario, immunosuppression is being evaluated as a therapeutic approach, as it may permit reconstitution of the marrow with the offspring of residual normal stem cells.

Immunohemolytic Anemia

Hemolytic anemias in this category are caused by extracorpuscular mechanisms. Although these disorders are commonly referred to as autoimmune hemolytic anemias, the designation *immunohemolytic anemias* is preferred because in some instances the immune reaction is initiated by drug ingestion.[31] The immunohemolytic disorders are classified in various ways, most centered on the characteristics of the responsible antibody (Table 13–4).

The diagnosis of immunohemolytic anemias requires the detection of antibodies and/or complement on patient red cells. This is done using the direct *Coombs antiglobulin test.* In

TABLE 13–4 Classification of Immunohemolytic Anemias

Warm Antibody Type
The antibody is of the IgG type, does not usually fix complement, and is active at 37°C.
Primary (idiopathic)
Secondary
Lymphomas and leukemias
Other neoplastic diseases
Autoimmune disorder (particularly systemic lupus erythematosus)
Drugs
Cold Agglutinin Type
The antibodies are IgM and most active in vitro at 0° to 4°C. Antibodies dissociate at 30°C or above; agglutination of cells by IgM and complement fixation occurs only in peripheral cool parts of the body (e.g., fingers, ears, and toes).
Acute (mycoplasmal infection, infectious mononucleosis)
Chronic
Idiopathic
Associated with lymphoma
Cold Hemolysins (Paroxysmal Cold Hemoglobinuria)
IgG antibodies bind red cells at low temperature, fix complement, and cause hemolysis when the temperature is raised above 30°C.

this test, patient red cells are mixed with heterologous antisera specific for human immunoglobulins or complement. If either is present, red cells are cross-linked by multivalent antibodies, causing clumping or agglutination. The indirect Coombs antiglobulin test, in which patient serum is tested for its ability to agglutinate defined test red cells, can then be used to characterize the target of the autoantibody. The temperature dependence of this reaction also helps to define the type of antibody responsible. Quantitative immunologic tests to measure such antibodies directly are also available.

Warm Antibody Immunohemolytic Anemia. This is the most common form (48% to 70%) of immune hemolytic anemia. About 50% of cases are idiopathic (primary); the remainder arise secondarily in the setting of a predisposing condition (see Table 13–4) or drug exposure. Most causative antibodies are of the immunoglobulin G (IgG) class; only sometimes are IgA antibodies culpable. Most red cell destruction in this form of hemolytic disease is extravascular. IgG-coated red cells bind Fc receptors on monocytes and splenic macrophages, which results in loss of red cell membrane during "partial" phagocytosis. As in hereditary spherocytosis, *the loss of cell membrane converts the red cells to spherocytes, which are sequestered and removed in the spleen, the major site of red cell destruction in this disorder. Thus, moderate splenomegaly is characteristic of this form of anemia.*

As with other forms of autoimmunity, the cause of autoantibody formation is largely unknown. In many cases, the antibodies are directed against the Rh blood group antigens. The mechanisms of drug-induced hemolysis are better understood. Two predominant immunologic mechanisms have been implicated.[31]

- *Hapten model.* The drugs—exemplified by penicillin and cephalosporins—act as haptens by binding to the red cell membrane. Antibodies directed against the cell-bound drug result in the destructive sequence cited before. This form of hemolytic anemia is usually caused by large intravenous doses of the antibiotic and occurs 1 to 2 weeks after onset of therapy. Sometimes the antibodies bind only to the offending drug, as in penicillin-induced hemolytic anemia. In other cases, such as quinidine-induced hemolysis, the antibodies recognize a complex of the drug and a membrane protein. In drug-induced hemolytic anemias, the destruction of red cells can occur intravascularly after fixation of complement or extravascularly in the mononuclear phagocyte system.
- *Autoantibody model.* These drugs, of which the antihypertensive agent α-methyldopa is the prototype, in some manner initiate the production of antibodies directed against intrinsic red cell antigens, in particular the Rh blood group antigens. Approximately 10% of patients taking α-methyldopa develop autoantibodies, as assessed by the direct Coombs test. However, only 1% develops clinically significant hemolysis.

Cold Agglutinin Immunohemolytic Anemia. This form of immunohemolytic anemia is caused by so-called *cold agglutinins,* IgM antibodies that bind and agglutinate red cells avidly at low temperatures (0° to 4°C).[32] It is less common than warm antibody immunohemolytic anemia, accounting for 16% to 32% of cases of immunohemolytic anemia. Such antibodies appear *acutely* during the recovery phase of certain infectious disorders, such as mycoplasma pneumonia and infectious mononucleosis. In these settings, the disorder is self-limited and rarely induces clinical manifestations of hemolysis. Other infectious agents associated with this form of anemia include cytomegalovirus, influenza virus, and human immunodeficiency virus (HIV). *Chronic* cold agglutinin immunohemolytic anemias occur in association with certain lymphoid neoplasms or as an idiopathic condition. Clinical symptoms result from binding of IgM to red cells at sites such as exposed fingers, toes, and ears where the temperature is below 30°C. IgM binding agglutinates red cells and rapidly fixes complement on their surface. As the blood recirculates and warms, IgM is rapidly released, usually before complement-mediated hemolysis can occur. However, the transient interaction with IgM is sufficient to deposit sublytic quantities of C3b, an excellent opsonin, leading to rapid removal of affected red cells by mononuclear phagocytes in the liver and spleen. The hemolysis is of variable severity. Vascular obstruction caused by red cell agglutinates results in pallor, cyanosis of the body parts exposed to cold temperatures, and Raynaud phenomenon (Chapter 11).

Cold Hemolysin Hemolytic Anemia. Cold hemolysins are autoantibodies responsible for an unusual entity known as *paroxysmal cold hemoglobinuria,* characterized by acute intermittent massive intravascular hemolysis, frequently with hemoglobinuria, after exposure to cold temperatures. This is the least common form of immunohemolytic anemia. Lysis is clearly complement dependent. The autoantibodies are IgGs that bind to the P blood group antigen on the red cell surface at low temperatures. Complement-mediated intravascular lysis does not occur until the cells recirculate to warm central regions, as the enzymes of the complement cascade function more efficiently at 37°C. The antibody, also known as the Donath-Landsteiner antibody, was first recognized in association with syphilis. Today, most cases of paroxysmal cold hemoglobinuria follow infections such as mycoplasma pneumonia, measles, mumps, and ill-defined viral and "flu" syndromes. The mechanisms responsible for production of such autoantibodies in these settings are unknown.

Hemolytic Anemia Resulting from Trauma to Red Cells

Red blood cells can be disrupted by physical trauma in a variety of circumstances. Of these, *hemolytic anemias caused by cardiac valve prostheses, or narrowing or obstruction of the microvasculature, are most important clinically.* Severe traumatic hemolytic anemia is more frequently associated with artificial mechanical valves than bioprosthetic porcine valves. Hemolysis in both instances stems from shear stresses produced by turbulent blood flow and abnormal pressure gradients. Microangiopathic hemolytic anemia, on the other hand, occurs when red cells are forced to squeeze through abnormally narrowed small vessels. Narrowing is most often caused by fibrin deposition in association with disseminated intravascular coagulation (discussed later in this chapter). Other causes of microangiopathic hemolytic anemia include malignant hypertension, systemic lupus erythematosus, thrombotic thrombocytopenic purpura (TTP), hemolytic-uremic syndrome (HUS), and disseminated cancer, most of which are discussed elsewhere in this book. The common feature among all these disorders is a microvascular lesion that causes mechanical injury to circulating red cells. This damage is evident in peripheral blood smears in the form of red cell fragments (schistocytes), "burr cells," "helmet cells," and "triangle cells" (Fig. 13–17). Except for TTP and HUS, hemolysis is not a major clinical problem in most instances.

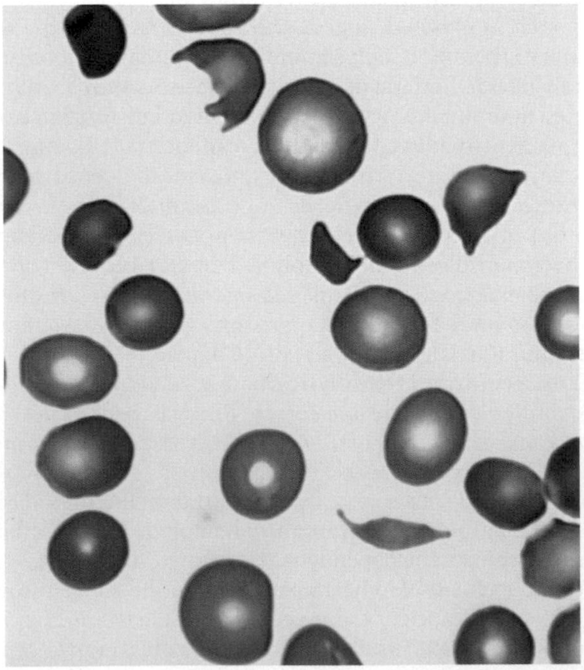

FIGURE 13–17 Microangiopathic hemolytic anemia. A peripheral blood smear from a patient with hemolytic-uremic syndrome shows several fragmented red cells. (Courtesy of Dr. Robert W. McKenna, Department of Pathology, University of Texas Southwestern Medical School, Dallas, TX.)

ANEMIAS OF DIMINISHED ERYTHROPOIESIS

Anemias often result from deficiencies of vital nutrients necessary for red cell formation. Included in this group are the anemias of vitamin B_{12} and folate deficiency, characterized by defective DNA synthesis (megaloblastic anemias), and iron deficiency anemias, in which heme synthesis is impaired. Other causes of decreased erythropoiesis include anemia of chronic disease, anemia of renal failure, and "marrow stem cell failure," which embraces such conditions as aplastic anemia and pure red cell aplasia.

Megaloblastic Anemias

The following discussion attempts first to characterize the major features of these anemias and then to discuss the two principal types of megaloblastic anemia: (1) pernicious anemia, the major form of vitamin B_{12} deficiency anemia, and (2) folate deficiency anemia.

The megaloblastic anemias constitute a diverse group of entities, having in common *impaired DNA synthesis* and distinctive morphologic changes in the blood and bone marrow. As the name implies, erythroid precursors and red cells are abnormally large due to defective cell maturation and division. The precise basis for these changes is not fully understood.

Some of the metabolic roles of vitamin B_{12} and folate are considered later, but for now it suffices that vitamin B_{12} and folic acid are coenzymes required for synthesis of thymidine, one of the four bases found in DNA. A deficiency of these vitamins or impairment in their metabolism results in defective nuclear maturation due to deranged or inadequate DNA synthesis, with an attendant delay or block in cell division. The synthesis of RNA and protein is relatively unaffected, however, so cytoplasmic maturation proceeds in advance of nuclear maturation, a situation described as nuclear/cytoplasmic asynchrony.

Morphology. Certain morphologic features are common to all forms of megaloblastic anemia. A peripheral blood examination usually reveals pancytopenia, as all myeloid lineages are affected. There is marked variation in the size and shape of red cells (anisocytosis), which nonetheless are normochromic. **Many red cells are macrocytic and oval (macro-ovalocytes), with mean corpuscular (cell) volumes above 100 fl (normal, 82 to 98).** Because they are thicker than normal and well-hemoglobinized, most macrocytes lack the central pallor of normal red cells and can even appear "hyperchromic," but the MCHC is not elevated. The reticulocyte count is low, and nucleated red cells occasionally appear in the circulating blood with severe anemia. **Neutrophils are also larger than normal (macropolymorphonuclear) and hypersegmented; that is, they have five to six or more nuclear lobules** (Fig. 13–18). The marrow is usually markedly hypercellular due to increased numbers of all types of myeloid precursors, which may completely replace the fatty marrow. Megaloblastic change is detected in all stages of red cell development. The most primitive cells (promegaloblasts) are large, with a deeply basophilic cytoplasm, prominent

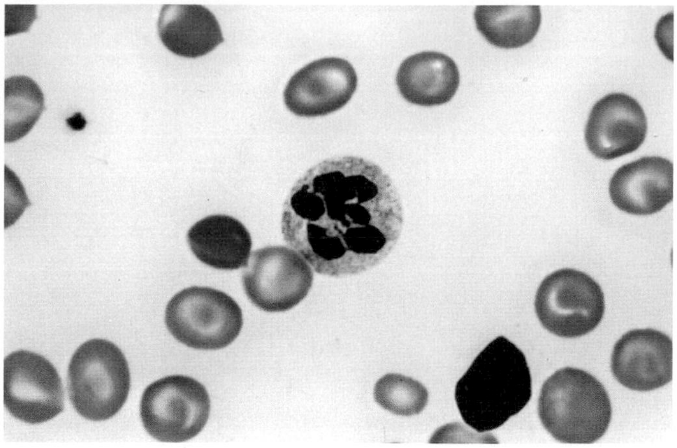

FIGURE 13–18 Megaloblastic anemia. A peripheral blood smear shows a hypersegmented neutrophil with a six-lobed nucleus. (Courtesy of Dr. Robert W. McKenna, Department of Pathology, University of Texas Southwestern Medical School, Dallas, TX.)

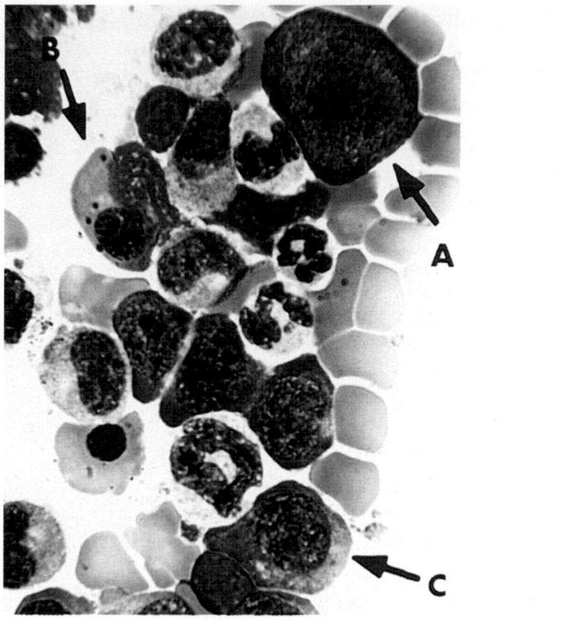

FIGURE 13–19 Megaloblastic anemia (bone marrow aspirate). *A* to *C*, Megaloblasts in various stages of differentiation. Note that the orthochromatic megaloblast *(B)* is hemoglobinized (as revealed by cytoplasmic color), but in contrast to normal orthochromatic normoblasts, the nucleus is not pyknotic. The granulocytic precursors are also large and have abnormally "immature" chromatin. (Courtesy of Dr. Jose Hernandez, Department of Pathology, University of Texas Southwestern Medical School, Dallas, TX.)

nucleoli, and a distinctive fine nuclear chromatin pattern (Fig. 13–19, cell A). As these cells differentiate and begin to accumulate hemoglobin, the nucleus retains its finely distributed chromatin and thus fails to undergo the chromatin clumping typical of the normoblast. For example, orthochromatic megaloblasts have a large amount of pink, well-hemoglobinized cytoplasm, but the nucleus, instead of becoming pyknotic, remains relatively large and immature. Because DNA synthesis is impaired in all proliferating cells, granulocytic precursors also display nuclear-cytoplasmic asynchrony in the form of giant metamyelocytes and band forms. Megakaryocytes, too, can be abnormally large and have bizarre, multilobate nuclei.

The marrow hyperplasia usually seen in megaloblastic anemias is a response to increased levels of growth factors such as erythropoietin. However, due to the derangement in DNA synthesis, most myeloid precursors undergo apoptosis in the marrow (another example of ineffective hematopoiesis), leading to pancytopenia. The anemia is further exacerbated by increased hemolytic destruction of red cells in the periphery. The basis for hemolysis is not entirely clear; both an acquired intracorpuscular defect and a poorly characterized plasma factor have been suggested to contribute. As in other states associated with ineffective erythropoiesis, if the deficiency persists enhanced uptake of iron in the gut can lead to anatomic signs of mild to moderate iron overload after several years (Chapter 18).

Anemias of Vitamin B_{12} Deficiency: Pernicious Anemia

The major causes of megaloblastic anemia are listed in Table 13–5. As mentioned at the outset, pernicious anemia is an important cause of vitamin B_{12} deficiency. *Pernicious anemia is a specific form of megaloblastic anemia caused by atrophic gastritis and an attendant failure of intrinsic factor production that leads to vitamin B_{12} deficiency.*

We first review vitamin B_{12} metabolism, as this helps to place pernicious anemia in perspective relative to the other causes of vitamin B_{12} deficiency anemia.

Normal Vitamin B_{12} Metabolism. Vitamin B_{12} is a complex organometallic compound known as cobalamin. Under normal circumstances, humans are totally dependent on dietary animal products for their vitamin B_{12} requirement. Microorganisms are the ultimate origin of cobalamin in the food chain. Plants and vegetables contain little cobalamin save that contributed by microbial contamination; strictly vegetarian or macrobiotic diets, then, do not provide adequate amounts of this essential nutrient. The daily requirement is 2 to 3 mg. A balanced diet contains significantly larger amounts and normally results in accumulation of vitamin B_{12} in sufficient quantities to last for several years.

Absorption of vitamin B_{12} requires intrinsic factor, which is secreted by the parietal cells of the fundic mucosa (Fig. 13–20). First, vitamin B_{12} is freed from binding proteins in food through the action of pepsin in the stomach. Free vitamin B_{12} then binds to salivary proteins called cobalophilins, or R-binders. In the duodenum, cobalophilin–vitamin B_{12} complexes are broken down by the action of pancreatic proteases, and released vitamin B_{12} then associates with intrinsic factor. This complex is transported to the ileum, where it is endocytosed by ileal enterocytes that express intrinsic factor–specific receptors on their surfaces. Within ileal cells, vitamin B_{12} associates with a major carrier protein, transcobalamin II, and is secreted into the plasma. Transcobalamin II delivers vitamin B_{12} to the liver and other cells of the body, particularly rapidly proliferating cells in the bone

TABLE 13–5 Causes of Megaloblastic Anemia

Vitamin B_{12} Deficiency
Decreased intake
Inadequate diet, vegetarianism
Impaired absorption
Intrinsic factor deficiency
Pernicious anemia
Gastrectomy
Malabsorption states
Diffuse intestinal disease, e.g., lymphoma, systemic sclerosis
Ileal resection, ileitis
Competitive parasitic uptake
Fish tapeworm infestation
Bacterial overgrowth in blind loops and diverticula of bowel
Increased requirement
Pregnancy, hyperthyroidism, disseminated cancer
Folic Acid Deficiency
Decreased intake
Inadequate diet—alcoholism, infancy
Impaired absorption
Malabsorption states
Intrinsic intestinal disease
Anticonvulsants, oral contraceptives
Increased loss
Hemodialysis
Increased requirement
Pregnancy, infancy, disseminated cancer, markedly increased hematopoiesis
Impaired use
Folic acid antagonists
Unresponsive to Vitamin B_{12} or Folic Acid Therapy
Metabolic inhibitors of DNA synthesis and/or folate metabolism, e.g., methotrexate

Modified from Beck WS: Megaloblastic anemias. In Wyngaarden JB, Smith LH (eds): Cecil Textbook of Medicine, 18th ed. Philadelphia, WB Saunders, 1988, p. 900.

marrow and mucosal lining of the gastrointestinal tract. In addition to the intrinsic-factor dependent pathway, evidence also supports the existence of an alternative mechanism that is not dependent on availability of intrinsic factor or intact terminal ileum. The mechanism involved is not entirely clear but up to 1% of a large oral dose can be absorbed by this pathway, thus making it feasible to treat pernicious anemia by oral vitamin B_{12} therapy.[33]

Etiology of Vitamin B_{12} Deficiency. With this background, we can consider the various causes of vitamin B_{12} deficiency (see Table 13–5). Inadequate diet is obvious but must be present for many years to deplete reserves. The absorption of vitamin B_{12} can be impaired by disruption of any one of the steps outlined earlier. With achlorhydria and loss of pepsin secretion (which occurs in some elderly individuals), vitamin B_{12} is not readily released from proteins in food. With gastrectomy and pernicious anemia, intrinsic factor is not available for transport to the ileum. With loss of exocrine pancreatic function, vitamin B_{12} cannot be released from R-binder–vitamin B_{12} complexes. Ileal resection or diffuse ileal disease can remove or damage the site of intrinsic factor–vitamin B_{12} complex absorption. Tapeworm infestation, by competing for the nutrient, can induce a deficiency state. Under some circumstances, for example, pregnancy, hyperthyroidism, disseminated cancer, and chronic infections,

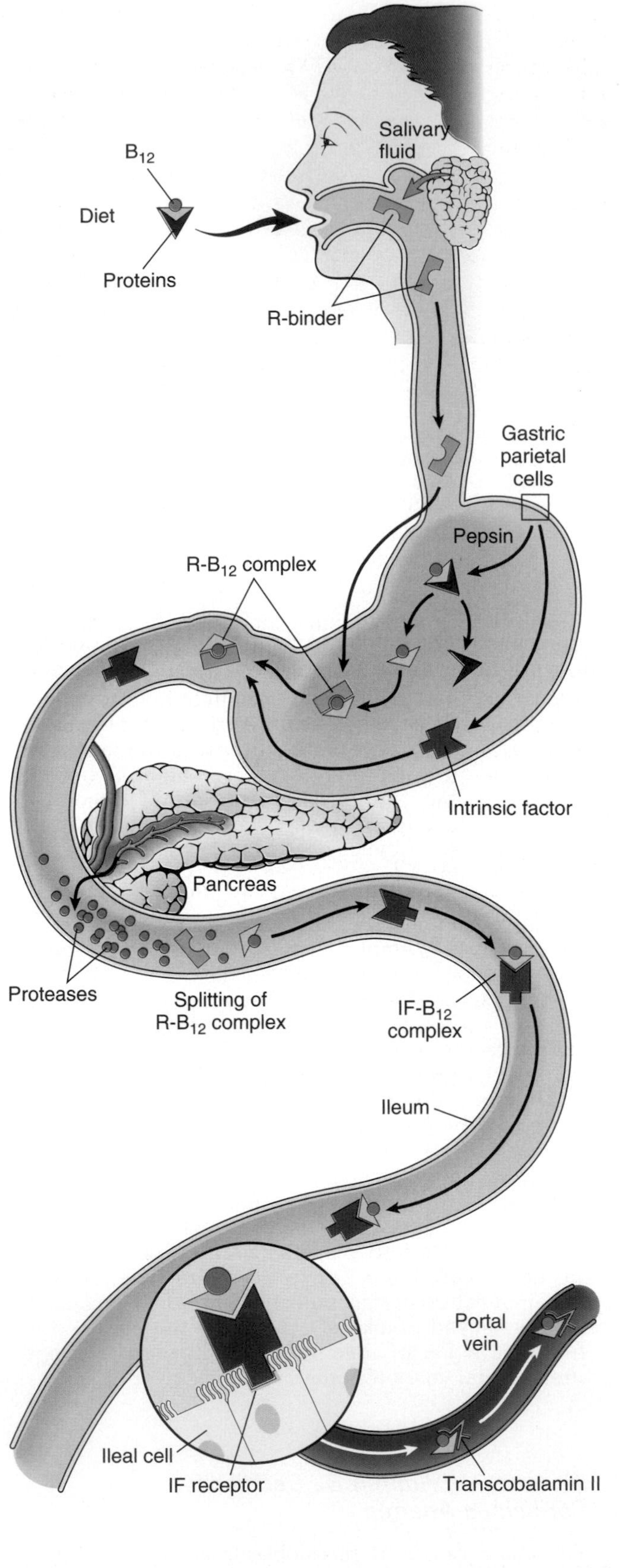

FIGURE 13–20 Schematic illustration of vitamin B_{12} absorption.

the demand for vitamin B_{12} can be so great as to produce a relative deficiency, even with normal absorption.

Biochemical Functions of Vitamin B_{12}. Two reactions in humans are known to require vitamin B_{12}. Methylcobalamin is an essential cofactor for methionine synthase, an enzyme involved in the conversion of homocysteine to methionine (Fig. 13–21). In the process, methylcobalamin yields a methyl group and is regenerated from N^5-methyltetrahydrofolic acid (N^5-methyl FH_4), the principal form of folic acid in plasma. In the same reaction, N^5-methyl FH_4 is converted to tetrahydrofolic acid (FH_4). FH_4 is crucial, since it is required (through its derivative $N^{5,10}$-methylene FH_4) for conversion of deoxyuridine monophosphate to deoxythymidine monophosphate, an immediate precursor of DNA. It has been postulated that the fundamental cause of impaired DNA synthesis in vitamin B_{12} deficiency is the reduced availability of FH_4, most of which is "trapped" as N^5-methyl FH_4.[34] In addition, the deficit in FH_4 can be exacerbated by an "internal" folate deficiency caused by a failure to synthesize metabolically active polyglutamylated forms.[35] This may stem from a requirement for vitamin B_{12} in synthesis of methionine, which contributes a carbon group needed in the metabolic reactions that create folate polyglutamates (see Fig. 13–21). Whatever the mechanism of internal folate deficiency, lack of folate is the proximate cause of anemia in vitamin B_{12} deficiency, as the anemia inevitably improves with administration of folic acid.

The neurologic complications associated with vitamin B_{12} deficiency are an enigma,[36] as treatment with folate fails to improve neurologic deficits. In addition to the transmethylation reaction discussed previously, the second reaction depending on cobalamin is the *isomerization of methylmalonyl coenzyme A to succinyl coenzyme A, which requires adenosylcobalamin as a prosthetic group on the enzyme methylmalonyl–coenzyme A mutase.* A deficiency of vitamin B_{12} thus leads to increased plasma and urine levels of methylmalonic acid. Interruption of the succinyl pathway and consequent build-up of methylmalonate and propionate (a precursor) could lead to the formation and incorporation of abnormal fatty acids into neuronal lipids. It has been suggested that this biochemical abnormality predisposes to myelin breakdown and thereby produces the neurologic complications of vitamin B_{12} deficiency (Chapter 28). However, rare individuals with hereditary deficiencies of methylmalonyl-coenzyme A mutase, while having complications related to methylmalonyl acidemia, do not suffer from the neurologic abnormalities seen in vitamin B_{12} deficiency,[37] casting doubt on this explanation.

With this overview of vitamin B_{12} metabolism, we can now turn our attention to pernicious anemia.

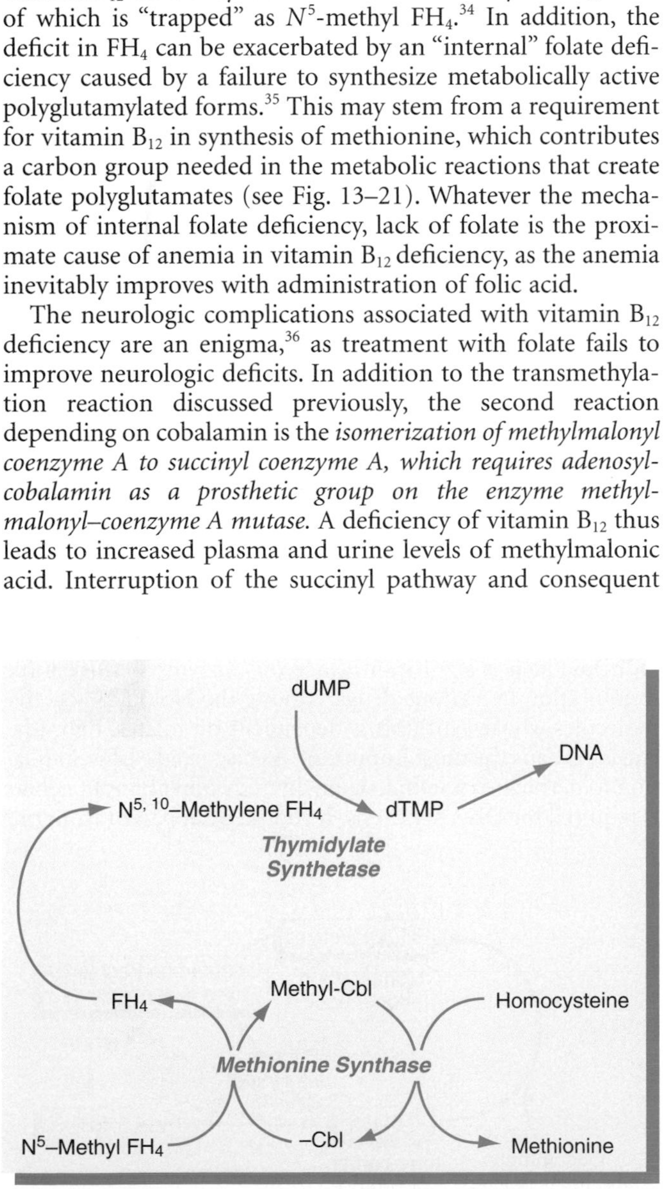

FIGURE 13–21 Relationship of N^5-methyl FH_4, methionine synthase, and thymidylate synthetase. In cobalamin deficiency, folate is sequestered as N^5-methyl FH_4. This ultimately deprives thymidylate synthetase of its folate coenzyme ($N^{5,10}$-methylene FH_4), thereby impairing DNA synthesis.

Incidence. Although somewhat more prevalent in Scandinavian and "English-speaking" populations, pernicious anemia occurs in all racial groups, including, in the United States, blacks and Hispanics. A disease of older age, it is generally diagnosed in the fifth to eighth decades of life. A genetic predisposition is strongly suspected, but no definable genetic pattern of transmission has been discerned. As described below, these patients probably have a tendency to form antibodies against multiple self-antigens.

Pathogenesis. Pernicious anemia is believed to result from immunologically mediated, possibly autoimmune, destruction of gastric mucosa. The resultant *chronic atrophic gastritis* is marked by a loss of parietal cells, a prominent infiltrate of lymphocytes and plasma cells, and megaloblastic changes in mucosal cells similar to those found in erythroid precursors. A number of immunologic reactions are associated with these morphologic changes. *Three types of antibodies are present in many but not all patients with pernicious anemia.* About 75% of patients have a type I antibody that blocks binding of vitamin B_{12} to intrinsic factor. Type I antibodies are found in both plasma and gastric juice. Type II antibodies prevent binding of the intrinsic factor–vitamin B_{12} complex to its ileal receptor. These immunoglobulins are also found in a large proportion of patients with pernicious anemia. The third type of antibodies, present in 85% to 90% of patients, recognize the α and β subunits of the gastric proton pump,[38] which is normally localized to the microvilli of the canalicular system of the gastric parietal cell. Type III antibodies are not specific for pernicious anemia or other autoimmune diseases, as they are found in up to 50% of elderly patients with idiopathic chronic gastritis not associated with pernicious anemia. As discussed next, they most likely result from gastric injury, rather than cause it.

Despite the presence of these autoantibodies, it is not established that they are the primary cause of gastric changes. It is believed that an autoreactive T-cell response initiates gastric mucosal injury, triggering the formation of autoantibodies, which may exacerbate epithelial injury. When the mass of intrinsic factor–secreting cells falls below a threshold (and reserves of stored vitamin B_{12} are depleted), anemia develops. In an animal model of autoimmune gastritis mediated by CD4+ T cells, a pattern of autoantibodies resembling that seen in pernicious anemia develops, thus supporting the primacy of T-cell autoimmunity.[38] An autoimmune basis is also supported by the association of pernicious anemia with other autoimmune disorders, particularly autoimmune thyroiditis and adrenalitis. Conversely, patients who present with other autoimmune diseases are predisposed to develop antibodies against intrinsic factor.

Morphology. The major specific changes in pernicious anemia are found in the bone marrow, alimentary tract, and central nervous system. The changes in the bone marrow and blood are similar to those described earlier for all megaloblastic anemias.

In the **alimentary system,** abnormalities are regularly found in the tongue and stomach. The tongue is shiny, glazed, and "beefy" **(atrophic glossitis).** The changes in the stomach are those of diffuse chronic gastritis (Chapter 17). The most characteristic histologic alteration is the atrophy of the fundic glands, affecting both chief cells and parietal cells, the latter being virtually absent. The glandular lining epithelium is replaced by mucus-secreting goblet cells that resemble those lining the large intestine, a form of metaplasia referred to as **intestinalization.** Some of the cells as well as their nuclei may increase to double the normal size, a form of "megaloblastic" change exactly analogous to that seen in the marrow. As will be seen, patients with pernicious anemia have a higher incidence of gastric cancer. The gastric atrophic and metaplastic changes are due to autoimmunity and not vitamin B_{12} deficiency; hence, parenteral administration of vitamin B_{12} corrects the bone marrow changes, but gastric atrophy and achlorhydria persist.

Central nervous system lesions are found in approximately three fourths of all cases of fulminant pernicious anemia, but in some instances neuronal involvement is seen in the absence of overt megaloblastic anemia. **The principal alterations involve the spinal cord, where there is degeneration of myelin in the dorsal and lateral tracts,** sometimes followed by loss of axons. These changes give rise to spastic paraparesis, sensory ataxia, and severe paresthesias in the lower limbs. Less frequently, degenerative changes occur in the ganglia of the posterior roots and in peripheral nerves (Chapter 28). Because both sensory and motor pathways are involved, the term "subacute combined degeneration" or "combined system disease" is sometimes used to describe the neurologic changes associated with vitamin B_{12} deficiency.

Clinical Course. Pernicious anemia is insidious in onset, so the anemia is often quite severe by the time the patient seeks medical attention. The course is progressive unless halted by therapy.

Diagnostic features include (1) a moderate to severe megaloblastic anemia, (2) leukopenia with hypersegmented granulocytes, (3) mild to moderate thrombocytopenia, (4) mild jaundice due to ineffective erythropoiesis and peripheral hemolysis of red cells, (5) neurologic changes related to involvement of the posterolateral spinal tracts, (6) achlorhydria even after histamine stimulation, (7) inability to absorb an oral dose of cobalamin (assessed by urinary excretion of radiolabeled cyanocobalamin given orally, called the Schilling test), (8) low serum levels of vitamin B_{12}, (9) elevated levels of homocysteine and methyl malonic acid in the serum (this is more sensitive than serum levels of vitamin B_{12}) (10) a striking reticulocytic response and improvement in hematocrit levels beginning about 5 days after parenteral administration of vitamin B_{12}. Serum antibodies to intrinsic factor are highly specific for pernicious anemia. Their presence attests to the cause of vitamin B_{12} deficiency, rather than the presence or absence of cobalamin deficiency.

As mentioned, serum homocysteine and methylmalonic acid levels are raised in patients with deficiency of vitamin B_{12}, and high levels of homocysteine are a risk factor for atherosclerosis and thrombosis. It is still not definite whether such an elevation in patients with folate or vitamin B_{12} deficiency increases the risk of vascular disease. The cytologic aberrations in the gastric mucosa are associated with an increased risk of gastric cancer (Chapter 17). With parenteral or high dose oral vitamin B_{12}, the anemia can be cured and the peripheral neurologic changes reversed, or at least halted in their progression, but the changes in the gastric mucosa are unaffected. Overall longevity can be restored virtually to normal.

Anemia of Folate Deficiency

A deficiency of folic acid, more properly pteroylmonoglutamic acid, results in a megaloblastic anemia having the same characteristics as that caused by vitamin B_{12} deficiency. However, the neurologic changes seen in vitamin B_{12} deficiency do not occur. Folic acid (or more specifically, tetrahydrofolate [FH_4] derivatives) acts as an intermediate in the transfer of one-carbon units such as formyl and methyl groups to various compounds (Fig. 13–22). In the process, FH_4 also serves as an acceptor of one-carbon fragments from compounds such as serine and formiminoglutamic acid (FIGlu). The FH_4 derivatives so generated in turn donate the acquired one-carbon fragments in reactions synthesizing various metabolites. FH_4, then, can be viewed as the biologic "middleman" in a series of swaps involving one-carbon moieties. The most important metabolic processes dependent on such one-carbon transfers are (1) purine synthesis; (2) conversion of homocysteine to methionine, a reaction also requiring vitamin B_{12}; and (3) deoxythymidylate monophosphate synthesis. In the first two reactions, FH_4 is regenerated from its one-carbon carrier derivatives and is available to accept another one-carbon fragment and re-enter the donor pool. In the synthesis of thymidylate, a dihydrofolate is produced that must be reduced by dihydrofolate reductase for reentry into the FH_4 pool. The reductase step is significant, since this enzyme is susceptible to inhibition by various drugs. Among the biologically active molecules whose synthesis is dependent on folates, thymidylate is perhaps the most important. As discussed earlier in relation to pernicious anemia, deoxythymidylate monophosphate is required for DNA synthesis. It should be apparent from our

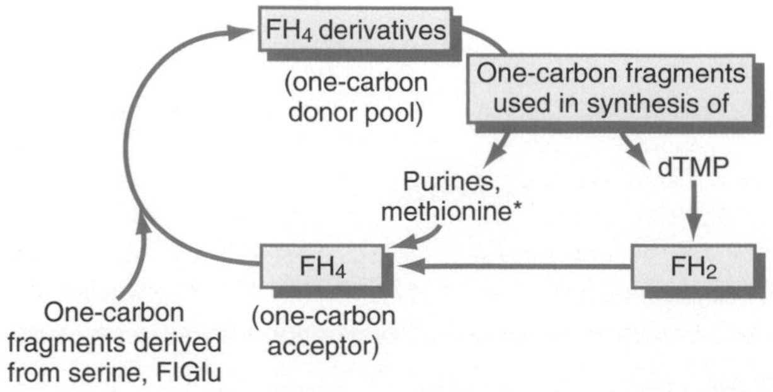

FIGURE 13–22 Role of folate derivatives in the transfer of one-carbon fragments for synthesis of biologic macromolecules. FH_4, tetrahydrofolic acid; FH_2, dihydrofolic acid; FIGlu, formiminoglutamate; dTMP, deoxythymidylate monophosphate. *Synthesis of methionine also requires vitamin B_{12}.

discussion that suppressed synthesis of DNA, the common denominator of folic acid and vitamin B_{12} deficiency, is the immediate cause of megaloblastosis.

Etiology. Humans are entirely dependent on dietary sources for their folic acid requirement, which is 50 to 200 mg daily. Most normal diets contain ample amounts. The richest sources are green vegetables such as lettuce, spinach, asparagus, and broccoli. Certain fruits (e.g., lemons, bananas, melons) and animal proteins (e.g., liver) contain lesser amounts. The folic acid in these foods is largely in the form of folylpolyglutamates. *Despite their abundance in raw foods, polyglutamates (depending on the specific form) are sensitive to heat; boiling, steaming, or frying of foods for 5 to 10 minutes destroys up to 95% of the folate content.* Intestinal conjugases split the polyglutamates into monoglutamates that are readily absorbed in the proximal jejunum. During intestinal absorption, they are modified to 5-methyltetrahydrofolate, the normal transport form of folate. The body's reserves of folate are relatively modest, and a deficiency can arise with months of a negative balance. There are three major causes of folic acid deficiency: (1) decreased intake, (2) increased requirements, and (3) impaired use (Table 13–5).

Decreased intake can result from either a nutritionally inadequate diet or impairment of intestinal absorption. A normal daily diet contains folate in excess of the minimal daily adult requirement. Inadequate dietary intakes are almost invariably associated with grossly deficient diets, particularly those lacking vitamins such as the "B group." *Such dietary inadequacies are most frequently encountered in chronic alcoholics, the indigent, and the very elderly.* In alcoholics with cirrhosis, other mechanisms of folate deficiency such as trapping of folate within the liver, excessive urinary loss, and disordered folate metabolism have also been implicated. Under these circumstances, the megaloblastic anemia is often accompanied by general malnutrition and manifestations of other avitaminoses, including cheilosis, glossitis, and dermatitis. Malabsorption syndromes such as nontropical and tropical sprue can lead to inadequate absorption of this nutrient, as can diffuse infiltrative diseases of the small intestine (e.g., lymphoma). In addition, certain drugs, particularly the anticonvulsant phenytoin and oral contraceptives, interfere with absorption.

Despite adequate intake of folic acid, a *relative deficiency* can be encountered in states of increased requirement, such as pregnancy, infancy, hematologic derangements associated with hyperactive hematopoiesis (hemolytic anemias), and disseminated cancer. In all these circumstances, the demands of active DNA synthesis render normal intake inadequate.

Folic acid antagonists, such as methotrexate, inhibit dihydrofolate reductase and lead to a deficiency of tetrahydrofolate. With inhibition of folate metabolism, all rapidly growing cells are affected, thus leading to ulcerative lesions within the gastrointestinal tract as well as megaloblastic anemia. Many other chemotherapeutic drugs damage DNA or inhibit DNA synthesis through other mechanisms; these can also cause megaloblastic changes in rapidly dividing cells. Owing to their growth inhibitory actions, antimetabolites are used in cancer therapy.

As mentioned at the outset, *megaloblastic anemia resulting from a deficiency of folic acid is identical to that encountered in vitamin B_{12} deficiency.* Thus, the diagnosis of folate deficiency can be made only by demonstration of decreased folate levels in the serum or red cells. As in vitamin B_{12} deficiency, serum homocysteine levels are increased.

Although prompt hematologic response heralded by reticulocytosis follows the administration of folic acid, it should be cautioned that the hematologic symptoms of a vitamin B_{12} deficiency anemia also respond to folate therapy. However, folate does not prevent (and may even exacerbate) the progression of the neurologic deficits typical of the vitamin B_{12} deficiency states. It is thus essential to exclude vitamin B_{12} deficiency in megaloblastic anemia before initiating therapy with folate.

Iron Deficiency Anemia

Deficiency of iron is probably the most common nutritional disorder in the world. Although the prevalence of iron deficiency anemia is higher in developing countries, this form of anemia is also common in the United States, particularly in toddlers, adolescent girls, and women of childbearing age.[39] The factors underlying the iron deficiency differ somewhat in various population groups and can be best considered in the context of normal iron metabolism.

Iron Metabolism. As might be expected given the very high prevalence of iron deficiency in human populations, evolutionary pressures have yielded iron metabolism pathways that are strongly biased toward the retention of iron. There is no regulated pathway for iron excretion, which is limited to the 1 to 2 mg per day lost by shedding of mucosal and skin epithelial cells. *Iron balance, therefore, is maintained largely by regulating the absorption of dietary iron.* The normal daily Western diet contains approximately 10 to 20 mg of iron, most in the form of heme contained in animal products, with the remainder being inorganic iron in vegetables. About 20% of heme iron (in contrast to 1% to 2% of nonheme iron) is absorbable, so the average Western diet contains sufficient iron to balance fixed daily losses. The total body iron content is normally about 2 gm in women and up to 6 gm in men. As indicated in Table 13–6, it is divided into functional and storage compartments. Approximately 80% of the functional iron is found in hemoglobin; myoglobin and iron-containing enzymes such as catalase and the cytochromes contain the rest. The storage pool represented by hemosiderin and ferritin contains approximately 15% to 20% of total body iron. Healthy young females have substantially smaller stores of iron than do males, primarily due to blood loss during menstruation. This precarious iron balance is easily tipped into deficiency by excessive losses or increased demands associated with menstruation and pregnancy, respectively.

TABLE 13–6 Iron Distribution in Healthy Young Adults (mg)

Pool	Men	Women
Total	3450	2450
Functional		
Hemoglobin	2100	1750
Myoglobin	300	250
Enzymes	50	50
Storage		
Ferritin, hemosiderin	1000	400

Free iron is highly toxic, and the pool of storage iron is tightly bound to either ferritin or hemosiderin.[40] *Ferritin is a protein–iron complex* found in all tissues but particularly in liver, spleen, bone marrow, and skeletal muscles. In the liver, most ferritin is stored within the parenchymal cells; in other tissues, such as spleen and bone marrow, it is mainly in the mononuclear phagocytic cells. Hepatocytic iron is derived from plasma transferrin, whereas storage iron in the mononuclear phagocytic cells (Kupffer cells) is derived from the breakdown of red cells (Fig. 13–23). Intracellular ferritin is located in both the cytosol and lysosomes, in which partially degraded protein shells of ferritin aggregate into *hemosiderin* granules. With a hematoxylin and eosin stain, hemosiderin appears in cells as golden yellow granules. The iron in hemosiderin is chemically reactive and turns blue-black when exposed to potassium ferrocyanide, which is the basis for the Prussian blue stain. With normal iron stores, only trace amounts of hemosiderin are found in the body, principally in mononuclear phagocytic cells in the bone marrow, spleen, and liver. In iron-overloaded cells, most iron is stored in hemosiderin.

Very small amounts of ferritin normally circulate in the plasma. *Since plasma ferritin is derived largely from the storage pool of body iron, its levels correlate well with body iron stores.* In iron deficiency, serum ferritin is always below 12 μg/L, whereas in iron overload, high values approaching 5000 μg/L can be seen. Of physiologic importance, the storage iron pool can be readily mobilized if iron requirements increase, as may occur after loss of blood.

Iron is transported in plasma by an iron-binding glycoprotein called *transferrin* (see Fig. 13–23), which is synthesized in the liver. In normal individuals, transferrin is about 33% saturated with iron, yielding serum iron levels that average 120 μg/dL in men and 100 μg/dL in women. Thus, the total iron-binding capacity of serum is in the range of 300 to 350 μg/dL. The major function of plasma transferrin is to deliver iron to cells, including erythroid precursors, where iron is required for hemoglobin synthesis. Immature red cells possess high-affinity receptors for transferrin, and iron is transported into erythroblasts by receptor-mediated endocytosis.

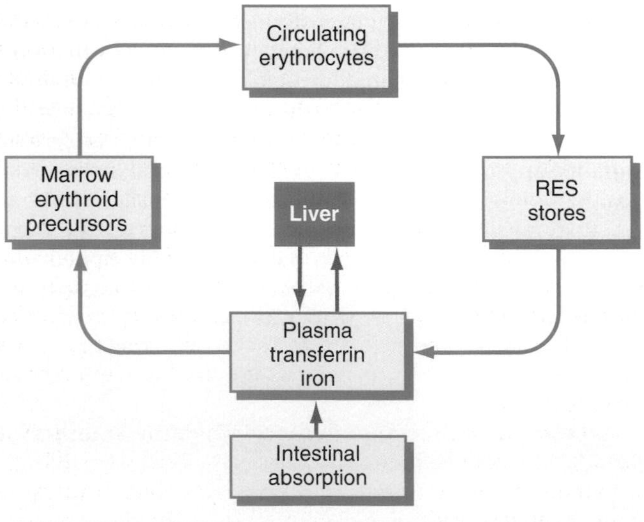

FIGURE 13–23 The internal iron cycle. Plasma iron bound to transferrin is transported to the marrow, where it is transferred to developing red cells and incorporated into hemoglobin. Mature red blood cells are released into the circulation and, after 120 days, are ingested by macrophages in the reticuloendothelial system (RES). Here iron is extracted from hemoglobin and returned to the plasma, completing the cycle. (From Wyngaarden JB, et al [eds]: Cecil Textbook of Medicine, 19th ed. Philadelphia, WB Saunders, 1992, p. 841.)

The absorption of iron and its regulation have become better understood over the last several years.[40] Most iron is absorbed in the duodenum, where uptake of heme and nonheme iron occurs through two distinct pathways (Fig. 13–24). Nonheme iron traverses the apical and basolateral membranes of villus enterocytes through the action of two distinct transporters. After reduction to ferrous (Fe^{++}) iron by a membrane-associated cytochrome B, divalent metal transporter 1 (DMT1) first moves nonheme iron across the apical membrane. At least two proteins are then required for the basolateral transfer of iron to transferrin in the plasma: ferroportin, a transporter, and hephaestin, an iron oxidase. Both DMT1 and ferroportin are widely distributed in the body, suggesting their involvement in iron transport in other tissues as well. For example, DMT1 also appears to be important in uptake of iron into erythroblasts. Dietary heme iron is absorbed through a different transporter that is not yet well characterized.

The efficacy of enterocyte uptake of heme and nonheme iron differs dramatically. Approximately 25% of the heme iron derived from hemoglobin, myoglobin, and other animal proteins is absorbed. The absorption of nonheme iron is more variable, being influenced by substances in the diet that inhibit (phytates, tannates, and phosphates) or enhance (ascorbic and amino acids) uptake, but frequently less than 5% of that consumed. After absorption, both heme and nonheme iron appear to enter a common pool in the mucosal cell. Normally, a fraction of the iron that enters the cell is rapidly delivered to plasma transferrin. Most, however, is deposited as ferritin, some to be transferred more slowly to plasma transferrin, and some to be lost with exfoliation of mucosal cells. The extent to which the mucosal iron is distributed along these various pathways depends on the body's iron requirements. When the body is replete with iron, formation of ferritin within the mucosal cells is maximal, whereas transport into plasma is enhanced in iron deficiency.

Since body losses of iron are limited, iron balance is maintained by regulating absorptive intake. The mechanisms that regulate the absorption of available iron into the mucosal cell are still incompletely understood.[41] Important clues come from observations demonstrating that the rate and level of absorption are dependent on total body iron content and erythropoietic activity, or more specifically the iron needs of the erythroid precursors. As body stores rise, the absorption of iron falls, and vice versa. With ineffective erythropoiesis, as may occur in β-thalassemias, iron absorption is increased despite an excess of stored body iron. Some signal must be delivered to the mucosal cell, modifying its uptake and transfer of iron. *An excellent candidate for a negative "iron metabolism regulatory hormone" is hepcidin, a small, liver-derived plasma peptide.* Hepcidin inhibits iron uptake in the duodenum and iron release from macrophages.[42] The concentration of hepcidin falls as iron stores become depleted, and hepcidin knockout mice develop hemochromatosis. Conversely, overexpression of hepcidin in transgenic mice causes an iron defi-

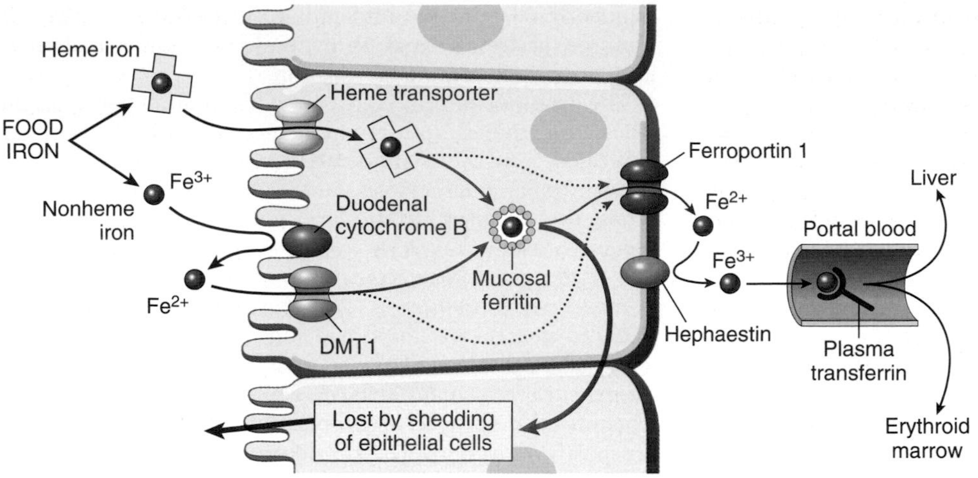

FIGURE 13–24 Diagrammatic representation of iron absorption. Mucosal uptake of heme and nonheme iron is depicted. When the storage sites of the body are replete with iron and erythropoietic activity is normal, most of the absorbed iron is lost into the gut by shedding of the epithelial cells. Conversely, when body iron needs increase or when erythropoiesis is stimulated, a greater fraction of the absorbed iron is transferred into plasma transferrin, with a concomitant decrease in iron loss through mucosal ferritin.

ciency anemia. These findings suggest the existence of a hepcidin receptor on duodenal enterocytes. The *HFE* gene, which encodes an HLA-like transmembrane protein, is also clearly involved in regulation of iron absorption.[41] As discussed in Chapter 18, mutation in this gene leads to excessive absorption of dietary iron and eventual hemochromatosis, a disease characterized by systemic iron overload.

Etiology. To maintain a normal iron balance, approximately 1 mg of iron must be absorbed from the diet every day. Because only 10% to 15% of ingested iron is absorbed, the daily iron requirement is 7 to 10 mg for adult men and 7 to 20 mg for adult women. Since the average daily dietary intake of iron in the Western world is about 15 to 20 mg, most men ingest more than adequate iron, whereas many women consume marginally adequate amounts of iron.

The bioavailability of dietary iron is as important as the overall content. Heme iron is much more absorbable than inorganic iron. The absorption of the latter is influenced by other dietary contents. Ascorbic acid, citric acid, amino acids, and sugars in the diet enhance absorption of inorganic iron, but tannates (as in tea), carbonates, oxalates, and phosphates inhibit its absorption.

An iron deficiency can result from (1) dietary lack, (2) impaired absorption, (3) increased requirement, or (4) chronic blood loss.

Dietary lack is a rare cause of iron deficiency in industrialized countries having abundant food supplies (including meat) where about two thirds of the dietary iron is in the readily assimilable heme form. The situation is different in developing countries, where food is less abundant and diets are predominantly vegetarian, containing poorly absorbable inorganic iron. Despite the availability of iron, dietary inadequacy still occurs in privileged societies in these groups:

- *Infants* are at high risk because milk diets contain very small amounts of iron. Human breast milk, for example, provides only about 0.3 mg/L of iron. Cow's milk contains about twice as much iron as human breast milk, but the iron in cow's milk has poor bioavailability.
- *Children,* especially during the early years of life, have increased dietary iron needs to accommodate growth, development, and the accompanying expansion of blood volume.
- *The impoverished,* at any age, can have suboptimal diets for socioeconomic reasons.
- *The elderly* often have restricted diets with little meat because of limited income or poor dentition.

Impaired absorption is found in sprue, other causes of intestinal steatorrhea, and chronic diarrhea. Gastrectomy impairs iron absorption by decreasing hydrochloric acid and transit time through the duodenum. Specific items in the diet, as is evident from the preceding discussion, can also affect absorption.

Increased requirement is an important potential cause of iron deficiency. Growing infants and children, adolescents, and premenopausal (particularly pregnant) women have a much greater requirement for iron than do nonmenstruating adults. Particularly at risk are economically deprived women having multiple, frequent pregnancies.

Chronic blood loss is the most common cause of iron deficiency in the Western world. If bleeding occurs into tissues or cavities of the body, the heme iron can be totally recovered and recycled. However, external hemorrhage, as can occur from the gastrointestinal tract (e.g., peptic ulcers, hemorrhagic gastritis, gastric carcinoma, colonic carcinoma, hemorrhoids, or hookworm or pinworm disease), the urinary tract (e.g., renal, pelvic, or bladder tumors), or the genital tract (e.g., menorrhagia, uterine cancer), depletes iron reserves.

When all the potential causes of an iron deficiency are taken into consideration, *deficiency in adult men and postmenopausal women in the Western world must be attributed to gastrointestinal blood loss until proven otherwise. To prematurely ascribe iron deficiency in such individuals to any other cause is to run the risk of missing an occult gastrointestinal cancer or other bleeding lesion.*

Whatever its basis, iron deficiency induces a hypochromic microcytic anemia. Simultaneously, depletion of essential iron-containing enzymes in cells throughout the body can cause other changes, including koilonychia, alopecia, atrophic changes in the tongue and gastric mucosa, and intestinal malabsorption. These changes are seen with severe and long-standing iron deficiency. Uncommonly, esophageal webs appear to complete the triad of major findings in the *Plummer-Vinson syndrome:* (1) microcytic hypochromic anemia, (2) atrophic glossitis, and (3) esophageal webs (Chapter 17).

At the outset of chronic blood loss or other states of negative iron balance, reserves in the form of ferritin and hemosiderin may be adequate to maintain normal hemoglobin and hematocrit levels as well as normal serum iron and transferrin saturation. Progressive depletion of these reserves first lowers serum iron and transferrin saturation levels, without producing anemia. In this early stage, there is increased erythroid activity in the bone marrow. Anemia only appears when iron stores are completely depleted, accompanied by low serum iron, serum ferritin, and transferrin saturation.

Morphology. The bone marrow reveals a mild to moderate increase in erythroid progenitors (normoblasts). A diagnostically significant finding is the disappearance of stainable iron from mononuclear phagocytic cells in the bone marrow, which is assessed by performing Prussian blue stains on aspirated or sectioned bone marrow. In the peripheral blood smear, red cells are small (microcytic) and pale (hypochromic). Normal well-hemoglobinized red cells have a zone of central pallor measuring about one third of the cell diameter. In established iron deficiency, the zone of pallor is enlarged; hemoglobin may be seen only in a narrow peripheral rim (Fig. 13–25). Poikilocytosis in the form of small, elongated red cells (pencil cells) is also characteristic.

The clinical manifestations of the anemia are nonspecific and were detailed earlier. The dominating signs and symptoms frequently relate to the underlying cause of the anemia, for example, gastrointestinal or gynecologic disease, malnutrition, pregnancy, and malabsorption.

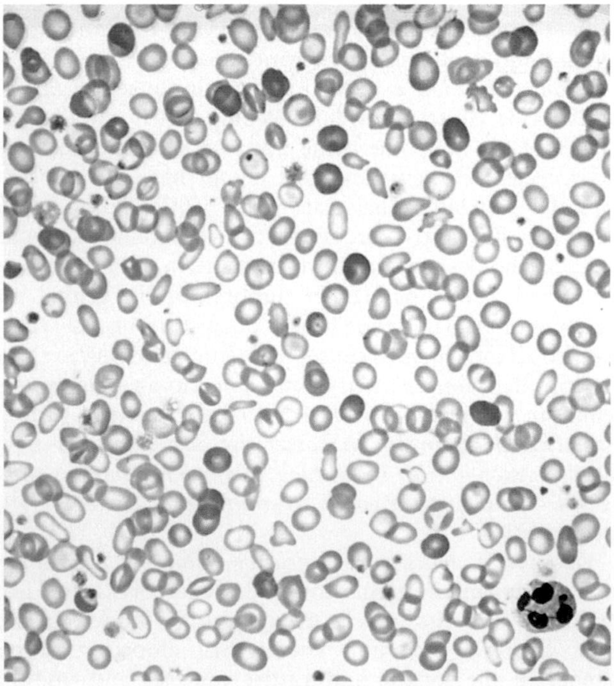

FIGURE 13–25 Hypochromic microcytic anemia of iron deficiency (peripheral blood smear). Note the small red cells containing a narrow rim of peripheral hemoglobin. Scattered fully hemoglobinized cells, present due to recent blood transfusion, stand in contrast. (Courtesy of Dr. Robert W. McKenna, Department of Pathology, University of Texas Southwestern Medical School, Dallas, TX.)

The diagnosis of iron deficiency anemia ultimately rests on laboratory studies. Both the hemoglobin and hematocrit are depressed, usually to moderate levels, in association with hypochromia, microcytosis, and some poikilocytosis. *The serum iron and ferritin are low, and the total plasma iron-binding capacity (reflecting transferrin concentration) is high. Low serum iron with increased iron-binding capacity results in a reduction of transferrin saturation levels to below 15%.* Reduced iron stores inhibit hepcidin synthesis and its serum levels fall. As mentioned earlier, transferrin receptor, expressed on the surface of many cells, is required for the transport of iron into cells. The level of soluble transferrin receptors, which are mostly derived from erythroid progenitors in the marrow, is elevated in iron deficiency due to a mild expansion of erythroid progenitors and an increased rate of transferrin receptor shedding. Reduced heme synthesis leads to elevation of free erythrocyte protoporphyrin. An alert clinician investigating unexplained iron deficiency anemia will occasionally discover an occult bleed or cancer and thereby save a life.

Anemia of Chronic Disease

Impaired red cell production associated with chronic diseases is perhaps the most common cause of anemia among hospitalized patients in the United States. It is associated with reduced erythroid proliferation and impaired iron utilization and can therefore mimic iron deficiency.[43] The chronic illnesses associated with this form of anemia can be grouped into three categories:

- Chronic microbial infections, such as osteomyelitis, bacterial endocarditis, and lung abscess
- Chronic immune disorders, such as rheumatoid arthritis and regional enteritis
- Neoplasms, such as Hodgkin lymphoma and carcinomas of the lung and breast

The common features characterizing anemia in these diverse clinical settings are *low serum iron and reduced total iron-binding capacity in association with abundant stored iron in the mononuclear phagocytic cells.* This combination suggests some impediment in the transfer of iron from the storage pool to the erythroid precursors. In addition, marrow erythroid progenitors do not proliferate adequately because erythropoietin levels are inappropriately low for the degree of anemia. The reduction in renal erythropoietin generation is caused by the action of interleukin-1, tumor necrosis factor (TNF), and interferon-γ, secretion of which is triggered by the underlying chronic inflammatory or neoplastic disease.[44] These cytokines also stimulate hepcidin synthesis in the liver, which in turn inhibits the release of iron from the storage pool.[42] The anemia is usually mild, and the dominant symptoms are those of the underlying disease. The red blood cells can be normocytic and normochromic or hypochromic and microcytic as in anemia of iron deficiency. *The presence of increased storage iron in the marrow macrophages, a high serum ferritin level, and reduced total iron-binding capacity readily rule out iron deficiency as the cause of anemia.* Only successful treatment of the underlying condition reliably corrects the anemia. However, many patients benefit from administration of erythropoietin.

Aplastic Anemia

Aplastic anemia is a somewhat misleading term applied to a syndrome of marrow failure associated with pancytopenia (anemia, neutropenia, and thrombocytopenia). The marrow failure stems from suppression or disappearance of multipotent myeloid stem cells.

Etiology. The major circumstances under which aplastic anemia can appear are listed in Table 13–7.

Most cases of aplastic anemia of "known" etiology follow exposure to chemicals and drugs. With some agents, marrow damage is predictable, dose related and, in most instances, reversible when exposure to the offending agent is stopped. Among the best-known dose-dependent myelotoxins are benzene, chloramphenicol, alkylating agents, and antimetabolites (e.g., 6-mercaptopurine, vincristine, and busulfan). In other instances, however, pancytopenia appears as an apparent idiosyncratic reaction to very small doses of known myelotoxins (e.g., chloramphenicol) or nonmyelotoxic drugs such as phenylbutazone, methylphenylethylhydantoin, streptomycin, and chlorpromazine. In such idiosyncratic reactions, the aplasia can be severe, irreversible, and fatal.

Whole-body *irradiation* is another insult that can destroy hematopoietic stem cells in a dose-dependent fashion. Persons who receive therapeutic irradiation or are exposed to radiation in nuclear accidents (e.g., Chernobyl) are at risk.

Aplastic anemia can appear after a variety of viral *infections,* most commonly viral hepatitis of the non-A, non-B, non-C, and non-G types. Why certain individuals develop this complication is not understood, but it is not related to the severity of infection.

Fanconi anemia is a rare autosomal recessive disorder caused by defects in a component of a multiprotein complex required for DNA repair[45] (Chapter 7). Marrow hypofunction in Fanconi anemia becomes evident early in life and is accompanied by multiple congenital anomalies, such as hypoplasia of the kidney and spleen and hypoplastic anomalies of bone, often involving the thumbs or radii.

Despite all these possible causes, no provocative factor can be identified in fully 65% of the cases, which are lumped into the *idiopathic* category.

Pathogenesis. The pathogenesis of aplastic anemia is not fully understood. Indeed, it is unlikely that a single mechanism underlies all cases. Two major etiologies have been invoked: an immunologically mediated suppression and an intrinsic abnormality of stem cells (Fig. 13–26).

Recent studies suggest that aplastic anemia results most commonly from suppression of stem cell function by activated T cells.[46] It is postulated that stem cells are first antigenically altered by exposure to drugs, infectious agents, or other unidentified environmental insults. This evokes a cellular immune response, during which activated T cells produce cytokines such as interferon-γ and TNF that prevent normal stem cell growth and development. This scenario is supported by several observations. Immunosuppressive therapy with antithymocyte globulin combined with drugs such as cyclosporine produces responses in 60% to 70% of patients, and successful bone marrow transplantation requires "conditioning" with high doses of myelotoxic drugs or radiation. In both instances, it is hypothesized these therapies work by suppressing or killing autoreactive T-cell clones. The target antigens for T-cell attack are not well defined. In some instances GPI-linked proteins may be the targets of sensitized T cells,

TABLE 13–7 Major Causes of Aplastic Anemia

Acquired
Idiopathic
Primary stem cell defect
Immune mediated
Chemical agents
Dose related
Alkylating agents
Antimetabolites
Benzene
Chloramphenicol
Inorganic arsenicals
Idiosyncratic
Chloramphenicol
Phenylbutazone
Organic arsenicals
Methylphenylethylhydantoin
Streptomycin
Chlorpromazine
Insecticides (e.g., DDT, parathion)
Physical agents (e.g., whole-body irradiation)
Viral infections
Hepatitis (unknown virus)
Cytomegalovirus infections
Epstein-Barr virus infections
Herpes varicella-zoster
Miscellaneous
Infrequently, many other drugs and chemicals
Inherited
Fanconi anemia

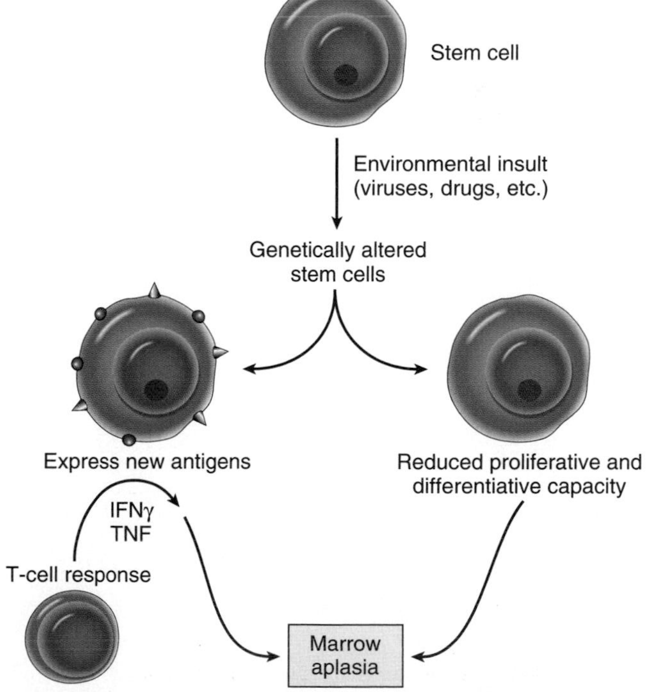

FIGURE 13–26 Pathophysiology of aplastic anemia. Damaged stem cells can produce progeny expressing neo-antigens that evoke an autoimmune reaction, or give rise to a clonal population with reduced proliferative capacity. Either pathway could lead to marrow aplasia.

possibly explaining why aplastic anemia sometimes evolves to paroxysmal nocturnal hemoglobinuria.

Alternatively, the notion that aplastic anemia results from a fundamental stem cell abnormality is supported by the presence of karyotypic aberrations in many cases and occasional transformation of aplasia to myeloid neoplasms, typically myelodysplasia or acute myelogenous leukemia.[46] Some marrow insult presumably causes genetic damage that limits the proliferative and differentiative capacity of stem cells. If the damage is extensive enough, aplastic anemia results. These two mechanisms are not mutually exclusive, as genetically altered stem cells might also express "neo-antigens" that could serve as targets for T-cell attack.

Morphology. The markedly hypocellular bone marrow is largely devoid of hematopoietic cells; often only fat cells, fibrous stroma, and scattered or clustered foci of lymphocytes and plasma cells remain. A marrow aspirate often yields little material (a "dry tap"). Hence, marrow aplasia is best appreciated in a bone marrow biopsy (Fig. 13–27). A number of additional pathologic changes commonly accompanying marrow failure are related to granulocytopenia and thrombocytopenia, such as mucocutaneous bacterial infections and abnormal bleeding, respectively. The toxic drug or agent sometimes injures other tissues as well. Benzene, for example, can cause fatty changes in the liver and kidneys. If the anemia necessitates multiple transfusions, systemic hemosiderosis can appear.

Clinical Course. Aplastic anemia can occur at any age and in either sex. The onset is usually insidious. Initial manifestations vary somewhat, depending on which cell line is predominantly affected. Anemia can cause progressive weakness, pallor, and dyspnea. Petechiae and ecchymoses can herald thrombocytopenia. Granulocytopenia can manifest as frequent and persistent minor infections or the sudden onset of chills, fever, and prostration. *Splenomegaly is characteristically absent; if present, the diagnosis of aplastic anemia should be seriously questioned.* The red cells are typically normocytic and normochromic, although slight macrocytosis is occasionally present. *Reticulocytopenia is the rule.*

The diagnosis rests on examination of bone marrow biopsy and peripheral blood. It is important to distinguish aplastic anemia from other causes of pancytopenia, such as "aleukemic" leukemia and myelodysplastic syndromes (Chapter 14), that can present with identical clinical manifestations. In aplastic anemia, the marrow is hypocellular (and usually markedly so), whereas myeloid neoplasms are associated with hypercellular marrow filled with abnormal myeloid progenitors. The prognosis of aplastic aplasia is unpredictable. As mentioned earlier, withdrawal of toxic drugs can lead to recovery in some cases. Spontaneous remission in idiopathic cases is unfortunately uncommon. In younger patients, allogeneic bone marrow transplantation offers a hope for cure. Older patients or those without suitable donors often respond well to immunosuppressive therapies (antithymocyte globulin and cyclosporine).

Pure Red Cell Aplasia

Pure red cell aplasia is a rare form of marrow failure characterized by a marked hypoplasia of marrow erythroid elements in the setting of normal granulopoiesis and thrombopoiesis.[47] Pure red cell aplasia can be primary, without any associated disease, or arise secondarily to neoplasms, particularly thymic tumors (thymomas) and large granular lymphocytic leukemia (Chapter 14), drug exposures, or autoimmune disorders. The association with thymoma raises the question of some thymus-related immunologic mechanism; indeed, in about half the patients, resection of the thymic tumor is followed by hematologic improvement. In all likelihood, the primary form is also related to autoimmunity against erythroid precursors, and immunosuppressive therapy can be beneficial in such patients. Plasmapheresis has also been used with some success in refractory cases.

Other Forms of Marrow Failure

Space-occupying lesions that destroy significant amounts of bone marrow or disturb the marrow architecture depress its productive capacity. This form of marrow failure is referred to as *myelophthisic anemia.* As you might anticipate, all formed blood elements are affected. Characteristically, immature erythroid and myeloid progenitors appear in the peripheral blood

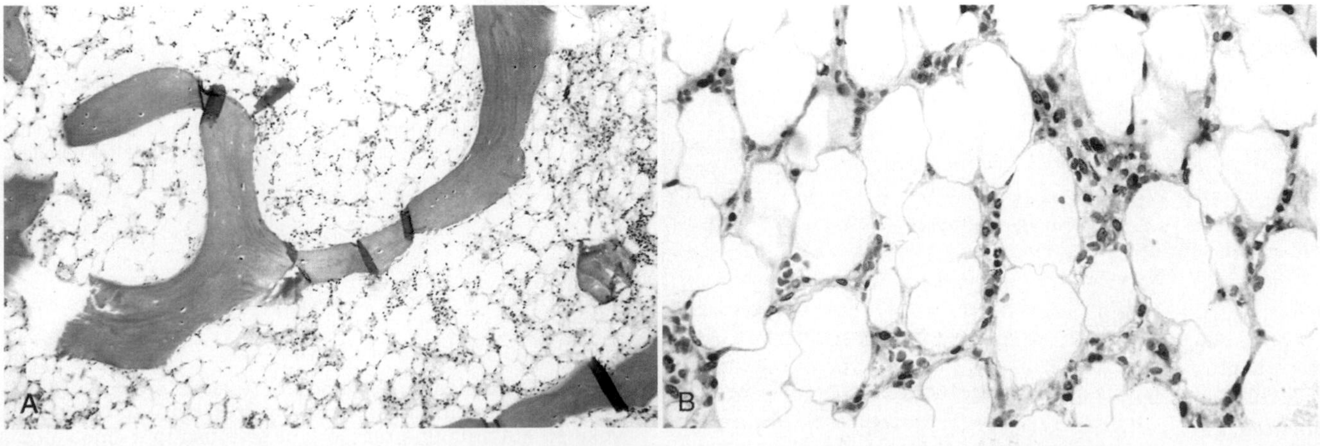

FIGURE 13–27 Aplastic anemia (bone marrow biopsy). Markedly hypocellular marrow contains mainly fat cells. *A,* Low power. *B,* High power. (Courtesy of Dr. Steven Kroft, Department of Pathology, University of Texas Southwestern Medical School, Dallas, TX.)

(leukoerythroblastosis). Infiltrative diseases of the marrow typically cause reactive fibrosis and distortion of the marrow architecture; presumably, this disturbs the normal mechanisms that restrict the release of immature erythroid and myeloid cells into the peripheral blood. The most common cause of myelophthisic anemia is metastatic cancer, most often carcinomas arising in the breast, lung, and prostate. However, any tumor or infiltrative process (e.g., granulomatous disease) involving the marrow can produce identical findings. Myelophthisic anemia is also observed in myelofibrosis and other myeloproliferative disorders (Chapter 14), all of which often cause marrow fibrosis.

Diffuse liver disease, whether toxic, infectious, or cirrhotic, is associated with an anemia attributed to hypofunction of the marrow. Concomitant folate deficiency and iron deficiency due to gastrointestinal blood loss (varices, hemorrhoids) can also contribute to the anemia. Most often, erythroid progenitors are preferentially affected; depression of the white cell count and platelets is less common, but has been described. The anemia is often slightly macrocytic due to lipid abnormalities associated with liver failure, which cause red cell membranes to acquire phospholipid and cholesterol in the periphery.

Chronic renal failure, whatever its cause, is almost invariably associated with anemia that tends to be roughly proportional to the severity of the uremia. The basis of the anemia is multifactorial. There is evidence of an extracorpuscular defect inducing chronic hemolysis. Some patients have an iron deficiency secondary to the bleeding tendency often encountered in uremia. Concomitantly, there is reduced red cell production, related to advanced destruction of the kidneys and inadequate synthesis of erythropoietin, which appears to be the dominant cause of anemia. Not surprisingly, therefore, administration of recombinant erythropoietin results in significant improvement of the anemia associated with renal failure,[48] although optimal response may require aggressive concomitant iron replacement therapy.

Polycythemia

Polycythemia, or *erythrocytosis,* denotes an abnormally high concentration of red cells, usually with a corresponding increase in hemoglobin level. The increase in red cells can be *relative,* when there is hemoconcentration due to decreased plasma volume, or *absolute,* when there is an increase in total red cell mass. *Relative polycythemia* results from any cause of dehydration, such as deprivation of water, prolonged vomiting, diarrhea, or excessive use of diuretics. It is also associated with an obscure condition of unknown etiology called stress polycythemia, or Gaisböck syndrome. Affected individuals are usually hypertensive, obese, and anxious ("stressed"). *Absolute polycythemia* is *primary* when it results from an intrinsic abnormality of the myeloid stem cells and *secondary* when the red cell progenitors are responding to increased levels of erythropoietin. Primary polycythemia (polycythemia vera) is one of several neoplasms originating from myeloid stem cells (considered in Chapter 14). Another much less common form of "primary" polycythemia results from mutations in the erythropoietin receptor that cause hyperresponsiveness to erythropoietin. Affected individuals have congenital polycythemia.[49] One such individual won an Olympic gold medal in cross-country skiing, having benefited from this natural form of blood doping![50] Secondary polycythemias can be caused by an increase in erythropoietin secretion that is physiologically appropriate (e.g., chronic hypoxia) or inappropriate (pathologic) (Table 13–8).

TABLE 13–8 Pathophysiologic Classification of Polycythemia

Relative		Reduced plasma volume (hemoconcentration)
Absolute		
	Primary	Polycythemia vera, rare erythropoietin receptor mutations (low erythropoietin)
	Secondary	High erythropoietin Appropriate: lung disease, high-altitude living, cyanotic heart disease Inappropriate: erythropoietin-secreting tumors (e.g., renal cell carcinoma, hepatocellular carcinoma, cerebellar hemangioblastoma)

Bleeding Disorders: Hemorrhagic Diatheses

Excessive bleeding can result from (1) increased fragility of vessels, (2) platelet deficiency or dysfunction, (3) derangement of coagulation, and (4) combinations of these.

Before discussing these specific bleeding disorders, it is helpful to review normal hemostasis (Chapter 4) and the common laboratory tests used in the evaluation of a bleeding diathesis. It should be recalled from the discussion in Chapter 4 that the normal hemostatic response involves the blood vessel wall, the platelets, and the clotting cascade. Tests used to evaluate different aspects of hemostasis are the following:

- *Bleeding time.* This measures the time taken for a standardized skin puncture to stop bleeding and provides an in vivo assessment of platelet response to limited vascular injury. The reference range depends on the actual method employed and varies from 2 to 9 minutes. Prolongation generally indicates a defect in platelet numbers or function. Bleeding time test is fraught with variability and poor reproducibility. Hence new instrument-based assay systems such as platelet function analyzer-100 (PFA-100) that provide a quantitative measure of platelet function under conditions of high shear stress are being evaluated as replacements for the bleeding time test.[51]
- *Platelet counts.* These are obtained on anticoagulated blood using an electronic particle counter. The reference range is 150 to 300 × $10^3/\mu L$. Counts well outside this range need to be confirmed by a visual inspection of a peripheral blood smear, as clumping of platelets can cause spurious "thrombocytopenia" during automated counting, and high counts may be indicative of a myeloproliferative disorder.
- *Prothrombin time (PT).* This assay tests the extrinsic and common coagulation pathways. The clotting of plasma after addition of an exogenous source of tissue thromboplastin (e.g., brain extract) and Ca^{2+} ions is measured in seconds. A prolonged PT can result from deficiency or dysfunction of factor V, factor VII, factor X, prothrombin, or fibrinogen.
- *Partial thromboplastin time (PTT).* This assay tests the intrinsic and common clotting pathways. The clotting of

plasma after addition of kaolin, cephalin, and calcium ions is measured in seconds. Kaolin serves to activate the contact-dependent factor XII, and cephalin substitutes for platelet phospholipids. Prolongation of the PTT can be due to deficiency or dysfunction of factor V, VIII, IX, X, XI, or XII, prothrombin, or fibrinogen.

More specialized tests are available to measure the levels of specific clotting factors, fibrinogen, fibrin split products, the presence of circulating anticoagulants, and platelet function. With this overview, we can turn to the various categories of bleeding disorders.

BLEEDING DISORDERS CAUSED BY VESSEL WALL ABNORMALITIES

Disorders within this category, sometimes called *nonthrombocytopenic purpuras,* are relatively common but do not usually cause serious bleeding problems. Most often, they induce small hemorrhages (petechiae and purpura) in the skin or mucous membranes, particularly the gingivae. On occasion, however, more significant hemorrhages can occur into joints, muscles, and subperiosteal locations or take the form of menorrhagia, nosebleeds, gastrointestinal bleeding, or hematuria. *The platelet count, bleeding time, and results of the coagulation tests (PT, PTT) are usually normal.*

The varied clinical conditions in which hemorrhages can be related to abnormalities in the vessel wall include the following:

- Many *infections* induce petechial and purpuric hemorrhages, but especially implicated are meningococcemia, other forms of septicemia, infective endocarditis, and several of the rickettsioses. The involved mechanism is presumably microbial damage to the microvasculature (vasculitis) or disseminated intravascular coagulation (DIC). Failure to recognize meningococcemia as a cause of petechiae and purpura can be catastrophic for the patient.
- *Drug reactions* sometimes induce cutaneous petechiae and purpura without causing thrombocytopenia. In many instances, the vascular injury is mediated by drug-induced antibodies and deposition of immune complexes in the vessel walls, leading to hypersensitivity (leukocytoclastic) vasculitis (Chapter 11).
- *Scurvy and the Ehlers-Danlos syndrome* are associated with microvascular bleeding resulting from impaired formation of collagens needed for support of vessel walls. The same mechanism may account for spontaneous purpura commonly seen in the very elderly. The predisposition to skin hemorrhages in *Cushing syndrome,* in which the protein-wasting effects of excessive corticosteroid production cause loss of perivascular supporting tissue, has a similar etiology.
- *Henoch-Schönlein purpura* is a systemic hypersensitivity disease of unknown cause characterized by a purpuric rash, colicky abdominal pain (presumably due to focal hemorrhages into the gastrointestinal tract), polyarthralgia, and acute glomerulonephritis (Chapter 20). All these changes result from the deposition of circulating immune complexes within vessels throughout the body and within the glomerular mesangial regions.
- *Hereditary hemorrhagic telangiectasia* is an autosomal dominant disorder characterized by dilated, tortuous blood vessels with thin walls that bleed readily. Bleeding can occur anywhere in the body but is most common under the mucous membranes of the nose (epistaxis), tongue, mouth, and eyes and throughout the gastrointestinal tract.
- *Amyloid infiltration of blood vessels.* Systemic amyloidosis is associated with perivascular deposition of amyloid and consequent weakening of blood vessel wall. This is most commonly observed in plasma cell dyscrasias (Chapter 14) and is manifested as mucocutaneous petechiae.

Bleeding in these conditions is rarely life threatening with the exception of some cases of hereditary telangiectasia. Recognition of the presenting symptoms should prompt further studies to establish a specific diagnosis.

BLEEDING RELATED TO REDUCED PLATELET NUMBER: THROMBOCYTOPENIA

Reduction in platelet number constitutes an important cause of generalized bleeding. Normal platelet counts range from 150,000 to 300,000/μL. A count below 100,000/μL is generally considered to constitute thrombocytopenia. However, spontaneous bleeding does not become evident until the count falls below 20,000/μL. Platelet counts in the range of 20,000 to 50,000/μL can aggravate post-traumatic bleeding. Bleeding resulting from thrombocytopenia alone is associated with a prolonged bleeding time and normal PT and PTT.

The important role of platelets in hemostasis is discussed in Chapter 4. It hardly needs reiteration that these cells are critical for hemostasis, as they form temporary plugs that quickly stop bleeding and promote key reactions in the clotting cascade. Spontaneous bleeding associated with thrombocytopenia most often involves small vessels. The common sites of such hemorrhage are the skin and the mucous membranes of the gastrointestinal and genitourinary tracts. Intracranial bleeding is a threat to any patient with a markedly depressed platelet count.

The many causes of thrombocytopenia can be classified into the four major categories listed in Table 13–9.

- *Decreased production of platelets.* This can accompany generalized diseases of bone marrow such as aplastic anemia and leukemias or result from diseases that affect the megakaryocytes somewhat selectively. In vitamin B_{12} or folic acid deficiency, there is poor development and accelerated destruction of megakaryocytes within the bone marrow (ineffective megakaryopoiesis) because DNA synthesis is impaired.
- *Decreased platelet survival.* This important cause of thrombocytopenia can have an *immunologic* or *nonimmunologic* etiology. In the immune conditions, platelet destruction is caused by circulating antiplatelet antibodies or, less often, immune complexes. The antiplatelet antibodies can be directed against a self-antigen on the platelets (autoantibodies) or against platelet antigens that differ among different individuals (alloantibodies). Common antigenic targets of both autoantibodies and alloantibodies are the platelet membrane glycoprotein complexes IIb-IIIa and Ib-IX. Autoimmune thrombocytopenias include idiopathic thrombocytopenic purpura, certain drug-induced thrombocytopenias, and HIV-associated thrombocytopenias. All of these are discussed later. Alloimmune thrombocytopenias arise when an individual is exposed to platelets

TABLE 13–9 Causes of Thrombocytopenia

Decreased production of platelets
Generalized diseases of bone marrow
Aplastic anemia: congenital and acquired (see Table 13–7)
Marrow infiltration: leukemia, disseminated cancer
Selective impairment of platelet production
Drug-induced: alcohol, thiazides, cytotoxic drugs
Infections: measles, human immunodeficiency virus (HIV)
Ineffective megakaryopoiesis
Megaloblastic anemia
Myelodysplastic syndromes
Decreased platelet survival
Immunologic destruction
Autoimmune: idiopathic thrombocytopenic purpura, systemic lupus erythematosus
Isoimmune: post-transfusion and neonatal
Drug-associated: quinidine, heparin, sulfa compounds
Infections: infectious mononucleosis, HIV infection, cytomegalovirus
Nonimmunologic destruction
Disseminated intravascular coagulation
Thrombotic thrombocytopenic purpura
Giant hemangiomas
Microangiopathic hemolytic anemias
Sequestration
Hypersplenism
Dilutional

of another person, as may occur after blood transfusion or during pregnancy. In the latter case, neonatal or even fetal thrombocytopenia occurs by a mechanism analogous to erythroblastosis fetalis.[52]

Nonimmunologic destruction of platelets may be caused by *mechanical injury*, in a manner analogous to red cell destruction in microangiopathic hemolytic anemia. The underlying conditions are also similar, including prosthetic heart valves and diffuse narrowing of the microvessels (e.g., malignant hypertension).

- *Sequestration.* Thrombocytopenia, usually moderate in severity, may develop in any patient with marked splenomegaly, a condition sometimes referred to as *hypersplenism* (Chapter 14). The spleen normally sequesters 30% to 40% of the body's platelets, which remain in equilibrium with the circulating pool. When necessary, hypersplenic thrombocytopenia can be ameliorated by splenectomy.
- *Dilutional.* Massive *transfusions* can produce a dilutional thrombocytopenia. Blood stored for longer than 24 hours contains virtually no viable platelets; thus, plasma volume and red cell mass are reconstituted by transfusion, but the number of circulating platelets is relatively reduced.

Immune Thrombocytopenic Purpura (ITP)

ITP can occur in the setting of a variety of conditions and exposures (secondary ITP) or in the absence of any known risk factors (primary or idiopathic ITP). There are two clinical subtypes of primary ITP, acute and chronic; both are autoimmune disorders in which platelet destruction results from the formation of antiplatelet autoantibodies. We first discuss the more common chronic form of primary ITP; acute ITP, a self-limited disease of children, is discussed later.

Immunologically mediated destruction of platelets (immune thrombocytopenia) occurs in many different settings, including systemic lupus erythematosus, acquired immunodeficiency syndrome (AIDS), after viral infections, and as a complication of drug therapy. These *secondary forms of immune thrombocytopenia can sometimes mimic the idiopathic autoimmune variety*, and hence the diagnosis of this disorder should be made only after exclusion of other known causes of thrombocytopenia. Particularly important in this regard is systemic lupus erythematosus, a multisystem autoimmune disease (Chapter 6) that can present with thrombocytopenia.

Pathogenesis. Chronic ITP is caused by the formation of autoantibodies against platelet membrane glycoproteins, most often IIb-IIIa or Ib-IX.[53] Antibodies reactive with these membrane glycoproteins can be demonstrated in the plasma as well as bound to the platelet surface (platelet-associated immunoglobulins) in approximately 80% of patients. In the overwhelming majority of cases, the antiplatelet antibodies are of the IgG class.

The mechanism of platelet destruction is similar to that seen in autoimmune hemolytic anemias. Opsonized platelets are rendered susceptible to phagocytosis by the cells of the mononuclear phagocyte system. About 75% to 80% of patients are remarkably improved after splenectomy, indicating that the spleen is the major site of removal of sensitized platelets. Since it is also an important site of autoantibody synthesis, the beneficial effects of splenectomy may in part derive from removal of the source of autoantibodies. Although destruction of sensitized platelets is the major mechanism responsible for thrombocytopenia, there is some evidence that megakaryocytes may be damaged by autoantibodies, leading to impairment of platelet production. In most cases, however, megakaryocyte injury is not significant enough to deplete their numbers.

Morphology. The principal morphologic lesions of thrombocytopenic purpura are found in the spleen and bone marrow but they are not diagnostic. Secondary changes related to the bleeding diathesis may be found in any tissue or structure in the body.

The spleen is normal in size. On histologic examination, there is congestion of the sinusoids and hyperactivity and enlargement of the splenic follicles, manifested by the formation of prominent germinal centers. In many instances, scattered megakaryocytes are found within the sinuses and sinusoidal walls. This may represent a very mild form of extramedullary hematopoiesis driven by elevated levels of thrombopoietin. These splenic findings are not sufficiently distinctive to be considered diagnostic.

Bone marrow reveals a modestly increased number of megakaryocytes. Some are apparently immature, with large, nonlobulated, single nuclei. These findings are not specific for autoimmune thrombocytopenic purpura but merely reflect accelerated thrombopoiesis, being found in most forms of thrombocytopenia resulting from increased platelet destruction. The importance of bone marrow examination is to rule out thrombocytopenias resulting from bone marrow failure. A decrease in the number of megakaryocytes argues against the diagnosis of ITP. The secondary changes relate to the hemorrhages that are dispersed throughout the body.

Clinical Features. Chronic ITP occurs most commonly in adult women younger than age 40 years. The female-to-male ratio is 3:1. This disorder is often insidious in onset and is characterized by bleeding into the skin and mucosal surfaces. Cutaneous bleeding is seen in the form of *pinpoint hemorrhages* (petechiae), especially prominent in the dependent areas where the capillary pressure is higher. Petechiae can become confluent, giving rise to *ecchymoses.* Often there is a history of easy bruising, nosebleeds, bleeding from the gums, and hemorrhages into soft tissues from relatively minor trauma. The disease may manifest first with melena, hematuria, or excessive menstrual flow. Subarachnoid hemorrhage and intracerebral hemorrhage are serious consequences of thrombocytopenic purpura but, fortunately, are rare in treated patients. Splenomegaly and lymphadenopathy are uncommon in primary ITP, and their presence should lead one to consider other possible diagnoses.

The clinical signs and symptoms associated with ITP are not specific for this condition but rather reflective of thrombocytopenia. Destruction of platelets as the cause of thrombocytopenia is supported by the findings of a low platelet count and normal or increased megakaryocytes in the bone marrow. Accelerated thrombopoiesis often leads to the formation of abnormally large platelets (megathrombocytes), detected easily in a blood smear. The bleeding time is prolonged, but PT and PTT are normal. Tests for platelet autoantibodies are not widely available. *Therefore, a diagnosis of ITP should be made only after other causes of platelet deficiencies, such as those listed in Table 13–9, have been ruled out.*

Almost all patients respond to immunosuppressive doses of glucocorticoids, but many eventually relapse and come to splenectomy. Most maintain safe platelet counts postsplenectomy and require no further therapy. A significant minority, however, have refractory forms of ITP that can be very difficult to treat. Various immunosuppressive approaches may be effective in such patients.

Acute Immune Thrombocytopenic Purpura

Like chronic ITP, this condition is caused by antiplatelet autoantibodies, but its clinical features and course are distinct. Acute ITP is a disease of childhood occurring with equal frequency in both sexes. The onset of thrombocytopenia is abrupt and is preceded in many cases by a viral illness. The usual interval between the infection and onset of purpura is 2 weeks. Unlike the adult chronic form of ITP, the childhood disease is self-limited, usually resolving spontaneously within 6 months. Steroid therapy is indicated only if thrombocytopenia is severe. Approximately 20% of the children, usually those without a viral prodrome, have persistent low platelet counts beyond 6 months and appear to have chronic ITP similar in most respects to the adult disease.

Drug-Induced Thrombocytopenia: Heparin-Induced Thrombocytopenia

Like hemolytic anemia, thrombocytopenia can result from immunologically mediated destruction of platelets after drug ingestion.[54] The drugs most commonly involved are quinine, quinidine, sulfonamide antibiotics, and heparin. Heparin-induced thrombocytopenia (HIT) is of particular importance because this anticoagulant is used widely and failure to make a correct diagnosis can have severe consequences. Thrombocytopenia occurs in approximately 5% of patients receiving heparin. Most develop so-called type I thrombocytopenia, which occurs rapidly after onset of therapy, is modest in severity and clinically insignificant, and may resolve despite continuation of heparin therapy. It most likely results from a direct platelet-aggregating effect of heparin.

Type II thrombocytopenia is more severe. It occurs 5 to 14 days after commencement of therapy (or sometimes sooner if the patient has been previously sensitized to heparin) and can, paradoxically, lead to life-threatening venous and arterial thrombosis.[54] HIT is caused by an immune reaction directed against a complex of heparin and platelet factor 4, a normal component of platelet granules that binds tightly to heparin. It appears that heparin binding modifies the conformation of platelet factor 4, making it susceptible to immune recognition.[55] *Binding of antibody to platelet factor 4 produces immune complexes that activate platelets, promoting thrombosis even in the setting of marked thrombocytopenia.* The mechanism of platelet activation is not understood. Unless therapy is immediately discontinued, clots within large arteries may lead to vascular insufficiency and limb loss, and emboli from deep venous thrombosis can cause fatal pulmonary thromboembolism.

HIV-Associated Thrombocytopenia

Thrombocytopenia is perhaps the most common hematologic manifestation of HIV infection. Both impaired platelet production and increased destruction are responsible. CD4, the receptor for HIV on T cells, has also been demonstrated on megakaryocytes, making it possible for these cells to be infected by HIV.[56] Infected megakaryocytes are prone to apoptosis and are impaired in terms of platelet production. HIV infection also causes hyperplasia and dysregulation of B cells, which predispose to the development of immune-mediated thrombocytopenia. Antibodies directed against platelet membrane glycoprotein IIb-III complexes are detected in some patients' sera. These autoantibodies, which sometimes cross-react with HIV-associated gp120, are believed to act as opsonins, thus promoting the phagocytosis of platelets by splenic phagocytes. Some studies also implicate nonspecific deposition of immune complexes on platelets as a factor in their premature destruction by the mononuclear phagocyte system.

Thrombotic Microangiopathies: Thrombotic Thrombocytopenic Purpura (TTP) and Hemolytic-Uremic Syndrome (HUS)

The term *thrombotic microangiopathy* encompasses a spectrum of clinical syndromes that includes TTP and HUS. TTP, as originally defined, is associated with the pentad of fever, thrombocytopenia, microangiopathic hemolytic anemia, transient neurologic deficits, and renal failure. HUS is also associated with microangiopathic hemolytic anemia and thrombocytopenia but is distinguished from TTP by the absence of neurologic symptoms, the prominence of acute renal failure, and frequent affliction of children. Recent studies, however, have tended to blur these clinical distinctions. Many adult patients with "TTP" lack one or more of the five criteria, and some patients with "HUS" have fever and neurologic dysfunction. The common fundamental feature in both of these conditions is widespread formation of hyaline thrombi, comprised primarily of platelet aggregates, in the microcirculation. Consumption of platelets leads to *thrombocytopenia,* and the intravascular thrombi provide a likely mechanism for the *microangiopathic hemolytic anemia* and widespread organ dysfunction. It is believed the varied clinical manifestations of TTP and HUS are related to differing proclivities for thrombus formation in specific microvascular beds.

For many years, the pathogenesis of TTP was enigmatic, although treatment with plasma exchange (initiated in the early 1970s) changed an almost uniformly fatal condition into one that is successfully treated in more than 80% of cases. Recently, the underlying cause of many, but not all, cases of TTP has been elucidated. In brief, symptomatic patients are often deficient in an enzyme called ADAMTS 13. This enzyme is designated "vWF metalloprotease" and it normally degrades very high molecular weight multimers of von Willebrand factor (vWF).[57] (ADAMTS 13 is unrelated to the other tissue metalloproteases that cleave extracellular matrix.) In the absence of this enzyme, very high molecular weight multimers of vWF accumulate in plasma and, under some circumstances, promote platelet microaggregate formation throughout the microcirculation, leading to the symptoms of TTP. Superimposition of endothelial cell injury (caused by some other condition) may further predispose a patient to microaggregate formation, thus initiating or exacerbating clinically evident TTP.

The deficiency of ADAMTS 13 may be inherited or acquired.[58] In many patients an antibody that inhibits vWF metalloprotease is detected.[57] Much less commonly the patients have inherited an inactivating mutation in the gene encoding this enzyme. Despite these advances, it is clear that factors other than vWF metalloprotease deficiency must be involved in triggering full-blown TTP, because symptoms are episodic even in those with hereditary deficiency of vWF metalloprotease. It is important to consider the possibility of TTP in any patient presenting with thrombocytopenia and microangiopathic hemolytic anemia, as any delay in diagnosis and treatment can be fatal. Plasma exchange can be life saving by providing the missing enzyme.

In contrast to TTP, most patients with HUS have normal levels of vWF metalloprotease, indicating that HUS usually has a different pathogenesis.[59] One important cause of HUS in children and the elderly is infectious gastroenteritis caused by *E. coli* strain 0157:H7.[60] This strain elaborates a Shiga-like toxin that is absorbed from the inflamed gastrointestinal mucosa. It binds to and damages endothelial cells in the glomerulus and elsewhere, thus initiating platelet activation and aggregation. Affected children present with bloody diarrhea, and a few days later HUS makes its appearance. With appropriate supportive care, affected children often recover completely, but irreversible renal damage and death can occur in more severe cases. HUS can also be seen in adults following exposures that damage endothelial cells (e.g., certain drugs, radiation therapy). The prognosis of adults with HUS is guarded, as it is most often seen in the setting of other chronic, life-threatening conditions.

While DIC and thrombotic microangiopathies share features such as microvascular occlusion and microangiopathic hemolytic anemia, they are pathogenetically distinct. In TTP and HUS (unlike DIC), activation of the coagulation cascade is not of primary importance, and hence results of laboratory tests of coagulation, such as PT and PTT, are usually normal.

BLEEDING DISORDERS RELATED TO DEFECTIVE PLATELET FUNCTIONS

Qualitative defects of platelet function can be congenital or acquired. Several congenital disorders characterized by prolonged bleeding time and normal platelet count have been described. A brief discussion of these rare diseases is warranted by the fact that they provide excellent models for investigating the molecular mechanisms of platelet function.[61]

Congenital disorders of platelet function can be classified into three groups on the basis of the specific functional abnormality: (1) *defects of adhesion,* (2) *defects of aggregation,* and (3) *disorders of platelet secretion (release reaction).*

- Bleeding resulting from defective adhesion of platelets to subendothelial matrix is best illustrated by the autosomal recessive disorder *Bernard-Soulier syndrome,* which is caused by an inherited deficiency of the platelet membrane glycoprotein complex Ib-IX. This glycoprotein is a receptor for vWF and is essential for normal platelet adhesion to subendothelial matrix (Chapter 4).
- Bleeding due to *defective platelet aggregation* is exemplified by *Glanzmann's thrombasthenia,* which is also transmitted as an autosomal recessive trait. Thrombasthenic platelets fail to aggregate in response to adenosine diphosphate (ADP), collagen, epinephrine, or thrombin owing to deficiency or dysfunction of glycoprotein IIb-IIIa, a protein complex that participates in the formation of "bridges" between platelets by binding fibrinogen and vWF.
- *Disorders of platelet secretion* are characterized by normal initial aggregation with collagen or ADP, but subsequent responses, such as secretion of thromboxanes and release of granule-bound ADP, are impaired. The underlying biochemical defects of these so-called *storage pool disorders* are varied, complex, and beyond the scope of our discussion.

Among the *acquired defects* of platelet function, two are clinically significant.[62] The first is *ingestion of aspirin* and other nonsteroidal anti-inflammatory drugs, which significantly prolongs the bleeding time. Aspirin is a potent, irreversible inhibitor of the enzyme cyclooxygenase, which is required for the synthesis of thromboxane A_2 and prostaglandins (Chapter 2). These mediators play important roles in platelet aggregation and subsequent release reactions (Chapter 4). The antiplatelet effects of aspirin form the basis for its use in the prophylaxis of thrombosis (Chapter 12). *Uremia* (Chapter 20) is the second condition exemplifying an acquired defect in platelet function. Although the pathogenesis of bleeding in uremia is complex and not fully understood, several abnormalities of platelet function are found.

HEMORRHAGIC DIATHESES RELATED TO ABNORMALITIES IN CLOTTING FACTORS

A deficiency of every clotting factor has been reported to be the cause of a bleeding disorder, with the exception of factor XII deficiency, which does not cause bleeding. The bleeding in factor deficiencies differs from platelet deficiencies in that spontaneous petechiae or purpura are uncommon. Rather, *the bleeding is manifested by large post-traumatic ecchymoses or hematomas, or prolonged bleeding after a laceration or any form of surgical procedure.* Bleeding into the gastrointestinal and urinary tracts, and particularly into weight-bearing joints, is common. Typical stories include the patient who continues to ooze for days after a tooth extraction or who develops a hemarthrosis after relatively trivial stress on a knee joint. The course of history may have been changed by a hereditary coagulation defect present in the intermarried royal families of Great Britain and other parts of Europe. Clotting abnormalities can also be acquired in many different conditions.

Acquired disorders are usually characterized by multiple clotting abnormalities. Vitamin K deficiency (Chapter 9) results in impaired synthesis of factors II, VII, IX, and X and protein C. Since the liver makes virtually all the clotting factors, severe parenchymal liver disease can be associated with a hemorrhagic diathesis. Disseminated intravascular coagulation produces a deficiency of multiple coagulation factors.

Hereditary deficiencies have been identified for each of the clotting factors. Deficiencies of factor VIII (hemophilia A) and of factor IX (Christmas disease, or hemophilia B) are transmitted as sex-linked recessive disorders. Most others follow autosomal patterns of transmission. *These hereditary disorders typically involve a single clotting factor.*

Deficiencies of Factor VIII–vWF Complex

Hemophilia A and von Willebrand disease, two of the most common inherited disorders of bleeding, are caused by qualitative or quantitative defects involving the factor VIII–vWF complex. Before we can discuss these disorders, it is essential to review the structure and function of these proteins.[63,64]

Plasma factor VIII–vWF is a complex made up of two separate proteins (factor VIII and vWF) that can be characterized according to functional, biochemical, and immunologic criteria. Factor VIII procoagulant protein, or factor VIII (Fig. 13–28; also see Chapter 4), is an intrinsic pathway component required for activation of factor X. Deficiency of factor VIII gives rise to hemophilia A. Circulating factor VIII is noncovalently associated with very large vWF multimers containing up to 100 subunits; the molecular mass of individual multimers can exceed 20×10^6 daltons. vWF also interacts with several other proteins involved in hemostasis, including collagen, heparin, and platelet membrane glycoproteins (Ib-IX and IIb-IIIa). Glycoprotein Ib-IX serves as the major receptor for vWF. The most important function of vWF in vivo is to promote the adhesion of platelets to subendothelial matrix, which is accomplished in two ways. Some vWF secreted by endothelial cells is normally deposited in the subendothelial matrix, where it promotes platelet adhesion should the endothelial lining be disrupted (see Fig. 13–28). Endothelial cells and platelets also release vWF into the circulation, and upon vascular injury this second pool of vWF is adsorbed to exposed subendothelial matrix and further augments platelet adhesion. vWF multimers can also promote platelet aggregation by binding to activated GpIIb/IIIa receptors; this activity may be of particular importance under conditions of high shear stress (such as occurs in small vessels). That vWF is crucial to the normal process of hemostasis (Chapter 4) is supported by the occurrence of a bleeding diathesis known as von Willebrand disease when there is deficiency of this factor.

vWF multimers also serve as a carrier for factor VIII and are important for its stability. The half-life of factor VIII in the circulation is 12 hours if vWF levels are normal but only 2.4 hours if it is deficient or abnormal (as in patients with von Willebrand disease).

vWF can be assayed by immunologic techniques or by the so-called *ristocetin agglutination test.* This assay, which can be

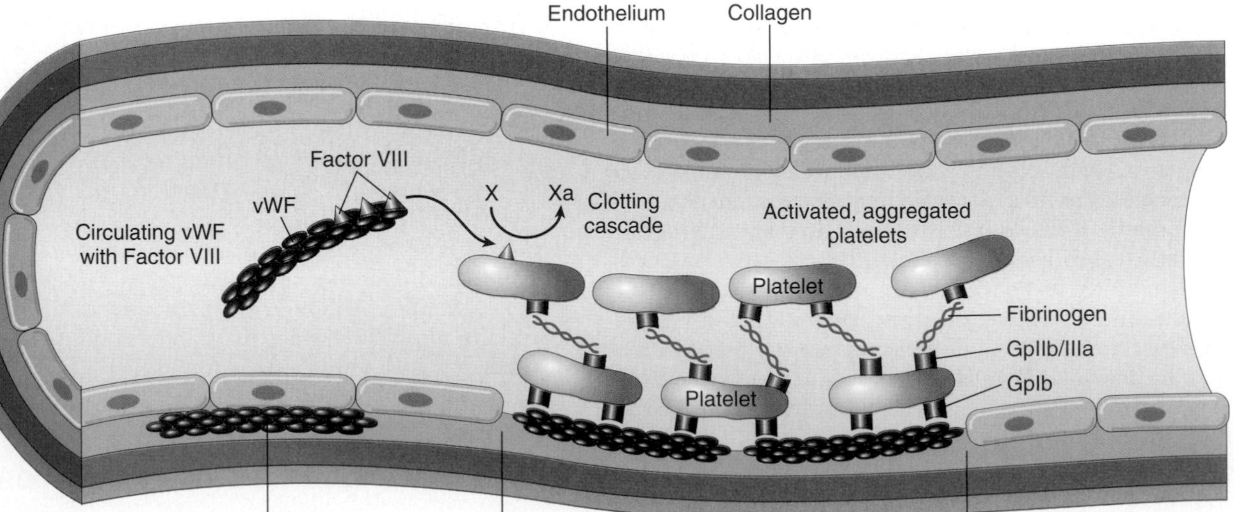

FIGURE 13–28 Structure and function of factor VIII–von Willebrand factor (vWF) complex. Factor VIII is synthesized in the liver and kidney, and vWF is made in endothelial cells and megakaryocytes. The two associate to form a complex in the circulation. vWF is also present in the subendothelial matrix of normal blood vessels and the alpha granules of platelets. Following endothelial injury, exposure of subendothelial vWF causes adhesion of platelets, primarily via glycoprotein Ib platelet receptor. Circulating vWF and vWF released from the alpha granules of activated platelets can bind exposed subendothelial matrix, further contributing to platelet adhesion and activation. Activated platelets form hemostatic aggregates; fibrinogen (and possibly vWF) participate in aggregation through bridging interactions with the platelet receptor GpIIb/III. Factor VIII takes part in the coagulation cascade as a cofactor in the activation of factor X on the surface of activated platelets.

performed with formalin-fixed platelets, measures the ability of ristocetin (developed as an antibiotic) to promote the interaction between vWF and platelet membrane glycoprotein Ib. Multivalent ristocetin-dependent binding of vWF creates interplatelet "bridges," leading to the formation of platelet clumps (agglutination), an event easily measured in a device called an *aggregometer.* Thus, the degree of ristocetin-dependent platelet agglutination caused by the addition of patient plasma provides a bioassay for vWF.

The two components of the factor VIII–vWF complex are encoded by separate genes and synthesized in different cells. vWF is produced by endothelial cells and megakaryocytes and can be demonstrated in platelet α-granules. *Endothelial cells are the major source of subendothelial and plasma vWF.* Factor VIII is made in several tissues; sinusoidal endothelial cells and Kupffer cells in the liver and glomerular and tubular epithelial cells in the kidney appear to be particularly important sites of synthesis. To summarize, *the two components of factor VIII–vWF complex, synthesized separately, come together and circulate in the plasma as a unit that serves to promote clotting as well as platelet–vessel wall interactions necessary to ensure hemostasis.* With this background, we can discuss the diseases resulting from deficiencies of factor VIII–vWF complex.

Von Willebrand Disease

With an estimated frequency of 1%, von Willebrand disease is believed to be one of the most common inherited disorders of bleeding in humans. Clinically, it is characterized by spontaneous bleeding from mucous membranes, excessive bleeding from wounds, menorrhagia, and a prolonged bleeding time in the presence of a normal platelet count. In most cases, it is transmitted as an autosomal dominant disorder, but several rare autosomal recessive variants have been identified.[65]

More than 20 variants of von Willebrand disease have been described, which can be grouped into two major categories:

- Type 1 and type 3 von Willebrand disease are associated with a *reduced quantity of circulating vWF.* Type 1, an autosomal dominant disorder, accounts for approximately 70% of all cases and is relatively mild. Reduced penetrance and variable expressivity characterize this type, and hence clinical manifestations are varied. Type 3 (an autosomal recessive disorder) is associated with extremely low levels of functional vWF, and the clinical manifestations are correspondingly severe. Because a severe deficiency of vWF has a marked affect on the stability of factor VIII, some of the bleeding characteristics resemble those seen in hemophilia. The nature of the mutations in the vast majority of patients with type 1 disease is poorly defined. In some cases missense mutations have been found. In others, it is suspected that both alleles are affected by distinct mutations (compound heterozygotes) producing an apparent dominant inheritance. Type 3 disease is associated with deletions or frameshift mutations.[66]
- Type 2 von Willebrand disease is characterized by qualitative defects in vWF; there are several subtypes, of which type 2A is the most common. It is inherited as an autosomal dominant disorder. Because of missense mutations, the vWF formed is abnormal, leading to defective multimer assembly. Large and intermediate multimers, representing the most active forms of vWF, are missing from plasma. Type 2 von Willebrand disease accounts for 25% of all cases and is associated with mild to moderate bleeding.

Patients with von Willebrand disease have *prolonged bleeding* time despite a *normal platelet count.* The plasma level of active vWF, measured as the *ristocetin cofactor activity, is reduced.* Because vWF stabilizes factor VIII by binding to it, a deficiency of vWF gives rise to a secondary decrease in factor VIII levels. This may be reflected by a prolongation of the PTT in von Willebrand disease types 1 and 3.

To summarize, patients with von Willebrand disease have a compound defect involving platelet function and the coagulation pathway. Even within families in which a single defective allele is segregating, there is often wide variability in the clinical expression of von Willebrand disease. This appears to be due to additional genetic factors that influence circulating levels of vWF, which vary greatly in normal populations.[67] However, except in the most severely affected type 3 patients, adverse complications of factor VIII deficiency, such as bleeding into the joints, are uncommon.

Hemophilia A (Factor VIII Deficiency)

Hemophilia A is the most common *hereditary disease associated with serious bleeding.* It is caused by a reduction in the amount or activity of factor VIII. This protein serves as a cofactor for factor IX in the activation of factor X in the coagulation cascade (Chapter 4). Hemophilia A is inherited as an X-linked recessive trait, and thus occurs in males and in homozygous females. However, excessive bleeding has been described in heterozygous females, presumably due to extremely unfavorable lyonization (inactivation of the normal X chromosome in most of the cells). Approximately 30% of patients have no family history; their disease is presumably caused by new mutations.

Hemophilia A exhibits a wide range of clinical severity that correlates well with the level of factor VIII activity. Those with less than 1% of normal activity develop severe disease; levels between 2% and 5% of normal are associated with moderate disease; and patients with 6% to 50% of activity develop mild disease. The variable degrees of factor VIII deficiency are largely explained by heterogeneity in the causative mutations.[68] As with β-thalassemias, several genetic lesions (deletions, nonsense mutations that create stop codons, splicing errors) have been documented. Most severe deficiencies result from an unusual inversion involving the X chromosome that completely abolishes the synthesis of factor VIII. Less commonly, severe hemophilia A is associated with point mutations in factor VIII that impair the function of the protein. In such cases, levels of factor VIII appear normal by immunoassay. Mutations permitting some active factor VIII to be synthesized are associated with mild to moderate disease. The disease in such patients may be modified by other genetic factors that influence factor VIII expression levels, which vary widely in normal individuals.[69]

In all symptomatic cases, there is a tendency toward easy bruising and massive hemorrhage after trauma or operative procedures. In addition, "spontaneous" hemorrhages frequently occur in regions of the body normally subject to trauma, particularly the joints, where they are known as *hemarthroses.* Recurrent bleeding into the joints leads to progressive deformities that can be crippling. *Petechiae are characteristically absent.*

Patients with hemophilia A typically have a normal bleeding time, platelet count, and PT, and a prolonged PTT. These tests point to an abnormality of the intrinsic coagulation pathway. Factor VIII–specific assays are required for diagnosis.

Given that one arm of the coagulation cascade, the extrinsic pathway, is intact in hemophilia A, it seems reasonable to ask, why do these patients bleed? Obviously, test tube assays of coagulation (discussed briefly below under DIC) are imperfect surrogates for what occurs in vivo, and it must be that in the face of factor VIII deficiency, fibrin deposition is inadequate to achieve hemostasis reliably. It is beyond our scope to discuss this issue in detail, but recent studies suggest the following.[70] First, it appears that the chief role of the extrinsic pathway in hemostasis is to produce a limited initial burst of thrombin activation upon tissue injury. This is reinforced and amplified by a critical feedback loop whereby thrombin activates factors XI and IX of the intrinsic pathway. In addition, high levels of thrombin are required to activate TAFI (thrombin activatable fibrinolysis inhibitor), a factor that augments fibrin deposition by inhibiting fibrinolysis. Thus, both inadequate coagulation (fibrinogenesis) and inappropriate clot removal (fibrinolysis) contribute to the bleeding diathesis in hemophilia. The precise explanation for the tendency of hemophiliacs to bleed at particular sites (joints, muscles, and the central nervous system) remains uncertain.

Treatment of hemophilia A involves infusion of recombinant factor VIII. Approximately 15% of patients with low or absent factor VIII develop antibodies that bind to and inhibit factor VIII. Inhibitors are most likely to develop in patients with severe factor VIII deficiency (possibly because the protein is perceived as foreign, having never been "seen" before by the immune system) and represent very difficult therapeutic challenges. There are other hazards of replacement therapy as well, the most serious of which has been the risk of transmission of viral diseases. Until the mid-1980s, before routine screening of blood for HIV antibodies was instituted, thousands of hemophiliacs received plasma-derived factor VIII concentrates containing HIV, and many developed AIDS (Chapter 6). With the availability of recombinant factor VIII, the risk of HIV transmission has been eliminated, but tragically too late for an entire generation of hemophiliacs. Efforts to develop somatic gene therapy for hemophilia are also under way.

Hemophilia B (Christmas Disease, Factor IX Deficiency)

Severe factor IX deficiency produces a disorder clinically indistinguishable from factor VIII deficiency (hemophilia A). This should not be surprising, given that factor VIII and IX function together to activate factor X. A wide spectrum of mutations involving the factor IX gene are found in hemophilia B.[68] Like hemophilia A, it is inherited as an X-linked recessive trait and shows variable clinical severity. In about 14% of these patients, factor IX is present but nonfunctional. As with hemophilia A, the PTT is prolonged and the PT is normal, as is the bleeding time. Identification of Christmas disease (named after the first patient with this condition and not the holiday) is possible only by assay of the factor levels. Recombinant factor IX is used for treatment.

DISSEMINATED INTRAVASCULAR COAGULATION (DIC)

DIC is an acute, subacute, or chronic thrombohemorrhagic disorder occurring as a secondary complication in a variety of diseases. It is characterized by activation of the coagulation sequence that leads to the formation of microthrombi throughout the microcirculation of the body, often in a quixotically uneven distribution. Sometimes the coagulopathy is localized to a specific organ or tissue. *As a consequence of the thrombotic diathesis, there is consumption of platelets, fibrin, and coagulation factors and, secondarily, activation of fibrinolytic mechanisms.* Thus, DIC can present with signs and symptoms relating to tissue hypoxia and infarction caused by the myriad microthrombi or as a hemorrhagic disorder related to depletion of the elements required for hemostasis (hence, the term "consumption coagulopathy" is sometimes used to describe DIC). Activation of the fibrinolytic mechanism aggravates the hemorrhagic diathesis.

Etiology and Pathogenesis. At the outset, it must be emphasized that DIC is not a primary disease. It is a coagulopathy that occurs in the course of a variety of clinical conditions. In discussing the general mechanisms underlying DIC, it is useful to briefly review the normal process of blood coagulation and clot removal. Clotting can be initiated by either of two pathways: (1) the *extrinsic pathway,* which is triggered by the release of tissue factor ("tissue thromboplastin"), and (2) the *intrinsic pathway,* which involves the activation of factor XII by surface contact with collagen or other negatively charged substances. Both pathways, through a series of intermediate steps, result in the generation of thrombin, which in turn converts fibrinogen to fibrin. Once activated at the site of injury, thrombin further augments local fibrin deposition through feedback activation of the intrinsic pathway and inhibition of fibrinolysis. Remarkably, as excess thrombin is swept away in the blood from sites of tissue injury it is converted to an anticoagulant. Upon binding a surface protein called *thrombomodulin* on intact endothelial cells, thrombin becomes capable of activating protein C, an inhibitor of the pro-coagulant factors V and VIII. Other important *clot-inhibiting factors* include the activation of fibrinolysis by plasmin and the clearance of activated clotting factors by the mononuclear phagocyte system and the liver. These and additional checks and balances normally ensure that just enough clotting occurs at the right place and time.

From this brief review, it should be clear that DIC could result from pathologic activation of the extrinsic and/or intrinsic pathways of coagulation or impairment of clot-inhibiting influences. Since the latter rarely constitute primary mechanisms of DIC, we focus our attention on the abnormal initiation of clotting.[71]

Two major mechanisms trigger DIC: (1) release of tissue factor or thromboplastic substances into the circulation and (2) widespread injury to the endothelial cells. Tissue thromboplastic substances can be derived from a variety of sources, such as the placenta in obstetric complications (Table 13–10) and the granules of leukemic cells in acute promyelocytic leukemia. Mucus released from certain adenocarcinomas can also act as a thromboplastic substance by directly activating factor X, independent of factor VII. In gram-negative sepsis (an important cause of DIC), bacterial endotoxins cause activated monocytes to release interleukin-1 and TNF, both of which

TABLE 13–10 Major Disorders Associated with Disseminated Intravascular Coagulation

Obstetric Complications
Abruptio placentae
Retained dead fetus
Septic abortion
Amniotic fluid embolism
Toxemia
Infections
Gram-negative sepsis
Meningococcemia
Rocky Mountain spotted fever
Histoplasmosis
Aspergillosis
Malaria
Neoplasms
Carcinomas of pancreas, prostate, lung, and stomach
Acute promyelocytic leukemia
Massive Tissue Injury
Traumatic
Burns
Extensive surgery
Miscellaneous
Acute intravascular hemolysis, snakebite, giant hemangioma, shock, heat stroke, vasculitis, aortic aneurysm, liver disease

increase the expression of tissue factor on endothelial cell membranes and simultaneously decrease the expression of thrombomodulin.[72] The net result is a shift in balance toward procoagulation.

Endothelial injury, the other major trigger, can initiate DIC by causing release of tissue factor, promoting platelet aggregation, and activating the intrinsic coagulation pathway. TNF is an extremely important mediator of endothelial cell inflammation and injury in septic shock. In addition to the effects previously mentioned, TNF up-regulates the expression of adhesion molecules on endothelial cells and thus favors adhesion of leukocytes, which in turn damage endothelial cells by releasing oxygen-derived free radicals and preformed proteases.[72] Even subtle endothelial injury can unleash procoagulant activity by enhancing membrane expression of tissue factor. Widespread endothelial injury may be produced by deposition of antigen–antibody complexes (e.g., systemic lupus erythematosus), temperature extremes (e.g., heat stroke, burns), or microorganisms (e.g., meningococci, rickettsiae).

Several disorders associated with DIC are listed in Table 13–10. Of these, DIC is most likely to follow *obstetric complications, malignant neoplasia, sepsis,* and *major trauma.* The initiating factors in these conditions are often multiple and interrelated. For example, particularly in infections caused by gram-negative bacteria, released endotoxins can activate both the intrinsic and extrinsic pathways by producing endothelial cell injury and release of thromboplastins from inflammatory cells; furthermore, endotoxins inhibit the anticoagulant activity of protein C by suppressing thrombomodulin expression on endothelium. Endothelial cell damage can also be produced directly by meningococci, rickettsiae, and viruses. Antigen–antibody complexes formed during the infection can activate the classical complement pathway, and complement fragments can secondarily activate both platelets and granulocytes. Endotoxins as well as other bacterial products are also capable of directly activating factor XII. In *massive trauma, extensive surgery,* and *severe burns,* the major mechanism of DIC is believed to be the release of tissue thromboplastins. In *obstetric* conditions, thromboplastins derived from the placenta, dead retained fetus, or amniotic fluid may enter the circulation. However, hypoxia, acidosis, and shock, which often coexist with the surgical and obstetric conditions, also cause widespread endothelial injury. Supervening infection can complicate the problems further. Among cancers, acute promyelocytic leukemia and carcinomas of the lung, pancreas, colon, and stomach are most frequently associated with DIC. These tumors release of a variety of thromboplastic substances, including tissue factors, proteolytic enzymes, mucin, and other undefined tumor products.

The consequences of DIC are twofold. First, there is *widespread deposition of fibrin* within the microcirculation. This can lead to ischemia of the more severely affected or more vulnerable organs and to a *hemolytic anemia* resulting from fragmentation of red cells as they squeeze through the narrowed microvasculature (microangiopathic hemolytic anemia). Second, a *hemorrhagic diathesis* can dominate the clinical picture. This results from consumption of platelets and clotting factors as well as activation of plasminogen. Plasmin can not only cleave fibrin, but also digest factors V and VIII, thereby reducing their concentration further. In addition, fibrinolysis leads to the formation of fibrin degradation products, which inhibit platelet aggregation and fibrin polymerization and have antithrombin activity. All these influences lead to the hemostatic failure seen in DIC (Fig. 13–29).

Morphology. In general, thrombi are found in the following sites in decreasing order of frequency: brain, heart, lungs, kidneys, adrenals, spleen, and liver. However, no tissue is spared, and thrombi are occasionally found in only one or several organs without affecting others. In giant hemangiomas, for example, thrombi are localized to the neoplasm, where they are believed to form due to local stasis and recurrent trauma to fragile blood vessels. The affected kidneys can reveal small thrombi in the glomeruli that may evoke only reactive swelling of endothelial cells or, in severe cases, microinfarcts or even bilateral renal cortical necrosis. Numerous fibrin thrombi may be found in alveolar capillaries, sometimes associated with pulmonary edema and fibrin exudation, creating "hyaline membranes" reminiscent of acute respiratory distress syndrome (Chapter 15). In the central nervous system, fibrin thrombi can cause microinfarcts, occasionally complicated by simultaneous hemorrhage. Such changes are the basis for the bizarre neurologic signs and symptoms sometimes observed in DIC. The manifestations of DIC in the endocrine glands are of considerable interest. In meningococcemia, fibrin thrombi within the microcirculation of the adrenal cortex are the likely basis for the massive adrenal hemorrhages seen in Waterhouse-Friderichsen syndrome (Chapter 24). Similarly, Sheehan postpartum pituitary necrosis (Chapter 24) is a form of DIC complicating labor and delivery. In toxemia of pregnancy (Chapter 22), the placenta exhibits widespread microthrombi, providing a plau-

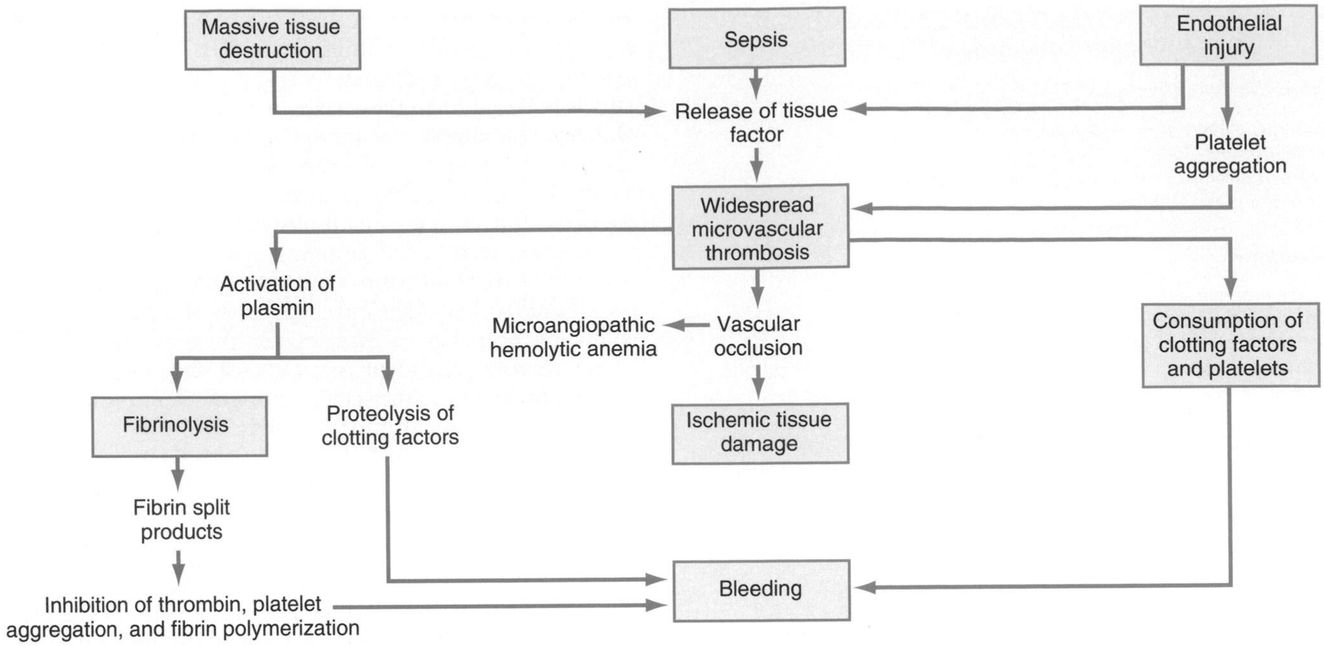

FIGURE 13–29 Pathophysiology of disseminated intravascular coagulation.

sible explanation for the premature atrophy of the cytotrophoblast and syncytiotrophoblast encountered in this condition.

The bleeding manifestations of DIC are not dissimilar to those encountered in the hereditary and acquired disorders affecting the hemostatic mechanisms discussed earlier.

Clinical Course. The onset can be fulminant, as in endotoxic shock or amniotic fluid embolism, or insidious and chronic, as in cases of carcinomatosis or retention of a dead fetus. Overall, about 50% of individuals with DIC are obstetric patients having complications of pregnancy. In this setting, the disorder tends to be reversible with delivery of the fetus. About 33% of the patients have carcinomatosis. The remaining cases are associated with the various entities previously listed.

It is almost impossible to detail all the potential clinical presentations, but a few common patterns are worthy of description. These include microangiopathic hemolytic anemia; dyspnea, cyanosis, and respiratory failure; convulsions and coma; oliguria and acute renal failure; and sudden or progressive circulatory failure and shock. In general, *acute DIC, associated with obstetric complications or major trauma, for example, is dominated by a bleeding diathesis, whereas chronic DIC, such as occurs in cancer patients, tends to present initially with thrombotic complications.* Accurate clinical observation and laboratory studies are necessary for the diagnosis. It is usually necessary to monitor fibrinogen, platelets, PT, PTT, and fibrin degradation products.

The prognosis is highly variable and depends, to a considerable extent, on the underlying disorder. The management of these cases requires meticulous maneuvering between the Scylla of thrombosis and the Charybdis of bleeding diathesis. Administration of anticoagulants or procoagulants has been advocated in specific settings, but not without controversy. The only definitive treatment is to remove or treat the inciting cause whenever possible.

REFERENCES

1. Dzierzak E: Embryonic beginnings of definitive hematopoietic stem cells. Ann NY Acad Sci 872:256, 1999.
2. Kondo M, et al: Identification of clonogenic common lymphoid progenitors in mouse bone marrow. Cell 91:661, 1997.
3. Akashi K, et al: A clonogenic common myeloid progenitor that gives rise to all myeloid lineages. Nature 404:193, 2000.
4. Orkin SH, Zon LL: Hematopoiesis and stem cells: plasticity versus developmental heterogeneity. Nature Immunol 3:323–328, 2002.
5. Clarke D, Frisen J: Differentiation potential of adult stem cells. Curr Opin Genet Dev 11:575, 2001.
6. Vogel G: Stem cell policy. Can adult stem cells suffice? Science 292:1820, 2001.
7. Wang X, et al: Cell fusion is the principal source of bone-marrow-derived hepatocytes. Nature 422:897–901, 2003.
8. Delaunay J: Molecular basis of red cell membrane disorders. Acta Haematol 108:210, 2002.
9. Eber SW, et al: Ankyrin-1 mutations are a major cause of dominant and recessive hereditary spherocytosis. Nat Genet 13:214, 1996.
10. Jarolim P, et al: Characterization of 13 novel band 3 gene defects in hereditary spherocytosis with band 3 deficiency. Blood 88:4366, 1996.
11. Jandl J, et al: Red cell filtration and the pathogenesis of certain hemolytic anemias. Blood 18:33, 1961.
12. Mehta A, Mason PJ, Vulliamy TJ: Glucose-6-phosphate dehydrogenase deficiency. Bailliers Best Pract Res Clin Hematol 13:21, 2000.
13. Tishkoff SA, et al: Haplotype diversity and linkage disequilibrium at human G6PD: recent origin of alleles that confer malarial resistance. Science 293:455, 2001.
14. Gomez-Gallego F, et al: Structural defects underlying protein dysfunction in human glucose-6-phosphate dehydrogenase A(−) deficiency. J Biol Chem 275:9256, 2000.
15. Aidoo M, et al: Protective effects of the sickle cell gene against malaria morbidity and mortality. Lancet 359:1311, 2002.
16. Brugnara C, et al: Erythrocyte-active agents and treatment of sickle cell disease. Semin Hematol 38:324, 2001.
17. Hebbel RP: Adhesive interactions of sickle erythrocytes with endothelium. J Clin Invest 100:S83, 1997.

18. Miller ST, et al: Prediction of adverse outcomes in children with sickle cell disease. N Engl J Med 342:83, 2000.
19. Zachlederora M, Jarolim, P: Gene expression profile of microvascular endothelial cells after stimuli implicated in pathogenesis of vaso-occlusion. Blood Cell Molecules Dis 30:71, 2003.
20. Frenette PS: Sickle cell vaso-occlusion: multistep and multicellular paradigm. Curr Opin Hematol 9:101, 2002.
21. Liao JC: Blood feud: keeping hemoglobin from nixing NO. Nature Med 8:1350, 2002.
22. Ballas SK: Sickle cell disease: current clinical management. Semin Hematol 38:307, 2001.
23. Smith J: Bone disorders in sickle cell disease. Hematol Oncol Clin North Am 10:1345, 1996.
24. Platt OS: The acute chest syndrome of sickle cell disease. N Engl J Med 342:1904, 2000.
25. Bunn HF: Pathogenesis and treatment of sickle cell disease. N Engl J Med 337:762, 1997.
26. Davies SC, Gilmore A: The role of hydroxyurea in the management of sickle cell disease. Blood Rev 17:99, 2003.
27. Ferster A, et al: Five years of experience with hydroxyurea in children and young adults with sickle cell disease. Blood 97:3628, 2001.
28. Olivieri NF: The β-thalassemias. N Engl J Med 341:99, 1999.
29. Rund D, Rachmilewitz E: Pathophysiology of α- and β-thalassemia: therapeutic implications. Semin Hematol 38:343, 2001.
30. Rosse WF: New insights into paroxysmal nocturnal hemoglobinuria. Curr Opin Hematol 8:61, 2001.
31. Wright MS: Drug-induced hemolytic anemias: increasing complications to therapeutic interventions. Clin Lab Sci 12:115, 1999.
32. Gehrs BC, Friedberg RC: Autoimmune hemolytic anemia. Am J Hematol 69:258, 2002.
33. Oh RC, Brown DL: Vitamin B_{12} deficiency. Am Fam Physican 67:979, 2003.
34. Hoffbrand AV,Jackson BF: Correction of the DNA synthesis defect in vitamin B12 deficiency by tetrahydrofolate: evidence in favour of the methyl-folate trap hypothesis as the cause of megaloblastic anaemia in vitamin B_{12} deficiency. Br J Haematol 83:643, 1993.
35. Chanarin I, et al: Cobalamin and folate: recent developments. J Clin Pathol 45:277, 1992.
36. Wickramasinghe SN: The wide spectrum and unresolved issues of megaloblastic anemia. Semin Hematol 36:3, 1999.
37. Shevell MI, et al: Varying neurological phenotypes among mut° and mut⁻ patients with methylmalonylCoA mutase deficiency. Am J Med Genet 45:619, 1993.
38. Toh BH, et al: Pernicious anemia. N Engl J Med 337:1441, 1997.
39. Looker AC, et al: Prevalence of iron deficiency in the United States. JAMA 277:973, 1997.
40. Andrews, NC: A genetic view of iron homeostasis. Semin Hematol 39:227, 2002.
41. Fleming RE, Sly WS: Mechanisms of iron accumulation in hereditary hemochromatosis. Annu Rev Physiol 64:663, 2002.
42. Ganz T: Hepcidin, a key regulator of iron metabolism and mediator of anemia of inflammation. Blood 102:783, 2003.
43. Means RT, Jr: Erythropoietin in the treatment of anemia in chronic infectious, inflammatory, and malignant diseases. Curr Opin Hematol 2:210, 1995.
44. Spivak J: Iron and anemia of chronic disease. Oncology (Huntingt) 16 (Suppl 10):25, 2002.
45. Dokal I: Inherited aplastic anemia. Hematol J 4:3, 2003.
46. Young NS: Acquired aplastic anemia. Ann Intern Med 136:534, 2002.
47. Erslev AJ, Soltan A: Pure red-cell aplasia: a review. Blood Rev 10:20, 1996.
48. Eschbach JW: Current concepts of anemia management in chronic renal failure. Semin Nephrol 20:320, 2000.
49. Gregg XT, Prchal JT: Erythropoietin receptor mutations and human disease. Semin Hematol 34:70, 1997.
50. Longmore GD: Erythropoietin receptor mutations and Olympic glory. Nat Genet 4:108, 1993.
51. Rand ML, Leung R, Packham MA: Platelet function assays. Trans Apher Sci 28:307, 2003.
52. Bussel JB: Alloimmune thrombocytopenia in the fetus and newborn. Semin Thromb Hemost 27:245, 2001.
53. Cines DB, Blanchette VS: Immune thrombocytopenic purpura. N Engl J Med 346:995, 2002.
54. Aster RH: Drug-induced immune thrombocytopenia: an overview of pathogenesis. Semin Hematol 36:2, 1999.
55. Visentin GP, et al: Heparin is not required for detection of antibodies associated with heparin-induced thrombocytopenia/thrombosis. J Lab Clin Med 138:22, 2001.
56. Scaradavou A: HIV-related thrombocytopenia. Blood Rev 16:73, 2002.
57 Tsai HM: Deficiency of *ADAMTS13* causes thrombotic thrombocytopenic purpura. Arterioscler Thromb Vasc Biol 23:388, 2003.
58. Levy GG, et al: Mutations in a member of the *ADAMTS* gene family cause thrombotic thrombocytopenic purpura. Nature 413:488, 2001.
59. Moake JL: Thrombotic thrombocytopenic purpura and the hemolytic uremic syndrome. Arch Pathol Lab Med 126:1430, 2002.
60. Zoja C, et al: The role of the endothelium in hemolytic uremic syndrome. J Nephrol 14(Suppl 4):S58, 2001.
61. Rao AK: Congenital disorders of platelet function: disorders of signal transduction and secretion. Am J Med Sci 316:69, 1998.
62. Bick RL: Platelet function defects associated with hemorrhage or thrombosis. Med Clin North Am 78:577, 1994.
63. Lenting PJ, et al: The life cycle of coagulation factor VIII in view of its structure and function. Blood 92:3983, 1998.
64. Ruggeri ZM: Structure of von Willebrand factor and its function in platelet adhesion and thrombus formation. Best Pract Res Clin Haematol 14:257, 2001.
65. Sadler JE, et al: Impact, diagnosis and treatment of von Willebrand disease. Thromb Haemost 84:160, 2000.
66. Castman G, et al: von Willebrand disease in year 2003: towards the complete identification of gene defects for correct diagnosis and treatment. Hematologica 88:94, 2003.
67. Levy G, Ginsburg D: Getting at the variable expressivity of von Willebrand disease. Thromb Haemost 86:144, 2001.
68. Bowen DJ: Haemophilia A and haemophilia B: molecular insights. Mol Pathol 55:1, 2002.
69. Lensen R, et al: High factor VIII levels contribute to the thrombotic risk in families with factor V Leiden. Br J Haematol 114:380, 2001.
70. Mosnier LO, et al: The defective down-regulation of fibrinolysis in haemophilia A can be restored by increasing the TAFI plasma concentration. Thromb Haemost 86:1035, 2001.
71. Bick RL: Disseminated intravascular coagulation: a review of etiology, pathophysiology, diagnosis, and management: guidelines for care. Clin Appl Thromb Hemost 8:1, 2002.
72. Esmon CT, et al: Inflammation, sepsis, and coagulation. Haematologica 84:254, 1999.

CHAPTER 14

Diseases of White Blood Cells, Lymph Nodes, Spleen, and Thymus

Jon C. Aster, MD, PhD

■ WHITE BLOOD CELLS AND LYMPH NODES

LEUKOPENIA

Neutropenia, Agranulocytosis

REACTIVE (INFLAMMATORY) PROLIFERATIONS OF WHITE CELLS AND NODES

Leukocytosis

Acute Nonspecific Lymphadenitis

Chronic Nonspecific Lymphadenitis

NEOPLASTIC PROLIFERATIONS OF WHITE CELLS

Etiological and Pathogenetic Factors in White Cell Neoplasia: Overview

Lymphoid Neoplasms

Definitions and Classifications

Precursor B-Cell and T-Cell Neoplasms

Peripheral B-Cell Neoplasms

Peripheral T-Cell and NK-Cell Neoplasms

Hodgkin Lymphoma

Myeloid Neoplasms

Acute Myelogenous Leukemia

Myelodysplastic Syndromes

Chronic Myeloproliferative Disorders

Langerhans Cell Histiocytosis

■ SPLEEN

SPLENOMEGALY

Nonspecific Acute Splenitis

Congestive Splenomegaly

Splenic Infarcts

NEOPLASMS

CONGENITAL ANOMALIES

RUPTURE

■ THYMUS

DEVELOPMENTAL DISORDERS

THYMIC HYPERPLASIA

THYMOMAS

WHITE BLOOD CELLS AND LYMPH NODES

Normal

The origin and differentiation of white blood cells (granulocytes, monocytes, and lymphocytes) were briefly discussed in Chapter 13. Lymphocytes and monocytes not only circulate in the blood and lymph but also accumulate in discrete, organized masses within lymph nodes, thymus, spleen, tonsils, adenoids, and Peyer patches. Less discrete collections of lymphoid cells occur in the bone marrow, lungs, gastrointestinal tract, and other tissues. Lymph nodes are the most widely distributed and easily accessible component of the lymphoid tissue and hence are frequently examined for diagnosis of lymphoreticular disorders. Before discussing these pathologic states, we will briefly review the normal morphology of lymph nodes (shown in Fig. 6–3, Chapter 6).

Lymph nodes are discrete structures surrounded by a capsule composed of connective tissue and a few elastic fibrils. The capsule is perforated by multiple afferent lymphatics that empty into a fenestrated subcapsular peripheral sinus. Lymph extravasates from this sinus and slowly percolates through the node, eventually collecting in medullary sinusoids and exiting through a single efferent lymphatic vessel in the hilus, which is the point of penetration by a single small artery and vein. Situated in the cortex subjacent to the peripheral sinus are spherical or egg-shaped aggregates of small lymphocytes, the so-called primary *follicles*, which contain numerous immunologically naïve B cells. The paracortical region lying between primary follicles is populated by numerous evenly dispersed small T lymphocytes. Deep to the cortex lies the medulla, which contains variable numbers of plasma cells and relatively few lymphocytes.

This morphologic description reflects the static organization of a lymph node that is not responding to a foreign invader. As secondary lines of defense, lymph nodes constantly respond to stimuli, particularly infectious microbes, even in the absence of clinical disease. Within several days of antigenic stimulation, primary follicles enlarge and are transformed into pale-staining *germinal centers*, highly dynamic structures in which B cells acquire the capacity to make high-affinity antibodies against specific antigens. Normal germinal centers are surrounded by a dark-staining mantle zone, which contains mainly small naïve B cells. In some reactive conditions, a rim of B cells with slightly more cytoplasm accumulates outside of the mantle zone; cells occupying this region are called *marginal zone B cells*. The paracortical T-cell zones also frequently undergo hyperplasia in immune reactions in which cellular immunity is particularly important, such as viral infections.

The degree and pattern of morphologic change are dependent on the inciting stimulus and the intensity of the immune response. Trivial injuries and infections induce subtle changes in lymph node histology, while more significant infections inevitably produce enlargement of nodes and sometimes leave residual scarring. For this reason, lymph nodes in adults are almost never "normal" or "resting," and it is often necessary to distinguish morphologic changes secondary to past experience from those related to present disease.

Pathology

Disorders of white blood cells can be classified into two broad categories: *proliferative disorders*, in which there is an expansion of leukocytes, and *leukopenias*, which are defined as a deficiency of leukocytes. Proliferations of white cells can be *reactive* or *neoplastic*. Since the major function of leukocytes is host defense, reactive proliferation in response to an underlying primary, often microbial, disease is fairly common. Neoplastic disorders, although less frequent, are much more important clinically. In the following discussion, we shall first describe the leukopenic states and summarize the common reactive disorders and then consider in some detail malignant proliferations of white cells.

Leukopenia

The number of circulating white cells may be markedly decreased in a variety of disorders. An abnormally low white cell count *(leukopenia)* usually results from reduced numbers of neutrophils *(neutropenia, granulocytopenia)*. *Lymphopenia* is less common; in addition to congenital immunodeficiency diseases (see Chapter 6), it is most commonly observed in specific settings, such as advanced HIV infection, following therapy with glucocorticoids or cytotoxic drugs, autoimmune disorders, malnutrition, and certain acute viral infections. Only the more common leukopenias involving granulocytes will be discussed further here.

NEUTROPENIA, AGRANULOCYTOSIS

Reduction in the number of granulocytes in the peripheral blood *(neutropenia)* can be seen in a wide variety of circumstances. A marked reduction in neutrophil count, referred to as *agranulocytosis*, has serious consequences by making individuals susceptible to infections.

Pathogenesis. A reduction in circulating granulocytes will occur if there is (1) reduced or ineffective production of neutrophils or (2) accelerated removal of neutrophils from the circulating blood. *Inadequate or ineffective granulopoiesis* is observed in the setting of:

- Suppression of myeloid stem cells, as occurs in aplastic anemia (see Chapter 13) and a variety of infiltrative marrow disorders (tumors, granulomatous disease, etc.); in these conditions, granulocytopenia is accompanied by anemia and thrombocytopenia.
- Suppression of committed granulocytic precursors due to exposure to certain drugs, as discussed below.

- Disease states associated with ineffective granulopoiesis, such as megaloblastic anemias due to vitamin B_{12} or folate deficiency (see Chapter 13) and myelodysplastic syndromes, where defective precursors are susceptible to death in the marrow.
- Rare inherited conditions (such as Kostmann syndrome) in which genetic defects in specific genes result in impaired granulocytic differentiation.

Accelerated removal or destruction of neutrophils occurs with:

- Immunologically mediated injury to the neutrophils, which may be idiopathic, associated with a well-defined immunologic disorder (e.g., systemic lupus erythematosus), or produced by exposure to drugs.
- Splenic sequestration, in which excessive destruction occurs secondary to enlargement of the spleen, usually associated with increased destruction of red cells and platelets as well.
- Increased peripheral utilization, as may occur in overwhelming bacterial, fungal, or rickettsial infections.

Drugs are responsible for most of the significant neutropenias (agranulocytoses). Certain drugs, such as alkylating agents and antimetabolites used in cancer treatment, produce agranulocytosis in a predictable, dose-related fashion. Because such drugs cause a generalized suppression of the bone marrow, production of erythrocytes and platelets is also affected. Agranulocytosis can also occur as an idiosyncratic reaction to a large variety of agents. The roster of implicated drugs includes aminopyrine, chloramphenicol, sulfonamides, chlorpromazine, thiouracil, and phenylbutazone. The neutropenia induced by chlorpromazine and related phenothiazines may result from a toxic effect on granulocytic precursors in the bone marrow. In contrast, agranulocytosis following administration of aminopyrine, thiouracil, and certain sulfonamides likely stems from immunologically mediated destruction of mature neutrophils through mechanisms similar to those involved in drug-induced hemolytic anemias (see Chapter 13).

In some patients with acquired idiopathic neutropenia, autoantibodies directed against neutrophil-specific antigens are detected.[1] Severe neutropenia can also occur in association with monoclonal proliferations of large granular lymphocytes (so-called LGL leukemia).[2] The mechanism of this neutropenia is not clear; suppression of marrow granulocytic progenitors is considered most likely.

Morphology. The anatomic alterations in the bone marrow vary according to the underlying cause. When neutropenia is caused by excessive destruction of mature neutrophils, the marrow is usually hypercellular owing to the presence of increased numbers of granulocytic precursors. Hypercellularity is also the rule in neutropenias associated with ineffective granulopoiesis, as occurs in megaloblastic anemias and myelodysplastic syndromes. Agranulocytosis caused by agents that suppress or destroy granulocytic precursors is understandably associated with marrow hypocellularity.

Infections (most often bacterial or fungal) are a common consequence of agranulocytosis. Ulcerating necrotizing lesions of the gingiva, floor of the mouth, buccal mucosa, pharynx, or anywhere within the oral cavity (agranulocytic angina) are quite characteristic. These ulcers are typically deep, undermined, and covered by gray to green-black necrotic membranes from which numerous bacteria or fungi can be isolated. Less frequently, similar ulcerative lesions occur in the skin, vagina, anus, or gastrointestinal tract. Severe life-threatening invasive bacterial or fungal infections can occur in the lungs, urinary tract, and kidneys. The neutropenic patient is at particularly high risk for deep fungal infections caused by organisms such as *Candida* and *Aspergillus*. Sites of infection often show a massive growth of organisms with little leukocytic response. In the most dramatic instances, bacteria grow in colonies (botryomycosis) resembling those seen on nutrient media. The regional lymph nodes draining these infections are enlarged and inflamed.

Clinical Course. The symptoms and signs of neutropenias are related to bacterial or fungal infections. They include malaise, chills, and fever, followed in sequence by marked weakness and fatigability. In severe agranulocytosis with virtual absence of neutrophils, these infections can be overwhelming and cause death within a few days.

A neutrophil count of less than 1000 cells per mm^3 of blood is worrisome, but most serious infections occur with counts below 500 per mm^3. Because infections are often fulminant, broad-spectrum antibiotics are given expeditiously whenever signs or symptoms appear. In some instances, such as following myelosuppressive chemotherapy, neutropenia is treated with granulocyte colony-stimulating factor (G-CSF), a growth factor that stimulates the production of granulocytes from marrow precursors.

Reactive (Inflammatory) Proliferations of White Cells and Lymph Nodes

LEUKOCYTOSIS

Leukocytosis refers to an increase in the number of blood leukocytes. It is a common reaction to a variety of inflammatory states and is sometimes the first indication of neoplastic growth of leukocytes.

Pathogenesis. The peripheral blood leukocyte count is influenced by several factors, including:

- The size of the myeloid (for granulocytes and monocytes) and lymphoid (for lymphocytes) precursor and storage cell pools in the bone marrow, circulation, and peripheral tissues
- The rate of release of cells from the storage pool into the circulation
- The proportion of cells that are adherent to blood vessel walls at any time (the marginating pool)
- The rate of extravasation of cells from the blood into tissues

As was discussed in Chapters 2 and 13, leukocyte homeostasis is maintained by cytokines, growth factors, and adhesion molecules through their effects on the commitment, proliferation, differentiation, and extravasation of leukocytes and their progenitors. The mechanisms of leukocytosis vary

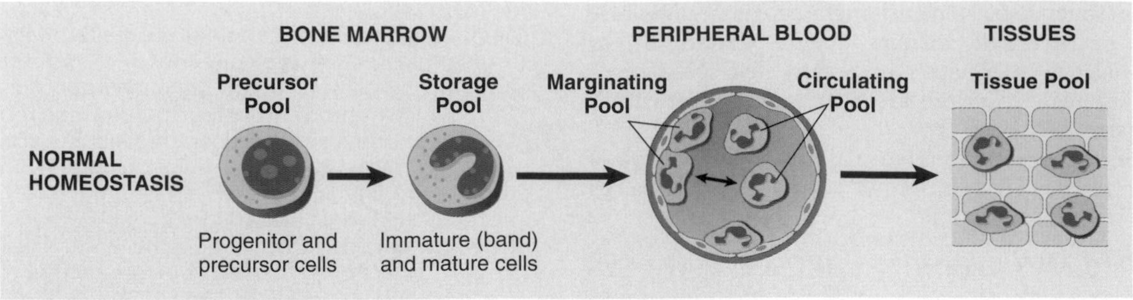

CAUSES OF LEUKOCYTOSIS	MECHANISMS
Endotoxemia Acute infection Hypoxia	Increased release from marrow stores
Exercise Epinephrine	Decreased margination
Glucocorticoids	Decreased extravasation into tissues
Chronic infection or inflammation Tumors Myeloproliferative disorders	Increased numbers of marrow precursors

FIGURE 14–1 Mechanisms of neutrophilic leukocytosis. Neutrophils and their precursors are distributed in five pools: a bone marrow precursor pool; a bone marrow storage pool, consisting of mature and slightly immature neutrophils (band forms); a peripheral blood marginating pool; a peripheral blood circulating pool; and a tissue pool. Sampling of the peripheral blood assesses only the circulating pool, which can be enlarged by increased release of neutrophils and band forms from the marrow storage pool, decreased margination, diminished extravasation into tissues, or expansion of the marrow precursor cell pool. Diverse stimuli that increase the circulating pool through various mechanisms are listed. It should be noted that certain stimuli (e.g., acute infection) cause changes in flux between multiple pools simultaneously.

depending on the affected leukocyte pool and the particular factor. In acute infection, there is a rapid increase in the egress of mature granulocytes from the bone marrow pool, which is roughly 50 times the size of the peripheral blood marginal pool. The release of IL-1, TNF, and other inflammatory cytokines stimulates bone marrow stromal cells and T cells to produce increased amounts of colony-stimulating factors (CSFs), which enhance the proliferation and differentiation of committed granulocytic progenitors and, over several days, cause a sustained increase in neutrophil production. Figure 14–1 summarizes the major mechanisms of neutrophilic leukocytosis and their causes.

Other growth factors preferentially stimulate other types of leukocytosis. For example, IL-5 causes eosinophilia by enhancing the growth, survival, and differentiation of eosinophils, while IL-7 plays a central role in lymphopoiesis. Such factors are differentially produced in response to various pathogenic stimuli, and as a result, the five principal types of leukocytosis (neutrophilic, eosinophilic, and basophilic leukocytosis, monocytosis, and lymphocytosis) each tend to be observed in particular clinical settings (summarized in Table 14–1).

In sepsis or severe inflammatory disorders (such as Kawasaki disease), leukocytosis is often accompanied by mor-

TABLE 14–1 Causes of Leukocytosis

Neutrophilic leukocytosis	Acute bacterial infections, especially those caused by pyogenic organisms; sterile inflammation caused by, for example, tissue necrosis (myocardial infarction, burns)
Eosinophilic leukocytosis (eosinophilia)	Allergic disorders such as asthma, hay fever, allergic skin diseases (e.g., pemphigus, dermatitis herpetiformis); parasitic infestations; drug reactions; certain malignancies (e.g., Hodgkin disease and some non-Hodgkin lymphomas); collagen vascular disorders and some vasculitides; atheroembolic disease (transient)
Basophilic leukocytosis (basophilia)	Rare, often indicative of a myeloproliferative disease (e.g., chronic myelogenous leukemia)
Monocytosis	Chronic infections (e.g., tuberculosis), bacterial endocarditis, rickettsiosis and malaria; collagen vascular diseases (e.g., systemic lupus erythematosus) and inflammatory bowel diseases (e.g., ulcerative colitis)
Lymphocytosis	Accompanies monocytosis in many disorders associated with chronic immunologic stimulation (e.g., tuberculosis, brucellosis); viral infections (e.g., hepatitis A, cytomegalovirus, Epstein-Barr virus); *Bordetella pertussis* infection

phologic changes in the neutrophils, such as toxic granulations, Döhle bodies, and cytoplasmic vacuoles (Fig. 14–2). *Toxic granules* are coarse and darker than the normal neutrophilic granules and are believed to represent abnormal azurophilic (primary) granules. *Döhle bodies* are patches of dilated endoplasmic reticulum that appear as sky-blue cytoplasmic "puddles" in smears stained with Wright-Giemsa stain.

In most instances, it is not difficult to distinguish reactive leukocytosis from leukocytosis caused by flooding of the peripheral blood by neoplastic white blood cells (leukemia), but uncertainties may arise in two settings. Particularly in children, acute viral infections can produce the appearance of activated lymphocytes in the peripheral blood and marrow that resemble neoplastic lymphoid cells. At other times, particularly in inflammatory states and severe chronic infections, many immature granulocytes appear in the blood, simulating a picture of myelogenous leukemia *(leukemoid reaction)*. Special laboratory studies (discussed later) are helpful in distinguishing reactive and neoplastic leukocytoses.

In addition to causing leukocytosis, infections and inflammatory stimuli often elicit immune reactions within lymph nodes. The infections that lead to lymphadenitis are numerous. Some that produce distinctive morphologic patterns are described in other chapters. Most, however, cause stereotypic patterns of lymph node reaction designated acute and chronic nonspecific lymphadenitis.

ACUTE NONSPECIFIC LYMPHADENITIS

Lymph nodes undergo reactive changes whenever they are challenged by microbiologic agents, cell debris, or foreign matter introduced into wounds or into the circulation. Acute lymphadenitis is most often seen in the cervical region due to microbial drainage from infections of the teeth or tonsils and in the axillary or inguinal regions secondary to infections in the extremities. Similarly, acute lymphadenitis often occurs in mesenteric lymph nodes draining acute appendicitis. Unfortunately, other self-limited infections can also cause mesenteric adenitis and induce abdominal symptoms mimicking acute appendicitis, a differential diagnosis that plagues the surgeon. Systemic viral infections (particularly in children) and bacteremia often produce generalized lymphadenopathy.

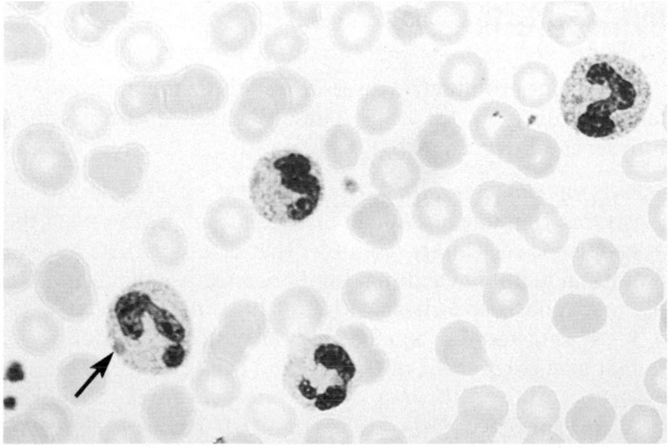

FIGURE 14–2 Reactive changes in neutrophils. Neutrophils containing coarse purple cytoplasmic granules (toxic granulations) and blue cytoplasmic patches of dilated endoplasmic reticulum (Döhle bodies, *arrow*) are observed in this peripheral blood smear taken from a patient with bacterial sepsis.

Morphology. Macroscopically, the nodes become swollen, gray-red, and engorged. Histologically, there is prominence of the lymphoid follicles, with large germinal centers containing numerous mitotic figures. Macrophages often contain particulate debris of bacterial origin or derived from necrotic cells. When pyogenic organisms are the cause of the reaction, the centers of the follicles may undergo necrosis; indeed, the entire node can sometimes be converted into a suppurative mass. With less severe reactions, there is sometimes a neutrophilic infiltrate about the follicles, and numerous neutrophils can be found within the lymphoid sinuses. The cells lining the sinuses become hypertrophied and cuboidal and often undergo hyperplasia.

Clinically, nodes with acute lymphadenitis are enlarged because of the cellular infiltration and edema. As a consequence of the distention of the capsule, they are tender to touch. When abscess formation is extensive, they become fluctuant. The overlying skin is frequently red, and sometimes penetration of the infection to the skin surface produces draining sinuses, particularly when the nodes have undergone suppurative necrosis. As might be expected, healing of such lesions is associated with scarring.

CHRONIC NONSPECIFIC LYMPHADENITIS

Chronic immunologic reactions can produce several different morphologic alterations, depending on the underlying stimulus.

Morphology

Follicular Hyperplasia. This is caused by stimuli that activate humoral immune responses. It is distinguished by the appearance of large, round or oblong B cell–rich germinal centers (secondary follicles) surrounded by a collar of small, resting naïve B lymphocytes (the mantle zone) (Fig. 14–3). Within germinal centers, two distinct regions are discernible: (1) a dark zone containing proliferating blast-like B cells (centroblasts) and (2) a light zone composed of B cells with irregular or cleaved nuclear contours (centrocytes). Also present throughout the follicle are phagocytic macrophages containing nuclear debris (tingible-body macrophages) and an inconspicuous network of follicular dendritic cells that function in antigen presentation. Plasma cells, macrophages, and occasionally neutrophils or eosinophils may be found in the parafollicular regions, and there is often striking hyperplasia of the mononuclear phagocytic cells lining the lymphatic sinuses. Some specific causes of follicular hyperplasia include rheumatoid arthritis, toxoplasmosis, and early stages of human immunodeficiency virus (HIV) infection. This form of lymphadenitis may be confused morphologically with

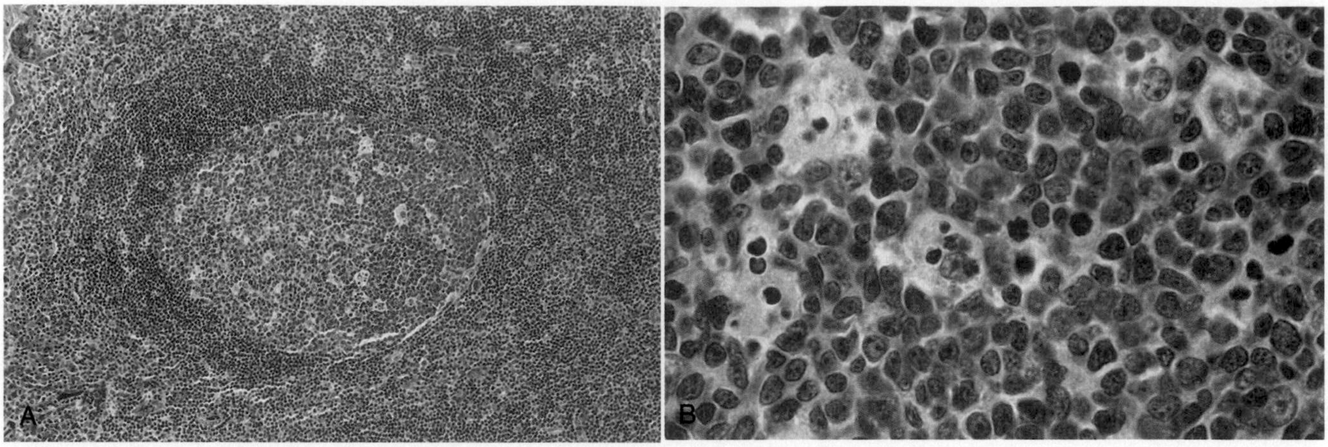

FIGURE 14–3 Follicular hyperplasia. *A,* Low-power view showing a reactive follicle and surrounding mantle zone. The dark-staining mantle zone is polarized, being much more prominent adjacent to the germinal center light zone in the left half of the follicle. The right half of the follicle consists of the dark zone. *B,* High-power view of the dark zone shows several mitotic figures and numerous macrophages containing phagocytosed apoptotic cells (tingible bodies).

follicular lymphomas (see later discussion of lymphoid neoplasms). It is beyond our scope to go into all the subtle morphologic features in this differential diagnosis, but several features favor reactive follicular hyperplasia: (1) preservation of the lymph node architecture, including interfollicular T-cell zones and the sinusoids, (2) marked variation in the shape and size of lymphoid nodules, and (3) the presence of frequent mitotic figures, phagocytic macrophages, and recognizable light and dark zones, all of which tend to be absent from neoplastic follicles.

Follicular hyperplasia is sometimes accompanied by **marginal zone B-cell hyperplasia.** In some immune reactions, particularly those caused by toxoplasmosis and early HIV infection, marginal zone B cells accumulate in a rim external to the mantle zone of germinal centers. These cells have moderately abundant pale cytoplasm and folded or reniform nuclei resembling those of monocytes, leading to the descriptive term **monocytoid B cells.** They appear to be memory B cells derived from antigen-stimulated germinal center B cells.

Paracortical Lymphoid Hyperplasia. This is caused by stimuli that trigger cellular immune responses. It is characterized by reactive changes within the T-cell regions of the lymph node that encroach on, and sometimes appear to efface, the B-cell follicles. Within interfollicular regions, activated T cells (immunoblasts) are observed. These cells are three to four times the size of resting lymphocytes and have round nuclei, open chromatin, several prominent nucleoli, and moderate amounts of pale cytoplasm. In addition, there is hypertrophy of sinusoidal and vascular endothelial cells and a mixed cellular infiltrate, principally of macrophages and sometimes of eosinophils. Such changes are encountered in immunologic reactions induced by drugs (especially Dilantin), in acute viral infections, particularly infectious mononucleosis, and following vaccination against certain viral diseases. In florid reactions, immunoblasts may be so numerous that special studies are needed to exclude a lymphoid neoplasm.

Sinus Histiocytosis (also called Reticular Hyperplasia). This refers to distention and prominence of the lymphatic sinusoids. Although nonspecific, this form of hyperplasia may be particularly prominent in lymph nodes draining cancers, such as carcinoma of the breast. The lining lymphatic endothelial cells are markedly hypertrophied, and macrophages are greatly increased in numbers, resulting in expansion and distension of sinuses. In the setting of cancer, this pattern of reaction has been thought to represent host immune response against the tumor or its products.

Characteristically, lymph nodes in chronic reactions are not tender, because their capsules are not under increased tension. Chronic lymphadenitis is particularly common in inguinal and axillary nodes, which drain relatively large areas of the body and are frequently challenged.

Neoplastic Proliferations of White Cells

Malignant proliferative diseases constitute the most important disorders of white cells. These diseases can be classified into several categories:

- *Lymphoid neoplasms* encompass a diverse group of entities. In many but not all instances, the phenotype of the neoplastic cell closely resembles that of a particular stage of normal lymphocyte differentiation, a feature that is used in the diagnosis and classification of these disorders.
- *Myeloid neoplasms* arise from hematopoietic stem cells that give rise to cells of the myeloid (i.e., erythroid, granulocytic, and/or thrombocytic) lineage. Three categories of myeloid neoplasia are recognized: *acute myelogenous leukemias,* in which immature progenitor cells accumulate in the bone marrow; *myelodysplastic syndromes,* which are associated with ineffective hematopoiesis and resultant peripheral blood cytopenias; and *chronic myeloproliferative disorders,* in which increased production of one or more ter-

minally differentiated myeloid elements (e.g., granulocytes) usually leads to elevated peripheral blood counts.

- The *histiocytoses* are uncommon proliferative lesions of macrophages and dendritic cells. Although "histiocyte" (literally, "tissue cell") is an archaic morphologic term, it is still often applied to cells of macrophage or dendritic-cell lineage. Rarely, "histiocytic" tumors present as masses resembling malignant lymphomas. A special category of immature dendritic cells referred to as Langerhans cells gives rise to a spectrum of neoplastic disorders, some of which behave as disseminated malignant tumors, and others as localized benign proliferations. This group is called Langerhans cell histiocytoses.

ETIOLOGICAL AND PATHOGENETIC FACTORS IN WHITE CELL NEOPLASIA: OVERVIEW

As we will see in the following sections, the neoplastic disorders of white cells are extremely varied. Before we delve into this complexity, it is worth considering a few themes of general relevance to their etiology and pathogenesis.

Chromosomal translocations and oncogenes. Nonrandom chromosomal abnormalities, most commonly translocations, are present in the majority of white cell neoplasms. As was discussed briefly in Chapter 7, many specific rearrangements are associated with particular neoplasms, suggesting a critical role in their genesis.

- In the case of lymphoid neoplasms, many of the oncogenic rearrangements stem from mistakes during the events that occur during antigen receptor gene expression. The normal immunoglobulin (Ig) and T-cell receptor gene diversity in B and T lymphocytes is produced by mechanisms relying on DNA breakage and rejoining. B- and T-cell progenitors express a V(D)J recombinase activity that cuts DNA at specific sequences within the immunoglobulin and T-cell receptor loci, and many pathogenic rearrangements seen in lymphoid neoplasms are caused by the inappropriate joining of these sites to sequences flanking proto-oncogenes. Mature, antigen-stimulated B cells undergo differentiation in the germinal centers of lymph nodes. There, immunoglobulin genes are further modified by class switching and somatic hypermutation, which are regulated forms of genomic instability. Like V(D)J recombination, class switching proceeds through a mechanism involving double-stranded DNA breaks, and mistakes during this process may account for some oncogenic rearrangements that are seen in certain B-cell malignancies. Although the mechanism is still unsettled, it appears that "misdirected" somatic hypermutation also causes mutations in oncogenes that are implicated in B-cell transformation.[3] The inherent genomic instability of germinal center B cells might explain why they are much more likely to give rise to lymphomas than are mature T cells,[4] which have fixed, stable T-cell receptor genes.
- Chromosomal translocations frequently occur in myeloid neoplasms, but the mechanisms underlying DNA breakage in these tumors are unknown.

Inherited genetic factors. As was discussed in Chapter 7, individuals with genetic diseases that promote genomic instability, such as Bloom syndrome, Fanconi anemia, and ataxia telangiectasia, are at increased risk for development of acute leukemia. In addition, both Down syndrome (trisomy 21) and neurofibromatosis type I are associated with an increased incidence of childhood leukemia.

Viruses. Three viruses—human T-cell leukemia virus-1 (HTLV-1), Epstein-Barr virus (EBV), and Kaposi sarcoma herpesvirus/human herpesvirus-8 (KSHV/HHV-8)—have been implicated as causative agents. The possible mechanisms of transformation by viral agents were discussed in Chapter 7. HTLV-1 has been associated only with adult T-cell leukemia/lymphoma. In contrast, clonal episomal EBV genomes are found in the tumor cells of a subset of Burkitt lymphoma, 30% to 40% of cases of Hodgkin lymphoma, many B-cell lymphomas occurring in the setting of T-cell immunodeficiency, and rare natural killer cell lymphomas. KSHV is uniquely associated with an unusual type of B-cell lymphoma that presents as a malignant effusion, often in the pleural cavity.[5]

Environmental agents. Several environmental agents that cause chronic inflammation predispose to lymphoid neoplasia. The most clear-cut associations are those of *Helicobacter pylori* infection with gastric B-cell lymphoma[6] (Chapter 17) and gluten-sensitive enteropathy with intestinal T-cell lymphoma.[7] In other instances, sustained B-cell stimulation due to immune dysregulation may increase the risk of oncogenic events. An important example is HIV infection, which leads to polyclonal B-cell activation and marked hyperplasia of germinal center B cells. HIV-infected individuals are at high risk for B-cell lymphomas derived from germinal center B cells, and most such tumors have oncogenic chromosomal translocations involving immunoglobulin loci. Diminished T cell–dependent immune surveillance may also contribute to this risk, particularly for B-cell lymphomas associated with EBV infection.

Iatrogenic factors. Ironically, radiotherapy and certain forms of chemotherapy used to treat cancer increase the risk of subsequent myeloid and lymphoid neoplasms. This association is believed to stem from mutagenic effects of ionizing radiation and chemotherapeutic drugs on hematolymphoid progenitor cells.

LYMPHOID NEOPLASMS

Definitions and Classifications

One of the confusing aspects of the lymphoid neoplasms concerns the use of the descriptive terms "lymphocytic leukemia" and "lymphoma." *Leukemia* is used for lymphoid neoplasms presenting with widespread involvement of the bone marrow, usually accompanied by the presence of large numbers of tumor cells in the peripheral blood. *Lymphoma*, on the other hand, is used to describe proliferations arising as discrete tissue masses. Traditionally, these terms were attached to what were felt to be distinct entities. However, the line between the "lymphocytic leukemias" and the "lymphomas" often blurs. Many types of "lymphoma" occasionally present with a leukemic peripheral blood picture accompanied by extensive marrow involvement, and evolution to "leukemia" is not unusual during progression of incurable "lymphomas." Conversely, tumors identical to "leukemias" sometimes arise as soft tissue masses without evidence of bone marrow disease. Hence, when applied to particular neoplasms, the terms "leukemia" and "lymphoma" merely describe the usual tissue distribution of the disease at the time of clinical presentation.

Within the broad group of lymphomas, *Hodgkin lymphoma* is segregated from all other forms, which constitute the *non-Hodgkin lymphomas (NHL).* As will be seen, Hodgkin lymphoma is clinically and histologically distinct from the NHLs. In addition, it is treated in a unique fashion, making the differentiation of Hodgkin lymphoma and NHL clinically important.

The other important category of lymphoid neoplasms encompasses the *plasma-cell neoplasms*, tumors composed of terminally differentiated B cells. Such tumors most commonly arise in the bone marrow, only rarely involving lymph nodes or producing a leukemic peripheral blood picture. In addition, as will be seen, much of their pathophysiology is related to the secretion of whole antibodies or immunoglobulin fragments by the tumor cells.

The clinical presentation of the various lymphoid neoplasms is dictated by the anatomic distribution of disease. Two-thirds of NHLs and virtually all cases of Hodgkin lymphoma present with nontender nodal enlargement (often greater than 2 cm) that can be localized or generalized. The remaining one-third of NHLs arise at extranodal sites (e.g., skin, stomach, or brain). In contrast, the leukemic forms (lymphocytic leukemia) most commonly come to clinical attention owing to signs and symptoms related to suppression of normal hematopoiesis by tumor cells in the bone marrow. Lymphocytic leukemias also characteristically infiltrate and enlarge the spleen and liver. Finally, plasma cell neoplasms involving the skeleton cause local bony destruction and hence often present with pain due to pathologic fractures.

Historically, few areas of pathology have evoked as much controversy and confusion as the classification of NHL and related lymphoid neoplasms. In some older classification schemes, more than two dozen types of B-cell lymphomas were listed—a nomenclature system that was a mind-numbing challenge for students and pathologists! This chaotic situation has improved greatly during the last decade. In 1994, a group of hematopathologists, oncologists, and molecular biologists came together to create the *Revised European-American Classification of Lymphoid Neoplasms* (REAL).[8] Of importance, this classification scheme incorporated objective criteria, such as immunophenotype and genetic aberrations, together with morphologic and clinical features, to define distinct clinicopathologic entities. Experience has shown that most entities in the REAL classification can be diagnosed reproducibly by experienced pathologists and stratify patients into good and bad prognosis groups.[9, 10] More recently, an international group of hematopathologists and oncologists convened by the World Health Organization (WHO) reviewed and updated the REAL classification, resulting in the inclusion of a number of additional rare entities.[11] Presented here is the WHO classification (Table 14–2), which sorts the lymphoid neoplasms into five broad categories, based on their cell of origin:

1. Precursor B-cell neoplasms (neoplasms of immature B cells)
2. Peripheral B-cell neoplasms (neoplasms of mature B cells)
3. Precursor T-cell neoplasms (neoplasms of immature T cells)
4. Peripheral T-cell and NK-cell neoplasms (neoplasms of mature T cells and natural killer cells)
5. Hodgkin lymphoma (neoplasms of Reed-Sternberg cells and variants).

Before we discuss the specific entities described in the WHO classification, some important principles relevant to the lymphoid neoplasms need to be emphasized.

- Lymphoid neoplasia can be suspected from the clinical features, but *histologic examination of lymph nodes or other involved tissues is required for diagnosis.*
- As will be recalled from Chapter 6, antigen receptor genes rearrange during normal B- and T-cell differentiation through a mechanism that ensures that each developing lymphocyte makes a single, unique antigen receptor. *In most lymphoid neoplasms, antigen receptor gene rearrangement*

TABLE 14–2 The WHO Classification of the Lymphoid Neoplasms

I. Precursor B-Cell Neoplasms	***IV. Peripheral T-Cell and NK-Cell Neoplasms***
Precursor-B lymphoblastic leukemia/lymphoma	T-cell prolymphocytic leukemia
	Large granular lymphocytic leukemia
II. Peripheral B-Cell Neoplasms	Mycosis fungoides/Sézary syndrome
Chronic lymphocytic leukemia/small lymphocytic lymphoma	Peripheral T-cell lymphoma, unspecified
B-cell prolymphocytic leukemia	Anaplastic large cell lymphoma
Lymphoplasmacytic lymphoma	Angioimmunoblastic T-cell lymphoma
Splenic and nodal marginal zone lymphomas	Enteropathy-associated T-cell lymphoma
Extranodal marginal zone lymphoma	Panniculitis-like T-cell lymphoma
Mantle cell lymphoma	Hepatosplenic $\gamma\delta$ T-cell lymphoma
Follicular lymphoma	Adult T-cell leukemia/lymphoma
Marginal zone lymphoma	NK/T-cell lymphoma, nasal type
Hairy cell leukemia	NK-cell leukemia
Plasmacytoma/plasma cell myeloma	***V. Hodgkin Lymphoma***
Diffuse large B-cell lymphoma	Classical subtypes
Burkitt lymphoma	Nodular sclerosis
	Mixed cellularity
III. Precursor T-Cell Neoplasms	Lymphocyte-rich
	Lymphocyte depletion
Precursor-T lymphoblastic leukemia/lymphoma	Lymphocyte predominance

precedes transformation; hence, the daughter cells derived from the malignant progenitor share the same antigen receptor gene configuration and sequence and synthesize identical antigen receptor proteins (either immunoglobulins or T-cell receptors). In contrast, normal immune responses are polyclonal and thus comprise populations of lymphocytes expressing many different antigen receptors. As a result, analyses of antigen receptor genes and/or their protein products can be used to distinguish reactive and malignant lymphoid proliferations. In addition, each antigen receptor gene rearrangement produces a unique DNA sequence that constitutes a highly specific clonal marker that can be used to detect small numbers of residual malignant cells after therapy.[12]

- *The vast majority of lymphoid neoplasms (80% to 85%) are of B-cell origin, most of the remainder being T-cell tumors; only rarely are tumors of NK origin encountered.* Most lymphoid neoplasms resemble some recognizable stage of B- or T-cell differentiation (Fig. 14–4), a feature that is used in their classification. Markers recognized by antibodies that are helpful in the characterization of lymphomas and leukemias are listed in Table 14–3.
- *As tumors of the immune system, lymphoid neoplasms often disrupt normal architecture and function of the immune system, leading to immune abnormalities.* Both a loss of vigilance (as evidenced by susceptibility to infection) and breakdown of tolerance (manifested by autoimmunity) can be seen, sometimes in the same patient. In a further, ironic twist, patients with inherited or acquired immunodeficiency are themselves at high risk of developing certain lymphoid neoplasms, particularly those caused by oncogenic viruses (e.g., EBV).
- *Neoplastic B and T cells tend to recapitulate the behavior of their normal counterparts.* Like normal lymphocytes, transformed B and T cells tend to home to particular tissue sites, leading to characteristic patterns of involvement. For example, follicular lymphomas proliferate in the B-cell areas of the lymph node, producing a nodular or follicular pattern of growth, whereas T-cell lymphomas typically grow in paracortical T-cell zones. As is true of their normal

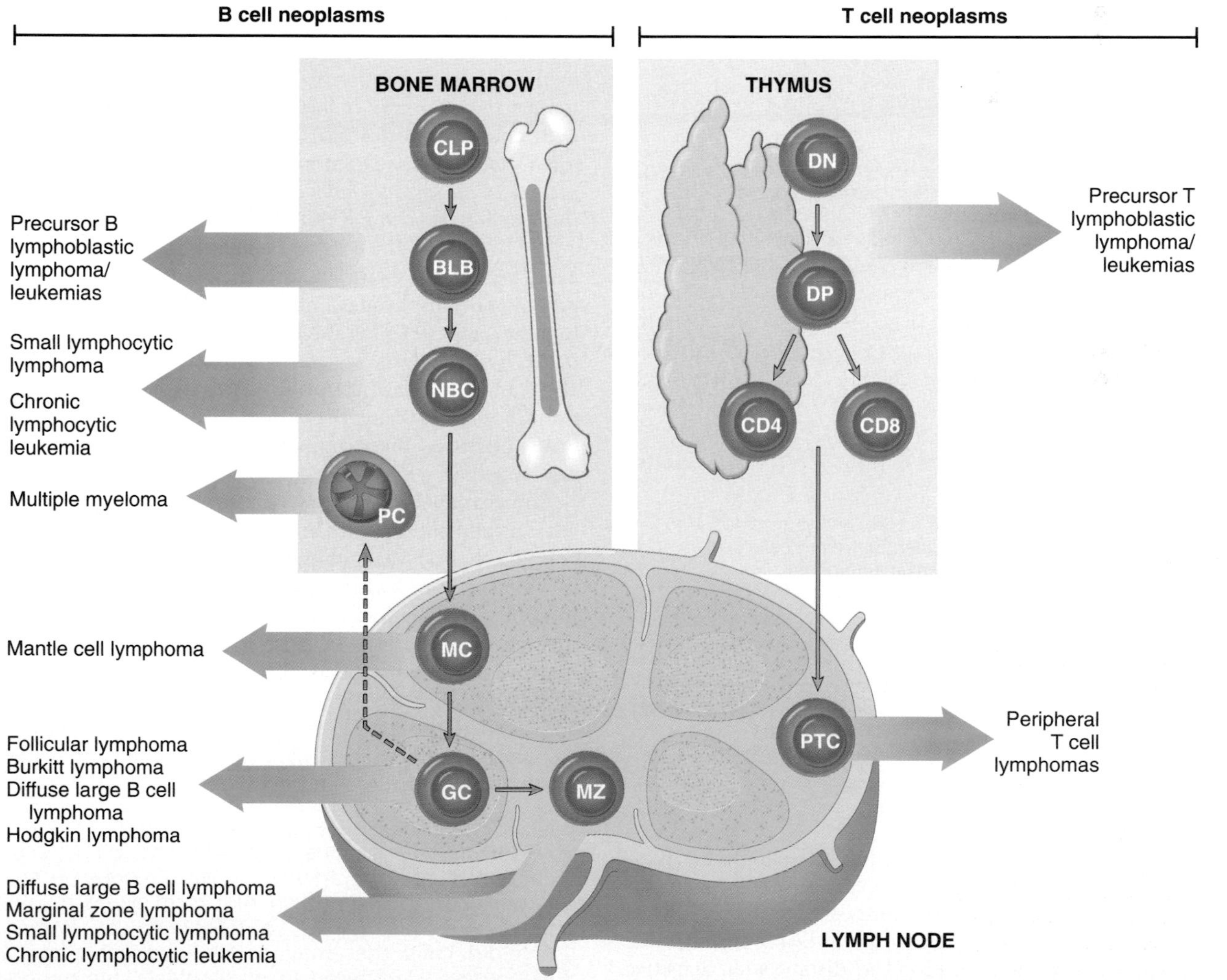

FIGURE 14–4 Origin of lymphoid neoplasms. Stages of B- and T-cell differentiation from which specific lymphoid tumors emerge are shown. Key: CLP, common lymphoid precursor; BLB, pre-B lymphoblast; NBC, naive B cell; MC, mantle B cell; GC, germinal center B cell; MZ, marginal zone B cell; DN, CD4/CD8 double negative pre-T cell; DP, CD4/CD8 double positive pre-T cell; PTC, peripheral T cell.

TABLE 14–3 Some Immune Cell Antigens Detected by Monoclonal Antibodies

Antigen Designation	Normal Cellular Distribution
Primarily T-Cell Associated	
CD1	Cortical thymocytes and Langerhans histiocytes
CD3	Thymocytes, peripheral T cells
CD4	Helper subset of peripheral T cells, single positive medullary thymocytes, and CD4/CD8 double positive thymocytes
CD5	T cells and a small subset of B cells
CD8	Cytotoxic subset of peripheral T cells, single positive medullary thymocytes, double positive cortical thymocytes, and some NK cells
Primarily B-Cell Associated	
CD10	Marrow pre-B cells and germinal center B cells; also called CALLA
CD19	Marrow pre-B cells and mature B cells but not plasma cells
CD20	Marrow pre-B cells after CD19 and mature B cells but not plasma cells
CD21	EBV receptor; present on mature B cells and follicular dendritic cells
CD23	Activated mature B cells
CD79a	Marrow pre-B cells and mature B cells.
Primarily Monocyte or Macrophage Associated	
CD11c	Granulocytes, monocytes, and macrophages; also expressed by hairy cell leukemias
CD13	Immature and mature monocytes and granulocytes
CD14	Monocytes
CD15	Granulocytes; also expressed by Reed-Sternberg cells and variants in classical Hodgkin lymphoma
CD33	Myeloid progenitors and monocytes
CD64	Mature myeloid cells
Primarily NK-Cell Associated	
CD16	NK cells and granulocytes
CD56	NK cells and a subset of T cells
Primarily Stem Cell and Progenitor Cell Associated	
CD34	Pluripotent hematopoietic stem cells and progenitor cells of many lineages
Activation Markers	
CD30	Activated B cells, T cells, and monocytes; also expressed by Reed-Sternberg cells and variants in classical Hodgkin lymphoma
Present on All Leukocytes	
CD45	All leukocytes; also known as leukocyte common antigen (LCA)

CD, cluster designation; NK, natural killer; CALLA, common acute lymphoblastic leukemia antigen; EBV, Epstein-Barr virus.

counterparts, lymph node homing of neoplastic lymphocytes is likely regulated by expression of particular chemokine receptors. Variable numbers of neoplastic B and T lymphoid cells also recirculate periodically through the lymphatics and peripheral blood to distant sites. Sensitive molecular techniques have shown that most lymphoid tumors are widely disseminated at the time of diagnosis. The most notable exception to this rule is Hodgkin lymphoma, which is sometimes restricted to one group of lymph nodes.

- *Hodgkin lymphoma spreads in an orderly fashion, and as a result staging is of importance in determining therapy.* In contrast, the spread of NHL is less predictable, and as was noted above, most patients are assumed to have systemic disease at the time of diagnosis. Hence, staging in particular NHLs provides useful prognostic information but is generally not as important in guiding therapy as is the case in Hodgkin lymphoma.

We now turn to the specific entities of the WHO classification. In the discussion that follows, only the most salient immunophenotypic and karyotypic features are included; this information is summarized in Table 14–4. We will begin with neoplasms of immature lymphoid cells and then move on to tumors of mature B cells, T cells, and NK cells. Within each immunophenotypic category, the most common (and thus most important) entities will be emphasized.

Precursor B- and T-Cell Neoplasms

Acute Lymphoblastic Leukemia/Lymphoma

Acute lymphoblastic leukemia/lymphoma (ALL) encompasses a group of neoplasms composed of immature, precursor B (pre-B) or T (pre-T) lymphocytes referred to as *lymphoblasts. The majority (~85%) of ALLs are precursor B-cell tumors that typically manifest as childhood acute "leukemias"* with extensive bone marrow and variable peripheral blood involvement. The less common *precursor T-cell ALLs tend to present in adolescent males as "lymphomas," often with thymic involvement.* It is worth noting, however, that there is considerable overlap in the clinical behavior of precursor B-cell and T-cell ALL; for example, pre-B cell tumors uncommonly present as "lymphomas," and many pre-T cell tumors evolve to a leukemic peripheral blood picture. Malignant pre-B and pre-T lymphoblasts are also morphologically indistinguishable, and subclassification of ALL is thus dependent on immunophenotyping. Because of their morphologic and clinical similarities, the various forms of ALL will be considered here together.

Approximately 2500 new cases of ALL are diagnosed each year in the United States, most cases occurring in individuals younger than 15 years of age. ALL is almost twice as common in whites as in nonwhites and is slightly more frequent in boys than in girls. The incidence of pre-B ALL is highest at about the age of 4, perhaps because the number of normal bone marrow pre-B lymphoblasts (the cell of origin) peaks in early childhood. Similarly, the peak incidence of pre-T ALL is in adolescence, the age when the thymus reaches its maximal size. Both pre-B and pre-T ALL occur in adults of all ages, but much less frequently than in children.

Morphology. Because of different responses to chemotherapeutic agents, it is of great practical importance to distinguish ALL from acute myelogenous leukemia (AML), a neoplasm of immature myeloid cells that may cause identical signs and symptoms. Compared to myeloblasts, lymphoblasts have condensed chromatin, inconspicuous nucleoli, and scant agranular cytoplasm (Fig. 14–5*A*). However,

TABLE 14–4 Summary of Major Types of Lymphoid Neoplasms

Diagnosis	Cell of Origin	Genotype	Salient Clinical Features
Neoplasms of immature B and T cells			
Precursor B-cell acute lymphoblastic leukemia/lymphoma	Bone marrow precursor B-cell expressing TdT and lacking surface Ig	Diverse chromosomal translocations; t(12;21) involving *CBFα* and *ETV6* most common rearrangement	Predominantly children with symptoms relating to pancytopenia secondary to marrow involvement; aggressive
Precursor T-cell acute lymphoblastic leukemia/lymphoma	Precursor T-cell (often of thymic origin) expressing TdT	Diverse chromosomal translocations, many involving T-cell receptor loci; rearrangements of *TAL1* most common	Predominantly adolescent males with thymic masses; variable splenic, hepatic, and bone marrow involvement; aggressive
Neoplasms of mature B cells			
Burkitt lymphoma	Germinal center B-cell; CD10 expression usually seen	Translocations involving c-myc and Ig loci; usually t(8;14), but also t(2;8) or t(8;22). African (endemic) cases latently infected with EBV	Adolescents or young adults with jaw or extranodal abdominal masses; uncommonly presents as a "leukemia"; aggressive
Diffuse large B-cell lymphoma	Germinal center or postgerminal center B-cell	Diverse chromosomal aberrations; ~30% have rearrangements of *BCL6*; ~10% contain the t(14;18); c*REL* amplification in a subset	All ages, but most common in adults; often appears as a single rapidly growing mass; 30% extranodal; aggressive
Extranodal marginal zone lymphoma	Postgerminal center memory B-cell	Trisomy 18, t(11;18), t(1;14); latter create *MALT1-IAP2* and *BCL10-IgH* fusion genes, respectively	Arises at extranodal sites in adults with chronic inflammatory diseases; may remain localized; indolent
Follicular lymphoma	Germinal center B-cell; typically expresses CD10, BCL2, and BCL6	t(14;18) involving the *BCL2* gene	Older adults with generalized lymphadenopathy and marrow involvement; indolent
Hairy cell leukemia	Postgerminal center memory B-cell	No specific chromosomal abnormality	Older males with pancytopenia and splenomegaly; indolent
Mantle cell lymphoma	Naïve B-cell; expresses cyclin D1 and (usually) CD5	t(11;14) involving *BCL1* (cyclin D1) and *IgH*	Older males with disseminated disease; moderately aggressive
Multiple myeloma/ solitary plasmacytoma	Plasma cell derived from a postgerminal center B-cell	Diverse rearrangements involving *IgH*	Myeloma: older adults with lytic bone lesions, pathologic fractures, hypercalcemia, renal failure, and primary amyloidosis. Plasmacytoma: isolated plasma cell masses in bone or soft tissue (e.g., oropharynx)
Small lymphocytic lymphoma/chronic lymphocytic leukemia	Naïve B-cell or postgerminal center memory B-cell; expresses CD5	Trisomy 12, deletions of 11q, 13q, and 17p	Older adults with bone marrow, lymph node, spleen and liver disease; most have peripheral blood involvement; autoimmune hemolysis and thrombocytopenia in a minority; indolent
Neoplasms of mature T-cells or NK-cells			
Adult T-cell leukemia/ lymphoma	Helper T-cell expressing CD25 (IL-2 receptor)	HTLV-1 provirus present in tumor cells	Adults with cutaneous lesions, marrow involvement, and hypercalcemia; Japan, West Africa, and the Caribbean; aggressive
Anaplastic large cell lymphoma	Cytotoxic T-cell	Rearrangements of *ALK*	Children and young adults, usually with lymph node and soft tissue disease; aggressive
Extranodal NK/T cell lymphoma	Natural killer cell (common) or cytotoxic T-cell (rare)	No specific chromosomal abnormality; uniformly EBV associated	Adults with destructive extranodal masses, most commonly sinonasal; often accompanied by hemophagocytic syndrome; aggressive
Mycosis fungoides/ Sézary syndrome	Helper T-cell	No specific chromosomal abnormality	Adult patients with cutaneous patches, plaques, nodules, or generalized erythema; indolent
T-cell granular lymphocytic leukemia	Two types: (1) CD8+ T-cell, (2) NK-cell	No specific chromosomal abnormality	Adult patients with splenomegaly, neutropenia, and anemia, sometimes, accompanied by autoimmune disease
Hodgkin lymphoma			
Hodgkin lymphoma, lymphocyte-depletion subtype	Germinal center or postgerminal center B-cell	No specific chromosomal abnormality; >70% EBV associated	More common in the elderly and in HIV+ individuals; moderately aggressive
Hodgkin lymphoma, lymphocyte-predominance subtype	Germinal center B-cell	No specific chromosomal abnormality; not associated with EBV	Young to middle-aged males with cervical or axillary lymphadenophathy; indolent
Hodgkin lymphoma, lymphocyte-rich subtype	Germinal center or postgerminal center B-cell	No specific chromosomal abnormality; 40% EBV associated	More common in males, usually presents with lymphadenopathy; moderately aggressive
Hodgkin lymphoma, mixed cellularity subtype	Postgerminal center memory B-cell	No specific chromosomal abnormality; 70% EBV associated	More common in males, usually presents with lymphadenopathy; moderately aggressive
Hodgkin lymphoma, nodular sclerosing subtype	Germinal center or postgerminal center B-cell	No specific chromosomal abnormality; rarely EBV associated	Commonly presents as a mediastinal mass in young females; moderately aggressive

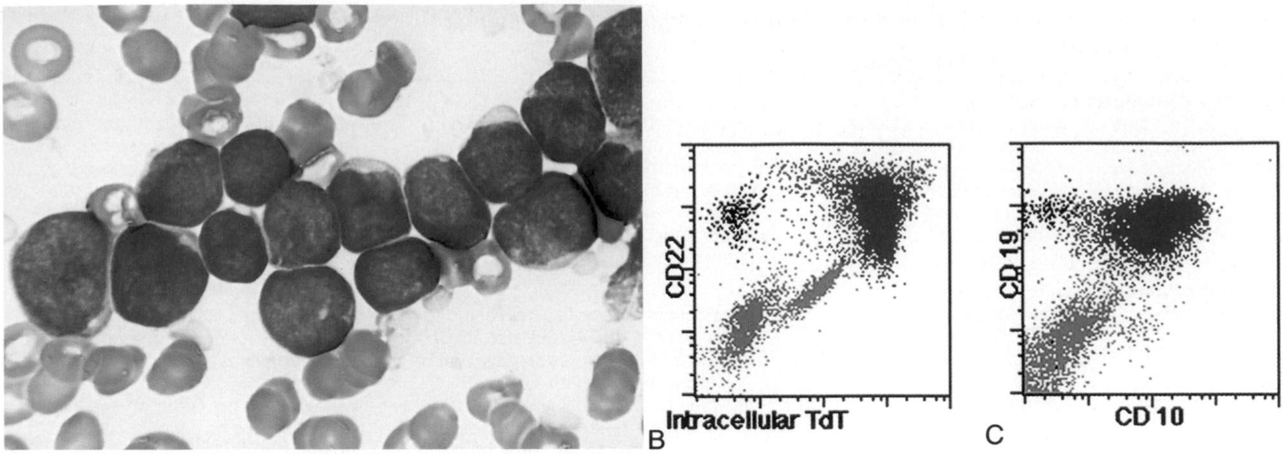

FIGURE 14–5 *A*, Acute lymphoblastic leukemia/lymphoma. Lymphoblasts with condensed nuclear chromatin, small nucleoli, and scant agranular cytoplasm. *B* and *C* represent the phenotype of the ALL shown in *A*, analyzed by flow cytometry. *B*, Note that the lymphoblasts represented by the red dots express TdT and the B-cell marker CD22. *C*, The same cells are positive for two other markers, CD10 and CD19, commonly expressed on pre-B lymphoblasts. Thus, this is a pre-B cell ALL. (*A*, courtesy of Dr. Robert W. McKenna; *B* and *C*, courtesy of Dr. Louis Picker, Oregon Health Science Center, Portland, OR.)

these morphologic distinctions are not absolute, and definitive diagnosis relies on detection of B and T lymphocyte–specific markers with antibodies (Figs. 14–5*B* and *C*). Histochemical stains can also be helpful, as lymphoblasts (in contrast to myeloblasts) lack peroxidase-positive granules and often contain cytoplasmic aggregates of periodic acid-Schiff (PAS)-positive material.

As has been noted, **ALLs with lymphomatous presentations are mostly of pre-T cell type.** Many pre-T ALLs (50% to 70%) are associated with mediastinal masses stemming from thymic involvement, and lymphadenopathy and splenomegaly are also more prevalent in this subtype.

Regardless of phenotype, the histologic appearance of ALL is similar. Normal tissue architecture is completely effaced by lymphoblasts having scant cytoplasm and nuclei somewhat larger than those of small lymphocytes. **The nuclear chromatin is delicate and finely stippled, and nucleoli are either absent or inconspicuous.** In many cases, the nuclear membrane shows deep subdivision, imparting a convoluted (lobulated) appearance. In keeping with its aggressive growth, the tumor shows a high rate of mitosis, and as with other tumors having a high mitotic rate (e.g., Burkitt lymphomas), a "starry sky" pattern can be produced by interspersed benign tingible body macrophages that have ingested the debris of dying neoplastic cells.

Immunophenotype. Immunostaining for terminal deoxynucleotidyltransferase (TdT), a specialized DNA polymerase that is expressed only by pre-B and pre-T lymphoblasts, is positive in >95% of cases (Fig. 14–5). Distinction between ALLs of precursor B- and T-cell origin requires staining for additional lineage-specific markers (summarized below):

- Precursor B ALL cells are arrested at stages preceding surface expression of Ig. The leukemic blasts almost always express the pan B-cell molecules CD19 and CD10. In very early pre-B cell ALL, CD19 is the only B cell–specific marker present. Early pre-B ALL is distinguished from late pre-B ALL by the absence of cytoplasmic IgM heavy chain (μ chain) in the former.
- Precursor T ALL cells are arrested at early stages of T-cell development. In most cases, the cells are CD1+, CD2+, CD5+, and CD7+. Early pre-T cell tumors are usually negative for surface CD3, CD4, and CD8, whereas late pre-T cell tumors are positive for these markers.

Cytogenetics and Molecular Genetics. *Approximately 90% of patients with ALL have numerical or structural changes in the chromosomes of the leukemic cells.*[13] Most common is hyperploidy (>50 chromosomes), but also polyploidy, and t(12;21), t(9;22) (Philadelphia chromosome) and t(4;11) translocations. These alterations correlate with immunophenotype and sometimes predict prognosis. It is noteworthy that pre-B and pre-T ALL are associated with distinct sets of translocations, suggesting that different molecular mechanisms underlie their pathogenesis. Recent studies of ALL using "gene chips," which determine the relative expression levels of thousands of genes simultaneously, have shown that the presence of certain chromosomal translocations also correlates with distinct patterns of gene expression.[14–16] Such studies promise to explain the basis for the correlation between specific chromosomal aberrations and outcome, and will likely identify additional patterns of gene expression that are independently predictive of clinical behavior.

Many of the chromosomal aberrations that are seen in ALL dysregulate the expression and function of transcription factors required for normal hematopoietic cell development. These derangements likely interfere with normal lymphoblast maturation, leading to arrested development and the accumulation of immature progenitors. As we will see, similar themes are relevant to the pathogenesis of AML as well.

Clinical Features. It should be emphasized that although ALL and AML are immunophenotypically and genotypically distinct, they usually present with very similar clinical features. In both diseases, an accumulation of neoplastic "blast" cells in the bone marrow suppresses normal hematopoiesis by physical crowding, competition for growth factors, and other poorly understood mechanisms. This results in anemia, neutropenia, and thrombocytopenia, which underlie the major clinical features of both ALL and AML. These common features and those more characteristic of ALL are listed below.

- *Abrupt stormy onset:* Patients present within days to a few weeks of the onset of symptoms.
- *Symptoms related to depression of normal marrow function:* fatigue due mainly to anemia; fever, reflecting infections due to absence of mature leukocytes; bleeding (petechiae, ecchymoses, epistaxis, gum bleeding) secondary to thrombocytopenia.
- *Bone pain and tenderness*, resulting from marrow expansion and infiltration of the subperiosteum.
- *Generalized lymphadenopathy, splenomegaly, and hepatomegaly* caused by neoplastic infiltration. Each is more common in ALL than in AML. In pre-T ALL presenting in the thymus, symptoms related to compression of large mediastinal vessels or airways may be seen. Testicular involvement is also common in ALL.
- *Central nervous system manifestations*, such as headache, vomiting, and nerve palsies resulting from meningeal spread, are also more common in ALL than in AML.

Prognosis. Dramatic advances have been made in the treatment of ALL. With aggressive chemotherapy (often given together with prophylactic treatment of the central nervous system), more than 90% of children with ALL achieve complete remission, and at least two thirds can be considered cured. *Several factors have been consistently associated with a worse prognosis: (1) age under 2,* possibly because of the strong association of infantile ALL with translocations involving the MLL gene on chromosome 11; *(2) presentation in adolescence or adulthood; (3) peripheral blood blast counts greater than 100,000,* which may reflect a high tumor burden; and *(4) the presence of unfavorable cytogenetic aberrations, such as the t(9;22) (the Philadelphia chromosome).*[13] The t(9;22) is present in only 3% of childhood ALL but up to 25% of adult cases, which could partially explain the poor outcome in adults. By contrast, favorable prognostic markers include age of 2 to 10 years, low white count, an early pre-B phenotype, and hyperploidy or t(12;21). Expression profiling shows promise as a means to identify additional subclasses of ALL of differing biology and clinical behavior.[14, 15] Allogeneic bone marrow transplantation also offers hope for those in poor prognostic categories.

Peripheral B-Cell Neoplasms

Chronic Lymphocytic Leukemia (CLL)/Small Lymphocytic Lymphoma (SLL)

These two disorders are morphologically, phenotypically, and genotypically indistinguishable, differing only in the degree of peripheral blood lymphocytosis. Most patients have sufficient lymphocytosis to fulfill the diagnostic requirement for CLL (absolute lymphocyte count >4000 per mm^3), which is the most common leukemia of adults in the Western world. In contrast, SLL constitutes only 4% of NHL. CLL/SLL is much less common in Japan and other Asian countries.

Morphology. Lymph node architecture is diffusely effaced by a predominant population of small lymphocytes 6 to 12 μm in diameter containing round to slightly irregular nuclei with condensed chromatin and scant cytoplasm (Fig. 14–6). These cells are mixed with variable numbers of larger cells called "prolymphocytes." In many cases, prolymphocytes gather together focally to form loose aggregates referred to as **proliferation centers,** so called because they contain relatively large numbers of mitotically active cells. When present, proliferation centers are pathognomonic for CLL/SLL.

In CLL, the peripheral blood contains increased numbers of small, round lymphocytes with scant cytoplasm (Fig. 14–7). These cells are fragile and are frequently disrupted in the process of making smears, producing so-called **smudge cells.** Involvement of the bone marrow is observed in all cases of CLL and most

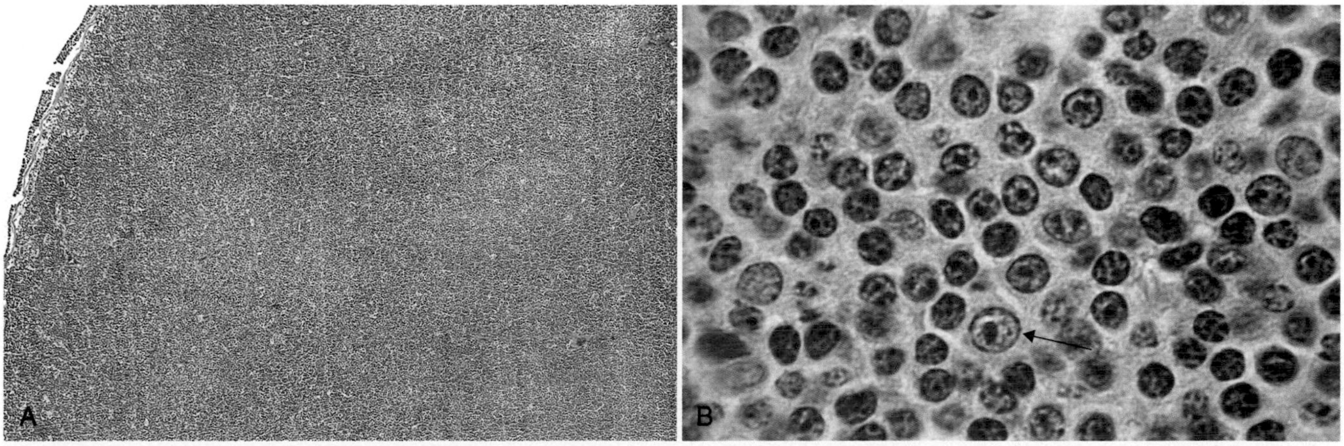

FIGURE 14–6 Small lymphocytic lymphoma/chronic lymphocytic leukemia (lymph node). *A,* Low-power view shows diffuse effacement of nodal architecture. *B,* At high power, the majority of the tumor cells are small round lymphocytes. A "pro-lymphocyte," a larger cell with a centrally placed nucleolus, is also present in this field (*arrow*). (*A,* courtesy of Dr. José Hernandez, Department of Pathology, University of Texas Southwestern Medical School, Dallas, TX.)

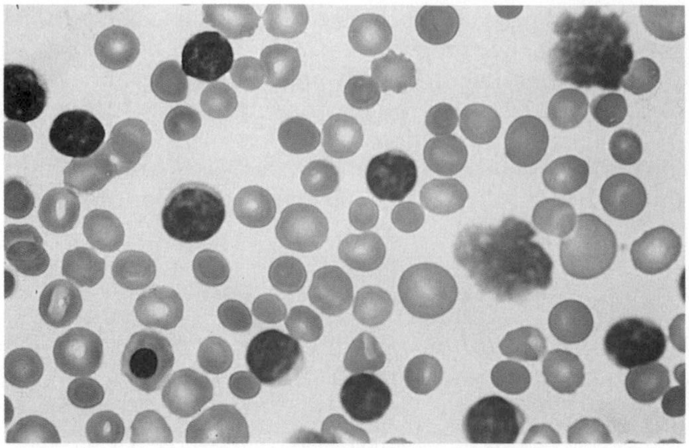

FIGURE 14–7 Chronic lymphocytic leukemia. This peripheral blood smear is flooded with small lymphocytes with condensed chromatin and scant cytoplasm. A characteristic finding is the presence of disrupted tumor cells (smudge cells). A coexistent autoimmune hemolytic anemia (see Chapter 13) explains the presence of spherocytes (hyperchromatic, round erythrocytes). A nucleated erythroid cell is present in the lower left-hand corner of the field. In this setting, circulating nucleated red cells could stem from premature release of progenitors in the face of severe anemia, marrow infiltration by tumor (leukoerythroblastosis), or both. (Courtesy of Dr. Jacqueline Mitus, Brigham and Women's Hospital, Boston, MA.)

cases of SLL, taking the form of interstitial infiltrates and/or non-paratrabecular aggregates of small lymphocytes. Tumor cells usually infiltrate the splenic white and red pulp and the hepatic portal tracts (Fig. 14–8), although the extent of involvement varies widely.

Immunophenotype. CLL/SLL has a distinctive immunophenotype. The tumor cells express the pan B-cell markers CD19 and CD20. In addition, CD23 and CD5, the latter a T-cell marker that is expressed on only a small subset of normal B cells, are present on the tumor cells. There is also typically low level expression of surface immunoglobulin heavy chain (usually IgM or IgM and IgD) and either κ or λ light chain.

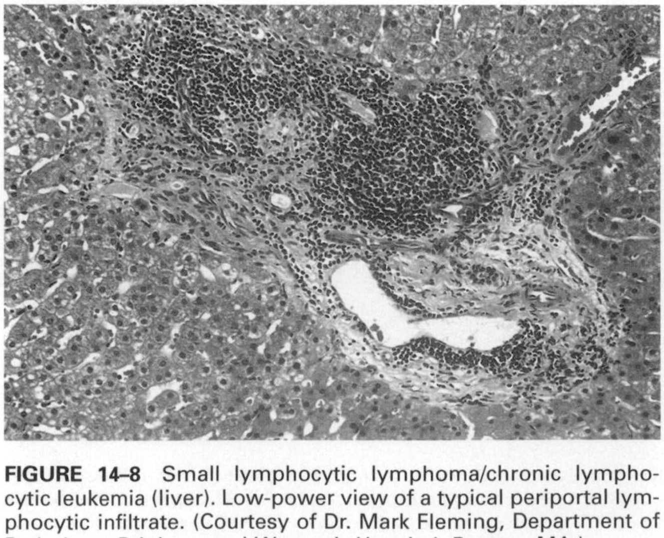

FIGURE 14–8 Small lymphocytic lymphoma/chronic lymphocytic leukemia (liver). Low-power view of a typical periportal lymphocytic infiltrate. (Courtesy of Dr. Mark Fleming, Department of Pathology, Brigham and Women's Hospital, Boston, MA.)

Chromosomal Abnormalities and Molecular Genetics. Unlike most other lymphoid malignancies, chromosomal translocations are rare in CLL/SLL. The most common findings are deletions of 13q12–14, deletions of 11q, trisomy 12q, and deletion of 17p.[17] DNA sequencing has revealed that the Ig genes of some CLL/SLL are somatically hypermutated, whereas others are not, suggesting that the cell of origin may be a postgerminal center memory B-cell or a naïve B-cell. For unclear reasons, tumors with unmutated Ig segments (those putatively of naïve B-cell origin) pursue a more aggressive course.

Clinical Features. Most patients present at ages over 50 (median age 60); a male predominance has been noted (M:F ratio of 2:1). *Patients with CLL/SLL are often asymptomatic.* When symptoms appear, they are nonspecific and include easy fatigability, weight loss, and anorexia. Generalized lymphadenopathy and hepatosplenomegaly are present in 50% to 60% of the cases. The total leukocyte count is highly variable. Patients with SLL and marrow involvement can be leukopenic, while patients with CLL and heavy tumor burdens can have leukocyte counts in excess of 200,000 per mm^3. A small monoclonal immunoglobulin "spike" is present in the serum of some patients.

CLL/SLL disrupts normal immune function through uncertain mechanisms. Hypogammaglobulinemia is common and contributes to increased susceptibility to infections. Conversely, some 10% to 15% of patients develop autoantibodies directed against red blood cells or platelets that produce autoimmune hemolytic anemia or thrombocytopenia. The pathogenic IgGs are produced by non-neoplastic, self-reactive B cells rather than tumor cells,[18] suggesting a systemic defect in immune regulation.

The course and prognosis of CLL/SLL are extremely variable and depend primarily on the clinical stage. Overall, the median survival is 4 to 6 years, but patients with minimal initial tumor burdens can survive for 10 years or more. The presence of deletions of 11q and 17p correlates with higher-stage disease and portends a worse prognosis.[17]

An additional important factor in patient survival is the tendency of CLL/SLL to transform to more aggressive lymphoid neoplasms. Most commonly, this takes the form of a *prolymphocytic transformation* (15% to 30% of patients) or a transformation to diffuse large B-cell lymphoma, so-called *Richter syndrome* (~10% of patients). Prolymphocytic transformation is marked by worsening of cytopenias, increasing splenomegaly, and the appearance in the peripheral blood of large numbers of "prolymphocytes," cells with a large nucleus containing a single prominent, centrally placed, nucleolus. Transformation to diffuse large B-cell lymphoma is often heralded by the appearance of a rapidly enlarging mass within a lymph node or the spleen. These transformations usually stem from tumor progression, as they retain B-cell phenotypes and are derived from the same clone as the underlying CLL/SLL. Both prolymphocytic and large-cell transformation are usually ominous events, most patients surviving less than 1 year.[19]

Follicular Lymphoma

Follicular lymphoma is the most common form of NHL in the United States, comprising about 45% of adult lymphomas.

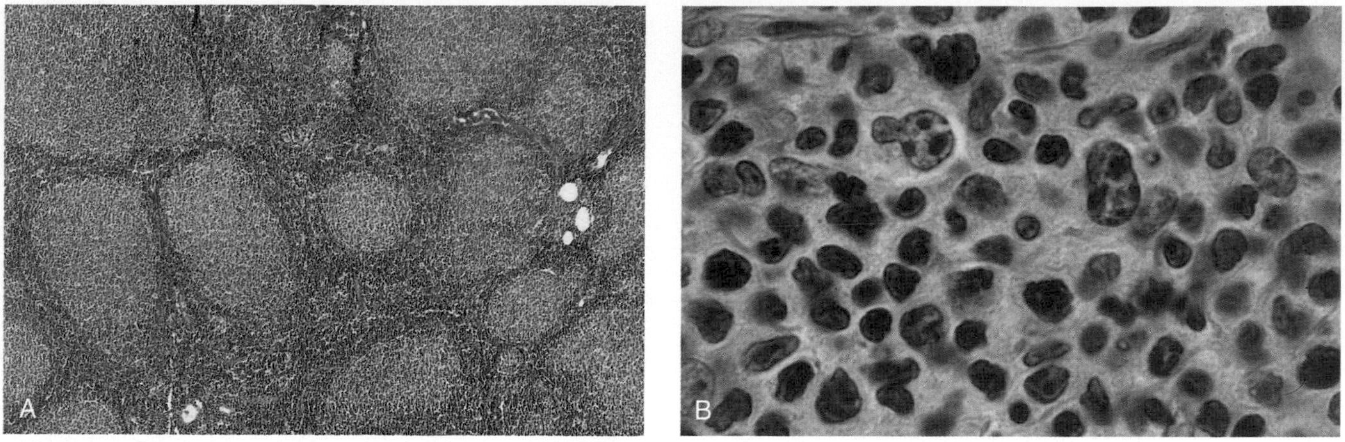

FIGURE 14–9 Follicular lymphoma (lymph node). *A*, Nodular aggregates of lymphoma cells are present throughout lymph node. *B*, At high magnification, small lymphoid cells with condensed chromatin and irregular or cleaved nuclear outlines (centrocytes) are mixed with a population of larger cells with nucleoli (centroblasts). (*A*, courtesy of Dr. Robert W. McKenna, Department of Pathology, University of Texas Southwestern Medical School, Dallas, TX.)

It usually presents in middle age and afflicts males and females equally. It is less common in Europe and rare in Asian populations. *The neoplastic cells closely resemble normal germinal center B cells.*

Morphology. In most cases, at low magnification, a predominantly nodular or nodular and diffuse growth pattern is observed in involved lymph nodes (Fig. 14–9). **Two principal cell types are observed in varying proportions: (1) small cells with irregular or cleaved nuclear contours and scant cytoplasm, referred to as centrocytes (small cleaved cells), and (2) larger cells with open nuclear chromatin, several nucleoli, and modest amounts of cytoplasm, referred to as centroblasts** (Fig. 14–9). In most follicular lymphomas, small cleaved cells make up the majority of the cells. Peripheral blood involvement sufficient to produce lymphocytosis (usually under 20,000 per mm^3) is seen in about 10% of patients. Bone marrow involvement occurs in 85% of patients and characteristically takes the form of paratrabecular lymphoid aggregates. Splenic white pulp (Fig. 14–10) and hepatic portal triads are also frequently involved.

Immunophenotype. The neoplastic cells resemble normal follicular center B cells, expressing CD19, CD20, CD10 (CALLA), and surface immunoglobulin. Unlike in CLL/SLL and mantle cell lymphoma, CD5 is not expressed. Follicular lymphoma cells also express BCL2 protein in more than 90% of cases, in distinction to normal follicular center B cells, which are BCL2 negative (Fig. 14–11). Almost all tumors also express BCL6, a transcriptional repressor that regulates germinal center B cell development.

Cytogenetics and Molecular Genetics. *The hallmark of typical follicular lymphoma is a (14;18) translocation that juxtaposes the* IgH *locus on chromosome 14 and the* BCL2 *locus on chromosome 18.* This translocation is seen in up to 90% of follicular lymphomas,[20] and leads to overexpression of BCL2 protein (Fig. 14–11). BCL2 is an antagonist of apoptotic cell death (Chapter 1) and appears to promote the survival of follicular lymphoma cells. Indeed, whereas reactive follicles contain numerous B cells undergoing apoptosis, neoplastic follicles are characteristically devoid of apoptotic cells. Uncommonly, follicular lymphomas lack the t(14;18) and instead have rearrangements of the *BCL6* gene on chromosome 3q27.

Clinical Features. Follicular lymphomas tend to present with painless, generalized lymphadenopathy. Involvement of extranodal sites, such as the gastrointestinal tract, central nervous system, or testis, is relatively uncommon. Although follicular lymphoma is incurable, it usually follows an indolent waxing and waning course. The overall median survival is 7 to 9 years and is not improved by aggressive therapy; hence, the usual clinical approach is to palliate patients with low-dose chemotherapy or radiation when they become symptomatic.

Histologic transformation occurs in 30% to 50% of follicular lymphomas, most commonly to diffuse large B-cell lymphoma. Rarely, follicular lymphoma transforms to an aggres-

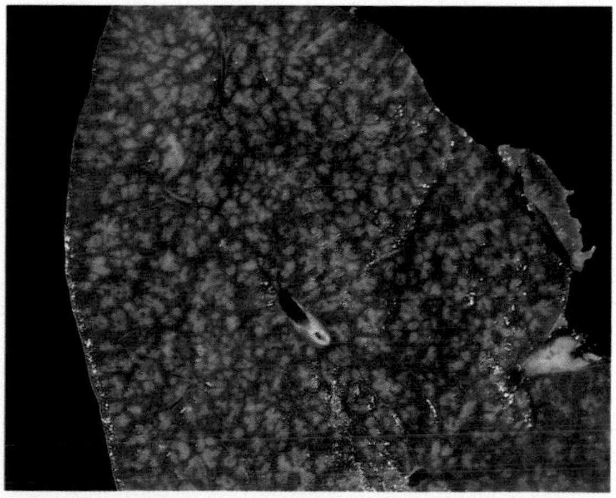

FIGURE 14–10 Follicular lymphoma (spleen). Prominent nodules represent white pulp follicles expanded by follicular lymphoma cells. Other indolent B-cell lymphomas (small lymphocytic lymphoma, mantle cell lymphoma, marginal zone lymphoma) can produce an identical pattern of involvement. (Courtesy of Dr. Jeffrey Jorgenson, Department of Pathology, Brigham and Women's Hospital, Boston, MA.)

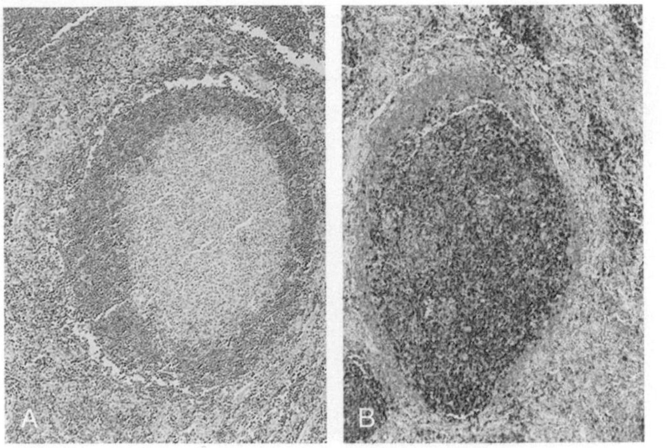

FIGURE 14–11 BCL2 expression in reactive and neoplastic follicles. BCL2 protein was detected by using an immunohistochemical technique that produces a brown stain. In reactive follicles (*A*), BCL2 is present in mantle zone cells but not follicular center B cells, whereas follicular lymphoma cells (*B*) exhibit strong BCL2 staining (Courtesy of Dr. Jeffrey Jorgenson, Department of Pathology, Brigham and Women's Hospital, Boston, MA.)

sive tumor resembling Burkitt lymphoma, an event usually associated with acquisition of a chromosomal translocation involving the *c-MYC* locus. These transformed tumors retain the t(14;18), proving a clonal relationship to the antecedent follicular lymphoma. Follicular lymphomas show evidence of ongoing somatic hypermutation, which may promote transformation by causing point mutations or DNA breakage that leads to chromosomal translocations.[3] Median survival is less than 1 year after transformation.

Diffuse Large B-Cell Lymphoma (DLBCL)

This important diagnostic category encompasses a heterogeneous group of tumors that together constitute about 20% of all NHL and 60% to 70% of aggressive lymphoid neoplasms. There is a slight male predominance, with a median age of about 60 years. However, the age range is wide, and diffuse large B-cell lymphoma constitutes about 5% of childhood lymphoma.

Morphology. The common morphologic features that unite this group of neoplasms are a relatively large cell size (usually four to five times the diameter of a small lymphocyte) and a diffuse pattern of growth (Fig. 14–12). In other respects, there is a fair degree of morphologic variation. Most commonly, the tumor cells have a round or oval nucleus that appears vesicular owing to margination of chromatin at the nuclear membrane, but large multilobated or cleaved nuclei are prominent in some cases. Nucleoli may be two to three in number and located adjacent to the nuclear membrane or single and centrally placed. The cytoplasm is usually moderately abundant and may be pale or basophilic. More anaplastic tumors may contain multinucleated cells with large, inclusionlike nucleoli that resemble Reed-Sternberg cells (the tumor cell of Hodgkin disease); in some difficult cases, immunophenotyping must be relied on to distinguish these two entities.

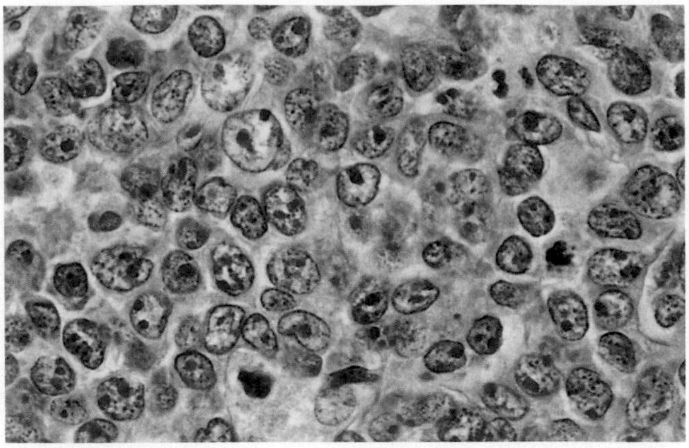

FIGURE 14–12 Diffuse large B-cell lymphoma. Tumor cells have large nuclei, open chromatin, and prominent nucleoli. (Courtesy of Dr. Robert W. McKenna, Department of Pathology, University of Texas Southwestern Medical School, Dallas, TX.)

Immunophenotype. These mature B-cell tumors express the B-cell markers CD19 and CD20, and they show variable expression of germinal center markers such as CD10 and BCL6. Most have surface Ig, and all are negative for TdT.

Cytogenetics and Molecular Profile. Cytogenetic and gene expression profiling studies indicate that diffuse large B-cell lymphomas are heterogeneous in terms of their pathogenesis. One frequent pathogenic event in these tumors is dysregulation of BCL6, a DNA-binding zinc-finger transcriptional regulator that is required for the formation of normal germinal centers.[21] About 30% of DLBCLs contain various translocations that have in common a breakpoint at chromosome 3q27 within the *BCL6* locus,[22] and tumors lacking 3q27 rearrangements often have acquired mutations in *BCL6* promoter sequences.[3] It is hypothesized that both of these genetic lesions are acquired in germinal center B cells undergoing somatic hypermutation.[23] Point mutations and possible DNA breakage in *BCL6* regulatory regions produced by somatic hypermutation provide plausible mechanisms for *BCL6* dysregulation and translocation. Curiously, *BCL6* is also subject to somatic hypermutation in normal germinal center B cells, explaining why abnormalities of this gene are so frequent in diffuse large B-cell lymphoma. Normally, BCL6 expression is downregulated when B cells leave the germinal center, but both 3q27 rearrangements and *BCL6* promoter mutations cause persistent and dysregulated expression of yet to be identified target genes.[24]

In addition to mutations in *BCL6* resembling those produced by somatic hypermutation, molecular analysis of DNA isolated from tumor cells has revealed similar mutations in the 5′ regions of multiple other genes, including oncogenes such as *c-MYC*.[3] Mutations in these genes are not seen in normal germinal center B cells, suggesting that ongoing somatic hypermutation in these tumors is aberrant and targets many different loci.

About 10% to 20% of tumors contain the t(14;18), the characteristic chromosomal abnormality of follicular lymphoma. Such tumors are considered to be of germinal center B-cell origin; indeed, some patients are found to have foci of follicular lymphoma comprising primarily small centrocytes (small, cleaved cells) at other sites, particularly the bone marrow. *Tumors with BCL2 rearrangements almost always lack BCL6 rearrangements, suggesting that there are at least two unique pathogenetic pathways.* The likelihood of pathogenetic heterogeneity is further supported by microarray analyses of gene expression profiles, which indicate the existence of several groups of tumors with distinctive patterns of gene expression.[25–27]

Special Subtypes Associated with Oncogenic Viruses. These distinctive subtypes of large B-cell lymphoma are of sufficient pathogenetic interest to merit a brief discussion.

- *Immunodeficiency-associated large B-cell lymphoma.* These occur in the setting of severe T-cell immunodeficiency (e.g., end-stage HIV infection, severe combined immunodeficiency, allogeneic bone marrow transplantation, and solid organ transplantation). *The neoplastic B cells are often latently infected with Epstein-Barr virus,* which is thought to play a critical pathogenic role. Restoration of T-cell immunity may lead to regression of such EBV-positive proliferations.
- *Body cavity large cell lymphoma.* These arise as malignant pleural or ascitic effusions, mostly in patients with advanced HIV infection, but occasionally in HIV-negative elderly adults. The tumor cells often fail to express surface B- or T-cell markers but have clonal IgH gene rearrangements. *In all cases, the tumor cells are infected with KSHV/HHV8,* which may play a causal role in the development of this tumor.[5] Among the malignant lymphomas, KSHV has been observed only in this particular subtype.

Clinical Course and Prognosis. In contrast to patients with low-grade lymphomas, who often present with generalized asymptomatic lymphadenopathy, *patients with diffuse large B-cell lymphoma typically present with a rapidly enlarging, often symptomatic, mass at a single nodal or extranodal site.* Large B-cell lymphomas can arise at virtually any site. Waldeyer ring, the oropharyngeal lymphoid tissues that include the tonsils and adenoids, is involved commonly. Primary or secondary involvement of the liver and spleen can take the form of large, destructive masses (Fig. 14–13). Extranodal disease can arise within the gastrointestinal tract, skin, bone, brain, and other sites. Bone marrow involvement usually occurs late in the disease; rarely a leukemic picture may emerge.

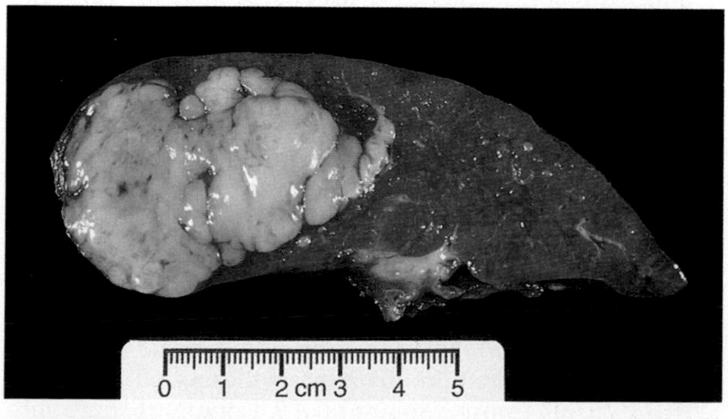

FIGURE 14–13 Diffuse large B-cell lymphoma (spleen). The presence of an isolated large mass is typical. In contrast, indolent B-cell lymphomas usually produce multifocal expansion of white pulp (see Fig. 14–10). (Courtesy of Dr. Mark Fleming, Department of Pathology, Brigham and Women's Hospital, Boston, MA.)

As a group, diffuse large B-cell lymphomas are aggressive tumors that are rapidly fatal if untreated. However, with intensive combination chemotherapy, complete remission can be achieved in 60% to 80% of patients, and approximately 50% remain free from disease for several years and may be considered cured. Patients with limited disease fare better than those with widespread disease or a large, bulky tumor mass.[28] Expression profiling shows promise in identifying distinct molecular subtypes with differing clinical outcomes.[25, 26]

Burkitt Lymphoma

Within this category fall (1) African (endemic) Burkitt lymphoma, (2) sporadic (nonendemic) Burkitt lymphoma, and (3) a subset of aggressive lymphomas occurring in individuals infected with HIV. Burkitt lymphomas occurring in each of these settings are histologically identical, but some clinical, genotypic, and virologic differences exist.

Morphology. Involved tissues are effaced by a diffuse infiltrate of intermediate-sized lymphoid cells, 10 to 25 μm in diameter, containing round or oval nuclei with coarse chromatin, several nucleoli, and a moderate amount of faintly basophilic or amphophilic cytoplasm (Fig. 14–14). The nuclear size approximates that of benign macrophages within the tumor. **A high mitotic index is typical, as is apoptotic tumor cell death,** accounting for the presence of numerous tissue macrophages with ingested nuclear debris. These benign macrophages are diffusely distributed among the tumor cells and have abundant clear cytoplasm, creating a characteristic **"starry sky" pattern.** In cases with bone marrow involvement, the tumor cells in marrow aspirates have slightly clumped nuclear chromatin, two to five distinct nucleoli, and royal blue cytoplasm containing multiple, clear cytoplasmic vacuoles.

Immunophenotype. These are tumors of mature B cells expressing surface IgM, monotypic κ or λ light chain, CD19, CD20, and CD10, and BCL6, a phenotype that closely resembles that of rapidly dividing B cells within the dark zones of normal germinal centers.

Cytogenetic and Molecular Genetic Features. *All forms of Burkitt lymphoma are associated with translocations of the* c-MYC *gene on chromosome 8.* The partner in the translocation is usually the IgH locus (t(8;14)) but may also be the κ (t(2;8)) or λ (t(8;22)) light chain locus. The chromosomal breakpoints in the IgH locus in sporadic BL usually occur in immunoglobulin class switch regions, whereas the breakpoints in endemic BL tend to lie within more 5′ V(D)J sequences, indicating subtle differences in underlying molecular mechanisms.[29] It is hypothesized that translocations involving switch regions result from errors during class switching, whereas those involving regions near V(D)J sequences may occur during attempted V(D)J joining or through breaks generated during somatic hypermutation of Ig genes. *Essentially all endemic tumors are latently infected with EBV,* which is also present in about 25% of HIV-associated tumors and 15% to 20% of sporadic cases. Molecular analysis has shown that the configura-

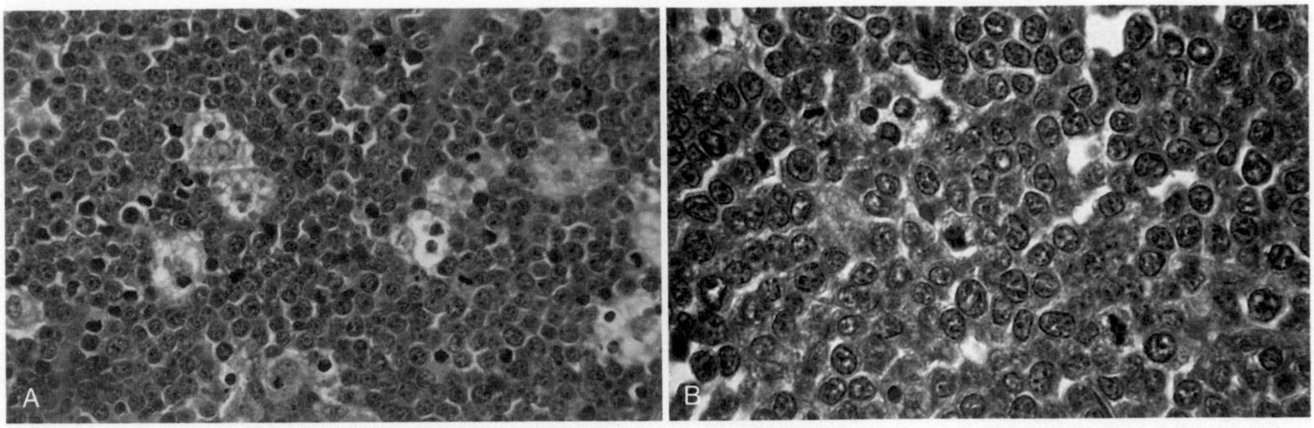

FIGURE 14–14 Burkitt lymphoma. *A*, At low power, numerous pale tingible body macrophages are evident, producing a "starry sky" appearance. *B*, At high power, tumor cells have multiple small nucleoli and high mitotic index. The lack of significant variation in nuclear shape and size lends a monotonous appearance. (*B*, courtesy of Dr. José Hernandez, Department of Pathology, University of Texas Southwestern Medical School, Dallas, TX.)

tion of the episomal EBV DNA is identical in all tumor cells within individual cases, indicating that infection precedes cellular transformation. While supporting a direct role for EBV in lymphomagenesis, this finding also raises interesting questions about the EBV-negative tumors: Is another infectious agent involved in such cases, or can mutations in critical genes in the host genome mimic the effects of the transforming proteins of EBV on cell growth and differentiation?

Clinical Features. Both the endemic and the sporadic cases are found largely in children or young adults, accounting for approximately 30% of childhood NHLs in the United States. Most tumors manifest at extranodal sites. Endemic Burkitt lymphoma often presents as a mass involving the mandible and shows an unusual predilection for involvement of abdominal viscera, particularly the kidneys, ovaries, and adrenal glands. In contrast, sporadic Burkitt lymphoma most often presents as an abdominal mass involving the ileocecum and peritoneum. Involvement of the bone marrow and peripheral blood is uncommon, especially in endemic cases. Burkitt lymphoma is very aggressive but responds well to short-term, high-dose chemotherapy. Most children and young adults can be cured, but the outcome is more guarded in older adults.

Plasma Cell Neoplasms and Related Disorders

The common feature of this collection of entities is the proliferation of a B-cell clone that synthesizes and secretes a single homogeneous immunoglobulin or its fragments. In many (but not all) cases, these proliferations (often referred to as dyscrasias) are malignant. Collectively, the plasma cell dyscrasias account for about 15% of deaths from white cell neoplasms.

The monoclonal immunoglobulin identified in the blood is referred to as an M component, in reference to myeloma. Since complete M components have molecular weights of 160,000 or higher, they are restricted to the plasma and extracellular fluid and are excluded from the urine in the absence of glomerular damage. However, unlike normal plasma cells, in which the production and coupling of heavy (H) and light (L) chains are tightly balanced, *neoplastic plasma cells often synthesize excess L or H chains along with complete immunoglobulins.* Occasionally, only L chains or H chains are produced. The free L chains, known as Bence Jones proteins, are small enough to be rapidly excreted in the urine. As a result, free L chains are detectable in the blood only in the setting of renal failure or very high levels of synthesis.

Designations applied to disorders associated with abnormal immunoglobulins include gammopathy, monoclonal gammopathy, dysproteinemia, and paraproteinemia. A variety of clinicopathologic entities are associated with monoclonal gammopathies.

- *Multiple myeloma (plasma cell myeloma)* is the most important and most common symptomatic monoclonal gammopathy. It is characterized by multiple tumorous masses of neoplastic plasma cells scattered throughout the skeletal system. *Solitary myeloma, or solitary plasmacytoma,* is an infrequent variant consisting of a solitary neoplastic mass of plasma cells found in bone or some soft tissue site.
- *Waldenström macroglobulinemia* is a syndrome caused by blood hyperviscosity due to high levels of IgM. It is seen most commonly in adults with lymphoplasmacytic lymphoma (and therefore is discussed later in more detail under this entity), but it can also occur in association with tumors morphologically resembling chronic lymphocytic leukemia/small lymphocytic lymphoma and with rare IgM-secreting myelomas.
- *Heavy-chain disease* is seen in a diverse group of disorders, including chronic lymphocytic leukemia/small lymphocytic lymphoma, lymphoplasmacytic lymphoma, and an unusual small bowel lymphoma that occurs in malnourished populations (so-called Mediterranean lymphoma). The common feature is synthesis and secretion of free H chain fragments.
- *Primary or immunocyte-associated amyloidosis* results from a monoclonal proliferation of plasma cells secreting free L chains (most commonly of λ isotype) that are subsequently processed and deposited as amyloid. While some patients with primary amyloidosis have overt multiple myeloma, others have only a minor clonal population of plasma cells in the marrow.

- *Monoclonal gammopathy of undetermined significance (MGUS)* refers to instances in which M components are identified in the blood of patients having no signs or symptoms. MGUS is very common in the elderly but progresses to a symptomatic monoclonal gammopathy (most often multiple myeloma) in only a small subset of patients.

Against this background, we can turn to some of the specific clinicopathologic entities. Primary amyloidosis was discussed along with other disorders of the immune system in Chapter 6.

Multiple Myeloma. *Multiple myeloma is a plasma cell neoplasm characterized by involvement of the skeleton at multiple sites.* Although bony disease dominates, it can also spread to lymph nodes and extranodal sites, such as the skin. Multiple myeloma causes 1% of all cancer deaths in Western countries. Its incidence is higher in men, people of African descent, and older adults.

Etiology and Pathogenesis. *The proliferation and survival of myeloma cells are dependent on several cytokines, most notably IL-6.*[30] IL-6 is produced by neoplastic plasma cells and normal stromal cells in the marrow. Serum levels of this cytokine are increased in patients with active disease, and high serum IL-6 levels are associated with a poor prognosis.

Factors produced by neoplastic plasma cells also mediate bone destruction, the major pathologic feature of multiple myeloma. A variety of cytokines produced by the tumor cells, particularly MIP1α and the receptor activator of NF-κB ligand (RANKL), serve as osteoclast-activating factors[31] and offer points of possible therapeutic intervention. For example, osteoprotegerin, a factor that regulates normal bone homeostasis by inhibiting RANKL, prevents bone resorption in an animal model of myeloma (see also Chapter 26).[32]

The most frequent karyotypic abnormalities are deletions of 13q and translocations involving the Ig heavy chain locus on 14q32. Common translocation partners with IgH are *FGFR3* (fibroblast growth factor receptor 3) on chromosome 4p16, a gene encoding a type of tyrosine kinase receptor implicated in control of cellular proliferation (see Chapter 7); the cell cycle regulatory genes cyclin D1 on chromosome 11q13 and cyclin D3 on chromosome 6p21; the gene for the transcription factor *cMAF* on chromosome 16 q23; and *MUM1/IRF4*, a gene for an interferon regulatory factor, on chromosome 6p25.[33] A comparison of mRNA expression profiles using gene chips suggests the existence of at least four subtypes with distinct patterns of gene expression.[34]

Morphology. Multiple myeloma presents most often as multifocal destructive bone tumors composed of plasma cells (plasmacytomas) throughout the skeletal system. Bones in the axial skeleton are affected most commonly. The following distribution was found in a large series of cases: vertebral column, 66%; ribs, 44%; skull, 41%; pelvis, 28%; femur, 24%; clavicle, 10%; and scapula, 10%. These focal lesions generally begin in the medullary cavity, erode cancellous bone, and progressively destroy the bony cortex, often leading to pathologic fractures. These are most common in the vertebral column but may occur in any affected bone. **The bone lesions appear radiographically as punched-out defects, usually 1 to 4 cm in diameter** (Fig. 14–15), and grossly consist of gelatinous, soft, red tumor masses. Less commonly, widespread myelomatous bone disease can produce diffuse demineralization (osteopenia) rather than focal defects.

Microscopic examination of the marrow reveals an increased number of plasma cells, which usually constitute more than 30% of the marrow cellularity. The plasma cells can infiltrate the marrow diffusely or be present in sheetlike masses that completely replace normal elements. Like their benign counterparts, neoplastic plasma cells usually have a perinuclear clearing (due to a prominent Golgi apparatus) and an eccentrically placed nucleus (Fig. 14–16). Relatively normal-appearing plasma cells, **plasmablasts**, with

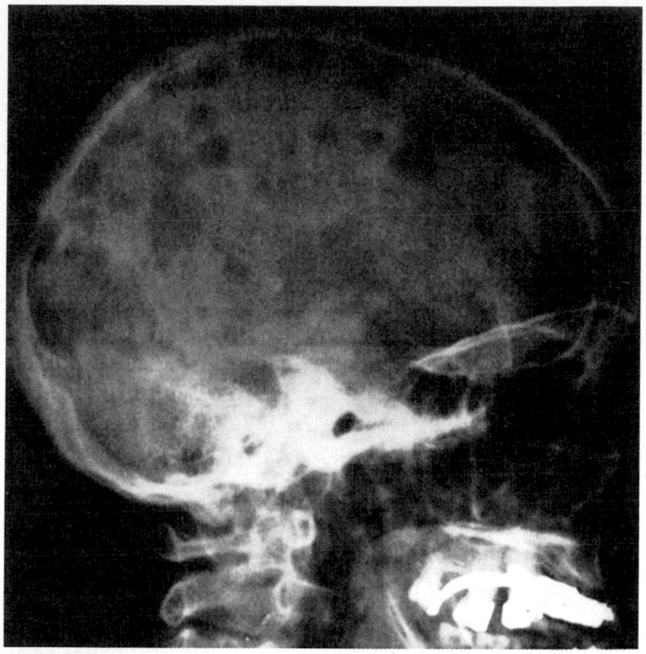

FIGURE 14–15 Multiple myeloma of the skull (radiograph, lateral view). The sharply punched-out bone lesions are most obvious in the calvarium.

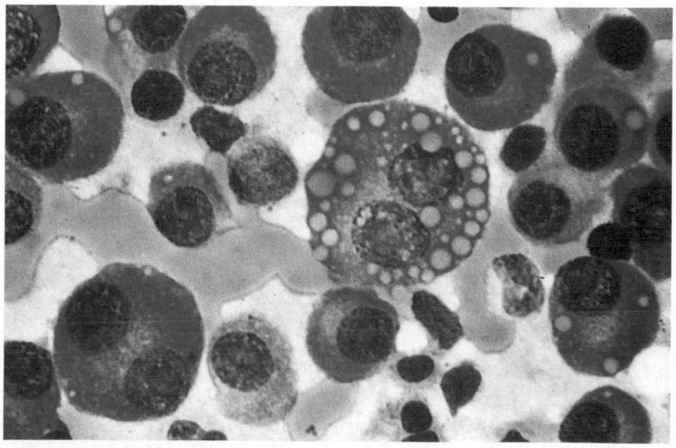

FIGURE 14–16 Multiple myeloma (bone marrow aspirate). Normal marrow cells are largely replaced by plasma cells, including forms with multiple nuclei, prominent nucleoli, and cytoplasmic droplets containing immunoglobulin.

vesicular nuclear chromatin and a prominent single nucleolus, or **bizarre multinucleated cells** may predominate. Other cytologic variants stem from the dysregulated synthesis and secretion of immunoglobulin, which sometimes leads to intracellular accumulation of intact or partially degraded Ig. Such variants include **flame cells,** with fiery red cytoplasm; **Mott cells** having multiple blue grapelike cytoplasmic droplets; and cells containing a variety of other inclusions, including **fibrils, crystalline rods, and globules,** sometimes **Russell bodies** (cytoplasmic) or **Dutcher bodies** (nuclear). With progressive disease, plasma cell infiltrations can be encountered in the spleen, liver, kidneys, lungs, lymph nodes, or other soft tissues.

Commonly, the high level of serum M proteins causes red cells in smears of peripheral blood to stick to one another in linear arrays, a finding referred to as **rouleaux formation**. Although characteristic, rouleaux formation is not specific, as it can be seen in other conditions in which immunoglobulin levels are elevated, such as lupus erythematosus and early HIV infection. Much more rarely, neoplastic plasma cells flood the peripheral blood, giving rise to **plasma cell leukemia**.

Bence Jones proteins are excreted in the kidney and contribute to a form of renal disease called *myeloma kidney* that is one of the more distinctive features of multiple myeloma. It is discussed in detail in Chapter 20.

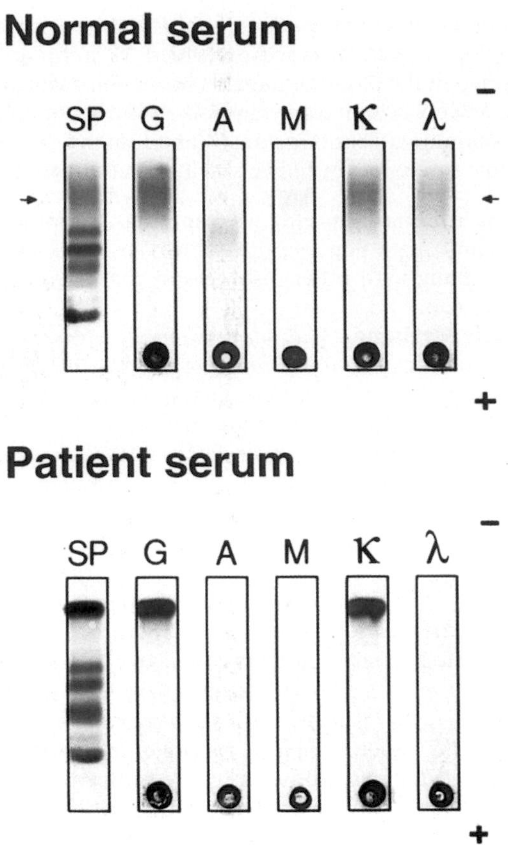

FIGURE 14–17 M protein detection, multiple myeloma. Serum protein electrophoresis (SP) is used to screen for a monoclonal immunoglobulin (M protein). Polyclonal IgG in normal serum (denoted by the *arrow*) appears as a broad band; in contrast, serum from a patient with multiple myeloma contains a single sharp protein band in this region of the electropherogram. The suspected monoclonal immunoglobulin is confirmed and characterized by immunofixation. In this procedure, proteins separated by electrophoresis within a gel are reacted with specific antisera. After extensive washing of the gel, only proteins that are cross-linked by antisera are retained. These are detected with a protein stain. Note the sharp band in the immunoglobulin region of the patient SP that is recognized by antisera against IgG heavy chain (G) and kappa light chain (κ), indicating the presence of a IgGκ M protein. Levels of polyclonal IgG, IgA (A), and lambda light chain (λ) are also decreased in the patient serum relative to normal, a common finding in multiple myeloma. (Courtesy of Dr. David Sacks, Department of Pathology, Brigham and Women's Hospital, Boston, MA.)

Clinical Course. The peak age of incidence of multiple myeloma is between 50 and 60 years. As was previously stated, the clinical features stem from the effects of (1) infiltration of organs, particularly bones, by the neoplastic plasma cells; (2) the production of excessive immunoglobulins, which often have abnormal physicochemical properties; and (3) the suppression of normal humoral immunity.

Bone resorption often leads to pathologic fractures and chronic pain. The attendant *hypercalcemia* can in turn give rise to neurologic manifestations such as confusion, weakness, lethargy, constipation, and polyuria and can contribute to renal disease. Decreased production of normal immunoglobulins sets the stage for *recurrent infections* with bacteria such as *Streptococcus pneumoniae, Staphylococcus aureus*, and *Escherichia coli*. Cellular immunity is relatively unaffected. *Of great significance is renal insufficiency, which is second only to infections as a cause of death.* The pathogenesis of the renal failure (discussed in detail in Chapter 20) that occurs in up to 50% of patients is multifactorial. However, the single most important factor appears to be *Bence Jones proteinuria*, as excreted light chains are toxic to renal tubular epithelial cells. *Amyloidosis* of the AL (amyloid light chain) type occurs in some patients owing to secretion of amyloidogenic Ig light chains (Chapter 6).

In 99% of patients with multiple myeloma, laboratory analyses reveal increased levels of immunoglobulins in the blood and/or light chains (Bence Jones proteins) in the urine. The monoclonal immunoglobulins are usually first detected as abnormal protein "spikes" in serum or urine electrophoresis and then further characterized by immunofixation (Fig. 14–17). Most myelomas are associated with more than 3 gm/dL of Ig in serum and/or more than 6 gm/dL of Bence Jones protein in urine. The most common serum monoclonal immunoglobulin ("M protein") is IgG, which is found in 55% of patients. An additional 25% of cases are associated with an IgA M protein. Myelomas expressing IgM, IgD, or IgE occur but are rare. Excessive production and aggregation of M proteins leads to the hyperviscosity syndrome (described under lymphoplasmacytic lymphoma) in approximately 7% of patients, mostly associated with tumors that secrete IgA and or IgG3.

Bence Jones proteinuria and a serum M protein are both observed in 60% to 70% of all myeloma patients. However, in approximately 20% of patients, Bence Jones proteinuria is present as an isolated finding. It is also notable that ~1% of myelomas are nonsecretory. Hence, the absence of serum and urine M proteins does not completely exclude myeloma.

The clinicopathologic diagnosis of multiple myeloma rests on radiographic and laboratory findings. The diagnosis can be strongly suspected when the distinctive radiographic changes are present, but definitive diagnosis requires a bone marrow examination. Extensive marrow involvement gives rise to a normocytic normochromic anemia, sometimes accompanied by moderate leukopenia and thrombocytopenia.

The prognosis for this condition is variable but generally poor. Patients with multiple bony lesions, if untreated, rarely survive for more than 6 to 12 months, whereas occasional patients with "indolent myeloma" can survive for many years. Chemotherapy with alkylating agents induces remission in 50% to 70% of patients, but the median survival is still a dismal 3 years. Biphosphonates, drugs that inhibit bone resorption, have shown some promise in reducing pathologic fractures and limiting hypercalcemia.[35] Multiple myeloma cells are unusually sensitive to inhibitors of the proteasome, a cellular organelle that specifically degrades unwanted and misfolded proteins, and proteasome inhibitor drugs have shown promise in patients.[36] A small subset of younger patients (less than age 50) receiving allogeneic bone marrow transplants have long-standing remissions.[37]

Solitary Myeloma (Plasmacytoma). About 3% to 5% of plasma cell neoplasms present as a solitary lesion of either bone or soft tissue. *The bony lesions tend to occur in the same locations as in multiple myeloma. Extraosseous lesions are often located in the lungs, oronasopharynx, or nasal sinuses.* Modest elevations of M proteins in the blood or urine may be found in a minority of patients.

Progression to classic multiple myeloma is common in patients with solitary osseous plasmacytoma, whereas extraosseous plasmacytomas disseminate in only a minor fraction of patients. It appears that the solitary plasmacytoma involving the bones often represents an early stage of multiple myeloma, but progression can take 10 to 20 years or longer. Extraosseous plasmacytomas, particularly those involving the upper respiratory tract, frequently represent limited disease that can be cured by local resection.

Monoclonal Gammopathy of Uncertain Significance. M proteins can be identified in the serum of 1% of asymptomatic healthy persons older than 50 years of age and in 3% of individuals older than 70 years of age. *This dysproteinemia without associated disease is called "monoclonal gammopathy of undetermined significance" (MGUS).* MGUS is the most common cause of monoclonal gammopathy.

Approximately 1% of patients with MGUS progress to an overt plasma cell dyscrasia (usually multiple myeloma) per year, a rate of conversion that remains roughly constant over up to 30 years.[38] Of pathogenic importance, the clonal plasma cells in MGUS often contain the same chromosomal aberrations (translocations involving the IgH locus and deletions of chromosome 13) that are seen in full-blown multiple myeloma,[39] further supporting the idea that MGUS is an early stage of myeloma development. The diagnosis of MGUS should be made only after careful exclusion of other causes of monoclonal gammopathy, particularly indolent multiple myeloma. In general, patients with MGUS have less than 3 gm/dL of monoclonal protein in the serum and no Bence Jones proteinuria.

Whether a given patient with MGUS will follow a benign course, as most do, or develop a well-defined plasma cell neoplasm cannot be predicted; hence, periodic assessment of serum M component levels and Bence Jones proteinuria is warranted.

Lymphoplasmacytic Lymphoma

Lymphoplasmacytic lymphoma is a B-cell neoplasm of older adults that usually presents in the sixth or seventh decade of life. It has gone by a variety of monikers, including small lymphocytic lymphoma with plasmacytic differentiation and immunocytoma. Although bearing a superficial resemblance to CLL/SLL, it differs in that a substantial fraction of the tumor cells undergo terminal differentiation to plasma cells. *Most commonly, the neoplastic plasma cells secrete monoclonal IgM, often in amounts sufficient to cause a hyperviscosity syndrome known as Waldenström macroglobulinemia.* Unlike multiple myeloma, heavy and light chain synthesis is usually balanced, and, therefore, complications stemming from the secretion of free light chains (e.g., renal failure and amyloidosis) are rare.

Morphology. Typically, the bone marrow contains a diffuse, sparse-to-heavy infiltrate of lymphocytes, plasma cells, and intermediate plasmacytoid lymphocytes, often accompanied by a reactive hyperplasia of mast cells (Fig. 14–18). The proportion of each of these cells may be quite variable, and some tumors also contain a population of larger lymphoid cells with more vesicular nuclear chromatin and prominent nucleoli. PAS-positive inclusions containing immunoglobulin are frequently seen in the cytoplasm (**Russell bodies**) or nucleus (**Dutcher bodies**) of plasmacytoid cells. Tumorous masses causing bony erosions, a hallmark of multiple myeloma, are absent. In addition to almost invariable involvement of marrow, the tumor is often disseminated to the lymph nodes, spleen, and liver at diagnosis. Infiltration of the nerve roots, meninges, and more rarely the brain can also occur with disease progression.

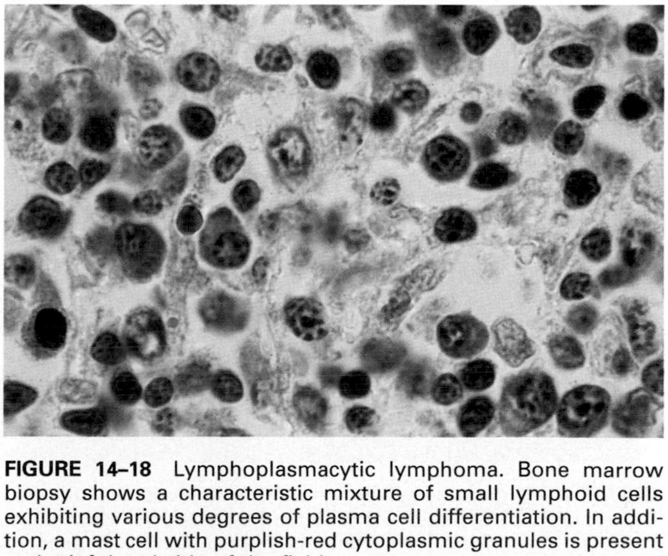

FIGURE 14–18 Lymphoplasmacytic lymphoma. Bone marrow biopsy shows a characteristic mixture of small lymphoid cells exhibiting various degrees of plasma cell differentiation. In addition, a mast cell with purplish-red cytoplasmic granules is present at the left-hand side of the field.

Immunophenotype and Molecular Genetics. The lymphocytic component of the tumor-cell infiltrate expresses B-cell markers such as CD20 and is usually negative for CD5 and CD10, whereas the plasma cell component expresses and secretes a monoclonal immunoglobulin. This tumor usually lacks chromosomal translocations or aberrant rearrangements involving the immunoglobulin loci; the most common cytogenetic abnormality is a deletion involving chromosome 6q.[40, 41]

Clinical Course. The dominant presenting complaints are weakness, fatigue, and weight loss—all nonspecific symptoms. Approximately half the patients have *lymphadenopathy, hepatomegaly*, and *splenomegaly.* Anemia caused by marrow infiltration is often present and can be exacerbated by *autoimmune hemolysis*, which is seen in about 10% of patients. Hemolysis is caused by *cold agglutinins*, IgM antibodies that bind to erythrocytes at temperatures of less than 37°C.

Patients with IgM-secreting tumors have additional complaints stemming from the physicochemical properties of macroglobulin. Because of its large size, at high concentrations IgM greatly increases the viscosity of the blood, giving rise to a *hyperviscosity syndrome* characterized by the following features:

- *Visual impairment* resulting from the striking tortuosity and distention of retinal veins; retinal hemorrhages and exudates can also contribute to the visual problems.
- *Neurologic problems* such as headaches, dizziness, deafness, and stupor, all stemming from sluggish blood flow and sludging.
- *Bleeding* related to the formation of complexes between macroglobulins and clotting factors as well as interference with platelet functions.
- *Cryoglobulinemia* resulting from precipitation of macroglobulins at low temperatures, producing symptoms such as Raynaud phenomenon and cold urticaria.

Lymphoplasmacytic lymphoma is an incurable progressive disease. Because most IgM is intravascular, symptoms caused by high IgM levels (such as hyperviscosity and hemolysis) can be alleviated by plasmapheresis. Transformation to large-cell lymphoma occurs uncommonly. Median survival is about 4 years.

Mantle Cell Lymphoma

Mantle cell lymphoma makes up about 3% of NHL in the United States and a somewhat higher fraction of NHL in Europe (7% to 9%). It usually presents in the fifth to sixth decades of life and shows a male predominance. As the name implies, *the tumor cells closely resemble the normal mantle zone B cells that surround germinal centers.*

Morphology. Tumor cells may surround reactive germinal centers, producing a vaguely nodular appearance at low power, or diffusely efface nodal architecture. **Typically, the proliferation consists of a homogeneous population of small lymphocytes with round to irregular to occasionally deeply clefted (cleaved) nuclear contours** (Fig. 14–19). Large cells resembling centroblasts are usually absent, as are proliferation centers, helping to distinguish mantle cell lymphoma from follicular lymphoma and chronic lymphocytic leukemia/small lymphocytic lymphoma, respectively. In most cases, the nuclear chromatin is condensed, nucleoli are inconspicuous, and the cytoplasm is scant. Occasionally, tumors composed of intermediate-sized cells with more open chromatin and a brisk mitotic rate are observed; immunophenotyping is necessary to distinguish these "blastic" mantle cell lymphoma variants from nodal acute lymphoblastic leukemia/lymphoma.

The majority of patients have generalized lymphadenopathy at diagnosis, with 20% to 40% having peripheral blood involvement. Frequent sites of extranodal involvement include the bone marrow, splenic white pulp zones, hepatic periportal areas, and the gut. Occasionally, multifocal mucosal involvement of the small bowel and colon produces "lymphomatoid polyposis"; of all forms of NHL, mantle cell lymphoma is most likely to spread in this fashion.

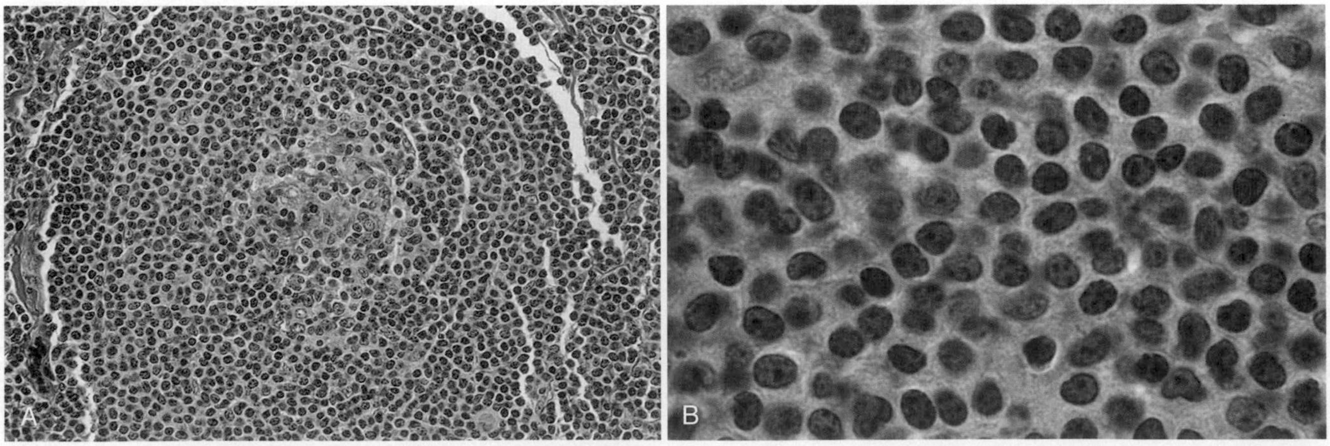

FIGURE 14–19 Mantle cell lymphoma. *A*, At low power, neoplastic lymphoid cells surround a small, atrophic germinal center, exhibiting a mantle zone pattern of growth. *B*, High-power view shows a homogeneous population of small lymphoid cells with somewhat irregular nuclear outlines, condensed chromatin, and scant cytoplasm. Large cells resembling prolymphocytes (seen in chronic lymphocytic leukemia) and centroblasts (seen in follicular lymphoma) are absent.

Immunophenotype. Mantle cell lymphoma expresses CD19, CD20, moderately high levels of surface immunoglobulin heavy chain (usually IgM and IgD), and either κ or λ light chain. It is usually CD5 positive and CD23 negative, which can help to distinguish it from chronic lymphocytic leukemia/small lymphocytic lymphoma. *It is also characteristically positive for cyclin D1 protein.* The rearranged IgH segments typically lack somatic mutations, supporting an origin from a naïve B cell.

Cytogenetic Abnormalities and Molecular Genetics. *Mantle cell lymphoma is associated with an (11;14) translocation involving the IgH locus on chromosome 14 and the cyclin D1 locus on chromosome 11.*[42] This translocation is detected in about 70% of cases by standard karyotyping and in an even higher fraction of tumors analyzed by fluorescence in situ hybridization. *The t(11;14) leads to increased expression of cyclin D1*, which promotes G1 to S phase progression during the cell cycle, as was described in Chapter 7.

Clinical Features. While the most common presentation is painless lymphadenopathy, symptoms related to splenomegaly (present in about 50% of cases) or involvement of the gastrointestinal tract are not unusual. The prognosis is generally poor, as the median survival is only 3 to 4 years. Mantle cell lymphoma is not curable with conventional chemotherapy, and most patients succumb eventually to organ dysfunction caused by tumor infiltration. For unclear reasons, histologic transformation is less frequent in mantle cell lymphoma than in other "indolent" B-cell lymphomas.

Marginal Zone Lymphomas

The category of marginal zone lymphoma encompasses a heterogeneous group of B-cell tumors that variously arise within the lymph nodes, spleen, or extranodal tissues. Because these tumors were initially recognized at mucosal sites, they have been referred to as tumors of mucosa-associated lymphoid tissues (or "maltoma"). In most cases, the predominant tumor cells resemble normal marginal zone B cells, which represent a postgerminal center memory B-cell population.

Although all marginal zone lymphomas share certain morphologic and immunophenotypic features, those occurring at extranodal sites deserve special attention because of their unusual pathogenesis. These tumors are exceptional in several regards: *(1) They often arise within tissues involved by chronic inflammatory disorders of autoimmune or infectious etiology.* Examples include tumors arising in the salivary gland in Sjögren disease, the thyroid gland in Hashimoto thyroiditis, and the stomach in *Helicobacter* gastritis. *(2) They remain localized for prolonged periods, spreading systemically only late in their course. (3) They may regress if the inciting agent (e.g.,* Helicobacter pylori*) is eradicated.*

The appearance of extranodal marginal zone lymphomas in chronically inflamed tissues has led to the suggestion that this neoplasm lies on a continuum between reactive lymphoid hyperplasia and full-blown B-cell lymphoma.[43] The process begins as a reactive, polyclonal immune reaction. With the acquisition of mutations and chromosomal aberrations over time, a monoclonal B-cell neoplasm emerges that is still dependent on reactive T-helper cells for growth and survival. In the case of gastric "maltomas," antibiotic therapy directed against *H. pylori* at this stage often leads to tumor regression. Some tumors acquire (11;18) or (1;14) chromosomal translocations, aberrations that are relatively specific for extranodal marginal zone lymphomas. "Maltomas" with the t(11;18) or t(1;14) no longer respond to antibiotic therapy, consistent with the idea that these mutations cause progression to a stage of tumor growth that is independent of extrinsic stimuli such as microbes and antigens. With further clonal evolution, spread to distant sites and transformation to diffuse large B-cell lymphoma may occur. This theme of polyclonal to monoclonal transition during lymphomagenesis is also applicable to the pathogenesis of EBV-induced lymphoma and was more fully discussed in Chapter 7.

Hairy Cell Leukemia

This rare but distinctive B-cell neoplasm constitutes about 2% of all leukemias. It is predominantly a disease of middle-aged Caucasian males (M:F ratio of 4:1).

Morphology. Hairy cell leukemia (HCL) derives its picturesque name from the appearance of the leukemic cells, which have fine hairlike projections that are best recognized under the phase-contrast microscope (Fig. 14–20). On routine peripheral blood smears, hairy cells have round, oblong, or reniform nuclei and modest amounts of pale blue cytoplasm, often with thread-like or bleb-like extensions. The number of circulating cells is highly variable. The bone marrow is always involved by a diffuse interstitial infiltrate of cells with oblong or reniform nuclei, condensed chromatin, and abundant pale cytoplasm. Because these cells are enmeshed in an extracellular matrix composed of reticulin fibrils, they usually cannot be aspirated from the bone marrow (a clinical difficulty referred to as a "dry tap"). The splenic red pulp is infiltrated preferentially, leading to a beefy red gross appearance and obliteration of white pulp. Hepatic portal triads are also involved frequently.

Immunophenotype and Molecular Characteristics. Hairy cells usually express the pan B-cell markers CD19 and CD20, surface IgH (usually IgG) and either κ or λ light chain, the monocyte-associated antigen CD11c, CD25 (the IL-2 receptor α chain), and CD103. Analysis of immunoglobulin gene sequences has revealed a high incidence of somatic hypermutation, suggesting a postgerminal center memory B-cell origin.

Clinical Features. Clinical manifestations result largely from infiltration of bone marrow, liver, and spleen. *Splenomegaly*, often massive, is the most common and sometimes the only abnormal physical finding. *Hepatomegaly* is less common and not as marked, and lymphadenopathy is distinctly rare. *Pancytopenia*, resulting from marrow failure and splenic sequestration, is seen in more than half the cases. About one third of those affected present with *infections.* There is an increased incidence of atypical mycobacterial infections,[44] possibly related in part to frequent monocytopenia.

HCL tends to follow an indolent course. For unclear reasons, the tumor cells are exceptionally sensitive to particular chemotherapeutic regimens, which produce long-lasting remissions in a majority of patients.[45] Whether such patients are truly cured is not yet known.

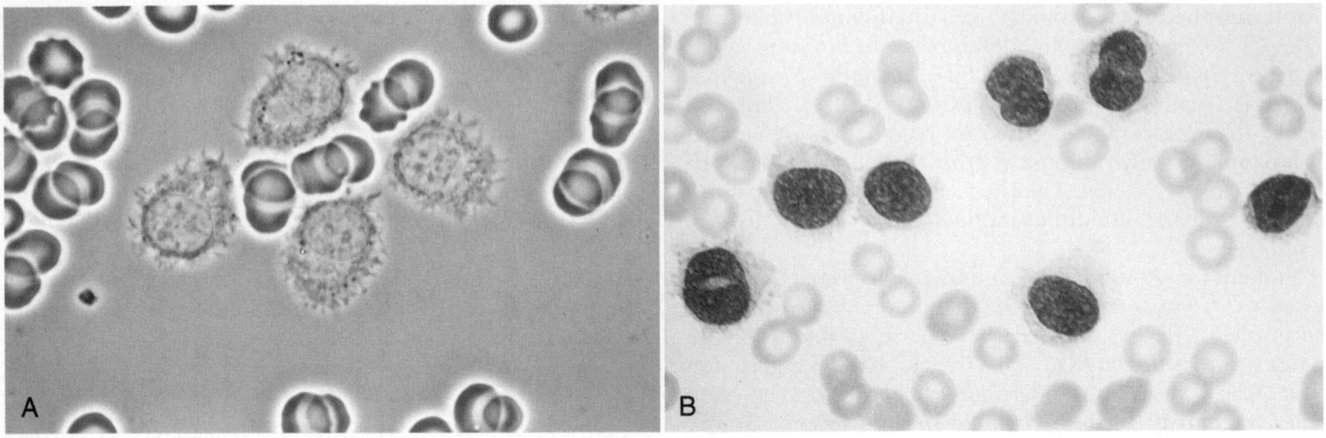

FIGURE 14–20 Hairy cell leukemia (peripheral blood smear). *A*, Phase-contrast microscopy shows tumor cells with fine hairlike cytoplasmic projections. *B*, In stained smears, these cells have round or folded nuclei and modest amounts of pale-blue, agranular cytoplasm. (Courtesy of Dr. David Weinberg, Department of Pathology, Brigham and Women's Hospital, Boston, MA.)

Peripheral T-Cell and NK-Cell Neoplasms

These categories include a heterogeneous group of neoplasms having phenotypes resembling mature T cells or natural killer (NK) cells, respectively. Peripheral T-cell tumors make up about 15% of NHLs in the United States and Europe but are substantially more common in Asia. NK-cell tumors are rare in the Western hemisphere but more common in the Far East. Only the more common entities and those of particular pathogenetic interest will be discussed.

Peripheral T-Cell Lymphoma, Unspecified

Although the WHO classification includes a number of distinct forms of peripheral T-cell neoplasia, peripheral T-cell lymphomas, as a group, are heterogeneous and not easily categorized. In recognition of this, a "wastebasket" diagnostic category, *peripheral T-cell lymphoma, unspecified*, has been created.

Although no morphologic feature is pathognomonic of peripheral T-cell lymphomas, certain findings are characteristic. The tumors diffusely efface the architecture of involved lymph nodes and are typically composed of a pleomorphic mixture of small, intermediate, and large-sized malignant T cells (Fig. 14–21). They can have a prominent infiltrate of reactive cells such as eosinophils and macrophages, probably attracted by T cell–derived cytokines. Prominent angiogenesis is also seen sometimes.

The diagnosis can be confirmed only by immunophenotyping. By definition, all peripheral T-cell lymphomas have a mature T-cell phenotype, lacking TdT and usually expressing CD2, CD5, surface CD3, and either $\alpha\beta$ or $\gamma\delta$ T-cell receptors. In some instances, expression of CD4 or CD8 is observed; such tumors are likely of helper T-cell or cytotoxic T-cell origin, respectively. However, many tumors have phenotypes that do not resemble any known normal peripheral T cell. DNA analyses usually reveal monoclonal rearrangements of at least one T-cell receptor locus.

Most patients present with generalized lymphadenopathy, sometimes accompanied by eosinophilia, pruritus, fever, and weight loss. Although cures of peripheral T-cell lymphoma have been reported, these tumors have a significantly worse prognosis than comparably aggressive mature B-cell neoplasms (e.g., diffuse large B-cell lymphoma).[9]

Anaplastic Large Cell Lymphoma

This entity merits brief mention because of its unique biology and strong association with rearrangements involving the *ALK* gene on chromosome 2p23.[46] Such rearrangements break the *ALK* locus and lead to the formation of chimeric genes encoding ALK fusion proteins, which behave as constitutively active tyrosine kinases. Among the lymphoid neoplasms, *ALK* rearrangements are specific for this entity.

As the name implies, this tumor often comprises large anaplastic cells, some of which typically contain horseshoe-shaped nuclei and voluminous cytoplasm (so-called hallmark cells) (Fig. 14–22*A*). The tumor cells sometimes cluster

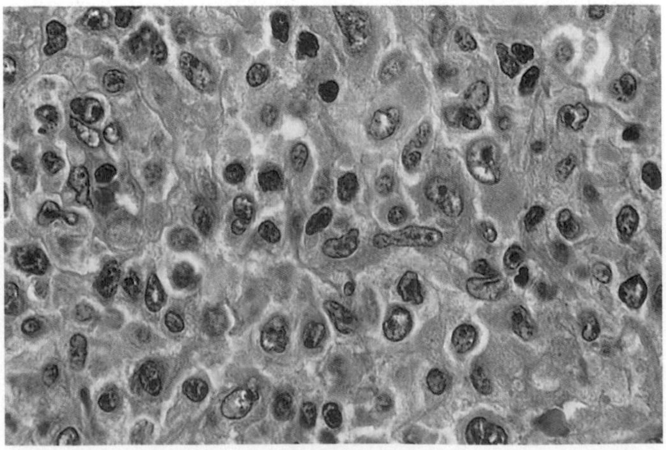

FIGURE 14–21 Peripheral T-cell lymphoma, unspecified (lymph node). A spectrum of small, intermediate, and large lymphoid cells, many with irregular nuclear contours, is seen.

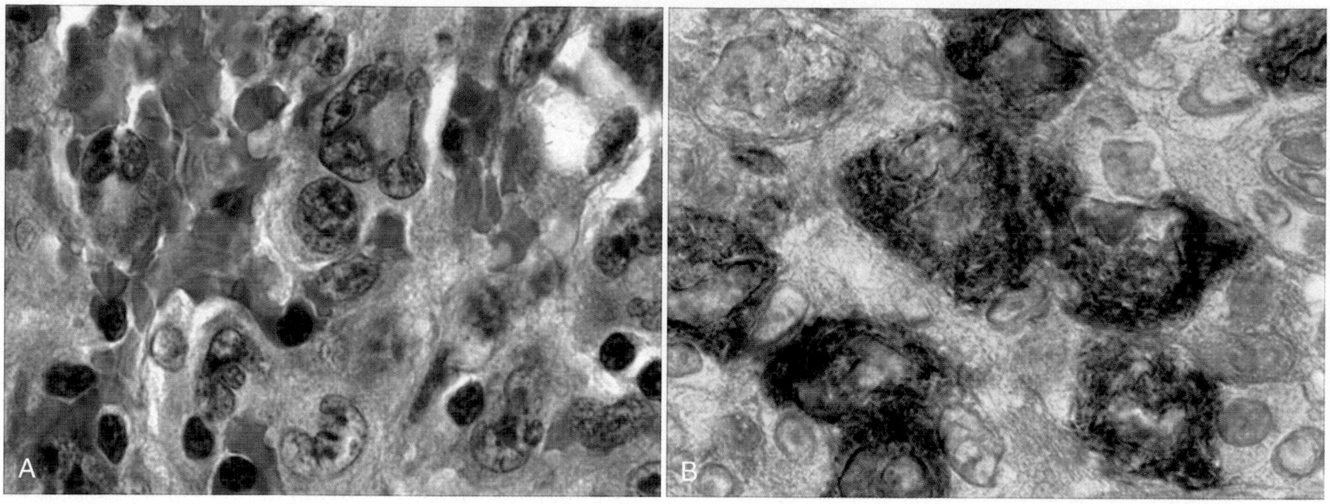

FIGURE 14–22 Anaplastic large cell lymphoma. *A*, Several "hallmark" cells with horseshoe-like or "embryo-like" nuclei and abundant cytoplasm lie near the center of the field. *B*, Immunohistochemical stain demonstrating expression of ALK protein. (Courtesy of Dr. Jeffrey Kutok, Department of Pathology, Brigham and Women's Hospital, Boston, MA.)

about venules and infiltrate lymphoid sinuses, mimicking the appearance of metastatic carcinoma.

It should be noted that only a subset of T-cell lymphomas with anaplastic morphology have *ALK* rearrangements or express ALK fusion proteins (Fig. 14–22*B*). Those with *ALK* rearrangements tend to occur in children or young adults, frequently involve soft tissues, and carry a very good prognosis (unlike other aggressive peripheral T-cell neoplasms), with a 75% to 80% cure rate with chemotherapy. Those lacking *ALK* rearrangements occur in older adults and have a poor prognosis, similar to that of peripheral T-cell lymphoma, not otherwise specified.

Adult T-Cell Leukemia/Lymphoma

This neoplasm of CD4+ T cells is observed in adults infected by *human T-cell leukemia virus type 1 (HTLV-1)*, as was discussed in Chapter 7. It is most frequent in regions where HTLV-1 is endemic (southern Japan, West Africa, and the Caribbean basin) and is characterized by skin lesions, generalized lymphadenopathy, hepatosplenomegaly, peripheral blood lymphocytosis, and hypercalcemia. The appearance of the tumor cells varies widely, but cells with multilobated nuclei, described as "cloverleaf" or "flower" cells, are frequently found in involved tissues and peripheral blood. Less commonly, multinucleated giant cells resembling Reed-Sternberg cells may be present. *The tumor cells contain clonal HTLV-1 provirus, compatible with direct pathogenic involvement of the virus in this neoplasm.*

Most patients present with rapidly progressive disease that is fatal within months to 1 year despite aggressive chemotherapy. Less commonly, the tumor primarily involves the skin and follows a much more indolent course resembling mycosis fungoides. It should be noted that, in addition to causing lymphoid malignancies, HTLV-1 infection can give rise to a progressive demyelinating disease affecting the central nervous system and the spinal cord (see Chapter 28).

Mycosis Fungoides/Sézary Syndrome

Mycosis fungoides and Sézary syndrome are different manifestations of a tumor of CD4+ helper T cells characterized by a marked predilection to involve the skin. Clinically, the cutaneous lesions of *mycosis fungoides* show three somewhat distinct stages, which are discussed in Chapter 25. Briefly, mycosis fungoides presents with an inflammatory *premycotic phase* and progresses through a *plaque phase* to a *tumor phase*. Histologically, there is infiltration of the epidermis and upper dermis by neoplastic T cells, which usually have nuclei with a cerebriform appearance due to marked infolding of the nuclear membrane. Disease progression is characterized by extracutaneous spread, most commonly to lymph nodes and bone marrow.

Sézary syndrome is a variant in which skin involvement is manifested as a *generalized exfoliative erythroderma*. In contrast to mycosis fungoides, the skin lesions rarely proceed to tumefaction. In addition, *there is an associated leukemia of "Sézary" cells* with characteristic cerebriform nuclei. Small numbers of circulating tumor cells can also be identified in peripheral smears in up to 25% of cases of mycosis fungoides in the plaque or tumor phase, emphasizing the overlap between mycosis fungoides and Sézary syndrome.

Although cutaneous disease dominates the clinical picture in these disorders, sensitive molecular analyses have shown that tumor cells are found early in the disease course in blood, bone marrow, and lymph nodes. The basis for the striking epidermotropism is uncertain; tumor cells may preferentially home to skin or be dependent on skin-specific factors for growth or survival. These are indolent tumors with a median survival rate of 8 to 9 years. Transformation to large cell lymphoma of T-cell type occasionally occurs as a terminal event.

Large Granular Lymphocytic Leukemia

This rare neoplasm has gone by a variety of names, including Tγ lymphoproliferative disease, CD8 lymphocytosis, and

CD8+ T-CLL. *Two variants are recognized, T cell and natural killer (NK) cell,* both of which occur mainly in adults.[2] Patients with T-cell disease usually present with mild to moderate lymphocytosis and splenomegaly; lymphadenopathy and hepatomegaly are usually absent. NK-cell disease often presents in an even more subtle fashion, with little or no lymphocytosis or splenomegaly.

The cytologic hallmark is the presence of lymphocytes in the peripheral blood and bone marrow with abundant blue cytoplasm containing scattered coarse azurophilic granules. Marrow involvement is usually focal, without physical displacement of normal hematopoietic elements. The splenic red pulp and hepatic sinusoids are also usually infiltrated.

Despite the relative paucity of marrow infiltration, neutropenia and anemia dominate the clinical picture. Neutropenia is often accompanied by a striking decrease in late myeloid forms in the bone marrow; the mechanism by which this occurs is uncertain. Less commonly, LGL is associated with pure red cell aplasia. *An increased incidence of rheumatologic disorders has also been observed in LGL.* Some patients with Felty syndrome, characterized by the triad of rheumatoid arthritis, splenomegaly, and neutropenia, have LGL as an underlying cause.

The course of LGL is variable, being largely dependent on the severity of the cytopenias and their responsiveness to low-dose chemotherapy or steroids. In general, LGLs of T-cell origin pursue an indolent course, whereas NK-cell tumors often behave in an aggressive fashion.

Extranodal NK/T-Cell Lymphoma

This neoplasm (previously called *lethal midline granuloma* and *midline malignant reticulosis*) is rare in the United States and Europe but constitutes up to 3% of NHLs in Asia. Most commonly presenting as a destructive midline mass involving the nasopharynx or, less commonly, the skin or other extranodal sites such as the testis, *the tumor cell infiltrate typically surrounds and invades small vessels, leading to extensive ischemic necrosis.* The neoplastic elements can consist of either a mixture of small and large lymphoid cells or predominantly large lymphoid cells. On touch preparations, the cytoplasm of the tumor cells contains *large azurophilic granules* resembling those observed in normal NK cells.

Most tumors express NK-cell markers, including a restricted set of killer cell immunoglobulin-like receptors,[47] and lack T-cell receptor rearrangements, supporting a NK-cell origin. Individual tumors contain identical EBV episomes, a finding indicative of an origin from a single EBV-infected cell. Acquired mutations in the *cKIT* proto-oncogene [48] and epigenetic silencing of the tumor suppressor gene *p73*,[49] a homologue of *p53*, have also been proposed to contribute to the pathogenesis of this neoplasm.

Although sinonasal NK/T-cell lymphomas sometimes follow an indolent course, most are aggressive and poorly responsive to therapy.

This ends the discussion of the lymphocytic leukemias and the NHLs, which are summarized in Table 14–4. We will now turn to the second major category of lymphoma: Hodgkin lymphoma.

Hodgkin Lymphoma

The term "Hodgkin lymphoma" (HL), previously known as Hodgkin disease, encompasses a group of lymphoid neoplasms that differ from NHL in several respects. While NHLs frequently occur at extranodal sites and spread in an unpredictable fashion, HL arises in a single node or chain of nodes and spreads first to the anatomically contiguous nodes. It is characterized morphologically by the presence of distinctive neoplastic giant cells called *Reed-Sternberg cells* that induce the accumulation of reactive lymphocytes, histiocytes (macrophages), and granulocytes. The neoplastic Reed-Sternberg cells typically make up a minor fraction (1% to 5%) of the total tumor cell mass, making HL more difficult to study than typical NHLs. However, it is now clear that in the vast majority of cases, the neoplastic Reed-Sternberg cells are derived from germinal center or post-germinal center B cells,[50] indicating that most HLs are unusual tumors of B-cell origin.

HL accounts for 0.7% of all new cancers in the United States, with approximately 7400 new cases reported per year. It is one of the most common forms of malignancy in young adults, with an average age at diagnosis of 32 years. Much progress has been made in the treatment of this disease in the last several decades, and it is now curable in most cases.

Classification. The WHO classification recognizes five subtypes of HL:

- Nodular sclerosis
- Mixed cellularity
- Lymphocyte-rich
- Lymphocyte depletion
- Lymphocyte predominance

In the first four subtypes—nodular sclerosis, mixed cellularity, lymphocyte-rich, and lymphocyte depletion—the Reed-Sternberg cells have a similar immunophenotype; as a result, these subtypes are often lumped together as *classical* forms of HL. In lymphocyte predominance HL, the Reed-Sternberg cells have a characteristic B-cell immunophenotype distinct from that of the classical HL subtypes.

Before describing the various subtypes of HL in detail, we will first review the morphology and immunophenotype of the Reed-Sternberg cell and its variants and the staging system used to characterize the extent of HL in the patient.

Morphology. Identification of Reed-Sternberg cells and their variants is essential for the histologic diagnosis. **Diagnostic Reed-Sternberg cells are large (15 to 45 μm in diameter) and have either multiple nuclei or a single nucleus with multiple nuclear lobes, each with a large inclusion-like nucleolus about the size of a small lymphocyte (5–7 μm in diameter)** (Fig. 14–23*A*). The cytoplasm is abundant. Several variants of Reed-Sternberg cells are also recognized. **Mononuclear variants** contain only a single round or oblong nucleus with a large inclusionlike nucleolus (Fig. 14–23*B*). **Lacunar cells**, seen predominantly in the nodular sclerosis subtype, have more delicate folded or multilobate nuclei surrounded by abundant pale cytoplasm that is often disrupted during the cutting of sections, leaving the nucleus sitting in an empty hole (the lacune) (Fig. 14–23*C*). In classical forms of HL, Reed-Sternberg cells undergo a peculiar form of cell death in which the cells shrink and become pyknotic,

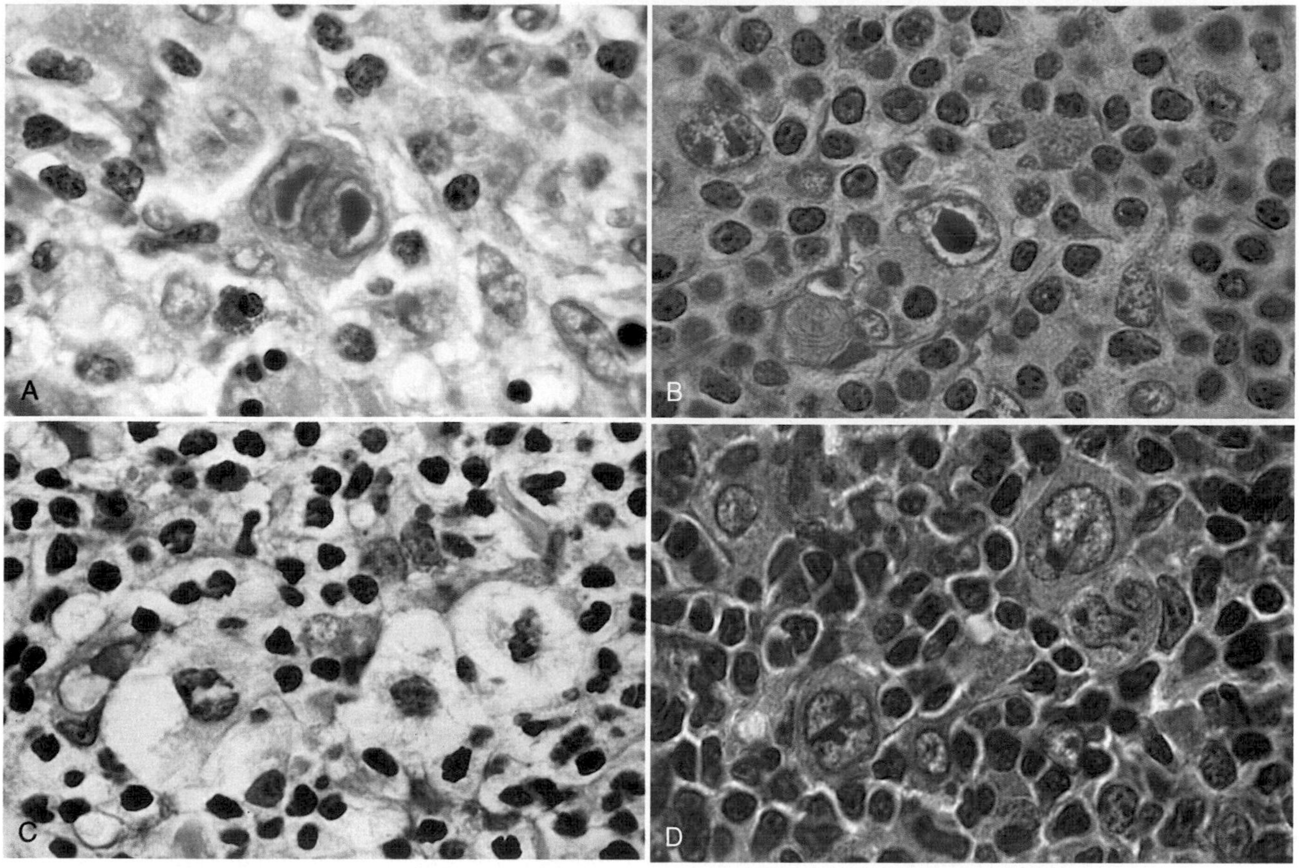

FIGURE 14–23 Reed-Sternberg cells and variants. *A*, Diagnostic Reed-Sternberg cell, with two nuclear lobes, large inclusion-like nucleoli, and abundant cytoplasm, surrounded by lymphocytes, macrophages, and an eosinophil. *B*, Reed-Sternberg cell, mononuclear variant. *C*, Reed-Sternberg cell, lacunar variant. This variant is characteristic of the nodular sclerosis subtype. It has a folded or multilobated nucleus lying within a clear space created by disruption of its cytoplasm during processing and cutting of the tissue. *D*, Reed-Sternberg cell, lymphohistiocytic (L&H) variant. Several such variants are present with complex nuclear irregularities, small nucleoli, fine chromatin, and abundant pale cytoplasm. (*A*, courtesy of Dr. Robert W. McKenna, Department of Pathology, University of Texas Southwestern Medical School, Dallas, TX.)

a process described as "mummification." **Lymphohistocytic variants (L&H cells)** with polypoid nuclei resembling popcorn kernels, inconspicuous nucleoli, and moderately abundant cytoplasm are specific to the lymphocyte predominance subtype (Fig. 14–23*D*).

The morphologic diagnosis of HL is complicated by the occasional presence of cells that are similar or identical in appearance to Reed-Sternberg cells in other conditions, such as infectious mononucleosis, solid tissue cancers, and NHL. **Thus, although Reed-Sternberg cells are requisite for the diagnosis, they must be present in an appropriate background of non-neoplastic inflammatory cells (lymphocytes, plasma cells, eosinophils).** In difficult cases, immunohistochemical markers and molecular genetic studies help in establishing the diagnosis.

The spread of HL is remarkably predictable: nodal disease first, then splenic disease, hepatic disease, and finally marrow involvement and extranodal disease. Because of this uniform pattern of spread, patients with limited disease may be cured with local radiotherapy. For this reason, the **staging of HL** (Table 14–5) is not only predictive of prognosis but also guides the choice of therapy. Staging involves careful physical examination and several investigative procedures, including radiologic imaging of the abdomen, pelvis, and chest and biopsy of the bone marrow. Systemic treatment is preferred whenever the staging is equivocal. The presence of constitutional symptoms (fever, night sweats, and weight loss) is characteristic of HL but can also be seen in other lymphoid neoplasms.

With this background, we can turn to the morphologic classification of HL into its subgroups and point out some of the salient immunophenotypic and clinical features of each (summarized in Table 14–6). The clinical manifestations common to all will be presented later.

Hodgkin Lymphoma, Nodular Sclerosis Type. This is the most common form of HL, constituting 65% to 70% of cases. It is characterized morphologically by the presence of (1) a particular variant of the Reed-Sternberg cell, the lacunar cell, and (2) collagen bands that divide the lymphoid tissue into circumscribed nodules (Fig. 14–24). The fibrosis can be scant or abundant, and the neoplastic cells are found in a polymorphous background of small T lymphocytes,

TABLE 14–5 Clinical Staging of Hodgkin and Non-Hodgkin Lymphomas (Ann Arbor Classification)

Stage	Distribution of Disease
I	Involvement of a single lymph node region (I) or involvement of a single extralymphatic organ or site (IE).
II	Involvement of two or more lymph node regions on the same side of the diaphragm alone (II) or with involvement of limited contiguous extralymphatic organ or tissue (IIE).
III	Involvement of lymph node regions on both sides of the diaphragm (III), which may include the spleen (IIIS) and/or limited contiguous extralymphatic organ or site (IIIE, IIIES).
IV	Multiple or disseminated foci of involvement of one or more extralymphatic organs or tissues with or without lymphatic involvement.

All stages are further divided on the basis of the absence (A) or presence (B) of the following systemic symptoms: significant fever, night sweats, and/or unexplained weight loss of greater than 10% of normal body weight.

Data from Carbone PT, et al: Symposium (Ann Arbor): Staging in Hodgkin's disease. Cancer Res 31:1707, 1971.

eosinophils, plasma cells, and macrophages. Diagnostic Reed-Sternberg cells are less frequent than in the mixed cellularity and lymphocyte depletion types. The tumor cells have a characteristic immunophenotype: positive for CD15 and CD30 and negative for CD45 and B-cell and T-cell markers. As in other forms of HL, involvement of the spleen, liver, bone marrow, and other organs and tissues can appear in due course and take the form of irregular tumor nodules resembling those present in the nodes.

The nodular sclerosis type occurs with equal frequency in males and females. It has a propensity to involve the lower cervical, supraclavicular, and mediastinal lymph nodes of adolescents or young adults and is only rarely associated with EBV. The prognosis is excellent.

Hodgkin Lymphoma, Mixed Cellularity Type. This form of HL constitutes about 20% to 25% of cases. Lymph node involvement by the mixed cellularity type takes the form of **diffuse effacement** by a heterogeneous cellular infiltrate, which includes small lymphocytes, eosinophils, plasma cells, and benign macrophages admixed with the neoplastic cells (Fig. 14–25). **Diagnostic Reed-Sternberg cells and mononuclear variants are usually plentiful.** The immunophenotype is identical to that observed in the nodular sclerosis type. Small lymphocytes in the background are predominantly T cells, and early nodal disease preferentially involves paracortical T-cell zones.

Mixed cellularity HL is more common in males and strongly associated with EBV, as the Reed-Sternberg cells contain EBV genomes in at least 70% of cases. Compared to the lymphocyte predominance and nodular sclerosis subtypes, it is more likely to be associated with older age, systemic symptoms such as night sweats and weight loss, and advanced tumor stage. Nonetheless, the prognosis is very good.

Hodgkin Lymphoma, Lymphocyte-Rich Type. This is an uncommon form of classical HL in which reac-

TABLE 14–6 Classification of Hodgkin Lymphoma

Subtype	Morphology and Immunophenotype	Typical Clinical Features
Nodular sclerosis	Frequent lacunar cells and occasional diagnostic R-S cells; background infiltrate composed of T lymphocytes, eosinophils, macrophages and plasma cells; fibrous bands dividing cellular areas into nodules. R-S cells CD15+, CD30+; EBV–.	Stage 1 or 2 disease most common. Frequent mediastinal involvement. F = M, most patients young adults
Mixed cellularity	Frequent mononuclear and diagnostic R-S cells; background infiltrate rich in T lymphocytes, eosinophils, macrophages, plasma cells. R-S cells CD15+, CD30+; 70% EBV+.	More than 50% present as stage 3 or 4 disease. M > F. Biphasic incidence, peaking in young adults and again in adults older than 55.
Lymphocyte-rich	Frequent mononuclear and diagnostic R-S cells; background infiltrate rich in T lymphocytes. R-S cells CD15+, CD30+; 40% EBV+.	Uncommon. M > F. Tends to be seen in older adults.
Lymphocyte depletion	Reticular variant: Frequent diagnostic R-S cells and variants with a paucity of background reactive cells; diffuse fibrosis variant; hypocellular fibrillar background with scattered diagnostic R-S cells and variants and few reactive cells. R-S cells CD15+, CD30+; most EBV+.	Uncommon. More common in older males, HIV-infected individuals, and in developing countries. More likely to present with advanced disease.
Lymphocyte predominance	Frequent L&H (popcorn cell) variants in a background of follicular dendritic cells and reactive B cells. R-S cells CD20+, CD15–, C30–; EBV–.	Uncommon. Young males with cervical or axillary lymphadenopathy. Mediastinal involvement rare.

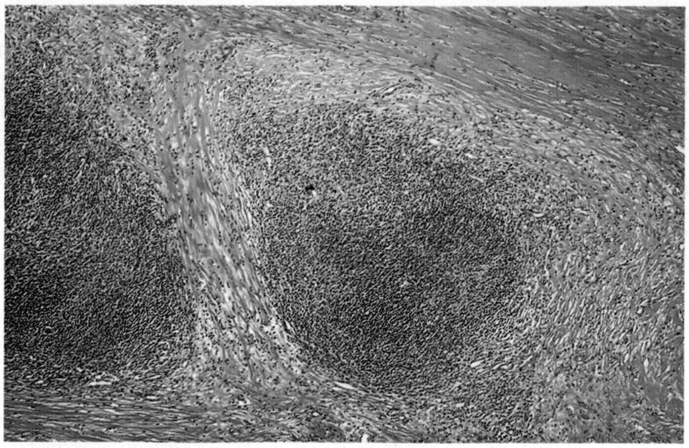

FIGURE 14–24 Hodgkin lymphoma, nodular sclerosis type. A low-power view shows well-defined bands of pink, acellular collagen that subdivide the tumor cells and associated reactive infiltrate into nodules. (Courtesy of Dr. Robert W. McKenna, Department of Pathology, University of Texas Southwestern Medical School, Dallas, TX.)

tive lymphocytes make up the vast majority of the cellular infiltrate. In most cases, lymph nodes are diffusely effaced, but vague nodularity due to the presence of residual B-cell follicles can sometimes be seen. This entity is distinguished from the lymphocyte predominance type by the presence of frequent mononuclear and diagnostic Reed-Sternberg cells with the characteristic CD45–, CD20–, CD15+, CD30+ immunophenotype. It is associated with EBV in about 40% of cases and also has a very good to excellent prognosis.

Hodgkin Lymphoma, Lymphocyte Depletion Type. This least common form of HL, amounting to less than 5% of cases, is characterized by a paucity of lymphocytes and a relative abundance of Reed-Sternberg cells or their pleomorphic variants. The phenotype of the tumor cells is identical to that observed in the nodular sclerosis and mixed cellularity types. Phenotyping is critical for the diagnosis, since most tumors suspected of being lymphocyte depletion HL actually prove to be large-cell non-Hodgkin lymphomas.

Lymphocyte depletion HL is observed predominantly in older patients, HIV-positive individuals, or patients in nonindustrialized countries and is often EBV-associated. Advanced stage and systemic symptoms are frequent, and the overall outcome is somewhat less favorable than with other subtypes.

Hodgkin Lymphoma, Lymphocyte Predominance Type. This uncommon variant, accounting for approximately 5% of all cases, is characterized by nodal effacement by a nodular infiltrate of small lymphocytes admixed with variable numbers of benign histiocytes (Fig. 14–26). Typical Reed-Sternberg cells are extremely difficult to find. More common are so-called lymphohistiocytic (L&H) variants that have a delicate, multilobed nucleus resembling a popcorn kernel ("popcorn cell"). Other cells such as eosinophils, neutrophils, and plasma cells are scanty or absent, and there is little evidence of necrosis or fibrosis.

Multiple features of L&H Reed-Sternberg variants point to an origin from germinal center B cells. In contrast to other forms of HL, L&H variants express B-cell markers (e.g., CD20) and the germinal center–specific transcription factor BCL6. The nodular pattern of nodal effacement is due to the presence of expanded B-cell follicles, which are populated not only with L&H variants, but also with numerous reactive B cells. Furthermore, L&H variants within individual tumors have identical IgH gene rearrangements and have V_H segments that show evidence of ongoing somatic hypermutation,[51] a modification that occurs only in

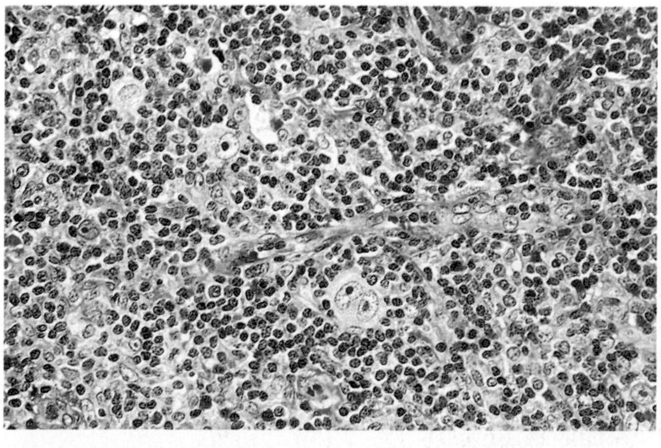

FIGURE 14–25 Hodgkin lymphoma, mixed cellularity type. A diagnostic, binucleate Reed-Sternberg cell is surrounded by reactive cells, including eosinophils (bright red cytoplasm), lymphocytes, and histiocytes. (Courtesy of Dr. Robert W. McKenna, Department of Pathology, University of Texas Southwestern Medical School, Dallas, TX.)

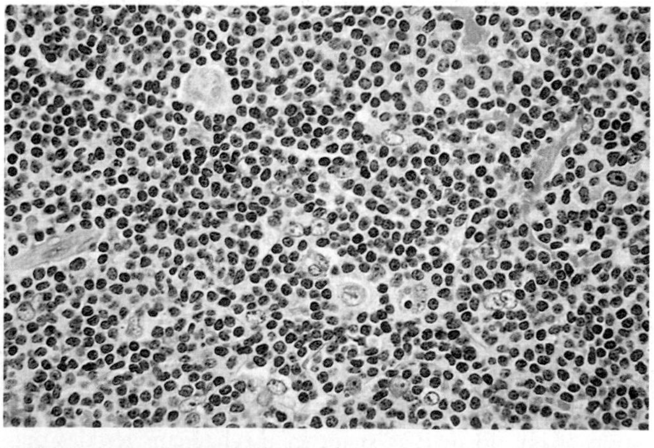

FIGURE 14–26 Hodgkin lymphoma, lymphocyte predominance type. Numerous mature-looking lymphocytes surround scattered, large, pale-staining L&H variants ("popcorn" cells). (Courtesy of Dr. Robert W. McKenna, Department of Pathology, University of Texas Southwestern Medical School, Dallas, TX.)

germinal center B cells. Finally, in 3% to 5% of cases the lymphocyte predominance type transforms to diffuse large B-cell lymphoma. EBV is not associated with this form of HL.

A majority of patients are males, usually younger than 35 years of age, who typically present with cervical or axillary lymphadenopathy. Mediastinal and bone marrow involvement is rare. In some series, this form of HL is more likely to recur than the classical subtypes, but the prognosis is excellent.

Etiology and Pathogenesis. The origin of the neoplastic Reed-Sternberg cells of classical HL has historically been extremely controversial, in large part because these cells fail to express many markers found on normal lymphocytes. This issue was settled only recently through elegant studies relying on the microdissection and analysis of single isolated Reed-Sternberg cells and variants. These studies have shown that within most individual cases, all Reed-Sternberg cells harbor identical rearranged immunoglobulin genes that show evidence of somatic hypermutation, establishing the cell of origin as a germinal center or post-germinal center B cell.[50] In a small proportion of cases (1% to 2%), Reed-Sternberg cells have immunoglobulin genes in the germ line configuration and instead have T-cell receptor rearrangements,[52, 53] suggesting that HL arises in rare instances from transformed T cells. Although of B-cell origin in the large majority of cases, Reed-Sternberg cells fail to express many genes that are normally turned on in germinal center or post-germinal center B cells, including the immunoglobulin genes themselves.[54, 55] The basis and significance of this wholesale reprogramming of gene expression are unknown but are likely key to understanding the biology of classical forms of HL.

Because Reed-Sternberg cells are difficult to study and animal models of HL do not yet exist, relatively little is known about the factors that contribute to their transformation. One important clue is the frequent presence of EBV episomes in the Reed-Sternberg cells of many cases of mixed cellularity HL.[56] Importantly, the configuration of the EBV DNA is the same in all tumor cells within a given case, indicating that infection occurs before cellular transformation. EBV-positive tumor cells express latent membrane protein-1 (LMP-1), a protein encoded by the EBV genome that has transforming activity.[57] LMP-1 transmits signals that upregulate NF-κB, a transcription factor of broad importance in lymphocyte activation. Of note, activation of NF-κB also occurs in EBV-negative tumors,[58] in some instances due to acquired mutations in a negative regulator of NF-κB, IκB.[59, 60] Hence, inappropriate activation of NF-κB appears to be a common event in classical HL.[61] In some cases of HL, the immunoglobulin genes of Reed-Sternberg cells contain "crippling" somatic mutations that prevent expression of surface immunoglobulin, which is normally needed for production of signals that permit the survival of germinal center B cells. It has been suggested that activation of NF-κB by EBV or other mechanisms rescues these doomed cells from apoptosis, somehow setting the stage for acquisition of other unknown mutations that collaborate to produce Reed-Sternberg cells.

The characteristic accumulation of reactive cells occurs in response to *cytokines* secreted by the Reed-Sternberg cells, such as IL-5, IL-6, IL-13, tumor necrosis factor (TNF), and GM-CSF. Once attracted by cytokines, the reactive infiltrate in turn supports the growth and survival of tumor cells. For example, reactive eosinophils and T cells express ligands for the CD30 and CD40 receptor, respectively, each of which produces signals that lead to the activation of NF-κB. Other factors, particularly chemokines and their cognate receptors, are also likely to be important in governing the interaction of Reed-Sternberg cells and surrounding reactive cells. Examples of proposed pathogenic "cross-talk" between Reed-Sternberg cells and surrounding reactive cells are summarized in Figure 14–27.

Reed-Sternberg cells are aneuploid and often possess diverse clonal chromosomal aberrations. Gains of chromosome 2p, the site of the *c-REL* proto-oncogene, are particularly common and may also act to upregulate NF-κB activity.[62, 63]

Clinical Course. HL, like NHL, usually presents with a painless enlargement of lymph nodes. Although the distinction between HL and NHL can be made only by examination of a lymph node biopsy, several clinical features favor the diagnosis of HL (Table 14–7). Younger patients with the more favorable histologic types tend to present with stage I or II disease and are usually free from systemic manifestations. Patients with disseminated disease (stages III and IV) or the mixed cellularity or lymphocyte depletion subtype are more likely to have systemic symptoms such as night sweats and weight loss. One rare paraneoplastic symptom specific to HL is pain in involved lymph nodes on consumption of alcohol. Cutaneous anergy resulting from depressed cell-mediated immunity is seen in most cases. The basis for immune dysfunction is not understood, but it tends to persist even in successfully treated patients, possibly indicating that HL arises in the background of an underlying immune abnormality.

With current treatment protocols, tumor stage rather than histologic type is the most important prognostic variable. The cure rate of patients with stages I and IIA is close to 90%. Even with advanced disease (stages IVA and IVB), 60% to 70% 5-year disease-free survival is obtained.

Progress in the treatment of HL has created a new set of problems. Long-term survivors of chemotherapy and radiotherapy have an increased risk of developing second cancers. Myelodysplastic syndromes, acute myelogenous leukemia (AML), and lung cancer lead the list of second malignancies, but also included are NHL, breast cancer, gastric cancer, sarcoma, and malignant melanoma.[64] The risk of breast cancer is particularly high in females treated with radiation to the chest during adolescence,[65] and the risk of other solid tumors also seems to correlate with radiotherapy, whereas alkylating chemotherapeutic drugs appear to be responsible for the increased risk of acute myelogenous leukemia and myelodysplasia. Non-neoplastic complications of radiotherapy include pulmonary fibrosis and accelerated atherosclerosis. New combinations of chemotherapeutic drugs and more judicious use of radiotherapy may avoid these complications and yet be equally curative.

MYELOID NEOPLASMS

The common feature that unites this heterogeneous group of neoplasms is an origin from hematopoietic progenitor cells capable of giving rise to terminally differentiated cells of the

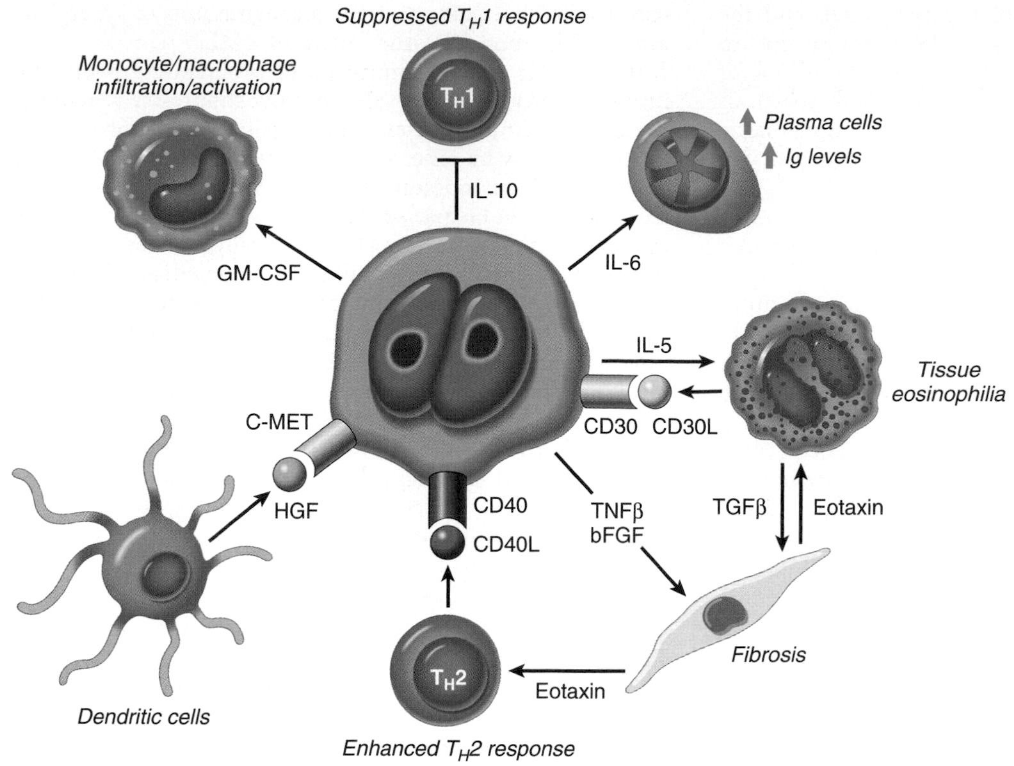

FIGURE 14–27 Proposed signals mediating "cross-talk" between Reed-Sternberg cells and surrounding normal cells in classical forms of Hodgkin lymphoma. bFGF, basic fibroblast growth factor; GM-CSF, granulocyte-macrophage colony-stimulating factor; HGF, hepatocyte growth factor (binds to the C-MET receptor); TNFβ, tumor necrosis factor β (lymphotoxin); TGFβ, transforming growth factor β.

TABLE 14–7 Clinical Differences Between Hodgkin and Non-Hodgkin Lymphomas

Hodgkin Lymphoma	Non-Hodgkin Lymphoma
More often localized to a single axial group of nodes (cervical, mediastinal, para-aortic)	More frequent involvement of multiple peripheral nodes
Orderly spread by contiguity	Noncontiguous spread
Mesenteric nodes and Waldeyer ring rarely involved	Waldeyer ring and mesenteric nodes commonly involved
Extranodal involvement uncommon	Extranodal involvement common

myeloid series (erythrocytes, granulocytes, monocytes, and platelets). These diseases primarily involve the bone marrow and to a lesser degree the secondary hematopoietic organs (the spleen, liver, and lymph nodes) and present with altered hematopoiesis. Three broad categories of myeloid neoplasia exist:

- *Acute myelogenous leukemias*, characterized by the accumulation of immature myeloid forms in the bone marrow and the suppression of normal hematopoiesis
- *Myelodysplastic syndromes*, associated with ineffective hematopoiesis and associated cytopenias
- *Chronic myeloproliferative disorders*, usually associated with an increased production of terminally differentiated myeloid cells

The pathogenesis of myeloid neoplasms is best understood in the context of normal hematopoiesis, which (you will remember from Chapter 13) involves a hierarchy of hematopoietic progenitor cells. At the top of the hierarchy sits the pluripotent stem cell, which gives rise to multipotent progenitor cells committed to lymphoid or myeloid differentiation. The latter in turn produce more committed progenitors, which eventually give rise to terminally differentiated cells of a single type (e.g., erythrocyte, monocyte). In addition to giving rise to committed daughter cells, hematopoietic progenitor cells must also replicate themselves without differentiating (or else they would eventually disappear), a process known as self-renewal.

Normal hematopoiesis is finely tuned by homeostatic feedback mechanisms involving cytokines and growth factors that modulate the marrow output of red cells, granulocytes, and platelets. These mechanisms are deranged in marrows involved by myeloid neoplasms, which "escape" from normal homeostatic controls on growth and survival, and suppress the function of residual normal stem cells. The specific manifestations of the different myeloid neoplasms are further influenced by *(1) the position of the transformed cell within the hierarchy of progenitors* and *(2) the effect of the transforming events on differentiation programs, which may be blocked or preferentially shunted toward one lineage at the expense of others.* We will return to these themes as each type of myeloid neoplasm is discussed.

Given that all myeloid neoplasms originate from a transformed hematopoietic progenitor cell, it should come as no surprise that divisions between these neoplasms are sometimes blurred. Myeloid neoplasms, like other malignancies, tend to evolve over time to more aggressive forms of disease.

In particular, both the myelodysplastic syndromes and the chronic myeloproliferative disorders often "transform" to acute myelogenous leukemias. In the specific case of one of the myeloproliferative disorders, chronic myelogenous leukemia, transformation to acute lymphoblastic leukemia/lymphoma is also seen, indicating a likely origin from a transformed pluripotent stem cell.

Acute Myelogenous Leukemia

Acute myelogenous leukemias affect primarily adults, peaking in incidence between the ages of 15 and 39 years, but are also observed in older adults and children. AML is quite heterogeneous, reflecting the complexities of myeloid cell differentiation.

Pathophysiology. Most AMLs are associated with acquired genetic alterations that inhibit terminal myeloid differentiation. As a result, normal marrow elements are replaced by relatively undifferentiated blasts exhibiting one or more types of early myeloid differentiation. The replication rate of these blasts is actually lower than that of normal myeloid progenitors, highlighting the pathogenic importance of blocked maturation and increased survival.

Specific recurrent chromosomal aberrations, including translocations, are seen in a high fraction of AMLs and tend to disrupt genes encoding transcription factors needed for normal myeloid differentiation. For example, the most common chromosomal rearrangements, t(8;21) and inv(16), involve genes that normally encode two subunits, CBF1α and CBF1β, of a single heterodimeric transcription factor. Both the t(8;21) and the inv(16) result in the formation of chimeric genes encoding fusion proteins with so-called dominant negative activity, meaning they interfere with the function of the normal CBF1α/CBF1β heterodimer. Myeloid progenitors harboring such aberrations thus give rise to daughter cells exhibiting a partial or complete block in terminal differentiation. A deficit of CBF1α/CBF1β activity is not sufficient to cause leukemia, however, as "knockout" mice lacking either CBF1α or CBF1β, or "knock-in" mice expressing the fusion proteins created by the t(8;21) or inv(16),[66] succumb to hematopoietic failure. In such animals, the "blocked" progenitors die rather than undergoing transformation, indicating that other aberrations must collaborate with defects in critical transcription factors to produce AML.

An example of such a pathogenic collaboration underlies a form of AML, acute promyeloctyic leukemia, associated with a (15;17) chromosomal translocation. This translocation produces a fusion gene encoding a portion of a transcription factor, retinoic acid receptor-α (RARα), fused to a portion of another protein, PML. RARα normally activates transcription, but when fused to PML, it is converted to a repressor that turns off genes required for full and complete myeloid differentiation. In addition to the t(15;17), acute promyelocytic leukemia cells also frequently acquire point mutations in FLT3, a tyrosine kinase, that result in its constitutive activation.[67] As you will recall from Chapter 3, tyrosine kinases produce signals that promote cellular proliferation and survival, activities that synergize with the block in differentiation produced by the RARα-PML fusion protein. This pathogenic collaboration has been proven in mouse models, in which coexpression of a RARα-PML fusion protein and activated forms of FLT3 produce the rapid onset of AML. It is believed that distinct, but pathogenically analogous, sets of synergistic genetic "hits" underlie other forms of AML.[68]

In all AMLs, the accumulation of proliferating neoplastic myeloid precursor cells in the marrow suppresses remaining normal hematopoietic progenitor cells by physical replacement as well as by other unknown mechanisms. The failure of normal hematopoiesis results in anemia, neutropenia, and thrombocytopenia, which cause most of the major clinical complications of AML. Therapeutically, the aim is to clear the bone marrow of the leukemic clone, thus permitting resumption of normal hematopoiesis. This can be accomplished by treatment with cytotoxic drugs or, in the specific case of acute promyelocytic leukemia, by overcoming the block in differentiation with pharmacologic doses of retinoic acid.

Classification. In the most widely used system in current use, the revised FAB classification (Table 14–8*A*), AML is divided into eight (M0 to M7) categories.[69] This scheme takes into account both the degree of maturation (M0 to M3) and the lineage of the leukemic blasts (M4 to M7). Histochemical stains for peroxidase, specific esterase, and nonspecific esterase, and immunostains for myeloid specific antigens (see Table 14–8A) play important roles in defining the type of myeloid differentiation that blasts exhibit.

A recently proposed WHO classification for AML (Table 14–8*B*) retains the FAB categories M0 to M7 but also creates special categories for AMLs associated with particular chromosomal aberrations (e.g., the t(15;17), t(8;21), inv(16), or 11q23 rearrangements), which arise after prior chemotherapy or follow a myelodysplastic syndrome.[11] This classification thus attempts to define forms of AML according to molecular pathogenesis and outcome. Given the increasing role of cytogenetic and molecular features in directing therapy, a further shift toward molecular genetic classifications of AML seems inevitable and desirable.

Morphology. The diagnosis of AML is based on finding that myeloid blasts make up more than 20% of the cells in the marrow. Several types of myeloid blasts are recognized, but more than one type of blast, or blasts with hybrid features, can be seen in individual patients. **Myeloblasts** have delicate nuclear chromatin, two to four nucleoli, and more voluminous cytoplasm than lymphoblasts (Fig. 14–28*A*). The cytoplasm often contains fine, azurophilic, peroxidase-positive granules. Distinctive red-staining peroxidase-positive structures called **Auer rods,** which represent abnormal azurophilic granules, are present in many cases and are particularly numerous in AML associated with the t(15;17) (acute promyelocytic leukemia) (Fig. 14–29*A*). The presence of Auer rods is taken to be definitive evidence of myeloid differentiation. **Monoblasts** (Fig. 14–29*B*) often have folded or lobulated nuclei, lack Auer rods, and are peroxidase negative and nonspecific esterase positive. In some AMLs, blasts exhibit megakaryocytic differentiation, which is often accompanied by marrow fibrosis caused by the release of fibrogenic cytokines. Rarely, the blasts of AML show evidence of erythroid differentiation (erythroblasts).

The number of leukemic cells in the peripheral blood is highly variable. Blast counts can be more than 100,000 cells per microliter but are under 10,000

TABLE 14–8A Revised FAB Classification of Acute Myelogenous Leukemias

Class	Incidence (% of AML)	Marrow Morphology/Comments
M0 Minimally differentiated AML	2–3%	Blasts lack definitive cytologic and cytochemical markers of myeloblasts (e.g., myeloperoxidase negative) but express myeloid lineage antigens and resemble myeloblasts ultrastructurally.
M1 AML without differentiation	20%	Very immature, but ≥3% of blasts are peroxidase positive; few granules or Auer rods and little maturation beyond the myeloblast stage.
M2 AML with maturation	30–40%	Full range of myeloid maturation through granulocytes; Auer rods present in most cases; often associated with the t(8;21).
M3 Acute promyelocytic leukemia	5–10%	Most cells are hypergranular promyelocytes, often with many Auer rods per cell; patients are younger (median age 35 to 40 years); high incidence of DIC; strong association with the t(15;17).
M4 Acute myelomonocytic leukemia	15–20%	Myelocytic and monocytic differentiation evident; myeloid elements show range of maturation; monoblasts are positive for nonspecific esterases; subset associated with the inv(16).
M5 Acute monocytic leukemia	10%	In M5a subtype, monoblasts (peroxidase-negative, nonspecific esterase-positive) and promonocytes predominate in marrow and blood; in M5b subtype, mature monocytes predominate in the peripheral blood; M5a and M5b occur in older patients; characterized by high incidence of organomegaly, lymphadenopathy, and tissue infiltration.
M6 Acute erythroleukemia	5%	Dysplastic erythroid precursors (some megaloblastoid, others with giant or multiple nuclei) predominate, and within the non-erythroid cells, >30% are myeloblasts; seen in advanced age; makes up 1% of de novo AML and 20% of therapy-related AML.
M7 Acute megakaryocytic leukemia	1%	Blasts of megakaryocytic lineage predominate; blasts react with platelet-specific antibodies directed against GPIIb/IIIa or vWF; myelofibrosis or increased marrow reticulin seen in most cases.

DIC, disseminated intravascular coagulation; vWF, von Willebrand factor.

TABLE 14–8B Proposed WHO Classification of Acute Myelogenous Leukemias

Class	Prognosis
I. AML with Recurrent Chromosomal Rearrangements	
AML with t(8;21)(q22;q22); *CBFα/ETO* fusion gene	Favorable
AML with inv(16)(p13;q22); *CBFβ/MYH11* fusion gene	Favorable
AML with t(15;17)(q22;11–12); *RARα/PML* fusion gene	Intermediate
AML with t(11q23;v); diverse *MML* fusion genes	Poor
II. AML with Multilineage Dysplasia	
With prior myelodysplastic syndrome	Very poor
Without prior myelodysplastic syndrome	Poor
III. AML, Therapy Related	
Alkylating agent related	Very poor
Epipodophyllotoxin related	Very poor
IV. AML, not Otherwise Specified	
Sub-classes defined by extent of differentiation and FAB classification (e.g., M0–M7)	Intermediate

cells per microliter in about 50% of the patients. **Occasionally, the peripheral smear might not contain any blasts** (aleukemic leukemia). For this reason, bone marrow examination is essential to exclude acute leukemia in pancytopenic patients.

Immunophenotype. Because it is difficult to distinguish myeloblasts and lymphoblasts morphologically in some cases, the diagnosis of AML is typically confirmed by staining cells for myeloid-specific surface markers (Fig. 14–28*B*, *C*).

Chromosomal Abnormalities. Special high-resolution banding techniques reveal chromosomal abnormalities in approximately 90% of all AML patients. In 50% to 70% of the cases, the karyotypic changes are detected by standard cytogenetic techniques.

Particular chromosomal abnormalities correlate with the clinical setting in which the tumor occurs. AML arising de novo in patients with no risk factors are often associated with balanced chromosomal translocations, particularly t(8;21), inv(16), and t(15;17). In contrast, AMLs following myelodysplastic syndromes or exposure to DNA-damaging agents (such as chemotherapy or radiation therapy) are commonly associated with deletions or monosomies involving chromosomes 5 and 7 and usually lack chromosomal translocations. The exception to this rule is AML occurring after treatment with topoisomerase II inhibitors, which is often associated with translocations involving the *MLL* gene on chromosome 11 at band q23.[70]

Clinical Features. The clinical findings in AML are similar to those in acute lymphoblastic leukemia/lymphoma (ALL). *Most patients present within weeks or a few months of the onset of symptoms related to anemia, neutropenia, and thrombocytopenia*, most notably fatigue, fever, and spontaneous mucosal and cutaneous bleeding. Often, the bleeding diathesis caused by thrombocytopenia is the most striking clinical feature.

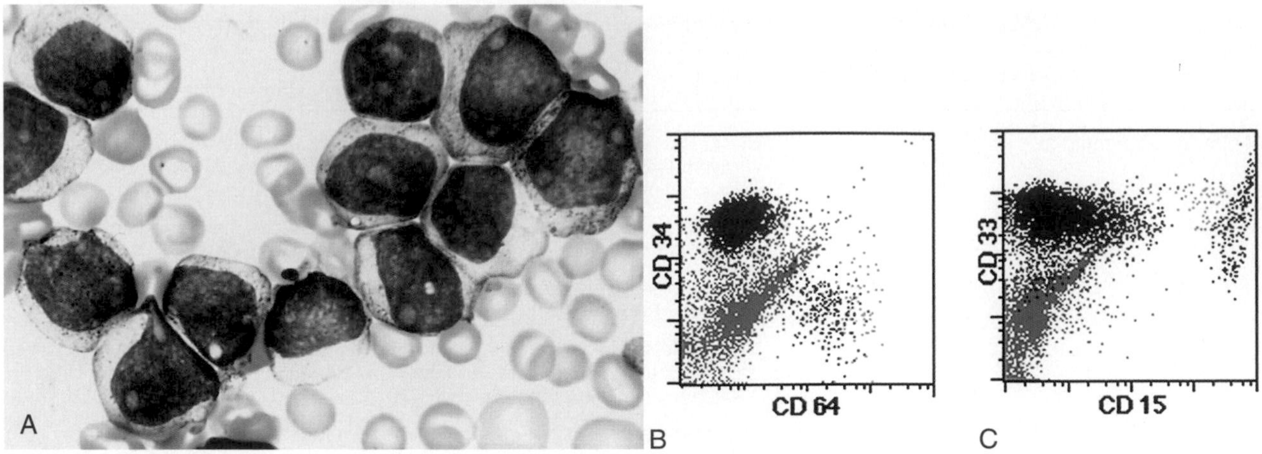

FIGURE 14–28 *A,* Acute myelogenous leukemia (FAB M1 subtype). Myeloblasts have delicate nuclear chromatin, prominent nucleoli, and fine azurophilic granules in the cytoplasm. *B,* In the flow cytometric analysis shown, the myeloid blasts, represented by the red dots, express CD34, a marker of multipotent stem cells, but do not express CD64, a marker of mature myeloid cells. *C,* The same myeloid blasts express CD33, a marker of immature myeloid cells, and a subset express CD15, a marker of more mature myeloid cells. Thus, these blasts are minimally differentiated myeloid cells. (*A,* courtesy of Dr. Robert W. McKenna Department of Pathology, University of Texas Southwestern Medical School, Dallas, TX; *B* and *C,* courtesy of Dr. Louis Picker, Oregon Health Science Center, Portland, OR.)

Cutaneous petechiae and ecchymoses, serosal hemorrhages into the linings of the body cavities and viscera, and mucosal hemorrhages into the gingivae and urinary tract are common. Procoagulants and fibrinolytic factors released by leukemic cells, especially in acute promyelocytic leukemia (M3), exacerbate the bleeding diathesis.[71] Infections are frequent, particularly in the oral cavity, skin, lungs, kidneys, urinary bladder, and colon, and are often caused by opportunists such as fungi, *Pseudomonas*, and commensals.

Signs and symptoms related to infiltration of tissues are usually less striking in AML than in ALL. Mild lymphadenopathy and organomegaly can occur. In tumors with monocytic differentiation (M4 and M5), infiltration of the skin (leukemia cutis) and the gingiva can be observed, likely reflecting the normal tendency of non-neoplastic monocytes to extravasate into tissues. Central nervous system spread is less common than in ALL but still seen. Quite uncommonly, patients present with localized masses composed of myeloblasts in the absence of marrow or peripheral blood involvement. These tumors, known variously as myeloblastomas, granulocytic sarcomas, or chloromas, inevitably progress to systemic AML over a period of up to several years.

Prognosis. AML is a difficult disease to treat. Approximately 60% of the patients achieve complete remission with chemotherapy, but only 15% to 30% remain free from disease for 5 years. AMLs associated with t(8;21) or inv(16) have a rel-

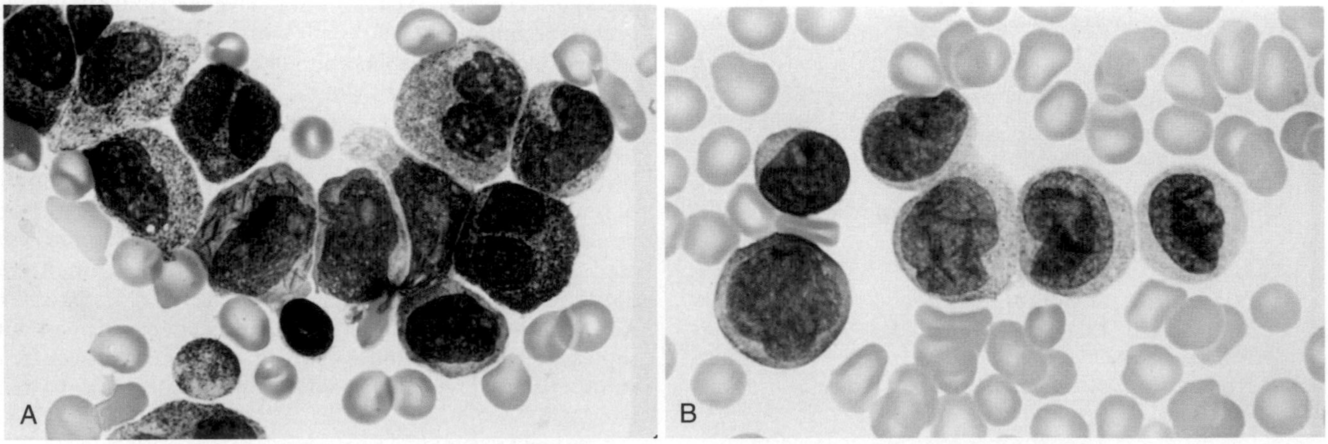

FIGURE 14–29 Acute myelogenous leukemia subtypes. *A,* Acute promyelocytic leukemia (FAB M3 subtype). Bone marrow aspirate shows neoplastic promyelocytes with abnormally coarse and numerous azurophilic granules. Other characteristic findings include the presence of several cells with bilobed nuclei and a cell in the center of the field that contains multiple needlelike Auer rods. *B,* Acute monocytic leukemia (FAB M5b subtype). Peripheral smear shows one monoblast and five promonocytes with folded nuclear membranes. (Courtesy of Dr. Robert W. McKenna, Department of Pathology, University of Texas Southwestern Medical School, Dallas, TX.)

atively good prognosis with conventional chemotherapy. In contrast, the prognosis is dismal for patients with AML with prior myelodysplastic syndrome or following genotoxic therapy, possibly because of damage to normal hematopoietic stem cells. These "high-risk" forms of AML, as well as relapsed AML of all types, are increasingly being treated with allogeneic bone marrow transplantation.

New approaches based on an improved understanding of the pathogenic basis of specific forms of AML promise to improve this situation. The best current example is AML associated with the t(15;17) and the presence of RARα-PML fusion proteins. The block in differentiation induced by this fusion protein is overcome by pharmacologic doses of the vitamin A derivative all-trans-retinoic acid, causing neoplastic promyelocytes to differentiate into neutrophils. Like their normal counterparts, neutrophils derived from the neoplastic clone are short-lived and rapidly die, thus clearing the marrow and allowing resumption of normal hematopoiesis. Remarkably, the same effect is also observed with arsenic trioxide, which somehow promotes the degradation of the PML-RARα fusion protein.[72]

Although retinoic acid "differentiation therapy" induces remissions in a high fraction of patients with acute promyelocytic leukemia, all patients ultimately relapse if treated with retinoic acid alone, probably because retinoic acid fails to prevent continued self-renewal of the neoplastic progenitor cell. Nonetheless, this was the first example in which an understanding of molecular pathogenesis led to a specific therapy directed at a tumor-specific aberration. Other therapies targeted at specific molecular lesions in AML (e.g., the activated FLT3 tyrosine kinase) are under development.

Myelodysplastic Syndromes

The term "myelodysplastic syndromes" (MDS) refers to a group of clonal stem cell disorders characterized by maturation defects associated with ineffective hematopoiesis and an increased risk of transformation to acute myelogenous leukemias (AML). In patients with MDS, the bone marrow is partly or wholly replaced by the clonal progeny of a mutant multipotent stem cell that retains the capacity to differentiate into red cells, granulocytes, and platelets but in an ineffective and disordered fashion. These disturbances usually manifest as peripheral blood cytopenias.

MDS arises in two distinct settings:

- *Idiopathic or primary MDS* occurs mainly at ages over 50 and often develops insidiously.
- *Therapy-related MDS (t-MDS)* is a complication of previous genotoxic drug or radiation therapy that appears 2 to 8 years after treatment.

All forms of MDS can transform to AML, but transformation occurs most rapidly and with highest frequency in t-MDS. Although characteristic morphologic changes are typically seen in the marrow and the peripheral blood, definitive diagnosis frequently requires correlation with other laboratory tests. Cytogenetic analysis is particularly helpful in confirming the diagnosis, as certain chromosomal aberrations (discussed below) are often observed.

Pathogenesis. The pathogenesis of MDS is unknown. Although the marrow is usually hypercellular at diagnosis, it can also be normocellular or, less commonly, hypocellular. Myelodysplastic bone marrow progenitors undergo apoptotic cell death at an increased rate, the hallmark of ineffective hematopoiesis. Given this, it is difficult to understand how myelodysplastic progenitors could displace any remaining normal marrow progenitors, suggesting that MDS arises within a background of stem cell damage or depletion. Both primary MDS and t-MDS occurring after exposure to radiation or alkylating chemotherapeutic drugs are associated with similar clonal chromosomal abnormalities, including monosomy 5 and monosomy 7, deletions of 5q and 7q, trisomy 8, and deletions of 20q.

Morphology. The most characteristic finding is disordered (dysplastic) differentiation affecting all non-lymphoid lineages (erythroid, granulocytic, monocytic, and megakaryocytic) (Fig. 14–30). Within the erythroid series, common abnormalities include: **ringed sideroblasts**, erythroblasts with iron-laden mitochondria visible as perinuclear granules in Prussian blue–stained aspirates or biopsies; **megaloblastoid maturation** resembling that seen in vitamin B_{12} and folate deficiency; and **nuclear budding abnormalities**, recognized as nuclei with misshapen, often polypoid, outlines. Neutrophils often contain decreased numbers of secondary granules, toxic granulations, and/or Döhle bodies. **Pseudo-Pelger-Hüet cells**, neutrophils with only two nuclear lobes, are frequently observed, and neutrophils may even be seen that completely lack nuclear segmentation. Megakaryocytes with single nuclear lobes or multiple separate nuclei **(pawn ball megakaryocytes)** are also characteristic. **Myeloblasts** may be increased but make up less than 20% of the overall marrow cellularity. The peripheral blood often contains pseudo-Pelger-Hüet cells, giant platelets, macrocytes, poikilocytes, and a relative or absolute monocytosis. Myeloblasts usually make up less than 10% of the peripheral leukocytes.

Clinical Course. Primary MDS affects mainly individuals older than 60 years of age. When symptomatic, it presents with weakness, infections, and hemorrhages, all due to pancytopenia. In up to half of the cases, MDS is discovered incidentally on routine blood testing.

On the basis of specific morphologic features in the marrow and peripheral blood, primary MDS is divided into five categories in the WHO classification, details of which are beyond our scope. Subtypes defined by having a higher proportion of blasts in the marrow or peripheral blood are associated with more severe cytopenias, an increased risk of progression to AML, and worse prognosis. The presence of multiple clonal chromosomal abnormalities and the severity of peripheral blood cytopenias are independent risk factors also portending a worse outcome.

The median survival in primary MDS varies from 9 to 29 months, but some individuals in good prognostic groups may live for 5 years or more. Overall, progression to AML occurs in 10% to 40% of individuals and is often accompanied by the appearance of additional clonal cytogenetic changes. Patients often succumb to the complications of thrombocytopenia

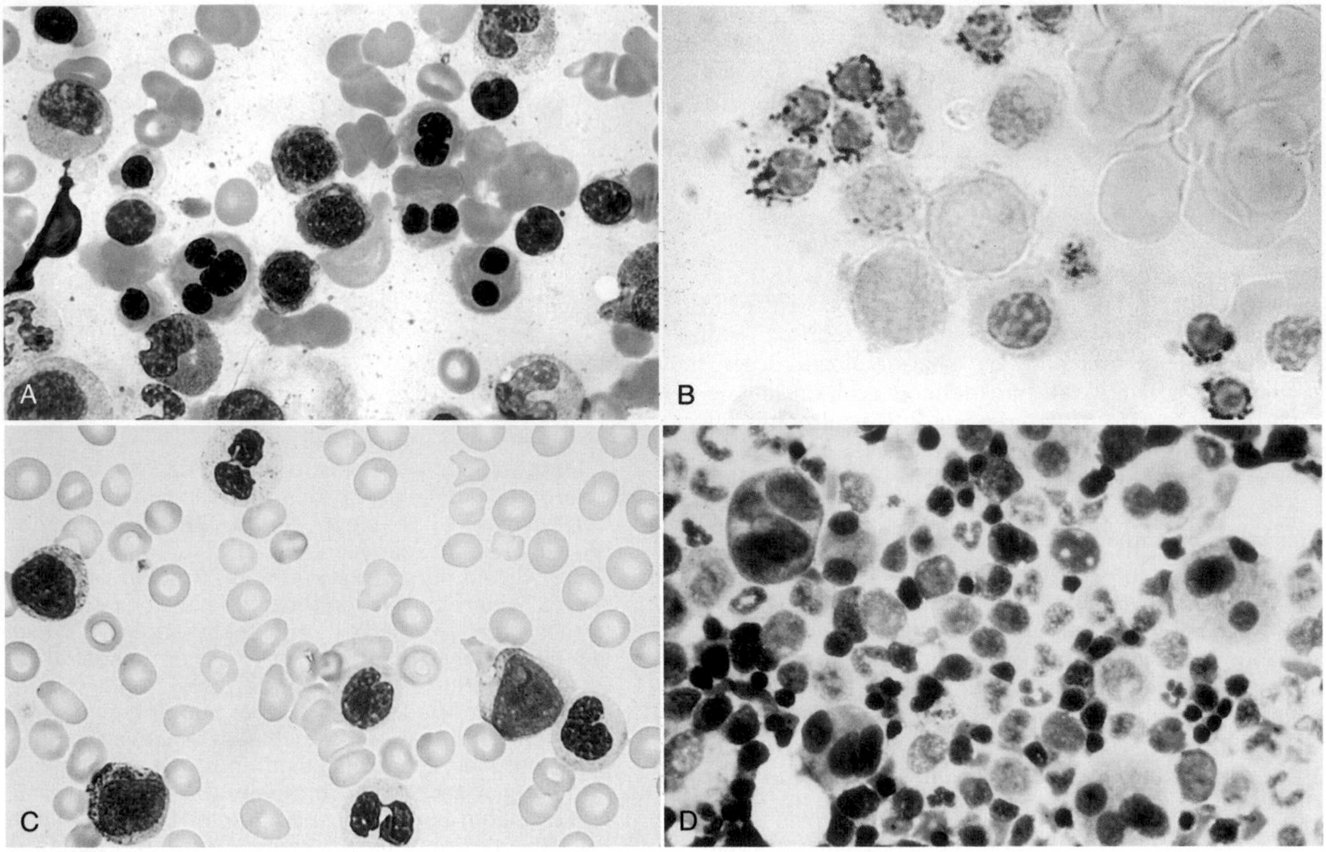

FIGURE 14–30 Myelodysplasia. Characteristic forms of dysplasia are shown. *A*, Nucleated red cell progenitors with multilobated or multiple nuclei. *B*, Ringed sideroblasts, erythroid progenitors with iron-laden mitochondria, seen as blue perinuclear granules (Prussian blue stain). *C*, Pseudo-Pelger-Hüet cells, neutrophils with only two nuclear lobes instead of the normal three to four, are observed at the top and bottom of this field. *D*, Megakaryocytes with multiple nuclei instead of the normal single multilobated nucleus. (*A*, *B*, *D*, marrow aspirates; *C*, peripheral blood smear.)

(bleeding) and neutropenia (infection). The outlook is even grimmer in t-MDS, which has an overall median survival of only 4 to 8 months. Cytopenias tend to be more severe than in primary MDS, and progression to AML is often rapid.

Treatment options in MDS are limited. In younger patients, allogeneic bone marrow transplantation offers some hope for reconstitution of normal hematopoiesis and long-term survival. Older patients with MDS are treated supportively with antibiotics and blood product transfusions.

Chronic Myeloproliferative Disorders

In most disorders of this group, the neoplastic cell is a multipotent progenitor cell that is capable of giving rise to mature erythrocytes, platelets, granulocytes, monocytes, and (in some cases) lymphocytes. The singular exception is chronic myelogenous leukemia, in which the pluripotent stem cell that gives rise to lymphoid and myeloid cells is affected. As in AML, the neoplastic cells and their offspring flood the bone marrow and suppress residual normal progenitor cells; however, in the chronic myeloproliferative disorders, terminal differentiation is relatively unaffected. This combination leads to marrow hypercellularity and increased hematopoiesis, often accompanied by elevated peripheral blood counts.

The four most common chronic myeloproliferative disorders (MPDs) are: (1) chronic myelogenous leukemia, (2) polycythemia vera, (3) essential thrombocytosis, and (4) primary myelofibrosis. All four have some similar features. The neoplastic stem cells have the capacity to circulate and home to secondary hematopoietic organs, particularly the spleen, where they give rise to extramedullary hematopoiesis. As a result, all chronic MPDs cause varying degrees of splenomegaly. They also share the propensity to terminate in a spent phase characterized by marrow fibrosis and peripheral blood cytopenias. Further, all can progress over time to acute leukemia, but only chronic myelogenous leukemia (CML) does so invariably.

Unlike the lymphoid neoplasms and AML, the pathologic findings in the chronic myeloproliferative disorders are not specific, having a considerable degree of overlap with one another and with some reactive conditions producing marrow hyperplasia. Diagnosis and classification depend on correlation of morphologic findings with other clinical and laboratory findings. Cytogenetic and molecular analyses also play an important role, as patients with chronic myelogenous leukemia uniformly possess the Philadelphia chromosome (Ph) or variants thereof, whereas other chronic MPDs lack the Ph.

Chronic Myelogenous Leukemia

Chronic myelogenous leukemia (CML) is a disease primarily of adults between the ages of 25 and 60 years, with the peak incidence in the fourth and fifth decades of life.

Pathophysiology. *CML is distinguished from other chronic MPDs by the presence of a distinctive molecular abnormality, namely, a translocation involving the* BCR *gene on chromosome 22 and the* ABL *gene on chromosome 9.* The resultant *BCR-ABL* fusion gene directs the synthesis of a 210-kDa fusion protein with tyrosine kinase activity. In more than 90% of CML cases, karyotyping reveals the so-called Philadelphia chromosome (Ph), which is created by a reciprocal (9;22)(q34;q11) translocation. However, in 5% to 10% of cases, the rearrangement is complex or cytogenetically cryptic; in such cases, other methods such as fluorescence in situ hybridization (FISH; shown in Fig. 14–31) or the reverse transcriptase–polymerase chain reaction (RT-PCR) can be used to detect the *BCR-ABL* fusion gene or transcript. Introduction of the *BCR-ABL* fusion gene into murine bone marrow cells gives rise to a syndrome resembling human CML;[73] hence, its acquisition is considered to be a critical pathogenetic event.

The activity of diverse tyrosine kinases is normally regulated by ligand-mediated dimerization, followed by the activation of multiple downstream pathways, which control cell survival and proliferation (discussed in Chapters 3 and 7). Detailed molecular dissection has shown that BCR contributes a dimerization domain that promotes self-association

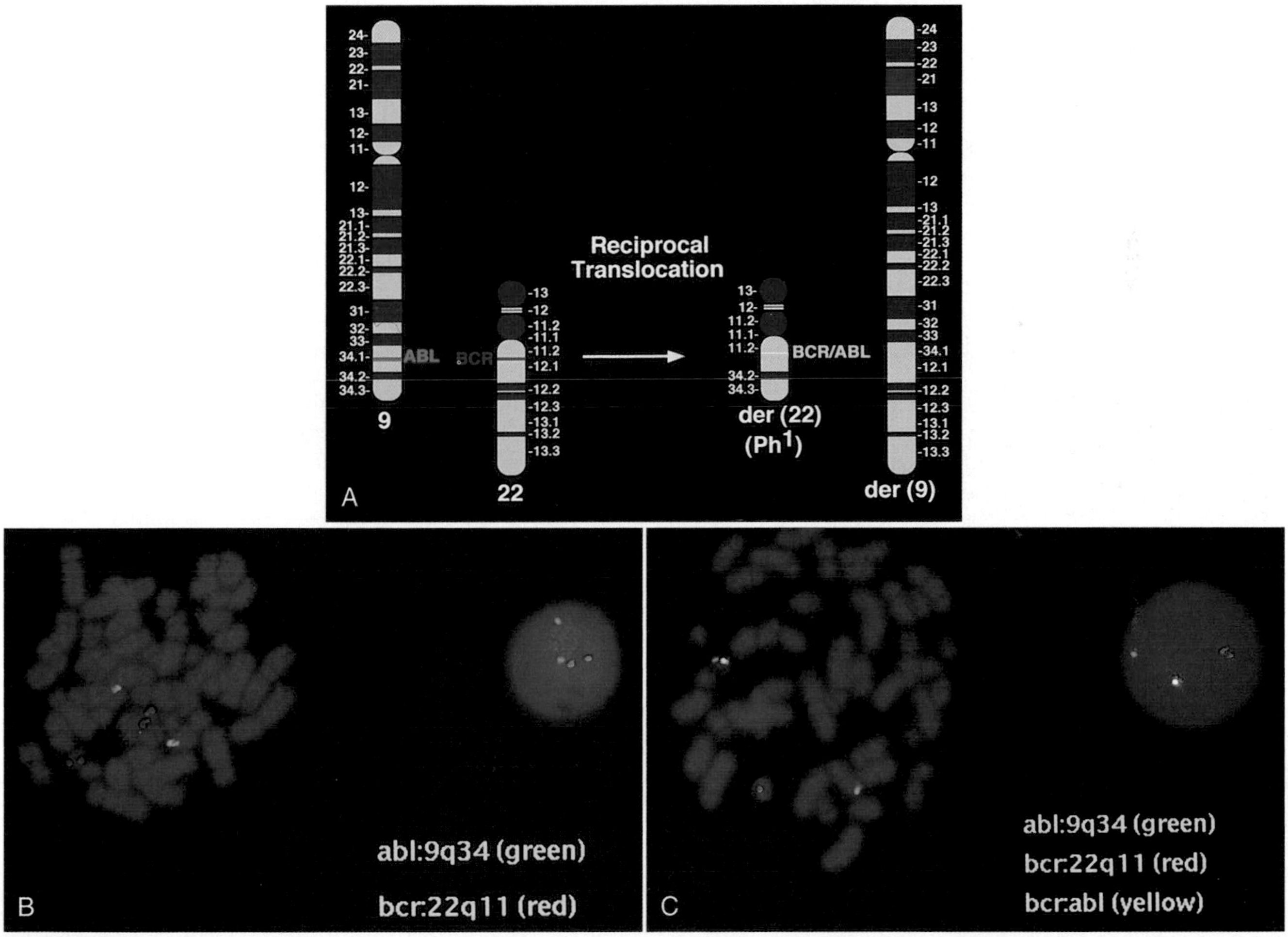

FIGURE 14–31 Detection of a *BCR-ABL* fusion gene by fluorescence in situ hybridization. *A,* An idiogram depicting chromosomes 9 and 22 and the position of the *ABL* and *BCR* genes. The Philadelphia chromosome (Ph) is created by a balanced chromosomal translocation that replaces the telomeric portion of 22q with the telomeric portion of 9q. At a molecular level, the breaking and rejoining of the DNA results in the formation of fusion gene on the Ph derived from the 5′ end of *BCR* and the 3′ end of *ABL* and hence brings *BCR* and *ABL* sequences that are normally far apart into close physical proximity. This abnormal colocalization of *BCR* and *ABL* can be detected by in situ hybridization with pairs of fluorescently tagged DNA probes complementary to genomic DNA sequences lying near the *BCR* and *ABL* breakpoints. *B,* A green *ABL* probe and a red *BCR* probe have been hybridized to metaphase chromosomes and interphase nuclei prepared from the peripheral blood cells of a normal individual. Because of the pairing of sister chromatids during mitosis, signals on metaphase chromosomes may be seen as a single dot or a pair of closely spaced dots. Two pairs of red signals and two green signals are seen on the metaphase chromosomes, while two red and two green signals are present in the interphase nucleus, indicating the presence of normal, spatially distant copies of *ABL* and *BCR,* respectively. *C,* In contrast, metaphase chromosomes and an interphase nucleus prepared from the bone marrow cells of a patient with CML show one normal *ABL* signal, one normal *BCR* signal, and an abnormal yellow signal created by superimposition of one *BCR* and one *ABL* signal, a finding indicative of the presence of a *BCR-ABL* fusion gene. (Courtesy of Dr. Cynthia Morton and Ms. Debbie Sandstrom, Department of Pathology, Brigham and Women's Hospital, Boston, MA.)

of the BCR-ABL fusion protein, resulting in constitutive BCR-ABL autophosphorylation and activation of downstream pathways. The net effect of these events is cell division and inhibition of apoptosis, independent of ligand binding. Such autonomous triggering contributes to unregulated myeloproliferation.

In CML, multiple myeloid lineages, B lymphoid cells and possibly T lymphoid cells express the BCR-ABL fusion protein, indicating that the target of transformation is a pluripotent stem cell. For unknown reasons, the effect of the constitutively active BCR-ABL kinase early in the course of CML is evident mainly in granulocytic progenitors and, to a lesser degree, in megakaryocytic progenitors.

Morphology. In contrast to normal bone marrow, which is usually about 50% cellular and 50% fat, CML marrows are usually 100% cellular, with maturing granulocytic precursors comprising most of the increased cellularity. Increased numbers of megakaryocytes, often including small dysplastic forms, are also frequently observed, whereas erythroid progenitors are usually present in normal or decreased numbers. A characteristic finding is the presence of scattered storage histiocytes with wrinkled, green-blue cytoplasm (sea-blue histiocytes). Increased deposition of reticulin fibers is typical, but overt marrow fibrosis is rare at presentation. Peripheral blood examination reveals a marked leukocytosis, often exceeding 100,000 cells per mm^3 (Fig. 14–32). The circulating cells are predominantly neutrophils, metamyelocytes, and myelocytes, with less than 10% myeloblasts. Peripheral blood eosinophilia and basophilia are also common, and up to 50% of patients have thrombocytosis early in the course of their disease. Neoplastic extramedullary hematopoiesis within the splenic red pulp produces marked splenomegaly (Fig. 14–33), often complicated by focal infarction. Extramedullary hematopoiesis can also lead to hepatomegaly and mild lymphadenopathy.

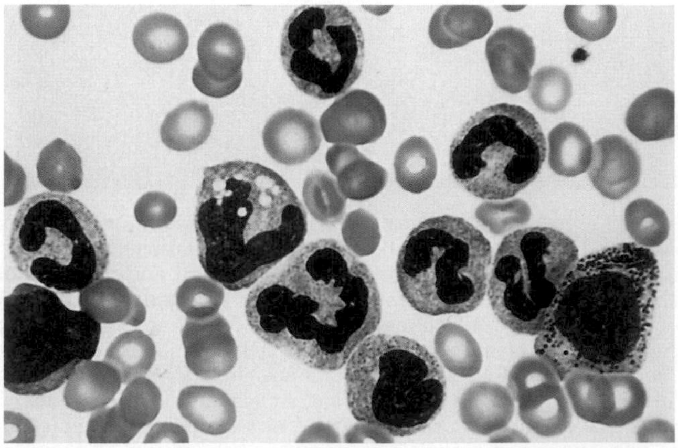

FIGURE 14–32 Chronic myelogenous leukemia. Peripheral blood smear shows many mature neutrophils, some metamyelocytes, and a myelocyte. (Courtesy of Dr. Robert W. McKenna, Department of Pathology, University of Texas Southwestern Medical School, Dallas, TX.)

FIGURE 14–33 Chronic myelogenous leukemia (spleen). Enlarged spleen (2630 gm; normal: 150 to 200 gm) with greatly expanded red pulp stemming from neoplastic hematopoiesis. (Courtesy of Dr. Daniel Jones, Department of Pathology, M.D. Anderson Cancer Center, Houston, TX.)

Clinical Features. The onset of CML is insidious. Mild-to-moderate anemia and hypermetabolism due to increased cell turnover lead to easy fatigability, weakness, weight loss, and anorexia. Sometimes the first symptom is a dragging sensation in the abdomen caused by the extreme splenomegaly, or acute onset of left upper quadrant pain due to splenic infarction. CML is best differentiated from other chronic myeloproliferative disorders by detection of the *BCR-ABL* fusion gene, through either chromosomal analysis or PCR-based molecular tests.

The natural history of CML is one of slow progression, and even without treatment, a median survival of 3 years can be expected. After a variable period averaging 3 years, approximately 50% of patients enter an "accelerated phase," during which there is increasing anemia and thrombocytopenia and sometimes striking peripheral blood basophilia. Additional clonal cytogenetic abnormalities, such as trisomy 8, isochromosome 17q, or duplication of the Ph, can also appear. Within 6 to 12 months, the accelerated phase terminates in a picture resembling acute leukemia (blast crisis). In the remaining 50%, blast crises occur abruptly without an intermediate accelerated phase. In 70% of blast crises, the blasts have the morphologic and cytochemical features of myeloblasts, whereas in most of the remainder, the blasts contain the enzyme TdT and express early B-lineage markers such as CD10 and CD19. Rarely, the blasts resemble precursor T cells. These observations further support the notion that the target cell for transformation is a pluripotent stem cell.

Understanding of the molecular pathogenesis of CML has led to the introduction of drugs that inhibit the BCR-ABL kinase, which induce complete hematologic remissions in more than 90% of patients.[74] This remarkable clinical success has rightfully created great excitement around the development of other drugs specifically targeting oncoproteins, particularly other oncogenic tyrosine kinases. However, BCR-ABL inhibitors suppress but do not extinguish the CML clone and, as a result, may not prevent progression to blast crisis. Moreover, while patients in blast crisis initially respond to BCR-ABL kinase inhibitors, they recur rapidly with refractory disease.[75] For these reasons, allogeneic bone marrow transplantation, which is most effective when performed in the stable phase, is the favored treatment in younger patients. Of those with a suitable donor, about 75% are cured.

Polycythemia Vera

Polycythemia vera is a neoplasm arising in a multipotent myeloid stem cell that is characterized by increased marrow production of erythroid, granulocytic, and megakaryocytic elements. This leads to erythrocytosis (polycythemia), granulocytosis, and thrombocytosis in the peripheral blood, the polycythemia being responsible for most of the clinical symptoms. Polycythemia vera must be differentiated from relative polycythemia resulting from hemoconcentration (see Chapter 13) and other causes of absolute polycythemia (defined as an increase in red cell mass).

Pathophysiology. Polycythemia vera progenitor cells have markedly decreased requirements for erythropoietin and other hematopoietic growth factors.[76] Accordingly, serum erythropoietin levels in polycythemia vera are very low, whereas almost all other forms of absolute polycythemia are caused by elevated erythropoietin levels. The causative molecular defect is unknown. A thorough search for erythropoietin receptor mutations, which cause rare forms of inherited polycythemia, has been unrevealing in polycythemia vera. Because polycythemia vera is characterized by panmyelosis (an increase in all three lineages), it seems likely that mutations in a factor or factors common to multiple hematopoietic growth factor signaling pathways are involved.

Morphology. The bone marrow is hypercellular, but some residual fat is often observed. The increase in erythroid progenitors can be quite subtle and is usually accompanied by increased numbers of maturing granulocytic precursors and megakaryocytes. At the time of diagnosis, a moderate to marked increase in marrow reticulin fibers is seen in approximately 10% of the patients. Mild organomegaly is common, being caused early in the course largely by congestion; at this stage, extramedullary hematopoiesis is minimal. The peripheral blood smear often shows increased basophils and abnormally large platelets.

Late in the course, polycythemia vera can progress to a spent phase characterized by extensive marrow fibrosis that displaces hematopoietic cells. This is accompanied by increased extramedullary hematopoiesis in the spleen and liver, which often leads to prominent organomegaly (Fig. 14–34). Uncommonly, transformation to AML also occurs.

Clinical Course. Polycythemia vera appears insidiously, usually in late middle age (median age at onset: 60 years). *Most symptoms are related to the increased red cell mass and hematocrit.* The elevation of hematocrit is usually accompanied by increased total blood volumes, and together these two promote abnormal blood flow, particularly on the low-pressure venous side of the circulation, which becomes greatly distended. Patients are plethoric and somewhat cyanotic owing to stagnation and deoxygenation of blood in peripheral vessels. Headache, dizziness, hypertension, and gastrointestinal symptoms are common. There is often intense pruritus and an increased likelihood of peptic ulceration, both possibly resulting from release of histamine from basophils. High cell turnover gives rise to hyperuricemia, and symptomatic gout is seen in 5% to 10% of cases.

More ominously, *the abnormal blood flow (and possibly the abnormal platelet function) leads to increased risk of both major bleeding and thrombotic episodes.* About 25% of patients first come to clinical attention with thrombotic episodes, often manifesting as deep venous thrombosis, myocardial infarction, and stroke. Other common sites for thromboses include the hepatic veins (producing Budd-Chiari syndrome), the portal and mesenteric veins (leading to bowel infarction), and the venous sinuses of the brain (leading to hemorrhagic strokes). Minor hemorrhages (epistaxis, bleeding gums) are also common; life-threatening hemorrhages occur in 5% to 10% of cases.

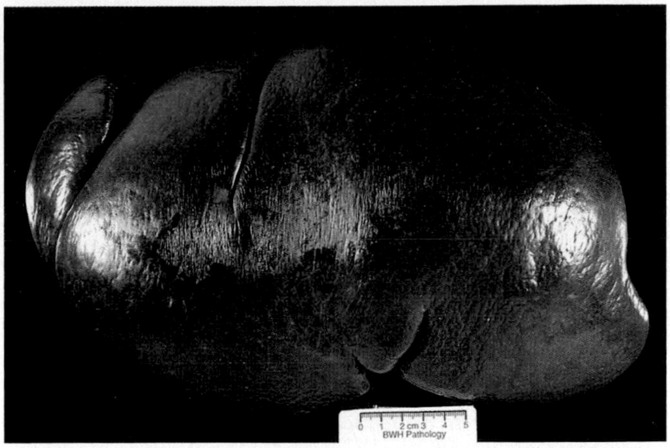

FIGURE 14–34 Polycythemia vera, spent phase. Massive splenomegaly (3020 gm; normal: 150 to 200 gm) largely owing to extramedullary hematopoiesis occurred in the setting of advanced marrow myelofibrosis. (Courtesy of Dr. Mark Fleming, Department of Pathology, Brigham and Women's Hospital, Boston, MA.)

The hemoglobin concentration ranges from 14 to 28 gm/dL with hematocrit values of 60% or more. Sometimes, chronic bleeding leads to iron deficiency, which can suppress erythropoiesis sufficiently to lower the hematocrit into the normal range, an example of two defects counteracting one another to "correct" a laboratory abnormality. The white cell count is elevated, ranging between 12,000 and 50,000 cells per mm^3, and the platelet count is often greater than 500,000 cells per mm^3. In contrast to CML, *BCR-ABL* fusion genes are not present. The platelets usually exhibit morphologic abnormalities, such as giant forms, and are often defective in functional aggregation studies.

Without treatment, death from bleeding or thrombosis occurs within months of diagnosis. However, simply maintaining the red cell mass at nearly normal levels by phlebotomies extends the median survival to about 10 years.

Extended survival with treatment has revealed that *polycythemia vera tends to evolve to a "spent phase," during which clinical and anatomic features of primary myelofibrosis develop.* Approximately 15% to 20% of patients undergo such a transformation after an average period of 10 years. This transition is brought about by obliterative fibrosis in the bone marrow (myelofibrosis) and marked by the appearance of extensive extramedullary hematopoiesis, principally in the spleen, which enlarges greatly. The pathogenetic basis for progression to the spent phase is not known.

Some patients develop terminal AML. Such transformation occurs in 2% of patients who are treated with phlebotomy alone but has been seen in up to 15% of those receiving myelosuppressive treatment with alkylating drugs or marrow irradiation with P^{32}, both of which are mutagenic. Because it is safe and effective, the current treatment of choice is phlebotomy. Unlike CML, transformation to ALL is rarely observed, possibly indicating that the target of neoplastic transformation is a progenitor cell committed to myeloid differentiation.

Essential Thrombocytosis

In this hematopoietic stem cell disorder, increased proliferation and production are largely confined to the megakaryocytic elements, most patients having platelet counts exceeding 600,000 per mm^3. *Since all chronic myeloproliferative disorders can be associated with thrombocytosis, essential thrombocytosis is a diagnosis of exclusion.* By definition, features that are characteristic of other chronic myeloproliferative disorders are absent. It must also be distinguished from reactive causes of thrombocytosis, including inflammatory disorders, asplenism, and iron deficiency.

The pathogenetic basis for essential thrombocytosis is unknown. This disorder bears some resemblance to polycythemia vera, in that the cells of the megakaryocytic series have a diminished requirement for growth factors. Dysfunctions of platelets derived from the neoplastic clone contribute to the major clinical features of bleeding and thrombosis.

Bone marrow examination is most helpful in excluding other chronic myeloproliferative disorders. Cellularity is usually increased mildly to moderately. Megakaryocytes are often markedly increased in number and include abnormally large forms. Deposition of delicate reticulin fibrils can be seen, but the overt fibrosis characteristic of primary myelofibrosis (see below) is absent. *Peripheral smears usually reveal abnormally large platelets* (Fig. 14–35), often accompanied by mild leukocytosis. Neoplastic extramedullary hematopoiesis can occur within the spleen and liver, producing mild organomegaly in about 50% of patients. Terminally, a spent phase of marrow fibrosis or transformation to AML can supervene.

Essential thrombocytosis is the least common of the chronic myeloproliferative disorders. It usually occurs past the age of 60, but it may also be seen in young adults. The major clinical manifestations are thrombosis and hemorrhage, probably reflecting both qualitative and quantitative abnormalities in platelets. The types of thrombotic events resemble those observed in polycythemia vera; they include deep venous thrombosis, portal and hepatic vein thrombosis, and myocardial infarction. One characteristic symptom is *erythromelalgia*, the throbbing and burning of hands and feet caused by occlusion of small arterioles by platelet aggregates. Erythromelalgia can also be seen in polycythemia vera patients with high platelet counts.

Essential thrombocytosis is an indolent disorder with long asymptomatic periods punctuated by occasional thrombotic or hemorrhagic crises. Median survival times are 12 to 15 years. For unclear reasons, both thrombosis and bleeding occur in those patients with very high platelet counts. To lower the risk of such complications, myelosuppressive alkylating drugs or other agents are used to lower platelet counts.

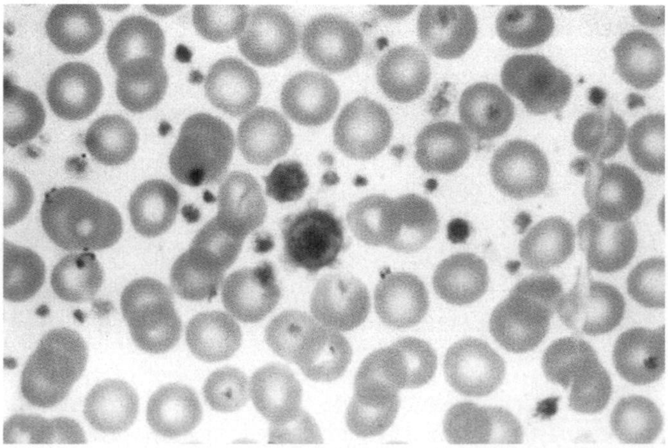

FIGURE 14–35 Essential thrombocytosis. Peripheral blood smear shows marked thrombocytosis, including giant platelets approximating the size of surrounding red cells. (Courtesy of Dr. Jacqueline Mitus, Brigham and Women's Hospital, Boston, MA.)

Primary Myelofibrosis

The hallmark of primary myelofibrosis is rapid development of obliterative marrow fibrosis. Histologically, the appearance is identical to the spent phase that occurs occasionally late in the course of other chronic myeloproliferative disorders. Myelofibrosis suppresses bone marrow hematopoiesis, leading to peripheral blood cytopenias and extensive neoplastic extramedullary hematopoiesis in the spleen, liver, and lymph nodes.

Pathophysiology. The pathologic features of primary myelofibrosis stem from extensive collagen deposition by nonneoplastic fibroblasts in the marrow.[77] Fibrosis inexorably displaces hematopoietic elements, including stem cells, from the marrow, leading to extensive extramedullary hematopoiesis in the spleen, the liver, and sometimes the lymph nodes. The marrow fibrosis is likely caused by the inappropriate release of fibrogenic factors from neoplastic megakaryocytes. Two factors synthesized by megakaryocytes have been implicated: platelet-derived growth factor (PDGF) and TGF-β. As you recall, PDGF and TGF-β are fibroblast mitogens. In addition, TGF-β promotes fibrosis and causes angiogenesis, both of which are observed in myelofibrosis. As marrow fibrosis progresses, circulating hematopoietic stem cells take up residence in secondary hematopoietic organs, such as the spleen, the liver, and the lymph nodes, which become the main sites of hematopoiesis. For incompletely understood reasons, in myelofibrosis blood cell production from sites of extramedullary hematopoiesis is disordered and ineffective, such that cytopenias persist.

Morphology. Early in the course, the marrow is often hypercellular owing to increases in maturing cells of all lineages. Morphologically, the erythroid and granulocytic precursors appear normal, but megakaryocytes are large, dysplastic, and abnormally clustered. During this cellular phase, fibrosis is minimal. With progression, the marrow becomes hypocellular and diffusely fibrotic. Even at this stage, clusters of atypical megakaryocytes can be found in the sea of fibrosis. Very late in the disease course, the fibrotic marrow space can be largely converted to bone, a development that is termed "osteosclerosis."

Myelofibrotic obliteration of the marrow space leads to extensive extramedullary hematopoiesis, principally in the spleen, which is usually markedly enlarged, sometimes up to 4000 gm. On section, such spleens are firm and diffusely red to gray. As in CML, subcapsular infarcts are common (see Fig. 14–39). Histologically, there is trilineage hematopoiesis, usually associated with a predominance of **large, clustered megakaryocytes**. Initially, extramedullary hematopoiesis is confined to the sinusoids, but later it extends to involve the cords. The **liver** can be enlarged moderately owing to sinusoidal foci of extramedullary hematopoiesis. Hematopoiesis can also appear within lymph nodes, but significant lymphadenopathy is uncommon.

The peripheral blood reveals a number of characteristic findings in full-blown myelofibrosis (Fig. 14–36). Fibrotic distortion of the marrow microenvironment leads to inappropriate release of nucleated erythroid progenitors and early granulocytes, and immature cells also enter the circulation from sites of extramedullary hematopoiesis. **The presence of erythroid and granulocytic precursors in the peripheral blood is termed leukoerythroblastosis.** In addition, the fibrotic marrow distorts and damages the membranes of erythroid progenitors in the marrow, leading to the appearance of teardrop-shaped erythrocytes (dacryocytes). Although characteristic of primary myelofibrosis, leukoerythroblastosis and dacryocytes can be observed in many infiltrative disorders of the bone marrow, including granulomatous diseases and metastatic tumors. Other common, albeit nonspecific, peripheral blood findings include abnormally large platelets and basophilia.

Clinical Course. Primary myelofibrosis is uncommon in individuals younger than 60 years of age. Except when preceded by polycythemia vera or CML, it usually comes to clinical attention because of either progressive anemia or marked splenic enlargement, producing a sensation of fullness in the left upper quadrant. Nonspecific symptoms such as fatigue, weight loss, and night sweats result from increased metabolism associated with the expanded mass of hematopoietic cells. Owing to a high rate of cell turnover, hyperuricemia and secondary gout can complicate the picture.

The laboratory findings include a moderate-to-severe normochromic normocytic anemia accompanied by leukoerythroblastosis. The white cell count is usually normal or reduced but can be markedly elevated (80,000 to 100,000 cells per mm^3) during the early cellular phase. The platelet count is usually normal or elevated at the time of diagnosis, but thrombocytopenia supervenes as the disease progresses. These peripheral blood findings are not specific, however, and bone marrow biopsy is essential for diagnosis.

The course of this disease is difficult to predict, but the median survival is in the range of 3 to 5 years.[78] Threats to life are intercurrent infections, thrombotic episodes or bleeding related to platelet abnormalities, and, in 5% to 20% of cases, transformation to AML. When marrow fibrosis is extensive, AML can arise at unusual extramedullary sites, including lymph nodes and soft tissues.

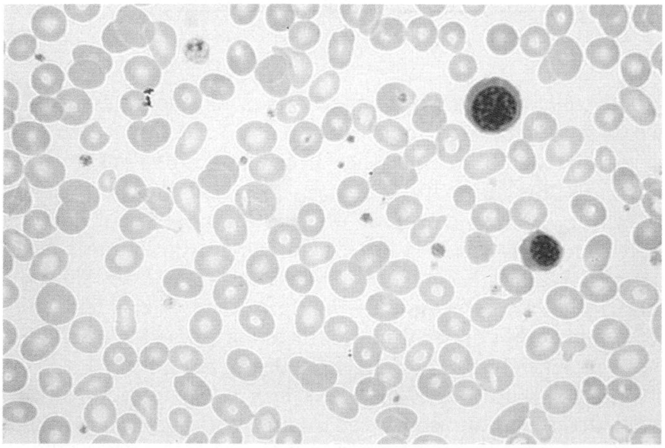

FIGURE 14–36 Primary myelofibrosis (peripheral blood smear). Two nucleated erythroid precursors and several teardrop-shaped red cells (dacryocytes) are evident. Immature myeloid cells were present in other fields. An identical picture can be seen in other diseases producing marrow distortion and fibrosis.

LANGERHANS CELL HISTIOCYTOSIS

The term *histiocytosis* is an "umbrella" designation for a variety of proliferative disorders of dendritic cells or macrophages. Some, such as the rare "histiocytic" lymphomas, are clearly malignant, whereas others, such as reactive proliferations of macrophages in lymph nodes, are clearly benign. Between these two extremes is a small cluster of conditions characterized by proliferation of a special type of immature dendritic cell (DC) called the Langerhans cell (see Chapter 6). In most instances, these proliferations are monoclonal and therefore likely to be neoplastic in origin.[79]

In the past, these disorders were referred to as histiocytosis X and were subdivided into three categories: *Letterer-Siwe syndrome*, *Hand-Schuller-Christian disease*, and *eosinophilic granuloma*. These three conditions are now considered different expressions of the same basic disorder. The tumor cells in each are derived from dendritic cells and express HLA-DR, S-100, and CD1a. They have abundant, often vacuolated cytoplasm and vesicular nuclei containing linear grooves or folds. *The presence of Birbeck granules in the cytoplasm is characteristic.* Under the electron microscope, Birbeck granules have a pentalaminar, rodlike, tubular appearance and sometimes a dilated terminal end (tennis-racket appearance) (Fig. 14–37). As Birbeck granules are not seen in all tumor cells by electron microscopy, the detection of S-100 and CD1a expression by immunohistochemical techniques aids in the diagnosis.

The distribution of neoplastic DCs in lymphoid tissues and viscera, characteristic of these disorders, is likely attributable to aberrant expression of chemokine receptors.[80] Whereas normal, skin resident DCs express CCR6, their neoplastic counterparts co-express CCR6 and CCR7, and this allows the abnormal DCs to migrate into tissues that express the relevant chemokines—CCL20 in skin and bone (the ligand for CCR6) and CCL19 and 21 in lymphoid organs (ligands for CCR7).

Langerhans cell histiocytosis presents as three clinicopathologic entities:

Multifocal multisystem Langerhans cell histiocytosis (Letterer-Siwe disease) occurs most frequently before 2 years of age but

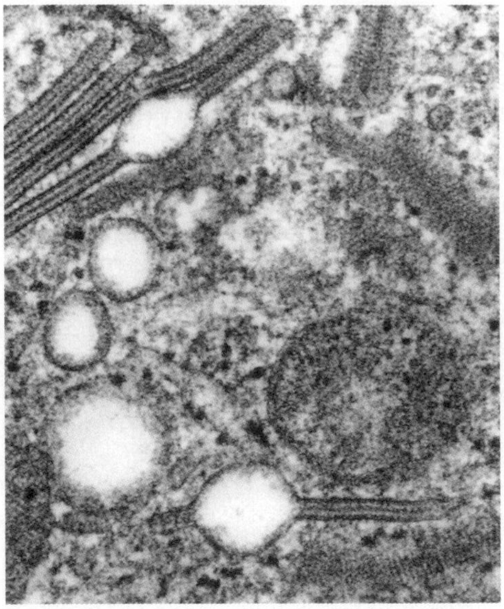

FIGURE 14–37 Langerhans cell histiocytosis. An electron micrograph shows rodlike Birbeck granules with characteristic periodicity and dilated terminal end. (Courtesy of Dr. George Murphy, University of Pennsylvania School of Medicine, Philadelphia, PA.)

occasionally affects adults. A dominant clinical feature is the development of cutaneous lesions resembling a seborrheic eruption, which is caused by infiltrates of Langerhans cells over the front and back of the trunk and on the scalp. Most of those affected have concurrent hepatosplenomegaly, lymphadenopathy, pulmonary lesions, and, eventually, destructive osteolytic bone lesions. Extensive infiltration of the marrow often leads to anemia, thrombocytopenia, and predisposition to recurrent infections such as otitis media and mastoiditis. The course of untreated disease is rapidly fatal. With intensive chemotherapy, 50% of patients survive 5 years.

Unifocal and multifocal unisystem Langerhans cell histiocytoses (eosinophilic granuloma) are characterized by expanding, erosive accumulations of Langerhans cells, usually within the medullary cavities of bones. Histiocytes are variably admixed with eosinophils, lymphocytes, plasma cells, and neutrophils. The eosinophilic infiltrate is usually prominent but is sparse in a subset of cases. Virtually any bone in the skeletal system can be involved, most commonly the calvarium, ribs, and femur. Less commonly, unisystem lesions of identical histology arise in the skin, lungs, or stomach.

Unifocal lesions usually affect the skeletal system in older children or adults. They can be asymptomatic, or they can cause pain, tenderness, and, in some instances, pathologic fractures. This is an indolent disorder that can heal spontaneously or be cured by local excision or irradiation.

Multifocal unisystem Langerhans cell histiocytosis usually affects young children, who present with multiple erosive bony masses that sometimes expand into adjacent soft tissue. In about 50% of patients, involvement of the posterior pituitary stalk of the hypothalamus leads to diabetes insipidus. The combination of calvarial bone defects, diabetes insipidus, and exophthalmos is referred to as the Hand-Schuller-Christian triad. Many patients experience spontaneous regression; others can be treated successfully with chemotherapy.

Pulmonary Langerhans cell histiocytosis represents a special category of disease most often seen in adult smokers. It can regress spontaneously on cessation of smoking and usually comprises a polyclonal population of Langerhans cells,[81] suggesting it is a reactive hyperplasia rather than a true neoplasm.

SPLEEN

Normal

The spleen is to the circulatory system as the lymph nodes are to the lymphatic system. Among its functions are filtration from the bloodstream of all foreign matter, including obsolescent and damaged blood cells, and participation in the immune response to blood-borne antigens. Designed ingeniously for these functions, the spleen is a major repository of mononuclear phagocytic cells in the red pulp and of lymphoid cells in the white pulp. Normally, in the adult, it weighs about 150 gm and measures some 12 cm in length, 7 cm in width, and 3 cm in thickness. It is enclosed within a thin, glistening, slate-gray connective tissue capsule, through which dusky red, friable splenic parenchyma is seen. The cut surface of the spleen is dotted with gray specks: the splenic, or Malpighian, white pulp follicles. The white pulp consists of aggregates of lymphoid cells that surround medium-sized splenic arteries. A cross-section of such an artery reveals an eccentric collar of T lymphocytes, the so-called periarteriolar lymphatic sheath. At intervals, this lymphatic sheath expands, usually on one side of the artery, to form lymphoid nodules composed principally of B lymphocytes (Fig. 14–38). On antigenic stimulation, typical germinal centers form within these B-cell areas. Eventually, the arterial system terminates in fine penicilliary arterioles enclosed within only a thin mantle of lymphocytes, which disappears entirely as these vessels enter the red pulp.

The red pulp of the spleen is traversed by numerous thin-walled vascular sinusoids, separated by the splenic cords, or "cords of Billroth." The endothelial lining of the sinusoid is of the open or discontinuous type, providing passage of blood cells between the sinusoids and cords. The splenic cords are spongelike and consist of a labyrinth of macrophages loosely connected through long dendritic processes to create both a

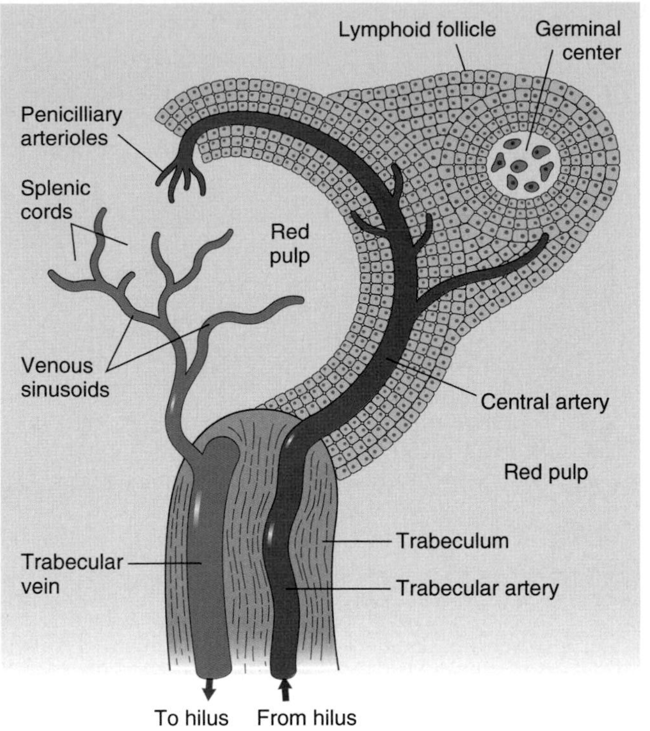

FIGURE 14–38 Normal splenic architecture. (Modified from Faller DV: Diseases of the spleen. In Wyngaarden JB, Smith LH (eds): Cecil Textbook of Medicine, 18th ed. Philadelphia, WB Saunders, 1988, p. 1036.)

physical and a functional filter through which blood slowly seeps.

As it traverses the red pulp, the blood likely takes two routes to reach the splenic veins. Some flows through capillaries into the splenic cords, from which it then gradually filters out into the surrounding splenic sinusoids to reach the veins; this is the so-called open circulation or slow compartment. In the other pathway, blood passes directly from the capillaries to the splenic veins. This "closed circuit" is understandably the compartment with the more rapid blood flow. Although only a small fraction of the blood entering the spleen at any given time pursues the "open" route, during the course of a day, the entire blood volume passes through the filtration beds of the splenic cords, where it is "screened" by the remarkably sensitive and effective sinusoidal macrophages.

Most anatomic alterations of the spleen are enlargements caused by systemic disorders that enhance some aspect of normal splenic function. These functions can be segregated into four categories:

1. *Removal of unwanted elements from the blood* by splenic phagocytosis in the cords is a major function. As you know, 1/120th of all red cells are removed daily by the phagocytes of the mononuclear phagocyte system. This amounts to removal of $\sim 2 \times 10^{11}$ red cells per day in a 70-kg adult, about 50% of which are phagocytosed in the spleen. Splenic phagocytes are also remarkably efficient in culling damaged red cells and leukocytes, red cells rendered foreign by antibody coating, and abnormal red cells encountered in several hereditary hemolytic anemias (e.g., hereditary spherocytosis). As was discussed earlier (see Chapter 13), red cells undergo extreme deformation during passage from the cords into the sinusoids. In conditions in which red cell elasticity is decreased, red cells become entrapped within the cords and are more readily phagocytosed by cordal macrophages. Splenic macrophages are also responsible for "pitting" of red cells, the process by which inclusions such as Heinz bodies are neatly excised from red cells. Splenic phagocytes also actively remove other particulate matter from the blood, such as bacteria, cell debris, and abnormal macromolecules produced in some inborn errors of metabolism (e.g., Gaucher disease, Niemann-Pick disease).
2. The spleen is a *major secondary organ of the immune system.* Dendritic cells in the periarterial lymphatic sheath trap antigens and present them to T lymphocytes. T and B cells interact at the edges of white pulp follicles, leading to the generation of antibody-secreting plasma cells, which are found mainly within the sinuses of the red pulp.
3. The spleen can be a *source of hematopoietic cells.* Splenic hematopoiesis normally ceases before birth, but in severe anemia, extramedullary splenic hematopoiesis can be reactivated.
4. Because of its rich vascularization and sluggish circulation, the spleen *sequesters a portion of the formed blood elements.* In animals with contractile spleens, such as the dog, these elements can be mobilized and thus constitute a reserve pool. The human spleen lacks contractility, however, limiting its function in this regard. In humans, the normal spleen contains only about 30 to 40 mL of red cells, but with splenomegaly, this is greatly increased. The normal spleen also harbors approximately 30% to 40% of the total platelet mass in the body. With splenomegaly, up to 80% to 90% of the total platelet mass can be sequestered in the interstices of the red pulp, producing thrombocytopenia. Similarly, the enlarged spleen can trap a sufficient number of white cells to induce leukopenia.

Despite the diverse functions of the spleen, deficient splenic function due to splenectomy or autoinfarction (as in sickle-cell disease) has a single major clinical manifestation: increased susceptibility to disseminated infection with encapsulated bacteria such as pneumococcus, meningococcus, and *Haemophilus influenzae.* The reduced filtering and antibody production functions of the spleen probably contribute to these infections, which often cause fatal sepsis in asplenic individuals.

Pathology

As the largest unit of the mononuclear phagocyte system, the spleen is involved in all systemic inflammations, generalized hematopoietic disorders, and many metabolic disturbances. In each of these disorders, the spleen undergoes enlargement, which is the major manifestation of disorders of this organ. It is rarely the primary site of disease.

Splenomegaly

Splenic enlargement can be an important diagnostic clue to the existence of an underlying disorder, but it can itself also cause problems. When sufficiently enlarged, the spleen causes a dragging sensation in the left upper quadrant and, through pressure on the stomach, discomfort after eating. In addition, its enlargement can lead to sequestration of significant numbers of blood elements. This gives rise to a syndrome known as *hypersplenism*, which is characterized by the triad of (1) splenomegaly; (2) anemia, leukopenia, thrombocytopenia, or any combination of these, in association with hyperplasia of the marrow precursors of the deficient cell type; and (3) correction of the blood cytopenia(s) by splenectomy. The likely cause of the cytopenias in this syndrome is increased sequestration of formed elements and the consequent enhanced phagocytosis by the splenic macrophages.

A listing, by no means exhaustive, of the disorders associated with splenomegaly is provided in Table 14–9. Splenomegaly in virtually all the conditions mentioned has been discussed elsewhere. There remain only a few disorders to consider.

TABLE 14–9 Disorders Associated with Splenomegaly

I. Infections
Nonspecific splenitis of various blood-borne infections (particularly infective endocarditis)
Infectious mononucleosis
Tuberculosis
Typhoid fever
Brucellosis
Cytomegalovirus
Syphilis
Malaria
Histoplasmosis
Toxoplasmosis
Kala-azar
Trypanosomiasis
Schistosomiasis
Leishmaniasis
Echinococcosis
II. Congestive States Related to Portal Hypertension
Cirrhosis of the liver
Portal or splenic vein thrombosis
Cardiac failure
III. Lymphohematogenous Disorders
Hodgkin lymphoma
Non-Hodgkin lymphomas and lymphocytic leukemias
Multiple myeloma
Myeloproliferative disorders
Hemolytic anemias
Thromobocytopenic purpura
IV. Immunologic-Inflammatory Conditions
Rheumatoid arthritis
Systemic lupus erythematosus
V. Storage Diseases
Gaucher disease
Niemann-Pick disease
Mucopolysaccharidoses
VI. Miscellaneous
Amyloidosis
Primary neoplasms and cysts
Secondary neoplasms

NONSPECIFIC ACUTE SPLENITIS

Enlargement of the spleen occurs in any blood-borne infection. The nonspecific splenic reaction in these infections is caused both by the microbiologic agents themselves and by cytokines that are released as part of the immune response.

Morphology. The spleen is enlarged (up to 200 to 400 gm) and soft. The splenic substance is often diffluent and can be so soft that it literally flows out from the cut surface. Microscopically, the major change is acute congestion of the red pulp, which can encroach on and sometimes virtually efface the lymphoid follicles. Neutrophils, plasma cells, and occasionally eosinophils are usually present throughout the white and red pulp. At times, there is acute necrosis of the centers of the splenic follicles, particularly when the causative agent is a hemolytic streptococcus. Rarely, abscess formation occurs.

CONGESTIVE SPLENOMEGALY

Chronic venous congestion can cause a form of splenic enlargement referred to as *congestive splenomegaly.* Venous congestion can be systemic in origin, caused by intrahepatic disorders that retard portal venous drainage, or may arise from extrahepatic disorders that directly obstruct the portal or splenic veins. All these disorders ultimately lead to portal or splenic vein hypertension. *Systemic, or central, venous congestion* is encountered in cardiac decompensation involving the right side of the heart, as can occur in tricuspid or pulmonic valvular disease, chronic cor pulmonale, or following left-sided heart failure. Systemic passive congestion produces only moderate enlargement of the spleen that rarely exceeds 500 gm in weight.

The only common causes of striking congestive splenomegaly are the various forms of cirrhosis of the liver. The "pipe-stem" hepatic fibrosis of schistosomiasis causes particularly severe congestive splenomegaly, while the diffuse fibrous scarring of alcoholic cirrhosis and pigment cirrhosis also evokes profound enlargements. Other forms of cirrhosis are less commonly implicated.

Congestive splenomegaly is also caused by obstruction of the extrahepatic portal vein or splenic vein. This can stem from *spontaneous portal vein thrombosis*, which is usually associated with some intrahepatic obstructive disease, or inflammation of the portal vein *(pylephlebitis)*, such as follows intraperitoneal infections. Thrombosis of the splenic vein itself can be initiated by compression by tumors in neighboring organs, for example, carcinoma of the stomach or pancreas.

Morphology. Long-standing congestion produces marked enlargement of the spleen (1000 gm or more); the organ is firm and becomes increasingly so the longer the congestion lasts. The weight can reach 5000 gm. The capsule is usually thickened and fibrous. The cut surface has a meaty appearance and varies from gray-red to deep red, depending on the amount of fibrosis. Often the white pulp is indistinct. Microscopically, the red pulp is congested in early chronic congestion but becomes increasingly more fibrous and cellular with time. The increased portal venous pressure causes deposition of collagen in the basement membrane of the sinusoids, which appear dilated owing to the rigidity of their walls. The resultant slowing of blood flow from the cords to the sinusoids prolongs the exposure of the blood cells to the cordal macrophages, resulting in excessive destruction (hypersplenism). Foci of recent or old hemorrhage are often present. Organization of these focal hemorrhages gives rise to Gandy-Gamma nodules: foci of fibrosis containing iron and calcium salts deposited on connective tissue and elastic fibers.

SPLENIC INFARCTS

Splenic infarcts are common lesions. Caused by occlusion of the major splenic artery or any of its branches, in normal-sized spleens they are most often due to emboli that arise from thrombi in the heart. The spleen, along with kidneys and brain, ranks as one of the most frequent sites within which emboli lodge. The resulting infarcts can be small or large, single or multiple or can even involve the entire organ. They are usually bland but can be septic when associated with infectious endocarditis of mitral and aortic valves. Infarcts are also common in markedly enlarged spleens, presumably because the blood supply cannot keep up with the increased demands of the organ.

Morphology. Bland infarcts are characteristically pale and wedge-shaped, with their bases at the periphery, where the overlying capsule is often covered with fibrin (Fig. 14–39). In septic infarcts, this appearance is modified by the development of suppurative necrosis. In the course of healing of splenic infarcts, large, depressed scars often develop.

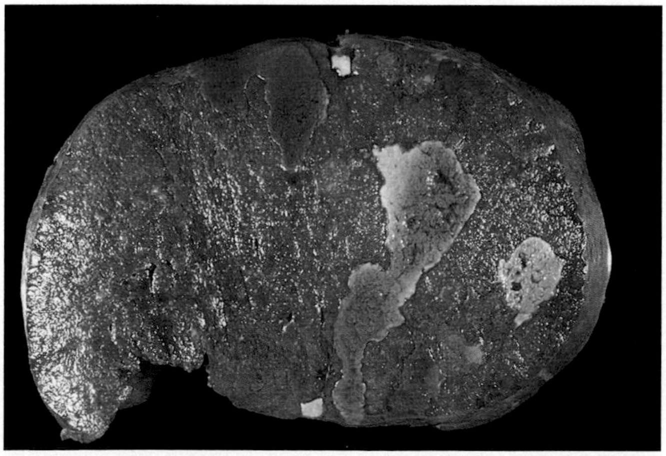

FIGURE 14–39 Splenic infarcts. Multiple well-circumscribed infarcts are present in this spleen, which is massively enlarged (2820 gm; normal: 150 to 200) by extramedullary hematopoiesis secondary to a chronic myeloproliferative disorder (myelofibrosis). Recent infarcts are hemorrhagic, whereas older, more fibrotic infarcts are a pale yellow-gray color.

Neoplasms

Neoplastic involvement of the spleen is rare except in tumors of the lymphohematopoietic system. When present, they induce splenomegaly. The following types of benign tumors may arise in the spleen: fibromas, osteomas, chondromas, lymphangiomas, and hemangiomas. The two last-named are the most common and are often cavernous in type. Some of the hemangiomas are probably more accurately classified as hamartomas than as neoplasms. Splenic involvement occurs in a variety of lymphoid and myeloid neoplasms, as has already been discussed.

Congenital Anomalies

Complete absence of the spleen is rare and is usually associated with other congenital abnormalities such as situs inversus and cardiac malformations. *Hypoplasia* is a more common finding.

Accessory spleens (spleniculi) are common and have been encountered singly or multiply in one-fifth to one-third of all postmortem examinations. They are small, spherical structures that are histologically and functionally identical to the normal spleen, reacting to various stimuli in the same manner. They are generally situated in the gastrosplenic ligament or the tail of the pancreas but are sometimes located in the omentum or mesenteries of the small or large intestine. Accessory spleens can have great clinical importance. In some hematologic disorders, such as hereditary spherocytosis and idiopathic thrombocytopenia purpura, splenectomy is a standard method of treatment. If an accessory spleen is overlooked, the benefit of removal of the definitive spleen can be lost.

Rupture

Splenic rupture is usually precipitated by a crushing injury or severe blow. Much less often, it occurs in the apparent absence of trauma. Such "spontaneous ruptures" never occur in truly normal spleens, but rather stem from some minor physical insult to a spleen that has been rendered fragile by an underlying condition. The most common predisposing conditions are infectious mononucleosis, malaria, typhoid fever, and lymphoid neoplasms. These diverse entities can all cause rapid splenic enlargement, producing a thin, tense splenic capsule that is susceptible to rupture. This dramatic event is usually followed by extensive, sometimes massive, intraperitoneal hemorrhage, which must be treated by prompt splenectomy to prevent death from loss of blood and shock. Spontaneous rupture of chronically enlarged spleens is less likely because of reactive fibrosis that toughens the capsule and pulp.

THYMUS

Normal

Once an organ buried in obscurity within the mediastinum, the thymus has risen to a starring role in cell-mediated immunity, as was detailed in Chapter 6. Here, our interest centers on the disorders of the gland itself.

The thymus, along with the lower pair of parathyroid glands, is embryologically derived from the third and, inconstantly, the fourth pair of pharyngeal pouches. Not surprisingly, one or two parathyroids occasionally become enclosed within the thymic capsule, an aberration that can plague the parathyroid surgeon. The thymus, or a portion of it, can be found in ectopic locations in the neck or on the pleural surface. At birth, the thymus weighs 10 to 35 gm; it continues to grow in size until puberty, when it achieves a maximum weight of 20 to 50 gm. Thereafter, it undergoes progressive atrophy to little more than 5 to 15 gm in the elderly. This age-related involution is accompanied by replacement of the thymic parenchyma by fibrofatty tissue. The rate of thymic growth in the child and involution in the adult is extremely variable, and so it is difficult to determine weight appropriate for age. The thymus can also involute in children and young adults in response to episodes of severe stress, including HIV infection.

The fully developed thymus is pyramid shaped, well encapsulated, and composed of two fused lobes. Fibrous extensions of the capsule divide each lobe into numerous lobules, each of which has an outer cortical layer enclosing the central medulla. A diversity of cell types populate the thymus, but thymic epithelial cells and immature lymphocytes of T-cell lineage predominate. Directly beneath the capsule, the epithelial cells are present in a near-continuous row, but deeper in the cortex, they are arranged in a loose meshwork within which lymphocytes develop and mature. These cortical epithelial cells have an abundant cytoplasm and pale vesicular nuclei with finely divided chromatin and only small nucleoli; cytoplasmic extensions contact adjacent cells. In contrast, the epithelial cells in the medulla are packed more densely; can be "spindled" with oval, darkly staining nuclei; and have only scant cytoplasm devoid of interconnecting processes. Whorls of these cells create *Hassall corpuscles*, with their characteristic keratinized cores.

As you know from the earlier consideration of the thymus in relation to immunity (see Chapter 6), progenitor cells of marrow origin migrate to the thymus and there give rise to mature T cells that are exported to the periphery. The thymic production of T cells slowly declines during adulthood as the organ atrophies.

In addition to thymocytes and epithelial cells, macrophages, dendritic cells, a minor population of B lymphocytes, rare neutrophils and eosinophils, and scattered myoid (muscle-like) cells are found within the thymus. The myoid cells are of particular interest because, as will be seen subsequently, the thymus in some obscure manner is related to myasthenia gravis, a musculoskeletal disorder of immune origin.

Pathology

Morphologic lesions in the thymus are associated with a variety of systemic conditions ranging from immunologic to hematologic to neoplastic. Fortunately, the changes within the thymus itself are relatively limited and can be adequately considered under the following headings: (1) developmental disorders, (2) thymic hyperplasia, and (3) thymomas. The changes associated with myasthenia gravis are considered in Chapter 27.

Developmental Disorders

Thymic hypoplasia or *aplasia* is seen in DiGeorge syndrome, accompanied by parathyroid developmental failures. As was detailed in Chapter 6, this condition is marked by severe deficits in cell-mediated immunity and variable hypoparathyroidism. As discussed in Chapter 5, DiGeorge syndrome is often associated with other developmental defects as part of the 22q11 deletion syndrome.

Isolated *thymic cysts* are uncommon lesions that are usually discovered incidentally postmortem or during surgery. They rarely exceed 4 cm in diameter, can be spherical or arborizing, and are lined by stratified to columnar epithelium. The fluid contents can be serous or mucinous and are often modified by hemorrhage.

While isolated cysts are not clinically significant, neoplastic thymic masses (whatever their origin) are often associated with cysts that presumably develop because of distortion and compression of adjacent normal thymus. Therefore, the presence of a cystic thymic lesion in a symptomatic patient should provoke a thorough search for a neoplasm, particularly a lymphoma or a thymoma.

Thymic Hyperplasia

The term "thymic hyperplasia" is a bit misleading, as it usually applies to the appearance of lymphoid follicles within the thymus, a state that is referred to as *thymic follicular hyperplasia.* The lymphoid follicles are similar to reactive germinal centers and contain predominantly B lymphocytes, which are present in only small numbers in the normal thymus. Although follicular hyperplasia can occur in a number of chronic inflammatory and immunologic states, it is most frequently encountered in myasthenia gravis, being present in about 65% to 75% of cases (see Chapter 27). Similar thymic changes are sometimes encountered in Graves disease, systemic lupus erythematosus, scleroderma, and rheumatoid arthritis as well as other autoimmune disorders.

Thymomas

A diversity of neoplasms may arise in the thymus—germ cell tumors, lymphomas, and carcinoids as well as others—but *the designation "thymoma" is restricted to tumors of thymic epithelial cells.* Such tumors typically have, in addition, a background of immature T cells (thymocytes).

Thymomas have been classified and reclassified in an effort to create subsets of clinical and prognostic usefulness. No effort will be made here to present these varied classifications; we shall resort to one that has the virtues of simplicity and clinical usefulness. According to this approach, thymomas can be divided into the following categories:

- Benign or encapsulated thymoma: cytologically and biologically benign
- Malignant thymoma
  - Type I, also called invasive thymoma: cytologically benign but biologically aggressive and capable of local invasion and, rarely, distant spread
  - Type II, also called "thymic carcinoma": cytologically malignant with all of the biologic features of cancer

All categories, benign and malignant, are tumors of adults, usually older than 40 years of age, and are rare in children. Males and females are affected equally. Most arise in the anterior superior mediastinum, but sometimes they occur in the neck, thyroid, pulmonary hilus, or elsewhere. They are uncommon in the posterior mediastinum. They account for only 20% to 30% of tumors in the anterosuperior mediastinum, as this is also a common location for the nodular sclerosis type of Hodgkin lymphoma and certain forms of non-Hodgkin lymphoma.

Morphology. Macroscopically, thymomas are lobulated, firm, gray-white masses up to 15 to 20 cm in the longest dimension. They sometimes have areas of cystic necrosis and calcification even in tumors that later prove to be biologically benign. The majority are encapsulated, but 20% to 25% of the tumors penetrate the capsule and infiltrate perithymic tissues and structures.

Thymomas typically consist of jigsaw puzzle–type lobules separated by fibrous bands. Microscopically, virtually all are made up of a mixture of epithelial cells and a variable infiltrate of non-neoplastic thymocytes. The relative proportions of the epithelial and thymocytic components are of little clinical significance but of some biologic interest, as the neoplastic thymic epithelial cells, even at metastatic sites, often support the homing and differentiation of T-cell progenitors.

Benign thymomas are most often composed of medullary-type epithelial cells or a mixture of medullary and cortical type epithelial cells. In medullary-type thymomas, the epithelial cells are elongated or spindle shaped (Fig. 14–40). There is usually a sparse infiltrate of thymocytes, which often recapitulate the phenotype of medullary T cells. In mixed thymomas, there is an admixture of plumper, rounder, cortical-type epithelial cells and a denser infiltrate of thymocytes. The medullary and mixed patterns together account for about 50% of all thymomas. Tumors that have a significant proportion of medullary-type epithelial cells are usually benign. Hassall corpuscles are rarely present with either pattern and, when found, often are poorly formed. They are of no diagnostic significance because they might represent residual normal thymic tissue.

The designation **malignant thymoma type I**, as used here, refers to a tumor that, although cytologically benign, is locally invasive and has the capacity for metastasis. The epithelial cells are most commonly of the cortical variety, with abundant cytoplasm and rounded vesicular nuclei (Fig. 14–40), and are usually accompanied by immature thymocytes expressing TdT. Palisading of epithelial cells about blood vessels is sometimes seen. Minor areas of spindled "medullary-type" epithelial cells are commonly present, and rarely medullary-type epithelial cells predominate. In other cases, the neoplastic cells ex-

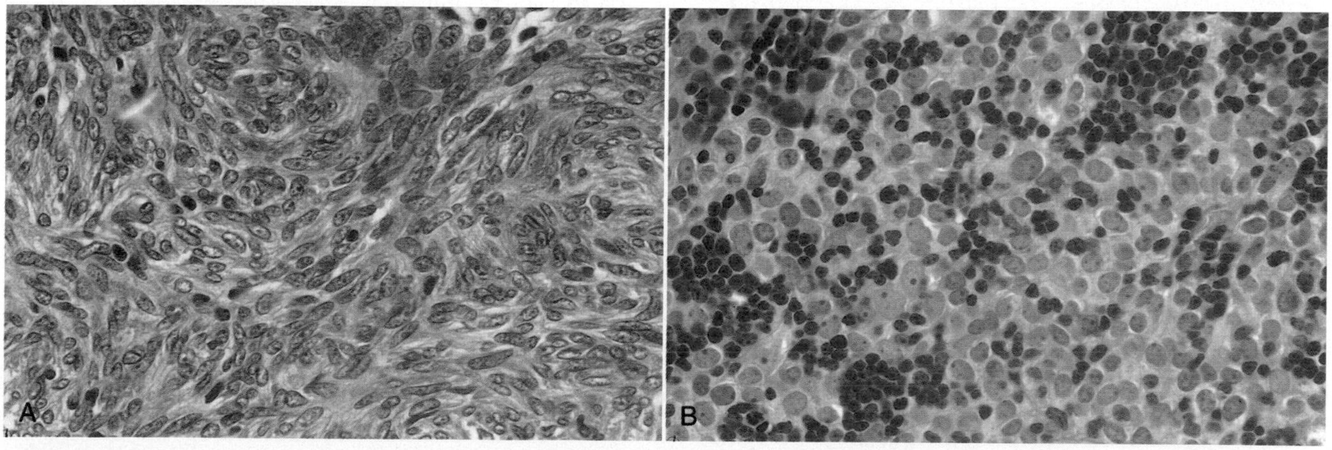

FIGURE 14–40 Thymoma. *A*, Benign thymoma (medullary type). The neoplastic epithelial cells are arranged in a swirling pattern and have bland, oval to elongated nuclei with inconspicuous nucleoli. Only a few small, reactive lymphoid cells are interspersed. *B*, Malignant thymoma, type I. The neoplastic epithelial cells are polygonal and have round to oval, bland nuclei with inconspicuous nucleoli. Numerous small, reactive lymphoid cells are interspersed. The morphologic appearance of this tumor is identical to that of benign thymomas of the cortical type. In this case, however, the tumor was locally aggressive, invading adjacent lung and pericardium.

hibit cytologic atypia, a feature that correlates with a propensity for more aggressive behavior. These tumors account for about 20% to 25% of all thymomas.

The critical feature of malignant thymoma type I is penetration of the capsule and invasion into surrounding structures. The extent of invasion has been subdivided into various stages, which are somewhat beyond our scope, but it suffices that with minimal invasion, complete excision yields a greater than 90% 5-year survival rate. Extensive invasion is often accompanied by metastasis and associated with a 5-year survival rate of less than 50%.

Malignant thymoma type II, perhaps better designated **"thymic carcinoma,"** represents about 5% of thymomas. In contrast to the type I malignant thymomas, these are cytologically malignant, having all of the anaplastic features seen in other carcinomas. Macroscopically, they are usually fleshy, obviously invasive masses sometimes accompanied by metastases to such sites as the lungs. Microscopically, most are **squamous cell carcinomas, either well or poorly differentiated**. The next most common variant is **lymphoepithelioma-like carcinoma**, a tumor composed of sheets of cells with indistinct borders that bears a close histologic resemblance to nasopharyngeal carcinoma. About 50% of lymphoepithelioma-like carcinomas contain monoclonal EBV genomes, suggesting a role for this virus in their pathogenesis. A variety of other histologic patterns of thymic carcinoma have been described, including sarcomatoid variants, basaloid carcinoma, and clear cell carcinoma. Curiously, thymic carcinomas tend to express CD5, a molecule that is normally restricted to T cells and a small subset of B cells, whereas cytologically benign thymomas and other carcinomas do not.[82]

Clinical Course. About 40% of thymomas present because of symptoms stemming from impingement on mediastinal structures, and another 30% to 45% present due to their association with myasthenia gravis. The remainder are discovered incidentally during imaging studies or cardiothoracic surgery. In addition to myasthenia gravis, other paraneoplastic syndromes, such as acquired hypogammaglobulinemia, pure red cell aplasia, Graves disease, pernicious anemia, dermatomyositis-polymyositis, and Cushing syndrome, can be seen. The basis for these associations is still obscure, but the thymocytes that arise within thymomas give rise to long-lived CD4+ and CD8+ cells,[83] and cortical thymomas rich in thymocytes are more likely to be associated with autoimmune disease.[84] Hence, it is possible that abnormalities in the selection or "education" of T cells within the disturbed environment of the neoplasm contribute to the development of autoimmune disorders.

REFERENCES

1. Dale DC: Immune and idiopathic neutropenia. Curr Opin Hematol 5:33, 1998.
2. Lamy T, Loughran TP, Jr: Current concepts: large granular lymphocyte leukemia. Blood Rev 13:230, 1999.
3. Pasqualucci L, et al: Hypermutation of multiple proto-oncogenes in B-cell diffuse large-cell lymphomas. Nature 412: 341, 2001.
4. Shaffer AL, et al: Lymphoid malignancies: the dark side of B-cell differentiation. Nat Rev Immunol 2:920, 2002.
5. Schulz TF: KSHV/HHV8-associated lymphoproliferations in the AIDS setting. Eur J Cancer 37:1217, 2001.
6. Wotherspoon AC, et al: Mucosa-associated lymphoid tissue lymphoma. Curr Opin Hematol 9:50, 2002.
7. Ryan BM, Kelleher D: Refractory celiac disease. Gastroenterology 119:243, 2000.
8. Harris NL, et al: A revised European-American classification of lymphoid neoplasms: a proposal from the International Lymphoma Study Group. Blood 84:1361, 1994.
9. Melnyk A, et al: Evaluation of the Revised European-American Lymphoma classification confirms the clinical relevance of immunophenotype in 560 cases of aggressive non-Hodgkin's lymphoma. Blood 89:4514, 1997.
10. A clinical evaluation of the International Lymphoma Study Group classification of non-Hodgkin's lymphoma. The Non-Hodgkin's Lymphoma Classification Project. Blood 89:3909, 1997.
11. Harris NL, et al: World Health Organization classification of neoplastic diseases of the hematopoietic and lymphoid tissues: report of the Clinical Advisory Committee meeting-Airlie House, Virginia, November 1997. J Clin Oncol 17:3835, 1999.
12. Dolken G: Detection of minimal residual disease. Adv Cancer Res 82:133, 2001.
13. Harrison CJ: The detection and significance of chromosomal abnormalities in childhood acute lymphoblastic leukaemia. Blood Rev 15:49, 2001.
14. Ferrando AA, et al: Gene expression signatures define novel oncogenic pathways in T cell acute lymphoblastic leukemia. Cancer Cell 1:75, 2002.
15. Yeoh E-J, et al: Classification, subtype discovery, and prediction of outcome in pediatric acute lymphoblastic leukemia by gene expression profiling. Cancer Cell 1:133, 2002.
16. Armstrong SA, et al: MLL translocations specify a distinct gene expression profile that distinguishes a unique leukemia. Nat Genet 30:41, 2002.
17. Dohner H, et al: Genomic aberrations and survival in chronic lymphocytic leukemia. N Engl J Med 343:1910, 2000.
18. Stahl D, et al: Broad alterations of self-reactive antibody-repertoires of plasma IgM and IgG in B-cell chronic lymphocytic leukemia (B-CLL) and B-CLL related target-restricted autoimmunity. Leuk Lymphoma 42:163, 2001.
19. O'Brien S, et al: Advances in the biology and treatment of B-cell chronic lymphocytic leukemia. Blood 85:307, 1995.
20. Aster JC, Longtine JA: Detection of BCL2 rearrangements in follicular lymphoma. Am J Pathol 160:759, 2002.
21. Ye BH, et al: The BCL-6 proto-oncogene controls germinal-centre formation and Th2-type inflammation. Nat Genet 16:161, 1997.
22. Chaganti SR, et al: Involvement of BCL6 in chromosomal aberrations affecting band 3q27 in B-cell non-Hodgkin lymphoma. Genes Chromosomes Cancer 23:323, 1998.
23. Papavasiliou FN, Schatz DG: Somatic hypermutation of immunoglobulin genes: merging mechanisms for genetic diversity. Cell 109:S35, 2002.
24. Capello D, et al: Distribution and pattern of BCL-6 mutations throughout the spectrum of B-cell neoplasia. Blood 95:651, 2000.
25. Alizadeh AA, et al: Distinct types of diffuse large B-cell lymphoma identified by gene expression profiling. Nature 403:503, 2000.
26. Staudt LM: Molecular diagnosis of the hematologic cancers. N Engl J Med 348:1777, 2003.
27. Rosenwald A, et al: The use of molecular profiling to predict survival after chemotherapy for diffuse large-B-cell lymphoma. N Engl J Med 346:1937, 2002.
28. Shipp MA: Prognostic factors in aggressive non-Hodgkin's lymphoma: who has "high-risk" disease? Blood 83:1165, 1994.
29. Hecht JL, Aster JC: Molecular biology of Burkitt's lymphoma. J Clin Oncol 18:3707, 2000.
30. Hussein MA, et al: Multiple myeloma: present and future. Curr Opin Oncol 14:31, 2002.
31. Callander NS, Roodman GD: Myeloma bone disease. Semin Hematol 38:276, 2001.
32. Croucher PI, et al: Osteoprotegerin inhibits the development of osteolytic bone disease in multiple myeloma. Blood 98:3534, 2001.
33. Kuehl WM, Bergsagel PL: Multiple myeloma: evolving genetic events and host interactions. Nat Rev Cancer 2:175, 2002.
34. Zhan F, et al: Global gene expression profiling of multiple myeloma, monoclonal gammopathy of undetermined significance, and normal bone marrow plasma cells. Blood 99:1745, 2002.

35. Berenson JR: New advances in the biology and treatment of myeloma bone disease. Semin Hematol 38:15, 2001.
36. Hideshima T, et al: Molecular mechanisms mediating antimyeloma activity of proteasome inhibitor PS-341. Blood 101:1530, 2003.
37. Huff CA, Jones RJ: Bone marrow transplantation for multiple myeloma: where we are today. Curr Opin Oncol 14:147, 2002.
38. Kyle RA, et al: A long-term study of prognosis in monoclonal gammopathy of undetermined significance. N Engl J Med 346:564, 2002.
39. Fonseca R, et al: Genomic abnormalites in monoclonal gammopathy of undetermined significance. Blood 100:1417, 2002.
40. Mansoor A, et al: Cytogenic findings in lymphoplasmacytic lymphoma/Waldenstrom macroglobulinemia. Am J Clin Pathol 116:543, 2001.
41. Schop RF, et al: Waldentrom macroglobulinemia neoplastic cells lack immunoglobulin heavy chain locus translocations but have frequent 6q deletions. Blood 100:2996, 2002.
42. Leonard JP, et al: Biology and management of mantle cell lymphoma. Curr Opin Oncol 13:342, 2002.
43. Du MQ, Isaacson PG: Gastric MALT lymphoma: from aetiology to treatment. Lancet Oncol 3:97, 2002.
44. Bennett C, et al: Disseminated atypical mycobacterial infection in patients with hairy cell leukemia. Am J Med 80:891, 1986.
45. Andrey J, Saven A: Therapeutic advances in the treatment of hairy cell leukemia. Leuk Res 25:361, 2001.
46. Kutok JL, Aster JC: ALK+ anaplastic large cell lymphoma. J Clin Oncol 20:3691, 2002.
47. Lin CW, et al: Restricted killer cell immunoglobulin-like receptor repertoire without T-cell receptor gamma rearrangement supports a true natural killer-cell lineage in a subset of sinonasal lymphomas. Am J Pathol 159:1671, 2001.
48. Hongyo T, et al: Specific c-kit mutations in sinonasal natural killer/T-cell lymphoma in China and Japan. Cancer Res 60:2345, 2000.
49. Ping Siu LL, et al: Specific patterns of gene methylation in natural killer cell lymphomas: p73 is consistently involved. Am J Pathol 160:59, 2002.
50. Kuppers R, et al: Biology of Hodgkin's lymphoma. Ann Oncol 13:S11, 2002.
51. Braeuninger A, et al: Hodgkin and Reed-Sternberg cells in lymphocyte predominant Hodgkin disease represent clonal populations of germinal center-derived tumor B cells. Proc Natl Acad Sci U S A 94:9337, 1997.
52. Seitz V, et al: Detection of clonal T-cell receptor gamma-chain gene rearrangements in Reed-Sternberg cells of classic Hodgkin disease. Blood 95:3020, 2000.
53. Muschen M, et al: Rare occurrence of classical Hodgkin's disease as a T cell lymphoma. J Exp Med 191:387, 2000.
54. Stein H, et al: Down-regulation of BOB.1/OBF.1 and Oct2 in classical Hodgkin disease but not in lymphocyte predominant Hodgkin disease correlates with immunoglobulin transcription. Blood 97:496, 2001.
55. Marafioti T, et al: Hodgkin and Reed-Sternberg cells represent an expansion of a single clone originating from a germinal center B-cell with functional immunoglobulin gene rearrangements but defective immunoglobulin transcription. Blood 95:1443, 200
56. Flavell KJ, Murray PG: Hodgkin's disease and the Epstein-Barr virus. Mol Pathol 53:262, 2000.
57. Knecht H, et al: The role of Epstein-Barr virus in neoplastic transformation. Oncology 60:289, 2001.
58. Bargou RC, et al: Constitutive nuclear factor-kappaB-RelA activation is required for proliferation and survival of Hodgkin's disease tumor cells. J Clin Invest 100:2961, 1997.
59. Cabannes E, et al: Mutations in the IkBa gene in Hodgkin's disease suggest a tumour suppressor role for IkappaBalpha. Oncogene 18:3063, 1999.
60. Jungnickel B, et al: Clonal deleterious mutations in the IkappaBalpha gene in the malignant cells in Hodgkin's lymphoma. J Exp Med 191:395, 2000.
61. Krappmann D, Emmerich F, Kordes U, Scharschmidt E, Dorken B, Scheidereit C: Molecular mechanisms of constitutive NF-κ B/Rel activation in Hodgkin/Reed-Sternberg cells. Oncogene 18:943–953, 1999.
62. Martin-Subero JI, et al: Recurrent involvement of the REL and BCL11A loci in classical Hodgkin lymphoma. Blood 99:1474, 2002.
63. Joos S, et al: Classical Hodgkin lymphoma is characterized by recurrent copy number gains of the short arm of chromosome 2. Blood 99:1381, 2002.
64. Tucker MA, et al: Risk of second cancers after treatment for Hodgkin's disease. N Engl J Med 318:76, 1988.
65. Deniz K, et al: Breast cancer in women after treatment for Hodgkin's disease. Lancet Oncol 4:207, 2003.
66. Yergeau DA, et al: Embryonic lethality and impairment of haematopoiesis in mice heterozygous for an AML1-ETO fusion gene. Nat Genet 15:303, 1997.
67. Kiyoi H, et al: Prognostic implication of FLT3 and N-RAS gene mutations in acute myeloid leukemia. Blood 93:3074, 1999.
68. Dash A, Gilliland DG: Molecular genetics of acute myeloid leukaemia. Best Pract Res Clin Haematol 14:49, 2001.
69. Bennett JM, et al: Proposal for the recognition of minimally differentiated acute myeloid leukemia. Br J Hematol 78:325, 1991.
70. Stanulla M, et al: DNA cleavage within the MLL breakpoint cluster region is a specific event which occurs as part of higher-order chromatin fragmentation during the initial stages of apoptosis. Mol Cell Biol 17:4070, 1997.
71. Tallman MS: The thrombophilic state in acute promyelocytic leukemia. Semin Thromb Hemost 25:209, 1999.
72. Tallman MS, et al: Acute promyelocytic leukemia: evolving therapeutic strategies. Blood 99: 759, 2002.
73. Daley GQ, et al: Induction of chronic myelogenous leukemia in mice by the P210bcr/abl gene of the Philadelphia chromosome. Science 247: 824, 1990.
74. Druker BJ, et al: Efficacy and safety of a specific inhibitor of the BCR-ABL tyrosine kinase in chronic myeloid leukemia. N Engl J Med 344:1031, 2001.
75. Druker BJ, et al: Activity of a specific inhibitor of the BCR-ABL tyrosine kinase in the blast crisis of chronic myeloid leukemia and acute lymphoblastic leukemia with the Philadelphia chromosome. N Engl J Med 344:1038, 2001.
76. Prchal JT: Pathogenetic mechanisms of polycythemia vera and congenital polycythemic disorders. Semin Hematol 38:10, 2001.
77. Tefferi A, Silverstein MN: Current perspective in agnogenic myeloid metaplasia. Leuk Lymphoma 22 (Suppl 1):169, 1996.
78. Dupriez B, et al: Prognostic factors in agnogenic myeloid metaplasia: a report on 195 cases with a new scoring system. Blood 88:1013, 1996.
79. Laman JD, et al: Langerhans-cell histocytosis "insight into DC biology." Trends Immunol 24: 190, 2003.
80. Fleming M, et al: Coincident expression of chemokine receptors CCR6 and CCR7 by pathologic Langerhans cells in Langerhans cell histiocytosis. Blood 101:2473, 2003.
81. Yousem SA, et al: Pulmonary Langerhans cell histiocytosis: molecular analysis of clonality. Am J Surg Pathol 25:630, 2001.
82. Dorfman DM, et al: Thymic carcinomas, but not thymomas and carcinomas of other sites, show CD5 immunoreactivity. Am J Surg Pathol 21:936, 1997.
83. Buckley C, et al: Mature, long-lived CD4+ and CD8+ T cells are generated by the thymoma in myasthenia gravis. Ann Neurol 50:64, 2001.
84. Okumura M, et al: Clinical and functional significance of WHO classification on human thymic epithelial neoplasms: a study of 146 consecutive tumors. Am J Surg Pathol 25:103, 2001.

CHAPTER 15

The Lung*

Aliya N. Husain MBBS • Vinay Kumar MD

CONGENITAL ANOMALIES

ATELECTASIS (COLLAPSE)

ACUTE LUNG INJURY

Pulmonary Edema

Hemodynamic Pulmonary Edema

Edema Caused by Microvascular Injury

Acute Repiratory Distress Syndrome (Diffuse Alveolar Damage)

Acute Interstitial Pneumonia

OBSTRUCTIVE VERSUS RESTRICTIVE PULMONARY DISEASES

OBSTRUCTIVE PULMONARY DISEASE

Emphysema

Chronic Bronchitis

Asthma

Bronchiectasis

DIFFUSE INTERSTITIAL (INFILTRATIVE, RESTRICTIVE) DISEASE

Fibrosing Diseases

Idiopathic Pulmonary Fibrosis

Nonspecific Interstitial Pneumonia

Cryptogenic Organizing Pneumonia

Pulmonary Involvement in Collagen Vascular Diseases

Pneumoconioses

Complications of Therapies

Granulomatous Diseases

Sarcoidosis

Hypersensitivity Pneumonitis

Pulmonary Eosinophilia

Smoking-Related Interstitial Diseases

Desquamative Interstitial Pneumonia (DIP)

Respiratory Bronchiolitis-Associated Interstitial Lung Disease

Pulmonary Alveolar Proteinosis

DISEASES OF VASCULAR ORIGIN

Pulmonary Embolism, Hemorrhage, and Infarction

Pulmonary Hypertension

Diffuse Pulmonary Hemorrhage Syndromes

Goodpasture Syndrome

Idiopathic Pulmonary Hemosiderosis

Wegener Granulomatosis

PULMONARY INFECTIONS

Community-Acquired Acute Pneumonias

Streptococcus Pneumoniae

Haemophilus Influenzae

Moraxella Catarrhalis

Staphylococcus Aureus

Klebsiella Pneumoniae

Pseudomonas Aeruginosa

Legionella Pneumophila

Community-Acquired Atypical (Viral and Mycoplasmal) Pneumonias

Influenza Infections

Severe Acute Respiratory Syndrome (SARS)

Nosocomial Pneumonia

Aspiration Pneumonia

Lung Abscess

Chronic Pneumonia

Histoplasmosis

Blastomycosis

*The contributions of Dr. Lester Kobzik to the previous editions of this text are gratefully acknowledged. Dr. Anirban Maitra is also acknowledged for his contributions to this chapter.

Coccidioidomycosis
Pneumonia in the Immunocompromised Host
Pulmonary Disease in Human Immunodeficiency Virus Infection
LUNG TRANSPLANTATION
TUMORS
Carcinomas
Neuroendocrine Proliferations and Tumors
Miscellaneous Tumors
Metastatic Tumors
PLEURA
Pleural Effusion
Inflammatory Pleural Effusions
Noninflammatory Pleural Effusions
Pneumothorax
Pleural Tumors
Solitary (Localized) Fibrous Tumors
Malignant Mesothelioma

Normal Lung

The lungs are ingeniously constructed to carry out their cardinal function: the exchange of gases between inspired air and blood. Developmentally, the respiratory system is an outgrowth from the ventral wall of the foregut. The midline trachea develops two lateral outpocketings, the lung buds. The right lung bud eventually divides into three branches—the main bronchi—and the left into two main bronchi, thus giving rise to three lobes on the right and two on the left. The lingula on the left is the middle lobe equivalent; however, the left lung is smaller than the right. The right main stem bronchus is more vertical and more directly in line with the trachea than is the left. Consequently, aspirated foreign material, such as vomitus, blood, and foreign bodies, tends to enter the right lung rather than the left. The main right and left bronchi branch dichotomously, giving rise to progressively smaller airways. Accompanying the branching airways is the double arterial supply to the lungs, that is, the pulmonary and bronchial arteries. In the absence of significant cardiac failure, the bronchial arteries of aortic origin can often sustain the vitality of the pulmonary parenchyma when pulmonary arterial supply is blocked, as by emboli.

Progressive branching of the bronchi forms *bronchioles*, which are distinguished from bronchi by the lack of cartilage and submucosal glands within their walls. Further branching of bronchioles leads to the *terminal bronchioles*, which are less than 2 mm in diameter. The part of the lung distal to the terminal bronchiole is called the *acinus*; it is approximately spherical, with a diameter of about 7 mm. As illustrated in Figure 15–5*A*, an acinus is composed of *respiratory bronchioles* (emanating from the terminal bronchiole), which give off several alveoli from their sides. These bronchioles then proceed into the *alveolar ducts*, which immediately branch into *alveolar sacs*, the blind ends of the respiratory passages, whose walls are formed entirely of alveoli, which are the site of gas exchange. The alveoli open into the ducts through large mouths. In the correct plane of section, therefore, all alveoli are open and have incomplete walls. A cluster of three to five terminal bronchioles, each with its appended acinus, is usually referred to as the pulmonary *lobule*. As will be seen subsequently, this lobular architecture assumes importance in distinguishing the major forms of emphysema.

From the microscopic standpoint, except for the vocal cords, which are covered by stratified squamous epithelium, the entire respiratory tree, including the larynx, trachea, and bronchioles, is lined by pseudostratified, tall, columnar, ciliated epithelial cells, heavily admixed in the cartilaginous airways with mucus-secreting goblet cells. The bronchial mucosa also contains neuroendocrine cells that exhibit neurosecretory-type granules and contain serotonin, calcitonin, and gastrin-releasing peptide (bombesin). Numerous submucosal, mucus-secreting glands are dispersed throughout the walls of the trachea and bronchi (but not the bronchioles).

The microscopic structure of the alveolar walls (or alveolar septa) consists, from blood to air, of the following (Fig. 15–1):

- The *capillary endothelium* lining the intertwining network of anastomosing capillaries.
- A *basement membrane and surrounding interstitial tissue* separating the endothelial cells from the alveolar lining

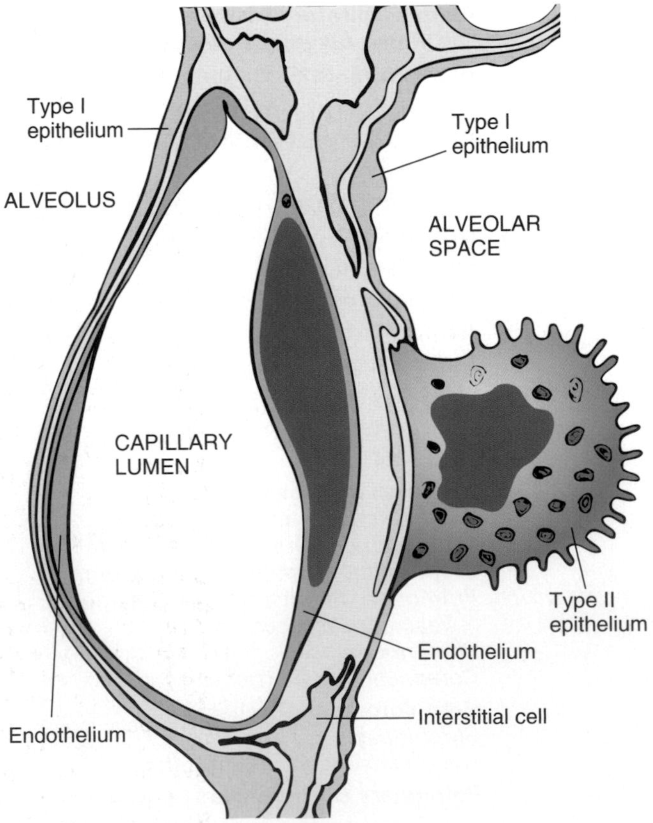

FIGURE 15–1 Microscopic structure of the alveolar wall. Note that the basement membrane (*yellow*) is thin on one side and widened where it is continuous with the interstitial space. Portions of interstitial cells are shown.

epithelial cells. In thin portions of the alveolar septum, the basement membranes of epithelium and endothelium are fused, whereas in thicker portions, they are separated by an interstitial space (*pulmonary interstitium*) containing fine elastic fibers, small bundles of collagen, a few fibroblast-like interstitial cells, smooth muscle cells, mast cells, and, rarely, lymphocytes and monocytes.

- *Alveolar epithelium*, which contains a continuous layer of two principal cell types: flattened, platelike *type I pneumocytes* (or membranous pneumocytes) covering 95% of the alveolar surface and rounded *type II pneumocytes*. Type II cells are important for at least two reasons: (1) They are the source of *pulmonary surfactant*, contained in osmiophilic *lamellar bodies* seen with electron microscopy, and (2) they are the main cell type involved in the repair of alveolar epithelium after destruction of type I cells.
- *Alveolar macrophages*, loosely attached to the epithelial cells or lying free within the alveolar spaces, derived from blood monocytes and belonging to the mononuclear phagocyte system. Often, they are filled with carbon particles and other phagocytosed materials.

The alveolar walls are not solid but are perforated by numerous *pores of Kohn*, which permit the passage of bacteria and exudate between adjacent alveoli (see Fig. 15–35*B*). Adjacent to the alveolar cell membrane is the pulmonary surfactant layer (discussed in Chapter 10 in the section on respiratory distress syndrome in newborns).

Pathology

The importance of lung disease in the overall perspective of pathology and clinical medicine cannot be overemphasized. Primary respiratory infections, such as bronchitis and pneumonia, are commonplace in clinical and pathologic practice. In these days of cigarette smoking, air pollution, and other environmental inhalants, chronic bronchitis and emphysema have become rampant. In men, malignancy of the lungs had been rising steadily but has now plateaued and is expected to decline in the future. Unfortunately, as more and more women are smoking, it has become the most common malignancy in women, surpassing even breast cancer. In both men and women, it is the most common lethal visceral malignancy. Moreover, the lungs are secondarily involved in almost all forms of terminal disease, so some degree of pulmonary edema, atelectasis, or bronchopneumonia is present in virtually every dying patient. In the present consideration of the lung, emphasis is placed on primary diseases that affect this important organ. For detailed descriptions of the less common conditions, the reader is referred to comprehensive texts on pulmonary disease.

Congenital Anomalies

Developmental defects of the lung include the following:[1]

- Agenesis or hypoplasia of both lungs, one lung, or single lobes
- Tracheal and bronchial anomalies (atresia, stenosis, tracheoesophageal fistula)
- Vascular anomalies
- Congenital lobar overinflation (emphysema)
- Foregut cysts
- Congenital pulmonary airway malformation
- Pulmonary sequestrations

Only the more common anomalies are discussed here. *Pulmonary hypoplasia* is the defective development of both lungs (one may be more affected than the other) resulting in decreased weight, volume, and acini compared to the body weight and gestational age. It is a common anomaly, seen in 10% of neonatal autopsies, and is most often secondary to space-occupying lesions in the uterus, oligohydramnios, or impaired fetal respiratory movements, as may occur in congenital diaphragmatic hernia, renal cystic diseases, renal agenesis, premature prolonged rupture of fetal membranes, and anencephaly.

Foregut cysts represent an abnormal detachment of primitive foregut and are most often located in the hilum or middle mediastinum. Depending on the wall structure, these cysts are classified into bronchogenic (most common), esophageal, or enteric cysts. A bronchogenic cyst is rarely connected to the tracheobroncheal tree. It presents in children and young adults as an incidental finding or with symptoms related to mass effect or secondary infection. Its size varies from 1 to 4 cm in diameter, but it may be larger in older patients. Microscopically, the cyst is lined by ciliated pseudostratified columnar epithelium with squamous metaplasia occurring in areas of inflammation. The wall contains bronchial glands, cartilage, and smooth muscle. Surgical resection is curative.

Congenital pulmonary airway malformation (CPAM) is a hamartomatous lesion of the lung, with an incidence of about 1 in 5,000 live births. It can be separated into five types based on clinical and pathologic features. CPAM type 1 is the most common with large cysts and good prognosis. CPAM type 2, with medium-sized cysts, often has a poor prognosis owing to its frequent association with other significant anomalies. Other types are rare.

Pulmonary sequestration refers to the presence of a discrete mass of lung tissue *without any normal connection to the airway system*. Blood supply to the sequestered area arises not from the pulmonary arteries but from the aorta or its branches. *Extralobar sequestrations* are external to the lung and may be found anywhere in the thorax or mediastinum. Found most commonly in infants as abnormal mass lesions, they may be associated with other congenital anomalies. *Intralobar sequestrations* are found within the lung substance and are usually associated with recurrent localized infection or bronchiectasis. Although a small percentage of these are clearly congenital in origin, the vast majority are probably acquired lesions formed through repeated episodes of pneumonia.

Atelectasis (Collapse)

Atelectasis refers either to incomplete expansion of the lungs (neonatal atelectasis) or to the collapse of previously inflated lung, producing areas of relatively airless pulmonary parenchyma. Acquired atelectasis, encountered principally in adults, may be divided into *resorption* (or *obstruction*), *compression*, and *contraction atelectasis* (Fig. 15–2).

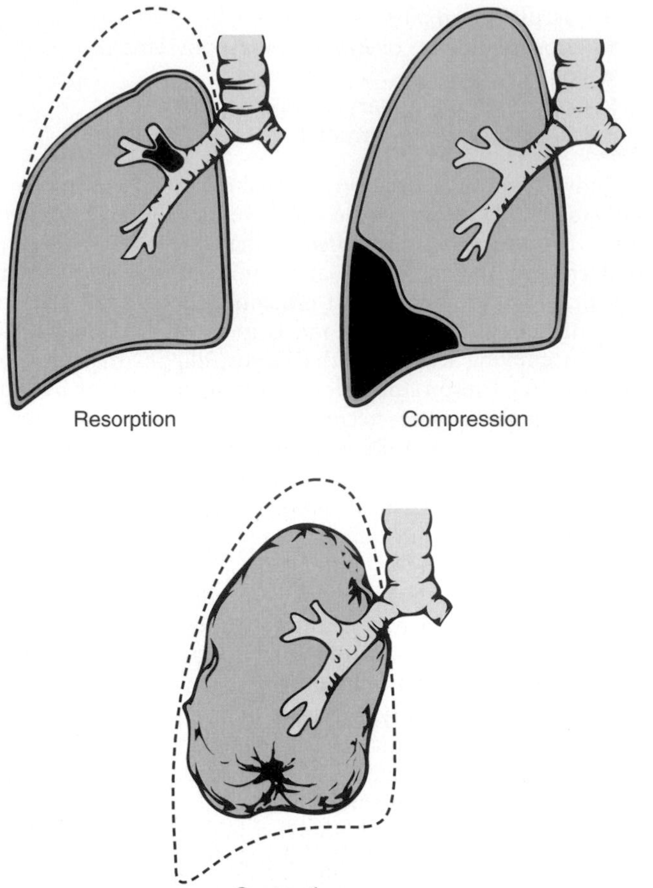

FIGURE 15–2 Various forms of atelectasis in adults.

Resorption atelectasis is the consequence of complete obstruction of an airway, which in time leads to *resorption* of the oxygen trapped in the dependent alveoli, without impairment of blood flow through the affected alveolar walls. Since lung volume is diminished, the mediastinum shifts *toward* the atelectatic lung. Resorption atelectasis is caused principally by excessive secretions (e.g., mucous plugs) or exudates within smaller bronchi and is therefore most often found in bronchial asthma, chronic bronchitis, bronchiectasis, and postoperative states and with aspiration of foreign bodies. Although bronchial neoplasms can cause atelectasis, in most instances they cause subtotal obstruction and produce localized emphysema.

Compression atelectasis results whenever the pleural cavity is partially or completely filled by fluid exudate, tumor, blood, or air (the last-mentioned constituting *pneumothorax*) or, with *tension pneumothorax*, when air pressure impinges on and threatens the function of the lung and mediastinum, especially the major vessels. Compression atelectasis is most commonly encountered in patients with cardiac failure who develop pleural fluid and in patients with neoplastic effusions within the pleural cavities. Similarly, abnormal elevation of the diaphragm, such as that which follows peritonitis or subdiaphragmatic abscesses or occurs in seriously ill postoperative patients, induces basal atelectasis. With compressive atelectasis, the mediastinum shifts *away* from the affected lung. *Contraction atelectasis* occurs when local or generalized fibrotic changes in the lung or pleura prevent full expansion.

Significant atelectasis reduces oxygenation and predisposes to infection. Because the collapsed lung parenchyma can be re-expanded, *atelectasis is a reversible disorder* (except that caused by contraction).

Acute Lung Injury

The term "acute lung injury" encompasses a spectrum of pulmonary lesions (endothelial and epithelial), which can be initiated by numerous factors. Susceptibility to lung injury appears to be heritable, and response and survival depend on the interaction of multiple loci on different chromosomes.[2] Mediators include cytokines, oxidants, and growth factors, such as tumor necrosis factor (TNF), interleukin (IL)-1, IL-6, IL-10, and transforming growth factor (TGF)-β. Lung injury may manifest as congestion, edema, surfactant disruption, and atelectasis, and these may progress to acute respiratory distress syndrome or acute interstitial pneumonia. Each of these forms of pulmonary injury is described below.

PULMONARY EDEMA

A general consideration of edema is in Chapter 4, and pulmonary congestion and edema are described briefly in the context of congestive heart failure (Chapter 12). Pulmonary edema can result from *hemodynamic* disturbances (*hemodynamic* or *cardiogenic pulmonary edema*) or from direct *increases in capillary permeability*, owing to microvascular injury (Table 15–1). Therapy and outcome depend on the underlying etiology.

Hemodynamic Pulmonary Edema

The most common *hemodynamic* mechanism of pulmonary edema is that attributable to *increased hydrostatic pressure*, as occurs in left-sided congestive heart failure. What-

TABLE 15–1 Classification and Causes of Pulmonary Edema

Hemodynamic Edema
Increased hydrostatic pressure (increased pulmonary venous pressure)
Left-sided heart failure (common)
Volume overload
Pulmonary vein obstruction
Decreased oncotic pressure (less common)
Hypoalbuminemia
Nephrotic syndrome
Liver disease
Protein-losing enteropathies
Lymphatic obstruction (rare)
Edema Due to Microvascular Injury (Alveolar Injury)
Infections: pneumonia, septicemia
Inhaled gases: oxygen, smoke
Liquid aspiration: gastric contents, near-drowning
Drugs and chemicals: chemotherapeutic agents (bleomycin), other medications (amphotericin B), heroin, kerosene, paraquat
Shock, trauma
Radiation
Transfusion related
Edema of Undetermined Origin
High altitude
Neurogenic (central nervous system trauma)

ever the clinical setting, pulmonary congestion and edema are characterized by heavy, wet lungs. Fluid accumulates initially in the basal regions of the lower lobes because hydrostatic pressure is greater in these sites (dependent edema). Histologically, the alveolar capillaries are engorged, and an intra-alveolar granular pink precipitate is seen. Alveolar microhemorrhages and hemosiderin-laden macrophages ("heart failure" cells) may be present. In long-standing cases of pulmonary congestion, such as those seen in mitral stenosis, hemosiderin-laden macrophages are abundant, and fibrosis and thickening of the alveolar walls cause the soggy lungs to become firm and brown (*brown induration*). These changes not only impair normal respiratory function, but also predispose to infection.

Edema Caused by Microvascular Injury

The second mechanism leading to pulmonary edema is *injury to the capillaries of the alveolar septa*. Here the pulmonary capillary hydrostatic pressure is usually not elevated, and hemodynamic factors play a secondary role. The edema results from primary injury to the vascular endothelium or damage to alveolar epithelial cells (with secondary microvascular injury). This results in leakage of fluids and proteins first into the interstitial space and, in more severe cases, into the alveoli. When the edema remains localized, as it does in most forms of pneumonia, it is overshadowed by the manifestations of infection. When diffuse, however, alveolar edema is an important contributor to a serious and often fatal condition, *acute respiratory distress syndrome*, discussed in the following section.

ACUTE RESPIRATORY DISTRESS SYNDROME (DIFFUSE ALVEOLAR DAMAGE)

Acute respiratory distress syndrome (ARDS) (synonyms include "shock lung," "diffuse alveolar damage," "acute alveolar injury," and "acute lung injury") is a clinical syndrome caused by diffuse alveolar capillary damage. It is characterized clinically by the rapid onset of severe life-threatening respiratory insufficiency, cyanosis, and severe arterial hypoxemia that is refractory to oxygen therapy and that may progress to extrapulmonary multisystem organ failure. Chest radiographs show diffuse alveolar infiltration. Diffuse alveolar damage (DAD) is the histologic manifestation.

ARDS is a well-recognized complication of numerous and diverse conditions, including both direct injuries to the lungs and systemic disorders (Table 15–2). In many cases, a combination of predisposing conditions is present (e.g., shock, oxygen therapy, and sepsis).

TABLE 15–2 Conditions Associated with Development of Acute Respiratory Distress Syndrome

Infection	***Chemical Injury***
Sepsis* Diffuse pulmonary infections* Viral, *Mycoplasma*, and *Pneumocystis* pneumonia; miliary tuberculosis Gastric aspiration*	Heroin or methadone overdose Acetylsalicylic acid Barbiturate overdose Paraquat
Physical/Injury	***Hematologic Conditions***
Mechanical trauma, including head injuries* Pulmonary contusions Near-drowning Fractures with fat embolism Burns Ionizing radiation	Multiple transfusions Disseminated intravascular coagulation ***Pancreatitis*** ***Uremia*** ***Cardiopulmonary Bypass***
Inhaled Irritants	***Hypersensitivity Reactions***
Oxygen toxicity Smoke Irritant gases and chemicals	Organic solvents Drugs

*More than 50% of cases of acute respiratory distress syndrome are associated with these four conditions.

Morphology. In the acute stage, the lungs are heavy, firm, red, and boggy. They exhibit congestion, interstitial and intra-alveolar edema, inflammation, and fibrin deposition. The alveolar walls become lined with waxy **hyaline membranes** (Fig. 15–3) that are morphologically similar to those seen in hyaline membrane disease of neonates (Chapter 10). Alveolar hyaline membranes consist of fibrin-rich edema fluid mixed with the cytoplasmic and lipid remnants of necrotic epithelial cells. In the organizing stage, type II epithelial cells undergo proliferation in an attempt to regenerate the alveolar lining. Resolution is unusual; more commonly, there is organization of the fibrin exudate, with resultant intra-alveolar fibrosis. Marked thickening of the alveolar septa ensues, caused by proliferation of interstitial cells and deposition of collagen. Fatal cases often have superimposed bronchopneumonia.

Pathogenesis. ARDS and DAD are best viewed as the clinical and pathologic end results, respectively, of acute alveolar injury caused by a variety of insults and initiated by different mechanisms.[3] Central to the causation of ARDS is *diffuse damage to the alveolar capillary walls*; this is followed by a relatively nonspecific, often predictable series of morphologic

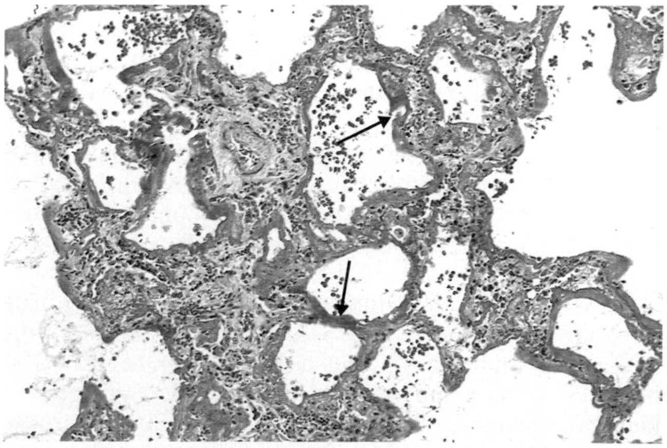

FIGURE 15–3 Diffuse alveolar damage (acute respiratory distress syndrome) shown in a photomicrograph. Some of the alveoli are collapsed; others are distended. Many contain dense proteinaceous debris, desquamated cells, and hyaline membranes (*arrows*).

and physiologic alterations leading to respiratory failure. *In contrast, the mechanism of the respiratory distress syndrome of newborns is a deficiency in pulmonary surfactant* (Chapter 10). In ARDS, the initial injury is to either capillary endothelium (most frequently) or alveolar epithelium (occasionally), but eventually both are clearly affected. The acute consequences of damage to the alveolar capillary membrane include increased vascular permeability and alveolar flooding, loss of diffusion capacity, and widespread surfactant abnormalities caused by damage to type II pneumocytes. Importantly, the exudate and diffuse tissue destruction that occur with ARDS cannot be easily resolved, and generally the result is organization with scarring, producing chronic disease. This is in contrast to the transudate of cardiogenic pulmonary edema, which usually resolves.

Acute lung injury occurs as a result of a cascade of cellular events initiated by either infectious or noninfectious inflammatory stimuli. An elevated level of pro-inflammatory mediators combined with a decreased expression of anti-inflammatory molecules is a critical component of lung inflammation. Expression of proinflammatory genes is regulated by transcriptional mechanisms, particularly NF-κ B, since it is required for maximal expression of many cytokines involved in the pathogenesis of acute lung injury. A complicated signaling cascade tightly controls activation and regulation of NF-κB. For example, in acute lung injury caused by bacterial infection, Toll-like receptors play a central role in triggering the innate immune system and activating NF-κB. NF-κB can interact with other transcription factors, and these interactions thereby lead to greater transcriptional selectivity. Anti-inflammatory cytokines such as IL-10 have been shown to suppress the inflammatory processes. Modification of such transcriptional cascade is likely to be a logical therapeutic target for acute lung injury.[4]

The most proximate signals leading to uncontrolled activation of the acute inflammatory response are not yet understood. However, as early as 30 minutes following an acute insult (e.g., acid aspiration, trauma, or exposure to bacterial lipopolysaccharide), there is increased synthesis of IL-8, a potent neutrophil chemotactic and activating agent, by pulmonary macrophages. Release of this and other cytokines, like IL-1 and TNF, leads to pulmonary microvascular sequestration and activation of neutrophils. *Neutrophils are thought to play an important role in the pathogenesis of acute lung injury and ARDS.* Histologic examination of lungs early in the disease process has shown increased numbers of neutrophils within the vascular space, the interstitium, and the alveoli. Activated neutrophils release a variety of products (such as oxidants, proteases, platelet-activating factor, and leukotrienes) that cause active tissue damage and maintain the inflammatory cascade. Release of macrophage inhibitory factor sustains the ongoing inflammatory response (Fig. 15–4).

Clinical Course. Patients who develop ARDS are usually hospitalized for one of the predisposing conditions listed earlier. Profound dyspnea and tachypnea herald ARDS, but the chest radiograph is initially normal. Subsequently, there are increasing cyanosis and hypoxemia, respiratory failure, and the appearance of diffuse bilateral infiltrates on radiographic examination. Hypoxemia can then become unresponsive to oxygen therapy, and respiratory acidosis can develop.

The functional abnormalities in ARDS are not homogeneously distributed throughout the lungs. The lungs are focally stiff and have a decrease in functional volume. In essence, patients' lungs can be divided into areas that are infiltrated, consolidated, or collapsed (and thus poorly aerated and poorly compliant) and regions that have nearly normal levels of compliance and ventilation. Lungs with ARDS continue to have perfusion of poorly aerated regions, contributing to ventilation-perfusion mismatching and hypoxemia. ARDS is a serious disorder. Despite improvements in supportive therapy, the mortality rate among the 150,000 ARDS cases seen yearly in the United States is still about 60%.

ACUTE INTERSTITIAL PNEUMONIA

"Acute interstitial pneumonia" is a clinicopathologic term that is used to describe widespread acute lung injury with a rapidly progressive clinical course similar to that seen in ARDS. Whereas ARDS is associated with known causes such as sepsis, pulmonary infection, gastric aspiration, and trauma, acute interstitial pneumonia is of unknown etiology. The mean age of patients is 50 years with no sex predilection. Patients present with acute respiratory failure often following an illness of less than 3 weeks' duration that resembles an upper respiratory tract infection. The radiographic and pathologic features are identical to that of ARDS. The mortality rate is about 50%, with most deaths occurring within 1 to 2 months. In the surviving patients, recurrences and chronic interstitial disease may develop.[5–7]

Obstructive Versus Restrictive Pulmonary Diseases

Although lung diseases can be classified and studied according to etiology, it is useful to segregate diffuse pulmonary diseases on the basis of deranged pulmonary physiology. Such a classification is based on pulmonary function tests, a critical part of the initial workup of patients. Based on the results of these tests, the patient with diffuse pulmonary disease can be put in one of two categories: (1) *obstructive disease* (or *airway disease*), characterized by an increase in resistance to airflow owing to partial or complete obstruction at any level, from the trachea and larger bronchi to the terminal and respiratory bronchioles, and (2) *restrictive disease*, characterized by reduced expansion of lung parenchyma, with decreased total lung capacity. Although many conditions have both obstructive and restrictive components, distinction between the two patterns of pulmonary dysfunction is useful in correlating the results of pulmonary function tests with the radiologic and histologic findings in individual patients.

The major diffuse obstructive disorders are *emphysema*, *chronic bronchitis*, *bronchiectasis*, and *asthma*. In patients with these diseases, pulmonary function tests show limitation of maximal airflow rates during forced expiration, usually measured by forced expiratory volume at 1 second. Expiratory airflow obstruction may result either from *anatomic airway narrowing*, such as is classically observed in asthma, or from *loss of elastic recoil of the lung*, which characteristically occurs in emphysema.

In contrast, restrictive diseases are identified by a reduced total lung capacity, while the expiratory flow rate is normal or

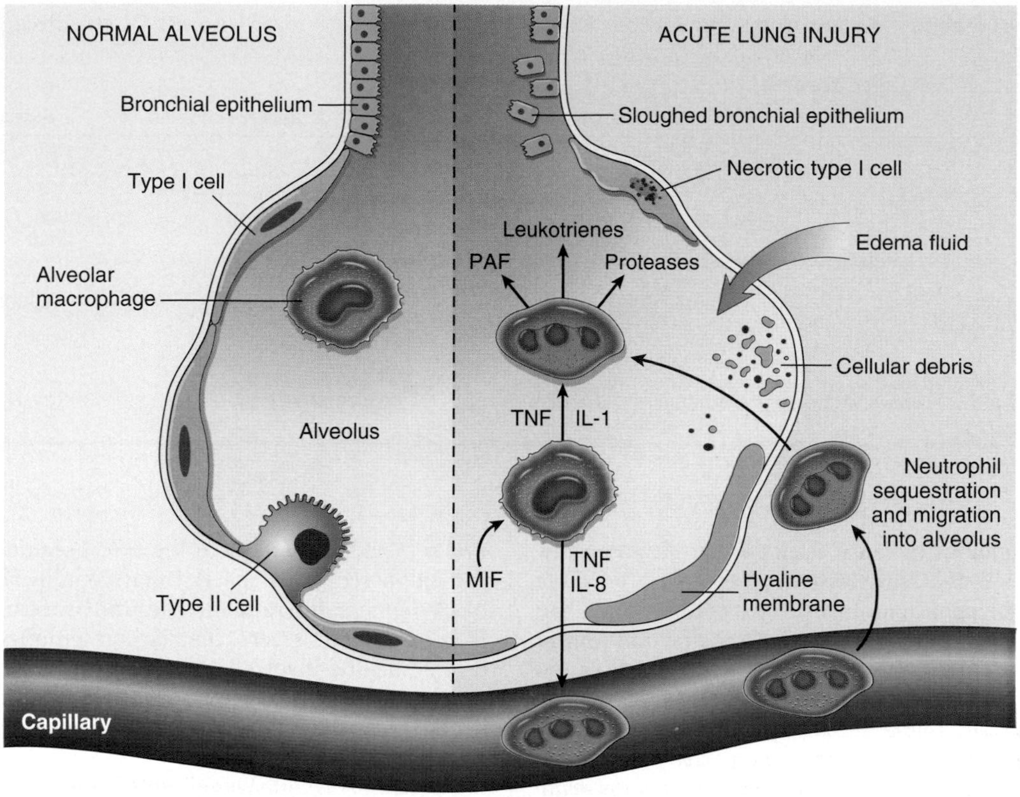

FIGURE 15–4 The normal alveolus (*left side*) compared with the injured alveolus in the early phase of acute lung injury and acute respiratory distress syndrome. Under the influence of proinflammatory cytokines such as interleukin 8 (IL-8), interleukin 1 (IL-1), and tumor necrosis factor (TNF) (released by macrophages), neutrophils initially undergo sequestration in the pulmonary microvasculature, followed by margination and egress into the alveolar space, where they undergo activation. Activated neutrophils release a variety of factors, such as leukotrienes, oxidants, proteases, and platelet-activating factor (PAF), which contribute to local tissue damage, accumulation of edema fluid in the airspaces, surfactant inactivation, and hyaline membrane formation. Macrophage inhibitory factor (MIF) released into the local milieu sustains the ongoing pro-inflammatory response. Subsequently, the release of macrophage-derived fibrogenic cytokines such as transforming growth factor β (TGF-β) and platelet-derived growth factor (PDGF) stimulate fibroblast growth and collagen deposition associated with the healing phase of injury. (Modified with permission from Ware LB, Matthay MA: The acute respiratory distress syndrome. N Engl J Med 342:1334, 2000.)

reduced proportionately. The restrictive defect occurs in two general conditions: (1) *chest wall disorders in the presence of normal lungs* (e.g., neuromuscular diseases such as poliomyelitis, severe obesity, pleural diseases, and kyphoscoliosis) and (2) *acute or chronic interstitial and infiltrative diseases.* The classic acute restrictive disease is ARDS (discussed earlier). Chronic restrictive diseases including the dust diseases, or pneumoconioses, interstitial fibrosis of unknown etiology, and most of the infiltrative conditions, are discussed later.

Obstructive Pulmonary Diseases

In their prototypical forms, these individual disorders—emphysema, chronic bronchitis, asthma, and bronchiectasis—have distinct anatomic and clinical characteristics (Table 15–3). Emphysema and chronic bronchitis are often clinically grouped together and referred to as *chronic obstructive pulmonary disease* (COPD), since many patients have overlapping features of damage at both the acinar level (emphysema) and bronchial level (bronchitis), almost certainly because one extrinsic trigger—cigarette smoking—is common to both. In most patients, COPD is the result of long-term heavy cigarette smoking; about 10% of patients are nonsmokers.[8,9] However, only a minority of smokers develop COPD, the reason for which is still unknown. Although asthma (reversible airway hyperreactivity) is a distinct disorder, it may be a component of COPD in some patients. Because of the increase in smoking, environmental pollutants, and other noxious exposures, the incidence of COPD has increased dramatically in the last few decades and now ranks fourth in the United States as a cause of morbidity and mortality.

EMPHYSEMA

Emphysema is a condition of the lung characterized by abnormal permanent enlargement of the airspaces distal to the terminal bronchiole, accompanied by destruction of their walls and without obvious fibrosis.[10] In contrast, the enlargement of airspaces unaccompanied by destruction is termed "overinflation," for example, the distention of airspaces that occurs in the remaining lung after unilateral pneumonectomy.

Types of Emphysema. Emphysema is classified according to its *anatomic distribution* within the lobule. Recall that the lobule is a cluster of acini, the alveolated terminal respiratory units. Although the term "emphysema" is sometimes loosely applied to diverse conditions, there are four major types: (1) *centriacinar*, (2) *panacinar*, (3) *paraseptal*, and (4) *irregular.*

TABLE 15–3 Disorders Associated with Airflow Obstruction: The Spectrum of Chronic Obstructive Pulmonary Disease

Clinical Term	Anatomic Site	Major Pathologic Changes	Etiology	Signs/Symptoms
Chronic bronchitis	Bronchus	Mucous gland hyperplasia, hypersecretion	Tobacco smoke, air pollutants	Cough, sputum production
Bronchiectasis	Bronchus	Airway dilation and scarring	Persistent or severe infections	Cough, purulent sputum, fever
Asthma	Bronchus	Smooth muscle hyperplasia, excess mucus, inflammation	Immunologic or undefined causes	Episodic wheezing, cough, dyspnea
Emphysema	Acinus	Airspace enlargement; wall destruction	Tobacco smoke	Dyspnea
Small airway disease,* bronchiolitis	Bronchiole	Inflammatory scarring/ obliteration	Tobacco smoke, air pollutants, miscellaneous	Cough, dyspnea

*A feature of chronic bronchitis (see text).

Of these, only the first two cause clinically significant airflow obstruction (Fig. 15–5). Centriacinar emphysema is far more common than the panacinar form, constituting more than 95% of cases. Clinical management does not rely on precise anatomic diagnosis and classification, which, however, do provide important clues to pathogenesis.

Centriacinar (Centrilobular) Emphysema. The distinctive feature of this type of emphysema is the pattern of involvement of the lobules; *the central or proximal parts of the acini, formed by respiratory bronchioles, are affected, whereas distal alveoli are spared* (Fig. 15–6*B*). Thus, both emphysematous and normal airspaces exist within the same acinus and lobule. The lesions are more common and usually more severe in the upper lobes, particularly in the apical segments. The walls of the emphysematous spaces often contain large amounts of black pigment. Inflammation around bronchi and bronchioles is common. In severe centriacinar emphysema, the distal acinus may be involved, and differentiation from panacinar emphysema becomes difficult. Centriacinar emphysema occurs predominantly in heavy smokers, often in association with chronic bronchitis.

Panacinar (Panlobular) Emphysema. In this type, the *acini are uniformly enlarged from the level of the respiratory bronchiole to the terminal blind alveoli* (Fig. 15–6*C*). The prefix "pan" refers to the entire acinus but not to the entire lung. In contrast to centriacinar emphysema, panacinar emphysema

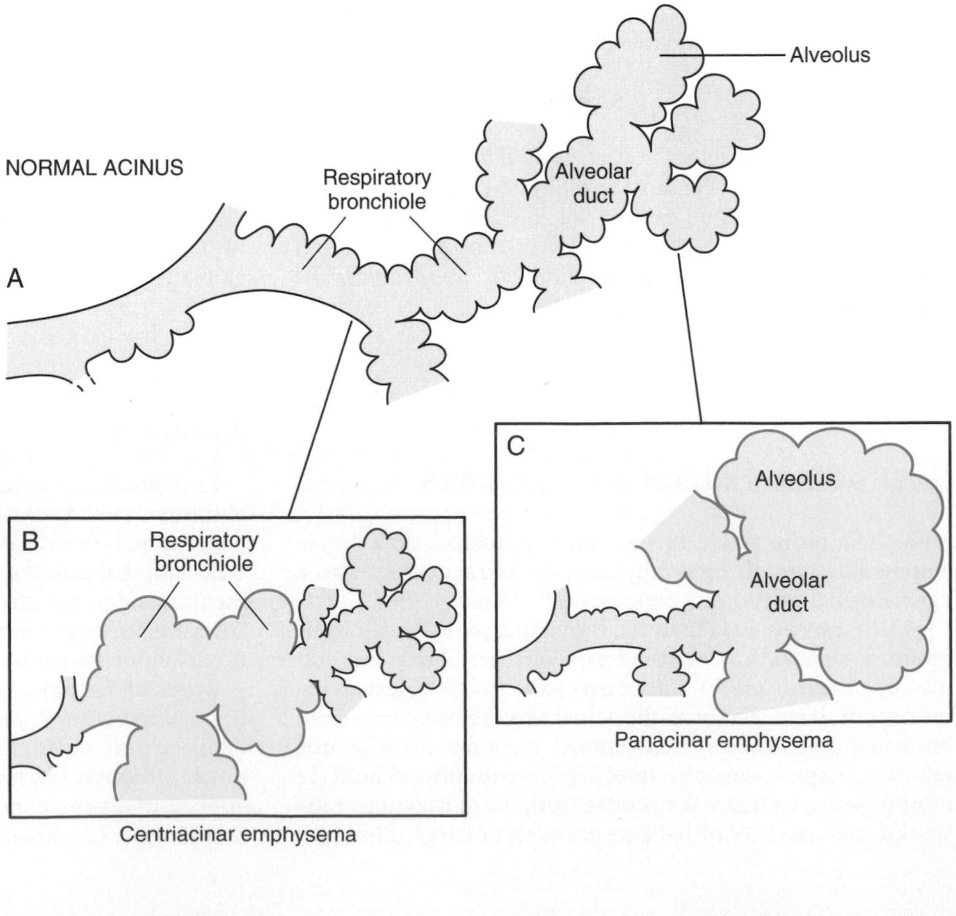

FIGURE 15–5 *A,* Diagram of normal structures within the acinus, the fundamental unit of the lung. A terminal bronchiole (*not shown*) is immediately proximal to the respiratory bronchiole. *B,* Centriacinar emphysema with dilation that initially affects the respiratory bronchioles. *C,* Panacinar emphysema with initial distention of the peripheral structures (i.e., the alveolus and alveolar duct); the disease later extends to affect the respiratory bronchioles.

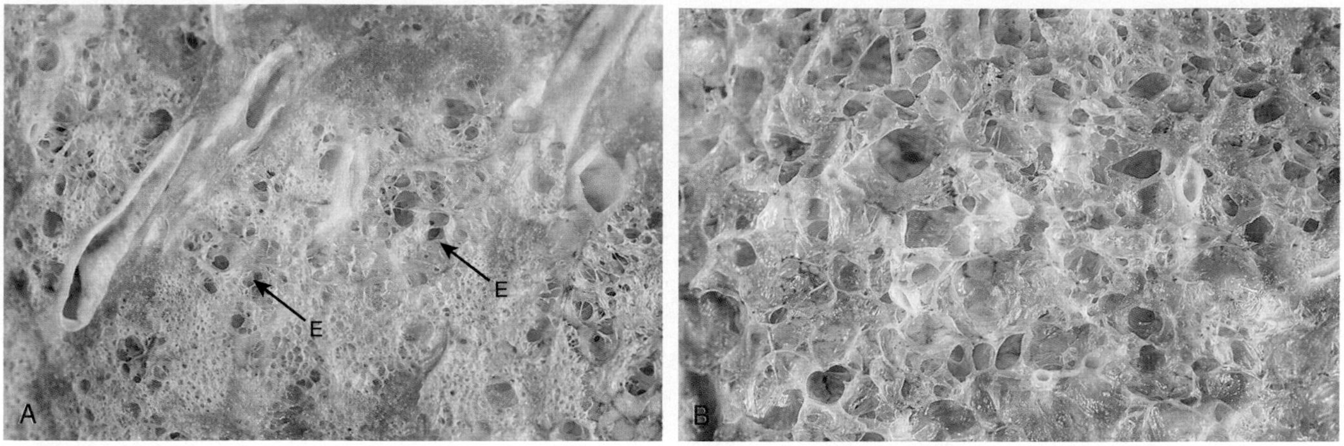

FIGURE 15–6 *A*, Centriacinar emphysema. Central areas show marked emphysematous damage (E), surrounded by relatively spared alveolar spaces. *B*, Panacinar emphysema involving the entire pulmonary architecture.

tends to occur more commonly in the lower zones and in the anterior margins of the lung, and it is usually most severe at the bases. This type of emphysema is associated with α_1-*antitrypsin (α_1-AT) deficiency* (Chapter 18).

Distal Acinar (Paraseptal) Emphysema. In this type, the *proximal portion of the acinus is normal, but the distal part is predominantly involved.* The emphysema is more striking adjacent to the pleura, along the lobular connective tissue septa, and at the margins of the lobules. It occurs adjacent to areas of fibrosis, scarring, or atelectasis and is usually more severe in the upper half of the lungs. The characteristic findings are of multiple, continuous, enlarged airspaces from less than 0.5 cm to more than 2.0 cm in diameter, sometimes forming cystlike structures. This type of emphysema probably underlies many of the cases of spontaneous pneumothorax in young adults.

Airspace Enlargement with Fibrosis (Irregular Emphysema). *Irregular emphysema, so named because the acinus is irregularly involved, is almost invariably associated with scarring.* Thus, it may be the most common form of emphysema because careful search of most lungs at autopsy shows one or more scars from a healed inflammatory process. In most instances, these foci of irregular emphysema are asymptomatic and clinically insignificant.

Incidence. COPD is a major public health problem. It is the fourth leading cause of morbidity and mortality in the United States[11] and is projected to rank fifth by 2020 as a worldwide burden of disease.[12] In one study, there was a 50% combined incidence of panacinar and centriacinar emphysema at autopsy, and the pulmonary disease was considered to be responsible for death in 6.5% of these patients.[13] *There is a clear-cut association between heavy cigarette smoking and emphysema,* and the most severe type occurs in men who smoke heavily.

Pathogenesis. COPD is characterized by mild chronic inflammation throughout the airways, parenchyma, and pulmonary vasculature. Macrophages, CD8+ T lymphocytes, and neutrophils are increased in various parts of the lung. Activated inflammatory cells release a variety of mediators, including leukotriene B_4, IL-8, TNF, and others, that are capable of damaging lung structures or sustaining neutrophilic inflammation.[14] Although details of the genesis of the two common forms of emphysema—centriacinar and panacinar—remain unsettled, *the most plausible hypothesis to account for the destruction of alveolar walls is the protease-antiprotease mechanism, aided and abetted by oxidant-antioxidant imbalance.*

The *protease-antiprotease theory* holds that alveolar wall destruction results from an imbalance between proteases (mainly elastase) and antiproteases in the lung (Fig. 15–7). It is based on two important observations, one clinical and one experimental. The first is that homozygous patients with a genetic deficiency of the protease inhibitor α_1-AT (see Chapter 18) have a markedly enhanced tendency to develop pulmonary emphysema, which is compounded by smoking.[15] α_1-AT (which is synthesized in the liver and is present in serum, tissue fluids, and macrophages) is a major inhibitor of proteases secreted by neutrophils during inflammation (Chapter 2). The normal α_1-AT phenotype, called *PiMM,* is present in 90% of the population. Of the several phenotypes associated with α_1-AT deficiency, PiZZ is the most common. More than 80% of PiZZ phenotypes develop symptomatic emphysema that occurs at an earlier age and with greater severity if the individual smokes. Therefore, the most important therapeutic intervention in α_1-AT deficiency is cessation of smoking. The second observation bearing on the protease-antiprotease hypothesis is experimental, in that intratracheal instillation of the proteolytic enzyme papain, which degrades elastin, causes emphysema in experimental animals.[16,17]

The principal antielastase activity in serum and interstitial tissue is α_1-AT (others are *secretory leukoprotease inhibitor* in bronchial mucus and serum *α_1-macroglobulin*), and the principal cellular elastase activity is derived from neutrophils (other elastases are formed by macrophages, mast cells, pancreas, and bacteria). Neutrophil elastase is capable of digesting human lung, and this digestion can be inhibited by α_1-AT. Thus, the following sequence is postulated to explain the effect of α_1-AT deficiency on the lung: Neutrophils are normally sequestered in the lung (more in the lower zones than in the upper), and a few gain access to the alveolar space. Any stimulus that increases either the number of leukocytes (neutrophils and macrophages) in the lung or the release of their elastase-containing granules increases elastolytic activity. Stimulated neutrophils also release oxygen free radicals, which

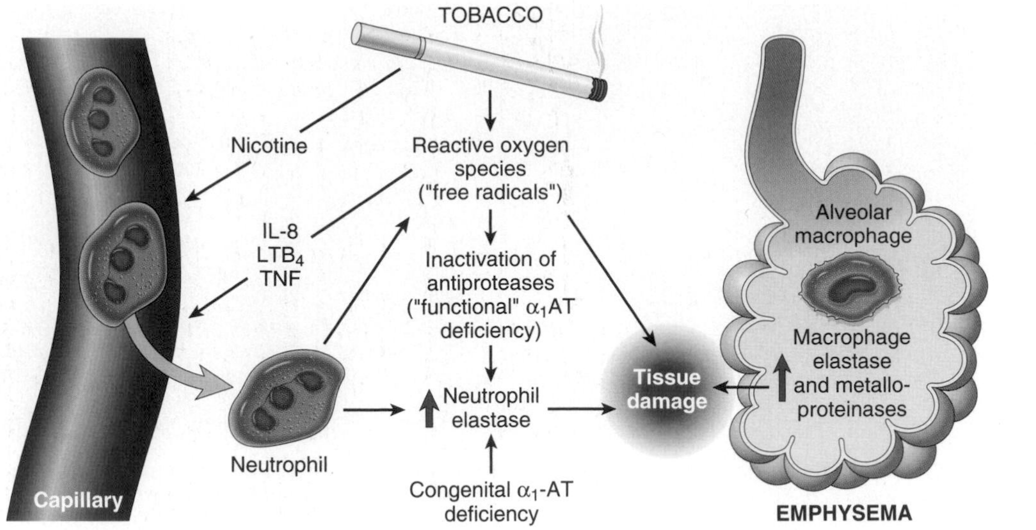

FIGURE 15–7 Pathogenesis of emphysema. The protease-antiprotease imbalance and oxidant-antioxidant imbalance are additive in their effects and contribute to tissue damage. α_1-antitrypsin (α_1-AT) deficiency can be either congenital or "functional" as a result of oxidative inactivation. See text for details. IL-8, interleukin 8; LTB_4, leukotriene B_4; TNF, tumor necrosis factor.

inhibit α_1-AT activity. With low levels of serum α_1-AT, the process of elastic tissue destruction is unchecked, with consequent emphysema. *Thus, emphysema is seen to result from the destructive effect of high protease activity in subjects with low antiprotease activity.* The primacy of the neutrophil is accepted for patients with α_1-AT deficiency, but in the more common smoking-related emphysema, both neutrophil and macrophage proteases play a role.[18] In addition, the accumulated CD8+ T cells may also participate either by causing apoptosis of alveolar epithelial cells or by recruiting macrophages.[19]

The protease-antiprotease hypothesis also explains the deleterious effect of cigarette smoking because both increased elastase availability and decreased antielastase activity occur in smokers (Fig. 15–7). In *smokers, neutrophils and macrophages accumulate in alveoli.* The mechanism of inflammation is not entirely clear but possibly involves the direct chemoattractant effects of nicotine as well as the effects of reactive oxygen species contained in smoke. Accumulated neutrophils are activated and release their granules, rich in a variety of cellular proteases (neutrophil elastase, proteinase 3, and cathepsin G), resulting in tissue damage. Smoking also enhances elastase activity in macrophages; macrophage elastase is not inhibited by α_1-antitrypsin and indeed can proteolytically digest this antiprotease. There is now increasing evidence that, in addition to elastase, matrix metalloproteinases derived from macrophages and neutrophils have a role in tissue destruction.

Smoking also plays a seminal role in perpetuating the *oxidant-antioxidant imbalance* in the pathogenesis of emphysema. Normally, the lung contains a healthy complement of antioxidants (superoxide dismutase, glutathione) that keep oxidative damage to a minimum. Tobacco smoke contains abundant reactive oxygen species ("free radicals"), which deplete these antioxidant mechanisms, thereby inciting tissue damage (see Chapter 1). Activated neutrophils also add to the pool of reactive oxygen species in the alveoli. A secondary consequence of oxidative injury is inactivation of native antiproteases, resulting in "functional" α_1-antitrypsin deficiency even in patients without enzyme deficiency.

In summary, it is likely that the impaction of smoke particles, predominantly at the bifurcation of respiratory bronchioles, results in the influx of neutrophils and macrophages, both of which secrete proteases. An increase in protease activity localized in the centriacinar region, together with the smoke-induced oxidative damage, causes the centriacinar pattern of emphysema that is seen in smokers. Tissue breakdown is enhanced as a consequence of inactivation of protective antiproteases by reactive oxygen species in cigarette smoke. This schema also explains the additive influence of smoking and α_1-antitrypsin deficiency in inducing serious obstructive airway disease.

In contrast to centriacinar emphysema, it is postulated that the panacinar emphysema of α_1-AT–deficient individuals reflects total lack of antiprotease throughout the acinus and susceptibility to chronic low-level proteolysis from neutrophils in transit through the lung circulation. The predominantly lower lung distribution (where perfusion and neutrophil numbers are greatest) of panacinar emphysema is also consistent with this postulate. Finally, some speculate that the upper lobe distribution of centriacinar emphysema (discussed later) also reflects a relative lack of serum α_1-AT delivery to this less perfused region.

Morphology. Panacinar emphysema, when well developed, produces voluminous lungs, often overlapping the heart and hiding it when the anterior chest wall is removed. The macroscopic features of centriacinar emphysema are less impressive. The lungs might not appear particularly pale or voluminous unless the disease is well advanced. Generally, the upper two thirds of the lungs are more severely affected. Large apical blebs or bullae are more characteristic of irregular emphysema secondary to scarring and of distal acinar emphysema. Large alveoli can easily be seen on the cut surface of formalin-inflated fixed lung (Fig. 15–6).

Microscopically, there are abnormally large alveoli separated by thin septa with only focal centriacinar fibrosis. There is loss of attachments of the alveoli to the outer wall of small airways. The pores of Kohn are so large that septa appear to be floating or protrude blindly into alveolar spaces with a club-shaped end.

With advance of the disease, there are even larger abnormal airspaces and possibly blebs or bullae. Often, the respiratory bronchioles and vasculature of the lung are deformed and compressed by the emphysematous distortion of the airspaces, and as has been mentioned, there is often chronic bronchitis or bronchiolitis.

Clinical Course. The clinical manifestations of emphysema do not appear until at least one third of the functioning pulmonary parenchyma is damaged. Dyspnea is usually the first symptom; it begins insidiously but is steadily progressive. In some patients, cough or wheezing is the chief complaint, easily confused with asthma. Cough and expectoration are extremely variable and depend on the extent of the associated bronchitis. Weight loss is common and can be so severe as to suggest a hidden malignant tumor. Classically, the patient is barrel-chested and dyspneic, with obviously prolonged expiration, sits forward in a hunched-over position, and breathes through pursed lips. *Expiratory airflow limitation, best measured through spirometry, is the key to diagnosis.*

In patients with severe emphysema, cough is often slight, overdistention is severe, diffusion capacity is low, and blood gas values are relatively normal at rest. Such patients may overventilate and remain well oxygenated and therefore are somewhat ingloriously designated as *pink puffers* (see Table 15–4). Patients with chronic bronchitis more often have a history of recurrent infection, abundant purulent sputum, hypercapnia, and severe hypoxemia, prompting the equally inglorious designation of *blue bloaters*. Development of cor pulmonale and eventual congestive heart failure, related to secondary pulmonary vascular hypertension, is associated with a poor prognosis. Death in most patients with COPD is due to (1) respiratory acidosis and coma, (2) right-sided heart failure, and (3) massive collapse of the lungs secondary to pneumothorax. Treatment options include bronchodilators, steroids, bullectomy, and, in selected patients, lung volume reduction surgery and lung transplantation.

Other Types of Emphysema. Now we come to some conditions in which the term "emphysema" is applied less stringently and to some closely related conditions.

TABLE 15–4 Emphysema and Chronic Bronchitis

	Predominant Bronchitis	Predominant Emphysema
Age (yr)	40–45	50–75
Dyspnea	Mild; late	Severe; early
Cough	Early; copious sputum	Late; scanty sputum
Infections	Common	Occasional
Respiratory insufficiency	Repeated	Terminal
Cor pulmonale	Common	Rare; terminal
Airway resistance	Increased	Normal or slightly increased
Elastic recoil	Normal	Low
Chest radiograph	Prominent vessels; large heart	Hyperinflation; small heart
Appearance	*Blue bloater*	*Pink puffer*

Compensatory Hyperinflation (Emphysema). The term *compensatory hyperinflation (emphysema)* is sometimes used to designate dilation of alveoli but not destruction of septal walls in response to loss of lung substance elsewhere. It is best exemplified by the hyperexpansion of the residual lung parenchyma that follows surgical removal of a diseased lung or lobe.

Obstructive Overinflation. *Obstructive overinflation refers to the condition in which the lung expands because air is trapped within it.* A common cause is subtotal obstruction by a tumor or foreign object. A classic example is *congenital lobar overinflation* in infants, probably resulting from hypoplasia of bronchial cartilage and sometimes associated with other congenital cardiac and lung abnormalities. Overinflation in obstructive lesions occurs either (1) because of a ball-valve action of the obstructive agent, so that air enters on inspiration but cannot leave on expiration, or (2) because the bronchus may be totally obstructed but ventilation through *collaterals* may bring in air from behind the obstruction. These collaterals are the *pores of Kohn* and other direct accessory *bronchioloalveolar connections* (the canals of Lambert). Obstructive overinflation can be a life-threatening emergency because the affected portion distends sufficiently to compress the remaining normal lung.

Bullous Emphysema. *Bullous emphysema* refers merely to any form of emphysema that produces large subpleural blebs or bullae (spaces more than 1 cm in diameter in the distended state) (Fig. 15–8). They represent localized accentuations of one of the four forms of emphysema, are most often subpleural, and occur near the apex, sometimes in relation to old tuberculous scarring. On occasion, rupture of the bullae may give rise to pneumothorax.

Interstitial Emphysema. *The entrance of air into the connective tissue stroma of the lung, mediastinum, or subcutaneous tissue is designated interstitial emphysema.* In most instances, alveolar tears in pulmonary emphysema provide the avenue of entrance of air into the stroma of the lung, but rarely, a wound of the chest that allows air to be sucked in or a fractured rib that punctures the lung substance may underlie this disorder. Alveolar tears usually occur when there is a combination

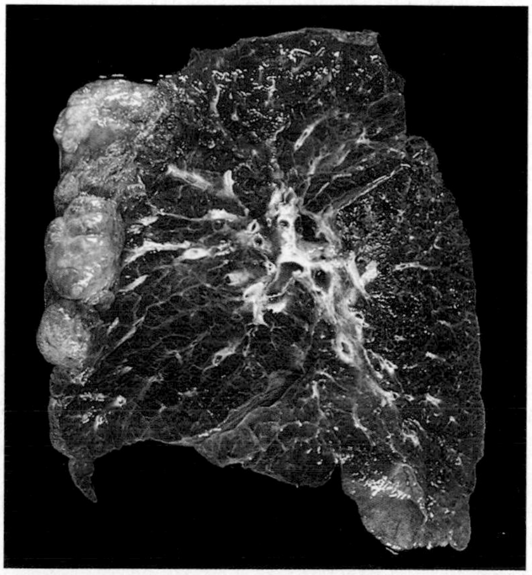

FIGURE 15–8 Bullous emphysema with large subpleural bullae (*upper left*).

of coughing plus some bronchiolar obstruction, producing sharply increased pressures within the alveolar sacs. Children with whooping cough and bronchitis, patients with obstruction to the airways (by blood clots, tissue, or foreign bodies) or who are being artificially ventilated, and individuals who suddenly inhale irritant gases provide classic examples.

CHRONIC BRONCHITIS

Chronic bronchitis, so common among habitual smokers and inhabitants of smog-laden cities, is not nearly as trivial as was once thought. When persistent for years, it may (1) progress to chronic obstructive airway disease, (2) lead to cor pulmonale and heart failure, or (3) cause atypical metaplasia and dysplasia of the respiratory epithelium, providing a rich soil for cancerous transformation. Important definitions in bronchitis include the following:

- *Chronic bronchitis per se is defined clinically*. It is present in any patient who has persistent cough with sputum production for at least 3 months in at least 2 consecutive years, in the absence of any other identifiable cause.
- In *simple chronic bronchitis*, patients have a productive cough but no physiologic evidence of airflow obstruction.
- Some individuals may demonstrate hyperreactive airways with intermittent bronchospasm and wheezing. This condition is called *chronic asthmatic bronchitis*.
- Finally, some patients, especially heavy smokers, develop chronic airflow obstruction, usually with evidence of associated emphysema, and are classified as showing *obstructive chronic bronchitis*.

Pathogenesis. The primary or initiating factor in the genesis of chronic bronchitis appears to be chronic irritation by inhaled substances such as tobacco smoke (90% of patients are smokers) and grain, cotton, and silica dust. Bacterial and viral infections are important in triggering acute exacerbation of the disease. Both sexes and all ages may be affected, but chronic bronchitis is most frequent in middle-aged men. Chronic bronchitis is 4 to 10 times more common in heavy smokers regardless of age, sex, occupation, and place of dwelling.

The earliest feature of chronic bronchitis is *hypersecretion of mucus* in the large airways, associated with hypertrophy of the submucosal glands in the trachea and bronchi.[20] Proteases released from neutrophils, such as neutrophil elastase and cathepsin, and matrix metalloproteinases, stimulate this mucus hypersecretion. As chronic bronchitis persists, there is also *a marked increase in goblet cells of small airways—small bronchi and bronchioles*—leading to excessive mucus production that contributes to airway obstruction. It is thought that both the submucosal gland hypertrophy and the increase in goblet cells are a protective metaplastic reaction against tobacco smoke or other pollutants (e.g., sulfur dioxide and nitrogen dioxide). Many of the respiratory epithelial effects of environmental irritants are believed to be mediated through the epidermal growth factor (EGF) receptor. For example, transcription of the mucin gene *MUC 5AC*, which is increased as a consequence of exposure to tobacco smoke in both in vitro and in vivo experimental models, is in part mediated by EGF receptor pathways.

Although mucus hypersecretion in large airways is the cause of sputum overproduction, it is now thought that accompanying *alterations in the small airways of the lung* (small bronchi and bronchioles, less than 2 to 3 mm in diameter) *can result in physiologically important and early manifestations of chronic airway obstruction.*[21,22] Histologic studies of the small airways in young smokers disclose (1) goblet cell metaplasia with mucus plugging of the lumen, (2) clustering of pigmented alveolar macrophages, (3) inflammatory infiltration, and (4) fibrosis of the bronchiolar wall (in a somewhat older group of patients).[23,24] Smoke and other irritants, which cause the hypertrophy of mucous glands, also result in *bronchiolitis*,[25] or *small airway disease*. Certain physiologic studies suggest that this respiratory bronchiolitis is an important component in early and relatively mild airflow obstruction. *When bronchitis is accompanied by moderate to severe airflow obstruction, however, coexistent emphysema is the dominant lesion.*[22]

The role of *infection* appears to be secondary. It is not responsible for the initiation of chronic bronchitis but is probably significant in maintaining it and may be critical in producing acute exacerbations. Cigarette smoke predisposes to infection in more than one way. It interferes with ciliary action of the respiratory epithelium, it may cause direct damage to airway epithelium, and it inhibits the ability of bronchial and alveolar leukocytes to clear bacteria. Viral infections can also cause exacerbations of chronic bronchitis.

Following this review of the pathogenesis of both emphysema and chronic bronchitis, the reader is referred to Figure 15–9, which follows the evolution of both conditions into chronic obstructive airway disease.

Morphology. Grossly, there may be hyperemia, swelling, and edema of the mucous membranes, frequently accompanied by excessive mucinous to mucopurulent secretions layering the epithelial surfaces. Sometimes, heavy casts of secretions and pus fill the bronchi and bronchioles. The characteristic histologic features of chronic bronchitis are chronic inflammation of the airways (predominantly lymphocytes) and enlargement of the mucus-secreting glands of the trachea and bronchi. Although the numbers of goblet cells increase slightly, the **major increase is in the size of the mucous glands**. This increase can be assessed by the ratio of the thickness of the mucous gland layer to the thickness of the wall between the epithelium and the cartilage (**Reid index**). The Reid index (normally 0.4) is increased in chronic bronchitis, usually in proportion to the severity and duration of the disease. The bronchial epithelium may exhibit squamous metaplasia and dysplasia. There is marked narrowing of bronchioles caused by goblet cell metaplasia, mucus plugging, inflammation, and fibrosis. In the most severe cases, there may be obliteration of lumen due to fibrosis (**bronchiolitis obliterans**). As was discussed earlier, these bronchiolar changes probably contribute to the obstructive features in bronchitis patients.

Clinical Features. The cardinal symptom of chronic bronchitis is a persistent cough productive of sputum. For many years, no other respiratory functional impairment is present, but eventually, dyspnea on exertion develops. With the passage of time, and usually with continued smoking, other elements of COPD may appear, including hypercapnia, hypoxemia, and

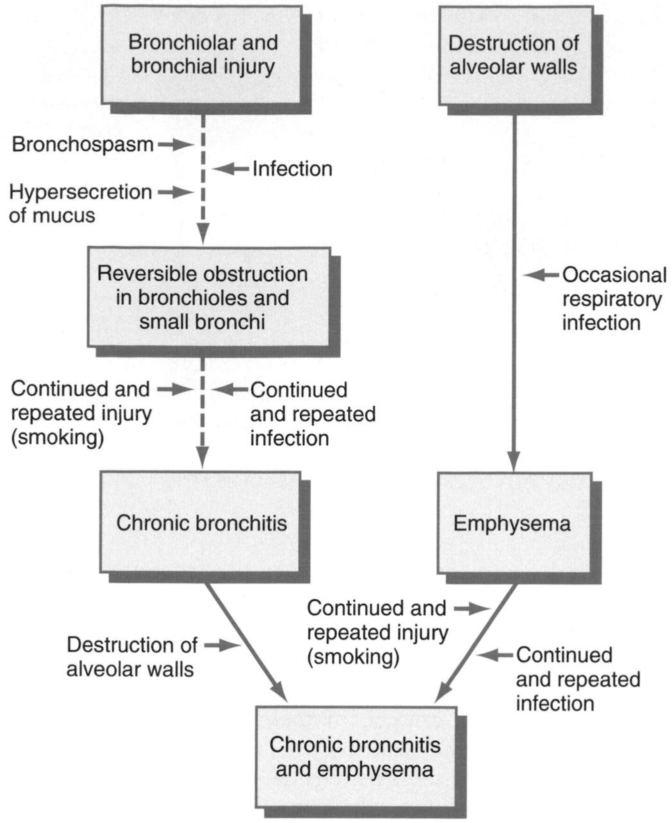

FIGURE 15–9 Schematic representation of evolution of chronic bronchitis (*left*) and emphysema (*right*). Although both can culminate in chronic bronchitis and emphysema, the pathways are different, and either one may predominate. The dashed arrows on the left indicate that in the natural history of chronic bronchitis, it is not known whether there is a predictable progression from obstruction in small airways to chronic (obstructive) bronchitis. (Redrawn from Fishman AP: The spectrum of chronic obstructive disease of the airways. In Fishman AP (ed): Pulmonary Diseases and Disorders, 2nd ed. New York, McGraw-Hill, 1988, p. 1164.)

mild cyanosis. Differentiation of pure chronic bronchitis from that associated with emphysema can be made in the classic case (see Table 15–4), but, as has been mentioned, many patients with COPD have both conditions. Long-standing severe chronic bronchitis commonly leads to cor pulmonale with cardiac failure. Death may also result from further impairment of respiratory function incident to acute intercurrent bacterial infections.

ASTHMA

Asthma is a chronic inflammatory disorder of the airways that causes recurrent episodes of wheezing, breathlessness, chest tightness, and cough, particularly at night and/or in the early morning. These symptoms are usually associated with widespread but variable bronchoconstriction and airflow limitation that is at least partly reversible, either spontaneously or with treatment. It is thought that inflammation causes an increase in airway responsiveness (bronchospasm) to a variety of stimuli. Some of these stimuli would have little or no effect on nonasthmatics with normal airways. Many cells play a role in the inflammatory response, in particular eosinophils, mast cells, macrophages, T lymphocytes, neutrophils, and epithelial cells.[26]

Patients with asthma experience disabling attacks of severe dyspnea, coughing, and wheezing triggered by sudden episodes of bronchospasm. Rarely, a state of unremitting attacks, called status asthmaticus, proves fatal; usually, such patients have had a long history of asthma. Between the attacks, patients may be virtually asymptomatic. In some cases, the attacks are triggered by exercise and cold or by exposure to an allergen to which the patient has previously been sensitized, but often no trigger can be identified. *There has been a significant increase in the incidence of asthma in the Western world in the past three decades.*

Asthma has such a wide spectrum of predisposing factors and clinical presentations that there is no uniform classification. Categorization into mild intermittent, mild, moderate, and severe persistent asthma, based on the frequency and severity of symptoms, is useful as a guide to therapy. Other clinical categories include steroid-dependent, steroid-resistant, difficult, and brittle asthma. Typically, asthma is categorized into *extrinsic* (initiated by a type I hypersensitivity reaction induced by exposure to an extrinsic antigen) and *intrinsic* (initiated by diverse, nonimmune mechanisms, including ingestion of aspirin; pulmonary infections, especially viral; cold; inhaled irritants; stress; and exercise). This distinction is useful from the point of pathophysiology; however, so many patients manifest overlapping characteristics and have elevated IgE levels that this classification is no longer clinically applicable. Other informal categories classify asthma according to the agents or events that trigger bronchoconstriction. These include seasonal, exercise-induced, drug-induced, and occupational asthma and asthmatic bronchitis in smokers. Allergic bronchopulmonary aspergillosis, which may complicate asthma, is partly an allergic reaction to fungus that has colonized the bronchial mucosa. Patients with this disease have very high serum IgE levels, eosinophilia, and serum antibodies to *Aspergillus*.

Pathogenesis. The major etiologic factors of asthma are genetic predisposition to type I hypersensitivity ("atopy"), acute and chronic airway inflammation, and bronchial hyperresponsiveness. *The inflammation involves many cell types and numerous inflammatory mediators,*[27] but the precise relationship of specific inflammatory cells and the mediators to airway hyperreactivity is not fully understood. Type 2 helper T (T_H2) cells, a type of CD4+ helper T cell, are prominent components of the bronchial inflammation. T_H2 cells secrete interleukins that promote allergic inflammation and stimulate B cells to produce IgE and other antibodies. In contrast, type 1 helper T (T_H1) cells, the other class of CD4+ T cells, produce interferon-γ and interleukin-2, which initiate the killing of viruses and other intracellular organisms by activating macrophages and cytotoxic T cells (Chapter 6). These two subgroups of helper T cells arise in response to different immunogenic stimuli and cytokines, and they constitute an immunoregulatory loop: cytokines from T_H1 cells inhibit T_H2 cells, and vice versa (Fig. 15–10).[28] An imbalance in this reciprocal arrangement may be the key to asthma: There is credible evidence that, when freed from the restraining influence of interferon-γ, T_H2 cells can provoke airway inflammation.[29] It appears that in patients with allergic asthma, T cell differentiation is skewed in the direction of T_H2. The molecular basis of such bias is not clear. Recent studies indicate that a

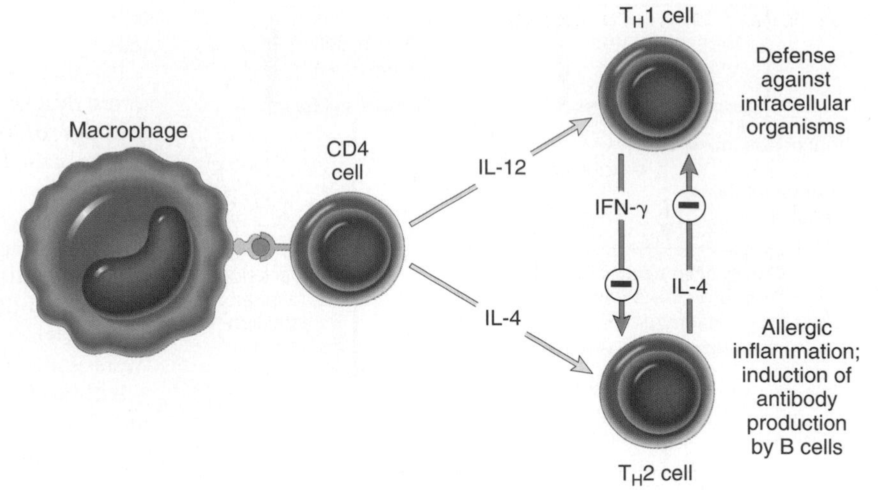

FIGURE 15–10 A simplified scheme of the system of type 1 helper T (T_H1) and type 2 helper (T_H2) cells. The differentiation of T_H1 and T_H2 cells depends on interleukin-12 and interleukin-4, cytokines produced by antigen-stimulated precursor CD4 T cells. In a regulatory loop, interferon-γ from T_H1 cells inhibits T_H2 cells and interleukin-4 from T_H2 cells inhibits T_H1 cells. An imbalance that favors T_H2 cells may be important in asthma. Bronchial lymphocytes from patients with asthma have been found to lack T-bet, a transcription factor required for the production of interferon-γ (IFN-γ) by T_H1 cells. (From Schwartz RS: A new element in the mechanism of asthma. N Engl J Med 346(11):857, 2002. Permission requested.)

transcription factor called T-bet is required for T_H1 cell differentiation, and immunohistochemical studies on lung tissues from asthmatics reveal absence of T-bet in lung lymphocytes. These studies suggest that therapeutic upregulation of T-bet might be an attractive molecular therapy for asthma.

In addition to the inflammatory responses mediated by T_H2 type cells, asthma is characterized by structural changes in the bronchial wall, referred to as "airway remodeling." These changes, described later in greater detail, include hypertrophy of bronchial smooth muscles and deposition of subepithelial collagen. Until recently, these changes were considered secondary to chronic inflammation occurring late in the disease. However, this view has been challenged,[30] since in some studies, airway remodeling has been seen several years before the onset of symptoms. According to some, therefore, an abnormal, perhaps genetically determined, microenvironment in the bronchial wall is an essential cofactor in the pathogenesis of asthma. This view has been bolstered by the recent linkage of the ADAM-33 gene to asthma.[31] ADAM-33 belongs to a subfamily of metalloproteinases related to the matrix metalloproteinases (MMPs) such as collagenases (Chapter 3). Although the precise function of ADAM-33 remains to be elucidated, it is known to be expressed by lung fibroblasts and bronchial smooth muscle cells. It is speculated that ADAM-33 polymorphisms accelerate proliferation of bronchial smooth muscle cells and fibroblasts, thus contributing to bronchial hyperreactivity and subepithelial fibrosis. Mast cells are also suspected to contribute to airway remodeling.[32] Bronchial biopsies of patients with asthma reveal heavy infiltration of smooth muscle cells by mast cells. When mast cells are triggered by IgE or other stimuli, they not only release vasoactive mediators and cytokines but also growth factors such as PDGF and proteases that can trigger smooth muscle proliferation. In a reciprocal action, activated smooth muscle cells secrete stem cell factor, which is a chemoattractant and growth factor for mast cells.

Atopic Asthma. This most common type of asthma usually begins in childhood. The disease is triggered by environmental antigens, such as dusts, pollens, animal dander, and foods, but potentially any antigen is implicated. A positive family history of atopy is common, and asthmatic attacks are often preceded by allergic rhinitis, urticaria, or eczema.

Candidate genes for predisposition to atopy and airway hyperresponsiveness are currently subjects of intensive search and include genes involved in antigen presentation (the HLA complex), T-cell activation (T-cell receptor complex, γ-interferon), regulation of cytokine production or function of relevant cytokines (IL-4, IL-5, IL-13), and receptors for bronchodilators (β_2-adrenergic receptors).[27] In any case, a skin test with the offending antigen in these patients results in an immediate wheal-and-flare reaction, a *classic example of type I IgE-mediated hypersensitivity reaction*, discussed in detail in Chapter 6. In the airways, the scene for the reaction is set in large part by initial sensitization to inhaled antigens (allergens), which stimulate induction of *T_H2-type cells* that release cytokines such as IL-4 and IL-5 (Fig. 15–11*A*). These cytokines, in turn, promote IgE production by B cells, growth of mast cells (IL-4), and growth and activation of eosinophils (IL-5). Subsequent IgE-mediated reaction to inhaled allergens elicits an *acute response and a late-phase reaction*.

Recall that exposure of presensitized IgE-coated mast cells to the same or a cross-reacting antigen stimulates cross-linking of IgE and the release of chemical mediators. In the case of airborne antigens, the reaction occurs first on sensitized mast cells *on the mucosal surface* (Fig. 15–11*B*); the resultant mediator release opens the mucosal intercellular tight junctions and enhances penetration of antigen to the more numerous submucosal mast cells. In addition, direct stimulation of *subepithelial vagal* (parasympathetic) *receptors* provokes bronchoconstriction through both central and local reflexes (including those mediated by unmyelinated sensory C fibers). This occurs within minutes after stimulation and is called the *acute*, or *immediate*, response, which consists of bronchoconstriction, edema (owing to increased vascular permeability), mucus secretion, and, in extreme instances, hypotension. Mast cells also release cytokines that cause the influx of other leukocytes, including neutrophils and monocytes, lymphocytes, basophils, and particularly eosinophils (IL-5). These inflammatory cells set the stage for the *late-phase reaction*, which starts 4 to 8 hours later and may persist for 12 to 24 hours or more (Fig. 15–11*C*).

The *late-phase reaction*, as was noted earlier, is mediated by the swarm of leukocytes recruited by the chemotactic factors and cytokines derived from mast cells during the acute-phase response.[33] However, mediators can also be produced by other cells in the affected bronchi, including (1) inflammatory cells that are *already present* in asthmatics suffering a recurrent attack, (2) *vascular endothelium*, or (3)

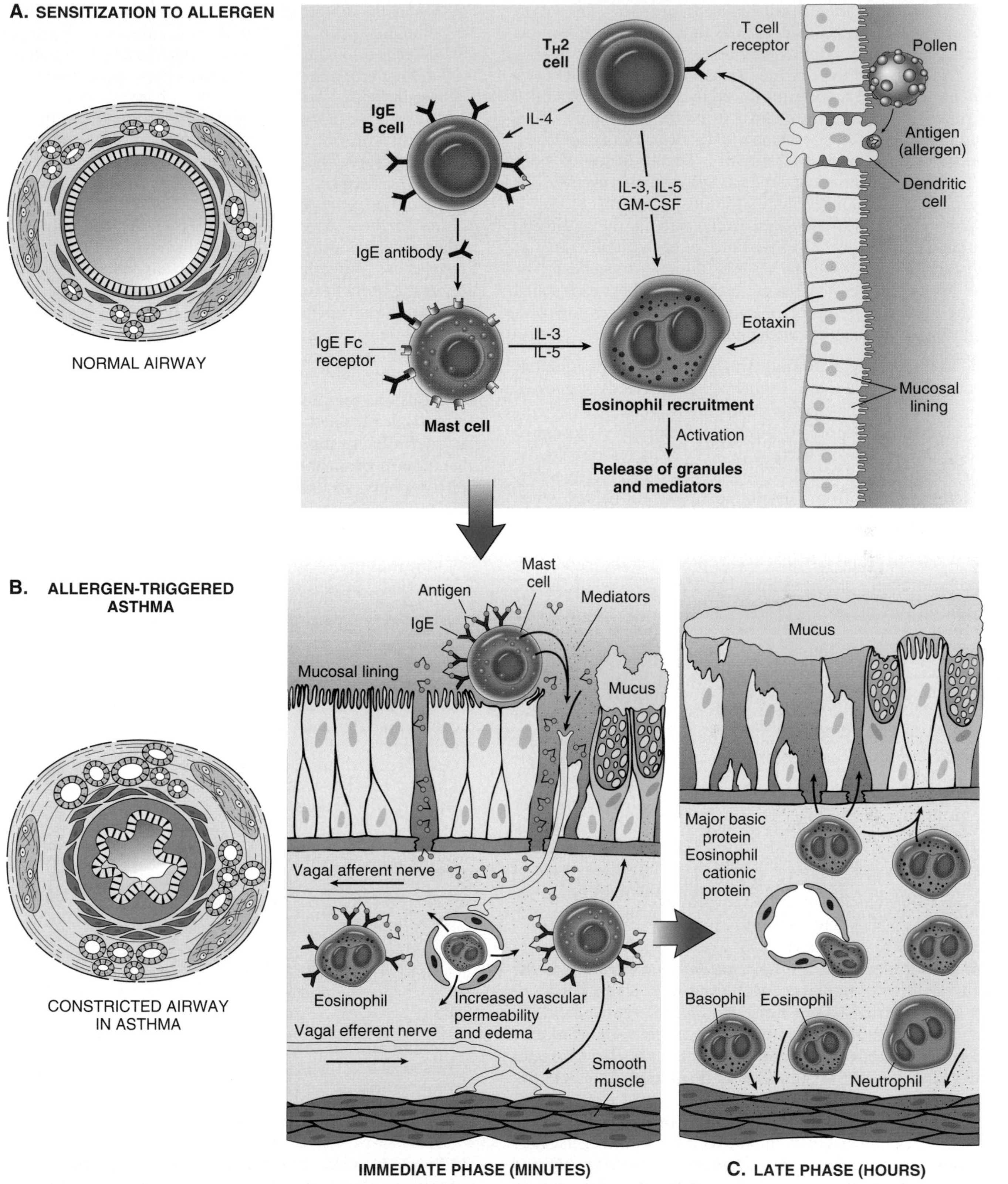

FIGURE 15–11 A model for allergic asthma. *A*, Inhaled allergens (antigen) elicit a T_H2-dominated response favoring IgE production and eosinophil recruitment (priming or sensitization). *B*, On re-exposure to antigen (Ag), the immediate reaction is triggered by Ag-induced cross-linking of IgE bound to IgE receptors on mast cells in the airways. These cells release preformed mediators that open tight junctions between epithelial cells. Antigen can then enter the mucosa to activate mucosal mast cells and eosinophils, which in turn release additional mediators. Collectively, either directly or via neuronal reflexes, the mediators induce bronchospasm, increased vascular permeability, and mucus production and recruit additional mediator-releasing cells from the blood. *C*, The arrival of recruited leukocytes (neutrophils, eosinophils, and basophils; also lymphocytes and monocytes [*not shown*]) signals the initiation of the late phase of asthma and a fresh round of mediator release from leukocytes, endothelium, and epithelial cells. Factors, particularly from eosinophils (e.g., major basic protein, eosinophil cationic protein), also cause damage to the epithelium.

airway epithelial cells. Epithelial cells are now known to produce a large variety of cytokines in response to infectious agents, drugs, and gases as well as to inflammatory mediators.[34] This second wave of mediators stimulates the late reaction. For example, *eotaxin*, produced by airway epithelial cells, is a potent chemoattractant and activator of eosinophils.[35] *The major basic protein of eosinophils, in turn, causes epithelial damage*[34] *and airway constriction.*[36] The presence of both immediate and delayed reactions in IgE-mediated events helps to explain the prolonged manifestations of asthma.

Many mediators have been implicated in the asthmatic response, but the relative importance of each putative mediator in actual human asthma has been difficult to establish. The long list of "suspects" in acute asthma can be subclassified by the clinical efficacy of pharmacologic intervention with inhibitors or antagonists of the mediators.

- The first (disappointingly small) group includes putative mediators whose role in bronchospasm is clearly supported by efficacy of pharmacologic intervention: (1) *leukotrienes* C_4, D_4, and E_4, extremely potent mediators that cause prolonged bronchoconstriction as well as increased vascular permeability and increased mucus secretion, and (2) *acetylcholine*, released from intrapulmonary motor nerves, which can cause airway smooth muscle constriction by directly stimulating muscarinic receptors.
- A second group includes agents present at the *scene of the crime* and with potent asthma-like effects but whose actual clinical role in acute allergic asthma appears relatively minor on the basis of lack of efficacy of potent antagonists or synthesis inhibitors: (1) *histamine*, a potent bronchoconstrictor; (2) *prostaglandin* D_2 (PGD_2), which elicits bronchoconstriction and vasodilation; and (3) *PAF*, which causes aggregation of platelets and release of histamine and serotonin from their granules. These mediators might yet prove important in other types of chronic or nonallergic asthma.
- Finally, a large third group comprises the *suspects* for whom specific antagonists or inhibitors are not available or have been insufficiently studied as yet. These include numerous cytokines, such as IL-1, TNF, and IL-6 (some of which exist in a preformed state within the mast cell granules),[37] chemokines (e.g., eotaxin), neuropeptides, nitric oxide, bradykinin, and endothelins.

It is thus clear that multiple mediators contribute to the acute asthmatic response. Moreover, the composition of this mediator *soup* might differ among different individuals or types of asthma. The appreciation of the importance of inflammatory cells and mediators in asthma has led to greater emphasis on anti-inflammatory therapeutics in clinical practice.

Nonatopic Asthma. The second large group is the *nonatopic*, or *nonreaginic*, variety of asthma, which is most frequently triggered by respiratory tract infection. Viruses (e.g., rhinovirus, parainfluenza virus) rather than bacteria are the most common provokers.[38] A positive family history is uncommon, serum IgE levels are normal, and there are no other associated allergies. In these patients, skin test results are usually negative, and although hypersensitivity to microbial antigens may play a role, present theories place more stress on hyperirritability of the bronchial tree. *It is thought that virus-induced inflammation of the respiratory mucosa lowers the threshold of the subepithelial vagal receptors to irritants.* Inhaled air pollutants, such as sulfur dioxide, ozone, and nitrogen dioxide, may also contribute to the chronic airway inflammation and hyperreactivity that are present in some cases.

Drug-Induced Asthma. Several pharmacologic agents provoke asthma. *Aspirin-sensitive asthma* is an uncommon yet fascinating type, occurring in patients with recurrent rhinitis and nasal polyps. These individuals are exquisitely sensitive to small doses of aspirin, and they experience not only asthmatic attacks but also urticaria. It is probable that aspirin triggers asthma in these patients by inhibiting the cyclooxygenase pathway of arachidonic acid metabolism without affecting the lipoxygenase route, thus tipping the balance toward elaboration of the bronchoconstrictor leukotrienes.

Occupational Asthma. This form of asthma is stimulated by fumes (epoxy resins, plastics), organic and chemical dusts (wood, cotton, platinum), gases (toluene), and other chemicals (formaldehyde, penicillin products). Minute quantities of chemicals are required to induce the attack, which usually occurs after repeated exposure. The underlying mechanisms vary according to stimulus and include type I reactions, direct liberation of bronchoconstrictor substances, and hypersensitivity responses of unknown origin.

Morphology. The morphologic changes in asthma have been described principally in patients dying of status asthmaticus, but it appears that the pathology in nonfatal cases is similar. Grossly, the lungs are overdistended because of overinflation, and there may be small areas of atelectasis. The most striking macroscopic finding is occlusion of bronchi and bronchioles by thick, tenacious **mucous plugs.** Histologically, the mucous plugs contain whorls of shed epithelium, which give rise to the well-known **Curschmann spirals.** Numerous eosinophils and Charcot-Leyden crystals are present; the latter are collections of crystalloid made up of eosinophil membrane protein. The other characteristic histologic findings of asthma, collectively called "airway remodeling" (Fig. 15–12), include:

- Thickening of the basement membrane of the bronchial epithelium
- Edema and an inflammatory infiltrate in the bronchial walls, with a prominence of eosinophils and mast cells
- An increase in size of the submucosal glands
- Hypertrophy of the bronchial wall muscle

While airflow obstruction is primarily attributed to muscular bronchoconstriction, the airway remodeling may contribute as well.

Clinical Course. The classic asthmatic attack lasts up to several hours and is followed by prolonged coughing; the raising of copious mucous secretions provides considerable relief of the respiratory difficulty. In some patients, these symptoms persist at a low level all the time. In its most severe form, *status asthmaticus*, the severe acute paroxysm persists for days and even weeks, and under these circumstances, ventilatory function might be so impaired as to cause severe cyanosis and even death. The clinical diagnosis is aided by the demon-

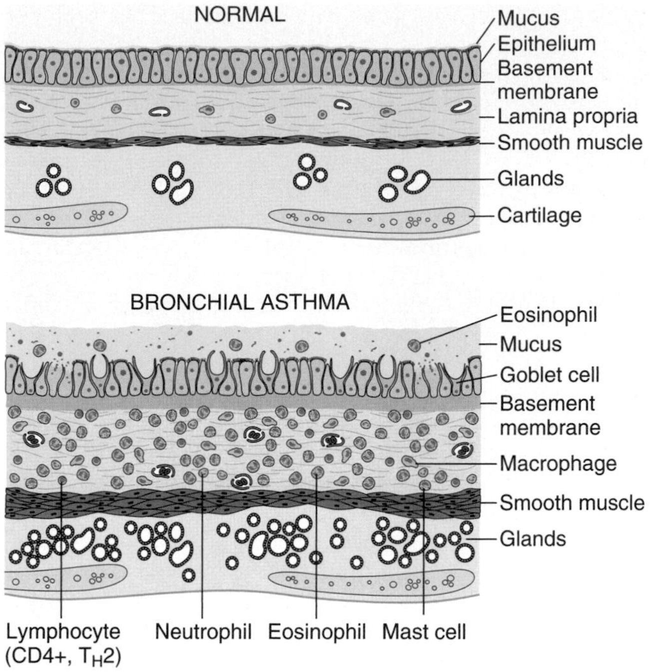

FIGURE 15–12 Comparison of a normal bronchiole with that in a patient with asthma. Note the accumulation of mucus in the bronchial lumen resulting from an increase in the number of mucus-secreting goblet cells in the mucosa and hypertrophy of submucosal mucus glands. In addition, there is intense chronic inflammation due to recruitment of eosinophils, macrophages, and other inflammatory cells. Basement membrane underlying the mucosal epithelium is thickened, and there is hypertrophy and hyperplasia of smooth muscle cells.

stration of an elevated eosinophil count in the peripheral blood and the finding of eosinophils, Curschmann spirals, and Charcot-Leyden crystals in the sputum. In the usual case, with intervals of freedom from respiratory difficulty, the disease is more discouraging and disabling than lethal. With appropriate therapy to relieve the attacks, patients with asthma are able to maintain a productive life. Occasionally, the disease disappears spontaneously.

BRONCHIECTASIS

Bronchiectasis is a disease characterized by permanent dilation of bronchi and bronchioles caused by destruction of the muscle and elastic tissue, resulting from or associated with chronic necrotizing infections. To be considered bronchiectasis, the dilation should be permanent; reversible bronchial dilation often accompanies viral and bacterial pneumonia. Because of better control of lung infections, bronchiectasis is now an uncommon condition. It is manifested clinically by cough, fever, and expectoration of copious amounts of foul-smelling, purulent sputum. Bronchiectasis develops in association with a variety of conditions, which include the following:[39,40]

- *Congenital* or *hereditary conditions,* including *cystic fibrosis* (Chapter 10), *intralobar sequestration of the lung* (discussed earlier in this chapter), *immunodeficiency states,* and *primary ciliary dyskinesia* and *Kartagener syndromes* (discussed later)
- *Postinfectious conditions,* including necrotizing pneumonia caused by bacteria (*Mycobacterium tuberculosis, Staphylococcus aureus, Haemophilus influenzae, Pseudomonas*), viruses (adenovirus, influenza virus, HIV), and fungi (*Aspergillus* species)
- *Bronchial obstruction,* owing to tumor, foreign bodies, and occasionally mucus impaction, in which the bronchiectasis is localized to the obstructed lung segment
- Other conditions, including rheumatoid arthritis, systemic lupus erythematosus, inflammatory bowel disease, and post-transplantation (chronic lung rejection, and chronic graft-versus-host disease after bone marrow transplantation)

Etiology and Pathogenesis. *Obstruction* and *infection* are the major influences associated with bronchiectasis, and it is likely that both are necessary for the development of full-fledged lesions, although either may come first. After bronchial obstruction (e.g., by mucus impaction, tumors, or foreign bodies), normal clearing mechanisms are impaired, there is pooling of secretions distal to the obstruction, and there is inflammation of the airway. Conversely, severe infections of the bronchi lead to inflammation, often with necrosis, fibrosis, and eventually dilatation of airways.

These mechanisms—infection and obstruction—are most readily apparent in the severe form of bronchiectasis associated with cystic fibrosis (Chapter 10). In this disorder, the primary defect in chloride transport leads to impaired secretion of chloride ions into mucus, low sodium and water content, defective mucociliary action, and accumulation of thick viscid secretions that obstruct the airways. This leads to a marked susceptibility to bacterial infections, which further damage the airways. With repeated infections, there is widespread damage to airway walls, with destruction of supporting smooth muscle and elastic tissue, fibrosis, and further dilatation of bronchi. The smaller bronchioles become progressively obliterated owing to fibrosis (bronchiolitis obliterans).

In *primary ciliary dyskinesia,* an autosomal-recessive syndrome with variable penetrance and a frequency of 1 in 15,000 to 40,000 births, poorly functioning cilia contribute to the retention of secretions and recurrent infections that in turn lead to bronchiectasis. There is an absence or shortening of the dynein arms that are responsible for the coordinated bending of the cilia. Approximately half of the patients with primary ciliary dyskinesia have *Kartagener syndrome* (bronchiectasis, sinusitis, and situs inversus or partial lateralizing abnormality).[40] The lack of ciliary activity interferes with bacterial clearance, predisposes the sinuses and bronchi to infection, and affects cell motility during embryogenesis, resulting in the situs inversus. Males with this condition tend to be infertile, owing to ineffective mobility of the sperm tail.

Allergic bronchopulmonary aspergillosis (ABPA) is a condition that results from a hypersensitivity reaction to the fungus *Aspergillus fumigatus.* ABPA is also an important complication of asthma and cystic fibrosis. It is characterized by an intense airway inflammation with eosinophils and the formation of mucus plugs, which play a primary role in its pathogenesis. There is evidence that neutrophil-mediated inflammation and the potential deficiency of anti-inflammatory cytokines such as IL-10 may also play a role.[41] Clinically, there are periods of exacerbation and remission that may lead to proximal bronchiectasis and fibrotic lung disease.

Morphology. Bronchiectasis usually affects the lower lobes bilaterally, particularly air passages that are vertical, and is most severe in the more distal bronchi and bronchioles. When tumors or aspiration of foreign bodies leads to bronchiectasis, the involvement may be sharply localized to a single segment of the lung. **The airways are dilated, sometimes up to four times normal size.** These dilations may produce long, tubelike enlargements (**cylindrical bronchiectasis**) or, in other cases, may cause **fusiform** or even sharply saccular distention (**saccular bronchiectasis**).

Characteristically, the bronchi and bronchioles are sufficiently dilated that they can be followed, on gross examination, directly out to the pleural surfaces. By contrast, in the normal lung, the bronchioles cannot be followed by ordinary gross dissection beyond a point 2 to 3 cm removed from the pleural surfaces. On the cut surface of the lung, the transected dilated bronchi appear as cysts filled with mucopurulent secretions (Fig. 15–13).

The histologic findings vary with the activity and chronicity of the disease. In the full-blown, active case, there is an intense acute and chronic inflammatory exudation within the walls of the bronchi and bronchioles, associated with desquamation of the lining epithelium and extensive areas of necrotizing ulceration. There may be pseudostratification of the columnar cells or squamous metaplasia of the remaining epithelium. In some instances, the necrosis completely destroys the bronchial or bronchiolar walls and forms a lung abscess. Fibrosis of the bronchial and bronchiolar walls and peribronchiolar fibrosis develop in the more chronic cases, leading to varying degrees of subtotal or total obliteration of bronchiolar lumina.

In the usual case of bronchiectasis, a mixed flora can be cultured from the involved bronchi, including staphylococci, streptococci, pneumococci, enteric organisms, anaerobic and microaerophilic bacteria, and (particularly in children) *Haemophilus influenzae* and *Pseudomonas aeruginosa*. In ABPA, a few fungal hypae can be seen on special stains within the muco-inflammatory contents of the cylindrically dilated segmental bronchi. In late stages, the fungus may infiltrate the bronchial wall.

Clinical Course. Bronchiectasis causes severe, persistent cough; expectoration of foul-smelling, sometimes bloody sputum; dyspnea and orthopnea in severe cases; and occasional life-threatening hemoptysis. A systemic febrile reaction may occur when powerful pathogens are present. These symptoms are often episodic and are precipitated by upper respiratory tract infections or the introduction of new pathogenic agents. In the full-blown case, the cough is paroxysmal in nature. Such paroxysms are particularly frequent when the patient rises in the morning, and changes in position lead to drainage into the bronchi of the collected pools of pus. Obstructive ventilatory insufficiency can lead to marked dyspnea and cyanosis. Cor pulmonale, metastatic brain abscesses, and amyloidosis are less frequent complications of bronchiectasis.

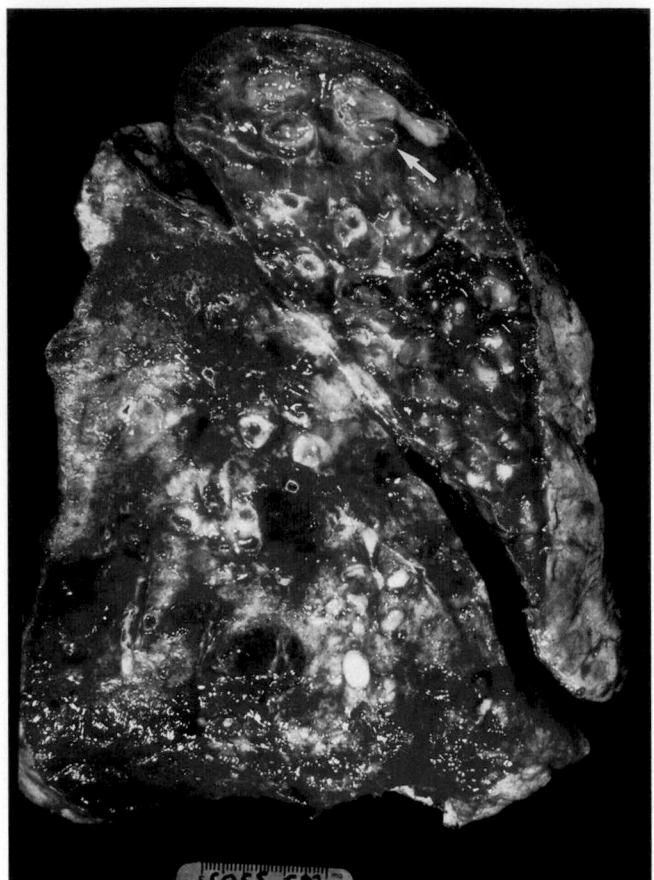

FIGURE 15–13 Bronchiectasis in a patient with cystic fibrosis, who underwent lung transplantation. Cut surface of lung shows markedly distended peripheral bronchi filled with mucopurulent secretions.

Diffuse Interstitial (Infiltrative, Restrictive) Diseases

Diffuse interstitial diseases are a heterogeneous group of disorders characterized predominantly by diffuse and usually chronic involvement of the pulmonary connective tissue, principally the most peripheral and delicate interstitium in the alveolar walls. The interstitium consists of the basement membrane of the endothelial and epithelial cells (fused in the thinnest portions), collagen fibers, elastic tissue, proteoglycans, fibroblasts, a few mast cells, and occasional lymphocytes and monocytes.

Many of the entities are of unknown cause and pathogenesis, some have an intra-alveolar as well as an interstitial component, and there is frequent overlap in histologic features among the different conditions. Nevertheless, their similar clinical signs, symptoms, radiologic alterations, and pathophysiologic changes justify their consideration as a group. These disorders account for about 15% of noninfectious diseases seen by pulmonary physicians.

In general, the clinical and pulmonary functional changes are those of *restrictive rather than obstructive lung disease* (see the previous section on obstructive versus restrictive pulmonary disease). Patients have dyspnea, tachypnea, end-inspiratory crackles, and eventual cyanosis, without wheezing or other evidence of airway obstruction. The classic physiologic features are reductions in carbon monoxide diffusing capacity, lung volume, and compliance. *Chest radiographs show diffuse infiltration by small nodules, irregular lines, or ground glass shadows*, hence the term *infiltrative*. Eventually, secondary pulmonary hypertension and right-sided heart failure with cor pulmonale may result. Although the entities can often be distinguished in the early stages, the advanced forms are hard to differentiate because they result in scarring and gross destruction of the lung, often referred to as *end-stage lung* or *honeycomb lung*.

Diffuse infiltrative diseases are categorized either as clinicopathologic syndromes or as having characteristic histology (Table 15–5).[42] Many of these entities are discussed in other sections of this book. Here, we briefly review current concepts of pathogenesis that may be common to all and discuss those in which lung involvement is the primary or a major problem. In terms of frequency, the most common associations are environmental diseases (approximately 25%), sarcoidosis (approximately 20%), idiopathic pulmonary fibrosis (approximately 15%), and the collagen vascular diseases (approximately 10%). The remaining interstitial diseases have more than 100 different causes and associations.

Pathogenesis. It is now thought that regardless of the type of interstitial disease or specific cause, the earliest common manifestation of most of the interstitial diseases is *alveolitis*,[43,44] that is, an accumulation of inflammatory and immune effector cells within the alveolar walls and spaces (Fig. 15–14). The accumulation of leukocytes has two consequences. It distorts the normal alveolar structures, and it results in the release of mediators that can injure parenchymal cells and stimulate fibrosis. These give rise to an end-stage fibrotic lung in which the alveoli are replaced by cystic spaces separated by thick bands of connective tissue interspersed with inflammatory cells.

The initial stimuli for alveolitis are as heterogeneous as the causes outlined in Table 15–5. Some of these stimuli, such as oxygen-derived free radicals and some chemicals, are directly toxic to endothelial cells, epithelial cells, or both. Beyond direct toxicity, a critical event is the *recruitment and activation of inflammatory and immune effector cells*. Neutrophil recruitment can be caused by complement activation in some disorders,[45] but in addition, the alveolar macrophages, which increase in number in all interstitial diseases, release *chemotactic factors* for neutrophils (e.g., IL-8,[46] leukotriene B_4[47]). In diseases such as sarcoidosis, *cell-mediated immune reactions* result in the accumulation of monocytes and T lymphocytes and in the formation of granulomas (Chapter 6). It is thought that interactions among lymphocytes and macrophages and the release of lymphokines and monokines are responsible for the slowly progressive pulmonary fibrosis that ensues. The alveolar macrophage, in particular, plays a central role in the development of fibrosis, as reviewed in the discussion of chronic inflammation (Chapter 2).

TABLE 15–5 Major Categories of Chronic Interstitial Lung Disease

Fibrosing
Usual interstitial pneumonia (idiopathic pulmonary fibrosis)
Nonspecific interstitial pneumonia
Cryptogenic organizing pneumonia
Associated with collagen vascular diseases
Pneumoconiosis
Drug reactions
Radiation pneumonitis
Granulomatous
Sarcoidosis
Hypersensitivity pneumonitis
Eosinophilic
Smoking-Related
Desquamative interstitial pneumonia
Respiratory bronchiolitis-associated interstitial lung disease
Other
Pulmonary alveolar proteinosis

FIBROSING DISEASES

Idiopathic Pulmonary Fibrosis

The term "idiopathic pulmonary fibrosis" (IPF) refers to a clinicopathologic syndrome with characteristic radiologic, pathologic, and clinical features. In Europe, the term "cryptogenic fibrosing alveolitis" is more popular. The histologic pattern of fibrosis is referred to as usual interstitial pneumonia (UIP), which is required for the diagnosis of IPF but can also be seen in other diseases, notably collagen vascular disorders and asbestosis. Desquamative interstitial pneumonia (DIP), previously considered an early form of IPF, has now been shown to be a smoking-related disorder. "Hamman-Rich syndrome" is a term that was used to describe a rapidly progressive type of IPF but is now considered a form of acute lung injury and is synonymous with acute interstitial pneumonia. The International Multidisciplinary Consensus Classification is an excellent reference for definitions and understanding of idiopathic interstitial pneumonias.[48,49]

Pathogenesis. While the causative agent(s) of IPF remain unknown, our concepts of pathogenesis have evolved over the past several years. The earlier view that IPF was initiated by an unidentified insult that gives rise to chronic inflammation resulting in fibrosis is probably not correct. According to this hypothesis, if the inflammatory response could be controlled before irreversible tissue injury occurs, fibrosis may be prevented. In clinical practice, however, anti-inflammatory therapy has failed to provide much benefit.[50] The current concept, therefore, is that IPF is caused by "repeated cycles" of acute lung injury (alveolitis) by some unidentified agent. "Wound healing" at these sites gives rise to exuberant fibroblastic proliferation, giving rise to the "fibroblastic foci" that are so characteristic of IPF. Mediators of wound healing such as TGF-β are expressed at these sites.

The inflammatory response in IPF may be modified by genetic or environmental factors and is thought to be of the T_H2 type. Thus, eosinophils, mast cells, and IL-4 and IL-13 are found in the lesions. Repeated cycles of injury and wound healing ultimately lead to widespread fibrosis and loss of lung function. Hence, one effective therapeutic strategy might be to reduce or prevent fibroblast replication. It is interesting to note in this connection that there is an abnormal activation of the Wnt-β-catenin signaling pathway (Chapter 7) within the mesenchymal cells of the fibroproliferative lesions of IPF.[51]

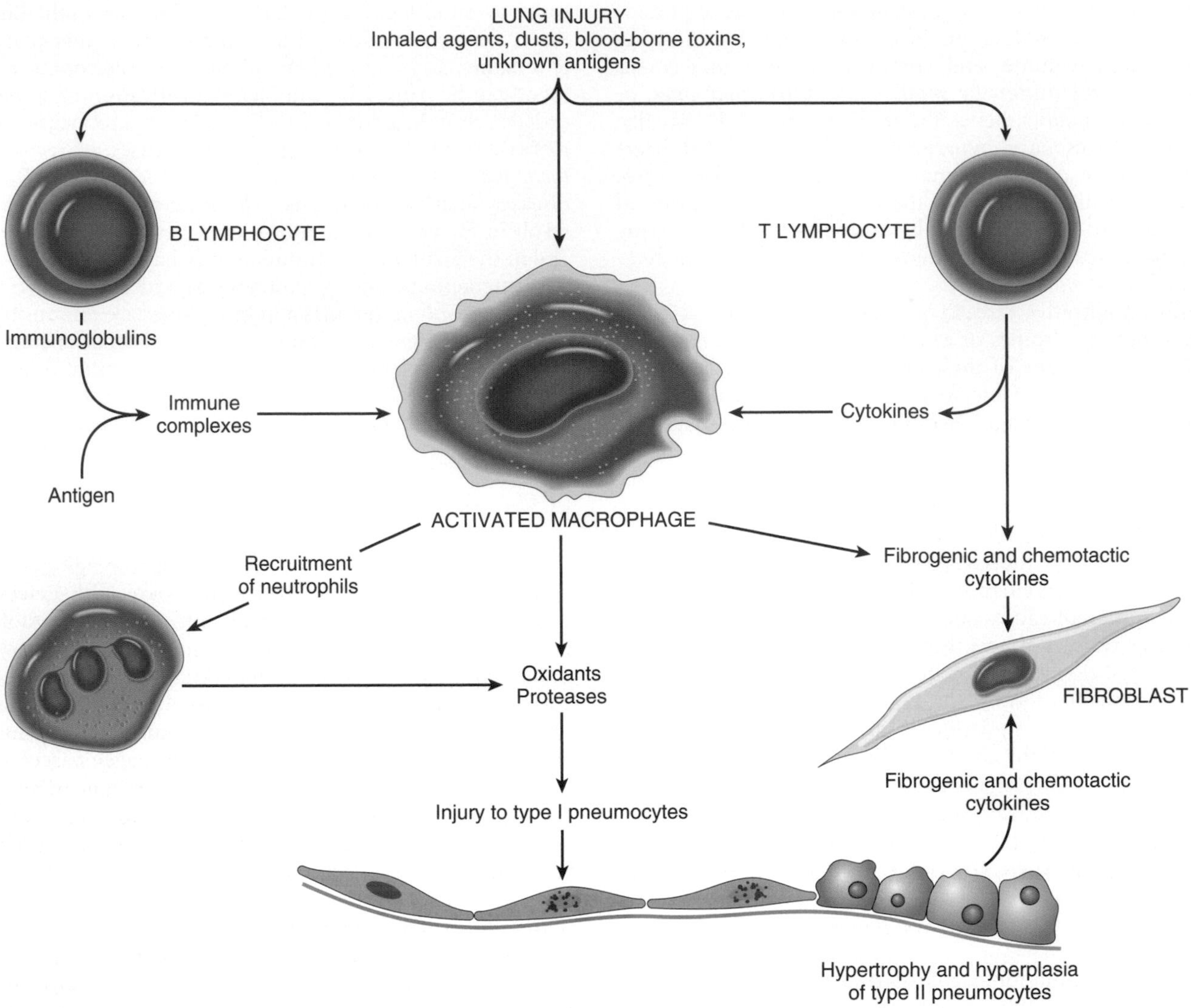

FIGURE 15–14 A possible schema of the pathogenesis of idiopathic pulmonary fibrosis.

This pathway, as is well known, is activated in several tumors, including colonic cancers. Hence, there is interest in identifying molecules that can inhibit the Wnt signaling pathway. These might become the "designer molecules" used to treat colonic tumors and IPF.

Morphology. Grossly, the pleural surfaces of the lung are cobblestoned owing to the retraction of scars along the interlobular septa. The cut surface shows fibrosis (firm, rubbery white areas) of the lung parenchyma with lower-lobe predominance and a distinctive distribution in the **subpleural regions** and along the **interlobular septa**. Microscopically, the hallmark of the UIP is **patchy interstitial fibrosis**, which varies in intensity (Fig. 15–15) and with time. The earliest lesions contain exhuberent fibroblastic proliferation and appear as **fibroblastic foci**. With time these areas become more collagenous and less cellular. Quite typical is the coexistence of both early and late lesions (Fig. 15–16). The dense fibrosis causes collapse of alveolar walls and formation of cystic spaces lined by hyperplastic type II pneumocytes or bronchiolar epithelium (**honeycomb fibrosis**). With adequate sampling, these diagnostic histologic changes (i.e., areas of dense collagenous fibrosis with relatively normal lung and fibroblastic foci) can be identified even in terminal IPF. There is mild to moderate inflammation within the fibrotic areas, consisting of mostly lymphocytes, with few plasma cells, neutrophils, eosinophils, and mast cells. Foci of squamous metaplasia and smooth muscle hyperplasia may be present. Secondary pulmonary hypertensive changes (intimal fibrosis and medial thickening of pulmonary arteries) are often present. Since the UIP pattern can be seen in other diseases, these must be excluded by taking into account clinical, radiographic, and laboratory findings.

Clinical Course. IPF begins insidiously, with gradually increasing dyspnea on exertion and dry cough. Most patients are 40 to 70 years old at the time of presentation. Hypoxemia, cyanosis, and clubbing occur late in the course. The progression in an individual patient is unpredictable. Most patients

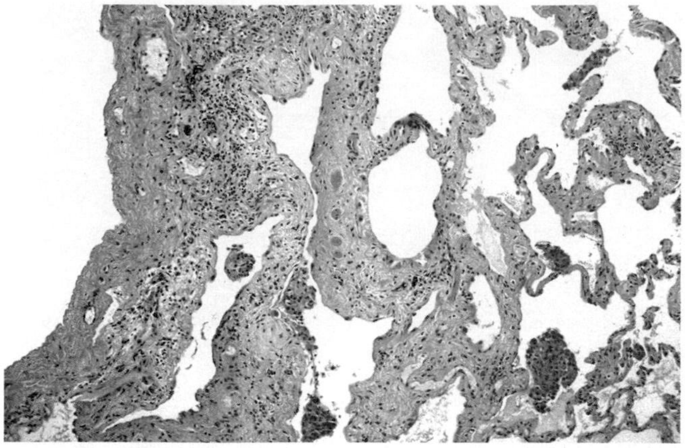

FIGURE 15–15 Usual interstitial pneumonia. The fibrosis, which varies in intensity, is more pronounced in the subpleural region.

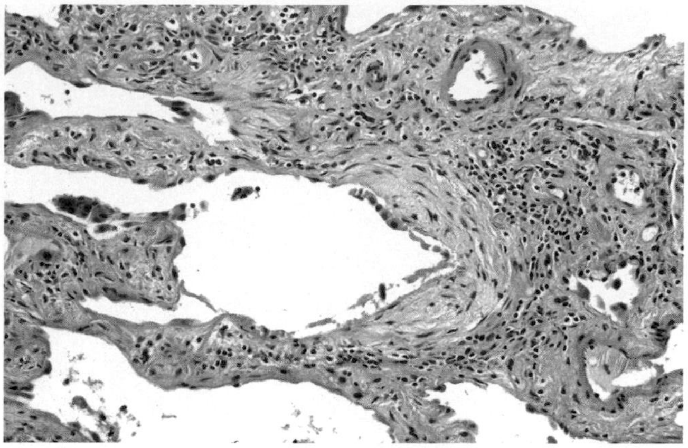

FIGURE 15–16 Usual interstitial pneumonia. Fibroblastic focus with fibers running parallel to surface and bluish myxoid extracellular matrix.

have a gradual deterioration of their pulmonary status, despite medical treatment (steroids, cyclophosphamide, or azathioprine). In some IPF patients, there is acute exacerbation of the underlying disease with a rapid downhill clinical course. The mean survival is 3 years or less. Lung transplantation is the only definitive therapy available.

Nonspecific Interstitial Pneumonia

The concept of nonspecific interstitial pneumonia (NSIP) emerged when it was realized that there is a group of patients with diffuse interstitial lung disease of unknown etiology whose lung biopsies fail to show diagnostic features of any of the other well-characterized interstitial diseases. Although this definition makes NSIP a "wastebasket" type of diagnosis, it is important to recognize it, since these patients have a much better prognosis than do those with UIP.[52]

Morphology. On the basis of its histology, NSIP is divided into cellular and fibrosing patterns. The cellular pattern consists primarily of mild to moderate chronic interstitial inflammation, containing lymphocytes and a few plasma cells, in a uniform or patchy distribution. The fibrosing pattern consists of diffuse or patchy, interstitial fibrosis without the temporal heterogeneity that is characteristic of UIP. Fibroblastic foci are absent. This suggests that NSIP is not caused by recurrent sequential bouts of alveolitis. Mild to moderate chronic inflammation and lymphoid aggregates may be present.

Clinical Course. Patients present with dyspnea and cough of several months' duration. They are typically between 46 and 55 years of age, those having the NSIP cellular pattern being somewhat younger than those with fibrosing pattern or UIP. Patients with cellular pattern have a better outcome than do those with fibrosing pattern and UIP.[53]

Cryptogenic Organizing Pneumonia

Cryptogenic organizing pneumonia (COP) is synonymous with the popular term "bronchiolitis obliterans organizing pneumonia"; however, the former is now preferred, since it conveys the essential features of a clinicopathologic syndrome of unknown etiology and avoids confusion with airway diseases such as bronchiolitis obliterans. Patients present with cough and dyspnea and have subpleural or peribronchial patchy areas of airspace consolidation radiographically. Histologically, COP is characterized by the presence of polypoid plugs of loose organizing connective tissue within alveolar ducts, alveoli (Fig. 15–17), and often bronchioles. The connective tissue is all of the same age, and the underlying lung architecture is normal. There is no interstitial fibrosis or honeycomb lung. Some patients recover spontaneously, but most need treatment with oral steroids for 6 months or longer for complete recovery.

It is important to recognize that organizing pneumonia with intra-alveolar fibrosis can also be seen as a response to infections or inflammatory injury of the lungs. These include viral and bacterial pneumonia, inhaled toxins, drugs, collagen vascular disease, and graft-versus-host disease in bone marrow transplant recipients. The prognosis for these patients is the same as that for the underlying disorder.

Pulmonary Involvement in Collagen Vascular Diseases

Many collagen vascular diseases, notably systemic lupus erythematosus, rheumatoid arthritis, progressive systemic sclerosis (scleroderma), dermatomyositis-polymyositis, and mixed connective tissue disease, can involve the lung to a lesser or greater degree at some time in their course. Pulmonary involvement can occur in different patterns, NSIP (more prevalent than UIP in systemic sclerosis), UIP-pattern (similar to that seen in IPF), vascular sclerosis, organizing pneumonia, and bronchiolitis (small airway disease, with or without fibrosis) being the most common. Diffuse interstitial fibrosis (NSIP pattern) occurs classically in progressive systemic sclerosis (*scleroderma*), discussed in Chapter 6. Less commonly, patchy, transient parenchymal infiltrates are noted in *lupus erythematosus*, and severe lupus pneumonitis may occasionally occur and can be one of the major clinical problems in such patients. In *rheumatoid arthritis*, pulmonary involvement is common and may occur in one of four forms: (1) chronic pleuritis, with or without effusion; (2) diffuse interstitial

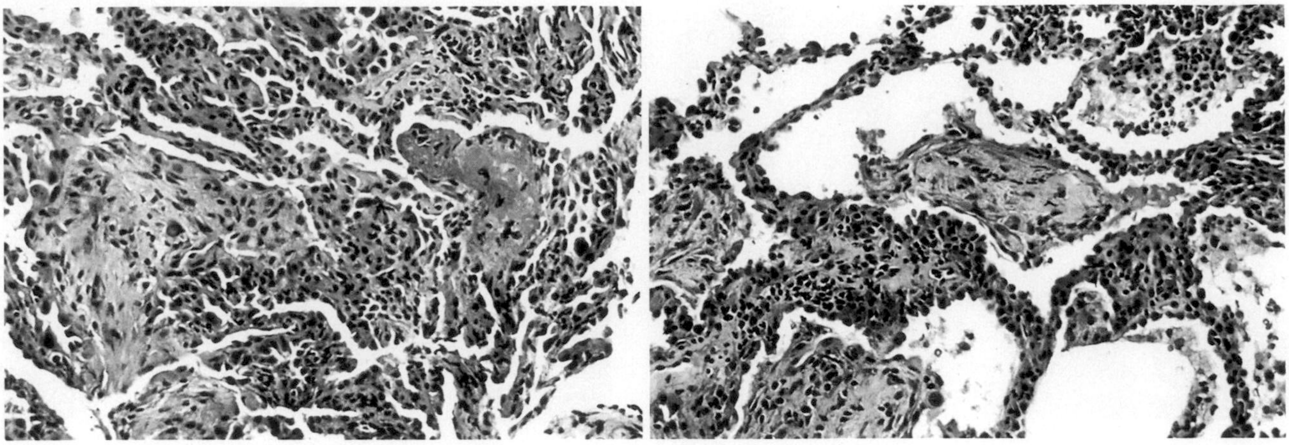

FIGURE 15–17 Cryptogenic organizing pneumonia (COP). Alveolar spaces are filled with balls of fibroblasts (Masson bodies), while the alveolar walls are relatively normal.

pneumonitis and fibrosis; (3) intrapulmonary rheumatoid nodules; and (4) pulmonary hypertension. Thirty per cent to 40% of patients with classic rheumatoid arthritis have abnormalities in pulmonary function. In certain patients, the disorder progresses to end-stage lung disease. Pleural involvement (pleuritis, pleural nodules, and pleural effusion) may also be present. Pulmonary involvement in these diseases is usually associated with a poor prognosis, although it is still better than that of idiopathic UIP.

Pneumoconioses

The term "pneumoconiosis" was originally coined to describe the non-neoplastic lung reaction to inhalation of mineral dusts encountered in the workplace. Now it also includes diseases induced by organic as well as inorganic particulates and chemical fumes and vapors. A simplified classification is presented in Table 15–6. Regulations limiting worker exposure have resulted in a marked decrease in dust-associated diseases.

Although the pneumoconioses result from well-defined occupational exposure to specific airborne agents, particulate air pollution also has deleterious effects on the general population, especially in urban areas. Studies have found increased morbidity (e.g., asthma incidence) and mortality rates in populations that are exposed to increased ambient air particulate levels,[54,55] leading to calls for greater efforts to reduce the levels of particulates in urban air.

General Pathogenesis. The specific changes caused by the more important dusts are presented in succeeding sections; however, certain pathogenetic principles apply to all. The development of a pneumoconiosis depends on (1) the amount of dust retained in the lung and airways; (2) the size, shape, and therefore buoyancy of the particles; (3) particle solubility and physiochemical reactivity; and (4) the possible additional effects of other irritants (e.g., concomitant tobacco smoking).

The amount of dust retained in the lungs is determined by the dust concentration in ambient air, the duration of exposure, and the effectiveness of clearance mechanisms. Any influence, such as cigarette smoking, that affects the integrity of the mucociliary apparatus significantly predisposes to the accumulation of dust. *The most dangerous particles range from 1 to 5 μm in diameter because they may reach the terminal small airways and air sacs and settle in their linings.* Under normal conditions, there is a small pool of intra-alveolar macrophages and this is expanded by recruitment of more macrophages when dust reaches the alveolar spaces. The protection provided by phagocytosis of particles, however, can be overwhelmed by the large dust burden deposited with occupational exposures and by specific chemical interactions of the particles with cells.

The *solubility and cytotoxicity of particles*, which are influenced to a considerable extent by their size, modify the nature of the pulmonary response. In general, the smaller the particle, the more likely it is to appear in the pulmonary fluids and reach toxic levels rapidly, depending, of course, on the solubility of the agent. Therefore, smaller particles tend to cause acute lung injury. Larger particles resist dissolution and so may persist within the lung parenchyma for years. These tend to evoke fibrosing collagenous pneumoconioses, such as is characteristic of silicosis. The reaction to crystalline silica illustrates how the *physiochemical reactivity* of particles contributes to pathogenesis. Quartz (a form of crystalline silica) can cause direct injury to tissue and cell membranes by interaction with free radicals and other chemical groups on the particle surface. The resulting membrane damage may ultimately cause cell death. Of more importance, however, is the ability of silica to trigger macrophages to release a number of products that mediate an inflammatory response and initiate fibroblast proliferation and collagen deposition.[56,57] Pro-inflammatory and fibrosing mediators are also critical in the pathogenesis of the pulmonary reaction to asbestos.[58]

Some of the particles may be taken up by epithelial cells or may cross the epithelial cell lining and interact directly with fibroblasts and interstitial macrophages. Some may reach the lymphatics either by direct drainage or within migrating macrophages and thereby initiate an immune response to components of the particulates or to self proteins modified by the particles, (or both). This response leads to an amplification and extension of the local reaction. Although tobacco smoking worsens the effects of all inhaled mineral dusts, the effects of asbestos are particularly magnified by smoking. Also, it has been recognized that the effects of inhaled particles are not confined to the lung alone, since particles can translocate to the blood and lung inflammation invokes systemic responses.[59]

TABLE 15–6 Lung Diseases Caused by Air Pollutants

Agent	Disease	Exposure
Mineral Dusts		
Coal dust	Anthracosis Macules Progressive massive fibrosis Caplan syndrome	Coal mining (particularly hard coal)
Silica	Silicosis Caplan syndrome	Foundry work, sandblasting, hardrock mining, stone cutting, others
Asbestos	Asbestosis Pleural plaques Caplan syndrome Mesothelioma Carcinoma of the lung, larynx, stomach, colon	Mining, milling, and fabrication; installation and removal of insulation
Beryllium	Acute berylliosis Beryllium granulomatosis Bronchogenic carcinoma (?)	Mining, fabrication
Iron oxide	Siderosis	Welding
Barium sulfate	Baritosis	Mining
Tin oxide	Stannosis	Mining
Organic Dusts That Induce Hypersensitivity Pneumonitis		
Moldy hay	Farmer's lung	Farming
Bagasse	Bagassosis	Manufacturing wallboard, paper
Bird droppings	Bird-breeder's lung	Bird handling
Organic Dusts That Induce Asthma		
Cotton, flax, hemp	Byssinosis	Textile manufacturing
Red cedar dust	Asthma	Lumbering, carpentry
Chemical Fumes and Vapors		
Nitrous oxide, sulfur dioxide, ammonia, benzene, insecticides	Bronchitis, asthma Pulmonary edema ARDS* Mucosal injury Fulminant poisoning	Occupational and accidental exposure

*Acute respiratory distress syndrome.

In general, only a small percentage of exposed people develop occupational respiratory diseases. In one study, genetic variation of serum and erythrocytic proteins was shown to correlate with susceptibility to developing silicosis, chronic bronchitis, and occupational asthma. Such studies could be useful for assessment and forecast of individual risk of occupational diseases.[60] Many of the diseases listed in Table 15–6 are quite uncommon. Hence only a selected few that cause fibrosis of the lung are presented next.

COAL WORKERS' PNEUMOCONIOSIS (CWP). Dust reduction measures in coal mines around the globe have drastically reduced the incidence of coal dust–induced disease. The spectrum of lung findings in coal workers is wide, varying from (1) asymptomatic anthracosis to (2) simple coal workers' pneumoconiosis (CWP) with little to no pulmonary dysfunction to (3) complicated CWP, or progressive massive fibrosis (PMF), in which lung function is compromised.[61] It should be noted that PMF is a generic term that applies to a confluent, fibrosing reaction in the lung that can be a complication of any pneumoconiosis, although it is more common in CWP and silicosis.

The pathogenesis of complicated CWP, particularly what causes the lesions of simple CWP to progress to PMF, is incompletely understood. Contaminating silica in the coal dust can favor progressive disease. In most cases, carbon dust itself is the major culprit, and studies have shown that complicated lesions contain considerably more dust than simple lesions do.

Morphology. Anthracosis is the most innocuous coal-induced pulmonary lesion in coal miners and is commonly seen in all urban dwellers and tobacco smokers. Inhaled carbon pigment is engulfed by alveolar or interstitial macrophages, which then accumulate in the connective tissue along the lymphatics, including the pleural lymphatics, or in organized lymphoid tissue along the bronchi or in the lung hilus. At autopsy, linear streaks and aggregates of anthracotic pigment readily identify pulmonary lymphatics and mark the pulmonary lymph nodes.

Simple CWP is characterized by **coal macules** (1 to 2 mm in diameter) and the somewhat larger **coal nodules**. The coal macule consists of carbon-laden macrophages; the nodule also contains small amounts of a delicate network of collagen fibers. Although these lesions are scattered throughout the lung, the upper lobes and upper zones of the lower lobes are more heavily involved. They are located primarily adjacent to respiratory bronchioles, the site of initial dust accumulation. In due course, dilation of adjacent alveoli occurs, a condition sometimes referred to as **centrilobular emphysema.**

Complicated CWP (PMF) occurs on a background of simple CWP and generally requires many years to develop. It is characterized by intensely blackened scars larger than 2 cm, sometimes up to 10 cm in greatest diameter. They are usually multiple (Fig. 15–18). Microscopically, the lesions consist of dense collagen and pigment. The center of the lesion is often necrotic, resulting most likely from local ischemia.

Clinical Course. CWP is usually a benign disease that causes little decrement in lung function. Even mild forms of complicated CWP fail to demonstrate abnormalities of lung function. In a minority of cases (fewer than 10%), PMF develops, leading to increasing pulmonary dysfunction, pulmonary hypertension, and cor pulmonale. Once PMF develops, it may become progressive even if further exposure to dust is prevented. Unlike silicosis (discussed later), there is no convincing evidence that coal dust increases susceptibility to tuberculosis. There is some evidence that exposure to coal dust increases the incidence of chronic bronchitis and emphysema, independent of smoking, thus complicating the management of the patient with CWP. To date, however, there is no compelling evidence that CWP in the absence of smoking predisposes to cancer.

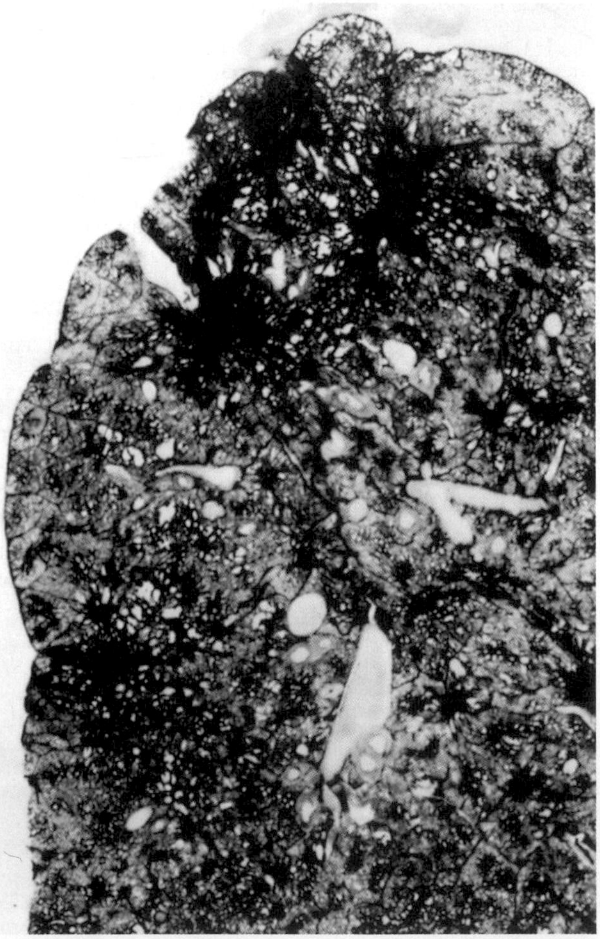

FIGURE 15–18 Progressive massive fibrosis superimposed on coal workers' pneumoconiosis. The large, blackened scars are located principally in the upper lobe. Note the extensions of scars into surrounding parenchyma and retraction of adjacent pleura. (Courtesy of Dr. Werner Laquer, Dr. Jerome Kleinerman, and the National Institute of Occupational Safety and Health, Morgantown, WV.)

SILICOSIS. Silicosis is a lung disease caused by inhalation of crystalline silicon dioxide (silica).[62] *Currently the most prevalent chronic occupational disease in the world,* silicosis usually presents, after decades of exposure, as a slowly progressing, nodular, fibrosing pneumoconiosis. As Table 15–6 shows, workers in a large number of occupations are at risk, especially sandblasters and many mine workers. Less commonly, heavy exposure over months to a few years can result in acute silicosis, a lesion characterized by the generalized accumulation of a lipoproteinaceous material within alveoli (identical morphologically to alveolar proteinosis, which is discussed later).

Pathogenesis. Silica occurs in both crystalline and amorphous forms, but crystalline forms (including quartz, crystobalite, and tridymite) are much more fibrogenic, revealing the importance of the physical form and surface properties in pathogenesis. Of these, quartz is most commonly implicated in silicosis. After inhalation, the particles interact with epithelial cells and macrophages. *Although lung macrophages that ingest the silica particles may ultimately succumb to its toxic effects, silica causes activation and release of mediators by viable macrophages.* Such mediators include IL-1, TNF, fibronectin, lipid mediators, oxygen-derived free radicals, and fibrogenic cytokines.[63,64] Especially compelling is evidence incriminating TNF since anti-TNF monoclonal antibodies can block lung collagen accumulation in mice that are given silica intratracheally. Animals exposed to silica demonstrate a steady recruitment of macrophages and lymphocytes to the alveoli and interstitium. These cells may further amplify the process.

It has been noted that when mixed with other minerals, quartz has a reduced fibrogenic effect. This phenomenon is of practical importance because quartz in the workplace is rarely pure. Thus, miners of the iron-containing ore hematite may have more quartz in their lungs than some quartz-exposed workers and yet have relatively mild lung disease because the hematite provides a protective effect. In the earth, much of the silica combines with oxygen and other elements to form silicates. Although amorphous silicates are biologically less active than crystalline silica, heavy lung burdens of these minerals may also produce lesions. Talc, vermiculite, and mica are examples of noncrystalline silicates that are less common causes of pneumoconioses.

Morphology. Silicosis is characterized grossly in its early stages by tiny, barely palpable, discrete pale to blackened (if coal dust is also present) nodules in the upper zones of the lungs. As the disease progresses, these nodules may coalesce into **hard, collagenous scars** (Fig. 15–19). Some nodules may undergo central softening and cavitation. This change may be due to superimposed tuberculosis or to ischemia. Fibrotic lesions may also occur in the hilar lymph nodes and pleura. Sometimes, thin sheets of calcification occur in the lymph nodes and are seen radiographically as **eggshell** calcification (i.e., calcium surrounding a zone lacking calcification). If the disease continues to progress, expansion and coalescence of lesions produce PMF. Histologically, the nodular lesions consist of concentric layers of hyalinized collagen sur-

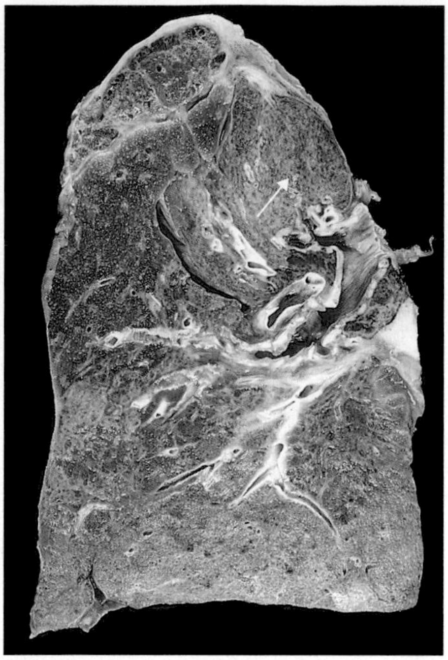

FIGURE 15–19 Advanced silicosis seen on transection of lung. Scarring has contracted the upper lobe into a small dark mass (*arrow*). Note the dense pleural thickening. (Courtesy of Dr. John Godleski, Brigham and Women's Hospital, Boston, MA.)

rounded by a dense capsule of more condensed collagen (Fig. 15–20). Examination of the nodules by polarized microscopy reveals the birefringent silica particles.

Clinical Course. The disease is usually detected when routine chest radiography is performed on an asymptomatic worker. The radiographs typically show a fine nodularity in the upper zones of the lung, but pulmonary functions are either normal or only moderately affected. Most patients do not develop shortness of breath until late in the course, after PMF is present. At this time, the disease may be progressive, even if the patient is no longer exposed. The disease is slow to

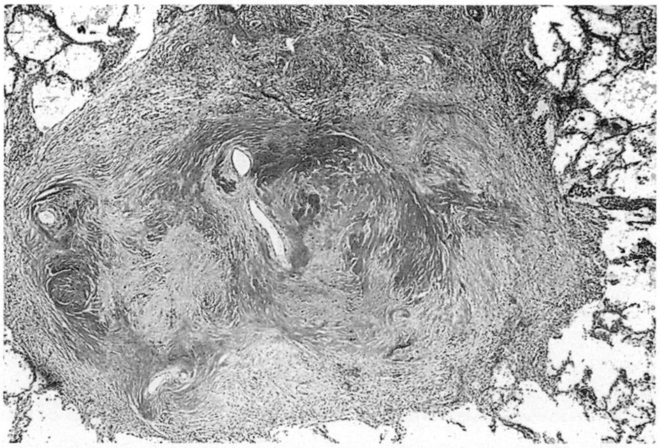

FIGURE 15–20 Several coalescent collagenous silicotic nodules. (Courtesy of Dr. John Godleski, Brigham and Women's Hospital, Boston, MA.)

kill, but impaired pulmonary function may severely limit activity. Silicosis is associated with an increased susceptibility to *tuberculosis*. It is postulated that silicosis results in a depression of cell-mediated immunity, and crystalline silica may inhibit the ability of pulmonary macrophages to kill phagocytosed mycobacteria. Nodules of silicotuberculosis often display a central zone of caseation. The relationship between silica and *lung cancer* has been a contentious issue. In 1997, the International Agency for Research on Cancer (IARC) concluded that *crystalline silica from occupational sources is carcinogenic in humans*. However, this subject continues to be controversial.

Asbestos-Related Diseases. Asbestos is a family of crystalline hydrated silicates that form fibers. On the basis of epidemiologic studies, *occupational exposure* to asbestos is linked to:

- Localized fibrous plaques or, rarely, diffuse pleural fibrosis
- Pleural effusions
- Parenchymal interstitial fibrosis (*asbestosis*)
- Lung carcinoma
- Mesotheliomas
- Laryngeal and perhaps other extrapulmonary neoplasms, including colon carcinomas

An increased incidence of asbestos-related cancer in family members of asbestos workers has alerted the general public to the potential hazards of asbestos in the environment. The proper public health policy toward low-level exposures that might be encountered in old buildings or schools is controversial; some experts question the wisdom of expensive asbestos abatement programs for environments with airborne fiber counts that are up to 100-fold lower than allowed by occupational standards.

Pathogenesis. Concentration, size, shape, and solubility of the different forms of asbestos dictate whether it causes disease.[65] There are two distinct geometric forms of asbestos: *serpentine* (curly and flexible fibers) and *amphibole* (straight, stiff, and brittle fibers). The serpentine chrysotile chemical form accounts for most of the asbestos used in industry. Amphiboles include crocidolite, amosite, tremolite, anthophyllite, and actinolyte. This confusing array of terms is important because amphiboles, even though less prevalent, are more pathogenic than chrysotiles, particularly with respect to induction of malignant pleural tumors (mesotheliomas).

The greater pathogenicity of amphiboles is apparently related to their aerodynamic properties and solubility. Chrysotiles, with their more flexible, curled structure, are likely to become impacted in the upper respiratory passages and removed by the mucociliary elevator. Furthermore, once trapped in the lungs, chrysotiles are gradually leached from the tissues because they are more soluble than amphiboles. In contrast, the straight, stiff amphiboles may align themselves in the airstream and thus be delivered deeper into the lungs, where they can penetrate epithelial cells and reach the interstitium. The length of amphibole fibers also plays a role in their pathogenicity, those longer than 8 μm and thinner than 0.5 μm being more injurious than shorter, thicker ones. Nevertheless, both amphiboles and serpentines are fibrogenic, and increasing doses are associated with a higher incidence of all asbestos-related disease except that only amphibole exposure correlates with mesothelioma.

In contrast to other inorganic dusts, asbestos can also act as a tumor initiator and a tumor promoter. Some of the oncogenic effects of asbestos are mediated by reactive free radicals generated by asbestos fibers, which preferentially localize in the distal lung, close to the mesothelial layers. Potentially toxic chemicals adsorbed onto the asbestos fibers, however, undoubtedly contribute to the oncogenicity of the fibers. For example, the adsorption of carcinogens in tobacco smoke onto asbestos fibers may well be important in the remarkable synergy between tobacco smoking and the development of lung carcinoma in asbestos workers. One study of asbestos workers found a fivefold increase of lung carcinoma for asbestos exposure alone, while asbestos exposure and smoking together led to a 55-fold increase in the risk of lung cancer.[66]

The occurrence of asbestosis, like the other pneumoconioses, depends on the interaction of inhaled fibers with lung macrophages and other parenchymal cells. The initial injury occurs at bifurcations of small airways and ducts, where the asbestos fibers land and penetrate. Macrophages, both alveolar and interstitial, attempt to ingest and clear the fibers and are activated to release chemotactic factors and fibrogenic mediators that amplify the response. Chronic deposition of fibers and persistent release of mediators eventually lead to generalized interstitial pulmonary inflammation and interstitial fibrosis. It is not completely understood why silicosis is a nodular fibrosing disease and asbestosis is a diffuse interstitial process. The more diffuse distribution may be related to the ability of asbestos to reach alveoli more consistently, its ability to penetrate epithelial cells, or both.

Morphology. Asbestosis is marked by **diffuse pulmonary interstitial fibrosis,** which is indistinguishable from diffuse interstitial fibrosis resulting from other causes, except for the presence of **asbestos bodies.** Asbestos bodies appear as **golden brown, fusiform or beaded rods with a translucent center and consist of asbestos fibers coated with an iron-containing proteinaceous material** (Fig. 15–21). They arise when macrophages attempt to phagocytose asbestos fibers; the iron is presumably derived from phagocyte ferritin. Other inorganic particulates may become coated with similar iron protein complexes and are called **ferruginous bodies.** Sometimes asbestos bodies can be found in the lungs of normal people, but usually in much lower concentrations and without interstitial fibrosis.

Asbestosis begins as fibrosis around respiratory bronchioles and alveolar ducts and extends to involve adjacent alveolar sacs and alveoli. The fibrous tissue distorts the native architecture, creating enlarged airspaces enclosed within thick fibrous walls; eventually, the affected regions become honeycombed. The pattern of fibrosis is similar to that seen in UIP, with fibroblastic foci and varying degrees of fibrosis, the only difference being the presence of numerous asbestos bodies. In contrast to CWP and silicosis, asbestosis begins in the lower lobes and subpleurally. The middle and upper lobes of the lungs become affected as fibrosis progresses. The scarring may trap and narrow pulmonary arteries and arterioles, causing pulmonary hypertension and cor pulmonale.

Pleural plaques, the most common manifestation of asbestos exposure, are well-circumscribed plaques of dense collagen (Fig. 15–22), often containing calcium. They develop most frequently on the anterior and posterolateral aspects of the **parietal pleura** and over the domes of the diaphragm. The size and number of pleural plaques do not correlate with the level of exposure to asbestos or the time since exposure.[67] They do not contain asbestos bodies, however, only rarely do they occur in individuals who have no history or evidence of asbestos exposure. Uncommonly, asbestos exposure induces pleural effusions, which are usually serous but may be bloody. Rarely, diffuse visceral pleural fibrosis may occur and, in advanced cases, bind the lung to the thoracic cavity wall.

Both lung carcinomas and mesotheliomas (pleural and peritoneal) develop in workers exposed to asbestos. The risk of lung carcinoma is increased about fivefold for asbestos workers; the relative risk of mesotheliomas, normally a rare tumor (2 to 17 cases per 1 million persons), is more than 1000-fold greater. Concomitant cigarette smoking greatly increases the risk of lung carcinoma but not that of mesothelioma. These asbestos-related tumors are morphologically indistinguishable from other forms of lung cancer that are described later.

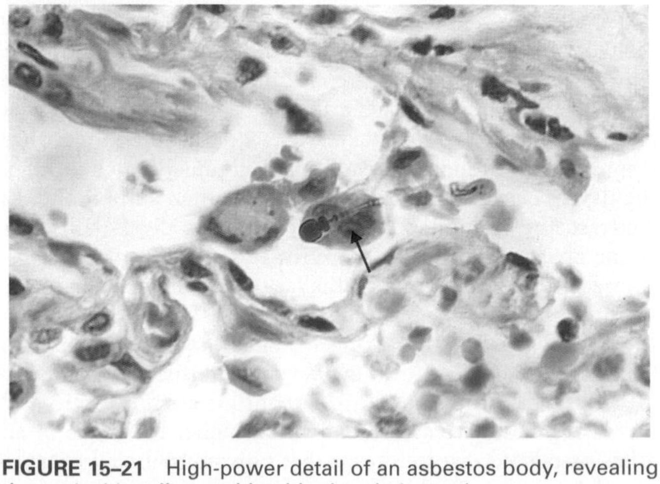

FIGURE 15–21 High-power detail of an asbestos body, revealing the typical beading and knobbed ends (*arrow*).

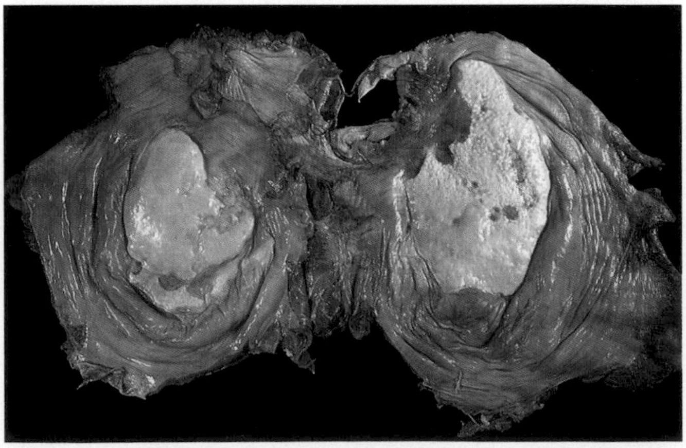

FIGURE 15–22 Asbestos exposure evidenced by severe, discrete, characteristic fibrocalcific plaques on the pleural surface of the diaphragm. (Courtesy of Dr. John Godleski, Brigham and Women's Hospital, Boston, MA.)

Clinical Course. The clinical findings in asbestosis are very similar to those caused by other diffuse interstitial lung disease (discussed earlier). Dyspnea is usually the first manifestation; at first, it is provoked by exertion, but later it is present even at rest. The dyspnea is usually accompanied by a cough associated with production of sputum. These manifestations rarely appear fewer than 10 years after first exposure and are more common after 20 years or more. The disease may remain static or progress to respiratory failure, cor pulmonale, and death. Chest films reveal irregular linear densities, particularly in both lower lobes. With advancement of the pneumoconiosis, a honeycomb pattern develops. Pleural plaques are usually asymptomatic and are detected on radiographs as circumscribed densities. Asbestosis complicated by lung or pleural cancer is associated with a particularly grim prognosis.

Complications of Therapies

Drug-Induced Lung Diseases. Drugs can cause a variety of both acute and chronic alterations in respiratory structure and function, including bronchospasm, pulmonary edema, diffuse alveolar damage, organizing pneumonia, interstitial fibrosis, bronchiolitis obliterans, and eosinophilic pneumonia (Table 15–7).[68] For example, cytotoxic drugs used in cancer therapy (e.g., bleomycin) cause pulmonary damage and fibrosis as a result of direct toxicity of the drug and by stimulating the influx of inflammatory cells into the alveoli. Amiodarone, a drug that controls resistant cardiac arrhythmias, is preferentially concentrated in the lung and causes significant pneumonitis in 5% to 15% of patients receiving it.

Radiation-Induced Lung Diseases. Radiation pneumonitis is a well-known complication of therapeutic radiation of pulmonary or other thoracic tumors (esophageal, breast, mediastinal).[69] It most often involves the lung within the radiation port but occasionally may extend to other areas of the same lung or even the contralateral lung. It occurs in acute and chronic forms. After clinical fractionated irradiation, *acute radiation pneumonitis* occurs in 10% to 20% of patients, 1 to 6 months after therapy, manifested by fever, dyspnea out of proportion to the volume of lung irradiated, pleural effusion, and radiologic infiltrates that usually correspond to an area of previous radiation. With steroid therapy, these symptoms may resolve completely in some patients without long-term effects,[70] while in others there is progression to *chronic radiation pneumonitis*. There is increasing evidence that irradiation of the lungs initially causes a lymphocytic alveolitis or hypersensitivity pneumonitis that can lead to pulmonary fibrosis (chronic radiation pneumonitis). The latter is a consequence of repair, which is initiated by direct tissue injury to endothelial and epithelial cells within the radiation portal.

TABLE 15–7 Examples of Drug-Induced Pulmonary Disease

Drug	Pulmonary Disease
Cytotoxic drugs	
Bleomycin	Pneumonitis and fibrosis
Methotrexate	Hypersensitivity pneumonitis
Amiodarone	Pneumonitis and fibrosis
Nitrofurantoin	Hypersensitivity pneumonitis
Aspirin	Bronchospasm
β-Antagonists	Bronchospasm

Morphologic changes are those of diffuse alveolar damage, including severe atypia of hyperplastic type II cells and fibroblasts. Epithelial cell atypia and foam cells within vessel walls are also characteristic of radiation damage.

GRANULOMATOUS DISEASES

Sarcoidosis

Sarcoidosis is a systemic disease of unknown cause characterized by noncaseating granulomas in many tissues and organs. Sarcoidosis presents many clinical patterns, but bilateral hilar lymphadenopathy or lung involvement is visible on chest radiographs in 90% of cases. Eye and skin lesions are next in frequency. Since other diseases, including mycobacterial or fungal infections and berylliosis, can also produce noncaseating (*hard*) granulomas, the histologic diagnosis of sarcoidosis is made by exclusion.

The prevalence of sarcoidosis is higher in women than in men but varies widely in different countries and populations. In the United States, the rates are highest in the Southeast; they are 10 times higher in American blacks than in whites. By contrast, among Chinese and Southeast Asians, the disease is rare.

Etiology and Pathogenesis. Although the etiology of sarcoidosis remains unknown, several lines of evidence suggest that it is a disease of disordered immune regulation in genetically predisposed individuals exposed to certain environmental agents.[71] The role of each of these three contributory factors is summarized below.

Immunologic Factors. There are several *immunologic abnormalities* in the local milieu of sarcoid granulomas that suggest the development of a cell-mediated response to an unidentified antigen. The process is driven by CD4+ helper T cells. These abnormalities include:[72]

- Intra-alveolar and interstitial accumulation of CD4+ T cells, resulting in CD4:CD8 T-cell ratios ranging from 5:1 to 15:1. There is oligoclonal expansion of T-cell subsets as determined by analysis of T-cell receptor rearrangement, suggesting an antigen-driven proliferation.
- Increased levels of T cell–derived T_H1 cytokines such as IL-2 and interferon-γ (IFN-γ), resulting in T-cell expansion and macrophage activation, respectively.
- Increased levels of several cytokines in the local environment (IL-8, TNF, macrophage inflammatory protein 1α [MIP-1α]) that favor recruitment of additional T cells and monocytes and contribute to the formation of granulomas. TNF in particular is released at high levels by activated alveolar macrophages, and the TNF level in the bronchoalveolar fluid is a marker of disease activity.

Additionally, there are *systemic immunologic abnormalities* in patients with sarcoidosis:

- Anergy to common skin test antigens such as *Candida* or purified protein derivative (PPD)
- Polyclonal hypergammaglobulinemia, another manifestation of helper T-cell dysregulation

Genetic Factors. Evidence of genetic influences can be seen:

- Familial and racial clustering of cases
- Association with certain HLA genotypes (e.g., class I HLA-A1 and HLA-B8)

Environmental Factors. These are possibly the most tenuous of all the associations in the pathogenesis of sarcoidosis. Several putative microbes have been proposed as the inciting agent for sarcoidosis (e.g., mycobacteria, *Propionibacterium acnes*, and *Rickettsia* species).[73] To date, *there is no unequivocal evidence to suggest that sarcoidosis is caused by an infectious agent.*

Morphology. Histologically, all involved tissues show the classic **noncaseating granulomas** (Fig. 15–23), each composed of an aggregate of tightly clustered epithelioid cells, often with Langhans or foreign body type giant cells. Central necrosis is unusual. With chronicity, the granulomas may become enclosed within fibrous rims or may eventually be replaced by hyaline fibrous scars. Two other microscopic features are often present in the granulomas: (1) laminated concretions composed of calcium and proteins known as Schaumann bodies and (2) stellate inclusions known as asteroid bodies enclosed within giant cells found in approximately 60% of the granulomas. Although characteristic, these microscopic features are not pathognomonic of sarcoidosis because asteroid and Schaumann bodies may be encountered in other granulomatous diseases (e.g., tuberculosis). Pathologic involvement of virtually every organ in the body has been cited at one time or another.

The **lungs** are common sites of involvement.[74] Macroscopically, there is usually no demonstrable alteration, although at times, the coalescence of granulomas may produce small nodules that are palpable or visible as 1- to 2-cm, noncaseating, noncavitated consolidations. Histologically, the lesions are distributed primarily along the lymphatics, around bronchi and blood vessels, although alveolar lesions are also seen. The relative frequency of granulomas in the bronchial submucosa accounts for the high diagnostic yield of bronchoscopic biopsies. A CD4/CD8 ratio >2.5 and the CD3/CD4 ratio <0.31 in bronchoalveolar lavage lymphocytes is commonly seen in sarcodosis.[75] There appears to be a strong tendency for lesions to heal in the lungs, so varying stages of fibrosis and hyalinization are often found. The pleural surfaces are sometimes involved.

Lymph nodes are involved in almost all cases, specifically the hilar and mediastinal nodes, but any other node in the body may be involved. Nodes are characteristically enlarged, discrete, and sometimes calcified. The tonsils are affected in about one quarter to one third of cases.

The **spleen** is affected microscopically in about three quarters of cases, but it is enlarged in only one fifth. On occasion, granulomas may coalesce to form small nodules that are barely visible macroscopically. The capsule is not involved. The **liver** is affected slightly less often than the spleen. It may also be moderately enlarged and may contain scattered granulomas, more in portal triads than in the lobular parenchyma. Needle biopsy may permit the identification of these focal lesions.

The **bone marrow** is an additional favored site of localization. Roentgenographic changes can be identified in about one fifth of cases of systemic involvement. The radiologically visible bone lesions have a particular tendency to involve phalangeal bones of the hands and feet, creating small circumscribed areas of bone resorption within the marrow cavity and a diffuse reticulated pattern throughout the cavity, with widening of the bony shafts or new bone formation on the outer surfaces.

Skin lesions are encountered in one third to one half of cases. Sarcoidosis of the skin assumes a variety of macroscopic appearances (e.g., discrete subcutaneous nodules; focal, slightly elevated, erythematous plaques; or flat lesions that are slightly reddened and scaling and resemble those of lupus erythematosus). Lesions may also appear on the mucous membranes of the oral cavity, larynx, and upper respiratory tract. The **eye, its associated glands, and the salivary glands** are involved in about one fifth to one half of cases. The ocular involvement takes the form of iritis or iridocyclitis, either bilaterally or unilaterally. Consequently, corneal opacities, glaucoma, and total loss of vision may occur. These ocular lesions are frequently accompanied by inflammation of the lacrimal glands, with suppression of lacrimation. Bilateral sarcoidosis of the parotid, submaxillary, and sublingual glands completes the combined uveoparotid involvement designated as Mikulicz syndrome (Chapter 16). **Muscle** involvement is often underdiagnosed, since it may be asymptomatic. Symptoms of muscle weakness, aches, tenderness, and fatigue should prompt consideration of occult sarcoid myositis.[76] In one study, 22 patients presenting with bilateral hilar adenopathy and a variety of symptoms underwent biopsies of asymptomatic gastrocnemius muscle. All 22 were found to have noncaseating granulomas. These findings suggest that muscle biopsy could be a useful tool in the diagnosis of sarcodosis.[77] Sarcoid granulomas occasionally occur in the heart, kidneys, central nervous system, and endocrine glands, particularly in the pituitary, as well as in other body tissues. Whereas presence of noncaseating granulomas is suggestive of sarcoidosis, other identifiable causes of granulomatous inflammation (e.g., tuberculosis, fungal infections) must be excluded before the diagnosis of sarcoidosis is made.

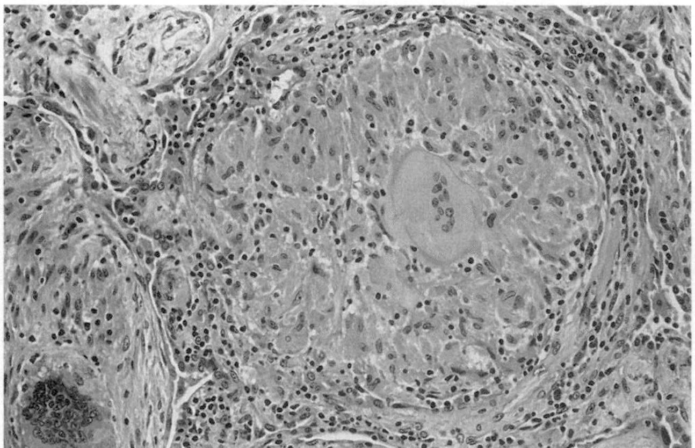

FIGURE 15–23 Characteristic sarcoid noncaseating granulomas in lung with many giant cells. (Courtesy of Dr. Ramon Blanco, Department of Pathology, Brigham and Women's Hospital, Boston, MA.)

Clinical Course. Because of its varying severity and the inconstant distribution of the lesions, sarcoidosis is a protean clinical disease. Sarcoidosis may be discovered unexpectedly on routine chest films as bilateral hilar adenopathy or may present with peripheral lymphadenopathy, cutaneous lesions, eye involvement, splenomegaly, or hepatomegaly. In the great majority of cases, however, patients seek medical attention because of the insidious onset of respiratory abnormalities (shortness of breath, cough, chest pain, hemoptysis) or of constitutional signs and symptoms (fever, fatigue, weight loss, anorexia, night sweats).

Sarcoidosis follows an unpredictable course characterized by either progressive chronicity or periods of activity interspersed with remissions, sometimes permanent, that may be spontaneous or induced by steroid therapy. Overall, 65% to 70% of affected patients recover with minimal or no residual manifestations. Twenty per cent have permanent loss of some lung function or some permanent visual impairment. Of the remaining 10% to 15%, some die of cardiac or central nervous system damage, but most succumb to progressive pulmonary fibrosis and cor pulmonale. Patients presenting with hilar lymphadenopathy alone have the best prognosis, followed by those with adenopathy and pulmonary infiltrates. Patients presenting with pulmonary disease and no adenopathy have few spontaneous remissions and are most likely to develop chronic pulmonary fibrosis.

Hypersensitivity Pneumonitis

The term "hypersensitivity pneumonitis" describes a spectrum of immunologically mediated, predominantly interstitial, lung disorders caused by intense, often prolonged exposure to inhaled organic dusts and related occupational antigens.[78] Affected individuals have an abnormal sensitivity or heightened reactivity to the antigen, which, in contrast to that occurring in asthma, involves primarily the *alveoli* (thus the synonym "allergic alveolitis"). *It is important to recognize these diseases early in their course because progression to serious chronic fibrotic lung disease can be prevented by removal of the environmental agent.*

Most commonly, hypersensitivity results from the inhalation of organic dust containing antigens made up of spores of thermophilic bacteria, true fungi, animal proteins, or bacterial products. Numerous specifically named syndromes are described, depending on the occupation or exposure of the individual. *Farmer's lung* results from exposure to dusts generated from harvested humid, warm hay that permits the rapid proliferation of the spores of thermophilic actinomycetes. *Pigeon breeder's lung* (bird fancier's disease) is provoked by proteins from serum, excreta, or feathers of birds. *Humidifier* or *air-conditioner lung* is caused by thermophilic bacteria in heated water reservoirs.

Several lines of evidence suggest that hypersensitivity pneumonitis is an immunologically mediated disease:

- Bronchoalveolar lavage specimens obtained during the acute phase show increased levels of proinflammatory chemokines such as MIP-1α and IL-8.
- Bronchoalveolar lavage specimens also consistently demonstrate increased numbers of T lymphocytes of both CD4+ and CD8+ phenotypes.
- Most patients have specific antibodies in their serum, a feature that is suggestive of type III (immune complex) hypersensitivity.
- Complement and immunoglobulins have been demonstrated within vessel walls by immunofluorescence, also indicating a type III hypersensitivity.

Finally, the presence of noncaseating granulomas in two thirds of the patients suggests the development of a T cell-mediated (type IV) delayed-type hypersensitivity against the implicated antigen(s).

In summary, hypersensitivity pneumonitis is an immunologically mediated response to an extrinsic antigen that involves both immune complex and delayed type hypersensitivity reactions.

Morphology. Histologic changes in subacute and chronic forms are characteristically centered on bronchioles. They include (1) interstitial pneumonitis consisting primarily of lymphocytes, plasma cells, and macrophages; (2) noncaseating granulomas in two thirds of patients (Fig. 15–24); and (3) interstitial fibrosis and obliterative bronchiolitis (in late stages). In more than half the patients, there is also evidence of an intra-alveolar infiltrate.

Clinical Features. The clinical manifestations are varied. Acute attacks, which follow inhalation of antigenic dust in sensitized patients, consist of recurring episodes of fever, dyspnea, cough, and leukocytosis. Diffuse and nodular infiltrates appear in the chest radiograph, and pulmonary function tests show an acute restrictive disorder. Symptoms usually appear 4 to 6 hours after exposure. If exposure is continuous and protracted, a chronic form of the disease supervenes that no longer features the acute exacerbations on antigen reexposure. Instead, there are signs of progressive respiratory failure, dyspnea, and cyanosis and a decrease in total lung capacity and compliance—a picture that is hard to differentiate from other forms of chronic interstitial disease.

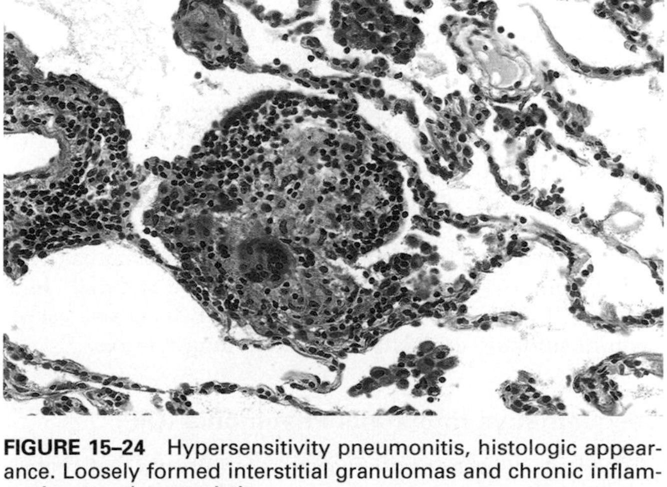

FIGURE 15–24 Hypersensitivity pneumonitis, histologic appearance. Loosely formed interstitial granulomas and chronic inflammation are characteristic.

PULMONARY EOSINOPHILIA

A number of clinical and pathologic pulmonary entities are characterized by an infiltration of eosinophils, recruited in part by elevated alveolar levels of eosinophil attractants such as IL-5.[79] These diverse diseases are generally of immunologic origin but are incompletely understood.[80]

Pulmonary eosinophila is divided into the following categories:

- Acute eosinophilic pneumonia with respiratory failure
- Simple pulmonary eosinophilia, or Löffler syndrome
- Tropical eosinophilia, caused by infection with microfilariae
- Secondary eosinophilia (which occurs in a number of parasitic, fungal, and bacterial infections; in hypersensitivity pneumonitis; in drug allergies; and in association with asthma, allergic bronchopulmonary aspergillosis, or vasculitis)
- So-called idiopathic chronic eosinophilic pneumonia

Acute eosinophilic pneumonia with respiratory failure is an acute illness of unknown cause. It has a rapid onset with fever, dyspnea, and hypoxemic respiratory failure. The chest X-ray shows diffuse infiltrates and bronchoalveolar lavage fluid contains more than 25% eosinophils. There is a prompt response to corticosteroids.

Simple pulmonary eosinophilia is characterized by transient pulmonary lesions, eosinophilia in the blood, and a benign clinical course. Roentgenograms are often quite striking, with shadows of varying size and shape in any of the lobes, suggesting irregular intrapulmonary densities. The alveolar septa are thickened by an infiltrate composed of eosinophils and occasional interspersed giant cells, but there is no vasculitis, fibrosis, or necrosis. In some cases, eosinophils are found in a background of diffuse alveolar damage.[81]

Chronic eosinophilic pneumonia is characterized by focal areas of cellular consolidation of the lung substance distributed chiefly in the periphery of the lung fields. Prominent in these lesions are heavy aggregates of lymphocytes and eosinophils within both the septal walls and the alveolar spaces. These patients have high fever, night sweats, and dyspnea, all of which respond to corticosteroid therapy. Chronic eosinophilic pneumonia is diagnosed when other causes of chronic pulmonary eosinophilia are excluded.

SMOKING-RELATED INTERSTITIAL DISEASES

Smoking-related diseases can be grouped into obstructive diseases (emphysema and chronic bronchitis, already discussed) and restrictive or interstitial diseases. A majority of patients with idiopathic interstitial fibrosis (IPF) are smokers; however, the role of cigarette smoking in its etiology has not been clarified yet. Desquamative interstitial pneumonia (DIP) and respiratory bronchiolitis–associated interstitial lung disease (RB-ILD) are thought to represent two ends of a spectrum of smoking-associated interstitial lung diseases.

Desquamative Interstitial Pneumonia (DIP)

The large collections of airspace macrophages that characterize this disease were originally thought to be desquamated pneumocytes, thus the misnomer "desquamative interstitial pneumonia." Also, it was thought that DIP was a precursor lesion or early phase of IPF, which is a fibrosing process with progressive destruction of alveoli and honeycombing. DIP, however, has minimal if any fibrosis and is nonprogressive in the vast majority of cases.

Morphology. The most striking histologic finding is the accumulation of a large number of macrophages with abundant cytoplasm containing dusty brown pigment (**smokers' macrophages**) in the airspaces. Finely granular iron may be seen in the macrophage cytoplasm. Some of the macrophages contain lamellar bodies (surfactant) within phagocytic vacuoles, presumably derived from necrotic type II pneumocytes. The alveolar septa are thickened by a sparse inflammatory infiltrate of lymphocytes that often includes plasma cells and occasional eosinophils (Fig. 15–25). The septa are lined by plump, cuboidal pneumocytes. Interstitial fibrosis, when present, is mild. Emphysema is often present.

DIP usually presents in the fourth or fifth decade of life, and it is more common in men than in women by a ratio of 2:1. Virtually all patients are cigarette smokers. Presenting symptoms include an insidious onset of dyspnea and dry cough over weeks or months, often associated with clubbing of digits. Pulmonary functions usually show a mild restrictive abnormality with a moderate reduction of the diffusing capacity of carbon dioxide. Patients with DIP typically have a good prognosis with excellent response to steroid therapy and cessation of smoking. Recent studies have shown a 100% survival rate.[82,83]

Respiratory Bronchiolitis–Associated Interstitial Lung Disease

Respiratory bronchiolitis is a common histologic lesion found in cigarette smokers. It is characterized by the presence of pigmented intraluminal macrophages within first- and second-order respiratory bronchioles. In its mildest form, it is

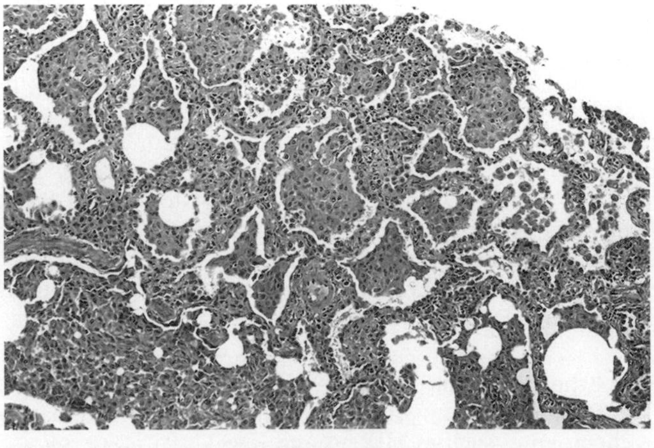

FIGURE 15–25 Desquamative interstitial pneumonia: medium-power detail of lung to demonstrate the accumulation of large numbers of mononuclear cells within the alveolar spaces with only mild fibrous thickening of the alveolar walls.

seen most often as an incidental histologic finding in the lungs of smokers or ex-smokers.[84] The term "respiratory bronchiolitis–associated interstitial lung disease" is used for patients who develop significant pulmonary symptoms, abnormal pulmonary function, and imaging abnormalities.

Morphology. The changes are patchy at low magnification and have a bronchiolocentric distribution. Respiratory bronchioles, alveolar ducts, and peribronchiolar spaces contain aggregates of dusty brown macrophages (**smokers' macrophages**) similar to those seen in DIP. There is a patchy submucosal and peribronchiolar infiltrate of lymphocytes and histiocytes. Mild peribronchiolar fibrosis is also seen, which expands contiguous alveolar septa. Centrilobular emphysema is common but not severe. Histologic overlap with DIP is often found in different parts of the same lung.

Symptoms are usually mild, consisting of gradual onset of dyspnea and cough in patients who are typically current smokers in the fourth or fifth decade of life with average exposures of over 30 pack-years of cigarette smoking. There is a 2:1 male predominance. Cessation of smoking usually results in improvement.[85,86]

PULMONARY ALVEOLAR PROTEINOSIS

Pulmonary alveolar proteinosis (PAP) is a rare disease that is characterized radiologically by bilateral patchy asymmetric pulmonary opacification and histologically by *accumulation of acellular surfactant in the intra-alveolar and bronchiolar spaces.* There are three distinct classes of this disease, namely, acquired, congenital, and secondary PAP, each with a different pathogenesis but with a similar spectrum of histologic changes.

Acquired PAP is of unknown etiology and without any familial predisposition; it represents 90% of all cases of PAP. Unexpectedly, researchers working with gene knockout mice lacking the hematopoietic growth factor GM-CSF ($GM^{-/-}$) found that these mice had impaired surfactant clearance by alveolar macrophages, leading to a condition that resembled human PAP. Subsequently, a GM-CSF–neutralizing autoantibody was found in the serum and bronchial fluid of patients with acquired PAP that was not present in patients with congenital or secondary PAP. Currently, it is thought that the anti–GM-CSF antibody is pathogenic in the development of the disease. These antibodies inhibit the activity of endogenous GM-CSF, leading to a state of functional GM-CSF deficiency, recapitulating the findings in the $GM^{-/-}$ mouse.[87] The systemic production of the antibody also provides an explanation for the recurrence of PAP following double-lung transplantation. Thus, acquired PAP can be considered an autoimmune disorder.

Congenital PAP is a rare cause of immediate-onset neonatal respiratory distress. To date, mutations have been identified in three genes, suggesting at least three different etiologies for congenital PAP: surfactant protein B (SP-B), GM-CSF, and GM receptor (GM/IL-3/IL-5) β chain. These represent only a small proportion of congenital PAP cases. In the majority, the genetic basis is as yet undefined.[88] SP-B deficiency is transmitted in an autosomal-recessive manner and is most often caused by homozygosity for a frameshift mutation in the *SP-B* gene. This leads to an unstable SP-B mRNA, reduced or absent SP-B, secondary disturbances of SP-C, and intra-alveolar accumulation of SP-A and SP-C.

Secondary PAP is uncommon. The underlying causes include lysinuric protein intolerance, acute silicosis and other inhalational syndromes, immunodeficiency disorders, malignancies, and hematopoietic disorders.

Morphology. The disease is characterized by a peculiar homogeneous, granular precipitate within the alveoli, causing focal-to-confluent consolidation of large areas of the lungs with minimal inflammatory reaction (Fig. 15–26). On section, turbid fluid exudes from these areas. As a consequence, there is a marked increase in the size and weight of the lung. The alveolar precipitate is PAS positive and also contains cholesterol clefts. Immunohistochemical stains show the presence of surfactant proteins A and C in congenital SP-B deficiency and all three proteins in the acquired form.

Adult patients, for the most part, present with nonspecific respiratory difficulty of insidious onset, cough, and abundant sputum that often contains chunks of gelatinous material. Some have symptoms lasting for years, often with febrile illnesses. These patients are at risk for developing secondary infections with a variety of organisms. Progressive dyspnea, cyanosis, and respiratory insufficiency may occur, but some patients tend to have a benign course, with eventual resolution of the lesions. Whole-lung lavage remains the current standard of care, with GM-CSF therapy still in study phase.

Congenital PAP is a fatal respiratory disorder that is usually immediately apparent in the newborn. Typically, the infant is full term and rapidly develops progressive respiratory distress shortly after birth. Without lung transplantation, death ensues between 3 and 6 months of age.

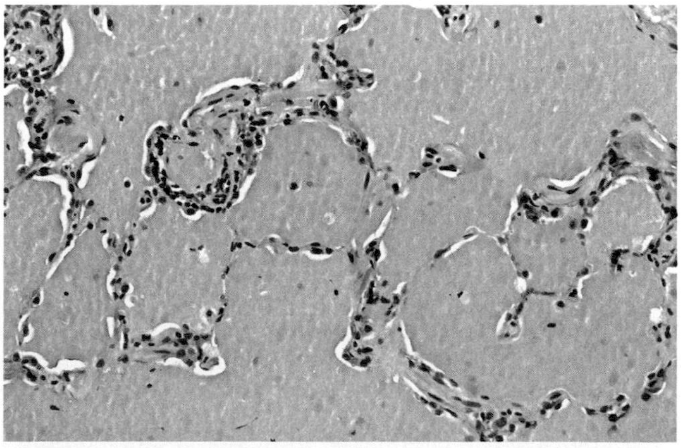

FIGURE 15–26 Pulmonary alveolar proteinosis, histologic appearance. The alveoli are filled with a dense, amorphous, protein-lipid granular precipitate, while the alveolar walls are normal.

Diseases of Vascular Origin

PULMONARY EMBOLISM, HEMORRHAGE, AND INFARCTION

Blood clots that occlude the large pulmonary arteries are almost always embolic in origin. Large-vessel in situ thromboses are rare and develop only in the presence of pulmonary hypertension, pulmonary atherosclerosis, and heart failure. The usual source of pulmonary emboli—thrombi in the deep veins of the leg in more than 95% of cases—and the magnitude of the clinical problem were discussed in Chapter 4, in which the disturbing frequency of pulmonary embolism and infarction was emphasized. Pulmonary embolism causes more than 50,000 deaths in the United States each year. Its incidence at autopsy has varied from 1% in the general population of hospital patients to 30% in patients dying after severe burns, trauma, or fractures to 65% of hospitalized patients in one study in which special techniques were applied to discover emboli at autopsy. It is the sole or a major contributing cause of death in about 10% of adults who die acutely in hospitals.

Pulmonary embolism is a complication principally in patients who are already suffering from some underlying disorder, such as cardiac disease or cancer, or who are immobilized for several days or weeks, those with hip fracture being at high risk. Hypercoagulable states, either *primary* (e.g., factor V Leiden, prothrombin 20210 A, hyperhomocysteinemia, and antiphospholipid syndrome) or *secondary* (e.g., obesity, recent surgery, cancer, oral contraceptive use, pregnancy), are frequent risk factors. Indwelling central venous lines can be a nidus for right atrial thrombus, which can be a source of pulmonary embolism.

The pathophysiologic response and clinical significance of pulmonary embolism depend on the extent to which the pulmonary artery blood flow is obstructed, the size of the occluded vessel(s), the number of emboli, the overall status of the cardiovascular system, and the release of vasoactive factors such as thromboxane A_2 from platelets that accumulate at the site of thrombus. Emboli result in two main pathophysiologic consequences: *respiratory compromise* owing to the nonperfused, although ventilated, segment and *hemodynamic compromise* owing to increased resistance to pulmonary blood flow engendered by the embolic obstruction. The latter leads to pulmonary hypertension and can cause acute right-sided heart failure.

Morphology. The morphologic consequences of embolic occlusion of the pulmonary arteries depend on the size of the embolic mass and the general state of the circulation. Large emboli may impact in the main pulmonary artery or its major branches or lodge at the bifurcation as a saddle embolus (Fig. 15–27). Sudden death often ensues, owing largely to the blockage of blood flow through the lungs. Death may also be caused by acute failure of the right side of the heart (**acute cor pulmonale**). Smaller emboli can travel out into the more peripheral vessels, where they may cause infarction. In patients with adequate cardiovascular function, the bronchial arterial supply can often sustain the lung parenchyma despite obstruction to the pulmonary arterial system. Under these circumstances, hemorrhages may occur, but there is no infarction of the underlying lung parenchyma. Only about 10% of emboli actually cause infarction. Although the underlying pulmonary architecture may be obscured by the suffusion of blood, hemorrhages are distinguished by the preservation of the pulmonary alveolar architecture; in such cases, resorption of the blood permits reconstitution of the preexisting architecture.

Pulmonary embolism usually causes infarction only when the circulation is already inadequate, as in patients with heart or lung disease. For this reason, pulmonary infarcts tend to be uncommon in the young. About three fourths of all infarcts affect the lower lobes, and in more than half, multiple lesions occur. They vary in size from lesions that are barely visible to the naked eye to massive involvement of large parts of an entire lobe. Characteristically, they extend to the periphery of the lung substance as a wedge with the apex pointing toward the hilus of the lung. In many cases, an occluded vessel can be identified near the apex of the infarct.

The pulmonary infarct is classically hemorrhagic and appears as a raised, red-blue area in the early stages (Fig. 15–28). Often, the apposed pleural surface is covered by a fibrinous exudate. The red cells begin

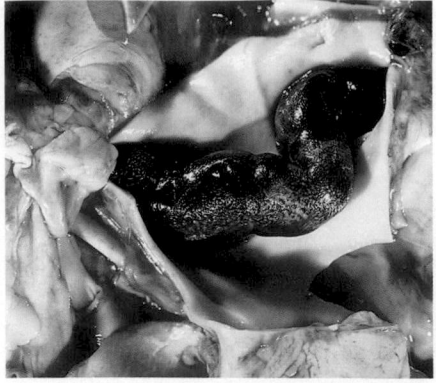

FIGURE 15–27 Large saddle embolus from the femoral vein lying astride the main left and right pulmonary arteries. (From the teaching collection of the Department of Pathology, University of Texas Southwestern Medical School, Dallas, TX.)

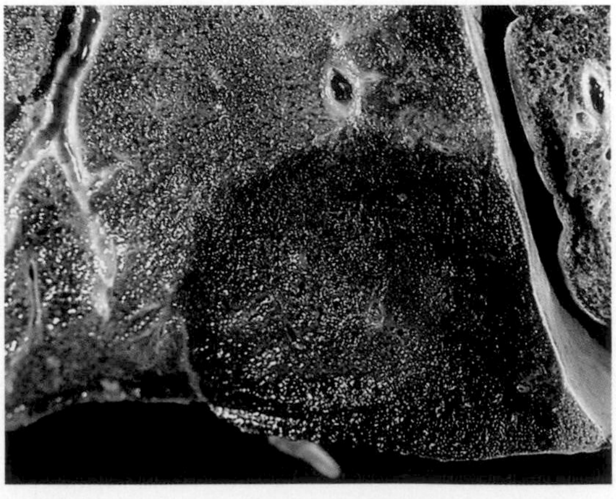

FIGURE 15–28 Recent, small, roughly wedge-shaped hemorrhagic pulmonary infarct.

to lyse within 48 hours, and the infarct becomes paler and eventually red-brown as hemosiderin is produced. With the passage of time, fibrous replacement begins at the margins as a gray-white peripheral zone and eventually converts the infarct into a contracted scar. Histologically, the diagnostic feature of acute pulmonary infarction is the ischemic necrosis of the lung substance within the area of hemorrhage, affecting the alveolar walls, bronchioles, and vessels. If the infarct is caused by an infected embolus, it is modified by a more intense neutrophilic exudation and more intense inflammatory reaction. Such lesions are referred to as **septic infarcts,** and some convert to abscesses.

Clinical Course. *A large pulmonary embolus is one of the few causes of virtually instantaneous death.* During cardiopulmonary resuscitation in such instances, the patient frequently is said to have *electromechanical dissociation*, in which the electrocardiogram has a rhythm but no pulses are palpated because of the massive blockage of blood in the systemic venous circulation. If the patient survives after a sizable pulmonary embolus, however, the clinical syndrome may mimic myocardial infarction, with severe chest pain, dyspnea, shock, elevation of temperature, and increased levels of serum lactic dehydrogenase. Usually, however, in individuals with a normal cardiovascular system *small emboli* induce only transient chest pain and cough or possibly pulmonary hemorrhages without infarction. Only in the predisposed, in whom the bronchial circulation itself is inadequate, do small emboli cause small infarcts. Such patients manifest dyspnea, tachypnea, fever, chest pain, cough, and hemoptysis. An overlying fibrinous pleuritis may produce a pleural friction rub.

The chest radiograph may disclose a pulmonary infarct, usually 12 to 36 hours after it has occurred, as a wedge-shaped infiltrate. Emboli can also be detected by spiral computed tomographic angiography and D-dimer testing. Pulmonary angiography is the most definitive diagnostic technique but entails more risk to the patient.

After the initial acute insult, emboli often resolve via contraction and fibrinolysis, particularly in the relatively young. Unresolved, multiple small emboli over the course of time may lead to pulmonary hypertension, pulmonary vascular sclerosis, and chronic cor pulmonale. Perhaps most important is the fact that a small embolus may presage a larger one. In the presence of an underlying predisposing factor, patients with a pulmonary embolus have a 30% chance of developing a second embolus.

Prevention of pulmonary embolism constitutes a major clinical problem for which there is no easy solution. Prophylactic therapy includes early ambulation in postoperative and postpartum patients, elastic stockings and graduated compression stockings for bedridden patients, and preventive anticoagulation in high-risk individuals. It is sometimes necessary to resort to insertion of a filter ("umbrella") into the inferior vena cava or to ligation of this vein, which are not minor procedures in an already seriously ill patient. Treatment of existing pulmonary embolism often includes anticoagulation, preceded by thrombolysis in some cases.

There are nonthrombotic forms of pulmonary emboli, which are uncommon but potentially lethal. These include air (may be iatrogenic), bone marrow (after trauma and bone marrow necrosis in sickle cell patients), fat (trauma and surgery), amniotic fluid (during parturition), and foreign bodies (in I/V drug abusers).

PULMONARY HYPERTENSION

The pulmonary circulation is normally one of low resistance, and pulmonary blood pressure is only about one eighth of systemic blood pressure. Pulmonary hypertension (when mean pulmonary pressure reaches one fourth of systemic levels) is most frequently *secondary* to structural cardiopulmonary conditions that increase pulmonary blood flow or pressure (or both), pulmonary vascular resistance, or left heart resistance to blood flow. These include the following:

- *Chronic obstructive or interstitial lung diseases:* Patients with these diseases have hypoxia as well as destruction of lung parenchyma and hence have fewer alveolar capillaries. This causes increased pulmonary arterial resistance and, secondarily, elevated pressure.
- *Antecedent congenital or acquired heart disease:* Pulmonary hypertension occurs in patients with mitral stenosis, for example, because of an increase in left atrial pressure that leads to an increase in pulmonary venous pressure and, consequently, to an increase in pulmonary artery pressure.
- *Recurrent thromboemboli:* Patients with recurrent pulmonary emboli may have pulmonary hypertension primarily owing to a reduction in the functional cross-sectional area of the pulmonary vascular bed brought about by the obstructing emboli, which, in turn, leads to an increase in pulmonary vascular resistance.
- *Autoimmune disorders:* Several of these disorders (most notably systemic sclerosis) involve the pulmonary vasculature, leading to inflammation, intimal fibrosis, medial hypertrophy, and pulmonary hypertension.

Uncommonly, pulmonary hypertension is encountered in patients in whom all known causes of increased pulmonary pressure are excluded; this is referred to as *primary*, or *idiopathic, pulmonary hypertension*. This condition is most commonly sporadic; only 6% of patients have the familial form with autosomal-dominant mode of inheritance. Within these families, there is incomplete penetrance, and only 10% to 20% of the family members actually develop overt disease.

Pathogenesis. As is often the case, much has been learned about the pathogenesis of pulmonary hypertension by investigating the molecular basis of the uncommon familial form of the disease. These studies have revealed that primary pulmonary hypertension is caused by mutations in the bone morphogenetic protein receptor type 2 (BMPR2) signaling pathway.[89]

To understand how such a mutation causes pulmonary hypertension, it is essential to review the vascular pathology of the disease and to understand the physiologic functions of the BMPR2 signaling. As will be described in greater detail below, pulmonary hypertension is associated with obstruction to the vasculature caused by proliferation of endothelial, smooth muscle, and intimal cells accompanied by concentric laminar intimal fibrosis. How does BMPR2 cause these changes?

BMPR2 is a cell-surface protein belonging to the TGF-β receptor superfamily, which binds a variety of cytokines, including TGF-β, bone morphogenetic protein (BMP), activin, and inhibin. Although originally described in the context of bone growth, BMP-BMPR2 signaling is now known to be important for embryogenesis, apoptosis and cell proliferation and differentiation. The specific effects depend on the tissue and its microenvironment. *In vascular smooth muscle cells, BMPR2 signaling causes inhibition of proliferation and favors apoptosis.* Thus, in the absence of such signaling, smooth muscle proliferation may be expected. In keeping with this, *inactivating germ line mutations in the BMPR2 gene are found in 50% of the familial (primary) cases of pulmonary hypertension and 26% of sporadic cases.* In many families, without mutations in the coding regions of the *BMPR2* gene, linkage to the *BMPR2* locus on 2q33 can be established, thus indicating that other possible lesions such as gene rearrangements, large deletions, or insertions could be involved.

Despite these discoveries, several questions remain unanswered. First, how does loss of a single allele of the BMPR2 lead to complete loss of signaling? Two possibilities exist: the mutation might act as a dominant negative (Chapter 5), or a secondary loss of the normal allele might occur in the vascular wall, thus leading to a homozygous loss of BMPR2. This is reminiscent of how germ line mutations in tumor suppressor genes give rise to neoplasia. Interestingly, in some studies, microsatellite instability has been reported in the proliferating endothelial cells within the vascular lesions. This could be a mechanism by which the normal allele is lost in the vasculature. Note that a similar mechanism can inactivate the TGF-β receptors in hereditary nonpolyposis colon cancer (Chapters 7 and 17). The second unanswered question is why the phenotypic disease occurs only in 10% to 20% of individuals with *BMPR2* mutations. This strongly suggests the existence of modifier genes and/or environmental triggers. Among the modifier genes are those that control vascular tone, e.g., endothelin, prostacyclin synthetase, and angiotensin-converting enzymes. The nature of the environmental factors remains unknown, but presumably, they cause dysfunction of vasoregulatory mechanisms. Thus, as with tumor suppressor genes, a two-hit model has been proposed whereby a genetically susceptible individual with *BMPR2* mutation requires additional genetic or environmental insults to develop the disease (Fig. 15–29).

In *secondary forms of pulmonary hypertension*, endothelial cell dysfunction is produced by the process that initiates the disorder, such as the increased shear and mechanical injury associated with left-to-right shunts or the biochemical injury produced by fibrin in thromboembolism. Decreased elaboration of prostacyclin, decreased production of nitric oxide, and increased release of endothelin all promote pulmonary vasoconstriction. Also, decreased elaboration of prostacyclin and nitric oxide promotes platelet adhesion and activation. Moreover, endothelial activation, as detailed in Chapters 2 and 11, makes endothelial cells thrombogenic and promotes the persistence of fibrin. Finally, production and release of growth factors and cytokines induce the migration and replication of vascular smooth muscle cells and elaboration of extracellular matrix.

Some patients with pulmonary hypertension have a vasospastic component; in such patients, pulmonary vascular resistance can be rapidly decreased with vasodilators. Pulmonary hypertension has also been reported after ingestion of certain plants or medicines, including the leguminous plant

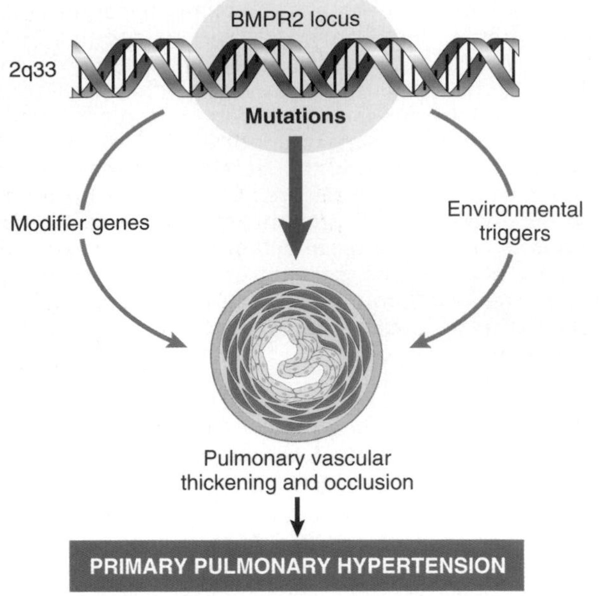

FIGURE 15–29 Pathogenesis of primary pulmonary hypertension.

Crotalaria spectabilis, which is indigenous to the tropics and used medicinally in *bush tea*; the appetite depressant agent *aminorex*; adulterated olive oil; and most recently the anti-obesity drugs fenfluramine and phentermine.[90] It has been suggested that such substances might act through effect on serotonin transporter expression or activity.

Morphology. A variety of vascular lesions occur in pulmonary hypertension.[91] Although they are not always specific and frequently overlap between primary and secondary forms, specific histologic appearances have diagnostic and prognostic implications.[92] The presence of many organizing or recanalized thrombi favors recurrent pulmonary emboli as the cause, and the coexistence of diffuse pulmonary fibrosis, or severe emphysema and chronic bronchitis, points to chronic hypoxia as the initiating event. The vessel changes can involve the entire arterial tree, from the main pulmonary arteries down to the arterioles (Fig. 15–30). In the most severe cases, atheromatous deposits form in the pulmonary artery and its major branches, resembling (but being lesser in degree than) systemic atherosclerosis. The arterioles and small arteries (40 to 300 μm in diameter) are most prominently affected, with striking increases in the muscular thickness of the media (medial hypertrophy) and intimal fibrosis, sometimes narrowing the lumina to pinpoint channels. These changes are present in all forms of pulmonary hypertension but are best developed in the primary form. One extreme in the spectrum of pathologic changes, present most prominently in primary pulmonary hypertension or congenital heart disease with left-to-right shunts, is **plexogenic pulmonary arteriopathy,** so called because a tuft of capillary formations is present, producing a network, or web, that spans the lumens of

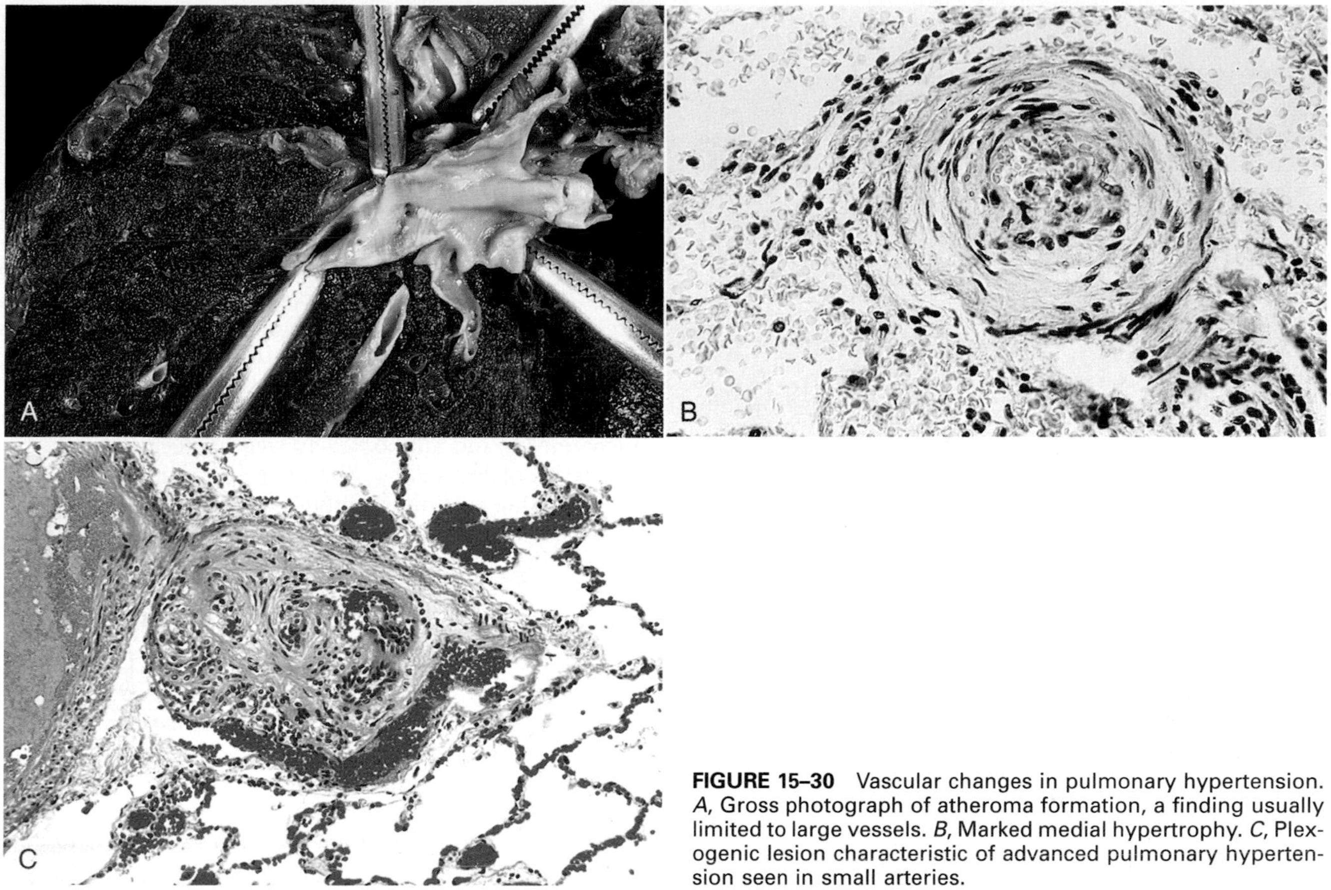

FIGURE 15–30 Vascular changes in pulmonary hypertension. *A*, Gross photograph of atheroma formation, a finding usually limited to large vessels. *B*, Marked medial hypertrophy. *C*, Plexogenic lesion characteristic of advanced pulmonary hypertension seen in small arteries.

dilated thin-walled, small, arteries. Biopsy of the lung may be done in some cases to grade the degree of pulmonary hypertensive vascular abnormalities and thereby aid therapeutic decision making, especially in congenital heart disease, in which severe secondary pulmonary vascular changes may preclude surgical repair of the underlying cardiac anomaly (Chapter 12).

Clinical Course. Although secondary forms can occur at any age, primary pulmonary hypertension is most common in women who are 20 to 40 years of age and is also seen occasionally in young children. Clinical signs and symptoms of both the primary and the secondary forms of vascular sclerosis become evident only with advanced arterial disease. In cases of primary disease, the presenting features are usually dyspnea and fatigue, but some patients have chest pain of the anginal type. In the course of time, severe respiratory distress, cyanosis, and right ventricular hypertrophy occur, and death from decompensated cor pulmonale, often with superimposed thromboembolism and pneumonia, usually ensues within 2 to 5 years in 80% of patients.[93] Continuous therapy with vasodilators (e.g., calcium channel blockers or inhaled nitric oxide) and antithrombotic medications (e.g., warfarin, prostacyclin, and thromboxane receptor blockers), however, appears to improve the outcome in many patients. Gene therapy has been successful in animals and may be possible for humans in the future.

DIFFUSE PULMONARY HEMORRHAGE SYNDROMES

Hemorrhage from the lung is a dramatic complication of some interstitial lung disorders.[94,95] Among these so-called *pulmonary hemorrhage syndromes* (Fig. 15–31) are (1) Goodpasture syndrome, (2) idiopathic pulmonary hemosiderosis, and (3) vasculitis-associated hemorrhage, which is found in conditions such as hypersensitivity angiitis, Wegener granulomatosis, and lupus erythematosus (Chapter 11).

Goodpasture Syndrome

Goodpasture syndrome is an uncommon autoimmune disease characterized by the presence of circulating autoantibodies targeted against the noncollagenous domain of the α-3 chain of collagen IV. The antibodies initiate an inflammatory destruction of the basement membrane in kidney glomeruli and lung alveoli,[96] giving rise to *proliferative, usually rapidly progressive glomerulonephritis and a necrotizing hemorrhagic interstitial pneumonitis.* Most cases occur in the teens or twenties, and in contrast to many other autoimmune diseases, there is a preponderance among men.

Pathogenesis. The evidence is quite substantial that the renal and pulmonary lesions are the consequence of antibody mediated injury to the glomerular and pulmonary basement membranes. The immunopathogenesis of the syndrome and the nature of the Goodpasture antigens are described in

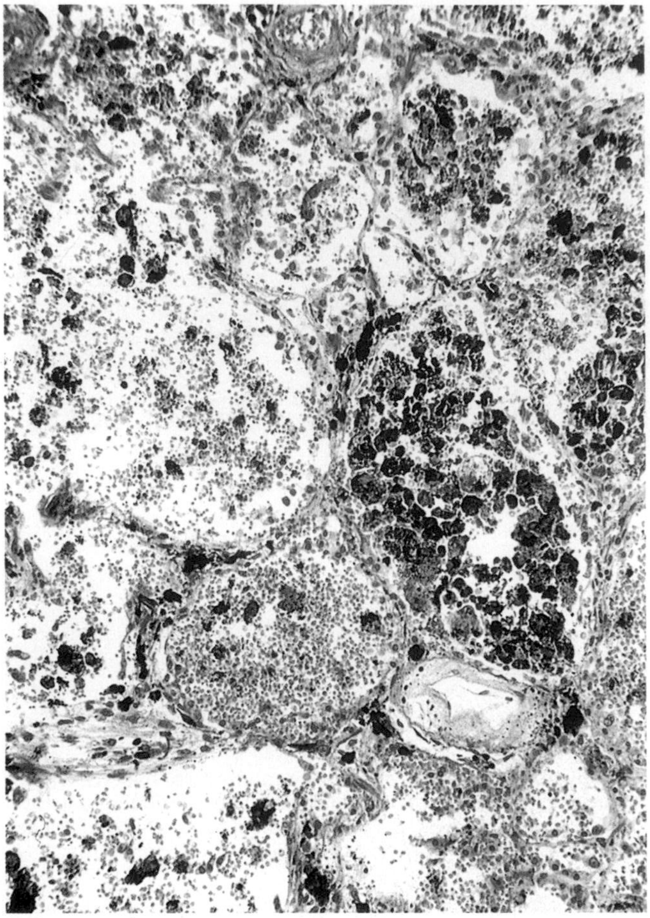

FIGURE 15–31 Acute intra-alveolar hemorrhage and hemosiderin-laden macrophages, reflecting previous hemorrhage, are common features of the diffuse pulmonary hemorrhage syndromes (Prussian blue stain for iron).

Chapter 20. The trigger that initiates the antibasement membrane antibodies is still unknown. Since the epitopes that evoke anti-collagen antibodies are normally hidden within the molecule, it is presumed that some environmental insult such as viral infection, exposure to hydrocarbon solvents (used in the dry cleaning industry), or smoking is required to unmask the cryptic epitopes. As in other autoimmune disorders, a genetic predisposition is indicated by association with certain HLA subtypes (e.g., HLA-DRB1*1501 and *1502).[94]

Morphology. In the classic case, the lungs are heavy, with areas of red-brown consolidation. Histologically, there is focal necrosis of alveolar walls associated with intra-alveolar hemorrhages. Often, the alveoli contain hemosiderin-laden macrophages (Fig. 15–31). In later stages there may be fibrous thickening of the septae, hypertrophy of type II pneumocytes, and organization of blood in alvelolar spaces. In many cases, immunofluorescence studies reveal linear deposits of immunoglobulins along the basement membranes of the septal walls. The kidneys have the characteristic findings of focal proliferative glomerulonephritis in early cases or crescentic glomerulonephritis in patients with rapidly progressive glomerulonephritis. Diagnostic linear deposits of immunoglobulins and complement are seen by immunofluorescence studies along the glomerular basement membranes, similar to those in the alveolar septa.

Clinical Features. Most cases begin clinically with respiratory symptoms, principally hemoptysis, and radiographic evidence of focal pulmonary consolidations. Soon, manifestations of glomerulonephritis appear, leading to rapidly progressive renal failure. The common cause of death is uremia. The once dismal prognosis for this disease has been markedly improved by intensive *plasma exchange*. This procedure is thought to be beneficial by removing circulating antibasement membrane antibodies as well as chemical mediators of immunologic injury. Simultaneous immunosuppressive therapy inhibits further antibody production. Both the lung hemorrhage and the glomerulonephritis improve with this form of therapy.

Idiopathic Pulmonary Hemosiderosis

Idiopathic pulmonary hemosiderosis is a rare disorder characterized by intermittent, diffuse alveolar hemorrhage. It usually presents with an insidious onset of productive cough, hemoptysis, anemia, and weight loss associated with diffuse pulmonary infiltrations similar to Goodpasture syndrome. Most cases occur in children, although the disease has been reported in adults as well.

Morphology. The lungs are moderately increased in weight, with areas of consolidation that are usually red-brown to red. The cardinal histologic features of pulmonary hemosiderosis are hemorrhage into the alveolar spaces, and hemosiderosis, both within the alveolar septa and in macrophages lying free within the pulmonary alveoli. These may also be hyperplasia of type II pneumocytes and varying degrees of interstitial fibrosis. Of note, there is no vasculitis, capillaritis, or inflammatory infiltration.

The cause and pathogenesis are unknown, and no antibasement membrane antibodies are detectable in serum or tissues. However, favorable response to long-term immunosuppression with prednisone and/or azathioprine indicates that an immunologic mechanism could be involved in the pulmonary capillary damage underlying alveolar bleeding. In addition, long-term follow-up of patients shows that some of them develop other immune disorders.

Wegener Granulomatosis

This autoimmune disease most often involves the upper respiratory tract and/or the lungs, with hemoptysis being the common presenting symptom. The general features are discussed in Chapter 11. Here, it is enough to emphasize that a transbronchial lung biopsy might be the only tissue available for diagnosis. Since the amount of tissue is small, necrosis and granulomatous vasculitis might not be present. Rather, the diagnostically important features are *capillaritis and scattered, poorly formed granulomas* (unlike those of sarcoidosis, which are rounded and well-defined).

Pulmonary Infections

Respiratory tract infections are more frequent than infections of any other organ and account for the largest number of workdays lost in the general population. The vast majority are upper respiratory tract infections caused by viruses (common cold, pharyngitis) but bacterial, viral, mycoplasmal, and fungal infections of the lung (pneumonia) still account for an enormous amount of morbidity and are responsible for one sixth of all deaths in the United States.[97] Pneumonia can be very broadly defined as any infection of the lung parenchyma (although the same term is used for many interstitial lung diseases that are not infectious in origin, such as usual interstitial pneumonia). Pneumonia can be caused by a wide variety of organisms, some of which produce distinctive features, as will be discussed later.

Pulmonary defense mechanisms were described in Chapter 8. Here we should reiterate that *pneumonia can result whenever these defense mechanisms are impaired or whenever the resistance of the host in general is lowered.* Factors that affect resistance in general include chronic diseases, immunologic deficiency, and treatment with immunosuppressive agents, leukopenia, and unusually virulent infections. The clearing mechanisms can be interfered with by many factors, such as the following:

- *Loss or suppression of the cough reflex,* as a result of coma, anesthesia, neuromuscular disorders, drugs, or chest pain. (This may lead to *aspiration* of gastric contents.)
- *Injury to the mucociliary apparatus,* by either impairment of ciliary function or destruction of ciliated epithelium, owing to cigarette smoke, inhalation of hot or corrosive gases, viral diseases, or genetic disturbances (e.g., the immotile cilia syndrome)
- *Interference with the phagocytic or bactericidal action of alveolar macrophages* by alcohol, tobacco smoke, anoxia, or oxygen intoxication
- *Pulmonary congestion and edema*
- *Accumulation of secretions* in conditions such as cystic fibrosis and bronchial obstruction

Defects in innate immunity (including neutrophil and complement defects) and humoral immunodeficiency typically lead to an increased incidence of infections with pyogenic bacteria. On the other hand, cell-mediated immune defects lead to increased infections with intracellular microbes such as mycobacteria and herpesviruses as well as with microorganisms of very low virulence, such as *Pneumocystis carinii.*

Several other points need to be emphasized. First, *one type of pneumonia sometimes predisposes to another, especially in debilitated patients.* For example, the most common cause of death in viral influenza epidemics is bacterial pneumonia. Second, although the portal of entry for most pneumonias is the respiratory tract, *hematogenous spread from one organ to other organs can occur,* and secondary seeding of the lungs may be difficult to distinguish from primary pneumonia. Finally, many *patients with chronic diseases acquire terminal pneumonias while hospitalized (nosocomial infection).* Bacteria common to the hospital environment may have acquired resistance to antibiotics; opportunities for spread are increased; invasive procedures, such as intubations and injections, are common; and bacteria may contaminate equipment used in respiratory care units.

Pneumonias are classified by the specific etiologic agent, which determines the treatment, or, if no pathogen can be isolated, by the clinical setting in which the infection occurs. Classifying by the clinical setting considerably narrows the list of suspected pathogens for administering empirical antimicrobial therapy. As Table 15–8 indicates, pneumonia can arise in seven distinct clinical settings ("pneumonia syndromes"), and the implicated pathogens are reasonably specific to each category.

TABLE 15–8 The Pneumonia Syndromes

Community-Acquired Acute Pneumonia
Streptococcus pneumoniae
Haemophilus influenzae
Moraxella catarrhalis
Staphylococcus aureus
Legionella pneumophila
Enterobacteriaceae (*Klebsiella pneumoniae*) and *Pseudomonas* spp.
Community-Acquired Atypical Pneumonia
Mycoplasma pneumoniae
Chlamydia spp. (*C. pneumoniae, C. psittaci, C. trachomatis*)
Coxiella burnetti (Q fever)
Viruses: respiratory syncytial virus, parainfluenza virus (children); influenza A and B (adults); adenovirus (military recruits); SARS* virus
Nosocomial Pneumonia
Gram-negative rods belonging to Enterobacteriaceae (*Klebsiella* spp., *Serratia marcescens, Escherichia coli*) and *Pseudomonas* spp.
Staphylococcus aureus (usually penicillin-resistant)
Aspiration Pneumonia
Anaerobic oral flora (*Bacteroides, Prevotella, Fusobacterium, Peptostreptococcus*), admixed with aerobic bacteria (*Streptococcus pneumoniae, Staphylococcus aureus, Haemophilas influenzae,* and *Pseudomonas aeruginosa*)
Chronic Pneumonia
Nocardia
Actinomyces
Granulomatous: *Mycobacterium tuberculosis* and atypical mycobacteria, *Histoplasma capsulatum, Coccidioides immitis, Blastomyces dermatitidis*
Necrotizing Pneumonia and Lung Abscess
Anaerobic bacteria (extremely common), with or without mixed aerobic infection
Staphylococcus aureus, Klebsiella pneumoniae, Streptococcus pyogenes, and type 3 pneumococcus (uncommon)
Pneumonia in the Immunocompromised Host
Cytomegalovirus
Pneumocystis carinii
Mycobacterium avium-intracellulare
Invasive aspergillosis
Invasive candidiasis
"Usual" bacterial, viral, and fungal organisms (listed above)

*SARS, Severe acute respiratory syndrome

COMMUNITY-ACQUIRED ACUTE PNEUMONIAS

Community-acquired pneumonias may be bacterial or viral. Here we discuss acute pneumonias caused by bacteria, viral pneumonias are considered later in the section on atypical pneumonias. Often, the bacterial infection follows an upper respiratory tract viral infection. Bacterial invasion of the lung parenchyma causes the alveoli to be filled with an inflammatory exudate, thus causing consolidation ("solidification") of the pulmonary tissue. Many variables, such as the specific etiologic agent, the host reaction, and the extent of involvement, determine the precise form of pneumonia. Predisposing conditions include extremes of age, chronic diseases (congestive heart failure, COPD, and diabetes), congenital or acquired immune deficiencies, and decreased or absent splenic function (sickle cell disease or post splenectomy, which puts the patient at risk for infection with encapsulated bacteria such as pneumococcus). First we describe pneumonias caused by various organisms and then the morphologic and clinical features common to most pneumonias.

Streptococcus Pneumoniae

Streptococcus pneumoniae, or *pneumococcus*, is the most common cause of community-acquired acute pneumonia. Examination of Gram-stained sputum is an important step in the diagnosis of acute pneumonia. The presence of numerous neutrophils containing the typical Gram-positive, lancet-shaped diplococci supports the diagnosis of pneumococcal pneumonia, but it must be remembered that *S. pneumoniae* is a part of the endogenous flora in 20% of adults, and therefore false-positive results may be obtained. Isolation of pneumococci from blood cultures is more specific but less sensitive (in the early phase of illness, only 20% to 30% of patients have positive blood cultures). Pneumococcal pneumonias respond readily to penicillin treatment, but there are increasing numbers of penicillin-resistant strains of pneumococci, so whenever possible, antibiotic sensitivity should be determined. Pneumococcal vaccines containing capsular polysaccharides from the common serotypes are available for use in patients at high risk.

Haemophilus Influenzae

Haemophilus influenzae is a pleomorphic, Gram-negative organism that is a major cause of life-threatening acute lower respiratory tract infections and meningitis in young children. In adults it is a very common cause of community-acquired acute pneumonia.[98] This bacterium is a ubiquitous colonizer of the pharynx, where it exists in two forms: encapsulated (5%) and unencapsulated (95%). Typically, the encapsulated form dominates the unencapsulated forms by secreting an antibiotic called haemocin that kills the unencapsulated *H. influenzae*.[99] Although there are six serotypes of the encapsulated form (types a to f), type b, which has a polyribosephosphate capsule, used to be the most frequent cause of severe invasive disease. With routine use of *H. influenzae* conjugate vaccines, the incidence of disease caused by the b serotype has declined significantly. By contrast, infections with nonencapsulated forms are increasing. Also called nontypable forms, they spread along the surface of the upper respiratory tract and produce otitis media (infection of the middle ear), sinusitis, and bronchopneumonia.

Pili on the surface of *H. influenzae* mediate adherence of the organisms to the respiratory epithelium.[100] In addition, *H. influenzae* secretes a factor that disorganizes ciliary beating and a protease that degrades IgA, the major class of antibody secreted into the airways. Survival of *H. influenzae* in the bloodstream correlates with the presence of the capsule, which, like that of pneumococcus, prevents opsonization by complement and phagocytosis by host cells. Antibodies against the capsule protect the host from *H. influenzae* infection, hence the capsular polysaccharide b is incorporated in the vaccine for children against *H. influenzae*.

H. influenzae pneumonia, which may follow a viral respiratory infection, is a pediatric emergency and has a high mortality rate. Descending laryngotracheobronchitis results in airway obstruction as the smaller bronchi are plugged by dense, fibrin-rich exudate of polymorphonuclear cells, similar to that seen in pneumococcal pneumonias. Pulmonary consolidation is usually lobular and patchy but may be confluent and involve the entire lung lobe. Before a vaccine became widely available, *H. influenzae* was a common cause of suppurative meningitis in children up to 5 years of age. *H. influenzae* also causes an acute, purulent conjunctivitis (pinkeye) in children and, in predisposed older patients, may cause septicemia, endocarditis, pyelonephritis, cholecystitis, and suppurative arthritis. *H. influenzae* is the most common bacterial cause of acute exacerbation of COPD.

Moraxella Catarrhalis

Moraxella catarrhalis is being increasingly recognized as a cause of bacterial pneumonia, especially in the elderly. It is the second most common bacterial cause of acute exacerbation of COPD. Along with *S. pneumoniae* and *H. influenzae*, *M. catarrhalis* constitutes one of the three most common causes of otitis media in children.

Staphylococcus Aureus

Staphylococcus aureus is an important cause of secondary bacterial pneumonia in children and healthy adults following viral respiratory illnesses (e.g., measles in children and influenza in both children and adults). Staphylococcal pneumonia is associated with a high incidence of complications, such as lung abscess and empyema. *Intravenous drug abusers* are at high risk of developing staphylococcal pneumonia in association with endocarditis. It is also an important cause of nosocomial pneumonia, as will be discussed later.

Klebsiella Pneumoniae

Klebsiella pneumoniae is the most frequent cause of Gram-negative bacterial pneumonia. It commonly afflicts debilitated and malnourished people, particularly *chronic alcoholics*. Thick and gelatinous sputum is characteristic because the organism produces an abundant viscid capsular polysaccharide, which the patient may have difficulty coughing up.

Pseudomonas Aeruginosa

Although *Pseudomonas aeruginosa* most commonly causes nosocomial infections, it is mentioned here because of its occurrence in cystic fibrosis patients. It is common in patients who are neutropenic and it has a propensity to invade blood vessels with consequent extrapulmonary spread. *Pseudomonas* septicemia is a very fulminant disease.

Legionella Pneumophila

Legionella pneumophila is the agent of Legionnaires disease, an eponym for the epidemic and sporadic forms of pneumonia caused by this organism. Pontiac fever is a related self-limited upper respiratory tract infection caused by *L. pneumophila*, without pneumonic symptoms. This organism flourishes in artificial aquatic environments, such as water-cooling towers and within the tubing system of domestic (potable) water supplies. The mode of transmission is thought to be either inhalation of aerosolized organisms or aspiration of contaminated drinking water. *Legionella* pneumonia is common in individuals with some predisposing condition such as cardiac, renal, immunologic, or hematologic disease. *Organ transplant recipients are particularly susceptible.* It can be quite severe, frequently requiring hospitalization, and immunosuppressed patients may have fatality rates of up to 50%. Rapid diagnosis is facilitated by demonstration of *Legionella* antigens in the urine or by a positive fluorescent antibody test on sputum samples; culture remains the gold standard of diagnosis.

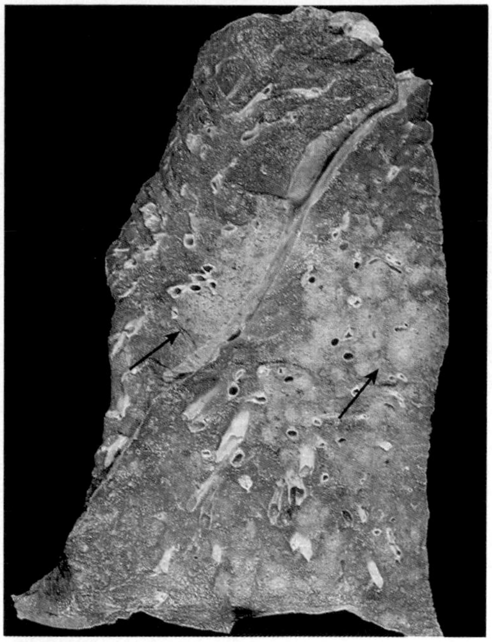

FIGURE 15–33 Bronchopneumonia. Gross section of lung showing patches of consolidation (*arrows*).

Morphology. Bacterial pneumonia has two gross patterns of anatomic distribution: lobular bronchopneumonia and lobar pneumonia (Fig. 15–32). Patchy consolidation of the lung is the dominant characteristic of **bronchopneumonia** (Fig. 15–33). **Lobar pneumonia** is an acute bacterial infection resulting in fibrinosuppurative consolidation of a large portion of a lobe or of an entire lobe (Fig. 15–34). These anatomic but still classic categorizations are often difficult to apply in the individual case because patterns overlap. The patchy involvement may become confluent, producing virtually total lobar consolidation; in contrast, effective antibiotic therapy for any form of pneumonia may limit involvement to a subtotal consolidation. Moreover, the same organisms may produce bronchopneumonia in one patient, whereas in the more vulnerable individual, a full-blown lobar involvement develops. **Most important from the clinical standpoint are identification of the causative agent and determination of the extent of disease.**

In **lobar pneumonia**, four stages of the inflammatory response have classically been described: congestion, red hepatization, gray hepatization, and resolution. Present-day effective antibiotic therapy frequently slows or halts the progression. In the first

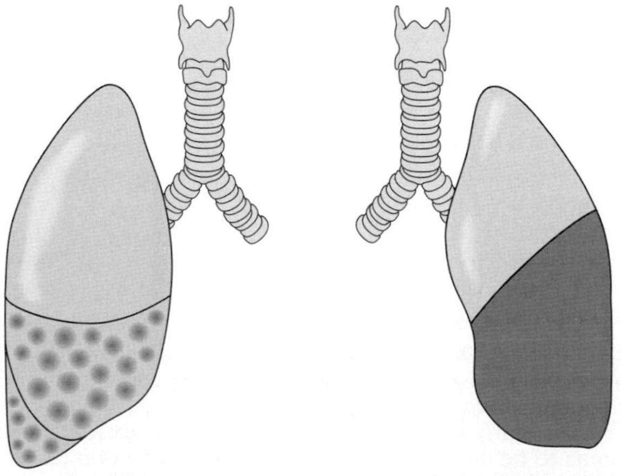

FIGURE 15–32 Comparison of bronchopneumonia and lobar pneumonia.

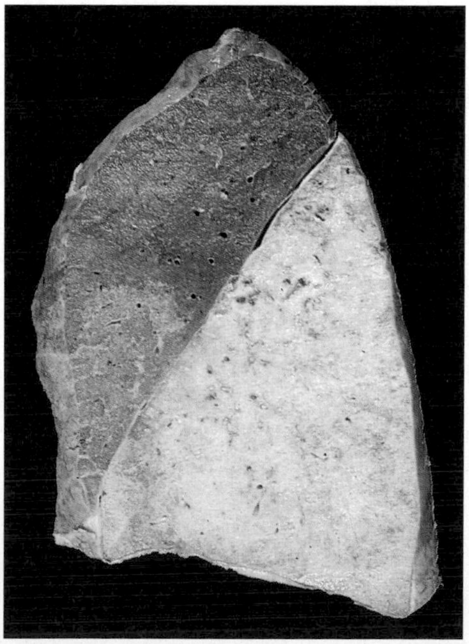

FIGURE 15–34 Lobar pneumonia—gray hepatization, gross photograph. The lower lobe is uniformly consolidated.

stage of **congestion,** the lung is heavy, boggy, and red. It is characterized by vascular engorgement, intra-alveolar fluid with few neutrophils, and often the presence of numerous bacteria. The stage of **red hepatization** that follows is characterized by massive confluent exudation with red cells (congestion), neutrophils, and fibrin filling the alveolar spaces (Fig. 15–35*A*). On gross examination, the lobe now appears distinctly red, firm, and airless, with a liver-like consistency, hence the term **hepatization.** The stage of **gray hepatization** follows with progressive disintegration of red cells and the persistence of a fibrinosuppurative exudate (Fig. 15–35*B*), giving the gross appearance of a grayish brown, dry surface. In the final stage of **resolution,** the consolidated exudate within the alveolar spaces undergoes progressive enzymatic digestion to produce a granular, semifluid, debris that is resorbed, ingested by macrophages, coughed up, or organized by fibroblasts growing into it (Fig. 15–35*C*). Pleural fibrinous reaction to the underlying inflammation, often present in the early stages if the consolidation extends to the surface (**pleuritis**), may similarly resolve. More often, it undergoes organization, leaving fibrous thickening or permanent adhesions.

Foci of **bronchopneumonia** are consolidated areas of acute suppurative inflammation. The consolidation may be patchy through one lobe but is more often multilobar and frequently bilateral and basal because of the tendency of secretions to gravitate into the lower lobes. Well-developed lesions are usually 3 to 4 cm in diameter, slightly elevated, dry, granular, gray-red to yellow, and poorly delimited at their margins (see Fig. 15–33). Histologically, the reaction usually elicits a suppurative, neutrophil-rich exudate that fills the bronchi, bronchioles, and adjacent alveolar spaces (see Fig. 15–35*A*).

Complications of pneumonia include (1) tissue destruction and necrosis, causing **abscess formation** (particularly common with type 3 pneumococci or *Klebsiella* infections); (2) spread of infection to the pleural cavity, causing the intrapleural fibrinosuppurative reaction known as **empyema;** (3) **organization** of the exudate, which may convert a portion of the lung into solid tissue (Fig. 15–35*C*); and (4) **bacteremic dissemination** to the heart valves, pericardium, brain, kidneys, spleen, or joints, causing metastatic abscesses, endocarditis, meningitis, or suppurative arthritis.

Clinical Course. The major symptoms of community-acquired acute pneumonia are abrupt onset of high fever, shaking chills, and cough productive of mucopurulent sputum; occasional patients may have hemoptysis. When fibrinosuppurative pleuritis is present, it is accompanied by pleuritic pain and pleural friction rub. The characteristic radiologic appearance of lobar pneumonia is that of a radio-opaque, usually well-circumscribed lobe, whereas bronchopneumonia shows focal opacities.

The clinical picture is dramatically modified by the administration of antibiotics. Treated patients may be relatively

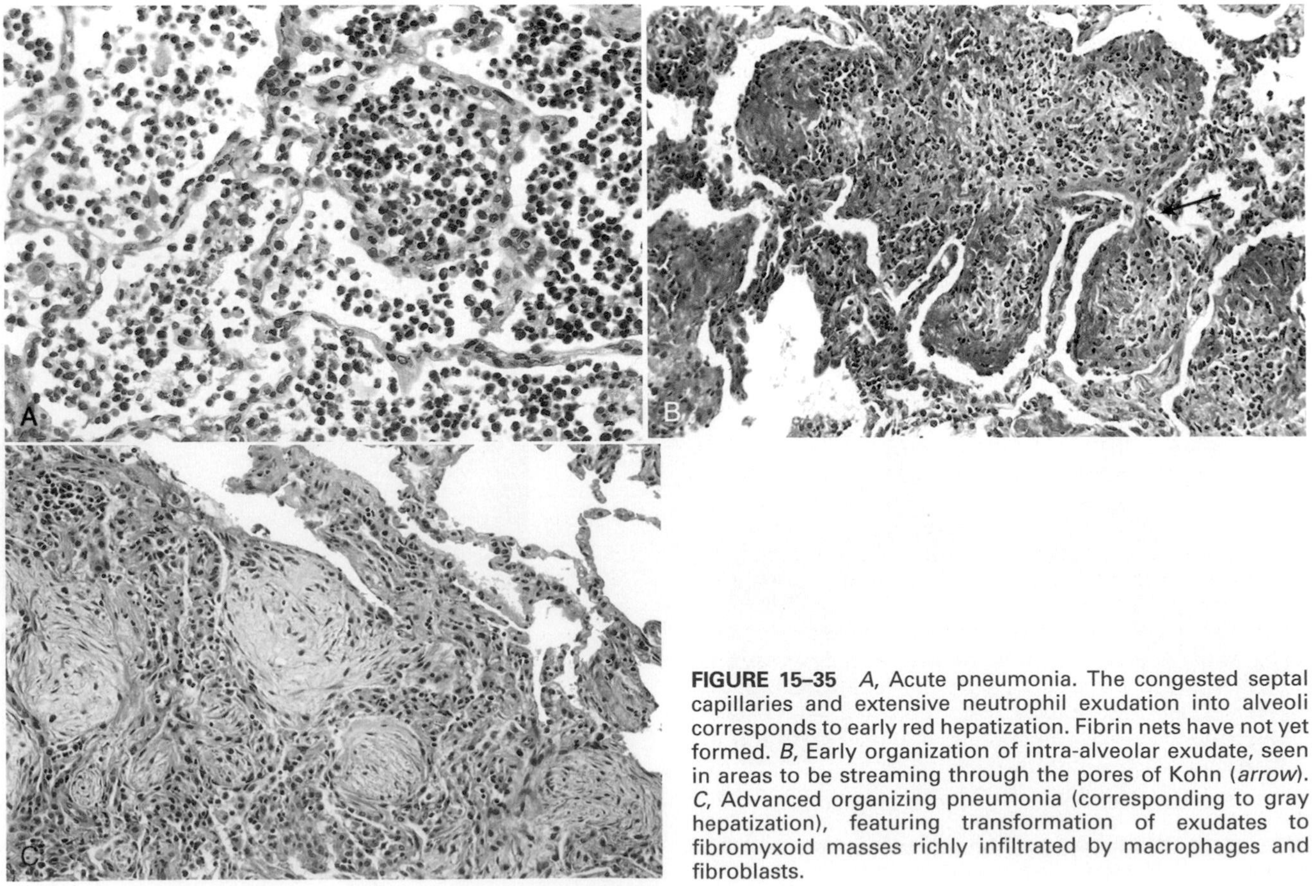

FIGURE 15–35 *A,* Acute pneumonia. The congested septal capillaries and extensive neutrophil exudation into alveoli corresponds to early red hepatization. Fibrin nets have not yet formed. *B,* Early organization of intra-alveolar exudate, seen in areas to be streaming through the pores of Kohn (*arrow*). *C,* Advanced organizing pneumonia (corresponding to gray hepatization), featuring transformation of exudates to fibromyxoid masses richly infiltrated by macrophages and fibroblasts.

afebrile with few clinical signs 48 to 72 hours after the initiation of antibiotics. The identification of the organism and the determination of its antibiotic sensitivity are the keystones to appropriate therapy. Fewer than 10% of patients with pneumonia severe enough to merit hospitalization now succumb, and in most such instances, death may be attributed either to a complication, such as empyema, meningitis, endocarditis, or pericarditis, or to some predisposing influence, such as debility or chronic alcoholism.

COMMUNITY-ACQUIRED ATYPICAL (VIRAL AND MYCOPLASMAL) PNEUMONIAS

The term "primary atypical pneumonia" was initially applied to an acute febrile respiratory disease characterized by patchy inflammatory changes in the lungs, largely confined to the alveolar septa and pulmonary interstitium. The term "atypical" denotes the moderate amount of sputum, no physical findings of consolidation, only moderate elevation of white cell count, and lack of alveolar exudate. The pneumonitis is caused by a variety of organisms, the most common being *Mycoplasma pneumoniae. Mycoplasma* infections are particularly common among children and young adults. They occur sporadically or as local epidemics in closed communities (schools, military camps, and prisons). Other etiologic agents are viruses, including influenza virus types A and B, the respiratory syncytial viruses, adenovirus, rhinoviruses, rubeola, and varicella viruses; *Chlamydia pneumoniae*; and *Coxiella burnetti* (Q fever).[100] In some cases, the cause cannot be determined. Any one of these agents can cause merely an upper respiratory tract infection, recognized as the common cold, or a more severe lower respiratory tract infection. The circumstances that favor such extension of the infection are often mysterious but include malnutrition, alcoholism, and underlying debilitating illnesses.

The common pathogenetic mechanism is attachment of the organisms to the upper respiratory tract epithelium followed by necrosis of the cells and an inflammatory response. When the process extends to the alveoli, there is usually interstitial inflammation, but there may also be some outpouring of fluid into alveolar spaces, so that on chest films the changes may mimic bacterial pneumonia. Damage to and denudation of the respiratory epithelium inhibit mucociliary clearance and predispose to secondary bacterial infections.

Morphology. All causal agents produce essentially similar morphologic patterns. The pneumonic involvement may be quite patchy or may involve whole lobes bilaterally or unilaterally. The affected areas are red-blue, congested, and subcrepitant. The pleura is smooth, and pleuritis or pleural effusions are infrequent.

The histologic pattern depends on the severity of the disease. **Predominant is the interstitial nature of the inflammatory reaction, virtually localized within the walls of the alveoli.** The alveolar septa are widened and edematous and usually have a mononuclear inflammatory infiltrate of lymphocytes, histiocytes, and occasionally plasma cells. In acute cases, neutrophils may also be present. The alveoli may be free from exudate, but in many patients, there is intraalveolar proteinaceous material, a cellular exudate, and characteristically pink hyaline membranes lining the alveolar walls, similar to those seen in hyaline membrane disease of infants. These changes reflect **alveolar damage** similar to that seen diffusely in ARDS (see Fig. 15–3). Eradication of the infection is followed by reconstitution of the normal architecture of the lung.

Superimposed bacterial infection modifies the histologic picture by causing ulcerative bronchitis and bronchiolitis and may yield the anatomic changes that were described in the section on bacterial pneumonia. Some viruses, such as herpes simplex, varicella, and adenovirus, may be associated with necrosis of bronchial and alveolar epithelium and acute inflammation. Epithelial giant cells with intranuclear or intracytoplasmic inclusions may be present in cytomegalic inclusion disease. Other viruses produce cytopathic changes, as described in Chapter 8.

Clinical Course. The clinical course is extremely varied. Many cases masquerade as severe upper respiratory tract infections or as *chest colds*. Even patients with well-developed atypical pneumonia have few localizing symptoms. Cough may well be absent, and the major manifestations may consist only of fever, headache, muscle aches, and pains in the legs. The edema and exudation are both strategically located to cause mismatching of ventilation and blood flow and thus evoke symptoms out of proportion to the scanty physical findings.

The ordinary sporadic form of the disease is usually mild with a low mortality rate, below 1%. Interstitial pneumonia, however, may assume epidemic proportions with intensified severity and greater mortality, as documented in the devestating influenzal pandemics of 1915 and 1918 and the many smaller epidemics since then. Secondary bacterial infection by staphylococci or streptococci is common in such circumstances.

Influenza Infections

The genome of influenza virus is composed of eight helices of single-stranded RNA, each encoding a single gene and each bound by a nucleoprotein that determines the type of influenza virus (A, B, or C). The spherical surface of influenza virus is a lipid bilayer (envelope) containing the viral hemagglutinin and neuraminidase, which determine the subtype of the virus (H1 to H3; N1 or N2). Host antibodies to the hemagglutinin and neuraminidase prevent and ameliorate, respectively, future infection with the influenza virus. Two mechanisms account for the clearance of primary influenza virus infection: cytotoxic T cells kill virus-infected cells, and an intracellular anti-influenza protein (called Mx1) is induced in macrophages by the cytokines interferon-α and interferon-β.[101]

Influenza viruses of type A infect humans, pigs, horses, and birds and are the major cause of pandemic and epidemic influenza infections. A single subtype of influenza virus A predominates throughout the world at a given time.[102] Epidemics of influenza occur through mutations of the hemagglutinin and neuraminidase that allow the virus to escape most host antibodies (*antigenic drift*). Pandemics, which are longer and more widespread than epidemics, may occur when both the hemagglutinin and the neuraminidase are replaced through recombination of RNA segments with those of animal viruses, making all individuals susceptible to the new influenza virus (*antigenic shift*). Polymerase chain reaction analysis of influenza virus from the lungs of a soldier who died in the 1918 influenza pandemic that killed between 20 million and 40 million people worldwide identified a swine influenza virus belonging to the same family of influenza viruses causing illness today.[103] Current antiviral drugs have been found to be effective against recombinant influenza viruses bearing the 1918 hemagglutinin, neuraminidase, and matrix genes.[104] Influenza virus types B and C, which do not show antigenic drift or shift, infect mostly children, who develop antibodies against reinfection in a manner similar to that of chickenpox, mumps, and other childhood viral illnesses. Rarely, influenza virus may cause interstitial myocarditis or, after aspirin therapy, Reye syndrome (Chapter 18).

Morphology. Viral upper respiratory infections are marked by mucosal hyperemia and swelling with a predominantly lymphomonocytic and plasmacytic infiltration of the submucosa accompanied by overproduction of mucus secretions. The swollen mucosa and viscid exudate may plug the nasal channels, sinuses, or the Eustachian tubes and lead to suppurative secondary bacterial infection. Virus-induced tonsillitis with enlargement of the lymphoid tissue within Waldeyer ring is frequent in children, although lymphoid hyperplasia is not usually associated with suppuration or abscess formation, such as is encountered with streptococci or staphylococci.

In **laryngotracheobronchitis** and **bronchiolitis,** there are vocal cord swelling and abundant mucous exudation. Impairment of bronchociliary function invites bacterial superinfection with more marked suppuration. Plugging of small airways may give rise to focal lung atelectasis. In the more severe bronchiolar involvement, widespread plugging of secondary and terminal airways by cell debris, fibrin, and inflammatory exudate may, when prolonged, cause organization and fibrosis, resulting in obliterative bronchiolitis and permanent lung damage. Viral pneumonias, like bacterial pneumonias, take a variety of anatomic forms as described above.

Severe Acute Respiratory Syndrome (SARS)

The severe acute respiratory syndrome first appeared in November of 2002 in the Guangdong Province of China and subsequently spread to Hong Kong, Taiwan, Singapore, Vietnam, and Toronto, where large outbreaks also occurred.[105] The ease of travel between continents clearly contributed to this pandemic. Between fall of 2002 and spring of 2003, there were more than 8,000 cases of SARS, including 774 deaths. After an incubation period of 2 to 10 days, SARS begins with a dry cough, malaise, myalgias, fever and chills. As compared to other atypical pneumonias caused, for example, by Mycoplasmas, SARS less commonly gives rise to symptoms related to the upper respiratory tract such as sore throat. A third of patients improve and resolve the infection, but the rest progress to severe respiratory disease with shortness of breath, tachypnea, and pleurisy and nearly 10% of patients die from the illness, for which there is no specific treatment.

The cause of SARS is a previously undiscovered coronavirus. Nearly a third of upper respiratory infections are caused by coronaviruses, however the SARS virus differs from previously known coronaviruses in that it infects the lower respiratory tract and spreads throughout the body. The SARS virus appears to have been first transmitted to humans through contact with wild masked palm civets that are eaten in China. Subsequent cases were spread person-to-person, mainly through infected respiratory secretions, although some cases may have been contracted from stool.

SARS can be diagnosed either by detection of the virus by PCR, or by detection of antibodies to the virus. Levels of the virus are low initially and peak 10 days after onset of illness, so testing of different specimens (respiratory secretions, blood, and stool) collected on several days may be needed to detect the virus. Detection of antibodies specific for the SARS virus is a very sensitive and specific test, however patients may not have a measurable antibody response for up to 28 days after infection.

The pathophysiology of SARS is not understood, nor is it known why the virus moved from animals to humans. The SARS coronavirus isolated from most human cases has a 29 nucleotide deletion in the RNA when compared to the virus found in wild animals, and this variation may enhance transmission or pathogenicity of the virus in humans. The lungs of patients who have died of SARS show diffuse alveolar damage and multinucleated giant cells. Coronaviruses can be seen within pneumocytes by electron microscopy.

NOSOCOMIAL PNEUMONIA

Nosocomial, or hospital-acquired, pneumonias are defined as pulmonary infections acquired in the course of a hospital stay. They are common in patients with severe underlying disease, immunosuppression, prolonged antibiotic therapy, or invasive access devices such as intravascular catheters. Patients on mechanical ventilation are at particularly high risk. Superimposed on an underlying disease (that caused hospitalization), nosocomial infections are serious and often life-threatening complications. Gram-negative rods (Enterobacteriaceae and *Pseudomonas* species) and *Staphylococcus aureus* are the most common isolates; unlike community-acquired pneumonias, *Streptococcus pneumoniae* is not a major pathogen in nosocomial infections.

ASPIRATION PNEUMONIA

Aspiration pneumonia occurs in markedly debilitated patients or those who aspirate gastric contents either while unconscious (e.g., after a stroke) or during repeated vomiting. These patients have abnormal gag and swallowing reflexes that predispose to aspiration. The resultant pneumonia is partly chemical, owing to the extremely irritating effects of the gastric acid, and partly bacterial (from the oral flora). Typically, more than one organism is recovered on culture, aerobes being more common than anaerobes. This type of pneumonia is often necrotizing, pursues a fulminant clinical course, and is a frequent cause of death. In those who survive, lung abscess formation is a common complication.

LUNG ABSCESS

The term "pulmonary abscess" describes a local suppurative process within the lung, characterized by necrosis of lung tissue. Oropharyngeal surgical procedures, sinobronchial infections, dental sepsis, and bronchiectasis play important roles in their development.

Etiology and Pathogenesis. Although under appropriate circumstances any pathogen can produce an abscess, the commonly isolated organisms include aerobic and anaerobic streptococci, *Staphylococcus aureus*, and a host of Gram-negative organisms. Mixed infections occur often because of the important causal role that inhalation of foreign material plays.[106] *Anaerobic organisms* normally found in the oral cavity, including members of the *Bacteroides*, *Fusobacterium*, and *Peptococcus* species, are the exclusive isolates in about 60% of cases. The causative organisms are introduced by the following mechanisms:

- *Aspiration of infective material* (the most frequent cause): This is particularly common in acute alcoholism, coma, anesthesia, sinusitis, gingivodental sepsis, and debilitation in which the cough reflexes are depressed. Aspiration of gastric contents is serious because the gastric acidity adds to the irritant role of the food particles, and in the course of aspiration, mouth organisms are inevitably introduced.
- *Antecedent primary bacterial infection*: Post-pneumonic abscess formations are usually associated with *S. aureus*, *Klebsiella pneumoniae*, and the type 3 pneumococcus. Fungal infections and bronchiectasis are additional antecedents to lung abscess formation. Post-transplant or otherwise immunosuppressed individuals are at special risk for this complication.
- *Septic embolism*: Infected emboli from thrombophlebitis in any portion of the systemic venous circulation or from the vegetations of infective bacterial endocarditis on the right side of the heart are trapped in the lung.
- *Neoplasia*: Secondary infection is particularly common in the bronchopulmonary segment obstructed by a primary or secondary malignancy (*postobstructive pneumonia*).
- *Miscellaneous*: Direct traumatic penetrations of the lungs; spread of infections from a neighboring organ, such as suppuration in the esophagus, spine, subphrenic space, or pleural cavity; and hematogenous seeding of the lung by pyogenic organisms all may lead to lung abscess formation.

When all these causes are excluded, there are still cases in which no reasonable basis for the abscess formation can be identified. These are referred to as *primary cryptogenic lung abscesses.*

Morphology. Abscesses vary in diameter from lesions of a few millimeters to large cavities of 5 to 6 cm. They may affect any part of the lung and may be single or multiple. Pulmonary abscesses due to aspiration are more common on the right (because of the more vertical right main bronchus) and are most often single. Abscesses that develop in the course of pneumonia or bronchiectasis are usually multiple, basal, and diffusely scattered. Septic emboli and pyemic abscesses, by the haphazard nature of their genesis, are multiple and may affect any region of the lungs.

The abscess cavity might or might not be filled with suppurative debris, depending on the presence or absence of a communication with one of the air passages. When such communications exist, the contained exudate may be partially drained to create an air-containing cavity. Superimposed saprophytic infections are prone to flourishing within the already necrotic debris of the abscess cavity. Continued infection leads to large, fetid, green-black, multilocular cavities with poor demarcation of their margins, designated **gangrene of the lung.** The **cardinal histologic change in all abscesses is suppurative destruction of the lung parenchyma within the central area of cavitation** (Fig. 15–36). In chronic cases, considerable fibroblastic proliferation produces a fibrous wall.

Clinical Course. The manifestations of pulmonary abscesses are much like those of bronchiectasis and are characterized principally by cough, fever, and copious amounts of foul-smelling purulent or sanguineous sputum. Fever, chest pain, and weight loss are common. Clubbing of the fingers and toes may appear within a few weeks after the onset of an abscess. Diagnosis of this condition can be only suspected from the clinical findings and must be confirmed by roentgenography. Whenever an abscess is discovered, it is important to rule out an underlying carcinoma because this is present in 10% to 15% of cases.

The course of abscesses is variable. With antimicrobial therapy, most resolve with no major sequelae. Complications include extension of the infection into the pleural cavity, hemorrhage, the development of *brain abscesses* or *meningitis* from septic emboli, and (rarely) secondary amyloidosis (type AA).

CHRONIC PNEUMONIA

Chronic pneumonia is most often a localized lesion in the immunocompetent patient, with or without regional lymph

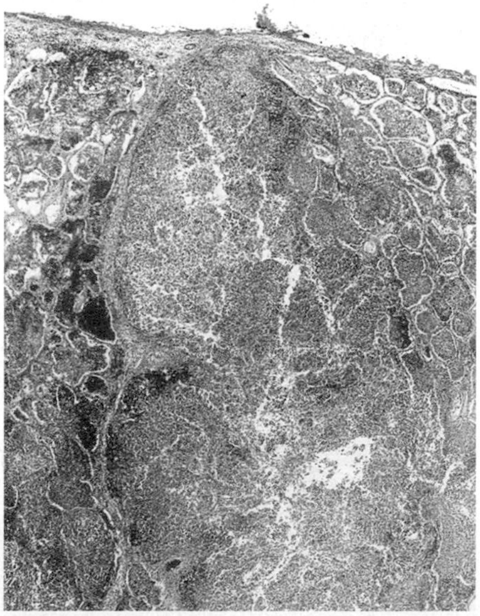

FIGURE 15–36 Pyemic lung abscess in the center of section with complete destruction of underlying parenchyma within the focus of involvement.

node involvement. There is granulomatous inflammation, which may be due to bacteria (e.g., *M. tuberculosis*) or fungi (e.g., *Histoplasma capsulatum*). Tuberculosis of the lung and other organs was described in Chapter 8. Here we will discuss chronic pneumonias caused by fungi.

Histoplasmosis, blastomycosis, and *coccidioidomycosis* are discussed together because (1) they are granulomatous diseases of the lungs that may resemble tuberculosis, (2) they are caused by fungi that are thermally dimorphic in that they grow as hyphae that produce spores at environmental temperatures but grow as yeasts (spherules or ellipses) at body temperature within the lungs, and (3) each fungus is geographic in that it causes disease primarily among immunocompetent individuals living along the Ohio and Mississippi rivers and in the Caribbean (*Histoplasma*), in the central and southeastern United States (*Blastomyces*), and in the Southwest and Far West of the United States and in Mexico (*Coccidioides*).

Histoplasmosis

Histoplasma capsulatum infection is acquired by inhalation of dust particles from soil contaminated with bird or bat droppings that contain small spores (microconidia), the infectious form of the fungus. Like *M. tuberculosis, H. capsulatum* is an intracellular parasite of macrophages. The clinical presentations and morphologic lesions of histoplasmosis also strikingly resemble those of tuberculosis, including (1) a self-limited and often latent primary pulmonary involvement, which may result in coin lesions on chest radiography; (2) chronic, progressive, secondary lung disease, which is localized to the lung apices and causes cough, fever, and night sweats; (3) localized lesions in extrapulmonary sites, including mediastinum, adrenals, liver, or meninges; and (4) a widely disseminated involvement, particularly in immunosuppressed patients.

The pathogenesis of histoplasmosis is incompletely understood. It is known that macrophages are the major target of infection. *H. capsulatum* may be internalized into macrophages after opsonization with antibody or by a distinct mechanism that appears unique to this fungus. The fungus expresses heat shock protein 60 (HSP60) on the cell surface that binds to the β_2 integrins on the surface of macrophages.[107] *Histoplasma* yeasts so phagocytosed by the unstimulated macrophages, multiply within the phagolysosome, and lyse the host cells. *Histoplasma* infections are controlled by helper T cells that recognize fungal cell wall antigens and heat-shock proteins and subsequently secrete interferon-γ, which activates macrophages to kill intracellular yeasts. In addition, *Histoplasma* induces macrophages to secrete TNF, which recruits and stimulates other macrophages to kill *Histoplasma*. Lacking cellular immunity, patients with AIDS are susceptible to disseminated infection with *Histoplasma*, which is a major opportunistic pathogen in this disease.

Morphology. In the lungs of otherwise healthy adults, *Histoplasma* infections produce epithelioid cell granulomas, which usually undergo coagulative necrosis and coalesce to produce large areas of consolidation but may also liquefy to form cavities. With spontaneous or drug control of the infection, these lesions undergo fibrosis and concentric calcification (tree-bark appearance) (Fig. 15–37). Histologic differentiation from tuberculosis, sarcoidosis, and coccidioidomycosis requires identification of the 3- to 5-μm thin-walled yeast forms (stained with methenamine silver) that may persist in tissues for years.

In **chronic histoplasmosis,** gray-white granulomas are usually present in the apices of the lungs with retraction and thickening of the pleura and in the hilar nodes. Further progression involves more and more of the lung parenchyma, with cavity formation less frequent than in tuberculosis.

In **fulminant disseminated histoplasmosis,** which occurs in immunosuppressed individuals, epithelioid cell granulomas are not formed; instead, there are focal accumulations of mononuclear phagocytes filled with fungal yeasts throughout the tissues and organs of the body (Fig. 15–38). The presence of macrophages stuffed with organisms resembles that found in severe cases of visceral leishmaniasis, described in Chapter 8.

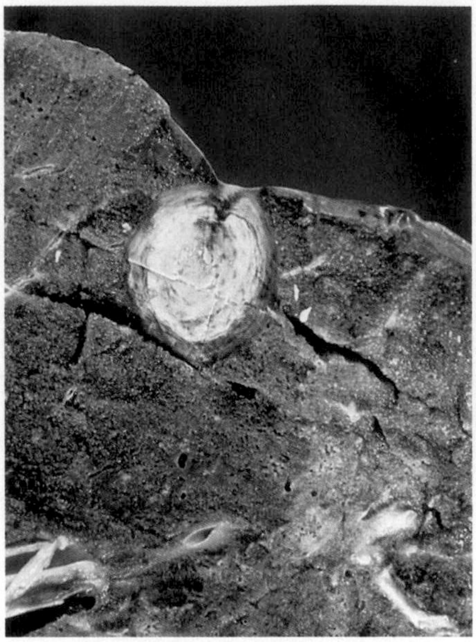

FIGURE 15–37 Laminated *Histoplasma* granuloma of the lung.

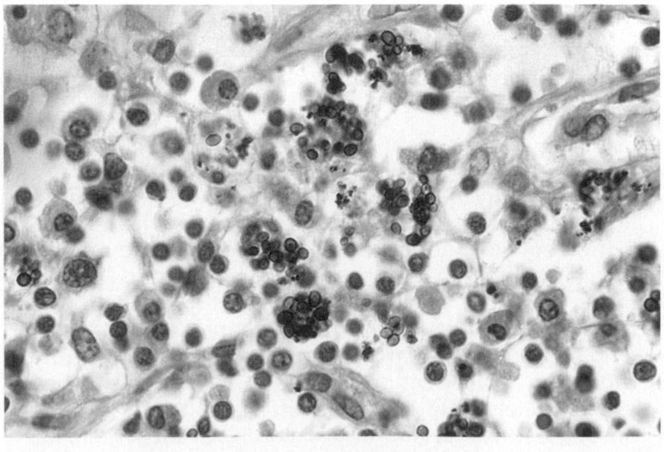

FIGURE 15–38 *Histoplasma capsulatum* yeast forms fill phagocytes in a lymph node of a patient with disseminated histoplasmosis.

The diagnosis of histoplasmosis is firmly established by culture of the fungus. Identification of the fungus in tissue lesions can also be useful. In addition, serologic tests for antibodies and antigen are also available. Antigen detection in body fluids is most useful in the early stages, because antibodies are formed two to six weeks after infection.[108]

Blastomycosis

Blastomyces dermatidis is a soil-inhabiting, dimorphic fungus that is remarkably difficult to isolate. It is a cause of disease in people living in or visiting the central and southeastern United States; infection also occurs in Canada, Mexico, the Middle East, Africa, and India. There are three clinical forms: pulmonary blastomycosis, disseminated blastomycosis, and a rare primary cutaneous form that results from direct inoculation of organisms into the skin. Pulmonary blastomycosis most often presents as an abrupt illness with productive cough, headache, chest pain, weight loss, fever, abdominal pain, night sweats, chills, and anorexia. Chest radiographs reveal lobar consolidation, multilobar infiltrates, perihilar infiltrates, multiple nodules, or miliary infiltrates. The upper lobes are most frequently involved. The process may resolve spontaneously, persist, or progress to a chronic lesion.

Morphology. In the normal host, the lung lesions of blastomycosis are suppurative granulomas. Macrophages have a limited ability to ingest and kill *B. dermatidis*, and the persistence of the yeast cells leads to continued recruitment of neutrophils. In tissue, *B. dermatidis* is a round, 5- to 15-μm yeast cell that divides by broad-based budding. It has a thick, double-contoured cell wall and multiple nuclei (Figs. 15–39*A* and 15–39*B*). Involvement of the skin and larynx is associated with marked epithelial hyperplasia, which may be mistaken for squamous cell carcinoma.

Coccidioidomycosis

Almost everyone who inhales the spores of *Coccidioides immitis* becomes infected and develops a delayed type hypersensitivity to the fungus, so more than 80% of people in endemic areas of the Southwest and western United States have a positive skin test reaction. Indeed, increases in populations in the West and construction projects that mobilize spores from the soil have caused *Coccidioides* to be classified as a reemerging pathogen.[109] One reason for the high rate of infectivity by *C. immitis* is that infective arthroconidia, when ingested by alveolar macrophages, block fusion of the phagosome and lysosome and so resist intracellular killing. As is the case with *Histoplasma*, most primary infections with *C. immitis* are asymptomatic, but 10% of people have lung lesions, fever, cough, and pleuritic pains, accompanied by erythema nodosum or erythema multiforme (the San Joaquin Valley fever complex). Fewer than 1% of people develop disseminated *C. immitis* infection, which frequently involves the skin and meninges.

Morphology. The primary and secondary lung lesions of *C. immitis* are similar to the granulomatous lesions of *Histoplasma*. Within macrophages or giant cells, *C. immitis* is present as thick-walled, nonbudding spherules 20 to 60 μm in diameter, often filled with small endospores (Fig. 15–40). A pyogenic reaction is superimposed when the spherules rupture to release the endospores, which are not infectious. In contrast, in infectious *C. immitis*, boxcar-like arthrospores produced in culture are easily detached and disseminated by air, so extreme caution is needed in handling this fungus in the laboratory. Rare progressive *C. immitis* disease involves the lungs, meninges, skin, bones, adrenals, lymph nodes, spleen, or liver. At all these sites, the inflammatory response may be purely granulomatous, pyogenic, or mixed. Purulent lesions dominate in patients with diminished resistance and with widespread dissemination.

PNEUMONIA IN THE IMMUNOCOMPROMISED HOST

The appearance of a pulmonary infiltrate and signs of infection (e.g., fever) is one of the most common and serious complications in patients whose immune and defense systems are suppressed by disease, immunosuppression for organ transplants and tumors, or irradiation.[110] A wide variety of so-

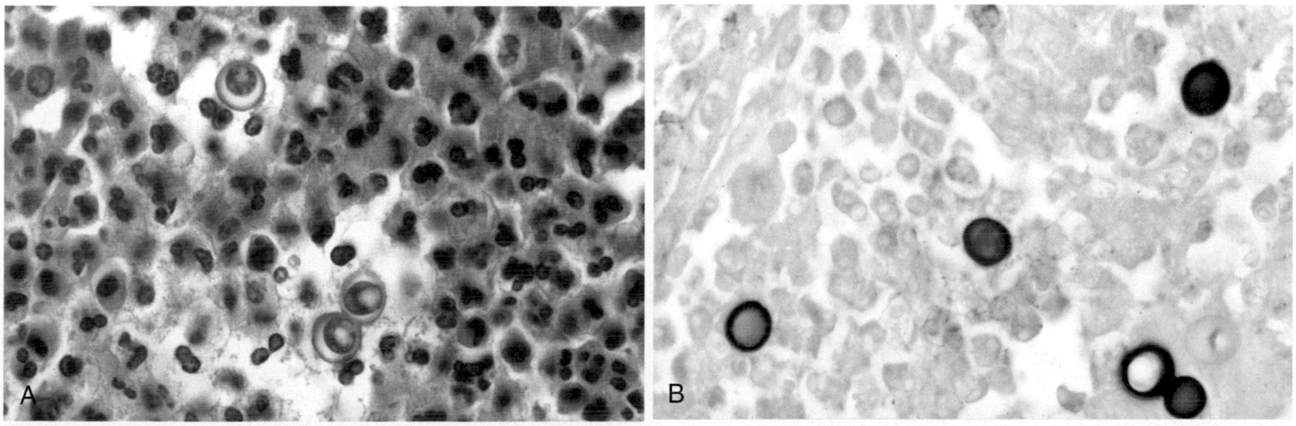

FIGURE 15–39 Blastomycosis. *A*, Rounded budding yeasts, larger than neutrophils, are present. Note the characteristic thick wall and nuclei (not seen in other fungi). *B*, Silver stain.

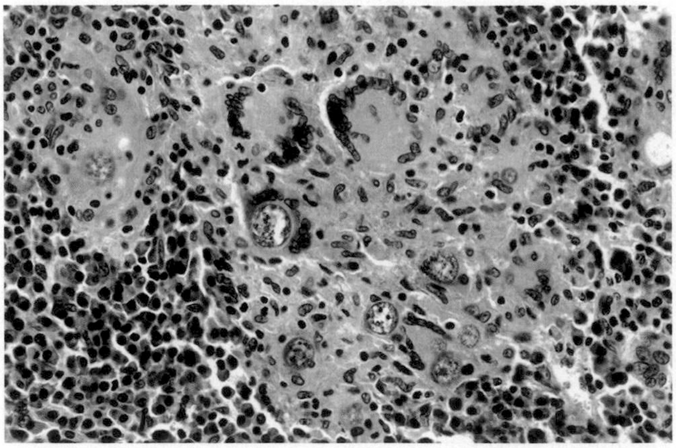

FIGURE 15–40 Coccidioidomycosis with intact spherules within multinucleated giant cells.

called opportunistic infectious agents, many of which rarely cause infection in normal hosts, can cause these pneumonias, and often, more than one agent is involved. Mortality from these opportunistic infections is high. In the case of AIDS, nearly 100% of patients suffer from an opportunistic infection, often caused by *P. carinii.*[111] Table 15–9 lists some of the opportunistic agents according to their prevalence and whether they cause local or diffuse pulmonary infiltrates. The differential diagnosis of such infiltrates includes drug reactions and involvement of the lung by tumor. The specific infections are discussed in Chapter 8. Of these, the ones that commonly involve the lung can be divided according to the etiologic agent: (1) bacteria (*Pseudomonas aeruginosa*, *Mycobacterium* species, *Legionella pneumophilia*, and *Listeria monocytogenes*), (2) viruses (CMV and herpesvirus), and (3) fungi (*Pneumocystis carinii*, *Candida* species, *Aspergillus* species, the Phycomycetes, and *Cryptococcus neoformans*).

PULMONARY DISEASE IN HUMAN IMMUNODEFICIENCY VIRUS INFECTION

Pulmonary disease continues to be the leading cause of morbidity and mortality in HIV-infected patients. Although the use of potent antiretroviral agents and effective chemoprophylaxis has dramatically altered the incidence and outcome of pulmonary disease in HIV-infected patients, the plethora of entities involved makes diagnosis and treatment a distinct challenge. Some of the individual microbial agents afflicting HIV-infected patients have already been discussed; this section will focus only on the general principles of HIV-associated pulmonary disease.

- Despite the emphasis on "opportunistic" infections, it must be remembered that bacterial lower respiratory tract infection caused by the "usual" pathogens is one of the most serious pulmonary disorders in HIV infection. The implicated organisms include *Streptococcus pneumoniae, Staphylococcus aureus, Haemophilus influenzae,* and Gram-negative rods. Bacterial pneumonias in HIV-infected patients are more common, more severe, and more often associated with bacteremia than in those without HIV infection.
- Not all pulmonary infiltrates in HIV-infected individuals are infectious in etiology. A host of noninfectious diseases, including Kaposi sarcoma (Chapters 6 and 11), pulmonary non-Hodgkin lymphoma (Chapter 14), and primary lung cancer, occur with increased frequency and need to be excluded.
- *The CD4+ T cell count can define the risk of infection with specific organisms.* As a rule of thumb, bacterial and tubercular infections are more likely at higher CD4+ counts (>200 cells/mm^3). Pneumocystis pneumonia usually strikes at CD4+ counts below 200 cells/mm^3, while cytomegalovirus and *Mycobacterium avium* complex infections are uncommon until the very late stages of immunosuppression (CD4+ counts <50 cells/mm^3).

Finally, it is useful to remember that pulmonary disease in HIV-infected patients may result from more than one cause, and even common pathogens may present with atypical manifestations. Therefore, the diagnostic workup of these patients may be more extensive (and expensive) than would be mandated in an immunocompetent individual.

TABLE 15–9 Causes of Pulmonary Infiltrates in Immunocompromised Hosts

Diffuse Infiltrate	Focal Infiltrate
Common	***Common***
Cytomegalovirus	Gram-negative rods
Pneumocystis carinii	*Staphylococcus aureus*
Drug reaction	*Aspergillus*
	Candida
	Malignancy
Uncommon	***Uncommon***
Bacteria	*Cryptococcus*
Aspergillus	*Mucor*
Cryptococcus	*Pneumocystis carinii*
Malignancy	*Legionella pneumophila*

Lung Transplantation

Indications for transplantation may include almost all non-neoplastic terminal lung diseases, provided that the patient does not have any other serious disease, which would preclude lifelong immunosuppressive therapy. The most common indications are end-stage emphysema, idiopathic pulmonary fibrosis, cystic fibrosis, and primary pulmonary hypertension. While bilateral lung and heart-lung transplants are possible, in many cases a single lung transplant is performed, offering sufficient improvement in pulmonary function for each of two recipients from a single (and all too scarce) donor. When bilateral chronic infection is present (e.g., cystic fibrosis, bronchiectasis), both lungs of the recipient must be replaced to remove the reservoir of infection.

Morphology. With improving surgical and organ preservation techniques, postoperative complications (e.g., anastomotic dehiscence, vascular thrombosis, primary graft dysfunction) are happily becoming rare. The transplanted lung is subject to two major complications: infection and rejection.

Pulmonary infections in lung transplant patients are essentially those of any immunocompromised host, discussed earlier. They include bacterial and viral (especially cytomegalovirus) pneumonias, *Pneumocystis carinii* pneumonia (PCP), and fungal infections. In the early posttransplant period (the first few weeks), bacterial infections are most common. With Gancyclovir prophylaxis and matching of donor-recipient CMV status, CMV pneumonia occurs less frequently and is less severe, although some resistant strains are emerging. Most cases occur in the third to twelfth month after transplant. PCP is rare, since almost all patients receive adequate prophylaxis (usually Bactrim™). Fungal infections are mostly due to *Candida* and *Aspergillus* species, and they involve the bronchial anastamotic site and/or the lung.

Acute rejection of the lung occurs to some degree in all patients despite routine immunosuppression postoperatively. It often occurs during the early weeks to months after surgery but may occur years later whenever immunosuppression is decreased. Patients present with fever, dyspnea, cough, and radiologic infiltrates. Since these are similar to the picture of infections, diagnosis often relies on transbronchial biopsy. The morphologic features of acute rejection are primarily those of inflammatory infiltrates (lymphocytes, plasma cells, and few neutrophils and eosinophils), either around small vessels, in the submucosa of airways, or both.[112]

Chronic rejection is a significant problem in at least half of all lung transplant patients by 3 to 5 years. It is manifested by cough, dyspnea, and an irreversible decrease in lung function tests. The major morphologic correlate of chronic rejection is **bronchiolitis obliterans,** the partial or complete occlusion of small airways by fibrosis, with or without active inflammation (Fig. 15–41). Bronchiolitis obliterans is patchy and therefore difficult to diagnose via transbronchial biopsy. Bronchiectasis may develop in long-standing cases.

The acute cellular airway rejection (the presumed forerunner of later, fibrous obliteration of these airways) is generally responsive to therapy, but the treatment of established bronchiolitis obliterans has been disappointing. Its progress may be slowed or even halted for some time, but it cannot be reversed. Infrequent complications of lung transplantation include accelerated pulmonary arteriosclerosis in the graft and lymphoproliferative disease. With continuing improvement in surgical, immunosuppressive, and antimicrobial therapies, the outcome of lung transplantation has improved considerably, although it is still not as good as that for renal or cardiac transplantation. One-year and 6-year survival rates are about 90% and 54%, respectively.[113,114]

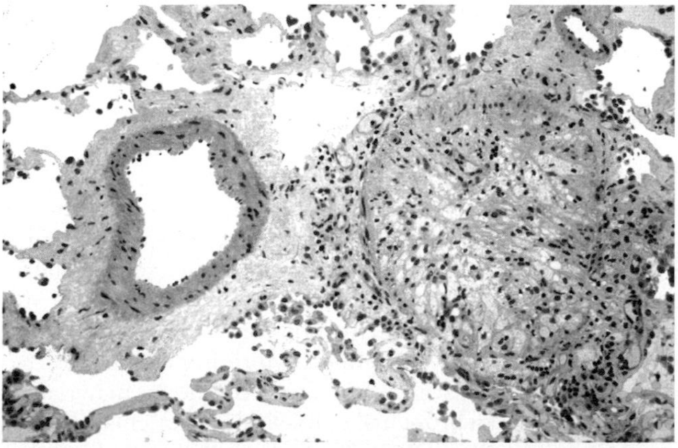

FIGURE 15–41 Chronic rejection of lung allograft, with total occlusion of bronchiole (bronchiolitis obliterans). Adjacent pulmonary artery branch is normal. (Courtesy of Dr. Thomas Krausz, Department of Pathology, The University of Chicago, Pritzker School of Medicine, Chicago, IL.)

Tumors

A variety of benign and malignant tumors may arise in the lung, but the vast majority (90% to 95%) are carcinomas, about 5% are bronchial carcinoids, and 2% to 5% are mesenchymal and other miscellaneous neoplasms.[42]

CARCINOMAS

Lung cancer is currently the most frequently diagnosed major cancer in the world and the most common cause of cancer mortality worldwide. This is largely due to the carcinogenic effects of cigarette smoke. Over the coming decades, changes in smoking habits will greatly influence lung cancer incidence and mortality as well as the prevalence of various histologic types of lung cancer.[115]

The number of new cases of lung cancer occurring in 2003 in the United States is estimated to be 171,900 (note that in 1950 it was 18,000), accounting for about 13% of cancer diagnoses. The incidence rate is declining significantly in men, from a high of 86.5 per 100,000 in 1984 to 69.8 in 1998. In the 1990s, the increase among women reached a plateau, with incidence in 1998 at 43.4 per 100,000. The annual number of deaths from lung cancer in the United States is estimated to be 157,200 in 2003. During 1992 to 1998, mortality from lung cancer declined significantly (1.9% per year) among men, while rates for women continued to increase but at a much slower pace (0.8% per year). Since 1987, more women have died each year of lung cancer than of breast cancer, which for over 40 years had been the major cause of cancer death in women. Decreasing lung cancer incidence and mortality rates have most likely resulted from the decreased smoking rates over the past 30 years. However, decreases in smoking patterns among women lag behind those of men. Declines in adult tobacco use have slowed, as have declines in mortality under 45 years old; tobacco use among youth increased considerably during the 1990s except in states with vigorous control programs.

Cancer of the lung occurs most often between ages 40 and 70 years, with a peak incidence in the fifties or sixties. Only 2% of all cases appear before the age of 40. The outlook for patients diagnosed with lung cancer is dismal. The 1-year relative survival rate has increased from 34% in 1975 to 41% in 1997, largely owing to improvements in surgical techniques. However, the 5-year rate for all stages combined is only 15%.

Etiology and Pathogenesis. Carcinomas of the lung, similar to cancer at other sites, arise by a stepwise accumulation of genetic abnormalities that transform benign bronchial epithelium to neoplastic tissue. Unlike many other cancers, however, the major environmental insult that inflicts genetic damage is known. We begin our discussion with the well known lung carcinogen—cigarette smoke.

Tobacco Smoking. The evidence provided by statistical and clinical observations establishing a positive relationship between tobacco smoking and lung cancer is overwhelming. Experimental data have also been pursued, but this approach is limited by species differences.

Statistical evidence is most compelling: 87% of lung carcinomas occur in active smokers or those who stopped recently. In numerous retrospective studies, there was an invariable statistical association between the frequency of lung cancer and (1) the amount of daily smoking, (2) the tendency to inhale, and (3) the duration of the smoking habit. Compared with nonsmokers, average smokers of cigarettes have a 10-fold greater risk of developing lung cancer, and heavy smokers (more than 40 cigarettes per day for several years) have a 60-fold greater risk. Women have a higher susceptibility to tobacco carcinogens than men do. Cessation of smoking for 10 years reduces risk but never to control levels. Epidemiologic studies also show an association between cigarette smoking and carcinoma of the mouth, pharynx, larynx, esophagus, pancreas, uterine cervix, kidney, and urinary bladder. Secondhand smoke, or environmental tobacco smoke, contains numerous human carcinogens for which there is no safe level of exposure. Each year, about 3000 nonsmoking adults die of lung cancer as a result of breathing secondhand smoke.[116] Cigar and pipe smoking also increase risk, although much more modestly than smoking cigarettes. The use of smokeless tobacco is not a safe substitute for smoking cigarettes or cigars, as these products cause oral cancers and can lead to nicotine addiction.

Clinical evidence is obtained largely through observations of histologic changes in the lining epithelium of the respiratory tract in habitual smokers. These sequential changes have been best documented for squamous cell carcinoma, but they may also be present in other histologic subtypes. In essence, there is a linear correlation between the intensity of exposure to cigarette smoke and the appearance of ever more worrisome epithelial changes that begin with squamous metaplasia and progress to squamous dysplasia, carcinoma in situ, and invasive carcinoma.

Experimental work has consisted mainly of attempts to induce cancer in experimental animals with extracts of tobacco smoke.[117] More than 1200 substances have been counted in cigarette smoke, many of which are potential carcinogens. They include both initiators (polycyclic aromatic hydrocarbons such as benzo[*a*]pyrene) and promoters, such as phenol derivatives. Radioactive elements may also be found (polonium-210, carbon-14, potassium-40) as well as other contaminants, such as arsenic, nickel, molds, and additives. Protracted exposure of mice to these additives induces skin tumors. Efforts to produce lung cancer by exposing animals to tobacco smoke, however, have been unsuccessful. The few cancers that have developed have been bronchioloalveolar carcinomas, a type of tumor that is not strongly associated with smoking in humans.

Industrial Hazards. Certain industrial exposures increase the risk of developing lung cancer. High-dose ionizing *radiation* is carcinogenic. There was an increased incidence of lung cancer among survivors of the Hiroshima and Nagasaki atomic bomb blasts. *Uranium* is weakly radioactive, but lung cancer rates among nonsmoking uranium miners are 4 times higher than those in the general population, and among smoking miners, they are about 10 times higher.

The risk of lung cancer is increased with *asbestos*. Lung cancer is the most frequent malignancy in individuals exposed to asbestos, which has become a universally recognized carcinogen, particularly when coupled with smoking.[66] Asbestos workers who do not smoke have a five times greater risk of developing lung cancer than do nonsmoking control subjects, and those who smoke have a 50 to 90 times greater risk . The latent period before the development of lung cancer is 10 to 30 years. Among asbestos workers, one death in five is due to lung carcinoma, 1 in 10 to pleural or peritoneal mesotheliomas (discussed later), and 1 in 10 to gastrointestinal carcinomas.

Air Pollution. Atmospheric pollutants may play some role in the increased incidence of lung carcinoma today. Attention has been drawn to the potential problem of *indoor* air pollution, especially by radon.[118,119] Radon is a ubiquitous radioactive gas that has been linked epidemiologically to increased lung cancer in miners exposed to relatively high concentrations. The pathogenetic mechanism is believed to be inhalation and bronchial deposition of radioactive decay products that become attached to environmental aerosols. These data have generated concern that low-level indoor exposure (e.g., in homes in areas of high radon in soil) could also lead to increased incidence of lung tumors; some attribute the bulk of lung cancers in nonsmokers to this insidious carcinogen (Chapter 9).[120]

Molecular Genetics. Ultimately, the exposures cited previously are thought to act by causing genetic alterations in lung cells, which accumulate and eventually lead to the neoplastic phenotype. It has been estimated that 10 to 20 genetic mutations have occurred by the time the tumor is clinically apparent.[121]

As will be discussed below, for all practical purposes, lung cancers can be divided into two clinical subgroups: *small cell carcinoma* and *non–small cell carcinoma*. Some molecular lesions are common to both types, whereas others are relatively specific. The dominant oncogenes that are frequently involved in lung cancer include *c-MYC*, *K-RAS*, *EGFR*, and *HER-2/neu*. The commonly deleted or inactivated tumor suppressor genes include *p53*, *RB*, *p16*^{INK4a}, and multiple loci on chromosome 3p. At this locale, there are numerous candidate tumor suppressor genes, such as *FHIT*, *RASSF1A*, and others that remain to be identified. Of the genetic alterations listed above, *p53* mutations are common to both small cell and non–small cell carcinomas. In contrast, small cell cancers harbor more frequent alterations in *c-MYC* and *RB*, whereas non–small cell tumors are associated with mutations in *RAS* and *p16*^{INK4a}. Some of these differences are further highlighted in the ensuing discussion.[122] Although certain genetic changes are known to be early (inactivation of chromosome 3p suppressor genes) or late (activation of *RAS*), the temporal sequence is not yet well defined. More importantly, certain genetic changes such as loss of chromosome 3p material can be found in benign bronchial epithelium of patients with lung cancer, as well as in the respiratory epithelium of smokers without lung cancers, suggesting that large areas of the respiratory mucosa are mutagenized after exposure to carcinogens ("field effect"). On this fertile soil, the cells that accumulate additional mutations ultimately develop into cancer.

Occasional familial clustering has suggested a genetic predisposition, as has the variable risk even among heavy smokers. Attempts at defining markers of genetic susceptibility are ongoing and have, for example, identified a role for polymorphisms in the cytochrome P-450 gene *CYP1A1* (Chapter 7). People with certain alleles of *CYP1A1* have an increased capacity to metabolize procarcinogens derived from cigarette smoke and, conceivably, incur the greatest risk of developing lung cancer. Similarly, individuals whose peripheral blood lymphocytes undergo chromosomal breakages following exposure to tobacco-related carcinogens (mutagen sensitivity genotype) have a greater than tenfold risk of developing lung cancer compared with controls.

Precursor Lesions. Three types of precursor epithelial lesions are recognized: (1) squamous dysplasia and carcinoma in situ, (2) atypical adenomatous hyperplasia, and (3) diffuse idiopathic pulmonary neuroendocrine cell hyperplasia. It should be noted that the term "precursor" does not imply that progression to invasion will occur in all cases. Currently, it is not possible to distinguish between preinvasive lesions that are likely to progress and those that will remain localized.

Classification. Tumor classification is important for consistency in patient treatment and because it provides a basis for epidemiologic and biological studies. The most recent classification of the World Health Organization[115] has gained wide acceptance (Table 15–10). Several histologic variants of each type of lung cancer are described; however, their clinical significance is still undetermined, except as mentioned below. The relative proportions of the major categories are:

- Squamous cell carcinoma (25% to 40%)
- Adenocarcinoma (25% to 40%)
- Small cell carcinoma (20% to 25%)
- Large cell carcinoma (10% to 15%)

The incidence of adenocarcinoma has increased significantly in the last two decades; it is now the most common form of lung cancer in women and, in many studies, men as well.[42,123] The basis for this change is unclear. A possible factor is the increase in women smokers, but this only highlights our lack of knowledge about why women tend to show more adenocarcinomas. One interesting postulate is that changes in cigarette type (filter tips, lower tar and nicotine) have caused smokers to inhale more deeply and thereby expose more peripheral airways and cells (with a predilection to adenocarcinoma) to carcinogens.[124] There may be mixtures of histologic patterns, even in the same cancer. Thus, combined types of squamous cell carcinoma and adenocarcinoma or of small cell and squamous cell carcinoma occur in about 10% of patients. For common clinical use, however, the various histologic types of lung cancer can be clustered into two groups on the basis of likelihood of metastases and response to available therapies: *small cell carcinomas* (most often metastatic, high initial response to chemotherapy) versus *non–small cell carcinomas* (less often metastatic, less responsive). The strongest relationship to smoking is with squamous cell and small cell carcinoma.

Morphology. Lung carcinomas arise most often in and about the hilus of the lung. About three fourths of the lesions take their origin from first-order, second-order, and third-order bronchi. A small number of primary carcinomas of the lung arise in the periphery of the lung substance from the alveolar septal cells or terminal bronchioles. These are predominantly adenocarcinomas, including those of the bronchioloalveolar type, to be discussed separately.

Squamous cell carcinoma of the lung begins as an area of in situ cytologic dysplasia that, over an unknown interval of time, yields a small area of thickening or piling up of bronchial mucosa. With progression, this small focus, usually less than 1 cm^2 in area, assumes the appearance of an irregular, warty excrescence that elevates or erodes the lining epithelium. The tumor may then follow a variety of paths. It may continue to fungate into the bronchial lumen to produce an intraluminal mass. It can also rapidly penetrate the wall of the bronchus to infiltrate along the peribronchial tissue (Fig. 15–42) into the adjacent region of the carina or mediastinum. In other instances, the tumor grows along a broad front to produce a cauliflower-like intraparenchymal mass

TABLE 15–10 Histologic Classification of Malignant Epithelial Lung Tumors

Squamous cell carcinoma
Small cell carcinoma Combined small cell carcinoma
Adenocarcinoma Acinar; papillary, bronchioloalveolar, solid, mixed subtypes
Large cell carcinoma Large cell neuroendocrine carcinoma
Adenosquamous carcinoma
Carcinomas with pleomorphic, sarcomatoid, or sarcomatous elements
Carcinoid tumor Typical, atypical
Carcinomas of salivary gland type
Unclassified carcinoma

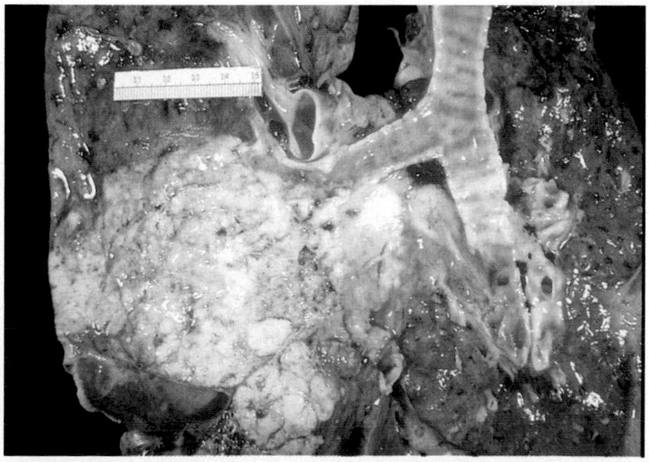

FIGURE 15–42 Lung carcinoma. The gray-white tumor tissue is seen infiltrating the lung substance. Histologically, this large tumor mass was identified as a squamous cell carcinoma.

that appears to push lung substance ahead of it. In almost all patterns, the neoplastic tissue is gray-white and firm to hard. Especially when the tumors are bulky, focal areas of hemorrhage or necrosis may appear to produce yellow-white mottling and softening. Sometimes these necrotic foci cavitate. Often these tumors erode the bronchial epithelium and can be diagnosed by cytologic examination of sputum, bronchoalveolar lavage fluid, or fine-needle aspiration (Figs. 15–43*A* and *B*).

Extension may occur to the pleural surface and then within the pleural cavity or into the pericardium. Spread to the tracheal, bronchial, and mediastinal nodes can be found in most cases. The frequency of nodal involvement varies slightly with the histologic pattern but averages greater than 50%.

Distant spread of lung carcinoma occurs through both lymphatic and hematogenous pathways. These tumors have a distressing habit of spreading widely throughout the body and at an early stage in their evolution except for squamous cell carcinoma, which metastasizes outside the thorax late. Often the metastasis presents as the first manifestation of the underlying occult pulmonary lesion. No organ or tissue is spared in the spread of these lesions, but the adrenals, for obscure reasons, are involved in more than half the cases. The liver (30% to 50%), brain (20%), and bone (20%) are additional favored sites of metastases.

Squamous Cell Carcinoma. Squamous cell carcinoma is most commonly found in men and is **closely correlated with a smoking history.** Histologically, this tumor is characterized by the presence of keratinization and/or intercellular bridges. Keratinization may take the form of squamous pearls or individual cells with markedly eosinophilic dense cytoplasm (Fig. 15–44*A*). These features are prominent in the well-differentiated tumors, are easily seen but not extensive in moderately differentiated tumors, and are focally seen in poorly differentiated tumors. Mitotic activity is higher in poorly differentiated tumors. In the past, most squamous cell carcinomas were seen to arise centrally from the segmental or subsegmental bronchi. However, the incidence of squamous cell carcinoma of the peripheral lung is increasing. Squamous metaplasia, epithelial dysplasia, and foci of frank carcinoma in situ may be seen in bronchial epithelium adjacent to the tumor mass.

Squamous cell carcinomas show the highest frequency of p53 mutations of all histologic types of lung carcinoma. An influence of p53 status on prognosis has not been demonstrated, except in very early stages. p53 protein overexpression and, less commonly, mutations may precede invasion. Abnormal p53 accumulation is reported in 10% to 50% of dysplasias. There is increasing frequency and intensity of p53 immunostaining with higher-grade dysplasia, and positivity can be seen in 60% to 90% of squamous cell carcinoma in situ. Loss of protein expression of the tumor suppressor gene *RB* is detected by immunohistochemistry in 15% of squamous cell carcinomas. The CDK-inhibitor $p16^{INK4}$ is inactivated, and its protein product is lost in 65% of tumors. Multiple allelic losses are observed in squamous cell carcinomas at locations bearing tumor suppressor genes. These losses, especially those involving 3p, 9p, and 17p, may precede invasion and be detected in histologically normal cells in smokers. Overexpression of epidermal growth-factor receptor has been detected in 80% of squamous cell carcinomas, but it is rarely mutated. HER-2/neu is highly expressed in 30% of these cancers, but unlike in breast cancer, gene amplification is not the underlying mechanism.[122]

Adenocarcinoma. This is a malignant epithelial tumor with glandular differentiation or mucin production by the tumor cells. Adenocarcinomas show various growth patterns, either pure or, more often, mixed. These patterns are acinar, papillary, bronchioloalveolar, and solid with mucin formation. Of these, only the pure bronchioloalveolar carcinoma has distinct gross, microscopic, and clinical features and will be discussed separately.

Adenocarcinoma is the most common type of lung cancer in women and nonsmokers. As compared to squamous cell cancers, the lesions are usually more peripherally located, and tend to be smaller. They vary histologically from well-differentiated tumors with obvious glandular elements (Fig. 15–44*B*) to papillary

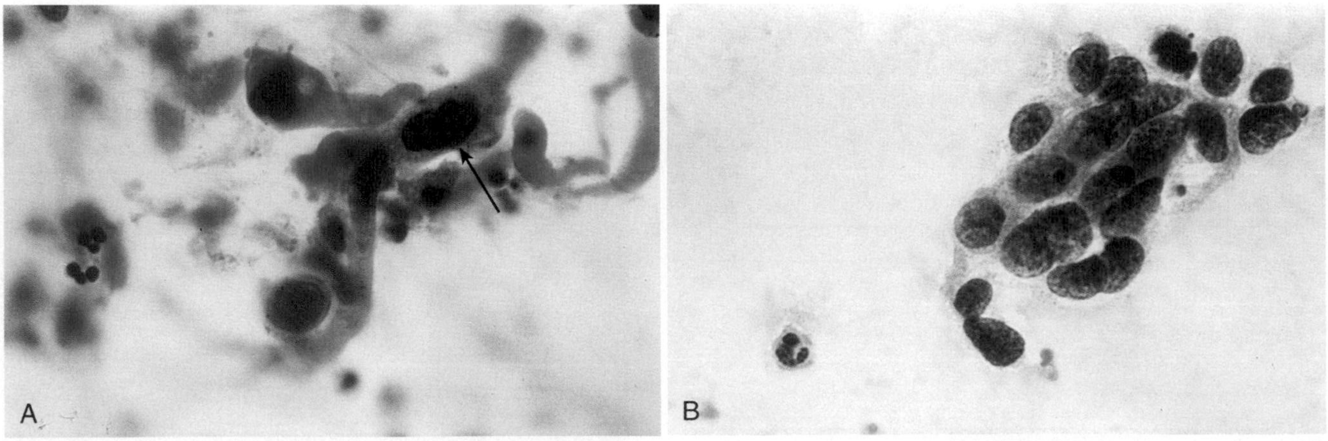

FIGURE 15–43 Cytologic diagnosis of lung cancer is often possible. *A*, A sputum specimen shows an orange-staining, keratinized squamous carcinoma cell with a prominent hyperchromatic nucleus (*arrow*). *B*, A fine-needle aspirate of an enlarged lymph node shows clusters of tumor cells from a small cell carcinoma, with molding and nuclear atypia characteristic of this tumor (see also Fig. 15–44*C*); note the size of the tumor cells compared with normal polymorphonuclear leukocytes in the left lower corner.

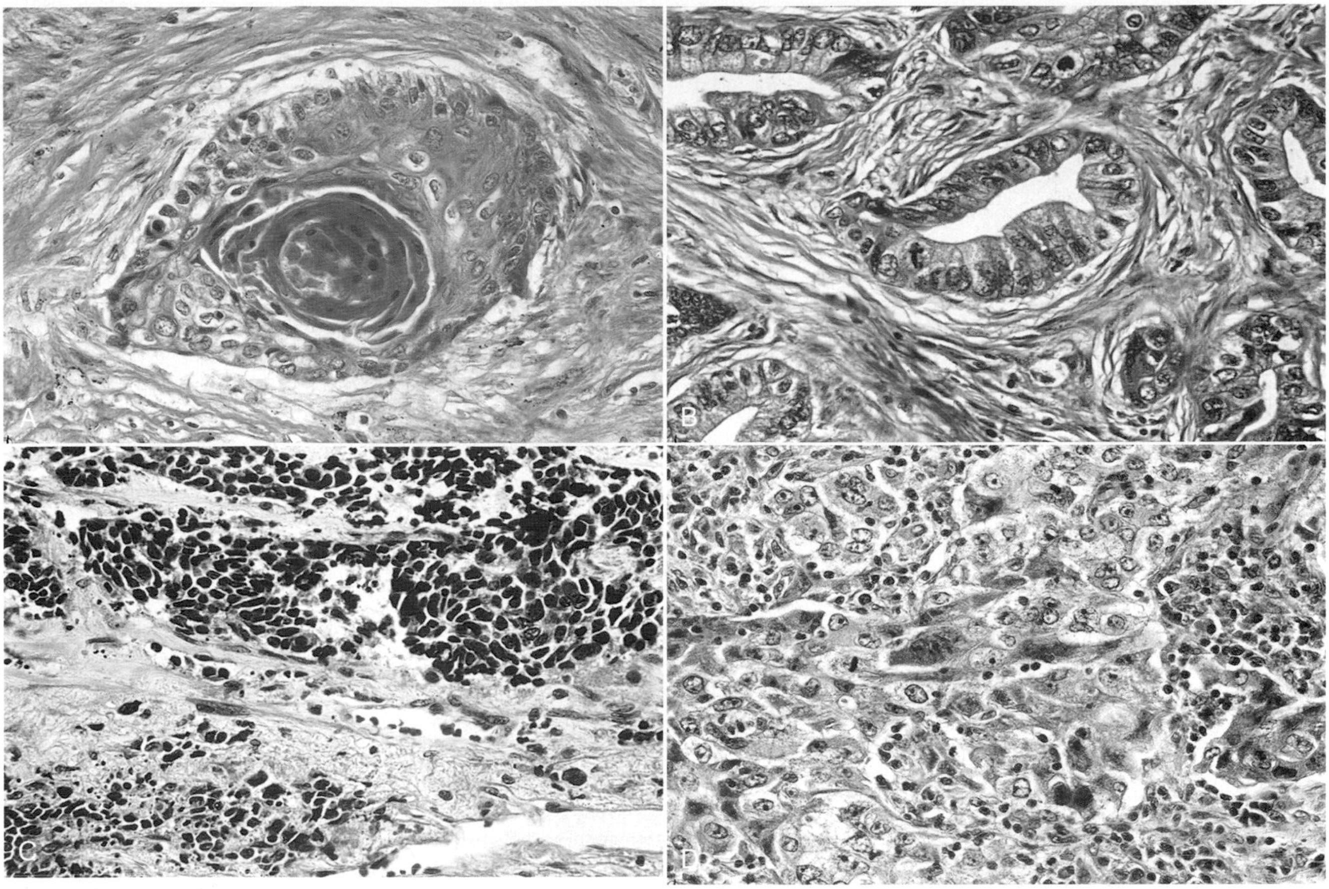

FIGURE 15–44 Histologic appearance of lung carcinoma. *A,* Well-differentiated squamous cell carcinoma showing keratinization. *B,* Gland-forming adenocarcinoma. *C,* Small cell carcinoma with islands of small deeply basophilic cells and areas of necrosis. *D,* Large cell carcinoma, featuring pleomorphic, anaplastic tumor cells and absence of squamous or glandular differentiation.

lesions resembling other papillary carcinomas to solid masses with only occasional mucin-producing glands and cells. About 80% contain mucin. At the periphery of the tumor, there is often a bronchioloalveolar pattern of spread (see below). Adenocarcinomas grow more slowly than squamous cell carcinomas but tend to metastasize widely and earlier. Peripheral adenocarcinomas are sometimes associated with areas of scarring. Adenocarcinomas, including bronchioloalveolar carcinomas, are less frequently associated with a history of smoking (still, greater than 75% are found in smokers) than are squamous or small cell carcinomas (>98%).

K-RAS mutations are seen primarily in adenocarcinoma, with a much lower frequency in nonsmokers (5%) than in smokers (30%). *p53, RB,* and *p16* mutations and inactivation have the same frequency in adenocarcinoma as in squamous cell carcinoma.

As the name implies, **bronchioloalveolar carcinoma** occurs in the pulmonary parenchyma in the terminal bronchioloalveolar regions. It represents, in various series, 1% to 9% of all lung cancers. Macroscopically, the tumor almost always occurs in the peripheral portions of the lung either as a single nodule or, more often, as multiple diffuse nodules that sometimes coalesce to produce a pneumonia-like consolidation. The parenchymal nodules have a mucinous, gray translucence when secretion is present but otherwise appear as solid, gray-white areas that can be confused with pneumonia on casual inspection. Because the tumor does not involve major bronchi, atelectasis and emphysema are infrequent.

Histologically, the tumor is characterized by a pure bronchioloalveolar growth pattern with no evidence of stromal, vascular, or pleural invasion. The key feature of bronchioloalveolar carcinomas is their growth along preexisting structures without destruction of alveolar architecture. This growth pattern has been termed "lepidic," an allusion to the neoplastic cells resembling butterflies sitting on a fence. It has two subtypes: nonmucinous and mucinous. The former has columnar, peg-shaped, or cuboidal cells, while the latter has distinctive, tall, columnar cells with cytoplasmic and intra-alveolar mucin, growing along the alveolar septa (Fig. 15–45). Ultrastructurally, bronchioloalveolar carcinomas are a heterogeneous group, consisting of mucin-secreting bronchiolar cells, Clara cells, or, rarely, type II pneumocytes.

Nonmucinous bronchioloalveolar carcinomas often consist of a peripheral lung nodule with only rare aerogenous spread and therefore are amenable to surgical resection. Mucinous bronchioloalveolar carcinomas, on the other hand, tend to spread aerogenously, forming satellite tumors. These may present as a solitary nodule or as multiple nodules, or an entire lobe may be consolidated by tumor, resembling

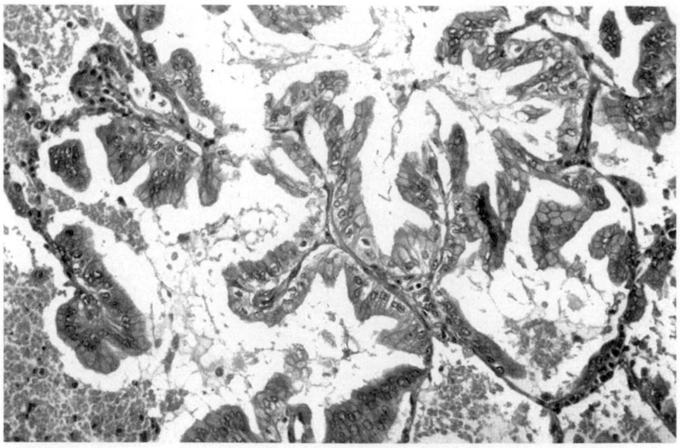

FIGURE 15–45 Bronchioloalveolar carcinoma with characteristic growth along pre-existing alveolar septa, without invasion. (Courtesy of Dr. Jerome B. Taxy, Department of Pathology, The University of Chicago, Pritzker School of Medicine, Chicago, IL.)

lobar pneumonia. Such lesions are less likely to be cured by surgery.

Analogous to the adenoma-carcinoma sequence in the colon, it is proposed that adenocarcinoma of the lung arises from **atypical adenomatous hyperplasia progressing to bronchioloalveolar carcinoma**, which then transforms into invasive adenocarcinoma. This is supported by the fact that lesions of atypical adenomatous hyperplasia are monoclonal and they share many molecular aberrations with invasive adenocarcinomas.[125] Microscopically, atypical adenomatous hyperplasia is recognized as a well-demarcated focus of epithelial proliferation composed of cuboidal to low columnar epithelium. These cells demonstrate some cytologic atypia but not to the extent seen in frank adenocarcinoma. It should be pointed out, however, that not all adenocarcinomas arise in this manner, nor do all bronchioloalveolar carcinomas become invasive if left untreated.

Small Cell Carcinoma. This highly malignant tumor has a distinctive cell type. The epithelial cells are small, with scant cytoplasm, ill-defined cell borders, finely granular nuclear chromatin (salt and pepper pattern), and absent or inconspicuous nucleoli (Fig. 15–44*C*). The cells are round, oval, and spindle-shaped, and nuclear molding is prominent. There is no absolute size for the tumor cells, but in general, they are smaller than small resting lymphocytes. The mitotic count is high. The cells grow in clusters that exhibit neither glandular nor squamous organization. Necrosis is common and often extensive. Basophilic staining of vascular walls due to encrustation by DNA from necrotic tumor cells is frequently present. Grading is inappropriate, since all small cell carcinomas are high grade. A single variant of small cell carcinoma is recognized: combined small cell carcinoma, in which there is a mixture of small cell carcinoma and any other non–small cell component, including large cell neuroendocrine carcinoma and sarcoma.

Electron microscopy shows dense-core neurosecretory granules 100 nm in diameter in two thirds of cases. The granules are similar to those found in the neuroendocrine argentaffin (Kulchitsky) cells present along the bronchial epithelium, particularly in the fetus and neonate. Although distinctive, electron microscopy is not needed for routine diagnosis. The occurrence of neurosecretory granules, the ability of some of these tumors to secrete polypeptide hormones, and the presence (ascertained by immunohistochemical stains) of neuroendocrine markers such as chromogranin, synaptophysin, and Leu-7 (in 75% of cases) and parathormone-like and other hormonally active products suggest derivation of this tumor from neuroendocrine progenitor cells of the lining bronchial epithelium. They are the most common pattern associated with ectopic hormone production (discussed later).

Small cell carcinomas have a strong relationship to cigarette smoking; only about 1% occur in nonsmokers. They occur both in major bronchi and in the periphery of the lung. There is no known preinvasive phase or carcinoma in situ. They are the most aggressive of lung tumors, metastasize widely, and are virtually incurable by surgical means.

p53 and *RB* tumor suppressor genes are frequently mutated (50% to 80% and 80% to 100% of small cell carcinomas, respectively). Immunohistochemistry demonstrates intense expression of the anti-apoptotic gene *BCL2* in 90% of tumors, in contrast with a low frequency of expression of the pro-apoptotic gene *BAX*.

Large Cell Carcinoma. This is an undifferentiated malignant epithelial tumor that lacks the cytologic features of small cell carcinoma and glandular or squamous differentiation. The cells typically have large nuclei, prominent nucleoli, and a moderate amount of cytoplasm (Fig. 15–44*D*). Large cell carcinomas probably represent squamous cell carcinomas and adenocarcinomas that are so undifferentiated that they can no longer be recognized by light microscopy. Ultrastructurally, however, minimal glandular or squamous differentiation is common. One histologic variant is large cell neuroendocrine carcinoma. This is recognized by such features as organoid nesting, trabecular, rosette-like and palisading patterns. These features suggest neuroendocrine differentiation, which can be confirmed by immunohistochemistry or electron microscopy. This tumor has the same molecular changes as small cell carcinoma.

Combined Carcinoma. Approximately 10% of all lung carcinomas have a combined histology, including two or more of the above types.

Secondary Pathology. Lung carcinomas cause related anatomic changes in the lung substance distal to the point of bronchial involvement. **Partial obstruction may cause marked focal emphysema; total obstruction may lead to atelectasis.** The impaired drainage of the airways is a common cause for **severe suppurative or ulcerative bronchitis or bronchiectasis. Pulmonary abscesses** sometimes call attention to a silent carcinoma that has initiated the chronic suppuration. Compression or invasion of the superior vena cava can cause venous congestion, dusky head and arm edema, and, ultimately, circulatory compromise—the **superior vena cava syndrome.** Extension to the pericardial or pleural sacs may cause **pericarditis** (Chapter 12) or **pleuritis** with significant effusions.

Staging. A uniform TNM system for staging cancer according to its anatomic extent at the time of diagnosis is extremely useful for many reasons, chiefly for comparing treatment results from different centers. The staging system in current use[126] is presented in Table 15–11.

Clinical Course. Lung cancer is one of the most insidious and aggressive neoplasms in the whole realm of oncology. In the usual case, it is discovered in patients in their fifties whose symptoms are of several months' duration. The major presenting complaints are cough (75%), weight loss (40%), chest pain (40%), and dyspnea (20%). Some of the more common local manifestations of lung cancer and their pathologic bases are listed in Table 15–12. Not infrequently, the tumor is discovered by its secondary spread during the course of investigation of an apparent primary neoplasm elsewhere. Bronchioloalveolar carcinomas, by definition, are noninvasive tumors and do not metastasize; rather, they kill by suffocation.

The outlook is poor for most patients with lung carcinoma. Despite all efforts at early diagnosis by frequent radioscopic examination of the chest, cytologic examination of sputum, and bronchial washings or brushings and the many improvements in thoracic surgery, radiotherapy, and chemotherapy, the overall 5-year survival rate is on the order of 15%. In many large clinics, not more than 20% to 30% of lung cancer patients have lesions sufficiently localized to permit even an attempt at resection. In general, the adenocarcinoma and squamous cell patterns tend to remain localized longer and have a slightly better prognosis than do the undifferentiated cancers, which usually are advanced lesions by the time they are discovered. The survival rate is 48% for cases detected when the disease is still localized. Only 15% of lung cancers are diagnosed at this early stage. Surgical resection for *small cell carcinoma* is so ineffective that the diagnosis essentially precludes surgery. Untreated, the survival time for patients with small cell cancer is 6 to 17 weeks. This cancer is particularly sensitive to radiation and chemotherapy, and potential cure rates of 15% to 25% for limited disease have been reported in some centers. Most patients have distant metastases on diagnosis. Thus, even with treatment, the mean survival after diagnosis is about 1 year.

Despite this discouraging outlook, some patients have been cured by lobectomy or pneumonectomy, emphasizing the continued need for early diagnosis and adequate prompt therapy.

Paraneoplastic Syndromes. Lung carcinoma can be associated with a number of paraneoplastic syndromes[127] (Chapter 7), some of which may antedate the development of a gross pulmonary lesion. The hormones or hormone-like factors elaborated include

- *Antidiuretic hormone* (ADH), inducing hyponatremia owing to inappropriate ADH secretion
- *Adrenocorticotropic hormone* (ACTH), producing Cushing syndrome
- *Parathormone, parathyroid hormone-related peptide, prostaglandin E, and some cytokines*, all implicated in the hypercalcemia often seen with lung cancer
- *Calcitonin*, causing hypocalcemia
- *Gonadotropins*, causing gynecomastia
- *Serotonin and bradykinin*, associated with the carcinoid syndrome

The incidence of clinically significant syndromes related to these factors ranges from 1% to 10% of all lung cancer

TABLE 15–12 Local Effects of Lung Tumor Spread

Clinical Feature	Pathologic Basis
Pneumonia, abscess, lobar collapse	Tumor obstruction of airway
Lipid pneumonia	Tumor obstruction; accumulation of cellular lipid in foamy macrophages
Pleural effusion	Tumor spread into pleura
Hoarseness	Recurrent laryngeal nerve invasion
Dysphagia	Esophageal invasion
Diaphragm paralysis	Phrenic nerve invasion
Rib destruction	Chest wall invasion
SVC syndrome	SVC compression by tumor
Horner syndrome	Sympathetic ganglia invasion
Pericarditis, tamponade	Pericardial involvement

SVC, superior vena cava.

TABLE 15–11 New International Staging System for Lung Cancer

T1	Tumor <3 cm without pleural or main stem bronchus involvement
T2	Tumor >3 cm or involvement of main stem bronchus 2 cm from carina, visceral pleural involvement, or lobar atelectasis
T3	Tumor with involvement of chest wall (including superior sulcus tumors), diaphragm, mediastinal pleura, pericardium, main stem bronchus 2 cm from carina, or entire lung atelectasis
T4	Tumor with invasion of mediastinum, heart, great vessels, trachea, esophagus, vertebral body, or carina or with a malignant pleural effusion
N0	No demonstrable metastasis to regional lymph nodes
N1	Ipsilateral hilar or peribronchial nodal involvement
N2	Metastasis to ipsilateral mediastinal or subcarinal lymph nodes
N3	Metastasis to contralateral mediastinal or hilar lymph nodes, ipsilateral or contralateral scalene, or supraclavicular lymph nodes
M0	No (known) distant metastasis
M1	Distant metastasis present

Stage Grouping			
Stage Ia	T1	N0	M0
Stage Ib	T2	N0	M0
Stage IIa	T1	N1	M0
Stage IIb	T2 T3	N1 N0	M0 M0
Stage IIIa	T1–3 T3	N2 N1	M0 M0
Stage IIIb	Any T T3 T4	N3 N2 Any N	M0 M0 M0
Stage IV	Any T	Any N	M1

Adapted from Mountain C: Revisions in the International System for Staging Lung Cancer. Chest 111:1710, 1997.

patients, although a much higher proportion of patients show elevated serum levels of these (and other) peptide hormones. Any one of the histologic types of tumors may occasionally produce any one of the hormones, but tumors that produce ACTH and ADH are predominantly small cell carcinomas, whereas those that produce hypercalcemia are mostly squamous cell tumors. The carcinoid syndrome is more common with the carcinoid tumor, described later, and is only rarely associated with small cell carcinoma. However, small cell carcinoma occurs much more commonly; therefore, one is much more likely to encounter carcinoid syndrome in these patients.

Other systemic manifestations of lung carcinoma include the *Lambert-Eaton myasthenic syndrome* (Chapter 27), in which muscle weakness is caused by auto-antibodies (possibly elicited by tumor ionic channels) directed to the neuronal calcium channel;[127] *peripheral neuropathy*, usually purely sensory; dermatologic abnormalities, including *acanthosis nigricans* (Chapter 25); hematologic abnormalities, such as *leukemoid reactions*; and finally, a peculiar abnormality of connective tissue called *hypertrophic pulmonary osteoarthropathy*, associated with clubbing of the fingers.

Apical lung cancers in the superior pulmonary sulcus tend to invade the neural structures around the trachea, including the cervical sympathetic plexus, and produce a group of clinical findings that includes severe pain in the distribution of the ulnar nerve and *Horner syndrome* (enophthalmos, ptosis, miosis, and anhidrosis) on the same side as the lesion. Such tumors are also referred to as *Pancoast tumors*.

NEUROENDOCRINE PROLIFERATIONS AND TUMORS

Neuroendocrine lesions share morphologic and biochemical features with cells of the *dispersed neuroendocrine cell system* (Chapter 24).[128] The normal lung contains neuroendocrine cells within the epithelium as single cells or as clusters, the neuroepithelial bodies. While virtually all pulmonary neuroendocrine cell hyperplasias are secondary to airway fibrosis and/or inflammation, a rare disorder called diffuse idiopathic pulmonary neuroendocrine cell hyperplasia appears to be a precursor to the development of multiple tumorlets and typical or atypical carcinoids.

Neoplasms of neuroendocrine cells in the lung include benign *tumorlets*, small, inconsequential hyperplastic neuroendocrine cells seen in areas of scarring or chronic inflammation; *carcinoids*; and the (already discussed) highly aggressive small cell carcinoma and large cell neuroendocrine carcinoma of the lung. Although neuroendocrine tumors share certain morphologic, ultrastructural, molecular genetic, and immunohistochemical characteristics, they are classified separately, since there are significant differences between them in incidence, clinical, epidemiologic, histologic, survival, and molecular characteristics. For example, in contrast to small cell and large cell neuroendocrine carcinomas, both typical and atypical carcinoids can occur in patients with multiple endocrine neoplasia type I. Also note that neuroendocrine differentiation can be demonstrated by immunohistochemistry in 10% to 20% of lung carcinomas that do not show neuroendocrine morphology by light microscopy, the clinical significance of which is uncertain.

Carcinoid Tumors. Carcinoid tumors represent 1% to 5% of all lung tumors. Most patients with these tumors are younger than 40 years of age, and the incidence is equal for both sexes. Approximately 20% to 40% of patients are nonsmokers. Carcinoid tumors are low-grade malignant epithelial neoplasms that are subclassified into *typical* and *atypical carcinoids* on the basis of morphologic criteria described below. Typical carcinoids have no *p53* mutations or *BCL2/BAX* imbalance, while atypical carcinoids show these changes in 20% to 40% and 10% to 20% of tumors, respectively. Some carcinoids also show loss of heterozygosty at 3p, 13q14 (RB), 9p, and 5q22, which are found in all neuroendocrine tumors with increasing frequency from typical to atypical carcinoid to large cell neuroendocrine and small cell carcinoma.

Morphology. Carcinoids may arise centrally or may be peripheral. On gross examination, the central tumors grow as finger-like or spherical polypoid masses that commonly project into the lumen of the bronchus and are usually covered by an intact mucosa (Fig. 15–46*A*). They rarely exceed 3 to 4 cm in diameter. Most are confined to the main stem bronchi.

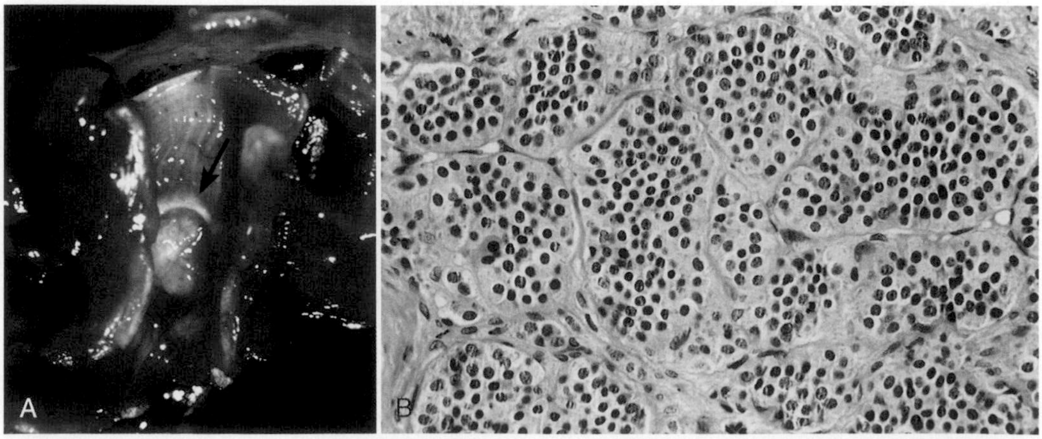

FIGURE 15–46 *A*, Bronchial carcinoid growing as a spherical, pale mass (*arrow*) protruding into the lumen of the bronchus. *B*, Histologic appearance of bronchial carcinoid, demonstrating small, rounded, uniform cells.

Others, however, produce little intraluminal mass but instead penetrate the bronchial wall to fan out in the peribronchial tissue, producing the so-called collar-button lesion. Peripheral tumors are solid and nodular. Spread to local lymph nodes at the time of resection is more likely with atypical carcinoid.

Histologically, the tumor is composed of organoid, trabecular, palisading, ribbon, or rosette-like arrangements of cells separated by a delicate fibrovascular stroma. In common with the lesions of the gastrointestinal tract, the individual cells are quite regular and have uniform round nuclei and a moderate amount of eosinophilic cytoplasm (Fig. 15–46*B*). On electron microscopy, the cells exhibit the dense-core granules characteristic of other neuroendocrine tumors and, by immunochemistry, are found to contain serotonin, neuron-specific enolase, bombesin, calcitonin, or other peptides. Typical carcinoids have fewer than two mitoses per 10 high-power fields and lack necrosis, while atypical carcinoids have between two and 10 mitoses per 10 high-power fields and/or foci of necrosis.[129] The atypical carcinoids tend to show more cellular atypia, increased cellularity, nucleoli, lymphatic invasion, and disorganized architecture.

Clinical Features. The clinical manifestations of bronchial carcinoids emanate from their intraluminal growth, their capacity to metastasize, and the ability of some of the lesions to elaborate vasoactive amines. Persistent cough, hemoptysis, impairment of drainage of respiratory passages with secondary infections, bronchiectasis, emphysema, and atelectasis all are byproducts of the intraluminal growth of these lesions.

Most interesting, albeit rare, are functioning lesions capable of producing the classic carcinoid syndrome, that is, intermittent attacks of diarrhea, flushing, and cyanosis. Overall, most bronchial carcinoids do not have secretory activity and do not metastasize to distant sites but follow a relatively benign course for long periods and are therefore amenable to resection. The reported 5- to 10-year survival rates are 87% and 87% for typical carcinoids, 56% and 35% for atypical carcinoids, 27% and 9% for large cell neuroendocrine carcinoma, and 9% and 5% for small cell carcinoma, respectively.[129]

MISCELLANEOUS TUMORS

Lesions of the complex category of benign and malignant mesenchymal tumors, such as inflammatory myofibroblastic tumor, fibroma, fibrosarcoma, lymphangioleiomyomatosis, leiomyoma, leiomyosarcoma, lipoma, hemangioma, hemangiopericytoma, and chondroma, may occur but are rare. Benign and malignant hematopoeitic tumors, similar to those described in other organs, may also affect the lung, either as isolated lesions or, more commonly, as part of a generalized disorder. These include Langerhans cell histiocytosis, non-Hodgkin and Hodgkin lymphomas, lymphomatoid granulomatosis (which are diffuse large B-cell and T-cell lymphomas), and low-grade marginal zone B-cell lymphoma of the mucosa-associated lymphoid tissue.

A lung *hamartoma* is a relatively common lesion that is usually discovered as an incidental, rounded focus of radio-opacity (*coin lesion*) on a routine chest film. The majority of the tumors are peripheral, solitary, less than 3 to 4 cm in diameter, and well circumscribed. Pulmonary hamartoma consists of nodules of connective tissue intersected by epithelial clefts. Cartilage is the most common connective tissue, but there may also be cellular fibrous tissue and fat. The epithelial clefts are lined by ciliated columnar epithelium or nonciliated epithelium and probably represent entrapment of respiratory epithelium. The traditional term "hamartoma" is retained for this lesion, but several features suggest that it is a neoplasm rather than a congenital lesion, such as its rarity in childhood, its increasing incidence with age, and the finding of chromosomal aberrations involving either 6p21 or 12q14–15, indicating a clonal origin.[115]

Inflammatory myofibroblastic tumor, although rare, is more common in children, with an equal male to female ratio. Presenting symptoms include fever, cough, chest pain, and hemoptysis. It may also be asymptomatic. Imaging studies show a single (rarely multiple) round, well-defined, usually peripheral mass with calcium deposits in about a quarter of cases. Grossly, the lesion is firm, 3 to 10 cm in diameter, and grayish white. Microscopically, there is proliferation of spindle-shaped fibroblasts and myofibroblasts, lymphocytes, plasma cells, and peripheral fibrosis. Clonal chromosomal aberrations have been demonstrated in a number of these tumors, indicating that these are neoplastic proliferations.

Tumors in the mediastinum either may arise in mediastinal structures or may be metastatic from the lung or other organs. They may also invade or compress the lungs. Table 15–13 lists the most common tumors in the various compartments of the mediastinum. Specific tumor types are discussed in appropriate sections of this book.

METASTATIC TUMORS

The lung is the most common site of metastatic neoplasms. Both carcinomas and sarcomas arising anywhere in the body may spread to the lungs via the blood or lymphatics or by direct continuity. Growth of contiguous tumors into the lungs

TABLE 15–13 Mediastinal Tumors and Other Masses

Superior Mediastinum
Lymphoma
Thymoma
Thyroid lesions
Metastatic carcinoma
Parathyroid tumors
Anterior Mediastinum
Thymoma
Teratoma
Lymphoma
Thyroid lesions
Parathyroid tumors
Posterior Mediastinum
Neurogenic tumors (schwannoma, neurofibroma)
Lymphoma
Gastroenteric hernia
Middle Mediastinum
Bronchogenic cyst
Pericardial cyst
Lymphoma

occurs most often with esophageal carcinomas and mediastinal lymphomas.

Morphology. The pattern of metastatic growth within the lungs is quite variable. In the usual case, multiple discrete nodules (cannonball lesions) are scattered throughout all lobes (Fig. 15–47). These discrete lesions tend to occur in the periphery of the lung rather than in the central locations of the primary lung carcinoma. Other patterns include solitary nodule, endobronchial, pleural, pneumonic consolidation, and mixtures of the above. Foci of lepidic growth similar to bronchioloalveolar carcinoma are seen occasionally with metastatic carcinomas and may be associated with any of the patterns listed above.

Metastatic growth may be confined to peribronchiolar and perivascular tissue spaces, presumably when the tumor has extended to the lung through the lymphatics. In these cases, the lung septa and connective tissue are diffusely infiltrated with the gray-white tumor. The subpleural lymphatics may be outlined by the contained tumor, producing a gross appearance referred to as lymphangitis carcinomatosa. Least commonly, the metastatic tumor is not apparent on gross examination and becomes evident only on histologic section as a diffuse intralymphatic dissemination dispersed throughout the peribronchial and perivascular channels. In certain instances, microscopic tumor emboli fill the small pulmonary vessels and may result in life-threatening pulmonary hypertension or hemorrhage and hemoptysis.

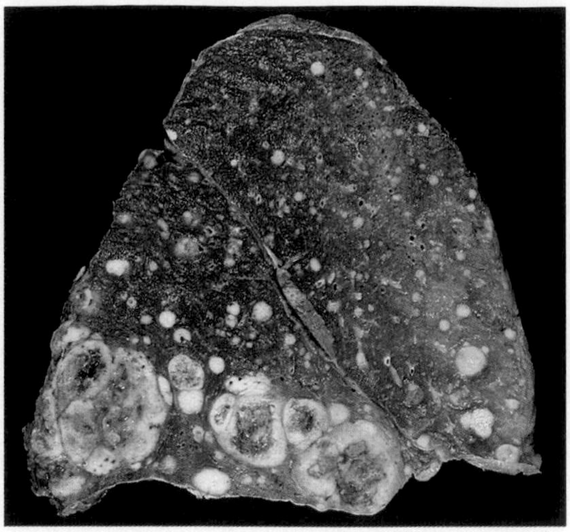

FIGURE 15–47 Numerous metastases from a renal cell carcinoma. (Courtesy of Dr. Michelle Mantel, Brigham and Women's Hospital, Boston, MA.)

Pleura

Pathologic involvement of the pleura is, with rare exceptions, a secondary complication of some underlying disease. Secondary infections and pleural adhesions are particularly common findings at autopsy. Occasionally, the secondary pleural disease assumes a dominant role in the clinical problem, as occurs in bacterial pneumonia with the development of empyema. Important primary disorders include (1) primary intrapleural bacterial infections that imply seeding of this space as an isolated focus in the course of a transient bacteremia and (2) a primary neoplasm of the pleura: mesothelioma (discussed later).

PLEURAL EFFUSION

Pleural effusion is a common manifestation of both primary and secondary pleural diseases. Normally, no more than 15 mL of serous, relatively acellular, clear fluid lubricates the pleural surface. Increased accumulation of pleural fluid occurs in the following settings:

- Increased hydrostatic pressure, as in congestive heart failure
- Increased vascular permeability, as in pneumonia
- Decreased osmotic pressure, as in nephrotic syndrome
- Increased intrapleural negative pressure, as in atelectasis
- Decreased lymphatic drainage, as in mediastinal carcinomatosis

The character of the pleural effusion can be divided, for convenience, into inflammatory or noninflammatory, as summarized in Table 15–14.

Inflammatory Pleural Effusions

Serous, *serofibrinous*, and fibrinous *pleuritis* all are caused by essentially the same processes. Fibrinous exudations generally reflect a later, more severe exudative reaction that, in an earlier developmental phase, might have presented as a serous or serofibrinous exudate.

The common causes of pleuritis are inflammatory diseases within the lungs, such as tuberculosis, pneumonia, lung infarcts, lung abscess, and bronchiectasis. Rheumatoid arthritis, disseminated lupus erythematosus, uremia, diffuse systemic infections, other systemic disorders, and metastatic

TABLE 15–14 Pleural Space Fluid Accumulations

Condition	Type of Fluid	Common Associations
Inflammatory		
Serofibrinous pleuritis	Serofibrinous exudate	Inflammation in adjacent lung Collagen vascular disease
Suppurative pleuritis (empyema)	Pus	Suppurative infection in adjacent lung
Hemorrhagic pleuritis	Bloody exudate	Tumor
Noninflammatory		
Hydrothorax	Transudate	Congestive heart failure
Hemothorax	Blood	Ruptured aortic aneurysm, trauma
Chylothorax	Chyle (lymph)	Tumor obstruction of normal lymphatics

involvement of the pleura can also cause serous or serofibrinous pleuritis. Radiation used in therapy for tumors in the lung or mediastinum often causes a serofibrinous pleuritis. In most instances, the serofibrinous reaction is only minimal, and the fluid exudate is resorbed with either resolution or organization of the fibrinous component. Accumulation of large amounts of fluid can sufficiently encroach on lung space to give rise to respiratory distress.

A purulent pleural exudate (*empyema*) usually results from bacterial or mycotic seeding of the pleural space. Most commonly, this seeding occurs by contiguous spread of organisms from intrapulmonary infection, but occasionally, it occurs through lymphatic or hematogenous dissemination from a more distant source. Rarely, infections below the diaphragm, such as the subdiaphragmatic or liver abscess, may extend by continuity through the diaphragm into the pleural spaces, more often on the right side.

Empyema is characterized by loculated, yellow-green, creamy pus composed of masses of neutrophils admixed with other leukocytes. Although it might be difficult to visualize microorganisms on smears of the exudate, it should be possible to demonstrate them by culture. Although empyema may accumulate in large volumes (up to 500 to 1000 mL), usually the volume is small, and the pus becomes localized. Empyema may resolve, but this outcome is less common than organization of the exudate, with the formation of dense, tough fibrous adhesions that frequently obliterate the pleural space or envelop the lungs; either can seriously embarrass pulmonary expansion.

True *hemorrhagic pleuritis* manifested by sanguineous inflammatory exudates is infrequent and is found in hemorrhagic diatheses, rickettsial diseases, and neoplastic involvement of the pleural cavity. The sanguineous exudate must be differentiated from hemothorax (discussed later). When hemorrhagic pleuritis is encountered, careful search should be made for the presence of exfoliated tumor cells.

Noninflammatory Pleural Effusions

Noninflammatory collections of serous fluid within the pleural cavities are called *hydrothorax*. The fluid is clear and straw colored. Hydrothorax may be unilateral or bilateral, depending on the underlying cause. The most common cause of hydrothorax is cardiac failure, and for this reason, it is usually accompanied by pulmonary congestion and edema. In cardiac failure, hydrothorax is usually, but not invariably, bilateral. Transudates may collect in any other systemic disease associated with generalized edema and are therefore found in renal failure and cirrhosis of the liver.

In most instances, hydrothorax is not loculated, but in the presence of preexistent pleural adhesions, local collections may be found walled off by bridging fibrous tissue. Except for these localized collections, the fluid usually collects basally, when the patient is in an upright position, and causes compression and atelectasis of the regions of the lung surrounded by fluid. If the underlying cause is alleviated, hydrothorax may be resorbed, usually leaving behind no permanent alterations. Relief of respiratory distress is accomplished by the withdrawal of large pleural transudates.

The escape of blood into the pleural cavity is known as *hemothorax*. It is almost invariably a fatal complication of a ruptured aortic aneurysm or vascular trauma. Pure hemothorax is readily identifiable by the large clots that accompany the fluid component of the blood. Because this calamity often leads to death within minutes to hours, it is uncommon to find any inflammatory response within the pleural cavity. Rarely, nonfatal leakage of smaller amounts can provide a stimulus to organization and the development of pleural adhesions.

Chylothorax is an accumulation of milky fluid, usually of lymphatic origin, in the pleural cavity. Chyle is milky white because it contains finely emulsified fats. When it is allowed to stand, a creamy, fatty, supernatant layer separates. True chyle should be differentiated from turbid serous fluid, which does not contain fat and does not separate into an overlying layer of high fat content. Chylothorax may be bilateral but is more often confined to the left side. The volume of fluid is variable but rarely assumes the massive proportions of hydrothorax.

Chylothorax is most often caused by thoracic duct trauma or obstruction that secondarily causes rupture of major lymphatic ducts. This disorder is encountered in malignant conditions arising within the thoracic cavity that cause obstruction of the major lymphatic ducts. More distant cancers may metastasize via the lymphatics and grow within the right lymphatic or thoracic duct to produce obstruction.

A pleural effusion, more commonly right-sided, may be associated with ascites from any cause. The pressure gradient between the peritoneal and pleural cavities favors movement of fluid into the thorax across lymphatics and, occasionally, diaphragmatic defects.

PNEUMOTHORAX

Pneumothorax refers to air or gas in the pleural cavities and may be spontaneous, traumatic, or therapeutic. Spontaneous pneumothorax may complicate any form of pulmonary disease that causes rupture of an alveolus. An abscess cavity that communicates either directly with the pleural space or with the lung interstitial tissue may also lead to the escape of air. In the latter circumstance, the air may dissect through the lung substance or back through the mediastinum (interstitial emphysema), eventually entering the pleural cavity. *Pneumothorax is most commonly associated with emphysema, asthma, and tuberculosis.* Traumatic pneumothorax is usually caused by some perforating injury to the chest wall, but sometimes the trauma pierces the lung and thus provides two avenues for the accumulation of air within the pleural spaces. Resorption of the pleural space air occurs slowly in spontaneous and traumatic pneumothorax, provided that the original communication seals itself.

Of the various forms of pneumothorax, the one that attracts greatest clinical attention is so-called *spontaneous idiopathic pneumothorax.* This entity is encountered in relatively young people; appears to be due to rupture of small, peripheral, usually apical subpleural blebs; and usually subsides spontaneously as the air is resorbed. Recurrent attacks are common and can be quite disabling.

Pneumothorax may have as much clinical significance as a fluid collection in the lungs because it also causes compression, collapse, and atelectasis of the lung and may be responsible for marked respiratory distress. Occasionally, the lung collapse is marked. When the defect acts as a flap valve and permits the entrance of air during inspiration but fails to permit its escape during expiration, it effectively acts as a pump that creates the progressively increasing pressures of *tension pneumothorax*, which may be sufficient to compress the vital mediastinal structures and the contralateral lung.

PLEURAL TUMORS

The pleura may be involved by primary or secondary tumors. Secondary metastatic involvement is far more common than are primary tumors. The most frequent metastatic malignancies arise from primary neoplasms of the lung and breast. In addition to these cancers, malignancy from any organ of the body may spread to the pleural spaces. Ovarian carcinomas, for example, tend to cause widespread implants in both the abdominal and thoracic cavities. In most metastatic involvements, a serous or serosanguineous effusion follows that often contains neoplastic cells. For this reason, careful cytologic examination of the sediment is of considerable diagnostic value.

Solitary (Localized) Fibrous Tumors

Previously called "benign mesothelioma" or "benign fibrous mesothelioma" in the pleura and "fibroma" in the lung, localized fibrous tumors are now recognized as soft tissue tumors with a propensity to occur in the pleura and, less commonly, in the lung, as well as other sites. The tumor is often attached to the pleural surface by a pedicle.[130] It may be small (1 to 2 cm in diameter) or may reach an enormous size, but it tends to remain confined to the surface of the lung. These tumors do not usually produce a pleural effusion. Grossly, they consist of dense fibrous tissue with occasional cysts filled with viscid fluid; microscopically, the tumors show whorls of reticulin and collagen fibers among which are interspersed spindle cells resembling fibroblasts. Rarely, these tumors may be malignant, with pleomorphism, mitotic activity, necrosis, and large size (>10 cm). The tumor cells are CD34+ and keratin-negative by immunostaining. This feature can be diagnostically useful in distinguishing these lesions from malignant mesotheliomas (which show the opposite phenotype). The solitary fibrous tumor has no relationship to asbestos exposure.

Malignant Mesothelioma

Malignant mesotheliomas in the thorax arise from either the visceral or the parietal pleura.[131,132] Although uncommon, they have assumed great importance in the past few years because of their increased incidence among people with heavy exposure to asbestos (see the earlier section on pneumoconioses). In coastal areas with shipping industries in the United States and Great Britain and in Canadian and South African mining areas, up to 90% of reported mesotheliomas are asbestos-related. The lifetime risk of developing mesothelioma in heavily exposed individuals is as high as 7% to 10%. There is a long latent period of 25 to 45 years for the development of asbestos-related mesothelioma, and there seems to be no increased risk of mesothelioma in asbestos workers who smoke. *This is in contrast to the risk of asbestos-related lung carcinoma, already high, and is markedly magnified by smoking. Thus, for asbestos workers (particularly those who are also smokers), the risk of dying of lung carcinoma far exceeds that of developing mesothelioma.*

Asbestos bodies (see Fig. 15–21) are found in increased numbers in the lungs of patients with mesothelioma. Another marker of *asbestos exposure*, the *asbestos plaque*, has been previously discussed.

Cytogenetic studies have shown that approximately 60% to 80% of malignant mesotheliomas have deletions in chromosomes 1p, 3p, 6q, 9p, or 22q. There is a low frequency of *p53* mutations, although *p53* accumulation can be detected immunohistochemically in 70% of malignant mesotheliomas. Some but not all studies have demonstrated the presence of SV40 (simian virus 40) viral DNA sequences in 60% to 80% of pleural malignant mesotheliomas and in a smaller fraction of peritoneal mesotheliomas. The SV40 T-antigen is a potent carcinogen that binds to and inactivates several critical regulators of growth, such as *p53* and *RB*. Whether SV40 is involved in the pathogenesis of mesothelioma remains controversial.

Morphology. Malignant mesothelioma is a diffuse lesion that spreads widely in the pleural space and is usually associated with extensive pleural effusion and direct invasion of thoracic structures. The affected lung gets ensheathed by a thick layer of soft, gelatinous, grayish pink tumor tissue (Fig. 15–48).

Microscopically, malignant mesotheliomas consist of a mixture of two types of cells, either one of which might predominate in an individual case. Mesothelial cells have the potential to develop as either epithelium-like lining cells or mesenchymal stromal cells. The **epithelioid type** of mesothelioma consists of cuboidal, columnar, or flattened cells forming tubular or papillary structures resembling adenocarcinoma (Fig. 15–49*A*). Epithelioid mesothelioma may at times be difficult to differentiate grossly and histologically from pulmonary adenocarcinoma. Features that favor mesothelioma include (1) positive staining for acid mucopolysaccharide, which is inhibited by previous digestion by hyaluronidase; (2) lack of staining for carcinoembryonic antigen (CEA) and other epithelial glycoprotein antigens, markers that are generally expressed by adenocarcinoma; (3) strong staining for keratin proteins, with accentuation of perinuclear

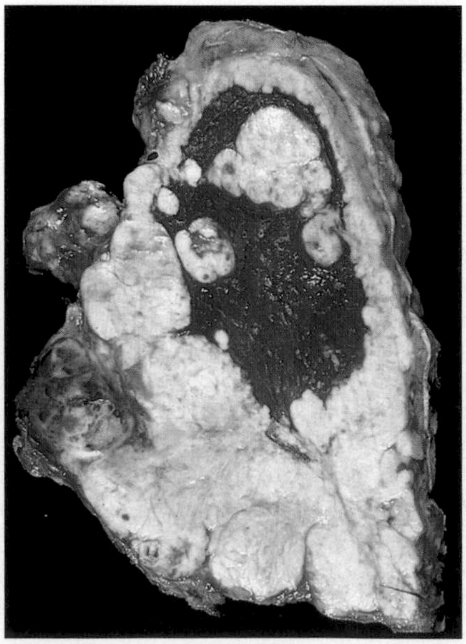

FIGURE 15–48 Malignant mesothelioma. Note the thick, firm, white pleural tumor tissue that ensheathes this bisected lung.

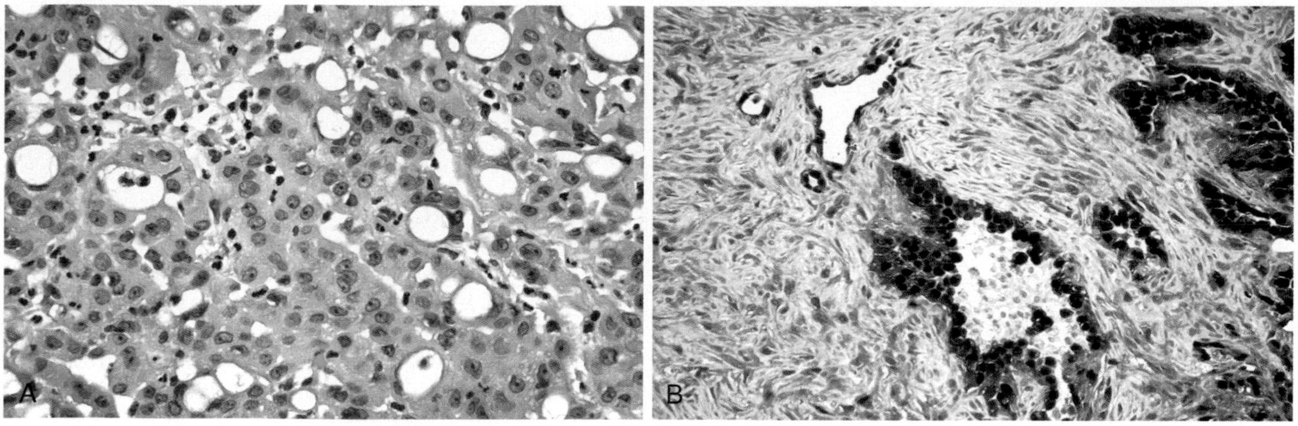

FIGURE 15–49 *A*, Malignant mesothelioma, epithelial type. *B*, Malignant mesothelioma, mixed type, stained for calretinin (immunoperoxidase method). The epithelial component is strongly positive (*dark brown*), while the sarcomatoid component is less so. (Courtesy of Dr. Thomas Krausz, Department of Pathology, The University of Chicago, Pritzker School of Medicine, Chicago, IL.)

rather than peripheral staining; (4) positive staining for calretinin (Fig. 15–49*B*), Wilms tumor 1 susceptibility gene product, cytokeratin 5/6, mesothelin, and thrombomodulin; and (5) on electron microscopy, the presence of long microvilli and abundant tonofilaments but absent microvillous rootlets and lamellar bodies (Fig. 15–50). The gold standard of diagnosis is electron microscopy. However, the panel of special stains is very helpful when interpreted in the context of morphology and clinical presentation. The mesenchymal type of mesothelioma appears as a spindle cell sarcoma, resembling fibrosarcoma (**sarcomatoid type**). The **mixed type** of mesothelioma contains both epithelioid and sarcomatoid patterns (Fig. 15–49*B*).

Clinical Course. The presenting complaints are chest pain, dyspnea, and, as noted, recurrent pleural effusions. Concurrent pulmonary asbestosis (fibrosis) is present in only 20% of patients with pleural mesothelioma. The lung is invaded directly, and there is often metastatic spread to the hilar lymph nodes and, eventually, to the liver and other distant organs. Fifty per cent of patients die within 12 months of diagnosis, and few survive longer than 2 years. Aggressive therapy (extrapleural pneumonectomy, chemotherapy, radiation therapy) appears to improve this poor prognosis in some patients.

Mesotheliomas also arise in the peritoneum, pericardium, tunica vaginalis, and genital tract (benign adenomatoid tumor; see Chapter 21). *Peritoneal mesotheliomas* are particularly related to heavy asbestos exposure; 50% of such patients also have pulmonary fibrosis. Although in about 50% of cases

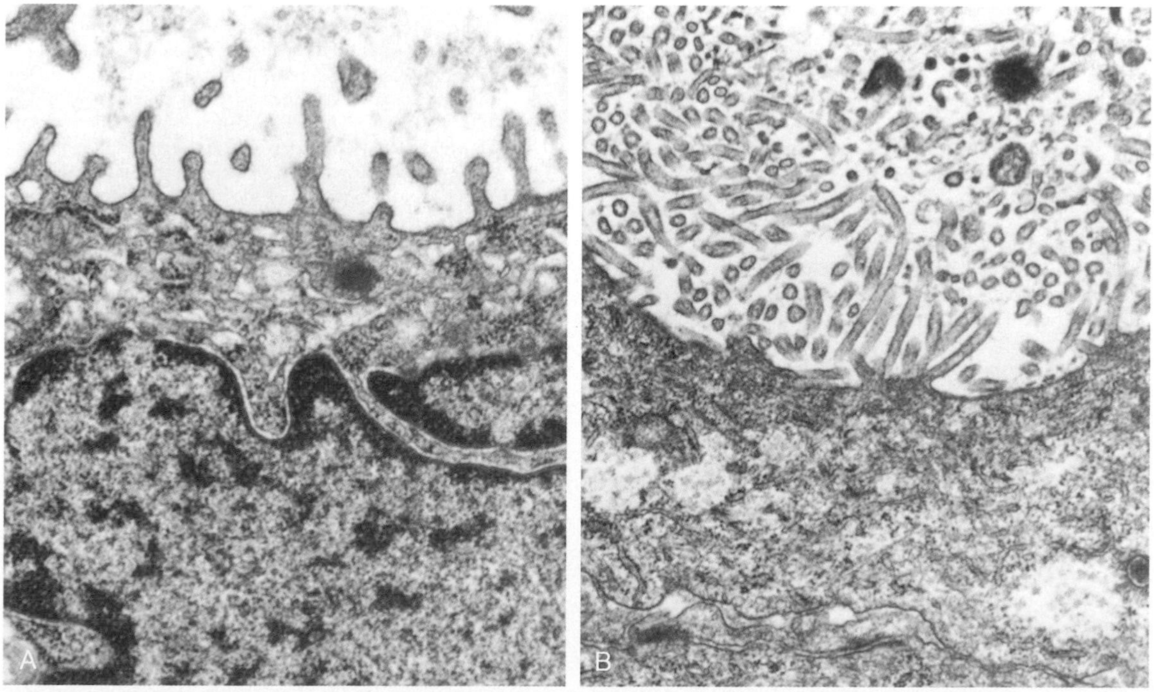

FIGURE 15–50 Ultrastructural features of pulmonary adenocarcinoma (*A*), characterized by short, plump microvilli, contrasted with those of mesothelioma (*B*), in which microvilli are numerous, long, and slender. (Courtesy of Dr. Noel Weidner, University of California, San Francisco, School of Medicine, San Francisco, CA.)

the disease remains confined to the abdominal cavity, intestinal involvement frequently leads to death from intestinal obstruction or inanition.

REFERENCES

1. Stocker JT: The respiratory tract. In Stocker JT, Dehner LP (eds): Pediatric Pathology, 2nd ed. Philadelphia, Lippincott Williams & Wilkins, 2001, pp 446–517.
2. Leikauf GD, McDowell SA, Wesselkamper SC, Hardie WD, Leikauf JE, Korfhagen TR, Prows DR: Acute lung injury: functional genomics and genetic susceptibility. Chest 121:70S, 2002.
3. Bigatello LM, Zapol WM: New approaches to acute lung injury. Br J Anaesth 77:99, 1996.
4. Fan J, Ye RD, Malik AB: Transcriptional mechanisms of acute lung injury. Am J Physiol Lung Cell Mol Physiol 281:L1037, 2001.
5. Katzenstein AL, Myers JL, Mazur MT: Acute interstitial pneumonia: a clinicopathologic, ultrastructural, and cell kinetic study. Am J Surg Pathol 10:256, 1986.
6. Bouros D, Nicholson AC, Polychronopoulos V, du Bois RM: Acute interstitial pneumonia. Eur Respir J 15:412, 2000.
7. Katzenstein AL, Askin FB (eds): Surgical Pathology of Non-Neoplastic Lung Disease. Philadelphia, WB Saunders, 1997.
8. Shaw RJ, Djukanovic R, Tashkin DP, Millar AB, du Bois RM, Orr PA: The role of small airways in lung disease. Respir Med 96:67, 2002.
9. Barnes PJ: Novel approaches and targets for treatment of chronic obstructive pulmonary disease. Am J Respir Crit Care Med 160:S72, 1999.
10. Snider G, et al: The definition of emphysema: report of the National Heart, Lung, and Blood Institute, Division of Lung Diseases Workshop. Am Rev Respir Dis 132:182, 1985.
11. National Heart Lung and Blood Institute. Morbidity and Mortality Chartbook on Cardiovascular Lung and Blood Disease. Bethesda, MD, US Department of Health and Human Services, National Institutes of Health, 1998.
12. World Health Report. Geneva, Switzerland, World Health Organization, 2000.
13. Wright JL: Emphysema: concepts under change: a pathologist's perspective. Mod Pathol 8:873, 1995.
14. Pauwels RA, Buist AS, Calverley PM, Jenkins CR, Hurd SS: Global strategy for the diagnosis, management, and prevention of chronic obstructive pulmonary disease. NHLBI/WHO Global Initiative for Chronic Obstructive Lung Disease (GOLD) Workshop summary. Am J Respir Crit Care Med 163:1256, 2001.
15. Lamb, D: Chronic bronchitis, emphysema, and the pathological basis of chronic obstsructive pulmonary disease. In Hasleton P (ed): Spencer's Pathology of the Lung. New York, McGraw-Hill, 1996, pp 597–630.
16. Gross P: Enzymatically produced pulmonary emphysema: a preliminary report. J Occup Med 6:481, 1964.
17. Senior RM, Tegner H, Kuhn C, Ohlsson K, Starcher BC, Pierce JAL: The induction of pulmonary emphysema with human leukocyte elastase. Am Rev Respir Dis 116:469, 1977.
18. Hautami R: Requirement for macrophage elastase for cigarette smoke-induced emphysema in mice. Science 277:2002, 1997.
19. Barnes PJ: New concepts in chronic obstructive pulmonary disease. Annu Rev Med 54:113, 2003.
20. DeMello D, Reid L: Chronic bronchitis. In Saldana M (ed): Pathology of Pulmonary Disease, Philadelphia, J.B. Lippincott, 1994, p 287.
21. Wright JL, Cagle P, Churg A, Colby TV, Myers J: Diseases of the small airways. Am Rev Respir Dis 146:240, 1992.
22. Thurlbeck WM: Pathology of chronic airflow obstruction. In Cherniack NS (ed): Chronic Obstructive Pulmonary Disease, Philadelphia, WB Saunders, 1991, p 3.
23. Hogg JC, Macklem PT, Thurlbeck WM: Site and nature of airway obstruction in chronic obstructive lung disease. N Engl J Med 278:1355, 1968.
24. Cosio M, Ghezzo H, Hogg JC, Corbin R, Lovel M, Dosman J, Macklem PT: The relations between structural changes in small airways and pulmonary-function tests. N Engl J Med 298:1277, 1978.
25. Colby TV: Bronchiolitis: pathologic considerations. Am J Clin Pathol 101–109, 1998.
26. Boushey HA, Corry DB, Fahy JV: Asthma. In Murray JF, Nadel JA (eds): Textbook of Respiratory Medicine, 3rd ed. Philadelphia, WB Saunders, 2000, p 1247.
27. Vogel G: New clues to asthma therapies. Science 276:1643, 1997.
28. Schwartz RS: A new element in the mechanism of asthma. N Engl J Med 346:857, 2002.
29. Busse WW, Lemanske RF Jr: Asthma N Engl J Med 344:350, 2001.
30. Davies D, et al: Airway remodeling in asthma: new insights. J Allergy Clin Immunol 111:215, 2003.
31. Shapiro S, Owen C: CA ADAM-33 surfaces as an asthma gene. N Engl J Med 347:936, 2002.
32. Black J: The role of mast cells in the pathophysiology of asthma. N Engl J Med 346:1742, 2002.
33. Galli SJ: The Paul Kallos Memorial Lecture: The mast cell: a versatile effector cell for challenging world. Intl Arch Allery Immunol 113:14, 1997.
34. Shelhamer JH, Levine SJ, Wu T, Jacoby DB, Kaliner MA, Rennard SI: NIH conference: airway inflammation. Ann Intern Med 123:288, 1995.
35. Lilly CM, Nakamura H, Kesselman H, Nagler-Anderson C, Asano K, Garcia-Zepeda EA, Rothenberg ME, Drazen JM, Luster AD: Expression of eotaxin by human lung epithelial cells: induction by cytokines and inhibition by glucocorticoids. J Clin Invest 99:1767, 1997.
36. Costa JJ, Weller PF, Galli SJ: The cells of the allergic response: mast cells, basophils, eosinophils. JAMA 278:1815, 1997.
37. Barnes P: Inflammatory mediators and neural mechanisms in severe asthma. In Szefler S, Leung D (eds): Severe Asthma: Pathogenesis and Clinical Management. New York, Marcel Dekker 1996, p 129.
38. Corne JM, Holgate ST: Mechanisms of virus induced exacerbations of asthma. Thorax 52:380, 1997.
39. Luce L: Bronchiectasis. In Murray J, Nadel J (eds): Textbook of Respiratory Medicine, vol 2. Philadelphia, WB Saunders, 1994, pp 1398–1417.
40. Barker A: Bronchiectasis. New Engl J Med 18:1383, 2002.
41. Wark PA, Gibson PG: Allergic bronchopulmonary aspergillosis: new concepts of pathogenesis and treatment. Respirology 6:1–7, 2001.
42. Colby V: Tumors of the Lower Respiratory Tract, 3rd series. Washington, DC, Armed Forces Institute of Pathology, 1995.
43. Chan-Yeung M, Muller NL: Cryptogenic fibrosing alveolitis. Lancet 350:651–656, 1997.
44. Kumar RK, Lykke AW: Messages and handshakes: cellular interactions in pulmonary fibrosis. Pathology 27:18–26, 1995.
45. Vaillant P, Menard O, Vignaud JM, Martinet N, Martinet Y: The role of cytokines in human lung fibrosis. Monaldi Arch Chest Dis 51:145–152, 1996.
46. Lynch JP 3rd, Standiford TJ, Rolfe MW, Kunkel SL, Strieter RM: Neutrophilic alveolitis in idiopathic pulmonary fibrosis: the role of interleukin-8. Am Rev Respir Dis 145:1433–1439, 1992.
47. Peters-Golden M: Lipid mediator synthesis by lung macrophages. In Lipscomb M, Russell S (eds): Lung Macrophages and Dendritic Cells in Health Disease. New York, Marcel Dekker, 1997, pp 151–182.
48. Collard HR, King TE Jr: Demystifying idiopathic interstitial pneumonia. Arch Intern Med 163:17–29, 2003.
49. ATS European Respiratory Society International Multidisclipinary Consensus: Classification of the idiopathic interstitial pneumonias Am J Respir Crit Care Med 165:277–304, 2002.
50. Gross, TJ, Hunninghake GW: Idiopathic pulmonary fibrosis. N Engl J Med 345:517–525, 2001.
51. Morrisey, E: Wnt signaling pulmonary fibrosis. Am J Pathol 162:1393, 2003.
52. Katzenstein AL, Fiorelli RF: Nonspecific interstitial pneumonia/fibrosis: histologic features and clinical significance. Am J Surg Pathol 18:136–147, 1994.
53. Travis WD, Matsu, K, Moss J, Ferrans, VJ: Idiopathic nonspecific interstitial pneumonia: prognostic significance of cellular and fibrosing patterns: survival comparison with usual interstitial pneumonia and desquamative interstitial pneumonia. Am J Surg Pathol 24:19–33, 2000.
54. Dockery DW, Pope CA 3rd, Xu X, Spengler JD, Ware JH, Fay ME, Ferris BG Jr, Speizer FE: An association between air pollution and mortality in six US cities. N Engl J Med 329:1753–1759, 1993.
55. Pope CA 3rd, Bates DV, Raizenne ME: Health effects of particulate air pollution: time for reassessment? Environ Health Perspect 103:472–480, 1995.
56. Vallyathan V, Shi X: The role of oxygen free radicals in occupational and environmental lung diseases. Environ Health Perspect 105 (Suppl 1):165–177, 1997.
57. Vallyathan V, Shi XL, Dalal NS, Irr W, Castranova V: Generation of free radicals from freshly fractured silica dust: potential role in

acute silica-induced lung injury. Am Rev Respir Dis 138:1213–1219, 1988.
58. Kamp DW, Weitzman SA: Asbestosis: clinical spectrum and pathogenic mechanisms. Proc Soc Exp Biol Med 214:12–26, 1997.
59. Borm PJ: Particle toxicology: from coal mining to nanotechnology. Inhal Toxicol 14:311–324, 2002.
60. Izmerov NF, Kuzmina LP, Tarasova LA: Genetic-biochemical criteria for individual sensitivity in development of occupational bronchopulmonary diseases. Cent Eur J Public Health 10:35–41, 2002.
61. Green F, Vallyathan V: Coal workers' pneumoconioses and pneumonoconiosis due to other carbonaceous dusts. In Churg A, Green F (eds): Pathology of Occupational Lung Disease. Philadelphia, JB Lippincott, 1998, p 387.
62. Godleski JJ: The pneumoconioses: silicosis and silicatosis. In Saldana M (ed): Pathology of Pulmonary Disease. Philadelphia, JB Lippincott, 1994, p 387.
63. Vanhee D, Gosset P, Boitelle A, Wallaert B, Tonnel AB: Cytokines and cytokine network in silicosis and coal workers' pneumoconiosis. Eur Respir J 8:834–842, 1995.
64. Ding M, et al: Diseases caused by silica: mechanisms of injury and disease development. Intl Immunopharmacol 2:173–182, 2002.
65. Kemp D, Wertzman S: The molecular basis of asbestos-induced lung injury. Thorax 54, 1999.
66. Hammond EC: Asbestos exposure, cigarette smoking and death rates. Ann N Y Acad Sci 330:473–490, 1979.
67. Van Cleemput J, De Raeve H, Verschakelen JA, Rombouts J, Lacquet LM, Nemery B: Surface of localized pleural plaques quantitated by computed tomography scanning: no relation with cumulative asbestos exposure and no effect on lung function. Am J Respir Crit Care Med 163:705–710, 2001.
68. Rossi SE, Erasmus JJ, McAdams HP, Sporn TA, Goodman PC: Pulmonary drug toxicity: radiologic and pathologic manifestations. Radiographics 20:1245–1259, 2000.
69. Movsas B, Raffin TA, Epstein AH, Link CJ Jr: Pulmonary radiation injury. Chest 111:1061–1076, 1997.
70. Abratt RP, Morgan GW: Lung toxicity following chest irradiation in patients with lung cancer. Lung Cancer 35:103–109, 2002.
71. Baughman RP, et al: Sarcoidosis. Lancet 361:1111, 2003.
72. Ziegenhagen M, Muller-Quernheim J: The cytokine network in sarcoidosis and its clinical relevance. J Internal Med 253:18, 2003.
73. du Bois RM, Goh N, McGrath D, Cullinan P: Is there a role for microorganisms in the pathogenesis of sarcoidosis? J Intern Med 253:4–17, 2003.
74. Gal AA, Koss MN: The pathology of sarcoidosis. Curr Opin Pulm Med 8:445, 2002.
75. Kolopp-Sarda MN, Kohler C, De March AK, Bene MC, Faure G: Discriminative immunophenotype of bronchoalveolar lavage CD4 lymphocytes in sarcoidosis. Lab Invest 80:1065–1069, 2000.
76. Barnard J, Newman, LS: Sarcoidosis: immunology, rheumatic involvement, and therapeutics. Curr Opin Rheumatol 13:84–91, 2001.
77. Andonopoulos AP, Papadimitriou C, Melachrinou M, Meimaris N, Vlahanastasi C, Bounas A, Georgiou P: Asymptomatic gastrocnemius muscle biopsy: an extremely sensitive and specific test in the pathologic confirmation of sarcoidosis presenting with hilar adenopathy. Clin Exp Rheumatol 19:569–572, 2001.
78. Sharma OP, Fujimura N: Hypersensitivity pneumonitis: a noninfectious granulomatosis. Semin Respir Infect 10:96–106, 1995.
79. Kita H, Sur S, Hunt LW, Edell ES, Weiler DA, Swanson MC, Samsel RW, Abrams JS, Gleich GJ: Cytokine production at the site of disease in chronic eosinophilic pneumonitis. Am J Respir Crit Care Med 153:1437–1441, 1996.
80. Douglas N, Goetzl E: Pulmonary eosinophilia and eosinophilic granuloma. In Murray J, Nadel J (eds): Textbook of Respiratory Medicine. Philadelphia, WB Saunders, 1994, p 1913.
81. Tazelaar HD, Linz LJ, Colby TV, Myers JL, Limper AH: Acute eosinophilic pneumonia: histopathologic findings in nine patients. Am J Respir Crit Care Med 155:296–302, 1997.
82. Nicholson AG, Colby TV, du Bois RM, Hansell DM, Wells AU: The prognostic significance of the histologic pattern of interstitial pneumonia in patients presenting with the clinical entity of cryptogenic fibrosing alveolitis. Am J Respir Crit Care Med 162:2213–2217, 2000.
83. Travis WD: Idiopathic nonspecific interstitial pneumonia: prognostic significance of cellular and fibosing patterns: survival comparison with usual interstitial pneumonia and desquamative interstitial pneumonia. Am J Surg Path 24:19, 2000.
84. Fraig M, Shreesha U, Savici D, Katzenstein AL: Respiratory bronchiolitis: a clinicopathologic study in current smokers, ex-smokers, and never-smokers. Am J Surg Pathol 26:647–653, 2002.
85. Heyneman LE, Ward S, Lynch DA, Remy-Jardin M, Johkoh T, Muller NL: Respiratory bronchiolitis, respiratory bronchiolitis-associated interstitial lung disease, and desquamative interstitial pneumonia: different entities or part of the spectrum of the same disease process? AJR Am J Roentgenol 173:1617–1622, 1999.
86. Moon J, du Bois RM, Colby TV, Hansell DM, Nicholson AG: Clinical significance of respiratory bronchiolitis on open lung biopsy and its relationship to smoking related interstitial lung disease. Thorax 54:1009–1014, 1999.
87. Seymour JF, Presneill JJ: Pulmonary alveolar proteinosis: progress in the first 44 years. Am J Respir Crit Care Med 166:215–235, 2002.
88. DeMello DE, Lin Z: Pulmonary alveolar proteinosis: a review. Pediatr Pathol Mol Med 20:413–432, 2001.
89. Runo J, Loyd J: Primary pulmonary hypertension. Lancet 361:1533, 2003.
90. Mark EJ, Patalas ED, Chang HT, Evans RJ, Kessler SC: Fatal pulmonary hypertension associated with short-term use of fenfluramine and phentermine. N Engl J Med 337:602–606, 1997.
91. Burke AP, Farb A, Virmani R: The pathology of primary pulmonary hypertension. Mod Pathol 4:269–282, 1991.
92. Pietra GG, Edwards WD, Kay JM, Rich S, Kernis J, Schloo B, Ayres SM, Bergofsky EH, Brundage BH, Detre KM, et al: Histopathology of primary pulmonary hypertension: a qualitative and quantitative study of pulmonary blood vessels from 58 patients in the National Heart, Lung, and Blood Institute, Primary Pulmonary Hypertension Registry. Circulation 80:1198–1206, 1989.
93. Fuster V, Steele PM, Edwards WD, Gersh BJ, McGoon MD, Frye RL: Primary pulmonary hypertension: natural history and the importance of thrombosis. Circulation 70:580–587, 1984.
94. Hudson BG, et al: Alport's syndrome, goat pasture syndrome, and type IV collagen. New Engl J Med 348:2543, 2003.
95. Travis WD, Fleming MV: Vasculitis of the lung. Pathology (Phila) 4:23–41, 1996.
96. Gunnarsson A, Hellmark T, Wieslander J: Molecular properties of the Goodpasture epitope. J Biol Chem 275:30844–30848, 2000.
97. Pennington JE: Respiratory Infections: Diagnosis and Management, 3rd ed. New York, Raven Press, 1994.
98. Bartlett JG, et al: The community-acquired pneumonias in adults: guidelines for management. Clin Infect Di 26:811, 1998.
99. Roche RJ, Moxon ER: Phenotypic variation of carbohydrate surface antigens and the pathogenesis of Haemophilus influenzae infections. Trends Microbiol 3:304–309, 1995.
100. Hasleton P: Atypical pnemonias. In Haselton P (ed): Spencer's Pathology of the Lung. New York, McGraw-Hill, 1996, p 179.
101. Arnheiter H, Skuntz S, Noteborn M, Chang S, Meier E: Transgenic mice with intracellular immunity to influenza virus. Cell 62:51–61, 1990.
102. Gorman OT, Bean WJ, Webster RG: Evolutionary processes in influenza viruses: divergence, rapid evolution, and stasis. Curr Top Microbiol Immunol 176:75–97, 1992.
103. Taubenberger JK, Reid AH, Krafft AE, Bijwaard KE, Fanning TG: Initial genetic characterization of the 1918 "Spanish" influenza virus. Science 275:1793–1796, 1997.
104. Tumpey TM, Garcia-Sastre A, Mikulasova A, Taubenberger JK Swayne DE, Palese P, Basler CF: Existing antivirals are effective against influenza viruses with genes from the 1918 pandemic virus. Proc Natl Acad Sci U S A 99:13849–13854, 2002.
105. Peiris JSM, Yuen KY, Osterhaus ADME, Stohr K: The severe acute respiratory syndrome. N Engl J Med 349(25):2431–2441, 2003.
106. Lomotan JR, George SS, Brandstetter RD: Aspiration pneumonia: strategies for early recognition and prevention. Postgrad Med 102:225–226, 229–231, 1997.
107. Woods JP: Knocking on the right door and making a comfortable home: histoplasma capsulatum intracellular pathogenesis. Curr Opin Microbiol 6:327, 2003.
108. Wheat JL: Current diagnosis of histoplasmoss. Trends in Microbiol 11:488, 2003.
109. Kirkland TN, Fierer J, Coccidioidomycosis: a reemerging infectious disease. Emerg Infect Dis 2:192–199, 1996.
110. Rosenow EC 3rd: Diffuse pulmonary infiltrates in the immunocompromised host. Clin Chest Med 11:55–64, 1990.
111. Nash G, Said JW, Nash SV, DeGirolami U: The pathology of AIDS. Mod Pathol 8:199–217, 1995.

112. Yousem SA, Berry GJ, Cagle PT, Chamberlain D, Husain AN, Hruban RH, Marchevsky A, Ohori NP, Ritter J, Stewart S, Tazelaar HD: Revision of the 1990 working formulation for the classification of pulmonary allograft rejection: Lung Rejection Study Group. J Heart Lung Transplant 15:1–15, 1996.
113. Izbicki G, Shitrit D, Aravot D, Sulkes J, Saute M, Sahar G, Kramer MR: Improved survival after lung transplantation in patients treated with tacrolimus/mycophenolate mofetil as compared with cyclosporine/azathioprine. Transplant Proc 34:3258–3259, 2002.
114. Johnson BA, Iacono AT, Zeevi A, McCurry KR, Duncan SR: Statin use is associated with improved function and survival of lung allografts. Am J Respir Crit Care Med 167:1271–1278, 2003.
115. Travis, WD, Colby TV, Corrin B, Shimosato Y, Brambilla E: Histological typing of lung and pleural tumours. In WHO International Histological Classifications of Tumours, 3rd ed. New York, Springer, 1999.
116. Respiratory Health Effects of Passive Smoking: Lung Cancer and Other Disorders. Washington DC: US Environmental Protection Agency, 1992.
117. Marchevsky A: Pathogenesis and experimental models of lung cancer. In Marchevsky AM (ed): Surgical Pathology of Lung Neoplasms. New York, Marcel Dekker, 1990, p 7.
118. Samet JM: Indoor radon and lung cancer: estimating the risks. West J Med 156:25–29, 1992.
119. Pershagen G, Akerblom G, Axelson O, Clavensjo B, Damber L, Desai G, Enflo A, Lagarde F, Mellander H, Svartengren M, et al: Residential radon exposure and lung cancer in Sweden. N Engl J Med 330:159–164, 1994.
120. Frumkin H, Samet JM: Radon. CA Cancer J Clin 51:337–344, 322; quiz 345–338, 2001.
121. Salgia R, Skarin AT: Molecular abnormalities in lung cancer. J Clin Oncol 16:1207–1217, 1998.
122. Sekido Y, Fong KM, Minna, JD: Molecular genetics of lung cancer. Annu Rev Med 54:73–87, 2003.
123. el-Torky M, el-Zeky F, Hall JC: Significant changes in the distribution of histologic types of lung cancer: a review of 4928 cases. Cancer 65:2361–2367, 1990.
124. Hoffmann D, Rivenson A, Hecht SS: The biological significance of tobacco-specific N-nitrosamines: smoking and adenocarcinoma of the lung. Crit Rev Toxicol 26:199–211, 1996.
125. Aoyagi Y, Yokose T, Minami Y, Ochiai A, Iijima T, Morishita Y, Oda T, Fukao K, Noguchi M: Accumulation of losses of heterozygosity and multistep carcinogenesis in pulmonary adenocarcinoma. Cancer Res 61:7950–7954, 2001.
126. Greene FL, Page DL, Fleming ID, et al: AJCC Cancer Staging Manual, 6th ed. New York, Springer-Verlag, 2002.
127. Patel AM, Davila DG, Peters SG: Paraneoplastic syndromes associated with lung cancer. Mayo Clin Proc 68:278–287, 1993.
128. Marchevsky AM: Neuroendocrine tumors of the lung. Pathology (Phila) 4:103–123, 1996.
129. Travis WD, Rush W, Flieder DB, Falk R, Fleming MV, Gal AA, Koss MN: Survival analysis of 200 pulmonary neuroendocrine tumors with clarification of criteria for atypical carcinoid and its separation from typical carcinoid. Am J Surg Pathol 22:934–944, 1998.
130. Gold JS, Antonescu CR, Hajdu C, Ferrone CR, Hussain M, Lewis JJ, Brennan MF, Coit DG: Clinicopathologic correlates of solitary fibrous tumors. Cancer 94:1057–1068, 2002.
131. Corson JM: Pathology of diffuse malignant pleural mesothelioma. Semin Thorac Cardiovasc Surg 9:347–355, 1997.
132. Churg A: Neoplastic asbestos-induced diseases. In Churg A, Green F (eds): Pathology of Occupational Lung Disease. Baltimore, Williams and Wilkins, 1998, p 328.

CHAPTER 16

Head and Neck

Mark W. Lingen, DDS, PhD • Vinay Kumar, MD

ORAL CAVITY

TEETH AND SUPPORTING STRUCTURES
Caries (Tooth Decay)
Gingivitis
Periodontitis
INFLAMMATORY/REACTIVE LESIONS
Fibrous Proliferative Lesions
Aphthous Ulcers (Canker Sores)
Glossitis
INFECTIONS
Herpes Simplex Virus Infections
Other Viral Infections
Oral Candidiasis (Thrush)
Deep Fungal Infections
ORAL MANIFESTATIONS OF SYSTEMIC DISEASE
Hairy Leukoplakia
TUMORS AND PRECANCEROUS LESIONS
Leukoplakia and Erythroplakia
Squamous Cell Carcinoma
ODONTOGENIC CYSTS AND TUMORS

UPPER AIRWAYS

NOSE
Inflammations
Necrotizing Lesions of the Nose and Upper Airways
NASOPHARYNX
Inflammations
TUMORS OF THE NOSE, SINUSES, AND NASOPHARYNX
LARYNX
Inflammations
Reactive Nodules (Vocal Cord Nodules and Polyps)
Carcinoma of the Larynx
Squamous Papilloma and Papillomatosis

EARS

INFLAMMATORY LESIONS
OTOSCLEROSIS
TUMORS

NECK

BRANCHIAL CYST (LYMPHOEPITHELIAL CYST)
THYROGLOSSAL TRACT CYST
PARAGANGLIOMA (CAROTID BODY TUMOR)

SALIVARY GLANDS

XEROSTOMIA
INFLAMMATION (SIALADENITIS)
NEOPLASMS
Pleomorphic Adenoma
Warthin Tumor (Papillary Cystadenoma Lymphomatosum)
Mucoepidermoid Carcinoma
Other Salivary Gland Tumors

Diseases of the head and neck range from the common cold to uncommon neoplasms of the nose. Those selected for discussion are assigned, sometimes arbitrarily, to one of the following anatomic sites: (1) oral cavity; (2) upper airways, including the nose, pharynx, larynx, and nasal sinuses; (3) ears; (4) neck; and (5) salivary glands.

ORAL CAVITY

The oral cavity is a fearsome orifice guarded by ranks of upper and lower "horns" (lamentably, quite subject to erosion), demanding constant gratification, and teeming with microorganisms, some of which are potentially harmful. Among the many disorders that affect its various parts, only the more important or frequent conditions involving the teeth and supporting structures, oral mucous membranes, lips, and tongue are considered.

Teeth and Supporting Structures

Teeth contribute to a number of important functions, including mastication and proper speech. It is useful to briefly review normal dental anatomy before we delve into the common pathologic conditions affecting teeth. As is well known, teeth are firmly implanted in the jaw and are surrounded by the gingival mucosa (Fig. 16–1). The anatomic crown of the tooth projects into the mouth and is covered by *enamel*, a hard, inert, acellular tissue—the most highly mineralized tissue in the body. The enamel rests upon *dentin*, which is a specialized form of connective tissue that makes up the remainder of the hard tissue portion of teeth. Unlike enamel, dentin is cellular and contains numerous dentinal tubules, which contain the cytoplasmic extensions of odontoblasts. These cells are present within the pulp and continually produce new (secondary) dentin within the interior of the tooth. The pulp chamber itself is surrounded by the dentin and consists of connective tissue stroma, nerve bundles, lymphatics, and capillaries.

To perform mastication, teeth must not only be composed of hard tissue, but they must also be firmly attached to the bones of the jaw. If this attachment were excessively firm, chewing would impose sufficient physical stress on the teeth to cause their loss or fracturing. Therefore, in mammals, teeth are attached to the alveolar ridge of the jaws by the *periodontal ligament*, which provides a strong yet flexible attachment that can withstand the forces of mastication. The periodontal ligament attaches to the alveolar bone of the jaw on one side and to *cementum*, present on the roots of the teeth, which acts as a "cement" to anchor the periodontal ligament to the tooth.

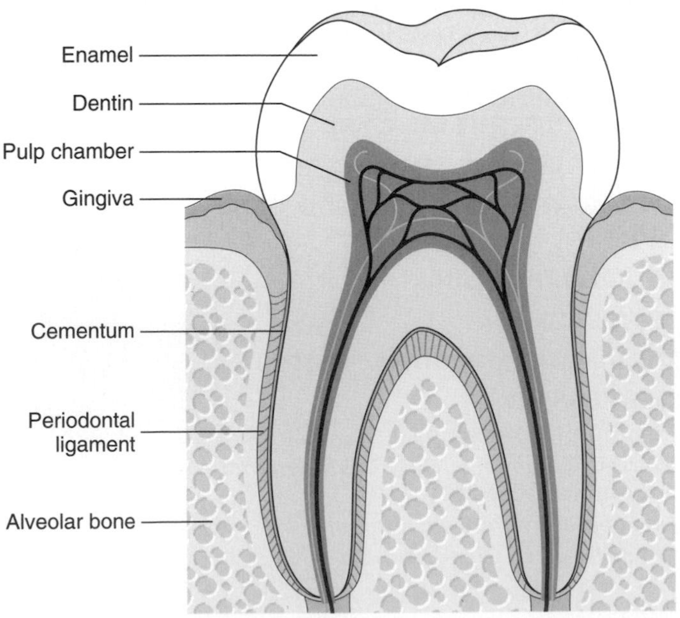

FIGURE 16–1 Schematic representation of the normal dental anatomy and surrounding supporting tissues.

CARIES (TOOTH DECAY)

Dental caries, caused by focal degradation of the tooth structure, is one of the most common diseases throughout the world and is the most common cause of tooth loss before age 35. Carious lesions are the result of mineral dissolution of tooth structure by acid metabolic end products from bacteria that are present in the oral cavity and are capable of fermenting sugars. Traditionally, the rate of caries has been higher in industrialized countries, where there is ready access to processed foods containing large amounts of carbohydrates. However, global trends may change these demographics. First of all, the rate of caries has dramatically dropped in countries such as the United States, where improved oral hygiene and fluoridation of the drinking water has become a standard practice. Fluoride incorporates into the crystalline structure of enamel, forming fluoroapatite, and contributes to resistance to degradation by bacterial acids. Secondly, with globalization of the world's economy, increased amounts of processed foods with high carbohydrate content are being imported into developing nations. With these trends, one can expect the rate of caries to dramatically increase in the less developed world over the next several decades.

GINGIVITIS

Gingivitis is a condition in which there is inflammation of the soft tissues that surround the teeth. Typically, the development of gingivitis is the result of a lack of proper oral hygiene, leading to an accumulation of dental plaque and calculus. *Dental plaque* is a complex mass of microorganisms from the normal oral flora, proteins from the saliva, and desquamated epithelial cells. *Calculus* consists of mineralized bacterial plaque and can form extensive deposits around the teeth. Chronic gingivitis is characterized by gingival redness, edema, bleeding, changes in contour, and loss of soft tissue adaptation to the teeth. Gingivitis can occur at any age but is most prevalent and severe in adolescence (ranging from 40% to 60%), after which the incidence tends to taper off. It is a reversible disease; therapy is primarily aimed at the reduction of the accumulation of plaque and calculus via brushing, flossing, and regular hygiene visits.[1] This allows the gingival tissues to heal.

PERIODONTITIS

Periodontitis refers to an inflammatory process that affects the supporting structures of the teeth: periodontal ligaments, alveolar bone, and cementum. With progression, periodontitis can lead to serious sequelae, including the loss of attachment caused by complete destruction of the periodontal ligament and alveolar bone. Loosening and eventual loss of teeth are possible. The pathogenesis of periodontal inflammation is not entirely clear. Until the 1960s, it was believed that longstanding gingivitis uniformly progressed to periodontal disease. However, this is no longer thought to be the case. Rather, the development of periodontal disease is now considered to be an independent process, which, for reasons that are still unclear, is associated with a dramatic shift in the types and proportions of bacteria along the gums.[2,3] This shift, along with other environmental conditions such as poor oral hygiene, is believed to be important in the pathogenesis of periodontitis. This view is supported by significant differences in the content of dental plaque in areas of healthy and diseased periodontium. For the most part, facultative gram-positive organisms colonize healthy sites, while plaque within areas of active periodontitis contains anaerobic and microaerophilic gram-negative flora. Although 300 types of bacteria reside in the oral cavity, adult periodontitis is associated primarily with *Actinobacillus actinomycetemcomitans*, *Porphyromonas gingivalis*, and *Prevotella intermedia*.

While it typically presents without any associated disorders, periodontal disease can also be a component of a number of different systemic diseases, including acquired immunodeficiency syndrome (AIDS), leukemia, Crohn disease, diabetes mellitus, Down syndrome, sarcoidosis, and syndromes associated with polymorphonuclear defects (Chédiak-Higashi syndrome, agranulocytosis, and cyclic neutropenia). In addition to being a component of certain systemic diseases, periodontal infections can also be etiologic factors in several important systemic diseases. These include, for example, infective endocarditis, pulmonary and brain abscesses, and increased adverse pregnancy outcomes.[4]

Inflammatory/Reactive Lesions

A number of soft tissue lesions of the oral cavity, which present as tumor masses or ulcerations, are indeed reactive in nature and represent inflammations induced by irritation or by unknown mechanisms. All suspicious lesions, however, should be examined by biopsy. Reactive nodules of the oral cavity are fairly common and are a diverse group. The most common fibrous proliferative lesions of the oral cavity are fibroma (61%), peripheral ossifying fibroma (22%), pyogenic granuloma (12%), and peripheral giant cell granuloma (5%).[5] The most common inflammatory/reactive ulcerations of the oral cavity are traumatic and aphthous ulcers.

FIBROUS PROLIFERATIVE LESIONS

The so-called *irritation fibroma* (Fig. 16–2) primarily occurs in the buccal mucosa along the bite line or at the gingivodental margin. It consists of a nodular mass of fibrous tissue, with few inflammatory cells, covered by squamous mucosa. Treatment is complete surgical excision.

The *pyogenic granuloma* (Fig. 16–3) is a highly vascular peduncular lesion, usually occurring in the gingiva of children, young adults, and, commonly, pregnant women (pregnancy tumor). The surface of the lesion is typically ulcerated and can be red to purple in color. In some cases, growth is alarmingly rapid, raising the fear of a malignant neoplasm. Histologically, these lesions demonstrate a highly vascular proliferation that is similar to granulation tissue. Because of this histologic picture, pyogenic granulomas can also be considered a form of capillary hemangioma (Chapter 11). They either regress, particularly after pregnancy, or undergo fibrous maturation, and they may develop into a peripheral ossifying fibroma. Treatment is complete surgical excision.

The *peripheral ossifying fibroma* is a relatively common growth of the gingiva that is considered to be reactive in nature rather than neoplastic. However, the specific etiology of the lesion is unknown. Some may arise as a result of the maturation of a long-standing pyogenic granuloma, while others do not. With a peak incidence in young and teenage females, peripheral ossifying fibromas appear as red, ulcer-

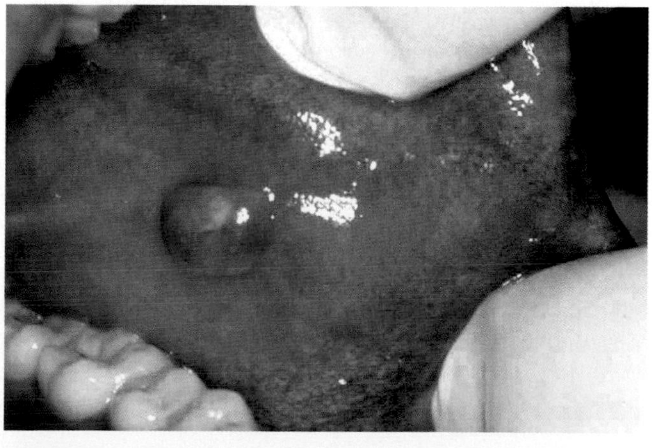

FIGURE 16–2 Fibroma. Smooth, pink, exophytic nodule on the buccal mucosa.

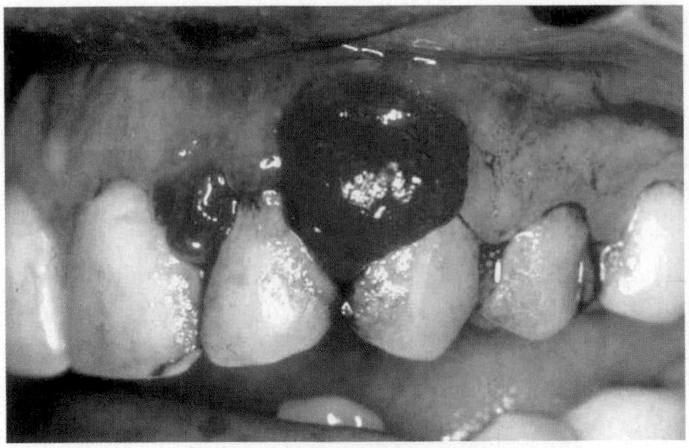

FIGURE 16–3 Pyogenic granuloma. Erythematous, hemorrhagic, and exophytic mass arising from the gingival mucosa.

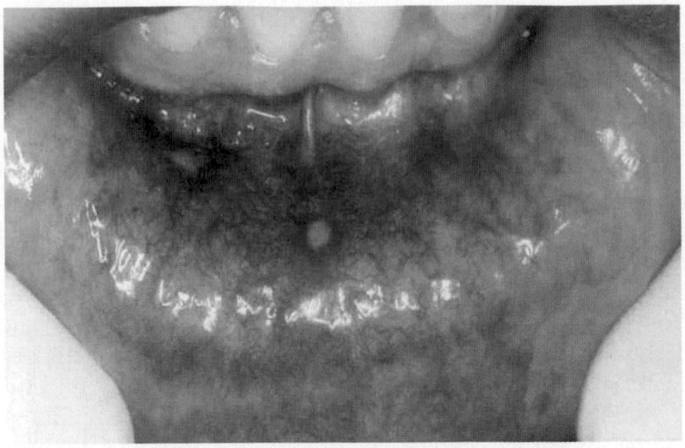

FIGURE 16–4 Aphthous ulcer. Single ulceration with an erythematous halo surrounding a yellowish fibrinopurulent membrane.

ated, and nodular lesions of the gingiva. They are often mistaken clinically for pyogenic granulomas. Complete surgical excision down to the periosteum is the treatment of choice, as these lesions have a recurrence rate of 15% to 20%.

The *peripheral giant cell granuloma (giant cell epulis)*, a relatively common lesion of the oral cavity, characteristically protrudes from the gingiva at some site of chronic inflammation. This lesion is generally covered by intact gingival mucosa, but it may be ulcerated. The clinical appearance of peripheral giant cell granuloma can be similar to that of pyogenic granuloma but, in general, this lesion is more bluish-purple in color while the pyogenic granuloma is more bright red. Histologically, however, these lesions are distinct. Peripheral giant cell granuloma is made up of a striking aggregation of multinucleate, foreign body–like giant cells separated by a fibroangiomatous stroma. Although not encapsulated, these lesions are usually well delimited and readily excised. They should be differentiated from central giant cell granulomas found within the maxilla or the mandible and from the histologically similar but frequently multiple reparative giant cell "brown tumors" seen in hyperparathyroidism (Chapter 24).

APHTHOUS ULCERS (CANKER SORES)

These extremely common superficial ulcerations of the oral mucosa affect up to 40% of the population in the United States.[6] They are more common in the first two decades of life, are painful and often recurrent, and tend to be prevalent within certain families.

The lesions appear as single or multiple, shallow, hyperemic ulcerations covered by a thin exudate and rimmed by a narrow zone of erythema (Fig. 16–4). The underlying inflammatory infiltrate is at first largely mononuclear, but secondary bacterial infection introduces numerous neutrophils. The lesions may spontaneously resolve in 7 to 10 days or be stubbornly persistent for weeks. The causation of these lesions is obscure. Most ulcers are more painful than serious and require only symptomatic treatment.

GLOSSITIS

Although the designation *glossitis* implies inflammation of the tongue, it is sometimes applied to the beefy-red tongue encountered in certain deficiency states; this change results from atrophy of the papillae of the tongue and thinning of the mucosa, exposing the underlying vasculature. In some instances, the atrophic changes do indeed lead to inflammation and even shallow ulcerations. Such changes may be encountered in deficiencies of vitamin B_{12} (pernicious anemia), riboflavin, niacin, or pyridoxine. Similar alterations are sometimes encountered with sprue and iron-deficiency anemia, possibly complicated by one of the vitamin B deficiencies. *The combination of iron-deficiency anemia, glossitis, and esophageal dysphagia usually related to webs is known as the Plummer-Vinson or Paterson-Kelly syndrome.* Glossitis, characterized by ulcerative lesions (sometimes along the lateral borders of the tongue), may also be seen with jagged carious teeth, ill-fitting dentures, and, rarely, with syphilis, inhalation burns, or ingestion of corrosive chemicals.

Infections

The oral mucosa is highly resistant to its indigenous flora, having many defenses, including the competitive suppression of potential pathogens by organisms of low virulence, the elaboration of secretory immunoglobulin A and other immunoglobulins by submucosal collections of lymphocytes and plasma cells, the antibacterial effects of saliva, and the diluting and irrigating effects of food and drink. Nonetheless, any lowering of these defenses, for example, with immunodeficiency or disruption of the microbiologic balance by antibacterial therapy, sets the stage for oral infection. Most of these infections are discussed in Chapter 8, and here we only briefly recapitulate the principal features of the oral lesions.

HERPES SIMPLEX VIRUS INFECTIONS

Most orofacial herpetic infections are caused by herpes simplex virus type 1 (HSV-1). However, owing to changes in sexual habits, an increase in HSV-2 (genital herpes) has been observed in the oral cavity. Primary HSV infection typically occurs in children age 2 to 4 years, is often asymptomatic, and does not cause significant morbidity. Approximately 10% to 20% of the time, primary infection presents as *acute herpetic gingivostomatitis,* in which there is an abrupt onset of vesicles and ulcerations throughout the oral cavity, especially in the gingiva. These lesions are also accompanied by lymphadenopathy, fever, anorexia, and irritability.

Morphology. The vesicles range from lesions of a few millimeters to large bullae and are at first filled with a clear, serous fluid, but they often rupture to yield extremely painful, red-rimmed, and shallow ulcerations. On microscopic examination, there is intracellular and intercellular edema (acantholysis), yielding clefts that may become transformed into macroscopic vesicles. Individual epidermal cells in the margins of the vesicle or lying free within the fluid sometimes develop eosinophilic **intranuclear viral inclusions,** or several cells may fuse to produce giant cells **(multinucleate polykaryons),** changes that are demonstrated by the diagnostic **Tzanck test**, based on microscopic examination of the vesicle fluid. The vesicles and shallow ulcers usually spontaneously clear within 3 to 4 weeks, but the virus treks along the regional nerves and eventually becomes dormant in the local ganglia (e.g., the trigeminal).

The great preponderance of adults harbor latent HSV-1, but in some individuals, usually young adults, the virus becomes reactivated to produce the common but usually mild *cold sore.* The influences predisposing to activation are poorly understood but are thought to include trauma, allergies, exposure to ultraviolet light, upper respiratory tract infections, pregnancy, menstruation, immunosuppression, and excessive exposure to heat or cold.

Recurrent herpetic stomatitis (in contrast to acute gingivostomatitis) occurs either at the site of primary inoculation or in adjacent mucosal areas that are associated with the same ganglion; it takes the form of groups of small (1 to 3 mm) vesicles. The lips *(herpes labialis),* nasal orifices, buccal mucosa, gingiva, and hard palate are the most common locations for recurrent lesions. They resemble those already described in the primary infections but are much more limited in duration, are milder, usually dry up in 4 to 6 days, and heal within a week to 10 days.

OTHER VIRAL INFECTIONS

Additional viral infections that can be seen in the oral cavity as well as the head and neck region include herpes zoster, Epstein-Barr virus (EBV; mononucleosis), cytomegalovirus, enterovirus (herpangina, hand-foot-and-mouth disease, acute lymphonodular pharyngitis), and rubeola (measles).

ORAL CANDIDIASIS (THRUSH)

The many localizations of candidal infection are fully described in Chapter 8, and so this discussion is limited to presentations in the oral cavity. Candidiasis is by far the most common fungal infection in the oral cavity. As is well known, *Candida albicans* is a normal component of the oral flora in approximately 50% of the population. As such, three factors appear to influence the likelihood of a clinical infection: (1) immune status of the individual; (2) the strain of *C. albicans* present; and (3) the composition of an individual's oral flora. There are three major clinical forms of oral candidiasis, including pseudomembranous (thrush), erythematous, and hyperplastic, with a number of different variations within these groups. Only the pseudomembranous form, the most common of these, is discussed here. Also known as "*thrush*," pseudomembranous candidiasis typically takes the form of a superficial, curdy, gray to white inflammatory membrane composed of matted organisms enmeshed in a fibrinosuppurative exudate that can be readily scraped off to reveal an underlying erythematous inflammatory base. This fungus is a normal inhabitant of the oral cavity and causes mischief only in individuals who have some form of immunosuppression, as occurs in patients with diabetes mellitus, organ or bone marrow transplant recipients, those with neutropenia, chemotherapy-induced immunosuppression, or AIDS. In addition, broad-spectrum antibiotics that eliminate or alter the normal bacterial flora of the mouth can result in the development of oral candidiasis.

DEEP FUNGAL INFECTIONS

In addition to their more common sites of infection, certain deep fungal infections have a rather significant predilection for the oral cavity and head and neck region. Such fungi include histoplasmosis, blastomycosis, coccidioidomycosis, cryptococcosis, zygomycosis, and aspergillosis. With an increasing number of patients who are immunocompromised as a result of diseases such as AIDS or therapies for cancer and organ transplantation, the prevalence of fungal infections of the oral cavity has also increased in recent years.

Oral Manifestations of Systemic Disease

As oral clinicians are at pains to emphasize, the mouth is a part of the body, and not merely a gateway for delicacies. Not surprisingly, then, many systemic diseases are associated with oral lesions. In fact, it is not uncommon for oral lesions to be the first sign of some underlying systemic condition. Some of the more common are cited in Table 16–1, with a few words about the associated oral changes. Only one—hairy leukoplakia—is characterized in more detail.

HAIRY LEUKOPLAKIA

Hairy leukoplakia is a distinctive oral lesion that is seen in immunocompromised patients. Approximately 80% of patients with hairy leukoplakia have been infected with the human immunodeficiency virus (HIV); the presence of this lesion sometimes calls attention to the existence of the infection. However, 20% of lesions are seen in patients who are immunocompromised for other reasons, such as cancer therapy or transplant immunosuppression. Hairy leukoplakia takes the form of *white, confluent patches of fluffy ("hairy"), hyperkeratotic thickenings, almost always situated on the lateral border of the tongue.* The distinctive microscopic appearance consists of *hyperparakeratosis* and *acanthosis with "balloon cells" in the upper spinous layer*. Sometimes there is koilocytosis of the superficial, nucleated epidermal cells, suggestive of human papillomavirus (HPV) infection, and HPV transcripts have occasionally been found. However, EBV is present in

TABLE 16–1 Oral Manifestations of Some Systemic Diseases

Infectious Diseases	
Scarlet fever	Fiery red tongue with prominent papillae (raspberry tongue); white coated tongue through which hyperemic papillae project (strawberry tongue)
Measles	A spotty enanthema in the oral cavity often precedes the rash; ulcerations on the buccal mucosa about Stensen duct produce Koplik spots
Infectious mononucleosis	An acute pharyngitis and tonsillitis that may cause coating with a gray-white exudative membrane; enlargement of lymph nodes in the neck
Diphtheria	A characteristic dirty white, fibrinosuppurative, tough, inflammatory membrane over the tonsils and retropharynx
Human immunodeficiency virus infection; AIDS	Predisposition to opportunistic oral infections, particularly with herpesvirus, *Candida*, and other fungi; sometimes oral lesions of Kaposi sarcoma and hairy leukoplakia (described in text)
Dermatologic Conditions*	
Lichen planus	Reticulate, lacelike, white keratotic lesions that rarely become bullous and ulcerated; seen in more than 50% of patients with cutaneous lichen planus; rarely, is the sole manifestation
Pemphigus	Usually vulgaris; vesicles and bullae prone to rupture, leaving hyperemic erosions covered with exudate
Bullous pemphigoid	Oral lesions resemble macroscopically those of pemphigus but can be differentiated histologically
Erythema multiforme	A maculopapular, vesiculobullous eruption that sometimes follows an infection elsewhere, ingestion of drugs, development of cancer, or a collagen vascular disease; when it involves the lips and oral mucosa, it is referred to as *Stevens-Johnson syndrome*
Hematologic Disorders	
Pancytopenia (agranulocytosis, aplastic anemia)	Severe oral infections in the form of gingivitis, pharyngitis, tonsillitis; may extend to cellulitis of the neck *(Ludwig angina)*
Leukemia	With depletion of functioning neutrophils, oral lesions may appear like those in pancytopenia
Monocytic leukemia	Leukemic infiltration and enlargement of the gingivae, often with accompanying periodontitis
Miscellaneous	
Melanotic pigmentation	May appear in Addison disease, hemochromatosis, fibrous dysplasia of bone (Albright syndrome), and Peutz-Jegher syndrome (gastrointestinal polyposis)
Phenytoin (Dilantin) ingestion	Striking fibrous enlargement of the gingivae
Pregnancy	A friable, red, pyogenic granuloma protruding from the gingiva ("pregnancy tumor")
Rendu-Osler-Weber syndrome	Autosomal dominant disorder with multiple aneurysmal telangiectasias from birth beneath the skin or mucosal surfaces of the oral cavity, lips, gastrointestinal tract, respiratory tract, and urinary tract as well as in internal viscera

*See Chapter 25 for details

most cells and is now accepted as the cause of the condition.[7] Sometimes there is superimposed candidal infection on the surface of the lesions, adding to the "hairiness." When the hairy leukoplakia is a harbinger of HIV infection, manifestations of AIDS generally appear within 2 or 3 years.

Tumors and Precancerous Lesions

A number of epithelial and soft tissue neoplasms can arise in the oral cavity. Many of these tumors (e.g., papillomas, hemangiomas, lymphomas) also occur elsewhere in the body and are described adequately in other chapters. Therefore, this discussion will consider only oral squamous cell carcinoma and its associated precancerous lesions.

LEUKOPLAKIA AND ERYTHROPLAKIA

As is discussed in more detail below, oral cancers are common worldwide, with a fairly high mortality. Screening and early detection in populations at risk have been proposed to decrease both the morbidity and mortality associated with oral cancer.[8,9] However, the visual detection of definitive premalignant oral lesions is problematic. This is in stark contrast to skin lesions, where visual screening for melanomas of the skin has been shown to have sensitivity and specificity rates of 93% and 98%.[10,11] One explanation for this discrepancy is that the early lesions frequently do not demonstrate any of the clinical characteristics observed in advanced oral cancer: ulceration, induration, pain, or associated cervical lymphadenopathy.[12] In addition, the clinical presentation of potentially premalignant lesions in the oral cavity is highly heterogeneous. We begin our discussion with two premalignant lesions—leukoplakia and erythroplakia.

The term *leukoplakia* is defined by the World Health Organization as "a white patch or plaque that cannot be scraped off and cannot be characterized clinically or pathologically as any other disease." Simply put, if a white lesion in the oral cavity can be given a specific diagnosis it is not a leukoplakia. This clinical term is reserved for lesions that are present in the oral cavity for no apparent reason. As such, white patches caused by entities such as lichen planus and candidiasis are not leukoplakias. Approximately 3% of the world's population have leukoplakic lesions, and somewhere between 5% and 25% of these lesions are premalignant.[13] *Thus, until it is proved otherwise via histologic evaluation, all leukoplakias must be considered precancerous.*

Related to leukoplakia, but much less common and much more ominous, is *erythroplakia.* It represents a red, velvety, possibly eroded area within the oral cavity that usually remains level with or may be slightly depressed in relation to the surrounding mucosa (Fig. 16–5). The epithelium in such

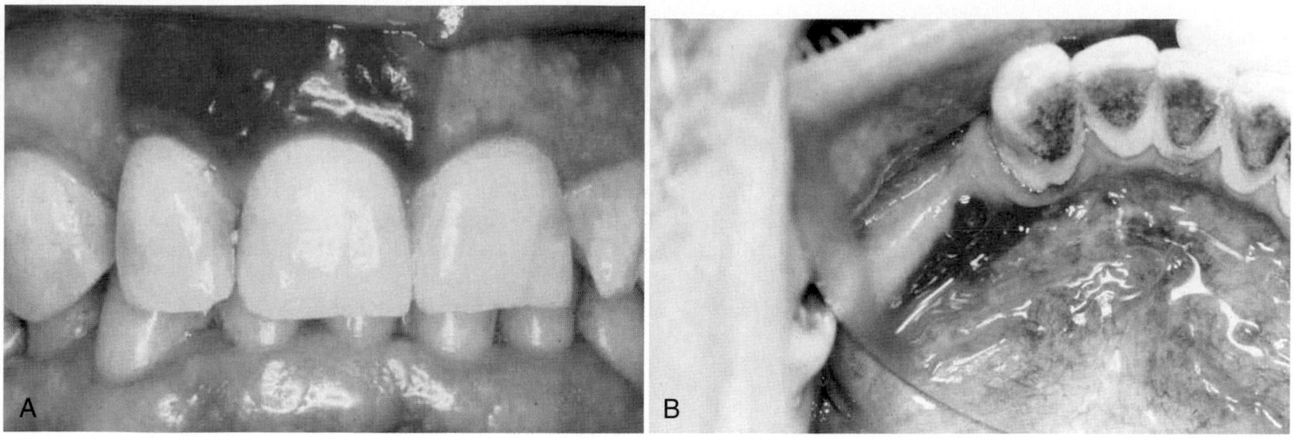

FIGURE 16–5 Erythroplakia. *A,* Lesion of the maxillary gingiva. *B,* Red lesion of the mandibular alveolar ridge. Biopsy of both lesions revealed carcinoma in situ.

lesions tends to be markedly atypical, incurring a much higher risk of malignant transformation than that seen with leukoplakia. Intermediate forms are occasionally encountered that have the characteristics of both leukoplakia and erythroplakia, termed *speckled leukoerythroplakia.*

Both leukoplakia and erythroplakia may be seen in adults at any age, but they are usually found between ages 40 and 70, with a 2:1 male preponderance. *Although these lesions have multifactorial origins, the use of tobacco (cigarettes, pipes, cigars, and chewing tobacco) is the most common antecedent.*

Morphology. Leukoplakias may occur anywhere in the oral cavity (favored locations are buccal mucosa, floor of the mouth, ventral surface of the tongue, palate, and gingiva). They appear as solitary or multiple white patches or plaques with indistinct or sharply demarcated borders. They may be slightly thickened and smooth or wrinkled and fissured, or they may appear as raised, sometimes corrugated, verrucous plaques (Fig. 16–6*A–D*). On histologic

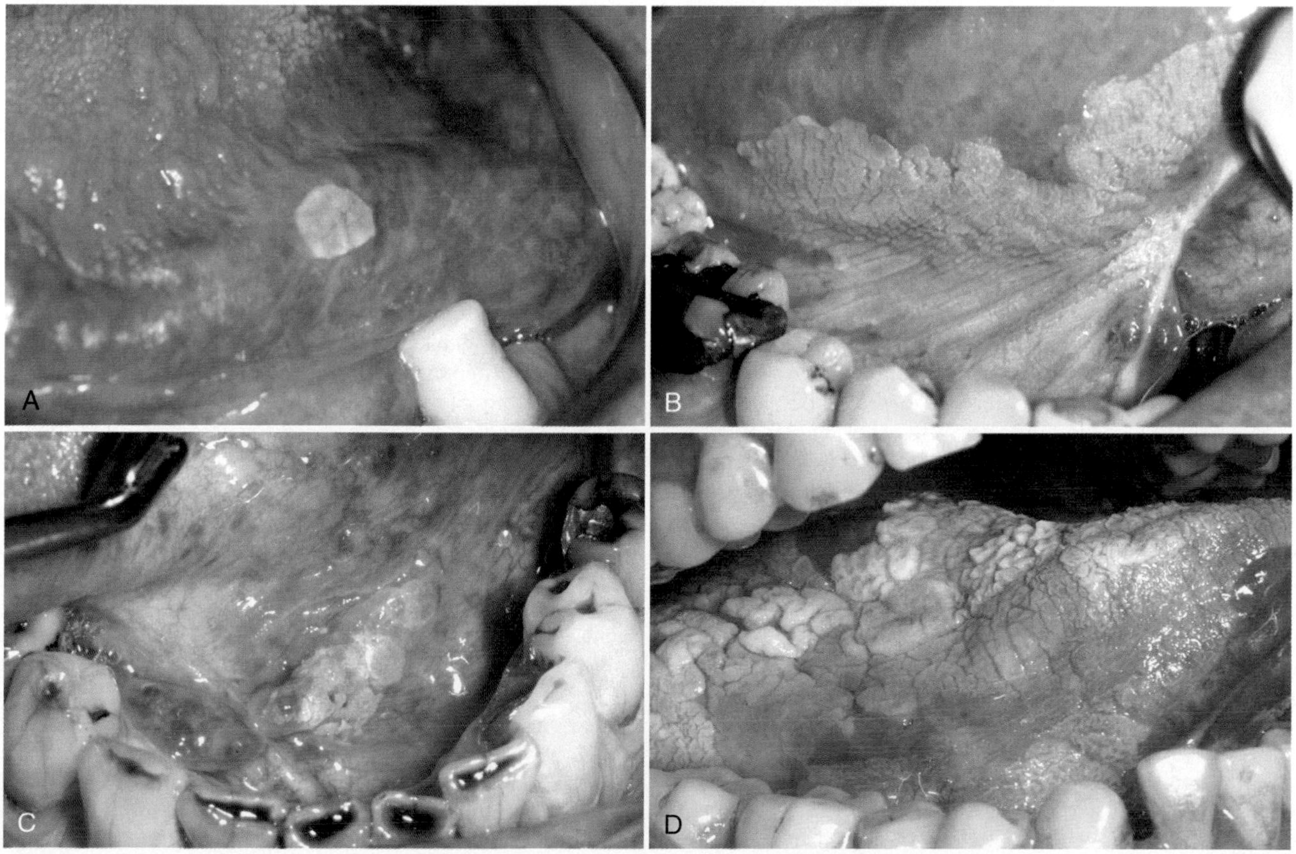

FIGURE 16–6 Leukoplakia. Clinical appearance of leukoplakias is highly variable and can range from *A,* smooth and thin with well-demarcated borders. *B,* diffuse and thick. *C,* irregular with a granular surface. *D,* diffuse and corrugated. (Courtesy of Drs. Neville, Damm, Allen, Bouquot [eds], Oral & Maxillofacial Pathology, Philadelphia, WB Saunders, 2002.)

examination, they present a spectrum of epithelial changes ranging from hyperkeratosis overlying a thickened, acanthotic but orderly mucosal epithelium (Fig. 16–7) to lesions with markedly dysplastic changes sometimes merging into carcinoma in situ. The more dysplastic or anaplastic the lesion, the more likely it is that a subjacent inflammatory infiltrate of lymphocytes and macrophages is present.

The histologic changes in **erythroplakia** only rarely consist of orderly epidermal thickening; virtually all (approximately 90%) disclose superficial erosions with dysplasia, carcinoma in situ, or already developed carcinoma in the surrounding margins. An intense subepithelial inflammatory reaction with vascular dilation accounts for the red appearance of the lesion.

SQUAMOUS CELL CARCINOMA

At least 95% of cancers of the head and neck are squamous cell carcinomas (HNSCC), arising most commonly in the oral cavity. The remainder includes adenocarcinomas (of salivary gland origin), melanomas, various carcinomas, and other rarities. Biologically, squamous cell carcinomas in the oral cavity are fairly similar to those elsewhere in the head and neck, hence they are described together here. Features that apply to squamous cell cancer at specific sites in the head and neck are mentioned in the following discussion. Laryngeal squamous cell cancers are described later.

HNSCC is an aggressive epithelial malignancy that is the sixth most common neoplasm in the world today. At current rates, approximately 40,000 cases in the United States and more than 500,000 cases worldwide will be diagnosed each year.[14] Despite numerous advances in treatment utilizing the most recent protocols for surgery, radiation, and chemotherapy, the long-term survival has remained at less than 50% for the past 50 years.[15,16] This dismal outlook is due to a number of factors. For example, oral cancer is often diagnosed when the disease has already reached an advanced stage. The 5-year survival rate of early-stage oral cancer is approximately 80%, while survival drops to 19% for late-stage disease.[17] In addition, the frequent development of multiple primary tumors markedly decreases survival. The rate of second primary tumors in these patients has been reported to be 3% to 7% per year, which is higher than for any other malignancy.[18,19] This observation has led to the concept of "field cancerization." It is postulated that multiple individual primary tumors develop independently in the upper aerodigestive tract as a result of years of chronic exposure of the mucosa to carcinogens.[20,21] Because of such field cancerization, an individual who is fortunate to live 5 years after the initial primary tumor has up to a 35% chance of developing at least one new primary tumor within that period of time. The occurrence of new primary tumors can be particularly devastating for individuals whose initial lesions are small. The 5-year survival rate for the first primary tumor is considerably better than 50%, but in such individuals, second primary tumors are the most common cause of death.[22] Therefore, the early detection of all premalignant lesions is critical for the long-term survival of these patients.

Pathogenesis. The pathogenesis of squamous cell carcinoma is multifactorial. Within North America and Europe, it has classically been considered to be a disease of middle-aged men who have been chronic abusers of smoked tobacco and alcohol. Not unexpectedly, therefore, and concurrent with increased cigarette usage, the incidence of oral cancer in women is on the rise. In addition, it is now known that at least 50% of oropharyngeal cancers, particularly those involving the tonsils and the base of tongue, harbor oncogenic variants of HPV.[23] (Interestingly, these patients have a better overall survival than do HPV-negative patients.) There is increasing epidemiologic evidence that a family history of head and neck cancer is a risk factor for the disease, and it is postulated that inherited genomic instability may make individuals more susceptible to developing cancer.[27] Finally, actinic radiation (sunlight) and, particularly, pipe smoking are known predisposing influences to cancer of the lower lip. Outside of North America and Europe, a major regional predisposing influence is the chewing of betel quid and paan in India and parts of Asia. The betel quid is a "witches brew" that contains various ingredients such as areca nut, slaked lime, and tobacco, which are wrapped in a betel leaf. While protracted irritation from ill-fitting dentures, jagged teeth, or chronic infections is no longer thought to be an important direct antecedent to oral cancer, chronic irritation of the mucosa could act as a "promoter" of cancer in much the same way as alcohol does. The incidence of oral cancer in individuals under age 40 who have no known risk factors has been on the rise for the past several years.[24–26] The basis of this is not understood.

Molecular Biology of Squamous Cell Carcinoma. Like all epithelial neoplasms, the development of squamous cell carcinoma is thought to be a multi-step process involving the sequential activation of oncogenes and inactivation of tumor suppressor genes in a clonal population of cells. A number of genetic alterations, some definitively identified and some inferred from tumor-specific chromosomal alterations, have been found in HNSCC. While not all of the specific mutations required for progression have been delineated, a working molecular model has been established (Fig. 16–7). The first reproducible change is the loss of chromosomal regions of 3p and 9p21.[28] Loss of heterozygosity (LOH) in conjunction with promoter hypermethylation at this locus results in the inactivation of the *p16* gene, an inhibitor of cyclin-dependent kinase (Chapter 7). This alteration is associated with the transition from normal to hyperplasia/hyperkeratosis and occurs prior to the development of histologic atypia, thus underscoring the histologic limitations for early diagnosis. Subsequent LOH at 17p with mutation of the *p53* tumor suppressor gene is associated with progression to dysplasia.[29] Recently, it has been demonstrated that gross genomic alterations as well as deletions on 4q, 6p, 8p, 11q, 13q, and 14q may act as predictors of progression to frank malignancy.[30] Ultimately, amplification and overexpression of the Cyclin D1 gene (located on chromosome 11q13), which constitutively activates cell cycle progression, is a common late event. Data suggest that alterations of this gene confer the ability to invade in certain clones.[31,32]

However, while this model is a good working draft of the molecular changes involved in development of HNSCC, it is incomplete. First, while some of the gross genomic alterations correlate with genes known to be important in HNSCC (such as *p16*, *p53*, and *CyclinD1*), many of the specific genes are still unknown. Second, this model does not take into account alterations to genes such as the epidermal growth factor re-

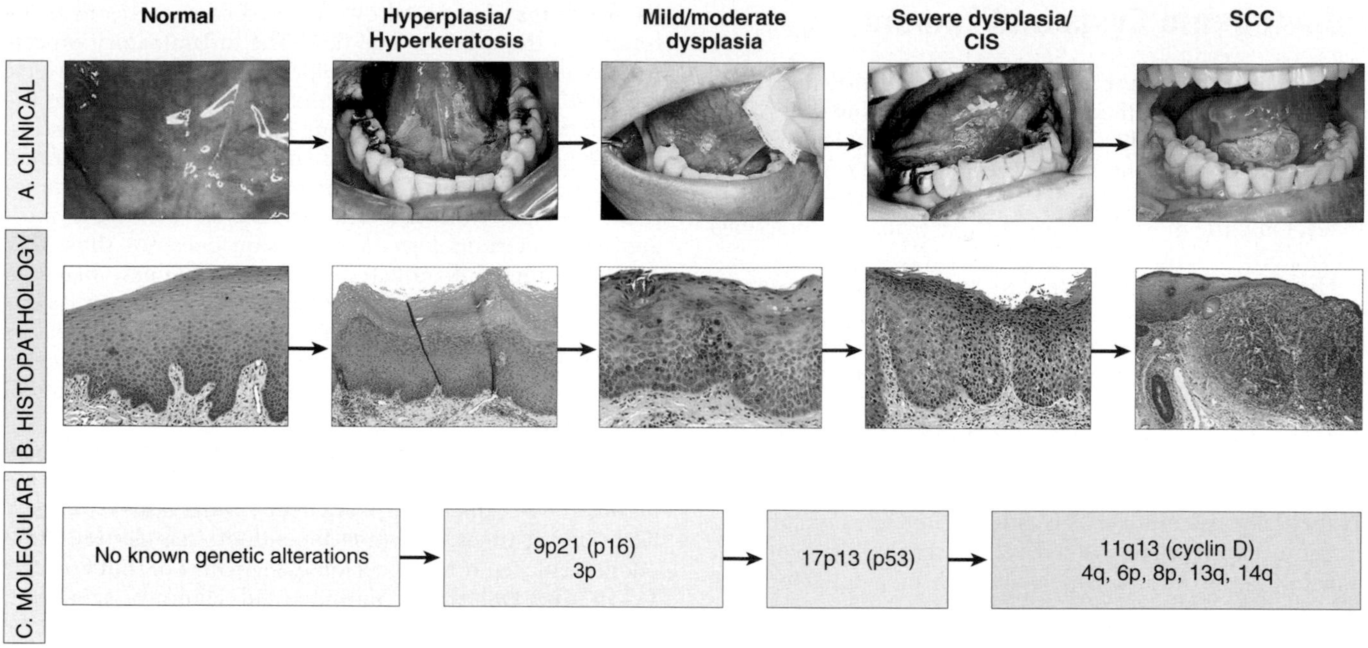

FIGURE 16–7 Clinical, histologic, and molecular progression of oral cancer. *A,* The typical clinical progression of oral cancer. *B,* The histologic progression of squamous epithelium from normal, to hyperkeratosis, to mild/moderate dysplasia, to severe dysplasia, to cancer. *C,* The sites of the most common genetic alterations identified as important for cancer development. (Clinical photographs courtesy of Sol Silverman, M.D., from the text Silverman S: Oral Cancer. Hamilton, Ontario, BD Dekker, 2003.)

ceptor (EGFR), which is overexpressed in a high percentage of HNSCC and has been successfully targeted in the treatment of this disease. Finally, as indicated above, it is increasingly clear that HNSCC is a heterogeneous disease in terms of etiology and therefore its molecular mechanisms of development.

Morphology. Squamous cell carcinoma may arise anywhere in the oral cavity, but the favored locations are the ventral surface of the tongue, floor of the mouth, lower lip, soft palate, and gingiva (Fig. 16–8). The malignancies themselves are typically preceded by the presence of premalignant lesions that can be very heterogeneous in presentation (see above).

In the early stages, cancers of the oral cavity appear either as raised, firm, pearly plaques or as irregular, roughened, or verrucous areas of mucosal thickening, possibly mistaken for leukoplakia. Either pattern may be superimposed on a background of apparent leukoplakia or erythroplakia. As these lesions enlarge, they typically create ulcerated and protruding masses that have irregular, firm, and indurated (rolled) borders.

On histologic examination, these cancers begin as dysplastic lesions, which may or may not progress to full-thickness dysplasia (carcinoma in situ) prior to invading the underlying connective tissue stroma. This difference in progression should be contrasted with cervical cancer (Chapter 22), in which, typically, full-thickness dysplasia, representing carcinoma in situ, develops prior to invasion. Squamous cell carcinomas range from well-differentiated keratinizing neoplasms to anaplastic, sometimes sarcomatoid, tumors, and from slowly to rapidly growing lesions. However, the degree of histologic differentiation, as determined by the relative degree of keratinization, is not correlated with behavior. As a group, these tumors tend, to infiltrate locally before they metastasize to other sites. The routes of extension depend on the primary site. The favored sites of local metastasis are the cervical lymph nodes, while the most common sites of distant metastasis are mediastinal lymph nodes, lungs, liver, and bones. Unfortunately, such distant metastases are often occult at the time of discovery of the primary lesion.

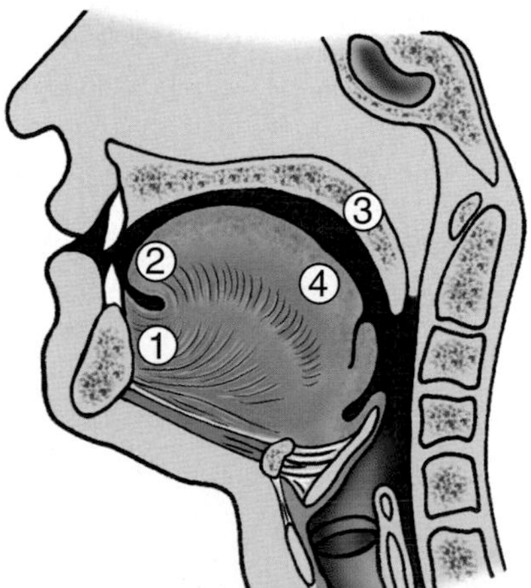

FIGURE 16–8 Schematic representation of the sites of origin of squamous cell carcinoma of the oral cavity, in numerical order of frequency.

Odontogenic Cysts and Tumors

In contrast to the rest of the skeleton, epithelial-lined cysts are quite common in the jaws. The overwhelming majority of these cysts are derived from remnants of odontogenic epithelium present within the jaws. In general, these cysts are subclassified as either inflammatory or developmental (Table 16–2). Only the most common of these lesions are described below.

The *dentigerous cyst* is defined as a cyst that originates around the crown of an unerupted tooth and is thought to be the result of a separation of the dental follicle. Radiographically, they are unilocular lesions and are most often associated with impacted third molar (wisdom) teeth. Histologically, they are lined by a thin layer of stratified squamous epithelium. Often, there is a very dense chronic inflammatory cell infiltrate in the connective tissue stroma. Complete removal of the lesion is curative. This is important since incomplete excision may result in recurrence or, very rarely, neoplastic transformation into an ameloblastoma or a squamous cell carcinoma.

The *odontogenic keratocyst (OKC)* is an important entity to differentiate from other odontogenic cysts because of its potential to be aggressive. OKCs can be seen at any age but are most often diagnosed in patients between ages 10 and 40. They occur most commonly in males within the posterior mandible. Radiographically, OKCs present as well-defined unilocular or multilocular radiolucencies. Histologically, the cyst lining consists of a thin layer of parakeratinized or orthokeratinized stratified squamous epithelium with a prominent basal cell layer and a corrugated appearance of the epithelial surface. Treatment requires aggressive and complete removal of the lesion, as recurrence rates for inadequately removed lesions can reach 60%. Multiple OKCs may occur; these patients should be evaluated for nevoid basal cell carcinoma syndrome (Gorlin syndrome), which, as we shall see, is related to mutations in the tumor suppressor gene *PTCH* (Chapter 25).

The *periapical cyst* (also called periapical granuloma), in contrast to the two lesions described above, is inflammatory in origin. These are extremely common lesions found at the apex of teeth. They develop as a result of longstanding pulpitis, which may be caused by advanced carious lesions or by trauma to the tooth in question. The inflammatory process may result in necrosis of the pulpal tissue, which can traverse the length of the root and exit the apex of the tooth into the surrounding alveolar bone giving rise to a periapical abscess. Over time, like any chronic inflammatory process, a lesion with granulation tissue (with or without an epithelial lining) may develop. While the term *granuloma* is not the most appropriate terminology (as the lesion does not show true granulomatous inflammation), old terminology, like bad habits, is difficult to shed. Periapical inflammatory lesions persist as a result of the continued presence of bacteria or other offensive agents in the area. Successful treatment therefore necessitates the complete removal of offending material and appropriate restoration of the tooth or extraction.

Odontogenic tumors are a complex group of lesions with diverse histology and clinical behavior.[33] Some are true neoplasms (both benign and malignant), while others are more likely hamartomas. Odontogenic tumors are derived from odontogenic epithelium, ectomesenchyme, or both (Table 16–3). The two most common and clinically significant tumors are:

Ameloblastoma, which arises from odontogenic epithelium and shows *no* ectomesenchymal differentiation. It is commonly cystic, slow growing, and locally invasive but has a benign course in most cases.

Odontoma, the most common type of odontogenic tumor, arises from epithelium but shows extensive depositions of enamel and dentin. Odontomas are probably hamartomas rather than true neoplasms and are cured by local excision.

TABLE 16–2 Histologic Classification of Odontogenic Cysts

1. Inflammatory
a. Periapical cyst
b. Residual cyst
c. Paradental cyst
2. Developmental
a. Dentigerous cyst
b. Odontogenic keratocyst
c. Gingival cyst of newborn
d. Gingival cyst of adult
e. Eruption cyst
f. Lateral periodontal cyst
g. Glandular odontogenic cyst
h. Calcifying epithelial odontogenic cyst (Gorlin cyst)

TABLE 16–3 Histologic Classification of Odontogenic Tumors

1. Tumors of Odontogenic Epithelium
Benign
a. Ameloblastoma
b. Calcifying epithelial odontogenic tumor (Pindborg tumor)
c. Squamous odontogenic tumor
Malignant
a. Ameloblastic carcinoma
b. Malignant ameloblastoma
c. Clear cell odontogenic carcinoma
2. Tumors of Odontogenic Ectomesenchyme
a. Odontogenic fibroma
b. Odontogenic myxoma
c. Cementoblastoma
3. Tumors of Odontogenic Epithelium and Ectomesenchyme
Benign
a. Ameloblastic fibroma
b. Ameloblastic fibro-odontoma
c. Ameloblastic fibrosarcoma
d. Adenomatoid odontogenic tumor
e. Odontoameloblastoma
f. Complex odontoma
g. Compound odontoma
Malignant
a. Ameloblastic fibrosarcoma

UPPER AIRWAYS

The term *upper airways* is used here to include the nose, pharynx, and larynx and their related parts. Disorders of these structures are among the most common afflictions of humans, but fortunately the overwhelming majority are more nuisances than threats.

Nose

Inflammatory diseases, mostly in the form of the common cold, as everyone knows, are the most common disorders of the nose and accessory air sinuses. Most of these inflammatory conditions are viral in origin, but they are often complicated by superimposed bacterial infections having considerably greater significance. Much less common are a few destructive inflammatory nasal diseases and tumors primary in the nasal cavity or paranasal sinuses.

INFLAMMATIONS

Infectious Rhinitis. Infectious rhinitis, the more elegant way of saying "common cold," is in most instances caused by one or more viruses. Major offenders are adenoviruses, echoviruses, and rhinoviruses. They evoke a profuse catarrhal discharge that is familiar to all and the bane of the kindergarten teacher. During the initial acute stages, the nasal mucosa is thickened, edematous, and red; the nasal cavities are narrowed; and the turbinates are enlarged. These changes may extend, producing a concomitant pharyngotonsillitis. Secondary bacterial infection enhances the inflammatory reaction and produces an essentially mucopurulent or sometimes frankly suppurative exudate. But as everyone knows, these infections soon clear up—as the saying goes, in a week if treated but after 7 days if ignored.

Allergic Rhinitis. Allergic rhinitis (hay fever) is initiated by sensitivity reactions to one of a large group of allergens, most commonly the plant pollens, fungi, animal allergens, and dust mites.[34] It affects 20% of the U.S. population. As is the case with asthma, allergic rhinitis is an immunoglobulin E–mediated immune reaction with an early- and late-phase response (see section on type I hypersensitivity in Chapter 6). The allergic reaction is characterized by marked mucosal edema, redness, and mucus secretion, accompanied by a leukocytic infiltration in which eosinophils are prominent.

Nasal Polyps. Recurrent attacks of rhinitis eventually lead to focal protrusions of the mucosa, producing so-called *nasal polyps,* which may reach 3 to 4 cm in length. On histologic examination, these polyps consist of edematous mucosa having a loose stroma, often harboring hyperplastic or cystic mucous glands and infiltrated with a variety of inflammatory cells, including prominently neutrophils, eosinophils, and plasma cells with occasional clusters of lymphocytes (Fig. 16–9). In the absence of bacterial infection, the mucosal covering of these polyps is intact, but with chronicity, it may become ulcerated or infected. When multiple or large, the polyps may encroach on the airway and impair sinus drainage. Although the features of nasal polyps point to an allergic etiology, most patients with nasal polyps are not atopic, and only 0.5% of atopic patients develop polyps.[35]

Chronic Rhinitis. Chronic rhinitis is a sequel to repeated attacks of acute rhinitis, whether microbial or allergic in origin, with the eventual development of superimposed bacterial infection. A deviated nasal septum or nasal polyps with impaired drainage of secretions contribute to the microbial invasion. Frequently, there is superficial desquamation or ulceration of the mucosal epithelium and a variable inflammatory infiltrate of neutrophils, lymphocytes, and plasma cells subjacent to the epithelium. These suppurative infections sometimes extend into the air sinuses.

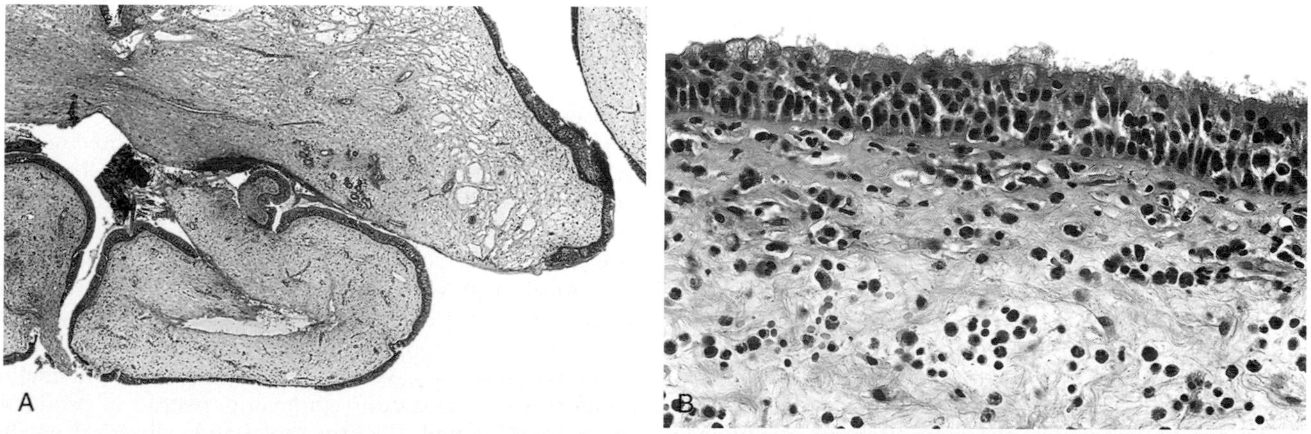

FIGURE 16–9 *A,* Nasal polyps. Low-power magnification showing edematous masses lined by epithelium. *B,* High-power view showing edema and eosinophil-rich inflammatory infiltrate.

Sinusitis. Acute sinusitis is most commonly preceded by acute or chronic rhinitis, but maxillary sinusitis occasionally arises by extension of a periapical infection through the bony floor of the sinus. The offending agents are usually inhabitants of the oral cavity, and the inflammatory reaction is entirely nonspecific. Impairment of drainage of the sinus by inflammatory edema of the mucosa is an important contributor to the process and, when complete, may impound the suppurative exudate, producing *empyema* of the sinus. Obstruction of the outflow, most often of the frontal and next most often of the anterior ethmoid sinuses, occasionally leads to an accumulation of mucous secretions in the absence of direct bacterial invasion, producing a so-called *mucocele.* Acute sinusitis may, in time, give rise to *chronic sinusitis,* particularly when there is interference with drainage. There is usually a mixed microbial flora, largely of normal inhabitants of the oral cavity. Particularly severe forms of chronic sinusitis are caused by fungi (e.g., mucormycosis), especially in diabetics. Uncommonly, sinusitis is a component of *Kartagener syndrome,* which also includes bronchiectasis and situs inversus (Chapter 15). All these features are secondary to defective ciliary action. Although most instances of chronic sinusitis are more uncomfortable than disabling or serious, the infections have the potential of spreading into the orbit or of penetrating into the enclosing bone and producing osteomyelitis or, even, of penetrating into the cranial vault, causing septic thrombophlebitis of a dural venous sinus.

NECROTIZING LESIONS OF THE NOSE AND UPPER AIRWAYS

Necrotizing ulcerating lesions of the nose and upper respiratory tract may be produced by

- Spreading fungal infections (principally mucormycosis [Chapter 8]), particularly in the diabetic
- Wegener granulomatosis (discussed in Chapter 11)
- A condition once called *lethal midline granuloma* or *polymorphic reticulosis* and now thought to represent, in most cases, a neoplasm of natural killer cells[36] (Chapter 14). Ulceration and superimposed bacterial infection frequently complicate the process, confusing the histologic changes by producing tumor-related granulomatous inflammation. Concomitant lymphomatous lesions may be found in other organs and sites. At one time, these lesions were highly fatal owing to uncontrolled growth of the lymphoma, possibly with penetration into the cranial vault, or because of tumor necrosis with secondary bacterial infection and blood-borne dissemination of the infection. Currently, the treatment of the lymphoma with the usual modalities has proved in many cases to be effective in bringing the destructive process under control.

Nasopharynx

Although the nasopharyngeal mucosa, related lymphoid structures, and glands may be involved in a wide variety of specific infections (e.g., diphtheria, infectious mononucleosis) as well as by neoplasms, the only disorders mentioned here are nonspecific inflammations; tumors are discussed separately.

INFLAMMATIONS

Pharyngitis and *tonsillitis* are frequent concomitants of the usual viral upper respiratory infections. Most often implicated are the multitudinous rhinoviruses, echoviruses, and adenoviruses, and, less frequently, respiratory syncytial viruses and the various strains of influenza virus. In the usual case, there is reddening and slight edema of the nasopharyngeal mucosa, with reactive enlargement of the related lymphoid structures. Bacterial infections may be superimposed on these viral involvements, or the bacteria may be primary invaders. The most common offenders are the β-hemolytic streptococci, but sometimes *Staphylococcus aureus* or other pathogens may be implicated. Particularly severe forms of pharyngitis and tonsillitis are seen in infants and children who have not yet developed any protective immunity to such agents and in adults rendered susceptible by neutropenia, some form of immunodeficiency, uncontrolled diabetes, or disruption of the normal oral flora by antibiotics. In these circumstances, microbial opportunists may be involved. The inflamed nasopharyngeal mucosa may be covered by an exudative membrane (pseudomembrane), and the nasopalatine and palatine tonsils may be enlarged and covered by exudate. A typical appearance is of enlarged, reddened tonsils (due to reactive lymphoid hyperplasia) dotted by pinpoints of exudate emanating from the tonsillar crypts, so-called *follicular tonsillitis.*

The major importance of streptococcal "sore throats" lies in the possible development of late sequelae, for example, rheumatic fever (Chapter 12) and glomerulonephritis (Chapter 20). Whether recurrent episodes of acute tonsillitis favor the development of chronic tonsillitis (true chronic tonsillitis is extremely rare) is open to debate, but they may leave residual enlargement of the lymphoid tissue, inviting the tender mercies of the otolaryngologist.

Tumors of the Nose, Sinuses, and Nasopharynx

Tumors in these locations are infrequent but include the entire category of mesenchymal and epithelial neoplasms.[36,37] Brief mention is made of somewhat distinctive types.

Nasopharyngeal Angiofibroma. This is a highly vascular tumor that occurs almost exclusively in adolescent males. Despite its benign nature, it may cause serious clinical problems because of its tendency to bleed profusely during surgery.

Sinonasal Papillomas. These are benign neoplasms arising from the sinonasal mucosa and are composed of squamous or columnar epithelium. Although their etiology is still unproven, HPV types 6 and 11 have been identified in the lesions. These occur in three forms: *septal* (most common), *inverted* (most important biologically), and *cylindrical.* Given its uniquely aggressive biologic behavior, only inverted papilloma is discussed here. Inverted papillomas are benign but locally aggressive neoplasms occurring in both the nose and the paranasal sinuses. As the name implies, the papillomatous proliferation of squamous epithelium, instead of producing an exophytic growth (like the septal and cylindrical papillomas), extends into the mucosa, that is, is it inverted (Fig. 16–10). If not adequately excised, it has a high rate of recur-

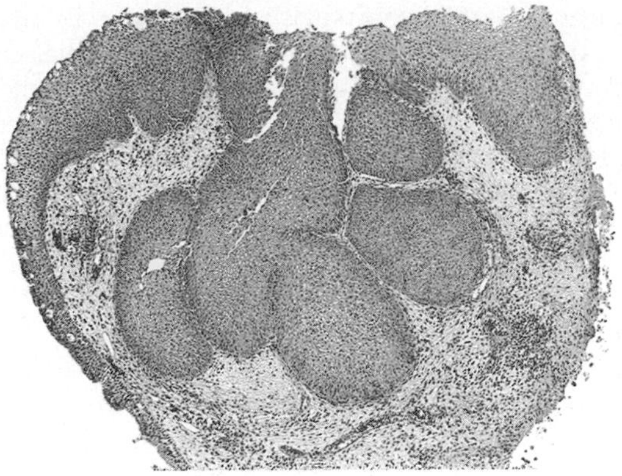

FIGURE 16–10 Inverted papilloma. The masses of squamous epithelium are growing inward; hence, the term inverted. (Courtesy of Dr. James Gulizia, Brigham and Women's Hospital, Boston, MA.)

rence, with the potentially serious complication of invasion of the orbit or cranial vault; rarely, frank carcinoma may also develop.

Isolated Plasmacytomas. These extramedullary plasmacytomas (Chapter 14) arise in the lymphoid structures adjacent to the nose and sinuses. The tumors may protrude within these cavities as polypoid growths, varying from 1 cm to several centimeters in diameter, covered usually by an intact overlying mucosa. The histology is that of a malignant plasma cell tumor and is identical to that described in Chapter 14. Only rarely do these lesions progress to multiple myeloma.

Olfactory Neuroblastomas (Esthesioneuroblastomas). These are uncommon, highly malignant tumors composed of small round cells resembling neuroblasts proliferating into lobular nests encircled by vascularized connective tissue. They arise most often superiorly and laterally in the nose from the neuroendocrine cells dispersed in the olfactory mucosa. The differential diagnosis of these neoplasms includes all other small cell tumors (Chapter 10), such as lymphoma, Ewing sarcoma, and embryonal rhabdomyosarcoma.[38] The cells are of neuroendocrine origin and thus exhibit membrane-bound secretory granules on electron microscopy and stain immunohistochemically for neuron-specific enolase, S-100 protein, and chromogranin. Although they are thus classifiable as primitive neuroectodermal tumors, many do not share the 11;22 translocation or fusion-gene products typical of Ewing sarcoma of bone (Chapter 26) and other primitive neuroectodermal tumors.[38] Some of these tumors also reveal trisomy 8. Olfactory neuroblastomas tend to metastasize widely. Combinations of surgery, radiation, and chemotherapy yield a 5-year survival rate of 50% to 70%.[39]

Nasopharyngeal Carcinomas. This tumor is characterized by a distinctive geographic distribution, a close anatomic relationship to lymphoid tissue, and an association with EBV infection.[40] It takes one of three patterns: (1) keratinizing squamous cell carcinomas, (2) nonkeratinizing squamous cell carcinomas, and (3) undifferentiated carcinomas that have an abundant non-neoplastic, lymphocytic infiltrate. This last pattern has often been called, erroneously, *lymphoepithelioma.*

Three sets of influences apparently affect the origins of these neoplasms: (1) heredity, (2) age, and (3) infection with EBV. Nasopharyngeal carcinomas are particularly common in parts of Africa, where they are the most frequent childhood cancer. In contrast, in southern China, they are very common in adults but rarely occur in children. In the United States, they are rare in both adults and children. Environment must play some role in this distribution, because migration from a high-incidence locale to a low-incidence locale is followed by a progressive decline in incidence over generations. The EBV genome has been identified in the tumor epithelial cells (not the lymphocytes) of most undifferentiated and nonkeratinizing squamous cell nasopharyngeal carcinomas.[41]

Morphology. On histologic examination, the keratinizing and nonkeratinizing squamous cell lesions more or less resemble usual well-differentiated and poorly differentiated squamous cell carcinomas arising in other locations. The undifferentiated variant is composed of large epithelial cells with oval or round vesicular nuclei, prominent nucleoli, and indistinct cell borders disposed in a syncytium-like array (Fig. 16–11). Admixed with the epithelial cells are abundant, mature, normal-appearing lymphocytes. The three histologic variants present as masses in the nasopharynx or sometimes in other locations, such as the tonsils, posterior tongue, or upper airways.

Nasopharyngeal carcinomas tend to grow silently until they have become unresectable and have often spread to cervical nodes or distant sites. Radiotherapy is the standard modality of treatment, yielding in most studies about a 50% to 70% 3-year survival rate. The undifferentiated carcinoma is the most radiosensitive and the keratinizing the least radiosensitive.

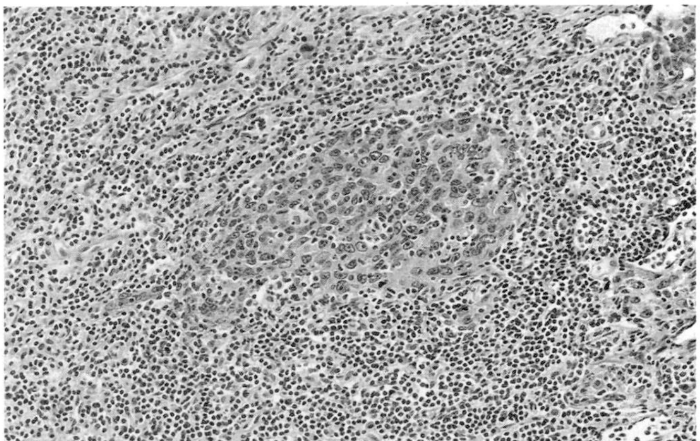

FIGURE 16–11 Nasopharyngeal carcinoma, lymphoepithelioma type. The syncytium-like nests of epithelium are surrounded by lymphocytes. (Courtesy of Dr. James Gulizia, Brigham and Women's Hospital, Boston, MA.)

Larynx

The most common disorders that affect the larynx are inflammations. Tumors are uncommon but are amenable to resection, although often at the price of loss of natural voice.

INFLAMMATIONS

Laryngitis may occur as the sole manifestation of allergic, viral, bacterial, or chemical insult, but it is more commonly part of a generalized upper respiratory tract infection or the result of heavy exposure to tobacco smoke. The larynx may also be affected in many systemic infectious diseases, such as tuberculosis and diphtheria. Although most infections are self-limited, they may at times be serious, especially in infancy or childhood, when mucosal congestion, exudation, or edema may cause laryngeal obstruction. In particular, laryngoepiglottitis, caused by *Haemophilus influenzae* or β-hemolytic streptococci in infants and young children with their small airways, may induce such sudden swelling of the epiglottis and vocal cords that a potentially lethal medical emergency is created. This form of disease is uncommon in adults owing to the larger size of the larynx and the stronger accessory muscles of respiration. *Croup* is the name given to laryngotracheobronchitis in children, in which the inflammatory narrowing of the airway produces the inspiratory stridor so frightening to parents. The most common form of laryngitis, encountered in heavy smokers, constitutes an important predisposition to the development of squamous epithelial changes in the larynx and sometimes overt carcinoma.

REACTIVE NODULES (VOCAL CORD NODULES AND POLYPS)

Reactive nodules, also called polyps, sometimes develop on the vocal cords, most often in heavy smokers or in individuals who impose great strain on their vocal cords *(singers' nodules)*. By convention, singers' nodules are bilateral lesions and polyps are unilateral. Adults, predominantly men, are most often affected. These nodules constitute smooth, rounded, sessile or pedunculated excrescences, generally only a few millimeters in greatest dimension, located usually on the true vocal cords. They are typically covered by squamous epithelium that may become keratotic, hyperplastic, or even slightly dysplastic. The core of the nodule is a loose myxoid connective tissue that may be variably fibrotic or punctuated by numerous vascular channels. When nodules on opposing vocal cords impinge on each other, the mucosa may undergo ulceration.

Because of their strategic location, with corresponding greater inflammatory infiltration of the core of the lesion, they characteristically change the character of the voice and often cause progressive hoarseness. They virtually never give rise to cancers.

CARCINOMA OF THE LARYNX

Sequence of Hyperplasia-Dysplasia-Carcinoma. A spectrum of epithelial alterations is seen in the larynx. These are termed, from one end of the spectrum to the other, hyperplasia, atypical hyperplasia, dysplasia, carcinoma in situ, and invasive carcinoma.[42] Macroscopically, the epithelial changes range from smooth, white or reddened focal thickenings, sometimes roughened by keratosis, to irregular verrucous or ulcerated, white-pink lesions looking like cancer.

When first seen, the orderly thickenings have almost no potential for malignant transformation, but the risk rises to 1% to 2% during the span of 5 to 10 years with mild dysplasia and 5% to 10% with severe dysplasia. In essence, *there are all gradations of epithelial hyperplasia of the true vocal cords, and the likelihood of the development of an overt carcinoma is directly proportional to the level of atypia when the lesion is first seen.* Only histologic evaluation can determine the gravity of the changes.

The various changes described are most often related to tobacco smoke, the risk being proportional to the level of exposure. Indeed, up to the point of frank cancer, the changes often regress after cessation of smoking. However, alcohol is also clearly a risk factor and other factors may contribute to increased risk, including nutritional factors, exposure to asbestos, and irradiation.[43,44] HPV sequences are present in about 5% of cases.

Morphology. About 95% of laryngeal carcinomas are typical squamous cell tumors. Rarely, adenocarcinomas are seen, presumably arising from mucous glands. The tumor usually develops directly on the vocal cords, but it may arise above or below the cords, on the epiglottis or aryepiglottic folds, or in the piriform sinuses. Those confined within the larynx proper are termed **intrinsic,** whereas those that arise or extend outside the larynx are called **extrinsic.** Squamous cell carcinomas of the larynx follow the growth pattern of all squamous cell carcinomas. They begin as in situ lesions that later appear as pearly gray, wrinkled plaques on the mucosal surface, ultimately ulcerating and fungating (Fig. 16–12). The degree of anaplasia of the laryngeal tumors is highly variable. Sometimes massive tumor giant cells and multiple bizarre mitotic figures are seen. As expected with lesions arising from recurrent exposure to environmental carcinogens, adjacent mucosa may demonstrate squamous cell hyperplasia with foci of dysplasia or even carcinoma in situ.

Carcinoma of the larynx manifests itself clinically by persistent hoarseness. At presentation, about 60% of these cancers are confined to the larynx; as a result, the prognosis is better than for those that have spread into adjacent structures. Later, laryngeal tumors may produce pain, dysphagia, and hemoptysis. Patients with this condition are extremely vulnerable to secondary infection of the ulcerating lesion. With surgery, radiation, or combination therapy, many patients can be cured, but about one third die of the disease. The usual cause of death is infection of the distal respiratory passages or widespread metastases and cachexia.

SQUAMOUS PAPILLOMA AND PAPILLOMATOSIS

Laryngeal squamous papillomas are benign neoplasms, usually on the true vocal cords, that form soft, raspberry-like

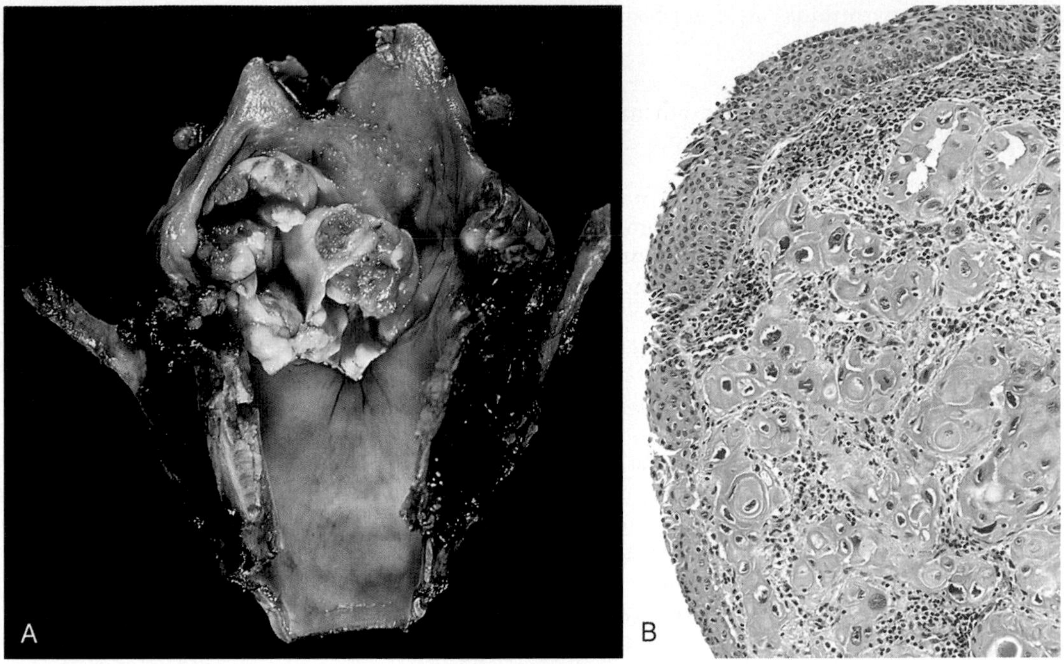

FIGURE 16–12 *A,* Laryngeal carcinoma. Note the large, ulcerated, fungating lesion involving the vocal cord and piriform sinus. *B,* Histologic appearance of laryngeal squamous cell carcinoma. Note the atypical lining epithelium and invasive keratinizing cancer cells in the submucosa.

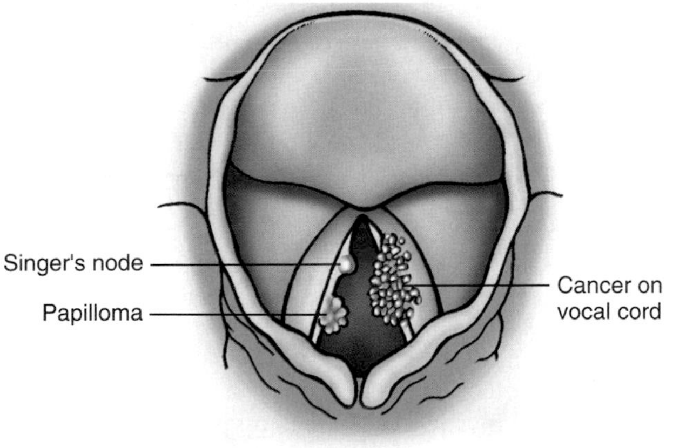

FIGURE 16–13 Diagrammatic comparison of a benign papilloma and an exophytic carcinoma of the larynx to highlight their quite different appearances.

excrescences rarely more than 1 cm in diameter (Fig. 16–13). On histologic examination, the papillomas are made up of multiple slender, finger-like projections supported by central fibrovascular cores and covered by an orderly, typical, stratified squamous epithelium. When the papillomas are on the free edge of the vocal cord, trauma may lead to ulceration that can be accompanied by hemoptysis.

Papillomas are usually single in adults but are often multiple in children, in whom they are referred to as *juvenile laryngeal papillomatosis.*[45] However, multiple recurring papillomas also occur in adults. *The lesions are caused by HPV types 6 and 11.* They do not become malignant, but they frequently recur. They often spontaneously regress at puberty, but some affected patients endure numerous surgeries before this occurs. Cancerous transformation is rare.

EARS

Although disorders of the ear rarely shorten life, many impair its quality. The most common aural disorders, in descending order of frequency, are (1) acute and chronic otitis (most often involving the middle ear and mastoid), sometimes leading to a cholesteatoma; (2) symptomatic otosclerosis; (3) aural polyps; (4) labyrinthitis; (5) carcinomas, largely of the external ear; and (6) paragangliomas, found mostly in the middle ear. Only those conditions that have distinctive morphologic features (save for labyrinthitis) are described. Paragangliomas are discussed later.

Inflammatory Lesions

Inflammations of the ear—*otitis media, acute or chronic*—occur mostly in infants and children. They usually produce a serous exudate (when viral in origin) but may become suppurative with superimposed bacterial infection. The most common offenders are *Streptococcus pneumoniae*, nontypeable *H. influenzae*, and *Moraxella catarrhalis*.[45a]

Repeated bouts of acute otitis media with failure of resolution lead to chronic disease. The causative agents of chronic disease are usually *Pseudomonas aeruginosa, Staphylococcus aureus*, or a fungus; sometimes, a mixed flora is the cause. Chronic infection has the potential to perforate the eardrum, encroaching on the ossicles or labyrinth, spreading into the mastoid spaces, and even penetrating into the cranial vault to produce a temporal cerebritis or abscess. Otitis media in the diabetic person, when caused by *P. aeruginosa*, is especially aggressive and spreads widely (destructive necrotizing otitis media).

Cholesteatomas, associated with chronic otitis media, are not neoplasms, nor do they always contain cholesterol. Rather, they are cystic lesions 1 to 4 cm in diameter, lined by keratinizing squamous epithelium or metaplastic mucus-secreting epithelium and filled with amorphous debris (derived largely from desquamated epithelium). Sometimes they contain spicules of cholesterol. The precise events involved in their development are not clear, but it is proposed that chronic inflammation and perforation of the eardrum with ingrowth of the squamous epithelium or metaplasia of the secretory epithelial lining of the middle ear are responsible for the formation of a squamous cell nest that becomes cystic. A chronic inflammatory reaction surrounds the keratinous cyst. Sometimes, the cyst ruptures, not only enhancing the inflammatory reaction, but also inducing the formation of giant cells that enclose partially necrotic squames and other particulate debris. These lesions, by progressive enlargement, can erode into the ossicles, the labyrinth, the adjacent bone, or the surrounding soft tissue and sometimes produce visible neck masses.

Otosclerosis

As the name implies, otosclerosis refers to abnormal bone deposition in the middle ear about the rim of the oval window into which the footplate of the stapes fits. Both ears are usually affected. At first there is fibrous ankylosis of the footplate, followed in time by bony overgrowth anchoring it into the oval window. The degree of immobilization governs the severity of the hearing loss. This condition usually begins in the early decades of life; minimal degrees of this derangement are exceedingly common in the United States in young to middle-aged adults, but fortunately more severe symptomatic otosclerosis is relatively uncommon. In most instances it is familial, following autosomal dominant transmission with variable penetrance. The basis for the osseous overgrowth is completely obscure, but it appears to represent uncoupling of normal bone resorption and bone formation. Thus, it begins with bone resorption, followed by fibrosis and vascularization of the temporal bone in the immediate vicinity of the oval window, in time replaced by dense new bone anchoring the footplate of the stapes. In most instances, the process is slowly progressive over the span of decades, leading eventually to marked hearing loss.

Tumors

The large variety of epithelial and mesenchymal tumors that arise in the ear—external, medial, internal—are rare save for basal cell or squamous cell carcinomas of the pinna (external ear). These carcinomas tend to occur in elderly men and are thought to be associated with actinic radiation. By contrast, those within the canal tend to be squamous cell carcinomas, which occur in middle-aged to elderly women and are not associated with sun exposure. Wherever they arise, they morphologically resemble their counterparts in other skin locations, beginning as papules that extend and eventually erode and invade locally. Neither the basal cell nor the squamous cell lesions of the pinna commonly extend beyond local invasion, but squamous cell carcinomas arising in the external canal may invade the cranial cavity or metastasize to regional nodes and, indeed, account for a 5-year mortality of about 50%.

NECK

Most of the conditions that involve the neck are described elsewhere (e.g., squamous cell and basal cell carcinomas of the skin, melanomas, lymphomas), or they are only a component of a systemic disorder (e.g., generalized rashes, the lymphadenopathy of infectious mononucleosis or tonsillitis). What remains for consideration here are a few uncommon lesions unique to the neck.

Branchial Cyst (Lymphoepithelial Cyst)

These benign cysts, usually appearing on the anterolateral aspect of the neck, arise either from remnants of the branchial arches or, as many believe, from developmental salivary gland inclusions within cervical lymph nodes.[46] Whatever their origin, they are circumscribed cysts, 2 to 5 cm in diameter, with fibrous walls usually lined by stratified squamous or pseudostratified columnar epithelium underlain by an intense lymphocytic infiltrate or, more often, well-developed lymphoid tissue with reactive follicles. The cystic contents may be clear, watery to mucinous fluid or may contain desquamated, granular cellular debris. The cysts enlarge only slowly, are rarely the site of malignant transformation, and generally are readily excised. Similar lesions sometimes appear in the parotid gland or in the oral cavity beneath the tongue.

Thyroglossal Tract Cyst

Embryologically, the thyroid anlage begins in the region of the foramen cecum at the base of the tongue; as the gland develops, it descends to its definitive location in the anterior neck. Remnants of this developmental tract may persist, producing cysts, 1 to 4 cm in diameter, that may be lined by stratified squamous epithelium, when the cyst is near the base of the tongue, or by pseudostratified columnar epithelium in lower locations. Obviously, transitional patterns are also encountered. The connective tissue wall of the cyst may harbor lymphoid aggregates or remnants of recognizable thyroid tissue. The treatment is excision, but if it is not complete, stubborn recurrence can be expected. Malignant transformation within the lining epithelium has been reported but is rare.

Paraganglioma (Carotid Body Tumor)

Paraganglia are clusters of neuroendocrine cells dispersed throughout the body, some connected with the sympathetic nervous system and others with the parasympathetic nervous system. The largest collection of these cells is found in the adrenal medulla, where they give rise to *pheochromocytomas* (Chapter 24). Tumors arising in extra-adrenal paraganglia are not surprisingly referred to as *paragangliomas.*[47] Paragangliomas develop in two general locations:

- Paravertebral paraganglia (e.g., organs of Zuckerkandl and, rarely, bladder). Such tumors have sympathetic connections and are chromaffin positive; about half elaborate catecholamines, as do pheochromocytomas.
- Paraganglia related to the great vessels of the head and neck, the so-called aorticopulmonary chain, including the *carotid bodies;* aortic bodies; jugulotympanic ganglia; ganglion nodosum of the vagus nerve; and clusters located about the oral cavity, nose, nasopharynx, larynx, and orbit. These are innervated by the parasympathetic nervous system, and their tumors are referred to as *nonchromaffin paragangliomas.* These tumors infrequently release catecholamines, but because the neuroendocrine cells that make up these lesions sense oxygen and carbon dioxide tensions within adjacent vessels, the tumors are also sometimes referred to as *chemodectomas.*

Morphology. The **carotid body tumor** is a prototype of a parasympathetic paraganglioma. It rarely exceeds 6 cm in diameter and arises close to or envelops the bifurcation of the common carotid artery. The tumor tissue is red-pink to brown. The microscopic features of all paragangliomas, wherever they arise, are remarkably uniform. They are composed of nests **(zellballen)** of polygonal chief cells enclosed by trabeculae of fibrous and sustentacular elongated cells.[48] The tumor cells have abundant, clear or granular, eosinophilic cytoplasm and uniform, round to ovoid, sometimes vesicular, nuclei (Fig. 16–14). In most tumors, there is little cellular pleomorphism, and mitoses are scant. Electron microscopy often discloses well-demarcated neuroendocrine granules in paravertebral tumors, but they tend to be scant in nonfunctioning tumors. However, the cells in most tumors are argyrophilic and stain positively for neuroendocrine markers by immunohistochemistry (nonspecific enolase; S-100; chromogranin) as well as possibly other bioactive products (e.g., serotonin, gastrin, somatostatin, bombesin).

Carotid body tumors (and paragangliomas in general) are rare. They usually arise in the sixth decade of life. They commonly occur singly and sporadically but may be familial, with autosomal dominant transmission in the multiple endocrine neoplasia 2 syndrome (Chapter 24); in this case, they are fre-

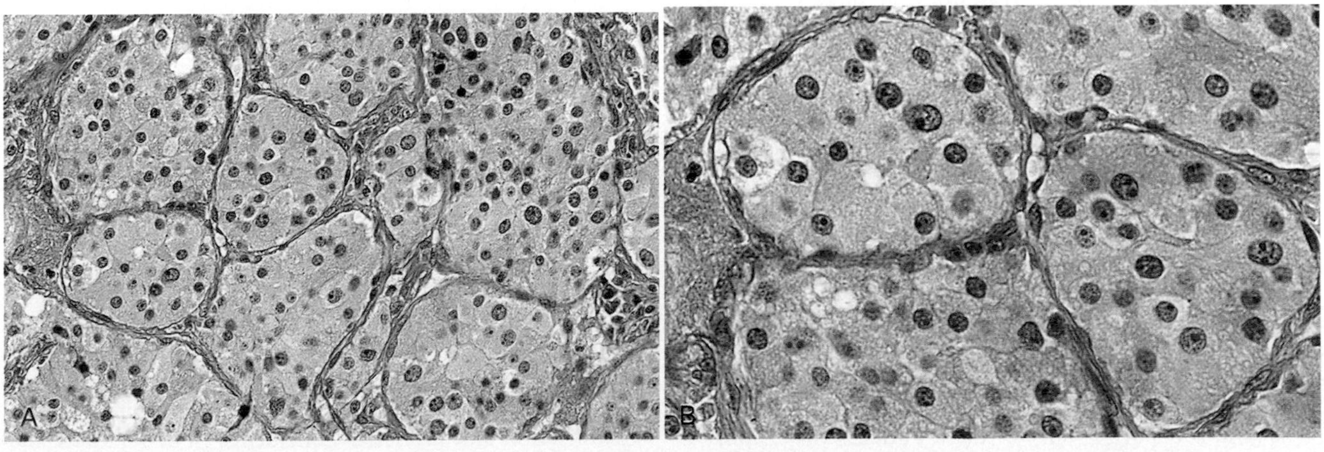

FIGURE 16–14 Carotid body tumor. *A,* Low-power view showing tumor clusters separated by septa (zellballen). *B,* High-power view of large, eosinophilic, slightly vacuolated tumor cells with elongated sustentacular cells in the septa.

quently multiple and sometimes bilaterally symmetric. Carotid body tumors frequently recur after incomplete resection and, despite their benign appearance, many metastasize to local and distant sites. About 50% ultimately prove fatal, largely because of infiltrative growth. Unfortunately, it is almost impossible histologically to judge the clinical course of a carotid body tumor—mitoses, pleomorphism, and even vascular invasion are unreliable.[47]

SALIVARY GLANDS

There are three major salivary glands—parotid, submandibular, and sublingual—as well as innumerable minor salivary glands distributed throughout the mucosa of the oral cavity. All these glands are subject to inflammation or to the development of neoplasms.

Xerostomia

Xerostomia refers to dry mouth; it is a major feature of the autoimmune disorder Sjögren syndrome, in which it is usually accompanied by dry eyes (Chapter 6). A lack of salivary secretions may also be a complication of radiation therapy. The oral cavity may merely reveal dry mucosa or atrophy of the papillae of the tongue, with fissuring and ulcerations, or in Sjögren syndrome, concomitant inflammatory enlargement of the salivary glands.

Inflammation (Sialadenitis)

Sialadenitis may be of traumatic, viral, bacterial, or autoimmune origin. Mucoceles are the most common type of inflammatory salivary gland lesion. The most common form of viral sialadenitis is mumps, in which usually the major salivary glands, particularly the parotids, are affected (epidemic parotitis; Chapter 8). Other glands (e.g., the pancreas and testes) may also be involved. Autoimmune disease underlies the inflammatory salivary changes of Sjögren syndrome, discussed in Chapter 6. In this condition, the widespread involvement of the salivary glands and the mucus-secreting glands of the nasal mucosa induces xerostomia. Associated involvement of the lacrimal glands produces dry eyes—*keratoconjunctivitis sicca.*

Mucocele. This is the most common lesion of the salivary glands and it results from either blockage or rupture of a salivary gland duct, with consequent leakage of saliva into the surrounding connective tissue stroma. Mucoceles are most often found on the lower lip and are the result of trauma. As such, they are typically seen in toddlers and young adults as well as the geriatric population (as a result of falling). Clinically, they present as fluctuant swellings of the lower lip and have a blue translucent hue to them. Patients may report a history of fluctuating size of the lesion, particularly in association with meals (Fig. 16–15*A*). Histologically, mucoceles demonstrate a cystlike space that is lined by inflammatory granulation tissue or by fibrous connective tissue. The cystic spaces are filled with mucin as well as inflammatory cells, particularly macrophages (Fig. 16–15*B*). Complete excision of the cyst with the minor salivary gland lobule of origin is required. Incomplete excision can result in recurrence.

A *ranula* is histologically identical to a mucocele. However, this term is reserved for mucoceles that arise when the duct of the sublingual gland has been damaged. A *ranula* can become extremely large and develop into a "plunging ranula" when it dissects its way through the connective tissue stroma connecting the two bellies of the mylohyoid muscle.

Sialolithiasis and Nonspecific Sialadenitis. Nonspecific bacterial sialadenitis, most often involving the major salivary glands, particularly the submandibular glands, is a common condition, usually secondary to ductal obstruction produced by stones *(sialolithiasis).* The common offenders are *S. aureus* and *Streptococcus viridans.* The stone formation is sometimes related to obstruction of the orifices of the salivary glands by impacted food debris or by edema about the orifice after some injury. Frequently, the stones are of obscure origin. Dehydration with decreased secretory function may also predispose to secondary bacterial invasion, as sometimes occurs in patients receiving long-term phenothiazines that suppress salivary secretion. Perhaps dehydration with decreased secretion explains the development of bacterial suppurative parotitis in elderly patients with a recent history of major thoracic or abdominal surgery.

Whatever the origin, the obstructive process and bacterial invasion lead to a nonspecific inflammation of the affected glands that may be largely interstitial or, when induced by staphylococcal or other pyogens, may be associated with overt suppurative necrosis and abscess formation. Unilateral involvement of a single gland is the rule. The inflammatory involvement causes painful enlargement and sometimes a purulent ductal discharge.

Neoplasms

Despite their relatively undistinguished normal morphology, the salivary glands give rise to no fewer than 30 histologically distinct benign and malignant tumors.[49–51] A classification and the relative incidence of benign and malignant tumors is shown in Table 16–4; not included are the rare benign and malignant mesenchymal tumors.

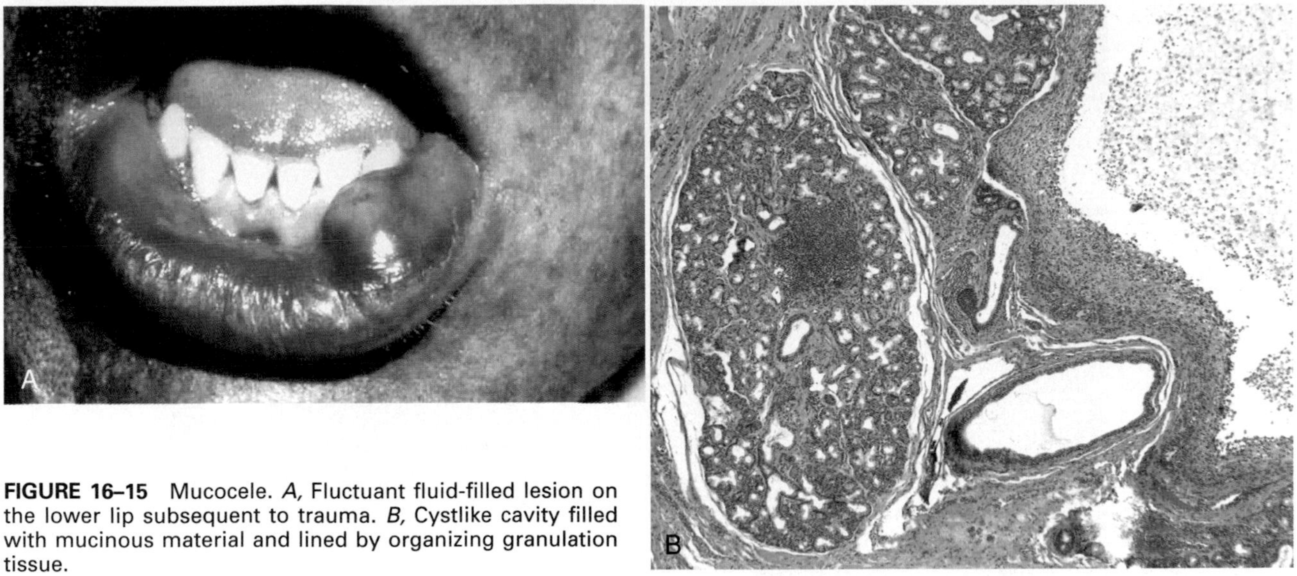

FIGURE 16–15 Mucocele. *A,* Fluctuant fluid-filled lesion on the lower lip subsequent to trauma. *B,* Cystlike cavity filled with mucinous material and lined by organizing granulation tissue.

As indicated in Table 16–4, a small number of neoplasms makes up more than 90% of salivary gland tumors, and so our consideration is restricted to these. Overall, these neoplasms are relatively uncommon and represent less than 2% of tumors in humans. About 65% to 80% arise within the parotid, 10% in the submandibular gland, and the remainder in the minor salivary glands, including the sublingual glands. Fifteen percent to 30% of tumors in the parotid glands are malignant, in contrast to about 40% in the submandibular glands, 50% in the minor salivary glands, and 70% to 90% of sublingual tumors. *The likelihood, then, of a salivary gland tumor being malignant is more or less inversely proportional to the size of the gland.*

These tumors usually occur in adults, with a slight female predominance, but about 5% occur in children younger than age 16 years. For unknown reasons, Warthin tumors occur much more often in males than in females. The benign tumors most often appear in the fifth to seventh decades of life. The malignant ones tend, on average, to appear somewhat later. Whatever the histologic pattern, neoplasms in the parotid glands produce distinctive swellings in front of and below the ear. In general, when they are first diagnosed, both benign and malignant lesions range from 4 to 6 cm in diameter and are mobile on palpation except in the case of neglected malignant tumors. Although benign tumors are known to have been present usually for many months to several years before coming to clinical attention, cancers seem to demand attention more promptly, probably because of their more rapid growth. Ultimately, however, there are no reliable criteria to differentiate, on clinical grounds, the benign from the malignant lesions, and morphologic evaluation is necessary.

TABLE 16–4 Histologic Classification and Approximate Incidence of Benign and Malignant Tumors of the Salivary Glands

Benign	Malignant
Pleomorphic adenoma (50%) (mixed tumor)	Mucoepidermoid carcinoma (15%)
Warthin tumor (5%–10%)	Adenocarcinoma (NOS) (10%)
Oncocytoma (1%)	Acinic cell carcinoma (5%)
Other adenomas (5%–10%)	Adenoid cystic carcinoma (5%)
Basal cell adenoma	Malignant mixed tumor (3%–5%)
Canalicular adenoma	Squamous cell carcinoma (1%)
Ductal papillomas	Other carcinomas (2%)

NOS, not otherwise specified. Data from Ellis GL, Auclair PL: Tumors of the Salivary Glands. Atlas of Tumor Pathology, Third Series. Washington, DC, Armed Forces Institute of Pathology, 1996.

PLEOMORPHIC ADENOMA

Because of their remarkable histologic diversity, these neoplasms have also been called *mixed tumors.* They represent about 60% of tumors in the parotid, are less common in the submandibular glands, and are relatively rare in the minor salivary glands. They are benign tumors that are derived from a mixture of ductal (epithelial) and myoepithelial cells, and therefore they show both epithelial and mesenchymal differentiation. They also reveal epithelial elements dispersed throughout a matrix along with varying degrees of myxoid, hyaline, chondroid (cartilaginous), and even osseous tissue. In some tumors, the epithelial elements predominate; in others, they are present only in widely dispersed foci.

Little is known about the origins of these neoplasms except that radiation exposure increases the risk. Equally uncertain is the histogenesis of the various components. A currently popular view is that all neoplastic elements, including those that appear mesenchymal, are of either myoepithelial or ductal reserve cell origin (hence the designation *pleomorphic adenoma*).

Morphology. Most pleomorphic adenomas present as rounded, well-demarcated masses rarely exceeding 6 cm in greatest dimension (Fig. 16–16). Although they are encapsulated, in some locations (particularly the palate) the capsule is not fully developed, and expansile growth produces tonguelike protrusions

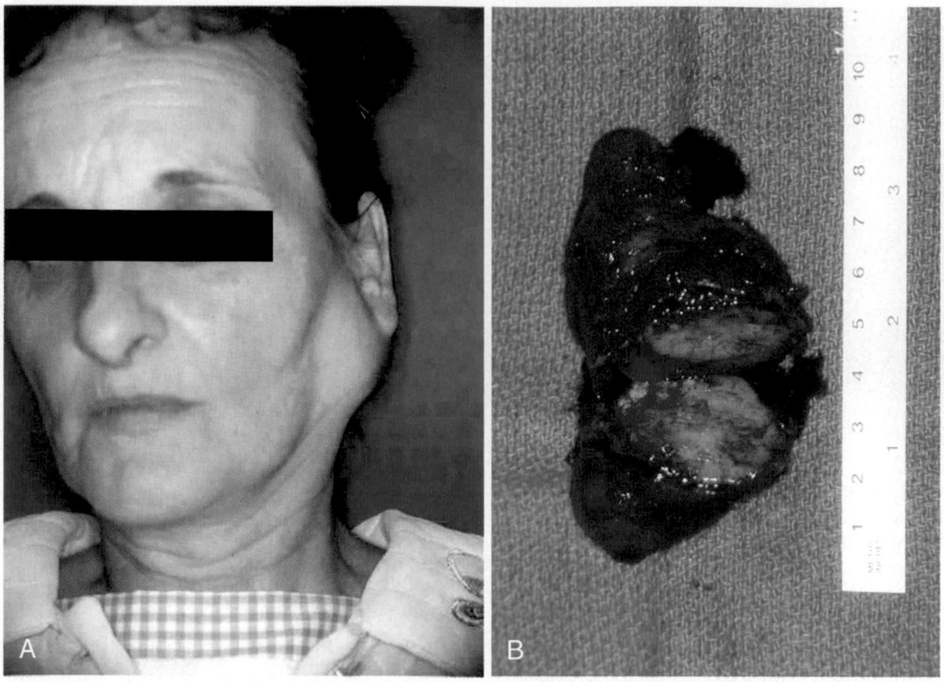

FIGURE 16–16 Pleomorphic adenoma. *A,* Slowly enlarging neoplasm in the parotid gland of many years duration. *B,* The bisected, sharply circumscribed, yellow-white tumor can be seen surrounded by normal salivary gland tissue.

into the surrounding gland, rendering enucleation of the tumor hazardous. The cut surface is gray-white with myxoid and blue translucent areas of chondroid.

The dominant histologic feature is the great heterogeneity mentioned. The epithelial elements resembling ductal cells or myoepithelial cells are disposed in duct formations, acini, irregular tubules, strands, or sheets of cells. These elements are typically dispersed within a mesenchyme-like background of loose myxoid tissue containing islands of chondroid and, rarely, foci of bone (Fig. 16–17). Sometimes the epithelial cells form well-developed ducts lined by cuboidal to columnar cells with an underlying layer of deeply chromatic, small myoepithelial cells. In other instances, there may be strands or sheets of myoepithelial cells. Islands of well-differentiated squamous epithelium may also occur. In most cases, there is no epithelial dysplasia or evident mitotic activity. There is no difference in biologic behavior between the tumors composed largely of epithelial elements and those composed only of seemingly mesenchymal elements.

Clinical Features. These tumors present as painless, slow-growing, mobile discrete masses within the parotid or submandibular areas or in the buccal cavity. The recurrence rate (perhaps months to years later) with adequate parotidectomy is about 4% but, with attempted enucleation, approaches 25% because of failure to recognize at surgery minute protrusions from the main mass.

A carcinoma arising in a pleomorphic adenoma is referred to variously as a *carcinoma ex pleomorphic adenoma* or a *malignant mixed tumor.* The incidence of malignant transformation increases with the duration of the tumor, being about 2% for tumors present less than 5 years and almost 10% for those of more than 15 years' duration. The cancer usually takes the form of an adenocarcinoma or undifferentiated carcinoma, and often it virtually completely overgrows the last vestiges of the pre-existing pleomorphic adenoma; but to substantiate the diagnosis of carcinoma ex pleomorphic adenoma, recognizable traces of the latter must be found. Regrettably, these cancers, when they appear, are among the most aggressive of all salivary gland malignant neoplasms, accounting for 30% to 50% mortality in 5 years.

WARTHIN TUMOR (PAPILLARY CYSTADENOMA LYMPHOMATOSUM)

This curious benign neoplasm with its intimidating histologic name is the second most common salivary gland neoplasm. It arises almost always in the parotid gland (the only

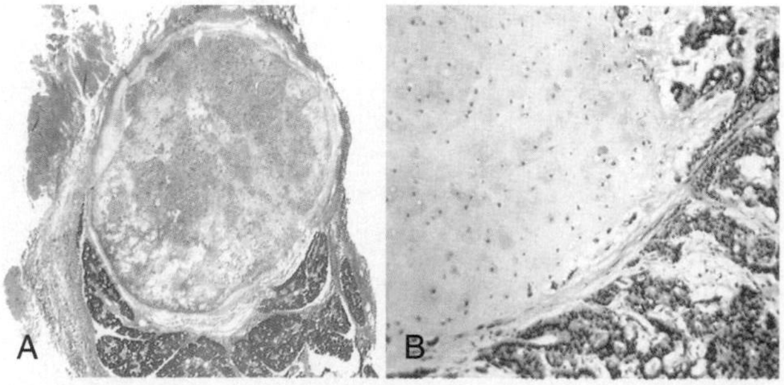

FIGURE 16–17 Pleomorphic adenoma. *A,* Low-power view showing a well-demarcated tumor with adjacent normal salivary gland parenchyma. *B,* High-power view showing epithelial cells as well as myoepithelial cells found within a chondroid matrix material.

tumor virtually restricted to the parotid) and occurs more commonly in males than in females, usually in the fifth to seventh decades of life. About 10% are multifocal and 10% bilateral. Smokers have eight times the risk of nonsmokers for developing these tumors.

Morphology. Most Warthin tumors are round to oval, encapsulated masses, 2 to 5 cm in diameter, arising in most cases in the superficial parotid gland, where they are readily palpable. Transection reveals a pale gray surface punctuated by narrow cystic or cleft-like spaces filled with a mucinous or serous secretion. On microscopic examination, these spaces are lined by a double layer of neoplastic epithelial cells resting on a dense lymphoid stroma sometimes bearing germinal centers (Fig. 16–18). The spaces are frequently narrowed by polypoid projections of the lymphoepithelial elements. The double layer of lining cells is distinctive, with a surface palisade of columnar cells having an abundant, finely granular, eosinophilic cytoplasm, imparting an oncocytic appearance, resting on a layer of cuboidal to polygonal cells. Oncocytes are epithelial cells stuffed with mitochondria that impart the granular appearance to the cytoplasm. Secretory cells are dispersed in the columnar cell layer, accounting for the secretion within the lumens. On occasion, there are foci of squamous metaplasia.

The histogenesis of these tumors has long been disputed. The occasional finding of small salivary gland rests in lymph nodes in the neck suggests that these tumors arise from the aberrant incorporation of similar inclusion-bearing lymphoid tissue in the parotids. Indeed, rarely, Warthin tumors have arisen within cervical lymph nodes, a finding that should not be misconstrued to imply a metastasis. These neoplasms are benign, with recurrence rates of only 2% after resection.

MUCOEPIDERMOID CARCINOMA

These neoplasms are composed of variable mixtures of squamous cells, mucus-secreting cells, and intermediate cells. They represent about 15% of all salivary gland tumors, and while they occur mainly (60% to 70%) in the parotids, they account for a large fraction of salivary gland neoplasms in the other glands, particularly the minor salivary glands. Overall, they are the most common form of primary *malignant* tumor of the salivary glands.

Morphology. Mucoepidermoid carcinomas can grow up to 8 cm in diameter and although they are apparently circumscribed, they lack well-defined capsules and are often infiltrative at the margins. Pale and gray-white on transection, they frequently reveal small, mucin-containing cysts. The basic histologic pattern is that of cords, sheets, or cystic configurations of squamous, mucous, or intermediate cells. The hybrid cell types often have squamous features, with small to large mucus-filled vacuoles, best seen when highlighted with mucin stains (Fig. 16–19*A,B*). The tumor cells may be regular and benign appearing or, alternatively, highly anaplastic and unmistakably malignant. Accordingly, mucoepidermoid carcinomas are subclassified into low, intermediate, or high grade.

The clinical course and prognosis depend on the grade of the neoplasm. Low-grade tumors may invade locally and recur in about 15% of cases, but only rarely do they metastasize and so yield a 5-year survival rate of more than 90%. By contrast, high-grade neoplasms and, to a somewhat lesser extent, intermediate-grade tumors are invasive and difficult to excise and so recur in about 25% to 30% of cases and, in 30% of cases, disseminate to distant sites. The 5-year survival rate of these tumors is only 50%.

OTHER SALIVARY GLAND TUMORS

Two less common neoplasms merit brief description: adenoid cystic carcinoma and acinic cell tumor.

Adenoid cystic carcinoma is a relatively uncommon tumor, which in approximately 50% of cases is found in the minor salivary glands (in particular the palate). Among the major salivary glands, the parotid and submandibular glands are the most common locations. Similar neoplasms have been

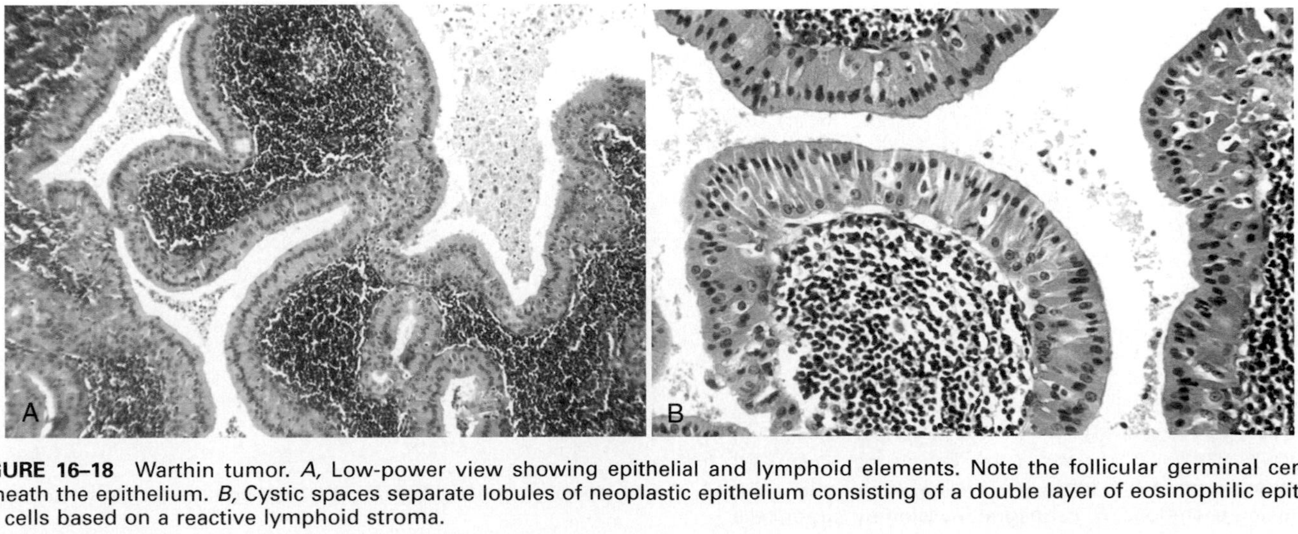

FIGURE 16–18 Warthin tumor. *A,* Low-power view showing epithelial and lymphoid elements. Note the follicular germinal center beneath the epithelium. *B,* Cystic spaces separate lobules of neoplastic epithelium consisting of a double layer of eosinophilic epithelial cells based on a reactive lymphoid stroma.

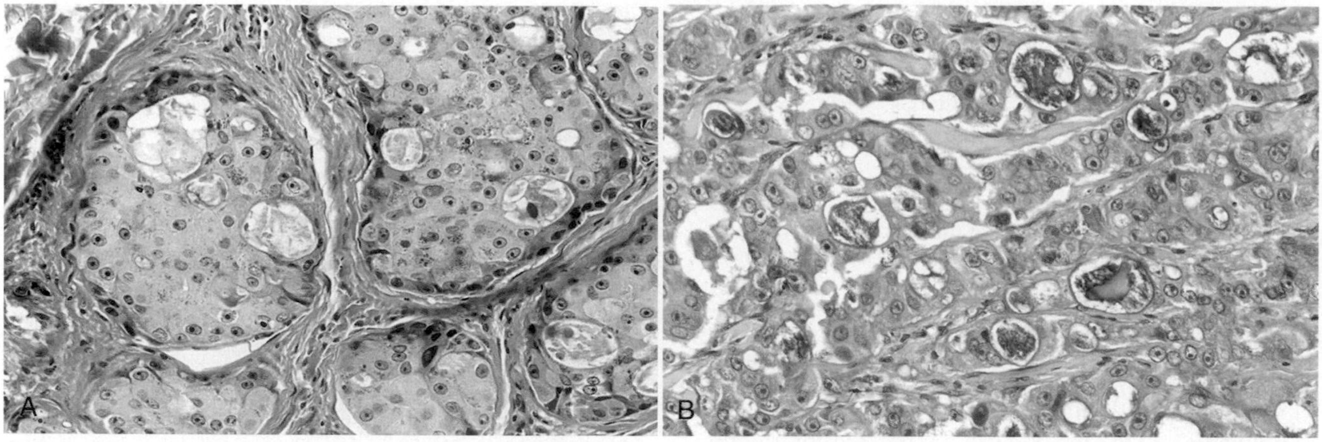

FIGURE 16–19 *A,* Mucoepidermoid carcinoma showing islands having squamous cells as well as clear cells containing mucin. *B,* Mucicarmine stains the mucin reddish-pink. (Courtesy of Dr. James Gulizia, Brigham and Women's Hospital, Boston.)

reported in the nose, sinuses, and upper airways and elsewhere.

Morphology. In gross appearance, they are generally small, poorly encapsulated, infiltrative, gray-pink lesions. On histologic evaluation, they are composed of small cells having dark, compact nuclei and scant cytoplasm. These cells tend to be disposed in tubular, solid, or cribriform patterns reminiscent of cylindromas arising in the adnexa of the skin. The spaces between the tumor cells are often filled with a hyaline material thought to represent excess basement membrane (Fig. 16–20*A*). Other less common histologic patterns have been designated as tubular and solid variants.

Although slow growing, these are relentless and unpredictable tumors with a tendency to invade perineural spaces (Fig. 16–20*B*), and they are stubbornly recurrent. Eventually, 50% or more disseminate widely to distant sites such as bone, liver, and brain, sometimes decades after attempted removal. Thus, although the 5-year survival rate is about 60% to 70%, it drops to about 30% at 10 years and 15% at 15 years. Neoplasms arising in the minor salivary glands have, on average, a poorer prognosis than those primary in the parotids.

The *acinic cell tumor* is composed of cells resembling the normal serous acinar cells of salivary glands. They are relatively uncommon, representing only 2% to 3% of salivary gland tumors. Most arise in the parotids; the small remainder arise in the submandibular glands. They rarely involve the minor glands, which normally have only a scant number of serous cells. Like Warthin tumor, they are sometimes bilateral or multicentric. They are generally small, discrete lesions that may appear encapsulated. On histologic examination, they reveal a variable architecture and cell morphology. Most characteristically, the cells have apparent cleared cytoplasm, but the cells are sometimes solid or at other times vacuolated. The cells are disposed in sheets or microcystic, glandular, follicular, or papillary patterns. There is usually little anaplasia and few mitoses, but some tumors are occasionally slightly more pleomorphic. Several histologic patterns of growth (*solid, microcystic, papillary-cystic,* and *follicular*) are recognized.

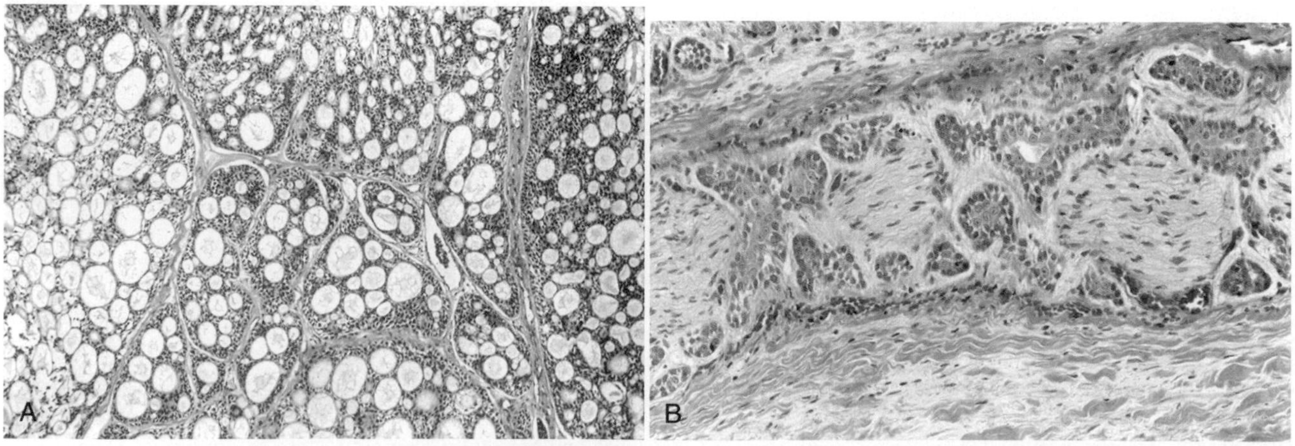

FIGURE 16–20 Adenoid cystic carcinoma in a salivary gland. *A,* Low-power view. The tumor cells have created a cribriform pattern enclosing secretions. *B,* Perineural invasion by tumor cells.

The clinical course of these neoplasms is somewhat dependent on the level of pleomorphism. Overall, recurrence after resection is uncommon, but about 10% to 15% of these neoplasms metastasize to lymph nodes. The survival rate is in the range of 90% at 5 years and 60% at 20 years.

REFERENCES

1. Research, Science and Therapy Committee of the American Academy of Periodontology: Treatment of plaque-induced gingivitis, chronic periodontitis, and other clinical conditions. J Periodontol 72:1790, 2001.
2. Research, Science and Therapy Committee of the American Academy of Periodontology: Epidemiology of periodontal disease. J Periodontol 67:935, 1996.
3. Research, Science and Therapy Committee of the American Academy of Periodontology: The pathogenesis of periodontal disease. J Periodontol 70:457, 1999.
4. Research, Science and Therapy Committee of the American Academy of Periodontology: Periodontal disease as a potential risk factor for systemic disease. J Periodontol 69:841, 1998.
5. Cawson RA, et al (eds): Lucas's Pathology of Tumors of the Oral Tissues. London, Churchill Livingstone, 1998.
6. Hutton KP, Rogers RS III: Recurrent aphthous stomatitis. Dermatol Clin 5:761, 1987.
7. Sciubba JJ: Opportunistic oral infections in the immunosuppressed patient: oral hairy leukoplakia and oral candidiasis. Adv Dent Res 10:69, 1996.
8. Silverman S: Early diagnosis of oral cancer. Cancer 62:1796, 1988.
9. Shugars DC, Patton LL: Detecting, diagnosing, and preventing oral cancer. Nurse Pract 22:109, 1997.
10. Whited JD, Grichnick JM: Does this patient have a mole or a melanoma? JAMA 279:696, 1998.
11. Rampen FH, et al: False-negative findings in skin cancer and melanoma screening. J Am Acad Dermatol 33:59, 1995.
12. Mashberg A, Feldman LJ: Clinical criteria for identifying early oral and oropharyngeal carcinoma: erythroplasia revisted. Am J Surg 156:273, 1988.
13. Neville BW, et al (eds): Oral and Maxillofacial Pathology. Philadelphia, WB Saunders, 1995.
14. Jemal A, et al: Cancer Statistics, 2004. CA Cancer J Clin 54:8, 2004.
15. Vokes EE, et al: Head and neck cancer. N Engl J Med 328:184, 1993.
16. Forastiere A, et al: Head and neck cancer. N Engl J Med 345:1890, 2001.
17. Murphy GP, Lawrence W, Lenhhartd RE: American Cancer Society Textbook of Clinical Oncology, 2nd ed. Atlanta: American Cancer Society, 1995.
18. Anderson WF, Hawk E, Berg CD: Secondary chemoprevention of upper aerodigestive tract tumors. Semin Oncol 28:106, 2001.
19. Day GL, Blot WJ: Second primary tumors in patients with oral cancer. Cancer 70:14, 1992.
20. Slaughter DP, Southwick HW, Smejkal W: "Field cancerization" in oral stratified squamous epithelium. Cancer 6:962, 1953.
21. Braakhuis BJM, et al: A genetic explanation of Slaughter's concept of field cancerization: evidence and clinical implications. Cancer Res 63:1727, 2003.
22. Lippman SM, Hong WK: Second malignant tumors in head and neck squamous cell carcinoma: the overshadowing threat for patients with early-stage disease. Int J Radiat Oncol Biol Phys 17:691, 1989.
23. Gillison ML, et al: Evidence for a causal association between human papillomavirus and a subset of head and neck cancers. JNCI 92:709, 2000.
24. Koch WM, et al: Head and neck cancer in nonsmokers: a distinct clinical and molecular entity. Laryngoscope 109:1544, 1999.
25. Lingen MW, et al: Overexpression of *p53* in squamous cell carcinoma of the tongue in young patients with no known risk factors is not associated with mutations in exons 5–9. Head Neck 22:328, 2000.
26. Schantz SP, Yu GP: Head and neck cancer incidence trends in young Americans, 1973–1997, with a special analysis for tongue cancer. Arch Otolaryngol Head Neck Surg 128:268, 2002.
27. Jefferies S, Foulkes WD: Genetic mechanisms in squamous cell carcinoma of the head and neck. Oral Oncol 37:115, 2001.
28. Mao L, et al: Frequent microsatellite alterations at chromosomes 9p21 and 3p14 in oral premalignant lesions and their value in cancer risk assessment. Nature Med 2:682, 1996.
29. Boyle JO, et al: The incidence of *p53* mutations increases with progression of head and neck cancer. Cancer Res 53:4477, 1993.
30. Rosin MP, et al: Use of allelic loss to predict malignant risk for low-grade oral epithelial dysplasia. Clin Cancer Res 6:357, 2000.
31. Michalides R, et al: Overexpression of cyclin D1 correlates with recurrence in a group of forty-seven operable squamous cell carcinomas of the head and neck. Cancer Res 55:975, 1995.
32. Izzo JG, et al: Dysregulated cyclin D1 expression early in head and neck tumorigenesis: in vivo evidence for an association with subsequent gene amplification. Oncogene 17:2313, 1998.
33. El-Mofty S (ed): Odontogenic tumors. Seminars in Diagnostic Pathology 16:269, 1999.
34. Naclerio R, Solomon W: Rhinitis and inhaled allergens. JAMA 278:1842, 1997.
35. Slavin RG: Nasal polyps and sinusitis. JAMA 278:1845, 1997.
36. Hyams VJ, et al: Tumors of the upper respiratory tract and ear. In Atlas of Tumor Pathology, Second Series. Washington, DC, Armed Forces Institute of Pathology, 1988.
37. Goodman ML, Pilch BZ: Tumors of the upper respiratory tract. In Fletcher DM (ed): Diagnostic Histopathology of Tumors. London, Churchill Livingstone, 1995, pp 79–126.
38. Argani P, et al: Olfactory neuroblastoma is not related to the Ewing family of tumors. Am J Surg Pathol 22:391, 1998.
39. Broich G, et al: Esthesioneuroblastoma: a general review of the cases published since the discovery of the tumour in 1924. Anticancer Res 17:2683, 1997.
40. Rabb-Traub N: Epstein-Barr virus in the pathogenesis of NPC. Semin Cancer Biol 12:431, 2002.
41. Hawkins EP, et al: Nasopharyngeal carcinoma in children — a retrospective review and demonstration of Epstein-Barr viral genomes in tumor cell cytoplasm: a report of the Pediatric Oncology Group. Hum Pathol 21:805, 1990.
42. Kristt D, et al: The spectrum of laryngeal neoplasia: the pathologist's view. Pathol Res Pract 198:709, 2002.
43. Cattaruzza MS, et al: Epidemiology of laryngeal cancer. Eur J Cancer B Oral Oncol 32B:293, 1996.
44. Koufman JA, Burke AJ: The etiology and pathogenesis of laryngeal carcinoma. Otolaryngol Clin North Am 30:1, 1997.
45. Bauman NM, Smith RJ: Recurrent respiratory papillomatosis. Pediatr Clin North Am 43:1385, 1996.

45a. Rovers MM, et al: Otitis media. Lancet 363:465, 2004.

46. Regauer S, et al: Lateral neck cysts — the branchial theory revisited. A critical review and clinicopathological study of 97 cases with special emphasis on cytokeratin expression. APMIS 105:623, 1997.
47. Capella C, et al: Histopathology, cytology, and cytochemistry of pheochromocytomas and paragangliomas including chemodectomas. Pathol Res Pract 186:176, 1988.
48. Wick MR, Rosai JR: Neuroendocrine tumors of the mediastinum. Semin Diagn Pathol 8:35, 1991.
49. Ellis GL, Auclair PL, Gnepp DR: Surgical Pathology of Salivary Glands. Philadelphia, WB Saunders, 1991.
50. Ellis GL, Auclair PL: Tumors of the salivary glands. In Atlas of Tumor Pathology, Third Series, Fascicle 17. Washington, DC, Armed Forces Institute of Pathology, 1996.
51. Dardick I: Color Atlas/Text of Salivary Gland Pathology. New York, Igaku-Shoin, 1996.

CHAPTER 17

The Gastrointestinal Tract

Chen Liu, MD, PhD • James M. Crawford, MD, PhD

ESOPHAGUS

CONGENITAL ANOMALIES

Atresia and Fistulas

Webs, Rings, and Stenosis

LESIONS ASSOCIATED WITH MOTOR DYSFUNCTION

Achalasia

Hiatal Hernia

Diverticula

Lacerations (Mallory-Weiss Syndrome)

ESOPHAGEAL VARICES

ESOPHAGITIS

Reflux Esophagitis (Gastroesophageal Reflux Disease)

Barrett Esophagus

Infectious and Chemical Esophagitis

TUMORS

Benign Tumors

Malignant Tumors

Squamous Cell Carcinoma

Adenocarcinoma

STOMACH

GASTRIC MUCOSAL PHYSIOLOGY

Acid Secretion

Mucosal Protection

CONGENITAL ANOMALIES

Pyloric Stenosis

GASTRITIS

Acute Gastritis

Chronic Gastritis

Special Forms of Gastritis

PEPTIC ULCER DISEASE

Peptic Ulcers

Acute Gastric Ulceration

MISCELLANEOUS CONDITIONS

Hypertrophic Gastropathy

Gastric Varices

TUMORS

Benign Tumors

Gastric Carcinoma

Less Common Gastric Tumors

SMALL AND LARGE INTESTINES

ANATOMY

VASCULATURE

SMALL INTESTINAL MUCOSA

COLONIC MUCOSA

ENDOCRINE CELLS

INTESTINAL IMMUNE SYSTEM

NEUROMUSCULAR FUNCTION

CONGENITAL ANOMALIES

Atresia and Stenosis

Meckel Diverticulum

Congenital Aganglionic Megacolon—Hirschsprung Disease

ENTEROCOLITIS

Diarrhea and Dysentery

Infectious Enterocolitis

Viral Gastroenteritis

Bacterial Enterocolitis

Bacterial Overgrowth Syndrome

Parasitic Enterocolitis

Necrotizing Enterocolitis

Collagenous and Lymphocytic Colitis

Miscellaneous Intestinal Inflammatory Disorders
Acquired Immunodeficiency Syndrome (AIDS)
Transplantation
Drug-Induced Intestinal Injury
Radiation Enterocolitis
Neutropenic Colitis (Typhlitis)
Diversion Colitis
Solitary Rectal Ulcer Syndrome

MALABSORPTION SYNDROMES
Celiac Disease
Tropical Sprue (Postinfectious Sprue)
Whipple Disease
Disaccharidase (Lactase) Deficiency
Abetalipoproteinemia

IDIOPATHIC INFLAMMATORY BOWEL DISEASE
Etiology and Pathogenesis
Crohn Disease
Ulcerative Colitis

VASCULAR DISORDERS
Ischemic Bowel Disease
Angiodysplasia
Hemorrhoids

DIVERTICULAR DISEASE

INTESTINAL OBSTRUCTION
Hernias
Adhesions
Intussusception
Volvulus

TUMORS OF THE SMALL AND LARGE INTESTINE
Tumors of the Small Intestine
Adenomas
Adenocarcinoma
Tumors of the Colon and Rectum
Non-Neoplastic Polyps
Adenomas
Familial Syndromes
Colorectal Carcinogenesis
Colorectal Carcinoma
Carcinoid Tumors
Gastrointestinal Lymphoma
Mesenchymal Tumors
Tumors of the Anal Canal

■ APPENDIX
ACUTE APPENDICITIS
TUMORS OF THE APPENDIX
Mucocele and Pseudomyxoma Peritonei

■ PERITONEUM
INFLAMMATION
Peritoneal Infection
Sclerosing Retroperitonitis
Mesenteric Cysts
TUMORS

ESOPHAGUS

Normal

The esophagus develops from the cranial portion of the foregut and is recognizable by the third week of gestation. The normal esophagus is a hollow, highly distensible muscular tube that extends from the epiglottis in the pharynx, at about the level of the C6 vertebra, to the gastroesophageal junction at the level of the T11 or T12 vertebra. Measuring between 10 and 11 cm in the newborn, it grows to a length of about 25 cm in the adult. For the endoscopist, the esophagus is recorded as the anatomic distance between 15 and 40 cm from the incisor teeth, with the gastroesophageal junction located at the 40-cm point. Several points of luminal narrowing can be identified along its course—proximally at the cricoid cartilage, midway in its course alongside the aortic arch and at the anterior crossing of the left main bronchus and left atrium, and distally where it pierces the diaphragm. Although the pressure in the esophageal lumen is negative compared with the atmosphere, manometric recordings of intraluminal pressures have identified two higher-pressure areas that remain relatively contracted in the resting phase. A 3-cm segment in the proximal esophagus at the level of the cricopharyngeus muscle is referred to as the upper esophageal sphincter (UES). The 2- to 4-cm segment just proximal to the anatomic gastroesophageal junction, at the level of the diaphragm, is referred to as the lower esophageal sphincter (LES). Both "sphincters" are physiologic, in that there are no anatomic landmarks that delineate these higher-pressure regions from the intervening esophageal musculature.

The wall of the esophagus consists of a mucosa, submucosa, muscularis propria, and adventitia, reflecting the general structural organization of the gastrointestinal tract.[1] The *mucosa* has a smooth, glistening, and pink-tan surface. It has three components: a nonkeratinizing stratified squamous epithelial layer, lamina propria, and muscularis mucosa. The epithelial layer has mature squamous cells overlying basal cells. The basal cells, constituting 10% to 15 % of the mucosal thickness, are reserve cells with great proliferative potential. A small number of specialized cell types, such as melanocytes, endocrine cells, dendritic cells, and lymphocytes, are present in the deeper portion of the epithelial layer. The lamina propria is the nonepithelial portion of the mucosa, above the muscularis mucosae. It consists of areolar connective tissue and contains vascular structures and scattered leukocytes. Finger-like extensions of the lamina propria, called *papillae,* extend into the epithelial layer. The muscularis mucosae is a delicate layer of longitudinally oriented smooth-muscle bundles.

The *submucosa* consists of loose connective tissue containing blood vessels, a rich network of lymphatics, a sprinkling of leukocytes with occasional lymphoid follicles, nerve fibers (including the ganglia of the Meissner plexus), and submucosal glands. Submucosal glands connected to the lumen by squamous epithelium–lined ducts are scattered along the entire esophagus but are more concentrated in the upper and lower portions. Their mucin-containing fluid secretions help lubricate the esophagus.

As is true throughout the alimentary tract, the *muscularis propria* consists of an inner circular and an outer longitudinal coat of smooth muscle with an intervening, well-developed myenteric plexus (Auerbach plexus). The muscularis propria of the proximal 6 to 8 cm of the esophagus also contains striated muscle fibers from the cricopharyngeus muscle. Besides creating a unique histologic interplay of smooth muscle and skeletal muscle fibers, this feature explains why skeletal muscle disorders can cause upper esophageal dysfunction.

In sharp contrast to the rest of the gastrointestinal tract, the esophagus is mostly devoid of a serosal coat. Only small segments of the intra-abdominal esophagus are covered by serosa; the thoracic esophagus is surrounded by fascia that condenses around the esophagus to form a sheathlike structure. In the upper mediastinum, the esophagus is supported by this fascial tissue, which forms a similar sheath around adjacent structures, the great vessels and the tracheobronchial tree. This intimate anatomic proximity to important thoracic viscera is of significance in permitting the ready and widespread dissemination of infections and tumors of the esophagus into the posterior mediastinum. The rich network of mucosal and submucosal lymphatics that runs longitudinally along the esophagus further facilitates spread.

The main functions of the esophagus are to conduct food and fluids from the pharynx to the stomach, to prevent passive diffusion of substances from the food into the blood, and to prevent reflux of gastric contents into the esophagus. These functions require motor activity coordinated with swallowing, namely a wave of peristaltic contraction, relaxation of the LES in anticipation of the peristaltic wave, and closure of the LES after the swallowing reflex. The mechanisms governing this motor function are complex, involving both extrinsic and intrinsic innervation, humoral regulation, and properties of the muscle wall itself.

The control of the lower esophageal sphincter (LES) is critical to esophageal function.[2] Maintenance of sphincter tone is necessary to prevent reflux of gastric contents, which are under positive pressure relative to the esophagus. During deglutition, both active inhibition of the muscularis propria muscle fibers by inhibitory nonadrenergic/noncholinergic neurons and cessation of tonic excitation by cholinergic neurons enable the LES to relax. Many chemical agents (e.g., gastrin, acetylcholine, serotonin, prostaglandin $F_{2\alpha}$, motilin, substance P, histamine, and pancreatic polypeptide) increase LES tone, while some agents (nitric oxide, vasoactive intestinal peptide) decrease the tone. However, their precise roles in normal esophageal function remain unclear.

Pathology

Lesions of the esophagus run the gamut from highly lethal cancers to the merely annoying "heartburn" that has affected many a partaker of a large, spicy meal. Esophageal varices, the result of cirrhosis and portal hypertension, are of major importance, since their rupture is frequently followed by massive hematemesis (vomiting of blood) and even death by exsanguination. Esophagitis and hiatal hernias are far more frequent and rarely threaten life. Distressing to the physician is that all disorders of the esophagus tend to produce similar symptoms, namely heartburn, dysphagia, pain, and/or hematemesis.

Heartburn (retrosternal burning pain) usually reflects regurgitation of gastric contents into the lower esophagus. *Dysphagia* (difficulty in swallowing) is encountered both with deranged esophageal motor function and with diseases that narrow or obstruct the lumen. *Pain* and *hematemesis* are sometimes evoked by esophageal disease, particularly by those lesions associated with inflammation or ulceration of the esophageal mucosa. The clinical diagnosis of esophageal disorders often requires specialized procedures such as esophagoscopy, radiographic barium studies, and manometry.

Congenital Anomalies

Ectopic tissue rests are not uncommon in the esophagus. The most common is ectopic gastric mucosa in the upper third of the esophagus ("inlet patch"), occurring in up to 2% of individuals. Sebaceous glands or ectopic pancreatic tissue are much less frequent. The acid secretions of the ectopic gastric mucosa or pancreatic enzymatic secretions can produce localized inflammation and discomfort.

Embryologic formation of the foregut can also give rise to *congenital cysts.* These are usually duplication cysts, containing double smooth muscle layers and derived from the lower esophagus in 60% of cases. Rarely, bronchial or parenchymal pulmonary tissue may arise from the upper gut and is denoted *bronchogenic cyst* or *pulmonary sequestration,* respectively. These lesions usually present as masses. Lastly, impaired formation of the diaphragm may permit herniation of abdominal viscera into the thorax. When severe, this lesion is incompatible with life, since the lungs are severely hypoplastic at the time of birth. This condition is to be distinguished from hiatal hernias, to be discussed presently.

ATRESIA AND FISTULAS

Although developmental defects in the esophagus are uncommon, they must be corrected early because they are incompatible with life. Because they cause immediate regurgitation when feeding is attempted, they are usually discovered soon after birth. *Absence* (agenesis) of the esophagus is extremely rare; much more common are *atresia* and *fistula formation* (Fig. 17–1). In atresia, a segment of the esophagus is represented by only a thin, noncanalized cord, with a proximal blind pouch connected to the pharynx and a lower pouch leading to the stomach. Atresia is most commonly located at or near the tracheal bifurcation. It rarely occurs alone, but is usually associated with a fistula connecting the lower or upper pouch with a bronchus or the trachea. Associated anomalies include congenital heart disease, neurologic disease, genitourinary disease, and other gastrointestinal malformations. Atresia sometimes is associated with the presence of a single umbilical artery.[3] Aspiration and paroxysmal suffocation from food are obvious hazards; pneumonia and severe fluid and electrolyte imbalances may also occur.

WEBS, RINGS, AND STENOSIS

Esophageal mucosal webs are uncommon ledgelike protrusions of the mucosa into the esophageal lumen. These are semicircumferential, eccentric, and most common in the upper esophagus. Well-developed webs rarely protrude more than 5 mm into the lumen, with a thickness of 2 to 4 mm. The webs consist of squamous mucosa and a vascularized submucosal core. Webs can be congenital in origin, or they may arise in association with long-standing reflux esophagitis, chronic graft-versus-host disease (GVHD), or blistering skin diseases. When an upper esophageal web is accompanied by an iron-deficiency anemia, glossitis, and cheilosis, the condition is referred to as the Paterson-Brown-Kelly or Plummer-Vinson syndrome, with an attendant risk for postcricoid esophageal carcinoma.

Esophageal rings are concentric plates of tissue protruding into the lumen of the distal esophagus. One occurring above the squamocolumnar junction of the esophagus and stomach is referred to as an *A ring.* One located at the squamocolumnar junction of the lower esophagus is designated a *Schatzki ring* or a *B ring.* Histologically, these rings consist of mucosa, submucosa, and sometimes a hypertrophied muscularis propria. Schatzki rings may have columnar gastric epithelium on their undersurface.

Esophageal webs and rings are encountered most frequently in women over age 40 and are of uncertain etiology. Episodic dysphagia is the main symptom associated with webs and rings, usually provoked when an individual bolts solid food. Pain is infrequent.

Esophageal stenosis consists of fibrous thickening of the esophageal wall, particularly the submucosa, with atrophy of the muscularis propria. The lining epithelium is usually thin and sometimes ulcerated. Although occasionally of congenital origin, stenosis is more frequently the result of severe esophageal injury with inflammatory scarring, as from gastroesophageal reflux, radiation, scleroderma, or caustic injury. Stenosis usually develops in adulthood and becomes manifest by progressive dysphagia, at first to solid foods only but eventually to all foods, which constitutes the major symptom. In severe stenosis, virtually total obstruction may result.

Lesions Associated with Motor Dysfunction

Coordinated motor function is critical to proper function of the esophagus; gravity alone is not sufficient to move food from the pharynx to the stomach, nor to prevent reflux of gastric contents—witness the blissful suckling of the supine infant. The major entities (achalasia, hiatal hernia, diverticulum and Mallory-Weiss tear) that are caused by or induce motor dysfunction of the esophagus are diagrammed in Figure 17–2.

ACHALASIA

Achalasia means "failure to relax." It is characterized by three major abnormalities: (1) aperistalsis, (2) partial or incomplete relaxation of the LES with swallowing, and (3) increased resting tone of the LES. The pathogenesis of primary

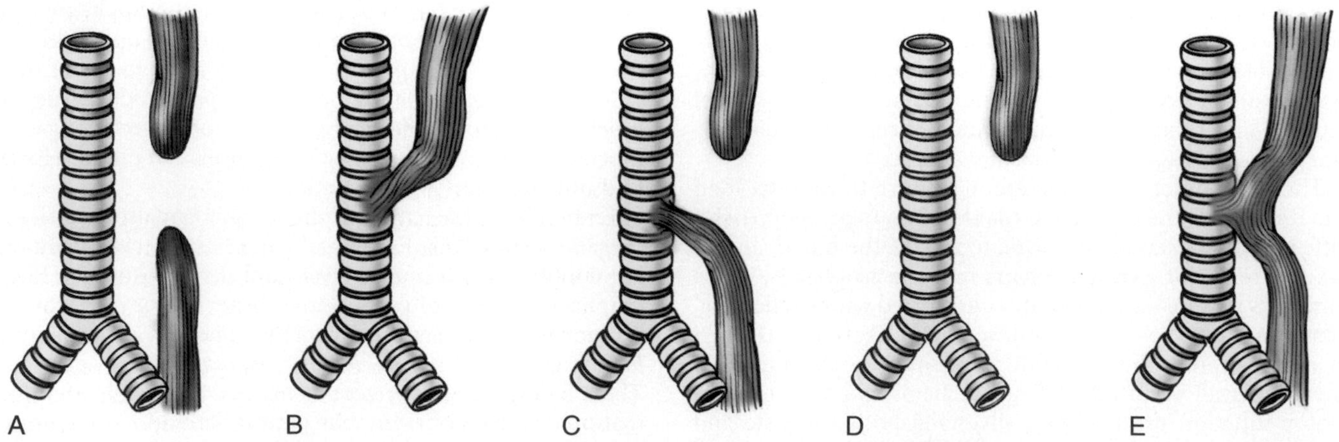

FIGURE 17–1 Esophageal atresia and tracheoesophageal fistula. *A,* Blind upper and lower esophageal segments. *B,* Fistula between blind upper segment and trachea. *C,* Blind upper segment, fistula between blind lower segment and trachea. *D,* Blind upper segment only. E, Fistula between patent esophagus and trachea. Type C is the most common variety. (Adapted from Morson BC, and Dawson IMP, eds., Gastrointestinal Pathology. Oxford, Blackwell Scientific Publications, 1972, p. 8.)

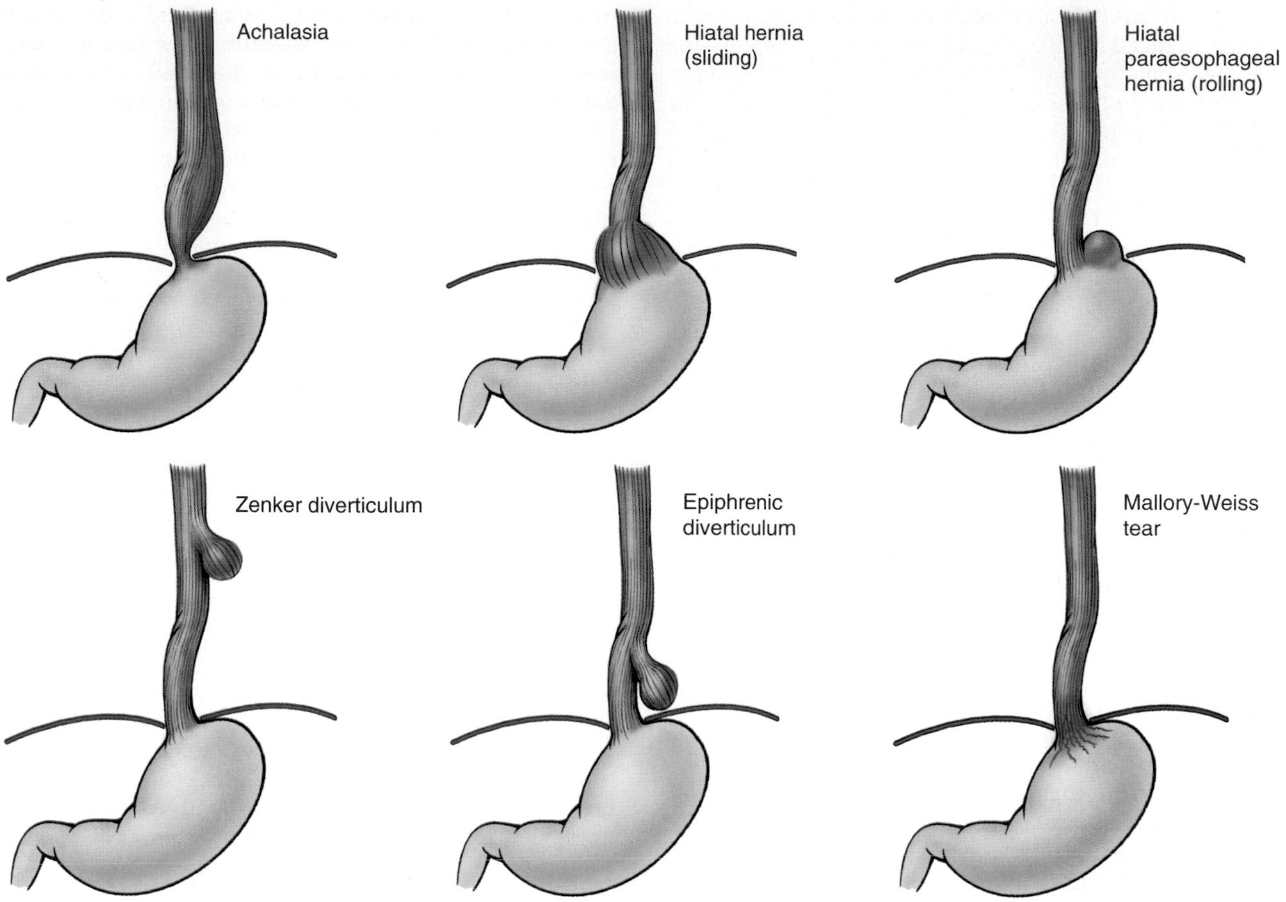

FIGURE 17–2 Major conditions associated with esophageal motor dysfunction.

achalasia is poorly understood. It is thought to involve dysfunction of inhibitory neurons containing nitric oxide and vasoactive intestinal polypeptide in the distal esophagus.[4,5] Degenerative changes in neural innervation, either intrinsic to the esophagus or in the extraesophageal vagus nerves and the dorsal motor nucleus of the vagus, may also occur. Secondary achalasia may arise in Chagas disease, in which *Trypanosoma cruzi* causes destruction of the myenteric plexus of the esophagus, duodenum, colon, and ureter, with resultant dilation of these viscera. Disorders of the dorsal motor nuclei, particularly polio or surgical ablation, can cause an achalasia-like illness, as can diabetic autonomic neuropathy and infiltrative disorders such as malignancy, amyloidosis, and sarcoidosis. *In most instances, however, achalasia occurs as a primary disorder of uncertain etiology.*

Morphology. In primary achalasia there is progressive dilation of the esophagus above the level of the LES. The wall of the esophagus may be of normal thickness, thicker than normal owing to hypertrophy of the muscularis, or markedly thinned by dilation. The myenteric ganglia are usually absent from the body of the esophagus, but may or may not be reduced in number in the region of the LES. The mucosal lining may be unaffected, but sometimes inflammation, ulceration, or fibrotic thickening may be evident just above the LES.

Clinical Features. Achalasia usually becomes manifest in young adulthood, but may appear in infancy or childhood. The classic clinical symptom of achalasia is progressive dysphagia. Nocturnal regurgitation and aspiration of undigested food may occur. The most serious aspect of this condition is the hazard of developing esophageal squamous cell carcinoma, said to occur in about 5% of patients, typically at an earlier age than those without this disease. Other complications include *Candida* esophagitis, lower esophageal diverticula (see below), and aspiration with pneumonia or airway obstruction.

HIATAL HERNIA

Hiatal hernia is characterized by separation of the diaphragmatic crura and widening of the space between the muscular crura and the esophageal wall. Two anatomic patterns are recognized (see Fig. 17–2): the axial, or *sliding hernia,* and the nonaxial, or *paraesophageal hiatal hernia.* The sliding hernia constitutes 95% of cases; protrusion of the stomach above the diaphragm creates a bell-shaped dilation, bounded below by the diaphragmatic narrowing. In paraesophageal hernias, a separate portion of the stomach, usually along the greater curvature, enters the thorax through the widened foramen.

The cause of hiatal hernia is unknown. It is not clear whether it is a congenital malformation or is acquired during life. Based on barographic studies, hiatal hernias are reported in 1% to 20% of adult subjects, with incidence increasing with age. However, hiatal hernias are well recognized in infants and children. Only about 9% of adults with a sliding hernia suffer from heartburn or regurgitation of gastric juices into the mouth. These symptoms are attributed to incompetence of the LES and are accentuated by positions favoring reflux (bending forward, lying supine) and obesity.

Complications of hiatal hernias are numerous. Both types may ulcerate, causing bleeding and perforation. Paraesophageal hernias can become strangulated or obstructed, and early surgical repair has been advocated. Reflux esophagitis (discussed later) is frequently seen in association with sliding hernias, but compromise of the LES with regurgitation of peptic juices into the esophagus is probably the result of, rather than the cause of, a sliding hernia. The uncommon paraesophageal hernias may be caused by previous surgery, including operations for sliding hernia.

DIVERTICULA

A *diverticulum* is an outpouching of the alimentary tract that contains all visceral layers; a false diverticulum denotes an outpouching of mucosa and submucosa only (Fig. 17–2). True diverticula are usually discovered in later life and may develop in three regions of the esophagus:

- *Zenker diverticulum (pharyngoesophageal diverticulum)* immediately above the UES
- *Traction diverticulum* near the midpoint of the esophagus
- *Epiphrenic diverticulum* immediately above the LES.

Disordered cricopharyngeal motor dysfunction with or without gastroesophageal reflux disease (GERD) and diminished luminal size of the UES are implicated in the genesis of Zenker diverticulum. Scarring resulting from mediastinal lymphadenitis (as from tuberculosis) was presumed to be a cause of traction on the esophagus that gave rise to midesophageal diverticula. However, arguments have been advanced in favor of traction diverticula actually arising from motor dysfunction or being a congenital lesion. Dyscoordination of peristalsis and LES relaxation are the proposed cause of epiphrenic diverticula.

Zenker diverticula may reach several centimeters in size and can accumulate significant amounts of food. Typical symptoms include dysphagia, food regurgitation, and a mass in the neck; aspiration with resultant pneumonia is a significant risk. While midesophageal diverticula are generally asymptomatic, epiphrenic diverticula can give rise to nocturnal regurgitation of massive amounts of fluid.

LACERATIONS (MALLORY-WEISS SYNDROME)

Longitudinal tears in the esophagus at the esophagogastric junction or gastric cardia are termed *Mallory-Weiss tears* and are believed to be the consequence of severe retching or vomiting.[6] They are encountered most commonly in alcoholics, in whom they are attributed to episodes of excessive vomiting in the setting of an alcoholic stupor. Normally, a reflex relaxation of the musculature of the gastrointestinal tract precedes the antiperistaltic wave of contraction. During episodes of prolonged vomiting, it is speculated that this reflex relaxation fails to occur. The refluxing gastric contents suddenly overwhelm the contraction of the musculature at the gastric inlet, and massive dilation with tearing of the stretched wall ensues. Since these tears may occur in persons who have no history of vomiting or alcoholism, other mechanisms must exist; underlying hiatal hernia is a known predisposing factor.

Morphology. The linear irregular lacerations are oriented in the axis of the esophageal lumen and are several millimeters to several centimeters in length. **They are usually found astride the esophagogastric junction or in the proximal gastric mucosa** (Fig. 17–3). The tears may involve only the mucosa or may penetrate deeply enough to perforate the wall. The histology is not distinctive and reflects trauma accompanied by fresh hemorrhage and a nonspecific inflammatory response. Infection of the mucosal defect may lead to an inflammatory ulcer or to mediastinitis.

Clinical Features. Esophageal lacerations account for 5% to 10% of bleeding episodes in the upper gastrointestinal tract. Most often, bleeding is not profuse and ceases without surgical intervention, although massive hematemesis may occur. Supportive therapy, such as vasoconstrictive medications and transfusions, and sometimes balloon tamponade, is usually all that is required. Healing tends to be prompt, with minimal to no residua. The rare instance of esophageal rupture is known as *Boerhaave syndrome* and may be a catastrophic event.

Esophageal Varices

Regardless of cause, portal hypertension, when sufficiently prolonged or severe, induces the formation of collateral bypass channels wherever the portal and caval systems communicate. The pathogenesis of portal hypertension and the

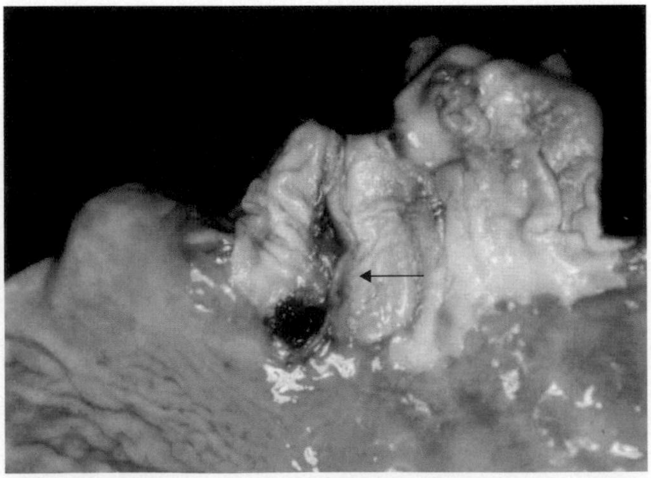

FIGURE 17–3 Esophageal laceration (Mallory-Weiss tears). Gross view demonstrating longitudinal lacerations extending from esophageal mucosa into stomach mucosa *(arrow)*. (Courtesy of Dr. Richard Harruff, King County Medical Examiner's Office, Seattle, WA.)

locations of these bypasses are considered in Chapter 18. Here we are concerned with the collaterals that develop in the region of the lower esophagus when portal blood flow is diverted through the coronary veins of the stomach into the plexus of esophageal subepithelial and submucosal veins, thence into the azygos veins, and eventually into the systemic circulation. The increased pressure in the esophageal plexus produces dilated tortuous vessels called *varices. Varices develop in 90% of cirrhotic patients and are most often associated with alcoholic cirrhosis.* Worldwide, hepatic schistosomiasis is the second most common cause of variceal bleeding.

Morphology. Varices appear as tortuous dilated veins lying primarily within the submucosa of the distal esophagus and proximal stomach; venous channels directly beneath the esophageal epithelium may also become massively dilated. The net effect is irregular protrusion of the overlying mucosa into the lumen, although varices are collapsed in surgical or postmortem specimens (Fig. 17–4*A*). When the varix is unruptured, the mucosa may be normal, but often it is eroded and inflamed because of its exposed position. **Variceal rupture produces massive hemorrhage into the lumen, as well as suffusion of the esophageal wall with blood.** In this instance the overlying mucosa appears ulcerated and necrotic (Fig. 17–4*B*). If rupture has occurred in the past, venous thrombosis and superimposed inflammation may be present. Varices can be detected by hepatic venogram (Fig. 17–4*C*).

Clinical Features. Varices usually produce no symptoms until they rupture, causing massive hematemesis. Among patients with advanced cirrhosis of the liver, half the deaths result from rupture of a varix. Some patients die as a direct consequence of the hemorrhage and others of the hepatic coma triggered by the hemorrhage. It must be remembered, however, that even when varices are present, they account for less than half of all episodes of hematemesis. Collectively, concomitant gastritis, esophageal laceration, or peptic ulcers are more common causes. Factors leading to rupture of a varix are unclear: silent inflammatory erosion of overlying thinned mucosa, increased tension in progressively dilated veins, and vomiting with increased vascular hydrostatic pressure are likely to play roles. Once begun, the hemorrhage rarely subsides spontaneously, and endoscopic injection of thrombotic agents ("sclerotherapy") or balloon tamponade is usually required. Forty to fifty percent of patients die in the first bleeding episode. Among those who survive, rebleeding occurs in over half within 1 year, with a similar rate of mortality for each episode.

Esophagitis

Inflammation of the esophageal mucosa is known as esophagitis. Injury to the esophageal mucosa with subsequent inflammation is common worldwide. In the United States and other Western countries, esophagitis is present in about 5% of the adult population; much higher prevalence is encountered in selected regions such as northern Iran and portions of China. Esophagitis may be caused by a variety of physical, chemical, or biologic agents. We review the common ones encountered in the clinical practice.

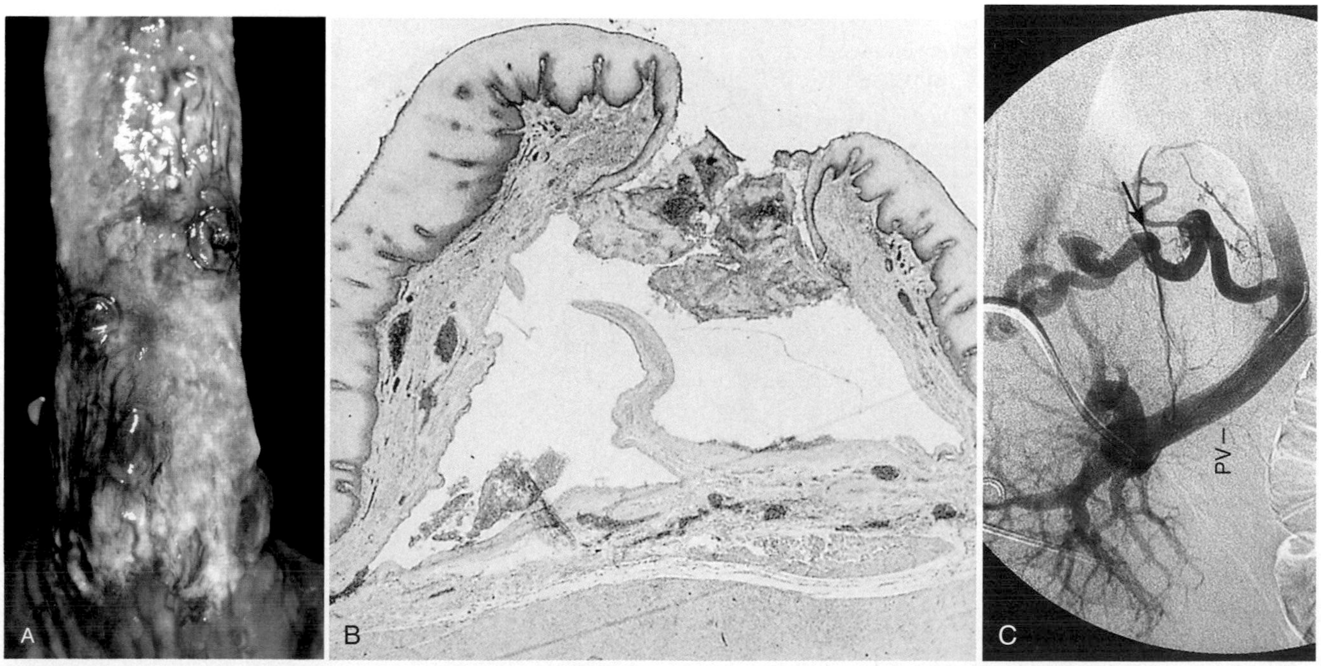

FIGURE 17–4 Esophageal varices. *A,* A view of the everted esophagus and gastroesophageal junction, showing dilated submucosal veins (varices). The blue-colored varices have collapsed in this postmortem specimen. *B,* Low-power cross-section of a dilated submucosal varix that has ruptured through the mucosa. A small amount of thrombus is present within the point of rupture. *C,* Hepatic venogram after injection of dye into portal veins (PV) to show a large tortuous gastroesophageal varix *(arrow)* extending superiorly from the patent main portal vein. (*C,* courtesy of Dr. Emily Sedgwick, Brigham and Women's Hospital, Boston, MA.)

REFLUX ESOPHAGITIS (GASTROESOPHAGEAL REFLUX DISEASE)

Reflux of gastric contents into the lower esophagus is the most important cause of esophagitis. Many causative factors are involved:[7]

- Decreased efficacy of esophageal antireflux mechanisms, particularly LES tone. Central nervous system depressants, hypothyroidism, pregnancy, systemic sclerosing disorders, alcohol or tobacco exposure, or the presence of a nasogastric tube may be contributing causes. However, in most instances no antecedent etiology is identified.
- Presence of a sliding hiatal hernia
- Inadequate or slowed esophageal clearance of refluxed material
- Delayed gastric emptying and increased gastric volume, contributing to the volume of refluxed material
- Reduction in the reparative capacity of the esophageal mucosa by protracted exposure to gastric juices.

Any one of these influences may assume primacy in an individual case, but more than one is likely to be involved in most instances. *The action of gastric juices is critical to the development of esophageal mucosal injury;* in severe cases refluxed bile from the duodenum also may contribute to the mucosal disruption.

Morphology. The anatomic changes depend on the causative agent and on the duration and severity of the exposure. Simple hyperemia ("redness") may be the only alteration. In uncomplicated reflux esophagitis, three histologic features are characteristic (Fig. 17–5):

- The presence of inflammatory cells, including eosinophils, neutrophils, and excessive numbers of lymphocytes, in the squamous epithelial layer
- Basal zone hyperplasia exceeding 20% of the epithelial thickness
- Elongation of lamina propria papillae with capillary congestion, extending into the top third of the epithelial layer.

Infiltrates of intraepithelial eosinophils are believed to be an early histologic abnormality, since they occur even in the absence of basal zone hyperplasia. Intraepithelial neutrophils, on the other hand, are markers of more severe injury such as ulceration rather than reflux esophagitis per se.

Clinical Features. Although largely limited to adults over age 40, reflux esophagitis is occasionally seen in infants and children. The clinical manifestations consist principally of dysphagia, heartburn, and sometimes regurgitation of a sour brash, hematemesis, or melena. *The severity of symptoms is not closely related to the presence or degree of histologic esophagitis;* most people experience reflux symptoms without damage to the distal esophageal mucosa, due to the short duration of the reflux. Anatomic damage appears best correlated with prolonged exposure of the lower esophagus to refluxed material. Rarely, chronic symptoms are punctuated by attacks of severe chest pain that may be mistaken for a "heart attack." The potential consequences of severe reflux esophagitis are bleeding, ulceration, development of stricture, and a tendency to develop Barrett esophagus, with its attendant risks.

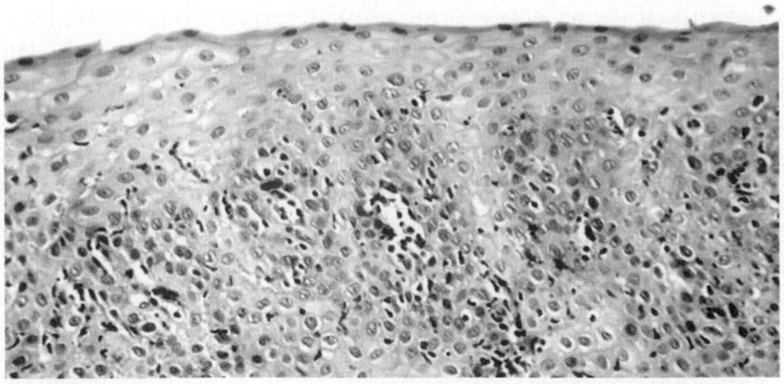

FIGURE 17–5 Reflux esophagitis. Low-power view of the superficial portion of the mucosa. Numerous eosinophils within the squamous epithelium, elongation of the lamina propria papillae, and basal zone hyperplasia are present.

BARRETT ESOPHAGUS

Barrett esophagus is a complication of long-standing gastroesophageal reflux, occurring over time in up to 10% of patients with symptomatic gastroesophageal reflux disease (GERD). *It is the single most important risk factor for esophageal adenocarcinoma. In Barrett esophagus, the distal squamous mucosa is replaced by metaplastic columnar epithelium, as a response to prolonged injury.* Two criteria are required for the diagnosis of Barrett esophagus: (1) endoscopic evidence of columnar epithelial lining above the gastroesophageal junction and (2) histologic evidence of intestinal metaplasia in the biopsy specimens from the columnar epithelium.[8] Barrett esophagus is further classified as long segment (extending cephalad more than 3 cm from the manometric gastroesophageal junction) or short segment (extending less than 3 cm cephalad). Barrett esophagus patients tend to have a long history of heartburn and other reflux symptoms and appear to have more massive reflux with more and longer reflux episodes than most reflux patients. It is unknown why the columnar epithelium develops in some patients with reflux and not in others.

The pathogenesis of Barrett esophagus remains unclear, but it appears to result from an alteration in the differentiation program of stem cells of the esophageal mucosa.[9] The concept of "intestinal metaplasia" in Barrett esophagus may be not entirely correct, since true absorptive enterocytes are not observed. Rather, admixed with intestinal mucin-secreting goblet cells are columnar cells exhibiting both secretory and absorptive ultrastructural features; this is a phenotype not observed elsewhere in the alimentary tract. Nevertheless the term "intestinal metaplasia" continues to be used to denote the altered histology of the mucosa.

Morphology. Barrett esophagus is recognized as a red, velvety mucosa located between the smooth, pale pink esophageal squamous mucosa and the lusher light brown gastric mucosa. It may exist as tongues or patches (islands) extending up from the gastroesophageal junction or as a broad irregular circumferential band displacing the squamocolumnar junction several centimeters cephalad (Fig. 17–6). A small zone of metaplastic mucosa may be present only at the esophagogastric junction (short-segment

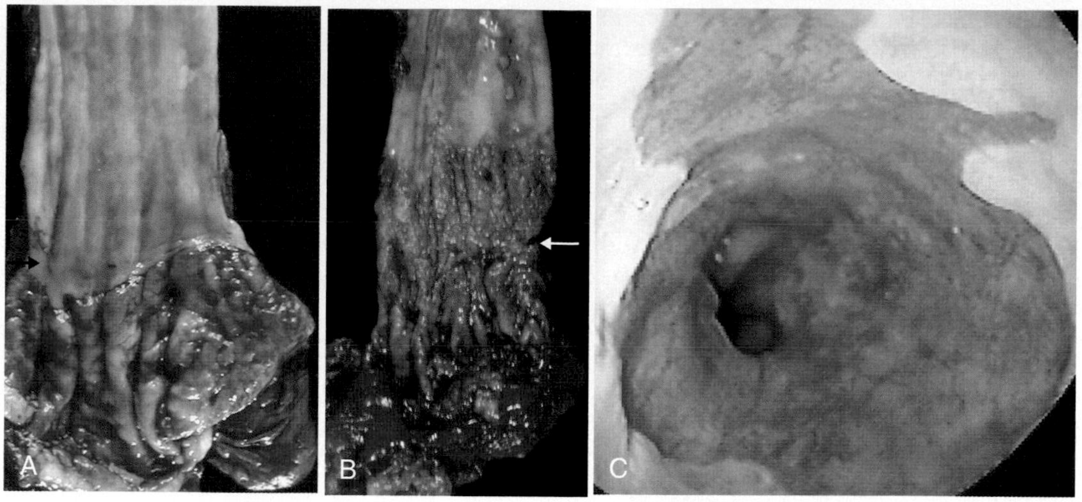

FIGURE 17–6 Barrett esophagus. *A, B,* Gross view of distal esophagus *(top)* and proximal stomach *(bottom)*, showing *A,* the normal gastroesophageal junction *(arrow)* and *B,* the granular zone of Barrett esophagus *(arrow). C,* Endoscopic view of Barrett esophagus showing red velvety gastrointestinal mucosa extending from the gastroesophageal orifice. Note the paler squamous esophageal mucosa.

Barrett mucosa), sometimes less than 0.5 cm in length. Microscopically, the esophageal squamous epithelium is replaced by metaplastic columnar epithelium, complete with surface epithelium and mucosal glands. The metaplastic mucosa may contain only gastric surface and glandular mucus-secreting cells, making clinical distinction from a hiatal hernia difficult. **Definitive diagnosis is made when the columnar mucosa contains intestinal goblet cells** (Fig. 17–7).

Critical to the pathologic evaluation of patients with Barrett mucosa is the search for dysplasia, the presumed precursor of malignancy, in columnar epithelium with intestinal metaplasia. Dysplasia is recognized by the presence of cytologic and architectural abnormalities in the columnar epithelium, consisting of enlarged, crowded, and stratified hyperchromatic nuclei and loss of intervening stroma between adjacent glandular structures.[10] Dysplasia is classified as low-grade or high-grade, with the predominant distinction being a basal orientation of all nuclei in low-grade dysplasia versus nuclei consistently reaching the apex of epithelial cells in high-grade dysplasia. Approximately 50% of patients with high-grade dysplasia may already have adjacent adenocarcinoma, according to some studies;[11] therefore, persistent high-grade dysplasia demands clinical intervention.

Clinical Features. Most of the patients with first diagnosis of Barrett esophagus are between ages 40 and 60, although children can also occasionally develop this condition. The incidence is highest among white males. In addition to the symptoms of reflux esophagitis, Barrett esophagus is clinically significant due to the secondary complications of local ulceration with bleeding and stricture. Of greatest importance is the development of adenocarcinoma, which, in patients with over 3 cm of Barrett mucosa, occurs at an estimated 30- to 40-fold increased rate over the general population. The presence of short-segment Barrett esophagus also appears to impart risk for adenocarcinoma, but at what rate is not yet known.

INFECTIOUS AND CHEMICAL ESOPHAGITIS

In addition to gastroesophageal reflux (which is, in fact, a chemical injury), esophageal inflammation may have many origins, as follows:

- Ingestion of mucosal irritants such as alcohol, corrosive acids or alkalis (in suicide attempts), excessively hot fluids (e.g., hot tea in Iran); or heavy smoking
- Cytotoxic anticancer therapy, with or without superimposed infection
- Infection following bacteremia or viremia; herpes simplex viruses and cytomegalovirus (CMV) are common offenders in immunosuppressed patients

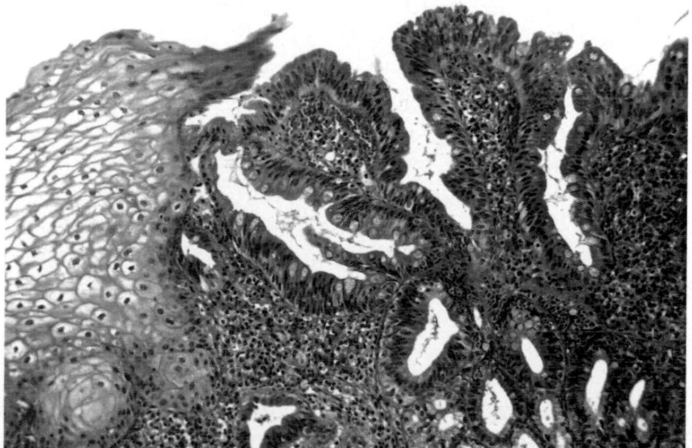

FIGURE 17–7 Barrett esophagus. Microscopic view showing squamous mucosa and intestinal-type columnar epithelial cells (goblet cells) in a glandular mucosa.

- Fungal infection in debilitated or immunosuppressed patients or during broad-spectrum antimicrobial therapy; candidiasis by far the most common; mucormycosis and aspergillosis may occur
- Uremia in the setting of renal failure.

Esophageal inflammation may also arise following radiation treatment and in association with systemic graft-versus-host disease (GVHD), autoimmune diseases, or the desquamative dermatologic conditions of pemphigoid and epidermolysis bullosa. On rare occasion, esophagitis occurs in the setting of Crohn disease.

Morphology. Esophagitis of different causes have their own characteristic features; the final common pathway for all is severe acute inflammation, superficial necrosis and ulceration with the formation of granulation tissue, and eventual fibrosis.

- In candidiasis, patches of the entire esophagus become covered by adherent, gray-white pseudomembranes teeming with densely matted fungal hyphae.
- Herpesviruses typically cause punched-out ulcers; the nuclear inclusions of herpesvirus are found in a narrow rim of degenerating epithelial cells at the margin of the ulcer. CMV causes liner ulceration of the esophageal mucosa; the histologic findings of CMV-associated change with both intranuclear and cytoplasmic inclusions are found in capillary endothelium and stromal cells in the base of the ulcer. In both forms of infection, immunohistochemical staining for virus-specific antigens provides a sensitive and specific diagnostic tool if routine histology is equivocal.
- Pathogenic bacteria account for 10% to 15% of cases of infectious esophagitis and exhibit bacterial invasion of the lamina propria with necrosis of the squamous epithelium.
- Injury induced by chemicals (lye, acids, detergents) may produce only mild erythema and edema, sloughing of the mucosa, or outright necrosis of the entire esophageal wall. Localized esophageal ulceration may result from pharmaceutical tablets or capsules "sticking" in the esophagus.
- Following irradiation of the esophagus, submucosal and mural blood vessels exhibit marked intimal proliferation with luminal narrowing. The submucosa becomes severely fibrotic, and the mucosa exhibits atrophy, with flattening of the papillae and thinning of the epithelium.
- GVHD shares features with the skin manifestations (e.g., apoptosis of basal epithelial cells, separation of epithelium and lamina propria, atrophy, and fibrosis of the lamina propria with minimal inflammation).

Clinical Features. Infections of the esophagus may occur in otherwise healthy individuals, but most often occur in the debilitated or immunosuppressed. Chemical injury in children is usually accidental, as opposed to attempted suicide, which is an adult phenomenon.

Tumors

BENIGN TUMORS

Benign tumors of the esophagus are mostly mesenchymal in origin and lie within the esophageal wall. Most common are benign tumors of smooth muscle origin, called *leiomyomas.* Fibromas, lipomas, hemangiomas, neurofibromas, and lymphangiomas may also arise. Mucosal polyps are usually composed of a combination of fibrous, vascular, or adipose tissue covered by an intact mucosa, known as *fibrovascular polyps* or *pedunculated lipomas. Squamous papillomas* are sessile lesions with a central core of connective tissue and a hyperplastic papilliform squamous mucosa. When the papilloma is associated with human papillomavirus (HPV) infection, the term *condyloma* applies. In rare instances a mesenchymal mass of inflamed granulation tissue, called an *inflammatory polyp,* may resemble a malignant lesion, hence its alternative name *inflammatory pseudotumor.*

MALIGNANT TUMORS

In the United States, carcinomas of the esophagus represent about 6% of all cancers of the gastrointestinal tract but cause a disproportionate number of cancer deaths. They remain asymptomatic during much of their development and are often discovered too late to permit cure. With rare exceptions, malignant esophageal tumors arise from the epithelial layer. In the United States, most esophageal cancers used to be of squamous cell origin, but the incidence of these tumors has declined with a steady increase of adenocarcinomas. Worldwide, squamous cell cancers constitute 90% of esophageal cancers, but in the United States squamous cell carcinoma and adenocarcinoma exhibit comparable incidence rates. Rare tumors (undifferentiated, carcinoid, malignant melanoma, lymphoma, sarcoma, and adenocarcinomas arising from the submucosal glands) are not discussed here.

Squamous Cell Carcinoma

Squamous cell carcinoma is the most common type of carcinoma in the esophagus. Most squamous cell carcinomas occur in adults over age 50. The male-to-female ratio varies, in different studies, from 2:1 to as high as 20:1. While squamous cell carcinoma of the esophagus occurs throughout the world, its incidence varies widely between countries and within regions of the same country. The regions with higher incidence are Iran, central China, South Africa, and southern Brazil, where annual incidence rates are as high as 100 per 100,000, with deaths from cancer of the esophagus constituting over 20% of all cancer deaths. Other areas of high incidence include Puerto Rico and Eastern Europe. In the United States, it affects from 2 to 8 persons per 100,000 yearly and is predominantly a disease of adult males (the male-to-female ratio is 4:1). Blacks throughout the world are at higher risk than are whites; incidence in this group in the United States is fourfold higher than for U.S. whites.

Etiology and Pathogenesis. The marked differences in epidemiology strongly implicate dietary and environmental factors (Table 17–1), with a contribution from genetic predisposition.[12] The majority of cancers in Europe and the United

TABLE 17–1 Factors Associated with the Development of Squamous Cell Carcinoma of the Esophagus

Dietary
Deficiency of vitamins (A, C, riboflavin, thiamine, pyridoxine)
Deficiency of trace elements (zinc, molybdenum)
Fungal contamination of foodstuffs
High content of nitrites/nitrosamines
Betel chewing
Lifestyle
Burning-hot beverages or food
Alcohol consumption
Tobacco use
Urban environment
Esophageal Disorders
Long-standing esophagitis
Achalasia
Plummer-Vinson syndrome
Genetic Predisposition
Long-standing celiac disease
Ectodermal dysplasia
Epidermolysis bullosa
Racial disposition

States are attributable to alcohol and tobacco usage. Some alcoholic drinks contain significant amounts of such carcinogens as polycyclic hydrocarbons, fuel oils, and nitrosamines, along with other mutagenic compounds. Nutritional deficiencies associated with alcoholism may contribute to the process of carcinogenesis.

Alcohol and tobacco cannot be invoked as risk factors in many high-incidence regions of the world. The presence of carcinogens, such as fungus-contaminated and nitrosamine-containing foodstuffs in China, may play a significant role in the extraordinary high incidence of carcinoma in this region. Dietary deficiencies in vitamins and essential metals have been documented in China and South Africa. Human papillomavirus DNA is found frequently in esophageal squamous cell carcinomas from high-incidence regions, but is infrequent in cancer-bearing patients in North America.[13]

Based on the above considerations, dietary and environmental factors have been proposed to increase risk, with nutritional deficiencies acting as promoters or potentiators of the tumorigenic effects of environmental carcinogens. For example, methylating nitroso compounds in the diet and in tobacco smoke may be the reason for the broad spectrum of *p53* point mutations present in over half of esophageal cancers. Other genetic alterations, such as mutations in *p16INK4*, and amplification of *CYCLIN D1*, *C-MYC*, and epithelial growth factor receptor *(EGFR)*, are prevalent in these cancers as well. This is in keeping with the concept that stepwise acquisition and accumulation of genetic alterations ultimately give rise to cancer.[14] Notably rare in esophageal squamous cell carcinomas are K-*RAS* and adenomatous polyposis coli *(APC)* mutations.

Finally, the chronic esophagitis so commonly observed in persons living in areas of high incidence may itself be the result of sustained exposure to the carcinogens listed earlier. This chronic esophagitis results in an increased epithelial cell turnover, which, over a length of time in a continuously carcinogenic environment, progresses to dysplasia and eventually to carcinoma. The rate of progression along the chronic esophagitis–dysplasia–cancer sequence may well be modified or modulated by genetic or racial factors.

Morphology. Like squamous cell carcinomas arising in other locations, those of the esophagus begin as apparent in situ lesions **(intraepithelial neoplasm or carcinoma in situ)**. When they become overt, about 20% of these tumors are located in the upper third, 50% in the middle third, and 30% in the lower third of the esophagus. Early lesions appear as small, gray-white, plaque-like thickenings or elevations of the mucosa. In months to years, these lesions become tumorous masses and may eventually encircle the lumen. Three morphologic patterns are described: (1) protruded (60%), a polypoid exophytic lesion that protrudes into the lumen; (2) flat (15%), a diffuse, infiltrative form that tends to spread within the wall of the esophagus, causing thickening, rigidity, and narrowing of the lumen; and (3) excavated (ulcerated, 25%; Fig. 17–8), a necrotic cancerous ulceration that excavates deeply into surrounding structures and may erode into the respiratory tree (with resultant fistula and pneumonia) or aorta (with catastrophic exsanguination) or may permeate the mediastinum and pericardium. The fortunate patient is found at the stage of superficial esophageal carcinoma, in which the malignant lesion is confined to the epithelial layer (in situ) or is superficially invading the lamina propria or submucosa (Fig. 17–9).

Most squamous cell carcinomas are moderately to well differentiated. Several histologic variants may be seen, such as verrucous squamous cell carcinoma, spindle cell carcinoma, and basaloid squamous cell carcinoma. Irrespective of their degree of differentiation, most symptomatic tumors are quite large by the time they are diagnosed and have already invaded the wall or beyond. The rich lymphatic network in the sub-

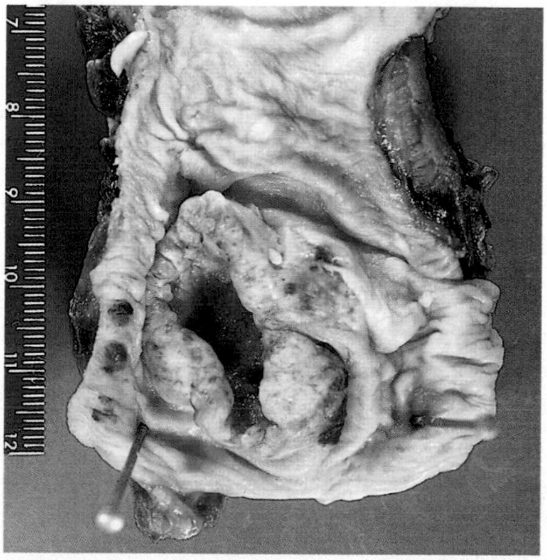

FIGURE 17–8 Large ulcerated squamous cell carcinoma of the esophagus.

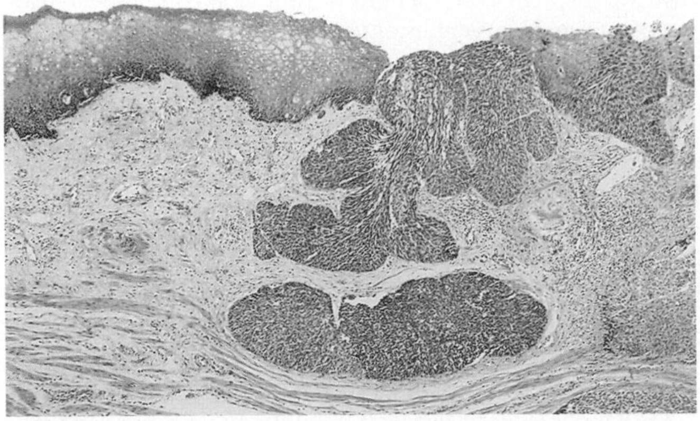

FIGURE 17–9 Squamous cell carcinoma of the esophagus: low-power microscopic view showing invasion into the submucosa.

mucosa promotes extensive circumferential and longitudinal spread, and intramural tumor cell clusters may often be seen several centimeters away from the main mass. Local extension into adjacent mediastinal structures occurs early and often in this disease, possibly due to the absence of serosa for most of the esophagus. Tumors located in the upper third of the esophagus also metastasize to cervical lymph nodes; those in the middle third to the mediastinal, paratracheal, and tracheobronchial nodes; and those in the lower third most often spread to the gastric and celiac groups of nodes.

Clinical Features. Esophageal carcinoma is insidious in onset and produces dysphagia and obstruction gradually and late. Patients subconsciously adjust to their increasing difficulty in swallowing by progressively altering their diet from solid to liquid foods. Extreme weight loss and debilitation result from both the impaired nutrition and the effects of the tumor itself. Hemorrhage and sepsis may accompany ulceration of the tumor. Occasionally, the first alarming symptom of this neoplasm is aspiration of food via a cancerous tracheoesophageal fistula. Although the insidious growth of these neoplasms often leads to large lesions by the time a diagnosis is established, resectability rates have improved modestly (from less than half to over 80%) with the advent of endoscopic screening in patient populations at risk and accurate staging by endoscopic ultrasonography. The five-year survival rate in patients with superficial esophageal carcinoma is about 75%, compared to 25% in patients who undergo "curative" surgery for more advanced disease and 9% for all patients with esophageal squamous cell carcinoma. Local and distant recurrence following surgery is common. The presence of lymph node metastases at the time of resection significantly reduces five-year survival.

Adenocarcinoma

Adenocarcinoma of the esophagus is a malignant epithelial tumor with glandular differentiation. Because of confusion in the past with gastric cancers arising at the gastroesophageal junction, true esophageal adenocarcinomas were thought to be unusual. With increasing recognition of Barrett mucosa, it is apparent that most adenocarcinomas in the lower third of the esophagus are true esophageal cancers, rather than gastric cancers straddling the esophagogastric junction. Accordingly, adenocarcinoma now represents up to half of all esophageal cancers reported in the United States, and the incidence has been increasing in recent decades, particularly among white men. *The majority of cases arise from the Barrett mucosa.* In rare instances, adenocarcinoma originates from heterotopic gastric mucosa or submucosal glands.

Etiology and Pathogenesis. The discussion of adenocarcinoma focuses on Barrett esophagus. The lifetime risk for cancer development from Barrett esophagus is approximately 10%. Tobacco exposure and obesity are risk factors, but there is no close association between alcohol ingestion and the development of adenocarcinoma of the esophagus. *Helicobacter pylori* infection may be a contributing factor, but there is no general agreement about this issue.

Molecular studies have suggested that the pathogenesis of adenocarcinoma from Barrett esophagus is a multistep process with a long latency period associated with many genetic changes. The development of dysplasia seems to be a critical step in this process (Fig. 17–10). Barrett epithelial cells have higher proliferative activity, and dysplastic epithelial cells have lost cell-cycle control. Several growth factors, oncogenes, and tumor suppressor genes are implicated in this process.[15] Overexpression of p53 and an increased proportion of cycling cells are present in the dysplastic epithelium, presumably the result of chronic cell and DNA damage induced by gastric reflux. In high-grade dysplasia, chromosomal abnormalities, such as chromosome 4 amplification, are generally present.[16] When the dysplastic epithelium develops into adenocarcinoma, additional genetic changes, including nuclear translocation of β-catenin and amplification of *c-ERB-B2*, are present. Although specific genetic abnormalities associated with the Barrett esophagus-carcinoma transition have not been identified, *p53* mutations, along with tetraploidy and aneuploidy, seem to occur early. These genetic alterations may be suitable biomarkers of disease progression.

Morphology. Adenocarcinomas arising in the setting of Barrett esophagus are usually located in the distal esophagus and may invade the adjacent gastric cardia. Initially appearing as flat or raised patches of an otherwise intact mucosa, they may develop into large nodular masses up to 5 cm in diameter or may exhibit diffusely infiltrative or deeply ulcerative features (Fig. 17–11*A*). Microscopically, most tumors are mucin-producing glandular tumors exhibiting intestinal-type features (Fig. 17–11*B*); less often they are made up of diffusely infiltrative signet-ring cells of a gastric type or even poorly differentiated small cell-type tumor. Multiple foci of dysplastic mucosa are frequently adjacent to the tumor, which is the basis for the recommendation of multisite biopsy when performing endoscopic screening for dysplasia and malignancy.

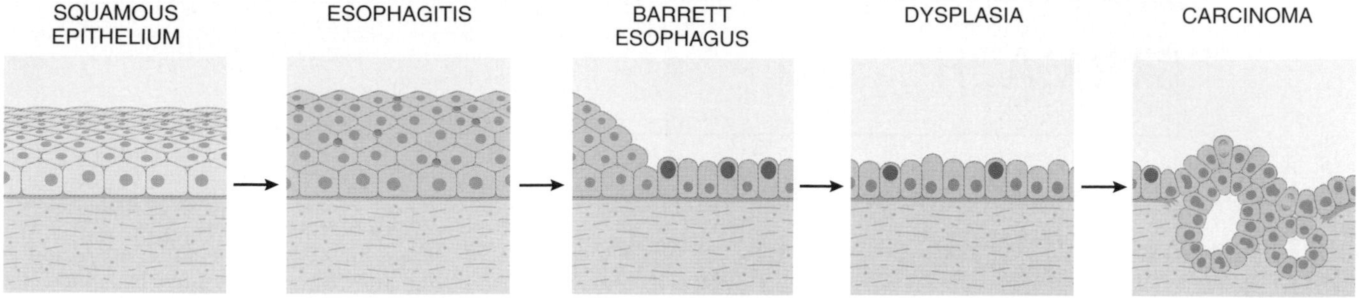

FIGURE 17–10 Transition from Barrett esophagus to adenocarcinoma.

Clinical Features. Adenocarcinomas arising in Barrett esophagus chiefly occur in patients over age 40, with a median age in the sixth decade. Similar to Barrett esophagus, adenocarcinoma is more common in men than in women, and whites are affected more frequently than blacks, in contrast to squamous cell carcinomas. As in other forms of esophageal carcinoma, patients usually present because of difficulty swallowing, progressive weight loss, bleeding, chest pain, and vomiting. Long-term symptoms of heartburn, regurgitation, and epigastric pain related to concurrent gastroesophageal reflux disease and sliding hiatal hernias are present in less than half of newly diagnosed patients.

The prognosis for esophageal adenocarcinoma is as poor as that for other forms of esophageal cancer, with under 20% overall five-year survival. Identification and resection of early cancers with invasion limited to the mucosa or submucosa improves five-year survival to over 80%. Although dysplasia appears to be a requisite for the development of adenocarcinoma, patients with low-grade dysplasia may not progress to cancer over long periods of follow-up, and apparent regression may occur. Regression or ablation of Barrett esophagus has not yet been shown to eliminate the risk for adenocarcinoma.

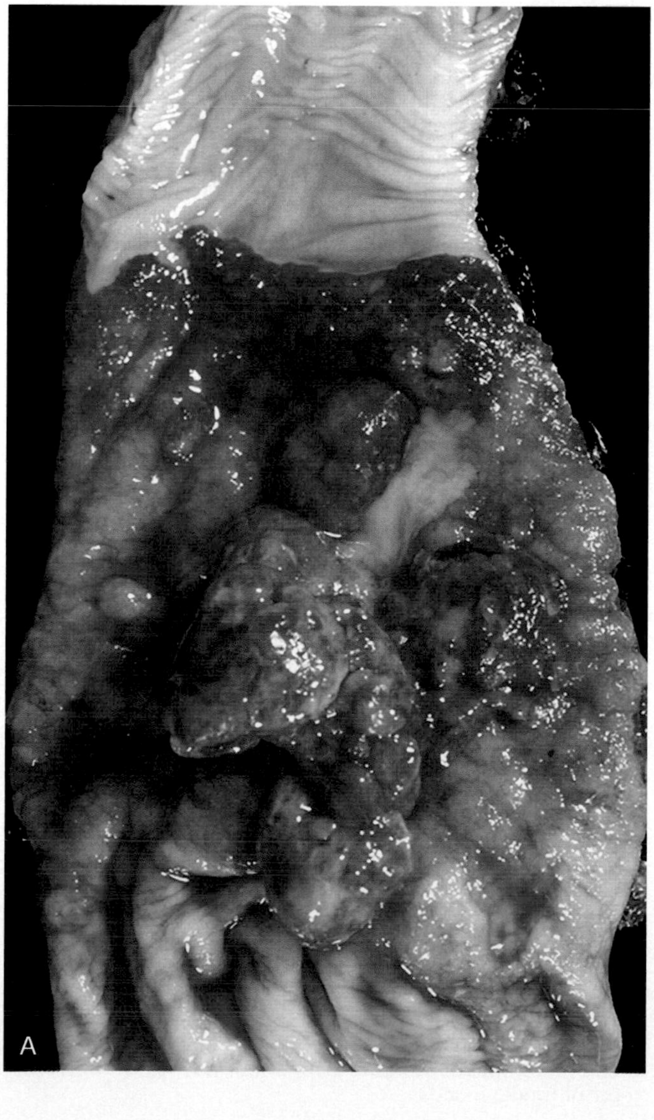

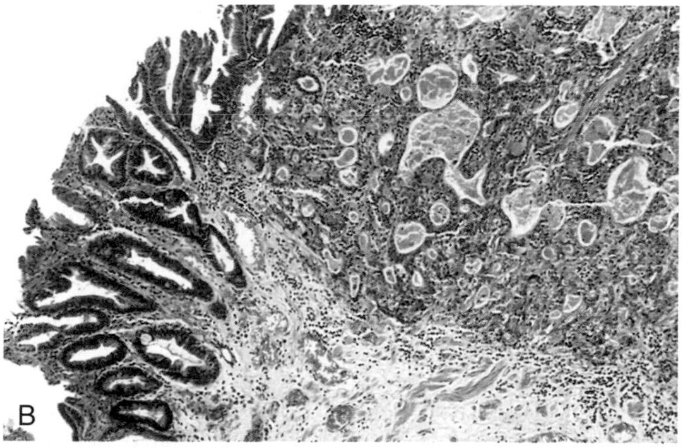

FIGURE 17–11 Adenocarcinoma of the esophagus. *A,* Gross view of an ulcerated, exophytic mass at the gastroesophageal junction, arising from the granular mucosa of Barrett esophagus. The gray-white esophageal mucosa is on the top, and the folds of gastric mucosa are below. (*A,* courtesy of Dr. James Gulizia, Brigham and Women's Hospital, Boston, MA.) *B,* Microscopic view of malignant intestinal-type glands in adenocarcinoma arising from Barrett esophagus.

STOMACH

Normal

The stomach develops from the distal part of the foregut. It is a saccular organ with a volume of 1200 to 1500 mL, but a capacity of over 3000 mL. It extends from just left of the midline where it is joined to the esophagus, to just right of the midline where it connects to the duodenum. The concavity of the right, inner curve is called the *lesser curvature,* and the convexity of the left, outer curve is the *greater curvature.* An angle along the lesser curve, the *incisura angularis,* marks the approximate point at which the stomach narrows prior to its junction with the duodenum. The entire stomach is covered by peritoneum; an exaggerated peritoneal fold, the greater omentum, extends beyond the greater curvature to the transverse colon.

The stomach is divided into five anatomic regions (Fig. 17–12*A*). The *cardia* is the narrow conical portion of the stomach immediately distal to the gastroesophageal junction. The *fundus* is the dome-shaped portion of the proximal stomach that extends superolateral to the gastroesophageal junction. The *body,* or *corpus,* comprises the remainder of the stomach proximal to the incisura angularis. The stomach distal to this angle is the *antrum,* demarcated from the duodenum by the muscular *pyloric sphincter.*

The gastric wall, like the rest of the gastrointestinal tract, consists of mucosa, submucosa, muscularis propria, and serosa. The interior surface of the stomach exhibits coarse *rugae* (meaning "folds"). These infoldings of mucosa and submucosa extend longitudinally and are most prominent in the proximal stomach, flattening out when the stomach is distended. A finer mosaic-like pattern is delineated by small furrows in the mucosa. The delicate texture of the mucosa is punctuated by millions of gastric foveolae, or *pits,* leading to the mucosal glands.

The normal gastric mucosa has two compartments: the superficial foveolar (meaning leaflike) compartment and the deeper glandular compartment. The foveolar compartment is relatively uniform throughout the stomach. In contrast, the glandular compartment exhibits major differences in thickness and in glandular composition in different regions of the stomach (Fig. 17–12*B, C*). The foveolar compartment consists of *surface epithelial cells (the foveolar cells) lining the entire mucosal surface as well as the gastric pits.* The lush undulation of the mucosal surface and pits imparts the leaflike texture to the gastric mucosa. The tall, columnar mucin-secreting foveolar cells have basal nuclei and crowded, small, relatively clear mucin-containing granules in the supranuclear region. Deeper in the gastric pits are so-called *mucous neck cells,* which have a lower content of mucin granules and are thought to be the progenitors of both the surface epithelium and the cells of the gastric glands.[17] Mitoses are extremely common in this region, as the entire gastric mucosal surface is totally replaced every 2 to 6 days. The glandular compartment consists of gastric glands, which vary between anatomic regions:

- *Cardia glands* contain mucus-secreting cells only.
- *Oxyntic (also called gastric or fundic) glands* are found in the fundus and body and contain parietal cells, chief cells, and scattered endocrine cells. The term *oxyntic* means acid-forming (derived from Greek, *oxynein).*
- *Antral* or *pyloric glands* contain mucus-secreting cells and endocrine cells.

The main cell types in these glands are the following:

- *Mucous cells* populate the glands of the cardia and antral regions and secrete mucus and pepsinogen II. The mucous neck cells in the glands of the body and fundus secrete mucus as well as group I and II pepsinogens.
- *Parietal cells* line predominantly the upper half of the oxyntic glands in the fundus and body. They are recogniz-

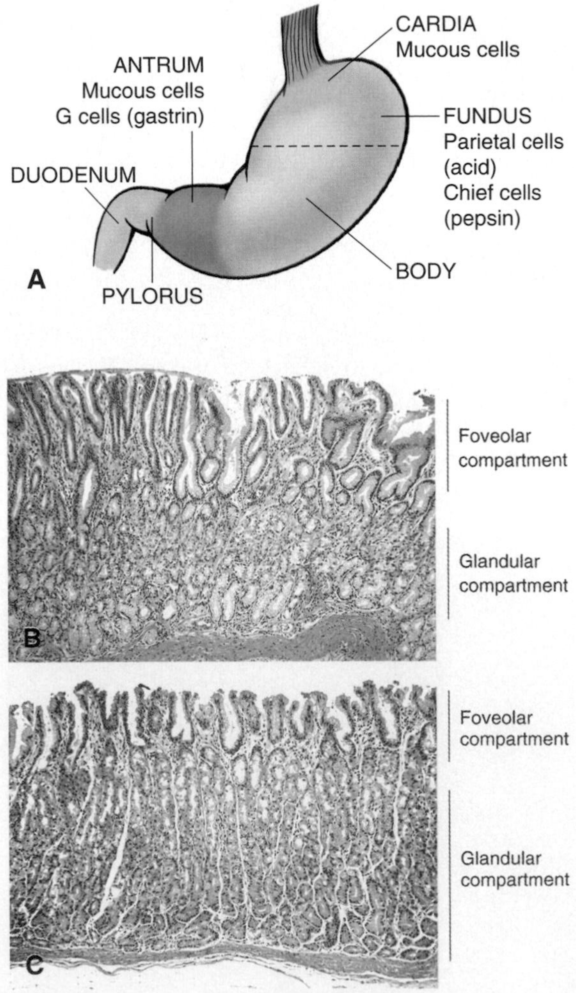

FIGURE 17–12 Anatomy and histology of the stomach. *A,* Gross anatomy. *B,* Microscopic view of antral mucosa. *C,* Microscopic view of fundic mucosa.

able by their bright eosinophilia on H & E stained preparations, which are attributable to their abundant mitochondria. The apical membrane of the parietal cell is invaginated, forming an extensive intracellular canalicular system complete with microvilli. In the resting state, vesicles lie in close approximation to the canalicular system. These vesicles contain the proton pump, a unique hydrogen-potassium-ATPase (H^+,K^+-ATPase) that pumps hydrogen across membranes in exchange for potassium ions. Within minutes of parietal cell stimulation, the vesicles fuse with the canalicular system, thereby creating an apically directed acid-secreting membrane of enormous surface area. Parietal cells also secrete *intrinsic factor,* which binds luminal *vitamin* B_{12} in the duodenum and permits its absorption in the ileum.

- *Chief cells,* concentrated more at the base of gastric glands, are responsible for the secretion of the proteolytic proenzymes *pepsinogen I and II.* Chief cells are notable for their basophilic cytoplasm, and ultrastructurally are classic protein-synthesizing cells, having an extensive rough endoplasmic reticulum, a prominent supranuclear Golgi apparatus, and numerous apical secretory granules. Upon stimulation of chief cells, the pepsinogens contained in the granules are released by exocytosis. The pepsinogens are activated to *pepsin* by the low luminal pH and inactivated above pH 6.0 upon entry into the duodenum.
- *Endocrine* or *enteroendocrine cells* are scattered among the epithelial cells of gastric and antral glands. The cytoplasm of these triangular cells contains small brightly eosinophilic granules, which are concentrated on the basal aspect of the cell. These cells can act in an endocrine mode, releasing their products into the circulation, or a paracrine mode, via secretion into the local tissue. In the antral mucosa, most of the endocrine cells are the gastrin-producing cells, or *G cells.* In the body (gastric) mucosa, the endocrine cells produce histamine, which binds the histamine-2 (H_2) receptor on the parietal cells to increase acid production. These cells are also referred as *enterochromaffin-like (ECL) cells.* Other ECL cells in the gastric mucosa include *D cells* (producing somatostatin) and *X cells* (producing endothelin). These cells play an important role in modulating acid production.

Gastric Mucosal Physiology

ACID SECRETION

The hallmark of gastric physiology is secretion of hydrochloric acid, divided into three phases.

- The *cephalic phase,* initiated by the sight, taste, smell, chewing, and swallowing of palatable food, is mediated by vagal activity.
- The *gastric phase* involves stimulation of stretch receptors by gastric distention and is mediated by vagal impulses; it also involves gastrin release from endocrine cells, the G cells, in the antral glands. Gastrin release is promoted by luminal amino acids and peptides and possibly by vagal stimulation.
- The *intestinal phase,* initiated when food containing digested protein enters the proximal small intestine, involves a number of polypeptides besides gastrin.

All signals converge on the gastric parietal cell to activate the *proton pump:*

- Acetylcholine released from cephalic-vagal or gastric-vagal afferents stimulates the parietal cell via the muscarine-3 cholinergic receptor, resulting in an increase in cytosolic Ca^{2+} and subsequent activation of the proton pump.
- Gastrin activates a gastrin receptor, resulting in an increase of cytosolic Ca^{2+} within the parietal cells.
- *An oxyntic gland ECL cell plays a central role:* gastrin and vagal afferents induce the release of histamine from the ECL cell, thereby stimulating the H_2 receptor on parietal cells. This pathway is considered to be the most important for activation of the proton pump.

Activation of some receptors on the parietal cell surface inhibit acid production. They include receptors for somatostatin, prostaglandins of the E series, and epidermal growth factor.

MUCOSAL PROTECTION

At maximal secretory rates the intraluminal concentration of hydrogen ion is *3 million times* greater than that of the blood and tissues. The "mucosal barrier" protects the gastric mucosa from autodigestion and consists of:

- *Mucus secretion:* The thin layer of surface mucus in the stomach and duodenum exhibits a diffusion coefficient for H^+ that is one quarter that of water. Acid- and pepsin-containing fluid exits the gastric glands as "jets" passing through the surface mucus layer, entering the lumen directly without contacting surface epithelial cells.
- *Bicarbonate secretion:* Surface epithelial cells in both the stomach and duodenum secrete bicarbonate into the boundary zone of adherent mucus, creating an essentially pH-neutral microenvironment immediately adjacent to the cell surface.
- *The epithelial barrier:* Intercellular tight junctions provide a barrier to the back-diffusion of hydrogen ions. Epithelial disruption is followed rapidly by *restitution,* in which existing cells migrate along the exposed basement membrane to fill in the defects and restore epithelial barrier integrity.
- *Mucosal blood flow:* The rich mucosal blood supply provides oxygen, bicarbonate, and nutrients to epithelial cells and removes back-diffused acid.
- *Prostaglandin synthesis:* Production of prostaglandins by the mucosal cells impacts on many other components of mucosal defense. For example, prostaglandins favor production of mucus and bicarbonates, and they inhibit acid secretion by parietal cells. In addition, by their vasodilatory action, prostaglandins E and I improve mucosal blood flow. Drugs that block prostaglandin synthesis reduce this cytoprotection and thus promote gastric mucosal injury and ulceration.

When the mucosal barrier is breached, the muscularis mucosa limits injury. Superficial damage limited to the mucosa can heal within hours to days. When damage extends into the submucosa, weeks are required for complete healing. Imperfect as our understanding of these defensive mechanisms may be, they are clearly a physiologic marvel, or our gastric walls would suffer the same fate as a piece of swallowed meat.

In addition to the well-characterized barrier function and digestive function of the gastric mucosa, mucosal endocrine cells also produce hormones that are involved in growth regulation. Ghrelin is a recently identified growth hormone that regulates body growth and appetite via a possible effect on the gastrointestinal-hypothalamic-pituitary axis.[18]

Pathology

Gastric lesions are frequent causes of clinical disease. In Western industrialized nations, peptic ulcers develop in up to 10% of the general population at some point during life. Chronic infection of the gastric mucosa by the bacterium *H. pylori* is the most common infection worldwide. Lastly, gastric cancer remains a leading cause of death in the United States, despite its decreasing incidence.

Congenital Anomalies

Heterotopic rests of normal tissue may be present in the stomach, and are usually asymptomatic. With *pancreatic heterotopia,* nodules of essentially normal pancreatic tissue up to 1 cm in diameter may be present in the gastric submucosa, muscle wall, or at a subserosal location. When in the pylorus, localized inflammation may lead to pyloric obstruction. With *gastric heterotopia,* small patches of ectopic gastric mucosa in the duodenum or in more distal sites may present as perplexing sources of bleeding, due to peptic ulceration of adjacent mucosa.

Defective closure of the diaphragm leads to weakness or partial to total absence of a region of the diaphragm, usually on the left. Resultant herniation of abdominal contents into the thorax in utero produces a *diaphragmatic hernia.* Usually, the stomach or a portion of it insinuates into the pouch, but occasionally small bowel and even a portion of the liver accompany it. The herniation may be asymptomatic or may engender potentially lethal respiratory problems in the newborn.

Rarely, and in keeping with the foregut origin of the stomach, a bud of pulmonary tissue complete with bronchial structures may be attached to the stomach. This pulmonary sequestrum may become infected or present as a mass lesion.

PYLORIC STENOSIS

Congenital hypertrophic pyloric stenosis is encountered in infants as a disorder that affects males three to four times more often than females, occurring in 1 in 300 to 900 live births. Familial occurrence implicates a multifactorial pattern of inheritance; monozygotic twins have a high rate of concordance of the condition. Pyloric stenosis also may occur in association with Turner syndrome, trisomy 18, and esophageal atresia. Regurgitation and persistent, projectile, nonbilious vomiting usually appear in the second or third week of life. Physical examination reveals visible peristalsis and a firm, ovoid palpable mass in the region of the pylorus or distal stomach, the result of hypertrophy, and possibly hyperplasia, of the muscularis propria of the pylorus. Edema and inflammatory changes in the mucosa and submucosa may aggravate the narrowing. Surgical muscle splitting is curative.

Acquired pyloric stenosis in adults is one of the long-term risks of antral gastritis or peptic ulcers close to the pylorus. Carcinomas of the pyloric region, lymphomas, or adjacent carcinomas of the pancreas are more ominous causes. In these cases, inflammatory fibrosis or malignant infiltration narrow the pyloric channel, producing pyloric outlet obstruction. In rare instances, hypertrophic pyloric stenosis is the result of prolonged pyloric spasm.

Gastritis

This diagnosis is both overused and often missed—overused when it is applied loosely to any transient upper abdominal complaint in the absence of validating evidence, and missed because most patients with chronic gastritis are asymptomatic. *Gastritis is simply defined as inflammation of the gastric mucosa.* It is a histologic diagnosis. Inflammation may be predominantly *acute,* with neutrophilic infiltration, or *chronic,* with lymphocytes and/or plasma cells predominating and associated intestinal metaplasia and atrophy.[19]

ACUTE GASTRITIS

Acute gastritis is an acute mucosal inflammatory process, usually of a transient nature. The inflammation may be accompanied by hemorrhage into the mucosa and, in more severe circumstances, by sloughing of the superficial mucosa (mucosal erosion). This severe erosive form of the disease is an important cause of acute gastrointestinal bleeding.

Pathogenesis. The pathogenesis is poorly understood, in part because the normal mechanisms for gastric mucosal protection are not entirely clear. Acute gastritis is frequently associated with:

- Heavy use of nonsteroidal anti-inflammatory drugs (NSAIDs), particularly aspirin
- Excessive alcohol consumption
- Heavy smoking
- Treatment with cancer chemotherapeutic drugs
- Uremia
- Systemic bacterial or viral infections (e.g., salmonellosis or CMV infection)
- Severe stress (e.g., trauma, burns, surgery)
- Ischemia and shock
- Suicidal attempts, as with acids and alkali
- Gastric irradiation or freezing
- Mechanical trauma (e.g., nasogastric intubation)
- Distal gastrectomy.

One or more of the following influences are thought to be operative in these varied settings: increased acid secretion with back-diffusion, decreased production of bicarbonate buffer, reduced blood flow, disruption of the adherent mucus layer, and direct damage to the epithelium. Not surprisingly, mucosal insults can act synergistically. Thus, ischemic injury worsens the effects of back-diffusion of hydrogen ions. Other mucosal insults have been identified, such as regurgitation of detergent bile acids and lysolecithins from the proximal duodenum, and inadequate mucosal synthesis of prostaglandins. It must be emphasized that a substantial portion of patients has idiopathic gastritis, with no associated disorders.

Morphology. In the mildest form of acute gastritis, the lamina propria exhibits only moderate edema and slight vascular congestion. The surface epithelium is intact, and scattered neutrophils are present among the surface epithelial cells or within the epithelial layer and lumen of mucosal glands. **The presence of neutrophils above the basement membrane (within the epithelial space) is abnormal and signifies active inflammation ("activity").** With more severe mucosal damage, erosion and hemorrhage develop. "**Erosion" denotes loss of the superficial epithelium, generating a defect in the mucosa that does not cross the muscularis mucosa.** It is accompanied by a robust acute inflammatory infiltrate and extrusion of a fibrin-containing purulent exudate into the lumen. Hemorrhage may occur independently, generating punctate dark spots in an otherwise hyperemic mucosa or in association with erosion. Concurrent erosion and hemorrhage is termed **acute erosive hemorrhagic gastritis** (Fig. 17–13*A*). Large areas of the gastric mucosa may be denuded, but the involvement is superficial and rarely affects the entire depth of the mucosa (Fig. 17–13*B*). These lesions are but one step removed from stress ulcers, to be described later.

Clinical Features. Depending on the severity of the anatomic changes, acute gastritis may be entirely asymptomatic; may cause variable epigastric pain, nausea, and vomiting; or may present with overt hemorrhage, massive hematemesis, melena, and potentially fatal blood loss. Overall, it is one of the major causes of massive hematemesis, as in alcoholics. In particular settings, the condition is quite common. As many as 25% of persons who take daily aspirin for rheumatoid arthritis develop acute gastritis, many with bleeding.

CHRONIC GASTRITIS

Chronic gastritis is defined as the presence of chronic mucosal inflammatory changes leading eventually to mucosal atrophy and intestinal metaplasia, usually in the absence of erosions. The epithelial changes may become dysplastic and constitute a background for the development of carcinoma. Chronic gastritis is notable for distinct causal subgroups and for patterns of histologic alterations that vary in different parts of the world. In the Western world, the prevalence of histologic changes indicative of chronic gastritis in the later decades of life is higher than 50%.

Pathogenesis. The major etiologic associations of chronic gastritis are:

- Chronic infection by *H. pylori*
- Immunologic *(autoimmune)*, in association with pernicious anemia
- Toxic, as with alcohol and cigarette smoking
- Postsurgical, especially following antrectomy with gastroenterostomy with reflux of bilious duodenal secretions
- Motor and mechanical, including obstruction, bezoars (luminal concretions), and gastric atony
- Radiation
- Granulomatous conditions (e.g., Crohn disease)
- Miscellaneous—amyloidosis, graft-versus-host disease, uremia.

***Helicobacter pylori* Infection and Chronic Gastritis.** By far the most important etiologic association with chronic gastritis is chronic infection by the bacillus *H. pylori*. The link was discovered in 1983, when the bacterium was called *Campylobacter pyloridis.*[20] Since then, studies on *H. pylori* have yielded tremendous knowledge on the property of the bacteria and their role in the pathogenesis of gastric diseases. The complete genome of this bacterium has now been sequenced.[21] Effective treatment with antibiotics has revolutionized the way chronic gastritis and peptic ulcer disease are managed.[22]

In addition to chronic gastritis, this organism plays a critical role in other major gastric and duodenal diseases (Table 17–2). Peptic ulcer disease is now approached as an infectious disease that can be treated by antibiotics. *H. pylori* is present in 90% of patients with chronic gastritis affecting the antrum. Colonization rates increase with age, reaching 50% in asymptomatic American adults over age 50. Prevalence of infection among adults in Puerto Rico exceeds 80%. In this and other

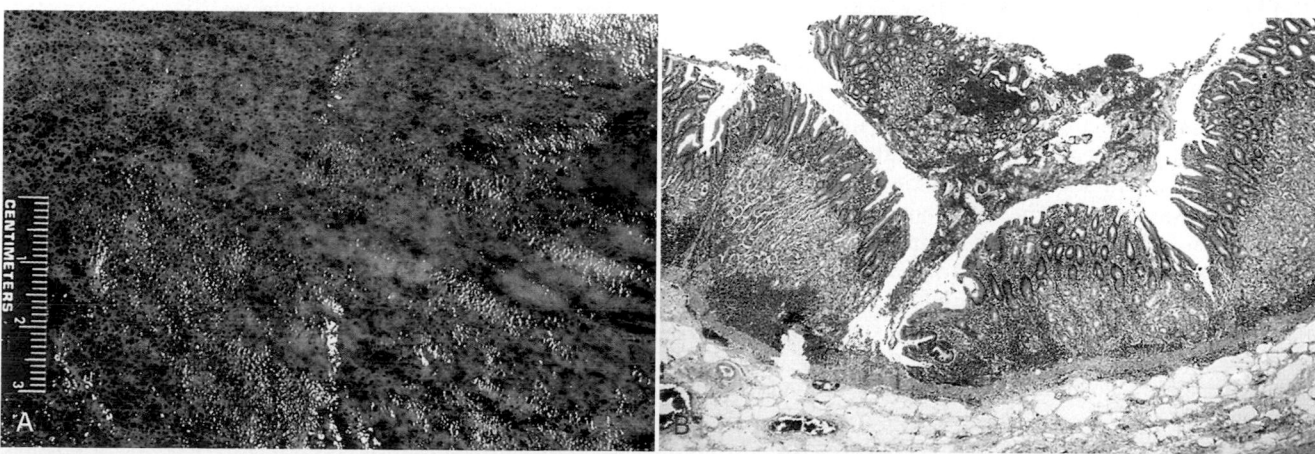

FIGURE 17–13 Acute gastritis. *A*, Gross view showing punctate erosions in an otherwise unremarkable mucosa; adherent blood is dark due to exposure to gastric acid. *B*, Low-power microscopic view of focal mucosal disruption with hemorrhage; the adjacent mucosa is normal.

TABLE 17–2 Diseases Associated with *Helicobacter pylori* Infection

Disease	Association
Chronic gastritis	Strong causal association
Peptic ulcer disease	Strong causal association
Gastric carcinoma	Strong causal association
Gastric MALT lymphoma*	Definitive etiologic role

* MALT, mucosa-associated lymphoid tissue

areas where infection is endemic, the organism seems to be acquired in childhood and persists for decades. The mode of transmission of *H. pylori* has not been well defined, although oral-oral transmission, fecal-oral transmission, and environmental spread are among the possible routes. *Most infected persons also have the associated gastritis but are asymptomatic.* Nevertheless, infected persons are at increased risk for the development of peptic ulcer disease and possibly gastric cancer.

H. pylori is a nonsporing, curvilinear gram-negative rod measuring approximately 3.5 × 0.5 μm. *H. pylori* is part of a genus of bacteria that have adapted to the ecologic niche provided by gastric mucus, which is lethal to most bacteria. The specialized traits that allow it to flourish include:

- Motility (via flagella), allowing it to swim through viscous mucus
- Elaboration of a *urease,* which produces ammonia and carbon dioxide from endogenous urea, thereby buffering gastric acid in the immediate vicinity of the organism
- Expression of *bacterial adhesins,* such as BabA, which binds to the fucosylated Lewis B blood-group antigens, enhances binding to blood group O antigen bearing cells.[23]
- Expression of bacterial toxins, such as cytotoxin association gene A *(CagA)* and vacuolating cytotoxin gene A *(VacA).*[24] These are discussed later under "Peptic Ulcer."

The *H. pylori* genome is 1.65 million base pairs and encodes approximately 1500 proteins. Extensive molecular studies suggest that the bacteria cause gastritis by stimulating production of pro-inflammatory cytokines and by directly injuring epithelial cells (discussed later).

After initial exposure to *H. pylori,* gastritis occurs in two patterns: a predominantly antral-type gastritis with high acid production and elevated risk for duodenal ulcer, and a pangastritis that is followed by multifocal atrophy (multifocal atrophic gastritis) with lower gastric acid secretion and higher risk for adenocarcinoma. The underlying mechanisms contributing to this difference are not completely clear, but host–microorganism interplay appears to be critical. IL-1β is a potent pro-inflammatory cytokine and a powerful gastric acid inhibitor. Patients who have higher IL-1β production in response to *H. pylori* infection tend to develop pangastritis, while patients who have lower IL-1β production exhibit antral-type gastritis.[25]

A number of diagnostic tests have been developed for the detection of *H. pylori.* Noninvasive tests include a serologic test for antibodies, fecal bacterial detection, and a urea breath test. The breath test is based on the generation of ammonia by bacterial urease. Invasive tests are based on the identification of *H. pylori* in gastric biopsy tissue. Detection methods in gastric tissue include visualization of the bacteria in histologic sections, bacterial culture, a rapid urease test, and bacterial DNA detection by the polymerase chain reaction.

Patients with chronic gastritis and *H. pylori* usually improve when treated with antibiotics. Relapses are associated with reappearance of the organism. The current treatment regimens include antibiotics and hydrogen pump inhibitors.[22] Prophylactic and therapeutic vaccine development is still in the early research stage, but it holds the promise to eradicate or at least greatly reduce the worldwide prevalence of *H. pylori* infection.

In addition to *H. pylori,* humans can also be infected by *Helicobacter heilmannii,* a spiral bacterium found in dogs, cats, and nonhuman primates.[26] This bacterium causes a relatively mild gastritis.

Autoimmune Gastritis. This form of gastritis accounts for less than 10% of cases of chronic gastritis. It results from the presence of autoantibodies to components of gastric gland parietal cells, including antibodies against the acid-producing enzyme H^+,K^+-ATPase,[27] gastrin receptor, and intrinsic factor. Gland destruction and mucosal atrophy lead to loss of acid production. In the most severe cases, production of intrinsic factor is lost, leading to pernicious anemia. This uncommon form of gastritis is seen in association with other autoimmune disorders such as Hashimoto thyroiditis, Addison disease, and type 1 diabetes. Patients with autoimmune gastritis have a significant risk for developing gastric carcinoma and endocrine tumors (carcinoid tumor).

Morphology. Chronic gastritis may affect different regions of the stomach and exhibit varying degrees of mucosal damage.[19] Autoimmune gastritis is characterized by diffuse mucosal damage of the body-fundic mucosa, with less intense to absent antral damage, probably due to the autoantibodies against parietal cells. Gastritis in the setting of environmental etiologies (including infection by *H. pylori*) tends to affect antral mucosa or both antral and body-fundic mucosa (pangastritis). The mucosa is usually reddened and has a coarser texture than normal. The inflammatory infiltrate may create a mucosa with thickened rugal folds, mimicking early infiltrative lesions. Alternatively, with long-standing atrophic disease, the mucosa may become thinned and flattened. Irrespective of cause or location, the histologic changes are similar. An inflammatory infiltrate of lymphocytes and plasma cells is present within the lamina propria (Fig. 17–14). **"Active" inflammation is signified by the presence of neutrophils within the glandular and surface epithelial layer.** Active inflammation may be prominent or absent. Lymphoid aggregates, some with germinal centers, are frequently observed within the mucosa. Several additional histologic features are characteristic:

- ***Regenerative Change.*** A proliferative response to the epithelial injury is a constant feature of chronic gastritis. In the neck region of the gastric glands mitotic figures are increased. Epithelial cells of the

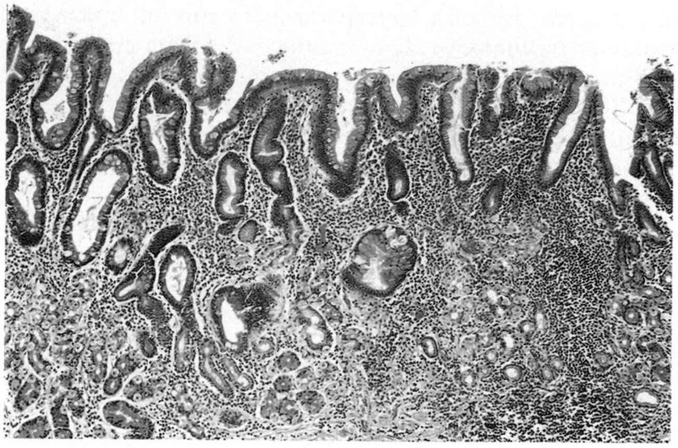

FIGURE 17–14 Chronic gastritis, showing partial replacement of the gastric mucosal epithelium by intestinal metaplasia (upper left) and inflammation of the lamina propria (right) containing lymphocytes and plasma cells.

surface mucosa, and to a lesser extent the glands, exhibit enlarged, hyperchromatic nuclei and a higher nuclear–cytoplasmic ratio. Mucus vacuoles are diminished or absent in the superficial cells. When regenerative changes are severe, particularly with ongoing active inflammation, distinguishing regenerative change from dysplasia may be difficult.

- ***Metaplasia.*** The antral, body, and fundic mucosa may become partially replaced by metaplastic columnar absorptive cells and goblet cells of intestinal morphology **(intestinal metaplasia),** both along the surface epithelium and in rudimentary glands. Occasionally, villus-like projections may appear. Although small intestinal features predominate, in some instances, features of colonic epithelium may be present.
- ***Atrophy.*** Atrophic change is evident by marked loss in glandular structures. **Atrophy is quite frequently associated with autoimmune gastritis and pangastritis caused by *H. pylori*.** Parietal cells, in particular, may be conspicuously absent in the autoimmune form. Persisting glands frequently undergo cystic dilatation. A particular feature of atrophic gastritis of autoimmune origin or chronic gastritis treated by inhibitors of acid secretion is hyperplasia of gastrin-producing G-cells in the antral mucosa. This is attributed to the hypochlorhydria or achlorhydria arising from severe parietal cell loss. The G-cell hyperplasia is responsible for the increased gastrinemia, which stimulates hyperplasia of enterochromaffin-like cells in the gastric body. As will be discussed later, the ECL cell hyperplasia is the frequent background for gastric carcinoid tumor formation.
- ***Dysplasia.*** With long-standing chronic gastritis, the epithelium develops cytologic alterations, including variation in size, shape, and orientation of epithelial cells, and nuclear enlargement and atypia. Intestinal metaplasia may precede the development of dysplasia. Dysplastic alterations may become so severe as to constitute in situ carcinoma. The development of dysplasia is thought to be a precursor lesion of gastric cancer in atrophic forms of gastritis, particularly in association with pernicious anemia (autoimmune gastritis) and *H. pylori*-associated chronic gastritis.

In those individuals infected by *H. pylori,* the organism lies in the superficial mucus layer and among the microvilli of epithelial cells. The distribution of organisms can be very patchy and irregular, with areas of heavy colonization adjacent to those with no organisms. In extreme cases, the organisms carpet the luminal surfaces of surface epithelial cells, the mucous neck cells, and the epithelial cells lining the gastric pits; they do not invade the mucosa. This is most easily demonstrated with silver stains (Fig. 17–15), although organisms can be seen on Giemsa- and routine H & E-stained tissue. Even in heavily colonized stomachs, **the organisms are absent from areas with intestinal metaplasia.** Conversely, organisms may be present in foci of pyloric metaplasia in an inflamed duodenum and in the gastric-type mucosa of Barrett esophagus.

Clinical Features. Chronic gastritis usually causes few symptoms. Nausea, vomiting, and upper abdominal discomfort may occur. Individuals with advanced gastritis from *H. pylori* or other environmental causes are often hypochlorhydric, owing to parietal cell damage and atrophy of body and fundic mucosa. However, since parietal cells are never completely destroyed, these patients do not develop achlorhydria or pernicious anemia. Serum gastrin levels are usually within the normal range or only modestly elevated.

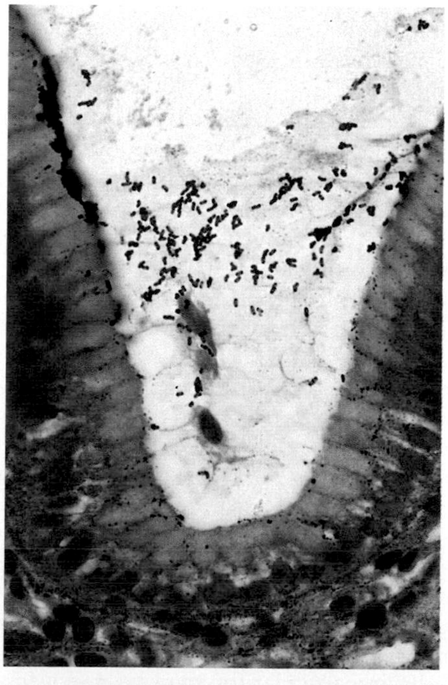

FIGURE 17–15 *Helicobacter pylori.* A Steiner silver stain demonstrates the numerous darkly stained *Helicobacter* organisms along the luminal surface of the gastric epithelial cells. Note that there is no tissue invasion by bacteria.

When severe parietal cell loss occurs in the setting of autoimmune gastritis, hypochlorhydria or achlorhydria and hypergastrinemia are characteristically present. Circulating autoantibodies to a diverse array of parietal cell antigens may be detected. A small subset of these patients (10%) may develop overt pernicious anemia after a period of years. The familial occurrence of pernicious anemia is well established; a high prevalence of gastric autoantibodies is also found in asymptomatic relatives of patients with pernicious anemia. The distribution suggests that the inheritance of autoimmune gastritis is autosomal dominant.

Most important is the relationship of chronic gastritis to the development of peptic ulcer and gastric carcinoma. Most patients with a peptic ulcer, whether duodenal or gastric, have *H. pylori* infection. *H. pylori* is thought to contribute to the pathogenesis of both gastric carcinoma and lymphoma. The long-term risk of gastric cancer in patients with autoimmune gastritis is 2% to 4%, which is considerably greater than that of the normal population.

SPECIAL FORMS OF GASTRITIS

Eosinophilic gastritis is an idiopathic condition that features a prominent eosinophilic infiltrate of the mucosa, muscle wall, or all layers of the stomach, usually in the antral or pyloric region. This disorder typically affects middle-aged women, and the primary symptom is abdominal pain, although swelling of the pylorus may produce gastric outlet obstruction. It may occur in association with *eosinophilic enteritis* and is often accompanied by a peripheral eosinophilia. Steroid therapy is usually effective.

Allergic gastroenteropathy is a disorder of children that may produce symptoms of diarrhea, vomiting, and growth failure. An infiltrate of eosinophils limited to the mucosa can usually be demonstrated in antral biopsies.

Lymphocytic gastritis is a condition in which lymphocytes densely populate the epithelial layer of the mucosal surface and gastric pits and suffuse the lamina propria. The intraepithelial lymphocytes are exclusively T lymphocytes, mostly CD8+ cells. The gastritis is generally restricted to the body of the stomach. This condition produces indistinct symptoms such as abdominal pain, anorexia, nausea, and vomiting. Although idiopathic in nature, 45% to 60% of cases are associated with celiac disease. Therefore, an immune-mediated pathogenesis is most likely.

Granulomatous gastritis. The presence of intramucosal epithelioid granulomas can usually be attributed to Crohn disease, sarcoidosis, infection (tuberculosis, histoplasmosis, anisakiasis), a systemic vasculitis, or as a reaction to foreign materials. *Granulomatous gastritis* is the term reserved for patients without these concurrent conditions. This idiopathic disorder is clinically benign. The predominant pathologic finding is narrowing and rigidity of the gastric antrum due to transmural granulomatous inflammation.

Graft-versus-Host Disease. Gastritis associated with GVHD can be encountered in the setting of bone marrow transplantation. Histologically, there is a relatively mild lymphocytic infiltrate in the lamina propria and apoptosis of glandular epithelial cells, in particular the mucous neck cells.

Reactive gastropathy is a group of disorders that exhibit characteristic mucosal histologic changes (Fig. 17–16) that may include: foveolar hyperplasia with loss of mucin and glandular regenerative changes, mucosal edema and dilation of mucosal capillaries, and smooth muscle fibers extending into the lamina propria between the glands. The key to the definition is the absence of active (neutrophilic) inflammation of the epithelium. Reactive gastropathy is fairly common. The etiology is related to chemical injury from cyclooxygenase inhibition (aspirin and NSAIDs) or bile reflux, and from mucosal trauma resulting from prolapse. In particular, gastric antral trauma or prolapse induce a characteristic lesion referred to as *gastric antral vascular ectasia*. Endoscopy shows longitudinal stripes of edematous erythematous mucosa alternating with less severely injured mucosa *(watermelon stomach)*. Histologically, the antral mucosa exhibits reactive gastropathy and dilated capillaries containing fibrin thrombi.

Peptic Ulcer Disease

Ulcers are defined histologically as a breach in the mucosa of the alimentary tract that extends through the muscularis mucosa into the submucosa or deeper. Although they may occur anywhere in the alimentary tract, none are as prevalent as the peptic ulcers that occur in the duodenum and stomach. Acute gastric ulcers may also appear under conditions of severe systemic stress or ingestion of NSAIDs. Ulcers are to be distinguished from *erosions,* in which there is epithelial disruption within the mucosa but no breach of the muscularis mucosa.

PEPTIC ULCERS

Peptic ulcers are chronic, most often solitary, lesions that occur in any portion of the gastrointestinal tract exposed to the aggressive action of acid/peptic juices. Peptic ulcers are usually solitary lesions less than 4 cm in diameter, located in the following sites, in order of decreasing frequency:[28]

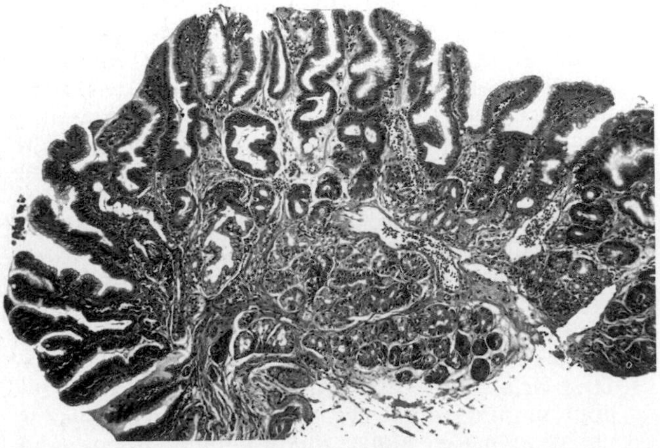

FIGURE 17–16 Reactive gastropathy. Gastric mucosa, showing hyperplasia of foveolar surface epithelial cells, glandular regenerative changes, and smooth muscle fibers extending into lamina propria.

- Duodenum, first portion
- Stomach, usually antrum
- At the gastroesophageal junction, in the setting of gastroesophageal reflux or Barrett esophagus
- Within the margins of a gastrojejunostomy
- In the duodenum, stomach, and/or jejunum of patients with Zollinger-Ellison syndrome
- Within or adjacent to an ileal Meckel diverticulum that contains ectopic gastric mucosa.

Epidemiology. In the United States, approximately 4 million people have peptic ulcers (duodenal and gastric), and 350,000 new cases are diagnosed each year. Around 180,000 patients are hospitalized yearly, and about 5000 people die each year as a result of peptic ulcer disease.[28] The lifetime likelihood of developing a peptic ulcer is about 10% for American males and 4% for females.

Peptic ulcers are relapsing lesions that are most often diagnosed in middle-aged to older adults, but they may first become evident in young adult life. They often appear without obvious precipitating conditions and may then, after a period of weeks to months of active disease, heal with or without therapy. *Even with healing, however, the tendency to develop peptic ulcers remains, in part because of recurrent infections with H. pylori.* Although it is difficult to obtain estimates of the prevalence of active disease, autopsy studies and population surveys indicate a prevalence of 6% to 14% for men and 2% to 6% for women. The male-to-female ratio for duodenal ulcers is about 3:1, and for gastric ulcers about 1.5 to 2:1. Women are most often affected at or after menopause. For unknown reasons, there has been a significant decrease in the prevalence of duodenal ulcers over the past decades but little change in the prevalence of gastric ulcers.

Pathogenesis. *Peptic ulcers are produced by an imbalance between gastroduodenal mucosal defense mechanisms and the damaging forces,[29] particularly gastric acid and pepsin* (Fig. 17–17). However, hyperacidity is not a prerequisite, as only a minority of patients with duodenal ulcers has hyperacidity, and it is even less common in those with gastric ulcers. Rather, gastric ulceration occurs when mucosal defenses fail, as when mucosal blood flow drops, gastric emptying is delayed, or epithelial restitution is impaired.

H. pylori infection is a major factor in the pathogenesis of peptic ulcer. It is present in virtually all patients with duodenal ulcers and in about 70% of those with gastric ulcers. Furthermore, antibiotic treatment of *H. pylori* infection promotes healing of ulcers and tends to prevent their recurrence. Hence, much interest is focused on the possible mechanisms by which this tiny spiral organism tips the balance of mucosal defenses. Some likely possibilities include:

- *Although H. pylori* does not invade the tissues, it induces an intense inflammatory and immune response. There is increased production of pro-inflammatory cytokines such as interleukin (IL)-1, IL-6, tumor necrosis factor (TNF), and, most notably, IL-8. This cytokine is produced by the mucosal epithelial cells, and it recruits and activates neutrophils.
- Several bacterial gene products are involved in causing epithelial cell injury and induction of inflammation. *H.*

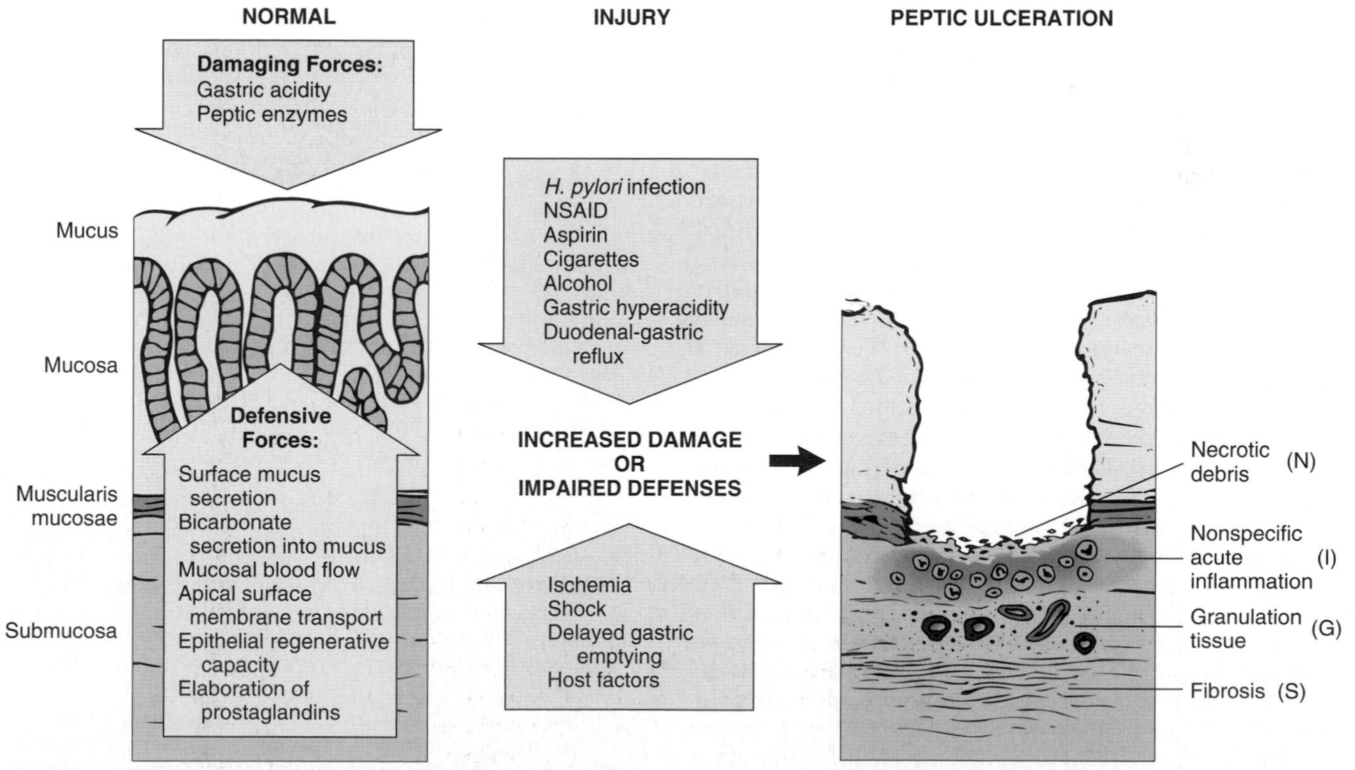

FIGURE 17–17 Diagram of causes of, and defense mechanisms against, peptic ulceration. Diagram of the base of a nonperforated peptic ulcer, demonstrating the layers of necrosis (N), inflammation (I), granulation tissue (G), and scar (S), moving from the luminal surface at the top to the muscle wall at the bottom.

pylori secretes a urease that breaks down urea to form toxic compounds such as ammonium chloride and monochloramine. The organisms also elaborate phospholipases that damage surface epithelial cells. Bacterial proteases and phospholipases break down the glycoprotein-lipid complexes in the gastric mucus, thus weakening the first line of mucosal defense.

- *H. pylori* enhances gastric acid secretion and impairs duodenal bicarbonate production, thus reducing luminal pH in the duodenum. This altered milieu seems to favor gastric metaplasia (the presence of gastric epithelium) in the first part of the duodenum. Such metaplastic foci provide areas for *H. pylori* colonization.
- Several *H. pylori* proteins are immunogenic, and they evoke a robust immune response in the mucosa. Both activated T cells and B cells can be seen in chronic gastritis caused by *H. pylori*. The B lymphocytes aggregate to form follicles. The role of T and B cells in causing epithelial injury is not established, but T-cell–driven activation of B cells may be involved in the pathogenesis of gastric lymphomas.
- Thrombotic occlusion of surface capillaries is promoted by a bacterial platelet-activating factor.
- Other antigens (including lipopolysaccharide) recruit inflammatory cells to the mucosa. The chronically inflamed mucosa is more susceptible to acid injury.
- Damage to the mucosa is thought to permit leakage of tissue nutrients into the surface microenvironment, thereby sustaining the bacillus.

With the unraveling of the *H. pylori* genome, the basis of the pathogenicity of this organism is beginning to be understood.[22,30] Over 80% of patients with duodenal ulcers are infected by strains that are cytotoxin-associated antigen (CagA) positive. This antigen elicits a strong serologic response, but more importantly it is a marker for the *Cag* pathogenicity island, a 37 kb DNA fragment that encodes 29 genes, some of which are involved in the pro-inflammatory and tissue damaging effects of *H. pylori*. In keeping with this, infection with *Cag* positive strains is associated with greater number of organisms in the tissue, more severe epithelial damage, greater acute and chronic inflammation, higher likelihood of peptic ulceration and an increased risk for gastric cancer (discussed later). One of the important genes regulated by CagA is the *vacuolating toxin* (VacA); the CagA gene is essential for the expression of VacA. This toxin causes cell injury (characterized by vacuole formation) in vitro and gastric tissue damage in vivo. VacA also behaves as a passive urea transporter thereby increasing the permeability of the epithelium to urea. As discussed above, urea is broken down into toxic intermediates by bacterial urease.

Only 10% to 20% of individuals worldwide infected with *H. pylori* actually develop peptic ulcer. Why most infected persons are spared and some are susceptible remains an enigma. Perhaps there are unknown interactions between *H. pylori* and the mucosa that occur only in some individuals. Another perplexing observation is that in patients with duodenal ulcer, the actual infection by *H. pylori* is limited to the stomach. Increased acid production by *H. pylori* infection seems to play a role. Suffice it to say that while the link between *H. pylori* infection and gastric and duodenal ulcers is well established, the interactions leading to ulceration remain to be defined.

Other events may act alone or in concert with *H. pylori* to promote peptic ulceration. Gastric hyperacidity, when present, may be strongly ulcerogenic. *Hyperacidity* may arise from increased parietal cell mass, increased sensitivity to secretory stimuli, increased basal acid secretory drive, or impaired inhibition of stimulatory mechanisms such as gastrin release. The classic example is *Zollinger-Ellison syndrome,* in which there are multiple peptic ulcerations in the stomach, duodenum, and even jejunum, owing to excess gastrin secretion by a tumor and, hence, excess gastric acid production.

Chronic use of NSAIDs suppresses mucosal prostaglandin synthesis; aspirin also is a direct irritant. *Cigarette smoking* impairs mucosal blood flow and healing. *Alcohol* has not been proved to directly cause peptic ulceration, but alcoholic cirrhosis is associated with an increased incidence of peptic ulcers. *Corticosteroids* in high dose and with repeated use promote ulcer formation. *In some patients with duodenal ulcers, there is too-rapid gastric emptying, exposing the duodenal mucosa to an excessive acid load.* Duodenal ulcer also is more frequent in patients with alcoholic cirrhosis, chronic obstructive pulmonary disease, chronic renal failure, and hyperparathyroidism. In the latter two conditions, hypercalcemia stimulates gastrin production and therefore acid secretion. Genetic influences appear to play no major role in peptic ulceration. Finally, there are compelling arguments that *personality* and *psychological stress* are important contributing factors, even though hard data on cause and effect are lacking. Indeed, we might develop ulcers by trying to fathom their cause(s).

Morphology. At least 98% of peptic ulcers are located in the first portion of the duodenum or in the stomach, in a ratio of about 4:1. Most duodenal ulcers occur within a few centimeters of the pyloric ring. The anterior wall of the duodenum is affected more often than the posterior wall. Gastric ulcers are predominantly located along the lesser curvature, in or around the border zone between the oxyntic mucosa and the antral mucosa. Less commonly, gastric ulcers may occur on the anterior or posterior walls, or along the greater curvature. Although the great majority of individuals have a single ulcer, in 10% to 20% of patients with gastric ulceration there may be a coexistent duodenal ulcer.

Wherever they occur, chronic peptic ulcers have a fairly standard, virtually diagnostic gross appearance (Fig. 17–18). Small lesions (<0.3 cm) are most likely to be shallow erosions; those over 0.6 cm are likely to be ulcers. Although over 50% of peptic ulcers have a diameter less than 2 cm, about 10% of benign ulcers are greater than 4 cm. Since carcinomatous ulcers may be less than 4 cm in diameter and may be located anywhere in the stomach, **size and location do not differentiate a benign from a malignant ulcer.**

The classic peptic ulcer is a round to oval, sharply punched-out defect with relatively straight walls. The mucosal margin may overhang the base slightly, particularly on the upstream portion of the circumference. The margins are usually level with the surrounding mucosa or only slightly elevated. Heaping-up of these margins is rare in the benign ulcer but is characteristic of the malignant lesion. The depth of these ulcers varies, from superficial lesions involving only the mucosa and muscularis mucosa to

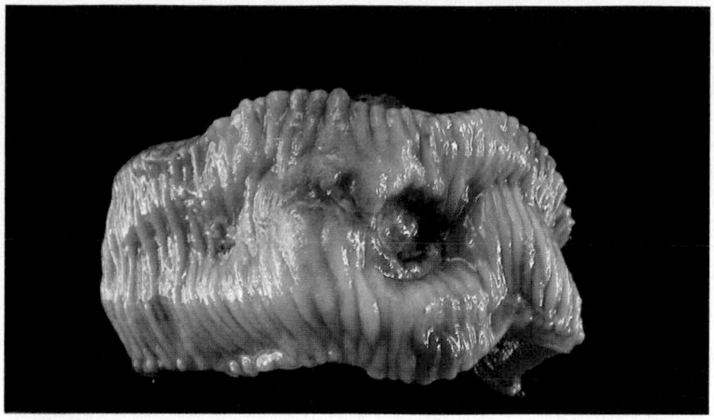

FIGURE 17–18 Peptic ulcer of the duodenum. Note that the ulcer is small (2 cm) with a sharply punched-out appearance. Unlike cancerous ulcers, the margins are not elevated. The ulcer base is clean. (Courtesy of Robin Foss, University of Florida, Gainesville, FL.)

deeply excavated ulcers having their bases on the muscularis propria. When the entire wall is penetrated, the base of the ulcer may be formed by adherent pancreas, omental fat, or liver. Free perforation into the peritoneal cavity may occur.

The base of a peptic ulcer is smooth and clean, owing to peptic digestion of any exudate that may form. At times, thrombosed or even patent blood vessels (the source of life-threatening hemorrhage) are evident in the base of the ulcer. Scarring may involve the entire thickness of the stomach; puckering of the surrounding mucosa creates mucosal folds that radiate from the crater in spokelike fashion. The gastric mucosa surrounding a gastric ulcer is somewhat edematous and reddened, owing to the almost invariable gastritis.

The histologic appearance varies from active necrosis, to chronic inflammation and scarring, to healing (see Fig. 2–26, Chapter 2). In active ulcers with ongoing necrosis, four zones are demonstrable: (1) the base and margins have a superficial thin layer of necrotic fibrinoid debris not visible to the naked eye; (2) beneath this layer is a zone of non-specific inflammatory infiltrate, with neutrophils predominating; (3) in the deeper layers, especially in the base of the ulcer, there is active granulation tissue infiltrated with mononuclear leukocytes; and (4) the granulation tissue rests on a more solid fibrous or collagenous scar. Vessel walls within the scarred area are typically thickened by the surrounding inflammation and are occasionally thrombosed.

Chronic gastritis is virtually universal among patients with peptic ulcer disease, occurring in 85% to 100% of patients with duodenal ulcers and in 65% with gastric ulcers. *H. pylori* infection is almost always demonstrable in patients with gastritis. Gastritis remains after the ulcer has healed; recurrence of the ulcer does not appear to be related to progression of the gastritis. This feature is helpful in distinguishing peptic ulcers from acute erosive gastritis or stress ulcers, since the adjacent mucosa is generally normal in the latter two conditions.

Clinical Features. The great majority of peptic ulcers cause epigastric gnawing, burning, or aching pain. A significant minority first comes to light with complications such as iron-deficiency anemia, frank hemorrhage, or perforation. The pain tends to be worse at night and occurs usually 1 to 3 hours after meals during the day. Classically, the pain is relieved by alkalis or food, but there are many exceptions. Nausea, vomiting, bloating, belching, and significant weight loss (raising the possibility of some hidden malignancy) are additional manifestations. With penetrating ulcers, the pain is occasionally referred to the back, the left upper quadrant, or chest. This type of pain may be misinterpreted as being of cardiac origin.

Peptic ulcers are notoriously chronic, recurring lesions. They more often impair the quality of life than shorten it. When untreated, it takes an average of 15 years for healing a duodenal or gastric ulcer. With present-day therapies aimed at neutralization of gastric acid, promotion of mucus secretion, inhibition of acid secretion (H_2 receptor antagonists and parietal cell H^+,K^+-ATPase pump inhibitors), and eradication of *H. pylori* infection, most ulcers heal within a few weeks, and victims usually escape the surgeon's knife.

The complications of peptic ulcer disease are listed in Table 17–3. Malignant transformation does not occur with duodenal ulcers and is extremely rare with gastric ulcers. When it occurs, it is always possible that a seemingly benign lesion was, from the outset, a deceptive ulcerative gastric carcinoma.

ACUTE GASTRIC ULCERATION

Focal, acutely developing gastric mucosal defects are a well-known complication of therapy with NSAIDs. Alternatively, they may appear following severe physiologic stress, whatever its nature—hence the term *stress ulcers.* Generally, there are multiple lesions located mainly in the stomach and occasionally in the duodenum. They range in depth from mere shedding of the superficial epithelium *(erosion)* to deeper lesions that involve the entire mucosal thickness *(ulceration).* The shallow erosions are, in essence, an extension of acute erosive gastritis. The deeper lesions comprise well-defined ulcerations, but they are not precursors of chronic peptic ulcers.

Stress erosions and ulcers are most commonly encountered in patients with shock, extensive burns, sepsis, or severe trauma; in any intracranial injury that raises intracranial pressure; and following intracranial surgery. Those occurring in the proximal duodenum and associated with severe burns or trauma are called *Curling ulcers.* Gastric, duodenal, and esophageal ulcers arising in patients with intracranial injury, operations, or

TABLE 17–3 Complications of Peptic Ulcer Disease

Bleeding
• Occurs in 15% to 20% of patients
• Most frequent complication
• May be life-threatening
• Accounts for 25% of ulcer deaths
• May be the first indication of an ulcer
Perforation
• Occurs in about 5% of patients
• Accounts for two thirds of ulcer deaths
• Rarely, is the first indication of an ulcer
Obstruction from edema or scarring
• Occurs in about 2% of patients
• Most often due to pyloric channel ulcers
• May also occur with duodenal ulcers
• Causes incapacitating, crampy abdominal pain
• Rarely, may lead to total obstruction with intractable vomiting

tumors are designated *Cushing ulcers* and carry a high incidence of perforation.

The genesis of the acute mucosal defects in these varied clinical settings is poorly understood. No doubt, many factors are shared with acute gastritis, such as impaired oxygenation. NSAID-induced ulcers are related to decreased prostaglandin production from the inhibition of cyclooxygenase. In the case of lesions associated with intracranial injury, the proposed mechanism involves the direct stimulation of vagal nuclei by increased intracranial pressure, leading to hypersecretion of gastric acid, which is common in these patients. Systemic acidosis, a frequent finding in these clinical settings, may contribute to mucosal injury by lowering the intracellular pH of mucosal cells. These cells are also hypoxic as a consequence of stress-induced splanchnic vasoconstriction.

Morphology. Acute stress ulcers are usually less than 1 cm in diameter and are circular and small. The ulcer base is frequently stained a dark brown by the acid digestion of extruded blood (Fig. 17–19). Unlike chronic peptic ulcers, acute stress ulcers are found anywhere in the stomach, the gastric rugal pattern is essentially normal and the margins and base of the ulcers are not indurated. While they may occur singly, more often there are multiple stress ulcers throughout the stomach and duodenum. Microscopically, acute stress ulcers are abrupt lesions, with essentially unremarkable adjacent mucosa. Depending on the duration of the ulceration, there may be a suffusion of blood into the mucosa and submucosa and some inflammatory reaction. Conspicuously absent are scarring and thickening of blood vessels, as seen in chronic peptic ulcers. Healing with complete re-epithelialization occurs after the causative factors are removed. The time required for complete healing varies from days to several weeks.

Clinical Features. Most critically ill patients admitted to hospital intensive care units develop histologic evidence of gastric mucosal damage. Bleeding from superficial gastric erosions or ulcers sufficient to require transfusion develops in 1% to 4% of these patients. Although prophylactic H_2-receptor antagonists and proton pump inhibitors may blunt the impact of stress ulceration, *the single most important determinant of clinical outcome is the ability to correct the underlying condition(s).* The gastric mucosa can recover completely if the patients do not succumb to their primary disease.

Miscellaneous Conditions

Gastric dilation may arise from gastric outlet obstruction (e.g., pyloric stenosis) or from the functional atony of the stomach and intestines (paralytic ileus) that may develop in patients with generalized peritonitis. The stomach may contain as much as 10 to 15 L of fluid; on rare occasion, *gastric rupture* may occur. This is a calamitous event followed rapidly by shock or death if not treated immediately. Rarely, spontaneous gastric perforation may occur in the newborn, during labor and delivery, severe vomiting, or cardiopulmonary resuscitation, and following ingestion of extreme amounts of carbonated beverages.

The stomach has the dubious privilege of being the major site for formation of luminal concretions of indigestible ingested material. *Phytobezoars* are derived from plant material, including fibers, leaves, roots, and skins of almost any plant matter. *Trichobezoars*, better known as "hairballs," consist of ingested hair within a mucoid coat containing decaying foodstuff (Fig. 17–20). The dysmotility following partial gastrectomy or partial gastric outlet obstruction is conducive to bezoar formation from more conventional ingested food. Bizarre bezoars have developed among partakers of illicit pharmaceuticals, glue swallowers, and children or patients with neuropsychiatric disorders, who have been known to ingest pins, nails, razor blades, coins, gloves, and even leather wallets.

HYPERTROPHIC GASTROPATHY

This designation includes a group of uncommon conditions, all characterized by giant cerebriform enlargement of the rugal folds of the gastric mucosa (Fig. 17–21). The rugal enlargement is caused by hyperplasia of the mucosal epithelial cells, without inflammation. Three variants are recognized:

- *Ménétrier disease,* resulting from profound hyperplasia of the surface mucous cells with accompanying glandular atrophy

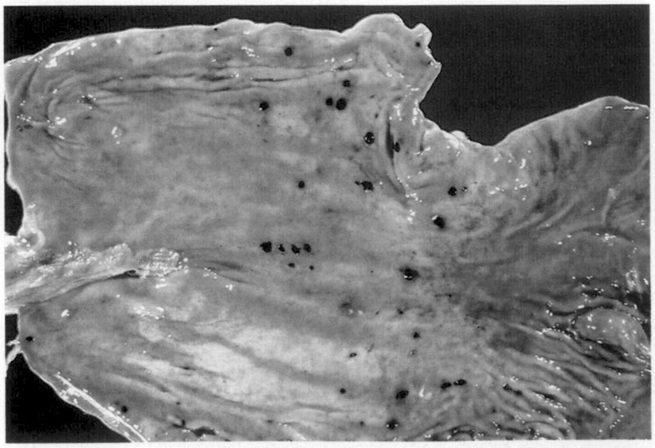

FIGURE 17–19 Multiple stress ulcers of the stomach, highlighted by dark digested blood on their surfaces.

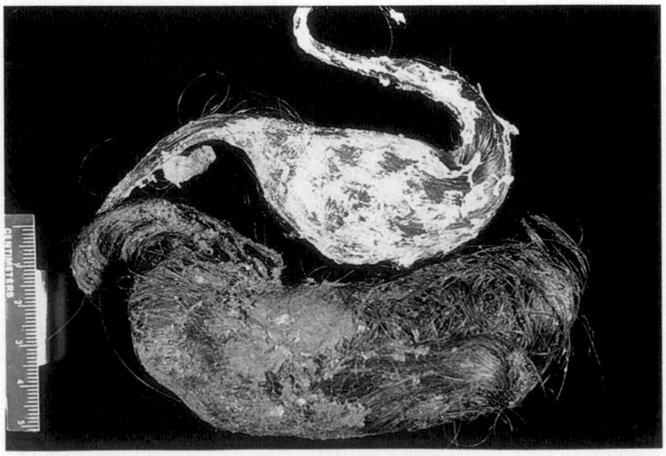

FIGURE 17–20 Trichobezoar, showing agglomeration of hair, food, and mucus that occurred within the gastric lumen.

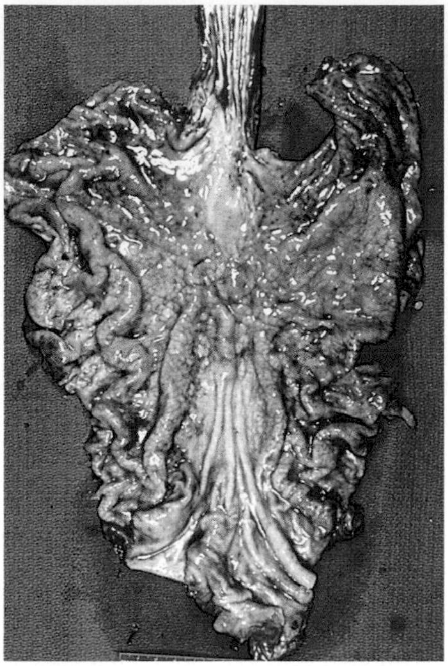

FIGURE 17–21 Hypertrophic gastropathy, showing markedly thickened gastric folds.

- *Hypertrophic-hypersecretory gastropathy,* associated with hyperplasia of the parietal and chief cells within gastric glands
- *Gastric gland hyperplasia secondary to excessive gastrin secretion,* in the setting of a gastrinoma *(Zollinger-Ellison syndrome).*

All three conditions are of clinical importance for two reasons: (1) *they may mimic infiltrative carcinoma or lymphoma of the stomach on endoscopic and radiographic examinations;* and (2) the enormous increase in acid secretions in hypertrophic-hypersecretory gastropathy and Zollinger-Ellison syndrome places patients at risk for peptic ulceration. A pure form of parietal cell hypertrophy, without hyperacidity, may occur in long-term takers of acid secretion inhibitors. Cessation of therapy may cause a transient rebound of excess acid secretion.

Ménétrier disease is most often encountered in males (male : female ratio 3 : 1) in the fourth to sixth decade of life but occasionally is seen in children. The etiology of this disease is unknown, but a role has been suggested for growth factor overexpression in superficial gastric epithelium. Transgenic mice with transforming growth factor-α (TGF-α) expressed in the stomach exhibit a disorder clinically and histologically similar to human Ménétrier disease. Although the disorder may be asymptomatic, it often produces epigastric discomfort, diarrhea, weight loss, and sometimes bleeding related to superficial rugal erosions. The hypertrophic change may predominantly involve the body-fundus or antrum or may affect the entire stomach. The gastric secretions contain excessive mucus and in many instances little to no hydrochloric acid due to glandular atrophy. In some patients, there may be sufficient protein loss in the gastric secretions to produce hypoalbuminemia and peripheral edema, thus constituting a form of *protein-losing gastroenteropathy.* Infrequently, the mucosal hyperplasia becomes metaplastic, providing a soil for the development of gastric carcinoma.

GASTRIC VARICES

Gastric varices develop in the setting of portal hypertension but less often than esophageal varices. Most gastric varices lie within 2 to 3 cm of the gastroesophageal junction, arising from longitudinally placed submucosal veins. They often appear as masslike nodular and tortuous winding elevations of the mucosa in the cardia or fundus. Due to their deep submucosal or subserosal location and the normal color of the overlying mucosa, it may be difficult to distinguish varices from enlarged rugae or even malignancy. Since they rarely occur in the absence of esophageal varices, diagnosis can usually be made without resorting to a potentially disastrous biopsy.

Tumors

As in the esophagus and intestines, tumors arising from the mucosa predominate over mesenchymal and stromal tumors. These can be classified as benign and malignant lesions.

BENIGN TUMORS

In the alimentary tract, the term polyp is applied to any nodule or mass that projects above the level of the surrounding mucosa. Use of the term is generally restricted to mass lesions arising in the mucosa, although occasionally a submucosal lipoma or leiomyoma may protrude, generating a polypoid lesion. The mucosal polyps are classified as non-neoplastic or neoplastic. Gastric polyps are uncommon.[31] Although they are usually found incidentally, dyspepsia or anemia resulting from blood loss may prompt the search for a gastrointestinal lesion.

Morphology. The great majority of gastric polyps (up to 90%) are **non-neoplastic** and appear to be of a **hyperplastic** nature. These polyps are composed of a variable mixture of hyperplastic surface epithelium (foveolar epithelium) and cystically dilated glandular tissue, with a lamina propria containing increased inflammatory cells and smooth muscle (Fig. 17–22). The surface epithelium may be regenerative in response to surface erosion and inflammation, but true dysplasia is not present. Most hyperplastic polyps are small and sessile and are commonly located in the antrum; some may approach several centimeters in diameter and have an apparent stalk. In about 20% to 25% of cases multiple polyps, sometimes more than twenty, are observed.

The adenoma of the stomach constitutes 5% to 10% of the polypoid lesions in the stomach. **By definition, an adenoma contains proliferative dysplastic epithelium and thereby has malignant potential.** Adenomatous polyps are much more common in the colon, and they are described in considerable detail in the discussion of the colon. Gastric adenomas may be **sessile** (without a stalk) or **pedunculated** (stalked). The most common location is the antrum. These lesions are usually single, and may grow up to 3 to 4 cm in size before detection (Fig. 17–23). In contrast to the colon, adenomatous change in the stomach may cover a large region of flat gastric mucosa without forming a mass lesion.

Other specific types of gastric polyps are relatively uncommon. Among these are **fundic gland polyps,**

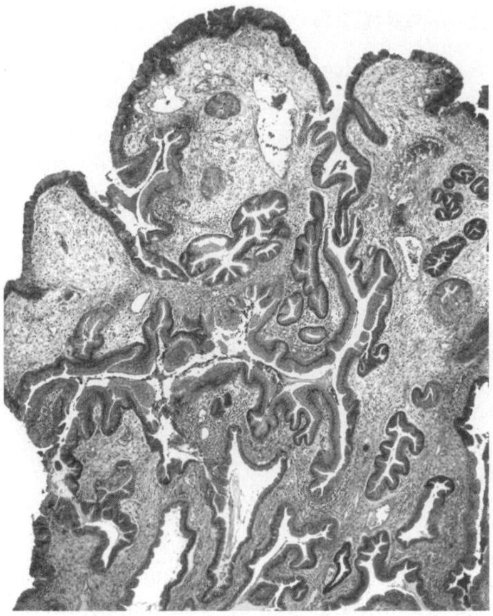

FIGURE 17–22 Gastric hyperplastic polyp. Low-power microscopic view of the polyp showing hyperplastic foveolar epithelium and inflammation.

hamartomatous **Peutz-Jeghers polyps,** and **juvenile polyps.** The fundic gland polyp is an innocuous cystic dilation of glands in the oxyntic mucosa. These polyps usually occur sporadically, but they can occur in the syndrome of familial adenomatous polyposis (FAP, described later). Curiously, sporadic fundic gland polyps also exhibit mutations in β-catenin with high frequency.[32] The hamartomatous polyps may occur in isolation, but gastric Peutz-Jeghers polyps are most commonly seen as part of the Peutz-Jeghers syndrome, and gastric juvenile polyps as part of the juvenile polyposis syndrome. All of these conditions will be discussed later.

The **inflammatory fibroid polyp (eosinophilic granuloma)** is a striking lesion in that it is a bulky submucosal growth composed of inflamed vascularized fibromuscular tissue with a prominent eosinophilic infiltrate and a tenuous mucosa stretched over the surface (Fig. 17–24). These polyps may occur anywhere in the alimentary tract but are found most frequently in the distal stomach. As they protrude into the lumen, they may occlude the pyloric channel and present abruptly as acute gastric outlet obstruction. Their origin is unknown. Whether these are inflammatory or neoplastic lesions is still debatable.

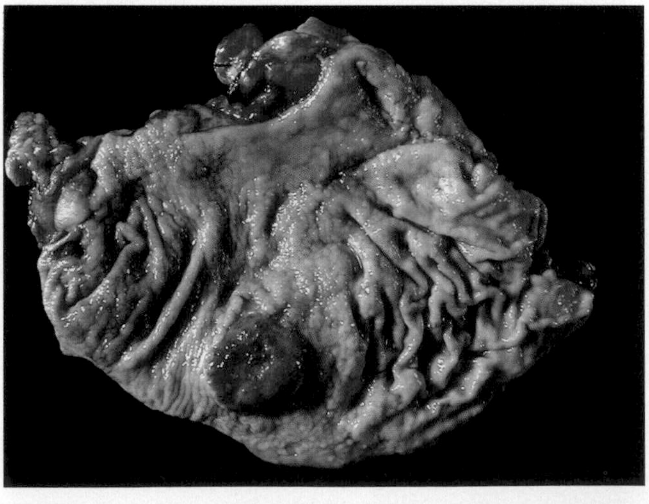

FIGURE 17–23 Gastric adenoma. Gross photograph showing a large polyp in the stomach.

Clinical Features. Hyperplastic polyps are seen most frequently in the setting of chronic gastritis. They are regarded as having no malignant potential as such but are nevertheless found in about 20% of stomachs resected for carcinoma. This is attributed to the tendency of chronically inflamed gastric mucosa both to form hyperplastic polyps and to develop into malignancy.

As with the colonic counterpart, the incidence of gastric adenomas increases with age, particularly into and beyond the seventh decade of life. The male-to-female ratio is 2:1. Up to 40% of gastric adenomas contain a focus of carcinoma at the time of diagnosis, particularly the larger lesions. The risk of cancer in the adjacent gastric mucosa may be as high as 30%. Unlike colonic adenomas, which usually arise from apparently normal mucosa, the usual substratum for gastric adenomas is chronic gastritis with intestinal metaplasia. Autoimmune gastritis can also lead to gastric adenoma formation.

Otherwise innocuous hyperplastic polyps may occasionally harbor foci of adenomatous epithelium. *As non-neoplastic and adenomatous polyps cannot reliably be distinguished endoscopically, histologic examination of gastric polyps is mandatory.*

GASTRIC CARCINOMA

Carcinoma is the most important and the most common (90% to 95%) of malignant tumors of the stomach. Next in order of frequency are lymphomas (4%), carcinoids (3%), and mesenchymal tumors (2%), which include gastrointestinal stromal tumors, leiomyosarcoma, and schwannoma.

Epidemiology. Gastric carcinoma is the second most common tumor in the world. Its incidence, however, varies widely, being particularly high in countries such as Japan, Chile, Costa Rica, Colombia, China, Portugal, Russia, and Bul-

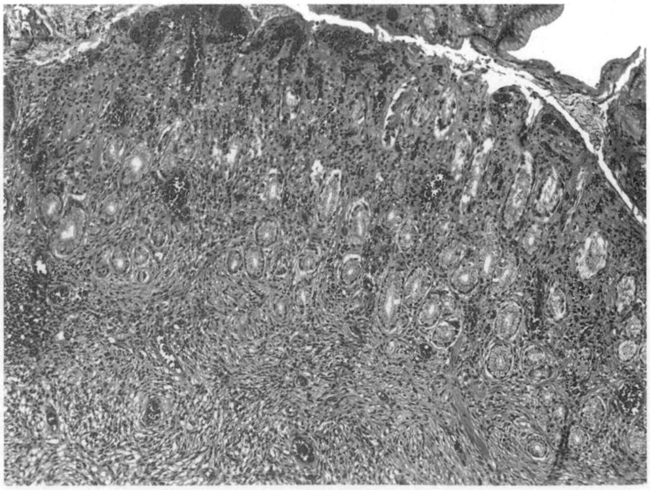

FIGURE 17–24 Inflammatory fibroid polyp; microscopic photograph showing submucosal growth of inflamed vascularized fibromuscular tissue with prominent eosinophilic infiltrate.

garia, and fourfold to sixfold less common in the United States, the United Kingdom, Canada, Australia, New Zealand, France, and Sweden. It is more common in lower socioeconomic groups and exhibits a male-to-female ratio of about 2:1. In most countries, there has been a steady decline in both the incidence and the mortality of gastric cancer over the past six decades. In 1930, gastric cancer was the most common cause of cancer death in the United States. Between 1930 and 1998, the annual mortality rate in the United States dropped from about 38 to 5 per 100,000 for men, and from 28 to 3 per 100,000 for women.[33] Yet it causes 2.5% of all cancer deaths in the United States and is the leading cause of cancer death worldwide. Although five-year survival rates have improved since the advent of endoscopy in the 1960s, they remain poor (about 20% in the United States).

There are several classification systems for gastric carcinoma. The most commonly used are the Laurén and the World Health Organization (WHO) classifications. In 1965, Laurén classified gastric carcinoma into two subtypes: those exhibiting an *intestinal* morphology with the formation of bulky tumors composed of glandular structures and those with *diffuse,* infiltrative growth of poorly differentiated discohesive malignant cells. *The intestinal and diffuse sub-types appear to have a different pathogenetic basis.* The intestinal type predominates in high-risk areas, and develops from precursor lesions. By contrast, the incidence of the diffuse type is relatively constant, and the tumors have no identifiable precursor lesions. The intestinal type exhibits a mean age of incidence of 55 years and a male-to-female ratio of 2:1. Diffuse gastric cancer occurs in slightly younger patients (mean age, 48), with an approximately equal male-to-female ratio. Although the intestinal type was far more common, the drop in incidence of gastric cancer has occurred only for this type. As a consequence, the incidence of intestinal and diffuse cancer is now approximately the same. The WHO classification system has been in use since 1977, is relatively simple, and has gained wide acceptance. It classifies the tumor based on histologic appearance alone (Table 17–4).

TABLE 17–4 WHO Histologic Classification of Gastric Tumors

Epithelial Tumors

Intraepithelial neoplasia: adenoma
Adenocarcinoma*
- Papillary adenocarcinoma
- Tubular adenocarcinoma
- Mucinous adenocarcinoma
- Signet-ring cell carcinoma
- Undifferentiated carcinoma
- Adenosquamous carcinoma

Small-cell carcinoma
Carcinoid tumor

Nonepithelial Tumors

Leiomyoma
Schwannoma
Granular cell tumor
Leiomyosarcoma
Gastrointestinal stromal tumor (GIST) (gradation from benign to malignant)
Kaposi sarcoma
Others

Malignant Lymphoma

*The Laurén classification subdivides adenocarcinomas into intestinal and diffuse types.

Pathogenesis. The major factors thought to affect the genesis of gastric cancer are summarized in Table 17–5. They apply more to the intestinal type, as the risk factors for diffuse gastric cancer are not as well defined.

Helicobacter pylori Infection. Chronic infection with *H. pylori* generally increases the risk for developing gastric carcinoma by five- to six-fold. The bacterial infection causes chronic gastritis, followed by atrophy, intestinal metaplasia, dysplasia, and carcinoma.[34] The sequential alterations depend on both the presence of bacterial proteins and the host immune response; the latter is influenced by the host genetic background. In particular, long-standing mucosal inflammation reduces acid secretion (hypochlorhydria) and pepsin secretion. This favors bacterial growth and perpetuation of chronic inflammation, sustained mucosal epithelial cell proliferation, and hence increased risk of genomic mutation. The increased oxidative stress further promotes DNA damage. *However, the vast majority of individuals infected with H. pylori will not develop cancer and not all H. pylori infections increase the risk of cancer.* Therefore, other factors must be involved in tumorigenesis. The risk for tumor development is greatly increased in patients in whom mucosal inflammation progresses to multifocal mucosal atrophy and intestinal metaplasia. Dysplasia of the gastric mucosa is the final common pathway by which intestinal-type gastric cancers develop. Adenomas containing mucosal dysplasia can also become malignant.

Environment. Environmental influences may be critical in gastric carcinogenesis.[35] When families migrate from high-risk to low-risk areas (or the reverse), successive generations acquire the level of risk that prevails in the new locales. The *diet*

TABLE 17–5 Factors Associated with Increased Incidence of Gastric Carcinoma

Environmental Factors

Infection by *H. pylori*
- Present in most cases of intestinal-type carcinoma

Diet
- Nitrites derived from nitrates (water, preserved food)
- Smoked and salted foods, pickled vegetables, chili peppers
- Lack of fresh fruit and vegetables

Low socioeconomic status

Cigarette smoking

Host Factors

Chronic gastritis
- Hypochlorhydria: favors colonization with *H. pylori*
- Intestinal metaplasia is a precursor lesion

Partial gastrectomy
- Favors reflux of bilious, alkaline intestinal fluid

Gastric adenomas
- 40% harbor cancer at time of diagnosis
- 30% have adjacent cancer at time of diagnosis

Barrett esophagus
- Increased risk of gastroesophageal junction tumors

Genetic Factors

Slightly increased risk with blood group A
Family history of gastric cancer
Hereditary nonpolyposis colon cancer syndrome
Familial gastric carcinoma syndrome (E-cadherin mutation)

is suspected to be a primary factor, and adherence to certain culinary practices is associated with a high risk of gastric carcinoma. Lack of refrigeration; consumption of preserved, smoked, cured, and salted foods; water contamination with nitrates; and lack of fresh fruit and vegetables are common themes in high-risk areas. The consumption of dietary carcinogens, such as N-nitroso compounds and benzopyrene, appears to be particularly important. Conversely, intake of green, leafy vegetables and citrus fruits, which contain antioxidants such as ascorbate (vitamin C), alpha-tocopherol (vitamin E), and beta-carotene, is negatively correlated with gastric cancer. A specific protective role for any one of these nutrients cannot be assumed, however, since intake of fresh food may simply displace consumption of preserved foods.

So far there is no conclusive evidence linking alcohol intake and cigarette smoking to the development of gastric cancer. Despite initial concern, *to date there appears to be no increased risk of stomach cancer from the use of antacid drug therapies.*

Host. *Autoimmune gastritis*, like *H. pylori* infection, increases the risk of gastric cancer, presumably due to chronic inflammation and intestinal metaplasia. It has been noted that blood group A patients have higher risk but it is not yet clear whether this is related to the binding of *H. pylori* to Lewis B antigen, or to other mechanisms.

Within the United States, blacks, Native Americans, and Hawaiians have a higher risk of developing gastric cancer. But since only about 8% to 10% of patients with gastric cancer have a family history of this disease, genetic factors are unlikely to be a major influence. Environmental factors mentioned above, are likely to play a major role in the higher incidence of gastric cancer among these various groups. Genetic traits play a critical role in some familial cases of gastric cancer, including gastric carcinoma occurring in the hereditary nonpolyposis colorectal cancer (HNPCC) syndrome. Recently, E-cadherin gene *(CDH1)* germ-line mutations have also been identified as the underlying genetic basis for another familial gastric cancer syndrome that is characterized by early occurrence of diffuse type adenocarcinoma.[36] These patients are also at risk for developing lobular breast cancer.[37]

Other Risk Factors. Peptic ulcer disease per se does not impart increased risk for development of gastric cancer. However, patients who have had *partial gastrectomies* for peptic ulcer disease have a slightly higher risk of gastric cancer in the residual gastric stump, attributed to the hypochlorhydria, bile reflux, and chronic gastritis that occur in the post-gastrectomy state. Ménétrier disease is also a risk factor for gastric carcinoma.

Multiple genetic alterations have been described in gastric cancers, mostly in studies involving intestinal-type cancers. Among these are allelic losses in various chromosomal loci, and microsatellite instability in several genes including *TGFβRII, BAX* and *IGFRII*.[36–38] Moreover, *p53* mutations are present in a majority of tumors, and abnormalities in E-cadherin expression are quite frequent. Nevertheless, it has not been possible so far to define a clear sequence of events in gastric tumorigenesis. It appears that intestinal and diffuse gastric cancers may develop through different genetic pathways.

Morphology. The location of gastric carcinomas within the stomach is as follows: pylorus and antrum, 50% to 60%; cardia, 25%; with the remainder in the body and fundus. The lesser curvature is involved in about 40% and the greater curvature in 12%. **Thus, a favored location is the lesser curvature of the antropyloric region.** Although less common, an ulcerative lesion on the greater curvature is more likely to be malignant.

Gastric carcinoma is classified on the basis of: (1) depth of invasion; (2) macroscopic growth pattern; and (3) histologic subtype. **The morphologic feature having the greatest impact on clinical outcome is the depth of invasion. Early gastric carcinoma is defined as a lesion confined to the mucosa and submucosa, regardless of the presence or absence of perigastric lymph node metastases.** Some early tumors cover large areas of the gastric mucosa (up to 10 cm in diameter) and yet show no invasion into the muscular wall. Early gastric carcinoma is not synonymous with carcinoma in situ, as the latter is confined to the surface epithelial layer. **Advanced gastric carcinoma is a neoplasm that has extended below the submucosa into the muscular wall** and has perhaps spread

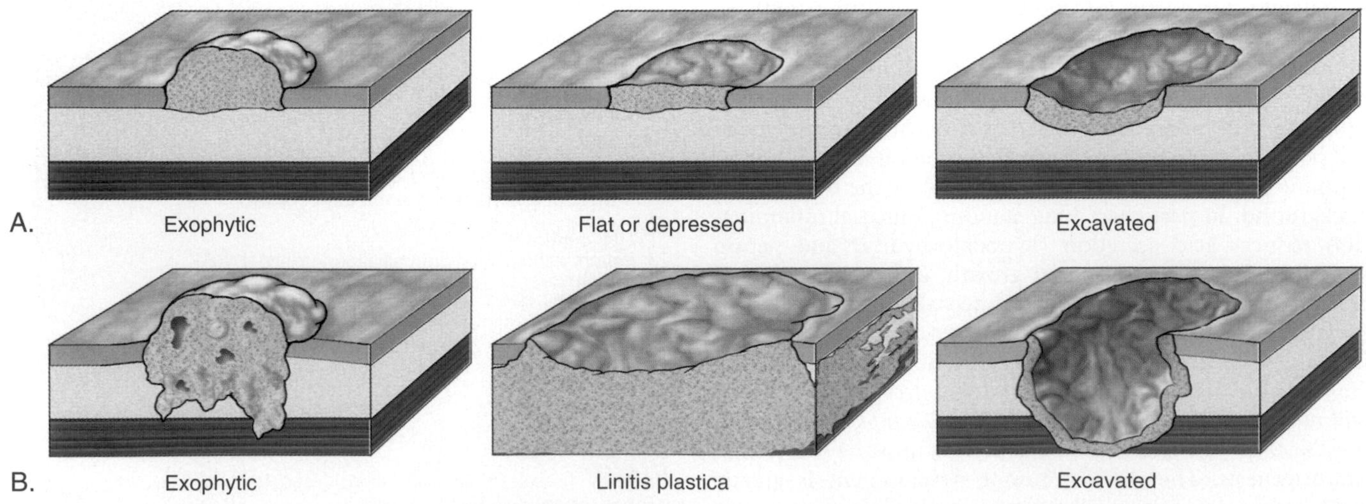

FIGURE 17–25 Diagram of growth patterns and spread of gastric carcinoma. In early gastric carcinoma (*A*), the tumor is confined to the mucosa and submucosa and may exhibit an exophytic, flat or depressed, or excavated conformation. Advanced gastric carcinoma (*B*) extends into the muscularis propria and beyond. Linitis plastica is an extreme form of flat or depressed advanced gastric carcinoma.

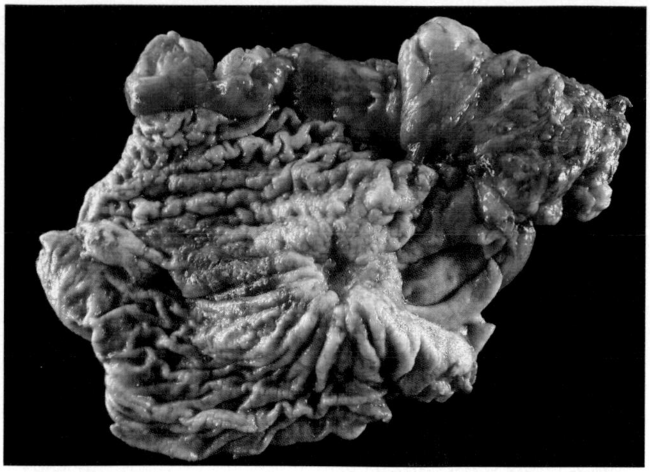

FIGURE 17–26 Gastric carcinoma. Gross photograph showing an ill-defined, excavated central ulcer surrounded by irregular, heaped-up borders.

more widely. All cancers presumably begin as "early" lesions, which develop over time into "advanced" lesions.

The three macroscopic growth patterns of gastric carcinoma, which may be evident at both the early and advanced stages, are: (1) **exophytic,** with protrusion of a tumor mass into the lumen; (2) **flat or depressed,** in which there is no obvious tumor mass within the mucosa; and (3) **excavated,** whereby a shallow or deeply erosive crater is present in the wall of the stomach (Fig. 17–25). Exophytic tumors are readily identified by radiographic techniques and at endoscopy and may contain portions of an adenoma. In contrast, flat or depressed malignancy may not be apparent to even the experienced eye, except as regional effacement of the normal surface mucosal pattern. Excavated cancers may closely mimic, in size and appearance, chronic peptic ulcers. In advanced cases, cancerous craters can be identified by their heaped-up, beaded margins and shaggy, necrotic bases, as well as by the overt neoplastic tissue extending into the surrounding mucosa and wall (Fig. 17–26).

Uncommonly, a broad region of the gastric wall or the entire stomach is extensively infiltrated by malignancy, creating a rigid, thickened "leather bottle," termed **linitis plastica.** Metastatic carcinoma, from the breast and lung, may generate a similar picture.

The histologic subtypes of gastric cancer have been variously subclassified, but the two most important types, as noted earlier, are the intestinal type and diffuse type of the Lauren classification (Fig. 17–27). The intestinal variant is composed of neoplastic intestinal glands resembling those of colonic adenocarcinoma (see Fig. 17–27*A*), which permeate the gastric wall but tend to grow along broad cohesive fronts in an "expanding" growth pattern. The neoplastic cells often contain apical mucin vacuoles, and abundant mucin may be present in gland lumens. The diffuse variant is composed of gastric-type mucous cells, which generally do not form glands, but rather permeate the mucosa and wall as scattered individual cells or small clusters in an "infiltrative" growth pattern. These cells appear to arise from the middle layer of the mucosa, and the presence of intestinal metaplasia is not a prerequisite. In this variant, mucin formation expands the malignant cells and pushes the nucleus to the periphery, creating a "signet ring" conformation (see Fig. 17–27*B*). If the signet-ring cells are more than 50% of the tumor, the tumor is classified as signet-ring cell carcinoma under the WHO classification. Regardless of cell type, the amount of mucin formation varies, and in poorly differentiated portions of the tumor it may be absent. Conversely, excessive mucin production may generate large mucinous lakes that dissect tissue planes; isolated tumor cells or glands may be difficult to identify in such areas. Infiltrative tumors often evoke a strong mural desmoplastic reaction, in which the scattered cells are embedded; the fibrosis creates local rigidity of the wall, which provides a valuable clue to the presence of an infiltrative lesion.

Whatever the classification and variant, all gastric carcinomas eventually penetrate the wall to involve the serosa and spread to regional and more distant lymph nodes. For obscure reasons, gastric carcinomas frequently metastasize to the supraclavicular sentinel (Virchow) node as the first clinical manifestation of an

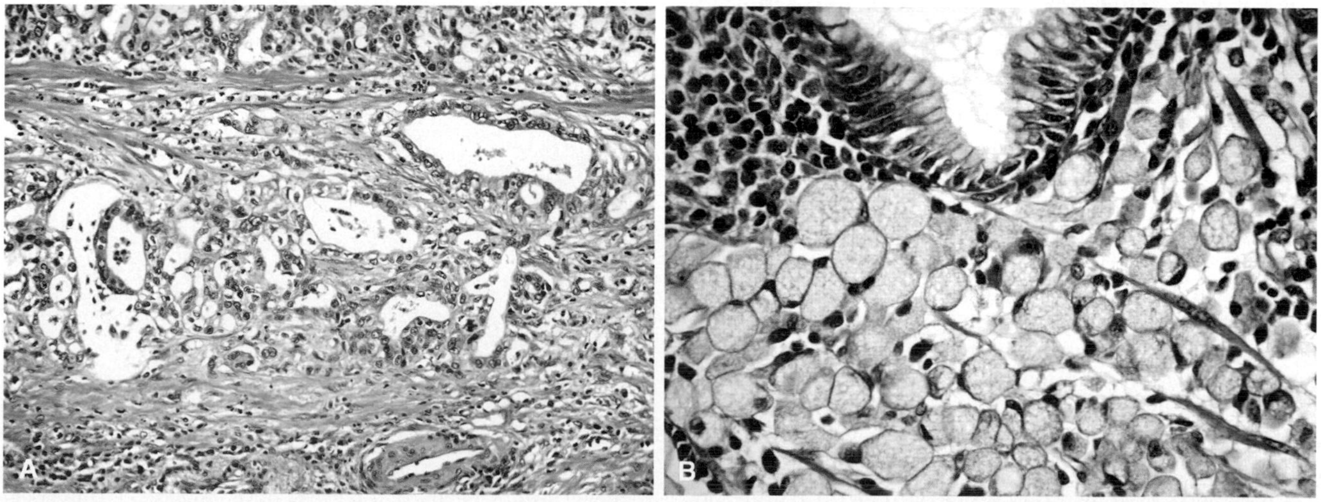

FIGURE 17–27 Gastric carcinoma. *A,* Intestinal type demonstrating gland formation by malignant cells, which are invading the muscular wall of the stomach. *B,* Diffuse type demonstrating signet-ring carcinoma cells.

occult neoplasm. The tumor can also metastasize to the periumbilical region to form a subcutaneous nodule. This nodule is called a **Sister Mary Joseph nodule,** after the nun who noted this lesion as a marker of metastatic carcinoma. Local invasion of gastric carcinoma into the duodenum, pancreas, and retroperitoneum also is characteristic. At the time of death, widespread peritoneal seeding and metastases to the liver and lungs are common. A notable site of visceral metastasis is to one or both ovaries. Although uncommon, metastatic adenocarcinoma to the ovaries (from stomach, breast, pancreas, and even gallbladder) is so distinctive as to be called **Krukenberg tumor.**

Clinical Features. Gastric carcinoma is an insidious disease that is generally asymptomatic until late in its course. The symptoms include weight loss, abdominal pain, anorexia, vomiting, altered bowel habits, and less frequently dysphagia, anemic symptoms, and hemorrhage. As these symptoms are essentially nonspecific, early detection of gastric cancer is difficult. The proportion of cancers diagnosed as early gastric carcinoma clearly depends on the intensity of the diagnostic effort to uncover asymptomatic disease. In Japan, where mass endoscopy screening programs are in place, early gastric cancer constitutes about 35% of all newly diagnosed gastric cancers. In Europe and the United States, this figure has remained at 10% to 15% over several decades.

The prognosis for gastric carcinoma depends primarily on the depth of invasion and the extent of nodal and distant metastasis at the time of diagnosis; histologic type has minimal independent prognostic significance. The prognostic value of biomarkers such as *p53* mutation and c-*ERB-B2* amplification remains to be determined. Clinical prognosis of gastric cancer largely depends on the depth of tumor invasion and the presence or absence of nodal or visceral metastasis. Surgical resection is still the standard treatment option, without or with adjuvant chemotherapy and radiation. The five-year survival rate of surgically treated early gastric cancer is 90% to 95%, with only a small negative increment if lymph node metastases are present. In contrast, the five-year survival rate for advanced gastric cancer remains below 15%.

LESS COMMON GASTRIC TUMORS

Gastric Lymphoma. Gastric lymphomas represent 5% of all gastric malignancies. However, the stomach is the most common site for extranodal lymphoma (20% of such cases). Nearly all gastric lymphomas are B-cell lymphomas of mucosa-associated lymphoid tissue (MALT lymphomas). Nodal-type lymphomas that may develop in the stomach are unrelated to MALT lymphomas and similar to lymphomas originating in lymph nodes (discussed in Chapter 14). While some gastric lymphomas appear to arise de novo, the majority (>80%) are associated with chronic gastritis and *H. pylori* infection. The role of *H. pylori* infection as an important etiologic factor for gastric lymphoma is supported by the elimination of about 50% of gastric lymphomas with antibiotic treatment for *H. pylori*. Tumors that do not regress with this type of treatment usually contain genetic abnormalities, particularly Trisomy 3 and t(11;18) translocation. This translocation brings together the *API2* (apoptosis-inhibitor 2) gene on chromosome 11 with the *MLT* (mutated in MALT lymphoma) gene on chromosome 18. The protein encoded by the fused genes is thought to inhibit apoptosis, but its precise contribution to the development of MALT lymphoma remains to be established.

Morphology. Gastric lymphoma commonly occurs in the mucosa or superficial submucosa. In the MALT lymphoma, a monomorphic lymphocytic infiltrate of the lamina propria surrounds gastric glands massively infiltrated with atypical lymphocytes and undergoing destruction (the "lymphoid epithelioid" lesion; Fig. 17–28). These gut-type lymphomas are usually CD5, CD10, and CD23 negative. In contrast, nodal-type lymphomas exhibit features characteristic of lymphomas arising de novo in lymph nodes, with frequently positive immunoreactivity for CD5, GYCLIN D1, CD10, or BCL-2. Rarely, Burkitt lymphoma, AIDS-associated lymphoma, and Hodgkin lymphoma may occur in the stomach.

Gastrointestinal Stromal Tumor. A wide variety of mesenchymal neoplasms may arise in the stomach. Those originating in nerve sheaths are known as schwannomas. All of these tumors are rare. Much more common are gastrointestinal stromal tumors, also called GISTs. It is thought that GISTs originate from the interstitial cells of Cajal, which control gastrointestinal peristalsis. These tumors have a special phenotype in that 95% of them stain with antibodies against c-KIT, and approximately 70% stain for CD34. Despite these phenotypic similarities, GISTs show different histological patterns, and can be sub-classified into spindle and epithelioid types. Tumors that show features of enteric plexus differentiation (called gastrointestinal autonomic nerve tumors or GANTs) are often classified among GISTs. On rare occasions, gastric GISTs occur as part of a tumor syndrome, such as *Carney's triad* (gastric GIST, paraganglioma and pulmonary chondroma), or neurofibromatosis type 1.

Morphology. GISTs can be solitary or multiple. The tumor can protrude into the lumen with an overlying attenuated mucosa or extrude on the serosal side of

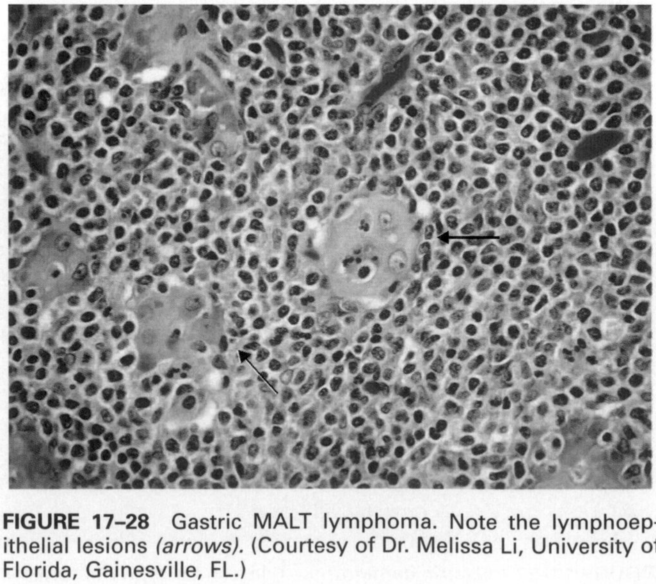

FIGURE 17–28 Gastric MALT lymphoma. Note the lymphoepithelial lesions *(arrows)*. (Courtesy of Dr. Melissa Li, University of Florida, Gainesville, FL.)

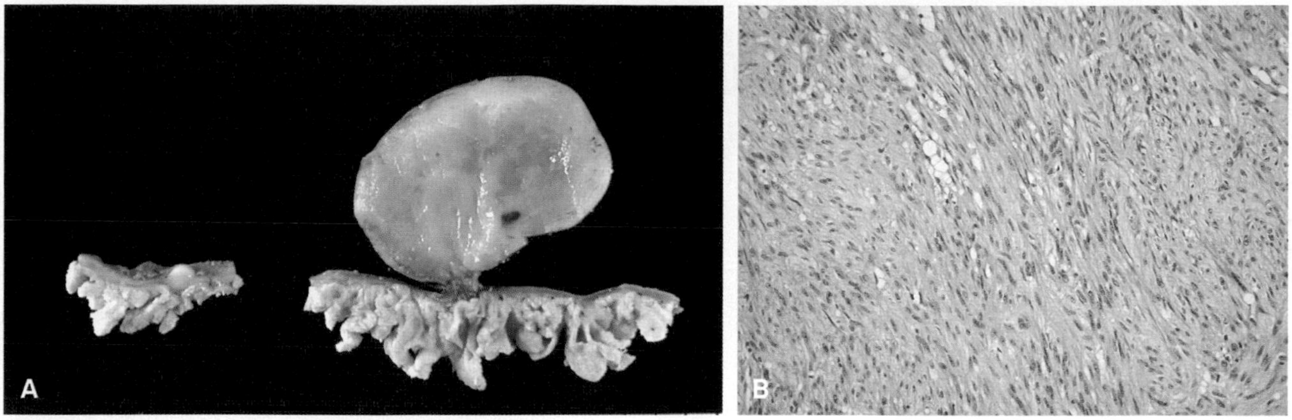

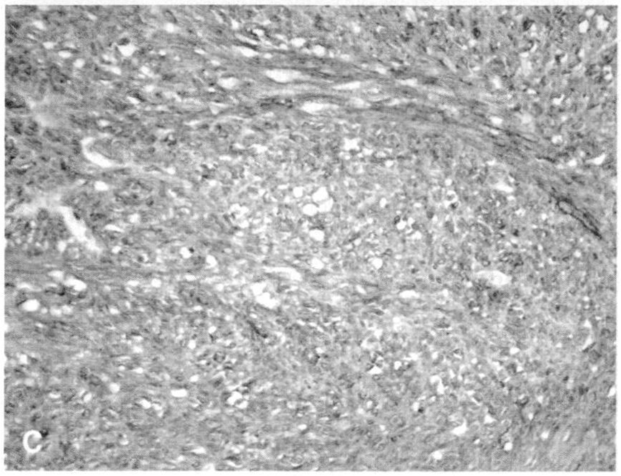

FIGURE 17–29 Gastrointestinal stromal tumor. *A,* Gross photograph of the tumor arising from the muscularis propria of the gastric wall. *B,* Microscopic view of the tumor showing spindle cell feature. *C,* Immunohistochemical stain showing the tumor cell c-*KIT* positivity.

the gastric wall (Fig. 17–29*A*). The cut surface of the tumor is tan and usually lacks the whirling smooth muscle pattern of leiomyomas or leiomyosarcomas. It varies from slightly firm to soft, and hemorrhagic changes are common. Necrosis or cystic changes can be seen in a large tumor. Microscopically, the tumor can exhibit spindle cells (Fig. 17–29*B*), plump "epithelioid" cells, or a mixture of both. Most of the tumors are quite cellular, and mitotic activity is variable. **The majority of the tumor cells are positive for c-KIT (CD117),** as demonstrated by positive immunohistochemical staining (Fig. 17–29*C*).

Pathogenesis. The identification of c-*KIT* mutations and platelet-derived growth factor receptor-α *(PDGFRA)* mutations in these tumors constitute significant progress in understanding the pathogenesis of GISTs.[39,40] c-KIT is the receptor for stem cell factor, and PDGFRA is a receptor for platelet-derived growth factor (PDGF). It is known that 85% of GISTs have *c-KIT* mutations and 35% of GISTs with normal *c-KIT* contain *PDGFRA* mutations.[41] Both c-KIT and PDGFRA have cytoplasmic tyrosine kinases that activate similar intracellular pathways. The mutations lead to constitutive activation of the tyrosine kinase signaling pathway, promoting cell proliferation and inhibiting apoptosis. *c-KIT* mutations and *PDGFRA* mutations appear to be mutually exclusive.

Based on these pathogenic insights, a newly designed tyrosine kinase inhibitor (STI571) has been shown to be effective against this tumor.[42] Recall that this drug is used to treat chronic myeloid leukemia, also associated with abnormal tyrosine kinase activity (Chapter 14). Currently, STI571 is widely used as an agent to treat GISTs; this demonstrates the application of a targeted therapeutic approach to the treatment of human malignancies.

Gastric Neuroendocrine Cell (Carcinoid) Tumors. Most gastric carcinoid tumors originate from the ECL cells in the oxyntic mucosa. The tumor can arise in the setting of chronic atrophic gastritis or multiple endocrine neoplasia type 1 (MEN1) and Zollinger-Ellison syndrome. The underlying pathogenesis is probably related to the *hypergastrinemic state,* resulting in *ECL cell hyperplasia,* a presumed pretumorous condition. Less common is the sporadic gastric carcinoid without a hypergastrinemic state, for which the pathogenesis is not known. Gastric carcinoid tumors exhibit similar histologic features to other carcinoid tumors. The clinical course is quite variable. To date, there are no reliable pathologic markers to predict the tumor behavior.

Lipomas. Lipomas are a benign neoplasm of adipose tissue, usually present in the submucosa.

Metastatic Cancer. Metastatic involvement of the stomach is unusual. The most common sources of gastric metastases are systemic lymphomas. Metastases of malignant melanoma and carcinomas tend to be multiple and may develop central ulceration. Breast and lung carcinoma may mimic diffuse gastric carcinoma by diffusely infiltrating the gastric wall to generate *linitis plastica,* as described earlier for primary gastric carcinoma.

SMALL AND LARGE INTESTINES

Normal

Anatomy

The *small intestine* in the human adult is approximately 6 meters in length, and the *colon* (large intestine) approximately 1.5 meters. The first 25 cm of the small intestine, the duodenum, are retroperitoneal; the jejunum marks the entry of the small intestine into the peritoneal cavity, terminating where the ileum enters the colon at the ileocecal valve. The demarcation between jejunum and ileum is not clearly defined; the jejunum arbitrarily constitutes the proximal third of the intraperitoneal portion and the ileum the remainder. The colon is subdivided into the cecum and the ascending, transverse, and descending colon. The sigmoid colon begins at the pelvic brim and loops within the peritoneal cavity, becoming the rectum at about the level of the third sacral vertebra. Halfway along its 15-cm length, the rectum passes between the crura of the peroneal muscles to become extraperitoneal. The reflection of the peritoneum from the rectum over the pelvic floor creates a cul de sac known as the *pouch of Douglas.*

Vasculature

The arterial supply of the intestine, from the proximal jejunum to the hepatic flexure of the colon, is derived from the superior mesenteric artery. The inferior mesenteric artery feeds the remainder of the colon to the level of the rectum. Each artery progressively divides as it approaches the gut, with rich arterial interconnections via arching mesenteric arcades. Numerous collaterals connect the mesenteric circulation with the celiac arterial axis proximally and the pudendal circulation distally. The lymphatic drainage essentially parallels the vascular supply but does not have the intricate patterns of arcades.

The upper rectum is supplied by the superior hemorrhoidal branch of the inferior mesenteric artery. The lower portion receives its blood supply from the hemorrhoidal branches of the internal iliac or internal pudendal artery. The venous drainage follows essentially the same distribution and is connected by an anastomotic capillary bed between the superior and inferior hemorrhoidal veins, providing a connection between the portal and systemic venous systems. Since the colon is a retroperitoneal organ in the ascending and descending portions, it derives considerable accessory arterial blood supply and lymphatic drainage from a wide area of the posterior abdominal wall.

Small Intestinal Mucosa

The most distinctive feature of the small intestine is its mucosal lining, which is studded with innumerable *villi* (Fig. 17–30*A*). These extend into the lumen as finger-like projections covered by epithelial lining cells. The central core of lamina propria contains blood vessels, lymphatics, a minimal population of lymphocytes, eosinophils and mast cells, and scattered fibroblasts and vertically oriented smooth muscle cells. Between the bases of the villi are the pitlike crypts of Lieberkühn, which contain stem cells that replenish and regenerate the epithelium. The crypts extend down to the muscularis mucosa. The muscularis mucosa is a smooth, continuous sheet, serving to anchor the configuration of villi and

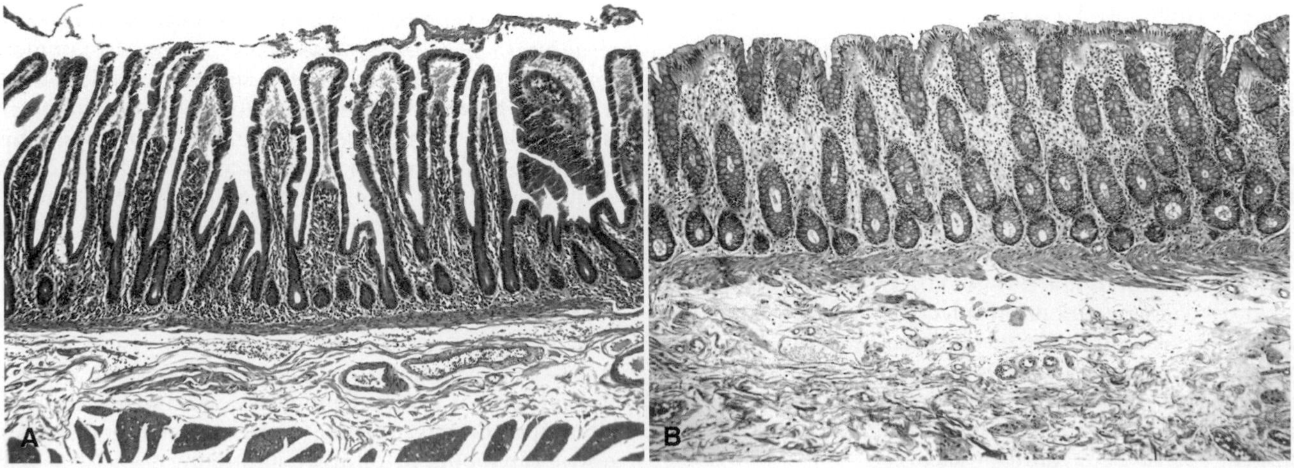

FIGURE 17–30 *A,* Normal small-bowel histology, showing mucosal villi and crypts, lined by columnar cells. *B,* Normal colon histology, showing flat mucosal surface and abundant vertically oriented crypts.

crypts alike. In normal individuals, the villus-to-crypt height ratio is about 4 to 5:1. Within the duodenum are abundant submucosal mucous glands, termed *Brunner glands.* These glands secrete bicarbonate ions, glycoproteins, and pepsinogen II and are virtually indistinguishable from the pyloric mucous glands.

The surface epithelium of the villi contains three cell types. *Columnar absorptive cells* are recognized by the dense array of *microvilli* on their luminal surface (the brush border) and the underlying mat of microfilaments (the terminal web). Interspersed regularly between the absorptive cells are mucin-secreting *goblet cells* and a few *endocrine cells,* described below. Within the crypts reside stem cells, goblet cells, more abundant endocrine cells, and scattered *Paneth cells.* Paneth cells have apically oriented bright eosinophilic granules containing a variety of antimicrobial proteins (such as *defensins*), which play a role in mucosal innate immunity against bacterial infection.[43]

The villi of the small intestinal mucosa are the site for terminal digestion and absorption of foodstuffs through the action of the columnar absorptive cells. The crypts secrete ions and water, deliver immunoglobulin A (IgA) and antimicrobial peptides to the lumen, and serve as the site for cell division and renewal. The mucous cells of both crypts and villi generate an adherent mucous coat, which both protects the surface epithelium and provides an ideal local milieu for uptake of nutrients. Specific receptors for uptake of macromolecules are also present on the surface epithelial cells, such as those in the ileum for intrinsic factor–vitamin B_{12} complexes.

Colonic Mucosa

The small intestine accomplishes its absorptive function with a highly liquid luminal stream. *The function of the colon is to reclaim luminal water and electrolytes.* Unlike the mucosa of the small intestine, *the colonic mucosa has no villi and is flat.* The mucosa is punctuated by numerous straight tubular crypts that extend down to the muscularis mucosa (Fig. 17–30*B*). The surface epithelium is composed of columnar absorptive cells, which have shorter and less abundant microvilli than found in the small intestine, and goblet mucous cells. The crypts contain abundant goblet cells, endocrine cells, and stem cells. Paneth cells are occasionally present at the base of crypts in the cecum and ascending colon. The intestinal mucosa, particularly in the ileum, is colonized by endogenous bacteria, particularly non-pathogenic strains of *E. coli* and organisms such as Proteus, Enterobacter, Serratia and Klebsiella. The components of the endogenous flora may be displaced by exogenous bacteria, such as pathogenic strains of *E. coli* that cause damage to the mucosa.

The regenerative capacity of the intestinal epithelium is remarkable. Cellular proliferation is confined to the crypts; differentiation and luminal migration serve to replenish superficial cells lost to senescence and surface abrasion. Within the small intestine, cells migrate out of the crypts and upward to the tips of the villi, where they are shed into the lumen. This journey normally takes between 96 and 144 hours, leading to normal renewal of the epithelial lining every 4 to 6 days. Turnover of the colonic surface epithelium takes 3 to 8 days. The rapid renewal of intestinal epithelium provides a remarkable capacity for repair but also renders the intestine particularly vulnerable to agents that interfere with cell replication, such as radiation and chemotherapy for cancer.

Endocrine Cells

A diverse population of *endocrine cells* is scattered among the epithelial cells lining the gastric glands, small intestinal villi, and small and large intestinal crypts. Comparable cells are present in the epithelia lining the pancreas, biliary tree, lung, thyroid, and urethra. As a population, gut endocrine cells exhibit characteristic morphologic features. In most cells, the cytoplasm contains abundant fine eosinophilic granules, which harbor secretory products. The main portion of the cell is at the base of the epithelium, and the nuclei reside on the luminal side of the cytoplasmic granules.

These cells exhibit a marked diversity of secretory peptides and distribution of cell subtypes. Secretory granules are released at the basal surface of the endocrine cell or along the basal part of its lateral surface; apical secretion (into the lumen) has not been observed. The various secretory products, some of which are also present in the mural autonomic neural plexus, act as chemical messengers and modulate normal digestive functions by a combination of endocrine, paracrine, and neurocrine mechanisms. Each endocrine cell type, therefore, exhibits a distribution tailored to meet the physiologic needs pertinent to a gut segment.

Intestinal Immune System

Humans are exposed to an enormous load of environmental antigens through the gastrointestinal tract. The surface area of the gastrointestinal tract through which ingested antigens may enter far exceeds that of the skin and pulmonary tract. The immune system must balance tolerance of harmless ingested substances against active defense reactions to potential microbial invaders. Dysfunction of this regulatory machinery may cause smoldering chronic disease and, occasionally, life-threatening acute conditions. Throughout the small intestine and colon are nodules of *lymphoid tissue,* which lie either within the mucosa or span the mucosa and a portion of the submucosa.[44] The lymphoid nodules distort the surface epithelium to produce broad domes rather than villi; within the ileum confluent lymphoid tissue becomes macroscopically visible as *Peyer patches.* The surface epithelium over lymphoid nodules contains both columnar absorptive cells and *M (membranous) cells,* the latter found only in small and large intestinal lymphoid sites. M cells are able to transcytose antigenic macromolecules intact from the lumen to antigen-presenting cells under the surface epithelium. Antigen-presenting cells include macrophages and dendritic cells. Throughout the intestines, T lymphocytes are scattered within the surface epithelium, usually at the basolateral aspects of the cell. These T cells are referred to as *intraepithelial lymphocytes* and include cytotoxic CD8+ cells. The lamina propria contains helper T cells (CD4+), activated B cells, and plasma cells. The lamina propria plasma cells secrete dimeric IgA, IgG, and IgM, which enter into the splanchnic circulation. IgA is transcytosed directly across enterocytes or across hepatocytes for secretion into bile; both are mechanisms for delivering IgA to the intestinal lumen. The intestinal lymphoid nodules, mucosal lymphocytes, and isolated lymphoid follicles in the appendix and mesenteric lymph nodes constitute the MALT, mentioned in the discussion of gastric tumors.

Neuromuscular Function

Small intestinal peristalsis, both *anterograde* and *retrograde,* mixes the food stream and promotes maximal contact of nutrients with the mucosa. Colonic peristalsis prolongs contact of the luminal contents with the mucosa. Although intestinal smooth muscle cells are capable of initiating contractions, *both small and large intestinal peristalsis is mediated by intrinsic (myenteric plexus) and extrinsic (autonomic innervation) neural control.* The myenteric plexus consists of two neural networks: *Meissner plexus* resides at the base of the submucosa, and *Auerbach plexus* lies between the inner circumferential and outer longitudinal muscle layers of the muscle wall; lesser neural twigs extend between smooth muscle cells and ramify within the submucosa.

Pathology

Many conditions, such as infections, inflammatory diseases, motility disorders, and tumors, affect both the small and large intestines. These two organs will therefore be considered together. Collectively, disorders of the intestines account for a large portion of human disease.

Congenital Anomalies

Rare anomalies of gut formation may occur.

- *Duplication* of the small intestine or colon, usually in the form of saccular to long, cystic structures
- *Malrotation* of the entire bowel, resulting from improper embryologic rotation of the gut
- *Omphalocele,* in which the abdominal musculature fails to form, leading to birth of an infant with herniation of abdominal contents into a ventral membranous sac
- *Gastroschisis,* in which a portion of the abdominal wall fails to form altogether, causing extrusion of the intestines.

The above lesions may be silent (malrotation) or catastrophic (gastroschisis). A far more common and innocuous lesion is *heterotopia* of normal pancreatic tissue but occasionally of gastric mucosa. Both heterotopias may occur anywhere in the intestine and usually are small, 1- to 2-cm nodules in the mucosa or intestinal wall.

ATRESIA AND STENOSIS

Congenital intestinal obstruction is an uncommon but dramatic lesion that may affect any level of the intestines. Duodenal atresia is most common; the jejunum and ileum are equally involved, but the colon is not involved. The obstruction may be complete *(atresia)* or incomplete *(stenosis).* Atresia may take the form of an imperforate mucosal diaphragm or a stringlike segment of bowel connecting intact proximal and distal intestine. Stenosis is less common and is due to a narrowed intestinal segment or a diaphragm with a narrow central opening. Single or multiple lesions appear to arise from developmental failure, intrauterine vascular accidents, or *intussusceptions* (telescoping of one intestinal segment within another) occurring after the intestine has developed. Failure of the cloacal diaphragm to rupture leads to an *imperforate anus.*

MECKEL DIVERTICULUM

Failure of involution of the vitelline duct, which connects the lumen of the developing gut to the yolk sac, produces a *Meckel diverticulum.* This solitary diverticulum lies on the antimesenteric side of the bowel, usually within 2 feet (85 cm) of the ileocecal valve (Fig. 17–31). *This is a true diverticulum, in that it contains all three layers of the normal bowel wall: mucosa, submucosa, and muscularis propria.* Meckel diverticula may take the form of only a small pouch, or of a blind segment having a lumen greater in diameter than that of the ileum and a length of up to 6 cm. Although the mucosal lining may be that of normal small intestine, *heterotopic rests of gastric mucosa or pancreatic tissue are found in about one half of these anomalies.* Meckel diverticula are present in an estimated 2% of the normal population, but most remain asymptomatic or are discovered incidentally. *When peptic ulceration occurs in the small intestinal mucosa adjacent to the gastric mucosa, intestinal bleeding or symptoms resembling those of an acute appendicitis may result.* Alternatively, presenting symptoms may be related to intussusception, incarceration, or perforation.

CONGENITAL AGANGLIONIC MEGACOLON—HIRSCHSPRUNG DISEASE

Hirschsprung disease is a congenital disorder characterized by aganglionosis of a portion of the intestinal tract. The enteric neuronal plexus develops from neural crest cells, which migrate into the bowel wall during development, mostly in a cephalad to caudad direction. Congenital megacolon, or

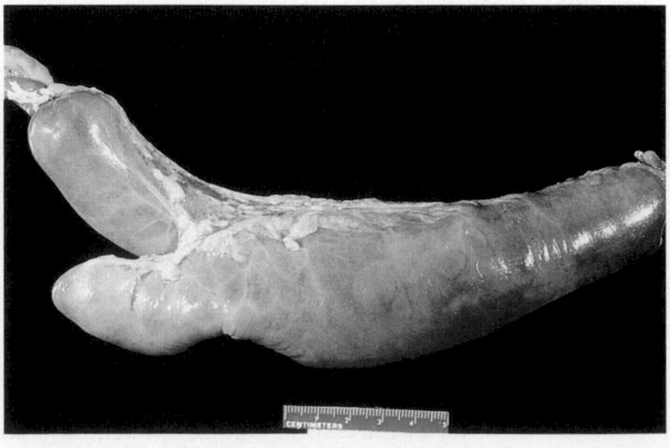

FIGURE 17–31 Meckel diverticulum. The blind pouch is located on the antimesenteric side of the small bowel.

Hirschsprung disease, results when the migration of neural crest cells arrests at some point before reaching the anus or when the ganglion cells undergo inappropriate premature death.[45] This produces an intestinal segment that lacks both Meissner submucosal and Auerbach myenteric plexuses. Depending on the severity of migration arrest, a variable length of the distal gut is not innervated. Loss of enteric neural coordination leads to functional obstruction and intestinal dilation proximal to the affected segment. Note that the dilated segment may contain normal ganglia; ganglia are absent or nearly so in the contracted region.

The cause of the developmental failure is unclear, but at least eight susceptibility genes have been identified. Mutations in these genes are associated with varying degrees of intestinal aganglionosis and other congenital anomalies. The phenotypic expression (penetrance) among these gene mutations varies. The long-segment and short-segment disease (see explanation under "Morphology") appear to have different modes of inheritance.[46–48] About 50% of familial cases and approximately 15% of sporadic cases are a consequence of mutations in the *RET* gene (Chapter 7) that inactivate the kinase activity of this receptor. A much smaller proportion of cases (3%–5%) may be caused by mutations in the endothelin/endothelin-receptor system. *RET* and its ligands (members of the Glial-Derived Neurotrophic Factor family) promote survival and growth of neurites, and provide direction to migrating neural crest cells. The endothelin system participates in the regulation of morphogenesis during embryonic development. Despite the identification of the involvement of these and other genes in Hirschprung disease pathogenesis, the genetic defect is unknown in a large number of cases.

Morphology. Hirschsprung disease is characterized by the absence of ganglion cells and ganglia in the muscle wall and submucosa of the affected segment. The rectum is always affected, with involvement of more proximal colon to variable extent. Most cases involve the rectum and sigmoid only (short-segment disease), with longer segments in a fifth of cases, and rarely the entire colon (long-segment disease). Absence of mural ganglion cells is sometimes accompanied by thickening and hypertrophy of nonmyelinated nerve fibers, representing ramifications of the lumbosacral preganglionic fibers. **Proximal to the aganglionic segment, the colon undergoes progressive dilation and hypertrophy, beginning with the descending colon. With time, the proximal innervated colon may become massively distended, sometimes achieving a diameter of 15 to 20 cm *(megacolon).*** When distention outruns the hypertrophy, the colonic wall becomes markedly thinned and may rupture, usually near the cecum. Mucosal inflammation or shallow, so-called **stercoral ulcers** may appear. Unequivocal diagnosis of Hirschsprung disease can be made histologically by the failure to detect ganglion cells in intestinal submucosa samples stained for acetylcholinesterase.

Clinical Features. Hirschsprung disease occurs in approximately 1 out of 5,000 live births and is present with increased frequency (3.6%) in siblings of index cases. Males predominate 4:1. Short-segment aganglionosis with megacolon is more common in males, whereas females predominate among patients with long affected segments. Ten percent of all cases of Hirschsprung disease occur in children with Down syndrome, and serious neurologic abnormalities are present in another 5%, raising the possibility that this disease is only one feature of more generalized abnormal development of the neural crest.[47,48]

Hirschsprung disease usually manifests itself in the immediate neonatal period by failure to pass meconium, followed by obstructive constipation. In those instances when only a few centimeters of the rectum are affected, the build-up of pressure may permit occasional passage of stools or even intermittent bouts of diarrhea. Abdominal distention develops if a sufficiently large segment of colon is involved. The major threats to life in this disorder are superimposed enterocolitis with fluid and electrolyte disturbances and perforation of the colon or appendix with peritonitis.

Acquired megacolon is a condition that may occur at any age and may result from: (1) *Chagas disease* (see Chapter 8), in which the trypanosomes directly invade the bowel wall to destroy the enteric plexuses; (2) organic obstruction of the bowel, by a neoplasm or inflammatory stricture; (3) *toxic megacolon* complicating ulcerative colitis or Crohn disease (see later); or (4) a functional psychosomatic disorder. Save for Chagas disease, where inflammatory involvement of the ganglia is evident, the remaining forms of megacolon are not associated with any deficiency of mural ganglia.

Enterocolitis

Diarrheal diseases of the bowel make up a veritable Augean stable of entities (a messy situation cleaned by the fifth task of Hercules). Many are caused by microbiologic agents; others arise in the setting of malabsorptive disorders and idiopathic inflammatory bowel disease. Consideration should first be given to the conditions known as *diarrhea* and *dysentery.*

DIARRHEA AND DYSENTERY

A healthy adult drinks 2 L of fluid per day, to which is added 1 L of saliva, 2 L of gastric juice, 1 L of bile, 2 L of pancreatic juice, and 1 L of intestinal secretions. Of these 9 L of fluid presented to the intestine, less than 200 gm of stool are excreted per day, of which 65% to 85% is water. Jejunal absorption of water amounts to 3 to 5 L/day, ileal absorption 2 to 4 L/day. The colon normally absorbs 1 to 2 L/day, but is capable of absorbing almost 6 L/day.

A precise definition of diarrhea is elusive, given the considerable variation in normal bowel habits. An increase in stool mass, stool frequency, and/or stool fluidity are perceived as diarrhea by most patients. For many individuals, this consists of daily stool production in excess of 250 gm, containing 70% to 95% water. However, over 14 L of fluid may be lost per day in severe cases of diarrhea (i.e., the equivalent of the circulating blood volume). Diarrhea is often accompanied by pain, urgency, perianal discomfort, and incontinence. Low-volume, painful, bloody diarrhea is known as *dysentery.*

The major causes of diarrhea are presented in Table 17–6. The principal mechanisms of diarrhea, one or more of which may be operative in any one patient, are as follows:

TABLE 17–6 Major Causes of Diarrheal Illnesses

Secretory Diarrhea
Infectious: viral damage to mucosal epithelium • Rotavirus • Caliciviruses • Enteric adenoviruses • Astroviruses
Infectious: enterotoxin mediated • *Vibrio cholerae* • *Escherichia coli* • *Bacillus cereus* • *Clostridium perfringens*
Neoplastic • Tumor elaboration of peptides, serotonin, prostaglandins • Villous adenoma in distal colon (nonhormone mediated)
Excess laxative use
Osmotic Diarrhea
Disaccharidase (lactase) deficiencies Lactulose therapy (for hepatic encephalopathy, constipation) Prescribed gut lavage for diagnostic procedures Antacids ($MgSO_4$ and other magnesium salts) Primary bile acid malabsorption
Exudative Diseases
Infectious: bacterial damage to mucosal epithelium • *Shigella* • *Salmonella* • *Campylobacter* • *Entamoeba histolytica*
Idiopathic inflammatory bowel disease
Typhlitis (neutropenic colitis in the immunosuppressed)
Malabsorption
Defective intraluminal digestion
Primary mucosal cell abnormalities
Reduced small intestinal surface area
Lymphatic obstruction
Infectious: impaired mucosal cell absorption • *Giardia lamblia* infection
Deranged Motility
Decreased intestinal transit time • Surgical reduction of gut length • Neural dysfunction, including irritable bowel syndrome • Hyperthyroidism • Diabetic neuropathy • Carcinoid syndrome
Decreased motility (increased intestinal transit time) • Small intestinal diverticula • Surgical creation of a "blind" intestinal loop • Bacterial overgrowth in the small intestine

- *Secretory diarrhea:* Net intestinal fluid secretion leads to the output of more than 500 mL of fluid stool per day, which is isotonic with plasma and persists during fasting.
- *Osmotic diarrhea:* Excessive osmotic forces exerted by luminal solutes lead to output of more than 500 mL of stool per day, which abates upon fasting. Stool exhibits an osmotic gap (stool osmolality exceeds plasma electrolyte concentration by ≥50 mOsm).
- *Exudative diseases:* Mucosal destruction leads to output of purulent, bloody stools that persist on fasting; stools are frequent but may be small or large volume.
- *Deranged motility:* Improper gut neuromuscular function may produce highly variable patterns of increased stool volume; other forms of diarrhea must be excluded.
- *Malabsorption:* Improper absorption of gut nutrients produces voluminous, bulky stools with increased osmolarity combined with excess stool fat (steatorrhea). The diarrhea usually abates on fasting.

INFECTIOUS ENTEROCOLITIS

Intestinal diseases of microbial origin are marked principally by diarrhea and sometimes ulcerative and inflammatory changes in the small and/or large intestine. *Infectious enterocolitis is a global problem of staggering proportions, causing more than 12,000 deaths per day among children in developing countries, and constituting one half of all deaths before age 5 worldwide.*[49] *Although far less prevalent in industrialized nations, these infections still have attack rates of one to two illnesses per person per year, second only to the common cold in frequency.* This results in an estimated 99 million acute cases of either vomiting or diarrhea per year in the United States, equivalent to 40% of the population. The infections are mainly associated with contaminated food and water.

Acute, self-limited infectious diarrhea, which is a major cause of morbidity among children, is most frequently caused by enteric viruses. In infants, infectious diarrhea may cause severe dehydration and metabolic acidosis, which may result in hospitalization in developed countries and death in developing countries. Bacterial infections, such as enterotoxigenic *Escherichia coli*, are also common offenders. However, *many pathogens can cause diarrhea*; the major offenders vary with the age, nutrition, immune status of the host, environment (living conditions, public health measures), and special predispositions, such as hospitalization, wartime dislocation, or foreign travel. In 40% to 50% of cases, the specific agent cannot be isolated.

Viral Gastroenteritis

Symptomatic human infection is caused by several distinct groups of viruses (Table 17–7). *Rotavirus* accounts for an estimated 140 million cases and 1 million deaths worldwide per year. The target population is children age 6 to 24 months, but young infants and debilitated adults are susceptible to symptomatic infection. This virus accounts for 25% to 65% of severe diarrhea in infants and young children.[50] Rotavirus is an encapsulated virus with a segmented double-stranded RNA genome. *Rotavirus selectively infects and destroys mature enterocytes in the small intestine, without infecting crypt cells.* The surface epithelium of the villus is repopulated by immature secretory cells. With the loss of absorptive function and excess of secretory cells, there is net secretion of water and electrolytes, compounded by an osmotic diarrhea from incompletely absorbed nutrients. The minimal infective inoculum is approximately 10 viral particles, whereas an individual with rotavirus gastroenteritis typically sheds up to 10^{12} particles/mL stool. Thus, outbreaks among pediatric populations in hospitals and day-care centers are very common. The clinical syndrome has an incubation period of approximately 2 days, which is followed by vomiting and watery diarrhea for several days. Viral infection can induce protective immunity, but the protection for reinfection is often short-lived. Antiro-

TABLE 17–7 Common Gastrointestinal Viruses

Virus	Genome	Size (nm)	% of U.S. Childhood Viral Enterocolitis	Host Age	Mode of Transmission	Prodrome/ Duration of Illness
Rotavirus (Group A)	dsRNA	70	60	6–24 months	Person-to-person, food, water	2 days/3–5 days
Caliciviruses Norwalk-like viruses Sapporo-like viruses	ssRNA	35–40	20	Child or adult	Person-to-person, water, cold foods, raw shellfish	1–3 days/4 days
Enteric adenoviruses	dsDNA	80	8	Child <2 years	Person-to-person	3–10 days/7+ days
Astroviruses	ssRNA	28	4	Child	Person-to-person, water, raw shellfish	24–36 hours/1–4 days

Data from Goodgame RW: Viral causes of diarrhea. Gastroenterol Clin North Am 30:779,2001.
ds, double-stranded; ss, single stranded.

tavirus antibodies are present in mother's milk, so rotavirus infection is most frequent at the time of weaning.

Among the numerous types of *adenovirus*, the subtypes (enteric serotypes) Ad40, Ad41, and Ad31 appear to be responsible for enteric infections and are a common cause of diarrhea among infants. They can be distinguished from adenoviruses that cause respiratory disease by their failure to grow easily in culture. Adenoviruses cause a moderate gastroenteritis with diarrhea and vomiting, lasting for a week to 10 days after an incubation period of approximately 1 week. In the small intestine, adenoviral infection causes atrophy of the villi and compensatory hyperplasia of the crypts similar to rotavirus, resulting in malabsorption and fluid loss. The virus can also cause colitis. Immunohistochemical stain of nuclear inclusions facilitates the diagnosis.

Caliciviruses include two major groups: the classic Caliciviruses (Sapporo-like viruses) and the Norwalk-like viruses (small round structured viruses). Sapporo-like viral infection is rare, while *Norwalk virus,* the prototype of Norwalk-like viruses, is responsible for the majority of cases of nonbacterial food-borne epidemic gastroenteritis in all age groups. Norwalk-like viruses are small icosahedral viruses containing a single-stranded RNA genome. They cause epidemic gastroenteritis with diarrhea, nausea, and vomiting among children. Outbreaks occur following exposure of multiple individuals to a common source. The clinical syndrome has an incubation period of 1 to 2 days, which is followed by 12 to 60 hours of nausea, vomiting, watery diarrhea, and abdominal pain.

Astrovirus is named after its starlike appearance. It primarily affects children, (it accounts for 4% of acute gastroenteritis in young children), and has a worldwide distribution. Those infected develop anorexia, headache, and fever. Other viruses such as enterotrophic coronaviruses and toroviruses are occasionally implicated in human diarrheal disease.

Despite the high incidence of viral gastroenteritis, insights into disease pathogenesis have been slow in coming.

Morphology. Although the enteric viruses are genetically and morphologically different from each other, the lesions they cause in the intestinal tract are similar. The small intestinal mucosa usually exhibits modestly shortened villi and infiltration of the lamina propria by lymphocytes. Vacuolization and loss of the microvillus brush border in surface epithelial cells may be evident, and the crypts become hypertrophied. Viral particles may be visualized by electron microscopy within surface epithelial cells. In infants, rotavirus can produce a flat mucosa resembling celiac sprue (discussed later).

Bacterial Enterocolitis

Diarrheal illness may be caused by numerous bacteria (Table 17–8). There are several pathogenic mechanisms for bacterial enterocolitis (also termed *food poisoning*):

- *Ingestion of preformed toxin,* present in contaminated food. Major offenders are *Staphylococcus aureus, Vibrio,* and *Clostridium perfringens.* Symptoms develop within a matter of hours; explosive diarrhea and acute abdominal distress herald an illness that passes within a day or so. Ingested systemic neurotoxins, as from *Clostridium botulinum,* may produce rapid, and fatal, respiratory failure.
- *Infection by toxigenic organisms,* which proliferate within the gut lumen and elaborate an enterotoxin. An incubation period of several hours to days is followed by *diarrhea and dehydration* if the primary pathogenic mechanism is a secretory enterotoxin, or *dysentery* if the primary mechanism is a cytotoxin. *Traveler's diarrhea* (Montezuma's revenge, turista) usually occurs following ingestion of fecally contaminated food or water; it begins abruptly and subsides within 2 to 3 days. It affects 20% to 50% of the 35 million people who travel worldwide from industrialized countries to developing countries each year.
- *Infection by enteroinvasive organisms,* which proliferate, invade, and destroy mucosal epithelial cells, also leading to dysentery. As with ingestion of toxigenic organisms, the incubation period is several hours to days.

The main properties of bacteria that contribute to the pathogenesis of enterocolitis are: *(1) the ability to adhere to the mucosal epithelial cells and replicate, (2) the ability to elaborate enterotoxins, and (3) the capacity to invade.*

Bacterial Adhesion and Replication. *In order to produce disease, ingested organisms must adhere to the mucosa; otherwise they will be swept away by the fluid stream.* Adherence of enterotoxigenic organisms such as *E. coli* and *Vibrio cholerae* is mediated by plasmid-encoded adhesins. These proteins are expressed on the surface of the organism, sometimes in the form of fimbriae or *pili,* which are rigid or wiry surface

TABLE 17–8 Major Causes of Bacterial Enterocolitis

Organism	Pathogenic Mechanism	Source	Clinical Features
Escherichia coli			Traveler's diarrhea, including:
• ETEC	Cholera-like toxin, no invasion	Food, water	Watery diarrhea
• EHEC	Shiga-like toxin, no invasion	Undercooked beef products	Hemorrhagic colitis, hemolytic-uremic syndrome
• EPEC	Attachment, enterocyte effacement, no invasion	Weaning foods, water	Watery diarrhea, infants and toddlers
• EIEC	Invasion, local spread	Cheese, water, person-to-person	Fever, pain, diarrhea, dysentery
Salmonella	Invasion, translocation, lymphoid inflammation, dissemination	Milk, beef, eggs, poultry	Fever, pain, diarrhea or dysentery, bacteremia, extraintestinal infection, common source outbreaks
Shigella	Invasion, local spread	Person-to-person, low-inoculum	Fever, pain, diarrhea, dysentery, epidemic spread
Campylobacter	Toxins, invasion	Milk, poultry, animal contact	Fever, pain, diarrhea, dysentery, food sources, animal reservoirs
Yersinia enterocolitica	Invasion, translocation, lymphoid inflammation, dissemination	Milk, pork	Fever, pain, diarrhea, mesenteric adenitis, extraintestinal infection, food sources
Vibrio cholerae, other *Vibrios*	Enterotoxin, no invasion	Water, shellfish, person-to-person spread	Watery diarrhea, cholera, pandemic spread
Clostridium difficile	Cytotoxin, local invasion	Nosocomial environmental spread	Fever, pain, bloody diarrhea, following antibiotic use, nosocomial acquisition
Clostridium perfringens	Enterotoxin, no invasion	Meat, poultry, fish	Watery diarrhea, food sources, "pigbel"
Mycobacterium tuberculosis	Invasion, mural inflammatory foci with necrosis and scarring	Contaminated milk, swallowing of coughed-up organisms	Chronic abdominal pain; complications of malabsorption, stricture, perforation, fistulae, hemorrhage

ETEC, enterotoxigenic *E. coli*; EHEC, enterohemorrhagic *E. coli*; EPEC, enteropathogenic *E. coli*; EIEC, enteroinvasive *E. coli*.

projections. Adherence of enteropathogenic and enterohemorrhagic organisms, including *E. coli* and *Shigella,* is also dependent on plasmid-encoded proteins, but the nature of these proteins is not known. Adherence causes effacement of the apical enterocyte membrane, with destruction of the microvillus brush border and changes in the underlying cell cytoplasm.[35] The factors regulating bacterial replication are not well understood, particularly since pathogenic organisms must compete with the normal bacterial flora to achieve a critical population density.

Bacterial Enterotoxins. *Bacterial enterotoxins are polypeptides that cause diarrhea.* Some *enterotoxins* cause intestinal secretion of fluid and electrolytes without causing tissue damage; this is accomplished by binding of the toxin to the epithelial cell membrane, entry of a portion of the toxin into the cell, and massive activation of electrolyte secretion accompanied by water. *Cholera toxin, elaborated by Vibrio cholerae, is the prototype secretagogue toxin.* The toxin causes increased levels of intracellular calcium, resulting in dysfunction of the fluid and electrolyte transport, as discussed below under Cholera. *Strains of E. coli (enterotoxigenic E. coli) that produce heat-labile (LT) and heat-stable (ST) secretagogue toxins are the major cause of traveler's diarrhea.* The LT toxin is similar to cholera toxin, and the ST toxin induces cyclic guanosine monophosphate, resulting in increased fluid excretion. Leukocytes are absent from the stool of patients with traveler's diarrhea. A second group of enterotoxins are *cytotoxins,* exemplified by Shiga toxin produced by *Shigella dysenteriae* and Shiga-like toxins produced by enterohemorrhagic *E. coli* (e.g., *E. coli O157:H7*). These toxins cause direct tissue damage through epithelial cell necrosis. *Staphylococcal enterotoxins,* which are major causes of food poisoning, represent yet another group of enterotoxins; are proteins that bind to the antigen receptors of large numbers of T cells and activate the lymphocytes to secrete cytokines. The cytokines stimulate intestinal motility and fluid secretion.

Bacterial Invasion. Both enteroinvasive *E. coli* and *Shigella* possess a large virulence plasmid that confers the capacity for epithelial cell invasion, apparently by microbe-stimulated endocytosis. This is followed by intracellular proliferation, cell lysis, and cell-to-cell spread. *Salmonella* quickly pass through intestinal epithelial cells via transcytosis with minimal epithelial damage; entry into the lamina propria leads to a 5% to 10% incidence of bacteremia, which can sometimes cause typhoid fever, meningitis, endocarditis, and osteomyelitis (commonly in the setting of sickle cell disease). *Yersinia enterocolitica* penetrates the ileal mucosa and multiplies within Peyer patches and regional lymph nodes. Bacteremia is rare and usually occurs in the setting of iron-overload disease, since iron is a growth factor for *Yersinia.*

Bacterial cytotoxins and invasion give rise to bacillary dysentery, which generates its own unique misery for its victims: abdominal cramping and tenesmus with loose stools containing blood, pus, and mucus. Bacillary dysentery, which results in as many as 500,000 deaths among children in developing countries each year, is caused by *Shigella dysenteriae, Shigella flexneri, Shigella boydii,* and *Shigella sonnei* as well as certain O type enterotoxic *E. coli.* (Amebic dysentery is caused by the protozoan parasite *Entamoeba histolytica,* discussed later in this chapter).

Shigella Bacillary Dysentery

Shigella species are gram-negative facultative anaerobes that infect only humans. *S. flexneri* is the major cause of endemic bacillary dysentery in locations of poor hygiene, including large regions of the developing world and institutions in the developed world. Epidemic shigellosis can occur when individuals consume uncooked foods at picnics or other events.

Pathogenesis. Transmission is fecal-oral and is remarkable for the small number of organisms that may cause disease (10 ingested organisms cause illness in 10% of volunteers, and 500 organisms cause disease in 50% of volunteers). *Shigella* bacteria invade the intestinal mucosal cells but do not usually go beyond the lamina propria. Dysentery is caused when the bacteria escape the epithelial cell phagolysosome, multiply within the cytoplasm, and destroy host cells. Shiga toxin causes hemorrhagic colitis and hemolytic-uremic syndrome by damaging endothelial cells in the microvasculature of the colon and the glomeruli, respectively (Chapter 20). In addition, chronic arthritis secondary to *S. flexneri* infection, called *Reiter syndrome,* may be caused by a bacterial antigen; the occurrence of this syndrome is strongly linked to HLA-B27 genotype, but the immunologic basis of this reaction is not understood.[51]

Salmonellosis and Typhoid Fever

Salmonellae are flagellated, gram-negative bacteria that cause a self-limited food-borne and water-borne gastroenteritis (*S. enteritidis, S. typhimurium,* and others) or a life-threatening systemic illness, typhoid fever, marked by fever and systemic symptoms *(S. typhi).* In the United States, *Salmonella* species cause approximately 500,000 reported cases of food poisoning, and many cases go unreported. Because *Salmonella* species other than *S. typhi* infect most commercially raised chickens and many cows, the major sources of *Salmonella* in the United States are feces-contaminated beef and chicken that are insufficiently washed and cooked. Stringent hygiene in the production plants and the home kitchen helps minimize risk of contamination. In contrast, humans are the only host of *S. typhi,* which is shed in the feces, urine, vomitus, and oral secretions by acutely ill persons and in the feces by chronic carriers without overt disease. Therefore, typhoid fever from *S. typhi* is a disease largely of developing countries, where sanitary conditions are insufficient to stop its spread. Typhoid fever is a protracted disease that is associated with bacteremia, fever, and chills during the first week; widespread mononuclear phagocyte involvement with rash, abdominal pain, and prostration in the second week; and ulceration of Peyer patches with intestinal bleeding and shock during the third week.

Pathogenesis. *Salmonella* invades intestinal epithelial cells as well as tissue macrophages. Invasion of intestinal epithelial cells is controlled by invasion genes that are induced by the low oxygen tension found in the gut. These genes encode proteins involved in adhesion and in recruitment of host cytoskeletal proteins that internalize the bacterium. Similarly, intramacrophage growth is important in pathogenicity, and this seems to be mediated by bacterial genes that are induced by the acid pH within the macrophage phagolysosome. The enteric nervous system also is a critical regulator of fluid secretion in the normal gut. Neural reflex pathways increase epithelial fluid secretion in response to enteric pathogens such as *Salmonella* and *Clostridium difficile.*[52]

Campylobacter Enterocolitis

This comma-shaped, flagellated, gram-negative organism was once classified with the vibrios. When special culture conditions permitted its isolation in the 1970s, it became apparent that *Campylobacter* was an important cause of enterocolitis and septicemia in humans. In the United States, *Campylobacter jejuni* is responsible for twice the enteric disease of *Salmonella* and four times that of *Shigella.* Most infections with *Campylobacter* are sporadic and are associated with ingestion of improperly cooked chicken, which may be contaminated with *Campylobacter* and/or *Salmonella.* Sporadic infections may also be associated with contact with infected dogs. Outbreaks of *Campylobacter* are usually associated with unpasteurized milk or contaminated water.

Pathogenesis. Invasiveness is strain dependent. Flagella of *Campylobacter,* which give the organism its comma shape and motility, are necessary for the bacterium to penetrate mucus covering epithelial surfaces. Three clinical outcomes of *Campylobacter* infection are possible: (1) diarrhea, which is independent of bacterial invasion; (2) dysentery with blood and mucus in the stool; and (3) enteric fever when bacteria proliferate within the lamina propria and mesenteric lymph nodes. Postinfectious complications of *Campylobacter* infections include reactive arthritis in HLA-B27 carriers (as with *Shigella* infection) and Guillain-Barré syndrome, a demyelinating disease of peripheral nerves due to autoantibodies against gangliosides G_{M1} and GQ1b, described in Chapter 27. Recently, *C. jejuni* was found to be associated with the development of immunoproliferative small intestinal disease (discussed later).

Cholera

Vibrio cholerae are comma-shaped, gram-negative bacteria that have been the cause of seven great long-lasting epidemics (pandemics) of diarrheal disease. Many of these pandemics began in the Ganges Valley of India and Bangladesh, which is never free from cholera, and then moved east. Although there are 140 serotypes of *V. cholerae,* until recently only the 01 serotype was associated with severe diarrhea. Beginning in 1992, a new *V. cholerae* serotype (0139, also known as Bengal) has been associated with severe, watery diarrhea.[53]

Pathogenesis. The vibrios never invade the epithelium but instead remain within the lumen and secrete an enterotoxin, which is encoded by a virulence phage. Flagellar proteins involved in motility and attachment are necessary for efficient bacterial colonization, as has been described for *Campylobacter.* (This is in contrast to *Shigella* species and certain *E. coli* strains, which are nonmotile and yet invasive.) The *Vibrio* hemagglutinin, which is a metalloprotease, is important for detachment of *Vibrio* from epithelial cells.

The secretory diarrhea characteristic of the disease is caused by release of *cholera toxin* (Fig. 17–32). Cholera toxin is composed of five binding peptides B and a catalytic peptide A. The B peptides, serving as a "landing pad," bind to carbohydrates on G_{M1} ganglioside on the surface of epithelial cells of the small intestine, enabling calveolar-mediated endosomal entry of toxin subunit A into the cell. Reverse transport of the subunit A from the endosome into the cell cytoplasm is followed by cleavage of the disulfide bond linking the two fragments of peptide A (A1 and A2). Catalytic peptide A1 is generated, leading to the following sequence:

- A1 interacts with 20-kD cytosolic proteins called ADP-ribosylation factors (ARF).
- The ARF–A1 complex catalyzes ADP-ribosylation of a 49-kD G-protein (called $G_{s\alpha}$).[54]
- Binding of NAD and GTP generates an activated $G_{s\alpha}$, which in turn binds to and stimulates adenylate cyclase. ADP-ribosylated $G_{s\alpha}$ is permanently in an active GTP-

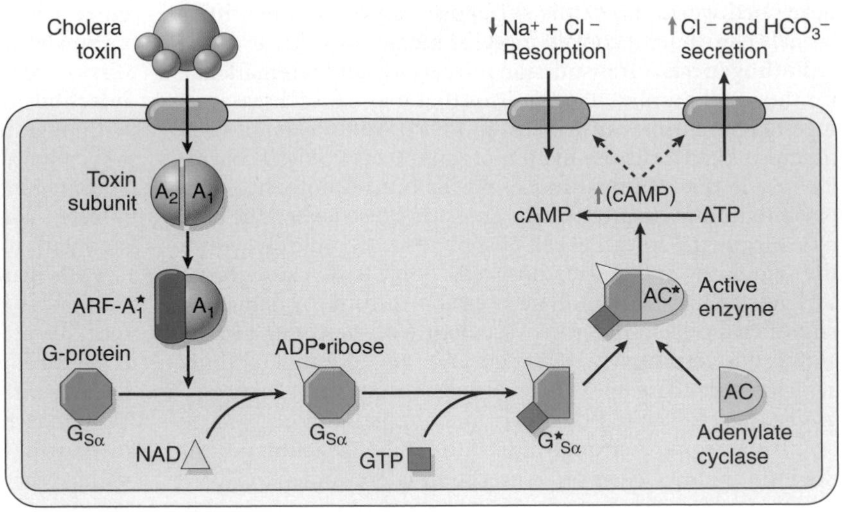

FIGURE 17–32 Mechanisms of cholera toxin action.

bound state, resulting in persistent activation of adenylate cyclase.

- The activated adenylate cyclase generates high levels of intracellular cAMP from ATP.
- Cyclic AMP stimulates secretion of chloride and bicarbonate, with associated sodium and water secretion. Chloride and sodium resorption are also inhibited.

The reabsorptive function of the colon is overwhelmed, and liters of dilute "rice water" diarrhea containing flecks of mucus—up to 14 L/day, equivalent to the circulating blood volume, causing dehydration and electrolyte imbalances. Because overall absorption in the gut remains intact, oral formulas can replace the massive sodium, chloride, bicarbonate, and fluid losses and reduce the mortality rate from 50% to less than 1%.

Antibiotic-Associated Colitis (Pseudomembranous Colitis)

This entity is an *acute colitis characterized by formation of an adherent layer of inflammatory cells and debris overlying sites of mucosal injury, a so-called pseudomembrane.* It is usually caused by toxins of *Clostridium difficile,* a normal gut commensal. The two major toxins produced by *C. difficile* are toxin A and toxin B, which modulate cellular signaling pathways, induce cytokine production, and cause host cell apoptosis.[55] The disease occurs most often in patients without a background of chronic enteric disease, following a course of broad-spectrum antibiotic therapy. Nearly all antibacterial agents have been implicated. Presumably toxin-forming strains flourish following alteration of the normal intestinal flora; factors favoring the initiation of toxin production are not understood. Rarely, the condition may appear in the absence of antibiotic therapy, typically after surgery or superimposed on a chronic debilitating illness. Infrequently, the small intestine is involved.

Antibiotic-associated colitis occurs primarily in adults as an acute or chronic diarrheal illness, although it has been recorded as a spontaneous infection in young adults without predisposing influences. Diagnosis is confirmed by the detection of the *C. difficile* cytotoxin in stool. Response to treatment is usually prompt, but relapse occurs in up to 25% of patients.

Morphology. Given the variety of bacterial pathogens, the pathologic manifestations of enteric bacterial disease are quite variable. Dramatic, even lethal, diarrhea may occur without a significant pathologic lesion, as in cholera resulting from *V. cholerae.* Alternatively, characteristic histology may enable diagnosis with reasonable certainty, as with *C. difficile*–induced pseudomembranous colitis. **Most bacterial infections exhibit a non-specific pattern of damage to the surface epithelium, decreased epithelial cell maturation and an increased mitotic rate ("regenerative change"), hyperemia and edema of the lamina propria, and variable neutrophilic infiltration into the lamina propria and epithelial layer.** In the small intestine, modest villus blunting may occur; in the colon, mucosal architecture is usually preserved. With recovery, epithelial damage and neutrophilic inflammation subside, leaving the residua of regenerative change and lymphoplasmacytic infiltration of the lamina propria. Alternatively, progressive destruction of the mucosa leads to erosion, ulceration, and severe submucosal inflammation. Notable features of particular infections are summarized below:

- *Shigella* primarily affects the distal colon, first with hyperemia and edema and enlargement of mucosal lymphoid nodules, creating small, projecting nodules. Within 24 hours, the acute mucosal inflammation and erosion generate a patchy and then confluent purulent exudate (Fig. 17–33). The mucosa then becomes soft and friable, and irregular ulcerations appear; severe infection generates large denuded tracts of mucosa. The recovery phase is marked by formation of mucosal granulation tissue and eventual regeneration of the mucosal epithelium.
- *Salmonella* (multiple species, including *S. typhimurium* and *S. paratyphi*) primarily affects the ileum and colon, generating blunted villi, vascular congestion, and mononuclear inflammation. Peyer patch involvement produces swelling, congestion, and eventual ulceration with linear ulcers. With *S. typhi,* bacteremia and systemic dissemination

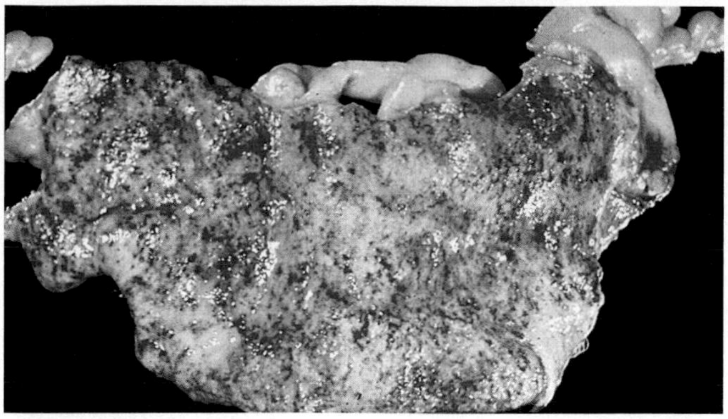

FIGURE 17–33 Shigella enterocolitis. Segment of colon showing pale, granular, inflamed mucosa with patches of coagulated exudate.

cause proliferation of phagocytes with enlargement of reticuloendothelial and lymphoid tissues throughout the body. Peyer patches in the terminal ileum become sharply delineated, plateau-like elevations up to 8 cm in diameter, with enlargement of draining mesenteric lymph nodes. Shedding of the mucosa and swollen lymphoid tissue creates oval ulcers with their long axes along the axis of the ileum. Microscopic examination reveals macrophages containing bacteria, red blood cells, and nuclear debris. Intermingled with the phagocytes are lymphocytes and plasma cells, whereas neutrophils are present near the ulcerated surface. The **spleen** is enlarged, soft, and bulging, with uniformly pale red pulp, obliterated follicular markings, and prominent sinus histiocytosis and reticuloendothelial proliferation. The **liver** shows small, randomly scattered foci of parenchymal necrosis in which the hepatocytes are replaced by a phagocytic mononuclear aggregate, called **a typhoid nodule**. These distinctive nodules also occur in the bone marrow and lymph nodes. **Gallbladder** colonization, which may be associated with gallstones, causes a chronic carrier state.

- *Campylobacter jejuni* and other species may involve the entire intestine from the jejunum to the anus. The small intestine exhibits a decrease in the villus-to-crypt ratio. In invasive colonic infection, the colonic mucosa appears friable and superficially eroded on proctoscopy. Histology reveals multiple superficial ulcers, mucosal inflammation, and a purulent exudate. The formation of colonic crypt abscesses and mucosal ulceration may be confused with those of ulcerative colitis (discussed later).
- *Yersinia enterocolitica* and *Y. pseudotuberculosis* involve ileum, appendix, and colon. They cause mucosal hemorrhage and ulceration, bowel wall thickening, Peyer patch and mesenteric lymph node hypertrophy with necrotizing granulomas, and systemic spread with peritonitis, pharyngitis, and pericarditis.
- *Vibrio cholerae* affects the small intestine, especially the more proximal segment. The mucosa essentially remains intact, with mucus-depleted crypts.
- *Clostridium perfringens* and *Clostridium difficile*. *C. perfringens* infection is usually similar to *V. cholerae,* but with some epithelial damage; some strains produce severe necrotizing enterocolitis (NEC) with perforation ("pigbel"). ***C. difficile*–induced pseudomembranous colitis** derives its name from the plaquelike adhesion of fibrinopurulent-necrotic debris and mucus to damaged colonic mucosa (Fig. 17–34*A*)—these are not true "membranes" since the coagulum is not an epithelial layer. Pseudomembrane formation is not restricted to *C. difficile*–induced colitis: It also may occur following any severe mucosal injury, as in ischemic colitis, volvulus, and with necrotizing infections (staphylococci, shigella, candida, NEC). What is striking about *C. difficile* toxin–induced colitis is the microscopic lesion (Fig. 17–34*B*). The surface epithelium is denuded, and the superficial lamina propria contains a dense infiltrate of neutrophils and occasional capillary fibrin thrombi. Superficially damaged crypts are distended by a mucopu-

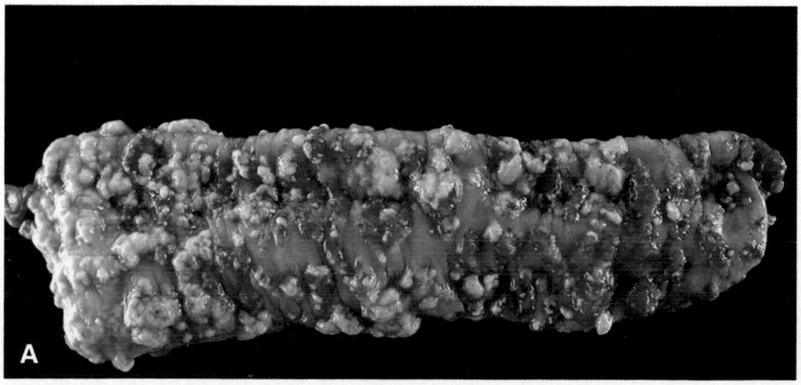

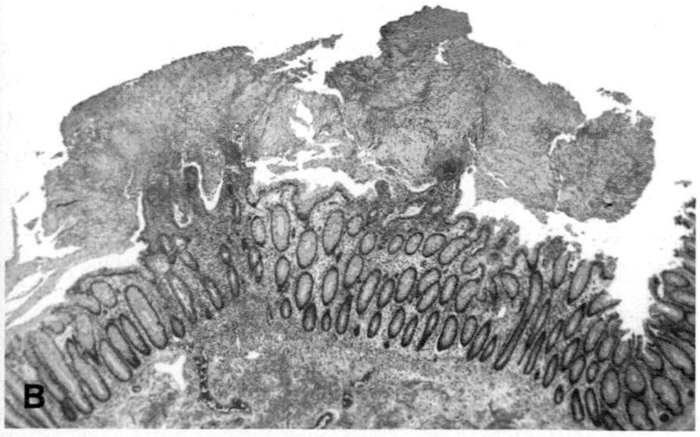

FIGURE 17–34 Pseudomembranous colitis from *C. difficile* infection. *A,* Gross photograph showing plaques of yellow fibrin and inflammatory debris adherent to a reddened colonic mucosa. *B,* Low-power micrograph showing superficial erosion of the mucosa and an adherent pseudomembrane of fibrin, mucus, and inflammatory debris.

rulent exudate, which erupts out of the crypt to form a mushrooming cloud that adheres to the damaged surface—the coalescence of this "cloud" forms the pseudomembrane.

- Enteropathogenic *E. coli:* At least four distinct types of pathogenic *E. coli* are known to cause significant diseases—the enterotoxigenic (ETEC), enterohemorrhagic (EHEC), enteroinvasive (EIEC), and enteroadherent (mainly, enteropathogenic, EPEC). In North America, the most important one is EHEC serotype *E. coli* O157:H7.[56] EHEC are intestinal commensals in many animals. Humans are usually infected by contaminated meat. These bacteria produce Shiga-like toxins, which damage enterocytes and vascular endothelial cells. In addition to abdominal pain and diarrhea, some patients, particularly children, may develop life-threatening hemolytic-uremic syndrome characterized by the clinical triad of hemolytic anemia, renal failure, and thrombocytopenia.

The complications of severe bacterial enterocolitis are the expected consequences of massive fluid loss or destruction of the intestinal mucosal barrier and include dehydration, sepsis, and perforation. Without quick intervention, death ensues rapidly, particularly in the very young. Alternatively, an infection may produce extreme discomfort without being life threatening. All enteroinvasive organisms can mimic acute onset of idiopathic inflammatory bowel disease.

Yersinia and *Mycobacterium tuberculosis* may also present as subacute diarrheal illnesses. Tuberculosis is covered in detail in Chapter 8.

Bacterial Overgrowth Syndrome

A key mechanism for clearing bacteria from the small intestine is the normal motility, which ensures that bacteria entering into the small intestine are propelled downstream before they can adhere to the mucosa and proliferate. Gastric hypoacidity, immunologic deficiencies, and intestinal dysmotility with intestinal stasis may enable bacteria to proliferate within the small bowel, so-called *bacterial overgrowth syndrome.* Surgical procedures in particular may set the stage for bacterial overgrowth. These include Billroth procedures, in which the gastric antrum is resected, thereby decreasing the time for exposure of ingested bacteria to gastric acid. Surgical creation of Roux-en-Y loops, as in the Billroth II procedure or in a pancreatoduodenectomy (Whipple) procedure, creates a blind intestinal loop that is a site for bacterial overgrowth. The bacterial populations are mixed enteric populations, without specific dominant species.

Patients usually present with chronic diarrhea, abdominal pain, malabsorption, and weight loss. The clinical diagnosis largely depends on the clinical history and demonstration of the presence of bacteria in the proximal segment of the small intestine by direct culture of an aspirate. Breath tests for volatile bacterial byproducts may be a noninvasive option for a presumptive diagnosis of bacterial overgrowth syndrome.

Parasitic Enterocolitis

Although viruses and bacteria are the predominant enteric pathogens in the United States, *parasitic disease and protozoal infection collectively affect over one half of the world's population on a chronic or recurrent basis.* The small intestine can harbor as many as 20 species of parasites, including nematodes (the roundworms *Ascaris* and *Strongyloides,* hookworms, pinworms), cestodes (flatworms, tapeworms), trematodes (flukes), and protozoa. Some of the parasitic infections are covered in Chapter 8. Here we will briefly discuss the common parasitic infections of the intestinal tract.

Nematodes

Ascaris lumbricoides is the most common nematode, infecting over a billion individuals worldwide. Infection occurs by ingestion of eggs as a result of human fecal-oral contamination. The ingested ova hatch in the intestine, and larvae penetrate the intestinal mucosa. The disease associated with this parasitic infection is related to larval migration from the splanchnic circulation to the systemic circulation (jejunum-to-liver-to-lung), with formation of hepatic abscess or *Ascaris* pneumonitis. Larvae migrate up the trachea, are swallowed, and arrive again in the intestine to mature into adult worms. Adult worm masses can physically obstruct the intestine or the biliary tree. Diagnosis is usually made by detection of the eggs in the feces.

Strongyloides larvae live in fecally contaminated ground soil and penetrate through unbroken skin. They migrate through the lungs, generating pulmonary infiltrates with eosinophilia, and arrive in the intestine to mature into adult worms. Unlike other intestinal worms, which require an ova or larval stage outside the human, the eggs of *Strongyloides* can hatch within the intestine and larvae can penetrate the mucosa, causing autoinfection. Hence, *Strongyloides* infection can persist in one individual for life; immunosuppressed individuals can have overwhelming autoinfection. *Strongyloides* incites a strong tissue eosinophilic reaction, causing eosinophilia as well.

Hookworm (*Necator duodenale* and *Ancylostoma duodenale*) infection affects an estimated 1 billion people worldwide and causes significant morbidity. The infection initiates from larva penetration through the skin. The larva develops further in the lungs and gains access to the duodenum by upward migration in the bronchial tree, followed by swallowing. The worms attach to the mucosa, suck blood, and reproduce. The small intestinal mucosa usually exhibits multiple superficial erosions, focal hemorrhage, and inflammatory infiltrates. Long-term infection causes iron deficiency anemia. Diagnosis can be made by detection of the eggs in fecal smear.

Enterobius vermicularis (pinworms) do not invade host tissue and live their entire life within the intestinal lumen. Pinworm infections occur in industrialized countries as well as developing countries; in the United States more than 60 million people have pinworms. Because these are noninvasive worms, they rarely cause serious illness. *Enterobius vermicularis* infection (enterobiasis) occurs in situations where fecal-oral contamination is common. Adult worms living in the intestine migrate to the anal orifice at night, where the female deposits eggs on the perirectal mucosa. As the eggs are quite irritative, rectal and perineal pruritus ensue. Human-to-human contact is aided by digital manipulation of the area. Both eggs and adult pinworms remain viable external to the body, and reinfection is common. Diagnosis is easily made by applying cellophane tape to the perianal skin and examining the tape for eggs under the microscope.

Trichuris trichiura (whipworm) is less common, occurring primarily in young children. Similar to *Enterobius vermicularis,* these worms do not penetrate the intestinal mucosa and rarely cause serious disease. Heavy infections, however, may cause bloody diarrhea and rectal prolapse. Diagnosis is established by finding the characteristic eggs in the stool.

Cestodes

The intestinal cestodes reside only within the intestinal lumen and never invade beyond the intestinal mucosa. Three species of cestodes (multisegmental flatworms, tapeworms) are *Diphyllobothrium latum* (fish tapeworm), *Taenia solium* (pork tapeworm), and *Hymenolepsis nana* (dwarf tapeworm). Infection occurs by ingestion of raw or undercooked meat that contains encysted larvae. Release of the larvae enables attachment to the intestinal mucosa through its head, or *scolex.* The worm derives its nutrients from the food stream and enlarges by formation of egg-filled proglottids (segments). Humans are generally infected by one worm only; since the worm does not penetrate the intestinal mucosa, eosinophilia does not generally occur. Nevertheless, the parasite burden can be staggering, as adult worms can grow to many meters in length. Shedding of proglottids or individual eggs produces copious fecal release of eggs. Diagnosis is established by examination of stool for the ova.

Amebiasis

Entamoeba histolytica (ameba) is a dysentery-causing protozoan parasite spread by fecal-oral transmission. This protozoan infects approximately 500 million persons in developing countries such as India, Mexico, and Colombia, resulting in approximately 40 million cases of dysentery and liver abscess.

Pathogenesis. *E. histolytica* cysts, which have a chitin wall and four nuclei, are the infectious form because they are resistant to gastric acid. Ingested quadrinucleate cysts colonize the surface of colonic mucin epithelial cells. Cysts release trophozoites, the ameboid forms, which reproduce under anaerobic conditions without harming the host. Because the parasites lack mitochondria or Krebs cycle enzymes, amebae are obligate fermenters of glucose to ethanol. Metronidazole, the best drug to treat invasive infections with entamoebae (as well as other parasites such as *Giardia* and trichomonads), targets ferridoxin-dependent pyruvate oxidoreductase, an enzyme critical in such fermentation that is present in these organisms but is absent in humans.

Amebae cause dysentery when they attach to the colonic epithelium, as they cause epithelial cell apoptosis, invade the crypts of colonic glands, and burrow into the lamina propria. The organisms then burrow laterally to create, with the accompanying inflammation and tissue necrosis, a flask-shaped ulcer with a narrow neck and broad base. Amebic proteins that may be involved in tissue invasion include: (1) cysteine proteinases, which are able to break down proteins of the extracellular matrix; (2) a lectin on the parasite surface that binds to carbohydrates on the surface of colonic epithelial cells and red blood cells; and (3) a channel-forming protein called the amebapore, which makes holes in the plasma membrane of host cells and lyses them. The presence in stool of trophozoites containing ingested red blood cells is indicative of tissue invasion by virulent organisms.

Morphology. Amebiasis most frequently involves the cecum and ascending colon, followed in order by the sigmoid, rectum, and appendix. In severe full-blown cases, however, the entire colon is involved. Amebae can mimic the appearance of macrophages because of their comparable size and large number of vacuoles; the parasites, however, have a smaller nucleus, which contains a large karyosome (Fig. 17–35). Amebae invade through the crypt epithelium and burrow into the mucosa and submucosa, eliciting a neutrophilic reaction. They are stopped by the muscularis propria and fan out laterally to create a flask-shaped ulcer with a narrow neck and broad base. These maturing ulcers contain few host inflammatory cells and exhibit extensive liquefactive necrosis. As the lesion progresses, the overlying surface mucosa is deprived of its blood supply and sloughs. The mucosa between ulcers is often normal or mildly inflamed. On occasion, the formation of profuse circumferential granulation tissue can create colonic stricture.

In about 40% of patients with amebic dysentery, parasites penetrate splanchnic vessels and embolize to the liver to produce solitary, or less often multiple, discrete abscesses, sometimes exceeding 10 cm in diameter. **Amebic liver abscesses** have a scant inflammatory reaction at their margins and a shaggy fibrin lining. Because of hemorrhage into the cavities, the abscesses are sometimes filled with a chocolate-colored, odorless, pasty material. Secondary bacterial infection may make these abscesses purulent.

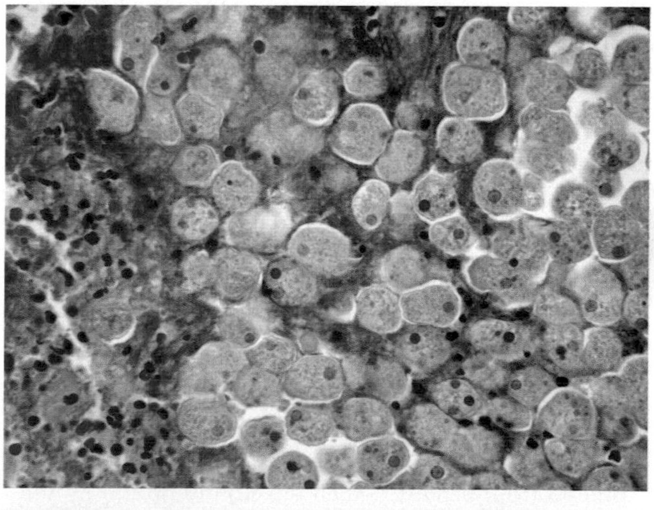

FIGURE 17–35 *Entamoeba histolytica* in colon. High-power view of the organisms. Note some of the organisms ingesting red blood cells.

Clinical Features. Clinically, the patient may present with abdominal pain, bloody diarrhea, or weight loss. Occasionally, acute necrotizing colitis and megacolon can occur, which carry significant mortality. Rarely, amebic abscesses reach the lung and the heart by direct extension from the liver or spread from the liver through the blood into the kidneys and brain. Such abscesses remain long after the acute intestinal illness has passed.

Giardiasis

Giardia lamblia is the most common pathogenic parasitic infection in humans.[57] It is an intestinal protozoan spread by fecally contaminated water or food. Infection may be subclinical or may cause acute or chronic diarrhea, steatorrhea, or constipation. Because *Giardia* cysts are not killed by chlorine, *Giardia* is endemic in public water supplies that are not filtered through sand and in contaminated streams accessed by campers.

Pathogenesis. In the United States, *Giardia* infections are especially frequent in institutions for the mentally ill and in day-care centers. *Giardia,* like *Entamoeba,* ferments glucose, lacks mitochondria, and exists in two forms: (1) a dormant but infectious cyst spread by the fecal-oral route from person to person (as well as from beavers to persons); and (2) trophozoites that multiply in the intestinal lumen. Transition from trophozoites to cysts is induced by decreases in availability of cholesterol as *Giardia* moves from duodenum to jejunum. In contrast to *Entamoeba, Giardia* trophozoites have two nuclei rather than one, are flagellated, reside in the duodenum rather than the colon, adhere to but do not invade the intestinal epithelial cells, and so cause diarrhea rather than dysentery.

Infection can occur by ingestion of as few as 10 cysts. *Giardia* trophozoites adhere to sugars on intestinal epithelial cells through a parasite lectin that is activated when it is cleaved by proteases, which are plentiful in the lumen of the duodenum. Tight contact between the parasite and the epithelial cell is made by a sucker-like disc, composed of cytoplasmic tubulin and unique intermediate filaments called *giardins.* Although *Giardia* does not secrete toxin, it contains a cystein-rich surface protein that resembles diarrhea-causing toxins secreted by certain snakes. The physical presence of rapidly proliferating trophozoites and their toxic proteins damages the microvillus brush border, causing a malabsorptive state.[52]

Immunity mediated by antibodies, including secretory IgA, is important in resistance to *Giardia,* because agammaglobulinemic individuals are severely affected by the parasite. Immunity to *Giardia,* however, is limited by the parasite's ability to vary its major surface proteins into antigenically distinct forms, encoded by more than 50 different genes.

Morphology. In stool smears, *G. lamblia* trophozoites are pear shaped and binucleate. Duodenal biopsy specimens are often teeming with sickle-shaped trophozoites, which are tightly bound by the concave attachment disc to the villus surface of the intestinal epithelial cells (Fig. 17–36). As *Giardia* does not actually invade the mucosa, small intestinal morphology may be virtually normal. However, many patients exhibit marked blunting of the small intestinal villi with a mixed inflammatory infiltrate in the lamina propria. The brush borders of the surface absorptive epithelial cells are irregular, and sometimes there is virtual absence of villi, resembling the atrophic stage of celiac disease.

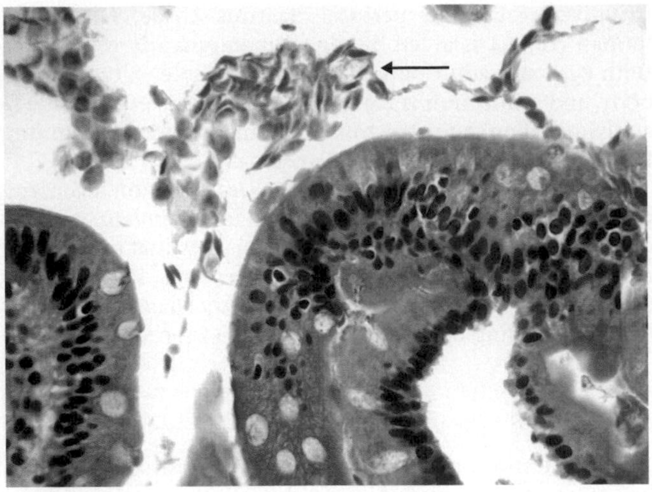

FIGURE 17–36 *Giardia lamblia.* Trophozoite *(arrow)* of the organism immediately adjacent to the duodenal surface epithelium.

Clinical Features. Infected patients exhibit a malabsorptive diarrhea, owing to mucosal epithelial cell injury. Functional lactase deficiency also occurs in 20% to 40% of chronically infected patients by mechanisms that are not understood. The infection can last for months or years. The symptoms may be severe in immunocompromised patients. Diagnosis is readily made by examination of stool for cysts; small intestinal biopsy or examination of a small intestinal aspirate also permits identification of the organisms. While giardiasis is responsive to oral antimicrobial therapy, recurrence is common following cessation of treatment.

Necrotizing Enterocolitis

Necrotizing enterocolitis (NEC) is an acute, necrotizing inflammation of the small and large intestines with the severe consequence of transmural necrosis of intestinal segments. While it can occur at any age, NEC is particularly devastating in the neonate.[58] It is the most common acquired gastrointestinal emergency of neonates, particularly those who are premature or of low birth weight. It may occur at any time in the first 3 months of life, but its peak incidence is around the time when infants are started on oral foods (2 to 4 days old). This condition is described in Chapter 10.

Collagenous and Lymphocytic Colitis

Collagenous colitis is a distinctive disorder of the colon characterized by chronic watery diarrhea and patches of bandlike collagen deposits directly under the surface epithelium. *Lymphocytic colitis* is characterized by chronic watery diarrhea and a prominent intraepithelial infiltrate of lymphocytes. Collagenous colitis occurs primarily in middle-aged and older women; lymphocytic colitis affects males and females equally. Both sets of patients can have between 3 to 20 nonbloody, watery bowel movements per day, accompanied by cramping abdominal pain. Radiographic studies are unremarkable, and endoscopy characteristically reveals normal mucosa. The pathogenesis of both these conditions remains unclear; they do appear to be separate conditions.[59] Lymphocytic colitis shows a strong association with autoimmune diseases, including celiac sprue, thyroiditis, arthritis, and autoimmune gastritis. Both diseases are benign in nature, with neither debilitating weight loss nor malignancy as potential outcomes. While collagenous colitis and lymphocytic colitis are uncommon, they must be considered in every adult patient who presents with a noninflammatory, watery diarrhea.

MISCELLANEOUS INTESTINAL INFLAMMATORY DISORDERS

Acquired Immunodeficiency Syndrome (AIDS)

Diarrheal illness occurs in 50% of AIDS patients in North America and may approach 100% in developing countries.[60] Some patients exhibit a malabsorptive syndrome with small intestinal villus atrophy or a colitic syndrome resembling ulcerative colitis in the absence of demonstrable pathogens. Although most cases are probably due to coexistent infections in these immunocompromised patients, the concept of *AIDS enteropathy,* attributable to direct mucosal damage by human immunodeficiency virus infection, has been proposed but remains unproven. The spectrum of infections occurring in AIDS is discussed in Chapter 6.

Transplantation

Diarrhea is a significant complication of bone marrow transplantation. Pretransplant conditioning may cause direct *toxic injury* to the small intestinal mucosa, evident as villus blunting, degeneration and flattening of crypt epithelial cells, decreased mitoses, and atypia of cell nuclei. Abrupt onset of severe watery diarrhea is a major feature of *acute GVHD.* A distinctive histologic lesion is focal crypt cell necrosis, in which debris from necrotic cells occupies lacunae within the epithelial layer, with minimal to absent inflammatory cell response in the lamina propria (Fig. 17–37).[61] In more advanced GVHD, necrosis may become so severe as to lead to total sloughing of the mucosa. In addition to fluid and electrolyte derangements, the life-threatening complications of sepsis and intestinal hemorrhage may ensue. Alimentary tract symptoms are less evident in chronic GVHD but may include dysphagia secondary to esophageal involvement and occasionally malabsorption due to chronic intestinal injury. *Small intestinal transplantation* also carries with it a spectrum of complications, including rejection and CMV infection.

Drug-Induced Intestinal Injury

When one considers the vast quantities of drugs ingested by humans, with or without the blessings of the medical profession, it is remarkable that the gastrointestinal tract escapes relatively unscathed. *Focal ulceration* can occur when a pill adheres to the mucosa and releases all of its contents locally, as may occur in the esophagus with "dry swallows." Drug-induced acute erosive gastritis has been mentioned earlier. The small intestine and colon are susceptible to drug-induced enterocolitis, most commonly associated with the use of *NSAIDs.*[62] A nonspecific pattern of small intestinal inflammation may lead to malabsorption. Colonic inflammation may produce an acute or chronic diarrheal illness; ulceration and stricture formation also occur. *Drug-induced gastrointestinal injury must be considered whenever abdominal illness is encountered.* Considering this possibility may, on occasion, spare patients from erroneous diagnosis of a chronic intestinal illness.

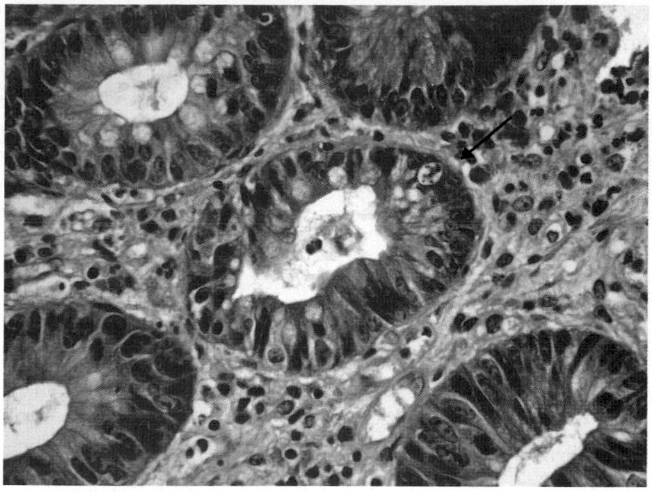

FIGURE 17–37 Graft-versus-host disease of the colon. Note the apoptotic cell in the crypt *(arrow).*

Radiation Enterocolitis

Abdominal irradiation may severely impair the normal proliferative activity of the small intestinal and colonic mucosal epithelia. *Acute radiation enteritis* manifests as anorexia, abdominal cramps, and a malabsorptive diarrhea, attributable to acute mucosal injury. *Chronic radiation enteritis* or *colitis* may exhibit more indolent symptoms than the acute form or may present as an inflammatory colitis. The mucosal damage may be perpetuated by radiation-induced vascular injury and may be accompanied by ischemic fibrosis and stricture.

Neutropenic Colitis (Typhlitis)

Typhlitis was a nineteenth-century term for severe acute and chronic inflammation of the cecal and appendiceal region, which in retrospect was probably the outcome of untreated acute appendicitis. The term is now used to describe a life-threatening acute inflammatory destruction of the mucosa of the cecal region occurring in neutropenic individuals. The presumed pathogenesis is impaired mucosal immunity in combination with compromised blood flow in the cecal region.

Diversion Colitis

Diversion colitis is an inflammatory mucosal lesion occurring in segments of the colon that have been surgically isolated. Colonic enterocytes derive a significant portion of their caloric supply from short-chain fatty acids present in the luminal stream. Surgical diversion of the stream, as through an ileostomy, renders the colonic mucosa susceptible to nutritional deprivation. The changes may range from very mild with increased lamina propria lymphocytes, to a severe exudative diarrheal disease that resembles ulcerative colitis. Restoration of fecal flow through the colon, or enemas containing short-chain fatty acids, permits mucosal recovery.

Solitary Rectal Ulcer Syndrome

Solitary rectal ulcer syndrome is an inflammatory condition of the rectum resulting from motor dysfunction of the anorectal musculature. Dysregulation of the anorectal sphincter, in particular impaired relaxation of the anorectal sling, may create sharp angulation of the anterior rectal shelf. Abrasion of the overlying rectal mucosa creates an oval ulcer and surrounding mucosal inflammation, frequently with the formation of an inflammatory polyp. Associated partial prolapse of the rectal mucosa is common. Patients experience a characteristic triad: rectal bleeding, mucus discharge from the anus, and superficial ulceration of the anterior rectal wall.

Malabsorption Syndromes

Malabsorption is characterized by defective absorption of fats, fat-soluble and other vitamins, proteins, carbohydrates, electrolytes and minerals, and water. The most common clinical presentation is chronic diarrhea, and the hallmark of malabsorption is steatorrhea (excessive fecal fat content). At the most basic level, malabsorption is the result of disturbance of at least one of these normal digestive functions:

1. *Intraluminal digestion,* in which proteins, carbohydrates and fats are broken down into assimilable forms. The process begins in the mouth with saliva, receives a major boost from gastric peptic digestion, and continues in the small intestine, assisted by the emulsive action of bile salts (see Chapter 18).
2. *Terminal digestion,* which involves the hydrolysis of carbohydrates and peptides by disaccharidases and peptidases, respectively, in the brush border of the small intestinal mucosa.
3. *Transepithelial transport,* in which nutrients, fluid, and electrolytes are transported across the epithelium of the small intestine for delivery to the intestinal vasculature. Absorbed fatty acids are converted to triglycerides and, with cholesterol, are assembled into chylomicrons for delivery to the intestinal lymphatic system.

The major diseases and disorders causing malabsorption are listed in Table 17–9. This classification is most helpful for diseases in which there is a single, clear-cut abnormality. In many malabsorptive disorders a defect in one pathophysiologic process predominates, but others may contribute or may be secondary outcomes of the primary cause. Although many causes of malabsorption can be established clinically, small intestinal mucosal biopsy may be required to satisfactorily identify or exclude celiac disease.

Clinically, the malabsorption syndromes resemble each other more than they differ. The consequences of malabsorption affect many organ systems:

TABLE 17–9 Major Malabsorption Syndromes

Defective Intraluminal Digestion
Digestion of fats and proteins • Pancreatic insufficiency, owing to pancreatitis or cystic fibrosis • Zollinger-Ellison syndrome, with inactivation of pancreatic enzymes by excess gastric acid secretion
Solubilization of fat, owing to defective bile secretion • Ileal dysfunction or resection, with decreased bile salt uptake • Cessation of bile flow from obstruction, hepatic dysfunction
Nutrient preabsorption or modification by bacterial overgrowth
Primary Mucosal Cell Abnormalities
Defective terminal digestion • Disaccharidase deficiency (lactose intolerance) • Bacterial overgrowth, with brush border damage
Defective epithelial transport • Abetalipoproteinemia • Primary bile acid malabsorption owing to mutations in the ileal bile acid transporter
Reduced Small Intestinal Surface Area
Gluten-sensitive enteropathy (celiac disease) Crohn disease
Lymphatic Obstruction
Lymphoma Tuberculosis and tuberculous lymphadenitis
Infection
Acute infectious enteritis Parasitic infestation Tropical sprue Whipple disease (*Tropheryma whippelii*)
Iatrogenic
Subtotal or total gastrectomy Short-gut syndrome, following extensive surgical resection Distal ileal resection or bypass

- *Alimentary tract:* diarrhea, both from nutrient malabsorption and excessive intestinal secretions, flatus, abdominal pain, weight loss, and mucositis resulting from vitamin deficiencies
- *Hematopoietic system:* anemia from iron, pyridoxine, folate, and/or vitamin B_{12} deficiency and bleeding from vitamin K deficiency
- *Musculoskeletal system:* osteopenia and tetany from calcium, magnesium, and vitamin D deficiency
- *Endocrine system:* amenorrhea, impotence, and infertility from generalized malnutrition; hyperparathyroidism from protracted calcium and vitamin D deficiency
- *Epidermis:* purpura and petechiae from vitamin K deficiency, edema from protein deficiency, dermatitis and hyperkeratosis from deficiencies of vitamin A, zinc, essential fatty acids and niacin
- *Nervous system:* peripheral neuropathy from vitamin A and B_{12} deficiencies.

The passage of abnormally bulky, frothy, greasy, yellow, or gray stools *(steatorrhea)* is a prominent feature of malabsorption, accompanied by weight loss, anorexia, abdominal distention, borborygmi, and muscle wasting. *The malabsorptive disorders most commonly encountered in the United States are celiac disease, pancreatic insufficiency, and Crohn disease.*

Pancreatic insufficiency, primarily from chronic pancreatitis or cystic fibrosis, is a major cause of *defective intraluminal digestion.* Typical features of defective intraluminal digestion are an osmotic diarrhea from undigested nutrients and steatorrhea. Excessive growth of normal bacteria within the proximal small intestine (*bacterial overgrowth,* discussed earlier) also impairs intraluminal digestion and can damage mucosal epithelial cells, causing impaired terminal digestion and epithelial absorption.

CELIAC DISEASE

Celiac disease (also referred to as celiac sprue, gluten-sensitive enteropathy) is a chronic disease, in which there is a characteristic mucosal lesion of the small intestine and impaired nutrient absorption, which improves on withdrawal of wheat gliadins and related grain proteins from the diet.[63] Celiac disease occurs largely in Caucasians and is rare or nonexistent among native Africans, Japanese, and Chinese. Its prevalence in the United States is somewhat difficult to define; in Europe the prevalence is in the range of 1:100 to 1:200.[64] The disease was first described more than a century ago, but its connection to gluten was not known until the 1940s, changing its clinical management.

Pathogenesis. *The fundamental disorder in celiac disease is a sensitivity to gluten, which is the alcohol-soluble, water-insoluble protein component (gliadin) of wheat and closely related grains (oat, barley, and rye).* The hallmark of this disease is a T-cell mediated chronic inflammatory reaction with an autoimmune component, which most likely develops as a consequence of a loss of tolerance to gluten. Interplay between genetic predisposing factors, the host immune response, and environmental factors is central to disease pathogenesis. The small intestinal mucosa, when exposed to gluten, accumulates intraepithelial CD8+ T cells and large numbers of lamina propria CD4+ T cells, which are sensitized to gliadin. The recognized epitopes are confined to residues 57–75 of gliadin.[65]

It has been long known that family history is important in celiac disease. Almost all individuals with celiac disease share the major histocompatibility complex class II HLA-DQ2 or HLA-DQ8 haplotype. It has been proposed that gliadin is deamidated by the enzyme transglutaminase and that deamidated gliadin peptides bind to DQ2 and DQ8. Recognition of these peptides by CD4+ T cells leads to secretion of interferon γ, which damages the intestinal wall. Although this is an attractive hypothesis, its key elements remain to be proven. It is also unclear how CD8+ T cells accumulate in the epithelium. They do not recognize gliadin, but seem to respond to stress-induced molecules on epithelial cells. The epithelial cells secrete large amounts of IL-15 that activates CD8+ T cells and increases the risk of lymphoma development.

Morphology. By endoscopy, the small intestinal mucosa appears flat or scalloped, or may be visually normal. Biopsies demonstrate **diffuse enteritis, with marked atrophy or total loss of villi.** The surface epithelium shows vacuolar degeneration, loss of the microvillus brush border, and an increased number of intraepithelial lymphocytes (Fig. 17–38). The crypts, on the other hand, exhibit increased mitotic activity and are elongated, hyperplastic, and tortuous, so that the overall mucosal thickness remains the same. The lamina propria has an overall increase in plasma cells, lymphocytes, macrophages, eosinophils, and mast cells. All these changes are usually more marked in the proximal small intestine than in the distal, since it is the duodenum and proximal jejunum that are exposed to the highest concentration of dietary gluten. Although these changes are characteristic of celiac disease, they can be mimicked by other diseases, most notably tropical sprue. Mucosal histology usually reverts to normal or near-normal following a period of gluten exclusion from the diet.

Clinical Features. The symptoms of celiac disease vary tremendously from patient to patient. Symptomatic diarrhea and failure to thrive may be evident during infancy, yet adults may seek attention only in their fifth decade of life. The classic presentation includes diarrhea, flatulence, weight loss, and fatigue. However, extraintestinal manifestations of malabsorption may overshadow the intestinal symptoms. A charac-

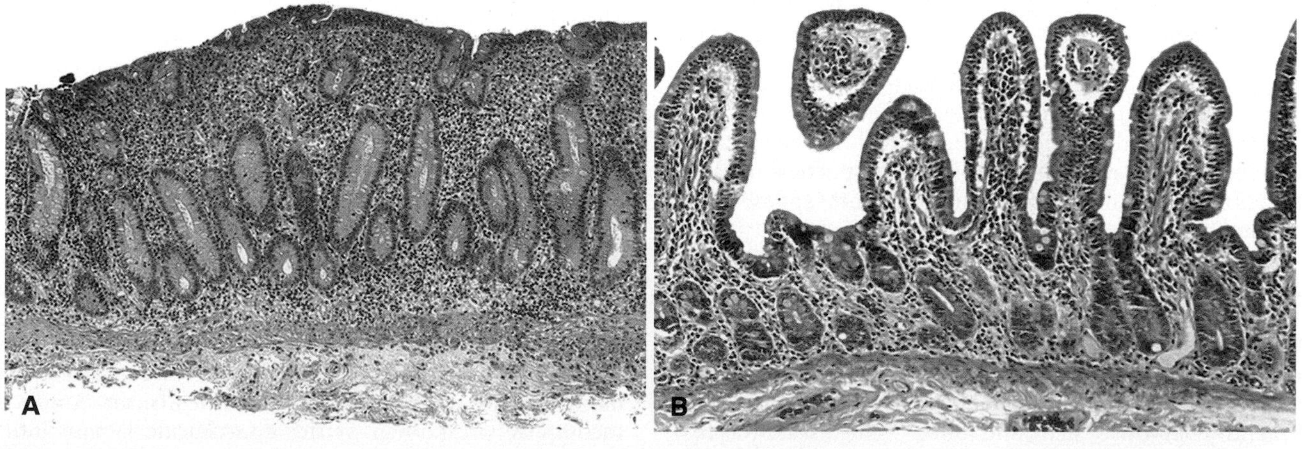

FIGURE 17–38 Celiac disease (gluten-sensitive enteropathy). *A,* A peroral jejunal biopsy specimen of diseased mucosa shows diffuse severe atrophy and blunting of villi, with a chronic inflammatory infiltrate of the lamina propria. *B,* A normal mucosal biopsy.

teristic skin blistering lesion, dermatitis herpetiformis, can occur in patients with celiac disease. Neurologic disorders are occasionally seen. Detection of circulating anti-gliadin or "anti-endomysial" antibodies strongly favors the diagnosis; antibodies against tissue transglutaminase also may be detected, as this is the autoantigen recognized by anti-endomysial antibody. *Definitive diagnosis rests on (1) clinical documentation of malabsorption; (2) demonstration of the intestinal lesion by small bowel biopsy; and (3) unequivocal improvement in both symptoms and mucosal histology on gluten withdrawal from the diet.* If there is doubt about the diagnosis, gluten challenge followed by rebiopsy has been advocated. Serologic tests used for screening or treatment follow-up include the detection of antibodies against tissue transglutaminase and gliadin.

Most patients with celiac disease who adhere to a gluten-free diet remain well indefinitely and ultimately die of unrelated causes. However, there is a long-term risk of malignant disease, which includes non-Hodgkin lymphoma (moderate risk), small intestinal adenocarcinoma, and esophageal squamous cell carcinoma (50- to 100-fold higher risk than the general population).

TROPICAL SPRUE (POSTINFECTIOUS SPRUE)

This condition is so named because it is a celiac-like disease that occurs almost exclusively in people living in or visiting the tropics. The distribution of the disease is curious: It is common in the Caribbean (but not in Jamaica), central and southern Africa, the Indian subcontinent and Southeast Asia, and portions of Central and South America. The disease may occur in endemic form, and epidemic outbreaks have occurred. No specific causal agent has been clearly associated with tropical sprue, but bacterial overgrowth by enterotoxigenic organisms (e.g., *E. coli* and *Hemophilus*) has been implicated.

Morphology. Intestinal changes are extremely variable, ranging from near normal to severe diffuse enteritis. Unlike celiac sprue, injury is seen at all levels of the small intestine. Patients frequently have folate and/or vitamin B_{12} deficiency, leading to markedly atypical enlargement of the nuclei of epithelial cells (megaloblastic change), reminiscent of the changes seen in pernicious anemia.

Malabsorption usually becomes apparent within days or a few weeks of an acute diarrheal enteric infection in visitors to endemic locales and may persist if untreated. The mainstay of treatment is broad-spectrum antibiotics, supporting an infectious etiology. Intestinal lymphoma does not appear to be associated with this disorder.

WHIPPLE DISEASE

Whipple disease is a rare disease caused by the bacterium *Tropheryma whippelii.* It is a systemic condition that may involve any organ of the body, but principally affects the intestine, central nervous system, and joints.[66] The disease was first described as intestinal lipodystrophy by George Whipple in 1907. The bacterial etiology was discovered in the 1960s on the basis of ultrastructural observations. The pathogenesis of Whipple disease is still not clear. The causal organism *T. whippelii* is a gram-positive actinomycete, named on the basis of molecular phylogenetic analysis. The bacteria proliferate preferentially within macrophages and invoke no significant host immune reaction.

Morphology. The hallmark of Whipple disease is a small-intestinal mucosa laden with distended macrophages in the lamina propria. The macrophages contain PAS-positive, diastase-resistant granules (which are lysosomes stuffed with partially digested microorganisms) and rod-shaped bacilli on electron microscopy (Fig. 17–39). The PAS stain is not specific for this bacterium. In untreated cases, bacilli can be seen as well in neutrophils, the extracellular space of the lamina propria, and even in epithelial cells. Expansion of the villi by the dense infiltrate of macrophages imparts a shaggy gross appearance to the intestinal mucosal surface; edema of the mucosa thickens the intestinal wall. Accompanying these changes is involvement of mesenteric lymph nodes by the same process and lymphatic dilation, suggesting lymphatic obstruction. The lymphatic blockade is believed to be responsible for lipid deposition in the villi, thus the original impression of *intestinal lipodystrophy.* Bacilli-laden macrophages also can be found in the synovial membranes of affected joints, the brain, cardiac valves, and elsewhere. At each of these sites, inflammation is essentially absent. Functional impairment nevertheless can be considerable at each affected site.

Clinical Features. Whipple disease is principally encountered in Caucasians in the fourth to fifth decades of life, with a strong male predominance of 10:1. Many of the published cases came from rural regions, suggesting an environmental influence. It usually presents as a form of malabsorption with diarrhea and weight loss, sometimes of years' duration. Arthropathy is often the initial presentation. Atypical presentations, with polyarthritis, obscure psychiatric complaints, cardiac abnormalities, and other symptom complexes, are common. Lymphadenopathy and hyperpigmentation are present in over half of patients. Currently, the diagnosis still rests on demonstration of small intestinal PAS-positive macrophages that contain rod-shaped organisms on electron microscopy. The culture of this bacterium in 1997 and the completion of its whole genome sequence in 2003 will most likely give rise to more specific molecular diagnosis of this disease.[67] Response to antibiotic therapy is usually prompt, although some patients have a protracted, refractory course.

DISACCHARIDASE (LACTASE) DEFICIENCY

The disaccharidases, of which the most important is lactase, are located in the apical cell membrane of the villous absorptive epithelial cells. Congenital lactase deficiency is a very rare condition, but acquired lactase deficiency is common, particularly among Native Americans and African Americans. Incomplete breakdown of the disaccharide lactose into its monosaccharides glucose and galactose leads to osmotic diarrhea from the unabsorbed lactose. Bacterial fermentation of

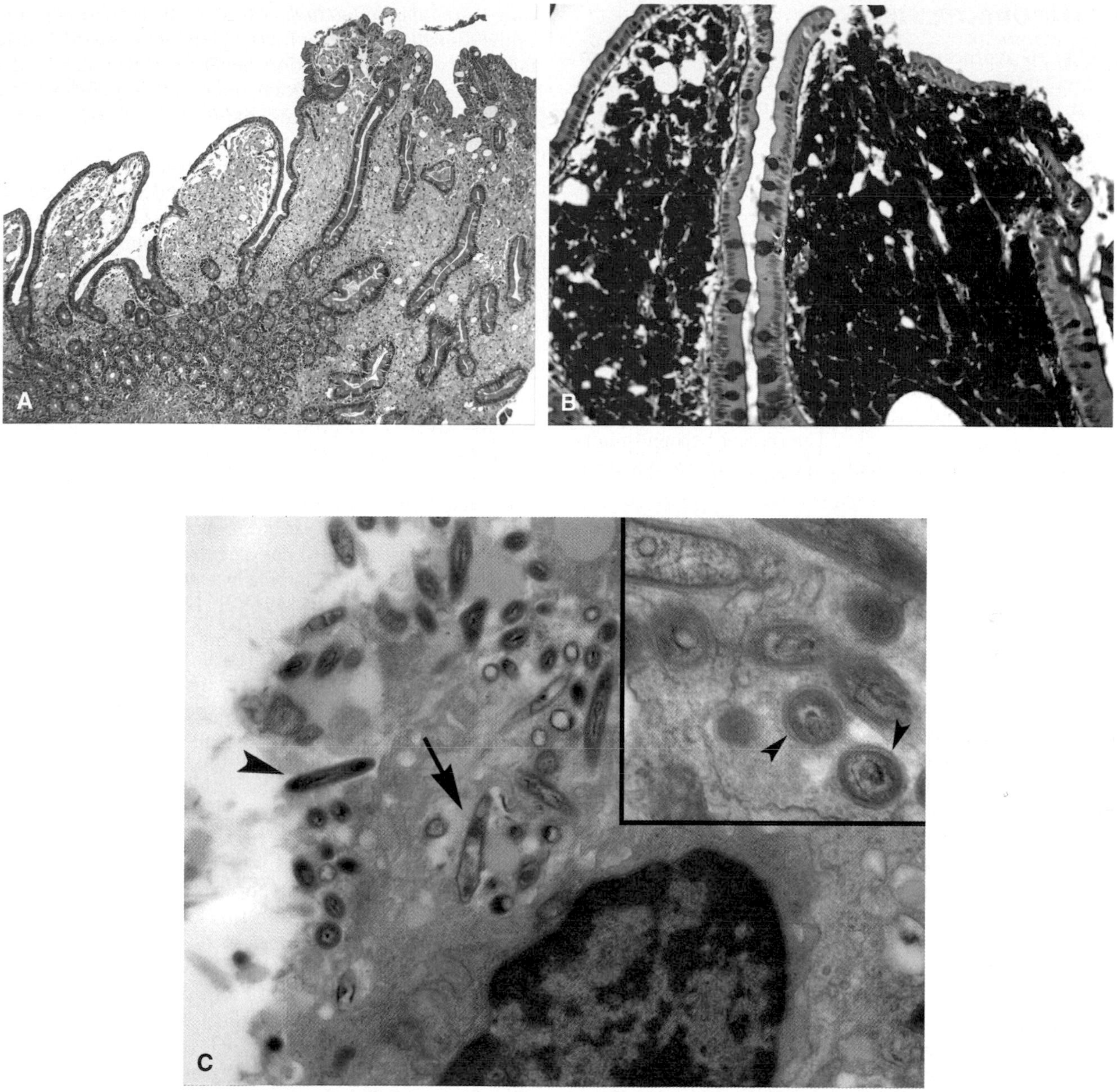

FIGURE 17–39 Whipple disease. *A,* Note foamy macrophages in the lamina propria. *B,* PAS stain showing the positive granules in the foamy macrophages. *C,* Electron micrograph of a lamina propria macrophage showing many bacilli within the cell (*arrow*) and in the extracellular space (*arrowhead*). *Inset,* Higher magnification of macrophage cytoplasm showing cross-sectional profiles of bacilli and their cell walls (small *arrows*). (*C,* courtesy of George Kasnic and Dr. William Clapp, University of Florida, Gainesville, FL.)

the unabsorbed sugars leads to increased hydrogen production, which is readily measured in exhaled air by gas chromatography.

When caused by an inherited enzyme deficiency, malabsorption becomes evident with the initiation of milk feeding. The infants develop explosive, watery, frothy stools and abdominal distention. Malabsorption is promptly corrected when exposure to milk and milk products is terminated. In the adult, lactase insufficiency apparently develops as an acquired disorder, sometimes in association with viral and bacterial enteric infections or other disorders of the gut. Neither light nor electron microscopy has disclosed abnormalities of the mucosal cells of the bowel in either the hereditary or acquired form of the disease.

ABETALIPOPROTEINEMIA

Inability to synthesize apolipoprotein B is a rare inborn error of metabolism transmitted by autosomal recessive inheritance. It is characterized by a defect in the synthesis and export of lipoproteins from intestinal mucosal cells. Free fatty acids and monoglycerides that are produced by hydrolysis of dietary fat enter the absorptive epithelial cells and are re-esterified in the normal fashion but cannot be assembled into chylomicrons. As a consequence, triglycerides are stored within the cells, creating lipid vacuolation that is readily evident under the light microscope, particularly with special fat stains. Concomitantly, there is complete absence in plasma of all lipoproteins containing apolipoprotein B (chylomicrons, very-low-density lipoproteins, and low-density lipoproteins). The failure to absorb certain essential fatty acids leads to lipid membrane defects, readily evident in the characteristic acanthocytic erythrocytes (burr cells). The disease becomes manifest in infancy and is dominated by failure to thrive, diarrhea, and steatorrhea.

Idiopathic Inflammatory Bowel Disease

Idiopathic inflammatory bowel disease is a set of chronic inflammatory conditions resulting from inappropriate and persistent activation of the mucosal immune system, driven by the presence of normal intraluminal flora.[68] The two disorders known as *inflammatory bowel disease* (IBD) are Crohn disease (CD) and ulcerative colitis (UC). These diseases share many common features but have distinctly different clinical manifestations. IBD is common in developed countries, with up to 1 in 200 of individuals of Northern European descent affected by these diseases. The annual incidence of IBD in the United States is approximately 3 to 10 new cases per 100,000 people.

Both CD and UC are chronic, relapsing inflammatory disorders of obscure origin. CD is an autoimmune disease that may affect any portion of the gastrointestinal tract from esophagus to anus, but most often involves the distal small intestine and colon. UC is a chronic inflammatory disease limited to the colon and rectum. Both exhibit extraintestinal inflammatory manifestations. Before considering these diseases separately, the pathogenesis of IBD is considered.

ETIOLOGY AND PATHOGENESIS

A remarkable attribute of the normal gastrointestinal tract is that the mucosal immune system is always poised to respond against ingested pathogens but is unresponsive to normal intestinal microflora.[69] In IBD, this state of homeostasis is disrupted, leading to two *key pathogenic abnormalities—strong immune responses against normal flora, and defects in epithelial barrier function*. The basis of these abnormalities is still not established, which is why both CD and UC are considered idiopathic diseases. However, recently, extensive investigations of animal models, and more limited analyses of lesions from patients, have led to some important conclusions about the pathogenesis of IBD.[70] It is postulated that *IBD results from unregulated and exaggerated local immune responses to commensal microbes in the gut, in genetically susceptible individuals*. Thus, as in many other autoimmune disorders (Chapter 6), the pathogenesis of IBD involves failure of immune regulation, genetic susceptibility, and environmental triggers, specifically microbial flora. Below we summarize some salient points about each of the factors that contribute to IBD.

Genetic Susceptibility. Fifteen percent of IBD patients have affected first-degree relatives, and the lifetime risk if either a parent or sibling is affected is 9%. Dizygotic twins have the concordance rates expected for siblings; monozygotic twins exhibit a 30% to 50% concordance rate for CD. These associations clearly indicate that genetic susceptibility plays an important role in the development of IBD. The disease is a complex multigenic trait, and is not inherited in Mendelian fashion. Many candidate genes are known to be associated with, and likely contribute to, the development of IBD. These include HLA associations; an HLA-DR1/DR1/DQw5 allelic combination has been observed in 27% of North American white patients with CD, whereas HLA-DR2 is increased in patients with UC. A gene called *NOD2* (so named because the encoded protein has a *n*ucleotide-binding *o*ligomerization *d*omain) has recently been shown to be associated with CD.[71] The NOD2 protein is expressed in many types of leukocytes as well as epithelial cells, and is thought to function as an intracellular receptor for microbes. Upon binding microbial components, it may trigger the NF-κB pathway; recall that NF-κB is a transcription factor that triggers the production of cytokines and other proteins involved in innate immune defense against infectious pathogens (Chapter 6). The *NOD2* mutations that are associated with Crohn disease may reduce the activity of the protein, resulting in the persistence of intracellular microbes and uncontrolled, prolonged immune responses. There is, however, no direct proof in support of this hypothesis. Other gene(s) associated with CD have been localized to chromosome 5q31; although a candidate gene in this locus has not been identified, this region is rich in genes encoding several cytokines that may contribute to IBD. Finally, it is worth mentioning that in inbred mice, the knockout of many different genes, individually, leads to the common pathologic manifestation of chronic inflammation in the intestine. It is, therefore, likely that immune dysregulations arising by multiple mechanisms may contribute to IBD in humans.

Role of Intestinal Flora. Animal studies have definitively established the importance of gut flora in IBD.[72] If gene-knockout mice that normally develop IBD are made germ-free, the disease disappears. However, the hunt for a specific microbe as the underlying cause has been largely fruitless. There is also no clear evidence that reducing intestinal flora has a beneficial effect on the course of IBD in humans. Microbes could exacerbate immune reactions by providing antigens and inducing costimulators and cytokines, all of which contribute to T-cell activation (Chapter 6). Defects in the barrier function of the intestinal epithelium could allow luminal flora to gain access to the mucosal lymphoid tissue, and thus trigger immune responses.

Abnormal T-Cell Responses. It is believed that the exaggerated local immune response in IBD is a consequence of too much T-cell activation and/or too little control by regulatory T lymphocytes. Both aspects have been clearly illustrated in animal models of the disease, and the lesions in humans show clear evidence of T-cell reactions (see below).

Thus, susceptibility genes, intestinal flora, and defective control of immune reactions all seem to play a role in the initiation and progression of IBD. One interesting, and largely unanswered question is, are these diseases caused by "true" autoimmunity, i.e. are the immune responses directed against self-antigens in the intestinal epithelium or only against the antigens of intestinal microbes. Regardless of the specificity of the pathogenic immune response, several features of the response and its role in the disease are known.

- In both CD and UC, the prime culprits appear to be T-cells, particularly CD4+ T-cells, and the lesions are likely caused by T-cells and their products. Although antibodies against certain self-antigens, such as tropomyosin, have been detected in some patients with UC, it is not clear that these autoantibodies play a pathogenic role.
- Crohn disease appears to be the result of a chronic delayed-type hypersensitivity reaction induced by IFN-γ-producing T_H1 cells. The nature of the inflammatory infiltrate, especially the presence of granulomas, is consistent with a T_H1 response.
- Although animal models suggest that ulcerative colitis is caused by excessive activation of T_H2 cells, in the human disease the signature T_H2 cytokine, IL-4, has not been found in the lesions. It may be that the lesions are caused by an atypical T_H2 response, or that there is no consistent pattern of T cell activation or dominant cytokine production.

Diagnosis of IBD. Since the exact etiology of IBD is not known, the diagnosis of IBD and the distinction between CD and UC are dependent on clinical history, radiographic examination, laboratory findings, and pathologic examination of tissue. There is no single test upon which a diagnosis is made. Even with the best efforts, the distinction between the two diseases still cannot be made in some cases. As discussed later, pathologic appearance, both macroscopic and microscopic, plays a central role in establishing a definitive diagnosis. In recent years, considerable effort has been given to developing accurate noninvasive laboratory tests.[73] The pANCA (perinuclear antineutrophilic cytoplasmic antibody) is positive in 75% of patients with UC and in only 11% with CD.[74] Another test detects an antibody against the cell wall mannan polysaccharide of *Saccharomyces cerevisiae* (ASCA). This antibody appears to be elevated in CD patients. The clinical utility of these tests remains to be proven.

CROHN DISEASE

When first described by Crohn, Ginsburg, and Oppenheimer in 1932, this idiopathic disorder was thought to be limited to the terminal ileum, hence the designation *terminal ileitis.* Recognition that sharply delineated bowel segments might be affected, with intervening unaffected ("skip") areas, led to the alternative name *regional enteritis.* Predominant involvement of the colon gave rise to the term *granulomatous colitis.* It is now clear that any level of the alimentary tract may be involved and that there are systemic manifestations; thus, the eponymic name *Crohn disease* is preferred. *When fully developed, Crohn disease is characterized pathologically by (1) sharply delimited and typically transmural involvement of the bowel by an inflammatory process with mucosal damage, (2) the presence of noncaseating granulomas, and (3) fissuring with formation of fistulae.*

Epidemiology. Crohn disease occurs throughout the world, but primarily in Western developed populations. Its annual incidence in the United States is around 3 per 100,000, with rates between 4 and 10 per 100,000 reported in Great Britain and Scandinavia. The incidence and prevalence of CD has been steadily rising in the United States and Northern Europe. It occurs at any age, from young childhood to advanced age, but peak ages of detection are the second and third decades of life with a minor peak in the sixth and seventh decades. Females are affected slightly more often than males. Whites appear to develop the disease two to five times more often than do nonwhites. In the United States, CD occurs three to five times more often among Jews than among non-Jews. Smoking is a strong exogenous risk factor.

Morphology. In CD, there is gross involvement of the small intestine alone in about 40% of cases, of small intestine and colon in 30%, and of the colon alone in about 30%. CD may involve the duodenum, stomach, esophagus, and even mouth, but these sites are distinctly uncommon. In diseased bowel segments, the serosa is granular and dull gray, and often the mesenteric fat wraps around the bowel surface (creeping fat). The mesentery of the involved segment is also thickened, edematous, and sometimes fibrotic. **The intestinal wall is rubbery and thick, as a consequence of edema, inflammation, fibrosis, and hypertrophy of the muscularis propria.** As a result, the lumen is almost always narrowed; in the small intestine this is evidenced on x-ray as the "string sign," a thin stream of barium passing through the diseased segment. Strictures may occur in the colon but are usually less severe. **A classic feature of CD is the sharp demarcation of diseased bowel segments from adjacent uninvolved bowel.** When multiple bowel segments are involved, the intervening bowel is essentially normal **("skip" lesions).**

A characteristic sign of early disease is focal mucosal ulcers resembling canker sores (aphthous ulcers), edema, and loss of the normal mucosal texture. With progressive disease, mucosal ulcers coalesce into long, serpentine linear ulcers, which tend to be oriented along the axis of the bowel (Fig. 17–40). As the intervening mucosa tends to be relatively spared, the mucosa acquires a coarsely tex-

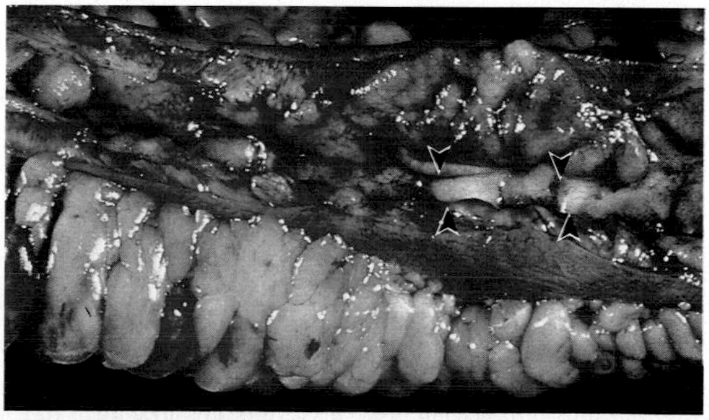

FIGURE 17–40 Crohn disease of ileum, showing narrowing of the lumen, bowel wall thickening, serosal extension of mesenteric fat ("creeping fat"), and linear ulceration of the mucosal surface *(arrowheads).*

tured, cobblestone appearance. **Narrow fissures develop between the folds of the mucosa,** often penetrating deeply through the bowel wall (Fig. 17–41) and leading to bowel adhesions and serositis. Further extension of fissures leads to **fistula or sinus tract formation,** either to an adherent viscus, to the outside skin, or into a blind cavity. Free perforation or localized abscesses may also develop.

The characteristic histologic features of CD are:

- ***Mucosal inflammation.*** The earliest lesion in CD appears to be focal neutrophilic infiltration into the epithelial layer, particularly overlying mucosal lymphoid aggregates. As the disease becomes more established, neutrophils infiltrate isolated crypts; when a sufficient number of neutrophils have traversed the epithelium of a crypt (both in the small and large intestines), a ***crypt abscess*** is formed, usually with ultimate destruction of the crypt.
- ***Chronic mucosal damage.*** **The hallmark of inflammatory bowel disease, both CD and UC, is chronic mucosal damage.** Architectural distortion is manifested in the small intestine as variable villus blunting; in the colon, crypts exhibit irregularity and branching. The degree of the glandular architectural distortion in CD is usually less severe than in UC. Crypt destruction leads to progressive atrophy, particularly in the colon. The mucosa may undergo metaplasia: This may take the form of gastric antral-type glands **(pyloric metaplasia)** or the development of Paneth cells in the distal colon, where they are normally absent (Paneth cell metaplasia).
- ***Ulceration.*** Ulceration is the usual outcome of severe active disease. Ulceration may be superficial, may undermine adjacent mucosa in a lateral fashion, or may penetrate deeply into underlying tissue layers. There is often an abrupt transition between ulcerated and adjacent normal mucosa.
- ***Transmural inflammation affecting all layers.*** Chronic inflammatory cells suffuse the affected mucosa and, to a lesser extent, all underlying tissue layers. Lymphoid aggregates are usually scattered throughout the bowel wall.
- ***Noncaseating granulomas.*** In about half of the cases, sarcoid-like granulomas may be present in all tissue layers, both within areas of active disease and in uninvolved regions of the bowel (Fig. 17–42). Granulomas have been documented throughout the alimentary tract, from mouth to rectum, in patients with CD limited to one bowel segment. Conversely, the absence of granulomas does not preclude the diagnosis of CD.
- ***Other mural changes.*** In diseased segments, the muscularis mucosa usually exhibits reduplication, thickening, and irregularity. Fibrosis of the submucosa, muscularis propria, and mucosa eventually leads to stricture formation. Less common findings are mucosal and submucosal lymphangiectasia, hypertrophy of mural nerve fibers, and localized vasculitis.

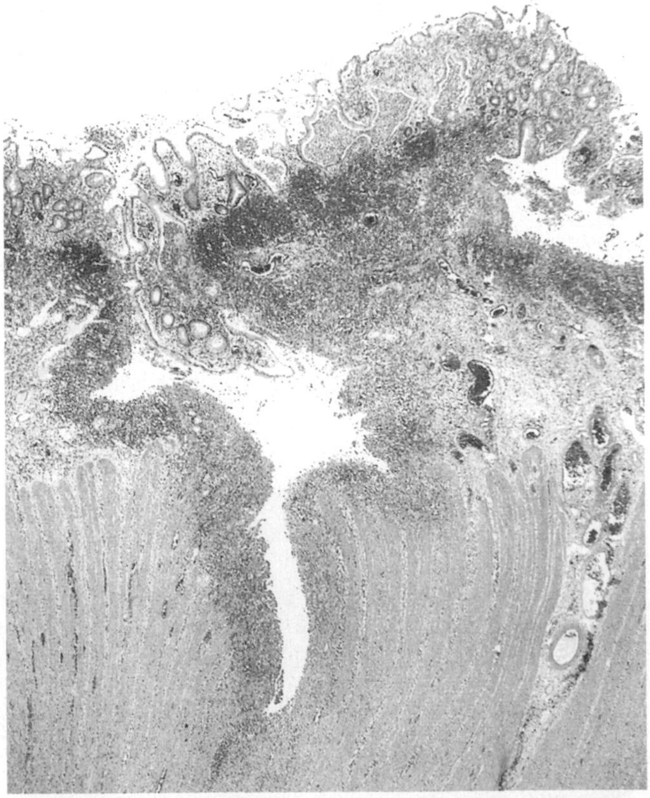

FIGURE 17–41 Crohn disease of the colon; a deep fissure extending into the muscle wall, a second, shallow ulcer (on the upper right), and relative preservation of the intervening mucosa. Abundant lymphocyte aggregates are present, evident as dense blue patches of cells at the interface between mucosa and submucosa.

Clinical Features. The clinical manifestations of Crohn disease are extremely variable. They are generally more subtle than those of UC. The disease usually begins with intermittent attacks of relatively mild diarrhea, fever, and abdominal pain, spaced by asymptomatic periods lasting for weeks to many months. Often the attacks are precipitated by periods of physical or emotional stress. Although emotional influences are thought not to have any direct role in the initiation of the disease, they may contribute to flare-ups. In those with colonic involvement, occult or overt fecal blood loss may lead to

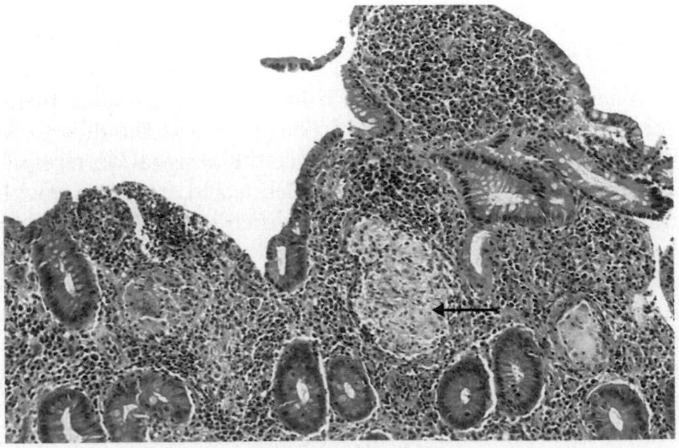

FIGURE 17–42 Crohn disease of the colon. A noncaseating granuloma is present in the lamina propria of an uninvolved region of colonic mucosa (*arrow*).

anemia over time, but massive bleeding is uncommon. In about one-fifth of patients the onset is more abrupt, with acute right lower quadrant pain, fever, and diarrhea sometimes suggesting acute appendicitis or an acute bowel perforation. The course of the disease includes bouts of diarrhea with fluid and electrolyte losses, weight loss, and weakness.

During this lengthy, chronic disease, complications may arise from *fibrosing strictures,* particularly of the terminal ileum, and *fistulas* to other loops of bowel, the urinary bladder, vagina, or perianal skin, or into a peritoneal abscess. Extensive involvement of the small bowel, including the terminal ileum, may cause *marked loss of albumin (protein-losing enteropathy), generalized malabsorption, specific malabsorption of vitamin B_{12}* (resulting in *pernicious anemia*), *or malabsorption of bile salts, leading to steatorrhea.*

Extraintestinal manifestations of this disease include migratory polyarthritis, sacroiliitis, ankylosing spondylitis, erythema nodosum, and clubbing of the fingertips. Hepatic primary sclerosing cholangitis (see Chapter 18) occurs, but the association is not as strong as in UC. Any of these manifestations can develop before onset of intestinal symptoms. Deranged systemic immunity is thought to underlie these related disorders. Uveitis, nonspecific mild hepatic pericholangitis, and renal disorders secondary to trapping of the ureters in the inflammatory process sometimes develop. Systemic amyloidosis is a rare late consequence.

There is an increased incidence of cancer of the gastrointestinal tract in patients with long-standing progressive CD, with a five- to six-fold increased risk over age-matched populations. However, the risk of cancer in CD is considerably less than in patients with chronic UC.

ULCERATIVE COLITIS

Ulcerative colitis is an ulceroinflammatory disease limited to the colon and affecting only the mucosa and submucosa except in the most severe cases. Unlike CD, *UC extends in a continuous fashion proximally from the rectum. Well-formed granulomas are absent.* Like CD, UC is a systemic disorder associated in some patients with migratory polyarthritis, sacroiliitis, ankylosing spondylitis, uveitis, hepatic involvement (pericholangitis and primary sclerosing cholangitis; Chapter 18), and skin lesions.

Epidemiology. UC is global in distribution and varies in incidence relative to CD, supporting the concept that they are separate diseases. In the United States, Great Britain, and Scandinavia the incidence is about 4 to 12 per 100,000 population, which is slightly greater than CD. As with CD, the incidence of this condition has risen in recent decades. In the United States it is more common among whites than among blacks, and females are affected more often than males. The onset of disease peaks between ages 20 and 25, but the condition may arise in both younger and considerably older individuals. Nonsmoking is associated with UC; ex-smokers are at higher risk for developing UC than never-smokers.

Morphology. Ulcerative colitis involves the rectum and extends proximally in a retrograde fashion to involve the entire colon ("pancolitis") in the more severe cases. It is a disease of continuity, and "skip" lesions such as occur in Crohn disease are not found (Fig. 17–43). In 10% of patients with severe pancolitis, the distal ileum may develop mucosal inflammation ("backwash ileitis"). This is probably due to the incompetence of the iliocecal valve, resulting in reflux of the inflammatory material from the colon. In contrast to CD, the ileitis is often diffuse and limited to within 25 cm from the ileocecal valve. The appendix may be involved with both CD and UC.

In the course of colonic involvement with UC, the mucosa may exhibit slight reddening and granularity with friability and easy bleeding. With fully developed severe, active inflammation, there may be extensive and broad-based **ulceration of the mucosa in the distal colon or throughout its length** (Fig. 17–44). Isolated islands of regenerating mucosa bulge upward to create **pseudopolyps.** Often the undermined edges of adjacent ulcers interconnect to create tunnels covered by tenuous mucosal bridges. As with CD, the ulcers of UC are frequently aligned along the axis of the colon, but rarely do they replicate the linear serpentine ulcers of CD. With indolent chronic disease or with healing of active disease, progressive mucosal atrophy leads to a flattened and attenuated mucosal surface (Fig. 17–45). Unlike CD, mural thickening does not occur in UC, and the serosal surface is usually completely normal. Only in the most severe cases of ulcerative disease (UC, CD, and other severe inflammatory diseases) does toxic damage to the muscularis propria and neural plexus lead to complete shutdown of neuromuscular function. In this instance the colon progressively swells and becomes gangrenous **(toxic megacolon)** (Fig. 17–46).

The mucosal alterations in UC are similar to those of colonic CD, with inflammation, chronic mucosal

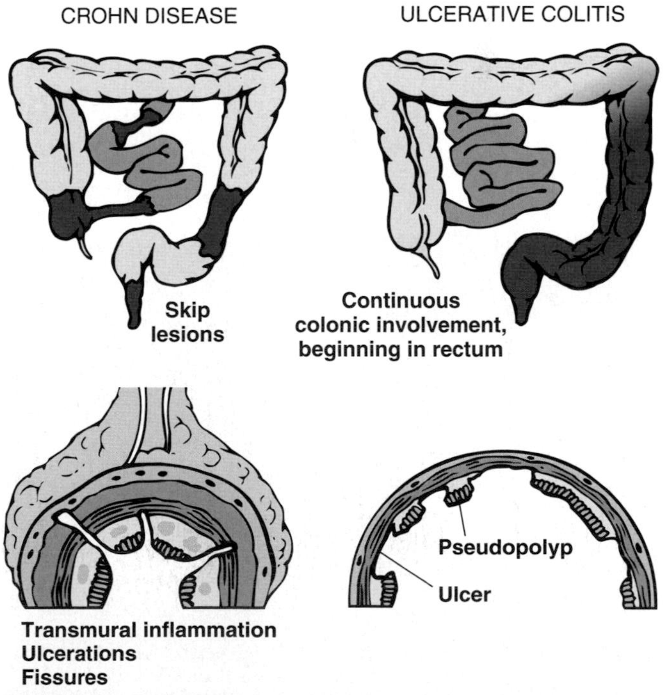

FIGURE 17–43 Comparison of the distribution patterns of Crohn disease and ulcerative colitis, as well as the different conformations of the ulcers and wall thickenings.

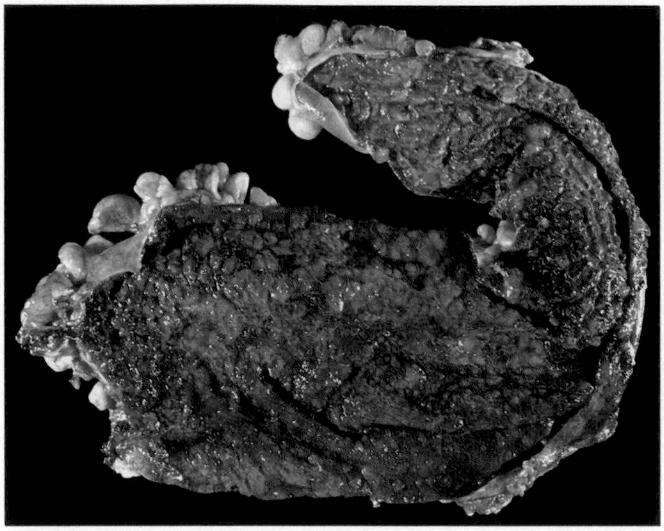

FIGURE 17–44 Ulcerative colitis. Ulcerated hemorrhagic surface with knobby pseudopolyps. (Courtesy of Dr. Kim Bechard, Brigham and Women's Hospital, Boston, MA.)

damage, and ulceration (Fig. 17–47). First, a diffuse, predominantly mononuclear inflammatory infiltrate in the lamina propria is almost universally present, even at the time of clinical presentation. Neutrophilic infiltration of the epithelial layer may produce collections of neutrophils in crypt lumina **(crypt abscesses).** These are not specific for UC and may be observed in CD or any active inflammatory colitis. Unlike CD, there are no granulomas, although rupture of crypt abscesses may incite a foreign body reaction in the lamina propria. Second, further destruction of the mucosa leads to outright ulceration, extending into the submucosa and sometimes leaving only the raw, exposed muscularis propria. Third, with remission of active disease, granulation tissue fills in the ulcer craters, followed by regeneration of the mucosal epithelium. Submucosal fibrosis and mucosal architectural disarray and atrophy remain as residua of healed disease.

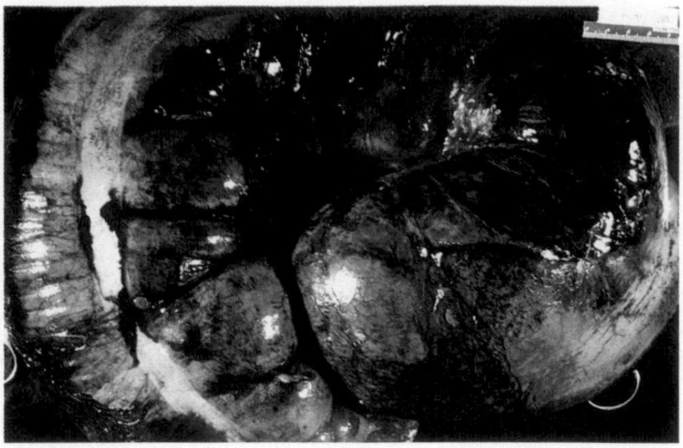

FIGURE 17–46 Toxic megacolon. Complete cessation of colon neuromuscular activity has led to massive dilatation of the colon and black-green discoloration signifying gangrene and impending rupture.

A key feature of UC is that the mucosal damage is continuous from the rectum and extending proximally. In CD, mucosal damage in the colon may be continuous but is just as likely to exhibit skip areas. It should be noted that quiescent UC, particularly treated disease in which active neutrophilic inflammation is not present, may appear virtually normal histologically. This does not preclude risk for dysplasia, as now described.

Particularly significant in ulcerative colitis is the spectrum of epithelial changes signifying dysplasia and the progression to frank carcinoma. Nuclear atypia and loss of cytoplasmic differentiation may be present in inflamed or uninflamed colonic mucosa. Epithelial dysplasia is referred to as being **low-grade** or **high-grade;**[75] cytologic features are the key to evaluating dysplasia. Distinguishing between regenerative changes and dysplasia can be very difficult and sometimes impossible. Pathologists are allowed some latitude in noting atypical changes that may not be definitive for a diagnosis of dysplasia.[76] Plaque-like dysplastic lesions, overt polypoid dysplasia (adeno-

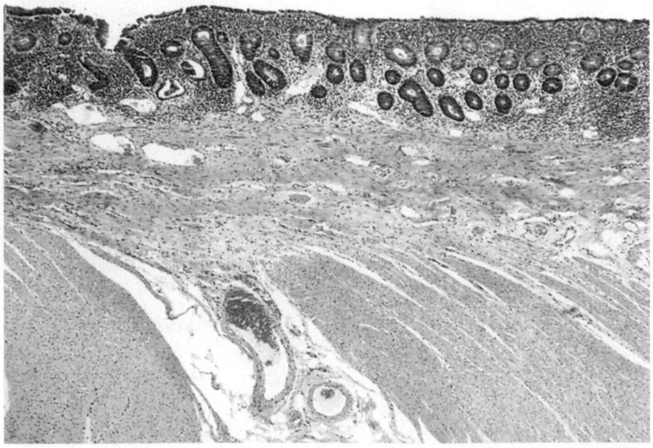

FIGURE 17–45 Ulcerative colitis. Low-power micrograph showing marked chronic inflammation of the mucosa with atrophy of colonic glands, moderate submucosal fibrosis, and a normal muscle wall.

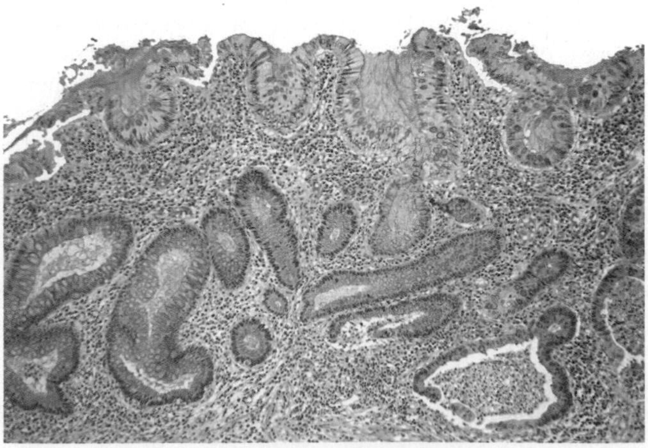

FIGURE 17–47 Ulcerative colitis. Microscopic view of the mucosa, showing diffuse active inflammation with crypt abscess and glandular architectural distortion.

mas), or invasive carcinoma are the ultimate lesions arising from flat dysplasia. It should be noted that elderly patients with UC are also at risk for sporadic adenomas. Distinction between IBD-associated dysplasia and a coexistent incidental adenoma may be difficult.

Clinical Features. Ulcerative colitis typically presents as a relapsing disorder marked by attacks of bloody mucoid diarrhea that may persist for days, weeks, or months and then subside, only to recur after an asymptomatic interval of months to years or even decades. In the fortunate patient, the first attack is the last. At the other end of the spectrum, the explosive initial attack may lead to such serious bleeding and fluid and electrolyte imbalance as to constitute a medical emergency. In most patients, bloody diarrhea containing stringy mucus, accompanied by lower abdominal pain and cramps usually relieved by defecation, is the first manifestations of the disease. In a small number of patients, constipation may appear paradoxically, due to disruption of normal peristalsis. Often the first attack is preceded by a stressful period in the patient's life. Spontaneously, or more often after appropriate therapy, these symptoms abate in the course of days to weeks. Flare-ups, when they do occur, may be precipitated by emotional or physical stress and rarely by concurrent intraluminal growth of enterotoxin-forming *C. difficile*. Sudden cessation of bowel function with toxic dilatation (toxic megacolon) rarely develops with severe acute attacks; perforation is a potentially lethal event.

The outlook for patients with UC depends on two factors: (1) the severity of active disease and (2) its duration. About 60% of patients have clinically mild disease. In these individuals, the bleeding and diarrhea are not severe, and systemic signs and symptoms are absent. However, almost all patients (97%) have at least one relapse during a 10-year period, and about 30% of patients require colectomy within the first 3 years of onset due to uncontrollable disease. On rare occasion, the disease runs a fulminant course; unless medically or surgically controlled, this toxic form of the disease can lead to death soon after onset.

The most feared long-term complication of UC is cancer. There is a tendency for dysplasia to arise in multiple sites, and the underlying inflammatory disease may mask the symptoms and signs of carcinoma. UC is characterized by DNA damage with microsatellite instability in mucosal cells. More recently, genomic instability was detected in non-dysplastic areas of patients with UC, suggesting that these patients have DNA repair deficiency and genomic instability throughout the intestinal tract.[77] *The associated carcinomas are often infiltrative without obvious exophytic masses, further underscoring the importance of early diagnosis.* Historically, the risk of cancer is highest in patients with pancolitis of 10 or more years' duration, in whom it is 20- to 30-fold higher than in a control population.[78] However, recent screening programs of patients with UC now indicate that the rate of progression to dysplasia and carcinoma is in fact quite low, provided that initial examinations were negative for dysplasia. Since great cost is involved in mass screening, the debate over the cost-effectiveness of repeated colonoscopies in patients with long-term inactive disease continues; the modest improvement in patient outcome may be related to better patient care, rather than identification of dysplasia per se.

The features of CD and UC are compared in Table 17–10.

Vascular Disorders

ISCHEMIC BOWEL DISEASE

Ischemic lesions may be restricted to the small or large intestine, or may affect both, depending on the particular vessel(s) affected. Acute occlusion of one of the three major supply trunks of the intestines—celiac, superior mesenteric, and inferior mesenteric arteries—may lead to infarction of several meters of intestine. However, insidious loss of one

TABLE 17–10 Distinctive Features of Crohn Disease and Ulcerative Colitis*

Feature	Crohn Disease - SI	Crohn Disease - C	Ulcerative Colitis
Macroscopic			
Bowel region	Ileum ± colon	Colon ± ileum	Colon only
Distribution	Skip lesions	Skip lesions	Diffuse
Stricture	Early	Variable	Late/rare
Wall appearance	Thickened	Thin	Thin
Dilation	No	Yes	Yes
Microscopic			
Inflammation	Transmural	Transmural	Limited in mucosa
Pseudopolyps	No to slight	Marked	Marked
Ulcers	Deep, linear	Deep, linear	Superficial
Lymphoid reaction	Marked	Marked	Mild
Fibrosis	Marked	Moderate	Mild
Serositis	Marked	Variable	Mild to none
Granulomas	Yes (50%)	Yes (50%)	No
Fistulae/sinuses	Yes	Yes	No
Clinical			
Fat/vitamin malabsorption	Yes	Yes, if ileum	No
Malignant potential	Yes	Yes	Yes
Response to surgery	Poor	Fair	Good

*SI, Crohn disease of the small intestine; C, Crohn disease of the colon. Features are often not all present in a single case.

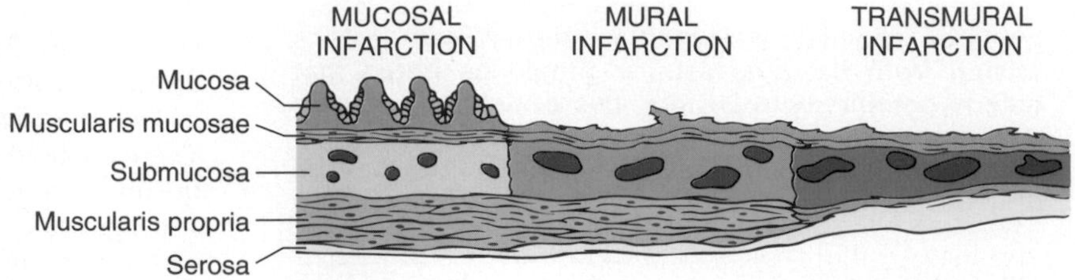

FIGURE 17–48 Acute ischemic bowel disease. Schematic of the three levels of severity, diagrammed for the small intestine.

vessel may be without effect, due to the rich anastomotic interconnections. Lesions within the end arteries, which penetrate the gut wall, produce small, focal ischemic lesions. As depicted in Figure 17–48, the severity of injury ranges from: (1) *transmural infarction* of the gut, involving all visceral layers; to (2) *mural infarction* of the mucosa and submucosa; to (3) *mucosal infarction*, if the lesion extends no deeper than the muscularis mucosae. *Almost always, transmural infarction is caused by mechanical compromise of the major mesenteric blood vessels. Mucosal or mural infarction more often results from hypoperfusion, either acute or chronic.* Mesenteric venous thrombosis is a less frequent cause of vascular compromise. The predisposing conditions for ischemia are as follows:

- *Arterial thrombosis:* severe atherosclerosis (usually at the origin of the mesenteric vessel), systemic vasculitis, dissecting aneurysm, angiographic procedures, aortic reconstructive surgery, surgical accidents, hypercoagulable states, and oral contraceptives
- *Arterial embolism:* cardiac vegetations, angiographic procedures, and aortic atheroembolism
- *Venous thrombosis:* hypercoagulable states, oral contraceptives, antithrombin III deficiency, intraperitoneal sepsis, the postoperative state, invasive neoplasms (particularly hepatocellular carcinoma), cirrhosis, and abdominal trauma
- *Nonocclusive ischemia:* cardiac failure, shock, dehydration, and vasoconstrictive drugs (e.g., digitalis, vasopressin, propranolol)
- *Miscellaneous:* radiation injury, volvulus, stricture, amyloidosis, diabetes mellitus, and internal or external herniation.

Embolic arterial occlusion most often involves the branches of the superior mesenteric artery. The origin of the inferior mesenteric artery from the artery is more oblique, and this may contribute to the relative sparing of this arterial axis from embolism. Despite the multiplicity of possible causes, there remains a significant percentage of cases in which no well-defined basis for the vascular insufficiency can be identified. Mesenteric vascular spasm has been invoked in some cases, without definitive proof.

Ischemic injury has two phases: the *initial hypoxic injury at* the onset of blood supply compromise and *secondary reperfusion injury* at the time of blood resupply to the hypoxic tissue. Most of the intestinal injury in ischemic bowel disease is actually caused by reperfusion. The underlying pathophysiology in reperfusion injury is a complex process. Among the most important factors in this process are the generation of oxygen free radicals, neutrophil infiltration, and the production of inflammatory mediators in tissue that has insufficient metabolic reserve to detoxify injurious free radicals and other mediators (Chapter 1).

Morphology. The severity of vascular compromise and the time frame during which it develops are major determinants of the morphology of ischemic bowel disease. The most severe, acute lesions are considered first.

Transmural Infarction. Small intestinal infarction following sudden and total occlusion of mesenteric arterial blood flow may involve only a short segment, but more often involves a substantial portion. The splenic flexure of the colon is at greatest risk of ischemic injury because it is the watershed between the distribution of the superior and inferior mesenteric arteries, but any portion of the colon may be affected. With mesenteric venous occlusion, anterograde and retrograde propagation of thrombus may lead to extensive involvement of the splanchnic bed. Regardless of whether the arterial or venous side is occluded, the infarction appears hemorrhagic because of blood reflow into the damaged area. In the early stages, the infarcted bowel appears intensely congested and dusky to purple-red (Fig. 17–49), with foci of subserosal and submucosal ecchymotic discoloration. With time, the wall becomes edematous, thickened, rubbery, and hemorrhagic. The lumen commonly contains sanguineous mucus or frank blood. In arterial occlusions the demarcation from normal bowel is usually sharply defined, but in venous occlusions the area of dusky cyanosis fades gradually into the adjacent normal bowel, having no clear-cut definition between viable and nonviable bowel. Histologically, there is obvious edema, interstitial hemorrhage, and sloughing necrosis of the mucosa. Normal features of the mural musculature, particularly cellular nuclei,

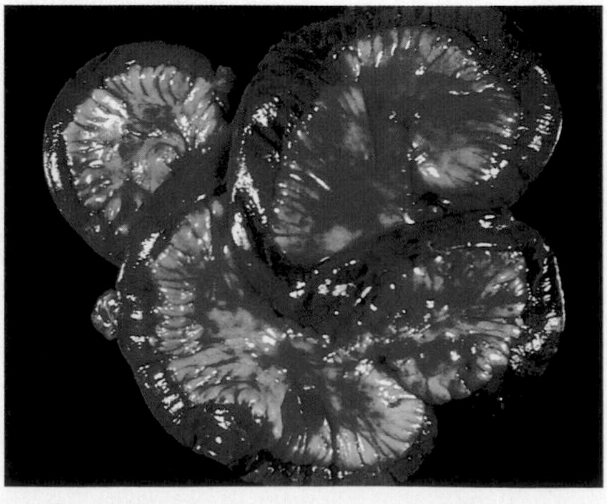

FIGURE 17–49 Infarcted small bowel, secondary to acute thrombotic occlusion of the superior mesenteric artery.

become indistinct. Within 1 to 4 days, intestinal bacteria produce outright gangrene and sometimes perforation of the bowel. There may be little inflammatory response.

Mucosal and Mural Infarction. Mucosal and mural infarction may involve any level of the gut from the stomach to the anus. The lesions may be multifocal or continuous and widely distributed. Affected areas of the bowel may appear dark red or purple, owing to the accumulated luminal hemorrhage. However, hemorrhage and an inflammatory exudate are absent from the serosal surface. On opening the bowel, there is hemorrhagic, edematous thickening of the mucosa, which may penetrate more deeply into the submucosa and muscle wall. Superficial ulceration may be present.

In the mildest form of ischemic injury, the superficial epithelium of the colon or the tips of small intestinal villi may be necrotic or sloughed. Inflammation is absent, and there may only be mild vascular dilation. With complete mucosal necrosis, epithelial sloughing leaves behind only the acellular scaffolding of the lamina propria (Fig. 17–50). When severe, there is extensive hemorrhage and necrosis of multiple tissue layers. Secondary acute and chronic inflammation is evident along the viable margins underlying and adjacent to the affected area. Bacterial superinfection and the formation of enterotoxic bacterial products may induce superimposed pseudomembranous inflammation, particularly in the colon. Thus, the mucosal changes may mimic enterocolitis of nonvascular origin.

Chronic Ischemia. With chronic vascular insufficiency to a region of intestine, mucosal inflammation and ulceration may develop, mimicking both acute enterocolitis from other causes and idiopathic IBD. Submucosal chronic inflammation and fibrosis may lead to stricture (Fig. 17–51). Although colonic strictures typically occur in the watershed area of the splenic flexure, both acute and chronic mucosal ischemia are notoriously segmental and patchy.

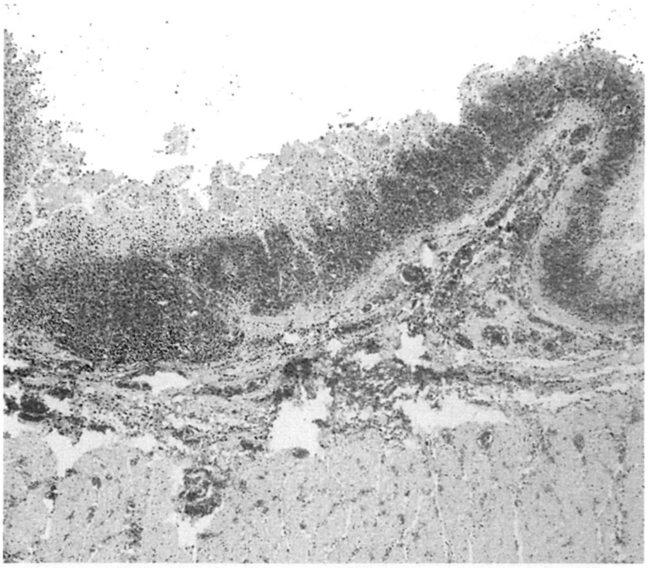

FIGURE 17–50 Mucosal infarction of the small bowel. The mucosa is hemorrhagic, and there is no epithelial layer. The remaining layers of the bowel are intact.

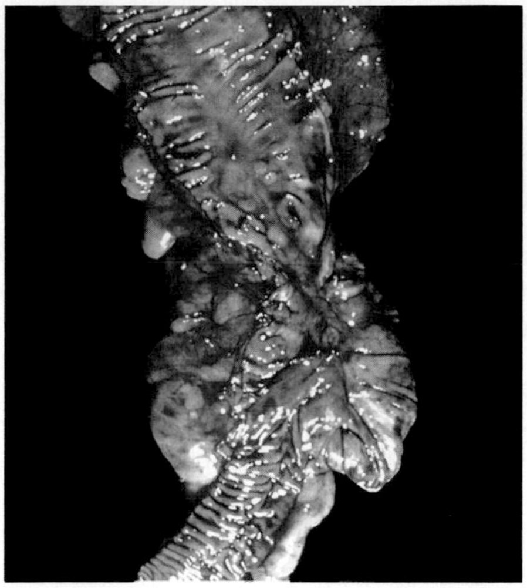

FIGURE 17–51 Chronic ischemia of the colon, resulting in chronic mucosal damage and a stricture.

Clinical Features. Bowel infarction is an uncommon but grave disorder that imposes a 50% to 75% death rate, largely because the window of time between onset of symptoms and perforation is small. It tends to occur in older individuals, when cardiac and vascular diseases are most prevalent. Preexistent abdominal disease also increases the risk of bowel infarction, due to adhesions and torsion. Severe abdominal pain and tenderness develop suddenly in the setting of transmural infarction, sometimes accompanied by nausea, vomiting, and bloody diarrhea or grossly melanotic stool. Patients may progress to shock and vascular collapse within hours. Peristaltic sounds diminish or disappear, and spasm creates board-like rigidity of the abdominal wall musculature. Because there are far more common causes of these physical signs, such as acute appendicitis, perforated peptic ulcer, and acute cholecystitis, the diagnosis of intestinal gangrene may be delayed or missed, with disastrous consequences.

Mucosal and mural infarction, by themselves, may not be fatal, particularly if the cause of vascular compromise is corrected. A confusing array of nonspecific abdominal complaints, combined with intermittent bloody diarrhea, may be the only indication of nonocclusive enteric ischemia. Nevertheless, bowel embarrassment may progress to more extensive infarction, and sepsis or serious blood loss may set in. Chronic ischemic colitis may present as an insidious inflammatory disease, with intermittent episodes of bloody diarrhea interspersed with periods of healing, mimicking IBD.

Several clinical conditions that cause ischemic intestinal injury merit emphasis. Ischemic bowel or infarction may occur in the setting of severe atherosclerosis of the aorta and mesenteric vasculature. Cholesterol emboli dislodged from large vessels occlude smaller vessels downstream, leading to regions of localized compromise. Second, vasculitis affecting the mesenteric vasculature may cause ischemic injury. The commonly seen vasculitides that affect the intestine are polyarteritis nodosum, Henoch-Schönlein disease, and Wegener granulomatosis. Third, amyloidosis often affects mesenteric blood vessels and may actually present as chronic intestinal ischemia.

ANGIODYSPLASIA

Angiodysplasia is a non-neoplastic intestinal lesion of vascular dilation and malformation. Tortuous dilations of submucosal and mucosal blood vessels are seen most often in the cecum or right colon, usually only after the sixth decade of life. Although the prevalence of these lesions is less than 1% in the adult population, *they account for 20% of significant lower intestinal bleeding; intestinal hemorrhage may be chronic and intermittent, or acute and massive.* Most angiodysplasias span the mucosa and submucosa and contain a small amount of smooth muscle, suggesting that they are ectatic nests of preexisting veins, venules, and capillaries. The vascular channels may be separated from the intestinal lumen by only the vascular wall and a layer of attenuated epithelial cells, explaining the propensity toward bleeding.

The pathogenesis of angiodysplasia remains speculative, but it is attributed to mechanical factors operative in the colonic wall, with possibly a congenital contribution. Normal distention and contraction may intermittently occlude the submucosal veins that penetrate through the muscle wall. This then leads to focal dilation and tortuosity of overlying submucosal and mucosal vessels. According to LaPlace's Law, tension in the wall of a cylinder is a function of intraluminal pressure and diameter. Because the cecum has the widest diameter of the colon, it develops the greatest wall tension, perhaps explaining the distribution of these lesions. Vascular degenerative changes related to aging may also play some role. The evidence to support a congenital cause is the association of angiodysplasia with other congenital abnormalities such as aortic stenosis and Meckel diverticulum.

HEMORRHOIDS

Hemorrhoids are variceal dilations of the anal and perianal venous plexuses. These extremely common lesions affect about 5% of the general population and develop secondary to persistently elevated venous pressure within the hemorrhoidal plexus. The most frequent predisposing influences are constipation with straining at stool and the venous stasis of pregnancy. Except for pregnant women, they are rarely encountered in persons under age 30. More rarely, but much more importantly, hemorrhoids may reflect collateral anastomotic channels that develop as a result of portal hypertension (Chapter 18).

Morphology. The varicosities may develop in the inferior hemorrhoidal plexus and thus are located below the anorectal line **(external hemorrhoids).** Alternatively, they may develop from dilation of the superior hemorrhoidal plexus and produce **internal hemorrhoids.** Commonly, both plexuses are affected, and the varicosities are referred to as **combined hemorrhoids.** Histologically, these lesions consist only of thin-walled, dilated, submucosal varices that protrude beneath the anal or rectal mucosa. In their exposed, traumatized position, they tend to become thrombosed and, in the course of time, recanalized. Superficial ulceration, fissure formation, and infarction with strangulation may develop.

Diverticular Disease

A diverticulum is a blind pouch leading off the alimentary tract, lined by mucosa that communicates with the lumen of the gut. Congenital diverticula involve all three layers of the bowel wall. The prototype is the *Meckel diverticulum,* discussed earlier; congenital diverticula are not uncommon in the ascending colon.

Virtually all other diverticula are *acquired* and either lack or have an attenuated muscularis propria. Acquired diverticula may occur in the esophagus, stomach, and duodenum, *but the most common site is the left side of the colon, with the majority in the sigmoid colon.* Acquired duodenal diverticula occur in over 1% of adults, possibly reflecting defects from healed peptic ulcer disease. Multiple diverticula of the jejunum and ileum are rare, occurring in the setting of abnormalities in the muscle wall or myenteric plexus.

Unless otherwise specified, diverticular disease refers to acquired outpouchings of the colonic mucosa and submucosa. *Colonic diverticula are rare in persons under age 30, but in Western adult populations over age 60 the prevalence approaches 50%. They generally occur multiply and are referred to as diverticulosis.* They are much less frequent in nonindustrialized tropical countries and in Japan.

Morphology. Most colonic diverticula are small, flask-like or spherical outpouchings, usually 0.5 to 1 cm in diameter and located in the sigmoid colon (Fig. 17–52*A*). However, the descending colon or entire colon may be affected. They tend to occur alongside the taeniae coli and are elastic, compressible, and easily emptied of fecal contents. As these sacs dissect into the fat-containing peritoneal pouches on the surface of the colon (epiploic appendices), they may be missed on casual inspection. Histologically, colonic diverticula have a thin wall composed of a flattened or atrophic mucosa, compressed submucosa, and attenuated or totally absent muscularis propria (Fig. 17–52*B*). Hypertrophy of the circular layer of the muscularis propria in the affected bowel segment is usually seen; the taeniae coli are also unusually prominent.

Obstruction and/or perforation of diverticula leads to inflammatory changes, producing peridiverticulitis and dissecting into the immediately adjacent pericolic fat. In time, the inflammation may lead to marked fibrotic thickening in and about the colonic wall, sometimes producing narrowing sufficient to resemble a colonic cancer. Extension of diverticular infection may lead to pericolic abscesses, sinus tracts, and sometimes pelvic or generalized peritonitis.

Pathogenesis. The morphology of colonic diverticula strongly suggests that *two factors are important in their genesis: (1) focal weakness in the colonic wall and (2) increased intraluminal pressure.* The colon is unique in that the longitudinal

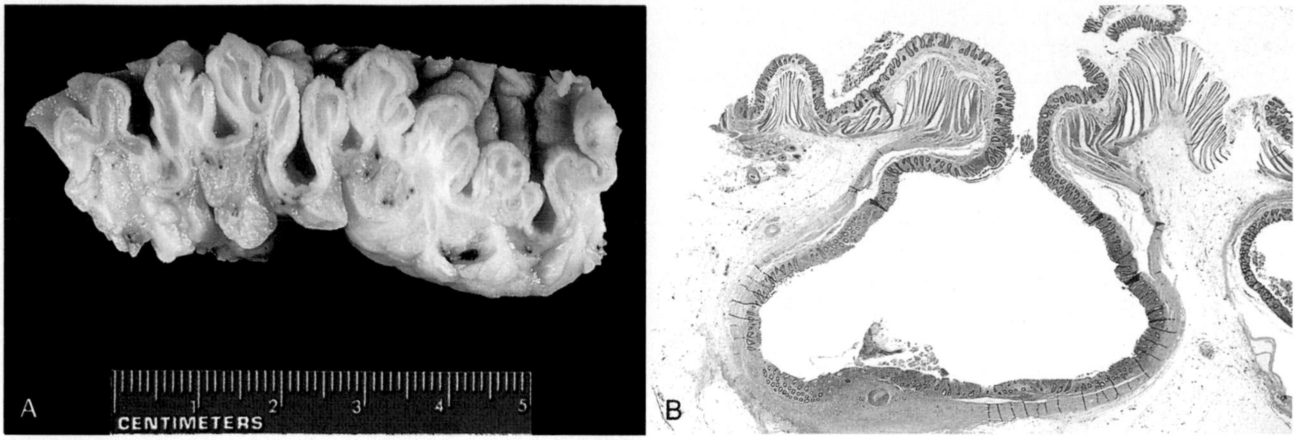

FIGURE 17–52 Diverticulosis. *A,* Section through the sigmoid colon, showing multiple sac-like diverticula protruding through the muscle wall into the mesentery. The muscularis propria in between the diverticular protrusions is markedly thickened. *B,* Low-power photomicrograph of diverticulum of the colon, showing protrusion of mucosa and submucosa through the muscle wall. A dilated blood vessel at the base of the diverticulum was a source of bleeding; some blood clot is present within the diverticular lumen.

muscle coat is not complete, but is gathered into three equidistant bands (the taeniae coli). Where nerves and arterial vasa recta penetrate the inner circular muscle coat alongside the taeniae, focal defects in the muscle wall are created. The connective tissue sheaths accompanying these perforating vessels provide points of weakness for herniations. *Exaggerated peristaltic contractions, with spasmodic sequestration of bowel segments, are the likely cause of increased intraluminal pressure.* It has been proposed that diets low in fiber reduce stool bulk, which in turn leads to increased peristaltic activity, particularly in the sigmoid colon. Exaggerated contractions sequester segments of bowel (segmentation); this deranged motility can lead to symptoms in the absence of inflammation.

Clinical Features. Most individuals with diverticular disease remain asymptomatic throughout their lives, and the lesions are most often discovered incidentally. Only about 20% of those affected ever develop manifestations. These may include intermittent cramping or continuous lower abdominal discomfort, constipation, distention, and a sensation of never being able to completely empty the rectum. Patients sometimes experience alternating constipation and diarrhea. Occasionally there may be minimal chronic or intermittent blood loss, or rarely massive hemorrhages.

Longitudinal studies have shown that diverticula can regress early in their development or may become more numerous and prominent with time. Whether a high-fiber diet prevents such progression or protects against superimposed diverticulitis is still unclear. Diets supplemented with high fiber may provide symptomatic improvement, but the treatment may seem worse than the disease. Even when diverticulitis supervenes, it most often resolves spontaneously. Relatively few patients require surgical intervention for obstructive or inflammatory complications.

Intestinal Obstruction

Obstruction of the gastrointestinal tract may occur at any level, but the small intestine is most often involved due to its narrow lumen. The causes of small and large intestinal obstruction are presented in Table 17–11. Tumors and infarction, although the most serious, account for only about 10% to 15% of small-bowel obstructions. Four of the entities—hernias, intestinal adhesions, intussusception, and volvulus—collectively account for 80% (Fig. 17–53). The clinical manifestations of intestinal obstruction include abdominal pain and distention, vomiting, constipation, and failure to pass flatus. If the obstruction is mechanical or vascular in origin, immediate surgical intervention is usually required.

HERNIAS

A weakness or defect in the wall of the peritoneal cavity may permit protrusion of a pouch-like, serosa-lined sac of peritoneum called a *hernial sac.* The usual sites of such weakness are anterior at the inguinal and femoral canals, umbilicus, and in surgical scars. Rarely, retroperitoneal hernias may occur, chiefly about the ligament of Trietz. *Hernias are of concern chiefly because segments of viscera frequently protrude and become trapped in them (external herniation).* This is particularly true with inguinal hernias, since they tend to have narrow orifices and large sacs. The most frequent intruders are small-bowel loops, but portions of omentum or large bowel also may

TABLE 17–11 Major Causes of Intestinal Obstruction

Mechanical Obstruction
Adhesions
Hernias, internal or external
Volvulus
Intussusception
Tumors
Inflammatory strictures
Obstructive gallstones, fecaliths, foreign bodies
Congenital strictures; atresias
Congenital bands
Meconium in mucoviscoidosis
Imperforate anus
Pseudo-obstruction
Paralytic ileus (e.g., postoperative)
Vascular—bowel infarction
Myopathies and neuropathies (e.g., Hirschsprung)

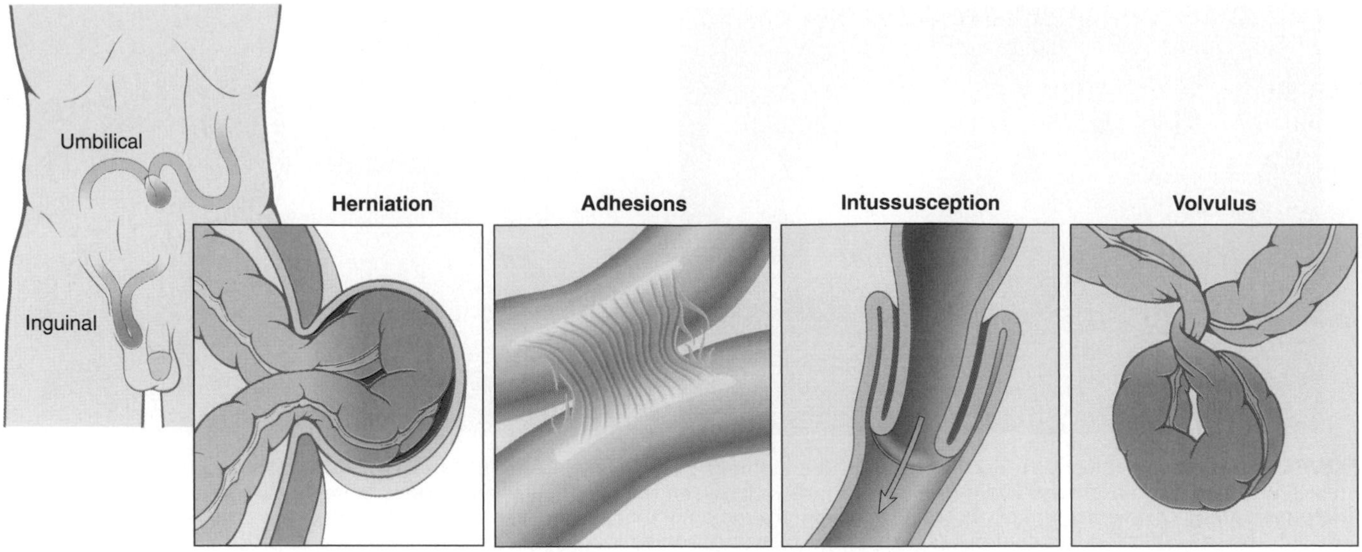

FIGURE 17–53 Schematic depicting the four major causes of intestinal obstruction: (1) Herniation of a segment in the umbilical or inguinal regions; (2) adhesion between loops of intestine; (3) intussusception; (4) volvulus formation.

become trapped. Pressure at the neck of the pouch may impair venous drainage of the trapped viscus. The resultant stasis and edema increase the bulk of the herniated loop, leading to permanent trapping, or *incarceration.* With time, compromise of arterial supply and venous drainage *(strangulation)* leads to infarction of the trapped segment.

ADHESIONS

Surgical procedures, infection, and even endometriosis often cause localized or more general peritoneal inflammation *(peritonitis).* As the peritonitis heals, adhesions may develop between bowel segments and/or the abdominal wall and operative site. These fibrous bridges can create closed loops through which other viscera may slide and eventually become trapped *(internal herniation).* The sequence of events following herniation—obstruction and strangulation—is much the same as with external hernias. Quite rarely, fibrous adhesions arise as congenital defects. Intestinal herniation must be considered, then, even without a previous history of peritonitis or surgery.

INTUSSUSCEPTION

Intussusception occurs when one segment of the intestine, constricted by a wave of peristalsis, suddenly becomes telescoped into the immediately distal segment of bowel. Once trapped, the invaginated segment is propelled by peristalsis farther into the distal segment, pulling its mesentery along behind it. When encountered in infants and children, there is usually no underlying anatomic lesion or defect in the bowel, and the patient is otherwise healthy. Some cases of intussusception are associated with rotavirus infection, suggesting that localized intestinal inflammation may serve as a traction point for the intussusception. However, intussusception in adults signifies an intraluminal mass or tumor as the point of traction. In both settings, intestinal obstruction ensues, and trapping of mesenteric vessels leads to infarction.

VOLVULUS

Complete twisting of a loop of bowel about its mesenteric base of attachment also produces intestinal obstruction and infarction. This lesion occurs most often in large redundant loops of sigmoid, followed in frequency by the cecum, small bowel (all or portions), stomach, or (rarely) transverse colon. Recognition of this seldom-encountered lesion demands constant awareness of its possible occurrence.

Tumors of the Small and Large Intestine

Epithelial tumors of the intestines are a major cause of morbidity and mortality worldwide. The colon (including the rectum) is host to more primary neoplasms than any other organ in the body. Colorectal cancer ranks second only to bronchogenic carcinoma among the cancer killers in North America. Adenocarcinomas constitute the vast majority of colorectal cancers and represent 70% of all malignancies arising in the gastrointestinal tract. Curiously, the small intestine is an uncommon site for benign or malignant tumors despite its great length and vast pool of dividing mucosal cells.

The classification of intestinal tumors is the same for the small intestine and colon and is summarized in Table 17–12. Although small intestinal tumors are addressed first, the bulk of our discussion is devoted to colorectal neoplasia.

TUMORS OF THE SMALL INTESTINE

While the small bowel represents 75% of the length of the alimentary tract, its tumors account for only 3% to 6% of gastrointestinal tumors, with a slight preponderance of benign tumors. The most common benign tumors in the small intestine are adenomas and mesenchymal tumors (see later discussion on gastrointestinal stromal tumors). Lipomas,

TABLE 17–12 Tumors of the Small Intestine and Colon

Non-neoplastic (Benign) Polyps
Hyperplastic polyps
Hamartomatous polyps • Juvenile polyps • Peutz-Jeghers polyps
Inflammatory polyps
Lymphoid polyps
Neoplastic Epithelial Lesions
Benign • Adenoma*
Malignant • Adenocarcinoma* • Carcinoid tumor • Anal zone carcinoma
Mesenchymal Lesions
Gastrointestinal stromal tumor (GIST) (gradation from benign to malignant)
Other benign lesions • Lipoma • Neuroma • Angioma
Kaposi sarcoma
Lymphoma

*Benign and malignant counterparts of the most common neoplasms in the intestines; virtually all lesions are in the colon.

angiomas, and rare hamartomatous mucosal lesions comprise the remainder. One of the enigmas of medicine is the rarity of malignant tumors of the small intestine—annual U.S. death rate is under 1000, representing only about 1% of gastrointestinal malignancies. Small intestinal adenocarcinomas and carcinoids have roughly equal incidence, followed in order by lymphomas and sarcomas. As the latter three exhibit a broader distribution than the small intestine, they are discussed later.

Adenomas

Adenomas account for approximately 25% of benign small intestinal tumors, with benign mesenchymal tumors (especially leiomyomas), lipomas, and neuromatous lesions following in frequency. *Most adenomas occur in the region of the ampulla of Vater.* The usual presentation is that of a 30- to 60-year-old patient with occult blood loss, rarely with obstruction or intussusception; some are discovered incidentally during radiographic investigation. Patients with familial polyposis coli (discussed later) are particularly prone to developing periampullary adenomas. Macroscopically, the ampulla of Vater is enlarged and exhibits a velvety surface (Fig. 17–54). Microscopically, these adenomas resemble their counterparts in the colon (discussed later). Frequently, there is extension of adenomatous tissue into the ampullary orifice, rendering surgical excision difficult, short of a pancreatoduodenectomy to remove the entire ampullary region. Like its counterpart in the colon, the small intestinal adenoma is a premalignant lesion. The adenoma-carcinoma sequence has been demonstrated in small intestinal tumors.

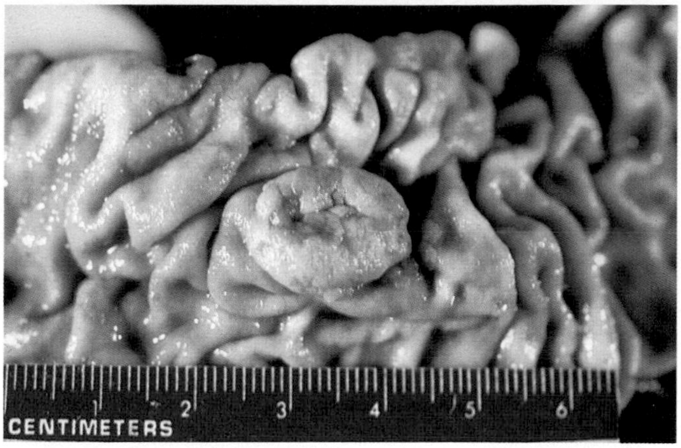

FIGURE 17–54 Adenoma of the ampulla of Vater, showing exophytic tumor at the ampullary orifice.

Adenocarcinoma

The large majority of small intestinal adenocarcinomas occur in the duodenum, usually in 40- to 70-year-old patients. These tumors grow in a napkin-ring encircling pattern or as polypoid exophytic masses, in a manner similar to colonic cancers. Tumors in the duodenum, particularly those involving the ampulla of Vater, may cause obstructive jaundice early in their course. More typically, intestinal obstruction is the presenting event, with symptoms of cramping pain, nausea, vomiting, and weight loss. As in patients with adenoma, fatigue from occult blood loss may be the only sign. Rarely, the tumorous mass is a lead point for intussusception.

A major risk factor for adenocarcinoma of the small intestine is the chronic inflammation associated with CD, although most tumors are sporadic and have no identifiable predisposing condition. Other conditions with increased risk for small intestinal adenocarcinoma are: celiac disease, familial adenomatous polyposis (FAP), hereditary nonpolyposis colorectal cancer (HNPCC) syndrome, and Peutz-Jeghers syndrome. From a broader epidemiologic perspective, alcohol and tobacco consumption are considered risk factors.

At the time of diagnosis, most tumors have already penetrated the bowel wall, invaded the mesentery or other segments of the gut, spread to regional nodes, and sometimes metastasized to the liver and even more widely. Despite these problems, wide en bloc excision of these cancers yields about a 70% five-year survival rate.

TUMORS OF THE COLON AND RECTUM

Colorectal carcinoma is one of the most common malignancies of Western countries. Consideration must first be given to the panoply of non-neoplastic and neoplastic but benign tumorous lesions of the colon and rectum. These are collectively known as *polyps.* Polyps of the colorectal mucosa are extraordinarily common in the older adult population. Several concepts pertaining to terminology must be emphasized (Fig. 17–55):

- A *polyp* is a tumorous mass that protrudes into the lumen of the gut. Presumably all polyps start as small, *sessile* lesions without a definable stalk. In many instances, traction on the mass may create a stalked, or *pedunculated* polyp.

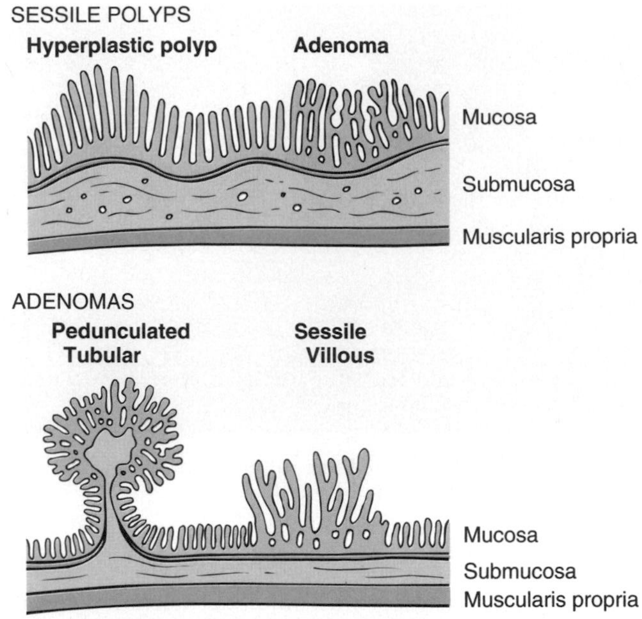

FIGURE 17–55 Diagrammatic representation of two forms of sessile polyp (hyperplastic polyp and adenoma) and of two types of adenoma (pedunculated and sessile). There is only a loose association between the tubular architecture for pedunculated adenomas and the villous architecture for sessile adenomas.

- Polyps may be formed as the result of abnormal mucosal maturation, inflammation, or architecture. These polyps are *non-neoplastic* and do not have malignant potential per se. An example is the *hyperplastic polyp.*
- Those epithelial polyps that arise as the result of proliferation and dysplasia are termed *adenomatous polyps, or adenomas. They are true neoplastic lesions and are precursors of carcinoma.*
- Some polypoid lesions may be caused by submucosal or mural tumors. However, as with the stomach and small intestine, unless otherwise specified the term polyp refers to lesions arising from the epithelium of the mucosa.

Non-Neoplastic Polyps

The overwhelming majority of intestinal polyps occur on a sporadic basis, particularly in the colon, and increase in frequency with age. Non-neoplastic polyps include the hyperplastic polyp, the hamartomatous polyp, the inflammatory polyp, and the lymphoid polyp. Hyperplastic polyps represent about 90% of all epithelial polyps in the large intestine. They may arise at any age but usually are discovered incidentally in the sixth and seventh decades. They are found in more than half of all persons age 60 and older. It is believed that the hyperplastic polyp results from decreased epithelial cell turnover and accumulation of mature cells on the surface. Harmatomatous polyps are malformations of the glands and the stroma. They can occur sporadically or occur in the setting of genetic syndromes (Table 17–13). Inflammatory polyps, also known as *pseudopolyps,* represent islands of inflamed regenerating mucosa surrounded by ulceration. These are seen primarily in patients with severe, active IBD. Lymphoid polyps are an essentially normal variant of the mucosal bumps containing intramucosal lymphoid tissue.

Morphology.

Hyperplastic Polyps. These are small (usually <5 mm in diameter) epithelial polyps that appear as nipple-like, hemispheric, smooth, moist protrusions of the mucosa, usually positioned on the tops of mucosal folds. They may occur singly but more often are multiple, and over half are found in the rectosigmoid colon. Histologically, they are composed of well-formed glands and crypts lined by non-neoplastic epithelial cells, most of which show differentiation into mature goblet or absorptive cells. The delayed shedding of surface epithelial cells leads to infoldings of the crowded epithelial cells and fission of the crypts, creating a serrated epithelial profile and an irregular crypt architecture (Fig. 17–56*A*). Although large hyperplastic polyps may rarely coexist with foci of adenomatous change, **the usual small, hyperplastic polyp is considered to have virtually no malignant potential.** However, the hyperplastic polyps occurring in the setting of the rare hyperplastic polyposis syndrome can harbor epithelial cell dysplasia (adenoma), and hence are considered at risk for carcinoma. The

TABLE 17–13 Hereditary Syndromes Involving the Gastrointestinal Tract

Syndromes	Altered Gene	Pathology in GI Tract
Familial adenomatous polyposis (FAP) • Classic FAP • Attenuated FAP • Gardner syndrome • Turcot syndrome	*APC*	Multiple adenomatous polyps
Peutz-Jeghers syndrome	*STK11*	Hamartomatous polyps
Juvenile polyposis syndrome	*SMAD4* *BMPRIA*	Juvenile polyps
Hereditary nonpolyposis colorectal carcinoma	Defects in mismatch DNA repair genes	Colon cancer
Tuberous sclerosis	*TSC1* *TSC2*	Inflammatory polyps
Cowden disease	*PTEN*	Hamartomatous polyps

underlying genetic basis for this syndrome is not known.

Hamartomatous Polyps. **Juvenile polyps** represent focal hamartomatous malformations of the mucosal epithelium and lamina propria. For the most part they are sporadic lesions, with the vast majority occurring in children younger than age 5. Isolated hamartomatous polyps may be identified in the colon of adults; these incidental lesions are referred to as **retention polyps.** In both age groups, nearly 80% of the polyps occur in the rectum, but they may be scattered throughout the colon. Juvenile polyps tend to be large (1 to 3 cm in diameter), rounded, smooth or slightly lobulated lesions with stalks up to 2 cm in length; retention polyps tend to be smaller (<1 cm diameter). Histologically, lamina propria comprises the bulk of the polyp, enclosing abundant cystically dilated glands. Inflammation is common, and the surface may be congested or ulcerated. In general they occur singly and being hamartomatous lesions have no malignant potential. However, the rare autosomal dominant **juvenile polyposis syndrome,** in which there are multiple (50 to 100) juvenile polyps in the gastrointestinal tract, does carry a risk of adenomas and hence adenocarcinoma. Mutations in the *SMAD4/DPC4* gene (which encodes a TGF-β signaling intermediate) account for some cases of juvenile polyposis syndrome.[79]

Peutz-Jeghers polyps are hamartomatous polyps that involve the mucosal epithelium, lamina propria, and muscularis mucosa. These hamartomatous lesions may also occur singly or multiply in the **Peutz-Jeghers syndrome.** This rare autosomal dominant syndrome is characterized by multiple hamartomatous polyps scattered throughout the entire gastrointestinal tract and melanotic mucosal and cutaneous pigmentation around the lips, oral mucosa, face, genitalia, and palmar surfaces of the hands. Patients with this syndrome are at risk for intussusception, which is a common cause of mortality. Peutz-Jeghers polyps tend to be large and pedunculated with a firm lobulated contour. Histologically, an arborizing network of connective tissue and well-developed smooth muscle extends into the polyp and surrounds normal abundant glands lined by normal intestinal epithelium rich in goblet cells (Fig. 17–56*B*). The distribution of polyps in patients is reported as follows: stomach, 25%; colon, 30%; and small bowel, 100%. **While these hamartomatous polyps themselves do not have malignant potential, patients with the syndrome have an increased risk of developing carcinomas of the pancreas, breast, lung, ovary, and uterus.** The well-documented and characteristic tumors include sex cord tumors of the ovary, adenoma malignum of the uterine cervix, and Sertoli cell tumors of the testis. When gastrointestinal adenocarcinoma occurs, it arises from concomitant adenomatous lesions. The underlying genetic basis for Peutz-Jeghers syndrome is the mutation of the gene *STK11 (LKB1)* located on chromosome 19. The gene encodes a protein with serine/threonine kinase activity.

Two other hamartomatous polyposis syndromes merit comment: Cowden syndrome and Cronkhite-Canada syndrome.

Cowden syndrome is an autosomal dominant genetic syndrome characterized by multiple hamartomas involving organs derived from all three germinal layers. The commonly involved sites are gastrointestinal tract and mucocutaneous locations. Intestinal hamartomatous polyps, facial trichilemmomas, acral keratoses, and oral papillomas are characteristic. While these hamartomas do not have malignant potential, the syndrome predisposes the patient to develop thyroid and breast cancers. The underlying genetic abnormality is the germ line mutation of the *PTEN* gene located on chromosome 10 (Chapter 7).

Cronkhite-Canada syndrome is a nonhereditary disorder characterized by the presence of gastrointestinal hamartomatous polyposis and ectodermal abnormalities (such as nail atrophy, skin pigmentation, and alopecia). The etiology of this disorder is currently unknown.

Adenomas

Adenomas (adenomatous polyps) are intraepithelial neoplasms that range from small, often pedunculated lesions to large neoplasms that are usually sessile. The prevalence of

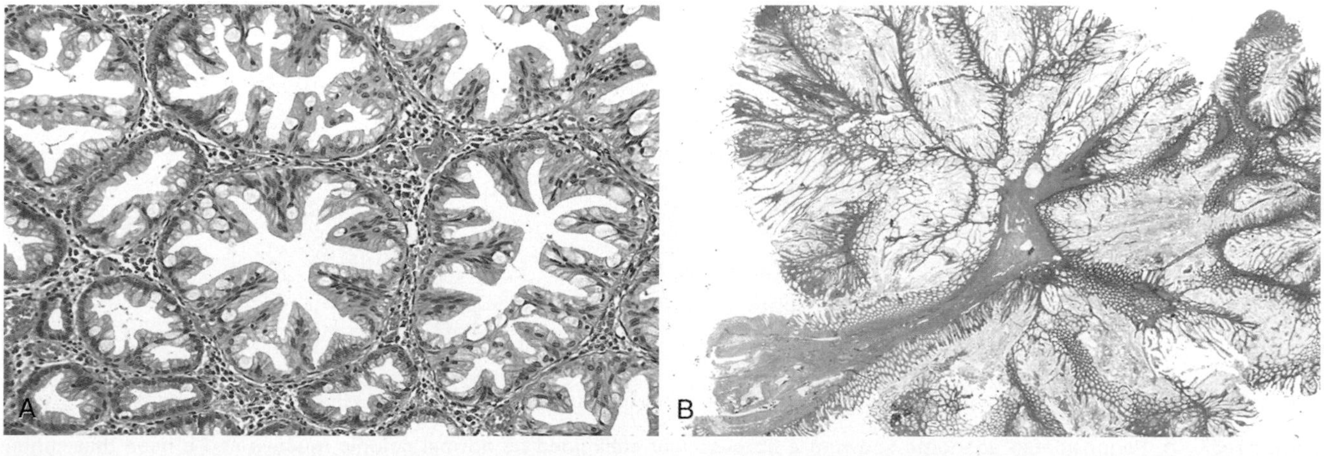

FIGURE 17–56 Non-neoplastic colonic polyps. *A,* Hyperplastic polyp; high-power view showing the serrated profile of the epithelial layer. *B,* Peutz-Jeghers polyp; low-power view showing the splaying of smooth muscle into the superficial portion of the pedunculated polyp.

colonic adenomas is about 20% to 30% before age 40, rising to 40% to 50% after age 60. Males and females are affected equally. There is a well-defined familial predisposition to sporadic adenomas, accounting for about a fourfold greater risk among first-degree relatives and also a fourfold greater risk of colorectal carcinoma.

Adenomatous polyps are segregated into three subtypes on the basis of the epithelial architecture:

- *Tubular adenomas:* tubular glands
- *Villous adenomas:* villous projections
- *Tubulovillous adenoma:* a mixture of the above.

There is considerable overlap among these categories, so by convention, tubular adenomas exhibit more than 75% tubular architecture, villous adenomas contain more than 50% villous architecture, and tubulovillous adenomas contain 25% to 50% villous architecture. Tubular adenomas are by far the most common; about 5% to 10% of adenomas are tubulovillous, and only 1% are villous.

All adenomatous lesions arise as the result of epithelial proliferative dysplasia, which may range from low-grade to high-grade dysplasia (carcinoma in situ). Furthermore, there is strong evidence that adenomas are a precursor lesion for invasive colorectal adenocarcinomas (discussed below).[80] The period required for an adenoma to double in size is estimated to be about 10 years. Thus, they are slow growing and must certainly have been present for many years before detection. The following concepts are pertinent:

- Most tubular adenomas are small and pedunculated; conversely, most pedunculated polyps are tubular.
- Villous adenomas tend to be large and sessile, and sessile polyps usually exhibit villous features.

The malignant risk with an adenomatous polyp is correlated with three interdependent features: polyp size, histologic architecture, and severity of epithelial dysplasia, as follows:

- Cancer is rare in tubular adenomas smaller than 1 cm in diameter.
- The risk of cancer is high (approaching 40%) in sessile villous adenomas more than 4 cm in diameter.
- Severe dysplasia, when present, is often found in villous areas.

Thus, the most worrisome lesions are villous adenomas greater than 4 cm in diameter. However, *since all degrees of dysplasia (low-grade and high-grade) and even invasive adenocarcinoma may be encountered in an adenoma of any subtype, it is impossible from gross inspection of a polyp to determine its clinical significance.*

It must be mentioned that not all adenomas are protuberant polyps. Some adenomas are essentially "flat" and can only be identified by histologic examination. These adenomas are referred to as flat adenoma, depressed adenoma, or microscopic adenoma.

Morphology. Most **tubular adenomas** (90%) are found in the colon, but they can occur in the stomach and small intestine, especially in the vicinity of the ampulla of Vater. About half the time they occur singly; in the remainder, two or more lesions are distributed at random. The smallest tubular adenomas are smooth-contoured and sessile; larger ones tend to be coarsely lobulated and have slender stalks (Fig. 17–57*A*). Uncommonly, they exceed 2.5 cm in diameter. Histologically, the stalk is composed of fibromuscular tissue and prominent blood vessels (derived from the submucosa) and it is usually covered by

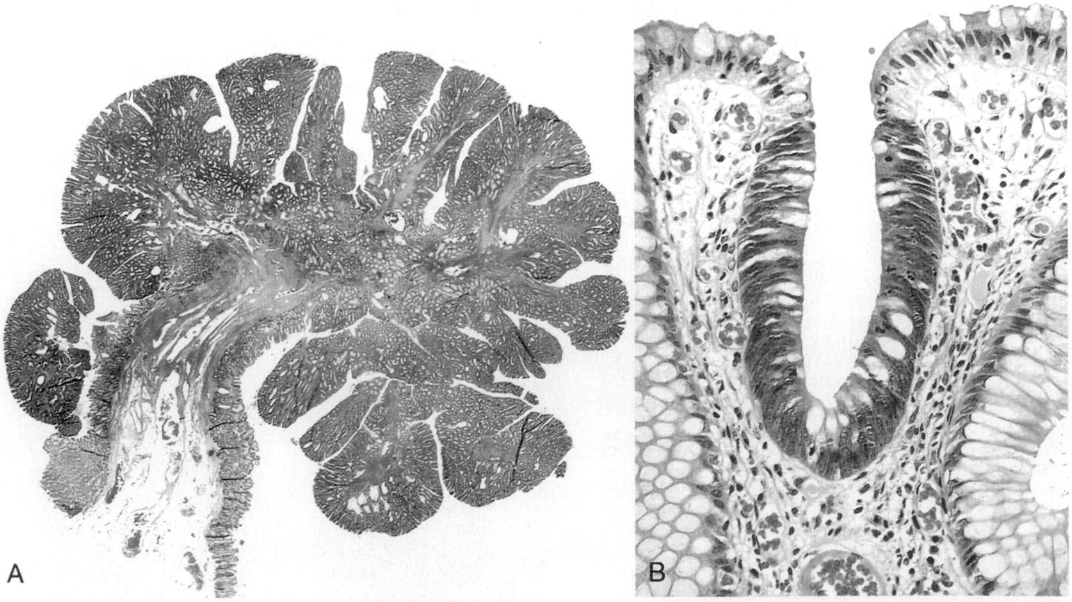

FIGURE 17–57 *A,* Pedunculated adenoma showing a fibrovascular stalk lined by normal colonic mucosa and a head that contains abundant dysplastic epithelial glands, hence the blue color with the H & E stain. *B,* A small focus of adenomatous epithelium in an otherwise normal (mucin-secreting, clear) colonic mucosa, showing how the dysplastic columnar epithelium (deeply stained) can populate a colonic crypt and create a tubular architecture.

normal, non-neoplastic mucosa. However, adenomatous epithelium may extend down the stalk and into adjacent regions of the mucosa, particularly in the stomach. Whether small or large, adenomatous lesions are composed of neoplastic (dysplastic) epithelium, which lines glands as a tall, hyperchromatic, somewhat disordered epithelium that may or may not show mucin vacuoles (Fig. 17–57*B*). In the clearly benign tubular adenoma, the branching glands are well separated by lamina propria and **the degree of dysplasia is low-grade.** However, **high-grade dysplasia may be present and may merge with areas of overt malignant change confined to the mucosa (intramucosal carcinoma).** Carcinomatous invasion into the submucosal stalk of the polyp constitutes invasive adenocarcinoma.

Villous adenomas are the larger and more ominous of the epithelial polyps. They tend to occur in older persons, most commonly in the rectum and rectosigmoid colon, but they may be located elsewhere. They generally are sessile, up to 10 cm in diameter, velvety or cauliflower-like masses projecting 1 to 3 cm above the surrounding normal mucosa. Their histology is that of frondlike villiform extensions of the mucosa (Fig. 17–58*A*), covered by dysplastic, sometimes very disorderly columnar epithelium (Fig. 17–58*B*). All degrees of dysplasia may be encountered. When invasive carcinoma occurs, there is no stalk as a buffer zone, and invasion is directly into the wall of the colon (submucosa or deeper).

Tubulovillous adenomas are typically intermediate between the tubular and villous lesions in terms of their frequency of having a stalk or being sessile, their size, and the general level of dysplasia found in such lesions. The risk of harboring in situ or invasive carcinoma generally correlates with the proportion of the lesion that is villous.

Clinical Features. Colorectal tubular (and tubulovillous) adenomas may be asymptomatic, but many are discovered during evaluation of anemia or occult bleeding. Villous adenomas are much more frequently symptomatic than the other patterns, and often are discovered because of overt rectal bleeding. Rarely, villous adenomas may hypersecrete copious amounts of mucoid material rich in protein and potassium, leading to either hypoproteinemia or hypokalemia. Notably, screening programs are intended to detect asymptomatic adenomas before they progress to malignancy.

The clinical impact of malignant change in an adenoma depends on the following:

- *High-grade dysplasia (carcinoma in situ)* has not yet acquired the ability to metastasize and is still a *clinically* benign lesion.
- Because lymphatic channels are largely absent in the colonic mucosa, being present erratically only at the very base of the lamina propria, *intramucosal carcinoma with lamina propria invasion* only is regarded also as having little or no metastatic potential.
- If the lesion penetrates through the muscularis mucosa into the submucosal space, the resultant *invasive adenocarcinoma* is a malignant tumor with metastatic potential. Nevertheless, *endoscopic removal of a pedunculated adenoma is regarded as an adequate excision provided that three histologic conditions are met:* (1) the adenocarcinoma is superficial and does not approach the margin of excision across the base of the stalk; (2) there is no vascular or lymphatic invasion; and (3) the carcinoma is not poorly differentiated.
- *Invasive adenocarcinoma arising in a sessile polyp cannot be adequately resected by polypectomy,* and further surgery may be required.
- Regardless of whether carcinoma is present, *the only adequate treatment for a pedunculated or sessile adenoma is complete resection.* If adenomatous epithelium remains behind the patient still has a premalignant lesion or may even be harboring invasive carcinoma in the residual lesion.

Familial Syndromes

Familial polyposis syndromes are uncommon autosomal dominant disorders. Their importance lies in the propensity for malignant transformation and in the insights that they have provided in unraveling the molecular basis of colorectal

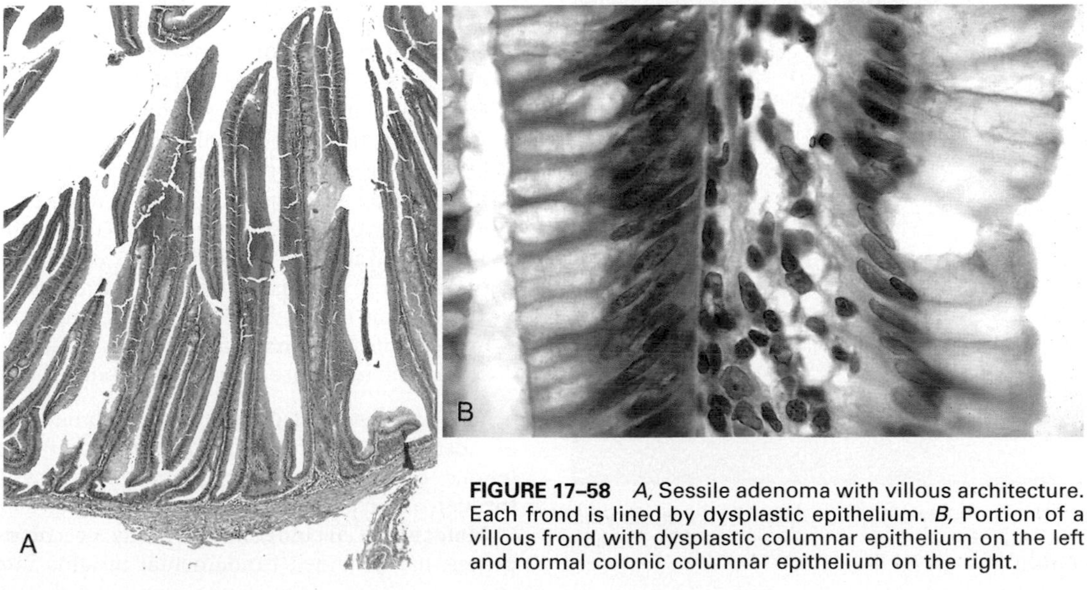

FIGURE 17–58 *A,* Sessile adenoma with villous architecture. Each frond is lined by dysplastic epithelium. *B,* Portion of a villous frond with dysplastic columnar epithelium on the left and normal colonic columnar epithelium on the right.

cancer. Peutz-Jeghers syndrome, described earlier, is characterized by hamartomatous polyps and a modestly increased risk of cancer, frequently in extragastrointestinal sites. Juvenile polyposis syndrome and Cowden syndrome have also been mentioned earlier. FAP exhibits innumerable adenomatous polyps and has a frequency of progression to colon adenocarcinoma approaching 100%. Hereditary nonpolyposis colorectal cancer syndrome (HNPCC or Lynch syndrome) is characterized by the development of colorectal carcinoma, endometrial carcinoma, and carcinoma of the small intestine, ureter, or renal pelvis. As we discuss later, many of the molecular events underlying these syndromes have been identified.

Familial Adenomatous Polyposis (FAP) Syndrome. *FAP is the archetype of the adenomatous polyposis syndromes.* It is caused by mutations of the adenomatous polyposis coli *(APC)* gene on chromosome 5q21 (Chapter 7).[81] The same gene mutations cause a broad spectrum of clinical manifestations. Based on the clinical presentation, FAP can be further classified as classic FAP, attenuated FAP, Gardner syndrome, and Turcot syndrome.

In the *classic FAP syndrome,* patients typically develop 500 to 2500 colonic adenomas that carpet the mucosal surface (Fig. 17–59). Occasionally as few as 150 polyps are present; a minimum of 100 polyps is necessary for a diagnosis of classic FAP. Multiple adenomas may also be present elsewhere in the alimentary tract, including the region of the ampulla of Vater. Histologically, the vast majority of polyps are tubular adenomas; occasional polyps may have villous features. Some patients already have cancer of the colon or rectum at the time of diagnosis. Cancer-prevention measures include early detection and prophylactic colectomy in siblings and first-degree relatives at risk. In addition to colonic polyps, FAP patients can have polyps in the stomach (adenomas or fundic gland polyps) and small intestine (especially around the ampulla of Vater).

In *attenuated FAP,* patients tend to develop fewer polyps (average, 30), and most of the polyps are located in the proximal colon. The lifetime risk of cancer development is usually around 50%.

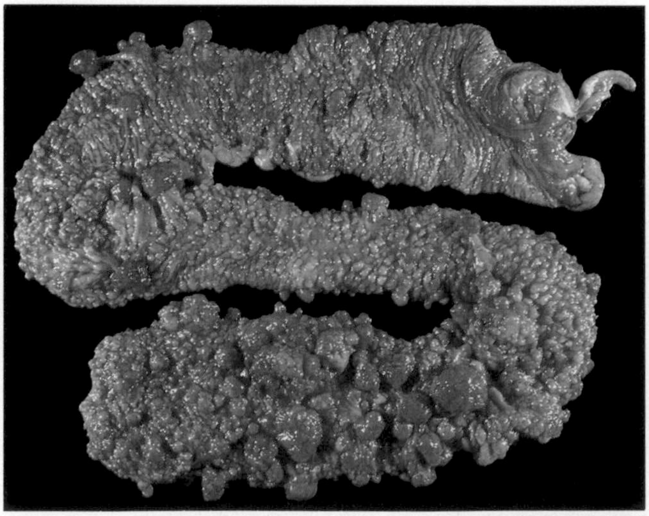

FIGURE 17–59 Familial adenomatous polyposis in an 18-year-old woman. The mucosal surface is carpeted by innumerable polypoid adenomas.

Patients with *Gardner syndrome* exhibit intestinal polyps identical to those in classic FAP, combined with multiple osteomas (particularly of the mandible, skull, and long bones), epidermal cysts, and fibromatosis. Less frequent are abnormalities of dentition, such as unerupted and supernumerary teeth, and a higher frequency of duodenal and thyroid cancer.

Turcot syndrome is a rare clinical syndrome marked by the combination of adenomatous colonic polyposis and tumors of the central nervous system. Two thirds of patients with Turcot syndrome have *APC* gene mutations and develop brain medulloblastomas. The remaining one third have mutations in one of the genes associated with HNPCC and develop brain glioblastomas.

Hereditary Nonpolyposis Colorectal Cancer (HNPCC) Syndrome. *HNPCC* is an autosomal dominant familial syndrome (extensively described by Henry Lynch, hence the alternative name of Lynch syndrome).[82] It is characterized by an increased risk of colorectal cancer and extraintestinal cancer, particularly of the endometrium. Adenomas occur in low numbers and considerably earlier than in the general adult population. However, the colonic malignancies that develop in this syndrome often are multiple and are not usually associated with pre-existing adenomas. The hallmark of HNPCC is mutations in DNA repair genes, leading to microsatellite instability, as discussed in Chapter 7.

Colorectal Carcinogenesis

Most colorectal carcinomas occur sporadically in the absence of well-defined familial syndromes. Like the majority of cancers in other organs, there are conditions associated with risk of tumor development. Regardless of the inciting event, a well-described set of genetic alterations occurs that ultimately leads to colorectal malignancy. The model proposed by Fearon and Vogelstein is widely accepted as the prototypical sequence for colorectal cancer development.[83] The pathologic basis for this model is *the adenoma-carcinoma sequence,* which has been documented by these observations:

- Populations that have a high prevalence of adenomas have a high prevalence of colorectal cancer, and vice versa.
- The distribution of adenomas within the colorectum is more or less comparable to that of colorectal cancer.
- The peak incidence of adenomatous polyps antedates by some years the peak for colorectal cancer.
- When invasive carcinoma is identified at an early stage, surrounding adenomatous tissue is often present
- The risk of cancer is directly related to the number of adenomas, and hence the virtual certainty of cancer in patients with familial polyposis syndromes.
- Programs that assiduously follow patients for the development of adenomas and remove all that are suspicious reduce the incidence of colorectal cancer.

The occurrence of colorectal carcinoma without evidence of adenomatous precursors suggests that some dysplastic lesions can degenerate into malignancy without passing through a polypoid stage.

Molecular Carcinogenesis. Study of colorectal carcinogenesis has provided fundamental insights into the general mechanisms of cancer evolution. Many of these principles were discussed in Chapter 7. Here we will discuss concepts specifically pertinent to carcinogenesis in the colon.

It is now believed that there are two pathogenetically distinct pathways for the development of colon cancer,[84] both of which involve the stepwise accumulation of multiple mutations. However, the genes involved and the mechanisms by which the mutations accumulate are different.

The first pathway, sometimes called the *APC/β-caterin pathway,* is characterized by chromosomal instability that results in stepwise accumulation of mutations in a series of oncogenes and tumor suppressor genes. The molecular evolution of colon cancer along this pathway occurs through a series of morphologically identifiable stages. Initially, there is localized colon epithelial proliferation. This is followed by the formation of small adenomas that progressively enlarge, become more dysplastic, and ultimately develop into invasive cancers. This is referred to as the adenoma-carcinoma sequence (Fig. 17–60). The genetic correlates of this pathway are as follows:

Loss of Adenomatous Polyposis Coli (APC) Gene. The *APC* gene has been mapped to 5q21. Its mutation is the genetic basis for FAP syndrome and fulfills the "first hit" concept advanced by Knudson in the 1970s.[85] Loss of this gene is believed to be the earliest event in the formation of adenomas. This dual-function tumor suppressor gene encodes a protein that binds to microtubule bundles and promotes cell migration and adhesion. APC also acts as a gatekeeper protein, as it regulates levels of β-catenin, an important mediator of the Wnt/β-catenin signaling pathway (see Fig. 7–38, Chapter 7). This signaling pathway plays a critical role in the normal intestinal epithelial development. It is also involved in development of colorectal carcinomas. More than 80% of colorectal carcinomas have inactivated APC, and 50% of cancers without *APC* mutations have β-catenin mutations. β-catenin is a member of the cadherin-based cell adhesive complex, which also acts as a transcription factor if the protein is translocated to the nucleus. When it is not bound to E-cadherin and participating in cell-to-cell adhesion, a cytoplasmic degradation complex (consisting of APC, Axin, GSK-3β, and β-catenin) leads to β-catenin phosphorylation and degradation. In the setting of *APC* mutations (loss of normal function), β-catenin accumulates in the cytoplasm and is translocated to the nucleus to bind to a family of transcription factors called T-cell factor or lymphoid enhancer factor (TCF or LEF) proteins. The TCF contributes a DNA-binding domain and β-catenin contributes a transactivation domain. Genes activated by the β-catenin–TCF complex are thought to include those regulating cell proliferation and apoptosis, such as *c-MYC* and *CYCLIN D1*. Hence, *normal APC function promotes cell adhesion and regulates cell proliferation; absence of APC function leads to decreased cell adhesion and increased cellular proliferation.*

Reported mutations in the *APC* gene include missense mutations and deletions, resulting in synthesis of truncated APC proteins. Mutant β-catenin loses binding affinity to GSK-3β, the kinase that phosphorylates and degrades β-catenin, in normal cells. APC mutations are present in 80% of sporadic carcinomas.

***Mutation of* K-RAS.** The *K-RAS* gene (Chapter 7) is the most frequently observed activated oncogene in adenomas and colon cancers. *K-RAS* plays a role in intracellular signal transduction and is mutated in fewer than 10% of adenomas less than 1 cm in size, in about 50% of adenomas larger than 1 cm, and in approximately 50% of carcinomas.

***Loss of* SMADs.** A common allelic loss in colon cancer is on 18q21. Initially, *DCC* (*d*eleted in *c*olon *c*ancer), was thought to be the suppressor gene involved in colorectal

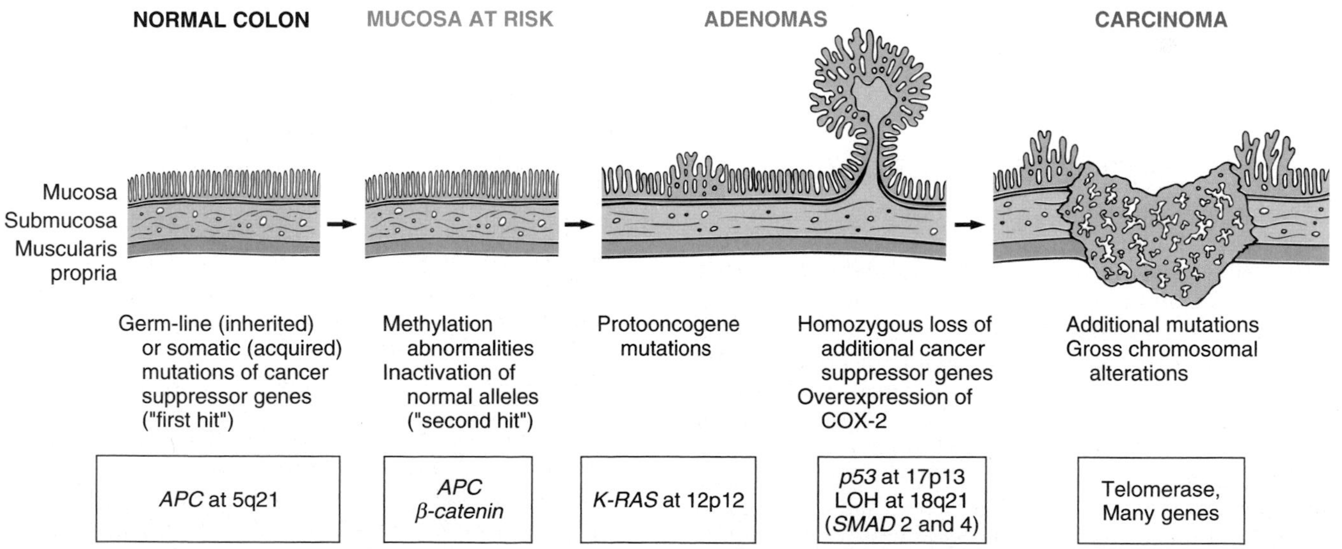

FIGURE 17–60 Schematic of the morphologic and molecular changes in the adenoma-carcinoma sequence. It is postulated that loss of one normal copy of the tumor suppressor gatekeeper gene *APC* occurs early. Indeed, individuals may be born with one mutant allele of APC, rendering them extremely likely to develop colon cancer. This is the "first hit," according to Knudson's hypothesis. The loss of the normal copy of the *APC* gene follows ("second hit"). Mutations of the oncogene *K-RAS* seem to occur next. Additional mutations or losses of heterozygosity inactivate the tumor suppressor gene *p53* (on chromosome 17p) and *SMAD*2 and *SMAD*4 on chromosome 18q, leading finally to the emergence of carcinoma, in which additional mutations occur. It is important to note that while there seems to be a temporal sequence of changes, as shown, the accumulation of mutations, rather than their occurrence in a specific order, is more important.

cancer, which was located in this region. However, the role of *DCC* in colorectal carcinogenesis has been questioned, since mutant mice lacking both alleles of *DCC* show no abnormalities.[88] *SMAD2* and *SMAD4* (Chapter 7), involved in TGF-β signaling, are located on 18q21. Lack of *SMAD4* increases gastrointestinal tumorigenesis.[89]

***Loss of* p53.** Losses at chromosome 17p have been found in 70% to 80% of colon cancers, yet comparable losses are infrequent in adenomas. These chromosomal deletions affect the *p53* gene, suggesting that mutations in *p53* occur late in colon carcinogenesis. The critical role of *p53* in cell-cycle regulation is discussed in Chapter 7.

***Activation of* Telomerase.** Telomeres plays a role in stabilizing the chromosome. They shorten with each cell division until cell senescence develops (Chapter 1). Telomerase is a ribonucleoprotein complex with telomeric reverse transcriptase (TERT) as the catalytic subunit. Telomerase activity is required to maintain telomere stability and hence cell immortality, a prerequisite for all cancer cells (Chapter 7). Most adenomas lack telomerase activity, but a majority of cancers in humans, including colorectal carcinoma, have increased telomerase activity.[90]

Although the sequence of events outlined above is common, it should be emphasized that the *accumulation of mutations is more important than their occurrence in a specific order.*

Microsatellite Instability Pathway. The second pathway is characterized by genetic lesions in *DNA mismatch repair genes* (Chapter 7). It is involved in 10% to 15% of sporadic cases and in the HNPCC syndrome. As in the *APC/β*-catenin schema, there is accumulation of mutations, but the involved genes are different, and, unlike in the adenoma-carcinoma sequence, there are no clearly identifiable morphologic correlates. Defective DNA repair caused by inactivation of DNA mismatch repair genes is the fundamental and the most likely initiating event in colorectal cancers that travel this road. Inherited mutations *(germ-line mutations)* in any of five genes that are involved in DNA repair are responsible for the familial syndrome of HNPCC. These human mismatch repair genes, *hMSH2* (chromosome 2p22), *hMLH1* (chromosome 3p21), *MSH6* (chromosome 2p21), *hPMS1* (chromosome 2q31-33), and *hPMS2* (chromosome 7p22), are involved in genetic "proofreading" during DNA replication and have earned the moniker of caretaker genes (Chapter 7).[86] The majority of the mutations (90%) involve *MSH2* and *MLH1*. Mutations in the mismatch repair genes cause alteration of microsatellites, leading to *microsatellite instability*. Microsatellites are fragments of repeat sequences in the human genome, which contains approximately 50,000 to 100,000 microsatellites. These sequences are prone to misalignment during DNA replication. In normal cells, the misalignment is repaired by the caretaker genes. Patients with HNPCC inherit one mutant DNA repair gene ("the first hit") and one normal allele. For unclear reasons, cells in some organs (colon, stomach, endometrium) are susceptible to a second, somatic mutation ("the second hit" of the Knudson hypothesis), which inactivates the normal allele (loss of heterozygosity or LOH). With homozygous loss of mismatch repair genes, mutation rates are up to 1000 times higher than normal, and most of the HNPCC tumors show microsatellite instability. About 10% to 15% of sporadic colon cancers have mutations in similar DNA repair genes, Most microsatellite sequences are in noncoding regions of the genes, and, hence, mutations in these genes are probably harmless. However, some microsatellite sequences are located in the coding or promoter region of genes involved in regulation of cell growth. Such genes include type II TGF-*β* receptor and *BAX*. TGF-*β* signaling inhibits the growth of colonic epithelial cells, and the *BAX* gene causes apoptosis. Loss of mismatch repair leads to the accumulation of mutations in these and other growth-regulating genes, culminating in the emergence of colorectal carcinomas.

Although there is no readily identifiable adenoma-carcinoma sequence that typifies tumors arising from defects in mismatch repair, it has been noted that some of the so-called hyperplastic polyps seen on the right side of the colon display microsatellite instability and may well be precancerous.[87] Fully developed tumors that arise via the mismatch repair pathway do show some distinctive morphologic features, including proximal colonic location, mucinous histology, and infiltration by lymphocytes. In general, these tumors have better prognosis than stage-matched tumors that arise by the APC pathway.

Colorectal Carcinoma

Virtually 98% of all cancers in the large intestine are adenocarcinomas. They represent one of the prime challenges to the medical profession, because they usually arise in polyps and produce symptoms relatively early and at a stage generally curable by resection. Yet, there are an estimated 148,300 new cases per year and about 56,600 deaths, accounting for 10% of all cancer-related deaths in the United States.[91]

Epidemiology, Etiology, and Pathogenesis. The peak incidence for colorectal carcinoma is between ages 60 and 79. Fewer than 20% of cases occur before age 50. When colorectal carcinoma is found in a young person, pre-existing ulcerative colitis or one of the polyposis syndromes must be suspected. With lesions in the rectum, the male-to-female ratio is 1.2:1; for more proximal tumors there is no gender difference. Colorectal carcinoma has a worldwide distribution, with the highest death rates in the United States, Australia, New Zealand, and Eastern European countries. Its incidence is substantially lower—up to 10-fold—in Mexico, South America, and Africa. Environmental factors, particularly dietary practices, are implicated in these striking geographic contrasts in incidence. Japanese and Polish families that have migrated from their low-risk areas to the United States have acquired, over the course of 20 years, the rate prevailing in the new environment. Both groups, for the most part, adopted the common dietary practices of the U.S. population. Other studies implicate obesity and physical inactivity as risk factors for colon cancer.[92,93]

The dietary factors receiving the most attention as predisposing to a higher incidence of cancer are (1) excess dietary caloric intake relative to requirements, (2) a low content of unabsorbable vegetable fiber, (3) a corresponding high content of refined carbohydrates, (4) intake of red meat, and (5) decreased intake of protective micronutrients. It is theorized that reduced fiber content leads to decreased stool bulk, increased fecal transit time in the bowel, and an altered bacterial flora of the intestine. Potentially toxic oxidative byproducts of carbohydrate degradation by bacteria are therefore present in higher concentrations in the stools and are held in contact with the colonic mucosa for longer periods of time. Moreover, high cholesterol intake in red meat enhances the synthesis of bile acids by the liver, which in turn may be converted into potential carcinogens by intestinal bacteria. Refined diets also contain less of vitamins A, C, and E, which may act as oxygen-radical scavengers (Chapter 1). Intriguing as these speculations may be, the putative mechanisms of dietary effects remain unproven. Indeed, recent studies have challenged the notion that low-fat, high-fiber diets protect against recurrence of colorectal adenomas, the precursors of colon cancer.

Several epidemiological studies suggest that use of aspirin and other NSAIDs exerts a protective effect against colon cancer. In the Nurses' Health Study, women who used four to six tablets of aspirin/day for 10 years or more had a decreased incidence of colon cancer. Two recent studies have revealed that aspirin reduces the risk of recurrent adenomas in patients with previous colorectal carcinomas or adenomas.[94] The mechanism of such chemoprevention is not fully understood, but it is likely mediated by inhibition of cyclooxygenase-2 (Chapter 2). This enzyme is overexpressed in neoplastic epithelium and seems to regulate angiogenesis and apoptosis. On the basis of these findings, the U.S. Food and Drug Administration has approved the use of COX-2 inhibitors as chemopreventive agents in patients with the familial adenomatous polyposis syndrome.

Morphology. The distribution of the cancers in the colorectum is as follows: cecum/ascending colon, 22%; transverse colon, 11%; descending colon, 6%; rectosigmoid colon, 55%; and other sites, 6%. The right-sided colon cancers tend to have greater microsatellite instability. Ninety-nine per cent of carcinomas occur singly, but when multiple carcinomas are present, they are often at widely disparate sites in the colon. While most cases occur sporadically, about 1% to 3% of colorectal carcinomas occur in patients with familial syndromes (i.e., FAP or HNPCC) or IBD.

Although all colorectal carcinomas begin as in situ lesions, they evolve into different morphologic patterns. Tumors in the proximal colon tend to grow as polypoid, exophytic masses that extend along one wall of the capacious cecum and ascending colon (Fig. 17–61). Obstruction is uncommon. When carcinomas in the distal colon are discovered, they tend to be annular, encircling lesions that produce so-called napkin-ring constrictions of the bowel (Fig. 17–62). The margins of the napkin ring are classically heaped up, beaded, and firm, and the midregion is ulcerated. The lumen is markedly narrowed, and the proximal bowel may be distended. Both forms of neoplasm directly penetrate the bowel wall over the course of time (probably years) and may appear as subserosal and serosal white, firm masses, frequently causing puckering of the serosal surface. Uncommonly, but particularly in association with ulcerative colitis, colorectal cancers are insidiously infiltrative and difficult to identify radiographically and macroscopically. Such lesions tend to be exceedingly aggressive, and spread at an early stage in their evolution.

Unlike the gross pathology, the microscopic characteristics of right- and left-sided colonic adenocarcinomas are similar. Differentiation may range from tall, columnar cells resembling their counterparts in adenomatous lesions, which now invade the submucosa and muscularis propria (Fig. 17–63), to undifferentiated, frankly anaplastic masses. **Invasive tumor incites a strong desmoplastic stromal response,** leading to the characteristic firm, hard consistency of most colonic carcinomas. Many tumors produce mucin, which is secreted into the gland lumina or into the interstitium of the gut wall. Because this secretion

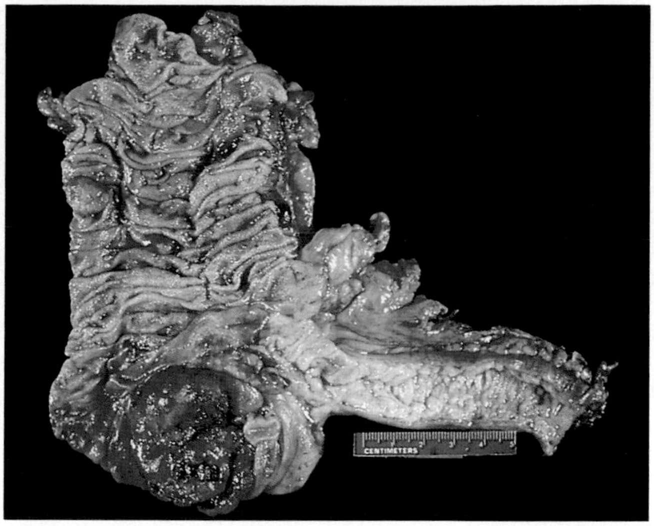

FIGURE 17–61 Carcinoma of the cecum. The fungating carcinoma projects into the lumen but has not caused obstruction.

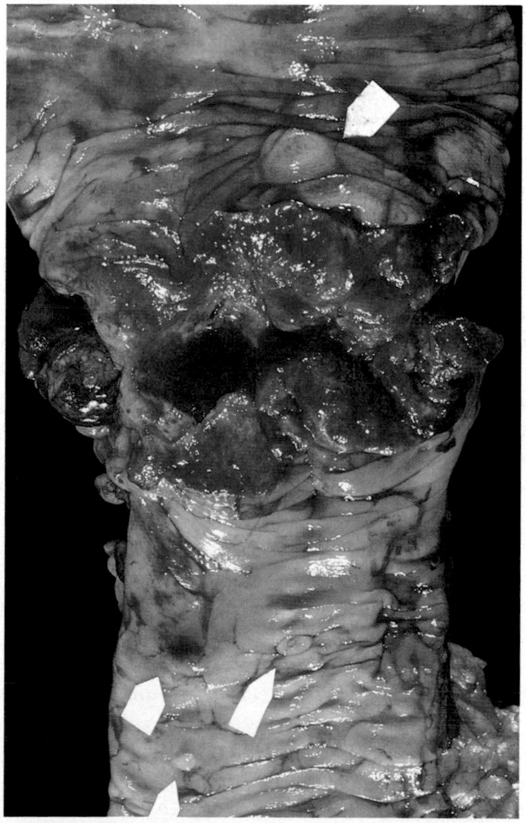

FIGURE 17–62 Carcinoma of the descending colon. This circumferential tumor has heaped-up edges and an ulcerated central portion. The arrows identify separate mucosal polyps.

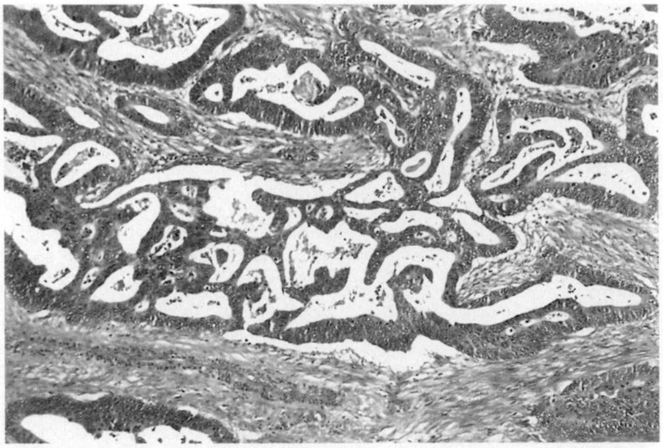

FIGURE 17–63 Invasive adenocarcinoma of colon, showing malignant glands infiltrating the muscle wall.

dissects through the gut wall, it aids the extension of the malignancy and worsens the prognosis.

Certain specific features should be noted. Foci of endocrine differentiation may be found in about 10% of colorectal carcinomas. Alternatively, in some cancers the cells take on a **signet-ring appearance.** The small-cell undifferentiated carcinoma appears to arise from endocrine cells per se and elaborates a variety of bioactive secretory products. Some cancers, particularly in the distal colon, have foci of squamous cell differentiation and are therefore referred to as adenosquamous carcinomas. In contrast, **carcinomas arising in the anorectal canal constitute a distinct subgroup of tumors,** dominated by squamous cell carcinoma. Tumors associated with HNPCC tend to be poorly differentiated and rich in mucin.

Clinical Features. Colorectal cancers remain asymptomatic for years; symptoms develop insidiously and frequently have been present for months, sometimes years, before diagnosis. Cecal and right colonic cancers are most often called to clinical attention by the appearance of fatigue, weakness, and iron-deficiency anemia. These bulky lesions bleed readily and may be discovered at an early stage, provided the colon is examined thoroughly radiographically and during colonoscopy. Left-sided lesions come to attention by producing occult bleeding, changes in bowel habit, or crampy left lower quadrant discomfort. In theory, the chance for early discovery and successful removal should be greater for patients with lesions on the left side, because these patients usually have prominent disturbances in bowel function such as melena, diarrhea, and constipation. However, cancers of the rectum and sigmoid tend to be more infiltrative at the time of diagnosis than proximal lesions, and therefore have a somewhat poorer prognosis. *It is a clinical maxim that iron-deficiency anemia in an older male means gastrointestinal cancer until proven otherwise.* In females the situation is less clear, since menstrual losses, multiple pregnancies, or abnormal uterine bleeding may underlie such an anemia. Systemic manifestations such as weakness, malaise, and weight loss are ominous, in that they usually signify more extensive disease.

All colorectal tumors spread by direct extension into adjacent structures and by metastasis through the lymphatics and blood vessels. In order of preference, the favored sites of metastatic spread are the regional lymph nodes, liver, lungs, and bones, followed by many other sites, including the serosal membrane of the peritoneal cavity, brain, and others. In general, the disease has spread beyond the range of curative surgery in 25% to 30% of patients. Anal region carcinomas are locally invasive and metastasize to regional lymph nodes and distant sites.

The single most important prognostic indicator of colorectal carcinoma is the extent of the tumor at the time of diagnosis, the so-called stage. A staging system formerly widely used is that described by Aster and Coller in 1954, which represents a modification of classifications proposed by Dukes and Kirklin. Currently, the system most widely used is the tumor-nodes-metastasis (TNM) classification and staging system from the American Joint Commission on Cancer (Table 17–14). The criteria for pathologic staging are shown in Figure 17–64. Regardless of the system used, survival at 1, 5, and 10 years is strongly correlated with the stage of disease at the time of surgical resection. Staging can be accurately applied only after the extent of spread is determined by surgical exploration and anatomic examination.

The overriding challenge is to discover these neoplasms when curative resection is possible, preferably when they are still adenomatous polyps. Indeed, each death from colonic cancer in the United States must be viewed as a preventable tragedy, but progress has been relatively slow in coming.

Carcinoid Tumors

The first carcinoid tumor was identified in the ileum by Lubarsch more than 100 years ago. The term *carcinoid* was used by Oberndorfer in 1907 because the tumor was described as a carcinoma-like lesion but with a much more indolent clinical course. Carcinoid tumor is derived from resident endocrine cells, with the gastrointestinal tract and lung as the predominant sites of occurrence.

TABLE 17–14 TNM Classification of Carcinoma of the Colon and Rectum

Tumor Stage	Histologic Features of the Neoplasm
Tis	Carcinoma in situ (high-grade dysplasia) or intramucosal carcinoma (lamina propria invasion)
T1	Tumor invades submucosa
T2	Extending into the muscularis propria but not penetrating through it
T3	Penetrating through the muscularis propria into subserosa
T4	Tumor penetrates through serosa and may directly invade other organs or structures
Nx	Regional lymph nodes cannot be assessed
N0	No regional lymph node metastasis
N1	Metastasis in 1 to 3 lymph nodes
N2	Metastasis in 4 or more lymph nodes
Mx	Distant metastasis cannot be assessed
M0	No distant metastasis
M1	Distant metastasis

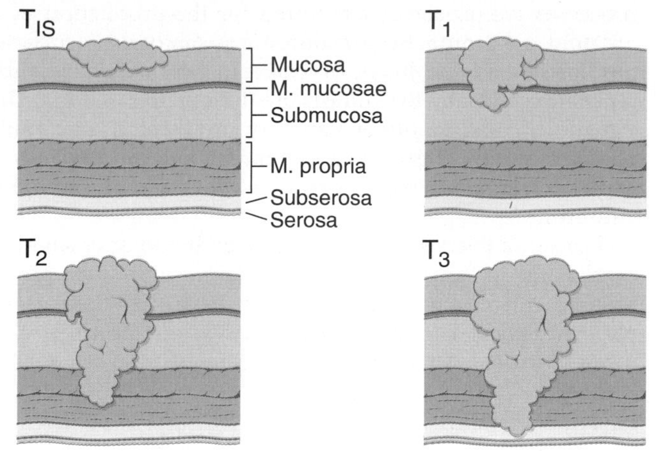

FIGURE 17–64 Pathologic staging of colorectal cancer. Staging is based on the depth of tumor invasion.

Mucosal endocrine cells generate bioactive compounds, particularly peptide and nonpeptide hormones, and play a major role in coordinated gut function. Although they are derived from epithelial stem cells in the mucosal crypts, they are designated *endocrine* cells because of their endocrine and paracrine function and their resemblance to endocrine cells elsewhere, as in the pancreas. Mucosal endocrine cells are abundant in other organs, including the lungs, but the great preponderance of carcinoid tumors arising from these cells are in the gut. A scattering of carcinoid tumors arises in the pancreas or peripancreatic tissue, lungs, biliary tree, and even liver. The peak incidence of these neoplasms is in the sixth decade, but they may appear at any age. They comprise less than 2% of colorectal malignancies but almost half of small intestinal malignant tumors.

The classification of carcinoid tumors is still controversial. The prevailing view is that carcinoid tumor may represent a well-differentiated neuroendocrine neoplasm, while at the poorly differentiated end of the spectrum is the small cell carcinoma. Carcinoid tumors may be confined to the mucosa and submucosa or may be malignant in behavior with deep invasion and metastatic spread to regional lymph nodes and the liver. Intriguingly, there is no reliable histologic difference between seemingly benign and obviously malignant carcinoid tumors. While there are no reliable molecular markers to predict tumor behavior, the tendency for aggressive behavior correlates with the site of origin, the depth of local penetration, the size of the tumor, and the histologic features of necrosis and mitosis. Hence, it is possible to establish a reasonable clinical assessment of these tumors. *Appendiceal and rectal carcinoids infrequently metastasize, even though they may show extensive local spread.* By contrast, 90% of ileal, gastric, and colonic carcinoids that have penetrated halfway through the muscle wall have spread to lymph nodes and distant sites such as the liver at the time of diagnosis. This is especially true for tumors greater than 2 cm in diameter.

Morphology. The appendix is the most common site of gut carcinoid tumors, followed by the small intestine (primarily ileum), rectum, stomach, and colon. However, the rectal tumors may represent up to half of tumors that come to clinical attention. Those that arise in the stomach and ileum are frequently multicentric, but the remainder tend to be solitary lesions. In the appendix they appear as bulbous swellings of the tip, which frequently obliterate the lumen. Elsewhere in the gut, they appear as intramural or submucosal masses that create small, polypoid or plateau-like elevations rarely more than 3 cm in diameter (Fig. 17–65*A*). The overlying mucosa may be intact or ulcerated, and the tumors may permeate the bowel wall to invade the mesentery. A characteristic feature is a solid, yellow-tan appearance on transection. The tumors are exceedingly firm owing to striking desmoplasia, and when these fibrosing lesions penetrate the mesentery of the small bowel they may cause angulation or kinking sufficient to cause obstruction. When present, visceral metastases are usually small, dispersed nodules and rarely achieve the size seen with the primary lesions. Notably, rectal and appendiceal carcinoids almost never metastasize.

Histologically, the neoplastic cells may form discrete islands, trabeculae, stands, glands, or undifferentiated sheets. Whatever their organization the tumor cells are monotonously similar, having a scant, pink granular cytoplasm and a round to oval stippled nucleus. In most tumors there is minimal variation in cell and nuclear size and mitoses are infrequent or absent (Fig. 17–65*B*). In unusual cases there may be more significant anaplasia and sometimes mucin

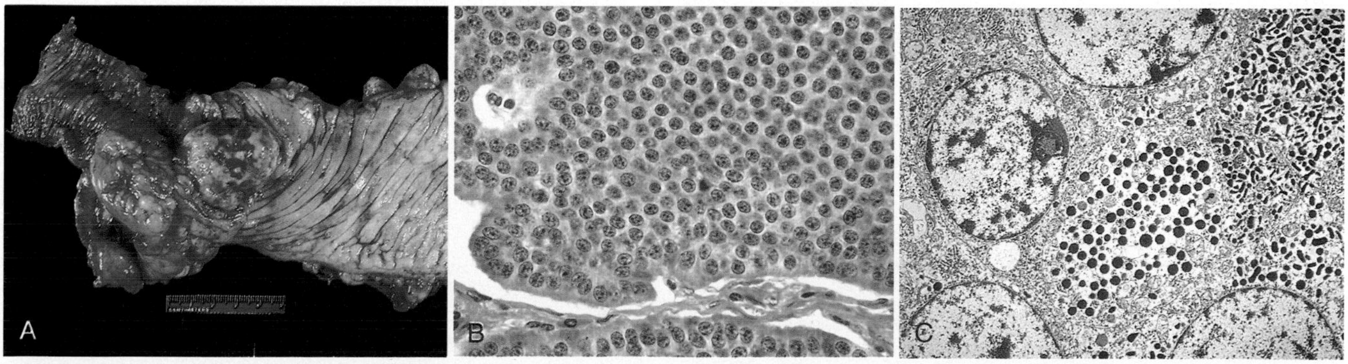

FIGURE 17–65 Carcinoid tumor. *A,* Multiple protruding tumors are present at the ileocecal junction. *B,* The tumor cells exhibit a monotonous morphology, with a delicate intervening fibrovascular stroma. *C,* Electron micrograph showing dense core bodies in the cytoplasm.

secretion within the cells and gland formations. Rarely, tumors arise resembling small-cell carcinomas of the lung (Chapter 15) or contain abundant psammoma bodies similar to those seen in thyroid carcinomas (Chapter 24). By electron microscopy (Fig. 17–65*C*), the cells in most tumors contain membrane-bound secretory granules with osmophilic centers (dense-core granules) in the cytoplasm. Most carcinoids contain chromogranin A, synaptophysin, and neuron-specific enolase. Specific hormonal peptides may occasionally be identified by immunocytochemical techniques.

Clinical Features. Gastrointestinal carcinoids only rarely produce local symptoms, which are caused by angulation or obstruction of the small intestine. Many (especially rectal and appendiceal) are asymptomatic and are found incidentally. However, the secretory products of some carcinoids may produce a variety of syndromes or endocrinopathies, depending on their anatomic site (Chapter 7). Gastric, peripancreatic, and pancreatic carcinoids can release their products directly into the systemic circulation, and can produce, for example, the *Zollinger-Ellison syndrome* related to excess elaboration of gastrin, Cushing syndrome associated with corticotropin secretion, and hyperinsulinism. In some instances, these tumors may be smaller than 1 cm and extremely difficult to find, even during surgical exploration.

Some neoplasms are associated with a distinctive *carcinoid syndrome* (Table 17–15). The syndrome occurs in about 1% of all patients with carcinoids and in 20% of those with widespread metastases. Uncertainties remain about the precise origin of the carcinoid syndrome, but most manifestations are thought to arise from excess elaboration of serotonin (*5-hydroxytryptamine,* 5-HT). Elevated levels of 5-HT and its metabolite, *5-hydroxyindoleacetic acid* (5-HIAA), are present in the blood and urine of most patients with the classic syndrome. 5-HT produced by gastrointesinal carcinoid tumors is degraded to functionally inactive 5-HIAA in the liver. Thus, hepatic metastases are usually present for the development of the syndrome from gastrointestinal carcinoids, because under these conditions, a sufficient amount of substances produced by the tumors can reach the systemic circulation without metabolic degradation by the liver. Not surprisingly, hepatic metastases are usually not required for the production of a carcinoid syndrome by extraintestinal carcinoids (such as those arising in the lungs or ovaries), because active substances produced by the tumors are directly released into the systemic circulation. Other secretory products of carcinoids such as histamine, bradykinin, kallikrein, and prostaglandins may also contribute to the manifestations of the carcinoid syndrome.

The overall five-year survival rate for carcinoids (excluding appendiceal) is approximately 90%. Even with small-bowel tumors with hepatic metastases, it is better than 50%. However, widespread disease will usually cause death.

TABLE 17–15 Clinical Features of the Carcinoid Syndrome

• Vasomotor distubances Cutaneous flushes and apparent cyanosis (most patients)
• Intestinal hypermotility Diarrhea, Cramps, nausea, vomiting (most patients)
• Asthmatic bronchoconstrictive attacks Couth, wheezing, dyspnea (about one third of patients)
• Hepatomegaly Nodular liver owing to hepatic metastases (some patients)
• Systemic fibrosis (some patients) Cardiac involvement Pulmonic and tricuspid valve thickening and stenosis Endocardial fibrosis, principally in the right ventricle (Bronchial carcinoids affect the left side) Retroperitoneal and pelvic fibrosis Collagenous pleural and intimal aortic plaques

GASTROINTESTINAL LYMPHOMA

Any segment of the gastrointestinal tract may be secondarily involved by systemic dissemination of non-Hodgkin lymphomas. However, up to 40% of lymphomas arise in sites other than lymph nodes, and the gut is the most common location. Conversely, about 1% to 4% of all gastrointestinal malignancies are lymphomas. *By definition, primary gastrointestinal lymphomas exhibit no evidence of liver, spleen, mediastinal lymph node, or bone marrow involvement at the time of diagnosis*—regional lymph node involvement may be present. *Primary gastrointestinal lymphomas usually arise as sporadic neoplasms but also occur more frequently in certain patient populations: (1) Chronic gastritis caused by H. pylori, (2) chronic spruelike syndromes, (3) natives of the Mediterranean region, (4) congenital immunodeficiency states, (5) infection with human immunodeficiency virus, and (6) following organ transplantation with immunosuppression.*

Intestinal tract lymphomas can be classified into B-cell and T-cell lymphomas. The B-cell lymphoma can be subdivided into MALT lymphoma, immunoproliferative small-intestinal disease (IPSID), and Burkitt lymphoma.

1. *MALT lymphoma is a sporadic lymphoma, which* arises from the B cells of MALT (mucosa-associated lymphoid tissue, described under gastric lymphoma). *This type of lymphoma is the most common form in the Western hemisphere.* The biologic features of these lymphomas are different from node-based lymphomas in that (1) many behave as focal tumors in their early stages and are amenable to surgical resection; (2) relapse may occur exclusively in the gastrointestinal tract; (3) genotypic changes are different than those observed in nodal lymphomas: the t(11;18) translocation is relatively common in MALT lymphoma; and (4) the cells are usually CD5- and CD10-negative. This type of gastrointestinal lymphoma usually affects adults, has no gender predilection, and may arise anywhere in the gut: stomach (55% to 60% of cases); small intestine (25% to 30%), proximal colon (10% to 15%), and distal colon (up to 10%). The appendix and esophagus are only rarely involved.

The pathogenesis of these lymphomas is under intense scrutiny. The concept has been advanced that lymphomas of MALT origin arise in the setting of mucosal lymphoid activation and that these lymphomas are the malignant counterparts of hypermutated, postgerminal-center memory B cells. As discussed earlier, *Helicobacter*-associated chronic gastritis, in particular, has been proposed as a driving force for the development of gastric MALT lymphoma, the result of antigen-driven somatic mutation of gastric lymphoid tissue. However, the etiologic factors for intestinal lymphoma are still unknown, although history of IBD appears to increase the risk.

2. *IPSID is also referred to as Mediterranean lymphoma.* It is an unusual intestinal B-cell lymphoma arising in patients with Mediterranean ancestry, having a background of chronic diffuse mucosal plasmacytosis. The plasma cells synthesize an abnormal Igα heavy chain, in which the variable portion has been deleted. A high proportion of patients have malabsorption and weight loss preceding the development of the lymphoma. The diagnosis is made most commonly in children and young adults, and both sexes appear to be affected equally. The exact etiology of this type of lymphoma is not known, although infection appears to play a role.[95]

3. *The intestinal T-cell lymphoma* is usually associated with a long-standing malabsorption syndrome (such as celiac disease) that may not constitute a true gluten-sensitive enteropathy. This lymphoma occurs in relatively young individuals (age 30 to 40), often following a 10- to 20-year history of symptomatic malabsorption. Alternatively, a diffuse enteropathy with malabsorption may accompany the development of a lymphoma. Intestinal T-cell lymphoma arises most often in the proximal small bowel, and its overall prognosis is poor (reported 11% five-year survival rate).

Morphology. Gastrointestinal lymphomas can assume a variety of gross appearances. Since all the gut lymphoid tissue is mucosal and submucosal, early lesions appear as plaque-like expansions of the mucosa and submucosa. Diffusely infiltrating lesions may produce full-thickness mural thickening, with effacement of the overlying mucosal folds and focal ulceration. Others may be polypoid, protruding into the lumen, or form large, fungating, ulcerated masses. Tumor infiltration into the muscularis propria splays the muscle fibers, gradually destroying them. Because of this feature, advanced lesions frequently cause motility problems with secondary obstruction. Large tumors sometimes perforate because of lack of stromal support; reduction in tumor bulk during chemotherapy also may lead to perforation.

In the earliest histologic lesions, atypical lymphoid cells may be seen infiltrating the mucosa, with effacement and loss of glands and massive expansion of lymphoid tissue. Extreme numbers of atypical lymphoid cells may populate the superficial or glandular epithelium (lymphoepithelial lesion). With established lymphomas, the mucosa, submucosa, and even muscle wall are replaced by a monotonous infiltrate of malignant cells, consisting of a mixture of small lymphocytes and immunoblasts in varying proportions. Lymphoid follicles are occasionally formed. Most gut lymphomas are of B-cell type (over 95%) and are evenly split between low- and high-grade tumors. The small fraction of T-cell lymphomas occurring in the intestine are commonly high-grade lesions.

Clinical Features. With the exception of T-cell lymphomas, primary gastrointestinal lymphomas generally have a better prognosis than do those arising in other sites. Ten-year survival for patients with localized mucosal or submucosal disease approaches 85%. Early discovery is key to survival; thus, gastric lymphomas generally have a better outcome than those of the small or large bowel. In general, the depth of local invasion, size of the tumor, the histologic grade of the tumor, and extension into adjacent viscera are important determinants of prognosis.

MESENCHYMAL TUMORS

Mesenchymal tumors may occur anywhere in the alimentary tract. The nomenclature for these tumors is largely based on the tumor cell phenotypes. Lipomas show a propensity for the submucosa of the small and large intestines, and lipomatous hypertrophy may occur in the ileocecal valve. A variety of spindle-cell lesions may arise in the muscle wall of any gut segment. The great majority of these tumors are of smooth muscle origin, and hence can be termed *leiomyomas* and *leiomyosarcomas.* Gastrointestinal stromal tumors (GISTs), are now considered to be a distinctive tumor type, characterized by c-KIT immunoreactivity, as discussed earlier (see "Gastric Tumors"). The small intestine is the second most common location for this tumor, (the stomach being the most common). Both benign and malignant versions of GIST may occur at any age and in either sex. Vascular tumors such as *Kaposi sarcomas* are considered elsewhere (see Chapter 11).

Morphology. Lipomas are usually well-demarcated, firm nodules (almost always less than 4 cm in diameter) arising within the submucosa or muscularis propria. The overlying mucosa is stretched and attenuated. Rarely, they grow to larger size and produce hemispheric elevation of the mucosa with ulceration over the dome of the tumor. Malignant stromal tumors (primarily leiomyosarcoma) tend to produce large, bulky, intramural masses that eventually fungate and ulcerate into the lumen or project subserosally into the abdominal space. Histologically, lipomas, leiomyomas, and leiomyosarcomas resemble their counterparts encountered elsewhere (Chapter 26). In the case of the stromal tumors (e.g., leiomyomas and leiomyosarcomas), large size and a high mitotic rate are correlated with an aggressive course.

Clinical Features. Most mesenchymal tumors are asymptomatic. In the stomach, larger lesions (benign or malignant) may produce symptoms resembling those of peptic ulcer, particularly bleeding that is sometimes massive. Intestinal lesions may present with bleeding, and for the small intestine, rare obstruction or intussusception. Benign lesions are easily resectable. Surgical removal is usually possible for the malignant lesions as well, since they tend to grow as cohesive masses. Five-year survival rate for leiomyosarcoma, for example, is 50% to 60%. Metastases, however, are present in about one third of cases.

TUMORS OF THE ANAL CANAL

The anal canal is the terminal portion of the large intestine. It is divided into three zones: the upper (covered with rectal mucosa), the middle (partially covered with a transitional mucosa), and the lower (covered by stratified squamous mucosa). The tumors located in this anatomic location are designated as carcinoma of the anal canal. Patterns of differentiation include a basaloid pattern, squamous cell carcinoma, and adenocarcinoma.

Anal canal carcinoma with basaloid differentiation is a tumor populated by immature proliferative cells derived from the basal layer of a stratified squamous epithelium. These tumors may occur sporadically and be uniform in their histologic features. Alternatively, basaloid differentiation may be a component of a tumor that exhibits more genuine squamous cell differentiation and/or the mucin vacuole-containing features of adenocarcinoma. All such tumors remain classified as anal canal carcinoma.

Pure squamous cell carcinomas of the anal canal are closely associated with chronic HPV infection.[96] Some rare cases are also related to immunosuppression, as encountered in renal transplantation and in AIDS patients. As with the genital tract, chronic HPV infection of the anal canal often causes precursor lesions such as condyloma acuminatum, squamous epithelium dysplasia, and carcinoma in situ.

Pure adenocarcinoma of the anal canal is often the extension of rectal adenocarcinoma. Rarely, other tumors may arise from the anal canal, notably *Paget disease*, small-cell carcinoma, and melanoma.

APPENDIX

Normal

The appendix is an underdeveloped residuum of the otherwise voluminous cecum. The adult appendix averages 6 to 7 cm in length, is partially anchored by a mesenteric extension from the adjacent ileum, and has no known function. The appendix has the same four layers as the remainder of the gut and possesses a colonic-type mucosa. A distinguishing feature of this organ is the extremely rich lymphoid tissue of the mucosa and submucosa, which in young individuals forms an entire layer of germinal follicles and lymphoid pulp. This lymphoid tissue undergoes progressive atrophy during life to the point of complete disappearance in advanced age. In the elderly the appendix, particularly the distal portion, sometimes undergoes fibrous obliteration.

Pathology

Diseases of the appendix loom large in surgical practice; appendicitis is the most common acute abdominal condition the surgeon is called on to treat. Appendicitis is one of the best-known medical entities and yet may be one of the most difficult diagnostic problems to confront the emergency physician. A differential diagnosis must include virtually every acute process that can occur within the abdominal cavity, as well as some emergent conditions affecting organs of the thorax.

Acute Appendicitis

Inflammation in the right lower quadrant was considered a nonsurgical disease of the cecum (typhlitis or perityphlitis) until Fitz recognized acute appendicitis as a distinct entity in 1886. Appendiceal inflammation is associated with obstruction in 50% to 80% of cases, usually in the form of a fecalith and, less commonly, a gallstone, tumor, or ball of worms *(oxyuriasis vermicularis).* Continued secretion of mucinous fluid in the obstructed viscus presumably leads to a progressive increase in intraluminal pressure sufficient to cause eventual collapse of the draining veins. Ischemic injury then favors bacterial proliferation with additional inflammatory edema and exudation, further embarrassing the blood supply. Nevertheless, a significant minority of inflamed appendices have no demonstrable luminal obstruction, and the pathogenesis of the inflammation remains unknown.

Morphology. At the earliest stages, only a scant neutrophilic exudate may be found throughout the mucosa, submucosa, and muscularis propria. Subserosal vessels are congested, and often there is a modest perivascular neutrophilic infiltrate. The inflammatory reaction transforms the normal glistening serosa into a dull, granular, red membrane; this transformation signifies **early acute appendicitis** for the operating surgeon. At a later stage, a prominent neutrophilic exudate generates a fibrinopurulent reaction over the serosa (Fig. 17–66). As the inflammatory process worsens, there is abscess formation within the wall, along with ulcerations and foci of suppurative necrosis in the mucosa. This state constitutes **acute suppurative appendicitis.** Further appendiceal compromise leads to large areas of hemorrhagic green ulceration of the mucosa and green-black gangrenous necrosis through the wall, extending to the serosa, creating **acute gangrenous appendicitis,** which is quickly followed by rupture and suppurative peritonitis.

The histologic criterion for the diagnosis of acute appendicitis is neutrophilic infiltration of the muscularis propria. Usually, neutrophils and ulcerations are also present within the mucosa. Since drainage of an exudate into the appendix from alimentary tract infection may also induce a mucosal neutrophilic infiltrate, evidence of muscular wall inflammation is requisite for the diagnosis.

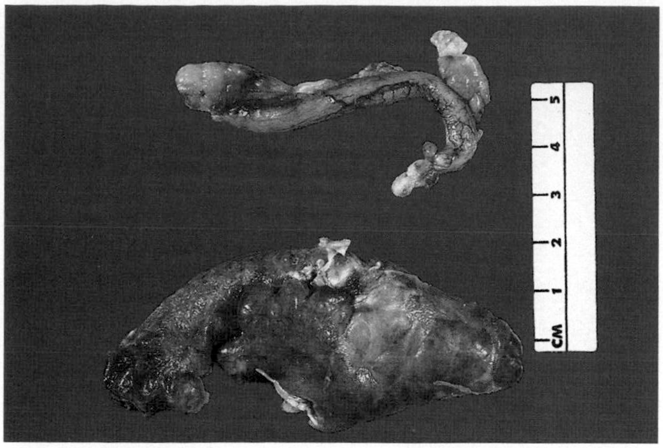

FIGURE 17–66 Acute appendicitis. The inflamed appendix shown below is red, swollen, and covered with a fibrinous exudate. For comparison, a normal appendix is shown above.

Clinical Features. Acute appendicitis is mainly a disease of adolescents and young adults, but it may occur in any age group and affects males slightly more often than females. The lifetime risk for appendicitis is 7%. Classically, acute appendicitis produces the following manifestations, in the sequence given: (1) pain, at first periumbilical but then localizing to the right lower quadrant; (2) nausea and/or vomiting; (3) abdominal tenderness, particularly in the region of the appendix; (4) mild fever; and (5) an elevation of the peripheral white blood cell count up to 15,000 to 20,000 cell/μL. Regrettably, this classic presentation is more often not present. While pain, nausea, and vomiting usually develop, tenderness may be deceptively absent or present in atypical locations. In some cases, a retrocecal appendix may generate right flank or pelvic pain, while a malrotated colon may give rise to appendicitis in the left upper quadrant. The peripheral leukocytosis may be minimal or so high as to suggest alternative diagnoses. Nonclassic presentations are encountered more often in young children and in the very elderly, populations with a host of other plausible abdominal emergencies.

There is general agreement that highly competent surgeons make false-positive diagnoses of acute appendicitis and remove normal appendices about 20% to 25% of the time. *The discomfort and risks associated with an exploratory laparotomy and discovery of "no disease" are far outweighed by the morbidity and mortality (about 2%) associated with appendiceal perforation.* Besides perforation, uncommon complications of appendicitis include pyelophlebitis with thrombosis of the portal venous drainage, liver abscess, and bacteremia. In instances when the appendix is normal, most often no disease of any kind is found during abdominal exploration. Definable conditions that mimic appendicitis are mesenteric lymphadenitis, usually secondary to an enterocolitis (often unrecognized) caused by *Yersinia* or a virus; systemic viral infection; acute salpingitis; ectopic pregnancy; mittelschmerz (pain caused by trivial pelvic bleeding at the time of ovulation); cystic fibrosis; and Meckel diverticulitis.

True *chronic inflammation* of the appendix is difficult to define as a pathologic entity, although occasionally granulation tissue and fibrosis associated with acute and chronic inflammation of the appendix suggest an organizing acute appendicitis. Much more frequently, recurrent acute attacks underlie a seemingly chronic condition. Since in some individuals the appendix is a mere fibrous cord from birth, it cannot be assumed that appendiceal fibrosis is the result of a previous inflammation.

Tumors of the Appendix

The most common appendiceal tumor is the carcinoid, discussed earlier. It is usually discovered incidentally at the time of surgery or examination of a resected appendix.[97] This neoplasm most frequently involves the distal tip of the appendix, where it produces a solid bulbous swelling up to 2 to 3 cm in diameter. Although intramural and transmural extension may be evident, nodal metastases are very infrequent, and distant spread is rare. One unique type of appendiceal carcinoid tumor is goblet cell carcinoid (adenocarcinoid). Histologically, the tumor shows a typical carcinoid pattern, but with plump mucin vacuole-containing cells. The biologic behavior of the tumor is between that of typical carcinoid and adenocarcinoma. Genetic alterations have been found in both typical carcinoid tumors and goblet cell carcinoids.[98]

Conventional adenomas or non–mucin-producing adenocarcinomas of the appendix may cause a typical neoplastic enlargement of this organ. Hyperplastic polyps may occur in this location as well. Benign and malignant mesenchymal growths resemble their counterparts in other areas.

MUCOCELE AND PSEUDOMYXOMA PERITONEI

Mucocele is the macroscopic description of a dilated appendix filled with mucin. The true pathologic nature of mucocele runs the gamut from an innocuous obstructed appendix containing inspissated mucin, to a mucin-secreting adenoma (mucinous cystadenoma) and adenocarcinoma (mucinous cystadenocarcinoma). In the last instance, invasion through the appendiceal wall with intraperitoneal seeding and spread of tumor may occur.

Morphology. All mucinous lesions are associated with appendiceal dilatation secondary to mucinous secretions. With the simple **mucocele,** globular enlargement of the appendix by inspissated mucus occurs, usually the result of obstruction by a fecalith or other lesion such as an inflammatory stricture. Eventually, the distention produces sufficient atrophy of the mucin-secreting mucosal cells and the secretions stop. Rarely, a focus of mucin-secreting hyperplastic epithelium appears to be the culprit. This condition is usually asymptomatic; rarely a mucocele ruptures, spilling otherwise innocuous mucus into the peritoneal cavity.

The most common mucinous neoplasm is the benign **mucinous cystadenoma,** which replaces the appendiceal mucosa and is histologically identical to analogous tumors in the ovary. The luminal dilation is associated with appendiceal perforation in 20% of instances, producing localized collections of mucus attached to the serosa of the appendix or lying free within the peritoneal cavity. Histologic examination of the mucus, however, reveals no malignant cells.

Malignant **mucinous cystadenocarcinomas** are one fifth as common as cystadenomas. Macroscopically they produce mucin-filled cystic dilatation of the appendix indistinguishable from that seen with benign cystadenomas. Penetration of the appendiceal wall by invasive cells and spread beyond the appendix in the form of localized or disseminated peritoneal implants, however, is frequently present (Fig. 17–67). In its fully developed state, continued cellular proliferation and mucin secretion fills the abdomen with tenacious, semisolid mucin—**pseudomyxoma peritoneii**. Anaplastic adenocarcinomatous cells can be found, distinguishing this process from mucinous spillage. Instances in which pseudomyxoma peritoneii is accompanied by both appendiceal and ovarian mucinous adenocarcinomas are usually ascribed to spread of an appendiceal primary lesion.

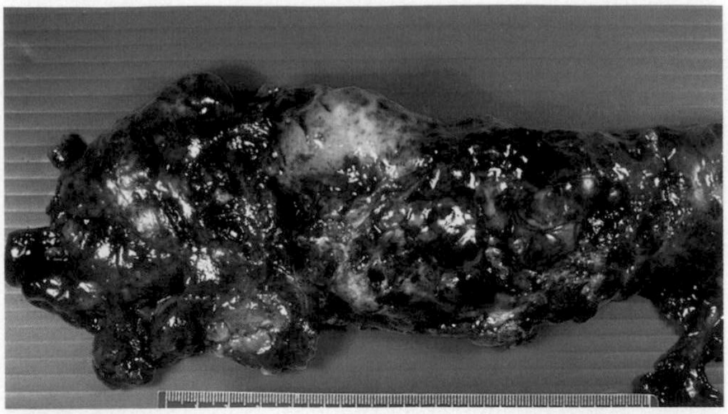

FIGURE 17–67 Mucinous cystadenocarcinoma of the appendix, with spread into the immediate periappendiceal tissues.

Mucoceles are generally encountered as an incidental lesion. Mucinous cystadenomas and adenocarcinomas may present with pain, attributable to distention of the viscus. Laparotomy for presumed acute appendicitis is a typical diagnostic setting. For lesions confined to the resected specimen (appendix or more radical excision), the outlook is excellent. Pseudomyxoma peritoneii may be held in check for years by repeated debulking procedures but in most instances eventually runs its inexorable fatal course.

PERITONEUM

Inflammation

Peritonitis may result from bacterial invasion or chemical irritation. The most common causes of peritonitis are as follows.

- *Sterile peritonitis* from mild leakage of bile or pancreatic enzymes
- *Perforation or rupture of the biliary system*, which evokes a highly irritating peritonitis, usually complicated by bacterial superinfection
- *Acute hemorrhagic pancreatitis* (see Chapter 19), with leakage of pancreatic enzymes and digestion of adipose tissue to produce fatty acids. These in turn precipitate with calcium to produce chalky white precipitates in areas of fat digestion and necrosis. Globules of free fat may be found floating in the peritoneal fluid, and bacterial permeation of the bowel wall leads to a frank suppurative exudate after 24 to 48 hours.
- *Surgical procedures.* The reaction to surgically introduced foreign material such as talc is usually localized and minimal, leaving residual foreign-body type granulomas and fibrous tissue. Abrasion of serosal surfaces during abdominal surgery may lead to fibrous adhesions between visceral structures. While usually asymptomatic, these occasionally are the points of internal herniation or intestinal obstruction.
- *Gynecologic conditions.* Endometriosis may introduce irritant blood into the peritoneal cavity, and ruptured dermoid cysts may invoke an intense peritoneal granulomatous reaction.

PERITONEAL INFECTION

Bacterial peritonitis is almost invariably secondary to extension of bacteria through the wall of a hollow viscus or to rupture of a viscus. The more common disorders leading to such bacterial disseminations are *appendicitis, ruptured peptic ulcer, cholecystitis, diverticulitis, strangulation of bowel, acute salpingitis, abdominal trauma,* and *peritoneal dialysis.* Virtually every bacterial organism has been implicated, most commonly *E. coli*, alpha- and beta-hemolytic streptococci, *Staphylococcus aureus,* enterococci, gram-negative rods, and *Clostridium perfringens.* The last organism is a frequent inhabitant of the gut and contributor to peritonitis but rarely causes gas gangrene in the abdominal cavity. Gynecologic infections may introduce gonococcus and Chlamydia.

Spontaneous bacterial peritonitis may develop in the absence of an obvious source of contamination. It is an uncommon disorder seen most often in children, particularly those with the nephrotic syndrome. Among adults, 10% of cirrhotic patients with ascites develop spontaneous bacterial peritonitis during the course of their illness. The usual causal agents of the latter are *E. coli* and pneumococci, but the manner by which they invade the peritoneal cavity is unknown, possibly blood-borne.

Morphology. Depending on the duration of the peritonitis, the membranes show the following changes. Approximately 2 to 4 hours after initiation, there is loss of the gray, glistening quality of the peritoneal surface, and it becomes dull and lusterless. At this time, there is a small accumulation of essentially serous or slightly turbid fluid. Later the exudate becomes creamy and obviously suppurative. In some cases, it may be extremely thick and plastic and even inspissated, especially in dehydrated patients. The volume of exudates varies enormously. In many cases, it may be localized by the omentum and viscera to a small area of the abdominal cavity. In generalized peritonitis, it is important to remember that an exudate may accumulate under and above the liver to form subhepatic and subdiaphragmatic abscesses. Collections in the lesser omental sac may likewise create residual persistent foci of infection.

The inflammatory process is typical of an acute bacterial infection anywhere and produces the characteristic neutrophilic infiltration with fibrinopurulent exudation. The reaction usually remains superficial and does not penetrate deeply into the visceral structures or abdominal wall. Tuberculous peritonitis tends to produce a plastic exudate studded with minute, pale granulomas.

These inflammatory processes can heal either spontaneously or with therapy. In the course of healing, the following may occur: (1) The exudate may be totally resolved, leaving no residual fibrosis; (2) residual, walled-off abscesses may persist, eventually to heal or serve as foci of new infection; or (3) organization of the exudate may occur, with the formation of fibrous adhesions, which may be delicate or quite dense.

SCLEROSING RETROPERITONITIS

Dense fibromatous overgrowth of the retroperitoneal tissues may sometimes develop, designated *sclerosing retroperitonitis* or *idiopathic retroperitoneal fibrosis* (also called *Ormond disease*). In some instances the mesentery is also involved. The fibrous overgrowth is entirely nondistinctive and, although infiltrative, does not display anaplasia. There is usually an accompanying inflammatory infiltrate of lymphocytes, plasma cells, and neutrophils, suggesting inflammatory rather than neoplastic disease. The fibrosis may encroach on the ureters to produce hydronephrosis. Alternatively, fibrous tissue may surround retroperitoneal organs and extend into the mesentery. In some ways this process is an analogue of the desmoid tumor. The cause of this curious condition is obscure; in some instances there is a history of intake of the drug methysergide, an ergot derivative used for migraine, or history of previous surgery or radiation therapy. However, most cases have no obvious cause. Similar fibrotic changes seen in other sites (mediastinal fibrosis, sclerosing cholangitis, and Riedel fibrosing thyroiditis) suggest that the disorder is autoimmune and systemic in origin, preferentially involving the retroperitoneum.

MESENTERIC CYSTS

Large to small cystic masses are sometimes found within the mesenteries in the abdominal cavity or attached to the peritoneal lining of the abdominal wall. These cysts sometimes offer difficult clinical problems because they present on palpation as abdominal masses. Many classifications have been attempted; the most widely used is based on pathogenetic origins: (1) those arising from sequestered lymphatic channels; (2) those derived from pinched-off enteric diverticula of the developing foregut and hindgut; (3) those derived from the urogenital ridge or its derivatives (i.e., the urinary tract and male and female genital tracts); (4) those derived from walled-off infections or following pancreatitis, more properly called *pseudocysts;* and (5) those of malignant origin, most often resulting from peritoneal involvement by intra-abdominal adenocarcinomas.

Tumors

Virtually all tumors of the peritoneum are malignant and can be divided into primary and secondary forms.

Primary tumors arising from the mesothelium of the peritoneum are extremely rare and are called *mesotheliomas.* These exactly duplicate mesotheliomas found in the pleura and the pericardium, but the prognosis is poor. Like the supradiaphragmatic tumors, peritoneal mesotheliomas are associated with asbestos exposure in at least 80% of cases. How inhaled asbestos induces a peritoneal neoplasm remains a mystery. It has been recently suggested that genetic factors or viral infections may play a role in the genesis of peritoneal mesothelioma. The histopathologic diagnosis of mesothelioma is not always straightforward. In many occasions, immunohistochemical stains are required to differentiate this tumor from forms of adenocarcinoma.

Desmoplastic small round cell tumor is a rare tumor arising from peritoneum. The exact histogenesis and pathogenesis of this tumor are still not known. Molecular marker studies have suggested that this tumor is in the family of small round cell tumors such as Ewing sarcoma, rhabdoid myosarcoma, and primitive neuroectodermal tumor. The characteristic genetic marker for this tumor is the reciprocal chromosome translocation t(11;22) (p13;q12) resulting in *EWS-WT1* fusion.[99]

Secondary tumors of the peritoneum are, in contrast, quite common. In any form of advanced cancer, penetration to the serosal membrane or metastatic seeding (peritoneal carcinomatosis) may occur. The most common tumors producing diffuse serosal implantation are ovarian and pancreatic. Appendiceal mucinous carcinomas may produce pseudomyxoma peritoneii, as described earlier. However, any type of intra-abdominal malignancy, and occasionally tumors from extra-abdominal locations, may be implicated in peritoneal seeding.

Additional mention might be made of the very uncommon tumors that may arise from retroperitoneal tissues (i.e., fat, fibrous tissue, blood vessels, lymphatics, nerves, and the lymph nodes alongside the aorta). These native structures may give rise to benign or malignant tumors derived from any of the indigenous mesenchymal cell types, resembling their counterparts arising elsewhere in the body.

REFERENCES

1. DeNardi FG, Riddell RH: The normal esophagus. Am J Surg Pathol 15:296, 1991.
2. Hornby PJ, Abrahams TP, Partosoedarso ER: Central mechanisms of lower esophageal sphincter control. Gastroenterol Clin North Am 31:S11, v–vi, 2002.
3. Rittler M, Paz JE, Castilla EE: VATERL: an epidemiologic analysis of risk factors. Am J Med Genet 73:162, 1997.
4. Hirano I: Pathophysiology of achalasia. Curr Gastroenterol Rep 1:198, 1999.
5. Richter JE: Oesophageal motility disorders. Lancet 358:823, 2001.
6. Weiss S, Mallory G: Lesions of cardiac orifice of the stomach produced vomiting. JAMA 98:1353, 1932.
7. Shaheen N, Ransohoff DF: Gastroesophageal reflux, Barrett esophagus, and esophageal cancer: scientific review. JAMA 287:1972, 2002.
8. Spechler SJ: Clinical practice. Barrett's esophagus. N Engl J Med 346:836, 2002.
9. Sbarbati A, et al: Ultrastructural phenotype of "intestinal-type" cells in columnar-lined esophagus. Ultrastruct Pathol 26:107, 2002.
10. Haggitt RC: Pathology of Barrett's esophagus. J Gastrointest Surg 4:117, 2000.
11. Jankowski JA, et al: Molecular evolution of the metaplasia-dysplasia-adenocarcinoma sequence in the esophagus. Am J Pathol 154:965, 1999.
12. Souza RF: Molecular and biologic basis of upper gastrointestinal malignancy—esophageal carcinoma. Surg Oncol Clin N Am 11:257, 2002.
13. Kok TC, et al: No evidence of known types of human papillomavirus in squamous cell cancer of the oesophagus in a low-risk area. Rotterdam Oesophageal Tumour Study Group. Eur J Cancer 33:1865, 1997.
14. Lam AK: Molecular biology of esophageal squamous cell carcinoma. Crit Rev Oncol Hematol 33:71, 2000.
15. Jenkins GJ, et al: Genetic pathways involved in the progression of Barrett's metaplasia to adenocarcinoma. Br J Surg 89:824, 2002.
16. Croft J, et al: Analysis of the premalignant stages of Barrett's oesophagus through to adenocarcinoma by comparative genomic hybridization. Eur J Gastroenterol Hepatol 14:1179, 2002.
17. Hanby AM, et al: The mucous neck cell in the human gastric corpus: a distinctive, functional cell lineage. J Pathol 187:331, 1999.
18. Kojima M, et al: Ghrelin is a growth-hormone-releasing acylated peptide from stomach. Nature 402:656, 1999.
19. Owen DA: Gastritis and carditis. Mod Pathol 16:325, 2003.
20. Moss SF, Sood S: *Helicobacter pylori*. Curr Opin Infect Dis 16:445, 2003.
21. Tomb JF, et al: The complete genome sequence of the gastric pathogen *Helicobacter pylori*. Nature 388:539, 1997.
22. Blaser MJ, Atherton JC: *Helicobacter pylori* persistence: biology and disease. J Clin Invest 113:321, 2004.
23. Covacci A, Rappuoli R: *Helicobacter pylori*: after the genomes, back to biology. J Exp Med 197:807, 2003.
24. Backert S, et al: Functional analysis of the cag pathogenicity island in *Helicobacter pylori* isolates from patients with gastritis, peptic ulcer, and gastric cancer. Infect Immun 72:1043, 2004.
25. Furuta T, et al: Interleukin 1β polymorphisms increase risk of hypochlorhydria and atrophic gastritis and reduce risk of duodenal ulcer recurrence in Japan. Gastroenterology 123:92, 2002.
26. Solnick JV, Schauer DB: Emergence of diverse *Helicobacter* species in the pathogenesis of gastric and enterohepatic diseases. Clin Microbiol Rev 14:59, 2001.
27. Toh BH, van Driel IR, Gleeson PA: Pernicious anemia. N Engl J Med 337:1441, 1997.
28. Sandler RS, et al: The burden of selected digestive diseases in the United States. Gastroenterology 122:1500, 2002.
29. Chan FK, Leung WK: Peptic-ulcer disease. Lancet 360:933, 2002.
30. Prinz C, Hafsi N, Voland P: *Helicobacter pylori* virulence factors and the host immune response: implications for therapeutic vaccination. Trends Microbiol 11:134, 2003.
31. Ming SC: Cellular and molecular pathology of gastric carcinoma and precursor lesions: a critical review. Gastric Cancer 1:31, 1998.
32. Abraham SC, et al: Sporadic fundic gland polyps: common gastric polyps arising through activating mutations in the β-catenin gene. Am J Pathol 158:1005, 2001.
33. Wingo PA, et al: Long-term trends in cancer mortality in the United States, 1930–1998. Cancer 97:3133, 2003.
34. Normark S, et al: Persistent infection with *Helicobacter pylori* and the development of gastric cancer. Adv Cancer Res 90:63, 2003.
35. Kelley JR, Duggan JM: Gastric cancer epidemiology and risk factors. J Clin Epidemiol 56:1, 2003.
36. Powell SM: Stomach cancer. In: Vogelstein B, Kinzler W (eds): The Genetic Basis of Human Cancer, 2nd Edition. New York: McGraw-Hill, 703, 2002.
37. Naumann M, Crabtree JE: *Helicobacter pylori*-induced epithelial cell signalling in gastric carcinogenesis. Trends Microbiol 12:29, 2004.
38. El-Rifai W, Powell SM: Molecular biology of gastric cancer. Semin Radiat Oncol 12:128, 2002.
39. Connolly EM, Gaffney E, Reynolds JV: Gastrointestinal stromal tumours. Br J Surg 90:1178, 2003.
40. Duffaud F, Blay JY: Gastrointestinal stromal tumors: biology and treatment. Oncology 65:187, 2003.
41. Heinrich MC, et al: *PDGFRA* activating mutations in gastrointestinal stromal tumors. Science 299:708, 2003.
42. Demetri GD, et al: Efficacy and safety of imatinib mesylate in advanced gastrointestinal stromal tumors. N Engl J Med 347:472, 2002.
43. Fellermann K, Stange EF: Defensins—innate immunity at the epithelial frontier. Eur J Gastroenterol Hepatol 13:771, 2001.
44. Gewirtz AT, et al: Intestinal epithelial pathobiology: past, present and future. Best Pract Res Clin Gastroenterol 16:851, 2002.
45. Bordeaux MC, et al: The *RET* proto-oncogene induces apoptosis: a novel mechanism for Hirschsprung disease. EMBO J 19:4056, 2000.
46. Martucciello G, et al: Pathogenesis of Hirschsprung's disease. J Pediatr Surg 35:1017, 2000.
47. Newgreen D, Young HM: Enteric nervous system: development and developmental disturbances–part 2. Pediatr Dev Pathol 5:329, 2002.
48. Bates MD, Deutsch GH: Molecular insights into congenital disorders of the digestive system. Pediatr Dev Pathol 6:284, 2003.
49. Guerrant RL, et al: Magnitude and impact of diarrheal diseases. Arch Med Res 33:351, 2002.
50. Goodgame RW: Viral causes of diarrhea. Gastroenterol Clin North Am 30:779, 2001.
51. Yu D, Kuipers JG: Role of bacteria and HLA-B27 in the pathogenesis of reactive arthritis. Rheum Dis Clin North Am 29:21, 2003.
52. Jones SL, Blikslager AT: Role of the enteric nervous system in the pathophysiology of secretory diarrhea. J Vet Intern Med 16:222, 2002.
53. Faruque SM, Albert MJ, Mekalanos JJ: Epidemiology, genetics, and ecology of toxigenic *Vibrio cholerae*. Microbiol Mol Biol Rev 62:1301, 1998.
54. Randazzo PA, et al: Molecular aspects of the cellular activities of ADP–ribosylation factors. Sci STKE 2000:RE1, 2000.
55. Borriello SP: Pathogenesis of *Clostridium difficile* infection. J Antimicrob Chemother 41 (suppl) C:13, 1998.
56. Procop GW: Gastrointestinal infections. Infect Dis Clin North Am 15:1073, 2001.
57. Katz DE, Taylor DN: Parasitic infections of the gastrointestinal tract. Gastroenterol Clin North Am 30:797, 2001.
58. Caplan MS, Jilling T: New concepts in necrotizing enterocolitis. Curr Opin Pediatr 13:111, 2001.
59. Pardi DS: Microscopic colitis. Mayo Clin Proc 78:614, 2003.
60. Cohen J, West AB, Bini EJ: Infectious diarrhea in human immunodeficiency virus. Gastroenterol Clin North Am 30:637, 2001.
61. Cruz-Correa M, et al: Endoscopic findings predict the histologic diagnosis in gastrointestinal graft-versus-host disease. Endoscopy 34:808, 2002.
62. Cipolla G, et al: Nonsteroidal anti-inflammatory drugs and inflammatory bowel disease: current perspectives. Pharmacol Res 46:1, 2002.
63. Farrell RJ, Kelly CP: Celiac sprue. N Engl J Med 346:180, 2002.
64. Catassi C, Fasano A: New developments in childhood celiac disease. Curr Gastroenterol Rep. 4:238, 2002.
65. Green PH, Jabri B: Celiac disease. Lancet 362:383, 2003.
66. Marth T, Raoult D: Whipple's disease. Lancet 361:239, 2003.
67. Bentley SD, et al: Sequencing and analysis of the genome of the Whipple's disease bacterium *Tropheryma whipplei*. Lancet 361:637, 2003.
68. Podolsky DK: Inflammatory bowel disease. N Engl J Med 347:417, 2002.
69. Mowat AM: Anatomical basis of tolerance and immunity to intestinal atigens. Nat Rev Immunol 3:331, 2003.
70. Bouma G, Strober W: The immunological and genetic basis of inflammatory bowel disease. Nat Rev Immunol 3:521, 2003.
71. Hugot JP, et al: Association of *NOD2* leucine-rich repeat variants with susceptibility to Crohn's disease. Nature 411:599, 2001.
72. McKay DM: Intestinal inflammation and the gut microflora. Can J Gastroenterol 13:509, 1999.

73. Dubinsky MC, et al: Clinical utility of serodiagnostic testing in suspected pediatric inflammatory bowel disease. Am J Gastroenterol 96:758, 2001.
74. Bansi DS, Chapman RW, Fleming KA: Prevalence and diagnostic role of antineutrophil cytoplasmic antibodies in inflammatory bowel disease. Eur J Gastroenterol Hepatol 8:881, 1996.
75. Greenson JK: Dysplasia in inflammatory bowel disease. Semin Diagn Pathol 2002;19:31.
76. McKenna BJ, Appelman HD: Dysplasia can be a pain in the gut. Pathology 34:518, 2002.
77. Chen R, et al: DNA fingerprinting abnormalities can distinguish ulcerative colitis patients with dysplasia and cancer from those who are dysplasia/cancer-free. Am J Pathol 162:665, 2003.
78. Eaden JA, Abrams KR, Mayberry JF: The risk of colorectal cancer in ulcerative colitis: a meta-analysis. Gut 48:526, 2001.
79. Miyaki M, Kuroki T: Role of Smad4 (DPC4) inactivation in human cancer. Biochem Biophys Res Commun 306:799, 2003.
80. Burgart LJ: Colorectal polyps and other precursor lesions. Need for an expanded view. Gastroenterol Clin North Am 31:959, 2002.
81. Bienz M: Apc. Curr Biol 13:R215, 2003.
82. Lynch HT, de la Chapelle A: Hereditary colorectal cancer. N Engl J Med 348:919, 2003.
83. Kinzler KW, Vogelstein B: Lessons from hereditary colorectal cancer. Cell 87:159, 1996.
84. Jass JR: Pathogenesis of colorectal cancer. Surg Clin N Am 82:891, 2002.
85. Knudson AG: Two genetic hits (more or less) to cancer. Nat Rev Cancer 1:157, 2001.
86. Kinzler KW, Vogelstein B: Colorectal tumors. In: Kinzler KW, Vogelstein B (eds): The Genetic Basis of Human Cancer, 2nd Edition. New York: McGraw-Hill 583, 2002.
87. Wynter CV, et al: Methylation patterns define two types of hyperplastic polyp associated with colorectal cancer. Gut 53:573, 2004.
88. Bader S, et al: MBD1, MBD2, and CGBP genes at chromosome 18q21 are infrequently mutated in human colon and lung cancers. Oncogene 22:3506, 2003.
89. Taketo MM, Takaku K: Gastro-intestinal tumorigenesis in Smad4 mutant mice. Cytokine Growth Factor Rev 11:147, 2000.
90. Rudolph KL, et al: Telomere dysfunction and evolution of intestinal carcinoma in mice and humans. Nat Genet 28:155, 2001.
91. Jemal A, et al: Cancer statistics, 2002. CA Cancer J Clin 52:23, 2002.
92. Wei EK, et al: Comparison of risk factors for colon and rectal cancer. Int J Cancer 108:433, 2004.
93. Lieberman DA, et al: Risk factors for advanced colonic neoplasia and hyperplastic polyps in asymptomatic individuals. JAMA 290:2959, 2003.
94. Imperiale TF: Aspirin and the prevention of colorectal cancer. N Engl J Med 348:879, 2003.
95. Parsonnet J, Isaacson PG: Bacterial infection and MALT lymphoma. N Engl J Med 350:213, 2004.
96. Matczak E: Human papillomavirus infection: an emerging problem in anal and other squamous cell cancers. Gastroenterology 120:1046, 2001.
97. Goede AC, Caplin ME, Winslet MC: Carcinoid tumour of the appendix. Br J Surg 90:1317, 2003.
98. Stancu M, et al: Genetic alterations in goblet cell carcinoids of the vermiform appendix and comparison with gastrointestinal carcinoid tumors. Mod Pathol 16:1189, 2003.
99. Reynolds PA, et al: Identification of a DNA-binding site and transcriptional target for the EWS-WT1 (+KTS) oncoprotein. Genes Dev 17:2094, 2003.

CHAPTER 18

Liver and Biliary Tract

James M. Crawford, MD, PhD

THE LIVER

GENERAL FEATURES OF HEPATIC DISEASE
- Patterns of Hepatic Injury
- Hepatic Failure
- Cirrhosis
- Portal Hypertension
- Jaundice and Cholestasis

INFECTIOUS DISORDERS
- Viral Hepatitis
- Bacterial, Parasitic, and Helminthic Infections

AUTOIMMUNE HEPATITIS

DRUG- AND TOXIN-INDUCED LIVER DISEASE
- Alcoholic Liver Disease

METABOLIC LIVER DISEASE
- Nonalcoholic Fatty Liver Disease and Steatohepatitis
- Hemochromatosis
- Wilson Disease
- α_1-Antitrypsin Deficiency
- Neonatal Cholestasis

INTRAHEPATIC BILIARY TRACT DISEASE
- Secondary Biliary Cirrhosis
- Primary Biliary Cirrhosis
- Primary Sclerosing Cholangitis
- Anomalies of the Biliary Tree (Including Liver Cysts)

CIRCULATORY DISORDERS
- Impaired Blood Flow into the Liver
- Impaired Blood Flow Through the Liver
- Hepatic Venous Outflow Obstruction

HEPATIC DISEASE ASSOCIATED WITH PREGNANCY
- Preeclampsia and Eclampsia
- Acute Fatty Liver of Pregnancy
- Intrahepatic Cholestasis of Pregnancy

HEPATIC COMPLICATIONS OF ORGAN OR BONE MARROW TRANSPLANTATION
- Drug Toxicity After Bone Marrow Transplantation
- Graft-Versus-Host Disease and Liver Rejection
- Nonimmunologic Damage to Liver Allografts

NODULES AND TUMORS
- Nodular Hyperplasias
- Benign Neoplasms
- Malignant Tumors

THE BILIARY TRACT

CONGENITAL ANOMALIES

DISORDERS OF THE GALLBLADDER
- Cholelithiasis (Gallstones)
- Cholecystitis

DISORDERS OF THE EXTRAHEPATIC BILE DUCTS
- Choledocholithiasis and Ascending Cholangitis
- Biliary Atresia
- Choledochal Cysts

TUMORS
- Carcinoma of the Gallbladder
- Carcinoma of the Extrahepatic Bile Ducts

IATROGENIC INJURY TO THE BILIARY TREE

THE LIVER

Normal

The liver and biliary tree and the gallbladder occupy the right upper quadrant of the abdomen. The liver resides between the digestive tract and the rest of the body and functions as a way station between the splanchnic and systemic circulation. As the headwater of the biliary tree, the liver sits astride the enterohepatic circulation. The liver has the critical job of maintaining the body's metabolic homeostasis. This includes the processing of dietary amino acids, carbohydrates, lipids, and vitamins; removal of microbes and toxins in splanchnic blood en route to the systemic circulation; synthesis of many plasma proteins; and detoxification and excretion into bile of endogenous waste products and pollutant xenobiotics. Hepatic disorders, therefore, have far-reaching consequences.

The mature liver lies in the right hypochondrium under the rib cage and extends from the right fifth intercostal space at the midclavicular line to just below the costal margin. It projects slightly below the costal margin at the right intercostal line and under the xyphoid process in the midline. The conventional division of the liver into the right, left, caudate, and quadrate lobes is a topographic classification that does not correspond to the functional lobes or segments of the liver. The physiologic or functional right and left lobes are defined by the distribution of the right and left portal vein systems. The watershed between these two vascular beds corresponds to a plane that passes superiorly through the left side of the sulcus of the inferior vena cava to the middle of the gallbladder fossa inferiorly. The quadrate lobe and the greater part of the caudate lobe on the posterior aspect of the liver belong functionally to the left hemiliver. Of greater significance to the surgeon is the functional organization of the liver into eight segments, numbered I to VIII, the caudate lobe being segment I and the remainder, II to VIII, moving roughly from left to right across the liver. Each segment has its own independent vascular and biliary pedicle and venous drainage. *This anatomic arrangement facilitates limited segmental resections of the liver* as is sometimes performed for partial hepatectomy.

The normal adult liver weighs 1400 to 1600 gm, representing 2.5% of body weight. Incoming blood—approximately 25% of total cardiac output—arrives via the portal vein (60% to 70% of hepatic blood flow) and the hepatic artery (30% to 40%) through the hilum, the "gateway" of the liver (*porta hepatis*). The major bile ducts exit in this same region. The initial right and left branches of the portal vein, hepatic artery, and bile duct lie just outside the liver. The remaining branches travel in parallel within the liver in *portal tracts*, ramifying variably through 17 to 20 orders of branches. The vast expanse of hepatic parenchyma is serviced via approximately 450,000 terminal branches of the portal tract system. Portal vein blood enters the parenchyma via penetrating *septal venules*; hepatic arteriolar twigs supply the parenchyma, the major bile ducts, the vasa vasorum of the major portal veins and hepatic veins, and the hepatic capsule. Blood from all sources is collected into ramifications of the hepatic vein, which exits by the "back door" of the liver into the closely apposed inferior vena cava.

Microarchitecture. Classically, the liver has been divided into 1- to 2-mm diameter hexagonal *lobules* oriented around the terminal tributaries of the hepatic vein (*terminal hepatic veins*), with portal tracts at the periphery of the lobule. Accordingly, the hepatocytes in the vicinity of the terminal hepatic vein are called "centrilobular" (or centrolobular); those near the portal tract are "periportal." However, since hepatocytes near the terminal hepatic veins are most remote from the blood supply, it has been argued that they are at the distal apices of roughly triangular *acini*, with the bases formed by penetrating septal venules from the portal vein extending out from the portal tracts (Fig. 18–1).[1] In the "acinus," the parenchyma is divided into three zones, zone 1 being closest to the vascular supply, zone 3 abutting the terminal hepatic venule, and zone 2 being intermediate. This zonation is of considerable metabolic consequence, since a lobular gradient of activity exists for many hepatic enzymes.[2] Moreover, many forms of hepatic injury exhibit a zonal distribution. While acinar architecture is of greater physiologic significance, the anatomic terminology of the liver remains anchored in the older lobular terminology.

The hepatic parenchyma is organized into cribiform, anastomosing sheets or "plates" of hepatocytes, seen in microscopic sections as cords of cells (Fig. 18–2). Hepatocytes immediately abutting the portal tract are referred to as the *limiting plate*, forming a discontinuous rim around the mesenchyme of the portal tract. There is a radial orientation of the hepatocyte cords around the terminal hepatic vein. Hepatocytes exhibit minimal variation in overall size, but nuclei may vary in size, number, and ploidy, particularly with advancing age. Uninucleate, diploid cells tend to be the rule, but with increasing age, a significant fraction are binucleate, and the karyotype may range up to octaploidy.

Between the cords of hepatocytes are vascular sinusoids. Blood traverses the sinusoids and exits into the terminal hepatic vein through innumerable orifices in the vein wall. Hepatocytes are thus bathed on two sides by well-mixed portal venous and hepatic arterial blood, placing hepatocytes among the most richly perfused cells in the body. The sinusoids are lined by fenestrated and discontinuous endothelial cells, which demarcate an extrasinusoidal *space of Disse*, into which protrude abundant microvilli of hepatocytes. Scattered *Kupffer cells* of the mononuclear phagocyte system are attached to the luminal face of endothelial cells, and scattered fat-containing *perisinusoidal stellate cells* are found in the space of Disse. These stellate cells play a role in the storage and metabolism of vitamin A and are transformed into collagen-producing myofibroblasts when there is inflammation of the liver.

Between abutting hepatocytes are *bile canaliculi*, which are channels 1 to 2 μm in diameter, formed by grooves in the

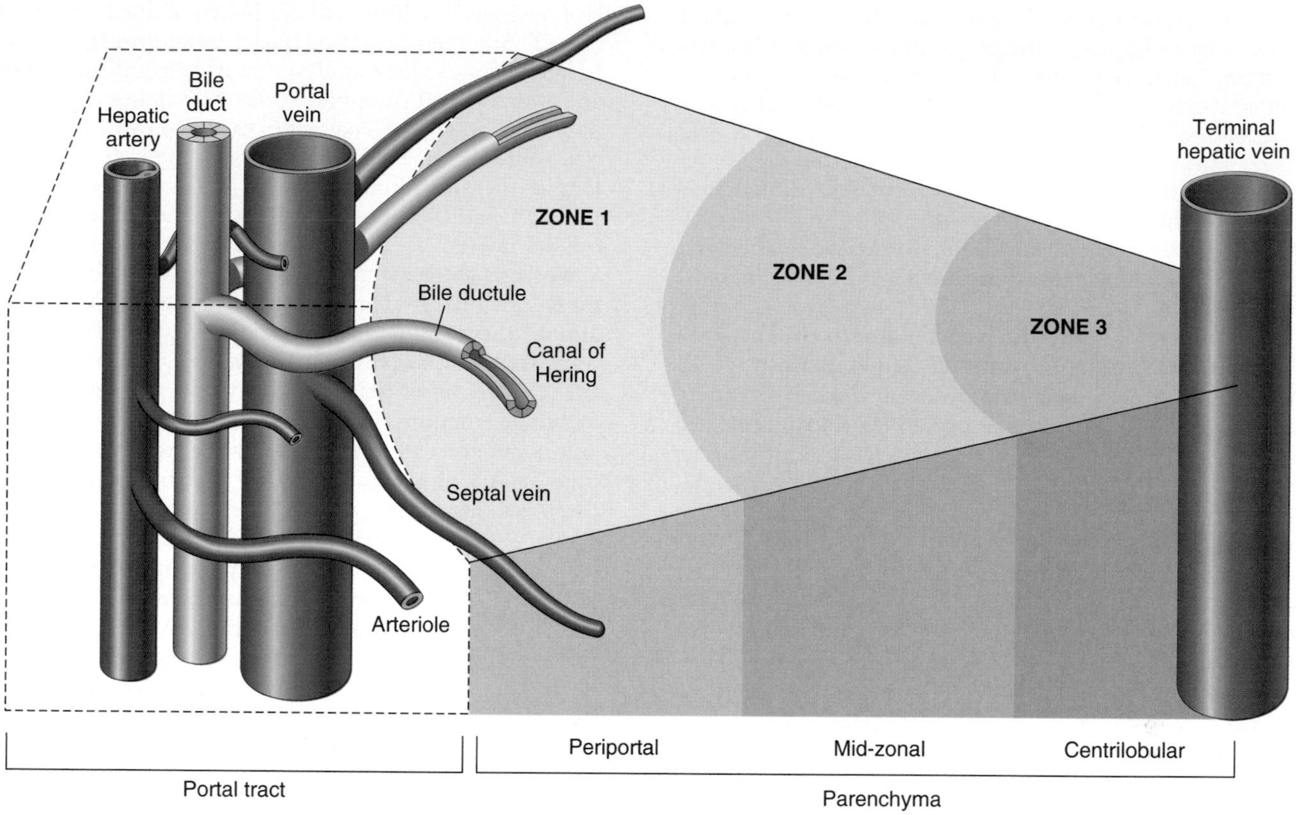

FIGURE 18–1 Microscopic anatomy of the liver. The portal tract carries branches of the portal vein, hepatic artery, and bile duct system. The portal vein gives rise to branching septal veins, which penetrate the hepatocellular parenchyma at regular intervals. Blood from the septal veins enters directly into the parenchymal sinusoids between hepatocytes. The hepatic artery gives off capillaries that supply the bile duct system; these capillaries usually dump into the portal vein but may deposit blood directly into sinusoids. Arterioles also occasionally convey blood directly to the sinusoids. The bile duct system gives off bile ductules, which traverse the mesenchyme of the portal tract to penetrate the parenchyma; at that point, they become hemicircular, abutting hepatocytes (not shown) to form the canals of Hering. Bile traveling through the bile canalicular system between hepatocytes enters into the biliary tree through these canals of Hering. Blood from the portal vein and hepatic artery travels through the sinusoids of the parenchyma toward the terminal hepatic vein, leaving the liver by this route. On the basis of blood flow, three zones can be defined, zone 1 being the closest to the blood supply and zone 3 being the farthest. Pathologists refer to the regions of the parenchyma as "periportal, midzonal, and centrilobular," the last term owing to the historical concept that the terminal hepatic vein was at the center of a "lobule."

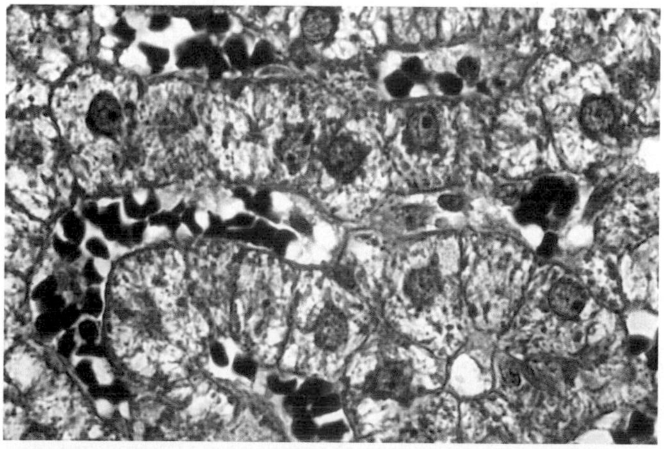

FIGURE 18–2 Photomicrograph of liver (trichrome stain). Note the blood-filled sinusoids and cords of hepatocytes; the delicate network of reticulin fibers in the subendothelial space of Disse stains light blue.

plasma membranes of the facing cells and delineated from the vascular space by tight junctions. Numerous microvilli extend into these intercellular spaces, which constitute the outermost reaches of the biliary tree. Hepatocellular actin and myosin microfilaments surrounding the canaliculus help propel secreted biliary fluid along the canaliculi. These channels drain into the *canals of Hering* in the periportal region. These canals are troughlike extensions of biliary epithelium into the periportal parenchyma, abutting with hepatocytes to form efficient channels for draining bile. Biliary fluid is conveyed through their lumina to *bile ductules,* which traverse the portal mesenchyme to empty into the *terminal bile ducts* within the portal tracts.[3]

Pathology

General Features of Hepatic Disease

The liver is vulnerable to a wide variety of metabolic, toxic, microbial, circulatory, and neoplastic insults. The dominant primary diseases of the liver are viral hepatitis, alcoholic liver disease, and hepatocellular carcinoma. More often, hepatic damage is secondary, to some of the most common diseases in humans, such as cardiac decompensation, disseminated cancer, and extrahepatic infections. The enormous functional reserve of the liver masks the clinical impact of early liver damage. However, with progression of diffuse disease or strategic disruption of bile flow, the consequences of deranged liver function become life-threatening.

With the rare exception of fulminant hepatic failure, liver disease is an insidious process in which symptoms of hepatic decompensation may occur weeks, months, or even years after the onset of injury. There is often a long time interval between disease onset (or initiation) and detection. Conversely, the liver may be injured and heal without clinical detection. Hence, patients with hepatic abnormalities who are referred to specialists in liver disease most frequently have chronic liver disease. Recent surveillance studies in the United States document an annual incidence of newly diagnosed chronic liver disease of 72.3 per 100,000 population.[4] Over half (57%) of patients have hepatitis C viral infection, followed by alcohol-induced liver disease (24%), nonalcoholic fatty liver disease (9%), and hepatitis B viral infection (4%). Liver disease accounts for over 44,000 deaths per year in the United States (1.9% of all deaths), placing it as the eighth leading cause of death, ranking between diabetes and suicide.

Before discussing specific disease processes, three general aspects of liver disease will be reviewed: (1) patterns of hepatic injury, (2) hepatic failure and cirrhosis, and (3) jaundice and cholestasis.

PATTERNS OF HEPATIC INJURY

From a morphologic standpoint, the liver is an inherently simple organ with a limited repertoire of responses to injurious events. Regardless of cause, five general responses are seen. These processes and the morphologic terms used to describe them are as follows:

- **Degeneration and Intracellular Accumulation.** Damage from toxic or immunologic insult may cause swelling of hepatocytes. Moderate cell swelling is reversible. With more severe damage (**ballooning degeneration**), swollen hepatocytes have irregularly clumped cytoplasmic organelles and large clear spaces. In cholestatic liver injury, retained biliary material may impart a diffuse, foamy appearance to the swollen hepatocyte (**feathery degeneration**). This lesion can be difficult to distinguish from ballooning degeneration, except for the variable yellow discoloration of the cytoplasm. Substances may accumulate in viable hepatocytes, including **iron** and **copper**. Accumulation of triglyceride fat droplets within hepatocytes is known as **steatosis** (see Chapter 1). Multiple tiny droplets that do not displace the nucleus are known as **microvesicular steatosis**, and appear in such conditions as acute fatty liver of pregnancy and valproic acid toxicity. A single large droplet that displaces the nucleus, **macrovesicular steatosis**, may be seen in hepatocytes throughout the livers of obese or diabetic individuals and, interestingly, in scattered hepatocytes in patients with hepatitis C viral infection. Both microvesicular and macrovesicular steatosis may be present in alcoholic fatty liver, affecting virtually every hepatocyte.
- **Necrosis and Apoptosis.** Any significant insult to the liver can cause hepatocyte **necrosis**. In **ischemic coagulative necrosis**, the liver cells are poorly stained and "mummified" and often have lysed nuclei. In **apoptotic cell death**, isolated hepatocytes round up to form shrunken, pyknotic, and intensely eosinophilic cells containing fragmented nuclei (Chapter 1). Hepatocytes may also osmotically swell and rupture, so-called **lytic necrosis,** the outcome of ballooning degeneration. Lytic necrosis leaves neither mummified hepatocytes nor pyknotic cells but rather shards of cellular debris.

  Necrosis frequently exhibits a zonal distribution. The most obvious is necrosis of hepatocytes immediately around the terminal hepatic vein (so-called **centrilobular necrosis,** using the historical terminology), an injury that is characteristic of ischemic injury and a number of drug and toxic reactions. Pure **midzonal** and **periportal necrosis** are rare; the latter may be seen in eclampsia. With most other causes of hepatic injury, a variable mixture of hepatocellular death through the parenchyma is encountered. The hepatocyte necrosis may be limited to scattered cells within hepatic lobules (**focal** or **spotty necrosis**) or to the interface between the periportal parenchyma and inflamed portal tracts (**interface hepatitis**). With more severe inflammatory injury, necrosis of contiguous hepatocytes may span adjacent lobules in a portal-to-portal, portal-to-central, or central-to-central fashion (**bridging necrosis**). Necrosis of entire lobules (**submassive necrosis**) or of most of the liver (**massive necrosis**) is usually accompanied by hepatic failure. With disseminated candidal or bacterial infection, macroscopic **abscesses** may occur.
- **Inflammation.** Injury to the liver associated with an influx of acute or chronic inflammatory cells is termed **hepatitis**. Direct toxic or ischemic hepatocyte necrosis incites an inflammatory reaction. With toxic damage, inflammation may also precede the onset of inflammation. Destruction of antigen-expressing liver cells by cytotoxic lymphocytes is a common mechanism of liver damage, especially during viral infection. In viral hepatitis, quiescent lymphocytes may collect in the portal tracts as a reflection of mild smoldering inflammation, spill over into the periportal parenchyma as activated lymphocytes (**interface hepatitis**) causing a moderately active hepatitis, or suffuse the entire parenchyma in severe hepatitis. Once killed, apoptotic hepatocytes do not incite an inflammatory reaction per se. However, scavenger macrophages (Kupffer cells and circulating monocytes recruited to the liver) engulf the apoptotic cell fragments within a few hours, generating clumps of inflammatory cells. Hence, identification of apoptotic hepatocytes is a sign of very recent hepatocyte destruction. Foreign bodies, organisms, and a variety of drugs may incite a granulomatous reaction.
- **Regeneration.** Hepatocytes have long life spans, and they proliferate in response to tissue resection or cell death (see Chapter 3). Regeneration occurs in all but the most fulminant hepatic diseases. Hepatocellular proliferation is marked by mitoses, thickening of the hepatocyte cords, and some disorganization of the parenchymal structure. The canal of Hering–bile ductule unit constitutes a reserve compartment for restitution of severe parenchymal injury; when it is activated, innumerable serpentine profiles resembling bile ductules appear—so-called **ductular reaction**. This compartment also proliferates during large bile duct obstruction. When hepatocellular necrosis occurs and

leaves the connective tissue framework intact, almost perfect restitution of liver structure can occur, even when the necrosis is submassive or massive.

- **Fibrosis.** Fibrous tissue is formed in response to inflammation or direct toxic insult to the liver. Unlike other responses, which are reversible, **fibrosis points toward generally irreversible hepatic damage**. However, there is now considerable debate about the irreversibility of liver fibrosis and even cirrhosis (see below). Deposition of collagen has lasting consequences on patterns of hepatic blood flow and perfusion of hepatocytes. In the initial stages, fibrosis may develop around portal tracts or the terminal hepatic vein or may be deposited directly within the space of Disse. **With continuing fibrosis, the liver is subdivided into nodules of proliferating hepatocytes surrounded by scar tissue, termed "cirrhosis."** This end-stage form of liver disease is discussed later in this section.

The ebb and flow of hepatic injury may be imperceptible to the patient and detectable only by abnormal laboratory tests (Table 18–1). Alternatively, hepatic function may be so impaired as to be life threatening. The major clinical consequences of liver disease are listed in Table 18–2 and are discussed next.

TABLE 18–2 Clinical Consequences of Liver Disease

Characteristic signs	Hepatic dysfunction: Jaundice and cholestasis Hypoalbuminemia Hyperammonemia Hypoglycemia Fetor hepaticus Palmar erythema Spider angiomas Hypogonadism Gynecomastia Weight loss Muscle wasting Portal hypertension from cirrhosis: Ascites Splenomegaly Hemorrhoids Caput medusae—abdominal skin
Life-threatening complications	Hepatic failure Multiple organ failure Coagulopathy Hepatic encephalopathy Hepatorenal syndrome Portal hypertension from cirrhosis Esophageal varices, risk of rupture Malignancy with chronic disease Hepatocellular carcinoma

HEPATIC FAILURE

The most severe clinical consequence of liver disease is *hepatic failure*. This may be the result of sudden and massive hepatic destruction, with about 2500 new cases per year in the United States. More often, it is the end point of progressive damage to the liver as part of chronic liver disease, either by insidious destruction of hepatocytes or by repetitive discrete waves of parenchymal damage. Whatever the sequence, 80% to 90% of hepatic functional capacity must be eroded before hepatic failure ensues. In many cases, the balance is tipped toward decompensation by intercurrent diseases that place demands on the liver. These include gastrointestinal bleeding, systemic infection, electrolyte disturbances, and severe stress such as major surgery or heart failure. In most cases of severe hepatic dysfunction, liver transplantation is the only hope for survival. Overall, mortality from hepatic failure without liver transplantation is 70% to 95%.

TABLE 18–1 Laboratory Evaluation of Liver Disease

Test Category	Serum Measurement
Hepatocyte integrity	Cytosolic hepatocellular enzymes *Serum aspartate aminotransferase* (AST)* *Serum alanine aminotransferase* (ALT)* Serum lactate dehydrogenase (LDH)*
Biliary excretory function	Substances normally secreted in bile *Serum bilirubin* *Total:* unconjugated plus conjugated* *Direct:* conjugated only* Delta: covalently linked to albumin* Urine bilirubin* Serum bile acids* Plasma membrane enzymes (from damage to bile canaliculus) *Serum alkaline phosphatase** Serum γ-glutamyl transpeptidase* Serum 5′-nucleotidase*
Hepatocyte function	Proteins secreted into the blood *Serum albumin*† *Prothrombin time** (factors V, VII, X, prothrombin, fibrinogen) Hepatocyte metabolism Serum ammonia* Aminopyrine breath test (hepatic demethylation)† Galactose elimination (intravenous injection)†

The most common tests are in italics.
*An elevation implicates liver disease.
†A decrease implicates liver disease.

The morphologic alterations that cause liver failure fall into three categories:

- *Massive hepatic necrosis.* This is most often drug- or toxin-induced, as from acetaminophen (38% of massive hepatic necrosis cases in the United States), halothane, antituberculosis drugs (rifampin, isoniazid), antidepressant monoamine oxidase inhibitors, industrial chemicals such as carbon tetrachloride, and mushroom poisoning (*Amanita phalloides*), collectively accounting for an additional 14% of cases. The mechanism may be direct toxic damage to hepatocytes (e.g., acetaminophen, carbon tetrachloride, mushroom toxins) but more often is a variable combination of toxicity and inflammation with immune-mediated hepatocyte destruction. Hepatitis A infection accounts for 4% of cases, hepatitis B infection accounts for 8%, and other causes (including unknown) account for 37%. Hepatitis C infection does not cause massive hepatic necrosis.
- *Chronic liver disease.* This is the most common route to hepatic failure and is the endpoint of relentless chronic hepatitis ending in cirrhosis. The many causes of cirrhosis will be discussed shortly.
- *Hepatic dysfunction without overt necrosis.* Hepatocytes may be viable but unable to perform normal metabolic function, as with Reye syndrome, tetracycline toxicity, and acute fatty liver of pregnancy.

Clinical Features. Regardless of cause, the clinical signs of hepatic failure are much the same. *Jaundice* is an almost invariable finding. *Hypoalbuminemia*, which predisposes to peripheral edema, and *hyperammonemia*, which may play a role in cerebral dysfunction, are extremely worrisome developments. *Fetor hepaticus* is a characteristic body odor that is variously described as "musty" or "sweet and sour" and occurs occasionally. It is related to the formation of mercaptans by the action of gastrointestinal bacteria on the sulfur-containing amino acid methionine and shunting of splanchnic blood from the portal into the systemic circulation (portosystemic shunting). Impaired estrogen metabolism and consequent hyperestrogenemia are the putative causes of *palmar erythema* (a reflection of local vasodilatation) and *spider angiomas* of the skin. Each angioma is a central, pulsating, dilated arteriole from which small vessels radiate. In the male, hyperestrogenemia also leads to *hypogonadism* and *gynecomastia*.

Hepatic failure is life-threatening because *with severely impaired liver function, patients are highly susceptible to failure of multiple organ systems*. Thus, respiratory failure with pneumonia and sepsis combine with renal failure to claim the lives of many patients with hepatic failure. A *coagulopathy* develops, attributable to impaired hepatic synthesis of blood clotting factors II, VII, IX, and X. The resultant bleeding tendency can lead to massive gastrointestinal bleeding as well as petechial bleeding elsewhere. Intestinal absorption of blood places a metabolic load on the liver, which worsens the extent of hepatic failure. The outlook of full-blown hepatic failure is grave: A rapid downhill course is usual, death occurring within weeks to a few months in about 80% of cases. A fortunate few can endure an acute episode until hepatocellular regeneration restores adequate hepatic function. Alternatively, liver transplantation might save the patient.

Two particular complications merit separate consideration, as they herald the most grave stages of hepatic failure.

Hepatic encephalopathy is manifested by a spectrum of disturbances in consciousness, ranging from subtle behavioral abnormalities to marked confusion and stupor to deep coma and death. These changes may progress over hours or days in fulminant hepatic failure or more insidiously in a patient with marginal hepatic function from chronic liver disease. Associated fluctuating neurologic signs include rigidity, hyperreflexia, and particularly *asterixis*: nonrhythmic, rapid extension-flexion movements of the head and extremities, best seen when the arms are held in extension with dorsiflexed wrists. *Hepatic encephalopathy is regarded as a disorder of neurotransmission in the central nervous system and neuromuscular system*[5] and appears to be associated with elevated blood ammonia levels, which impair neuronal function and promote generalized brain edema. *In the great majority of instances, there are only minor morphologic changes in the brain, such as edema and an astrocytic reaction*, and the encephalopathy is reversible if the underlying hepatic condition can be corrected.

Hepatorenal syndrome refers to the appearance of renal failure in patients with severe chronic liver disease, in whom there are no intrinsic morphologic or functional causes for the renal failure. Sodium retention, impaired free-water excretion, and decreased renal perfusion and glomerular filtration rate are the main renal functional abnormalities.[6] Several factors are involved in its development, including a decreased renal perfusion pressure due to systemic vasodilation, activation of the renal sympathetic nervous system with vasoconstriction of the afferent renal arteriolae, and increased synthesis of renal vasoactive mediators, which further decrease glomerular filtration. Onset of this syndrome is typically heralded by a drop in urine output, associated with rising blood urea nitrogen and creatinine. *The ability to concentrate urine is retained, producing a hyperosmolar urine devoid of proteins and abnormal sediment, and surprisingly low in sodium* (unlike renal tubular necrosis). Rapid development of renal failure is usually associated with a precipitating stress factor such as infection, gastrointestinal hemorrhage, or a major surgical procedure. Insidious development of renal failure is the result of progressive destabilization of circulatory physiology, frequently in the setting of severe refractory ascites. The prognosis is poor, with a median survival of only 2 weeks in the rapid-onset form and 6 months with the insidious-onset form.

CIRRHOSIS

Cirrhosis is among the top 10 causes of death in the Western world. The chief worldwide contributors are alcohol abuse and viral hepatitis. Other causes include biliary disease, and iron overload. An example of the progression to cirrhosis is given under the subsequent discussion on alcohol. Cirrhosis as the end-stage of chronic liver disease is defined by three characteristics:

- Bridging *fibrous septae* in the form of delicate bands or broad scars linking portal tracts with one another and portal tracts with terminal hepatic veins
- *Parenchymal nodules* containing proliferating hepatocytes encircled by fibrosis, with diameters varying from very small (<3 mm, micronodules) to large (several centimeters, macronodules)
- *Disruption of the architecture of the entire liver*

Several features of cirrhosis should be underscored:

- *The parenchymal injury and consequent fibrosis are diffuse*, extending throughout the liver. Focal injury with scarring does not constitute cirrhosis, nor does diffuse nodular transformation without fibrosis.
- *Nodularity is part of the diagnosis* and reflects the balance between regenerative activity and constrictive scarring. It should be noted that rapid development of fibrosis, as in alcoholic hepatitis, may leave little time for the development of spherical nodules.
- *Vascular architecture is reorganized* by the parenchymal damage and scarring, with the formation of abnormal interconnections between vascular inflow and hepatic vein outflow channels. As a result, portal vein and arterial blood partially bypasses the functional hepatocyte mass through these abnormal channels.
- *Fibrosis is the key feature of progressive damage to the liver.* With cessation of the causal injury, slow regression of fibrosis may occur. Once cirrhosis has developed, reversal is thought to be rare. However, the liver contains abundant metalloproteinases and collagenases that are capable of degrading extracellular matrix. Collagen degradation is a slow process, since collagen I sustains extensive cross-linking after its deposition and hence becomes more resistant to collagenases over time. Nevertheless, there are a sufficient number of clinical reports of patients whose full-blown cirrhosis has subsided to a form of incomplete septation of the liver or apparent absence of fibrosis, to raise

hopes that even patients with cirrhosis may improve without resorting to liver transplantation.

The only satisfactory classification of cirrhosis is based on the presumed underlying etiology. The descriptive terms "micronodular" and "macronodular" should not be used as primary classifications. Many forms of cirrhosis (particularly alcoholic cirrhosis) are initially micronodular, but there is a tendency for nodules to increase in size with time, counterbalanced by the constraints imposed by fibrous scarring.

The etiology of cirrhosis varies both geographically and socially. The following is the approximate frequency of etiologic categories in the Western world, most of which are discussed in detail later:

Alcoholic liver disease	60% to 70%
Viral hepatitis	10%
Biliary diseases	5% to 10%
Primary hemochromatosis	5%
Wilson disease	Rare
α_1-Antitrypsin deficiency	Rare
Cryptogenic cirrhosis	10% to 15%

Infrequent types of cirrhosis also include the cirrhosis developing in infants and children with galactosemia and tyrosinosis (Chapter 10), and drug-induced cirrhosis, as with α-methyldopa. Severe fibrosis can occur in the setting of cardiac disease (sometimes called "cardiac cirrhosis," discussed later). After all the categories of cirrhosis of known causation have been excluded, a substantial number of cases remain. Referred to as *cryptogenic cirrhosis*, the magnitude of this "wastebasket" category speaks eloquently to the difficulties in discerning the many origins of cirrhosis. A growing concern is that many of these cases are due to undiagnosed *nonalcoholic fatty liver disease*, to be discussed. *Once cirrhosis is established, it is usually impossible to establish an etiologic diagnosis on morphologic grounds alone.*

Pathogenesis. The central pathogenetic processes in cirrhosis are progressive fibrosis and reorganization of the vascular microarchitecture of the liver.[7] In the normal liver, interstitial collagens (types I and III) are concentrated in portal tracts and around central veins, with occasional bundles in the space of Disse. The collagen (reticulin) coursing alongside hepatocytes is composed of delicate strands of type IV collagen in the space of Disse. In cirrhosis, types I and III collagen are deposited in the lobule, creating delicate or broad septal tracts. New vascular channels in the septae connect the vascular structures in the portal region (hepatic arteries and portal veins) and terminal hepatic veins, shunting blood around the parenchyma. Continued deposition of collagen in the space of Disse within preserved parenchyma is accompanied by the loss of fenestrations in the sinusoidal endothelial cells. In the process, the sinusoidal space comes to resemble a capillary rather than a channel for exchange of solutes between hepatocytes and plasma. In particular, hepatocellular secretion of proteins (e.g., albumin, clotting factors, lipoproteins) is greatly impaired.

The major source of excess collagen in cirrhosis is the perisinusoidal stellate cells, which lie in the space of Disse. Although normally functioning as vitamin A fat-storing cells, during the development of cirrhosis they become activated, a process that includes (1) robust mitotic activity in areas developing new parenchymal fibrosis, (2) a shift from the resting-state lipocyte phenotype to a transitional myofibroblast phenotype, and (3) increased capacity for synthesis and secretion of extracellular matrix. It is predominantly the cytokines secreted by activated Kupffer cells and other inflammatory cells that stimulate perisinusoidal stellate cells to divide and to produce large amounts of extracellular matrix. Moreover, the greatest activation of stellate cells is in areas of severe hepatocellular necrosis and inflammation. As depicted in Figure 18–3, the stimuli for stellate cell activation may come from several sources:

- Chronic inflammation, with production of inflammatory cytokines such as tumor necrosis factor (TNF), lymphotoxin, and interleukin-1 (IL-1).
- Cytokine production by activated endogenous cells (Kupffer cells, endothelial cells, hepatocytes, and bile duct epithelial cells), including transforming growth factor-β (TGF-β), platelet-derived growth factor (PDGF), and lipid peroxidation products.
- Disruption of the extracellular matrix, as stellate cells are extraordinarily responsive to the status of their substrate.
- Direct stimulation of stellate cells by toxins.

Acquisition of myofibers by perisinusoidal stellate cells also increases vascular resistance within the liver parenchyma, since tonic contraction of these "myofibroblasts" constricts the sinusoidal vascular channels.

Throughout the process of liver damage and fibrosis, remaining hepatocytes are stimulated to regenerate and proliferate as spherical nodules within the confines of the fibrous septae. The net outcome is a fibrotic, nodular liver in which delivery of blood to hepatocytes is severely compromised, as is the ability of hepatocytes to secrete substances into plasma. Disruption of the interface between the parenchyma and portal tracts obliterates biliary channels as well. Thus, *the cirrhotic patient may develop jaundice and even hepatic failure, despite having a liver of normal mass.*

Clinical Features. All forms of cirrhosis may be clinically silent. When symptomatic they lead to nonspecific clinical manifestations: anorexia, weight loss, weakness, osteoporosis, and, in advanced disease, frank debilitation. Incipient or overt hepatic failure may develop, usually precipitated by a superimposed metabolic load on the liver, as from systemic infection or a gastrointestinal hemorrhage. Imbalances of pulmonary blood flow, which are poorly understood, may lead to severely impaired oxygenation (*hepatopulmonary syndrome*), further stressing the patient. *The ultimate mechanism of most cirrhotic deaths is (1) progressive liver failure (discussed earlier), (2) a complication related to portal hypertension, or (3) the development of hepatocellular carcinoma.*

PORTAL HYPERTENSION

Increased resistance to portal blood flow may develop in a variety of circumstances, which can be divided into *prehepatic, intrahepatic, and posthepatic causes*. The major *prehepatic conditions* are obstructive thrombosis and narrowing of the portal vein before it ramifies within the liver. Massive splenomegaly may also shunt excessive blood into the splenic vein. The major *posthepatic causes* are severe right-sided heart failure, constrictive pericarditis, and hepatic vein outflow obstruction. *The dominant intrahepatic cause is cirrhosis, accounting for most cases of portal hypertension.* Far less frequent are schistosomiasis, massive fatty change, diffuse fibrosing granulomatous disease such as sarcoidosis and miliary

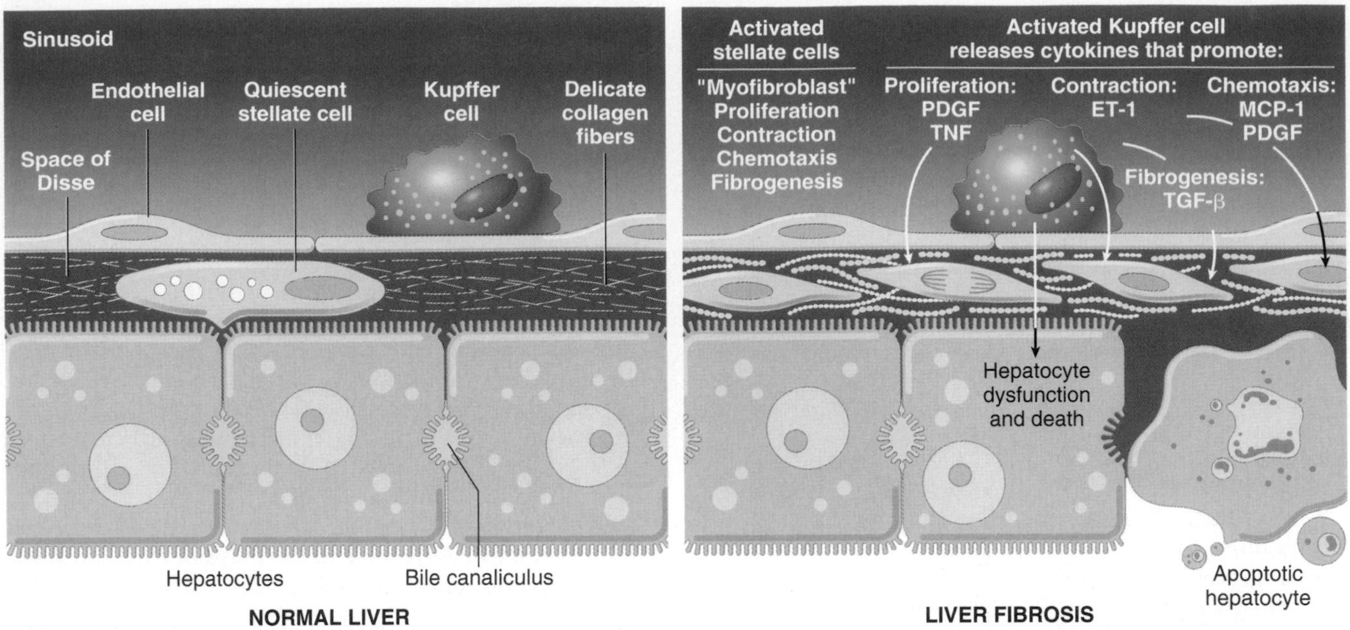

FIGURE 18–3 Schematic of stellate cell activation and liver fibrosis in comparison to the normal liver. Kupffer cell activation leads to secretion of multiple cytokines; cytokines also may be released by endothelial cells, hepatocytes, and inflammatory cells entering the liver (not shown). These cytokines "activate" stellate cells, whereby they loose their lipid droplets (which are present in the quiescent state) and acquire a myofibroblastic state. Stellate cell proliferation is stimulated in particular by platelet-derived growth factor (PDGF); tumor necrosis factor (TNF) is a potent stimulant of the change to a myofibroblastic phenotype. Contraction of the activated stellate cells is stimulated by endothelin-1 (ET-1). Deposition of extracellular matrix (fibrogenesis) is stimulated especially by transforming growth factor β (TGF-β). Chemotaxis of activated stellate cells to areas of injury, such as where hepatocytes have undergone apoptosis, is promoted by PDGF and monocyte chemotactic protein-1 (MCP-1). Kupffer cells also are a major source of TNF released into the system circulation. (Schematic based on concepts presented in Friedman SL: Molecular regulation of hepatic fibrosis: an integrated cellular response to tissue injury. J Biol Chem 275:2247–2250, 2000; and Crawford JM: Cellular and molecular biology of the liver. Curr Op Gastroenterol 13:175–185, 1997.)

tuberculosis, and diseases affecting the portal microcirculation, exemplified by nodular regenerative hyperplasia (discussed later).

Portal hypertension in cirrhosis results from increased resistance to portal flow at the level of the sinusoids, and compression of terminal hepatic veins by perivenular scarring and expansile parenchymal nodules. Anastomoses between the arterial and portal systems in the fibrous septa also contribute to portal hypertension by imposing arterial pressure on the low-pressure hepatic venous system. *The four major clinical consequences are (1) ascites, (2) the formation of portosystemic venous shunts, (3) congestive splenomegaly, and (4) hepatic encephalopathy (discussed earlier).* These are illustrated in Figure 18–4.

Ascites

Ascites refers to the collection of excess fluid in the peritoneal cavity. It usually becomes clinically detectable when at least 500 mL has accumulated, but many liters may collect and cause massive abdominal distention. It is generally a serous fluid having less than 3 gm/dL of protein (largely albumin) as well as the same concentrations of solutes such as glucose, sodium, and potassium as in the blood. The fluid may contain a scant number of mesothelial cells and mononuclear leukocytes. Influx of neutrophils suggests secondary infection, whereas red cells point to possible disseminated intra-abdominal cancer. With long-standing ascites, seepage of peritoneal fluid through transdiaphragmatic lymphatics may produce hydrothorax, more often on the right side.

The *pathogenesis of ascites* is complex, involving the following mechanisms:[8]

- *Sinusoidal hypertension*, altering Starling's forces and driving fluid into the space of Disse, which is then removed by hepatic lymphatics; this movement of fluid is also promoted by *hypoalbuminemia*.
- *Percolation of hepatic lymph into the peritoneal cavity*: Normal thoracic duct lymph flow approximates 800 to 1000 mL/day. With cirrhosis, hepatic lymphatic flow may approach 20 L/day, exceeding thoracic duct capacity. Hepatic lymph is rich in proteins and low in triglycerides, which is reflected in the protein-rich ascitic fluid.
- *Intestinal fluid leakage*: Portal hypertension also causes increased perfusion pressure in intestinal capillaries. The osmotic action of the protein-rich ascitic fluid promotes movement of additional fluid out of intestinal capillaries into the abdomen.
- *Renal retention of sodium and water* due to secondary hyperaldosteronism (Chapter 24).

Portosystemic Shunts

With the rise in portal system pressure, bypasses develop wherever the systemic and portal circulation share common capillary beds. Principal sites are veins around and within

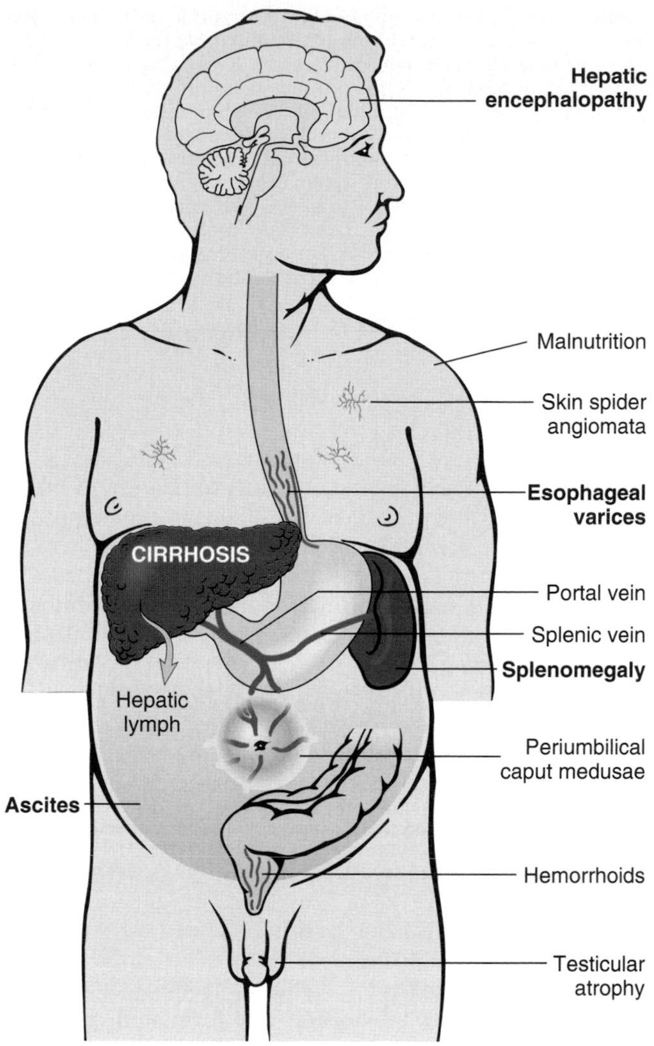

FIGURE 18–4 The major clinical consequences of portal hypertension in the setting of cirrhosis, shown for the male. In women, oligomenorrhea, amenorrhea, and sterility are frequent, owing to hypogonadism.

the rectum (manifest as hemorrhoids), the cardioesophageal junction (producing esophagogastric varices), the retroperitoneum, and the falciform ligament of the liver (involving periumbilical and abdominal wall collaterals). Although hemorrhoidal bleeding may occur, it is rarely massive or life-threatening. *Much more important are the esophagogastric varices that appear in about 65% of patients with advanced cirrhosis of the liver and cause massive hematemesis and death in about half of them.* Abdominal wall collaterals appear as dilated subcutaneous veins extending from the umbilicus towards the rib margins (*caput medusae*) and constitute an important clinical hallmark of portal hypertension.

Splenomegaly

Long-standing congestion may cause congestive splenomegaly. The degree of enlargement varies widely up to 1000 gm and is not necessarily correlated with other features of portal hypertension. Massive splenomegaly may secondarily induce a variety of hematologic abnormalities attributable to hypersplenism.

JAUNDICE AND CHOLESTASIS

Hepatic bile formation serves two major functions: (1) the emulsification of dietary fat in the lumen of the gut through the detergent action of bile salts and (2) the elimination of systemic waste products. Bile constitutes the primary pathway for elimination of bilirubin, excess cholesterol, and xenobiotics that are insufficiently water-soluble to be excreted into urine. Because bile formation requires well-functioning hepatocytes, it is readily disrupted. Such disruption becomes clinically evident as yellow discoloration of the skin and sclerae (*jaundice* and *icterus*, respectively) due to retention of pigmented bilirubin, and as *cholestasis*, characterized by systemic retention of not only bilirubin but also other solutes eliminated in bile.

Bilirubin and Bile Formation

Bilirubin is the end product of heme degradation (Fig. 18–5). The majority of daily production (0.2 to 0.3 gm) is derived from breakdown of senescent erythrocytes by the mononuclear phagocytic system, especially in the spleen, liver, and bone marrow. Most of the remainder of bilirubin is derived from the turnover of hepatic heme or hemoproteins (e.g., the P-450 cytochromes) and from premature destruction of newly formed erythrocytes in the bone marrow. The latter pathway is important in hematologic disorders associated with excessive intramedullary hemolysis of defective erythrocytes (ineffective erythropoiesis; Chapter 13).

Whatever the source, heme oxygenase oxidizes heme to biliverdin (step 1 in Fig. 18–5), which is then reduced to bilirubin by biliverdin reductase. Bilirubin thus formed outside the liver is released and bound to serum albumin (step 2). Albumin binding is necessary, since bilirubin is virtually insoluble in aqueous solutions at physiologic pH. The very small fraction of unbound bilirubin in plasma may increase in severe hemolytic disease or when protein-binding drugs displace bilirubin from albumin.

Hepatic processing of bilirubin involves carrier-mediated uptake at the sinusoidal membrane (step 3), conjugation with one or two molecules of glucuronic acid by bilirubin UDP-glucuronyltransferase (UGT1A1, step 4) in the endoplasmic reticulum, and excretion of the water-soluble, nontoxic bilirubin glucuronides into bile. Most bilirubin glucuronides are deconjugated by bacterial β-glucuronidases and degraded to colorless urobilinogens (step 5). The urobilinogens and the residue of intact pigment are largely excreted in feces. Approximately 20% of the urobilinogens formed are reabsorbed in the ileum and colon, returned to the liver, and promptly re-excreted into bile. The small amount that escapes this enterohepatic circulation is excreted in urine.

The hepatic conjugating enzyme, UGT1A1, is a product of the *UGT1* gene located on chromosome 2q37. It is a member of a family of UGTs that catalyze the glucuronidation of an array of substrates such as steroid hormones, carcinogens, and drugs. The various UGTs are distributed in a wide range of tissues, including the liver, kidney, intestine, skin, lung, olfactory epithelium, and testis. UGT1A1 is located primarily in the smooth and rough endoplasmic reticulum of hepatocytes, as

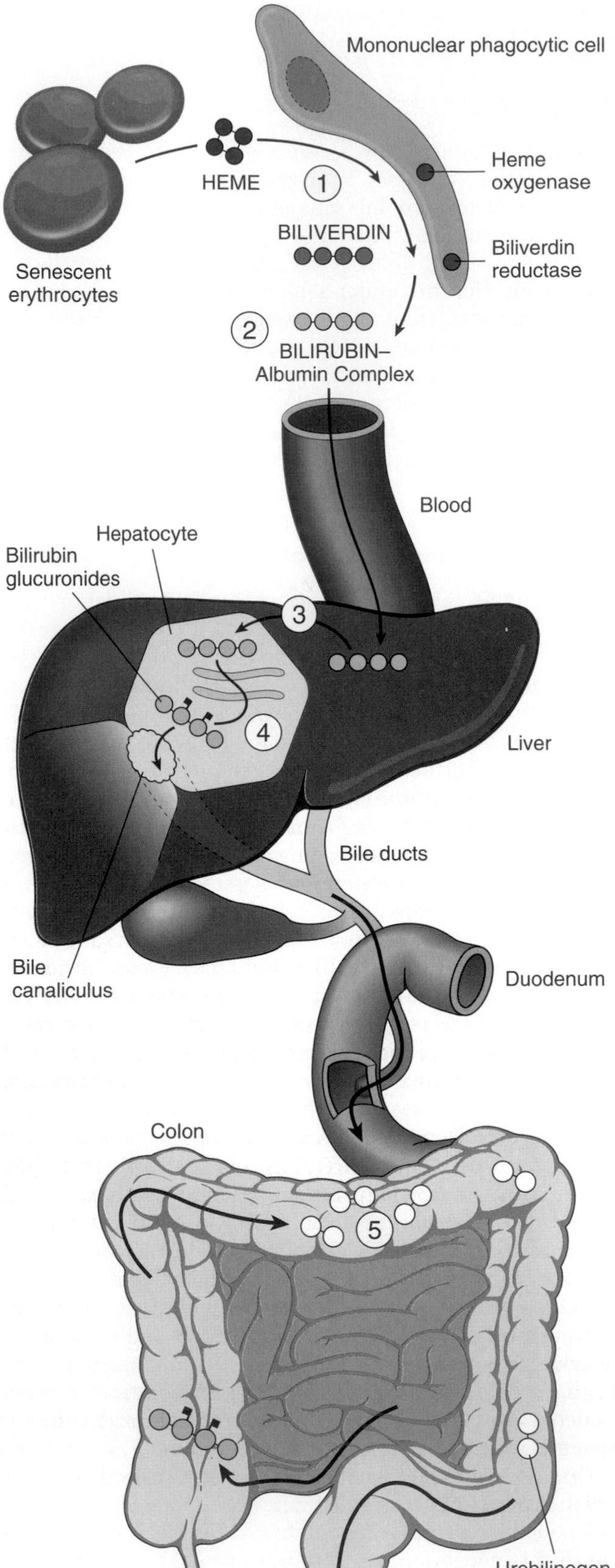

FIGURE 18–5 Bilirubin metabolism and elimination. 1, Normal bilirubin production from heme (0.2 to 0.3 gm/day) is derived primarily from the breakdown of senescent circulating erythrocytes, with a minor contribution from degradation of tissue heme-containing proteins. 2, Extrahepatic bilirubin is bound to serum albumin and delivered to the liver. 3, Hepatocellular uptake and (4) glucuronidation in the endoplasmic reticulum generate bilirubin monoglucuronides and diglucuronides, which are water soluble and readily excreted into bile. 5, Gut bacteria deconjugate the bilirubin and degrade it to colorless urobilinogens. The urobilinogens and the residue of intact pigments are excreted in the feces, with some reabsorption and excretion into urine.

a single isoform that catalyzes the glucuronidation of bilirubin to its monoglucuronidated and diglucuronidated forms. The sequence of the human *UGT1* gene shows that there are 13 isoform sequences in a tandem array for exon 1, each of which possesses a unique promoter and undergoes differential splicing to four common exons (exons 2 through 5). This differential splicing leads to the generation of different mRNAs that encode the different UGT isoforms. Following translation into a polypeptide, the unique amino terminus specifies acceptor–substrate selection, and the common carboxy terminus specifies the enzyme interaction with the common donor substrate, UDP-glucuronic acid. In humans, two members of the UGT1 family possess the capability to glucuronidate bilirubin in vitro, but only one isoform is physiologically relevant in vivo. This bilirubin glucuronidating isoform is termed UGT1A1, as it is generated from the exon 1A of the *UGT1* gene locus.

The brilliant yellow color of bilirubin makes it an easily identified component of hepatic bile formation. However, bilirubin metabolism and excretion are but minor cogs in the hepatic machinery that secretes approximately 0.5 to 1.0 L of bile daily. Newly secreted bile is a bicarbonate-rich fluid containing by weight about 3% organic solutes. Two thirds of the organic material in bile are bile salts: bile acids conjugated with taurine or glycine to form bile salts. Bile acids are the major catabolic products of cholesterol and are a family of water-soluble sterols with carboxylated side chains.[9]

The primary human bile acids are cholic acid and chenodeoxycholic acid. *Bile acids and their taurine- or glycine-conjugated salts act as highly effective detergents. Their primary physiologic role is solubilizing water-insoluble lipids secreted by hepatocytes into bile, and solubilizing dietary lipids within the gut lumen.* The principal secreted lipids (>95%) are *lecithins* (phosphatidylcholine), which are very hydrophobic and have no appreciable aqueous solubility of their own. However, these insoluble amphiphiles enhance the limited cholesterol-solubilizing capacity of bile salts in bile. *Cholesterol* is a negligibly soluble steroid molecule with a single polar hydroxyl group, whose *solubility in bile is increased several million-fold by the presence of bile salts and lecithin.*

Ten percent to 20% of secreted bile salts are deconjugated in the intestines by bacterial action. Ninety-five percent of secreted bile acids, conjugated or unconjugated, are reabsorbed, primarily through the action of a sodium–bile acid cotransporter in the apical membrane of ileal enterocytes and are returned to the liver via portal blood for uptake, reconjugation with taurine or glycine, and resecretion. The *enterohepatic circulation* of bile acids provides an efficient mechanism for maintaining a large endogenous pool of bile acids for digestive and excretory purposes.

Fecal loss of bile acids (0.2 to 0.6 gm per day) is matched by their daily de novo hepatic synthesis from cholesterol. This obligatory fecal loss of sterols in the form of bile salts and residual free cholesterol constitutes the only effective mechanism for elimination of excess cholesterol from the body.

Pathophysiology of Jaundice

Both unconjugated bilirubin and bilirubin glucuronides may accumulate systemically and deposit in tissues, giving rise to the yellow discoloration of jaundice. This is particularly evident in the yellowing of the sclerae (icterus). There are two important pathophysiologic differences between the two forms of bilirubin. *Unconjugated bilirubin is virtually insoluble in water at physiologic pH and is tightly complexed to serum albumin. This form cannot be excreted in the urine even when blood levels are high.* Normally, a very small amount of unconjugated bilirubin is present as an albumin-free anion in plasma. This fraction of unbound bilirubin may diffuse into tissues, particularly the brain in infants, and produce toxic injury. The unbound plasma fraction may increase in severe hemolytic disease or when protein-binding drugs displace bilirubin from albumin. Hence, *hemolytic disease of the newborn (erythroblastosis fetalis) may lead to accumulation of unconjugated bilirubin in the brain, which can cause severe neurologic damage, referred to as kernicterus* (Chapter 10). In contrast, *conjugated bilirubin is water soluble, nontoxic, and only loosely bound to albumin. Because of its solubility and weak association with albumin, excess conjugated bilirubin in plasma can be excreted in urine.* With prolonged conjugated hyperbilirubinemia, a portion of circulating pigment may become covalently bound to albumin (the *delta* fraction).

In the normal adult, serum bilirubin levels vary between 0.3 and 1.2 mg/dL, and the rate of systemic bilirubin production is equal to the rates of hepatic uptake, conjugation, and biliary excretion. Jaundice becomes evident when the serum bilirubin levels rise above 2.0 to 2.5 mg/dL; levels as high as 30 to 40 mg/dL can occur with severe disease. *Jaundice occurs when the equilibrium between bilirubin production and clearance is disturbed* by one or more of the following mechanisms (Table 18–3): *(1) excessive production of bilirubin, (2) reduced hepatocyte uptake, (3) impaired conjugation, (4) decreased hepatocellular excretion, and (5) impaired bile flow (both intrahepatic and extrahepatic).* The first three mechanisms produce unconjugated hyperbilirubinemia, and the latter two produce predominantly conjugated hyperbilirubinemia. More than one mechanism may operate to produce jaundice, especially hepatitis, which can produce unconjugated and conjugated hyperbilirubinemia. Generally speaking, however, one mechanism predominates, so knowledge of the major form of plasma bilirubin is of value in evaluating possible causes of hyperbilirubinemia.

Of the various causes of jaundice listed in Table 18–3, the most common are due to bilirubin overproduction (as from hemolytic anemias and resorption of major hemorrhages), hepatitis, and obstruction to the flow of bile (considered later in this chapter). Several particular conditions merit consideration.

TABLE 18–3 Causes of Jaundice

Predominantly Unconjugated Hyperbilirubinemia
Excess production of bilirubin
Hemolytic anemias
Resorption of blood from internal hemorrhage (e.g., alimentary tract bleeding, hematomas)
Ineffective erythropoiesis syndromes (e.g., pernicious anemia, thalassemia)
Reduced hepatic uptake
Drug interference with membrane carrier systems
Some cases of Gilbert syndrome
Impaired bilirubin conjugation
Physiologic jaundice of the newborn (decreased UGT1A1 activity, decreased excretion)
Breast milk jaundice (β-glucuronidases in milk)
Genetic deficiency of UGT1A1 activity (Crigler-Najjar syndrome types I and II)
Gilbert syndrome (mixed etiologies)
Diffuse hepatocellular disease (e.g., viral or drug-induced hepatitis, cirrhosis)
Predominantly Conjugated Hyperbilirubinemia
Deficiency of canalicular membrane transporters (Dubin-Johnson syndrome, Rotor syndrome)
Impaired bile flow

UGT, uridine diphosphate–glucuronyltransferase.

Neonatal Jaundice. Because the hepatic machinery for conjugating and excreting bilirubin does not fully mature until about 2 weeks of age, almost every newborn develops transient and mild unconjugated hyperbilirubinemia, termed neonatal jaundice or *physiologic jaundice of the newborn.* Breast-fed infants tend to exhibit jaundice with greater frequency, possibly the result of β-glucuronidases present in maternal milk. These enzymes deconjugate bilirubin glucuronides in the gut, increasing intestinal reabsorption of unconjugated bilirubin. Sustained jaundice in the newborn is indicative of a disease condition, discussed later under *neonatal hepatitis.*

Hereditary Hyperbilirubinemias. *In rare instances, there may be a genetic lack of UGT1A1* (Table 18–4). In *Crigler-Najjar syndrome type I*, the enzyme is completely absent. Multiple genetic defects in the locus coding for UGT1A1 may give rise to this disorder.[10] The liver is incapable of synthesizing a functional enzyme, and the colorless bile contains only trace amounts of unconjugated bilirubin. The liver is morphologically normal by light and electron microscopy. However, serum unconjugated bilirubin reaches very high levels, producing severe jaundice and icterus. Without liver transplantation, this condition is invariably fatal, causing death within 18 months of birth secondary to kernicterus.

Crigler-Najjar syndrome type II is a less severe, nonfatal disorder in which UGT1A1 enzyme activity is greatly reduced, and the enzyme is capable of forming only monoglucuronidated bilirubin. Unlike Crigler-Najjar syndrome type I, the only major consequence is extraordinarily yellow skin from moderate to high levels of circulating unconjugated bilirubin; phenobarbital treatment can improve bilirubin glucuronidation by inducing hypertrophy of the hepatocellular endoplasmic reticulum. Mutations either reduce the affinity of UGT1A1 toward bilirubin or reduce enzyme activity.[11] Almost

TABLE 18–4 Hereditary Hyperbilirubinemias

Disorder	Inheritance	Defects in Bilirubin Metabolism	Liver Pathology	Clinical Course
Unconjugated Hyperbilirubinemia				
Crigler-Najjar syndrome type I	Autosomal recessive	Absent UGT1A1 activity	Normal	Fatal in neonatal period
Crigler-Najjar syndrome type II	Autosomal dominant with variable penetrance	Decreased UGT1A1 activity	Normal	Generally mild, occasional kernicterus
Gilbert syndrome	Autosomal dominant?	Decreased UGT1A1 activity	Normal	Innocuous
Conjugated Hyperbilirubinemia				
Dubin-Johnson syndrome	Autosomal recessive	Impaired biliary excretion of bilirubin glucuronides due to mutation in canalicular multidrug resistance protein 2 (MRP2)	Pigmented cytoplasmic globules; ?epinephrine metabolites	Innocuous
Rotor syndrome	Autosomal recessive	Decreased hepatic uptake and storage? Decreased biliary excretion?	Normal	Innocuous

UGT, uridine diphosphate–glucuronyltransferase.

all patients develop normally, but there is a risk for some neurologic damage from kernicterus.

Gilbert syndrome is a relatively common, benign, somewhat heterogeneous inherited condition presenting with mild, fluctuating hyperbilirubinemia. The primary cause is reduction in hepatic bilirubin glucuronidating activity to about 30% of normal levels. In most patients, two extra bases (TA) are found in the TATAA element of the 5′ promoter region (creating an $A(TA)_7TAA$ element rather than the normal $A(TA)_6TAA$, resulting in reduced expression of UGT1A1. Alternatively, patients may be heterozygous for missense mutations in the *UGT1A1* gene. Affecting some 6% of the population, the mild hyperbilirubinemia may go undiscovered for years and is not associated with functional derangements. When detected in adolescence or adult life, it is typically in association with stress, such as an intercurrent illness, strenuous exercise, or fasting. Gilbert syndrome has no clinical consequence except for the anxiety that a jaundiced sufferer might justifiably experience with this otherwise innocuous condition.

Dubin-Johnson syndrome results from a hereditary defect in hepatocellular excretion of bilirubin glucuronides across the canalicular membrane. The defect is due to absence of the canalicular protein, the *multidrug resistance protein 2* (MRP2; located on chromosome 10q24), that is responsible for transport of bilirubin glucuronides and related organic anions into bile.[12] The liver is darkly pigmented owing to coarse pigmented granules within the cytoplasm of hepatocytes (Fig. 18–6). Electron microscopy reveals that the pigment is located in lysosomes, and it appears to be composed of polymers of epinephrine metabolites, not bilirubin pigment. The liver is otherwise normal. Apart from chronic or recurrent jaundice of fluctuating intensity, most patients are asymptomatic and have a normal life expectancy.

Rotor syndrome is a rare form of asymptomatic conjugated hyperbilirubinemia with multiple defects in hepatocellular uptake and excretion of bilirubin pigments. The liver is not pigmented. As with Dubin-Johnson syndrome, patients with Rotor syndrome exhibit jaundice but otherwise live normal lives.

Cholestasis

Cholestatic conditions, which result from hepatocellular dysfunction or intrahepatic or extrahepatic biliary obstruction, also may present with jaundice. Alternatively, *pruritus* is a presenting symptom, related to the elevation in plasma bile acids and their deposition in peripheral tissues, particularly skin. *Skin xanthomas* (focal accumulations of cholesterol) sometimes appear, the result of hyperlipidemia and impaired excretion of cholesterol. *A characteristic laboratory finding is elevated serum alkaline phosphatase*, an enzyme present in bile duct epithelium and in the canalicular membrane of hepatocytes that is released into the circulation because of the detergent action of retained bile salts on hepatocyte membranes. An isozyme derived from posttranscriptional changes is normally present in many other tissues such as bone, so the increased levels must be verified as being hepatic in origin. Another canalicular ectoenzyme, *γ-glutamyl transpeptidase*, is also released into the circulation. The elevated levels of these

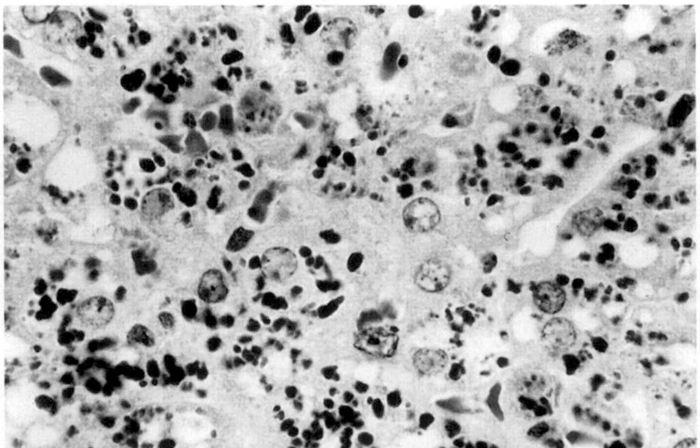

FIGURE 18–6 Dubin-Johnson syndrome, showing abundant pigment inclusions in otherwise normal hepatocytes (H&E).

enzymes in the circulation reflects the detergent action of bile salts retained in the luminal space of the bile canaliculus on the apical membranes of hepatocytes and bile duct epithelial cells, with solubilization of these membrane ectoenzymes. Other manifestations of reduced bile flow relate to intestinal malabsorption, including nutritional deficiencies of the fat-soluble vitamins A, D, or K.

Morphology. The morphologic features of cholestasis depend on its severity, duration, and underlying cause. **Common to both obstructive and nonobstructive cholestasis is the accumulation of bile pigment within the hepatic parenchyma** (Fig. 18–7). Elongated green-brown plugs of bile are visible in dilated bile canaliculi. Rupture of canaliculi leads to extravasation of bile, which is quickly phagocytosed by Kupffer cells. Droplets of bile pigment also accumulate within hepatocytes, which can take on a fine, foamy appearance (**feathery degeneration**).

Obstruction of the biliary tree, either intrahepatic or extrahepatic, induces distention of upstream bile ducts and ductules by bile. The bile stasis and back-pressure induce proliferation of the duct epithelial cells and looping and reduplication of ducts and ductules. Unlike the extensive ductular reaction in the setting of massive hepatic necrosis, in obstruction, the ductular proliferation is confined to portal tracts. The labyrinthine ductules reabsorb secreted bile salts, serving to protect the downstream obstructed bile ducts from the toxic detergent action of bile salts. Associated histologic findings include portal tract edema and periductular infiltrates of neutrophils. Prolonged obstructive cholestasis leads not only to feathery change of hepatocytes, but also to focal detergent dissolution of hepatocytes, giving rise to **bile lakes** filled with cellular debris and pigment. **Unrelieved obstruction leads to portal tract fibrosis**, which initially extends into and subdivides the parenchyma with relative preservation of hepatic architecture. Ultimately, an end-stage bile-stained, cirrhotic liver is created (biliary cirrhosis, discussed later).

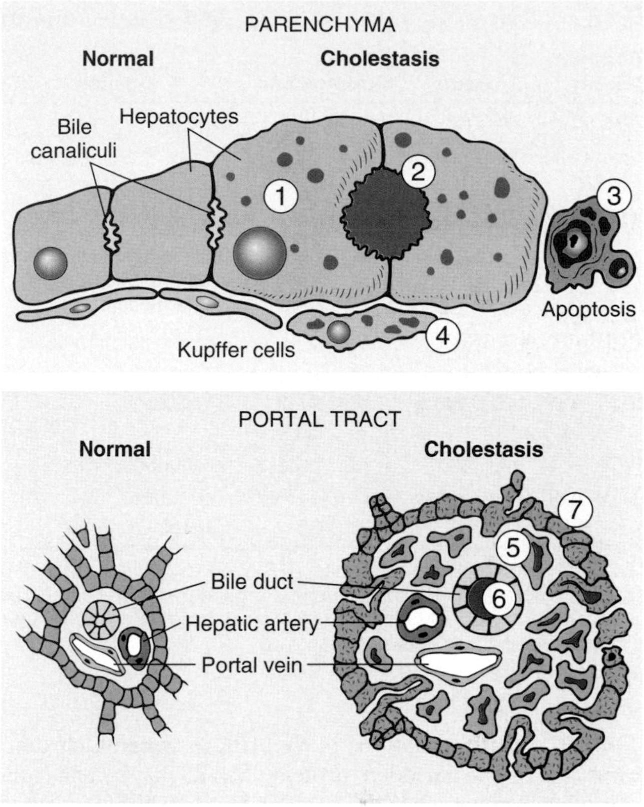

FIGURE 18–7 Illustration of the morphologic features of cholestasis (*right*) and comparison with normal liver (*left*). In the parenchyma (*upper panel*), cholestatic hepatocytes (1) are enlarged with dilated canalicular spaces (2). Apoptotic cells (3) may be seen, and Kupffer cells (4) frequently contain regurgitated bile pigments. In the portal tracts of obstructed liver (*lower panel*), there is also bile ductular proliferation (5), edema, bile pigment retention (6), and eventually neutrophilic inflammation (not shown). Surrounding hepatocytes (7) are swollen and undergoing degeneration.

Extrahepatic biliary obstruction is frequently amenable to surgical alleviation; correct and prompt diagnosis is imperative. In contrast, cholestasis due to diseases of the intrahepatic biliary tree or hepatocellular secretory failure (collectively termed *intrahepatic cholestasis*) cannot be benefited by surgery (short of transplantation), and the patient's condition may be worsened by an operative procedure. *There is thus some urgency in making a correct diagnosis of the cause of jaundice and cholestasis.*

Familial Intrahepatic Cholestasis. Mention should be made of a striking but heterogeneous group of autosomal-recessively inherited cholestatic conditions (Table 18–5).[13]

One group of disorders is characterized by low bile salt secretion into bile. Because luminal bile salts within the canaliculus are required for elution of phosphatidylcholines and cholesterol from hepatocytes and serve as an osmotic stimulus for biliary fluid secretion, there is severe impairment of bile formation. However, unlike many other cholestatic conditions, the virtual absence of bile salts within the canalicular lumen between hepatocytes means that serum γ-glutamyl transpeptidase (GGT) levels are low for the degree of hyperbilirubinemia. In *benign recurrent intrahepatic cholestasis (BRIC)*, there are intermittent attacks of cholestasis over life without progression to chronic liver disease. In *progressive familial intrahepatic cholestasis 1 (PFIC-1)*, cholestasis begins in infancy with severe pruritus due to high serum bile acid levels and relentlessly progresses to liver failure before adulthood. The first major characterized family with the latter syndrome are descendants of Jacob Byler, an Amish patient. Affected members of this particular family are designated as having *Byler syndrome*; unrelated individuals with different mutations have *Byler disease.* These conditions encompass a spectrum arising usually from mutations in the *ATP8B1* gene on chromosome 18q21. The encoded protein is a canalicular P-type ATPase of uncertain function, possibly playing a role in secretion of bile salts indirectly through maintenance of aminophospholipid polarity in the canalicular membrane. Mutations in the canalicular bile salt export pump (BSEP, encoded by the *ABCB11* gene on chromosome 2q24), are the cause of *progressive familial intrahepatic cholestasis 2 (PFIC-2).* This cholestatic disorder features severely impaired bile salt secretion into bile, with extreme pruritus, growth failure, and progression to cirrhosis in the first decade of life.

An autosomal-recessive cholestatic disorder with high serum GGT is *progressive familial intrahepatic cholestasis 3*

TABLE 18–5 Inherited Cholestatic Conditions

Common Names	Gene	Chromosome	Ligands	Location	Diseases
ABC1	ABCAI	9q22–q31	Lipids? Cholesterol?	Many tissues	Tangier disease type 1
MDR3	ABCB4	7q21	Phosphatidylcholine	Hepatocyte apical (canalicular) membrane	PFIC-3
BSEP	ABCB11	2q24	Bile Salts	Hepatocyte apical (canalicular) membrane	PFIC-2
MRP2 (cMOAT)	ABCC2	10q24	Anionic conjugates with glutathione, sulfate, and glucuronate	Liver, intestine, kidney apical membranes	Dubin-Johnson Syndrome
CFTR	ABCC7	7q31–2	Organic anions? GSH?	Lung, intestine (crypt), cholangiocytes: apical membranes	Cystic Fibrosis
IBST	SLC10A2	13q33	Bile Salts	Cholangiocytes, intestine: apical membranes	PBAM
FIC1	ATP8B1	18q21–22	Aminophospholipid?	Cholangiocytes, hepatoctyes: apical membranes	PFIC-1, BRIC, Byler disease, Byler syndrome
ATP7B	ATP7B	13q14.3	Copper	Hepatocyte endoplasmic reticulum	Wilson disease

ABC, of the ABC transporter family; ATP, adenosine triphospatase; BRIC, benign recurrent intrahepatic cholestasis; BSEP, bile salt export pump; CFTR, cystic fibrosis transmembrane regulator; cMOAT, canalicular multiple organic anion transporter; PFIC, progressive familial intrahepatic cholestasis; IBST, intestinal bile salt transporter; MRP, multidrug resistant protein; PBAM, primary bile acid malabsorption; PFIC, progressive familial intrahepatic cholestasis.

(PFIC-3), due to mutations in the *ABCB4* gene on chromosome 7q21. The encoded protein, MDR3, is a canalicular transport protein that is responsible for flipping phosphatidylcholine from the internal to the external hemileaflet of the canalicular membrane. In patients with this disorder, the absence of secreted phosphatidylcholine in bile leaves the apical surfaces of the biliary tree epithelia subject to the full detergent action of secreted bile salts, with resultant toxic destruction of these epithelia and release of GGT into the circulation.

Children with severe cholestasis but with absence of elevated serum GGT and absence of pruritus may also have inherited defects in bile acid synthesis. The most common condition is a deficiency of *3β-hydroxysteroid dehydrogenase*, an enzyme located early in the pathway for bile acid synthesis from cholesterol.

Infectious Disorders

Inflammatory disorders of the liver dominate the clinical practice of hepatology. This is due in part to the fact that virtually any insult to the liver can kill hepatocytes and recruit inflammatory cells, but also because inflammatory diseases are frequently long-term chronic conditions that must be managed medically. Among inflammatory disorders, infection is by far the most frequent. The liver is almost inevitably involved in blood-borne infections, whether systemic or arising within the abdomen. The foremost hepatic infections are viral in origin. Other infections in which the hepatic lesion is prominent include miliary tuberculosis, malaria, staphylococcal bacteremia, the salmonelloses, candida, and amebiasis.

VIRAL HEPATITIS

Unless otherwise specified, the term "viral hepatitis" is reserved for infection of the liver caused by a group of viruses having a particular affinity for the liver (Table 18–6).[14, 15] Systemic viral infections that can involve the liver include (1) infectious mononucleosis (Epstein-Barr virus), which may cause a mild hepatitis during the acute phase; (2) cytomegalovirus, particularly in the newborn or immunosuppressed patient; and (3) yellow fever, which has been a major and serious cause of hepatitis in tropical countries. Infrequently, in children and immunosuppressed patients, the liver is affected in the course of rubella, adenovirus, herpesvirus, or enterovirus infections. Hepatotropic viruses cause overlapping patterns of disease. Each hepatotropic virus and the disease conditions it causes will be introduced before a general discussion of hepatitis.

Hepatitis A Virus

Hepatitis A virus (HAV), the scourge of military campaigns since antiquity, is a benign, self-limited disease with an incubation period of 2 to 6 weeks.[16] *HAV does not cause chronic hepatitis or a carrier state and only rarely causes fulminant hepatitis, so the fatality rate associated with HAV is about 0.1%.* The outcome of HAV infection may be more severe if it is superimposed on chronic hepatitis due to Hepatitis B virus (HBV), Hepatitis C virus (HCV), or alcohol. HAV occurs throughout the world and is endemic in countries with substandard hygiene and sanitation, so populations there may have detectable anti-HAV by the age of 10 years. Clinical disease tends to be mild or asymptomatic and rare after childhood. In developed countries, the prevalence of seropositivity increases gradually with age, reaching 50% by age 50 years in the United States. In this population, acute HAV tends to be a sporadic febrile illness. Overall, HAV accounts for about 25% of clinically evident acute hepatitis worldwide and an estimated 270,000 new cases per year in the United States.[4]

HAV is a small, nonenveloped, single-stranded RNA picornavirus that occupies its own genus, *Hepatovirus*. Ultrastructurally, HAV is an icosahedral capsid 27 nm in diameter. HAV

TABLE 18–6 The Hepatitis Viruses

	Hepatitis A Virus	Hepatitis B Virus	Hepatitis C Virus	Hepatitis D Virus	Hepatitis E Virus	Hepatitis G Virus*
Agent	Icosahedral capsid, ssRNA	Enveloped dsDNA	Enveloped ssRNA	Enveloped ssRNA	Unenveloped ssRNA	ssRNA virus
Transmission	Fecal-oral	Parenteral; close contact	Parenteral; close contact	Parenteral; close contact	Waterborne	Parenteral
Incubation period	2–6 wk	4–26 wk	2–26 wk	4–7 wk	2–8 wk	Unknown
Carrier state	None	0.1–1.0% of blood donors in U.S. and Western world	0.2–1.0% of blood donors in U.S. and Western world	1–10% in drug addicts and hemophiliacs	Unknown	1–2% of blood donors in U.S.
Chronic hepatitis	None	5–10% of acute infections	>50%	<5% coinfection, 80% upon superinfection	None	None
Hepatocellular carcinoma	No	Yes	Yes	No increase above HBV	Unknown, but unlikely	None

*At present, hepatitis G virus is not considered pathogenic.

is spread by ingestion of contaminated water and foods and is shed in the stool for 2 to 3 weeks before and 1 week after the onset of jaundice. Thus, close personal contact with an infected individual or fecal-oral contamination during this period accounts for most cases and explains the outbreaks in institutional settings such as schools and nurseries and the waterborne epidemics in places where people live in overcrowded, unsanitary conditions. HAV is not shed in any significant quantities in saliva, urine, or semen. In developed countries, sporadic infections may be contracted by the consumption of raw or steamed shellfish (oysters, mussels, clams), which concentrate the virus from seawater contaminated with human sewage. Infected workers in the food industry may also be the source of outbreaks. Outbreaks of the disease in September and November, 2003, in the United States involved more than 600 infected persons and caused at least three deaths. Consumption of raw green onions contaminated with HAV was the most likely cause of these outbreaks. *Because HAV viremia is transient, blood-borne transmission of HAV occurs only rarely; therefore, donated blood is not specifically screened for this virus.*

Serologic Diagnosis. Specific antibody against HAV of the immunoglobulin (Ig) M type appears in blood at the onset of symptoms, constituting a reliable marker of acute infection (Fig. 18–8). Fecal shedding of the virus ends as the IgM titer rises. The IgM response usually begins to decline in a few months and is followed by the appearance of IgG anti-HAV. The latter persists for years, perhaps for life, providing protective immunity against reinfection by all strains of HAV. Hence, the HAV vaccine is effective.

Hepatitis B Virus

Hepatitis B virus (HBV) can produce (1) acute hepatitis with resolution, (2) chronic hepatitis, which may evolve to cirrhosis, (3) fulminant hepatitis with massive liver necrosis, and (4) the backdrop for hepatitis D virus infection. Patients with chronic hepatitis represent carriers of actively replicating virus and hence are a source of infection to other individuals.[17] HBV also plays an important role in the development of hepatocellular carcinoma. The approximate frequencies of clinical outcomes of HBV infection are depicted in Figure 18–9.

Liver disease due to HBV is an enormous problem globally, with an estimated worldwide carrier rate of 350 million. It is estimated that HBV has infected over 2 billion of the individuals alive today at some point in their lives. Seventy-five percent of all chronic carriers live in Asia and the Western Pacific rim. The global prevalence of chronic hepatitis B infection varies widely, from high (>8%) in Africa, Asia, and the Western Pacific to intermediate (2% to 7%) in Southern and Eastern Europe to low (<2%) in Western Europe, North America, and Australia. In the United States alone, there are

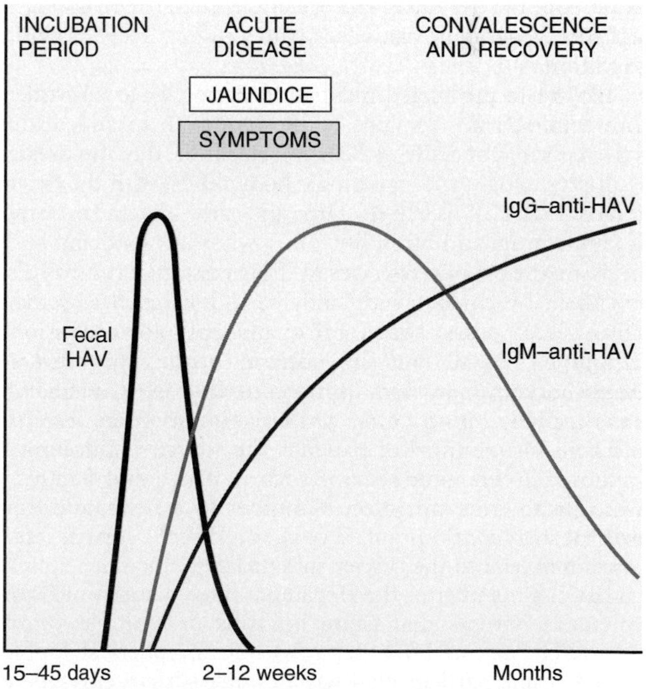

FIGURE 18–8 Sequence of serologic markers in acute hepatitis A viral hepatitis.

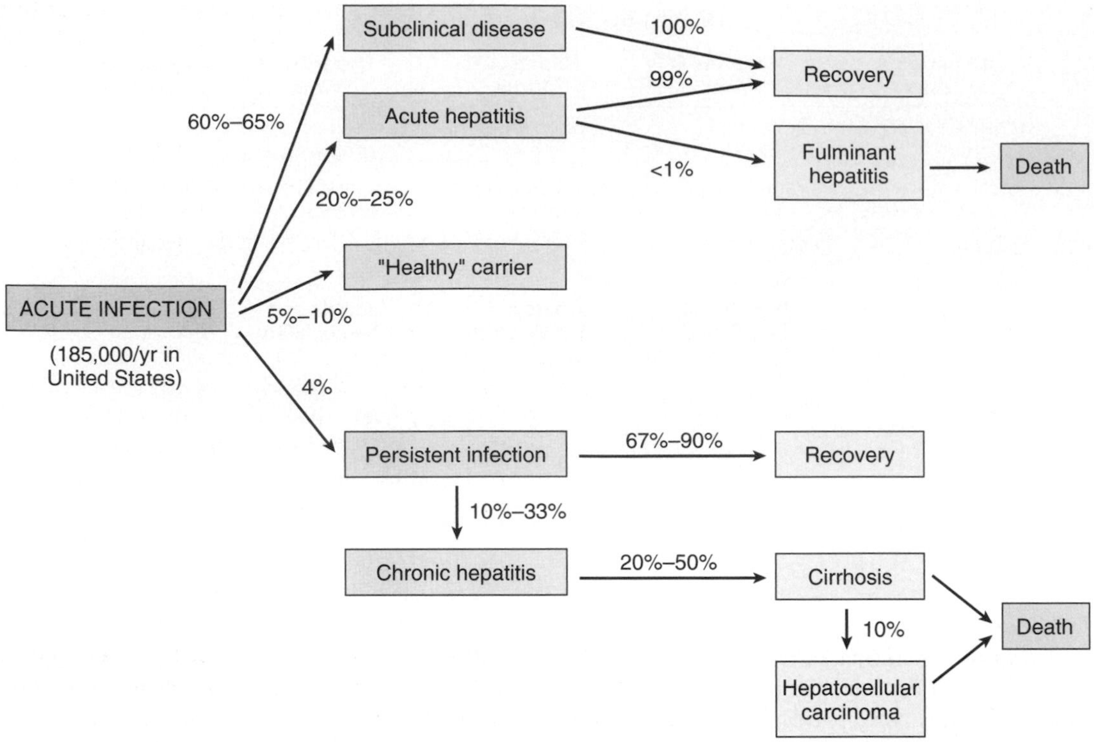

FIGURE 18–9 Schematic of the potential outcomes of hepatitis B infection in adults, with their approximate frequencies in the United States.

an estimated 185,000 new infections per year.[4] Because circulating host IgG antibodies effectively neutralize HBV, the HBV vaccine has been highly effective in reducing the prevalence of HBV in endemic areas, particularly in a mass vaccination program in Taiwan. As a public health measure, vaccination against HBV thus offers the hope that a viral vaccine may reduce the risk of malignancy, hepatocellular carcinoma, in high-risk geographic areas (see below under "Hepatocellular Carcinoma").

HBV has a prolonged incubation period (4 to 26 weeks). Unlike HAV, HBV remains in the blood up to and during active episodes of acute and chronic hepatitis. It is also present in all physiologic and pathologic body fluids, with the exception of stool. HBV is a hardy virus and can withstand extremes of temperature and humidity. Thus, whereas blood and body fluids are the primary vehicles of transmission, virus may also be spread by contact with body secretions such as semen, saliva, sweat, tears, breast milk, and pathologic effusions. *Transfusion, blood products, dialysis, needle-stick accidents among health care workers, intravenous drug abuse, and homosexual activity constitute the primary risk categories for HBV infection.* In one third of patients, the source of infection is unknown. In endemic regions such as Africa and Southeast Asia, spread from an infected mother to a neonate during birth (*vertical transmission*) is common. These neonatal infections often lead to the carrier state for life.

HBV is a member of the Hepadnaviridae, a family of DNA-containing viruses that cause hepatitis in multiple animal species. The mature HBV virion is a 42-nm, spherical double-layered "Dane particle" that has an outer surface envelope of protein, lipid, and carbohydrate enclosing an electron-dense, 28-nm, slightly hexagonal core. The genome of HBV is a partially double-stranded circular DNA molecule having 3200 nucleotides (Fig. 18–10). All regions of the HBV genome encode protein sequences:[18]

- A nucleocapsid "core" protein (HBcAg, hepatitis B core antigen) and a longer polypeptide transcript with a precore and core region, designated HBeAg (hepatitis B "e" antigen). The precore region directs the HBeAg polypeptide toward secretion into blood, whereas HBcAg remains in hepatocytes for the assembly of complete virions.
- Envelope glycoprotein (HBsAg, hepatitis B surface antigen). Infected hepatocytes are capable of synthesizing and secreting massive quantities of noninfective surface protein (HBsAg), over and above HBcAg synthesis. HBsAg appears in cells and the serum as spheres and tubules approximately 22 nm in diameter.
- A DNA polymerase that exhibits reverse transcriptase activity; genomic replication occurs via an intermediate RNA template.
- A protein from the X region, HBx, which is necessary for virus replication and acts as a transcriptional transactivator of the viral genes and a wide variety of host genes. HBx modulation of gene transcription affects viral replication and the function of hepatocyte cell cycle checkpoints. HBx may play a role in deregulation of hepatocyte replication and development of hepatocellular carcinoma in HBV-infected patients.

HBV infection of a hepatocyte passes through two phases. During the *proliferative phase*, HBV-DNA is present in episomal form, with formation of complete virions and all associated antigens. Cell surface expression of viral HBsAg and

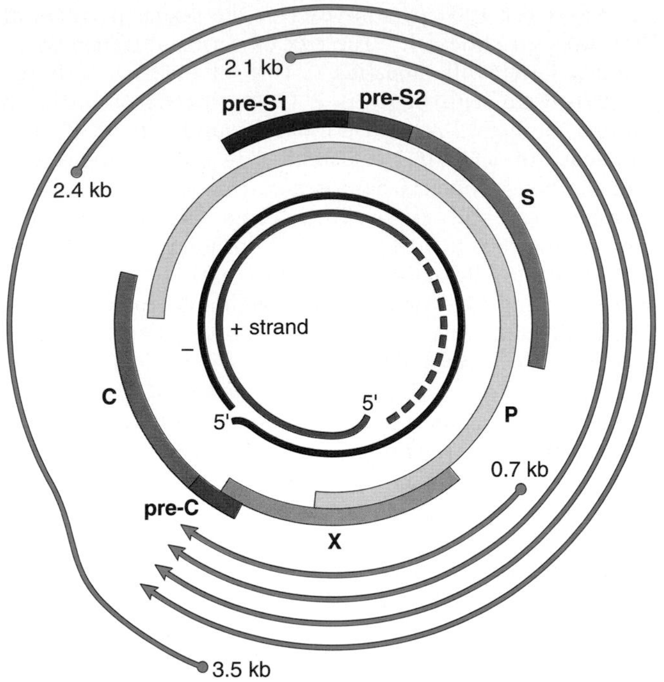

FIGURE 18–10 Diagrammatic representation of genomic structure and transcribed components of the hepatitis B virion. The innermost circles represent the DNA (+) strand and the DNA (–) strand of the virion. The thick bars labeled "P," "X," "pre-C," "C," "pre-SI," "pre-S2," and "S" denote the peptides derived from the virion. The outermost lines denote the mRNA transcripts of the virion. (After Kidd-Ljunggren K, Myakawa Y, Kidd AH: J Gen Virol 83:1267–1280, 2002.)

HBcAg in association with MHC class I molecules leads to activation of CD8+ cytotoxic T lymphocytes. Hepatocyte destruction occurs if a cytotoxic T lymphocyte interacts with the infected hepatocyte. For the infected hepatocytes that are not destroyed by the immune system, an *integrative phase* may occur in which viral DNA is incorporated into the host genome.

With cessation of viral replication within hepatocytes and the appearance of antiviral antibodies, infectivity ends and liver damage subsides. However, because of the HBV DNA integrated into the host genome, the risk of hepatocellular carcinoma persists.

There is little doubt that HBV is not directly toxic to liver cells; instead it is the immune response to viral antigens, expressed on infected hepatocytes, that cause liver cell injury. In keeping with this, patients with immune defects suffer relatively mild liver injury (but are more prone to develop a carrier state, discussed later). HBV evokes both a humoral and cellular immune response, the latter involving both CD4+ helper T cells and CD8+ cytotoxic T cells. Whereas on one hand, cytotoxic T cells mediate hepatocellular injury (by lysis of infected liver cells), on the other hand, they also help clear the infection by destroying the intracellular reservoirs of HBV. Recent studies suggest that some of the anti-viral effects of T cells may also be mediated by the secretion of γ-interferon. The antibody response can confer long-term protection against HBV, as is discussed next.

Serologic Diagnosis. After exposure to HBV, the long asymptomatic 4- to 26-week incubation period (mean: 6 to 8 weeks) is followed by acute disease lasting many weeks to months (Fig. 18–11*A*). Most patients experience a self-limited illness:

- HBsAg appears before the onset of symptoms, peaks during overt disease, and then declines to undetectable levels in 3 to 6 months.
- HBeAg, HBV-DNA, and DNA polymerase appear in the serum soon after HBsAg, and all signify active viral replication.
- IgM anti-HBc becomes detectable in serum shortly before the onset of symptoms, concurrent with the onset of elevation of serum aminotransferases. Over months, the IgM antibody is replaced by IgG anti-HBc.
- Anti-HBe is detectable shortly after the disappearance of HBeAg, implying that the acute infection has peaked and the disease is on the wane.

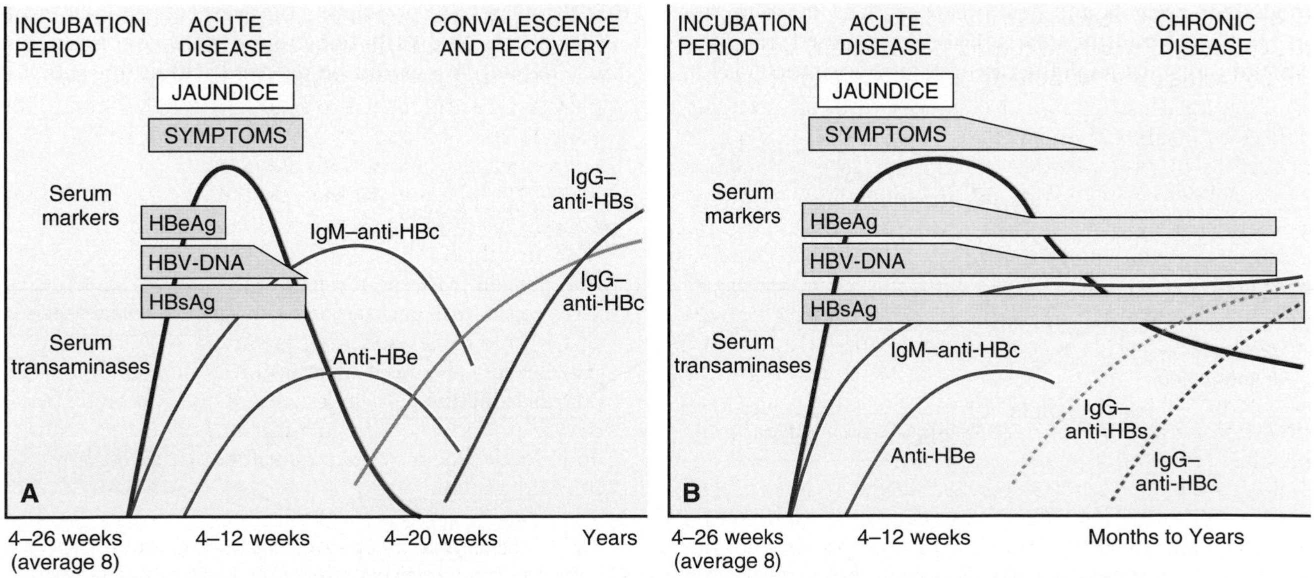

FIGURE 18–11 Sequence of serologic markers for hepatitis B viral hepatitis demonstrating *(A)* acute infection with resolution and *(B)* progression to chronic infection.

- IgG anti-HBs does not rise until the acute disease is over and is usually not detectable for a few weeks to several months after the disappearance of HBsAg. Anti-HBs may persist for life, conferring protection; this is the basis for current vaccination strategies using noninfectious HBsAg.

The carrier state is defined by the presence of HBsAg in serum for 6 months or longer after initial detection. The presence of HBsAg alone does not necessarily indicate replication of complete virions, and patients may be asymptomatic and without liver damage. In contrast, *chronic replication of HBV virions is characterized by persistence of circulating HBsAg, HBeAg, and HBV DNA, usually with anti-HBc and occasionally with anti-HBs* (Fig. 18–11*B*). In these patients, progressive liver damage may occur.

Hepatitis C Virus

Hepatitis C virus (HCV) is a major cause of liver disease worldwide. Forty thousand new infections of HCV are estimated to occur annually in the United States. Approximately 3.9 million Americans, or 1.8% of the population, have antibodies against HCV. Fully 70% of these individuals, or 2.7 million, have evidence of chronic infection as determined by the presence of viral DNA in the serum. This makes HCV the most common chronic blood-borne infection and accounts for almost half of all patients in the United States with chronic liver disease.[4] There has been a slight decrease in seropositivity since the peak of slightly over 2.0% in the mid-1990s. Notably, there also has been a decrease in the annual incidence of infection from its mid-1980s peak of over 150,000 new infections per year to a current 40,000 new infections per year. Nevertheless, the number of patients with long-standing infection is projected to increase fourfold over the 25 years from 1990 to 2015. Hence, the prevalence of life-limiting chronic liver disease and the risk of hepatocellular carcinoma are only expected to increase.

The major routes of transmission are inoculations and blood transfusions. Intravenous drug use accounts for 60% of cases, transfusions prior to 1991 account for 10%, and hemodialysis patients and health care workers make up less than 5%. Sexual transmission is the only presumed risk factor in 15% of cases, although the case risk for transmission is low (12 events per 1000 person-years in the sexual partners of HCV-infected patients).[19] The risk of perinatal transmission is much lower with hepatitis C (6% of births to infected mothers) than with hepatitis B (20% to 60% of births to infected mothers).[4] Against the background anti-HCV seroprevalence of 1.8% in the United States, the prevalence is higher in house contacts, homosexuals, hemodialysis patients, hemophiliacs, and intravenous drug abusers (the last approaching 50% to 90%). Patients with unexplained cirrhosis and hepatocellular carcinoma have anti-HCV prevalence rates exceeding 50%. Acute HCV infection is generally undetected clinically. *In contrast to HBV, progression to chronic disease occurs in the majority of infected individuals, and cirrhosis eventually occurs in approximately 20% of patients with chronic HCV infection* (Fig. 18–12). *Thus, over the next decade, HCV could become the leading cause of chronic liver disease in the Western world, as there is a substantial reservoir of individuals at risk for progression to cirrhosis.*

HCV, and the closely related hepatitis G virus, is a hepacivirus and occupies a genus in the Flaviviridae family. HCV is a small, enveloped, single-stranded RNA virus, with a 9-kb genome that codes for single polyprotein of approximately 3010 amino acids in one single open reading frame (Fig. 18–13). This protein is subsequently processed into functional proteins. The 5′ end of the genome encodes a highly conserved nucleocapsid core protein, followed by envelope proteins E1 and E2. Two hypervariable regions (HVR 1 and 2) are present in the E2 sequence. A protein of uncertain function, p7, is coded next. Toward the 3′ end are six less conserved nonstructural proteins: NS2, NS3, NS4A, NS4B, NS5A, and NS5B. NS5B is the viral RNA-dependent RNA polymerase. The 3′ sequences of both the positive- and negative-strand RNAs contribute cis-acting functions that are essential for viral replication. The secondary structure and protein-binding properties of these highly conserved nontranslated regions are thought to promote HCV RNA synthesis and genome stability through the binding of various host and viral proteins.

Owing to the poor fidelity of the HCV RNA polymerase (NS5B), the virus is inherently unstable, giving rise to multiple genotypes and subtypes. Indeed, within any given patient, HCV circulates as a population of divergent genomes exhibiting a quasispecies distribution.[20] Specifically, over time, several dozen mutant strains can be detected within one individual

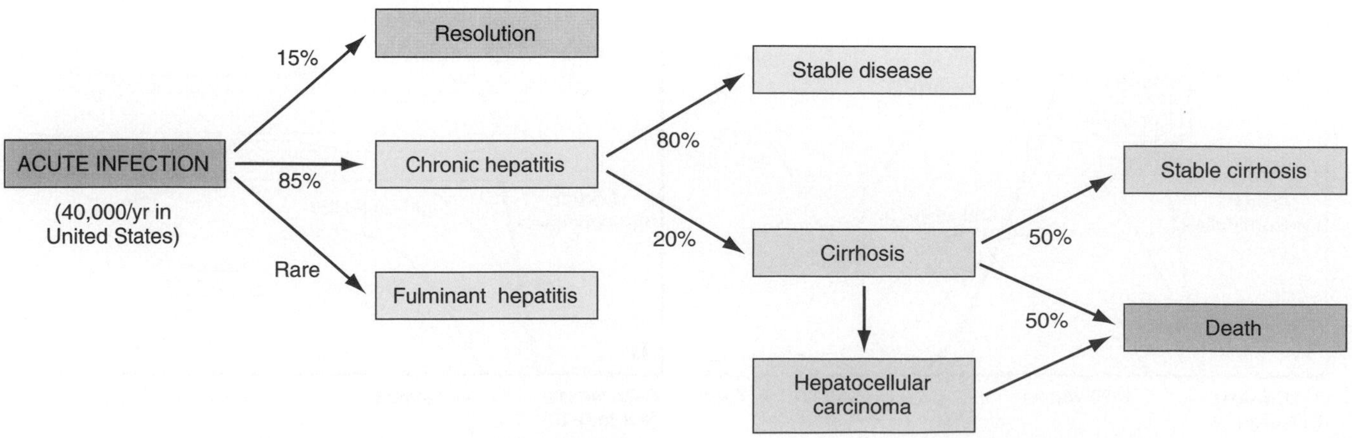

FIGURE 18–12 Schematic of the potential outcomes of hepatitis C infection in adults, with their approximate frequencies in the United States.

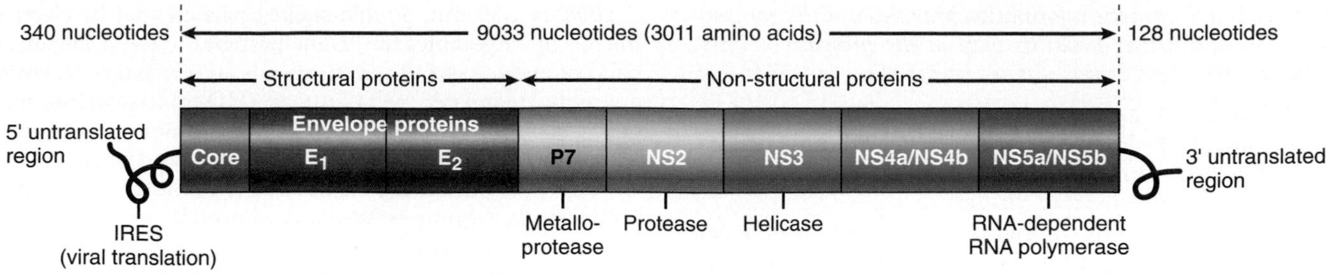

FIGURE 18–13 Diagrammatic representation of the genomic structure and transcribed components of the hepatitis C virion. The hepatitis C virion is transcribed in one single transcript, as depicted in the top line; 340 nucleotides at the 5′ end and 128 nucleotides at the 3′ end are not translated into protein. The protein products cleaved from the single translated peptide are shown in the bottom bar.

and mapped as derivative strains of the original HCV strain infecting that individual. The E2 protein of the envelope is the target of many anti-HCV antibodies but is also the most variable region of the entire viral genome, enabling emergent virus strains to escape from neutralizing antibodies. This genomic instability and antigenic variability have seriously hampered efforts to develop an HCV vaccine. In particular, *elevated titers of anti-HCV IgG occurring after an active infection do not confer effective immunity.* Moreover, HCV is able to actively evade the interferon (IFN)-mediated cellular antiviral response, because E2 and NS5A inhibit the interferon-induced double-stranded RNA-activated protein kinase, which is involved in the antiviral response to IFN.[21] A characteristic feature of HCV infection, therefore, is repeated bouts of hepatic damage, the result of reactivation of a preexisting infection or emergence of an endogenous, newly mutated strain. *Persistent infection and chronic hepatitis are the hallmarks of HCV infection,* despite the generally asymptomatic nature of the acute illness. *Cirrhosis may develop over 5 to 20 years after acute infection.*

Serologic Diagnosis. The incubation period for HCV hepatitis ranges from 2 to 26 weeks, with a mean between 6 and 12 weeks. HCV RNA is detectable in blood for 1 to 3 weeks, coincident with elevations in serum transaminases (Fig. 18–14*A*). In symptomatic acute HCV infection, anti-HCV antibodies are detected in only 50% to 70% of patients; in the remaining patients, the anti-HCV antibodies emerge after 3 to 6 weeks. The clinical course of acute HCV hepatitis is milder than that of HBV; rare cases may be severe and indistinguishable from HAV or HBV hepatitis.

In chronic HCV infection, circulating HCV RNA persists in many patients despite the presence of neutralizing antibodies, including more than 90% of patients with chronic disease (Fig. 18–14*B*). Hence, in patients with symptoms of chronic hepatitis, HCV RNA testing must be performed to assess viral replication and to confirm the diagnosis of HCV infection. *A clinical feature that is quite characteristic of chronic HCV infection is episodic elevations in serum aminotransferases, with intervening normal or near-normal periods.*

Hepatitis D Virus

Also called "hepatitis delta virus," hepatitis D virus (HDV) is a unique RNA virus that is replication defective, causing infection only when it is encapsulated by HBsAg. Thus, *although taxonomically distinct from HBV, HDV is absolutely*

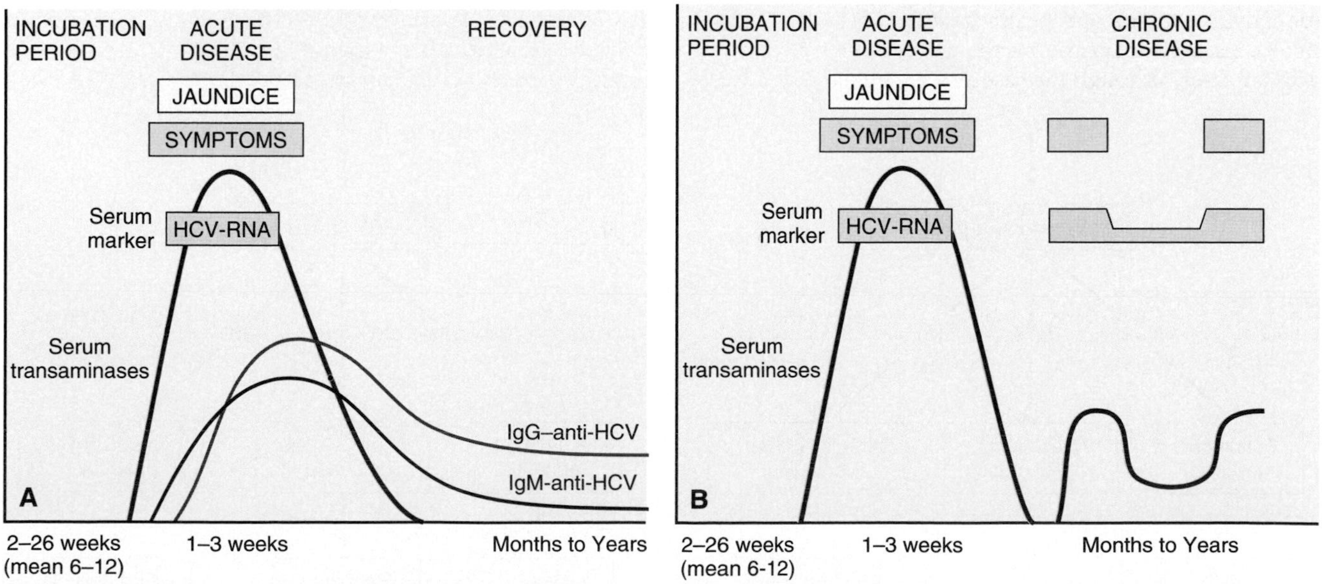

FIGURE 18–14 Sequence of serologic markers for hepatitis C viral hepatitis demonstrating (*A*) acute infection with resolution and (*B*) progression to chronic relapsing infection.

dependent on the genetic information provided by HBV for multiplication and causes hepatitis only in the presence of HBV. Delta hepatitis thus arises in two settings (Fig. 18–15):[22]

- Acute *coinfection* occurs following exposure to serum containing both HDV and HBV. The HBV must become established first to provide the HBsAg necessary for development of complete HDV virions.
- *Superinfection* of a chronic carrier of HBV with a new inoculum of HDV (and HBV) results in disease about 30 to 50 days later. The carrier may have been previously "healthy" or may have had underlying chronic hepatitis.

Simultaneous coinfection with HBV and HDV results in hepatitis ranging from mild to fulminant, fulminant disease being more likely (about 3% to 4%) than with HBV alone. Chronicity rarely develops. When HDV is superimposed on chronic HBV infection, there are three possible outcomes: (1) acute, severe hepatitis may erupt in a previously healthy HBV carrier; (2) mild HBV hepatitis may be converted into fulminant disease; and/or (3) chronic, progressive disease may develop (in 80% of patients), often culminating in cirrhosis.

Infection by the delta agent is worldwide, but the prevalence varies greatly. In Africa, the Middle East, and southern Italy, 20% to 40% of HBsAg carriers have anti-HDV antibody. In the United States, delta infection is uncommon and is largely restricted to drug addicts and hemophiliacs, who exhibit prevalence rates of 1% to 10%. Other groups at high risk for HBV, such as homosexual men and health care workers, are at low risk for HDV infection, for unclear reasons. Surprisingly, delta infection is uncommon in the large population of HBsAg carriers in Southeast Asia and China.

HDV is a 35-nm, double-shelled particle that by electron microscopy resembles the "Dane particle" of HBV. The external coat antigen of HBsAg surrounds an internal polypeptide assembly, designated delta antigen (HDAg). Associated with HDAg is a small (1689 base pairs), circular molecule of single-stranded RNA, whose length is smaller than the genome of any known animal virus.[23] This RNA is considered "genomic," but HDAg is the only HDV-encoded protein product that has been detected to date.

Serologic Diagnosis. HDV RNA is detectable in the blood and liver just prior to and in the early days of acute symptomatic disease (Fig. 18–16). IgM anti-HDV is the most reliable indicator of recent HDV exposure, although its appearance is late and frequently short-lived. Nevertheless, acute coinfection by HDV and HBV is best indicated by detection of IgM against both HDAg and HBcAg (denoting new infection with hepatitis B). With chronic delta hepatitis arising from HDV superinfection, HBsAg is present in serum, and IgM anti-HDV persists for months or longer.

Hepatitis E Virus

Hepatitis E virus (HEV) hepatitis is an enterically transmitted, water-borne infection that occurs primarily in young to middle-aged adults; sporadic infection and overt illness in children are rare. Epidemics have been reported from Asia and the Indian subcontinent, sub-Saharan Africa, and Mexico. Sporadic infection seems to be uncommon and is seen mainly in travelers. Indeed, HEV accounts for over 50% of cases of sporadic acute hepatitis in India, exceeding the frequency of HAV. *A characteristic feature of HEV infection is the high*

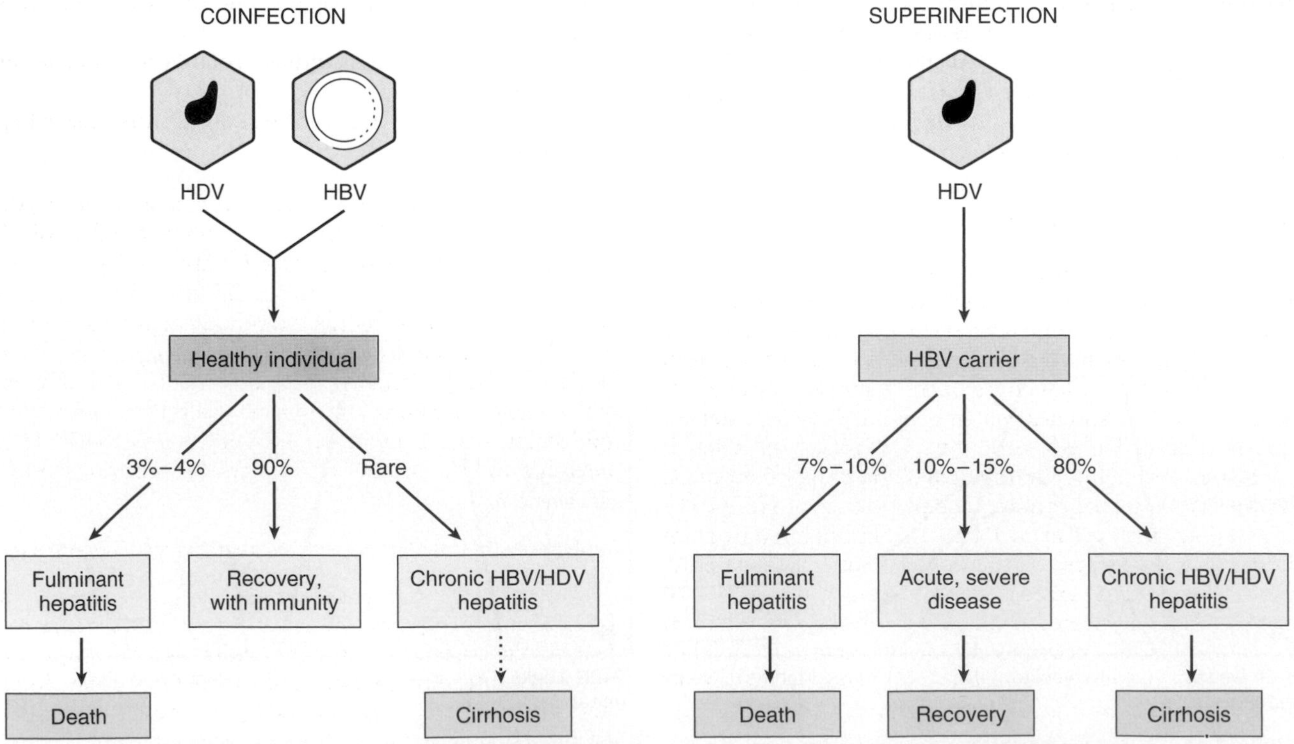

FIGURE 18–15 Differing clinical consequences of two patterns of combined hepatitis D virus and hepatitis B virus infection.

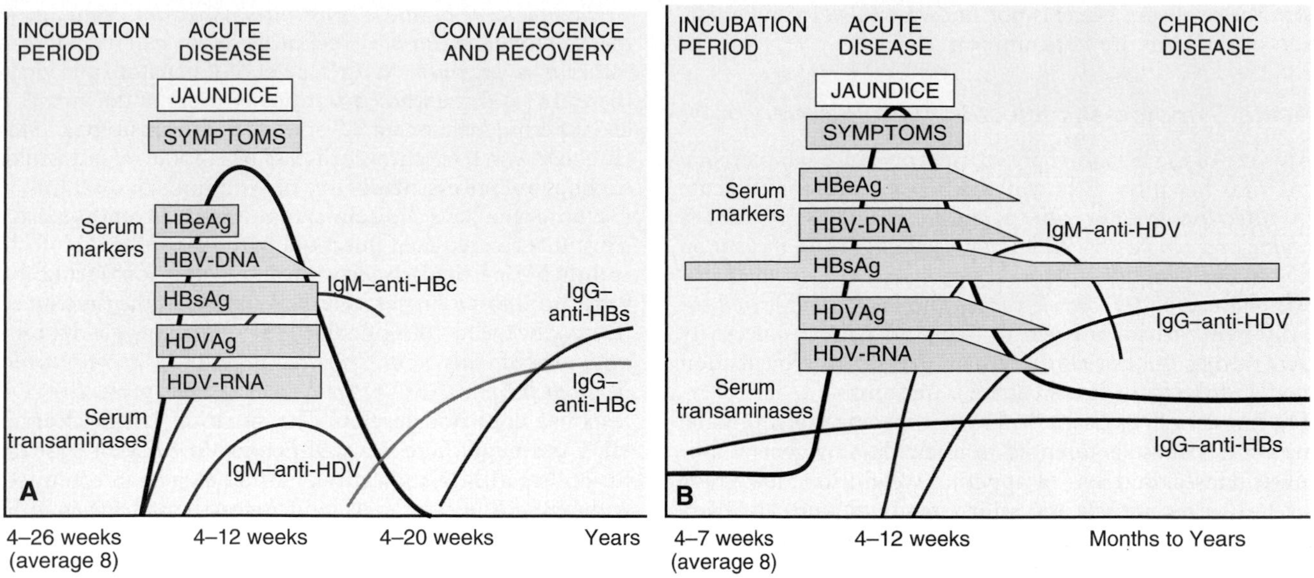

FIGURE 18–16 Sequence of serologic markers for hepatitis D viral hepatitis depicting (*A*) coinfection with hepatitis B virus (HBV) and (*B*) superinfection of an HBV carrier.

mortality rate among pregnant women, approaching 20%. In most cases, the disease is self-limiting; HEV is not associated with chronic liver disease or persistent viremia. The average incubation period following exposure is 6 weeks.

HEV is an unenveloped, single-stranded RNA virus that is structurally similar to the Caliciviridae.[24] Viral particles are 32 to 34 nm in diameter, and the RNA genome is approximately 7.6 kb in size. A specific antigen (HEV Ag) can be identified in the cytoplasm of hepatocytes during active infection, and virions are shed in stool during the acute illness.

Serologic Diagnosis. Before the onset of clinical illness, HEV RNA and HEV virions can be detected in stool and liver. The onset of rising serum aminotransferases, clinical illness, and elevated IgM anti-HEV titers are virtually simultaneous. Symptoms resolve in 2 to 4 weeks, during which time the IgM is replaced with a persistent IgG anti-HEV titer.

Other Hepatitis Viruses

Epidemiologic studies have established that some cases of hepatitis are caused by infectious agents other than those listed earlier. The epidemiologic event that was ascribed to a putative "F" has not been repeated, and no F agent has been identified. However, a flavivirus bearing similarities to HCV was cloned in 1995 and designated hepatitis G virus. Later, an identical virus called GB virus type C (GBC) was isolated. HGV is transmitted by contaminated blood or blood products and possibly via sexual contact. The prevalence of HGV RNA in blood donors ranges from 1% to 4%; and in a report from Taiwan, the incidence of new HGV infections among hemodialysis patients exceeds 2% per year. In up to 75% of infections, HGV is cleared from plasma; in the remainder of cases, HGV infection becomes chronic. *The site of HGV replication is most likely in mononuclear cells; hence, HGV is inappropriately named, as it is not hepatotropic and does not cause elevations in serum aminotransferases. Extensive data do not indicate any pathologic effects of HGV, and the blood supply does not appear to need screening for HGV RNA. This virus commonly co-infects patients with HIV, and curiously this dual infection is somewhat protective against HIV disease.*[24a]

Clinicopathologic Syndromes

A number of clinical syndromes may develop following exposure to hepatitis viruses:

- Acute asymptomatic infection with recovery: serologic evidence only
- Acute symptomatic hepatitis with recovery: anicteric or icteric
- Chronic hepatitis: without or with progression to cirrhosis
- Fulminant hepatitis: with massive to submassive hepatic necrosis

Each of the hepatotropic viruses can cause acute asymptomatic or symptomatic infection. A small number of HBV-infected patients develop chronic hepatitis; HCV is notorious for chronic infection. With rare exceptions, HAV and HEV do not cause chronic hepatitis. Fulminant hepatitis is unusual, and almost unheard of with HCV. *Other infectious or noninfectious causes, particularly drugs and toxins, can lead to essentially identical clinical syndromes.* Therefore, serologic and molecular studies are essential for the diagnosis of viral hepatitis and the distinction between the various types.

Acute Asymptomatic Infection with Recovery

Patients in this group are identified only incidentally on the basis of minimally elevated serum transaminases or, after the fact, by the presence of antiviral antibodies. Worldwide, HAV and HBV infection are frequently subclinical events in childhood, verified only in adulthood by the presence of anti-HAV or anti-HBV antibodies. Although asymptomatic acute infection is most often the case for HCV-infected patients for whom the exposure event is not known, recovery and eradication of the virus are not common.

Acute Symptomatic Infection with Recovery

Any one of the hepatotropic viruses can cause symptomatic acute viral hepatitis, although this is uncommon for acute HCV infection. Whatever the agent, *the disease is more or less the same and can be divided into four phases: (1) an incubation period, (2) a symptomatic preicteric phase, (3) a symptomatic icteric phase, and (4) convalescence.* The *incubation period* for the different viruses is given in Table 18–6. Peak infectivity occurs during the last asymptomatic days of the incubation period and the early days of acute symptoms.

The *preicteric phase* is marked by nonspecific, constitutional symptoms. Malaise is followed in a few days by general fatigability, nausea, and loss of appetite. Weight loss, low-grade fever, headaches, muscle and joint aches, and pains and diarrhea are inconstant symptoms. About 10% of patients with acute hepatitis, most often those with hepatitis B, develop a serum sickness–like syndrome. This consists of fever, rash, and arthralgias, attributable to circulating immune complexes. The true origin of all these symptoms is suggested by elevated serum aminotransferase levels. Physical examination reveals a mildly enlarged, tender liver. In some patients, the nonspecific symptoms are more severe, with higher fever, shaking chills, and headache, sometimes accompanied by right upper quadrant pain and tender liver enlargement.

The *icteric phase*, if it appears, is caused mainly by conjugated hyperbilirubinemia. *Icteric hepatitis is usual in adults (but not children) with acute HAV infection, but it is absent in about half the cases of HBV and in the majority of cases of HCV.* Curiously, as jaundice appears and these patients enter the icteric phase, other symptoms begin to abate and the patient feels better. Although not the result of biliary obstruction, the jaundice is nevertheless caused predominantly by conjugated hyperbilirubinemia and hence is accompanied by dark-colored urine related to the presence of conjugated bilirubin. The stools may become lighter owing to cholestasis. Retention of bile acids can cause distressing pruritus. The liver may be mildly enlarged and moderately tender to percussion. Laboratory findings include prolonged prothrombin time and hyperglobulinemia; the serum alkaline phosphatase is usually only mildly elevated. In a few weeks to perhaps several months, the jaundice and most of the other systemic symptoms clear as convalescence begins. Recovery is heralded by the generation of strong T cell responses against viral antigens expressed on infected liver cells.

Chronic Hepatitis

Chronic hepatitis is defined as symptomatic, biochemical, or serologic evidence of continuing or relapsing hepatic disease for more than 6 months, with histologically documented inflammation and necrosis. Although the hepatitis viruses (HBV, HCV, and HBV + HDV) are responsible for most cases of chronic hepatitis, there are many other causes of chronic hepatitis (described later). They include chronic alcoholism, Wilson disease, α_1-antitrypsin deficiency, drugs (e.g., isoniazid, α-methyldopa, methotrexate), and autoimmunity. *In all instances of chronic hepatitis, etiology is the single most important indicator of likelihood to progress to cirrhosis.*

Chronic viral hepatitis constitutes a "carrier" state, in that these individuals harbor replicating virus and therefore can transmit an organism. With "carriers" of hepatotropic viruses, there are (1) those who harbor one or more of the viruses but are suffering little or no adverse clinical or histologic effects, (2) those who have chronic disease by laboratory or histologic findings but are essentially free of symptoms or disability, and (3) those who have clinically symptomatic chronic disease. All constitute reservoirs of infection. In the case of HBV, infection early in life, particularly via vertical transmission during childbirth, produces a carrier state 90% to 95% of the time. In contrast, only 1% to 10% of adult HBV infections yield a carrier state. *Individuals with impaired immunity are particularly likely to become HBV carriers*, because the protective T cell response does not develop. The situation is less clear with HDV, although there is a well-defined low risk of posttransfusion hepatitis D, indicative of a carrier state in conjunction with HBV. HCV can clearly induce a carrier state given its high rate of chronicity.

The clinical features of chronic hepatitis are extremely variable and are not predictive of outcome. In some patients, the only signs of chronic disease are persistent elevations of serum transaminases. The most common symptom is fatigue; less common symptoms are malaise, loss of appetite, and occasional bouts of mild jaundice. Physical findings are few, the most common being spider angiomas, palmar erythema, mild hepatomegaly, hepatic tenderness, and mild splenomegaly. Laboratory studies may reveal prolongation of the prothrombin time and, in some instances, hyperglobulinemia, hyperbilirubinemia, and mild elevations in alkaline phosphatase levels. Occasionally, in cases of HBV and HCV, immune complex disease may develop secondary to the presence of circulating antibody–antigen complexes, in the form of vasculitis (subcutaneous or visceral, Chapter 11) and glomerulonephritis (Chapter 20). Cryoglobulinemia is found in about 35% of patients with chronic HCV hepatitis.

Morphology of Acute and Chronic Hepatitis. The general morphologic features of viral hepatitis are given in Table 18–7 and are depicted schematically in Figure 18–17.[14] **The morphologic changes in acute and chronic viral hepatitis are shared among the hepatotropic viruses and can be mimicked by drug reactions.** Tissue alterations caused by acute infection with HAV, HBV, HCV, and HEV are similar, as is the chronic hepatitis caused by HBV, HCV, and HBV + HDV. A few histologic changes may be indicative of a particular type of virus. HBV-infected hepatocytes may exhibit a cytoplasm packed with spheres and tubules of HBsAg, producing a finely granular eosinophilic cytoplasm (**"ground glass hepatocytes,"** Fig. 18–18). HCV-infected livers frequently show lymphoid aggregates within portal tracts and focal sublobular regions of hepatocyte macrovesicular steatosis, which are to be distinguished from the extensive panlobular microvesicular and macrovesicular steatosis seen in many forms of toxic hepatitis (e.g., alcohol-induced).

Acute Hepatitis. With acute hepatitis (Figs. 18–17*A* and 18–19), hepatocyte injury takes the form of diffuse swelling (**"ballooning degeneration"**), so the cytoplasm looks empty and contains only scattered eosinophilic remnants of cytoplasmic organelles. An inconstant finding is **cholestasis**, with bile plugs in canaliculi and brown pigmentation of hepatocytes.

TABLE 18–7 Key Morphologic Features of Viral Hepatitis

Acute Hepatitis

Enlarged, reddened liver; greenish if cholestatic
Parenchymal changes:
- Hepatocyte injury: swelling (ballooning degeneration)
  - Cholestasis: canalicular bile plugs
  - HCV: mild focal fatty change of hepatocytes
- Hepatocyte necrosis: isolated cells or clusters
  - Cytolysis (rupture) or apoptosis (shrinkage)
  - If severe: bridging necrosis (portal-portal, central-central, portal-central)
  - Lobular disarray: loss of normal architecture
- Regenerative changes: hepatocyte proliferation
- Sinusoidal cell reactive changes:
  - Accumulation of phagocytosed cellular debris in Kupffer cells
  - Influx of mononuclear cells into sinusoids
- Portal tracts:
  - Inflammation: predominantly mononuclear
  - Inflammatory spillover into adjacent parenchyma, with hepatocyte necrosis

Chronic Hepatitis

Changes shared with acute hepatitis:
- Hepatocyte injury, necrosis, and regeneration
- Sinusoidal cell reactive changes

Portal tracts:
- Inflammation:
  - Confined to portal tracts, *or*
  - Spillover into adjacent parenchyma, with necrosis of hepatocytes ("interface hepatitis"), *or*
  - Bridging inflammation and necrosis
- Fibrosis:
  - Portal deposition, *or*
  - Portal and periportal deposition, *or*
  - Formation of bridging fibrous septa

HBV: "ground-glass" hepatocytes, "sanded" nuclei
HCV: bile duct epithelial cell proliferation, lymphoid aggregate formation

Cirrhosis: The end-stage outcome

The canalicular bile plugs result from cessation of the contractile activity of the hepatocyte pericanalicular actin microfilament web. Two patterns of hepatocyte cell death are seen. In the first, rupture of cell membranes leads to cytolysis and focal loss of hepatocytes. The sinusoidal collagen reticulin framework collapses where the cells have disappeared, and scavenger **macrophage aggregates** mark sites of hepatocyte loss. The second pattern of cell death, **apoptosis**, is more conspicuous. It is caused by anti-viral cytotoxic T cells. Apoptotic hepatocytes shrink, become intensely eosinophilic, and have fragmented nuclei; effector T cells may still be present in the immediate vicinity. Apoptotic cells also are phagocytosed within hours by macrophages and hence might be difficult to find despite a brisk rate of hepatocyte injury. In severe cases of acute hepatitis (not depicted in Fig. 18–17*A*), confluent necrosis of hepatocytes may lead to **bridging necrosis** connecting portal-to-portal, central-to-central, or portal-to-central regions of adjacent lobules. Hepatocyte swelling and regeneration compress sinusoids, and the more or less radial array of the parenchyma is lost.

Inflammation is a characteristic and usually prominent feature of acute hepatitis. **Kupffer cells undergo hypertrophy and hyperplasia** and are often laden with lipofuscin pigment due to phagocytosis of hepatocellular debris. **The portal tracts are usually infiltrated with a mixture of inflammatory cells.** The inflammatory infiltrate may spill over into the adjacent parenchyma to cause necrosis of periportal hepatocytes; this **"interface hepatitis"** can occur in both acute and chronic hepatitis. Finally, bile duct epithelia may become reactive and even proliferate to form poorly defined ductular structures (ductular reaction), particularly in cases of HCV hepatitis.

Chronic Hepatitis. The histologic features of chronic hepatitis (Figs. 18–17*B* and 18–20) range from exceedingly mild to severe. In the mildest forms, significant inflammation is limited to portal tracts and consists of lymphocytes, macrophages, occasional plasma cells, and rare neutrophils or eosinophils. Liver architecture is usually well preserved, but smoldering hepatocyte necrosis throughout the lobule may occur in all forms of chronic hepatitis. Even in mild chronic hepatitis due to HCV infection, common findings are **lymphoid aggregates** and **bile duct damage** in the portal tracts and focally mild to moderate macrovesicular **steatosis**. In all forms of chronic hepatitis, continued **interface hepatitis** and **bridging necrosis** are harbingers of progressive liver damage. **The hallmark of irreversible liver damage is the deposition of fibrous tissue.** At first, only portal tracts exhibit increased fibrosis, but with time, **periportal** septal **fibrosis** occurs, followed by linking of fibrous septa between lobules (**bridging fibrosis**).

Continued loss of hepatocytes and fibrosis results in cirrhosis, with fibrous septae and hepatocyte regenerative nodules. This pattern of cirrhosis is characterized by irregularly sized nodules separated by variable but mostly broad scars (Fig. 18–21). Historically, this pattern of cirrhosis has been termed **postnecrotic cirrhosis**, but it should be noted that the term "postnecrotic cirrhosis" has been applied to all forms of cirrhosis in which the liver shows large, irregular-sized nodules with broad scars, regardless of etiology. Autoimmune hepatitis, hepatotoxins (carbon tetrachloride, mushroom poisoning), pharmaceutical drugs (acetaminophen, α-methyldopa), and even alcohol (discussed later) may give rise to a cirrhotic liver with irregular-sized large nodules. In some cases that come to autopsy, the inciting cause of the so-called postnecrotic cirrhosis cannot be determined at all ("cryptogenic cirrhosis"). In essence, the morphology of the end-stage cirrhotic liver is neither helpful in determining the basis of the liver injury, nor can it be easily related to any specific set of clinical circumstances.

The clinical course of viral hepatitis is unpredictable. Patients may experience spontaneous remission or may have indolent disease without progression for many years. Conversely, some patients have rapidly progressive disease and develop cirrhosis within a few years. The major causes of death are cirrhosis, with liver failure and hepatic encephalopathy or massive hematemesis from esophageal varices, and hepatocellular carcinoma in those with long-standing HBV (particularly neonatal) or HCV infection.

Fulminant Hepatitis

When hepatic insufficiency progresses from onset of symptoms to hepatic encephalopathy within 2 to 3 weeks, it is

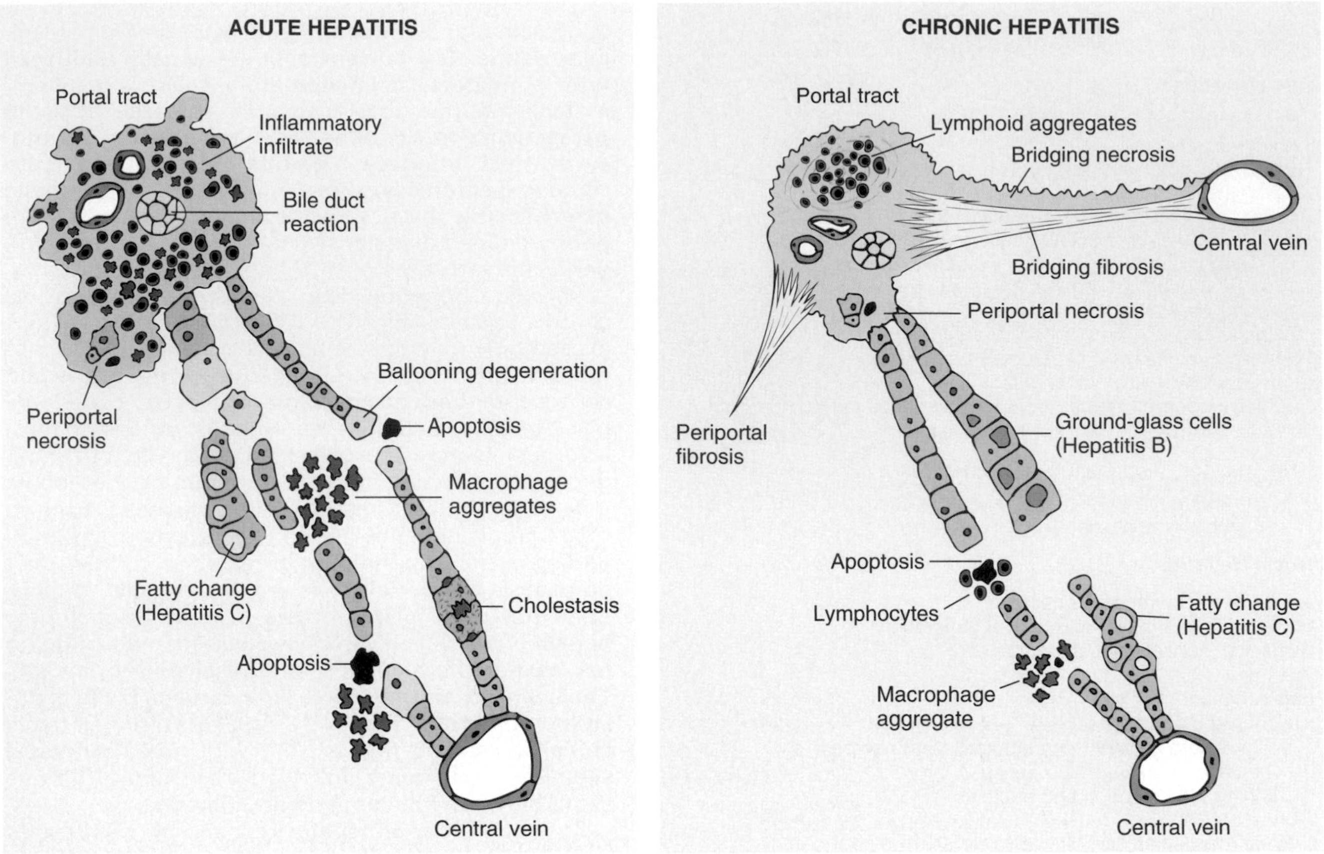

FIGURE 18–17 Diagrammatic representations of the morphologic features of acute and chronic hepatitis. Bridging necrosis (and fibrosis) is shown only for chronic hepatitis; bridging necrosis may also occur in acute hepatitis (not shown).

termed *fulminant hepatic failure.* A less rapid course, extending up to 3 months, is called *subfulminant failure.* Causes of fulminant hepatitis include:

- *In the United States, fulminant viral hepatitis is responsible for about 12% of cases of fulminant hepatic failure; almost all due to HAV or HBV.* Sometimes, reactivation of chronic hepatitis B or acute herpesvirus infection is the cause.
- Drug and chemical toxicity account for a substantial remainder (52%), acting either as direct hepatotoxins or via idiosyncratic inflammatory reactions. Principally implicated are acetaminophen (in suicidal doses), other drugs such as isoniazid, antidepressants (particularly monoamine oxidase inhibitors), halothane, and methyldopa.
- Miscellaneous other causes such as exposure to the mycotoxins of the mushroom *Amanita phalloides* account

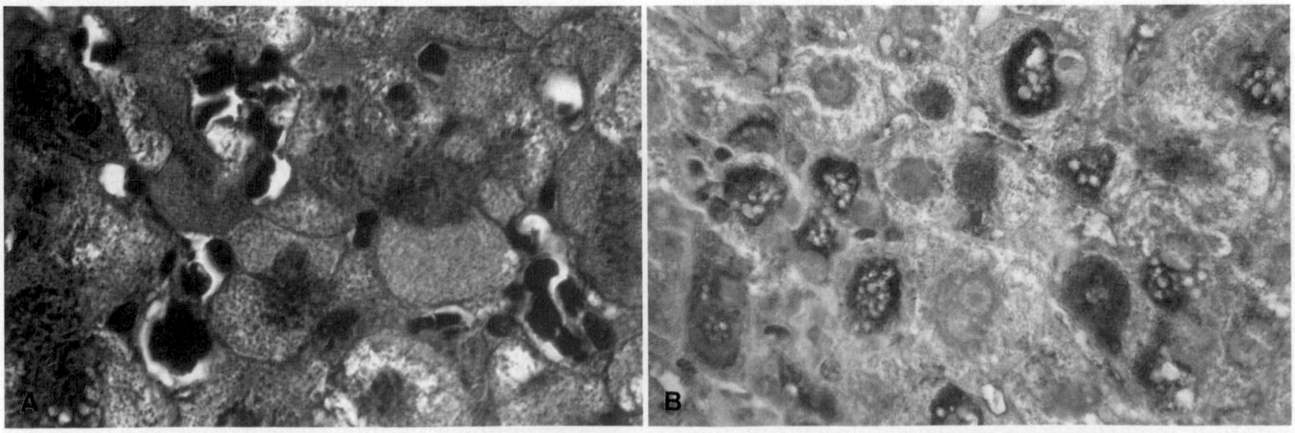

FIGURE 18–18 Hepatitis B viral infection. *A,* Liver parenchyma showing hepatocytes with diffuse granular cytoplasm, so-called ground glass hepatocytes. (H&E) *B,* Immunoperoxidase stain for HBsAg from the same case, showing cytoplasmic inclusions of viral particles.

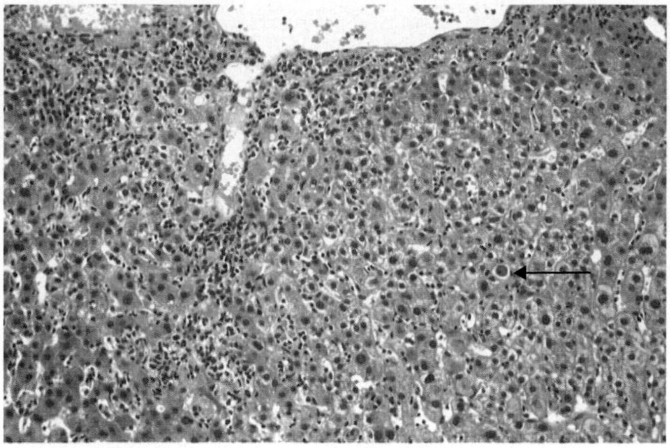

FIGURE 18–19 Acute viral hepatitis showing disruption of lobular architecture, inflammatory cells in the sinusoids, and hepatocellular apoptosis (*arrow*).

for the remainder. In about 18% of cases, the cause of fulminant hepatic failure is unknown.

Much rarer causes, but just as life-threatening, are ischemic hepatic necrosis, obstruction of the hepatic veins, massive malignant infiltration of the liver, Wilson disease, hyperthermia (heat stroke), and microvesicular steatosis syndromes, particularly acute fatty liver of pregnancy. The evolution of hepatic failure is extremely variable and is significantly influenced by the previous status of the liver and patient age (younger patients fare better).

Morphology. All causative agents produce essentially identical morphologic changes that vary with the severity of the necrotizing process. With all, the distribution of liver destruction is extremely capricious: **The entire liver may be involved or only random areas.** With massive loss of substance, the liver may shrink to as little as 500 to 700 gm. In so doing, it is transformed into a limp, red organ covered by a wrinkled, too-large capsule. On transection (Fig. 18–22*A*), necrotic areas have a muddy red, mushy appearance with blotchy bile staining. Microscopically, complete destruction of hepatocytes in contiguous lobules leaves only a collapsed reticulin framework and preserved portal tracts. There may be surprisingly little inflammatory reaction. Alternatively, with survival for several days, there is a massive influx of inflammatory cells to begin the phagocytic cleanup process (Fig. 18–22*B*).

Patient survival for more than a week also permits secondary regenerative activity of surviving hepatocytes and bile ducts. The bipotential proliferative compartment linking hepatocytes with the biliary tree—the canal of Hering—also is a major site of the regenerative response, giving rise to poorly formed ductular structures. A dormant stem cell population lying alongside the bile ductules and canals of Hering also proliferates, generating a population of small cells with a high nuclear:cytoplasmic ratio (so-called oval cells) interspersed with surviving hepatocytes (see Chapter 3).[25] Given sufficient time (i.e., survival of the patient beyond the first several weeks), the liver can recover completely with maturation of all proliferating cell populations into morphologically normal hepatocytes and bile duct epithelial cells.

With centrilobular zonal necrosis caused by direct hepatotoxins (acetaminophen, carbon tetrachloride) or ischemia, the parenchymal framework is preserved. Regeneration is directly from hepatocytes, and native liver architecture is restored in time. With more massive destruction of confluent lobules, regeneration is disorderly, yielding nodular masses of liver cells that produce a more irregular liver on healing.

Fibrous scarring may occur in patients with a protracted course of submassive or patchy necrosis, representing a route for developing so-called postnecrotic cirrhosis, as noted earlier.

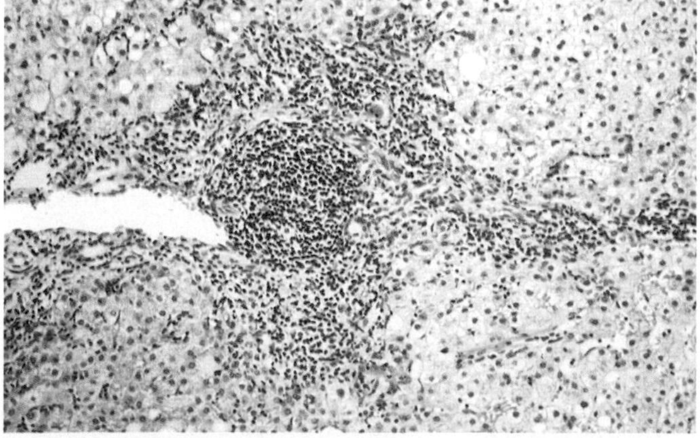

FIGURE 18–20 Chronic viral hepatitis due to hepatitis C virus, showing portal tract expansion with inflammatory cells and fibrous tissue and interface hepatitis with spillover of inflammation into the adjacent parenchyma. A lymphoid aggregate is present.

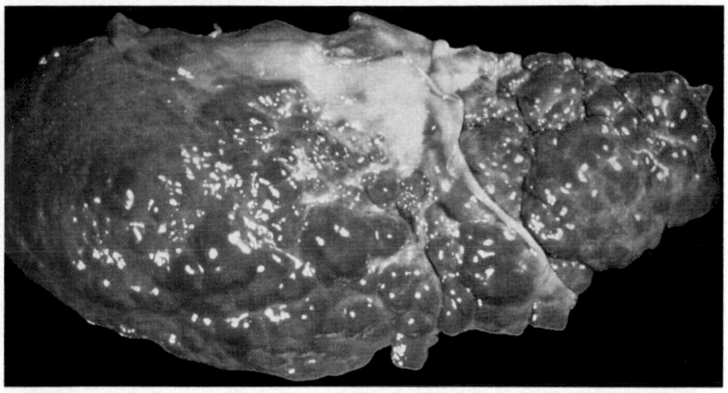

FIGURE 18–21 Cirrhosis resulting from chronic viral hepatitis. Note the broad scar and coarse nodular surface.

Fulminant hepatic failure may present as jaundice, encephalopathy, and fetor hepaticus, as described previously. Notably absent on physical examination are stigmata of chronic liver disease (e.g., gynecomastia, spider angiomas). Life-threatening extrahepatic complications include coagulopathy and bleeding, cardiovascular instability, renal failure, adult respiratory distress syndrome, electrolyte and acid-base

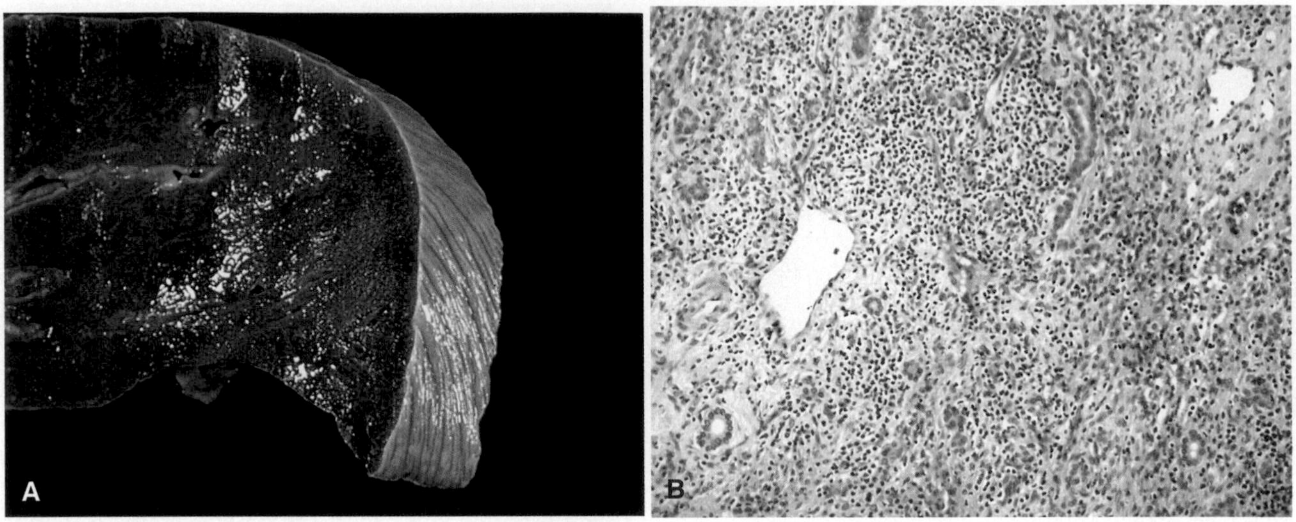

FIGURE 18–22 Massive necrosis. *A*, Cut section of liver. The liver is small (700 gm), bile-stained, and soft. The capsule is wrinkled. *B*, Microscopic section. Portal tracts and terminal hepatic veins are closer together than normal, owing to necrosis and collapse of the intervening parenchyma. The rudimentary ductal structures are the result of early ductular regeneration. An infiltrate of mononuclear inflammatory cells is present.

disturbances, and sepsis. The overall mortality rate ranges from 25% to 90% in the absence of liver transplantation.

BACTERIAL, PARASITIC, AND HELMINTHIC INFECTIONS

Extrahepatic bacterial infections, particularly sepsis, can induce mild hepatic inflammation and varying degrees of hepatocellular cholestasis. The latter effect is attributable to the effects of pro-inflammatory cytokines released by Kupffer cells and endothelial cells in response to circulating endotoxin. A number of bacteria can infect the liver directly, including *Staphylococcus aureus* in the setting of toxic shock syndrome, *Salmonella typhi* in the setting of typhoid fever, and secondary or tertiary syphilis. Alternatively, bacteria may proliferate in a biliary tree that is compromised by partial or complete obstruction. The bacterial composition reflects the gut flora, and the severe acute inflammatory response within the intrahepatic biliary tree is called *ascending cholangitis*.

Parasitic and helminthic infections are major causes of morbidity worldwide, and the liver is frequently involved. Diseases with liver involvement are discussed in Chapter 8; these diseases include malaria, schistosomiasis, strongyloidiasis, cryptosporidiosis, leishmaniasis, echinococcus, and infections by the liver flukes *Fasciola hepatica*, *Clonorchis sinensis*, and *Opisthorchis viverrini*.

A form of liver infection that deserves special mention is the *liver abscess*. In developing countries, liver abscesses are common. Most represent parasitic infections, for example, amebic, echinococcal, and (less commonly) other protozoal and helminthic organisms. In developed countries, liver abscesses are uncommon; the incidence of amebic infections is low, usually in immigrants from endemic regions. Most abscesses are pyogenic, representing a complication of a bacterial infection elsewhere. The organisms reach the liver by (1) the portal vein, (2) arterial supply, (3) ascending infection in the biliary tract (ascending cholangitis), (4) direct invasion of the liver from a nearby source, or (5) a penetrating injury. The majority of hepatic abscesses used to result from portal spread of intra-abdominal infections (e.g., appendicitis, diverticulitis, colitis). With improved management of these conditions, spread now occurs primarily through the biliary tree or the arterial supply in patients suffering from some form of immune deficiency (e.g., old age with debilitating disease, immunosuppression, or cancer chemotherapy with marrow failure). In these settings, abscesses may develop without a primary focus elsewhere.

Morphology. Liver abscesses may occur as solitary or multiple lesions, ranging in size from millimeters to massive lesions many centimeters in diameter. Bacteremic spread through the arterial or portal system tends to produce multiple small abscesses, whereas direct extension and trauma usually cause solitary large abscesses. Biliary abscesses, which are usually multiple, may contain purulent material from adjacent bile ducts. Gross and microscopic features are those to be seen in any abscess. The causative organism can occasionally be identified in the case of fungal or parasitic abscesses (Chapter 2). On rare occasion, abscesses located in the subdiaphragmatic region, particularly amebic, may burrow into the thoracic cavity to produce empyema or a lung abscess. Rupture of subcapsular liver abscesses has also led to peritonitis or localized peritoneal abscesses.

Liver abscesses are associated with fever and, in many instances, right upper quadrant pain and tender hepatomegaly. Jaundice may result from extrahepatic biliary obstruction. Although antibiotic therapy may control smaller lesions, surgical drainage is often necessary for the larger lesions. Because diagnosis is frequently delayed and because patients are often elderly and have serious coexistent disease, the mortality rate with large liver abscesses ranges from 30% to 90%. With early recognition and management, up to 80% of patients can survive.

Autoimmune Hepatitis

Autoimmune hepatitis is a chronic hepatitis with histologic features that may be indistinguishable from those of chronic viral hepatitis. This disease may run an indolent or severe course; salient features include the following:[26]

- Female predominance (78%), particularly in young and perimenopausal women. The annual incidence is highest among white Northern Europeans at 1.9 per 100,000, but all ethnic groups are susceptible.
- The absence of viral serologic markers
- Elevated serum IgG and γ-globulin levels (>1.5 times normal)
- High serum titers of autoantibodies in 80% of cases, including antinuclear (ANA), antismooth muscle (SMA), and/or antiliver/kidney microsomes (anti-LKM1) antibodies
- Negative antimitochondrial antibody (AMA)

Other forms of autoimmune disease are present in up to 60% of patients with autoimmune hepatitis, including rheumatoid arthritis, thyroiditis, Sjögren syndrome, and ulcerative colitis. Subgroups of autoimmune hepatitis have been noted, the most common, type 1, exhibiting ANA and/or SMA serum markers. The type 2 subgroup of younger patients exhibits antibodies to liver/kidney microsomes (anti-LKM1). Such subclassification is currently of uncertain value, since there are no distinctive etiologies or differences in treatment responses.

The entire histologic spectrum of chronic hepatitis may be seen in autoimmune hepatitis, marked by prominent inflammatory infiltrates of lymphocytes and plasma cells (prominent plasma cell infiltrates are generally not seen in other forms of chronic hepatitis). Clinical presentation is often similar to other forms of chronic hepatitis, and autoimmune hepatitis may even progress to cirrhosis without clinical diagnosis. However, symptomatic patients tend to exhibit substantial liver destruction and scarring at the time of diagnosis. Autoimmune hepatitis may present in an atypical fashion with symptoms primarily from involvement of other organ systems, hampering diagnostic efforts. An acute appearance of clinical illness is common (40%), and a fulminant presentation with onset of hepatic encephalopathy within 8 weeks of disease onset is possible. In a small subset of patients, autoimmune hepatitis by clinical criteria may exhibit histologic destruction of bile ducts ("autoimmune cholangitis"), making distinction from primary biliary cirrhosis or primary sclerosing cholangitis (discussed later) quite difficult.

In untreated severe disease, as many as 40% of patients die within 6 months of diagnosis, and cirrhosis develops in at least 40% of survivors. Patients with less severe disease fare better. This disease is responsive to immunosuppressive therapy, and liver transplantation offers excellent prospects for treatment of patients with severe disease.

Drug- and Toxin-Induced Liver Disease

As the major drug metabolizing and detoxifying organ in the body, the liver is subject to potential damage from an enormous array of pharmaceutical and environmental chemicals.[27] Injury may result (1) from direct toxicity, (2) via hepatic conversion of a xenobiotic to an active toxin, or (3) through immune mechanisms, usually by a drug or a metabolite acting as a hapten to convert a cellular protein into an immunogen.

Principles of drug and toxic injury are discussed in Chapter 9. Here it suffices to recall that drug reactions may be *predictable (intrinsic)* or *unpredictable (idiosyncratic)* ones. Predictable drug reactions can occur in anyone who accumulates a sufficient dose. Unpredictable reactions depend on idiosyncracies of the host, particularly the rate at which the host metabolizes the agent and the host's propensity to mount an immune response to the antigenic stimulus. Important examples include chlorpromazine, an agent that causes cholestasis in patients who are slow to metabolize it to an innocuous byproduct, and halothane, which can cause a fatal immune-mediated hepatitis in some patients who are exposed to this anesthetic on multiple occasions. Table 18–8 lists offending agents, grouped according to the type of morphologic injury. It should be noted that:

- The injury may be immediate or may take weeks to months to develop, presenting only after severe liver damage has developed.
- The injury may take the form of *hepatocyte necrosis*, *cholestasis*, or *insidious onset of liver dysfunction.*
- *Drug-induced chronic hepatitis is clinically and histologically indistinguishable from chronic viral hepatitis; hence, serologic markers of viral infection are critical for making the distinction.*
- In alcohol-induced liver disease (discussed later), the microvesicular and macrovesicular steatosis both arise from the same etiology: the production of excess reducing

TABLE 18–8 Drug- and Toxin-Induced Hepatic Injury

Hepatocellular Damage	Examples
Microvesicular fatty change	• Tetracycline, salicylates, yellow phosphorus, ethanol
Macrovesicular fatty change	• Ethanol, methotrexate, amiodarone
Centrilobular necrosis	• Bromobenzene, CCl_4, acetaminophen, halothane, rifampin
Diffuse or massive necrosis	• Halothane, isoniazid, acetaminophen, methyldopa, trinitrotoluene, *Amanita phalloides* (mushroom) toxin
Hepatitis, acute and chronic	• Methyldopa, isoniazid, nitrofurantoin, phenytoin, oxyphenisatin
Fibrosis-cirrhosis	• Ethanol, methotrexate, amiodarone, most drugs that cause chronic hepatitis
Granuloma formation	• Sulfonamides, methyldopa, quinidine, phenylbutazone, hydralazine, allopurinol
Cholestasis (with or without hepatocellular injury)	• Chlorpromazine, anabolic steroids, erythromycin estolate, oral contraceptives, organic arsenicals

equivalents (NADH + H^+) owing to the metabolism of ethanol. With some hepatotoxins, such as valproic acid, the microvesicular steatosis is the result of direct mitochondrial injury and impaired oxidative metabolism. This latter form of injury is an ominous harbinger of hepatic failure.

Among the agents listed in Table 18–8, hepatic injury is considered predictable from overdoses of acetaminophen (also called phenacetin or paracetamol) and exposure to *Amanita phalloides* toxin, carbon tetrachloride, and, to a certain extent, alcohol. However, individual genetic differences in the hepatic metabolism of xenobiotics through activating and detoxification pathways play a major role in individual susceptibility to "predictable" hepatotoxins. Many other xenobiotics, such as sulfonamides, α-methyldopa, and allopurinol, cause idiosyncratic reactions. *Reye syndrome*, a potentially fatal syndrome of mitochondrial dysfunction in liver, brain, and elsewhere, occurs predominantly in children who are given acetylsalicylic acid (aspirin) for the relief of virus-induced fever. This disease, which features extensive accumulation of fat droplets within hepatocytes (microvesicular steatosis), is exceedingly rare. A causal relationship with use of salicylates was never established, but a national campaign in the 1970s and 1980s warning against the use of aspirin in children with febrile illness might have served to break the Reye syndrome epidemic.

Drug-induced liver disease is usually followed by recovery upon removal of the drug. *Exposure to a toxin or therapeutic agent should always be included in the differential diagnosis of liver disease.*

ALCOHOLIC LIVER DISEASE

Excessive alcohol (ethanol) consumption is the leading cause of liver disease in most Western countries. These U.S. statistics attest to the magnitude of the problem:[4,28]

- Currently, 67% of the population 18 years of age or older drink alcohol. A subset of these individuals suffer serious health consequences associated with alcoholism.
- More than 14 million Americans meet criteria for alcohol abuse and/or dependence, corresponding to a prevalence of 7.4%. This is higher in men (11%) than in women (4%).
- Alcohol abuse causes 200,000 deaths annually, the fifth-leading cause of death, many related to automobile accidents. Approximately 40% of deaths from cirrhosis are attributed to alcohol-induced liver disease.
- Twenty-five percent to 30% of hospitalized patients have problems related to alcohol abuse, 1.5% as the first-listed diagnosis.

Chronic alcohol consumption has a variety of adverse effects, as was pointed out in Chapter 9. Of greatest impact, however, are the three distinctive, albeit overlapping, forms of liver disease: (1) hepatic steatosis, (2) alcoholic hepatitis, and (3) cirrhosis, collectively referred to as alcoholic liver disease. Because the first two conditions may develop independently, they do not necessarily represent a continuum of changes. The morphology of the three forms of alcoholic liver disease is presented first, because this facilitates consideration of their pathogenesis. The various forms of alcoholic liver disease are depicted in Figure 18–23.

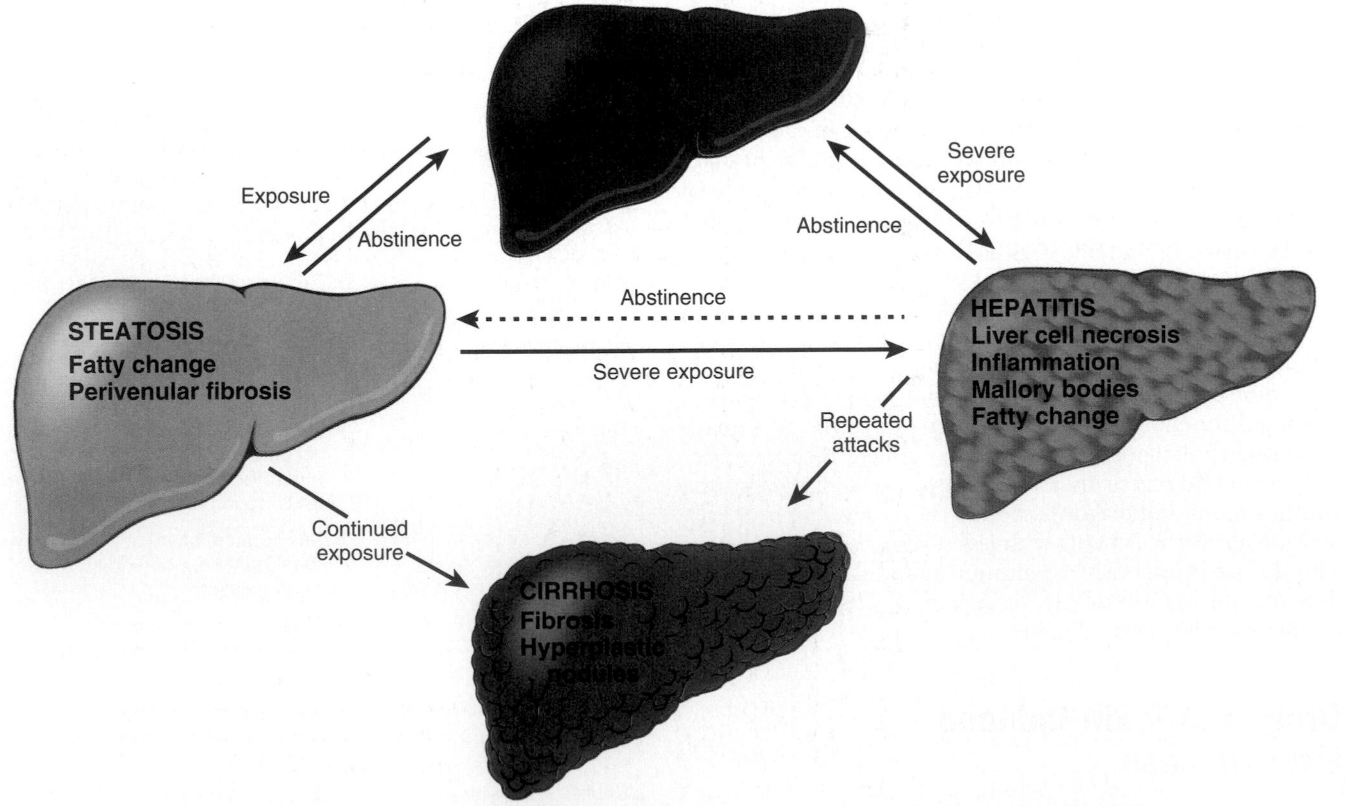

FIGURE 18–23 Alcoholic liver disease. The interrelationships among hepatic steatosis, hepatitis, and cirrhosis are shown, along with a depiction of key morphologic features at the morphologic level.

Morphology

Hepatic Steatosis (Fatty Liver). Following even moderate intake of alcohol, small (**microvesicular**) lipid droplets accumulate in hepatocytes. With chronic intake of alcohol, lipid accumulates to the point of creating large, clear **macrovesicular** globules, compressing and displacing the nucleus to the periphery of the hepatocyte. This transformation is initially centrilobular, but in severe cases, it may involve the entire lobule (Fig. 18–24). Macroscopically, the fatty liver of chronic alcoholism is a large (up to 4 to 6 kg), soft organ that is yellow and greasy. Although there is little or no fibrosis at the outset, with continued alcohol intake, fibrous tissue develops around the terminal hepatic veins and extends into the adjacent sinusoids. **The fatty change is completely reversible if there is abstention from further intake of alcohol.**

Alcoholic Hepatitis. Alcoholic hepatitis is characterized by the following:

- **Hepatocyte swelling and necrosis**: Single or scattered foci of cells undergo swelling (ballooning) and necrosis. The swelling results from the accumulation of fat and water, as well as proteins that normally are exported. In some cases, there is cholestasis in surviving hepatocytes and mild deposition of hemosiderin (iron) in hepatocytes and Kupffer cells.
- **Mallory bodies**: Scattered hepatocytes accumulate tangled skeins of cytokeratin intermediate filaments and other proteins, visible as eosinophilic cytoplasmic inclusions in degenerating hepatocytes (Fig. 18–25). These inclusions are a characteristic but not specific feature of alcoholic liver disease, as they also are seen in primary biliary cirrhosis, Wilson disease, chronic cholestatic syndromes, and hepatocellular tumors.
- **Neutrophilic reaction**: Neutrophils permeate the lobule and accumulate around degenerating hepatocytes, particularly those having Mallory bodies. Lymphocytes and macrophages also enter portal tracts and spill into the parenchyma.
- **Fibrosis**: Alcoholic hepatitis is almost always accompanied by prominent activation of sinusoidal stellate cells and portal tract fibroblasts, giving rise to fibrosis. This is most frequently in the form of sinusoidal and perivenular fibrosis that splits apart the parenchyma; occasionally, periportal fibrosis may predominate, particularly with repeated bouts of heavy alcohol intake.

Although steatotic hepatocytes are present, they are interspersed with the inflammatory cells and activated stellate cells. In macroscopic appearance, the liver is mottled red with bile-stained areas. Although the liver may be of normal or increased size, it often contains visible nodules and fibrosis, indicative of evolution to cirrhosis.

Alcoholic Cirrhosis. The final and irreversible form of alcoholic liver disease usually evolves slowly and insidiously. At first, the cirrhotic liver is yellow-tan, fatty, and enlarged, usually weighing over 2 kg. Over the span of years, it is transformed into a brown, shrunken, nonfatty organ, sometimes less than 1 kg in weight. Cirrhosis may develop more rapidly in the setting of alcoholic hepatitis, within 1 to 2 years. Initially, the developing fibrous septae are delicate and extend through sinusoids from central to portal

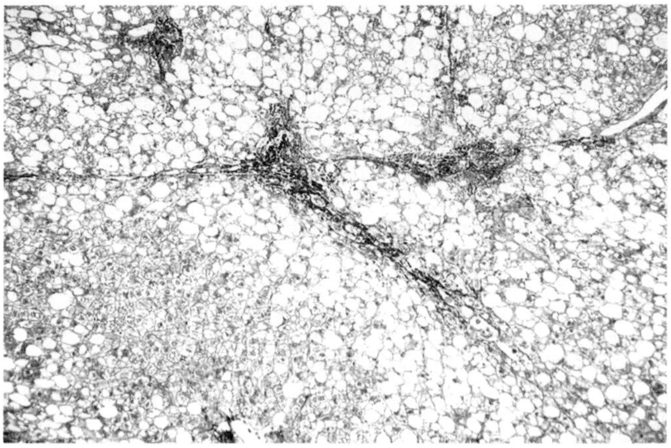

FIGURE 18–24 Alcoholic liver disease: macrovesicular steatosis, involving most regions of the hepatic lobule. The intracytoplasmic fat is seen as clear vacuoles. Some early fibrosis (stained blue) is present (Masson trichrome).

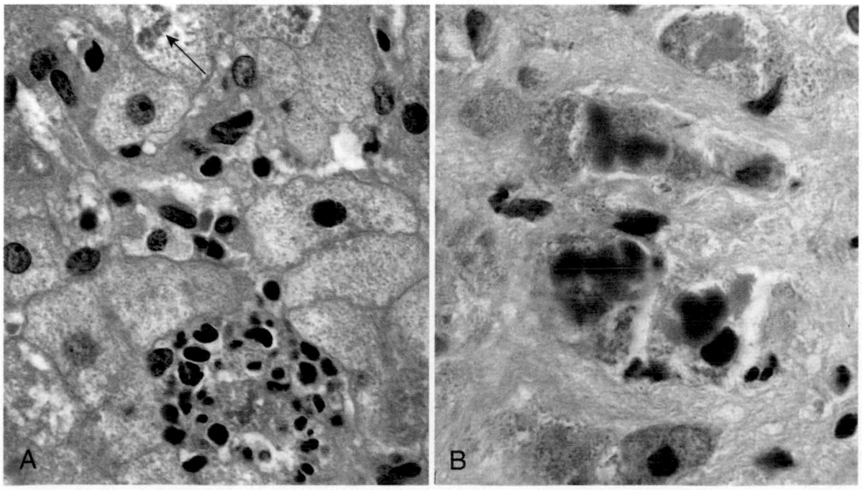

FIGURE 18–25 Alcoholic hepatitis. *A,* The cluster of inflammatory cells marks the site of a necrotic hepatocyte. A Mallory body is present in a second hepatocyte (*arrow*). *B,* Eosinophilic Mallory bodies are seen in hepatocytes, which are surrounded by fibrous tissue (H&E).

regions as well as from portal tract to portal tract. Regenerative activity of entrapped parenchymal hepatocytes generates fairly uniformly sized "micronodules." With time, the nodularity becomes more prominent; scattered larger nodules create a "hobnail" appearance on the surface of the liver (Fig. 18–26*A*). As fibrous septae dissect and surround nodules, the liver becomes more fibrotic, loses fat, and shrinks progressively in size. Parenchymal islands are engulfed by ever wider bands of fibrous tissue, and the liver is converted into a mixed micronodular and macronodular pattern (Fig. 18–26*B*). Ischemic necrosis and fibrous obliteration of nodules eventually create broad expanses of tough, pale scar tissue ("Laennec cirrhosis"). Bile stasis often develops; Mallory bodies are only rarely evident at this stage. Thus, **end-stage alcoholic cirrhosis comes to resemble, both macroscopically and microscopically, the cirrhosis developing from viral hepatitis and other causes.**

Pathogenesis. Short-term ingestion of up to 80 gm of alcohol (eight beers or 7 ounces of 80-proof liquor) over one to several days generally produces mild, reversible hepatic changes, such as fatty liver. Daily intake of 80 gm or more of ethanol generates significant risk for severe hepatic injury, and daily ingestion of 160 gm or more for 10 to 20 years is associated more consistently with severe injury. *Only 10% to 15% of alcoholics, however, develop cirrhosis.* For reasons that might relate to decreased gastric metabolism of ethanol and differences in body mass, women appear to be more susceptible to hepatic injury than men are. Individual, possibly genetic, susceptibility must exist, current attention being given to genetic polymorphisms in detoxifying enzymes and cytokine promoters. However, no reliable genetic markers of susceptibility have been identified yet. In addition, the relationship between hepatic steatosis and alcoholic hepatitis as precursors to cirrhosis, both causally and temporally, is not yet clear. Cirrhosis may develop without antecedent evidence of steatosis or alcoholic hepatitis. *In the absence of a clear understanding of the pathogenetic factors influencing liver damage, no "safe" upper limit for alcohol consumption can be proposed* (despite the current popularity of red wines for amelioration of coronary vascular disease).

The pharmacokinetics and metabolism of alcohol were described in Chapter 9. Pertinent to our discussion are the detrimental effects of alcohol and its byproducts on hepatocellular function:[29]

- Hepatocellular steatosis results from (1) shunting of normal substrates away from catabolism and toward lipid biosynthesis, owing to generation of excess reduced nicotinamide-adenine dinucleotide (NADH + H^+) by the two major enzymes of alcohol metabolism: alcohol dehydrogenase and acetaldehyde dehydrogenase; (2) impaired assembly and secretion of lipoproteins; and (3) increased peripheral catabolism of fat.
- Alcohol-induced impaired hepatic metabolism of methionine leads to decreased intrahepatic glutathione (GSH) levels, thereby sensitizing the liver to oxidative injury.
- Induction of cytochromes P-450, especially CYP2E1, increases catabolism of alcohol in the endoplasmic reticulum, and increases the conversion of other drugs (e.g., acetaminophen) to toxic metabolites. Cytochrome P-450 metabolism produces reactive oxygen species that react with cellular proteins, damage membranes, and alter hepatocellular function.
- As a solute at millimolar concentrations, alcohol directly affects microtubular and mitochondrial function and membrane fluidity.
- Acetaldehyde (the major intermediate metabolite of alcohol en route to acetate production) induces lipid peroxidation and acetaldehyde-protein adduct formation, further disrupting cytoskeletal and membrane function.
- Alcohol-induced and acetaldehyde-induced changes in hepatocellular proteins create new epitopes to which the immune system reacts, producing inflammation and immune-mediated hepatocellular injury.

In addition, alcohol is food and can become a major caloric source in the diet of an alcoholic, displacing other nutrients

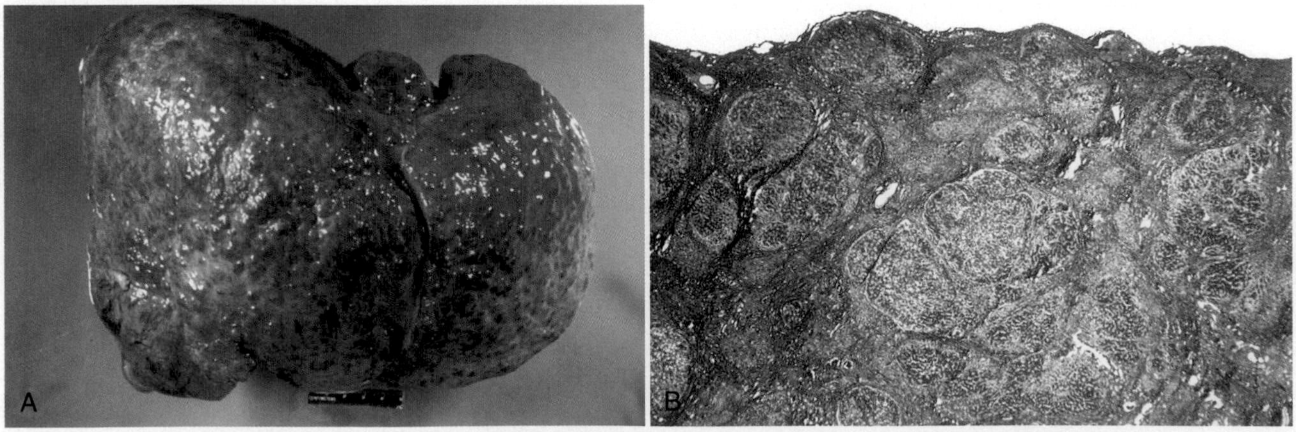

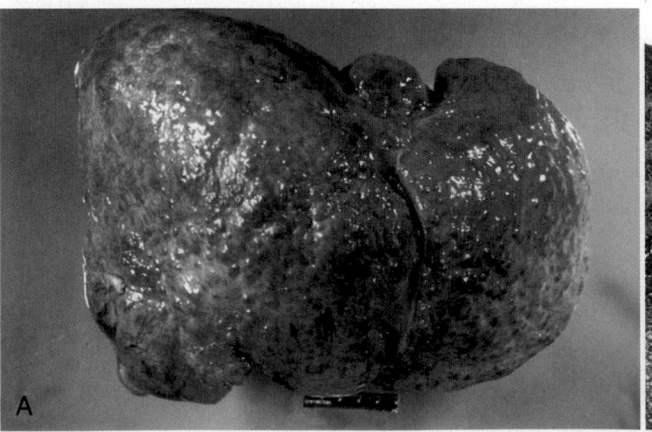

FIGURE 18–26 Alcoholic cirrhosis. *A*, The characteristic diffuse nodularity of the surface reflects the interplay between nodular regeneration and scarring. The greenish tint of some nodules is due to bile stasis. A hepatocellular carcinoma is present as a budding mass at the lower edge of the right lobe (lower left of figure). *B*, The microscopic view shows nodules of varying sizes entrapped in blue-staining fibrous tissue. The liver capsule is at the top (Masson trichrome).

and leading to malnutrition and deficiencies of vitamins (such as vitamin B_{12}). This is compounded by impaired digestive function, primarily related to chronic gastric and intestinal mucosal damage, and pancreatitis.

Interestingly, alcohol induces release of bacterial endotoxin into the portal circulation from the gut, which in itself activates inflammatory events within the liver. Alcohol also induces release of endothelins from sinusoidal endothelial cells. Endothelins are potent vasoconstrictors, and they induce the myofibroblast-like perisinusoidal stellate cells to contract, decreasing hepatic sinusoidal perfusion and causing regional hypoxia.

Alcoholic liver disease, thus, is a chronic disorder featuring steatosis, hepatitis, progressive fibrosis, cirrhosis, and marked derangement of vascular perfusion. In essence, alcoholic liver disease can be regarded as a maladaptive state in which cells in the liver respond in an increasingly pathologic manner to a stimulus (alcohol) that originally was only marginally harmful.

Clinical Features. *Hepatic steatosis* may become evident as hepatomegaly with mild elevation of serum bilirubin and alkaline phosphatase levels. Alternatively, there might be no clinical or biochemical evidence of liver disease. Severe hepatic dysfunction is unusual. Alcohol withdrawal and the provision of an adequate diet are sufficient treatment.

In contrast, *alcoholic hepatitis* tends to appear relatively acutely, usually following a bout of heavy drinking. Symptoms and laboratory manifestations may be minimal or those of fulminant hepatic failure. Between these two extremes are the nonspecific symptoms of malaise, anorexia, weight loss, upper abdominal discomfort, tender hepatomegaly, and the laboratory findings of hyperbilirubinemia, elevated alkaline phosphatase, and often, a neutrophilic leukocytosis. An acute cholestatic syndrome may appear, resembling large bile duct obstruction. The outlook is unpredictable; each bout of hepatitis incurs about a 10% to 20% risk of death. With repeated bouts, cirrhosis appears in about one third of patients within a few years. Alcoholic hepatitis also may be superimposed on established cirrhosis. With proper nutrition and total cessation of alcohol consumption, the alcoholic hepatitis may clear slowly. However, in some patients, the hepatitis persists despite abstinence and progresses to cirrhosis.

The manifestations of *alcoholic cirrhosis* are similar to those of other forms of cirrhosis, presented earlier. Commonly, the first signs of cirrhosis relate to complications of portal hypertension, including life-threatening variceal hemorrhage. Alternatively, malaise, weakness, weight loss, and loss of appetite precede the appearance of jaundice, ascites, and peripheral edema, the latter due to impaired synthesis of albumin. The stigmata of cirrhosis (e.g., grossly distended abdomen, wasted extremities, caput medusae) may be dramatically evident. Laboratory findings reflect the developing hepatic compromise, with elevated serum aminotransferase, hyperbilirubinemia, variable elevation of serum alkaline phosphatase, hypoproteinemia (globulins, albumin, and clotting factors), and anemia. In some instances, liver biopsy may be indicated, since experience teaches that in about 10% to 20% of cases of presumed alcoholic cirrhosis, another disease process is found on biopsy. Finally, cirrhosis may be clinically silent, discovered only at autopsy or when stress such as infection or trauma tips the balance toward hepatic insufficiency.

The long-term outlook for alcoholics with liver disease is variable. Five-year survival approaches 90% in abstainers who are free of jaundice, ascites, or hematemesis; it drops to 50% to 60% in those who continue to imbibe. In the end-stage alcoholic, the proximate causes of death are (1) hepatic coma, (2) a massive gastrointestinal hemorrhage, (3) an intercurrent infection (to which these patients are predisposed), (4) hepatorenal syndrome following a bout of alcoholic hepatitis, and (5) hepatocellular carcinoma in 3% to 6% of cases.

Metabolic Liver Disease

A distinct group of liver diseases is attributable to disorders of metabolism. These range from acquired disorders of metabolism to inherited disorders, of which hemochromatosis, Wilson disease, and α_1-antitrypsin deficiency are most prominent. We must also consider here neonatal hepatitis, a broad disease category encompassing rare inherited diseases and neonatal infections.

NONALCOHOLIC FATTY LIVER DISEASE AND STEATOHEPATITIS

Nonalcoholic fatty liver disease (NAFL) is a condition that resembles alcohol-induced liver disease but occurs in patients who are not heavy drinkers.[30] Men and women are equally affected, and there are strong associations with obesity, dyslipidemia, hyperinsulinemia and insulin resistance, and overt type 2 diabetes. Although NAFL is a diagnosis of exclusion (especially of excessive alcohol intake), it is the most likely explanation for the elevated serum aminotransferases and/or gamma glutamyl transpeptidase values documented in 24% of the general U.S. adult population. It is estimated that 31% of men and 16% of women have NAFL, representing approximately 31 million Americans.

Morphology. This condition features liver biopsy findings of *steatosis.* Large and small vesicles of fat, predominantly triglycerides, accumulate within hepatocytes. At the most clinically benign end of the spectrum, there is no appreciable hepatic inflammation, hepatocyte death, or scarring (despite persistent elevation of serum liver enzymes). **Steatohepatitis** (also called **nonalcoholic steatohepatitis,** or *NASH*) is an intermediate form of liver damage. Liver biopsy shows steatosis, multifocal parenchymal inflammation, Mallory hyaline, hepatocyte death (both ballooning degeneration and apoptosis), and sinusoidal fibrosis. **Cirrhosis** may occur, presumably the result of years of subclinical progression of the inflammatory and fibrotic processes.

Patients are largely asymptomatic, with abnormalities only in biochemical laboratory tests. Hence, there is debate as to whether NAFL actually represents a well-defined disease. With increasing recognition of this condition, however, NAFL is thought to account for up to 70% of the cases of chronic hepatitis of "unknown" cause. Studies also suggest that 10% to 30% of patients with NAFL eventually develop cirrhosis.

Hence, NAFL is now considered to be the most common cause of "cryptogenic" cirrhosis, with its attendant morbidity and mortality. There is also growing evidence that NAFL contributes to the progression of other liver diseases such as hepatitis C viral infection. The incidence of hepatocellular carcinoma in NAFL is unknown at this time.

The epidemic of obesity in the United States heightens concern that NAFL will increase in prevalence. Lifestyle modifications, especially diet and exercise, are a starting point for treatment. Additional recommendations for treating this condition are likely to be forthcoming in the near future.

HEMOCHROMATOSIS

Hemochromatosis is characterized by the excessive accumulation of body iron, most of which is deposited in parenchymal organs such as the liver and pancreas. Because humans do not have a major excretory pathway for iron, hemochromatosis results either from a genetic defect causing excessive iron absorption or as a consequence of parenteral administration of iron (usually in the form of transfusions). *Hereditary hemochromatosis* is a homozygous-recessive inherited disorder. Acquired forms of hemochromatosis with known sources of excess iron are called *secondary hemochromatosis* (Table 18–9).

As was discussed in Chapter 13, the total body iron pool ranges from 2 to 6 gm in normal adults; about 0.5 gm is stored in the liver, 98% of which is in hepatocytes. In hereditary hemochromatosis, total iron accumulation may exceed 50 gm, over one third of which accumulates in the liver. The following features characterize this disease:[31]

- Fully developed cases exhibit (1) *micronodular cirrhosis* in all patients; (2) *diabetes mellitus* in 75% to 80% of patients; and (3) *skin pigmentation* in 75% to 80% of patients.
- Iron accumulation is lifelong; symptoms usually first appear in the fifth to sixth decades of life.
- The hemochromatosis gene is located on the short arm of chromosome 6 at 6p21.3, close to the *HLA* gene locus. This gene, called *HFE*, encodes an HLA class I–like molecule that regulates intestinal absorption of dietary iron.[32] The most common *HFE* mutation is a cysteine-to-tyrosine substitution at amino acid 282 (called C282Y), which inactivates this 343-amino-acid protein. This is due to a single G → A transition at nucleotide 845 (G845A), present in 70% to 100% of the diagnosed patients with hereditary hemochromatosis. The *HFE* gene is in linkage disequilibrium with HLA-A3, thus accounting for the association of this haplotype with hereditary hemochromatosis.
- Males predominate (5 to 7:1) with slightly earlier clinical presentation, partly because physiologic iron loss (menstruation, pregnancy) delays iron accumulation in women.

TABLE 18–9 Classification of Iron Overload

I. Hereditary Hemochromatosis	
II. Secondary Hemochromatosis	
A. Parenteral iron overload	
Transfusions	
Long-term hemodialysis	
Aplastic anemia	
Sickle cell disease	
Myelodysplastic syndromes	
Leukemias	
Iron-dextran injections	
B. Ineffective erythropoiesis with increased erythroid activity	
β-Thalassemia	
Sideroblastic anemia	
Pyruvate kinase deficiency	
C. Increased oral intake of iron	
African iron overload (Bantu siderosis)	
D. Congenital atransferrinemia	
E. Chronic liver disease	
Chronic alcoholic liver disease	
Porphyria cutanea tarda	

In white populations of northern European extraction, the frequency of the C282Y mutation is estimated at 6.4% to 9.5%.[4] The frequency of homozygosity is 0.45% (1 of every 220 persons), and that for heterozygosity is 11% (1 of every 9 persons), making hereditary hemochromatosis one of the most common genetic disorders in humans. However, the penetrance of this disorder is only about 20% in patients with the homozygous C282Y mutation, so the genetic condition does not lead to disease in all individuals.

Pathogenesis. It may be recalled that the total body content of iron is tightly regulated, as the limited daily losses of iron are matched by gastrointestinal absorption. *In hereditary hemochromatosis, regulation of intestinal absorption of dietary iron is lost, leading to net iron accumulation of 0.5 to 1.0 gm/year.* The disease manifests itself typically after 20 gm of storage iron have accumulated.

The critical site for HFE expression appears to be the basolateral surface of the small intestinal crypt epithelial cell, where it is prominently expressed. According to the current hypothesis (Fig. 18–27),[32,33] HFE complexes with the transferrin receptor, TfR, enabling the binding of plasma transferrin and its bound iron. The TfR-Tf-iron complex is endocytosed into the crypt enterocyte; acidification of the endosome releases iron into the regulatory iron pool of the crypt cell. This is a sensing mechanism for the systemic iron balance, as increased levels of circulating iron bound to transferrin will lead to an increased iron regulatory pool in enterocytes. This pool "sets" the level of expression of apical iron uptake systems. *Crypt cells with mutant HFE lack the facilitating effect on TfR-dependent iron uptake, thus decreasing the regulatory iron pool in the crypt cell.* As small intestinal crypt cells are the progenitors of villus absorptive cells, these cells are preprogrammed to absorb dietary iron regardless of the systemic iron overload.

Excessive iron appears to be directly toxic to host tissues, by the following mechanisms: (1) lipid peroxidation via iron-catalyzed free radical reactions, (2) stimulation of collagen formation, and (3) interactions of reactive oxygen species and of iron itself with DNA, leading to lethal injury or predisposition to hepatocellular carcinoma. Whatever the actions of iron, they are reversible in cells that are not fatally injured, and removal of excess iron during therapy promotes recovery of tissue function.

The most common causes of secondary hemochromatosis are the hemolytic anemias associated with ineffective erythropoiesis, discussed in Chapter 13. In these disorders, the excess iron may result not only from transfusions, but also from increased absorption. Transfusions alone, as in aplastic

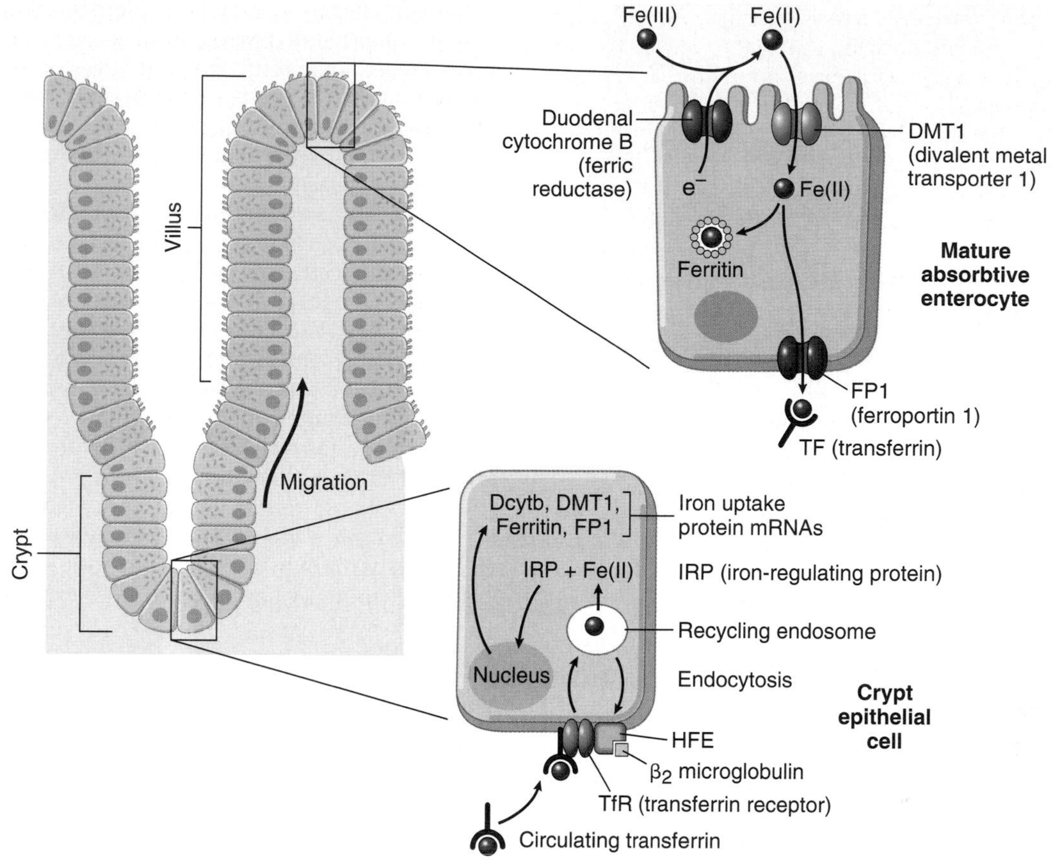

FIGURE 18–27 Schematic diagram of HFE function in the intestine. The *crypt epithelial cell* expresses HFE on its basolateral surface; complexing of HFE with β_2-microglobulin is required for its expression on the cell surface. HFE-β_2-microglobulin complexes with the transferrin receptor (TfR) to bind circulating transferrin (Tf). Endocytosis ensues; on acidification of the recycling endosome, transferrin-bound iron (Fe(II)) is released and enters into the cytoplasm. High levels of cytoplasmic iron downregulate levels of the iron-regulatory proteins (IRP), a family of proteins with potent effects on nuclear transcription. With low levels of cytoplasmic iron, the IRP content of the cell remains high. IRPs upregulate nuclear transcription of the genes for several proteins required for intestinal absorption of dietary iron: Dcytb (duodenal cytochrome B), DMT1 (divalent metal transporter 1), ferritin (a cytoplasmic iron-binding protein), and FP1 (ferroportin 1). *A mutation in HFE prevents "sensing" of circulating iron levels by the crypt epithelial cell, leading to unregulated expression of these four proteins.* The crypt epithelial cell is the precursor cell of the *mature absorptive enterocyte* on the tip of the villus, through migration up the villus axis. On the apical membrane of the absorptive enterocyte, Dcytb reduces dietary ferric iron (Fe(III)) to ferrous iron (Fe(II)). Fe(II) is then taken up by DMT1 into the enterocyte. Iron can be bound to ferritin (and hence sloughed back into the gut lumen) or transported across the basolateral plasma membrane by FP1 for binding to transferrin and entry into the systemic circulation. *In the patient with mutant HFE, the inability to downregulate expression of these four proteins leads to lifelong excessive absorption of dietary iron.*

anemias, lead to systemic hemosiderosis in which parenchymal organ injury tends to occur only in extreme cases. *Alcoholic cirrhosis* is often associated with a modest increase in stainable iron within liver cells. However, this represents alcohol-induced redistribution of iron, since total body iron is not significantly increased. A rather unusual form of iron overload resembling hereditary hemochromatosis occurs in sub-Saharan Africa, the result of ingesting large quantities of alcoholic beverages fermented in iron utensils (Bantu siderosis). Home brewing in steel drums continues to this day, and a genetic susceptibility has been identified in this population.[34]

Morphology. The morphologic changes in hereditary hemochromatosis are characterized principally by (1) the **deposition of hemosiderin** in the following organs (in decreasing order of severity): liver, pancreas, myocardium, pituitary gland, adrenal gland, thyroid and parathyroid glands, joints, and skin (detected by the Prussian blue histologic reaction or by atomic absorption analysis of tissue); (2) **cirrhosis;** (3) **pancreatic fibrosis.** In the liver, iron becomes evident first as golden-yellow hemosiderin granules in the cytoplasm of periportal hepatocytes, which stain blue with the Prussian blue stain (Fig. 18–28). With increasing iron load, there is progressive involvement of the rest of the lobule, along with bile duct epithelium and Kupffer cell pigmentation. Iron is a direct hepatotoxin, and inflammation is characteristically absent. At this stage, the liver is typically slightly larger than normal, dense, and chocolate brown. Fibrous septa develop slowly, leading ultimately to a micronodular pattern of cirrhosis in an intensely pigmented liver.

Biochemical determination of hepatic iron concentration in unfixed tissue is the standard for

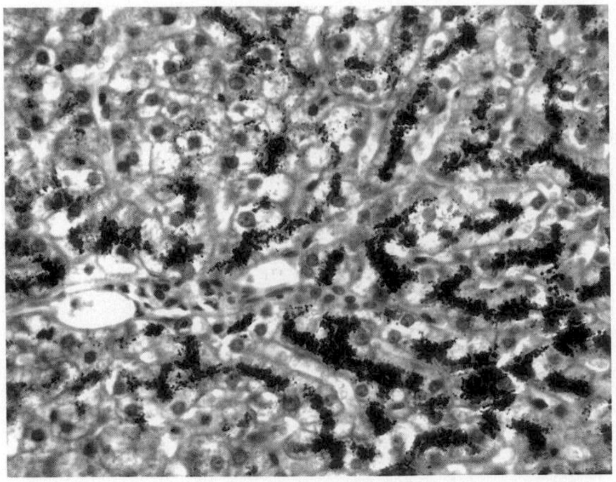

FIGURE 18–28 Hereditary hemochromatosis. Hepatocellular iron deposition is blue in this Prussian blue–stained section of an early stage of the disease, in which parenchymal architecture is normal.

quantitating hepatic iron content. In normal individuals, the iron content of unfixed liver tissue is less than 1000 μg per gram dry weight of liver. Adult patients with hereditary hemochromatosis exhibit over 10,000 μg iron per gram dry weight; hepatic iron concentrations in excess of 22,000 μg per gram dry weight are associated with the development of fibrosis and cirrhosis.

The **pancreas** becomes intensely pigmented, has diffuse interstitial fibrosis, and may exhibit some parenchymal atrophy. Hemosiderin is found in both the acinar and the islet cells, and sometimes in the interstitial fibrous stroma. The **heart** is often enlarged and has hemosiderin granules within the myocardial fibers, producing a striking brown coloration to the myocardium. A delicate interstitial fibrosis may appear. Although **skin** pigmentation is partially attributable to hemosiderin deposition in dermal macrophages and fibroblasts, most of the pigmentation results from increased epidermal melanin production. The combination of these pigments imparts a characteristic slate-gray color to the skin. With hemosiderin deposition in the **joint synovial linings**, an acute synovitis may develop. Excessive deposition of calcium pyrophosphate damages the articular cartilage, producing a disabling polyarthritis referred to as **pseudo-gout**. The **testes** may be small and atrophic but are not usually significantly pigmented. It is thought that the atrophy is secondary to a derangement in the hypothalamic-pituitary axis.

Clinical Features. Hereditary hemochromatosis is more often a disease of males and rarely becomes evident before age 40. The principal manifestations include hepatomegaly, abdominal pain, skin pigmentation (particularly in sun-exposed areas), deranged glucose homeostasis or frank diabetes mellitus due to destruction of pancreatic islets, cardiac dysfunction (arrhythmias, cardiomyopathy), and atypical arthritis. In some patients, the presenting complaint is hypogonadism (e.g., amenorrhea in the female and impotence and loss of libido in the male). The classic triad of pigment cirrhosis with hepatomegaly, skin pigmentation, and diabetes mellitus might not develop until late in the course of the disease. Death may result from cirrhosis or cardiac disease. A significant cause of death is hepatocellular carcinoma; the risk is 200-fold greater than in the general population, and treatment for iron overload does not remove the risk for this aggressive neoplasm.

Fortunately, hereditary hemochromatosis can be diagnosed long before irreversible tissue damage has occurred. Screening involves demonstration of very high levels of serum iron and ferritin, exclusion of secondary causes of iron overload, and liver biopsy if indicated. *Screening of family members of probands is important.* Heterozygotes for hereditary hemochromatosis also accumulate excessive iron, but not to the degree required to cause significant tissue damage. Homozygotes may be identified before onset of clinical disease. *The identification of the HFE gene opens the way for genetic screening, limited by the heterogeneity of mutations in this disease.* Patients with hereditary hemochromatosis diagnosed in the subclinical, precirrhotic stage and treated by regular phlebotomy have a normal life expectancy.

WILSON DISEASE

This autosomal-recessive disorder is marked by *the accumulation of toxic levels of copper in many tissues and organs, principally the liver, brain and eye.* Normally, 40% to 60% of daily ingested copper (2 to 5 mg) is absorbed in the stomach and duodenum and transported to the liver loosely complexed with albumin. Free copper dissociates and is taken up into hepatocytes, where it is incorporated into an α_2-globulin synthesized in the endoplasmic reticulum to form ceruloplasmin (a copper-containing metallothionein) and resecreted into plasma. Ceruloplasmin accounts for 90% to 95% of plasma copper, although its biologic role is unknown, since the six to seven atoms of copper in each protein molecule are not readily exchangeable. Circulating ceruloplasmin is desialylated as part of normal plasma protein aging; desialylated ceruloplasmin is endocytosed by the liver, degraded within lysosomes, and its copper is excreted into bile. This degradation/excretion pathway is the primary route for copper elimination. Estimated total body copper is only 50 to 150 mg.

The gene for Wilson disease, designated *ATP7B*, is on chromosome 13 and encodes a 7.5-kB transcript for a transmembrane copper-transporting ATPase, located on the hepatocyte canalicular membrane.[35] Over 30 mutations in this gene have been identified. *The overwhelming majority of patients are compound heterozygotes containing different mutations of the Wilson disease gene on each allele.* The overall frequency of mutated alleles is 1:200, engendering a prevalence of the disease of approximately 1:30,000 to 1:50,000. Defective biliary excretion leads to copper accumulation in the liver in excess of the metallothionein-binding capacity, causing toxic liver injury through copper-catalyzed formation of reactive oxygen species. Although there is a latent period of variable duration for the disease, once the hepatic capacity for incorporating copper into ceruloplasmin is exceeded, there may be sudden onset of critical illness. It is usually by 5 years of age that non-ceruloplasmin–bound copper spills over from the liver into the circulation, causing hemolysis and pathologic changes at other sites such as the brain, corneas, kidneys, bones, joints, and parathyroids. Concomitantly, urinary excretion of copper markedly increases from its normal miniscule levels.

Morphology. The liver often bears the brunt of injury in Wilson disease, with hepatic changes ranging from relatively minor to massive damage. **Fatty change** may be mild to moderate, with vacuolated nuclei (glycogen or water) and occasionally, focal hepatocyte necrosis. An **acute hepatitis** can exhibit features mimicking acute viral hepatitis, except possibly for the accompanying fatty change. The **chronic hepatitis** of Wilson disease exhibits moderate to severe inflammation and hepatocyte necrosis, with the particular features of macrovesicular steatosis, vacuolated hepatocellular nuclei, and Mallory bodies. With progression of chronic hepatitis, **cirrhosis** will develop. **Massive liver necrosis** is a rare manifestation that is indistinguishable from that caused by viruses or drugs. Excess copper deposition can often be demonstrated by special stains (rhodanine stain for copper, orcein stain for copper-associated protein). Because copper also accumulates in chronic obstructive cholestasis and because histology cannot reliably distinguish Wilson disease from viral- and drug-induced hepatitis (and vice versa), demonstration of hepatic copper content in excess of 250 μg per gram dry weight is most helpful for making a diagnosis.

In the **brain**, toxic injury primarily affects the basal ganglia, particularly the putamen, which demonstrates atrophy and even cavitation. Nearly all patients with neurologic involvement develop **eye lesions** called **Kayser-Fleischer rings:** green to brown deposits of copper in Desçemet's membrane in the limbus of the cornea.

Clinical Features. The age at onset and the clinical presentation of Wilson disease are extremely variable, but the disorder rarely manifests before 6 years of age. The most common presentation is acute or chronic liver disease. Neuropsychiatric manifestations, including mild behavioral changes, frank psychosis, or a Parkinson disease–like syndrome, are the initial features in most of the remaining cases. The biochemical diagnosis of Wilson disease is based on *a decrease in serum ceruloplasmin, an increase in hepatic copper content, and increased urinary excretion of copper.* Serum copper levels are of no diagnostic value, since they may be low, normal, or elevated, depending on the stage of evolution of the disease. Demonstration of Kayser-Fleischer rings further favors the diagnosis. Early recognition and long-term copper chelation therapy (as with D-penicillamine) have dramatically altered the usual progressive downhill course. Fulminant hepatitis or unmanageable cirrhosis necessitate liver transplantation.

α_1-ANTITRYPSIN DEFICIENCY

α_1-Antitrypsin deficiency is an autosomal-recessive disorder marked by abnormally low serum levels of this important protease inhibitor. The major function of this protein is the inhibition of proteases, particularly elastase, cathepsin G, and proteinase 3, which are normally released from neutrophils at sites of inflammation. α_1-antitrypsin deficiency leads to the development of pulmonary emphysema, because a relative lack of this protein permits tissue-destructive enzymes to run amok (discussed in Chapter 15). It also causes liver disease, mainly in neonates and young adults, by a distinct mechanism.

α_1-Antitrypsin is a small, 394-amino-acid plasma glycoprotein synthesized predominantly by hepatocytes. The gene, located on human chromosome 14, is very polymorphic, and at least 75 α_1-antitrypsin forms have been identified, denoted alphabetically by their relative migration on an isoelectric gel. The general notation is "Pi" for "protease inhibitor" and an alphabetic letter for the position on the gel; two letters denote the genotype of the two alleles. The most common genotype is PiMM, occurring in 90% of individuals (in the traditional sense, this would be the wild-type genotype). Most allelic variants exhibit conservative substitutions in the polypeptide chain and produce normal functioning levels of α_1-antitrypsin. Some *deficiency variants,* including the PiS variant, result in a reduction in serum concentrations of α_1-antitrypsin without clinical manifestations. Rare variants termed Pi-null have no detectable serum α_1-antitrypsin. The most common clinically significant mutation is PiZ; homozygotes for the PiZZ protein have circulating α_1-antitrypsin levels that are only 10% of normal. These individuals are at high risk for developing clinical disease. Expression of alleles is autosomal codominant, and consequently, PiMZ heterozygotes have intermediate plasma levels of α_1-antitrypsin. The gene frequency of PiZ is 0.0122 in the North American white population, yielding a PiZZ genotype frequency of approximately 1:7000. However, because of its early presentation, α_1-antitrypsin deficiency is the most commonly diagnosed genetic liver disease in infants and children.

Pathogenesis. With most allelic variants, the mRNA is translated, and the protein is synthesized and secreted normally. Deficiency variants exhibit a selective defect in migration of this secretory protein from the endoplasmic reticulum (ER) to Golgi apparatus; this is most marked for the PiZ polypeptide, attributable to a single amino acid substitution of Glu_{342} to Lys_{342}. *The mutant polypeptide (α_1AT-Z) is abnormally folded, and polymerizes, causing its retention in the ER.* All individuals with the PiZZ genotype accumulate α_1AT-Z in the ER of hepatocytes.

However, only 10% of PiZZ individuals develop clinical liver disease. This subgroup of susceptible individuals exhibit lags in the ER protein degradation pathway, a fundamental quality control apparatus of the normal cell that is designed to degrade abnormally folded or unassembled polypeptides. The accumulated α_1AT-Z is not toxic per se, nor does the liver suffer from a lack of protease inhibitor activity (since α_1-antitrypsin is secreted from the liver into the circulation). Rather, it is the intense autophagocytic response stimulated within hepatocytes, as an alternative degradative pathway, that appears to be the chief cause of liver injury, possibly by autophagocytosis of mitochondria.[36,37] It is worth noting that there are many syndromes in which misfolded proteins are retained within the hepatocyte ER. In most of them, there is little evidence for hepatotoxicity. It is still an open question why accumulation of α_1-antitrypsin causes severe damage to hepatocytes.

Morphology. α_1-Antitrypsin deficiency is characterized by the presence of round-to-oval cytoplasmic globular inclusions in hepatocytes, which in routine H and E stains are acidophilic and indistinctly demarcated from the surrounding cytoplasm. They are strongly PAS-positive and diastase-resistant (Fig. 18–29). The globules are also present in diminished size and number in intermediate deficiency states. The hepatic syndromes associated with PiZZ homozygosity are extremely varied, ranging from neonatal hepatitis without or with cholestasis and fibrosis (discussed shortly) to childhood cirrhosis to a smoldering chronic inflammatory hepatitis or cirrhosis that becomes apparent only late in life. For the most part, the only distinctive feature of the hepatic disease is the PAS-positive globules; infrequently, fatty change and Mallory bodies are present. The diagnostic α_1-antitrypsin globules may be absent in the young infant; steatosis may be present as a tip-off to the possibility of α_1-antitrypsin deficiency.

Clinical Features. Neonatal hepatitis with cholestatic jaundice appears in 10% to 20% of newborns with the deficiency. In adolescence, presenting symptoms may be related to hepatitis or cirrhosis. Attacks of hepatitis may subside with apparent complete recovery, or they may become chronic and lead progressively to cirrhosis. Finally, the disease may remain silent until cirrhosis appears in middle to later life. Hepatocellular carcinoma develops in 2% to 3% of PiZZ adults, usually but not always in the setting of cirrhosis. The treatment, and the cure, for severe hepatic disease is orthotopic liver transplantation. In patients with pulmonary disease, the single most important treatment is avoidance of cigarette smoking, since this behavior markedly accelerates the destructive lung disease associated with α_1-antitrypsin deficiency.

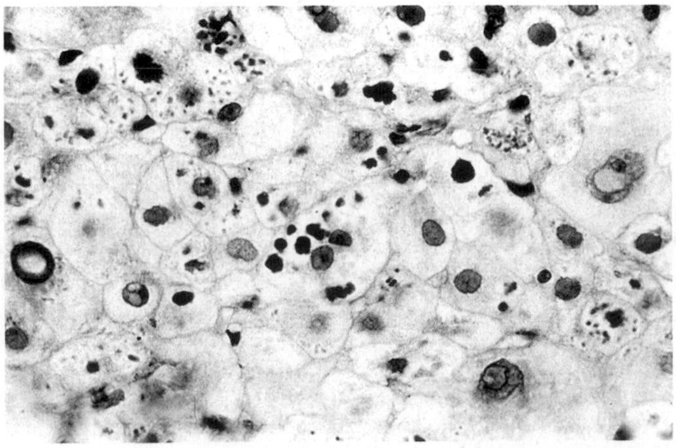

FIGURE 18–29 α_1-Antitrypsin deficiency. Periodic acid-Schiff stain of the liver, highlighting the characteristic red cytoplasmic granules. (Courtesy of Dr. I. Wanless, Toronto General Hospital, Toronto, Ontario, Canada.)

TABLE 18–10 Major Causes of Neonatal Cholestasis

Bile duct obstruction
Extrahepatic biliary atresia
Neonatal infection
Cytomegalovirus
Bacterial sepsis
Urinary tract infection
Syphilis
Toxic
Drugs
Parenteral nutrition
Metabolic disease
Tyrosinemia
Niemann-Pick disease
Galactosemia
Defective bile acid synthetic pathways
α_1-Antitrypsin deficiency
Cystic fibrosis
Miscellaneous
Shock/hypoperfusion
Indian childhood cirrhosis
Alagille syndrome (paucity of bile ducts)
Idiopathic neonatal hepatitis

NEONATAL CHOLESTASIS

Prolonged conjugated hyperbilirubinemia in the neonate, termed *neonatal cholestasis*, affects approximately 1 in 2500 live births. The major conditions causing it are (1) cholangiopathies, primarily *biliary atresia* (discussed later) and (2) a variety of disorders causing conjugated hyperbilirubinemia in the neonate, collectively referred to as *neonatal hepatitis. Neonatal cholestasis and hepatitis are not specific entities, nor are the disorders necessarily inflammatory.* Instead, the finding of "neonatal cholestasis" should evoke a diligent search for recognizable toxic, metabolic, and infectious liver diseases, the more common of which are listed in Table 18–10.[38] Once identifiable causes have been excluded, one is left with the syndrome of "idiopathic" neonatal hepatitis, which shows considerable clinical overlap with biliary atresia.

Affected infants have jaundice, dark urine, light or acholic stools, and hepatomegaly. Variable degrees of hepatic synthetic dysfunction may be identified, such as hypoprothrombinemia. Thus, liver biopsy is critical in distinguishing neonatal hepatitis from an identifiable cholangiopathy.

Morphology. The morphologic features of neonatal hepatitis are:

- Lobular disarray with focal liver cell necrosis
- Panlobular giant cell transformation of hepatocytes and formation of hepatocyte "rosettes": radially arrayed hepatocytes
- Prominent hepatocellular and canalicular cholestasis
- Mild mononuclear infiltration of the portal areas
- Reactive changes in the Kupffer cells
- Extramedullary hematopoiesis

This predominantly parenchymal pattern of injury may blend imperceptibly into a ductal pattern of injury, with bile ductular proliferation and fibrosis of portal tracts. Clear distinction from an obstructive cholangiopathy may therefore be impossible. Specific features that point toward a particular etiology include the inclusions of cytomegalovirus, or fatty change with cirrhosis in galactosemia and tyrosinemia. Electron microscopy may be helpful, for example, by showing phospholipid whorls in Neimann-Pick disease.

Despite the long list of disorders associated with neonatal cholestasis, most are quite rare. "Idiopathic" neonatal hepatitis represents up to 50% of cases, biliary atresia represents another 20%, and α_1-antitrypsin deficiency represents 15%. Differentiation of biliary atresia from nonobstructive neonatal cholestasis assumes great importance, since definitive treatment of biliary atresia requires surgical intervention, whereas surgery may adversely affect the clinical course of a child with other disorders. Fortunately, discrimination can be made with clinical data, without or with liver biopsy, in about 90% of cases.

Intrahepatic Biliary Tract Disease

In this section, we discuss three disorders of intrahepatic bile ducts: secondary biliary cirrhosis, primary biliary cirrhosis, and primary sclerosing cholangitis, (summarized in Table 18–11). Secondary biliary cirrhosis is a condition resulting most often from uncorrected obstruction of the extrahepatic biliary tree. Primary biliary cirrhosis is a destructive disorder of the intrahepatic biliary tree. Primary sclerosing cholangitis involves both the extrahepatic and intrahepatic biliary tree. It should also be noted (although not discussed here) that intrahepatic bile ducts are frequently damaged as part of more general liver disease, as in drug toxicity, viral hepatitis, and transplantation—both orthotopic liver transplantation and graft-versus-host disease after bone marrow transplantation.

SECONDARY BILIARY CIRRHOSIS

Prolonged obstruction of the extrahepatic biliary tree results in profound alteration of the liver itself. The most common cause of obstruction in adults is extrahepatic cholelithiasis (gallstones, described later), followed by malignancies of the biliary tree or head of the pancreas and strictures resulting from previous surgical procedures. Obstructive conditions in children include biliary atresia, cystic fibrosis, choledochal cysts (a cystic anomaly of the extrahepatic biliary tree, see later), and syndromes in which there are insufficient intrahepatic bile ducts (paucity of bile duct syndromes).[39] The initial morphologic features of *cholestasis* were described earlier and are entirely reversible with correction of the obstruction. However, secondary inflammation resulting from biliary obstruction initiates periportal fibrosis, which eventually leads to hepatic scarring and nodule formation, generating secondary biliary cirrhosis. Subtotal obstruction may promote secondary bacterial infection of the biliary tree (*ascending cholangitis*), which aggravates the inflammatory injury. Enteric organisms such as coliforms and enterococci are common culprits.

Morphology. The end-stage obstructed liver exhibits extraordinary yellow-green pigmentation and is accompanied by marked icteric discoloration of body tissues and fluids. On cut surface, the liver is hard, with a finely granular appearance (Fig. 18–30). The histology is characterized by coarse fibrous septae that subdivide the liver in a jigsaw-like pattern. Embedded in the septa are distended small and large bile ducts, which frequently contain inspissated pigmented material. There is extensive proliferation of smaller bile ductules and edema, particularly at the interface between septa (formerly portal tracts) and the parenchyma. Cholestatic features in the parenchyma may be severe, with extensive feathery degeneration and formation of bile lakes. However, once regenerative nodules have formed, bile stasis

TABLE 18–11 Distinguishing Features of the Major Intrahepatic Bile Duct Disorders

	Secondary Biliary Cirrhosis	Primary Biliary Cirrhosis	Primary Sclerosing Cholangitis
Etiology	Extrahepatic bile duct obstruction: biliary atresia, gallstones, stricture, carcinoma of pancreatic head	Possibly autoimmune	Unknown, possibly autoimmune; 50–70% associated with inflammatory bowel disease
Sex predilection	None	Female to male: 6:1	Female to male: 1:2
Symptoms and signs	Pruritus, jaundice, malaise, dark urine, light stools, hepatosplenomegaly	Same as secondary biliary cirrhosis; insidious onset	Same as secondary biliary cirrhosis; insidious onset
Laboratory findings	Conjugated hyperbilirubinemia, increased serum alkaline phosphatase, bile acids, cholesterol	Same as secondary biliary cirrhosis, plus elevated serum IgM autoantibodies (especially M2 form of antimitochondrial antibody-AMA)	Same as secondary biliary cirrhosis, plus elevated serum IgM, hypergammaglobulinemia
Important pathologic findings before cirrhosis develops	Prominent bile stasis in bile ducts, bile ductular proliferation with surrounding neutrophils, portal tract edema	Dense lymphocytic infiltrate in portal tracts with granulomatous destruction of bile ducts	Periductal portal tract fibrosis, segmental stenosis of extrahepatic and intrahepatic bile ducts

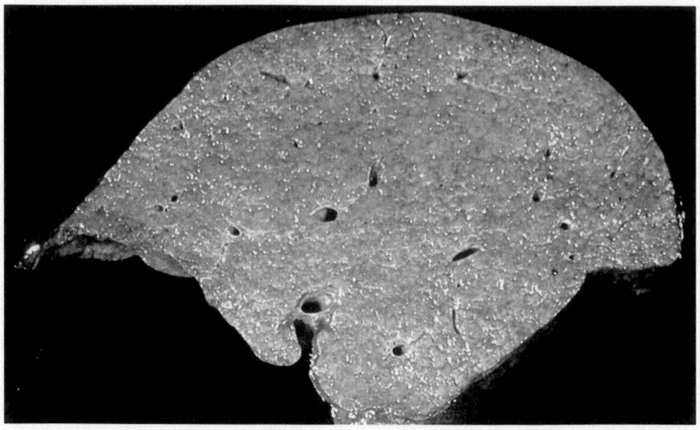

FIGURE 18–30 Biliary cirrhosis. Sagittal section through the liver demonstrates the fine nodularity and bile staining of end-stage biliary cirrhosis.

may become less conspicuous. Ascending bacterial infection incites a robust neutrophilic infiltration of bile ducts; severe pylephlebitis and cholangitic abscesses may develop.

PRIMARY BILIARY CIRRHOSIS

Primary biliary cirrhosis is a chronic, progressive, and often fatal cholestatic liver disease, characterized by the destruction of intrahepatic bile ducts, portal inflammation and scarring, and the eventual development of cirrhosis and liver failure. *The primary feature of this disease is a nonsuppurative, inflammatory destruction of medium-sized intrahepatic bile ducts.* Because cirrhosis develops only after many years, the disease name is somewhat misleading for patients diagnosed early in their course.

This is primarily a disease of middle-aged women, with a female:male predominance in excess of 6:1. Age of onset is between 20 and 80 years, with peak incidence between 40 and 50 years of age. The onset is insidious, usually presenting with pruritus. Jaundice develops late in the course. Hepatomegaly is typical. Xanthomas and xanthelasmas arise owing to cholesterol retention. Stigmata of chronic liver disease are late features. Over a period of two or more decades, patients develop hepatic decompensation, including portal hypertension with variceal bleeding and hepatic encephalopathy.

Serum alkaline phosphatase and cholesterol are almost always elevated; hyperbilirubinemia is a late development and usually signifies incipient hepatic decompensation. Present in 90% of patients with primary biliary cirrhosis are circulating "antimitochrondrial antibodies." These antibodies are against the E2 subunit of the pyruvate dehydrogenase complex (PDC-E2), dihydrolipoamide acetyltransferase. This enzyme complex is located on the inner face of the inner mitochondrial membrane and hence is well shielded from circulating antibodies in undamaged hepatocytes. Whether the formation of antimitochondrial antibodies is a causal event or an epiphenomenon remains a continued enigma. 5% to 10% of patients with otherwise diagnostic primary biliary cirrhosis do not exhibit antimitochondrial antibodies.

Pathogenesis. Many lines of evidence indicate an autoimmune etiology for primary biliary cirrhosis, including aberrant expression of MHC class II molecules on bile duct epithelial cells and accumulation of autoreactive T cells around bile ducts.[40] In addition to antimitochondrial antibodies, antibodies against other cellular components (nuclear pore proteins, centromeric proteins, among others) are also produced, demonstrating the autoimmune nature of the disease.[41] Moreover, there are extrahepatic manifestations of autoimmunity, including the sicca complex of dry eyes and mouth (Sjögren syndrome; from the Latin *sicca,* meaning dryness), scleroderma, thyroiditis, rheumatoid arthritis, Raynaud phenomenon, membranous glomerulonephritis, and celiac disease. However, despite insights gained into general mechanisms for immunologic destruction of bile ducts and the molecular pathology of the PDC-E2 protein, the etiology and inciting triggers of primary biliary cirrhosis are not clear.

Morphology. Primary biliary cirrhosis is the prototype of conditions leading to small-duct biliary fibrosis and cirrhosis. Primary biliary cirrhosis is a focal and variable disease, exhibiting different degrees of severity in different portions of the liver. During the precirrhotic stage, portal tracts are infiltrated by a dense accumulation of lymphocytes, macrophages, plasma cells, and occasional eosinophils. Terminal and conducting bile ducts are infiltrated by lymphocytes and may exhibit noncaseating granulomatous inflammation (Fig. 18–31) and undergo progressive destruction. With time, the obstruction to intrahepatic bile flow leads to progressive secondary hepatic damage. Portal tracts upstream from damaged bile ducts exhibit bile ductular proliferation, inflammation, and necrosis of the adjacent periportal hepatic parenchyma. The parenchyma develops generalized cholestasis. Over years to decades, relentless portal tract scarring and bridging fibrosis lead to cirrhosis.

Macroscopically, the liver does not at first appear abnormal, but as the disease progresses, bile stasis stains the liver green. The capsule remains smooth and glistening until a fine granularity appears, culminating in a well-developed, uniform micronodularity.

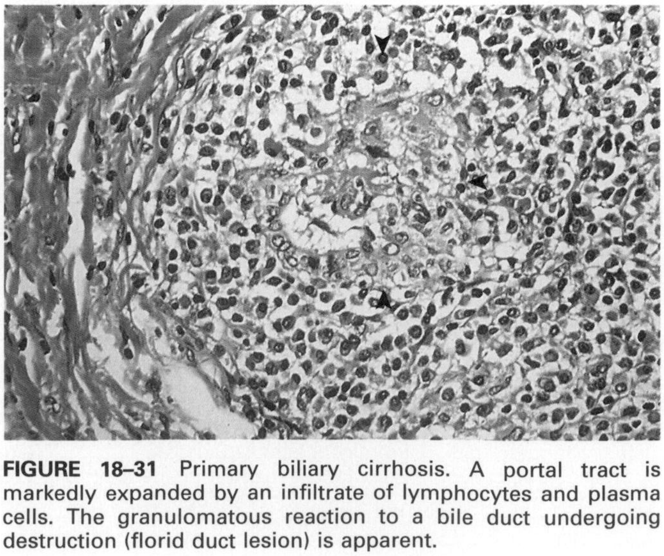

FIGURE 18–31 Primary biliary cirrhosis. A portal tract is markedly expanded by an infiltrate of lymphocytes and plasma cells. The granulomatous reaction to a bile duct undergoing destruction (florid duct lesion) is apparent.

Liver weight is at first normal to increased (owing to inflammation); ultimately, liver weight is slightly decreased. **In most cases, the end-stage picture is indistinguishable from secondary biliary cirrhosis or the cirrhosis that follows chronic hepatitis from other causes.**

Clinical Features. The onset is extremely insidious, and patients may be symptom free for many years. Eventually, pruritus, fatigue, and abdominal discomfort develop, followed in time by secondary features: xanthomas and xanthelasmas, steatorrhea, and malabsorption-related osteomalacia and/or osteoporosis. More general features of jaundice and hepatic decompensation, including portal hypertension and variceal bleeding, mark entry into the end-stages of the disease. The major cause of death is liver failure, followed in order by massive variceal hemorrhage and intercurrent infection.

PRIMARY SCLEROSING CHOLANGITIS

Primary sclerosing cholangitis is characterized by inflammation and obliterative fibrosis of intrahepatic and extrahepatic bile ducts, with dilation of preserved segments. Characteristic "beading" of a barium column in radiographs of the intrahepatic and extrahepatic biliary tree is attributable to the irregular strictures and dilations of affected bile ducts. *Primary sclerosing cholangitis is commonly seen in association with inflammatory bowel disease* (see Chapter 17), particularly chronic ulcerative colitis, which coexists in approximately 70% of primary sclerosing cholangitis patients. Conversely, the prevalence of primary sclerosing cholangitis in ulcerative colitis patients is about 4%. Primary sclerosing cholangitis tends to occur in the third through fifth decades of life, and males predominate 2:1 (see Table 18–11).

Pathogenesis. The cause of primary sclerosing cholangitis is unknown, despite its clear association with inflammatory bowel disease. Key events appear to be secretion of proinflammatory cytokines by activated hepatic macrophages followed by infiltration of T cells into the stroma immediately around bile ducts.[42] The stimuli that initiate and perpetuate the characteristic periductal fibrosis remain unknown. Since hepatic artery infusions with 5-fluorodeoxyuridine and hepatic artery thrombosis after liver transplantation can generate a primary sclerosing cholangitis–like picture, an ischemic contribution to bile duct loss in primary sclerosing cholangitis patients has also been postulated.

Morphology. Primary sclerosing cholangitis is a fibrosing cholangitis of bile ducts, with a lymphocytic infiltrate, progressive atrophy of the bile duct epithelium, and obliteration of the lumen (Fig. 18–32). The concentric periductal fibrosis around affected ducts ("onion-skin fibrosis") is followed by their disappearance, leaving behind a solid, cordlike fibrous scar. In between areas of progressive stricture, bile ducts become ectatic and inflamed, presumably the result of downstream obstruction. As the disease progresses, the liver becomes markedly cholestatic, culminating in biliary cirrhosis much like that seen with primary and secondary biliary cirrhosis.

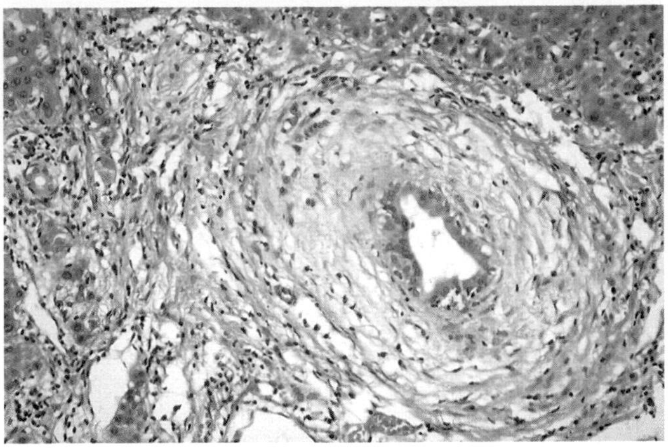

FIGURE 18–32 Primary sclerosing cholangitis. A bile duct undergoing degeneration is entrapped in a dense, "onion-skin" concentric scar.

Clinical Features. Asymptomatic patients may come to attention only because of persistent elevation of serum alkaline phosphatase. Alternatively, progressive fatigue, pruritus, and jaundice may develop. Unlike primary biliary cirrhosis, autoantibodies are present in less than 10% of patients. Severely afflicted patients exhibit symptoms associated with chronic liver disease, including weight loss, ascites, variceal bleeding, and encephalopathy. This disease also follows a protracted course over many years. There does appear to be an increased risk for cholangiocarcinoma. As with primary biliary cirrhosis, liver transplantation is the definitive treatment.

ANOMALIES OF THE BILIARY TREE (INCLUDING LIVER CYSTS)

A heterogeneous group of lesions exist in which the primary abnormality is altered architecture of the intrahepatic biliary tree. Lesions may be found incidentally during radiographic studies or at autopsy or may become manifest as hepatosplenomegaly and portal hypertension in the absence of hepatic dysfunction, typically in late childhood or adolescence or during the adult years. Four distinct lesions have been described (Fig. 18–33). Although one pattern usually predominates, it is not uncommon to find features of more than one pattern in the same liver.

Morphology.

Von Meyenburg Complexes. Close to or within portal tracts, these are small clusters of modestly dilated bile ducts embedded in a fibrous, sometimes hyalinized stroma. Although these "bile duct microhamartomas" may communicate with the biliary tree, they generally are free of pigmented material. They presumably arise from residual embryonic bile duct remnants.[43] Occasionally, a triangular bile duct hamartoma may lie just under Glisson's capsule.

Polycystic Liver Disease. The liver contains multiple diffuse cystic lesions, numbering from a scattered few to hundreds. The cysts are lined by cuboidal or

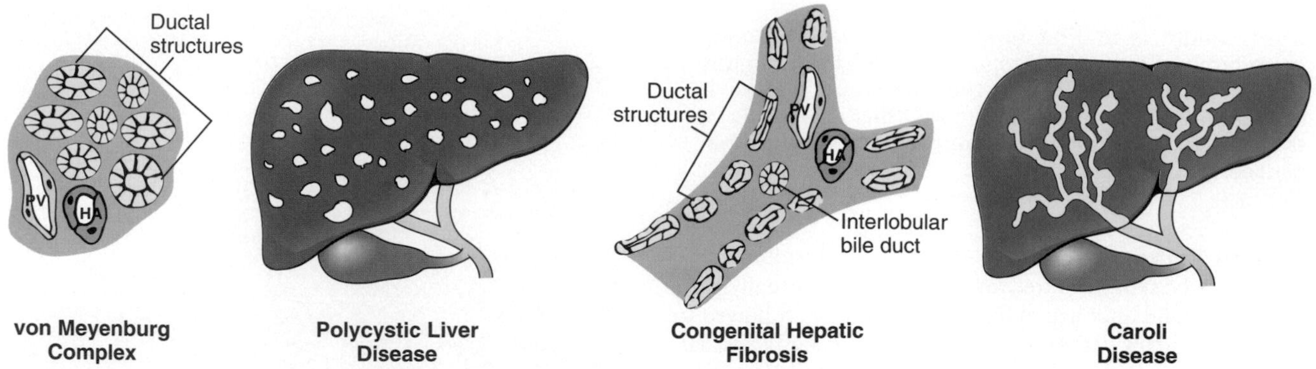

	von Meyenburg Complex	Polycystic Liver Disease	Congenital Hepatic Fibrosis	Caroli Disease
INHERITANCE:	Sporadic	Autosomal Dominant	Autosomal Recessive	Autosomal Recessive
ASSOCIATION WITH POLYCYSTIC KIDNEY DISEASE (PKD)				
Autosomal dominant PKD:	+	+ + +	+	+
Autosomal recessive PKD:	-	-	+ + +	+

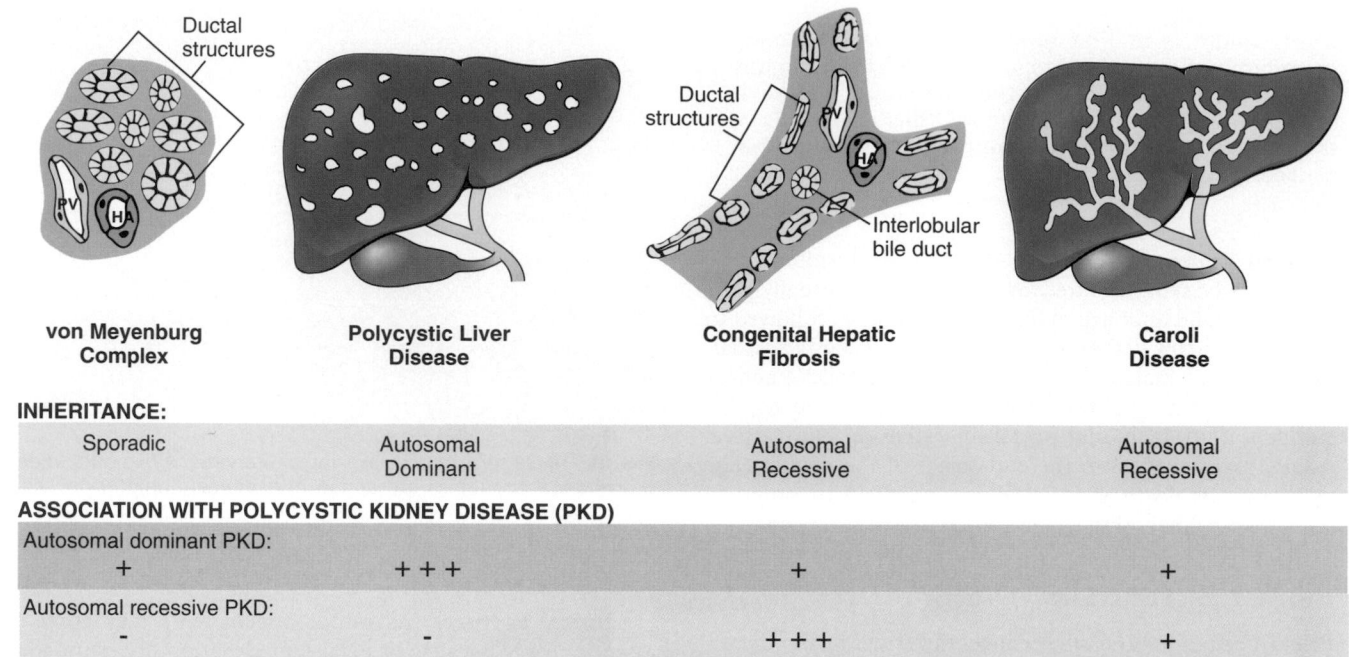

FIGURE 18–33 Bile duct anomalies. The morphologic features of the four major groups are diagrammed, along with apparent patterns of inheritance and associations with polycystic kidney disease. PV, portal vein. HA, hepatic artery.

flattened biliary epithelium and contain straw-colored fluid. They do not contain pigmented material and appear to be detached from the biliary tree. Occasionally, solitary liver cysts of biliary origin are identified, more commonly in women than in men (4:1).

Congenital Hepatic Fibrosis. The portal tracts are enlarged by irregular and broad bands of collagenous tissue, forming septa and dividing the liver into irregular islands. Variable numbers of abnormally shaped bile ducts are embedded in the fibrous tissue, and bile duct remnants are distributed along the septal margins. Sometimes curved bile duct profiles are arranged in a concentric circle around portal tracts. The increased number of bile duct profiles are in continuity with the biliary tree. This anomaly arises because of persistence of a malformed embryonic form of the biliary tree, with ensuing portal tract fibrosis over the individual's lifetime.

Caroli Disease. The larger ducts of the intrahepatic biliary tree are segmentally dilated and may contain inspissated bile. Pure forms are rare; this disease is usually associated with portal tract fibrosis of the congenital hepatic fibrosis type.

Clinical Features. *Von-Meyenburg complexes* are rather common and are usually without clinical significance, save to avoid mistaking lesions radiographically for metastatic carcinoma. Patients with *polycystic liver disease* may develop abdominal tenderness or pain on stooping, occasionally requiring surgical intervention. There is a slight female predilection, with presentation common during pregnancy. Although patients with *congenital hepatic fibrosis* rarely develop cirrhosis, they may still face complications of portal hypertension, particularly bleeding varices. *Caroli disease* is frequently complicated by intrahepatic cholelithiasis (see later), cholangitis, and hepatic abscesses, as well as by portal hypertension. There is an increased risk of cholangiocarcinoma with Caroli disease and congenital hepatic fibrosis. Each of these four conditions exhibits some association with polycystic kidney disease and appears to arise from intrinsic anomalies in the development of the smaller to larger portions of the intrahepatic biliary tree.

As shown in Figure 18–33, there is a well-documented association of autosomal-dominant polycystic kidney disease with polycystic liver disease. Liver cysts in isolation or in abundance represent the most frequent extra-renal manifestation of autosomal-dominant polycystic kidney disease (see Chapter 20) and occur in most patients. Congenital hepatic fibrosis is strongly associated with the autosomal-recessive form of polycystic kidney disease. The exact pathogenesis of these biliary lesions and their association with mutations described for the polycystic disorders remains unclear.[44]

Alagille syndrome (syndromatic paucity of bile ducts) is an uncommon autosomal-dominant condition in which *the liver is almost normal, but portal tract bile ducts are completely absent.*[45] The syndrome is caused by mutations in the gene Jagged1 on chromosome 20p, a cell-surface protein that functions as a ligand for the Notch transmembrane receptors. The Jagged1:Notch signaling pathway regulates cell fate and is involved in the development of the organ systems affected in Alagille syndrome: liver, heart, skeleton, eye, face, and kidney. Patients exhibit a number of extrahepatic features, including a peculiar facies, vertebral anomalies, and cardiovascular defects. Patients can survive into adulthood but are at risk for hepatic failure and hepatocellular carcinoma.

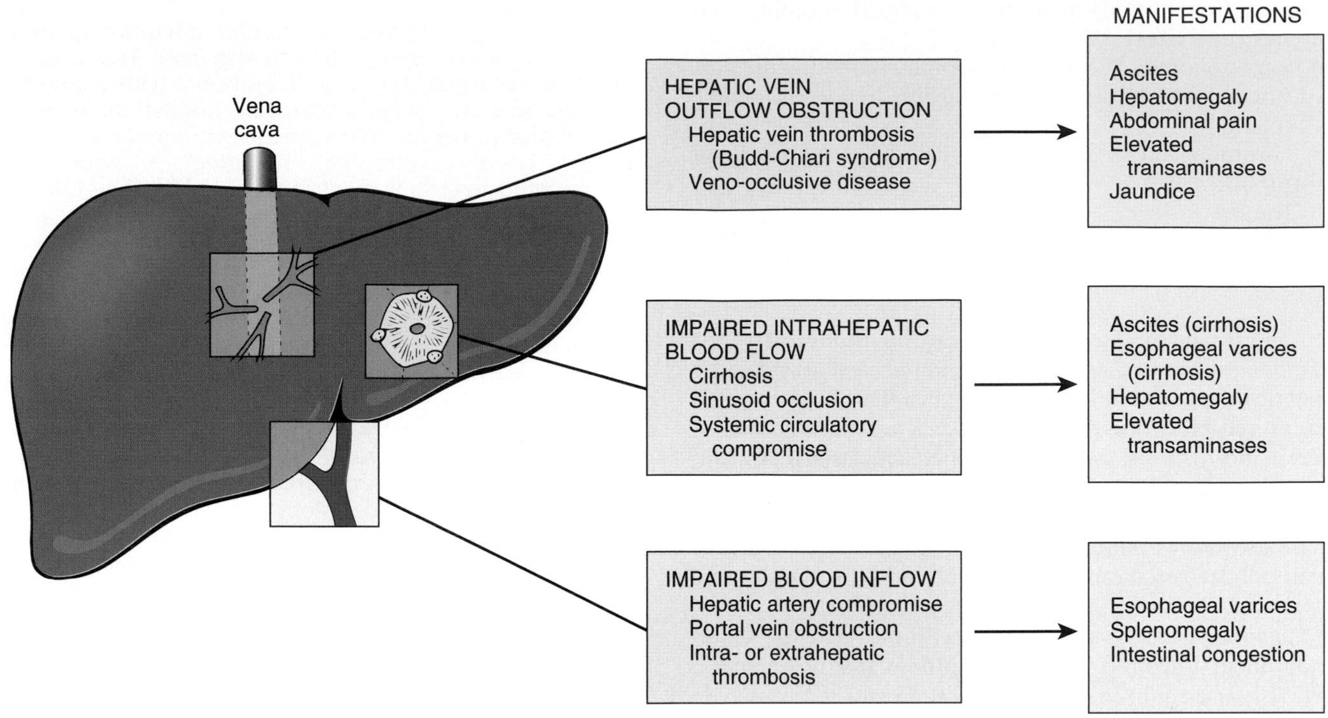

FIGURE 18–34 Hepatic circulatory disorders. The forms and clinical manifestations of impaired blood flow are contrasted.

Circulatory Disorders

Given the enormous flow of blood through the liver, it is not surprising that circulatory disturbances have considerable impact on the liver. In most instances, however, clinically significant abnormalities of liver function do not develop, but hepatic morphology may be strikingly affected. These disorders can be grouped according to whether blood flow into, through, or from the liver is impaired (Fig. 18–34).

IMPAIRED BLOOD FLOW INTO THE LIVER

Hepatic Artery Compromise

Liver infarcts are rare, thanks to the double blood supply to the liver. Nonetheless, thrombosis or compression of an intrahepatic branch of the hepatic artery by embolism (Fig. 18–35), neoplasia, polyarteritis nodosa (Chapter 11), or sepsis may result in a localized infarct that is usually anemic and pale-tan, or sometimes hemorrhagic, owing to suffusion of portal blood. Interruption of the main hepatic artery does not always produce ischemic necrosis of the organ, particularly if the liver is otherwise normal. Retrograde arterial flow through accessory vessels, when coupled with the portal venous supply, is usually sufficient to sustain the liver parenchyma. The one exception is hepatic artery thrombosis in a transplanted liver, which generally leads to infarction of the major ducts of the biliary tree and loss of the organ.

Portal Vein Obstruction and Thrombosis

Blockage of the extrahepatic portal vein may be insidious and well tolerated or may be a catastrophic and potentially lethal event; most cases fall somewhere in between.[46] Occlusive disease of the portal vein or its major radicles typically produces abdominal pain and, in most instances, ascites and other manifestations of portal hypertension, principally esophageal varices which are prone to rupture. The ascites, when present, is often massive and intractable. Acute impairment of visceral blood flow leads to profound congestion and bowel infarction.

Extrahepatic portal vein obstruction may arise from:

- *Banti syndrome,* in which subclinical occlusion of the portal vein (as from neonatal umbilical sepsis or umbilical

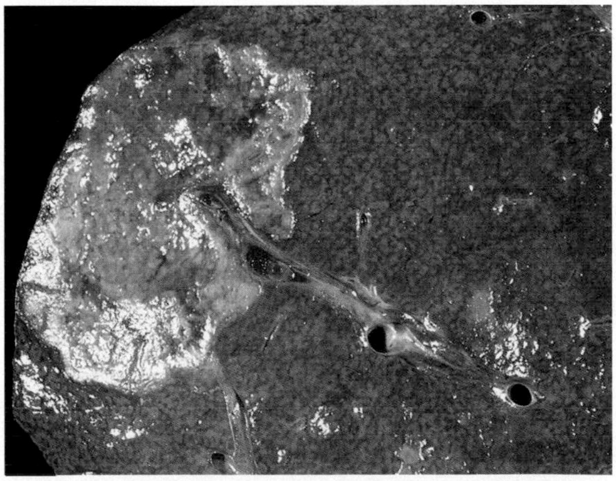

FIGURE 18–35 Liver infarct. A thrombus is lodged in a peripheral branch of the hepatic artery and compresses the adjacent portal vein; the distal hepatic tissue is pale, with a hemorrhagic margin.

vein catheterization) presents as variceal bleeding and ascites years later

- Intra-abdominal sepsis, for example, acute diverticulitis or appendicitis leading to *pylephlebitis* in the splanchnic circulation
- Thrombogenic disorders, including postsurgical thromboses
- Trauma
- Pancreatitis that initiates splenic vein thrombosis which propagates into the portal vein

In about half of cases, no cause can be implicated. *Acute thrombosis of an intrahepatic portal vein radicle* does not cause ischemic infarction but instead results in a sharply demarcated area of red-blue discoloration (so-called *infarct of Zahn*). There is no necrosis, only severe hepatocellular atrophy and marked hemostasis in distended sinusoids. Invasion of the portal vein system by primary or secondary cancer in the liver can progressively occlude portal inflow to the liver; tongues of hepatocellular carcinoma can even occlude the extrahepatic portal vein.

Idiopathic portal hypertension is a chronic, generally bland condition of impaired portal vein inflow and noncirrhotic portal hypertension. In those instances in which a cause can be identified, it may be associated with hypercoagulability of the blood, myeloproliferative disorders, peritonitis, or chronic exposure to arsenicals. The histologic manifestation is termed *hepatoportal sclerosis*, owing to dense fibrosis of intrahepatic portal tracts with obliteration of portal vein channels. Whether this histology represents a late stage of healed liver injury or a primary progressive disorder is unclear.

IMPAIRED BLOOD FLOW THROUGH THE LIVER

The most common *intrahepatic cause* of blood flow obstruction is *cirrhosis*, as described earlier.

In addition, physical occlusion of the *sinusoids* occurs in a small but striking group of diseases. In *sickle cell disease*, the hepatic sinusoids may become packed with sickled erythrocytes, both free within the vascular space and phagocytosed by Kupffer cells. This leads to panlobular parenchymal necrosis. *Disseminated intravascular coagulation (DIC)* may occlude sinusoids. This is usually inconsequential except for the periportal sinusoidal occlusion and parenchymal necrosis that may arise in pregnancy as part of *eclampsia* (discussed shortly). Finally, metastatic tumor cells (e.g., breast carcinoma, lymphoma, malignant melanoma) may fill the hepatic sinusoids in the absence of a mass lesion. The attendant obstruction to blood flow and massive necrosis of hepatocytes can lead to fulminant hepatic failure.

Passive Congestion and Centrolobular Necrosis

These hepatic manifestations of systemic circulatory compromise are considered together because they represent a morphologic continuum. Both changes are commonly seen at autopsy because there is an element of preterminal circulatory failure with virtually every death.

Morphology. Right-sided cardiac decompensation leads to passive congestion of the liver. The liver is slightly enlarged, tense, and cyanotic, with rounded edges. Microscopically, there is congestion of centrolobular sinusoids. With time, centrolobular hepatocytes become atrophic, resulting in markedly attenuated liver cell cords. **Left-sided cardiac failure** or **shock** may lead to hepatic hypoperfusion and hypoxia. In this instance, hepatocytes in the central region of the lobule undergo ischemic coagulative necrosis (**centrolobular necrosis**).

The combination of hypoperfusion and retrograde congestion acts synergistically to generate **centrolobular hemorrhagic necrosis**. The liver takes on a variegated mottled appearance reflecting hemorrhage and necrosis in the centrilobular regions, known traditionally as the **nutmeg liver** (Fig. 18–36). By microscopy, there is a sharp demarcation of viable periportal and necrotic pericentral hepatocytes, with suffusion of blood through the centrilobular region. An uncommon complication of sustained chronic severe congestive heart failure is so-called **cardiac sclerosis.** The pattern of liver fibrosis is distinctive, inasmuch as it is mostly centrilobular. The damage rarely fulfills the criteria for the diagnosis of cirrhosis, but the historically sanctified term **cardiac cirrhosis** cannot easily be dislodged.

In most instances, the only clinical evidence of centrilobular necrosis or its variants is mild to moderate transient elevation of serum aminotransferases. The parenchymal damage may be sufficient to induce mild to moderate jaundice.

Peliosis Hepatis

Sinusoidal dilation occurs in any condition in which efflux of hepatic blood is impeded. *Peliosis hepatitis* is a rare condition in which the dilation is primary. It is most commonly associated with exposure to anabolic steroids and, rarely, oral contraceptives and danazol, although the pathogenesis is not known. Clinical signs are generally absent even in advanced peliosis, but potentially fatal intra-abdominal hemorrhage or

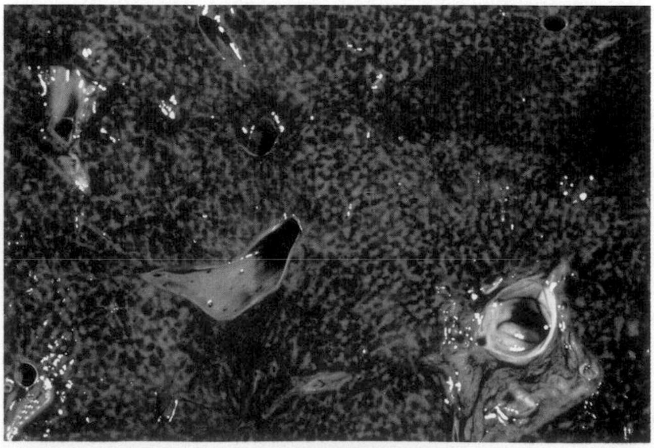

FIGURE 18–36 Centrolobular hemorrhagic necrosis. The cut liver section, in which major blood vessels are visible, is notable for a variegated, mottled, red appearance (nutmeg liver).

hepatic failure may occur. Peliotic lesions usually disappear after cessation of drug treatment.

HEPATIC VENOUS OUTFLOW OBSTRUCTION

Hepatic Vein Thrombosis and Inferior Vena Cava Thrombosis

Obstruction of a single main hepatic vein by thrombosis is clinically silent. The obstruction of two or more major hepatic veins produces liver enlargement, pain, and ascites (so-called *Budd-Chiari syndrome*), the result of increased intrahepatic blood pressure and an inability of the massive hepatic blood flow to shunt around the blocked outflow tract. *Hepatic vein thrombosis* is associated with primary myeloproliferative disorders (including polycythemia vera), inherited disorders of coagulation (e.g., deficiencies in antithrombin, protein S, or protein C, or mutations of factor V; see Chapter 4), antiphospholipid syndrome, paroxysmal nocturnal hemoglobinuria, and intra-abdominal cancers, particularly hepatocellular carcinoma. The occurrence of hepatic vein thrombosis in the setting of pregnancy or oral contraceptive use is usually through interaction with an underlying thrombogenic disorder. About 10% of cases are idiopathic in origin, presumably unrecognized thrombogenic disorders.

A separate distinction is made for *inferior vena cava thrombosis at its hepatic portion (obliterative hepatocavopathy)*. While inferior vena cava thrombosis may arise from the same thrombogenic disorders as for hepatic vein thrombosis, it is frequently idiopathic. In Nepal, it is endemic, with a suspected association with infections.

Morphology. With acutely developing thrombosis of the major hepatic veins or hepatic portion of the inferior vena cava, the liver is swollen and red-purple and has a tense capsule (Fig. 18–37). Microscopically, the affected hepatic parenchyma reveals severe centrilobular congestion and necrosis. Centrilobular fibrosis develops in instances in which the thrombosis is more slowly developing. The major veins may contain totally occlusive fresh thrombi, subtotal occlusion, or, in chronic cases, organized adherent thrombi. Unlike hepatic vein thrombosis, which heals leaving extensive scarring of the hepatic parenchyma, the thrombosis of obliterative hepatocavopathy may heal to leave only an incomplete membranous web protruding into the lumen of the inferior vena cava.

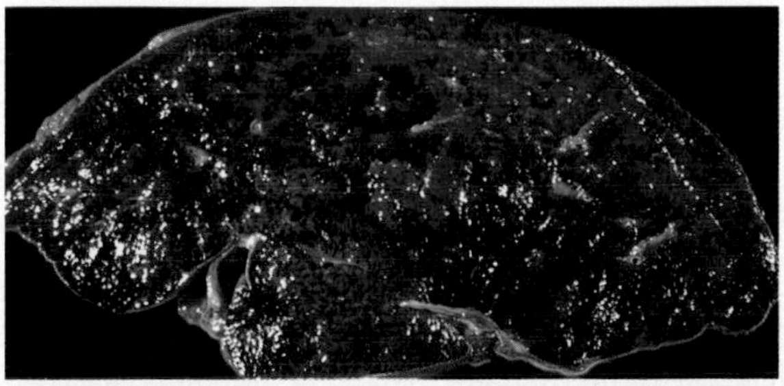

FIGURE 18–37 Budd-Chiari syndrome. Thrombosis of the major hepatic veins has caused extreme blood retention in the liver.

The mortality of untreated acute hepatic vein thrombosis is high. Prompt surgical creation of a portosystemic venous shunt permits reverse flow through the portal vein and considerably improves the prognosis. In the case of vena caval thrombosis, direct dilation of caval obstruction may be possible during angiography. The chronic forms of these thrombotic syndromes are far less lethal, and over two thirds of patients are alive after 5 years.

Veno-Occlusive Disease (Sinusoidal Obstruction Syndrome)

Originally described in Jamaican drinkers of pyrrolizidine alkaloid–containing bush tea, veno-occlusive disease now occurs primarily in the immediate weeks following bone marrow transplantation. The incidence approaches 25% in recipients of allogeneic marrow transplants, with mortality rates of over 30%. A diagnosis of veno-occlusive disease is frequently made on clinical grounds only (tender hepatomegaly, ascites, weight gain, and jaundice), owing to the high risk of liver biopsy in these patients.

Morphology. Veno-occlusive disease is characterized by obliteration of hepatic vein radicles by varying amounts of subendothelial swelling and fine reticulated collagen. In acute disease, there is striking centrolobular congestion with hepatocellular necrosis and accumulation of hemosiderin-laden macrophages. As the disease progresses, obliteration of the lumen of the venule is easily identified by using special stains for connective tissue (Fig. 18–38). With chronic or healed veno-occlusive disease, dense perivenular fibrosis radiating out into the parenchyma may be present, frequently with total obliteration of the venule; hemosiderin deposition is evident in the scar tissue, and congestion is minimal.

Veno-occlusive disease presumably arises from toxic injury to the sinusoidal endothelium.[47] The cells round up and slough off the sinusoidal wall, embolizing downstream and obstructing sinusoidal blood flow. This is accompanied by passage of erythrocytes into the space of Disse and down-

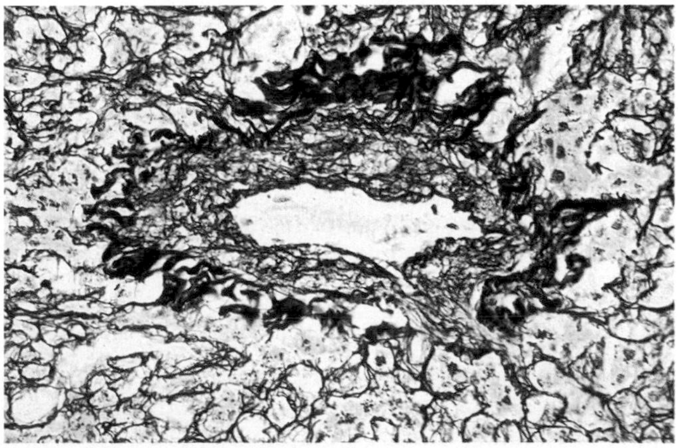

FIGURE 18–38 Veno-occlusive disease. A reticulin stain reveals the parenchyma framework of the lobule and the marked deposition of collagen within the lumen of the central vein.

stream accumulation of cellular debris in the terminal hepatic vein. Proliferation of perisinusoidal stellate cells and subendothelial fibroblasts in the terminal hepatic vein follows, with deposition of extracellular matrix. The obliterative changes in the terminal hepatic vein are thus secondary to sinusoidal damage, hence the recommended alternative name of *sinusoidal obstruction syndrome.* Seventy percent to 85% of patients recover spontaneously; the remainder spiral toward a fatal outcome. Treatment of veno-occlusive disease is largely supportive.

Hepatic Disease Associated with Pregnancy

Women with chronic liver disease may become pregnant, or liver diseases can become manifest during pregnancy. Viral hepatitis (HAV, HBV, HCV, and even HBV+HDV) is the most common cause of jaundice in pregnancy. While these women require careful clinical management, pregnancy does not specifically alter the course of the liver disease. The one exception is hepatitis E viral infection (HEV), which, for unknown reasons, runs a more severe course in pregnant patients, with fatality rates of 10% to 20%.

A unique and very small subgroup of pregnant patients (0.1%) develop hepatic complications directly attributable to pregnancy: preeclampsia, acute fatty liver of pregnancy, and intrahepatic cholestasis of pregnancy. In extreme cases of the first two conditions, the outcome is fatal.

PREECLAMPSIA AND ECLAMPSIA

Preeclampsia affects 7% to 10% of pregnancies and is characterized by maternal hypertension, proteinuria, peripheral edema, coagulation abnormalities, and varying degrees of disseminated intravascular coagulation. When hyperreflexia and convulsions occur, the condition is called *eclampsia* and may be life threatening. Alternatively, subclinical hepatic disease may be the primary manifestation of preeclampsia, as part of a syndrome of hemolysis, elevated liver enzymes, and low platelets, dubbed the *HELLP syndrome.*[48]

Morphology. The affected liver in preeclampsia is normal in size, firm, and pale, with small red patches due to hemorrhage. Occasionally, yellow or white patches of ischemic infarction can be seen. Microscopically, **the periportal sinusoids contain fibrin deposits with hemorrhage into the space of Disse,** leading to periportal hepatocellular coagulative necrosis. Blood under pressure may coalesce and expand to form a **hepatic hematoma; dissection of blood under Glisson's capsule may lead to catastrophic hepatic rupture** (Fig 18–39).

Patients with hepatic involvement in preeclampsia may exhibit modest to severe elevation of serum aminotransferases and mild elevation of serum bilirubin. Hepatic dysfunction sufficient to cause a coagulopathy signifies far-advanced and potentially lethal disease. *Definitive treatment in severe cases requires termination of the pregnancy.* In mild cases, patients

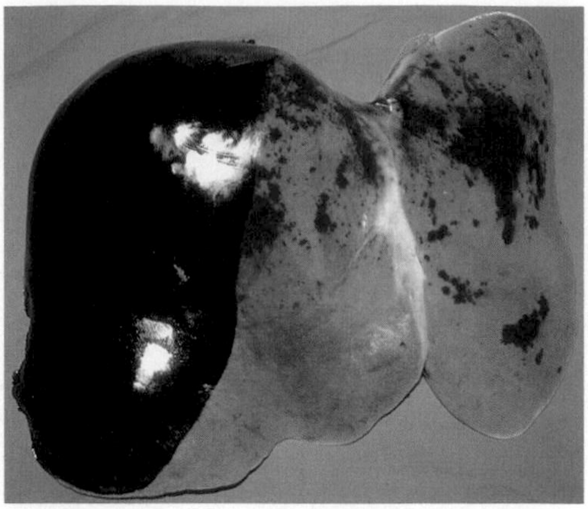

FIGURE 18–39 Eclampsia. Subcapsular hematoma dissecting under Glisson's capsule in a fatal case of eclampsia. (Courtesy of Dr. Brian Blackbourne, Office of the Medical Examiner, San Diego, CA.)

may be managed conservatively. Patients who survive mild or severe preeclampsia recover without sequelae.

ACUTE FATTY LIVER OF PREGNANCY

Acute fatty liver of pregnancy (AFLP) exhibits a spectrum ranging from modest or even subclinical hepatic dysfunction (evidenced by elevated serum aminotransferase levels) to hepatic failure, coma, and death. Affected women present in the latter half of pregnancy, usually in the third trimester. Symptoms are directly attributable to incipient hepatic failure, including bleeding, nausea and vomiting, jaundice, and coma. In 20% to 40% of cases, the presenting symptoms may be those of coexistent preeclampsia.

Morphology. The diagnosis of acute fatty liver rests on biopsy identification of the characteristic microvesicular fatty transformation of hepatocytes. In severe cases, there may be lobular disarray with hepatocyte dropout, reticulin collapse, and portal tract inflammation, making distinction from viral hepatitis difficult. **Diagnosis depends on (1) a high index of suspicion and (2) confirmation of microvesicular steatosis using special stains for fat (oil-red-O or Sudan black) on frozen tissue sections;** electron microscopy may also be used to demonstrate the steatosis.

While this condition most commonly runs a mild course, patients with AFLP can progress within days to hepatic failure and death. *The primary treatment for AFLP is termination of the pregnancy.* Multiple metabolic defects are likely to underlie this condition. In one striking example, both mother and father carry a heterozygous deficiency in mitochondrial long chain 3-hydroxyacyl CoA dehydrogenase. The homozygously deficient fetuses fare well during pregnancy but cause hepatic dysfunction in the heterozygous mother because long chain 3-hydroxylacyl metabolites produced by the fetus or placenta are washed away into the maternal circulation and cause hepatic toxicity. This is a rare instance of a fetus causing metabolic disease in the mother.[49]

INTRAHEPATIC CHOLESTASIS OF PREGNANCY

The onset of pruritus in the third trimester, followed by darkening of the urine and occasionally light stools and jaundice, heralds the development of this enigmatic syndrome. Serum bilirubin (mostly conjugated) rarely exceeds 5 mg/dL; alkaline phosphatase may be slightly elevated. Liver biopsy reveals mild cholestasis without necrosis. The altered hormonal state of pregnancy appears to combine with biliary secretion defects, as in secretion of bile salts or sulfated progesterone metabolites, to engender cholestasis.[50] Although this is generally a benign condition, the mother is at risk for gallstones and malabsorption, and the incidence of fetal distress, stillbirths, and prematurity is modestly increased.

Hepatic Complications of Organ or Bone Marrow Transplantation

The increasing use of transplantation for bone marrow, renal, hepatic and other organ disorders has generated a challenging group of hepatic complications. For patients undergoing bone marrow transplantation, the liver may be damaged by toxic drugs or graft-versus-host disease, whereas patients receiving a liver transplant may encounter graft failure or graft rejection. Although the clinical settings are obviously different for each patient population, the common themes of toxic or immunologically mediated liver damage, infection of immunosuppressed hosts, recurrent disease, and posttransplant lymphoproliferative disorder are readily apparent. The following focuses on lesions peculiar to the liver.

DRUG TOXICITY AFTER BONE MARROW TRANSPLANTATION

"Liver toxicity" describes a syndrome of hepatic dysfunction following the cytotoxic therapy administered to patients just prior to bone marrow transplantation. It affects up to one half of such patients and is characterized by weight gain, tender hepatomegaly, edema, ascites, hyperbilirubinemia and a fall in urinary sodium excretion. The onset is typically on the days immediately following the donor marrow transplantation. A spectrum of centrolobular necrosis and inflammatory changes is encountered, culminating in veno-occlusive disease (sinusoidal obstruction syndrome, described earlier). Clinical outcome is directly related to the severity of liver toxicity. Persistent severe liver dysfunction is a harbinger of a fatal outcome, with patients succumbing to septicemia, pneumonia, bleeding, and/or multiorgan failure. A form of vascular injury evolving over weeks to several months, nodular regenerative hyperplasia, is discussed under the section on tumors.

GRAFT-VERSUS-HOST DISEASE AND LIVER REJECTION

The liver has the unenviable position of being attacked by graft-versus-host and host-versus-graft mechanisms, in the setting of bone marrow transplantation and liver transplantation, respectively. These processes are discussed in detail in Chapter 6. More than other solid organs, liver transplants are reasonably well tolerated by recipients. In some cases, minimal immunosuppression is sufficient to prevent rejection.[51] One explanation for this apparent tolerance is that the transplanted liver carries many donor lymphocytes, establishing a state of chimerism in the recipient. This prevents the recipient's immune system from reacting against donor alloantigens. That being said, the hepatic morphologic features that are peculiar to graft-versus-host disease after transplantation deserve comment.

Morphology. Liver damage in **acute graft-versus-host disease** (10 to 50 days after bone marrow transplantation) is dominated by direct attack of donor lymphocytes on epithelial cells of the liver. This results in a hepatitis with necrosis of hepatocytes and bile duct epithelial cells and inflammation of the parenchyma and portal tracts. In **chronic hepatic graft-versus-host disease** (usually more than 100 days after transplantation), there is portal tract inflammation, selective **bile duct destruction**, and eventual fibrosis. Portal vein and hepatic vein radicles may exhibit **endotheliitis**, a process in which a subendothelial lymphocytic infiltrate lifts the endothelium from its basement membrane. Cholestasis may be observed in both acute and chronic graft-versus-host disease. **Acute cellular rejection** of transplanted livers is characterized by infiltration of a mixed population of inflammatory cells into portal tracts, bile duct and hepatocyte injury, and endothelitis. With **chronic rejection**, a severe obliterative arteritis of small and larger arterial vessels results in ischemic changes in the liver parenchyma. Alternatively, bile ducts are progressively occluded, due to either direct attack or obliteration of their arterial supply. Both may lead to loss of the graft.

NONIMMUNOLOGIC DAMAGE TO LIVER ALLOGRAFTS

Besides technical problems in the surgical procedure and the very rare *hyperacute rejection*, revascularization and perfusion of the donor liver (which may have been kept outside of the body for many hours) may result in *preservation injury*, attributable to the generation of oxygen radicals in a hypoxic organ with insufficient reserves of oxygen scavengers to prevent damage. This leads to *sinusoidal endothelial injury and Kupffer cell activation, neutrophil adhesion, platelet aggregation, and local cytokine release*. Hepatocyte ballooning and cholestasis follow, with variable degrees of centrilobular necrosis.[52] With severe injury, the portal tracts also are damaged, resulting in inflammation, bile duct proliferation, and fibrosis. These histologic features may take weeks to months to resolve.

In the days to weeks following transplantation, other complications can threaten the viability of the graft. Unlike in the native liver, *hepatic artery thrombosis* is a sufficiently severe vascular insult to cause severe compromise in the transplanted liver. Alternatively, *portal vein thrombosis* may be insidious and present only as variceal hemorrhage weeks to months later. *Bile duct obstruction*, particularly from stricture at the anastomosis with the native common bile duct, presents in the expected fashion.

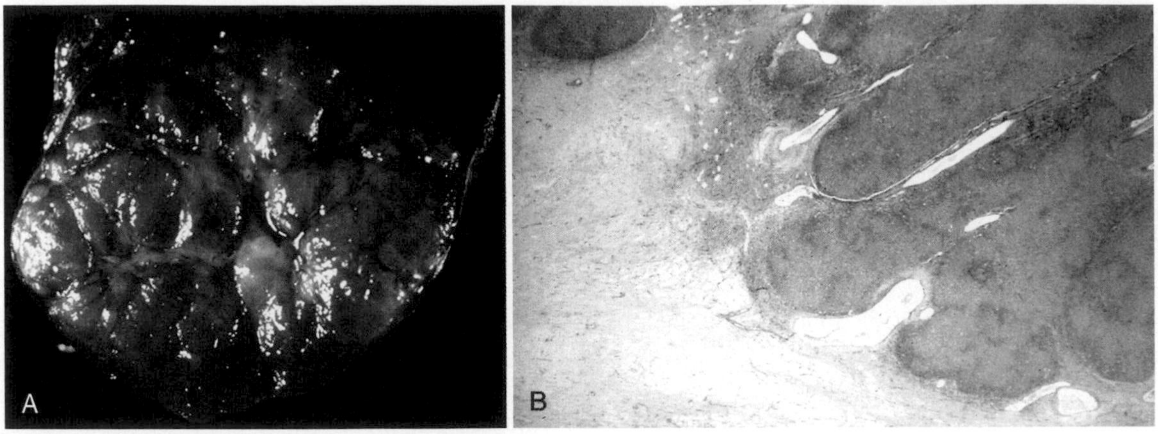

FIGURE 18–40 Focal nodular hyperplasia. *A*, Resected specimen showing lobulated contours and a central stellate scar. *B*, Low-power photomicrograph showing a broad fibrous scar with hepatic arterial and bile duct elements and chronic inflammation, present within hepatic parenchyma that lacks the normal sinusoidal plate architecture (H&E).

Nodules and Tumors

Hepatic masses may come to attention for a variety of reasons. They may generate epigastric fullness and discomfort or be detected by routine physical examination or radiographic studies for other indications. Nodular hyperplasias are not neoplasms, nor are cysts of biliary origin (addressed previously). The remaining lesions are true neoplasms.

NODULAR HYPERPLASIAS

Solitary or multiple hyperplastic hepatocellular nodules may develop in the noncirrhotic liver. Two such conditions, having confusingly overlapping names, are *focal nodular hyperplasia* and *nodular regenerative hyperplasia*.

Morphology. Focal nodular hyperplasia appears as a well-demarcated but poorly encapsulated nodule, ranging up to many centimeters in diameter (Fig. 18–40*A*). The lesion is generally lighter than the surrounding liver and is sometimes yellow. Typically, there is a central gray-white, depressed stellate scar from which fibrous septa radiate to the periphery (Fig. 18–40*B*). The central scar contains large vessels, usually arterial, that typically exhibit fibromuscular hyperplasia with eccentric or concentric narrowing of the lumen. The radiating septa exhibit foci of intense lymphocytic infiltrates and exuberant bile duct proliferation along septal margins. The parenchyma between the septa exhibits essentially normal hepatocytes but with a thickened plate architecture characteristic of regeneration.

Nodular regenerative hyperplasia affects the entire liver with roughly spherical nodules, in the absence of fibrosis (Fig. 18–41). Microscopically, plump hepatocytes are surrounded by rims of atrophic cells. The variation in parenchymal architecture may be missed on a hematoxylin and eosin stain, and reticulin staining is required to appreciate the changes in hepatocellular architecture.

Focal nodular hyperplasia presents as a spontaneous mass lesion, most frequently in young to middle-aged adults, with a female preponderance. Nodular regenerative hyperplasia is associated with the development of portal hypertension with its attendant clinical manifestations. This latter lesion occurs in association with conditions affecting intrahepatic blood flow, including solid organ (particularly renal) transplantation, bone marrow transplantation, and vasculitic conditions. The common factor in both lesions appears to be heterogeneity in hepatic blood supply, arising from focal obliteration of portal vein radicles with compensatory augmentation of arterial blood supply.[53]

BENIGN NEOPLASMS

The most common benign lesions are *cavernous hemangiomas*, blood vessel tumors identical to those occurring elsewhere (see Chapter 11). They appear as discrete red-blue, soft nodules, usually less than 2 cm in diameter, and often occur directly beneath the capsule. Their chief clinical significance is that they not be mistaken for metastatic tumors and that blind percutaneous biopsies not be performed on them.

Benign neoplasms developing from hepatocytes are called *liver cell adenomas*. These tend to occur in young women who

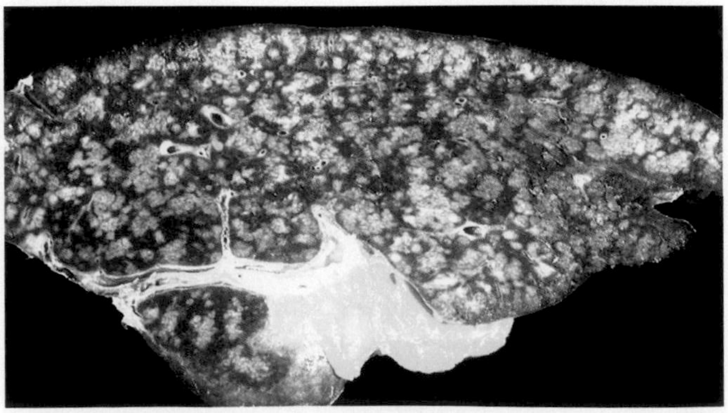

FIGURE 18–41 Nodular regenerative hyperplasia. Autopsied liver showing diffuse nodular transformation.

have used oral contraceptives and regress on discontinuance of their use. Liver cell adenomas have clinical significance for three reasons:

- When they present as an intrahepatic mass, they may be mistaken for the more ominous hepatocellular carcinoma.
- Subcapsular adenomas have a tendency to rupture, particularly during pregnancy (under estrogen stimulation), causing severe intraperitoneal hemorrhage.
- Rarely, they may harbor hepatocellular carcinoma.

Morphology. Liver cell adenomas are pale, yellow-tan, and frequently bile-stained nodules, found anywhere in the hepatic substance but often beneath the capsule (Fig. 18–42*A*). They may reach 30 cm in diameter. Although they are usually well demarcated, encapsulation might not be present. On microscopic examination, liver cell adenomas are composed of sheets and cords of cells that may resemble normal hepatocytes or have some variation in cell and nuclear size (Fig. 18–42*B*). Abundant glycogen may generate a clear cytoplasm. Portal tracts are absent; instead, prominent arterial vessels and draining veins are distributed through the substance of the tumor.

MALIGNANT TUMORS

The liver and lungs share the dubious distinction of being the visceral organs that are most often involved in the metastatic spread of cancers. Primary carcinomas of the liver are relatively uncommon in North America and Western Europe (0.5% to 2% of all cancers) but represent 20% to 40% of cancers in many other countries. Most arise from hepatocytes and are termed *hepatocellular carcinoma* (HCC). Much less common are carcinomas of bile duct origin, *cholangiocarcinomas*. Before embarking on a discussion of the major forms of malignancy affecting the liver, two rare forms of primary liver cancer deserve brief mention: hepatoblastomas and angiosarcomas.

Hepatoblastoma is the most common liver tumor of young childhood, usually fatal within a few years if not resected. This tumor has two anatomic variants:

- The *epithelial type*, composed of small, polygonal fetal cells or even smaller embryonal cells forming acini, tubules, or papillary structures vaguely recapitulating liver development.
- The *mixed epithelial and mesenchymal type*, which contains foci of mesenchymal differentiation that may consist of primitive mesenchyme, osteoid, cartilage, or striated muscle.

A striking feature of hepatoblastomas is the frequent activation of the Wnt/β-catenin signaling pathway by stabilizing mutations of β-catenin, contributing to the process of carcinogenesis (Chapter 7). Approximately 80% of hepatoblastomas exhibit this change, with chromosomal deletions constituting more than half of such mutations.[54]

Angiosarcoma resembles those occurring elsewhere. The primary liver form is of interest because of its association with exposure to vinyl chloride, arsenic, or Thorotrast (Chapters 9 and 11). The latency period after exposure to the putative carcinogen may be several decades. These highly aggressive neoplasms metastasize widely and generally kill within a year.

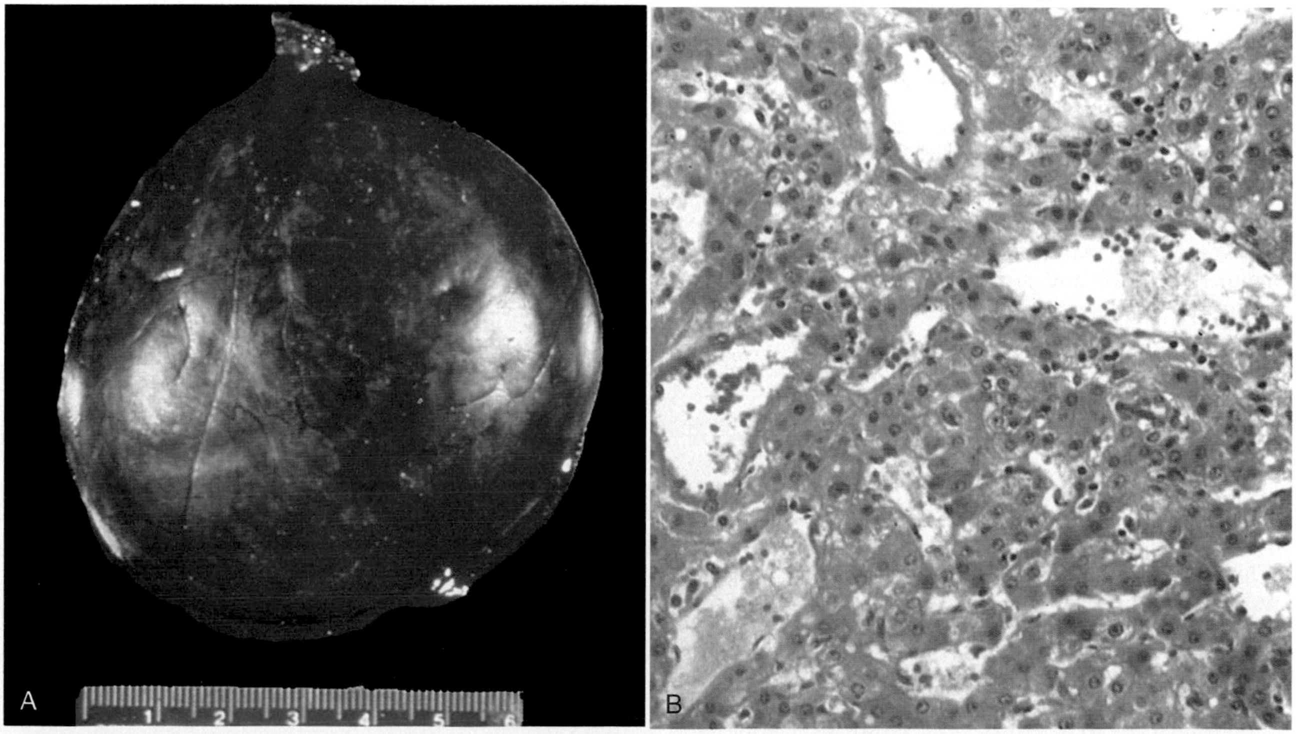

FIGURE 18–42 Liver cell adenoma. *A*, Resected specimen presenting as a pendulous mass arising from the liver. *B*, Microscopic view showing cords of hepatocytes, with an arterial vascular supply and no portal tracts.

Hepatocellular Carcinomas

On a global basis, primary liver cancer—almost entirely HCC—constitutes approximately 5.4% of cancers and in some populations is the most common cancer.[55, 56] The largest numbers of cases are found in Asia (76% of all HCC), followed by Africa. Annual incidence rates for hepatocellular carcinoma are below five cases per 100,000 population in North and South America, North and Central Europe, and Australia, with intermediate rates of up to 15 cases per 100,000 in countries bordering the Mediterranean. The highest annual incidence rates are found in Korea, Taiwan, Mozambique, and Southeast China, approaching 36 per 100,000. Within each geographic area (low or high incidence), blacks have attack rates approximately threefold higher than Caucasians. Worldwide, there is a clear predominance of males, ranging from 1.5:1 in countries with a low incidence of hepatocellular carcinoma to approximately 3:1 in populations with a high frequency.

More than 85% of cases of HCC occur in countries with high rates of chronic HBV infection. In these regions, the HBV carrier state begins in infancy following vertical transmission of virus from infected mothers, conferring a 200-fold increased risk for HCC by adulthood. Cirrhosis may be absent in up to half of these patients, and the cancer often occurs between 20 and 40 years of age. In the Western world where HBV is not prevalent, cirrhosis is present in 85% to 90% of cases of HCC, usually in the setting of other chronic liver diseases; this cancer is seldom encountered before age 60. The documented incidence of HCC is rising in the United States, tripling from 1.4 per 100,000 during 1976 to 1980 to 4.7 per 100,000 during 1996 to 1997. An increase in the prevalence of viral-induced cirrhosis especially from hepatitis C virus is the likely explanation. This trend may continue, owing to the large pool of chronically HCV-infected persons.

Pathogenesis. Several factors relevant to the pathogenesis of HCC were discussed in Chapter 7. Several points deserve emphasis at this time.

Three major etiologic associations have been established: viral infection (HBV, HCV), chronic alcoholism, and food contaminants (primarily aflatoxins). Other conditions include tyrosinemia and hereditary hemochromatosis.

- Many factors, including age, sex, chemicals, viruses, hormones, alcohol, and nutrition, interact in the development of HCC. For example, the disease that is most likely to give rise to HCC is, in fact, the extremely rare hereditary tyrosinemia, in which almost 40% of patients develop this tumor despite adequate dietary control.
- The pathogenesis of HCC may be different in high-incidence, HBV-prevalent populations versus low-incidence Western populations, in which other chronic liver diseases such as alcoholism, HCV, and hereditary hemochromatosis are more common.
- The development of cirrhosis appears to be an important, but not requisite, contributor to the emergence of HCC.

Extensive epidemiologic studies link chronic HBV and chronic HCV infection with liver cancer. The following factors have been implicated:[57, 58]

- Repeated cycles of cell death and regeneration, as occurs in chronic hepatitis from any cause, are important in the pathogenesis of hepatocellular carcinomas.
- Preneoplastic changes such as hepatocyte dysplasia can result from point mutations in selected cellular genes, loss of heterozygosity in tumor suppressor genes, DNA methylation changes, and constitutive expression of hepatocyte growth factor (HGF) and transforming growth factor alpha (TGF-α). These changes and possibly the effect of some viral proteins act to further stimulate the replication of hepatocytes.
- The accumulation of mutations during continuous cycles of cell division may damage DNA repair mechanisms and eventually transform hepatocytes. The molecular changes observed in different HCC nodules within one liver are often distinct, suggesting individual mutational events throughout the liver. Indeed, molecular analysis of tumor cells in HBV-infected individuals reveals that each case is clonal with respect to HBV DNA integration pattern, suggesting that viral integration precedes or accompanies a transforming event.
- For reasons that are not clear, genomic instability is more likely in the presence of integrated HBV DNA, giving rise to chromosomal aberrations such as deletions, translocations, and duplications.
- The HBV genome encodes a regulatory element, the X-protein, that is a transcriptional activator of many genes and is present in most tumors with integrated HBV DNA. It is conceivable that in liver cells infected with HBV, the X-protein disrupts normal growth control by activation of host cell proto-oncogenes and disruption of cell cycle control. The core protein of HCV may have oncogenic potential as well, although the pathways through which HBx and HCV core proteins operate may differ. As yet, there is no evidence for an ordered sequence of genomic events leading to hepatocarcinogenesis.

In certain regions of the world, such as China and South Africa, where HBV is endemic, there is also high exposure to dietary aflatoxins derived from the fungus *Aspergillus flavus*. These highly carcinogenic toxins are found in "moldy" grains and peanuts. Animal studies reveal that aflatoxin can bind covalently with cellular DNA and cause mutations in proto-oncogenes or tumor suppressor genes, particularly *p53* (Chapter 7). However, carcinogenesis does not occur unless the liver is mitotically active, as is the case in chronic viral hepatitis with recurrent bouts of injury and regeneration.

Despite our incomplete understanding of hepatocellular carcinogenesis, one fact is clear: *Universal vaccination of children against HBV in endemic areas may dramatically decrease the incidence of hepatocellular carcinoma.* Such a program was begun in Taiwan in 1984 and reduced HBV infection rates from 10% to 1.3% in 10 years. A randomized trial of vaccination in Gambia demonstrated 83% protection against primary infection and 95% against development of a carrier state.[58a] However, because of the latency period for hepatocellular carcinoma, three to four decades will be needed to fully determine the impact of HBV control on hepatocellular carcinoma incidence.

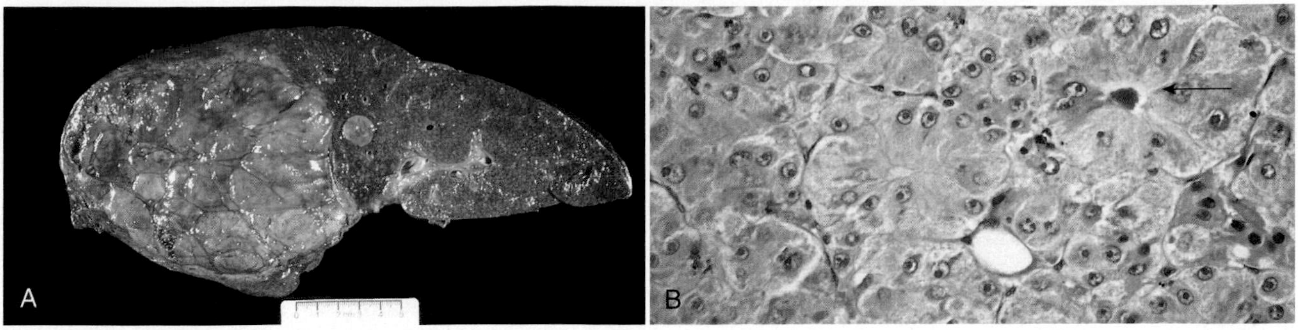

FIGURE 18–43 Hepatocellular carcinoma. *A,* Autopsied liver showing a unifocal, massive neoplasm replacing most of the right hepatic lobe in a noncirrhotic liver; a satellite tumor nodule is directly adjacent. *B,* In this microscopic view of a well-differentiated lesion, tumor cells are arranged in nests, sometimes with a central lumen, one of which contains bile (*arrow*). Other tumor cells contain intracellular bile pigment.

Morphology. Hepatocellular carcinoma may appear grossly as (1) a **unifocal** (usually large) mass (Fig. 18–43*A*); (2) **multifocal,** widely distributed nodules of variable size; or (3) a **diffusely infiltrative** cancer, permeating widely and sometimes involving the entire liver. All three patterns may cause liver enlargement, particularly the unifocal massive and multinodular patterns. The diffusely infiltrative tumor may blend imperceptibly into a cirrhotic liver background.

Hepatocellular carcinomas are usually paler than the surrounding liver substance and sometimes take on a green hue when composed of well-differentiated hepatocytes capable of secreting bile. **All patterns of hepatocellular carcinomas have a strong propensity for invasion of vascular channels.** Extensive intrahepatic metastases ensue, and occasionally, long, snakelike masses of tumor invade the portal vein (with occlusion of the portal circulation) or inferior vena cava, extending even into the right side of the heart.

Hepatocellular carcinomas range from well-differentiated to highly anaplastic undifferentiated lesions. In well-differentiated and moderately well-differentiated tumors, cells that are recognizable as hepatocytic in origin are disposed either in a trabecular pattern (recapitulating liver cell plates) or in an acinar, pseudoglandular pattern (Fig. 18–43*B*). In poorly differentiated forms, tumor cells can take on a pleomorphic appearance with numerous anaplastic giant cells, can become small and completely undifferentiated cells, or may even resemble a spindle cell sarcoma.

A distinctive variant of hepatocellular carcinoma is the **fibrolamellar carcinoma.** This tumor occurs in young male and female adults (20 to 40 years of age) with equal incidence, has no association with HBV or cirrhosis risk factors, and often has a better prognosis. It usually presents as single large, hard "scirrhous" tumor with fibrous bands coursing through it. On microscopic examination, it is composed of well-differentiated polygonal cells growing in nests or cords and separated by parallel lamellae of dense collagen bundles (Fig. 18–44).

Hepatocellular carcinoma spreads extensively within the liver by obvious contiguous growth and by the development of satellite nodules, which can be shown by molecular methods to be derived from the parent tumor. Metastasis outside the liver is primarily via venous invasion, especially into the hepatic vein system. However, hematogenous metastases,

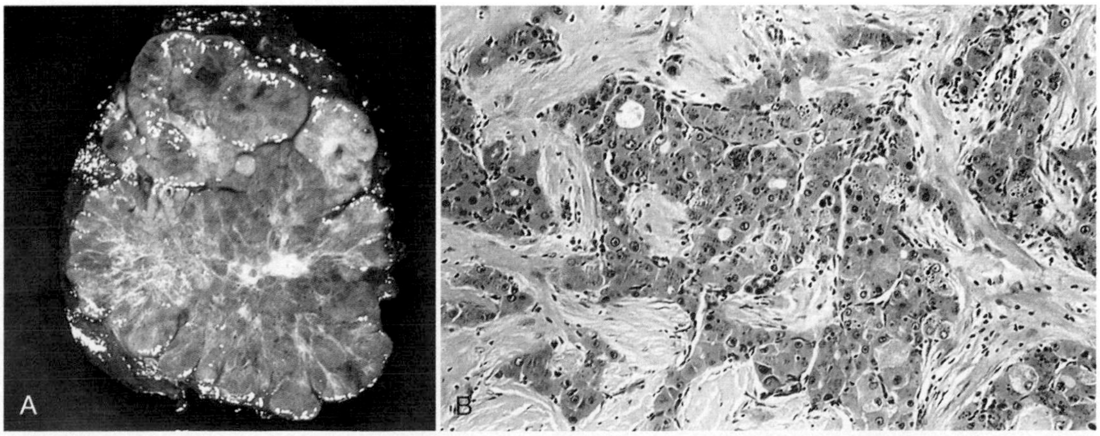

FIGURE 18–44 Fibrolamellar carcinoma. *A,* Resected specimen showing a demarcated nodule in an otherwise normal liver. *B,* Microscopic view showing nests and cords of malignant-appearing hepatocytes separated by dense bundles of collagen.

especially to the lung, tend to occur late in the disease. Lymph node metastases to the perihilar, peripancreatic, and para-aortic nodes above and below the diaphragm are found in less than half of hepatocellular carcinomas that spread beyond the liver. If hepatocellular carcinoma with venous invasion is identified in explanted livers at the time of liver transplantation, tumor recurrence is likely to occur in the transplanted donor liver.

Clinical Features. The clinical manifestations of HCC are seldom characteristic and, in the Western population, often are masked by those related to the background cirrhosis or chronic hepatitis. In areas of high incidence such as tropical Africa, patients usually have no clinical history of liver disease, although cirrhosis may be detected at autopsy. In both populations, most patients have ill-defined upper abdominal pain, malaise, fatigue, weight loss, and sometimes awareness of an abdominal mass or abdominal fullness. In many cases, the enlarged liver can be felt on palpation, with sufficient irregularity or nodularity to permit differentiation from cirrhosis. Jaundice, fever, and gastrointestinal or esophageal variceal bleeding are inconstant findings.

Laboratory studies may be helpful but are rarely conclusive. Elevated levels of serum α-fetoprotein are found in 50% to 75% of patients with HCC. However, false-positive results are encountered with yolk-sac tumors and many non-neoplastic conditions, including cirrhosis, massive liver necrosis, chronic hepatitis, normal pregnancy, fetal distress or death, and fetal neural tube defects such as anancephaly and spina bifida. This and other biochemical tests (such as serum carcinoembryonic antigen levels) often fail to detect small lesions, when curative resection might be possible. Most valuable for small tumors are radiologic studies: ultrasonography, hepatic angiography, computed tomography, and magnetic resonance imaging.[59]

The natural course of HCC is progressive enlargement of the primary mass until it encroaches on hepatic function or metastasizes, generally first to the lungs and then to other sites. Overall, death usually occurs from (1) cachexia, (2) gastrointestinal or esophageal variceal bleeding, (3) liver failure with hepatic coma, or, rarely, (4) rupture of the tumor with fatal hemorrhage.

The fibrolamellar variant of HCC is associated with a more favorable outlook. It arises in otherwise healthy young adults and may be discovered while still amenable to surgical resection.

Cholangiocarcinoma

Cholangiocarcinoma is a malignancy of the biliary tree, arising from bile ducts within and outside of the liver. The incidence is approximately 0.6 case per 100,000 in North America, with essentially equal rates for Caucasians and non-Caucasians and for men and women. The risk conditions for development of cholangiocarcinoma include primary sclerosing cholangitis, congenital fibropolycystic diseases of the biliary system (particularly Caroli disease and choledochal cysts, discussed later), and previous exposure to Thorotrast (formerly used in radiography of the biliary tract). Most cholangiocarcinomas in the Western world, however, arise without evidence of antecedent risk conditions. In the Orient, where the incidence rates are higher, a major risk condition is chronic infection of the biliary tract by the liver fluke *Opisthorchis sinensis* and its close relatives.

Morphology. Intrahepatic cholangiocarcinomas occur in the non-cirrhotic liver and may track along the intrahepatic portal tract system to create a treelike tumorous mass within a portion of the liver. Alternatively, a massive tumor nodule may develop. In either instance, lymphatic and vascular invasion may be prominent features, giving rise to extensive intrahepatic metastasis (Fig. 18–45*A*). By microscopy, cholangiocarcinomas resemble adenocarcinomas arising in other parts of the body, and they may exhibit the full range of morphologic variation. Most are well to moderately differentiated sclerosing adenocarcinomas with clearly defined glandular and tubular structures lined by cuboidal-to-low columnar epithelial cells (Fig. 18–45*B*). These neoplasms are usually markedly desmoplastic, with dense collagenous stroma separating the glandular elements. As a result, the tumor substance is extremely firm and gritty. **Cholangiocarcinomas are rarely bile stained**, because differentiated bile duct epithelium does not synthesize bile.

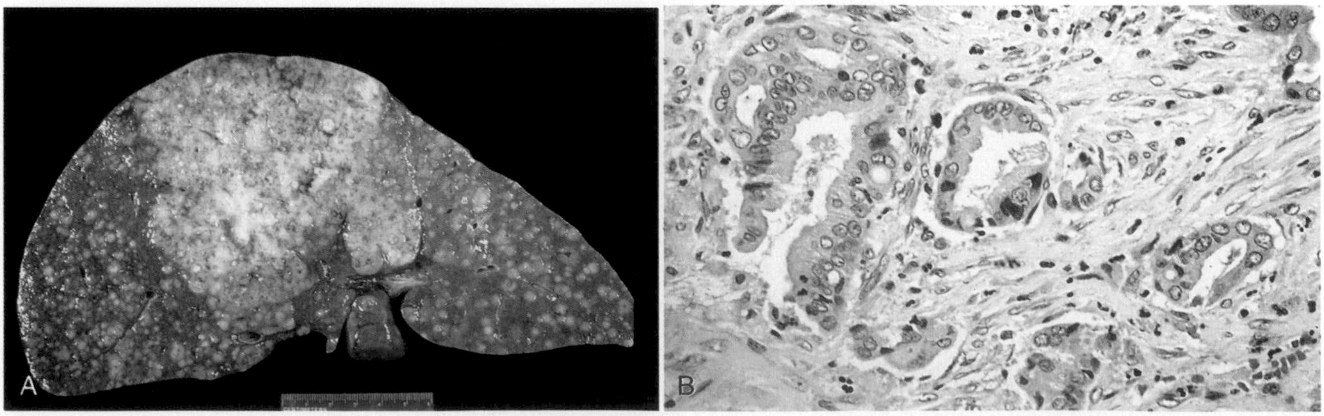

FIGURE 18–45 Cholangiocarcinoma. *A*, Autopsied liver showing a massive neoplasm in the right hepatic lobe and innumerable metastases permeating the entire liver. *B*, Microscopic view showing tubular glandular structures embedded in a dense sclerotic stroma.

Mixed variants occur, in which elements of both hepatocellular carcinoma and cholangiocarcinoma are present. Three forms are recognized: (1) separate tumor masses of HCC and cholangiocarcinoma within the same liver; (2) "collision tumors," in which tumorous masses of HCC and cholangiocarcinoma comingle at an identifiable interface; and (3) tumors in which elements of HCC and cholangiocarcinoma are intimately mixed at the microscopic level. These "mixed tumors" are infrequent, but careful microscopic examination of cholangiocarcinomas can often reveal small foci of hepatocellular differentiation. The HCC/cholangiocarcinoma may be generated from a common bipotential precursor cell (oval cells, Chapter 3) capable of producing both hepatocytes and bile duct epithelial cells (cholangiocytes).

Hematogenous metastases to the lungs, bones (mainly vertebrae), adrenals, brain, or elsewhere are present at autopsy in about 50% of cases of cholangiocarcinoma. Lymph node metastases to the regional lymph nodes are also found in about half of all cholangiocarcinomas.

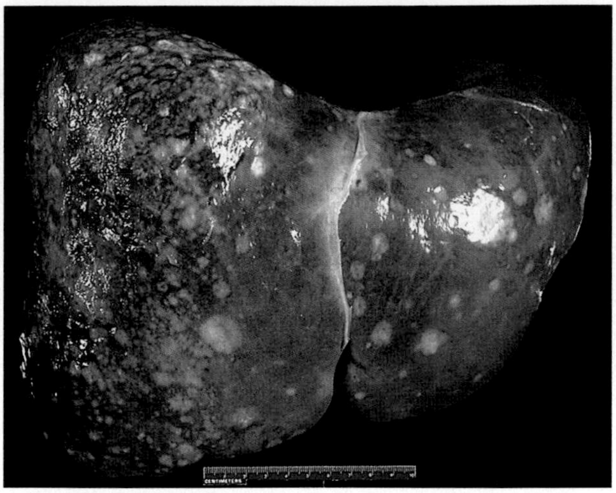

FIGURE 18–46 Multiple hepatic metastases from a primary colon adenocarcinoma.

Clinical Features. Intrahepatic cholangiocarcinoma is not usually detected until late in its course, either as the result of obstruction to bile flow through the hilum of the liver or as a symptomatic liver mass. The clinical outlook is dismal, with 1- and 2-year survival rates of 25% and 13%, respectively. The median time from diagnosis to death is 6 months. Aggressive surgery remains the only treatment offering hope for long-term survival.

Metastatic Tumors

Metastatic involvement of the liver is far more common than primary neoplasia. Although the most common primaries producing hepatic metastases are those of the breast, lung, and colon, any cancer in any site of the body may spread to the liver, including leukemias and lymphomas. Typically, multiple nodular metastases are found that often cause striking hepatomegaly and may replace over 80% of existent hepatic parenchyma (Fig. 18–46). The liver weight can exceed several kilograms. There is a tendency for metastatic nodules to outgrow their blood supply, producing central necrosis and umbilication when viewed from the surface of the liver. Always surprising is the amount of metastatic involvement that may be present in the absence of clinical or laboratory evidence of hepatic functional insufficiency. Often, the only telltale clinical sign is hepatomegaly, sometimes with nodularity of the free edge. However, with massive destruction of liver substance or direct obstruction of major bile ducts, jaundice and abnormal elevations of liver enzymes may appear.

THE BILIARY TRACT

Disorders of the biliary tract affect a significant portion of the world's population. Over 95% of biliary tract disease is attributable to cholelithiasis (gallstones). In the United States, the annual cost of cholelithiasis and its complications was $6 billion to $8 billion in 1998, representing 1% of the national health care budget.

Normal

Up to 1 liter of bile is secreted by the liver per day. Between meals, bile is stored in the gallbladder, which in the adult has a capacity of about 50 mL. Storage is facilitated by fivefold to tenfold concentration of bile through the coupled active absorption of electrolytes, coupled with passive movement of water. In preparation for fat digestion, the gallbladder releases stored bile into the gut. This organ is not essential for biliary function, since humans do not suffer from maldigestion or malabsorption of fat after cholecystectomy.

Unlike the rest of the gastrointestinal tract, the gallbladder lacks a muscularis mucosae and submucosa and consists only of (1) a mucosal lining with a single layer of columnar cells; (2) a fibromuscular layer; (3) a layer of subserosal fat with arteries, veins, lymphatics, nerves, and paraganglia; and (4) a peritoneal covering, except where the gallbladder lies adjacent

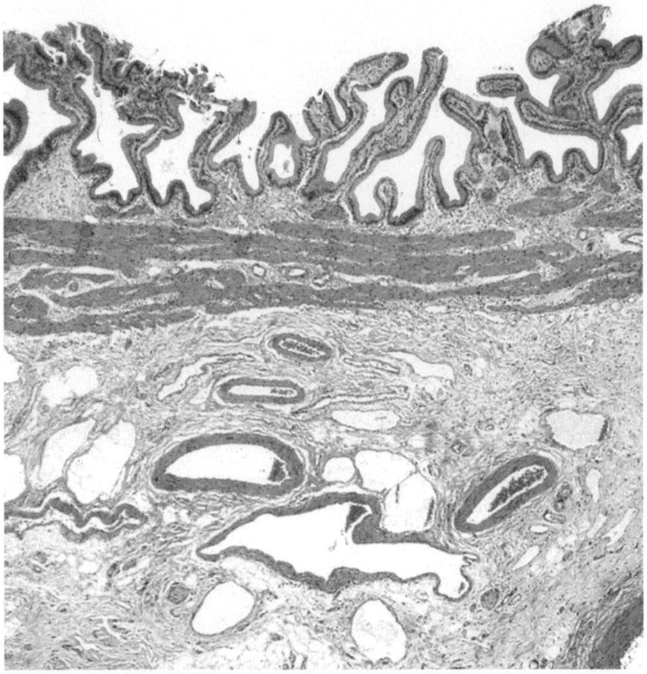

FIGURE 18–47 Normal gallbladder histology. The undulating mucosal epithelium overlies a delicate lamina and only one smooth muscle layer. This is different from elsewhere in the gut, where two muscle layers exist (muscularis mucosa and muscularis propria).

to, or is even embedded, in the liver (Fig. 18–47). The mucosal epithelium takes the form of numerous interlacing tiny folds, creating a honeycombed surface. In the neck of the gallbladder, these folds coalesce to form the *spiral valves of Heister*, which extend into the cystic duct. In combination with muscle action, these "valves" may assist in retaining bile between meals. The rapid taper of the gallbladder neck just proximal to the cystic duct is the site at which gallstones become impacted.

Small tubular channels (*ducts of Luschka*) are sometimes found buried within the gallbladder wall adjacent to the liver. The channels communicate with the intrahepatic biliary tree but only rarely form patent accessory bile ducts that directly enter the gallbladder lumen. Small outpouchings of the gallbladder mucosa may penetrate into and through the muscle wall (*Rokitansky-Aschoff sinuses*); their prominence in the settings of inflammation and gallstone formation suggests that they are acquired herniations.

The confluence of the biliary tree is the common bile duct, which courses through the head of the pancreas for about 2 cm before disgorging its contents through the *ampulla of Vater* into the duodenal lumen. In approximately 60% to 70% of individuals, the main pancreatic duct joins the common bile duct to drain through a common channel; in the remainder, the two ducts run in parallel without joining. Scattered along the length of both the intrahepatic and extrahepatic biliary tree are mucin-secreting submucosal glands. These become prominent near the terminus of the common bile duct, appearing as microscopic outpouchings that interdigitate with the spiraling smooth muscle of the ampullary sphincter. The unwary can mistake these embedded glands for invasive cancer.

Pathology

Congenital Anomalies

Although major developmental anomalies of the gallbladder and bile ducts are rare, anatomic variation is sufficiently common as to present occasional surprises during surgery. The more distinctive variations, which also may be appreciated during ultrasonography, computed tomography, and magnetic resonance imaging scans, merit comment. The gallbladder may be *congenitally absent*, or there may be gallbladder *duplication* with conjoined or independent cystic ducts. A longitudinal or transverse septum may create a *bilobed gallbladder*. *Aberrant locations* of the gallbladder occur in 5% to 10% of the population, most commonly partial or complete embedding in the liver substance. A *folded fundus* is the most common anomaly, creating the so-called *phrygian cap* (Fig. 18–48). *Agenesis* of all or any portion of the hepatic or common bile ducts and *hypoplastic* narrowing of biliary channels (true "biliary atresia") represent a spectrum of hepatobiliary malformations.

Disorders of the Gallbladder

CHOLELITHIASIS (GALLSTONES)

Gallstones afflict 10% to 20% of adult populations in developed countries. It is estimated that over 20,000,000 persons in the United States have gallstones,[4] totaling some 25 to 50 tons in weight! About 1,000,000 new patients annually are found to have gallstones, of whom half undergo surgery. Nevertheless, the vast majority of gallstones (>80%) are "silent," and most individuals remain free of biliary pain or stone complications for decades. There are two main types of gallstones. In the West, *about 80% are cholesterol stones, containing more than 50% of crystalline cholesterol monohydrate. The remainder are composed predominantly of bilirubin calcium salts and are designated pigment stones.*

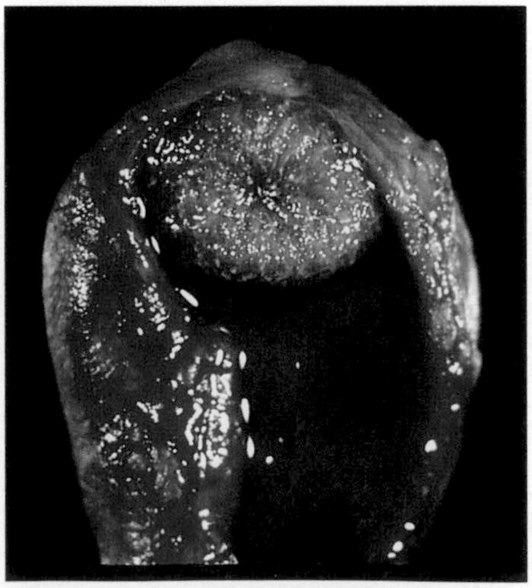

FIGURE 18–48 Phrygian cap of the gallbladder; the fundus is folded inward.

Prevalence and Risk Factors. Certain populations are far more prone than others to develop gallstones. The major risk factors are cited in Table 18–12. The following applies to cholesterol gallstones.

Ethnic-Geographic. The prevalence rates of cholesterol gallstones approach 75% in Native Americans of the first migration from Asia, which includes the Pima, Hopi, and Navajo;[60] pigment stones are rare. Cholesterol gallstones are more prevalent in industrialized societies and uncommon in developing societies. The predominant type of gallstones in non-Western populations, when they occur, is pigment gallstones, primarily arising in the setting of bacterial infections of the biliary tree and parasitic infestations.

Age and Sex. The prevalence of gallstones increases throughout life. In the United States, less than 5% to 6% of the population under age 40 have stones, in contrast to 25% to 30% of those over age 80. The prevalence in Caucasian women is about twice as high as in men. With both aging and gender, hypersecretion of biliary cholesterol appears to play the major role.

Environmental Factors. Estrogenic influence, including oral contraceptives and pregnancy, increases the expression of hepatic lipoprotein receptors and stimulates hepatic HMG-CoA reductase activity. Thus, both cholesterol uptake and biosynthesis, respectively, are increased. Clofibrate, used to lower blood cholesterol, increases hepatic HMG-CoA reductase and decreases conversion of cholesterol to bile acids by reducing cholesterol 7α-hydroxylase activity. The net result of these influences is excess biliary secretion of cholesterol. Obesity and rapid weight loss also are strongly associated with increased biliary cholesterol secretion.

Acquired Disorders. Although gastrointestinal conditions may severely impair intestinal resorption of bile salts, there is compensatory enhanced hepatic conversion of cholesterol to bile salts, leading to less cholesterol excretion, and no particular tendency to cholesterol stone formation. However, gallbladder stasis, either neurogenic or hormonal, fosters a local environment that is favorable for both cholesterol and pigment gallstone formation.

TABLE 18–12 Risk Factors for Gallstones

Cholesterol Stones
Demography: Northern Europe, North and South America, Native Americans, Mexican Americans
Advancing age
Female sex hormones
Female gender
Oral contraceptives
Pregnancy
Obesity
Rapid weight reduction
Gallbladder stasis
Inborn disorders of bile acid metabolism
Hyperlipidemia syndromes
Pigment Stones
Demography: Asian more than Western, rural more than urban
Chronic hemolytic syndromes
Biliary infection
Gastrointestinal disorders: ileal disease (e.g., Crohn disease), ileal resection or bypass, cystic fibrosis with pancreatic insufficiency

Hereditary Factors. In addition to ethnicity, family history alone imparts increased risk, as do a variety of inborn errors of metabolism that (1) lead to impaired bile salt synthesis and secretion or (2) generate increased serum and biliary levels of cholesterol, such as defects in lipoprotein receptors (hyperlipidemia syndromes), which engender marked increases in cholesterol biosynthesis. Animal studies strongly implicate specific genetic susceptibilities, many attributable to aberrant regulation of the transport proteins responsible for the secretion of biliary solutes into bile.[61]

Certain risk factors are well established for the development of pigment stones. Disorders that are associated with elevated levels of unconjugated bilirubin in bile include hemolytic syndromes, severe ileal dysfunction (or bypass), and bacterial contamination of the biliary tree.

Pathogenesis of Cholesterol Stones. Cholesterol is rendered soluble in bile by aggregation with water-soluble bile salts and water-insoluble lecithins, both of which act as detergents. *When cholesterol concentrations exceed the solubilizing capacity of bile (supersaturation), cholesterol can no longer remain dispersed and nucleates into solid cholesterol monohydrate crystals. Cholesterol gallstone formation involves four simultaneous defects* (Fig. 18–49):

- Bile must be supersaturated with cholesterol.
- Gallbladder hypomotility promotes nucleation.
- Cholesterol nucleation in bile is accelerated.
- Mucus hypersecretion in the gallbladder traps the crystals, permitting their aggregation into stones.

Supersaturation of bile with cholesterol is the result of hepatocellular hypersecretion of cholesterol. This appears to be a primary defect, mediated by abnormal regulation of hepatic mechanisms for delivering cholesterol to bile.[62] The abundant free cholesterol is toxic to the gallbladder, penetrating the wall and exceeding the ability of the mucosa to detoxify it by esterification. *Gallbladder hypomotility ensues.* Muscular stasis appears to result both from intrinsic neuromuscular dysmotility and from diminished muscular responsiveness to cholecystokinin, the hormone secreted by the gut that promotes gallbladder contraction. The relative composition of trace proteins in bile also may be altered, such that the balance of antinucleating and pronucleating proteins shifts in favor of *accelerated nucleation of cholesterol crystals.* Nucleation is further promoted by the presence of microprecipitates of inorganic or organic calcium salts. As a result of these events, supersaturated bile is sequestered in a hypomotile gallbladder under favorable nucleating conditions. *Hypersecretion of gallbladder mucus completes the tetralogy, as the cholesterol crystals are trapped for sustained periods, enabling their growth into macroscopic concretions.* Superimposed conditions exacerbate defective gallbladder emptying and the likelihood of forming cholesterol stones: prolonged fasting, pregnancy, rapid weight loss, total parenteral nutrition, and spinal cord injury.

Pathogenesis of Pigment Stones. Pigment gallstones are complex mixtures of abnormal insoluble calcium salts of unconjugated bilirubin along with inorganic calcium salts.[63] Unconjugated bilirubin is normally a minor component of bile but increases when infection of the biliary tract leads to release of microbial β-glucuronidases, which hydrolyze bilirubin glucuronides. Thus, infection of the biliary tract, as with *Escherichia coli* or *Ascaris lumbricoides* or by the liver fluke *Opisthorchis sinensis*, increases the likelihood of pigment stone

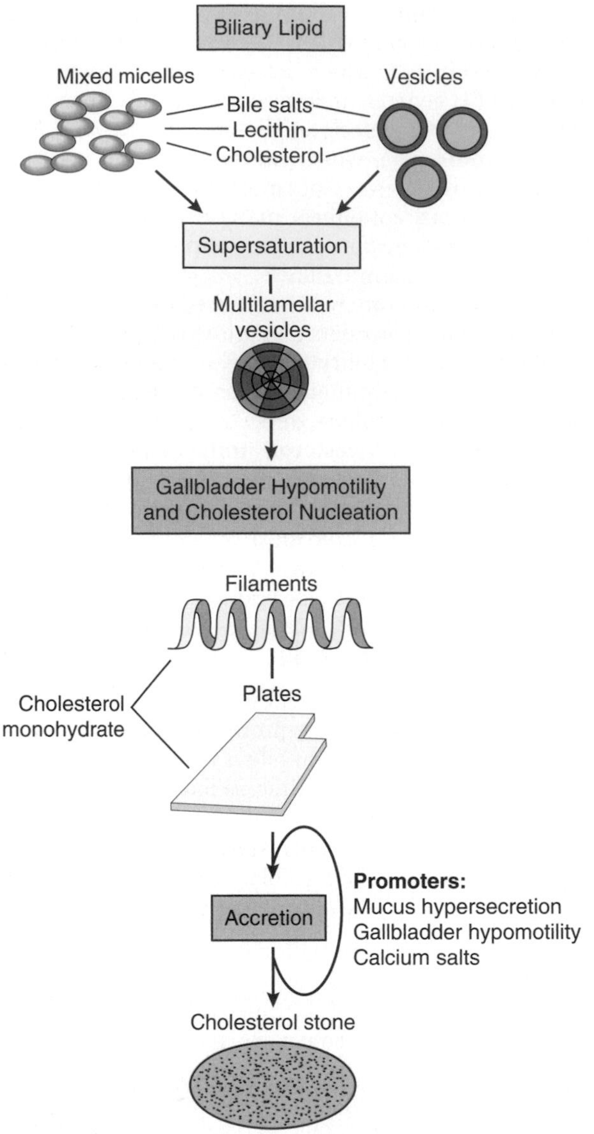

FIGURE 18–49 Schematic representation of the four contributing factors for cholelithiasis: supersaturation, gallbladder hypomotility, crystal nucleation, and accretion within the gallbladder mucous layer.

formation. Alternatively, intravascular hemolysis leads to increased hepatic secretion of conjugated bilirubin. Since a low level (about 1%) of bilirubin glucuronides are deconjugated in the biliary tree even normally, the aqueous solubility of free bilirubin may easily be exceeded under hemolytic conditions.

Morphology. Cholesterol stones arise exclusively in the gallbladder and are composed of cholesterol ranging from 100% pure (which is rare) down to around 50%. **Pure cholesterol stones** are pale yellow, round to ovoid, and have a finely granular, hard external surface (Fig. 18–50), which on transection reveals a glistening radiating crystalline palisade. With increasing proportions of calcium carbonate, phosphates, and bilirubin, the stones exhibit discoloration and may be lamellated and gray-white to black on transection. Most often, multiple stones are present that range up to several centimeters in diameter. Rarely, there is a single much larger stone that may virtually fill the fundus. Surfaces of multiple stones may be rounded or faceted, owing to tight apposition. **Stones composed largely of cholesterol are radiolucent; sufficient calcium carbonate is found in 10% to 20% of cholesterol stones to render them radio-opaque.**

Pigment gallstones are trivially classified as "black" and "brown." In general, black pigment stones are found in sterile gallbladder bile, and brown stones are found in infected intrahepatic or extrahepatic ducts. "Black" pigment stones contain oxidized polymers of the calcium salts of unconjugated bilirubin; lesser amounts of calcium carbonate, calcium phosphate, and mucin glycoprotein; and a modicum of cholesterol monohydrate crystals. "Brown" pigment stones contain pure calcium salts of unconjugated bilirubin, mucin glycoprotein, a substantial cholesterol fraction, and calcium salts of palmitate and stearate. The black stones are rarely greater than 1.5 cm in diameter, are almost invariably present in great number (with an inverse relationship between size and number; Fig. 18–51), and may crumble to the touch. Their contours are usually spiculated and molded. Brown stones tend to be laminated and soft and may have a soaplike or greasy consistency. Because of calcium carbonates and phosphates, **approximately 50% to 75% of black stones are radio-opaque.** Brown stones, which contain calcium soaps, are radiolucent. Mucin glycoproteins constitute the scaffolding and interparticle cement of all stones, whether pigment or cholesterol.

An incidental finding, pertinent to cholesterol biology, but not directly related to gallstone formation, is **cholesterolosis** (Chapter 1, Fig. 1–37). Cholesterol normally entering the gallbladder mucosa by free exchange with the lumen may be esterified by acyl CoA:cholesterol acyltransferase. Cholesterol hypersecretion by the liver promotes excessive accumulation of cholesterol esters within the lamina

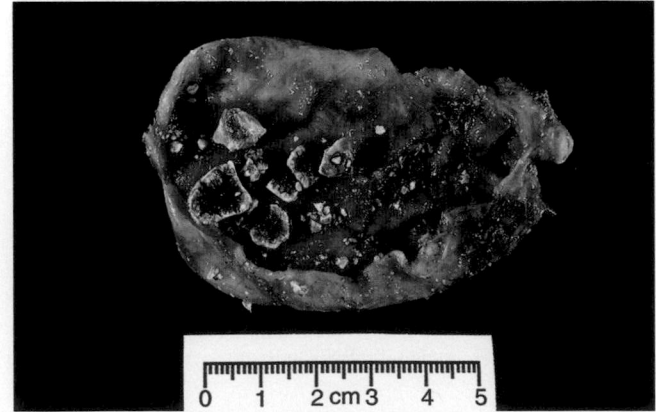

FIGURE 18–50 Cholesterol gallstones. Mechanical manipulation during laparoscopic cholecystectomy has caused fragmentation of several cholesterol gallstones, revealing interiors that are pigmented because of entrapped bile pigments. The gallbladder mucosa is reddened and irregular as a result of coexistent chronic cholecystitis.

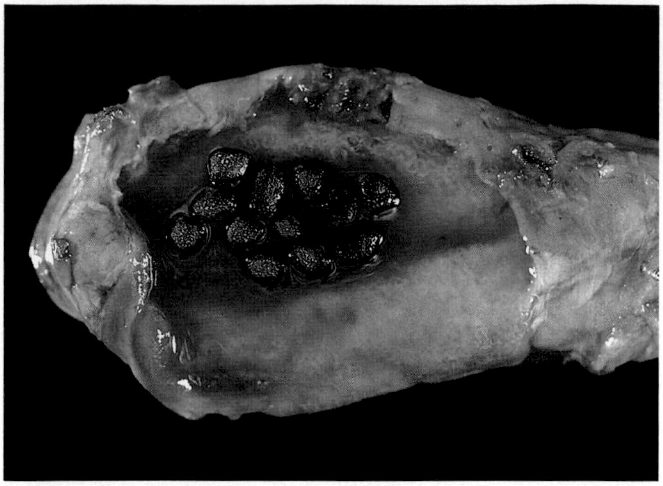

FIGURE 18–51 Pigment gallstones. Several faceted black gallstones are present in this otherwise unremarkable gallbladder from a patient with a mechanical mitral valve prosthesis, leading to chronic intravascular hemolysis.

propria of the gallbladder. The mucosal surface is studded with minute yellow flecks, producing the "strawberry gallbladder."

Clinical Features. Gallstones may be present for decades before symptoms develop, and 70% to 80% of patients remain asymptomatic throughout their lives. *It appears that asymptomatic patients convert to symptomatic ones at the rate of 1% to 3% per year, and the risk diminishes with time.*[64] Prominent among symptoms is biliary pain, which tends to be excruciating and constant or "colicky" (spasmodic), owing to the obstructive nature of gallstones in the biliary tree and perhaps in the gallbladder itself. Inflammation of the gallbladder (cholecystitis, discussed below), in association with stones, also generates pain. More severe complications include empyema, perforation, fistulae, inflammation of the biliary tree (cholangitis), and obstructive cholestasis or pancreatitis with ensuing problems. The larger the calculi, the less likely they are to enter the cystic or common ducts to produce obstruction; it is the very small stones, or "gravel," that are the more dangerous. Occasionally, a large stone may erode directly into an adjacent loop of small bowel, generating intestinal obstruction ("gallstone ileus"). Most notable is the increased risk for carcinoma of the gallbladder, discussed later.

CHOLECYSTITIS

Inflammation of the gallbladder may be acute, chronic, or acute superimposed on chronic. It almost always occurs in association with gallstones. In the United States, cholecystitis is one of the most common indications for abdominal surgery. Its epidemiologic distribution closely parallels that of gallstones.

Acute Cholecystitis

Acute calculous cholecystitis is an acute inflammation of the gallbladder, precipitated 90% of the time by obstruction of the neck or cystic duct. It is the primary complication of gallstones and the most common reason for emergency cholecystectomy. Acute acalculous cholecystitis occurs in the absence of gallstones, generally in the severely ill patient. Most cases of cholecystitis without gallstones occur in the following circumstances: (1) the postoperative state after major, nonbiliary surgery; (2) severe trauma (motor vehicle accidents, war injuries); (3) severe burns; (4) multisystem organ failure; (5) sepsis; (6) prolonged intravenous hyperalimentation; and (7) the postpartum state.

Pathogenesis. Acute calculous cholecystitis results from chemical irritation and inflammation of the obstructed gallbladder. The action of mucosal phospholipases hydrolyzes luminal lecithins to toxic lysolecithins. The normally protective glycoprotein mucus layer is disrupted, exposing the mucosal epithelium to the direct detergent action of bile salts. Prostaglandins released within the wall of the distended gallbladder contribute to mucosal and mural inflammation. Gallbladder dysmotility develops; distention and increased intraluminal pressure compromise blood flow to the mucosa. *These events occur in the absence of bacterial infection*; only later in the course may bacterial contamination develop.

Acute acalculous cholecystitis is thought to result from ischemia. The cystic artery is an end artery with essentially no collateral circulation. Contributing factors may include:[65]

- Dehydration and multiple blood transfusions, leading to a pigment load
- Gallbladder stasis, as may occur with hyperalimentation and assisted ventilation
- Accumulation of microcrystals of cholesterol (biliary sludge), viscous bile, and gallbladder mucus, causing cystic duct obstruction in the absence of frank stone formation
- Inflammation and edema of the wall, compromising blood flow
- Bacterial contamination and generation of lysolecithins

Morphology. In **acute cholecystitis**, the gallbladder is usually enlarged and tense, and it may assume a bright red or blotchy, violaceous to green-black discoloration, imparted by subserosal hemorrhages (Fig. 18–52). The serosal covering is frequently layered by fibrin and, in severe cases, by a definite suppurative, coagulated exudate. There are no specific morphologic differences between acute acalculous and calcu-

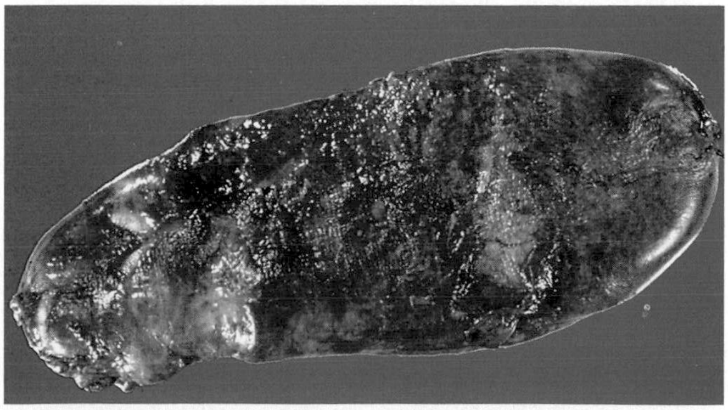

FIGURE 18–52 Acute calculous cholecystitis; the stone was not photographed.

lous cholecystitis, except for the absence of macroscopic stones in the former. In the latter instance, an obstructing stone is usually present in the neck of the gallbladder or the cystic duct. In addition to one or more stones, the gallbladder lumen is filled with a cloudy or turbid bile that may contain large amounts of fibrin and frank pus, as well as hemorrhage. When the contained exudate is virtually pure pus, the condition is referred to as **empyema of the gallbladder**. In mild cases, the gallbladder wall is thickened, edematous, and hyperemic. In more severe cases, it is transformed into a green-black necrotic organ, termed **gangrenous cholecystitis**, with small-to-large perforations. The inflammatory reactions are not histologically distinctive and consist of the usual patterns of acute inflammation, that is, edema, leukocytic infiltration, vascular congestion, frank abscess formation, or gangrenous necrosis.

Clinical Features. An attack of acute cholecystitis begins with progressive right upper quadrant or epigastric pain, frequently associated with mild fever, anorexia, tachycardia, sweating, and nausea and vomiting. The upper abdomen is tender, but a distended tender gallbladder is not usually evident. Most patients are free of jaundice; the presence of hyperbilirubinemia suggests obstruction of the common bile duct. Mild to moderate leukocytosis may be accompanied by mild elevations in serum alkaline phosphatase values.

Patients with acute calculous cholecystitis usually, but not always, have experienced previous episodes of biliary pain. *Acute calculous cholecystitis may appear with remarkable suddenness and constitute an acute surgical emergency or may present with mild symptoms that resolve without medical intervention.* In the absence of medical attention, the attack usually subsides in 7 to 10 days and frequently within 24 hours. However, up to 25% of patients develop progressively more severe symptoms, requiring immediate surgical intervention. In patients who recover, recurrence is common.

Clinical symptoms of acute acalculous cholecystitis tend to be more insidious, since symptoms are obscured by the underlying conditions precipitating the attacks. A higher proportion of patients have no symptoms referable to the gallbladder; diagnosis therefore rests on a high index of suspicion. In the severely ill patient, early recognition of this condition is crucial, since failure to do so almost ensures a fatal outcome. As a result of either delay in diagnosis or the disease itself, the incidence of gangrene and perforation is much higher than in calculous cholecystitis. In rare instances, primary bacterial infection can give rise to acute acalculous cholecystitis, including agents such as *Salmonella typhi* and staphylococci. The invasion of gas-forming organisms, notably clostridia and coliforms, may cause an acute "emphysematous" cholecystitis. A more indolent form of acute acalculous cholecystitis may occur in the outpatient population in the setting of systemic vasculitis, severe atherosclerotic ischemic disease in the elderly, and acquired immunodeficiency syndrome with biliary tract infection.[66]

Chronic Cholecystitis

Chronic cholecystitis may be a sequel to repeated bouts of mild to severe acute cholecystitis, but in many instances, it develops in the apparent absence of antecedent attacks. Since it is associated with cholelithiasis in over 90% of cases, the patient populations are the same as those for the latter condition. The evolution of chronic cholecystitis is obscure, in that it is not clear that gallstones play a direct role in the initiation of inflammation or the development of pain, particularly since chronic acalculous cholecystitis exhibits symptoms and histology similar to those of the calculous form. Rather, supersaturation of bile predisposes to both chronic inflammation and, in most instances, stone formation. Microorganisms, usually *E. coli* and enterococci, can be cultured from the bile in about one third of cases. Unlike acute calculous cholecystitis, obstruction of gallbladder outflow is not a requisite. Nevertheless, the symptoms of calculous chronic cholecystitis are similar to those of the acute form and range from biliary colic to indolent right upper quadrant pain and epigastric distress. Since most gallbladders that are removed at elective surgery for gallstones exhibit features of chronic cholecystitis, one must conclude that biliary symptoms often emerge following long-term coexistence of gallstones and low-grade inflammation.

Morphology. The morphologic changes in chronic cholecystitis are extremely variable and sometimes minimal. The serosa is usually smooth and glistening but may be dulled by subserosal fibrosis. Dense fibrous adhesions may remain as sequelae of preexistent acute inflammation. On sectioning, the wall is variably thickened, rarely to more than three times normal. The wall has an opaque gray-white appearance and may be less flexible than normal. In the uncomplicated case, the lumen contains fairly clear, green-yellow, mucoid bile and usually stones (Fig. 18–53). The mucosa itself is generally preserved.

On histologic examination, the degree of inflammation is variable. In the mildest cases, only scattered lymphocytes, plasma cells, and macrophages are found in the mucosa and in the subserosal fibrous tissue. In more developed cases, there is marked subepithelial and subserosal fibrosis, accompanied by

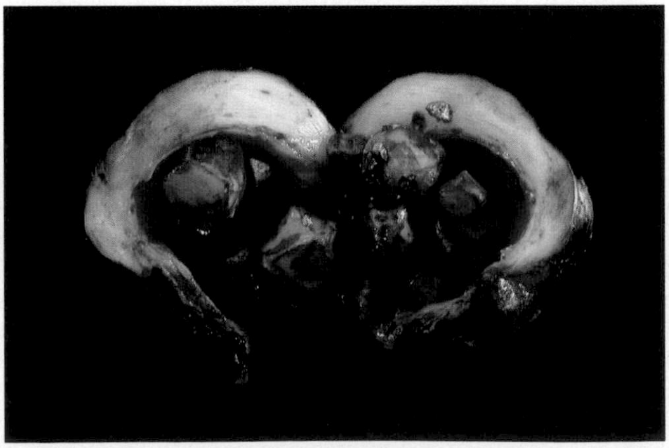

FIGURE 18–53 Chronic cholecystitis with cholesterol stones. The gallbladder wall is thickened and gray-white, owing to fibrosis and inflammation. The mucosa is effaced. Multiple faceted cholesterol gallstones are present within the lumen. The exterior of the specimen is black as a result of India ink application.

mononuclear cell infiltration. Reactive proliferation of the mucosa and fusion of the mucosal folds may give rise to buried crypts of epithelium within the gallbladder wall. Outpouchings of the mucosal epithelium through the wall (**Rokitansky-Aschoff sinuses**) may be quite prominent. Superimposition of acute inflammatory changes imply acute exacerbation of a previously chronically injured gallbladder.

In rare instances, extensive dystrophic calcification within the gallbladder wall may yield a **porcelain gallbladder**, notable for a markedly increased incidence of associated cancer. **Xanthogranulomatous cholecystitis** is also a rare condition in which the gallbladder is shrunken, nodular, and chronically inflamed with foci of necrosis and hemorrhage. Abundant macrophages packed with lipids are admixed with an exuberant fibrous tissue response, resulting in a massively thickened wall. Gallstones are usually present. This rare condition can be confused macroscopically with a malignant neoplasm. Finally, an atrophic, chronically obstructed gallbladder may contain only clear secretions, a condition known as **hydrops of the gallbladder**.

Clinical Features. Chronic cholecystitis does not have the striking manifestations of the acute forms and is usually characterized by recurrent attacks of either steady or colicky epigastric or right upper quadrant pain. Nausea, vomiting, and intolerance for fatty foods are frequent accompaniments.

Diagnosis of both acute and chronic cholecystitis is important because of the following complications:

- Bacterial superinfection with cholangitis or sepsis
- Gallbladder perforation and local abscess formation
- Gallbladder rupture with diffuse peritonitis
- Biliary enteric (cholecystenteric) fistula, with drainage of bile into adjacent organs, entry of air and bacteria into the biliary tree, and potentially gallstone-induced intestinal obstruction (ileus)
- Aggravation of pre-existing medical illness, with cardiac, pulmonary, renal, or liver decompensation

Disorders of the Extrahepatic Bile Ducts

CHOLEDOCHOLITHIASIS AND ASCENDING CHOLANGITIS

These conditions are considered together, since they frequently go hand in hand. *Choledocholithiasis is defined as the presence of stones within the bile ducts of the biliary tree*, as opposed to cholelithiasis (stones in the gallbladder). In Western nations, almost all biliary tract stones are derived from the gallbladder, although both cholesterol and pigmented stones can form de novo anywhere in the biliary tree. In Asia, there is a much higher incidence of primary stone formation within the biliary tree, usually pigmented as a result of the biliary tract infections noted earlier in the discussion of gallstones. Choledocholithiasis may be asymptomatic or may cause symptoms from (1) obstruction, (2) pancreatitis, (3) cholangitis, (4) hepatic abscess, (5) secondary biliary cirrhosis, and (6) acute calculous cholecystitis.

Cholangitis is the term used for bacterial infection of the bile ducts. Cholangitis can result from any lesion that creates obstruction to bile flow, most commonly choledocholithiasis. Uncommon causes include indwelling stents or catheters, tumors, acute pancreatitis, benign strictures, and rarely fungi, viruses, or parasites. Bacteria most likely enter the biliary tract through the sphincter of Oddi; infection of intrahepatic biliary radicals is termed *ascending cholangitis*. Bacteria (causing cholangitis) are usually enteric Gram-negative aerobes such as E. Coli, Klebsiella, Bacteroides or Enterobacter, Group D streptococci, and in some cases gram positive microbes like Clostridia. Cholangitis usually presents with fever, chills, abdominal pain, and jaundice, accompanied by acute inflammation of the wall of the bile ducts with entry of neutrophils into the luminal space. Intermittence of symptoms suggests bouts of partial obstruction. The most severe form of cholangitis is suppurative cholangitis, in which purulent bile fills and distends bile ducts. Since sepsis rather than cholestasis tends to dominate the picture, prompt diagnostic evaluation and intervention are imperative in these seriously ill patients.

BILIARY ATRESIA

The infant presenting with neonatal cholestasis has been discussed previously in the context of intrahepatic disorders. A major contributor to neonatal cholestasis is *biliary atresia*, representing one third of infants with neonatal cholestasis and occurring in approximately 1:10,000 live births. *Biliary atresia is defined as a complete obstruction of the lumen of the extrahepatic biliary tree within the first 3 months of life.*[67] It is the single most frequent cause of death from liver disease in early childhood and accounts for 50% to 60% of children referred for liver transplantation, owing to the rapidly progressing secondary biliary cirrhosis.

Pathogenesis. Two major forms of biliary atresia are recognized; they are based on the presumed timing of luminal obliteration. The *fetal form* accounts for up to 20% of cases and is commonly associated with other anomalies resulting from ineffective establishment of laterality of thoracic and abdominal organ development. These include malrotation of abdominal viscera, interrupted inferior vena cava, polysplenia, and congenital heart disease. The presumed cause is aberrant intrauterine development of the extrahepatic biliary tree. Much more common is the *perinatal form* of biliary atresia, in which a presumed normally developed biliary tree is destroyed following birth. Although the cause of perinatal biliary atresia remains unknown, viral infection has long been implicated, particularly reovirus and rotavirus. Genetic inheritance is also under scrutiny, given reports of biliary atresia occurring in twins and in families with anomalies of the intrahepatic biliary tree. Regardless, a "multihit" process is proposed in which viral or toxic insult to the biliary epithelium leads to destruction of the biliary tree.

Morphology. The salient features of biliary atresia include inflammation and fibrosing stricture of the hepatic or common bile ducts, periductular inflammation of intrahepatic bile ducts, and progressive destruction of the intrahepatic biliary tree (Fig. 18–54). On liver biopsy, florid features of extrahepatic biliary

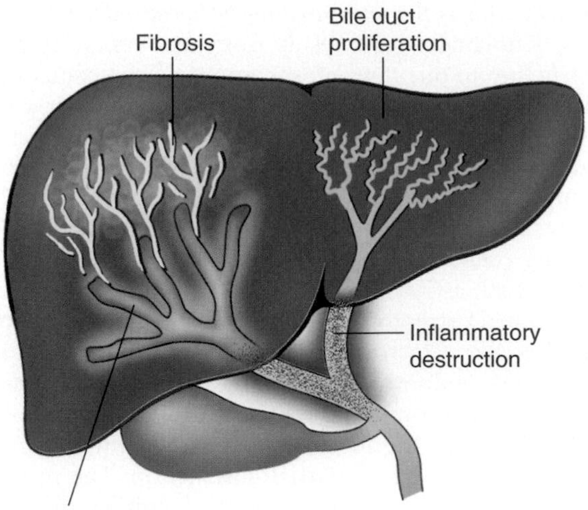

FIGURE 18–54 Biliary atresia, schematized to show the pattern of biliary tract injury.

obstruction are evident in about two thirds of cases, that is, marked bile ductular proliferation, portal tract edema and fibrosis, and parenchymal cholestasis. In the remainder, inflammatory destruction of intrahepatic ducts leads to paucity of bile ducts and absence of edema or bile ductular proliferation on liver biopsy. When biliary atresia is unrecognized or uncorrected, cirrhosis develops within 3 to 6 months of birth.

There is considerable variability in the anatomy of biliary atresia. When the disease is limited to the common (type I) or hepatic bile ducts (type II) with patent proximal branches, the disease is surgically correctable. Unfortunately, 90% of patients have type III biliary atresia, in which there also is obstruction of bile ducts at or above the porta hepatis. These cases are noncorrectable, since there are no patent bile ducts amenable to surgical anastomosis. Moreover, in most patients, bile ducts within the liver are initially patent but are progressively destroyed.

Clinical Features. Infants with biliary atresia present with neonatal cholestasis, discussed previously. These infants exhibit normal birth weight and postnatal weight gain, a slight female preponderance, and the progression of initially normal stools to acholic stools as the disease evolves. At the time of presentation, serum bilirubin values are usually in the 6 to 12 mg/dL range, with only moderately elevated aminotransferase and alkaline phosphatase levels. The success of surgical resection and bypass of the biliary tree is limited by subsequent bacterial contamination of the intrahepatic biliary tree and intrahepatic progression of the disease. Liver transplantation with accompanying donor bile ducts remains the primary hope for salvage of these young patients. Without surgical intervention, death usually occurs within 2 years of birth.

CHOLEDOCHAL CYSTS

Choledochal cysts are congenital dilations of the common bile duct, presenting most often in children before age 10 with the nonspecific symptoms of jaundice and/or recurrent abdominal pain that are typical of biliary colic. Approximately 20% of cases become symptomatic only in adulthood; these sometimes occur in conjunction with cystic dilation of the intrahepatic biliary tree (Caroli disease, discussed earlier). The female to male ratio is 3 to 4:1.[68] These uncommon cysts may take the form of segmental or cylindrical dilation of the common bile duct, diverticuli of the extrahepatic ducts, or choledochoceles, which are cystic lesions that protrude into the duodenal lumen. Choledochal cysts predispose to stone formation, stenosis and stricture, pancreatitis, and obstructive biliary complications within the liver. In the older patient, the risk of bile duct carcinoma is elevated.

Tumors

Although heterotopic tissues and carcinoids, fibromas, myomas, neuromas, hemangiomas, and their malignant counterparts have been described in the biliary tract, the neoplasms of primary clinical importance are those derived from the epithelium lining the biliary tree.[69] Adenomas are benign epithelial tumors, representing localized neoplastic growth of the lining epithelium. Adenomas are classified as tubular, papillary, and tubulopapillary and are similar to adenomas found elsewhere in the alimentary tract. *Inflammatory polyps* are sessile mucosal projections with a surface stroma infiltrated with chronic inflammatory cells and lipid-laden macrophages. These lesions may be difficult to differentiate from neoplasms on imaging studies. *Adenomyosis* of the gallbladder is characterized by hyperplasia of the muscularis, containing intramural hyperplastic glands.

CARCINOMA OF THE GALLBLADDER

Carcinoma of the gallbladder is slightly more common in women and occurs most frequently in the seventh decade of life. Only rarely is it discovered at a resectable stage, and the mean 5-year survival rate has remained for many years at about 1%, despite surgical intervention.[70] Gallstones are present in 60% to 90% of cases. In Asia, where pyogenic and parasitic diseases of the biliary tree are common, the coexistence of gallstones is much lower. Presumably, gallbladders containing stones or infectious agents develop cancer as a result of irritative trauma and chronic inflammation. Carcinogenic derivatives of bile acids also may play a role.

Morphology. Carcinomas of the gallbladder exhibit two patterns of growth: **infiltrating** and **exophytic**. The infiltrating pattern is more common and usually appears as a poorly defined area of diffuse thickening and induration of the gallbladder wall that may cover several square centimeters or may involve the entire gallbladder. Deep ulceration can cause direct penetration of the gallbladder wall or fistula formation to adjacent viscera into which the neoplasm has grown. These tumors are scirrhous and have a very firm consistency. The exophytic pattern grows into the lumen as an irregular, cauliflower mass but at the same time invades the underlying wall. The luminal portion may be necrotic, hemorrhagic, and ulcerated (Fig. 18–55*A*). The most common sites of involvement are the fundus and the neck; about 20% involve the lateral walls.

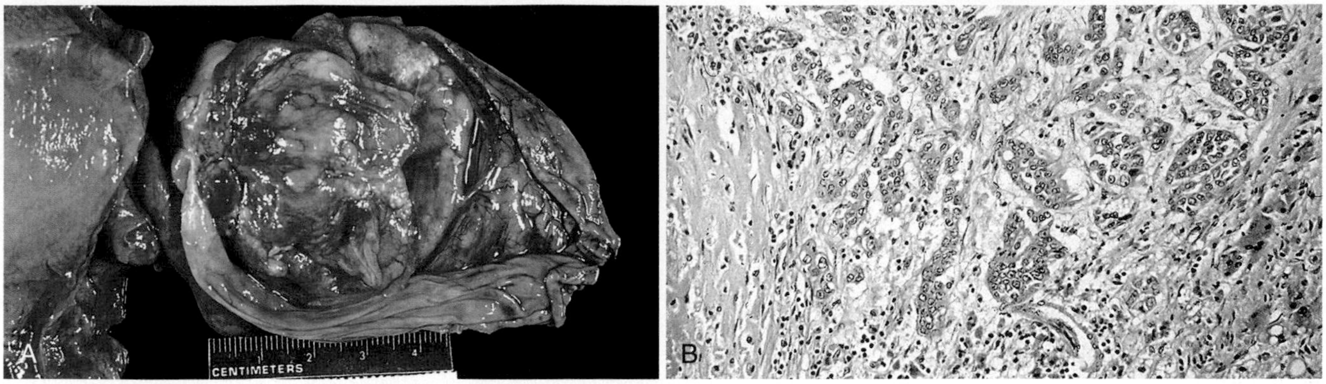

FIGURE 18–55 Gallbladder adenocarcinoma. *A,* The opened gallbladder contains a large, exophytic tumor that virtually fills the lumen. *B,* Malignant glandular structures are present within a densely fibrotic gallbladder wall.

Most carcinomas of the gallbladder are adenocarcinomas. Some are papillary in architecture and are well to moderately differentiated; others are infiltrative and poorly differentiated to undifferentiated (Fig. 18–55*B*). About 5% are squamous cell carcinomas or have adenosquamous differentiation. A minority may exhibit carcinoid or a variety of mesenchymal features. By the time these neoplasms are discovered, **most have invaded the liver centrifugally**, and many have extended to the cystic duct and adjacent bile ducts and portahepatic lymph nodes. The peritoneum, gastrointestinal tract, and lungs are common sites of seeding.

Clinical Features. Preoperative diagnosis of carcinoma of the gallbladder is the exception rather than the rule, occurring in fewer than 20% of patients. Presenting symptoms are insidious and typically indistinguishable from those associated with cholelithiasis: abdominal pain, jaundice, anorexia, and nausea and vomiting. The fortunate patient will develop a palpable gallbladder and acute cholecystitis before extension of the tumor into adjacent structures or will have incidental carcinoma at the time of cholecystectomy for symptomatic gallstones.

CARCINOMA OF THE EXTRAHEPATIC BILE DUCTS

Carcinomas of the extrahepatic biliary tree, down to the level of the ampulla of Vater, are uncommon tumors. They are extremely insidious tumors and generally produce painless, progressively deepening jaundice. They occur in older individuals and, unlike cancers of the gallbladder, occur slightly more frequently in men. Gallstones are present in only about a third of cases. As with intrahepatic biliary tract carcinomas (cholangiocarcinoma), risk is increased in patients with primary sclerosing cholangitis, ulcerative colitis, and cystic liver diseases (especially Caroli disease and choledochal cysts) and, in Asia, from biliary tree fluke infections (such as *Clonorchis sinensis*).

A subgroup of biliary tree carcinomas are those arising in the immediate vicinity of the ampulla of Vater. Tumors of this region also include adenomas of the duodenal mucosa and pancreatic carcinoma (discussed in Chapters 17 and 19, respectively). Collectively, these tumors are referred to as periampullary carcinomas, and all are treated by surgical resection.

Morphology. Because partial or complete obstruction of bile ducts rapidly leads to jaundice, these tumors are generally small lesions at the time of diagnosis. Most tumors appear as firm, gray nodules within the bile duct wall; some may be diffusely infiltrative lesions; others are papillary, polypoid lesions. Most bile duct tumors are adenocarcinomas that may or may not be mucin-secreting. Uncommonly, squamous features are present. For the most part, an abundant fibrous stroma accompanies the epithelial proliferation. Tumors arising from the part of the common bile duct between the cystic duct junction and the confluence of the right and left hepatic ducts at the liver hilus are called **Klatskin tumors.**[71] These tumors are notable for their slow-growing behavior, marked sclerosing characteristics, and the infrequent occurrence of distal metastases.

Clinical Features. Jaundice generally arises because of obstruction, often preceded by decolorization of the stools, nausea and vomiting, and weight loss. Hepatomegaly is present in about 50%, and a palpable gallbladder is present in about 25%. Associated changes are elevated levels of serum alkaline phosphatase and aminotransferases and bile-stained urine. Differentiation of obstructive jaundice due to calculous disease or other benign conditions versus neoplasia is a major clinical problem, since the presence of stones does not preclude the existence of concomitant malignancy. The majority of ductal cancers are not surgically resectable at the time of diagnosis, despite their small size. Mean survival times range from 6 to 18 months.

Iatrogenic Injury to the Biliary Tree

As a hollow viscus lying adjacent to the liver, the gallbladder is the occasional recipient of a needle thrust from percutaneous liver biopsy or transhepatic cholangiography. Needles are also intentionally introduced for diagnostic and therapeutic procedures. Reconstruction of the biliary tree following liver transplantation, particularly using the living-related specimens, might not be entirely free of bile leakage. In each instance, leaks of irritant bile into the peritoneum can give rise to chemically induced inflammation, so-called *bile peritonitis*.

Repeated infusion of chemotherapeutic agents into the hepatic artery for metastatic liver disease can cause iatrogenic *drug injury*. Since the intrahepatic and extrahepatic bile ducts and gallbladder are sustained by branches of this artery, chemically induced arterial obliteration can lead to a sclerosing cholangitis-like picture in the biliary tree with loss of intrahepatic bile ducts or to an acute cholecystitis progressing to chronic fibrosis.[72] *Biliary stricture* most commonly follows operative trauma, involving iatrogenic injury to the biliary tree or the feeding vasculature. This is a particular concern with laparoscopic cholecystectomy, in which the common bile duct may be compromised during mobilization and resection of the gallbladder. Fewer than 10% of strictures of the common bile duct are caused by pancreatitis, external trauma, and other rare causes. Strictures of the common hepatic duct proximal to the cystic duct are usually malignant.

REFERENCES

1. Saxena R, Theise ND, Crawford JM: Microanatomy of the human liver: exploring the hidden interfaces. Hepatology 30:1339–1346, 1999.
2. Jungermann K, Kietzmann T: Zonation of parenchymal and non-parenchymal metabolism in liver. Annu Rev Nutr 16:179–203, 1996.
3. Crawford JM: Development of the intrahepatic biliary tree. Semin Liver Dis 22:213–226, 2002.
4. Kim WR, Brown RS, Terrault NA, El-Serag HH: Burden of liver disease in the United States: summary of a workshop. Hepatology 36:227–242, 2002.
5. Butterworth RF: Complications of cirrhosis. III: Hepatic encephalopathy. J Hepatol 32 (Suppl 1):171–180, 2000.
6. Arroyo V, Guevara M, Gines P: Hepatorenal syndrome in cirrhosis: pathogenesis and treatment. Gastroenterology 122:1658–1676, 2002.
7. Crawford JM: Cirrhosis. In MacSween RNM, Anthony PP, Scheuer PJ, Burt AD, Portmann BC (eds): Pathology of the Liver, 4th ed. Philadelphia,WB Saunders, 2001, pp 575–619.
8. Wong F, Blendis L: The pathophysiologic basis for the treatment of cirrhotic ascites. Clin Liver Dis 10:819–832, 2001.
9. Van Erpecum KJ, van Berge Henegouwen GP: Intestinal aspects of cholesterol formation. Dig Liver Dis 35:58, 2003.
10. Crawford JM: Bilirubin metabolism and the pathophysiology of jaundice. In Maddrey WC, Sorrell MF, Schiff ER (eds): Diseases of the Liver, 9th ed. Philadelphia, WB Saunders, 2002, pp 167–220.
11. Kadakol A, Ghosh SS, Sappal BS, Sharma G, Chowdhury JR, Chowdhury NR: Genetic lesions of bilirubin uridine-diphosphoglucuronate glucuronosyltransferase (UGT1A1) causing Crigler-Najjar and Gilbert syndromes: correlation of genotype to phenotype. Hum Mutat 16:297–306, 2000.
12. Toh S, Wada M, Uchiumi T, Inokuchi A, Makino Y, Horie Y, Adachi Y, Sakisaka S, Kuwano M: Genomic structure of the canalicular multispecific organic anion-transporter gene (*MRP2/cMOAT*) and mutations in the ATP-binding-cassette region in Dubin-Johnson syndrome. Am J Hum Genet 64:739–746, 1999.
13. Sokol RJ, Feranchak AP: Genetic and metabolic basis of pediatric liver diseases. Semin Liver Dis 21:469–571, 2001.
14. Ishak KG: Pathologic features of chronic hepatitis: a review and update. Am J Clin Pathol 113:40–55, 2000.
15. Pawlotsky JM: Molecular diagnosis of viral hepatitis. Gastroenterology 122:1554–1568, 2002.
16. Cuthbert JA: Hepatitis A: old and new. Clin Microbiol Rev 14:38–58, 2001.
17. Ganem D, Prince AM: Hepatitis B virus infection—natural history and clinical consequences. N Engl J Med 350:11, 2004.
18. Chisari FV: Viruses, immunity and cancer: lessons from hepatitis B. Am J Pathol 156:1118–1132, 2000.
19. Rooney G, Gilson RJC: Sexual transmission of hepatitis C virus infection. Sex Transm Infect 1998; 74:399–404.
20. Farci P, Purcell RH: Clinical significance of hepatitis C virus genotypes and quasispecies. Semin Liver Dis 20:103–126, 2000.
21. Taylor DR: Hepatitis C virus: evasion of the interferon-induced antiviral response. J Mol Med 78:182–190, 2000.
22. Hoofnagle JH: Type D (delta) hepatitis. JAMA 261:1321–1325, 1989.
23. Lai MMC: The molecular biology of hepatitis delta virus. Annu Rev Biochem 64:259–286, 1995.
24. Mast EE, Krawczynski K: Hepatitis E: An overview. Annu Rev Med 47:257–266, 1996.
24a. Pomerantz RJ, Nunnari G: HIV and GB virus C—can two viruses be better than one? N Engl J Med 350:963, 2004.
25. Sell S. Heterogeneity and plasticity of hepatocyte lineage cells. Hepatology 33:38–50, 2001.
26. Czaja AJ, Freese DK: Diagnosis and treatment of autoimmune hepatitis. Hepatology 36:479–497, 2002.
27. Farrell GC, Liddle C: Hepatotoxicity in the twenty-first century. Semin Liver Dis 22:109–206, 2002.
28. Carithers RL Jr: Alcoholic hepatitis and cirrhosis. In Kaplowitz N (ed): Liver and Biliary Diseases. Baltimore, Williams and Wilkins, 1992, pp 334–346.
29. Tsukamoto H, Lu SC: Current concepts in the pathogenesis of alcoholic liver injury. FASEB J 15:1335–1349, 2001.
30. Clark JM, Brancati FL, Diehl AM: Nonalcoholic fatty liver disease. Gastroenterology 122:1649–1657, 2002.
31. Fletcher LM, Halliday JW: Haemochromatosis: understanding the mechanism of disease and implications for diagnosis and patient management following the recent cloning of novel genes involved in iron metabolism. J Intern Med 251:181–192, 2002.
32. Philpott CC: Molecular aspects of iron absorption: insights into the role of HFE in hemochromatosis. Hepatology 35:993–1001, 2002.
33. Pietrangelo A: Physiology of iron transport and the hemochromatosis gene. Am J Physiol 282:G403–G414, 2001.
34. Moyo VM, Mandishona E, Hasstedt SJ, et al: Evidence of genetic transmission in African iron overload. Blood 91:1076–1082, 1998.
35. Llanos RM, Mercer JF: The molecular basis of copper homeostasis copper-related disorders. DNA Cell Biol 21:259–270, 2002.
36. Teckman JH, An JK, Loethen S, Perlmutter DH: Fasting in alpha1-antitrypsin deficient liver: consultative activation of autophagy. Am J Physiol 283:G1156–G1165, 2002.
37. Perlmutter DH: Liver injury in alpha1-antitrypsin deficiency: an aggregated protein induces mitochondrial injury. J Clin Invest 110:1579, 2002.
38. Andres JM: Neonatal hepatobiliary disorders. Clin Perinatol 23:321–352, 1996.
39. McEvoy CF, Suchy FJ: Biliary tract disease in children. Pediatr Clin North Am 43:75–98, 1996.
40. Kita H, Nalbandian G, Keeffe EB, Coppel RL: Gershwin: Pathogenesis of primary biliary cirrhosis. Clin Liver Dis 7:821, 2003.
41. Mackay IR, Whittingham S, Fida S, et al: The peculiar autoimmunity of primary biliary cirrhosis. Immunol Rev 174:226, 2000.
42. Vierling JM: Animal models for primary sclerosing cholangitis. Best Pract Res Clin Gastroenterol 15:591–610, 2001.
43. Desmet VJ: Pathogenesis of ductal plate abnormalities. Mayo Clin Proc 73:80–89, 1998.
44. Onuchic LF, Furu L, Nagasawa I, et al: PKHD1, the polycystic kidney and hepatic disease 1 gene, encodes a novel large protein containing multiple immunoglobulin-like plexin-transcription-factor domains and parallel beta-helix 1 repeats. Am J Hum Genet 70:1305–1317, 2002.
45. Piccoli DA, Spinner NB: Alagille syndrome and the Jagged1 gene. Semin Liver Dis 21:525–534, 2001.
46. Sarin SK, Agarwal SR: Extrahepatic portal vein obstruction. Semin Liver Dis 22:43–58, 2002.
47. DeLeve LD, Shulman HM, McDonald GB: Toxic injury to hepatic sinusoids: sinusoidal obstruction syndrome (veno-occlusive disease). Semin Liver Dis 22:27–41, 2002.
48. Rychel V, Williams KP: Correlation of platelet count changes with liver cell destruction in HELLP syndrome. Hypertens Pregnancy 22:57, 2003.
49. Maitra A, Domiati-Saad R, Yost N, et al: Absence of the G1528C (E474Q) mutation in the alpha-subunit of the mitochondrial trifunctional protein in women with acute fatty liver of pregnancy. Pediatr Res 51:658–661, 2002.
50. Reyes H, Sjovall J: Bile acids and progesterone metabolites in intrahepatic cholestasis of pregnancy. Ann Med 32:94–106,2000.
51. Starzl TE, Murase N, Demetris A, Trucco M, Fung J: The mystique of hepatic tolerogenicity. Semin Liver Dis 2000; 20:497–510.

52. Ng IOL, Burroughs AK, Rolles K, Belli LS, Scheuer PJ: Hepatocellular ballooning after liver transplantation: a light and electronmicroscopic study with clinicopathological correlation. Histopathology 18:323–330, 1991.
53. Wanless IR: Benign liver tumors. Clin Liver Dis 6:513, 2002.
54. Taniguchi K, Roberts LR, Aderca IN, Dong X, Qian C, Murphy LM, Nagorney DM, Burgart LJ, Roche PC, Smith DI, Ross JA, Liu W: Mutational spectrum of beta-catenin, AXIN1, and AXIN2 in hepatocellular carcinomas and hepatoblastomas. Oncogene 21:4863–4871, 2002.
55. Monto A, Wright TL: The epidemiology and prevention of hepatocellular carcinoma. Semin Oncol 28:441–449, 2001.
56. El-Serag HB: Hepatocellular carcinoma: an epidemiologic view. J Clin Gastroenterology 35 (5, Suppl 2):S72–S78, 2002.
57. Koike K, Tsutsumi T, Fujie H, et al: Molecular mechanism of viral hepatocarcinogenesis. Oncology 62 (Suppl 1):29–37, 2002.
58. Feitelson MA, Sun B, Satiroglu NL, et al: Genetic mechanisms of hepatocarcinogenesis. Oncogene 21:2593–2604, 2002.
58a. Montesano R: Hepatitis B immunization and hepatocellular carcinoma: the Gambia Hepatitis Intervention Study. J Med Virol 67:444, 2002.
59. Llovet JM, Beaugrand M: Hepatocellular carcinoma: present status and future prospects. J Hepatol 38:S136, 2003.
60. Gibbons A: Geneticists trace the DNA trail of the first Americans. Science 259:312–313, 1993.
61. Lamert F, Carey MC, Paigen B: Chromosomal organization of candidate genes involved in cholesterol gallstone formation: a murine gallstone map. Gastroenterology 120:221–238, 2001.
62. Ko CW, Lee SP: Epidemiology and natural history of common bile duct stones and prediction of disease. Gastrointest Endosc 56:S165, 2002.
63. Stewart L, Oesterle Al, Erdan I, Griffiss JM, Way LW: Pathogenesis of pigment gallstones in Western societies: the central role of bacteria. J Gastrointest Surg 6:891, 2002.
64. Malet PF: Complications of cholelithiasis. In Kaplowitz N (ed): Liver and Biliary Diseases, 2nd ed. Baltimore, Williams and Wilkins, 1996, pp 673–691.
65. Barie PS, Eachempati SP: Acute acalculous cholecystitis. Curr Gastroenterol Rep 5:302, 2003.
66. Ryu JK, Ryu KH, Kim KH: Clinical features of acute acalculous cholecystitis. J Clin Gastroenterol 36:166, 2003.
67. Sokol RJ, Mack C: Etiopathogenesis of biliary atresia. Semin Liver Dis 21: 517–524, 2001.
68. Oldham KT, Hart MJ, White TT: Choledochal cysts presenting in late childhood and adulthood. Am J Surg 141:568–571, 1981.
69. Albores-Saavedra J, Henson DE, Sobin LH: The WHO Histological Classification of Tumors of the Gallbladder and Extrahepatic Bile Ducts: a commentary on the second edition. Cancer 70:410–414, 1992.
70. Misra S, Chaturvedi A, Misra NC, Sharma ID: Carcinoma of the gallbladder. Lancet Oncol 4:167, 2003.
71. Knoefel WT, Prenzel KL, Peiper M, et al.: Klatskin tumors and Klatskin mimicking lesions of the biliary tree. Eur J Surg Oncol 29:658, 2003.
72. Barnett KT, Malafa MP: Complications of hepatic artery infusion: a review of 4580 reported cases. Int J Gastrointest Cancer 30:147, 2001.

CHAPTER 19

The Pancreas

Ralph H. Hruban, MD • Robb E. Wilentz, MD

CONGENITAL ANOMALIES
Agenesis
Pancreas Divisum
Annular Pancreas
Ectopic Pancreas
PANCREATITIS
Acute Pancreatitis
Chronic Pancreatitis
NON-NEOPLASTIC CYSTS
Congenital Cysts
Pseudocysts
NEOPLASMS
Cystic Neoplasms
Pancreatic Carcinoma
Precursors to Pancreatic Cancer
Molecular Carcinogenesis
Pancreatoblastoma

Normal

The pancreas has important endocrine and exocrine functions, and diseases of the pancreas cause significant morbidity and mortality. Despite the physiologic importance of the pancreas, the retroperitoneal location of the gland and the vague signs and symptoms associated with injury to the gland allow many diseases to progress relatively unnoticed for extended periods of time. Diseases of the pancreas thus remain a continuing source of frustration in modern medicine.

The adult pancreas is a transversely oriented retroperitoneal organ extending from the "C" loop of the duodenum to the hilum of the spleen (Fig. 19–1). On average, the pancreas measures 20 cm in length and weighs 90 gm in men and 85 gm in women.[1] Although the pancreas does not have well-defined anatomic subdivisions, the adjacent vasculature can be used to separate the pancreas into three parts: the head, body, and tail.

The pancreatic duct system is highly variable. The main pancreatic duct, also known as the duct of Wirsung, most commonly drains into the duodenum at the papilla of Vater, whereas the accessory pancreatic duct, also known as the duct of Santorini, most often drains into the duodenum through a separate minor papilla approximately 2 cm cephalad (proximal) to the major papilla of Vater (Fig. 19–2*A*). In many adults, the main pancreatic duct merges with the common bile duct proximal to the papilla of Vater, thus creating the ampulla of Vater, a common channel for biliary and pancreatic drainage. Owing to developmental variability, however, this ductal architecture can differ tremendously from patient to patient.

Embryologically, the pancreas arises from the fusion of dorsal and ventral outpouchings of the foregut.[1] During early embryonic development, the dorsal and ventral pancreatic primordia rotate and fuse at approximately the seventh week of gestation to form a single gland.[2] The majority of the gland, including the body, the tail, the superior/anterior aspect of the head, and the accessory duct of Santorini, is derived from the dorsal primordium. Although the ventral primordium gives rise only to the posterior/inferior part of the head of the pancreas, the ventral primordium is important because it drains into the papilla of Vater. Fusion of the dorsal and ventral duct systems allows the majority of the gland to drain through the larger Vaterian papilla.

Although the organ gets its name from the Greek *pankreas*, meaning "all flesh," the pancreas is, in fact, a complex lobulated organ with distinct exocrine and endocrine components. The exocrine portion of the gland, which produces digestive

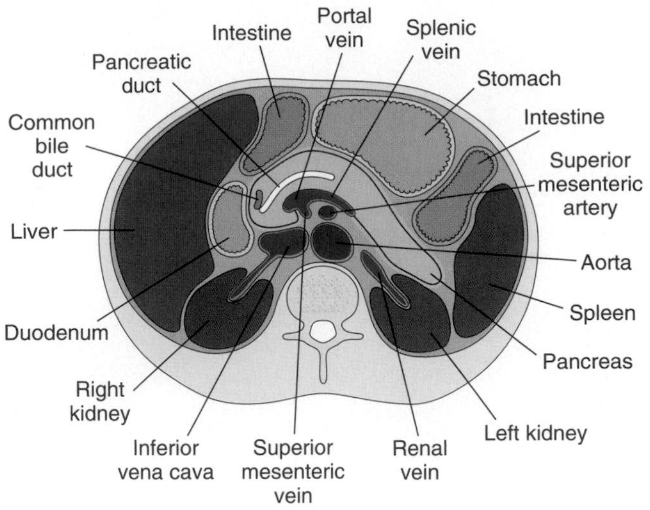

FIGURE 19–1 Anatomic relationships of the pancreas seen in a cross-section of the abdomen at the level of the upper lumbar vertebrae. (From Go VW, et al (eds): The Pancreas: Biology, Pathobiology, and Disease, 2nd ed. New York, Raven Press, 1993.)

enzymes, constitutes 80% to 85% of the pancreas. The endocrine portion is composed of about 1 million clusters of cells, the islets of Langerhans. The islet cells secrete insulin, glucagon, and somatostatin and constitute only 1% to 2% of the organ. Diseases of the endocrine pancreas are described in detail in Chapter 24.

The exocrine pancreas is composed of acinar cells, which produce the enzymes needed for digestion, and a series of ductules and ducts to convey the secretions to the duodenum.[1] Acinar cells are pyramidally shaped epithelial cells that are radially oriented around a central lumen (Fig. 19–3). The basal portion of acinar cells is deeply basophilic and contains abundant endoplasmic reticulum. Acinar cells also contain a well-developed supranuclear Golgi complex that is part of an apically (luminally) oriented secretory pathway that forms membrane-bound zymogen granules containing the digestive enzymes. The zymogen granules impart a distinctive eosinophilic granular appearance to the apices of acinar cells. When the acinar cells are stimulated to secrete, the zymogen-containing granules migrate apically, fuse with the apical plasma membrane, and release their contents into the central acinar lumen.

These secretions are then transported to the duodenum through a series of anastomosing ducts. Interestingly, the epithelial cells lining the ducts are also active participants in pancreatic secretion. Smaller ductules lined by cuboidal epithelial cells secrete a fluid rich in bicarbonate. The epithelial cells lining the larger ducts are more columnar and can produce mucin. In addition, the epithelial cells of the larger pancreatic ducts express the cystic fibrosis transmembrane conductance regulator, which plays a significant role in the pathophysiology of pancreatic disease in patients with cystic fibrosis (Chapter 10).

The pancreas secretes 2 to 2.5 liters per day of a bicarbonate-rich fluid containing digestive enzymes and proenzymes. Regulation of this secretion involves both neural stimulation mediated by vagal nerves (acetylcholine) and humoral factors. The most important of the latter are the hormones *secretin* and *cholecystokinin*, produced in the duodenum. Secretin stimulates water and bicarbonate secretion by duct cells, and cholecystokinin promotes the discharge of digestive proenzymes by acinar cells. The primary stimulants of duodenal secretin production are an acid load from the gastric effluent and the presence of luminal fatty acids. Cholecystokinin is

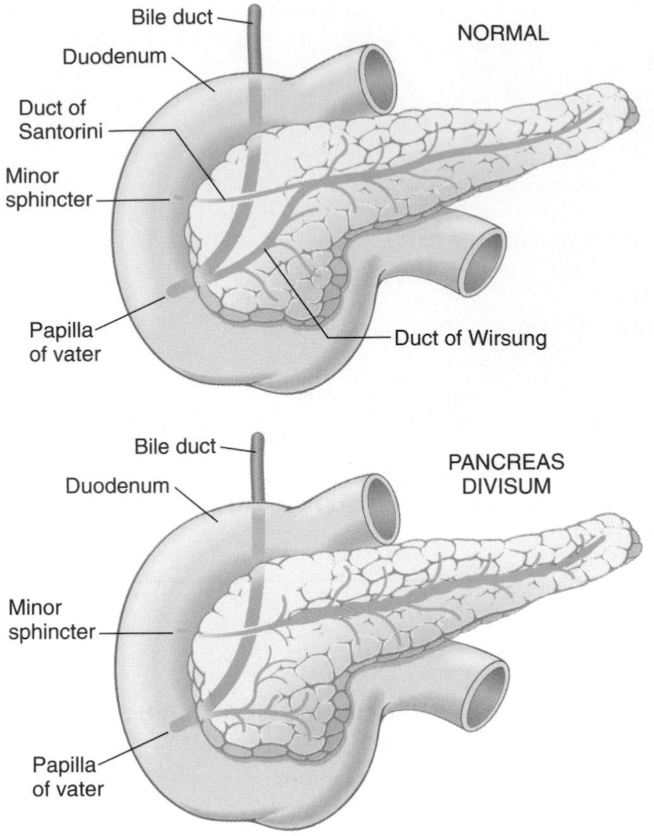

FIGURE 19–2 Pancreatic ductal anatomy. *A*, The normal ductal anatomy. *B*, The ductal anatomy in pancreatic divisum. (Adapted from Gregg JA, Monaco AP, McDermott WV: Pancreas divisum: results of surgical intervention. Am J Surg 145:488–492, 1983.)

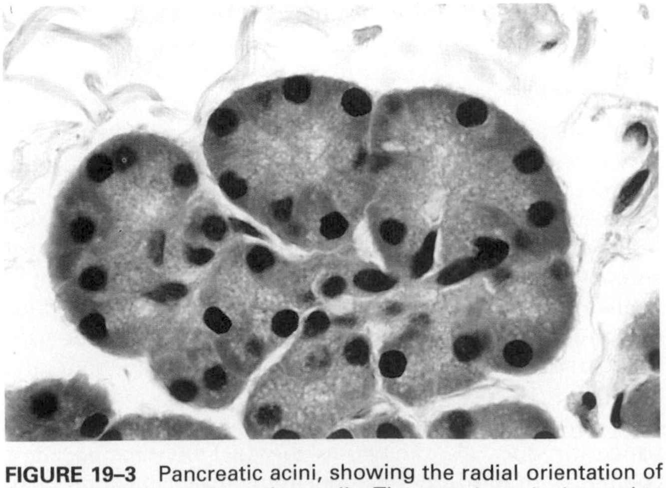

FIGURE 19–3 Pancreatic acini, showing the radial orientation of the pyramidal exocrine acinar cells. The cytoplasm is devoted to the synthesis and packaging of digestive enzymes for secretion into a central lumen.

released from the duodenal mucosa predominantly in response to fatty acids and protein digestive products: peptides and amino acids.

In general, the pancreas secretes its exocrine products as enzymatically inert proenzymes both to prevent self-digestion and to efficiently utilize the enzymes within the lumen of the duodenum. The proenzymes produced by the pancreas include trypsinogen, chymotrypsinogen, procarboxypeptidase, proelastase, kallikreinogen, and prophospholipase A and B.[1] These proenzymes remain inactive until they reach the lumen of the duodenum, where the brush border enzyme, enteropeptidase, cleaves trypsinogen into its active form trypsin. Activated trypsin then plays a key role in catalyzing the cleavage of the other proenzymes to yield active chymotrypsin, carboxypeptidase, elastase, kallikrein, and phospholipase A and B. The enzymes amylase and lipase, however, do not require trypsin activation and are secreted in an active form. The self-digestion of the pancreas is thus prevented at a number of levels:

- The majority of the enzymes are synthesized as inactive proenzymes (with the exception of amylase and lipase).
- The enzymes are sequestered in membrane-bound zymogen granules in the acinar cells.
- Activation of proenzymes requires conversion of inactive trypsinogen to active trypsin by duodenal enteropeptidase (enterokinase).
- Trypsin inhibitors including serine protease inhibitor Kazal type l (SPINK1 or PSTI) are present within acinar and ductal secretions.
- Trypsin contains a critical self-recognition cleavage site that allows trypsin to inactivate itself.
- Lysosomal hydrolases are capable of degrading zymogen granules when normal acinar secretion is impaired or blocked.
- Acinar cells are remarkably resistant to the action of trypsin, chymotrypsin, and phospholipase A_2.

Pathology

The most significant disorders of the *endocrine* pancreas include diabetes mellitus and neoplasms (Chapter 24). Diseases of *exocrine* pancreas include cystic fibrosis, congenital anomalies, acute and chronic pancreatitis, and neoplasms. Cystic fibrosis is discussed in detail in Chapter 10. The remainder of this chapter will discuss the other pathologic processes specific to the exocrine pancreas.

Congenital Anomalies

The complex process by which the dorsal and ventral pancreatic primordia fuse during pancreatic development frequently gives rise to congenital variations in pancreatic anatomy. Most of these do not directly cause disease; however, such variations, especially in ductal anatomy, may present particular problems to the endoscopist and surgeons. For example, failure to recognize aberrant ductal anatomy may lead to the inadvertent severance of a pancreatic duct during surgery, causing serious sequelae such as pancreatitis.

AGENESIS

Very rarely, the pancreas may be totally absent (agenesis), a condition associated with widespread severe malformations that are usually incompatible with life. The homeodomain transcription factor IPF1 (PDX1) is critical for the development of the pancreas, and germ line (inherited) homozygous mutations in the *IPF1* gene on chromosome 13q12.1 have been reported in a patient with pancreatic agenesis.[3]

PANCREAS DIVISUM

Pancreas divisum is the most common clinically significant congenital anomaly of the pancreas, with an incidence of 3% to 10%.[4] This anomaly is caused by a failure of the fetal duct systems of the dorsal and ventral pancreatic primordia to fuse.[5] As a result, the bulk of the pancreas (formed by the dorsal pancreatic primordium) drains through the dorsal pancreatic duct and the *diminutive minor papilla* (Fig. 19–2*B*).[5] The duct of Wirsung, normally the main pancreatic duct, is very short (1 to 2 cm) and drains only a small portion of the head of the gland through the larger major papilla of Vater. The relative stenosis caused by the bulk of the pancreatic secretions passing through the minor papilla predisposes patients with pancreatic divisum to the development of chronic pancreatitis.[5,6]

ANNULAR PANCREAS

Annular pancreas is a relatively uncommon condition and is often associated with other anomalies.[7] It develops embryologically when one portion of the ventral pancreatic primordium becomes fixed, while the other portion of this primordium is drawn around the duodenum. When this portion of the ventral primordium fuses with the head of the pancreas, it forms a bandlike ring of normal pancreatic tissue that completely encircles the second portion of the duodenum.[8] Annular pancreas may present early in life or in adults with signs and symptoms of duodenal obstruction such as gastric distention and vomiting.

ECTOPIC PANCREAS

Aberrantly situated, or *ectopic*, pancreatic tissue is found in about 2% of careful routine postmortem examinations. The favored sites for ectopia are the stomach and duodenum, followed by the jejunum, Meckel diverticula, and ileum. Usually, these embryologic rests are a few millimeters to centimeters in diameter and are located in the submucosa. Histologically, they are composed of normal-appearing pancreatic acini and glands with the occasional presence of islets of Langerhans. Although usually incidental, ectopic pancreas may be visualized as a sessile mass, may cause pain from localized inflammation, or, rarely, may incite mucosal bleeding. Approximately 2% of islet cell tumors (Chapter 24) arise in ectopic pancreatic tissue.

Pancreatitis

Pancreatitis encompasses a group of disorders characterized by inflammation of the pancreas. The clinical manifestations can range in severity from a mild, self-limited disease to a life-threatening acute inflammatory process, and the duration of the disease can range from a transient attack to an irreversible loss of function.[9–11] By definition, in *acute pancreatitis*, the gland can return to normal if the underlying cause of the pancreatitis is removed.[12] By contrast, *chronic pancreatitis* is defined by the presence of irreversible destruction of exocrine pancreatic parenchyma.[10]

ACUTE PANCREATITIS

Acute pancreatitis is a group of reversible lesions characterized by inflammation of the pancreas ranging in severity from edema and fat necrosis to parenchymal necrosis with severe hemorrhage. Acute pancreatitis is relatively common, with an annual incidence rate in Western countries of 10 to 20 cases per 100,000 people. Approximately 80% of cases in Western countries are associated with one of two conditions: biliary tract disease or alcoholism (Table 19–1).[11,13] Gallstones are present in 35% to 60% of cases of acute pancreatitis, and about 5% of patients with gallstones develop pancreatitis. The proportion of cases of acute pancreatitis caused by excessive alcohol intake varies from 65% in the United States to 20% in Sweden to 5% or less in southern France and the United Kingdom.[14] The male-female ratio is 1:3 in the group with biliary tract disease and 6:1 in those with alcoholism.

Less common causes of acute pancreatitis include the following:

- Obstruction of the pancreatic duct system. Reasons for obstruction other than gallstones described above include periampullary tumors, pancreas divisum, choledochoceles (congenital cystic dilatation of the common bile duct), biliary "sludge," and parasites (particularly *Ascariasis lumbricoides* and *Clonorchis sinensis* organisms).[15,16]
- Medications. More than 85 drugs have been reported to cause acute pancreatitis. These include thiazide diuretics, azathioprine, estrogens, sulfonamides, furosemide, methyldopa, pentamidine, and procainamide.[17]
- Infections with mumps, coxsackieviruses, and *Mycoplasma pneumoniae*
- Metabolic disorders, including hypertriglyceridemia, hyperparathyroidism, and other hypercalcemic states
- Acute ischemia induced by vascular thrombosis, embolism, vasculitis (polyarteritis nodosa, systemic lupus erythematosus, Henoch-Schönlein purpura), and shock
- Trauma, both blunt trauma and iatrogenic injury during surgery or endoscopic retrograde cholangiopancreatography
- Inherited alterations in genes encoding pancreatic enzymes and their inhibitors, including germ line mutations in the cationic trypsinogen (*PRSS1*) and trypsin inhibitor (*SPINK1*) genes.[18–21] These are discussed below.

TABLE 19–1 Etiologic Factors in Acute Pancreatitis

Metabolic
Alcoholism
Hyperlipoproteinemia
Hypercalcemia
Drugs (e.g., thiazide diuretics)
Genetic
Mechanical
Trauma
Gallstones
Iatrogenic injury
Perioperative injury
Endoscopic procedures with dye injection
Vascular
Shock
Atheroembolism
Polyarteritis nodosa
Infectious
Mumps
Coxsackievirus
Mycoplasma pneumoniae

Of note, 10% to 20% of patients with acute pancreatitis have no known associated processes. Although this condition is currently termed *idiopathic*, a growing body of evidence suggests that many, in fact, have a genetic basis. The genetic alterations associated with the development of pancreatitis therefore deserve special note.[22]

Cationic Trypsinogen (PRSS1). Hereditary pancreatitis is an autosomal-dominant disease with an 80% penetrance characterized by recurrent attacks of severe pancreatitis usually beginning in childhood.[19] This disorder is caused by germ line (inherited) mutations in the *cationic trypsinogen* gene (also known as *PRSS1*).[18] Most are point mutations, with G to A transitions, that result in an arginine (R) to histidine (H) substitution (called R122H).[19] This mutation abrogates a critical failsafe mechanism, by affecting a site on the cationic trypsinogen molecule that is essential for the cleavage (inactivation) of trypsin by trypsin itself.[23] When this site is mutated, trypsinogen and trypsin become resistant to inactivation, and the abnormally active trypsin activates other digestive proenzymes, resulting in the development of pancreatitis.

Serine Protease Inhibitor, Kazal Type 1 (SPINK1). The *SPINK1* gene codes for a pancreatic secretory trypsin inhibitor that, as the name suggests, inhibits trypsin activity, helping to prevent the autodigestion of the pancreas by activated trypsin.[20] As one might suspect, inherited homozygous inactivating mutations in the *SPINK1* gene can also lead to the development of pancreatitis.

Morphology. The morphology of acute pancreatitis ranges from trivial inflammation and edema to severe extensive necrosis and hemorrhage. The basic alterations are **(1) microvascular leakage causing edema, (2) necrosis of fat by lipolytic enzymes, (3) an acute inflammatory reaction, (4) proteolytic destruction of pancreatic parenchyma, and (5) destruction of blood vessels with subsequent interstitial hemorrhage**. The extent and predominance of each of these alterations depend on the duration and severity of the process.

In the milder form, acute interstitial pancreatitis, histologic alterations are limited to interstitial edema and focal areas of fat necrosis in the pancreatic substance and peripancreatic fat (Fig. 19–4). Fat necrosis, as we have seen, results from enzymatic destruction of fat cells. The released fatty acids combine with calcium to form insoluble salts that precipitate in situ (Chapter 1).

In the more severe form, **acute necrotizing pancreatitis**, necrosis of pancreatic tissue affects acinar and

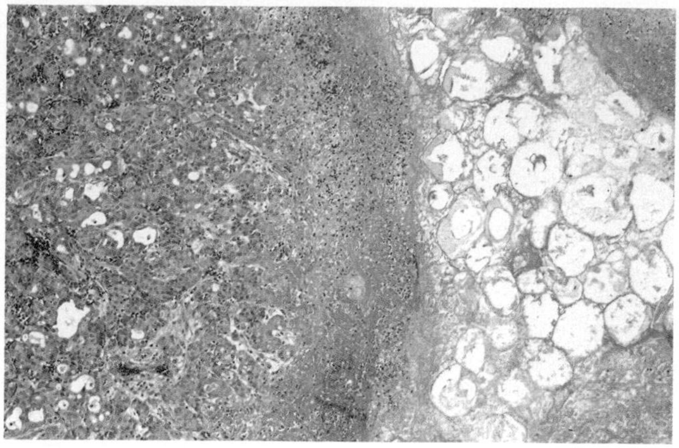

FIGURE 19–4 Acute pancreatitis. The microscopic field shows a region of fat necrosis on the right and focal pancreatic parenchymal necrosis (*center*).

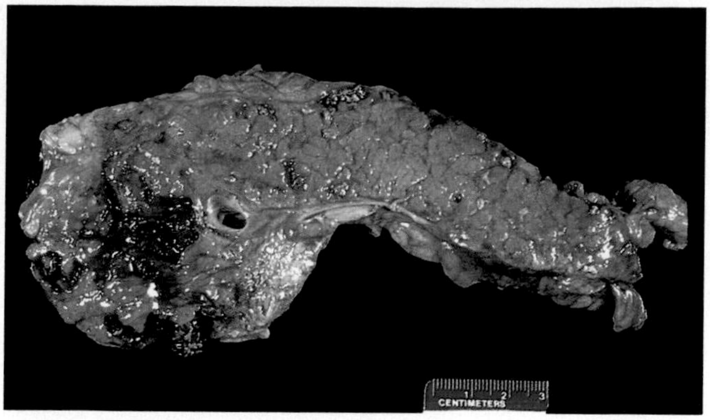

FIGURE 19–5 Acute pancreatitis. The pancreas has been sectioned across to reveal dark areas of hemorrhage in the head of the pancreas and a focal area of pale fat necrosis in the peripancreatic fat (*upper left*).

ductal tissues as well as the islets of Langerhans. There may be sufficient damage to the vasculature to cause hemorrhage into the parenchyma of the pancreas. Macroscopically, the pancreatic substance exhibits areas of red-black hemorrhage interspersed with foci of yellow-white, chalky fat necrosis (Fig. 19–5). Foci of fat necrosis may also be found in extrapancreatic fat depots, such as the omentum and the mesentery of the bowel, and even outside the abdominal cavity, such as in the subcutis. In most cases, the peritoneal cavity contains a serous, slightly turbid, brown-tinged fluid in which globules of fat (derived from the action of enzymes on adipose tissue) can be identified. In its most severe form, **hemorrhagic pancreatitis**, extensive parenchymal necrosis is accompanied by diffuse hemorrhage within the substance of the gland.[24]

Pathogenesis. The anatomic changes of acute pancreatitis strongly suggest *autodigestion of the pancreatic substance by inappropriately activated pancreatic enzymes.* This hypothesis is supported by the hereditary forms of pancreatitis described above. Here we focus on the more common, acquired forms of acute pancreatitis.

As has been discussed, pancreatic enzymes are present in acinar cells in the proenzyme form and have to be activated to fulfill their enzymatic potential. A major role is attributed to trypsin, which itself is synthesized as the proenzyme trypsinogen. Once trypsin is generated, it can in turn activate other proenzymes such as prophospholipase and proelastase, which then take part in the process of autodigestion.[12] The activated enzymes that are so generated cause disintegration of fat cells and damage the elastic fibers of blood vessels, respectively. Trypsin also converts prekallikrein to its activated form, thus bringing into play the kinin system and, by activation of Hageman factor, the clotting and complement systems as well (Chapters 2 and 4). In this way, inflammation and small-vessel thromboses (which may lead to congestion and rupture of already weakened vessels) are amplified. Thus, *activation of trypsinogen is an important triggering event in acute pancreatitis.*

The mechanisms by which activation of pancreatic enzymes is initiated are not entirely clear, but there is evidence for three possible pathways (Fig. 19–6):

1. *Pancreatic duct obstruction.* Regardless of whether the common bile duct and pancreatic duct share a common channel or separate channels, impaction of a gallstone or biliary sludge in the region of the ampulla of Vater raises intrapancreatic ductal pressure. Blockage to ductal flow favors the accumulation of an enzyme-rich interstitial fluid. Since lipase is one of the few enzymes secreted in an active form, this can cause local fat necrosis. Injured tissues, periacinar myofibroblasts, and leukocytes then release proinflammatory cytokines including interleukin-1β (IL-1β), interleukin-6 (IL-6), tumor necrosis factor (TNF), platelet-activating factor (PAF), and substance P, initiating local inflammation and promoting the development of interstitial edema through a leaky microvasculature.[25–30] According to one hypothesis, edema further compromises local blood flow, causing vascular insufficiency and ischemic injury to acinar cells.[31]
2. *Primary acinar cell injury.* This mechanism is most clearly involved in the pathogenesis of acute pancreatitis caused by certain viruses (e.g., mumps), drugs, and direct trauma to the pancreas, as well as that following ischemia or shock.
3. *Defective intracellular transport of proenzymes within acinar cells.* Aberrant acinar cell packaging of digestive enzymes has been shown to occur when there is either pancreatic duct obstruction or exposure to alcohol. It also occurs in animal models of metabolic pancreatic injury.[32] In normal acinar cells, digestive enzymes and the lysosomal hydrolases are transported in separate pathways after being synthesized in the endoplasmic reticulum and packaged in the Golgi apparatus. The digestive enzymes make their way through zymogen granules to the apical cell surface, while lysosomal hydrolases are transported into the lysosomes. In animal models of acinar injury, the pancreatic proenzymes are delivered to an intracellular compartment containing lysosomal hydrolases, thereby permitting proenzyme activation, rupture of the lysosomes, and local release of activated enzymes.[33] The role of this mechanism in human acute pancreatitis is less clear.[34]

The manner by which alcohol causes pancreatitis is unknown. Transient increases in pancreatic exocrine secretion, contraction of the sphincter of Oddi (the muscle at the ampulla of Vater), and direct toxic effects on acinar cells have

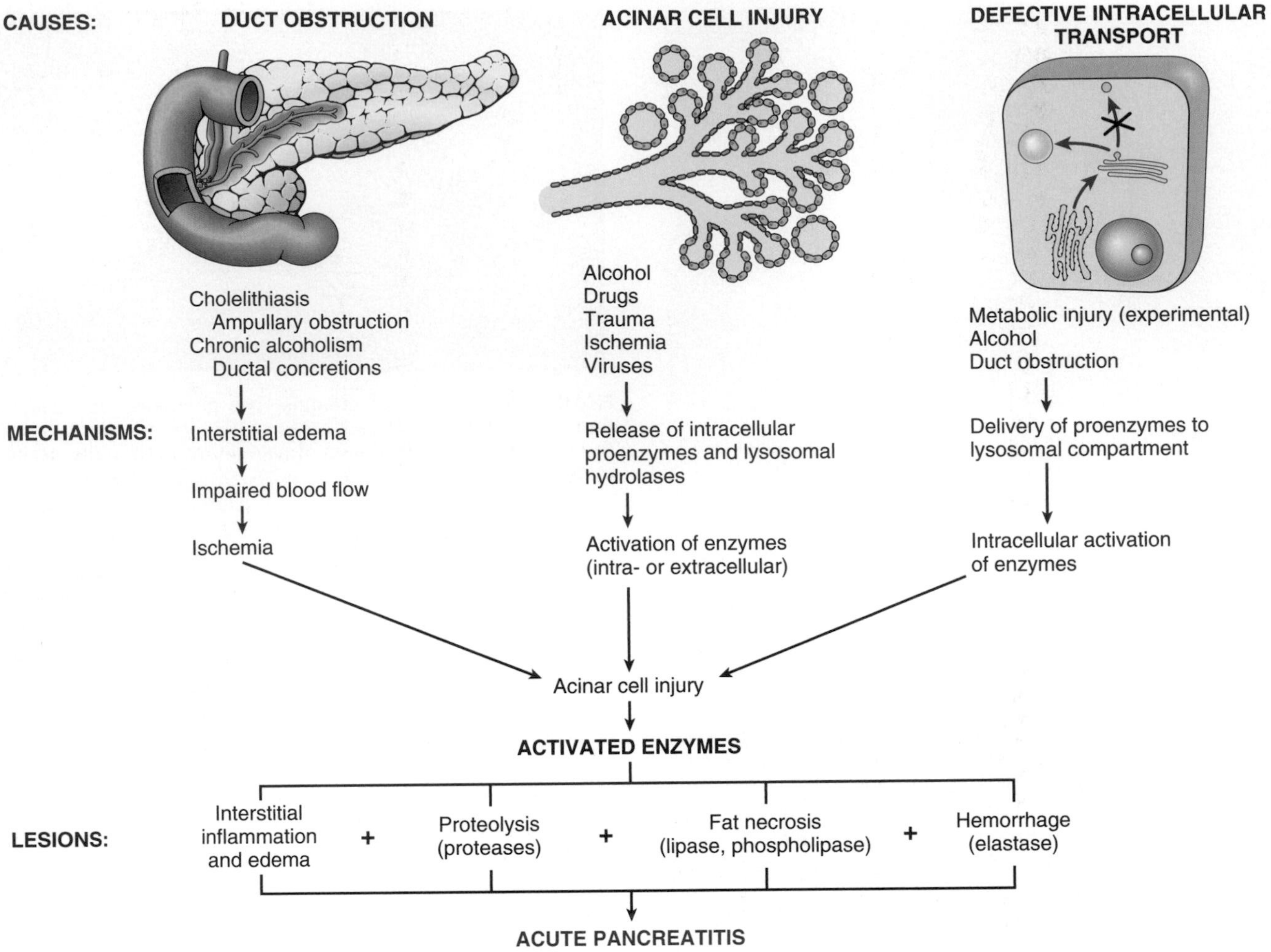

FIGURE 19–6 Three proposed pathways in the pathogenesis of acute pancreatitis.

all been postulated from experimental studies. *Many authorities think that most cases of alcoholic pancreatitis are sudden exacerbations of chronic pancreatitis, presenting as apparent de novo acute pancreatitis.*[35] According to this view, chronic alcohol ingestion causes secretion of protein-rich pancreatic fluid, leading to deposition of inspissated protein plugs and obstruction of small pancreatic ducts, followed by the train of events described above.

Clinical Features. *Abdominal pain* is the cardinal manifestation of acute pancreatitis. Its severity varies from mild and uncomfortable to severe and incapacitating. Suspected acute pancreatitis is primarily diagnosed by the presence of elevated plasma levels of amylase and lipase and the exclusion of other causes of abdominal pain.

Full-blown acute pancreatitis is a medical emergency of the first magnitude. These patients usually have the sudden calamitous onset of an "acute abdomen" that must be differentiated from diseases such as ruptured acute appendicitis, perforated peptic ulcer, acute cholecystitis with rupture, and occlusion of mesenteric vessels with infarction of the bowel. Characteristically, the pain is constant and intense and is often referred to the upper back.

Many of the systemic features of severe acute pancreatitis can be attributed to release of toxic enzymes, cytokines, and other mediators into the circulation and explosive activation of the systemic inflammatory response, resulting in *leukocytosis, hemolysis, disseminated intravascular coagulation, fluid sequestration, acute respiratory distress syndrome, and diffuse fat necrosis. Peripheral vascular collapse and shock with acute renal tubular necrosis may occur* (Fig. 19–7). Explanations for the rapid development of shock include loss of blood volume and electrolyte disturbances, endotoxemia, and the release of cytokines and vasoactive agents such as bradykinin, prostaglandins, nitric oxide (NO), and platelet-activating factor.[36]

Laboratory findings include marked elevation of serum amylase levels during the first 24 hours, followed within 72 to 96 hours by a rising serum lipase level. Glycosuria occurs in 10% of cases. Hypocalcemia may result from precipitation of calcium soaps in the fat necrosis; if persistent, it is a poor prognostic sign. Direct visualization of the enlarged inflamed pancreas by radiographic means is useful in the diagnosis of pancreatitis.

The key to the management of acute pancreatitis is "resting" the pancreas by total restriction of food and fluids and by supportive therapy. Although most patients with acute pancreatitis recover fully, about 5% die from shock during the first week of illness. Acute respiratory distress syndrome and acute renal failure are ominous complications.[37] In surviving patients, sequelae include a sterile *pancreatic abscess* and a

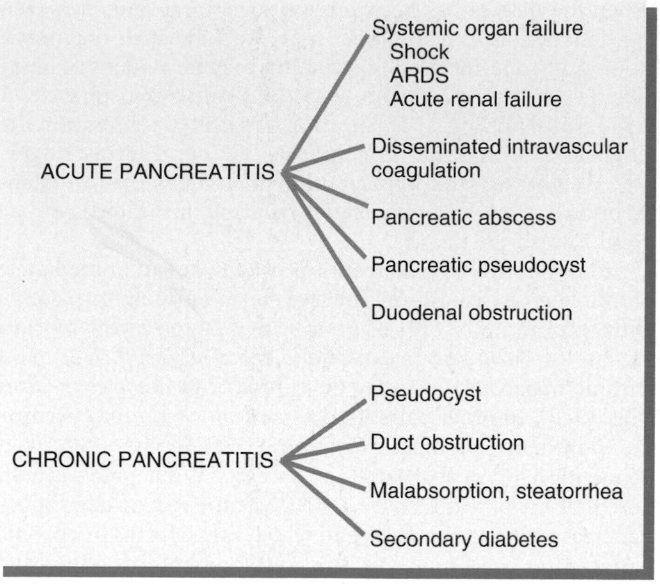

FIGURE 19–7 Comparison of the sequelae of acute and chronic pancreatitis. (ARDS = acute respiratory distress syndrome)

pancreatic pseudocyst (discussed later). In 40% to 60% of patients with acute necrotizing pancreatitis, the necrotic debris becomes infected, usually by Gram-negative organisms from the alimentary tract, further complicating the clinical course.[11]

CHRONIC PANCREATITIS

Chronic pancreatitis is characterized by inflammation of the pancreas with destruction of exocrine parenchyma, fibrosis, and, in the late stages, the destruction of endocrine parenchyma.[10,38] Although chronic pancreatitis may present as repeated bouts of acute pancreatitis, the chief distinction between acute and chronic pancreatitis is the irreversible impairment in pancreatic function that is characteristic of chronic pancreatitis. The prevalence of chronic pancreatitis is hard to determine, but it probably ranges between 0.04% and 5%.[10] There is significant overlap in the causes of acute and chronic pancreatitis. By far *the most common cause of chronic pancreatitis is long-term alcohol abuse*, and these patients are usually middle-aged males.

Less common causes of chronic pancreatitis include the following:

- Long-standing *obstruction* of the pancreatic duct by pseudocysts, calculi, trauma, neoplasms, or pancreas divisum. There is often dilation of the pancreatic duct.
- *Tropical pancreatitis*, which is a poorly characterized heterogeneous disease seen in Africa and Asia.[39] It has been attributed to malnutrition.
- *Hereditary pancreatitis*, which is caused by germ line mutations in the *PRSS1* or *SPINK1* genes and which is associated with the development of both acute and chronic pancreatitis.[18,20]
- *Idiopathic chronic pancreatitis*. As was discussed in detail in Chapter 10, cystic fibrosis is caused by mutations in the cystic fibrosis transmembrane conductance regulator *(CFTR)* gene. *CFTR* is expressed in pancreatic ducts. Mutations in *CFTR* decrease bicarbonate secretion, thereby promoting protein plugging and the development of chronic pancreatitis.[21,40] *CFTR*-related pancreatitis is seen in individuals who inherit two distinct *CFTR* gene mutations (compound heterozygous).[21] It is interesting to note that *in patients with idiopathic chronic pancreatitis associated with CFTR mutations, other clinical features of cystic fibrosis are typically absent, and the sweat chloride level is normal.* The mutations of the *CFTR* gene in such patients are distinct from those associated with cystic fibrosis. In typical cystic fibrosis, the secretory defects in the pancreatic ducts are much more severe, giving rise to pancreatic atrophy early in the course of the disease, rather than to chronic pancreatitis.

Up to 40% of patients with chronic pancreatitis have no recognizable predisposing factor, but as is true for acute pancreatitis, a growing number of these "idiopathic" cases can now be shown to be caused by inherited mutations in pancreatitis-associated genes.[21]

Pathogenesis. The pathogenesis of chronic pancreatitis is not well defined. Four hypotheses have been proposed to account for the development of chronic pancreatitis.[41–43] These include:

1. *Ductal obstruction by concretions.* Some of the inciting agents responsible for the development of chronic pancreatitis, such as alcohol, are believed to increase protein concentrations in the pancreatic juice. These proteins form ductal plugs. Such plugs are observed in most forms of chronic pancreatitis and are particularly prominent in alcoholic chronic pancreatitis.[44] The ductal plugs may calcify, forming calculi composed of calcium carbonate precipitates, and these calculi can further obstruct the pancreatic ducts and contribute to the development of chronic pancreatitis.
2. *Toxic-metabolic.* Toxins, including alcohol and its metabolites, can exert a direct toxic effect on acinar cells. This may lead to the accumulation of lipids in acinar cells, acinar cell loss, and eventually parenchymal fibrosis.
3. *Oxidative stress.* Alcohol-induced oxidative stress may generate free radicals in acinar cells, leading to membrane lipid oxidation and the activation of transcription factors, including AP1 and NFκB, which in turn induce the expression of chemokines that attract mononuclear cells.[42] Oxidative stress thereby promotes the fusion of lysosomes and zymogen granules, acinar cell necrosis, inflammation, and fibrosis.
4. *Necrosis-fibrosis.* It has been proposed that acute pancreatitis initiates a sequence of perilobular fibrosis, duct distortion, and altered pancreatic secretions. Over time and with multiple episodes, this can lead to loss of pancreatic parenchyma and fibrosis.[41] Perhaps the strongest support for this hypothesis comes from observations made in patients with hereditary pancreatitis. As was discussed earlier, some cases of hereditary pancreatitis are caused by inherited mutations in the *PRSS1* gene. These mutations produce an autolysis-resistant trypsin molecule that causes acute pancreatitis. Patients with repeated episodes of acute pancreatitis almost all later develop chronic pancreatitis.[19] This suggests that activated trypsin, in and of itself, can cause chronic pancreatitis.

A variety of chemokines have been identified in chronic pancreatitis, including interleukin-8 (IL-8) and monocyte chemoattractant protein (MCP-1).[45] In addition, transforming growth factor-β (TGF-β) and platelet-derived growth factor induce the activation and proliferation of periacinar myofibroblasts (pancreatic stellate cells), resulting in the deposition of collagen and ultimately fibrosis.[19, 46–48]

Morphology. Chronic pancreatitis is characterized by parenchymal fibrosis, reduced number and size of acini with relative sparing of the islets of Langerhans, and variable dilation of the pancreatic ducts (Fig. 19–8*A*). These changes are usually accompanied by a chronic inflammatory infiltrate around lobules and ducts. The interlobular and intralobular ducts are frequently dilated and contain protein plugs in their lumens. The ductal epithelium may be atrophied or hyperplastic or may show squamous metaplasia, and ductal concretions may be evident (Fig. 19–8*B*). Acinar loss is a constant feature. The remaining islets of Langerhans become embedded in the sclerotic tissue and may fuse and appear enlarged. Eventually, they too disappear. Grossly, the gland is hard, sometimes with extremely dilated ducts and visible calcified concretions.

Clinical Features. Chronic pancreatitis may present in many different forms. It may be associated with repeated attacks of moderately severe abdominal pain, recurrent attacks of mild pain, or persistent abdominal and back pain. The disease may be entirely silent until pancreatic insufficiency and diabetes mellitus develop, the latter from associated destruction of islets of Langerhans. In still other instances, recurrent attacks of jaundice or vague attacks of indigestion may hint at pancreatic disease. Attacks may be precipitated by alcohol abuse, overeating (which increases demand on the pancreas), or the use of opiates and other drugs that increase the tone of the sphincter of Oddi.

The diagnosis of chronic pancreatitis requires a high degree of suspicion. During an attack of abdominal pain, there may be mild fever and mild-to-moderate elevations of serum amylase. When the disease has been present for a long time, however, the destruction of acinar cells may preclude such diagnostic clues. Gallstone-induced obstruction may be evident as jaundice or elevations in serum levels of alkaline phosphatase. A very helpful finding is visualization of calcifications within the pancreas by computed tomography (CT) and ultrasonography. Weight loss and hypoalbuminemic edema from malabsorption caused by pancreatic exocrine insufficiency may point toward the disease.

Although chronic pancreatitis is usually not an immediately life-threatening condition, the long-term outlook for patients with chronic pancreatitis is poor, with a 20 to 25 year mortality rate of 50%. Severe *pancreatic exocrine insufficiency* and chronic malabsorption may develop, as can *diabetes mellitus* (Fig. 19–7). In other patients, *severe chronic pain* may become the dominant problem. *Pancreatic pseudocysts* (described below) develop in about 10% of patients. While patients with hereditary pancreatitis have a 40% lifetime risk of developing pancreatic cancer, the degree to which other forms of chronic pancreatitis predispose to the development of pancreatic cancer is unclear.[49,50]

Non-Neoplastic Cysts

A variety of cysts can arise in the pancreas. Most are non-neoplastic pseudocysts (discussed later), but congenital cysts and neoplastic cystic tumors also occur. In general, unilocular cysts tend to be benign, while multilocular cysts are more often neoplastic and possibly malignant.

CONGENITAL CYSTS

Congenital cysts are believed to result from anomalous development of the pancreatic ducts. Cysts in the kidney, liver, and pancreas frequently coexist in *polycystic disease* (discussed in Chapter 20). The pancreatic cysts range from microscopic lesions to those 3 to 5 cm in diameter. They are lined by a glistening, duct type cuboidal epithelium or by a completely attenuated cell layer; they are enclosed in a thin, fibrous capsule and are filled with a clear-to-turbid mucoid or serous

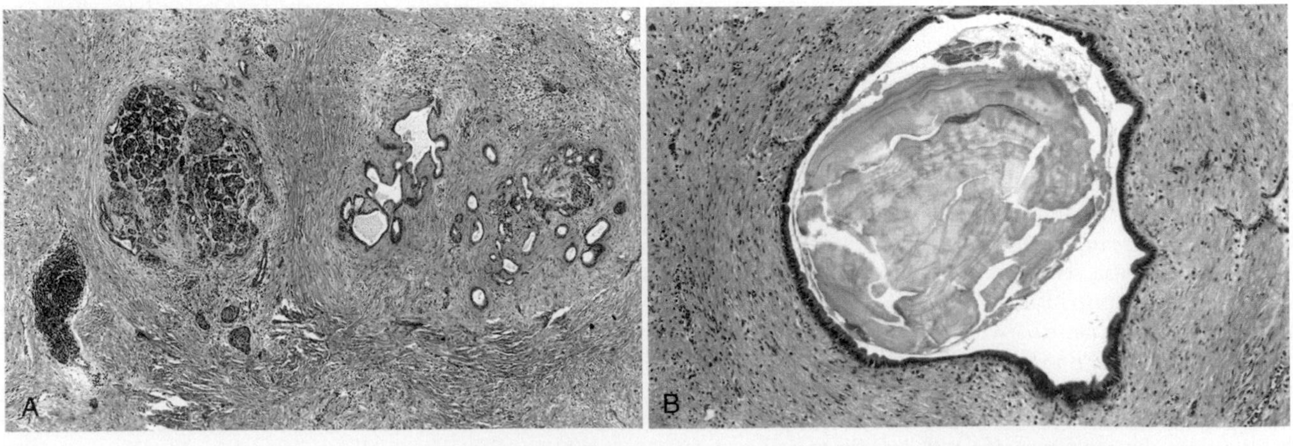

FIGURE 19–8 Chronic pancreatitis. *A*, Extensive fibrosis and atrophy has left only residual islets (*left*) and ducts (*right*), with a sprinkling of chronic inflammatory cells and acinar tissue. *B*, A higher-power view demonstrating dilated ducts with inspissated eosinophilic ductal concretions in a patient with alcoholic chronic pancreatitis.

fluid. In *von Hippel-Lindau disease* (Chapter 20), vascular neoplasms are found in the retina and cerebellum or brain stem in association with congenital cysts (and also neoplasms) in the pancreas, liver, and kidney.

PSEUDOCYSTS

Pseudocysts are localized collections of necrotic-hemorrhagic material rich in pancreatic enzymes.[49] Such cysts lack an epithelial lining (hence the prefix "pseudo"), and they account for approximately 75% of cysts in the pancreas.[51] Pseudocysts usually arise after an episode of acute pancreatitis, often in the setting of chronic alcoholic pancreatitis. Traumatic injury to the abdomen can also give rise to pseudocysts.

Morphology. Pseudocysts are usually solitary and may be situated within the substance of the pancreas, or, more commonly, they are attached to the surface of the gland and involve peripancreatic tissues (Fig. 19–9). They are formed by the walling off of areas of peripancreatic hemorrhagic fat necrosis with fibrous tissue. As such, they usually are composed of central necrotic-hemorrhagic material rich in pancreatic enzymes surrounded by nonepithelial lined fibrous walls of granulation tissue (Fig. 19–9).[51] Pseudocysts can range in size from 2 to 30 cm in diameter, and they often involve the lesser omental sac or lie in the retroperitoneum between the stomach and transverse colon or between the stomach and liver. They can even be subdiaphragmatic.[51]

While many pseudocysts spontaneously resolve, they may become secondarily infected, and larger pseudocysts may compress or even perforate into adjacent structures.

Neoplasms

A broad spectrum of exocrine neoplasms can arise in the pancreas. They may be cystic or solid; some are benign, while others are among the most lethal of all malignancies.

CYSTIC NEOPLASMS

Only 5% to 15% of all pancreatic cysts are neoplastic (most cysts are pseudocysts; see the previous section), and cystic neoplasms make up fewer than 5% of all pancreatic neoplasms. While some, such as the serous cystadenoma, are entirely benign, others, such as mucinous cystic neoplasms, can be benign, borderline malignant, or malignant. Borderline malignant neoplasms have some, but not all, of the features of a fully malignant neoplasm.

Serous cystadenomas are benign cystic neoplasms composed of glycogen-rich low-cuboidal cells surrounding small cysts containing clear, thin, straw-colored fluid (Fig. 19–10).[52] They account for about 25% of all cystic neoplasms of the pancreas. These tumors arise twice as often in women as in men and typically present in the seventh decade of life with nonspecific symptoms such as abdominal pain. They may also present as palpable abdominal masses. Serous cystadenomas are almost always benign, and surgical resection is curative in the vast majority of patients.

Mucinous cystic neoplasms almost always arise in women, and in contrast to serous cystadenomas, they can be benign, borderline malignant, or malignant.[53,54] Mucinous cystic neoplasms usually arise in the body or tail of the pancreas and present as painless, slow-growing masses. The cystic spaces are filled with thick, tenacious mucin, and the cysts are lined by a columnar mucinous epithelium with an associated dense stroma similar to ovarian stroma (Fig. 19–11).[54] The only way to distinguish the entirely benign form (cystadenoma) from its malignant counterpart (cystadenocarcinoma) is pathologic assessment after complete surgical removal, usually by distal pancreatectomy.[55] Benign mucinous cystadenomas lack significant cytologic or architectural atypia, while borderline mucinous cystic neoplasms show significant cytologic and architectural atypia but no tissue invasion. Malignant mucinous cystadenocarcinomas have an associated invasive carcinoma.

Intraductal papillary mucinous neoplasms (IPMNs) also produce cysts containing mucin, and like mucinous cystic neoplasms, IPMNs can be benign, borderline malignant, or malignant.[56] In contrast to mucinous cystic neoplasms, IPMNs arise more frequently in men than in women, and they involve the head of the pancreas more often than the tail. Two

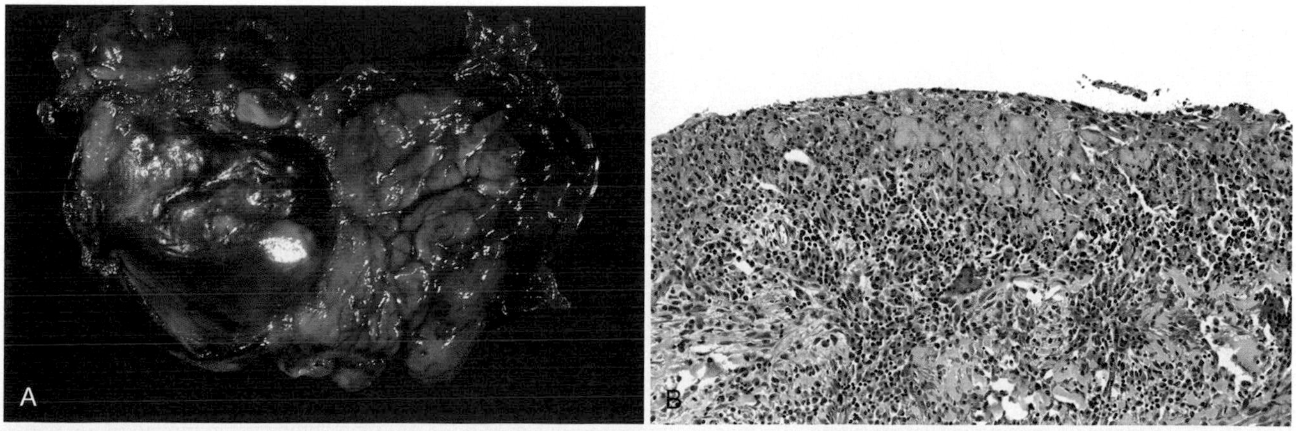

FIGURE 19–9 Pancreatic pseudocyst. *A*, Cross-section through this previously bisected lesion revealing a poorly defined cyst with a necrotic brown-black wall. *B*, Histologically, the cyst lacks a true epithelial lining and instead is lined by fibrin and granulation tissue.

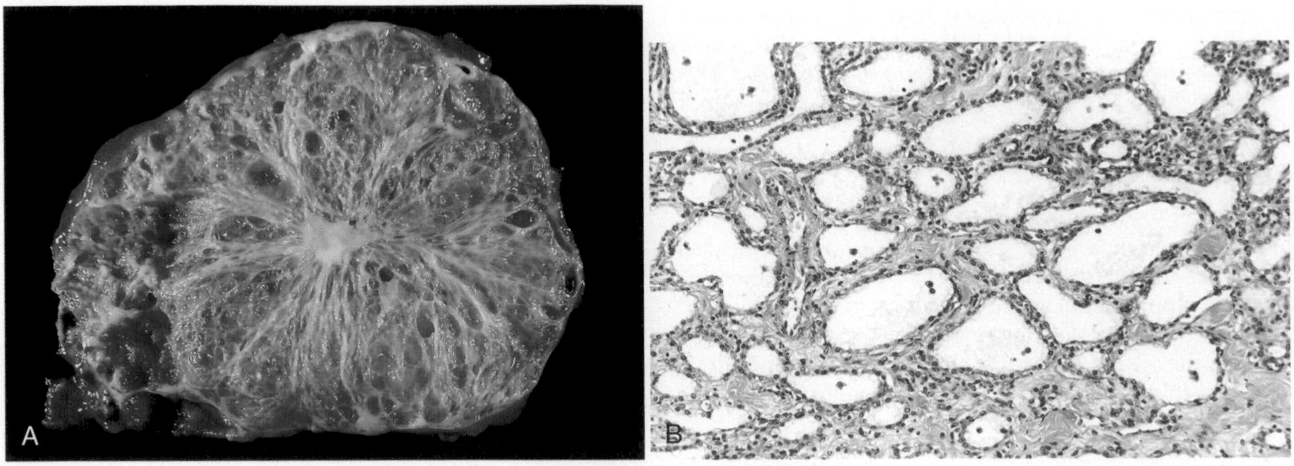

FIGURE 19–10 Serous cystadenoma. *A,* Cross-section through a serous cystadenoma. Only a thin rim of normal pancreatic parenchyma remains. The cysts are relatively small and contain clear, straw-colored fluid. *B,* The cysts are lined by cuboidal epithelium without atypia.

features are useful in distinguishing IPMNs from mucinous cystic neoplasms: IPMNs lack the dense "ovarian" stroma seen in mucinous cystic neoplasms, and IPMNs arise in the main pancreatic ducts (Fig. 19–12), while mucinous cystic neoplasms do not connect to the main pancreatic duct system. Just as with mucinous cystic neoplasms, benign IPMNs are distinguished from malignant IPMNs by the lack of tissue invasion.

The unusual *solid-pseudopapillary tumor* is seen mainly in adolescent girls and young women.[57] These large, well-circumscribed masses have solid and cystic zones. The cystic areas are filled with hemorrhagic debris, and histologically, the neoplastic cells grow in solid sheets or, as the name suggests, as papillary projections. These tumors often cause abdominal discomfort because of their large size, and they are usually cured by resection. Of note, the β-catenin/adenomatous polyposis coli genetic pathway (Chapter 7) appears to be almost universally altered in these neoplasms.[57] Surgical resection is the treatment of choice, and although some solid-pseudopapillary tumors are locally aggressive, most pursue a benign course if they are completely resected.

PANCREATIC CARCINOMA

Infiltrating ductal adenocarcinoma of the pancreas, more commonly known as "pancreatic cancer," is the fourth leading cause of cancer death in the United States, preceded only by lung, colon, and breast cancers.[58] Pancreatic cancer has one of the highest mortality rates of any cancer. It is estimated that in 2004, approximately 30,000 Americans will be diagnosed with pancreatic cancer, and virtually all of them will die from it. The 5-year survival rate is a dismal, less than 5%.

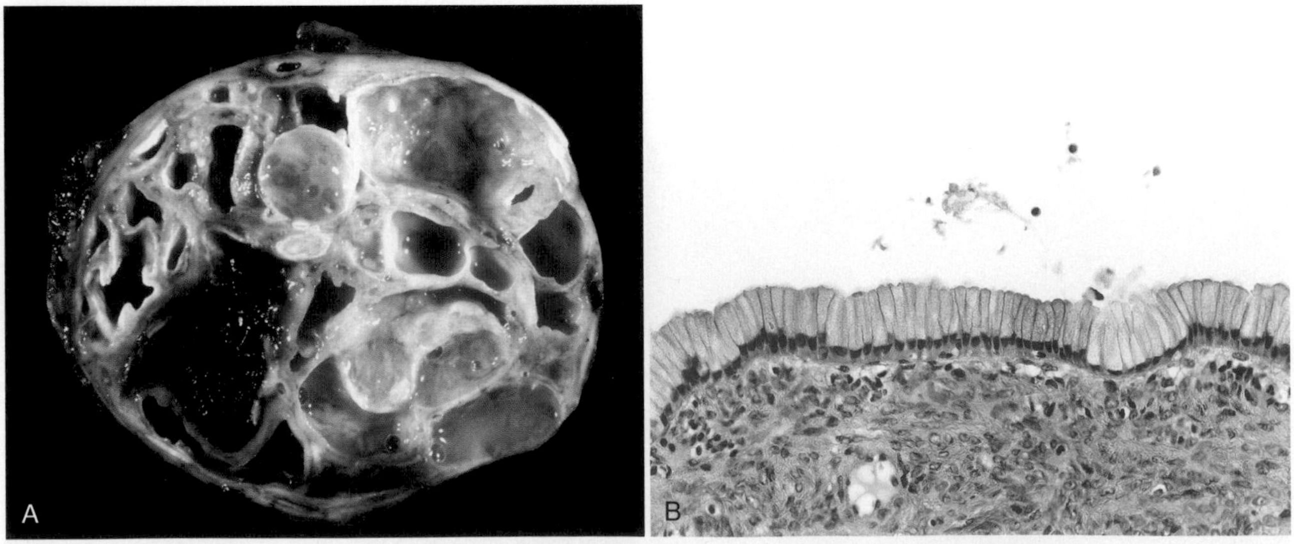

FIGURE 19–11 Pancreatic mucinous cystadenoma. *A,* Cross-section through a mucinous multiloculated cyst in the tail of the pancreas. The cysts are large and filled with tenacious mucin. *B,* The cysts are lined by columnar mucinous epithelium, and a dense "ovarian" stroma is noted.

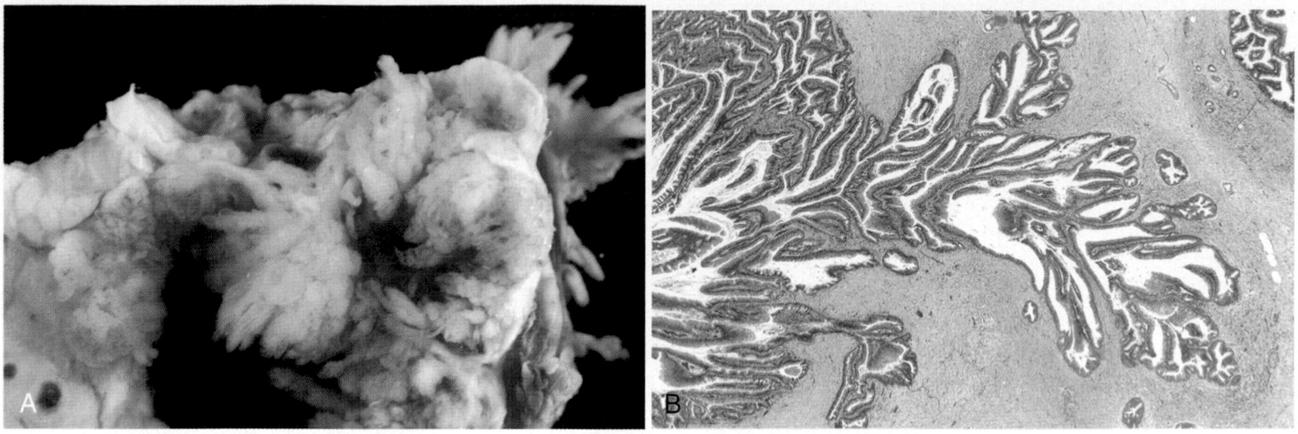

FIGURE 19–12 Intraductal papillary mucinous neoplasm. *A,* Cross-section through the head of the pancreas showing a prominent papillary neoplasm distending the main pancreatic duct. *B,* The papillary mucinous neoplasm involved the main pancreatic duct (*left*) and extending down into the smaller ducts and ductules (*right*).

Precursors to Pancreatic Cancer

Just as there is a progression in the colorectum from non-neoplastic epithelium to adenoma to invasive carcinoma (Chapter 7), there is a progression in the pancreas from non-neoplastic epithelium to histologically well-defined noninvasive lesions in small ducts and ductules to invasive carcinoma.[59] These precursor lesions are called "pancreatic intraepithelial neoplasias" (PanINs). The PanIN-invasive carcinoma sequence is supported by the following observations:

- The distribution of PanINs within the pancreas parallels that of invasive cancer.
- PanINs are often found in pancreatic parenchyma adjacent to infiltrating carcinomas.
- Isolated case reports have documented patients with PanINs who later developed an invasive pancreatic cancer.
- The genetic alterations identified in PanINs are similar to those present in invasive cancers.
- The epithelial cells in PanINs show dramatic telomere shortening. A critical shortening of telomere length in PanINs may predispose these lesions to accumulate progressive chromosomal abnormalities and to develop invasive carcinoma.[60]

Based on these observations, a model for progression of PanINs has been proposed (Fig. 19–13).

Molecular Carcinogenesis

Like all cancers, pancreatic cancer is fundamentally a genetic disease—a disease of inherited and acquired mutations in cancer-associated genes. Multiple genes are often altered in a single pancreatic cancer, and the patterns of genetic alterations differ from those seen in other malignancies.[61] Molecular alterations in pancreatic carcinogenesis are summarized in Table 19–2 and include the following genetic alterations.

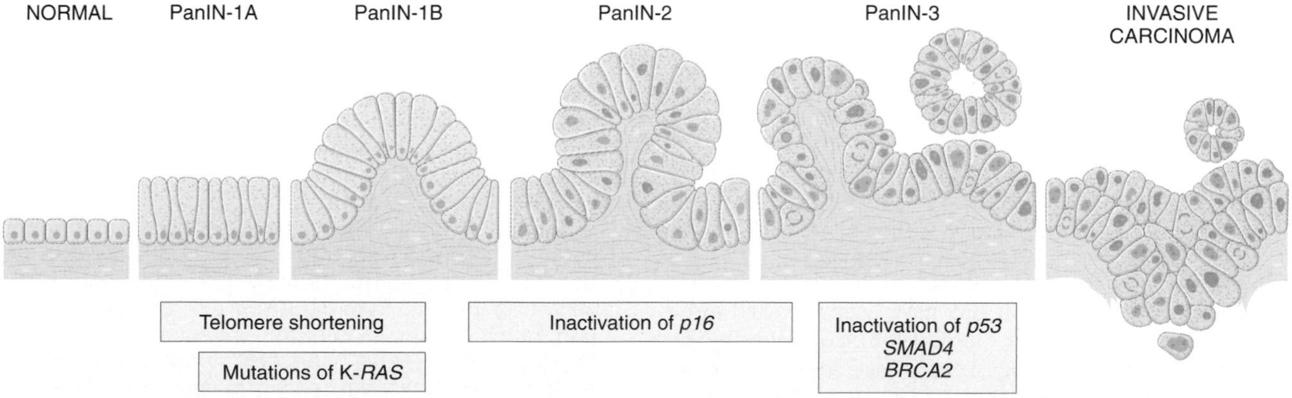

FIGURE 19–13 Progression model for the development of pancreatic cancer. It is postulated that telomere-shortening, and mutations of the oncogene *K-RAS* occur at early stages, that inactivation of the *p16* tumor suppressor gene occurs at intermediate stages, and the inactivation of the *p53*, *SMAD4* (*DPC4*), and *BRCA2* tumor suppressor genes occur at late stages. It is important to note that while there is a general temporal sequence of changes, the accumulation of multiple mutations is more important than their occurrence in a specific order. (Adapted from Wilentz RE, Iacobuzio-Donahue CA, et al: Loss of expression of DPC4 in pancreatic intraepithelial neoplasia: evidence that *DPC4* inactivation occurs late in neoplastic progression. Cancer Res 2000; 60:2002.)

TABLE 19–2 Molecular Alterations in Invasive Pancreatic Adenocarcinoma

Gene (Chromosomal Region)	Percent of Tumors with Genetic Alteration
K-ras (12p)	>90%
p16 CDKN2A (9p)	>95%
p53 (17p)	50–70%
SMAD4 (18q)	55%
AKT2 (19q)	10–20%
MYB (6q)	10%
AIB1 (20q)	10%
BRCA2 (13q)	7–10%
LKB1/STK11 (19p)	<5%
MKK4 (17p)	<5%
TGFβ-R1 (9q) or *TGFβ-R2* (3p)	<5%
RB1 (13q)	<5%

K-RAS. The *K-RAS* gene (chromosome 12p) is the most frequently altered oncogene in pancreatic cancer. This oncogene is activated by point mutation in 80% to 90% of pancreatic cancers. These point mutations impair the intrinsic GTPase activity of the K-*ras* gene product, resulting in a protein that is constitutively active. Ras in turn activates several intracellular signal transduction pathways that, among other effects, culminate in the activation of the transcription factors fos and jun.

p16. The *p16* gene (chromosome 9p) is the most frequently inactivated tumor suppressor gene in pancreatic cancer.[62] It is inactivated in 95% of cases. The *p16* gene product, p16, plays a critical role in the control of the cell cycle, and inactivation of p16 abrogates an important cell cycle checkpoint.

SMAD4. The *SMAD4* tumor suppressor gene (chromosome 18q) is inactivated in 55% of pancreatic cancers.[63] *SMAD4*, also known as *DPC4*, codes for a protein that plays an important role in signal transduction from the transforming growth factor-β (TGF-β) family of cell-surface receptors. The normal function of *SMAD4* is most likely to suppress growth and promote apoptosis. Loss of *SMAD4* therefore abrogates two important controls on cell population. *SMAD4* is only rarely inactivated in other cancer types.

p53. Inactivation of the *p53* tumor suppressor gene (chromosome 17p) is seen in 50% to 70% of pancreatic cancers.[64] The *p53* gene product is a nuclear DNA-binding protein that acts both as a cell cycle checkpoint and as an inducer of cell death (apoptosis).

Other Genes. A growing number of less common, but nonetheless important, genetic loci have been reported to be damaged in pancreatic cancer (Table 19–2). For example, the *AKT2* gene (chromosome 19q) is amplified in 10% to 20%, the *MYB* gene (6q) in 10%, and the *AIB1* gene (chromosome 20q) in 10%. The *BRCA2* (chromosome 13q), *LKB1/STK11* (chromosome 19p), *MKK4* (chromosome 17p), *TGFβ-R1* (chromosome 9q), *TGFβ-R2* (chromosome 3p), and *RB1* (chromosome 13q) tumor suppressor genes are inactivated in fewer than 10% of pancreatic cancers.

Methylation Abnormalities. A number of methylation abnormalities also occur in pancreatic cancer. Hypermethylation of the promoter of a number of tumor suppressor genes is associated with transcriptional silencing of the genes.

Gene Expression. In addition to DNA alterations, global analyses of gene expression have identified a number of genes that are highly overexpressed in pancreatic cancers.[65,66] These overexpressed genes are potential targets for novel therapeutics and may form the basis of future screening tests. For example the hedgehog signaling pathway has recently been shown to be activated in pancreatic cancer. Inhibition of this pathway with the drug cyclopamine blocks growth of pancreatic cancers in experimental systems.[67]

Epidemiology, Etiology, and Pathogenesis. Unlike other cancers of the alimentary tract, little is known about the cause of pancreatic cancer. Pancreatic cancer is primarily a disease in the elderly, 80% of cases occurring between the ages of 60 and 80.[68] It is more common in blacks than in whites, and it is slightly more common in individuals of Jewish decent.

The strongest environmental influence is *smoking*, which is believed to double the risk of pancreatic cancer.[68] Even though the magnitude of this increased risk is not great, the impact of smoking on pancreatic cancer is significant because of the large number of people who smoke. Consumption of a diet rich in fats has also been implicated but less consistently. Chronic pancreatitis and diabetes mellitus have both been associated with an increased risk of pancreatic cancer. Pancreatic cancer arises with greater frequency in patients with chronic pancreatitis,[50] but a causal role for pancreatitis, with the exception of hereditary pancreatitis, is not well established. Smoking and alcohol use in patients with chronic pancreatitis may underlie some of the association.[50] It is also hard to sort out whether chronic pancreatitis is the cause of pancreatic cancer or an effect of the disease, since small pancreatic cancers may block the pancreatic duct and produce chronic pancreatitis. A similar argument applies to the association of diabetes mellitus with pancreatic cancer, since diabetes may develop as a consequence of pancreatic cancer.

Familial clustering of pancreatic cancer has been reported, and a growing number of inherited genetic syndromes are now recognized that increase pancreatic cancer risk (Table 19–3).[69]

Morphology. Approximately 60% of cancers of the pancreas arise in the head of the gland, 15% in the body, and 5% in the tail; in 20%, the neoplasm diffusely involves the entire gland. Carcinomas of the pancreas are usually hard, stellate, gray-white, poorly defined masses (Fig. 19–14*A*).

The vast majority of carcinomas are ductal adenocarcinomas that recapitulate to some degree the normal ductal epithelium by forming glands and secreting mucin. Two features are characteristic of pancreatic cancer: It is highly invasive (even "early" invasive pancreatic cancers extensively invade peripancreatic tissues), and it elicits an intense non-neoplastic host reaction composed of fibroblasts, lymphocytes, and extracellular matrix (called a "desmoplastic response").

Most carcinomas of the head of the pancreas obstruct the distal common bile duct as it courses

TABLE 19–3 Familial Syndromes Predisposing to Pancreatic Cancer

Disorder	Gene (Chromosome Location)	Increased Risk of Pancreatic Cancer
Hereditary nonpolyposis colorectal cancer (Lynch II variant)	*hMSH2* (2p22), *hMLH1* (3p21)	?
Hereditary breast and ovarian cancer	*BRCA2* (13q12–q13)	4–10×
Familial atypical multiple mole melanoma syndrome (FAMMM)	*p16* (9p21)	20–35×
Hereditary pancreatitis	*PRSS1* (7q35)	50–80×
Peutz-Jeghers syndrome	*STK11/LKB1* (19p13)	130×

through the head of the pancreas. As a consequence, there is marked distention of the biliary tree in about 50% of patients with carcinoma of the head of the pancreas, and most develop jaundice. In marked contrast, **carcinomas of the body and tail of the pancreas do not impinge on the biliary tract and hence remain silent for some time. They may be quite large and widely disseminated by the time they are discovered.** Pancreatic cancers often extend through the retroperitoneal space, entrapping adjacent nerves, and occasionally invade the spleen, adrenals, vertebral column, transverse colon, and stomach. Peripancreatic, gastric, mesenteric, omental, and portahepatic lymph nodes are frequently involved, and the liver is often enlarged owing to metastatic deposits. Distant metastases occur, principally to the lungs and bones.

Microscopically, there is no difference between carcinomas of the head of the pancreas and those of the body and tail of the pancreas. The appearance is usually that of a **moderately to poorly differentiated adenocarcinoma forming abortive tubular structures or cell clusters and exhibiting an aggressive, deeply infiltrative growth pattern** (Fig. 19–14*B*). Dense stromal fibrosis accompanies tumor invasion, and there is a proclivity for perineural invasion within and beyond the organ. Lymphatic invasion is also commonly seen. The malignant glands are atypical, irregular, small, and bizarre and are usually lined by anaplastic cuboidal-to-columnar epithelial cells. Well-differentiated tumors are the exception.

Less common variants of pancreatic cancer include **acinar cell carcinomas, adenosquamous carcinomas,** and **undifferentiated carcinomas with osteoclast-like giant cells.** Acinar cell carcinomas, by definition, show prominent acinar cell differentiation, including the formation of zymogen granules and the production of exocrine enzymes including trypsin and lipase.[70] Adenosquamous carcinomas have focal squamous differentiation in addition to glandular differentiation, and undifferentiated carcinomas may contain large multinucleated osteoclast-like giant cells.[71]

Clinical Features. From the preceding discussion, it should be evident that *carcinomas of the pancreas remain silent until their extension impinges on some other structure.* Pain is usually the first symptom, but by the time pain appears, these cancers are usually beyond cure. *Obstructive jaundice* is associated with most cases of carcinoma of the head of the pancreas, but it rarely draws attention to the invasive cancer soon enough. Weight loss, anorexia, and generalized malaise and weakness tend to be signs of advanced disease. *Migratory thrombophlebitis,* known as the *Trousseau sign,* occurs in about 10% of patients and is attributable to the elaboration of platelet-aggregating factors and procoagulants from the

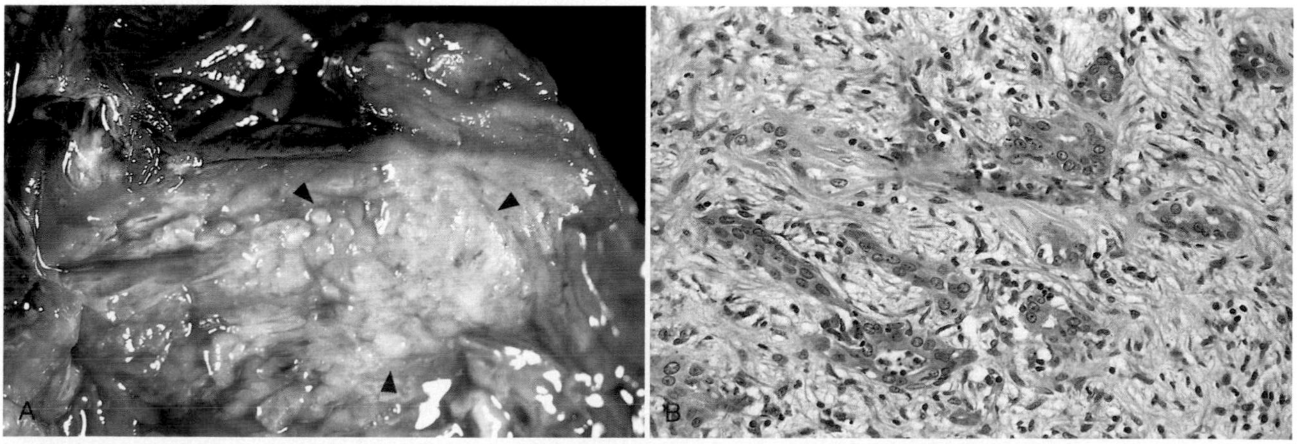

FIGURE 19–14 Carcinoma of the pancreas. *A,* A cross-section through the head of the pancreas and adjacent common bile duct showing both an ill-defined mass in the pancreatic substance (*arrowheads*) and the green discoloration of the duct resulting from total obstruction of bile flow. *B,* Poorly formed glands are present in densely fibrotic stroma within the pancreatic substance; there are some inflammatory cells.

tumor or its necrotic products (Chapter 4). Ironically, Trousseau diagnosed his own fatal disease as cancer of the pancreas when he developed these spontaneously appearing and disappearing thromboses.

The symptomatic course of pancreatic carcinoma is typically brief and progressive. Despite the tendency of lesions of the head of the pancreas to obstruct the biliary system, fewer than 20% of pancreatic cancers overall are resectable at the time of diagnosis. There has long been a search for biochemical tests that could be useful in the early detection of pancreatic cancer. The *K-RAS* oncogene is mutated in 90% of pancreatic cancers; however, the utility of screening tests for *K-RAS* mutations remains unproven. Serum levels of many enzymes and antigens (e.g., carcinoembryonic antigen and CA19–9 antigen) have been found to be elevated, but these markers are not specific nor are they sensitive enough to be used as screening tests. Several imaging techniques, such as endoscopic ultrasonography and CT, have proved of great value in diagnosis and the performance of percutaneous needle biopsy. Both of these techniques, while useful in establishing a diagnosis, are not useful as screening tests.

PANCREATOBLASTOMA

Pancreatoblastomas are rare neoplasms that occur primarily in children aged 1 to 15 years.[72] They have a distinct microscopic appearance with squamous islands admixed with undifferentiated cells. These are fully malignant neoplasms, although survival may be better than that for pancreatic ductal adenocarcinomas.

REFERENCES

1. Solcia E, Capella C, Klöppel G: Atlas of Tumor Pathology: Tumors of the Pancreas, 3rd series ed. Washington, DC: Armed Forces Institute of Pathology, 1997.
2. Oertel JE: The pancreas: nonneoplastic alterations. Am J Surg Pathol 13:50, 1989.
3. Stoffers DA, Zinkin NT, Stanojevic V, Clarke WL, Habener JF: Pancreatic agenesis attributable to a single nucleotide deletion in the human IPF1 gene coding sequence. Nat Genet 15:106, 1997.
4. Gregg JA: Pancreas divisum: its association with pancreatitis. Am J Surg 134:539, 1977.
5. Gregg JA, Monaco AP, McDermott WV: Pancreas divisum: results of surgical intervention. Am J Surg 145:488, 1983.
6. Richter JM, Schapiro RH, Mulley AG, Warshaw AL: Association of pancreas divisum and pancreatitis and its treatment by sphincteroplasty of the accessory ampulla. Gastroenterology 81:1104, 1981.
7. Kiernan PD, ReMine SG, Kiernan PC, ReMine WH: Annular pancreas. Arch Surg 1980;115:46–50.
8. Benger JR, Thompson MH. Annular pancreas and obstructive jaundice. Am J Gastroenterol 92:713, 1997.
9. Ashizawa N, Niigaki M, Hamamoto N, Niigaki M, Kaji T, Katsube T, Sato S, Endoh H, Hidaka K, Watanabe M, et al: The morphological changes of exocrine pancreas in chronic pancreatitis. Histol Histopathol 14:539, 1999.
10. Mitchell RMS, Byrne MF, Baillie J: Pancreatitis. Lancet 361:1447, 2003.
11. Steinberg W, Tenner S: Acute pancreatitis. N Engl J Med 330:1198, 1994.
12. Marshall JB: Acute pancreatitis: a review with an emphasis on new developments. Arch Intern Med 153:1185, 1993.
13. Beger HG, Rau B, Mayer J, Pralle U: Natural course of acute pancreatitis. World J Surg 21:130, 1997.
14. Ranson J: Risk factors in acute pancreatitis. Hosp Pract 20:69, 1985.
15. Lee SP, Nicholls JF, Park HZ: Biliary sludge as a cause of acute pancreatitis. N Engl J Med 326:589, 1992.
16. Bank S, Indaram A: Causes of acute and recurrent pancreatitis: clinical considerations and clues to diagnosis. Gastroenterol Clin North Am 28:571, 1999.
17. Scarpelli DG: Toxicology of the pancreas. Toxicol Appl Pharmacol 101:543, 1989.
18. Whitcomb DC, Gorry MC, Preston RA, Furey W, Sossenheimer MJ, Ulrich C, Martin SP, Gates LK, Amann ST, Toskes PP, et al: Hereditary pancreatitis is caused by a mutation in the cationic trypsinogen gene. Nat Genet 14:141, 1996.
19. Whitcomb DC: Hereditary pancreatitis: new insights into acute and chronic pancreatitis. Gut 45:317, 1999.
20. Witt H, Luck W, Hennies HC, Classen M, Kage A, Lass U, Landt O, Becker M: Mutations in the gene encoding the serine protease inhibitor, Kazal type 1 are associated with chronic pancreatitis. Nat Genet 25:213, 2000.
21. Noone PG, Zhou Z, Silverman LM, Jowell PS, Knowles MR, Cohn JA: Cystic fibrosis gene mutations and pancreatitis risk: relation to epithelial ion transport and trypsin inhibitor gene mutations. Gastroenterology 121:1310, 2001.
22. Grendell JH: Genetic factors in pancreatitis. Curr Gastroenterol Rep 5:105, 2003.
23. Chen JM, Montier T, Ferec C: Molecular pathology and evolutionary and physiological implications of pancreatitis-associated cationic trypsinogen mutations. Hum Genet 109:245, 2001.
24. Phat VN, Guerrieri MT, Alexandre JH, Camilleri JP: Early histological changes in acute necrotizing hemorrhagic pancreatitis. Pathol Res Pract 178:273, 1984.
25. Norman J: The role of cytokines in the pathogenesis of acute pancreatitis. Am J Surg 175:76, 1998.
26. Saluja AK, Steer MLP: Pathophysiology of pancreatitis: role of cytokines and other mediators of inflammation. Digestion 60 (Suppl 1):27, 1999.
27. Rau B, Paszkowski A, Lillich S, Baumgart K, Moller P, Beger HG: Differential effects of caspase-1/interleukin-1beta-converting enzyme on acinar cell necrosis and apoptosis in severe acute experimental pancreatitis. Lab Invest 81:1001, 2001.
28. Shimada M, Andoh A, Hata K, Tasaki K, Araki Y, Fujiyama Y, Bamba T: IL-6 secretion by human pancreatic periacinar myofibroblasts in response to inflammatory mediators. J Immunol 168:861, 2002.
29. Kusske AM, Rongione AJ, Reber HA: Cytokines and acute pancreatitis. Gastroenterology 110:639, 1996.
30. Kingsnorth A: Role of cytokines and their inhibitors in acute pancreatitis. Gut 40:1, 1997.
31. Blackstone MO: Hypothesis: vascular compromise is the central pathogenic mechanism for acute hemorrhagic pancreatitis. Perspect Biol Med 39:56, 1995.
32. Steer ML: Pathogenesis of acute pancreatitis. Digestion 58 (Suppl 1):46, 1997.
33. Steer ML, Meldolesi J: The cell biology of experimental pancreatitis. N Engl J Med 316:144, 1987.
34. Whitcomb DC. Early trypsinogen activation in acute pancreatitis. Gastroenterology 116:770, 1999.
35. Pitchumoni CS, Bordalo O: Evaluation of hypotheses on pathogenesis of alcoholic pancreatitis. Am J Gastroenterol 91:637, 1996.
36. Karne S, Gorelick FS: Etiopathogenesis of acute pancreatitis. Surg Clin North Am 79:699, 1999.
37. Watanabe S: Acute pancreatitis: overview of medical aspects. Pancreas 16:307, 1998.
38. Sarles H: Definitions and classifications of pancreatitis. Pancreas 6:470, 1991.
39. Chari ST, Mohan V, Pitchumoni CS, Viswanathan M, Madanagopalan N, Lowenfels AB: Risk of pancreatic carcinoma in tropical calcifying pancreatitis: an epidemiologic study. Pancreas 9:62, 1994.
40. Witt H: Chronic pancreatitis and cystic fibrosis. Gut 52 (Suppl 2): ii31, 2003.
41. Klöppel G: Progression from acute to chronic pancreatitis: a pathologist's view. Surg Clin North Am 79:801, 1999.
42. Adler G, Schmid RM: Chronic pancreatitis: still puzzling? Gastroenterology 112:1762, 1997.
43. Pitchumoni CS: Pathogenesis of alcohol-induced chronic pancreatitis: facts, perceptions, and misperceptions. Surg Clin North Am 81:379, 2001.
44. Suda K, Mogaki M, Oyama T, Matsumoto Y: Histopathologic and immunohistochemical studies on alcoholic pancreatitis and chronic obstructive pancreatitis: a special emphasis on ductal obstruction and genesis of pancreatitis. Am J Gastroenterol 85:271, 1990.

45. Saurer L, Reber P, Schaffner T, Buchler MW, Buri C, Kappeler A, Walz A, Friess H, Mueller C: Differential expression of chemokines in normal pancreas and in chronic pancreatitis. Gastroenterology 118:356, 2000.
46. Bachem MG, Schneider E, Gross H, Weidenbach H, Schmid RM, Menke A, Siech M, Beger H, Grunert A, Adler G: Identification, culture, and characterization of pancreatic stellate cells in rats and humans. Gastroenterology 115:421, 1998.
47. Luttenberger T, Schmid-Kotsas A, Menke A, Siech M, Beger H, Adler G, Grunert A, Bachem MG: Platelet-derived growth factors stimulate proliferation and extracellular matrix synthesis of pancreatic stellate cells: implications in pathogenesis of pancreas fibrosis. Lab Invest 80:47, 2000.
48. Van Laethem JL, Deviere J, Resibois A, Rickaert F, Vertongen P, Ohtani H, Cremer M, Miyazono K, Robberecht P: Localization of transforming growth factor beta 1 and its latent binding protein in human chronic pancreatitis. Gastroenterology 108:1873, 1995.
49. Lowenfels AB, Maisonneuve EP, Dimagno YE, Gates LK, Perrault J, Whitcomb DC: International Hereditary Pancreatitis Study Group. Hereditary pancreatitis and the risk of pancreatic cancer. J Natl Cancer Inst 89:442, 1997.
50. Lowenfels AB, Maisonneuve P, Cavallini G, Ammann RW, Lankisch PG, Andersen JR, Dimango EP, Andren-Sandberg A, Domellof L: Pancreatitis and the risk of pancreatic cancer. N Engl J Med 328:1433, 1993.
51. Klöppel G: Pseudocysts and other non-neoplastic cysts of the pancreas. Semin Diagn Pathol 17:7, 2000.
52. Compagno J, Oertel JE: Microcystic adenomas of the pancreas (glycogen-rich cystadenomas): a clinicopathologic study of 34 cases. Am J Clin Pathol 69:289, 1978.
53. Compagno J, Oertel JE: Mucinous cystic neoplasms of the pancreas with overt and latent malignancy (cystadenocarcinoma and cystadenoma): a clinicopathologic study of 41 cases. Am J Clin Pathol 69:573, 1978.
54. Wilentz RE, Albores-Saavedra J, Hruban RH: Mucinous cystic neoplasms of the pancreas. Semin Diagn Pathol 17:31, 2000.
55. Wilentz RE, Albores-Saavedra J, Zahurak M, Talamini MA, Yeo CJ, Cameron JL, Hruban RH: Pathologic examination accurately predicts prognosis in mucinous cystic neoplasms of the pancreas. Am J Surg Pathol 23:1320, 1999.
56. Sohn TA, Yeo CJ, Cameron JL, Iacobuzio-Donahue CA, Hruban RH, Lillemoe KD: Intraductal papillary mucinous neoplasms of the pancreas: an increasingly recognized clinicopathologic entity. Ann Surg 234:313, 2001.
57. Abraham SC, Klimstra DS, Wilentz RE, Wu T-T, Cameron JL, Yeo CJ, Hruban RH: Solid-pseudopapillary tumors of the pancreas almost always harbor mutations in the beta-catenin gene. Am J Pathol 160:1361, 2002.
58. American Cancer Society: Cancer facts and figures 2004. American Cancer Society, 2004.
59. Hruban RH, Wilentz RE, Kern SE: Genetic progression in the pancreatic ducts. Am J Pathol 156:1821, 2000.
60. van Heek NT, Meeker AK, Kern SE, Yeo CJ, Lillemoe KD, Cameron JL, Offerhaus GJ, Hicks JL, Wilentz, RE, Goggins MG, De Marzo AM, Hruban RH, Maitra A: Telomere shortening is nearly universal in pancreatic intraepithelial neoplasia. Am J Pathol 161:1541, 2002.
61. Bardeesy N, DePinho RA: Pancreatic cancer biology and genetics. Nat Rev Cancer 2:897, 2002.
62. Caldas C, Hahn SA, da Costa LT, Redston MS, Schutte M, Seymour AB, Weinstein CL, Hruban RH, Yeo CJ, Kern SE: Frequent somatic mutations and homozygous deletions of the *p16* (*MTS1*) gene in pancreatic adenocarcinoma. Nat Genet 8:27, 1994.
63. Hahn SA, Schutte M, Hoque ATMS, Moskaluk CA, daCosta LT, Rozenblum E, Weinstein CL, Fischer A, Yeo CJ, Hruban RH, et al: *DPC4*, a candidate tumor suppressor gene at human chromosome 18q21.1. Science 271:350, 1996.
64. Redston MS, Caldas C, Seymour AB, Hruban RH, da Costa L, Yeo CJ, Kern SE: *p53* mutations in pancreatic carcinoma and evidence of common involvement of homocopolymer tracts in DNA microdeletions. Cancer Res 54:3025, 1994.
65. Ryu B, Jones J, Blades NJ, Parmigiani G, Hollingsworth MA, Hruban RH, Kern SE: Relationships and differentially expressed genes among pancreatic cancers examined by large-scale serial analysis of gene expression. Cancer Res 62:819, 2002.
66. Iacobuzio-Donahue CA, Maitra A, Shen-Ong GL, van Heek T, Ashgaq R, Meyer R, Walter K, Berg K, Hollingsworth MA, Cameron JL, et al: Discovery of novel tumor markers of pancreatic cancer using global gene expression technology. Am J Pathol 160:1239, 2002.
67. Berman DM, et al: Widespread requirement for hedgehog ligand stimulation in growth of digestive tract tumors. Nature 425:846, 2003.
68. Gold EB, Goldin SB: Epidemiology of and risk factors for pancreatic cancer. Surg Oncol Clin N Am 7:67, 1998.
69. Hruban RH, Petersen GM, Ha PK, Kern SE: Genetics of pancreatic cancer: from genes to families. Surg Oncol Clin N Am 7:1, 1998.
70. Klimstra DS, Heffess CS, Oertel JE, Rosai J: Acinar cell carcinoma of the pancreas: a clinicopathologic study of 28 cases. Am J Surg Pathol 16:815, 1992.
71. Westra WH, Sturm PJ, Drillenburg P, Choti MA, Klimstra DS, Abores-Saavedra J, Montag A, Offerhaus GJA, Hruban RH: K-*ras* oncogene mutations in osteoclast-like giant-cell tumors of the pancreas and liver: genetic evidence to support origin from the duct epithelium. Am J Surg Pathol 22:1247, 1998.
72. Klimstra DS, Wenig BM, Adair CF, Heffess CS: Pancreatoblastoma: a clinicopathologic study and review of the literature. Am J Surg Pathol 19:1371, 1995.

CHAPTER 20

The Kidney

Charles E. Alpers, MD

CLINICAL MANIFESTATIONS OF RENAL DISEASES

CONGENITAL ANOMALIES

CYSTIC DISEASES OF THE KIDNEY

Cystic Renal Dysplasia

Autosomal-Dominant (Adult) Polycystic Kidney Disease

Autosomal-Recessive (Childhood) Polycystic Kidney Disease

Cystic Diseases of Renal Medulla

Medullary Sponge Kidney

Nephronophthisis–Medullary Cystic Disease Complex

Acquired (Dialysis-Associated) Cystic Disease

Simple Cysts

GLOMERULAR DISEASES

Clinical Manifestations

Histologic Alterations

Pathogenesis of Glomerular Injury

In Situ Immune Complex Deposition

Circulating Immune Complex Nephritis

Antibodies to Glomerular Cells

Cell-Mediated Immunity in Glomerulonephritis

Activation of Alternative Complement Pathway

Epithelial Cell Injury

Mediators of Glomerular Injury

Mechanisms of Progression in Glomerular Diseases

Acute Glomerulonephritis

Acute Proliferative (Poststreptococcal, Postinfectious) Glomerulonephritis

Rapidly Progressive (Crescentic) Glomerulonephritis

Nephrotic Syndrome

Membranous Glomerulopathy (Membranous Nephropathy)

Minimal Change Disease (Lipoid Nephrosis)

Focal Segmental Glomerulosclerosis

Membranoproliferative Glomerulonephritis

IgA Nephropathy (Berger Disease)

Hereditary Syndromes of Isolated Hematuria

Alport Syndrome

Thin Basement Membrane Disease (Benign Familial Hematuria)

Chronic Glomerulonephritis

Glomerular Lesions Associated with Systemic Diseases

Systemic Lupus Erythematosus

Henoch-Schönlein Purpura

Bacterial Endocarditis

Diabetic Glomerulosclerosis

Amyloidosis

Fibrillary and Immunotactoid Glomerulonephritis

Other Systemic Disorders

DISEASES AFFECTING TUBULES AND INTERSTITIUM

Acute Tubular Necrosis

Tubulointerstitial Nephritis

Pyelonephritis and Urinary Tract Infection

Acute Pyelonephritis

Chronic Pyelonephritis and Reflux Nephropathy

Tubulointerstitial Nephritis Induced by Drugs and Toxins

Other Tubulointerstitial Diseases

DISEASES OF BLOOD VESSELS

Benign Nephrosclerosis

Malignant Hypertension and Accelerated Nephrosclerosis

Renal Artery Stenosis
Thrombotic Microangiopathies
Classic (Childhood) Hemolytic-Uremic Syndrome
Adult Hemolytic-Uremic Syndrome
Familial HUS
Idiopathic TTP
Other Vascular Disorders
Atherosclerotic Ischemic Renal Disease
Atheroembolic Renal Disease
Sickle Cell Disease Nephropathy
Diffuse Cortical Necrosis
Renal Infarcts
URINARY TRACT OBSTRUCTION (OBSTRUCTIVE UROPATHY)
UROLITHIASIS (RENAL CALCULI, STONES)
TUMORS OF THE KIDNEY
Benign Tumors
Renal Papillary Adenoma
Renal Fibroma or Hamartoma (Renomedullary Interstitial Cell Tumor)
Angiomyolipoma
Oncocytoma
Malignant Tumors
Renal Cell Carcinoma (Adenocarcinoma of the Kidney)
Urothelial Carcinomas of the Renal Pelvis

Normal

What is a human but an ingenious machine designed to turn, with "infinite artfulness, the red wine of Shiraz into urine"? So said the storyteller in Isak Dinesen's *Seven Gothic Tales.*[1] More accurately but less poetically, human kidneys serve to convert more than 1700 liters of blood per day into about 1 liter of a highly specialized concentrated fluid called urine. In so doing, the kidney excretes the waste products of metabolism, precisely regulates the body's concentration of water and salt, maintains the appropriate acid balance of plasma, and serves as an endocrine organ, secreting such hormones as erythropoietin, renin, and prostaglandins. The physiologic mechanisms that the kidney has evolved to carry out these functions require a high degree of structural complexity.

Each human adult kidney weighs about 150 gm. As the ureter enters the kidney at the hilum, it dilates into a funnel-shaped cavity, the *pelvis*, from which derive two or three main branches, the *major calyces*; each of these subdivides again into three or four *minor calyces*. There are about 12 minor calyces in the human kidney. On the cut surface, the kidney is made up of a *cortex* and a *medulla*, the former 1.2 to 1.5 cm in thickness. The medulla consists of *renal pyramids*, the apices of which are called *papillae*, each related to a calyx. Cortical tissue extends into spaces between adjacent pyramids as the *renal columns of Bertin*. From the standpoint of its diseases, the kidney can be divided into four components: blood vessels, glomeruli, tubules, and interstitium.

Blood Vessels. The kidney is richly supplied by blood vessels, and although both kidneys make up only 0.5% of the total body weight, they receive about 25% of the cardiac output. The cortex is by far the most richly vascularized part of the kidney, receiving 90% of the total renal blood supply. The main renal artery divides into anterior and posterior sections at the hilum. From these, *interlobar arteries* emerge, course between lobes, and give rise to the *arcuate arteries*, which arch between cortex and medulla, in turn giving rise to the *interlobular arteries*. From the interlobular arteries, *afferent arterioles* enter the glomerular tuft, where they progressively subdivide into 20 to 40 capillary loops arranged in several units or lobules architecturally centered by a supporting mesangial stalk. Capillary loops merge to exit from the glomerulus as *efferent arterioles*. In general, efferent arterioles from superficial nephrons form a rich vascular network that encircles cortical tubules (*peritubular vascular network*), and deeper juxtamedullary glomeruli give rise to the *vasa recta*, which descend as straight vessels to supply the outer and inner medulla. These descending arterial vasa recta then make several loops in the inner medulla and ascend as the *venous vasa recta*.

The anatomy of renal vessels has several important implications. First, because the arteries are largely end-arteries, *occlusion of any branch usually results in infarction of the specific area it supplies*. Glomerular disease that interferes with blood flow through the glomerular capillaries has profound effects on the tubules, within both the cortex and the medulla, because *all tubular capillary beds are derived from the efferent arterioles*. The peculiarities of the blood supply to the renal medulla render them especially vulnerable to ischemia; *the medulla does not have its own arterial blood supply but is dependent on the blood emanating from the glomerular efferent arterioles*. The blood in the capillary loops in the medulla has a remarkably low level of oxygenation. Thus, minor interference with the blood supply of the medulla may result in medullary necrosis from ischemia.

Glomeruli. The glomerulus consists of an anastomosing network of capillaries lined by fenestrated endothelium invested by two layers of epithelium (Fig. 20–1). The visceral epithelium is incorporated into and becomes an intrinsic part of the capillary wall, separated from endothelial cells by a basement membrane. The parietal epithelium, situated on Bowman's capsule, lines the urinary space, the cavity in which plasma filtrate first collects.

The glomerular capillary wall is the filtering membrane and consists of the following structures[2] (Fig. 20–2):

- A thin layer of fenestrated *endothelial cells*, each fenestrum being about 70 to 100 nm in diameter.
- A *glomerular basement membrane* (GBM) with a thick electron-dense central layer, the *lamina densa*, and thinner electron-lucent peripheral layers, the *lamina rara interna* and *lamina rara externa*. The GBM consists of collagen (mostly type IV), laminin, polyanionic proteoglycans (mostly heparan sulfate), fibronectin, entactin, and several other glycoproteins. Type IV collagen forms a network

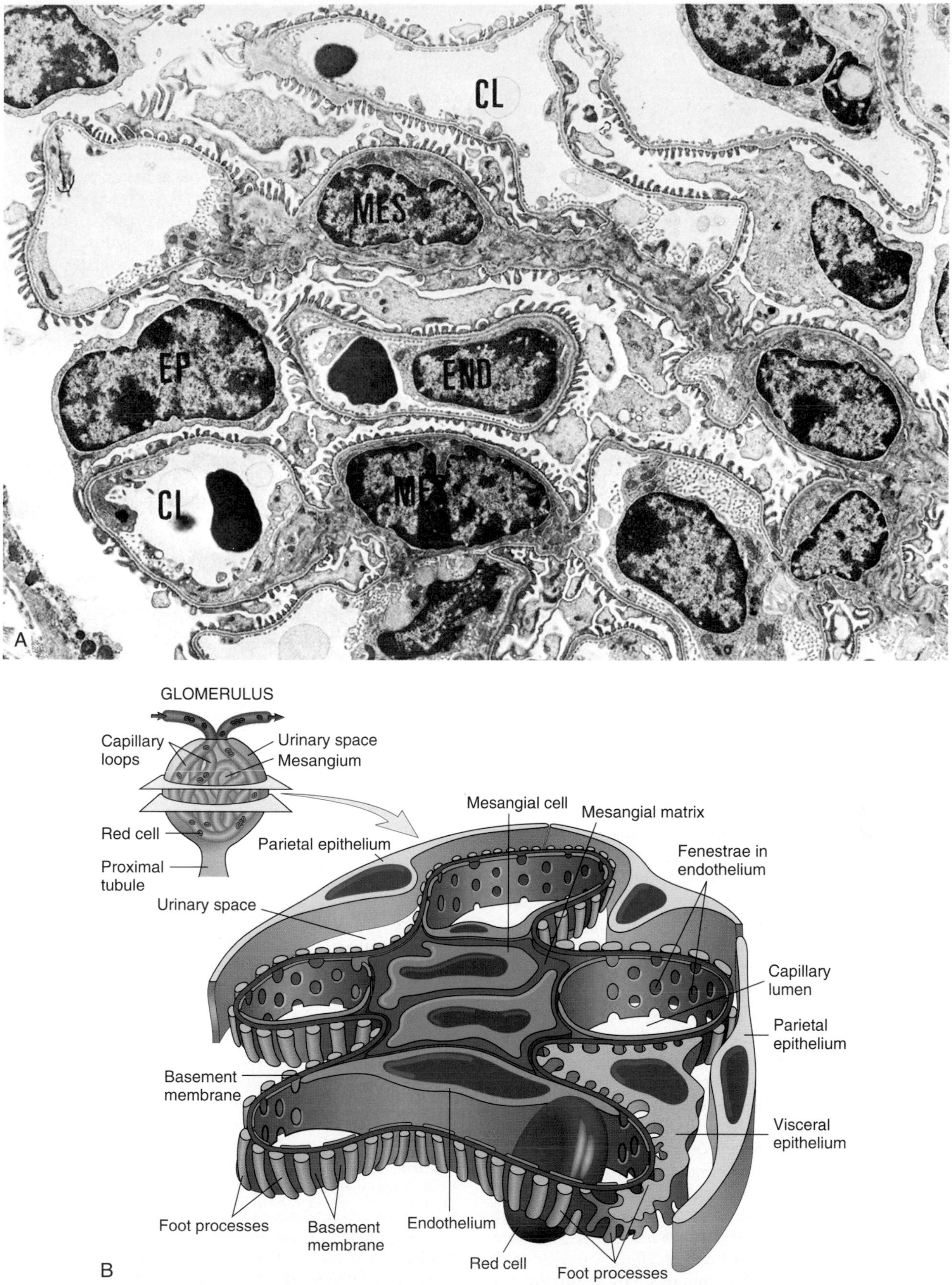

FIGURE 20–1 *A*, Low-power electron micrograph of renal glomerulus. CL, capillary lumen; MES, mesangium; END, endothelium; EP, visceral epithelial cells with foot processes. (Courtesy of Dr. Vicki Kelley, Brigham and Women's Hospital, Boston, MA.) *B*, Schematic representation of a glomerular lobe.

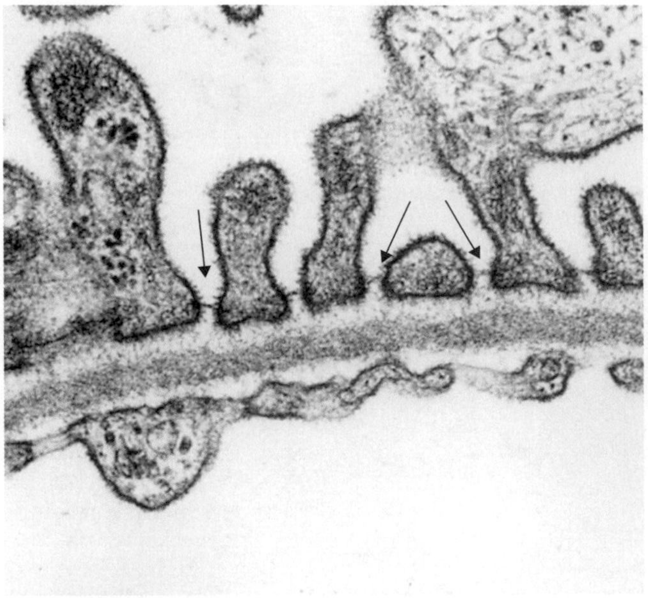

FIGURE 20–2 Glomerular filter consisting, from bottom to top, of fenestrated endothelium, basement membrane, and foot processes of epithelial cells. Note the filtration slits (*arrows*) and diaphragm. Note also that the basement membrane consists of a central lamina densa, sandwiched between two looser layers, the lamina rara interna and lamina rara externa. (Courtesy of Dr. Helmut Rennke, Brigham and Women's Hospital, Boston, MA.)

suprastructure to which other glycoproteins attach. The building block (monomer) of this network is a triple-helical molecule made up of three α-chains, composed of one or more of six types of α-chains (α_1 to α_6 or COL4A1 to COL4A6), the most common consisting of α_1, α_2, α_1 (Fig. 20–3).[3] Each molecule consists of a 7S domain at the amino terminus, a triple-helical domain in the middle, and a globular noncollagenous domain (NC1) at the carboxyl terminus. The NC1 domain is important for helix formation and for assembly of collagen monomers into the basement membrane suprastructure. Glycoproteins (laminin, entactin) and acidic proteoglycans (heparan sulfate, perlecan) attach to the collagenous suprastructure[3–5] (Fig. 20–4). *These biochemical determinants are critical to understanding glomerular diseases.* For example, as we shall see, the antigens in the NC1 domain are the targets of antibodies in anti-GBM nephritis; genetic defects in the α-chains underlie some forms of hereditary nephritis; and the acidic porous nature of the GBM determines its permeability characteristics.

- The *visceral epithelial cells* (podocytes), are structurally complex cells that possess interdigitating processes embedded in and adherent to the lamina rara externa of the basement membrane. Adjacent *foot processes* (pedicels) are separated by 20- to 30-nm–wide *filtration slits,* which are bridged by a thin diaphragm (see Fig. 20–2).
- The entire glomerular tuft is supported by *mesangial cells* lying between the capillaries. Basement membrane–like *mesangial matrix* forms a meshwork through which the mesangial cells are centered (Fig. 20–1). These cells, of mesenchymal origin, are contractile, phagocytic, and capable of proliferation, of laying down both matrix and collagen, and of secreting a number of biologically active mediators. Biologically, they are most akin to vascular smooth muscle cells and pericytes. They are, as we shall see, important players in many forms of human glomerulonephritis.

The major characteristics of normal glomerular filtration are an extraordinarily high permeability to water and small solutes, because of the highly fenestrated nature of the endothelium, and impermeability to proteins, such as molecules of the size of albumin (+3.6-nm radius; 70 kilodaltons [kDa] molecular weight) or larger. The latter property, called

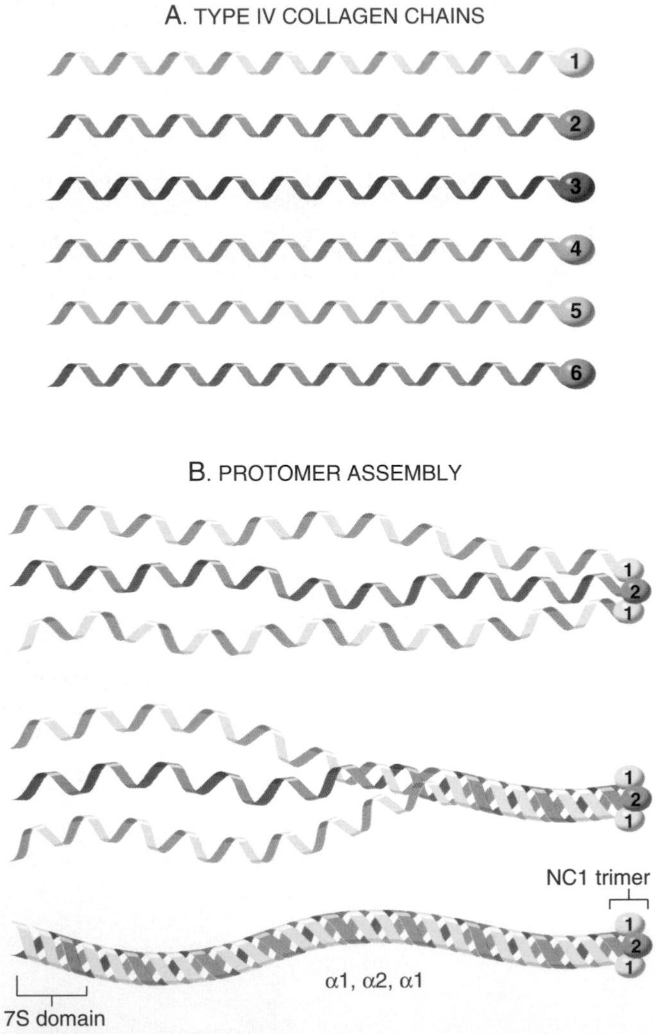

FIGURE 20–3 Schematic illustration of type IV collagen supramolecular network assembly. *A,* Six genetically distinct α-chains (α1 to α6) assemble into three distinct protomers. The protomers are characterized by a long central collagen triple helix, the 7S domain at the N terminus, and a globular NC1 trimer at the C terminus. *B,* NC1 domains provide specificity for chain association, alignment, registration, and propagation from the C- to N-terminal direction. This sequence of events, shown for the α1, α2 protomer, is true for other protomers also. (Courtesy of Dr. Billy Hudson, Vanderbilt University, Nashville, TN, reprinted with permission.)

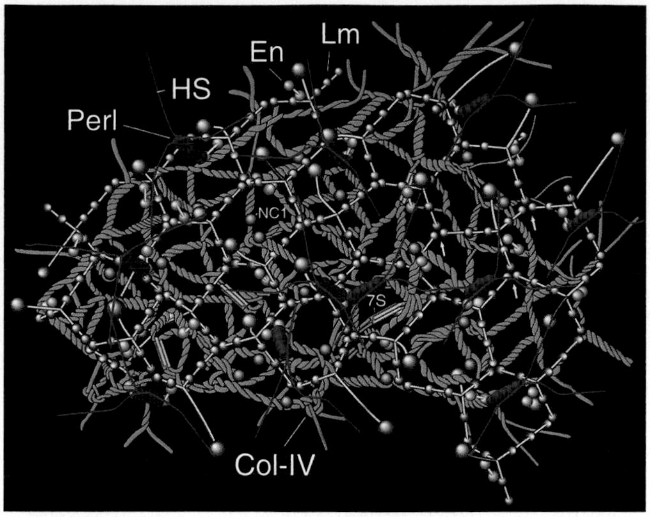

FIGURE 20–4 A proposed model of the GBM molecular architecture in which type IV collagen monomers (*gray*) form a stable network through their NC1 domains (dimeric interactions, gray spheres) and 7S domains (tetrameric interactions) and intertwine along the triple-helical domains. Laminin monomers (*red*) separately form a reversible meshwork. Entactin (*green*) connects laminin to the collagen network and binds to perlecan (*blue*), an anionic heparan sulfate proteoglycan. This anionic suprastructure determines the charged porous nature of the GBM. (Courtesy of Dr. Peter Yurchenco, Robert W. Johnson Medical School, Piscataway, NJ.)

glomerular barrier function, discriminates among various protein molecules, depending on their size (the larger, the less permeable) and charge (the more cationic, the more permeable). This size- and charge-dependent barrier function is accounted for by the complex structure of the capillary wall, the collagenous porous and charged structure of the GBM, and the many anionic moieties present within the wall, including the acidic proteoglycans of the GBM (Fig. 20–4) and the sialoglycoproteins of epithelial and endothelial cell coats. The charge-dependent restriction is important in the virtually complete exclusion of albumin from the filtrate, because

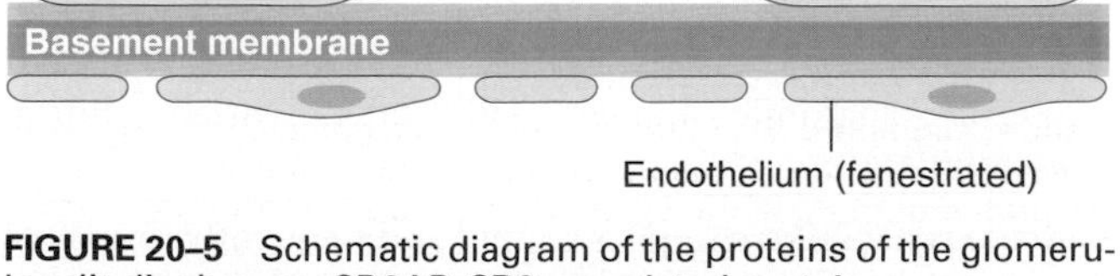

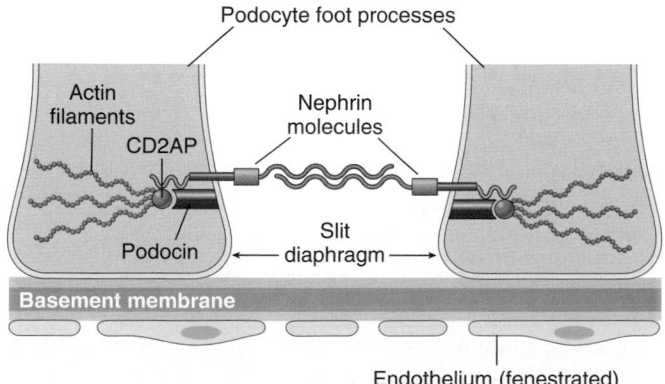

FIGURE 20–5 Schematic diagram of the proteins of the glomerular slit diaphragm. CD2AP, CD2-associated protein.

albumin is an anionic molecule of a pI 4.5. The *visceral epithelial cell*, also known as a podocyte, is important for the maintenance of glomerular barrier function; its slit diaphragm presents a size-selective distal diffusion barrier to the filtration of proteins, and it is the cell type that is largely responsible for synthesis of GBM components. Proteins located in the slit diaphragm control glomular permeability. While the details are imcomplete, three important proteins have been identified (Fig. 20–5). Nephrin is a transmembrane protein with a large extracellular portion made up of immunoglobulin (Ig)-like domains. Nephrin molecules extend towards each other from neighboring foot processes and dimerize across the slit diaphragm. Within the cytoplasm of the foot processes, nephrin forms molecular connections with podocin, CD2-associated protein, and ultimately the actin cytoskeleton. The importance of these proteins in maintaining glomerular permeability is demonstrated by the observation that mutations in the genes encoding them give rise to nephrotic syndrome (discussed later). This has resulted in renewed appreciation of the importance of the slit diaphragm in glomerular barrier function and its contribution to protein leakage in disease states.[6]

Tubules. The structure of renal tubular epithelial cells varies considerably at different levels of the nephron and, to a certain extent, correlates with function. For example, the highly developed structure of the *proximal tubular cells*, with their abundant long microvilli, numerous mitochondria, apical canaliculi, and extensive intercellular interdigitations, is correlated with their major functions: reabsorption of two-thirds of filtered sodium and water as well as glucose, potassium, phosphate, amino acids, and proteins. The proximal tubule is particularly vulnerable to ischemic damage. Furthermore, toxins are frequently reabsorbed by the proximal tubule, rendering it also susceptible to chemical injury.

The *juxtaglomerular apparatus* snuggles closely against the glomerulus where the afferent arteriole enters it. The juxtaglomerular apparatus consists of (1) the *juxtaglomerular cells*, modified granulated smooth muscle cells in the media of the afferent arteriole that contain renin; (2) the *macula densa*, a specialized region of the distal tubule as it returns to the vascular pole of its parent glomerulus, where the tubular cells are more crowded and the cells are somewhat shorter and possess distinct patterns of interdigitation between adjacent membranes; and (3) the *lacis cells* or *nongranular cells*, which reside in the area bounded by the afferent arteriole, the macula densa, and the glomerulus. They resemble mesangial cells and appear to be continuous with them. The juxtaglomerular apparatus is a small endocrine organ, the juxtaglomerular cells being the principal sources of renin production in the kidney.

Interstitium. In the normal cortex, the interstitial space is compact, being occupied by the fenestrated peritubular capillaries and a small number of fibroblast-like cells. Any obvious expansion of the cortical interstitium is usually abnormal; this expansion can be due to edema or infiltration by acute inflammatory cells, as in acute interstitial diseases, or it may be caused by accumulation of chronic inflammatory cells and fibrous tissue, as in chronic interstitial diseases. The amounts of proteoglycans in the interstitial tissue of the medulla increase with age and in the presence of ischemia.

Pathology

Renal diseases are responsible for a great deal of morbidity but, fortunately, are not equally major causes of mortality. To place the problem in some perspective, approximately 70,000 deaths are attributed yearly to renal disease in the United States,[7] in contrast to about 700,000 to heart disease, 550,000 to cancer, and 170,000 to stroke.[8] Morbidity, however, is by no means insignificant. Millions of people are affected annually by nonfatal kidney diseases, most notably infections of the kidney or lower urinary tract, kidney stones, and urinary obstruction. Twenty per cent of all women suffer from infection of the urinary tract or kidney at some time in their lives, and as many as 5% of the U.S. population develops renal stones. Similarly, dialysis and transplantation keep many patients alive who would formerly have died of renal failure, adding to the pool of renal morbidity. The cost of such programs now exceeds several billion dollars annually.

Diseases of the kidney are as complex as its structure, but their study is facilitated by dividing them into those that affect the four basic morphologic components: glomeruli, tubules, interstitium, and blood vessels. This traditional approach is useful, since the early manifestations of disease affecting each of these components tend to be distinct. Further, some components appear to be more vulnerable to specific forms of renal injury; for example, most glomerular diseases are immunologically mediated, whereas tubular and interstitial disorders are frequently caused by toxic or infectious agents. Nevertheless, some agents affect more than one structure. In addition, the anatomic and functional interdependence of the components of the kidney implies that damage to one almost always secondarily affects the others. Disease primarily in the blood vessels, for example, inevitably affects all the structures that depend on this blood supply. Severe glomerular damage impairs the flow through the peritubular vascular system and also delivers potentially toxic products to tubules; conversely, tubular destruction, by increasing intraglomerular pressure, may induce glomerular atrophy. Thus, whatever the origin, there is a tendency for all forms of chronic renal disease ultimately to destroy all four components of the kidney, culminating in chronic renal failure and what has been called end-stage kidneys. The functional reserve of the kidney is large, and much damage may occur before there is evident functional impairment. For these reasons, the early signs and symptoms are particularly important clinically.

In this chapter, we review the clinical manifestations, pathogenesis, and pathology of the major renal diseases.

Clinical Manifestations of Renal Diseases

The clinical manifestations of renal disease can be grouped into reasonably well-defined syndromes. Some are peculiar to glomerular diseases, and others are present in diseases that affect any one of the components. Before we list the syndromes, a few terms must be clarified.

Azotemia is a biochemical abnormality that refers to an elevation of the blood urea nitrogen (BUN) and creatinine levels and is related largely to a decreased glomerular filtration rate (GFR). Azotemia is produced by many renal disorders, but it also arises from extrarenal disorders. *Prerenal azotemia* is encountered when there is hypoperfusion of the kidneys (e.g., in hemorrhage, shock, volume depletion, and congestive heart failure) that impairs renal function in the absence of parenchymal damage. Similarly, *postrenal azotemia* is seen whenever urine flow is obstructed below the level of the kidney. Relief of the obstruction is followed by correction of the azotemia.

When azotemia becomes associated with a constellation of clinical signs and symptoms and biochemical abnormalities, it is termed *uremia*. Uremia is characterized not only by failure of renal excretory function, but also by a host of metabolic and endocrine alterations resulting from renal damage. There is, in addition, secondary involvement of the gastrointestinal system (e.g., uremic gastroenteritis), peripheral nerves (e.g., peripheral neuropathy), and heart (e.g., uremic fibrinous pericarditis), which is usually necessary for the diagnosis of uremia.

We can now turn to a brief description of the clinical presentations of renal disease:

- *Acute nephritic syndrome* is a glomerular syndrome dominated by the acute onset of usually grossly visible hematuria (red blood cells in urine), mild to moderate proteinuria, and hypertension; it is the classic presentation of acute poststreptococcal glomerulonephritis.
- The *nephrotic syndrome* is characterized by heavy proteinuria (more than 3.5 gm/day), hypoalbuminemia, severe edema, hyperlipidemia, and lipiduria (lipid in the urine).
- Asymptomatic hematuria or proteinuria, or a combination of these two, is usually a manifestation of subtle or mild glomerular abnormalities.
- *Acute renal failure* is dominated by oliguria or anuria (reduced or no urine flow), with recent onset of azotemia. It can result from glomerular, interstitial, or vascular injury or acute tubular necrosis.
- *Chronic renal failure*, characterized by prolonged symptoms and signs of uremia, is the end result of all chronic renal parenchymal diseases.
- Renal tubular defects are dominated by polyuria (excessive urine formation), nocturia, and electrolyte disorders (e.g., metabolic acidosis). They are the result of either diseases that directly affect tubular structure (e.g., medullary cystic disease) or defects in specific tubular functions. The latter can be inherited (e.g., familial nephrogenic diabetes, cystinuria, renal tubular acidosis) or acquired (e.g., lead nephropathy).
- Urinary tract infection is characterized by bacteriuria and pyuria (bacteria and leukocytes in the urine). The infection may be symptomatic or asymptomatic, and it may affect the kidney (pyelonephritis) or the bladder (cystitis) only.
- Nephrolithiasis (renal stone) is manifested by renal colic, hematuria, and recurrent stone formation.
- Urinary tract obstruction and renal tumors represent specific anatomic lesions with often varied clinical manifestations.

Acute renal failure implies a rapid and frequently reversible deterioration of renal function. It is discussed in the section on acute tubular necrosis because it frequently occurs in this disorder. Here, the discussion is limited to chronic renal failure, which is the end result of a variety of renal diseases and is the major cause of death from renal disease.

Although exceptions abound, the evolution from normal renal function to symptomatic **chronic renal failure** progresses through four stages that merge into one another.

1. In **diminished renal reserve**, the GFR is about 50% of normal. Serum BUN and creatinine values are normal, and the patients are asymptomatic. However, they are more susceptible to developing azotemia with an additional renal insult.
2. In **renal insufficiency**, the GFR is 20% to 50% of normal. Azotemia appears, usually associated with anemia and hypertension. Polyuria and nocturia can occur as a result of decreased concentrating ability. Sudden stress (e.g., with nephrotoxins) may precipitate uremia.
3. In **renal failure**, the GFR is less than 20% to 25% of normal. The kidneys cannot regulate volume and solute composition, and patients develop edema, metabolic acidosis, and hypocalcemia. Overt uremia may ensue, with neurologic, gastrointestinal, and cardiovascular complications.
4. In **end-stage renal disease**, the GFR is less than 5% of normal; this is the terminal stage of uremia.

The details of the pathophysiology of chronic renal failure are beyond the scope of this book and are well covered in various nephrology texts. Table 20–1 lists the major systemic abnormalities in uremic renal failure.

TABLE 20–1 Principal Systemic Manifestations of Chronic Renal Failure and Uremia

Fluid and Electrolytes
Dehydration
Edema
Hyperkalemia
Metabolic acidosis
Calcium Phosphate and Bone
Hyperphosphatemia
Hypocalcemia
Secondary hyperparathyroidism
Renal osteodystrophy
Hematologic
Anemia
Bleeding diathesis
Cardiopulmonary
Hypertension
Congestive heart failure
Pulmonary edema
Uremic pericarditis
Gastrointestinal
Nausea and vomiting
Bleeding
Esophagitis, gastritis, colitis
Neuromuscular
Myopathy
Peripheral neuropathy
Encephalopathy
Dermatologic
Sallow color
Pruritus
Dermatitis

Congenital Anomalies

About 10% of all people are born with potentially significant malformations of the urinary system. Renal dysplasias and hypoplasias account for 20% of chronic renal failure in children. Autosomal-dominant polycystic kidney disease, a congenital anomaly that becomes apparent in adults, is responsible for about 10% of chronic renal failure in humans.

Congenital renal disease can be hereditary but is most often the result of an acquired developmental defect that arises during gestation. As was discussed in Chapter 10, defects in genes involved in development, including the Wilms tumor (WT1)–associated genes, cause urogenital anomalies. As a rule, developmental abnormalities involve structural components of the kidney and urinary tract. However, genetic abnormalities also cause enzymatic or metabolic defects in tubular transport, such as cystinuria and renal tubular acidosis. Here, we restrict the discussion to structural anomalies involving primarily the kidney. All except horseshoe kidney are uncommon. Anomalies of the lower urinary tract are discussed in Chapter 21.

Agenesis of the Kidney. Total bilateral agenesis, which is incompatible with life, is usually encountered in stillborn infants. It is often associated with many other congenital disorders (e.g., limb defects, hypoplastic lungs) and leads to early death. Unilateral agenesis is an uncommon anomaly that is compatible with normal life if no other abnormalities exist. The opposite kidney is usually enlarged as a result of compensatory hypertrophy. Some patients eventually develop progressive glomerular sclerosis in the remaining kidney as a result of the adaptive changes in hypertrophied nephrons, discussed later in the chapter, and in time, chronic renal failure ensues.

Hypoplasia. Renal hypoplasia refers to failure of the kidneys to develop to a normal size. This anomaly may occur bilaterally, resulting in renal failure in early childhood, but it is more commonly encountered as a unilateral defect. True renal hypoplasia is extremely rare; most cases reported probably represent acquired scarring due to vascular, infectious, or other parenchymal diseases rather than an underlying developmental failure. Differentiation between congenital and acquired atrophic kidneys may be impossible, but *a truly hypoplastic kidney shows no scars and has a reduced number of renal lobes and pyramids*, usually six or fewer. In one form of hypoplastic kidney, *oligomeganephronia*, the kidney is small but the nephrons are markedly hypertrophied.

Ectopic Kidneys. The development of the definitive metanephros may occur in ectopic foci, usually at abnormally low levels. These kidneys lie either just above the pelvic brim or sometimes within the pelvis. They are usually normal or slightly small in size but otherwise are not remarkable. Because of their abnormal position, kinking or tortuosity of the ureters may cause some obstruction to urinary flow, which predisposes to bacterial infections.

Horseshoe Kidneys. Fusion of the upper or lower poles of the kidneys produces a horseshoe-shaped structure that is continuous across the midline anterior to the great vessels. This anatomic anomaly is common and is found in about 1 in 500 to 1000 autopsies. Ninety per cent of such kidneys are fused at the lower pole, and 10% are fused at the upper pole.

Cystic Diseases of the Kidney

Although not all cysts of the kidney are congenital, all types of cysts are discussed here for convenience.

Cystic diseases of the kidney are a heterogeneous group comprising hereditary, developmental but nonhereditary, and acquired disorders. As a group, they are important for several reasons: (1) they are reasonably common and often represent diagnostic problems for clinicians, radiologists, and pathologists; (2) some forms, such as adult polycystic disease, are major causes of chronic renal failure; and (3) they can occasionally be confused with malignant tumors. A useful classification of renal cysts is as follows:[9]

1. Cystic renal dysplasia
2. Polycystic kidney disease
   a. Autosomal-dominant (adult) polycystic disease
   b. Autosomal-recessive (childhood) polycystic disease
3. Medullary cystic disease
   a. Medullary sponge kidney
   b. Nephronophthisis
4. Acquired (dialysis-associated) cystic disease
5. Localized (simple) renal cysts
6. Renal cysts in hereditary malformation syndromes (e.g., tuberous sclerosis)
7. Glomerulocystic disease
8. Extraparenchymal renal cysts (pyelocalyceal cysts, hilar lymphangitic cysts)

Only the more important of the cystic diseases are discussed below. Table 20–2 summarizes the characteristic features of the principal renal cystic diseases.

CYSTIC RENAL DYSPLASIA

This sporadic disorder is due to an abnormality in metanephric differentiation *characterized histologically by the persistence in the kidney of abnormal structures—cartilage, undifferentiated mesenchyme, and immature collecting ductules—and by abnormal lobar organization.* Most cases are associated with ureteropelvic obstruction, ureteral agenesis or atresia, and other anomalies of the lower urinary tract.

Dysplasia can be unilateral or bilateral and is almost always cystic. In gross appearance, the kidney is usually enlarged, extremely irregular, and multicystic (Fig. 20–6*A*). The cysts vary in size from microscopic structures to some that are several centimeters in diameter. On histologic examination, they are lined by flattened epithelium. Although normal nephrons are present, many have immature ducts. The characteristic histologic feature is the *presence of islands of undifferentiated mesenchyme, often with cartilage, and immature collecting ducts* (Fig. 20–6*B*).

When unilateral, the dysplasia is discovered by the appearance of a flank mass that leads to surgical exploration and nephrectomy. The function of the opposite kidney is normal, and such patients have an excellent prognosis after surgical removal of the affected kidney. In bilateral renal dysplasia, renal failure may ultimately result.

AUTOSOMAL-DOMINANT (ADULT) POLYCYSTIC KIDNEY DISEASE

Autosomal-dominant (adult) polycystic kidney disease (ADPKD) is a hereditary disorder characterized by multiple expanding cysts of both kidneys that ultimately destroy the renal parenchyma and cause renal failure.[10] It is a common condition affecting roughly 1 of every 400 to 1000 live births and accounting for about 5% to 10% of cases of chronic renal failure requiring transplantation or dialysis. The pattern of inheritance is *autosomal dominant*, with high penetrance. The disease is universally bilateral; reported unilateral cases probably represent multicystic dysplasia. The cysts initially involve only portions of the nephrons, so renal function is retained until about the fourth or fifth decade of life. ADPKD is genet-

TABLE 20–2 Summary of Renal Cystic Diseases

	Inheritance	Pathologic Features	Clinical Features or Complications	Typical Outcome	Diagrammatic Representation
Adult polycystic kidney disease	Autosomal dominant	Large multicystic kidneys, liver cysts, berry aneurysms	Hematuria, flank pain, urinary tract infection, renal stones, hypertension	Chronic renal failure beginning at age 40–60 yr	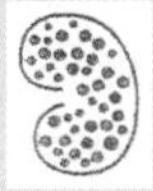
Childhood polycystic kidney disease	Autosomal recessive	Enlarged, cystic kidneys at birth	Hepatic fibrosis	Variable, death in infancy or childhood	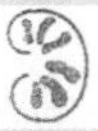
Medullary sponge kidney	None	Medullary cysts on excretory urography	Hematuria, urinary tract infection, recurrent renal stones	Benign	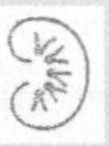
Familial juvenile nephronophthisis	Autosomal recessive	Corticomedullary cysts, shrunken kidneys	Salt wasting, polyuria, growth retardation, anemia	Progressive renal failure beginning in childhood	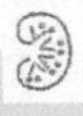
Adult-onset medullary cystic disease	Autosomal dominant	Corticomedullary cysts, shrunken kidneys	Salt wasting, polyuria	Chronic renal failure beginning in adulthood	
Simple cysts	None	Single or multiple cysts in normal-sized kidneys	Microscopic hematuria	Benign	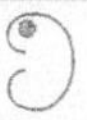
Acquired renal cystic disease	None	Cystic degeneration in end-stage kidney disease	Hemorrhage, erythrocytosis, neoplasia	Dependence on dialysis	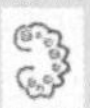

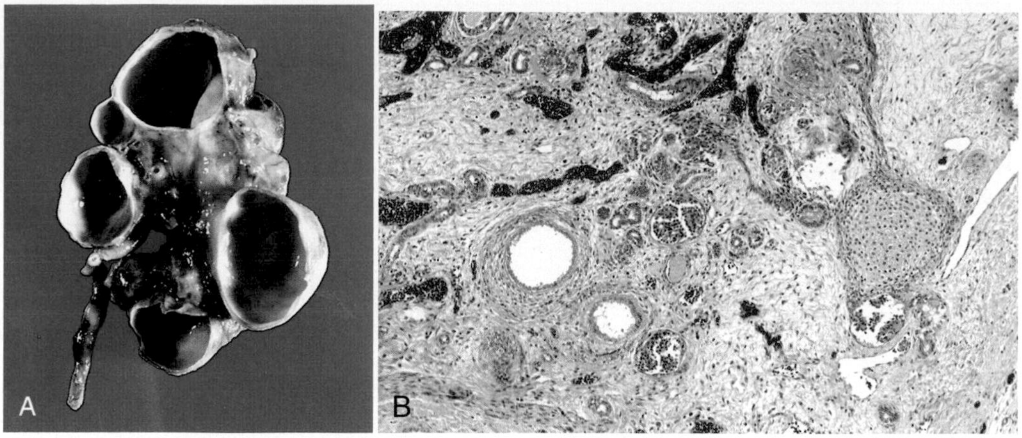

FIGURE 20–6 Renal dysplasia. *A,* Gross appearance. *B,* Histologic section showing disorganized architecture, dilated tubules with cuffs of primitive stroma, and an island of cartilage (H&E stain). (*A,* courtesy of Dr. D. Schofield, Children's Hospital, Los Angeles, CA; *B,* courtesy of Dr. Laura Finn, Children's Hospital, Seattle, WA.)

ically heterogeneous. Family studies show that the disease is caused by mutations in genes located on chromosome 16p13.3 (*PKD1*) and 4q21 (*PKD2*), and rare unlinked families suggest the presence of at least one additional disease-associated gene. Mutations of *PKD1* account for about 85% of cases (most of the remainder involving *PKD2*) and are associated with a more severe disease, end-stage renal disease or death occurring at an average age of 53 years, compared to 69 years for *PKD2*.[11] For *PKD1* mutations, the likelihood of developing renal failure is less than 5% by 40 years of age, rising to more than 35% by 50 years, more than 70% at 60 years of age, and more than 95% by 70 years of age.[12] Corresponding figures for *PKD2* are less than 5% at 50 years of age, about 15% at 60 years of age, and about 45% at 70 years of age.[10] Although the major pathologic process is in the kidneys, adult polycystic kidney disease is a systemic disorder in which cysts and other anomalies also arise in other organs (discussed later).

Genetics and Pathogenesis. A wide range of different mutations in *PKD1* and *PKD2* has been described, and this allelic heterogeneity has complicated genetic diagnosis of this disorder.

- The *PKD1* gene encodes a large (460-kDa) integral membrane protein named *polycystin-1*, which has a large extracellular region, multiple transmembrane domains, and a short cytoplasmic tail.[13,14] It has been localized to tubular epithelial cells, particularly those of the distal nephron.[14] At present, its precise function is not known, but it contains domains that are usually involved in cell–cell and cell–matrix interactions.
- The *PKD2* gene product *polycystin-2* is an integral membrane protein.[15] It has been localized to all segments of the renal tubules and is also expressed in many extrarenal tissues. Recent evidence indicates that polycystin-2 may act as a Ca^{2+}-permeable cation channel and that a basic defect in ADPKD is a disruption in the regulation of intracellular Ca^{2+} levels.[16] Details of the cellular location of polycystin-2 remain controversial, with an endoplasmic reticulum location likely, consistent with a role in the release of intracellular Ca^{2+} stores.[16] Another leading possibility is that polycystin-2 may also occupy a plasma membrane position, where it may form a complex with polycystin-1.[17]

Any hypothesis to explain the pathogenesis of this disease has to ultimately account for global processes of cyst formation, progressive cyst expansion, and progressive renal damage. Current thought has focused on links between the polycystins and *cell–cell* and *cell–matrix interactions important in tubular epithelial cell growth and differentiation.*

It has long been known that epithelial cells lining the cysts of ADPKD have a high proliferation rate, and that the nonproliferating cells in cysts exhibit abnormally simplified structure, with a relatively immature phenotype. Cysts are frequently detached from adjacent tubules and enlarge by active *fluid secretion* from the lining epithelial cells. In addition, the extracellular matrix (ECM) produced by cyst-lining cells is abnormal. These findings have led to the hypothetical scenario (Fig. 20–7) that cysts develop as a result of an abnormality in cell differentiation, associated with sustained cellular proliferation and some degree of increased apoptosis, transepithelial fluid secretion, and remodeling of the ECM.[10] The increase in cells caused by abnormal proliferation, and the expanding volume of intraluminal fluid caused by abnormal secretion from epithelial cells lining the cysts, result in progressive cyst enlargement. In addition, cyst fluids have been shown to harbor mediators, derived from epithelial cells, that enhance fluid secretion and induce inflammation. These abnormalities contribute to further enlargement of cysts and the interstitial fibrosis characteristic of progressive polycystic kidney disease.[11]

The distribution of polycystin-1 in developing renal tubules in fetal life is consistent with a role in the cell–cell and cell–matrix interactions critical to cell growth and differentiation. Indeed, targeted *PKD1* mutations in mice interfere with nephrogenesis and result in cyst formation.[18] Recent molecular analyses of *PKD* gene alleles in single cysts suggest that the *PKD1* gene serves a suppressor function: its loss leads to hyperplasia of epithelial cells.[19] Akin to tumor-suppressor genes (Chapter 7), a second somatic mutation is necessary for

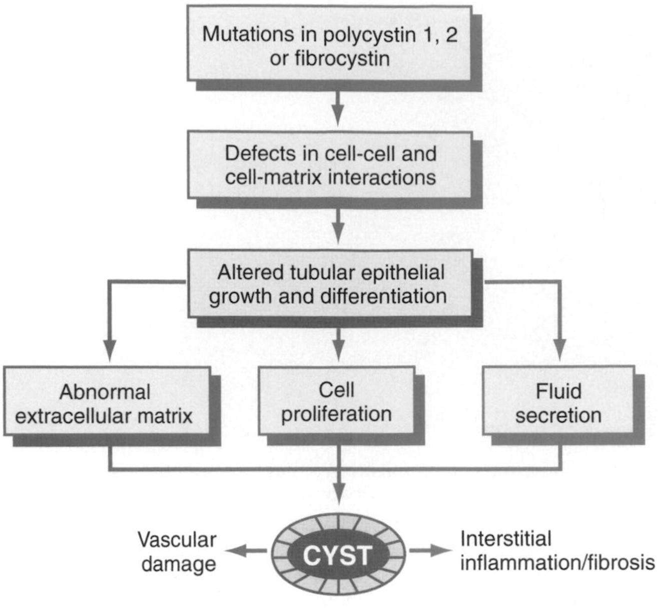

FIGURE 20–7 Possible mechanisms of cyst formation in polycystic kidney disease (see text).

full expression of the defect. This intriguing speculation is thought to explain the variable phenotypic expression and focal nature of the initial cyst formation.

The molecular mechanisms by which mutations in *PKD1* and *PKD2* lead to the multiple cellular changes associated with cyst development remain uncertain. A current working hypothesis can be formulated in which polycystin-1 and polycystin-2 form components of a polycystin complex, which acts to regulate intracellular Ca^{2+}.[14,19] The extracellular region of polycystin-1 may be the binding site for one or more ligands that modulate the activity of the channel. Mutation of either of these genes may lead to loss of the polycystin complex or the formation of an aberrant complex. The consequent disruption of normal polycystin activity may lead to changes in intracellular Ca^{2+} levels and, given the second messenger effects of Ca^{2+}, to changes in *cellular proliferation, abnormal extracellular matrix,* and the *secretory function of the epithelia* that together result in the characteristic features of ADPKD. The interaction of *PKD1* and *PKD2* gene products probably accounts for the similar phenotype in the disease induced by mutations in the two different genes.[11,14]

Morphology. In gross appearance, the kidneys are usually bilaterally enlarged and may achieve enormous sizes; weights up to 4 kg for each kidney have been reported. The external surface appears to be composed solely of a mass of cysts, up to 3 to 4 cm in diameter, with no intervening parenchyma (Fig. 20–8). However, microscopic examination reveals functioning nephrons dispersed between the cysts. The cysts may be filled with a clear, serous fluid or, more usually, with turbid, red to brown, sometimes hemorrhagic fluid. As these cysts enlarge, they may encroach on the calyces and pelvis to produce pressure defects. The cysts arise from the tubules throughout the nephron and therefore have variable lining epithelia. On occasion, papillary epithelial formations and polyps project into the lumen. Bowman capsules are occasionally involved in cyst formation, and glomerular tufts may be seen within the cystic space.

Clinical Features. Many of these patients remain asymptomatic until indications of renal insufficiency announce the presence of the underlying kidney disease. In others, hemorrhage or progressive dilation of cysts may produce pain. Excretion of blood clots causes renal colic. The larger masses, usually apparent on abdominal palpation, may induce a dragging sensation. The disease occasionally begins with the insidious onset of hematuria, followed by other features of progressive chronic renal disease, such as proteinuria (rarely more than 2 gm/day), polyuria, and hypertension. Patients with *PKD2* mutations tend to have an older age at onset and later development of renal failure. Progression is accelerated in blacks (largely correlated with sickle cell trait), in males compared with females, and in the presence of hypertension.

Patients with polycystic kidney disease also tend to have extrarenal congenital anomalies.[20] *About 40% have one to several cysts in the liver (polycystic liver disease) that are usually asymptomatic.* The cysts are derived from biliary epithelium. Cysts occur much less frequently in the spleen, pancreas, and lungs. *Intracranial berry aneurysms, presumably from altered expression of polycystin in vascular smooth muscle, arise in the circle of Willis,* and subarachnoid hemorrhages from these[21] account for death in about 4% to 10% of patients with polycystic kidney disease. *Mitral valve prolapse* and other cardiac valvular anomalies occur in 20% to 25% of patients, but most are asymptomatic. The clinical diagnosis is made by radiologic imaging techniques.

This form of chronic renal failure is remarkable in that patients may survive for many years with azotemia slowly progressing to uremia. Dialysis prolongs life further. Ultimately, about 40% of adult patients die of coronary or hypertensive heart disease, 25% of infection, 15% of a ruptured berry aneurysm or hypertensive intracerebral hemorrhage, and the rest of other causes.

AUTOSOMAL-RECESSIVE (CHILDHOOD) POLYCYSTIC KIDNEY DISEASE

Autosomal-recessive (childhood) polycystic kidney disease (ARPKD), a rare developmental anomaly, is genetically distinct from adult polycystic kidney disease, having an *autosomal-recessive* type of inheritance. *Perinatal, neonatal, infantile,* and *juvenile* subcategories have been defined, depending on the time of presentation and presence of associated hepatic lesions. The first two are the most common; serious manifestations are usually present at birth, and the young infant might succumb rapidly to renal failure.

From linkage studies, the disease appears to be genetically homogeneous, being associated with a gene, *PKHD1*, that maps to chromosome region 6p21–23. The *PKHD1* gene encodes a large novel protein, *fibrocystin*.[22] The gene is highly expressed in adult and fetal kidney and also in liver and pancreas. Fibrocystin is a 447-kDa integral membrane protein

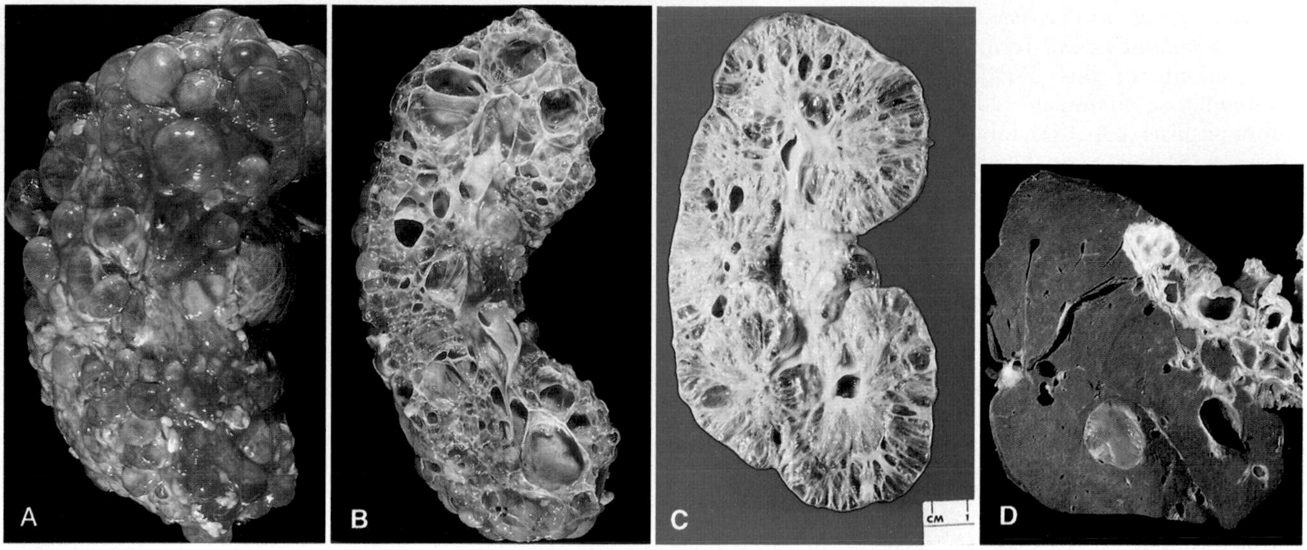

FIGURE 20–8 *A* and *B*, Autosomal-dominant adult polycystic kidney disease (ADPKD) viewed from the external surface and bisected. The kidney is markedly enlarged with numerous dilated cysts. *C*, Autosomal-recessive childhood polycystic kidney disease, showing smaller cysts and dilated channels at right angles to the cortical surface. *D*, Liver with cysts in adult PKD.

with a large extracellular region, a single transmembrane component and a short cytoplasmic tail. The extracellular region contains multiple copies of a domain forming an immunoglobulin-like fold.[14] The function of fibrocystin is unknown but its putative conformational structure indicates it may be a cell surface receptor with a role in collecting-duct and biliary differentiation.

Analysis of ARPKD patients has revealed a wide range of different mutations. All cases characterized thus far are compound heterozygotes, which complicates molecular diagnosis of ARPKD.

Morphology. The kidneys are enlarged and have a smooth external appearance. On cut section, numerous small cysts in the cortex and medulla give the kidney a spongelike appearance. Dilated elongated channels are present at right angles to the cortical surface, completely replacing the medulla and cortex (Fig. 20–8*C*). On microscopic examination, there is cylindrical or, less commonly, saccular dilation of all collecting tubules. The cysts have a uniform lining of cuboidal cells, reflecting their origin from the collecting tubules. The disease is invariably bilateral. In almost all cases, the liver has cysts with portal fibrosis (Fig. 20–8*D*) as well as proliferation of portal bile ducts.

Patients who survive infancy (infantile and juvenile forms) may develop a peculiar type of hepatic fibrosis characterized by bland periportal fibrosis and proliferation of well-differentiated biliary ductules, a condition now termed *congenital hepatic fibrosis*. In older children, the hepatic picture in fact predominates. Such patients may develop portal hypertension with splenomegaly. Curiously, congenital hepatic fibrosis sometimes occurs in the absence of polycystic kidneys and has been reported occasionally in the presence of adult polycystic kidney disease.

CYSTIC DISEASES OF RENAL MEDULLA

The two major types of medullary cystic disease are *medullary sponge kidney*, a relatively common and usually innocuous structural change, and *nephronophthisis–medullary cystic disease complex*, which is almost always associated with renal dysfunction.

Medullary Sponge Kidney

The term "medullary sponge kidney" should be restricted to lesions consisting of multiple cystic dilations of the collecting ducts in the medulla. The condition occurs in adults and is usually discovered radiographically, either as an incidental finding or sometimes in relation to secondary complications. The latter include calcifications within the dilated ducts, hematuria, infection, and urinary calculi. Renal function is usually normal. On gross inspection, the papillary ducts in the medulla are dilated, and small cysts may be present. The cysts are lined by cuboidal epithelium or occasionally by transitional epithelium. Unless there is superimposed pyelonephritis, cortical scarring is absent. The pathogenesis is unknown.

Nephronophthisis–Medullary Cystic Disease Complex

This is a group of progressive renal disorders that usually have their onset in childhood. The common characteristic is the presence of a variable number of *cysts in the medulla, usually concentrated at the corticomedullary junction.* Initial injury likely involves the distal tubules with tubular basement membrane disruption, followed by chronic and progressive tubular atrophy involving both medulla and cortex and interstitial fibrosis. Although the presence of medullary cysts is important, the *cortical tubulointerstitial damage is the cause of the eventual renal insufficiency,* and some prefer the term *hereditary tubulointerstitial nephritis* for this group.[9]

Four variants of this disease complex are recognized: (1) sporadic, nonfamilial (20%); (2) familial juvenile nephronophthisis (40–50%), inherited as an autosomal recessive disease; (3) renal-retinal dysplasia (15%), also an autosomal recessive disease, in which the kidney disease is accompanied by ocular lesions; and (4) adult-onset medullary cystic disease (15%), which shows an autosomal dominant inheritance. As a group, this complex is now thought to be the most common genetic cause of end-stage renal disease in children and young adults.

Affected children present first with polyuria and polydipsia, which reflect a marked defect in the concentrating ability of renal tubules. Sodium wasting and tubular acidosis are also prominent. Some variants of juvenile nephronophthisis can have extrarenal associations, including ocular motor abnormalities, retinitis pigmentosa, liver fibrosis, and cerebellar abnormalities. The expected course is progression to terminal renal failure during a period of 5 to 10 years.

Pathogenesis. At least five gene loci have been identified for this complex, with both autosomal dominant and recessive modes of inheritance. Three genes, *NPH1*, *NPH2*, and *NPH3*, define the juvenile forms of nephronophthisis and cause autosomal recessive disease.[23] The protein product of NPH1 has recently been identified (nephrocystin), but its function is not yet known. Two genes (*MCKD1* and *MCKD2*), with autosomal dominant transmission, have been identified as causing medullary cystic disease that is characterized by progression to endstage kidney disease in adult life.[23]

Morphology. In gross appearance, the kidneys are small, have contracted granular surfaces, and show cysts in the medulla, most prominently at the corticomedullary junction (Fig. 20–9). Small cysts are also seen in the cortex. The cysts are lined by flattened or cuboidal epithelium and are usually surrounded by either inflammatory cells or fibrous tissue. In the cortex, there is widespread atrophy and thickening of the basement membranes of proximal and distal tubules, together with interstitial fibrosis. Some glomeruli may be hyalinized, but in general, glomerular structure is preserved.

There are few specific clues to diagnosis because the medullary cysts might be too small to be visualized radiographically. The disease should be strongly considered in children or adolescents with otherwise unexplained chronic renal failure, a positive family history, and chronic tubulointerstitial nephritis on biopsy.

ACQUIRED (DIALYSIS-ASSOCIATED) CYSTIC DISEASE

The kidneys from patients with end-stage renal disease who have undergone prolonged dialysis sometimes exhibit numerous cortical and medullary cysts. The cysts measure 0.5 to 2 cm in diameter, contain clear fluid, are lined by either hyperplastic or flattened tubular epithelium, and often contain calcium oxalate crystals. They probably form as a result of obstruction of tubules by interstitial fibrosis or by oxalate crystals.

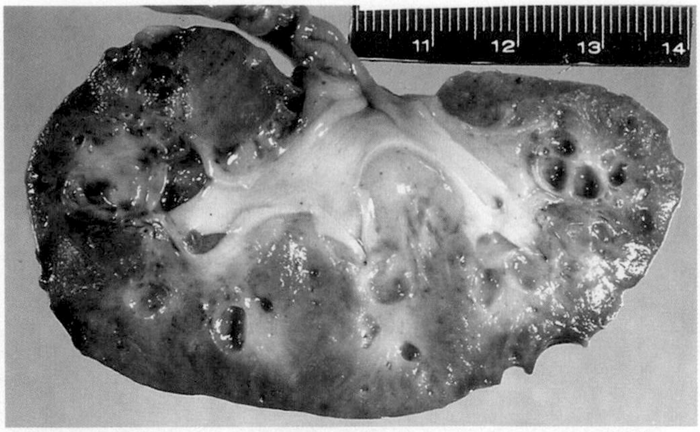

FIGURE 20–9 Uremic medullary cystic disease. Cut section of kidney showing cysts at the corticomedullary junction and in the medulla.

Most are asymptomatic, but sometimes the cysts bleed, causing hematuria. The most ominous complication is the development of renal cell carcinoma in the walls of these cysts, occurring in 7% of dialyzed patients observed for 10 years.

SIMPLE CYSTS

These occur as multiple or single, usually cortical, cystic spaces that vary widely in diameter. They are commonly 1 to 5 cm but may reach 10 cm or more in size. They are translucent; lined by a gray, glistening, smooth membrane; and filled with clear fluid. On microscopic examination, these membranes are composed of a single layer of cuboidal or flattened cuboidal epithelium, which in many instances may be completely atrophic.

Simple cysts are common postmortem findings without clinical significance. On occasion, hemorrhage into them may cause sudden distention and pain, and calcification of the hemorrhage may give rise to bizarre radiographic shadows. The main importance of cysts lies in their differentiation from kidney tumors when they are discovered either incidentally or because of hemorrhage and pain. Radiologic studies show that in contrast to renal tumors, renal cysts have smooth contours, are almost always avascular, and give fluid rather than solid signals on ultrasonography.

Glomerular Diseases

Glomerular diseases constitute some of the major problems in nephrology; indeed, chronic glomerulonephritis is one of the most common causes of chronic renal failure in humans. Glomeruli may be injured by a variety of factors and in the course of a number of systemic diseases. Systemic immunologic diseases such as systemic lupus erythematosus (SLE), vascular disorders such as hypertension and polyarteritis nodosa, metabolic diseases such as diabetes mellitus, and some purely hereditary conditions such as Fabry disease often affect the glomerulus. These are termed *secondary glomerular diseases* to differentiate them from disorders in which the kidney is the only or predominant organ involved. The latter constitute the various types of *primary glomerulonephritis* or, because some do not have a cellular inflammatory component, *glomerulopathy. However, both the clinical manifestations and glomerular histologic changes in primary and secondary forms can be similar.*

Here we discuss the various types of primary glomerulonephritis and briefly review the secondary forms covered in other parts of this book. Table 20–3 lists the most common forms of glomerulonephritis that have reasonably well defined morphologic and clinical characteristics.

CLINICAL MANIFESTATIONS

The clinical manifestations of glomerular disease are clustered into the five major glomerular syndromes summarized in Table 20–4. Both the primary glomerulonephritides and the systemic diseases affecting the glomerulus can result in these syndromes. Because glomerular diseases are often associated with systemic disorders, mainly *diabetes mellitus, SLE, vasculitis,* and *amyloidosis,* in any patient with manifestations of glomerular disease, it is essential to consider these systemic syndromes.

HISTOLOGIC ALTERATIONS

Various types of glomerulonephritis are characterized by one or more of four basic tissue reactions.

Hypercellularity. Some *inflammatory diseases* of the glomerulus are characterized by an increase in the number of cells in the glomerular tufts. This hypercellularity is characterized by one or more combinations of the following:

- *Cellular proliferation* of mesangial or endothelial cells
- *Leukocytic infiltration,* consisting of neutrophils, monocytes, and, in some diseases, lymphocytes
- *Formation of crescents.* These are accumulations of cells composed of proliferating parietal epithelial cells and infiltrating leukocytes. The epithelial cell proliferation that characterizes crescent formation occurs following an immune/inflammatory injury (see later). Fibrin, which leaks into the urinary space, often through ruptured basement membranes, has been long thought to be the molecule that elicits the crescentic response. In support of this, fibrin can be demonstrated immunohistochemically in the glomerular tufts and urinary spaces of glomeruli that contain crescents. Mice that are deficient in fibrin are protected to a degree from crescent formation, and mice that are deficient in molecules important in fibrinolysis (e.g., plasminogen activators) develop exacerbated crescent formation in anti-GBM antibody models of crescentic glomerulonephritis.[24] Other molecules that have been implicated in crescent formation and recruitment of leukocytes into crescents include precoagulants such as tissue factor and cytokines such as interleukin-1, tumor necrosis factor, and interferon-γ.

Basement Membrane Thickening. By light microscopy, this change appears as thickening of the capillary walls, best seen in sections stained with periodic acid-Schiff (PAS). By electron microscopy, such thickening can be resolved as one of two alterations: (1) deposition of amorphous electron-dense material, most often immune complexes, on the endothelial or epithelial side of the basement membrane or within the GBM itself. Fibrin, amyloid, cryoglobulins, and abnormal fibrillary proteins may also deposit in the GBM; or (2) thickening of the basement membrane proper, as occurs in diabetic glomerulosclerosis.

Hyalinization and Sclerosis. Hyalinization, or hyalinosis, as applied to the glomerulus, denotes the accumulation of material that is homogeneous and eosinophilic by light microscopy. By electron microscopy, the hyalin is extracellular and consists of amorphous substance, made up of plasma proteins that have exuded from circulating plasma into glomerular structures. This change contributes to obliteration of capillary lumina of the glomerular tuft (a feature of sclerosis). Hyalinosis is usually a consequence of endothelial or capillary wall injury and typically is the end result of various forms of glomerular damage. Additional alterations include *intraglomerular thrombosis* or *accumulation of lipid* or other metabolic materials.

Because many of the primary glomerulonephritides are of unknown cause, they are often classified by their histology, as

TABLE 20–4 The Glomerular Syndromes

Acute nephritic syndrome	• Hematuria, azotemia, variable proteinuria, oliguria, edema, and hypertension
Rapidly progressive glomerulonephritis	• Acute nephritis, proteinuria, and acute renal failure
Nephrotic syndrome	• >3.5 gm proteinuria, hypoalbuminemia, hyperlipidemia, lipiduria
Chronic renal failure	• Azotemia → uremia progressing for years
Asymptomatic hematuria or proteinuria	• Glomerular hematuria; subnephrotic proteinuria

TABLE 20–3 Glomerular Diseases

Primary Glomerulopathies

Acute diffuse proliferative glomerulonephritis
  Poststreptococcal
  Non-poststreptococcal
Rapidly progressive (crescentic) glomerulonephritis
Membranous glomerulopathy
Minimal change disease
Focal segmental glomerulosclerosis
Membranoproliferative glomerulonephritis
IgA nephropathy
Chronic glomerulonephritis

Systemic Diseases with Glomerular Involvement

Systemic lupus erythematosus
Diabetes mellitus
Amyloidosis
Goodpasture syndrome
Microscopic polyarteritis/polyangiitis
Wegener granulomatosis
Henoch-Schönlein purpura
Bacterial endocarditis

Hereditary Disorders

Alport syndrome
Thin basement membrane disease
Fabry disease

can be seen in Table 20–3. The histologic changes can be further subdivided into *diffuse*, involving all glomeruli; *global*, involving the entire glomerulus; *focal*, involving only a proportion of the glomeruli; *segmental*, affecting a part of each glomerulus; and *mesangial*, affecting predominantly the mesangial region. These terms are sometimes appended to the histologic classifications.

PATHOGENESIS OF GLOMERULAR INJURY

Although we know little of etiologic agents and triggering events, it is clear that immune mechanisms underlie most forms of primary glomerulonephritis and many of the secondary glomerular disorders[25,26] (Table 20–5). Glomerulonephritis can be readily induced experimentally by antigen-antibody reactions. Furthermore, glomerular deposits of immunoglobulins, often with various components of complement, are found in the majority of patients with glomerulonephritis. Cell-mediated immune reactions also clearly play a role, usually in concert with antibody-mediated events. We therefore begin this discussion with a review of antibody-instigated injury.

Two forms of antibody-associated injury have been established: (1) injury by *antibodies reacting in situ within the glomerulus, either with insoluble fixed (intrinsic) glomerular antigens or with molecules planted within the glomerulus,* and (2) injury resulting from *deposition of circulating antigen–antibody complexes* in the glomerulus. In addition, there is experimental evidence that *cytotoxic antibodies* directed against glomerular cell components may cause glomerular injury. These pathways are not mutually exclusive, and in humans, all may contribute to injury.

In Situ Immune Complex Deposition

In this form of injury, antibodies react directly with intrinsic tissue antigen, or antigens "planted" in the glomerulus from the circulation. There are two well-established experimental models for anti–tissue antibody-mediated glomerular injury, for which there are counterparts in human disease: antiglomerular basement membrane (anti-GBM) antibody–induced nephritis and Heymann nephritis.

TABLE 20–5 Immune Mechanisms of Glomerular Injury

Antibody-Mediated Injury
In Situ Immune Complex Deposition
Fixed intrinsic tissue antigens
NC1 domain of collagen type IV antigen (anti-GBM nephritis)
Heymann antigen (membranous glomerulopathy)
Mesangial antigens
Others
Planted antigens
Exogenous (infectious agents, drugs)
Endogenous (DNA, nuclear proteins, immunoglobulins, immune complexes, IgA)
Circulating Immune Complex Deposition
Endogenous antigens (e.g., DNA, tumor antigens)
Exogenous antigens (e.g., infectious products)
Cytotoxic Antibodies
Cell-Mediated Immune Injury
Activation of Alternative Complement Pathway

Anti-GBM Antibody–Induced Nephritis

In this type of injury, *antibodies are directed against intrinsic fixed antigens that are normal components of the GBM proper.* It has its experimental counterpart in so-called Masugi or nephrotoxic nephritis, produced in rats by injections of anti–rat kidney antibodies prepared in rabbits by immunization with rat kidney tissue. The injected antibodies bind along the entire length of the GBM, *resulting in a diffuse linear pattern of staining for the antibodies by immunofluorescent techniques* (Figs. 20–10*B* and *E*). This is contrasted with the granular lumpy pattern of immunofluorescent staining seen in other in situ models, such as the Heymann model of membranous glomerulopathy, or after deposition of circulating immune complexes.

In the Masugi model, the injected anti-GBM antibody is rabbit immunoglobulin, which is foreign to the host and thus acts as an antigen eliciting anti-Ig antibody in the rat. The rat antibodies then react with the rabbit immunoglobulin deposited in the basement membrane, leading to further glomerular injury. Thus, experimental anti-GBM antibody–mediated glomerulonephritis consists of an initial *heterologous phase* caused by the injected anti-GBM antibody, and a subsequent, more injurious, *autologous phase* caused by host antibodies against the injected Ig. Often the anti-GBM antibodies cross-react with other basement membranes, especially those in the lung alveoli, resulting in simultaneous lung and kidney lesions (*Goodpasture syndrome*). *The GBM antigen that is responsible for classic anti-GBM antibody–induced nephritis and Goodpasture syndrome is a component of the noncollagenous domain (NC1) of the α_3-chain of collagen type IV,* which, as was discussed earlier (see Fig. 20–3), is critical for maintenance of GBM superstructure.[3–5,27] Anti-GBM antibody–induced nephritis accounts for fewer than 5% of cases of human glomerulonephritis. It is solidly established as the cause of injury in Goodpasture syndrome, discussed later. Most instances of anti-GBM antibody–induced nephritis are characterized by severe crescentic glomerular damage and the clinical syndrome of rapidly progressive glomerulonephritis.

Heymann Nephritis

The Heymann model of rat glomerulonephritis is induced by immunizing animals with an antigen contained within preparations of proximal tubular brush border (Fig. 20–10*C*). The rats develop antibodies to this antigen, and a membranous glomerulopathy, resembling human membranous glomerulopathy, develops (discussed later; see also Fig. 20–19). On electron microscopy, the glomerulopathy is characterized by the presence of numerous electron-dense deposits (made up largely of immune reactants) along the *subepithelial aspect* of the basement membrane. The pattern of immune deposition by immunofluorescence microscopy is *granular* rather than linear (Fig. 20–10*C*). It is now clear that this type of disease results largely from the reaction of antibody with an antigen complex located on the basal surface of visceral epithelial cells and cross-reacting with the brush

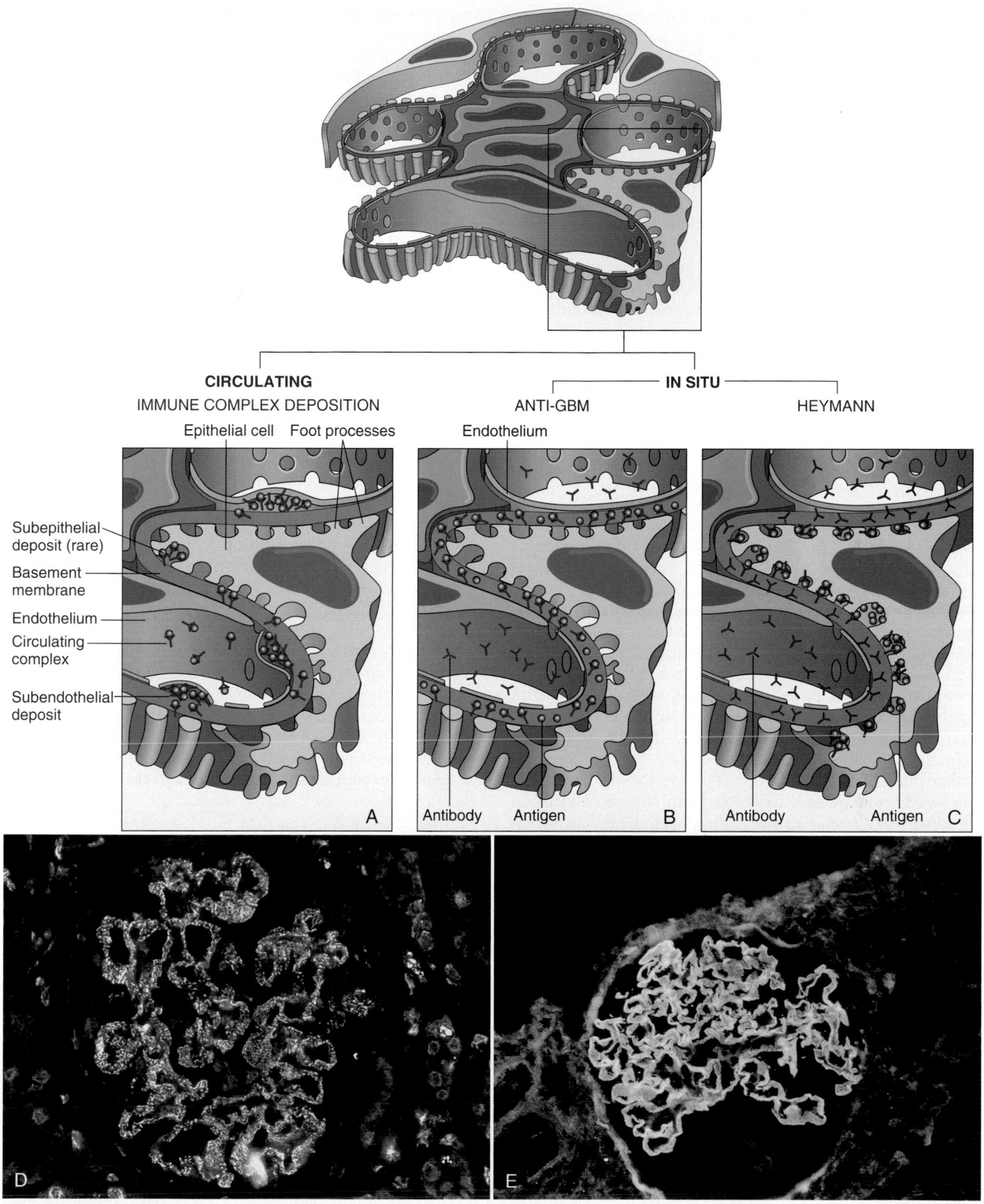

FIGURE 20–10 Antibody-mediated glomerular injury can result either from the deposition of circulating immune complexes (*A*) or, more commonly, from in situ formation of complexes exemplified by anti-GBM disease (*B*) or Heymann nephritis (*C*). *D* and *E*, Two patterns of deposition of immune complexes as seen by immunofluorescence microscopy: granular, characteristic of circulating and in situ immune complex nephritis (*D*) and linear, characteristic of classic anti-GBM disease (*E*) .

border antigen used in the original experiments. This so-called Heymann antigen in rats is a large 330-kDa protein called *megalin*, having homology to the low-density lipoprotein receptor (Chapter 5), but the corresponding antigen in human membranous glomerulopathy has not yet been identified.[28] Antibody binding to glomerular epithelial cell membrane is followed by complement activation and then shedding of the immune aggregates from the cell surface to form the characteristic subepithelial deposits (Fig. 20–10*C*).

In humans, anti-GBM antibody–induced disease and membranous glomerulopathy are autoimmune diseases, caused by antibodies to endogenous tissue components. What triggers these autoantibodies is unclear, but any one of the several mechanisms responsible for autoimmunity, discussed in Chapter 6, may be involved. Several forms of autoimmune glomerulonephritis can be experimentally induced by drugs (e.g., mercuric chloride), infectious products (endotoxin), and the graft-versus-host reaction (Chapter 6). In such models, there is an alteration of immune regulation associated with B-cell activation and the induction of an array of autoantibodies that react with renal antigens.

Antibodies Against Planted Antigens

Antibodies can react in situ with antigens that are not normally present in the glomerulus but are "planted" there. There is increasing experimental support for such a mechanism of glomerulonephritis. Such antigens may localize in the kidney by interacting with various intrinsic components of the glomerulus. Planted antigens include cationic molecules that bind to glomerular capillary anionic sites; DNA, nucleosomes, and other nuclear proteins, which have an affinity for GBM components; bacterial products; large aggregated proteins (e.g., aggregated immunoglobulins [Ig], which deposit in the mesangium because of their size; and immune complexes themselves, since they continue to have reactive sites for further interactions with free antibody, free antigen, or complement. There is no dearth of other possible planted antigens, including viral, bacterial, and parasitic products and drugs. Antibodies that bind to most of these planted antigens induce a discrete pattern of immunoglobulin deposition detected as granular staining by immunofluorescence microscopy, similar to the pattern found in circulating immune complex nephritis.

Circulating Immune Complex Nephritis

In this type of nephritis, glomerular injury is caused by the trapping of circulating antigen–antibody complexes within glomeruli. The antibodies have no immunologic specificity for glomerular constituents, and the complexes localize within the glomeruli because of their physicochemical properties and the hemodynamic factors peculiar to the glomerulus (Fig. 20–10*A*).

The pathogenesis of immune complex diseases was discussed in Chapter 6. Here, we briefly review the salient features that relate to glomerular injury.

The antigens that trigger the formation of circulating immune complexes may be of endogenous origin, as in the glomerulonephritis associated with SLE, or they may be exogenous, as is likely in the glomerulonephritis that follows certain infections. Microbial antigens that are implicated include bacterial products (streptococci), the surface antigen of hepatitis B virus (HBsAg), hepatitis C virus antigen, and antigens of *Treponema pallidum*, *Plasmodium falciparum*, and several viruses. Some tumor antigens are also thought to cause immune complex–mediated nephritis. In many cases, the inciting antigen is unknown.

Whatever the antigen may be, antigen–antibody complexes are formed in the circulation and then trapped in the glomeruli, where they produce injury. It has long been thought that this injury is mediated and amplified by the binding of complement, but recent studies in knockout mice also point to the importance of engagement of Fc receptors on leukocytes and perhaps intrinsic renal cells as mediators of the injury process.[29] The glomerular lesions usually consist of leukocytic infiltration in glomeruli and proliferation of mesangial and endothelial cells. Electron microscopy reveals the immune complexes as electron-dense deposits that lie in the mesangium, between the endothelial cells and the GBM (subendothelial deposits), or between the outer surface of the GBM and the podocytes (subepithelial deposits). Deposits may be located at more than one site in a given case. By immunofluorescence microscopy, the immune complexes are seen as granular deposits along the basement membrane, in the mesangium, or in both locations. Once deposited in the kidney, immune complexes may eventually be degraded, mostly by infiltrating neutrophils and monocytes/macrophages, mesangial cells, and endogenous proteases, and the inflammatory reaction may then subside. Such a course occurs when the exposure to the inciting antigen is short-lived and limited, as in most cases of poststreptococcal glomerulonephritis. However, if a continuous shower of antigens is provided, as may be seen in SLE or viral hepatitis, repeated cycles of immune complex formation, deposition, and injury may occur, leading to a more chronic membranous or membranoproliferative type of glomerulonephritis.

Several factors affect glomerular localization of antigen, antibody, or complexes. The molecular charge and size of these reactants are clearly important. Highly cationic immunogens tend to cross the GBM, and the resultant complexes eventually achieve a subepithelial location. Highly anionic macromolecules are excluded from the GBM and either are trapped subendothelially or may, in fact, not be nephritogenic at all. Molecules with more neutral charge and immune complexes containing these molecules tend to accumulate in the mesangium. Large circulating complexes are not usually nephritogenic because they are cleared by the mononuclear phagocyte system and do not enter the GBM in sufficient quantities. The pattern of localization is also affected by changes in glomerular hemodynamics, mesangial function, and integrity of the charge-selective barrier in the glomerulus. These influences may underlie the variable pattern of immune reactant deposition and histologic change in various forms of glomerulonephritis, as shown in Figure 20–11.

Antibodies to Glomerular Cells

In addition to causing immune deposits, antibodies against glomerular cell antigens may react with cellular components and cause injury by cytotoxic or other mechanisms. Antibodies to mesangial cell antigens, for example, can cause mesangiolysis followed by mesangial cell proliferation; antibodies to

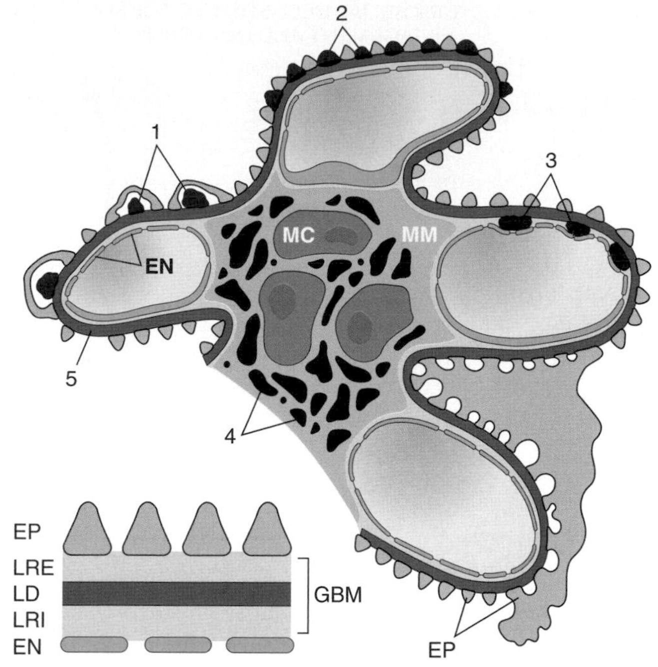

FIGURE 20–11 Localization of immune complexes in the glomerulus: (1) subepithelial humps, as in acute glomerulonephritis; (2) epimembranous deposits, as in membranous and Heymann glomerulonephritis; (3) subendothelial deposits, as in systemic lupus erythematosus and membranoproliferative glomerulonephritis; (4) mesangial deposits, as in IgA nephropathy; (5) basement membrane. LRE, lamina rara externa; LRI, lamina rara interna; LD, lamina densa; EP, epithelium; EN, endothelium; MC, mesangial cell; MM, mesangial matrix. (Modified from Couser WG: Mediation of immune glomerular injury. J Am Soc Nephrol 1:13, 1990.)

endothelial cell antigens cause endothelial injury and intravascular thrombosis; and antibodies to certain visceral epithelial cell components cause proteinuria in experimental animals. This mechanism may well play a role in certain human immune disorders that are not associated with demonstrable immune deposits.

To conclude the discussion of antibody-mediated injury, it must be stated that *in the largest proportion of cases of human glomerulonephritis, the pattern of immune deposition is granular and along the basement membrane or in the mesangium.* However, it may be difficult to determine whether the deposition has occurred in situ, by circulating complexes, or by both mechanisms because, as was discussed earlier, trapping of circulating immune complexes can initiate further in situ complex formation. Single etiologic agents, such as hepatitis B and C viruses, can cause either a membranous pattern of glomerulonephritis, suggesting in situ deposition, or a membranoproliferative pattern, more indicative of circulating complexes. It is best then to consider that *antigen–antibody deposition in the glomerulus is a major pathway of glomerular injury and that in situ immune reactions, trapping of circulating complexes, interactions between these two events, and local hemodynamic and structural determinants in the glomerulus all contribute to the diverse morphologic and functional alterations in glomerulonephritis.*

Cell-Mediated Immunity in Glomerulonephritis

Although antibody-mediated mechanisms may initiate many forms of glomerulonephritis, there is now considerable evidence that sensitized T cells cause some forms of glomerular injury and are involved in the progression of many glomerulonephritides.[30,31] Clues to the role of cellular immunity include the presence of activated macrophages and T cells and their products in the glomerulus in some forms of human and experimental glomerulonephritis;[32] in vitro and in vivo evidence of lymphocyte activation on exposure to antigen in human and experimental glomerulonephritis;[33] abrogation of glomerular injury by lymphocyte depletion; and successful attempts to induce glomerular injury by transfer of T cells in experimental models. The evidence is most compelling for certain types of experimental crescentic glomerulonephritis in which antibodies to GBM may initiate or facilitate glomerular injury by activated T lymphocytes.[34,35]

Activation of Alternative Complement Pathway

Alternative complement pathway activation occurs in the clinicopathologic entity called dense-deposit disease, also referred to as *membranoproliferative glomerulonephritis (MPGN type II)*. It may also occur in some forms of proliferative glomerulonephritis. This mechanism is discussed later, in the discussion of MPGN.

Epithelial Cell Injury

This can be induced by antibodies to visceral epithelial cell antigens; by toxins, as in an experimental model of proteinuria induced by puromycin aminonucleoside; conceivably by certain cytokines; or by still poorly characterized factors, as in the case of human minimal change disease and focal segmental glomerulosclerosis, discussed later. Such injury is reflected morphologically by changes in the visceral epithelial cells, which include effacement of foot processes, vacuolization, retraction, and detachment of cells from the GBM, and functionally by proteinuria. It is hypothesized that the detachment of visceral epithelial cells is caused by loss of adhesive interactions with the basement membrane and that this detachment contributes to protein leakage (Fig. 20–12).

Mediators of Glomerular Injury

Once immune reactants or sensitized T cells have localized in the glomerulus, how does the glomerular damage ensue? The mediators—both cells and molecules—are the usual suspects involved in acute and chronic inflammation, described in Chapter 2, and only a few are highlighted here (Fig. 20–13).

Cells

- *Neutrophils* and *monocytes* infiltrate the glomerulus in certain types of glomerulonephritis, largely owing to activation of complement, resulting in generation of chemotactic agents (mainly C5a), but also by Fc-mediated adherence and activation. Neutrophils release proteases,

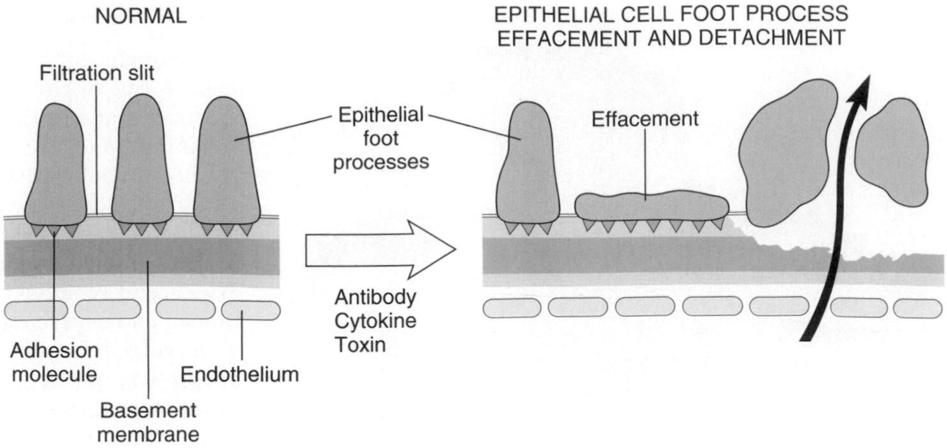

FIGURE 20–12 Epithelial cell injury. The postulated sequence is a consequence of antibodies against epithelial cell antigens, toxins, cytokines, or other factors causing injury with foot process effacement and sometimes detachment of epithelial cells and protein leakage through defective GBM and filtration slits.

which cause GBM degradation; oxygen-derived free radicals, which cause cell damage; and arachidonic acid metabolites, which contribute to the reductions in glomerular filtration rate (GFR).

- *Macrophages, T lymphocytes,* and *natural killer (NK) cells,* which infiltrate the glomerulus in antibody- and cell-mediated reactions, when activated release a vast number of biologically active molecules.
- *Platelets* aggregate in the glomerulus during immune-mediated injury. Their release of eicosanoids and growth factors may contribute to the manifestations of glomerulonephritis. Antiplatelet agents have beneficial effects in both human and experimental glomerulonephritis.
- *Resident glomerular cells,* particularly mesangial cells, can be stimulated to produce several inflammatory mediators, including reactive oxygen species, cytokines, chemokines, growth factors, eicosanoids, nitric oxide, and endothelin. In the absence of leukocytic infiltration, they may initiate inflammatory responses in the glomerulus.

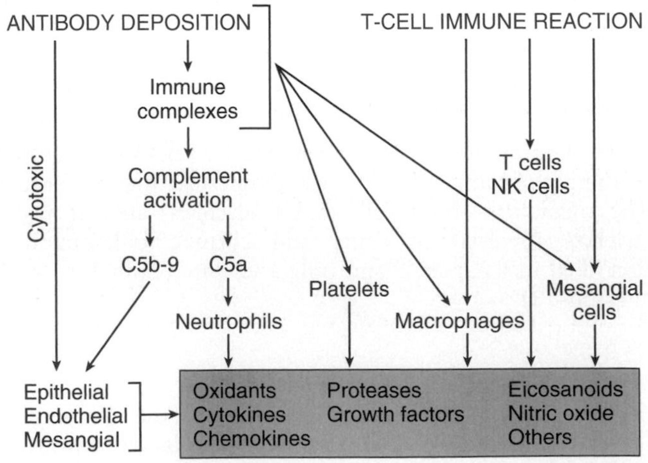

FIGURE 20–13 Mediators of immune glomerular injury including cells and soluble mediators (see text). (Modified from Couser WG: Mediation of immune glomerular injury. J Am Soc Nephrol 1:13, 1990.)

Soluble Mediators

Virtually all the known inflammatory chemical mediators have been implicated in glomerular injury.

- The *chemotactic complement components* induce leukocyte influx (complement-neutrophil–dependent injury) and lead to formation of C5b–C9, the lytic component. C5b–C9 causes cell lysis but, in addition, stimulates mesangial cells to produce oxidants, proteases, and other mediators. Thus, even in the absence of neutrophils, C5b–C9 can cause proteinuria, as has been postulated in membranous glomerulopathy.
- *Eicosanoids, nitric oxide, angiotensin,* and *endothelin* are involved in the hemodynamic changes.
- *Cytokines,* particularly interleukin-1 and tumor necrosis factor, which may be produced by infiltrating leukocytes and resident glomerular cells, induce leukocyte adhesion and a variety of other effects.
- *Chemokines* such as monocyte chemoattractant protein 1 (MCP-1) and RANTES promote monocyte and lymphocyte influx. *Growth factors,* such as platelet-derived growth factor, are involved in mesangial cell proliferation.[36] Transforming growth factor (TGF)-β and fibroblast growth factor appear to be critical in the ECM deposition and hyalinization leading to glomerulosclerosis in chronic injury.[37] Vascular endothelial growth factor appears to maintain endothelial integrity and may help regulate capillary permeability.
- The *coagulation system* is also a mediator of glomerular damage. Fibrin is frequently present in the glomeruli in glomerulonephritis, and fibrin may leak into Bowman space, serving as a stimulus for parietal epithelial cell proliferation (crescent formation). Fibrin deposition is mediated largely by stimulation of macrophage procoagulant activity. Plasminogen activator inhibitor-1 (PAI-1) is linked to increased thrombosis and fibrosis by inhibiting degradation of fibrin and matrix proteins.

MECHANISMS OF PROGRESSION IN GLOMERULAR DISEASES

Thus far, we have discussed the immunologic mechanisms and mediators that *initiate* glomerular injury. The outcome of such injury depends on several factors, including the initial severity of renal damage, the nature and persistence of the antigens, and the immune status, age, and genetic predisposition of the host.

It has long been known that once any renal disease, glomerular or otherwise, destroys functioning nephrons and reduces the GFR to about 30% to 50% of normal, progression to end-stage renal failure proceeds at a relatively constant rate, independent of the original stimulus or activity of the underlying disease. The secondary factors that lead to progression are of great clinical interest, since they can be targets of therapy that delays or even prevents the inexorable journey to dialysis or transplantation.

The two major histologic characteristics of such progressive renal damage are *focal segmental glomerulosclerosis* and *tubulointerstitial fibrosis*; we discuss these separately.[38–40]

Focal Segmental Glomerulosclerosis (FSGS). Patients with this secondary change develop proteinuria, even if the primary disease was nonglomerular. The glomerulosclerosis appears to be initiated by the *adaptive change* that occurs in the relatively unaffected glomeruli of diseased kidneys.[40,41] Such a mechanism is suggested by experiments in rats subjected to ablation of renal mass by subtotal nephrectomy. *Compensatory hypertrophy* of the remaining glomeruli serves to maintain renal function in these animals, but proteinuria and glomerulosclerosis soon develop, leading eventually to total glomerular sclerosis and uremia. The glomerular hypertrophy is associated with *hemodynamic changes*, including increases in glomerular blood flow, filtration, and transcapillary pressure (capillary hypertension), and often with systemic hypertension. The sequence of events (Fig. 20–14) that is thought to lead to sclerosis in this setting entails endothelial and epithelial cell injury, increased glomerular permeability to proteins, and accumulation of proteins in the mesangial matrix. This is followed by proliferation of mesangial cells, infiltration by macrophages, increased accumulation of extracellular matrix, and segmental and eventually global sclerosis of glomeruli (renal ablation FSGS). This results in further reductions in nephron mass and a vicious circle of continuing glomerulosclerosis. Most of the mediators of chronic inflammation and fibrosis, particularly TGF-β, play a role in the induction of sclerosis. Currently, the most successful interventions to interrupt these mechanisms of progressive glomerulosclerosis involve treatment with inhibitors of the renin-angiotensin system, which not only reduce intraglomerular hypertension, but also have direct effects on each of the mechanisms identified above.[40] Importantly, these agents have been shown to ameliorate progression of FSGS in both animal and human studies.[40,42]

Contributing to the progressive injury of focal and segmental glomerulosclerosis is the inability of mature visceral epithelial cells (podocytes) to proliferate after injury. This can lead to a decrease in glomerular podocyte number after a severe injury resulting in loss of some of these cells, leading in turn to a process whereby remaining podocytes are either abnormally stretched to maintain an appropriate filtration barrier or portions of the glomerular basement membranes become denuded of the overlying podocyte foot processes. These alterations lead to abnormal protein filtration as well as loss of structural support for the glomerular capillary walls. This latter alteration in turn may lead to segmental loop dilatation because of now incompletely opposed intracapillary pressures, with subsequent formation of a fibrous attachment to Bowman capsule by the bulging capillary segment, and eventual sclerosis of this segment.[43]

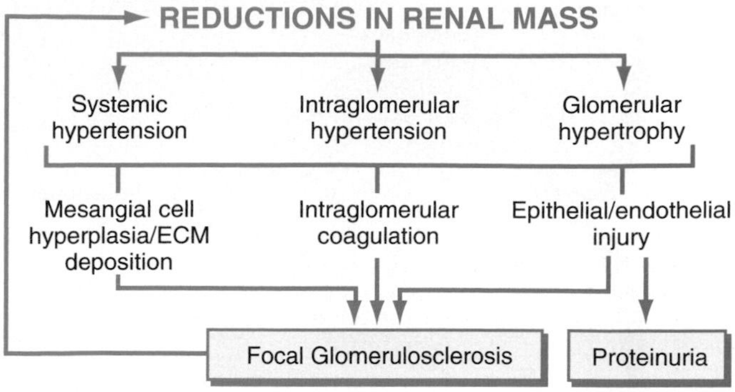

FIGURE 20–14 Renal ablation focal segmental glomerulosclerosis. The adaptive changes in glomeruli (hypertrophy and glomerular capillary hypertension), as well as systemic hypertension, cause epithelial and endothelial injury and resultant proteinuria. The mesangial response, involving mesangial cell proliferation and extracellular matrix (ECM) production together with intraglomerular coagulation, causes the glomerulosclerosis. This results in further loss of functioning nephrons and a vicious circle of progressive glomerulosclerosis.

Tubulointerstitial Fibrosis. Tubulointerstitial injury, manifested by tubular damage and interstitial inflammation, is a component of many acute and chronic glomerulonephritides. Tubulointerstitial fibrosis contributes to progression in both immune and nonimmune glomerular diseases, for example, diabetic nephropathy. *Indeed, there is often a much better correlation of decline in renal function with the extent of tubulointerstitial damage than with the severity of glomerular injury.*[44] Many factors may lead to such tubulointerstitial injury, including ischemia of tubule segments downstream from sclerotic glomeruli, acute and chronic inflammation in the adjacent interstitium, and damage or loss of the peritubular capillary blood supply. Current work also points to the effects of *proteinuria* on tubular cell structure and function[45] (Fig. 20–15). On the basis of in vitro and animal studies, proteinuria is thought to cause *direct injury to and activation of tubular cells.* Activated tubular cells in turn express adhesion molecules and elaborate pro-inflammatory cytokines, chemokines, and growth factors that contribute to interstitial fibrosis.[46] Components of the filtered protein that may produce these tubular effects include cytokines, complement products, the iron in transferrin, immunoglobulins, lipid moieties, and oxidatively modified plasma proteins.

Having discussed factors in the initiation and progression of glomerular injury, we now turn to a discussion of individual glomerular diseases. Table 20–6 summarizes the main clinical and histologic features of the major forms of primary glomerulonephritis.

ACUTE GLOMERULONEPHRITIS

This group of glomerular diseases is *characterized anatomically by inflammatory alterations in the glomeruli and clinically by the syndrome of acute nephritis.* The nephritic patient usually presents with hematuria, red cell casts in the urine, azotemia,

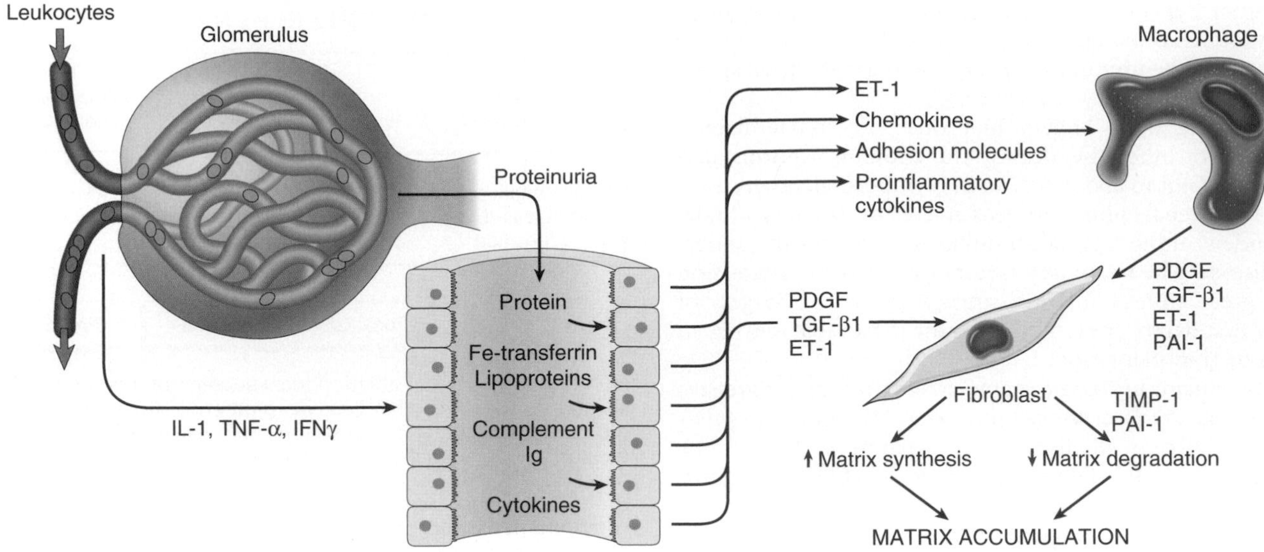

FIGURE 20–15 Mechanisms of chronic tubulointerstitial injury in glomerulonephritis (see text). Various components of the protein-rich filtrate and cytokines derived from leukocytes cause tubular cell activation and secretion of cytokines, growth factors, and other mediators. These, together with products of macrophages, incite interstitial inflammation and fibrosis. ET-1, endothelin-1, PAI-1, plasminogen activator inhibitor-1; TIMP-1, tissue inhibitor of metalloproteinases. (Adapted and modified from Remuzzi G, Ruggenenti P, Benigni A: Understanding the nature of renal disease progression. Kidney Int 51:2, 1997; Schena FP, et al: Progression of renal damage in human glomerulonephritis. Kidney Int 52:1439, 1997; Fogo AB: Progression and potential regression of glomerulosclerosis. Kidney Int 59:804, 2001.)

oliguria, and mild to moderate hypertension. The patient also commonly has proteinuria and edema, but these are not as severe as those encountered in the nephrotic syndrome, discussed later. The acute nephritic syndrome may occur in such multisystem diseases as SLE and microscopic polyarteritis. Typically, however, it is characteristic of acute proliferative glomerulonephritis and is an important component of crescentic glomerulonephritis, which is described later.

Acute Proliferative (Poststreptococcal, Postinfectious) Glomerulonephritis

As the name implies, this cluster of diseases is characterized histologically by diffuse proliferation of glomerular cells, associated with influx of leukocytes. These lesions are typically caused by immune complexes. The inciting antigen may be exogenous or endogenous. The prototypic exogenous antigen–induced disease pattern is postinfectious glomerulonephritis, whereas that produced by an endogenous antigen is the nephritis of systemic lupus erythematosus, described in Chapter 6. The most common infections are streptococcal, but the disorder has also been associated with other infections.

Poststreptococcal Glomerulonephritis

This glomerular disease is decreasing in frequency in the United States but continues to be a fairly common disorder worldwide.[47] It usually appears 1 to 4 weeks after a streptococcal infection of the pharynx or skin (impetigo). Skin infections are commonly associated with overcrowding and poor hygiene. Poststreptococcal glomerulonephritis occurs most frequently in children 6 to 10 years of age, but adults of any age can be affected.

Etiology and Pathogenesis. Only certain strains of group A β-hemolytic streptococci are nephritogenic, more than 90% of cases being traced to types 12, 4, and 1, which can be identified by typing of M protein of the cell wall.

Poststreptococcal glomerulonephritis is an immunologically mediated disease. The latent period between infection and onset of nephritis is compatible with the time required for the production of antibodies and the formation of immune complexes. Elevated titers of antibodies against one or more streptococcal antigens are present in a great majority of patients. Serum complement levels are low, compatible with activation of the complement system and consumption of complement components. The presence of granular immune deposits in the glomeruli demonstrates an immune complex–mediated mechanism, and so does the finding of electron-dense deposits. The streptococcal antigenic component responsible for the immune reaction has eluded identification for years. A cytoplasmic antigen called *endostreptosin* and several *cationic antigens*, including a proteinase (nephritis strain–associated protein, NSAP) related to streptokinase and unique to nephritogenic strains of streptococci, can be present in affected glomeruli. It is not known if these represent planted antigens, part of circulating immune complexes, or both. GBM proteins altered by streptococcal enzymes have also been implicated as antigens at one time or another.

Morphology. The classic diagnostic picture is one of **enlarged, hypercellular glomeruli** (Fig. 20–16). The hypercellularity is caused by (1) infiltration by leukocytes, both neutrophils and monocytes; (2) proliferation of endothelial and mesangial cells; and (3) in severe cases by crescent formation. The proliferation and leukocyte infiltration are diffuse, that is, involving

TABLE 20–6 Summary of Major Primary Glomerulonephritides

Disease	Most Frequent Clinical Presentation	Pathogenesis	Glomerular Pathology		
			Light Microscopy	*Fluorescence Microscopy*	*Electron Microscopy*
Poststreptococcal glomerulonephritis	Acute nephritis	Antibody mediated; circulating or planted antigen	Diffuse proliferation; leukocytic infiltration	Granular IgG and C3 in GBM and mesangium	Subepithelial humps
Goodpasture syndrome	Rapidly progressive glomerulonephritis	Anti-GBM COL4-A3 antigen	Proliferation; crescents	Linear IgG and C3; fibrin in crescents	No deposits; GBM disruptions; fibrin
Idiopathic RPGN	Rapidly progressive glomerulonephritis	Anti-GBM antibody Immune complex ANCA-associated	Proliferation; focal necrosis; crescents	Linear IgG and C3 Granular IgG or IgA or IgM Negative or equivocal	No deposits Deposits may be present No deposits
Membranous glomerulopathy	Nephrotic syndrome	In situ antibody-mediated; antigen unknown	Diffuse capillary wall thickening	Granular IgG and C3; diffuse	Subepithelial deposits
Minimal change disease	Nephrotic syndrome	Unknown, loss of glomerular polyanion; podocyte injury	Normal; lipid in tubules	Negative	Loss of foot processes; no deposits
Focal segmental glomerulosclerosis	Nephrotic syndrome; non-nephrotic proteinuria	Unknown, Ablation nephropathy Plasma factor(?); podocyte injury	Focal and segmental sclerosis and hyalinosis	Focal; IgM and C3	Loss of foot processes; epithelial denudation
Membranoproliferative glomerulonephritis (MPGN) Type I	Nephrotic syndrome	(I) Immune complex	Mesangial proliferation; basement membrane thickening; splitting	(I) IgG + C3; C1q + C4	(I) Subendothelial deposits
Dense deposit disease (MPGN Type II)	Hematuria Chronic renal failure	(II) Autoantibody: alternative complement pathway		(II) C3 ± IgG; no C1q or C4	(II) Dense deposits
IgA nephropathy	Recurrent hematuria or proteinuria	Unknown; see text	Focal proliferative glomerulonephritis; mesangial widening	IgA +/– IgG, IgM, and C3 in mesangium	Mesangial and paramesangial dense deposits
Chronic glomerulonephritis	Chronic renal failure	Variable	Hyalinized glomeruli	Granular or negative	

ANCA, antineutrophil cytoplasmic antibody; GBM, glomerular basement membrane; RPGN, rapidly progressive glomerulonephritis.

all lobules of all glomeruli. There is also swelling of endothelial cells, and the combination of proliferation, swelling, and leukocyte infiltration obliterates the capillary lumens. There may be interstitial edema and inflammation, and the tubules often contain red cell casts.

By **immunofluorescence microscopy,** there are granular deposits of IgG, IgM, and C3 in the mesangium and along the basement membrane. Although almost universally present, they are often focal and sparse. The characteristic **electron microscopic findings** are discrete, amorphous, electron-dense deposits on the epithelial side of the membrane, often having the appearance of "humps" (Fig. 20–16*C),* presumably representing the antigen–antibody complexes at the epithelial cell surface. Subendothelial and intramembranous deposits are also commonly seen, and mesangial deposits may be present. There is often swelling of endothelial and mesangial cells.

Clinical Course. In the classic case, a young child abruptly develops malaise, fever, nausea, oliguria, and hematuria (smoky or cocoa-colored urine) 1 to 2 weeks after recovery from a sore throat. The patients exhibit red cell casts in the urine, mild proteinuria (usually less than 1 gm/day), periorbital edema, and mild to moderate hypertension. In adults, the onset is more likely to be atypical, with the sudden appearance of hypertension or edema, frequently with elevation of BUN. During epidemics caused by nephritogenic streptococcal infections, glomerulonephritis may be asymptomatic, discovered only on screening for microscopic hematuria. Important laboratory findings include elevations of antistreptococcal antibody (ASO) titers and a decline in the serum concentration of C3 and other components of the complement cascade and the presence of cryoglobulins in the serum.

More than 95% of affected children eventually recover totally with conservative therapy aimed at maintaining sodium and water balance. A small minority of children (perhaps less than 1%) do not improve, become severely oliguric, and develop a rapidly progressive form of glomeru-

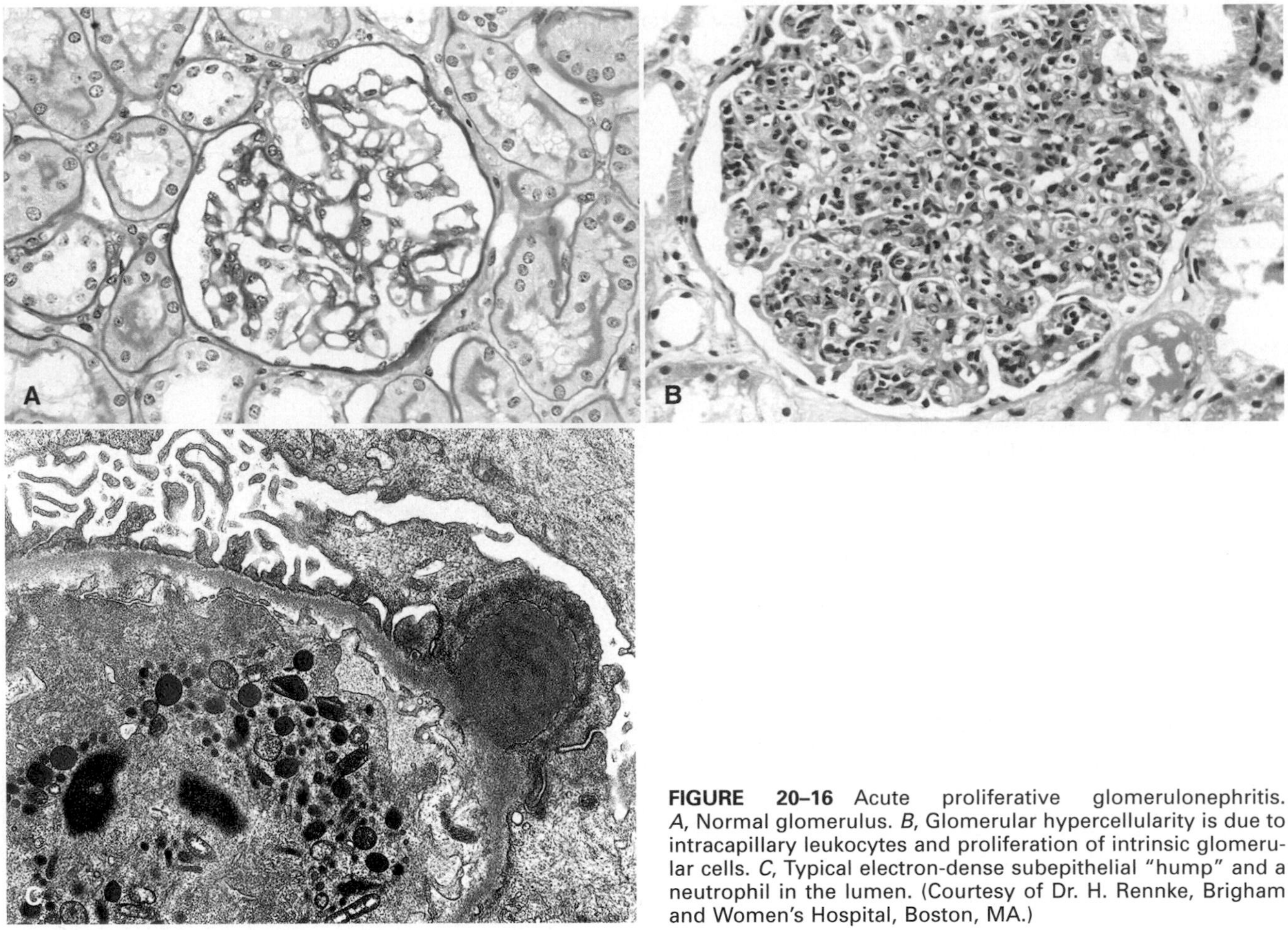

FIGURE 20–16 Acute proliferative glomerulonephritis. *A,* Normal glomerulus. *B,* Glomerular hypercellularity is due to intracapillary leukocytes and proliferation of intrinsic glomerular cells. *C,* Typical electron-dense subepithelial "hump" and a neutrophil in the lumen. (Courtesy of Dr. H. Rennke, Brigham and Women's Hospital, Boston, MA.)

lonephritis (described later). Some of the remaining patients may undergo slow progression to chronic glomerulonephritis with or without recurrence of an active nephritic picture. Prolonged and persistent heavy proteinuria and abnormal GFR mark patients with an unfavorable prognosis.

In adults, the disease is less benign. Although the overall prognosis in epidemics is good, in only about 60% of *sporadic cases* do the patients recover promptly. In the remainder, the glomerular lesions fail to resolve quickly, as manifested by persistent proteinuria, hematuria, and hypertension. In some of these patients, the lesions eventually clear totally, but others develop chronic glomerulonephritis. Some patients will develop a syndrome of rapidly progressive glomerulonephritis.

Nonstreptococcal Acute Glomerulonephritis (Postinfectious Glomerulonephritis)

A similar form of glomerulonephritis occurs sporadically in association with other bacterial infections (e.g., staphylococcal endocarditis, pneumococcal pneumonia, and meningococcemia), viral disease (e.g., hepatitis B, hepatitis C, mumps, human immunodeficiency virus [HIV] infection, varicella, and infectious mononucleosis), and parasitic infections (malaria, toxoplasmosis). In this setting, granular immunofluorescent deposits and subepithelial humps characteristic of immune complex nephritis are present.

RAPIDLY PROGRESSIVE (CRESCENTIC) GLOMERULONEPHRITIS

Rapidly progressive glomerulonephritis (RPGN) is a syndrome associated with severe glomerular injury and does not denote a specific etiologic form of glomerulonephritis. It is characterized clinically by rapid and progressive loss of renal function associated with severe oliguria and (if untreated) death from renal failure within weeks to months. *Regardless of the cause, the classic histologic picture is characterized by the presence of crescents in most of the glomeruli* (crescentic glomerulonephritis). As discussed earlier, these are produced in part by proliferation of the parietal epithelial cells lining Bowman capsule and in part by infiltration of monocytes and macrophages.

Classification and Pathogenesis. RPGN may be caused by a number of different diseases, some restricted to the kidney and others systemic. Although no single mechanism can explain all cases, there is little doubt that in most cases, the glomerular injury is immunologically mediated. Thus, a practical classification divides RPGN into three groups on the basis of immunologic findings (Table 20–7). In each group, the disease may be associated with a known disorder, or it may be idiopathic.

The first type of *RPGN* is best remembered as *anti-GBM antibody–induced disease* and hence is characterized by linear deposits of IgG and, in many cases, C3 in the GBM, as

TABLE 20–7 Rapidly Progressive Glomerulonephritis (RPGN)

Type I RPGN (Anti-GBM Antibody)
Idiopathic
Goodpasture syndrome
Type II RPGN (Immune Complex)
Idiopathic
Postinfectious
Systemic lupus erythematosus
Henoch-Schönlein purpura (IgA)
Others
Type III RPGN (Pauci-Immune)
ANCA associated
Idiopathic
Wegener granulomatosis
Microscopic polyarteritis nodosa/microscopic polyangiitis

previously described.[48] In some of these patients, the anti-GBM antibodies cross-react with pulmonary alveolar basement membranes to produce the clinical picture of pulmonary hemorrhage associated with renal failure (*Goodpasture syndrome*). Plasmapheresis to remove the pathogenic circulating antibodies is usually part of the treatment, which also includes therapy to suppress the underlying immune response.

The Goodpasture antigen, as was noted earlier, is a peptide within the noncollagenous portion of the α_3-chain of collagen type IV.[27] What triggers the formation of these antibodies is unclear in most patients. Exposure to viruses or hydrocarbon solvents (found in paints and dyes) has been implicated in some patients, as have various drugs and cancers. There is a high prevalence of certain HLA subtypes and haplotypes (e.g., HLA-DRB1) in affected patients, a finding consistent with the genetic predisposition to autoimmunity.[49]

The second type of *RPGN* is the result of *immune complex–mediated disease.* It can be a complication of any of the immune complex nephritides, including postinfectious glomerulonephritis, SLE, IgA nephropathy, and Henoch-Schönlein purpura. In all of these cases, immunofluorescence studies reveal the granular pattern of staining characteristic of immune complex deposition. These patients cannot usually be helped by plasmapheresis, and they require treatment for the underlying disease.

The third type of *RPGN*, also called *pauci-immune type*, is defined by the lack of anti-GBM antibodies or immune complexes by immunofluorescence and electron microscopy. Most patients with this type of RPGN have *antineutrophil cytoplasmic antibodies* (ANCA), of cytoplasmic (C) or perinuclear (P) patterns, in the serum, which, as we have seen (Chapter 11), play a role in some vasculitides. Hence, in some cases, this type of RPGN is a component of a systemic vasculitis such as Wegener granulomatosis or microscopic polyarteritis. In many cases, however, pauci-immune crescentic glomerulonephritis is isolated and hence *idiopathic*. More than 90% of such idiopathic cases have c-ANCA or p-ANCA in the sera.[50] The presence of circulating ANCAs in both idiopathic RPGN and cases of RPGN that occur as a component of systemic vasculitis, and the similar pathologic features in either setting, have led to the idea that these disorders are pathogenetically related. According to this concept, all cases of RPGN of the pauci-immune type are manifestations of small vessel vasculitis or polyangiitis, which is limited to glomerular and perhaps peritubular capillaries in cases of idiopathic crescentic glomerulonephritis.[51] The clinical distinction between systemic vasculitis with pauci-immune renal involvement and idiopathic crescentic glomerulonephritis accordingly has become deemphasized, as these entities are viewed as part of a spectrum of vasculitic disease. ANCAs have proved to be invaluable as a highly sensitive diagnostic marker for pauci-immune RPGN, but proof of their role as a direct cause of RPGN has been elusive. Recent strong evidence of their pathogenic potential has been obtained by studies in which antibodies against myeloperoxidase (the target antigen of most p-ANCAs) are transferred into mice.[52]

To summarize, all three types of RPGN may be associated with a well-defined renal or extrarenal disease, but in many cases (approximately 50%), the disorder is idiopathic. Of the patients with this syndrome, about one fifth have anti-GBM antibody–induced disease without lung involvement; another one fourth have immune complex–mediated disease RPGN; and the remainder are of the pauci-immune type. *The common denominator in all types of RPGN is severe glomerular injury.*

Morphology. The kidneys are enlarged and pale, often with petechial hemorrhages on the cortical surfaces. Depending on the underlying cause, the glomeruli may show focal necrosis, diffuse or focal endothelial proliferation, and mesangial proliferation. The histologic picture, however, is dominated by the formation of distinctive **crescents** (Fig. 20–17). Crescents are formed by proliferation of parietal cells and by migration of monocytes and macrophages into the urinary space. Neutrophils and lymphocytes may be present. The crescents eventually obliterate Bowman space and compress the glomerular tuft. **Fibrin strands are prominent between the cellular layers in the crescents;** indeed, as discussed earlier, the escape of fibrin into Bowman space is an important

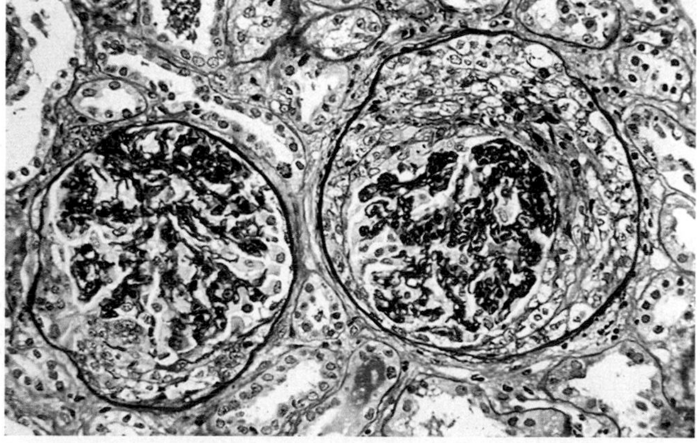

FIGURE 20–17 Crescentic glomerulonephritis (PAS stain). Note the collapsed glomerular tufts and the crescent-shaped mass of proliferating cells and leukocytes internal to Bowman capsule. (Courtesy of Dr. M.A. Venkatachalam, University of Texas Health Sciences Center, San Antonio, TX.)

contributor to crescent formation. Electron microscopy may, as expected, disclose subepithelial deposits in some cases, but in many cases, it shows distinct **ruptures in the GBM**, the severe injury that allows leukocytes, proteins, and inflammatory mediators into the urinary space, where they trigger the crescent formation (Fig. 20–18). In time, most crescents undergo sclerosis, but restoration of normal glomerular architecture marks a successful clinical outcome in some patients, particularly those with an infection-associated immune complex etiology.

By immunofluorescence microscopy, postinfectious cases exhibit granular immune deposits; Goodpasture syndrome cases show linear fluorescence for immunoglobulin and complement, and pauci-immune cases have little or no deposition of immune reactants.

Clinical Course. The renal manifestations of all forms include hematuria with red cell casts in the urine, moderate proteinuria occasionally reaching the nephrotic range, and variable hypertension and edema. In Goodpasture syndrome, the course may be dominated by recurrent hemoptysis or even life-threatening pulmonary hemorrhage. Serum analyses for anti-GBM antibodies, antinuclear antibodies, and ANCA are helpful in the diagnosis of specific subtypes. Although milder forms of glomerular injury may subside, the renal involvement is usually progressive over a matter of weeks and culminates in severe oliguria. Recovery of renal function may follow early intensive plasmapheresis (plasma exchange) combined with steroids and cytotoxic agents in Goodpasture syndrome. This therapy appears to reverse both pulmonary hemorrhage and renal failure. Other forms of RPGN also respond well to steroids and cytotoxic agents. Despite therapy, patients may eventually require chronic dialysis or transplantation.

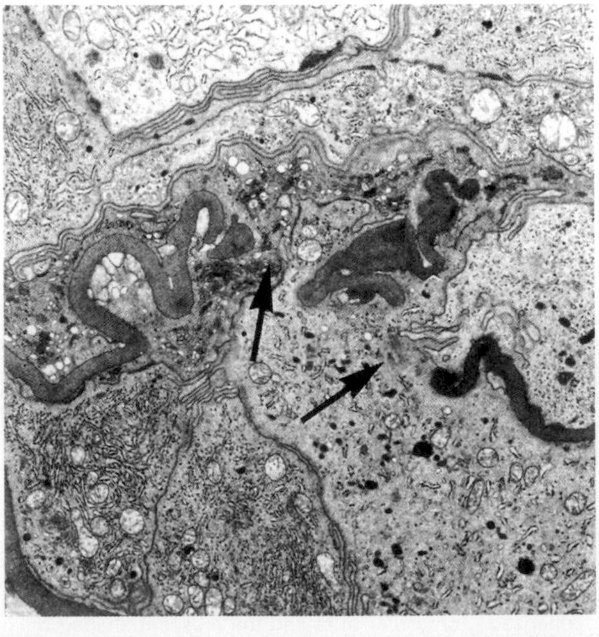

FIGURE 20–18 Rapidly progressive glomerulonephritis. Electron micrograph showing characteristic wrinkling of GBM with focal disruptions in its continuity (*arrows*).

NEPHROTIC SYNDROME

Certain glomerular diseases virtually always produce the nephrotic syndrome. In addition, many other forms of primary and secondary glomerulonephritis discussed in this chapter may underlie the syndrome. Before the major diseases associated with nephrotic syndrome are presented, the pathophysiology of this clinical complex is briefly discussed, and the causes are listed.

Pathophysiology. The manifestations of the nephrotic syndrome include:

1. *Massive proteinuria*, with the daily loss of 3.5 gm or more of protein (less in children)
2. *Hypoalbuminemia*, with plasma albumin levels less than 3 gm/dL
3. *Generalized edema*
4. *Hyperlipidemia and lipiduria*

The various components of nephrotic syndrome bear a logical relationship to one another. The initial event is a derangement in glomerular capillary walls resulting in *increased permeability to plasma proteins.* It will be remembered that the glomerular capillary wall, with its endothelium, GBM, and visceral epithelial cells, acts as a size and charge barrier through which the glomerular filtrate must pass. Increased permeability resulting from either structural or physicochemical alterations allows protein to escape from the plasma into the glomerular filtrate. *Massive proteinuria results.*

The heavy proteinuria leads to depletion of serum albumin levels below the compensatory synthetic abilities of the liver, with consequent hypoalbuminemia and a reversed albumin-globulin ratio. Increased renal catabolism of filtered albumin also contributes to the hypoalbuminemia. The generalized edema is, in turn, the consequence of the loss of colloid osmotic pressure of the blood with subsequent accumulation of fluid in the interstitial tissues. There is also *sodium and water retention*, which aggravates the edema (Chapter 4). This appears to be due to several factors, including compensatory secretion of aldosterone, mediated by the hypovolemia-enhanced antidiuretic hormone secretion; stimulation of the sympathetic system; and a reduction in the secretion of natriuretic factors such as atrial peptides. Edema is characteristically soft and pitting, most marked in the periorbital regions and dependent portions of the body. It may be massive, with pleural effusions and ascites.

The largest proportion of protein lost in the urine is albumin, but globulins are also excreted in some diseases. The ratio of low- to high-molecular-weight proteins in the urine in various cases of nephrotic syndrome is a manifestation of the *selectivity* of proteinuria. A *highly selective proteinuria* consists mostly of low-molecular-weight proteins (albumin: 70 kDa; transferrin: 76 kDa molecular weight), whereas a *poorly selective proteinuria* consists of higher-molecular-weight globulins in addition to albumin.

The genesis of the *hyperlipidemia* is complex. Most patients have increased blood levels of cholesterol, triglyceride, very-low-density lipoprotein, low-density lipoprotein, Lp(a) lipoprotein, and apoprotein, and there is a decrease in high-density lipoprotein concentration in some patients. These defects seem to be due in part to *increased synthesis of lipoproteins in the liver, abnormal transport of circulating lipid particles, and decreased catabolism. Lipiduria* follows the hyperlipidemia because not only albumin molecules but also lipoproteins leak across the glomerular capillary wall. The lipid appears in the urine either as free fat or as *oval fat bodies*, representing lipoprotein resorbed by tubular epithelial cells and then shed along with the degenerated cells.

These patients are particularly vulnerable to *infection*, especially with staphylococci and pneumococci. This vulnerability could be related to loss of immunoglobulins or low-molecular-weight complement components in the urine. *Thrombotic and thromboembolic complications* are also common in nephrotic syndrome, owing in part to loss of anticoagulant factors (e.g., antithrombin III) and antiplasmin activity through the leaky glomerulus. *Renal vein thrombosis*, once thought to be a cause of nephrotic syndrome, is most often a *consequence* of this hypercoagulable state.

Causes. The relative frequencies of the several causes of the nephrotic syndrome vary according to age and geography. In children younger than 17 years in North America, for example, the nephrotic syndrome is almost always caused by a lesion primary to the kidney; whereas among adults, it may often be associated with a systemic disease. Table 20–8 represents a composite derived from several studies of the causes of the nephrotic syndrome and is therefore only approximate. As Table 20–8 indicates, the most frequent *systemic causes* of the nephrotic syndrome are diabetes, amyloidosis, and SLE. The most important of the *primary glomerular lesions* are *minimal change disease*, *membranous glomerulopathy*, and *focal segmental glomerulosclerosis*. The first is most common in children in North America, the second is most common in older adults, but focal segmental glomerulosclerosis occurs at all ages.[53] These three lesions, as well as a fourth, less common disorder, membranoproliferative glomerulonephritis, are discussed individually in the following sections. Other primary causes, the various proliferative glomerulonephritides, frequently present as a mixed syndrome with nephrotic and nephritic features.

TABLE 20-8 Causes of Nephrotic Syndrome

	Prevalence (%)*	
	Children	Adults
Primary Glomerular Disease		
Membranous glomerulopathy	5	30
Minimal change disease	65	10
Focal segmental glomerulosclerosis	10	35
Membranoproliferative glomerulonephritides	10	10
Other proliferative glomerulonephritis (focal, "pure mesangial," IgA nephropathy)	10	15
Systemic Diseases		
Diabetes mellitus		
Amyloidosis		
Systemic lupus erythematosus		
Drugs (nonsteroidal anti-inflammatory, penicillamine, "street heroin")		
Infections (malaria, syphilis, hepatitis B and C, acquired immunodeficiency syndrome)		
Malignant disease (carcinoma, lymphoma)		
Miscellaneous (bee-sting allergy, hereditary nephritis)		

*Approximate prevalence of primary disease = 95% in children, 60% in adults. Approximate prevalence of systemic disease = 5% in children, 40% in adults.

MEMBRANOUS GLOMERULOPATHY (MEMBRANOUS NEPHROPATHY)

Membranous glomerulopathy is the most common cause of the nephrotic syndrome in adults. It is characterized by diffuse thickening of the glomerular capillary wall and the accumulation of electron-dense, immunoglobulin-containing deposits along the subepithelial side of the basement membrane.[54]

Membranous glomerulopathy occurring in association with other systemic diseases and a variety of identifiable etiologic agents is referred to as secondary membranous glomerulopathy. The most notable such associations are as follows:

- *Drugs* (penicillamine, captopril, gold, nonsteroidal anti-inflammatory drugs [NSAIDs]): 1% to 7% of patients with rheumatoid arthritis treated with penicillamine or gold (drugs now used infrequently for this purpose) develop membranous glomerulopathy. NSAIDs, as we shall see, also cause minimal change disease.
- *Underlying malignant tumors*, particularly carcinoma of the lung and colon and melanoma. According to some investigators, these are present in up to 5% to 10% of adults with membranous glomerulopathy.[55]
- *SLE.* About 15% of glomerulonephritis in SLE is of the membranous type.
- *Infections* (chronic hepatitis B, hepatitis C, syphilis, schistosomiasis, malaria)
- *Other autoimmune disorders*, such as thyroiditis

In about 85% of patients, no associated condition can be uncovered, and the disease is considered idiopathic.

Etiology and Pathogenesis. Membranous glomerulopathy is a form of chronic immune complex–mediated disease. In secondary membranous glomerulopathy, particular antigens can sometimes be identified in the immune complexes. For example, membranous glomerulopathy in SLE is associated with deposition of autoantigen–antibody complexes. Exogenous (hepatitis B, *Treponema* antigens) or endogenous (thyroglobulin) antigens have been identified within deposits in some patients.

The lesions bear a striking resemblance to those of experimental Heymann nephritis, which, as you might recall, is induced by antibodies to a *megalin* antigenic complex. A similar but still unidentified antigen is presumed to be present in most cases of idiopathic membranous glomerulopathy in humans. Susceptibility to Heymann nephritis in rats and membranous glomerulopathy in humans is linked to the MHC locus, which influences the ability to produce antibodies to the nephritogenic antigen. Thus, idiopathic membranous glomerulopathy, like Heymann nephritis, is considered *an autoimmune disease linked to susceptibility genes and caused by antibodies to a renal autoantigen.*

How does the glomerular capillary wall become leaky in membranous glomerulopathy? There is a paucity of neutrophils, monocytes, or platelets in glomeruli and the virtually uniform presence of complement, and experimental work suggests a direct action of C5b–C9, the pathway leading to the formation of the membrane attack complex. C5b–C9 causes activation of glomerular epithelial and mesangial cells, inducing them to liberate proteases and oxidants, which cause capillary wall injury and increased protein leakage.

Morphology. By light microscopy, the glomeruli either appear normal in the early stages of the disease or exhibit **uniform, diffuse thickening of the glomerular capillary wall** (Fig. 20–19*A*). By electron microscopy, the thickening is seen to be caused by irregular dense deposits between the basement membrane and the overlying epithelial cells, the latter having effaced foot processes (Figs. 20–19*B* and 20–19*D*). Basement membrane material is laid down between these deposits, appearing as irregular spikes protruding from the GBM. These spikes are best seen by silver stains, which color the basement membrane black. In time, these spikes thicken to produce dome-like protrusions and eventually close over the immune

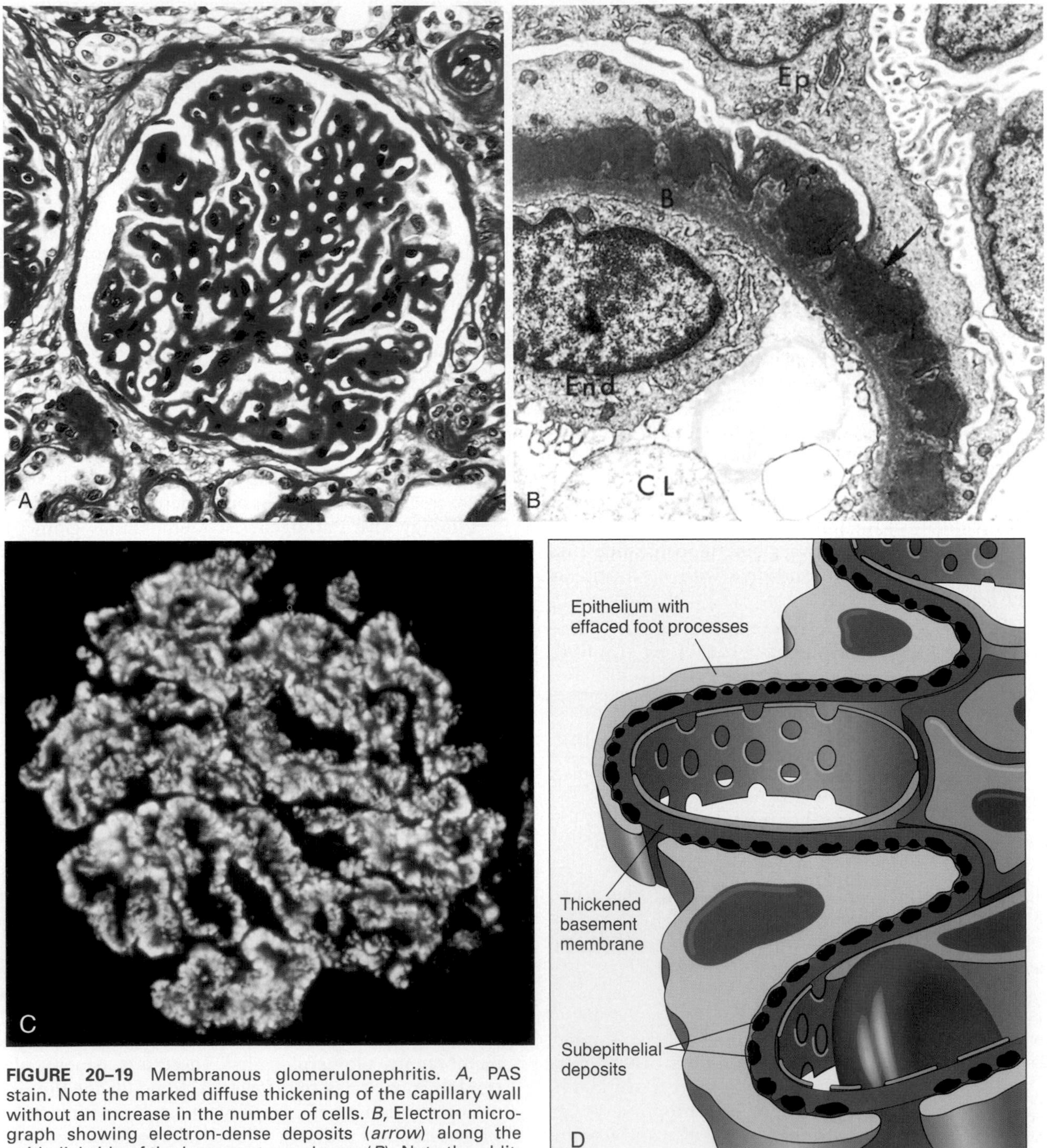

FIGURE 20–19 Membranous glomerulonephritis. *A*, PAS stain. Note the marked diffuse thickening of the capillary wall without an increase in the number of cells. *B*, Electron micrograph showing electron-dense deposits (*arrow*) along the epithelial side of the basement membrane (*B*). Note the obliteration of foot process overlying deposits. CL, capillary lumen; End, endothelium; Ep, epithelium. *C*, Characteristic granular immunofluorescent deposits of IgG along GBM. *D*, Diagrammatic representation of membranous glomerulonephritis.

deposits, burying them within a markedly thickened, irregular membrane. Immunofluorescence microscopy demonstrates that the granular deposits contain both immunoglobulins and various amounts of complement (Fig. 20–19*C*). As the disease advances, the membrane thickening progressively encroaches on the capillary lumens, and sclerosis of the mesangium may occur; in the course of time, glomeruli may become totally sclerosed. The epithelial cells of the proximal tubules contain protein reabsorption droplets, and there may be considerable mononuclear cell interstitial inflammation.

Clinical Course. In a previously healthy individual, this disorder usually begins with the insidious onset of the nephrotic syndrome or, in 15% of patients, with non-nephrotic proteinuria. Hematuria and mild hypertension are present in 15% to 35% of cases. It is necessary in any patient to first rule out the secondary causes described earlier, since treatment of the underlying condition (malignant neoplasm, infection, or SLE) or discontinuance of the offending drug can reverse progression.

The course of the disease is variable but generally indolent. In contrast to minimal change disease, described later, the proteinuria is nonselective and does not usually respond well to corticosteroid therapy. Progression is associated with increasing sclerosis of glomeruli, rising BUN reflecting renal insufficiency, and development of hypertension. Although proteinuria persists in more than 60% of patients, only about 10% die or progress to renal failure within 10 years, and no more than 40% eventually develop renal insufficiency. Concurrent sclerosis of glomeruli in the renal biopsy at the time of diagnosis is a predictor of worse prognosis. Spontaneous remissions and a relatively benign outcome occur more commonly in women and in those with proteinuria in the non-nephrotic range. Because of the variable course of the disease, it has been difficult to evaluate the overall effectiveness of corticosteroids or other immunosuppressive therapy in controlling the proteinuria or progression.

MINIMAL CHANGE DISEASE (LIPOID NEPHROSIS)

This relatively benign disorder is the *most frequent cause of nephrotic syndrome in children*, but it is less common in adults (Table 20–8). *It is characterized by diffuse effacement of foot processes of epithelial cells in glomeruli that appear virtually normal by light microscopy.* The peak incidence is between 2 and 6 years of age. The disease sometimes follows a respiratory infection or routine prophylactic immunization. *Its most characteristic feature is its usually dramatic response to corticosteroid therapy.*[56]

Etiology and Pathogenesis. Although the absence of immune deposits in the glomerulus excludes classic immune complex mechanisms, several features of the disease point to an immunologic basis,[31,56] including (1) the clinical association with respiratory infections and prophylactic immunization; (2) the response to corticosteroids and/or other immunosuppressive therapy; (3) the association with other atopic disorders (e.g., eczema, rhinitis); (4) the increased prevalence of certain HLA haplotypes in patients with minimal change disease associated with atopy (suggesting a genetic predisposition); (5) the increased incidence of minimal change disease in patients with Hodgkin disease, in whom defects in T cell–mediated immunity are well recognized; and (6) reports of proteinuria-inducing factors in the plasma or lymphocyte supernatants of patients with minimal change disease and focal glomerulosclerosis.

The current leading hypothesis is that minimal change disease involves some immune dysfunction, eventually resulting in the elaboration of a cytokine that damages visceral epithelial cells and causes proteinuria. The ultrastructural changes point to a primary *visceral epithelial cell injury*, and studies in animal models suggest the loss of glomerular polyanions. Thus, defects in the charge barrier may contribute to the proteinuria. The actual route by which protein traverses the epithelial cell portion of the capillary wall remains an enigma. Possibilities include transcellular passage through the epithelial cells, passage through residual spaces between remaining but damaged foot processes, or leakage through foci in which the epithelial cells have become detached from the basement membrane.

Additional insight into mechanisms by which epithelial cell injury results in proteinuria in minimal change disease, focal and segmental glomerulosclerosis, and related entities should come from the recent discovery of mutations in several glomerular proteins, including *nephrin*, discussed in the section on focal glomerulosclerosis below. A mutation in the nephrin gene causes a hereditary form of congenital nephrotic syndrome (Finnish type) with minimal change glomerular morphology.[57] Such mutations and the proteinuria they engender demonstrate that at least some cases of nephrotic syndrome with minimal change disease morphology can occur in the absence of abnormal responses of the immune system.

Morphology. The glomeruli are normal by light microscopy (Fig. 20–20). By electron microscopy, the basement membrane appears normal, and no electron-dense material is deposited. **The principal lesion is in the visceral epithelial cells, which show a**

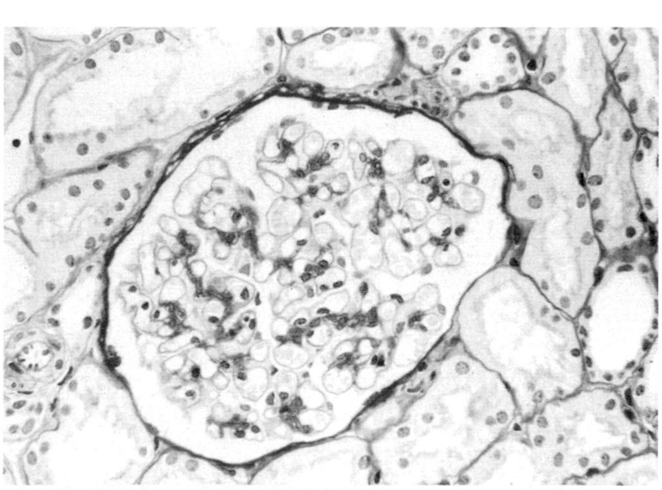

FIGURE 20–20 Minimal change disease. Glomerulus stained with PAS. Note normal basement membrane and absence of proliferation. Compare with membranous glomerulopathy in Figure 20–19*A*.

uniform and diffuse effacement of foot processes, these being replaced by a rim of cytoplasm often showing vacuolization, swelling, and hyperplasia of villi (Fig. 20–21). This change, often incorrectly termed "fusion" of foot processes, actually represents simplification of the epithelial cell architecture with flattening, retraction, and swelling of foot processes. Foot process effacement is also present in other proteinuric states (e.g., membranous glomerulopathy, diabetes); it is only when effacement is associated with normal glomeruli by light microscopy that the diagnosis of minimal change disease can be made. The visceral epithelial changes are completely reversible after corticosteroid therapy, concomitant with remission of the proteinuria. The cells of the proximal tubules are often laden with lipid and protein, reflecting tubular reabsorption of lipoproteins passing through diseased glomeruli (thus, the historical term **lipoid nephrosis**). Immunofluorescence studies show no immunoglobulin or complement deposits.

Clinical Course. Despite massive proteinuria, renal function remains good, and there is commonly no hypertension or hematuria. The proteinuria usually is highly selective, most of the protein consisting of albumin. Most children (more than 90%) with minimal change disease respond rapidly to corticosteroid therapy. However, the nephrotic phase may recur, and some patients may become steroid dependent or resistant. Nevertheless, the long-term prognosis for patients is excellent, and even steroid-dependent disease resolves when children reach puberty. Although adults are slower to respond, the long-term prognosis is also excellent.

As has been noted, minimal change disease in adults can be associated with Hodgkin disease and, less frequently, other lymphomas and leukemias. In addition, secondary minimal change disease may follow NSAID therapy, usually in association with acute interstitial nephritis, to be described later in this chapter.

FOCAL SEGMENTAL GLOMERULOSCLEROSIS

As the name implies, *this lesion is characterized by sclerosis of some, but not all, glomeruli (thus, it is focal); and in the affected glomeruli, only a portion of the capillary tuft is involved (thus, it is segmental).* Focal segmental glomerulosclerosis is frequently accompanied clinically by the nephrotic syndrome or heavy proteinuria.

Classification and Types. Focal segmental glomerulosclerosis (FSGS) occurs in the following settings:[58]

- In association with other known conditions, such as HIV infection (HIV nephropathy), heroin addiction (heroin nephropathy), sickle cell disease, and massive obesity
- As a secondary event, reflecting glomerular scarring, in cases of focal glomerulonephritis (e.g., IgA nephropathy)
- As a component of the adaptive response to loss of renal tissue (renal ablation, described earlier) in advanced stages of other renal disorders, such as reflux nephropathy, hypertensive nephropathy, or with unilateral renal agenesis
- In certain inherited forms of nephrotic syndrome where the disease, in some pedigrees, has been linked to mutations in genes encoding nephrin, podocin, or α-actinin 4
- As a primary disease (idiopathic focal segmental glomerulosclerosis)

Idiopathic focal segmental glomerulosclerosis accounts for up to 10% and 35% of cases of nephrotic syndrome in children and adults in many series, respectively. FSGS (both primary and secondary forms) has increased in incidence and is now the most common cause of nephrotic syndrome in adults in the United States.[53] It is a particularly common cause of

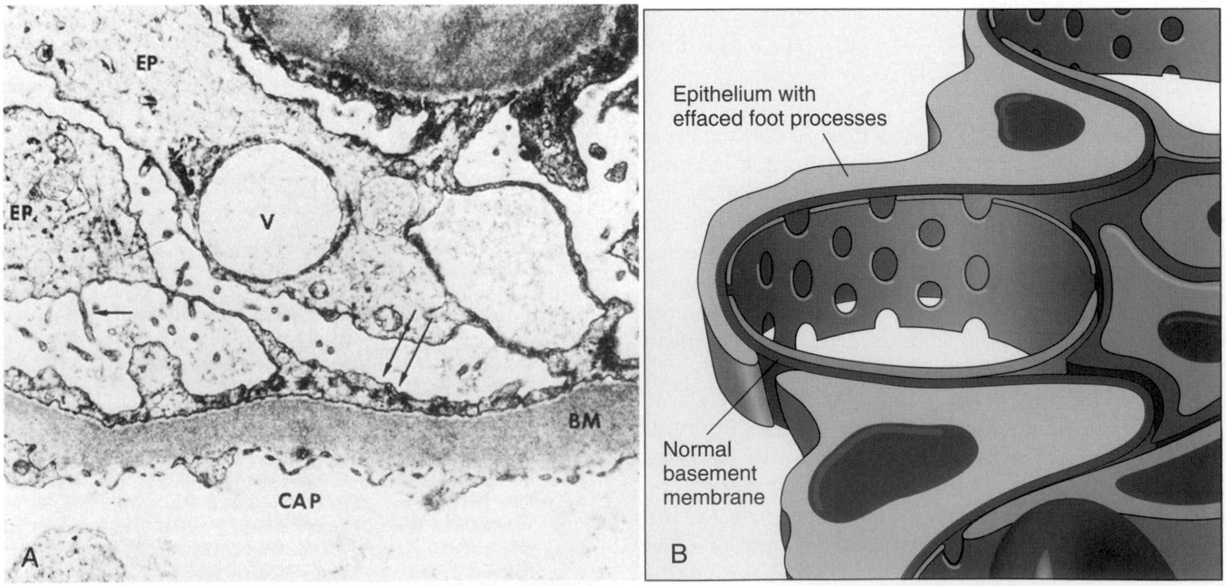

FIGURE 20–21 *A*, Ultrastructural characteristics of minimal change disease: effacement of foot processes (*double arrows*), absence of deposits, vacuoles (V), and microvilli in visceral epithelial cells (*single arrow*). *B*, Schematic representation of minimal change disease, showing diffuse effacement of foot processes.

nephrotic syndrome in Hispanic and African American patients. The clinical signs differ from those of minimal change disease in the following respects: (1) there is a higher incidence of hematuria, reduced GFR, and hypertension; (2) proteinuria is more often nonselective; (3) there is poor response to corticosteroid therapy; (4) there is progression to chronic glomerulosclerosis, with at least 50% developing end-stage renal disease within 10 years; and (5) immunofluorescence microscopy may show nonspecific deposition ("trapping") of IgM and C3 in the sclerotic segment.

Morphology. By light microscopy, the segmental lesions may involve only a minority of the glomeruli and may be missed if the biopsy specimen contains an insufficient number of glomeruli (Fig. 20–22*A*). The lesions initially tend to involve the juxtamedullary glomeruli, although they subsequently become more generalized. In the sclerotic segments, there is collapse of basement membranes, increase in matrix, and segmental insudation of plasma proteins along the capillary wall (hyalinosis), which may extend to aggregates within glomerular capillaries that occlude the lumina. Lipid droplets and foam cells are often present (Fig. 20–22*B*). Glomeruli that do not exhibit segmental lesions either appear normal on light microscopy or may show increased mesangial matrix and mesangial proliferation. On electron microscopy, both sclerotic and nonsclerotic areas show the diffuse effacement of foot processes characteristic of minimal change disease, but in addition, there may be focal detachment of the epithelial cells with denudation of the underlying GBM. By immunofluorescence microscopy, IgM and C3 may be present in the sclerotic areas and/or in the mesangium. In addition to the focal sclerosis, there may be pronounced hyalinosis and thickening of afferent arterioles. With the progression of the disease, increased numbers of glomeruli become involved, sclerosis spreads within each glomerulus, and there is an increase in mesangial matrix. In time, this leads to total sclerosis of glomeruli, with pronounced tubular atrophy and interstitial fibrosis.

A morphologic variant of focal segmental glomerulosclerosis, called **collapsing glomerulopathy**, is characterized by collapse and sclerosis of the entire glomerular tuft in addition to the usual focal segmental glomerulosclerosis lesions. A characteristic feature is proliferation and hypertrophy of glomerular visceral epithelial cells. This lesion may be seen in situations in which it is idiopathic, but it is the most characteristic lesion of HIV-associated nephropathy. In both cases, there is associated prominent tubular injury with formation of microcysts. It has a particularly poor prognosis.[59]

Pathogenesis. Whether idiopathic focal segmental glomerulosclerosis represents a distinct disease or is simply a phase in the evolution of a subset of patients with minimal change disease remains unresolved. The characteristic degeneration and focal disruption of visceral epithelial cells are thought to represent an accentuation of the diffuse epithelial cell change typical of minimal change disease. *It is this epithelial damage that is the hallmark of focal segmental glomerulosclerosis.* The hyalinosis and sclerosis represent entrapment of plasma proteins in extremely hyperpermeable foci with increased ECM deposition. The recurrence of proteinuria, sometimes within 24 hours after transplantation, suggests that a circulating factor, perhaps a cytokine, may be the cause of the epithelial damage. An approximately 50-kDa nonimmunoglobulin factor causing proteinuria has been isolated from sera of such patients.[60]

The recent discovery of a genetic basis for some cases of FSGS has improved the understanding of the pathogenesis of proteinuria in the nephrotic syndrome and has provided new methods for diagnosis and prognosis of affected patients. The first relevant gene to be identified, *NPHS1*, maps to chromosome 19q13 and encodes the protein *nephrin*.[43,57] Nephrin is a key component of the slit diaphragm (Fig. 20–5), the zipper-like structure between podocyte foot processes that might control glomerular permeability.[43] Several types of mutations of the *NPHS1* gene have been identified, and they give rise to

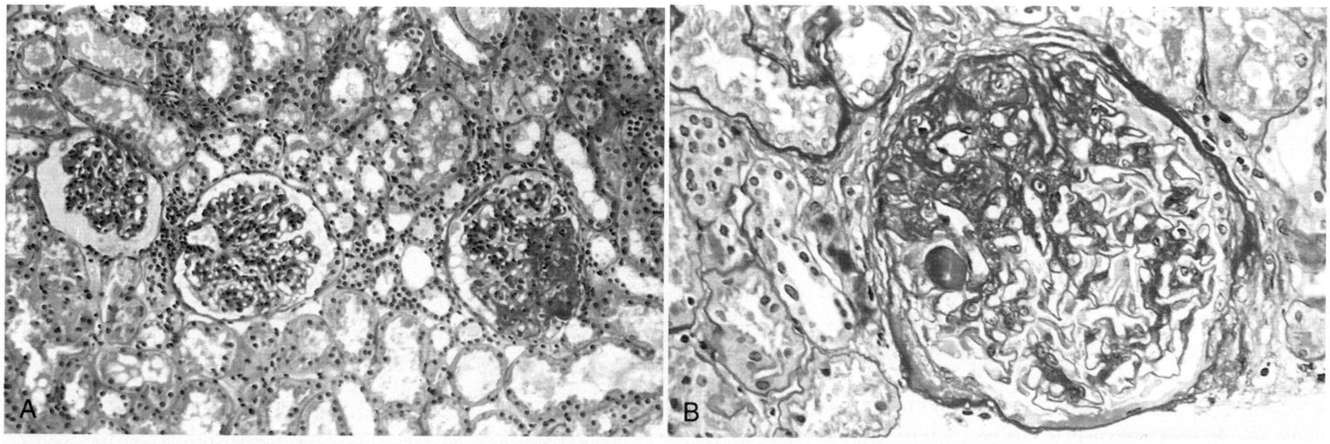

FIGURE 20–22 Focal segmental glomerulosclerosis, PAS stain. *A*, Low-power view showing segmental sclerosis in one of three glomeruli (at 3 o'clock). *B*, High-power view showing hyaline insudation and lipid (small vacuoles) in sclerotic area.

congenital nephrotic syndrome of the Finnish type. Prenatal diagnosis of CNF is now possible based on analysis of the *NPHS1* gene.

A distinctive pattern of autosomal recessive FSGS results from mutations in the *NPHS2* gene, which maps to chromosome 1q25–31 and encodes the protein product *podocin.* Podocin has also been localized to the slit diaphragm. Mutations in *NPHS2* result in a syndrome of steroid-resistant nephrotic syndrome of childhood onset. Affected children usually show pathologic features of FSGS but sometimes of minimal change disease. Podocin mutations may account for up to 30% of cases of steroid-resistant nephrotic syndrome in children.[61] A third set of mutations in the gene encoding the podocyte actin-binding protein α-actinin 4 underlies some cases of autosomal dominant FSGS, which can be insidious in onset but has a high rate of progression to renal insufficiency.[62]

What these proteins have in common is their localization to the slit diaphragm and to adjacent podocyte cytoskeletal structures such as actin. Their specific functions and interactions are incompletely understood, but it is clear that the integrity of each is necessary to maintain the normal glomerular filtration barrier. Additional components of the podocyte/slit diaphragm apparatus, such as CD2-associated protein (CD2AP), have been identified that may also contribute to proteinuria, as has been suggested in studies of knockout mice (but not yet demonstrated in humans).[63] While identification of these genetic defects has clarified the pathogenesis of some cases of the so-called idiopathic nephrotic syndrome, many other factors contribute to permeability defects. These include cell–cell and cell–matrix interactions, particularly those mediated by $\alpha_3\beta_1$ integrins and dystroglycans. Defects in these interactions may also cause a loss of podocyte adhesion to the glomerular basement membrane.

Renal ablation focal segmental glomerulosclerosis occurs as a complication of glomerular and nonglomerular diseases causing reduction in functioning renal tissue, particularly reflux nephropathy and unilateral agenesis. These may lead to progressive glomerulosclerosis and renal failure. The pathogenesis of focal segmental glomerulosclerosis in this setting has been described earlier in this chapter.

Clinical Course. There is little tendency for spontaneous remission in idiopathic focal segmental glomerulosclerosis, and responses to corticosteroid therapy are variable. In general, children have a better prognosis than adults do. Progression of renal failure occurs at variable rates. About 20% of patients follow an unusually rapid course, with intractable massive proteinuria ending in renal failure within 2 years. Recurrences are seen in 25% to 50% of patients receiving allografts.

HIV-Associated Nephropathy

HIV infection can result directly or indirectly in a number of renal complications, including acute renal failure and/or acute interstitial nephritis induced by drugs or infection, thrombotic microangiopathies, postinfectious glomerulonephritis, and, *most commonly, a severe form of the collapsing variant of focal segmental glomerulosclerosis.*[64] The last occurs in 5% to 10% of HIV-infected patients in some series, more frequently in blacks than in whites. In rare cases, the nephrotic syndrome may precede the development of acquired immunodeficiency syndrome. The morphologic features are characterized by:

- A high frequency of the *collapsing variant of focal segmental glomerulosclerosis,* with global involvement of the tuft
- A striking focal cystic dilation of tubule segments, which are filled with proteinaceous material, and inflammation and fibrosis
- The presence of large numbers of *tubuloreticular inclusions* in endothelial cells, detected by electron microscopy. Such inclusions, also present in SLE, have been shown to be induced by circulating interferon-α. They are not present in idiopathic focal segmental glomerulosclerosis and therefore may have diagnostic value in a biopsy specimen.

The pathogenesis of HIV-related focal segmental glomerulosclerosis is unclear. It might be due to infection of glomerular and tubular cells by HIV, which has been detected in a few cases by very sensitive PCR methods, or it might be a consequence of altered systemic or local release of cytokines.[65,66]

MEMBRANOPROLIFERATIVE GLOMERULONEPHRITIS

Membranoproliferative glomerulonephritis (MPGN) is characterized histologically by *alterations in the basement membrane, proliferation of glomerular cells, and leukocyte infiltration.* Because the proliferation is predominantly in the mesangium, a frequently used synonym is *mesangiocapillary glomerulonephritis.* MPGN accounts for 10% to 20% of cases of nephrotic syndrome in children and young adults. Some patients present only with hematuria or proteinuria in the non-nephrotic range, and others have a combined nephrotic–nephritic picture. Like many other glomerulonephritides, MPGN either can be associated with other systemic disorders and known etiologic agents (secondary MPGN) or may be idiopathic (primary MPGN).[67]

Primary MPGN is divided into two major types on the basis of distinct ultrastructural, immunofluorescent, and pathologic findings: type I and type II MPGN (dense-deposit disease).

Morphology. By light microscopy, both types are similar. The glomeruli are large and hypercellular. The hypercellularity is produced both by proliferation of cells in the mesangium and so-called endocapillary cell proliferation involving capillary endothelium and infiltrating leukocytes. Parietal epithelial crescents are present in many cases. The glomeruli have a "lobular" appearance accentuated by the proliferating mesangial cells and increased mesangial matrix (Fig. 20–23). The GBM is clearly thickened, often focally; this is most evident in the peripheral capillary loops. The glomerular capillary wall often shows a "double-contour" or "tram-track" appearance, especially evident in silver or PAS stains. This is caused by "duplication" of the basement membrane, usually as the result of new basement membrane synthesis. Within the besement membrane there is inclusion or interposition of cellular elements, which can be of mesangial, endothelial, or leukocytic origin. Such interposition gives rise to the appearance of "split" basement membranes (see Fig. 20–24*C*).

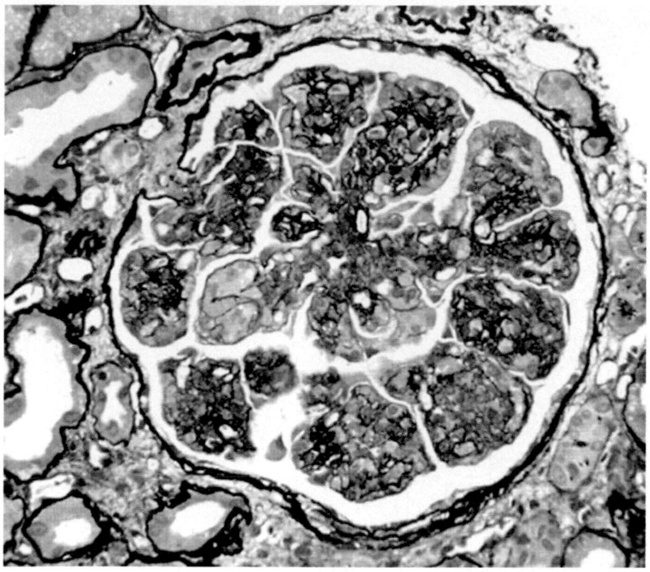

FIGURE 20–23 Membranoproliferative glomerulonephritis, showing mesangial cell proliferation, increased mesangial matrix (staining black with silver stain), basement membrane thickening and focal splitting, accentuation of lobular architecture, swelling of cells lining peripheral capillaries, and influx of leukocytes.

Types I and II MPGN differ in their ultrastructural and immunofluorescent features (Fig. 20–24).

Type I MPGN (the great majority of cases) is characterized by the presence of **subendothelial electron-dense deposits.** Mesangial and occasional subepithelial deposits may also be present (Fig. 20–24*A*). By immunofluorescence, C3 is deposited in a granular pattern, and IgG and early complement components (C1q and C4) are often also present, suggesting an immune complex pathogenesis.

In **dense-deposit disease (type II MPGN)** (Fig. 20–24*B*), a relatively rare entity, the lamina densa of the GBM is transformed into an irregular, ribbon-like, extremely electron-dense structure because of the **deposition of dense material** of unknown composition in the GBM proper, giving rise to the term dense-deposit disease. C3 is present in irregular granular or linear foci in the basement membranes on either side but not within the dense deposits. C3 is also present in the mesangium in characteristic circular aggregates (mesangial rings). IgG is usually absent, as are the early-acting complement components (C1q and C4).

Pathogenesis. *In most cases of type I MPGN there is evidence of immune complexes in the glomerulus and activation of both classical and alternative complement pathways.* The antigens involved in idiopathic MPGN are unknown. In many cases, they are believed to be proteins derived from infectious agents such as hepatitis C and B viruses, which presumably behave either as "planted" antigens after first binding to or becoming trapped within glomerular structures or are contained in preformed immune complexes deposited from the circulation.

Most patients with dense-deposit disease (type II MPGN) have abnormalities that suggest activation of the alternative complement pathway. These patients have a consistently *decreased serum C3* but normal C1 and C4, the immune complex–activated early components of complement. They also have diminished serum levels of factor B and properdin, components of the alternative complement pathway. In the glomeruli, C3 and properdin are deposited, but IgG is not. Recall that in the alternative complement pathway, C3 is directly cleaved to C3b (Fig. 20–25; see also Chapter 2, Fig. 2–14). The reaction depends on the initial interaction of C3 with such substances as bacterial polysaccharides, endotoxin, and aggregates of IgA in the presence of factors B and D. This leads to the generation of C3bBb, the alternative pathway C3 convertase. This C3 convertase is labile, being degraded by factors I and H, but it can be stabilized by properdin. More than 70% of patients with dense-deposit disease have a circulating antibody termed *C3 nephritic factor (C3NeF)*, which is an autoantibody that binds to the alternative pathway C3 convertase (Fig. 20–25). Binding of the antibody stabilizes the convertase, protecting it from enzymatic degradation and thus favoring persistent C3 degradation and hypocomplementemia. There is also decreased C3 synthesis by the liver, further contributing to the profound hypocomplementemia. Precisely how C3NeF is related to glomerular injury and the nature of the dense deposits is unknown. C3NeF activity also occurs in some patients with a genetically determined disease, *partial lipodystrophy*, some of whom develop dense-deposit disease (type II MPGN).

Clinical Course. The principal mode of presentation is the nephrotic syndrome occurring in older children or young adults (idiopathic MPGN type I and cases of type II), but usually with a nephritic component manifested by hematuria or, more insidiously, as mild proteinuria. Few remissions occur spontaneously in either type, and the disease follows a slowly progressive but unremitting course. Some patients develop numerous crescents and a clinical picture of RPGN. About 50% develop chronic renal failure within 10 years. Treatments with steroids, immunosuppressive agents, and antiplatelet drugs have not been proved to be materially effective. There is a high incidence of recurrence in transplant recipients, particularly in dense-deposit disease; dense deposits may recur in 90% of such patients, although renal failure in the allograft is much less common.

Secondary MPGN

Secondary MPGN (invariably type I) is more common in adults and arises in the following settings:[67]

- Chronic immune complex disorders, such as SLE; hepatitis B infection; hepatitis C infection, usually with cryoglobulinemia; endocarditis; infected ventriculoatrial shunts; chronic visceral abscesses; HIV infection; and schistosomiasis
- α_1-Antitrypsin deficiency
- Malignant diseases (chronic lymphocytic leukemia and lymphoma)
- Hereditary deficiencies of complement regulatory proteins

The mechanisms underlying the process of immune complex deposition in the last three categories above remain unknown.

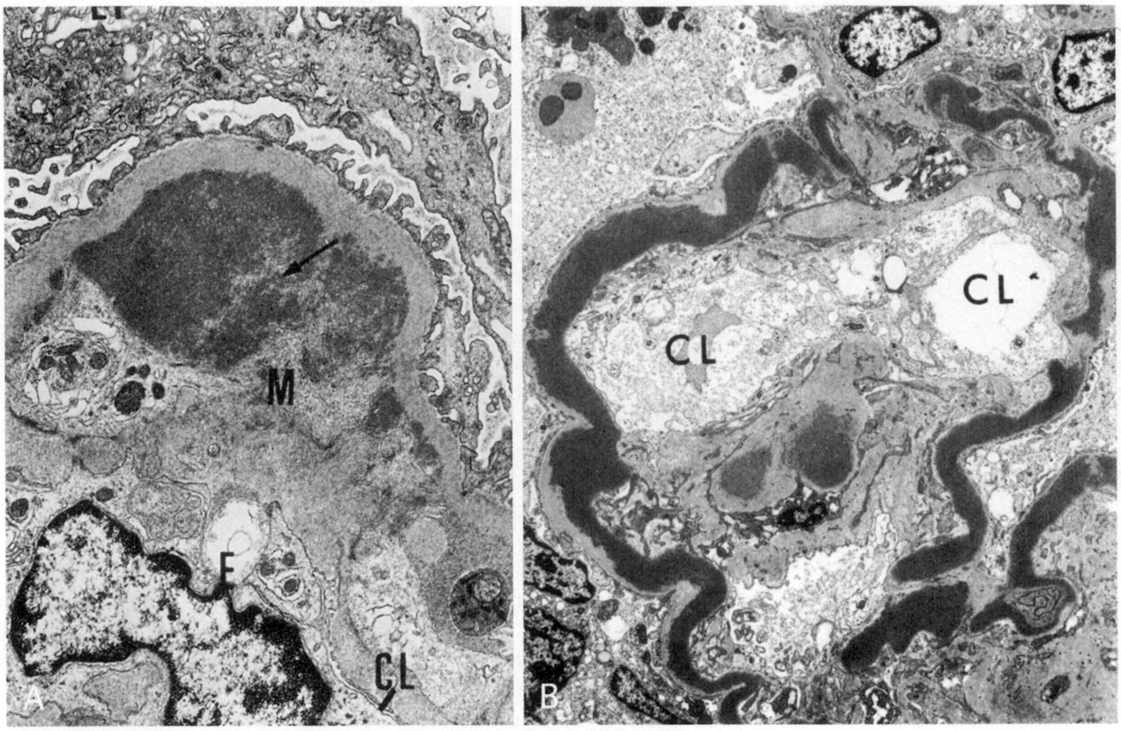

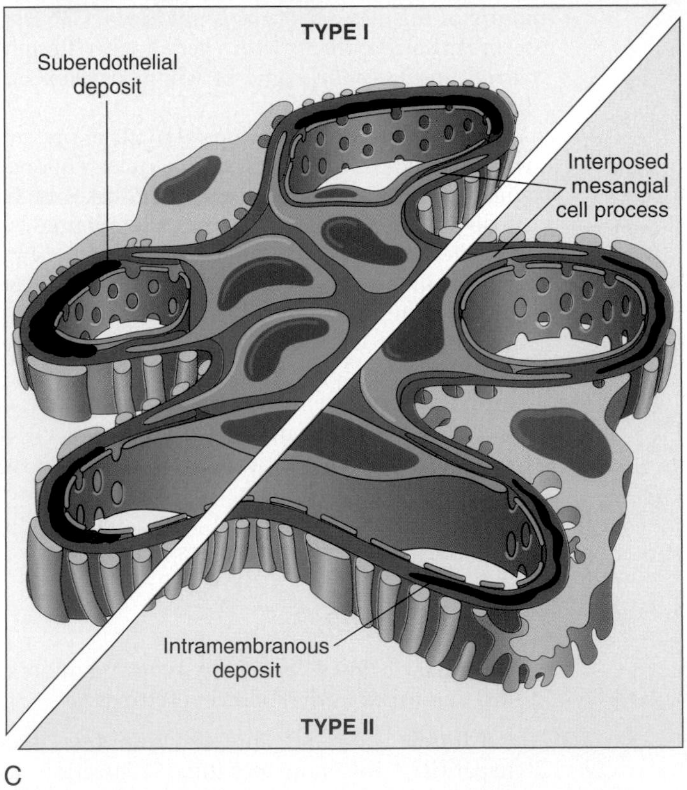

FIGURE 20–24 *A*, Membranoproliferative glomerulonephritis, type I. Note the large subendothelial deposit (*arrow*) incorporated into mesangial matrix (M). E, endothelium; EP, epithelium; CL, capillary lumen. *B*, Type II membranoproliferative glomerulonephritis, dense-deposit disease. There are markedly dense homogeneous deposits within the basement membrane proper. CL, capillary lumen. *C*, Schematic representation of patterns in the two types of membranoproliferative GN. In type I there are subendothelial deposits; type II is characterized by intramembranous dense deposits (dense-deposit disease). In both, mesangial interposition gives the appearance of split basement membranes when viewed in the light microscope.

IgA NEPHROPATHY (BERGER DISEASE)

This form of glomerulonephritis is characterized by the presence of prominent IgA deposits in the mesangial regions, detected by immunofluorescence microscopy. The disease can be suspected by light microscopic examination, but diagnosis is made only by immunocytochemical techniques (Fig. 20–26). *IgA nephropathy is a frequent cause of recurrent gross or microscopic hematuria* and is probably the most common type of glomerulonephritis worldwide.[68] Mild proteinuria is usually present, and the nephrotic syndrome may occasionally develop. Rarely, patients may present with rapidly progressive crescentic glomerulonephritis.

Whereas IgA nephropathy is typically an isolated renal disease, similar IgA deposits are present in a systemic disorder of children, *Henoch-Schönlein purpura*, to be discussed later,

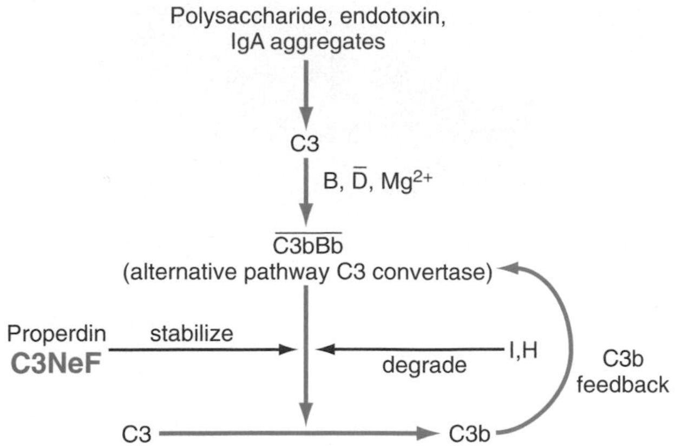

FIGURE 20–25 The alternative complement pathway. Note that C3NeF, present in the serum of patients with membranoproliferative glomerulonephritis, acts at the same step as properdin, serving to stabilize the alternative pathway C3 convertase, thus enhancing C3 breakdown and causing hypocomplementemia.

which has many overlapping features with IgA nephropathy. In addition, *secondary IgA nephropathy* occurs in patients with liver and intestinal diseases, as discussed in the section on pathogenesis.

Pathogenesis. IgA, the main immunoglobulin in mucosal secretions, is at low levels in normal serum, where it is present mostly in monomeric form, the polymeric forms being catabolized in the liver. In patients with IgA nephropathy, serum polymeric IgA is increased, and circulating IgA-containing immune complexes are present in some patients. However, it is clear that increased production of IgA cannot itself cause this disease. Although there are two subclasses of IgA molecules in humans (IgA1 and IgA2), only IgA1 forms the nephritogenic deposits of IgA nephropathy. A genetic influence is suggested by the occurrence of this condition in families and in HLA-identical brothers and the increased frequency of certain HLA and complement phenotypes in some populations. The prominent mesangial deposition of IgA suggests entrapment of IgA immune complexes in the mesangium, and the presence of C3 combined with the absence of C1q and C4 in glomeruli points to activation of the alternative complement pathway.

Taken together, these clues suggest a genetic or acquired abnormality of immune regulation leading to increased mucosal IgA synthesis in response to respiratory or gastrointestinal exposure to environmental agents (e.g., viruses, bacteria, food proteins). IgA1 and IgA1-containing immune complexes are then trapped in the mesangium, where they activate the alternative complement pathway and initiate glomerular injury. In support of this scenario, IgA nephropathy occurs with increased frequency in patients with *gluten enteropathy* (celiac disease), in whom intestinal mucosal defects are well defined, and in *liver disease*, in which there is defective hepatobiliary clearance of IgA complexes (*secondary IgA nephropathy*).

The nature of the initiating antigens is unknown, and several infectious agents and food products have been implicated. The deposited IgA appears to be polyclonal, and it may be that a variety of antigens are involved in the course of the disease. Alternatively, there is evidence that qualitative alterations in the IgA1 molecule itself, specifically a defect in normal galactosylation, make it more likely to bind to mesangial antigens or form mesangial deposits owing to other as yet unidentified mechanisms.

Morphology. On histologic examination, the lesions vary considerably. The glomeruli may be normal or may show mesangial widening and proliferation (mesangioproliferative glomerulonephritis), segmental proliferation confined to some glomeruli (focal proliferative glomerulonephritis), or rarely, overt crescentic glomerulonephritis. The presence of leukocytes within glomerular capillaries is a variable feature. The mesangial widening may be the result of cell proliferation, accumulation of matrix, or both. Healing of the focal proliferative lesion may lead to focal segmental sclerosis. The characteristic immunofluorescent picture is of **mesangial deposition of IgA** (Fig. 20–26), often with C3 and properdin and lesser amounts of IgG or IgM. Early complement components are usually absent. Electron microscopy confirms the presence of electron-dense deposits in the mesangium.

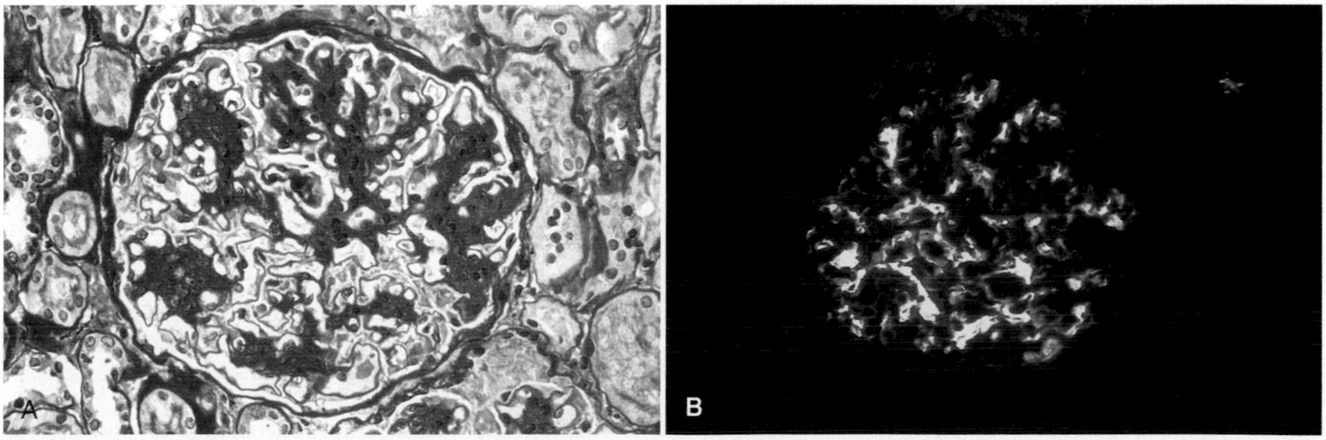

FIGURE 20–26 IgA nephropathy. *A*, Light microscopy showing mesangial proliferation and matrix increase. *B*, Characteristic deposition of IgA, principally in mesangial regions, detected by immunofluorescence.

Clinical Course. The disease affects people of any age, but older children and young adults are most commonly affected. Many patients present with gross hematuria after an infection of the respiratory or, less commonly, gastrointestinal or urinary tract; 30% to 40% have only microscopic hematuria, with or without proteinuria; and 5% to 10% develop a typical acute nephritic syndrome. The hematuria typically lasts for several days and then subsides, only to return every few months. The subsequent course is highly variable.[67] Many patients maintain normal renal function for decades. Slow progression to chronic renal failure occurs in 15% to 40% of cases over a period of 20 years. Onset in old age, heavy proteinuria, hypertension, and the extent of glomerulosclerosis on biopsy are clues to an increased risk of progression. Recurrence of IgA deposits in transplanted kidneys is frequent. In approximately 15% of those with recurrent IgA deposits, there is resulting clinical disease, which most frequently runs the same indolent, slowly progressive course as that of the primary IgA nephropathy.[68]

HEREDITARY SYNDROMES OF ISOLATED HEMATURIA

Hereditary nephritis refers to a group of heterogeneous familial renal diseases associated primarily with glomerular injury. Two deserve discussion: *Alport syndrome*, because the lesions and genetic defects have been well studied,[69] and *thin basement membrane disease*, the most common cause of *benign familial hematuria.*[70]

Alport Syndrome

Alport syndrome, when fully developed, is manifest by nephritis progressing to chronic renal failure, accompanied by nerve deafness and various eye disorders, including lens dislocation, posterior cataracts, and corneal dystrophy.[69] In the most common X-linked form, males express the full syndrome, and females are carriers in whom manifestations of disease are typically limited to hematuria. Rare autosomal-recessive and autosomal-dominant pedigrees also exist, in which males and females are equally susceptible to the full syndrome.

Morphology. On histologic examination, the glomeruli are always involved. The early lesion is detectable only by electron microscopy and consists of diffuse glomerular basement membrane thinning. In some kidneys, interstitial cells acquire a foamy appearance owing to accumulation of neutral fats and mucopolysaccharides (foam cells). As the disease progresses, there is development of focal segmental and global glomerulosclerosis and other changes of progressive renal injury, including vascular sclerosis, tubular atrophy, and interstitial fibrosis.

The characteristic findings of fully developed disease are seen with the electron microscope and are found in most patients with hereditary nephritis. The GBM shows irregular foci of thickening alternating with attenuation (thinning), with pronounced splitting and lamination of the lamina densa, often with a distinctive basket-weave appearance (Fig. 20–27). Similar alterations can be found in the tubular basement membranes. Although such basement membrane changes may be seen focally in diseases other than hereditary nephritis, they are most widespread and pronounced in patients with this disorder.

Immunohistochemistry can be helpful in cases with absent or borderline basement membrane lesions, because antibodies to α_3, α_4, and α_5 collagen fail to stain both glomerular and tubular basement membranes in the classic X-linked form. There is also absence of α_5 staining in skin biopsy specimens.

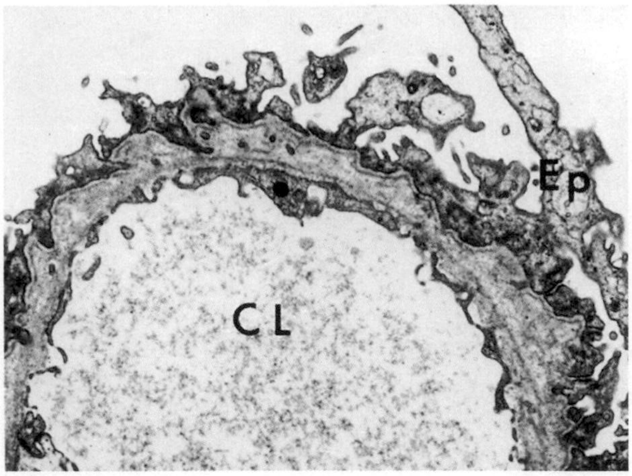

FIGURE 20–27 Hereditary nephritis. Electron micrograph of glomerulus with irregular thickening of the basement membrane, lamination of the lamina densa, and foci of rarefaction. Such changes may be present in other diseases but are most pronounced and widespread in hereditary nephritis. CL, capillary lumen; Ep, epithelium.

Pathogenesis. *Defective GBM synthesis because of the production of abnormal collagen type IV underlies the renal lesions.* In patients with X-linked disease, the defect is caused by *mutations in the gene encoding the α_5-chain of collagen type IV (COL4A5)*, a component of the GBM[27,70] (see Fig. 20–3). The mutations are heterogeneous and affect all domains of the α_5-chain. This is thought to interfere with the assembly and architecture of collagen type IV and thus the structure and function of the GBM.[27,70] In addition, probably as a result of this defect, patients synthesize lesser amounts of other collagen components, including the α_3-chain, which, as you recall, includes the Goodpasture antigen, and the α_4-chain. Indeed, glomeruli from patients with Alport syndrome who lack the α_3-chain fail to react with anti-GBM antibodies from patients with Goodpasture syndrome. In the autosomal-recessive pedigrees, mutations in the α_3- and α_4-chains have been reported.

Clinical Course. The most common presenting sign is gross or microscopic hematuria, frequently accompanied by erythrocyte casts. Proteinuria may occur, and rarely, the nephrotic syndrome develops. Symptoms appear at ages 5 to 20 years, and the onset of overt renal failure is between ages 20 and 50 years in men. The auditory defects may be subtle, requiring sensitive testing.

Thin Basement Membrane Disease (Benign Familial Hematuria)

This is a fairly common entity manifested *clinically by familial asymptomatic hematuria*—usually uncovered on routine urinalysis—*and morphologically by diffuse thinning of the GBM* to between 150 and 250 nm (compared with 300 to 400 nm in normal adult individuals). Although mild or moderate proteinuria may also be present, renal function is normal and prognosis is excellent.

The disorder should be distinguished from IgA nephropathy, another common cause of hematuria, and X-linked Alport syndrome. In contrast to Alport syndrome, hearing loss, ocular abnormalities, and a family history of renal failure are absent, and skin biopsy specimens show presence of the α_5-chain of collagen type IV by immunohistochemistry.[70]

The anomaly in thin basement membrane disease has also been traced to genes encoding α_3- or α_4-chains type IV collagen.[27,71] Most patients are heterozygous for the defective gene. The disorder in homozygotes resembles autosomal-recessive Alport disease and may progress to renal failure, even in women. Thus, these diseases illustrate a continuum of changes resulting from mutations in collagen type IV genes.

CHRONIC GLOMERULONEPHRITIS

Chronic glomerulonephritis is best considered a pool of end-stage glomerular disease fed by a number of streams of specific types of glomerulonephritis. Most of these diseases were described earlier in this chapter (Fig. 20–28). Poststreptococcal glomerulonephritis is a rare antecedent of chronic glomerulonephritis, except in adults. Patients with RPGN, if they survive the acute episode, usually progress to chronic glomerulonephritis. Membranous glomerulonephritis, MPGN, IgA nephropathy, and focal segmental glomerulosclerosis all may progress to chronic renal failure. *Nevertheless, in any series of patients with chronic glomerulonephritis, a variable percentage of cases arise mysteriously with no antecedent history of any of the well-recognized forms of acute glomerulonephritis.* These cases must represent the end result of relatively asymptomatic forms of glomerulonephritis, either known or still unrecognized, that progress to uremia. Clearly, the proportion of such unexplained cases depends on the availability of renal biopsy material from patients early in their disease.

Morphology. The kidneys are symmetrically contracted and have diffusely granular, cortical surfaces. On section, **the cortex is thinned**, and there is an increase in peripelvic fat. The glomerular histology depends on the stage of the disease. In early cases, the glomeruli may still show evidence of the primary disease (e.g., membranous glomerulopathy or MPGN). However, there eventually ensues **hyaline obliteration of glomeruli**, transforming them into acellular eosinophilic masses. The hyalin represents a combination of trapped plasma proteins, increased mesangial matrix, basement membrane–like material, and collagen (Fig. 20–29). Because hypertension is an accompaniment of chronic glomerulonephritis, **arterial and arteriolar sclerosis may be conspicuous. Marked atrophy of associated tubules**, irregular interstitial fibrosis, and mononuclear leukocytic infiltration of the interstitium also occur.

Dialysis Changes. Kidneys from patients with end-stage disease on long-term dialysis exhibit a variety of changes that are unrelated to the primary disease. These include **arterial intimal thickening** caused by accumulation of smooth muscle–like cells and a loose, proteoglycan-rich stroma; focal calcification, usually within residual tubular segments; **extensive deposition of calcium oxalate crystals** in tubules and interstitium; **acquired cystic disease,** discussed earlier; and increased numbers of renal adenomas and adenocarcinomas.

Uremic Complications. Patients dying with chronic glomerulonephritis also exhibit pathologic changes outside the kidney that are related to the uremic state and are also present in other forms of chronic renal failure. Often clinically important, these include uremic **pericarditis**, uremic gastroenteritis, **secondary hyperparathyroidism** with nephrocalcinosis and renal

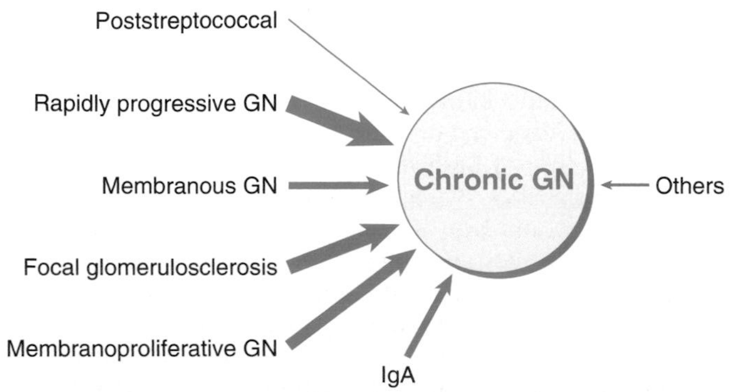

FIGURE 20–28 Primary glomerular diseases leading to chronic glomerulonephritis (GN). The thickness of the arrows reflects the approximate proportion of patients in each group who progress to chronic glomerulonephritis: poststreptococcal (1% to 2%); rapidly progressive (crescentic) (90%), membranous (30% to 50%), focal glomerulosclerosis (50% to 80%), membranoproliferative glomerulonephritis (50%), IgA nephropathy (30% to 50%).

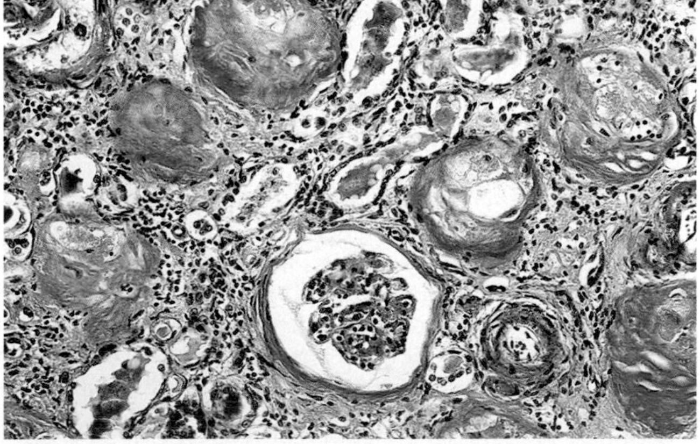

FIGURE 20–29 Chronic glomerulonephritis. A Masson trichrome preparation shows complete replacement of virtually all glomeruli by blue-staining collagen. (Courtesy of Dr. M.A. Venkatachalam, Department of Pathology, University of Texas Health Sciences Center, San Antonio, TX.)

osteodystrophy, **left ventricular hypertrophy** due to hypertension, and pulmonary changes of diffuse alveolar damage often ascribed to uremia (uremic pneumonitis).

Clinical Course. In most patients, chronic glomerulonephritis develops insidiously and slowly progresses to renal insufficiency or death from uremia during a span of years or possibly decades (see the discussion of chronic renal failure). Not infrequently, patients present with such nonspecific complaints as loss of appetite, anemia, vomiting, or weakness. In some, the renal disease is suspected with the discovery of proteinuria, hypertension, or azotemia on routine medical examination. In others, the underlying renal disorder is discovered in the course of investigation of edema. *Most patients are hypertensive, and sometimes the dominant clinical manifestations are cerebral or cardiovascular.* In all, the disease is relentlessly progressive, although at widely varying rates. In nephrotic patients, as glomeruli become obliterated, the protein loss in the urine diminishes. If patients with chronic glomerulonephritis are not maintained with continued dialysis or if they do not receive a renal transplant, the outcome is invariably death.

GLOMERULAR LESIONS ASSOCIATED WITH SYSTEMIC DISEASES

Many immunologically mediated, metabolic, or hereditary systemic disorders are associated with glomerular injury; in some (e.g., SLE and diabetes mellitus), the glomerular involvement is a major clinical manifestation. Most of these diseases are discussed elsewhere in this book. Here we briefly recall some of the lesions and discuss only those not considered in other sections.

Systemic Lupus Erythematosus

The various types of lupus nephritis were described and illustrated in Chapter 6. As discussed, SLE gives rise to a heterogeneous group of lesions and clinical presentations. The clinical manifestations can include recurrent microscopic or gross hematuria, acute nephritis, the nephrotic syndrome, chronic renal failure, and hypertension.

Henoch-Schönlein Purpura

This syndrome consists of *purpuric skin lesions characteristically involving the extensor surfaces of arms and legs as well as buttocks; abdominal manifestations including pain, vomiting, and intestinal bleeding; nonmigratory arthralgia; and renal abnormalities.* The renal manifestations occur in one-third of patients and include gross or microscopic hematuria, proteinuria, and nephrotic syndrome. A small number of patients, mostly adults, develop a rapidly progressive form of glomerulonephritis with many crescents. Not all components of the syndrome need to be present, and individual patients may have purpura, abdominal pain, or urinary abnormalities as the dominant feature. The disease is most common in children 3 to 8 years old, but it also occurs in adults, in whom the renal manifestations are usually more severe. There is a strong background of atopy in about one-third of patients, and onset often follows an upper respiratory infection. IgA is deposited in the glomerular mesangium in a distribution similar to that of IgA nephropathy. This has led to the concept that *IgA nephropathy and Henoch-Schönlein purpura are spectra of the same disease.*[68]

Morphology. On histologic examination, the renal lesions vary from mild focal mesangial proliferation to diffuse mesangial proliferation to crescentic glomerulonephritis. Whatever the histologic lesions, the prominent feature by fluorescence microscopy is the **deposition of IgA, sometimes with IgG and C3, in the mesangial region.** The skin lesions consist of subepidermal hemorrhages and a necrotizing vasculitis involving the small vessels of the dermis. IgA is also present in such vessels. Vasculitis also occurs in other organs, such as the gastrointestinal tract, but is rare in the kidney.

The course of the disease is variable, but recurrences of hematuria may persist for many years after onset. Most children have an excellent prognosis. Patients with the more diffuse lesions, crescents, or the nephrotic syndrome have a somewhat poorer prognosis.

Bacterial Endocarditis

Glomerular lesions occurring in the course of bacterial endocarditis represent a type of immune complex nephritis initiated by complexes of bacterial antigen and antibody. Hematuria and proteinuria of various degrees characterize this entity clinically, but an acute nephritic presentation is not uncommon, and even RPGN may occur in rare instances. The histologic lesions, when present, generally reflect these clinical manifestations. Milder forms have a more focal and segmental necrotizing glomerulonephritis, whereas more severe ones exhibit a diffuse proliferative glomerulonephritis, and the rapidly progressive forms show large numbers of crescents.

Diabetic Glomerulosclerosis

Diabetes mellitus is a major cause of renal morbidity and mortality, and diabetic nephropathy is one of the leading causes of chronic kidney failure in the United States (see Chapter 24). Advanced or end-stage kidney disease occurs in as many as 40% of both insulin-dependent type 1 diabetics and type 2 diabetics. By far the most common lesions involve the glomeruli and are associated clinically with three glomerular syndromes: non-nephrotic proteinuria, nephrotic syndrome, and chronic renal failure.[72] However, diabetes also affects the arterioles, causing *hyalinizing arteriolar sclerosis*; increases susceptibility to the development of pyelonephritis and particularly *papillary necrosis*; and causes a variety of tubular lesions. The term *diabetic nephropathy* is applied to the conglomerate of lesions that often occur concurrently in the diabetic kidney.

Proteinuria, sometimes in the nephrotic range, occurs in about 50% of both type 1 and type 2 diabetics. It is usually discovered 12 to 22 years after the clinical appearance of diabetes and often heralds the progressive development of chronic renal failure ending in death or end-stage disease within a period of 4 to 5 years. Overt proteinuria is preceded by the development of lesser degrees of protein leakage into the urine, termed "microalbuminuria," which may occur within a few years of the onset of diabetes. The morphologic changes in the glomeruli include (1) capillary basement membrane thickening, (2) diffuse mesangial sclerosis, and (3) nodular glomerulosclerosis. The morphologic manifestations of diabetic nephropathy are identical in type 1 and type 2 diabetes and are described below as a single entity.[73]

Pathogenesis. The pathogenesis of diabetic glomerulosclerosis is intimately linked with that of generalized diabetic microangiopathy, discussed in Chapter 24. The principal points are as follows:[74,75]

- The bulk of the evidence suggests that diabetic glomerulosclerosis *is caused by the metabolic defect*, that is, the insulin deficiency, the resultant hyperglycemia, or some other aspects of glucose intolerance. These metabolic defects are responsible for biochemical alterations in diabetic GBM, including increased amount and synthesis of collagen type IV and fibronectin and decreased synthesis of the heparan sulfate proteoglycan.
- *Nonenzymatic glycosylation* of proteins, which is known to occur in diabetics and gives rise to advanced glycosylation end products, may contribute to the glomerulopathy. The mechanisms by which advanced glycosylation end products cause their effects are discussed in Chapter 24.
- One hypothesis implicates *hemodynamic changes* in the initiation and progression of diabetic glomerulosclerosis. It is well known that the early stages of diabetic nephropathy are characterized by an increased GFR with increased glomerular capillary pressure and *glomerular hypertrophy* with increased glomerular filtration area.[73,76] Hemodynamic alterations and glomerular hypertrophy also occur in experimental streptozotocin-induced diabetes in rats, in which they are associated with proteinuria and can be reversed or inhibited by diabetic control and angiotensin inhibition. It has been speculated that the subsequent morphologic alterations discussed above are somehow influenced by the glomerular hypertrophy and hemodynamic changes, akin to the adaptive responses to ablation of renal mass, discussed earlier.

To sum up, two processes seem to play a role in the fully developed diabetic glomerular lesions: a metabolic defect, possibly linked to advanced glycosylation end products, that accounts for the thickened GBM and increased mesangial matrix that occur in patients; and hemodynamic effects, associated with glomerular hypertrophy, which also contributes to the development of glomerulosclerosis.

Morphology

Capillary Basement Membrane Thickening. Widespread thickening of the glomerular capillary basement membrane (GBM) occurs in virtually all diabetics, irrespective of the presence of proteinuria, and is part and parcel of the diabetic microangiopathy. Pure capillary basement membrane thickening can be detected only by electron microscopy. Careful morphometric studies demonstrate that this thickening begins as early as 2 years after the onset of type I diabetes and by 5 years amounts to about a 30% increase.[77] The thickening continues progressively and usually concurrently with mesangial widening (Fig. 20–30). Simultaneously, there is thickening of the tubular basement membranes.

Diffuse Mesangial Sclerosis. This lesion consists of diffuse increase in mesangial matrix. There can be mild proliferation of mesangial cells early in the disease process, but cell proliferation is not a prominent part of this injury. The mesangial increase is typically associated with the overall thickening of the GBM. The matrix depositions are PAS-positive (Fig. 20–31). As the disease progresses, the expansion of mesangial areas can extend to nodular configurations. The progressive expansion of the mesangium has been shown to correlate well with measures of deteriorating renal function such as increasing proteinuria.

Nodular Glomerulosclerosis. This is also known as **intercapillary glomerulosclerosis or Kimmelstiel-Wilson disease**. The glomerular lesions take the form of ovoid or spherical, often laminated, nodules of matrix situated in the periphery of the glomerulus. The nodules are PAS-positive. They lie within the mesangial core of the glomerular lobules and can be surrounded by patent peripheral capillary loops (Fig. 20–31) or loops that are markedly dilated. The nodules often exhibit features of mesangiolysis with fraying of the mesangial/capillary lumen interface, disruption of sites at which the capillaries are anchored into the mesangial stalks, and resultant capillary microaneurysm formation as the untethered capillaries distend outward as a result of intracapillary pressures and flows. Usually, not all the lobules in the individ-

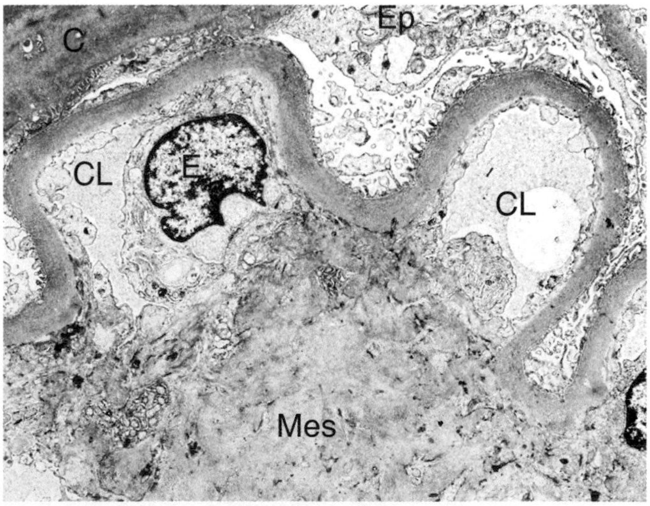

FIGURE 20–30 Electron micrograph of advanced diabetic glomerulosclerosis. Note the massive increase in mesangial matrix (Mes) encroaching on the glomerular capillary lumina (CL). The GBM and Bowman capsule (C) are markedly thickened. Ep, epithelium; E, endothelium.

ual glomerulus are involved by nodular lesions, but even uninvolved lobules and glomeruli show striking diffuse mesangial sclerosis. As the disease advances, the individual nodules enlarge and may eventually compress and engulf capillaries, obliterating the glomerular tuft. These nodular lesions are frequently accompanied by prominent accumulations of hyaline material in capillary loops ("fibrin caps") or adherent to Bowman's capsules ("capsular drops"). As a consequence of the glomerular and arteriolar lesions, the kidney suffers from ischemia, develops tubular atrophy and interstitial fibrosis, and usually undergoes overall contraction in size.

Nodular glomerulosclerosis and diffuse mesangial sclerosis are fundamentally similar lesions of the mesangium. The nodular lesion, however, is highly but not completely specific for diabetes, as long as care is taken to exclude membranoproliferative (lobular) glomerulonephritis, the glomerulopathy associated with light-chain and monoclonal immunoglobulin deposition disease, amyloidosis, and a few rare entities, which can have a similar appearance. Approximately 15% to 30% of patients with long-term diabetes develop nodular glomerulosclerosis, and in most instances it is associated with renal failure.

Clinical Course. The clinical manifestations of diabetic glomerulosclerosis are linked to those of diabetes. The increased GFR typical of early-onset type 1 diabetics is associated with *microalbuminuria*, which is defined as urinary albumin excretion of 30 to 300 mg/day of albumin. Microalbuminuria and increased GFR are important predictors of future overt diabetic nephropathy in these patients. Overt proteinuria then develops, which may be mild and asymptomatic initially but gradually increases to nephrotic levels in some patients. This is followed by progressive loss of GFR, leading to end-stage renal failure within a period of 5 years.

Systemic hypertension may precede the development of proteinuria and renal insufficiency. Indeed, the risk of renal disease in type 1 diabetics is associated with a genetic predisposition to hypertension, possibly related to polymorphisms in the genes encoding proteins of the renin-angiotensin system (Chapter 11). Hypertension in turn increases the susceptibility to developing diabetic nephropathy in the presence of poor hyperglycemic control.

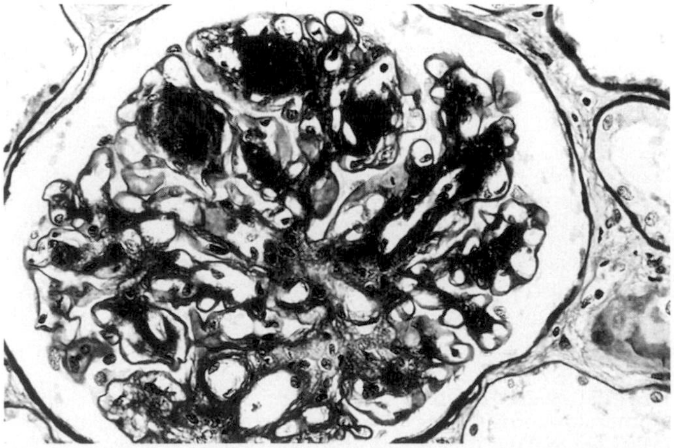

FIGURE 20–31 Diffuse and nodular diabetic glomerulosclerosis (PAS stain). Note the diffuse increase in mesangial matrix and characteristic acellular PAS-positive nodules.

At present, most patients with end-stage diabetic nephropathy are maintained on long-term dialysis, and many undergo renal transplantation. Diabetic lesions may recur in the renal allografts. Several studies have now shown that precise control of the blood glucose level in diabetics delays or prevents the progression of glomerulopathy. Most exciting is the recent demonstration that achievement of good glycemic homeostasis by pancreatic transplantation in patients with diabetic nephropathy can actually reverse the nephropathy when the glycemic control is maintained for periods of 10 years or more.[78] Inhibition of angiotensin by converting enzyme inhibitors or angiotensin receptor blockers also has a beneficial effect on progression, possibly by reversing the increased intraglomerular capillary pressure.

Amyloidosis

The various forms of amyloidosis and their pathogenesis are discussed in Chapter 6. Most types of disseminated amyloidosis may be associated with deposits of amyloid within the glomeruli; most commonly renal amyloid is of light-chain (AL) or AA type. The typical Congo red amyloid-positive fibrillary deposits are present within the mesangium and capillary walls and rarely are localized to the subepithelial space. Eventually, they obliterate the glomerulus completely. Recall that deposits of amyloid also appear in blood vessel walls and in the kidney interstitium. Patients with glomerular amyloid may present with the nephrotic syndrome and later, owing to destruction of the glomeruli, die of uremia. Characteristically, kidney size tends to be either normal or increased.

Fibrillary and Immunotactoid Glomerulonephritis

Fibrillary glomerulonephritis is a morphologic variant of glomerulonephritis associated with characteristic fibrillar deposits in the mesangium and glomerular capillary walls that resemble amyloid fibrils in appearance but differ from amyloid fibrils when measured ultrastructurally and in that they do not stain with Congo red. The fibrils are typically 18 to 24 nm in diameter and hence are larger than the 10 to 12 nm characteristic of amyloid. The glomerular lesions usually exhibit membranoproliferative or mesangioproliferative patterns by light microscopy, and by immunofluorescence microscopy, there is selective deposition of IgG, often of IgG4 subclass, with complement C3 and Ig κ and λ light chains also present. Clinically, patients develop nephrotic syndrome, hematuria, and progressive renal insufficiency. The disease is found in about 1% of cases in large renal biopsy series. The disease recurs in kidney transplants.

In *immunotactoid glomerulopathy*, a much rarer condition, the deposits are microtubular in structure and 30 to 50 nm in width. Patients often have circulating paraproteins and/or monoclonal immunoglobulin deposition in glomeruli.[79]

The pathogenesis of both of these entities is unknown.

Other Systemic Disorders

Goodpasture syndrome (Chapter 15), *microscopic polyarteritis*, and *Wegener granulomatosis* (Chapter 11) are commonly associated with glomerular lesions, as described in the discussion of these diseases. Suffice it to say here that the glomerular lesions in these three conditions can be histologically similar and are principally characterized by foci of glomerular necrosis and crescent formation. In the early or mild forms of involvement, there is focal and segmental, sometimes necrotizing, glomerulonephritis, and most of these patients will have hematuria with mild decline in GFR. In the more severe cases associated with RPGN, there is more extensive necrosis, fibrin deposition, and extensive formation of epithelial (cellular) crescents, which can become organized to form fibrocellular and fibrous crescents if the glomerular injury evolves into segmental or global scarring (sclerosis).

Essential mixed cryoglobulinemia is another systemic condition in which deposits of cryoglobulins composed principally of IgG-IgM complexes induce cutaneous vasculitis, synovitis, and a proliferative glomerulonephritis, typically membranoproliferative glomerulonephritis. Most cases of essential mixed cryoglobulinemia have been associated with infection with hepatitis C virus, and this condition in particular is associated with glomerulonephritis, usually of the MPGN type.

Plasma cell dyscrasias may also induce glomerular lesions. *Multiple myeloma* and other dyscrasias producing circulating monoclonal immunoglobulins are associated with (1) amyloidosis, in which the fibrils are usually composed of monoclonal lambda light chains, (2) deposition of monoclonal immunoglobulins or light chains in glomerular basement membranes, and (3) distinctive nodular glomerular lesions resulting from the deposition of *nonfibrillar* light chains. This so-called *light-chain* or *monoclonal immunoglobulin deposition disease* sometimes occurs in the absence of overt myeloma and is usually characterized by deposition of Ig κ light chains in glomeruli. The glomeruli show PAS-positive mesangial nodules, lobular accentuation, and mild mesangial hypercellularity. These lesions need to be differentiated from diabetic nodular glomerulosclerosis and other glomerulopathies that can cause nodular mesangial expansion, such as membranoproliferative GN. These patients usually present with proteinuria or the nephrotic syndrome, hypertension, and progressive azotemia. Other renal manifestations of multiple myeloma are discussed later.

Diseases Affecting Tubules and Interstitium

Most forms of tubular injury involve the interstitium as well; therefore, diseases affecting these two components are discussed together. Under this heading, we consider two major groups of processes: (1) ischemic or toxic tubular injury, leading to *acute tubular necrosis (ATN)* and acute renal failure, and (2) inflammatory reactions of the tubules and interstitium (*tubulointerstitial nephritis*).

ACUTE TUBULAR NECROSIS

ATN is a clinicopathologic entity characterized morphologically by destruction of tubular epithelial cells and clinically by acute diminution or loss of renal function. It is the most common cause of acute renal failure,[80] which signifies rapid reduction of renal function and urine flow, falling within 24 hours to less than 400 mL per day. It can be caused by a variety of conditions, including:

- *Ischemia, due to decreased or interrupted blood flow*, examples of which include diffuse involvement of the intrarenal blood vessels such as in polyarteritis nodosa, malignant hypertension, or the hemolytic-uremic syndrome, or decreased effective circulating blood volume
- *Direct toxic injury to the tubules* (e.g., by drugs, radiocontrast dyes, myoglobin, hemoglobin, radiation)
- *Acute tubulointerstitial nephritis*, most commonly occurring as a hypersensitivity reaction to drugs
- *Disseminated intravascular coagulation*
- *Urinary obstruction* by tumors, prostatic hypertrophy, or blood clots (so-called postrenal acute renal failure)

ATN accounts for some 50% of cases of acute renal failure in hospitalized patients. Other causes of acute renal failure are discussed elsewhere in this chapter.

ATN is a reversible renal lesion that arises in a variety of clinical settings. Most of these, ranging from severe trauma to acute pancreatitis, have in common a period of inadequate blood flow to the peripheral organs, usually accompanied by marked hypotension and shock. This pattern of ATN is called *ischemic ATN*. Mismatched blood transfusions and other hemolytic crises causing *hemoglobinuria* and skeletal muscle injuries causing *myoglobinuria* also produce a picture resembling ischemic ATN. The second pattern, called *nephrotoxic ATN*, is caused by a multitude of drugs, such as gentamicin and other antibiotics; radiographic contrast agents; poisons, including heavy metals (e.g., mercury); and organic solvents (e.g., carbon tetrachloride). In addition to its frequency, the potential reversibility of ATN adds to its clinical importance. Proper management means the difference between full recovery and death.

Pathogenesis. The critical events in both ischemic and nephrotoxic ATN are believed to be (1) tubular injury and (2) persistent and severe disturbances in blood flow[81] (Fig. 20–32).

- *Tubule cell injury:* Tubular epithelial cells are particularly sensitive to ischemia and are also vulnerable to toxins. Several factors predispose the tubules to toxic injury, including a vast charged surface for tubular reabsorption, active transport systems for ions and organic acids, a high metabolic rate and oxygen consumption requirement in order to perform these transport and reabsorption functions, and the capability for effective concentration.

  Ischemia causes numerous structural and functional alterations in epithelial cells, as discussed in Chapter 1. The structural changes include those of reversible injury (such as cellular swelling, loss of brush border, blebbing, loss of polarity, and cell detachment) and those associated with lethal injury (necrosis and apoptosis). Biochemically, there is depletion of adenosine triphosphate; accumulation of intracellular calcium; activation of proteases (e.g., calpain), which cause cytoskeletal disruption, and phospholipases, which damage membranes; generation of reactive oxygen species; and activation of caspases, which induce apoptotic cell death. One early reversible result of ischemia is *loss of*

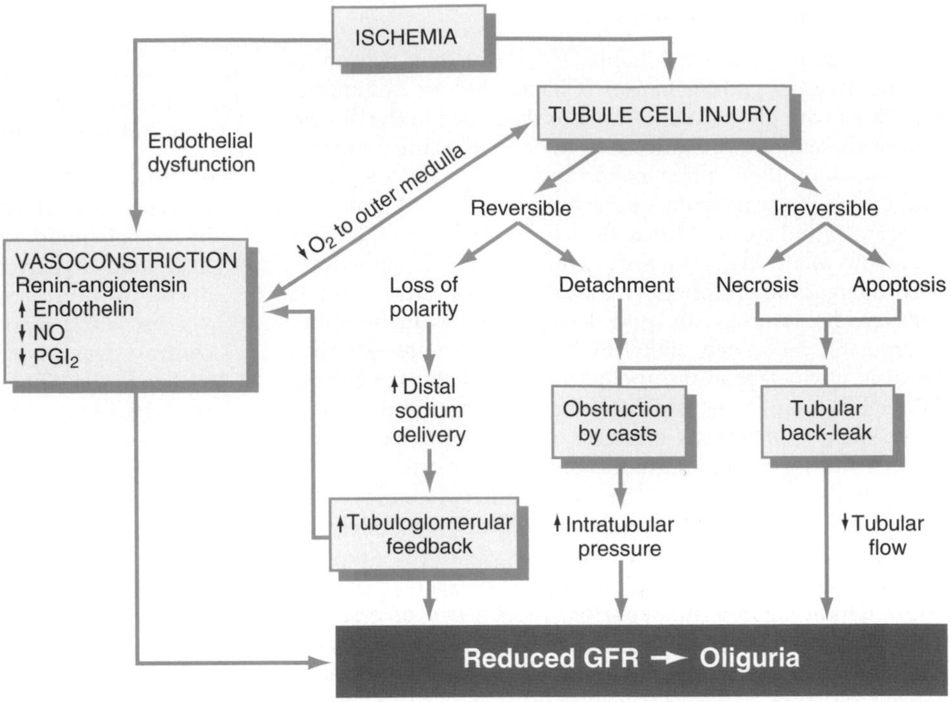

FIGURE 20–32 Possible pathogenetic mechanisms in ischemic acute renal failure (see text).

cell polarity due to redistribution of membrane proteins (e.g., the enzyme Na^+K^+-ATPase) from the basolateral to the luminal surface of the tubular cells, resulting in abnormal ion transport across the cells, and *increased sodium delivery to distal tubules.* The latter incites vasoconstriction via *tubuloglomerular feedback*, which will be discussed below.[82] In addition, ischemic tubular cells express cytokines and adhesion molecules (such as ICAM-1), thus recruiting leukocytes that appear to participate in the subsequent injury.[83] In time, injured cells detach from the basement membranes and cause *luminal tubule obstruction*, increased intratubular pressure, and decreased GFR. In addition, fluid from the damaged tubules can leak into the interstitium, resulting in interstitial edema, increased interstitial pressure, and further damage to the tubule. All these effects, as shown in Figure 20–32, contribute to the decreased GFR.

- *Disturbances in blood flow:* Ischemic renal injury is also characterized by *hemodynamic alterations* that cause reduced GFR. The major one is *intrarenal vasoconstriction*, which results in both reduced glomerular plasma flow and reduced oxygen delivery to the functionally important tubules in the outer medulla (thick ascending limb and straight segment of the proximal tubule). A number of vasoconstrictor pathways have been implicated, including the renin-angiotensin mechanism, stimulated by increased distal sodium delivery (via *tubuloglomerular feedback*), and *sublethal endothelial injury*, leading to increased release of the vasoconstrictor *endothelin* and decreased production of the vasodilators *nitric oxide* and PGI_2. Finally, there is also some evidence of a direct effect of ischemia or toxins on the glomerulus, causing a reduced glomerular ultrafiltration coefficient, possibly due to mesangial contraction.

The patchiness of tubular necrosis and maintenance of the integrity of the basement membrane along many segments allow ready repair of the necrotic foci and recovery of function if the precipitating cause is removed. This repair is dependent on the capacity of reversibly injured epithelial cells to proliferate and differentiate. Re-epithelialization is mediated by a variety of growth factors and cytokines produced locally by the tubular cells themselves (autocrine stimulation) or by inflammatory cells in the vicinity of necrotic foci (paracrine stimulation).[84] Of these, epidermal growth factor (EGF), TGF-α, insulin-like growth factor type I, and hepatocyte growth factor have been shown to be particularly important in renal tubular repair. Growth factors, indeed, are being explored as possible therapeutic agents to enhance re-epithelialization in ATN.[84]

Morphology. Ischemic ATN is characterized by focal tubular epithelial necrosis at multiple points along the nephron, with large skip areas in between, often accompanied by rupture of basement membranes (tubulorrhexis) and occlusion of tubular lumens by casts[85] (Figs. 20–33 and 20–34). The straight portion of the proximal tubule and the ascending thick limb in the renal medulla are especially vulnerable, but focal lesions may also occur in the distal tubule, often in conjunction with casts. Paradoxically, the clinical syndrome of ATN is not manifest by overt tubular cell necrosis, but often lesser degrees of tubular injury. This includes attenuation or loss of proximal tubule brush borders, simplification of cell structure, cell swelling and vacuolization, and sloughing of nonnecrotic tubular cells into the tubular lumina (Fig. 20–34). The severity of the morphologic findings often does not correlate well with the severity of the clinical findings.

Eosinophilic hyaline casts, as well as pigmented granular casts, are common, particularly in distal tubules and collecting ducts. These casts consist principally of Tamm-Horsfall protein (a urinary glycoprotein normally secreted by the cells of ascending thick limb and distal tubules) in conjunction with hemoglobin, myoglobin, and other plasma proteins. Other findings in ischemic ATN are interstitial edema and accumulations of leukocytes within dilated vasa recta. There is also evidence of epithelial regeneration: Flattened epithelial cells with hyperchromatic nuclei and mitotic figures are often present. In the course of time, this regeneration repopulates the tubules so that if survival occurs, no residual evidence of damage can be seen.

Toxic ATN is manifested by acute tubular injury, most obvious in the proximal convoluted tubules. On histologic examination, the tubular necrosis may be entirely nonspecific, but it is somewhat distinctive in poisoning with certain agents. With mercuric chloride, for example, severely injured cells that are not yet dead might contain large acidophilic inclusions. Later, these cells become totally necrotic, are desquamated into the lumen, and may undergo calcification. Carbon tetrachloride poisoning, in contrast, is characterized by the accumulation of neutral lipids in injured cells, but again, such fatty change is followed by necrosis. Ethylene glycol produces marked ballooning and hydropic or vacuolar degeneration of proximal convoluted tubules. Calcium oxalate crystals are often found in the tubular lumens in such poisoning.

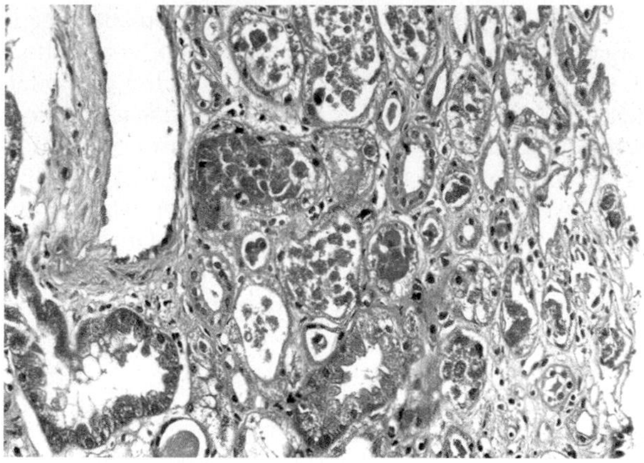

FIGURE 20–34 Acute tubular necrosis. Some of the tubular epithelial cells in the tubules are necrotic, and many have become detached (from their basement membranes) and been sloughed into the tubular lumina, whereas others are swollen, vacuolated, and regenerating. (Courtesy of Dr. Agnes Fogo, Vanderbilt University, Nashville, TN.)

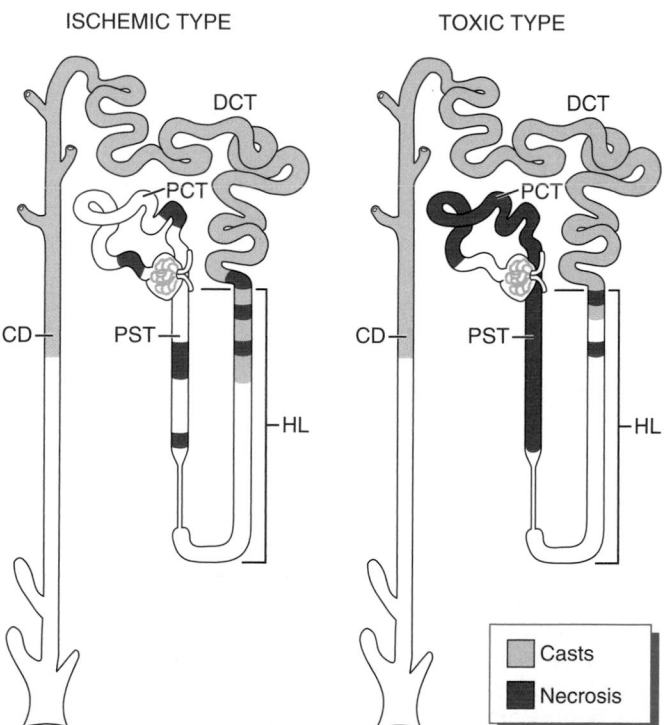

FIGURE 20–33 Patterns of tubular damage in ischemic and toxic acute tubular necrosis. In the ischemic type, tubular necrosis is patchy, relatively short lengths of tubules are affected, and straight segments of proximal tubules (PST) and ascending limbs of Henle's loop (HL) are most vulnerable. In toxic acute tubular necrosis, extensive necrosis is present along the proximal tubule segments (PCT) with many toxins (e.g., mercury), but necrosis of the distal tubule, particularly ascending Henle's loop, also occurs. In both types, lumens of the distal convoluted tubules (DCT) and collecting ducts (CD) contain casts.

Clinical Course. The clinical course of ATN is highly variable, but the classic case may be divided into *initiation*, *maintenance*, and *recovery* stages. The *initiation phase*, lasting for about 36 hours, is dominated by the inciting medical, surgical, or obstetric event in the ischemic form of ATN. The only indication of renal involvement is a slight decline in urine output with a rise in BUN. At this point, oliguria could be explained on the basis of a transient decrease in blood flow to the kidneys.

The *maintenance phase* is characterized by sustained decreases in urine output to between 40 and 400 mL/day (oliguria), with salt and water overload, rising BUN concentrations, hyperkalemia, metabolic acidosis, and other manifestations of uremia dominating this phase. With appropriate attention to the balance of water and blood electrolytes, including dialysis, the patient can be carried over this oliguric crisis.

The *recovery phase* is ushered in by a steady increase in urine volume that may reach up to 3 L/day. The tubules are still damaged, so large amounts of water, sodium, and potassium are lost in the urinary flood. *Hypokalemia, rather than hyperkalemia, becomes a clinical problem.* There is a peculiar increased vulnerability to infection at this stage. Eventually, renal tubular function is restored, with improvement in concentrating ability. At the same time, BUN and creatinine levels begin to return to normal. Subtle tubular functional impairment may persist for months, but most patients who reach this phase eventually recover completely.

The prognosis of ATN depends on the clinical setting surrounding its development. Recovery is expected with nephrotoxic ATN when the toxin has not caused serious damage to other organs, such as the liver or heart. With modern methods of care, 95% of those who do not succumb to the precipitating cause have a chance of recovery. Conversely, in shock related to sepsis, extensive burns, or other causes of multiorgan failure, the mortality rate can rise to more than 50%.

Up to 50% of patients with ATN might not have oliguria and might in fact have increased urine volumes. This so-called *nonoliguric ATN* occurs particularly often with nephrotoxins, and it generally tends to follow a more benign clinical course.

TUBULOINTERSTITIAL NEPHRITIS

This group of renal diseases is characterized by histologic and functional alterations that involve predominantly the tubules and interstitium. We have previously seen that chronic tubulointerstitial injury may occur in diseases that primarily affect the glomerulus (see Fig. 20–15) and indeed that such injury may be an important cause of progression in these diseases.[43] This *secondary tubulointerstitial nephritis* is also present in a variety of vascular, cystic (polycystic kidney disease), metabolic (diabetes), and renal disorders, in which it may also contribute to progressive damage. Here we discuss disorders in which tubulointerstitial injury appears to be a primary event. *These disorders have diverse causes and different pathogenetic mechanisms* (Table 20–9). Thus, the disorders are identified by cause or by associated disease (e.g., analgesic nephropathy, radiation nephropathy). Glomerular and vascular abnormalities may also be present but either are mild or occur only in advanced stages of these diseases.

TABLE 20–9 Causes of Tubulointerstitial Nephritis

Infections
Acute bacterial pyelonephritis
Chronic pyelonephritis (including reflux nephropathy)
Other infections (e.g., viruses, parasites)
Toxins
Drugs
Acute hypersensitivity interstitial nephritis
Analgesic nephropathy
Heavy metals
Lead, cadmium
Metabolic Diseases
Urate nephropathy
Nephrocalcinosis (hypercalcemic nephropathy)
Hypokalemic nephropathy
Oxalate nephropathy
Physical Factors
Chronic urinary tract obstruction
Radiation nephropathy
Neoplasms
Multiple myeloma (cast nephropathy)
Immunologic Reactions
Transplant rejection
Sjögren syndrome
Sarcoidosis
Vascular Diseases
Miscellaneous
Balkan nephropathy
Nephronophthisis–medullary cystic disease complex
"Idiopathic" interstitial nephritis

Tubulointerstitial nephritis can be acute or chronic. Acute tubulointerstitial nephritis has a rapid clinical onset and is characterized histologically by interstitial edema, often accompanied by leukocytic infiltration of the interstitium and tubules, and focal tubular necrosis. In *chronic interstitial nephritis*, there is infiltration with predominantly mononuclear leukocytes, prominent interstitial fibrosis, and widespread tubular atrophy. Morphologic features that are helpful in separating acute from chronic tubulointerstitial nephritis include edema and, when present, eosinophils and neutrophils in the acute form, contrasted with fibrosis and tubular atrophy in the chronic form.

These conditions are distinguished clinically from the glomerular diseases by the absence, in early stages, of such hallmarks of glomerular injury as nephritic or nephrotic syndromes and by the presence of defects in tubular function. The latter may be subtle and include impaired ability to concentrate urine, evidenced clinically by polyuria or nocturia; salt wasting; diminished ability to excrete acids (metabolic acidosis); and isolated defects in tubular reabsorption or secretion. The advanced forms, however, may be difficult to distinguish clinically from other causes of renal insufficiency.

Some of the specific conditions listed in Table 20–9 are discussed elsewhere in this book. In this section, we deal principally with pyelonephritis and interstitial diseases induced by drugs.

Pyelonephritis and Urinary Tract Infection

Pyelonephritis is a renal disorder affecting the tubules, interstitium, and renal pelvis and is one of the most common diseases of the kidney. It occurs in two forms. *Acute pyelonephritis* is caused by bacterial infection and is the renal lesion associated with urinary tract infection. *Chronic pyelonephritis* is a more complex disorder: bacterial infection plays a dominant role, but other factors (vesicoureteral reflux, obstruction) are involved in its pathogenesis. Pyelonephritis is a serious complication of an extremely common clinical spectrum of *urinary tract infections* that affect the urinary bladder (cystitis), the kidneys and their collecting systems (pyelonephritis), or both. Bacterial infection of the lower urinary tract may be completely asymptomatic (asymptomatic bacteriuria) and most often remains localized to the bladder without the development of renal infection. However, lower urinary tract infection always carries the potential of spread to the kidney.

Etiology and Pathogenesis. The dominant etiologic agents, accounting for more than 85% of cases of urinary tract infection, are the Gram-negative bacilli that are normal inhabitants of the intestinal tract.[86] By far the most common is *Escherichia coli*, followed by *Proteus*, *Klebsiella*, and *Enterobacter*. *Streptococcus faecalis*, also of enteric origin, staphylococci, and virtually every other bacterial and fungal agent can also cause lower urinary tract and renal infection. In immunocompromised patients, particularly those with transplanted organs, viruses such as polyoma virus, cytomegalovirus, and adenovirus can also be a cause of renal infection.

In most patients with urinary tract infection, the infecting organisms are derived from the patient's own fecal flora. This is thus a form of *endogenous infection*. There are two routes by which bacteria can reach the kidneys: (1) through the bloodstream (hematogenous infection) and (2) from the lower urinary tract (ascending infection) (Fig. 20–35). Although the hematogenous route is the less common of the two, acute pyelonephritis does result from seeding of the kidneys by bacteria from distant foci in the course of septicemia or infective endocarditis. Hematogenous infection is more likely to occur in the presence of ureteral obstruction, in debilitated patients, in patients receiving immunosuppressive therapy, and with nonenteric organisms, such as staphylococci and certain fungi and viruses.

Ascending infection is the most common cause of clinical pyelonephritis. Normal human bladder and bladder urine are sterile; therefore, a number of steps must occur for renal infection to occur:

- The first step in the pathogenesis of ascending infection appears to be the *colonization of the distal urethra and introitus* (in the female) by coliform bacteria. This colonization is influenced by the ability of bacteria to adhere to urethral mucosal cells. Such bacterial adherence, as discussed in Chapter 8, involves adhesive molecules (adhesins) on the P-fimbriae (pili) of bacteria that interact with receptors on the surface of uroepithelial cells. Specific adhesins (e.g., the *pap* variant) are associated with infection. In addition, certain types of fimbriae promote renal tropism, or persistence of infection, or an enhanced inflammatory response to bacteria.[87]
- *From the urethra to the bladder*, organisms gain entrance during urethral catheterization or other instrumentation. Long-term catheterization, in particular, carries a risk of infection. In the absence of instrumentation, *urinary infections are much more common in females*, and this has been variously ascribed to the shorter urethra in females, the absence of antibacterial properties such as are found in prostatic fluid, hormonal changes affecting adherence of bacteria to the mucosa, and urethral trauma during sexual intercourse or a combination of these factors.
- *Multiplication in the bladder.* Ordinarily, organisms introduced into the bladder are cleared by the continual flushing of voiding and by antibacterial mechanisms. However, outflow obstruction or bladder dysfunction results in incomplete emptying and increased residual volume of urine. In the presence of stasis, bacteria introduced into the bladder can multiply unhindered without being flushed out or destroyed in the bladder wall. Accordingly, urinary tract infection is particularly frequent among patients with lower urinary tract obstruction, such as may occur with benign prostatic hypertrophy, tumors, or calculi or with neurogenic bladder dysfunction caused by diabetes or spinal cord injury.
- *Vesicoureteral reflux.* Although obstruction is an important predisposing factor in the pathogenesis of ascending infection, *it is incompetence of the vesicoureteral valve* that allows bacteria to ascend the ureter into the renal pelvis. The normal ureteral insertion into the bladder is a competent one-way valve that prevents retrograde flow of urine, especially during micturition, when the intravesical pressure rises. An incompetent vesicoureteral orifice allows the reflux of bladder urine into the ureters (*vesicoureteral reflux*) (Fig. 20–36). Reflux is most often due to a congenital absence or shortening of the intravesical portion of the ureter (Fig. 20–37), such that the ureter is not compressed during micturition. In addition, bladder infection itself, probably as a result of the action of bacterial or inflammatory products on ureteral contractility, can cause or accentuate vesicoureteral reflux, particularly in children. *Acquired vesicoureteral reflux* in adults can result from persistent bladder atony caused by spinal cord injury. The effect of

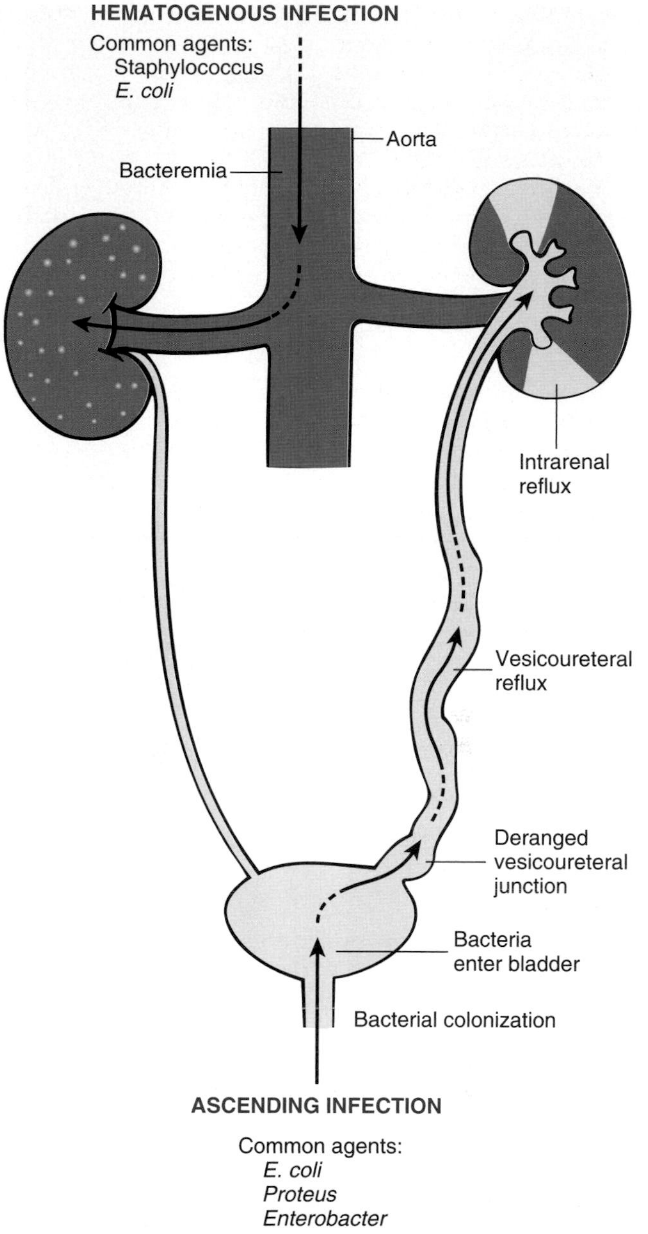

FIGURE 20–35 Schematic representation of pathways of renal infection. Hematogenous infection results from bacteremic spread. More common is ascending infection, which results from a combination of urinary bladder infection, vesicoureteral reflux, and intrarenal reflux.

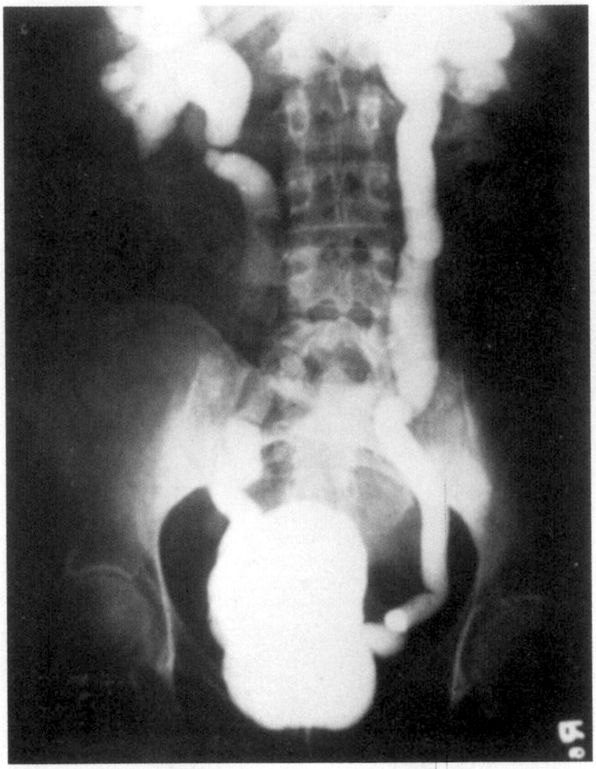

FIGURE 20–36 Vesicoureteral reflux demonstrated by a voiding cystourethrogram. Dye injected into the bladder refluxes into both dilated ureters, filling the pelvis and calyces.

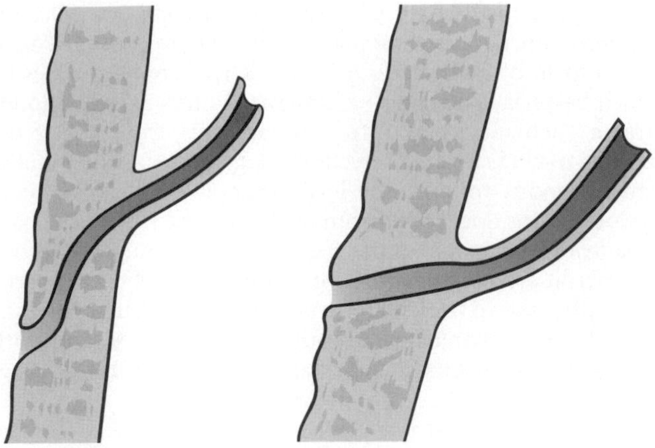

FIGURE 20–37 The vesicoureteral junction. In normal individuals (*A*), the intravesical portion of the ureter is oblique, such that the ureter is closed by muscle contraction during micturition. The most common cause of reflux is congenital complete or partial absence of the intravesical ureter (*B*).

vesicoureteral reflux is similar to that of an obstruction in that after voiding, there is residual urine in the urinary tract, which favors bacterial growth.

- *Intrarenal reflux.* Vesicoureteral reflux also affords a ready mechanism by which the infected bladder urine can be propelled up to the renal pelvis and deep into the renal parenchyma through open ducts at the tips of the papillae (intrarenal reflux). Intrarenal reflux is most common in the upper and lower poles of the kidney, where papillae tend to have flattened or concave tips rather than the convex pointed type present in the midzones of the kidney (and depicted in most textbooks). Reflux can be demonstrated radiographically by a voiding cystourethrogram: The bladder is filled with a radio-opaque dye, and films are taken during micturition. Vesicoureteral reflux can be demonstrated in about 30% of infants and children with urinary tract infection (see Fig. 20–36).

In the absence of vesicoureteral reflux, infection usually remains localized in the bladder. Thus, the majority of patients with repeated or persistent bacterial colonization of the urinary tract suffer from cystitis and urethritis (*lower urinary tract infection*) rather than pyelonephritis.

Acute Pyelonephritis

Acute pyelonephritis is an acute suppurative inflammation of the kidney caused by bacterial and sometimes viral (e.g., polyoma virus) infection, whether hematogenous and induced by septicemic spread or ascending and associated with vesicoureteral reflux.

Morphology. The hallmarks of acute pyelonephritis are **patchy interstitial suppurative inflammation, intratubular aggregates of neutrophils, and tubular necrosis.** The suppuration may occur as discrete focal abscesses involving one or both kidneys, which can extend to large wedge-shaped areas of suppuration (Fig. 20–38). The distribution of these lesions is unpredictable and haphazard, but in pyelonephritis associated with reflux, damage occurs most commonly in the lower and upper poles.

In the early stages, the neutrophilic infiltration is limited to the interstitial tissue. Soon, however, the reaction involves tubules and produces a characteristic abscess with the destruction of the engulfed tubules (Fig. 20–39). Since the tubular lumens present a ready pathway for the extension of the infection, large masses of intraluminal neutrophils frequently extend along the involved nephron into the collecting tubules. Characteristically, the glomeruli appear to be resistant to the infection. Large areas of severe necrosis, however, eventually destroy the glomeruli, and fungal pyelonephritis (e.g., *Candida*) often affects glomeruli.

Three complications of acute pyelonephritis are encountered in special circumstances.

- **Papillary necrosis** is seen mainly in diabetics and in those with urinary tract obstruction. Papillary necrosis is usually bilateral but may be unilateral. One or all of the pyramids of the affected kidney may be involved. On cut section, the tips or distal two-thirds of the pyramids have areas of gray-white to yellow necrosis (Fig. 20–40). On microscopic examination, the necrotic tissue shows characteristic coagulative necrosis, with preservation of outlines of tubules. The leukocytic response is limited to the junctions between preserved and destroyed tissue.
- **Pyonephrosis** is seen when there is total or almost complete obstruction, particularly when it is high in the urinary tract. The suppurative exudate is unable

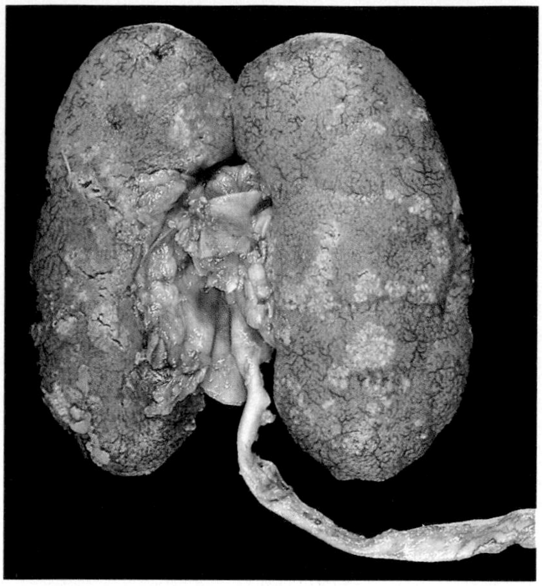

FIGURE 20–38 Acute pyelonephritis. Cortical surface exhibits grayish white areas of inflammation and abscess formation.

to drain and thus fills the renal pelvis, calyces, and ureter, producing pyonephrosis.

- **Perinephric abscess** implies extension of suppurative inflammation through the renal capsule into the perinephric tissue.

After the acute phase of pyelonephritis, healing occurs. The neutrophilic infiltrate is replaced by one that is predominantly mononuclear, with macrophages, plasma cells, and (later) lymphocytes. The inflammatory foci are eventually replaced by scars that can be seen on the cortical surface as fibrous depressions. Such scars are characterized microscopically by atrophy of tubules, interstitial fibrosis, and lymphocyte infiltrate and may resemble scars produced by ischemic or other types of injury to the kidney. **However, the pyelonephritic scar is almost always associated with inflammation, fibrosis, and deformation of the underlying calyx and pelvis,** reflecting the role of ascending infection and vesicoureteral reflux in the pathogenesis of the disease.

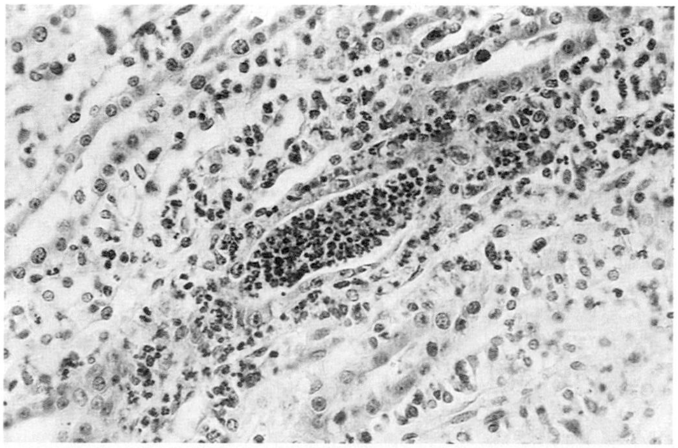

FIGURE 20–39 Acute pyelonephritis marked by an acute neutrophilic exudate within tubules and the renal substance.

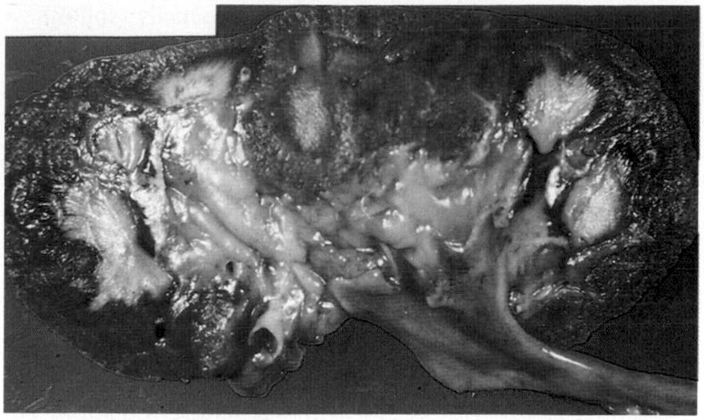

FIGURE 20–40 Papillary necrosis. Areas of pale gray necrosis are limited to the papillae.

Clinical Course. Acute pyelonephritis is often associated with predisposing conditions, some of which were mentioned in the discussion of pathogenetic mechanisms. These include the following:

- *Urinary tract obstruction,* either congenital or acquired
- *Instrumentation* of the urinary tract, most commonly catheterization
- *Vesicoureteral reflux*
- *Pregnancy.* Four percent to 6% of pregnant women develop bacteriuria sometime during pregnancy, and 20% to 40% of these eventually develop symptomatic urinary infection if not treated.
- *Patient's sex and age.* After the first year of life (when congenital anomalies in males commonly become evident) and up to around age 40 years, infections are much more frequent in females. With increasing age, the incidence in males rises owing to the development of prostatic hypertrophy and frequent instrumentation.
- *Preexisting renal lesions,* causing intrarenal scarring and obstruction
- *Diabetes mellitus,* in which acute pyelonephritis is caused by more frequent instrumentation, the general susceptibility to infection, and the neurogenic bladder dysfunction exhibited by patients
- *Immunosuppression and immunodeficiency*

When acute pyelonephritis is clinically apparent, the onset is usually sudden, with pain at the costovertebral angle and systemic evidence of infection, such as fever and malaise. There are usually indications of bladder and urethral irritation, such as dysuria, frequency, and urgency. The urine contains many leukocytes (pyuria) derived from the inflammatory infiltrate, but pyuria does not differentiate upper from lower urinary tract infection. The finding of leukocyte *casts,* typically filled with neutrophils (pus casts), indicates renal involvement, because casts are formed only in tubules. The diagnosis of infection is established by quantitative urine culture.

Uncomplicated acute pyelonephritis usually follows a benign course, and the symptoms disappear within a few days after the institution of appropriate antibiotic therapy. Bacteria, however, may persist in the urine, or there may be recurrence of infection with new serologic types of *E. coli* or other organisms. Such bacteriuria then either disappears or may persist, sometimes for years. In the presence of unrelieved urinary obstruction, diabetes mellitus, or immunodeficiency, acute pyelonephritis may be more serious, leading to repeated septicemic episodes. The superimposition of *papillary necrosis* may lead to acute renal failure.

An emerging viral pathogen causing pyelonephritis in kidney allografts is *polyoma virus*. Latent infection with polyoma virus is widespread in the general population, but immunosuppression of the allograft recipient can lead to reactivation of latent infection and the development of a nephropathy resulting in allograft failure in up to 1% to 5% of kidney transplant recipients.[88] This form of pyelonephritis is characterized by viral infection of tubular epithelial cell nuclei, leading to nuclear enlargement and intranuclear inclusions visible by light microscopy (viral cytopathic effect). The inclusions are composed of viral structures arrayed in distinctive crystalline-like lattices when visualized by electron microscopy (Fig. 20–41). An interstitial inflammatory response is invariably present. Treatment is reduction in immunosuppression.

Chronic Pyelonephritis and Reflux Nephropathy

Chronic pyelonephritis is a chronic tubulointerstitial renal disorder in which *chronic tubulointerstitial inflammation and renal scarring are associated with pathologic involvement of the calyces and pelvis* (Fig. 20–42). Pelvocalyceal damage is important in that virtually all the diseases listed in Table 20–9 produce chronic tubulointerstitial alterations, but except for chronic pyelonephritis and analgesic nephropathy, none affects the calyces. Chronic pyelonephritis is an important cause of end-stage kidney disease; at one time, it accounted for up to 10% to 20% of patients in renal transplant or dialysis units, until predisposing conditions such as reflux became better recognized and diligently evaluated. This condition remains an important cause of kidney destruction in children with severe lower urinary tract abnormalities.

Chronic pyelonephritis can be divided into two forms: chronic reflux-associated and chronic obstructive.

Reflux Nephropathy. This is by far the more common form of chronic pyelonephritic scarring. Renal involvement in reflux nephropathy occurs early in childhood as a result of superimposition of a urinary infection on congenital vesicoureteral reflux and intrarenal reflux, the latter conditioned by the number of potentially refluxing papillae. Reflux may be unilateral or bilateral; thus, the resultant renal damage either may cause scarring and atrophy of one kidney or may involve both and lead to chronic renal insufficiency. Vesicoureteral reflux occasionally causes renal damage in the absence of infection (sterile reflux) but only in the presence of severe obstruction.

Chronic Obstructive Pyelonephritis. We have seen that obstruction predisposes the kidney to infection. Recurrent infections superimposed on diffuse or localized obstructive lesions lead to recurrent bouts of renal inflammation and scarring, resulting in a picture of chronic pyelonephritis. In this condition, the effects of obstruction contribute to the parenchymal atrophy; indeed, it is sometimes difficult to differentiate the effects of bacterial infection from those of obstruction alone. The disease can be bilateral, as with obstructive anomalies of the urinary tract (e.g., posterior urethral valves), resulting in renal insufficiency unless the anomaly is corrected, or unilateral, such as occurs with calculi and unilateral obstructive anomalies of the ureter.

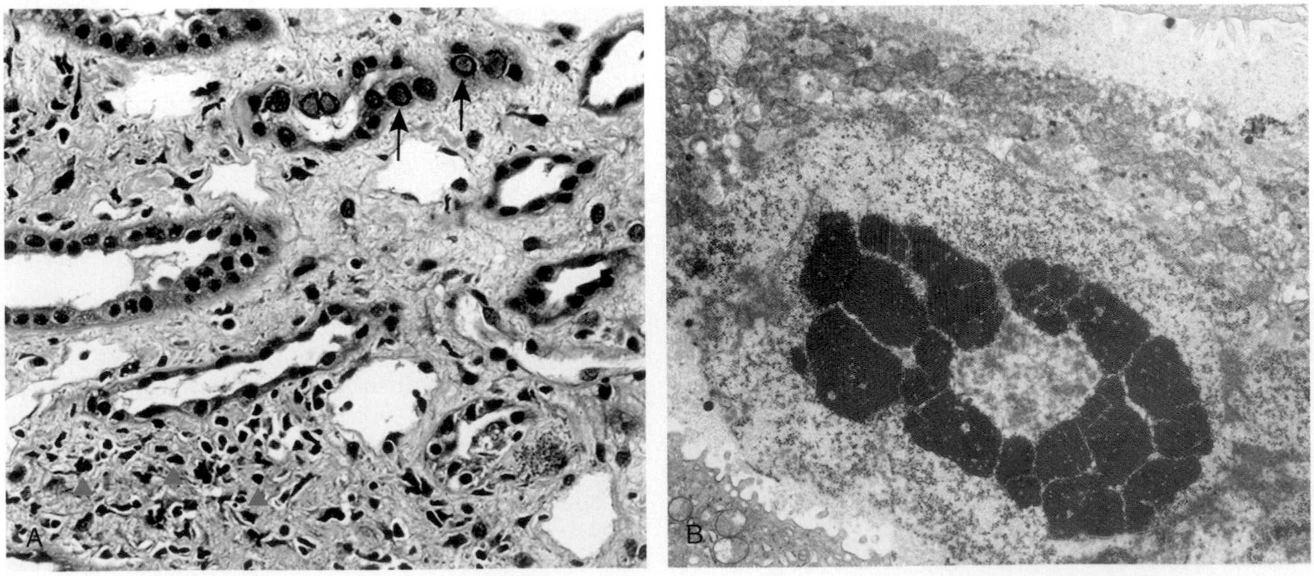

FIGURE 20–41 Polyoma virus nephropathy. *A,* The kidney shows enlarged tubular epithelial cells with nuclear inclusions (*arrow*) and interstitial inflammation (*arrowheads*). *B,* Intranuclear viral inclusions visualized by electron microscopy. (Courtesy of Dr. Jean Olson, Department of Pathology, University of California San Francisco, San Francisco, CA.)

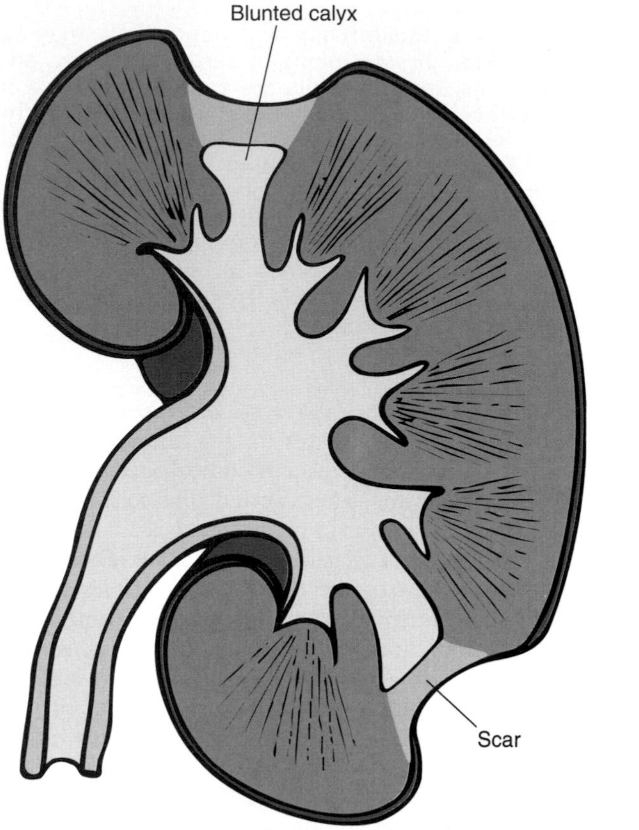

FIGURE 20–42 Typical coarse scars of chronic pyelonephritis associated with vesicoureteral reflux. The scars are usually polar and are associated with underlying blunted calyces.

Morphology. The characteristic changes of chronic pyelonephritis are seen on gross examination (Figs. 20–42 and 20–43). The kidneys usually are irregularly scarred; if bilateral, the involvement is asymmetric. This contrasts with chronic glomerulonephritis, in which the kidneys are diffusely and symmetrically scarred. The hallmark of chronic pyelonephritis is the coarse, discrete, corticomedullary scar overlying a dilated, blunted, or deformed calyx (Fig. 20–43). The scars can vary from one to several in number and may affect one or both kidneys. Most are in the upper and lower poles, consistent with the frequency of reflux in these sites.

The microscopic changes involve predominantly tubules and interstitium. The tubules show atrophy in some areas and hypertrophy or dilation in others. Dilated tubules with flattened epithelium may be filled with colloid casts (thyroidization). There are varying degrees of chronic interstitial inflammation and fibrosis in the cortex and medulla. In the presence of active infection, there may be neutrophils in the interstitium and pus casts in the tubules. Arcuate and interlobular vessels demonstrate obliterative intimal sclerosis in the scarred areas; and in the presence of hypertension, hyaline arteriosclerosis is seen in the entire kidney. There is often fibrosis around the calyceal epithelium as well as a marked chronic inflammatory infiltrate. Glomeruli may appear normal except for periglomerular fibrosis, but a variety of glomerular changes may be present, including ischemic fibrous obliteration as well as secondary changes related to hypertension. Patients with chronic pyelonephritis and reflux nephropathy who develop proteinuria in advanced stages exhibit secondary focal segmental glomerulosclerosis, as described later.

Xanthogranulomatous pyelonephritis is an unusual and relatively rare form of chronic pyelonephritis characterized by accumulation of foamy macrophages intermingled with plasma cells, lymphocytes, polymorphonuclear leukocytes, and occasional giant cells. Often associated with *Proteus* infections and obstruction, the lesions sometimes produce large, yellowish orange nodules that may be confused with renal cell carcinoma.

Clinical Course. Chronic obstructive pyelonephritis may be insidious in onset or may present with clinical manifestations of acute recurrent pyelonephritis with back pain, fever, frequent pyuria, and bacteriuria. Chronic pyelonephritis asso-

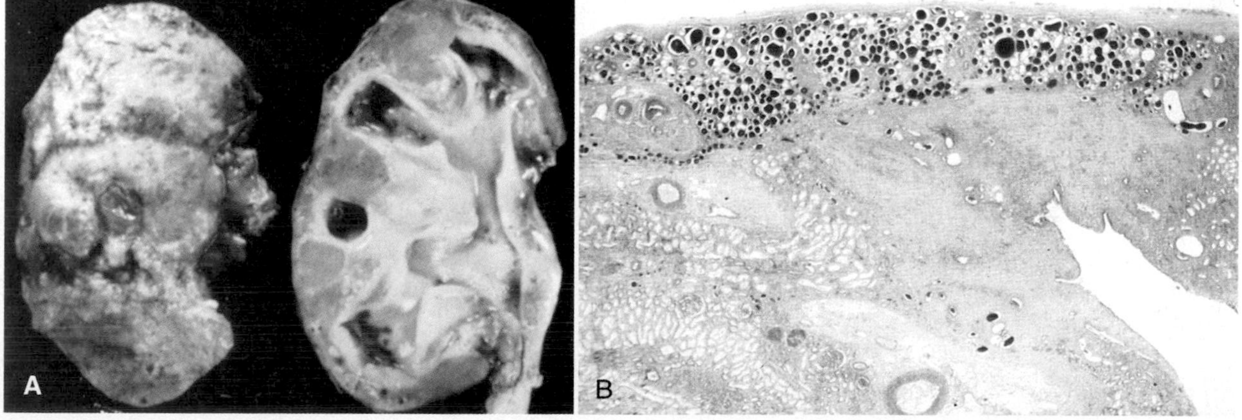

FIGURE 20–43 *A*, Chronic pyelonephritis. The surface (*left*) is irregularly scarred. The cut section (*right*) reveals characteristic dilation and blunting of calyces. The ureter is dilated and thickened, a finding that is consistent with chronic vesicoureteral reflux. *B*, Low-power view showing a corticomedullary renal scar with an underlying dilated deformed calyx. Note the thyroidization of tubules in the cortex.

ciated with reflux may have a silent onset. These patients come to medical attention relatively late in the course of their disease because of the gradual onset of renal insufficiency and hypertension or because of the discovery of pyuria or bacteriuria on routine examination. Reflux nephropathy is often discovered when the etiology of hypertension in children is investigated. Loss of tubular function—in particular of concentrating ability—gives rise to polyuria and nocturia. Radiographic studies show asymmetrically contracted kidneys with characteristic coarse scars and blunting and deformity of the calyceal system. Significant bacteriuria may be present, but it is often absent in the late stages.

Although proteinuria is usually mild, some patients with pyelonephritic scars develop *focal segmental glomerulosclerosis* with significant proteinuria, even in the nephrotic range, usually several years after the scarring has occurred and often in the absence of continued infection or persistent vesicoureteral reflux. The appearance of proteinuria and focal segmental glomerulosclerosis is a poor prognostic sign, and patients with these findings may proceed to chronic or end-stage renal failure. The glomerulosclerosis, as we have discussed, may be attributable to the adaptive glomerular alterations secondary to loss of renal mass caused by pyelonephritic scarring (renal ablation nephropathy).

Tubulointerstitial Nephritis Induced by Drugs and Toxins

Toxins and drugs can produce renal injury in at least three ways: (1) They may trigger an interstitial immunologic reaction, exemplified by the acute hypersensitivity nephritis induced by such drugs as methicillin; (2) they may cause acute renal failure, as described earlier; and (3) they may cause subtle but cumulative injury to tubules that takes years to become manifest, resulting in chronic renal insufficiency.[89] The last type of damage is especially treacherous because it may be clinically unrecognized until significant renal damage has occurred. Such is the case with analgesic abuse nephropathy, which is usually detected only after the onset of chronic renal insufficiency.

Acute Drug-Induced Interstitial Nephritis

This is a well-recognized adverse reaction to a constantly increasing number of drugs. First reported after the use of sulfonamides, acute tubulointerstitial nephritis most frequently occurs with synthetic penicillins (methicillin, ampicillin), other synthetic antibiotics (rifampin), diuretics (thiazides), NSAIDs, and miscellaneous drugs (allopurinol, cimetidine). The disease begins about 15 days (range: 2 to 40) after exposure to the drug and is characterized by *fever*, *eosinophilia* (which may be transient), *a rash* in about 25% of patients, and *renal abnormalities.* The last include hematuria, mild proteinuria, and leukocyturia (often including eosinophils). A *rising serum creatinine level or acute renal failure with oliguria develops in about 50% of cases,* particularly in older patients.

Morphology. On histologic examination, the abnormalities are in the interstitium, which shows variable but frequently pronounced edema and infiltration by mononuclear cells, principally lymphocytes and macrophages. Eosinophils and neutrophils may be present (Fig. 20–44), often in large numbers, and plasma cells and basophils are sometimes found in small numbers. With some drugs (e.g., methicillin, thiazides), interstitial granulomas with giant cells may be seen. "Tubulitis," the infiltration of tubules by lymphocytes, is common. Variable degrees of tubular necrosis and regeneration are present. The glomeruli are normal except in some cases caused by NSAIDs, when minimal change disease and the nephrotic syndrome develop concurrently (see the discussion of NSAIDs later in the chapter).

Pathogenesis. Many features of the disease suggest an immune mechanism. The basis for the immune response is idiosyncratic and not dose related. Clinical evidence of hypersensitivity includes the latent period, the eosinophilia and rash, the fact that the onset of nephropathy is not dose related, and the recurrence of hypersensitivity after re-exposure to the same or a cross-reactive drug. Serum IgE levels are increased in some patients, and IgE-containing plasma cells and basophils are sometimes present in the lesions, suggesting that the *late-phase reaction of an IgE-mediated (type I) hypersensitivity* may be involved in the pathogenesis (Chapter 6). The mononuclear or granulomatous infiltrate, together with positive results of skin tests to drug haptens, suggests a delayed hypersensitivity type reaction (type IV).

The most likely sequence of events is that the drugs act as haptens, which, during secretion by tubules, covalently bind to some cytoplasmic or extracellular component of tubular cells and become immunogenic. The resultant injury is then due to IgE and/or cell-mediated immune reactions to tubular cells or their basement membranes.

Clinical Features. It is important to recognize drug-induced renal failure because withdrawal of the offending drug is followed by recovery, although it may take several months for renal function to return to normal, and irreversible damage may occur occasionally in older subjects. It is also important to remember that while drugs are the leading identifiable cause of acute interstitial nephritis, in many

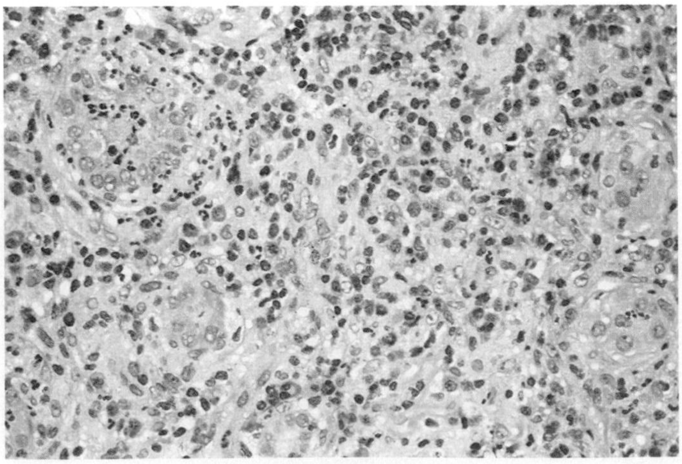

FIGURE 20–44 Drug-induced interstitial nephritis, with prominent eosinophilic and mononuclear cell infiltrate. (Courtesy of Dr. H. Rennke, Brigham and Women's Hospital, Boston, MA.)

affected patients (approximately 30% to 40%) an offending drug or mechanism for nephritis cannot be identified.

Analgesic Nephropathy

This is a form of chronic renal disease caused by excessive intake of analgesic mixtures and characterized morphologically by chronic tubulointerstitial nephritis with renal papillary necrosis.[90]

The incidence of analgesic nephropathy reflects the consumption of analgesics in various populations throughout the world. In some parts of Australia, it ranked as one of the most common causes of chronic renal insufficiency until public health measures described below reduced its incidence. Its incidence in the United States is relatively low but varies among states, being highest in the Southeast. Overall, it accounted for 9%, 3%, and 1% of patients undergoing dialysis in Australia, Europe, and the United States, respectively, before the recent surge in end-stage renal disease attributable to diabetes reduced these relative percentages. The renal damage was first ascribed to phenacetin, but the analgesic mixtures that are consumed often contain, in addition, aspirin, caffeine, acetaminophen (a metabolite of phenacetin), and codeine. Patients who develop this disease usually ingest large quantities of mixtures of at least two antipyretic analgesics. Most patients consume phenacetin-containing mixtures, and cases ascribed to ingestion of aspirin, phenacetin, or acetaminophen alone are uncommon. In most countries, restriction of over-the-counter sale of phenacetin or analgesic mixtures has reduced the incidence of the disorder but has not eradicated it, presumably because non–phenacetin-containing mixtures are available.

Pathogenesis. Papillary necrosis is readily induced experimentally by a mixture of aspirin and phenacetin, usually combined with water depletion. It is now clear that in the sequence of events leading to renal damage, *papillary necrosis occurs first, and cortical tubulointerstitial nephritis is a secondary phenomenon.* The phenacetin metabolite acetaminophen injures cells by both *covalent binding and oxidative damage.* Aspirin induces its potentiating effect by inhibiting the vasodilatory effects of prostaglandin, predisposing the papillae to ischemia. Thus, the papillary damage may be due to a combination of direct toxic effects of phenacetin metabolites and ischemic injury to both tubular cells and vessels.

Morphology. In gross appearance, the kidneys are either normal or slightly reduced in size, and the cortex exhibits depressed and raised areas; the depressed areas represent cortical atrophy overlying necrotic papillae. The papillae show various stages of necrosis, calcification, fragmentation, and sloughing. This gross appearance contrasts with the papillary necrosis seen in diabetic patients, in which all papillae are at the same stage of acute necrosis. On microscopic examination, the papillary changes may take one of several forms: In early cases, there is patchy necrosis; but in the advanced form, the entire papilla is necrotic, often remaining in place as a structureless mass with ghosts of tubules and foci of dystrophic calcification (Fig. 20–45). Segments of entire portions of the papilla may then be sloughed and excreted in the urine.

The cortical changes consist of loss and atrophy of tubules and interstitial fibrosis and inflammation. These changes are mainly due to obstructive atrophy caused by the tubular damage in the papillae. The cortical columns of Bertin are characteristically spared from this atrophy.

Clinical Course. Analgesic nephropathy is more common in women than in men and is particularly prevalent in individuals with recurrent headaches and muscle pain, in psychoneurotic patients, and in factory workers. Early renal findings include inability to concentrate the urine, as would be expected with lesions in the papillae. Acquired distal renal tubular acidosis contributes to the development of renal

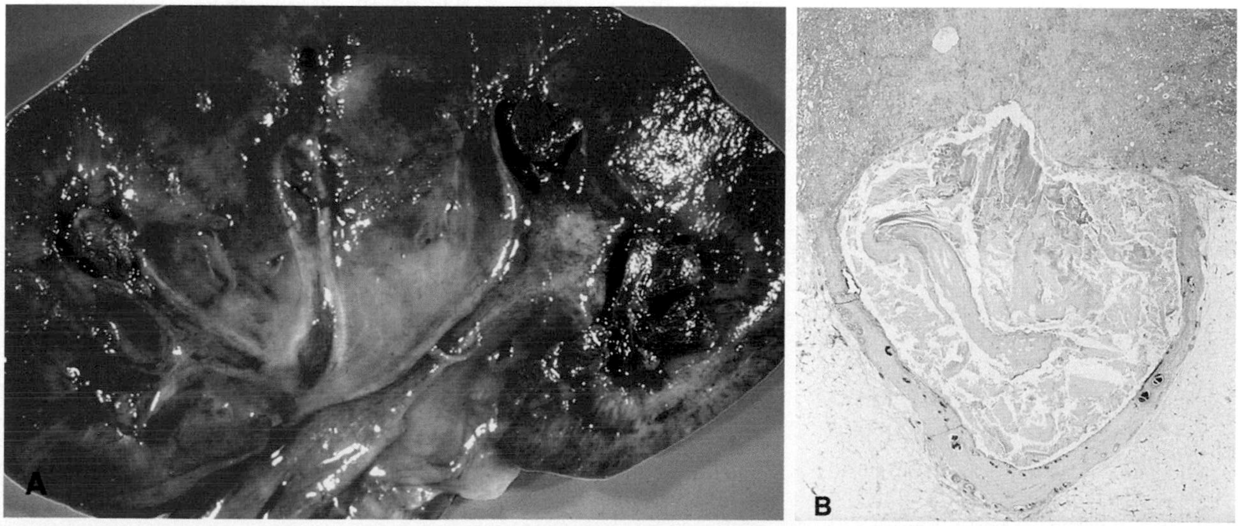

FIGURE 20–45 Analgesic nephropathy. *A,* The brownish necrotic papilla, transformed to a necrotic, structureless mass, fills the pelvis. *B,* Microscopic view. Note the fibrosis in the medulla. (Courtesy of Dr. F.J. Gloor, Institut für Pathologie, Kantonsspital, St. Gallen, Switzerland.)

stones. Headache, anemia, gastrointestinal symptoms, and hypertension are common accompaniments of analgesic nephropathy. The anemia, in particular, is out of proportion to the renal insufficiency, owing to damage to red cells by the phenacetin metabolites. Urinary tract infection complicates about 50% of cases. On occasion, entire tips of necrotic papillae are excreted, and these may cause gross hematuria or renal colic due to obstruction of the ureter by necrotic fragments. Magnetic resonance and computed tomographic imaging are helpful in detecting papillary necrosis and calcifications. Progressive impairment of renal function may lead to chronic renal failure, but with *drug withdrawal, renal function may either stabilize or actually improve.*

Unfortunately, a small percentage of patients with analgesic nephropathy develop *transitional papillary carcinoma of the renal pelvis*. Whether the carcinogenic effect is due to a metabolite of phenacetin or to some other component of the analgesic compounds is unsettled.

Papillary necrosis is not specific for analgesic nephropathy. It is also seen in diabetes mellitus, as was mentioned earlier, as well as in urinary tract obstruction, sickle cell anemia or trait, and focally in renal tuberculosis. Table 20–10 lists certain features of papillary necrosis in these conditions.

Nephropathy Associated with Nonsteroidal Anti-Inflammatory Drugs (NSAIDs)

NSAIDs are one of the most common classes of drugs currently in use and produce several forms of renal injury. Although these complications are fortunately uncommon, they need to be kept in mind, since NSAIDs are frequently administered to patients with other potential causes of renal disease. Many NSAIDs in common use are non-selective cyclooxygenase inhibitors, and their adverse renal effects are related to their ability to inhibit cyclooxygenase-dependent prostaglandin synthesis. The selective COX-2 inhibitors, while sparing the gastrointestinal tract, do affect the kidneys because COX-2 is expressed quite well in human kidneys.[91] NSAID-associated renal syndromes include:

- Hemodynamically induced *acute renal failure*, due to the inhibition of vasodilatory prostaglandin synthesis by NSAIDs. This is particularly likely to occur in the setting of other renal diseases or conditions causing volume depletion.
- Acute hypersensitivity interstitial nephritis, resulting in acute renal failure, as described earlier.
- Acute interstitial nephritis and minimal change disease. This curious association of two diverse renal conditions, one leading to renal failure and the other to nephrotic syndrome, suggests a hypersensitivity reaction affecting the interstitium and possibly the glomeruli but also is consistent with injury to podocytes mediated by cytokines released as part of the inflammatory process.
- Membranous glomerulonephritis, with the nephrotic syndrome, is a recently appreciated association, also of unclear pathogenesis.

Chinese Herbs Nephropathy

A syndrome of chronic tubulointerstitial nephritis caused by aristolochic acid, a supplement found in some formulations of herbal remedies, has been recognized recently. The drug causes a distinctive picture of renal failure with histopathologic features of interstitial fibrosis with a relative paucity of infiltrating interstitial leukocytes. As with analgesic nephropathy, there is an increased incidence of carcinoma in the kidney and urinary tract.

Other Tubulointerstitial Diseases

Urate Nephropathy

Three types of nephropathy can occur in patients with hyperuricemic disorders:

- *Acute uric acid nephropathy* is caused by the precipitation of uric acid crystals in the renal tubules, principally in collecting ducts, leading to obstruction of nephrons and the development of acute renal failure. This type is particularly likely to occur in patients with leukemias and lymphomas who are undergoing chemotherapy; the drugs increase the death of tumor cells, and uric acid is released as the nuclei of these cells disintegrate. Precipitation of uric acid is favored by the acidic pH in collecting tubules.
- *Chronic urate nephropathy*, or gouty nephropathy, occurs in patients with more protracted forms of hyperuricemia. The lesions are ascribed to the deposition of monosodium urate crystals in the acidic milieu of the distal tubules and collecting ducts as well as in the interstitium. *These deposits have a distinct histologic appearance and may form birefringent needle-like crystals either in the tubular lumina or in the interstitium* (Fig. 20–46). The urates induce a *tophus* consisting of foreign body giant cells, other

TABLE 20–10 Causes of Papillary Necrosis

	Diabetes Mellitus	Analgesic Nephropathy	Sickle Cell Disease	Obstruction
Male-to-female ratio	1:3	1:5	1:1	9:1
Time course	10 years	7 years of abuse	Variable	Variable
Infection	80%	25%	±	90%
Calcification	Rare	Frequent	Rare	Frequent
Number of papillae affected	Several; all of same stage	Almost all; different stages of necrosis	Few	Variable

Data from Seshan S, et al (eds): Classification and Atlas of Tubulointerstitial and Vascular Diseases. Baltimore, Williams & Wilkins, 1999.

mononuclear cells, and a fibrotic reaction (Chapter 26). Tubular obstruction by the urates causes cortical atrophy and scarring. Arterial and arteriolar thickening is common in these kidneys, owing to the relatively high frequency of hypertension in patients with gout. Clinically, urate nephropathy is a subtle disease associated with tubular defects that may progress slowly. Patients with gout who actually develop a chronic nephropathy commonly have evidence of increased exposure to lead, sometimes by way of drinking "moonshine" whiskey contaminated with lead.

- The third renal syndrome in hyperuricemia is *nephrolithiasis*; uric acid stones are present in 22% of patients with gout and 42% of those with secondary hyperuricemia (see later discussion of renal stones).

Hypercalcemia and Nephrocalcinosis

Disorders characterized by hypercalcemia, such as hyperparathyroidism, multiple myeloma, vitamin D intoxication, metastatic bone disease, or excess calcium intake (milk-alkali syndrome), may induce the formation of calcium stones and deposition of calcium in the kidney (nephrocalcinosis). Extensive degrees of calcinosis, under certain conditions, may lead to a form of chronic tubulointerstitial disease and renal insufficiency. The first damage induced by the hypercalcemia is at the *intracellular level*, in the tubular epithelial cells, resulting in mitochondrial distortion and evidence of cell injury. Subsequently, calcium deposits can be demonstrated within the mitochondria, cytoplasm, and basement membrane. Calcified cellular debris contributes to obstruction of tubular lumens and causes obstructive atrophy of nephrons with interstitial fibrosis and nonspecific chronic inflammation. Atrophy of entire cortical areas drained by calcified tubules may occur, and this accounts for the alternating areas of normal and scarred parenchyma seen in such kidneys.

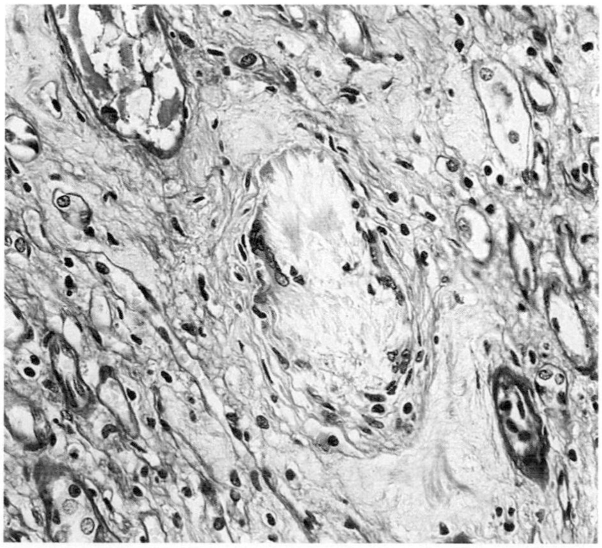

FIGURE 20–46 Urate crystals in the renal medulla. Note the giant cells and fibrosis around the crystals.

The earliest functional defect is an inability to elaborate a concentrated urine. Other tubular defects, such as tubular acidosis and salt-losing nephritis, may also occur. With further damage, a slowly progressive renal insufficiency develops. This is usually due to nephrocalcinosis, but many of these patients also have calcium stones and secondary pyelonephritis.

Multiple Myeloma

Nonrenal malignant tumors, particularly those of hematopoietic origin, affect the kidneys in a number of ways (Table 20–11). The most common involvements are tubulointerstitial, caused by complications of the tumor (hypercalcemia, hyperuricemia, obstruction of ureters) or therapy (irradiation, hyperuricemia, chemotherapy, infections in immunosuppressed patients). As the survival rate of patients with malignant neoplasms increases, so do these renal complications. We limit the discussion to the renal lesions in *multiple myeloma* that sometimes dominate the clinical picture in patients with this disease.

Renal involvement is a sometimes ominous manifestation of multiple myeloma; overt renal insufficiency occurs in half the patients with this disease. Several factors contribute to renal damage:

- *Bence Jones proteinuria and cast nephropathy*. The main cause of renal dysfunction is related to Bence Jones (light-chain) proteinuria, because renal failure correlates well with the presence and amount of such proteinuria and is uncommon in its absence. Two mechanisms appear to account for the renal toxicity of Bence Jones proteins. First, some light chains are directly toxic to epithelial cells; different light chains may have different nephrotoxic potential. Second, Bence Jones proteins combine with the urinary glycoprotein (Tamm-Horsfall protein) under acidic conditions to form large, histologically distinct tubular casts that obstruct the tubular lumina and also induce a characteristic inflammatory reaction around the casts (cast nephropathy).
- *Amyloidosis*, formed by accumulations of light chains with a predisposition to form amyloid fibrils, which occurs in 6% to 24% of patients with myeloma

TABLE 20–11 Renal Involvement in Nonrenal Neoplasms

Direct tumor invasion of renal parenchyma
  Ureters (obstruction)
  Artery (renovascular hypertension)

Hypercalcemia
Hyperuricemia
Amyloidosis
Excretion of abnormal proteins (multiple myeloma)

Glomerulopathy
  Immune complex glomerulonephritis (carcinomas)
  Minimal change disease (Hodgkin disease)
  Membranoproliferative glomerulonephritis (leukemias and lymphomas)

Effects of radiotherapy, chemotherapy, secondary infection

- *Light-chain deposition disease.* In some patients, light chains deposit in glomerular basement membranes and mesangium in nonfibrillar forms, causing a glomerulopathy (described earlier), or in tubular basement membranes, which may cause tubulointerstitial nephritis.
- *Hypercalcemia and hyperuricemia,* which are often present in these patients

Morphology. The tubulointerstitial changes in multiple myeloma are fairly characteristic. The Bence Jones tubular casts appear as pink to blue amorphous masses, sometimes concentrically laminated, often with a fractured appearance, filling and distending the tubular lumens. Some of the casts are surrounded by multinucleate giant cells that are derived from mononuclear phagocytes (Fig. 20–47). The adjacent interstitial tissue usually shows a nonspecific inflammatory response and fibrosis. On occasion, the casts erode their way from the tubules into the interstitium and here evoke a granulomatous inflammatory reaction. The histologic features of amyloidosis, light-chain deposition disease and nephrocalcinosis and infection, may also be present.

Clinically, the renal manifestations are of several types. In the most common form, *chronic renal failure* develops insidiously and usually progresses slowly during a period of several months to years. Another form occurs suddenly and is manifested by *acute renal failure* with oliguria. Precipitating factors in these patients include dehydration, hypercalcemia, acute infection, and treatment with nephrotoxic antibiotics. *Bence Jones proteinuria* occurs in 70% of patients with myeloma; the presence of significant non–light-chain proteinuria (e.g., albumin) suggests secondary amyloidosis or light-chain deposition disease.

Diseases of Blood Vessels

Nearly all diseases of the kidney involve the renal blood vessels secondarily. Systemic vascular diseases, such as various forms of vasculitis, also affect renal vessels, and often their effects on the kidney are clinically important. Hypertension, as we discussed in Chapter 11, is intimately linked with the kidney, because kidney disease can be both the cause and consequence of increased blood pressure.[92,93] In this chapter, we discuss benign and malignant nephrosclerosis and renal artery stenosis, lesions associated with hypertension, and sundry lesions involving mostly smaller vessels of the kidney.

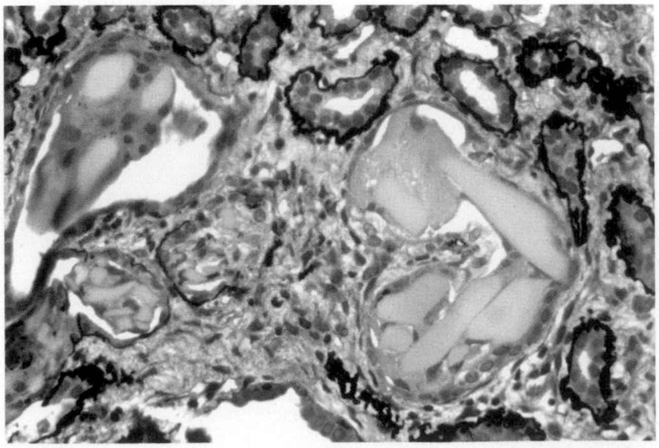

FIGURE 20–47 Myeloma kidney. Note the angulated and tubular casts with macrophages, including multinucleate cells, engulfing them.

BENIGN NEPHROSCLEROSIS

Benign nephrosclerosis is the term used for the renal pathology associated with sclerosis of renal arterioles and small arteries. The resultant effect is focal ischemia of parenchyma supplied by vessels with thickened walls and consequent narrowed lumens. Some degree of nephrosclerosis is present at autopsy with increasing age, more in blacks than whites, preceding or in the absence of hypertension.[94] Hypertension and diabetes mellitus, however, increase the incidence and severity of the lesions.

Pathogenesis. Two processes participate in inducing the arterial lesions:

- Medial and intimal thickening, as a response to hemodynamic changes, aging, genetic defects, or some combination of these
- Hyaline deposition in arterioles, caused partly by extravasation of plasma proteins through injured endothelium and partly by increased deposition of basement membrane matrix

Morphology. In gross appearance, the kidneys are either normal in size or moderately reduced, with average weights between 110 and 130 gm. The cortical surfaces have a fine, even granularity that resembles grain leather (Fig. 20–48). The loss of mass is due mainly to cortical scarring and shrinking.

On histologic examination, there is narrowing of the lumens of arterioles and small arteries, caused by thickening and hyalinization of the walls **(hyaline arteriolosclerosis)** (Fig. 20–49).

In addition to arteriolar hyalinization, the interlobular and arcuate arteries exhibit a characteristic lesion that consists of medial hypertrophy, reduplication of the elastic lamina, and increased myofibroblastic tissue in the intima, with consequent narrowing of the lumen. This change, called fibroelastic hyperplasia, often accompanies hyaline arteriolosclerosis and increases in severity with age and in the presence of hypertension.

Consequent to the vascular narrowing, there is patchy ischemic atrophy, which consists of (1) foci of tubular atrophy and interstitial fibrosis and (2) a variety of glomerular alterations. The latter include collapse of GBMs, deposition of collagen within the Bowman space, periglomerular fibrosis, and total sclerosis of glomeruli. When the ischemic changes are pronounced and affect large areas of parenchyma, they can produce regional scars and histologic alterations that may resemble those seen in renal ablation injury, mentioned earlier.

Clinical Features. It is unusual for uncomplicated benign nephrosclerosis alone to cause renal insufficiency or uremia.

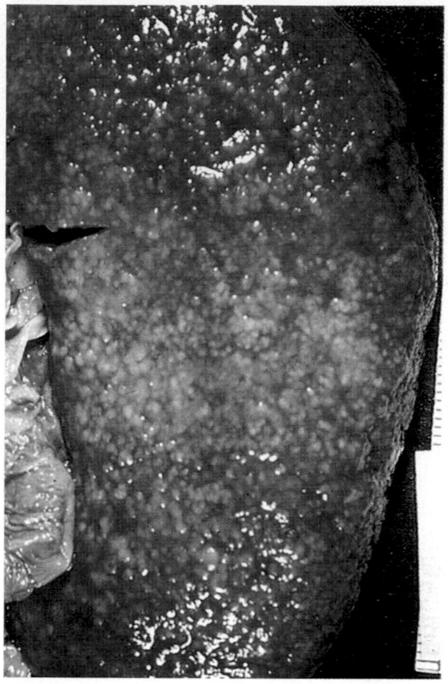

FIGURE 20–48 Close-up of the gross appearance of the cortical surface in benign nephrosclerosis illustrating the fine, leathery granularity of the surface.

There are usually moderate reductions in renal plasma flow, but the GFR is normal or only slightly reduced. On occasion, there is mild proteinuria. However, three groups of hypertensives with benign nephrosclerosis are at increased risk of developing renal failure: blacks, patients with more severe blood pressure elevations, and patients with a second underlying disease, especially diabetes. In these groups, renal insufficiency may supervene after prolonged benign hypertension, but more rapid renal failure results from the development of the malignant or accelerated phase of hypertension, discussed next.

MALIGNANT HYPERTENSION AND ACCELERATED NEPHROSCLEROSIS

Malignant nephrosclerosis is the form of renal disease associated with the malignant or accelerated phase of hypertension.[94,95] This dramatic pattern of hypertension may occasionally develop in previously normotensive individuals but often is superimposed on pre-existing essential benign hypertension, secondary forms of hypertension, or an underlying chronic renal disease, particularly glomerulonephritis or reflux nephropathy (Table 20–12). It is also a frequent cause of death from uremia in patients with scleroderma. Malignant hypertension is relatively uncommon, occurring in 1% to 5% of all patients with elevated blood pressure. In its pure form, it usually affects younger individuals, with a high preponderance in men and in blacks.

Pathogenesis. The basis for this turn for the worse in hypertensive subjects is unclear, but the following sequence of events is suggested. The initial insult appears to be some form of vascular damage to the kidneys. This might result from long-standing benign hypertension, with eventual injury to the arteriolar walls, or the initiating injury may spring de novo from arteritis or a coagulopathy or some injury causing acute exacerbation of the hypertension. In any case, the result is increased permeability of the small vessels to fibrinogen and other plasma proteins, endothelial injury, focal death of cells of the vascular wall, and platelet deposition. This leads to the appearance of *fibrinoid necrosis* of arterioles and small arteries, swelling of the vascular intima, and intravascular thrombosis. Mitogenic factors from platelets (e.g., platelet-derived growth factor [PDGF]), plasma, and other cells cause hyperplasia of intimal smooth muscle of vessels, resulting in the

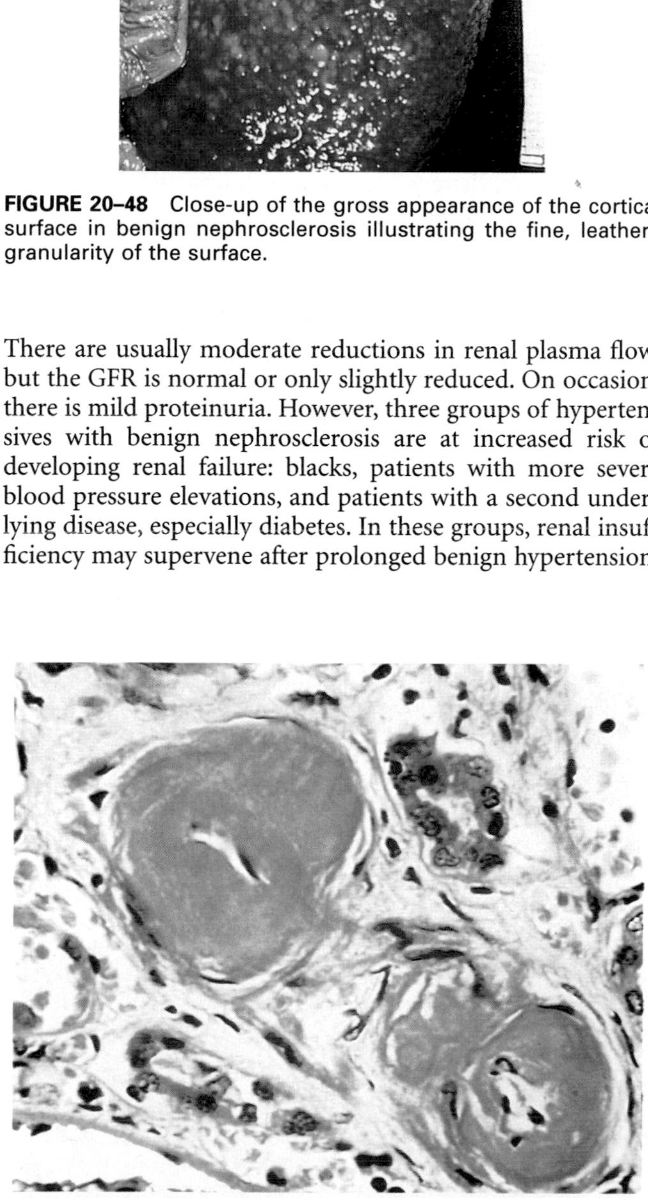

FIGURE 20–49 Hyaline arteriolosclerosis. High-power view of two arterioles with hyaline deposition, marked thickening of the walls, and a narrowed lumen. (Courtesy of Dr. M.A. Venkatachalam, Department of Pathology, University of Texas Health Sciences Center, San Antonio, TX.)

TABLE 20–12 Types of Hypertension

Primary or Essential Hypertension
Secondary Hypertension
Renal
Acute glomerulonephritis
Chronic renal disease
Renal artery stenosis
Renal vasculitis
Renin-producing tumors
Endocrine
Adrenocortical hyperfunction (Cushing syndrome)
Oral contraceptives
Pheochromocytoma
Acromegaly
Myxedema
Thyrotoxicosis (systolic hypertension)
Vascular
Coarctation of aorta
Polyarteritis nodosa
Aortic insufficiency (systolic hypertension)
Neurogenic
Psychogenic
Increased intracranial pressure
Polyneuritis, bulbar poliomyelitis, others

hyperplastic arteriolosclerosis that is typical of malignant hypertension and further narrowing of the lumens. The kidneys become markedly ischemic. With severe involvement of the renal afferent arterioles, the renin-angiotensin system receives a powerful stimulus; indeed, *patients with malignant hypertension have markedly elevated levels of plasma renin.* This then sets up a self-perpetuating cycle in which angiotensin II causes intrarenal vasoconstriction, and the attendant renal ischemia perpetuates renin secretion. Other vasoconstrictors (e.g., endothelin) and loss of vasodilators (nitric oxide) may also contribute to vasoconstriction. Aldosterone levels are also elevated, and salt retention undoubtedly contributes to the elevation of blood pressure. The consequences of the markedly elevated blood pressure on the blood vessels throughout the body are known as *malignant arteriosclerosis,* and the renal disorder is malignant nephrosclerosis.

Morphology. On gross inspection, the kidney size depends on the duration and severity of the hypertensive disease. Small, pinpoint petechial hemorrhages may appear on the cortical surface from rupture of arterioles or glomerular capillaries, giving the kidney a peculiar "flea-bitten" appearance.

Two histologic alterations characterize blood vessels in malignant hypertension (Fig. 20–50):

- **Fibrinoid necrosis of arterioles.** This appears as an eosinophilic granular change in the blood vessel wall, which stains positively for fibrin by histochemical or immunofluorescence techniques. This change represents an acute event, and it may be accompanied by limited inflammatory infiltrate within the wall. However, usually this pattern of necrosis is not accompanied by prominent inflammation.
- In the interlobular arteries and arterioles, there is intimal thickening caused by a proliferation of elongated, concentrically arranged smooth muscle cells, together with fine concentric layering of collagen and accumulation of pale staining material that likely represents accumulations of proteoglycans and plasma proteins. This alteration has been referred to as **onion-skinning** because of its concentric appearance. The lesion, also called hyperplastic arteriolitis, correlates well with renal failure in malignant hypertension. Sometimes the glomeruli become necrotic and infiltrated with neutrophils, and the glomerular capillaries may thrombose. The arteriolar and arterial lesions result in considerable narrowing of all vascular lumens, with ischemic atrophy and, at times, infarction distal to the abnormal vessels.

Clinical Course. The full-blown syndrome of malignant hypertension is characterized by diastolic pressures greater than 130 mm Hg, papilledema retinopathy, encephalopathy, cardiovascular abnormalities, and renal failure. Most often, the early symptoms are related to increased intracranial pressure and include headaches, nausea, vomiting, and visual impairments, particularly the development of scotomas or spots before the eyes. "Hypertensive crises" are sometimes encountered, characterized by episodes of loss of consciousness or even convulsions. At the onset of rapidly mounting blood pressure, there is marked proteinuria and microscopic or sometimes macroscopic hematuria but no significant alteration in renal function. Soon, however, renal failure makes its appearance. The syndrome is a true medical emergency requiring the institution of aggressive and prompt antihypertensive therapy before the development of irreversible renal lesions. Before the introduction of current antihypertensive drugs, malignant hypertension was associated with a 50% mortality rate within 3 months of onset, progressing to 90% within a year. At present, however, about 75% of patients will survive 5 years, and 50% survive with pre-crisis renal function.

RENAL ARTERY STENOSIS

Unilateral renal artery stenosis is a relatively uncommon cause of hypertension, responsible for 2% to 5% of cases, but it is of importance because it is a potentially curable form of hypertension; surgical treatment is successful in 70% to 80%

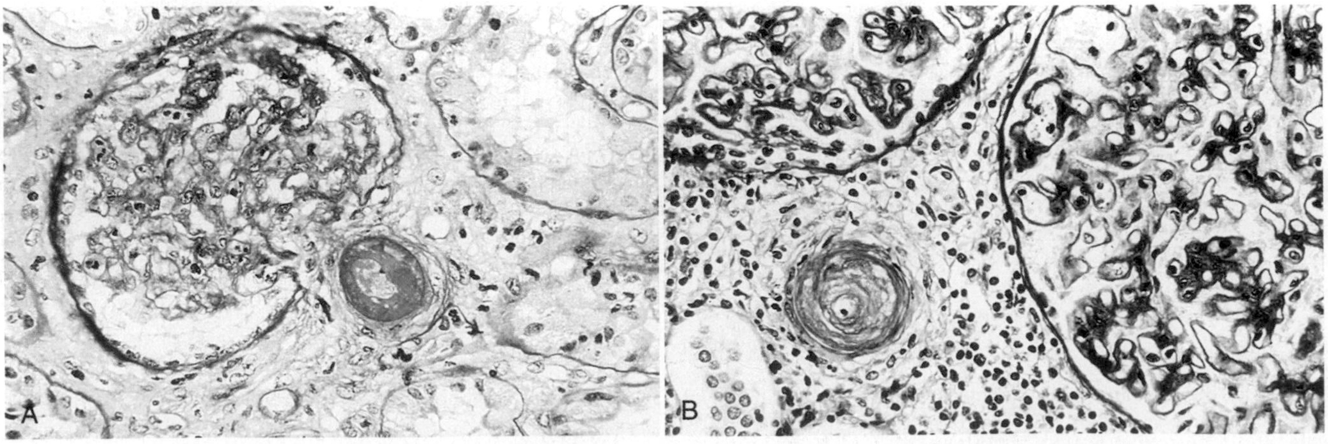

FIGURE 20–50 Malignant hypertension. *A,* Fibrinoid necrosis of afferent arteriole (PAS stain). *B,* Hyperplastic arteriolitis (onion-skin lesion). (Courtesy of Dr. H. Rennke, Brigham and Women's Hospital, Boston, MA.)

of carefully selected cases in humans.[96] Furthermore, much early knowledge of renal mechanisms in hypertension has come from studies of experimental and human renal artery stenosis.

Pathogenesis. The classic experiments of Goldblatt and colleagues[97] in 1934 showed that constriction of one renal artery in dogs results in hypertension and that the magnitude of the effect is roughly proportional to the amount of constriction. Later experiments in rats confirmed these results, and in time it was shown that the hypertensive effect, at least initially, is due to stimulation of renin secretion by cells of the juxtaglomerular apparatus and the subsequent production of the vasoconstrictor angiotensin II. *A large proportion of patients with renovascular hypertension have elevated plasma or renal vein renin levels*, and almost all show a reduction of blood pressure when given competitive antagonists of angiotensin II. Further, unilateral renal renin hypersecretion can be normalized after renal revascularization, usually resulting in a decrease in blood pressure. Other factors, however, may contribute to the maintenance of renovascular hypertension after the renin-angiotensin system has initiated it, including *sodium retention* and possibly endothelin and loss of nitric oxide.

Morphology. The most common cause of renal artery stenosis (70% of cases) is occlusion by an atheromatous plaque at the origin of the renal artery. This lesion occurs more frequently in men, and the incidence increases with advancing age and diabetes mellitus. The plaque is usually concentrically placed, and superimposed thrombosis often occurs.

The second type of lesion leading to stenosis is so-called **fibromuscular dysplasia** of the renal artery. This is a heterogeneous group of lesions characterized by fibrous or fibromuscular thickening and may involve the intima, the media, or the adventitia of the artery. These lesions are thus subclassified into **intimal**, **medial**, and **adventitial hyperplasia**, the medial type being by far the most common (Fig. 20–51). The stenoses, as a whole, are more common in women and tend to occur in younger age groups (i.e., in the third and fourth decades). The lesions may consist of a single well-defined constriction or a series of narrowings, usually in the middle or distal portion of the renal artery. They may also involve the segmental branches and may be bilateral.

The ischemic kidney is usually reduced in size and shows signs of diffuse ischemic atrophy, with crowded glomeruli, atrophic tubules, interstitial fibrosis, and focal inflammatory infiltrates. The arterioles in the ischemic kidney are usually protected from the effects of high pressure, thus showing only mild arteriolosclerosis. In contrast, the contralateral nonischemic kidney may exhibit more severe arteriolosclerosis, depending on the severity of the hypertension.

Clinical Course. Few distinctive features suggest the presence of renal artery stenosis, and in general, these patients resemble those presenting with essential hypertension. On occasion, a bruit can be heard on auscultation of the kidneys. Elevated plasma or renal vein renin, response to angiotensin-converting enzyme inhibitor, renal scans, and intravenous pyelography may aid with diagnosis, but arteriography is required to localize the stenotic lesion. As was noted, the cure rate after surgery is 70% to 80% in well-selected cases.

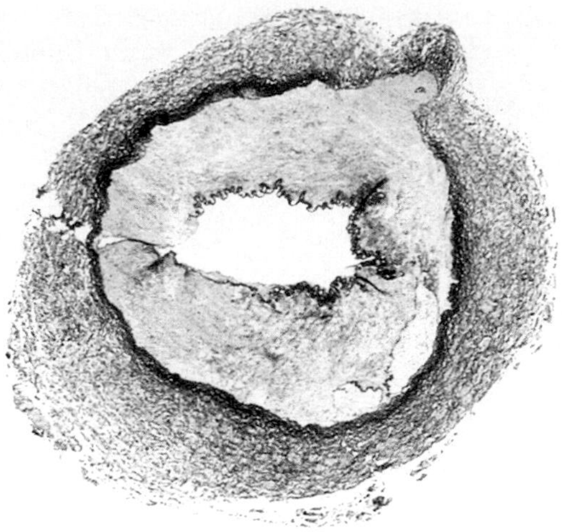

FIGURE 20–51 Fibromuscular dysplasia of the renal artery, medial type (elastic tissue stain). The medium shows marked fibrous thickening, and the lumen is stenotic. (Courtesy of Dr. Seymour Rosen, Beth Israel Hospital, Boston, MA.)

THROMBOTIC MICROANGIOPATHIES

As was described in Chapter 13, these represent a group of disorders with overlapping clinical manifestations that are *characterized morphologically by thrombosis in capillaries and arterioles throughout the body* (Fig. 20–52) *and clinically by microangiopathic hemolytic anemia, thrombocytopenia, and, in certain conditions, renal failure.*[98,99] The renal failure is associated with platelet or platelet-fibrin thrombi in the interlobular renal arteries, arterioles, and glomeruli (Fig. 20–52), together with necrosis and thickening of the vessel walls.

The classification of these diseases is somewhat muddied by the fact that two of the conditions, hemolytic-uremic syndrome (HUS) and thrombotic thrombocytopenic purpura (TTP), show considerable overlap even though they are pathogenetically distinct; indeed, they are often considered as a HUS/TTP syndrome.[98] A useful categorization by cause and condition is as follows:

1. *Classic childhood HUS*, most frequently associated with bloody diarrhea caused by intestinal infection by verocytotoxin-releasing bacteria
2. *Adult HUS*, associated with
   a. Infection
   b. Antiphospholipid antibodies
   c. Complications of pregnancy and contraceptives
   d. Vascular renal diseases such as scleroderma and hypertension
   e. Chemotherapeutic and immunosuppressive drugs
   f. Radiation
3. *Familial HUS*
4. *Idiopathic TTP*

The morphologic changes may be similar to those seen in malignant hypertension; but in these conditions, they may precede development of hypertension or may be seen in its absence.

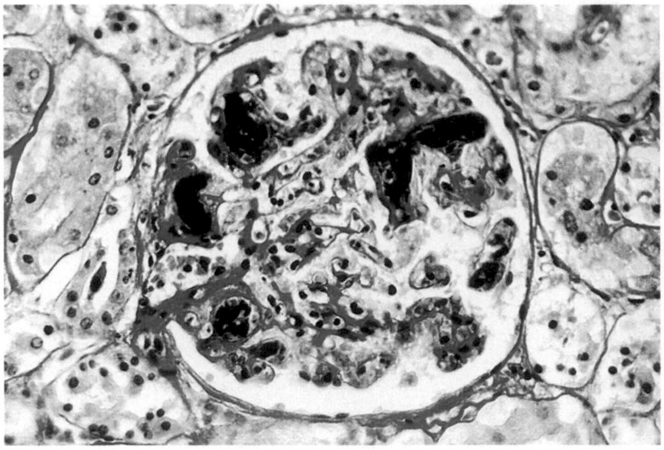

FIGURE 20–52 Fibrin stain showing platelet-fibrin thrombi (*red*) in the glomerular capillaries, characteristic of microangiopathic disorders.

Pathogenesis. Although these disorders may have diverse causes, two processes dominate the pathogenetic sequence of events: (1) *endothelial injury and activation*, with subsequent intravascular thrombosis, and (2) *platelet aggregation*. Both of these events cause *vascular obstruction* and *vasoconstriction* and thus precipitate distal ischemia.[99]

Endothelial Injury. The triggers for endothelial injury and activation, as described in Chapter 2 and Chapter 11 can be bacterial endotoxins and cytotoxins, cytokines, viruses, drugs, antiendothelial antibodies, and abnormal multimers or inhibitors of the von Willebrand coagulation factor. In childhood HUS associated with diarrheal infections, *verocytotoxin*, as we shall see, is clearly the culprit. But in many cases, the proximate endothelial toxin is unknown.

Endothelial injury may mediate the microangiopathy in several ways:

- Endothelial denudation exposes a potentially thrombogenic subendothelial connective tissue.
- Reduced production of prostaglandin I_2 and nitric oxide (both of which normally cause vasodilation and inhibit platelet aggregation) enhances platelet aggregation and causes vasoconstriction. Vasoconstriction can also be induced by endothelial-derived endothelin. Endothelial cells may also be *activated*, increasing their adhesivity to leukocytes, which themselves contribute to thrombosis, as described in Chapter 4.
- Endothelial cells elaborate multimers of von Willebrand factor that remain abnormally large, causing platelet aggregation (see below).

Platelet Aggregation. Because many thrombi in HUS/TTP are composed largely of aggregated platelets with scant fibrin, serum factors causing platelet aggregation have been sought. These include unusually large von Willebrand factor multimers that are secreted by endothelial cells. Normally, they are degraded into smaller multimers by the action of ADAMTS-13, a von Willebrand factor (vWF)-cleaving metalloprotease. With congenital or acquired loss of ADAMTS-13 activity, very large vWF multimers persist in the circulation and induce aggregation by activating platelet surface glycoproteins (Chapter 4).[99,100]

Classic (Childhood) Hemolytic-Uremic Syndrome

This is the most well characterized of the hemolytic-uremic syndromes, since as many as 75% of cases occur in children after intestinal infection with verocytotoxin-producing *E. coli* (e.g., type O157:H7).[101] Verocytotoxins (so called because they cause damage to *Vero* cells in culture) are similar to *Shiga* toxins produced by *Shigella* (Chapter 17). Some epidemics have been traced to ingestion of infected ground meat (as in hamburgers).

The disease is one of the main causes of acute renal failure in children. It is characterized by the *sudden onset, usually after a gastrointestinal or influenza-like prodromal episode, of bleeding manifestations* (especially hematemesis and melena), *severe oliguria, hematuria, a microangiopathic hemolytic anemia, and (in some patients) prominent neurologic changes.* Hypertension is present in about half the patients.

The *pathogenesis* of this syndrome is clearly related to the Shiga-like toxin. The toxin has a variety of effects on endothelium, causing increased adhesion of leukocytes; increased endothelin production and loss of endothelial nitric oxide (both favoring vasoconstriction); and in the presence of cytokines, such as tumor necrosis factor, endothelial lysis. The resultant endothelial effects enhance both thrombosis and vasoconstriction, resulting in the characteristic microangiopathy. Verocytotoxin also binds to platelets and can directly activate them.

Morphology. In gross appearance, the kidneys may show patchy or diffuse renal cortical necrosis (described later). On microscopic examination, the glomeruli show thickening and sometimes splitting of capillary walls, due largely to endothelial and subendothelial swelling, and deposits of fibrin-related materials in the capillary lumens, subendothelially, and in the mesangium. Mesangiolysis is a common finding. Interlobular and afferent arterioles show fibrinoid necrosis and intimal hyperplasia and are often occluded by thrombi.

If the renal failure is managed properly with dialysis, most patients recover in a matter of weeks. However, the long-term (15 to 25 years) prognosis is not uniformly favorable. In one study, only 10 of 25 patients had normal renal function, and seven had chronic renal failure.[102]

Adult Hemolytic-Uremic Syndrome

HUS occurs in adults under a variety of settings by mechanisms that are unclear:

1. *In association with infection*, such as typhoid fever, *E. coli* septicemia, viral infections, and shigellosis (postinfectious HUS). *Endotoxin*, or *Shiga toxin* (from *Shigella* species), plays a role in the pathogenesis of such cases.
2. In the *antiphospholipid syndrome*, either primary or secondary to SLE (lupus anticoagulant). The syndrome is described in detail in Chapter 4. The microangiopathic changes in the kidney tend to be more chronic, and healing of the thrombotic changes in glomeruli can result in changes mimicking membranoproliferative glomerulonephritis by light microscopy but without evidence of immune complex deposition.

3. As complications of pregnancy (placental hemorrhage) or the postpartum period. So-called *postpartum renal failure* usually occurs after an uneventful pregnancy, 1 day to several months after delivery, and is characterized by microangiopathic hemolytic anemia, oliguria, anuria, and initially mild hypertension. The condition has a grave prognosis, although recovery can occur in milder cases.
4. Associated with *vascular renal diseases*, such as systemic sclerosis and malignant hypertension.
5. In patients treated with chemotherapeutic and immunosuppressive drugs, such as mitomycin, cyclosporine, bleomycin, cisplatin, and radiation.

Familial HUS

About 5%–10% of cases of HUS present with recurrent thromboses, and have a much higher mortality rate (about 50%) than classical childhood HUS (less than 5%).[99] Most patients with familial HUS have an inherited deficiency of the complement regulatory protein Factor H, which normally breaks down the alternative pathway C3 convertase and protects cells from damage by uncontrolled complement activation (Chapter 2).

Idiopathic TTP

Idiopathic TTP is manifested by fever, neurologic symptoms, hemolytic anemia, thrombocytopenic purpura, and the presence of thrombi in glomerular capillaries and afferent arterioles.[99] As discussed in Chapter 13, it is caused by an acquired or genetic defect in ADAMTS-13, the protease that cleaves large von Willebrand factor (vWF) multimers.[100] The abnormal (noncleaved) forms of vWF promote platelet aggregation. The disease is more common in women, and most patients are younger than 40 years. Idiopathic TTP and various forms of HUS overlap considerably, both clinically and morphologically. In classic TTP, however, central nervous system involvement is the dominant feature, whereas renal involvement occurs in only about 50% of patients. In the kidney, eosinophilic granular thrombi are present predominantly in the terminal part of the interlobular arteries, afferent arterioles, and glomerular capillaries. Other glomerular changes are similar to those described for HUS. The thrombi are composed of platelets and fibrin and are found in arterioles of many organs throughout the body. Untreated, the disease was once highly fatal, but exchange transfusions and corticosteroid therapy have reduced mortality to less than 50%.

OTHER VASCULAR DISORDERS

Atherosclerotic Ischemic Renal Disease

We have seen that atherosclerotic unilateral artery stenosis can lead to hypertension. *Bilateral* disease, usually diagnosed definitively by arteriography, now appears to be a fairly common cause of chronic ischemia with renal insufficiency in older individuals, sometimes in the absence of hypertension.[103] The importance of recognizing this condition is that surgical revascularization is beneficial in reversing further decline in renal function.

Atheroembolic Renal Disease

Embolization of fragments of atheromatous plaques from the aorta or renal artery into intraparenchymal renal vessels occurs in elderly patients with severe atherosclerosis, especially after surgery on the abdominal aorta, aortography, or intra-aortic cannulization. These emboli can be recognized in the lumens and walls of arcuate and interlobular arteries by their content of cholesterol crystals, which appear as rhomboid clefts (Fig. 20–53). The clinical consequences of atheroemboli vary according to the number of emboli and the preexisting state of renal function. Frequently, they have no functional significance. However, acute renal failure may develop in elderly patients in whom renal function is already compromised, principally after abdominal surgery on atherosclerotic aneurysms.

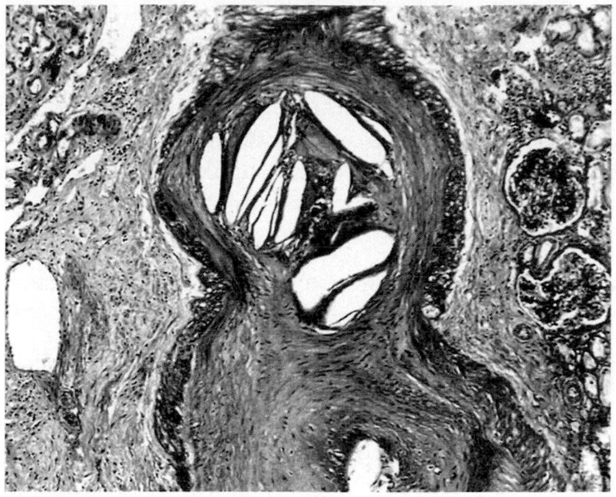

FIGURE 20–53 Atheroemboli with typical cholesterol clefts in an interlobar artery.

Sickle Cell Disease Nephropathy

Sickle cell disease in both the homozygous and the heterozygous forms may lead to a variety of alterations in renal morphology and function, some of which, fortunately uncommonly, produce clinically significant abnormalities. The various manifestations are termed sickle cell nephropathy.

The most common clinical and functional abnormalities are *hematuria* and a *diminished concentrating ability*. These are thought to be due largely to accelerated sickling in the hypertonic hypoxic milieu of the renal medulla, which increases the viscosity of the blood during its passage through the vasa recta, leading to plugging of vessels and decreased flow. Patchy *papillary necrosis* may occur in both homozygotes and heterozygotes; this is sometimes associated with cortical scarring. *Proteinuria* is also common in sickle cell disease, occurring in about 30% of patients. It is usually mild to moderate, but on occasion, the overt nephrotic syndrome arises, associated with sclerosing glomerular lesions.

Diffuse Cortical Necrosis

This is an uncommon condition that occurs most frequently after an obstetric emergency, such as abruptio placentae (premature separation of the placenta), septic shock, or extensive surgery. When bilateral and symmetric, it can be fatal in the absence of supportive therapy, but patchy cortical necrosis may permit survival. The cortical destruction has the features of ischemic necrosis. Glomerular and arteriolar microthrombi are found in most cases; they clearly contribute to the necrosis and renal damage. The morphologic features have considerable overlap with thrombotic microangiopathy and disseminated intravascular coagulation, but the pathogenetic sequence of events in this injury remains obscure.

Morphology. The gross alterations of massive ischemic necrosis are sharply limited to the cortex (Fig. 20–54). The histologic appearance is that of acute ischemic infarction. The lesions may be patchy, with areas of coagulative necrosis and apparently better-preserved cortex. Intravascular and intraglomerular thromboses may be prominent but are usually focal, and acute necroses of small arterioles and capillaries may occasionally be present. Hemorrhages occur into the glomeruli, together with the formation of fibrin plugs in the glomerular capillaries.

Massive acute cortical necrosis is of grave significance, since it gives rise to sudden anuria, terminating rapidly in uremic death. Instances of unilateral or patchy involvement are compatible with survival.

Renal Infarcts

The kidneys are favored sites for the development of infarcts. Contributing to this predisposition is the extensive blood flow to the kidneys (one fourth of the cardiac output), but likely more important is the "end-organ" nature of the arterial blood supply with extremely limited collateral circulation from extrarenal sites (essentially small blood vessels penetrating from the renal capsule). Although thrombosis in advanced atherosclerosis and the acute vasculitis of polyarteritis nodosa may occlude arteries, most infarcts are due to embolism. A major source of such emboli is mural thrombosis in the left atrium and ventricle as a result of myocardial infarction. Vegetative endocarditis, thrombosis in aortic aneurysms, and aortic atherosclerosis are less frequent sites for the origin of emboli.

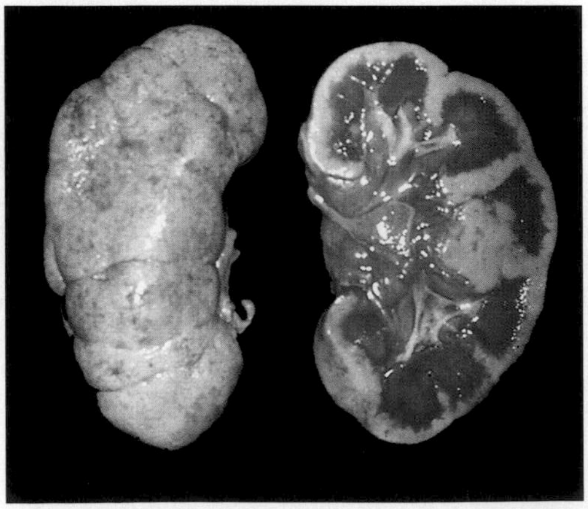

FIGURE 20–54 Diffuse cortical necrosis. The pale ischemic necrotic areas are confined to the cortex and columns of Bertin.

Morphology. Because the arterial supply to the kidney is of the end-organ type, most infarcts are of the "white" anemic type. They may occur as solitary lesions or may be multiple and bilateral. Within 24 hours, infarcts become sharply demarcated, pale, yellow-white areas that may contain small irregular foci of hemorrhagic discoloration. They are usually ringed by a zone of intense hyperemia.

On section, the infarcts are wedge-shaped, with the base against the cortical surface and the apex pointing toward the medulla. There may be a narrow rim of preserved subcortical tissue that has been spared by the collateral capsular circulation. In time, these acute areas of ischemic necrosis undergo progressive fibrous scarring, giving rise to depressed, pale, gray-white scars that assume a V shape on section. The histologic changes in renal infarction are those of ischemic coagulation necrosis, described in Chapter 1.

Many renal infarcts are clinically silent. Sometimes, pain with tenderness localized to the costovertebral angle occurs, and this is associated with showers of red cells in the urine. Large infarcts of one kidney are likely associated with narrowing of the renal artery or one of its major branches, which in turn may be a cause of hypertension.

Urinary Tract Obstruction (Obstructive Uropathy)

Recognition of urinary obstruction is important because *obstruction increases susceptibility to infection and to stone formation, and unrelieved obstruction almost always leads to permanent renal atrophy*, termed *hydronephrosis* or *obstructive uropathy*. Fortunately, many causes of obstruction are surgically correctable or medically treatable.

Obstruction may be sudden or insidious, partial or complete, unilateral or bilateral; it may occur at any level of the urinary tract from the urethra to the renal pelvis. It can be caused by lesions that are *intrinsic* to the urinary tract or *extrinsic* lesions that compress the ureter.[104] The common causes are as follows (Fig. 20–55):

1. *Congenital anomalies:* posterior urethral valves and urethral strictures, meatal stenosis, bladder neck obstruction; ureteropelvic junction narrowing or obstruction; severe vesicoureteral reflux
2. *Urinary calculi*
3. *Benign prostatic hypertrophy*
4. *Tumors:* carcinoma of the prostate, bladder tumors, contiguous malignant disease (retroperitoneal lymphoma), carcinoma of the cervix or uterus
5. *Inflammation:* prostatitis, ureteritis, urethritis, retroperitoneal fibrosis
6. *Sloughed papillae or blood clots*
7. *Normal pregnancy*
8. *Uterine prolapse and cystocele*
9. *Functional disorders:* neurogenic (spinal cord damage or diabetic nephropathy) and other functional abnormal-

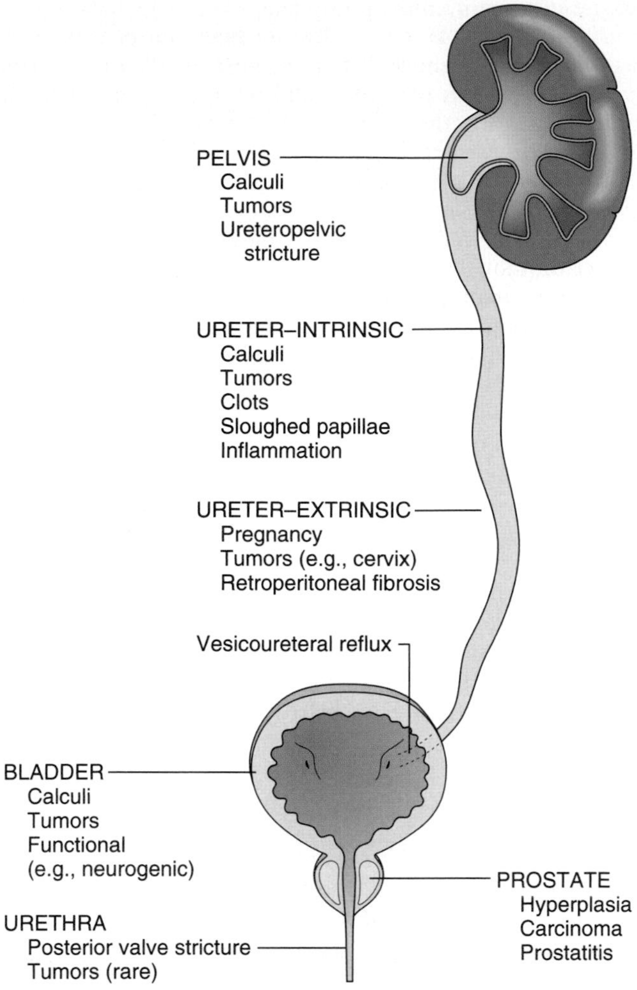

FIGURE 20–55 Obstructive lesions of the urinary tract.

ities of the ureter or bladder (often termed *dysfunctional obstruction*)

Hydronephrosis is the term used to describe dilation of the renal pelvis and calyces associated with progressive atrophy of the kidney due to obstruction to the outflow of urine. Even with complete obstruction, glomerular filtration persists for some time because the filtrate subsequently diffuses back into the renal interstitium and perirenal spaces, where it ultimately returns to the lymphatic and venous systems. Because of this continued filtration, the affected calyces and pelvis become dilated, often markedly so. The high pressure in the pelvis is transmitted back through the collecting ducts into the cortex, causing renal atrophy, but it also compresses the renal vasculature of the medulla, causing a diminution in inner medullary plasma flow. The medullary vascular defects are reversible, but if they are protracted, obstruction will lead to medullary functional disturbances. Accordingly, the initial functional alterations are largely tubular, manifested primarily by impaired concentrating ability. Only later does the GFR begin to diminish. *Obstruction also triggers an interstitial inflammatory reaction, leading eventually to interstitial fibrosis,* by mechanisms similar to those discussed earlier (see Fig. 20–15).[104]

Morphology. When the obstruction is sudden and complete, the reduction of glomerular filtration usually leads to mild dilation of the pelvis and calyces but sometimes to atrophy of the renal parenchyma. When the obstruction is subtotal or intermittent, glomerular filtration is not suppressed, and progressive dilation ensues. Depending on the level of urinary block, the dilation may affect first the bladder or ureter and then the kidney.

In gross appearance, the kidney may have slight to massive enlargement. The earlier features are those of simple dilation of the pelvis and calyces, but in addition, there is often significant interstitial inflammation, even in the absence of infection. In chronic cases, the picture is one of cortical tubular atrophy with marked diffuse interstitial fibrosis. Progressive blunting of the apices of the pyramids occurs, and these eventually become cupped. In far-advanced cases, the kidney may become transformed into a thin-walled cystic structure having a diameter of up to 15 to 20 cm (Fig. 20–56) with striking parenchymal atrophy, total obliteration of the pyramids, and thinning of the cortex.

Clinical Course. *Acute obstruction* may provoke pain attributed to distention of the collecting system or renal capsule. Most of the early symptoms are produced by the underlying cause of the hydronephrosis. Thus, calculi lodged in the ureters may give rise to renal colic, and prostatic enlargements may give rise to bladder symptoms.

Unilateral, complete, or partial hydronephrosis may remain silent for long periods, since the unaffected kidney can maintain adequate renal function. Sometimes its existence first

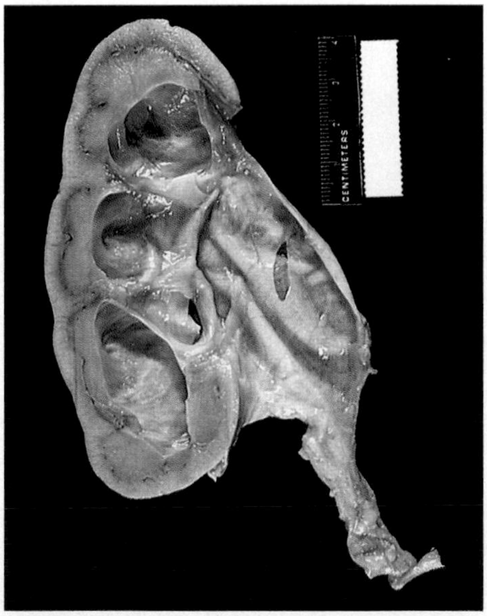

FIGURE 20–56 Hydronephrosis of the kidney, with marked dilation of the pelvis and calyces and thinning of the renal parenchyma.

becomes apparent in the course of intravenous pyelography. It is regrettable that this disease tends to remain asymptomatic, because it has been shown that in its early stages, perhaps the first few weeks, relief of obstruction leads to reversion to normal function. *Ultrasonography* is a useful noninvasive technique in the diagnosis of obstructive uropathy.

In *bilateral partial obstruction,* the earliest manifestation is inability to concentrate the urine, reflected by polyuria and nocturia. Some patients have acquired distal tubular acidosis, renal salt wasting, secondary renal calculi, *and a typical picture of tubulointerstitial nephritis* with scarring and atrophy of the papilla and medulla. Hypertension is common in such patients.

Complete bilateral obstruction results in oliguria or anuria and is incompatible with long survival unless the obstruction is relieved. Curiously, after relief of complete urinary tract obstruction, postobstructive *diuresis* occurs. This can often be massive, with the kidney excreting large amounts of urine that is rich in sodium chloride.

Urolithiasis (Renal Calculi, Stones)

Stones may form at any level in the urinary tract, but most arise in the kidney. Urolithiasis is a frequent clinical problem, affecting 5% to 10% of Americans in their lifetime.[105] Men are affected more often than women are, and the peak age at onset is between 20 and 30 years. Familial and hereditary predisposition to stone formation has long been known. Many of the inborn errors of metabolism, such as gout, cystinuria, and primary hyperoxaluria, provide good examples of hereditary disease characterized by excessive production and excretion of stone-forming substances.

Cause and Pathogenesis. There are four main types of calculi[106,107] (Table 20–13): (1) *most stones (about 70%) are calcium containing,* composed largely of calcium oxalate or calcium oxalate mixed with calcium phosphate; (2) another 15% are so-called *triple stones* or *struvite stones,* composed of magnesium ammonium phosphate; (3) *5% to 10% are uric acid stones;* and (4) *1% to 2% are made up of cystine.* An organic matrix of mucoprotein, making up 1% to 5% of the stone by weight, is present in all calculi. Although there are many causes for the initiation and propagation of stones, *the most important determinant is an increased urinary concentration of the stones' constituents, such that it exceeds their solubility in urine (supersaturation). A low urine volume* in some metabolically normal patients may also favor supersaturation.

TABLE 20–13 Prevalence of Various Types of Renal Stones

	Percentage of All Stones
Calcium Oxalate and Phosphate	70

Idiopathic hypercalciuria (50%)
Hypercalciuria and hypercalcemia (10%)
Hyperoxaluria (5%)
  Enteric (4.5%)
  Primary (0.5%)
Hyperuricosuria (20%)
Hypocitraturia
No known metabolic abnormality (15–20%)	

Magnesium Ammonium Phosphate (Struvite)	15–20
Uric Acid Associated with hyperuricemia Associated with hyperuricosuria Idiopathic (50% of uric stones)	5–10
Cystine	1–2
Others or Unknown	±5

Calcium oxalate stones (Table 20–13) are associated in about 5% of patients with both *hypercalcemia* and *hypercalciuria,* caused by hyperparathyroidism, diffuse bone disease, sarcoidosis, and other hypercalcemic states. About 55% have *hypercalciuria without hypercalcemia.* This is caused by several factors, including hyperabsorption of calcium from the intestine (absorptive hypercalciuria), an intrinsic impairment in renal tubular reabsorption of calcium (renal hypercalciuria), or idiopathic fasting hypercalciuria with normal parathyroid function. As many as 20% of calcium oxalate stones are associated with increased uric acid secretion (*hyperuricosuric calcium nephrolithiasis*), with or without hypercalciuria. The mechanism of stone formation in this setting involves "nucleation" of calcium oxalate by uric acid crystals in the collecting ducts. Five per cent are associated with *hyperoxaluria,* either hereditary (primary oxaluria) or, more commonly, acquired by intestinal overabsorption in patients with enteric diseases. The latter, so-called enteric hyperoxaluria, also occurs in vegetarians, because much of their diet is rich in oxalates. *Hypocitraturia* associated with acidosis and chronic diarrhea of unknown cause may produce calcium stones. *In a variable proportion of patients with calcium stones,* no cause can be found (idiopathic calcium stone disease).

Magnesium ammonium phosphate stones are formed largely after infections by urea-splitting bacteria (e.g., *Proteus* and some staphylococci), which convert urea to ammonia. The resultant alkaline urine causes the precipitation of magnesium ammonium phosphate salts. These form some of the largest stones, as the amounts of urea excreted normally are huge. Indeed, so-called *staghorn calculi* occupying large portions of the renal pelvis are almost always a consequence of infection.

Uric acid stones are common in patients with hyperuricemia, such as gout, and diseases involving rapid cell turnover, such as the leukemias. However, *more than half of all patients with urate calculi have neither hyperuricemia nor increased urinary excretion of uric acid.* In this group, it is thought that an unexplained tendency to excrete urine of pH below 5.5 may predispose to uric acid stones, because uric acid is insoluble in relatively acidic urine. In contrast to the radio-opaque calcium stones, uric acid stones are radiolucent.

Cystine stones are caused by genetic defects in the renal reabsorption of amino acids, including cystine, leading to cystinuria. Stones form at low urinary pH.

It can therefore be appreciated that increased concentration of stone constituents, changes in urinary pH, decreased urine volume, and the presence of bacteria influence the formation of calculi. *However, many calculi occur in the absence of these factors; conversely, patients with hypercalciuria, hyperoxaluria, and hyperuricosuria often do not form stones.* It has therefore been postulated that stone formation is enhanced by a *deficiency in inhibitors of crystal formation in urine.* The list of such inhibitors is long, including pyrophosphate, diphosphonate, citrate, glycosaminoglycans, osteopontin, and a glycoprotein called *nephrocalcin*.

Morphology. Stones are unilateral in about 80% of patients. The favored sites for their formation are within the renal calyces and pelves (Fig. 20–57) and in the bladder. If formed in the renal pelvis, they tend to remain small, having an average diameter of 2 to 3 mm. These may have smooth contours or may take the form of an irregular, jagged mass of spicules. Often, many stones are found within one kidney. On occasion, progressive accretion of salts leads to the development of branching structures known as staghorn stones, which create a cast of the pelvic and calyceal system.

Clinical Course. Stones are of importance when they obstruct urinary flow or produce ulceration and bleeding. They may be present without producing any symptoms or significant renal damage. In general, smaller stones are most hazardous, because they may pass into the ureters, producing pain referred to as colic (one of the most intense forms of pain) as well as ureteral obstruction. Larger stones cannot enter the ureters and are more likely to remain silent within the renal pelvis. Commonly, these larger stones first manifest themselves by hematuria. Stones also predispose to superimposed infection, both by their obstructive nature and by the trauma they produce.

Tumors of the Kidney

Both benign and malignant tumors occur in the kidney.[108,109] With the exception of oncocytoma, the benign tumors rarely cause clinical problems. Malignant tumors, on the other hand, are of great importance clinically and deserve considerable emphasis. By far the most common of these malignant tumors is renal cell carcinoma, followed by Wilms tumor, which is found in children and is described in Chapter 10, and finally urothelial tumors of the calyces and pelves.

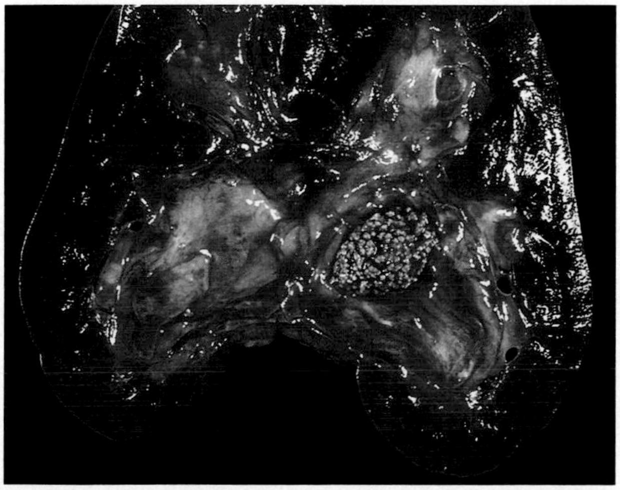

FIGURE 20–57 Nephrolithiasis. A large stone impacted in the renal pelvis. (Courtesy of Dr. E. Mosher, Brigham and Women's Hospital, Boston, MA.)

BENIGN TUMORS

Renal Papillary Adenoma

Small, discrete adenomas arising from the renal tubular epithelium are found commonly (7% to 22%) at autopsy. They are most frequently papillary and are therefore called *papillary adenomas* in the most recent international classifications.[108]

Morphology. These are small tumors, usually less than 5 mm in diameter.[108] They are present invariably within the cortex and appear grossly as pale yellow-gray, discrete, well-circumscribed nodules. On microscopic examination, they are composed of complex, branching, papillomatous structures with numerous complex fronds. Cells may also grow as tubules, glands, cords, and sheets of cells. The cells are cuboidal to polygonal in shape and have regular, small central nuclei, scanty cytoplasm, and no atypia.

By histologic criteria, these tumors do not differ from low-grade papillary renal cell adenocarcinoma and indeed share some immunohistochemical and cytogenetic features (trisomies 7 and 17) with papillary cancers, to be discussed later, although less extensively. The size of the tumor was once used as a prognostic feature, with a cutoff of 3 cm separating those that metastasize from those that rarely do. However, because tumors of relatively small size, 1 to 3 cm in diameter, are increasingly being detected during X-ray procedures performed for nonrenal symptoms and because of occasional reports of small tumors that have metastasized, the current view is to consider and treat all adenomas, regardless of size, as early cancers until an unequivocal marker of benignity is discovered.

Renal Fibroma or Hamartoma (Renomedullary Interstitial Cell Tumor)

On occasion, at autopsy, small foci of gray-white firm tissue, usually less than 1 cm in diameter, are found within the pyramids of the kidneys. Microscopic examination of these nodules discloses fibroblast-like cells and collagenous tissue. Ultrastructurally, the cells have features of renal interstitial cells. The tumors have no malignant propensities.

Angiomyolipoma

This is a benign tumor consisting of vessels, smooth muscle, and fat. *Angiomyolipomas are present in 25% to 50% of patients with tuberous sclerosis,* a disease characterized by lesions of the cerebral cortex that produce epilepsy and mental retardation as well as a variety of skin abnormalities (Chapter 25).

Oncocytoma

This is an epithelial tumor composed of large, eosinophilic cells having small, round, benign-appearing nuclei that have large nucleoli. It is thought to arise from the intercalated cells of collecting ducts. It is not an uncommon tumor, accounting for approximately 5% to 15% of surgically resected renal neoplasms. *Ultrastructurally, the eosinophilic cells have numerous mitochondria.* In gross appearance, the tumors are tan or mahogany brown, relatively homogeneous, and usually well encapsulated. However, they may achieve a large size (up to 12 cm in diameter). Although anecdotal cases with metastases have been reported, the tumor is considered benign. There are some familial cases in which these tumors are multicentric rather than solitary.

MALIGNANT TUMORS

Renal Cell Carcinoma (Adenocarcinoma of the Kidney)

Renal cell carcinomas represent about 1% to 3% of all visceral cancers and account for 85% of renal cancers in adults. There are 30,000 new cases per year and 12,000 deaths from the disease.[110] The tumors occur most often in older individuals, usually in the sixth and seventh decades of life, showing a male preponderance in the ratio of 2 to 3:1. Because of their gross yellow color and the resemblance of the tumor cells to clear cells of the adrenal cortex, they were at one time called *hypernephroma*. It is now clear that all these tumors arise from tubular epithelium and are therefore renal adenocarcinomas.

Epidemiology. Tobacco is the most significant risk factor. Cigarette smokers have double the incidence of renal cell carcinoma than do non-smokers, and pipe and cigar smokers are also more susceptible. An international study has identified additional risk factors, including obesity (particularly in women); hypertension; unopposed estrogen therapy; and exposure to asbestos, petroleum products, and heavy metals.[110] There is also increased incidence in patients with chronic renal failure and acquired cystic disease (see earlier) and in tuberous sclerosis.

Most renal cancer is sporadic, but unusual forms of autosomal-dominant familial cancers occur, usually in younger individuals. Although they account for only 4% of renal cancers, familial variants have been enormously instructive in studying renal carcinogenesis.

- *Von Hippel-Lindau (VHL) syndrome:* Half to two-thirds of patients with VHL (Chapter 28), characterized by hemangioblastomas of the cerebellum and retina, develop renal cysts and bilateral, often multiple, renal cell carcinomas (nearly all, if they live long enough). As we shall see, *current studies implicate the VHL gene in the development of both familial and sporadic clear cell tumors.*
- *Hereditary (familial) clear cell carcinoma*, confined to the kidney, without the other manifestations of VHL but with abnormalities involving the same or a related gene.
- *Hereditary papillary carcinoma.* This autosomal-dominant form is manifested by multiple bilateral tumors with papillary histology. These tumors exhibit a series of cytogenetic abnormalities and, as will be described, mutations in the *MET* protooncogene.

Classification of Renal Cell Carcinoma: Histology, Cytogenetics, and Genetics. The classification of renal cell carcinoma has recently undergone revision, based on correlative cytogenetic, genetic, and histologic studies of both familial and sporadic tumors.[109,111] The major types of tumor are as follows (Fig. 20–58):

1. *Clear cell carcinoma.* This is the most common type, accounting for 70% to 80% of renal cell cancers. On histologic examination, the tumors are made up of cells with clear or granular cytoplasm and are *nonpapillary*. They can be familial, associated with VHL disease, or in most cases (95%) sporadic. In 98% of these tumors, *whether familial, sporadic, or associated with VHL*, there is loss of sequences on the short arm of chromosome 3. This occurs by deletion (3p–) or by unbalanced chromosomal translocation (3;6, 3;8, 3;11) resulting in loss of chromosome 3 spanning 3p12 to 3p26. This region harbors the *VHL* gene (3p25.3).[111] A second nondeleted allele of the *VHL* gene shows somatic mutations or hypermethylation-induced inactivation in about 80% of clear cell cancers, indicating that the *VHL* gene acts as a tumor-suppressor gene in both sporadic and familial cancers (Chapter 7). The *VHL* gene encodes a protein that is part of a ubiquitin ligase complex involved in targeting other proteins for degradation.[112] Important among the targets of the VHL protein is hypoxia-inducible factor-1 (HIF-1). When VHL is mutated, HIF-1 levels remain high, and this constitutively active protein increases the transcription and production of hypoxia-inducible, pro-angiogenic proteins such as VEGF and TGF-β1. In addition, insulin-like growth factor-1, another VHL target, is upregulated. Thus, both cell growth and angiogenesis are stimulated. At least two other tumor-suppressor genes have also been mapped to 3p.[113]
2. *Papillary carcinoma* accounts for 10% to 15% of renal cancers.[108] It is characterized by a papillary growth pattern and also occurs in both familial and sporadic forms. These tumors are not associated with 3p deletions. The most common cytogenetic abnormalities are trisomies 7, 16, and 17 and loss of Y in male patients in the sporadic form, and trisomy 7 in the familial form. The gene for the familial form has been mapped to a locus on chromosome 7, encompassing the locus for *MET*, a protooncogene that serves as the tyrosine kinase receptor for *hepatocyte growth factor*. This gene has also been shown to be mutated in a proportion of the sporadic cases of papillary carcinoma. Described in Chapter 3, hepatocyte growth factor (also called scatter factor) mediates growth, cell mobility, invasion, and morphogenetic differentiation.[111] Both germline and somatic mutations in the tyrosine kinase domain of the *MET* gene have been identified, making mutated *MET* a likely candidate oncogene in these cancers. A second gene, called *PRCC* (for papillary renal cell carcinoma), on chromosome 1, has also been implicated in sporadic tumors, largely in children, exhibiting characteristic t (X;1) translocations.[114] This causes PRCC to fuse with a gene called TFE-3 on the X chromosome, and the fusion protein dysregulates mitotic checkpoints, allowing abnormal segregation of chromosomes. Unlike clear cell carcinomas, papillary carcinomas are frequently multifocal in origin.
3. *Chromophobe renal carcinoma* represents 5% of renal cell cancers and is composed of cells with prominent cell membranes and pale eosinophilic cytoplasm, usually with a halo around the nucleus. On cytogenetic examination, these tumors exhibit multiple chromosome losses and extreme hypodiploidy. They are, like the benign oncocytoma,

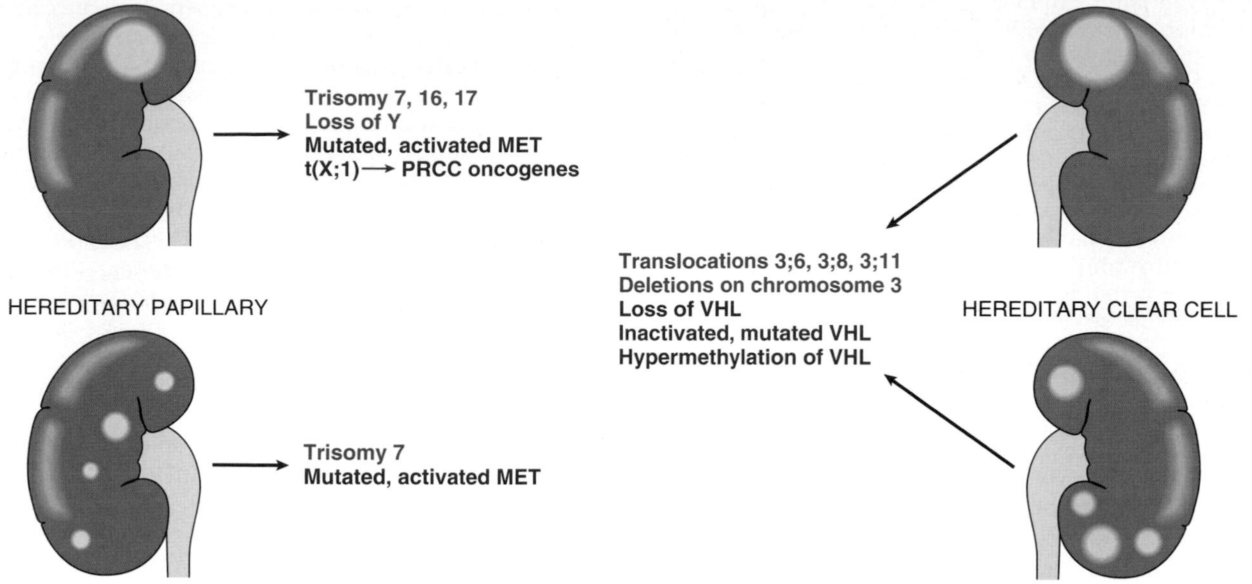

FIGURE 20–58 Cytogenetics (*blue*) and genetics (*red*) of clear cell versus papillary renal cell carcinoma. (Courtesy of Dr. Keith Ligon, Brigham and Women's Hospital, Boston, MA.)

thought to grow from intercalated cells of collecting ducts and have an excellent prognosis compared with that of the clear cell and papillary cancers. Histologic distinction from oncocytoma can be difficult.

4. Collecting duct (Bellini duct) carcinoma represents approximately 1% or less of renal epithelial neoplasms. They arise from collecting duct cells in the medulla. A number of chromosomal losses and deletions have been described for this tumor, but a distinct pattern has not been identified. Histologically, these tumors are characterized by nests of malignant cells enmeshed within a prominent fibrotic stroma, typically in a medullary location.

Morphology. Renal cell carcinomas have a characteristic macroscopic appearance. The tumor may arise in any portion of the kidney, but more commonly, it affects the poles, particularly the upper one. Clear cell neoplasms arise most likely from proximal tubular epithelium, and occur as solitary unilateral lesions. They are spherical masses, which can vary in size, composed of bright yellow-gray-white tissue that distorts the renal outline. The yellow color is a consequence of the prominent lipid accumulations in tumor cells. There are commonly large areas of ischemic, opaque, gray-white necrosis, foci of hemorrhagic discoloration, and areas of softening. The margins are usually sharply defined and confined within the renal capsule (Fig. 20–59). **Papillary tumors**, thought to arise from distal convoluted tubules, can be multifocal and bilateral. They are typically hemorrhagic and cystic, especially when large. Papillary carcinomas are the most common type of renal cancer in patients who develop dialysis-associated cystic disease.

As tumors enlarge, they may bulge into the calyces and pelvis and eventually may fungate through the walls of the collecting system to extend even into the ureter. One of the striking characteristics of this tumor is its tendency to invade the renal vein (Fig. 20–59) and grow as a solid column of cells within this vessel. Further extension produces a continuous cord of tumor in the inferior vena cava and even in the right side of the heart.

In **clear cell carcinoma,** the growth pattern varies from solid to trabecular (cordlike) or tubular (resembling tubules). The tumor cells have a rounded or polygonal shape and abundant clear or granular cyto-

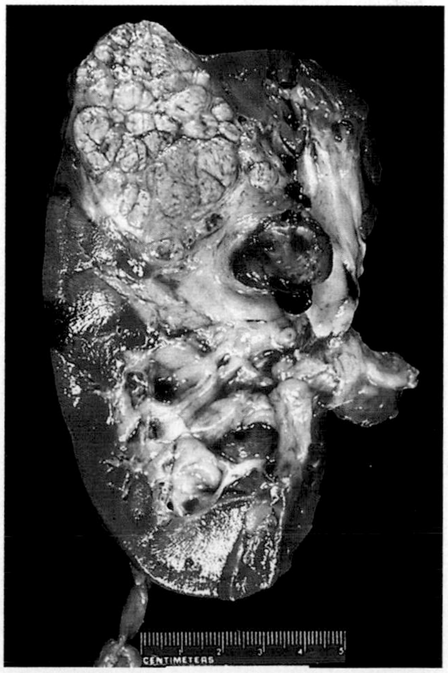

FIGURE 20–59 Renal cell carcinoma. Typical cross-section of yellowish, spherical neoplasm in one pole of the kidney. Note the tumor in the dilated thrombosed renal vein.

plasm; the latter on special stains contains glycogen and lipids (Fig. 20–60*A*). The tumors have delicate branching vasculature and may exhibit cystic as well as solid areas. Most tumors are well differentiated, but some show marked nuclear atypia with formation of bizarre nuclei and giant cells. **Papillary carcinoma** is composed of cuboidal or low columnar cells arranged in papillary formations. Interstitial foam cells are common in the papillary cores (Fig. 20–60*B*). Psammoma bodies may be present. The stroma is usually scanty but highly vascularized. **Chromophobe renal carcinoma** is made up of pale eosinophilic cells, often with a perinuclear halo, arranged in solid sheets with a concentration of the largest cells around blood vessels (Fig. 20–60*C*). **Collecting duct carcinoma** is a rare variant showing irregular channels lined by highly atypical epithelium with a hobnail pattern. Sarcomatoid changes arise infrequently in all types of renal cell carcinoma and are a decidedly ominous feature of these tumors.

Clinical Course. The three classic diagnostic features of renal cell carcinoma are *costovertebral pain, palpable mass,* and *hematuria,* but these are seen in only 10% of cases. The most reliable of the three is hematuria, but it is usually intermittent and may be microscopic; thus, the tumor may remain silent until it attains a large size. At this time, it gives rise to generalized constitutional symptoms, such as fever, malaise, weakness, and weight loss. This pattern of asymptomatic growth occurs in many patients, so the tumor may have reached a diameter of more than 10 cm when it is discovered. In current times, however, many of these tumors are being discovered in the asymptomatic state by incidental radiologic studies (e.g., computed tomographic scan or magnetic resonance imaging) usually performed for nonrenal indications.

Renal cell carcinoma is classified as one of the great mimics in medicine because it tends to produce a diversity of systemic symptoms not related to the kidney. In addition to the fever and constitutional symptoms mentioned earlier, renal cell carcinomas produce a number of paraneoplastic syndromes (Chapter 7), ascribed to abnormal hormone production, including *polycythemia, hypercalcemia, hypertension, hepatic dysfunction, feminization or masculinization, Cushing syndrome, eosinophilia, leukemoid reactions, and amyloidosis.*

One of the common characteristics of this tumor is its *tendency to metastasize widely before giving rise to any local symptoms or signs.* In 25% of new patients with renal cell carcinoma, there is radiologic evidence of metastases at the time of presentation. The most common locations of metastasis are the lungs (more than 50%) and bones (33%), followed in order by the regional lymph nodes, liver and adrenals, and brain.

The average 5-year survival rate of patients with renal cell carcinoma is about 45% and up to 70% in the absence of distant metastases. With renal vein invasion or extension into the perinephric fat, the figure is reduced to approximately 15% to 20%. Nephrectomy has been the treatment of choice, but partial nephrectomy to preserve renal function is being done with increasing frequency and similar outcome.

Urothelial Carcinomas of the Renal Pelvis

Approximately 5% to 10% of primary renal tumors originate from the urothelium of the renal pelvis (Fig. 20–61).

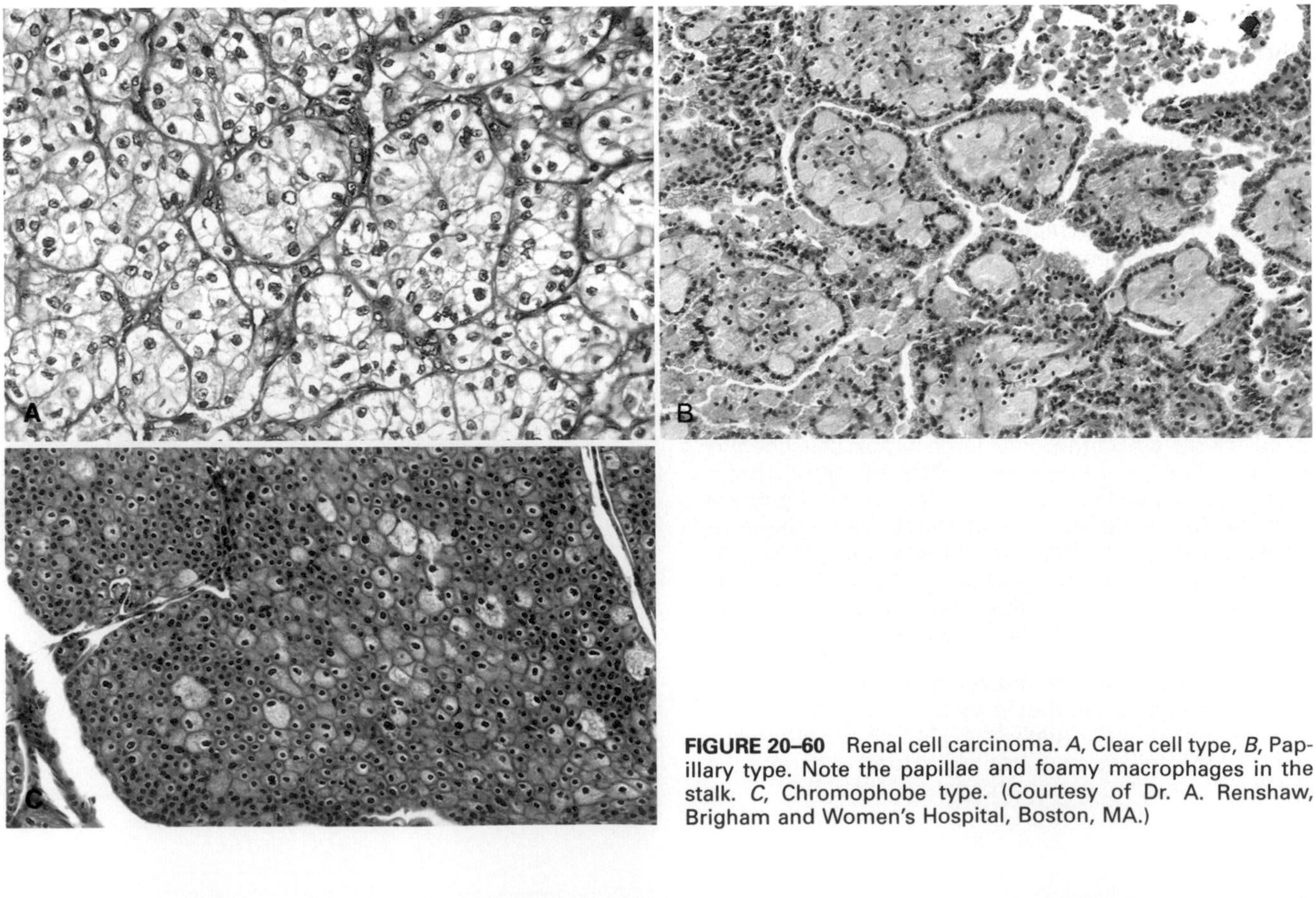

FIGURE 20–60 Renal cell carcinoma. *A,* Clear cell type, *B,* Papillary type. Note the papillae and foamy macrophages in the stalk. *C,* Chromophobe type. (Courtesy of Dr. A. Renshaw, Brigham and Women's Hospital, Boston, MA.)

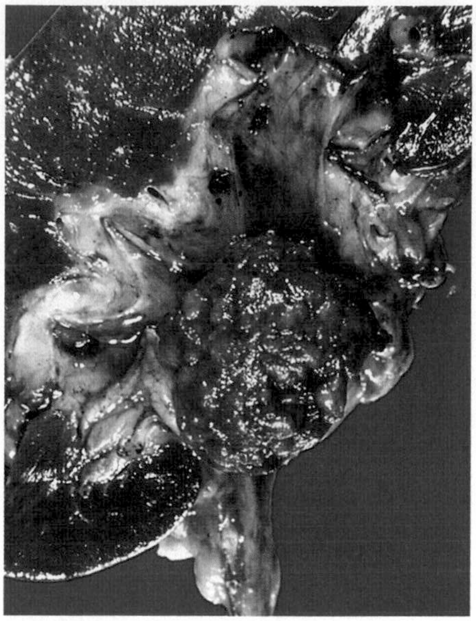

FIGURE 20–61 Urothelial carcinoma of the renal pelvis. The pelvis has been opened to expose the nodular irregular neoplasm, just proximal to the ureter.

These tumors span the range from apparently benign papillomas to invasive urothelial (transitional cell) carcinomas.

Renal pelvic tumors usually become clinically apparent within a relatively short time because they lie within the pelvis and, by fragmentation, produce noticeable hematuria. They are almost invariably small when discovered. These tumors are almost never palpable clinically; however, they may block the urinary outflow and lead to palpable hydronephrosis and flank pain. On histologic examination, pelvic tumors are the exact counterpart of those found in the urinary bladder; further details are in Chapter 21.

Urothelial tumors may occasionally be multiple, involving the pelvis, ureters, and bladder. In 50% of renal pelvic tumors, there is a preexisting or concomitant bladder urothelial tumor. On histologic examination, there are also foci of atypia or carcinoma in situ in grossly normal urothelium remote from the pelvic tumor. There is an increased incidence of urothelial carcinomas of the renal pelvis and bladder in patients with analgesic nephropathy.

Infiltration of the wall of the pelvis and calyces is common. For this reason, despite their apparently small, deceptively benign appearance, the prognosis for these tumors is not good. Five-year survival rates vary from 50% to 70% for low-grade superficial lesions to 10% with high-grade infiltrating tumors.

REFERENCES

1. Dinesen I: Seven Gothic Tales. New York, Modern Library, 1939.
2. Kanwar YS, Venkatachalam MA: Morphology of the glomerulus and juxtaglomerular apparatus. In Handbook of Physiology, Section of Renal Physiology, 2nd ed. Washington, DC, American Physiological Society, 1990.
3. Miner JH: Renal basement membrane components. Kidney Int 56:2016, 1999.
4. Timpl R, Brown JC: Supramolecular assembly of basement membranes. Bioassays 18:123, 1997.
5. Sundaramoorthy M, Meiyappan M, Todd P, Hudson BG: Crystal structure of NC1 domains. J Biol Chem 277:31142, 2002.
6. Tryggvason K, Wartiovaara J: Molecular basis of glomerular permselectivity. Curr Opin Nephrol Hypertens 10:543, 2001.
7. US Renal Data System, USRDS 2002 Annual Data Report: Atlas of End Stage Renal Disease in the United States. Bethesda, MD, National Institutes of Health, National Institute of Diabetes and Digestive and Kidney Diseases, 2002.
8. National Center for Health Statistics: National Vital Statistics Report, vol 50, no 15, 2002.
9. Gardner KD Jr, Bernstein J: The Cystic Kidney. Dordrecht, Kluwer Academic Publishers, 1990.
10. Grantham JJ: The pathogenesis, etiology and treatment of autosomal dominant polycystic kidney disease. Am J Kidney Dis 28:788, 1996.
11. Hateboer N, et al: Comparison of phenotypes of polycystic kidney disease types 1 and 2. Lancet 353:103, 1999.
12. Rossetti S, et al: The position of the polycystic kidney disease 1 (PKD1) gene mutation correlates with the severity of renal disease. J Am Soc Nephrol 13:1230, 2002.
13. The International Polycystic Kidney Disease Consortium: Polycystic kidney disease: the complete structure of the PKD1 gene and its protein. Cell 81:289, 1995.
14. Wilson PD: Polycystic kidney disease. N Engl J Med 350:151, 2004.
15. Mochizuki T, et al: PKD2, a gene for polycystic kidney disease that encodes an integral membrane protein. Science 272:1339, 1996.
16. Koulen P, et al: Polycystin-2 is an intracellular calcium release channel. Nat Cell Biol 4:191, 2002.
17. Hanaoka K, et al: Co-assembly of polycystin-1 and -2 produces unique cation-permeable currents. Nature 408:990, 2000.
18. Lu W, et al: Perinatal lethality with kidney and pancreas defects in mice with a targeted PKD-1 mutation. Nat Gen 17:179, 1997.
19. Qian F, et al: The molecular basis of focal cyst formation in human autosomal dominant polycystic kidney disease type I. Cell 87:979, 1996.
20. Watson MC: Complications of APKD. Kidney Int 51:353, 1997.
21. Griffin MD, et al: Vascular expression of polycystin. J Am Soc Nephrol 8:616, 1997.
22. Ward CJ, et al: The gene mutated in autosomal recessive polycystic kidney disease encodes a large, receptor-like protein. Nat Genet 30:259, 2002.
23. Hildebrandt F, Omram H: New insights: nephronophthisis-medullary cystic kidney disease. Pediatr Nephrol 16:168–176, 2001.
24. Drew AF, et al: Crescentic glomerulonephritis is diminished in fibrinogen-deficient mice. Am J Physiol Renal Physiol 281:F1157, 2001.
25. Nielsen EG, Couser WG: Immunologic Renal Diseases, 2nd ed. New York, Lippincott-Raven, 2001.
26. Wilson CB: Renal response to immunological injury. In Brenner BM, Rector F (eds): The Kidney, 5th ed. Philadelphia, WB Saunders, 1996, pp 1253–1391.
27. Hudson BG, Tryggvason K, Sundaramoorthy M, Neilson EG: Alport's syndrome, Goodpasture's syndrome, and type IV collagen. N Engl J Med 348:2543, 2003.
28. Farquhar M, et al: The Heymann nephritis antigenic complex: megalin (gp330) and RAP. J Am Soc Nephrol 6:35, 1996.
29. Ravetch JV, Lanier LL: Immune inhibitory receptors. Science 290:84, 2000.
30. Couser WG: Sensitized cells come of age: a new era in renal immunology with important therapeutic implications. J Am Soc Nephrol 10:664, 1999.
31. Cunard R, Kelly CJ: T cells and minimal change disease. J Am Soc Nephrol 13:1409, 2002.
32. Cunningham MA, et al: Prominence of cell-mediated immunity effectors in "pauci-immune" glomerulonephritis. J Am Soc Nephrol 10:499, 1999.
33. Rennke HG, et al: Cell-mediated immune injury in the kidney: acute nephritis induced in the rat by azobenzenearsonate. Kidney Int 45:1044, 1994.
34. Kalluri R, et al: Susceptibility to anti-glomerular basement membrane disease and Goodpasture syndrome is linked to MHC class II genes and emergence of T cell-mediated immunity in mice. J Clin Invest 100:2263, 1997.
35. Tipping PG, et al: Crescentic glomerulonephritis in CD4- and CD8-deficient mice: requirement for CD4 but not CD8 cells. Am J Pathol 152:1541, 1998.
36. Johnson RJ: Cytokines, growth factors and renal injury. Kidney Int 52:S2, 1997.

37. Border WA, Noble NA: TGF-β in kidney fibrosis: a target for gene therapy. Kidney Int 51:1389, 1997.
38. Remuzzi G, Ruggenenti P, Benigni A: Understanding the nature of renal disease progression. Kidney Int 51:2, 1997.
39. Schena FP, et al: Progression of renal damage in human glomerulonephritis. Kidney Int 52:1439, 1997.
40. Fogo AB: Progression and potential regression of glomerulosclerosis. Kidney Int 59:804, 2001.
41. Rennke HG, et al: The progression of renal disease: structural and functional correlations. In Tisher CC, Brenner B (eds): Renal Pathology, 2nd ed. Philadelphia, JB Lippincott, 1994, pp 116–139.
42. Brenner BM: Remission of renal disease: recounting the challenge, acquiring the goal. J Clin Invest 110:1753, 2003.
43. Mundel P, Shankland SJ: Podocyte biology and response to injury. J Am Soc Nephrol 13:3005, 2002.
44. Bohle A, et al: Pathogenesis of chronic renal failure in the primary glomerulopathies, renal vasculopathies, and chronic interstitial nephritides. Kidney Int Suppl 54:S2, 1996.
45. Abbate M, et al: Proteinuria as a mediator of tubulointerstitial injury. Kidney Blood Press Res 22:37, 1999.
46. Eddy AA: Molecular basis of renal fibrosis. Pediatr Nephrol 15:290, 2000.
47. Couser WG, et al: Postinfectious glomerulonephritis. In Neilson EG, Couser WG (eds): Immunologic Renal Diseases, 2nd ed. Philadelphia, Lippincott Williams & Wilkins, 2001, pp 899–929.
48. Kluth DC, et al: Anti-glomerular basement membrane disease. J Am Soc Nephrol 10:2446, 1999.
49. Phelps RG, et al: The HLA complex in Goodpasture's disease: a model for analyzing susceptibility to autoimmunity. Kidney Int 56:1638, 1999.
50. Savige J, et al: Antineutrophil cytoplasmic antibodies and associated diseases: a review of the clinical and laboratory features. Kidney Int 57:846, 2000.
51. Jennette JC, et al: Small-vessel vasculitis. N Engl J Med 337:1512, 1997.
52. Xiao H, et al: Antineutrophil cytoplasmic autoantibodies specific for myeloperoxidase cause glomerulonephritis and vasculitis in mice. J Clin Invest 110:955, 2002.
53. Haas M, et al: Changing etiologies of unexplained adult nephrotic syndrome. Am J Kidney Dis 30:621, 1997.
54. Wasserstein AG: Membranous glomerulonephritis. J Am Soc Nephrol 8:664, 1997.
55. Burstein DM, et al: Membranous glomerulonephritis and malignancy. Am J Kidney Dis 22:5, 1993.
56. Schnaper HW: Primary nephrotic syndrome of childhood. Curr Opin Pediatr 8:141, 1996.
57. Tryggvason K: Unraveling the mechanisms of glomerular ultrafiltration: nephrin, a key component of the slit diaphragm. J Am Soc Nephrol 10:2440, 1999.
58. D'Agati V: The many masks of focal segmental glomerulosclerosis. Kidney Int 46:1223, 1994.
59. Laurinavicius A, Rennke HG: Collapsing glomerulopathy: a new pattern of renal injury. Semin Diagn Pathol 19:106, 2002.
60. Sharma M, et al: "The FSGS factor": enrichment and in vivo effect of activity from focal segmental glomerulosclerosis plasma. J Am Soc Nephrol 10:552, 1999.
61. Antignac C: Genetic models: clues for understanding the pathogenesis of idopathic nephrotic syndrome. J Clin Invest 109:447, 2002.
62. Pollak MR: Inherited podocytopathies: FSGS and nephrotic syndrome from a genetic viewpoint. J Am Soc Nephrol 13:3016, 2002.
63. Shaw AS, Miner JH: CD2-associated protein and the kidney. Curr Opin Nephrol Hypertens 10:19, 2001.
64. D'Agati V, Appel GB: HIV infection and the kidney. J Am Soc Nephrol 8:139, 1997.
65. Ross MJ, et al: Recent progress in HIV-associated nephropathy. J Am Soc Nephrol 13:2997, 2002.
66. Marras D, et al: Replication and compartmentalization of HIV-1 in kidney epithelium of patients with HIV-associated nephropathy. Nat Med 8:522, 2002.
67. Rennke HG: Secondary MPGN. Kidney Int 47:643, 1995.
68. Donadio JV, Grande JP: IgA nephropathy. N Engl J Med 347:738, 2002.
69. Kashtan CE: Alport syndrome: an inherited disorder of renal, ocular, and cochlear basement membranes. Medicine (Baltimore) 78:338, 1999.
70. Kashtan CE: Alport syndromes: phenotypic heterogeneity of progressive hereditary nephritis. Pediatr Nephrol 14:502, 2000.
71. Badenas C, et al: Mutations in the COLA4A4 and COLA4A3 genes cause familial benign hematuria. J Am Soc Nephrol 13:1248, 2002.
72. Ibrahim HN, Hostetter TH: Diabetic nephropathy. J Am Soc Nephrol 8:487, 1997.
73. Dalla Vestra M, et al: Structural involvement in type 1 and type 2 diabetic nephropathy. Diabetes Metab 26 (Suppl 4):8, 2000.
74. Sharma K, Ziyadeh FN: Biochemical events and cytokine interactions linking glucose metabolism to the development of diabetic nephropathy. Semin Nephrol 17:80, 1997.
75. Sheetz MJ, King GL: Molecular understanding of hyperglycemia's adverse effects for diabetic complications. JAMA 288:2579, 2002.
76. Wolf G, Ziyadeh FN: Molecular mechanisms of diabetic renal hypertrophy. Kidney Int 56:393, 1999.
77. Drummond K, Mauer M: The early natural history of nephropathy in type 1 diabetes: II. Early renal structural changes in type 1 diabetes. Diabetes 51:1580, 2002.
78. Fioretto P, et al: Reversal of lesions of diabetic nephropathy after pancreas transplantation. N Engl J Med 339:69, 1998.
79. Rosenstock JL, et al: Fibrillary and immunotactoid glomerulonephritis: distinct entities with different clinical and pathologic features. Kidney Int 63:1450, 2003.
80. Lieberthal WL: Biology of acute renal failure. Kidney Int 52:1102, 1997.
81. Lameire N, Vanholder R: Pathophysiologic features and prevention of human and experimental acute tubular necrosis. J Am Soc Nephrol 12 (Suppl 17):S20, 2001.
82. Edelstein CL, et al: The nature of renal cell injury. Kidney Int 51:341, 1997.
83. Rabb H, et al: Leukocytes, cell adhesion molecules and ischemic renal failure. Kidney Int 51:1463, 1997.
84. Humes DH, et al: Acute renal failure: growth factors, cell therapy and gene therapy. Proc Am Assoc Physicians 109:547, 1997.
85. Oliver J, et al: The pathogenesis of acute renal failure associated with traumatic and toxic injury, renal ischemia, nephrotoxic damage, and the ischemic episode. J Clin Invest 30:1307, 1951.
86. Ronald A: The etiology of urinary tract infection: traditional and emerging pathogens. Am J Med 113 (Suppl 1A):14S, 2002.
87. Langermann S, et al: Prevention of mucosal *Escherichia coli* infection by FimH-adhesin-based systemic vaccination. Science 276:607, 1997.
88. Hirsch HH: Polyomavirus BK nephropathy: a (re-)emerging complication in renal transplantation. Am J Transplant 2:25, 2002.
89. Michel DM, Kelly CJ: Acute interstitial nephritis. J Am Soc Nephrol 9:506, 1998.
90. De Broe ME, Elseveirs MM: Analgesic nephropathy. N Engl J Med 338:446, 1998.
91. Gambaro G, Perazella MA: Adverse renal effects of anti-inflammatory agents: evaluation of selective and non-selective cyclooxygenase inhibitors. J Intern Med 253:643, 2003.
92. Kurokawa K, et al (eds): Hypertension: causes and consequences of renal injury. Kidney Int 49 (Suppl 55):S1, 1997.
93. Preston RA, et al: Renal parenchymal hypertension: present concepts. Arch Intern Med 156:602, 1996.
94. Meyrier A, et al: Ischemic renal diseases: new insights into old entities. Kidney Int 54:2, 1998.
95. Kitiyakara C, Guzman NJ: Malignant hypertension and hypertensive emergencies. J Am Soc Nephrol 9:128, 1998.
96. Safian RD, Textor SC: Renal-artery stenosis. N Engl J Med 344:431, 2001.
97. Goldblatt H, et al: Studies on experimental hypertension: I. Production of persistent elevation of systolic blood pressure by means of renal ischemia. J Exp Med 59:347, 1934.
98. Elliott MA, Nichols WL: Thrombotic thrombocytopenic purpura and hemolytic uremic syndrome. Mayo Clin Proc 76:1154, 2001.
99. Moake JL: Thrombotic microangiopathies. N Engl J Med 347:589, 2002.
100. Chung DW, Fujikawa K: Processing of von Willebrand factor by ADAMTS-13. Biochemistry 41:11065, 2002.
101. Grabowski EF: The hemolytic-uremic syndrome—toxin, thrombin and thrombosis. New Engl J Med 346:58, 2002.
102. Gagnuandou MF, et al: Long-term (15–25 years) prognosis of hemolytic-uremic syndrome. J Am Soc Nephrol 4:275, 1993.
103. Textor SC, Wilcox CS: Ischemic nephropathy/azotemic renovascular disease. Semin Nephrol 20:489, 2000.
104. Klahr S: Obstructive nephropathy. Kidney Int 54:286, 1998.
105. Scheinman SJ: Nephrolithiasis. Semin Nephrol 19:381, 1999.

106. Coe FL, Parks JH: New insights into the pathophysiology and treatment of nephrolithiasis: new research venues. J Bone Miner Res 12:522, 1997.
107. Pak CY: Kidney stones. Lancet 351:1797, 1998.
108. Eble JN (ed): Tumors of the kidney. Semin Diagn Pathol 15:1–81, 1998.
109. Reuter VE, Presti JC, Jr.: Contemporary approach to the classification of renal epithelial tumors. Semin Oncol 27:124, 2000.
110. McLaughlin JK, Lipworth L: Epidemiologic aspects of renal cell cancer. Semin Oncol 27:115, 2000.
111. Bodmer D, et al: Understanding familial and non-familial renal cell cancer. Hum Mol Genet 11:2489, 2002.
112. Karumanchi SA, Merchan J, Sukhatme VP: Renal cancer: molecular mechanisms and newer therapeutic options. Curr Opin Nephrol Hypertens 11:37, 2002.
113. Pavlovich CP, Schmidt LS, Phillips JL: The genetic basis of renal cell carcinoma. Urol Clin North Am 30:437, 2003.
114. Weterman MA, et al: Impairment of MAD2B-PRCC interaction in mitotic checkpoint defective t(X;1)-positive renal cell carcinomas. Proc Natl Acad Sci U S A 98:13808, 2001.

CHAPTER 21

The Lower Urinary Tract and Male Genital System

Jonathan I. Epstein, MD

THE LOWER URINARY TRACT

URETERS

Congenital Anomalies

Inflammations

Tumors and Tumor-Like Lesions

Obstructive Lesions

URINARY BLADDER

Congenital Anomalies

Inflammations

Acute and Chronic Cystitis

Special Forms of Cystitis

Metaplastic Lesions

Neoplasms

Urothelial (Transitional Cell) Tumors

Other Types of Carcinoma

Mesenchymal Tumors

Secondary Tumors

Obstruction

URETHRA

Inflammations

Tumors and Tumor-Like Lesions

THE MALE GENITAL TRACT

PENIS

Congenital Anomalies

Hypospadias and Epispadias

Phimosis

Inflammations

Tumors

Benign Tumors

Malignant Tumors

TESTIS AND EPIDIDYMIS

Congenital Anomalies

Cryptorchidism

Regressive Changes

Atrophy

Findings Associated with Decreased Fertility

Inflammations

Non-Specific Epididymitis and Orchitis

Granulomatous (Autoimmune) Orchitis

Specific Inflammations

Vascular Disturbances

Torsion

Spermatic Cord and Paratesticular Tumors

Testicular Tumors

Germ Cell Tumors

Tumors of Sex Cord–Gonadal Stroma

Gonadoblastoma

Testicular Lymphoma

Miscellaneous Lesions of Tunica Vaginalis

PROSTATE

Inflammations

Benign Enlargement

Nodular Hyperplasia (Benign Prostatic Hypertrophy or Hyperplasia)

Tumors

Adenocarcinoma

Miscellaneous Tumors and Tumor-Like Conditions

THE LOWER URINARY TRACT

NORMAL

Despite differing embryonic origins, the various components of the lower urinary tract come to have many morphologic similarities. The renal pelves, ureters, bladder, and urethra (except for its terminal portion) are lined by a special form of transitional epithelium (urothelium) that is two to three cells thick in the pelvis, three to five cells thick in the ureters, and three to seven cells thick in the bladder. The surface layer consists of large, flattened "umbrella cells" that cover several underlying cells. The umbrella cells have a trilaminar asymmetric unit membrane and possess apical plaques composed of specific proteins called *uroplakins*. Toward the basal layer, the cells become smaller or more cylindrical (particularly in contracted bladders), but they are capable of some flattening when the underlying wall is stretched. This epithelium rests on a well-developed basement membrane, beneath which there is a lamina propria. The lamina propria in the urinary bladder contains wisps of smooth muscle that form a discontinuous muscularis mucosae. It is important to differentiate the muscularis mucosae from the deeper well-defined larger muscle bundles of the detrusor muscle (muscularis propria), since bladder cancers are staged on the basis of invasion of the latter. The bladder musculature is capable of great thickening if there is obstruction to the flow of urine.

Several variants of the normal epithelial patterns may be encountered. Nests of urothelium or inbudding of the surface epithelium may be found occasionally in the mucosa lamina propria; these are referred to as *Brunn nests*.

The ureters lie throughout their course in a retroperitoneal position. Retroperitoneal tumors or fibrosis may trap the ureters in neoplastic or dense, fibrous tissue, sometimes obstructing them. As ureters enter the pelvis, they pass anterior to either the common iliac or the external iliac artery. In the female pelvis, they lie close to the uterine arteries and are therefore vulnerable to injury in operations on the female genital tract. There are three points of slight narrowing: at the ureteropelvic junction, where they enter the bladder, and where they cross the iliac vessels, all providing loci where renal calculi may become impacted when they pass from the kidney to the bladder. As the ureters enter the bladder, they pursue an oblique course, terminating in a slitlike orifice. The obliquity of this intramural segment of the ureteral orifice permits the enclosing bladder musculature to act like a sphincteric valve, blocking the upward reflux of urine even in the presence of marked distention of the urinary bladder. As discussed in Chapter 20, a defect in the intravesical portion of the ureter leads to vesicoureteral reflux. The orifices of the ureters demarcate an area at the base of the bladder known as the trigone. In women, the trigone is frequently covered by glycogenated squamous epithelium, a normal finding, not metaplasia resulting from injury.

The close relationship of the female genital tract to the bladder makes possible the spread of disease from one tract to the other. In middle-aged and elderly women, relaxation of pelvic support leads to prolapse (descent) of the uterus, pulling with it the floor of the bladder. In this fashion, the bladder protrudes into the vagina, creating a pouch (*cystocele*) that fails to empty readily with micturition. In men, the seminal vesicles and prostate have similar close relationships, being situated just posterior and inferior to the neck of the bladder. Thus, enlargement of the prostate, so common in middle to later life, constitutes an important cause of urinary tract obstruction. In the subsequent sections, we discuss the major pathologic lesions in the ureters, urinary bladder, and urethra separately.[1,2]

Ureters

CONGENITAL ANOMALIES

Congenital anomalies of the ureters occur in about 2% or 3% of all autopsies. Although most have little clinical significance, certain anomalies may contribute to obstruction to the flow of urine and thus cause clinical disease. Anomalies of the ureterovesical junction, potentiating reflux, are discussed with pyelonephritis in Chapter 20.

Double ureters (derived from a double or split ureteral bud) are almost invariably associated either with totally distinct double renal pelves or with the anomalous development of a large kidney having a partially bifid pelvis terminating in separate ureters. Double ureters may pursue separate courses to the bladder but commonly are joined within the bladder wall and drain through a single ureteral orifice. The majority of double ureters are unilateral and of no clinical significance.

Ureteropelvic junction obstruction, a congenital disorder, results in hydronephrosis. It usually presents in infants or children, much more commonly in boys, usually in the left ureter. However, it is bilateral in 20% of cases and may be associated with other congenital anomalies. *It is the most common cause of hydronephrosis in infants and children.* In adults, ureteropelvic junction obstruction is more common in women and is most often unilateral. There is agenesis of the kidney on the opposite side in a significant number of cases, probably resulting from obstructive lesions in utero.

Diverticula, saccular outpouchings of the ureteral wall, are uncommon lesions that are usually asymptomatic and found incidentally on imaging studies. They appear as congenital or acquired defects and are of importance as pockets of stasis and secondary infections. Dilation (*hydroureter*), elongation, and tortuosity of the ureters may occur as congenital anomalies or as acquired defects. Congenital hydroureter is thought to reflect some neurogenic defect in the innervation of the ureteral musculature. Massive enlargement of the ureter is known as *megaloureter* and is probably due to a functional defect of ureteral muscle. Hydronephrosis and decreased renal function results if the lesion goes untreated. These anomalies are sometimes associated with some congenital defect of the kidney.

INFLAMMATIONS

Ureteritis may develop as one component of urinary tract infections. The morphologic changes are entirely nonspecific. Only infrequently does such ureteritis make a significant contribution to the clinical problem. Persistence of infection or repeated acute exacerbations may give rise to chronic inflammatory changes within the ureters.

Morphology. In certain cases of long-standing chronic ureteritis, specialized reaction patterns are sometimes observed. The accumulation or aggregation of lymphocytes in the subepithelial region may cause slight elevations of the mucosa and produce a fine granular mucosal surface (**ureteritis follicularis**). At other times, the mucosa may become sprinkled with fine cysts varying in diameter from 1 to 5 mm (**ureteritis cystica**). These changes are also found in the bladder (described in greater detail later, in the section on the urinary bladder). The cysts may aggregate to form small, grapelike clusters (Fig. 21–1). Histologic sections through such cysts demonstrate a lining of modified transitional epithelium with some flattening of the superficial layer of cells.

TUMORS AND TUMOR-LIKE LESIONS

Primary neoplasia of the ureter is rare. Small *benign tumors* of the ureter are generally of mesenchymal origin. The two most common are fibroepithelial polyps and leiomyomas. The *fibroepithelial polyp* is a tumor-like lesion that grossly presents as a small mass projecting into the lumen. The lesion occurs more commonly in the ureters (left more often than right) but may also appear in the bladder, renal pelves, and urethra. The polyp presents as a loose, vascularized connective tissue mass lying beneath the mucosa.

Primary *malignant tumors* of the ureter follow patterns similar to those arising in the renal pelvis, calyces, and bladder, and the majority are transitional cell carcinomas (Fig. 21–2).

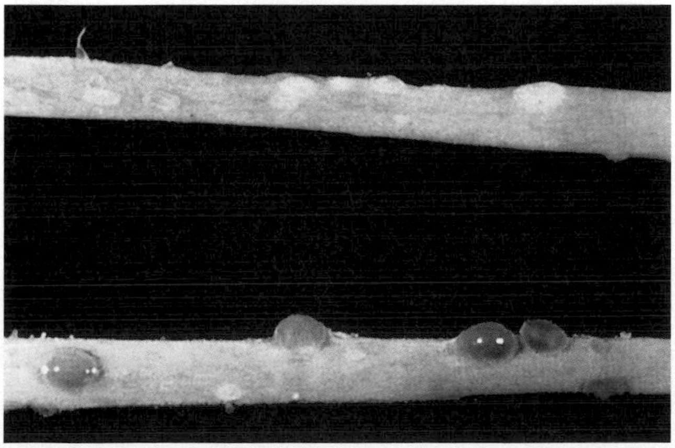

FIGURE 21–1 Opened ureters showing ureteritis cystica. Note the smooth cysts projecting from the mucosa.

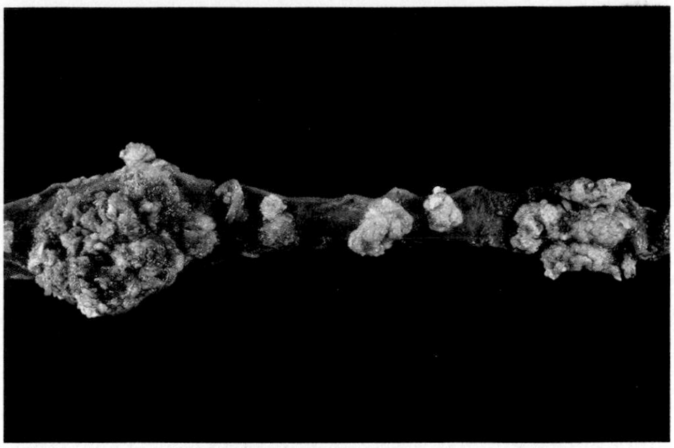

FIGURE 21–2 Papillary transitional cell carcinoma extensively involving the ureter. (Courtesy of Dr. Cristina Magi-Galluzzi, The Johns Hopkins Hospital, Baltimore, MD.)

They cause obstruction of the ureteral lumen and are found most frequently during the sixth and seventh decades of life. They are sometimes multiple and occasionally occur concurrently with similar neoplasms in the bladder or renal pelvis.

OBSTRUCTIVE LESIONS

A great variety of pathologic lesions may obstruct the ureters and give rise to hydroureter, hydronephrosis, and sometimes pyelonephritis (Chapter 20). Obviously, it is not the ureteral dilation that is of significance in these cases, but the consequent involvement of the kidneys. The more important causes, divided into those of intrinsic and those of extrinsic origin, are cited in Table 21–1. Unilateral obstruction

TABLE 21–1 Major Causes of Ureteral Obstruction

Intrinsic	
Calculi	Of renal origin, rarely more than 5 mm in diameter Larger renal stones cannot enter ureters Impact at loci of ureteral narrowing—ureteropelvic junction, where ureters cross iliac vessels, and where they enter bladder—and cause excruciating "renal colic"
Strictures	Congenital or acquired (inflammations)
Tumors	Transitional cell carcinomas arising in ureters Rarely, benign tumors or fibroepithelial polyps
Blood clots	Massive hematuria from renal calculi, tumors, or papillary necrosis
Neurogenic	Interruption of the neural pathways to the bladder
Extrinsic	
Pregnancy	Physiologic relaxation of smooth muscle or pressure on ureters at pelvic brim from enlarging fundus
Periureteral inflammation	Salpingitis, diverticulitis, peritonitis, sclerosing retroperitoneal fibrosis
Endometriosis	With pelvic lesions, followed by scarring
Tumors	Cancers of the rectum, bladder, prostate, ovaries, uterus, cervix, lymphomas, sarcomas

typically results from proximal causes, whereas bilateral obstruction arises from distal causes, such as nodular hyperplasia of the prostate. Only sclerosing retroperitoneal fibrosis is discussed further.

Sclerosing Retroperitoneal Fibrosis. This refers to an uncommon cause of ureteral narrowing or obstruction characterized by a *fibrous proliferative inflammatory process encasing the retroperitoneal structures and causing hydronephrosis.*[3] The disorder occurs in middle to late age. In some cases, specific causes can be identified, such as drugs (ergot derivatives, β-adrenergic blockers), adjacent inflammatory conditions (vasculitis, diverticulitis, Crohn disease), or malignant disease (lymphomas, urinary tract carcinomas). However, 70% of cases have no obvious cause and are considered primary or idiopathic (Ormond disease). Several cases have been reported with similar fibrotic changes in other sites (referred to as mediastinal fibrosis, sclerosing cholangitis, and Riedel fibrosing thyroiditis), suggesting that the disorder is systemic in distribution but preferentially involves the retroperitoneum. Thus, an autoimmune reaction, sometimes triggered by drugs, has been proposed.

On microscopic examination, the inflammatory fibrosis is marked by a prominent inflammatory infiltrate of lymphocytes, often with germinal centers, plasma cells, and eosinophils. Sometimes, foci of fat necrosis and granulomatous inflammation are seen in and about the fibrosis.

Urinary Bladder

Diseases of the bladder, particularly inflammation (cystitis), constitute an important source of clinical signs and symptoms. Usually, however, these disorders are more disabling than lethal. Cystitis is particularly common in young women of reproductive age and in older age groups of both sexes. Tumors of the bladder are an important source of both morbidity and mortality.

CONGENITAL ANOMALIES

Diverticula. A bladder or vesical diverticulum consists of a pouchlike eversion or evagination of the bladder wall. Diverticula may arise as congenital defects but more commonly are acquired lesions from persistent urethral obstruction.

Congenital diverticula may be due to a focal failure of development of the normal musculature or to some urinary tract obstruction during fetal development. *Acquired diverticula* are most often seen with prostatic enlargement (hyperplasia or neoplasia), producing obstruction to urine outflow and marked muscle thickening of the bladder wall. The increased intravesical pressure causes outpouching of the bladder wall and the formation of diverticula. They are frequently multiple and have narrow necks located between the interweaving hypertrophied muscle bundles. In both the congenital and acquired forms, the diverticulum usually consists of a round to ovoid, saclike pouch that varies from less than 1 cm to 5 to 10 cm in diameter.

Although most diverticula are small and asymptomatic, they may be clinically significant, as they constitute sites of urinary stasis and predispose to infection and the formation of bladder calculi. They may also predispose to vesicoureteral reflux as a result of impingement on the ureter. Rarely, carcinomas may arise in bladder diverticuli. When invasive cancers arise in diverticula, they tend to be more advanced in stage as a result of diverticula's thin or absent muscle wall.

Exstrophy. Exstrophy of the bladder implies the presence of a developmental failure in the anterior wall of the abdomen and in the bladder, so that the bladder either communicates directly through a large defect with the surface of the body or lies as an opened sac (Fig. 21–3). These lesions are amenable to surgical correction, and long-term survival is possible. The exposed bladder mucosa may undergo colonic glandular metaplasia and is subject to the development of infections that often spread to upper levels of the urinary system. In the course of persistent chronic infections, the mucosa often becomes converted into an ulcerated surface of granulation tissue, and the preserved marginal epithelium becomes transformed into a stratified squamous type. There is an increased tendency toward the development of carcinoma later in life, mostly adenocarcinoma of the colon.[4] Patients also have an increased risk of adenocarcinoma arising from the bladder remnant.

Miscellaneous Anomalies. *Vesicoureteral reflux* is the most common and serious anomaly. As a major contributor to renal infection and scarring, it was discussed earlier in Chapter 20 in the consideration of pyelonephritis. Abnormal connections between the bladder and the vagina, rectum, or uterus may create *congenital fistulas.*

Rarely, the *urachus* may remain patent in part or in whole (persistent urachus). When it is totally patent, a fistulous urinary tract is created that connects the bladder with the umbilicus. At times, the umbilical end or the bladder end remains patent, while the central region is obliterated. A sequestered umbilical epithelial rest or bladder diverticulum is formed that may provide a site for the development of infection. At other times, only the central region of the urachus persists, giving rise to *urachal cysts,* lined by either transitional or metaplastic epithelium. *Carcinomas,* mostly glandular tumors resembling colonic adenocarcinomas, may arise in such cysts. These account for only a minority of all bladder cancers (0.1% to 0.3%) but 20% to 40% of bladder adenocarcinomas.[2]

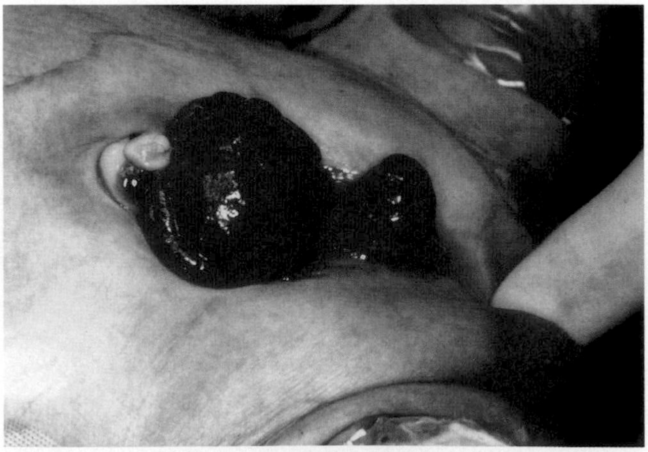

FIGURE 21–3 Exstrophy of the bladder in a newborn boy. The tied umbilical cord is seen above the hyperemic mucosa of the everted bladder. Below is an incompletely formed penis with marked epispadias. (Courtesy of Dr. John Gearhart, The Johns Hopkins Hospital, Baltimore, MD.)

INFLAMMATIONS

Acute and Chronic Cystitis

The pathogenesis of cystitis and the common bacterial etiologic agents are discussed in Chapter 20 in the consideration of urinary tract infections. As was emphasized earlier, bacterial pyelonephritis is frequently preceded by infection of the urinary bladder, with retrograde spread of microorganisms into the kidneys and their collecting systems. The common etiologic agents of cystitis are the coliforms: *Escherichia coli*, followed by *Proteus*, *Klebsiella*, and *Enterobacter*. Women are more likely to develop cystitis as a result of their shorter urethras. *Tuberculous cystitis* is almost always a sequel to renal tuberculosis. *Candida albicans (Monilia)* and, much less often, cryptococcal agents cause cystitis, particularly in immunosuppressed patients or those receiving long-term antibiotics. Schistosomiasis (*Schistosoma haematobium*) is rare in the United States but is common in certain Middle Eastern countries, notably Egypt. Viruses (e.g., adenovirus), *Chlamydia*, and *Mycoplasma* may also be causes of cystitis. Predisposing factors include bladder calculi, urinary obstruction, diabetes mellitus, instrumentation, and immune deficiency. Patients receiving *cytotoxic antitumor drugs*, such as cyclophosphamide, sometimes develop hemorrhagic cystitis.[5] Finally, radiation of the bladder region gives rise to *radiation cystitis*.

Morphology. Most cases of cystitis take the form of nonspecific acute or chronic inflammation of the bladder. In gross appearance, there is hyperemia of the mucosa, sometimes associated with exudate. When there is a hemorrhagic component, the cystitis is designated **hemorrhagic cystitis.** This form of cystitis sometimes follows radiation injury or antitumor chemotherapy and is often accompanied by epithelial atypia. Adenovirus infection also causes a hemorrhagic cystitis.

The accumulation of large amounts of suppurative exudate may merit the designation of **suppurative cystitis.** When there is ulceration of large areas of the mucosa, or sometimes the entire bladder mucosa, this is known as ulcerative cystitis.

Persistence of the infection leads to **chronic cystitis,** which differs from the acute form only in the character of the inflammatory infiltrate. There is more extreme heaping up of the epithelium with the formation of a red, friable, granular, sometimes ulcerated surface. Chronicity of the infection gives rise to fibrous thickening in the muscularis propria and consequent thickening and inelasticity of the bladder wall. Histologic variants include **follicular cystitis,** characterized by the aggregation of lymphocytes into lymphoid follicles within the bladder mucosa and underlying wall, and **eosinophilic cystitis,** manifested by infiltration with submucosal eosinophils together with fibrosis and occasionally giant cells. Most cases of eosinophilic cystitis represent nonspecific subacute inflammation, although, rarely, these lesions are manifestations of a systemic allergic disorder. The ubiquitous presence of mild chronic inflammation in the bladder unaccompanied by clinical symptoms should not be glorified with the diagnosis of chronic cystitis.

All forms of clinical cystitis are characterized by a triad of symptoms: (1) frequency, which in acute cases may necessitate urination every 15 to 20 minutes; (2) lower abdominal pain localized over the bladder region or in the suprapubic region; and (3) dysuria—pain or burning on urination. Associated with these localized changes, there may be systemic signs of inflammation such as elevation of temperature, chills, and general malaise. In the usual case, the bladder infection does not give rise to such a constitutional reaction.

The local symptoms of cystitis may be disturbing, but these infections are also important as antecedents to pyelonephritis. Cystitis is sometimes a secondary complication of some underlying disorder such as prostatic enlargement, cystocele of the bladder, calculi, or tumors. These primary diseases must be corrected before the cystitis can be relieved.

Special Forms of Cystitis

Several special variants of cystitis are distinctive by either their morphologic appearance or their causation.

Interstitial Cystitis (Hunner Ulcer). This is a *persistent, painful form of chronic cystitis occurring most frequently in women and associated with inflammation and fibrosis of all layers of the bladder wall.*[6] It is characterized clinically by intermittent, often severe, suprapubic pain, urinary frequency, urgency, hematuria, and dysuria without evidence of bacterial infection, and cystoscopic findings of fissures and punctate hemorrhages (glomerulations) in the bladder mucosa after luminal distention. Some but not all patients exhibit morphologic features of chronic mucosal ulcers (*Hunner ulcers*), which is termed *the late (classic, ulcerative) phase*. Inflammatory cells and granulation tissue may involve the mucosa, lamina propria, and muscularis, and *mast cells* may be particularly prominent. In the early (nonclassic, nonulcerative) form of interstitial cystitis, recent submucosal hemorrhages are noted. Although mast cells are characteristic of this disease, there is no uniformity in the literature as to their specificity and diagnostic utility. The major role of biopsy is not to specifically diagnose the disease as much as it is to rule out flat carcinoma in situ, which may clinically mimic interstitial cystitis. The condition is of unknown etiology but is thought by some to be of autoimmune origin, particularly because it is sometimes associated with lupus erythematosus and other autoimmune disorders.

Malacoplakia. This designation refers to a *peculiar pattern of vesical inflammatory reaction characterized macroscopically by soft, yellow, slightly raised mucosal plaques 3 to 4 cm in diameter* (Fig. 21–4) and *histologically by infiltration with large, foamy macrophages with occasional multinucleate giant cells and interspersed lymphocytes.*[7] The macrophages have an abundant granular cytoplasm. The granularity is periodic acid–Schiff positive and due to phagosomes stuffed with particulate and membranous debris of bacterial origin. In addition, laminated mineralized concretions resulting from deposition of calcium in enlarged lysosomes, known as *Michaelis-Gutmann bodies*, are typically present, both within the macrophages and between cells (Fig. 21–5). Similar lesions have been described in the colon, lungs, bones, kidneys, prostate, and epididymis.

Malacoplakia is clearly related to chronic bacterial infection, mostly by *E. coli* or occasionally *Proteus* species. It occurs with increased frequency in immunosuppressed transplant recipients. The unusual-appearing macrophages and giant phagosomes point to defects in phagocytic or degradative

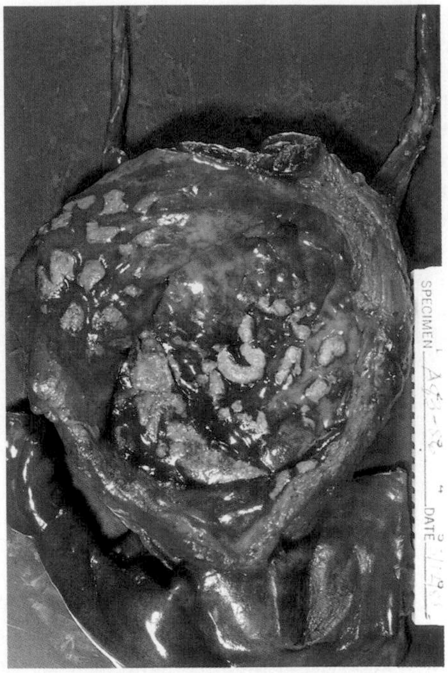

FIGURE 21–4 Cystitis with malacoplakia of bladder showing inflammatory exudate and broad, flat plaques.

function of macrophages such that phagosomes become overloaded with undigested bacterial products.

Polypoid Cystitis. Polypoid cystitis is an inflammatory condition resulting from irritation to the bladder mucosa.[8] Although indwelling catheters are the most commonly cited culprits, any injurious agent may give rise to this lesion. The urothelium is thrown into broad, bulbous, polypoid projections as a result of marked submucosal edema. Polypoid cystitis may be confused with papillary urothelial carcinoma both clinically and histologically.

METAPLASTIC LESIONS

Cystitis Glandularis and Cystitis Cystica. These terms refer to common lesions of the urinary bladder in which nests of transitional epithelium (Brunn nests) grow downward into the lamina propria and undergo transformation of their central epithelial cells into cuboidal or columnar epithelium lining (*cystitis glandularis*) or cystic spaces lined by urothelium (*cystitis cystica*). As the two processes often coexist, the condition is typically referred to as *cystitis cystica et glandularis.* In a variant of cystitis glandularis, goblet cells are present, and the epithelium resembles intestinal mucosa (*intestinal or colonic metaplasia*). Both variants are common microscopic incidental findings in relatively normal bladders. In contrast to earlier reports, lesions exhibiting extensive intestinal metaplasia have recently been shown not to be associated with an increased risk for the development of adenocarcinoma.[9]

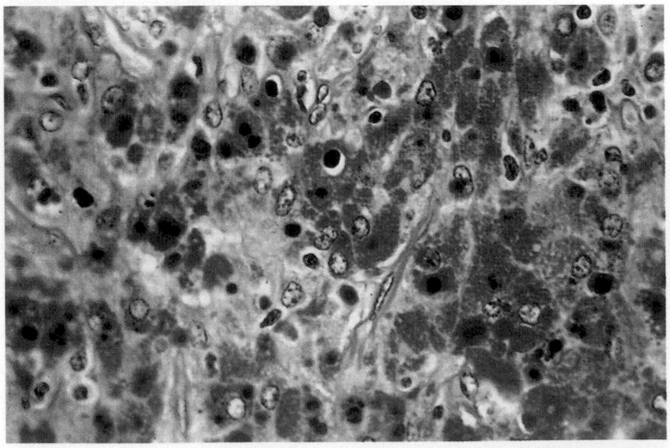

FIGURE 21–5 Malacoplakia, PAS stain. Note the large macrophages with granular PAS-positive cytoplasm and several dense, round Michaelis-Gutmann bodies surrounded by artifactual cleared holes in the upper middle field.

In *cystitis cystica*, the cysts are usually 0.1 to 1 cm in diameter, filled with clear fluid, and lined by cuboidal or urothelial cells. As was noted, similar cysts occur in the pelvis and ureter (ureteritis and pyelitis cystica).

Squamous Metaplasia. As a response to injury, the urothelium often converts to squamous epithelium, which is a more durable lining. This contrasts with the normal finding of glycogenated squamous epithelium commonly found in women at the trigone.

Nephrogenic Metaplasia (Nephrogenic Adenoma). Nephrogenic metaplasia also represents a reaction of the urothelium to injury.[10,11] The overlying urothelium may be focally replaced by cuboidal epithelium, which can assume a papillary growth pattern. In addition, a tubular proliferation in the underlying lamina propria and superficial detrusor muscle may produce lesions that histologically mimic a carcinoma. Although typically less than a centimeter in diameter, they may be sizable, and thus, they may also clinically resemble cancer.

NEOPLASMS

Neoplasms of the bladder pose biologic and clinical challenges. Despite significant inroads into their origins and improved methods of diagnosis and treatment, they continue to exact a high toll in morbidity and mortality. The incidence of bladder epithelial tumors in the United States has been steadily increasing during the past years and is now more than 57,000 new cases annually.[12] Despite improvements in detection and management of these neoplasms, the death toll remains at about 12,000 annually because the increased prevalence offsets such gains as have been made.

About 95% of bladder tumors are of epithelial origin, the remainder being mesenchymal tumors (Table 21–2). Most epithelial tumors are composed of urothelial (transitional) type cells and are thus interchangeably called urothelial or transitional tumors, but squamous and glandular carcinomas also occur. Here, we discuss the urothelial cell tumors in some detail and only touch on the others.

Urothelial (Transitional Cell) Tumors

These represent about 90% of all bladder tumors and run the gamut from small, benign lesions that might never recur to aggressive cancers associated with a high risk of death.[13] Many of these tumors are multifocal at presentation. Although most commonly seen in the bladder, any of the lesions

TABLE 21–2 Tumors of the Urinary Bladder
Urothelial (transitional cell) tumors
Inverted papilloma
Papilloma (exophytic)
Urothelial tumors of low malignant potential
Papillary urothelial carcinoma
Carcinoma in situ
Squamous cell carcinoma
Mixed carcinoma
Adenocarcinoma
Small cell carcinoma
Sarcomas

described below may be seen at any site where there is urothelium, from the renal pelvis to the distal urethra.

There are two distinct precursor lesions to invasive urothelial carcinoma. The more common are noninvasive papillary tumors, which appear to arise from papillary urothelial hyperplasia.[14] These lesions demonstrate a range of atypia, and several grading systems exist to reflect their biologic behavior. The other precursor lesion is flat urothelial carcinoma, which is simply referred to as carcinoma in situ (CIS). This lesion is by definition high grade and hence not assigned a grade. In about half the patients with invasive bladder cancer, at the time of presentation the tumor has already invaded the bladder wall, and there is no associated precursor lesion. In these cases, it is presumed that the precursor lesion has been destroyed by the high-grade invasive component, which typically appears as a large mass that is often ulcerated. Although invasion into the lamina propria worsens the prognosis, the major decrease in survival is associated with tumor invading the muscularis propria (detrusor muscle). Once muscularis propria invasion occurs, there is a 50% 5-year mortality rate.

Table 21–3 lists two of many systems of grading these tumors.[15–18] The World Health Organization (WHO) 1973 classification grades tumors into a rare totally benign papilloma and three grades of transitional cell carcinoma (grades I, II, and III). A more recent classification, based on a consensus reached at a conference by the International Society of Urological Pathology (ISUP) in 1998, recognizes a rare benign papilloma, a group of papillary urothelial neoplasms of low malignant potential, and two grades of carcinoma (low and high grade). This system was adopted by the WHO in 2004.

TABLE 21–3 Grading of Urothelial (Transitional Cell) Tumors
WHO/ISUP Grades*
Urothelial papilloma
Urothelial neoplasm of low malignant potential
Papillary urothelial carcinoma, low grade
Papillary urothelial carcinoma, high grade
***WHO Grades*†**
Urothelial papilloma
Urothelial neoplasm of low malignant potential
Papillary urothelial carcinoma, Grade 1
Papillary urothelial carcinoma, Grade 2
Papillary urothelial carcinoma, Grade 3

WHO, World Health Organization; ISUP, International Society of Urological Pathology.

*Adopted as the WHO System in 2004.

†The 1973 WHO grades.

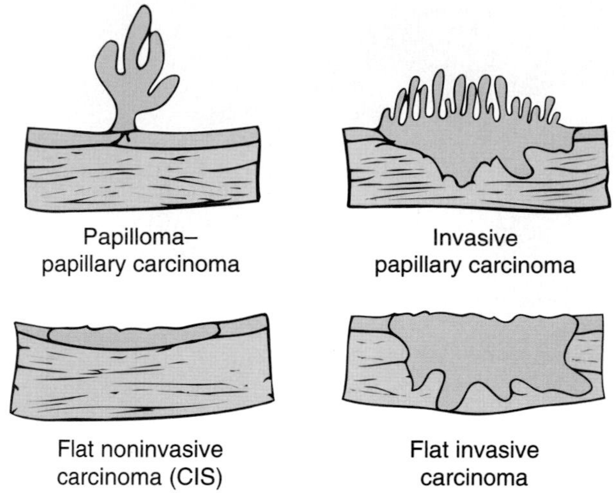

FIGURE 21–6 Four morphologic patterns of bladder tumors.

Morphology. The gross patterns of urothelial cell tumors vary from purely papillary to nodular or flat. The tumors may also be invasive or noninvasive (Fig. 21–6). Papillary lesions appear as red, elevated excrescences varying in size from less than 1 cm in diameter to large masses up to 5 cm in diameter (Fig. 21–7). Multicentric origins may produce separate tumors. As was noted, the histologic changes encompass a spectrum from benign papilloma to highly aggressive anaplastic cancers. Overall, the majority of papillary tumors are low grade. Most arise from the lateral or posterior walls at the bladder base.

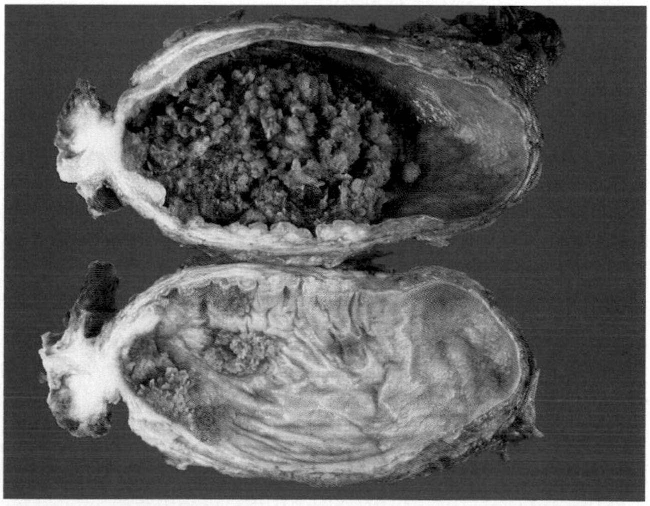

FIGURE 21–7 Cross-section of bladder with upper section showing a large papillary tumor. The lower section demonstrates multifocal smaller papillary neoplasms. (Courtesy of Dr. Fred Gilkey, Sinai Hospital, Baltimore, MD.)

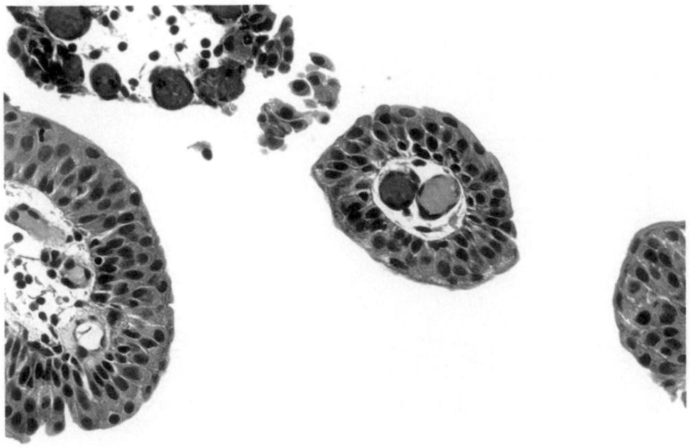

FIGURE 21–8 Papilloma consisting of small papillary fronds lined by normal-appearing urothelium.

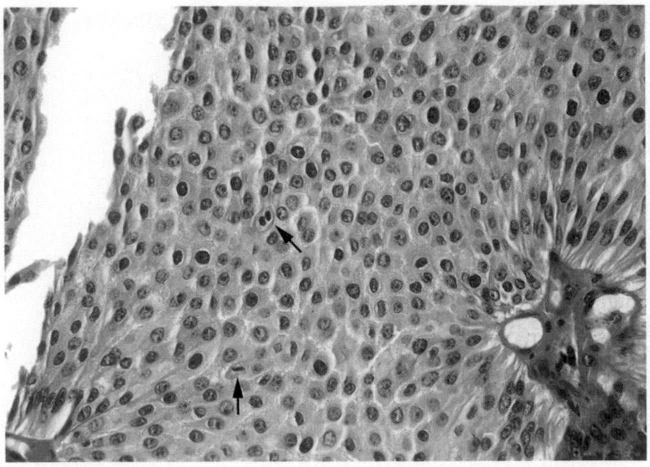

FIGURE 21–9 Low-grade papillary urothelial carcinoma with an overall orderly appearance, a thicker lining than papilloma, and scattered hyperchromatic nuclei and mitotic figures (*arrows*).

Papillomas represent 1% or fewer of bladder tumors, most commonly seen in younger patients. The tumors usually arise singly as small (0.5 to 2.0 cm), delicate, structures, superficially attached to the mucosa by a stalk. The individual finger-like papillae have a central core of loose fibrovascular tissue covered by transitional epithelial cells that are **histologically identical to normal urothelium** (Fig. 21–8). True recurrences rarely if ever occur. In contrast to the above described exophytic papilloma, **inverted papillomas** are benign lesions consisting of inter-anastomosing cords of cytologically bland urothelium extending down into the lamina propria.[19,20]

Papillary urothelial neoplasms of low malignant potential (PUNLMP) share many histologic features with papilloma, the only differences being either thicker urothelium or diffuse nuclear enlargement in PUNLMP. Mitotic figures are rare. At cystoscopy, PUNLMP tend to be larger than papillomas and may be indistinguishable from low- and high-grade papillary cancers. PUNLMP may recur with the same morphology, are not associated with invasion, and only rarely recur as higher-grade tumors associated with invasion and progression.

Low-grade papillary urothelial carcinomas are characterized by an orderly appearance both architecturally and cytologically. The cells are evenly spaced (i.e., maintain polarity) and cohesive. There is minimal but definite evidence of nuclear atypia consisting of scattered hyperchromatic nuclei, infrequent mitotic figures predominantly towards the base, and mild variation in nuclear size and shape (Fig. 21–9). Low-grade cancers can recur and, although infrequent, can invade. Only rarely do these tumors pose a threat to the patient's life.

High-grade papillary urothelial cancers contain cells that may be dyscohesive and have large hyperchromatic nuclei. Some of the tumor cells show frank anaplasia (Fig. 21–10). Mitotic figures, including atypical ones, are frequent. Architecturally, there is disarray with loss of polarity. These tumors have a much higher incidence of invasion into the muscular layer, a higher risk of progression than low-grade lesions, and significant metastatic potential.

In most analyses, less than 10% of low-grade cancers invade, but as many as 80% of high-grade papillary urothelial cell carcinomas are invasive.[21,22] Aggressive tumors may not only extend into the bladder wall but, with progression, invade the adjacent prostate, seminal vesicles, ureters, and retroperitoneum. Some produce fistulous communications to the vagina or rectum. About 40% of these deeply invasive tumors metastasize to regional lymph nodes. Hematogenous dissemination, principally to the liver, lungs, and bone marrow, generally occurs late, and only with highly anaplastic tumors.

Carcinoma in situ (CIS) is defined by the presence of any cytologically malignant cells within a flat urothelium.[15,23–26] CIS may range from full-thickness cytologic atypia to scattered malignant cells in an otherwise normal urothelium, the latter termed pagetoid spread (Fig. 21–11). A common feature shared with high-grade papillary urothelial carcinoma is the lack of cohesiveness, which leads to the shedding of malignant cells into the urine. This may give rise to denuded urothelium with only a few CIS cells clinging to the basement membrane. Grossly, CIS usually appears as an area of mucosal reddening, granularity, or thickening without an intraluminal mass. It is com-

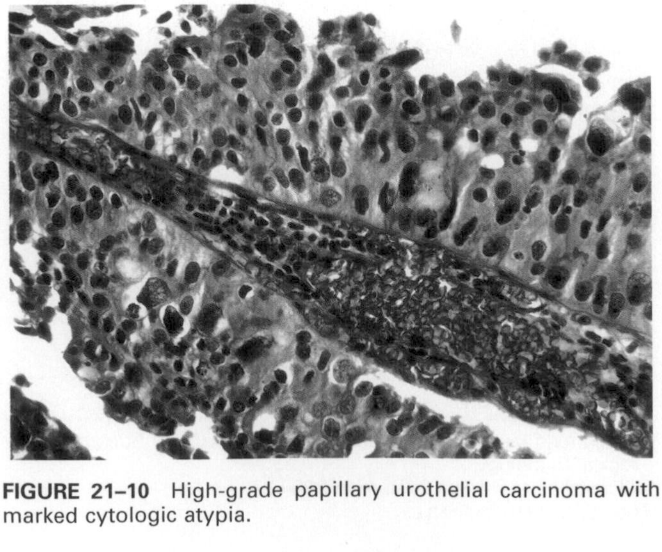

FIGURE 21–10 High-grade papillary urothelial carcinoma with marked cytologic atypia.

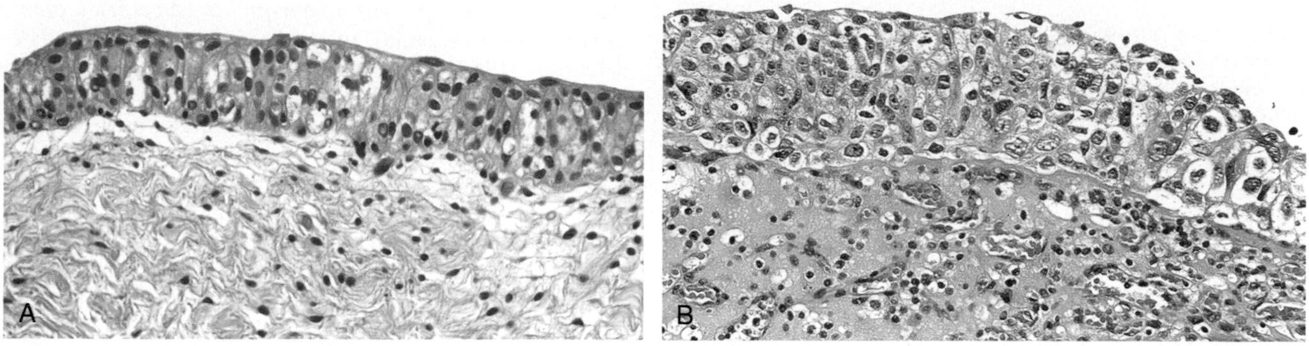

FIGURE 21–11 *A,* Normal urothelium with uniform nuclei and well-developed umbrella cell layer. *B,* Flat carcinoma in situ with numerous cells having enlarged and pleomorphic nuclei.

monly multifocal and may involve most of the bladder surface and extend into the ureters and urethra. Although carcinoma in situ is most often found in bladders harboring other patterns of transitional cell carcinoma, about 1% to 5% of cases occur in the absence of such tumors. If untreated, 50% to 75% of CIS cases progress to muscle-invasive cancer.

Invasive urothelial cancer, which is detected early, may be superficial in the lamina propria and can be associated with either papillary urothelial cancer, usually high grade, or with CIS. The extent of the invasion is of prognostic significance. Understaging on biopsy is a significant problem; on resection, there may be cancer invading the muscularis propria (Fig. 21–12). The extent of spread at the time of initial diagnosis is the most important factor in determining the outlook for a patient. Thus, **staging,** in addition to grade, is critical in the assessment of bladder neoplasms. The staging system most commonly used is given in Table 21–4.

Unusual variants of urothelial cancer include the nested variant with deceptively bland cytology lymphoepithelioma-like carcinoma and small cell carcinoma.[27–29]

Other Types of Carcinoma

Squamous cell carcinomas represent about 3% to 7% of bladder cancers in the United States, but in countries endemic for urinary schistosomiasis, they occur much more frequently.[30,31] Pure squamous cell carcinomas are nearly always associated with chronic bladder irritation and infection. **Mixed urothelial cell carcinomas with areas of squamous carcinoma** are more frequent than pure squamous cell carcinomas. Most are invasive, fungating tumors or infiltrative and ulcerative. True papillary patterns are almost never seen. The level of cytologic differentiation varies widely, from the highly differentiated lesions producing abundant keratohyaline pearls to anaplastic giant

TABLE 21–4 Pathologic T (Primary Tumor) Staging of Bladder Carcinoma

AJCC/UICC	Depth of Invasion
Noninvasive, papillary	Ta
Carcinoma in situ (noninvasive, flat)	Tis
Lamina propria invasion	T1
Muscularis propria invasion	T2
Microscopic extravesicle invasion	T3a
Grossly apparent extravesicle invasion	T3b
Invades adjacent structures	T4

AJCC/UICC, American Joint Commission on Cancer/Union Internationale Contre le Cancer.

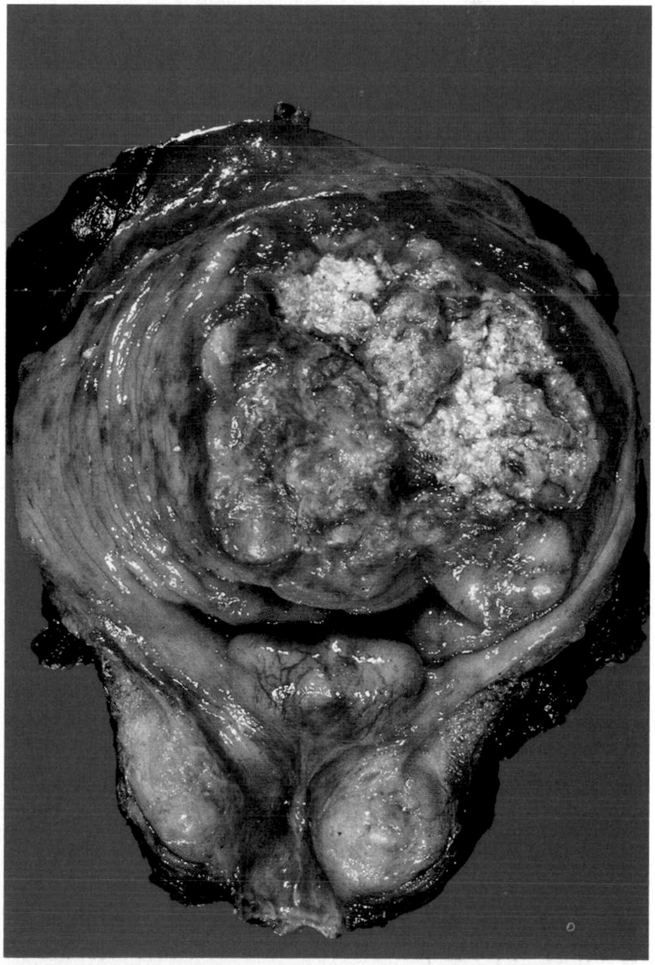

FIGURE 21–12 Opened bladder showing a high-grade invasive urothelial cell carcinoma at an advanced stage. The aggressive multinodular neoplasm has fungated into the bladder lumen and spread over a wide area. The yellow areas represent areas of ulceration and necrosis.

cell tumors showing little evidence of squamous differentiation. They often cover large areas of the bladder and are deeply invasive by the time of discovery.

Adenocarcinomas of the bladder are rare and they are histologically identical to adenocarcinomas seen in the gastrointestinal tract.[32,33] Some arise from urachal remnants or in association with extensive intestinal metaplasia (discussed earlier). Urachal tumors occur in the dome or anterior wall, arise within the wall rather than from the mucosa, and extend out of the bladder towards the umbilicus. Rare variants of adenocarcinoma are the highly malignant **signet-ring cell carcinoma, and mixed adenocarcinoma** and urothelial cell carcinomas.

Epidemiology and Pathogenesis. The epidemiology of carcinoma of the bladder resembles that of bronchogenic carcinoma, being more common in men than in women, in industrialized than in developing nations, and in urban than in rural dwellers. The male to female ratio for transitional cell tumors is approximately 3:1. About 80% of patients are between the ages of 50 and 80 years. Bladder cancer, with rare exception, is not familial.

A number of factors have been implicated in the causation of transitional cell carcinoma. Some of the more important contributors include the following:

- *Cigarette smoking* is clearly the most important influence, increasing the risk threefold to sevenfold, depending on the pack-years and smoking habits. Fifty per cent to 80% of all bladder cancers among men are associated with the use of cigarettes. Cigars, pipes, and smokeless tobacco invoke a much smaller risk.
- *Industrial exposure to arylamines,* particularly 2-naphthylamine as well as related compounds, as was pointed out in the earlier discussion of chemical carcinogenesis (Chapter 7). The cancers appear 15 to 40 years after the first exposure.
- *Schistosoma haematobium* infections in areas where these are endemic (Egypt, Sudan) are an established risk. The ova are deposited in the bladder wall and incite a brisk chronic inflammatory response that induces progressive mucosal squamous metaplasia and dysplasia and, in some instances, neoplasia. Seventy per cent of the cancers are squamous, the remainder being urothelial cell carcinoma.
- Long-term use of analgesics, implicated also in analgesic nephropathy (Chapter 20).
- Heavy long-term exposure to cyclophosphamide, an immunosuppressive agent, induces, as noted, hemorrhagic cystitis and increases the risk of bladder cancer.
- Prior exposure of the bladder to radiation, often performed for other pelvic malignancies, increases the risk of urothelial carcinoma. In this setting, bladder cancer occurs many years after the radiation.

How these influences induce cancer is unclear, but a number of genetic alterations have been observed in urothelial cell carcinoma.[34–39] The cytogenetic and molecular alterations are heterogeneous. Particularly common (occurring in 30% to 60% of tumors studied) are chromosome 9 monosomy or deletions of 9p and 9q as well as deletions of 17p, 13q, 11p, and 14q.[38] The *chromosome 9 deletions are the only genetic changes that are present frequently in superficial papillary tumors and occasionally in noninvasive flat tumors.* The 9p deletions (9p21) involve the tumor-suppressor gene *p16INK4a,* which encodes an inhibitor of a cyclin-dependent kinase (Chapter 7). The 9q deletion includes numerous other potential tumor-suppressor loci, but their identity is not yet known. On the other hand, many invasive urothelial cell carcinomas show *deletions of 17p,* including the region of the *p53* gene, as well as mutations in the *p53* gene, suggesting that these contribute to the progression of urothelial cell carcinoma. Mutations in *p53* are also found in flat in situ cancer lesions. The *13q* deletion involves the *retinoblastoma gene* and is also present in invasive tumors. Deletions of *14q* are seen exclusively in flat lesions or invasive tumors but not in papillary tumors, and a putative tumor-suppressor gene is being pursued. Increased expression of *RAS* and epidermal growth factor receptors is also seen in some bladder cancers.

On the basis of these findings, a model for bladder carcinogenesis has been proposed. In this two-pathway model,[35] the first pathway is *initiated by deletions of tumor-suppressor genes* on 9p and 9q, leading to superficial papillary tumors, a few of which may then acquire *p53* mutations and progress to invasion; a second pathway, possibly *initiated by p53 mutations,* leads to CIS and, with loss of chromosome 9, progresses to invasion.

Clinical Course. Bladder tumors classically produce painless hematuria. This is their dominant and sometimes only clinical manifestation. Frequency, urgency, and dysuria occasionally accompany the hematuria. When the ureteral orifice is involved, pyelonephritis or hydronephrosis may follow. About 60% of neoplasms, when first discovered, are single, and 70% are localized to the bladder.

Patients with urothelial tumors, whatever the grade, have a tendency to develop new tumors after excision, and recurrences may exhibit a higher grade. The risk of recurrence and progression is related to several factors, including tumor size, stage, grade, multifocality, prior recurrence rate, and associated dysplasia and/or carcinoma in situ in the surrounding mucosa.[40–45] Although the term "recurrence" is used, most of the subsequent tumors arise at different sites from the original lesion. Recurrent tumors reflect new tumors in some cases, and in other instances, they share the same clonal abnormalities as the initial tumor and represent a true recurrence of the initial lesion as a result of shedding and implantation of the original tumor cells.

The most important factors for progression-free survival are grade, presence of lamina propria invasion, and associated carcinoma in situ. Papillomas, papillary urothelial neoplasms of low malignant potential, and low-grade papillary urothelial cancer yield a 98% 10-year survival rate regardless of the number of recurrences; only a few patients (<10%) experience progression of their disease to higher-grade lesions. In contrast, only about 40% of individuals with a high-grade cancer survive 10 years; the tumor is progressive in 65%. Approximately 70% of patients with squamous cell carcinomas are dead within the year.

The clinical challenge with these neoplasms is early detection and adequate follow-up. Although cystoscopy and biopsy are the mainstays of diagnosis, carcinoma in situ that produces no or only subtle gross mucosal changes and early small papillary lesions may be difficult to detect. Of value in these circumstances are *cytologic examinations* and tests that detect the presence of various urine markers such as human complement factor H–related protein, telomerase, fibrin-fibrinogen degradation products, mucins, CEA, hyaluronic acid, hyaluronidase, nuclear matrix proteins, and DNA content.[46–49] The major deficiency with cytologic examination is the underrecognition of low-grade papillary neoplasms. The predominant limitation of many of the tests measuring urine markers is their relatively low specificity, because positive test results may occur in conditions associated with injured urothelium.

The treatment for bladder cancer depends on the grade, the stage, and whether the lesion is flat or papillary. For small, localized papillary tumors that are not high grade, the initial diagnostic transurethral resection is all that is done. Patients are closely followed with periodic cystoscopies and urine cytology for the rest of their life for tumor recurrence. Research is ongoing as to whether less invasive urine marker studies can be substituted for some of the follow-up tests so as to lengthen the intervals between the more invasive cystoscopic procedures. When a patient presents with multifocal bladder tumors, instillation of topical chemotherapy into the bladder, in the immediate postoperative period, can reduce the likelihood of tumor recurrence. After the biopsy site has healed, patients who are at high risk of recurrence and/or progression (CIS; papillary tumors that are high-grade, multifocal, have a history of rapid recurrence, or are associated with lamina propria invasion) receive topical immunotherapy consisting of intravesical installation of an attenuated strain of *Mycobacterium tuberculosis* called Bacillus Calmette-Guérin (BCG).[50] The therapy presumably works by eliciting a local cell-mediated immune reaction that destroys tumor cells. Radical cystectomy is typically performed for (1) tumor invading the muscularis propria, (2) CIS or high-grade papillary cancer refractory to BCG, and (3) CIS extending into the prostatic urethra and extending down the prostatic ducts beyond the reach of BCG. Advanced bladder cancer is treated by chemotherapy.

Mesenchymal Tumors

Benign. A great variety of benign mesenchymal tumors may arise in the bladder. Collectively, they are rare. The most common is *leiomyoma*. They all tend to grow as isolated, intramural, encapsulated, oval to spherical masses, varying in diameter up to several centimeters. On occasion, they assume submucosal pedunculated positions. They have the histologic features of their counterparts elsewhere.

Sarcomas. True sarcomas are distinctly uncommon in the bladder. Inflammatory pseudotumors, postoperative spindle cell nodules, and various carcinomas may assume sarcomatoid growth patterns and be mistaken histologically for sarcomas.[51,52] As a group, sarcomas tend to produce large masses (varying up to 10 to 15 cm in diameter) that protrude into the vesical lumen. Their soft, fleshy, gray-white gross appearance suggests their sarcomatous nature. The most common sarcoma in infancy or childhood is *embryonal rhabdomyosarcoma*. In some cases, they present as a polypoid, grapelike mass (*sarcoma botryoides*). The most common sarcoma in the bladder in adults is *leiomyosarcoma*.

Secondary Tumors

Secondary malignant involvement of the bladder is most often by direct extension from primary lesions in nearby organs, cervix, uterus, prostate, and rectum. On casual inspection of the bladder, secondary tumors may appear as primary carcinomas of this organ. Hemorrhage, ureteral obstruction, and vesicovaginal fistulas are the common sequelae. Distinction between primary adenocarcinoma of the bladder (urethral or otherwise) from local extension of colorectal cancer can be difficult. Lymphomas may also involve the bladder as a component of systemic disease but also, rarely, as primary bladder lymphoma.[53]

OBSTRUCTION

Obstruction to the bladder neck is of major clinical importance, not only for the changes that are induced in the bladder, but also because of its eventual effect on the kidney. A great variety of intrinsic and extrinsic diseases of the bladder can narrow the urethral orifice and cause partial or complete vesical obstruction. In males, the most important lesion is enlargement of the prostate gland due either to nodular hyperplasia or to carcinoma (Fig. 21–13). Outlet obstruction is somewhat less common in females and is most often caused by cystocele of the bladder. The other, less frequent, causes are: (1) congenital narrowings or strictures of the urethra; (2) inflammatory strictures of the urethra; (3) inflammatory fibrosis and contraction of the bladder after varying types of cystitis; (4) bladder tumors, either benign or malignant, when strategically located; (5) secondary invasion of the bladder neck by growths arising in perivesical structures, such as the cervix, vagina, prostate, and rectum; (6) mechanical obstructions caused by foreign bodies and calculi; and (7) injury to the innervation of the bladder, causing neurogenic bladder.

Morphology. In the early stages, there is only some thickening of the bladder wall, presumably due to hypertrophy of the smooth muscle. The mucosal surface at this time may be entirely normal. With progressive hypertrophy of the muscle coat, the individual muscle bundles greatly enlarge and produce trabeculation of the bladder wall. In the course of time, crypts form and may then become converted into true acquired diverticula.

In some cases of acute obstruction or in terminal disease, when the patient's normal reflex mechanisms are depressed, the bladder may become extremely

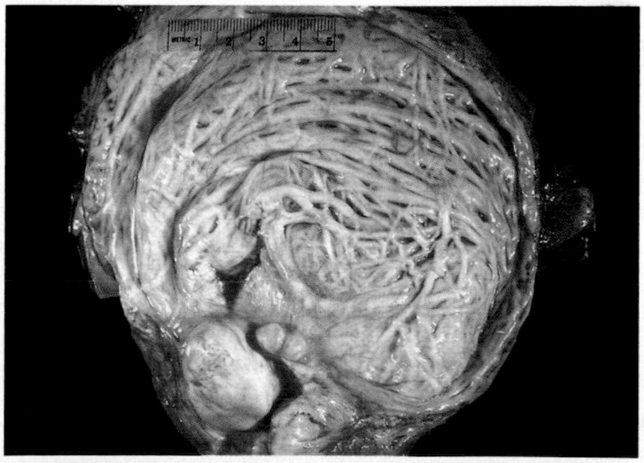

FIGURE 21–13 Hypertrophy and trabeculation of bladder wall secondary to polypoid hyperplasia of the prostate.

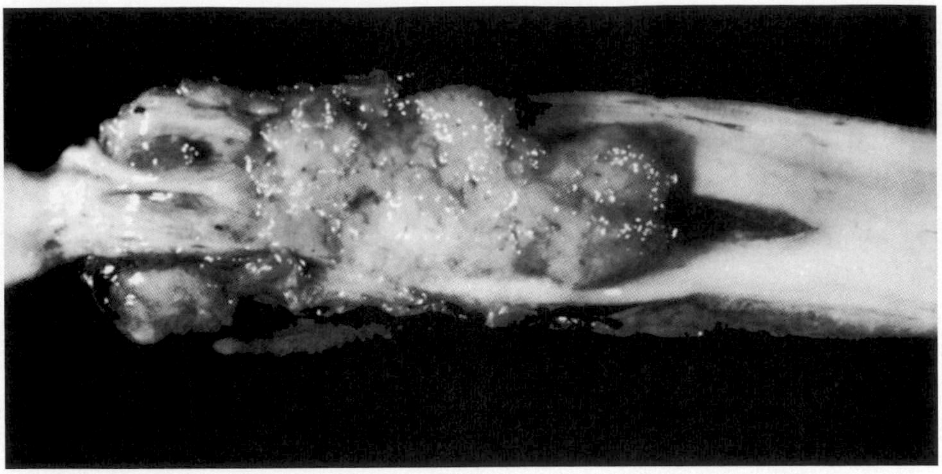

FIGURE 21–14 Carcinoma of urethra with typical fungating growth.

dilated. The enlarged bladder may reach the brim of the pelvis or even the level of the umbilicus. In these cases, the bladder wall is markedly thinned, and the trabeculation becomes totally unapparent.

Urethra

INFLAMMATIONS

Urethritis is classically divided into gonococcal and nongonococcal urethritis. Gonococcal urethritis is one of the earliest manifestations of this venereal infection. Nongonococcal urethritis is common and can be caused by a variety of bacteria, among which *E. coli* and other enteric organisms predominate. Urethritis is often accompanied by cystitis in women and by prostatitis in men. In many instances, bacteria cannot be isolated. Various strains of *Chlamydia* (e.g., *C. trachomatis*) are the cause of 25% to 60% of nongonococcal urethritis in men and about 20% in women. *Mycoplasma (Ureaplasma urealyticum)* also accounts for the symptoms of urethritis in many cases. Urethritis is also one component of *Reiter syndrome*, which comprises the clinical triad of arthritis, conjunctivitis, and urethritis.

The morphologic changes are entirely typical of inflammation in other sites within the urinary tract. The urethral involvement is not itself a serious clinical problem but may cause considerable local pain, itching, and frequency and may represent a forerunner of more serious disease at higher levels of the urogenital tract.

TUMORS AND TUMOR-LIKE LESIONS

Urethral caruncle is an inflammatory lesion presenting as a small, red, painful mass about the external urethral meatus in the female patient. Caruncles may be found at any age but are more common in later life. The lesion consists of a hemispheric, friable, 1- to 2-cm nodule that occurs singly, either just outside or just within the external urethral meatus. It may be covered by an intact mucosa but is extremely friable, and the slightest trauma may cause ulceration of the surface and bleeding. On histologic examination, it is composed of a *highly vascularized, young, fibroblastic connective tissue, usually heavily infiltrated with leukocytes.* The overlying epithelium, where present, is either transitional or squamous cell in type. Surgical excision affords prompt relief and cure.

Benign epithelial tumors of the urethra include squamous and transitional cell papillomas, inverted papillomas, and condylomas.

Primary *carcinoma of the urethra* is an uncommon lesion (Fig. 21–14). It tends to occur in advanced age in women. Tumors arising within the proximal urethra tend to show urothelial differentiation and are analogous to those occurring within the bladder. Those lesions found within the distal urethra are more typically squamous carcinomas. Glandular carcinomas less frequently occur in the urethra as primary tumors, and are also more frequent in women. Some lesions are similar to those described in the bladder, arising through metaplasia or less commonly from periurethral glands. The other, rarer, variant of urethral adenocarcinoma is clear cell adenocarcinoma. Cancers arising within the prostatic urethra are dealt with in the section on the prostate.

THE MALE GENITAL TRACT

Penis

The penis can be affected by congenital anomalies, inflammations, and tumors, the most important of which are inflammations and tumors. The venereal infections (e.g., syphilis and gonorrhea) usually begin with penile lesions. Carcinoma of the penis, although not one of the more common neoplasms in North America, accounts for about 1% of cancers in men.

CONGENITAL ANOMALIES

The penis is the site of many varied forms of congenital anomalies, only some of which have clinical significance. These range from congenital absence and hypoplasia to hyperplasia, duplication, and other aberrations in size and form. Most of these deviations are extremely uncommon and are readily apparent on inspection. Certain other anomalies are more frequent and therefore have greater clinical significance.

Hypospadias and Epispadias

Malformation of the urethral groove and urethral canal may create abnormal openings either on the *ventral surface of the penis (hypospadias)* or on the *dorsal surface (epispadias)*.[54] Although more frequent with epispadias, either of these two anomalies may be associated with failure of normal descent of the testes and with malformations of the urinary tract. Hypospadias, the more common of the two, occurs in approximately 1 in 300 live male births.[55] Even when isolated, these urethral defects may have clinical significance because often the abnormal opening is constricted, resulting in urinary tract obstruction and an increased risk of ascending urinary tract infections. When the orifices are situated near the base of the penis, normal ejaculation and insemination are hampered or totally blocked. These lesions therefore are possible causes of sterility in men.

Phimosis

When the orifice of the prepuce is too small to permit its normal retraction, the condition is designated *phimosis*. Such an abnormally small orifice may result from anomalous development but is more frequently the result of repeated attacks of infection that cause scarring of the preputial ring.[56] Phimosis is important because it interferes with cleanliness and permits the accumulation of secretions and detritus under the prepuce, favoring the development of secondary infections and possibly carcinoma. When a phimotic prepuce is forcibly retracted over the glans penis, marked constriction and subsequent swelling may block the replacement of the prepuce, creating what is known as *paraphimosis*. Not only is this condition extremely painful, but also it may be a potential cause of urethral constriction and serious acute urinary retention.

INFLAMMATIONS

Inflammations of the penis almost invariably involve the glans and prepuce and include a wide variety of specific and nonspecific infections. The specific infections—syphilis, gonorrhea, chancroid, granuloma inguinale, lymphopathia venerea, genital herpes—are sexually transmitted and are discussed in Chapters 8 and 22. Only the nonspecific infections causing so-called balanoposthitis need description here.

Balanoposthitis refers to infection of the glans and prepuce caused by a wide variety of organisms. Among the more common agents are *Candida albicans*, anaerobic bacteria, *Gardnerella*, and pyogenic bacteria.[57] Most cases occur as a consequence of poor local hygiene in uncircumcised males, with accumulation of desquamated epithelial cells, sweat, and debris, termed *smegma*, acting as local irritant. Persistence of such infections leads to inflammatory scarring and, as was mentioned earlier, is a common cause of phimosis.

TUMORS

Tumors of the penis are, on the whole, uncommon. The most frequent neoplasms are carcinomas and a benign epithelial tumor: condyloma acuminatum. In addition to the clearly defined benign and malignant categories, however, there are several forms of carcinoma in situ, exemplified by Bowen disease.

Benign Tumors

Condyloma Acuminatum

Condyloma acuminatum is a benign tumor caused by human papillomavirus (HPV). It is related to the common wart (verruca vulgaris) and may occur on any moist mucocutaneous surface of the external genitals in either sex. There is ample evidence that HPV and associated diseases are sexually transmitted. Of the various antigenically and genetically distinct types of HPV that have been identified, type 6 and, less frequently, type 11 have been clearly associated with condylomata acuminata. The antigens and genomes of these HPV types can be demonstrated in most lesions by immunoperoxidase and DNA hybridization techniques, respectively.

Morphology. Condylomata acuminata may occur on the external genitalia or perineal areas. On the penis, these lesions occur most often about the coronal sulcus and inner surface of the prepuce. They consist of single or multiple sessile or pedunculated, red papillary excrescences that vary from 1 mm to several millimeters in diameter (Fig. 21–15). Histologically, a branching, villous, papillary connective tissue stroma is covered by epithelium that may have considerable superficial hyperkeratosis and thickening of the underlying epidermis (acanthosis) (Fig. 21–16).

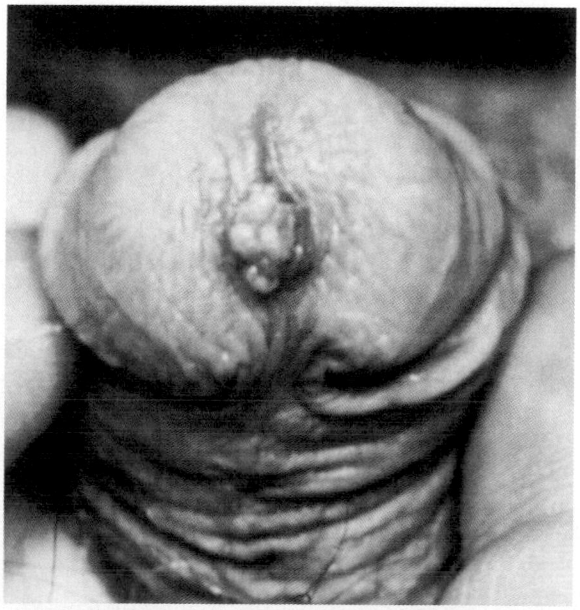

FIGURE 21–15 Condyloma acuminatum of the penis.

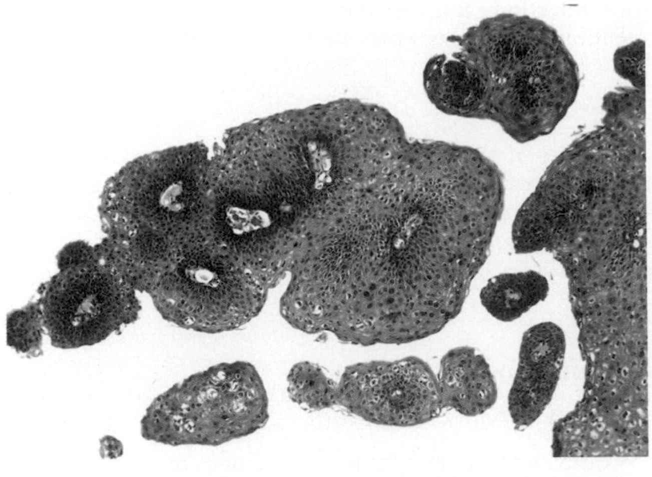

FIGURE 21–16 Condyloma acuminatum of the penis. Low magnification reveals the papillary (villous) architecture.

The normal orderly maturation of the epithelial cells is preserved. Clear vacuolization of the prickle cells (koilocytosis), characteristic of HPV infection, is noted in these lesions (Fig. 21–17). The basement membrane is intact, and there is no evidence of invasion of the underlying stroma. Condylomata acuminata tend to recur but do not evolve into invasive cancers.

Malignant Tumors

Carcinoma in Situ

As discussed in Chapters 7 and 22, *carcinoma in situ* (high-grade squamous intraepithelial neoplasia) is a histologic term used to describe epithelial lesions in which the cytologic changes of malignancy are confined to the epithelium, with no evidence of local invasion or distant metastases. It is considered a precancerous condition because of its potential to evolve into invasive cancer. In the external male genitalia, two distinct lesions that display histologic features of carcinoma in situ have been described: *Bowen disease* and *bowenoid papulosis*. All these lesions have a strong association with infection by HPV. Data compiled from a large number of studies reveal that HPV DNA, most commonly type 16, is found in approximately 80% of cases.[58]

Bowen disease occurs in the genital region of both men and women, usually in those over the age of 35 years. In men, it is prone to involve the skin of the shaft of the penis and the scrotum. Grossly, it appears as a solitary, thickened, gray-white, opaque plaque with shallow ulceration and crusting. It can also manifest on the glans and prepuce as single or multiple shiny red, sometimes velvety, plaques where it is clinically referred to as *Erythroplasia of Queyrat*. Histologically, the epidermis shows proliferation with numerous mitoses, some atypical. The cells are markedly dysplastic with large hyperchromatic nuclei and lack of orderly maturation (Fig. 21–18). Nevertheless, *the dermal-epidermal border is sharply delineated by an intact basement membrane.* Over the span of years, Bowen disease may transform into infiltrating squamous cell carcinoma in approximately 10% of patients. Another feature that is said to be associated with Bowen disease is the occurrence of visceral cancer in approximately one third of the patients. However, in the absence of long-term studies, this issue remains unresolved.

Bowenoid papulosis occurs in sexually active adults. Clinically, it differs from Bowen disease by the younger age of patients and the presence of multiple (rather than solitary) pigmented (reddish brown) papular lesions. In some cases, the lesions may be verrucoid and readily mistaken for condyloma acuminatum. Histologically, bowenoid papulosis is indistinguishable from Bowen disease and is also related to HPV 16. In contrast to Bowen disease, bowenoid papulosis virtually never develops into an invasive carcinoma, and in many cases, it spontaneously regresses.

Invasive Carcinoma

Squamous cell carcinoma of the penis is an uncommon malignancy in the United States, accounting for less than 1% of cancers in males.[59] By contrast, the incidence of squamous cell carcinoma of the penis ranges from 10% to 20% of male

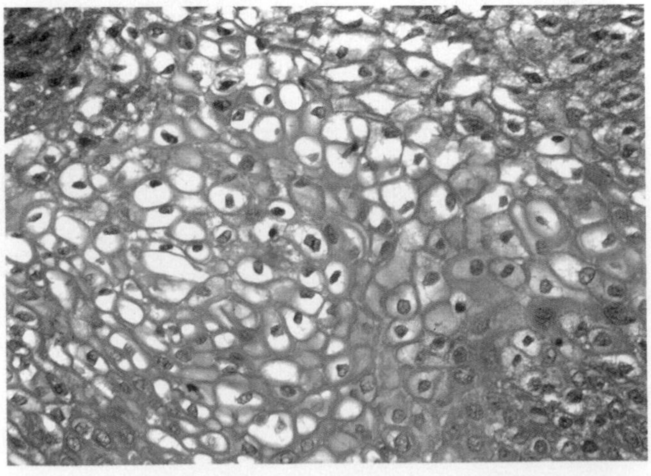

FIGURE 21–17 Condyloma acuminatum of the penis. The epithelium shows vacuolization (koilocytosis), characteristic of human papillomavirus (HPV) infection.

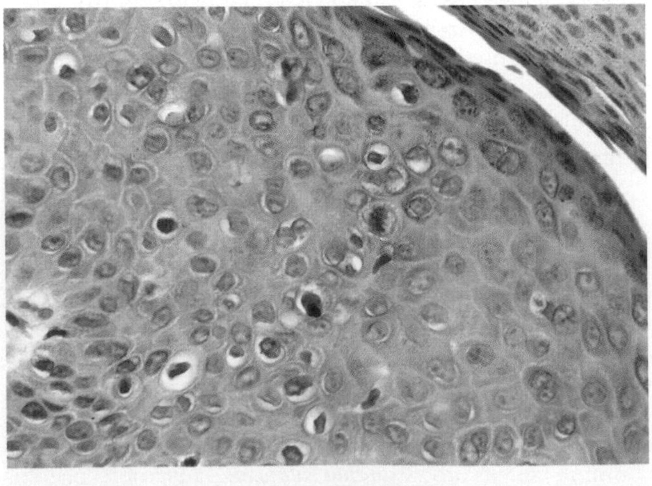

FIGURE 21–18 Bowen disease (carcinoma in situ) of the penis. The epithelium above the intact basement membrane (*not seen in this picture*) shows hyperchromatic, dysplastic dyskeratotic epithelial cells with scattered mitoses above the basal layer.

malignancies in some parts of Asia, Africa, and South America. A striking correlation exists between the practice of circumcision and the occurrence of penile cancer. Circumcision confers protection; hence, this cancer is extremely rare among Jews and Moslems and is correspondingly more common in populations in which circumcision is not routinely practiced. It is postulated that circumcision is associated with better genital hygiene, which, in turn, reduces exposure to carcinogens that may be concentrated in smegma and decreases the likelihood of infection with potentially oncogenic human papillomavirus (HPV). This notion is supported by the observation that HPV DNA can be detected in the cancer cells in approximately 50% of patients.[58] HPV type 16 is the most frequent culprit, but as with other genitourinary malignancies, HPV 18 is also implicated. Carcinoma in situ (Bowen disease), the presumed precursor lesion of invasive squamous cell carcinoma of the penis, has a much stronger association with HPV, being detected in 80% of lesions. This disparity suggests that infection with HPV is not sufficient for transformation and that it probably acts in concert with other carcinogenic influences. These may include carcinogens in cigarette smoke, which elevates the risk of developing cancer of the penis.[59] Carcinomas are usually found in patients between the ages of 40 and 70.

Morphology. Squamous cell carcinoma of the penis usually begins on the glans or inner surface of the prepuce near the coronal sulcus. Two macroscopic patterns are seen: papillary and flat. The papillary lesions simulate condylomata acuminata and may produce a cauliflower-like fungating mass. Flat lesions appear as areas of epithelial thickening accompanied by graying and fissuring of the mucosal surface. With progression, an ulcerated papule develops (Fig. 21–19). Histologically, both the papillary and the flat lesions are squamous cell carcinomas with varying degrees of differentiation. **Verrucous carcinoma** is an uncommon, well-differentiated variant of squamous cell carcinoma that has low malignant potential. These tumors are locally invasive, but they rarely metastasize. As the name indicates, these tumors have a verrucous (papillary) appearance, similar to condylomata acuminata, but they are larger than the usual condylomata. In contrast to condylomata acuminata, however, verrucous carcinomas can invade the underlying tissues. Other, less common, subtypes of penile squamous carcinoma include basaloid, warty, and papillary variants.[60,61]

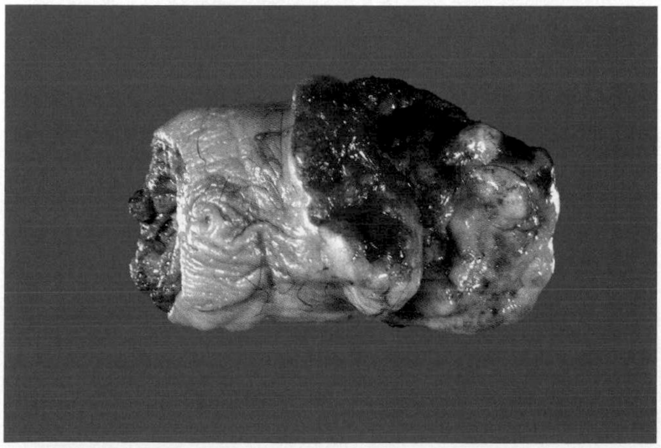

FIGURE 21–19 Carcinoma of the penis. The glans penis is deformed by a firm, ulcerated, infiltrative mass.

Clinical Course. Invasive squamous cell carcinoma of the penis is a slowly growing, locally invasive lesion[62] that often has been present for a year or more before it is brought to medical attention. The lesions are not painful until they undergo secondary ulceration and infection. Frequently, they bleed. Metastases to inguinal and iliac lymph nodes characterize the early stage, but widespread dissemination is extremely uncommon until the lesion is far advanced. Clinical assessment of regional lymph node involvement is notoriously inaccurate; 50% of men with penile squamous cell carcinoma and clinically enlarged inguinal nodes have only reactive lymphoid hyperplasia when examined histologically. The prognosis is related to the stage of the tumor. In persons with limited lesions without involvement of the inguinal lymph nodes, there is a 66% 5-year survival rate, whereas metastasis to the lymph nodes carries a grim 27% 5-year survival.

Testis and Epididymis

The major pathologic involvements of the testis and epididymis are quite distinct. In the case of the epididymis, the most important and frequent involvements are inflammatory diseases, whereas in the testis, the major lesions are tumors. Their close anatomic relationship, however, permits the extension of any of these processes from one organ to the other.

CONGENITAL ANOMALIES

With the exception of incomplete descent of the testes (cryptorchidism), congenital anomalies are extremely rare and include absence of one or both testes, fusion of the testes (so-called *synorchism*), and the formation of clinically insignificant cysts within the testis.

Cryptorchidism

Cryptorchidism is synonymous with undescended testes and is found in approximately 1% of 1-year-old boys.[63] This anomaly represents a complete or incomplete failure of the intra-abdominal testes to descend into the scrotal sac. It usually occurs as an isolated anomaly but may be accompanied by other malformations of the genitourinary tract, such as hypospadias.

Testicular descent occurs in two morphologically and hormonally distinct phases.[64] During the first, transabdominal, phase, the testis comes to lie within the lower abdomen or brim of the pelvis. This phase is believed to be controlled by a hormone called *müllerian-inhibiting substance.* In the second, or inguinoscrotal, phase, the testes descend through the inguinal canal into the scrotal sac. This phase is androgen dependent and is possibly mediated by androgen-induced release of calcitonin gene-related peptide from the genitofemoral nerve. Although testes may be arrested anywhere along their pathway of descent, defects in transabdominal descent are uncommon, accounting for approximately 5% to 10% of cases. In most patients, the undescended testis is palpable in the inguinal canal. The precise cause of cryptorchidism is still poorly understood. Despite the fact that testicular descent is controlled by hormonal factors, cryptorchidism is only rarely associated with hormonal disorders. It may be one of several congenital defects in chromosomal disorders, such as trisomy 13. The condition is completely asymptomatic, and it is found by the patient or the examining physician only when the scrotal sac is discovered not to contain the testis.

Morphology. Cryptorchidism is unilateral in most cases, but it may be bilateral in 25% of patients. Histologic changes in the malpositioned testis begin as early as 2 years of age. They are characterized by an arrest in the development of germ cells associated with marked hyalinization and thickening of the basement membrane of the spermatic tubules (Fig. 21–20). Eventually, the tubules appear as dense cords of hyaline connective tissue outlined by prominent basement membranes. There is concomitant increase in interstitial stroma. Because Leydig cells are spared, they appear to be prominent. As might be expected with progressive tubular atrophy, the cryptorchid testis is small in size and firm in consistency, owing to fibrotic changes. Histologic deterioration, leading to a paucity of germ cells, has also been noted in the contralateral (descended) testis in patients with unilateral cryptorchidism, supporting a hormonal basis for the development of this condition.

Cryptorchidism is of more than academic interest for many reasons. When the testis lies in the inguinal canal, it is particularly exposed to trauma and crushing against the ligaments and bones. A concomitant inguinal hernia accompanies such malposition of the testis in about 10% to 20% of cases. From the morphologic changes, it is apparent that bilateral cryptorchidism may result in sterility. Infertility, however, is also noted in a significant number of cases with uncorrected unilateral cryptorchidism because, as was mentioned earlier, the contralateral descended testis may also be deficient in germ cells. In addition, the undescended testis is at a greater risk of developing testicular cancer than is the descended testis.[65] During the first year of life, the majority of inguinal cryptorchid testes will descend spontaneously into the scrotum. Persistently undescended testes require surgical correction, preferably before histologic deterioration sets in at around 2 years of age.[63] Orchiopexy (placement in the scrotal sac) does not guarantee fertility; deficient spermatogenesis has been reported in 10% to 60% of patients in whom surgical repositioning was performed.[63,66] To what extent the risk of cancer is reduced after orchiopexy is also unclear. According to some studies, orchiopexy of unilateral cryptorchidism before 10 years of age protects against cancer development.[67] This is not universally accepted, however.[68] Malignant change may occur in the contralateral, normally descended testis. These observations suggest that cryptorchidism is associated with an intrinsic defect in testicular development and cellular differentiation that is unrelated to anatomic position.

REGRESSIVE CHANGES

Atrophy

Atrophy is a regressive change that affects the scrotal testis, and it may have a number of causes, including (1) progressive atherosclerotic narrowing of the blood supply in old age; (2) the end stage of an inflammatory orchitis, whatever the etiologic agent; (3) cryptorchidism; (4) hypopituitarism; (5) generalized malnutrition or cachexia; (6) irradiation; (7) prolonged administration of female sex hormones, as in treatment of patients with carcinoma of the prostate; and (8) exhaustion atrophy, which may follow the persistent stimulation produced by high levels of follicle-stimulating pituitary hormone. The gross and microscopic alterations follow the pattern already described for cryptorchidism. When the process is bilateral, as it frequently is, sterility results. Atrophy or sometimes improper development of the testes occasionally occurs as a primary failure of genetic origin. The resulting condition, called *Klinefelter syndrome*, represents a sex chromosomal disorder (discussed in detail in Chapter 5, along with other cytogenetic diseases).

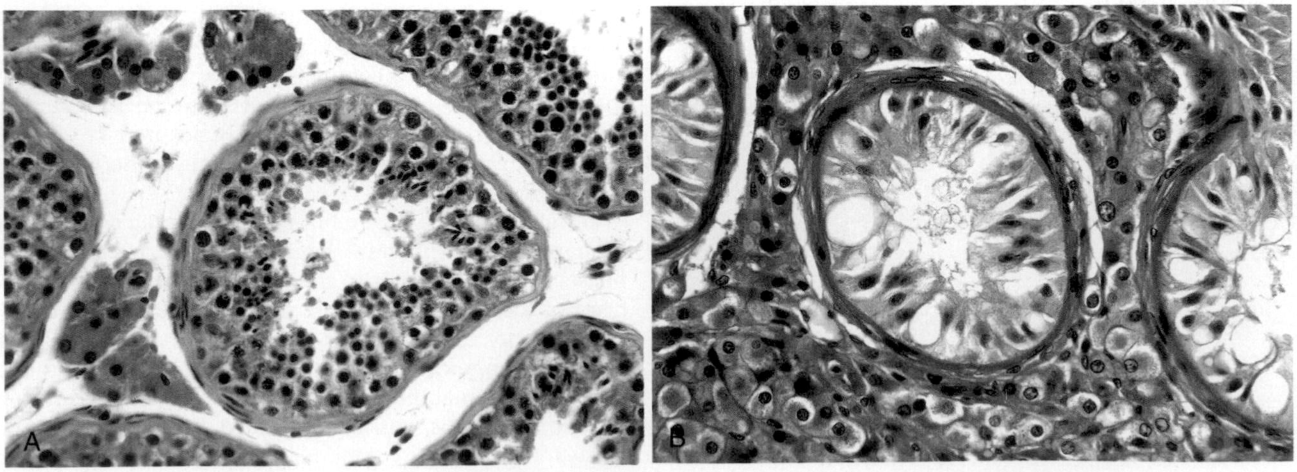

FIGURE 21–20 *A,* Normal testis shows tubules with active spermatogenesis. *B,* Testicular atrophy. The tubules show Sertoli cells but no spermatogenesis. There is thickening of basement membranes and an apparent increase in interstitial Leydig cells.

Findings Associated with Decreased Fertility

Atrophy represents the end-stage of many forms of testicular injury. Prior to this terminal nonspecific histologic appearance, several other patterns are recognized that are associated with decreased fertility.[69] These include hypospermatogenesis, maturation arrest, and findings associated with vas deferens obstruction. In some instances, a specific cause for the testicular injury can be found, and if it can be removed prior to the development of atrophy, testicular function can be restored.

INFLAMMATIONS

Inflammations are distinctly more common in the epididymis than in the testis. It is classically taught that, of the three major specific inflammatory states, *gonorrhea and tuberculosis almost invariably arise in the epididymis, whereas syphilis affects the testis first.*

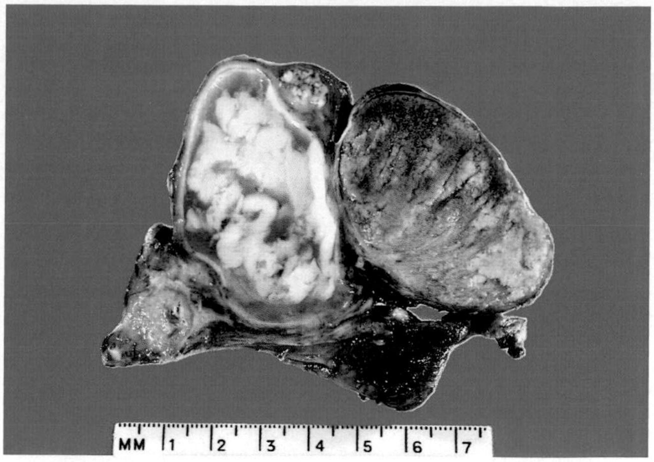

FIGURE 21–21 Acute epididymitis caused by gonococcal infection. The epididymis is replaced by an abscess. A normal testis is seen on the right.

Non-Specific Epididymitis and Orchitis

Epididymitis and possible subsequent orchitis are commonly related to infections in the urinary tract (cystitis, urethritis, genitoprostatitis), which presumably reach the epididymis and the testis through either the vas deferens or the lymphatics of the spermatic cord.

The cause of epididymitis varies with the age of the patient. Although uncommon in children, epididymitis in childhood is usually associated with a congenital genitourinary abnormality and infection with Gram-negative rods. In sexually active men younger than age 35 years, the sexually transmitted pathogens *Chlamydia trachomatis* and *Neisseria gonorrhoeae* are the most frequent culprits. In men older than age 35, the common urinary tract pathogens, such as *Escherichia coli* and *Pseudomonas*, are responsible for most infections.

Morphology. The bacterial invasion sets up a nonspecific acute inflammation characterized by congestion, edema, and infiltration by neutrophils, macrophages, and lymphocytes. Although the infection, in the early stage, is more or less limited to the interstitial connective tissue, it rapidly extends to involve the tubules and may progress to frank abscess formation or complete suppurative necrosis of the entire epididymis (Fig. 21–21). Usually, having involved the epididymis, the infection extends into the testis to evoke a similar inflammatory reaction. Such inflammatory involvement of the epididymis and testis is often followed by fibrous scarring, which, in many cases, leads to sterility. Usually, the interstitial cells of Leydig are not totally destroyed, so sexual activity is not disturbed.

Granulomatous (Autoimmune) Orchitis

Among middle-aged men, a rare cause of unilateral testicular enlargement is nontuberculous, granulomatous orchitis. It usually presents as a moderately tender testicular mass of sudden onset sometimes associated with fever. It may appear insidiously, however, as a painless testicular mass mimicking a testicular tumor, hence its importance. Histologically, the orchitis is distinguished by granulomas that are seen restricted within spermatic tubules. The lesions closely resemble tubercles but differ in that the granulomatous reaction is present diffusely throughout the testis and is confined to the seminiferous tubules. Although an autoimmune basis is suspected, the cause of these lesions remains unknown.

Specific Inflammations

Gonorrhea

Extension of infection from the posterior urethra to the prostate to the seminal vesicles and then to the epididymis is the usual course of a neglected gonococcal infection. Inflammatory changes similar to those described in the nonspecific infections occur, with the development of frank abscesses in the epididymis, resulting in extensive destruction of this organ. In the more neglected cases, the infection can then spread to the testis and produce a suppurative orchitis.

Mumps

Mumps is a systemic viral disease that most commonly affects school-age children. Testicular involvement is extremely uncommon in this age group. In postpubertal males, however, orchitis may develop and has been reported in 20% to 30% of male patients. Most often, the acute interstitial orchitis develops about 1 week after onset of swelling of the parotid glands. Rarely, cases of orchitis precede the parotitis or may be unaccompanied by parotid gland involvement.

Tuberculosis

Tuberculosis almost invariably begins in the epididymis and may spread to the testis. In many of these cases, there is associated tuberculous prostatitis and seminal vesiculitis, and it is believed that epididymitis usually represents a secondary spread from these other involvements of the genital tract. The infection invokes the classic morphologic reactions of caseating granulomatous inflammation that are characteristic of tuberculosis elsewhere.

Syphilis

The testis and epididymis are affected in both acquired and congenital syphilis, but *almost invariably, the testis is involved first by the infection.* In many cases, the orchitis is not accompanied by epididymitis. The morphologic pattern of the reaction takes two forms: the production of gummas or a diffuse interstitial inflammation characterized by edema and lymphocytic and plasma cell infiltration with the characteristic hallmark of all syphilitic infections (i.e., obliterative endarteritis with perivascular cuffing of lymphocytes and plasma cells).

VASCULAR DISTURBANCES

Torsion

Twisting of the spermatic cord may cut off the venous drainage and the arterial supply to the testis. Usually, however, the thick-walled arteries remain patent, so intense vascular engorgement and venous infarction follow. There are two types of testicular torsion. Neonatal torsion occurs either in utero or shortly after birth. It lacks any associated anatomic defect to account for its occurrence. Adult torsion is typically seen in adolescence, presenting as sudden onset of testicular pain. In contrast to neonatal torsion, adult torsion results from a bilateral anatomic defect in which the testis has increased mobility, giving rise to what is termed the bell-clapper abnormality. It often occurs without any inciting injury; sudden pain heralding the torsion may even occur during sleep. Torsion is one of the few urologic emergencies. If the testis is explored surgically and manually untwisted within approximately 6 hours after the onset of torsion, there is a good chance that the testis will remain viable. To prevent the catastrophic occurrence of subsequent torsion in the contralateral testis, the testis that is unaffected by torsion is surgically fixed to the scrotum (orchiopexy).

Morphology. Depending on the duration of the process, the morphologic changes range from intense congestion to widespread extravasation of blood into the interstitial tissue of the testis and epididymis. Eventually, hemorrhagic infarction of the entire testis occurs (Fig. 21–22). In the late stages, the testis is markedly enlarged and is converted virtually into a sac of soft, necrotic, hemorrhagic tissue.

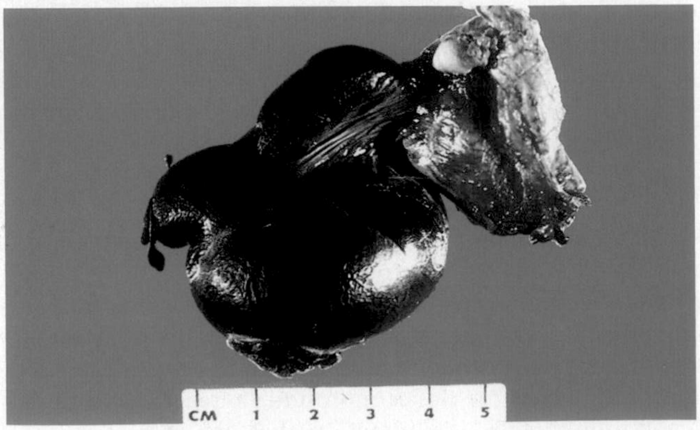

FIGURE 21–22 Torsion of the testis.

Spermatic Cord and Paratesticular Tumors

Lipomas are common lesions involving the proximal spermatic cord. They are often identified at the time of inguinal hernia repair. Although diagnosed as "lipomas," many of these lesions probably represent retroperitoneal adipose tissue that has been pulled into the inguinal canal along with the hernia sac, rather than a true neoplasm.

The most common benign paratesticular tumor is *adenomatoid tumor*. Although these lesions are mesothelial in nature, they are not referred to as mesotheliomas, in order to distinguish them from other mesothelial lesions that may occur at this site. Adenomatoid tumors are usually small nodules that typically occur near the upper pole of the epididymis. Although they are grossly well circumscribed, microscopically they may be minimally invasive into the surrounding tissue, including the adjacent testis. The importance of this lesion is that it is one of the few benign tumors seen near the testis. If the urologist can identify the nature of this lesion with the aid of intraoperative frozen sections, local excision of the adenomatoid tumor can spare the patient orchiectomy.

The most common malignant paratesticular tumors located at the distal end of the spermatic cord are rhabdomyosarcomas in children and liposarcomas in adults.

TESTICULAR TUMORS

Testicular neoplasms span an amazing gamut of anatomic types.[70–72] They are divided into two major categories: germ cell tumors and nongerminal tumors derived from stroma or sex cord. Approximately 95% arise from germ cells. Most of these germinal tumors are highly aggressive cancers that are capable of rapid, wide dissemination, although with current therapy, most can be cured.[73] Nongerminal tumors, in contrast, are generally benign, but some elaborate steroids, leading to interesting endocrinologic syndromes.

Germ Cell Tumors

Approximately 8000 cases of testicular tumors are diagnosed per year in the United States, resulting in about 400 deaths per year. For unexplained reasons, there is a worldwide increase in the incidence of these tumors. In the 15- to 34-year age group, when these neoplasms have a peak incidence, they constitute the most common tumor of men and cause approximately 10% of all cancer deaths. In the United States, these tumors are much more common in whites than in blacks (ratio 5:1).

Classification and Histogenesis. As one might guess, germ cells are multipotential, and once they become cancerous, they are not inhibited in their lines of differentiation. Table 21–5 lists the most common germ cell tumors and the classification system that is most widely used in the United States.

Testicular germ cell tumors may be divided into two categories on the basis of whether they are composed of a single histologic pattern or more than one. Tumors with a single histologic pattern constitute about 40% of all testicular neoplasms and are listed in Table 21–5. In approximately 60% of the tumors, there is a *mixture of two or more of the histologic patterns.*

TABLE 21–5 Pathologic Classification of Common Testicular Tumors

Germ Cell Tumors
Seminoma
Spermatocytic seminoma
Embryonal carcinoma
Yolk sac (endodermal sinus) tumor
Choriocarcinoma
Teratoma
Sex Cord–Stromal Tumors
Leydig cell tumor
Sertoli cell tumor

Most tumors in this group originate from intratubular germ cell neoplasia (ITGCN).[74,75] ITGCN is seen adjacent to all germ cell tumors in adults except for spermatocytic seminoma and epidermoid and dermoid cysts. With rare exceptions, it is also not seen in pediatric tumors (teratomas, yolk sac tumors). ITCGN is encountered with a high frequency in the following conditions, listed in order of increasing risk: cryptorchidism, prior germ cell tumors, strong family history of germ cell tumor, androgen insensitivity syndrome, and gonadal dysgenesis syndrome. Untreated ITGCN progresses to invasive germ cell tumor in approximately 50% of cases over 5 years of follow-up. Thus its significance is similar to carcinoma in situ in other organs. If ITGCN is identified, it is treated by low-dose radiotherapy, which destroys the germ cells yet maintains the androgen production of the Leydig cells.

Neoplastic germ cells may differentiate along gonadal lines to give rise to *seminoma* or transform into a totipotential cell population that gives rise to *nonseminomatous tumors.* Such totipotential cells may remain largely undifferentiated to form embryonal carcinoma or may differentiate along extraembryonic lines to form *yolk sac tumors* or *choriocarcinomas.* Teratoma results from differentiation of the embryonic carcinoma cells along the lines of all three germ cell layers. Some studies suggest that seminomas are not end-stage neoplasms. Similar to embryonal carcinomas, seminomas may also act as precursors from which other forms of testicular germ cell tumors originate. This view is supported by the fact that cells that form intratubular germ cell neoplasias (the presumed precursors of all types of germ cell tumors) share morphologic and molecular characteristics with tumor cells in seminomas. Despite the fascination of pathologists with the heterogeneity of testicular tumors, from a *clinical standpoint the most important distinction in germ cell tumors is between seminomas and nonseminomatous tumors.* As will be discussed later, this clinical distinction has important bearings on treatment and prognosis.

Pathogenesis As with all neoplasms, little is known about the ultimate cause of germ cell tumors. Several predisposing influences, however, are important: (1) cryptorchidism, (2) testicular dysgenesis, and (3) genetic factors, all of which may contribute to a common denominator: germ cell maldevelopment. Reference has already been made to the increased incidence of neoplasms in *undescended testes.* In most large series of testicular tumors, approximately 10% are associated with cryptorchidism. The higher the location of the undescended testicle (intra-abdominal versus inguinal), the greater is the risk of developing cancer.

Patients with disorders of testicular development (testicular dysgenesis), including testicular feminization and Klinefelter syndrome, harbor an increased risk of developing germ cell tumors. The risk is highest in patients with testicular feminization. In cryptorchid and dysgenetic testes, foci of intratubular germ cell neoplasms can be detected at a high frequency before the development of invasive tumors.

Genetic predisposition also seems to be important, although no well-defined pattern of inheritance has been identified. In support, striking racial differences in the incidence of testicular tumors can be cited. Blacks in Africa have an extremely low incidence of these neoplasms, which is unaffected by migration to the United States. Familial clustering has been reported, and according to one study, sibs of affected individuals have a tenfold higher risk of developing testicular cancer than does the general population.

As with all tumors, genomic changes are undoubtedly important in the pathogenesis of testicular cancers. An *isochromosome of the short arm of chromosome 12,* i(*12p*), *is found in virtually all germ cell tumors,* regardless of their histologic type. In the approximately 10% of cases in which i(12p) is not detected, extra genetic material derived from 12p is found on other chromosomes. Obviously, dosage of genes located on 12p is critical for the pathogenesis of germ cell tumors, and several candidate genes have been identified, including a novel gene, called *DAD-R,* that prevents apoptosis.[76,77] It is of interest that i(12p) is also noted in ovarian germ cell neoplasms, suggesting that the events leading to this alteration may be critical to the molecular pathogenesis of all germ cell neoplasms.

With this background of pathogenesis, we can discuss the morphologic patterns of germ cell tumors, followed by the clinical features that are common to most germinal tumors.

Seminoma

Seminomas are the most common type of germinal tumor (50%) and the type most likely to produce a uniform population of cells. They almost never occur in infants; they peak in the thirties. An identical tumor arises in the ovary, where it is called *dysgerminoma* (Chapter 22).

Morphology. If not otherwise specified, the term "seminoma" refers to "classic" or "typical" seminoma. Spermatocytic seminoma, despite its nosologic similarity, is actually a distinct tumor; it has been segregated into a separate category and will be discussed later.

Seminomas produce bulky masses, sometimes 10 times the size of the normal testis. The typical seminoma has a homogeneous, gray-white, lobulated cut surface, usually devoid of hemorrhage or necrosis (Fig. 21–23). In more than half of cases, the entire testis is replaced. Generally, the tunica albuginea is not penetrated, but occasionally, extension to the epididymis, spermatic cord, or scrotal sac occurs.

Microscopically, the typical seminoma presents sheets of uniform cells divided into poorly demarcated lobules by delicate septa of fibrous tissue (Fig. 21–24*A*). **The classic seminoma cell is large and round to polyhedral and has a distinct cell membrane; a clear or watery-appearing cytoplasm; and a large,**

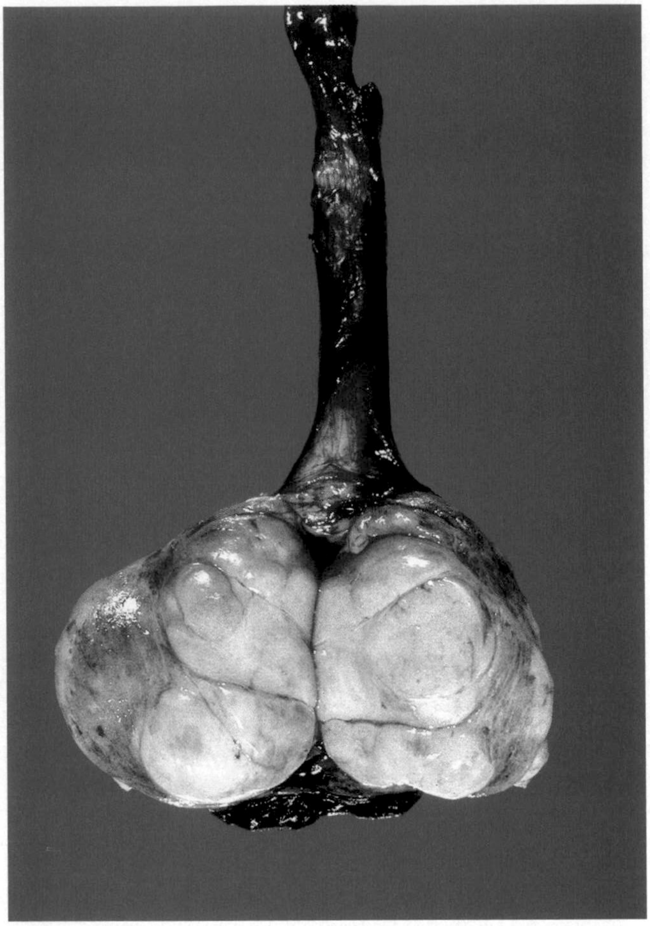

FIGURE 21–23 Seminoma of the testis appears as a fairly well circumscribed, pale, fleshy, homogeneous mass.

central nucleus with one or two prominent nucleoli (Fig. 21–24*B*). Mitoses vary in frequency. The cytoplasm contains varying amounts of glycogen. Classic seminoma cells do not contain α-fetoprotein (AFP) or human chorionic gonadotropin (HCG). The tumor cells stain positively for placental alkaline phosphatase, and scattered cells may be keratin positive.

Approximately 15% of seminomas contain syncytiotrophoblasts. In this subset of patients, serum HCG levels are also elevated, although not to the extent seen in patients with choriocarcinoma. The amount of stroma in typical seminomas varies greatly. Sometimes it is scant; at other times, it is abundant. Usually, well-defined fibrous strands are present, creating lobules of neoplastic cells. The septa are usually infiltrated with T lymphocytes, and in some tumors, they also bear prominent granulomas.

The term "anaplastic seminoma" is used by some to indicate greater cellular and nuclear irregularity with more frequent tumor giant cells and many mitoses. However, because "anaplastic seminoma" is not associated with a worse prognosis when matched for stage with classic seminoma, and is not treated differently, most authorities do not recognize "anaplastic seminoma" as a distinct entity.

Spermatocytic Seminoma

Although related by name to seminoma, spermatocytic seminoma is a distinctive tumor both clinically and histologically.[78] It is one of the two variants of germ cell tumors that do not arise from an intratubular germ cell neoplasia, the other being teratomas of children. Spermatocytic seminoma is an uncommon tumor, representing 1% to 2% of all testicular germ cell neoplasms. The age of involvement is much later than for most testicular tumors: Affected individuals are generally over the age of 65 years. In contrast to classic seminoma, it is a slow-growing tumor that rarely if ever produces metastases; hence, the prognosis is excellent.

Morphology. Grossly, spermatocytic seminoma tends to be larger than classic seminoma and presents with a pale gray, soft, cut surface sometimes with mucoid cysts. Spermatocytic seminomas have three cell populations, all intermixed: (1) medium-sized cells (15 to 18 μm), which are the most numerous, containing a round nucleus and eosinophilic cytoplasm; (2) smaller cells (6 to 8 μm), with a narrow rim of eosinophilic cytoplasm resembling secondary spermatocytes; and (3) scattered giant cells (50 to 100 μm), either uninucleate or multinucleate. In some intermediate-sized cells, chromatin is similar to that seen in

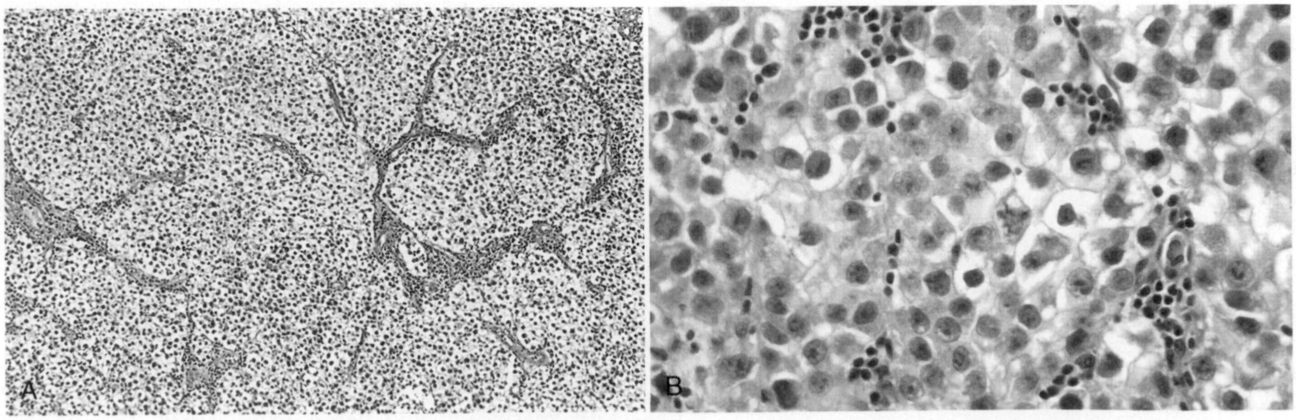

FIGURE 21–24 Seminoma. *A*, Low magnification shows clear seminoma cells divided into poorly demarcated lobules by delicate septa. *B*, Microscopic examination reveals large cells with distinct cell borders, pale nuclei, prominent nucleoli, and a sparse lymphocytic infiltrate.

the meiotic phase of non-neoplastic spermatocytes (spireme chromatin), thus justifying the term *spermatocytic seminoma.*

Embryonal Carcinoma

Embryonal carcinomas occur mostly in the 20- to 30-year age group. These tumors are more aggressive than seminomas.

Morphology. Grossly, the tumor is smaller than seminoma and usually does not replace the entire testis. On cut surfaces, the mass is often variegated, poorly demarcated at the margins, and punctuated by foci of hemorrhage or necrosis (Fig. 21–25). Extension through the tunica albuginea into the epididymis or cord is not infrequent. **Histologically, the cells grow in alveolar or tubular patterns, sometimes with papillary convolutions** (Fig. 21–26). Embryonal carcinomas lack the well-formed glands with basally situated nuclei and apical cytoplasm seen in teratomas. **More undifferentiated lesions may present sheets of cells.** The neoplastic cells have an epithelial appearance and are large and anaplastic, with hyperchromatic nuclei having prominent nucleoli. In contrast to seminoma, the cell borders are usually indistinct, and there is considerable variation in cell and nuclear size and shape. Mitotic figures and tumor giant cells are frequent. **Within this background, syncytial cells containing HCG, cells containing AFP, or both may be detected by immunoperoxidase techniques.** Most authorities allow for focal AFP positivity within an embryonal carcinoma without classifying the tumor as a mixed tumor. However, some purists designate any AFP positivity in an embryonal carcinoma, even if unaccompanied by yolk sac differentiation on the H&E stained section, as focal yolk sac tumor in a mixed tumor.

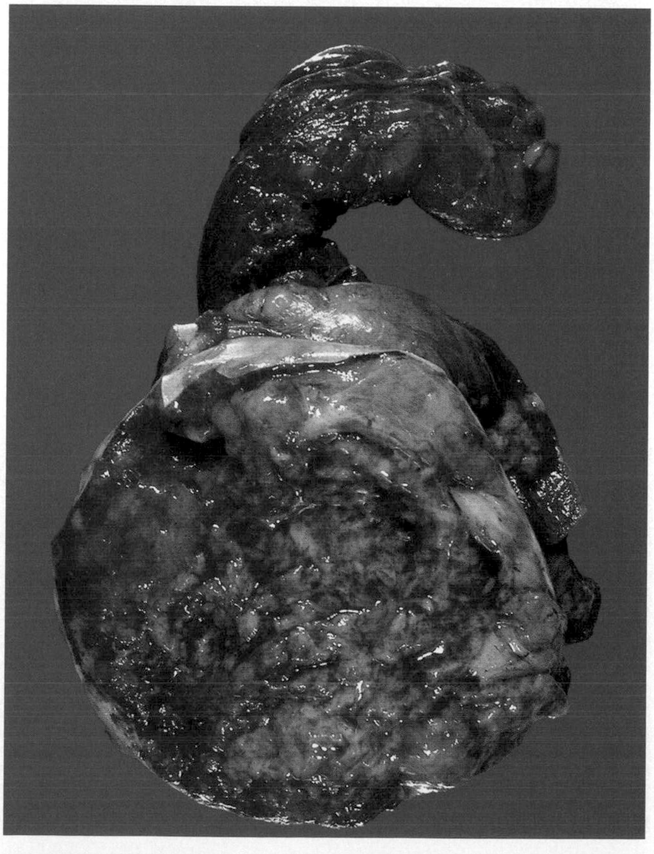

FIGURE 21–25 Embryonal carcinoma. In contrast to the seminoma illustrated in Figure 21–23, the embryonal carcinoma is a hemorrhagic mass.

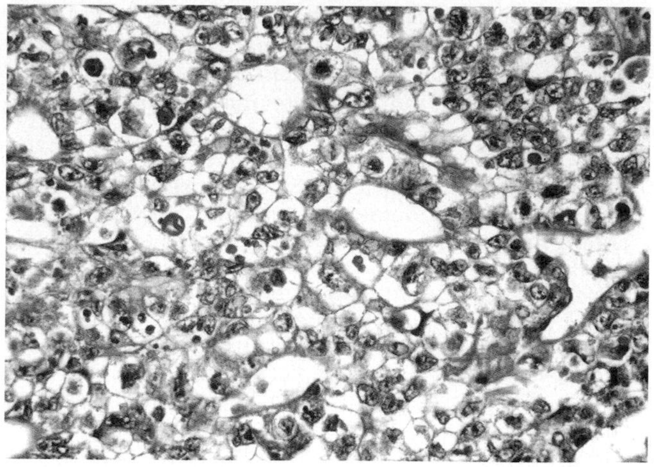

FIGURE 21–26 Embryonal carcinoma shows sheets of undifferentiated cells as well as primitive glandular differentiation. The nuclei are large and hyperchromatic.

Yolk Sac Tumor

Also known as *infantile embryonal carcinoma* or *endodermal sinus tumor*, the yolk sac tumor is of interest because it is the most common testicular tumor in infants and children up to 3 years of age, and in this age group, it has a very good prognosis. In adults, the pure form of this tumor is rare; instead, yolk sac elements frequently occur in combination with embryonal carcinoma.

Morphology. Grossly, the tumor is nonencapsulated, and on cross-section, it presents a homogeneous, yellow-white, mucinous appearance. Characteristic on microscopic examination is a lacelike (reticular) network of medium-sized cuboidal or elongated cells. In addition, papillary structures or solid cords of cells may be found. In approximately 50% of tumors, structures resembling endodermal sinuses (Schiller-Duval bodies) may be seen; these consist of a mesodermal core with a central capillary and a visceral and parietal layer of cells resembling primitive glomeruli. Present within and outside the cytoplasm are eosinophilic, hyalin-like globules in which AFP and α_1-antitrypsin can be demonstrated by immunocytochemical staining. The presence of AFP in the tumor cells is highly characteristic, and it underscores their differentiation into yolk sac cells.

Choriocarcinoma

Choriocarcinoma is a highly malignant form of testicular tumor that is composed of both cytotrophoblastic and syncytiotrophoblastic cells. Identical tumors may arise in the placental tissue, ovary, or sequestered rests of totipotential cells (e.g., in the mediastinum or abdomen). In its "pure" form, choriocarcinoma is rare, constituting fewer than 1% of all germ cell tumors. As will be emphasized later, foci of choriocarcinoma are much more common in mixed patterns.

Morphology. Despite their aggressive behavior, pure choriocarcinomas are usually small lesions. **Often, they cause no testicular enlargement and are detected only as a small palpable nodule.** Because they are rapidly growing, they may outgrow their blood supply, and sometimes the primary testicular focus is replaced by a small fibrous scar, leaving only widespread metastases. Typically, these tumors are small, rarely larger than 5 cm in diameter. Hemorrhage and necrosis are extremely common. Histologically, the tumors contain two cell types (Fig. 21–27). The syncytiotrophoblastic cell is large and has many irregular or lobular hyperchromatic nuclei and an abundant eosinophilic vacuolated cytoplasm. As might be expected, HCG can be readily demonstrated in the cytoplasm of syncytiotrophoblastic cells. The cytotrophoblastic cells are more regular and tend to be polygonal with distinct cell borders and clear cytoplasm; they grow in cords or masses and have a single, fairly uniform nucleus. More anatomic details are available in the discussion of these neoplasms in the female genital tract (Chapter 22).

Teratoma

The designation *teratoma* refers to a group of complex tumors having various cellular or organoid components reminiscent of normal derivatives from more than one germ layer. They may occur at any age from infancy to adult life. Pure forms of teratoma are fairly common in infants and children, second only in frequency to yolk sac tumors. In adults, pure teratomas are rare, constituting 2% to 3% of germ cell tumors. As with embryonal carcinomas, their frequency in combination with other histologic types is about 45%.

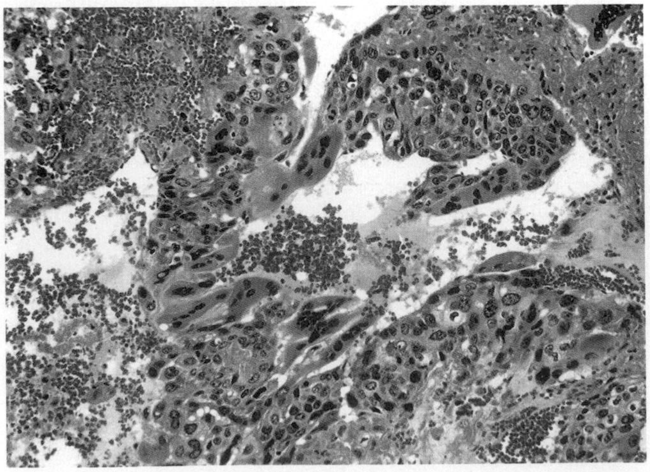

FIGURE 21–27 Choriocarcinoma shows clear cytotrophoblastic cells with central nuclei and syncytiotrophoblastic cells with multiple dark nuclei embedded in eosinophilic cytoplasm. Hemorrhage and necrosis are prominent.

Morphology. Grossly, teratomas are usually large, ranging from 5 to 10 cm in diameter. Because they are composed of various tissues, the gross appearance is heterogeneous, with solid, sometimes cartilaginous and cystic areas (Fig. 21–28). Hemorrhage and necrosis usually indicate admixture with embryonal carcinoma, choriocarcinoma, or both.

Teratomas are composed of a heterogeneous, helter-skelter collection of differentiated cells or organoid structures, such as neural tissue, muscle bundles, islands of cartilage, clusters of squamous epithelium, structures reminiscent of thyroid gland, bronchial or bronchiolar epithelium, and bits of intestinal wall or brain substance, all embedded in a fibrous or myxoid stroma (Fig. 21–29). Elements may be mature (resembling various tissues within the adult) or immature (sharing histologic features with fetal or embryonal tissue). Dermoid cysts and epidermoid cysts, common in the ovary (Chapter 22), are rare in the testis. These cysts should not be considered teratomas, since they have a uniformly benign behavior regardless of the patient's age.

Rarely, non–germ cell tumors may arise in a teratoma.[79] These tumors are referred to as "teratoma with malignant transformation," and they reveal malignancy in derivatives of one or more germ cell layers. Thus, there may be a focus of squamous cell carcinoma, mucin-secreting adenocarcinoma, or sarcoma. The importance of recognizing a non–germ cell malignancy arising in a teratoma is that when the non–germ cell component spreads outside of the testis it does not respond to chemotherapy, and the only hope for cure resides in the local resection of the tumor. These non–germ cell malignancies have some of the same chromosome abnormalities (isochromosome 12p) as the germ cell tumors from which they arose.

In children, differentiated mature teratomas may be expected to behave as benign tumors, and almost all these patients have a good prognosis. *In the postpubertal male, all teratomas are regarded as malignant and capable of metastatic behavior, regardless of whether the elements are mature or immature.* Consequently, it is not critical to note histologic differentiation in a postpubertal male with a testicular teratoma.

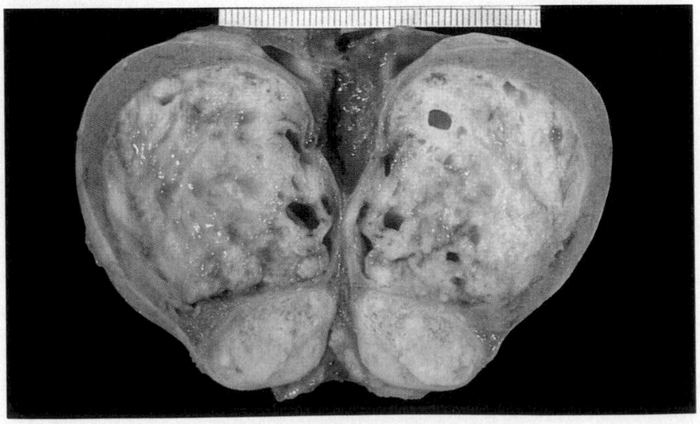

FIGURE 21–28 Teratoma of the testis. The variegated cut surface with cysts reflects the multiplicity of tissue found histologically.

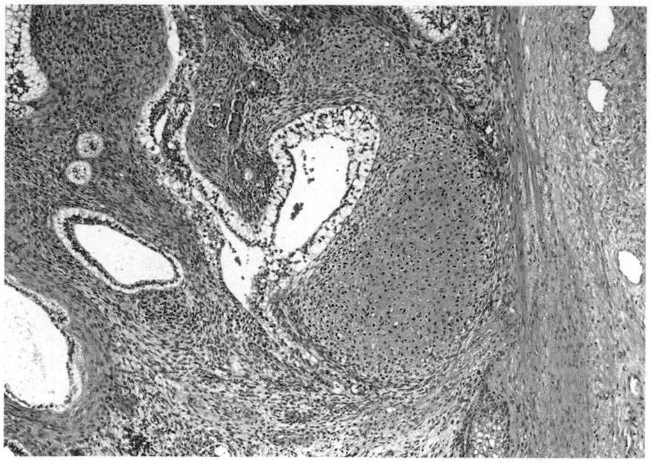

FIGURE 21–29 Teratoma of the testis consisting of a disorganized collection of glands, cartilage, smooth muscle, and immature stroma.

Mixed Tumors

About 60% of testicular tumors are composed of more than one of the "pure" patterns. Common mixtures include teratoma, embryonal carcinoma, and yolk sac tumor; seminoma with embryonal carcinoma; and embryonal carcinoma with teratoma (*teratocarcinoma*). In most instances, the prognosis is worsened by the inclusion of more aggressive elements.

Clinical Features of Testicular Tumors. From a clinical standpoint, tumors of the testis are segregated into two broad categories: *seminoma* and *nonseminomatous* germ cell tumors (NSGCT). *NSGCT* is an umbrella designation that includes tumors of one histologic type, such as embryonal cell carcinoma, as well as those with more than one histologic pattern. As is evident from the later discussion, seminomas and NSGCT not only present with somewhat distinctive clinical features, but they also differ with respect to therapy and prognosis. First we offer some general comments on the clinical manifestations of testicular tumors as a group. Although *painless enlargement of the testis* is a characteristic feature of germ cell neoplasms, any testicular mass should be considered neoplastic unless proved otherwise. Biopsy of a testicular neoplasm is associated with a risk of tumor spillage, which would necessitate excision of the scrotal skin in addition to orchiectomy. Consequently, the standard management of a solid testicular mass is radical orchiectomy based on the presumption of malignancy.

Testicular tumors have a characteristic mode of spread, the knowledge of which is helpful in treatment. Lymphatic spread is common to all forms of testicular tumors, and in general, retroperitoneal para-aortic nodes are the first to be involved. Subsequent spread may occur to mediastinal and supraclavicular nodes. Hematogenous spread is primarily to the lungs, but liver, brain, and bones may also be involved. Although most testicular tumors metastasize "true," the histology of metastases may sometimes be different from that of the testicular lesion. Thus, an embryonal carcinoma may present a teratomatous picture in the secondary deposits. Conversely, a teratoma may show foci of choriocarcinoma in the lymph nodes. As was discussed earlier, because all these tumors are derived from totipotential germ cells, the apparent "forward" and "backward" differentiation that is seen in different locations is not entirely surprising. Another explanation for the differing morphologic patterns at metastatic sites is that the primary tumor is mixed, and that minor components in the primary lesion, that were unresponsive to chemotherapy survived, resulting in the dominant metastatic pattern.

With this background, we now highlight the clinical differences between seminoma and NSGCT. Seminomas tend to remain localized to the testis for a long time; hence, approximately 70% present in clinical stage I (discussed later). In contrast, approximately 60% of patients with NSGCT present with advanced clinical disease (stages II and III). Metastases from seminomas typically involve lymph nodes. Hematogenous spread occurs later in the course of dissemination. NSGCT not only metastasize earlier but also use the hematogenous route more frequently. The rare pure choriocarcinoma is the most aggressive of the NSGCT. It might not cause any testicular enlargement but instead spreads predominantly and rapidly by the bloodstream. Therefore, lungs and liver are involved early in virtually every case. From a therapeutic viewpoint, seminomas are extremely radiosensitive, whereas NSGCT are relatively radioresistant. To summarize, as compared with seminomas, NSGCT are biologically more aggressive and in general have a poorer prognosis.

In the United States, three clinical stages of testicular tumors are defined:

- Stage I: Tumor confined to the testis, epididymis, or spermatic cord
- Stage II: Distant spread confined to retroperitoneal nodes below the diaphragm
- Stage III: Metastases outside the retroperitoneal nodes or above the diaphragm

Stages II and III are further subdivided ("early" or "advanced") on the basis of tumor burden in the secondary deposits.

Germ cell tumors of the testis often secrete polypeptide hormones and certain enzymes that can be detected in blood by sensitive assays. Such *biologic markers* include α-fetoprotein (AFP), human chorionic gonadotrophin (HCG), placental alkaline phosphatase, placental lactogen, and lactate dehydrogenase (LDH). HCG, AFP, and LDH are widely used clinically and have proved to be valuable in the diagnosis and management of testicular cancer.[80] Recent studies suggest that certain molecular markers may be of value in diagnosis of germ cell tumors.[81] For example, the transcription factor encoded by *OCT3/4* gene is expressed in primordial germ cells, as well as in seminomas and embryonal carcinomas, and testicular germ cell tumors reveal inactivation of the X-chromosome. These can be detected by immunoperoxidase and PCR techniques, respectively.

LDH is produced in many tissues, including skeletal and cardiac muscles; hence, elevations of this enzyme are not specific for testicular tumors. The degree of LDH elevation correlates with the mass of tumor cells, however, and the levels of this enzyme provide a tool to assess tumor burden.

AFP is the major serum protein of the early fetus and is synthesized by the fetal gut, liver cells, and yolk sac. One year after birth, the serum levels of AFP fall to less than 16 ng/mL, which is undetectable except by the most sensitive assays. HCG is a glycoprotein consisting of two dissimilar polypeptide units called α and β. It is normally synthesized and secreted by the placental syncytiotrophoblast. The β subunit of HCG has unique sequences that are not shared with other human glycoprotein hormones; therefore, the detection of HCG in the serum is based on a radioimmunoassay using antibodies to its β chain. As might be expected from the histogenesis and morphology, elevated levels of these markers are most often associated with nonseminomatous tumors. Marked elevation of serum AFP or HCG levels is produced by yolk sac tumor and choriocarcinoma elements, respectively. Both these markers are elevated in more than 80% of patients with NSGCT at the time of diagnosis. In the context of testicular tumors, the value of serum markers is fourfold:

- In the evaluation of testicular masses
- In the staging of testicular germ cell tumors. For example, after orchiectomy, persistent elevation of HCG or AFP indicates stage II disease even if the lymph nodes appear of normal size by computed tomography scanning.
- In assessing tumor burden. The levels of LDH in particular are related to tumor mass and provide an independent prognostic marker in patients with these tumors.
- In monitoring the response to therapy. After eradication of tumors, there is a rapid fall in serum level of AFP and HCG. With serial measurements, it is often possible to predict recurrence before the patients become symptomatic or develop any other clinical signs of relapse.

As was stated earlier, approximately 15% of seminomas have syncytiotrophoblastic giant cells and an associated relatively minimal elevation of HCG levels. The prognosis of these tumors, however, is no different than those without HCG elevation.

The therapy and prognosis of testicular tumors depend largely on clinical stage and on the histologic type. Seminoma, which is extremely radiosensitive and tends to remain localized for long periods, has the best prognosis. More than 95% of patients with stage I and II disease can be cured. Among nonseminomatous tumors, the histologic subtype does not influence the prognosis significantly; hence, these tumors are treated as a group. Although they do not share the excellent prognosis of seminoma, approximately 90% of patients with nonseminomatous tumors can achieve complete remission with aggressive chemotherapy, and most can be cured. Pure choriocarcinoma has a dismal prognosis. However, when it is a minor component of a mixed germ cell tumor, the prognosis is not so adversely affected. With all testicular tumors, distant metastases, if present, usually occur within the first 2 years after treatment.

Tumors of Sex Cord–Gonadal Stroma

As is indicated in Table 21–5, sex cord–gonadal stroma tumors are subclassified on the basis of their presumed histogenesis and differentiation. The two most important members of this group—Leydig cell tumors (derived from the stroma) and Sertoli cell tumors (derived from the sex cord)—are described here. Details of these tumors and others not described can be found in a review.[82]

Leydig (Interstitial) Cell Tumors

Tumors of Leydig cells are particularly interesting because they may elaborate androgens or combinations of androgens and estrogens, and some have also elaborated corticosteroids.[83,84] They arise at any age, although most of the reported cases have been noted between 20 and 60 years of age. As with other testicular tumors, the most common presenting feature is testicular swelling, but in some patients, gynecomastia may be the first symptom. In children, hormonal effects, manifested primarily as sexual precocity, are the dominating features.

Morphology. These neoplasms form circumscribed nodules, usually less than 5 cm in diameter. They have a distinctive golden brown, homogeneous cut surface. Histologically, tumorous Leydig cells usually are remarkably similar to their normal forebears in that they are large and round or polygonal, and they have an abundant granular eosinophilic cytoplasm with a round central nucleus. Cell boundaries are often indistinct. The cytoplasm frequently contains lipid granules, vacuoles, or lipofuscin pigment, but most characteristically, rod-shaped crystalloids of Reinke occur in about 25% of the tumors. Approximately 10% of the tumors in adults are invasive and produce metastases; most are benign.

Sertoli Cell Tumors (Androblastoma)

These tumors may be composed entirely of Sertoli cells or may have a component of granulosa cells.[85] Some induce endocrinologic changes. Either estrogens or androgens may be elaborated but only infrequently in sufficient quantity to cause precocious masculinization or feminization. Occasionally, as with Leydig cell tumors, gynecomastia appears.

Morphology. These neoplasms appear as firm, small nodules with a homogeneous gray-white to yellow cut surface. Histologically, the tumor cells are arranged in distinctive trabeculae with a tendency to form cordlike structures resembling immature seminiferous tubules. Most Sertoli cell tumors are benign, but occasional tumors (approximately 10%) are more anaplastic and pursue a malignant course.

Gonadoblastoma

Gonadoblastomas are rare neoplasms containing a mixture of germ cells and gonadal stromal elements, almost always arising in dysgenetic gonads. In some cases, the germ cell component becomes malignant, giving rise to an invasive seminoma.

Testicular Lymphoma

Although not primarily a tumor of the testis, testicular lymphoma is included here because affected patients present with only a testicular mass.[86] *Lymphomas account for 5% of testicular neoplasms and constitute the most common form of testicular neoplasm in men over the age of 60.* In most cases, disseminated disease is already present at the time of detection of the testicular mass; only rarely does it remain confined to the testis. The histologic type in almost all cases is the diffuse large cell lymphoma (see non-Hodgkin lymphomas, Chapter 14). The prognosis is extremely poor.

MISCELLANEOUS LESIONS OF THE TUNICA VAGINALIS

Brief mention should be made of the tunica vaginalis. As a serosa-lined sac immediately proximal to the testis and epididymis, it may become involved by any lesion arising in these two structures. Clear serous fluid may accumulate from neighboring infections or tumors, often spontaneously and without apparent cause (*hydrocele*). Considerable enlargement of the scrotal sac is produced, which can be readily mistaken for testicular enlargement. By transillumination, however, it is usually possible to define the clear, translucent character of the contained substance, and many times the opaque testis can be outlined within this fluid-filled space. Hydrocele sacs frequently contain benign mesothelial proliferations. Rarely, malignant mesotheliomas also can be seen arising from the tunica vaginalis.

Hematocele indicates the presence of blood in the tunica vaginalis. It is an uncommon condition that is usually encountered only when there has been either direct trauma to the testis or torsion of the testis with hemorrhagic suffusion into the surrounding tunica vaginalis or in hemorrhagic diseases associated with widespread bleeding diatheses.

Chylocele refers to the accumulation of lymph in the tunica and is almost always found in patients with elephantiasis who have widespread, severe lymphatic obstruction. For clarity's sake, mention should be made of the *spermatocele* and *varicocele*, which refer to a small cystic accumulation of semen in dilated efferent ducts or ducts of the rete testis (spermatocele) or to a dilated vein in the spermatic cord (varicocele), respectively. Varicoceles may be asymptomatic but have also been implicated in some men as a contributing factor to infertility, whereby they may be repaired surgically.

Prostate

In the normal adult, the prostate weighs approximately 20 grams. The prostate is a retroperitoneal organ encircling the neck of the bladder and urethra and is devoid of a distinct capsule. In the adult, prostatic parenchyma can be divided into four biologically and anatomically distinct zones or regions: the peripheral, central, and transitional zones and the region of the anterior fibromuscular stroma (Fig. 21–30).[87] The types of proliferative lesions are different in each region. For example, *most hyperplasias arise in the transitional zone, whereas most carcinomas originate in the peripheral zone.*

Histologically, the prostate is a compound tubuloalveolar organ, which, in one plane of section, presents small to fairly large glandular spaces lined by epithelium. Characteristically, the glands are lined by two layers of cells: a basal layer of low cuboidal epithelium covered by a layer of columnar secretory cells (Fig. 21–31). In many areas, there are small papillary inbuddings of the epithelium. These glands all have a distinct basement membrane and are separated by an abundant fibromuscular stroma. Testicular androgens are clearly of prime importance in controlling prostatic growth because castration leads to atrophy of the prostate.

Only three pathologic processes affect the prostate gland with sufficient frequency to merit discussion: inflammation, benign nodular enlargement, and tumors. Of these three, the benign nodular enlargements are by far the most common and

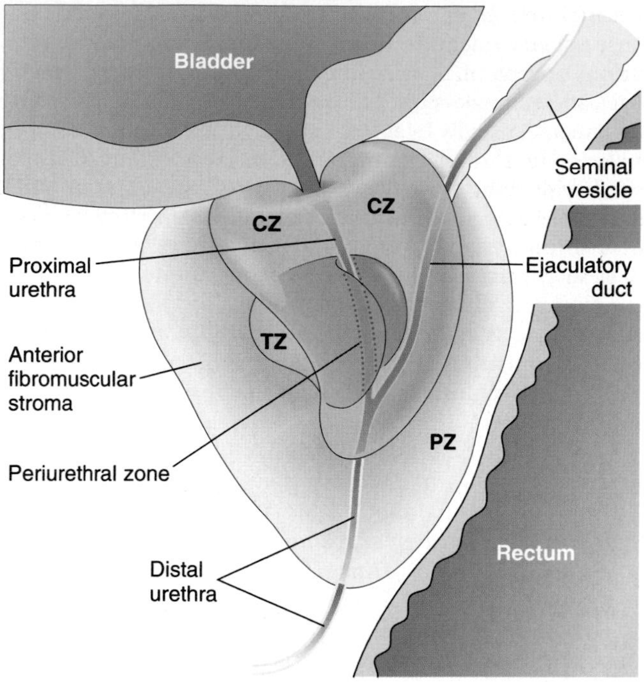

FIGURE 21–30 Adult prostate. The normal prostate contains several distinct regions, including a central zone (CZ), a peripheral zone (PZ), a transitional zone (TZ), and a periurethral zone. Most carcinomas arise from the peripheral glands of the organ and may be palpable during digital examination of the rectum. Nodular hyperplasia, in contrast, arises from more centrally situated glands and is more likely to produce urinary obstruction early on than is carcinoma.

occur so often in advanced age that they can almost be construed as a "normal" aging process. Prostatic carcinoma is also an extremely common lesion in men and therefore merits careful consideration. The inflammatory processes are, for the most part, of less clinical significance and can be treated briefly.

INFLAMMATIONS

Prostatitis may be divided into several categories: *acute and chronic bacterial prostatitis* and *chronic abacterial prostatitis and granulomatous prostatitis.*[88,89]

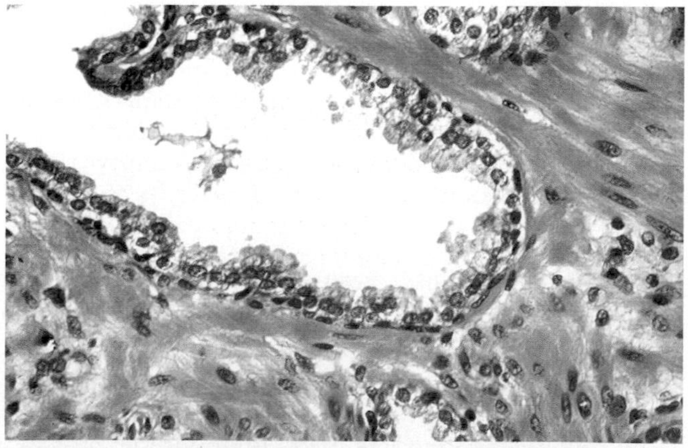

FIGURE 21–31 Benign prostate gland with basal cell and secretory cell layer.

Acute bacterial prostatitis typically results from bacteria that cause urinary tract infections. Thus, most cases are caused by various strains of *E. coli*, other Gram-negative rods, enterococci, and staphylococci. The organisms become implanted in the prostate, usually by intraprostatic reflux of urine from the posterior urethra or from the urinary bladder, but occasionally, they seed the prostate by the lymphohematogenous routes from distant foci of infection. Prostatitis sometimes follows some surgical manipulation on the urethra or prostate gland itself, such as catheterization, cystoscopy, urethral dilation, or resection procedures on the prostate. Clinically, acute bacterial prostatitis is associated with fever, chills, and dysuria. On rectal examination, the prostate is exquisitely tender and boggy. The diagnosis can be established by urine culture and clinical features.

Chronic bacterial prostatitis is difficult to diagnose and treat. It may present with low back pain, dysuria, and perineal and suprapubic discomfort. Alternatively, it may be virtually asymptomatic. *A common clinical setting is recurrent urinary tract infections (cystitis, urethritis) caused by the same organism.* Because most antibiotics penetrate the prostate poorly, bacteria find safe haven in the parenchyma and constantly seed the urinary tract. Diagnosis of chronic bacterial prostatitis depends on documentation within the expressed prostatic secretions of leukocytosis and positive bacterial cultures of the prostatic secretions. In most cases, there is no antecedent acute attack, and the disease appears insidiously and without obvious provocation. The implicated organisms are the same as those cited as causes of acute prostatitis.

Chronic abacterial prostatitis is the most common form of prostatitis seen today. *Clinically, it is indistinguishable from chronic bacterial prostatitis. There is no history, however, of recurrent urinary tract infection.* Expressed prostatic secretions contain more than 10 leukocytes per high-power field, but bacterial cultures are uniformly negative.

Granulomatous prostatitis may be specific, where an etiologic infectious agent may be identified.[90] In the United States, the most common cause is related to instillation within the bladder of Bacillus Calmette-Guérin (BCG) for treatment of superficial bladder cancer. BCG is an attenuated tuberculous strain that gives rise to a histologic picture in the prostate indistinguishable from that seen with systemic tuberculosis. However, in this setting, the finding of granulomas in the prostate is of no clinical significance, requiring no treatment. Fungal granulomatous prostatitis is typically seen only in immunocompromised hosts. Nonspecific granulomatous prostatitis is relatively common and represents a reaction to secretions from ruptured prostatic ducts and acini. Although some of these men have a recent history of urinary tract infection, bacteria are not seen within the tissue in these cases.

Morphology. Acute prostatitis may appear as minute, disseminated abscesses; as large, coalescent focal areas of necrosis; or as a diffuse edema, congestion, and boggy suppuration of the entire gland. When these reactions are fairly diffuse, they cause an overall soft, spongy enlargement of the gland.

In men with symptoms of acute or chronic prostatitis, surgical specimens are uncommonly examined under the microscope, as the disease is treated medically. In fact, biopsy of the prostate in a patient with acute prostatitis is contraindicated, as it may lead to sepsis. It is common in prostate specimens removed surgically (for other reasons) to find histologic evidence of acute or chronic inflammation in the absence of clinical symptoms of prostatitis. In these instances, the etiologic infectious agents have yet to be identified. In the absence of clinical features of prostatitis, these prostate specimens are diagnosed in descriptive terms as showing "acute inflammation" or "chronic inflammation."

The histologic diagnosis of **"chronic prostatitis,"** both bacterial and abacterial, should be restricted to those cases of inflammatory reaction in the prostate characterized by the aggregation of numerous lymphocytes, plasma cells, and macrophages as well as neutrophils within the prostatic substance only if accompanied by clinical signs and symptoms of chronic prostatitis.

BENIGN ENLARGEMENT

Nodular Hyperplasia (Benign Prostatic Hyperplasia)

Nodular hyperplasia, still referred to by the term *benign prostatic hyperplasia* (BPH), is an extremely common disorder in men over age 50.[91,92] It is characterized by hyperplasia of prostatic stromal and epithelial cells, resulting in the formation of large, fairly discrete nodules in the periurethral region of the prostate. When sufficiently large, the nodules compress and narrow the urethral canal to cause partial, or sometimes virtually complete, obstruction of the urethra.

Incidence. Histologic evidence of nodular hyperplasia can be seen in approximately 20% of men 40 years of age, a figure that increases to 70% by age 60 and to 90% by age 70. There is no direct correlation, however, between histologic changes and clinical symptoms. Only 50% of those who have microscopic evidence of nodular hyperplasia have clinically detectable enlargement of the prostate, and of these individuals, only 50% develop clinical symptoms. Nodular hyperplasia of the prostate is a problem of enormous magnitude, approximately 30% of white American males over 50 years of age have moderate to severe symptoms.

Etiology and Pathogenesis. Much has been learned about the origins of prostatic hyperplasia. There is little doubt that this form of prostatic enlargement is related to the action of androgens. For example, prepubertal castration prevents the development of nodular hyperplasia. Dihydrotestosterone (DHT), a metabolite of testosterone, is the ultimate mediator of prostatic growth (Fig. 21–32). It is synthesized in the prostate from circulating testosterone by the action of the enzyme 5α-reductase, type 2. This enzyme is localized principally in the stromal cells; hence, these cells are the main site for the synthesis of DHT. Once synthesized, DHT can act in an autocrine fashion on the stromal cells or in paracrine fashion by diffusing into nearby epithelial cells. In both of these cell types, DHT binds to nuclear androgen receptors and signals the transcription of growth factors that are mitogenic to the epithelial and stromal cells. Although testosterone can also bind to the androgen receptors and cause growth stimu-

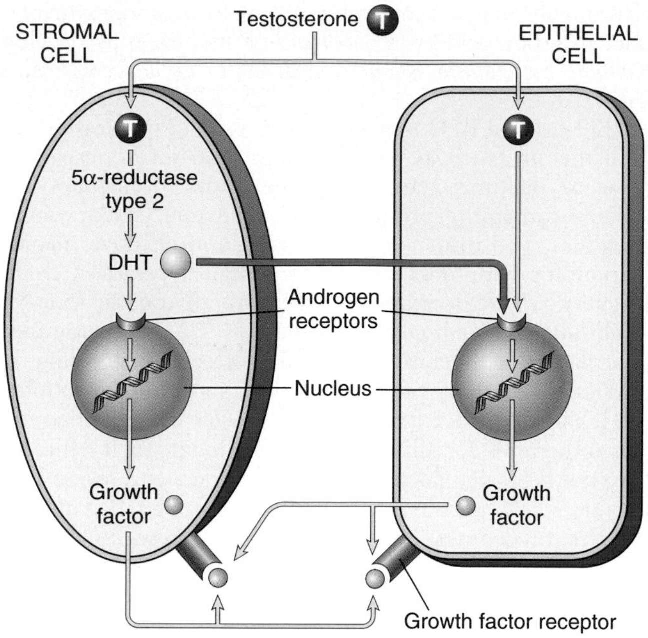

FIGURE 21–32 Simplified scheme of the pathogenesis of prostatic hyperplasia. The central role of the stromal cells in generating dihydrotestosterone should be noted.

lation, DHT is 10 times more potent because it dissociates from the androgen receptor more slowly. While DHT appears to be the major trophic factor mediating prostatic hyperplasia, estrogens also appear to play a role, perhaps by rendering cells more susceptible to the action of DHT. Stromal–epithelial interactions mediated by peptide growth factors are also integral to the process.[93] In addition to the mechanical effects of the enlarged prostate, clinical symptoms of lower urinary tract obstruction are also due to smooth muscle–mediated contraction of the prostate. The tension of prostate smooth muscle is mediated by the α_1-adrenoreceptor localized to the prostatic stroma. This is the basis of the common use of α-adrenergic receptor antagonists for the relief of urinary obstruction in patients with BPH.

The importance of DHT in causing nodular hyperplasia is supported by clinical observations in which an inhibitor of 5α-reductase is given to men with this condition. Therapy with 5α-reductase inhibitor markedly reduces the DHT content of the prostate, and in a proportion of cases, there is a decrease in prostatic volume and urinary obstruction.[94] The fact that not all patients benefit from androgen-depriving therapy suggests that prostatic hyperplasia may be etiologically heterogeneous, and in some cases, factors other than androgens may be more important.

Morphology. In the usual case of prostatic enlargement, the prostate weighs between 60 and 100 gm. Careful studies have demonstrated that nodular hyperplasia of the prostate originates almost exclusively in the inner aspect of the prostate gland, in the transition zone (see Fig. 21–33*A*). The first nodules are composed almost entirely of stromal cells; later, predominantly epithelial nodules arise. From their origin in this strategic location, the nodular enlargements may encroach on the lateral walls of the urethra to compress it to a slitlike orifice. In some cases, nodular enlargement may project up into the floor of the urethra as a hemispheric mass directly beneath the mucosa of the urethra, which is termed "median lobe hypertrophy" by clinicians.

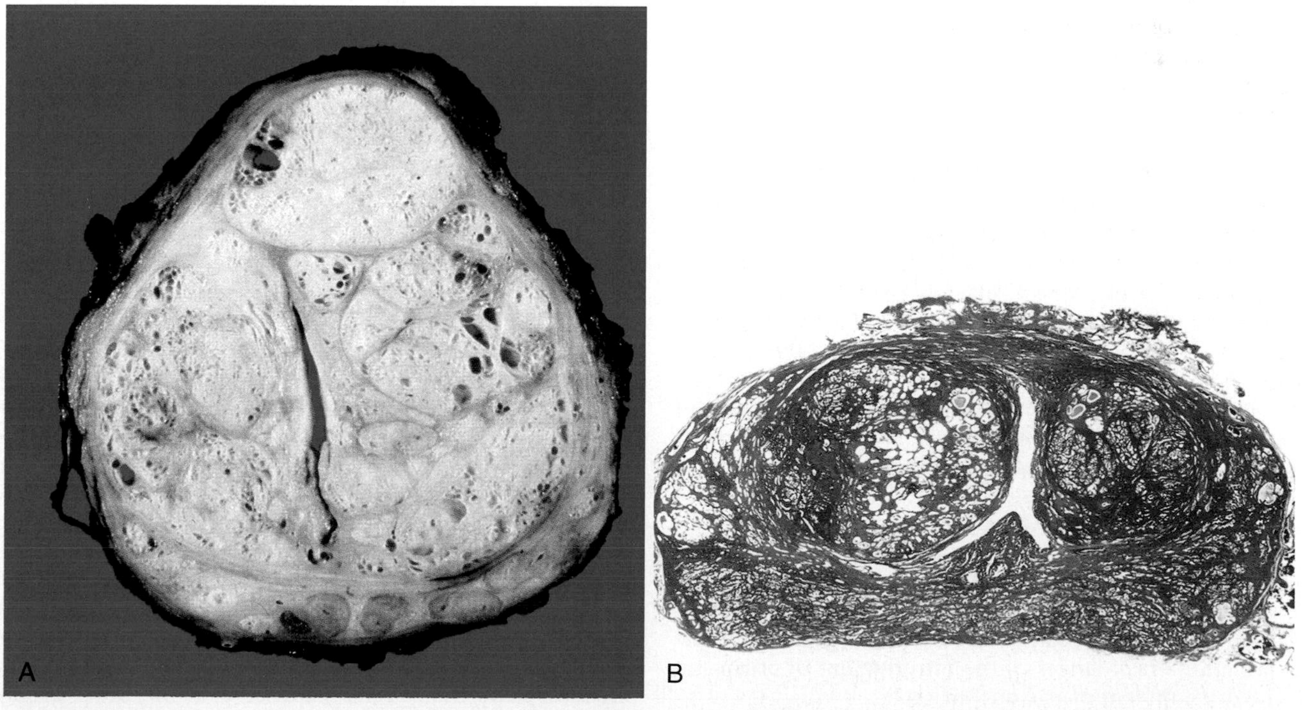

FIGURE 21–33 Nodular prostatic hyperplasia. *A*, Well-defined nodules of BPH compress the urethra into a slitlike lumen. *B*, A microscopic view of a whole mount of the prostate shows nodules of hyperplastic glands on both sides of the urethra.

On cross-section of the affected prostate, the nodules usually are fairly readily identified. They vary in color and consistency. In nodules with primarily glandular proliferation, the tissue is yellow-pink with a soft consistency, and a milky white prostatic fluid oozes out of these areas. In those primarily due to fibromuscular involvement, each nodule is pale gray, tough, does not exude fluid, and is less clearly demarcated from the surrounding prostatic capsule. Although the nodules do not have true capsules, the compressed surrounding prostatic tissue creates a plane of cleavage about them, which the surgeon uses in the enucleation of prostatic masses as a treatment for very large growths of BPH.

Microscopically, the hallmark of BPH is nodularity due to glandular proliferation or dilation and to fibrous or muscular proliferation of the stroma (Fig. 21–33*B*). The proportion of these elements varies from nodule to nodule, ranging from purely stromal fibromuscular nodules to fibroepithelial nodules with a glandular predominance. Glandular proliferation takes the form of aggregations of small to large to cystically dilated glands, lined by two layers, an inner columnar and an outer cuboidal or flattened epithelium, based on an intact basement membrane. Although the epithelium is characteristically thrown up into numerous papillary buds and infoldings, this finding is not specific for BPH. The diagnosis of BPH cannot usually be made on needle biopsy, as the histology of glandular or mixed glandular-stromal nodules of BPH cannot be appreciated on this limited sampling. Also, needle biopsies do not typically sample the transition zone where BPH occurs, and with the exception of stromal nodules, the histology of the prostate glands on needle biopsy does not correlate with gland size or lower urinary tract obstructive symptoms. Two other histologic changes associated with BPH are (1) foci of squamous metaplasia and (2) small areas of infarction. The former tend to occur in the margins of the foci of infarction as nests of metaplastic reactive squamous cells that can be confused with adenocarcinoma of the prostate or urothelial carcinoma involving the prostate.

Clinical Course. Symptoms of nodular hyperplasia, when present, relate to two secondary effects: (1) compression of the urethra with difficulty in urination and (2) retention of urine in the bladder with subsequent distention and hypertrophy of the bladder, infection of the urine, and development of cystitis and renal infections. Patients experience frequency, nocturia, difficulty in starting and stopping the stream of urine, overflow dribbling, and dysuria (painful micturition). In many cases, sudden, acute urinary retention appears for unknown reasons and persists until the patient receives emergency catheterization. In addition to these difficulties in urination, prostatic enlargement results in the inability to empty the bladder completely. Presumably, this inability is due to the raised level of the urethral floor so that, at the conclusion of micturition, a considerable amount of residual urine is left. This residual urine provides a static fluid that is vulnerable to infection. On this basis, catheterization or surgical manipulation provides a real danger of the introduction of organisms and the development of pyelonephritis.

Many secondary changes occur in the bladder, such as hypertrophy, trabeculation, and diverticulum formation. Hydronephrosis or acute retention, with secondary urinary tract infection and even azotemia or uremia, may develop. *Nodular hyperplasia is not considered to be a premalignant lesion.*

Mild cases of BPH may be treated without medical or surgical therapy, such as by decreasing fluid intake, especially prior to bedtime; moderating the intake of alcohol and caffeine-containing products; and following timed voiding schedules. The most commonly used and effective medical therapy for symptoms relating to benign hyperplasia are α-blockers, which decrease prostate smooth muscle tone via inhibition of α_1-adrenergic receptors.[94–96] Another common pharmacologic therapy aims to decrease symptoms by physically shrinking the prostate with an agent that inhibits DHT. Various plant extracts are also in wide use as a treatment (phytotherapy) for this condition, although their efficacies have not been well documented. For moderate to severe cases that are recalcitrant to medical therapy, a wide range of more invasive procedures exists. Transurethral resection of the prostate (TURP) is effective in reducing symptoms, improving flow rates, and decreasing postvoid residual urine. It is indicated as a first line of therapy in certain circumstances, such as recurrent urinary retention. Owing to its morbidity and cost, alternative procedures have been developed. These include high-intensity focused ultrasound, laser therapy, hyperthermia, transurethral electrovaporization, intraurethral stents, and transurethral needle ablation using radiofrequency.

TUMORS

Adenocarcinoma

Adenocarcinoma of the prostate is the most common form of cancer in men and the second leading cause of cancer death.[97] In 2003, approximately 220,900 new cases were detected, of which approximately 29,000 are likely to be lethal. In addition to these lethal neoplasms, there is an even more frequent anatomic form of prostatic cancer in which a microscopic focus of cancer is discovered as an incidental finding, either at postmortem examination or in a surgical specimen that was removed for other reasons (e.g., nodular hyperplasia).

Incidence. Cancer of the prostate is typically a disease of men over age 50. However, in men who are at increased risk (see the discussion of etiology), recommendations are for screening for prostate cancer to begin at age 40. Even for men without increased risk factors, consideration has been given to screening, initially at age 40 and again at age 45, to detect uncommon cases of prostate cancer before they become incurable.

The age-adjusted incidence of prostate cancer in the United States is 69 per 100,000. The incidence of latent prostatic cancer is even higher. It increases from 20% in men in their fifties to approximately 70% in men between the ages of 70 and 80 years. There are some remarkable and puzzling national and racial differences in the incidence of this disease.[98] Prostatic cancer is uncommon in Asians. The age-adjusted incidence per 100,000 among Japanese is in the range of 3 to 4 and that for the Chinese in Hong Kong is only 1, compared with a rate of 50 to 60 among whites in the United States. The disease is even more prevalent among blacks in the

United States, who have the highest rate among 24 countries having reasonably accurate mortality data. Despite the greater than tenfold differences in the incidence of clinically evident cancers, the age-adjusted incidence of the so-called latent or histologic form of prostate cancer is virtually identical in Japanese and U.S. white populations. Assuming that prostate cancer, similar to other cancers, arises from accumulation of multiple genetic events, these observations indicate that whereas the initial molecular events that give rise to latent cancers occur at the same rate in Japanese and American men, the probability of acquiring additional mutations, presumably environmentally induced, is lower in Japanese men. This notion is supported by the fact that in Japanese immigrants to the United States, the incidence of the disease seems to have risen, but not nearly to the level of that of native-born Americans. Also, as the diet in Asia becomes more Westernized, the incidence of clinical prostate cancer in this region of the world appears to be increasing.

Etiology. Little is known about the causes of prostatic cancer. Several risk factors, such as age, race, family history, hormone levels, and environmental influences, are suspected of playing roles.[99–102] The association of this form of cancer with advancing age and the enigmatic differences among races have already been mentioned. The tendency for the incidence of this disease to rise among those having a low-incidence rate when they migrate to a high-incidence locale is consistent with a role for environmental influences. There are many candidate environmental factors, but none has been proven to be causative. For example, increased consumption of fats has been implicated. Other dietary products, for which there is evidence that they may prevent, inhibit, or delay progression of prostate cancer, include lycopenes (found in tomatoes), vitamin A, vitamin E, selenium, and soy products.

As with nodular hyperplasia of the prostate, androgens are believed to play a role in the pathogenesis of prostate cancer. Support for this general thesis lies in the inhibition of these tumors that can be achieved with orchiectomy. Neoplastic epithelial cells, similar to their normal counterparts, possess androgen receptors. No significant or consistent alterations in the levels or metabolism of testosterone, however, have been disclosed in any studies. It seems more likely, therefore, that the role of hormones in this malignancy is essentially permissive because androgens are required for the maintenance of the prostatic epithelium. Androgen receptor (*AR*) gene mutations have been reported in only a minority of prostate cancers. However, *AR* gene amplification may also influence androgen-sensitivity of prostatic epithelium. The *AR* gene is polymorphic, with individuals having variable lengths of CAG repeats. Studies have shown that prostate cells with short CAG repeats have an increased sensitivity to androgens. The shortest CAG repeats on average are found in African Americans, Caucasians have an intermediate length, and Asians have the longest. Correspondingly, African Americans have the highest incidence and mortality of prostate cancer, and Asians have much lower risk.

Much interest has focused on the genetics and molecular pathogenesis of prostate cancer.[103–108] In approximately 10% of white American men, the development of prostate cancer has been linked to germ line inheritance of prostate cancer susceptibility genes. In one third of these familial cases, a susceptibility gene has been mapped to chromosome 1q24–25. Subsequently, numerous other chromosomal loci have been linked to prostate cancer. Men with one first-degree relative with prostate cancer have a twofold higher risk, and those with two first-degree relatives have a fivefold greater risk of developing prostate cancer compared with men with no family history. Men with a strong family history of prostate cancer also tend to develop the disease at an earlier age.

In addition, putative cancer-suppressor genes that are lost early in prostate carcinogenesis have been localized to chromosomes 8p, 10q, 13q, and 16q. In most instances, the identity of the relevant genes at these loci is unknown. *p53* mutations in primary prostate cancer are relatively low and are more frequently seen in metastatic disease, suggesting that *p53* mutations are late events in prostate carcinogenesis. Other tumor-suppressor genes that are thought to play a role in prostate cancer include *PTEN* and *KAI1*. Prostate cancers also show a relatively frequent loss of E-cadherin and CD44.

Although there are conflicting studies concerning *HER-2/neu* overexpression in prostate cancer, the prevailing view is that levels are relatively low; therefore, it is unlikely that prostate cancer will benefit from therapy with currently available antibodies to *HER-2/neu*. Using cDNA microarray technology, a number of studies have identified cohorts of genes that are specifically overexpressed in prostate cancer, including hepsin, a transmembrane serine protease, and α-methylacyl COA racemase, an enzyme involved in the breakdown of branched fatty acids. Using similar genomic approaches, the transcription factor EZH2 has been shown to be consistently overexpressed in locally aggressive and metastatic prostate cancer.[107]

One of the most common genetic alterations in prostate cancer is hypermethylation of glutathione S-transferase (GSTP1) gene promoter. More than 90% of prostate cancers show hypermethylation of the gene, which turns off its expression. The *GSTP1* gene is located on chromosome 11q13, and it is an important part of the pathway that prevents damage from a wide range of carcinogens.

Morphology. The terms "prostate cancer" and "prostate adenocarcinoma," when used without qualifications, refer to the common or acinar variant of prostate cancer. Our discussion here is focused on this variant. Other forms are briefly discussed later.

In approximately 70% of cases, carcinoma of the prostate arises in the peripheral zone of the gland, classically in a posterior location, often rendering it palpable on rectal examination (Fig. 21–34).[109] Characteristically, on cross-section of the prostate, **the neoplastic tissue is gritty and firm, but when embedded within the prostatic substance, it may be extremely difficult to visualize and be more readily apparent on palpation**. Spread of prostate cancer occurs by direct local invasion and through the bloodstream and lymph. Local extension most commonly involves the seminal vesicles and the base of the urinary bladder, which may result in ureteral obstruction.[110] Hematogenous spread occurs chiefly to the bones, particularly the axial skeleton, but some lesions spread widely to viscera.[111] Massive visceral dissemination is an exception rather than the rule. The bony metastases are typically osteoblastic and, in men, point strongly to prostatic cancer (Fig. 21–35). The bones that are commonly involved, in descending order of frequency, are lumbar spine, proximal

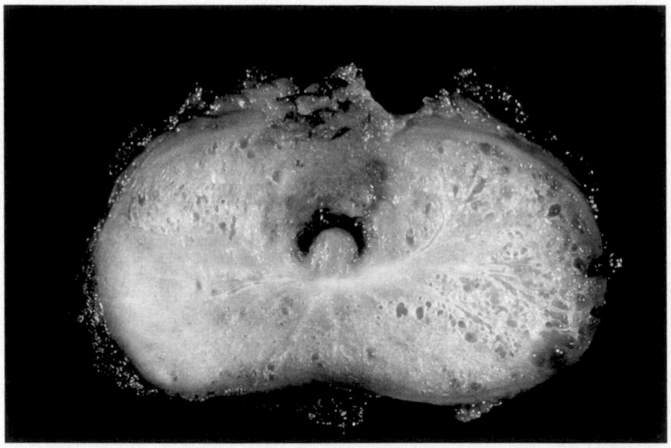

FIGURE 21–34 Adenocarcinoma of the prostate. Carcinomatous tissue is seen on the posterior aspect (*lower left*). Note the solid whiter tissue of cancer in contrast to the spongy appearance of the benign peripheral zone on the contralateral side.

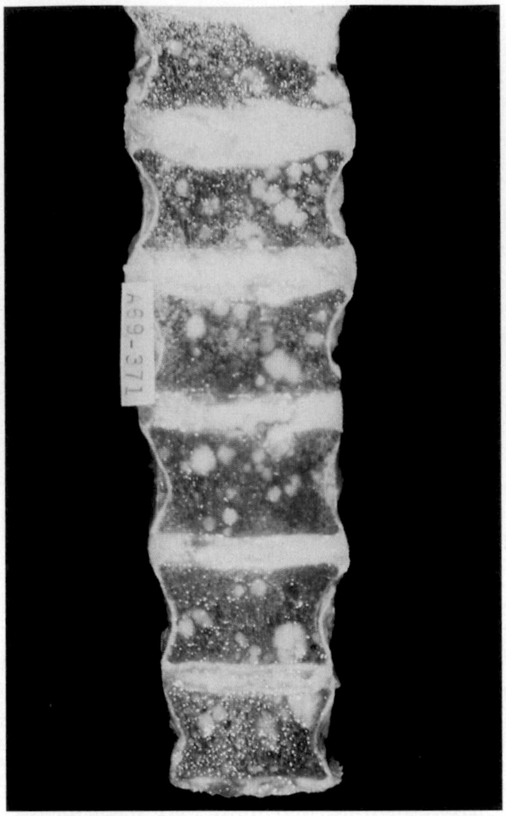

FIGURE 21–35 Metastatic osteoblastic prostatic carcinoma within vertebral bodies.

femur, pelvis, thoracic spine, and ribs. Lymphatic spread occurs initially to the obturator nodes followed by perivesical, hypogastric, iliac, presacral, and para-aortic nodes. Lymph node spread occurs frequently and often precedes spread to the bones.

Histologically, most lesions are adenocarcinomas that produce well-defined, readily demonstrable gland patterns.[112–114] The neoplastic glands are typically smaller than benign glands and are lined by a single uniform layer of cuboidal or low columnar epithelium. In contrast to benign glands, prostate cancer glands are more crowded, characteristically lacking branching and papillary infolding. The outer basal layer of cells typical of normal and hyperplastic glands is absent. The cytoplasm of the tumor cells ranges from pale to clear, as is seen in benign glands, to a distinctive amphophilic appearance. Nuclei are large and often contain one or more large nucleoli. There is some variation in nuclear size and shape, but in general, pleomorphism is not marked. Mitotic figures are extremely uncommon.

The histologic diagnosis of prostate cancer on biopsy specimens is one of the more difficult challenges for pathologists. In part, the difficulty stems from the scant amount of tissue available for histologic examination removed by the needle biopsy; in addition, biopsy often samples only a few malignant glands among many benign glands (Fig. 21–36). The histologic clues to malignancy may be subtle, thus

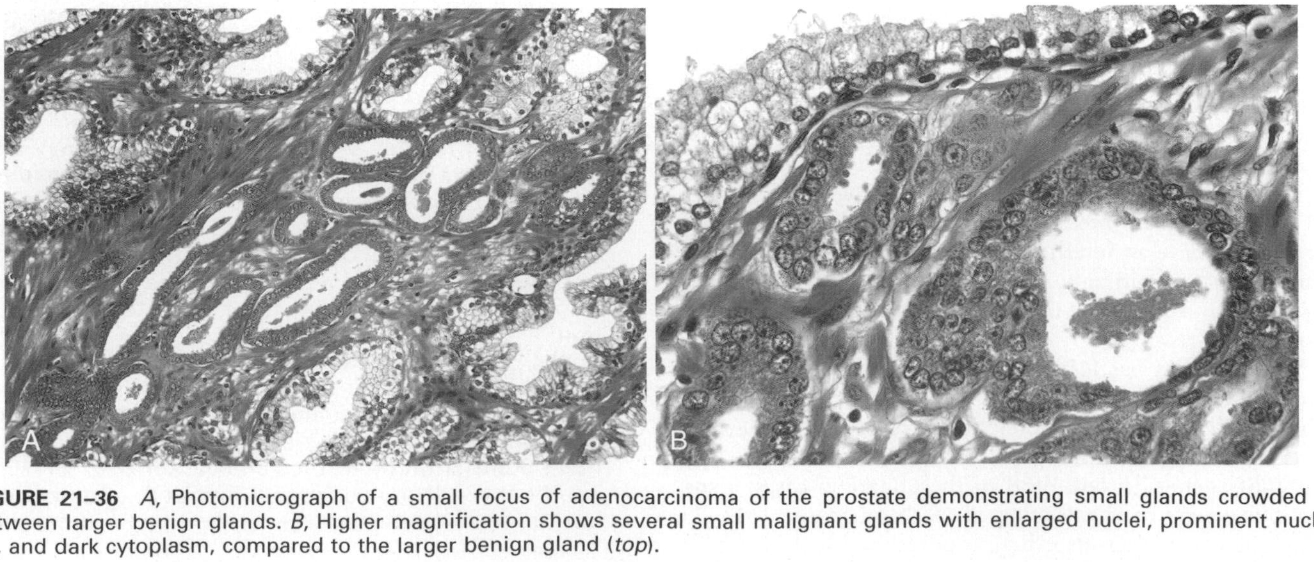

FIGURE 21–36 *A*, Photomicrograph of a small focus of adenocarcinoma of the prostate demonstrating small glands crowded in between larger benign glands. *B*, Higher magnification shows several small malignant glands with enlarged nuclei, prominent nucleoli, and dark cytoplasm, compared to the larger benign gland (*top*).

increasing the likelihood of underdiagnosis. There are a few histologic findings that are specific for prostate cancer, such as perineural invasion; in general the diagnosis is made on the basis of a constellation of architectural, cytological, and ancillary findings (Fig. 21–37). As was discussed earlier in the chapter, one feature that distinguishes benign and malignant prostate glands is that benign glands contain basal cells that are absent in cancer. Pathologists have exploited this finding by using various immunohistologic markers to label basal cells. Using cDNA microarrays, markers have also been found that are relatively specific for prostate cancer.[115] These markers, while improving the accuracy of the diagnosis of prostate cancer, have their limitations and must be used in conjunction with routine H&E-stained sections.

In approximately 80% of cases, prostatic tissue removed for carcinoma also harbors presumptive precursor lesions, referred to as **high-grade prostatic intraepithelial neoplasia (PIN)**.[115–119] These lesions consist of benign glands with intra-acinar proliferations of cells that demonstrate nuclear anaplasia. High-grade PIN consists of more widely separated, larger branching glands with papillary infolding, in contrast to invasive cancer, which is typically characterized by small, crowded glands with straight luminal borders. Cytologically, the two processes may be identical. PIN glands are surrounded by a patchy layer of basal cells and an intact basement membrane. There are several lines of evidence that link high-grade PIN to invasive cancer. First, both high-grade PIN and cancer typically predominate in the peripheral zone and are relatively uncommon in other zones. If one compares prostates without cancer to those with cancer, prostates containing cancer have a higher frequency and a greater extent of high-grade PIN. High-grade PIN is also often seen in proximity to cancer, with the cancer in some cases appearing to bud off of the high-grade PIN. Studies have revealed that many of the molecular changes that are seen in invasive cancers are also present in PIN. Such data strongly support the notion that PIN is an intermediate lesion between normal glands and invasive cancer.

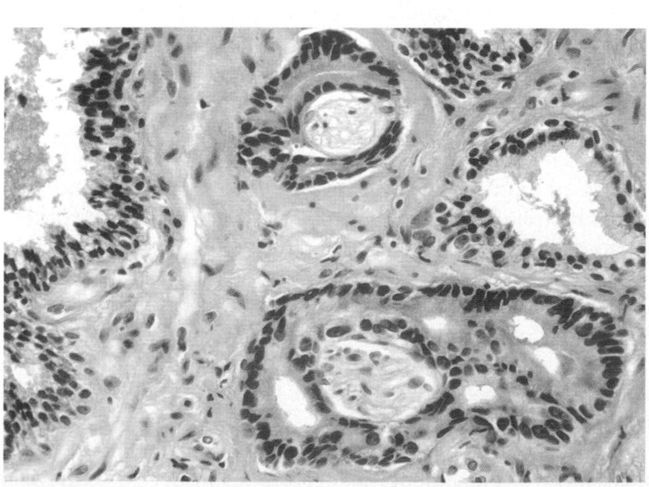

FIGURE 21–37 Carcinoma of the prostate showing perineural invasion by malignant glands. Compare to a benign gland (*left*).

Given the above findings, one might wonder why the term "carcinoma in situ" of the prostate is not used for lesions categorized as "high-grade PIN." What is lacking in our knowledge of high-grade PIN is its natural history. How often does untreated high-grade PIN progress to invasive cancer, and if it does progress, how long does it take to do so? What is known is that men with high-grade PIN found on biopsy are at increased risk of having prostate cancer, so repeat biopsy is often performed to look for cancer that might have been missed initially.

Grading and Staging. Several grading systems have been described, of which the Gleason system is the best known.[120–123] According to the Gleason system, prostate cancers are stratified into five grades on the basis of glandular patterns and degree of differentiation as seen under low magnification. Grade 1 represents the most well-differentiated tumors, in which the neoplastic glands are uniform and round in appearance and are packed into well-circumscribed nodules (Fig. 21–38). By contrast, grade 5 tumors show no glandular differentiation, and the tumor cells infiltrate the stroma in the form of cords, sheets, and nests. The other grades fall in between. Most tumors contain more than one pattern, in which case one assigns a primary grade to the dominant pattern and a secondary grade to the subdominant pattern. The two numeric grades are then added to obtain a combined Gleason grade or score. Thus, for example, a tumor with a dominant grade 3 and a secondary grade 4 would achieve a Gleason score of 7. Tumors with only one pattern are treated as if their primary and secondary grades are the same; hence, the number is doubled. Thus, under this schema the most well-differentiated tumors have a Gleason score of 2 (1 + 1) and the least-differentiated tumors merit a score of 10 (5 + 5). Gleason scores are often combined into groups with similar biologic behavior: 2 to 4 representing well-differentiated cancer, 5 to 6 representing intermediate-grade cancer, 7 representing moderate to poorly differentiated cancer, and 8 to 10 representing high-grade cancer. Gleason scores of 2 to 4 are typically found in small tumors within the transition zone. In surgical specimens, such low-grade cancer is typically an incidental finding on transurethral resection performed for symptoms of BPH. The majority of potentially treatable cancers that are detected on needle biopsy have Gleason scores of 5 to 7. Tumors with Gleason scores 8 to 10 tend to be advanced cancers that are unlikely to be curable. While there is some evidence that certain prostate cancers may become less differentiated over time, in general the Gleason score remains stable over a period of several years. *Grading is of particular importance in prostatic cancer because it is the best marker, along with the stage, for predicting prognosis.*

Staging of prostatic cancer is also important in the selection of the appropriate form of therapy. The most common staging system is the TNM system. Stage T1 refers to cancer found incidentally either on trans-urethral resection done for BPH symptoms (T1a and T1b depending on the extent and grade) or on needle biopsy, typically performed for elevated serum PSA levels (stage T1c).[124,125] Stage T2 is organ-confined cancer. Stage T3a and T3b tumors show extraprostatic extension, with and without seminal vesicle invasion, respectively. Stage T4 reflects direct invasion of contiguous organs. Any spread of

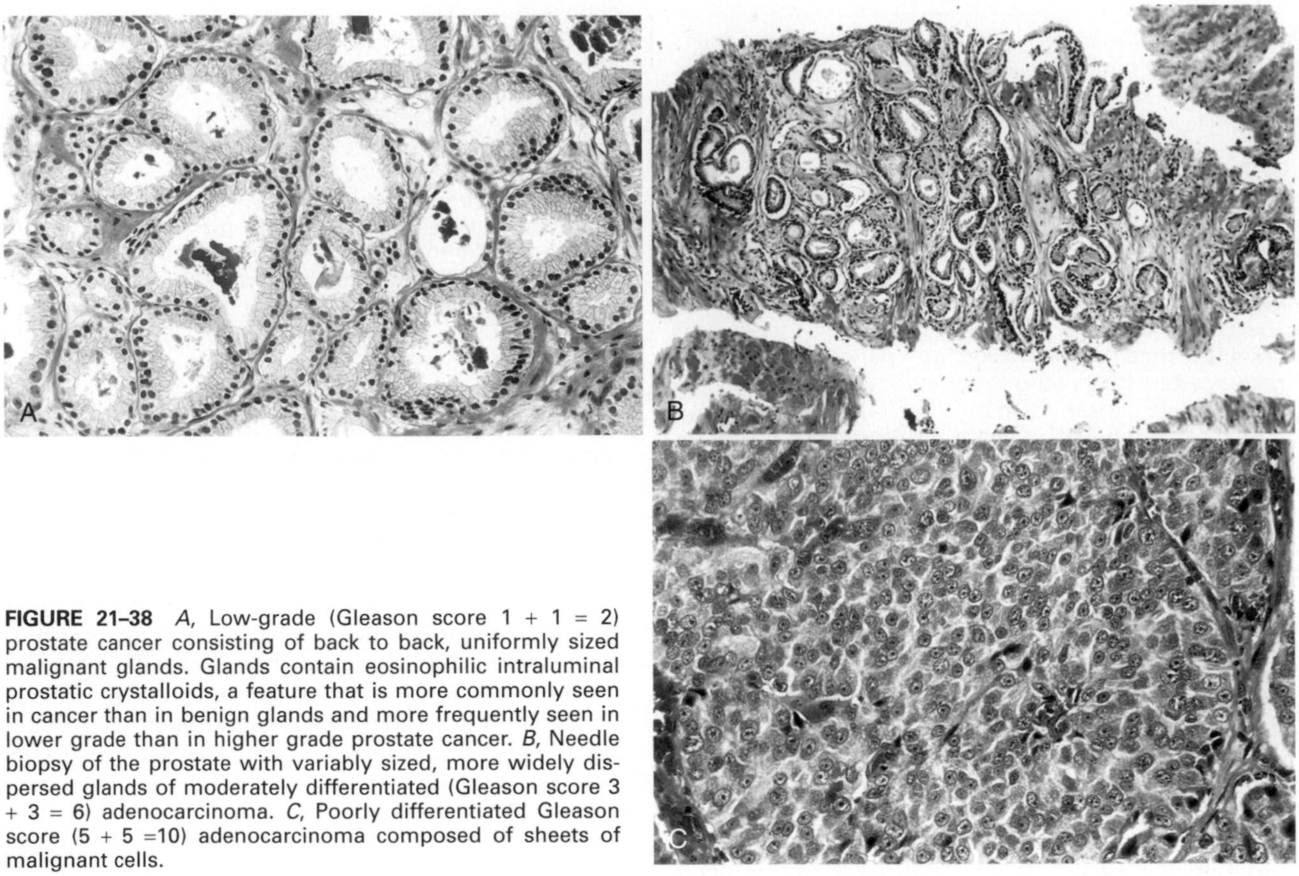

FIGURE 21–38 *A,* Low-grade (Gleason score 1 + 1 = 2) prostate cancer consisting of back to back, uniformly sized malignant glands. Glands contain eosinophilic intraluminal prostatic crystalloids, a feature that is more commonly seen in cancer than in benign glands and more frequently seen in lower grade than in higher grade prostate cancer. *B,* Needle biopsy of the prostate with variably sized, more widely dispersed glands of moderately differentiated (Gleason score 3 + 3 = 6) adenocarcinoma. *C,* Poorly differentiated Gleason score (5 + 5 =10) adenocarcinoma composed of sheets of malignant cells.

tumor to the lymph nodes, regardless of extent, is eventually associated with a fatal outcome, such that the staging system merely records the presence or absence of this finding (N0/N1).

Clinical Course. As was discussed earlier, the incidence of cancers found incidentally increases with age, approaching 70% or more in men past the age of 80 years. These microscopic cancers are asymptomatic and are discovered incidentally at autopsy or in tissue removed for nodular hyperplasia of the prostate. The long-term significance of these lesions is still not entirely clear. It is generally accepted that most patients with stage T1a cancer do not show evidence of progressive disease when followed for 10 or more years. Five per cent to 25% of patients, however, do develop local or distant spread. This is more likely in younger patients (less than 60 years), who have a longer life expectancy. For patients in this age group, most authorities recommend careful follow-up studies so that if progression occurs, the cancer can be detected early, at a stage amenable to surgical cure. Stage T1b lesions are more ominous. Approximately 30% to 50% can be expected to progress over a period of 5 years, with a mortality of 20% if left untreated.

Patients with clinically localized disease do not have urinary symptoms, and the lesion is discovered by the finding of a suspicious nodule on rectal examination or elevated serum prostate-specific antigen level (discussed later). Most prostatic cancers arise peripherally, away from the urethra; therefore, urinary symptoms occur late. Patients with clinically advanced prostatic cancer may present with urinary symptoms, such as difficulty in starting or stopping the stream, dysuria, frequency, or hematuria. Some patients come to attention because of back pain caused by vertebral metastases. *The finding of osteoblastic metastases in bone is virtually diagnostic of this form of cancer in men.* The outlook for these patients is universally fatal.

Careful digital rectal examination may detect some early prostatic carcinomas because of their posterior location, although the test suffers from both low sensitivity and low specificity. While there are characteristic findings of prostate cancer on transrectal ultrasonography (TRUS) and other imaging modalities, the poor sensitivity and specificity of these tests also limit their diagnostic utility. The major role of TRUS in the diagnosis of prostate cancer is in guiding the placement of the needle biopsies to thoroughly sample the gland. A transperineal or transrectal *biopsy is required to confirm the diagnosis.* Several procedures are used to determine the extent of disease. The involvement of lymph nodes is poorly detected by computed tomography scans or magnetic resonance imaging. Because microscopic metastases may be missed by either of these two procedures, many centers use pelvic lymphadenectomy as a staging procedure. Some centers forgo pelvic lymphadenectomy prior to surgery in men who are predicted to have a low risk of metastatic disease based on serum PSA levels, clinical stage, and biopsy findings. If pelvic lymph nodes are involved, curative surgery (radical prostatectomy) will often be abandoned. Osseous metastases may be detected by skeletal surveys or the much more sensitive radionuclide bone scanning.

Prostate-specific antigen (PSA) has been used in the diagnosis and management of prostate cancer.[126–131] PSA is a product of prostatic epithelium and is normally secreted in the semen. It is a serine protease whose function is to cleave and liquefy the seminal coagulum formed after ejaculation. In normal men, only minute amounts of PSA circulate in the serum. Elevated blood levels of PSA occur in association with localized as well as advanced cancer. In most laboratories, a serum level of 4 ng/mL as reported on laboratory reports is a cut-off point between normal and abnormal. However, as will be discussed below, this simplified approach to serum PSA tests is dangerous and has led to the delay in diagnosis of many prostate cancers.

PSA is organ specific but not cancer specific. Although serum levels of PSA are elevated to a lesser extent in benign nodular hyperplasia, as compared to cancer, there is considerable overlap. Other factors such as benign prostatic hyperplasia, prostatitis, infarct, instrumentation of the prostate, and ejaculation also increase serum PSA levels. Furthermore, 20% to 40% of patients with organ-confined prostate cancer have a PSA value of 4.0 ng/mL or less.

Whereas most readers of this text will not directly practice pathology, almost all will be confronted with evaluation of a serum PSA test, either as a treating primary care physician, in addressing the results of a family member's or friend's test or, for the male readers, reviewing their own test results. The widespread use of this test, along with its complexity and the corresponding increased risk of it being interpreted incorrectly, warrants greater coverage of this topic. This test differs from most other laboratory tests that a physician can order in that it is a cancer detection test. Consequently, physicians should adopt foolproof mechanisms to ensure that tests come back from the lab, abnormal values are recorded, and patients are contacted for follow-up of elevated levels. Numerous medical malpractice cases result from the mishandling of serum PSA test results and the subsequent delay in diagnosis.

Several refinements in the estimation and interpretation of PSA values have been proposed. These include the ratio between the serum PSA value and volume of prostate gland (*PSA density*), the rate of change in PSA value with time (PSA velocity), the use of *age-specific reference ranges*, and the *ratio of free and bound PSA* in the serum. Men with enlarged hyperplastic prostate glands will have higher total serum PSA levels than will men with small glands. The measurement of serum PSA density factors out the contribution of benign prostatic tissue to serum PSA levels. Serum PSA density reflects the PSA produced per gram of prostate tissue. It is calculated by dividing the total serum PSA level by the estimated gland volume (usually determined by transrectal ultrasound measurements), with an upper normal value of approximately 0.15. As men age, their prostates tend to enlarge with benign prostatic hyperplasia. One would then anticipate that, overall, older men would have higher serum PSA levels than younger men. Derived from measurements of serum PSA levels in a large group of men of varying ages without prostate cancer, the recommended age-specific upper reference ranges for serum PSA are 2.5 ng/mL for men 40 to 49 years of age, 3.5 ng/mL for men 50 to 59 years, 4.5 ng/mL for men 60 to 69 years, and 6.5 ng/mL for men 70 to 79 years. Consequently, a serum PSA value of 3.5 might appear as "normal" on a lab test, yet would be a worrisome finding in a man in his forties, warranting additional evaluation. Another way of interpreting serum PSA tests is to assess *PSA velocity*, also referred to as the rate of change of PSA. Men with prostate cancer demonstrate an increased rate of rise in PSA compared to men who do not have prostate cancer. The rate of change in PSA that best distinguishes between men with and without prostate cancer is 0.75 ng/mL per year. For this test to be valid, it requires that there be at least three PSA measurements over a period of 1.5 to 2 years. That is because there is substantial short-term variability (up to 20%) between repeat PSA measurements. A significant rise in serum PSA levels, despite the latest serum PSA test being below the normal cutoff (<4 ng/mL), is abnormal and should prompt a work-up.

Studies have revealed that immunoreactive PSA (the form that is detected by the widely used antibody test) exists in two forms: a major fraction bound to α_1-antichymotrypsin and a minor free fraction. The percentage of free PSA (free PSA ÷ total PSA × 100) is lower in men with prostate cancer than in men with benign prostatic diseases. Furthermore, it appears that per cent free PSA is most valuable in discriminating between benign and malignant disease when the total PSA level is in the "gray zone" of 4 to 10 ng/mL. When per cent free PSA is higher than 25%, it indicates a lower risk of cancer, whereas per cent free PSA values of less than 10% are worrisome for cancer. *Until the value of these refinements in the estimation and interpretations of PSA levels is better established, serum PSA by itself cannot be used for detection of early cancer.* When combined with rectal examination and transrectal ultrasonography, however, measurement of PSA levels is useful in detection of early-stage cancers. Because many small cancers localized to the prostate may never progress to clinically significant invasive cancers, there is considerable uncertainty about the management of small lesions that are detected because of an elevated PSA level. This has resulted in some controversy regarding the role of widespread screening for prostate cancer. Much effort is therefore being focused on devising criteria by which the localized lesions that are most likely to progress can be distinguished from those that may remain innocuous.

Although serum PSA levels are less than perfect for detection of early prostate cancer, there is little doubt that *serial measurements of PSA are of great value in assessing the response to therapy.* For example, a rising PSA level after radical prostatectomy or radiotherapy for localized disease is indicative of recurrent or disseminated disease. Immunohistochemical localization of PSA on tissue sections can also help the pathologist in determining whether a metastatic tumor originated in the prostate.[132]

Cancer of the prostate is treated by surgery, radiotherapy, and hormonal manipulations. More than 90% of patients who are treated by any of these methods can expect to live for 15 years. Currently, the most common treatment for clinically localized prostate cancer is radical prostatectomy. Major improvements in surgical technique, reducing the risk of intra-operative blood loss and postoperative impotence and incontinence, have popularized this procedure. The prognosis following radical prostatectomy is based on the pathologic stage, margin status, and Gleason grade. Alternative treatments for localized prostate cancer are external beam radiotherapy or interstitial radiotherapy, the latter consisting of placing radioactive seeds throughout the prostate (brachytherapy). External beam radiotherapy is also used to treat prostate cancer that is too locally advanced to be cured by surgery. The Gleason grade along with clinical stage and serum PSA values are important factors to predict the outcome following radiotherapy. Because some prostate cancers have a relatively indolent course, it can take as much as 10 years to see benefit from surgery or radiotherapy. Thus, watchful waiting is an appropriate treatment for many older men or those with significant comorbidity. Even some younger men with prostate cancer may elect watchful waiting if they present with low serum PSA values and limited cancer on biopsy that is not high grade. In these men, the risk of missing more extensive, higher-grade cancer on initial biopsy or progression of cancer that is truly limited at presentation, even with close follow-up and repeat biopsies, must be balanced against the potential morbidity of definitive therapy. Endocrine therapy is the mainstay for treatment of advanced, metastatic carcinoma. Because prostatic cancer cells depend on androgens for their sustenance, the aim of endocrine manipulations is to deprive the tumor cells of testosterone. This can be achieved by orchiectomy or by administration of synthetic agonists of luteinizing hormone–releasing hormone. Long-term administration of luteinizing hormone–releasing hormone agonists (after an initial transient increase in luteinizing hormone secretion) suppresses luteinizing hormone release, achieving in effect a pharmacologic orchiectomy. Although antiandrogen therapy does induce remissions, tumor progression leads to emergence of testosterone-insensitive clones; hence, despite all forms of treatment, patients with disseminated cancers have a poor prognosis. Both antiandrogen therapy and radiation induce morphologic changes in the prostate that alter both the non-neoplastic and cancerous tissue.[133,134]

Miscellaneous Tumors and Tumor-Like Conditions

Although acinar adenocarcinoma of the prostate is the most common tumor within the prostate, brief mention of other, less frequent variants and types is warranted. Prostate adenocarcinomas may also arise from prostatic ducts. Ductal adenocarcinomas arising in peripheral ducts may present in a fashion similar to that of ordinary prostate cancer, whereas those arising in the larger periurethral ducts present with signs and symptoms similar to urothelial cancer (hematuria and urinary obstructive symptoms).[135] Ductal adenocarcinomas are associated with a relatively poor prognosis, although early detection and treatment may be curative with surgery or radiation. Prostate cancer may show squamous differentiation, either following hormone therapy or de novo, resulting in either adenosquamous or pure squamous cancer.[136] Prostate cancers that reveal abundant mucinous secretions are termed *colloid carcinoma of the prostate.*[137] The most aggressive variant of prostate cancer is small cell cancer.[138] In some cases, the small cell cancer represents dedifferentiation of recurrent acinar adenocarcinoma; in other cases, men present with de novo small cell carcinoma of the prostate. Almost all such cases are rapidly fatal.

The most common tumor to secondarily involve the prostate is urothelial cancer.[139–141] Two distinct patterns of involvement exist. Large, invasive urothelial cancers can directly invade from the bladder into the prostate. Alternatively, carcinoma in situ of the bladder can extend into the prostatic urethra and down into the prostatic ducts and acini. The implications of this were discussed earlier in this chapter.

The same mesenchymal tumors that involve the bladder, described earlier, may also manifest in the prostate.[142–144] In addition, there exist unique mesenchymal tumors of the prostate derived from the prostatic stroma.[145,146] Although lymphomas may appear to first arise in the prostate, most patients demonstrate systemic disease.

REFERENCES

1. Bostwick DG, Eble JN (eds): Urologic Surgical Pathology. St. Louis, Mosby, 1997.
2. Murphy WM (ed): Urologic Pathology, 2nd ed. Philadelphia, WB Saunders, 1997.
3. Kottra JJ, Dunnick NR: Retroperitoneal fibrosis. Radiol Clin North Am 34:1259, 1996.
4. Smeulders N, Woodhouse CRJ: Neoplasia in adult extrophy patients. BJU Int 87:623, 2001.
5. de Vries CR, Freiha FS: Hemorrhagic cystitis: a review. J Urol 143:1, 1990.
6. Nickel JC: Interstitial cystitis: etiology, diagnosis, and treatment. Can Fam Physician 46:2430, 2000.
7. Long JR Jr, Althausen AF: Malacoplakia: a 25-year experience with a review of the literature. J Urol 141:1328, 1989.
8. Young RH.: Papillary and polypoid cystitis: a report of eight cases. Am J Surg Pathol 12:542, 1988.
9. Corica FA, et al: Intestinal metaplasia is not a strong risk factor for bladder cancer: study of 53 cases with long-term follow-up. Urol 50:427, 1997.
10. Young RH, Scully RE: Nephrogenic adenoma. Am J Surg Pathol 10:268, 1986.
11. Ford TF, et al: Adenomatous metaplasia (nephrogenic adenoma) of urothelium: an analysis of 70 cases. Br J Urol 57:427, 1985.
12. American Cancer Society: Cancer Facts and Figures. Atlanta, GA: American Cancer Society, 2003.
13. Murphy WM, et al: Tumors of the kidney, bladder, and related urinary structures. In Atlas of Tumor Pathology, 3rd series, fascicle 11. Washington, DC, Armed Forces Institute of Pathology, 1994.
14. Taylor DC, et al: Papillary urothelial hyperplasia: a precursor to papillary neoplasms. Am J Surg Pathol 20:1481, 1996.
15. Epstein JI, et al: The World Health Organization/International Society of Urological Pathology consensus classification of urothelial (transitional cell) neoplasms of the urinary bladder. Am J Surg Path 22:1435, 1998.
16. Bergkvist A, et al: Classification of bladder tumours based on the cellular pattern. Acta Chir Scand 130:371, 1965.
17. Mostofi FK, et al: Histological typing of urinary bladder tumours. In International Classification of Tumors, Vol. 19. Geneva, World Health Organization, 1973.
18. Jordan AM, et al: Transitional cell neoplasms of the urinary bladder: can biologic potential be predicted from histologic grading? Cancer 60:2766, 1987.
19. Cheville JC, et al: Inverted urothelial papilloma: is ploidy, MIB-1 proliferative activity, or p53 protein accumulation predictive of urothelial carcinoma? Cancer 88:632, 2000.
20. Witjes JA, et al: The prognostic value of a primary inverted papilloma of the urinary tract. J Urol 158:1500, 1997.
21. Gilbert HA, et al: The natural history of papillary transitional cell carcinoma of the bladder and its treatment in an unselected population on the basis of histologic grading. J Urol 119:488, 1978.
22. Heney NM, et al: Superficial bladder cancer: progression and recurrence. J Urol 130:1083, 1983.
23. Melamed MR, et al: Natural history and clinical behavior of in situ carcinoma of the human urinary bladder. Cancer 17:1533, 1964.
24. Melicow MM, Hollowell JW: Intra-urothelial cancer-carcinoma in situ. Bowen's disease of the urinary system: Discussion of thirty cases. J Urol 68:763, 1952.
25. Farrow GM, et al: Clinical observations on 69 cases of in situ carcinoma of the urinary bladder. Cancer Res 32:2794, 1977.
26. Elliot GB, et al: "Denuding cystitis" and in situ urothelial carcinoma. Arch Pathol 96:91, 1973.
27. Drew PA, et al: The nested variant of transitional cell carcinoma: an aggressive neoplasm with innocuous histology. Mod Pathol 9:898, 1996.
28. Talbert ML, Young RH: Carcinomas of the urinary bladder with deceptively benign-appearing foci. Am J Surg Pathol 13:374, 1989.
29. Amin MB, et al: Lymphoepithelioma-like carcinoma of the urinary bladder. Am J Surg Pathol 18:466, 1994.

30. Sakamoto N, et al: Urinary bladder carcinoma with neoplastic squamous component: a mapping study of 31 cases. Histopathology 21:135, 1992.
31. El-Bolkainy MN, et al: The impact of schistosomiasis on the pathology of bladder carcinoma. Cancer 48:2643, 1981.
32. Grignon DJ, et al: Primary adenocarcinoma of the urinary bladder: a clinicopathologic analysis of 72 cases. Cancer 67:2165, 1991.
33. Xiaoxu L, et al: Bladder adenocarcinoma: 31 reported cases. Can J Urol 8:1380, 2001.
34. Brandau S, Böhle A: Bladder: Molecular and genetic basis of carcinogenesis. Eur Urol 39:491, 2001.
35. Jung I, Messing E: Molecular mechanisms and pathways in bladder cancer development and progression. Cancer Control 7:325, 2000.
36. Cordon-Cardo C, et al: *P53* mutations in human bladder cancer: genotypic versus phenotypic patterns. Cancer 56:347, 1994.
37. Gibas C, Gibas L: Cytogenetics of bladder cancer. Cancer Genet Cytogenet 95:108, 1997.
38. Cairns P, Sidransky D: Bladder cancer. In Vogelstein B, Kinzler A (eds): Genetic Basis of Human Cancer. New York, McGraw-Hill, 1998, pp 639–645.
39. Spruck CH, et al: Two molecular pathways for transitional carcinoma of the bladder. Cancer Res 54:784, 1994.
40. Holmang S, et al: Stage progression in Ta papillary urothelial tumors: relationship to grade, immunohistochemical expression of tumor markers, mitotic frequency and DNA ploidy. J Urol 165:1124, 2001.
41. Malmström P-U, et al: Recurrence, progression, and survival in bladder cancer: a retrospective analysis of 232 patients with 5-year follow-up. Scand J Urol Nephrol 21:185, 1987.
42. Smith G, et al: Prognostic significance of biopsy results of normal-looking mucosa in cases of superficial bladder cancer. Br J Urol 55:665, 1983.
43. Melicow MM: Histological study of vesical urothelium intervening between gross neoplasms in total cystectomy. J Urol 68:261, 1952.
44. Murphy WM, Soloway MS. Developing carcinoma (dysplasia) of the urinary bladder. Pathol Annu 17:197, 1982.
45. Koss LG. Mapping of the urinary bladder: its impact on the concepts of bladder cancer. Hum Pathol 10:533, 1979.
46. Murphy WM, et al: Urinary cytology and bladder cancer: the cellular features of transitional cell neoplasms. Cancer 53:1555, 1984.
47. Murphy WM: Current status of urinary cytology in the evaluation of bladder neoplasms. Hum Pathol 21:886, 1990.
48. Koss LG: Diagnostic Cytology and Its Histopathologic Bases, 4th ed. Philadelphia, Lippincott Raven, 1992, p 890.
49. Koss LG: Diagnostic cytology of the urinary tract with histopathologic with histopathologic and clinical correlations. Philadelphia, Lippincott, 1995.
50. Herr HW, et al: Bacillus Calmette-Guérin therapy for special bladder cancer: a 10-year followup. J Urol 147:1020, 1992.
51. Lopez-Beltran A, et al: Carcinosarcoma and sarcomatoid carcinoma of the bladder: clinicopathological study of 41 cases. J Urol 159:1497, 1998.
52. Jones EC, et al: Inflammatory pseudotumor of the urinary bladder. Am J Surg Pathol 17:264, 1993.
53. Kempton CL, et al: Malignant lymphoma of the bladder: evidence from 36 cases that low-grade lymphoma of the MALT-type is the most common primary bladder lymphoma. Am J Surg Pathol 21:1324, 1997.
54. Diamond DA, Ransley PG: Male epispadias. J Urol 154:2150, 1995.
55. Belman AB: Hypospadias update. Urology 49:166, 1997.
56. Davenport M: ABC of general surgery in children: problems with penis and prepuce. BMJ 312:299, 1996.
57. Edwards S: Balanitis and balanoposthitis: a review. Genitourin Med 72:155, 1996.
58. Cupp MR, et al: The detection of human papilloma virus deoxyribonucleic acid in intraepithelial, in situ, verrucous and invasive carcinoma of the penis. J Urol 154:1024, 1995.
59. Dillner J, et al: Etiology of squamous cell carcinoma of the penis. Scand J Urol Nephrol Suppl 205:189, 2000.
60. Cubilla AL, et al: Histologic classification of penile carcinoma and its relation to outcome in 61 patients with primary resection. Int J Surg Pathol 9:111, 2001.
61. Cubilla AL, et al: Morphological features of epithelial abnormalities and precancerous lesions of the penis. Scand J Urol Nephrol Suppl 205:215, 2000.
62. Burgers JK, et al: Penile cancer: clinical presentation, diagnosis, and staging. Urol Clin North Am 19:267, 1992.
63. Rozanski TA, Bloom D: The undescended testis: theory and management. Urol Clin North Am 22:107, 1995.
64. Hutson J, et al: Normal testicular descent and the etiology of cryptorchidism. Adv Anal Embryol Cell Biol 132:1, 1996.
65. Swerdlow AJ, et al: Risk of testicular cancer in cohort of boys with cryptorchidism. BMJ 314:1507, 1997.
66. Davenport M: ABC of general pediatric surgery: inguinal hernia, hydrocele, and the undescended testis. BMJ 312:564, 1996.
67. Forman D, et al: Aetiology of testicular cancer: association with congenital abnormalities, age at puberty, infertility and exercise. BMJ 308:1393, 1994.
68. Beutow SA: Epidemiology of testicular cancer. Epidemiol Rev 17:433, 1995.
69. Nistal M, Paniagua R: Testicular biopsy: contemporary interpretation. Urol Clin N Am 26:555, 1999.
70. Ulbright TM, et al: Tumors of the testis, adnexa, spermatic cord, and scrotum. In Atlas of Tumor Pathology, 3rd series, fascicle 25. Washington, DC: Armed Forces Institute of Pathology, 1999.
71. Ulbright TM: Testis risk and prognostic factors: the pathologist's perspective. Urol Clin North Am 26:611, 1999.
72. Ulbright TM: Germ cell neoplasms of the testis. Am J Surg Pathol 17:1075, 1993.
73. Bosl GJ, Motzer RJ: Testicular germ-cell cancer. N Engl J Med 337:242, 1997.
74. Rorth M, et al: Carcinoma in situ in the testis. Scand J Urol Nephrol Suppl 205:166, 2000.
75. Looijenga LH, Oosterhuis JW: Pathogenesis of testicular germ cell tumours. Rev Reprod 4:90, 1999.
76. Looijenga LH, et al: Role of gain of 12p in germ cell tumor development. APMIS 111:161, 2003.
77. Rodriguez S, et al: Expression profile of genes from 12p in testicular germ cell tumors of adolescents and adults associated with I(12p) and amplification of 12p11.2-p12.1. Oncogene 22:1880, 2003.
78. Eble JN: Spermatocytic seminoma. Hum Pathol 25:1035, 1994.
79. Motzer RJ, et al: Teratoma with malignant transformation: diverse malignant histologies arising in men with germ cell tumors. J Urol 159:133, 1998.
80. Doherty AP, et al: The role of tumor markers in the diagnosis and treatment of testicular germ cell cancers. Br J Urol 79:247, 1997.
81. Leendert HJL, Oosterhuis JW: Clinical value of the x chromosome in testicular germ cell tumors. Lancet 363:6, 2004.
82. Dilworth JP, et al: Non-germ cell tumors of testis. Urology 37:399, 1991.
83. Kim I, et al: Leydig cell tumors of the testis: a clinicopathological analysis of 40 cases and review of the literature. Am J Surg Pathol 9:177, 1985.
84. Cheville JC, et al: Leydig cell tumor of the testis: a clinicopathologic, DNA content, and MIB-1 comparison of nonmetastasizing and metastasizing tumors. Am J Surg Pathol 22:1361, 1998.
85. Young RH, et al: Sertoli cell tumors of the testis, not otherwise specified: a clinicopathologic analysis of 60 cases. Am J Surg Pathol 22:709, 1998.
86. Ferry, JA, et al: Malignant lymphoma of the testis, epididymis, and spermatic cord: a clinicopathologic study of 69 cases with immunophenotypic analysis. Am J Surg Pathol 18:376, 1994.
87. McNeal JE: Normal and pathologic anatomy of prostate. Urology 17 (suppl):11, 1981.
88. Nickel JC: Prostatitis: Evolving management strategies. Urol Clin North Am 26:737, 1999.
89. Lipsky BA: Prostatitis and urinary tract infection in men: what's new; what's true? Am J Med 106:327, 1999.
90. Wise GJ, Silver DA: Fungal infections of the genitourinary system. J Urol 149:1377, 1993.
91. Foster CS: Pathology of benign prostatic hyperplasia. Prostate 9 (suppl):4, 2000.
92. Ramsey EW: Benign prostatic hyperplasia: a review. Can J Urol 7:1135, 2000.
93. Wong YC, Wang YZ: Growth factors and epithelial–stromal interactions in prostate cancer development. Int Rev Cytol 199:65, 2000.
94. McConnell JD, et al: The long-term effect of Doxazosin, Finasteride, and combination therapy on clinical progression of benign prostatic hyperplasia. New Engl J Med 349:2387, 2003.
95. Droller MJ: Medical approaches to the management of prostate disease. Br J Urol 79:42, 1997.

96. Walsh PC: Treatment of benign prostatic hyperplasia. N Engl J Med 335:586, 1996.
97. American Cancer Society: Cancer Facts and Figures. Atlanta, GA: American Cancer Society, 2004.
98. Ekman P: Genetic and environmental factors in prostate cancer genesis: identifying high-risk cohorts. Eur Urol 35:362, 1999.
99. Gronberg H: Prostate cancer epidemiology. Lancet 361:859, 2003.
100. Nelson WG, DeMarzo AM, Isaccs WB: Prostate cancer. New Engl J Med 349:366, 2003.
101. Yip I, et al: Nutrition and prostate cancer. Urol Clin North Am 26:403, 1999.
102. Boyle P, Severi G, and Giles GG: The epidemiology of prostate cancer. Urol Clin North Am 30:209, 2003.
103. Isaacs JT: Molecular markers of prostate cancer metastases. Am J Pathol 150:1511, 1997.
104. Ruijter E, et al: Molecular changes associated with prostate cancer development. Anal Quant Cytol Histol 23:67, 2001.
105. Primo NR Jr, et al: Molecular biology of prostate carcinogenesis. Crit Rev Oncol Hematol 32:197, 1999.
106. Jussi PE, Visakorpi T: Molecular genetics of prostate cancer. Ann Med 33:130, 2001.
107. Rhodes DR, et al: Multiplex biomarker approach for determining risk of prostate-specific antigen-defined recurrence of prostate cancer. J Natl Cancer Inst 95:661, 2003.
108. DeMarzo AM, et al: Pathologic and molecular aspects of prostate cancer. Lancet 361:955, 2003.
109. Byar DP, et al: Carcinoma of the prostate: prognostic evaluation of certain pathologic features in 208 radical prostatectomies. Cancer 30:5, 1972.
110. Potter SR, et al: Seminal vesicle invasion by prostate cancer: prognostic significance and therapeutic implications. Rev Urol 2:190, 2000.
111. Saitoh H, et al: Metastatic patterns of prostatic cancer: correlation between sites and number of organs involved. Cancer 54:3078, 1984.
112. Epstein JI: Diagnostic criteria of limited adenocarcinoma of the prostate on needle biopsy. Hum Pathol 26:223, 1995.
113. Epstein JI: Interpretation of Prostate Biopsies, 3rd ed. Philadelphia, Lippincott Williams & Wilkins, 2002.
114. Young RH, et al: Tumors of the prostate gland, seminal vesicles, male urethra, and penis. In Atlas of Tumor Pathology, 3rd series, fascicle 28. Washington, DC: Armed Forces Institute of Pathology, 2000.
115. Rubin MA, et al: α-Methylacyl coenzyme A racemase as a tissue biomarker for prostate cancer. JAMA 287:1662–1670, 2002.
116. Haggman MJ, et al: The relationship between prostatic intraepithelial neoplasia and prostate cancer: critical issues. J Urol 158:12, 1997.
117. McNeal JE, Bostwick DG. Intraductal dysplasia: a pre-malignant lesion of the prostate. Hum Pathol 17:64, 1986.
118. Kronz JD, et al: Predicting cancer following a diagnosis of high grade prostatic intraepithelial neoplasia on needle biopsy: data on men with more than one follow-up biopsy. Am J Surg Pathol 25:1079, 2001.
119. McNeal JE. Origin and development of carcinoma in the prostate. Cancer 23:24, 1969.
120. Epstein JI: Pathological assessment of the surgical specimen. Urol Clin North Am 28:567, 2001.
121. Gleason DF, et al: Prediction of prognosis for prostatic adenocarcinoma by combined histologic grading and clinical staging. J Urol 111:58, 1974.
122. Epstein JI, et al: The pathologic interpretation and significance of prostate biopsy findings: implications and current controversies. J Urol 166:402, 2001.
123. McNeal JE, et al: Histologic differentiation, cancer volume, and pelvic lymph node metastasis in adenocarcinoma of the prostate. Cancer 66:1225, 1990.
124. Epstein JI, et al: Pathological and clinical findings to predict tumor extent of non-palpable (stage T1c) prostate cancer. JAMA 271:368, 1994.
125. Matzkin H, et al: Stage T1a carcinoma of the prostate. Urology 43:11–21, 1994.
126. Sokoll LJ, Chan DW: Prostate-specific antigen: its discovery and biochemical characteristics. Urol Clin North Am 24:253, 1997.
127. Gretzer MD, Partin AW: PSA markers in prostate cancer. Urol Clin N Am 30:677, 2003.
128. Arcangeli CG, et al: Prostate-specific antigen as a screening test for prostate cancer: the United States experience. Urol Clin North Am 24:299, 1997.
129. Catalona WJ: Clinical utility of measurements of free and total prostate-specific antigen (PSA): a review. Prostate 7 (suppl):64, 1996.
130. Vashi AR, Oesterling JE: Percent free prostate-specific antigen: entering a new era in the detection of prostate cancer. Mayo Clin Proc 72:337, 1997.
131. Catalona WJ, et al: Use of the percentage of free prostate-specific antigen to enhance differentiation of prostate cancer from benign prostatic disease: a prospective multicenter clinical trial. JAMA 279:1542, 1998.
132. Epstein JI: PSAP and PSA as immunohistochemical markers. Urol Clin North Am 20:757, 1993.
133. Armas OA, et al: Clinical and pathobiological effects of neoadjuvant total androgen ablation therapy on clinically localized prostatic adenocarcinoma. Am J Surg Pathol 18:979, 1994.
134. Bostwick DG, et al: Radiation injury of the normal and neoplastic prostate. Am J Surg Pathol 6:501, 1982.
135. Brinker DA, et al. Ductal adenocarcinoma of the prostate diagnosed on needle biopsy: correlation with clinical and radical prostatectomy findings and progression. Am J Surg Pathol 23:1471, 1999.
136. Little NA, et al: Squamous cell carcinoma of the prostate: 2 cases of a rare malignancy and review of the literature. J Urol 149:137, 1993.
137. Ro JY, et al: Mucinous adenocarcinoma of the prostate: histochemical and immunohistochemical studies. Hum Pathol 21:593, 1990.
138. Tetu B, et al: Small cell carcinoma of prostate. Part 1: a clinicopathologic study of 20 cases. Cancer 59:1803, 1987.
139. Wood DP, et al: Transitional cell carcinoma of the prostate in cystoprostatectomy specimens removed for bladder cancer. J Urol 141:346, 1989.
140. Oliai BR, et al: A clinicopathologic analysis of urothelial carcinomas diagnosed on prostate needle biopsy. Am J Surg Pathol 25:794, 2001.
141. Esrig D, et al: Transitional cell carcinoma involving the prostate with a proposed staging classification for stromal invasion. J Urol 156:1071, 1996.
142. Proppe KH, et al: Postoperative spindle cell nodules of genitourinary tract resembling sarcoma. Am J Surg Pathol 8:101, 1984.
143. Sahin AA, et al: Pseudosarcomatous fibromyxoid tumor of the prostate: a case report with immunohistochemical, electron microscopic, and DNA flow cytometric analysis. Am J Clin Pathol 96:253, 1991.
144. Cheville JC, et al: Leiomyosarcoma of the prostate: report of 23 cases. Cancer 76:1422, 1995.
145. Gaudin PB, et al: Sarcomas and related proliferative lesions of specialized prostatic stroma. Am J Surg Pathol 22:148, 1998.
146. Lauwers GY, et al: Carcinosarcoma of the prostate. Am J Surg Pathol 17:342, 1993.

CHAPTER 22

The Female Genital Tract

Christopher P. Crum, MD

EMBRYOLOGY

ANATOMY

INFECTIONS OF THE FEMALE GENITAL TRACT

Infections Confined to the Lower Genital Tract

Infections Involving the Lower and Upper Genital Tract

Pelvic Inflammatory Disease (PID)

VULVA

BARTHOLIN CYST

VULVAR VESTIBULITIS

NON-NEOPLASTIC EPITHELIAL DISORDERS

Lichen Sclerosus

Lichen Simplex Chronicus

NEOPLASMS

Benign Tumors

Papillary Hidradenoma

Condyloma Acuminatum

Premalignant and Malignant Neoplasms

Carcinoma and Vulvar Intraepithelial Neoplasia

Extramammary Paget Disease

Malignant Melanoma

VAGINA

CONGENITAL ANOMALIES

PREMALIGNANT AND MALIGNANT NEOPLASMS

Vaginal Intraepithelial Neoplasia and Squamous Cell Carcinoma

Adenocarcinoma

Embryonal Rhabdomyosarcoma

CERVIX

INFLAMMATIONS

Acute and Chronic Cervicitis

Endocervical Polyps

INTRAEPITHELIAL AND INVASIVE SQUAMOUS NEOPLASIA

Cervical Intraepithelial Neoplasia

Squamous Cell Carcinoma

BODY OF UTERUS AND ENDOMETRIUM

ENDOMETRIAL HISTOLOGY IN THE MENSTRUAL CYCLE

FUNCTIONAL ENDOMETRIAL DISORDERS (DYSFUNCTIONAL UTERINE BLEEDING)

Anovulatory Cycle

Inadequate Luteal Phase

Endometrial Changes Induced by Oral Contraceptives

Menopausal and Postmenopausal Changes

INFLAMMATION

Chronic Endometritis

ENDOMETRIOSIS AND ADENOMYOSIS

ENDOMETRIAL POLYPS

ENDOMETRIAL HYPERPLASIA (ENDOMETRIAL INTRAEPITHELIAL NEOPLASIA)

MALIGNANT TUMORS OF THE ENDOMETRIUM

Carcinoma of the Endometrium

TUMORS OF THE ENDOMETRIUM WITH STROMAL DIFFERENTIATION
Carcinosarcomas
Adenosarcomas
Stromal Tumors
TUMORS OF THE MYOMETRIUM
Leiomyomas
Leiomyosarcomas
■ FALLOPIAN TUBES
INFLAMMATIONS
TUMORS AND CYSTS
■ OVARIES
NON-NEOPLASTIC AND FUNCTIONAL CYSTS
Follicular and Luteal Cysts
Polycystic Ovaries and Stromal Hyperthecosis
OVARIAN TUMORS
Tumors of Müllerian Epithelium
Serous Tumors
Mucinous Tumors
Endometrioid Tumors
Clear Cell Adenocarcinoma
Cystadenofibroma
Brenner Tumor
Clinical Course, Detection, and Prevention of Surface Epithelial Tumors
Germ Cell Tumors
Teratomas
Dysgerminoma
Endodermal Sinus (Yolk Sac) Tumors
Choriocarcinoma
Other Germ Cell Tumors
Sex Cord–Stromal Tumors
Granulosa-Theca Cell Tumors
Fibroma-Thecomas
Sertoli-Leydig Cell Tumors (Androblastomas)
Other Sex Cord–Stromal Tumors
Metastatic Tumors
■ GESTATIONAL AND PLACENTAL DISORDERS
DISORDERS OF EARLY PREGNANCY
Spontaneous Abortion
Ectopic Pregnancy
DISORDERS OF LATE PREGNANCY
Placental Abnormalities and Twin Placentas
Placental Inflammations and Infections
Toxemia of Pregnancy (Preeclampsia and Eclampsia)
Intrauterine Growth Restriction
GESTATIONAL TROPHOBLASTIC DISEASE
Hydatidiform Mole (Complete and Partial)
Invasive Mole
Choriocarcinoma
Placental Site Trophoblastic Tumor

NORMAL

Embryology

The embryology of the female genital tract is relevant to both anomalies in this region and the histogenesis of various tumors. The primordial germ cells arise in the wall of the yolk sac by the fourth week of gestation; by the fifth or sixth week, they migrate into the urogenital ridge. The mesodermal epithelium of the urogenital ridge then proliferates, eventually to produce the epithelium and stroma of the gonad. The dividing germ cells—of endodermal origin—are incorporated into these proliferating epithelial cells to form the ovary.[1] Failure of germ cells to develop may result in either absence of ovaries or premature ovarian failure. Disruption of normal migration may account for extragonadal distribution of germ cell midline structures (retroperitoneum, mediastinum, and even pineal gland) and may rarely lead to tumors in these sites.

A second component of female genital development is the müllerian duct. At about the sixth week, invagination and subsequent fusion of the coelomic lining epithelium form the lateral müllerian (or paramesonephric) ducts. Müllerian ducts progressively grow caudally to enter the pelvis, where they swing medially to fuse with the urogenital sinus at the müllerian tubercle (Fig. 22–1A). Further caudal growth brings these fused ducts into contact with the urogenital sinus, formed when the cloaca is subdivided by the urorectal septum. The urogenital sinus eventually becomes the vestibule of the external genitalia (Fig. 22–1*B*). Normally, the unfused portions mature into the fallopian tubes, the fused caudal portion developing into the uterus and upper vagina and the urogenital sinus forming the lower vagina and vestibule (Fig. 22–1*C*). Consequently, the entire lining of the uterus and tubes as well as the ovarian surface is ultimately derived from coelomic epithelium (mesothelium). This close embryologic relationship between the mesothelium and müllerian system may be reflected in adult life in the form of benign (endometriosis) and malignant (endometrioid and serous neoplasia) lesions, which may arise in both the surface mesothelium of the ovaries and the peritoneal surfaces.

The epithelium of the vagina, cervix, and urinary tract is formed by induction of basal cells from the underlying stroma, which undergo squamous and urothelial differentiation.[2] A portion of these cells remains uncommitted, forming the reserve cells of the cervix. The latter are capable of both squamous and columnar cell differentiation.[3]

In males, müllerian inhibitory substance[4] from the developing testis causes regression of the müllerian ducts, and the paired wolffian (or mesonephric) ducts form the epididymis and the vas deferens. Normally, the mesonephric duct regresses in the female, but remnants may persist into adult life as epithelial inclusions adjacent to the ovaries, tubes, and uterus. In the cervix and vagina, these rests may be cystic and are termed Gartner duct cysts. Many of the events in the

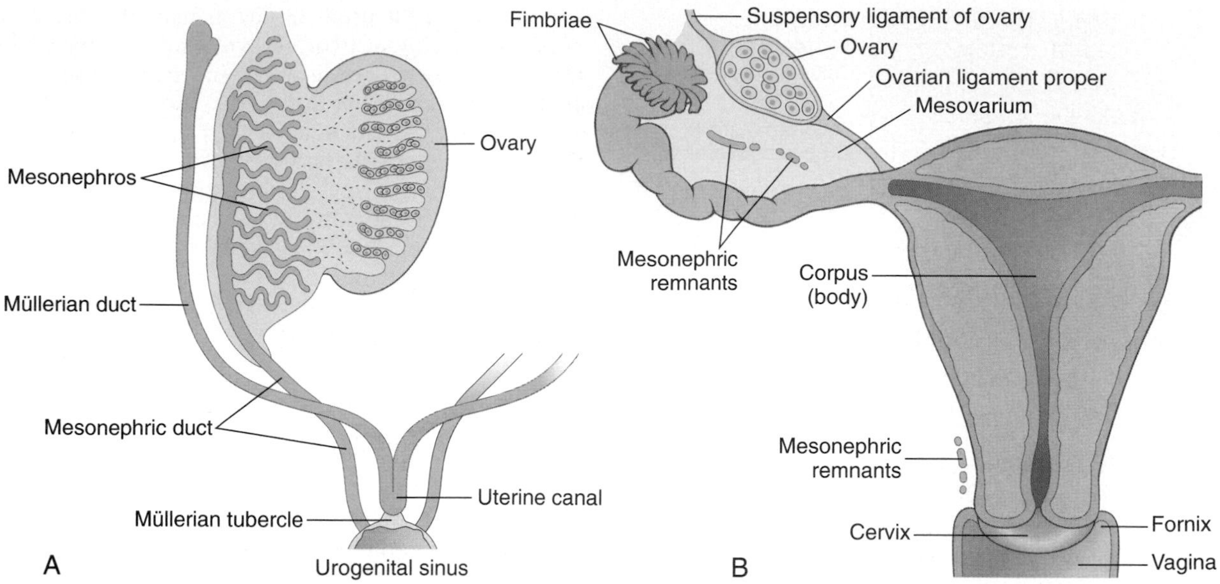

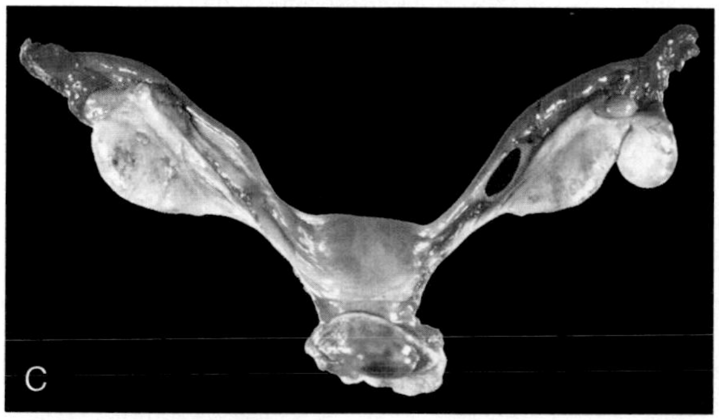

FIGURE 22–1 Embryology and anatomy of the female genital tract. *A*, Early in development the mesonephric (*red*) and müllerian (*blue*) ducts merge at the urogenital sinus to form the müllerian tubercle. *B*, By birth the müllerian ducts have fused to form the fallopian tubes, uterus and endocervix (*blue*) merging with the vaginal squamous mucosa. The mesonephric ducts regress but may be found as a remnant in the ovary, adnexa and cervix (Gartner duct). (Adapted from Langman J: Medical Embryology. Baltimore, Williams and Wilkins, 1981.) *C*, Normal adult genital tract, with cervix, uterus, fallopian tubes, and ovaries. A small paratubal cyst is present on the right.

formation of the internal and external genitalia and their epithelial coverings result from reciprocal epithelial-stromal signaling, leading to mesenchymal remodeling and changes in epithelial cell fate.[2,5]

Anatomy

During active reproductive life, the ovaries measure about 4 × 2.5 × 1.5 cm in dimension. The ovary is divided into a cortex and a medulla. The cortex consists of a layer of closely packed stromal cells and a thin covering of relatively acellular collagenous connective tissue. Follicles in varying stages of maturation are found within the outer cortex. With each menstrual cycle, one follicle develops into a graafian follicle, which is transformed into a corpus luteum following ovulation. Corpora lutea ranging from recent to senescent (corpora albicantia) may be found in the cortex of the adult ovary.

The medulla of the ovary consists of loosely arranged mesenchymal tissue and contains remnants of both wolffian duct (rete ovarii) and small clusters of round to polygonal, epithelioid cells around vessels and nerves. These “hilus” cells are vestigial remains of the gonad from its primitive “ambisexual” phase, are steroid producing, and resemble the interstitial cells of the testis. Rarely, these cells give rise to masculinizing tumors (hilar cell tumors).

The fallopian tube mucosa is composed of numerous delicate papillary folds (plica) consisting of three cell types: ciliated columnar cells; nonciliated, columnar secretory cells; and so-called intercalated cells, which may simply represent inactive secretory cells.

The uterus varies in size depending on the age and parity of the individual. It weighs about 50 gm and measures about 8.0 × 6.0 × 3.0 cm in nulliparous reproductive age women. Following pregnancies, uteri are slightly larger (up to 70 gm in weight), then diminish to half their weight and dimension following menopause.

The uterus has three distinctive anatomic and functional regions: the cervix, the lower uterine segment, and the corpus. The cervix is further divided into the vaginal portio (ectocervix) and the endocervix. The portio is visible to the naked eye on vaginal examination and is covered by a stratified nonkeratinizing squamous epithelium continuous with the vaginal vault. The squamous epithelium converges centrally at a small opening termed the *external os*. In the nulliparous woman, this os is virtually closed. Just cephalad to the os is the endocervix, which is lined by columnar, mucus-secreting epithelium that dips down into the underlying stroma to produce crypts (endocervical “glands”). The point at which the squamous and müllerian columnar epithelium meet is the squamocolumnar junction (Fig. 22–2). The position of the junction is variable due to both the cervical anatomy and the distribution of the basal and subcolumnar reserve cells that exist just cephalad of this junction. It is the progressive differentiation of these basal/reserve cells that governs the microanatomy of this region, ultimately resulting in the

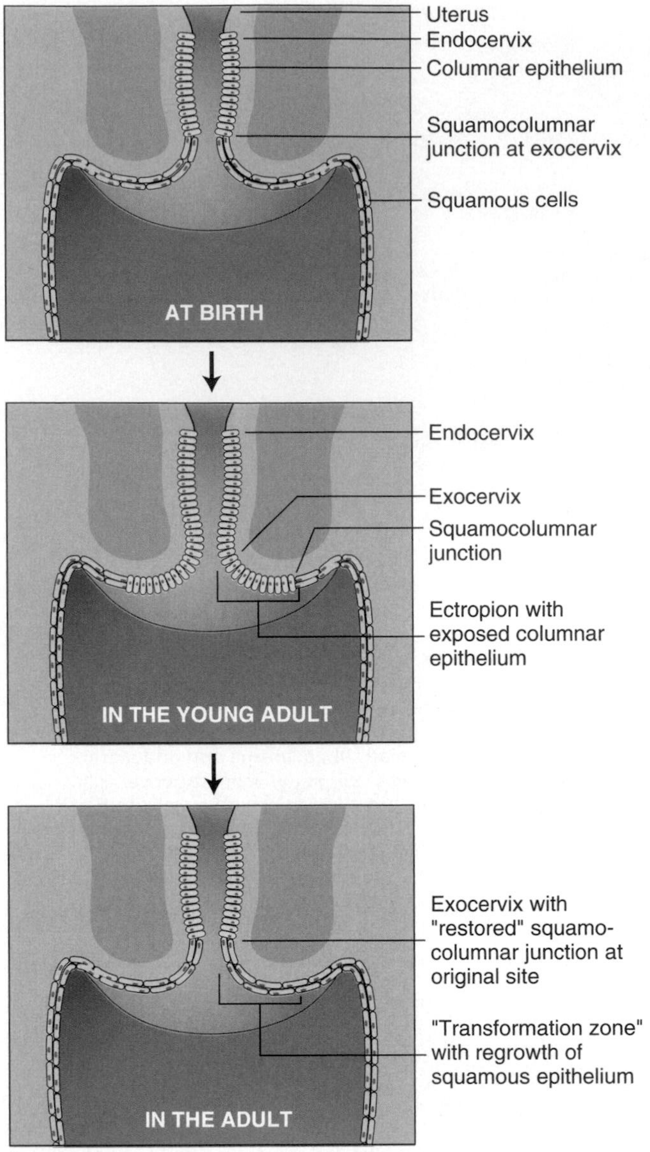

FIGURE 22–2 Schematic of the development of the cervical transformation zone.

cephalad migration of the squamocolumnar junction. The portion of the columnar epithelium that is ultimately replaced by squamous epithelium is termed the "*transformation zone*" (Figs. 22–2 and 22–3). As we shall see, it is in this transformation zone, including the squamocolumnar junction, where precancerous lesions and squamous carcinomas develop.[6]

The endometrial changes that occur during the menstrual cycle are keyed to the rise and fall in the levels of ovarian hormones, and the reader should be familiar with the complex but fascinating interactions among hypothalamic, pituitary, and ovarian factors underlying maturation of ovarian follicles, ovulation, and the menstrual cycle. It is also important to know that the hormonal patterns of most women differ from the "standard" as depicted diagrammatically (discussed later; see Fig. 22–25).[7] Under the influence of the pituitary follicle-stimulating hormone and luteinizing hormone, development and ripening of a single ovum occur, and estrogen production by the enlarging ovarian follicle progressively rises during the first 2 weeks of the usual 28-day menstrual cycle. It reaches a peak, presumably just before ovulation, and then falls. After ovulation, the estrogen levels again begin to rise to a plateau at about the end of the third week, but these levels are never as high as the preovulatory peak. The level of this hormone then progressively falls, beginning 3 to 4 days before the onset of menstruation. Progesterone, produced by the corpus luteum, rises throughout the last half of the menstrual cycle and falls to basal levels just before the onset of menstrual bleeding. The histology of the normal and abnormal endometrial cycle is discussed later in the section on the endometrium.

Pathology

Diseases of the female genital tract are extremely common in clinical and pathology practice and include complications of pregnancy, inflammations, tumors, and hormonally induced effects. The following discussion presents the pathology of the majority of clinical problems. Details can be found in current books of obstetric and gynecologic pathology and medicine.[8–11] The pathologic conditions peculiar to each segment of the female genital tract are discussed separately, but first we briefly review pelvic inflammatory disease (PID) and other infections because they can affect many of the segments concomitantly.

Infections of the Female Genital Tract

A large variety of organisms can infect the female genital tract and, in total, account for considerable suffering and morbidity (Table 22–1). Some, such as *Candida* infections, trichomoniasis, and *Gardnerella* infections, are extremely common and may cause significant discomfort with no serious sequelae. Others, such as gonorrhea and *Chlamydia* infection, are major causes of female infertility, and others still, such as *Mycoplasma* infections, are implicated in spontaneous abortions. Viruses, principally the human papillomaviruses (HPV), appear to be involved in the pathogenesis of vulvar and cervical cancer.

Many of these infections are sexually transmitted, including trichomoniasis, gonorrhea, chancroid, granuloma inguinale, lymphogranuloma venereum, syphilis, mycoplasmal infection, chlamydial infection, herpes, and HPV infection.[12] Most of these conditions have been considered in Chapters 6 and 8. Here we touch only on selected aspects relevant to the female genital tract, including pathogens confined to the lower genital tract (vulva, vagina, and cervix) and those that involve the entire genital tract and are implicated in PID. Papillomaviruses are discussed subsequently under tumors.

INFECTIONS CONFINED TO THE LOWER GENITAL TRACT

Herpes simplex infection is common and usually involves the vulva, vagina, and cervix.[12] In sexually transmitted disease clinics, approximately half of patients have current or prior

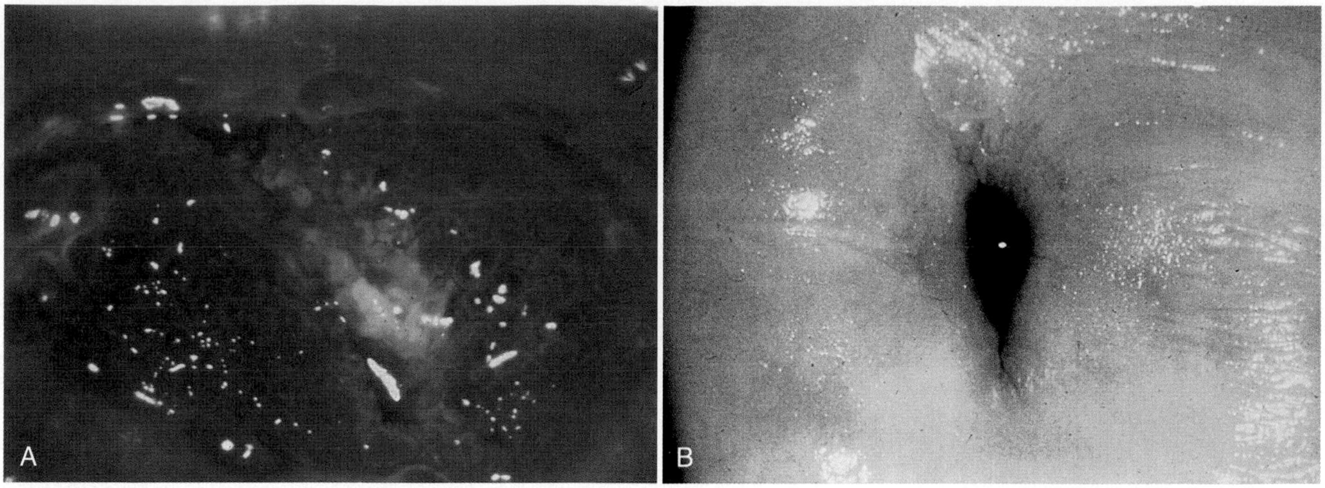

FIGURE 22–3 *A*, Colposcopic view of the cervix in a reproductive age woman. The portio epithelium (peripheral) merges with (at dotted boundary) and eventually replaces the endocervical columnar epithelium (red and grapelike) to form the transformation zone. The os is in the center. *B*, The postmenopausal cervix. The epithelial surface is smooth and completely covered by squamous epithelium. The squamocolumnar junction is not visible and is inside the endocervical canal. (*A* and *B*, courtesy of Dr. Alex Ferenczy, McGill University, Montreal, Quebec.)

evidence of infection compared to less than 10% of unselected women.[13] The frequency of genital herpes has increased dramatically in the past two decades, particularly in teenagers and young women. Herpes simplex virus type 2 (HSV-2) infection is now one of the major sexually transmitted diseases. Clinical symptoms are seen in about one third of infected individuals.[13] The lesions begin 3 to 7 days after sexual relations and consist of painful red papules in the vulva that progress to vesicles and then to coalescent ulcers. Cervical or vaginal involvement causes severe leukorrhea (genital discharge), and the initial infection produces systemic symptoms such as fever, malaise, and tender inguinal lymph nodes. The vesicles and ulcers contain numerous virus particles, accounting for the high transmission rate during active infection. The lesions heal spontaneously in 1 to 3 weeks, but as with herpetic infections elsewhere, latent infection of regional nerve ganglia persists. About two thirds of affected women suffer recurrences, which are less painful. Transmission may occur during active or inactive (latent) phases, although it is much less likely in asymptomatic carriers. The gravest consequence of HSV infection is transmission to the neonate during birth. This risk is highest if the infection is active during delivery and particularly if it is a primary (initial) infection in the mother.[14]

Mycotic and *yeast (Candida) infections* are common; about 10% of women are thought to be carriers of vulvovaginal fungi. Diabetes mellitus, oral contraceptives, and pregnancy may enhance the development of infection, which manifests as small white surface patches similar to monilial lesions elsewhere. It is accompanied by leukorrhea and pruritus. The diagnosis is made by finding the organism in wet mounts of the lesions.

Trichomonas vaginalis is a large, flagellated ovoid protozoan that can be readily identified in wet mounts of vaginal discharge in infected patients (Fig. 22–4). Infections may occur at any age and are seen in about 15% of women in sexually transmitted disease clinics.[15] They are associated with a purulent vaginal discharge and discomfort; the underlying vaginal and cervical mucosa typically has a characteristic fiery red appearance, called strawberry cervix. On histologic examination, the inflammatory reaction is usually limited to the mucosa and immediately subjacent lamina propria.

TABLE 22–1 Anatomic Distribution of Common Female Genital Infections

		Location and Manifestations of Infection				
Organism	**Source**	***Vulva***	***Vagina***	***Cervix***	***Corpus***	***Adnexa***
Herpesvirus	STD	Herpetic ulcers				
Molluscum contagiosum	STD	Molluscum lesions				
HPV	STD	Genital warts, intrapeithelial neoplasia, invasive carcinoma				
Chlamydia trachomatis	STD		Follicular cervicitis, endometritis, salpingo-oophoritis			
Neisseria gonorrhoeae	STD	Skene gland adenitis	Vaginitis in children	Acute cervicitis	Acute endometritis and salpingitis	
Candida	Endogenous	Vulvovaginitis				
Trichomonas	STD		Cervicovaginitis			

HPV, human papillomavirus; STD, sexually transmitted disease.

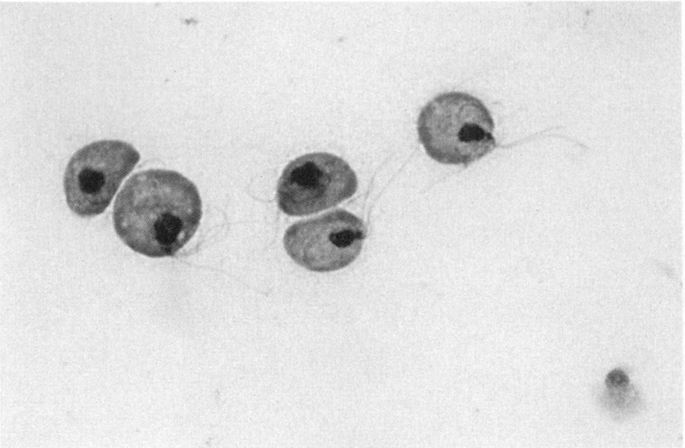

FIGURE 22–4 Flagellated trophozoites of *Trichomonas vaginalis.*

Mycoplasma species account for some cases of vaginitis and cervicitis and have been implicated in spontaneous abortion and chorioamnionitis. *Gardnerella* is a gram-negative, small bacillus that is implicated in cases of vaginitis when other organisms *(Trichomonas*, fungi) cannot be found.

INFECTIONS INVOLVING THE LOWER AND UPPER GENITAL TRACT

Pelvic Inflammatory Disease (PID)

PID is a common disorder characterized by pelvic pain, adnexal tenderness, fever, and vaginal discharge; it results from infection by one or more of the following groups of organisms: gonococci, chlamydiae, and enteric bacteria. The gonococcus continues to be a common cause of PID, the most serious complication of gonorrhea in women. *Chlamydia* infection is now another well-recognized cause of PID. Besides these two, infections after spontaneous or induced abortions and normal or abnormal deliveries (called puerperal infections) are important in the production of PID. Such PID is polymicrobial and is caused by staphylococci, streptococci, coliform bacteria, and *Clostridium perfringens.*

Gonococcal inflammation usually begins in the Bartholin gland and other vestibular glands or periurethral glands; cervix involvement is common and frequently asymptomatic. From any of these sites, the organisms may spread upward to involve the tubes and tubo-ovarian region. The adult vagina is remarkably resistant to the gonococcus, but in the child, presumably because of a more delicate lining mucosa, vulvovaginitis may develop. The nongonococcal bacterial infections that follow induced abortion, dilation and curettage of the uterus, and other surgical procedures on the female genital tract are thought to spread from the uterus upward through the lymphatics or venous channels rather than on the mucosal surfaces. These infections therefore tend to produce less mucosal involvement but more reaction within the deeper layers.

Morphology. With the gonococcus, inflammatory changes appear in the affected glands approximately 2 to 7 days after inoculation of the organism. Wherever it occurs, gonococcal disease is characterized by an acute suppurative reaction with inflammation largely confined to the superficial mucosa and underlying submucosa. Smears of the inflammatory exudate should disclose the intracellular gram-negative diplococcus, but absolute confirmation requires culture. If spread occurs, the endometrium is usually spared, for obscure reasons. Once it is within the tubes, an **acute suppurative salpingitis** ensues. The tubal serosa becomes hyperemic and layered with fibrin, the tubal fimbriae are similarly involved, and the lumen fills with purulent exudate that may leak out of the fimbriated end. In days or weeks, the fimbriae may seal or become plastered against the ovary to create a **salpingo-oophoritis**. Collections of pus within the ovary and tube **(tubo-ovarian abscesses)** or tubal lumen **(pyosalpinx)** may occur. Adhesions of the tubal plica may produce glandlike spaces (follicular salpingitis) (Fig. 22–5). In the course of time, the infecting organisms may disappear, the pus undergoing proteolysis to a thin, serous fluid, to produce a **hydrosalpinx** or hydrosalpinx follicularis.

PID caused by staphylococci, streptococci, and the other puerperal invaders tends to have less exudation

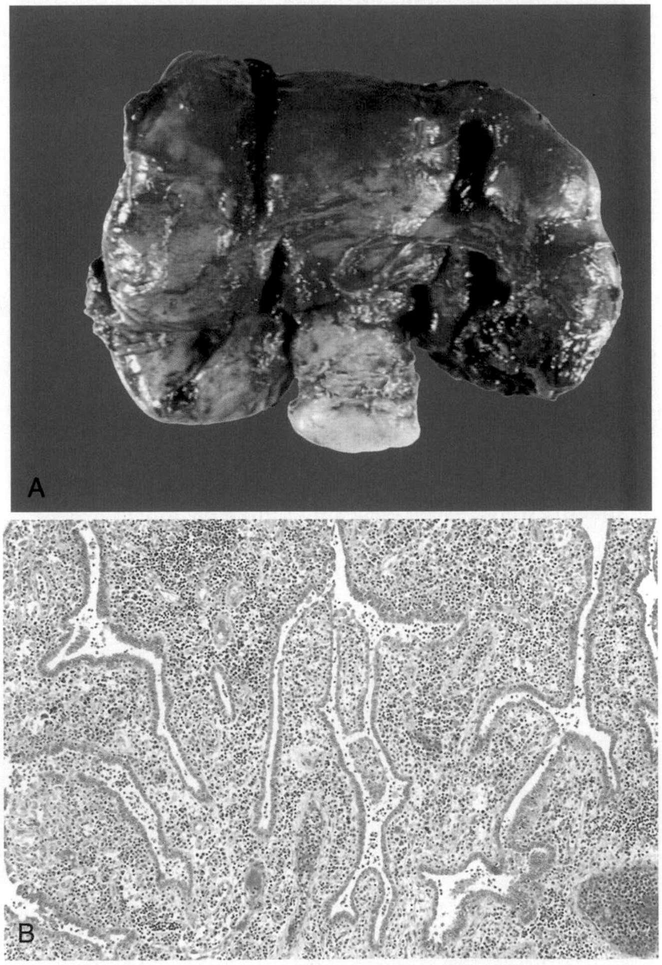

FIGURE 22–5 *A*, Acute salpingo-oophoritis, with tubo-ovarian abscess. The fallopian tube and ovaries have coalesced into an inflammatory mass adherent to the uterus. (Compare with Figure 22–1.) *B*, Chronic salpingitis with fusion of the tubal plicae and inflammatory cell infiltrates.

within the lumens of the tube and less involvement of the mucosa, with a greater inflammatory response within the deeper layers. The infection tends to spread throughout the wall to involve the serosa and may often involve the broad ligaments, pelvic structures, and peritoneum. Bacteremia is a more frequent complication of streptococcal or staphylococcal PID than of gonococcal infections.

The complications of PID include:

- Peritonitis
- Intestinal obstruction due to adhesions between the small bowel and the pelvic organs
- Bacteremia, which may produce endocarditis, meningitis, and suppurative arthritis
- Infertility, one of the most commonly feared consequences of long-standing chronic PID

In the early stages, gonococcal infections are readily controlled with antibiotics, although penicillin-resistant strains have regrettably emerged. When the infection becomes walled off in suppurative tubes or tubo-ovarian abscesses, it is difficult to achieve a sufficient level of antibiotic within the centers of such suppuration to control these infections effectively. Postabortion and postpartum PIDs are also amenable to antibiotics but are far more difficult to control than the gonococcal infections. It sometimes becomes necessary to remove the organs surgically.

VULVA

Diseases of the vulva in the aggregate constitute only a small fraction of gynecologic practice. Many inflammatory dermatologic diseases that affect hair-bearing skin elsewhere on the body may also occur on the vulva, so vulvitis may be encountered in psoriasis, eczema, and allergic dermatitis. The vulva is prone to skin infections because it is constantly exposed to secretions and moisture. Nonspecific vulvitis is particularly likely to occur in blood dyscrasias, uremia, diabetes mellitus, malnutrition, and avitaminoses. Most skin cysts (epidermal inclusion cysts) and tumors can also occur in the vulva. Here we discuss disorders peculiar to the vulva, including Bartholin cyst, vestibular adenitis, vulvar dystrophies, and tumors of the vulva.

Bartholin Cyst

Acute infection of the Bartholin gland produces an acute inflammation of the gland (adenitis) and may result in a Bartholin abscess. Bartholin cysts are relatively common, occur at all ages, and result from obstruction of the Bartholin duct, usually by a preceding infection. These cysts may become large, up to 3 to 5 cm in diameter. The cyst is lined by either the transitional epithelium of the normal duct or squamous metaplasia. The cysts produce pain and local discomfort; the cysts are either excised or opened permanently (marsupialization).

Vulvar Vestibulitis

The vulvar vestibule is located in the posterior introitus at the entrance to the vagina and contains small glands in the submucosa (vestibular glands). A variety of disorders cause chronic pain in this area, known as *vulvodynia*. Chief among them are inflammation of the surface mucosa and vestibular glands associated with a chronic, recurrent, and exquisitely painful condition known as vulvar vestibulitis. The inflammatory condition, which involves the glands and mucosa, produces small ulcerations, which account for extreme point tenderness in the vestibule. The cause of the condition is unknown, and the condition is relieved, in some but not in all cases, by surgical removal of the inflamed mucosa.[16]

Non-Neoplastic Epithelial Disorders

A spectrum of inflammatory lesions of the vulva is characterized by opaque, white, scaly, plaquelike mucosal thickenings that produce vulvar discomfort and itching (pruritus). Because of their white appearance, these disorders have traditionally been termed leukoplakia by clinicians. This is a clinical descriptive term because *white plaques may indicate a variety of benign, premalignant, or malignant lesions.*[17] In fact, a biopsy of "leukoplakia" may reveal one of several conditions: (1) vitiligo (loss of pigment); (2) inflammatory dermatoses (e.g., psoriasis, chronic dermatitis [Chapter 25]); (3) vulvar intraepithelial neoplasia, Paget disease, or even invasive carcinoma; and (4) a variety of alterations of unknown etiology that elude proper classification. To eliminate the confusion generated by using multiple terms to characterize white vulvar lesions (e.g., kraurosis vulvae, leukoplakia, atrophic vulvitis), clinical descriptive terminology has been separated from histologic diagnosis. Excluding neoplasms and specific disease entities, nonspecific inflammatory alterations of the vulva are now classified using accepted dermatologic diagnoses or are placed within two additional categories: (1) *lichen sclerosus*, a characteristic disorder manifested by subepithelial fibrosis, and (2) *lichen simplex chronicus*, manifested by epithelial thickening (acanthosis) and hyperkeratosis (Fig. 22–6). The two forms may coexist in different areas of the same vulva, and the lesions are often multiple, making their clinical management particularly difficult.[18]

LICHEN SCLEROSUS

Lichen sclerosus, also called chronic atrophic vulvitis, leads to atrophy, fibrosis, and scarring.[18] The skin becomes pale gray and parchment-like, the labia are atrophied, and the introitus is narrowed (Fig. 22–7). The four cardinal histologic features are 1) atrophy (thinning) of the epidermis, with disappearance of the rete pegs, 2) hydropic degeneration of the basal cells, 3) replacement of the underlying dermis by dense collagenous fibrous tissue, and 4) a monoclonal bandlike lymphocytic infiltrate (Fig. 22–6). Lichen sclerosus occurs in all age groups but is most common after menopause. The pathogenesis is unclear, but it has many features of an autoimmune disorder.[19] At all ages, the disorder tends to be slow in developing, insidious, and progressive. Lichen sclerosus is not recognized as a precancerous condition, but it has been associated with genetic alterations and confers a greater than expected risk of subsequent carcinoma, which may occur in 1% to 4% of cases.[19,20]

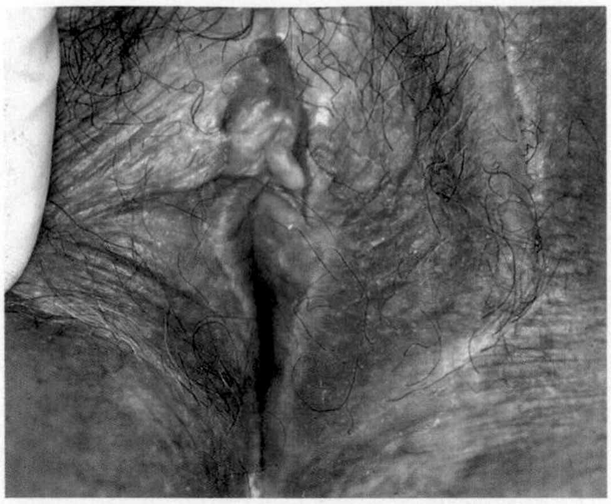

FIGURE 22–7 Lichen sclerosus, exhibiting the white parchment-like patches of the skin of the vulva and labial atrophy.

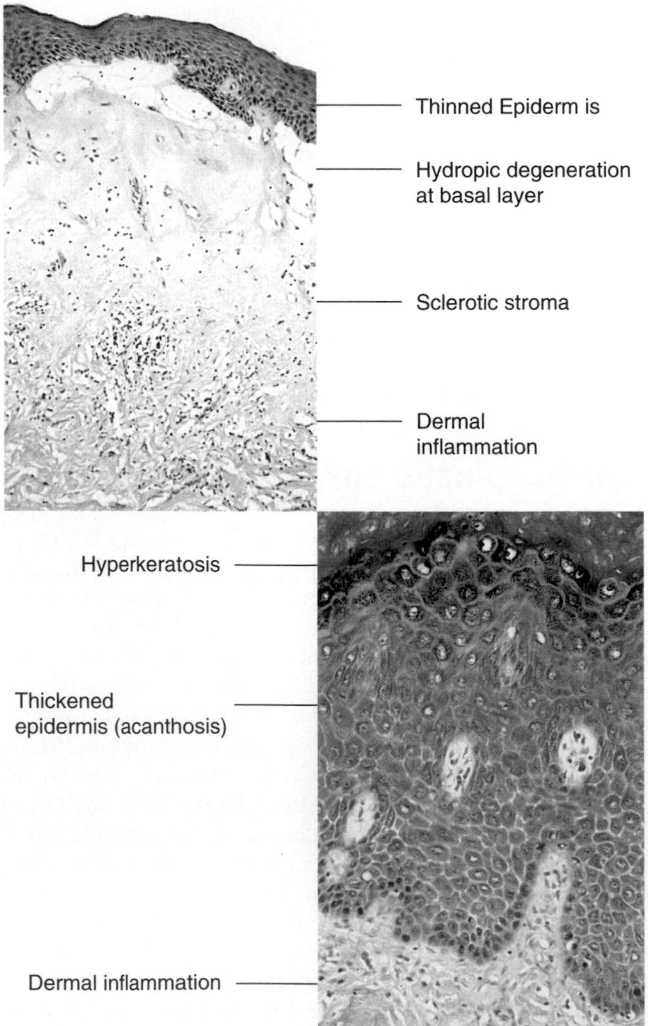

FIGURE 22–6 Inflammatory vulvar disorders. Lichen sclerosus (*upper panel*). Lichen simplex chronicus (*lower panel*). The main features of the lesions are indicated in the figures.

LICHEN SIMPLEX CHRONICUS

Previously called hyperplastic dystrophy, lichen simplex chronicus is a non-specific condition resulting from rubbing or scratching the skin to relieve pruritus. The latter may result from known or unknown irritants. Lichen simplex chronicus is characterized by acanthosis of the vulvar squamous epithelium, frequently with hyperkeratosis. The epithelium is thickened and may show increased mitotic activity in both the basal and prickle cell layers (Fig. 22–6) with variable leukocytic infiltration of the dermis. Similar to lichen sclerosus, lichen simplex chronicus is sometimes associated with carcinoma. It is not, however, considered a significant cancer precursor unless there is coexisting epithelial atypia, in which case it is classified as a precancerous lesion (vulvar intraepithelial neoplasia).[21]

Because lichen simplex chronicus is secondary to pruritus, it is, by definition, non-specific. Its causes include specific infections (tinea, candida, etc.), mucosal irritations secondary to chemical exposures, and unknown causes of pruritus. Because the lesions may present as white vulvar plaques, they may be indistinguishable clinically from more serious disorders. Thus, biopsy is indicated in all lesions, even those that are remotely suspicious. Disturbances in cellular differentiation, nuclear atypia, and verrucous growth may signify the onset of squamous neoplasia.

Neoplasms

Tumors of the vulva are the most important lesions to affect this region. Many types have been recorded, both benign and malignant, including neoplasms of the adnexal glands, epithelium, and underlying soft tissue. Many of these tumors are uncommon and are histologically similar to tumors occurring elsewhere in the body. Attention will be focused on the more common tumors unique to the vulva.

BENIGN TUMORS

Papillary Hidradenoma

Like the breast, the vulva contains modified apocrine sweat glands. In fact, the vulva may contain tissue closely resembling breast ("ectopic breast") and develop two tumors with counterparts in the breast. One of these, papillary hidradenoma, is identical in appearance to intraductal papillomas of the breast. The other, Paget disease, is discussed later. Hidradenoma presents as a sharply circumscribed nodule, most commonly on the labia majora or interlabial folds, and may be confused clinically with carcinoma because of its tendency to ulcerate. On histologic examination, hidradenomas consist of tubular ducts lined by a single or double layer of nonciliated columnar cells, with a layer of flattened "myoepithelial cells" underlying the epithelium. These myoepithelial elements are characteristic of sweat glands and sweat gland tumors.

Condyloma Acuminatum

Benign raised or wartlike (verrucous) conditions of the vulva occur in three forms: (1) Condyloma acuminatum, a papillomavirus-induced squamous lesion also called venereal wart, is, by far, the most common; (2) mucosal polyps, which are benign stromal proliferations covered with squamous epithelium; and (3) syphilitic condyloma latum, described in Chapter 8.

Condylomata acuminata are sexually transmitted, benign tumors that have a distinctly verrucous gross appearance[22] (Fig. 22–8*A*). Although they may be solitary, they are more frequently multiple and often coalesce; they involve perineal, vulvar, and perianal regions as well as the vagina and, less commonly, the cervix. The lesions are identical to those found on the penis and around the anus in males (Chapter 21). On histologic examination, they consist of a branching, treelike proliferation of stratified squamous epithelium supported by a fibrous stroma (Fig. 22–8*B*). Acanthosis, parakeratosis, hyperkeratosis, and, most specifically, nuclear atypia in the surface cells with perinuclear vacuolization (called *koilocytosis*) are present. Condylomata are caused by HPV, principally types 6 and 11,[23] which are associated with benign genital lesions and replicate in the squamous epithelium. The virus life cycle is completed in the mature superficial cells of the epithelium. This dependence of viral growth on squamous maturation is typical of HPV and produces a distinct cytologic change in the mature cells—*koilocytotic atypia* (nuclear atypia and perinuclear vacuolization)—that is considered a viral "cytopathic" effect. Except in immunosuppressed individuals, condylomata acuminata frequently regress spontaneously, and are not considered to be precancerous lesions. They are, however, a marker for sexually transmitted disease.[23]

PREMALIGNANT AND MALIGNANT NEOPLASMS

Carcinoma and Vulvar Intraepithelial Neoplasia

Carcinoma of the vulva is an uncommon malignant neoplasm (approximately one eighth as frequent as cervical cancer) representing about 3% of all genital cancers in the female; approximately two thirds occur in women older than 60 years.[24] *Eighty-five per cent of these malignant tumors are squamous cell carcinomas*, the remainder being basal cell carcinomas, melanomas, or adenocarcinomas. In terms of etiology, pathogenesis, and clinical presentation, vulvar squamous cell carcinomas may be divided into two general groups.

The first group is associated with cancer-related (high-risk) HPV, and frequently coexists with or is preceded by a classic and easily recognized precancerous change called vulvar intraepithelial neoplasia (VIN). This form of VIN includes lesions classified as carcinoma in situ or Bowen disease.[25] VIN is characterized by nuclear atypia in the epithelial cells, increased mitoses, and lack of surface differentiation (Fig. 22–9*A*). It is analogous to high-grade squamous intraepithelial lesions of the cervix (see under cervix). These lesions usually present as white or pigmented plaques on the vulva. VIN is appearing with increasing frequency in women younger than 40 years of age. With or without associated invasive carcinoma, *VIN is frequently multicentric*, and 10% to 30% are associated with another primary squamous neoplasm in the vagina or cervix. This association indicates a common etiologic agent. Indeed, 90% of cases of VIN and associated cancers contain HPV DNA, specifically types 16, 18, and other cancer-associated (high-risk) types.[20] Spontaneous regression of VIN lesions has been reported, usually in younger women; the risk of progression to invasive cancer increases in older (older than 45 years of age) or immunosuppressed women.[25]

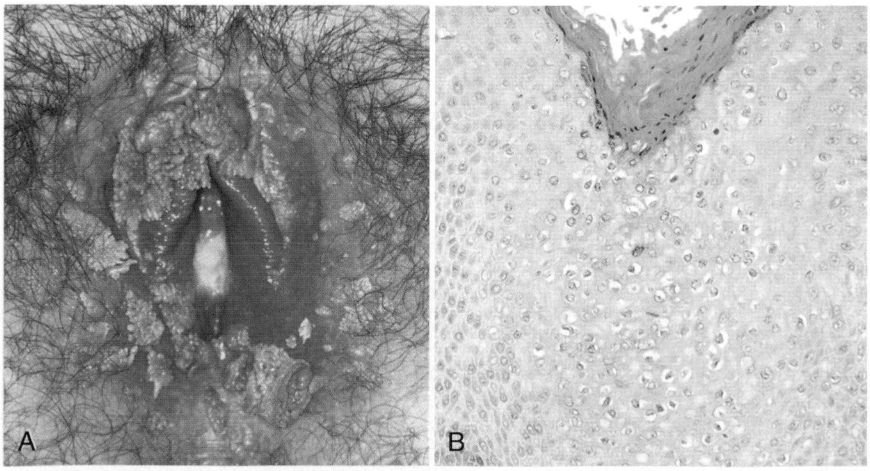

FIGURE 22–8 *A*, Numerous condylomas of the vulva encircling the introitus. (Courtesy of Dr. Alex Ferenczy, McGill University, Montreal, Quebec.) *B*, Histopathology of condyloma acuminatum showing acanthosis, hyperkeratosis, and cytoplasmic vacuolation (koilocytosis, *center*).

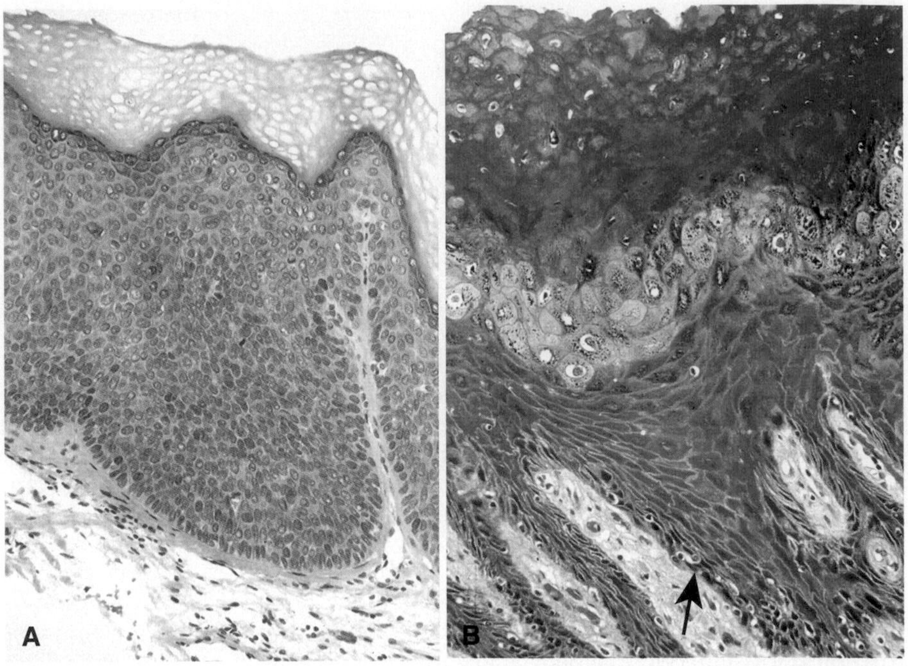

FIGURE 22–9 *A*, Histopathology of classic (HPV positive) vulvar intraepithelial neoplasia with diffuse cellular atypia, nuclear crowding, and increased mitotic index. *B*, differentiated (HPV negative) VIN, showing maturation, hyperkeratosis and basal cell atypia (*arrow*).

The second group of squamous cell carcinomas is associated with squamous cell hyperplasia and lichen sclerosus. The etiology of this group of carcinomas is unclear, and they are not typically associated with HPV. In one scenario, genetic alterations arise in lichen sclerosus or hyperplasia, leading directly to invasion, or by an intermediate step in which atypia develops within hyperplasia or lichen sclerosus, leading to an unusual form of VIN termed differentiated (simplex) VIN (Fig. 22–9*B*).[26,27] These tumors have also been associated with increased accumulation of p53 protein.[27] (Mutations of the *p53* gene increase its half-life and hence it is possible to detect the mutant p53 protein readily by immunohistochemistry.) A variety of chromosome abnormalities are linked to invasive vulvar cancer, some of which may be specific for HPV-positive tumors.[28]

Morphology. HPV-associated vulvar squamous cell carcinomas begin as classic VIN lesions, which present as discrete flesh-colored or pigmented, slightly raised lesions that may be hyperkeratotic. Coexisting carcinomas may be exophytic or indurated, frequently with ulceration. Carcinomas associated with lichen sclerosus, lichen simplex chronicus, and differentiated VIN may develop quickly as nodules in a background of vulvar inflammation. The often subtle emergence of the latter may be misinterpreted as dermatitis, eczema, or leukoplakia for long periods. The clinical manifestations are chiefly non-specific, including local discomfort, itching, and exudation because of superficial secondary infection, and underscore the importance of repeated examination in women with vulvar inflammatory disorders.

On histologic examination, tumors associated with HPV or VIN frequently exhibit invasive growth patterns that mimic intraepithelial neoplasia. These "intraepithelial-like" patterns may be well differentiated (warty) or poorly differentiated (basaloid)[25,29] (Fig. 22–10*A*). HPV-negative tumors, which at times arise from lichen sclerosus or squamous hyperplasia, typically exhibit an invasive pattern with prominent keratinization (Fig. 22–10*B*).

Risk of cancer development in VIN is principally a function of age, extent of tumor, and immune status.[30,31] Once invasive cancer develops, metastatic spread is linked to the size of tumor, depth of invasion, and involvement of lymphatic vessels. The inguinal, pelvic, iliac, and periaortic lymph nodes are most commonly involved. Ultimately, lymphohematogenous dissemination involves the lungs, liver, and other internal organs. Patients with lesions less than 2 cm in diameter have a 60% to 80% 5-year survival rate after treatment with one-stage vulvectomy and lymphadenectomy; larger lesions with lymph node involvement yield a less than 10% 5-year survival rate.

Rare variants of squamous cell carcinoma include *verrucous carcinomas*, which are fungating tumors resembling condyloma acuminatum, and *basal cell carcinomas*, which are identical to their counterparts on the skin (Fig. 22–11). Neither tumor is associated with papillomaviruses. Both tumors rarely metastasize and can usually be cured by wide excision.[32,33]

Extramammary Paget Disease

This curious and rare lesion of the vulva, and sometimes the perianal region, is similar in its skin manifestations to Paget disease of the breast[24] (Chapter 23). As a vulvar neoplasm, it manifests as a pruritic, red, crusted, sharply demarcated, maplike area, occurring usually on the labia majora. It may be accompanied by a palpable submucosal thickening or tumor.

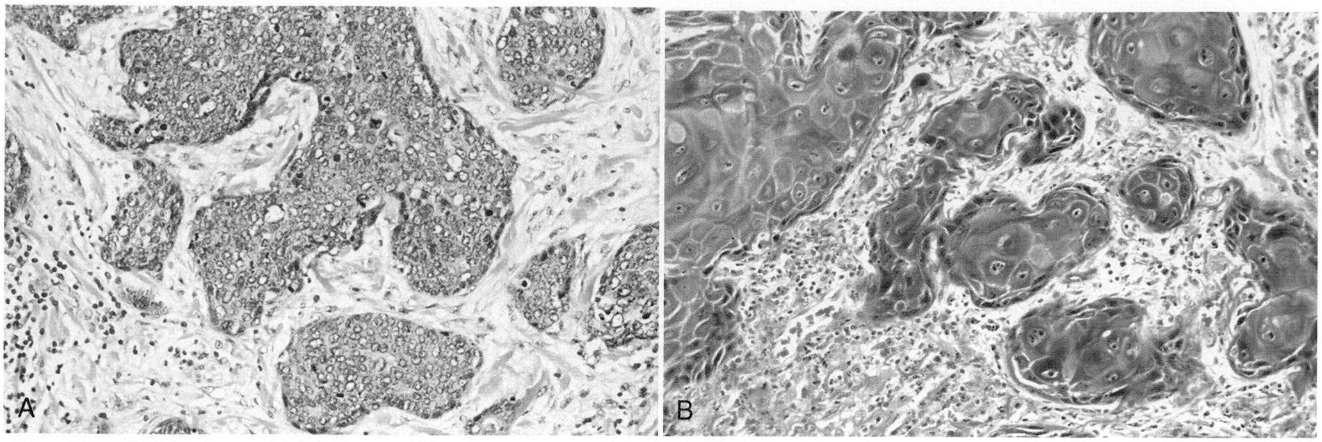

FIGURE 22–10 *A,* Poorly differentiated vulvar carcinoma associated with human papillomaviruses (HPV). *B,* Well-differentiated keratinizing vulvar carcinoma, typically HPV negative.

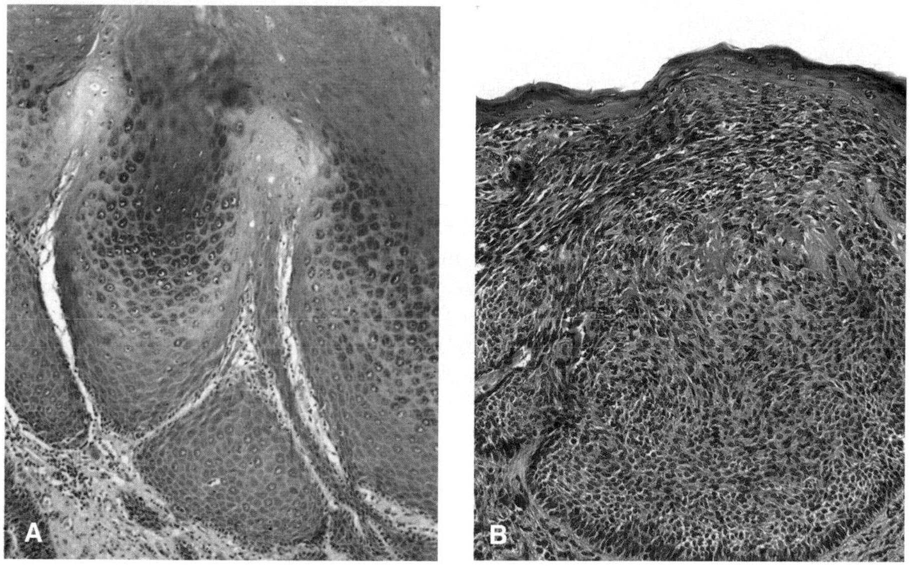

FIGURE 22–11 *A,* Verrucous carcinoma of the vulva. *B,* Basal cell carcinoma of the vulva.

Morphology. The diagnostic microscopic feature of this lesion is the presence of large tumor cells lying singly or in small clusters within the epidermis and its appendages. These cells are distinguished by a clear separation ("halo") from the surrounding epithelial cells (Fig. 22–12) and a finely granular cytoplasm containing mucopolysaccharide that stains with periodic acid-Schiff, Alcian blue or mucicarmine. Ultrastructurally, Paget cells display apocrine, eccrine, and keratinocyte differentiation and presumably arise from primitive epithelial progenitor cells.

In contrast to Paget disease of the nipple, in which 100% of patients show an underlying ductal breast carcinoma, vulvar lesions are most frequently confined to the epidermis of the skin and adjacent hair follicles and sweat glands. The prognosis of Paget disease is poor in the uncommon cases with associated carcinoma, but intraepidermal Paget disease may persist for many years, even decades, without the development of invasion. However, because Paget cells may extend beyond the confines of the grossly visible lesion, often into skin appendages, they are prone to recurrence.

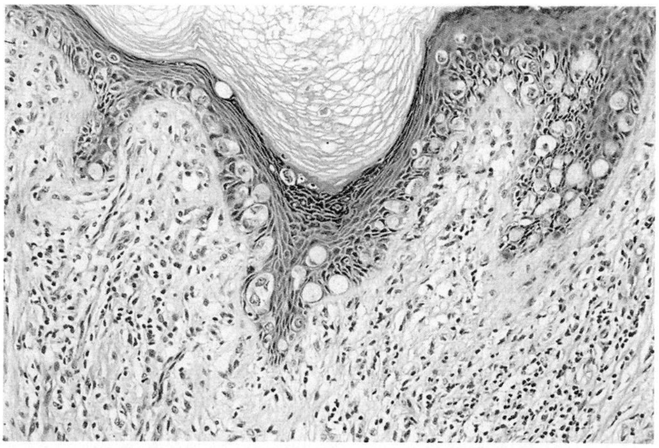

FIGURE 22–12 Paget disease of the vulva with a cluster of large clear tumor cells within the squamous epithelium.

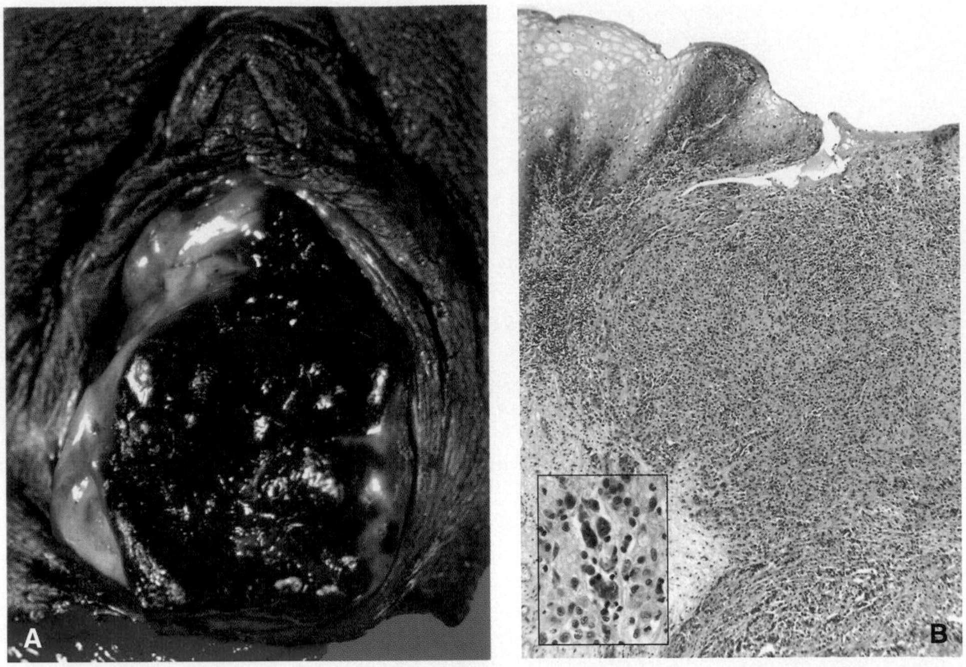

FIGURE 22–13 *A,* Malignant melanoma involving the vaginal introitus and labia minora. *B,* Histology of invasive melanoma with melanin production (*inset*).

Malignant Melanoma

Melanomas of the vulva are rare, representing less than 5% of all vulvar cancers and 2% of all melanomas in women. Their peak incidence is in the sixth or seventh decade; they tend to have the same biologic and histologic characteristics as melanomas occurring elsewhere and are capable of widespread metastatic dissemination (Fig. 22–13). The 5-year survival rate is less than 32%, presumably owing to delays in detection and the fact that the majority of these tumors rapidly enter a vertical growth phase following inception (Chapter 25). Prognosis is linked principally to depth of invasion, with greater than 60% mortality for lesions invading deeper than 1 mm.[34] Because it is initially confined to the epithelium, melanoma may resemble Paget disease, both grossly and histologically. It can usually be differentiated by its uniform reactivity with antibodies to S100 protein, absence of reactivity with antibodies to carcinoembryonic antigen, and lack of mucopolysaccharides, both of which are present in Paget disease.

VAGINA

The vagina is a portion of the female genital tract that is remarkably free from primary disease. In the adult, inflammations often affect the vulva and perivulvar structures and spread to the cervix without significant involvement of the vagina. The major serious primary lesion of this structure is the uncommon primary carcinoma. The remaining entities can therefore be cited briefly.

Congenital Anomalies

Atresia and total absence of the vagina are both extremely uncommon. The latter usually occurs only when there are severe malformations of the entire genital tract. Septate, or double, vagina is also an uncommon anomaly that arises from failure of total fusion of the müllerian ducts and accompanies double uterus (uterus didelphys). These and other anomalies of the external genitalia, including genital hypoplasia, may be the manifestations of genetic syndromes or other disturbances associated with abnormalities in reciprocal epithelial-stromal signaling during fetal development.[4,35]

Gartner duct cysts are relatively common lesions found along the lateral walls of the vagina and derived from wolffian duct rests. They are 1- to 2-cm fluid-filled cysts that occur submucosally. Other cysts include mucous cysts, which occur in the proximal vagina, are derived from müllerian epithelium, and often contain squamous metaplasia. Another müllerian-derived lesion (endometriosis, described later) may occur in the vagina and simulate a neoplasm.

Premalignant and Malignant Neoplasms

Most benign tumors of the vagina occur in reproductive-age women and are skeletal muscle tumors (rhabdomyomas) or stromal tumors (stromal polyps). The latter may exhibit cellular atypia but are benign, localized, and self-limited. Others include benign leiomyomas, hemangiomas, and rare mixed tumors.[36] Clinically important malignant tumors in terms of frequency and biologic behavior are carcinoma and embryonal rhabdomyosarcoma (sarcoma botryoides).

VAGINAL INTRAEPITHELIAL NEOPLASIA AND SQUAMOUS CELL CARCINOMA

Primary carcinoma of the vagina is an extremely uncommon cancer (about 0.6 per 100,000 women yearly) accounting for about 1% of malignant neoplasms in the female genital tract, and of these, 95% are squamous cell carcinomas. Most are associated with HPV. The greatest risk factor is a previous carcinoma of the cervix or vulva; 1% to 2% of patients with an invasive cervical carcinoma eventually develop a vaginal squamous carcinoma.

Morphology. Most often, the tumor affects the upper posterior vagina, particularly along the posterior wall at the junction with the ectocervix. It begins as a focus of epithelial thickening, often in association with dysplastic changes, progressing to a plaquelike mass that extends centrifugally and invades, by direct continuity, the cervix and perivaginal structures. The lesions in the lower two-thirds metastasize to the inguinal nodes, whereas upper lesions tend to involve the regional iliac nodes.

These tumors first come to the patient's attention by the appearance of irregular spotting or the development of a frank vaginal discharge (leukorrhea). At other times, they remain totally silent and become clinically manifest only with the onset of urinary or rectal fistulas.

ADENOCARCINOMA

Adenocarcinomas are rare but have received attention because of the increased frequency of clear cell adenocarcinomas in young women whose mothers had been treated with diethylstilbestrol (DES) during pregnancy (for a threatened abortion).[37] Fortunately, less than 0.14% of such DES-exposed young women develop adenocarcinoma.

Morphology. The tumors are most often located on the anterior wall of the vagina, usually in the upper third, and vary in size from 0.2 to 10 cm in greatest diameter. They are usually discovered between the ages of 15 and 20 years and are often composed of vacuolated, glycogen-containing cells, hence the term clear cell carcinoma (Fig. 22–14). These cancers can also arise in the cervix. A probable precursor of the tumor is **vaginal adenosis**, a condition in which glandular columnar epithelium of müllerian type either appears beneath the squamous epithelium or replaces it.[38] Adenosis presents clinically as red, granular foci contrasting with the normal pale pink, opaque vaginal mucosa. On microscopic examination, the glandular epithelium may be either mucus secreting, resembling endocervical mucosa, or so-called tuboendometrial, often containing cilia. Adenosis has been reported in 35% to 90% of the offspring of estrogen-treated mothers, but as mentioned earlier, malignant transformation is extremely rare.

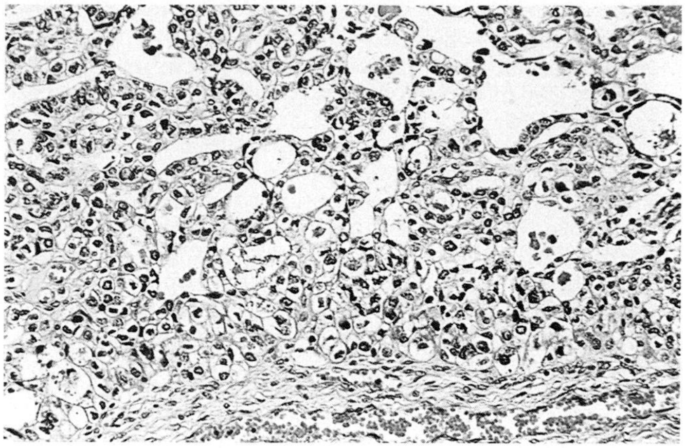

FIGURE 22–14 Clear cell adenocarcinoma of the vagina showing vacuolated tumor cells in clusters and glandlike structures.

Because of its insidious, invasive growth, vaginal cancer (squamous and adenocarcinomatous) is difficult to cure. Thus, early detection by careful follow-up is mandatory in DES-exposed women. Surgery and irradiation have successfully eradicated DES-related tumors in up to 80% of patients. Extension of cervical carcinoma to the vagina is much more common than are primary malignant neoplasms of the vagina. Accordingly, before a diagnosis of primary vaginal carcinoma can be made, a preexisting cervical lesion must be ruled out.

EMBRYONAL RHABDOMYOSARCOMA

Also called *sarcoma botryoides*, this is an interesting but uncommon vaginal tumor most frequently found in infants and in children younger than 5 years of age. The tumor consists predominantly of malignant embryonal rhabdomyoblasts and is thus a type of rhabdomyosarcoma.[39]

Morphology These tumors tend to grow as polypoid, rounded, bulky masses that sometimes fill and project out of the vagina; they have the appearance and consistency of grapelike clusters (hence the designation botryoides, meaning grapelike) (Fig. 22–15). On histologic examination, the tumor cells are small and have oval nuclei, with small protrusions of cytoplasm from one end, so they resemble a tennis racket. Rarely, striations can be seen within the cytoplasm. Beneath the vaginal epithelium, the tumor cells are crowded in a so-called cambium layer; but in the deep regions, they lie within a loose fibromyxomatous stroma that is edematous and may contain many inflammatory cells. For this reason, the lesions can be mistaken for benign inflammatory polyps, leading to unfortunate delays in diagnosis and treatment. These tumors tend to invade locally and cause death by penetration into the peritoneal cavity or by obstruction of the urinary tract.

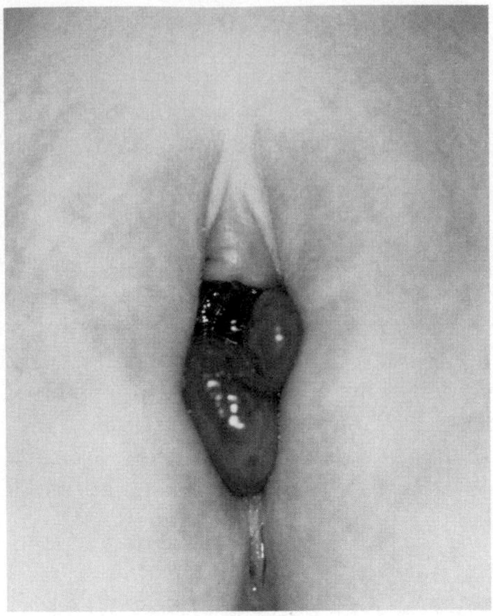

FIGURE 22–15 Sarcoma botryoides (embryonal rhabdomyosarcoma) of the vagina appearing as a polypoid mass protruding from the vagina. (Courtesy of Dr. Michael Donovan, Children's Hospital, Boston, MA.)

Conservative surgery, coupled with chemotherapy, appears to offer the best results in cases diagnosed sufficiently early.[40]

CERVIX

The cervix is both a sentinel for potentially serious upper genital tract infections and a target for viral and other carcinogens, which may lead to invasive carcinoma. Infection constitutes one of the most common clinical complaints in gynecologic practice and frequently vexes both patient and clinician. The potential threat of cancer, however, is central to Papanicolaou smear screening programs and histologic interpretation of biopsy specimens by the pathologist. Worldwide, cervical carcinoma alone is responsible for about 5% of all cancer deaths in women.

Inflammations

ACUTE AND CHRONIC CERVICITIS

At the onset of menarche, the production of estrogens by the ovary stimulates maturation (glycogen uptake) of cervical and vaginal squamous mucosa. As these cells are shed, the glycogen provides a substrate for endogenous vaginal aerobes and anaerobes, streptococci, enterococci, *Escherichia coli*, and staphylococci. The bacterial growth produces a drop in vaginal pH. The exposed endocervix is sensitive to these changes in chemical environment and bacterial flora and responds by undergoing a variety of changes including proliferation of reserve cells leading to squamous metaplasia. This process of transformation from a columnar to a squamous lining is also hastened by trauma and other infections occurring in the reproductive years. As the squamous epithelium overgrows and obliterates the surface columnar papillae, it covers and obstructs crypt openings, with the accumulation of mucus in deeper crypts (glands) to form mucous (nabothian) cysts. This process is invariably associated with an inflammatory infiltrate composed of a mixture of polymorphonuclear leukocytes and mononuclear cells, and if the inflammation is severe, it may be associated with loss of the epithelial lining (erosion or ulceration) and epithelial repair (reparative atypia or anaplasia of repair). All of these components characterize what is known as *chronic cervicitis* (Fig. 22–16).

Some degree of cervical inflammation may be found in virtually all multiparous and in many nulliparous adult women, and it is usually of little clinical consequence. Principal concerns include the potential presence of organisms, which may be clinically important. Specific infections by gonococci, chlamydiae, mycoplasmas, and herpes simplex virus (mostly type 2) may produce significant acute or chronic cervicitis and should be identified for their relevance to upper genital tract disease, pregnancy complications, or sexual transmission.

Morphology. The pathologic correlates of acute and chronic cervicitis include epithelial spongiosis (intercellular edema), submucosal edema, and a combination of epithelial and stromal changes. Acute cervicitis is characterized by acute inflammatory cells,

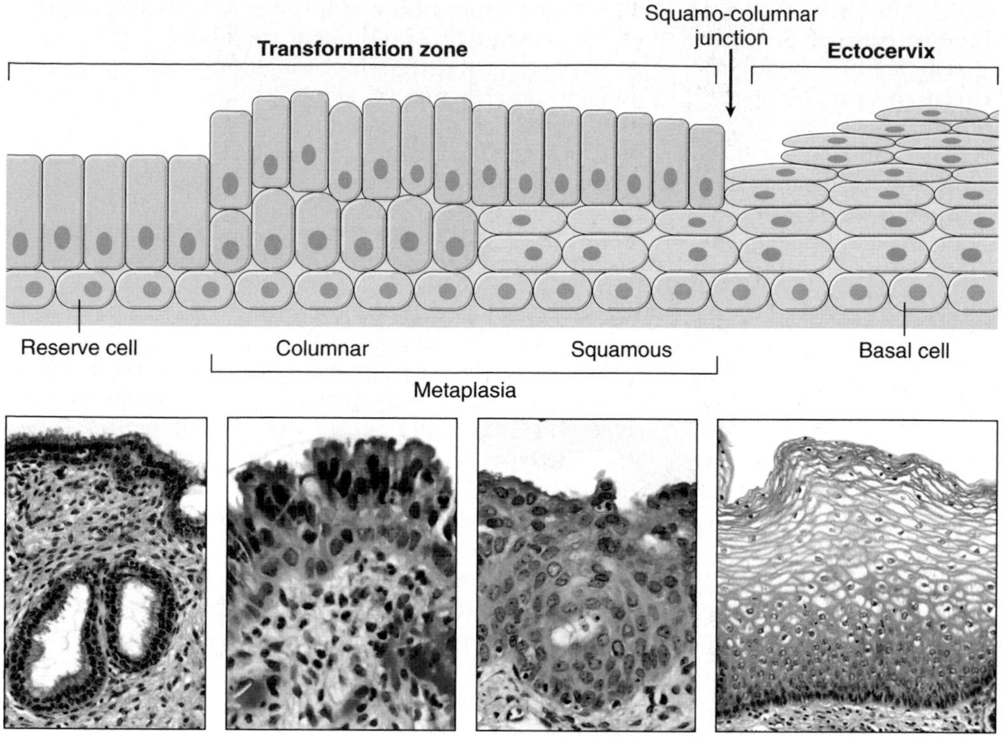

FIGURE 22–16 In the diagram (*upper*), reserve cells in the transformation zone are continuous with the basal cells of the ectocervix (*right*) and may undergo columnar and squamous differentiation (metaplasia). Photomicrographs at bottom depict (*from left to right*) quiescent subcolumnar reserve cells, reserve cells undergoing columnar differentiation (*second from left*), reserve cells undergoing squamous metaplasia (*second from right*) and ectocervical squamous epithelium (*right*).

erosion, and reactive or reparative epithelial change. Chronic cervicitis includes inflammation, usually mononuclear, with lymphocytes, macrophages, and plasma cells. Necrosis and granulation tissue may also be present. Although the inflammation alone is not specific, some patterns are associated with certain organisms. HSV is most strongly associated with epithelial ulcers (often with intranuclear inclusions in epithelial cells) and a lymphocytic infiltrate, and *C. trachomatis* with lymphoid germinal centers and a prominent plasmacytic infiltrate.[41] Epithelial spongiosis is associated with *T. vaginalis* infection.[42]

All the aforementioned changes are more pronounced in patients with clinical symptoms (mucopurulent cervicitis) or in whom specific organisms can be identified. These changes, however, may be observed in culture-negative or asymptomatic women, underscoring the importance of combined culture, clinical evaluation, and Papanicolaou smear examination. Severe reparative changes may shed atypical-appearing squamous cells that mimic precancerous lesions, because cells undergoing repair are depleted of their normal content of glycogen and may have nuclear atypia.

ENDOCERVICAL POLYPS

Endocervical polyps are relatively innocuous, inflammatory tumors that occur in 2% to 5% of adult women. Perhaps the major significance of polyps lies in their production of irregular vaginal "spotting" or bleeding that arouses suspicion of some more ominous lesion. Most polyps arise within the endocervical canal and vary from small and sessile to large, 5-cm masses that may protrude through the cervical os. All are soft, almost mucoid, and are composed of a loose fibromyxomatous stroma harboring dilated, mucus-secreting endocervical glands, often accompanied by inflammation and squamous metaplasia (Fig. 22–17). In almost all instances, simple curettage or surgical excision effects a cure.

Intraepithelial and Invasive Squamous Neoplasia

No form of cancer better documents the remarkable effects of prevention, early diagnosis, and curative therapy on the mortality rate than does cancer of the cervix. Fifty years ago, carcinoma of the cervix was the leading cause of cancer deaths in women in the United States, but the death rate has declined by two-thirds to its present rank as the eighth leading cause of cancer mortality. Cancer of the cervix causes about 4500 deaths annually (behind cancers of the lung, breast, colon,

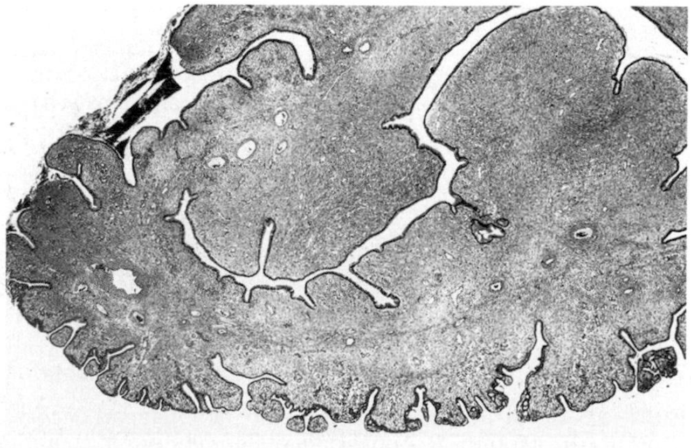

FIGURE 22–17 Endocervical polyp composed of a dense fibrous stroma covered with endocervical columnar epithelium.

pancreas, ovary, lymph nodes, and blood).[43] In sharp contrast to this reduced mortality, the detection frequency of early cancers and precancerous conditions is high. Much credit for these dramatic gains belongs to the effectiveness of the Papanicolaou cytologic test in detecting cervical precancers and to the accessibility of the cervix to colposcopy and biopsy. There are an estimated 13,000 new cases of invasive cancer annually and nearly 1 million precancerous conditions (squamous intraepithelial lesions) of varying grade. Thus, it is evident that Papanicolaou smear screening has increased the detection of potentially curable cancers and the detection and eradication of preinvasive lesions, some of which would progress to cancer if not discovered.

Pathogenesis. To understand the pathogenesis of cervical cancer, it is important to know the factors involved in its development, which have been identified from a series of clinical, epidemiologic, pathologic, and molecular studies. Epidemiologic data have long implicated a sexually transmitted agent, which is now established to be the human papillomavirus. HPV is currently considered to be the most important agent in cervical oncogenesis. As noted earlier, this virus is the known cause of the sexually transmitted vulvar condyloma acuminatum and has been isolated from vulvar and vaginal squamous cell carcinomas; it is also suspected of being an oncogenic agent in a variety of other squamous tumors or proliferative lesions of skin and mucous membranes, as detailed in Chapter 7.[43]

A wealth of molecular epidemiologic data has established the following risk factors for cervical neoplasia, all of which indicate a complex interaction between host and virus.[43,44]

- Early age at first intercourse
- Multiple sexual partners
- Increased parity
- A male partner with multiple previous sexual partners
- The presence of a cancer-associated HPV
- The persistent detection of a high-risk HPV, particularly in high concentration (viral load)
- Certain HLA and viral subtypes
- Exposure to oral contraceptives and nicotine
- Genital infections (chlamydia)

There is mounting molecular evidence linking HPV to cancer in general and cervical cancer in particular.

1. HPV DNA is detected by hybridization techniques in over 95% of cervical cancers.[23]
2. Specific HPV types are associated with cervical cancer (high risk) versus condylomata (low risk); low (include types 6, 11, 42, 44, 53, 54, 62, and 66) and high-risk types (include types 16, 18, 31, 33, 35, 39, 45, 51, 52, 56, 58, 59, and 68) (Fig. 22–18*A*).[23]
3. Experimental data indicate that viral (*E6* and *E7*) genes of high risk HPVs can disrupt the cell cycle via binding to RB with up-regulation of Cyclin E (E7) and p16INK4; interrupt cell death pathways by binding to p53 (E6); induce centrosome duplication and genomic instability (E6, E7); and prevent replicative senescence by up-regulation of telomerase (E6) (Chapter 7).[45–48] HPV E6 induces rapid degradation of p53 via ubiquitin-dependent proteolysis, reducing p53 levels by two- to three-fold. E7 complexes with the hypophosphorylated (active) form of RB, promoting its proteolysis via the proteosome pathway. Because hypophosphorylated RB normally inhibits S-phase entry via binding to the E2F transcription factor, the two viral oncogenes cooperate to promote DNA synthesis while interrupting p53-mediated growth arrest and apoptosis of genetically altered cells. Thus, the viral oncogenes are criti-

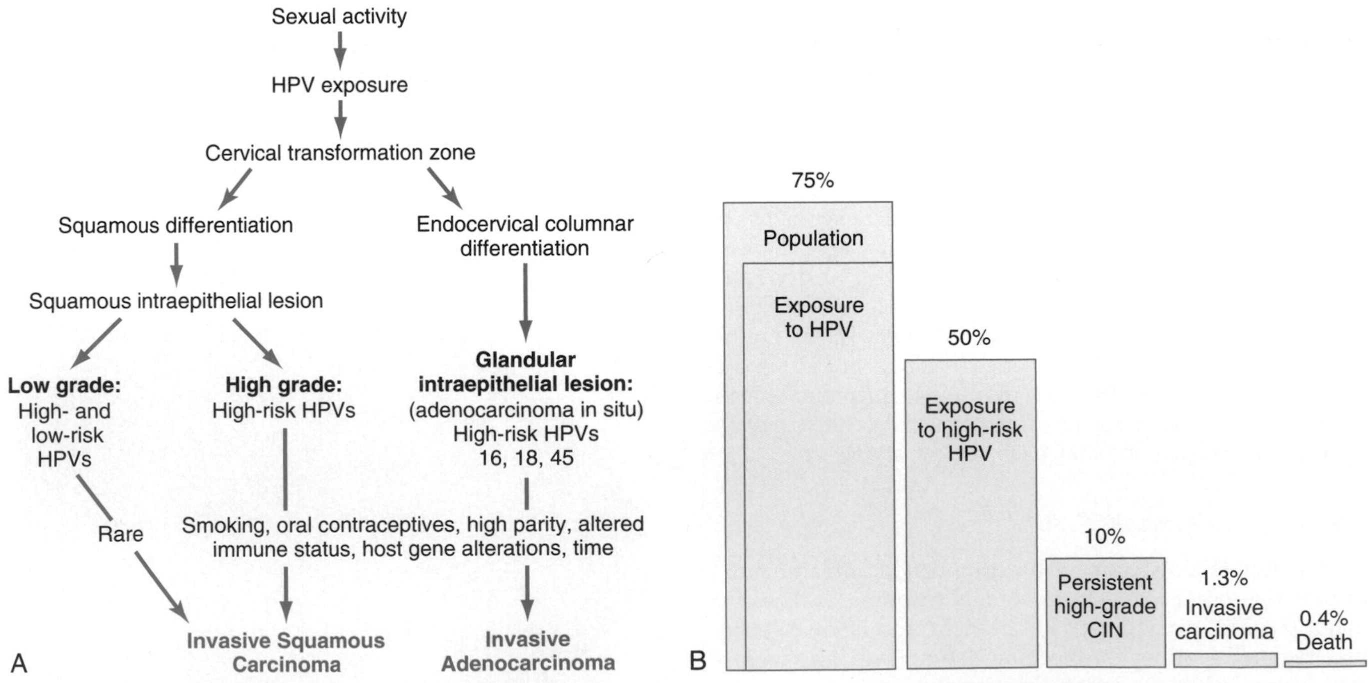

FIGURE 22–18 *A*, Postulated steps in the pathogenesis of cervical neoplasia. Conditions influencing progression are listed at the lower center of the diagram. *B*, Approximate lifetime risks of acquiring HPV infection (*left*) and dying of cervical cancer (*right*). The intermediate steps include risks of infection with high-risk HPV types, development of advanced cervical intraepithelial neoplasia (CIN), and progression to invasive carcinoma.

cal in extending the life span of genital epithelial cells—a necessary component of tumor development.[45]

4. The physical state of the virus differs in different lesions, being integrated into the host DNA in cancers, and present as free (episomal) viral DNA in condylomata and most precancerous lesions.[44]

5. Certain chromosome abnormalities, including deletions at 3p and amplifications of 3q, have been associated with cancers containing specific (HPV-16) papillomaviruses.[48,49]

6. Most compelling, recent data indicate that vaccines directed against papillomaviruses can prevent infection and the development of precancerous disorders.[50,51]

However, the evidence does not implicate HPV as the only factor. A high percentage of young women are infected with one or more HPV types during their reproductive years, and only a few develop cancer. Other cocarcinogens, the immune status of the individual, nutrition, and many other factors influence whether the HPV infection remains subclinical (latent), turns into a precancer, or eventually progresses to cancer. Figure 22–18 presents an attempt to explain the role of HPV in cervical carcinogenesis and its impact on the population in the United States.

CERVICAL INTRAEPITHELIAL NEOPLASIA

The reason that Papanicolaou smear screening is so effective in preventing cervical cancer is that the majority of cancers are preceded by a precancerous lesion. This lesion may exist in the noninvasive stage for as long as 20 years and shed abnormal cells that can be detected on cytologic examination.[52] These precancerous changes should be viewed with the following in mind: (1) they represent a continuum of morphologic change with indistinct boundaries; (2) they do not invariably progress to cancer and may spontaneously regress, with the risk of persistence or progression to cancer increasing with the severity of the precancerous change; (3) they are associated with papillomaviruses, and high-risk HPV types are found in increasing frequency in the higher-grade precursors.[53]

Cervical precancers have been classified in a variety of ways. The oldest is the *dysplasia/carcinoma in situ* system with mild dysplasia on one end and severe dysplasia/carcinoma in situ on the other. Another is the *cervical intraepithelial neoplasia* (CIN) classification, with mild dysplasias termed CIN grade I and carcinoma in situ lesions termed CIN III. Still another reduces these entities to two, terming them *low-grade and high-grade intraepithelial lesions*.[53] Because these systems describe noninvasive lesions of indeterminate biology that are usually easily treated, none of these classifications is indispensable to clinical management or immune to revision. In this chapter, we refer to lesions by the CIN terminology.[54]

Morphology. Figures 22–19 and 22–20 illustrate a spectrum of morphologic alterations that range from normal to the highest-grade precancer, and the host cell genes involved in this process.

On the extreme low end of the spectrum are lesions that are often indistinguishable histologically from condylomata acuminata and may be either raised (acuminatum) or macular (flat condyloma) in appearance (Figs. 22–19 and 22–20*A*). These lesions typically exhibit nuclear enlargement and hyperchromasia in the superficial epithelial cells, signifying the effects of active viral replication in the maturing cells (viral cytopathic effect). The nuclear changes may be accompanied by cytoplasmic halos (koilocytotic atypia) with few alterations in the lower epithelial cells. Such changes fall within the range of CIN I. CIN I often contains abundant papillomavirus nucleic acids (Fig. 22–20*B*). Raised lesions (acuminatum) often contain low-risk HPVs. Flat CIN usually contain high-risk HPVs. However, they have a low rate of progression to cancer, underscoring the fact that the sequence of molecular events required for lesion progression often does not transpire or is interrupted by the host immune system.

The next change in the spectrum consists of the appearance of atypical cells in the lower layers of the

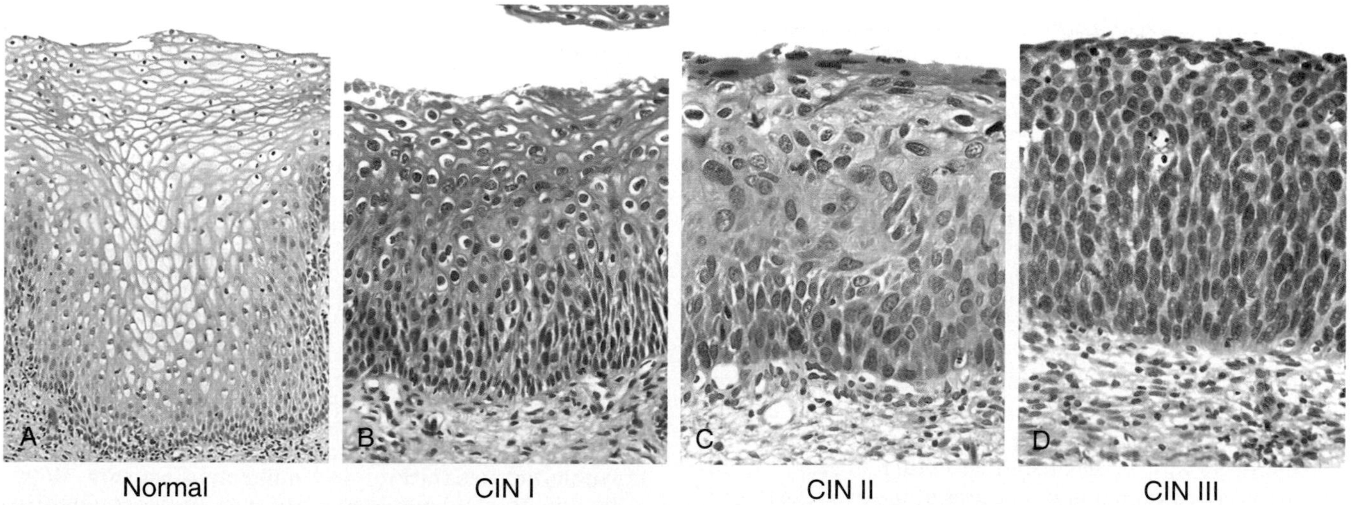

FIGURE 22–19 Spectrum of cervical intraepithelial neoplasia: normal squamous epithelium for comparison; CIN I with koilocytotic atypia; CIN II with progressive atypia in all layers of the epithelium; CIN III (carcinoma in situ) with diffuse atypia and loss of maturation.

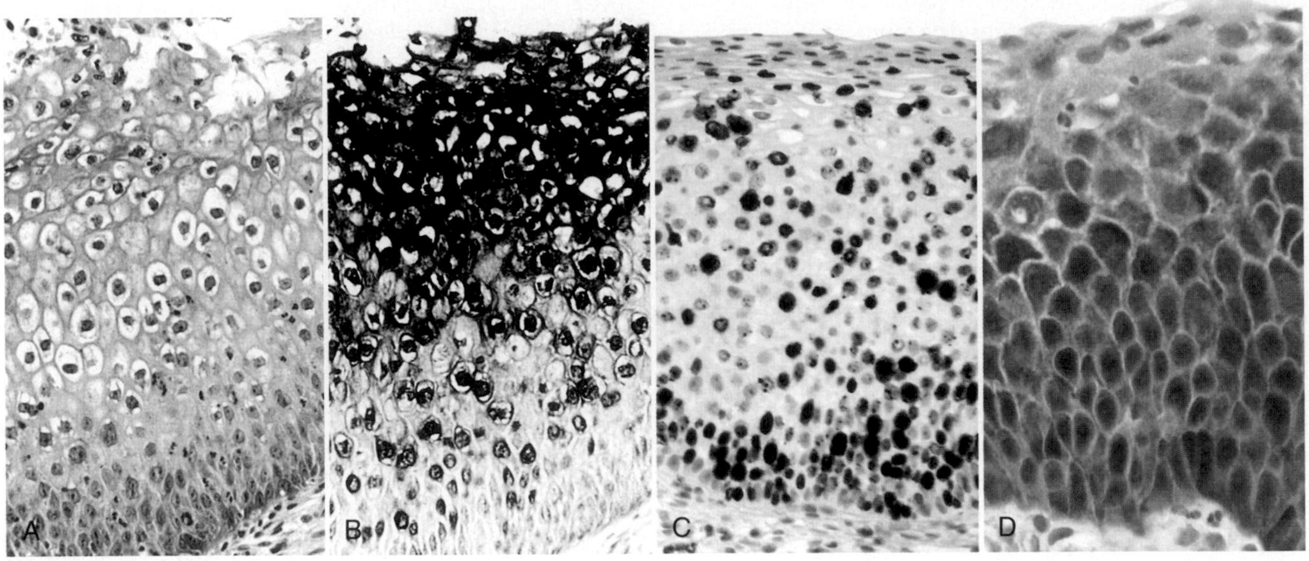

FIGURE 22–20 *A*, Histology of CIN I (flat condyloma), illustrating the prominent koilocytotic atypia in the upper epithelial cells, as evidenced by the prominent perinuclear halos. *B*, Nucleic acid in situ hybridization of the same lesion for HPV nucleic acids. The blue staining denotes HPV DNA, which is typically most abundant in the koilocytes. *C*, Diffuse immunostaining of CIN II for Ki-67, illustrating widespread deregulation of cell cycle controls. *D*, Up-regulation of p16INK4 (seen as intense immunostaining) characterizes high-risk HPV infections.

squamous epithelium but nonetheless with persistent (but abnormal) differentiation toward the prickle and keratinizing cell layers. The atypical cells show changes in nucleo-cytoplasmic ratio; variation in nuclear size; loss of polarity; increased mitotic figures, including abnormal mitoses; and hyperchromasia—in other words, they take on some of the characteristics of malignant cells. These lesions fall within the range of CIN II (see Fig. 22–19). These features have been associated with aneuploid cell populations and correlate strongly with high-risk HPV types. Presumably they reflect early changes in the replicating (basal/parabasal) cell population associated with the effects of the E6/E7 oncogenes on cell cycle and genomic stability. These include cell cycle disregulation and up-regulation of *p16INK4*[55] (Fig. 22–20*C* and *D*). Increased expression of *p16*, a cyclin-dependent kinase inhibitor, is possibly a compensatory response to cell disturbances brought on by the viral oncogenes. As the lesion evolves, there is progressive loss of differentiation accompanied by greater atypia in more layers of the epithelium, until it is totally replaced by immature atypical cells, exhibiting no surface differentiation (CIN III) (Fig. 22–19).[54] The cellular changes on Papanicolaou smear that correspond to this histologic spectrum are illustrated in Figure 22–21.

Although often illustrated as a simple progression from CIN I to cancer, the spectrum of precursor lesions is quite complex owing to its origins in a site (transformation zone) that supports a wide range of epithelial differentiation, including squamous, columnar and mixtures of the two. The lowest-grade CIN lesions, including condylomata, most likely do not progress, whereas lesions containing greater degrees of cellular atypia are at greater risk. *Not all lesions begin as condylomata or as CIN I, and they may enter at any point in the sequence*, depending on the associated HPV type and other host factors, including the type of cell (mature squamous, immature metaplastic, columnar, etc.) infected by the virus.[3] The rates of progression are by no means uniform, and although HPV type is a potential predictor of lesion behavior, it is difficult to predict the outcome in an individual patient. These findings underscore that *risk of cancer is conferred only in part by HPV type* and may depend on both host–virus interactions and environmental factors to bring about the evolution of a precancer. Predictably, lesions that have completely evolved (CIN III) constitute the greatest cancer risk. CIN III is most frequently associated with invasive cancer when the latter is identified. Progression to invasive carcinoma, when it occurs, may develop in a few months to more than 20 years.[56]

SQUAMOUS CELL CARCINOMA

Squamous cell carcinoma may occur at any age from the second decade of life to senility. The peak incidence is occurring at an increasingly younger age: 40 to 45 years for invasive cancer and about 30 years for high-grade precancers. This represents the combination of earlier onset of sexual activity (i.e., earlier acquisition of HPV infection) and active Papanicolaou smear screening programs in the United States, which detect either cancers or precancerous lesions at an earlier point in life.

Morphology. Invasive cervical carcinoma manifests in three somewhat distinctive patterns: **fungating (or exophytic), ulcerating, and infiltrative cancers**. With the advent of widespread screening, many squamous cell carcinomas are detected at a subclinical stage, often during evaluation of an abnormal Papanicolaou

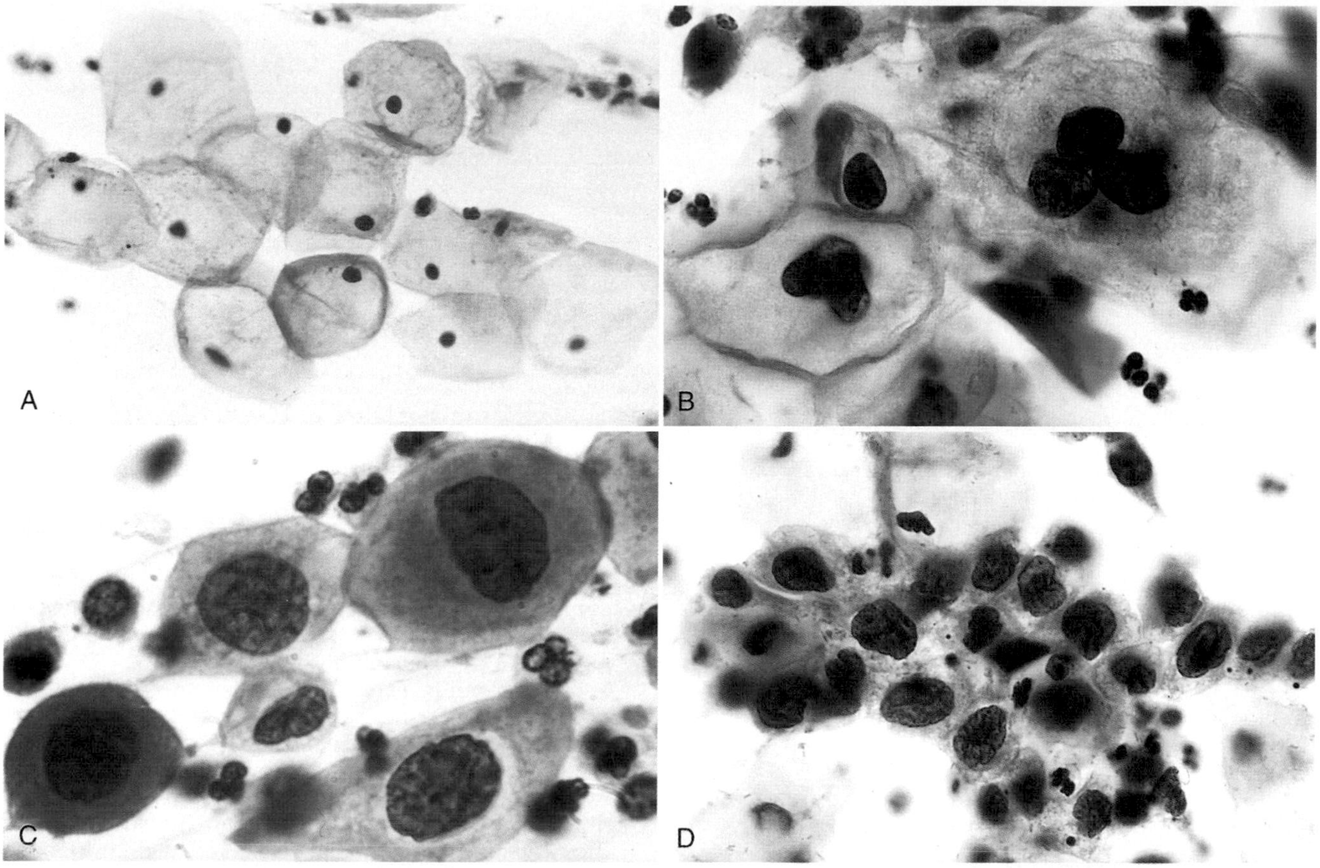

FIGURE 22–21 The cytology of cervical intraepithelial neoplasia as seen on the Papanicolaou smear. Cytoplasmic staining in superficial cells (*A*&*B*) may be either red or blue. *A*, Normal exfoliated superficial squamous epithelial cells. *B*, CIN I. *C*, CIN II. *D*, CIN III. Note the reduction in cytoplasm and the increase in the nucleus to cytoplasm ratio, which occurs as the grade of the lesion increases. This reflects the progressive loss of cellular differentiation on the surface of the lesions from which these cells are exfoliated (see Figure 22–19). (Courtesy of Dr. Edmund S. Cibas, Brigham and Women's Hospital, Boston, MA.)

smear. When obvious to the naked eye, the most common variant is the fungating tumor, which produces an obviously neoplastic mass that projects above the surrounding mucosa (Fig. 22–22*A*). Advanced cervical carcinoma extends by direct spread to involve every contiguous structure, including the peritoneum, urinary bladder, ureters, rectum, and vagina. Local and distant lymph nodes are also involved. Distant metastasis occurs to the liver, lungs, bone marrow, and other structures.

On histologic examination, about 95% of squamous carcinomas are composed of relatively large cells, either keratinizing (well-differentiated) or nonkeratinizing (moderately differentiated) patterns. A small subset of tumors (less than 5%) are poorly differentiated small cell squamous or, more rarely, small cell undifferentiated carcinomas (neuroendocrine or oat cell carcinomas) (Fig. 22–23). The latter closely resemble oat cell carcinomas of the lung and have an unusually poor prognosis owing to early spread by lymphatics and systemic spread. These tumors are also frequently associated with a specific high-risk HPV, type 18.[57]

Cervical cancer is staged as follows:

Stage 0. Carcinoma in situ (CIN III)
Stage I. Carcinoma confined to the cervix
Ia. Preclinical carcinoma, that is, diagnosed only by microscopy
Ia1. Stromal invasion no greater than 3 mm and no wider than 7 mm (so-called **microinvasive carcinoma**) (Fig. 22–22*B*).
Ia2. Maximum depth of invasion of stroma greater than 3 mm and no greater than 5 mm taken from base of epithelium, either surface or glandular, from which it originates; horizontal invasion not more than 7 mm
Ib. Histologically invasive carcinoma confined to the cervix and greater than stage Ia2
Stage II. Carcinoma extends beyond the cervix but not onto the pelvic wall. Carcinoma involves the vagina but not the lower third.
Stage III. Carcinoma has extended onto pelvic wall. On rectal examination, there is no cancer-free space between the tumor and the pelvic wall. The tumor involves the lower third of the vagina.
Stage IV. Carcinoma has extended beyond the true pelvis or has involved the mucosa of the bladder or rectum. This stage obviously includes those with metastatic dissemination.

Ten per cent to 25% of cervical carcinomas are **adenocarcinomas, adenosquamous carcinomas,**

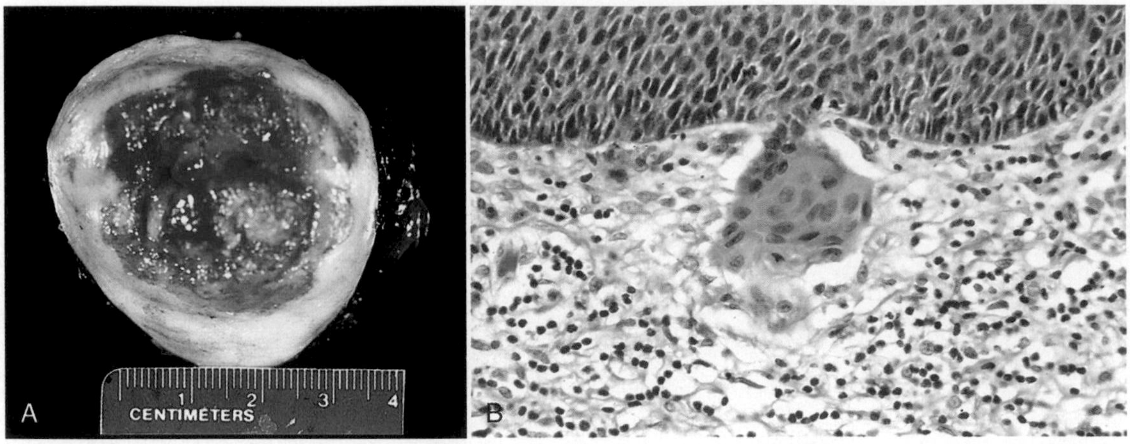

FIGURE 22–22 The spectrum of invasive cervical cancer. *A*, Carcinoma of the cervix, well advanced. *B*, Early stromal invasion occurring in a cervical intraepithelial neoplasm.

undifferentiated carcinomas, or other rare histologic types. The adenocarcinomas presumably arise in the endocervical glands and are often preceded by an intraepithelial glandular neoplasm (precancer) termed adenocarcinoma in situ that is approximately one fifth as common as its squamous counterpart. Once invasion develops, adenocarcinomas appear grossly and behave like the squamous cell lesions, with the exception of association with HPV type 18.[58] The **adenosquamous carcinomas** have mixed glandular and squamous patterns and are thought to arise from the multipotent reserve cells in the basal layers of the endocervical epithelium. They tend to have a less favorable prognosis than does squamous cell carcinoma of similar stage. Clear cell adenocarcinomas of the cervix in DES-exposed women are similar to those occurring in the vagina, described earlier. Their relationship to papillomaviruses is uncertain.

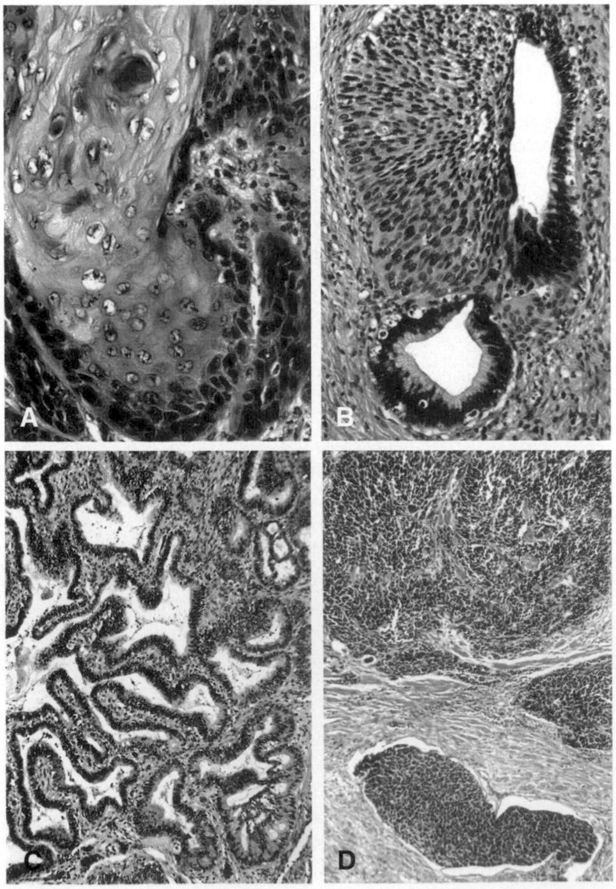

FIGURE 22–23 Morphology of cervical cancers. *A*, Squamous carcinoma. *B*, Adenocarcinoma in situ (*lower*), associated with CIN 3 (*upper*). *C*, Adenocarcinoma. *D*, Neuroendocrine carcinoma.

Clinical Course and Management. Cervical cancer prevention and control can be divided into several components. One includes cytologic screening and management of Papanicolaou smear abnormalities, both of which may entail the use of HPV testing. Another is the histologic diagnosis and removal of precancers. Still another component is surgical removal of invasive cancers, with adjunctive radiation and chemotherapy. A final aspect that is currently under investigation is the use of vaccines, either for preventing HPV infection or treating existing disease.

It is apparent from the preceding discussion that cancer of the cervix evolves slowly over many years. During this interval, the only sign of disease may be the shedding of abnormal cells from the cervix. Therefore, periodic Papanicolaou smears should be performed on all women after they become sexually active. Reduction in cervical cancer deaths would theoretically be greatest if all women were screened and if the accuracy of detecting Papanicolaou smear abnormalities was maximized. Once a cytologic abnormality is detected, management is predicated on whether the abnormality is clear-cut (CIN) or of uncertain significance (atypical cells). The former requires further examination by colposcopy. In the latter instance, HPV testing has been shown to aid in identifying which patients are amenable to yearly follow-up (HPV negatives, with a less than 1% risk of high-grade CIN) or merit colposcopy (HPV positives, with a 15% to 20% risk of high-grade CIN I).[59,60] At some point in the future, HPV testing may be used for primary screening of women over the age of 30.

However, the specificity of the test in the general population is low, and it needs to be used in conjunction with the Papanicolaou smear.[61]

Because most Papanicolaou smear abnormalities do not signify a serious precancerous or cancerous condition, treatment requires first that the abnormalities be visualized by colposcopic examination of the cervix. CIN lesions are characterized on colposcopic exam by white patches on the cervix after the application of acetic acid.[62] In addition, distinct vascular mosaic or punctuation patterns can be observed. Highly abnormal vascular patterns regularly accompany invasive cervical cancer. If abnormalities are visualized, they must be confirmed by histologic examination of a punch biopsy. This is facilitated by both the application of morphologic criteria and also, recently, the immunohistochemical identification of increased expression of host cell biomarkers (such as *p16INK4*, cyclin E, and Ki-67).[63] These markers are expressed in a greater proportion of cells in precancerous lesions (due to cell cycle disturbances) and will frequently distinguish these from non-neoplastic epithelial changes.

Once CIN is confirmed histologically, modes of treatment depend on the stage of the neoplasm; treatment of precursor lesions includes Papanicolaou smear follow-up for CIN I, and cryotherapy, laser, loop electrical excision procedures (LEEP), and cone biopsy for CIN II or CIN III. Rarely (approximately 1 in 500) a patient with a treated CIN III eventually develops an invasive cancer. The risk is minimized by follow-up pap smears. Although very early invasive cancers (microinvasive carcinomas) may be treated by cone biopsy alone, most invasive cancers are managed by hysterectomy with lymph node dissection and, for advanced lesions, radiation. The prognosis and survival for invasive carcinomas depend largely on the stage at which cancer is first discovered and to some degree on the cell type, with small cell neuroendocrine tumors having a poor prognosis. Approximately one half of cervical cancers develop in women who were not screened.

With current methods of treatment, there is a 5-year survival rate of at least 95% for stage IA (including microinvasive) carcinomas, about 80% to 90% with stage IB, 75% with stage II, and less than 50% for stage III and higher. Most patients with stage IV cancer die as a consequence of local extension of the tumor (e.g., into and about the urinary bladder and ureters, leading to ureteral obstruction, pyelonephritis, and uremia) rather than distant metastases. However, as mentioned above, early detection has reduced the number of patients with stage IV cancer by over two-thirds in the past 50 years.

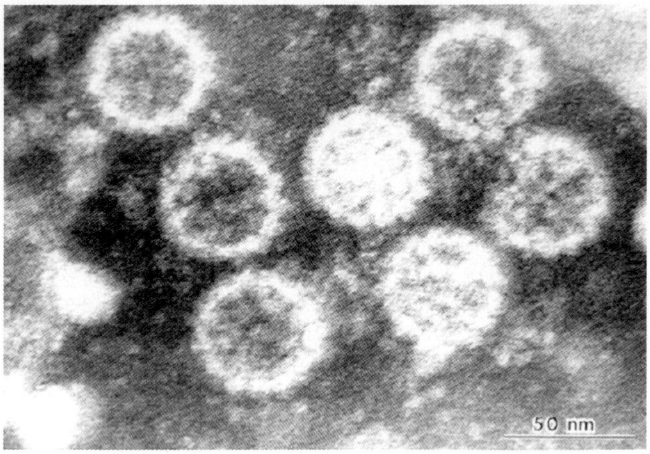

FIGURE 22–24 Electron micrograph of virus-like papillomavirus particles (VLPs) produced in eukaryotic cells by expression of the late region and used as vaccines. (Courtesy of Ian Frazer, MD, Princess Alexandra Hospital, University of Queensland, Australia.)

Beginning in 1991 a series of publications described the production in vitro of papillomavirus-like particles (VLPs) by transfecting eukaryotic cells with vector-driven HPV DNA (Fig. 22–24).[50] This discovery provided the unique opportunity to manipulate the viral genome to produce reagents that could be used to study—and ultimately generate—host immunity to HPVs. Studies have shown that vaccination with VLPs and similar reagents generates protective immunity in animals and strong host response in humans. Recent publications have shown that HPV vaccines may prevent cervical HPV infection and, by inference, cervical cancer.[51] Assuming vaccination trials against cervical papillomaviruses bear fruit, it is conceivable that the next 20 years will witness the beginning of a significant and sustained reduction in not only cervical cancer incidence but also of other papillomavirus-related diseases in both men and women.

BODY OF UTERUS AND ENDOMETRIUM

The uterus is composed principally of smooth muscle (myometrium), which encases the endometrial cavity. The latter is composed of a mucosa made up of endometrial glands and surrounding stroma. The uterus is stimulated continually by hormones, denuded monthly of its endometrial mucosa, and transiently inhabited by fetuses. It is subject to a variety of disorders, the most common of which result from endocrine imbalances, complications of pregnancy, and neoplastic proliferation. Together with the lesions that affect the cervix (causing abnormal pap smears), the lesions of the corpus of the uterus and the endometrium (causing abnormal vaginal bleeding) account for most patient visits to gynecologic practices.

Endometrial Histology in the Menstrual Cycle

"Dating" the endometrium by its histologic appearance is helpful clinically to assess hormonal status, document ovulation, and determine causes of endometrial bleeding and infertility. We can begin with the shedding of the upper half to two-thirds of the endometrium during the menstrual period (Fig. 22–25). The basal third does not respond to ovarian steroids and is retained at the conclusion of the menstrual flow. From the basal third of this preovulatory proliferative phase of the cycle, there is extremely rapid growth of both glands and stroma (*proliferative phase*). The glands are straight, tubular structures lined by regular, tall, pseudostratified columnar cells. Mitotic figures are numerous, and there is no evidence of mucus secretion or vacuolation (Fig. 22–26*A*). The endometrial stroma is composed of thickly compacted spindle cells that have scant cytoplasm but abundant mitotic activity.

At the time of ovulation, the endometrium slows in its growth, and it ceases apparent mitotic activity within days after ovulation. The postovulatory endometrium is initially marked by basal secretory vacuoles beneath the nuclei in the

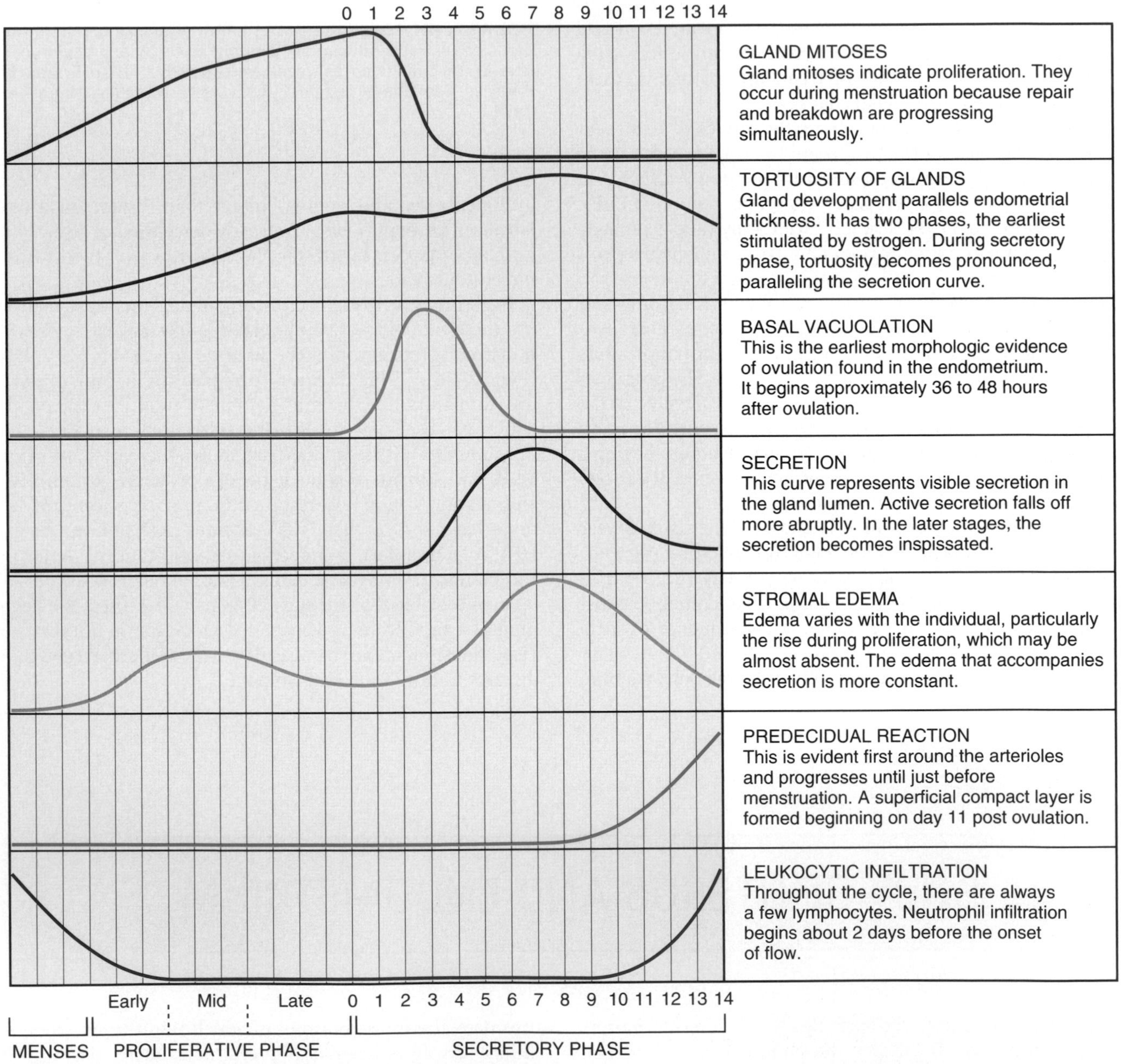
0 1 2 3 4 5 6 7 8 9 10 11 12 13 14
GLAND MITOSES
Gland mitoses indicate proliferation. They occur during menstruation because repair and breakdown are progressing simultaneously.
TORTUOSITY OF GLANDS
Gland development parallels endometrial thickness. It has two phases, the earliest stimulated by estrogen. During secretory phase, tortuosity becomes pronounced, paralleling the secretion curve.
BASAL VACUOLATION
This is the earliest morphologic evidence of ovulation found in the endometrium. It begins approximately 36 to 48 hours after ovulation.
SECRETION
This curve represents visible secretion in the gland lumen. Active secretion falls off more abruptly. In the later stages, the secretion becomes inspissated.
STROMAL EDEMA
Edema varies with the individual, particularly the rise during proliferation, which may be almost absent. The edema that accompanies secretion is more constant.
PREDECIDUAL REACTION
This is evident first around the arterioles and progresses until just before menstruation. A superficial compact layer is formed beginning on day 11 post ovulation.
LEUKOCYTIC INFILTRATION
Throughout the cycle, there are always a few lymphocytes. Neutrophil infiltration begins about 2 days before the onset of flow.
Early
Mid
Late
0 1 2 3 4 5 6 7 8 9 10 11 12 13 14
MENSES
PROLIFERATIVE PHASE
SECRETORY PHASE

FIGURE 22–25 Approximate quantitative changes in seven morphologic criteria found to be most useful in dating human endometrium. (Modified from Noyes RW: Normal phases of the endometrium. In Norris HJ, et al (eds): The Uterus. Baltimore, Williams & Wilkins, 1973.)

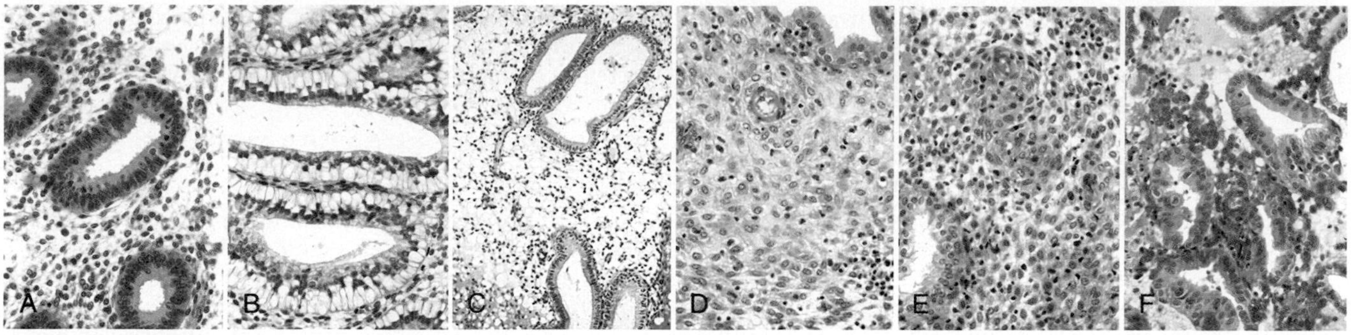

FIGURE 22–26 Histology of the menstrual cycle, including the proliferative phase with mitoses (*A*), the early secretory phase with subnuclear vacuoles (*B*) followed by secretory exhaustion (*C*), predecidual changes (*D*), stromal granulocytes (*E*), and stromal breakdown at the onset of menses (*F*) (see text).

glandular epithelium (Fig. 22–26*B*). This *secretory activity* is most prominent during the third week of the menstrual cycle, when the basal vacuoles progressively push past the nuclei. By the fourth week, the secretions are discharged into the gland lumens. When secretion is maximal, between 18 and 24 days, the glands are dilated. By the fourth week, the glands are tortuous, producing a serrated appearance when they are cut in their long axis. This serrated or "saw-toothed" appearance is accentuated by secretory exhaustion and shrinking of the glands.

The stromal changes in late secretory phase are important for dating the endometrium and consist of the development of prominent spiral arterioles by days 21 to 22. A considerable increase in ground substance and edema between the stromal cells occurs (Fig. 22–26*C*) and is followed in days 23 to 24 by stromal cell hypertrophy with accumulation of cytoplasmic eosinophilia (predecidual change) and resurgence of stromal mitoses (Fig. 22–26*D*). Predecidual changes spread throughout the functionalis (the hormonally responsive upper zone) during days 24 to 28 and are accompanied by scattered neutrophils and occasional lymphocytes (Fig. 22–26*E*), which here do not imply inflammation. This is followed by disintegration of the functionalis and escape of blood into the stroma, which marks the beginning of menstrual shedding (Fig. 22–26*F*).

The proliferative phase exhibits mitotic activity in glandular and stromal cells; ovulation is confirmed by prominent basal vacuolation of glandular epithelial cells, secretory exhaustion, or predecidual changes. Obviously, ovulation cannot be confirmed during the proliferative phase or in the late stages of endometrial shedding when only the basalis is present.[64]

Functional Endometrial Disorders (Dysfunctional Uterine Bleeding)

During active reproductive life, the endometrium is constantly engaged in the dynamics of shedding and regrowth. It is controlled by the rise and fall of pituitary and ovarian hormones, and this control is executed by proper timing of hormonal release in both absolute and relative amounts. Alterations in this fine-tuning mechanism may result in a spectrum of disturbances, including atrophy, abnormal proliferative or secretory patterns, and hyperplasia.[64]

By far the most common problem is the occurrence of excessive bleeding during or between menstrual periods. The causes of abnormal bleeding from the uterus are many and vary among women of different age groups (Table 22–2). In some instances, bleeding is the result of a well-defined organic abnormality, such as chronic endometritis, submucosal leiomyomas, endometrial polyp, or endometrial neoplasms. However, the largest single group encompasses functional disturbances (so-called dysfunctional uterine bleeding) due to abnormalities in the menstrual cycle or systemic diseases.[64]

ANOVULATORY CYCLE

In most instances, dysfunctional bleeding is due to the occurrence of an anovulatory cycle, which results in excessive and prolonged estrogenic stimulation without the development of the progestational phase that regularly follows ovulation. Less commonly, lack of ovulation is the result of (1) an endocrine disorder, such as thyroid disease, adrenal disease, or

TABLE 22–2 Causes of Abnormal Uterine Bleeding by Age Group

Age Group	Causes
Prepuberty	Precocious puberty (hypothalamic, pituitary, or ovarian origin)
Adolescence	Anovulatory cycle, coagulation disorders
Reproductive age	Complications of pregnancy (abortion, trophoblastic disease, ectopic pregnancy) Organic lesions (leiomyoma, adenomyosis, polyps, endometrial hyperplasia, carcinoma) Anovulatory cycle Ovulatory dysfunctional bleeding (e.g., inadequate luteal phase)
Perimenopausal	Anovulatory cycle Irregular shedding Organic lesions (carcinoma, hyperplasia, polyps)
Postmenopausal	Organic lesions (carcinoma, hyperplasia, polyps) Endometrial atrophy

pituitary tumors; (2) a primary lesion of the ovary, such as a functioning ovarian tumor (granulose-theca cell tumors) or polycystic ovaries (see section on ovaries); or (3) a generalized metabolic disturbance, such as marked obesity, severe malnutrition, or any chronic systemic disease. In most patients, however, anovulatory cycles are unexplainable, probably occurring because of subtle hormonal imbalances. Anovulatory cycles are most common at menarche and the perimenopausal period.

Failure of ovulation results in prolonged, excessive endometrial stimulation by estrogens. Under these circumstances, the endometrial glands undergo mild architectural changes, including cystic dilation (persistent proliferative endometrium). Unscheduled breakdown of the stroma may also occur ("anovulatory menstruation"), with no evidence of endometrial secretory activity (Fig. 22–27*A*). More severe consequences of anovulation are discussed under endometrial hyperplasia.

INADEQUATE LUTEAL PHASE

This term refers to the occurrence of inadequate corpus luteum function and low progesterone output, with an irregular ovulatory cycle. The condition often manifests clinically as infertility, with either increased bleeding or amenorrhea. Endometrial biopsy performed at an estimated postovulatory date shows secretory endometrium, which, however, lags in its secretory characteristics with respect to the expected date.

ENDOMETRIAL CHANGES INDUCED BY ORAL CONTRACEPTIVES

As might be suspected, oral contraceptives containing synthetic or derivative ovarian steroids induce a wide variety of endometrial changes, depending on the steroid used and the dose. A common response pattern is a discordant appearance between glands and stroma, usually with inactive glands amid a stroma showing large cells with abundant cytoplasm reminiscent of the decidua of pregnancy. When such therapy is discontinued, the endometrium reverts to normal. All these changes have been minimized with the newer low-dose contraceptives.

MENOPAUSAL AND POSTMENOPAUSAL CHANGES

Because the menopause is characterized by anovulatory cycles, architectural alterations in the endometrial glands may be present transiently, followed by ovarian failure and atrophy of the endometrium. As discussed next, a component of

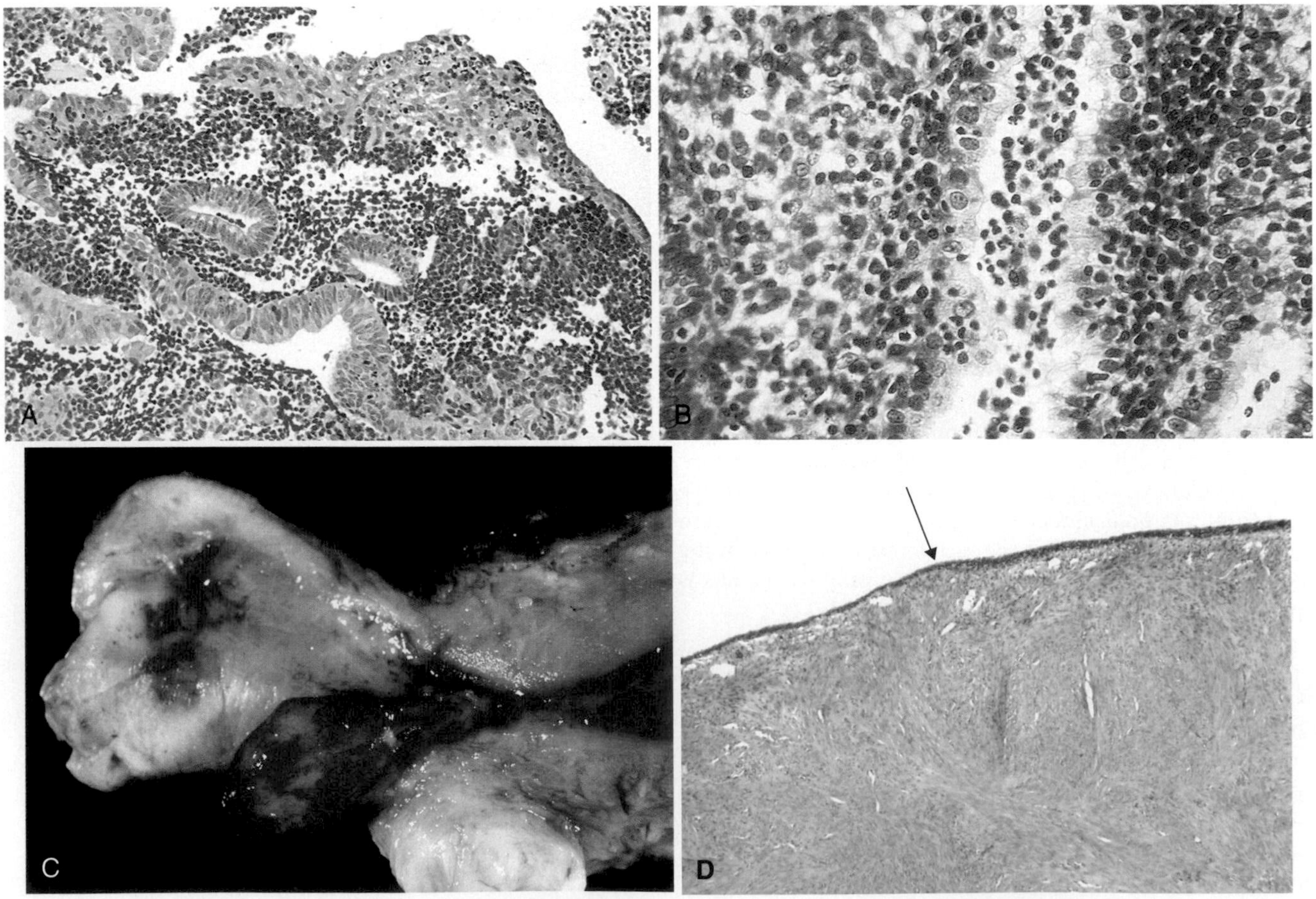

FIGURE 22–27 Common causes of abnormal uterine bleeding. *A*, The most common is dysfunctional uterine bleeding, seen here as anovulatory endometrium with stromal breakdown. Note breakdown associated with proliferative glands. *B*, Chronic endometritis. *C*, Endometrial polyp. *D*, Submucosal leiomyoma (*lower*) with attenuation of the endometrial lining (*arrow*).

anovulatory cycles and uninterrupted estrogen production includes mild hyperplasias with cystic dilation of glands. If this is followed by complete ovarian atrophy and loss of stimulus, the cystic dilation may remain, while the ovarian stroma and gland epithelium undergo atrophy. In this case, so-called cystic atrophy results. Such cystic changes should not be confused with more active cystic hyperplasia, which exhibits evidence of glandular and stromal proliferation.

Inflammation

The endometrium and myometrium are relatively resistant to infections, primarily because the endocervix normally forms a barrier to ascending infection. Thus, although chronic inflammation in the cervix is an expected and frequently insignificant finding, it is a concern in the endometrium, excluding the menstrual phase. Acute endometritis is uncommon and limited to bacterial infections that arise after delivery or miscarriage. Retained products of conception are the usual predisposing influence, causative agents including group A hemolytic streptococci, staphylococci, and other bacteria. The inflammatory response is chiefly limited to the interstitium and is entirely non-specific. Removal of the retained gestational fragments by curettage is promptly followed by remission of the infection.

CHRONIC ENDOMETRITIS

Chronic inflammation of the endometrium occurs in the following settings: (1) in patients suffering from chronic PID; (2) in patients with postpartal or postabortal endometrial cavities, usually due to retained gestational tissue; (3) in patients with intrauterine contraceptive devices; and (4) in patients with tuberculosis, either from miliary spread or, more commonly, from drainage of tuberculous salpingitis. The last is distinctly rare in Western countries. The chronic endometritis in all these cases represents a secondary disease, and under these circumstances there is a plausible cause.

In about 15% of cases, no such primary cause is obvious, yet plasma cells (which are not present in normal endometrium) are seen together with macrophages and lymphocytes (Fig. 22–27*B*). Some women with this so-called non-specific chronic endometritis have gynecologic complaints such as abnormal bleeding, pain, discharge, and infertility. *Chlamydia* may be involved and is commonly associated with both acute (e.g., polymorphonuclear leukocytes) and chronic (e.g., lymphocytes, plasma cells) inflammatory cell infiltrates. The organisms may or may not be successfully cultured.[65] Importantly, antibiotic therapy is indicated because it may prevent other sequelae (e.g., salpingitis).

Endometriosis and Adenomyosis

Endometriosis is the term used to describe the *presence of endometrial glands or stroma in abnormal locations outside the uterus.* It occurs in the following sites, in descending order of frequency: (1) ovaries; (2) uterine ligaments; (3) rectovaginal septum; (4) pelvic peritoneum; (5) laparotomy scars; and (6) rarely in the umbilicus, vagina, vulva, or appendix.

A closely related disorder, *adenomyosis*, is defined as the *presence of endometrial tissue in the uterine wall* (myometrium). Adenomyosis remains in continuity with the endometrium, presumably signifying downgrowth of endometrial tissue into and between the smooth muscle fascicles of the myometrium. Adenomyosis occurs in up to 20% of uteri. On microscopic examination, irregular nests of endometrial stroma, with or without glands, are arranged within the myometrium, separated from the basalis by at least 2 to 3 mm. In some patients, the most important consequence of adenomyosis is shedding of the endometrium during the menstrual cycle (Fig. 22–28). Hemorrhage within these small adenomyotic nests results in menorrhagia, colicky dysmenorrhea, dyspareunia, and pelvic pain, particularly during the premenstrual period.

Endometriosis is an important clinical condition; it often causes *infertility, dysmenorrhea, pelvic pain*, and other problems. The disorder is principally a disease of women in active reproductive life, most often in the third and fourth decades, and afflicts approximately 10% of women.

Three potential explanations exist regarding the origin of these dispersed lesions; they are not mutually exclusive (Fig. 22–29).

1. *The regurgitation/implantation theory.* Retrograde menstruation through the fallopian tubes occurs regularly even in normal women and could mediate spread of endometrial tissue to the peritoneal cavity. Endometriosis is common in the cervical mucosa, particularly following surgical procedures, supporting implantation from above.
2. *The metaplastic theory.* Endometrium could arise directly from coelomic epithelium, from which the müllerian ducts and ultimately the endometrium itself originate during embryonic development.
3. *The vascular or lymphatic dissemination theory.* Dissemination through pelvic veins and lymphatics would explain the presence of endometriotic lesions in the lungs or lymph nodes, a phenomenon not readily explainable by the first two theories.

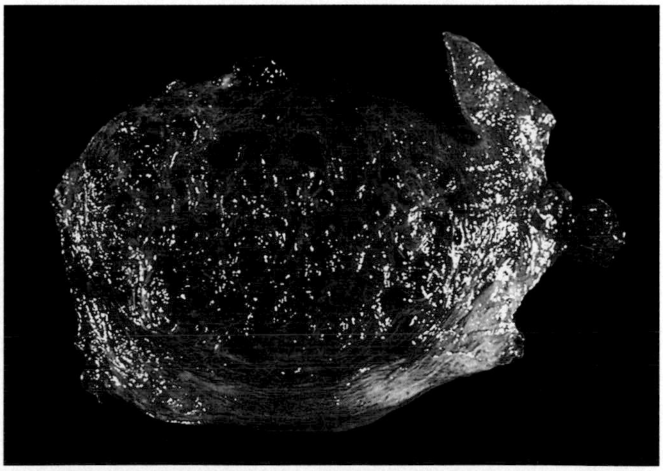

FIGURE 22–28 Adenomyosis. This disorder is characterized by functional endometrial nests within the myometrium, producing foci of hemorrhagic cysts within the uterine wall.

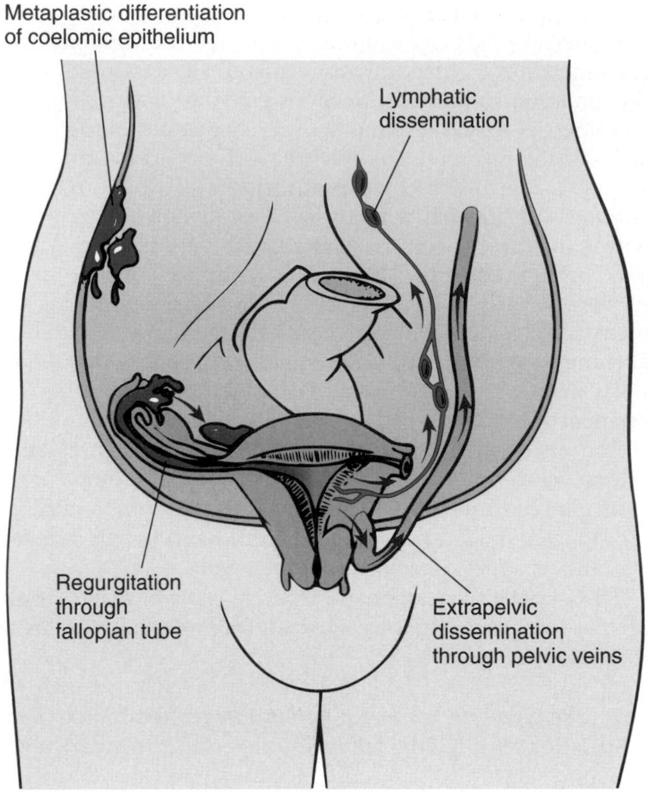

FIGURE 22–29 The potential origins of endometriosis.

The regurgitation implantation theory is the most reasonable explanation for endometriosis seen in the cervix or pelvic sites, whereas the metaplastic theory is an attractive explanation for other sites such as the ovary. Genetic, hormonal, and immune factors have also been postulated to increase susceptibility of some women to endometriosis.[66] Based on the finding of aromatase cytochrome P450 in endometriotic tissue but not in normal endometrium, it has been suggested that the endometriotic tissue possesses the capacity to produce its own estrogens via this enzyme.[67] Other reports indicate that endometriosis is clonal in origin, suggesting important biochemical differences between endometriotic tissue and normal uterine endometrium.

Morphology. The foci of endometrium respond to both extrinsic cyclic (ovarian) and intrinsic hormonal stimulation with periodic bleeding. This produces nodules with a red-blue to yellow-brown appearance on or just beneath the serosal surfaces in the site of involvement. When the disease is extensive, organizing hemorrhage causes extensive fibrous adhesions between tubes, ovaries, and other structures and obliteration of the pouch of Douglas. The ovaries may become markedly distorted by large cystic masses (3 to 5 cm in diameter) filled with brown blood debris (chocolate cysts) (Fig. 22–30*A*).

The histologic diagnosis of endometriosis is usually straightforward but may be difficult in long-standing cases in which the endometrial tissue is obscured by the fibro-obliterative response. A histologic diagnosis of endometriosis is satisfied if endometrial stroma is present, or in its absence, müllerian epithelium with subjacent hemosiderin pigment (Fig. 22–30*B*).

Clinical Course. Clinical signs and symptoms usually consist of severe dysmenorrhea, dyspareunia, and pelvic pain due to the intrapelvic bleeding and periuterine adhesions. Pain on defecation indicates rectal wall involvement, and dysuria reflects involvement of the serosa of the bladder. Intestinal disturbances may appear when the small intestine is affected. Menstrual irregularities are common, and infertility is the presenting complaint in 30% to 40% of women. Malignancies may develop in endometriotic lesions at any site, prompting theories that endometriosis is an "at-risk" epithelium.[68]

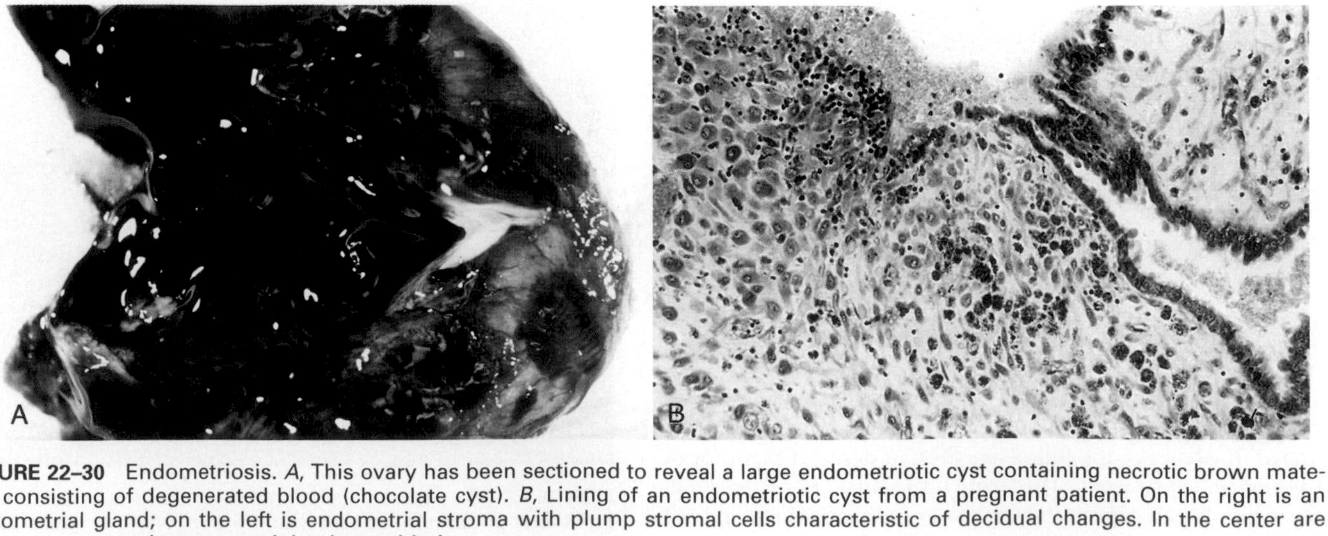

FIGURE 22–30 Endometriosis. *A*, This ovary has been sectioned to reveal a large endometriotic cyst containing necrotic brown material consisting of degenerated blood (chocolate cyst). *B*, Lining of an endometriotic cyst from a pregnant patient. On the right is an endometrial gland; on the left is endometrial stroma with plump stromal cells characteristic of decidual changes. In the center are numerous macrophages containing hemosiderin.

Endometrial Polyps

Endometrial polyps are sessile masses of variable size that project into the endometrial cavity. They may be single or multiple and are usually 0.5 to 3 cm in diameter but occasionally large and pedunculated. Polyps may be asymptomatic or may cause abnormal bleeding if they ulcerate or undergo necrosis. They are generally of two histologic types, made up of (1) functional endometrium, paralleling the adjacent cycling endometrium, or (2) more commonly, hyperplastic endometrium, mostly of the cystic variety. Such polyps may develop in association with generalized endometrial hyperplasia and are responsive to the growth effect of estrogen but exhibit no progesterone response (Fig. 22–27*C*). Rarely, adenocarcinomas may arise within endometrial polyps. Endometrial polyps have been observed in association with the administration of tamoxifen, an antiestrogen frequently used in the therapy of breast cancer.[69] Cytogenetic studies indicate that the stromal cells in endometrial polyps are clonal, with chromosome (6p21) rearrangements, indicating that genetic alterations may play a role in their development.[70]

Endometrial Hyperplasia (Endometrial Intraepithelial Neoplasia)

Endometrial hyperplasia—recently termed *endometrial intraepithelial neoplasia*—is another cause of abnormal bleeding that differs from typical anovulation by an increased gland to stroma ratio and abnormalities in epithleial growth relative to normal endometrium. Endometrial hyperplasia deserves special attention because of its relationship with endometrial carcinoma. Numerous studies have largely confirmed the malignant potential of certain endometrial hyperplasias and the concept of a continuum of glandular atypia culminating, in some cases, in carcinoma.[71]

Endometrial hyperplasia is linked to prolonged estrogen stimulation of the endometrium by anovulation or increased estrogen production. Conditions promoting hyperplasia include menopause, polycystic ovarian disease (including Stein-Leventhal syndrome), functioning granulosa cell tumors of the ovary, excessive cortical function (cortical stroma hyperplasia), and prolonged administration of estrogenic substances (estrogen replacement therapy). These are the same influences postulated to be of pathogenetic significance in some endometrial carcinomas, discussed later.

A key factor in the development of endometrial hyperplasia and related cancers is inactivation of the *PTEN* tumor suppressor gene through deletion and/or inactivation. It encodes a phosphatase with dual lipid and protein specificity (Chapter 7). Its most important function is as a lipid phosphatase blocking Akt phosphorylation in the P13K pathway. Unopposed estrogens normally increase native endometrial gland PTEN protein production, which is constantly expressed during the proliferative phase but is absent during the secretory phase. In the absence of PTEN endometrial cells become more sensitive to stimulation by estrogens, and this may be integral to the development of hyperplasias and subsequent cancer.[72,73] *PTEN* inactivation is seen in 63% of premalignant endometrial hyperplasias and 50% to 80% of endometrial carcinomas. It should also be noted that PTEN loss has been documented in some normal-appearing endometrial glands of 43% of premenopausal women. The latter observation suggests that loss of PTEN expression may be an early step in endometrial carcinogenesis.

Morphology. Endometrial hyperplasia has traditionally been subdivided into lower grade (simple) and higher grade (atypical) subgroups. Currently the lower-grade hyperplasias include both anovulatory epithelium and, less commonly, subtle endometrial intraepithelial neoplasms (EIN). In contrast, higher-grade hyperplasias, also termed atypical hyperplasias, typically have the morphologic features (gland crowding and cytologic atypia) and genetic characteristics (*PTEN* mutations) of intraepithelial neoplasia.[71,72]

Simple non-atypical hyperplasias, also known as cystic or mild hyperplasias, are characterized by architectural changes in glands of various sizes, producing irregularity in gland shape, with cystic alterations. The epithelial growth pattern and cytology are similar to those of proliferative endometrium, although mitoses are not as prominent (Fig. 22–31*A*). These lesions uncommonly progress to adenocarcinoma and largely reflect a response to persistent estrogen stimulation. These simple cystic "hyperplasias" frequently evolve into cystic atrophy in which both the epithelium and stroma become atrophic.

Complex atypical hyperplasias (endometrial intraepithelial neoplasias) exhibit an increase in the number and size of endometrial glands, with gland crowding, enlargement, and irregular shape. The latter is principally a manifestation of increased cell stratification and nuclear enlargement and may demonstrate complexity of the lining epithelium with scalloped or tufted surface. The glands remain distinct and non-confluent, characteristic of an intraepithelial neoplasm (Fig. 22–31*B*). Mitotic figures are common. Predictably, in the most severe forms, cytologic and architectural atypia may border on adenocarcinoma, and an accurate distinction between atypical hyperplasia and cancer may not be made without hysterectomy.

The shift in gland morphology from benign to precancerous is often highlighted by a loss of *PTEN* gene expression (Fig. 22–31*C*), although this is not invariable, and the diagnosis of hyperplasia is made on histologic grounds. In one study, 23% of patients with atypical hyperplasias eventually developed adenocarcinoma.[71] In another study, in which atypical hyperplasias were treated with progestin therapy alone, 50% persisted despite therapy, 25% recurred, and 25% progressed to carcinoma.[74] Currently endometrial intraepithelial neoplasias are managed by hysterectomy or, in young women, a trial of progestin therapy and close follow-up. Nevertheless, the low rate of regression usually requires eventual removal of the uterus.

A proportion of endometrial hyperplasias are less easily classified, including complex lesions without cellular atypia

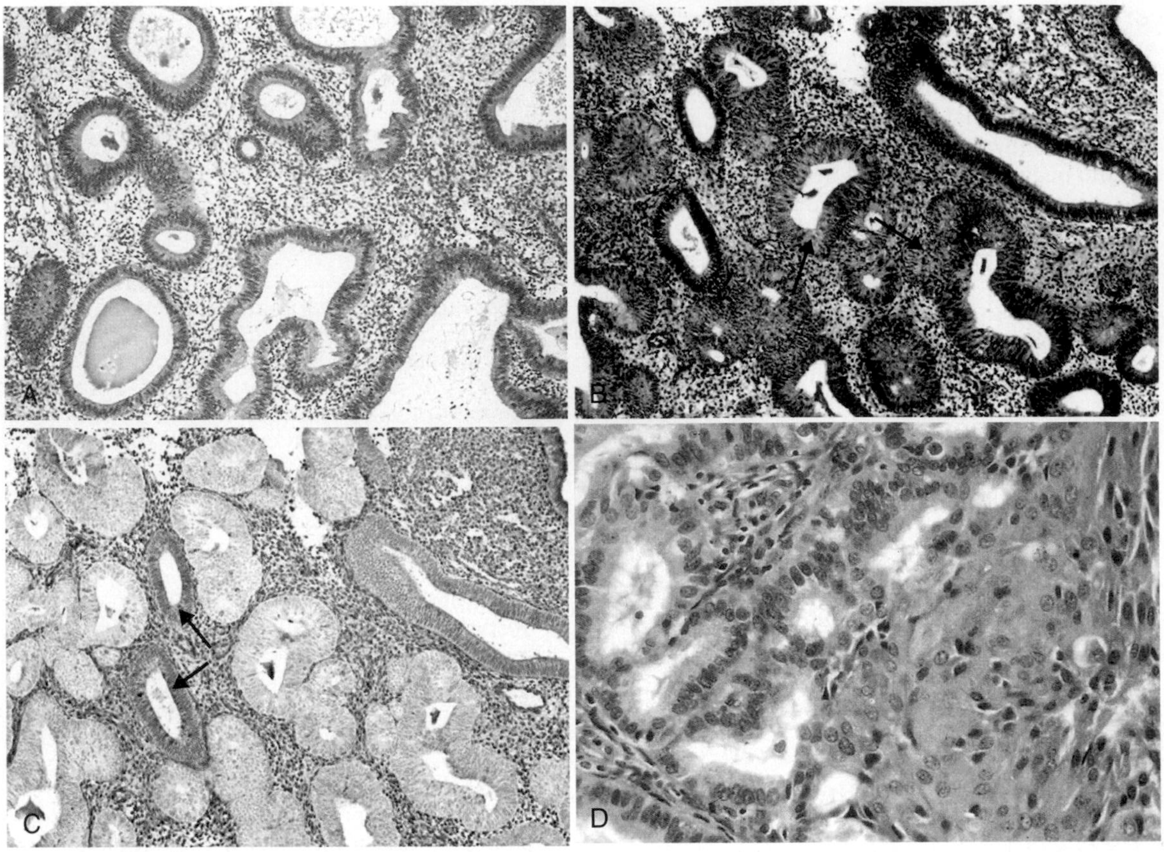

FIGURE 22–31 *A*, Lower-grade hyperplasias of the endometrium show principally architectural glandular changes with cystic glandular dilatation and are synonymous with anovulatory changes. *B*, Atypical hyperplasias (endometrial intraepithelial neoplasia) exhibit increased gland/stroma ratio (gland crowding) and epithelial stratification (*arrows*). *C*, Loss of *PTEN* gene expression in intraepithelial neoplasia, seen here as absence of staining. Compare to normal glands (*arrows*), which express the gene (Courtesy of Dr. George L. Mutter, Brigham and Women's Hospital, Boston, MA.) *D*, Endometrial hyperplasia with squamous metaplasia.

(uncommon) and those with altered cellular differentiation (metaplasia), including the presence of squamous, ciliated cell, and mucinous metaplasia (Fig. 22–31*D*). The latter may result from alterations in epithelial-stromal relationships inducing the basal endometrial cells to follow different differentiation pathways.[75] Because of these nuances of cell growth and differentiation, interpretation of endometrial hyperplasia may be highly subjective, and thus precise classification of every change is not possible. Any assessment of a suspected hyperplasia should include the degree of atypia in a manner clearly understandable by the clinician. The selection of diagnostic terminology may mean the difference between cyclic progestin therapy on one hand and continuous high-dose progestin therapy or hysterectomy (or both) on the other.

Malignant Tumors of the Endometrium

CARCINOMA OF THE ENDOMETRIUM

Endometrial carcinoma is the most common invasive cancer of the female genital tract and accounts for 7% of all invasive cancer in women, excluding skin cancer. At one time, it was far less common than cancer of the cervix, but earlier detection and eradication of CIN and an increase in endometrial carcinomas in younger age groups have reversed this ratio. There are now 34,000 new endometrial cancers per year, compared with 13,000 new invasive cervical cancers. Despite their high frequency, endometrial cancers arise mainly in postmenopausal women, causing abnormal (postmenopausal) bleeding. This permits early detection and cure at an early stage.

Incidence and Pathogenesis. Carcinoma of the endometrium is uncommon in women younger than 40 years of age. The peak incidence is in the 55- to 65-year-old woman. A higher frequency of this form of neoplasia is seen with (1) obesity, (2) diabetes (abnormal glucose tolerance is found in more than 60%), (3) hypertension, and (4) infertility (women who develop cancer of the endometrium tend to be single and nulliparous and to have a history of functional menstrual irregularities consistent with anovulatory cycles). Infrequently, both endometrial and breast carcinomas arise in the same patient.[76]

In terms of potential pathogenesis, two general groups of endometrial cancer can be identified. The first develops on a background of prolonged estrogen stimulation and *endometrial hyperplasia*.[77] The close relationship between hyperplasia and cancer of the endometrium in this setting is supported by the following:

- Both hyperplasia and cancer are also linked with obesity and anovulatory cycles.
- Women with ovarian estrogen-secreting tumors have a higher risk of endometrial cancer.

- Endometrial cancer is extremely rare in women with ovarian agenesis and in those castrated early in life.
- Estrogen replacement therapy is associated with increased risk.
- Prolonged administration of DES to laboratory animals may produce endometrial polyps, hyperplasia, and carcinoma.
- In postmenopausal women, there is greater synthesis of estrogens in body fat from adrenal and ovarian androgen precursors, a finding that may partly explain why there is increased risk of endometrial cancer with age and obesity.
- As discussed previously, inactivation of the *PTEN* gene is common to endometrial hyperplasia and cancer, as is microsatellite instability.[72,73,78,79]

Endometrial carcinomas that are associated with hyperplasia and the aforementioned risk factors tend either to be well differentiated, mimicking normal endometrial glands (*endometrioid*) in histologic appearance, or to display altered differentiation (mucinous, tubal, squamous differentiation). This latter group of tumors is associated with a more favorable prognosis than tumors without hyperplasia.[77] Although endometrial carcinomas may be associated with separate primary neoplasms arising in ovarian endometriosis, they tend to not spread to the peritoneal surfaces.

A second subset of patients with endometrial cancer less commonly exhibits the stigmata of hyperestrinism or preexisting hyperplasia, and acquires the disease at a somewhat older average age. In this group, tumors are generally more poorly differentiated, including tumors that resemble subtypes of ovarian carcinomas (*serous carcinomas*).[79] Overall, these tumors have a poorer prognosis than estrogen-related cancers do. In contrast to endometrioid tumors, serous subtypes infrequently display microsatellite instability and are linked to mutation of *p53*.[78,79] They presumably begin as surface epithelial neoplasms that extend into adjacent gland structures and later invade endometrial stroma. Their generally poorer prognosis is a consequence of their propensity to exfoliate, undergo transtubal spread, and implant on peritoneal surfaces like their ovarian counterparts.

Morphology. In gross appearance, endometrial carcinoma presents either as a localized polypoid tumor or as a diffuse tumor involving the entire endometrial surface (Fig. 22–32*A*). Spread generally occurs by direct myometrial invasion with eventual extension to the periuterine structures by direct continuity. Spread into the broad ligaments may create a clinically palpable mass. Dissemination to the regional lymph nodes eventually occurs, and in the late stages, the tumor may metastasize to the lungs, liver, bones, and other organs. In certain types, specifically papillary serous carcinoma, relatively superficial endometrial involvement may be associated with extensive peritoneal disease, suggesting spread by routes (i.e., tubal or lymphatic transmission) other than direct invasion.

On histologic examination, most endometrial carcinomas (about 85%) are **adenocarcinomas** characterized by more or less well-defined gland patterns closely resembling normal endometrial epithelium (Fig. 22–32*B*). A three-step grading system is applied to endometrioid tumors and includes well differentiated (grade 1), with easily recognizable glandular patterns; moderately differentiated (grade 2), showing well-formed glands mixed with solid sheets of malignant cells; or poorly differentiated (grade 3), characterized by solid sheets of cells with barely recognizable glands and a greater degree of nuclear atypia and mitotic activity (see below).

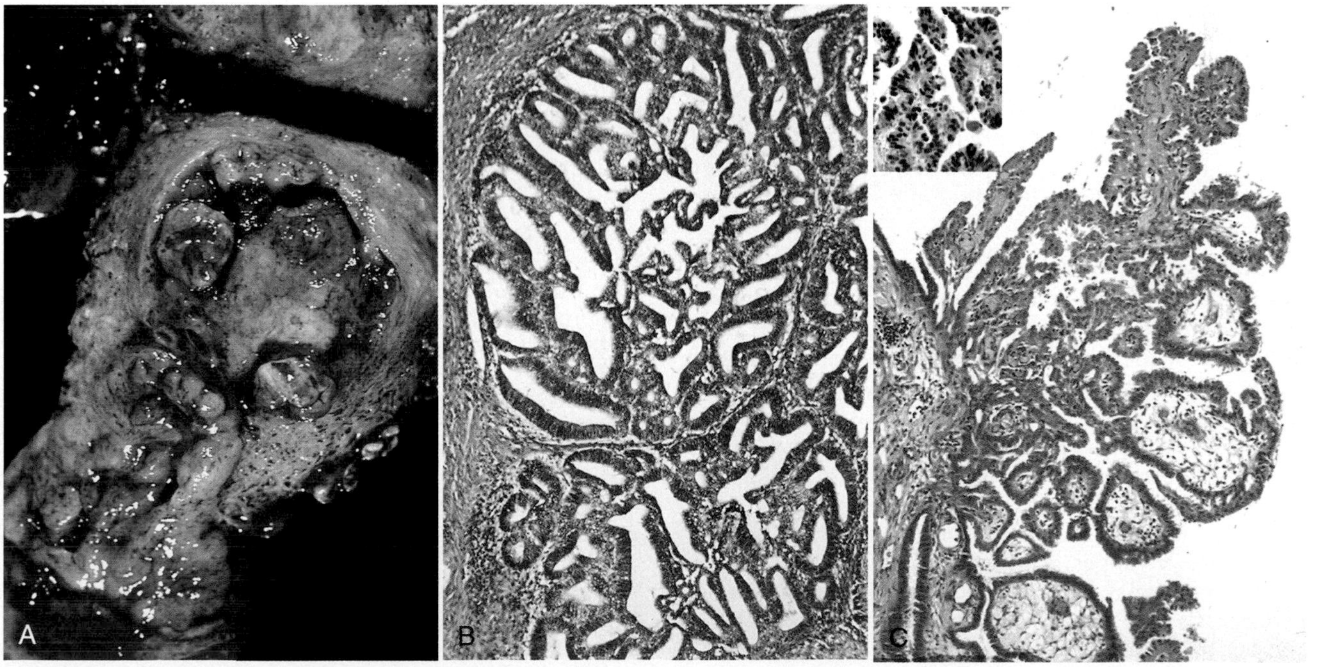

FIGURE 22–32 *A,* Endometrial adenocarcinoma presenting as a fungating mass in the fundus of the uterus. *B,* Well-differentiated endometrial adenocarcinoma. Glandular architecture is preserved but the tissue is confluent without intervening stroma, which distinguishes carcinoma from hyperplasia. *C,* Papillary serous carcinoma of the endometrium, with accumulation of nuclear p53 protein as seen by immunohistochemistry (*inset upper left*).

Up to 20% of endometrioid carcinomas contain foci of squamous differentiation. Squamous elements may be histologically benign-appearing when they are associated with well-differentiated adenocarcinomas. Less commonly, moderately or poorly differentiated endometrioid carcinomas contain squamous elements that appear frankly malignant. Terms such as adenoacanthoma and adenosquamous carcinoma were previously assigned to these tumors. Current classification systems grade the carcinomas based on glandular differentiation alone and use the term squamous differentiation for tumors falling into these categories.[77,80]

As mentioned earlier, a subset of endometrial cancers resemble serous carcinomas of the ovary. They comprise approximately 20% of endometrial carcinomas. Grading of these non-endometrioid carcinomas is unnecessary due to the poor prognosis conferred by these tumor types. **Papillary serous carcinomas and clear cell carcinomas** are managed as grade 3 carcinomas irrespective of histologic pattern (Fig. 22–32*C*). Serous tumors in particular are a highly aggressive form of uterine cancer, 80% of which harbor *p53* mutations and accumulate p53 protein (Fig. 22-32*C* inset).[79,81]

Staging of endometrial adenocarcinoma is as follows:[80]

Stage I. Carcinoma is confined to the corpus uteri itself.
Stage II. Carcinoma has involved the corpus and the cervix.
Stage III. Carcinoma has extended outside the uterus but not outside the true pelvis.
Stage IV. Carcinoma has extended outside the true pelvis or has obviously involved the mucosa of the bladder or the rectum.

Cases in various stages can also be subgrouped with reference to the three grades described above:

G1. Well-differentiated adenocarcinoma
G2. Differentiated adenocarcinoma with partly solid (less than 50%) areas
G3. Predominantly solid or entirely undifferentiated carcinoma. Serous and clear cell carcinomas are automatically classified as grade 3.

Clinical Course. Carcinoma of the endometrium may be asymptomatic for periods of time but usually produces irregular vaginal bleeding with excessive leukorrhea. Uterine enlargement in the early stages may be deceptively absent. Cytologic detection on Papanicolaou smears is variable and most likely associated with serous carcinomas, which produce easily detached clusters of cells that are sampled in pap smears. Exclusion of a cervical adenocarcinoma can usually be based on cervix exam and the fact that older age groups are much more susceptible to primary endometrial (versus cervical) cancer. However, upper genital tract carcinomas (fallopian tube and ovary) may be associated with abnormal cytology. The diagnosis of endometrial cancer must ultimately be established by curettage and histologic examination of the tissue.

As would be anticipated, the prognosis depends heavily on the clinical stage of the disease when it is discovered, and its histologic grade and type. In the United States, most women (about 80%) have stage I disease clinically and have well-differentiated or moderately well-differentiated endometrioid carcinomas. Surgery, alone or in combination with irradiation, gives about 90% 5-year survival in stage I (grade 1 or 2) disease. This rate drops to approximately 75% for grade 3/stage I and to 50% or less for stage II and III endometrial carcinomas.

As mentioned, uterine papillary serous and clear cell carcinomas have a propensity for extrauterine (lymphatic or transtubal) spread, even when confined to the endometrium or its surface epithelium. Overall, fewer than 50% of patients with these tumors are alive 3 years after diagnosis and 35% after 5 years. If peritoneal cytology and adnexal histologic exam are negative, the five year survival of stage I disease is approximately 80% to 85%.[82] The additional advantage of prophylactic radiation or chemotherapy in early-stage disease is unclear.[83,84]

Tumors of the Endometrium with Stromal Differentiation

A proportion of endometrial adenocarcinomas undergo stromal differentiation and are termed carcinosarcomas. A second group is composed of stromal neoplasias in association with benign glands (adenosarcomas). A third group consists of pure stromal neoplasms, ranging from benign (stromal nodule) to malignant (stromal sarcoma). Together, these tumors comprise less than 5% of endometrial cancers.

CARCINOSARCOMAS

Carcinosarcomas (formerly termed malignant mixed müllerian tumors) consist of endometrial adenocarcinomas in which malignant stromal differentiation takes place.[85] The stroma tends to differentiate into a variety of malignant mesodermal components, including muscle, cartilage, and even osteoid. The epithelial and stromal components are presumably derived from the same cell, a concept supported by the observation that the stromal cells often stain positive for epithelial cell markers. Carcinosarcomas occur in postmenopausal women and manifest, similarly to adenocarcinoma, with postmenopausal bleeding. Many affected patients give a history of previous radiation therapy.

Morphology. In gross appearance, such tumors are somewhat more fleshy than adenocarcinomas, may be bulky and polypoid, and sometimes protrude through the cervical os. On histology, the tumors consist of adenocarcinoma mixed with the stromal (sarcoma) elements (Fig. 22–33*A*); alternatively, the tumor may contain two distinct and separate epithelial and mesenchymal components. Sarcomatous components may mimic extrauterine tissues (i.e., striated muscle cells, cartilage, adipose tissue, and bone).

Outcome is determined primarily by depth of invasion and stage. As with endometrial carcinomas, the prognosis may be influenced by the grade and type of the adenocarcinoma, being poorest with serous differentiation. It is noteworthy that carcinosarcomas usually metastasize as adenocarcinomas. The tumors are highly malignant, and patients have a 5-year survival rate of 25% to 30%.[85]

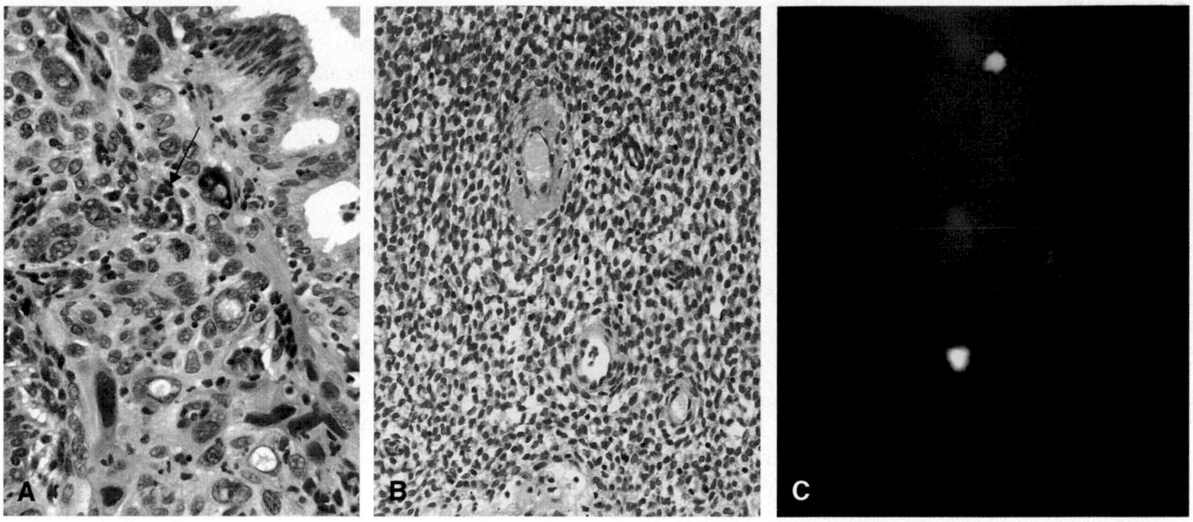

FIGURE 22–33 *A*, Carcinosarcoma, showing both epithelial (*upper right*) and stromal (*arrow*) differentiation. *B*, Endometrial stromal sarcoma infiltrating myometrium. *C*, Fluorescent in situ hybridization using two fluorescently labeled probes (*green and red*) that flank the breakpoint of the gene involved in the chromosomal translocation t(7;17) in endometrial stromal sarcoma. The yellow signal is indicative of the normal copy of chromosome 7. A separate green and red signal indicates that the gene on chromosome 7 has been redistributed. (Courtesy of Dr. Marisa R. Nucci, Brigham and Women's Hospital, Boston, MA.)

ADENOSARCOMAS

Adenosarcomas present most commonly as large broad-based endometrial polypoid growths, and may prolapse through the cervical os. The diagnosis is based on malignant appearing stroma, which coexists with benign but abnormally shaped endometrial glands. These tumors predominate in women between the fourth and fifth decades and are generally considered to be of low grade malignancy; recurrences develop in one-fourth and are nearly always confined to the pelvis.[86] The principal diagnostic dilemma is distinguishing these tumors from large benign polyps. The distinction is important because oophorectomy is typically performed in cases of adenosarcoma since they are estrogen sensitive.

STROMAL TUMORS

The endometrial stroma occasionally gives rise to neoplasms that may resemble normal stromal cells. Similar to most neoplasms, they may be well or poorly differentiated. Stromal neoplasms are divided into two categories: (1) benign stromal nodules and (2) endometrial stromal sarcomas.

Morphology. Stromal nodule is a well-circumscribed aggregate of endometrial stromal cells in the myometrium that does not penetrate the myometrium and is of little consequence. **Stromal sarcoma** consists of neoplastic endometrial stroma lying between muscle bundles of the myometrium and is distinguished from stromal nodules by either diffuse infiltration of myometrial tissue or the penetration of lymphatic channels (previously termed **endolymphatic stromal myosis**) (Fig. 22–33*B*).

About half of these tumors recur, with relapse rates of 36% to over 80% for Stage I and Stage III/IV tumor, respectively; relapse cannot be predicted by either mitotic index or degree of cytologic atypia.[87] Distant metastases, which sometimes may occur decades after initial diagnosis, and death from metastatic tumor occur in about 15% of cases. Five-year survival rates average 50%. Recent studies indicate that a recurrent chromosomal translocation, t(7;17)(p15;q21), occurs in endometrial stromal sarcoma. As a consequence of this translocation, the fusion of two previously unknown genes, *JAZF1* and *JJAZ1* occurs, with production of a fusion transcript and protein (Fig. 22–33*C*).[88]

Tumors of the Myometrium

LEIOMYOMAS

Uterine leiomyomas (commonly called *fibroids*) are perhaps the most common tumor in humans. These benign tumors may be present in about 75% of females of reproductive age, and each uterus harbors an average of 6.5 tumors. Each uterine leiomyoma is a unique clonal neoplasm. Most leiomyomas have normal karyotypes, but approximately 40% have a simple chromosomal abnormality. Six cytogenetic subgroups have been recognized: a balanced translocation between chromosomes 12 and 14 (i.e., t(12;14)(q14–15;q23–24)), partial deletions of the long arm of chromosome 7 (i.e., del(7)(q22q32)), trisomy 12, and rearrangements of 6p, 3q and 10q. The number and variety of cytogenetic abnormalities suggest that more than one genetic mechanism can lead to leiomyoma growth.[89,90]

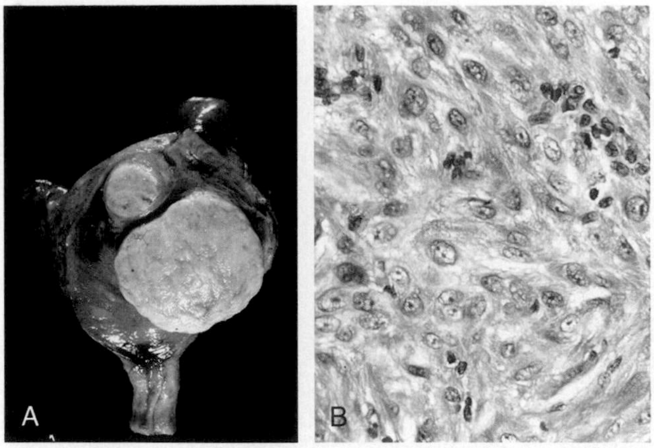

FIGURE 22–34 *A,* Leiomyomas of the myometrium. The uterus is opened to reveal the tumors bulging into the endometrial cavity and displaying a firm white appearance on sectioning. *B,* Leiomyoma showing well-differentiated, regular, spindle-shaped smooth muscle cells.

Morphology. Leiomyomas are sharply circumscribed, discrete, round, firm, gray-white tumors varying in size from small, barely visible nodules to massive tumors that fill the pelvis. Except in rare instances, they are found within the myometrium of the corpus. Only infrequently do they involve the uterine ligaments, lower uterine segment, or cervix. They can occur within the myometrium (intramural), just beneath the endometrium (submucosal) (Fig. 22–34*A* and Fig. 22–27*D*), or beneath the serosa (subserosal).

Whatever their size, the characteristic whorled pattern of smooth muscle bundles on cut section usually makes these lesions readily identifiable on gross inspection. Large tumors may develop areas of yellow-brown to red softening (red degeneration).

On histologic examination, the leiomyoma is composed of whorled bundles of smooth muscle cells that resemble the uninvolved myometrium (Fig. 22–34*B*). Usually, the individual muscle cells are uniform in size and shape and have the characteristic oval nucleus and long, slender bipolar cytoplasmic processes. Mitotic figures are scarce. Benign variants of leiomyoma include atypical or bizarre (symplastic) tumors with nuclear atypia and giant cells and cellular leiomyomas. Importantly, both have a low mitotic index. An extremely rare variant, **benign metastasizing leiomyoma**, consists of a uterine tumor that extends into vessels and migrates to other sites, most commonly the lung. Another variant, **disseminated peritoneal leiomyomatosis**, presents as multiple small nodules on the peritoneum. Both are considered benign despite their unusual behavior.

Leiomyomas of the uterus, even when they are extensive, may be asymptomatic. The most important symptoms are produced by submucosal leiomyomas (abnormal bleeding), compression of the bladder (urinary frequency), sudden pain if disruption of blood supply occurs, and impaired fertility. Myomas in pregnant women increase the frequency of spontaneous abortion, fetal malpresentation, uterine inertia, and postpartum hemorrhage. Malignant transformation (leiomyosarcoma) within a leiomyoma is extremely rare.

LEIOMYOSARCOMAS

These uncommon malignant neoplasms arise de novo directly from the myometrium or endometrial stroma undergoing smooth muscle differentiation. In contrast to leiomyomas, leiomyosarcomas have karyotypes that are complex and more random relative to those described above for leiomyomas. These include deletions identified on a number of chromosomes that are not seen in the benign tumors.[91]

Morphology. Leiomyosarcomas grow within the uterus in two somewhat distinctive patterns: bulky, fleshy masses that invade the uterine wall, or polypoid masses that project into the uterine lumen (Fig. 22–35*A*). On histologic examination, they contain a wide range of atypia, from those that are extremely well differentiated to anaplastic lesions that have the cytologic abnormalities of wildly growing sarcomas (Fig. 22–35*B*). The distinction of leiomyosarcomas from leiomyomas is based on the combination of degree of nuclear atypia, mitotic index, and zonal necrosis. With few exceptions, the presence of ten or more mitoses per ten high-power (×400) fields indicates malignancy, with or without cellular atypism. If the tumor contains nuclear atypia or large (epithelioid) cells, five mitoses per ten high-power fields are sufficient to justify a diagnosis of malignancy.[92] Rare exceptions include mitotically active leiomyomas in young or pregnant women, and caution should be exercised in interpreting such neoplasms as malignant. A proportion of smooth muscle neoplasms may be impossible to classify and are termed smooth muscle tumors of "uncertain malignant potential."[92]

Leiomyosarcomas are equally common before and after menopause, with a peak incidence at 40 to 60 years of age. These tumors have a striking tendency to recur after removal, and more than half the cases eventually metastasize through the bloodstream to distant organs, such as lungs, bone, and brain. Dissemination throughout the abdominal cavity is also encountered. The 5-year survival rate averages about 40%. The well-differentiated lesions have a better prognosis than the anaplastic lesions, which have a low 5-year survival rate of about 10% to 15%.[92]

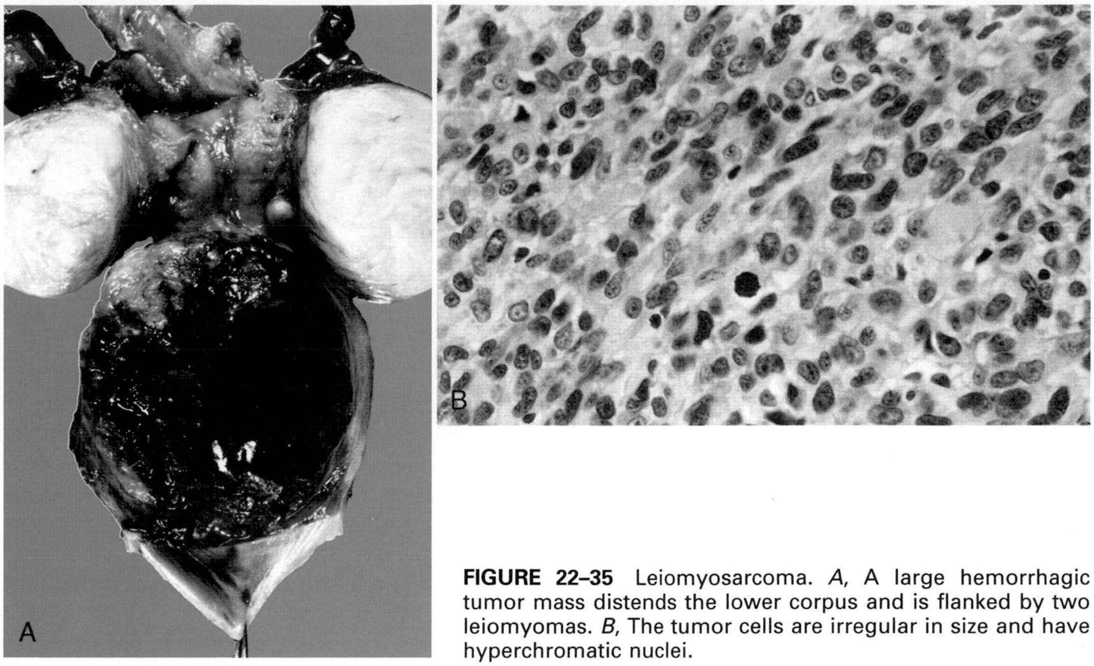

FIGURE 22–35 Leiomyosarcoma. *A,* A large hemorrhagic tumor mass distends the lower corpus and is flanked by two leiomyomas. *B,* The tumor cells are irregular in size and have hyperchromatic nuclei.

FALLOPIAN TUBES

The most common disorders in these structures are inflammations, followed in frequency by ectopic (tubal) pregnancy (see discussion later in this chapter) and endometriosis.

Inflammations

Suppurative salpingitis may be caused by any of the pyogenic organisms, and often more than one is involved. The gonococcus still accounts for more than 60% of cases of suppurative salpingitis, with chlamydiae less often a factor. These tubal infections are a part of PID described earlier in this chapter

Tuberculous salpingitis is extremely uncommon in the United States and accounts for probably not more than 1% to 2% of all forms of salpingitis. It is more common, however, in parts of the world where tuberculosis is prevalent and is an important cause of infertility in these areas.

Tumors and Cysts

The most common primary lesions of the fallopian tube (excluding endometriosis) are minute, 0.1- to 2-cm translucent cysts filled with clear serous fluid, called *paratubal cysts*. Larger varieties are found near the fimbriated end of the tube or in the broad ligaments and are referred to as *hydatids of Morgagni*. These cysts are presumed to arise in remnants of the müllerian duct and are of little significance.

Tumors of the fallopian tube are uncommon. Benign tumors include *adenomatoid tumors* (mesotheliomas), which occur subserosally on the tube or sometimes in the mesosalpinx. These small nodules are the exact counterparts of those already described in relation to the testes or epididymus (Chapter 21) and are benign. Primary *adenocarcinoma* of the fallopian tubes is rare and is defined as an adenocarcinoma with a dominant tubal mass and luminal and mucosal involvement. These tumors are detected by pelvic exam, abnormal discharge or bleeding, and occasionally, cervical cytology. Approximately one half are stage I at diagnosis, but nearly 40% of these patients will not survive 5 years. Higher stage tumors have a poor prognosis.[93] Patients are typically managed with ovarian cancer chemotherapy protocols. Recently, occult carcinoma of the fallopian tube has been associated with *BRCA* mutations, requiring attention to this site as a potential source of tumors in patients with *BRCA* germ-line mutations.[94]

OVARIES

The most common types of lesions encountered in the ovary include functional or benign cysts and tumors. Intrinsic inflammations of the ovary (oophoritis) are uncommon, usually accompanying tubal inflammation. Rarely, a primary inflammatory disorder involving ovarian follicles (autoimmune oophoritis) occurs and is associated with infertility.

Non-Neoplastic and Functional Cysts

FOLLICULAR AND LUTEAL CYSTS

Cystic follicles in the ovary are so common as to be virtually physiologic. They originate in unruptured graafian follicles or in follicles that have ruptured and immediately sealed.

Morphology. These cysts are usually multiple. They range in size up to 2 cm in diameter, are filled with a clear serous fluid, and are lined by a gray, glistening membrane. On occasion, larger cysts exceeding 2 cm (follicular cysts) may be diagnosed by palpation or ultrasonography and cause pelvic pain. Granulosa lining cells can be identified histologically if the intraluminal pressure has not been too great. The outer theca cells may be conspicuous with increased cytoplasm and a pale appearance (luteinized). As discussed subsequently, when this alteration is pronounced (hyperthecosis), it may ultimately result in increased estrogen production and endometrial abnormalities.

Granulosa **luteal cysts** (corpora lutea) are normally present in the ovary. These cysts are lined by a rim of bright yellow luteal tissue containing luteinized granulosa cells. They occasionally rupture and cause a peritoneal reaction. When advanced, the combination of old hemorrhage and fibrosis may make their distinction from endometriotic cysts difficult.

POLYCYSTIC OVARIES AND STROMAL HYPERTHECOSIS

Polycystic ovarian disease (PCOD, formerly termed *Stein-Leventhal syndrome*) affects 3% to 6% of reproductive-age women. The central pathologic abnormality is numerous cystic follicles or follicle cysts, often associated with oligomenorrhea. Patients with PCOD have persistent anovulation, obesity (40%), hirsutism (50%), and, rarely, virilism.[95,96]

Morphology. The ovaries are usually twice normal size, gray-white with a smooth outer cortex, and are studded with subcortical cysts 0.5 to 1.5 cm in diameter. On histologic examination, there is a thickened superficial cortex beneath which are innumerable follicle cysts with hyperplasia of the theca interna (follicular hyperthecosis) (Fig. 22–36*A–D*). Corpora lutea are frequently but not invariably absent.

The initiating event in polycystic ovarian disease is not clear. Increased secretion of luteinizing hormone may stimulate the theca-lutein cells of the follicles, with excessive production of androgen (androstenedione), which is converted to estrone. For years, these endocrine abnormalities were attributed to primary ovarian dysfunction because large wedge resections of the ovaries sometimes restored fertility. It is now believed that a variety of enzymes involved in androgen biosynthesis are poorly regulated in polycystic ovarian disease. Recent studies link polycystic ovarian disease, like type II diabetes, to insulin resistance. Administration of insulin mediators has been associated with resumption of ovulation.[97]

Stromal hyperthecosis, also called cortical stromal hyperplasia, is a disorder of ovarian stroma most commonly seen in postmenopausal women, but it may blend with polycystic ovarian disease in younger women. The disorder is characterized by uniform enlargement of the ovary (up to 7 cm) with a white to tan appearance on sectioning. The involvement is usually bilateral and microscopically consists of hypercellular stroma with luteinization of the stromal cells, which are visible as discrete nests with vacuolated cytoplasm. The clinical presentation and effects on the endometrium are similar to those of polycystic ovarian disease, although virilization may be striking.[95]

A physiologic condition mimicking the above syndromes is *theca lutein hyperplasia of pregnancy*. In response to pregnancy

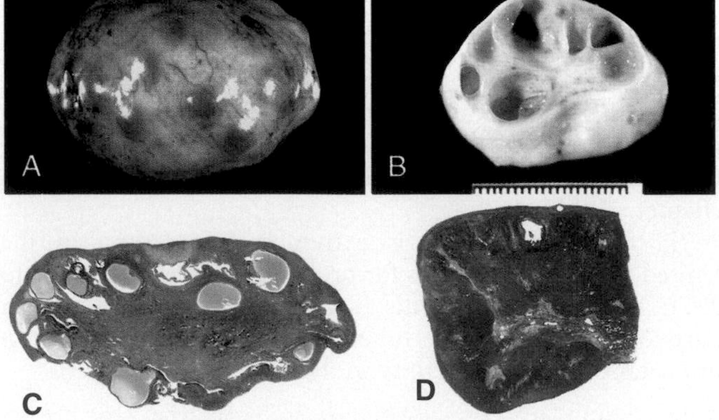

FIGURE 22–36 Polycystic ovarian disease and cortical stromal hyperplasia. *A,* The ovarian cortex reveals numerous clear cysts. *B,* Sectioning of the cortex reveals several subcortical cystic follicles. *C,* Cystic follicles seen in a low-power microphotograph. *D,* Cortical stromal hyperplasia manifests as diffuse stromal proliferation with symmetrical enlargement of the ovary.

hormones (gonadotropins), proliferation of theca cells with expansion of the perifollicular zone occurs. As the follicles regress, the concentric theca-lutein hyperplasia may appear nodular. This change is not to be confused with true luteomas of pregnancy (see below).

Ovarian Tumors

Tumors of the ovary are common forms of neoplasia in women.[98] Among cancers of the female genital tract, the incidence of ovarian cancer ranks below only carcinoma of the cervix and the endometrium. Ovarian cancer accounts for 6% of all cancers in the female and is the fifth most common form of cancer in women in the United States (excluding skin cancer). In addition, because many of these ovarian neoplasms cannot be detected early in their development, they account for a disproportionate number of fatal cancers, being responsible for almost half of the deaths from cancer of the female genital tract. There are numerous types of ovarian tumors, both benign and malignant. About 80% are benign, and these occur mostly in young women between the ages of 20 and 45 years. The malignant tumors are more common in older women between the ages of 40 and 65 years.

Pathogenesis. Risk factors for ovarian cancer are much less clear than for other genital tumors, but nulliparity, family history, and heritable mutations play a role in tumor development.[94,99] There is a higher frequency of carcinoma in unmarried women and in married women with low parity. Gonadal dysgenesis in children is associated with a higher risk of ovarian cancer. Women 40 to 59 years of age who have taken oral contraceptives or undergone tubal ligation have a reduced risk of developing ovarian cancer.[100,101] The most intriguing risk factors are genetic.[102] As discussed in Chapters 7 and 23, mutations in both *BRCA1* and *BRCA2* increase susceptibility to ovarian cancer.[94,99] *BRCA1* mutations occur in about 5% of patients younger than 70 years of age with ovarian cancer. The estimated risk of ovarian cancer in women bearing *BRCA1* or *BRCA2* mutations is 20% to 60% by the age of 70 years.[99] Most of these cancers are serous cystadenocarcinomas. Approximately 30% of ovarian adenocarcinomas express high levels of *HER2/neu* (ERB-B2) oncogene, which correlates with a poor prognosis. Mutations in the tumor-suppressor gene *p53* are found in 50% of ovarian carcinomas.[99]

TABLE 22–3 Ovarian Neoplasms (1993 WHO Classification)

Surface Epithelial-Stromal Tumors

- Serous tumors
  - Benign (cystadenoma)
  - Cystadenoma of borderline malignancy
  - Malignant (serous cystadenocarcinoma)
- Mucinous tumors, endocervical-like and intestinal type
  - Benign
  - Of borderline malignancy
  - Malignant
- Endometrioid tumors
  - Benign
  - Of borderline malignancy
  - Malignant
  - Epithelial-stromal
    - Adenosarcoma
    - Mesodermal (müllerian) mixed tumor
  - Clear cell tumors
    - Benign
    - Of borderline malignancy
    - Malignant
  - Transitional cell tumors
    - Brenner tumor
    - Brenner tumor of borderline malignancy
    - Malignant Brenner tumor
    - Transitional cell carcinoma (non-Brenner type)

Sex Cord–Stromal Tumors

- Granulosa-stromal cell tumors
  - Granulosa cell tumors
  - Tumors of the thecoma-fibroma group
- Sertoli-stromal cell tumors; androblastomas
- Sex cord tumor with annular tubules
- Gynandroblastoma
- Steroid (lipid) cell tumors

Germ Cell Tumors

- Teratoma
  - Immature
  - Mature (adult)
    - Solid
    - Cystic (dermoid cyst)
  - Monodermal (e.g., struma ovarii, carcinoid)
- Dysgerminoma
- Yolk sac tumor (endodermal sinus tumor)
- Mixed germ cell tumors

Malignant, Not Otherwise Specified

Metastatic Nonovarian Cancer (from Nonovarian Primary)

Data from the WHO Classification. (Courtesy Dr. Robert Scully, Massachusetts General Hospital, Boston, MA.)

Classification. The classification of ovarian tumors given in Table 22–3 and Figure 22–37 is a simplified version of the World Health Organization Histological Classification, which separates ovarian neoplasms according to the most probable tissue of origin. It is now believed that tumors of the ovary arise ultimately from one of three ovarian components: (1) surface epithelium derived from either the coelomic epithelium or ectopic endometrial epithelium (see endometriosis, later). The former gives rise to the müllerian epithelium during embryonic development. From it are derived the fallopian tubes (ciliated columnar serous cells), the endometrial lining (nonciliated, columnar cells), or the endocervical glands (mucinous nonciliated cells); (2) the germ cells, which migrate to the ovary from the yolk sac and are totipotential; and (3) the stroma of the ovary, which includes the sex cords, forerunners of the endocrine apparatus of the postnatal ovary. There is, as usual, a group of tumors that defy classification, and finally there are secondary or metastatic tumors, the ovary being a common site of metastases from a variety of other cancers.

Although some of the specific tumors have distinctive features and are hormonally active, most are nonfunctional and tend to produce relatively mild symptoms until they have reached a large size. Malignant tumors have usually spread outside the ovary by the time a definitive diagnosis is made. Some of these tumors, principally epithelial tumors, tend to be bilateral. Table 22–4 lists these tumors and their subtypes and shows the frequency of bilateral occurrence. Abdominal pain and distention, urinary and gastrointestinal tract symptoms due to compression by tumor or cancer invasion, and abdominal and vaginal bleeding are the most common symptoms. The benign forms may be entirely asymptomatic and occasionally are unexpected findings on abdominal or pelvic examination or during surgery.

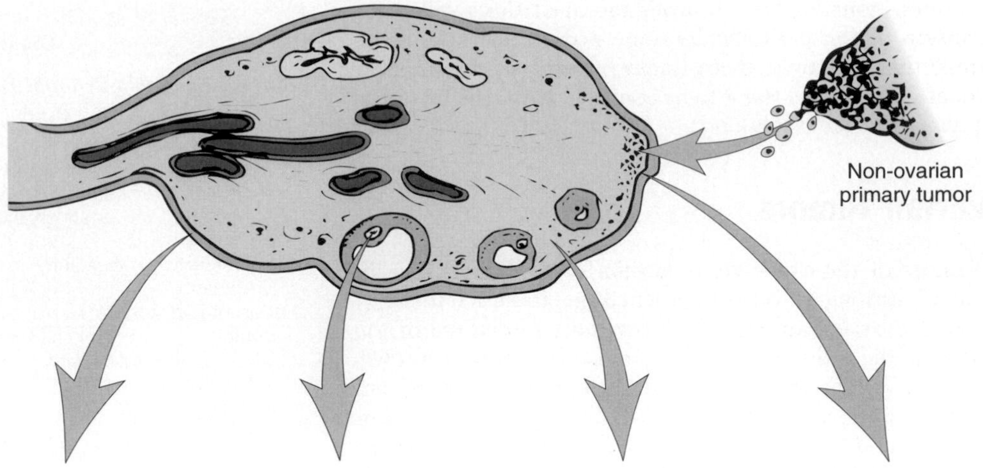

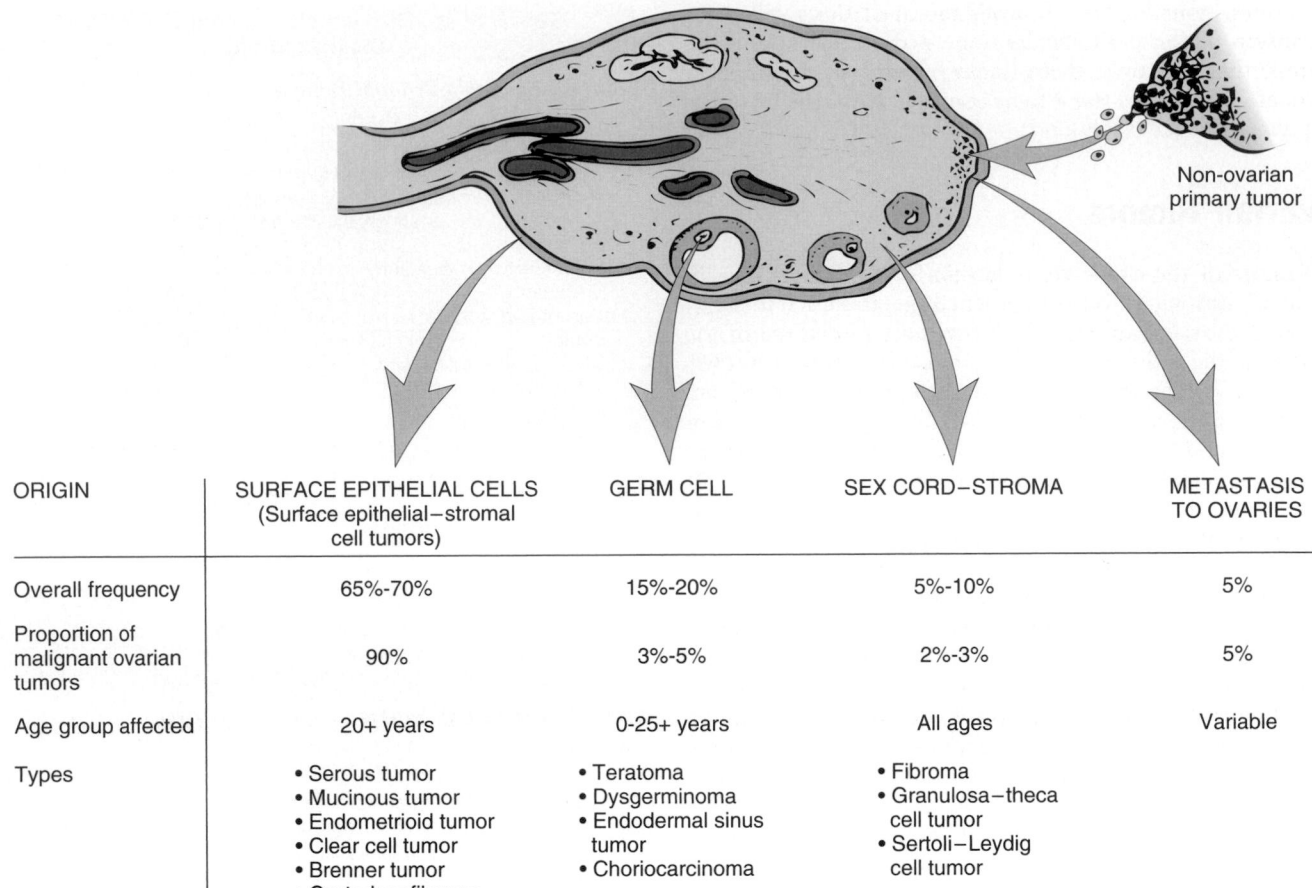

ORIGIN	SURFACE EPITHELIAL CELLS (Surface epithelial–stromal cell tumors)	GERM CELL	SEX CORD–STROMA	METASTASIS TO OVARIES
Overall frequency	65%-70%	15%-20%	5%-10%	5%
Proportion of malignant ovarian tumors	90%	3%-5%	2%-3%	5%
Age group affected	20+ years	0-25+ years	All ages	Variable
Types	• Serous tumor • Mucinous tumor • Endometrioid tumor • Clear cell tumor • Brenner tumor • Cystadenofibroma	• Teratoma • Dysgerminoma • Endodermal sinus tumor • Choriocarcinoma	• Fibroma • Granulosa–theca cell tumor • Sertoli–Leydig cell tumor	

FIGURE 22–37 Derivation of various ovarian neoplasms and some data on their frequency and age distribution.

TABLE 22–4 Frequency of Major Ovarian Tumors

Type	Percentage of Malignant Ovarian Tumors	Percentage That Are Bilateral
Serous	40	
Benign (60%)		25
Borderline (15%)		30
Malignant (25%)		65
Mucinous	10	
Benign (80%)		5
Borderline (10%)		10
Malignant (10%)		<5
Endometrioid carcinoma	20	40
Undifferentiated carcinoma	10	—
Clear cell carcinoma	6	40
Granulosa cell tumor	5	5
Teratoma		15
Benign (96%)		
Malignant (4%)	1	Rare
Metastatic	5	>50
Others	3	—

TUMORS OF MÜLLERIAN EPITHELIUM

Most primary neoplasms in the ovary fall within this category. There are three major types of such tumors: serous, endometrioid and mucinous tumors.[98] These neoplasms range in size and composition. Tumors may be small and grossly imperceptible or massive, filling the pelvis and even the abdominal cavity. Components of the tumors may include cystic areas (cystadenomas), cystic and fibrous areas (cystadenofibromas), and predominantly fibrous areas (adenofibromas). On gross examination, *the risk of malignancy increases as a function of the amount of discernible solid epithelial growth,* including papillary projections of soft tumor, thickened tumor lining the cyst spaces, or solid necrotic friable tissue depicting necrosis.

The most widely accepted theory for the derivation of müllerian epithelial tumors is through the transformation of coelomic mesothelium. This view is based on the embryologic pathway by which the müllerian *ducts are formed and evolve into serous (tubal), endometrioid (endometrium), and mucinous (cervix)* epithelia present in the normal female genital tract (see the section on anatomy). Such tumors occur predominantly in the ovary because coelomic epithelium is incorporated into the ovarian cortex to form mesothelial inclusion cysts. This incorporation occurs by the formation of surface adhesions, atrophy with epithelial infolding, and repair of ovulation sites. The close association of ovarian carcinomas with either the ovarian surface mesothelium or inclusion cysts may explain the development of extraovarian carcinomas of similar histology from similar coelomic epithelial rests (so-called endosalpingiosis) in the mesentery.[98] However, this is clearly an oversimplification of the pathogenesis of ovarian cancer. For example, endometrioid carcinomas may be derived from transplanted endometriosis, and some ovarian serous and mucinous (müllerian mucinous) tumors arise in association with endometriosis.[98] The origin of most mucinous tumors is unclear. Some arise within endometriosis; other proposed origins include teratomatous epithelium.

An intriguing question is the origin of the cortical müllerian inclusion cyst (CIC) and its relationship to serous carcinomas (Fig. 22–38). The continuity of pelvic mesothelium with these müllerian cysts suggests that the former gives rise to the latter. However, similarities between some of these cysts and endometrial or tubal epithelium raise the possibility of a uterine or tubal origin for the epithelium. Direct links between CICs and serous carcinoma are not common and studies of ovaries from women with *BRCA* mutations have not disclosed premalignant changes in these cysts.[100] Regardless of their specific origin(s), ovarian epithelial tumors composed of serous, mucinous, and endometrioid cell types are emblematic of the plasticity of müllerian epithelium and range from clearly benign, to tumors of borderline malignancy, to malignant tumors.[98]

Serous Tumors

These common cystic neoplasms are lined by tall, columnar, ciliated epithelial cells and are filled with clear serous fluid. Although the term serous appropriately describes the cyst fluid, it has become synonymous with the tubal-like epithelium in these tumors. Together the benign, borderline, and malignant types account for about 30% of all ovarian tumors. About 75% are benign or of borderline malignancy, and 25% are malignant. Serous cystadenocarcinomas account for approximately 40% of all cancers of the ovary and are the most common malignant ovarian tumors. Benign and borderline tumors are most common between the ages of 20 and 50 years. Cystadenocarcinomas occur later in life on average, although somewhat earlier in familial cases.

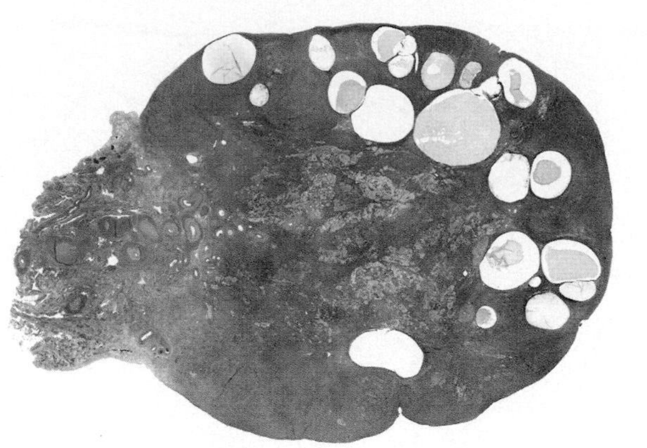

FIGURE 22–38 Cortical inclusion cysts of the ovary. These cysts appear to arise from the overlying mesothelium and are presumed to be the site of origin for many ovarian epithelial neoplasms. Another source of ovarian epithelium neoplasia is endometriosis (see Figure 22–29).

Morphology. The characteristic serous tumor may present on gross examination as either a cystic lesion in which the papillary epithelium is contained within a few fibrous walled cysts (intracystic) (Fig. 22–39*A*), or projecting from the ovarian surface. Benign tumors typically present with a smooth glistening cyst wall with no epithelial thickening or with small papillary projections (i.e., papillary cystadenoma). Borderline tumors contain an increased number of papillary projections (Fig. 22–39*A* and *B*). Larger amounts of solid or papillary tumor mass, irregularity in the tumor mass, and fixation or nodularity of the capsule are all important indicators of probable malignancy (Fig. 22–39*B*). Bilaterality is common, occurring in 20% of benign cystadenomas, 30% of borderline tumors, and approximately 66% of cystadenocarcinomas. A significant proportion of both borderline and malignant serous tumors involve (or originate from) the surface of the ovary (Fig. 22–39*C*). On histologic examination, the lining epithelium is composed of columnar epithelium with abundant cilia in benign tumors (Fig. 22–40). Microscopic papillae may be found. Tumors of borderline malignancy contain increased complexity of

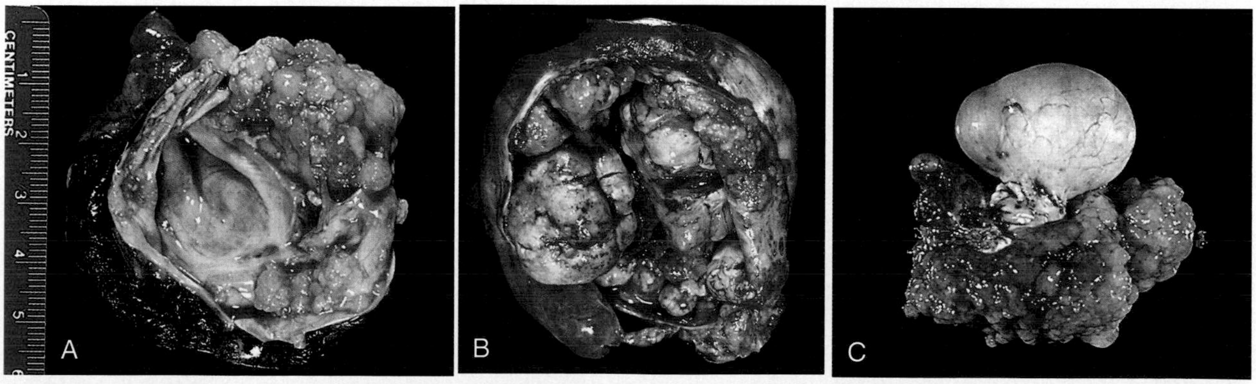

FIGURE 22–39 *A*, Borderline serous cystadenoma opened to display a cyst cavity lined by delicate papillary tumor growths. *B*, Cystadenocarcinoma. The cyst is opened to reveal a large, bulky tumor mass. *C*, Another borderline tumor growing on the ovarian surface (*lower*).

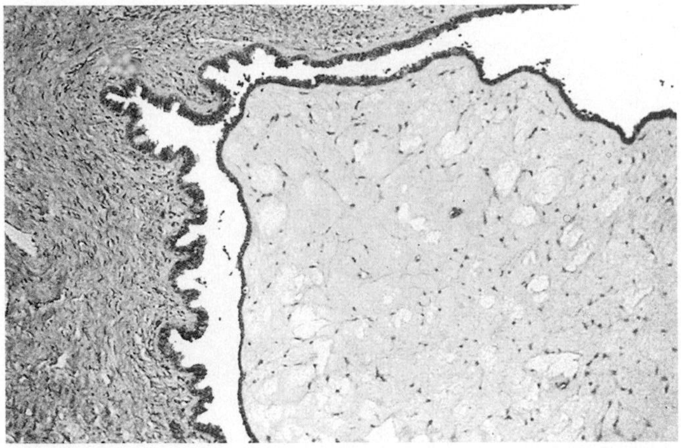

FIGURE 22–40 Papillary serous cystadenoma revealing stromal papillae with a columnar epithelium.

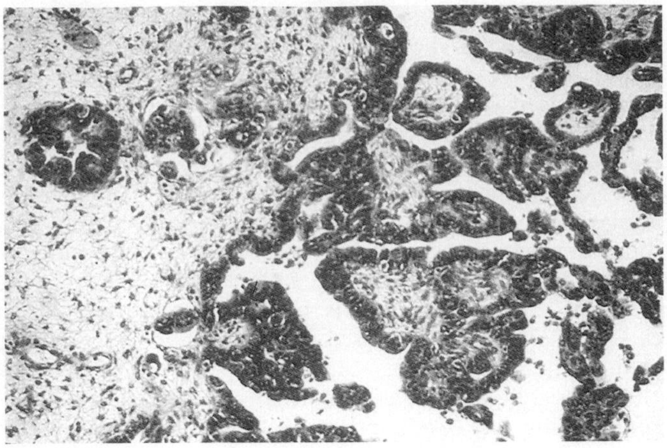

FIGURE 22–42 Papillary serous cystadenocarcinoma of the ovary with invasion of underlying stroma.

the stromal papillae with stratification of the epithelium and nuclear atypia, but destructive infiltrative growth into the stroma is not seen (Fig. 22–41).[98] Cystadenocarcinomas exhibit even more complex growth with infiltration or frank effacement of the underlying stroma by solid tumor (Fig. 22–42). The individual tumor cells in the carcinomatous lesions display the usual features of all malignant neoplasia, and with the more extreme degrees of atypia, the cells may become undifferentiated. Concentric calcifications (psammoma bodies) characterize serous tumors, although they are not specific for neoplasia when they are found alone.

A small number of tumors have been described that share features of both borderline and malignant serous neoplasms, exhibiting epithelial complexity and a greater risk of invasive peritoneal implants (Fig. 22–43). These so-called micropapillary serous carcinomas may account in part for the occasional aggressive behavior of "borderline" serous cystadenomas.[103]

Is there a relationship between borderline and malignant serous neoplasia? Studies of women with *BRCA* mutations have not shown an increase in risk of borderline neoplasms, underscoring differences in pathogenesis for these two histologically similar but biologically distinct tumors.[104]

The biologic behavior of serous tumors depends on degree of differentiation, distribution, and characteristics of the peritoneal implants, if present. Importantly, serous tumors may occur on the surface of the ovaries and, rarely, as primary tumors of the peritoneal surface (Fig. 22–39*B*). Predictably, unencapsulated serous tumors of the ovarian surface are more likely to extend to the peritoneal surfaces, and prognosis is closely related to the histologic appearance of the tumor and its growth pattern on the peritoneum. Peritoneal spread may manifest as noninvasive or invasive implants, the latter signifying malignancy. Borderline tumors may arise from or extend to the peritoneal surfaces as noninvasive implants, remaining localized and causing no symptoms, or slowly spread, producing intestinal obstruction or other complications after many years. Implants of carcinomas invade the adjacent stroma inducing desmoplasia (invasive implants) and may form large intra-abdominal masses with rapid clinical deterioration.[98] Consequently, careful pathologic classification of the tumor, even if it has extended to the peritoneum, is rele-

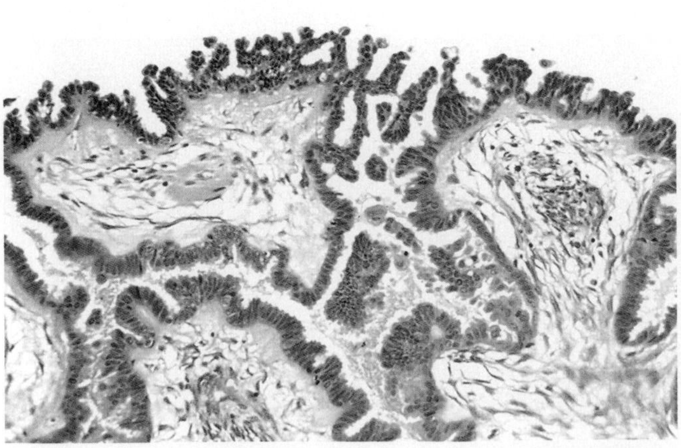

FIGURE 22–41 Borderline serous cystadenoma exhibiting increased architectural complexity and epithelial cell stratification.

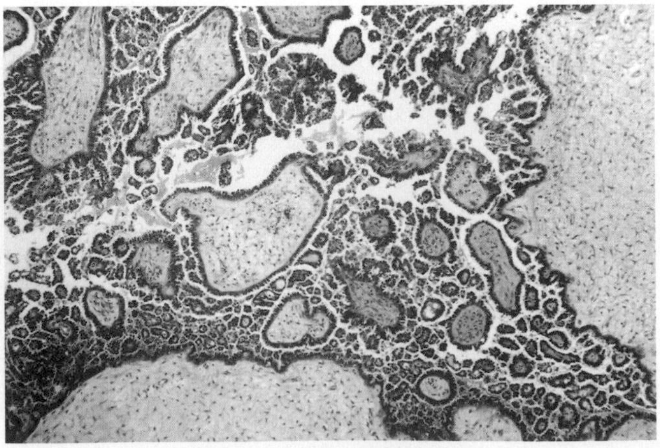

FIGURE 22–43 Complex micropapillary growth defines a low grade "micropapillary" serous carcinoma.

vant to both prognosis and selection of therapy.[98,104] The 5-year survival rate for borderline and malignant tumors confined within the ovarian mass is, respectively, 100% and 70%, whereas the 5-year survival rate for the same tumors involving the peritoneum is about 90% and 25%, respectively. Because of their protracted course, borderline tumors may recur after many years, and 5-year survival is not synonymous with cure.[98]

Mucinous Tumors

These tumors closely resemble their serous counterparts. They are somewhat less common, accounting for about 25% of all ovarian neoplasms. They occur principally in middle adult life and are rare before puberty and after menopause. Eighty per cent are benign or borderline, and about 15% are malignant. Mucinous cystadenocarcinomas are relatively uncommon and account for only 10% of all ovarian cancers.

Morphology. In gross appearance, the mucinous tumors differ from the serous variety in several ways. They are characterized by more cysts of variable size and a rarity of surface involvement. They are less frequently bilateral. Approximately 5% of primary mucinous cystadenomas and mucinous cystadenocarcinomas are bilateral. Mucinous tumors tend to produce larger cystic masses, and some have been recorded with weights of more than 25 kg. They appear grossly as multiloculated tumors filled with sticky, gelatinous fluid rich in glycoproteins (Fig. 22–44*A*).

On histologic examination, benign mucinous tumors are characterized by a lining of tall columnar epithelial cells with apical mucin and the absence of cilia, akin to benign cervical or intestinal epithelia (Fig. 22–44*B*). One group of typically benign or borderline mucinous tumors arises in endometriosis and is termed "müllerian mucinous" cystadenoma, resembling endometrial or cervical epithelium.[98] These tumors are uncommonly malignant. The second, more common group includes tumors exhibiting abundant gland-like or papillary growth with nuclear atypia and stratification and is strikingly similar to tubular adenomas or villous adenomas of the intestine. These tumors are presumed precursors to most cystadenocarcinomas. Cystadenocarcinomas contain more solid growth with conspicuous epithelial cell atypia and stratification, loss of gland architecture, and necrosis, and are similar to colonic cancer in appearance. Because both borderline and malignant mucinous cystadenomas form complex glands in the stroma, the documentation of clear-cut stromal invasion, which is easily ascertained in serous tumors, is more difficult. Some authors describe a category of "noninvasive" mucinous carcinomas (intraepithelial carcinomas) for those tumors with marked epithelial atypia without obvious stromal alterations.[105] Approximate 10-year survival rates for stage I borderline, noninvasive malignant, and frankly invasive malignant tumors are greater than 95%, 90%, and 66%, respectively.[106]

A condition associated with mucinous ovarian neoplasms is *pseudomyxoma peritonei.* This disorder consists of an ovarian tumor with extensive mucinous ascites, cystic epithelial implants on the peritoneal surfaces, and adhesions (Fig. 22–45*A* and *B*). Pseudomyxoma peritonei, if extensive, may result in intestinal obstruction and death. Recent evidence points to the presence of, in most cases, extraovarian (usually appendiceal) primary mucinous tumor with secondary ovarian and peritoneal spread[107] (Chapter 17). Bilateral presentation of mucinous tumors always requires exclusion of a non-ovarian origin.

Endometrioid Tumors

These neoplasms account for approximately 20% of all ovarian cancers, excluding endometriosis, which is considered non-neoplastic. Most endometrioid tumors are carcinomas. Less commonly, benign forms—usually cystadenofibromas—

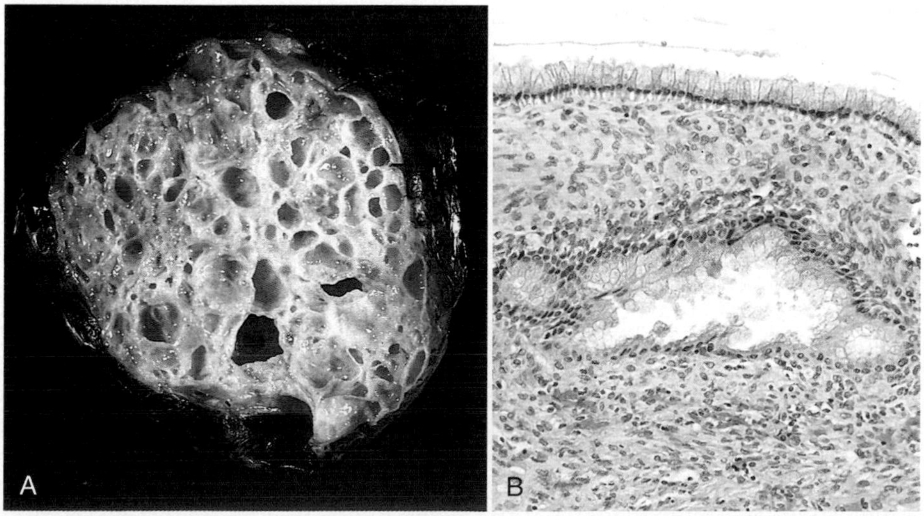

FIGURE 22–44 *A*, A mucinous cystadenoma with its multicystic appearance and delicate septa. Note the presence of glistening mucin within the cysts. *B*, Columnar cell lining of mucinous cystadenoma.

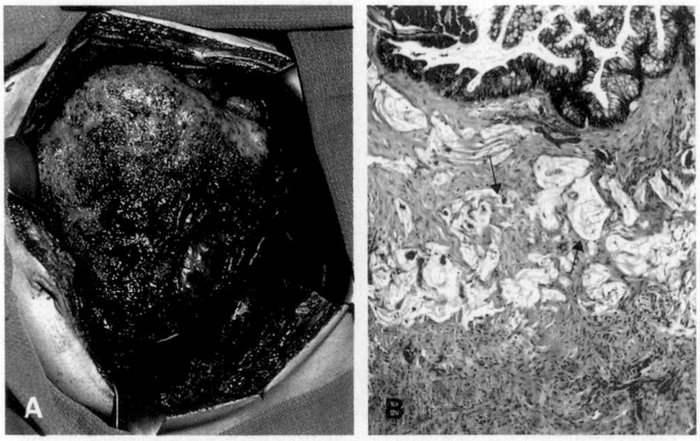

FIGURE 22–45 *A*, Pseudomyxoma peritonei viewed at laparotomy revealing massive overgrowth of a gelatinous metastatic tumor originating from the appendix. (Courtesy of Dr. Paul H. Sugarbaker, Washington Hospital Cancer Center, Washington, DC.). *B*, Histology of peritoneal implants from an appendiceal tumor, showing mucin-producing epithelium and free mucin (*arrows*).

are encountered.[108] They are distinguished from serous and mucinous tumors by the presence of tubular glands bearing a close resemblance to benign or malignant endometrium. Fifteen per cent to 30% of endometrioid carcinomas are accompanied by a carcinoma of the endometrium, and the relatively good prognosis in such cases suggests that the two may arise independently rather than by metastatic spread from one another.[109] About 15% of cases with endometrioid carcinoma coexist with endometriosis, although an origin directly from ovarian coelomic epithelium is also possible.

Morphology. In gross appearance, endometrioid carcinomas present as a combination of solid and cystic areas, similar to other cystadenocarcinomas. Forty per cent involve both ovaries, and such bilaterality usually, although not always, implies extension of the neoplasm beyond the genital tract. On histologic examination, glandular patterns bearing a strong resemblance to those of endometrial origin are seen. The 5-year survival rate for patients with stage I tumors is approximately 75%.

Clear Cell Adenocarcinoma

This uncommon pattern of surface epithelial tumor of the ovary is characterized by large epithelial cells with abundant clear cytoplasm. Because these tumors sometimes occur in association with endometriosis or endometrioid carcinoma of the ovary and resemble clear cell carcinoma of the endometrium, they are now thought to be of müllerian duct origin and variants of endometrioid adenocarcinoma.[98] The clear cell tumors of the ovary can be predominantly solid or cystic. In the solid neoplasm, the clear cells are arranged in sheets or tubules. In the cystic variety, the neoplastic cells line the spaces. The 5-year survival rate is approximately 65% when the tumors are confined to the ovaries; however, these tumors tend to be aggressive, and with spread beyond the ovary, a survival of 5 years is exceptional.

Cystadenofibroma

Cystadenofibromas are variants in which there is more pronounced proliferation of the fibrous stroma that underlies the columnar lining epithelium. These benign tumors are usually small and multilocular and have simple papillary processes that do not become so complicated and branching as those found in the ordinary cystadenoma. They may be composed of mucinous, serous, endometrioid, and transitional (Brenner tumors) epithelium. Borderline lesions with cellular atypia and, rarely, tumors with focal carcinoma occur, but metastatic spread of either is extremely uncommon.

Brenner Tumor

Brenner tumors are uncommon adenofibromas in which the epithelial component consists of nests of transitional cells resembling those lining the urinary bladder. Less frequently, the nests contain microcysts or glandular spaces lined by columnar, mucin-secreting cells. For unknown reasons, Brenner tumors are occasionally encountered in mucinous cystadenomas.

Morphology. These neoplasms may be solid or cystic, are usually unilateral (approximately 90%), and vary in size from small lesions less than 1 cm in diameter to massive tumors up to 20 and 30 cm (Fig. 22–46*A*). The fibrous stroma, resembling that of the normal ovary, is marked by sharply demarcated nests of epithelial cells resembling the epithelium of the urinary tract, often with mucinous glands in their center (Fig. 22–46*B*). Infrequently, the stroma is composed of somewhat plump fibroblasts resembling theca cells, and such neoplasms may have hormonal activity. Most Brenner tumors are benign, but borderline (proliferative Brenner tumor) and malignant counterparts have been reported.

Several reports have emphasized the occurrence of ovarian tumors that are composed in part or all of neoplastic epithelium similar to transitional carcinoma of the bladder but without a coexisting Brenner component. Although often referred to as *transitional cell carcinoma*, these tumors are frequently seen in association with conventional serous or endometrioid carcinomas and likely represent altered differentiation patterns of the tumor cells.

Clinical Course, Detection, and Prevention of Surface Epithelial Tumors

All ovarian epithelial carcinomas produce similar clinical manifestations, most commonly lower abdominal pain and abdominal enlargement. Gastrointestinal complaints, urinary frequency, dysuria, pelvic pressure, and many other symptoms may appear. Benign lesions are easily resected, with cure. The malignant forms, however, tend to cause the progressive weakness, weight loss, and cachexia characteristic of all malignant neoplasms. If the carcinomas extend through the capsule of the tumor to seed the peritoneal cavity, massive ascites is common. Characteristically, the ascitic fluid is filled with diagnostic exfoliated tumor cells. The peritoneal seeding that these

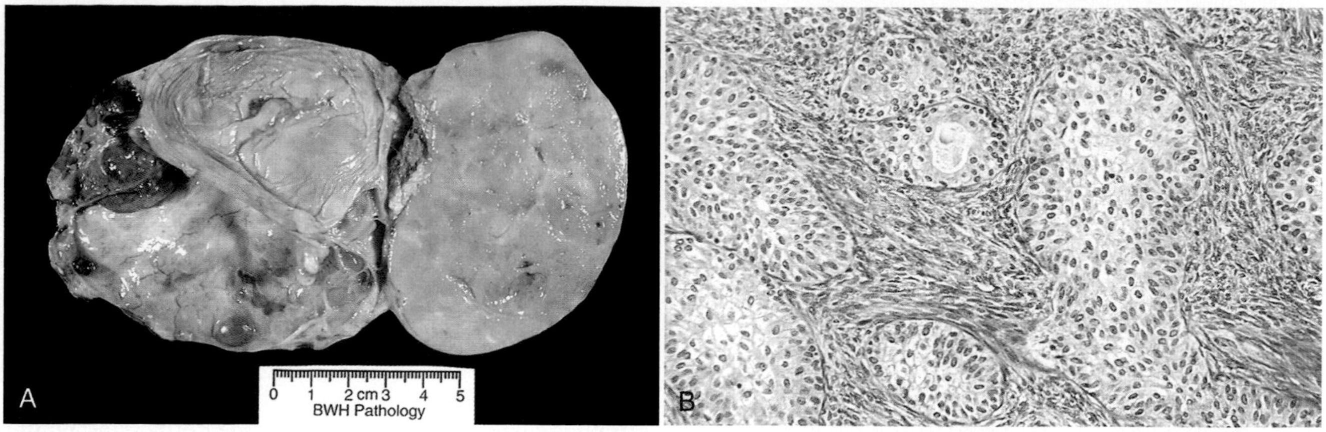

FIGURE 22–46 *A*, Brenner tumor (*right*) associated with a benign cystic teratoma (*left*). *B*, Histologic detail of characteristic epithelial nests within the ovarian stroma. (Courtesy of Dr. M. Nucci, Brigham and Women's Hospital, Boston, MA.)

malignant neoplasms produce is distinctive: they tend to seed all serosal surfaces diffusely with 0.1 to 0.5 cm nodules of tumor. These surface implants rarely invade deeply into the underlying parenchyma of the organ. The regional nodes are often involved, and metastases may be found in the liver, lungs, gastrointestinal tract, and elsewhere. Metastasis across the midline to the opposite ovary is discovered in about half the cases by the time of laparotomy and heralds a progressive downhill course to death within a few months or years.

Because ovarian carcinomas often remain undiagnosed until they are large, or originate on the ovarian surface from where they readily spread to the pelvis, many patients are first seen with lesions that are no longer confined to the ovary. This is perhaps the primary reason for the relatively poor 5- and 10-year survival rates for these patients, compared with rates in cervical and endometrial carcinoma. For these reasons, both early diagnosis and prevention are top priorities. Specific biochemical markers for tumor antigens or tumor products in the plasma of these patients are being sought vigorously. One such marker is a high-molecular-weight glycoprotein present in more than 80% of serous and endometrioid carcinomas, known as CA-125. Whether its use will influence outcome is unproven.[110] Newly identified biomarkers such as osteopontin, which is expressed at significantly higher levels in ovarian cancer patients, may improve early detection.[111] Assays based on proteomics attempt to distinguish cancer patients from non-affected individuals through patterns of circulating proteins generated by mass spectroscopic analysis of patient sera.[112] These and other approaches may, in the future, create a more cost-effective, noninvasive approach to ovarian cancer screening, but still need to be validated.

Prevention of ovarian cancer remains an elusive goal, but both fallopian tubal ligation and oral contraceptive therapy are associated with significant reductions in relative risk. Long-term contraceptive use has reduced risk by half in patients with a family history of ovarian cancer.[100] Tubal ligation reduces risk by more than half and may be effective in subsets of women with *BRCA* mutations and family history of ovarian cancer.[99,101,113] Screening strategies based on identifying women at risk (positive for *BRCA* mutations) and employing prophylactic oophorectomy are currently standard, but the long-term impact of these approaches on ovarian cancer death rates remains to be determined.

GERM CELL TUMORS

Germ cell tumors constitute 15% to 20% of all ovarian tumors.[98] Most are benign cystic teratomas, but the remainder, which are found principally in children and young adults, have a higher incidence of malignant behavior and pose problems in histologic diagnosis and in therapy. They bear a remarkable homology to germ cell tumors in the male testis, (Chapter 21) and arise from germ cell differentiation in a similar manner (Fig. 22–47).

Teratomas

Teratomas are divided into three categories: (1) mature (benign), (2) immature (malignant), and (3) monodermal or highly specialized.

Mature (Benign) Teratomas. Most benign teratomas are cystic and are better known in clinical parlance as *dermoid cysts*. These neoplasms are presumably derived from the ectodermal differentiation of totipotential cells. Cystic teratomas are usually found in young women during the active reproductive years.[98]

Morphology. Benign teratomas are bilateral in 10% to 15% of cases. Characteristically, they are unilocular cysts containing hair and cheesy sebaceous material (Fig. 22–48). On section, they reveal a thin wall lined by an opaque, gray-white, wrinkled, apparent epider-

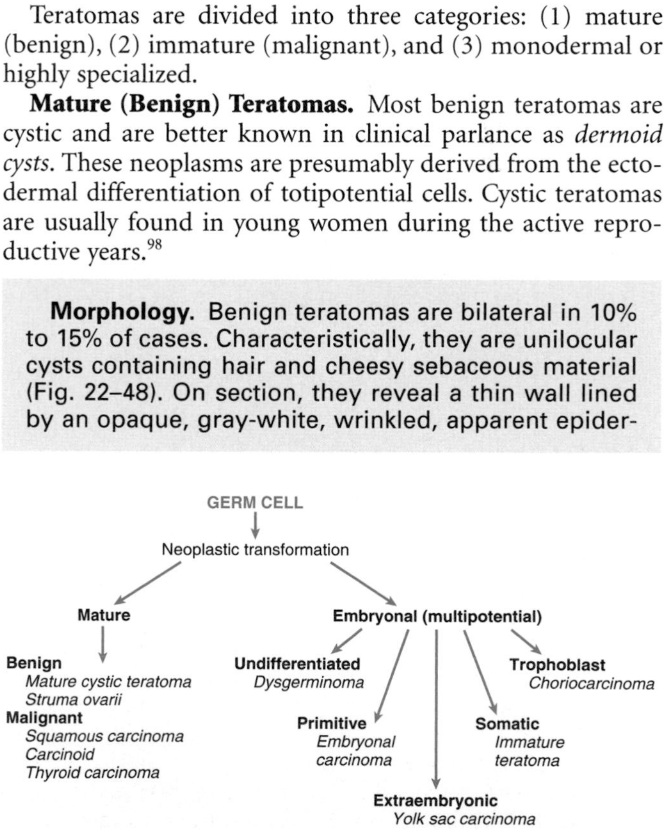

FIGURE 22–47 Histogenesis and interrelationships of tumors of germ cell origin.

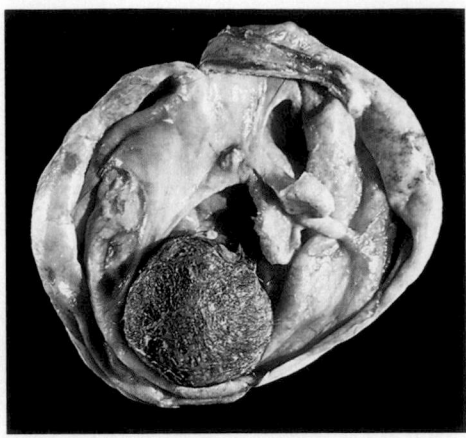

FIGURE 22–48 Opened mature cystic teratoma (dermoid cyst) of the ovary. Hair (*bottom*) and a mixture of tissues are evident.

mis. From this epidermis, hair shafts frequently protrude. Within the wall, it is common to find tooth structures and areas of calcification.

On histologic examination, the cyst wall is composed of stratified squamous epithelium with underlying sebaceous glands, hair shafts, and other skin adnexal structures (Fig. 22–49). In most cases, structures from other germ layers can be identified, such as cartilage, bone, thyroid tissue, and other organoid formations. Dermoid cysts are sometimes incorporated within the wall of a mucinous cystadenoma. **About 1% of the dermoids undergo malignant transformation of any one of the component elements (e.g., thyroid carcinoma, melanoma, but most commonly, squamous cell carcinoma).**

In rare instances, a teratoma is solid but is composed entirely of benign-looking heterogeneous collections of tissues and organized structures derived from all three germ layers. These tumors presumably have the same histogenetic origin as dermoid cysts but lack preponderant differentiation into ectodermal derivatives. These neoplasms may be initially difficult to differentiate from the malignant, immature teratomas, which almost always are largely solid.

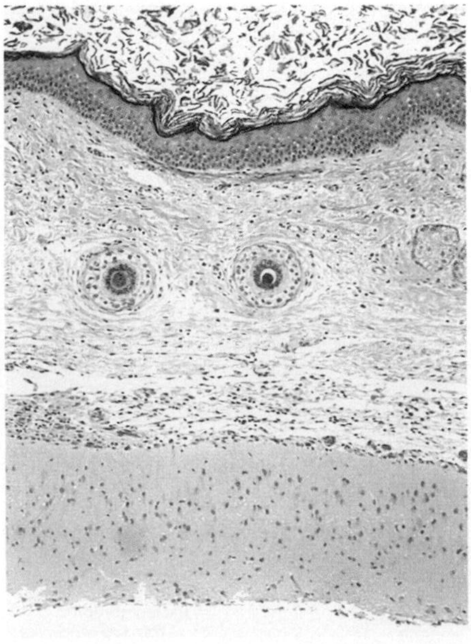

FIGURE 22–49 Benign cystic teratoma. Low-power view of skin (*top*), beneath which there is brain tissue (*bottom*).

The origin of teratomas has been a matter of fascination for centuries. Some common beliefs blamed witches, nightmares, or adultery with the devil. The current parthenogenetic theory suggests origin from a meiotic germ cell. The karyotype of all benign ovarian teratomas is 46,XX. From the results of chromosome banding techniques and the distribution of electrophoretic variants of enzymes in the normal and teratoma cells, Linder and coworkers suggested that tumors arise from an ovum after the first meiotic division.[114] Other derivations have been proposed.[115]

Monodermal or Specialized Teratomas. The specialized teratomas are a remarkable, rare group of tumors, the most common of which are struma ovarii and carcinoid. They are always unilateral, although a contralateral teratoma may be present. Struma ovarii is composed entirely of mature thyroid tissue. Interestingly, these thyroidal neoplasms may hyperfunction, causing hyperthyroidism. The ovarian carcinoid, which presumably arises from intestinal epithelium in a teratoma, might in fact be functioning, particularly in large (greater than 7 cm) tumors, producing 5-hydroxytryptamine and the carcinoid syndrome. Primary ovarian carcinoid can be distinguished from metastatic intestinal carcinoid, the latter virtually always bilateral. Even more rare is the strumal carcinoid, a combination of struma ovarii and carcinoid in the same ovary. Primary carcinoids are uncommonly (less than 2%) malignant.

Immature Malignant Teratomas. These are rare tumors that differ from benign teratomas in that the component tissue resembles that observed in the fetus or embryo rather than in the adult. The tumor is found chiefly in prepubertal adolescents and young women, the mean age being 18 years.[116]

Morphology. The tumors are bulky and have a smooth external surface. On section, they have a solid (or predominantly solid) structure. There are areas of necrosis and hemorrhage. Hair, grumous material, cartilage, bone, and calcification may be present. On microscopic examination, there are varying amounts of immature tissue differentiating toward cartilage, glands, bone, muscle, nerve, and others. An important risk for subsequent extraovarian spread is the histologic grade of tumor (I through III), which is based on the proportion of tissue (in histologic sections) containing immature neuroepithelium (Fig. 22–50).

Immature teratomas grow rapidly and frequently penetrate the capsule with local spread or metastases. Stage I tumors, however, particularly those with low-grade (grade 1) histology, have an excellent prognosis. Higher-grade tumors confined to the ovary are generally treated with prophylactic chemotherapy. Most recurrences develop in the first 2 years, and absence of disease beyond this period carries an excellent chance of cure.

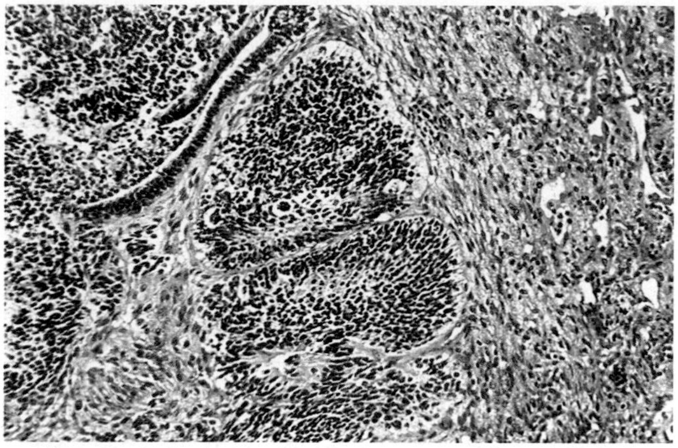

FIGURE 22–50 Immature teratoma of the ovary illustrating primitive neuroepithelium.

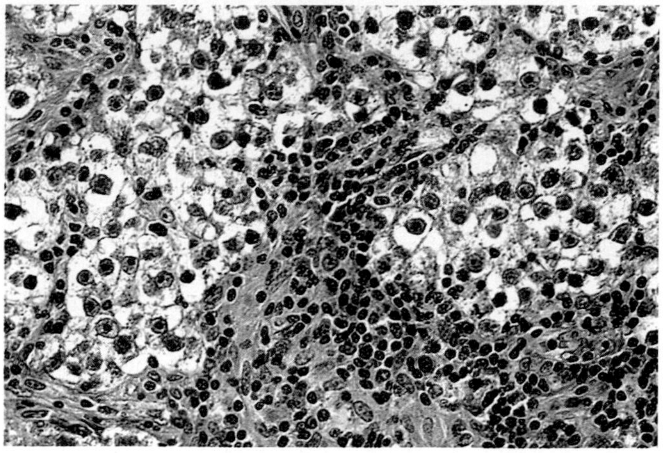

FIGURE 22–51 Dysgerminoma showing polyhedral tumor cells with round nuclei and adjacent inflammation.

Dysgerminoma

The dysgerminoma[117] is best considered as the ovarian counterpart of the seminoma of the testis. Similar to the seminoma, it is composed of large vesicular cells having a clear cytoplasm, well-defined cell boundaries, and centrally placed regular nuclei. Relatively uncommon tumors, the dysgerminomas account for about 2% of all ovarian cancers yet form about half of malignant germ cell tumors. They may occur in childhood, but 75% occur in the second and third decades. Some occur in patients with gonadal dysgenesis, including pseudohermaphroditism. Most of these tumors have no endocrine function. A few produce elevated levels of chorionic gonadotropin and may have syncytiotrophoblastic giant cells on histologic examination.

Morphology. Usually unilateral (80% to 90%), they most frequently are solid tumors ranging in size from barely visible nodules to masses that virtually fill the entire abdomen. On cut surface, they have a yellow-white to gray-pink appearance and are often soft and fleshy. On histologic examination, the dysgerminoma cells are dispersed in sheets or cords separated by scant fibrous stroma (Fig. 22–51). As in the seminoma, the fibrous stroma is infiltrated with mature lymphocytes and occasional granulomas. On occasion, small nodules of dysgerminoma are encountered in the wall of an otherwise benign cystic teratoma; conversely, a predominantly dysgerminomatous tumor may contain a small cystic teratoma.

All dysgerminomas are malignant, but the degree of histologic atypia is variable, and only about one third are aggressive. Thus, a unilateral tumor that has not broken through the capsule and has not spread has an excellent prognosis (up to 96% cure rate) after simple salpingo-oophorectomy. These neoplasms are extremely radiosensitive, and even those that have extended beyond the ovary can generally be controlled by radiotherapy. Overall survival exceeds 80%.

Endodermal Sinus (Yolk Sac) Tumor

This tumor is rare but is the second most common malignant tumor of germ cell origin. It is thought to be derived from differentiation of malignant germ cells toward extraembryonic yolk sac structure (Fig. 22–47). Similar to the yolk sac, the tumor is rich in α-fetoprotein and α_1-antitrypsin. Its characteristic histologic feature is a glomerulus-like structure composed of a central blood vessel enveloped by germ cells within a space lined by germ cells (Schiller-Duval body) (Fig. 22–52). Similar structures are observed in the yolk sac of the rat placenta. Conspicuous intracellular and extracellular hyaline droplets are present in all tumors, and some of these can be stained for α-fetoprotein by immunoperoxidase techniques.

Most patients are children or young women presenting with abdominal pain and a rapidly developing pelvic mass. The tumors usually appear to involve a single ovary but grow rapidly and aggressively. These tumors were once almost uniformly fatal within 2 years of diagnosis, but combination chemotherapy has measurably improved the outcome.

Choriocarcinoma

More commonly of placental origin, the choriocarcinoma, similar to the endodermal sinus tumor, is an example of extraembryonic differentiation of malignant germ cells. It is

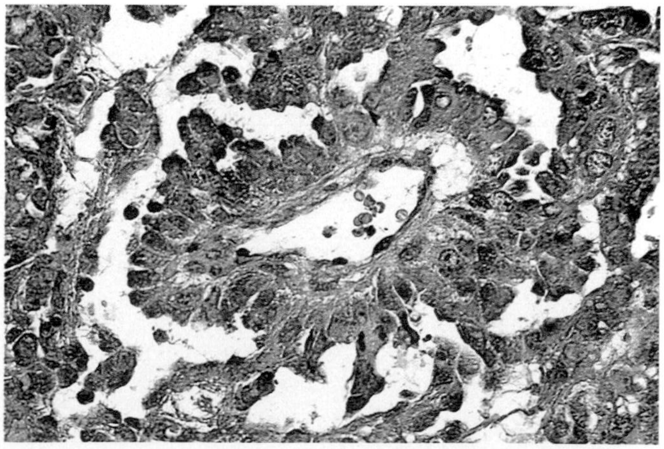

FIGURE 22–52 A Schiller-Duval body in yolk sac carcinoma.

generally held that a germ cell origin can be confirmed only in the prepubertal girl because after this age, an origin from an ovarian ectopic pregnancy cannot be excluded.

Most ovarian choriocarcinomas exist in combination with other germ cell tumors, and pure choriocarcinomas are extremely rare. They are histologically identical with the more common placental lesions, described later. The ovarian primaries are aggressive tumors that generally have metastasized widely through the bloodstream to the lungs, liver, bone, and other viscera by the time of diagnosis. Like all choriocarcinomas, they elaborate high levels of chorionic gonadotropins that are sometimes helpful in establishing the diagnosis or detecting recurrences. In contrast to choriocarcinomas arising in placental tissue, those arising in the ovary are generally unresponsive to chemotherapy and are often fatal.

Other Germ Cell Tumors

These include (1) embryonal carcinoma, another highly malignant tumor of primitive embryonal elements, histologically similar to tumors arising in the testes (Chapter 21);[98] (2) polyembryoma, a malignant tumor containing so-called embryoid bodies; and (3) mixed germ cell tumors containing various combinations of dysgerminoma, teratoma, endodermal sinus tumor, and choriocarcinoma.

SEX CORD–STROMAL TUMORS

These ovarian neoplasms are derived from the ovarian stroma, which in turn is derived from the sex cords of the embryonic gonad. Because the undifferentiated gonadal mesenchyme eventually produces structures of specific cell type in both male (Sertoli and Leydig) and female (granulosa and theca) gonads, tumors resembling all of these cell types can be identified in the ovary.[118] Moreover, because some of these cells normally secrete estrogens (theca cells) or androgens (Leydig cells), their corresponding tumors may be either feminizing (granulosa-theca cell tumors) or masculinizing (Leydig cell tumors).

Granulosa-Theca Cell Tumors

This designation embraces ovarian neoplasms composed of varying proportions of granulosa and theca cell differentiation. These tumors are composed almost entirely of granulosa cells or a mixture of granulosa and theca cells. Collectively, these neoplasms account for about 5% of all ovarian tumors. Although they may be discovered at any age, approximately two thirds occur in postmenopausal women.

Morphology. Granulosa cell tumors are usually unilateral and vary from microscopic foci to large, solid, and cystic encapsulated masses. Tumors that are hormonally active have a yellow coloration to their cut surfaces, produced by contained lipids. The pure thecomas are solid, firm tumors.

The granulosa cell component of these tumors takes one of many histologic patterns. The small, cuboidal to polygonal cells may grow in anastomosing cords, sheets, or strands (Fig. 22–53). In occasional cases, small, distinctive, glandlike structures filled with an acidophilic material recall immature follicles (Call-Exner bodies). When these structures are evident, the diagnosis is considerably more simple. The thecoma component consists of clusters or sheets of cuboidal to polygonal cells. In some tumors, the granulosa or theca cells may appear more plump with ample cytoplasm characteristic of luteinization (i.e., luteinized granulosa-theca cell tumors).

Granulosa-theca cell tumors have clinical importance for two reasons: (1) their potential elaboration of large amounts of estrogen and (2) the small but distinct hazard of malignancy in the granulosa cell forms. Functionally active tumors in young girls (juvenile granulosa cell tumors) may produce precocious sexual development in prepubertal girls. In adult women, they may be associated with endometrial hyperplasia, cystic disease of the breast, and endometrial carcinoma. About 10% to 15% of patients with steroid-producing tumors eventually develop an endometrial carcinoma. Occasional granulosa cell tumors produce androgens, masculinizing the patient.

The additional clinical significance of these tumors lies in the fact that all are potentially malignant. It is difficult, from the histologic evaluation of granulosa cell tumors, to predict their biologic behavior.[118] The estimates of clinical malignancy (recurrence, extension) range from 5% to 25%. In general,

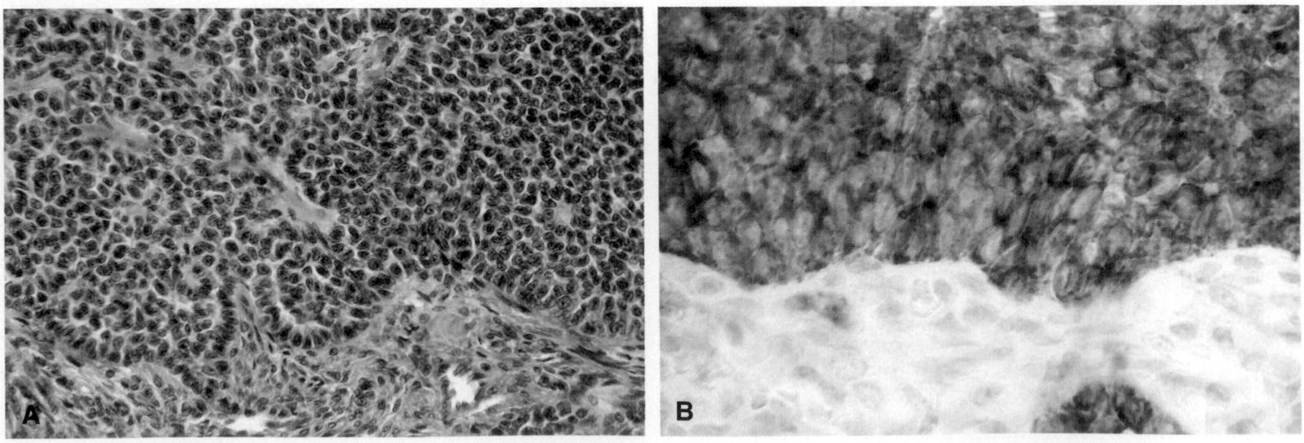

FIGURE 22–53 Granulosa cell tumor. *A*, The tumor cells are arranged in sheets punctuated by small follicle-like structures (Call-Exner bodies). *B*, Strong immunohistochemical positivity with an antibody to inhibin characterizes these tumors.

malignant tumors pursue an indolent course in which local recurrences may be amenable to surgical therapy. Recurrences within the pelvis and abdomen may appear many years (10 to 20) after removal of the original tumor. The 10-year survival rate is approximately 85%. Tumors composed predominantly of theca cells are almost never malignant.

Recently, elevated tissue and serum levels of *inhibin*, an ovarian product, have been associated with granulosa cell tumors. This biomarker may be useful for identifying granulosa and other sex cord stromal tumors, and for monitoring patients under therapy for these neoplasms (Fig. 22–53*B*).[119]

Fibroma-Thecomas

Tumors arising in the ovarian stroma that are composed of either fibroblasts (fibromas) or more plump spindle cells with lipid droplets (thecomas) are relatively common and account for about 4% of all ovarian tumors (Fig. 22–54*A*). Because many tumors contain a mixture of these cells, they are termed *fibroma-thecomas*. Pure thecomas are rare, but tumors in which these cells predominate may be hormonally active. Most are composed principally of fibroblasts and are hormonally inactive.

Fibroma-thecomas of the ovary are unilateral in about 90% of cases and are usually solid, spherical or slightly lobulated, encapsulated, hard, gray-white masses covered by glistening, intact ovarian serosa (Fig. 22–54*B*). On histologic examination, they are composed of well-differentiated fibroblasts with a more or less scant collagenous connective tissue interspersed between the cells. Areas of thecal differentiation may be identified and can be confirmed by fat stains. This step, however, is considered unnecessary on clinical grounds.

In addition to the relatively non-specific findings of pain and pelvic mass, the tumors may be accompanied by two curious associations. The first is ascites, found in about 40% of cases, in which the tumors measure more than 6 cm in diameter. Uncommonly, there is also hydrothorax, usually only of the right side. This combination of findings (i.e., ovarian tumor, hydrothorax, and ascites) is designated Meigs syndrome. Its genesis is unknown. The second association is with the basal cell nevus syndrome, described in Chapter 25. Rarely, cellular tumors with mitotic activity and increased nuclear: cytoplasmic ratio are identified; because they may pursue a malignant course, they are termed fibrosarcomas.[120]

Sertoli-Leydig Cell Tumors (Androblastomas)

These tumors recapitulate, to a certain extent, the cells of the testis at various stages of development.[121] They commonly produce masculinization or at least defeminization, but a few have estrogenic effects. They occur in women of all ages, although the peak incidence is in the second and third decades. The embryogenesis of such male-directed stromal cells remains a puzzle. These tumors are unilateral and resemble granulosa-theca cell neoplasms.

Morphology. The cut surface is usually solid and varies from gray to golden brown in appearance (Fig. 22–55*A*). On histologic examination, the well-differentiated tumors exhibit tubules composed of Sertoli cells or Leydig cells interspersed with stroma (Fig. 22–55*B*). The intermediate forms show only outlines of immature tubules and large eosinophilic Leydig cells. The poorly differentiated tumors have a sarcomatous pattern with a disorderly disposition of epithelial cell cords. Leydig cells may be absent. Heterologous elements, such as mucinous glands, bone, and cartilage, may be present in some tumors.

The incidence of recurrence or metastasis by Sertoli-Leydig cell tumors is less than 5%. These neoplasms may block normal female sexual development in children and may cause defeminization of women, manifested by atrophy of the breasts, amenorrhea, sterility, and loss of hair. The syndrome may progress to striking virilization, that is, hirsutism, male distribution of hair, hypertrophy of the clitoris, and voice changes.

Other Sex Cord–Stromal Tumors

The ovarian hilum normally contains clusters of polygonal cells arranged around vessels (hilar cells). *Hilus cell tumors (pure Leydig cell tumor)* are derived from these cells and are rare, unilateral, and characterized histologically by large lipid-laden cells with distinct borders. A typical cytoplasmic structure characteristic of Leydig cells (Reinke crystalloids) is usually present. Typically, patients with hilus cell tumors present with evidence of masculinization, hirsutism, voice changes, and clitoral enlargement. The tumors are unilateral. The most consistent laboratory finding is an elevated 17-ketosteroid excretion level unresponsive to cortisone suppres-

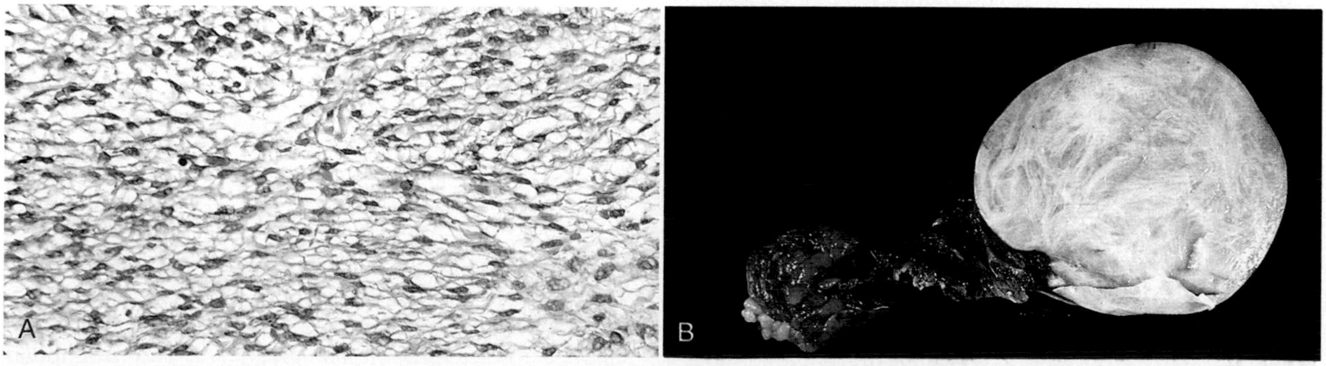

FIGURE 22–54 *A*, Thecoma-fibroma composed of plump, differentiated stromal cells with thecal appearance. *B*, Large bisected fibroma of the ovary apparent as a white, firm mass (*right*). The fallopian tube is attached.

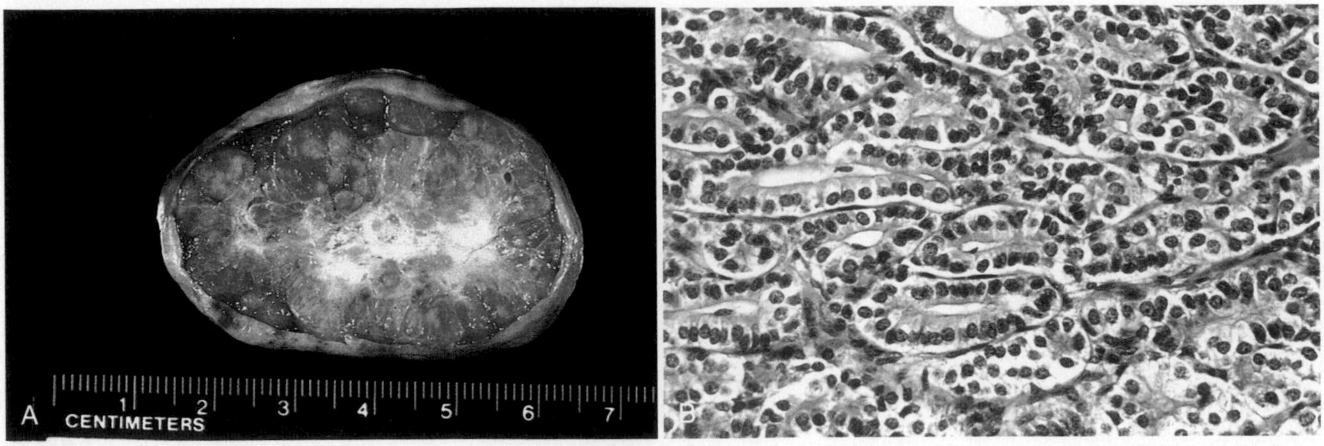

FIGURE 22–55 Sertoli cell tumor. *A,* Gross photograph illustrating characteristic golden yellow appearance of the tumor. *B,* Photomicrograph showing well-differentiated Sertoli cell tubules. (Courtesy of Dr. William Welch, Brigham and Women's Hospital, Boston, MA.)

sion. Treatment is surgical excision. True hilus cell tumors are almost always benign. On occasion, histologically identical tumors occur in the cortical stroma (*nonhilar Leydig cell tumors*).

In addition to Leydig cell tumors, the stroma may rarely give rise to tumors composed of pure luteinized cells, producing small benign tumors generally less than 3 cm in diameter. The tumor may produce the clinical effects of androgen, estrogen, or progestogen stimulation.

As mentioned previously, the ovary in pregnancy may exhibit microscopic nodular proliferation of theca cells in response to gonadotropins. Rarely, a frank tumor may develop (termed *pregnancy luteoma*) that closely resembles a corpus luteum of pregnancy. These tumors have been associated with virilization in pregnant patients and in their respective female infants.

Gonadoblastoma is an uncommon tumor thought to be composed of germ cells and sex cord-stroma derivatives. It occurs in individuals with abnormal sexual development and in gonads of indeterminate nature. Eighty per cent of patients are phenotypic females, and 20% are phenotypic males with undescended testicles and female internal secondary organs. On microscopic examination, the tumor consists of nests of a mixture of germ cells and sex cord derivatives resembling immature Sertoli and granulosa cells. A coexistent dysgerminoma occurs in 50% of the cases. The prognosis is excellent if the tumor is completely excised.[122]

Another tumor of possible stromal origin is small cell carcinoma of the ovary. These malignant tumors occur predominantly in young women and may be associated with hypercalcemia.[123]

Metastatic Tumors

The most common "metastatic" tumors of the ovary are probably derived from tumors of müllerian origin: the uterus, fallopian tube, contralateral ovary, or pelvic peritoneum. The most common extramüllerian primaries are the breast and gastrointestinal tract, including colon, stomach, biliary tract, and pancreas. Also included in this group are the rare cases of pseudomyxoma peritonei, derived from appendiceal tumors. A classic example of metastatic gastrointestinal neoplasia to the ovaries is termed Krukenberg tumor, characterized by bilateral metastases composed of mucin-producing, signet-ring cancer cells, most often of gastric origin.[124]

GESTATIONAL AND PLACENTAL DISORDERS

Diseases of pregnancy and pathologic conditions of the placenta are important causes of intrauterine or perinatal death, congenital malformations, intrauterine growth retardation, maternal death, and a great deal of morbidity for both mother and child.[10] Here we discuss only a limited number of disorders in which knowledge of the morphologic lesions contributes to an understanding of the clinical problem. This discussion is divided into selected disorders of early pregnancy, complications of late pregnancy, and trophoblastic neoplasia.

Disorders of Early Pregnancy

SPONTANEOUS ABORTION

Ten per cent to 15% of recognized pregnancies terminate in spontaneous abortion. However, studies using highly sensitive immunoassay of chorionic gonadotropin to detect pregnancy identified an additional 22% loss of presumably fertilized and implanted ova in otherwise healthy women.[125] The mechanisms leading to early loss of pregnancy are still mysterious.

The causes of recognized spontaneous abortion are both fetal and maternal. Defective implantation inadequate to support fetal development and death of the ovum or fetus in utero because of some genetic or acquired abnormality constitute the major origins of spontaneous abortion. Numerous studies have indicated chromosome abnormalities in more than half of spontaneous abortuses.[126]

Maternal influences, which are less well understood, include inflammatory diseases, both localized to the placenta and systemic; uterine abnormalities; and possibly trauma. The role of trauma is generally overemphasized and must be considered a rare to exceptional trigger of spontaneous abortion. *Toxoplasma*, *Mycoplasma*, *Listeria*, and viral infections have also been implicated as causes of abortion.[10]

The morphologic changes usually seen in endometrial curettage specimens depend, of course, on the interval between fetal death and passage of the products of conception.[127] In general, there are focal areas of decidual necrosis with intense neutrophilic infiltration, thrombi within decidual blood vessels, and considerable amounts of hemorrhage, both recent and old, within the necrotic decidua. Placental villi may be markedly edematous and devoid of blood vessels. The changes encountered in the ovum or fetus are highly variable. In many spontaneous abortions, no fetal products can be identified, but when they are present, they should be carefully examined for anomalies that would suggest specific genetic or karyotypic defects. Chromosomal studies are recommended (1) in habitual or recurrent abortion and (2) when there is a malformed fetus.

ECTOPIC PREGNANCY

Ectopic pregnancy is the term applied to implantation of the fetus in any site other than a normal uterine location. The most common site is within the tubes (approximately 90%).[128] The other sites are the ovary, the abdominal cavity, and the intrauterine portion of the fallopian tube (cornual pregnancy). Ectopic pregnancies occur about once in every 150 pregnancies. The most important predisposing condition in 35% to 50% of patients is PID with chronic salpingitis. Other factors are peritubal adhesions due to appendicitis or endometriosis, leiomyomas, and previous surgery. Fifty per cent, however, occur in tubes that are apparently normal. Intrauterine devices may also increase risk.

Ovarian pregnancy is presumed to result from the rare fertilization and trapping of the ovum within the follicle just at the time of its rupture. Abdominal pregnancies may develop when the fertilized ovum drops out of the fimbriated end of the tube. In all these abnormal locations, the fertilized ovum undergoes its usual development with the formation of placental tissue, amniotic sac, and fetus, and the host implantation site develops decidual changes.

Morphology. In tubal pregnancy, the placenta is poorly attached to the wall of the tube. Intratubal hemorrhage may thus occur from partial placental separation without tubal rupture (Fig. 22–56). Tubal pregnancy is the most common cause of hematosalpinx and should always be suspected when a tubal hematoma is present. More often, the placental tissue invades the tubal wall and causes tubal rupture and intraperitoneal hemorrhage. Less commonly, the tubal pregnancy may undergo spontaneous regression and resorption of the entire gestation. Still less commonly, the tubal pregnancy is extruded through the fimbriated end into the abdominal cavity (tubal abortion).

The clinical course of ectopic pregnancy is punctuated by the onset of severe abdominal pain about 6 weeks after a previous normal menstrual period, when rupture of the tube leads to pelvic hemorrhage. In such cases, the patient may rapidly develop a shocklike state with signs of an acute abdomen, and early diagnosis becomes critical. Chorionic gonadotropin assays, ultrasound studies, and laparoscopy may be helpful. Endometrial biopsy specimens may or may not disclose decidual changes but, excluding the extremely rare dual pregnancy, do not exhibit chorionic villi. Rupture of a tubal pregnancy constitutes a medical emergency.

Disorders of Late Pregnancy

The multitude of disorders that may occur in the third trimester reflect the complex anatomy of the maturing placenta (Fig. 22–57). Any interruption of blood flow through the umbilical cord (such as constricting knots or compression) will be lethal to the fetus. Ascending infections involving the chorioamnionic membranes may lead to premature rupture and delivery. Retroplacental hemorrhage at the interface of placenta and myometrium (abruptio placentae) will threaten both mother and fetus. Rupture of the fetal vessels in terminal villi (intervillous hemorrhage) may produce a sudden drop in fetal blood volume, with fetal stress or death. Uteroplacental insufficiency can be precipitated by abnormal placentation, altered placental development, or maternal vascular thrombosis, and the effects may range from mild intrauterine growth retardation to severe uteroplacental ischemia and maternal toxemia. The more common of these conditions are discussed.

PLACENTAL ABNORMALITIES AND TWIN PLACENTAS

Abnormalities in placental shape, structure, and implantation are not uncommon. Accessory placental lobes, bipartite placenta (placenta made up of two equal segments), and circumvallate placenta (having an extrachorial part) are examples of abnormalities that have limited clinical significance.

Placenta accreta is caused by partial or complete absence of the decidua with adherence of the placenta directly to the myometrium. It is important for two reasons: (1) postpartum bleeding, often life-threatening, occurs because of failure of placental separation; (2) in up to 60% of cases, it is associated

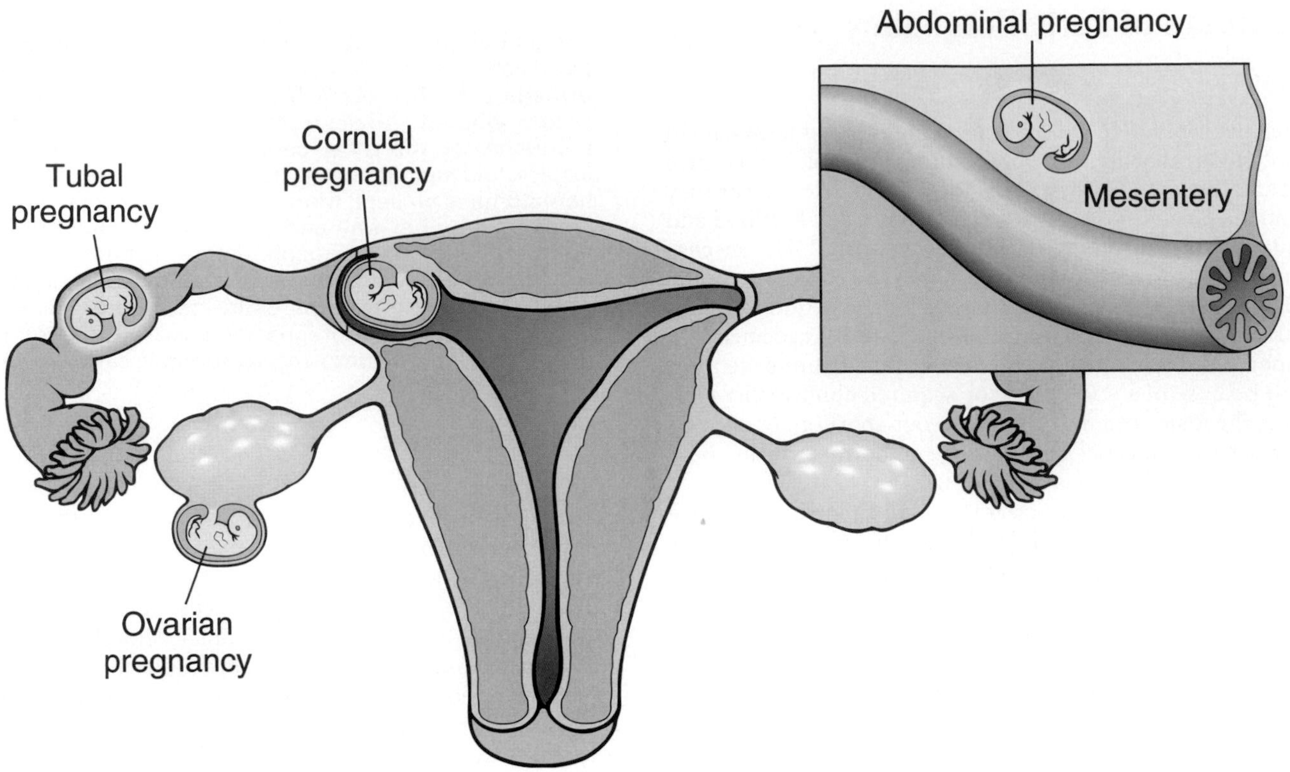

FIGURE 22–56 Potential sites for ectopic pregnancy, including the fallopian tube, ovary, cornu, and (rarely) abdominal viscera.

with placenta previa, a condition in which the placenta implants in the lower uterine segment or cervix, often with serious antepartum bleeding and premature labor. Many cases of placenta previa–associated accreta occur in patients with cesarean section scars.

Twin pregnancies arise from fertilization of two ova (dizygotic) or from division of one fertilized ovum (monozygotic). There are three basic types of twin placentas[129] (Fig. 22–58): dichorionic diamnionic (which may be fused), monochorionic diamnionic, and monochorionic monoamnionic. Monochorionic placentas imply monozygotic (identical) twins, and the time at which splitting occurs determines whether one or two amnions are present. Dichorionic gestation may occur with either monozygotic or dizygotic twins and is not specific.

One complication of twin pregnancy is twin-twin transfusion, in which placental vascular anastomoses (connections) create an abnormal sharing of fetal circulations through shunting. If an imbalance in blood flow occurs, a marked disparity in fetal blood volumes may result in the death of one or both fetuses (Fig. 22–59).

PLACENTAL INFLAMMATIONS AND INFECTIONS

Infections may occur in the placenta (placentitis, villitis), in the fetal membranes (chorioamnionitis), and in the umbilical cord (funisitis).[130] They reach the placenta by two pathways: (1) ascending infection through the birth canal and (2) hematogenous (transplacental) infection. Ascending infections are by far the most common and are most often bacterial; in many such instances, localized infection of the membranes by an organism produces premature rupture of membranes and entry of the organisms. Sexual intercourse has been implicated in enhancing ascending infections. The amniotic fluid may be cloudy with purulent exudate, and the chorion-amnion histologically contains a leukocytic polymorphonuclear infiltration with accompanying edema and congestion of the vessels (Fig. 22–60*A* and *B*). The infection frequently elicits a fetal response with umbilical cord vasculitis.

Uncommonly, bacterial infections of the placenta and fetal membranes may arise by the hematogenous spread of bacteria directly to the placenta. The villi are most often affected histologically (villitis) (Fig. 22–60*C*). Classically, TORCH (toxoplasmosis and others [syphilis, tuberculosis, listeriosis], rubella, cytomegalovirus, herpes simplex) should be considered, although the cause is usually obscure and may involve immunologic phenomena.[10] (See also Chapter 10.)

TOXEMIA OF PREGNANCY (PREECLAMPSIA AND ECLAMPSIA)

Toxemia of pregnancy refers to a symptom complex characterized by hypertension, proteinuria, and edema (preeclampsia). It occurs in about 6% of pregnant women, usually in the last trimester and more commonly in primiparas than in multiparas. Certain of these patients become more seriously ill, developing convulsions; this more severe form of toxemia is termed eclampsia. Patients with eclampsia develop disseminated intravascular coagulation (DIC) with lesions in the liver, kidneys, heart, placenta, and sometimes the brain. There is no absolute correlation between the severity of eclampsia and the magnitude of the anatomic changes.

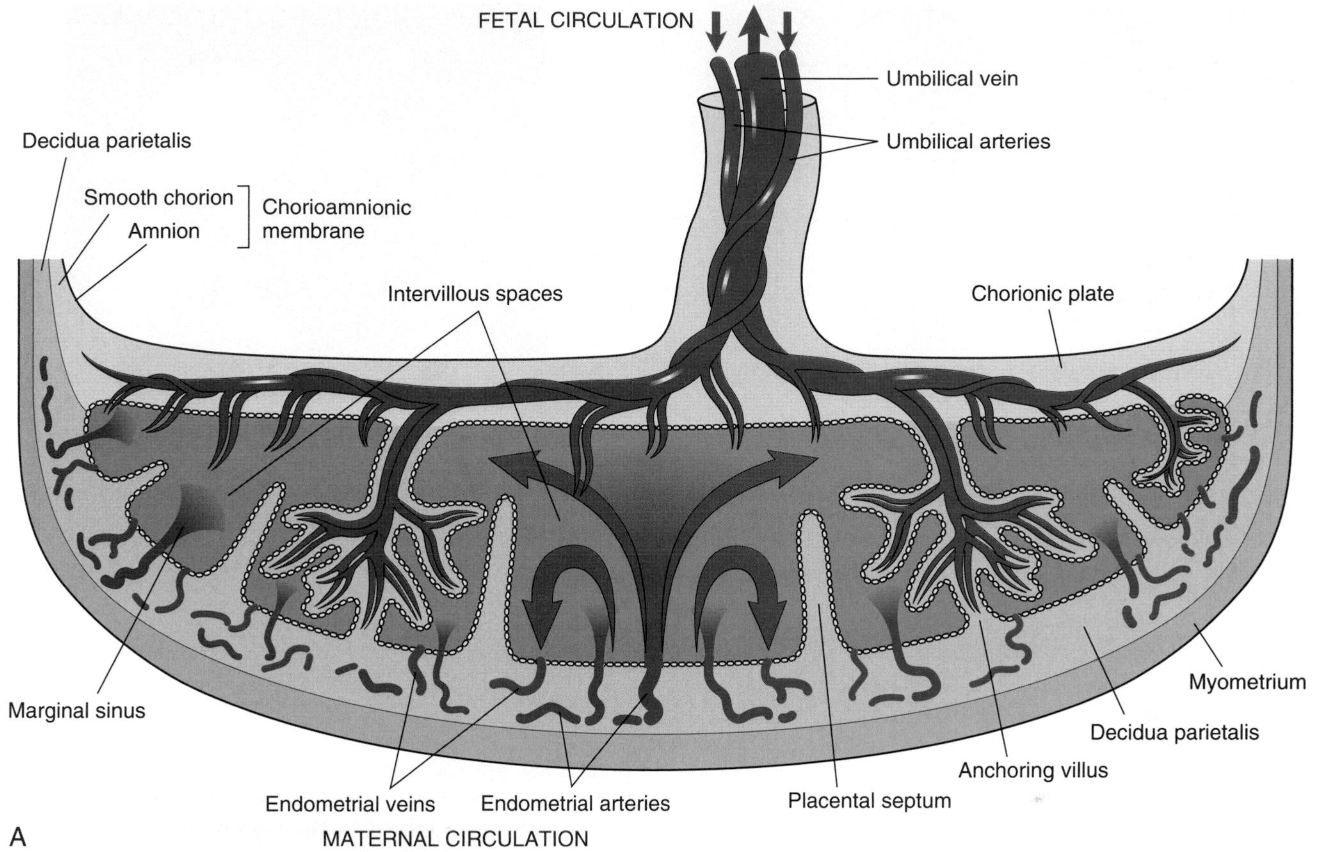

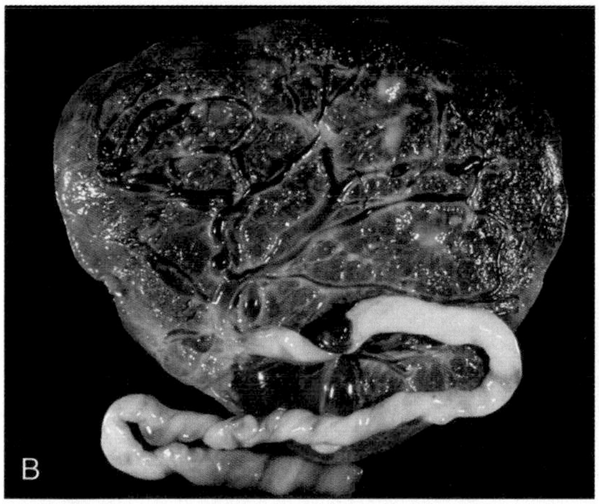

FIGURE 22–57 *A,* Diagram of placental anatomy. Within the outer boundary of myometrium is a layer of decidua, from which the maternal vessels originate and deliver blood to and from the intervillous spaces. Umbilical vessels branch and terminate in placental villi, where nutrient exchange takes place. *B,* Normal term placenta (fetal surface) with umbilical cord.

Pathogenesis. The many theories on the nature of toxemia of pregnancy[131–136] are beyond our scope, but three events that seem to be of prime importance in this disorder are addressed: placental ischemia, hypertension, and DIC (Fig. 22–61).

The causes of the initial events of toxemia are unknown, but evidence points to an abnormality of placentation, leading to *placental ischemia.* This may involve defects in both trophoblast invasion and the development of the physiologic alterations in the placental vessels required to perfuse the placental bed adequately. Immunologic, genetic, and other factors have been postulated as causes of these abnormalities. The net effect is a *shallow implantation* with incomplete conversion of decidual vessels to vessels adequate for the pregnancy state.[132] Investigators have hypothesized that an intrinsic *defect in the invading trophoblast* may contribute to altered vascular flow. This abnormality is manifest by the inability of the invading cytotrophoblast to assume the phenotype of normal endothelial cells, which normally includes the expression of adhesion receptors. These defects in trophoblastic conversion may further influence remodeling of uterine vasculature, reducing blood flow and leading to *placental ischemia, the basis for the toxemic placenta.*[133,134] It is thought that this decreased uteroplacental perfusion induces stimulation of vasoconstrictor substances (thromboxane, angiotensin, endothelin) and the inhibition of vasodilator influences (prostaglandin I_2, prostaglandin E_2, nitric oxide) from the ischemic placenta. DIC, hypertension, and organ damage then develop (Fig. 22–61).

As to the pathogenesis of DIC in toxemia, endothelial damage, abnormalities in the level and activities of coagula-

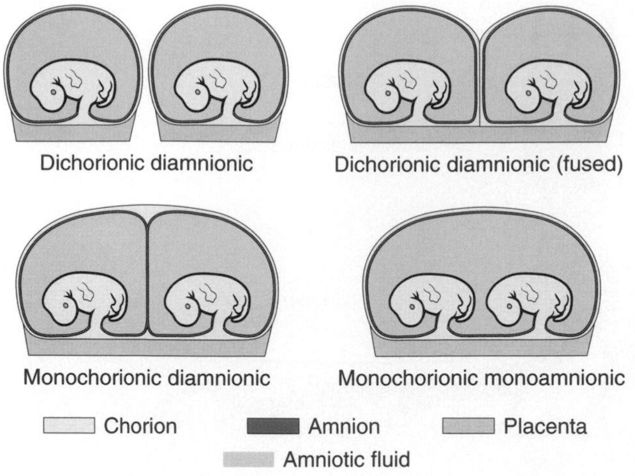

FIGURE 22–58 Diagrammatic representation of the various types of twin placentation and their membrane relationships. (Adapted from Gersell D, et al: Diseases of the placenta. In Kurman, R (ed): Blaustein's Pathology of the Female Genital Tract. New York, Springer-Verlag, 1994.)

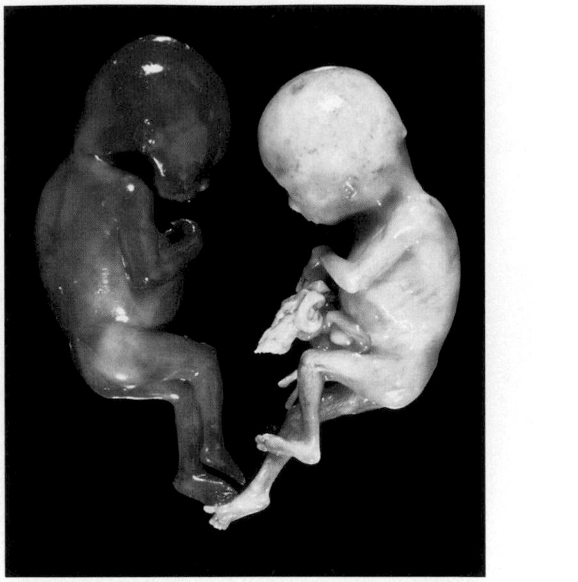

FIGURE 22–59 Twin-twin transfusion syndrome resulting in the death of both fetuses because of excessive (*left*) or deficient (*right*) blood volume.

tion factors, and primary platelet alteration may play a role.[135] For example, during toxemia, the placental ischemia leads to a higher output of thromboplastic substances, and antithrombin III levels are reduced. The characteristic lesions in eclampsia are in large part due to thrombosis of arterioles and capillaries throughout the body, particularly in the liver, kidneys, brain, pituitary, and placenta.

Several mechanisms have been proposed to explain toxemic hypertension. One mechanism involves renin-angiotensin and prostaglandins.[136] Normal pregnant women develop a resistance to the vasoconstrictive and hypertensive effects of angiotensin, but women with toxemia lose such resistance, developing a tendency to hypertension. Prostaglandins of the E series, produced in the uteroplacental vascular bed during pregnancy, are thought to mediate the normal resistance of pregnant women to angiotensin, and prostaglandin production is indeed decreased in the placenta of toxemic women. Thus, the increase in angiotensin hypersensitivity, characteristic of toxemia, may be due to decreased synthesis of prostaglandin by the toxemic placenta. There is also evidence that renin production by the toxemic placenta is increased, another potentially vasoconstrictive event. Figure 22–61 presents a hypothetical schema for the pathogenesis of eclampsia. An additional mechanism recently proposed involves circulating soluble fms-like tyrosine kinase (sFlt1), which

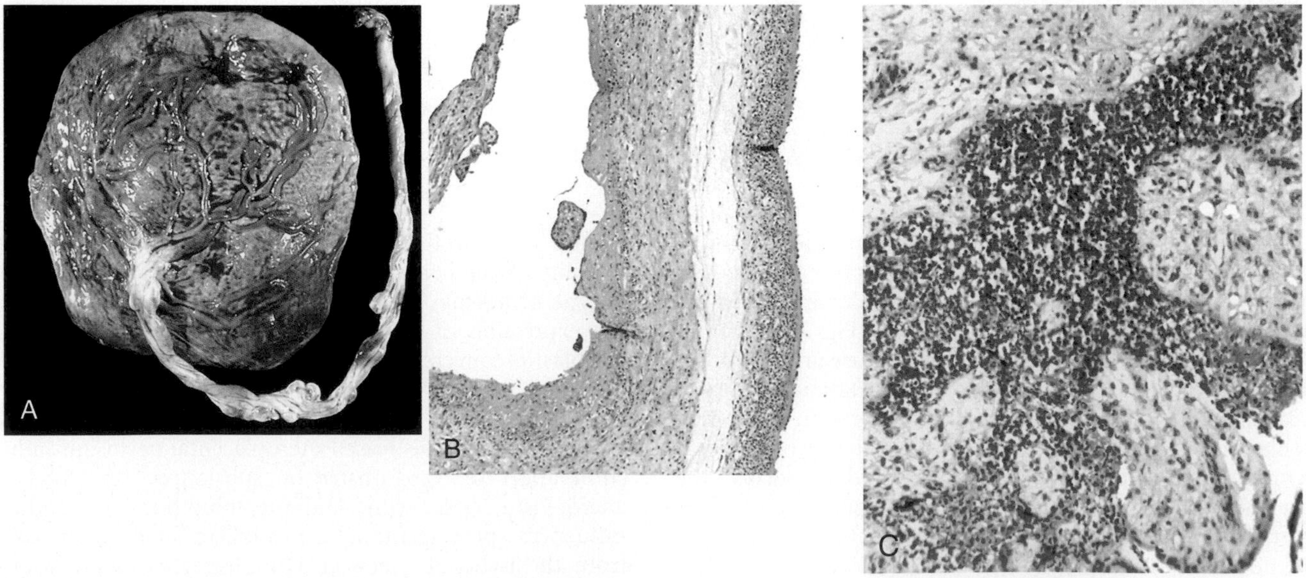

FIGURE 22–60 Placental infections derived from ascending and blood-borne routes. Acute chorioamnionitis. *A*, On gross examination, the placenta contains greenish opaque membranes. Compare with Figure 22–55*B*. *B*, A photomicrograph illustrates a dense band-like inflammatory exudate on the amniotic surface (*top*). *C*, Acute necrotizing intervillositis, from a fetal-maternal infection by listeria.

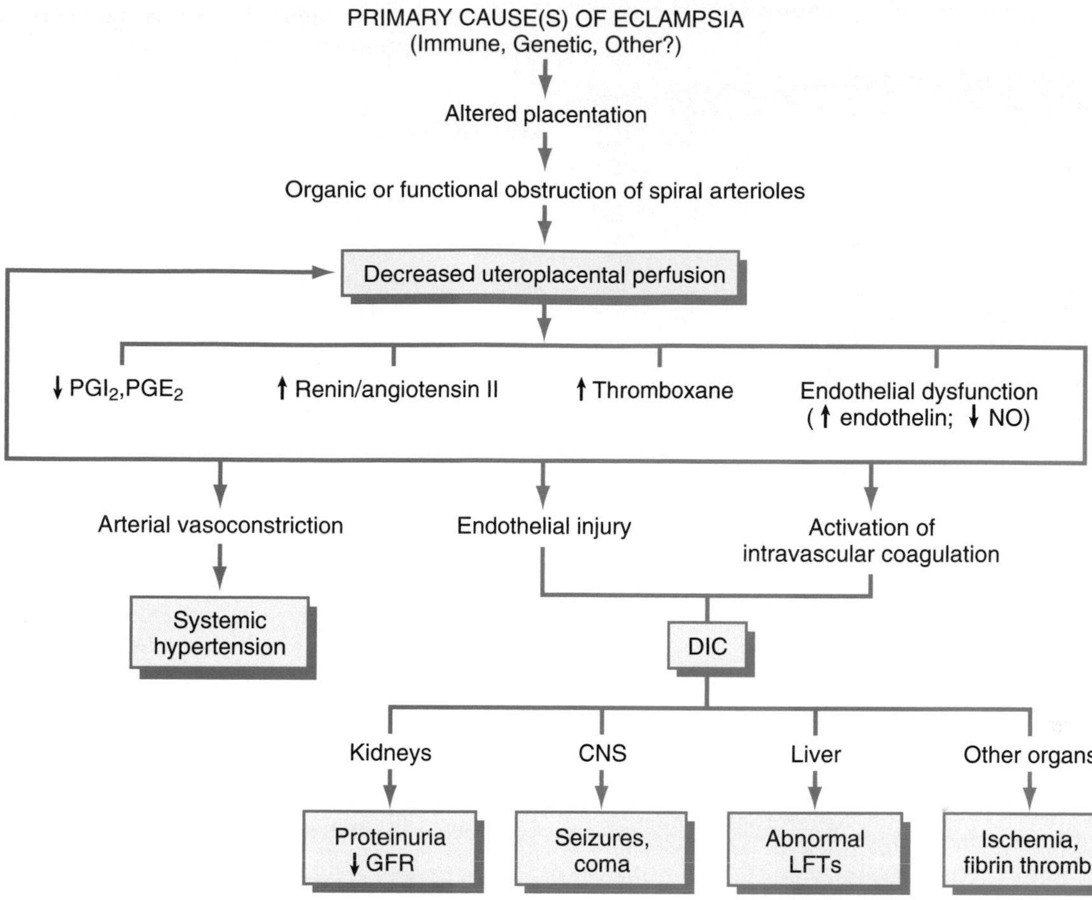

FIGURE 22–61 Proposed sequence of events in the pathogenesis of toxemia of pregnancy. The main features are (1) decreased uteroplacental perfusion; (2) increased vasoconstrictors and decreased vasodilators, resulting in local and systemic vasoconstriction; and (3) disseminated intravascular coagulation (DIC). (Adapted from Friedman SA: Pre-eclampsia: a review of the role of prostaglandins. Obstet Gynecol 71:122, 1988. Reprinted by permission of the American College of Obstetricians and Gynecologists; and Khong TY, et al: Inadequate maternal vascular response to placentation in pregnancies complicated by pre-eclampsia and by small for gestational age infants. Br J Obstet Gynecol 93:1049, 1986.)

binds both placental growth factor (PIGF) and vascular endothelial growth factor (VEGF). Normally, serum sFlt1 increases, and PIGF and VEGF decrease near term, reflecting a reduction in angiogenic activity. In preeclampsia, decreased angiogenesis occurs much earlier than in normal pregnancy. The premature application of an antiangiogenic "brake" may, thus, be a key factor in the initiation of preeclampsia.[136a] Administration of sFlt1 to pregnant rats produces the characteristic systemic and renal abnormalities seen in human preeclampsia.[136b]

Morphology. The **placenta** is the site of variable changes, most of which reflect ischemia and vessel injury. (1) Placental infarcts, which occur in normal full-term placentas, are larger and more numerous. (2) There is increased frequency of retroplacental hematomas. (3) There is evidence of increased villous ischemia; formation of prominent syncytial knots, thickening of trophoblastic basement membrane, and villous hypovascularity. (4) A characteristic finding in the walls of uterine vessels is striking fibrinoid necrosis and intramural lipid deposition (acute atherosis) (Fig. 22–62).

The **liver** lesions, when present, take the form of irregular, focal, subcapsular, and intraparenchymal hemorrhages. On histologic examination, there are fibrin thrombi in the portal capillaries with foci of characteristic peripheral hemorrhagic necrosis.

The **kidney** lesions are variable. Glomerular lesions are diffuse, when assessed by electron microscopy. They consist of striking swelling of endothelial cells, the deposition of fibrinogen-derived amorphous dense deposits on the endothelial side of the basement membrane, and mesangial cell hyperplasia. Immunofluorescent studies confirm the abundance of

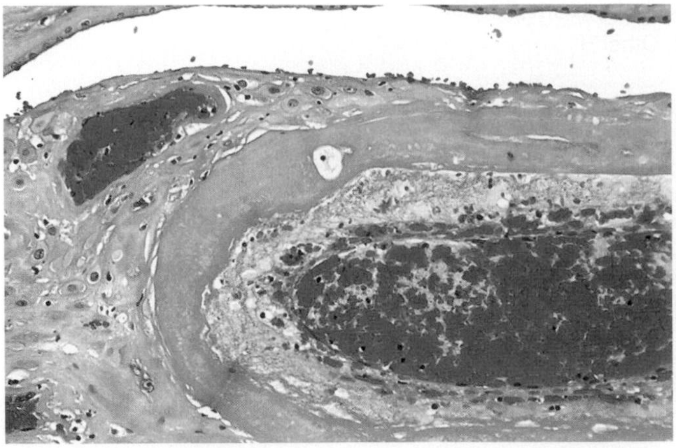

FIGURE 22–62 Acute atherosis of uterine vessels in eclampsia. Note fibrinoid necrosis of the vessel walls, subendothelial macrophages and perivascular lymphocytic infiltrate. (Courtesy of Dr. Drucilla J. Roberts, Massachusetts General Hospital, Boston, MA.)

fibrin in glomeruli. In the more well-defined cases, fibrin thrombi are present in the glomeruli and capillaries of the cortex. When the lesion is far advanced, it may produce complete destruction of the cortex in the pattern referred to as bilateral renal cortical necrosis (Chapter 20). The **brain** may have gross or microscopic foci of hemorrhage along with small-vessel thromboses. Similar changes are often found in the **heart** and the **anterior pituitary**.

Clinical Course. Preeclampsia usually starts after the 32nd week of pregnancy but begins earlier in patients with hydatidiform mole (discussed below) or pre-existing kidney disease or hypertension. The onset is typically insidious, characterized by hypertension and edema, with proteinuria following within several days. Headaches and visual disturbances are common. Eclampsia is heralded by central nervous system involvement, including convulsions and eventual coma. Mild and moderate forms of toxemia can be controlled by bed rest, a balanced diet, and antihypertensive agents, but induction of delivery is the only definitive treatment of established preeclampsia and eclampsia. Proteinuria and hypertension usually disappear within 1 or 2 weeks after delivery except in patients in whom these findings predate the pregnancy.

INTRAUTERINE GROWTH RESTRICTION

Intrauterine growth restriction is an important cause of infant mortality and morbidity and is defined as a birth weight below the 10th percentile (Chapter 10). Major causes include obvious fetal disorders such as chromosomal abnormalities and malformations (20%), and maternal vascular disease, including toxemia (30%). Other causes include thrombolytic disorders, maternal and fetal infections, autoimmune disorders (chronic villitis), fetal vascular disorders (fetal thrombosis), and other metabolic disorders.[137] In over one-third the placenta is small for date, implying poor perfusion. Management of these disorders, particularly when the fetus is otherwise normal, requires careful monitoring of fetal and placental development and rapid delivery if placental blood flow appears compromised.

Gestational Trophoblastic Disease

Gestational trophoblastic disease constitutes a spectrum of tumors and tumor-like conditions characterized by proliferation of pregnancy-associated trophoblastic tissue of progressive malignant potential. The lesions include the hydatidiform mole (complete and partial), the invasive mole, and the frankly malignant choriocarcinoma.[138] Gestational trophoblastic disease is important for the following reasons:

- The hydatidiform mole is a common complication of gestation, occurring about once in every 1000 to 2000 pregnancies in the United States and, curiously, far more commonly in the Far East.
- It has become possible, by monitoring the circulating levels of human chorionic gonadotropin, to determine the early development of persistent trophoblastic disease.
- Choriocarcinoma, once a dreaded and uniformly fatal complication, is now highly responsive to chemotherapy.[139]

HYDATIDIFORM MOLE (COMPLETE AND PARTIAL)

Hydatidiform mole is characterized by cystic swelling of the chorionic villi, accompanied by variable trophoblastic proliferation. The most important reason for the correct recognition of true moles is that they may precede choriocarcinoma.[138] Most patients present in the fourth or fifth month of pregnancy with vaginal bleeding and with a uterus that is usually, but not always, larger than expected for the duration of pregnancy. These moles can occur at any age during active reproductive life, but the risk is higher in pregnant women in their teens or between the ages of 40 and 50 years. For poorly explained reasons, the incidence varies considerably in different regions of the world: 1 in 1000 pregnancies in the United States but 10 in 1000 in Indonesia.[140]

Types and Pathogenesis. Two types of benign, noninvasive moles—complete and partial—can be identified by histologic, cytogenetic, and flow cytometric studies[141] (Table 22–5). In complete (or classic) mole, all or most of the villi are edematous, and there is diffuse trophoblast hyperplasia. Cyto-

TABLE 22–5 Features of Complete Versus Partial Hydatidiform Mole

Feature	Complete Mole	Partial Mole
Karyotype	46,XX (46,XY)	Triploid
Villous edema	All villi	Some villi
Trophoblast proliferation	Diffuse; circumferential	Focal; slight
Atypia	Often present	Absent
Serum hCG	Elevated	Less elevated
HCG in tissue	++++	+
Behavior	2% choriocarcinoma	Rare choriocarcinoma

HCG, human chorionic gonadotropin.

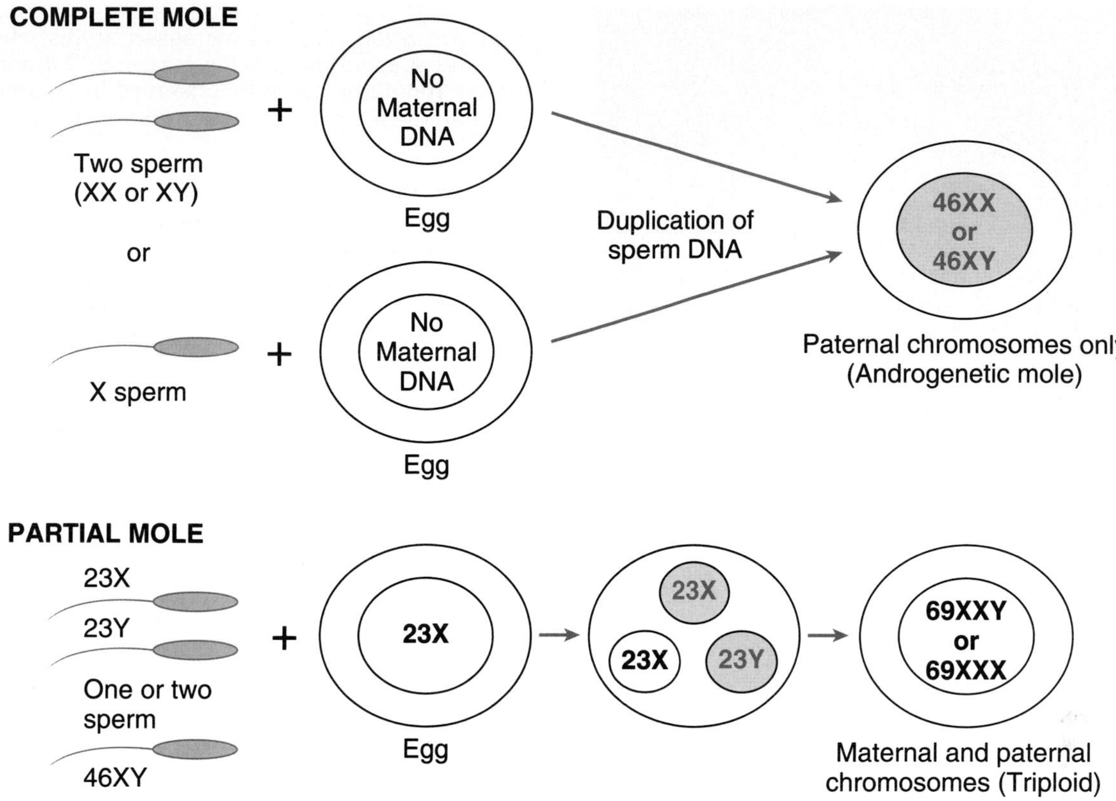

FIGURE 22–63 Patterns of fertilization to account for chromosomal origin of complete (46,XX) and triploid partial moles (XXY). In a complete mole, one or two sperm fertilize an egg that has lost its chromosomes. Partial moles are due to fertilization of an egg by one diploid, or two haploid sperm, depicted in this example as one 23,X and one 23,Y.

genetic studies of these moles show that more than 90% have a 46,XX diploid pattern, all derived from the sperm (a phenomenon called androgenesis). They are presumed to result from fertilization by a single sperm of an egg that has lost its chromosomes (Fig. 22–63). The remaining 10% are from the fertilization of such an empty egg by two sperm (46,XX and 46,XY). In both circumstances, embryonic development does not occur, and thus complete moles show no fetal parts.

In partial moles, some of the villi are edematous, and other villi show only minor changes; the trophoblastic proliferation is focal. In these moles, the karyotype is triploid (e.g., 69,XXY) or even occasionally tetraploid (92,XXXY). The moles result from fertilization of an egg with one or two sperm (Fig. 22–63). The embryo is viable for weeks, and thus fetal parts may be present when the resultant mole is aborted. In contrast to complete moles, partial moles are rarely followed by choriocarcinoma.

Only a portion of triploid gestations result in partial moles. A recent study showed that partial moles were significantly more likely when the gestation was *diandric*, that is, two of the three haploid chromosomal sets were derived from the male (via dispermy). This is in contrast to *digynic* triploid gestations, in which two haploid sets develop due to errors in meiosis.[142]

Morphology. In most instances, moles develop within the uterus, but they may occur in any site, including ectopic pregnancies. Timing of discovery is related to type of mole (partial versus complete, and level of pregnancy surveillance). Partial moles may be diagnosed in early spontaneous abortions or later, following fetal development. Careful dissection may disclose a small, usually collapsed amniotic sac. Fetal parts are frequently seen in partial moles but are never found in complete moles (unless there is a twin pregnancy). Currently, complete moles are being diagnosed and removed at an earlier mean gestational age (8.5 versus 17.0 weeks) due to routine ultrasound and close monitoring of early pregnancy, combined with more efficient histologic recognition of early complete hydatidiform mole.[143,144] The classic presentation is a uterine cavity filled with a delicate, friable mass of thin-walled, translucent, cystic, grape-like structures consisting of swollen edematous (hydropic) villi (Fig. 22–64).

On histologic examination, **partial moles** (Fig. 22–65*A*) demonstrate villous hydrops and architectural disturbances in only a proportion of villi. The trophoblastic proliferation is minimal and limited to the syncitiotrophoblast. In contrast, **complete moles** show hydropic swelling of most chorionic villi and

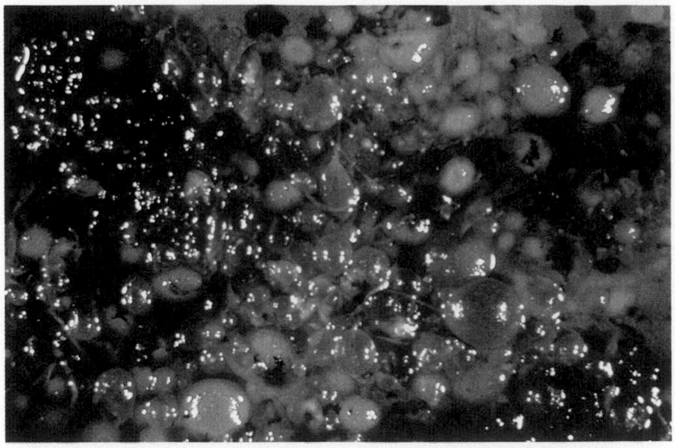

FIGURE 22–64 Complete hydatidiform mole suspended in saline showing numerous swollen (hydropic) villi.

virtual absence or inadequate development of vascularization of villi. Early complete moles exhibit subtle conformational changes in the villi accompanied by stromal cell karryorrhexis and modest syncytial and cytotrophoblastic hyperplasia. More advanced complete moles exhibit the classic spectrum of diffuse villous swelling, central cavitation (cisterns) and extensive concentric villous and extravillous trophoblastic proliferation (Fig. 22–65*B*). The implantation site often displays increased atypia. Histologic grading does not predict the outcome;[145] therefore, all moles should be carefully observed by monitoring of the human chorionic gonadotropin levels.

Clinical Course. Most patients with partial and early complete moles present with spontaneous pregnancy loss or undergo curettage due to abnormalities in ultrasound. Watery fluid and bits of tissue seen as small, grapelike masses may be seen in the uterine contents. Ultrasound examination will confirm the diffuse villous enlargement. In complete moles, quantitative analysis of human chorionic gonadotropin shows levels of hormone greatly exceeding those produced by a normal pregnancy of similar age. Serial hormone determination indicates a rapidly mounting level that climbs faster than for the usual normal single or even multiple pregnancy.

The vast majority of moles are removed by thorough curettage. Virtually no partial and only 2.5% of complete moles evolve into a malignant trophoblastic neoplasm (choriocarcinoma). Ten per cent of complete moles develop into invasive moles.[146] Because unattended complete moles may persist and recur, distinction of these moles from non-molar hydropic and partial molar gestations is important. A strongly paternally imprinted gene, the cell cycle inhibitor, p57, may be used to identify complete moles by absence of expression in the syncytial trophoblast and stromal cells of molar villi (Fig. 22–65*C* and *D*). Because *p57* is paternally imprinted, and both the X chromosomes in complete moles are derived from the father, there is no expression of p57 protein.[147]

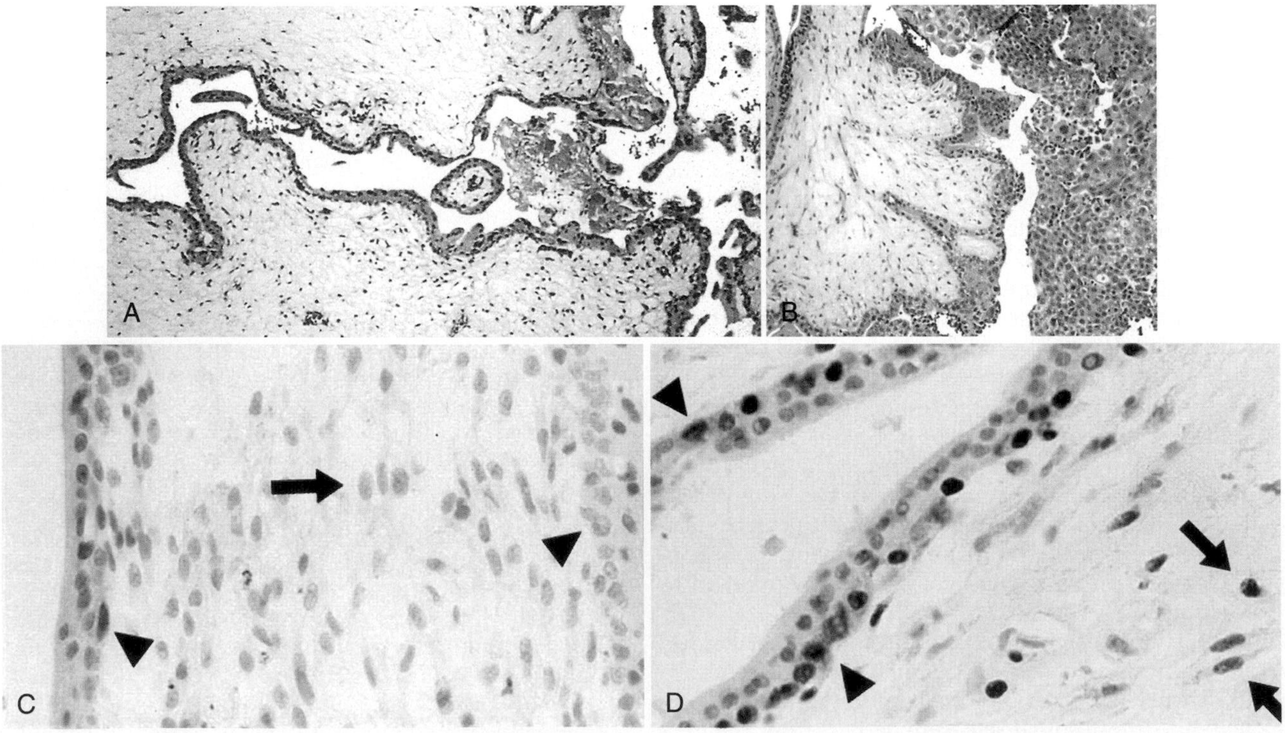

FIGURE 22–65 *A*, Photomicrograph of partial hydatidiform mole revealing swollen villi and slight hyperplasia of the surface trophoblast. *B*, Complete hydatidiform mole with extensive cytotrophoblastic hyperplasia (*lower field*) (Courtesy of Dr. David R. Genest, Brigham and Women's Hospital, Boston, MA.). *C*, Complete moles lack expression of *p57* in the cytotrophoblast (*arrowheads*) and villous stroma (*arrow*). *D*, Normal placenta immunostained for *p57* exhibits staining in both stromal (*arrows*) and cytotrophoblast (*arrowheads*) nuclei. (Courtesy of Dr. Diego C. Castrillon, Brigham and Women's Hospital, Boston, MA.)

INVASIVE MOLE

This is defined as a mole that penetrates and may even perforate the uterine wall. There is invasion of the myometrium by hydropic chorionic villi, accompanied by proliferation of both cytotrophoblast and syncytiotrophoblast (Fig. 22–66). The tumor is locally destructive and may invade parametrial tissue and blood vessels. Hydropic villi may embolize to distant sites, such as lungs and brain, but do not grow in these organs as true metastases, and even before the advent of chemotherapy, they eventually regressed unless fatal hemorrhage occurred. The tumor is manifested clinically by vaginal bleeding and irregular uterine enlargement. It is always associated with a persistent elevated human chorionic gonadotropin level and varying degrees of luteinization of the ovaries. The tumor responds well to chemotherapy but may result in uterine rupture and necessitate hysterectomy.

CHORIOCARCINOMA

Gestational choriocarcinoma is an epithelial malignant neoplasm of trophoblastic cells derived from any form of previously normal or abnormal pregnancy.[105] Although most cases arise in the uterus, ectopic pregnancies provide extrauterine sites of origin. Choriocarcinoma is a rapidly invasive, widely metastasizing malignant neoplasm, but once it is identified, it responds well to chemotherapy.

Incidence. This is an uncommon condition that arises in 1 in 20,000 to 30,000 pregnancies in the United States. It is much more common in some African countries; for example, it occurs in 1 in 2500 pregnancies in Ibadan, Nigeria. It is preceded by several conditions: 50% arise in hydatidiform moles, 25% in previous abortions, approximately 22% in normal pregnancies (intraplacental choriocarcinoma). The remainder occur in ectopic pregnancies and genital and extragenital teratomas. About 1 in 40 hydatidiform moles may be expected to give rise to a choriocarcinoma, in contrast to 1 in approximately 150,000 normal pregnancies.

Morphology. The choriocarcinoma is classically a soft, fleshy, yellow-white tumor with a marked tendency to form large pale areas of ischemic necrosis, foci of cystic softening, and extensive hemorrhage (Fig. 22–67*A*). On histologic examination, it is a purely epithelial tumor that does not produce chorionic villi and that grows by the abnormal proliferation of both cytotrophoblast and syncytiotrophoblast (Fig. 22–67*B*).

It is sometimes possible to identify anaplasia within such abnormal proliferation, replete with abnormal mitoses. The tumor invades the underlying myometrium, frequently penetrates blood vessels and lymphatics, and in some cases extends out onto the uterine serosa and adjacent structures. In its rapid growth, it is subject to hemorrhage, ischemic necrosis, and secondary inflammation.

In fatal cases, metastases are found in the lungs, brain, bone marrow, liver, and other organs. On occasion, metastatic choriocarcinoma is discovered without a detectable primary in the uterus (or ovary), presumably because the primary has undergone total necrosis.

Clinical Course. The uterine choriocarcinoma does not classically produce a large, bulky mass. It becomes manifest only by irregular spotting of a bloody, brown, sometimes foul-smelling fluid. This discharge may appear in the course of an apparently normal pregnancy, after a miscarriage, or after a curettage. Sometimes the tumor does not appear until months after these events. Usually, by the time the tumor is discovered locally, radiographs of the chest and bones already disclose the presence of metastatic lesions. The titers of human chorionic gonadotropin are elevated to levels above those encountered in hydatidiform moles. Occasional tumors, however, produce little hormone, and some tumors have become so necrotic as to become functionally inactive.

Widespread metastases are characteristic of these tumors. Favored sites of involvement are the lungs (50%) and vagina (30% to 40%), followed in descending order of frequency by the brain, liver, and kidney.

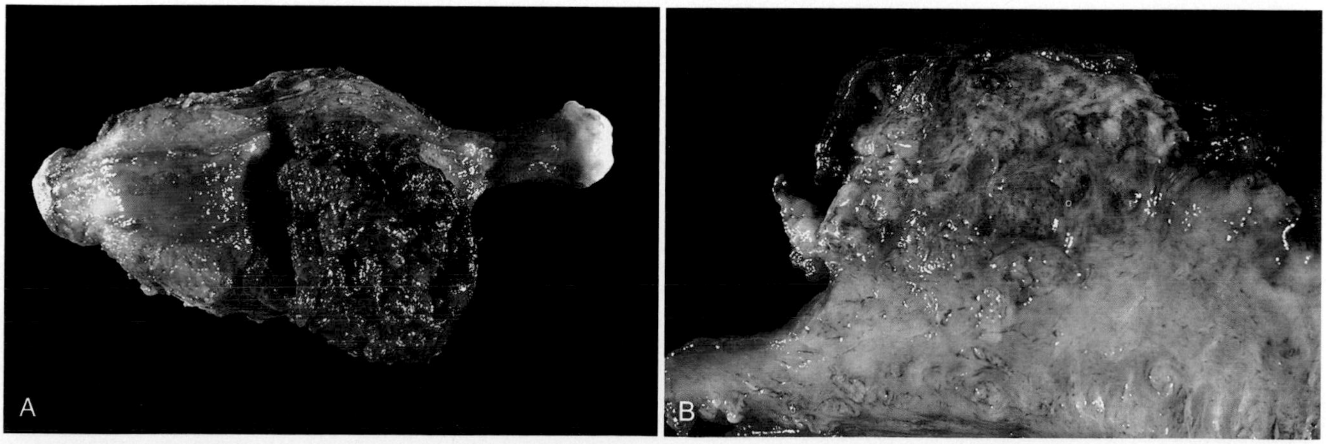

FIGURE 22–66 *A*, Invasive mole presenting as a hemorrhagic mass adherent to the uterine wall. *B*, On cross-section, the tumor invades into the myometrium. (Courtesy of Dr. David R. Genest, Brigham and Women's Hospital, Boston, MA.)

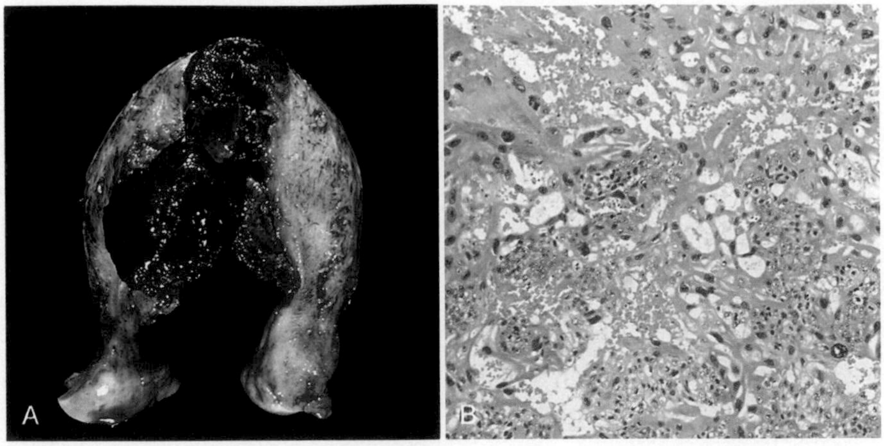

FIGURE 22–67 *A*, Choriocarcinoma presenting as a bulky hemorrhagic mass invading the uterine wall. *B*, Photomicrograph of choriocarcinoma illustrating both neoplastic cytotrophoblast and syncytiotrophoblast. (Courtesy of Dr. David R. Genest, Brigham and Women's Hospital, Boston, MA.)

The treatment of trophoblastic neoplasms depends on the type and stage of tumor and includes evacuation of the contents of the uterus, surgery, and chemotherapy. Chemotherapy consists of the administration of one or more of a group of drugs including methotrexate, actomycin D, and etoposide. The results of chemotherapy for gestational choriocarcinoma are spectacular and have resulted in up to 100% cure or remission in all patients except some who had high-risk metastatic trophoblastic disease. Many of the cured patients have had normal subsequent pregnancies and deliveries. By contrast, nongestational choriocarcinomas are much more resistant to therapy.[138–140]

PLACENTAL SITE TROPHOBLASTIC TUMOR

In contrast to syncytial cytotrophoblast, which is present on the chorionic villi, intermediate trophoblast is found in the implantation site and placental membranes. Intermediate trophoblast is composed of mononuclear cells with abundant cytoplasm that distinguish them from the syncytial cytotrophoblast. In contrast to syncytiotrophoblasts (which produce human chorionic gonadotropin), intermediate trophoblast cells are weakly immunoreactive for human placental lactogen. Intermediate trophoblasts compose the placental site trophoblast and residual placental site (implantation site nodule) following pregnancy, and may give rise to *placental site trophoblastic tumors* (PSTTs) (Fig. 22–68).

PSTTs comprise less than 2% of gestational trophoblastic neoplasms and present as neoplastic polygonal cells infiltrating the endomyometrium. PSTTs may be preceded by a normal pregnancy (one-half), spontaneous abortion (one-sixth), or hydatidiform mole (one-fifth).[149,150] Beta human chorionic gonadotropin levels may be high. Patients with localized (Stage I or II) disease or a less than 2-year interval from the prior pregnancy to diagnosis have an excellent prognosis. Tumors diagnosed 4 or more years following pregnancy, with lung involvement or with advanced stage have a poor prognosis. Overall, about 10% result in disseminated metastases and death.[151] Distinction of PSTTs from normal exaggerated placental implantation site trophoblast may be difficult and can be achieved by using biomarkers (Mel-Cam and Ki-67) that detect increased proliferation in the trophoblastic cells.[152]

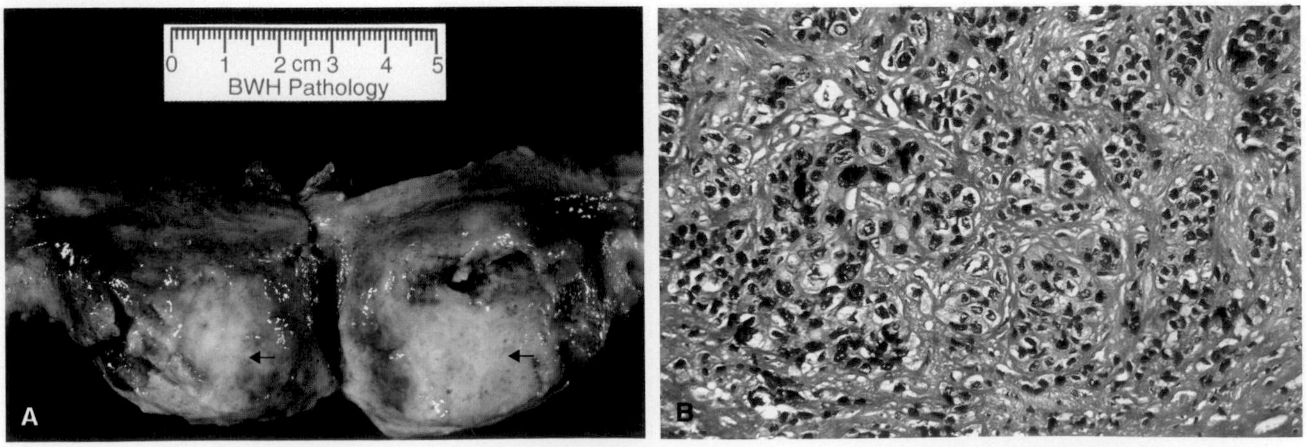

FIGURE 22–68 *A*, Placental site trophoblastic tumor, presenting as a discrete mass in the myometrium. *B*, Histology of PSTT. (Courtesy of Dr. Bradley J. Quade, Brigham and Women's Hospital, Boston, MA.)

REFERENCES

1. Robboy SJ, et al: Embryology of the female genital tract. In Kurman R (ed): Blaustein's Pathology of the Female Genital Tract, 4th ed. New York, Springer-Verlag, 1994, pp 3–31.
2. Kurita T, Cooke PS, Cunha GR. Epithelial-stromal tissue interaction in paramesonephric (Müllerian) epithelial differentiation. Dev Biol 240:194, 2001.
3. Quade BJ, Yang A, Wang Y, Sun D, Park J, Sheets EE, Cviko A, Federschneider JM, Peters R, McKeon FD, Crum CP: Expression of the p53 homologue p63 in early cervical neoplasia. Gynecol Oncol 80:24, 2001.
4. Malasanos TH: Sexual development of the fetus and pubertal child. Clin Obstet Gynecol 40:153, 1997.
5. Ince T, Cviko A, Quade BJ, Yang A, McKeon F, Mutter GL, Crum CP: P63 coordinates anogenital modeling and epithelial differentiation in the developing female urogenital tract. Am J Pathol 161:1111, 2002.
6. Richart RM: Cervical intraepithelial neoplasia. Pathol Annu 8:301, 1973.
7. Alliende ME: Mean versus individual hormonal profiles in the menstrual cycle. Fertil Steril 78:90, 2002.
8. Kurman R (ed): Blaustein's Pathology of the Female Genital Tract, 4th ed. New York, Springer-Verlag, 1994.
9. Fox H (ed): Haines and Taylor's Obstetrical and Gynaecologic Pathology, 4th ed. Edinburgh, Churchill Livingstone, 1987.
10. Benirschke K, Kaufmann P: Pathology of the Human Placenta, 3rd ed. New York, Springer-Verlag, 1995.
11. Robboy SJ, Anderson MC, Russell P: Pathology of the female reproductive tract. London, Churchill Livingstone, 2002.
12. Holmes KK, et al (eds): Sexually Transmitted Diseases, 2nd ed. New York, McGraw-Hill, 1990.
13. Brugha R, et al: Genital herpes infection: a review. Int J Epidemiol 26:698, 1997.
14. Prober CG: Herpetic vaginitis in 1993. Clin Obstet Gynecol 36:177, 1993.
15. Heine P, McGregor JA: Trichomonas vaginalis: a reemerging pathogen. Clin Obstet Gynecol 36:137, 1993.
16. Rosenman SD: Vulvar vestibulitis: a reappraisal. Conn Med. 66:589, 2002.
17. Wilkinson EJ: Normal histology, and nomenclature of the vulva and malignant neoplasms, including VIN. Dermatol Clin 10:283, 1992.
18. Wilkinson EJ, Stone KI: Atlas of Vulvar Disease. Baltimore, Williams & Wilkins, 1995.
19. Regauer S, Reich O, Beham-Schmid C: Monoclonal gamma-T-cell receptor rearrangement in vulvar lichen sclerosus and squamous cell carcinomas. Am J Pathol 160:1035, 2002.
20. Pinto AP, Lin MC, Sheets EE, Muto MG, Sun D, Crum CP: Allelic imbalance in lichen sclerosus, hyperplasia, and intraepithelial neoplasia of the vulva. Gynecol Oncol 77:171, 2000.
21. Crum CP: Vulvar intraepithelial neoplasia: histology and associated viral changes. Contemp Issues Surg Pathol 9:119,1987.
22. Sykes NL: Condyloma Acuminatum: Int J Dermatol 34:297, 1995.
23. zur Hausen H: Papillomavirus infections: a major cause of human cancers. Biochim Biophys Acta 1288:F55, 1996.
24. Kurman RJ, et al: Tumors of the cervix, vagina, and vulva. Atlas of Tumor Pathology, 3rd series, fascicle 4. Washington, DC, Armed Forces Institute of Pathology, 1992, p 191.
25. Crum CP: Carcinoma of the vulva: epidemiology and pathogenesis. Obstet Gynecol 79:3, 1992.
26. Leibowitch M, et al: The epithelial changes associated with squamous cell carcinoma of the vulva: a review of the clinical, histological and viral findings in 78 women. Br J Obstet Gynaecol 97:1135, 1990.
27. Hart WR: Vulvar intraepithelial neoplasia: historical aspects and current status. Int J Gynecol Pathol 20:16, 2001.
28. Worsham MJ, et al: Consistent chromosome abnormalities in squamous cell carcinoma of the vulva. Genes Chromosomes Cancer 3:420, 1991.
29. Kurman RJ, et al: Basaloid and warty carcinomas of the vulva. Distinctive types of squamous cell carcinoma frequently associated with human papillomaviruses. Am J Surg Pathol 17:133, 1993. [Published erratum appears in Am J Surg Pathol 17:536, 1993].
30. Jones RW: The natural history of vulvar intraepithelial neoplasia. Br J Obstet Gynaecol 102:764, 1995.
31. Jones RW, Rowan DM: Spontaneous regression of vulvar intraepithelial neoplasia 2-3. Obstet Gynecol 96:470, 2000.
32. Robertson DI, Maung R, Duggan MA: Verrucous carcinoma of the genital tract: is it a distinct entity? Can J Surg 36:147, 1993.
33. Gibson GE, Ahmed I: Perianal and genital basal cell carcinoma: A clinicopathologic review of 51 cases. J Am Acad Dermatol 45:68, 2001.
34. Ragnarsson-Olding BK, Kanter-Lewensohn LR, Lagerlof B, Nilsson BR, Ringborg UK: Malignant melanoma of the vulva in a nationwide, 25-year study of 219 Swedish females: clinical observations and histopathologic features. Cancer 86:1273, 1999.
35. van Bokhoven H, McKeon F: Mutations in the p53 homolog p63: allele-specific developmental syndromes in humans. Trends Mol Med 8:133, 2002.
36. Nucci MR, Fletcher CD: Vulvovaginal soft tissue tumours: update and review. Histopathology 36:97, 2000.
37. Mittendof R, Herbst AL: DES exposure: an update. Contemp Pediatr 11:59, 1994.
38. Scully RE, Welch WR: Pathology of the female genital tract after prenatal exposure to diethylstilbestrol. In Herbst AL, Bern HA (eds): Developmental Effects of Diethylstilbestrol in Pregnancy. New York, Thieme-Stratton, 1981, pp 26–45.
39. Copeland LJ, et al: Sarcoma botryoides of the female genital tract. Obstet Gynecol 66:262, 1985.
40. Andrassy RJ, et al: Conservative surgical management of vaginal and vulvar pediatric rhabdomyosarcoma: a report from the Intergroup Rhabdomyosarcoma Study III. J Pediatr Surg 30:1034, 1995.
41. Winkler B, Crum CP: *Chlamydia trachomatis* infection of the female genital tract. Pathogenetic and clinicopathologic correlations. Pathol Annu 5:193, 1984.
42. Kiviat NB, et al: Histopathology of endocervical infection by *Chlamydia trachomatis*, herpes simplex virus, *Trichomonas vaginalis*, and *Neisseria gonorrhoeae*. Hum Pathol 21:831, 1990.
43. Koutsky L: Epidemiology of genital human papillomavirus infection. Am J Med 102:3, 1997.
44. Crum CP: Human papillomaviruses: applications, caveats and prevention. J Repro Med 47:519, 2002.
45. Munger K, Howley PM: Human papillomavirus immortalization and transformation functions. Virus Res 89:213, 2002.
46. Klingelhutz AJ, Foster SA, McDougall JK: Telomerase activation by the E6 gene product of human papillomavirus type 16. Nature 380:79, 1996.
47. Duensing S, Lee LY, Duensing A, Basile J, Piboonniyom S, Gonzalez S, Crum CP, Munger K: The human papillomavirus type 16 E6 and E7 oncoproteins cooperate to induce mitotic defects and genomic instability by uncoupling centrosome duplication from the cell division cycle. Proc Natl Acad Sci U S A 97:10002, 2000.
48. Heselmeyer K, et al: Gain in chromosome 3q defines the transition from severe dysplasia to invasive carcinoma of the uterine cervix. Proc Natl Acad Sci U S A 93:479, 1996.
49. Rader JS, Gerhard DS, O'Sullivan MJ, Li Y, Li L, Liapis H, Huettner PC: Cervical intraepithelial neoplasia III shows frequent allelic loss in 3p and 6p. Genes Chromosomes Cancer 22:57, 1998.
50. Zhou J, Sun XY, Stenzel DJ, Frazer IH: Expression of vaccinia recombinant HPV 16 L1 and L2 ORF proteins in epithelial cells is sufficient for assembly of HPV virion-like particles. Virology 185:251, 1991.
51. Koutsky LA, Ault KA, Wheeler CM, Brown DR, Barr E, Alvarez FB, Chiacchierini LM, Jansen KU: A controlled trial of a human papillomavirus type 16 vaccine. N Engl J Med. 347:1645, 2002.
52. Wright T, et al: Precancerous lesions of the cervix. In Kurman R (ed): Blaustein's Pathology of the Female Genital Tract, 4th ed. New York, Springer-Verlag, 1994, p 229.
53. The Bethesda System for reporting cervical/vaginal cytologic diagnoses: Report of the 1991 Bethesda Workshop. Am J Surg Pathol 16:914, 1992.
54. Crum CP, et al: Pathology of Early Cervical Neoplasia. New York, Churchill Livingstone, 1996.
55. Sano T, Oyama T, Kashiwabara K, Fukuda T, Nakajima T: Expression status of p16 protein is associated with human papillomavirus oncogenic potential in cervical and genital lesions. Am J Pathol 153:1741, 1998.
56. Ostor AG: Natural history of cervical intraepithelial neoplasia: a critical review. Int J Gynaecol Pathol 12:186, 1993.
57. Stoler MH, et al: Small-cell neuroendocrine carcinoma of the cervix. A human papillomavirus type-18 associated tumor. Am J Surg Pathol 15:28, 1991.
58. Pirog EC, Kleter B, Olgac S, Bobkiewicz P, Lindeman J, Quint WG, Richart RM, Isacson C: Prevalence of human papillomavirus DNA in

different histological subtypes of cervical adenocarcinoma. Am J Pathol 157:1055, 2000.
59. Solomon D, Schiffman M, Tarone R: Comparison of three management strategies for patients with atypical squamous cells of undetermined significance: baseline results from a randomized trial. J Natl Cancer Inst 93:293, 2001.
60. Wright TC Jr, Cox JT, Massad LS, Twiggs LB, Wilkinson EJ: 2001 Consensus Guidelines for the management of women with cervical cytological abnormalities. JAMA 287:2120, 2002.
61. Denny L, Kuhn L, Risi L, Richart RM, Pollack A, Lorincz A, Kostecki F, Wright TC Jr: Two-stage cervical cancer screening: an alternative for resource-poor settings. Am J Obstet Gynecol 183:383, 2000.
62. Flowers LC, McCall MA: Diagnosis and management of cervical intraepithelial neoplasia. Obstet Gynecol Clin North Am 28:667, 2001.
63. Keating JT, Ince T, Crum CP: Surrogate biomarkers of HPV infection in cervical neoplasia screening and diagnosis. Adv Anat Pathol 8:83, 2001.
64. Dahlenbach-Hellweg G: Histopathology of the Endometrium, 4th ed. New York, Springer-Verlag, 1993.
65. Kiviat NB, et al: Endometrial histopathology in patients with culture-proved upper genital tract infection and laparoscopically diagnosed acute salpingitis. Am J Surg Pathol 14:167, 1990.
66. Simpson JL, Bischoff FZ: Heritability and molecular genetic studies of endometriosis. Ann N Y Acad Sci 955:239, 2002.
67. Noble LS, et al: Prostaglandin E2 stimulates aromatase expression in endometriosis-derived stromal cells. J Clin Endocrinol Metab 82:600, 1997.
68. Simpson JL, Bischoff FZ: Heritability and molecular genetic studies of endometriosis. Ann N Y Acad Sci 955:239, 2002.
69. Corley D, et al: Postmenopausal bleeding from unusual endometrial polyps in women on chronic tomoxifen therapy. Obstet Gynecol 79:111, 1992.
70. Fletcher JA, et al: Clonal 6p21 rearrangement is restricted to the mesenchymal component of an endometrial polyp. Genes Chromosomes Cancer 5:260, 1992.
71. Kurman RJ, et al: The behavior of endometrial hyperplasia: a long-term study of untreated hyperplasia in 170 patients. Cancer 56:403, 1985.
72. Mutter GL, Lin MC, Fitzgerald JT, Kum JB, Baak JP, Lees JA, Weng LP, Eng C: Altered PTEN expression as a diagnostic marker for the earliest endometrial precancers. J Natl Cancer Inst 92:924, 2000.
73. Mutter G, Nogales F, Kurman R, Silverberg S, Tavassoli F, et al: Endometrial Cancer. In Tavassoli FA, Stratton MR (eds): WHO Classification of Tumors: Pathology and Genetics, Tumors of the Breast and Female Genital Organs. Lyon, France, IARC Press, 2002.
74. Ferenczy A, Gelfand M: The biologic significance of cytologic atypia in progestogen-treated endometrial hyperplasia. Am J Obstet Gynecol 160:126, 1989.
75. O'Connell JT, Mutter GL, Cviko A, Nucci M, Quade BJ, Kozakewich HP, Neffen E, Sun D, Yang A, McKeon FD, Crum CP: Identification of a basal/reserve cell immunophenotype in benign and neoplastic endometrium: a study with the p53 homologue p63. Gynecol Oncol 80:30, 2001.
76. Brinton LA, et al: Reproductive, menstrual, and medical risk factors for endometrial cancer: results from a case-control study. Am J Obstet Gynecol 167:1317, 1992.
77. Silverberg SG, Kurman RJ: Tumors of the uterine corpus and gestational trophoblastic disease. Atlas of Tumor Pathology, 3rd series, fascicle 3. Washington, DC, Armed Forces Institute of Pathology, 1991, pp 219–287.
78. Mutter GL, et al: Allelotype mapping of unstable microsatellites establishes direct lineage continuity between endometrial precancers and cancer. Cancer Res 56:4483, 1996.
79. Sherman ME: Theories of endometrial carcinogenesis: a multidisciplinary approach. Mod Pathol. 13:295, 2000.
80. Rose PG: Endometrial carcinoma. N Engl J Med 335:640, 1997.
81. Nicklin JL, Copeland LJ: Endometrial papillary serous carcinoma: patterns of spread and treatment. Clin Obstet Gynecol 39:686, 1996.
82. Grice J, Ek M, Greer B, Koh WJ, Muntz HG, Cain J, Tamimi H, Stelzer K, Figge D, Goff BA: Uterine papillary serous carcinoma: evaluation of long-term survival in surgically staged patients. Gynecol Oncol 69:69, 1998.
83. Lim P, Al Kushi A, Gilks B, Wong F, Aquino-Parsons C: Early stage uterine papillary serous carcinoma of the endometrium: effect of adjuvant whole abdominal radiotherapy and pathologic parameters on outcome. Cancer 91:752, 2001.
84. Tay EH, Ward BG: The treatment of uterine papillary serous carcinoma (UPSC): are we doing the right thing? Int J Gynecol Cancer 9:463, 1999.
85. Silverberg SG, et al: Carcinosarcoma (malignant mixed mesodermal tumor of the uterus). Int J Gynaecol Pathol 9:1, 1990.
86. Clement PB, Scully RE: Müllerian adenosarcoma of the uterus: a clinicopathologic analysis of 100 cases with a review of the literature. Hum Pathol 21:363, 1990.
87. Chang KL, Crabtree GS, Lim-Tan SK, Kempson RL, Hendrickson MR: Primary uterine endometrial stromal neoplasms: a clinicopathologic study of 117 cases. Am J Surg Pathol 14:415, 1990.
88. Koontz JI, Soreng AL, Nucci M, Kuo FC, Pauwels P, van Den Berghe H, Cin PD, Fletcher JA, Sklar J: Frequent fusion of the JAZF1 and JJAZ1 genes in endometrial stromal tumors. Proc Natl Acad Sci U S A 98:6348, 2001.
89. Quade BJ: Pathology, cytogenetics, and molecular biology of uterine leiomyomas and other smooth muscle lesions. Curr Opin Obstet Gynecol 7:35, 1995.
90. Ligon AH, Morton CC: Genetics of uterine leiomyomata. Genes Chromosomes Cancer 28:235, 2000.
91. Quade BJ, Pinto AP, Howard DR, Peters WA 3rd, Crum CP: Frequent loss of heterozygosity for chromosome 10 in uterine leiomyosarcoma in contrast to leiomyoma. Am J Pathol 154:945, 1999.
92. Bell SW, et al: Problematic uterine smooth muscle neoplasms: a clinicopathologic study of 213 cases. Am J Surg Pathol 18:535, 1994.
93. Obermair A, Taylor KH, Janda M, Nicklin JL, Crandon AJ, Perrin L: Primary fallopian tube carcinoma: the Queensland experience. Int J Gynecol Cancer 11:69, 2001.
94. Aziz S, Kuperstein G, Rosen B, Cole D, Nedelcu R, McLaughlin J, Narod SA: A genetic epidemiological study of carcinoma of the fallopian tube. Gynecol Oncol. 80:341, 2001.
95. Young RH, Scully RE: Ovarian pathology in infertility. In Kraus FT (ed): Pathology of Reproductive Failure. Baltimore, Williams & Wilkins, 1991, pp 104–139.
96. Homburg R: Polycystic ovary syndrome: from gynaecological curiosity to multisystem endocrinopathy. Hum Reprod 11:29, 1996.
97. Ovalle F, Azziz R: Insulin resistance, polycystic ovary syndrome, and type 2 diabetes mellitus. Fertil Steril 77:1095, 2002.
98. Young RH, et al: The ovary. In Sternberg S, et al (eds): Diagnostic Surgical Pathology. New York, Raven Press, 1994, p 2195.
99. Narod SA, Boyd J: Current understanding of the epidemiology and clinical implications of BRCA1 and BRCA2 mutations for ovarian cancer. Curr Opin Obstet Gynecol. 14:19, 2002.
100. Narod SA, Sun P, Ghadirian P, Lynch H, Isaacs C, Garber J, Weber B, Karlan B, Fishman D, Rosen B, Tung N, Neuhausen SL: Tubal ligation and risk of ovarian cancer in carriers of BRCA1 or BRCA2 mutations: a case-control study. Lancet 357:1467, 2001.
101. Ness RB, Grisso JA, Vergona R, Klapper J, Morgan M, Wheeler JE: Study of Health and Reproduction (SHARE) Study Group 1: Oral contraceptives, other methods of contraception, and risk reduction for ovarian cancer. Epidemiology 12:307, 2001.
102. Werness BA, Afify AM, Eltabbakh GH, Huelsman K, Piver MS, Paterson JM: p53, c-erbB, and Ki-67 expression in ovaries removed prophylactically from women with a family history of ovarian cancer. Int J Gynecol Pathol 18:338, 1999.
103. Singer G, Kurman RJ, Chang HW, Cho SK, Shih IeM: Diverse tumorigenic pathways in ovarian serous carcinoma. Am J Pathol 160:1223, 2002.
104. Werness BA, Ramus SJ, Whittemore AS, Garlinghouse-Jones K, Oakley-Girvan I, Dicioccio RA, Tsukada Y, Ponder BA, Piver MS: Histopathology of familial ovarian tumors in women from families with and without germline BRCA1 mutations. Hum Pathol 31:1420, 2000.
105. Lee KR, Scully RE: Mucinous tumors of the ovary: a clinicopathologic study of 196 borderline tumors (of intestinal type) and carcinomas, including an evaluation of 11 cases with 'pseudomyxoma peritonei'. Am J Surg Pathol 24:1447, 2000.
106. Watkin W, et al: Mucinous carcinoma of the ovary. Cancer 69:208, 1992.
107. Young RH, et al: Mucinous tumors of the appendix associated with mucinous tumors of the ovary and pseudomyxoma peritonei: a clinicopathologic analysis of 22 cases supporting an origin in the appendix. Am J Surg Pathol 15:415, 1991.

108. Snyder RR, et al: Endometrial proliferative and low malignant potential tumors of the ovary. Am J Surg Pathol 12:661, 1988.
109. Eifel P, et al: Simultaneous presentation of carcinoma involving the ovary and uterine corpus. Cancer 50:163, 1982.
110. Berek JS, Bast RC Jr: Ovarian cancer screening: the use of serial complementary tumor markers to improve sensitivity and specificity for early detection. Cancer 76 (suppl):2092, 1995.
111. Kim JH, Skates SJ, Uede T, Wong KK, Schorge JO, Feltmate CM, Berkowitz RS, Cramer DW, Mok SC: Osteopontin as a potential diagnostic biomarker for ovarian cancer. JAMA 287:1671, 2002.
112. Petricoin EF, Ardekani AM, Hitt BA, Levine PJ, Fusaro VA, Steinberg SM, Mills GB, Simone C, Fishman DA, Kohn EC, Liotta LA: Use of proteomic patterns in serum to identify ovarian cancer. Lancet 359:572, 2002.
113. Hankinson SE, Hunter DJ, Colditz GA, Willett WC, Stampfer MJ, Rosner B, Hennekens CH, Speizer FE: Tubal ligation, hysterectomy, and risk of ovarian cancer: a prospective study. JAMA 270:2813, 1993.
114. Linder D, et al: Pathogenetic origin of benign ovarian teratomas. N Engl J Med 292:63, 1975.
115. Mutter GL: Teratoma genetics and stem cells: a review. Obstet Gynecol Surv 42:661, 1987.
116. O'Connor DM, Norris HJ: The influence of grade on the outcome of stage I ovarian immature (malignant) teratomas: the reproducibility of grading. Int J Gynecol Pathol 13:283, 1994.
117. Gordon T, et al: Dysgerminoma: a review of 158 cases from the Emil Novak ovarian tumor registry. Obstet Gynecol 58:497, 1981.
118. Young RH, Scully R: Ovarian sex cord-stromal tumors: recent progress. Int J Gynaecol Pathol 1:101, 1982.
119. Robertson DM, Stephenson T, Pruysers E, Burger HG, McCloud P, Tsigos A, Groome N, Mamers P, McNeilage J, Jobling T, Healy D: Inhibins/activins as diagnostic markers for ovarian cancer. Mol Cell Endocrinol 191:97, 2002.
120. Prat J, Scully RE: Cellular fibromas and fibrosarcomas of the ovary. Cancer 47:2663, 1981.
121. Roth LM, et al: Sertoli-Leydig cell tumors: a clinicopathologic study of 34 cases. Cancer 48:187, 1981.
122. Hart WR, Burkons DM: Germ cell neoplasms arising in gonadoblastomas. Cancer 43:669, 1979.
123. Eichhorn JH, et al: DNA content and proliferative activity in ovarian small cell carcinomas of the hypercalcemic type: implications for diagnosis, prognosis and histogenesis. Am J Clin Pathol 98:579, 1992.
124. Russell, P, Robboy SJ and Anderson, MC: Ovary: miscellaneous and metastatic tumors. In Robboy SJ, Anderson MC, Russell P: Pathology of the Female Reproductive Tract. London, Churchill Livingstone, 2002, p 691.
125. Wilcox AJ: Incidence of early loss of pregnancy. N Engl J Med 319:189, 1988.
126. Kalousek DK, Lau AE: Pathology of spontaneous abortion. In Dimmick JE, Kalousek DK (eds): Developmental Pathology of the Embryo and Fetus. Philadelphia, JB Lippincott, 1992, p 62.
127. Rushton DI: Examination of products of conception from previable human pregnancies. J Clin Pathol 34:819, 1981.
128. Saxon D, et al: A study of ruptured tubal ectopic pregnancy. Obstet Gynecol 90:46, 1997.
129. Gersell DJ, Kraus FT: Diseases of the placenta. In Kurman RJ (ed): Blaustein's Pathology of the Female Genital Tract. New York, Springer-Verlag, 1994, p 975.
130. Grossman JH: Infections affecting the placenta. In Lavery JP (ed): The Placenta. Rockville, MD, Aspen Publishing, 1987, pp 131–134.
131. Weiner GP: The clinical spectrum of preeclampsia. Am J Kidney Dis 9:312, 1987.
132. Khong TY, et al: Inadequate maternal vascular response to placentation in pregnancies complicated by preeclampsia and by small for gestational age infants. BMJ 93:1049, 1986.
133. Waite LL, Atwood AK, Taylor RN: Preeclampsia, an implantation disorder. Rev Endocr Metab Disord 3:151, 2002.
134. Zhou Y, et al: Preeclampsia is associated with failure of human cytotrophoblasts to mimic a vascular adhesion phenotype: one cause of defective endovascular invasion in this syndrome? J Clin Invest 99:2152, 1997.
135. Ferris TF: Pregnancy, preeclampsia and the endothelial cell. N Engl J Med 325:1439, 1991.
136. Friedman SA: Preelampsia: a review of the role of prostaglandins. Obstet Gynecol 71:122, 1988.
136a. Levine RJ, Maynard SE, Qian C, et al: Circulating angiogenic factors and the risk of preeclampsia. N Engl J Med 350:672, 2004.
136b. Maynard SE, Min JY, Merchan J, et al: Excess soluble fms-like tyrosine kinase (sFlt1) may contribute to endothelial dysfunction, hypertension, and proteinuria in preeclampsia. J Clin Invest 111:649, 2003.
137. Resnick R: Intrauterine fetal growth restriction. Obstet Gynecol 2002, 99:490–496.
138. Redline RW, Abdul-Karim FW: Pathology of gestational trophoblastic disease. Semin Oncol 22:96, 1995.
139. Berkowitz RS, Goldstein DP: Management of molar pregnancy and gestational trophoblastic tumors. In Knapp RC, Berkowitz RS (eds): Gynecologic Oncology. New York, McGraw-Hill, 1993, p 328.
140. Bracken MB, et al: Epidemiology of hydatidiform mole and choriocarcinoma. Epidemiol Rev 6:52, 1984.
141. Lage JM: Gestational trophoblastic tumors: refining histologic diagnosis by using DNA flow and image cytometry. Curr Opin Obstet Gynecol 6:359, 1994.
142. Zaragoza MV, Surti U, Redline RW, Millie E, Chakravarti A, Hassold TJ: Parental origin and phenotype of triploidy in spontaneous abortions: predominance of diandry and association with the partial hydatidiform mole. Am J Hum Genet 66:1807, 2000.
143. Keep D, Zaragoza MV, Hassold T, Redline RW: Very early complete hydatidiform mole. Hum Pathol 27:708, 1996.
144. Mosher R, Goldstein DP, Berkowitz R, Bernstein M, Genest DR: Complete hydatidiform mole: comparison of clinicopathologic features, current and past. J Reprod Med 43:21, 1998.
145. Genest DR, et al: A clinico-pathologic study of 153 cases of complete hydatidiform mole (1980–1990): histologic grade lacks prognostic significance. Obstet Gynecol 78:402, 1991.
146. Lurain JR, et al: Natural history of hydatidiform mole after primary evacuation. Am J Obstet Gynecol 145:591, 1983.
147. Castrillon DH, Sun D, Weremowicz S, Fisher RA, Crum CP, Genest DR: Discrimination of complete hydatidiform mole from its mimics by immunohistochemistry of the paternally imprinted gene product p57KIP2. Am J Surg Pathol 25:1225, 2001.
148. Chilosi M, Piazzola E, Lestani M, et al: Differential expression of p57kip2, a maternally imprinted cdk inhibitor, in normal human placenta and gestational trophoblastic disease. Lab Invest 1998;78:269–276.
149. Papadopoulos AJ, Foskett M, Seckl MJ, McNeish I, Paradinas FJ, Rees H, Newlands ES: Twenty-five years' clinical experience with placental site trophoblastic tumors. J Reprod Med 47:460, 2002.
150. Chang YL, Chang TC, Hsueh S, Huang KG, Wang PN, Liu HP, Soong YK: Prognostic factors and treatment for placental site trophoblastic tumor: report of 3 cases and analysis of 88 cases. Gynecol Oncol 73:216, 1999.
151. Finkler NJ, et al: Clinical experience with placental site trophoblastic tumors at the New England Trophoblastic Disease Center. Obstet Gynecol 71:854, 1988.
152. Shih IM, Kurman RJ: The pathology of intermediate trophoblastic tumors and tumor-like lesions. Int J Gynecol Pathol 20:31, 2001.

CHAPTER 23

The Breast

Susan C. Lester, MD, PhD

THE FEMALE BREAST

LIFE CYCLE CHANGES

DISORDERS OF DEVELOPMENT

CLINICAL PRESENTATIONS OF BREAST DISEASE

INFLAMMATIONS

Acute Mastitis

Periductal Mastitis

Mammary Duct Ectasia

Fat Necrosis

Lymphocytic Mastopathy (Sclerosing Lymphocytic Lobulitis)

Granulomatous Mastitis

BENIGN EPITHELIAL LESIONS

Non-Proliferative Breast Changes (Fibrocystic Changes)

Proliferative Breast Disease without Atypia

Proliferative Breast Disease with Atypia

Clinical Significance of Benign Epithelial Changes

CARCINOMA OF THE BREAST

Incidence and Epidemiology

Etiology and Pathogenesis

Hereditary Breast Cancer

Sporadic Breast Cancer

Mechanisms of Carcinogenesis

Classification of Breast Carcinoma

Carcinoma in Situ

Invasive (Infiltrating) Carcinoma

Invasive Carcinoma, No Special Type (NST; Invasive Ductal Carcinoma)

Invasive Lobular Carcinoma

Medullary Carcinoma

Mucinous (Colloid) Carcinoma

Tubular Carcinoma

Invasive Papillary Carcinoma

Metaplastic Carcinoma

Prognostic and Predictive Factors

Stromal Tumors

Fibroadenoma

Phyllodes Tumor

Sarcomas

Other Stromal Lesions

Other Malignant Tumors of the Breast

THE MALE BREAST

GYNECOMASTIA

CARCINOMA

THE FEMALE BREAST

Normal

The class Mammalia is remarkable for the evolution of modified skin appendages that provide complete nourishment and immunologic protection for the young. In humans, paired mammary glands rest on the pectoralis muscle on the upper chest wall. The breast is composed of specialized epithelium and stroma that give rise to both benign and malignant lesions specific to the organ (Fig. 23–1).

Six to ten major ductal systems originate at the nipple. The keratinizing squamous epithelium of the overlying skin continues into the ducts and then abruptly changes to a double-layered cuboidal epithelium. A small keratin plug is often found at the duct orifice. The surrounding areolar skin is pigmented and supported by smooth muscle.

Successive branching of the large ducts eventually leads to the terminal duct lobular unit (TDLU). In the adult woman, the terminal duct branches into a grapelike cluster of small acini to form a lobule (Figs. 23–1 and 23–2*B*). Each ductal system typically occupies over a quarter of the breast, and the systems extensively overlap each other. In some women, ducts extend into the subcutaneous tissue of the chest wall and into the axilla.

In the normal breast, ducts and lobules are lined by two cell types. A low, flattened discontinuous layer of contractile cells containing myofilaments (myoepithelial cells) lies on the basement membrane. These cells assist in milk ejection during lactation and have an important role in maintenance of the normal structure and function of the lobule and the basement membrane.[1] A second layer of epithelial cells lines the lumens. The luminal cells of the terminal duct and the lobule produce milk, but those lining the large duct system do not. A committed stem cell in the terminal duct is postulated to give rise to both luminal and myoepithelial cells.[2]

The majority of breast stroma consists of dense fibrous connective tissue admixed with adipose tissue (interlobular stroma). Lobules are enclosed by a breast-specific hormonally responsive, delicate, myxomatous stroma that contains a scattering of lymphocytes (intralobular stroma).

Life Cycle Changes

The breast is a unique organ in that it is not fully formed at birth, undergoes cyclic changes during reproductive life, and starts to involute long before menopause.

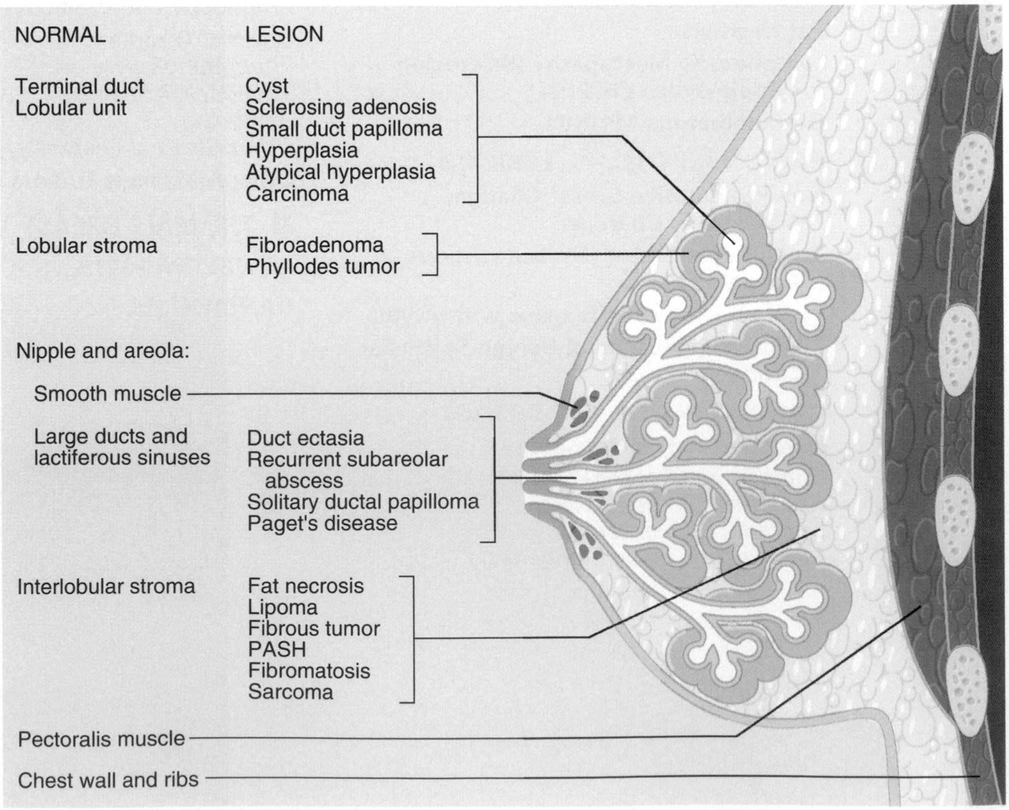

FIGURE 23–1 Normal breast anatomy and anatomical location of common breast lesions.

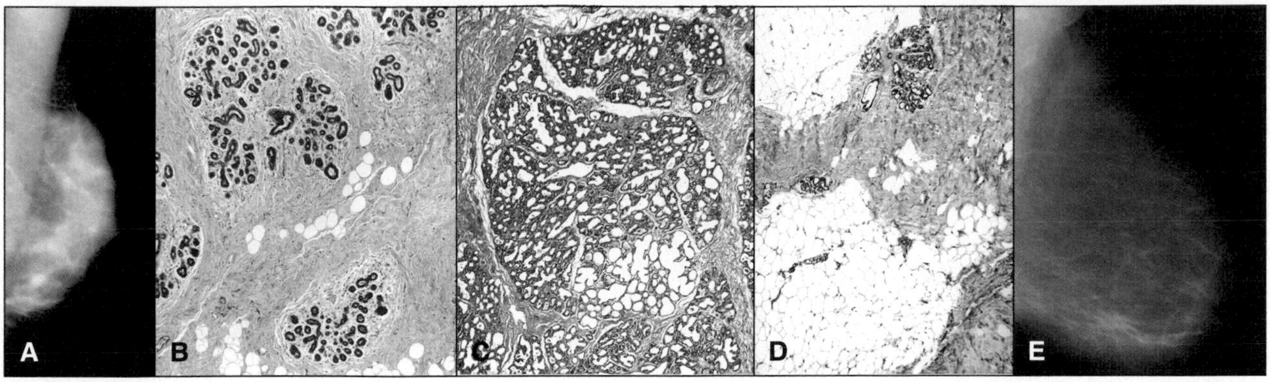

FIGURE 23–2 Lifecycle changes. *A*, Mammograms in young women are typically "dense" or white in appearance. In this setting, mass-forming lesions or calcifications can be difficult to detect. (Courtesy of Dr. Darrell Smith, Brigham and Women's Hospital, Boston, MA.) *B*, The density of a young woman's breast is due to the predominance of fibrous interlobular stroma and the paucity of adipose tissue (normally radiolucent or black). Prior to pregnancy, the terminal duct lobular units (TDLUs) are small and are invested by loose cellular intralobular stroma. Larger ducts interconnect the TDLUs. *C*, During pregnancy, branching of terminal ducts results in more numerous TDLUs, and the number of acini per TDLU increases. Luminal cells within TDLUs (but not the large duct system) undergo lactational change in preparation for milk production. *D*, With increasing age, the TDLUs decrease in size and number, and the interlobular stroma is replaced by adipose tissue. An older woman's breast typically consists of small ducts and atrophic lobules in adipose tissue. *E*, Mammograms become more radiolucent (darker) with age owing to the increase in adipose tissue. Radio-dense mass-forming lesions, and calcifications become easier to detect. (Courtesy of Dr. Darrell Smith, Brigham and Women's Hospital, Boston, MA.)

During midembryogenesis, the specialized mesenchyme of the breast fat pad condenses around the epithelium of the breast bud. Via a complex interaction between stromal and epithelial cells, cords of cells "invade" the stroma to form the rudimentary ductal system. The continuing cross-talk between epithelium and stroma promotes normal tissue structure and function throughout life.

The prepubertal breast in males and females consists of the large duct system ending in terminal ducts with minimal lobule formation. At the beginning of menarche in women, the terminal ducts give rise to lobules, and the interlobular stroma increases in volume. There is a paucity of adipose tissue, and hence the breast appears radio-dense (Fig. 23–2*A*, *B*). Just as the endometrium grows and ebbs with each menstrual cycle, so does the breast.[3] In the first half, or follicular, phase of the menstrual cycle, the lobules are relatively quiescent. After ovulation, under the influence of estrogen and rising progesterone levels, cell proliferation increases, as does the number of acini per lobule, and there is vacuolization of epithelial cells. Intralobular stroma becomes markedly edamatous. This combined stimulatory effect of estrogen and progesterone on the breast accounts for the sense of fullness commonly experienced by women during the premenstrual phase of the cycle. When menstruation occurs, the fall in estrogen and progesterone levels is followed by epithelial cell apoptosis, disappearance of the stromal edema, and overall regression in the size of the lobules.

It is only with the onset of pregnancy that the breast assumes its complete morphologic maturation and functional activity. Lobules increase both in number and in size. As a consequence, there is a reversal of the usual stromal-epithelial relationship so that, by the end of the pregnancy, the breast is composed almost entirely of lobules separated by a relatively scant amount of stroma (Fig. 23–2*C*). Numerous dermal glands in the areola (Montgomery tubercles) become more prominent and function in nipple lubrication. By the third trimester, secretory vacuoles of lipid material are found within the epithelial cells of the TDLU (Fig. 23–2*C*), but milk production is inhibited by the high levels of progesterone.

Immediately after birth, the breast produces colostrum (high in protein), which changes to milk (higher in fat and calories) within the first 10 days as progesterone levels drop. Just as the health of the mother and that of the infant are intricately linked during pregnancy, so too are they during breastfeeding. Breast milk not only provides complete nourishment from birth until several years of age, but also provides protection against infection and allergies. Maternal antibodies (chiefly secretory IgA), cells (neutrophils, lymphocytes, and macrophages), and other mediators (e.g., cytokines, fibronectin, and lysozyme) augment the infant's own developing defenses.[4,5] Some drugs, radioactive compounds given during diagnostic procedures, and viruses also pass into breast milk.[6] Thus, the postpartum health of the nursing mother continues to influence that of her infant.

After cessation of lactation, the lobules regress and atrophy, and the total breast size diminishes markedly. However, complete regression to the appearance of the normal nulliparous breast does not occur, and there is a permanent increase in the size and number of lobules.

After the third decade, long before menopause, lobules and their specialized stroma start to involute. The lobules may almost totally disappear in the very aged, leaving only ducts to create a morphologic pattern that closely resembles that of the male breast (Fig. 23–2*D*). However, in most women, there is sufficient persistent estrogenic stimulation, possibly of adrenal origin or from stores of body fat, to maintain the vestigial remnants of lobules that differentiate even the very aged female breast from the male breast. The radio-dense fibrous interlobular stroma of the young female breast (Fig. 23–2*A*) is progressively replaced by radiolucent adipose tissue (Fig. 23–2*E*).

Pathology

Disorders of Development

Milkline Remnants. Supernumerary nipples or breasts result from the persistence of epidermal thickenings along the milk line, extending from the axilla to the perineum, both below the adult breast and above it in the anterior axillary fold. The disorders that affect the normally situated breast may rarely arise in these heterotopic foci; occasionally, the cyclic changes of the menstrual cycle cause painful premenstrual enlargements.

Accessory Axillary Breast Tissue. In some women, the normal ductal system extends into subcutaneous tissue of the chest wall and into the axillary fossa. A mastectomy might remove the entire breast but not remove all breast epithelium. Therefore, prophylactic mastectomies markedly reduce but do not completely eliminate the risk of developing breast cancer. Breast epithelium outside of the breast proper might undergo lactational changes or give rise to tumors that appear to be outside the breast and therefore might be misidentified as lesions of the axillary lymph nodes or metastases from an occult breast cancer.

Congenital Nipple Inversion. The failure of the nipple to evert during development is common and may be unilateral. Inversion is usually spontaneously corrected during the growth activity of pregnancy, or it can sometimes be corrected by simple traction on the nipples. Nipple inversion is of clinical significance, since it may be confused with acquired retraction of the nipple, which is sometimes associated with an invasive cancer or inflammatory diseases of the nipple (e.g., recurrent subareolar abscess or duct ectasia).

Macromastia. The appropriate breast size is subjective and influenced by cultural norms. However, some women develop severe back pain and disability because of very large breasts. The large size may be due to variations in body habitus or to an unusual tissue response to hormonal changes during puberty resulting in massive rapid breast growth (juvenile hypertrophy). Reduction mammoplasty removes breast tissue but preserves the nipple.

Reconstruction or Augmentation. Breast tissue can be replaced or augmented by skin and muscle flaps or with synthetic breast prostheses. In the past, numerous types of materials were injected directly into the breast to increase volume but this was associated with a high incidence of complications due to an inflammatory response and the shift of these materials within the breast tissue. Silicone breast implants were developed in the early 1960s. Silicone, a polymer of silica, oxygen, and hydrogen, can be produced in liquid, gel, and solid forms by varying the length of the polymer. Silicone implants consist of a rubbery silicone shell filled with either silicone gel or saline.

The most common complication associated with breast implants is the formation of a thick fibrous capsule that causes cosmetic deformity. The typical histologic response is a chronic inflammatory infiltrate of lymphocytes, macrophages, and giant cells with associated fibrosis. Silicone gel seeps ("bleeds") through intact shells and is frequently seen in the surrounding tissue. The fibrous capsule can limit the spread of silicone after implant rupture. However, if the capsule is also ruptured, silicone gel can escape into surrounding tissues and be transported into axillary lymph nodes. Migration to more distant sites from implants has been demonstrated in animals but not definitively in humans. After long periods of implantation, the outer shell can weaken and rupture. Some implants become heavily calcified. The presence of implants, particularly if calcified, complicates the mammographic examination of the breast. Special techniques are necessary to visualize the breast tissue and avoid rupturing the implant.

Case reports have suggested linkage of implants to "human adjuvant disease," a proposed autoimmune-like illness in response to foreign material. However, multiple large epidemiologic studies have failed to show a connection between implants and objective evidence of rheumatologic disease or cancer.[7, 8] Nevertheless, the very long-term consequences of implants are unknown. There are approximately 2 million women in the United States with implants, and the number of women bearing implants for more than 20 years will rapidly increase in the next three decades. Current information from the U.S. Food and Drug Administration can be obtained at http://www.fda.gov/cdrh/breastimplants/.

Clinical Presentations of Breast Disease

An overall perspective of the frequency of various breast problems can be gained from analyzing a large series of patients with breast symptoms who were seen at a health maintenance organization (HMO)[9] (Fig. 23–3) and women undergoing diagnostic breast biopsies (Fig. 23–4). Three general points can be made. First, breast symptoms and signs are common problems in clinical practice. In the first group, 16% of women enrolled in the HMO presented with a breast symptom over a 10-year period. In the second group, diagnostic breast biopsies made up 5% of all surgical pathology specimens. Second, it is fortunate that the majority of breast symptoms or lesions will prove to have a benign etiology. Only 4% of outpatient visits for breast symptoms resulted in a diagnosis of breast cancer.[9] Of patients proceeding to surgery, only 26% proved to have cancer (Fig. 23–4). Finally, the physical, psychological, and financial costs of investigating benign breast disease, primarily to exclude malignancy, are substantial.

The most common symptoms reported by women are pain, a palpable mass, or nipple discharge (Fig. 23–3). In addition, women with abnormal findings on mammographic screening require further evaluation but are, by definition, asymptomatic. All other clinical presentations of breast disease are unusual. About 10% of the clinic visits in the HMO study were for other findings (such as "lumpy" breasts) that were considered normal by the doctor but had provoked enough concern for the woman to schedule an appointment.[9] Inflammatory conditions, as a group, account for less than 1% of breast symptoms.

Pain (mastalgia or mastodynia) is the most common breast symptom (Fig. 23–3) and may be cyclical with menses or noncyclical. Diffuse cyclical pain has no pathologic correlate, and most effective treatments target hormone levels. Noncyclical pain is usually associated with a focal site in the breast. Causes include ruptured cysts or areas of prior injury or infections, but more often, no specific lesion can be identified. Although

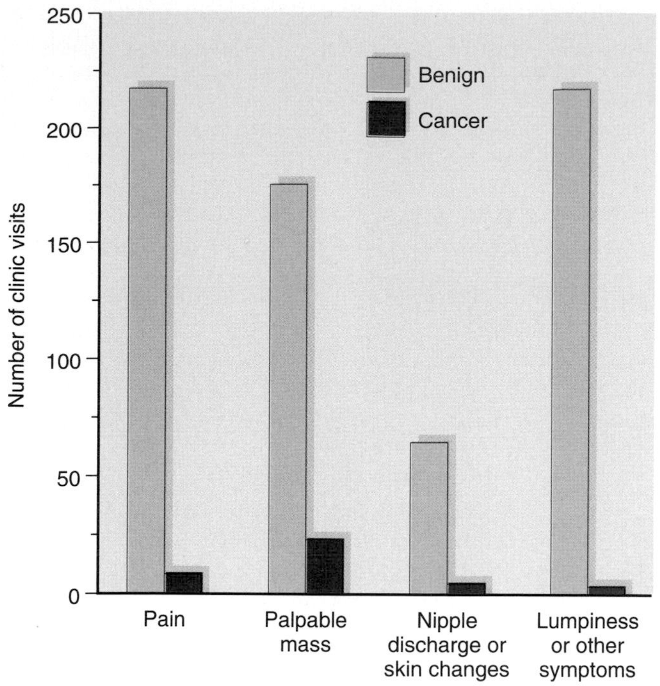

FIGURE 23–3 Common clinical presentations of breast disease. Over a 10-year period, 372 women over the age of 40 made 539 visits to a health maintenance organization for the listed breast symptoms.[9] Some women had more than one symptom and/or made more than one visit. In 10% of cases, the visit led to the performance of a biopsy.

the great majority of painful masses are benign, about 10% of breast cancers present with pain, and all masses need to be investigated. In the outpatient study, four of 221 (1.8%) women presenting with breast pain were diagnosed with cancer.[9] Three of the four women also had an associated palpable mass.

Discrete *palpable masses* are the second most common breast symptom (Fig. 23–3) and must be distinguished from the normal nodularity of the breast. A breast mass usually does not become palpable until it is about 2 cm in diameter (Table 23–1). These masses are most common in premenopausal women and become less frequent with age (Fig. 23–4). However, the likelihood that a palpable mass is malignant increases with the age of the patient. For example, only 10% of breast masses in women under age 40 proved to be malignant compared to 60% of masses in women over age 50 (Fig. 23–4). The most commonly encountered lesions are invasive carcinomas, fibroadenomas, and cysts. Approximately 50% of carcinomas arise in the upper outer quadrant, 10% in each of the remaining quadrants, and about 20% in the central or subareolar region.

Nipple discharge is a less common presenting symptom but is of concern when it is spontaneous and unilateral. A discharge produced by manipulating the breast is normal and unlikely to be associated with a pathologic lesion. A milky discharge (galactorrhea) is associated with increased production of prolactin (e.g., by a pituitary adenoma), hypothyroidism, or endocrine anovulatory syndromes. It can also occur in patients taking oral contraceptives, tricyclic antidepressants, methyldopa, or phenothiazines. Repeated nipple stimulation can also induce lactation (e.g., this method is sometimes used by women who wish to breast-feed adopted infants). Milky discharge has not been associated with malignancy. Bloody or serous discharges are most commonly associated with benign lesions but, rarely, can be due to a malignancy. A normal bloody discharge can also occur during pregnancy, possibly due to the rapid formation of new lobules. The risk of malignancy with discharge increases with age. Discharge is associated with carcinoma in 7% of women younger than 60 years and in 30% of women older than 60 years. The most common etiologies for discharge are a solitary large duct papilloma, cysts, or carcinoma (Fig. 23–4). Carcinomas presenting as nipple discharge not associated with a palpable mass are equally divided between invasive and in situ carcinomas.[10] There is considerable interest in developing the cytologic examination of induced nipple discharge into a screening test for breast cancer.

Mammographic screening was introduced in the 1980s as a means to detect small, nonpalpable breast carcinomas not associated with breast symptoms. The sensitivity and specificity of mammography increase with age. As the dense, fibrous interlobular tissue of the young woman is replaced by the fatty tissue of the older woman, it becomes easier to detect small masses and calcifications. Also, with increasing age, benign lesions become less frequent and malignant lesions become more frequent. Screening is generally recommended to start at age 40. Younger women usually undergo mammography only if they are at high risk for developing carcinoma, owing either to a prior palpable cancer or to a strong family history. Despite the screening of women at high risk of breast cancer, only 12% of mammographic lesions in women

TABLE 23–1 Characteristics of Breast Carcinomas by Clinical Presentation

Clinical Presentation	Invasive Carcinoma (% of Carcinomas)	Average Size of Invasive Carcinomas	Carcinomas with Lymph Node Metastases	DCIS (% of Carcinomas)	LCIS (% of Carcinomas)
Palpable mass	94%	2.4 cm	58%	2%	4%
Mammographic density	94%	1.1 cm	14%	4%	2%
Mammographic calcifications	26%	0.6 cm	6%	71%	3%

Based on the results of 235 carcinomas diagnosed in 914 women undergoing diagnostic biopsies at Brigham and Women's Hospital over a 6-month period in 2001.
Mammographic lesions were nonpalpable.
DCIS, ductal carcinoma in situ; LCIS, lobular carcinoma in situ.

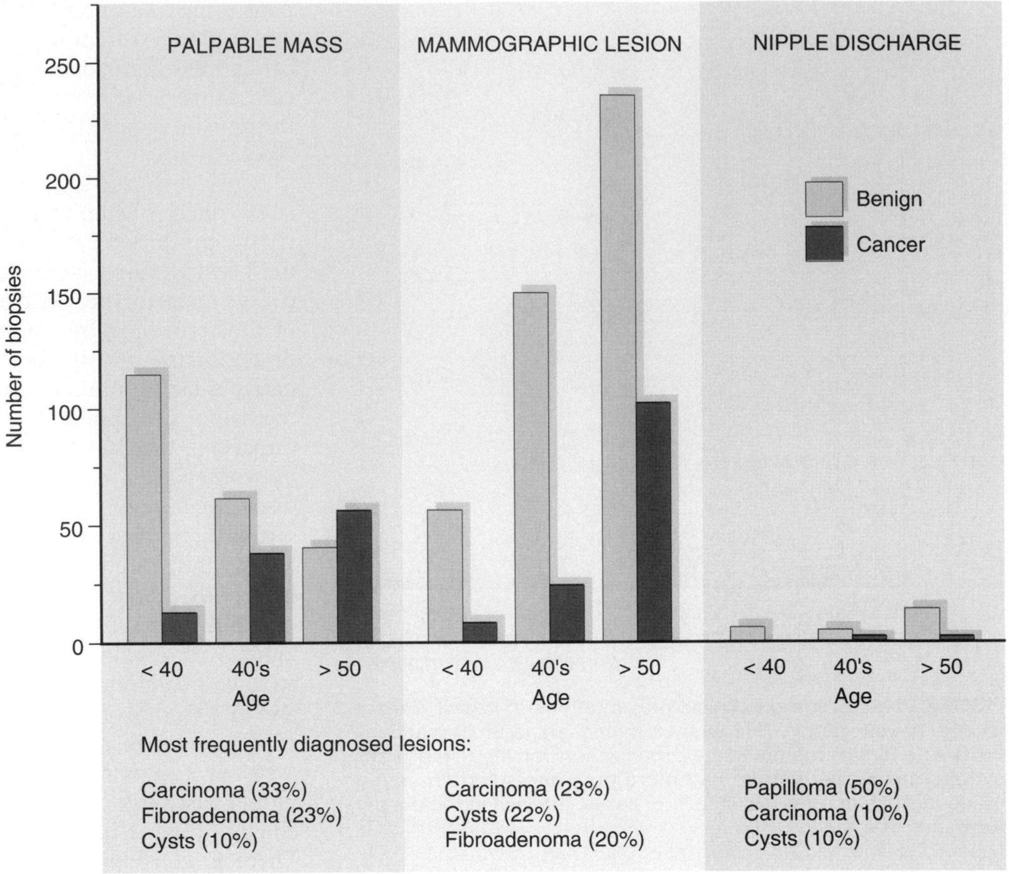

FIGURE 23–4 Frequency of benign and malignant breast lesions diagnosed after biopsy by clinical presentation and age. (Based on 914 women who underwent diagnostic breast surgery at Brigham and Women's Hospital, Boston, from January to June 2001.)

under age 40 proved malignant compared to 30% of lesions in women over age 50 (Fig. 23–4). *The principal mammographic signs of breast carcinoma are densities and calcifications:*

- *Densities.* Most neoplasms grow as solid masses and are radiologically denser than the intermingled connective and adipose tissue of the normal breast. Mammography can detect masses before they become palpable. For example, the average size of an invasive carcinoma that is detected as a mammographic density is only half that of carcinomas detected by palpation (Table 23–1). The most common lesions that are detected as densities are invasive carcinomas, fibroadenomas, and cysts (Fig. 23–4). Ductal carcinoma in situ (DCIS, or carcinoma limited to the ductal system) rarely presents as a density (Table 23–1).
- *Calcifications.* Calcifications are associated with secretory material, necrotic debris, and hyalinized stroma. Calcifications associated with malignancy are commonly small, irregular, numerous, and clustered or linear and branching. DCIS is the most common malignancy associated with calcifications (Table 23–1). Invasive carcinomas presenting as calcifications are quite small and are rarely associated with lymph node metastases. Benign calcifications are usually associated with clusters of apocrine cysts, hyalinized fibroadenomas, and sclerosing adenosis.

About 10% of carcinomas, even if they are palpable, are not detectable by mammography. The principal reasons are surrounding dense tissue (especially in younger women), absence of calcifications, small size, or location close to the chest wall or in the periphery of the breast. The inability to image a palpable mass does not indicate benignity, and all palpable masses require further investigation.

Other imaging modalities are useful adjuncts. Ultrasonography can distinguish solid and cystic lesions and can define more precisely the borders of solid lesions. Most palpable masses that cannot be imaged by mammography are detectable by ultrasound. Magnetic resonance imaging (MRI) detects cancers by the rapid uptake of contrast agents due to increased tumor vascularity. It has been most useful in detecting cancer in women with dense breasts, in determining the extent of chest wall invasion in locally advanced cancers, for detection of mammographically occult cancers, and for the evaluation of breast implant rupture.

Inflammations

Inflammatory diseases of the breast are rare; they often present as an erythematous swollen painful breast. Of these, the most important is acute mastitis, which is virtually confined to the lactating period. "Inflammatory breast cancer" mimics inflammation by obstructing dermal vasculature with tumor emboli, resulting in an enlarged erythematous breast, and should always be suspected in a nonlactating woman with the clinical appearance of mastitis.

ACUTE MASTITIS

Almost all cases of acute mastitis occur during lactation; most of these arise during the first month of nursing. During the early weeks of nursing, the breast is vulnerable to bacterial infection because of the development of cracks and fissures in the nipples. From this portal of entry, usually *Staphylococcus aureus* or, less commonly, streptococci invade the breast tissue. Women present with an erythematous painful breast, usually accompanied by fever. At the outset, only one duct system or sector of the breast is involved. If not treated, the infection may spread to the entire breast.

Morphology. Staphylococcal infections tend to produce a localized area of acute inflammation that may progress to the formation of single or multiple abscesses. Streptococcal infections tend to cause, as they do in all tissues, a diffuse spreading infection that eventually involves the entire breast. The involved breast tissue may be necrotic and is infiltrated by neutrophils.

Most cases of lactational mastitis are easily treated with appropriate antibiotics and complete drainage of milk from the breast. Rarely, surgical drainage may be required.

PERIDUCTAL MASTITIS

In this condition, known by a variety of names (recurrent subareolar abscess, squamous metaplasia of lactiferous ducts, Zuska disease), women, as well as men, present with a painful erythematous subareolar mass, which is usually clinically thought to be an infectious process.[11] More than 90% of patients with periductal mastitis are smokers.[12] This condition is not associated with lactation, a specific reproductive history, or age. In recurrent cases, a fistula tract often tunnels under the smooth muscle of the nipple and opens onto the skin at the edge of the areola. Many women with this condition have an inverted nipple secondary to fibrosis and scarring, and it has been suggested that this condition might contribute to the squamous metaplasia of the ducts. However, in most women, the inversion is more likely a secondary phenomenon due to the inflammatory response. The strong association with cigarette smoking is intriguing. It has been suggested that the vitamin A deficiency associated with smoking or toxic substances in tobacco smoke alter the differentiation of the ductal epithelium.[12]

Morphology. The main histologic feature is keratinizing squamous epithelium extending to an abnormal depth into the orifices of the nipple ducts (Fig. 23–5). Keratin is trapped within the ductal system and causes dilation and eventually rupture of the duct. An intense chronic and granulomatous inflammatory response develops to keratin spilled into periductal tissue. If secondary infections with skin bacteria or with mixed anaerobes occur, acute inflammation is also present.

Appropriate clinical management requires removing the involved duct and fistula tract in continuity, which, in most cases, is curative.[12] Incision drains the abscess cavity, but the offending keratinizing epithelium remains and recurrences are common. If a superimposed infection is present, antibiotic therapy must be directed toward the bacteria present, as standard staphylococcal therapy is usually ineffective.

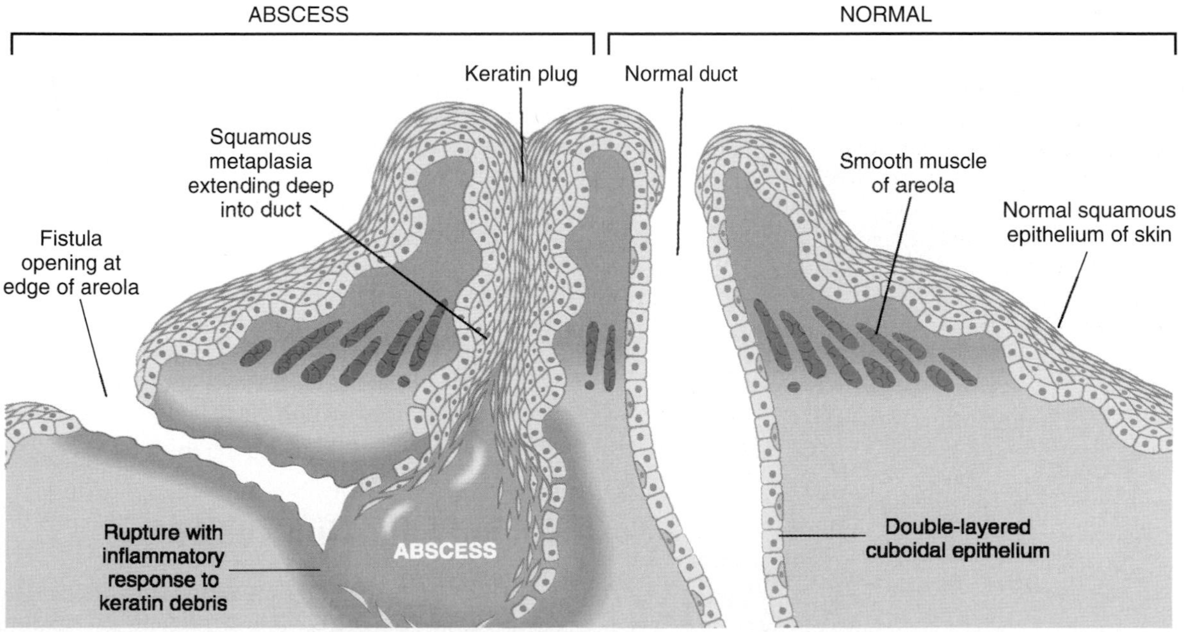

FIGURE 23–5 Recurrent subareolar abscess. When squamous metaplasia extends deep into a duct, keratin becomes trapped and accumulates. If the duct ruptures, the ensuing intense inflammatory response to keratin results in an erythematous painful mass. A fistula tract may burrow beneath the smooth muscle of the nipple to open at the edge of the areola.

MAMMARY DUCT ECTASIA

This disorder tends to occur in the fifth or sixth decade of life, usually in multiparous women, and, unlike periductal mastitis, is not associated with cigarette smoking. Patients present with a poorly defined palpable periareolar mass, sometimes with skin retraction, often accompanied by thick, white nipple secretions. Pain and erythema are uncommon.

Morphology. This lesion is characterized chiefly by dilation of ducts, inspissation of breast secretions, and a marked periductal and interstitial chronic granulomatous inflammatory reaction (Fig. 23–6). The dilated ducts are filled by granular debris that contains principally lipid-laden macrophages. The periductal and interductal inflammation is manifested by heavy infiltrates of lymphocytes and macrophages, with a striking predominance of plasma cells in some cases. On occasion, granulomatous inflammation forms around cholesterol deposits. Fibrosis may eventually produce skin and nipple retraction. Squamous metaplasia of nipple ducts is not a feature of this disorder.

This lesion is of clinical significance because the formation of an irregular mass can be mistaken for a carcinoma by palpation and by mammographic examination.

FAT NECROSIS

Fat necrosis can present as a painless palpable mass, skin thickening or retraction, a mammographic density, or mammographic calcifications. The majority of women will give a history of trauma or prior surgery.

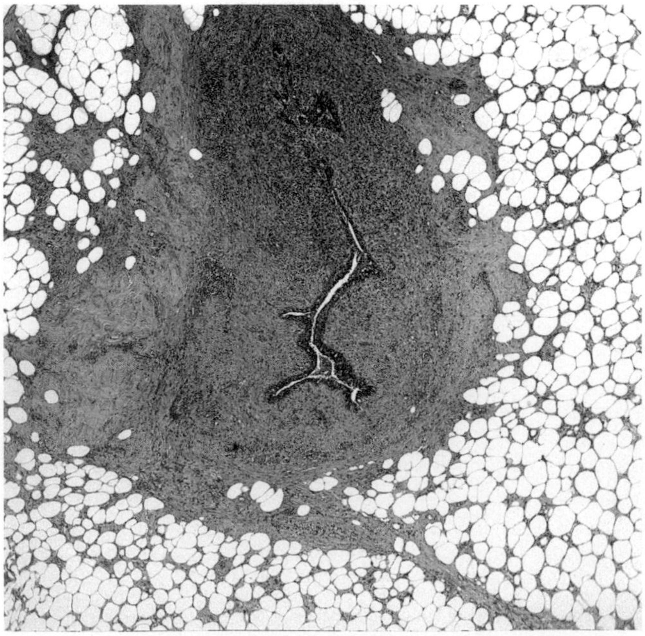

FIGURE 23–6 Mammary duct ectasia. Chronic inflammation and fibrosis surround an ectatic duct filled with inspissated debris. The fibrotic response can mimic the irregular shape of malignant carcinomas on palpation or mammogram.

Morphology. Grossly, the lesion may consist of hemorrhage in the early stages and, later, central liquefactive necrosis of fat. Still later, it may appear as an ill-defined nodule of gray-white, firm tissue containing small foci of chalky white or hemorrhagic debris. The central focus of necrotic fat cells is initially surrounded by macrophages and an intense neutrophilic infiltration. Then, during the next few days, progressive fibroblastic proliferation, increased vascularization, and lymphocytic and histiocytic infiltration wall off the focus. Subsequently, foreign body giant cells, calcifications, and hemosiderin make their appearance, and eventually, the focus is replaced by scar tissue or is encysted and walled off by collagenous tissue.

The major clinical significance of the condition is its possible confusion with breast carcinoma as a palpable mass or mammographic calcifications.

LYMPHOCYTIC MASTOPATHY (SCLEROSING LYMPHOCYTIC LOBULITIS)

This condition presents with single or multiple hard palpable masses. In some cases, the masses are bilateral or are detected as mammographic densities. The lesions are so hard that it can be difficult to obtain tissue with a needle biopsy. Microscopically, they show collagenized stroma surrounding atrophic ducts and lobules. The epithelial basement membrane is often thickened. A prominent lymphocytic infiltrate surrounds epithelium and blood vessels. This condition is most common in women with type 1 (insulin-dependent) diabetes or autoimmune thyroid disease. Therefore, it is hypothesized that this is an autoimmune disease of the breast. The only clinical significance is to distinguish this condition from carcinoma.

GRANULOMATOUS MASTITIS

Granulomas in the breast are caused by a wide variety of diseases, all of them rare, and are present in fewer than 1% of all breast biopsies. Systemic granulomatous diseases (e.g., Wegener granulomatosis, sarcoidosis) may involve the breast; on occasion, the breast may be the presenting site of involvement. Infections (mycobacterial, fungal) occur, most commonly in immunocompromised patients or in the setting of a breast prosthesis or nipple piercing. Granulomatous lobular mastitis is an uncommon breast-limited disease distinguished by granulomas involving lobular epithelium. Only parous women are affected, and it is hypothesized that the disease is a hypersensitivity reaction mediated by prior alterations in lobular epithelium during lactation.

Benign Epithelial Lesions

A wide variety of benign alterations in ducts and lobules are observed in the breast. Most present as mammographic lesions or as incidental findings. Less commonly, they present as palpable masses. These changes have been divided into three groups, according to the subsequent risk of developing breast cancer: (1) nonproliferative breast changes, (2) proliferative breast disease, and (3) atypical hyperplasia.

NONPROLIFERATIVE BREAST CHANGES (FIBROCYSTIC CHANGES)

This group includes a miscellany of alterations in the female breast that are often grouped under the term "fibrocystic changes." To the clinician, the term might mean "lumpy bumpy" breasts on palpation; to the radiologist, a dense breast with cysts; and to the pathologist, benign morphologic changes. These changes are termed "nonproliferative" to distinguish them from the "proliferative" changes associated with an increased risk of breast cancer.

These lesions might come to clinical attention when they mimic carcinoma by producing palpable lumps, mammographic densities or calcifications, or nipple discharge. The involved areas, by palpation, may have an ill-defined diffuse increase in consistency as well as discrete nodularities that can make detection of other breast masses more difficult. Cysts are the most common cause of a palpable mass and are alarming when they are solitary, firm, and unyielding. They can usually be diagnosed by disappearance of the mass after fine-needle aspiration of the contents. Calcifications are commonly found in cysts and adenosis and often form mammographically suspicious clusters. Cystic changes can also be associated with spontaneous unilateral nipple discharge.

Morphology. There are three principal patterns of morphologic change: (1) cyst formation, often with apocrine metaplasia; (2) fibrosis; and (3) adenosis.

- ***Cysts.*** Small cysts form by the dilation and unfolding of lobules. When cystic lobules coalesce, larger cysts are formed. Unopened cysts are brown to blue (blue-dome cysts) owing to the contained semi-translucent, turbid fluid. Cysts are lined either by a flattened atrophic epithelium or by cells altered by apocrine metaplasia. Metaplastic cells have an abundant granular, eosinophilic cytoplasm, with round nuclei, resembling the apocrine epithelium of sweat glands (Fig. 23–7). Papillary projections may be present in cysts and calcifications are common. "Milk of calcium" is a term radiologists use to describe calcifications in large cysts that look as if they are lining the bottom of a rounded cyst on mammography.
- ***Fibrosis.*** Cysts frequently rupture, with release of secretory material into the adjacent stroma. The resulting chronic inflammation and fibrous scarring contribute to the palpable firmness of the breast.
- ***Adenosis.*** Adenosis is defined as an increase in the number of acini per lobule. A normal physiologic adenosis occurs during pregnancy throughout the breast. In nonpregnant women, adenosis can occur as a focal change. The acini are often enlarged (blunt duct adenosis) and are not distorted as is seen in sclerosing adenosis, described later. Calcifications are occasionally present within lumens.

Lactational adenomas present as palpable masses in pregnant or lactating women. They are formed by normal-appearing breast tissue with physiologic adenosis and epithelial lactational changes. These lesions are probably not true neoplasms but an exaggerated focal response to hormonal influences.

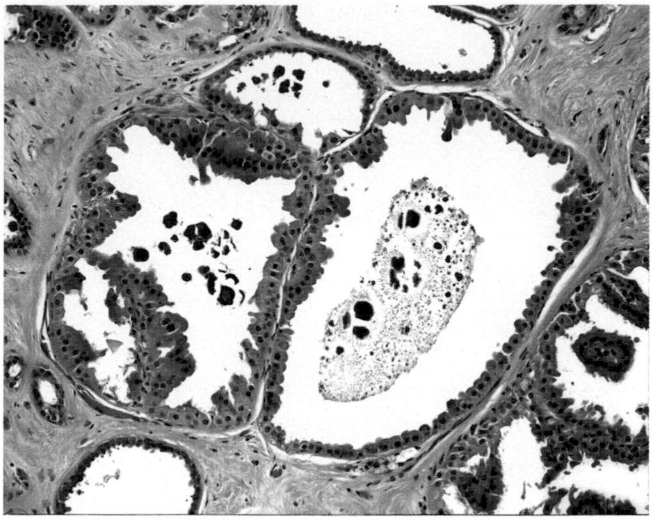

FIGURE 23–7 Apocrine cysts. Cells with round nuclei and abundant granular eosinophilic cytoplasm, resembling the cells of normal apocrine sweat glands, line the walls of a cluster of small cysts. Secretory debris, frequently with calcifications, is often present. Groups of cysts are common findings associated with clustered mammographic calcifications.

In a study of normal breasts in unselected forensic postmortem cases, grossly evident cysts and fibrosis were found in 20% and histologic changes were present in 59% of women.[13] Therefore, nonproliferative changes are most likely part of the spectrum of histologic features that can be observed in the normal breast.

PROLIFERATIVE BREAST DISEASE WITHOUT ATYPIA

These changes rarely form palpable masses. More commonly, they are detected as mammographic densities (e.g., complex sclerosing lesions or sclerosing adenosis), as calcifications (e.g., sclerosing adenosis), or as incidental findings in biopsies performed for other reasons (e.g., hyperplasia). More than 80% of large duct papillomas present as nipple discharge, the remainder as small palpable masses or mammographic densities. A large papilloma can spontaneously infarct, possibly because of torsion on the stalk, resulting in a bloody discharge. Non-bloody discharge probably results from intermittent blockage and release of normal breast secretions or irritation of the duct by the papilloma. Small papillomas occur deep within the breast and are usually incidental findings although they can be associated with calcifications. Although each of these lesions can be found in isolation, more commonly, more than one lesion is present, not infrequently in association with nonproliferative breast changes.

This group of disorders is characterized by proliferation of ductal epithelium and/or stroma without cellular abnormalities suggestive of malignancy. The following entities are included in this category: (1) moderate or florid epithelial hyperplasia, (2) sclerosing adenosis, (3) complex sclerosing

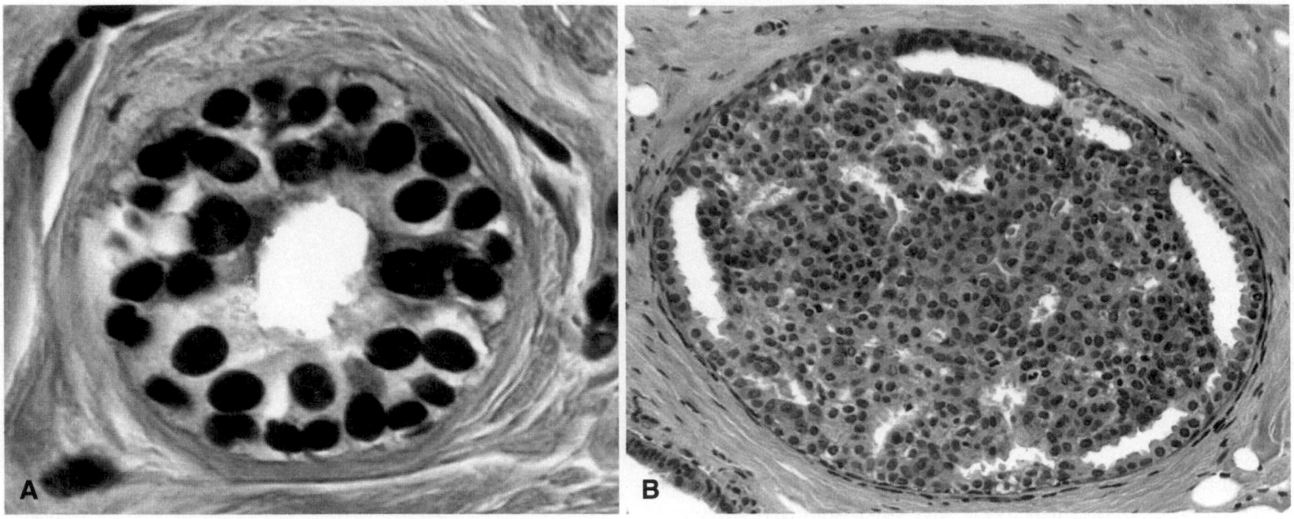

FIGURE 23–8 *A*, Normal. A normal duct or acinus has a single basally located myoepithelial cell layer (cells with dark, compact nuclei and scant cytoplasm) and a single luminal cell layer (cells with larger open nuclei, small nucleoli, and more abundant cytoplasm). *B*, Epithelial hyperplasia. The lumen is filled with a heterogeneous population of cells of different morphologies, often including both luminal and myoepithelial cell types. Irregular slitlike fenestrations are prominent at the periphary.

lesions, (4) papillomas, and (5) fibroadenoma with complex features.

Morphology.

Epithelial Hyperplasia. In the normal breast, only myoepithelial cells and a single layer of luminal cells are present above the basement membrane (Fig. 23–8*A*). Epithelial hyperplasia is defined by the presence of more than two cell layers. Hyperplasia is moderate to florid when there are more than four cell layers. The proliferating epithelium, often including both luminal and myoepithelial cells, fills and distends the ducts and lobules. Irregular lumens (fenestrations) can usually be discerned at the periphery of the cellular masses (Fig. 23–8*B*).

Sclerosing Adenosis. The number of acini per terminal duct is increased to at least twice the number found in uninvolved lobules. The normal lobular arrangement is maintained. The acini are compressed and distorted in the central portions of the lesion but characteristically dilated at the periphery. Myoepithelial cells are usually prominent. On occasion, stromal fibrosis may completely compress the lumens to create the appearance of solid cords or double strands of cells lying within dense stroma, a histologic pattern that at times closely mimics the appearance of invasive carcinoma (Fig. 23–9). Calcifications are frequently present within the lumens of the acini.

Complex Sclerosing Lesion (Radial Scar). Radial scars are stellate lesions characterized by a central nidus of entrapped glands in a hyalinized stroma (Fig. 23–10). These lesions can resemble irregular invasive carcinomas mammographically or on gross examination. The term "scar" refers to the morphologic appearance, as these lesions are not associated with prior trauma or surgery. A more general term is "complex sclerosing lesion," which includes not only radial scars but also related lesions with components of sclerosing adenosis, papilloma formation, and epithelial hyperplasia.

Papillomas. Papillomas are composed of multiple branching fibrovascular cores, each having a connective tissue axis lined by luminal and myoepithelial cells (Fig. 23–11). Growth occurs within a dilated duct. Epithelial hyperplasia and apocrine metaplasia are

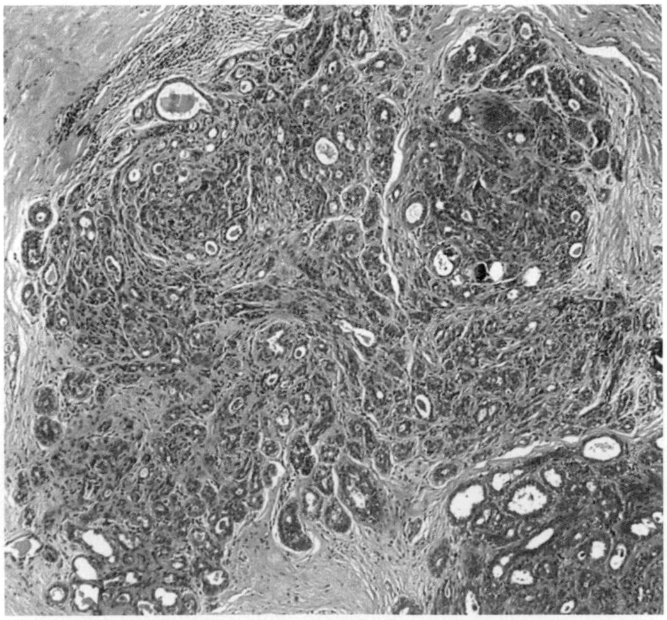

FIGURE 23–9 Sclerosing adenosis. The involved terminal duct lobular unit is enlarged, and the acini are compressed and distorted by the surrounding dense stroma. Calcifications are often present within the lumens. Although this lesion is frequently mistaken for an invasive carcinoma, unlike carcinomas, the acini are arranged in a swirling pattern, and the outer border is usually well circumscribed.

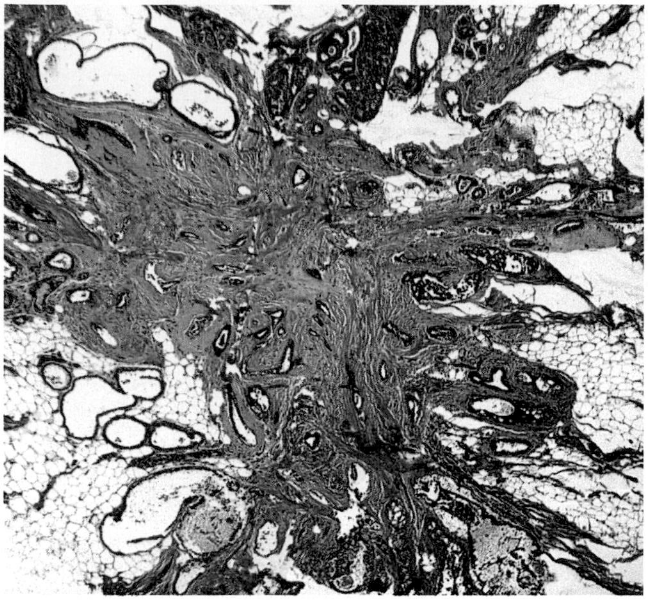

FIGURE 23–10 Complex sclerosing lesion (radial scar). There is a central nidus consisting of small tubules entrapped in a densely fibrotic stroma surrounded by radiating arms of epithelium with varying degrees of cyst formation and hyperplasia. These lesions typically present as an irregular mammographic density and closely mimic an invasive carcinoma.

frequently present. Large duct papillomas are usually solitary and situated in the lactiferous sinuses of the nipple. Small duct papillomas are commonly multiple and located deeper within the ductal system.

Small duct papillomas have been shown to be a component of proliferative breast disease and increase the risk of subsequent carcinoma. It is less clear whether or not large duct papillomas carry the same risk.

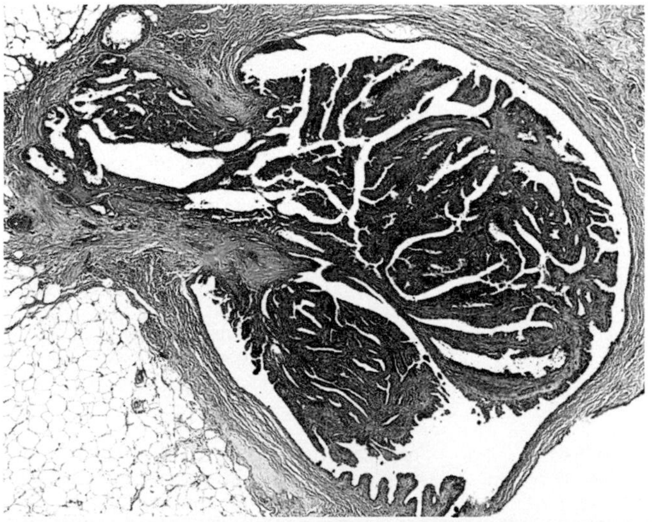

FIGURE 23–11 Intraductal papilloma. A central fibrovascular core extends from the wall of a duct. The papillae arborize within the lumen and are lined by myoepithelial and luminal cells.

Fibroadenomas will be discussed in the section devoted to stromal lesions.

PROLIFERATIVE BREAST DISEASE WITH ATYPIA

Proliferative disease with atypia includes atypical ductal hyperplasia (ADH) and atypical lobular hyperplasia (ALH). ADH is present in 5% to 17% of biopsies performed for calcifications and is found less frequently in biopsies for mammographic densities or palpable masses. Occasionally, ADH is associated with radiologic calcifications; more commonly, it is adjacent to another calcifying lesion. ALH is an incidental finding and is found in fewer than 5% of biopsies done for any reason.

Morphology. Atypical hyperplasia is a cellular proliferation resembling ductal carcinoma in situ (DCIS) or lobular carcinoma in situ (LCIS) but lacking sufficient qualitative or quantitative features for a diagnosis of carcinoma in situ.

ADH is recognized by its histologic resemblance to ductal carcinoma in situ, including a monomorphic cell population, regular cell placement, and round lumina. However, the lesions are characteristically limited in extent, and the cells are not completely monomorphic in type or they fail to completely fill ductal spaces (Fig. 23–12*A*).

ALH refers to a proliferation of cells identical to those of LCIS (described later), but the cells do not fill or distend more than 50% of the acini within a lobule (Fig. 23–12*B*). ALH can also extend into ducts, and this finding is associated with an increased risk of developing invasive carcinoma.

CLINICAL SIGNIFICANCE OF BENIGN EPITHELIAL CHANGES

Multiple epidemiologic studies have classified benign histologic changes in the breast and determined the subsequent risk these changes confer for the later development of invasive cancer (Table 23–2).[14–16] Nonproliferative changes do not increase the risk of cancer. Proliferative disease is associated with a mild increase in risk. Proliferative disease with atypia (ADH and ALH) confers a moderate increase in risk. Carcinoma in situ (DCIS and LCIS) is associated with a substantial risk if untreated and will be discussed later. The magnitude of risk may be modified by the woman's menopausal status, family history, and time since the biopsy (Table 23–2).

Carcinoma of the Breast

Carcinoma is the most common malignancy of the breast, and breast cancer is the most common non-skin malignancy in women. A woman who lives to age 90 has a one in eight chance of developing breast cancer. In 2001, almost 240,000 women were diagnosed with breast cancer, and over 40,000 died of the disease. As the demographic bulge of the "baby boomers" continues to grow older, the absolute number of women with breast cancer is expected to increase by about a third over the

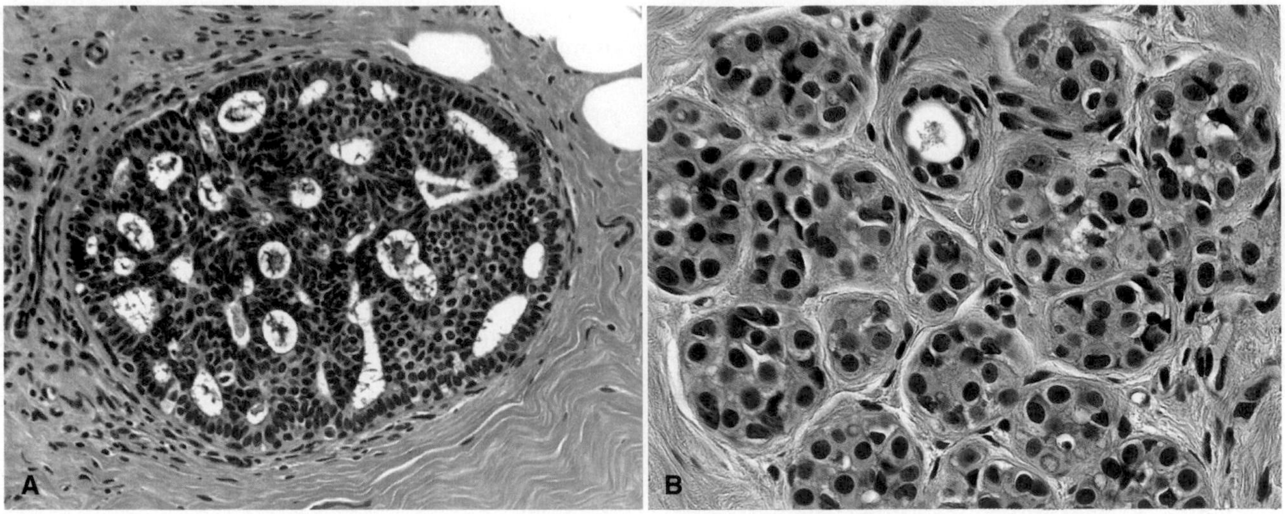

FIGURE 23–12 *A,* Atypical ductal hyperplasia. A duct is filled with a mixed population of cells consisting of oriented columnar cells at the periphery and more rounded cells within the central portion. Although some of the spaces are round and regular, the peripheral spaces are irregular and slitlike. These features are highly atypical but fall short of a diagnosis of DCIS. *B,* Atypical lobular hyperplasia. A population of monomorphic small, rounded, loosely cohesive cells partially fill a lobule. Some intracellular lumina can be seen. Although the cells are morphologically identical to the cells of LCIS, the extent of involvement is not sufficient for this diagnosis.

next 20 years, just because of the effect of the aging of the population. It is both ironic and tragic that a neoplasm arising in an exposed organ, readily accessible to self-examination and clinical diagnosis, continues to exact such a heavy toll. Only lung cancer causes more cancer deaths in women living in the United States.

INCIDENCE AND EPIDEMIOLOGY

After remaining constant for many years (except for a transient rise in 1974 attributed to increased awareness after the publicity surrounding Betty Ford and Happy Rockefeller developing breast cancer), the incidence of breast cancer

TABLE 23–2 Breast Lesions and Relative Risk of Developing Invasive Carcinoma

Pathologic Lesion	Relative Risk of Developing Invasive Carcinoma	Breast at Risk	Modifiers of Risk
Nonproliferative Breast Changes	1.0	Neither	
Duct ectasia Cysts Apocrine change Mild hyperplasia Adenosis Fibroadenoma without complex features			
Proliferative Disease Without Atypia	1.5–2.0	Both breasts	Increased risk if there is a family history of breast carcinoma Decreased risk 10 years after biopsy
Moderate or florid hyperplasia Sclerosing adenosis Papilloma Complex sclerosing lesion (radial scar) Fibroadenoma with complex features			
Proliferative Disease with Atypia	4.0–5.0	Both breasts	Increased risk if there is a family history of breast carcinoma Increased risk if premenopausal Decreased risk 10 years after biopsy for ALH
Atypical ductal hyperplasia Atypical lobular hyperplasia			
Carcinoma in Situ	8.0–10.0		
Lobular carcinoma in situ		Both breasts	Treatment (tamoxifen, bilateral mastectomy)
Ductal carcinoma in situ*		Ipsilateral breast	Treatment (tamoxifen, surgery to eradicate the lesion, radiation therapy)

*This risk applies to low-grade DCIS originally misdiagnosed as benign disease and followed without treatment. The risk for progression of high-grade DCIS is presumed to be greater than this.

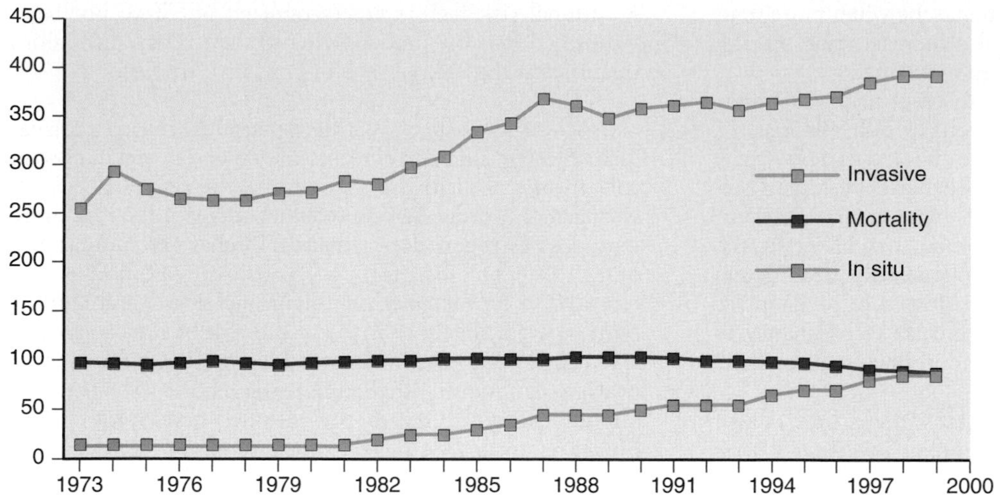

FIGURE 23–13 Breast cancer incidence and mortality rates for women over 50 years of age. Rates are per 100,000 women and are age-adjusted to the 2000 U.S. standard million population. (SEER Cancer Statistics Review 1973–1999; http://seer.cancer.gov/.)

began to increase in older women, raising concern that there was an unidentified environmental cause (Fig. 23–13). During this same period of time, starting in the early 1980s, mammographic screening was introduced, and the number of women of appropriate age undergoing screening increased steadily to current reported rates of 60% to 80%.[18] Screening results in the increased detection of small invasive carcinomas and in situ carcinomas. Since DCIS is almost exclusively detected by mammography (Table 23–1), this effect is shown by the accompanying increase in in situ carcinomas in this group of women (Fig. 23–13). During this period, the number of women presenting with large or locally advanced carcinomas decreased, whereas the number of women with only in situ carcinoma or small node-negative carcinomas markedly increased (Fig. 23–14). Over the same time period, the incidence of breast carcinoma in younger women, who have a much lower risk of breast cancer and for whom screening is not recommended, did not increase. In retrospect, the increase in incidence in older women can be explained primarily by the influence of screening.

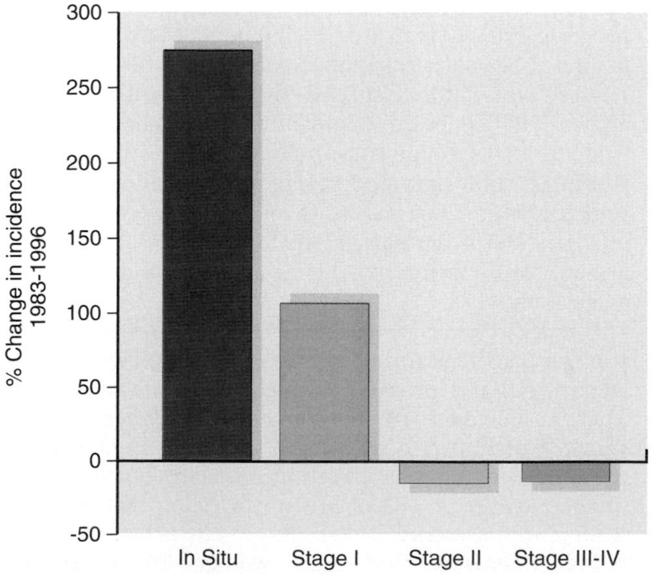

FIGURE 23–14 Change in stage of breast cancer at presentation from 1983 to 1996. (SEER Cancer Statistics Review, http://seer.cancer.gov/.)

Until recently, about one third of women diagnosed with breast cancer eventually succumbed to the disease. During the 1980s, the number of women dying of breast cancer remained constant, despite the increase in the incidence of breast cancer (Fig. 23–13). One possible explanation is that screening was detecting clinically insignificant cancers. In 1994, after a lag time of about 10 years, the mortality rate started to decline (Fig. 23–13). If screening is detecting clinically significant cancers at a curable stage, this downward trend will continue. Better treatment modalities should also contribute to this hopeful trend. Currently, only 20% of women with breast cancer are expected to die of the disease.

The frequency of this disease in women has prompted an intensive study of risk factors for developing breast cancer to gain clues as to its etiology as well as to identify modifiable risk factors that would be helpful for prevention strategies.

Risk Factors. The most common risk factors for the development of breast cancer, identified by epidemiologic studies, have been combined into a statistical model to calculate the absolute risk of an individual woman developing cancer within the next 5 years or by age 90.[19] A modified interactive version of this model is available at http://bcra.nci.nih.gov/brc/. It is designed for women over the age of 35 without a prior diagnosis of LCIS or DCIS and without a family history suggestive of a single gene mutation.[20] The model incorporates the following risk factors.

- ***Age.*** Breast cancer is rarely found before the age of 25 years except in certain familial cases. The incidence rises throughout a woman's lifetime. Seventy-seven per cent of cases occur in women over 50 years of age. The average age at diagnosis is 64 years.
- ***Age at Menarche.*** Women who reach menarche when younger than 11 years of age have a 20% increased risk

compared to women who reach menarche when more than 14 years of age. Late menopause also increases risk, but the magnitude of the risk has not been quantified.

■ ***First Live Birth.*** Women with a first full-term pregnancy at younger than 20 years of age have half the risk of nulliparous women or women over the age of 35 at their first birth. It is hypothesized that pregnancy results in terminal differentiation of epithelial cells, removing them from the potential pool of cancer precursors. However, the biologic basis of such differentiation has not been determined. This effect might be overshadowed in pregnancies in older women by the proliferation early in pregnancy of cells that might have already undergone preneoplastic changes.

■ ***First-Degree Relatives with Breast Cancer.*** The risk of breast cancer increases with the number of affected first-degree relatives (mother, sister, or daughter). However, the majority of cancers occur in women without such a history, as only 13% of women with breast cancer have one affected first-degree relative, and only 1% have two or more.[21] In turn, over 87% of women with a family history will not develop breast cancer. This model is not designed to calculate the risk for women in families with a high likelihood of a single gene mutation such as *BRCA1* or *BRCA2* (see the section on hereditary breast cancer below).

■ ***Breast Biopsies.*** Increased risk is associated with prior breast biopsies showing atypical hyperplasia. This model does not adjust for the mild increase in risk associated with proliferative breast changes without atypia (Table 23–2).

■ ***Race.*** Although the overall incidence of breast cancer is lower in women of African-American ancestry, women in this group present at a more advanced stage and have an increased mortality rate compared with white women.[22, 23] Social factors such as decreased access to health care and lower use of mammography account for some of the difference, but genetic factors also play a role. A greater number of breast cancers are diagnosed in black women than in white women younger than 40 years of age, and breast carcinomas in black women have a higher nuclear grade, more frequently lack hormone receptors, and have different types of sporadic *p53* mutations. Caucasian women generally have the highest rates of breast cancer. The risk of developing an invasive carcinoma within the next 20 years at age 50 is 1 in 15 for Caucasians, 1 in 20 for African Americans, 1 in 26 for Asian/Pacific Islanders, and 1 in 27 for Hispanics.[24]

Absolute risk for individual women, either for the next 5 years or lifetime risk, can be calculated by using this model. For example, a 60-year-old woman who first gave birth when she was more than 30 years of age (but with no other factors that would increase her risk) has a 2% risk of developing breast cancer over the next 5 years, compared to the 1% risk for a similar 60-year-old woman who had her first child when she was under the age of 20. Although all women are at high enough risk to undergo breast examination and screening mammography at the appropriate age, certain very high-risk women can consider other interventions such as chemoprevention or prophylactic mastectomy (discussed below). A risk of 1.7% of developing breast cancer in the next 5 years was used as the entry criterion for the chemoprevention trials.

Additional risk factors are recognized but have not been incorporated into the model owing to their rarity, difficulties in quantifying the risk, or lack of definitive studies.

■ ***Estrogen Exposure.*** Postmenopausal hormone replacement therapy slightly increases the risk of breast cancer in current users but might not increase the risk of death.[25,26] Estrogen and progesterone together increase the risk more than does estrogen alone. Invasive lobular carcinomas and other estrogen receptor (ER)–positive carcinomas are reported to be increased in this group does. Oral contraceptives are unlikely to increase the risk of breast cancer[27] and can decrease the risk of other malignancies such as ovarian carcinoma. Reducing endogenous estrogens by oophorectomy decreases the risk of developing breast cancer by up to 75%.

■ ***Radiation Exposure.*** Women who have been exposed to therapeutic radiation or radiation after atom bomb exposure have a higher rate of breast cancer. Risk increases with younger age and higher radiation doses. Women in their teens and twenties (but not at older ages) undergoing mantle radiation for Hodgkin disease have a 20% to 30% risk of developing breast cancer 10 to 30 years after treatment.[28] Modern mammographic screening uses low doses of radiation and is unlikely to have an effect on the risk of breast cancer.

■ ***Carcinoma of the Contralateral Breast or Endometrium.*** Increased risk is associated with carcinoma of the contralateral breast or endometrium, probably owing to the shared hormonal risk factors for these tumors.

■ ***Geographic Influence.*** Breast cancer incidence rates in the United States and Europe are four to seven times higher than those in other countries. The risk of breast cancer increases in immigrants to the United States during several generations. The specific factors have not been identified but have received considerable attention in the attempt to identify modifiable risk factors. Diet, physical activity, breast-feeding, and environmental factors have been investigated.

■ ***Diet.*** Various items in diet, in particular dietary fat, have been suggested to increase risk, but large studies have failed to find a strong correlation. Some studies have shown a reduced risk with increased β-carotene intake. Coffee addicts will be pleased to know that there is no substantial evidence that caffeine consumption increases the risk, but studies do show that moderate or heavy alcohol consumption confers an increased risk of breast cancer.[29] Higher estrogen levels and lower folate levels associated with alcohol consumption may be mechanisms underlying this association.

■ ***Obesity.*** There is decreased risk in obese women younger than 40 years owing to the association with anovulatory cycles and lower progesterone levels late in the cycle. There is increased risk in postmenopausal obese women, which is attributed to synthesis of estrogens in fat depots.

■ ***Exercise.*** Studies have been inconsistent, but some have shown a decreased risk of breast cancer in premenopausal women who exercise.

■ ***Breast-Feeding.*** The longer women breast-feed, the greater is the reduction in the risk of breast cancer.[30] The lower incidence of breast cancer in developing countries may be largely explained by the more frequent and longer nursing of infants.

- ***Environmental Toxins.*** There is concern that environmental contaminants such as organochlorine pesticides could have estrogenic effects on humans. The possible effect of environmental toxins on breast cancer risk is being intensively investigated. No specific substances have been definitively associated with an increased risk.
- ***Tobacco.*** Cigarette smoking is not associated with breast cancer but is associated with the development of periductal mastitis or a subareolar abscess (discussed earlier).

Treatment of Women at High Risk for Developing Breast Cancer. With the exception of DCIS, all other risk factors for the development of invasive breast cancer affect both breasts equally. Therefore, strategies to prevent cancer must treat both breasts.

Bilateral prophylactic mastectomy can prevent the development of 89% of breast cancers in women who are at moderate risk for the disease owing to a family history. However, prevention can come at a high cost. In one study, at least 12 women who were at risk owing to their family history underwent the procedure for every one case of cancer prevented.[31]

Chemoprevention is another option for women who are at risk for developing invasive breast cancer. Tamoxifen is a drug that competes for binding to the ER and has both estrogenic and antiestrogenic effects. It is the most widely used endocrine therapy for the treatment of breast cancer. In selected groups of women, tamoxifen has been shown to reduce the incidence of breast cancer.[32] However, tamoxifen also increased the risk of venous thromboembolism, endometrial cancer, and cataracts. Current clinical trials are attempting to identify other selective estrogen receptor modulators (SERMs) that have the same benefit but fewer side effects.

ETIOLOGY AND PATHOGENESIS

The major risk factors for the development of breast cancer are hormonal and genetic (family history). Breast carcinomas can, therefore, be divided into sporadic cases, possibly related to hormonal exposure, and hereditary cases, associated with family history or germ-line mutations. Hereditary carcinoma has received intense scrutiny in the hopes that the specific genetic mutations can be identified and that these alterations will illuminate the causes of all breast cancer. Recent studies have borne out these hopes. We begin our discussion with hereditary breast cancer and follow with sporadic breast cancer.

Hereditary Breast Cancer

A family history of breast cancer in a first-degree relative is reported in 13% of women with the disease.[21] However, only 1% of women have multiple affected relatives, a history suggestive of a highly penetrant germ-line mutation.

About 25% of familial cancers (or around 3% of all breast cancers) can be attributed to two highly penetrant autosomal-dominant genes: BRCA1 and BRCA2 (Table 23–3). The probability of breast cancer associated with a mutation in these genes increases if there are multiple affected first-degree relatives, if individuals are affected before menopause and/or

TABLE 23–3 *BRCA1* and *BRCA2*

	BRCA1	***BRCA2***
Chromosome	17q21	13q12.3
Gene size	81 kb	84 kb
Protein size	1863 amino acids	3418 amino acids
Function	Tumor suppressor Transcriptional regulation Role in DNA repair	Tumor suppressor Transcriptional regulation Role in DNA repair
Mutations	>500 identified	>300 identified
Mutations in population	about 0.1%	about 0.1%
Risk of breast cancer	60–80%	60–80%
Age at onset	Younger age (40s to 50s)	50 years
Families with breast cancer due to a single gene (%) Families with breast and ovarian cancer (%) Families with male and female breast cancer Risk of other tumors (varies with specific mutation)	52% 81% (20–40% risk) <20% Prostate, colon, pancreas	32% 14% (10–20% risk) 76% Prostate, pancreas, stomach, melanoma, colon
Mutations in sporadic breast cancer	Very rare (<5%)	Very rare (<5%)
Epidemiology	Specific mutations are found in certain ethnic groups	Specific mutations are found in certain ethnic groups
Pathology of breast cancers	Greater incidence of medullary carcinomas (13%), poorly differentiated carcinomas, ER-, PR-, and *Her2/neu*-negative carcinomas, carcinomas with *p53* mutations	Similar to sporadic breast cancers

Additional information about these genes can be found at http://www.ncbi.nlm.nih.gov/.

have multiple cancers, if there is a case of male breast cancer, or if family members also develop ovarian cancer. The general lifetime breast cancer risk for female carriers is 60% to 85%, and the median age at diagnosis is about 20 years earlier compared to women without these mutations. The penetrance (i.e., the number of carriers who actually develop breast cancer) can vary with the specific type of mutation present. Mutated *BRCA1* also markedly increases the risk of developing ovarian carcinoma, which is as high as 20% to 40%. *BRCA2* confers a smaller risk for ovarian carcinoma (10% to 20%) but is associated more frequently with male breast cancer. *BRCA1* and *BRCA2* carriers are also susceptible to other cancers, such as colon, prostate, and pancreas, but to a lesser extent.

Although BRCA1 and BRCA2 do not show sequence homology, they function in similar pathways and interact with the same multiprotein complexes. Both act as tumor suppressors, as it is a loss of function that confers the risk of malignancy. A wide variety of functions have been suggested for these proteins, including transcriptional regulation, cell-cycle control, ubiquitin-mediated protein degradation pathways, and chromatin remodeling. A key function for both appears to be their role in protecting the genome from damage by halting the cell cycle and promoting DNA damage repair in a complex process that is not yet fully understood. BRCA1 is phosphorylated in response to damage and may transduce DNA damage signals from checkpoint kinases to effector proteins. BRCA1 is also bound with BRCA2 and RAD51 in a nuclear dot complex—presumably the site of DNA repair.[33] BRCA2 can bind directly to DNA and functions in homologous recombination for the error-free repair of double-strand DNA breaks.[34] Why loss of these functions specifically affects the breast is unclear. Perhaps the intermittent proliferation of breast epithelium (as opposed to the constitutive proliferation of other epithelia such as colon or skin) makes this organ more susceptible to the accumulation of genetic damage, or possibly, other cell types have additional mechanisms for DNA repair that the breast lacks. BRCA1, but not BRCA2, interacts with the ER and is involved in X chromosome inactivation—two features that may be related to its gender-specific risk.[35] Interestingly, male breast cancers are markedly increased only in families carrying *BRCA2* mutations.

Both genes have a total length of over 80 kb, and hundreds of different mutations distributed throughout the coding region have been reported for each one. The frequency of mutations is only 0.1% to 0.2% in the general population. Some mutations diminish the function of the genes and increase cancer risk, whereas others might be unimportant sequence variants. Genetic testing is difficult and often inconclusive unless several family members are affected or unless the individual belongs to an ethnic group with a known high incidence of specific mutations.[36] For example, people of Ashkenazi Jewish descent have a 2% to 3% risk of three specific mutations. Identification of carriers of clinically significant mutations is important, as prophylactic mastectomy and/or oophorectomy can reduce the risk of cancer mortality.[31,37,38]

In hereditary carcinomas, one mutant *BRCA* allele is inherited, and the second allele is inactivated by somatic mutation. Although *BRCA1* and *BRCA2* mutations are rarely found in sporadic tumors, about 50% of such tumors have decreased or absent expression of BRCA1. In most cases, this is accomplished by a combination of loss of heterozygosity (LOH) and methylation of the promoter to inactivate both alleles.[39] Hypermethylation of the promoter is detected in 13% of unselected carcinomas but is more common in medullary carcinomas (67% of tumors) and mucinous carcinomas (55% of tumors)—histologic subtypes that are more commonly found in *BRCA1* carriers. A similar mechanism has not yet been described for *BRCA2*.

BRCA1-associated breast cancers are more commonly poorly differentiated, have a syncytial growth pattern with pushing margins, have a lymphocytic response, and do not express hormone receptors or overexpress HER2/neu (an epidermal growth factor receptor that is commonly overexpressed in breast cancer, to be discussed later), as compared to sporadic breast carcinomas. *BRCA2*-associated breast carcinomas do not have a distinct morphologic appearance. Initial results using gene expression RNA profiling have revealed that *BRCA1*, *BRCA2*, and subtypes of sporadic cancers can be recognized by their gene expression patterns[40,41] (Box 23–1). Sporadic carcinomas with an mRNA profile similar to *BRCA1* carcinomas have been termed "basal-like" carcinomas owing to the expression of genes that are characteristic of myoepithelial or possible breast progenitor cells. These results demonstrate that a subset of sporadic carcinomas have biologic similarities to hereditary carcinomas.

Genetic susceptibility due to other known genes is much less common, and together this group accounts for fewer than 10% of hereditary breast carcinomas.[42] Only five have been studied sufficiently to be worth noting. Mutations in the cell-cycle checkpoint kinase gene (*CHEK2*), which is an important component of the recognition and repair of DNA damage and which activates *BRCA1*, may account for 5% of familial cases.[43] The risk for a mutation carrier may be as low as 20%. Women with the Li-Fraumeni syndrome (due to a germ-line mutation in the *p53* gene) have an 18-fold higher risk of developing breast cancer before the age of 45. Mutations in *p53* also occur in 19% to 57% of sporadic breast carcinomas. Cowden syndrome ("multiple hamartoma syndrome" due to a mutation of the *PTEN* gene on chromosome 10q) confers a 25% to 50% lifetime risk of breast cancer in affected women. Mutations in the *PTEN* gene are rare in sporadic carcinomas, but LOH is found in 11% to 41%. Further studies will be necessary to determine whether the function of the other allele is altered (e.g., by methylation). Women with Peutz-Jeghers syndrome (caused by truncating mutations in the *LKBI* gene) are at increased risk for breast cancer. There is, as yet, no evidence that this gene plays a role in sporadic carcinoma. The role of the *ATM* gene in breast cancer susceptibility in ataxia telangiectasia carriers has been intensively studied owing to the high frequency of carriers in the population (approximately 7%) and the increased sensitivity to radiation exposure leading to concerns about screening mammography. Studies have had mixed results, some showing an increased risk and others not showing an association. The risk might be dependent on the type of germ-line mutation (e.g., truncating versus missense). Mutations in the *ATM* gene in sporadic carcinomas are rare.

All of these genes considered together still leave at least two-thirds of familial risk unexplained. The search for a putative "*BRCA3*" gene of high penetrance has, as yet, been unsuccessful, and such a gene might not exist.[44] A polygenic model in which many weakly penetrant genes (perhaps dozens or hundreds) act in combination to create a spectrum of risk could explain the majority of familial breast cancers, as well as risk in the general population.[45–47] This model suggests that most breast cancers arise in a minority of women carrying combinations of these susceptibility genes. The identification of these genes might allow better stratification of women into low-risk and high-risk groups, which would help to focus efforts toward prevention and early detection in these women. Yet to be determined are the number of genes that could be involved, the nature of interactions among these genes (e.g., additive or multiplicative), the interaction with environmental factors, and the possible role of protective alleles. Candidates for such genes have been identified by their ability to modify the expression of known genes such as *BRCA1*.

Genome-wide approaches (e.g., microarray technology; Box 23–1) could play an important role in identifying this potentially very large group of susceptibility genes. One current approach classifies hereditary cancers by mRNA profiling in the hopes that cancers arising due to the same germ-line mutation (or mutations) will have similar patterns, as has been demonstrated with *BRCA1* and *BRCA2*.[48] If true, this would simplify linkage analysis by identifying groups of families likely to carry similar mutations.

Many studies have confirmed that some of the genes involved in hereditary breast cancer (e.g., *BRCA1* and *p53*) are also important in many sporadic cancers. It is hoped that the continued investigation of the wide variety of naturally occurring mutations and combinations of mutations will provide important clues to breast cancer pathogenesis.

Sporadic Breast Cancer

The major risk factors for sporadic breast cancer are related to hormone exposure: gender, age at menarche and menopause, reproductive history, breast-feeding, and exogenous estrogens. The majority of these cancers occur in postmenopausal women and overexpress ER. Estrogen itself has at least two major roles in the development of breast cancer. Metabolites of estrogen can cause mutations or generate DNA-damaging free radicals.[49] Via its hormonal actions, estrogens drive the proliferation of premalignant lesions as well as cancers. However, other mechanisms also undoubtedly play a role, as a significant subset of breast carcinomas are ER-negative or occur in women without increased estrogen exposure.

Mechanisms of Carcinogenesis

The vast array of histologic appearances of proliferative and atypical breast disease, as well as carcinomas, are the outward manifestations of the dozens or hundreds of biologic changes taking place within these lesions and point to the complex and variable pathways to carcinogenesis. Indeed, not one common genetic or functional change can be found in every breast cancer. Most reported changes occur in only a subset of carcinomas and usually in highly variable combinations with other changes.

A general model for carcinogenesis postulates that a normal cell must achieve seven new capabilities, including genetic instability, to become malignant[50,51] (see Chapter 7) (Fig. 23–15). In hereditary carcinoma, one or more of these alterations is facilitated by the inheritance of germ-line mutations. Each of the new capabilities can be achieved by a change in one of many genes. For example, changes in *ER*, *EGF-R*, *RAS*, or *HER2/neu* may result in self-sufficiency in growth signals. On the other hand, one cellular alteration (e.g., a change in a gene such as *p53* that has a central role in controlling the cell cycle, DNA repair, and apoptosis) can affect more than one of these capabilities.

The morphologic changes in the breast associated with the smallest increased risk of cancer are lesions with increased numbers of epithelial cells (proliferative changes). This suggests that these early changes are related to evasion of growth-inhibiting signals, evasion of apoptosis, and self-sufficiency in growth signals. There is evidence that even at this early stage, there is abnormal expression of hormone receptors and abnormal regulation of proliferation in association with hormone receptor positivity.[52]

Genetic instability, in the form of LOH, appears to be a later change, as it is rarely detected in proliferative changes but becomes more frequent in atypical hyperplasias and is almost universally present in carcinoma in situ. Frank aneuploidy, as observed by nuclear enlargement, irregularity, and hyperchromasia, or image analysis to measure DNA content, is seen only in high-grade DCIS and some invasive carcinomas. Limitless replicative potential is suggested by the ability of clonal populations of the cells of DCIS to completely fill a ductal system in the breast. Increased angiogenesis is evident surrounding the basement membrane of some ducts that are involved by some types of DCIS. This might be due to direct stimulation by the malignant cells, secondary stimulatory effects on stromal cells, or the loss of inhibition of angiogenesis by myoepithelial cells.

The morphologic and biologic features of carcinomas are usually established at the in situ stage, as in the majority of cases, the in situ lesion closely resembles the accompanying invasive carcinoma. For example, lobular carcinomas are associated with LCIS, well-differentiated carcinomas with low-grade DCIS, and high-grade carcinomas with high-grade DCIS. Recurrent carcinomas generally have the appearance of the original carcinoma. Breast carcinomas do not generally "dedifferentiate," or become more poorly differentiated over time.

This view of oncogenesis focuses on the malignant epithelial cell and does not take into account the other tissue components. The structure and function of the normal breast require complex interactions between luminal cells, myoepithelial cells, and stromal cells. The same functions that allow for normal formation of new ductal branch points and lobules during puberty and pregnancy—abrogation of the basement membrane, increased proliferation, escape from growth inhibition, angiogenesis, and invasion of stroma—can be co-opted during carcinogenesis by abnormal epithelial cells, stromal cells, or both.[53] While the changes described above are accumulating in the luminal cells (or, less commonly, myoepithelial cells), parallel changes also occur due to mutation or epigenetic changes (e.g., DNA methylation) or via abnormal signaling pathways in these other cell types, resulting in the loss of normal cellular interactions and tissue structure.[54] Loss of these normal functions also occurs with age, and this loss might contribute to the increased risk of breast cancer in older women.

The final step of carcinogenesis, the transition of carcinoma limited by the basement membrane to ducts and lobules (car-

Box 23-1 GENE EXPRESSION PORTRAITS OF BREAST CARCINOMAS

Until recently, changes occurring in cancer cells were studied one at a time or in small groups in small sets of tumors. New microarray technologies ("gene chips") have enabled investigators to simultaneously detect and quantify the expression of large numbers of genes (potentially all genes) in different tumors (see Box 7–1, Chapter 7).

A major advantage of gene arrays is the ability to analyze a multitude of changes in cancer cells (i.e., a "molecular portrait") to discern overall patterns that would not be possible to detect by conventional techniques. An example of the type of data that may be generated from such assays is illustrated in a simplified form in the figure on the facing page. The results for 26 breast carcinomas (each corresponding to one column) for 28 genes (represented by each row) are displayed. A relative increased quantity of mRNA (relative to a reference standard) is shown by red, a relative decreased quantity by green, and an average amount by black. Also shown in the figure are the histology of the different tumor types and the expression of selected proteins detected by immunohistochemistry (ER, HER2, e-cadherin, and basal keratin).

Microarray studies, such as this one and others, have identified breast cancer subtypes previously identified by morphology (e.g., lobular carcinomas), by protein expression (e.g., ER-positive and HER2/neu-positive carcinomas), and by germ-line mutations (e.g., *BRCA1* and *BRCA2* carcinomas). In addition, new subtypes that were not previously well defined have been identified (e.g., the basal-like carcinomas). In the figure, results are not shown for many other tumor subtypes, such as tubular, mucinous, and medullary carcinomas, because these are relatively rare and too few cases have been examined to allow firm conclusions.

mRNA levels do not always correspond to changes in protein expression. The quantity of protein within a cell depends not only on the amount and rate of transcription and translation, but also on protein degradation and the rate of transport out of the cell. Therefore, other assays are necessary to determine actual protein content. Immunohistochemistry (IHC) uses antibodies to detect proteins on tissue sections. Whereas tissue used for mRNA profiling may include both tumor and stromal cells, IHC has the advantage of being able to identify the cell type expressing the protein and the specific cellular location of the protein.

Estrogen Receptor–Positive Carcinomas. Seventy per cent to 80% of breast carcinomas express ER and are thought to arise from intrinsically ER-positive luminal cells. ER-positive ductal carcinomas ("no special type") are usually well to moderately differentiated and often show tubule formation. Most special types of breast cancer (i.e. lobular, tubular, mucinous, and papillary) are also ER-positive. In the microarray data illustrated, the group of ductal carcinomas, in general, show normal or overexpression of the ER-related gene cluster and luminal keratins, and exhibit low levels of mRNAs from the groups of genes characteristic of the other tumor types. In the lower part of the figure, IHC on one representative ductal carcinoma demonstrates that ER is present in the nucleus, e-cadherin on the cell membrane, and that HER2/neu and basal keratins are undetectable.

In contrast to traditional IHC assays that determine the expression of only ER and a single gene under its regulation, PR, mRNA profiling provides information about many other ER-regulated genes. Using this type of assay, it might be possible to identify the cancers that express ER but fail to respond to hormonal treatments due to disruption of the signaling pathway, resulting in low expression of other ER-regulated genes.

Lobular carcinomas can be identified by the distinctive morphologic pattern of infiltration as single cells or loosely cohesive cell clusters. This appearance has been linked to the loss of the normal cell adhesion molecule e-cadherin, which is retained in most other carcinomas within the ER-positive group. By expression profiling, the lobular carcinomas cluster together and are most closely related to the other ER-positive carcinomas. The absence of e-cadherin can be seen by both diminished mRNA and the absence of the protein by IHC.

Estrogen Receptor–Negative Carcinomas. These carcinomas may arise owing to loss of ER expression or from normally ER-negative cells. Expression profiling identifies two major types of ER-negative carcinomas.

HER2-Positive Carcinomas. This group of carcinomas was previously identified by overexpression of the HER2/neu protein. In the majority of carcinomas, the mechanism of overexpression is amplification of the gene resulting in increased transcription into mRNA and protein translation. Breast cancers are routinely assayed for *HER2/neu* gene and protein using FISH or IHC (Figs. 23–27*C* and *B*, respectively) in order to predict clinical responses to antibodies targeted to the protein. These carcinomas tend to be poorly differentiated.

The expression profile reveals not only increased copies of *HER2/neu* mRNA, but also increased transcription of other adjacent genes that are amplified within this segment of DNA. These carcinomas do not overexpress the genes that are characteristic of the other subtypes of cancers in this array (e.g. ER and basal keratins), but do express e-cadherin.

Basal-like Carcinomas. This group of carcinomas is distinguished by the expression of keratins that are more typical of myoepithelial cells or potential breast progenitor cells; it has not been previously well characterized. Because the myoepithelial cell is located in the basal area of the lobules and ducts, in the absence of knowing the specific cell of origin, this group of carcinomas was termed *basal-like*. In addition to the expression of specific keratins, they also show expression of other genes in common with myoepithelial cells (e.g., p-cadherin) as well as numerous genes related to cell proliferation. This group of carcinomas does not express ER or ER-related genes or *HER2/neu*, as can be seen by the array data and by IHC.

Carcinomas arising in women with *BRCA1* mutations also cluster with this group. *BRCA1* carcinomas are similar to basal-like carcinomas in being poorly differentiated, lacking ER and HER2/neu expression, and expressing basal-like keratins. However, most women with basal-like carcinomas do not have germ-line *BRCA1* mutations.

Conclusions. mRNA expression profiling is a powerful tool for investigating breast carcinomas. Analogous arrays to analyze DNA and protein expression profiles are under development. In addition to identifying tumor types, as in this example, mRNA arrays have been used for predicting prognosis and response to therapy, examining tumor changes after therapy, and classifying hereditary carcinomas. Although it might not be feasible to perform transcriptional profiling on every clinical case of breast cancer, these studies will generate information that will lead to better diagnostic, prognostic, and therapeutic tests that are applicable to all patients.

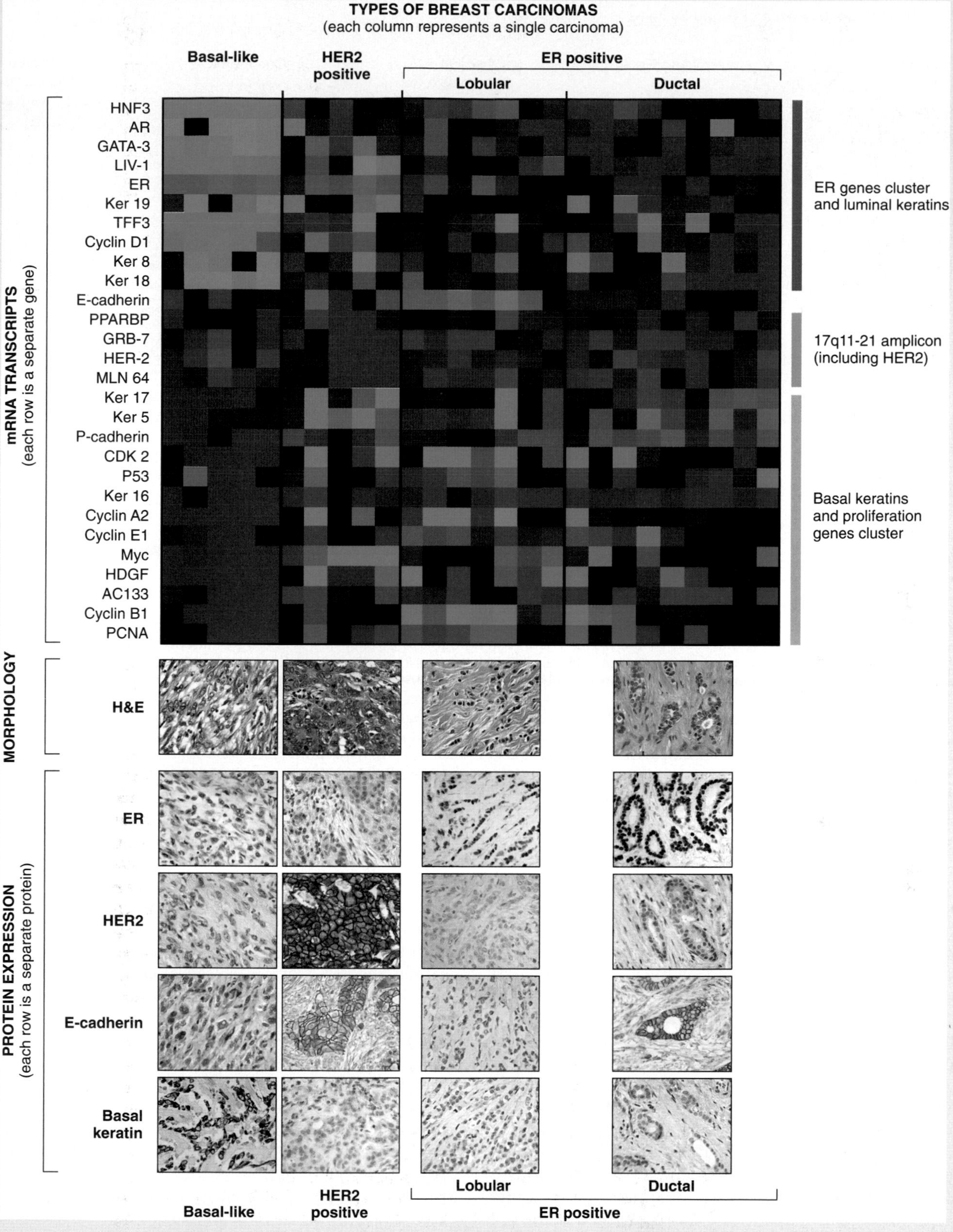

Selected data from mRNA expression profiling (26 carcinomas and 28 genes) are shown in the top half of the figure. Each vertical column represents one carcinoma (and shows information acquired from one "gene chip") and each horizontal row represents the data for a gene (identified at the left). Red indicates an increase, green a decrease, and black no change in mRNA relative to a standard. Cluster analysis was used to group carcinomas with similar expression patterns and the groups are identified as basal-like, *HER2* positive, and the ER-positive lobular and ductal carcinomas. The most important gene clusters are identified on the right. These carcinomas have typical morphologic appearances as shown in the middle row of images (H&E).

In the lower half of the figure, mRNA expression patterns are correlated with changes in protein expression by using antibodies to detect antigens within tissues. The presence of a protein is indicated by a brown reaction product within the tumor cells and can be localized to a subcellular site (estrogen receptor–nuclear; HER2/neu and e-cadherin–membrane; basal keratin–cytoplasmic). The array data are courtesy of Dr. Andrea Richardson, Brigham and Women's Hospital, Boston, MA, as modified from Signoretti S, Di Marcotullio L, Richardson A, et al.: Oncogenic role of the ubiquitin ligase subunit Skp2 in human breast cancer, J Clin Invest 110:633–641, 2002.

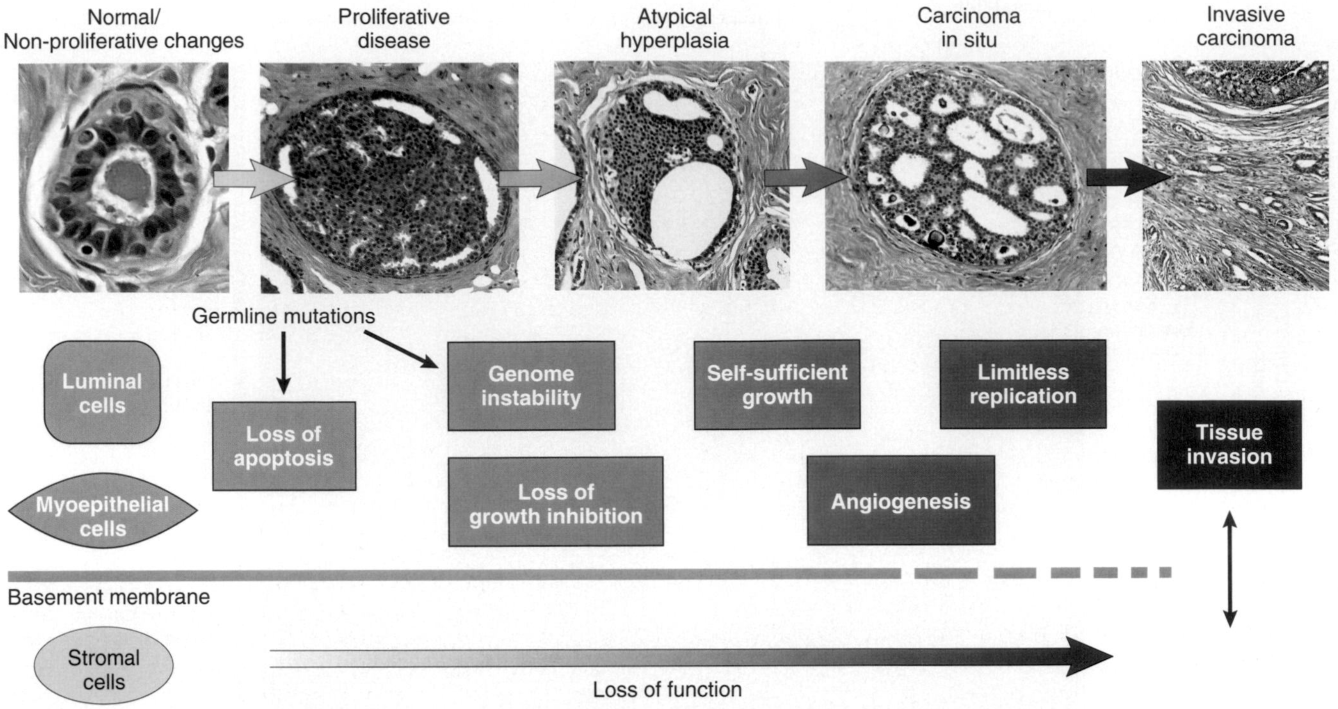

FIGURE 23–15 The normal breast is maintained by a complex set of interactions among luminal cells, myoepithelial cells, the basement membrane, and stromal cells (illustrated to the left of the figure). Morphologic changes are displayed according to the risk for subsequent invasive carcinoma (top row of pictures). The seven categories of changes in biologic functions that must occur in successful malignant cells are shown in colored boxes. The changes need not occur in a specific order but accumulate until cells acquire malignant potential. The association of these changes with premalignant breast lesions suggests that the earliest events are related to evasion of growth-inhibiting signals, evasion of apoptosis, and self-sufficiency in growth signals. Hereditary carcinomas arise from cells that have germ line mutations that alter DNA repair and/or normal signals for apoptosis and therefore require fewer acquired changes. Luminal cells likely give rise to the majority of cancers, but myoepithelial cells can also undergo malignant transformation. Changes in the malignant cells are accompanied by alterations in the supporting myoepithelial and stromal cells due to a combination of genetic and epigenetic events and disruption of the normal intercellular signaling pathways. The final alteration, invasion of stroma, is the least well understood. It has been difficult to identify biologic changes that are specific to invasive carcinomas. It is possible that invasion is a result of the loss of the ability of myoepithelial and stromal cells to maintain the basement membrane rather than a gain of function by the malignant cells.

cinoma in situ) to invasive carcinoma, is the least understood. Specific gene functions necessary for invasion have been difficult to identify.[55] It is possible that this transition is primarily due to the loss of the basement membrane and tissue integrity caused by the abnormal function of myoepithelial and stromal cells rather than to the gain of the ability of malignant cells to invade through the basement membrane and into stroma (Fig. 23–15).

New techniques that survey hundreds to thousands of changes in the DNA, RNA, and proteins of carcinomas have provided the first glimpses of the overall biologic diversity of invasive breast carcinomas[40,41,56,57] (Box 23–1). Not surprisingly, ER-positive and negative carcinomas segregate into separate groups. Dozens to hundreds of genes may be under transcriptional control by ER, and this is reflected by a set of common genes showing increased transcription in these carcinomas. In fact, the expression of these downstream genes in ER-positive tumors might ultimately be more predictive of tumor behavior and response to estrogen blocking agents than is the presence of the receptor itself. ER-positive carcinomas without this pattern have gene expression profiles that are more like the profiles of ER-negative carcinomas. ER-positive carcinomas also show increased transcription of so-called luminal type genes, thought to be characteristic of normal luminal cells and possibly related to the overall better differentiation seen in these carcinomas. The ER-negative tumors fall into two major groups. The basal-like carcinomas have features suggestive of myoepithelial cell differentiation (e.g., basal keratins, p-cadherin, and laminin expression). *BRCA1* carcinomas cluster with this group. A second ER-negative group is characterized by amplification of *Her2/neu*. Additional subgroups have also been identified.

Some of the important components of these gene expression profiles are thought to be derived from stromal cells intermingled with the cancer cells, again supporting the importance of nonepithelial cells in the overall behavior of cancer.

CLASSIFICATION OF BREAST CARCINOMA

Almost all breast malignancies are adenocarcinomas, all other types (i.e., squamous cell carcinomas, phyllodes tumors, sarcomas, and lymphomas) making up fewer than 5% of the total.

Carcinomas are divided into in situ carcinomas and invasive carcinomas. Carcinoma in situ refers to a neoplastic population of cells limited to ducts and lobules by the basement membrane. In some cases, the cells can extend to the overlying skin without crossing the basement membrane and appear clinically as Paget disease. However, carcinoma in situ does not invade into lymphatics and blood vessels and cannot metastasize. Invasive carcinoma (synonymous with "infiltrating" carcinoma) has invaded beyond the basement membrane into stroma. Here, the cells might also invade into the vasculature and thereby reach regional lymph nodes and distant sites. Even the smallest invasive breast carcinomas have some capacity to metastasize.

Carcinoma in situ was originally classified as ductal or lobular on the basis of the resemblance of the involved spaces to ducts and lobules. Invasive ductal and lobular carcinomas were named by their association with the characteristic in situ component. Although these descriptive terms are still used, all carcinomas are thought to arise from the terminal duct lobular unit, and the terms "ductal" and "lobular" do not imply a site or cell type of origin.[58]

Carcinoma in Situ

Ductal Carcinoma in Situ (DCIS; Intraductal Carcinoma)

The number of cases of DCIS has rapidly increased in the past two decades from fewer than 5% of all carcinomas before mammographic screening to 15% to 30% of carcinomas in well-screened populations (Fig. 23–13). Among mammographically detected cancers, almost half are DCIS. DCIS most frequently presents as mammographic calcifications (Fig. 23–16*A*). Less typically, DCIS presents as a mammographic density or a vaguely palpable mass or nipple discharge or is incidental in a biopsy for another lesion.

DCIS consists of a malignant population of cells limited to ducts and lobules by the basement membrane. The myoepithelial cells are preserved, although they may be diminished in number. DCIS is a clonal proliferation and usually involves only a single ductal system. However, the cells can spread throughout ducts and lobules and produce extensive lesions involving an entire sector of a breast. When DCIS involves lobules, the acini are often distorted and unfolded and take on the appearance of small ducts.

Morphology. Historically, DCIS has been divided into five architectural subtypes: comedocarcinoma, solid, cribriform, papillary, and micropapillary. Some cases of DCIS will have a single growth pattern, but the majority have a mixture of patterns.

Comedocarcinoma is characterized by solid sheets of pleomorphic cells with high-grade nuclei and central necrosis (Fig. 23–16*B*). The necrotic cell membranes commonly calcify and are detected on mammography as clusters or linear and branching microcalcifications (Fig. 23–16*A*). Periductal concentric fibrosis and chronic inflammation are common, and extensive lesions are sometimes palpable as an area of vague nodularity.

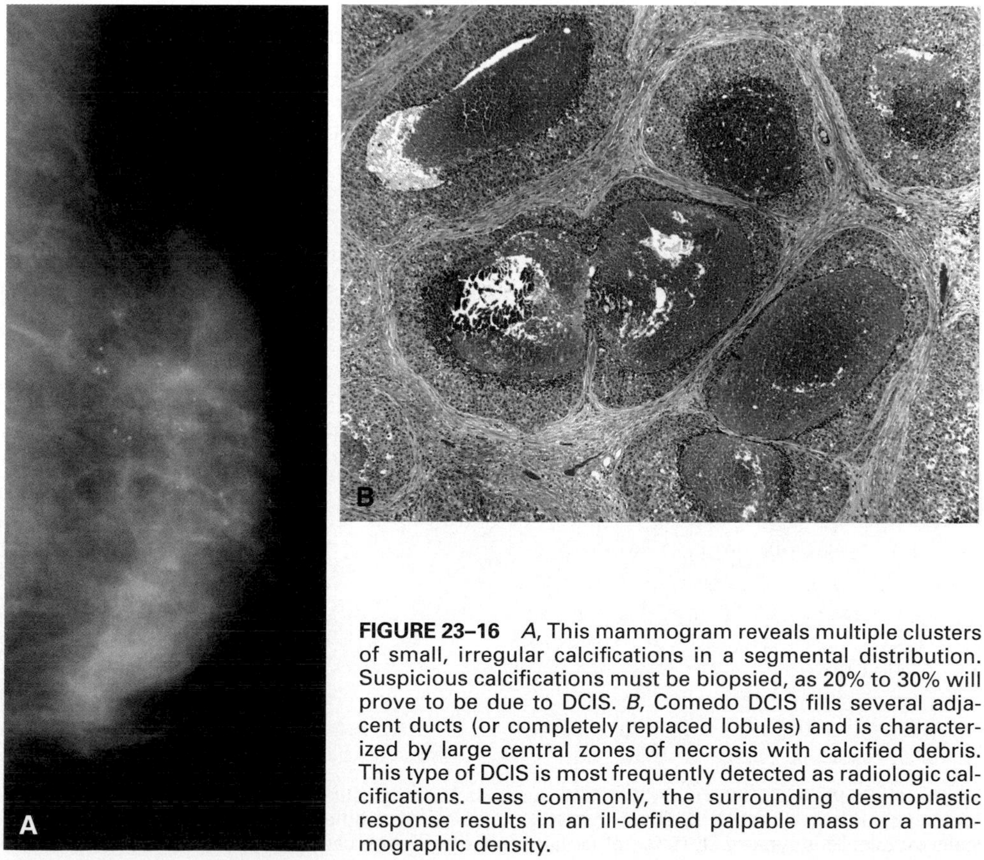

FIGURE 23–16 *A*, This mammogram reveals multiple clusters of small, irregular calcifications in a segmental distribution. Suspicious calcifications must be biopsied, as 20% to 30% will prove to be due to DCIS. *B*, Comedo DCIS fills several adjacent ducts (or completely replaced lobules) and is characterized by large central zones of necrosis with calcified debris. This type of DCIS is most frequently detected as radiologic calcifications. Less commonly, the surrounding desmoplastic response results in an ill-defined palpable mass or a mammographic density.

Noncomedo DCIS consists of a monomorphic population of cells with nuclear grades ranging from low to high. In cribriform DCIS, intraepithelial spaces are evenly distributed and regular in shape (cookie cutter–like) (Fig. 23–17*A*). Solid DCIS completely fills the involved spaces (Fig. 23–17*B*). Papillary DCIS grows into spaces and lines fibrovascular cores typically lacking the normal myoepithelial cell layer (Fig. 23–18*A*). Micropapillary DCIS is recognized by bulbous protrusions without a fibrovascular core, often forming complex intraductal patterns (Fig. 23–18*B*). Calcifications may be associated with central necrosis but more commonly form in intraluminal secretions (Fig. 23–17*A*).

Paget disease of the nipple is a rare manifestation of breast cancer (1% to 2% of cases) and presents as a unilateral erythematous eruption with a scale crust. Pruritus is common, and the lesion might be mistaken for eczema. Malignant cells, referred to as Paget cells, extend from DCIS within the ductal system into nipple skin without crossing the basement membrane (Fig. 23–19). The tumor cells disrupt the normal epithelial barrier, and this allows extracellular fluid to seep out onto the nipple surface. The Paget cells are easily detected by nipple biopsy or cytologic preparations of the exudate.

A palpable mass is present in 50% to 60% of women with Paget disease, and almost all of these women will have an underlying invasive carcinoma. In contrast, fewer than half of women without a palpable mass will have invasive carcinoma. The carcinomas are usually poorly differentiated and overexpress *HER2/neu*. The production by keratinocytes of heregulin-α, which acts via the HER2/neu receptor, may play a role in the pathogenesis of this disease.[59]

Prognosis depends on the extent of the underlying carcinoma and is not affected by the presence or absence of DCIS involving the skin when matched for age, tumor size, grade, *HER2/neu* status, and nodal status.[60]

DCIS with microinvasion is defined by foci of tumor cells less than 0.1 cm in diameter invading the stroma. Microinvasion is most commonly seen in association with comedocarcinoma.

The majority of cases of DCIS cannot be detected by either palpation or visual inspection of the involved tissue. Occasional cases of comedocarcinoma are associated with sufficient periductal fibrosis to produce a thickening of the tissue, and punctate areas of necrosis ("comedone"-like) can be seen grossly.

The natural history of DCIS has been difficult to determine because in the past, all women were treated with mastectomy, and the current practice of surgical excision usually followed by radiation is largely curative. The consensus seems to be that many cases of small, low-grade DCIS, and probably most cases of high-grade and extensive DCIS, progress to invasive carcinoma,[61] emphasizing the importance of proper diagnosis and appropriate therapy for this condition.

Mastectomy for DCIS is curative in over 95% of cases. Rare recurrence and/or death are usually due to residual DCIS in ducts in subcutaneous adipose tissue that was not removed during surgery, or occult foci of invasion that were not detected at the time of diagnosis.

Breast conservation is appropriate for most women with DCIS but results in a slightly higher risk of recurrence and therefore death from breast cancer. The major risk factors for recurrence are (1) grade, (2) size, and (3) margins.

Details of algorithms based on these features are beyond our scope. Suffice it to say that these three risk factors were combined to create a prognostic index that can be used to divide women with DCIS treated with breast conservation into three groups.[62] DCIS with the lowest scores rarely recurred, and radiation therapy did not appear to have an additional effect. DCIS with the highest scores recurred in over half of women despite radiation. In the intermediate group, about 20% of women had a recurrence, but radiation

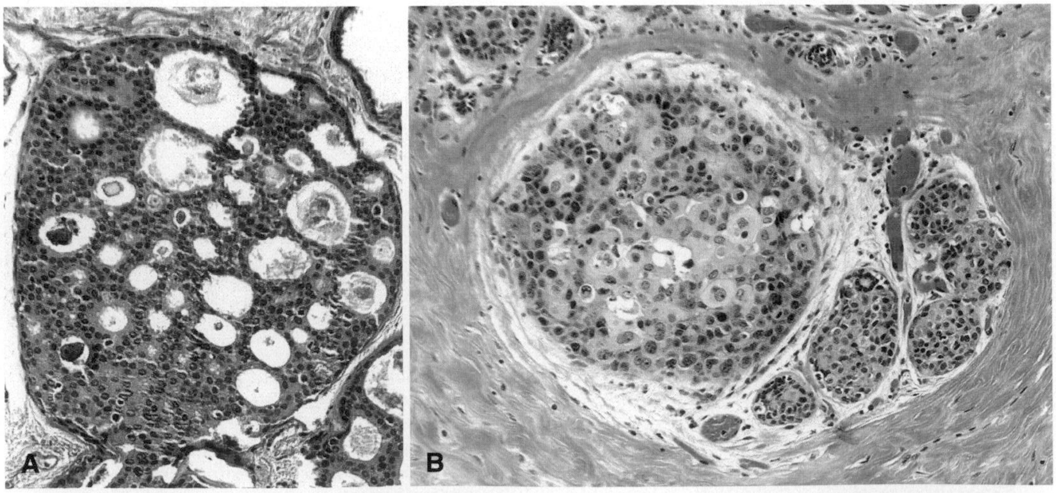

FIGURE 23–17 Noncomedo DCIS. *A*, Cribriform DCIS comprises cells forming round, regular ("cookie cutter") spaces. The lumens are often filled with calcifying secretory material. *B*, This solid DCIS has almost completely filled and distorted this lobule with only a few remaining luminal cells visible. This type of DCIS is not usually associated with calcifications and may be clinically occult.

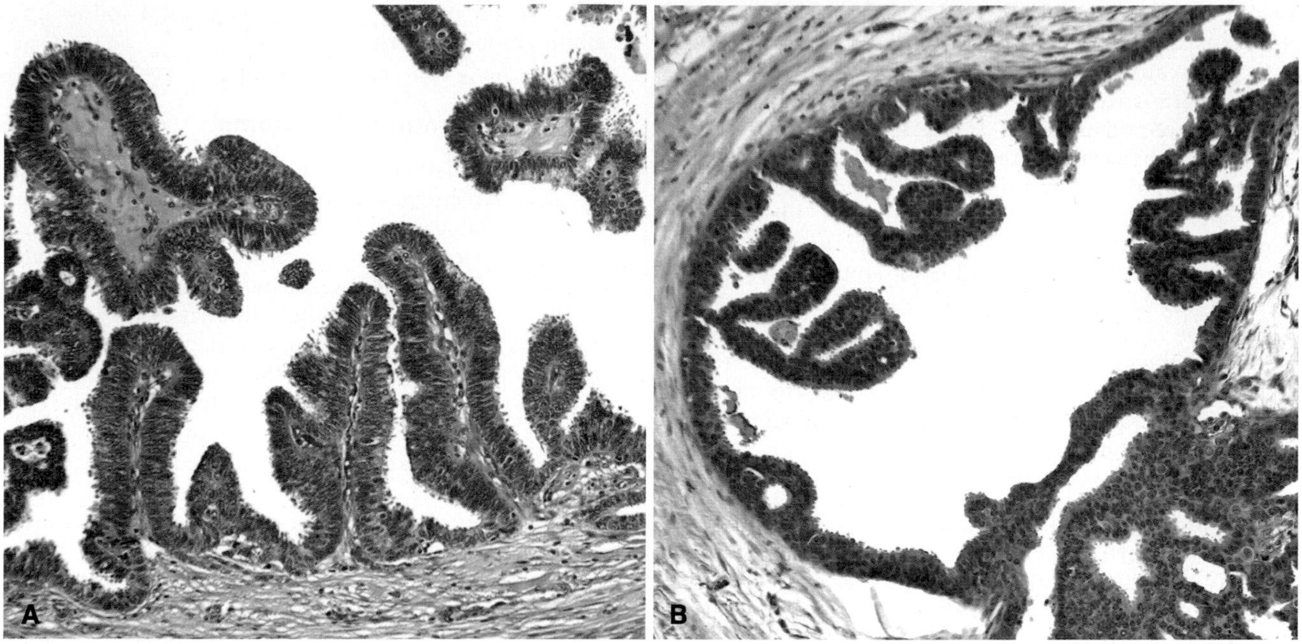

FIGURE 23–18 Noncomedo DCIS. *A*, Papillary DCIS. Delicate fibrovascular cores extend into a duct and are lined by a monomorphic population of tall columnar cells. Myoepithelial cells are absent. *B*, Micropapillary DCIS. The papillae are connected to the duct wall by a narrow base and often have bulbous or complex outgrowths. The papillae are solid and do not have fibrovascular cores.

appeared to reduce the risk. Although this index requires validation in prospective studies, it does suggest that pathologic features can be used to select women who can be safely treated with breast conservation. Tamoxifen also reduces the risk of local and distant recurrence, but the benefit is probably restricted to women with ER-positive DCIS.[63] Deaths from breast cancer in women with treated DCIS are very rare (<2% of women with DCIS), even when the breast is preserved.

Lobular Carcinoma in Situ (LCIS)

LCIS is always an incidental finding in a biopsy performed for another reason, as LCIS is not associated with calcifications or a stromal reaction that would form a density. Therefore, it remains infrequent (1% to 6% of all carcinomas) with or without mammographic screening (Table 23–1). LCIS is bilateral in 20% to 40% of women when both breasts are biopsied,

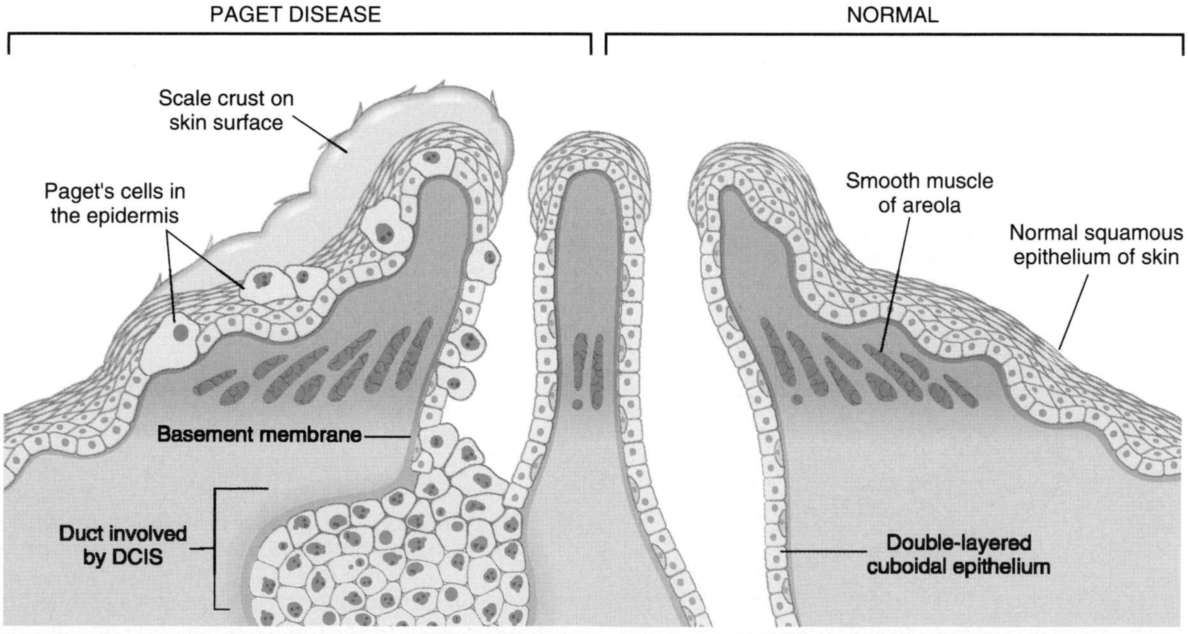

FIGURE 23–19 Paget disease of the nipple. DCIS arising within the ductal system of the breast can extend up the lactiferous ducts into nipple skin without crossing the basement membrane. The malignant cells disrupt the normally tight squamous epithelial cell barrier, allowing extracellular fluid to seep out and form an oozing scaly crust over the nipple skin.

compared to 10% to 20% of cases of DCIS. LCIS is more common in young women, 80% to 90% of cases occurring prior to menopause.

Because LCIS is frequently multicentric and bilateral and subsequent carcinomas occur at equal frequency in both breasts, it has been suggested that LCIS is not a true neoplasm but rather is a marker of breast cancer risk. However, the cells of LCIS and invasive lobular carcinoma are identical in appearance, and both lack expression of e-cadherin, the transmembrane protein that is responsible for epithelial cell adhesion.[64] The loss of expression correlates with the histologic appearance of lobular carcinomas as single detached cells. LCIS can have the same genetic changes (such as LOH on *16q*, the site of the gene for e-cadherin) as an adjacent area of invasive carcinoma, supporting its role as a true precursor of invasive carcinoma in some cases.[65]

Morphology. The abnormal cells of atypical lobular hyperplasia (ALH), LCIS, and invasive lobular carcinoma are identical and consist of small cells that have oval or round nuclei with small nucleoli that do not adhere to one another (Fig. 23–20). Signet-ring cells containing mucin are present commonly. LCIS rarely distorts the underlying architecture, and the involved acini remain recognizable as lobules. LCIS almost always expresses estrogen and progesterone receptors, and overexpression of *HER2/neu* is not observed.

Women with LCIS develop invasive carcinomas at a frequency similar to that of women with untreated DCIS. In patients observed for more than 20 years, invasive carcinoma develops in 25% to 35%, or at about 1% per year. Older studies indicated that both breasts were at equal risk, but a recent report suggests that the ipsilateral breast may be at greater risk in women with lobular neoplasia.[17] Invasive carcinomas developing in women after a diagnosis of LCIS are threefold more likely to be of lobular type compared with carcinomas overall, but the majority do not show specific lobular morphology. Treatment choices include bilateral prophylactic mastectomy, tamoxifen, or, more typically, close clinical follow-up and mammographic screening.

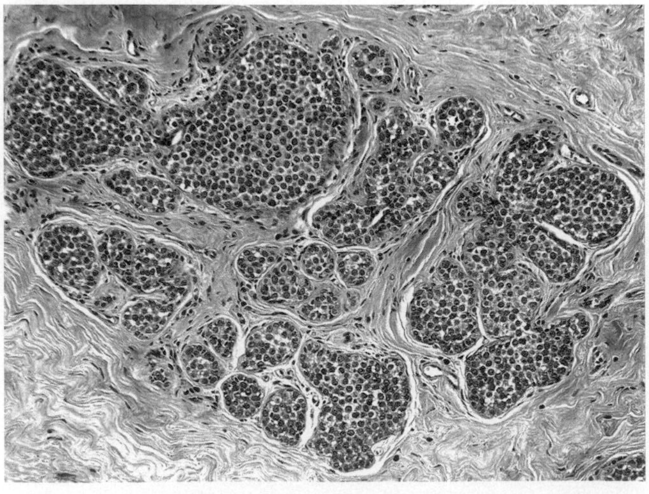

FIGURE 23–20 Lobular carcinoma in situ. A monomorphic population of small, rounded, loosely cohesive cells fills and expands the acini of a lobule. The underlying lobular architecture can still be recognized.

Invasive (Infiltrating) Carcinoma

In young women or in older women not undergoing mammographic screening, invasive carcinoma almost always presents as a palpable mass. *By the time a cancer becomes palpable, over half the patients will have axillary lymph node metastases* (Table 23–1). Larger carcinomas may be fixed to the chest wall or cause dimpling of the skin. Lymphatics may become so involved as to block the local area of skin drainage and cause lymphedema and thickening of the skin, a change referred to as *peau d'orange*. Tethering of the skin to the breast by Cooper ligaments mimics the appearance of an orange peel. When the tumor involves the central portion of the breast, retraction of the nipple may develop.

In older women undergoing mammography, invasive carcinomas most commonly present as a density (Fig. 23–21*A*) and are, on average, half the size of a palpable cancer (Table 23–1). Fewer than 20% will have nodal metastases. Invasive carcinomas presenting as mammographic calcifications without an associated density are very small in size, and metastases are unusual (Table 23–1).

The term "inflammatory carcinoma" refers to the clinical presentation of a carcinoma extensively involving dermal lymphatics, resulting in an enlarged erythematous breast. The underlying carcinoma usually has a diffuse infiltrative pattern and typically does not form a discrete palpable mass. This can result in confusion with inflammatory conditions and delay in diagnosis. The diagnosis is made on clinical grounds and does not correlate with a specific histologic type of carcinoma.

Rarely, breast cancer presents as an axillary nodal metastasis or distant metastasis. In most cases, the primary carcinoma is either small or obscured by dense breast tissue. The number of primary carcinomas that remain occult in such cases is small with the use of mammography, ultrasound, and MRI to examine the breast.

The most common histologic types of breast adenocarcinoma are listed in Table 23–4. These types are important to recognize owing to their specific clinical associations. Other rare types of adenocarcinoma (e.g., apocrine carcinomas, carcinomas with neuroendocrine differentiation, and clear cell carcinomas) are similar to carcinomas of no special type in behavior and prognosis.

Invasive Carcinoma, No Special Type (NST; Invasive Ductal Carcinoma)

Invasive carcinomas of no special type include the majority of carcinomas (70% to 80%) that cannot be classified as any other subtype.

Morphology. On gross examination, most carcinomas are firm to hard and have an irregular border (Fig. 23–21*B*). Within the center of the carcinoma, there are small pinpoint foci or streaks of chalky white elastotic stroma and occasionally small foci of calcification. There is a characteristic grating sound (similar to cutting a water chestnut) when cut or scraped. Less

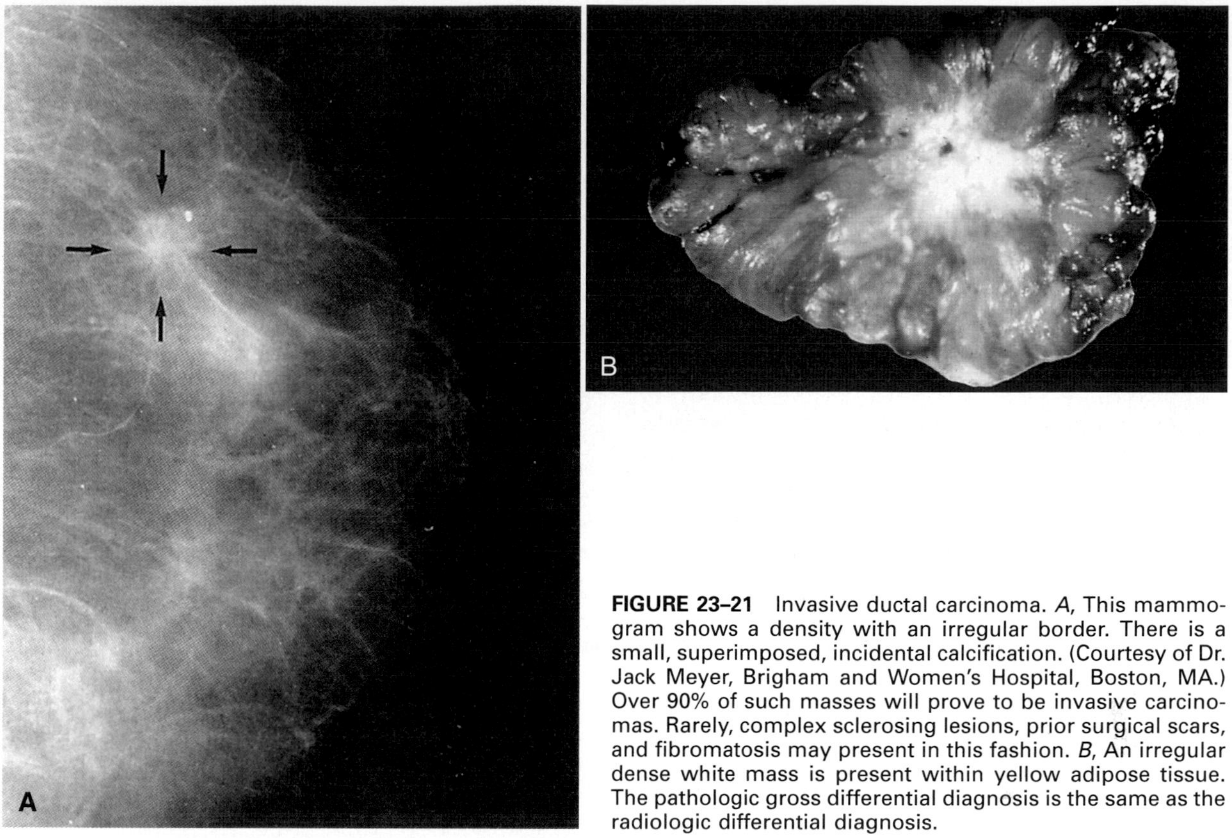

FIGURE 23–21 Invasive ductal carcinoma. *A*, This mammogram shows a density with an irregular border. There is a small, superimposed, incidental calcification. (Courtesy of Dr. Jack Meyer, Brigham and Women's Hospital, Boston, MA.) Over 90% of such masses will prove to be invasive carcinomas. Rarely, complex sclerosing lesions, prior surgical scars, and fibromatosis may present in this fashion. *B*, An irregular dense white mass is present within yellow adipose tissue. The pathologic gross differential diagnosis is the same as the radiologic differential diagnosis.

frequently, carcinomas have a well-circumscribed border and may be soft to firm in consistency.

These carcinomas display a wide spectrum of appearances. Well-differentiated tumors consist of tubules lined by minimally atypical cells and can occasionally be difficult to distinguish from benign sclerosing lesions (Fig. 23–22*A*). Such cancers typically express hormone receptors and do not overexpress *HER2/neu*. Others are composed of anastomosing sheets of pleomorphic cells (Fig. 23–22*B*) and are less likely to express hormone receptors and more likely to overexpress *HER2/neu*. The majority of invasive ductal carcinomas lie between these two extremes. Most carcinomas induce a marked increase in dense, fibrous desmoplastic stroma, giving the tumor a hard consistency on palpation and replace fat, resulting in a mammographic density (scirrhous carcinoma).

Carcinomas of NST are accompanied by varying amounts of DCIS. The grade of the DCIS usually correlates with the grade of the invasive carcinoma. For example, comedo DCIS is usually associated with poorly differentiated carcinomas, and low-grade DCIS is usually associated with well-differentiated carcinomas. Carcinomas associated with a large amount of DCIS require large excisions with wide margins to reduce local recurrences.

TABLE 23–4 Distribution of Histologic Types of Breast Cancer

Total Cancers	Per Cent
In Situ Carcinoma*	***15–30***
Ductal carcinoma in situ	80
Lobular carcinoma in situ	20
Invasive Carcinoma	***70–85***
No special type carcinoma ("ductal")	79
Lobular carcinoma	10
Tubular/cribriform carcinoma	6
Mucinous (colloid) carcinoma	2
Medullary carcinoma	2
Papillary carcinoma	1
Metaplastic carcinoma	<1

*The proportion of in situ carcinomas detected depends on the number of women undergoing mammographic screening and ranges from less than 5% in unscreened populations to almost 50% in patients with screen-detected cancers. Current observed numbers are between these two extremes.

The data on invasive carcinomas are modified from Dixon JM, et al: Long-term survivors after breast cancer. Br J Surg 72:445, 1985.

Morphologic analysis of this large group of carcinomas has not identified tumor types of significant clinical relevance beyond the specialized types to be described below. Recent studies using microarrays to analyze the transcriptional profile of these cancers have identified additional subgroups. (Box 23–1)[41,56,57] The challenge of future studies will be to show the clinical relevance of subtypes identified by gene expression profiling (e.g., with respect to etiology, presentation, prognosis, or response to treatment) and, if found, to determine whether these carcinomas can be recognized by more widely

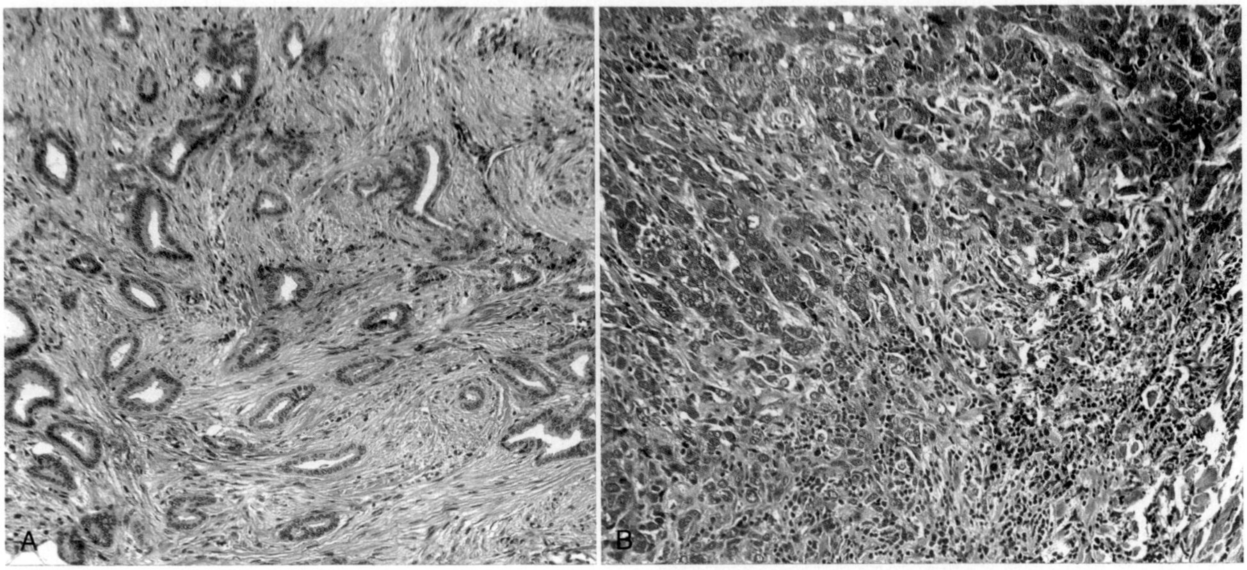

FIGURE 23–22 *A,* Well-differentiated invasive carcinoma of no special type. Well-formed tubules and nests of cells with small monomorphic nuclei invade into the stroma with a surrounding desmoplastic response. *B,* Poorly differentiated invasive carcinoma of no special type. Ragged sheets of pleomorphic cells without tubule formation infiltrate into the adjacent stroma.

available means of evaluation (e.g., by refined morphologic criteria or immunoperoxidase studies for protein expression).

Invasive Lobular Carcinoma

Invasive lobular carcinomas usually present like carcinomas of NST as a palpable mass or mammographic density. However, about one-fourth of cases have a diffuse pattern of invasion without prominent desmoplasia and might produce only a vaguely thickened area of the breast or subtle architectural changes on mammography. Metastases can also be difficult to detect clinically and radiologically owing to this type of invasion.

Lobular carcinomas have been reported to have a greater incidence of bilaterality. However, many studies have been biased owing to the greater likelihood of performing contralateral surgery in women with lobular carcinoma. The actual number of women who develop subsequent clinically detected invasive carcinomas is only 5% to 10%, similar to the number of women with NST carcinomas.

The incidence of lobular carcinomas has been reported to be increasing among postmenopausal women.[66] It has been suggested that this increase may be related to the use of postmenopausal hormone replacement therapy.[67]

Morphology. Grossly, most tumors are firm to hard with an irregular margin. Occasionally, the tissue may feel diffusely thickened and a discrete tumor mass cannot be defined. The histologic hallmark of lobular carcinomas is the pattern of single infiltrating tumor cells, often only one cell in width (in the form of a single file) or in loose clusters or sheets (Fig. 23–23). The desmoplastic response may be minimal or absent. The cells have the same cytologic features as LCIS and lack cohesion, without formation of tubules or papillae. Signet-ring cells are common. Tumor cells are frequently arranged in concentric rings surrounding normal ducts. Several variants, including tumors with large nests of cells and a high degree of pleomorphism, have been described.

Well-differentiated and moderately differentiated invasive lobular carcinomas are usually diploid, express hormone receptors, and are associated with LCIS in the majority of cases. *HER2/neu* overexpression is very rare. In contrast, poorly differentiated lobular carcinomas are usually aneuploid, often lack hormone receptors, and may overexpress

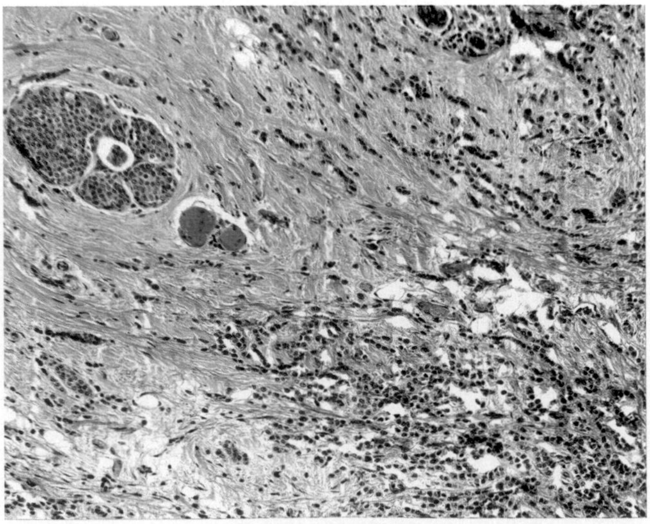

FIGURE 23–23 Invasive lobular carcinoma. Parallel arrays of small, regular cells with scant cytoplasm infiltrate singly in linear arrays or as small clusters of cells. There is often associated LCIS.

HER2/neu. If matched by grade and stage, lobular carcinomas have the same prognosis as carcinomas of NST.

Most lobular carcinomas show a loss of a region on chromosome 16 (16q22.1) that includes a cluster of at least eight genes responsible for cell adhesion, including e-cadherin and β-catenin.[68] The gene for e-cadherin on the opposite chromosome is inactivated by mutations, methylation of the promoter, or decreased expression of transcription factors. These changes are also found in LCIS.

Lobular carcinomas have a different pattern of metastasis compared to other breast cancers. Metastases to the peritoneum and retroperitoneum, the leptomeninges (carcinomatous meningitis), the gastrointestinal tract, and the ovaries and uterus are more frequently observed. These carcinomas are less likely to metastasize to the lungs and pleura.

Medullary Carcinoma

Medullary carcinoma presents as a well-circumscribed mass and may be mistaken clinically and radiologically for a fibroadenoma (described later). There is sometimes a history of rapid, almost explosive, growth.

Morphology. These tumors do not have the striking desmoplasia of the usual carcinoma and therefore are distinctly more yielding on external palpation and on cut section. The tumor has a soft, fleshy consistency (*medulla* is Latin for "marrow") and is well circumscribed. The carcinoma is characterized by (1) solid, syncytium-like sheets (occupying more than 75% of the tumor) of large cells with vesicular, pleomorphic nuclei, containing prominent nucleoli and frequent mitoses; (2) a moderate to marked lymphoplasmacytic infiltrate surrounding and within the tumor; and (3) a pushing (noninfiltrative) border (Fig. 23–24). All medullary carcinomas are poorly differentiated. DCIS is minimal or absent. Lymphatic or vascular invasion is never seen.

Medullary carcinomas have a slightly better prognosis than do carcinomas of no special type, despite the almost universal presence of poor prognostic factors, including high nuclear grade, aneuploidy, absence of hormone receptors, and high proliferative rates. However, *HER2/neu overexpression is not observed*. Lymph node metastases are infrequent and rarely involve multiple nodes. The syncytial growth pattern and pushing borders may reflect retention or overexpression of adhesion molecules that could potentially limit metastatic potential.

Among women carrying the *BRCA1* gene, 13% of cancers are reported to be of this type (Table 23–4). However, the majority of medullary carcinomas (or medullary-like carcinomas) are not associated with germ-line *BRCA1* mutations. Interestingly, hypermethylation of the *BRCA1* promoter is observed in 67% of medullary carcinomas, suggesting an association of this morphology with underlying gene expression.

Mucinous (Colloid) Carcinoma

This unusual type (1% to 6% of all breast carcinomas) also commonly presents as a circumscribed mass. It tends to occur in older women and may grow slowly during the course of many years.

Morphology. The tumor is extremely soft and has the consistency and appearance of pale gray-blue gelatin. The tumor cells are seen as clusters and small islands of cells within large lakes of mucin that push into the adjacent stroma (Fig. 23–25).

Mucinous carcinomas are usually diploid, and the majority express hormone receptors. The overall prognosis is slightly better than that of carcinomas of no special type.

The incidence of mucinous carcinomas is also slightly higher in women with *BRCA1* mutations. Similar to the observations in medullary carcinoma, hypermethylation of

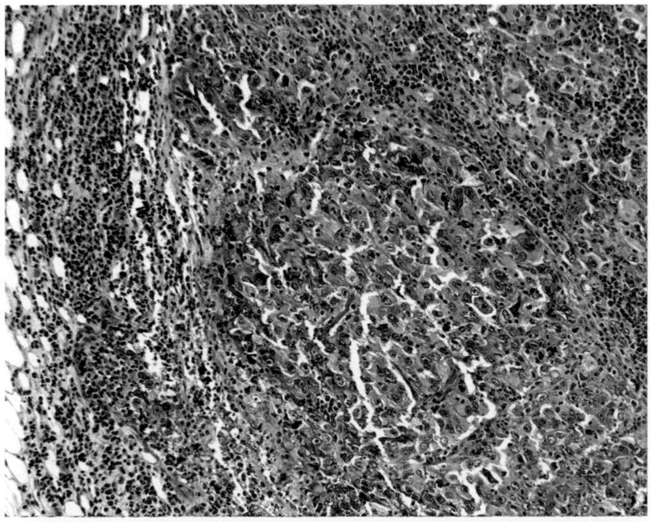

FIGURE 23–24 Medullary carcinoma. The cells are highly pleomorphic with frequent mitoses and grow as sheets of cohesive cells. A lymphoplasmacytic infiltrate is prominent.

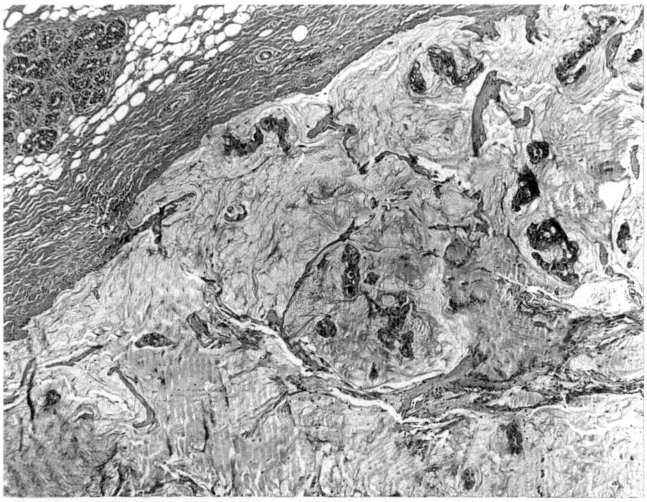

FIGURE 23–25 Mucinous (colloid) carcinoma. The tumor cells are present as small clusters within large pools of mucin. The borders are typically well circumscribed, and these cancers often mimic benign masses.

the *BRCA1* promoter has been observed in 55% of mucinous carcinomas not associated with *BRCA1* germ line mutations.

Tubular Carcinoma

Tubular carcinomas accounted for only 2% of all breast carcinomas before mammographic screening but have increased in frequency and represent up to 10% of carcinomas less than 1 cm in diameter. Tubular carcinomas are typically detected as irregular mammographic densities. Women usually present in their late forties. Tumors are multifocal within one breast in 10% to 56% of cases and bilateral in 9% to 38%.

Morphology. These tumors consist exclusively of well-formed tubules and are sometimes mistaken for benign sclerosing lesions (Fig. 23–26). However, a myoepithelial cell layer is absent, and tumor cells are in direct contact with stroma. Cribriform spaces may also be present. Apocrine snouts are typical, and calcifications may be present within the lumens. LCIS is frequently present, but this association has not been explained.

More than 95% of all tubular carcinomas are diploid and express hormone receptors. By definition, all are well differentiated. Axillary metastases occur in fewer than 10% of cases unless multiple foci of invasion are present. This subtype is important to recognize because of its excellent prognosis.

Invasive Papillary Carcinoma

Invasive carcinomas with a papillary architecture are rare and represent 1% or fewer of all invasive cancers. Papillary architecture is more commonly seen in DCIS. The clinical presentation is similar to that of carcinomas of NST, but the overall prognosis is better.

Metaplastic Carcinoma

"Metaplastic carcinoma" includes a wide variety of rare types of breast cancer (<1% of all cases), including conventional adenocarcinomas with a chondroid stroma, squamous cell carcinomas, and carcinomas with a prominent spindle cell component that might be difficult to distinguish from sarcomas. Some of these carcinomas express genes in common with myoepithelial cells and likely arise from this cell type.[69] Given the heterogeneity of tumor types and their rarity, little is firmly established with regard to clinical features and prognosis.

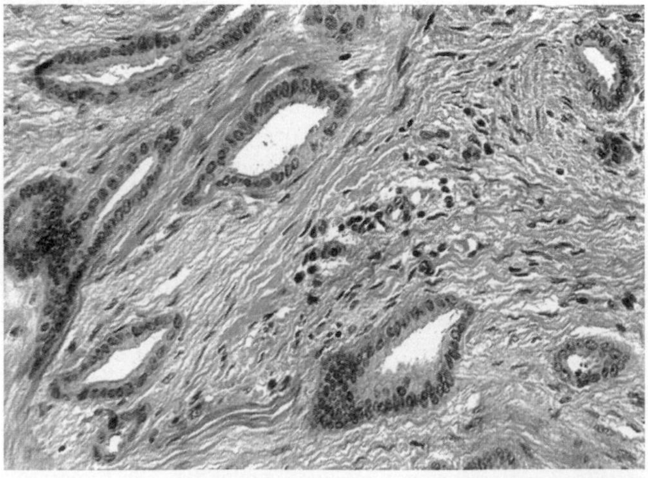

FIGURE 23–26 Tubular carcinoma. The carcinoma must be completely composed of well-formed tubules lined by a single layer of well-differentiated cells.

PROGNOSTIC AND PREDICTIVE FACTORS

The outcome for women with breast cancer varies widely. Some women have the same life expectancy as women without breast cancer. Other women have only a 13% chance of being alive in 5 years. Except for the few women (<10%) with distant metastases at presentation or with inflammatory carcinoma, *prognosis is determined by the pathologic examination of the primary carcinoma and the axillary lymph nodes.* This information is important for counseling patients about the likely outcome of their disease, for choosing appropriate treatment, and for accurately classifying groups of similar patients for clinical trials (e.g., see http://www.nci.nih.gov/search/clinical_trials/ for information about ongoing protocols for women with cancer at different stages).

Major prognostic factors are the strongest predictors of death from breast cancer and are incorporated into the American Joint Committee on Cancer (AJCC) staging system.[70] Predictive factors are used to determine the likelihood of response to a particular therapy.

The major prognostic factors are as follows:

1. **Invasive carcinoma or in situ disease**. By definition, in situ carcinoma is confined to the ductal system and cannot metastasize. Breast cancer deaths associated with DCIS are due to the subsequent development of invasive carcinoma or areas of invasion undetected at the time of diagnosis. The great majority of women with adequately treated DCIS will be cured. In contrast, at least half of invasive carcinomas will have metastasized locally or distantly at the time of diagnosis.
2. **Distant metastases**. Once distant metastases are present, cure is unlikely, although long-term remissions and palliation can be achieved, especially for women with hormonally responsive tumors. Favored sites for dissemination are the lungs, bones, liver, adrenals, brain, and meninges. The potential for metastasis can be reflected by gene expression patterns in the primary carcinoma.[71] The pattern associated with axillary lymph node metastasis may be different from that associated with distant metastasis.[72] The metastatic cells may be directed to specific sites by the expression of chemokine receptors in the cancer cells and the respective chemokines in target organs.[73]
3. **Lymph node metastases.** *Axillary lymph node status is the most important prognostic factor for invasive carcinoma in the absence of distant metastases.* The clinical assessment of nodal involvement is very inaccurate, with both false-positive findings (e.g., palpable reactive nodes) and false-negative findings (e.g., lymph nodes with small metastatic deposits). Therefore, biopsy is necessary for accurate assessment.

With no involvement, the 10-year disease-free survival rate is close to 70% to 80%; the rate falls to 35% to 40%

with one to three positive nodes and 10% to 15% in the presence of more than 10 positive nodes.

Most breast carcinomas drain to one or two *sentinel nodes* that can be identified by radiotracer, colored dye, or both. The sentinel node is highly predictive of the status of the remaining nodes. Sentinel node biopsy can spare women the increased morbidity of a complete axillary dissection. In some women, particularly those with medial tumors, the sentinel node may be an internal mammary node. These nodes are generally not biopsied owing to the morbidity associated with the procedure.

Macrometastases (>0.2 cm) are of proven prognostic importance. Because sentinel nodes often undergo more intense scrutiny with additional sections through the tissue, and immunohistochemistry or reverse transcriptase-polymerase chain reaction (RT-PCR) to detect rare tumor cells, increased numbers of women with minute metastatic deposits in lymph nodes are being identified. The clinical significance of small micrometastases is unclear and is being addressed by current clinical trials.

4. **Tumor size**. The size of the carcinoma is the second most important prognostic factor and is independent from lymph node status. However, the risk of axillary lymph node metastases does increase with the size of the carcinoma. Women with node-negative carcinomas under 1 cm in diameter have a prognosis approaching that of women without breast cancer. The 10-year survival rate of such women without treatment is approximately 90%. On the other hand, over half of women with cancers over 2 cm in diameter present with lymph node metastases, and many of these women will eventually succumb to breast cancer.
5. **Locally advanced disease**. Tumors invading into skin or skeletal muscle are frequently associated with concurrent or subsequent distant disease. With increased awareness of breast cancer detection, such cases have fortunately decreased in frequency and are now rare at initial presentation.
6. **Inflammatory carcinoma**. Women presenting with the clinical appearance of breast swelling and skin thickening have a particularly poor prognosis with a 3-year survival rate of only 3% to 10%.

The major prognostic factors are used by the American Joint Committee on Cancer to divide breast carcinomas into clinical stages as follows:[70]

- Stage 0. DCIS or LCIS (5-year survival rate: 92%).
- Stage I. Invasive carcinoma 2 cm or less in diameter (including carcinoma in situ with microinvasion) without nodal involvement (or only metastases < 0.02 cm in diameter) (5-year survival rate: 87%).
- Stage II. Invasive carcinoma 5 cm or less in diameter with up to three involved axillary nodes or invasive carcinoma greater than 5 cm without nodal involvement (5-year survival rate: 75%).
- Stage III. Invasive carcinoma 5 cm or less in diameter with four or more involved axillary nodes; invasive carcinoma greater than 5 cm in diameter with nodal involvement; invasive carcinoma with 10 or more involved axillary nodes; invasive carcinoma with involvement of the ipsilateral internal mammary lymph nodes; or invasive carcinoma with skin involvement (edema, ulceration, or satellite skin nodules), chest wall fixation, or clinical inflammatory carcinoma (5-year survival rate: 46%).
- Stage IV. Any breast cancer with distant metastases (5-year survival rate: 13%).

Minor Prognostic Factors. Most women with nodal involvement and/or carcinomas over 1 cm in diameter will benefit from some form of systemic therapy. In this group, minor prognostic factors can be used to decide among chemotherapy regimens and/or hormonal therapies. For node-negative women with small carcinomas, minor prognostic factors are used to identify the women most likely to benefit from systemic therapy and those who might not need any additional treatment.[74] Three of these factors—estrogen receptor, progesterone receptor, and *HER2/neu*—are most useful as predictive factors for response to specific therapeutic agents.

1. **Histologic subtypes.** The 30-year survival rate of women with special types of invasive carcinomas (tubular, mucinous, medullary, lobular, and papillary) is greater than 60%, compared with less than 20% for women with cancers of no special type.[75]
2. **Tumor grade.** The most commonly used grading system to assess the degree of tumor differentiation (*Scarff Bloom Richardson*) combines nuclear grade, tubule formation, and mitotic rate. Eighty-five per cent of women with well-differentiated grade I tumors, 60% of women with moderately differentiated grade II tumors, and 15% of women with poorly differentiated grade III tumors survive for 10 years.
3. **Estrogen and progesterone receptors.** Current assays use immunohistochemistry to detect the receptors in the nucleus (Fig. 23–27*A*). Fifty per cent to 85% of carcinomas express estrogen receptors, and such tumors are more common in postmenopausal women. Women with hormone receptor–positive cancers have a slightly better prognosis than do women with hormone receptor–negative carcinomas. The evaluation of hormone receptors is most valuable to predict response to therapy. Eighty per cent of tumors with estrogen receptors and progesterone receptors respond to hormonal manipulation, whereas only about 40% of those with only one type of receptor respond. Tumors with neither estrogen nor progesterone receptors have a less than 10% likelihood of responding.
4. *HER2/neu*. *HER2* (human epidermal growth factor receptor 2 or c-*erb B2* or *neu*) is a transmembrane glycoprotein involved in cell growth control.[76, 77] It does not appear to have a specific ligand but acts as a coreceptor for multiple growth factors. *HER2/neu* is overexpressed in 20% to 30% of breast carcinomas. In over 90% of cases, overexpression is associated with amplification of the gene on 17q21, and this can be determined either by evaluating protein content using immunohistochemistry or by determining gene copy number by using FISH (Figs. 23–27*B* and *C*). Although not all studies have come to the same conclusion, many have shown that overexpression of *HER2/neu* is associated with a poor prognosis. In addition, ongoing studies are addressing the possibility that *HER2/neu*-overexpressing tumors respond differently to hormonal or anthracycline chemotherapy regimens. However, evaluation of HER2/neu is most important to determine response to therapy targeted to this protein.

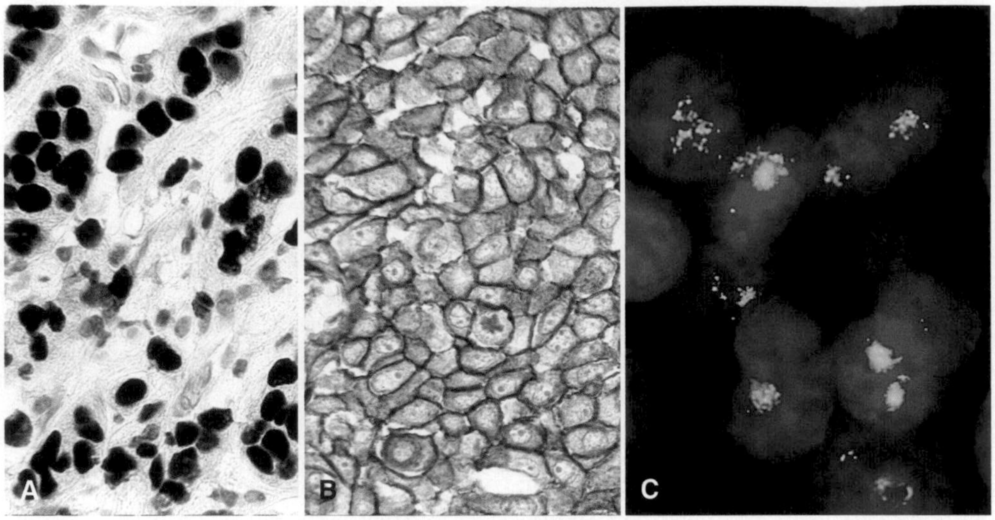

FIGURE 23–27 Predictive markers. *A,* Estrogen receptor is detected in the nucleus by immunohistochemical studies. Progesterone receptor has the same appearance. *B, HER2/neu* overexpression is detected on the cell membrane by immunohistochemistry. *C,* Amplification of the *HER2/neu* gene can be detected by FISH analysis with a fluorescent probe for the gene. A normal cell has two copies of the gene. These tumor cells have over 25 signals, indicating amplification of the gene for *HER2/neu.* (Courtesy of Dr. Jonathan Fletcher, Brigham and Women's Hospital, Boston, MA.)

Trastuzumab (Herceptin) is a humanized monoclonal antibody to HER2/neu developed to specifically target tumor cells and, it is hoped, spare normal cells. In clinical trials, the combination of Trastuzumab with chemotherapy improved response in patients with carcinomas overexpressing *HER2/neu.* Unfortunately, cardiac toxicity, due to an unknown mechanism, could limit its usefulness. However, as the first gene-targeted therapeutic agent for a solid tumor, the results have been very promising.

5. **Lymphovascular invasion (LVI).** Tumor cells may be seen within vascular spaces (either lymphatics or small capillaries) surrounding tumors. This finding is strongly associated with the presence of lymph node metastases and is a poor prognostic factor in women without lymph node metastases. The presence of tumor cells in lymphatics of the dermis is strongly associated with the clinical appearance of inflammatory cancer and bodes a very poor prognosis. LVI must be strictly defined to have prognostic significance.

6. **Proliferative rate.** Proliferation can be measured by flow cytometry (as the S-phase fraction), by thymidine labeling index, by mitotic counts, or by immunohistochemical detection of cellular proteins (e.g., cyclins, Ki-67) produced during the cell cycle. Cyclin E content, when both full-length and low-molecular-weight isoforms are detected, is a very strong predictor of survival.[78] Tumors with high proliferation rates have a worse prognosis, but the most reliable method to assess proliferation has not yet been established. Mitotic counts are included as part of the standard grading system.

7. **DNA content.** The amount of DNA per tumor cell can be determined by flow cytometric analysis or by image analysis of tissue sections. Tumors with a DNA index of 1 have the same total amount of DNA as normal diploid cells, although marked karyotypic changes may be present. Aneuploid tumors are those with abnormal DNA indices and have a slightly worse prognosis.

A new approach to prognosis, mentioned previously, is gene expression profiling. For example, changes in 70 marker genes were used to classify tumors according to a good or poor prognosis signature and were shown to be more predictive of outcome than the use of traditional indicators.[79] Currently, this method requires the use of rapidly frozen tissue and therefore cannot be used to evaluate most breast cancers. However, techniques for gene expression profiling on paraffin-embedded tissues are being developed.

Despite the numerous prognostic indicators currently in use or under investigation, it is impossible in an individual case to predict the outcome. Sadly, only time tells this story. For this reason, there are continuing searches for better or more refined biologic markers of prognosis and more effective treatment modalities.

A diagnosis of breast cancer is not a medical emergency. Most cancers have been present for many years prior to detection, and survival time, even for advanced cancer, is usually measured in years. Women can take the necessary time to make informed choices among the many, often equivalent, treatment options.

Current therapeutic approaches include local and regional control, using combinations of surgery (mastectomy or breast conservation) and postoperative radiation, and systemic control, using hormonal treatment or chemotherapy or both. Axillary node dissection or sentinel node sampling is performed for prognostic purposes, but the axilla can also be treated with radiation alone. Newer therapeutic strategies include inhibition (by pharmacologic agents or specific antibodies) of membrane-bound growth factor receptors (e.g., HER2/neu), stromal proteases, and angiogenesis.

Such therapies are based on models of breast cancer dissemination that have evolved as our understanding of its biology has changed. Earlier models proposed that breast cancer spreads in a contiguous fashion by direct extension from breast to nodes and could therefore be cured by en bloc surgical resection. However, radical surgery, including mastectomies with removal of pectoralis muscles, internal mammary nodes, and even supraclavicular nodes, failed to decrease mortality. A subsequent model, based on studies demonstrating that lumpectomy (removal of the breast mass) and radiation were equivalent to mastectomy, postulated that all cancers had spread systemically by the time of diagnosis and that local or regional treatment was unimportant for overall survival. In the current era of increased detection of early-stage carcinomas by mammography, a third model that combines the first two is thought to be more appropriate to guide therapy.[80] Although some women already have systemic involvement at first presentation and cannot be cured by local and regional control, in situ and small invasive carcinomas, especially those detected by mammography, are often limited to the breast, and local and regional treatment with intent to cure must be the goal for such cancers.[81] For more advanced cancers that have metastasized beyond the breast, newer therapies, such as Herceptin, and better hormonal therapies hold out the hope of sustained remission and longer survival.

STROMAL TUMORS

The two types of stroma in the breast, intralobular and interlobular (see the section on the normal breast), give rise to distinct types of neoplasms. The breast-specific biphasic tumors fibroadenoma and phyllodes tumor arise in the intralobular stroma. This specialized stroma may elaborate growth factors for epithelial cells, resulting in the proliferation of the non-neoplastic epithelial component of these tumors. Interlobular stroma is the source of the same types of tumors found in connective tissue in other sites of the body (e.g., lipomas and angiosarcomas) as well as tumors arising more commonly in the breast (e.g., pseudoangiomatous stromal hyperplasia and fibrous tumors).

Fibroadenoma

This is the most common benign tumor of the female breast. Occurring at any age within the reproductive period of life, fibroadenomas are somewhat more common before age 30. They are frequently multiple and bilateral. Young women usually present with a palpable mass and older women with a mammographic density (Fig. 23–28*A*) or mammographic calcifications. The epithelium of the fibroadenoma is hormonally responsive, and a slight increase in size may occur during the late phase of each menstrual cycle. An increase in size due to lactational changes or, not uncommonly, infarction and inflammation may lead to a fibroadenoma mimicking carcinoma during pregnancy. Regression usually occurs after menopause. The stroma often becomes densely hyalinized and may calcify. Large lobulated ("popcorn") calcifications have a characteristic mammographic appearance, but small calcifications may appear clustered and require biopsy to exclude carcinoma.

Morphology. Fibroadenomas grow as spherical nodules that are usually sharply circumscribed and freely movable in the surrounding breast substance. They vary in size from less than 1 cm in diameter to large tumors that can replace most of the breast. Grossly, the tumors are well-circumscribed, rubbery,

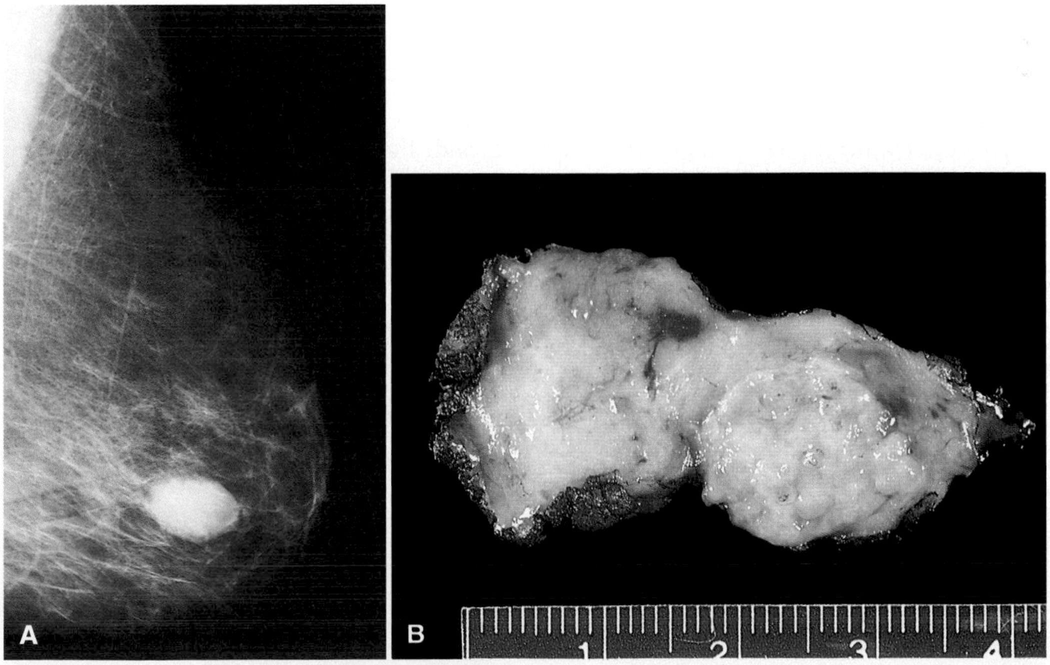

FIGURE 23–28 *A*, This mammogram shows a well-circumscribed mass. (Courtesy of Dr. Jack Meyer, Brigham and Women's Hospital, Boston, MA.) Although the most common lesion would be a fibroadenoma, other benign (e.g., fibrous lesions or PASH) and malignant (e.g., medullary or mucinous carcinomas) lesions can also have this appearance. *B*, Fibroadenoma. A rubbery, white, well-circumscribed mass is clearly demarcated from the surrounding yellow adipose tissue. The fibroadenoma does not contain adipose tissue and therefore appears denser than the surrounding normal tissue on mammogram.

grayish white nodules that bulge above the surrounding tissue and often contain slitlike spaces (Fig. 23–28*B*).

The stroma is usually delicate, cellular, and often myxoid, resembling intralobular stroma, enclosing glandular and cystic spaces lined by epithelium. The epithelium may be surrounded by stroma or compressed and distorted by it (Fig. 23–29). In older women, the stroma typically becomes densely hyalinized and the epithelium atrophic.

Some fibroadenomas are polyclonal in origin and are probably due to focal hyperplasia of lobular stroma. For example, almost half of women receiving cyclosporin A after renal transplantation develop fibroadenomas.[82] The tumors are frequently multiple and bilateral and are likely to be due to drug-related growth stimulation. On the other hand, there is a subset of fibroadenomas that are benign neoplasms of stromal cells. Multiple studies have shown that in some tumors, the fibrous (stromal) component is clonal and may have cytogenetic aberrations, but the epithelial component is polyclonal. No consistent cytogenetic changes have been found.[83,84]

Fibroadenomas were originally grouped with other "proliferative changes without atypia" in conferring a mild increase in the risk of subsequent cancer. However, in one study, only fibroadenomas associated with cysts larger than 0.3 cm, sclerosing adenosis, epithelial calcifications, or papillary apocrine change ("complex fibroadenomas") conferred a mild increase in the risk of subsequent breast cancer[85] (Table 23–2). It is hoped that future studies will better define the risk associated with these lesions.

Phyllodes Tumor

Phyllodes tumors, like fibroadenomas, arise from intralobular stroma. Although they can occur at any age, most present in the sixth decade, 10 to 20 years later than the average presentation of a fibroadenoma.[86] Most present as palpable masses, but a few are detected mammographically. The term "cystosarcoma phyllodes" is sometimes used for these lesions. However, the term "phyllodes tumor" is preferred, as the majority of these tumors behave in a relatively benign fashion, and most are not cystic.

Morphology. The tumors vary in size from a few centimeters in diameter to massive lesions involving the entire breast. The larger lesions often have bulbous protrusions (*phyllodes* is Greek for "leaflike") due to the presence of nodules of proliferating stroma covered by epithelium (Fig. 23–30). In some tumors, these protrusions extend into a cystic space. This growth pattern can also occasionally be seen in larger fibroadenomas and is not an indication of malignancy. Phyllodes tumors are distinguished from the more common fibroadenomas on the basis of cellularity, mitotic rate, nuclear pleomorphism, stromal overgrowth, and infiltrative borders. Low-grade lesions resemble fibroadenomas but with increased cellularity and mitotic figures. High-grade lesions may be difficult to distinguish from other types of soft tissue sarcomas and may have foci of mesenchymal differentiation (e.g., rhabdomyosarcoma or liposarcoma). These tumors not uncommonly recur with a higher grade.

Phyllodes tumors must be excised with wide margins or by mastectomy to avoid the high risk of local recurrences. Axillary lymph node dissection is not indicated because the incidence of nodal metastases, as for other stromal malignancies, is exceedingly small. The majority are low-grade tumors that may recur locally but only rarely metastasize. Rare high-grade lesions behave aggressively, with frequent local recurrences and distant hematogenous metastases in about one third of cases.[87] Only the stromal component metastasizes.

Sarcomas

Tumors of the extrinsic connective tissue of the breast include the same types of benign and malignant lesions that are seen elsewhere in the body. Malignant lesions include

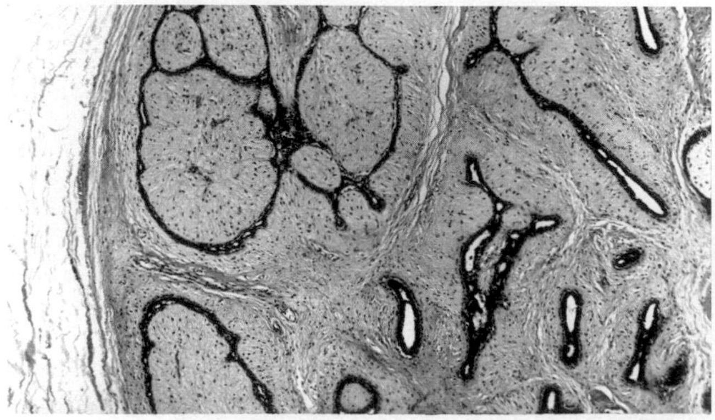

FIGURE 23–29 Fibroadenoma. The lesion consists of a proliferation of intralobular stroma surrounding and often pushing and distorting the associated epithelium. The border is sharply delimited from the surrounding tissue.

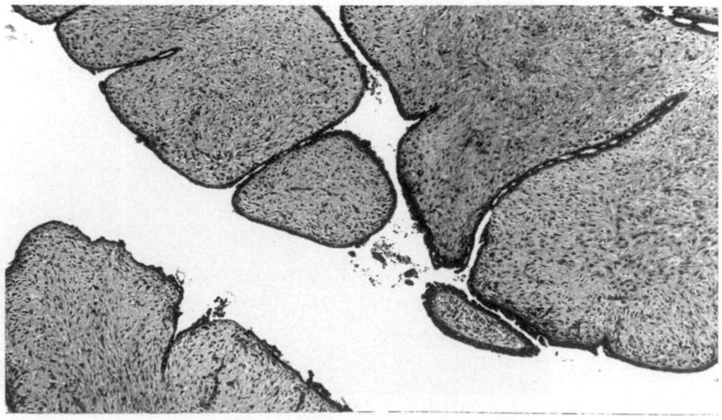

FIGURE 23–30 Phyllodes tumor. Compared to a fibroadenoma, there is increased stromal cellularity, cytologic atypia, and stromal overgrowth, giving rise to the typical leaflike architecture.

angiosarcoma, rhabdomyosarcoma, liposarcoma, leiomyosarcoma, chondrosarcoma, and osteosarcoma. Sarcomatous differentiation also occurs in phyllodes tumors and in carcinomas ("metaplastic carcinomas"). Sarcomas usually present as bulky palpable masses. Lymph node metastases are rare; hematogenous spread to the lung is commonly seen.

Angiosarcomas of the breast arise spontaneously or as a complication of radiation therapy.[88] There is a 0.3% to 4% risk of angiosarcoma after radiation therapy for breast cancer, most cases arising 5 to 10 years after treatment. Most of these tumors arise in the skin of the breast. Angiosarcomas can also arise in the skin of a chronically edematous arm after mastectomy (Stewart-Treves syndrome), but this complication has become much less common with greater attention to surgical techniques and more limited axillary dissections.

Other Stromal Lesions

Pseudoangiomatous stromal hyperplasia (PASH) and fibrous tumors commonly present as circumscribed palpable masses or mammographic densities in premenopausal women or older women on hormone replacement therapy. Histologically, they are benign proliferations of interlobular stroma. Lipomas and hamartomas are often palpable but can also be detected mammographically as fat-containing lesions. All are benign and require diagnosis only to distinguish them from malignancies.

Fibromatosis is due to a clonal proliferation of fibroblasts and myofibroblasts. It presents as an irregular mass that can involve both skin and muscle and closely mimics invasive carcinoma. Wide excision is mandatory, as recurrences are common and may be difficult to control. Although locally aggressive, this lesion does not metastasize. Most cases are sporadic, but some occur as part of familial adenomatous polyposis (FAP), hereditary desmoid syndrome, and Gardner syndrome. Mutations in the adenomatosis polyposis coli (APC) gene are found in patients with FAP as well as in sporadic cases of breast fibromatosis.[89]

OTHER MALIGNANT TUMORS OF THE BREAST

Malignant tumors may arise from the skin of the breast, sweat glands, sebaceous glands, and hair shafts; these tumors are identical to their counterparts found in other sites of the body. Lymphomas may arise primarily in the breast, or the breasts may be secondarily involved by a systemic lymphoma. Most are of large cell type of B-cell origin. Young women with Burkitt lymphoma may present with massive bilateral breast involvement and are often pregnant or lactating. Metastases to the breast are rare and most commonly arise from a contralateral breast carcinoma. The most frequent nonmammary metastases are from melanomas and lung cancers.

THE MALE BREAST

Pathology

The normal male breast consists of the nipple and a rudimentary duct system ending in terminal buds without lobule formation. Only two processes occur with sufficient frequency to merit consideration.

Gynecomastia

Gynecomastia (enlargement of the male breast) may be unilateral or bilateral and presents as a button-like subareolar enlargement. In advanced cases, the swelling can simulate the adolescent female breast. The lesion must be differentiated only from the rare carcinoma of the male breast. Gynecomastia is chiefly of importance as an indicator of hyperestrinism, suggesting cirrhosis of the liver or the possible existence of a functioning testicular tumor.

Morphology. There is proliferation of a dense collagenous connective tissue, but more striking are the changes in the epithelium of the ducts. Marked micropapillary hyperplasia of the ductal linings occurs (Fig. 23–31). The individual cells are fairly regular, columnar to cuboidal cells with regular nuclei. Lobule formation is rare.

Like the female breast, the male breast is subject to hormonal influences, and gynecomastia may occur as a result of an imbalance between estrogens, which stimulate breast tissue, and androgens, which counteract these effects. It is encountered under a variety of normal and abnormal circumstances. It may be found at the time of puberty, in the very aged, or at any time during adult life when there is cause for hyperestrinism. The most important of these is cirrhosis of the liver, since the liver is responsible for metabolizing estrogen. In older males, gynecomastia may occur owing to a relative increase in adrenal estrogens as the androgenic function

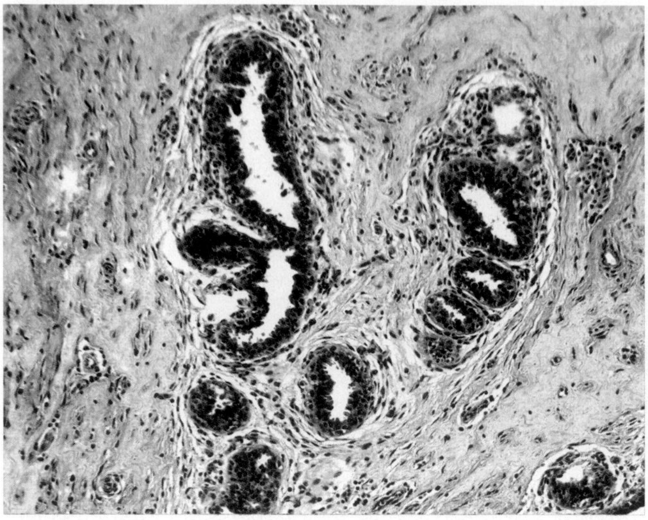

FIGURE 23–31 Gynecomastia. Terminal ducts (without lobule formation) are lined by a multilayered epithelium with small papillary tufts. There is typically surrounding periductal hyalinization and fibrosis.

of the testis fails. Drugs such as alcohol, marijuana, heroin, antiretroviral therapy, anabolic steroids used by some athletes and body builders, and some psychoactive agents have also been associated with gynecomastia.[90] Rarely, gynecomastia may occur as part of Klinefelter syndrome (XXY karyotype) or in association with functioning testicular neoplasms, such as Leydig cell and, rarely, Sertoli cell tumors.

Carcinoma

Carcinoma arising in the male breast is a rare occurrence, with a frequency ratio to breast cancer in the female of less than 1:100 or a lifetime risk of 0.11% compared to about 13% in women.[91] There are about 1500 cases and 400 deaths each year. Risk factors are similar to those in women and include first-degree relatives with breast cancer, decreased testicular function (e.g., Klinefelter syndrome), exposure to exogenous estrogens, increasing age, infertility, obesity, prior benign breast disease, exposure to ionizing radiation, and residency in Western countries. Gynecomastia does not appear to be a risk factor. Four per cent to 14% of cases in males are attributed to germ line *BRCA2* mutations. A breast cancer family with at least one affected male has a 60% to 76% chance of having a *BRCA2* mutation. Male breast cancer is less commonly observed in *BRCA1* families. Three per cent to 8% of cases are associated with Klinefelter syndrome.

The pathology of male breast cancer is remarkably similar to that of cancers seen in women. The same histologic subtypes of invasive cancer are present, although papillary carcinomas (both invasive and in situ) are more common and lobular carcinomas are less common. The expression of molecular markers is similar with the one exception that ER positivity is more common in male breast cancer (81% of tumors). Unlike in women, the incidence of ER-positive tumors does not increase with age. Prognostic factors are similar in men and women.

Because breast epithelium in men is limited to large ducts near the nipple, carcinomas usually present as a palpable subareolar mass, 2 to 3 cm in diameter. Nipple discharge is a common symptom. The carcinoma is situated close to the overlying skin and underlying thoracic wall, and even small carcinomas can invade these structures. Ulceration through the skin is more common than in women. Dissemination follows the same pattern as in women, and axillary lymph node involvement is present in about half of cases at the time of discovery of the lesion. Distant metastases to the lungs, brain, bone, and liver are common. Although men present at higher stages, prognosis is similar in men and women when they are matched by stage. Most cancers are treated locally with mastectomy and axillary node dissection. The same systemic treatment guidelines are used for men and women, and response rates are similar.

REFERENCES

1. Lakhani SR, O'Hare MJ: The mammary myoepithelial cell: Cinderella or ugly sister? Breast Cancer Res 3:1, 2001.
2. Bocker W, Moll R, Poremba C, Holland R, van Diest PJ, Dervan P, Burger H, Wai D, Diallo RI, Brandt B, Herbst H, Schmidt A, Lerch MM, Buchwallow IB: Common adult stem cells in the human breast give rise to glandular and myoepithelial cell lineages: a new cell biological concept. Lab Invest 82:737, 2002.
3. Longacre TA, Bartow SA: A correlative morphologic study of human breast and endometrium in the menstrual cycle. Am J Surg Pathol 10:382, 1986.
4. Neville MC, Morton J, Umemura S: Lactogenesis: the transition from pregnancy to lactation. Pediatr Clin North Am 48:35, 2001.
5. Zinkernagel RM: Maternal antibodies, childhood infections, and autoimmune diseases. N Engl J Med 345:1331, 2001.
6. Committee on Drugs: The transfer of drugs and other chemicals into human milk. Pediatrics 93:137, 1994.
7. Tugwell P, Wells G, Peterson J, et al: Do silicone implants cause rheumatologic disorders? a systematic review for a court-appointed science panel. Arthritis Rheum 44:2477, 2001.
8. Muzzaffar AR, Rohrich RJ: The silicone gel-filled breast implant controversy: an update. Plast Reconstr Surg 109:742, 2002.
9. Barton MB, Elmore JG, Fletcher, SW: Breast symptoms among women enrolled in a health maintenance organization: frequency, evaluation, and outcome. Ann Intern Med 130:651, 1999.
10. Ito Y, Tamaki Y, Nakano Y, Kobayashi T, Takeda T, Wakasugi E, Miyashiro I, Komoike Y, Miyazaki M, Nakayama T, Kano T, Monden M: Nonpalpable breast cancer with nipple discharge: how should it be treated? Anticancer Res 17:791, 1997.
11. Lester S: Subareolar abscess (Zuska's disease): a specific disease entity with specific treatment and prevention strategies. Pathol Case Rev 4:189, 1999.
12. Meguid M, et al: Pathogenesis-based treatment of recurring subareolar breast abscesses. Surgery 118:775, 1995.
13. Bartow SA, et al: Fibrocystic disease: a continuing enigma. Pathol Annu 17:93, 1982.
14. Fitzgibbons PL, Henson DE, Hutter RVP: Benign breast changes and the risk for subsequent breast cancer: an update of the 1985 consensus statement. Arch Pathol Lab Med 122:1053, 1998.
15. Jacobs TW, Byrne C, Colditz G, et al: Radial scars and breast cancer risk: a case-control study. N Engl J Med 340:430, 1999.
16. Schnitt SJ: Benign breast disease and breast cancer risk: morphology and beyond. Am J Surg Pathol 27:836, 2003.
17. Page DL, Schuyler PA, DuPont WD, Jensen RA, Plummer WD Jr, Simpson JF: Atypical lobular hyperplasia as a unilateral predictor of breast cancer risk: a retrospective cohort study. Lancet 361:125, 2003.
18. Coughlin SS, Thompson TD, Hall HI, Logan P, Uhler RJ: Breast and cervical carcinoma screening practices among women in rural and nonrural areas of the United States, 1998–1999. Cancer 94:2801, 2002.
19. Gail MH, Brinton LA, Byar DP, et al: Projecting individualized probabilities of developing breast cancer for white females who are being examined annually. J Natl Cancer Inst 81:1879, 1989.
20. Rhodes DJ: Identifying and counseling women at increased risk for breast cancer. Mayo Clin Proc 77:355, 2002.

21. Collaborative Group on Hormonal Factors in Breast Cancer: Familial breast cancer: collaborative reanalysis of individual data from 52 epidemiological studies including 58,209 women with breast cancer and 101,986 women without the disease. Lancet 358:1389, 2001.
22. Newman LA, Mason J, Cote D, Vin Y, Carolin K, Bouwman D, Colditz GA: African-American ethnicity, socioeconomic status, and breast cancer survival. Cancer 94:2844, 2002.
23. Shavers VL, Brown ML: Racial and ethnic disparities in the receipt of cancer treatment. J Natl Cancer Inst 94:334, 2002.
24. Morris CR, Wright WE, Schlag RD: The risk of developing breast cancer within the next 5, 10, or 20 years of a woman's life. Am J Prev Med 20:214, 2001.
25. Mahavani V, Sood AK: Hormone replacement therapy and cancer risk. Curr Opin Oncol 13:384, 2001.
26. Nelson HD, Humphrey LL, Nygren P, Teutsch SM, Allan JD: Postmenopausal hormone replacement therapy: scientific review. JAMA 288:872, 2002.
27. Marchbanks PA, McDonald JA, Wilson HG, et al: Oral contraceptives and the risk of breast cancer. N Engl J Med 346:2025, 2002.
28. Clemons M, Loijens L, Goss P: Breast cancer risk following irradiation for Hodgkin's disease. Cancer Treat Rev 26:291, 2000.
29. Hamajima N, et al: Alcohol, tobacco and breast cancer: collaborative reanalysis of individual data from 53 epidemiological studies, including 58,515 women with breast cancer and 95,067 women without the disease. Br J Cancer 87:1234, 2002.
30. Collaborative Group on Hormonal Factors in Breast Cancer, Beral V: Breast cancer and breastfeeding: collaborative reanalysis of individual data from 47 epidemiological studies in 30 countries, including 50302 women with breast cancer and 96973 women without the disease. Lancet 360:187, 2002.
31. Hartmann LC, Schaid DJ, Woods JE, et al: Efficacy of bilateral prophylactic mastectomy in women with a family history of breast cancer. N Engl J Med 340:77, 1999.
32. Cuzick J, Powles T, Veronesi U, Forbes J, Edwards R, Ashley S, Boyle, P: Overview of the main outcomes in breast-cancer prevention trials. Lancet 361:296, 2003.
33. Venkitaraman AR: Cancer susceptibility and the functions of BRCA1 and BRCA2. Cell 108:171, 2002.
34. Yang H, Jeffrey PD, Miller J, Kinnucan E, Sun Y, Thoma NH, Zheng N, Chen P-L, Lee W-H, Pavletich NP: BRCA2 function in DNA binding and recombination from a BRCA2-DSS1-ssDNA structure. Science 297:1837, 2002.
35. Ganesan S, Silver DP, Greenberg RA, Avni D, Drapkin R, Miron A, et al: BRCA1 supports XIST RNA concentration on the inactive X chromosome. Cell 111:393, 2002.
36. Carter RF: BRCA1, BRCA2 and breast cancer: a concise clinical review. Clin Invest Med 24:147, 2001.
37. Kauff ND, Satagopan JM, Robson ME, et al: Risk-reducing salpingo-oophorectomy in women with a BRCA1 or BRCA2 mutation. N Engl J Med 346:1609, 2002.
38. Rebbeck TR, Lynch HT, Neuhausen SL, et al: Prophylactic oophorectomy in carriers of BRCA1 or BRCA2 mutations. N Engl J Med 346:1616, 2002.
39. Esteller M, Herman JG: Cancer as an epigenetic disease: DNA methylation and chromatin alterations in human tumours. J Pathol 196:1, 2002.
40. Hedenfalk, I, Duggan, D, et al: Gene-expression profiles in hereditary breast cancer. N Engl J Med 344:539, 2001.
41. van't Veer LJ, Dai H, van de Vijver MJ, et al: Gene expression profiling predicts clinical outcome of breast cancer. Nature 415:530, 2002.
42. de Jong MM, Nolte IM, te Meerman GJ, van der Graaf WTA, Oosterwijk JC, Kleibeuker JH, Schaapveld M, de Vries EGE: Genes other than BRCA1 and BRCA2 involved in breast cancer suseptibility. J Med Genet 39:225, 2002.
43. Meijers-Heijboer, H, van den Ouweland A, Klijn, J, et al: Low-penetrance susceptibility to breast cancer due to CHEK2 (*) 1100delC in noncarriers of BRCA1 or BRCA2 mutations. Nat Genet 31:55, 2002.
44. Wooster R, Weber BL: Breast and ovarian cancer. N Engl J Med 348:2339, 2003.
45. Pharoah PDP, Antoniou A, Bobrow M, Zimmern RL, Easton DF, Ponder BAJ: Polygenic susceptibility to breast cancer and implications for prevention. Nat Genet 31:33, 2002.
46. Antoniou AC, Pharoah PD, McMullan G, Day NE, Stratton MR, Peto J, Ponder BJ, Easton DF: A comprehensive model for familial breast cancer incorporating BRCA1, BRCA2 and other genes. Br J Cancer 86:76, 2002.
47. Peto J: Breast cancer susceptibility: a new look at an old model. Cancer Cell 1:411, 2002.
48. Hedenfalk I, Ringner M, Ben-Dor A, et al: Molecular classification of familial non-BRCA1/BRCA2 breast cancer. Proc Natl Acad Sci U S A 100:2532, 2003.
49. Miller K: Estrogen and DNA damage: the silent source of breast cancer? J Natl Cancer Inst 95:100, 2003.
50. Hanahan D, Weinberg RA: The hallmarks of cancer. Cell 100:57, 2000.
51. Hahn WC, Weinberg RA: Rules for making human tumor cells. N Engl J Med 347:1593, 2002.
52. Iqbal M, Davies MP, Shoker BS, Jarvis C, Sibson DR, Sloane JP: Subgroups of non-atypical hyperplasia of breast defined by proliferation of oestrogen receptor-positive cells. J Pathol 193:333, 2001.
53. Wiseman BS, Werb Z: Stromal effects on mammary gland development and breast cancer. Science 296:1046, 2002.
54. Tlsty TD, Hein PW: Know thy neighbor: stromal cells can contribute oncogenic signals. Curr Opin Genet Dev 11:54, 2001.
55. Porter D, Lahti-Domenici J, Keshaviah A, Bae YK, et al: Molecular markers in ductal carcinoma in situ of the breast. Mol Cancer Res 1:362, 2003.
56. Sorlie T, Perou CM, Tibshirani R, et al: Gene expression patterns of breast carcinomas distinguish tumor subclasses wth potential clinical implications. Proc Natl Acad Sci U S A 98:10869, 2001.
57. West M, Blanchette C, Dressman H, et al: Predicting the clinical status of human breast cancer by using gene expression profiles. Proc Natl Acad Sci U S A 98:11462, 2001.
58. Wellings SR: A hypothesis of the origin of human breast cancer from the terminal ductal lobular unit. Pathol Res Pract 166:515, 1980.
59. Schelfhout VR, Coene ED, Delaey B, Thys S, Page DL, De Potter CR: Pathogenesis of Paget's disease: epidermal heregulin-alpha, motility factor, and the HER receptor family. J Natl Cancer Inst 92:622, 2000.
60. Kothari AS, Beechey-Newman N, Hamed H, Fentiman IS, D'Arrigo C, Hanby AM, Ryder K: Paget disease of the nipple: a multifocal manifestation of higher-risk disease. Cancer 95:1, 2002.
61. Page DL, et al: Continued local recurrence of carcinoma 15–25 years after a diagnosis of low grade ductal carcinoma in situ of the breast treated only by biopsy. Cancer 76:1197, 1995.
62. Silverstein MJ: Ductal carcinoma in situ of the breast. Annu Rev Med 51:17, 2000.
63. Vogel VG, Costantino JP, Wickerman DL, Cronin WM: National surgical adjuvant breast and bowel project update: prevention trials and endocrine therapy of ductal carcinoma in situ. Clin Cancer Res 9:495S, 2003.
64. Hajra KM, Fearon ER: Cadherin and catenin alterations in human cancer. Genes Chromosomes Cancer 34:255, 2002.
65. Lakhani SR: Molecular genetics of solid tumors: translating research into clinical practice. What we could do now: breast cancer. Mol Pathol 54:281, 2001.
66. Li CI, Anderson BO, Porter P, Holt SK, Daling JR, Moe RE: Changing incidence rate of invasive lobular breast carcinoma among older women. Cancer 88:2561, 2000.
67. Li CI, Weiss NS, Stanford JL, Daling JR: Hormone replacement therapy in relation to risk of lobular and ductal breast carcinoma in middle-aged women. Cancer 88:2570, 2000.
68. Berx G, Van Roy F: The E-cadherin/catenin complex: an important gatekeeper in breast cancer tumorigenesis and malignant progression. Breast Cancer Res 3:289, 2001.
69. Reis-Filho, JS, Milanezi, F, Paredes, J, et al: Novel and classic myoepithelial/stem cell markers in metaplastic carcinomas of the breast. Appl Immunohistochem Mol Morphol 11:1, 2003.
70. AJCC Cancer Staging Manual, 6th ed. New York, Springer, 2002.
71. Ramaswamy S, Ross KN, Lander, ES, Golub TR: A molecular signature of metastasis in primary solid tumors. Nat Genet 33:49, 2003.
72. Huang E, Cheng SH, Dressman H, et al: Gene expression predictors of breast cancer outcomes, Lancet 361:1590, 2003.
73. Muller A, Homey B, Soto H, Ge N, et al: Involvement of chemokine receptors in breast cancer metastasis. Nature 410:50, 2001.
74. Mirza AN, Mirza NQ, Vlastos G, Singletary SE: Prognostic factors in node-negative breast cancer: a review of studies with sample size more than 200 and follow-up more than 5 years. Ann Surg 235:10, 2001.
75. Simpson JF, Page DL: Prognostic value of histopathology in the breast. Semin Oncol 19:254, 1992.
76. Hayes DF, Thor AD: c-erbB-2 in breast cancer: development of a clinically useful marker. Semin Oncol 29:231, 2002.

77. Shawver LK, Slamon D, Ullrich A: Smart drugs: tyrosine kinase inhibitors in cancer therapy. Cancer Cell 1:117, 2002.
78. Keyomarsi K, et al: Cyclin E and survival in patients with breast cancer. N Engl J Med 346:1566, 2002.
79. van de Vijer MJ, He, YD, van't Veer LJ, Dai H, Hart AA, Voskuil DW, Schreiber GJ, et al: A gene-expression signature as a predictor of survival in breast cancer. N Engl J Med 347:1999, 2002.
80. Hellman S: Natural history of small breast cancers. J Clin Oncol 12:2229, 1994.
81. Goldhirsch A, Glick JH, Gelber RD, Coates AS, Senn H-J: Meeting highlights: international consensus panel on the treatment of primary breast cancer. J Clin Oncol 19:3817, 2001.
82. Baildam AD, et al: Cyclosporin A and multiple fibroadenomas of the breast. Br J Surg 83:1755, 1996.
83. Cavalli LR, Cornelio DA, Wuicik L, Bras ATS, Ribeiro EMSF, Lima RS, Urban CA, Rogatto SR, Cavalli IJ: Clonal chromosomal alterations in fibroadenomas of the breast. Cancer Genet Cytogenet 131:120, 2001.
84. Ojopi EP, Rogatto SR, Caldeira JR, Barbieri-Neto J, Squire JA: Comparative genomic hybridization detects novel amplifications in fibroadenomas of the breast. Genes Chromosomes Cancer 30:25, 2001.
85. Dupont WD, Page DL, Parl FE, et al: Long-term risk of breast cancer in women with fibroadenoma. N Engl J Med 331:10, 1994.
86. Parker SJ, Harries SA: Phyllodes tumours. Postgrad Med J 77:428, 2001.
87. Cohn-Cedermark G, et al: Prognostic factors in cystosarcoma phyllodes. Cancer 68:2017, 1991.
88. Yap J, Chuba PJ, Thomas R, Aref A, Lucas D, Severson RK, Hamre M: Sarcoma as a second malignancy after treatment for breast cancer. Int J Radiat Oncol Biol Phys 52:1231, 2002.
89. Abraham SC, Reynolds C, Lee JH, Montgomery EA, Baisden BL, Krasinskas AM, Wu TT: Fibromatosis of the breast and mutations involving the APC/beta-catenin pathway. Hum Pathol 33:39, 2002.
90. Braunstein GD: Gynecomastia. N Engl J Med 328:490, 1993.
91. Giordano SH, Buzdar AU, Hortobagyi GN: Breast cancer in men. Ann Intern Med 137:678, 2002.

CHAPTER 24

The Endocrine System

Anirban Maitra, MBBS • Abul K. Abbas, MBBS

■ PITUITARY GLAND

PITUITARY ADENOMAS AND HYPERPITUITARISM

Prolactinomas

Growth Hormone (Somatotroph Cell) Adenomas

Corticotroph Cell Adenomas

Other Anterior Pituitary Adenomas

HYPOPITUITARISM

POSTERIOR PITUITARY SYNDROMES

HYPOTHALAMIC SUPRASELLAR TUMORS

■ THYROID GLAND

HYPERTHYROIDISM

HYPOTHYROIDISM

Cretinism

Myxedema

THYROIDITIS

Hashimoto Thyroiditis

Subacute (Granulomatous) Thyroiditis

Subacute Lymphocytic (Painless) Thyroiditis

GRAVES DISEASE

DIFFUSE AND MULTINODULAR GOITER

Diffuse Nontoxic (Simple) Goiter

Multinodular Goiter

NEOPLASMS OF THE THYROID

Adenomas

Other Benign Tumors

Carcinomas

Papillary Carcinoma

Follicular Carcinoma

Medullary Carcinoma

Anaplastic Carcinoma

CONGENITAL ANOMALIES

■ PARATHYROID GLANDS

HYPERPARATHYROIDISM

Primary Hyperparathyroidism

Secondary Hyperparathyroidism

HYPOPARATHYROIDISM

PSEUDOHYPOPARATHYROIDISM

■ THE ENDOCRINE PANCREAS

DIABETES MELLITUS

Diagnosis

Classification

Normal Insulin Phsyiology

Regulation of Insulin Release

Insulin Action and Insulin-Signaling Pathways

Pathogenesis of Type 1 Diabetes Mellitus

Mechanisms of β-Cell Destruction

Genetic Susceptibility

Environmental Factors

Pathogenesis of Type 2 Diabetes Mellitus

Insulin Resistance

β-Cell Dysfunction

Monogenic Forms of Diabetes

Pathogenesis of Complications of Diabetes

Morphology of Diabetes and Its Late Complications

Clinical Features of Diabetes

PANCREATIC ENDOCRINE NEOPLASMS

Hyperinsulinism (Insulinoma)

Zollinger-Ellison Syndrome (Gastrinomas)

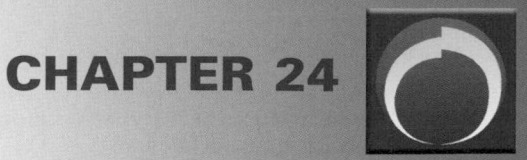

Other Rare Pancreatic Endocrine Neoplasms

ADRENAL GLANDS

ADRENAL CORTEX

Adrenocortical Hyperfunction (Hyperadrenalism)

Hypercortisolism (Cushing Syndrome)

Primary Hyperaldosteronism

Adrenogenital Syndromes

Adrenal Insufficiency

Primary Acute Adrenocortical Insufficiency

Waterhouse-Friderichsen Syndrome

Primary Chronic Adrenocortical Insufficiency (Addison Disease)

Secondary Adrenocortical Insufficiency

Adrenocortical Neoplasms

Other Lesions of the Adrenal

ADRENAL MEDULLA

Pheochromocytoma

Tumors of Extra-Adrenal Paraganglia

Neuroblastoma

MULTIPLE ENDOCRINE NEOPLASIA SYNDROMES

Multiple Endocrine Neoplasia, Type 1

Multiple Endocrine Neoplasia, Type 2

PINEAL GLAND

Pinealomas

The endocrine system contains a highly integrated and widely distributed group of organs that orchestrates a state of metabolic equilibrium, or homeostasis, among the various organs of the body. Signaling by extracellular secreted molecules can be classified into three types—autocrine, paracrine, or endocrine—on the basis of the distance over which the signal acts. In endocrine signaling, the secreted molecules, which are frequently called *hormones*, act on target cells that are distant from their site of synthesis. An endocrine hormone is frequently carried by the blood from its site of release to its target. Increased activity of the target tissue often down-regulates the activity of the gland that secretes the stimulating hormone, a process known as *feedback inhibition*.

Hormones can be classified into several broad categories on the basis of the nature of their receptors. Cellular receptors and signaling pathways were discussed in Chapter 3, and only a few comments about signaling by hormone receptors follow:

- *Hormones that trigger biochemical signals upon interacting with cell-surface receptors:* This large class of compounds is composed of two groups: (1) peptide hormones, such as growth hormone and insulin, and (2) small molecules, such as epinephrine. Binding of these hormones to cell-surface receptors leads to an increase in intracellular signaling molecules, termed *second messengers*, such as cyclic adenosine monophosphate (cAMP); production of mediators from membrane phospholipids, such as inositol 1,4,5-trisphosphate or IP_3; and shifts in the intracellular levels of ionized calcium. The elevated levels of one or more of these can control proliferation, differentiation, survival, and functional activity of cells, mainly by regulating the expression of specific genes.
- *Hormones that diffuse across the plasma membrane and interact with intracellular receptors:* Many lipid-soluble hormones diffuse across the plasma membrane and interact with receptors in the cytosol or the nucleus. The resulting hormone-receptor complexes bind specifically to recognition elements in DNA, thereby affecting the expression of specific target genes. Hormones of this type include the steroids (e.g., estrogen, progesterone, and glucocorticoids), and thyroxine.

A number of processes can disturb the normal activity of the endocrine system, including impaired synthesis or release of hormones, abnormal interactions between hormones and their target tissues, and abnormal responses of target organs. Endocrine diseases can be generally classified as (1) diseases of *underproduction or overproduction* of hormones and their resulting biochemical and clinical consequences and (2) diseases associated with the development of *mass lesions.* Such lesions might be nonfunctional, or they might be associated with overproduction or underproduction of hormones. The study of endocrine diseases requires integration of morphologic findings with biochemical measurements of the levels of hormones, their regulators, and other metabolites.

PITUITARY GLAND

Normal

The pituitary is a small bean-shaped organ that measures about 1 cm in greatest diameter and weighs about 0.5 gm, although it enlarges during pregnancy. Its small size belies its great functional significance. It is located at the base of the brain, where it lies nestled within the confines of the sella turcica in close proximity to the optic chiasm and the cavernous sinuses. The pituitary is attached to the hypothalamus by the pituitary stalk, which passes out of the sella through an opening in the dura mater surrounding the brain. Along with the hypothalamus, the pituitary gland plays a critical role in

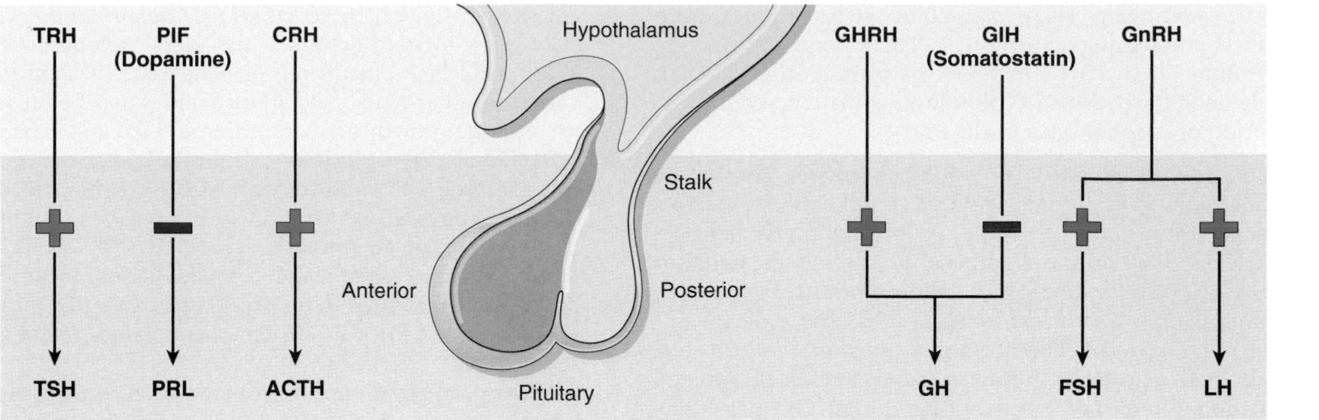

FIGURE 24–1 Hormones released by the anterior pituitary. The adenohypophysis (anterior pituitary) releases five hormones that are in turn under the control of various stimulatory and inhibitory hypothalamic releasing factors. TSH, thyroid-stimulating hormone (thyrotropin); PRL, prolactin; ACTH, adrenocorticotrophic hormone (corticotropin); GH, growth hormone (somatotropin); FSH, follicle-stimulating hormone; LH, luteinizing hormone. The stimulatory releasing factors are TRH (thyrotropin-releasing factor), CRH (corticotropin-releasing factor), GHRH (growth hormone–releasing factor), GnRH (gonadotropin-releasing factor). The inhibitory hypothalamic influences are comprised of PIF (prolactin inhibitory factor or dopamine) and growth hormone inhibitory factor (GIH or somatostatin).

the regulation of most of the other endocrine glands. The pituitary is composed of two morphologically and functionally distinct components: the anterior lobe (adenohypophysis) and the posterior lobe (neurohypophysis).

The *anterior pituitary*, or adenohypophysis, constitutes about 80% of the gland. It is derived embryologically from Rathke pouch, which is an extension of the developing oral cavity. It is eventually cut off from its origins by the growth of the sphenoid bone, which creates a saddle-like depression, the sella turcica. The anterior pituitary has a portal vascular system that is the conduit for the transport of hypothalamic releasing hormones from the hypothalamus to the pituitary. Hypothalamic neurons have terminals in the median eminence where the hormones are released into the portal system, from where they traverse the pituitary stalk and enter the anterior pituitary gland. The production of most pituitary hormones is controlled predominantly by positive-acting releasing factors from the hypothalamus (Fig. 24–1). Prolactin is the major exception, since its primary hypothalamic control is inhibitory, through the action of dopamine, while pituitary growth hormone receives both stimulatory and inhibitory influences via the hypothalamus. In routine histologic sections of the anterior pituitary, a colorful array of cells is present that contain eosinophilic cytoplasm (acidophil), basophilic cytoplasm (basophil), or poorly staining cytoplasm (chromophobe) cells (Fig. 24–2). Specific antibodies against the pituitary hormones identify five cell types:

1. *Somatotrophs*, producing growth hormone (GH): These acidophilic cells constitute half of all the hormone-producing cells in the anterior pituitary.
2. *Lactotrophs* (mammotrophs), producing prolactin: These acidophilic cells secrete prolactin, which is essential for lactation.
3. *Corticotrophs:* These basophilic cells produce adrenocorticotropic hormone (ACTH), pro-opiomelanocortin (POMC), melanocyte-stimulating hormone (MSH), endorphins, and lipotropin.
4. *Thyrotrophs:* These pale basophilic cells produce thyroid-stimulating hormone (TSH).

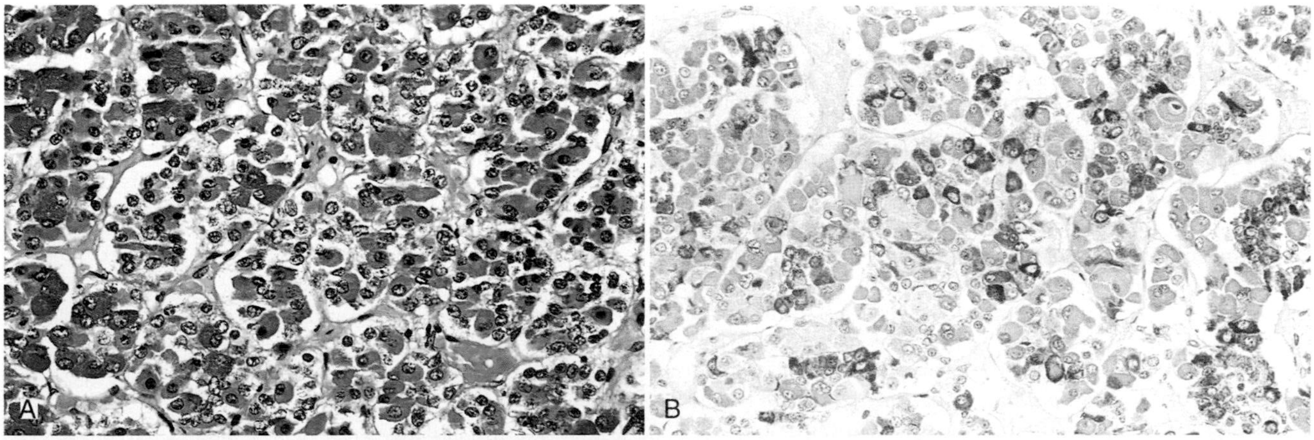

FIGURE 24–2 *A*, Photomicrograph of normal pituitary. The gland is populated by several distinct cell populations containing a variety of stimulating (trophic) hormones. *B*, Each of the hormones has different staining characteristics, resulting in a mixture of cell types in routine histologic preparations. Immunostain for human growth hormone.

5. *Gonadotrophs:* These basophilic cells produce both follicle-stimulating hormone (FSH) and luteinizing hormone (LH). FSH stimulates the formation of graafian follicles in the ovary, and LH induces ovulation and the formation of corpora lutea in the ovary.

The *posterior pituitary*, or neurohypophysis, consists of modified glial cells (termed *pituicytes*) and axonal processes extending from nerve cell bodies in the supraoptic and paraventricular nuclei of the hypothalamus, through the pituitary stalk to the posterior lobe. These neurons produce two peptide hormones, *anti-diuretic hormone* (ADH, also called *vasopressin*) and *oxytocin*. The hormones are stored in axon terminals in the posterior pituitary and are released into the circulation in response to appropriate stimuli. Oxytocin stimulates contraction of the smooth muscle cells in the gravid uterus and cells surrounding the lactiferous ducts of the mammary glands. ADH is a nonapeptide hormone synthesized predominantly in the supraoptic nucleus. In response to a number of different stimuli, including increased plasma osmotic pressure, left atrial distention, exercise, and certain emotional states, ADH is released from the axon terminals in the neurohypophysis into the general circulation. The posterior pituitary is derived embryologically from an outpouching of the floor of the third ventricle, which grows downward alongside the anterior lobe. In contrast to the anterior lobe, the posterior lobe of the pituitary is supplied by an artery and drains into a vein, where its hormones are released directly into the systemic circulation. Thus, the pituitary has a *dual circulation*, composed of arteries and veins and a portal venous system linking the hypothalamus and the anterior lobe.

Pathology

Clinical Manifestations of Pituitary Disease

The manifestations of pituitary disorders are as follows:

- *Hyperpituitarism:* Arising from excess secretion of trophic hormones. The causes of hyperpituitarism include pituitary adenoma, hyperplasia and carcinomas of the anterior pituitary, secretion of hormones by nonpituitary tumors, and certain hypothalamic disorders. The symptoms of hyperpituitarism are discussed in the context of individual tumors below.
- *Hypopituitarism:* Arising from deficiency of trophic hormones. This may be caused by destructive processes, including *ischemic injury, surgery or radiation*, and *inflammatory reactions*. In addition, *nonfunctional pituitary adenomas* may encroach upon and destroy adjacent normal anterior pituitary parenchyma and cause hypopituitarism.
- *Local mass effects:* Among the earliest changes referable to mass effect are *radiographic abnormalities of the sella turcica*, including sellar expansion, bony erosion, and disruption of the diaphragma sella. Because of the close proximity of the optic nerves and chiasm to the sella, expanding pituitary lesions often compress decussating fibers in the optic chiasm. This gives rise to *visual field abnormalities*, classically in the form of defects in the lateral (temporal) visual fields, so-called *bitemporal hemianopsia*. In addition, a variety of other visual field abnormalities may be caused by asymmetric growth of many tumors. Like any expanding intracranial mass, pituitary adenomas can produce signs and symptoms of *elevated intracranial pressure*, including headache, nausea, and vomiting. On occasion, acute hemorrhage into an adenoma is associated with clinical evidence of rapid enlargement of the lesion, a situation appropriately termed *pituitary apoplexy*. Acute pituitary apoplexy is a neurosurgical emergency, since it can cause sudden death (see below).
- Diseases of the posterior pituitary often come to clinical attention because of increased or decreased secretion of one of its products, ADH.

Pituitary Adenomas and Hyperpituitarism

The most common cause of hyperpituitarism is an adenoma arising in the anterior lobe. Other, less common, causes include hyperplasia and carcinomas of the anterior pituitary, secretion of hormones by some extrapituitary tumors, and certain hypothalamic disorders. Pituitary adenomas can be *functional* (i.e., associated with hormone excess and clinical manifestations thereof) or *silent* (i.e., immunohistochemical and/or ultrastructural demonstration of hormone production at the tissue level only, without clinical symptoms of hormone excess). Both functional and silent pituitary adenomas are usually composed of a single cell type and produce a single predominant hormone, although exceptions are known to occur. *Pituitary adenomas are classified on the basis of hormone(s) produced by the neoplastic cells detected by immunohistochemical stains performed on tissue sections* (Table 24–1). Some pituitary adenomas can secrete two hormones (GH and prolactin being the most common combination), and rarely, pituitary adenomas are plurihormonal. Finally, pituitary adenomas may be *hormone-negative*, based on absence of immunohistochemical reactivity and ultra-

TABLE 24–1 Classification of Pituitary Adenomas

Prolactin cell (lactotroph) adenoma
Growth hormone cell (somatotroph) adenoma Densely granulated GH cell adenoma Sparsely granulated GH cell adenoma with fibrous bodies
Thyroid-stimulating hormone cell (thyrotroph) adenomas
ACTH cell (corticotroph) adenomas
Gonadotroph cell adenomas Silent gonadotroph adenomas include most so-called null cell and oncocytic adenomas
Mixed growth hormone-prolactin cell (mammosomatotroph) adenomas
Other plurihormonal adenomas
Hormone-negative adenomas

ACTH, adrenocorticotropic hormone.

structural demonstration of lineage-specific differentiation. Both silent and hormone-negative pituitary adenomas may cause hypopituitarism as they encroach on and destroy adjacent anterior pituitary parenchyma.

Clinically diagnosed pituitary adenomas are responsible for about 10% of intracranial neoplasms; they are discovered incidentally in up to 25% of routine autopsies. In fact, using high-resolution computed tomography or magnetic resonance imaging suggest that approximately 20% of "normal" adult pituitary glands harbor an incidental lesion measuring 3 mm or more in diameter, usually a silent adenoma.[1] Pituitary adenomas are usually found in adults, with a peak incidence from the thirties to the fifties. Most pituitary adenomas occur as isolated lesions. In about 3% of cases, however, adenomas are associated with *multiple endocrine neoplasia (MEN) type 1* (discussed later). Pituitary adenomas are designated, somewhat arbitrarily, *microadenomas* if they are less than 1 cm in diameter and *macroadenomas* if they exceed 1 cm in diameter. Silent and hormone-negative adenomas are likely to come to clinical attention at a later stage than those associated with endocrine abnormalities and are therefore more likely to be macroadenomas.

With recent advances in molecular techniques, substantial insight has been gained into *the genetic abnormalities associated with pituitary adenomas*:[2]

- The great majority of pituitary adenomas are monoclonal in origin, even those that are plurihormonal, suggesting that most arise from a single somatic cell. Some plurihormonal tumors may arise from clonal expansion of primitive stem cells, which then differentiate in several directions simultaneously.
- G-protein mutations are possibly the best-characterized molecular abnormalities in pituitary adenomas. G-proteins are described in Chapter 3; here we will review their function in the context of endocrine neoplasms. G-proteins play a critical role in signal transduction, transmitting signals from *cell-surface receptors* (e.g., GHRH receptor) to *intracellular effectors* (e.g., adenyl cyclase), which then generate *second messengers* (e.g., cyclic AMP, cAMP). These are heterotrimeric proteins, composed of a specific α-subunit that binds guanine nucleotide and interacts with both cell surface receptors and intracellular effectors (Fig. 24–3); the β- and γ-subunits are noncovalently bound to the specific α-subunit. G_s is a stimulatory G-protein that has a pivotal role in signal transduction in several endocrine organs, including the pituitary. The α-subunit of G_s ($G_s\alpha$) is encoded by the *GNAS1* gene, located on chromosome 20q13. In the basal state, G_s exists as an inactive protein, with GDP bound to the guanine nucleotide-binding site of the α-subunit of G_s. On interaction with the ligand-bound cell-surface receptor, GDP dissociates, and GTP binds to $G_s\alpha$, activating the G-protein. The activation of $G_s\alpha$ results in the generation of cAMP, which acts as a potent mitogenic stimulus for a variety of endocrine cell types (such as pituitary somatotrophs and corticotrophs, thyroid follicular cells, parathyroid cells), promoting cellular proliferation and hormone synthesis and secretion. The activation of $G_s\alpha$, and resultant generation of cAMP, are *transient* because of an intrinsic GTPase activity in the α-subunit, which hydrolyzes GTP into GDP. *A mutation in the α-subunit that interferes with its intrinsic GTPase activity will therefore result in constitutive activation of $G_s\alpha$, persistent generation of cAMP, and unchecked cellular proliferation* (Fig. 24–3). Approximately 40% of somatotroph cell adenomas bear *GNAS1* mutations that abrogate the GTPase activity of $G_s\alpha$. The mutant form of *GNAS1* is also known as the *gsp oncogene* because of its effects on tumorigenesis. In addition, *GNAS1* mutations have also been described in a minority of corticotroph adenomas; in contrast, *GNAS1* mutations are absent in thyrotroph, lactotroph, and gonadotroph adenomas, since their respective hypothalamic release hormones do not mediate their action via cAMP-dependent pathways.
- Multiple endocrine neoplasia (MEN) syndrome (discussed in detail below) is a familial disorder associated with tumors and hyperplasias of multiple endocrine organs, including the pituitary. A subtype of MEN syndrome, known as MEN-1, is caused by germ line mutations of the gene *MEN1*, on chromosome 11q13. While *MEN1* mutations are, by definition, present in pituitary adenomas arising in context of the MEN-1 syndrome, they are uncommon in sporadic pituitary adenomas.
- Additional molecular abnormalities present in *aggressive or advanced pituitary adenomas* include activating mutations of the *RAS* oncogene and overexpression of the *c-MYC* oncogene, suggesting that these genetic events are linked to disease progression.[3]

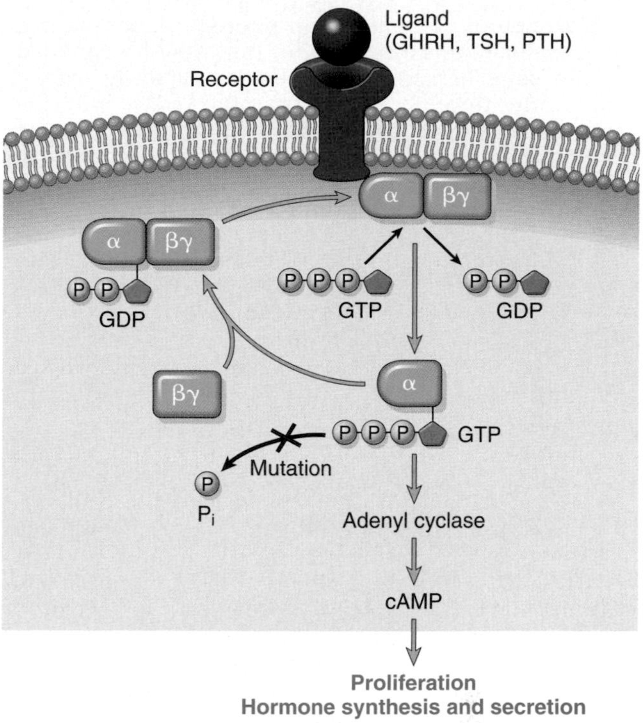

FIGURE 24–3 The mechanism of G-protein mutations in endocrine neoplasia. Mutations in the G-protein–signaling pathway are seen in a variety of endocrine neoplasms, including pituitary, thyroid, and parathyroid adenomas. G-proteins play a critical role in signal transduction, transmitting signals from cell-surface receptors (GHRH, TSH, or PTH receptor) to intracellular effectors (e.g., adenyl cyclase), which then generate second messengers (cAMP).

Morphology. The common pituitary adenoma is a soft, well-circumscribed lesion that may be confined to the sella turcica. Larger lesions typically extend superiorly through the diaphragm sella into the suprasellar region, where they often compress the optic chiasm and adjacent structures, such as some of the cranial nerves (Fig. 24–4). As these adenomas expand, they frequently erode the sella turcica and anterior clinoid processes. They may also extend locally into the cavernous and sphenoid sinuses. In up to 30% of cases, the adenomas are not grossly encapsulated and infiltrate adjacent bone, dura, and (rarely) brain, but they do not demonstrate the ability for distant metastasis. Such lesions are termed **invasive adenomas**. Foci of hemorrhage and necrosis are common in larger adenomas.

Histologically, pituitary adenomas are composed of relatively uniform, polygonal cells arrayed in sheets or cords. Supporting connective tissue, or reticulin, is sparse, accounting for the soft, gelatinous consistency of many of these lesions. The nuclei of the neoplastic cells may be uniform or pleomorphic. Mitotic activity is usually modest. The cytoplasm of the constituent cells may be acidophilic, basophilic, or chromophobic, depending on the type and amount of secretory product within the cells, but it is generally uniform throughout the cytoplasm. **This cellular monomorphism and the absence of a significant reticulin network distinguish pituitary adenomas from non-neoplastic anterior pituitary parenchyma** (Fig. 24–5). The functional status of the adenoma cannot be reliably predicted from its histologic appearance.

Clinical Course. The signs and symptoms of pituitary adenomas include endocrine abnormalities and mass effects. The abnormalities associated with the secretion of excessive quantities of anterior pituitary hormones are mentioned below, when we describe the specific types of pituitary adenoma. Local mass effects may be encountered in any type of pituitary tumor and have been discussed previously under clinical manifestations of pituitary disease. Briefly, these include *radiographic abnormalities of the sella turcica*, *visual field abnormalities*, signs and symptoms of elevated *intracranial pressure*, and occasionally *hypopituitarism*. Acute hemorrhage into an adenoma is sometimes associated with *pituitary apoplexy*, as was noted previously.

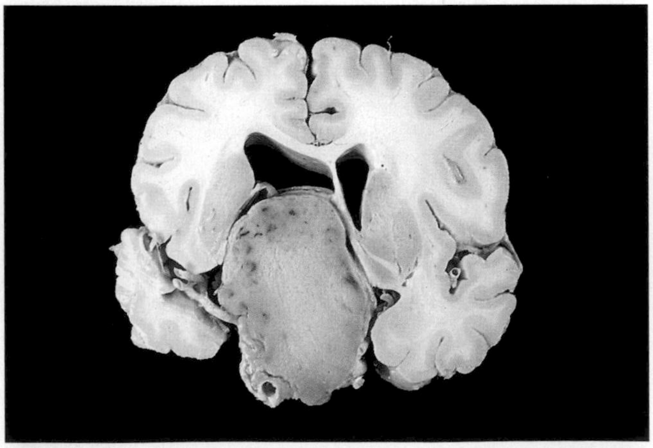

FIGURE 24–4 Pituitary adenoma. This massive, nonfunctional adenoma has grown far beyond the confines of the sella turcica and has distorted the overlying brain. Nonfunctional adenomas tend to be larger at the time of diagnosis than those that secrete a hormone.

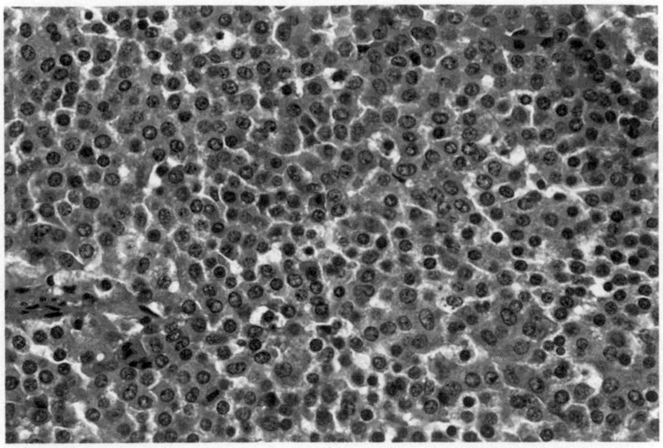

FIGURE 24–5 Pituitary adenoma. The monomorphism of these cells contrasts markedly with the mixture of cells seen in the normal anterior pituitary. Note also the absence of reticulin network.

With this general introduction to pituitary adenomas, we proceed to a discussion of the individual types of tumors.

PROLACTINOMAS

Prolactinomas (lactotroph adenomas) are the most frequent type of hyperfunctioning pituitary adenoma, accounting for about 30% of all clinically recognized pituitary adenomas. These lesions range from small microadenomas to large, expansile tumors associated with substantial mass effect. Microscopically, the overwhelming majority of prolactinomas are composed of weakly acidophilic or chromophobic cells (*sparsely granulated prolactinoma*); rare prolactinomas are strongly acidophilic (*densely granulated prolactinoma*) (Fig. 24–6). Prolactin can be demonstrated within the secretory granules in the cytoplasm of the cells using immunohistochemical approaches. Prolactinomas have a propensity to undergo dystrophic calcification, ranging from isolated psammoma bodies to extensive calcification of virtually the entire tumor mass ("pituitary stone"). Prolactin secretion by functioning adenomas is characterized by its *efficiency*—even microadenomas secrete sufficient prolactin to cause hyperprolactinemia—and by its *proportionality*, in that serum prolactin concentrations tend to correlate with the size of the adenoma.

Increased serum levels of prolactin, or *prolactinemia*, cause amenorrhea, galactorrhea, loss of libido, and infertility. The diagnosis of an adenoma is made more readily in women than in men, especially between the ages of 20 and 40 years, presumably because of the sensitivity of menses to disruption by hyperprolactinemia. This tumor underlies almost a quarter of cases of amenorrhea. In contrast, in men and older women, the hormonal manifestations may be subtle, allowing the tumors to reach considerable size (macroadenomas) before being detected clinically.

Hyperprolactinemia may result from causes other than prolactin-secreting pituitary adenomas. Physiologic hyperprolactinemia occurs in pregnancy; serum prolactin levels

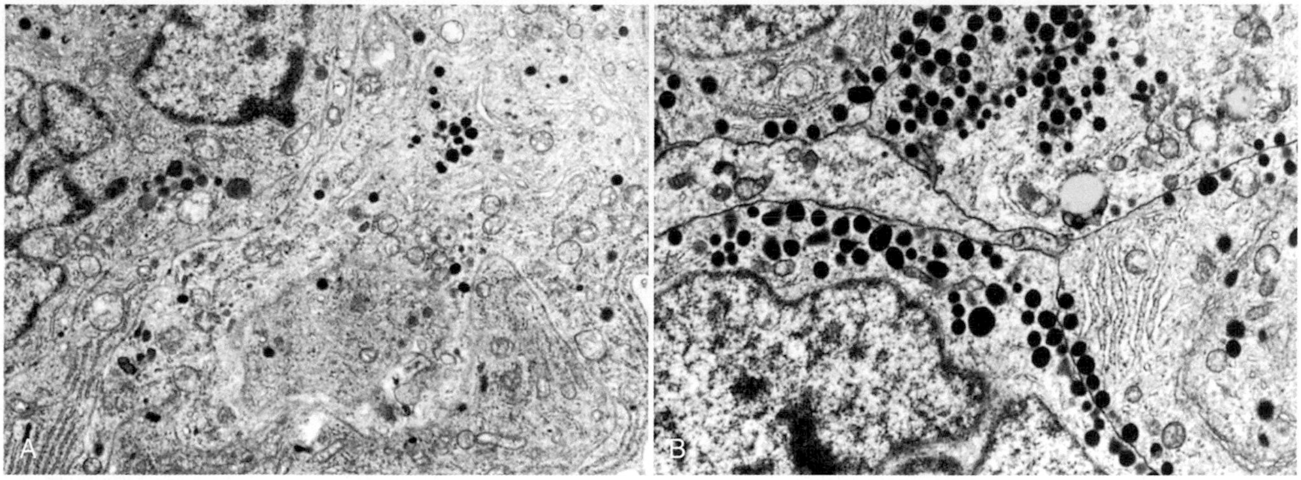

FIGURE 24–6 Ultrastructural features of prolactinomas. *A*, Electron micrograph of a sparsely granulated prolactinoma. The tumor cells contain abundant granular endoplasmic reticulum (indicative of active protein synthesis) and small numbers of secretory granules (6000×). *B*, Electron micrograph of densely granulated growth hormone–secreting adenoma. The tumor cells are filled with large, membrane-bound secretory granules (6000×). (Courtesy of Dr. Eva Horvath, St. Michael's Hospital, Toronto, Ontario, Canada.)

increase throughout pregnancy, reaching a peak at delivery. Prolactin levels are also elevated by nipple stimulation, as occurs during suckling in lactating women, and as a response to many types of stress. Pathologic hyperprolactinemia can also result from *lactotroph hyperplasia*, such as when there is interference with normal dopamine inhibition of prolactin secretion. This may occur as a result of damage to the dopaminergic neurons of the hypothalamus, pituitary stalk section (e.g., owing to head trauma), or drugs that block dopamine receptors on lactotroph cells. Any mass in the suprasellar compartment may disturb the normal inhibitory influence of the hypothalamus on prolactin secretion, resulting in hyperprolactinemia, a phenomenon called the stalk effect. *Therefore, a mild elevation in serum prolactin in a patient with a pituitary adenoma does not necessarily indicate a prolactin-secreting tumor.* Several classes of drugs can cause hyperprolactinemia, including dopamine receptor antagonists such as the neuroleptic drugs (phenothiazines, haloperidol) and older antihypertensive drugs, such as reserpine, which inhibit dopamine storage. Other causes of hyperprolactinemia include estrogens, renal failure, and hypothyroidism. Prolactinomas are treated by surgery or, more commonly, with bromocriptine, a dopamine receptor agonist, which causes the lesions to diminish in size.

GROWTH HORMONE (SOMATOTROPH CELL) ADENOMAS

GH-secreting tumors are the second most common type of functioning pituitary adenoma. As we have mentioned, 40% of somatotroph cell adenomas express a mutant GTPase-deficient α-subunit of the G-protein, G_s. Somatotroph cell adenomas may be quite large by the time they come to clinical attention because the manifestations of excessive GH may be subtle. Histologically, GH-containing adenomas are also classified into two subtypes: *densely granulated* and *sparsely granulated*. The densely granulated adenomas are composed of cells that are monomorphic and acidophilic in routine sections, retain strong cytoplasmic GH reactivity on immunohistochemistry, and demonstrate cytokeratin staining in a perinuclear distribution. In contrast, the sparsely granulated variants are composed of chromophobe cells with considerable nuclear and cytologic pleomorphism, and retain focal and weak GH reactivity.[4] Bihormonal *mammosomatotroph* adenomas that are reactive for both GH and prolactin are being increasingly recognized with the availability of better reagents for immunohistochemical analysis; morphologically, most bihormonal adenomas resemble the densely granulated pure somatotroph adenomas.

Persistent hypersecretion of GH stimulates the hepatic secretion of insulin-like growth factor I (IGF-I or somatomedin C), which causes many of the clinical manifestations. If a somatotrophic adenoma appears in children before the epiphyses have closed, the elevated levels of GH (and IGF-1) result in *gigantism*. This is characterized by a generalized increase in body size with disproportionately long arms and legs. If the increased levels of GH are present after closure of the epiphyses, patients develop *acromegaly*. In this condition, growth is most conspicuous in skin and soft tissues; viscera (thyroid, heart, liver, and adrenals); and bones of the face, hands, and feet. Bone density may be increased (hyperostosis) in both the spine and the hips. Enlargement of the jaw results in protrusion (prognathism) with broadening of the lower face. The hands and feet are enlarged with broad, sausage-like fingers. In most instances, gigantism is also accompanied by evidence of acromegaly. These changes develop for decades before being recognized, hence the opportunity for the adenomas to reach substantial size. GH excess is also correlated with a variety of other disturbances, including gonadal dysfunction, diabetes mellitus, generalized muscle weakness, hypertension, arthritis, congestive heart failure, and an increased risk of gastrointestinal cancers.

The diagnosis of pituitary GH excess relies on documentation of elevated serum GH and IGF-1 levels. *In addition, failure to suppress GH production in response to an oral load of glucose is one of the most sensitive tests for acromegaly.* The goals of treatment are to restore GH levels to normal and to decrease symptoms referable to a pituitary mass lesion while not causing hypopituitarism. To achieve these goals, the tumor can be removed surgically or destroyed by radiation therapy, or GH secretion can be reduced by drug therapy. When effective control of GH hypersecretion is achieved, the characteristic tissue overgrowth and related symptoms gradually recede, and the metabolic abnormalities improve.

CORTICOTROPH CELL ADENOMAS

Corticotroph adenomas are usually small microadenomas at the time of diagnosis. These tumors are most often basophilic (*densely granulated*) and occasionally chromophobic (*sparsely granulated*). Both variants stain positively with periodic acid–Schiff (PAS) because of the presence of carbohydrate in pre-opiomelanocorticotropin (POMC), the ACTH precursor molecule; in addition, they demonstrate variable immunoreactivity for POMC and its derivatives, including ACTH and β-endorphin.

Excess production of ACTH by the corticotroph adenoma leads to adrenal hypersecretion of cortisol and the development of *hypercortisolism* (also known as *Cushing syndrome*). This syndrome is discussed in more detail later with the diseases of the adrenal gland. It can be caused by a wide variety of conditions in addition to ACTH-producing pituitary tumors. When the hypercortisolism is due to excessive production of ACTH by the pituitary, the process is designated *Cushing disease*. Large destructive adenomas can develop in patients after surgical removal of the adrenal glands for treatment of Cushing syndrome. This condition, known as *Nelson syndrome*, occurs most often because of a loss of the inhibitory effect of adrenal corticosteroids on a pre-existing corticotroph microadenoma. Because the adrenals are absent in patients with this disorder, hypercortisolism does not develop. In contrast, patients present with mass effects of the pituitary tumor. In addition, there can be hyperpigmentation because of the stimulatory effect of other products of the ACTH precursor molecule on melanocytes.

OTHER ANTERIOR PITUITARY ADENOMAS

Pituitary adenomas may elaborate more than one hormone. For example, prolactin may be demonstrable by immunolabeling of somatotroph adenomas. In other cases, unusual plurihormonal adenomas are capable of secreting multiple hormones; these tumors are usually aggressive. A few comments are made about several of the less frequent functioning tumors.

Gonadotroph (LH-producing and FSH-producing) adenomas can be difficult to recognize because they secrete hormones inefficiently and variably, and the secretory products usually do not cause a recognizable clinical syndrome. Gonadotroph adenomas are most frequently found in middle-aged men and women when they become large enough to cause neurologic symptoms, such as impaired vision, headaches, diplopia, or pituitary apoplexy. Pituitary hormone deficiencies can also be found, most commonly impaired secretion of LH. This causes decreased energy and libido in men (due to reduced testosterone) and amenorrhea in premenopausal women. Thus, gonadotroph adenomas are paradoxically associated with secondary gonadal hypofunction. Most gonadotroph adenomas are large and composed of chromophobic cells. The neoplastic cells usually demonstrate immunoreactivity for the common gonadotropin α-subunit and the specific β-FSH and β-LH subunits; FSH is usually the predominant secreted hormone. The availability of reliable immunoassays for the gonadotropin β-subunit and the recognition of gonadotroph-specific transcription factors has led to the reclassification of many previously hormone-negative adenomas ("*null cell adenomas*") as silent gonadotroph adenomas[5] (see below).

Thyrotroph (TSH-producing) adenomas are rare, accounting for approximately 1% of all pituitary adenomas. Thyrotroph adenomas are chromophobic or basophilic and are a rare cause of hyperthyroidism.

Nonfunctioning pituitary adenomas comprise both clinically silent counterparts of the functioning adenomas described above (for example, a *silent somatotroph adenoma*) and true *hormone-negative adenomas*. Nonfunctioning adenomas constitute approximately 25% of all pituitary tumors. In the past, the majority of nonfunctioning adenomas were classified as "null cell adenomas" because of the inability to demonstrate markers of differentiation. *It is now known that most null cell adenomas have biochemical and ultrastructural features that allow their characterization as silent tumors of gonadotrophic lineage.*[5] *True hormone-negative adenomas are therefore unusual.* Not surprisingly, the typical presentation of nonfunctioning adenomas is mass effects. These lesions may also compromise the residual anterior pituitary sufficiently to cause hypopituitarism. This may occur as a result of gradual enlargement of the adenoma or after abrupt enlargement of the tumor because of acute hemorrhage (pituitary apoplexy).

Pituitary carcinomas are quite rare, and most are not functional. These malignant tumors range from well differentiated, resembling somewhat atypical adenomas, to poorly differentiated, with variable degrees of pleomorphism and the features that are characteristic of carcinomas in other locations. The diagnosis of carcinoma requires the demonstration of metastases, usually to lymph nodes, bone, liver, and sometimes elsewhere.

Hypopituitarism

Hypopituitarism refers to decreased secretion of pituitary hormones, which can result from diseases of the hypothalamus or of the pituitary. Hypofunction of the anterior pituitary occurs when approximately 75% of the parenchyma is lost or absent. This may be congenital or the result of a variety of acquired abnormalities that are intrinsic to the pituitary. *Hypopituitarism accompanied by evidence of posterior pituitary dysfunction in the form of diabetes insipidus (see below) is almost always of hypothalamic origin.* Most cases of hypofunction arise from destructive processes directly involving the anterior pituitary, although other mechanisms have been identified:

- *Tumors and other mass lesions:* Pituitary adenomas, other benign tumors arising within the sella, primary and metastatic malignancies, and cysts can cause hypopituitarism. Any mass lesion in the sella can cause damage by exerting pressure on adjacent pituitary cells.
- *Pituitary surgery or radiation:* Surgical excision of a pituitary adenoma may inadvertently extend to the nonadenomatous pituitary. Radiation of the pituitary, used to prevent

regrowth of residual tumor after surgery, can damage the nonadenomatous pituitary.

- *Pituitary apoplexy:* As has been mentioned, this is a sudden hemorrhage into the pituitary gland, often occurring into a pituitary adenoma. In its most dramatic presentation, apoplexy causes the sudden onset of excruciating headache, diplopia owing to pressure on the oculomotor nerves, and hypopituitarism. In severe cases, it can cause cardiovascular collapse, loss of consciousness, and even sudden death. Thus, pituitary apoplexy is a true neurosurgical emergency.
- *Ischemic necrosis of the pituitary and Sheehan syndrome:* Ischemic necrosis of the anterior pituitary is an important cause of pituitary insufficiency. *Sheehan syndrome*, or postpartum necrosis of the anterior pituitary, is the most common form of clinically significant ischemic necrosis of the anterior pituitary.[6] During pregnancy, the anterior pituitary enlarges to almost twice its normal size. This physiologic expansion of the gland is not accompanied by an increase in blood supply from the low-pressure venous system; hence, there is relative anoxia of the pituitary. Further reduction in blood supply caused by obstetric hemorrhage or shock may precipitate infarction of the anterior lobe. The posterior pituitary, because it receives its blood directly from arterial branches, is much less susceptible to ischemic injury in this setting and is therefore usually not affected. Pituitary necrosis may also be encountered in other conditions, such as disseminated intravascular coagulation and (more rarely) sickle cell anemia, elevated intracranial pressure, traumatic injury, and shock of any origin. Whatever the pathogenesis, the ischemic area is resorbed and replaced by a nubbin of fibrous tissue attached to the wall of an empty sella.
- *Rathke cleft cyst:* These cysts, lined by ciliated cuboidal epithelium with occasional goblet cells and anterior pituitary cells, can accumulate proteinaceous fluid and expand, compromising the normal gland.
- *Empty sella syndrome:* Any condition that destroys part or all of the pituitary gland, such as ablation of the pituitary by surgery or radiation, can result in an *empty sella*. The *empty sella syndrome* refers to the presence of an enlarged, empty sella turcica that is not filled with pituitary tissue. There are two types: (1) In a *primary* empty sella, there is a defect in the diaphragma sella that allows the arachnoid mater and cerebrospinal fluid to herniate into the sella, resulting in expansion of the sella and compression of the pituitary. Classically, affected patients are obese women with a history of multiple pregnancies. The empty sella syndrome may be associated with visual field defects and occasionally with endocrine anomalies, such as *hyperprolactinemia*, owing to interruption of inhibitory hypothalamic effects. Loss of functioning parenchyma can be severe enough to result in hypopituitarism. (2) In a *secondary* empty sella, a mass, such as a pituitary adenoma, enlarges the sella, but then it is either surgically removed or undergoes spontaneous necrosis, leading to loss of pituitary function. Hypopituitarism can result from the treatment or spontaneous infarction.
- *Genetic defects:* Rare congenital deficiencies of one or more pituitary hormones have been recognized in children. For example, mutations in *pit-1*, a pituitary transcription factor, result in combined deficiency of GH, prolactin, and TSH.[7]

Less frequently, disorders that interfere with the delivery of pituitary hormone–releasing factors from the *hypothalamus*, such as hypothalamic tumors, may also cause hypofunction of the anterior pituitary. Any disease involving the hypothalamus can alter secretion of one or more of the hypothalamic hormones that influence secretion of the corresponding pituitary hormones. In contrast to diseases that involve the pituitary directly, any of these conditions can also diminish the secretion of ADH, resulting in diabetes insipidus (discussed later). Hypothalamic lesions that cause hypopituitarism include:

- *Tumors*, including benign lesions that arise in the hypothalamus, such as craniopharyngiomas, and malignant tumors that metastasize to that site, such as breast and lung carcinomas. Hypothalamic hormone deficiency can ensue when brain or nasopharyngeal tumors are treated with radiation.
- *Inflammatory disorders and infections*, such as sarcoidosis or tuberculous meningitis, can cause deficiencies of anterior pituitary hormones and diabetes insipidus.

The clinical manifestations of anterior pituitary hypofunction depend on the specific hormone(s) that are lacking. Children can develop growth failure (*pituitary dwarfism*) due to growth hormone deficiency. Gonadotropin (GnRH) deficiency leads to amenorrhea and infertility in women and decreased libido, impotence, and loss of pubic and axillary hair in men. TSH and ACTH deficiencies result in symptoms of hypothyroidism and hypoadrenalism, respectively, and are discussed later in the chapter. Prolactin deficiency results in failure of postpartum lactation. The anterior pituitary is also a rich source of melanocyte-stimulating hormone (MSH), synthesized from the same precursor molecule that produces ACTH; therefore, one of the manifestations of hypopituitarism includes pallor due to a loss of stimulatory effects of MSH on melanocytes.

Posterior Pituitary Syndromes

The clinically relevant posterior pituitary syndromes involve ADH and include *diabetes insipidus and secretion of inappropriately high levels of ADH*.

- **Diabetes insipidus.** ADH deficiency causes diabetes insipidus, a condition characterized by excessive urination (polyuria) owing to an inability of the kidney to resorb water properly from the urine. It can result from a variety of processes, including head trauma, tumors, and inflammatory disorders of the hypothalamus and pituitary as well as surgical procedures involving these organs. The condition can also arise spontaneously, in the absence of an underlying disorder. Diabetes insipidus from ADH deficiency is designated as *central* to differentiate it from *nephrogenic* diabetes insipidus, which is a result of renal tubular unresponsiveness to circulating ADH. The clinical manifestations of the two diseases are similar and include the excretion of large volumes of dilute urine with an inappropriately low specific gravity. Serum sodium and osmolality are increased owing to excessive renal loss of free water, resulting in thirst and polydipsia. Patients who can drink water can generally compensate for urinary losses; patients who are obtunded, bedridden, or otherwise limited in their ability to obtain water may develop life-threatening dehydration.

- **Syndrome of inappropriate ADH (SIADH) secretion.** ADH excess causes resorption of excessive amounts of free water, resulting in *hyponatremia*. The most frequent causes of SIADH include the secretion of ectopic ADH by malignant neoplasms (particularly small cell carcinomas of the lung), non-neoplastic diseases of the lung, and local injury to the hypothalamus or posterior pituitary (or both). The clinical manifestations of SIADH are dominated by hyponatremia, cerebral edema, and resultant neurologic dysfunction. Although total body water is increased, blood volume remains normal, and peripheral edema does not develop.

Hypothalamic Suprasellar Tumors

Neoplasms in this location may induce hypofunction or hyperfunction of the anterior pituitary, diabetes insipidus, or combinations of these manifestations. The most commonly implicated lesions are *gliomas* (sometimes arising in the chiasm; see Chapter 28) and *craniopharyngiomas*. The craniopharyngioma is thought to be derived from vestigial remnants of Rathke pouch. These slow-growing tumors account for 1% to 5% of intracranial tumors; a small minority of these lesions arise within the sella, but most are suprasellar, with or without an intrasellar extension. A bimodal age distribution is observed, with one peak in childhood (5 to 15 years) and a second peak in adults in the sixth decade or older. Children usually come to clinical attention because of endocrine deficiencies such as growth retardation, whereas adults usually present with visual disturbances. Pituitary hormonal deficiencies, including diabetes insipidus, are common.

Morphology. Craniopharyngiomas average 3 to 4 cm in diameter; they may be encapsulated and solid, but more commonly, they are cystic and sometimes multiloculated. In their strategic location, they often encroach on the optic chiasm or cranial nerves, and not infrequently, they bulge into the floor of the third ventricle and base of the brain. Two distinct pathologic variants are recognized: **adamantinomatous craniopharyngioma** and **papillary craniopharyngioma**. The adamantinomatous type frequently contains radiologically demonstrable calcifications; the papillary variant is calcified only rarely.

Adamantinomatous craniopharyngioma consists of nests or cords of stratified squamous epithelium embedded in a spongy "reticulum" that becomes more prominent in the internal layers. Peripherally, the nests of squamous cells gradually merge into a layer of columnar cells, forming a palisade resting on a basement membrane. Compact, lamellar keratin formation ("wet keratin") is a diagnostic feature of this tumor. As was previously mentioned, dystrophic calcification is a frequent finding. Additional features include cyst formation, fibrosis, and chronic inflammatory reaction. The cysts of adamantinomatous craniopharyngiomas often contain a cholesterol-rich, thick brownish yellow fluid that has been compared to "machinery oil." These tumors extend fingerlets of epithelium into adjacent brain, where they elicit a brisk glial reaction.

Papillary craniopahryngiomas contain both solid sheets and papillae lined by well-differentiated squamous epithelium. These tumors usually lack keratin, calcification, and cysts. The squamous cells of the solid sections of the tumor do not have the peripheral palisading and do not typically generate a spongy reticulum in the internal layers.

Patients with craniopharyngiomas have an excellent recurrence-free and overall survival. Tumors greater than 5 cm in diameter are associated with a significantly higher recurrence rate. Adamantinomatous tumors are associated with a higher frequency of brain invasion, but this does not necessarily correlate with an adverse prognosis. Malignant transformation of craniopharyngiomas into squamous carcinomas is exceptionally rare and usually occurs postradiation.

THYROID GLAND

Normal

The thyroid gland consists of two bulky lateral lobes connected by a relatively thin isthmus, usually located below and anterior to the larynx. Normal variations in the structure of the thyroid gland include the presence of a pyramidal lobe, a remnant of the thyroglossal duct above the isthmus.

The thyroid gland develops from an evagination of the developing pharyngeal epithelium that descends as part of the thyroglossal duct from the foramen cecum at the base of the tongue to its normal position in the anterior neck. This pattern of descent explains the occasional presence of *ectopic thyroid tissue*, most commonly located at the base of the tongue (*lingual thyroid*) or at other sites abnormally high in the neck. Excessive descent leads to substernal thyroid glands. The clinical significance of these lesions lies in distinguishing them from metastatic thyroid carcinomas and the extremely rare occasions on which these ectopic sites can develop a primary thyroid malignancy.[8] Patients with lingual thyroids present an additional problem in that the ectopic thyroid tissue is sometimes the *only* thyroid tissue (total migration failure), and removal of the lingual thyroid results in symptomatic hypothyroidism. Malformations of branchial pouch differentiation may result in intrathyroidal sites of the thymus or parathyroid glands. The implication of these deviations becomes evident in the patient who has a total thyroidectomy and subsequently develops hypoparathyroidism.

The weight of the normal adult thyroid is approximately 15 to 25 gm. The thyroid has a rich intraglandular capillary network that is supplied by the superior and inferior thyroidal arteries. Nerve fibers from the cervical sympathetic ganglia indirectly influence thyroid secretion by acting on the blood vessels. The thyroid is divided by thin fibrous septae into lobules composed of about 20 to 40 evenly dispersed follicles. Normal follicles range from 50 to 500 μm in size, are lined by cuboidal to low columnar epithelium, and are filled with periodic acid Schiff (PAS)-positive thyroglobulin.

In response to trophic factors from the hypothalamus, TSH (*thyrotropin*) is released by thyrotrophs in the anterior pituitary into the circulation. The binding of TSH to its receptor on the thyroid follicular epithelium results in activation and conformational change in the receptor, allowing it to associate with a stimulatory G-protein (Fig. 24–7). Activation of the G-protein eventually results in an increase in intracellular cAMP levels, which stimulates thyroid growth, and hormone synthesis and release via cAMP-dependent protein kinases. The dissociation of thyroid hormone synthesis and release from the controlled influence of TSH-signaling pathways results in so-called *thyroid autonomy* and hyperfunction (see below).

Thyroid follicular epithelial cells convert thyroglobulin into *thyroxine* (T_4) and lesser amounts of *triiodothyronine* (T_3). T_4 and T_3 are released into the systemic circulation, where most of these peptides are reversibly bound to circulating plasma proteins, such as thyroxine-binding globulin (TBG) and transthyretin, for transport to peripheral tissues. The binding proteins serve to maintain the serum unbound ("free") T_3 and T_4 concentrations within narrow limits yet ensure that the hormones are readily available to the tissues. In the periphery, the majority of free T_4 is deiodinated to T_3; the latter binds to thyroid hormone nuclear receptors in target cells with tenfold greater affinity than does T_4 and has proportionately greater activity. *The interaction of thyroid hormone with its nuclear thyroid hormone receptor (TR) results in the formation of a multi-protein hormone-receptor complex that binds to thyroid hormone response elements (TREs) in target genes, regulating their transcription* (see Fig. 24–7).[9] Thyroid hormone has diverse cellular effects, including up-regulation of carbohydrate and lipid catabolism and stimulation of protein synthesis in a wide range of cells. The net result of these processes is an increase in the basal metabolic rate. One of the most important functions of thyroid hormone is its critical role in brain development, since absence of thyroid hormone during the fetal and neonatal periods may profoundly interfere with intellectual growth (see below).

The thyroid gland is one of the most responsive organs in the body and contains the largest store of hormones of any endocrine gland. The gland responds to many stimuli and is in a constant state of adaptation. During puberty, pregnancy, and physiologic stress from any source, the gland increases in size and becomes more active. This functional lability is reflected in transient hyperplasia of the thyroidal epithelium. At this time, thyroglobulin is resorbed, and the follicular cells become tall and more columnar, sometimes forming small, infolded buds or papillae. When the stress abates, involution occurs; that is, the height of the epithelium falls, colloid accumulates, and the follicular cells resume their normal size and architecture. Failure of this normal balance between hyperplasia and involution can produce major or minor deviations from the usual histologic pattern.

The function of the thyroid gland can be inhibited by a variety of chemical agents, collectively referred to as *goitrogens*. Because they suppress T_3 and T_4 synthesis, the level of TSH increases, and subsequent hyperplastic enlargement of the gland (goiter) follows. The antithyroid agent *propylthiouracil* inhibits the oxidation of iodide and blocks production

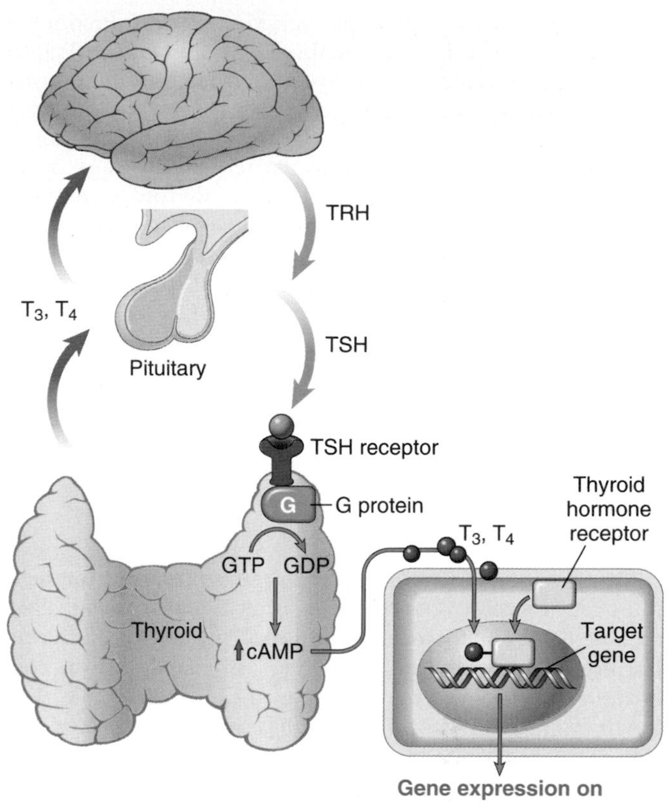

FIGURE 24–7 Homeostasis in the hypothalamus-pituitary-thyroid axis and mechanism of action of thyroid hormones. Secretion of thyroid hormones (T_3 and T_4) is controlled by trophic factors secreted by both the hypothalamus and the anterior pituitary. Decreased levels of T_3 and T_4 stimulate the release of thyrotropin-releasing hormone (TRH) from the hypothalamus and thyroid-stimulating hormone (TSH) from the anterior pituitary, causing T_3 and T_4 levels to rise. Elevated T_3 and T_4 levels, in turn, suppress the secretion of both TRH and TSH. This relationship is termed a negative-feedback loop. TSH binds to the TSH receptor on the thyroid follicular epithelium, which causes activation of G proteins, and cyclic AMP (cAMP)-mediated synthesis and release of thyroid hormones (T3 and T4). In the periphery, T_3 and T_4 interact with the thyroid hormone receptor (TR) to form a hormone-receptor complex that translocates to the nucleus and binds to so-called thyroid response elements (TREs) on target genes initiating transcription.

of the thyroid hormones; parenthetically, propylthiouracil also inhibits the peripheral deiodination of circulating T_4 into T_3, thus ameliorating symptoms of thyroid hormone excess (see below). Iodide, when given to patients with thyroid hyperfunction, also blocks the release of thyroid hormones but through different mechanisms. Iodides in large doses inhibit proteolysis of thyroglobulin. Thus, thyroid hormone is synthesized and incorporated within increasing amounts of colloid, but it is not released into the blood.

The thyroid gland follicles also contain a population of *parafollicular cells*, or C cells, which synthesize and secrete the hormone *calcitonin*. This hormone promotes the absorption of calcium by the skeletal system and inhibits the resorption of bone by osteoclasts.

Pathology

Diseases of the thyroid are of great importance because most are amenable to medical or surgical management. They include conditions associated with excessive release of thyroid hormones (hyperthyroidism), those associated with thyroid hormone deficiency (hypothyroidism), and mass lesions of the thyroid. We first consider the clinical consequences of disturbed thyroid function, then focus on the disorders that generate these problems.

Hyperthyroidism

Thyrotoxicosis is a hypermetabolic state caused by elevated circulating levels of free T_3 and T_4. Because it is caused most commonly by hyperfunction of the thyroid gland, it is often referred to as *hyperthyroidism*. However, in certain conditions the oversupply is related to either excessive release of preformed thyroid hormone (e.g., in thyroiditis) or to an extrathyroidal source, rather than hyperfunction of the gland (Table 24–2). *Thus, strictly speaking, hyperthyroidism is only one (albeit the most common) cause of thyrotoxicosis.* The terms *primary* and *secondary hyperthyroidism* are sometimes used to designate hyperthyroidism arising from an intrinsic thyroid abnormality and that arising from processes outside of the thyroid, such as a TSH-secreting pituitary tumor. With this disclaimer, we will follow the common practice of using the terms *thyrotoxicosis* and *hyperthyroidism* interchangeably. The three most common causes of thyrotoxicosis are also associated with hyperfunction of the gland and include the following:

- *Diffuse hyperplasia* of the thyroid associated with Graves disease (accounts for 85% of cases)
- Hyperfunctional *multinodular goiter*
- Hyperfunctional *adenoma* of the thyroid

TABLE 24–2 Disorders Associated with Thyrotoxicosis

Associated with Hyperthyroidism
Primary
Diffuse toxic hyperplasia (Graves disease)
Hyperfunctioning ("toxic") multinodular goiter
Hyperfunctioning ("toxic") adenoma
Hyperfunctioning thyroid carcinoma
Iodine-induced hyperthyroidism
Neonatal thyrotoxicosis associated with maternal Graves disease
Secondary
TSH-secreting pituitary adenoma (rare)*
Not Associated with Hyperthyroidism
Subacute granulomatous thyroiditis (*painful*)
Subacute lymphocytic thyroiditis (*painless*)
Struma ovarii (ovarian teratoma with ectopic thyroid)
Factitious thyrotoxicosis (exogenous thyroxine intake)

*Associated with increased TSH; all other causes of thyrotoxicosis associated with decreased TSH.

Clinical Course. The clinical manifestations of hyperthyroidism are protean and include changes referable to the *hypermetabolic state* induced by excess thyroid hormone as well as those related to overactivity of the *sympathetic nervous system* (i.e., an increase in the β-adrenergic "tone").

Excessive levels of thyroid hormone result in *an increase in the basal metabolic rate.* The *skin* of thyrotoxic patients tends to be soft, warm, and flushed because of increased blood flow and peripheral vasodilation to increase heat loss. *Heat intolerance* is common. Sweating is increased because of higher levels of calorigenesis. Increased basal metabolic rate also results in characteristic *weight loss despite increased appetite.*

Cardiac manifestations are among the earliest and most consistent features of hyperthyroidism. Patients with hyperthyroidism can have an increase in cardiac output, owing to both increased cardiac contractility and increased peripheral oxygen requirements. Tachycardia, palpitations, and cardiomegaly are common. Arrhythmias, particularly atrial fibrillation, occur frequently and are more common in older patients. Congestive heart failure may develop, particularly in elderly patients with pre-existing cardiac disease. Myocardial changes, such as foci of lymphocytic and eosinophilic infiltration, mild fibrosis in the interstitium, fatty changes in myofibers, and an increase in size and number of mitochondria, have been described. Some patients with thyrotoxicosis develop a reversible *diastolic dysfunction* and a "low-output" failure, so-called *thyrotoxic dilated cardiomyopathy.*

In the *neuromuscular system*, overactivity of the sympathetic nervous system produces tremor, hyperactivity, emotional lability, anxiety, inability to concentrate, and insomnia. Proximal muscle weakness is common with decreased muscle mass (*thyroid myopathy*).

Ocular changes often call attention to hyperthyroidism. A wide, staring gaze and lid lag are present because of sympathetic overstimulation of the levator palpebrae superioris (Fig. 24–8). However, true *thyroid ophthalmopathy* associated with proptosis is a feature seen only in Graves disease (see below).

In the *gastrointestinal system*, sympathetic hyperstimulation of the gut results in hypermotility, malabsorption, and diarrhea.

The *skeletal system* is also affected in hyperthyroidism. Thyroid hormone stimulates bone resorption, resulting in increased porosity of cortical bone and reduced volume of trabecular bone. The net effect is osteoporosis and an increased risk of fractures in patients with chronic hyperthyroidism.

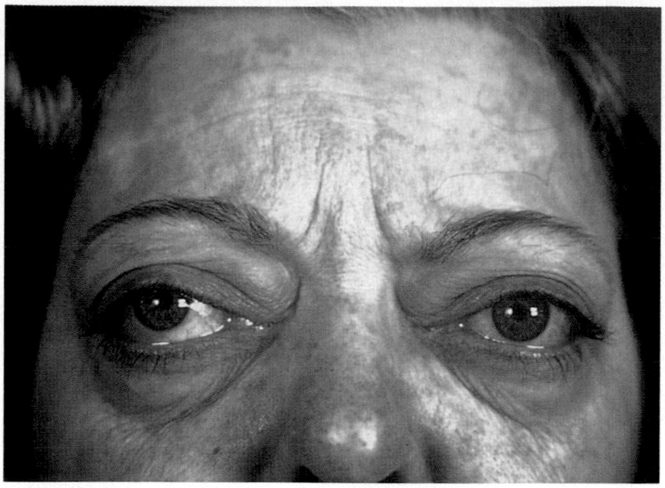

FIGURE 24–8 A patient with hyperthyroidism. A wide-eyed, staring gaze, caused by overactivity of the sympathetic nervous system, is one of the features of this disorder. In Graves disease, one of the most important causes of hyperthyroidism, accumulation of loose connective tissue behind the eyeballs also adds to the protuberant appearance of the eyes.

Other findings throughout the body include atrophy of skeletal muscle, with fatty infiltration and focal interstitial lymphocytic infiltrates; minimal liver enlargement due to fatty changes in the hepatocytes; and generalized lymphoid hyperplasia with lymphadenopathy in patients with Graves disease.

Thyroid storm is used to designate the abrupt onset of severe hyperthyroidism. This condition occurs most commonly in patients with underlying Graves disease and probably results from an acute elevation in catecholamine levels, as might be encountered during infection, surgery, cessation of antithyroid medication, or any form of stress. Patients are often febrile and present with tachycardia out of proportion to the fever. Thyroid storm is a medical emergency: A significant number of untreated patients die of cardiac arrhythmias.

Apathetic hyperthyroidism refers to thyrotoxicosis occurring in the elderly, in whom old age and various comorbidities may blunt the typical features of thyroid hormone excess seen in younger patients. The diagnosis of thyrotoxicosis in these patients is often made during laboratory work-up for unexplained weight loss or worsening cardiovascular disease.

A diagnosis of hyperthyroidism is made using both clinical and laboratory findings. *The measurement of serum TSH concentration using sensitive TSH (sTSH) assays provides the most useful single screening test for hyperthyroidism*, as its levels are decreased even at the earliest stages, when the disease may still be subclinical.[10] A low TSH value is usually confirmed with measurement of free T_4, which is expectedly increased. In an occasional patient, hyperthyroidism results predominantly from increased circulating levels of T_3 ("T_3 toxicosis"). In these cases, free T_4 levels may be decreased, and direct measurement of serum T_3 may be useful. In rare cases of pituitary-associated (secondary) hyperthyroidism, TSH levels are either normal or raised. Determining TSH levels after the injection of TRH (*TRH stimulation test*) is used in the evaluation of cases of suspected hyperthyroidism with equivocal changes in the baseline serum TSH level. A normal rise in TSH after administration of TRH excludes secondary hyperthyroidism. Once the diagnosis of thyrotoxicosis has been confirmed by a combination of sTSH assays and free thyroid hormone levels, measurement of radioactive iodine uptake by the thyroid gland may be valuable in determining the etiology. For example, there may be diffusely increased uptake in the whole gland (Graves disease), increased uptake in a solitary nodule (toxic adenoma), or decreased uptake (thyroiditis). The therapeutic options for hyperthyroidism include multiple medications, each of which has a different mechanism of action. Typically, these include a β-blocker to control symptoms induced by increased adrenergic tone, a thionamide to block new hormone synthesis, an iodine solution to block the release of thyroid hormone, and agents that inhibit peripheral conversion of T_4 to T_3. Radioiodine, which is incorporated into thyroid tissues, resulting in ablation of thyroid function over a period of 6 to 18 weeks, may also be used.

Hypothyroidism

Hypothyroidism is caused by any structural or functional derangement that interferes with the production of adequate levels of thyroid hormone. It can result from a defect anywhere in the hypothalamic-pituitary-thyroid axis. As in the case of hyperthyroidism, this disorder is divided into *primary* and *secondary* categories, depending on whether the hypothyroidism arises from an intrinsic abnormality in the thyroid or occurs as a result of pituitary disease; rarely, hypothalamic failure is a cause of *tertiary* hypothyroidism (Table 24–3). Primary hypothyroidism accounts for the vast majority of cases of hypothyroidism. Primary hypothyroidism can be *thyroprivic* (due to absence or loss of thyroid parenchyma) or *goitrous* (due to enlargement of the thyroid gland under the influence of TSH). The causes of primary hypothyroidism include the following.

Surgical or radiation-induced ablation of thyroid parenchyma can cause hypothyroidism. A large resection of the gland (total thyroidectomy) for the treatment of hyperthyroidism of a primary neoplasm can lead to hypothyroidism. The gland may also be ablated by radiation, whether in the form of radioiodine administered for the treatment of hyperthyroidism, or

TABLE 24–3 Causes of Hypothyroidism

Primary
Developmental (thyroid dysgenesis: *PAX-8, TTF-2, TSH-receptor* mutations)
Thyroid hormone resistance syndrome (TRβ mutations)
Postablative
Surgery, radioiodine therapy, or external radiation
Autoimmune hypothyroidism
Hashimoto thyroiditis*
Iodine deficiency*
Drugs (lithium, iodides, *p*-aminosalicylic acid)*
Congenital biosynthetic defect (dyshormonogenetic goiter)*
Secondary
Pituitary failure
Tertiary
Hypothalamic failure (rare)

*Associated with enlargement of thyroid ("goitrous hypothyroidism"). Hashimoto thyroiditis and postablative hypothroidism account for the majority of cases.

exogenous irradiation, such as external radiation therapy to the neck.

Autoimmune hypothyroidism is the most common cause of goitrous hypothyroidism in iodine-sufficient areas of the world. The vast majority of cases of autoimmune hypothyroidism are due to Hashimoto thyroiditis. Circulating autoantibodies, including *anti–TSH receptor autoantibodies*, are commonly found in Hashimoto thyroiditis. Some patients with hypothyroidism have circulating anti-TSH antibodies, but they usually do not have the goitrous enlargement or lymphocytic infiltrate characteristic of Hashimoto thyroiditis. In the past, many of these patients were classified as having primary "idiopathic" hypothyroidism, but the disease is now recognized as a type of autoimmune disorder of the thyroid, occurring either in isolation or in conjunction with other autoimmune endocrine manifestations.

Drugs given intentionally to decrease thyroid secretion (e.g., methimazole and propylthiouracil) can cause hypothyroidism, as can agents used to treat nonthyroid conditions (e.g., lithium, *p*-aminosalicylic acid).

Inborn errors of thyroid metabolism are an uncommon cause of goitrous hypothyroidism (*dyshormonogenetic goiter*). Any one of the multiple steps leading to thyroid hormone synthesis may be deficient: (1) iodide transport defect, (2) organification defect, (3) dehalogenase defect, and (4) iodotyrosine coupling defect. Organification of iodine involves binding of oxidized iodide with tyrosyl residues in thyroglobulin, and this process is deficient in patients with *Pendred syndrome*, wherein goitrous hypothyroidism is accompanied by sensorineural deafness.

Thyroid hormone resistance syndrome is a rare autosomal-dominant disorder caused by inherited mutations in the thyroid hormone receptor (TR), which abolish the ability of the receptor to bind thyroid hormones.[11] Patients demonstrate a generalized resistance to thyroid hormone, despite high circulating levels of T_3 and T_4. Since the pituitary is also resistant to feedback from thyroid hormones, TSH levels tend to be high as well. In rare instances, there may be complete absence of thyroid parenchyma (*thyroid agenesis*), or the gland may be greatly reduced in size (*thyroid hypoplasia*). Mutations in the *TSH receptor* are a newly recognized cause of congenital hypothyroidism associated with a hypoplastic thyroid gland.[12] Recently, mutations in two transcription factors that are expressed in the developing thyroid and regulate follicular differentiation—*thyroid transcription factor-2* (*TTF-2*)[13] and *Paired Homeobox-8* (*PAX-8*)[14]—have been reported in patients with thyroid agenesis. Thyroid agenesis caused by TTF-2 mutations is usually associated with a cleft palate.

Secondary hypothyroidism is caused by TSH deficiency, and tertiary (central) hypothyroidism is caused by TRH deficiency. Secondary hypothyroidism can result from any of the causes of hypopituitarism. Frequently, the cause is a pituitary tumor; other causes include postpartum pituitary necrosis, trauma, and nonpituitary tumors, as was previously discussed. *Tertiary* (central) hypothyroidism can be caused by any disorder that damages the hypothalamus or interferes with hypothalamic-pituitary portal blood flow, thereby preventing delivery of TRH to the pituitary. This can result from hypothalamic damage from tumors, trauma, radiation therapy, or infiltrative diseases. Classic clinical manifestations of hypothyroidism include cretinism and myxedema.

CRETINISM

Cretinism refers to hypothyroidism that develops in infancy or early childhood. The term *cretin* was derived from the French *chrétien*, meaning Christian or Christlike, and was applied to these unfortunates because they were considered to be so mentally retarded as to be incapable of sinning. In the past, this disorder occurred fairly commonly in areas of the world where dietary iodine deficiency is endemic, such as the Himalayas, inland China, Africa, and other mountainous areas. It has become much less frequent in recent years, owing to the widespread supplementation of foods with iodine. On rare occasions, cretinism may also result from inborn errors in metabolism (e.g., enzyme deficiencies) that interfere with the biosynthesis of normal levels of thyroid hormone (*sporadic* cretinism).

Clinical features of cretinism include impaired development of the skeletal system and central nervous system, manifested by severe mental retardation, short stature, coarse facial features, a protruding tongue, and umbilical hernia. The severity of the mental impairment in cretinism appears to be related to the time at which thyroid deficiency occurs in utero. Normally, maternal hormones, including T_3 and T_4, cross the placenta and are critical to fetal brain development. If there is maternal thyroid deficiency before the development of the fetal thyroid gland, mental retardation is severe. In contrast, reduction in maternal thyroid hormones later in pregnancy, after the fetal thyroid has developed, allows normal brain development.

MYXEDEMA

The term *myxedema* is applied to hypothyroidism developing in the older child or adult. Myxedema, or Gull disease, was first linked with thyroid dysfunction in 1873 by Sir William Gull in a paper addressing the development of a "cretinoid state" in adults. The clinical manifestations vary with the age of onset of the deficiency. The older child shows signs and symptoms intermediate between those of the cretin and those of the adult with hypothyroidism. In the adult, the condition appears insidiously and may take years to reach the level of clinical suspicion.

Clinical features of myxedema are characterized by a slowing of physical and mental activity. The initial symptoms include generalized fatigue, apathy, and mental sluggishness, which may mimic depression in the early stages of the disease. Speech and intellectual functions become slowed. Patients with myxedema are listless, cold-intolerant, and frequently overweight. Reduced cardiac output probably contributes to shortness of breath and decreased exercise capacity, two frequent complaints in patients with hypothyroidism. Decreased sympathetic activity results in constipation and decreased sweating. The skin in these patients is cool and pale because of decreased blood flow. Histologically, there is an accumulation of matrix substances, such as glycosaminoglycans and hyaluronic acid, in skin, subcutaneous tissue, and a number of visceral sites. This results in edema, a broadening and coarsening of facial features, enlargement of the tongue, and deepening of the voice.

Laboratory evaluation plays a vital role in the diagnosis of suspected hypothyroidism because of the nonspecific nature of symptoms. *Measurement of the serum TSH level is the most sensitive screening test for this disorder.* The TSH level is increased in primary hypothyroidism due to a loss of feedback inhibition of TRH and TSH production by the hypothalamus and pituitary, respectively. The TSH level is not increased in patients with hypothyroidism due to primary hypothalamic or pituitary disease. *T_4 levels are decreased* in patients with hypothyroidism of any origin.

Thyroiditis

Thyroiditis, or inflammation of the thyroid gland, encompasses a diverse group of disorders characterized by some form of thyroid inflammation. These diseases include conditions that result in acute illness with severe thyroid pain (e.g., infectious thyroiditis, subacute granulomatous thyroiditis) and disorders in which there is relatively little inflammation and the illness is manifested primarily by thyroid dysfunction (subacute lymphocytic thyroiditis and fibrous [Reidel] thyroiditis).

Infectious thyroiditis may be either acute or chronic. Acute infections can reach the thyroid via hematogenous spread or through direct seeding of the gland, such as via a fistula from the piriform sinus adjacent to the larynx. Other infections of the thyroid, including mycobacterial, fungal, and *Pneumocystis* infections, are more chronic and frequently occur in immunocompromised patients. Whatever the cause, the inflammatory involvement may cause sudden onset of neck pain and tenderness in the area of the gland and is accompanied by fever, chills, and other signs of infection. Infectious thyroiditis can be self-limited or can be controlled with appropriate therapy. Thyroid function is usually not significantly affected, and there are few residual effects except for possible small foci of scarring. This section focuses on the more common and clinically significant types of thyroiditis: (1) Hashimoto thyroiditis (or chronic lymphocytic thyroiditis), (2) subacute granulomatous thyroiditis, and (3) subacute lymphocytic thyroiditis.

HASHIMOTO THYROIDITIS

Hashimoto thyroiditis (or chronic lymphocytic thyroiditis) is the most common cause of hypothyroidism in areas of the world where iodine levels are sufficient. It is characterized by gradual thyroid failure because of autoimmune destruction of the thyroid gland. The name *Hashimoto thyroiditis* is derived from the 1912 report by Hashimoto describing patients with goiter and intense lymphocytic infiltration of the thyroid (*struma lymphomatosa*). This disorder is most prevalent between 45 and 65 years of age and is more common in women than in men, with a female predominance of 10:1 to 20:1. Although it is primarily a disease of older women, it can occur in children and is a major cause of nonendemic goiter in children.

Epidemiologic studies have demonstrated a significant *genetic component* to Hashimoto thyroiditis, although, as in most other autoimmune disorders, the pattern of inheritance is non-Mendelian and likely to be influenced by subtle variations in the functions of multiple genes. The concordance rate in monozygotic twins is 30% to 60%, and up to 50% of asymptomatic first-degree relatives of Hashimoto patients demonstrate circulating antithyroid antibodies.[15] Several chromosomal abnormalities have been associated with thyroid autoimmunity. For example, adults with Turner syndrome (see Chapter 5) have a high prevalence of circulating antithyroid antibodies, and a substantial minority (~20%) develops subclinical or clinical hypothyroidism that is indistinguishable from Hashimoto thyroiditis. Similarly, adults with trisomy 21 (Down syndrome, see Chapter 5) are also at an increased risk for developing Hashimoto thyroiditis and hypothyroidism. There are reports that polymorphisms in the HLA locus, specifically the HLA-DR3 and HLA-DR5 alleles, are linked to Hashimoto thyroiditis, but the association is weak. Finally, genomewide linkage analyses in families with Hashimoto thyroiditis have provided evidence for several susceptibility loci, such as on chromosomes 6p and 12q, that may harbor genes predisposing to this disorder.[16]

Pathogenesis. Hashimoto thyroiditis is an autoimmune disease in which the immune system reacts against a variety of thyroid antigens. The overriding feature of Hashimoto thyroiditis is progressive depletion of thyroid epithelial cells (thyrocytes), which are gradually replaced by mononuclear cell infiltration and fibrosis. Multiple immunologic mechanisms may contribute to the death of thyrocytes (Fig. 24–9).[17,18] Sensitization of autoreactive CD4+ T-helper cells to thyroid antigens appears to be the initiating event. The effector mechanisms for thyrocyte death include the following:

- *CD8+ cytotoxic T cell–mediated cell death:* CD8+ cytotoxic T cells may cause thyrocyte destruction by one of two pathways: exocytosis of perforin/granzyme granules or engagement of death receptors, specifically CD95 (also known as Fas) on the target cell (Chapter 6).
- *Cytokine-mediated cell death:* CD4+ T cells produce inflammatory cytokines such as IFN-γ in the immediate thyrocyte milieu, with resultant recruitment and activation of macrophages and damage to follicles.
- Binding of antithyroid antibodies (anti–TSH receptor antibodies, antithyroglobulin, and antithyroid peroxidase antibodies) followed by antibody-dependent cell-mediated cytotoxicity (ADCC) (Chapter 6).

Morphology. The thyroid is often diffusely enlarged, although more localized enlargement may be seen in some cases. The capsule is intact, and the gland is well demarcated from adjacent structures. The cut surface is pale, yellow-tan, firm, and somewhat nodular. Microscopic examination reveals extensive infiltration of the parenchyma by a **mononuclear inflammatory infiltrate** containing small lymphocytes, plasma cells, and well-developed **germinal centers** (Fig. 24–10). The thyroid follicles are atrophic and are lined in many areas by epithelial cells distinguished by the presence of abundant eosinophilic, granular cytoplasm, termed **Hürthle** cells. This is a metaplastic response of the normally low cuboidal follicular epithelium to ongoing injury. In fine-needle aspiration biopsies, the presence of Hürthle cells in conjunction with a heterogeneous population of lymphocytes is characteristic of Hashimoto thyroiditis. In "classic" Hashimoto thyroiditis, interstitial connective tissue is increased and may be abundant. A **fibrous variant** is

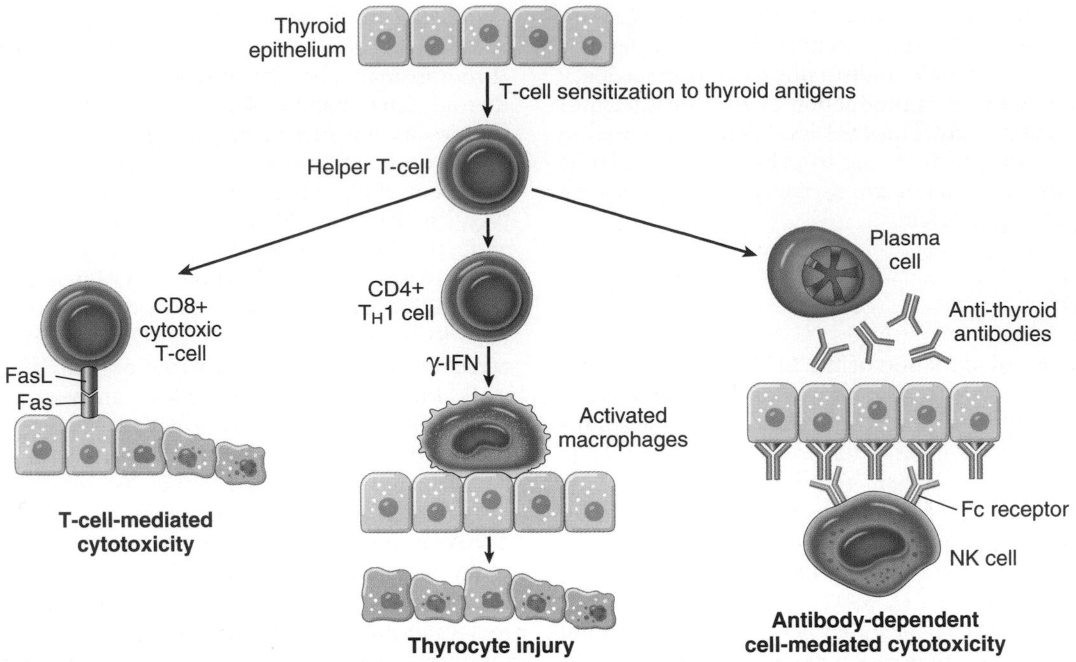

FIGURE 24–9 Pathogenesis of Hashimoto thyroiditis. Three proposed models for mechanism of thyrocyte destruction in Hashimoto disease. Sensitization of autoreactive CD4+ T cells to thyroid antigens appears to be the initiating event for all three mechanisms of thyroid cell death. See the text for details.

characterized by severe thyroid follicular atrophy and dense "keloid-like" fibrosis, with broad bands of acellular collagen encompassing residual thyroid tissue. Unlike Reidel thyroiditis (see below), the fibrosis does not extend beyond the capsule of the gland. The remnant thyroid parenchyma demonstrates features of chronic lymphocytic thyroiditis.

Clinical Course. Hashimoto thyroiditis comes to clinical attention as painless enlargement of the thyroid, usually associated with some degree of hypothyroidism, in a middle-aged woman. The enlargement of the gland is usually symmetric and diffuse, but in some cases, it may be sufficiently localized to raise a suspicion of neoplasm. In the usual clinical course, hypothyroidism develops gradually. In some cases, however, it may be preceded by transient thyrotoxicosis caused by disruption of thyroid follicles, with secondary release of thyroid hormones ("hashitoxicosis"). During this phase, free T_4 and T_3 levels are elevated, TSH is diminished, and radioactive iodine uptake is decreased. As hypothyroidism supervenes, T_4 and T_3 levels progressively fall, accompanied by a compensatory increase in TSH. Patients with Hashimoto thyroiditis are at increased risk for developing other concomitant autoimmune diseases, both endocrine (type 1 diabetes, autoimmune adrenalitis), and nonendocrine (systemic lupus erythematosus, myasthenia gravis, and Sjögren syndrome; see Chapter 6), and also at increased risk for the development of B-cell non-Hodgkin lymphomas. However, there is no established risk for developing thyroid epithelial neoplasms.

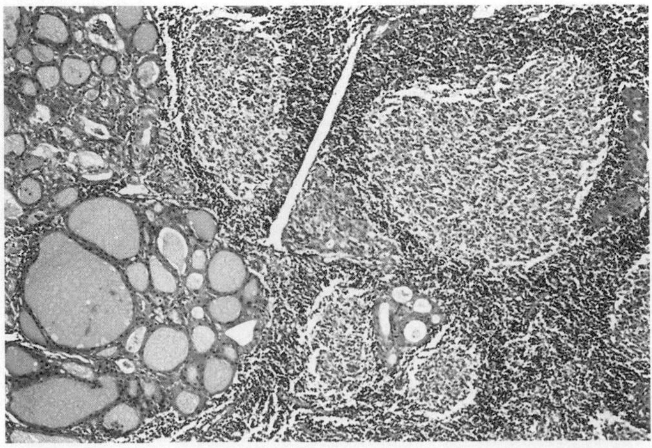

FIGURE 24–10 Hashimoto thyroiditis. The thyroid parenchyma contains a dense lymphocytic infiltrate with germinal centers. Residual thyroid follicles lined by deeply eosinophilic Hürthle cells are also seen.

SUBACUTE (GRANULOMATOUS) THYROIDITIS

Subacute thyroiditis, which is also referred to as *granulomatous thyroiditis* or *De Quervain thyroiditis*, occurs much less frequently than does Hashimoto disease. The disorder is most common between the ages of 30 and 50 and, like other forms of thyroiditis, affects women considerably more often than men (3:1 to 5:1).

Pathogenesis. Subacute thyroiditis is believed to be caused by a *viral infection* or a postviral inflammatory process. The majority of patients have a history of an upper respiratory infection just before the onset of thyroiditis. The disease has a seasonal incidence, with occurrences peaking in the summer, and clusters of cases have been reported in association with coxsackievirus, mumps, measles, adenovirus, and other viral illnesses. Although the pathogenesis of the disease is unclear, one model suggests that it results from a viral infection that provides an antigen, either viral or a thyroid antigen that is released secondary to virus-induced host tissue damage. This antigen stimulates cytotoxic T lymphocytes, which then damage thyroid follicular cells. In contrast to autoimmune thyroid disease, the immune response is virus-initiated and not self-perpetuating, so the process is limited.

Morphology. The gland may be unilaterally or bilaterally enlarged and firm, with an intact capsule. It may be slightly adherent to surrounding structures. On cut section, the involved areas are firm and yellow-white and stand out from the more rubbery, normal brown thyroid substance. Histologically, the changes are patchy and depend on the stage of the disease. Early in the active inflammatory phase, scattered follicles may be entirely disrupted and replaced by neutrophils forming microabscesses. Later, the more characteristic features appear in the form of aggregations of lymphocytes, histiocytes, and plasma cells about collapsed and damaged thyroid follicles. **Multinucleate giant cells** enclose naked pools or fragments of colloid (Fig. 24–11), hence the designation **granulomatous thyroiditis.** In later stages of the disease, a chronic inflammatory infiltrate and fibrosis may replace the foci of injury. Different histologic stages are sometimes found in the same gland, suggesting waves of destruction over a period of time.

Clinical Course. The presentation of subacute thyroiditis may be sudden or gradual. It is characterized by pain in the neck, which may radiate to the upper neck, jaw, throat, or ears, particularly when swallowing. Fever, fatigue, malaise, anorexia, and myalgia accompany a variable enlargement of the thyroid. The resultant thyroid inflammation and hyperthyroidism are transient, usually diminishing in 2 to 6 weeks, even if the patient is not treated. It may be followed by a period of transient, usually asymptomatic hypothyroidism lasting from 2 to 8 weeks, but recovery is virtually always complete.

The transient hyperthyroidism, as in other cases of thyroiditis, is due to disruption of thyroid follicles and release of excessive thyroid hormone. Nearly all patients have high serum T_4 and T_3 levels and low serum TSH levels. Radioactive iodine uptake is low because of suppression of TSH. The serum T_4 and T_3 levels are only modestly elevated. However, unlike in hyperthyroid states such as Graves disease, radioactive iodine uptake is diminished. After recovery, generally in 6 to 8 weeks, normal thyroid function returns.

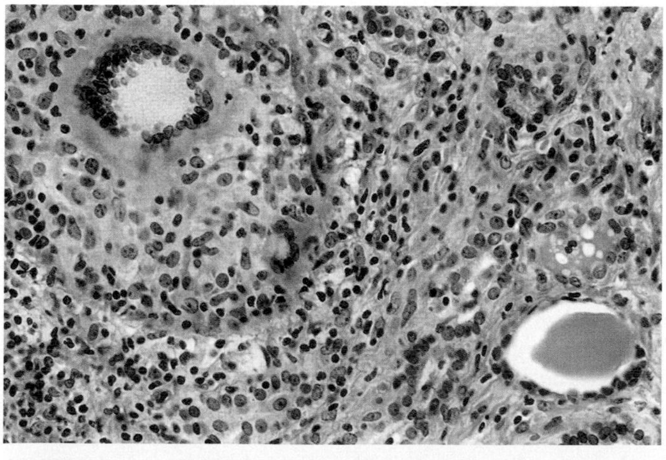

FIGURE 24–11 Subacute thyroiditis. The thyroid parenchyma contains a chronic inflammatory infiltrate with a multinucleate giant cell (*above left*) and a colloid follicle (*bottom right*).

SUBACUTE LYMPHOCYTIC (PAINLESS) THYROIDITIS

Subacute lymphocytic thyroiditis, which is also referred to as *painless thyroiditis or silent thyroiditis*, is an uncommon cause of hyperthyroidism. It usually comes to clinical attention because of mild hyperthyroidism, goitrous enlargement of the gland, or both. Although it can occur at any age, it is most often seen in middle-aged adults and is more common in women, especially during the postpartum period (*postpartum thyroiditis*), than in men.[19] Depending on the study, the frequency of this form of thyroiditis varies considerably, from 1% to about 10% of cases of hyperthyroid patients. The pathogenesis of this disorder is unknown. An autoimmune basis has been suggested because some patients have elevated levels of antibodies to thyroglobulin and thyroid peroxidase or a family history of thyroid autoimmune disease, and occasionally the disease evolves into overt chronic autoimmune thyroiditis several years later. There is no evidence that points toward a particular viral or other agent.

Morphology. Except for possible mild symmetric enlargement, the thyroid appears normal on gross inspection. The most specific histologic features consist of lymphocytic infiltration with hyperplastic germinal centers within the thyroid parenchyma and patch disruption and collapse of thyroid follicles. Unlike in Hashimoto thyroiditis, fibrosis and Hürthle cell metaplasia are not commonly seen.

Clinical Course. The principal clinical manifestation of painless thyroiditis is hyperthyroidism. Symptoms usually develop over 1 to 2 weeks and last from 2 to 8 weeks before subsiding. The patient may have any of the common findings of hyperthyroidism (e.g., palpitations, tachycardia, tremor, weakness, and fatigue). The thyroid gland is not usually tender but is minimally and diffusely enlarged. Infiltrative ophthalmopathy and other manifestations of Graves disease (see below) are not present. Patients with one episode of postpartum thyroiditis are at an increased risk of recurrence following subsequent pregnancies. A minority of affected individuals eventually progress to hypothyroidism. Some patients have no signs or symptoms, and the disorder is detected incidentally during routine thyroid testing.

Laboratory findings during periods of thyrotoxicosis include *elevated levels of T_4 and T_3* and *depressed levels of TSH.*

Other, less common forms of thyroiditis include *Riedel thyroiditis*, a rare disorder of unknown etiology characterized by extensive fibrosis involving the thyroid and contiguous neck structures. The presence of a hard and fixed thyroid mass clinically simulates a thyroid carcinoma. It may be associated with idiopathic fibrosis in other sites in the body, such as the retroperitoneum. The presence of circulating antithyroid antibodies in most patients suggests an autoimmune etiology. *Pal-*

pation thyroiditis, caused by vigorous clinical palpation of the thyroid gland, results in multifocal follicular disruption associated with chronic inflammatory cells and occasional giant cell formation. Unlike De Quervain thyroiditis, abnormalities of thyroid function are not present, and this is usually an incidental finding in specimens resected for other reasons.

Graves Disease

Graves reported in 1835 his observations of a disease characterized by "violent and long continued palpitations in females" associated with enlargement of the thyroid gland. *Graves disease is the most common cause of endogenous hyperthyroidism.* It is characterized by a *triad* of clinical findings:

1. *Hyperthyroidism* owing to hyperfunctional, diffuse enlargement of the thyroid
2. Infiltrative *ophthalmopathy* with resultant exophthalmos
3. Localized, infiltrative *dermopathy*, sometimes called *pretibial myxedema*, which is present in a minority of patients

Graves disease has a peak incidence between the ages of 20 and 40, *women being affected up to seven times more frequently than men.* This disorder is said to be present in 1.5% to 2.0% of women in the United States. Genetic factors are important in the etiology of Graves disease. An increased incidence of Graves disease occurs among family members of affected patients, and the concordance rate in monozygotic twins is as high as 60%. A recurring theme, as with other autoimmune disorders, is a genetic susceptibility to Graves disease associated with the presence of certain major histocompatibility haplotypes, specifically HLA-B8 and -DR3. Polymorphisms in the cytotoxic T-lymphocyte-associated-4 (*CTLA-4*) gene are also linked to Graves disease.[20,21] Recall that the HLA proteins are a critical component of antigen presentation to T cells, while CTLA-4 is an inhibitory receptor that prevents T-cell responses to self-antigens (Chapter 6). Genomewide linkage analyses have revealed additional susceptibility loci localized to chromosome 6p (also linked to Hashimoto thyroiditis) and to chromosome 20q, among others.[16]

Pathogenesis. *Graves disease is an autoimmune disorder* in which a variety of antibodies may be present in the serum, including antibodies to the TSH receptor, thyroid peroxisomes, and thyroglobulin. Of these, *autoantibodies to the TSH receptor are central to disease pathogenesis*, although the specific effects of the antibodies vary depending on which TSH receptor epitope they are directed against:

- *Thyroid-stimulating immunoglobulin (TSI):* Almost 50 years ago, serum from patients with Graves disease was found to contain a long-acting thyroid stimulator (LATS), so named because it stimulated thyroid function more slowly than TSH. LATS proved to be an IgG antibody that binds to the TSH receptor and mimics the action of TSH, stimulating adenyl cyclase, with resultant increased release of thyroid hormones. Almost all patients with Graves disease have detectable levels of this autoantibody to the TSH receptor. TSI is relatively specific for Graves disease, in contrast to thyroglobulin and thyroid peroxidase antibodies.
- *Thyroid growth-stimulating immunoglobulins* (*TGI*): Also directed against the TSH receptor, thyroid growth-stimulating immunoglobulins have been implicated in the proliferation of thyroid follicular epithelium.
- *TSH-binding inhibitor immunoglobulins* (*TBII*): These anti–TSH receptor antibodies prevent TSH from binding normally to its receptor on thyroid epithelial cells. In so doing, some forms of TSH-binding inhibitor immunoglobulins mimic the action of TSH, resulting in the stimulation of thyroid epithelial cell activity, whereas other forms may actually *inhibit* thyroid cell function. It is not unusual to find the coexistence of stimulating *and* inhibiting immunoglobulins in the serum of the same patient, a finding that could explain why some patients with Graves disease spontaneously develop episodes of hypothyroidism.

The key role of anti–TSH receptor antibodies in the pathogenesis of hyperthyroidism is underscored by animal models that recapitulate human Graves disease.[22] Immunization of mice with the TSH receptor results in generation of antibodies that cause thyroid stimulation, thyroid enlargement with lymphocytic infiltration, elevated thyroxine levels, and, in a subset of mice, ocular signs reminiscent of Graves ophthalmopathy (see below). Similar to the human disease, a gender predisposition as well as a genetic predisposition are seen in these animal models—females are affected more frequently than males and only certain inbred strains of mice demonstrate signs and symptoms of the disease. The trigger for the initiation of the autoimmune reaction in Graves disease remains uncertain, although the underlying mechanism is likely to be breakdown in helper T-cell tolerance, resulting in the production of anti-TSH autoantibodies.

A T cell–mediated autoimmune phenomenon also plays a role in the development of the *infiltrative ophthalmopathy* that is characteristic of Graves disease.[23] In Graves ophthalmopathy, the volume of the retro-orbital connective tissues and extraocular muscles is increased owing to several causes, including (1) marked infiltration of the retro-orbital space by mononuclear cells, predominantly T cells; (2) inflammatory edema and swelling of extraocular muscles; (3) accumulation of extracellular matrix components, specifically hydrophilic glycosaminoglycans (GAGs) such as hyaluronic acid and chondroitin sulfate; and (4) increased numbers of adipocytes (fatty infiltration). These changes displace the eyeball forward and can interfere with the function of the extraocular muscles. Recent evidence suggests that *orbital preadipocyte fibroblasts* express the TSH receptor and thus become targets of an autoimmune attack. T cells reactive against these fibroblasts secrete cytokines, which stimulate fibroblast proliferation and synthesis of extracellular matrix proteins (GAGs) and increase surface TSH receptor expression, perpetuating the autoimmune response.[22] The result is progressive infiltration of the retro-orbital space and ophthalmopathy.

Autoimmune disorders of the thyroid thus span a continuum in which Graves disease, characterized by hyperfunction of the thyroid, lies at one extreme and Hashimoto disease, manifesting as hypothyroidism, occupies the other end. Sometimes hyperthyroidism may supervene on pre-existing Hashimoto thyroiditis (*hashitoxicosis*); at other times, patients with Graves disease may spontaneously develop thyroid hypofunction; occasionally, there are families with coexistence of Hashimoto and Graves disease within the affected kindred. Not surprisingly, there is also an element of histologic overlap between the autoimmune thyroid disorders (most characteristically, prominent intrathyroidal lymphoid cell infiltrates with germinal center formation; see below). In both disorders, the frequency of other autoimmune diseases, such as systemic lupus erythematosus, pernicious anemia, type I diabetes, and Addison disease, is increased.

Morphology. The thyroid gland is usually symmetrically enlarged because of **diffuse hypertrophy and hyperplasia** of thyroid follicular epithelial cells. Increases in weight to over 80 gm are not uncommon. The gland is usually smooth and soft, and its capsule is intact. On cut section, the parenchyma has a soft, meaty appearance resembling normal muscle. Histologically, the dominant feature is **too many cells**. The follicular epithelial cells in untreated cases are tall and more crowded than usual. This crowding often results in the formation of small papillae, which project into the follicular lumen and encroach on the colloid, sometimes filling the follicles (Fig. 24–12). Such papillae lack fibrovascular cores, in contrast to those of papillary carcinoma (see below). The colloid within the follicular lumen is pale, with scalloped margins. Lymphoid infiltrates, consisting predominantly of T cells, with fewer B cells and mature plasma cells, are present throughout the interstitium; germinal centers are common.

Preoperative therapy alters the morphology of the thyroid in Graves disease. Preoperative administration of iodine causes involution of the epithelium and the accumulation of colloid by blocking thyroglobulin secretion. Treatment with the antithyroid drug propylthiouracil exaggerates the epithelial hypertrophy and hyperplasia by stimulating TSH secretion. Thus, in pre-treated patients it is impossible from histologic examination of surgical specimens to evaluate the functional activity of the gland.

Changes in extrathyroidal tissue include generalized lymphoid hyperplasia. The heart may be hypertrophied, and ischemic changes may be present, particularly in patients with preexisting coronary artery disease. In patients with ophthalmopathy, the tissues of the orbit are edematous because of the presence of hydrophilic mucopolysaccharides. In addition, there is infiltration by lymphocytes and fibrosis. Orbital muscles are edematous initially but may undergo fibrosis late in the course of the disease. The dermopathy, if present, is characterized by thickening of the dermis due to deposition of glycosaminoglycans and lymphocyte infiltration.

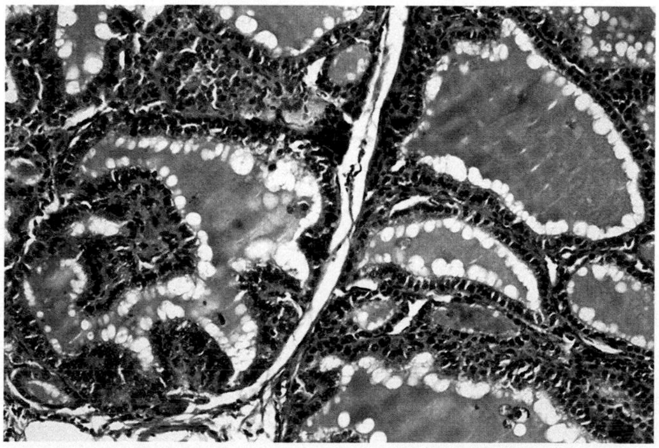

FIGURE 24–12 Diffusely hyperplastic thyroid in a case of Graves disease. The follicles are lined by tall, columnar epithelium. The crowded, enlarged epithelial cells project into the lumens of the follicles. These cells actively resorb the colloid in the centers of the follicles, resulting in the scalloped appearance of the edges of the colloid.

Clinical Course. The clinical findings in Graves disease include changes referable to *thyrotoxicosis* as well as those associated uniquely with Graves disease: *diffuse hyperplasia of the thyroid*, *ophthalmopathy*, and *dermopathy*. The degree of thyrotoxicosis varies from case to case and is sometimes less conspicuous than other manifestations of the disease. Diffuse enlargement of the thyroid is present in all cases of Graves disease. The *thyroid enlargement* may be accompanied by increased flow of blood through the hyperactive gland, often producing an audible bruit. Sympathetic overactivity produces a characteristic wide, staring gaze and lid lag. The ophthalmopathy of Graves disease results in abnormal protrusion of the eyeball (exophthalmos). The extraocular muscles are often weak. The exophthalmos may persist or progress despite successful treatment of the thyrotoxicosis, sometimes resulting in corneal injury. The infiltrative dermopathy, or *pretibial myxedema*, is most common in the skin overlying the shins, where it presents as scaly thickening and induration of the skin. However, it is present only in a minority of patients. The skin lesions may be slightly pigmented papules or nodules and often have an orange peel texture.

Laboratory findings in Graves disease include *elevated free T_4 and T_3* levels and *depressed TSH* levels. Because of ongoing stimulation of the thyroid follicles by thyroid-stimulating immunoglobulins, *radioactive iodine uptake is increased, and radioiodine scans show a diffuse uptake of iodine.*

Treatment of Graves disease consists of decreasing the symptoms of hyperthyroidism that are induced by increased β-adrenergic tone (e.g., tachycardia, palpitations, tremulousness, and anxiety) and measures aimed at decreasing thyroid hormone synthesis, such as the administration of thionamides (e.g., propylthiouracil), radioiodine ablation, and surgical intervention.

Diffuse and Multinodular Goiters

Enlargement of the thyroid, or *goiter*, is the most common manifestation of thyroid disease. *Diffuse and multinodular goiters reflect impaired synthesis of thyroid hormone,* most often caused by dietary iodine deficiency. Impairment of thyroid hormone synthesis leads to a compensatory rise in the serum TSH level, which, in turn, causes hypertrophy and hyperplasia of thyroid follicular cells and, ultimately, gross enlargement of the thyroid gland. The compensatory increase in functional mass of the gland is able to overcome the hormone deficiency, ensuring an *euthyroid* metabolic state in the vast majority of individuals. If the underlying disorder is sufficiently severe (e.g., a congenital biosynthetic defect or endemic iodine deficiency, see below), the compensatory responses may be inadequate to overcome the impairment in hormone synthesis, resulting in *goitrous hypothyroidism*. The degree of thyroid enlargement is proportional to the level and duration of thyroid hormone deficiency.

DIFFUSE NONTOXIC (SIMPLE) GOITER

Diffuse nontoxic (simple) goiter specifies a form of goiter that diffusely involves the entire gland without producing nodularity. Because the enlarged follicles are filled with colloid, the term *colloid goiter* has been applied to this condition. This disorder occurs in both an endemic and a sporadic distribution.

Endemic goiter occurs in geographic areas where the soil, water, and food supply contain only low levels of iodine. The term *endemic* is used when goiters are present in more than 10% of the population in a given region. Such conditions are particularly common in mountainous areas of the world, including the Alps, Andes, and Himalayas, where iodine deficiency is widespread. The lack of iodine leads to decreased synthesis of thyroid hormone and a compensatory increase in TSH, leading to follicular cell hypertrophy and hyperplasia and goitrous enlargement. With increasing dietary iodine supplementation, the frequency and severity of endemic goiter have declined significantly.

Variations in the prevalence of endemic goiter in regions with similar levels of iodine deficiency point to the existence of other causative influences, particularly dietary substances, referred to as *goitrogens.* The ingestion of substances that interfere with thyroid hormone synthesis at some level, such as excessive calcium and vegetables belonging to the *Brassica* and *Cruciferae* families (e.g., cabbage, cauliflower, Brussels sprouts, turnips, and cassava), has been documented to be goitrogenic. Native populations subsisting on cassava root are particularly at risk. Cassava contains a thiocyanate that inhibits iodide transport within the thyroid, worsening any possible concurrent iodine deficiency.

Sporadic goiter occurs less frequently than does endemic goiter. There is a striking female preponderance and a peak incidence at puberty or in young adult life. Sporadic goiter can be caused by a number of conditions, including the ingestion of substances that interfere with thyroid hormone synthesis. In other instances, goiter may result from hereditary enzymatic defects that interfere with thyroid hormone synthesis, all transmitted as autosomal-recessive conditions (dyshormonogenetic goiter; see above). In most cases, however, the cause of sporadic goiter is not apparent.

Morphology. Two phases can be identified in the evolution of diffuse nontoxic goiter: the **hyperplastic phase** and the phase of **colloid involution.** In the hyperplastic phase, the thyroid gland is diffusely and symmetrically enlarged, although the increase is usually modest, and the gland rarely exceeds 100 to 150 gm. The follicles are lined by crowded columnar cells, which may pile up and form projections similar to those seen in Graves disease. The accumulation is not uniform throughout the gland, and some follicles are hugely distended, whereas others remain small. If dietary iodine subsequently increases or if the demand for thyroid hormone decreases, the stimulated follicular epithelium involutes to form an enlarged, colloid-rich gland **(colloid goiter)**. In these cases, the cut surface of the thyroid is usually brown, somewhat glassy, and translucent. Histologically, the follicular epithelium is flattened and cuboidal, and colloid is abundant during periods of involution.

Clinical Course. The vast majority of patients with simple goiters are clinically euthyroid. Therefore, the clinical manifestations are primarily related to *mass effects* from the enlarged thyroid gland (discussed in detail with multinodular goiter; see below). Although serum T_3 and T_4 levels are normal, the serum TSH is usually elevated or at the upper range of normal, as is expected in marginally euthyroid individuals. In children, dyshormonogenetic goiter, caused by a congenital biosynthetic defect, may induce cretinism.

MULTINODULAR GOITER

With time, recurrent episodes of hyperplasia and involution combine to produce a more irregular enlargement of the thyroid, termed *multinodular goiter.* Virtually all long-standing simple goiters convert into multinodular goiters. They may be nontoxic or may induce thyrotoxicosis (toxic multinodular goiter). *Multinodular goiters produce the most extreme thyroid enlargements and are more frequently mistaken for neoplastic involvement than any other form of thyroid disease.* Because they derive from simple goiter, they occur in both sporadic and endemic forms, having the same female-to-male distribution and presumably the same origins but affecting older individuals because they are late complications.

It is believed that multinodal goiters may arise because of variations among follicular cells in responses to external stimuli, such as trophic hormones. If some cells in a follicle have a growth advantage, perhaps because of intrinsic genetic abnormalities similar to those that give rise to adenomas, those cells will develop into clones of proliferating cells. This may result in the formation of a nodule whose continued growth could even be autonomous, without the external stimulus. Consistent with this model, both polyclonal and monoclonal nodules coexist within the same multinodular goiter, the latter presumably having arisen owing to the acquisition of a genetic abnormality favoring growth.[24] Not surprisingly, *mutations in proteins of the TSH-signaling pathway that lead to constitutive activation of this pathway have been identified in a subset of autonomous thyroid nodules.* (TSH signaling pathway mutations and their implications are discussed in the section on follicular adenomas.)[25] With uneven follicular hyperplasia, generation of new follicles, and uneven accumulation of colloid, tensions and stresses are produced that lead to rupture of follicles and vessels followed by hemorrhages, scarring, and sometimes calcifications. The scarring adds to the tensions, and in this cyclical manner, nodularity appears. Moreover, the preexisting stromal framework of the gland may more or less enclose areas of expanded parenchyma, contributing to the nodularity.

Morphology. Multinodular goiters are multilobulated, asymmetrically enlarged glands that can achieve a weight of more than 2000 gm (Fig. 24–13). The pattern of enlargement is quite unpredictable and

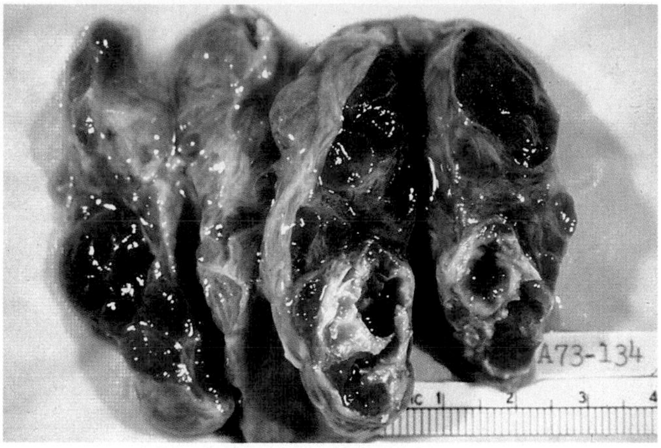

FIGURE 24–13 Nodular goiter. The gland is coarsely nodular and contains areas of fibrosis and cystic change.

may involve one lobe far more than the other, producing lateral pressure on midline structures, such as the trachea and esophagus. In other instances, the goiter grows behind the sternum and clavicles to produce the so-called **intrathoracic** or **plunging goiter**. Occasionally, most of it is hidden behind the trachea and esophagus; in other instances, one nodule may so stand out as to impart the clinical appearance of a solitary nodule. On cut section, irregular nodules containing variable amounts of brown, gelatinous colloid are present. Regressive changes occur frequently, particularly in older lesions, and include areas of hemorrhage, fibrosis, calcification, and cystic change. The microscopic appearance includes colloid-rich follicles lined by flattened, inactive epithelium and areas of follicular epithelial hypertrophy and hyperplasia, accompanied by the degenerative changes noted previously.

Clinical Course. The dominant clinical features of goiter are those caused by the *mass effects* of the enlarged gland. In addition to the obvious cosmetic effects of a large neck mass, goiters may cause airway obstruction, dysphagia, and compression of large vessels in the neck and upper thorax. Most patients are euthyroid, but in a substantial minority of patients, a hyperfunctioning nodule may develop within a long-standing goiter, resulting in *hyperthyroidism* (toxic multinodular goiter). This condition, known as *Plummer syndrome*, is not accompanied by the infiltrative ophthalmopathy and dermopathy of Graves disease. As was previously mentioned, goiter may be associated with clinical evidence of *hypothyroidism* in specific clinical settings. Radioiodine uptake is uneven, reflecting varied levels of activity in different regions. Hyperfunctioning nodules concentrate radioiodine and appear "hot." Goiters are also of clinical significance because of their ability to mask or to mimic neoplastic diseases arising in the thyroid.

Neoplasms of the Thyroid

The solitary thyroid nodule is a palpably discrete swelling within an otherwise apparently normal thyroid gland. The estimated incidence of solitary palpable nodules in the adult population of the United States varies between 1% and 10%, although it is significantly higher in endemic goitrous regions. Single nodules are about four times more common in women than in men. The incidence of thyroid nodules increases throughout life.

From a clinical standpoint, the possibility of neoplastic disease is of major concern in patients who present with thyroid nodules. Fortunately, the overwhelming majority of solitary nodules of the thyroid prove to be localized, non-neoplastic conditions (e.g., nodular hyperplasia, simple cysts, or foci of thyroiditis) or benign neoplasms such as follicular adenomas. In fact, benign neoplasms outnumber thyroid carcinomas by a ratio of nearly 10:1. Carcinomas of the thyroid are thus uncommon, accounting for well under 1% of solitary thyroid nodules and representing about 15,000 new cancer cases each year. Moreover, as will be seen subsequently, most are indolent, permitting a 90% survival at 20 years. Several clinical criteria might provide a clue to the nature of a given thyroid nodule:

- *Solitary nodules,* in general, are more likely to be neoplastic than are multiple nodules.
- *Nodules in younger patients* are more likely to be neoplastic than are those in older patients.
- *Nodules in males* are more likely to be neoplastic than are those in females.
- A history of *radiation* treatment to the head and neck region is associated with an increased incidence of thyroid malignancy.
- Nodules that take up radioactive iodine in imaging studies (*hot nodules*) are more likely to be benign than malignant.

Such general trends and statistics, however, are of little significance in the evaluation of a given patient, in whom the timely recognition of a malignancy, however uncommon, can be life-saving. Ultimately, it is the morphologic evaluation of a given thyroid nodule, in the form of fine-needle aspiration biopsy and histologic study of surgically resected thyroid parenchyma, that provides the most definitive information about its nature. In the following sections, we consider the major thyroid neoplasms, including adenoma and carcinoma in its various forms.

ADENOMAS

Adenomas of the thyroid are typically discrete, solitary masses. With rare exception, they are derived from follicular epithelium and so might all be called *follicular adenomas*. A variety of terms have been proposed for classifying adenomas on the basis of degree of follicle formation and the colloid content of the follicles. Simple colloid adenomas (macrofollicular adenomas), a common form, resemble normal thyroid tissue; others recapitulate stages in the embryogenesis of the normal thyroid (fetal or microfollicular, embryonal or trabecular). There is limited utility in these classifications because mixed patterns are common, and most of these benign tumors are nonfunctional. Clinically, follicular adenomas can be difficult to distinguish from dominant nodules of follicular hyperplasia or from the less common follicular carcinomas. Numerous studies have made it clear that adenomas are *not* forerunners of cancer except in rare instances. Although the vast majority of adenomas are nonfunctional, a small proportion produce thyroid hormones and cause clinically apparent thyrotoxicosis. Hormone production in functional adenomas ("toxic adenomas") occurs independent of TSH stimulation and represents another example of *thyroid autonomy*, analogous to toxic multinodular goiters.

Pathogenesis. The *TSH receptor signaling pathway* plays an important role in the pathogenesis of toxic adenomas. *Activating ("gain of function") somatic mutations in one of two components of this signaling system*—most often the TSH receptor itself or the α-subunit of G_s—cause chronic overproduction of cAMP, generating cells that acquire a growth advantage (see Fig. 24–3).[26] This results in clonal expansion of follicular epithelial cells that can autonomously produce thyroid hormone and cause symptoms of thyroid excess. Overall, mutations leading to constitutive activation of the cAMP pathway appear to be the cause of a proportion (10% to 75%) of autonomously functioning thyroid adenomas. However, the molecular pathogenesis of a significant proportion of thyroid tumors remains to be defined, especially the pathogenesis of nonfunctioning adenomas.

Morphology. The typical thyroid adenoma is a solitary, spherical, encapsulated lesion that is well demarcated from the surrounding thyroid parenchyma (Fig. 24–14). Follicular adenomas average about 3 cm in diameter, but some are smaller and others are much larger (up to 10 cm in diameter). In freshly resected specimens, the adenoma bulges from the cut surface and compresses the adjacent thyroid. The color ranges from gray-white to red-brown, depending on the cellularity of the adenoma and its colloid content. The neoplastic cells are demarcated from the adjacent parenchyma by a well-defined, intact capsule. **These features are important in making the distinction from multinodular goiters**, which contain multiple nodules on their cut surface (even though the patient may present clinically with a solitary dominant nodule), produce less compression of the adjacent thyroid parenchyma, and lack a well-formed capsule. Areas of hemorrhage, fibrosis, calcification, and cystic change, similar to those encountered in multinodular goiters, are common in follicular adenomas, particularly within larger lesions.

Microscopically, the constituent cells often form uniform-appearing follicles that contain colloid (Fig. 24–15). The follicular growth pattern within the adenoma is usually quite distinct from the adjacent non-neoplastic thyroid. This is another feature distinguishing adenomas from multinodular goiters, in which nodular and uninvolved thyroid parenchyma may have similar growth patterns. The epithelial cells composing the follicular adenoma reveal little variation in cell and nuclear morphology. Mitotic figures are rare, and extensive mitotic activity warrants careful examination of the capsule to exclude follicular carcinoma. Similarly, papillary change is not a typical feature of adenomas and, if extensive, should raise the suspicion of an encapsulated papillary carcinoma (see below). Occasionally, the neoplastic cells acquire brightly eosinophilic granular cytoplasm (oxyphil or Hürthle cell change) (Fig. 24–16); the clinical presentation and behavior of a follicular adenoma with oxyphilia **(Hürthle cell adenoma)** is no different from that of a conventional adenoma. Other variants of follicular adenomas include extensive clear cell change of the cytoplasm (clear cell follicular adenoma) and adenomas with "signet-ring" features (signet-ring cell follicular adenoma). Similar to endocrine tumors at other anatomic sites, even benign follicular adenomas may, on occasion, exhibit focal nuclear pleomorphism, atypia, and prominent nucleoli **(endocrine atypia)**; this by itself does not con-

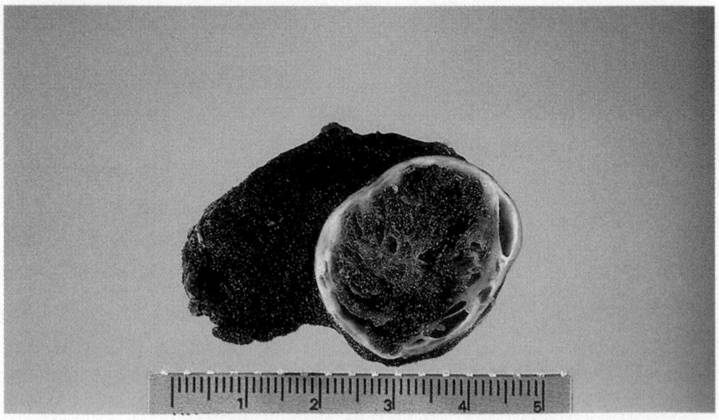

FIGURE 24–14 Follicular adenoma of the thyroid. A solitary, well-circumscribed nodule is seen.

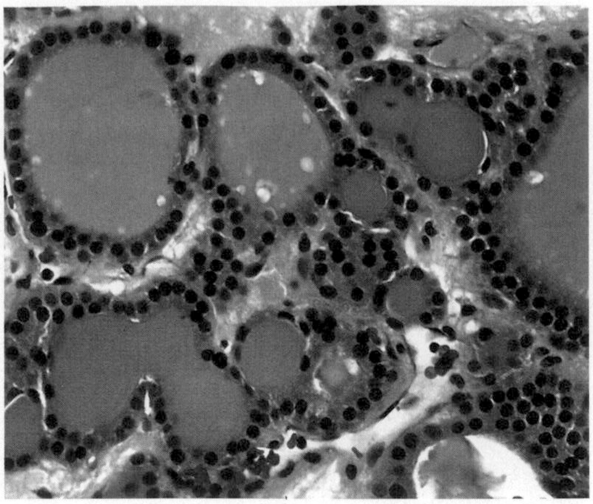

FIGURE 24–15 Follicular adenoma. The photomicrograph shows well-differentiated follicles resembling normal thyroid parenchyma.

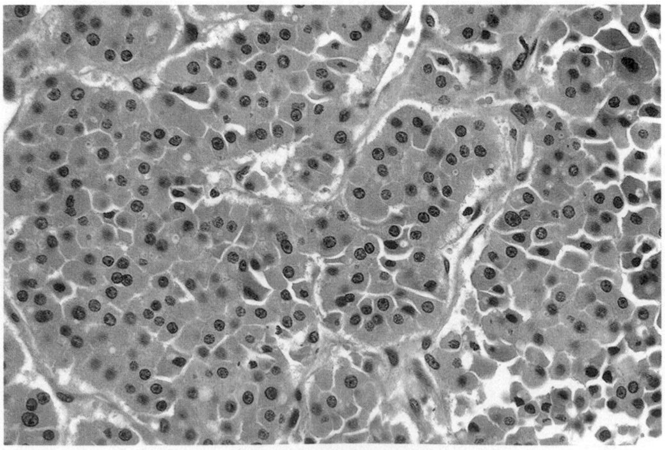

FIGURE 24–16 Hürthle cell tumor. A high-power view showing that the tumor is composed of cells with abundant eosinophilic cytoplasm and small regular nuclei. (Courtesy of Dr. Mary Sunday, Brigham and Women's Hospital, Boston, MA.)

stitute a feature of malignancy. Infrequently, adenomas can demonstrate increased cellularity, more extensive variation in cellular size and nuclear morphology, and even mitotic activity. These adenomas have been called **atypical follicular adenomas** and warrant careful examination of the tumor capsule to exclude capsular and/or vascular invasion.[27] The hallmark of all follicular adenomas is the presence of an intact, well-formed capsule encircling the tumor. **Careful evaluation of the integrity of the capsule is therefore critical in distinguishing follicular adenomas from follicular carcinomas,** which demonstrate capsular and/or vascular invasion (see below).

Clinical Features. Many thyroid adenomas present as a unilateral painless mass, often discovered during a routine physical examination. Larger masses may produce local symptoms, such as difficulty in swallowing.

Most adenomas take up less radioactive iodine than does normal thyroid parenchyma. On radionuclide scanning, therefore, adenomas usually appear as *cold* nodules relative to the adjacent thyroid tissue. Up to 10% of cold nodules eventually prove to be malignant on histologic analysis. By contrast, malignancy is rare in *hot* nodules. In a minority of cases, adenomas may be hyperfunctional, producing signs and symptoms of hyperthyroidism (toxic adenomas). On radionuclide imaging, hyperfunctioning adenomas appear hot compared with the paranodular thyroid tissue, which is deprived of thyrotropin stimulation. Hot adenomas occasionally have some dependence on TSH and may be induced to regress by the administration of thyroid hormones, which suppress TSH secretion.

Other techniques used in the preoperative evaluation of suspected adenomas are ultrasonography and fine-needle aspiration biopsy. *Owing to the need for evaluating capsular integrity, the definitive diagnosis of adenomas can be made only after careful histologic examination of the resected specimen.* Suspected adenomas of the thyroid are therefore removed surgically to exclude malignancy. Thyroid adenomas, including atypical adenomas, have an excellent prognosis and do not recur or metastasize. About 20% of follicular adenomas have point mutations in the *RAS* family of oncogenes, which have also been identified in 30% to 40% of follicular carcinomas. This finding raises the possibility that some adenomas may progress to carcinomas.

OTHER BENIGN TUMORS

Solitary nodules of the thyroid gland may also prove to be cysts. The great preponderance of these lesions represent cystic degeneration of a follicular adenoma; the remainder probably arise in multinodular goiters. They are often filled with a brown, turbid fluid containing blood, hemosiderin pigment, and cell debris. Additional benign rarities include dermoid cysts, lipomas, hemangiomas, and teratomas (seen mainly in infants).

CARCINOMAS

Carcinomas of the thyroid are relatively uncommon in the United States, accounting for about 1.5% of all cancers. Most cases occur in adults, although some forms, particularly papillary carcinomas, may present in childhood. A female predominance has been noted among patients who develop thyroid carcinoma in the early and middle adult years, perhaps related to the expression of estrogen receptors on neoplastic thyroid epithelium. In contrast, cases presenting in childhood and late adult life are distributed equally among males and females. Most thyroid carcinomas are well-differentiated lesions. The major subtypes of thyroid carcinoma and their relative frequencies include the following:

- Papillary carcinoma (75% to 85% of cases)
- Follicular carcinoma (10% to 20% of cases)
- Medullary carcinoma (5% of cases)
- Anaplastic carcinoma (<5% of cases)

Most thyroid carcinomas are derived from the follicular epithelium, except for medullary carcinomas; the latter are derived from the parafollicular or C cells. Because of the unique clinical and biologic features associated with each variant of thyroid carcinoma, these subtypes are described separately.

Pathogenesis

There are several factors, genetic and environmental, implicated in the pathogenesis of thyroid cancers.

Genetic Factors. Genetic factors are important in both familial and nonfamilial ("sporadic") forms of thyroid cancer. Familial medullary cancers account for most inherited cases of thyroid cancer. Familial nonmedullary thyroid cancers (papillary and follicular variants) are very rare. Distinct genes are involved in the histologic variants of thyroid cancer.

Follicular Thyroid Carcinomas. Approximately half of follicular thyroid carcinomas harbor mutations in the *RAS* family of oncogenes (*HRAS*, *NRAS*, and *KRAS*) (Chapter 7), *NRAS* mutations being the most common. Recently, a unique translocation has been described between *PAX8*, a paired homeobox gene that is important in thyroid development (see above), and the peroxisome proliferator-activated receptor $\gamma 1$ (*PPAR*γ*1*), a nuclear hormone receptor implicated in terminal differentiation of cells.[28] The *PAX8-PPAR*γ*1* fusion is present in approximately one-third of follicular thyroid carcinomas, specifically those cancers with a t(2;3)(q13;p25) translocation, which permits juxtaposition of portions of both genes. Follicular carcinomas appear to arise by at least two distinct and virtually nonoverlapping molecular pathways:[29] Tumors carry either a *RAS* mutation or a *PAX8-PPAR*γ*1* fusion, and rarely are both genetic abnormalities present in the same case. Fewer than 10% of follicular adenomas harbor a *PAX8-PPAR*γ*1* fusion transcript, and this translocation has not been documented to date in other thyroid neoplasms.[30]

Papillary Thyroid Carcinomas. Like follicular thyroid carcinomas, papillary carcinomas also appear to arise by multiple distinct, nonoverlapping molecular pathways. One pathway involves rearrangements of the tyrosine kinase receptors *RET* or *NTRK1* (neurotrophic tyrosine kinase receptor 1) and another involves activating mutations in the *BRAF* oncogene. A third pathway involves *RAS* mutations (10% to 20% of papillary carcinomas), suggesting that some of these cancers are related to follicular adenomas. *RET*, located on chromosome 10q11, and *NTRK1*, located on chromosome 1q21, belong to the family of receptor tyrosine kinases that transduce extracellular signals for cell growth and differentiation and exert many of their downstream effects through the ubiquitous MAP kinase signaling pathway (Chapter 7). Neither receptor is normally expressed on the surface of thyroid follicular cells. In papillary thyroid cancers, either a paracentric inversion of chromosome 10 or a reciprocal translocation between chromosomes 10 and 17 places the tyrosine kinase domain of *RET* under the transcriptional control of constitutively active genes on these two chromosomes. The novel fusion genes that are so formed are known as *ret/PTC* (ret/papillary thyroid carcinoma) and are present in approximately one-fifth of papillary thyroid cancers.[31] The frequency of *ret/PTC* rearrangements is significantly higher in papillary cancers arising in children and in the backdrop of radiation exposure. Similarly, paracentric inversions or translocations of *NTRK1* that constitutively activate its tyrosine kinase domain are present in 5% to 10% of papillary thyroid cancers.[32] One-third to one-half of papillary thyroid carcinomas harbor an activating mutation in the *BRAF* gene, which encodes a signaling intermediary in the MAP kinase pathway.[33,34] Since chromosomal rearrangements of the *RET* or *NTRK1* genes and mutations of *BRAF* have redundant effects on the thyroid epithelium (recall that both mechanisms result in activation of the MAP kinase signaling pathway), papillary thyroid carcinomas demonstrate either one or the other molecular abnormality, but not both.[35]

Medullary Thyroid Carcinomas. Medullary carcinomas arise from the parafollicular C cells in the thyroid. Familial medullary thyroid carcinomas occur in multiple endocrine neoplasia type 2 (MEN-2, see below) and are associated with germ-line *RET* protooncogene mutations that affect residues in the cysteine-rich extracellular or the intracellular tyrosine kinase domains, leading to constitutive activation of the receptor.[36] *RET* mutations are detectable in approximately 95% of families with MEN-2; in the remaining few cases, the mutations may arise in hard-to-detect promoter sequences or intronic sites. *RET* mutations are also seen in nonfamilial (sporadic) medullary thyroid cancers.[37] Chromosomal rearrangements involving *RET*, such as the *ret/PTC* translocations reported in papillary cancers, are not seen in medullary carcinomas.

Anaplastic Carcinomas. These highly aggressive and lethal tumors can arise de novo or by "dedifferentiation" of a well-differentiated papillary or follicular carcinoma. Inactivating point mutations in the *p53* tumor suppressor gene are rare in well-differentiated thyroid carcinomas but common in anaplastic tumors.[38]

Environmental Factors. The major risk factor predisposing to thyroid cancer is exposure to *ionizing radiation*, particularly during the first two decades of life. In the past, radiation therapy was liberally employed in the treatment of a number of head and neck lesions in infants and children, including reactive tonsillar enlargement, acne, and tinea capitis. Up to 9% of people receiving such treatment during childhood have subsequently developed thyroid malignancies, usually several decades after exposure. The importance of radiation as a risk factor for thyroid carcinoma was highlighted by the increased incidence of papillary thyroid carcinomas in children in the Marshall Islands after atomic bomb testing and, more recently, by the dramatic rise in the incidence of pediatric thyroid carcinoma among children exposed to ionizing radiation after the Chernobyl nuclear disaster in the Ukraine in 1986. More than 400 cases of pediatric thyroid carcinoma have been observed in this region of Belarus between the time of the incident and the present, a number far in excess of the usual incidence for this area.[39] More than half of the children lived in areas that had the highest radiation exposure.

Long-standing multinodular goiter has been suggested as a predisposing factor in some cases, since areas with iodine deficiency–related endemic goiter have a higher prevalence of follicular carcinomas. While most, if not all, thyroid lymphomas arise from pre-existing Hashimoto thyroiditis, there is no conclusive evidence to suggest that thyroiditis is associated with an increased risk of thyroid epithelial carcinomas.

Papillary Carcinoma

Papillary carcinomas are the most common form of thyroid cancer. They occur at any age but most often in the twenties to forties, and account for the majority of thyroid carcinomas associated with previous exposure to ionizing radiation.

Morphology. Papillary carcinomas are solitary or multifocal lesions. Some tumors may be well-circumscribed and even encapsulated; others may infiltrate the adjacent parenchyma with ill-defined margins. The lesions may contain areas of fibrosis and calcification and are often cystic. On the cut surface, they may appear granular and may sometimes contain grossly discernible papillary foci. The definitive diagnosis of papillary carcinoma can be made only after microscopic examination. The characteristic hallmarks of papillary neoplasms include the following (Fig. 24–17):

- Papillary carcinomas can contain branching **papillae** having a fibrovascular stalk covered by a single to multiple layers of cuboidal epithelial cells. In most neoplasms, the epithelium covering the papillae consists of well-differentiated, uniform, orderly, cuboidal cells, but at the other extreme are those with fairly anaplastic epithelium showing considerable variation in cell and nuclear morphology. When present, the papillae of papillary carcinoma differ from those seen in areas of hyperplasia. In contrast to hyperplastic papillary lesions, the neoplastic papillae are more complex and have dense fibrovascular cores.
- The nuclei of papillary carcinoma cells contain finely dispersed chromatin, which imparts an **optically clear** or **empty** appearance, giving rise to the designation **ground glass** or **Orphan Annie eye** nuclei. In addition, invaginations of the cytoplasm may in cross-sections give the appearance of intranuclear inclusions ("pseudo-inclusions") or intranuclear grooves. As currently used, *the diagnosis of papillary carcinoma is based on these nuclear features* even in the absence of papillary architecture.
- Concentrically calcified structures termed **psammoma bodies** are often present within the lesion, usually within the cores of papillae. These structures are almost never found in follicular and medullary carcinomas, and so, when present, they are a strong indication that the lesion is a papillary carcinoma. It is said that whenever a psammoma body is found within a lymph node or perithyroidal tissues, a **hidden** papillary carcinoma must be considered.[40]

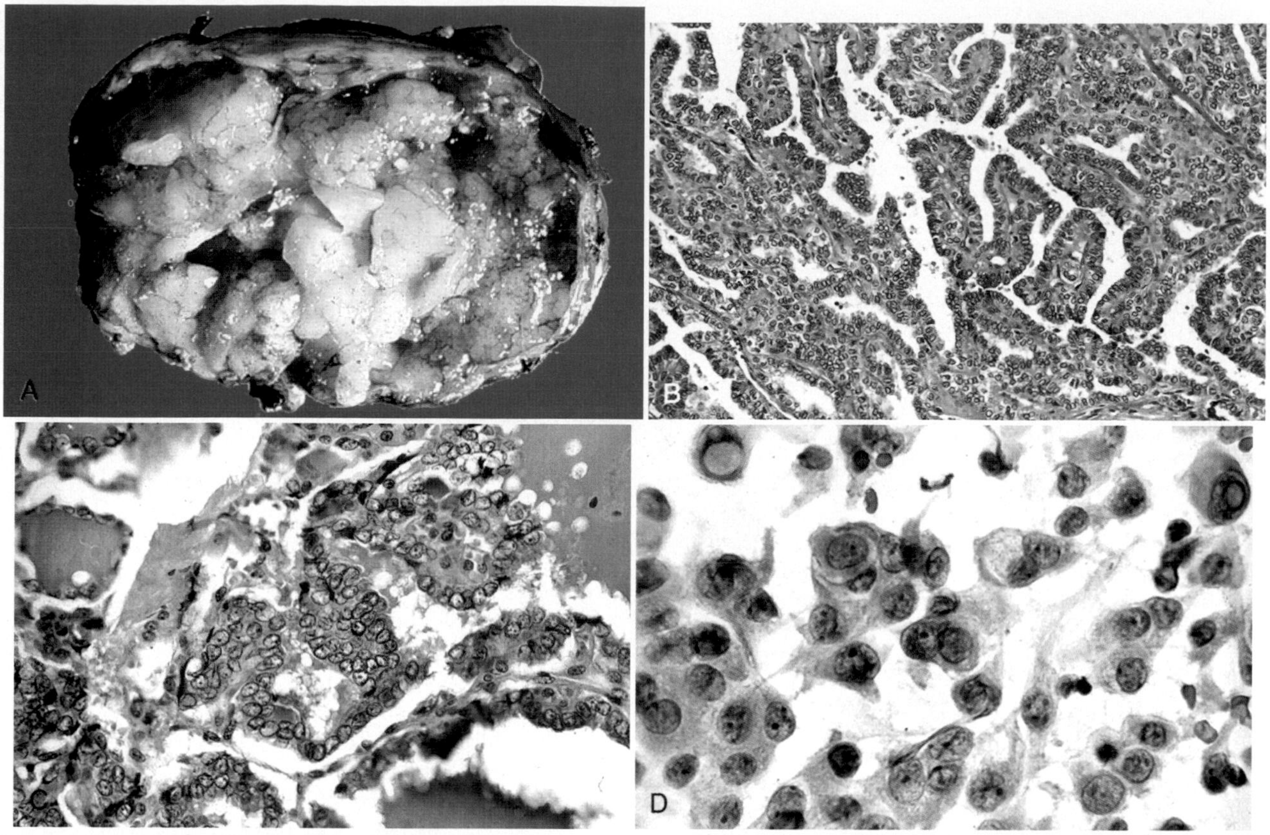

FIGURE 24–17 Papillary carcinoma of the thyroid. *A,* The macroscopic appearance of a papillary carcinoma with grossly discernible papillary structures. This particular example contains well-formed papillae (*B*), lined by cells with characteristic empty-appearing nuclei, sometimes termed "Orphan Annie eye" nuclei (*C*). *D,* Cells obtained by fine-needle aspiration of a papillary carcinoma. Characteristic intranuclear inclusions are visible in some of the aspirated cells.

- Foci of lymphatic invasion by tumor are often present, but involvement of blood vessels is relatively uncommon, particularly in smaller lesions. Metastases to adjacent cervical lymph nodes are estimated to occur in up to half the cases.

There are variant forms of papillary carcinoma that are important to recognize because they can resemble other lesions and have unique clinical features. The **encapsulated variant** constitutes about 10% of all papillary neoplasms. It is usually confined to the thyroid gland, is well encapsulated, and rarely presents with vascular or lymph node dissemination, and so it can easily be confused with a benign adenoma. In most cases, this variant has an excellent prognosis.

The **follicular variant** has the characteristic nuclei of papillary carcinoma but has an almost totally follicular architecture.[41] Grossly, the tumor may be encapsulated, and focally, psammoma bodies may be seen. These follicular variants still behave biologically as usual papillary carcinomas as long as they meet the nuclear criteria for diagnosis of papillary cancers (see above). The true follicular carcinoma, in contrast, lacks these nuclear features, frequently demonstrates capsular and vascular invasion, and has a less favorable prognosis. A differential diagnosis of thyroid lesions with a follicular architecture is summarized in Table 24–4.

A **tall cell variant** is marked by tall columnar cells with intensely eosinophilic cytoplasm lining the papillary structures. Typically, the cells are at least twice as tall as they are wide (hence the eponym "tall cell" variant). These tumors tend to occur in older individuals and are usually large with prominent vascular invasion, extrathyroidal extension, and cervical and distant metastases. It has been recently demonstrated that more than half the tall cell variants harbor a *ret/PTC* translocation that confers greater mitogenic

TABLE 24–4 Thyroid Lesions with a Follicular Architecture

Non-Neoplastic
Hyperplastic nodule in goiter
Neoplastic
Follicular adenoma*
Follicular carcinoma*
Follicular variant of papillary carcinoma†

*Differentiating follicular carcinoma from follicular adenoma requires histologic evidence of *capsular or blood vessel invasion*, or *documented metastasis*.

†The diagnosis of papillary carcinoma is rendered on the presence of *characteristic nuclear features*, irrespective of the presence or absence of papillae.

potential than the *ret/PTC* observed in usual papillary thyroid cancers. The presence of this genetic abnormality might result in more aggressive behavior.[42,43]

An unusual **diffuse sclerosing variant** of papillary carcinoma occurs in younger individuals, including children. These tumors do not present with a mass, but rather with a bilateral goiter. There is a characteristic "gritty" sensation to the cut surface of the lesion due to the presence of abundant psammoma bodies. The tumor demonstrates a prominent papillary growth pattern, intermixed with solid areas containing nests of squamous cells (squamous morules). The neoplastic cells exhibit classic nuclear features of a papillary neoplasm. As the name suggests, there is extensive, diffuse fibrosis throughout the thyroid gland, often associated with a prominent lymphocytic infiltrate, simulating Hashimoto thyroiditis. The neoplastic cells have a peculiar propensity to invade intrathyroidal lymphatic channels; hence, nodal metastases are present in almost all cases.

Hyalinizing trabecular tumors, a group that includes both adenomas and carcinomas, have recently been reconsidered as a variant of papillary carcinomas, based on the presence of *ret/PTC* gene rearrangements in 30% to 60% of these tumors.[44] They are characterized by an "organoid" growth pattern, with nests and trabeculae of elongated tumor cells within a fibrovascular stroma; at first glance, the tumor may resemble an extra-adrenal paraganglioma (see below). Both intracellular and extracellular hyalinization are prominent and confer a pink hue on the tumor on low-power microscopic examination. The nuclear features resemble those seen in classic papillary carcinomas, and psammoma bodies may be present. Hyalinizing trabecular adenomas are well encapsulated, while carcinomas demonstrate capsular and/or vascular invasion.

Clinical Course. Most papillary carcinomas present as asymptomatic thyroid nodules, but the first manifestation may be a mass in a cervical lymph node. Interestingly, the presence of isolated cervical nodal metastases does not appear to have a significant influence on the generally good prognosis of these lesions. The carcinoma, which is usually a single nodule, moves freely during swallowing and is not distinguishable from a benign nodule. Hoarseness, dysphagia, cough, or dyspnea suggests advanced disease. In a minority of patients, hematogenous metastases are present at the time of diagnosis, most commonly in the lung.

A variety of diagnostic tests have been employed to help separate benign from malignant thyroid nodules, including radionuclide scanning and fine-needle aspiration. Most papillary lesions are *cold* masses on scintiscans. Improvements in cytologic analysis have made fine-needle aspiration cytology a reliable test for distinguishing between benign and malignant nodules. The nuclear features are often nicely demonstrable in aspirated specimens.

Papillary thyroid cancers have an excellent prognosis, with a 10-year survival rate in excess of 95%. Five per cent to 20% of patients have local or regional recurrences, and 10% to 15% have distant metastases. The prognosis of a patient with papillary thyroid cancers is dependent on several factors including age (in general, the prognosis is less favorable among patients older than 40 years), the presence of extrathyroidal extension, and presence of distant metastases (stage).

Follicular Carcinoma

Follicular carcinomas are the second most common form of thyroid cancer, accounting for 10% to 20% of all thyroid cancers. They tend to present in women, and at an older age than do papillary carcinomas, with a peak incidence in the forties and fifties. The incidence of follicular carcinoma is increased in areas of dietary iodine deficiency, suggesting that in some cases, nodular goiter may predispose to the development of the neoplasm. The high frequency of *RAS* mutations in follicular adenomas and carcinomas suggests that the two may be related tumors.

Morphology. Follicular carcinomas are single nodules that may be well circumscribed or widely infiltrative (Fig. 24–18). Sharply demarcated lesions may be exceedingly difficult to distinguish from follicular adenomas by gross examination. Larger lesions may penetrate the capsule and infiltrate well beyond the thyroid capsule into the adjacent neck. They are gray to tan to pink on cut section and, on occasion, are somewhat translucent when large, colloid-filled follicles are present. Degenerative changes, such as central fibrosis and foci of calcification, are sometimes present.

Microscopically, most follicular carcinomas are composed of fairly uniform cells forming small follicles containing colloid, quite reminiscent of normal thyroid (Fig. 24–19). In other cases, follicular differentiation may be less apparent, and there may be nests

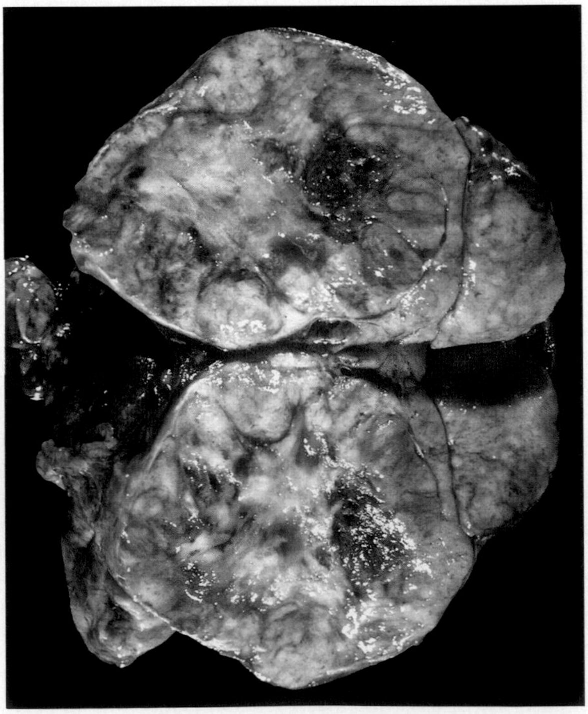

FIGURE 24–18 Follicular carcinoma. Cut surface of a follicular carcinoma with substantial replacement of the lobe of the thyroid. The tumor has a light-tan appearance and contains small foci of hemorrhage.

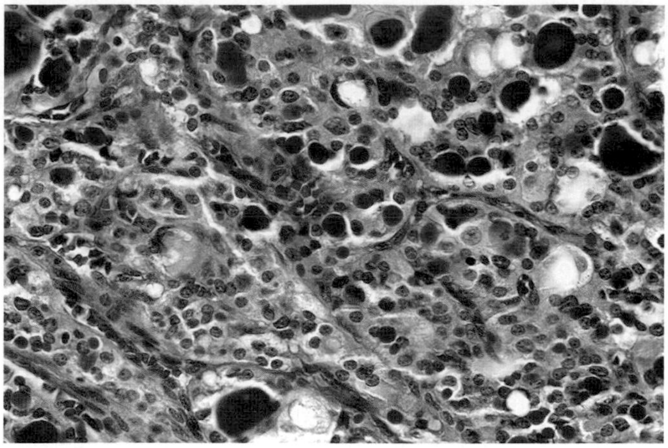

FIGURE 24–19 Follicular carcinoma of the thyroid. A few of the glandular lumens contain recognizable colloid.

or sheets of cells without colloid. Occasional tumors are dominated by cells with abundant granular, eosinophilic cytoplasm (Hürthle cells). Whatever the pattern, the nuclei lack the features typical of papillary carcinoma, and psammoma bodies are not present. It is important to note the absence of these details because some papillary carcinomas may appear almost entirely follicular (see Table 24–4). Follicular lesions in which the nuclear features are typical of papillary carcinomas should be treated as papillary cancers. While nuclear features are helpful in distinguishing papillary from follicular neoplasms, they are of little value in distinguishing follicular adenomas from **minimally invasive follicular carcinomas**. This distinction requires extensive histologic sampling of the tumor-capsule–thyroid interface to exclude capsular and/or vascular invasion (Fig. 24–20). The criterion for vascular invasion is applicable only to capsular vessels and vascular spaces beyond the capsule; **the presence of tumor plugs within intratumoral blood vessels has little prognostic significance.** Unlike in papillary cancers, lymphatic spread is distinctly uncommon in follicular cancers.

In contrast to minimally invasive follicular cancers, extensive invasion of adjacent thyroid parenchyma or extrathyroidal tissues makes the diagnosis of carcinoma obvious in **widely invasive follicular carcinomas.** Histologically, these cancers tend to have a greater proportion of solid or trabecular growth pattern, less evidence of follicular differentiation, and increased mitotic activity.

Clinical Course. Follicular carcinomas present as slowly enlarging painless nodules. Most frequently, they are *cold* nodules on scintigrams, although in rare cases, the better-differentiated lesions may be hyperfunctional, take up radioactive iodine, and appear *warm* on scintiscan. Follicular carcinomas have little propensity for invading lymphatics; therefore, regional lymph nodes are rarely involved, but vascular invasion is common, with spread to bone, lungs, liver, and elsewhere. The prognosis is largely dependent on the extent of invasion and stage at presentation. Widely invasive follicular carcinomas not infrequently develop metastases, and up to half succumb to their disease within 10 years. This is in stark contrast to minimally invasive follicular carcinoma, which has a 10-year survival rate greater than 90%. Most follicular carcinomas are treated with total thyroidectomy followed by the administration of radioactive iodine, the rationale being that metastases are likely to take up the radioactive element, which can be used to identify and ablate such lesions. In addition, because any residual follicular carcinoma may respond to TSH stimulation, patients are usually treated with thyroid hormone after surgery to suppress endogenous TSH.

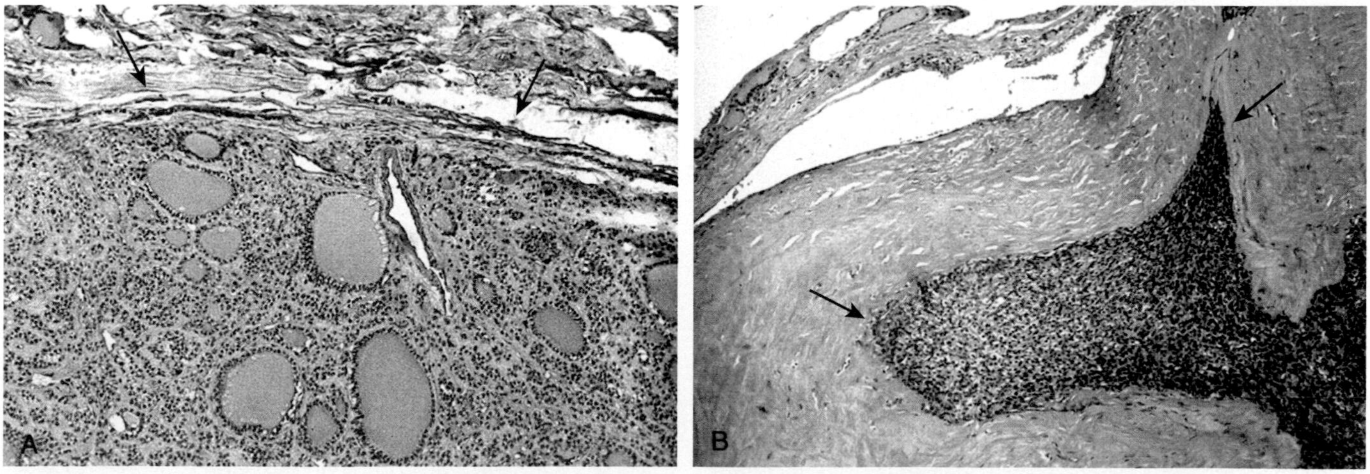

FIGURE 24–20 Capsular integrity in follicular neoplasms. Evaluating the integrity of the capsule is critical in distinguishing follicular adenomas from follicular carcinomas. In adenomas (*A*), a fibrous capsule, usually thin but occasionally more prominent, circumferentially surrounds the neoplastic follicles and no capsular invasion is seen (*arrowheads*); compressed normal thyroid parenchyma is usually present external to the capsule (*top of the panel*). In contrast, follicular carcinomas demonstrate capsular invasion (*B, arrowheads*) that may be minimal, as in this case, or widespread with extension into local structures of the neck. The presence of vascular invasion is another feature of follicular carcinomas.

Medullary Carcinoma

Medullary carcinomas of the thyroid are *neuroendocrine* neoplasms derived from the parafollicular cells, or C cells, of the thyroid.[45] The cells of medullary carcinomas, similar to normal C cells, secrete *calcitonin*, the measurement of which plays an important role in the diagnosis and postoperative follow-up of patients. In some instances, the tumor cells elaborate other polypeptide hormones, such as somatostatin, serotonin, and vasoactive intestinal peptide (VIP). The tumors arise sporadically in about 80% of cases. The remainder occurs in the setting of MEN syndrome 2A or 2B or as familial tumors without an associated MEN syndrome (familial medullary thyroid carcinoma, or FMTC; discussed later). Recall that activating point mutations in the *RET* protooncogene play an important role in the development of both familial and sporadic medullary carcinomas. Cases associated with MEN-2 occur in younger patients and may even arise during childhood. In contrast, sporadic medullary carcinomas as well as FMTC are lesions of adulthood, with a peak incidence in the forties and fifties.

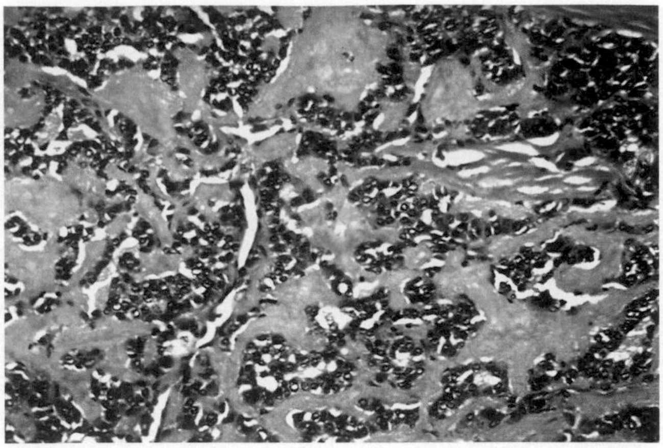

FIGURE 24–22 Medullary carcinoma of the thyroid. These tumors typically contain amyloid, visible here as homogeneous extracellular material, derived from calcitonin molecules secreted by the neoplastic cells.

Morphology. Medullary carcinomas can arise as a solitary nodule or may present as multiple lesions involving both lobes of the thyroid. The sporadic neoplasms tend to originate in one lobe (Fig. 24–21). In contrast, bilaterality and **multicentricity** are common in familial cases. Larger lesions often contain areas of necrosis and hemorrhage and may extend through the capsule of the thyroid. The tumor tissue is firm, pale gray to tan, and infiltrative. There may be foci of hemorrhage and necrosis in the larger lesions.

Microscopically, medullary carcinomas are composed of polygonal to spindle-shaped cells, which may form nests, trabeculae, and even follicles. Small, more anaplastic cells are present in some tumors and may be the predominant cell type. Acellular **amyloid deposits,** derived from altered calcitonin molecules, are present in the adjacent stroma in many cases (Fig. 24–22). Calcitonin is readily demonstrable within the cytoplasm of the tumor cells as well as in the stromal amyloid by immunohistochemical methods. Electron microscopy reveals variable numbers of membrane-bound electron-dense granules within the cytoplasm of the neoplastic cells (Fig. 24–23). One of the peculiar features of familial medullary cancers is the presence of multicentric **C-cell hyperplasia** in the surrounding thyroid parenchyma, a feature that is usually absent in sporadic lesions.[46] While the precise criteria for defining C-cell hyperplasia are not establisted, the presence of multiple prominent clusters of C cells scattered throughout the parenchyma should raise the specter of a familial tumor, even if that history is not explicitly present. Foci of C-cell hyperplasia are believed to represent the precursor lesions from which medullary carcinomas arise.

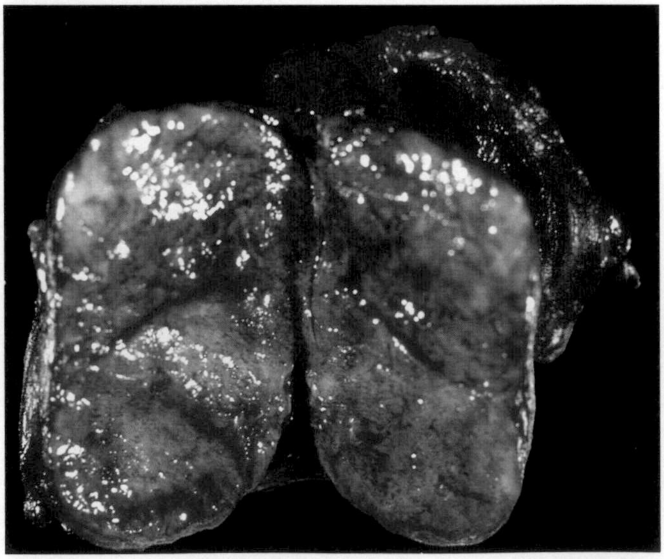

FIGURE 24–21 Medullary carcinoma of thyroid. These tumors typically show a solid pattern of growth and do not have connective tissue capsules. (Courtesy of Dr. Joseph Corson, Brigham and Women's Hospital, Boston, MA.)

Clinical Course. Sporadic cases of medullary carcinoma come to medical attention most often as a mass in the neck, sometimes associated with local effects such as dysphagia or

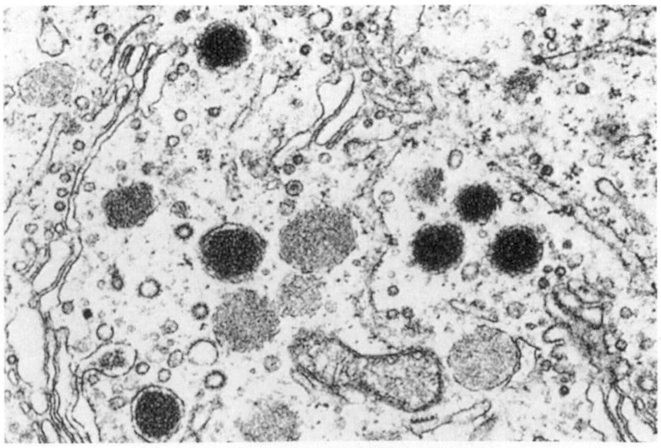

FIGURE 24–23 Electron micrograph of medullary thyroid carcinoma. These cells contain membrane-bound secretory granules that are the sites of storage of calcitonin and other peptides (30,000×).

hoarseness. In some instances, the initial manifestations are those of a paraneoplastic syndrome, caused by the secretion of a peptide hormone (e.g., diarrhea owing to the secretion of VIP). Notably, hypocalcemia is not a prominent feature, despite the presence of raised calcitonin levels. Screening of relatives for elevated calcitonin levels or *RET* mutations permits early detection of tumors in familial cases. As will be discussed later, all MEN-2 kindred carrying *RET* mutations are offered prophylactic thyroidectomy to preclude the development of medullary carcinomas, the major risk factor for poor outcome in these families. Sometimes, the only histologic finding in the resected thyroid of asymptomatic carriers is the presence of C-cell hyperplasia or small (<1 cm) "micromedullary" carcinomas.[47] Recent studies have shown that specific *RET* mutations correlate with the aggressiveness of medullary carcinomas and the propensity of MEN-2 patients to develop other coincident endocrine tumors.[48,49]

Anaplastic Carcinoma

Anaplastic carcinomas of the thyroid are undifferentiated tumors of the thyroid follicular epithelium. In striking contrast to the differentiated thyroid carcinomas, anaplastic carcinomas are aggressive tumors, with a mortality rate approaching 100%. These tumors account for fewer than 5% of all thyroid cancers. Patients with anaplastic carcinoma are older than those with other types of thyroid cancer, with a mean age of 65 years. About half of the patients have a history of multinodular goiter, whereas 20% of the patients with these tumors have a history of differentiated carcinoma, and another 20% to 30% have a concurrent differentiated thyroid tumor, frequently a papillary carcinoma. These findings have led to the proposal that anaplastic carcinoma develops by so-called dedifferentiation from more differentiated tumors as a result of one or more genetic changes, including the loss of the *p53* tumor suppressor gene.

Morphology. Microscopically, these neoplasms are composed of highly anaplastic cells, which may take one of several histologic patterns: (1) large, pleomorphic **giant** cells, including occasional osteoclast-like multinucleate giant cells; (2) **spindle** cells with a sarcomatous appearance; (3) **mixed** spindle and giant cells; and (4) **small** cells resembling those seen in small cell carcinomas arising at other sites. It is unlikely that a true small cell carcinoma exists in the thyroid, and a significant number of such "small cell" tumors have ultimately proven to be medullary carcinomas (discussed previously) or malignant lymphomas, which may also occur in the thyroid but have a much better prognosis. Foci of papillary or follicular differentiation may be present in some tumors, suggesting origin from a better differentiated carcinoma.

Clinical Course. Anaplastic carcinomas usually present as a rapidly enlarging bulky neck mass. In most cases, the disease has already spread beyond the thyroid capsule into adjacent neck structures or has metastasized to the lungs at the time of presentation. Compression and invasion symptoms, such as dyspnea, dysphagia, hoarseness, and cough, are common. There is no effective therapy for anaplastic thyroid carcinoma, and the disease is almost uniformly fatal. Although metastases to distant sites are common, in most cases death occurs in less than 1 year as a result of aggressive growth and compromise of vital structures in the neck.

Congenital Anomalies

Thyroglossal duct or cyst is the most common clinically significant congenital anomaly of the thyroid. A persistent sinus tract may remain as a vestigial remnant of the tubular development of the thyroid gland. Parts of this tube may be obliterated, leaving small segments to form cysts. These occur at any age and might not become evident until adult life. Mucinous, clear secretions may collect within these cysts to form either spherical masses or fusiform swellings, rarely over 2 to 3 cm in diameter. These are present in the midline of the neck anterior to the trachea. Segments of the duct and cysts that occur high in the neck are lined by stratified squamous epithelium, which is essentially identical with that covering the posterior portion of the tongue in the region of the foramen cecum. The anomalies that occur in the lower neck more proximal to the thyroid gland are lined by epithelium resembling the thyroidal acinar epithelium. Characteristically, subjacent to the lining epithelium, there is an intense lymphocytic infiltrate. Superimposed infection may convert these lesions into abscess cavities, and rarely, they give rise to cancers.

PARATHYROID GLANDS

Normal

The *parathyroid glands* are derived from the developing pharyngeal pouches that also give rise to the thymus. The four glands normally lie in close proximity to the upper and lower poles of each thyroid lobe but may also be found anywhere along the pathway of descent of the pharyngeal pouches, including the carotid sheath, the thymus, and elsewhere in the anterior mediastinum. Of note, 10% of individuals have only two or three glands.

In the adult, the parathyroid is a yellow-brown, ovoid encapsulated nodule weighing approximately 35 to 40 mg.

Most of the gland is composed of *chief cells*. The chief cells vary from light to dark pink with hematoxylin and eosin stains, depending on their glycogen content. They are polygonal; are 12 to 20 mm in diameter; and have central, round, uniform nuclei. In addition, they contain secretory granules of *parathyroid hormone (PTH)*. Sometimes, these cells have a *water-clear* appearance owing to lakes of glycogen. *Oxyphil cells* and transitional oxyphils are found throughout the normal parathyroid, either singly or in small clusters. They are slightly larger than the chief cells, have acidophilic cytoplasm, and are tightly packed with mitochondria. Glycogen granules are also present in these cells, but secretory granules are sparse or absent. In early infancy and childhood, the parathyroid glands are composed almost entirely of solid sheets of chief cells. The amount of stromal fat increases up to age 25, reaching a maximum of approximately 30% of the gland, and then plateaus. The precise proportion of fat is determined largely by constitutional factors; for instance, obese individuals have more adipose tissue in their glands.

The activity of the parathyroid glands is controlled by the level of free (ionized) calcium in the bloodstream rather than by trophic hormones secreted by the hypothalamus and pituitary. Normally, decreased levels of free calcium stimulate the synthesis and secretion of *PTH*. Circulating PTH is an 84-amino-acid linear polypeptide derived by sequential cleavage in the chief cell of a larger pre-pro form. Its biologic activity resides within the 34 residues at the amino terminus. Smaller nonfunctional fragments of the hormone, apparently lacking the critical amino-terminal domain, also circulate. These assume importance because, although they are biologically inert, they contain epitopes that react in certain radioimmunoassays for PTH.

The PTH receptor is a seven-transmembrane G-protein–coupled receptor. Binding of the hormone leads to activation of the stimulatory G-protein, G_s, causing adenylate cyclase–mediated generation of cAMP. *This pathway assumes clinical significance when abnormalities of the* G_s *protein result in either hyperactivity or hypoactivity of the parathyroid gland* (see below). The metabolic functions of PTH in supporting serum calcium levels can be summarized as follows:

- PTH activates osteoclasts, thereby mobilizing calcium from bone.
- It increases the renal tubular reabsorption of calcium, thereby conserving free calcium.
- It increases the conversion of vitamin D to its active dihydroxy form in the kidneys.
- It increases urinary phosphate excretion, thereby lowering serum phosphate levels.
- It augments gastrointestinal calcium absorption.

The net result of these activities is an increase in the level of free calcium, which, in turn, inhibits further PTH secretion in a classic feedback loop.

Hypercalcemia is one of a number of changes induced by elevated levels of PTH. As was discussed in Chapter 7, hypercalcemia is a relatively common complication of malignancy, occurring both with solid tumors, such as lung, breast, head and neck, and renal cancers, and with hematologic malignancies, notably multiple myeloma. In fact, *malignancy is the most common cause of clinically apparent hypercalcemia,* while primary hyperparathyroidism (see below) is a more common cause of asymptomatic elevated blood calcium. The prognosis of patients with malignancy-associated hypercalcemia is generally poor, in that it more frequently occurs in individuals with advanced cancers. Hypercalcemia of malignancy is due to increased bone resorption and subsequent release of calcium. There are two major mechanisms by which this can occur: (1) *osteolytic metastases and local release of cytokines* and (2) *release of PTH-related protein (PTHrP)*.

- *Osteolytic metastases:* Metastatic tumor cells, as well as stromal cells in the vicinity of the metastases, release a variety of soluble mediators that induce local osteolysis by promoting differentiation of committed osteoclast precursors into mature cells. Recently, a critical osteoclastogenic pathway has been discovered that involves the osteoblast cell-surface receptor *RANK* (receptor activator of nuclear factor κB), its ligand, *RANKL*, and a decoy receptor for RANKL, *osteoprotegerin*. (A *decoy receptor* is a soluble receptor that competes with the true receptor, in this case RANK, for binding the ligand of interest, in this case RANKL;[50] see Chapter 26.) RANKL is also known as "osteoclast differentiation factor," and by binding with the RANK receptor, it promotes all aspects of osteoclast function, including proliferation, differentiation, fusion, and activation. RANKL is secreted by tumor cells and peritumoral stromal cells in metastatic foci and causes osteolysis. Osteoprotegerin inhibits this pathway of osteoclastogenesis and has emerged as a possible therapeutic agent in cancer patients with hypercalcemia of malignancy.
- *PTH-related protein:* The most frequent cause of hypercalcemia in nonmetastatic solid tumors—particularly squamous cell cancers—is the release of PTHrP. This protein is immunologically distinct from PTH yet it is similar enough in structure to permit binding to identical receptors and simulation of second messengers, notably cAMP. This accounts for the ability of PTHrP to induce most of the actions of PTH, including increases in bone resorption and inhibition of proximal tubule phosphate transport.[51] Classically, PTHrP-induced hypercalcemia was known as "humoral hypercalcemia of malignancy" to distinguish it from hypercalcemia arising from osteolytic metastases. It is now recognized that a significant proportion of cancer patients with osteolytic metastases also have circulating PTHrP; therefore, PTHrP contributes to hypercalcemia of malignancy irrespective of the presence or absence of metastases.

Pathology

Similar to the other endocrine organs, abnormalities of the parathyroid glands include both hyperfunction and hypofunction. Tumors of the parathyroid glands, in contrast to thyroid tumors, usually come to attention because of excessive secretion of PTH rather than because of mass effects.

Hyperparathyroidism

Hyperparathyroidism occurs in two major forms—*primary* and *secondary*—and, less commonly, *tertiary*. The first condition represents an autonomous, spontaneous overproduction of PTH; the latter two conditions typically occur as secondary phenomena in patients with chronic renal insufficiency.

PRIMARY HYPERPARATHYROIDISM

Primary hyperparathyroidism is one of the most common endocrine disorders, and it is an important cause of *hypercalcemia*. The frequency of the various parathyroid lesions underlying the hyperfunction is as follows:

- Adenoma: 75% to 80%
- Primary hyperplasia (diffuse or nodular): 10% to 15%
- Parathyroid carcinoma: less than 5%

Primary hyperparathyroidism is usually a disease of adults and is more common in women than in men by a ratio of nearly 3:1. The annual incidence is now estimated to be about 25 cases per 100,000 in the United States and Europe; more cases are being detected due to the greater availability and use of advanced analyzers for measuring serum electrolytes.[52] Most cases occur in the fifties or later in life.

Studies have begun to provide a molecular understanding of the pathogenesis of primary hyperparathyroidism. *In more than 95% of cases, the disorder is caused by sporadic parathyroid adenomas or sporadic hyperplasia* (Fig. 24–24). Although familial syndromes are a distant second, they have provided a unique insight into the pathogenesis of primary hyperparathyroidism. The genetic syndromes associated with *familial primary hyperparathyroidism* include the following:

- *Multiple endocrine neoplasia-1 (MEN-1):* The *MEN1* gene on chromosome 11q13 is a tumor suppressor gene inactivated in a variety of MEN-1–related parathyroid lesions, including parathyroid adenomas and hyperplasia. In addition to familial cases, *MEN1* mutations have also been described in sporadic parathyroid tumors. The MEN-1 syndrome is discussed in further detail below.
- *Multiple endocrine neoplasia-2 (MEN-2):* The MEN-2 syndrome is caused by activating mutations in the tyrosine kinase receptor, *RET*, on chromosome 10q. Primary hyperparathyroidism occurs as a component of MEN-2A, which is discussed in further detail below. *RET* mutations have not been described in sporadic parathyroid lesions outside the context of MEN-2.
- *Familial hypocalciuric hypercalcemia* (FHH) is an autosomal-dominant disorder characterized by enhanced parathyroid function due to decreased sensitivity to extracellular calcium. Mutations in the parathyroid calcium-sensing receptor gene (*CASR*) on chromosome 3q are a primary cause for this disorder.[53] Patients with homozygous *CASR* mutations present in the neonatal period with severe hyperparathyroidism. *CASR* mutations have not been described in sporadic parathyroid tumors.

Most, if not all, *sporadic parathyroid adenomas* are monoclonal, suggesting that they are true neoplastic outgrowths from a single abnormal progenitor cell. Sporadic parathyroid hyperplasia is also monoclonal in many instances, particularly when associated with a persistent stimulus for parathyroid growth (refractory secondary or tertiary parathyroidism; see below). Among the sporadic adenomas, there are two molecular defects that have an established role in pathogenesis:[54]

- *Parathyroid adenoma 1 (PRAD1): PRAD1* encodes cyclin D1, a major regulator of the cell cycle. A pericentromeric inversion on chromosome 11 results in relocation of the *PRAD1* protooncogene (normally on 11q) so that it is positioned adjacent to the 5' flanking region of the *PTH* gene (on 11p). As a consequence of these changes, a regulatory element from the *PTH* gene 5' flanking sequence directs overexpression of cyclin D1 protein, forcing the cells to proliferate. Ten per cent to 20% of adenomas have this clonal genetic defect. In addition, cyclin D1 is overexpressed in approximately 40% of parathyroid adenomas, suggesting that mechanisms other than *PRAD1* inversion can lead to its activation.
- *MEN1:* Approximately 20% to 30% of parathyroid tumors not associated with the MEN-1 syndrome demonstrate mutations in both copies of the *MEN1* gene. The spectrum of *MEN1* mutations in the sporadic tumors is virtually identical to that in familial parathyroid adenomas.

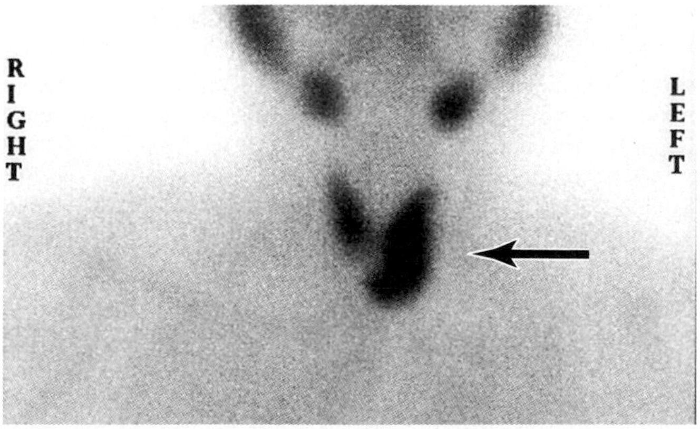

FIGURE 24–24 Parathyroid adenomas are almost always solitary lesions. Technetium-99m-sestamibi radionuclide scan demonstrates an area of increased uptake corresponding to the left inferior parathyroid gland *(arrow)*. This patient had a parathyroid adenoma. Preoperative scintigraphy is useful in localizing and distinguishing adenomas from parathyroid hyperplasia, where more than one gland would demonstrate increased uptake.

Morphology. The morphologic changes seen in primary hyperparathyroidism include those in the parathyroid glands as well as those in other organs affected by elevated levels of calcium. Parathyroid **adenomas** are almost always solitary and, similar to the normal parathyroid glands, may lie in close proximity to the thyroid gland or in an ectopic site (e.g., the mediastinum). The typical parathyroid adenoma averages 0.5 to 5.0 gm; is a well-circumscribed, soft, tan to reddish-brown nodule; and is invested by a delicate capsule (Fig. 24–25). In contrast to primary hyperplasia, the glands outside the adenoma are usually normal in size or somewhat shrunken because of feedback inhibition by elevations in serum calcium. Microscopically, parathyroid adenomas are often composed predominantly of fairly uniform, polygonal chief cells with small, centrally placed nuclei (see Fig. 24–25). In most cases, at least a few nests of larger cells containing oxyphil cells are present as well; uncommonly, entire adenomas may be composed of this cell type (**oxyphil adenomas**). The chief cells are

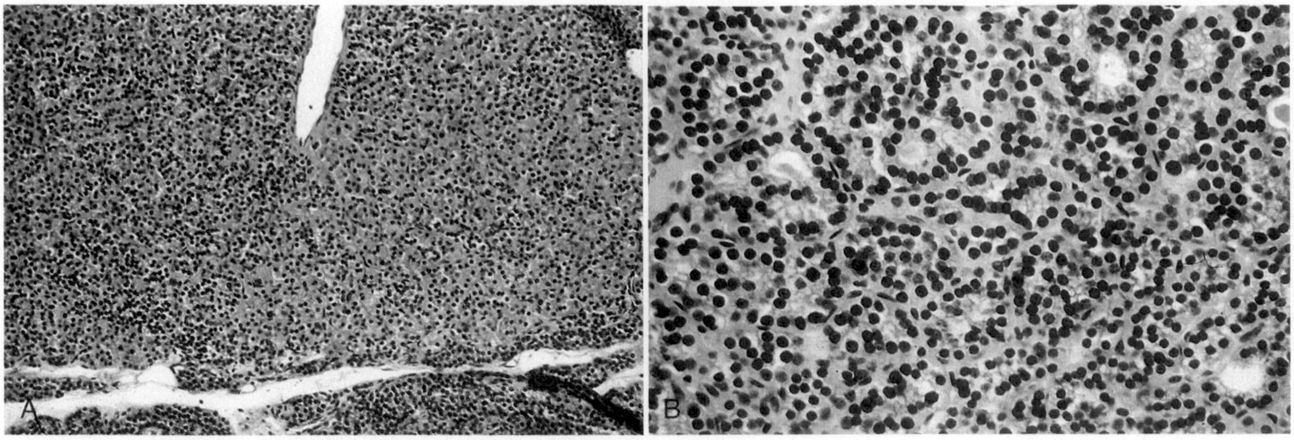

FIGURE 24–25 Parathyroid adenoma. *A*, Solitary chief cell parathyroid adenoma (low-power photomicrograph) revealing clear delineation from the residual gland below. *B*, High-power detail of a chief cell parathyroid adenoma. There is some slight variation in nuclear size but no anaplasia and some slight tendency to follicular formation.

arranged in a variety of patterns; follicles reminiscent of those seen in the thyroid are present in some cases. Mitotic figures are rare. A rim of compressed, non-neoplastic parathyroid tissue, generally separated by a fibrous capsule, is often visible at the edge of the adenoma. It is not uncommon to find bizarre and pleomorphic nuclei even within adenomas (so-called endocrine atypia), and this should not be used as a criterion for defining malignancy. In contrast to the normal parathyroid parenchyma, adipose tissue is inconspicuous within the adenoma.

Primary hyperplasia may occur sporadically or as a component of MEN syndrome. Although classically all four glands are involved, there is frequently asymmetry with apparent sparing of one or two glands, making the distinction between hyperplasia and adenoma difficult. The combined weight of all glands rarely exceeds 1.0 gm and is often less. Microscopically, the most common pattern seen is that of chief cell hyperplasia, which may involve the glands in a diffuse or multinodular pattern. Less commonly, the constituent cells contain abundant water-clear cells ("water-clear cell hyperplasia"). In many instances, there are islands of oxyphils, and poorly developed, delicate fibrous strands may envelop the nodules. As in the case of adenomas, stromal fat is inconspicuous within the foci of hyperplasia.

Parathyroid carcinomas may be fairly circumscribed lesions that are difficult to distinguish from adenomas, or they may be clearly invasive neoplasms. These tumors enlarge one parathyroid gland and consist of gray-white, irregular masses that sometimes exceed 10 gm in weight. The cells of parathyroid carcinomas are usually uniform and resemble normal parathyroid cells. They are arrayed in nodular or trabecular patterns with a dense, fibrous capsule enclosing the mass. There is general agreement that a **diagnosis of carcinoma based on cytologic detail is unreliable, and invasion of surrounding tissues and metastasis are the only reliable criteria of malignancy.** Local recurrence occurs in one third of cases, and more distant dissemination occurs in another third.

Morphologic changes in other organs deserving special mention include skeletal and renal lesions. **Skeletal changes** include prominence of osteoclasts, which, in turn, erode bone matrix and mobilize calcium salts, particularly in the metaphyses of long tubular bones (Chapter 26). Bone resorption is accompanied by increased osteoblastic activity and the formation of new bone trabeculae. In many cases, the resultant bone contains widely spaced, delicate trabeculae reminiscent of those seen in osteoporosis. In more severe cases, the cortex is grossly thinned, and the marrow contains increased amounts of fibrous tissue accompanied by foci of hemorrhage and cyst formation **(osteitis fibrosa cystica)**. Aggregates of osteoclasts, reactive giant cells, and hemorrhagic debris occasionally form masses that may be mistaken for neoplasms (**brown tumors** of hyperparathyroidism). PTH-induced hypercalcemia favors formation of **urinary tract stones** (nephrolithiasis) as well as calcification of the renal interstitium and tubules (nephrocalcinosis). Metastatic calcification secondary to hypercalcemia may also be seen in other sites, including the stomach, lungs, myocardium, and blood vessels.

Clinical Course. Primary hyperparathyroidism presents in one of two general ways: (1) It may be asymptomatic and be identified after a routine chemistry profile, or (2) patients may have the classic clinical manifestations of primary hyperparathyroidism.[52]

Asymptomatic Hyperparathyroidism. Because serum calcium levels are routinely assessed in the work-up of most patients who need blood tests for unrelated conditions, clinically silent hyperparathyroidism is often detected early. Hence, many of the classic clinical manifestations, particularly those referable to bone and renal disease, are now seen infrequently in clinical practice. The *most common manifestation of primary hyperparathyroidism is an increase in the level of serum ionized calcium*; in fact, primary hyperparathyroidism is the most common cause of *asymptomatic* hypercalcemia. It should be recalled that other conditions also produce hypercalcemia (Table 24–5). Malignancy, in particular, is the most common cause of *clinically apparent* hypercalcemia in adults and must be excluded by appropriate clinical and laboratory investigations in patients with suspected hyperparathy-

TABLE 24–5 Causes of Hypercalcemia

Raised PTH	Decreased PTH
Hyperparathyroidism Primary (adenoma > hyperplasia)* Secondary† Tertiary†	Hypercalcemia of malignancy Osteolytic metastases (RANKL-mediated) PTH-rP–mediated Vitamin D toxicity
Familial hypocalciuric hypercalcemia	Immobilization Thiazide diuretics Granulomatous disease (sarcoidosis)

*Primary hyperparathyroidism is the most common cause of hypercalcemia overall. Malignancy is the most common cause of *symptomatic* hypercalcemia. Primary hyperparathyroidism and malignancy account for nearly 90% of cases of hypercalcemia.

†Secondary and tertiary hyperparathyroidism are most commonly associated with progressive renal failure.

PTH-rP, Parathyroid hormone–related protein. RANKL, Receptor activator of nuclear factor κB ligand.

roidism. *In patients with primary hyperparathyroidism, serum PTH levels are inappropriately elevated for the level of serum calcium, whereas PTH levels are low to undetectable in hypercalcemia because of nonparathyroid diseases* (see Table 24–5). In patients with hypercalcemia caused by secretion of PTHrP by certain nonparathyroid tumors, radioimmunoassays specific for PTH and PTHrP can distinguish between the two molecules. Other laboratory alterations referable to PTH excess include hypophosphatemia and increased urinary excretion of both calcium and phosphate. Secondary renal disease may lead to phosphate retention with normalization of serum phosphates.

Symptomatic Primary Hyperparathyroidism. The signs and symptoms of hyperparathyroidism reflect the combined effects of increased PTH secretion and hypercalcemia. Primary hyperparathyroidism has been traditionally associated with a constellation of symptoms that included "painful bones, renal stones, abdominal groans, and psychic moans" (Fig. 24–26). The symptomatic presentation involves a diversity of clinical manifestations:

- *Bone disease* includes bone pain secondary to fractures of bones weakened by osteoporosis or osteitis fibrosa cystica.
- *Nephrolithiasis* (renal stones) occurs in 20% of newly diagnosed patients, with attendant pain and obstructive uropathy. Chronic renal insufficiency and a variety of abnormalities in renal function are found, including polyuria and secondary polydipsia.
- Gastrointestinal disturbances include constipation, nausea, peptic ulcers, pancreatitis, and gallstones.
- Central nervous system alterations include depression, lethargy, and eventually seizures.
- Neuromuscular abnormalities include complaints of weakness and fatigue.
- Cardiac manifestations include aortic or mitral valve calcifications (or both).

The abnormalities most directly related to hyperparathyroidism are nephrolithiasis and bone disease, whereas those attributable to hypercalcemia include fatigue, weakness, and constipation. The pathogenesis of many of the other manifestations of the disorder remains poorly understood.

SECONDARY HYPERPARATHYROIDISM

Secondary hyperparathyroidism is caused by any condition associated with a chronic depression in the serum calcium level because low serum calcium leads to compensatory overactivity of the parathyroid glands.[55] *Renal failure is by far the most common cause of secondary hyperparathyroidism,* although a number of other diseases, including inadequate dietary intake of calcium, steatorrhea, and vitamin D deficiency, may also cause this disorder. The mechanisms by which

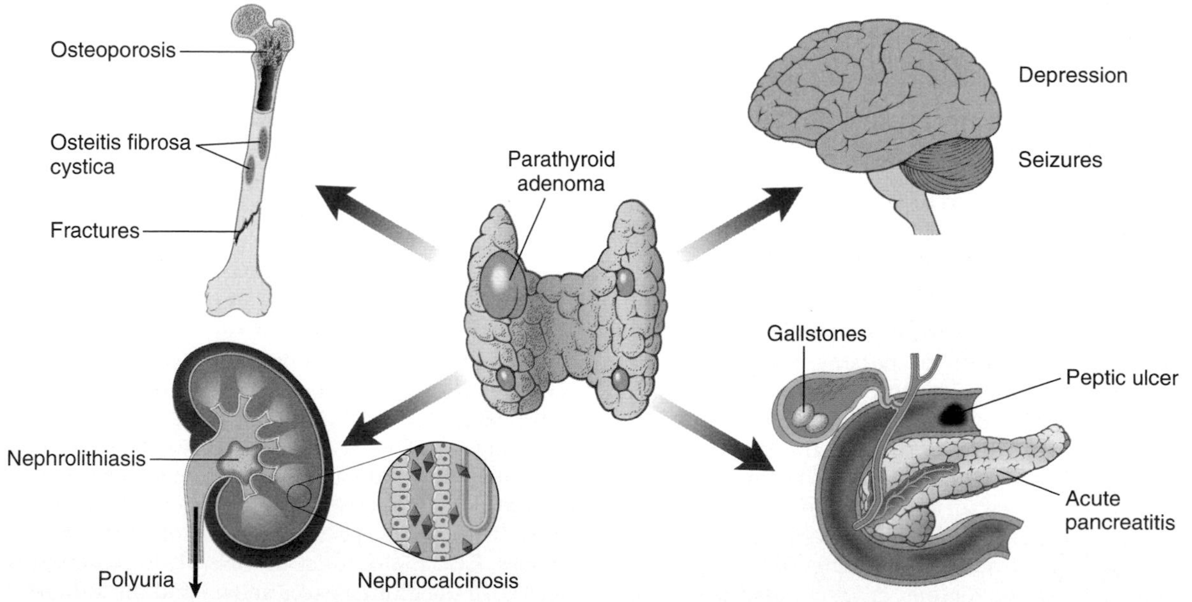

FIGURE 24–26 Cardinal features of hyperparathyroidism. With routine evaluation of calcium levels in most patients, primary hyperparathyroidism is often detected at a clinically silent stage. Hypercalcemia from any other cause can also give rise to the same symptoms.

chronic renal failure induces secondary hyperparathyroidism are complex and not fully understood. Chronic renal insufficiency is associated with decreased phosphate excretion, which in turn results in hyperphosphatemia. The elevated serum phosphate levels directly depress serum calcium levels and thereby stimulate parathyroid gland activity. In addition, loss of renal substance reduces the availability of α-1-hydroxylase necessary for the synthesis of the active form of vitamin D, which in turn reduces intestinal absorption of calcium (Chapter 9).

Morphology. The **parathyroid glands in secondary hyperparathyroidism are hyperplastic.** As in the case of primary hyperplasia, the degree of glandular enlargement is not necessarily symmetric. Microscopically, the hyperplastic glands contain an increased number of chief cells, or cells with more abundant, clear cytoplasm (so-called water-clear cells) in a diffuse or multinodular distribution. Fat cells are decreased in number. **Bone changes** similar to those seen in primary hyperparathyroidism may also be present. **Metastatic calcification** may be seen in many tissues, including lungs, heart, stomach, and blood vessels.

Clinical Course. The clinical features of secondary hyperparathyroidism are usually dominated by those associated with chronic renal failure. Bone abnormalities (renal osteodystrophy) and other changes associated with PTH excess are, in general, less severe than are those seen in primary hyperparathyroidism. The vascular calcification associated with secondary hyperparathyroidism may occasionally result in significant ischemic damage to skin and other organs, a process sometimes referred to as *calciphylaxis*. In a minority of patients, parathyroid activity may become autonomous and excessive, with resultant hypercalcemia, a process that is sometimes termed *tertiary hyperparathyroidism*. Parathyroidectomy may be necessary to control the hyperparathyroidism in such patients.

Hypoparathyroidism

Hypoparathyroidism is far less common than is hyperparathyroidism. There are many possible causes of deficient PTH secretion resulting in hypoparathyroidism:

- *Surgically induced* hypoparathyroidism occurs with inadvertent removal of all the parathyroid glands during thyroidectomy, excision of the parathyroid glands in the mistaken belief that they are lymph nodes during radical neck dissection for some form of malignant disease, or removal of too large a proportion of parathyroid tissue in the treatment of primary hyperparathyroidism.
- *Congenital absence* of all glands, as in certain developmental abnormalities, such as thymic aplasia and cardiac defects (22q11.2 syndrome) (see Chapter 5).
- *Familial hypoparathyroidism* is often associated with chronic mucocutaneous candidiasis and primary adrenal insufficiency; this syndrome is known as autoimmune polyendocrine syndrome type 1 (APS1) and is caused by mutations in the *autoimmune regulator* (*AIRE*) gene.[56] The syndrome typically presents in childhood with the onset of candidiasis, followed several years later by hypoparathyroidism and then adrenal insufficiency during adolescence. APS1 is discussed further in the section on adrenal glands.
- *Idiopathic hypoparathyroidism* most likely represents an autoimmune disease with isolated atrophy of the glands. Sixty per cent of the patients with this disorder have autoantibodies directed against the calcium-sensing receptor (CASR) in the parathyroid gland.[57] Antibody binding to the receptor may prevent the release of PTH.

The major clinical manifestations of hypoparathyroidism are referable to hypocalcemia and are related to the severity and chronicity of the hypocalcemia.

- The hallmark of hypocalcemia is *tetany*, which is characterized by *neuromuscular irritability*, resulting from decreased serum ionized calcium concentration. These findings can range from circumoral numbness or paresthesias (tingling) of the distal extremities and carpopedal spasm, to life-threatening laryngospasm and generalized seizures. The classic findings on physical examination of patients with neuromuscular irritability are *Chvostek sign* and *Trousseau sign*. Chvostek sign is elicited in subclinical disease by tapping along the course of the facial nerve, which induces contractions of the muscles of the eye, mouth, or nose. Occluding the circulation to the forearm and hand by inflating a blood pressure cuff about the arm for several minutes induces carpal spasm, which disappears as soon as the cuff is deflated (Trousseau sign).
- *Mental status changes* can include emotional instability, anxiety and depression, confusional states, hallucinations, and frank psychosis.
- *Intracranial manifestations* include calcifications of the basal ganglia, parkinsonian-like movement disorders, and increased intracranial pressure with resultant papilledema.
- *Ocular disease* results in calcification of the lens leading to cataract formation.
- *Cardiovascular manifestations* include a conduction defect, which produces a characteristic prolongation of the QT interval in the electrocardiogram.
- *Dental abnormalities* occur when hypocalcemia is present during early development. These findings are highly characteristic of hypoparathyroidism and include dental hypoplasia, failure of eruption, defective enamel and root formation, and abraded carious teeth.

Pseudohypoparathyroidism

In this condition, hypoparathyroidism occurs because of end-organ resistance to the actions of PTH. Indeed, serum PTH levels are normal or elevated. Central to the understanding of PTH resistance are two key concepts: (1) G-proteins, principally G_s, mediate the cellular actions of PTH on bone and kidney, and (2) *GNAS1* is a selectively imprinted gene, with tissue-specific patterns of imprinting.[58] In most tissues, $G_s\alpha$, the product of GNAS1, is expressed from both alleles. In the pituitary (see above) and the kidneys, GNAS1 is expressed only from the maternally inherited chromosome, owing to paternal imprinting (silencing) of the gene. As a result, a mutation that affects the maternal allele results in complete loss of $G_s\alpha$ expression in the kidney, while a mutation in the normally unexpressed paternal allele has no effect on $G_s\alpha$ levels; in contrast, a mutation of either allele will produce a 50% decrease in $G_s\alpha$ in tissues other than the kidneys and pituitary, since GNAS1 is expressed from both copies of the gene. Two types of pseudohypoparathyroidism have been identified depending on the parent of origin of the mutant allele:

1. *Pseudohypoparathyroidism type 1A* is associated with multihormone resistance and Albright hereditary osteodystrophy (AHO), a syndrome characterized by skeletal and developmental defects. Patients with AHO often have short stature, obesity, short metacarpal and metatarsal bones, and variable mental deficits. *The multihormone resistance involves three hormones (PTH, TSH, and LH/FSH), all of which activate $G_s\alpha$-mediated pathways in target tissues.* The PTH resistance is the most obvious clinical manifestation, presenting as hypocalcemia, hyperphosphatemia, and elevated circulating PTH. TSH resistance is generally mild, while LH/FSH resistance manifests as hypergonadotropic hypogonadism in females. *The mutation in this disorder is inherited on the maternal allele,* severely impeding the actions of PTH on the kidney in maintaining calcium homeostasis.
2. *Pseudopseudohypoparathyroidism:* In this disorder, *the mutation is inherited on the paternal allele,* and it is characterized by AHO *without* accompanying multihormonal resistance. As a result, serum calcium, phosphate and PTH levels are normal.

THE ENDOCRINE PANCREAS

Normal

The endocrine pancreas consists of about 1 million microscopic clusters of cells, the islets of Langerhans. The first evidence of islet formation in the human fetus is seen at 9 to 11 weeks. Embryologically, both endocrine and exocrine components of the pancreas are endodermal derivatives. Several transcription factors have now been identified that determine lineage specification (i.e., endocrine versus exocrine) in the developing pancreas. For example, expression of the transcription factor *neurogenin 3* (*Ngn3*) delineates endocrine progenitors that eventually give rise to mature islet cells.[59]

In aggregate, the islets in the adult human weigh only 1 to 1.5 gm; individually, most islets measure 100 to 200 μm and consist of four major and two minor cell types. The four main types are β, α, δ, and PP (pancreatic polypeptide) cells. These make up about 68%, 20%, 10%, and 2%, respectively, of the adult islet cell population. They can be differentiated morphologically by their staining properties, by the ultrastructural characteristics of their granules, and by their hormone content (see Fig. 24–27).

The β cell produces insulin, as will be detailed in the discussion of diabetes. The insulin-containing intracellular granules contain a crystalline matrix with a rectangular profile, surrounded by a halo. *The α cell secretes glucagon,* inducing hyperglycemia by its glycogenolytic activity in the liver. α-cell granules are round, with closely applied membranes and a dense center. *δ cells contain somatostatin,* which suppresses both insulin and glucagon release; they have large, pale granules with closely applied membranes. *PP cells contain a unique pancreatic polypeptide* that exerts a number of gastrointestinal effects, such as stimulation of secretion of gastric and intestinal enzymes and inhibition of intestinal motility. These cells have small, dark granules and not only are present in islets, but also are scattered in the exocrine pancreas.

The two rare cell types are *D1 cells* and *enterochromaffin cells.* D1 cells elaborate *vasoactive intestinal polypeptide (VIP),* a hormone that induces glycogenolysis and hyperglycemia; it also stimulates gastrointestinal fluid secretion and causes secretory diarrhea. *Enterochromaffin cells synthesize serotonin* and are the source of pancreatic tumors that cause the carcinoid syndrome (Chapter 17).

Pathology

We now turn to the two main disorders of islet cells: diabetes mellitus and pancreatic endocrine tumors.

Diabetes Mellitus

Diabetes mellitus (DM) is not a single disease entity, but rather a *group of metabolic disorders sharing the common underlying feature of hyperglycemia.* Hyperglycemia in diabetes results from defects in insulin secretion, insulin action, or, most commonly, both. The chronic hyperglycemia and attendant metabolic dysregulation may be associated with secondary damage in multiple organ systems, especially the kidneys, eyes, nerves, and blood vessels. Diabetes affects an estimated 16 million people in the United States, as many as half of whom are undiagnosed. Each year, an additional 800,000 individuals develop diabetes in this country, and 54,000 die from diabetes-related causes. Diabetes is a leading cause of end-stage renal disease, adult-onset blindness, and nontraumatic lower extremity amputations in the United States. For individuals born in the United States in 2000, the estimated lifetime risk of being diagnosed with diabetes mellitus is 1 in 3 for males and 2 in 5 for females.[60] The risk is 2 to 5 times higher in the African-American, Hispanic, and Native American communities, compared to non-Hispanic whites. Worldwide, more than 140 million people suffer from diabetes, making this one of the most common noncommunicable diseases.[61] The number of affected individuals with diabetes is expected to double by 2025. The countries with the largest number of diabetics are India, China, and the United States.

DIAGNOSIS

Blood glucose values are normally maintained in a very narrow range, usually 70 to 120 mg/dL. The diagnosis of diabetes is established by noting elevation of blood glucose by any one of three criteria:

1. A random glucose > 200 mg/dL, with classical signs and symptoms (discussed below)
2. A fasting glucose > 126 mg/dL on more than one occasion
3. An abnormal oral glucose tolerance test (OGTT), in which the glucose is > 200 mg/dL 2 hours after a standard carbohydrate load

Levels of blood glucose proceed along a continuum. Individuals with fasting glucoses less than 110 mg/dL, or less than 140 mg/dL following an OGTT, are considered to be euglycemic. However, those with fasting glucoses greater than 110 but less than 126, or OGTT values greater than 140 but less than 200, are considered to have impaired glucose tolerance (IGT).[62] Individuals with IGT have a significant risk of progressing to overt diabetes over time, with up to 5% to 10% advancing to DM per year. In addition, those with IGT are at risk for cardiovascular disease, due to the abnormal carbohydrate metabolism as well as the co-existence of other risk factors such as low HDL, hypertriglyceridemia, and increased plasminogen activator inhibitor-1 (PAI-1) (see Chapter 11).

CLASSIFICATION

Although all forms of diabetes mellitus share hyperglycemia as a common feature, the pathogenic processes involved in the development of hyperglycemia vary widely. The previous classification schemes of diabetes mellitus were based on the age at onset of the disease or on the mode of therapy; in contrast, the recently revised classification reflects our greater understanding of the pathogenesis of each variant (Table 24–6).[62] *The vast majority of cases of diabetes fall into one of two broad classes:*

Type 1 diabetes is characterized by an absolute deficiency of insulin caused by pancreatic β-cell destruction. It accounts for approximately 10% of all cases.

Type 2 diabetes is caused by a combination of peripheral resistance to insulin action and an inadequate secretory response by the pancreatic β-cells ("relative insulin deficiency"). Approximately 80% to 90% of patients have type 2 diabetes.

A variety of monogenic and secondary causes are responsible for the remaining cases, and these will be discussed later. It should be stressed that while the major types of diabetes have different pathogenic mechanisms, *the long-term complications in kidneys, eyes, nerves, and blood vessels are the same, as are the principal causes of morbidity and death.* The pathogenesis of the two major types is discussed separately, but first we briefly review normal insulin secretion and the mechanism of insulin signaling, since these aspects are critical to understanding the pathogenesis of diabetes.

TABLE 24–6 Classification of Diabetes Mellitus

1. Type 1 diabetes (β-cell destruction, leads to absolute insulin deficiency)
Immune-mediated
Idiopathic
2. Type 2 diabetes (insulin resistance with relative insulin deficiency)
3. Genetic defects of β-cell function
Maturity-onset diabetes of the young (MODY), caused by mutations in:
Hepatocyte nuclear factor 4α [HNF-4α] (MODY1)
Glucokinase (MODY2)
Hepatocyte nuclear factor 1α [HNF-1α] (MODY3)
Insulin promoter factor [IPF-1] (MODY4)
Hepatocyte nuclear factor 1β [HNF-1β] (MODY5)
Neurogenic differentiation factor 1 [Neuro D1] (MODY6)
Mitochondrial DNA mutations
4. Genetic defects in insulin processing or insulin action
Defects in proinsulin conversion
Insulin gene mutations
Insulin receptor mutations
5. Exocrine pancreatic defects
Chronic pancreatitis
Pancreatectomy
Neoplasia
Cystic fibrosis
Hemachromatosis
Fibrocalculous pancreatopathy
6. Endocrinopathies
Acromegaly
Cushing syndrome
Hyperthyroidism
Pheochromocytoma
Glucagonoma
7. Infections
Cytomegalovirus
Coxsackie virus B
8. Drugs
Glucocorticoids
Thyroid hormone
α-interferon
Protease inhibitors
β-adrenergic agonists
Thiazides
Nicotinic acid
Phenytoin
9. Genetic syndromes associated with diabetes
Down syndrome
Kleinfelter syndrome
Turner syndrome
10. Gestational diabetes mellitus

Data from the Report of the Expert Committee on the Diagnosis and Classification of Diabetes Mellitus. Diabetic Care 25 (suppl. 1):S5—S20, 2002.

NORMAL INSULIN PHYSIOLOGY

Normal glucose homeostasis is tightly regulated by three interrelated processes: glucose production in the liver; glucose uptake and utilization by peripheral tissues, chiefly skeletal muscle; and actions of insulin and counter-regulatory hormones, including glucagon, on glucose.

Insulin and glucagon have opposing regulatory effects on glucose homeostasis. During fasting states, low insulin and high glucagon levels facilitate hepatic gluconeogenesis and glycogenolysis (glycogen breakdown) while decreasing glycogen synthesis, thereby preventing hypoglycemia. Thus, fasting plasma glucose levels are determined primarily by hepatic glucose output. Following a meal, insulin levels rise and glucagon levels fall in response to the large glucose load. Insulin promotes glucose uptake and utilization in tissues (discussed later). The skeletal muscle is the major insulin-responsive site for postprandial glucose utilization, and is critical for preventing hyperglycemia and maintaining glucose homeostasis.

Regulation of Insulin Release

The insulin gene is expressed in the β cells of the pancreatic islets (Fig. 24–27). Preproinsulin is synthesized in the rough endoplasmic reticulum from insulin mRNA and delivered to the Golgi apparatus. There, a series of proteolytic cleavage steps generate the mature insulin and a cleavage peptide, C-peptide. Both insulin and C-peptide are then stored in secretory granules and secreted in equimolar quantities after physiologic stimulation; increasingly, C-peptide levels are being used as a clinical assay to measure endogenous insulin secretion.

The most important stimulus that triggers insulin synthesis and release is glucose itself. A rise in blood glucose levels results in glucose uptake into pancreatic β cells, facilitated by an insulin-independent, glucose-transporting protein, GLUT-2 (Fig. 24–28).[63] Metabolism of glucose via glycolysis generates ATP, resulting in increase in cytoplasmic ATP/ADP ratios. This inhibits the activity of the ATP-sensitive K^+-channel on the β-cell membrane, leading to membrane depolarization and the influx of extracellular Ca^{2+} through voltage-dependent Ca^{2+}-channels.[64] The resultant increase in intracellular Ca^{2+} stimulates secretion of insulin, presumably from stored hormone within the β-cell granules. This is the phase of *immediate release of insulin.* If the secretory stimulus persists, a delayed and protracted response follows that involves *active synthesis of insulin.* Other agents, including intestinal hormones and certain amino acids (leucine and arginine), stimulate insulin release but not synthesis.

Insulin Action and Insulin Signaling Pathways

Insulin is the most potent anabolic hormone known, with multiple synthetic and growth-promoting effects (Fig. 24–29). *Its principal metabolic function is to increase the rate of glucose transport into certain cells in the body.* These are the *striated*

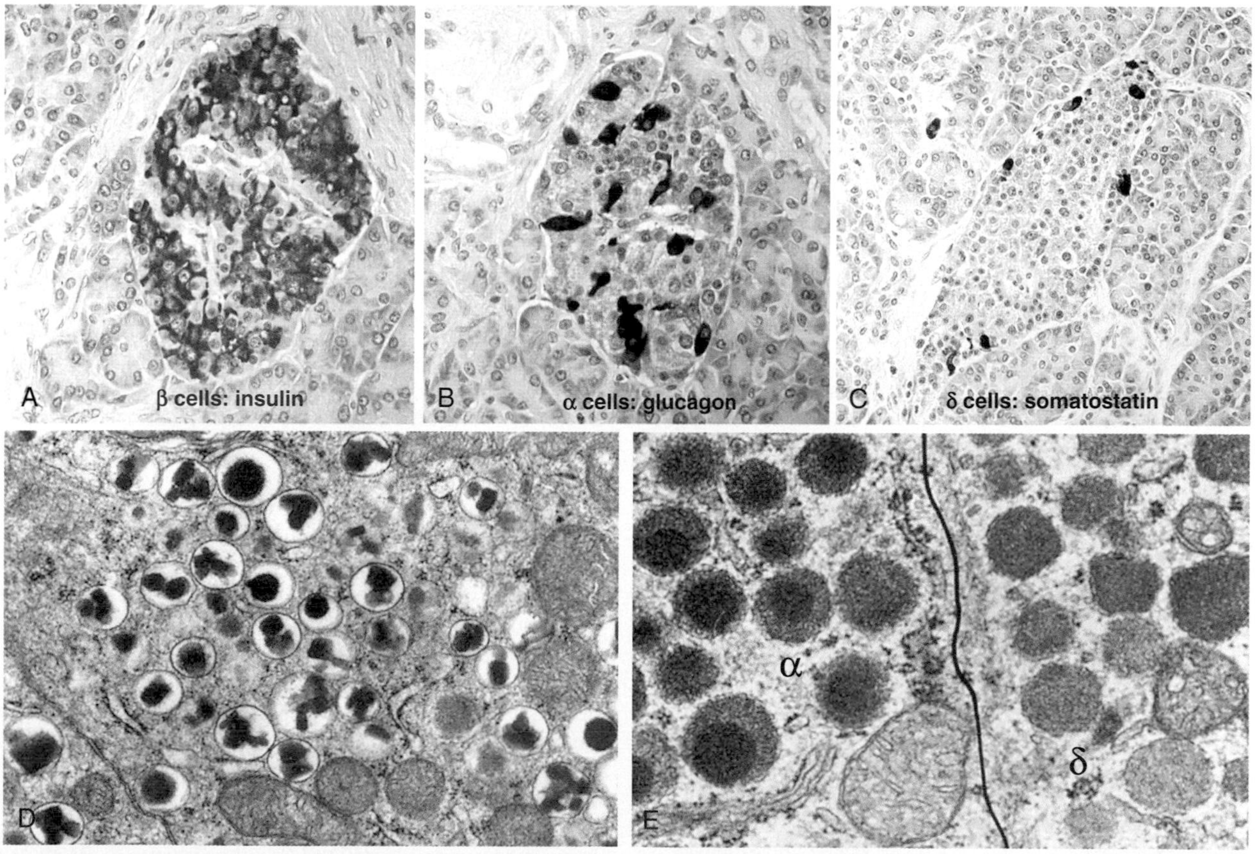

FIGURE 24–27 Hormone production in pancreatic islet cells. Immunoperoxidase staining shows a dark reaction product for insulin in β cells (*A*), glucagon in α cells (*B*), and somatostatin in δ cells (*C*). *D*, Electron micrograph of a β cell shows the characteristic membrane-bound granules, each containing a dense, often rectangular core and distinct halo. *E*, Portions of an α cell (*left*) and a δ cell (*right*) also exhibit granules, but with closely apportioned membranes. The α-cell granule exhibits a dense, round center. (Electron micrographs courtesy of Dr. A. Like, University of Massachusetts Medical School, Worcester, MA.)

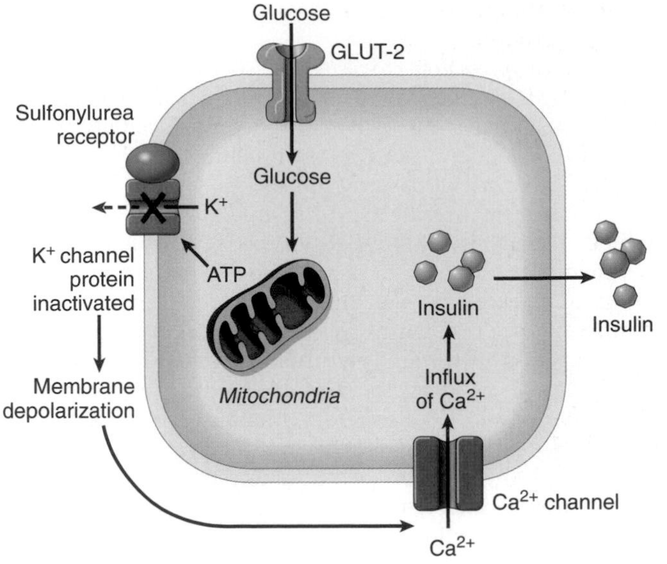

FIGURE 24–28 Insulin synthesis and secretion. Intracellular transport of glucose is mediated by GLUT-2, an insulin-independent glucose transporter in β cells. Glucose undergoes oxidative metabolism in the β cell to yield ATP. ATP inhibits an inward rectifying potassium channel receptor on the β-cell surface; the receptor itself is a dimeric complex of the sulfonylurea receptor and a K^+-channel protein. Inhibition of this receptor leads to membrane depolarization, influx of Ca^{2+} ions, and release of stored insulin from β cells.

muscle cells (including myocardial cells) and to a lesser extent, *adipocytes*, representing collectively about two thirds of the entire body weight. Glucose uptake in other peripheral tissues, most notably the brain, is insulin-independent. In muscle cells, glucose is then either stored as glycogen or oxidized to generate ATP. In adipose tissue, glucose is primarily stored as lipid. Besides promoting lipid synthesis, insulin also inhibits lipid degradation in adipocytes. Similarly, insulin promotes amino acid uptake and protein synthesis, while inhibiting protein degradation. *Thus, the anabolic effects of insulin are attributable to increased synthesis and reduced degradation of glycogen, lipids, and proteins.* In addition, insulin has several *mitogenic* functions, including initiation of DNA synthesis in certain cells and stimulation of their growth and differentiation.

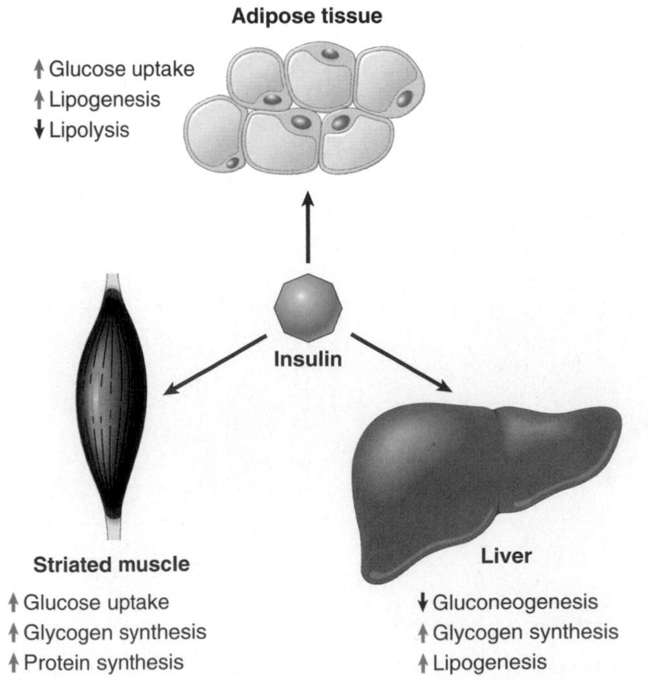

FIGURE 24–29 Metabolic actions of insulin in striated muscle, adipose tissue, and liver.

The binding of insulin to its receptor triggers a complex signaling cascade of *protein phosphorylation* and *dephosphorylation* culminating in the metabolic and mitogenic effects of insulin described above. Elucidation of the insulin signaling pathway has been central to our understanding of the mechanisms underlying insulin resistance in diabetes (see below). The complete description of this intricate network is beyond the scope of this book,[65] and we will only summarize some of the more pertinent mediators (Fig. 24–30). The *insulin receptor* is a tetrameric protein composed of two α- and two β-subunits. The β-subunit cytosolic domain possesses tyrosine kinase activity. Insulin binding to the α-subunit extracellular domain activates the β-subunit tyrosine kinase, resulting in both autophosphorylation of the receptor and phosphorylation of downstream signal transduction elements. For the sake of simplicity, we can separate the signaling pathways into two broad functional categories, *mitogenic* and *metabolic*, with the understanding that there may be considerable cross-talk between the protein intermediaries. The mitogen-activated protein kinase (MAPK) pathway[66] is responsible for the *mitogenic effects* of insulin (and insulin-like growth factors), promoting cellular proliferation and growth. The *metabolic effects* of insulin are principally mediated by phosphatidylinositol-3-kinase (PI-3K). PI-3K-dependent signaling mediates several of the cellular effects of insulin described above and summarized in Figure 24–30.[67,68]

PATHOGENESIS OF TYPE 1 DIABETES MELLITUS

This form of diabetes results from a severe lack of insulin caused by an immunologically mediated destruction of β cells. Type 1 diabetes most commonly develops in childhood, becomes manifest at puberty, and progresses with age. Since the disease can develop at any age, including late adulthood, the appellation "juvenile diabetes" is now considered obsolete. Similarly, the older moniker "insulin-dependent diabetes mellitus" (IDDM) has been excluded from the recent classification of diabetes to reflect the emphasis on pathogenic mechanisms rather than mode of therapy.[62] Nevertheless, most patients depend on insulin for survival; without insulin, they develop serious metabolic complications such as acute ketoacidosis and coma. A rare form of "idiopathic" type 1 diabetes has been described in which the evidence for autoimmunity is not definitive. Here we will focus on the typical immune-mediated type 1 diabetes.

Type 1 diabetes is an autoimmune disease in which islet destruction is caused primarily by T lymphocytes reacting against as yet poorly defined β-cell antigens. As in all autoimmune diseases, genetic susceptibility and environmental factors play important roles in the pathogenesis (Chapter 6). We first describe the mechanisms of β-cell destruction and

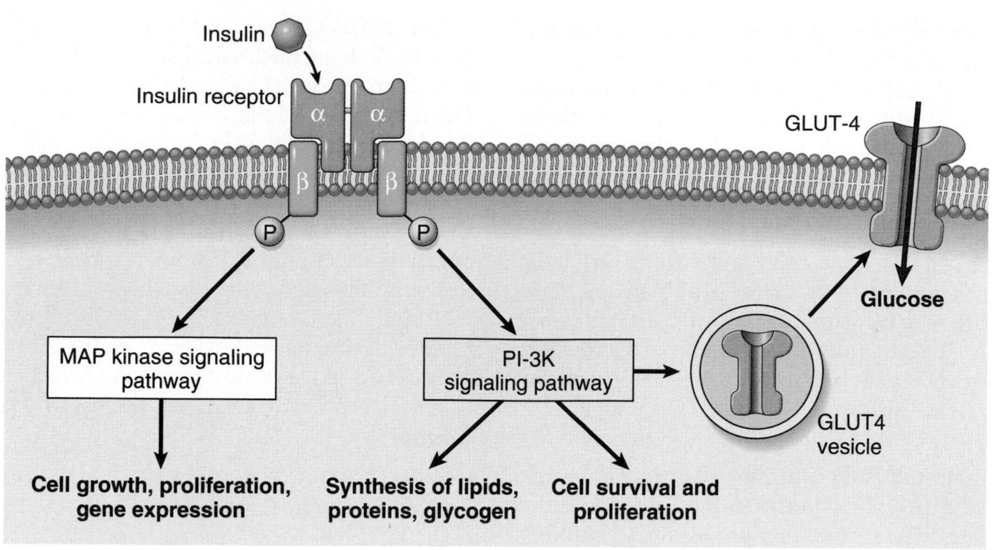

FIGURE 24–30 Insulin action on a target cell. Insulin binds to the α subunit of insulin receptor, leading to activation of the kinase activity in the β-subunit, and sets in motion a phosphorylation (i.e., activation) cascade of multiple downstream target proteins. The mitogenic functions of insulin (and the related insulin-like growth factors) are mediated via the mitogen-activated protein kinase (MAP kinase) pathway. The metabolic actions of insulin are mediated primarily by activation of the phosphatidylinositol-3-kinase (PI-3K) pathway. The PI-3K–signaling pathway is responsible for a variety of effects on target cells, including translocation of GLUT-4 containing vesicles to the surface; increasing GLUT-4 density on the membrane and rate of glucose influx; promoting glycogen synthesis via activation of glycogen synthase; and promoting protein synthesis and lipogenesis, while inhibiting lipolysis. The PI-3K pathway also promotes cell survival and proliferation.

then discuss the current ideas about the factors that trigger autoimmune attack against these cells.

Mechanisms of β Cell Destruction

Although the clinical onset of type 1 diabetes is abrupt, this disease in fact results from a chronic autoimmune attack on β cells that usually starts many years before the disease becomes evident (Fig. 24–31). The classic manifestations of the disease (hyperglycemia and ketosis) occur late in its course, after more than 90% of the β cells have been destroyed.

Several mechanisms contribute to β cell destruction:[69]

- *T lymphocytes* react against β-cell antigens and cause cell damage. These T cells include (1) CD4+ T cells of the T_H1 subset, which cause tissue injury by activating macrophages, and (2) CD8+ cytotoxic T lymphocytes, which directly kill β cells and also secrete cytokines that activate macrophages. In the rare cases in which the pancreatic lesions have been examined at the early active stages of the disease, the islets show cellular necrosis and lymphocytic infiltration. This lesion is called *insulitis*. The infiltrates consist of both $CD4^+$ and $CD8^+$ T cells. Surviving β cells often express class II MHC molecules, probably an effect of local production of the cytokine IFN-γ by the T cells. The specificity of these T cells is largely unknown.[70] Various studies have implicated a β-cell enzyme, glutamic acid decarboxylase (GAD), and insulin itself as autoantigens, but the evidence supporting their importance is mainly circumstantial or based on mouse models of the disease. Also, the key question of why tolerance to these self-antigens breaks down has not been answered.[70]

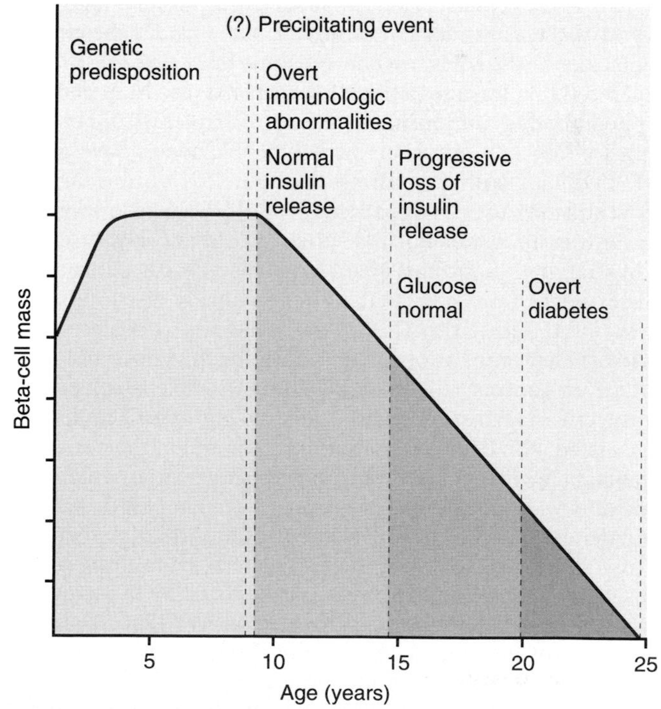

FIGURE 24–31 Stages in the development of type 1 diabetes mellitus. The stages are listed from left to right, and hypothetical β-cell mass is plotted against age. (From Eisenbarth GE: Type 1 diabetes: a chronic autoimmune disease. N Engl J Med 314:1360, 1986. Copyright © 1986, Massachusetts Medical Society. All rights reserved.)

- Locally produced *cytokines* damage β cells. Among the cytokines implicated in the cell injury are IFN-γ, produced by T cells, and TNF and IL-1, produced by macrophages that are activated during the immune reaction. All these cytokines have been shown to induce β-cell apoptosis in culture; in mouse models of the disease, β-cell destruction can be reduced by treatment with antagonists against these cytokines.
- *Autoantibodies* against islet cells and insulin are also detected in the blood of 70% to 80% of patients. The autoantibodies are reactive with a variety of β-cell antigens, including GAD. These antibodies may participate in causing the disease or may be a result of T cell–mediated cell injury and release of normally sequestered antigens.[71]

It is likely that many of these immune mechanisms work together to produce progressive destruction of β cells, resulting in clinical diabetes. The factors that predispose to autoimmunity are discussed next.

Genetic Susceptibility

Type 1 diabetes has a complex pattern of genetic associations, and putative susceptibility genes have been mapped to at least 20 loci.[72] Many of these associations are with chromosomal regions, and the particular genes involved are not known yet. Of the multiple loci that are associated with the disease, by far the most important is the class II MHC (HLA) locus; according to some estimates, the MHC contributes about half the genetic susceptibility, and all the other genes combined make up the other half.

The MHC Locus. The principal susceptibility locus for type 1 diabetes resides in the region that encodes the class II molecules of the MHC on chromosome 6p21 (HLA-D).[73] You will recall that linkage to the HLA locus has also been demonstrated in other autoimmune diseases (Chapter 6). Ninety per cent to 95% of Caucasians with type 1 diabetes have HLA-DR3, DR4, or both, in contrast to about 40% of normal subjects; and 40% to 50% of patients are DR3/DR4 heterozygotes, in contrast to 5% of normal subjects. Interestingly, susceptibility to type 1 diabetes is actually associated with a linked DQ allele called DQB1*0302 that is often in linkage disequilibrium with DR4. Thus, the DQB1*0302 allele is considered the primary determinant of susceptibility for the HLA-DR4 haplotype; in contrast, the HLA-DQB1*0602 allele is considered "protective" against diabetes.[74] Sequencing of DQ molecules associated with diabetes, both in humans and in the nonobese diabetic (NOD) mouse strain, suggests that an asparagine at position 57 in the DQβ chain protects against type 1 diabetes and that its absence increases susceptibility. Although there are many exceptions to this finding, a general hypothesis is that development of type 1 diabetes is influenced by the structure of the entire DQ peptide-binding cleft, with residue 57 playing a significant but not exclusive role. Despite the high relative risk of type 1 diabetes in individuals with particular class II alleles, most individuals who inherit these alleles do not develop the disease. We still do not know precisely how the MHC contributes to autoimmunity in this or in any other autoimmune disease (Chapter 6). Since MHC molecules normally function to display peptides to T cells, these associations clearly point to an important role of T cells in the disease.

Non-MHC Genes. The first disease-associated non-MHC gene to be identified was *insulin*, with tandem repeats in the promoter region being associated with disease susceptibility. The mechanism of this association is unknown. It may be that the disease-associated polymorphism makes the protein less functional or stable and thus compromises the functional reserve. Alternatively, these polymorphisms may influence the level of expression of insulin in the thymus, thus altering the negative selection of insulin-reactive T cells (Chapter 6). Recently, another gene has been shown to be associated with the disease, encoding the T-cell inhibitory receptor CTLA-4. Patients with type 1 diabetes show increased frequency of a splice variant that may abrogate the normal ability of this receptor to keep self-reactive T lymphocytes under control.[21]

Environmental Factors

There is evidence that environmental factors, especially infections, are involved in triggering autoimmunity in type 1 diabetes and other autoimmune diseases (Chapter 6). Epidemiologic studies suggest a role of viruses.[75] Seasonal trends that often correspond to the prevalence of common viral infections have long been noted in the diagnosis of new cases, as has the association between coxsackieviruses of group B and pancreatic diseases, including diabetes. Other implicated viral infections include mumps, measles, cytomegalovirus, rubella, and infectious mononucleosis. In all these cases, the viruses are not thought to cause diabetes by directly damaging β cells. Rather, as was discussed in Chapter 6, two mechanisms, which are not mutually exclusive, have been proposed to explain how infections can trigger autoimmunity.[76] One is that the infections induce tissue damage and inflammation, leading to the release of β-cell antigens and the recruitment and activation of lymphocytes and other inflammatory leukocytes in the tissue. The other possibility is that the viruses produce proteins that mimic self-antigens and the immune response to the viral protein cross-reacts with the self tissue.[77] Although there is experimental evidence in support of both possibilities, neither has been established as being actually involved. It should also be pointed out that recent epidemiologic studies have shown that in the United States, the incidence of type 1 diabetes in children under 15 years of age has tripled since the 1960s. Similar trends are seen in Western Europe. These findings are often interpreted as suggesting that infections may actually be protective in this disease and the increased incidence reflects the reduction in common infections. Consistent with this possibility, infections also prevent disease development in the nonobese diabetic mouse model.

PATHOGENESIS OF TYPE 2 DIABETES MELLITUS

While much has been learned in recent years, the pathogenesis of type 2 diabetes remains enigmatic. Environmental factors, such as a sedentary life style and dietary habits, clearly play a role, as will become evident when obesity is considered. Nevertheless, *genetic factors are even more important than in type 1 diabetes*. Among identical twins, the concordance rate is 50% to 90%, while among first-degree relatives with type 2 diabetes (and in fraternal twins), the risk of developing the disease is 20% to 40%, compared to 5% to 7% in the population at large. Unlike type 1 diabetes, however, the disease is not linked to genes involved in immune tolerance and regulation, and there is no evidence to suggest an autoimmune basis for type 2 diabetes.

The two metabolic defects that characterize type 2 diabetes are (1) a decreased ability of peripheral tissues to respond to insulin (insulin resistance) and (2) β-cell dysfunction that is manifested as inadequate insulin secretion in the face of insulin resistance and hyperglycemia. In most cases, insulin resistance is the primary event, and is followed by increasing degrees of β-cell dysfunction (Fig. 24–32).

Insulin Resistance

Insulin resistance is defined as resistance to the effects of insulin on glucose uptake, metabolism, or storage.[78] Insulin resistance is a characteristic feature of most patients with type 2 diabetes and is an almost universal finding in diabetic individuals who are obese. The role of insulin resistance in the pathogenesis of type 2 diabetes can be gauged from the findings that (1) insulin resistance is often detected 10 to 20 years before the onset of diabetes in predisposed individuals (e.g., offspring of type 2 diabetics) and (2) in prospective studies, insulin resistance is the best predictor for subsequent progression to diabetes.[79] Insulin resistance leads to decreased uptake of glucose in muscle and adipose tissues and an inability of the hormone to suppress hepatic gluconeogenesis. *Functional studies in individuals with insulin resistance have demonstrated numerous quantitative and qualitative abnormalities of the insulin signaling pathway*, including down-regulation of the insulin receptor; decreased insulin receptor phosphorylation and tyrosine kinase activity; reduced levels of active intermediates in the insulin signaling pathway; and impairment of translocation, docking, and fusion of GLUT-4–containing vesicles with the plasma membrane.[65]

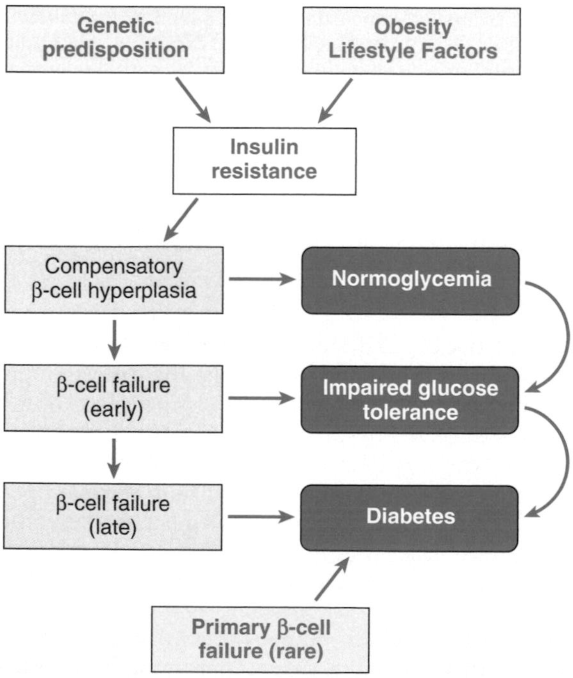

FIGURE 24–32 Metabolic staging of type 2 diabetes mellitus. Genetic predisposition and environmental influences converge to cause insulin resistance. Compensatory β-cell hyperplasia can maintain normoglycemia, but eventually, β-cell secretory dysfunction sets in, leading to impaired glucose tolerance and eventually frank diabetes. Rare instances of primary β-cell failure can directly lead to type 2 diabetes without a state of insulin resistance.

It is recognized that insulin resistance is a complex phenomenon. Here we discuss some of the likely culprits responside for decreased sensitivity to insulin in diabetic individuals.

Genetic Defects of the Insulin Receptor and Insulin Signaling Pathway. Loss-of-function abnormalities of either the insulin receptor or its downstream intermediates are obvious candidates for mediating insulin resistance in type 2 diabetes. In mice, tissue-specific knockout of genes encoding various insulin signaling proteins has resulted in insulin resistance, hyperinsulinemia and hyperglycemia, recapitulating human type 2 diabetes.[80] Unfortunately, the extrapolation of these single-gene knockout models to human disease has been less than gratifying. Point mutations of the insulin receptor are relatively rare, accounting for no more than 1% to 5% of patients with insulin resistance (see the section entitled "Monogenic Forms of Diabetes"). Analysis of candidate genes involved in insulin secretion or insulin action, as well as whole genome linkage studies of affected families, have yielded many polymorphisms that associate with the type 2 diabetic phenotype, but in most cases, the associations have been weak, or the studies were not reproducible.[81] From these analyses, it appears that while the *population* risk associated with any particular genetic variant (polymorphism) may be significant, the increased risk for developing diabetes for a given *individual* harboring that variant is small at best. Suffice it to say that while no one questions a genetic component to insulin resistance, the high "noise" to signal ratio has hampered identification of the genes involved. The genetic basis of insulin resistance, and by extension type 2 diabetes, therefore, remains an enigma.

Obesity and Insulin Resistance. The association of obesity with type 2 diabetes has been recognized for decades, visceral obesity being a common phenomenon in the majority of type 2 diabetics. *The link between obesity and diabetes is mediated via effects on insulin resistance.*[82] Insulin resistance is present even in simple obesity unaccompanied by hyperglycemia, indicating a fundamental abnormality of insulin signaling in states of fatty excess. The risk for diabetes increases as the body mass index (a measure of body fat content) increases. It is not only the absolute amount but also the distribution of body fat that has an effect on insulin sensitivity: Central obesity (abdominal fat) is more likely to be linked with insulin resistance than are peripheral (gluteal/subcutaneous) fat depots. Although many details of the so-called adipo-insulin axis remain to be elucidated, following are some of the putative pathways leading to insulin resistance:

- *Role of free fatty acids (FFAs)*: Cross-sectional studies have demonstrated an inverse correlation between fasting plasma FFAs and insulin sensitivity. Furthermore, the level of intracellular triglycerides is often markedly increased in muscle and liver tissues in obese individuals, presumably because excess circulating FFAs are deposited in these organs. Intracellular triglycerides and products of fatty acid metabolism are potent inhibitors of insulin signaling and result in an acquired insulin resistance state.[79] These "lipotoxic" effects of FFAs are most likely mediated through a decrease in activity of key insulin-signaling proteins.

- *Role of adipokines in insulin resistance:* It is increasingly recognized that adipose tissue is not merely a passive storage depot for fat, but can also operate as a functional endocrine organ, releasing hormones in response to changes in the metabolic status. A variety of proteins released into the systemic circulation by adipose tissue have been identified, and these are collectively termed adipokines (or adipose cytokines).[83] Dysregulation of adipokine secretion (either abnormally increased or decreased levels) may be one of the mechanisms by which insulin resistance is tied to obesity. Several adipokines have been implicated in insulin resistance, including *leptin,*[84] *adiponectin*[85] and *resistin.*[86] For brevity, only the first will be discussed. Leptin acts on central nervous system receptors and other sites to reduce food intake and induce satiety (Chapter 9). Leptin-deficient animals demonstrate severe insulin resistance that is reversed by administration of leptin.[87] Whereas many of leptin's insulin-sensitizing actions are mediated by central nervous system receptors, some effects may be exerted directly at the level of insulin target tissues. The role of leptin in states of insulin resistance in humans is an area of active investigation.
- *Role of the peroxisome proliferator–activated receptor gamma (PPARγ) and thiazolidinediones (TZDs):* TZDs are a class of antidiabetic compounds that were developed in the early 1980s as antioxidants. The target receptor for TZDs has been identified as peroxisome proliferator–activated receptor gamma (PPARγ), a nuclear receptor and transcription factor.[88] PPARγ is most highly expressed in adipose tissue, and activation of the receptor by TZDs results in modulation of gene expression in adipocytes, eventually leading to reduction of insulin resistance. The targets of PPARγ activation include several of the adipokines discussed above. PPARγ activation also decreases levels of free fatty acids, which, as mentioned earlier, contributes to insulin resistance in obesity.

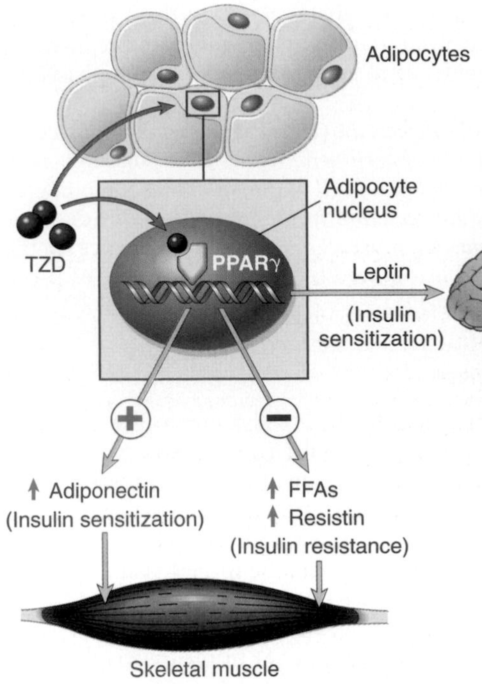

FIGURE 24–33 Obesity and insulin resistance: the missing links? Adipocytes release a variety of factors (free fatty acids and adipokines) that may play a role in modulating insulin resistance in peripheral tissues (illustrated here is striated muscle). Excess free fatty acids (FFAs) and resistin are associated with insulin resistance; in contrast, adiponectin, whose levels are decreased in obesity, is an insulin-sensitizing adipokine. Leptin is also an insulin-sensitizing agent, but it acts via central receptors (in the hypothalamus). The peroxisome proliferator–activated receptor gamma (PPARγ) is an adipocyte nuclear receptor that is activated by a class of insulin-sensitizing drugs called thiazolidinediones (TZDs). The mechanism of action of TZDs may eventually be mediated through modulation of adipokine and FFA levels that favor a state of insulin sensitivity.

To summarize, insulin resistance in type 2 diabetes is a complex and multifactorial phenomenon. Genetic defects in the insulin signaling pathway are not common and, when present, are more likely polymorphisms with subtle effects rather than inactivating mutations. Insulin resistance is acquired in the overwhelming majority of individuals, and obesity is central to this phenomenon. Figure 24–33 illustrates the links between obesity and insulin resistance.

β-Cell Dysfunction

β-cell dysfunction in type 2 diabetes reflects the inability of these cells to adapt themselves to the long-term demands of peripheral insulin resistance and increased insulin secretion. In states of insulin resistance, insulin secretion is initially higher for each level of glucose than in controls. This hyperinsulinemic state is a compensation for peripheral resistance and can often maintain normal plasma glucose for years. Eventually, however, β-cell compensation becomes inadequate, and there is progression to overt diabetes. The underlying basis for failure of β-cell adaptation is not known, although it is postulated that several mechanisms, including adverse effects of high circulating free fatty acids ("lipotoxicity") or chronic hyperglycemia ("glucotoxicity"), may play a role. *β-cell dysfunction in type 2 diabetes manifests itself as both qualitative and quantitative defects:*

- Qualitative β-cell dysfunction is initially subtle, and seen as loss of the normal pulsatile, oscillating pattern of insulin secretion and attenuation of the rapid first phase of insulin secretion triggered by an elevation in plasma glucose. Over time, the secretory defect affects all phases of insulin secretion, and even though some basal insulin secretion persists in type 2 diabetes, it is grossly inadequate to overcome the insulin resistance.
- Quantitative β-cell dysfunction is reflected by a *decrease in β-cell mass, islet degeneration, and deposition of islet amyloid.* Islet amyloid protein (amylin) is a characteristic finding in patients with type 2 diabetes and is present in more than 90% of diabetic islets examined. Islet amyloidosis is associated with a decrease in β-cell mass, although it is uncertain whether the amyloid is involved in or merely a consequence of the β-cell decrease. Although there are scant data in humans, studies from animal models of diabetes support the aforementioned sequence of events wherein β-

cell hyperplasia in the prediabetic state is followed by a decrease in β-cell mass that coincides with clinical progression to diabetes. In this context, it is important to note that even a "normal" β-cell mass in diabetic individuals may in fact indicate a relative reduction for the degree of insulin resistance.

MONOGENIC FORMS OF DIABETES

Although genetically defined causes of diabetes are uncommon, they have been intensively studied in the hope of gaining insights into the disease. As Table 24–6 illustrates, monogenic forms of diabetes are classified separately from types 1 and 2. Monogenic causes of diabetes result from either a primary defect in β-cell function or a defect in insulin/insulin receptor signaling, as described below.

Maturity-Onset Diabetes of the Young (MODY). Two per cent to 5% of diabetic patients do not fall clearly into either the type 1 or type 2 diabetes phenotype and are said to have "maturity-onset diabetes of the young." In these patients, there is a *primary defect in β-cell function that occurs without β-cell loss, affecting either β-cell mass and/or insulin production.*[89] It now appears that MODY is the outcome of a heterogeneous group of genetic defects characterized by (1) autosomal-dominant inheritance as a monogenic defect, with high penetrance; (2) early onset, usually before age 25, as opposed to after age 40 for most patients with type 2 diabetes; (3) absence of obesity; and (4) lack of islet cell autoantibodies and insulin resistance syndrome.

Six distinct genetic defects have been identified thus far (see Table 24–6). Glucokinase, implicated in MODY2, catalyzes the transfer of phosphate from ATP to glucose, which is the first and rate-limiting step in glucose metabolism. Glucokinase expressed in the pancreatic β-cell controls the influx of glucose by controlling its entry into the glycolytic cycle, which in turn is coupled to insulin secretion. Inactivating mutations of this enzyme increase the threshold for insulin release, such that insulin secretion is low for the degree of hyperglycemia present, causing modest increases in blood glucose. Activating mutations have been described that shift the enzyme activity in the opposite direction, with increased insulin secretion at a lower glucose level, resulting in states of chronic hypoglycemia with hyperinsulinism. The remaining five genes associated with MODY are transcription factors controlling insulin expression in β-cells and β-cell mass; IPF-1 also plays a central role in the development of the pancreas. In addition to genetic heterogeneity, MODY is characterized by clinical heterogeneity. Some forms (MODY1, MODY3, and MODY5) are associated with severe β-cell insulin secretory defects with the full range of diabetic complications, while others (MODY2) feature mild chronic hyperglycemia that typically does not worsen over time.

Up to 50% of carriers of glucokinase mutations develop gestational diabetes mellitus, defined as any degree of glucose intolerance with onset or first recognition during pregnancy;[90] conversely, approximately 5% of women with gestational diabetes mellitus and a first-degree relative with diabetes carry a mutation in the glucokinase gene. It is important to emphasize that *mutations or polymorphisms in the six known MODY genes do not appear to contribute to the development of late-onset (classic) type 2 diabetes in the vast majority of patients.*

Mitochondrial Diabetes. Mitochondrial DNA is inherited maternally and encodes several genes in the oxidative phosphorylation pathway, ribosomal RNAs, and 22 transfer RNAs (tRNAs). In rare cases, (<1%), diabetes is associated with point mutations in a mitochondrial tRNA gene, $tRNA^{Leu(UUR)}$.[91] Mitochondrial diabetes is caused by a primary defect in β-cell function. Recall that ATP is required for insulin secretion in β cells (Fig. 24–29), and impairment of mitochondrial ATP synthesis results in decreased insulin secretion.

Diabetes Associated with Insulin Gene or Insulin Receptor Mutations. Mutations that affect *insulin processing* from its precursor (proinsulin) or those that affect *insulin structure* and binding to its receptor are a rare cause of diabetes.[92] The metabolic impairment in most cases is mild, since these patients are heterozygous for their mutations. *Insulin receptor* mutations that affect either receptor synthesis, insulin binding, or receptor tyrosine kinase activity can, in rare cases, result in mild to severe insulin resistance and type 2 diabetes. Neither insulin gene nor insulin receptor mutations contribute significantly to the incidence of type 2 diabetes.

PATHOGENESIS OF THE COMPLICATIONS OF DIABETES

The morbidity associated with long-standing diabetes of either type results from a number of serious complications, involving both large- and medium-sized muscular arteries (*macrovascular disease*), as well as capillary dysfunction in target organs (*microvascular disease*). Macrovascular disease causes *accelerated atherosclerosis* among diabetics, resulting in increased risk of myocardial infarction, stroke, and lower-extremity gangrene. The effects of microvascular disease are most profound in the retina, kidneys, and peripheral nerves, resulting in *diabetic retinopathy*, *nephropathy*, and *neuropathy*, respectively. Diabetes is the leading cause of blindness and end-stage renal disease in the Western hemisphere, besides contributing substantially to the incidence of cardiovascular events each year. Hence, the basis of long-term complications of diabetes is the subject of a great deal of research. *Most of the available experimental and clinical evidence suggests that the complications of diabetes are a consequence of the metabolic derangements, mainly hyperglycemia.* For example, when kidneys are transplanted into diabetics from nondiabetic donors, the lesions of diabetic nephropathy may develop within 3 to 5 years after transplantation. Conversely, kidneys with lesions of diabetic nephropathy demonstrate a reversal of the lesion when transplanted into normal recipients. Two large multicenter trials to evaluate the effects of plasma glucose concentrations on long-term complications of diabetes—the Diabetes Control and Complication Trial (DCCT)[93] and the United Kingdom Prospective Diabetes Study (UKPDS)[94]—have convincingly demonstrated delayed progression of microvascular complications by strict control of the hyperglycemia. It is important to stress, however, that not all diabetics have long-term complications, irrespective of the level of blood glucose control over time, indicating that there are additional factors that modulate an individual's risk for microvascular disease. It is likely that such disease-modifying elements are genetic, and there is an ongoing search to identify these additional genes.

At least three distinct metabolic pathways appear to be involved in the pathogenesis of long-term diabetic complications, although the primacy of any one has not been established.[95] These pathways include the following.

Formation of Advanced Glycation End Products. Advanced glycation end products (AGEs) are formed as a result of nonenzymatic reactions between intracellular glucose-derived dicarbonyl precursors (glyoxal, methylglyoxal, and 3-deoxyglucosone) with the amino group of both intracellular and extracellular proteins.[96] AGEs have a number of chemical and biologic properties that are detrimental to extracellular matrix components and the target cells of diabetic complications (e.g., endothelial cells) (Table 24–7):

- *On extracellular matrix components*, such as collagen or laminin, the formation of AGEs causes cross-linking between polypeptides, resulting in abnormal matrix–matrix and matrix–cell interactions. For example, cross-linking between collagen type I molecules in large vessels decreases their elasticity, which may predispose these vessels to shear stress and endothelial injury (Chapter 11). Similarly, AGE-induced cross-linking of type IV collagen in basement membrane decreases endothelial cell adhesion and increases fluid filtration. *AGE cross-linked proteins are resistant to proteolytic digestion.* Thus, cross-linking decreases protein removal while enhancing protein deposition. AGE-modified matrix components also *trap nonglycated plasma or interstitial proteins.* In large vessels, trapping low-density lipoprotein (LDL), for example, retards its efflux from the vessel wall and enhances the deposition of cholesterol in the intima, thus accelerating atherogenesis (Chapter 11). In capillaries, including those of renal glomeruli, plasma proteins such as albumin may bind to the glycated basement membrane, accounting in part for the increased basement membrane thickening characteristic of diabetic microangiopathy.
- *Circulating plasma proteins* are modified by addition of AGE residues; these proteins, in turn, bind to *AGE receptors* on several cell types (endothelial cells, mesangial cells, macrophages). The AGE-receptor ligation results in activation and nuclear translocation of the pleotropic transcription factor NF-κB, generating a variety of cytokines, growth factors and other pro-inflammatory molecules.[97] The biologic effects of AGE-receptor signaling include (1) release of *cytokines and growth factors* from macrophages and mesangial cells (insulin-like growth factor-1, TGF-β, platelet-derived growth factor, VEGF); (2) increased *endothelial permeability*; (3) increased *procoagulant activity* on endothelial cells and macrophages (induction of thrombomodulin and tissue factor); and (4) enhanced *proliferation of and synthesis of extracellular matrix* by fibroblasts and smooth muscle cells.

TABLE 24–7 Effects of Advanced Glycation End Products (AGEs)

Extracellular Matrix Components
Abnormal matrix-matrix and matrix-cell interactions
Corss-linking of polypeptides of same protein (e.g., collagen)
Trapping of nonglycated proteins (e.g., LDL, albumin)
Resistance to proteolytic digestion
Intracellular and Plasma Proteins
AGE receptor ligation leads to generation of reactive oxygen species and NF-κB activation
Target cells (endothelium, mesangial cells, macrophages) respond by:
Cytokines and growth factor secretion
Induction of procoagulant activity
Increased vascular permeability
Enhanced ECM production

ECM, extracellular matrix; LDL, low-density lipoprotein.

You will recall from the discussion of atherosclerosis (Chapter 11) that *endothelial dysfunction*, particularly endothelial activation, is a critical process in vascular injury and atherogenesis. AGEs, by virtue of their ability to modify extracellular matrix components, as well as to activate NF-κB and its downstream targets in the vascular endothelium, are postulated to play a central role in the accelerated atherogenesis characteristic of diabetes. In addition to large vessel disease, AGEs also contribute to microvascular injury in diabetes. The AGE inhibitor aminoguanidine has recently been shown to retard the progression of nephropathy in type 1 diabetics.

Activation of Protein Kinase C. Activation of intracellular protein kinase C (PKC) by calcium ions and the second messenger diacylglycerol (DAG) is an important signal transduction pathway in many cellular systems. Intracellular hyperglycemia can stimulate the de novo synthesis of DAG from glycolytic intermediates and hence cause activation of PKC. The downstream effects of PKC activation are numerous and include the following:[97]

- Production of the proangiogenic molecule vascular endothelial growth factor (VEGF), implicated in the neovascularization characterizing diabetic retinopathy (Chapter 29)
- Increased activity of the vasoconstrictor endothelin-1 and decreased activity of the vasodilator endothelial nitric oxide synthase (eNOS)
- Production of profibrogenic molecules like transforming growth factor-β (TGF-β), leading to increased deposition of extracellular matrix and basement membrane material
- Production of the procoagulant molecule plasminogen activator inhibitor-1 (PAI-1), leading to reduced fibrinolysis and possible vascular occlusive episodes
- Production of pro-inflammatory cytokines by the vascular endothelium.

It should be evident that some effects of AGEs and activated PKCs (e.g., activation of NF-κB) are overlapping. Not surprisingly, therefore, therapeutic inhibition of PKC can retard the progression of diabetic retinopathy.[98]

Intracellular Hyperglycemia with Disturbances in Polyol Pathways. In some tissues that do not require insulin for glucose transport (e.g., nerves, lenses, kidneys, blood vessels), hyperglycemia leads to an increase in intracellular glucose that is then metabolized by the enzyme *aldose reductase* to sorbitol, a polyol, and eventually to fructose. In this process, intracellular NADPH is used as a cofactor. NADPH is also required as a cofactor by the enzyme glutathione reductase for regenerating reduced glutathione (GSH). You will recall that GSH is one of the important antioxidant mechanisms in the cell (Chapter 1), and a reduction in GSH levels increases cellular susceptibility to oxidative stress.[99] In the face of sustained hyperglycemia, progressive depletion of intracellular NADPH by aldol reductase leads to a compromise of

GSH regeneration. Thus, the deleterious consequences of the aldose reductase pathway arise primarily by increasing cellular susceptibility to oxidative stress. The importance of this pathway in human diabetes was best exemplified in clinical trials using an aldose reductase inhibitor, which significantly ameliorated the development of diabetic neuropathy. Unfortunately, the effects of these inhibitors on other long-term complications have been less promising.

MORPHOLOGY OF DIABETES AND ITS LATE COMPLICATIONS

Pathologic findings in the pancreas are variable and not necessarily dramatic. The important morphologic changes are related to the many late systemic complications of diabetes. There is extreme variability among patients in the time of onset of these complications, their severity, and the particular organ or organs involved. In individuals with tight control of diabetes, the onset might be delayed. In most patients, however, morphologic changes are likely to be found in arteries (*macrovascular disease*), basement membranes of small vessels (*microangiopathy*), kidneys (*diabetic nephropathy*), retina (*retinopathy*), nerves (*neuropathy*), and other tissues. These changes are seen in both type 1 and type 2 diabetes. A schematic overview is provided in Figure 24–34.

Morphology.

Pancreas. Lesions in the pancreas are inconstant and rarely of diagnostic value. Distinctive changes are more commonly associated with type 1 than with type 2 diabetes. One or more of the following alterations may be present:

- **Reduction in the number and size of islets.** This is most often seen in type 1 diabetes, particularly with rapidly advancing disease. Most of the islets are small and inconspicuous, and not easily detected.
- **Leukocytic infiltration of the islets** (insulitis) principally composed of T lymphocytes similar to that in animal models of autoimmune diabetes (Fig. 24–35*A*). This may be seen in type 1 diabetics at the time of clinical presentation. The distribution of insulitis may be strikingly uneven. Eosinophilic infiltrates may also be found, particularly in diabetic infants who fail to survive the immediate postnatal period.

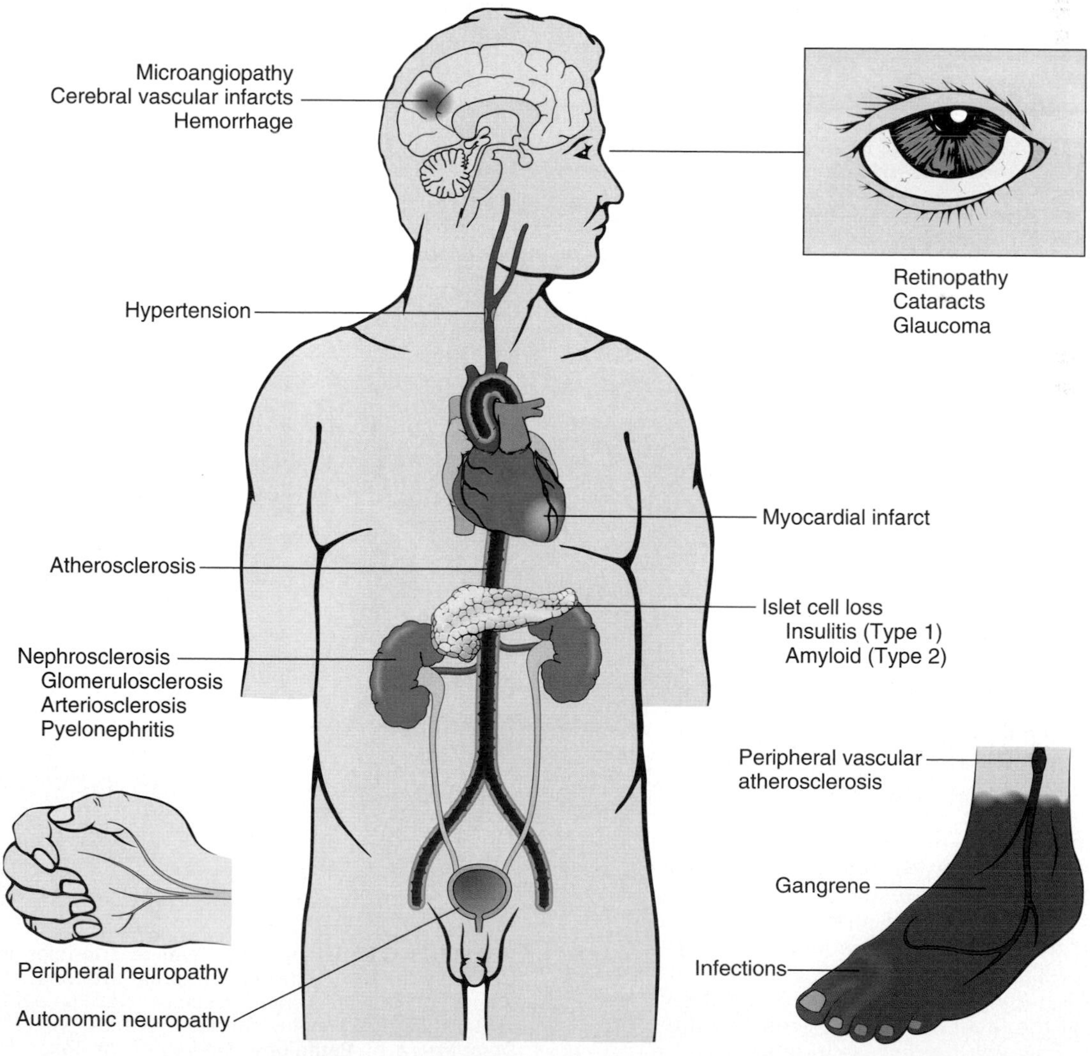

FIGURE 24–34 Long-term complications of diabetes.

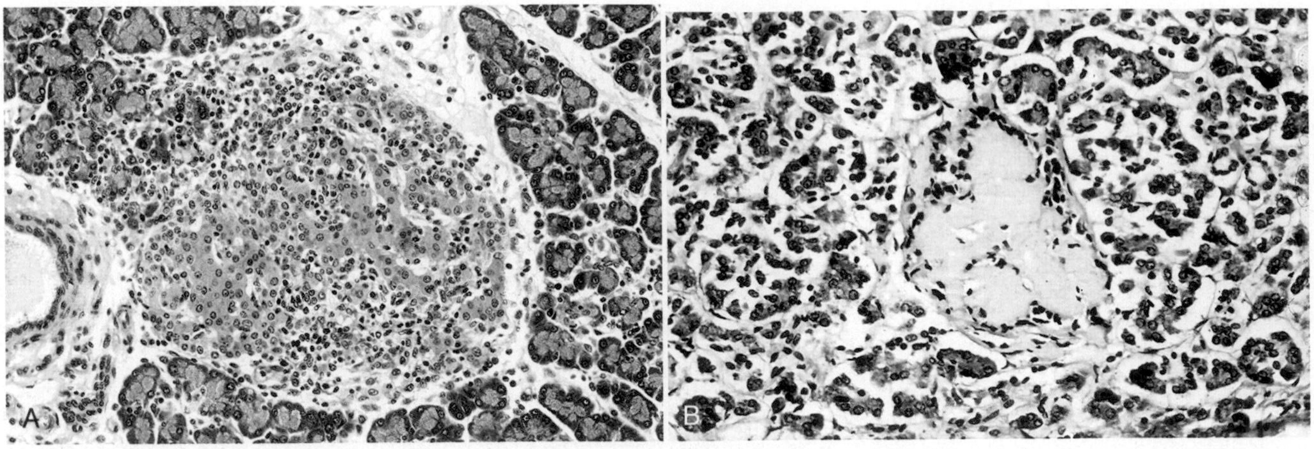

FIGURE 24–35 *A*, Insulitis, shown here from a rat (BB) model of autoimmune diabetes, also seen in type 1 human diabetes. (Courtesy of Dr. Arthur Like, University of Massachusetts, Worchester, MA.) *B*, Amyloidosis of a pancreatic islet in type 2 diabetes.

- By electron microscopy, **β-cell degranulation** may be observed, reflecting depletion of stored insulin in already damaged β cells. This is more commonly seen in patients with newly diagnosed type 1 disease, when some β cells are still present.
- **In type 2 diabetes, there may be a subtle reduction in islet cell mass,** demonstrated only by special morphometric studies.
- **Amyloid replacement of islets in type 2 diabetes** appears as deposition of pink, amorphous material beginning in and around capillaries and between cells. At advanced stages, the islets may be virtually obliterated (Fig. 24–35*B*); fibrosis may also be observed. This change is often seen in long-standing cases of type 2 diabetes. Similar lesions may be found in elderly nondiabetics, apparently as part of normal aging.
- An increase in the number and size of islets is especially characteristic of nondiabetic newborns of diabetic mothers. Presumably, fetal islets undergo hyperplasia in response to the maternal hyperglycemia.

Diabetic Macrovascular Disease. Diabetes exacts a heavy toll on the vascular system. **The hallmark of diabetic macrovascular disease is accelerated atherosclerosis** involving the aorta and large- and medium-sized arteries. Except for its greater severity and earlier age at onset, atherosclerosis in diabetics is indistinguishable from that in nondiabetics (Chapter 11). **Myocardial infarction, caused by atherosclerosis of the coronary arteries, is the most common cause of death in diabetics.** Significantly, it is almost as common in diabetic women as in diabetic men. In contrast, myocardial infarction is uncommon in nondiabetic women of reproductive age. **Gangrene of the lower extremities,** as a result of advanced vascular disease, is about 100 times more common in diabetics than in the general population. The larger renal arteries are also subject to severe atherosclerosis, but the most damaging effect of diabetes on the kidneys is exerted at the level of the glomeruli and the microcirculation. This will be discussed later.

Hyaline arteriolosclerosis, the vascular lesion associated with hypertension (Chapters 11 and 20), is both more prevalent and more severe in diabetics than in nondiabetics, but it is not specific for diabetes and may be seen in elderly nondiabetics without hypertension. It takes the form of an amorphous, hyaline thickening of the wall of the arterioles, which causes narrowing of the lumen (Fig. 24–36). Not surprisingly, in diabetics, it is related not only to the duration of the disease, but also to the level of blood pressure.

Diabetic Microangiopathy. One of the most consistent morphologic features of diabetes is **diffuse thickening of basement membranes**. The thickening is most evident in the capillaries of the skin, skeletal muscle, retina, renal glomeruli, and renal medulla. However, it may also be seen in such nonvascular structures as renal tubules, the Bowman capsule, peripheral nerves, and placenta. By both light and electron microscopy, the basal lamina separating parenchymal or endothelial cells from the surround-

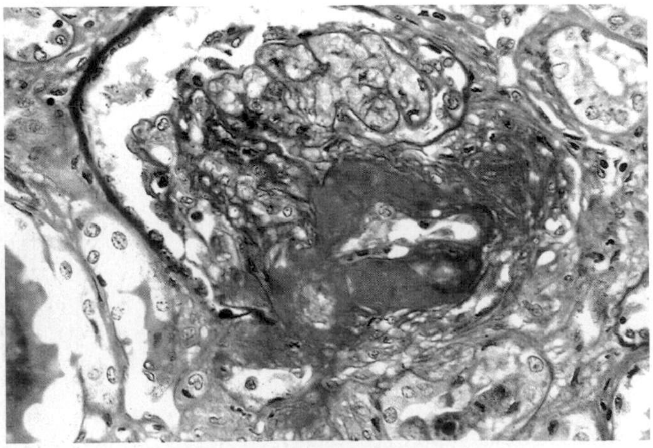

FIGURE 24–36 Severe renal hyaline arteriolosclerosis. Note a markedly thickened, tortuous afferent arteriole. The amorphous nature of the thickened vascular wall is evident. (Periodic acid–Schiff [PAS] stain; courtesy of M.A. Venkatachalam, MD, Department of Pathology, University of Texas Health Science Center at San Antonio, TX.)

ing tissue is markedly thickened by concentric layers of hyaline material composed predominantly of type IV collagen (Figs. 24–37 and 24–38). It should be noted that despite the increase in the thickness of basement membranes, **diabetic capillaries are more leaky than normal to plasma proteins. The microangiopathy underlies the development of diabetic nephropathy, retinopathy, and some forms of neuropathy.** An indistinguishable microangiopathy can be found in aged nondiabetic patients but rarely to the extent seen in patients with long-standing diabetes.

Diabetic Nephropathy. The kidneys are prime targets of diabetes. (See also Chapter 20.) Renal failure is second only to myocardial infarction as a cause of death from this disease. **Three lesions are encountered: (1) glomerular lesions; (2) renal vascular lesions, principally arteriolosclerosis; and (3) pyelonephritis, including necrotizing papillitis.**

The most important glomerular lesions are capillary basement membrane thickening, diffuse mesangial sclerosis, and nodular glomerulosclerosis. These are described in detail in Chapter 20. The glomerular capillary basement membranes are thickened throughout their entire length (see Fig. 24–38). This change can be detected by electron microscopy within a few years of the onset of diabetes, sometimes without any associated change in renal function.

Diffuse mesangial sclerosis consists of a diffuse increase in mesangial matrix and is always associated with basement membrane thickening. It is found in most patients with disease of more than 10 years' duration. When glomerulosclerosis becomes marked, patients manifest the nephrotic syndrome (Chapter 20), characterized by proteinuria, hypoalbuminemia, and edema.

Nodular glomerulosclerosis describes a glomerular lesion made distinctive by ball-like deposits of a laminated matrix situated in the periphery of the glomerulus. These nodules are PAS positive and usually contain trapped mesangial cells. This distinctive change has been called the **Kimmelstiel-Wilson lesion**, after the pathologists who described it. Nodular glomerulosclerosis is encountered in approximately 15% to 30% of long-term diabetics and is a major cause of morbidity and mortality. Diffuse mesangial sclerosis may also be seen in association with old age and hypertension; on the contrary, the nodular form of glomerulosclerosis, once certain unusual forms of nephropathies have been excluded (see Chapter 20), is essentially pathognomonic of diabetes. Both the diffuse and nodular forms of glomerulosclerosis induce sufficient ischemia to cause overall fine scarring of the kidneys, marked by a finely granular cortical surface (Fig. 24–39).

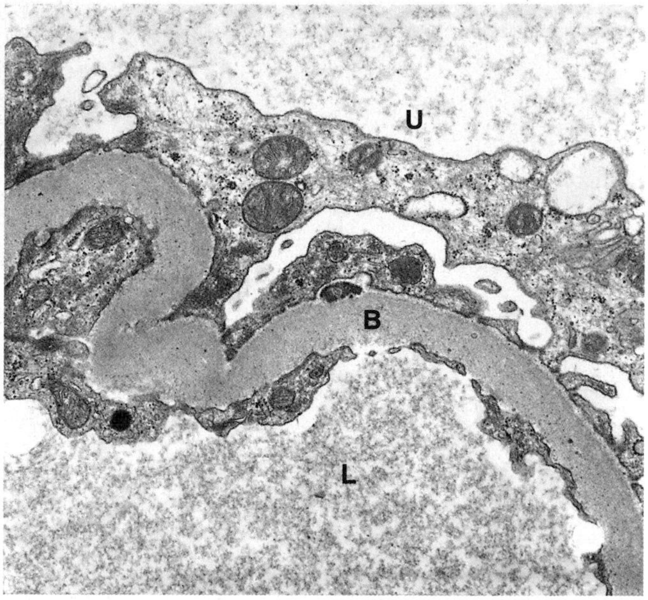

FIGURE 24–38 Electron micrograph of a renal glomerulus showing markedly thickened glomerular basement membrane (B) in a diabetic. L, glomerular capillary lumen; U, urinary space. (Courtesy of Dr. Michael Kashgarian, Department of Pathology, Yale University School of Medicine, New Haven, CT.)

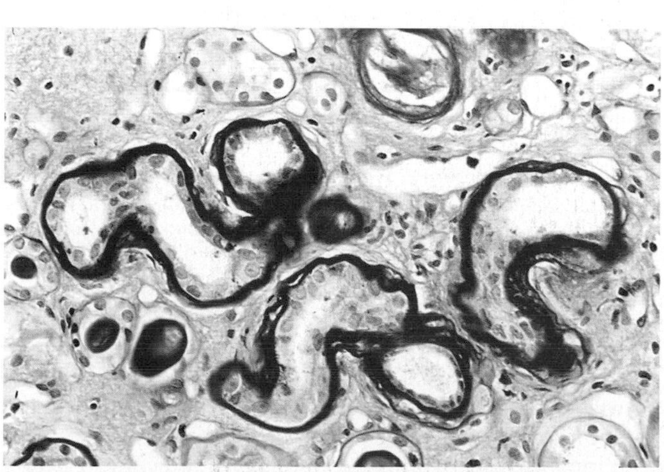

FIGURE 24–37 Renal cortex showing thickening of tubular basement membranes in a diabetic patient (PAS stain).

Renal atherosclerosis and arteriolosclerosis constitute part of the macrovascular disease in diabetics. The kidney is one of the most frequently and severely affected organs; however, the changes in the arteries and arterioles are similar to those found throughout the body. Hyaline arteriolosclerosis affects not only the afferent but also the efferent arteriole. Such efferent arteriolosclerosis is rarely, if ever, encountered in individuals who do not have diabetes.

Pyelonephritis is an acute or chronic inflammation of the kidneys that usually begins in the interstitial tissue and then spreads to affect the tubules. Both the acute and chronic forms of this disease occur in nondiabetics as well as in diabetics but are more common in diabetics than in the general population, and, once affected, diabetics tend to have more severe involvement. One special pattern of acute pyelonephritis, **necrotizing papillitis** (or papillary necrosis), is much more prevalent in diabetics than in nondiabetics.

Diabetic Ocular Complications. The ocular involvement may take the form of retinopathy, cataract formation, or glaucoma. The morphologic features are discussed further in Chapter 29.

Diabetic Neuropathy. The central and peripheral nervous systems are not spared by diabetes. The effects of diabetes on the nervous system are described further in Chapters 27 and 28.

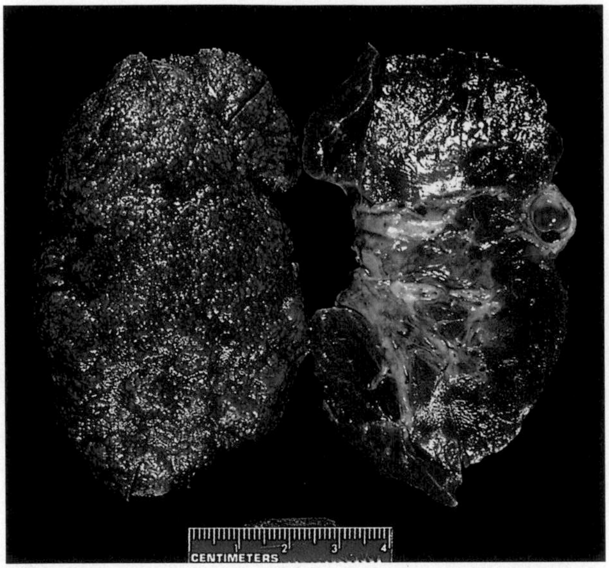

FIGURE 24–39 Nephrosclerosis in a patient with long-standing diabetes. The kidney has been bisected to demonstrate both diffuse granular transformation of the surface *(left)* and marked thinning of the cortical tissue *(right)*. Additional features include some irregular depressions, the result of pyelonephritis, and an incidental cortical cyst *(far right)*.

CLINICAL FEATURES OF DIABETES

It is difficult to sketch with brevity the diverse clinical presentations of diabetes mellitus. Only a few characteristic patterns will be presented.

Type 1 diabetes was traditionally thought to occur primarily in those under age 18 but is now known to occur at any age. In the initial 1 or 2 years following manifestation of overt type 1 diabetes, the exogenous insulin requirements may be minimal because of ongoing endogenous insulin secretion (referred to as the *honeymoon period*), but shortly thereafter, any residual β-cell reserve is exhausted and insulin requirements increase dramatically. Although β-cell destruction is a long-standing process, the transition from impaired glucose tolerance to overt diabetes may be abrupt, heralded by an event with increased insulin requirements, such as infection.

The onset is marked by polyuria, polydipsia, polyphagia, and, with extreme derangement, ketoacidosis, all resulting from metabolic derangements. As insulin is a major anabolic hormone in the body, *deficiency of insulin results in a catabolic state that affects not only glucose metabolism but also fat and protein metabolism.* Unopposed secretion of counter-regulatory hormones (glucagon, growth hormone, epinephrine) also plays a role in these metabolic derangements. The assimilation of glucose into muscle and adipose tissue is sharply diminished or abolished. Not only does storage of glycogen in liver and muscle cease, but also reserves are depleted by glycogenolysis. The resultant hyperglycemia exceeds the renal threshold for reabsorption, and glycosuria ensues. The glycosuria induces an osmotic diuresis and thus *polyuria*, causing a profound loss of water and electrolytes (Fig. 24–40). The obligatory renal water loss combined with the hyperosmolarity resulting from the increased levels of glucose in the blood tends to deplete intracellular water, triggering the osmoreceptors of the thirst centers of the brain. In this manner, intense thirst (*polydipsia*) appears. With a deficiency of insulin, the scales swing from insulin-promoted anabolism to catabolism of proteins and fats. Proteolysis follows, and the gluconeogenic amino acids are removed by the liver and used as building blocks for glucose. The catabolism of proteins and fats tends to induce a negative energy balance, which in turn leads to increasing appetite (*polyphagia*), thus completing the classic triad of diabetes: *polyuria*, *polydipsia*, and *polyphagia*. Despite the increased appetite, catabolic effects prevail, resulting in weight loss and muscle weakness. *The combination of polyphagia and weight loss is paradoxical and should always raise the suspicion of diabetes.*

Diabetic ketoacidosis (DKA) is a serious complication of type 1 diabetes but may also occur in type 2 diabetes, though not as commonly and not to as marked an extent. These patients have marked insulin deficiency, and the release of the catecholamine hormone *epinephrine* blocks any residual insulin action and stimulates the release of glucagon. The insulin deficiency coupled with glucagon excess decreases peripheral utilization of glucose while increasing gluconeogenesis, severely exacerbating hyperglycemia (the plasma glucose levels are usually in the range of 500 to 700 mg/dL). The hyperglycemia causes an osmotic diuresis and dehydration characteristic of the ketoacidotic state. The second major effect of an alteration in the insulin:glucagon ratio is activation of the ketogenic machinery. Insulin deficiency stimulates lipoprotein lipase, with resultant excessive breakdown of adipose stores, and an increase in levels of free fatty acids. When these free fatty acids reach the liver, they are esterified to fatty acyl CoA. Oxidation of fatty acyl CoA molecules within the hepatic mitochondria produces *ketone bodies* (acetoacetic acid and β-hydroxybutyric acid). The rate at which ketone bodies are formed may exceed the rate at which acetoacetic acid and β-hydroxybutyric acid can be utilized by peripheral tissues, leading to *ketonemia* and *ketonuria*. If the urinary excretion of ketones is compromised by dehydration, the plasma hydrogen ion concentration increases, and systemic *metabolic ketoacidosis* results. Release of ketogenic amino acids by protein catabolism aggravates the ketotic state.

Type 2 diabetes mellitus may also present with polyuria and polydipsia, but unlike in type 1 diabetes, patients are often older (over 40 years) and frequently obese. However, with the increase in obesity and sedentary lifestyle in our society, type 2 diabetes is now seen in children and adolescents with increasing frequency. In some cases, medical attention is sought because of unexplained weakness or weight loss. *Most frequently, however, the diagnosis is made after routine blood or urine testing in asymptomatic persons.* The absence of ketoacidosis and milder presentation in type 2 diabetes is presumably because of higher portal vein insulin levels in these patients than in type 1 diabetics, which prevents unrestricted hepatic fatty acid oxidation and keeps the formation of ketone bodies in check. In the decompensated state, these patients may develop *hyperosmolar nonketotic coma*, a syndrome engendered by the severe dehydration resulting from sustained osmotic diuresis in patients who do not drink enough water to compensate for urinary losses from chronic hyperglycemia. Typically, the patient is an elderly diabetic who is disabled by a stroke or an infection and is unable to maintain adequate water intake. Furthermore, the absence of ketoacidosis and its symptoms (nausea, vomiting, respiratory difficulties) delays the seeking of medical attention until severe dehydration and coma occur. In Table 24–8, we have summarized some of the

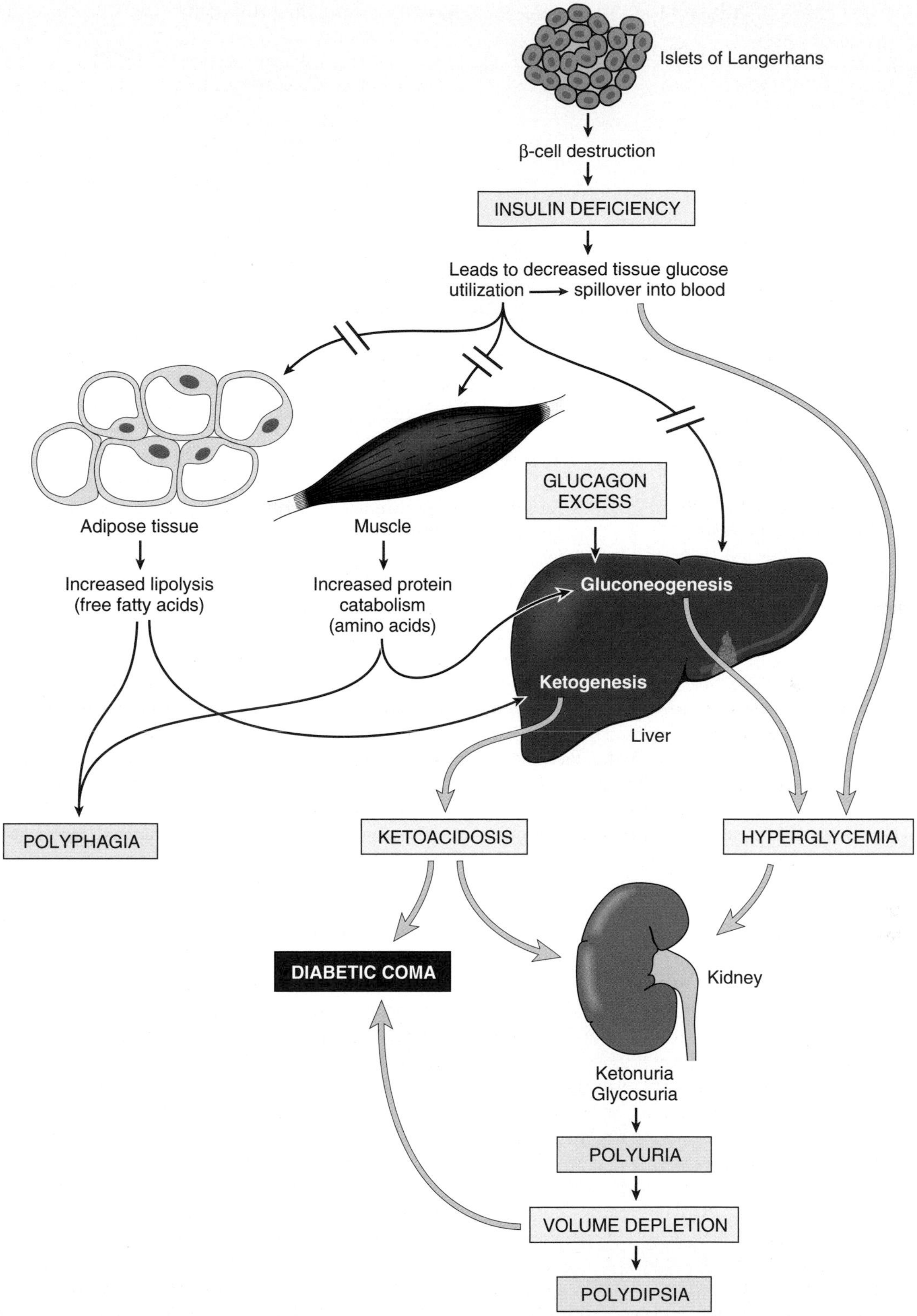

FIGURE 24–40 Sequence of metabolic derangements leading to diabetic coma in type 1 diabetes mellitus. An absolute insulin deficiency leads to a catabolic state, eventuating in ketoacidosis and severe volume depletion. These cause sufficient central nervous system compromise to lead to coma and eventual death if left untreated.

TABLE 24–8 Type 1 Versus Type 2 Diabetes Mellitus (DM)

	Type 1 DM	Type 2 DM
Clinical	Onset: <20 years Normal weight Markedly decreased blood insulin Anti-islet cell antibodies Ketoacidosis common	Onset: >30 years Obese Increased blood insulin (early);normal to moderate decreased insulin (late) No anti-islet cell antibodies Ketoacidosis rare; nonketotic hyperosmolar coma
Genetics	30–70% concordance in twins Linkage to MHC Class II HLA genes	50–90% concordance in twins No HLA linkage Linkage to candidate diabetogenic genes (PPARγ, calpain 10)
Pathogenesis	Autoimmune destruction of β-cells mediated by T cells and humoral mediators (TNF, IL-1, NO) Absolute insulin deficiency	Insulin resistance in skeletal muscle, adipose tissue and liver β-cell dysfunction and relative insulin deficiency
Islet cells	Insulitis early Marked atrophy and fibrosis β-cell depletion	No insulitis Focal atrophy and amyloid deposition Mild β-cell depletion

pertinent clinical, genetic, and histopathologic features that distinguish type 1 and type 2 diabetes.

In both forms, it is the long-term effects of diabetes, more than the acute metabolic complications, that are responsible for the overwhelming proportion of morbidity and mortality. In most instances, these complications appear approximately 15 to 20 years after the onset of hyperglycemia. *Cardiovascular events such as myocardial infarction, renal vascular insufficiency, and cerebrovascular accidents are the most common causes of mortality in long-standing diabetics.* The impact of cardiovascular disease can be gauged from the fact that it accounts for up to 80% of deaths in type 2 diabetes; in fact, diabetics have a 3 to 7.5 times greater incidence of death from cardiovascular causes compared to the nondiabetic population[100] (Fig. 24–41). The hallmark of cardiovascular disease is *accelerated atherosclerosis* of the large and medium-sized arteries (i.e., macrovascular disease). *The pathogenesis of accelerated atherosclerosis involves multiple factors.* We have previously

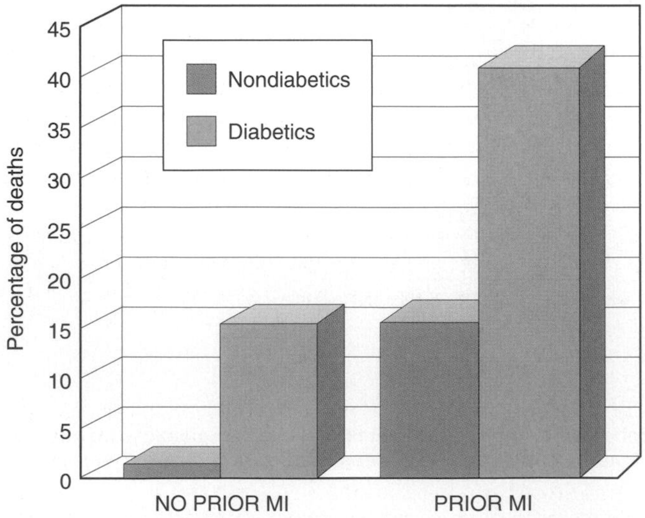

FIGURE 24–41 Incidence of death from cardiovascular causes in diabetic and nondiabetic individuals after a 7-year follow up. MI, myocardial infarction. (Reproduced with permission from Haffner et al: Mortality from coronary heart disease in subjects with type 2 diabetes and in nondiabetic subjects with and without myocardial infarction. N Engl J Med 339:229, 1998.)

mentioned the contribution of AGEs to endothelial dysfunction and vascular disease in diabetes. You will recall that the *binding of AGE-modified plasma proteins to AGE receptors on endothelial and vascular smooth muscle leads to generation of a variety of proatherogenic cytokines and growth factors.* Blockade of one such receptor—receptor for AGE, or RAGE—suppressed macrovascular disease in an atherosclerosis-prone animal model, underscoring the importance of this pathway in atherogenesis.[101] *Activation of protein kinase C,* with resultant impairment of vasodilation and increased procoagulant PAI-1 activity, may also contribute to the endothelial injury and accelerated atherosclerosis in diabetes.

The importance of *obesity* in the pathogenesis of insulin resistance has already been discussed, but it is also an independent risk factor for development of atherosclerosis (Chapter 11). Additional risk factors for atherosclerosis that are present in many type 2 diabetics include *hypertension, dyslipidemia,* and *platelet dysfunction.*[102] *Hypertension* is approximately twice as frequent in diabetics as in those without the disease. Similar to atherosclerosis, the increased frequency of hypertension may be a manifestation of hyperglycemia-induced endothelial dysfunction. *Dyslipidemias* include both increased triglycerides and LDL levels and decreased levels of the "protective" lipoprotein, HDL (Chapter 11); hepatic insulin resistance combined with peripheral activation of lipoprotein lipase plays a key role in maintaining a "proatherogenic" lipoprotein profile in diabetic individuals. Finally, increased *platelet adhesiveness* to the vessel wall is observed in states of insulin resistance, possibly owing to increased thromboxane A_2 synthesis and reduced prostacyclin.

Diabetic nephropathy is a leading cause of end-stage renal disease in the United States.[103] Approximately 30% to 40% of all diabetics develop clinical evidence of nephropathy, but a considerably smaller fraction of patients with type 2 diabetes progress to end-stage renal disease. However, because of the much greater prevalence of type 2 diabetes, these patients constitute slightly over half the diabetic patients starting dialysis each year. The frequency of diabetic nephropathy is greatly influenced by the genetic makeup of the population in question; for example, Native Americans, Hispanics, and African Americans have a greater risk of developing end-stage renal disease than do non-Hispanic whites with type 2 diabetes. The earliest manifestation of diabetic nephropathy is the appearance of low amounts of albumin in the urine (>30 mg/day, but <300 mg/day), that is, *microalbuminuria.* Of note, microalbuminuria is also a marker for greatly increased cardiovascular morbidity and mortality for patients with either type 1 or type 2 diabetes. Therefore, all patients with microalbuminuria should be screened for macrovascular disease, and aggressive intervention should be undertaken to reduce cardiovascular risk factors. Without specific interventions, approximately 80% of type 1 diabetics and 20% to 40% of type 2 diabetics will develop *overt nephropathy with macroalbuminuria* (>300 mg of urinary albumin per day) over 10 to 15 years, usually accompanied by the appearance of hypertension. The progression from overt nephropathy to end-stage renal disease can be highly variable. By 20 years, more than 75% of type 1 diabetics and approximately 20% of type 2 diabetics with overt nephropathy will develop end-stage renal disease, requiring dialysis or renal transplantation. Diabetic nephropathy is also discussed in Chapter 20.

Visual impairment, sometimes even total blindness, is one of the more feared consequences of long-standing diabetes. This disease is currently the fourth leading cause of acquired blindness in the United States. Approximately 60% to 80% of patients develop some form of *diabetic retinopathy* approximately 15 to 20 years after diagnosis (Chapter 29). As was previously stated, the fundamental lesion of retinopathy—neovascularization—is probably attributable to VEGF signaling in the retina.[104] In addition to retinopathy, diabetics also have an increased propensity for *glaucoma* and *cataract formation*, both of which contribute to visual impairment in diabetes. *Diabetic neuropathy* can elicit a variety of clinical syndromes, afflicting the central nervous system, peripheral sensorimotor nerves, and the autonomic nervous system; these are discussed further in Chapters 27 and 28.

Diabetics are plagued by enhanced susceptibility to infections of the skin and to tuberculosis, pneumonia, and pyelonephritis. Such infections cause the deaths of about 5% of diabetic patients. In an individual with diabetic neuropathy, a trivial infection in a toe may be the first event in a long succession of complications (gangrene, bacteremia, pneumonia) that may ultimately lead to death.

In recent years, increasingly sedentary lifestyles and poor eating habits have contributed to the simultaneous escalation of diabetes and obesity worldwide, which some have termed as "diabesity."[105] Sadly, this "epidemic" of diabetes and obesity has percolated even to children. As the incidence of communicable diseases has declined and expected life span has increased, diabetes has become a major public health problem, and it continues to be one of the top 10 "killers" in the United States. There is hope, however, since the role of primary prevention of type 2 diabetes by lifestyle and dietary alterations and secondary prevention of diabetic complications by strict glycemic control has become increasingly recognized. It is also hoped that islet cell transplantation will result in a cure for those afflicted with type 1 diabetes.

Pancreatic Endocrine Neoplasms

The preferred term for tumors of the pancreatic islet cells, referred to as "islet cell tumors" in common medical parlance, is *pancreatic endocrine neoplasms.*[106] They are rare in comparison with tumors of the exocrine pancreas, accounting for only 2% of all pancreatic neoplasms. They are most common in adults and can occur anywhere along the length of the pancreas, embedded in the substance of the pancreas or arising in the immediate peripancreatic tissues. They resemble in appearance their counterparts, carcinoid tumors, found elsewhere in the alimentary tract (Chapter 17). Pancreatic endocrine neoplasms may be single or multiple and benign or malignant, the latter metastasizing to lymph nodes and liver. When multiple, each tumor may be composed of a different cell type. Pancreatic endocrine neoplasms have a propensity to elaborate pancreatic hormones, but some may be totally nonfunctional.

Like any other endocrine neoplasms in the body (see below), it is difficult to predict the biologic behavior of a pancreatic endocrine neoplasm based on light microscopic criteria alone. *Unequivocal criteria for malignancy* include (1) metastases to regional lymph nodes or distant organs (including the liver), (2) vascular invasion, and (3) gross invasion of adjacent viscera. Other *features suggestive of malignancy* include infiltration beyond the tumor capsule into the pancreatic parenchyma, a high mitotic index, tumor necrosis, and significant cellular atypia. In general, tumors less than 2 cm in diameter tend to behave in an indolent manner, but there are significant exceptions to this rule. Finally, the functional status of the tumor might have some import on prognosis, as approximately 90% of insulinomas are benign, while 60% to 90% of other functioning and nonfunctioning pancreatic endocrine neoplasms tend to be malignant.[107] Fortunately, insulinomas are also the most common subtype of pancreatic endocrine neoplasms.

The three most common and distinctive clinical syndromes associated with functional pancreatic endocrine neoplasms are (1) *hyperinsulinism*, (2) *hypergastrinemia and the Zollinger-Ellison syndrome*, and (3) *multiple endocrine neoplasia* (the last is described in detail later).

HYPERINSULINISM (INSULINOMA)

β-cell tumors (insulinomas) are the most common of pancreatic endocrine neoplasms and may be responsible for the elaboration of sufficient insulin to induce clinically significant hypoglycemia. There is a characteristic clinical triad resulting from these pancreatic lesions: (1) Attacks of hypoglycemia occur with blood glucose levels below 50 mg/dL of serum; (2) the attacks consist principally of such central nervous system manifestations as confusion, stupor, and loss of consciousness; and (3) the attacks are precipitated by fasting or exercise and are promptly relieved by feeding or parenteral administration of glucose.

Morphology. Insulinomas are most often found within the pancreas and are generally benign. Most are solitary lesions, although multiple tumors or tumors ectopic to the pancreas may be encountered. Bona fide carcinomas, making up only about 10% of cases, are diagnosed on the basis of criteria for malignancy listed above. On rare occasions, an insulinoma may arise in ectopic pancreatic tissue.

Solitary tumors are usually small (often less than 2 cm in diameter) and are encapsulated, pale to red-brown nodules located anywhere in the pancreas. Histologically, these benign tumors look remarkably like giant islets, with preservation of the regular cords of monotonous cells and their orientation to the vasculature. Not even the malignant lesions present much evidence of anaplasia (Fig. 24–42*A*), and they may be deceptively encapsulated. By immunocytochemistry, insulin can be localized in the tumor cells (Fig. 24–42*B*). Under the electron microscope, neoplastic β cells, like their normal counterparts, display distinctive round granules that contain polygonal or rectangular dense crystals separated from the enclosing membrane by a distinct halo. It should be cautioned that granules may be present in the absence of clinically significant hormone activity.

Hyperinsulinism may also be caused by *diffuse hyperplasia of the islets.*[108] This change is found occasionally in adults but is usually encountered in neonates and infants. Several clinical scenarios may result in diffuse islet hyperplasia (previously known as *nesidioblastosis*), including maternal diabetes, Beckwith-Wiedemann syndrome (Chapter 10), and rare metabolic disorders. In maternal diabetes, the fetus, long exposed to the hyperglycemia of maternal blood, responds by an increase in the size and number of its islets. In the postnatal period, these hyperactive islets may be responsible for serious episodes of hypoglycemia. This phenomenon is usually transient, although persisting problems may result from mutations in the glucose-sensing mechanism or insulin-secreting mechanisms within the β cell.

While up to 80% of islet cell tumors may demonstrate excessive insulin secretion, the hypoglycemia is mild in all but about 20%, and many cases never become clinically symptomatic. The critical laboratory findings in insulinomas are high circulating levels of insulin and a high insulin-glucose ratio. Surgical removal of the tumor is usually followed by prompt reversal of the hypoglycemia.

It is important to note that *there are many other causes of hypoglycemia besides insulinomas.* The differential diagnosis of this frequently obscure metabolic abnormality includes such conditions as abnormal insulin sensitivity, diffuse liver disease, inherited glycogenoses, and ectopic production of insulin by certain retroperitoneal fibromas and fibrosarcomas.

ZOLLINGER-ELLISON SYNDROME (GASTRINOMAS)

Marked hypersecretion of gastrin usually has its origin in gastrin-producing tumors (*gastrinomas*), which are just as likely to arise in the duodenum and peripancreatic soft tissues as in the pancreas (so-called gastrinoma triangle).[109] There has been lack of agreement regarding the cell of origin for these tumors, although it appears likely that endocrine cells of either the gut or the pancreas could be the source. Zollinger and Ellison first called attention to the *association of pancreatic islet cell lesions with hypersecretion of gastric acid and severe peptic ulceration,*[110] which are present in 90% to 95% of patients.

Morphology. Gastrinomas may arise in the pancreas, the peripancreatic region, or the wall of the duodenum. **Over half of gastrin-producing tumors are locally invasive or have already metastasized at the time of diagnosis.** In approximately 25% of patients, gastrinomas arise in conjunction with other endocrine tumors, thus conforming to the MEN-1 syndrome (see below); MEN-1-associated gastrinomas are frequently multifocal, while sporadic gastrinomas are usually single. As with insulin-secreting tumors of the pancreas, gastrin-producing tumors are histologically bland and rarely exhibit marked anaplasia.

In the Zollinger-Ellison syndrome, hypergastrinemia from a pancreatic or duodenal tumor stimulates extreme gastric acid secretion, which in turn causes *peptic ulceration*. The duodenal and gastric ulcers are often *multiple*; although they are identical to those found in the general population, they are often unresponsive to usual modalities of therapy. In addition, ulcers may also occur in *unusual locations* such as the jejunum;

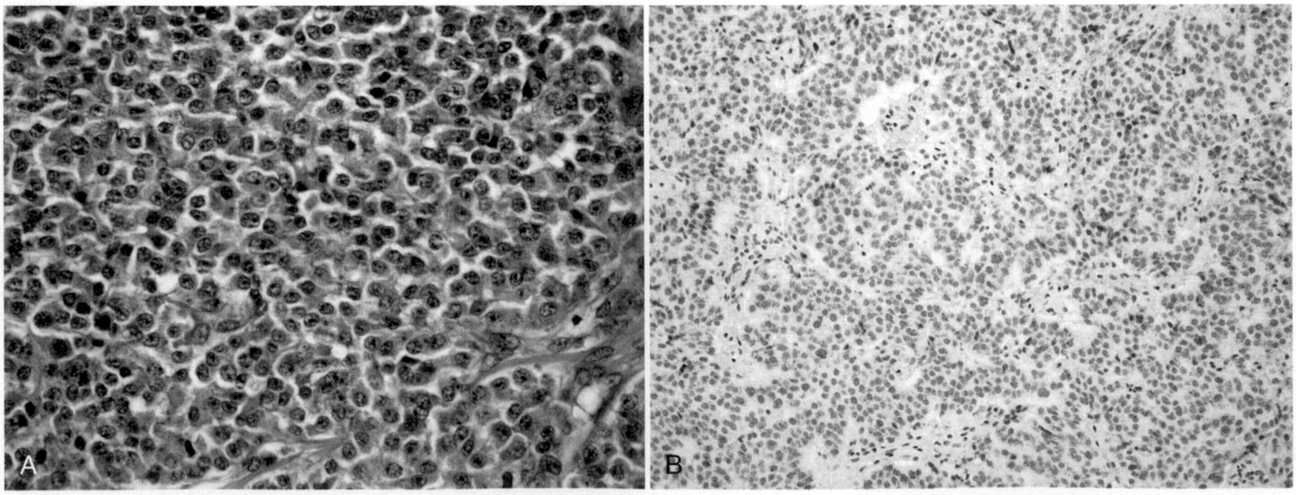

FIGURE 24–42 Pancreatic endocrine tumor ("islet cell tumor"). *A,* The neoplastic cells are monotonous and demonstrate minimal pleomorphism or mitotic activity (H & E stain). *B,* Immunoreactivity for insulin confirms the neoplasm is an insulinoma. Clinically, the patient had episodic hypoglycemia.

when intractable jejunal ulcers are found, Zollinger-Ellison syndrome should be considered. More than 50% of the patients have diarrhea; in 30%, it is the presenting symptom.

Treatment of Zollinger-Ellison syndrome involves control of gastric acid secretion by use of H^+/K^+-ATPase inhibitors (Chapter 17) and excision of the neoplasm. Total resection of the neoplasm, when possible, eliminates the syndrome. Patients with hepatic metastases have a significantly shortened life expectancy, with progressive tumor growth leading to liver failure usually within 10 years.

OTHER RARE PANCREATIC ENDOCRINE NEOPLASMS

α-cell tumors (glucagonomas) are associated with increased serum levels of glucagon and a syndrome consisting of mild diabetes mellitus, a characteristic skin rash (necrolytic migratory erythema), and anemia. They occur most frequently in perimenopausal and postmenopausal women and are characterized by extremely high plasma glucagon levels.

δ-cell tumors (somatostatinomas) are associated with diabetes mellitus, cholelithiasis, steatorrhea, and hypochlorhydria. They are exceedingly difficult to localize preoperatively. High plasma somatostatin levels are required for diagnosis.

VIPoma (watery diarrhea, hypokalemia, achlorhydria, or WDHA syndrome) is an endocrine tumor that induces a characteristic syndrome, caused by release of vasoactive intestinal peptide (VIP) from the tumor. Some of these tumors are locally invasive and metastatic. A VIP assay should be performed on all patients with severe secretory diarrhea. Neural crest tumors, such as neuroblastomas, ganglioneuroblastomas, and ganglioneuromas (Chapter 10) and pheochromocytomas (see below) can also be associated with the VIPoma syndrome.

Pancreatic carcinoid tumors producing serotonin and an atypical carcinoid syndrome are exceedingly rare. *Pancreatic polypeptide-secreting endocrine tumors* are endocrinologically asymptomatic, despite the presence of high levels of the hormone in plasma.

Some pancreatic and extrapancreatic endocrine tumors produce two or more hormones, usually simultaneously and occasionally in sequence. In addition to insulin, glucagon, and gastrin, pancreatic endocrine tumors may produce adrenocorticotropic hormone, melanocyte-stimulating hormone, vasopressin, serotonin, and norepinephrine. These *multihormonal tumors* are to be distinguished from the multiple endocrine neoplasias (see below), in which a multiplicity of hormones is produced by tumors in several different glands.

ADRENAL GLANDS

Adrenal Cortex

Normal

The *adrenal glands* are paired endocrine organs consisting of both cortex and medulla, which differ in their development, structure, and function. In the adult, the normal adrenal gland weighs about 4 gm; but with *acute* stress, lipid depletion may reduce the weight, or *prolonged* stress, such as dying after a long chronic illness, can induce hypertrophy and hyperplasia of the cortical cells and more than double the weight of the normal gland. Beneath the capsule of the adrenal is the narrow layer of zona glomerulosa. An equally narrow zona reticularis abuts the medulla. Intervening is the broad zona fasciculata, which makes up about 75% of the total cortex. The *adrenal cortex* synthesizes three different types of steroids: (1) *glucocorticoids* (principally cortisol), which are synthesized primarily in the zona fasciculata with a small contribution from the zona reticularis; (2) *mineralocorticoids*, the most important being aldosterone, which is generated in the zona glomerulosa; and (3) *sex steroids* (estrogens and androgens), which are produced largely in the zona reticularis. The *adrenal medulla* is composed of chromaffin cells, which synthesize and secrete *catecholamines*, mainly epinephrine. Catecholamines have many effects that allow rapid adaptations to changes in the environment.

Pathology

Diseases of the adrenal cortex can be conveniently divided into those associated with cortical hyperfunction and those characterized by cortical hypofunction.

ADRENOCORTICAL HYPERFUNCTION (HYPERADRENALISM)

Just as there are three basic types of corticosteroids elaborated by the adrenal cortex (glucocorticoids, mineralocorticoids, and sex steroids), so there are three distinctive hyperadrenal clinical syndromes: (1) *Cushing syndrome*, characterized by an excess of cortisol; (2) *hyperaldosteronism*; and (3) *adrenogenital* or virilizing syndromes caused by an excess of androgens. The clinical features of these syndromes overlap somewhat because of the overlapping functions of some of the adrenal steroids.

Hypercortisolism (Cushing Syndrome)

Pathogenesis. This disorder is caused by any condition that produces an elevation in glucocorticoid levels.[111] There are four possible sources of excess cortisol (Fig. 24–43). In clinical practice, *most causes of Cushing syndrome are the result of the administration of exogenous glucocorticoids.* The other

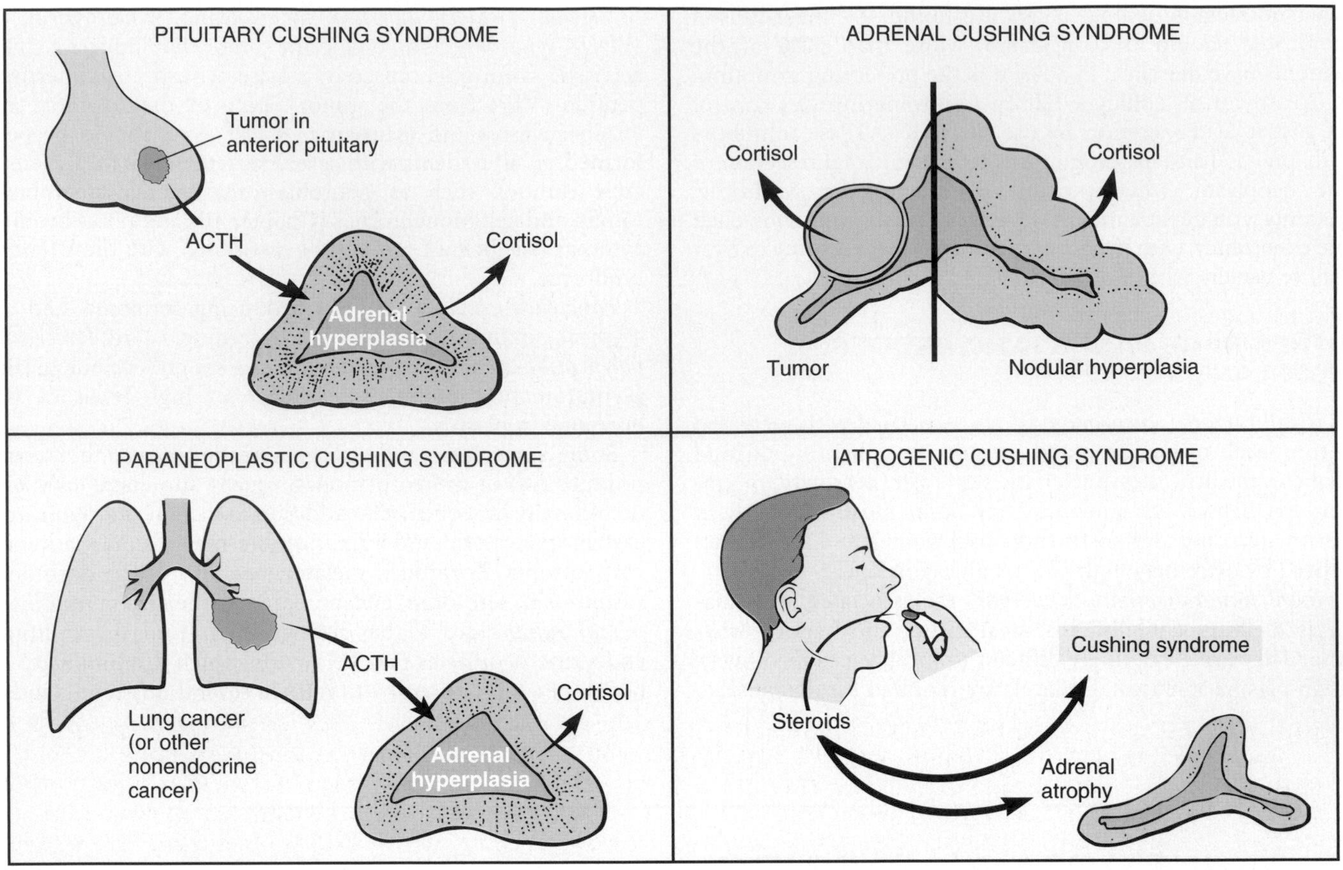

FIGURE 24–43 A schematic representation of the various forms of Cushing syndrome, illustrating the three endogenous forms as well as the more common exogenous (iatrogenic) form. ACTH, adrenocorticotropic hormone.

three sources of the hypercortisolism can be categorized as *endogenous* Cushing syndrome:

- Primary hypothalamic-pituitary diseases associated with hypersecretion of ACTH
- Hypersecretion of cortisol by an adrenal adenoma, carcinoma, or nodular hyperplasia
- The secretion of ectopic ACTH by a nonendocrine neoplasm

Primary hypersecretion of ACTH accounts for 70% to 80% of cases of endogenous hypercortisolism. In recognition of the neurosurgeon who first published the full description of this syndrome and related it to a pituitary lesion,[112] this pituitary form of Cushing syndrome is referred to as *Cushing disease.* The disorder affects women about five times more frequently than men, and it occurs most frequently during the twenties and thirties. In the vast majority of cases, the pituitary gland contains an *ACTH-producing microadenoma* that does not produce mass effects in the brain; some corticotroph tumors qualify as macroadenomas (>10 mm). In most of the remaining cases, the anterior pituitary contains areas of *corticotroph cell hyperplasia* without a discrete adenoma. Corticotroph cell hyperplasia may be primary or may arise secondarily from excessive stimulation of ACTH release by a hypothalamic corticotropin releasing hormone (CRH)–producing tumor. The adrenal glands in patients with Cushing disease are characterized by variable degrees of nodular cortical hyperplasia (discussed later), caused by the elevated levels of ACTH. The cortical hyperplasia, in turn, is responsible for hypercortisolism.

Primary adrenal neoplasms, such as adrenal adenoma and carcinoma, and *primary cortical hyperplasia* are responsible for about 10% to 20% of cases of endogenous Cushing syndrome. This form of Cushing syndrome is also designated *ACTH-independent Cushing syndrome* or adrenal Cushing syndrome because the adrenals function autonomously. The biochemical sine qua non of adrenal Cushing syndrome is elevated serum levels of cortisol with low levels of ACTH.

- Adenomas and carcinomas are about equally common in adults; in children, carcinomas predominate. The cortical carcinomas tend to produce more marked hypercortisolism than the adenomas or hyperplastic processes. In instances of a unilateral neoplasm, the uninvolved adrenal cortex and that in the opposite gland undergo atrophy because of suppression of ACTH secretion.
- The overwhelming majority of hyperplastic adrenals arise from secondary influences, and *primary cortical hyperplasia is uncommon.* Two types of primary bilateral adrenocortical hyperplasia have been described in association with Cushing syndrome. In *massive macronodular adrenocortical disease (MMAD)*, the nodules are usually greater than 3 mm in diameter.[113] MMAD affects older adults, and there is no known genetic component. The second variant of primary nodular hyperplasia, seen more often in children than in adults, is a familial condition known as *primary pigmented nodular adrenal disease (PPNAD).*[114] The adrenal glands

in PPNAD demonstrate diffuse bilateral micronodules (<3 mm in diameter) that are usually darkly pigmented (brown to black).

Secretion of ectopic ACTH by nonpituitary tumors accounts for most of the remaining cases (~10%) of Cushing syndrome. In many instances, the responsible tumor is a *small cell carcinoma of the lung*, although other neoplasms, including carcinoid tumors, medullary carcinomas of the thyroid, and islet cell tumors of the pancreas, have been associated with the syndrome. In addition to tumors that elaborate ectopic ACTH, an occasional neuroendocrine neoplasm produces ectopic corticotropin-releasing hormone, which, in turn, causes ACTH secretion and hypercortisolism. As in the pituitary variant, the adrenal glands undergo bilateral cortical hyperplasia, but often the rapid downhill course of the patients with these cancers cuts short the adrenal enlargement. This variant of Cushing syndrome is more common in men and usually occurs in the forties and fifties.

Morphology. The main lesions of Cushing syndrome are found in the pituitary and adrenal glands. The **pituitary** in Cushing syndrome shows changes regardless of the cause. The most common alteration, resulting from high levels of endogenous or exogenous glucocorticoids, is termed **Crooke hyaline change.** In this condition, the normal granular, basophilic cytoplasm of the ACTH-producing cells in the anterior pituitary is replaced by homogeneous, lightly basophilic material. This alteration is the result of the accumulation of intermediate keratin filaments in the cytoplasm.

The morphology of the **adrenal glands** depends on the cause of the hypercortisolism. The adrenals have one of the following abnormalities: (1) cortical atrophy; (2) diffuse hyperplasia; (3) nodular hyperplasia; and (4) an adenoma, rarely a carcinoma. In patients in whom the syndrome results from exogenous glucocorticoids, suppression of endogenous ACTH results in bilateral **cortical atrophy,** due to a lack of stimulation of the zonae fasciculata and reticularis by ACTH. The zona glomerulosa is of normal thickness in such cases because this portion of the cortex functions independently of ACTH. In cases of endogenous hypercortisolism, in contrast, the adrenals either are hyperplastic or contain a cortical neoplasm. **Diffuse hyperplasia** is found in 60% to 70% of cases of Cushing syndrome. Both glands are enlarged, either subtly or markedly, weighing up to 25 to 40 gm. The adrenal cortex is diffusely thickened and yellow, owing to an increase in the size and number of lipid-rich cells in the zonae fasciculata and reticularis. Some degree of nodularity is common but is pronounced in **nodular hyperplasia.** This takes the form of bilateral, 0.5- to 2.0-cm, yellow nodules scattered throughout the cortex, separated by intervening areas of widened cortex. The uninvolved cortex and nodules are composed of a mixture of lipid-laden clear cells and lipid-poor compact cells showing some variability in cell and nuclear size with occasional binucleate forms. The combined adrenals may weigh up to 30 to 50 gm. Most cases of hyperplasia are associated with elevated serum levels of ACTH, whether of pituitary or ectopic origin. **Primary adrenocortical neoplasms** causing Cushing syndrome may be malignant or benign. Adenomas or carcinomas of the adrenal cortex as the source of cortisol secretion are not macroscopically distinctive from nonfunctioning adrenal neoplasms to be described later. Both the benign and the malignant lesions are more common in women in their thirties to fifties. The adrenocortical **adenomas** are yellow tumors surrounded by thin or well-developed capsules, and most weigh less than 30 gm. Microscopically, they are composed of cells that are similar to those encountered in the normal zona fasciculata. Their morphology is identical to that of nonfunctional adenomas and of adenomas associated with hyperaldosteronism (see below). The **carcinomas** associated with Cushing syndrome, by contrast, tend to be larger than the adenomas. These tumors are unencapsulated masses frequently exceeding 200 to 300 gm in weight, having all of the anaplastic characteristics of cancer, as will be detailed later. With functioning tumors, both benign and malignant, the adjacent adrenal cortex and that of the contralateral adrenal gland are atrophic, owing to suppression of endogenous ACTH by high cortisol levels.

Clinical Course. Developing slowly over time, Cushing syndrome, similar to many other endocrine abnormalities, can be quite subtle in its early manifestations. Early stages of the disorder may present with hypertension and weight gain (Table 24–9). With time, the more characteristic central pattern of adipose tissue deposition becomes apparent, with resultant truncal obesity, moon facies, and accumulation of fat in the posterior neck and back (*buffalo hump*). Hypercortisolism causes selective atrophy of fast-twitch (type 2) myofibers, resulting in decreased muscle mass and proximal limb weakness. Glucocorticoids induce gluconeogenesis and inhibit the uptake of glucose by cells, with resultant *hyperglycemia, glucosuria,* and *polydipsia*; Cushing syndrome is an important cause of secondary diabetes. The catabolic effects on proteins cause loss of collagen and resorption of bones. Consequently, the *skin is thin, fragile, and easily bruised*; wound healing is poor; and cutaneous striae are particularly common in the abdominal area. Bone resorption results in the development of *osteoporosis,* with consequent backache and increased susceptibility to fractures. Patients with Cushing syndrome are at increased risk for a variety of infections

TABLE 24–9 Major Features of Cushing Syndrome with Approximate Frequency

Clinical Features	Percentages
Central obesity (about trunk and upper back)	85–90%
Moon facies	85%
Weakness and fatigability	85%
Hirsutism	75%
Hypertension	75%
Plethora	75%
Glucose intolerance/diabetes	75/20%
Osteoporosis	75%
Neuropsychiatric abnormalities	75–80%
Menstrual abnormalities	70%
Skin striae (sides of lower abdomen)	50%

because glucocorticoids suppress the immune response. Additional manifestations include a number of *mental disturbances*, including mood swings, depression, and frank psychosis, as well as *hirsutism* and *menstrual abnormalities*.

Cushing syndrome is diagnosed in the laboratory with the following: (1) the 24–hour urine free cortisol level, which is increased, and (2) loss of normal diurnal pattern of cortisol secretion. Determining the cause of Cushing syndrome depends on the level of serum ACTH and measurement of urinary steroid excretion after administration of dexamethasone. Three general patterns can be obtained:[111]

1. In pituitary Cushing syndrome, the most common form, ACTH levels are elevated and cannot be suppressed by the administration of a low dose of dexamethasone. Hence, there is no reduction in urinary excretion of 17-hydroxycorticosteroids. After higher doses of injected dexamethasone, however, the pituitary responds by reducing ACTH secretion, which is reflected by suppression of urinary steroid secretion.
2. Ectopic ACTH secretion results in an elevated level of ACTH, but its secretion is completely insensitive to low or high doses of exogenous dexamethasone.
3. When Cushing syndrome is caused by an adrenal tumor, the ACTH level is quite low because of feedback inhibition of the pituitary. As with ectopic ACTH secretion, both low-dose and high-dose dexamethasone fail to suppress cortisol excretion.

Primary Hyperaldosteronism

Hyperaldosteronism is the generic term for a small group of closely related, uncommon syndromes, all characterized by chronic excess aldosterone secretion. *Excessive levels of aldosterone cause sodium retention and potassium excretion, with resultant hypertension and hypokalemia.* Hyperaldosteronism may be primary, or it may be a secondary event resulting from an extra-adrenal cause.

Primary hyperaldosteronism indicates an autonomous overproduction of aldosterone, with resultant suppression of the renin-angiotensin system and decreased plasma renin activity. Primary hyperaldosteronism is caused by one of three mechanisms[115] (Fig. 24–44):

- *Adrenocortical neoplasm*, either an aldosterone-producing adrenocortical adenoma (the most common cause) or, rarely, an adrenocortical carcinoma. In approximately 80% of cases, primary hyperaldosteronism is caused by a solitary aldosterone-secreting adenoma, a condition referred to as *Conn syndrome*. This syndrome occurs most frequently in adult middle life and is more common in women than in men (2:1). Multiple adenomas may be present in an occasional patient.
- *Primary adrenocortical hyperplasia (idiopathic hyperaldosteronism)*, characterized by bilateral nodular hyperplasia of the adrenal glands, highly reminiscent of those found in the nodular hyperplasia of Cushing syndrome. The genetic basis of idiopathic hyperaldosteronism is not clear, although it is possibly caused by an overactivity of the aldosterone synthase gene, *CYP11B2*.[116]
- *Glucocorticoid-remediable hyperaldosteronism* is an uncommon cause of primary hyperaldosteronism that is familial and genetic. In some families, it is caused by a chimeric gene resulting from fusion between *CYP11B1* (the 11β-hydroxylase gene) and *CYP11B2* (the aldosterone synthase gene).[117] This leads to a sustained production of hybrid steroids in addition to both cortisol and aldosterone. The activation of aldosterone secretion is under the influence of ACTH and hence is suppressible by exogenous administration of dexamethasone.

In *secondary hyperaldosteronism*, in contrast, aldosterone release occurs in response to activation of the renin-angiotensin system (Chapter 4). It is characterized by increased levels of plasma renin and is encountered in conditions such as the following:

- Decreased renal perfusion (arteriolar nephrosclerosis, renal artery stenosis)
- Arterial hypovolemia and edema (congestive heart failure, cirrhosis, nephrotic syndrome)
- Pregnancy (due to estrogen-induced increases in plasma renin substrate).

Morphology. Aldosterone-producing adenomas are almost always solitary, small (<2 cm in diameter), well-circumscribed lesions, more often found on the left than on the right. They tend to occur in the thirties and forties, and in women more often than in men. These lesions are often buried within the gland and do not produce visible enlargement, a point to be remembered in interpreting sonographic or scanning images. They are bright yellow on cut section (Fig. 24–45) and, surprisingly, are composed of lipid-laden cortical cells that more closely resemble fasciculata cells than glomerulosa cells (the normal source of aldosterone). In general, the cells tend to be uniform in size and shape and resemble mature cortical cells; occasionally, there is some nuclear and cellular pleomorphism but no evidence of anaplasia (Fig. 24–46). A characteristic feature of aldesterone-producing adenomas is the presence of eosinophilic, laminated cytoplasmic inclusions, known as **spironolactone bodies**, found after treatment with the antihypertensive drug spironolactone. In contrast to cortical adenomas associated with Cushing syndrome, those associated with hyperaldosteronism do not usually suppress ACTH secretion. Therefore, the adjacent adrenal cortex and that of the contralateral gland are not atrophic.

Bilateral idiopathic hyperplasia (Fig. 24–47) is marked by diffuse and focal hyperplasia of cells resembling those of the normal zona glomerulosa. The hyperplasia is often wedge-shaped, extending from the periphery toward the center of the gland. Bilateral enlargement can be subtle in idiopathic hyperplasia, and as a rule, an adrenocortical adenoma should be carefully excluded as the cause for hyperaldosteronism.

Clinical Course. *The clinical manifestations of primary hyperaldosteronism are hypertension and hypokalemia.* Serum renin, as was mentioned previously, is low. Hypokalemia results from renal potassium wasting and can cause a variety of neuromuscular manifestations, including weakness, paresthesias, visual disturbances, and occasionally frank tetany. Sodium retention increases the total body sodium and

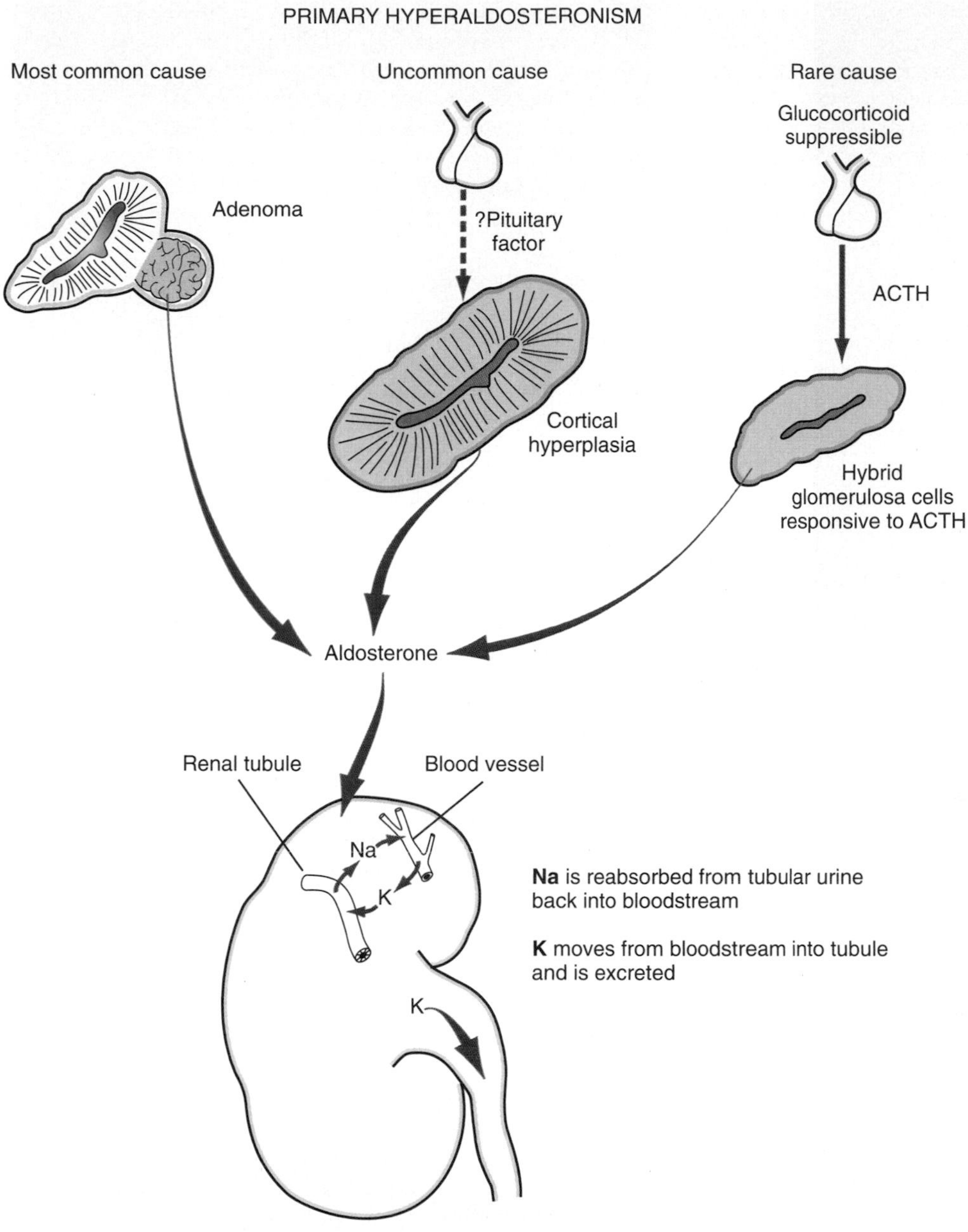

FIGURE 24–44 The major causes of primary hyperaldosteronism and its principal effects on the kidney.

expands the extracellular fluid volume, leading to elevation of the serum sodium concentration and an increase in intracellular sodium with increased vascular reactivity. The hypertension is, in part, a result of the sodium retention. The expanded extracellular fluid volume and hypokalemia both impose a burden on the heart, sometimes causing electrocardiographic changes and cardiac decompensation. The diagnosis of primary hyperaldosteronism is confirmed by the elevated levels of aldosterone and depressed levels of renin in the circulation. Even when the diagnosis of primary hyperaldosteronism is made, it is necessary to distinguish among the various causes, particularly the differentiation of an adenoma, which is amenable to surgical excision. Primary adrenal hyperplasia associated with hyperaldosteronism occurs more often in children and young adults than in older adults; surgical intervention is not very beneficial in these patients, who are best managed with medical therapy with an aldosterone antagonist such as spironolactone. Uncommon as primary hyperaldosteronism is, it should not be overlooked clinically, because it provides an opportunity to cure a form of hypertension. The treatment of secondary hyperaldosteronism rests on correcting the underlying cause stimulating the renin-angiotensin system.

Adrenogenital Syndromes

Disorders of sexual differentiation, such as virilization or feminization, can be caused by primary gonadal disorders (Chapter 22) and several primary adrenal disorders. The adrenal cortex secretes two compounds—dehydroepiandrosterone and androstenedione—that require conversion to testosterone in peripheral tissues for their androgenic effects. Unlike gonadal androgens, ACTH regulates adrenal androgen formation (Fig. 24–48); thus, excess secretion can occur either as a "pure" syndrome or as a component of Cushing disease. The adrenal causes of androgen excess include *adrenocortical*

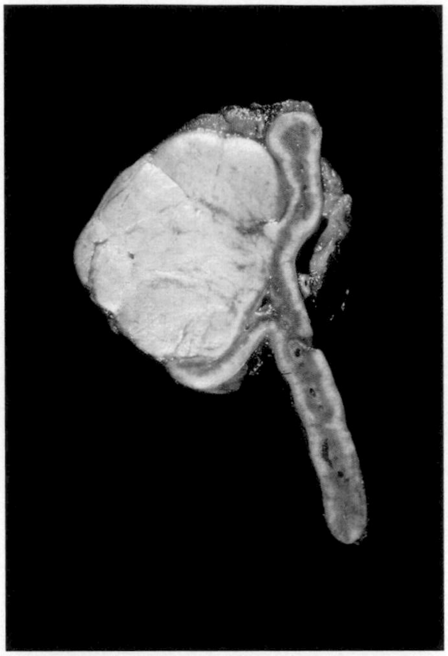

FIGURE 24–45 Adrenal cortical adenoma. The adenoma is distinguished from nodular hyperplasia by its solitary, circumscribed nature. The functional status of an adrenal cortical adenoma cannot be predicted from its gross or microscopic appearance.

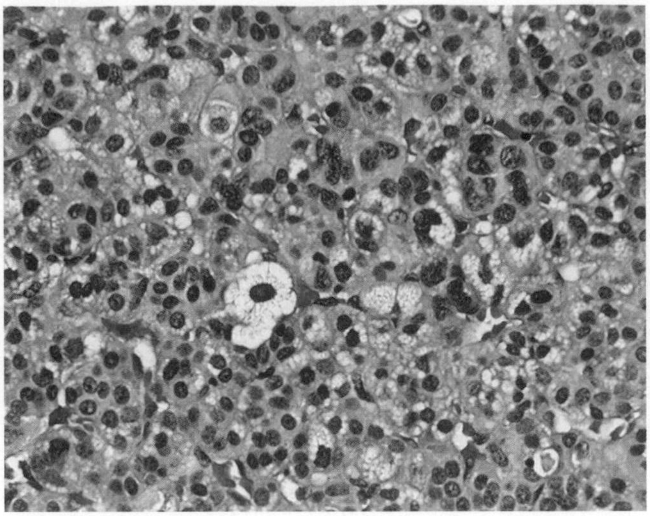

FIGURE 24–46 Histologic features of an adrenal cortical adenoma. The neoplastic cells are vacuolated because of the presence of intracytoplasmic lipid. There is mild nuclear pleomorphism. Mitotic activity and necrosis are not seen.

neoplasms and a group of disorders that have been designated *congenital adrenal hyperplasia.*

Adrenocortical neoplasms associated with virilization are more likely to be *androgen-secreting adrenal carcinomas* than adenomas. Conversely, functioning adrenal cortical carcinomas are most often associated with a virilization syndrome, usually in combination with hypercortisolism ("mixed syndrome"). These tumors are morphologically identical to other cortical neoplasms and will be discussed later.

Congenital adrenal hyperplasia (CAH) represents a group of autosomal-recessive, inherited metabolic errors, each characterized by a deficiency or total lack of a particular enzyme involved in the biosynthesis of cortical steroids, particularly cortisol.[118] Steroidogenesis is then channeled into other pathways, leading to increased production of androgens, which accounts for virilization. Simultaneously, the deficiency of cortisol results in increased secretion of ACTH, resulting in adrenal hyperplasia. Certain enzyme defects may also impair aldosterone secretion, adding *salt wasting* to the virilizing syndrome. Other enzyme deficiencies may be incompatible with life or, in rare instances, may involve only the aldosterone pathway without involving cortisol synthesis. Thus, there is a spectrum of these syndromes, and with each one, there may be a total lack of a particular enzyme or a mutation that only mildly impairs the effectiveness of the enzyme. The following remarks focus on the most common of these disorders.

21-Hydroxylase Deficiency. Defective conversion of progesterone to 11-deoxycorticosterone by 21-hydroxylase (*CYP21B*) accounts for over 90% of cases of congenital adrenal hyperplasia.[119] Figure 24–48 illustrates normal adrenal steroidogenesis and the consequences of 21-hydroxylase deficiency. 21-Hydroxylase deficiency may range from a total lack to a mild loss, depending on the nature of the *CYP21B* mutation. Three distinctive syndromes have been described: (1) salt-wasting (classic) adrenogenitalism, (2) simple virilizing adrenogenitalism, and (3) nonclassic adrenogenitalism, which implies mild disease that may be entirely asymptomatic or associated only with symptoms of androgen excess during childhood or puberty.

The carrier frequency of the classic form is approximately 1 in 60, while the carrier frequency of the nonclassic or mild form is 1 in 5 to 1 in 50, depending on the ethnic group; Hispanics and Ashkenazi Jewish populations have the highest carrier frequencies. The incidence of classic 21-hydroxylase deficiency varies somewhat between populations, with a

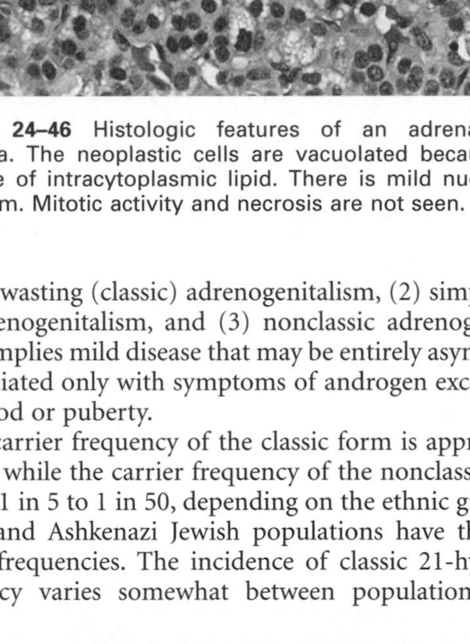

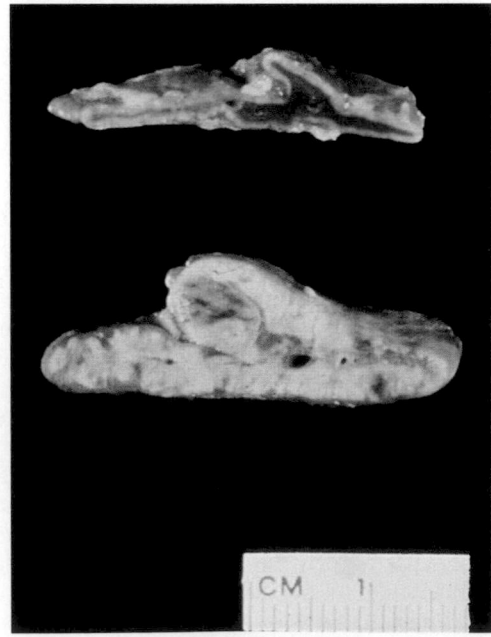

FIGURE 24–47 Nodular hyperplasia of the adrenal contrasted with normal adrenal gland. In cross-section, the adrenal cortex is yellow, thickened, and multinodular, owing to hypertrophy and hyperplasia of the lipid-rich zonae fasciculata and reticularis.

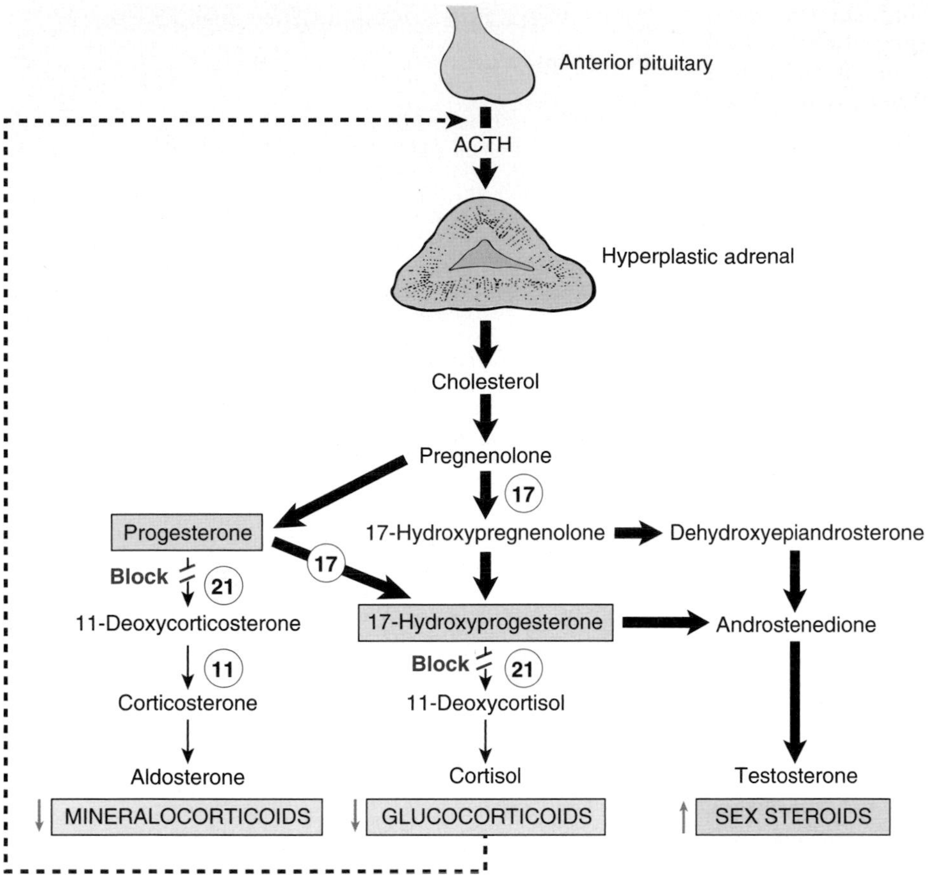

FIGURE 24–48 Consequences of C-21 hydroxylase deficiency. 21-Hydroxylase deficiency impairs the synthesis of both cortisol and aldosterone. The resultant decrease in feedback inhibition *(dashed line)* causes increased secretion of adrenocorticotropic hormone, resulting ultimately in adrenal hyperplasia and increased synthesis of testosterone. The sites of action of 11-, 17-, and 21-hydroxylase are shown by the numbers in circles.

worldwide mean of around 1 in 13,000 newborns. The mechanism of *CYP21B* gene inactivation in 21-hydroxylase deficiency involves recombination with a neighboring pseudogene on chromosome 6p21 called *CYP21A* (a *pseudogene* is an inactive homologous gene created by ancestral duplication in a localized region of the genome). In the majority of cases of CAH, portions of the *CYP21A* pseudogene replace all or part of the active *CYP21B* gene. The introduction of nonfunctional sequences from *CYP21A* into the *CYP21B* sequence has the same effect as inactivating mutations in *CYP21B*.

The *salt-wasting syndrome* results from an inability to convert progesterone into deoxycorticosterone because of a total lack of the hydroxylase. Thus, there is virtually no synthesis of mineralocorticoids, and concomitantly, there is a block in the conversion of hydroxyprogesterone into deoxycortisol with deficient cortisol synthesis. This pattern usually comes to light soon after birth because in utero the electrolytes and fluids can be maintained by the maternal kidneys. There is *salt wasting*, *hyponatremia*, and *hyperkalemia*, which induce acidosis, *hypotension*, cardiovascular collapse, and possibly death. The concomitant block in cortisol synthesis and excess production of androgens, however, lead to virilization, which is easily recognized in the female at birth or in utero but is difficult to recognize in the male. Various degrees of virilization are encountered, ranging from mild clitoral enlargement to complete labioscrotal fusion to marked clitoral enlargement enclosing the urethra, thus producing a phalloid organ. Males with this disorder are generally unrecognized at birth but come to clinical attention 5 to 15 days later because of some salt-losing crisis.

Simple virilizing adrenogenital syndrome without salt wasting (presenting as genital ambiguity) may occur in individuals with a less than total 21-hydroxylase defect because with less severe deficiencies the level of mineralocorticoid, although reduced, is sufficient for salt reabsorption, but the lowered glucocorticoid level fails to cause feedback inhibition of ACTH secretion. Thus, the level of aldosterone is mildly reduced, testosterone is increased, and ACTH is elevated, with resultant adrenal hyperplasia.

Nonclassic or late-onset adrenal virilism is much more common than the classic patterns already described. Patients with this syndrome may be virtually asymptomatic or have mild manifestations, such as hirsutism. The diagnosis can be made only by demonstration of biosynthetic defects in steroidogenesis and by genetic studies.

Morphology. In all cases of CAH, the adrenals are bilaterally hyperplastic, sometimes expanding to 10 to 15 times their normal weights because of the sustained elevation in ACTH. The adrenal cortex is thickened and nodular, and on cut section, the widened cortex appears brown, owing to total depletion of all lipid. The proliferating cells are mostly compact, eosinophilic, lipid-depleted cells, intermixed with lipid-laden clear cells. Hyperplasia of corticotroph (ACTH-producing) cells is present in the anterior pituitary in most CAH patients.

Clinical Course. The clinical features of these disorders are determined by the specific enzyme deficiency and include abnormalities related to *androgen excess* and *aldosterone* and *glucocorticoid deficiency*. CAH affects not only adrenal cortical enzymes, but also products synthesized in the medulla. High levels of intra-adrenal glucocorticoids are required to facilitate medullary catecholamine (epinephrine and norepinephrine) synthesis. In patients with severe salt-wasting 21-hydroxylase deficiency, a combination of low cortisol levels and developmental defects of the medulla (*adrenomedullary dysplasia*) profoundly affects catecholamine secretion, further predisposing these individuals to hypotension and circulatory collapse.[120]

Depending on the nature and severity of the enzymatic defect, the onset of clinical symptoms may occur in the perinatal period, later childhood, or, less commonly, adulthood. For example, in 21-hydroxylase deficiency, excessive androgenic activity causes signs of masculinization in females, ranging from clitoral hypertrophy and pseudohermaphroditism in infants, to oligomenorrhea, hirsutism, and acne in postpubertal females. In males, androgen excess is associated with enlargement of the external genitalia and other evidence of precocious puberty in prepubertal patients and oligospermia in older males.

CAH should be suspected in any neonate with ambiguous genitalia; severe enzyme deficiency in infancy can be a life-threatening condition with vomiting, dehydration, and salt wasting. In the milder variants, women may present with delayed menarche, oligomenorrhea, or hirsutism. Patients with congenital adrenal hyperplasia are treated with exogenous glucocorticoids, which, in addition to providing adequate levels of glucocorticoids, also suppress ACTH levels and thus decrease the excessive synthesis of the steroid hormones responsible for many of the clinical abnormalities. Mineralocorticoid supplementation is required in the salt-wasting variants of CAH. With the availability of routine neonatal metabolic screens for CAH and the feasibility of molecular testing for antenatal detection of 21-hydroxylase mutations, the outcome for even the most severe variants has improved significantly.

ADRENAL INSUFFICIENCY

Adrenocortical insufficiency, or hypofunction, may be caused by either primary adrenal disease (primary hypoadrenalism) or decreased stimulation of the adrenals owing to a deficiency of ACTH (secondary hypoadrenalism) (Table 24–10). The patterns of adrenocortical insufficiency can be considered under the following headings: (1) primary *acute* adrenocortical insufficiency (adrenal crisis), (2) primary *chronic* adrenocortical insufficiency (*Addison disease*), and (3) secondary adrenocortical insufficiency.

TABLE 24–10 Adrenocortical Insufficiency

Primary Insufficiency
Loss of cortex
Congential adrenal *hypo*plasia
X-linked adrenal hypoplasia (*DAX-1* gene on Xp21)
"Miniature" type adrenal hypoplasia (unknown cause)
Adrenoleukodystrophy (*ALD* gene on Xq28)
Autoimmune adrenal insufficiency
Autoimmune polyendocrinopathy syndrome type 1 (*AIRE-1* gene on 21q22)
Autoimmune polyendocrinopathy syndrome type 2 (polygenic)
Isolated autoimmune adrenalitis (polygenic)
Infection
Acquired immune deficiency syndrome
Tuberculosis
Fungi
Acute hemorrhagic necrosis (*Waterhouse-Friderichsen syndrome)*
Amyloidosis, sarcoidosis, hemochromatosis
Metastatic carcinoma
Metabolic failure in hormone production
Congenital adrenal *hyper*plasia (cortisol and aldosterone deficiency with virlization)
Drug- and steroid-induced inhibition of adrenocorticotropic hormone or cortical cell function
Secondary Insufficiency
Hypothalamic pituitary disease
Neoplasm, inflammation (sarcoidosis, tuberculosis, pyogens, fungi)
Hypothalamic pituitary suppression
Long-term steroid administration
Steroid-producing neoplasms

Primary Acute Adrenocortical Insufficiency

Acute adrenal cortical insufficiency occurs in a variety of clinical settings (see Table 24–10):

- As a *crisis* in patients with chronic adrenocortical insufficiency precipitated by any form of stress that requires an immediate increase in steroid output from glands incapable of responding
- In patients maintained on exogenous corticosteroids, in whom rapid withdrawal of steroids or failure to increase steroid doses in response to an acute stress may precipitate an adrenal crisis, owing to the inability of the atrophic adrenals to produce glucocorticoid hormones
- As a result of massive adrenal hemorrhage, which destroys the adrenal cortex sufficiently to cause acute adrenocortical insufficiency. This occurs in newborns following prolonged and difficult delivery with considerable trauma and hypoxia, leading to extensive adrenal hemorrhages beginning in the medulla and extending into the cortex. Newborns are particularly vulnerable because they are often deficient in prothrombin for at least several days after birth. It also occurs in some patients maintained on anticoagulant therapy, in postsurgical patients who develop disseminated intravascular coagulation with consequent hemorrhagic infarction of the adrenals, and when massive adrenal hemorrhage complicates a bacteremic infection; in this last setting, it is called *Waterhouse-Friderichsen syndrome.*

Waterhouse-Friderichsen Syndrome

This uncommon but catastrophic syndrome is characterized by the following:

- An overwhelming bacterial infection, which is classically associated with *Neisseria meningitidis* septicemia but occasionally is caused by other highly virulent organisms, such as *Pseudomonas* species, pneumococci, *Haemophilus influenzae*, or staphylococci
- Rapidly progressive hypotension leading to shock
- Disseminated intravascular coagulation with widespread purpura, particularly of the skin

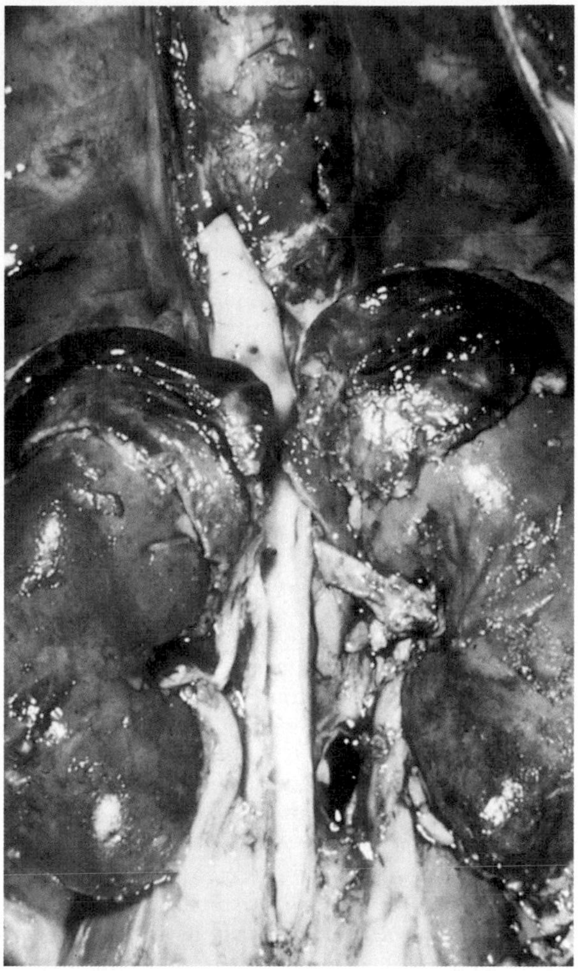

FIGURE 24–49 Waterhouse-Friderichsen syndrome in a child. The dark, hemorrhagic adrenal glands are distended with blood.

- Rapidly developing adrenocortical insufficiency associated with massive bilateral adrenal hemorrhage

Waterhouse-Friderichsen syndrome can occur at any age but is somewhat more common in children. The basis for the adrenal hemorrhage is uncertain but could be attributable to direct bacterial seeding of small vessels in the adrenal, the development of disseminated intravascular coagulation, endotoxin-induced vasculitis, or some form of hypersensitivity vasculitis. *Whatever the basis, the adrenals are converted to sacs of clotted blood virtually obscuring all underlying detail* (Fig. 24–49). Histologic examination reveals that the hemorrhage starts within the medulla in relationship to thin-walled venous sinusoids, then suffuses peripherally into the cortex, often leaving islands of recognizable cortical cells (Fig. 24–50). When it is recognized promptly and treated effectively with antibiotics, recovery is possible, but the clinical course is usually devastatingly abrupt, and prompt recognition and appropriate therapy must be instituted immediately, or death follows within hours to a few days.

Primary Chronic Adrenocortical Insufficiency (Addison Disease)

In a paper published in 1855, Thomas Addison described a group of patients suffering from a constellation of symptoms, including "general languor and debility, remarkable feebleness of the heart's action, and a peculiar change in the color of the skin" associated with disease of the "suprarenal capsules" or, in more current terminology, the adrenal glands. Addison disease, or chronic adrenocortical insufficiency, is an uncommon disorder resulting from progressive destruction of the adrenal cortex. In general, clinical manifestations of adrenocortical insufficiency do not appear until at least 90% of the adrenal cortex has been compromised. The causes of chronic adrenocortical insufficiency are listed in Table 24–10. Although all races and both sexes may be affected, certain causes of Addison disease (such as autoimmune adrenalitis) are much more common in whites, particularly in women.

Pathogenesis. A large number of diseases may attack the adrenal cortex, including lymphomas, amyloidosis, sarcoidosis, hemochromatosis, fungal infections, and adrenal hemorrhage, but more than 90% of all cases are attributable to one of four disorders: *autoimmune adrenalitis, tuberculosis, the acquired immune deficiency syndrome (AIDS), or metastatic cancers.*

Autoimmune adrenalitis accounts for 60% to 70% of cases, and it is by far the most common cause of primary adrenal insufficiency in developed countries.[121] As the name implies, there is autoimmune destruction of steroidogenic cells, and autoantibodies to several key steroidogenic enzymes (21-hydroxylase, 17-hydroxylase) have been detected in these patients. Autoimmune adrenalitis can occur in one of three clinical settings:

- *Autoimmune polyendocrine syndrome type 1* (APS1) is also known as autoimmune polyendocrinopathy, candidiasis, and ectodermal dystrophy (APECED). APS1 is characterized by chronic mucocutaneous candidiasis and abnormalities of skin, dental enamel, and nails (ectodermal dystrophy) occurring in association with a combination of organ-specific autoimmune disorders (autoimmune adrenalitis, autoimmune hypoparathyroidism, idiopathic hypogonadism, pernicious anemia) that result in immune destruction of target organs.[122] APS1 is caused by mutations in the autoimmune regulator (*AIRE*) gene on chromosome

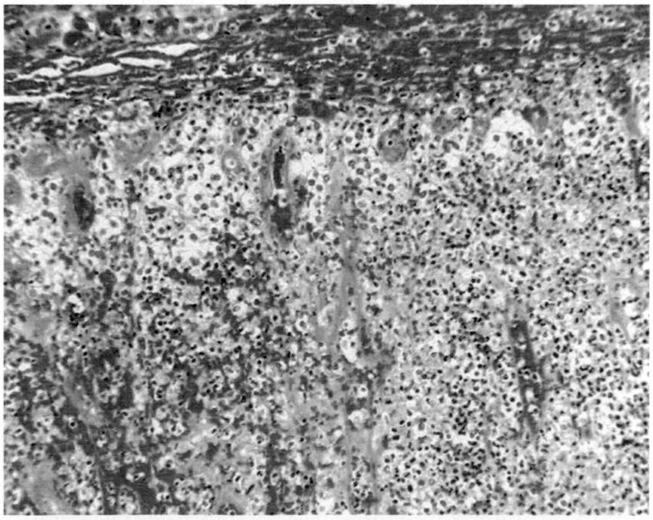

FIGURE 24–50 Waterhouse-Friderichsen syndrome. At autopsy, the adrenals were grossly hemorrhagic and shrunken; microscopically, little residual cortical architecture is discernible.

21q22. The expression of AIRE protein is primarily in the thymus, where it appears to function as a transcription factor that promotes the expression of many self-antigens, leading to negative selection (death) of self-reactive T cells[54] (Chapter 6).

- *Autoimmune polyendocrine syndrome type 2* (APS2) usually starts in early adulthood and presents as a combination of adrenal insufficiency with autoimmune thyroiditis or type 1 diabetes. Unlike in APS1, mucocutaneous candidiasis, ectodermal dysplasia, and autoimmune hypoparathyroidism do not occur. APS2, unlike APS1, is not a monogenic disorder, although some studies have suggested a possible association with polymorphisms in the HLA loci.[123]
- *Isolated autoimmune Addison disease* presents with autoimmune destruction restricted to the adrenal glands. However, in terms of age at presentation and linkage to HLA and other susceptibility loci, isolated autoimmune adrenalitis overlaps with APS2, suggesting that the former may be a variant of the latter.

Infections, particularly tuberculosis and those produced by fungi, may also cause primary chronic adrenocortical insufficiency. Tuberculous adrenalitis, which once accounted for as much as 90% of Addison disease, has become less common with the development of antituberculous agents. With the resurgence of tuberculosis in most urban centers and the persistence of the disease in developing countries, however, this cause of adrenal insufficiency must be kept in mind. When present, tuberculous adrenalitis is usually associated with active infection in other sites, particularly in the lungs and genitourinary tract. Among the fungi, disseminated infections caused by *Histoplasma capsulatum* and *Coccidioides immitis* may also result in chronic adrenocortical insufficiency. Patients with AIDS are at risk for developing adrenal insufficiency from several infectious (cytomegalovirus, *Mycobacterium avium-intercellulare*) and noninfectious complications (Kaposi sarcoma).

Metastatic neoplasms involving the adrenals are another potential cause of adrenal insufficiency. The adrenals are a fairly common site for metastases in patients with disseminated carcinomas. Although adrenal function is preserved in most such patients, the metastatic tumors occasionally destroy enough adrenal cortex to produce a degree of adrenal insufficiency. Carcinomas of the lung and breast are the source of a majority of metastases in the adrenals, although many other neoplasms, including gastrointestinal carcinomas, malignant melanoma, and hematopoietic neoplasms, may also metastasize to this organ.

Genetic disorders of adrenal insufficiency include adrenal hypoplasia congenital (AHC) and adrenoleukodystrophy. Technically, these disorders are also associated with chronic adrenal insufficiency, although they are not commonly included in the causes of Addison disease. Adrenoleukodystrophy is described in Chapter 28. Congenital adrenal hypoplasia is rare, and will not be discussed further.[124,125]

Morphology. The anatomic changes in the adrenal glands depend on the underlying disease. **Primary autoimmune adrenalitis** is characterized by irregularly shrunken glands, which may be difficult to identify within the suprarenal adipose tissue. Histologically, the cortex contains only scattered residual cortical cells in a collapsed network of connective tissue. A variable lymphoid infiltrate is present in the cortex and may extend into the subjacent medulla, although the medulla is otherwise preserved (Fig. 24–51). In cases of **tuberculous and fungal disease,** the adrenal architecture is effaced by a granulomatous inflammatory reaction identical to that encountered in other sites of infection. When hypoadrenalism is caused by **metastatic carcinoma,** the adrenals are enlarged, and their normal architecture is obscured by the infiltrating neoplasm.

Clinical Course. Addison disease begins insidiously and does not come to attention until at least 90% of the cortex of both glands is destroyed and the levels of circulating glucocorticoids and mineralocorticoids are significantly decreased. The initial manifestations include *progressive weakness and easy fatigability*, which may be dismissed as nonspecific complaints. *Gastrointestinal* disturbances are common and include anorexia, nausea, vomiting, weight loss, and diarrhea. In patients with primary adrenal disease, increased circulating levels of ACTH precursor hormone stimulate melanocytes, with resultant *hyperpigmentation* of the skin, particularly of sun-exposed areas and at pressure points, such as the neck, elbows, knees, and knuckles. By contrast, hyperpigmentation is not seen in patients with adrenocortical insufficiency caused by primary pituitary or hypothalamic disease. Decreased mineralocorticoid activity in patients with primary adrenal insufficiency results in potassium retention and sodium loss, with consequent *hyperkalemia, hyponatremia, volume depletion, and hypotension.* Hypoglycemia may occasionally occur as a result of glucocorticoid deficiency and impaired gluconeogenesis. Stresses such as infections, trauma, or surgical procedures in such patients can precipitate an acute adrenal crisis, manifested by intractable vomiting, abdominal pain, hypotension, coma, and vascular collapse. Death occurs rapidly unless corticosteroid therapy begins immediately.

Secondary Adrenocortical Insufficiency

Any disorder of the hypothalamus and pituitary, such as metastatic cancer, infection, infarction, or irradiation, that

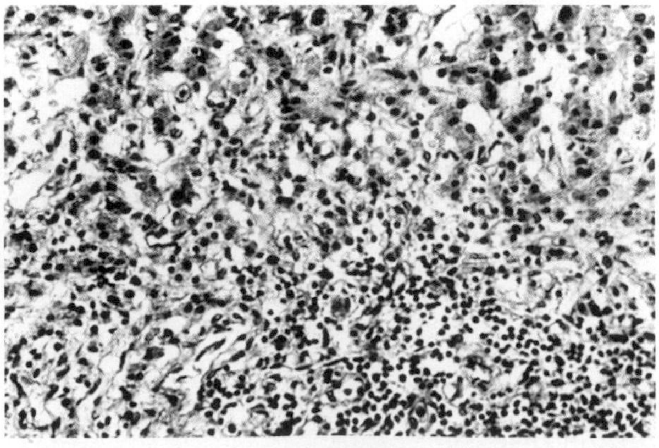

FIGURE 24–51 Autoimmune adrenalitis. In addition to loss of all but a subcapsular rim of cortical cells, there is an extensive mononuclear cell infiltrate.

reduces the output of ACTH leads to a syndrome of hypoadrenalism that has many similarities to Addison disease. Analogously, prolonged administration of exogenous glucocorticoids suppresses the output of ACTH and adrenal function. *With secondary disease, the hyperpigmentation of primary Addison disease is lacking because melanotropic hormone levels are low.* The manifestations also differ in that secondary hypoadrenalism is characterized by deficient cortisol and androgen output but normal or near-normal aldosterone synthesis. Thus, in adrenal insufficiency secondary to pituitary malfunction, marked hyponatremia and hyperkalemia are not seen.

ACTH deficiency can occur alone, but in some instances, it is only one part of panhypopituitarism, associated with multiple primary trophic hormone deficiencies. The differentiation of secondary disease from Addison disease can be confirmed with demonstration of low levels of plasma ACTH in the former. In patients with primary disease, the destruction of the adrenal cortex does not permit a response to exogenously administered ACTH in the form of increased plasma levels of cortisol, whereas in those with secondary hypofunction, there is a prompt rise in plasma cortisol levels.

Morphology. In cases of hypoadrenalism secondary to hypothalamic or pituitary disease (**secondary hypoadrenalism**), depending on the extent of ACTH lack, the adrenals may be moderately to markedly reduced in size. They are reduced to small, flattened structures that usually retain their yellow color owing to a small amount of residual lipid. The cortex may be reduced to a thin ribbon composed largely of zona glomerulosa. The medulla is unaffected.

ADRENOCORTICAL NEOPLASMS

It should be evident from the preceding sections that functional adrenal neoplasms may be responsible for any of the various forms of hyperadrenalism. While functional adenomas are most commonly associated with hyperaldosteronism and Cushing syndrome, a virilizing neoplasm is more likely to be a carcinoma. However, not all adrenocortical neoplasms elaborate steroid hormones. Determination of whether a cortical neoplasm is functional or not is based on clinical evaluation and measurement of the hormone or its metabolites in the laboratory. In other words, *functional and nonfunctional adrenocortical neoplasms cannot be distinguished on the basis of morphologic features.*

Morphology. Most **adrenocortical adenomas** are clinically silent and are usually encountered as incidental findings at the time of autopsy or during abdominal imaging for an unrelated cause (see the discussion of adrenal incidentalomas below). Some experts believe that all adrenal adenomas should, by definition, demonstrate clinical or biochemical evidence of hyperfunction and that the incidentally discovered "tumors" are best classified as hyperplastic nodules.[126] In either case, the typical cortical adenoma is a well-circumscribed, nodular lesion up to 2.5 cm in diameter that expands the adrenal. In contrast to functional adenomas, which are associated with atrophy of the adjacent cortex, the cortex adjacent to nonfunctional adenomas is of normal thickness. On cut surface, adenomas are usually yellow to yellow-brown because of the presence of lipid within the tumor cells. Microscopically, adenomas are composed of cells similar to those populating the normal adrenal cortex. The nuclei tend to be small, although some degree of pleomorphism may be encountered even in benign lesions ("endocrine atypia"). The cytoplasm of the neoplastic cells ranges from eosinophilic to vacuolated, depending on their lipid content (Fig. 24–46). Mitotic activity is generally inconspicuous.

Adrenocortical carcinomas are rare neoplasms that can occur at any age, including childhood. They are more likely to be functional than adenomas are, and carcinomas are therefore often associated with virilism or other clinical manifestations of hyperadrenalism. Two rare inherited causes of adrenal cortical carcinomas are Li-Fraumeni syndrome (Chapter 7) and Beckwith-Wiedemann syndrome (Chapter 10). In most cases, adrenocortical carcinomas are large, invasive lesions, many exceeding 20 cm in diameter, that efface the native adrenal gland. The less common, smaller, and better-circumscribed lesions may be difficult to distinguish from an adenoma. On cut surface, adrenocortical carcinomas are typically variegated, poorly demarcated lesions containing areas of necrosis, hemorrhage, and cystic change (Fig. 24–52). Invasion of contiguous structures, including the adrenal vein and inferior vena cava, is common. Microscopically, adrenocortical carcinomas may be composed of well-differentiated cells resembling those seen in cortical adenomas or bizarre, monstrous giant cells (Fig. 24–53), which may be difficult to distinguish from those of an undifferentiated carcinoma metastatic to the adrenal. Between these extremes are found cancers with moderate degrees of anaplasia, some composed predominantly of spindle cells. Carcinomas, particularly those of bronchogenic origin, may metastasize to the adrenals, and they may be extremely difficult to differentiate from primary cortical carcinomas. Adrenal cancers have a strong tendency to invade the adrenal vein, vena cava, and lymphatics. Metastases to regional and periaortic nodes are common, as is distant hematogenous

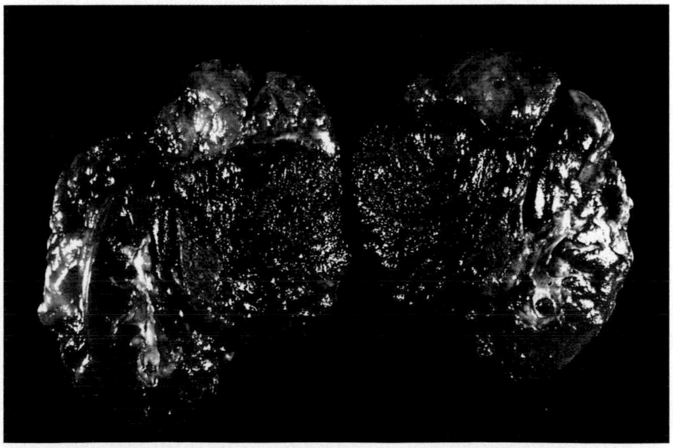

FIGURE 24–52 Adrenal carcinoma. The hemorrhagic and necrotic tumor dwarfs the kidney and compresses the upper pole.

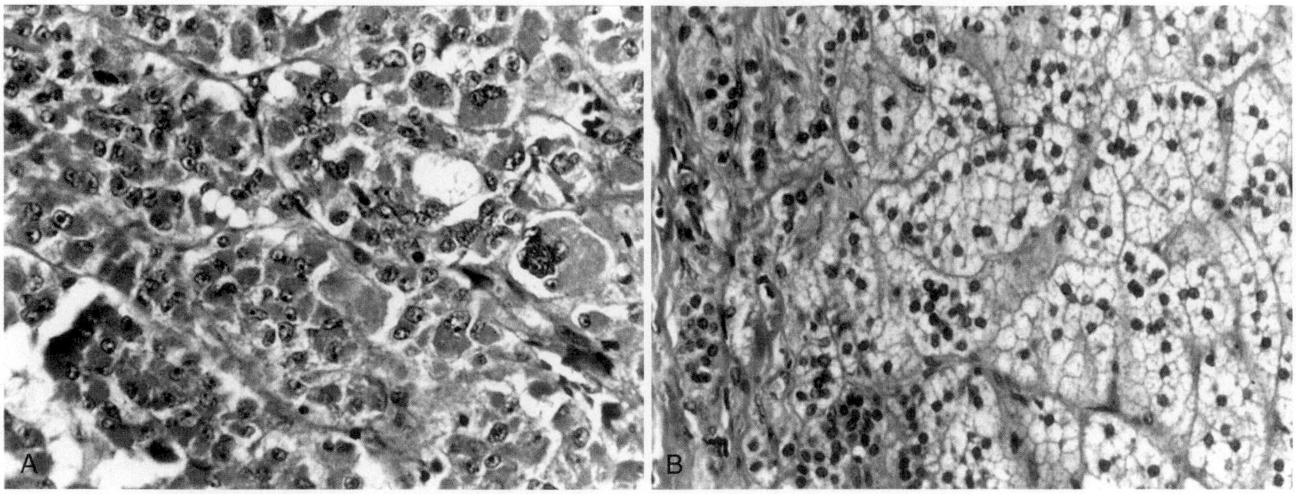

FIGURE 24–53 Adrenal carcinoma *(A)* revealing marked anaplasia, contrasted with normal cortical cells (*B*).

spread to the lungs and other viscera. Bone metastases are unusual. The median patient survival is about 2 years.

OTHER LESIONS OF THE ADRENAL

Adrenal cysts are relatively uncommon lesions; however, with the use of sophisticated abdominal imaging techniques, the frequency of detection of these lesions appears to be increasing. The larger cysts may produce an abdominal mass and flank pain. Both cortical and medullary neoplasms may undergo necrosis and cystic degeneration and may present as "nonfunctional" cysts.

Adrenal myelolipomas are unusual benign lesions composed of mature fat and hematopoietic cells. Although most of these lesions represent incidental findings, occasional myelolipomas may reach massive proportions. Histologically, mature adipocytes are admixed with aggregates of hematopoietic cells belonging to all three lineages. Foci of myelolipomatous change may be seen in cortical tumors and in adrenals with cortical hyperplasia.

The term *adrenal incidentaloma* is a half-facetious moniker that has crept into the medical lexicon as advancements in medical imaging have led to the incidental discovery of adrenal masses in asymptomatic individuals or in individuals in whom the presenting complaint is not directly related to the adrenal gland.[127] Fortunately, *the vast majority of adrenal incidentalomas are nonsecreting cortical adenomas,* but in effect, any adrenal cortical or medullary neoplasm or hyperplasia, metastatic cancer, or a non-neoplastic disease (abscess, amyloidosis, sarcoid) can result in an incidentally discovered adrenal mass.

Adrenal Medulla

Normal

The adrenal medulla is developmentally, functionally, and structurally distinct from the adrenal cortex. It is composed of specialized neural crest (neuroendocrine) cells, termed *chromaffin* cells, and their supporting (sustentacular) cells. The chromaffin cells are round to oval, have prominent cytoplasmic membrane–bound granules of stored catecholamines, and are supported by a richly vascularized scant stroma of spindled and sustentacular cells. These cells, so named because of their brown-black color after exposure to potassium dichromate (e.g., Zenker fixative), synthesize and secrete catecholamines in response to signals from preganglionic nerve fibers in the sympathetic nervous system. The adrenal medulla is the major source of catecholamines (epinephrine, norepinephrine) in the body. Norepinephrine functions as a local neurotransmitter, chiefly of sympathetic postganglionic neurons. Only small amounts reach the circulation. Epinephrine (adrenaline) is secreted into the vascular system. It interacts with α-adrenergic and β-adrenergic receptors in various cells, which then activate second messengers and a cascade of enzymatic reactions mediating the systemic actions of epinephrine, for example, increasing the force and rate of myocardial contractions and causing vasoconstriction of most vascular beds. Because the secretory cells are a part of the neuroendocrine system, they are also capable of synthesizing a variety of bioactive amines and peptides, such as histamine, serotonin, renin, chromogranin A, and neuropeptide hormones.

Neuroendocrine cells similar to chromaffin cells are widely dispersed in an extra-adrenal system of clusters and nodules that, together with the adrenal medulla, make up the *paraganglion system.* These extra-adrenal paraganglia are closely associated with the autonomic nervous system and can be divided into three groups based on their anatomic distribution: (1) branchiomeric, (2) intravagal, and (3) aorticosympathetic (Fig. 24–54). The branchiomeric and intravagal paraganglia associated with the parasympathetic system are located close to the major arteries and cranial nerves of the head and neck and include the carotid bodies (Chapter 16). The intravagal paraganglia, as the term implies, are distributed along the vagus nerve. The aorticosympathetic chain is found in association with segmental ganglia of the sympathetic system and therefore is distributed mainly alongside of the abdominal aorta. The organs of Zuckerkandl, close to the aortic bifurcation, belong to this group. The visceral paraganglia, as the term implies, are located within organs such as the urinary bladder. They are described in Chapter 16.

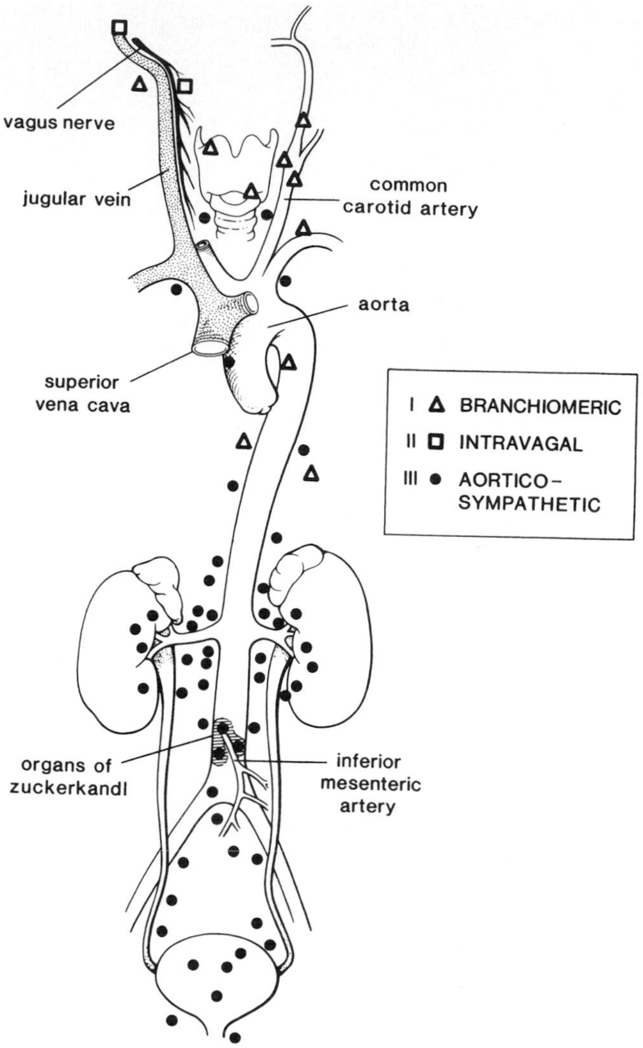

FIGURE 24–54 The paraganglion system. This schematic representation of the paraganglion system demonstrates sites of paraganglion cell nests, in which neoplasms may form. The extra-adrenal portion of the paraganglion system is grouped into three families based on anatomic distribution, innervation, and microscopic structure: (1) branchiomeric, (2) intravagal, and (3) aorticosympathetic. (From Whalen RK, et al: Extra-adrenal pheochromocytoma. J Urol 147:1–10, 1992; copyright Williams & Wilkins, 1992.)

Pathology

The most important diseases of the adrenal medulla are neoplasms, which include neoplasms of chromaffin cells (pheochromocytomas) and neuronal neoplasms (including neuroblastomas and more mature ganglion cell tumors).

PHEOCHROMOCYTOMA

Pheochromocytomas are uncommon neoplasms composed of chromaffin cells, which synthesize and release catecholamines and in some instances peptide hormones. These tumors are important because they (similar to aldosterone-secreting adenomas) give rise to surgically correctable forms of hypertension. Although only about 0.1% to 0.3% of hypertensive patients have an underlying pheochromocytoma, the hypertension can be fatal when the pheochromocytoma goes unrecognized. Occasionally, one of these tumors produces other steroids or peptides and so may be associated with Cushing syndrome or some other endocrinopathy.

Pheochromocytomas usually subscribe to a convenient *"rule of 10s"*:

- *10% of pheochromocytomas arise in association with one of several familial syndromes* (Table 24–11). These include the MEN-2A and MEN-2B syndromes (described later), type I neurofibromatosis (Chapter 5), von Hippel-Lindau syndrome (Chapter 28), and Sturge-Weber syndrome (Chapter 16).
- *10% of pheochromocytomas are extra-adrenal*, occurring in sites such as the organ of Zuckerkandl and the carotid body, where these chromaffin-negative tumors are usually called *paragangliomas* to distinguish them from pheochromocytomas.
- *10% of nonfamilial adrenal pheochromocytomas are bilateral*; this figure may rise to 70% in cases that are associated with familial syndromes.
- *10% of adrenal pheochromocytomas are biologically malignant*, although the associated hypertension represents a serious and potentially lethal complication of even "benign" tumors. Frank malignancy is somewhat more common (20% to 40%) in tumors arising in extra-adrenal sites.
- *10% of adrenal pheochromocytomas arise in childhood*, usually the familial subtypes, and with a strong male preponderance. The nonfamilial pheochromocytomas most

TABLE 24–11 Familial Syndromes Associated with Pheochromocytoma

Syndrome	Components
MEN, type 2A	Medullary thyroid carcinomas and C-cell hyperplasia Pheochromocytomas and adrenal medullary hyperplasia Parathyroid hyperplasia
MEN, type 2B	Medullary thyroid carcinomas and C-cell hyperplasia Pheochromocytomas and adrenal medullary hyperplasia Mucosal neuromas Marfanoid features
von Hippel-Lindau	Renal, hepatic, pancreatic, and epididymal cysts Renal cell carcinomas Pheochromocytomas Angiomatosis Cerebellar hemangioblastomas
von Recklinghausen	Neurofibromatosis Café au lait skin spots Schwannomas, meningiomas, gliomas Pheochromocytomas
Sturge-Weber	Cavernous hemangiomas of fifth cranial nerve distribution Pheochromocytomas

MEN, multiple endocrine neoplasia.
Data from Silverman ML, Lee AK: Anatomy and pathology of the adrenal glands. Urol Clin North Am 16:417, 1989.

often occur in adults between 40 and 60 years of age, with a slight female preponderance.

Morphology. Pheochromocytomas range from small, circumscribed lesions confined to the adrenal (Fig. 24–55) to large hemorrhagic masses weighing kilograms. The average weight of a pheochromocytoma is 100 gm, but variations from just over 1 gm to almost 4000 gm have been reported. The larger tumors are well demarcated by either connective tissue or compressed cortical or medullary tissue. Richly vascularized fibrous trabeculae pass into the tumor and produce a lobular pattern. In many tumors, remnants of the adrenal gland can be seen, stretched over the surface or attached at one pole. On section, the cut surfaces of smaller pheochromocytomas are yellow-tan. Larger lesions tend to be hemorrhagic, necrotic, and cystic and typically efface the adrenal gland. Incubation of fresh tissue with a potassium dichromate solution turns the tumor a dark brown color owing to oxidation of stored catecholamines, thus the term *chromaffin.*

The histologic pattern in pheochromocytoma is quite variable. The tumors are composed of polygonal to spindle-shaped chromaffin cells or chief cells, clustered with the sustentacular cells into small nests or alveoli (**zellballen**) by a rich vascular network (Fig. 24–56). Uncommonly, the dominant cell type is a spindle or small cell; various patterns can be found in any one tumor. The cytoplasm has a finely granular appearance, best demonstrated with silver stains, owing to the appearance of granules containing catecholamines. The nuclei are usually round to ovoid, with a stippled "salt and pepper" chromatin that is characteristic of most neuroendocrine tumors. Electron microscopy reveals variable numbers of membrane-bound, electron-dense granules, representing catecholamines and sometimes other peptides (Fig. 24–57). Immunoreactivity for neuroendocrine markers (chromogranin and synaptophysin) is present in the chief cells, while the peripheral sustentacular cells label with S-100, a calcium-binding protein expressed by a variety of mesenchymal cell types.

The criteria for determining malignancy in pheochromocytomas can be a vexing issue. **There is no single histologic feature that can reliably predict clinical behavior in pheochromocytomas.** Tumors with "benign" histologic features may metastasize, while bizarrely pleomorphic tumors may remain confined to the adrenal gland. In fact, cellular and nuclear pleomorphism, including the presence of giant cells, and mitotic figures are often seen in benign pheochromocytomas, while cellular monotony is paradoxically associated with an aggressive behavior (see below).

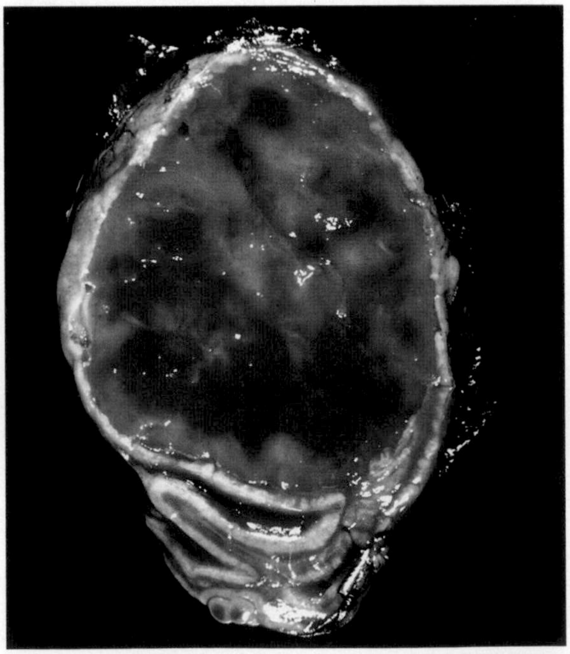

FIGURE 24–55 Pheochromocytoma. The tumor is enclosed within an attenuated cortex and demonstrates areas of hemorrhage. The comma-shaped residual adrenal is seen below.

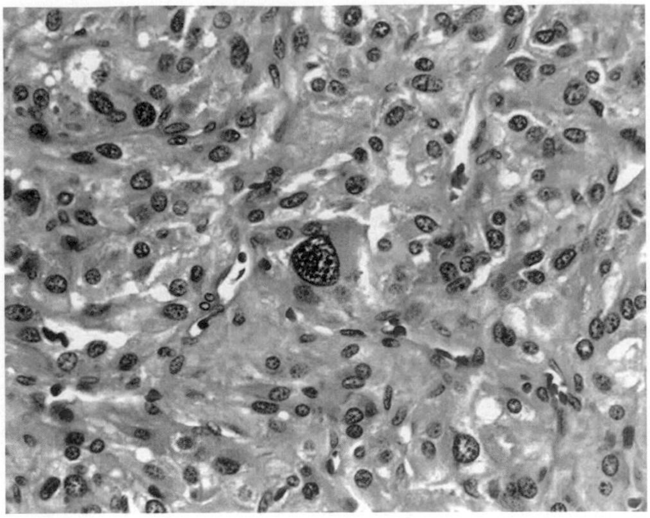

FIGURE 24–56 Pheochromocytoma demonstrating characteristic nests of cells ("zellballen") with abundant cytoplasm. Granules containing catecholamine are not visible in this preparation. It is not uncommon to find bizarre cells even in pheochromocytomas that are biologically benign, and this criterion by itself should not be used to diagnose malignancy.

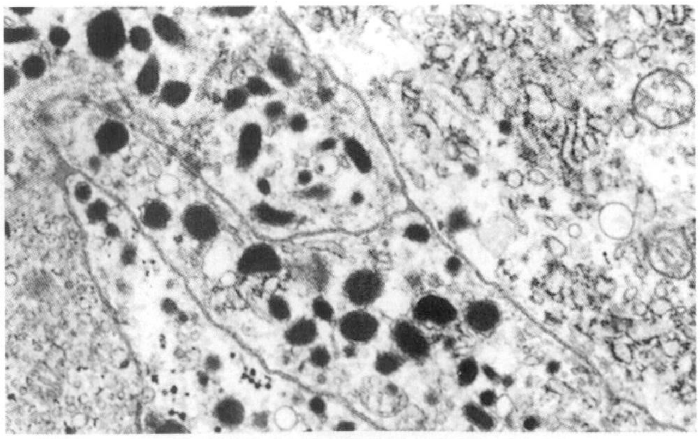

FIGURE 24–57 Electron micrograph of pheochromocytoma. This tumor contains membrane-bound secretory granules in which catecholamines are stored (30,000×).

Even capsular and vascular invasion may be encountered in benign lesions. **Therefore, the definitive diagnosis of malignancy in pheochromocytomas is based exclusively on the presence of metastases.** These may involve regional lymph nodes as well as more distant sites, including liver, lung, and bone. Several histologic features, such as numbers of mitoses, confluent tumor necrosis, and spindle cell morphology, have been associated with an aggressive behavior and increased risk of metastasis, but in and of itself, no single criterion is entirely reliable.[128]

Clinical Course. The dominant clinical feature in patients with pheochromocytoma is *hypertension*. Classically, this is described as an abrupt, precipitous elevation in blood pressure, associated with tachycardia, palpitations, headache, sweating, tremor, and a sense of apprehension. These episodes may also be associated with pain in the abdomen or chest, nausea, and vomiting. In practice, isolated paroxysmal episodes of hypertension occur in fewer than half of patients. In about two-thirds of patients, the hypertension occurs in the form of chronic, sustained elevation in blood pressure, although an element of labile hypertension is also present. The paroxysms may be precipitated by emotional stress, exercise, changes in posture, and palpation in the region of the tumor. The elevations of pressure are induced by the sudden release of catecholamines that may acutely precipitate congestive heart failure, pulmonary edema, myocardial infarction, ventricular fibrillation, and cerebrovascular accidents. The cardiac complications have been attributed to what has been called *catecholamine cardiomyopathy*, or catecholamine-induced myocardial instability and ventricular arrhythmias. Nonspecific myocardial changes, such as focal necrosis, mononuclear infiltrates, and interstitial fibrosis, have been attributed to ischemic damage secondary to the catecholamine-induced vasomotor constriction of the myocardial circulation or to direct catecholamine toxicity. In some cases, pheochromocytomas secrete other hormones, such as ACTH and somatostatin, and may therefore be associated with clinical features related to the secretion of these or other peptide hormones.

The laboratory diagnosis of pheochromocytoma is based on the demonstration of increased urinary excretion of free catecholamines and their metabolites, such as vanillylmandelic acid (VMA) and metanephrines. Isolated benign tumors are treated with surgical excision, after preoperative and intraoperative medication of patients with adrenergic-blocking agents to prevent a hypertensive crisis. Multifocal lesions require long-term medical treatment for hypertension.

TUMORS OF EXTRA-ADRENAL PARAGANGLIA

Pheochromocytomas that develop in paraganglia other than the adrenal medulla are often designated *paragangliomas*. Paragangliomas may arise in any organ that contains paraganglionic tissue. Tumors arising in the carotid body are designated carotid body tumors, whereas those originating in the jugulotympanic body are sometimes referred to as *chemodectomas* because these paraganglia sense the oxygen and carbon dioxide levels of the blood. The *carotid body tumor* is a typical paraganglioma, forming a palpable mass in the neck enveloping the carotid vessels. Paragangliomas are uncommon and occur about one tenth as frequently as adrenal pheochromocytomas. They are described in Chapter 16.

NEUROBLASTOMA

Neuroblastoma is the most common extracranial solid tumor of childhood. These neoplasms occur most commonly during the first 5 years of life and may arise during infancy. Neuroblastomas may occur anywhere in the sympathetic nervous system and occasionally within the brain, but they are most common in the abdomen; most cases arise in either the adrenal medulla or the retroperitoneal sympathetic ganglia. Most neuroblastomas are sporadic, although familial cases also occur. These tumors were discussed in Chapter 10, along with other pediatric neoplasms.

Multiple Endocrine Neoplasia Syndromes

The multiple endocrine neoplasia (MEN) syndromes are a group of genetically inherited diseases resulting in proliferative lesions (hyperplasia, adenomas, and carcinomas) of multiple endocrine organs. Like other inherited cancer disorders (Chapter 7), endocrine tumors arising in the context of MEN syndromes have certain distinct features that contrast with their sporadic counterparts:

- These tumors occur at a *younger age* than sporadic cancers.
- They arise in *multiple endocrine organs*, either *synchronously* (at the same time) or *metachronously* (at different times).
- Even in one organ, the tumors are often *multifocal*.
- The tumors are usually preceded by an *asymptomatic stage of endocrine hyperplasia* involving the cell of origin of the tumor. For example, patients with MEN-1 syndrome develop varying degrees of islet cell hyperplasia, some of which progress to pancreatic tumors.
- These tumors are usually *more aggressive* and *recur* in a higher proportion of cases than do similar endocrine tumors that occur sporadically.

The salient features of the MEN syndromes are summarized in Table 24–12 and discussed below.

MULTIPLE ENDOCRINE NEOPLASIA, TYPE 1

MEN-1, or *Wermer syndrome*, is a rare heritable disorder with a prevalence of about 2 per 100,000. It is characterized by abnormalities involving the *parathyroid, pancreas,* and *pituitary glands*; thus the mnemonic device, the *3Ps:*

- Parathyroid: *Primary hyperparathyroidism* is the most common manifestation of MEN-1 (80% to 95% of patients) and is the initial manifestation of the disorder in most patients, appearing in almost all patients by age 40 to 50. Parathyroid abnormalities include both hyperplasia and adenomas. Hyperplasias arising in the context of MEN-1 are monoclonal.

TABLE 24–12 **Multiple Endocrine Neoplasia (MEN) Syndromes**

	MEN-1	MEN-2A	MEN-2B
Pituitary	Adenomas		
Parathyroid	Hyperplasia +++ Adenomas +	Hyperplasia +	
Pancreatic islets	Hyperplasia ++ Adenomas ++ Carcinomas +++		
Adrenal	Cortical hyperplasia	Pheochromocytoma ++	Pheochromocytoma +++
Thyroid		C-cell hyperplasia +++ Medullary carcinoma +++	C-cell hyperplasia +++ Medullary carcinoma +++
Extraendocrine changes			Mucocutaneous ganglioneuromas Marfanoid habitus
Mutant gene locus	*MEN1*	*RET*	*RET*

Relative frequency: +, uncommon; +++, common.

- Pancreas: *Endocrine tumors of the pancreas* are a leading cause of morbidity and mortality in MEN-1 patients.[129] These tumors are usually aggressive and often present with metastatic disease. It is not uncommon to find multiple "microadenomas" scattered throughout the pancreas in conjunction with one or two dominant lesions. Pancreatic endocrine tumors are often functional; however, since pancreatic polypeptide is the most commonly secreted product, these tumors might not be accompanied by an endocrine hypersecretion syndrome. Among symptomatic pancreatic tumors, gastrinomas associated with Zollinger-Ellison syndrome and insulinomas associated with hypoglycemia and neurologic manifestations are the most common subtypes.
- Pituitary: The most frequent anterior pituitary tumor encountered in MEN-1 is a *prolactinoma*; some patients develop acromegaly from somatotrophin-secreting tumors.
- The spectrum of this disease has been expanded beyond the *3Ps*. The *duodenum is the most common site of gastrinomas in individuals with MEN-1* (far in excess of the frequency of pancreatic gastrinomas),[130] and synchronous duodenal and pancreatic tumors may be present in the same individual. In addition, carcinoid tumors, thyroid and adrenocortical adenomas, and lipomas are more frequent than in the general population.

MEN-1 syndrome is caused by germ-line mutations in the *MEN1* gene at 11q13. This gene encodes a 610–amino acid product known as menin, which localizes primarily to the nucleus. *MEN1* is a classic tumor suppressor gene (Chapter 7) in that both alleles are inactivated in the MEN-1–associated tumors.[131] The precise role of menin in tumor suppression remains elusive, although recent studies have shown that it may be important in regulating the cell cycle and transcription.[132]

The dominant clinical manifestations of MEN-1 are usually defined by the peptide hormones that are overproduced and include such abnormalities as recurrent hypoglycemia due to insulinomas, intractable peptic ulcers in patients with Zollinger-Ellison syndrome, nephrolithiasis caused by PTH-induced hypercalcemia, or symptoms of prolactin excess from a pituitary tumor. As expected, malignant behavior by one or more of the endocrine tumors arising in these patients is often the proximate cause of death.

MULTIPLE ENDOCRINE NEOPLASIA, TYPE 2

MEN-2 is subclassified into three distinct syndromes: MEN-2A, MEN-2B, and familial medullary thyroid cancer.

- *MEN-2A*, or *Sipple syndrome*, is characterized by *pheochromocytoma*, *medullary carcinoma*, and *parathyroid hyperplasia*. Medullary carcinomas of the thyroid occur in almost 100% of patients. They are usually multifocal and are virtually always associated with foci of C-cell hyperplasia in the adjacent thyroid. The medullary carcinomas may elaborate calcitonin and other active products and are usually clinically aggressive. Forty per cent to 50% of patients with MEN-2A have pheochromocytomas, which are often bilateral and may arise in extra-adrenal sites. As in the case of pheochromocytomas in general, they may be benign or malignant. Ten per cent to 20% of patients have parathyroid hyperplasia and evidence of hypercalcemia or renal stones. MEN-2A is clinically and genetically distinct from MEN-1 and has been linked to germ-line mutations in the *RET* (rearranged during transfection) protooncogene on chromosome 10q11.2. As was noted earlier, the *RET* protooncogene is a receptor tyrosine kinase that binds *glial-derived neurotrophic factor* (GDNF) and other ligands in the GDNF family and transmits growth and differentiation signals (Chapter 7). *Loss of function* mutations in *RET* result in intestinal aganglionosis and Hirschsprung disease (Chapter 17). In contrast, in MEN-2A (as well as in MEN-2B), germ-line mutations constitutively activate the *RET* receptor, resulting in *gain of function*.[133] This scenario is different from most other inherited predispositions to neoplasia, which are due to heritable loss of function mutations that inactivate tumor-suppressor proteins (Chapter 7).
- *MEN-2B* has significant clinical overlap with MEN-2A. Patients develop medullary thyroid carcinomas, which are usually multifocal and more aggressive than in MEN-2A, and pheochromocytomas. However, unlike in MEN-2A, primary hyperparathyroidism is not present. In addition, MEN-2B is accompanied by *neuromas* or ganglioneuromas involving the skin, oral mucosa, eyes, respiratory tract, and gastrointestinal tract, and a *marfanoid habitus*, with long axial skeletal features and hyperextensible joints. A single amino acid change in *RET* ($RET^{Met918Thr}$), distinct from the

mutational spectra that are seen in MEN-2A, appears to be responsible for virtually all cases of MEN-2B and affects a critical region of the tyrosine kinase catalytic domain of the protein.[134]

- *Familial medullary thyroid cancer* is a variant of MEN-2A, in which there is a strong predisposition to medullary thyroid cancer but not the other clinical manifestations of MEN-2A or MEN-2B. A substantial majority of cases of medullary thyroid cancer are sporadic, but as many as 20% may be familial. Familial medullary thyroid cancers develop at an older age than those occurring in the full-blown MEN-2 syndrome and follow a more indolent course.

In contrast to MEN-1, in which the long-term benefit of early diagnosis via genetic screening is not well established, diagnosis via screening of at-risk family members in MEN-2A kindred is important because medullary thyroid carcinoma is a life-threatening disease that can be prevented by early thyroidectomy. Prior to the advent of genetic testing, family members of patients with the MEN-2 syndrome were screened with annual biochemical tests, which often lacked sensitivity. Now, routine genetic testing identifies *RET* mutation carriers earlier and more reliably in MEN-2 kindred; *all individuals carrying germ-line RET mutations are advised to undergo prophylactic thyroidectomy to prevent the inevitable development of medullary carcinomas.*

PINEAL GLAND

Normal

The rarity of clinically significant lesions (virtually only tumors) justifies brevity in the consideration of the pineal gland. It is a minute, pinecone-shaped organ (hence its name), weighing 100 to 180 mg and lying between the superior colliculi at the base of the brain. It is composed of a loose, neuroglial stroma enclosing nests of epithelial-appearing *pineocytes*, cells with photosensory and neuroendocrine functions (hence the designation of the pineal gland as the "third eye"). Silver impregnation stains reveal that these cells have long, slender processes reminiscent of primitive neuronal precursors intermixed with the processes of astrocytic cells.

Pathology

All tumors involving the pineal are rare; most (50% to 70%) arise from sequestered embryonic germ cells. They most commonly take the form of so-called *germinomas*, resembling testicular seminoma (Chapter 21) or ovarian dysgerminoma (Chapter 22). Other lines of germ cell differentiation include embryonal carcinomas; choriocarcinomas; mixtures of germinoma, embryonal carcinoma, and choriocarcinoma; and, uncommonly, typical teratomas (usually benign). Whether to characterize these germ cell neoplasms as pinealomas is still a subject of debate, but most "pinealophiles" favor restricting the term *pinealoma* to neoplasms arising from the pineocytes.

PINEALOMAS

These neoplasms are divided into two categories, pineoblastomas and pineocytomas, based on their level of differentiation, which, in turn, correlates with their neoplastic aggressiveness.[135]

Morphology. Pineoblastomas are encountered mostly in the first two decades of life and appear as soft, friable, gray masses punctuated with areas of hemorrhage and necrosis. They typically invade surrounding structures, such as the hypothalamus, midbrain, and lumen of the third ventricle. Histologically, they are composed of masses of pleomorphic cells two to four times the diameter of an erythrocyte. Large hyperchromatic nuclei appear to occupy almost the entire cell, and mitoses are frequent. The cytology is that of **primitive embryonal tumor** ("small blue cell neoplasm") similar to medulloblastoma (Chapter 28) or retinoblastoma (Chapter 29).

Pineoblastomas, like medulloblastomas, tend to spread via the cerebrospinal fluid. As might be expected, the enlarging mass may compress the aqueduct of Sylvius, giving rise to internal hydrocephalus and all its consequences. Survival beyond 1 or 2 years is rare.

In contrast, **pineocytomas** occur mostly in adults and are much slower-growing than pineoblastomas. They tend to be well-circumscribed, gray, or hemorrhagic masses that compress but do not infiltrate surrounding structures. **Histologically, the tumors may be pure pineocytomas or exhibit divergent glial, neuronal, and retinal differentiation.** The tumors are composed largely of pineocytes having darkly staining, round-to-oval, fairly regular nuclei. Necrosis is unusual, and mitoses are virtually absent. The neoplastic cells resemble normal pineocytes in their strong immunoreactivity for neuro-specific enolase and synaptophysin. Particularly distinctive are the **pineocytomatous pseudorosettes** rimmed by rows of pineocytes. The centers of these rosettes are filled with eosinophilic cytoplasmic material representing tumor cell processes. These cells are set against a background of thin, fibrovascular, anastomosing septa, which confer a lobular growth pattern to the tumor. Glial and retinal differentiation is detectable by immunoreactivity for glial fibrillary acidic protein and retinal S-antigen, respectively.

The clinical course of patients with pineocytomas is prolonged, averaging 7 years. The manifestations are the consequence of their pressure effects and consist of visual disturbances, headache, mental deterioration, and sometimes dementia-like behavior. The lesions being located where they are, it is understandable that successful excision is at best difficult.

REFERENCES

1. Elster AD: Modern imaging of the pituitary. Radiology 187(1):1–14, 1993.
2. Asa SL, Ezzat S: The pathogenesis of pituitary tumours. Nat Rev Cancer 2(11):836–849, 2002.
3. Suhardja A, Kovacs K, and Rutka J: Genetic basis of pituitary adenoma invasiveness: a review. J Neurooncol 52(3):195–204, 2001.
4. Yamada S, et al: Growth hormone-producing pituitary adenomas: correlations between clinical characteristics and morphology. Neurosurgery 33(1):20–27, 1993.
5. Asa SL, Ezzat S: The cytogenesis and pathogenesis of pituitary adenomas. Endocr Rev 19(6):798–827, 1998.
6. Sheehan HL: The recognition of chronic hypopituitarism resulting from postpartum pituitary necrosis. Am J Obstet Gynecol, 111(6):852–854, 1971.
7. Rodriguez R, Andersen B: Cellular determination in the anterior pituitary gland: PIT-1 and PROP-1 mutations as causes of human combined pituitary hormone deficiency. Minerva Endocrinol 28(2):123–133, 2003.
8. LiVolsi VA, Perzin KH, Savetsky L: Carcinoma arising in median ectopic thyroid (including thyroglossal duct tissue). Cancer 34(4):1303–1315, 1974.
9. Cheng SY: Multiple mechanisms for regulation of the transcriptional activity of thyroid hormone receptors. Rev Endocr Metab Disord 1(1–2):9–18, 2000.
10. Helfand M, Redfern CC: Clinical guideline. Part 2: screening for thyroid disease: an update. American College of Physicians. Ann Intern Med 129(2):144–158, 1998.
11. Refetoff S: Resistance to thyroid hormone with and without receptor gene mutations. Ann Endocrinol (Paris) 64(1):23–25, 2003.
12. Yen PM: Thyrotropin receptor mutations in thyroid diseases. Rev Endocr Metab Disord 1(1–2):123–129, 2000.
13. Clifton-Bligh RJ, et al: Mutation of the gene encoding human TTF-2 associated with thyroid agenesis, cleft palate and choanal atresia. Nat Genet 19(4):399–401, 1998.
14. Macchia PE, et al: PAX8 mutations associated with congenital hypothyroidism caused by thyroid dysgenesis. Nat Genet 19(1):83–86, 1998.
15. Barbesino G, Chiovato L: The genetics of Hashimoto's disease. Endocrinol Metab Clin North Am 29(2):357–374, 2000.
16. Tomer Y, et al: Common and unique susceptibility loci in Graves and Hashimoto diseases: results of whole-genome screening in a data set of 102 multiplex families. Am J Hum Genet 73(4):736–747, 2003.
17. Stassi G, De Maria R: Autoimmune thyroid disease: new models of cell death in autoimmunity. Nat Rev Immunol 2(3):195–204, 2002.
18. Pearce EN, Farwell AP, Braverman LE: Thyroiditis. N Engl J Med 348:2646, 2003.
19. Muller AF, Drexhage HA, Berghout A: Postpartum thyroiditis and autoimmune thyroiditis in women of childbearing age: recent insights and consequences for antenatal and postnatal care. Endocr Rev 22(5):605–630, 2001.
20. Kouki T, et al: Relation of three polymorphisms of the CTLA-4 gene in patients with Graves' disease. J Endocrinol Invest 25(3):208–213, 2002.
21. Ueda H, et al: Association of the T-cell regulatory gene CTLA4 with susceptibility to autoimmune disease. Nature 423(6939):506–511, 2003.
22. Weetman AP: Grave's disease 1835–2002. Horm Res 59 (suppl 1):114–118, 2003.
23. Heufelder AE: Pathogenesis of ophthalmopathy in autoimmune thyroid disease. Rev Endocr Metab Disord 1(1–2):87–95, 2000.
24. Apel RL, et al: Clonality of thyroid nodules in sporadic goiter. Diagn Mol Pathol 4(2):113–121, 1995.
25. Siegel RD, Lee SL: Toxic nodular goiter: toxic adenoma and toxic multinodular goiter. Endocrinol Metab Clin North Am 27(1)151–168, 1998.
26. Rodien P, et al: Activating mutations of TSH receptor. Ann Endocrinol (Paris) 64(1):12–16, 2003.
27. Lang W, et al: The differentiation of atypical adenomas and encapsulated follicular carcinomas in the thyroid gland. Virchows Arch 385(2):125–141, 1980.
28. Kroll TG, et al: PAX8-PPARgamma1 fusion oncogene in human thyroid carcinoma [corrected]. Science 289(5483):1357–1360, 2000.
29. Nikiforova MN, et al: RAS point mutations and PAX8-PPAR gamma rearrangement in thyroid tumors: evidence for distinct molecular pathways in thyroid follicular carcinoma. J Clin Endocrinol Metab 88(5):2318–2326, 2003.
30. Nikiforova MN, et al: PAX8-PPARgamma rearrangement in thyroid tumors: RT-PCR and immunohistochemical analyses. Am J Surg Pathol 26(8):1016–1023, 2002.
31. Nikiforov YE: RET/PTC rearrangement in thyroid tumors. Endocr Pathol 13(1):3–16, 2002.
32. Pierotti MA, Vigneri P, Bongarzone I: Rearrangements of RET and NTRK1 tyrosine kinase receptors in papillary thyroid carcinomas. Recent Results Cancer Res, 154:237–247, 1998.
33. Xu X, et al: High prevalence of BRAF gene mutation in papillary thyroid carcinomas and thyroid tumor cell lines. Cancer Res 63(15):4561–4567, 2003.
34. Cohen Y, et al: BRAF mutation in papillary thyroid carcinoma. J Natl Cancer Inst 95(8):625–627, 2003.
35. Kimura ET, et al: High prevalence of BRAF mutations in thyroid cancer: genetic evidence for constitutive activation of the RET/PTC-RAS-BRAF signaling pathway in papillary thyroid carcinoma. Cancer Res 63(7):1454–1457, 2003.
36. Eng C, et al: The relationship between specific RET proto-oncogene mutations and disease phenotype in multiple endocrine neoplasia type 2: International RET Mutation Consortium analysis. JAMA 276(19):1575–1579, 1996.
37. Marsh DJ, et al: Somatic mutations in the RET proto-oncogene in sporadic medullary thyroid carcinoma. Clin Endocrinol (Oxf) 44(3):249–257, 1996.
38. Ito T, et al: Unique association of p53 mutations with undifferentiated but not with differentiated carcinomas of the thyroid gland. Cancer Res 52(5):1369–1371, 1992.
39. Rybakov SJ, et al: Thyroid cancer in children of Ukraine after the Chernobyl accident. World J Surg 24(11):1446–1449, 2000.
40. LiVolsi VA: Surgical Pathology of the Thyroid: Major Problems in Pathology. Philadelphia, WB Saunders, 1990.
41. Baloch ZW, Livolsi VA: Follicular-patterned lesions of the thyroid: the bane of the pathologist. Am J Clin Pathol 117(1):143–150, 2002.
42. Ruter A, Nishiyama R, Lennquist S: Tall-cell variant of papillary thyroid cancer: disregarded entity? World J Surg 21(1):15–20; discussion: 20–21, 1997.
43. Basolo F, et al: Potent mitogenicity of the RET/PTC3 oncogene correlates with its prevalence in tall-cell variant of papillary thyroid carcinoma. Am J Pathol 160(1):247–254, 2002.
44. Cheung CC, et al: Hyalinizing trabecular tumor of the thyroid: a variant of papillary carcinoma proved by molecular genetics. Am J Surg Pathol 24(12):1622–1626, 2000.
45. Wells SA Jr, Franz C: Medullary carcinoma of the thyroid gland. World J Surg 24(8):952–956, 2000.
46. Perry A, Molberg K, Albores-Saavedra J: Physiologic versus neoplastic C-cell hyperplasia of the thyroid: separation of distinct histologic and biologic entities. Cancer 77(4):750–756, 1996.
47. Krueger JE, Maitra A, Albores-Saavedra J: Inherited medullary microcarcinoma of the thyroid: a study of 11 cases. Am J Surg Pathol 24(6):853–858, 2000.
48. Machens A, et al: Early malignant progression of hereditary medullary thyroid cancer. N Engl J Med 349:1517, 2003.
49. Yip L, et al: Multiple endocrine neoplasia type 2: evaluation of the genotype–phenotype relationship. Arch Surg 138:409, 2003.
50. Boyle WJ, Simonet WS, Lacey DL: Osteoclast differentiation and activation. Nature 423:337, 2003.
51. Fiaschi-Taesch NM, Stewart AF: Minireview: parathyroid hormone-related protein as an intracrine factor: trafficking mechanisms and functional consequences. Endocrinology 144(2):407–411, 2003.
52. Bilezikian JP, Silverberg SJ: Clinical spectrum of primary hyperparathyroidism. Rev Endocr Metab Disord 1(4):237–245, 2000.

53. Fuleihan Gel H: Familial benign hypocalciuric hypercalcemia. J Bone Miner Res 17 (suppl 2):N51–N56, 2002.
54. Arnold A., et al: Molecular pathogenesis of primary hyperparathyroidism. J Bone Miner Res 17 (suppl 2):N30–N36, 2002.
55. Silver J, Kilav R, Naveh-Many T: Mechanisms of secondary hyperparathyroidism. Am J Physiol Renal Physiol 283(3):F367–F376, 2002.
56. Anderson MS, et al: Projection of an immunological self shadow within the thymus by the aire protein. Science 298(5597):1395–1401, 2002.
57. Li Y, et al: Autoantibodies to the extracellular domain of the calcium sensing receptor in patients with acquired hypoparathyroidism. J Clin Invest 97(4):910–914, 1996.
58. Weinstein LS, et al: Endocrine manifestations of stimulatory G protein alpha-subunit mutations and the role of genomic imprinting. Endocr Rev 22(5):675–705, 2001.
59. GuG, Brown JR, Melton DA: Direct lineage tracing reveals the ontogeny of pancreatic cell fates during mouse embryogenesis. Mech Dev 120(1):35–43, 2003.
60. Narayan KM, et al: Lifetime risk for diabetes mellitus in the United States. JAMA 290(14):1884–1890, 2003.
61. Zimmet P, Alberti KG, Shaw J: Global and societal implications of the diabetes epidemic. Nature 414(6865):782–787, 2001.
62. Report of the Expert Committee on the Diagnosis and Classification of Diabetes Mellitus. Diabetes Care 25 (suppl 1):S5–S20, 2002.
63. Thorens B: GLUT2 in pancreatic and extra-pancreatic gluco-detection (review). Mol Membr Biol 18(4):265–273, 2001.
64. Reis AF, Velho G: Sulfonylurea receptor-1 (SUR1): genetic and metabolic evidences for a role in the susceptibility to type 2 diabetes mellitus. Diabetes Metab 28(1):14–19, 2002.
65. Saltiel AR, Kahn CR: Insulin signalling and the regulation of glucose and lipid metabolism. Nature 414(6865):799–806, 2001.
66. Avruch J, et al: Ras activation of the Raf kinase: tyrosine kinase recruitment of the MAP kinase cascade. Recent Prog Horm Res 56:127–155, 2001.
67. Shepherd PR, Kahn BB: Glucose transporters and insulin action: implications for insulin resistance and diabetes mellitus. N Engl J Med 341(4):248–257, 1999.
68. Kozma SC, Thomas G: Regulation of cell size in growth, development and human disease: PI3K, PKB and S6K. Bioessays 24(1):65–71, 2002.
69. Mathis D, Vence L, Benoist C: Beta-cell death during progression to diabetes. Nature 414(6865):792–798, 2001.
70. Bach JF, Chatenoud L: Tolerance to islet autoantigens in type 1 diabetes. Annu Rev Immunol 19:131–161, 2001.
71. Pietropaolo M, Eisenbarth GS: Autoantibodies in human diabetes. Curr Dir Autoimmun 4:252–282, 2001.
72. Todd JA, Wicker LS: Genetic protection from the inflammatory disease type 1 diabetes in humans and animal models. Immunity 15(3):387–395, 2001.
73. McDevitt H: The role of MHC class II molecules in the pathogenesis and prevention of Type I diabetes. Adv Exp Med Biol 490:59–66, 2001.
74. Pugliese A, et al: HLA-DQB1*0602 is associated with dominant protection from diabetes even among islet cell antibody-positive first-degree relatives of patients with IDDM. Diabetes 44(6):608–613, 1995.
75. Jaeckel E, Manns M, Von Herrath M: Viruses and diabetes. Ann N Y Acad Sci 958:7–25, 2002.
76. Horwitz MS, Sarvetnick N: Viruses, host responses, and autoimmunity. Immunol Rev 169:241, 1999.
77. Benoist C, Mathis D: Autoimmunity provoked by infection: how good is the case for T cell epitope mimicry? Nat Immunol 2(9):797–801, 2001.
78. Saltiel AR: Series introduction: the molecular and physiological basis of insulin resistance: emerging implications for metabolic and cardiovascular diseases. J Clin Invest 106(2):163–164, 2000.
79. Shulman GI: Cellular mechanisms of insulin resistance. J Clin Invest 106(2):171–176, 2000.
80. Kadowaki T: Insights into insulin resistance and type 2 diabetes from knockout mouse models. J Clin Invest 106(4):459–465, 2000.
81. Elbein SC: Perspective: the search for genes for type 2 diabetes in the post-genome era. Endocrinology 143(6):2012–2018, 2002.
82. Kahn BB, Flier, JS: Obesity and insulin resistance. J Clin Invest 106(4):473–481, 2000.
83. Saltiel AR: You are what you secrete. Nat Med 7(8):887–888, 2001.
84. Flier, JS: Diabetes. The missing link with obesity? Nature 409(6818):292–293, 2001.
85. Yamauchi T, et al: The fat-derived hormone adiponectin reverses insulin resistance associated with both lipoatrophy and obesity. Nat Med 7(8):941–946, 2001.
86. Steppan CM, et al: The hormone resistin links obesity to diabetes. Nature 409(6818):307–312, 2001.
87. Shimomura I, et al: Leptin reverses insulin resistance and diabetes mellitus in mice with congenital lipodystrophy. Nature 401(6748): 73–76, 1999.
88. Celi FS, Shuldiner AR: The role of peroxisome proliferator-activated receptor gamma in diabetes and obesity. Curr Diab Rep 2(2):179–185, 2002.
89. Fajans SS, Bell GI, Polonsky KS: Molecular mechanisms and clinical pathophysiology of maturity-onset diabetes of the young. N Engl J Med 345(13):971–980, 2001.
90. Ellard S, et al: A high prevalence of glucokinase mutations in gestational diabetic subjects selected by clinical criteria. Diabetologia 43(2):250–253, 2000.
91. Maechler P, Wollheim CB: Mitochondrial function in normal and diabetic beta-cells. Nature 414(6865):807–812, 2001.
92. Saltiel AR: New perspectives into the molecular pathogenesis and treatment of type 2 diabetes. Cell 104(4):517–529, 2001.
93. The Diabetes Control and Complications Trial Research Group: The effect of intensive treatment of diabetes on the development and progression of long-term complications in insulin-dependent diabetes mellitus. N Engl J Med 329(14):977–986, 1993.
94. UK Prospective Diabetes Study (UKPDS) Group: Intensive blood-glucose control with sulphonylureas or insulin compared with conventional treatment and risk of complications in patients with type 2 diabetes (UKPDS 33). Lancet 352(9131):837–853, 1998.
95. Sheetz MJ, King GL: Molecular understanding of hyperglycemia's adverse effects for diabetic complications. JAMA 288(20):2579–2588, 2002.
96. Stitt AW, Jenkins AJ, Cooper ME: Advanced glycation end products and diabetic complications. Expert Opin Investig Drugs 11(9):1205–1223, 2002.
97. Brownlee M: Biochemistry and molecular cell biology of diabetic complications. Nature 414(6865):813–820, 2001.
98. Frank RN: Potential new medical therapies for diabetic retinopathy: protein kinase C inhibitors. Am J Ophthalmol 133(5):693–698, 2002.
99. Lee AY, Chung SS: Contributions of polyol pathway to oxidative stress in diabetic cataract. FASEB J 13(1):23–30, 1999.
100. Haffner SM, et al: Mortality from coronary heart disease in subjects with type 2 diabetes and in nondiabetic subjects with and without prior myocardial infarction. N Engl J Med 339(4):229–234, 1998.
101. Wendt T, et al: Receptor for advanced glycation endproducts (RAGE) and vascular inflammation: insights into the pathogenesis of macrovascular complications in diabetes. Curr Atheroscler Rep 4(3):228–237, 2002.
102. Eckel RH, et al: Prevention Conference VI: Diabetes and Cardiovascular Disease: Writing Group II: pathogenesis of atherosclerosis in diabetes. Circulation 105(18):E138–E143, 2002.
103. Diabetic nephropathy. Diabetes Care 25 (suppl 1):S85–S89, 2002.
104. Frank RN: Diabetic retinopathy. N Engl J Med 350:48, 2004.
105. Astrup A, Finer N: Redefining type 2 diabetes: "diabesity" or "obesity dependent diabetes mellitus"? Obesity Rev 1:57–59, 2000.
106. Rindi G, Capella C, Solcia E: Cell biology, clinicopathological profile, and classification of gastro-enteropancreatic endocrine tumors. J Mol Med 76(6):413–420, 1998.
107. Solcia E, Capella C, Kloppel G: Tumors of the endocrine pancreas. In Rosai J (ed): Atlas of Tumor Pathology: Tumors of the Pancreas. Washington, DC, AFIP, 1997.
108. Goossens A, Heitz P, Kloppel G: Pancreatic endocrine cells and their non-neoplastic proliferations. In Dayal Y (ed): Endocrine Pathology of the Gut and Pancreas. Boca Raton, FL, CRC Press, 1991, pp 69–104.
109. Komminoth P, Heitz PU, Kloppel G: Pathology of MEN-1: morphology, clinicopathologic correlations and tumour development. J Intern Med 243(6):455–464, 1998.
110. Zollinger RM, Ellison EH: Primary peptic ulcerations of the jejunum associated with islet cell tumors of the pancreas: 1955. CA Cancer J Clin 39(4):231–247, 1989.
111. Newell-Price J, et al: The diagnosis and differential diagnosis of Cushing's syndrome and pseudo-Cushing's states. Endocr Rev 19(5):647–672, 1998.
112. Cushing HW: The basophil adenomas of the pituitary body and their clinical manifestations (pituitary basophilism). Bull Johns Hopkins Hosp 50:137–195, 1932.

113. Stratakis CA, Kirschner LS: Clinical and genetic analysis of primary bilateral adrenal diseases (micro- and macronodular disease) leading to Cushing syndrome. Horm Metab Res 30(6–7):456–463, 1998.
114. Groussin L, et al: Mutations of the PRKAR1A gene in Cushing's syndrome due to sporadic primary pigmented nodular adrenocortical disease. J Clin Endocrinol Metab 87(9):4324–4329, 2002.
115. Fardella CE, Mosso L: Primary aldosteronism. Clin Lab 48(3–4):181–190, 2002.
116. Takeda Y: Genetic alterations in patients with primary aldosteronism. Hypertens Res 24(5):469–474, 2001.
117. Dluhy RG, Lifton RP: Glucocorticoid-remediable aldosteronism. J Clin Endocrinol Metab 84(12):4341–4344, 1999.
118. Speiser PW, White PC: Congenital adrenal hyperplasia. N Engl J Med 349:776, 2003.
119. Merke DP, et al: NIH conference. Future directions in the study and management of congenital adrenal hyperplasia due to 21-hydroxylase deficiency. Ann Intern Med 136(4):320–334, 2002.
120. Merke DP, et al: Adrenomedullary dysplasia and hypofunction in patients with classic 21-hydroxylase deficiency. N Engl J Med 343(19):1362–1368, 2000.
121. Peterson P, Uibo R, Krohn KJ: Adrenal autoimmunity: results and developments. Trends Endocrinol Metab 11(7):285–290, 2000.
122. Pitkanen J, Peterson P: Autoimmune regulator: from loss of function to autoimmunity. Genes Immun 4(1):12–21, 2003.
123. Vaidya B, Pearce S, Kendall-Taylor P: Recent advances in the molecular genetics of congenital and acquired primary adrenocortical failure. Clin Endocrinol (Oxf) 53(4):403–418, 2000.
124. Meeks JJ, Weiss J, Jameson JL: Dax1 is required for testis determination. Nat Genet 34(1):32–33, 2003.
125. Burke BA, et al: Congenital adrenal hypoplasia and selective absence of pituitary luteinizing hormone: a new autosomal recessive syndrome. Am J Med Genet 31(1):75–97, 1988.
126. Wenig BM, Heffess CS, Adair CF: Neoplasms of the adrenal gland. In Wenig BM, et al (ed): Atlas of Endocrine Pathology. Philadelphia, WB Saunders, 1997, pp 288–329.
127. Brunt LM, Moley JF: Adrenal incidentaloma. World J Surg 25(7):905–913, 2001.
128. Thompson LD: Pheochromocytoma of the adrenal gland scaled score (PASS) to separate benign from malignant neoplasms: a clinicopathologic and immunophenotypic study of 100 cases. Am J Surg Pathol 26(5):551–566, 2002.
129. Brandi ML: Multiple endocrine neoplasia type 1. Rev Endocr Metab Disord 1(4):275–282, 2000.
130. Mignon M, Cadiot G: Diagnostic and therapeutic criteria in patients with Zollinger-Ellison syndrome and multiple endocrine neoplasia type 1. J Intern Med 243(6):489–494, 1998.
131. Chandrasekharappa SC, et al: Positional cloning of the gene for multiple endocrine neoplasia-type 1. Science 276(5311):404–407, 1997.
132. Poisson A, Zablewska B, Gaudray P: Menin interacting proteins as clues toward the understanding of multiple endocrine neoplasia type 1. Cancer Lett 189(1):1–10, 2003.
133. Santoro M, et al: Different mutations of the RET gene cause different human tumoral diseases. Biochimie 81(4):397–402, 1999.
134. Salvatore D, et al: Increased in vivo phosphorylation of ret tyrosine 1062 is a potential pathogenetic mechanism of multiple endocrine neoplasia type 2B. Cancer Res 61(4):1426–1431, 2001.
135. Mena H, et al: Pineal parenchymal tumors. In Cavanee WK (ed): World Health Organization Classification of Tumors: Pathology and Genetics of Tumors of the Nervous System. Lyon, France, IARC Press, 2000, pp 115–121.

CHAPTER 25

The Skin

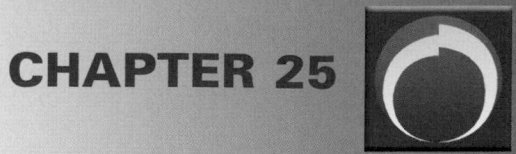

George F. Murphy, MD • Klaus Sellheyer, MD •
Martin C. Mihm, Jr., MD

THE SKIN: MORE THAN A MECHANICAL BARRIER
Definitions of Macroscopic Terms
Definitions of Microscopic Terms

DISORDERS OF PIGMENTATION AND MELANOCYTES
Vitiligo
Freckle (Ephelis)
Melasma
Lentigo
Melanocytic Nevus (Pigmented Nevus, Mole)
Dysplastic Nevi
Malignant Melanoma
Diagnostic Criteria and Prognostic Attributes

BENIGN EPITHELIAL TUMORS
Seborrheic Keratoses
Acanthosis Nigricans
Fibroepithelial Polyp
Epithelial Cyst (Wen)
Adnexal (Appendage) Tumors
Keratoacanthoma

PREMALIGNANT AND MALIGNANT EPIDERMAL TUMORS
Actinic Keratosis
Squamous Cell Carcinoma
Basal Cell Carcinoma
Merkel Cell Carcinoma
Molecular Genetics of Skin Cancers

TUMORS OF THE DERMIS
Benign Fibrous Histiocytoma (Dermatofibroma)
Dermatofibrosarcoma Protuberans
Xanthomas
Dermal Vascular Tumors

TUMORS OF CELLULAR IMMIGRANTS TO THE SKIN
Langerhans Cell Histiocytosis
Mycosis Fungoides (Cutaneous T-Cell Lymphoma)
Mastocytosis

DISORDERS OF EPIDERMAL MATURATION
Ichthyosis

ACUTE INFLAMMATORY DERMATOSES
Urticaria
Acute Eczematous Dermatitis
Erythema Multiforme

CHRONIC INFLAMMATORY DERMATOSES
Psoriasis
Seborrheic Dermatitis
Lichen Planus
Lupus Erythematosus

BLISTERING (BULLOUS) DISEASES
Pemphigus
Bullous Pemphigoid
Dermatitis Herpetiformis
Noninflammatory Blistering Diseases: Epidermolysis Bullosa, Porphyria

DISORDERS OF EPIDERMAL APPENDAGES
Acne Vulgaris

PANNICULITIS
Erythema Nodosum and Erythema Induratum
INFECTION AND INFESTATION
Verrucae (Warts)
Molluscum Contagiosum
Impetigo
Superficial Fungal Infections
Arthropod Bites, Stings, and Infestations

Normal

The Skin: More Than a Mechanical Barrier

Little more than 100 years ago, the noted pathologist Rudolph Virchow understood the skin as a protective covering for more delicate and functionally sophisticated internal viscera.[1] Then, and for the century that followed, the skin was considered primarily a passive barrier to fluid loss and mechanical injury. During the past three decades, however, enormously productive avenues of scientific inquiry have demonstrated the skin to be a complex organ in which precisely regulated cellular and molecular interactions govern many crucial responses to our environment.

We now know that skin is composed of a number of interdependent cell types and structures that work toward a common protective goal (Fig. 25–1). *Squamous epithelial cells (keratinocytes),* in addition to production of keratin protein, are major sites for the biosynthesis of soluble molecules (cytokines) that are important in the regulation of adjacent epidermal cells as well as cells in the dermis, as illustrated in Figure 25–2.[2] *Melanocytes* within the epidermis are cells responsible for the production of a brown pigment (melanin) that represents an important endogenous screen against harmful ultraviolet (UV) rays in sunlight. *Langerhans cells* are epidermal dendritic cells that take up and process antigens and communicate critical information to lymphoid cells. *Neural end-organs* and *axonal processes* warn of potentially damaging

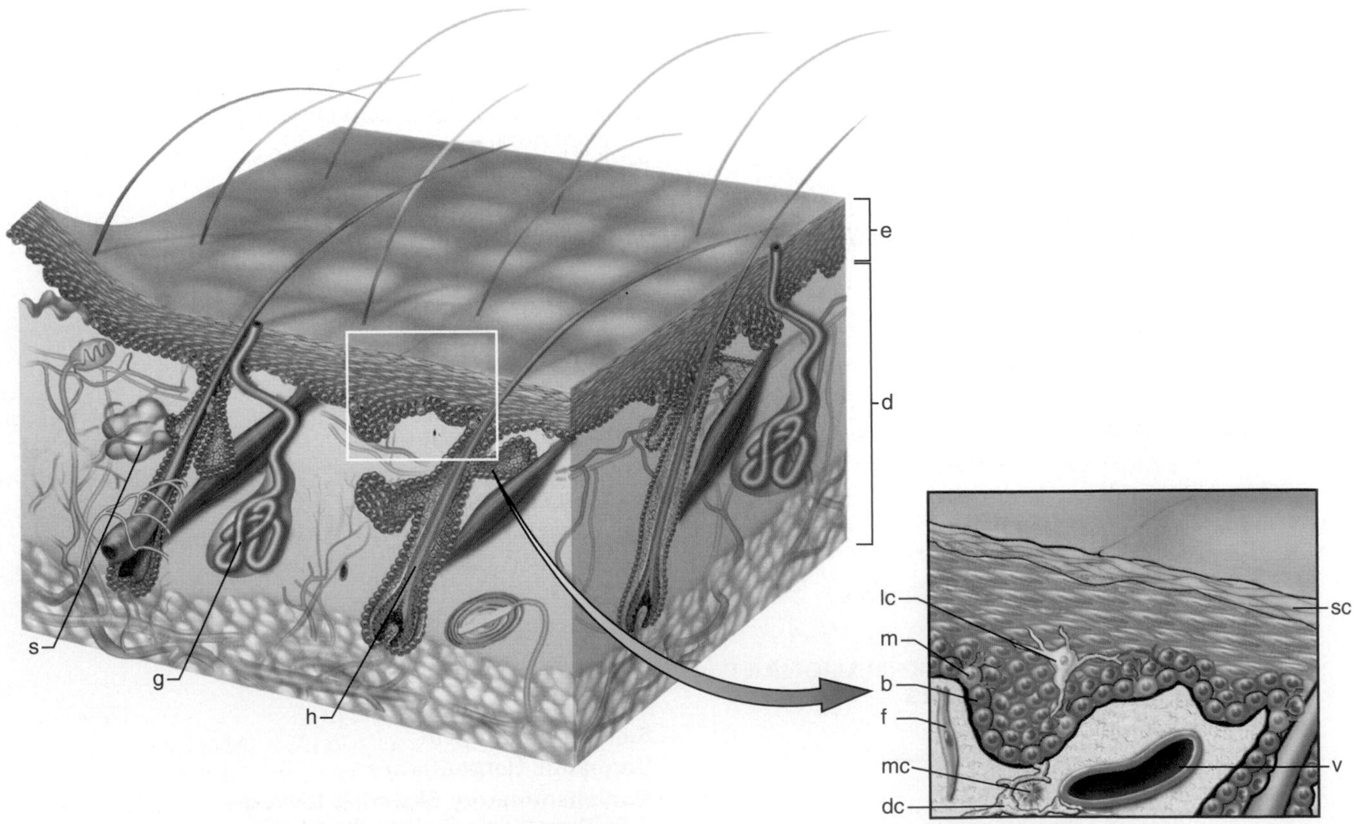

FIGURE 25–1 *A,* The skin is composed of an epidermal layer (e) from which specialized adnexa (hair follicles, h; sweat glands, g; and sebaceous glands, s) descend into the underlying dermis (d). *B,* This projection of the epidermal layer (e) and underlying superficial dermis demonstrates the progressive upward maturation of basal cells (b) into cornified squamous epithelial cells of the stratum corneum (sc). Melanin-containing dendritic melanocytes (m) (and rare Merkel cells containing neurosecretory granules) and midepidermal dendritic Langerhans cells (lc) are also present. The underlying dermis contains small vessels (v), fibroblasts (f), perivascular mast cells (mc), and dendrocytes (dc), potentially important in dermal immunity and repair.

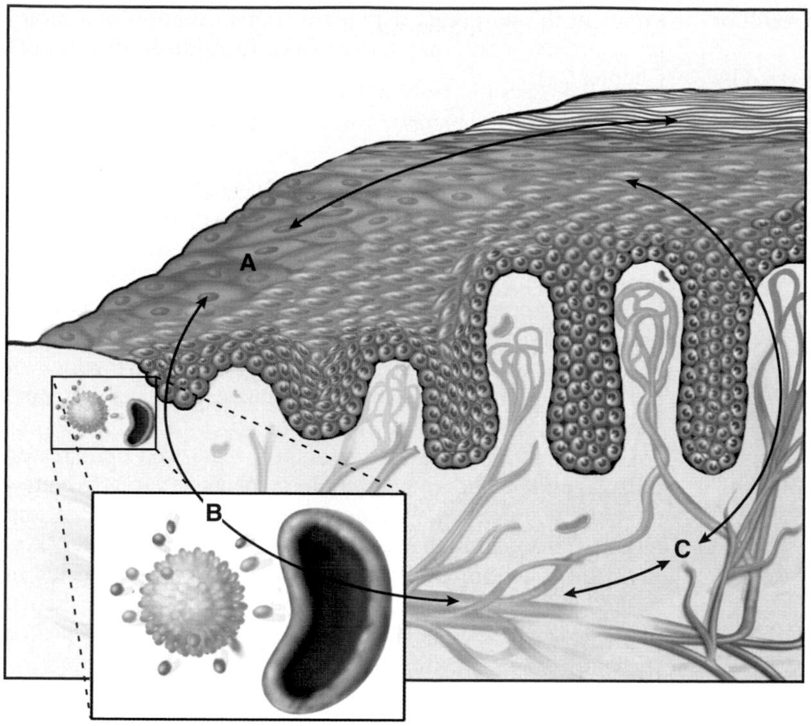

FIGURE 25–2 Schematic representation of dynamic interaction between the epidermal layer and the dermal layer. Keratinocytes at the edge of an ulcer *(A)* produce cytokines and factors that influence both keratinization and the function of underlying dermal cells *(B)*. In turn, dermal cells *(B)*, such as mast cells, also release cytokines *(green granules)* and proteases *(red granules)*, which may regulate both endothelial cells and overlying keratinocytes. Perturbations in these interactions between epidermal cells and dermal cells may contribute to pathologic processes, such as psoriasis *(C)*, in which both compartments become morphologically abnormal.

physical factors in the environment and have recently been found to assist in regulation of immunocompetent cells.[3] Among the neural network are *Merkel cells* that reside within the basal cell layer and, like melanocytes and Langerhans cells, are distinguishable from keratinocytes by light microscopy only with the aid of special immunohistochemical stains. Although their function in humans remains unclear, Merkel cells may serve as mechanoreceptors or may provide neuroendocrine function in skin.[4] *Sweat glands* guard against deleterious variations in body temperature, and *hair follicles*, in addition to manufacturing hair shafts, harbor protected repositories of epithelial stem cells[5] capable of regenerating superficial skin layers that have been disrupted by various hostile external and internal agents. Specialized dermal cells *(dendrocytes)* are probably engineered for antigen presentation as well as for production of molecules (e.g., factor XIIIa) capable of coordinating the assembly of macromolecular complexes important in the early stages of healing of wounds affecting the deeper cutaneous layers.[6] Although the human integument may appear drab compared with the skin and pelage of certain other members of the animal kingdom, it is indeed extraordinarily vibrant with regard to the diversity and complexity of protective functions that it serves.

Imbalances in factors affecting the delicate homeostasis that exists among skin cells may result in conditions as diverse as wrinkles and hair loss, blisters and rashes, and even life-threatening cancers and disorders of immune regulation. For example, chronic exposure to sunlight fosters premature cutaneous aging, blunting of immunologic responses to environmental antigens, and the development of a variety of premalignant and malignant cutaneous neoplasms. Ingested agents, such as therapeutic drugs, can cause an enormous number of rashes or exanthems. Internal disorders, such as diabetes mellitus, amyloidosis, and lupus erythematosus, may also have important manifestations in the skin.

Pathology

Accurate description of the clinical appearance of the skin at a macroscopic level is critical, since lesions before biopsy are, in effect, the gross pathology. Correlation between the gross and histologic appearances is often essential in formulating diagnoses and in understanding pathogenesis. Accordingly, efforts are made in the following pages to depict and describe clinical lesions whenever possible and to relate these findings to the microscopic appearance of lesions.

DEFINITIONS OF MACROSCOPIC TERMS

Macule Circumscribed lesion of up to 5 mm* in diameter characterized by flatness and usually distinguished from surrounding skin by its coloration.

Patch Circumscribed lesion of more than 5 mm in diameter characterized by flatness and usually distinguished from surrounding skin by its coloration.

Papule Elevated dome-shaped or flat-topped lesion 5 mm or less across.

Nodule Elevated lesion with spherical contour greater than 5 mm across.

Plaque Elevated flat-topped lesion, usually greater than 5 mm across (may be caused by coalescent papules).

Vesicle Fluid-filled raised lesion 5 mm or less across.

Bulla Fluid-filled raised lesion greater than 5 mm across.

Blister Common term used for vesicle or bulla.

Pustule Discrete, pus-filled, raised lesion.

Wheal Itchy, transient, elevated lesion with variable blanching and erythema formed as the result of dermal edema.

* Some sources use 10 mm as the size boundary between different lesions.

Scale Dry, horny, platelike excrescence; usually the result of imperfect cornification.
Lichenification Thickened and rough skin characterized by prominent skin markings; usually the result of repeated rubbing in susceptible persons.
Excoriation Traumatic lesion characterized by breakage of the epidermis, causing a raw linear area (i.e., a deep scratch); often self-induced.
Onycholysis Separation of nail plate from nail bed.

DEFINITIONS OF MICROSCOPIC TERMS

Hyperkeratosis Thickening of the stratum corneum, often associated with a qualitative abnormality of the keratin.
Parakeratosis Modes of keratinization characterized by the retention of the nuclei in the stratum corneum. On mucous membranes, parakeratosis is normal.
Hypergranulosis Hyperplasia of the stratum granulosum, often due to intense rubbing.
Acanthosis Diffuse epidermal hyperplasia.
Papillomatosis Surface elevation caused by hyperplasia and enlargement of contiguous dermal papillae.
Dyskeratosis Abnormal keratinization occurring prematurely within individual cells or groups of cells below the stratum granulosum.
Acantholysis Loss of intercellular connections resulting in loss of cohesion between keratinocytes.
Spongiosis Intercellular edema of the epidermis.
Hydropic swelling (ballooning) Intracellular edema of keratinocytes, often seen in viral infections.
Exocytosis Infiltration of the epidermis by inflammatory or circulating blood cells.
Erosion Discontinuity of the skin exhibiting incomplete loss of the epidermis.
Ulceration Discontinuity of the skin exhibiting complete loss of the epidermis and often of portions of the dermis and even subcutaneous fat.
Vacuolization Formation of vacuoles within or adjacent to cells; often refers to basal cell–basement membrane zone area.
Lentiginous Referring to a linear pattern of melanocyte proliferation within the epidermal basal cell layer. Lentiginous melanocytic hyperplasia can occur as a reactive change or as part of a neoplasm of melanocytes.

Disorders of Pigmentation and Melanocytes

Skin pigmentation has historically had major societal implications. Cosmetic desire for increased pigmentation (tanning) has resulted in many deleterious alterations that are described in the pages that follow. Focal or widespread loss of normal protective pigmentation not only renders individuals extraordinarily vulnerable to the harmful effects of sunlight (as in albinism), but has also resulted in severe emotional stress and, in some cultures, profound social and economic discrimination (as in vitiligo). Change in preexisting skin pigmentation may signify important primary events in the skin (e.g., malignant transformation of a mole) or disorders of internal viscera (e.g., in Addison disease, see Chapter 24).

VITILIGO

Vitiligo is a common disorder characterized by partial or complete loss of pigment-producing melanocytes within the epidermis. All ages and races are affected, but lesions are most noticeable in darkly pigmented individuals. Vitiligo may be entirely unapparent in lightly pigmented skin until tanning occurs in the surrounding normal skin. In darkly pigmented individuals with extensive involvement, residual zones of normal skin may at first appear to represent hyperpigmented lesions (Fig. 25–3*A*).

Clinical lesions are asymptomatic, flat, well-demarcated macules and patches of pigment loss; their size varies from few to many centimeters. Vitiligo often involves the hands and wrists; axillae; and perioral, periorbital, and anogenital skin. A curious phenomenon called *koebnerization* often occurs in vitiligo (as well as in certain other conditions; see lichen planus), where lesions develop primarily at sites of repeated trauma.

Morphology. On histologic examination, vitiligo usually appears indistinguishable from normal skin. However, it is characterized by loss of melanocytes, as revealed by electron microscopy; it also may be diagnosed by immunohistochemistry for melanocyte-associated proteins (e.g., tyrosinase or Melan-A, or S-100; Fig. 25–3*B*). This is in contrast to some forms of **albinism,** in which melanocytes are present but melanin pigment is not produced because of a lack of or defect in tyrosinase. There are other causes of hypopigmentation that are unrelated to diminished expression of melanin or melanocytes (e.g., post-inflammatory hypopigmentation, which represents redistribution of existing pigment within skin possibly coupled with diminished transfer of pigment to keratinocytes).

Pathogenesis. Why are melanocytes progressively lost or destroyed in vitiligo? Theories of pathogenesis include (1) autoimmunity, (2) neurohumoral factors toxic to melanocytes and released by nearby nerve endings, and (3) self-destruction of melanocytes by toxic intermediates of melanin synthesis. Most evidence supports autoimmune causation, focusing on the presence of circulating antibodies against melanocytes[7] and the association of vitiligo with other autoimmune disorders, such as pernicious anemia, Addison disease, and autoimmune thyroiditis. Abnormalities in macrophages,[8] and in T lymphocytes in skin[9] and in the peripheral blood have been described recently, suggesting that aberrations in cell-mediated immunity may also be operative in the pathogenesis of vitiligo. Another interesting facet of vitiligo is its response to therapy with UV light of the A wavelength coupled with use of the photosensitizing drug, psoralen (a therapy known as *PUVA*). Lesions so treated may regain pigment initially at the ostia of hair follicles, suggesting that melanocyte precursors harbored within the uppermost follicular epithelium are stimulated by this therapeutic approach.

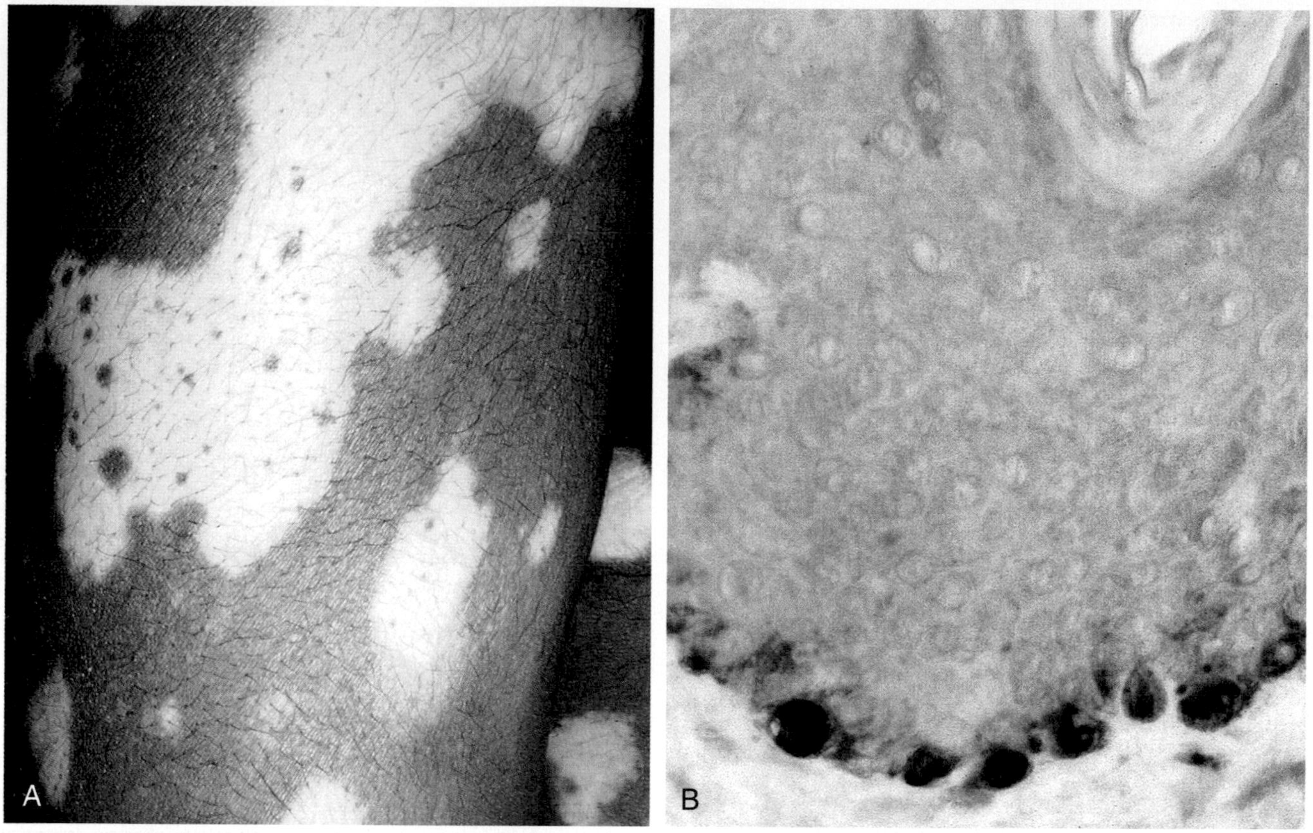

FIGURE 25–3 *A,* Clinical appearance of vitiligo. Well-demarcated zones of pigment loss result from depletion of melanocytes that produce small melanin granules. Note small macules of normal pigment within the patches of vitiligo; Some of these appear to surround follicular ostia. *B,* Immunochemistry for S-100 protein revealing positively stained melanocytes within the basal cell layer of the epidermis; these cells are decreased or absent in vitiligo.

FRECKLE (EPHELIS)

Freckles are the most common pigmented lesions of childhood in lightly pigmented individuals. They are generally small (1 to several mm in diameter), tan-red or light brown macules that first appear in early childhood after sun exposure. Once present, freckles will fade and intensify in a cyclic fashion with winter and summer, respectively. This feature separates them from a lentigo, which maintains stable coloration independent of sun exposure.

Morphology. The clinical hyperpigmentation of the freckle is the result of increased amounts of melanin pigment within basal keratinocytes; melanocytes are relatively normal in number, although they may be slightly enlarged. It is unclear whether the freckle represents a focal abnormality in pigment production by a discrete field of melanocytes, enhanced pigment donation to adjacent basal keratinocytes, or both. The café au lait spots seen in neurofibromatosis (Chapter 5) are histologically indistinguishable from freckles, but the former evolve independent from sun exposure and often contain aggregated melanosomes (macromelanosomes) within the cytoplasm of melanocytes.

MELASMA

Melasma is a mask-like zone of facial hyperpigmentation commonly seen in association with pregnancy—hence its designation as the "mask of pregnancy." It also may occur in some individuals taking oral contraceptives. It presents as poorly defined, blotchy, tan-brown macules and patches involving the cheeks, temples, and forehead bilaterally. Sunlight may accentuate this pigmentation, which often resolves spontaneously, particularly with cessation of hormonal stimulation.

Morphology. Three histologic patterns have been recognized: an **epidermal type,** in which there is increased melanin deposition in the basal layers; a **dermal type,** characterized by macrophages in the superficial (papillary) dermis that have phagocytosed melanin from the adjacent epidermal layer (a process referred to as **melanin pigment incontinence**); and a mixed type, characterized by a combination of the changes seen in the epidermal and dermal types. These three types may be distinguished by the use of a Wood's light ("black light"), which permits distinction between epidermal versus dermal pigmentation on clinical inspection. This is important because melasma of the epidermal type, and partially of the mixed type, may respond to the topical bleaching agent hydroquinone.

The pathogenesis of melasma appears to relate to functional alterations in melanocytes resulting in enhanced pigment transfer to basal keratinocytes or to dermal macrophages. Apart from its association with pregnancy and oral contraceptives, melasma may occur during the administration of hydantoins, or it may be idiopathic.

LENTIGO

Until now, we have been addressing disorders of pigmentation that do not involve proliferation of melanocytes. The term *lentigo* (plural, *lentigines*) refers to a common benign localized hyperplasia of melanocytes occurring at all ages but often in infancy and childhood. There is no sex or racial predilection, and the cause and pathogenesis are unknown. These lesions may involve mucous membranes as well as the skin, and they appear as small (5 to 10 mm across), oval, tan-brown patches. Unlike freckles, lentigines do not darken when they are exposed to sunlight.

Morphology. The essential histologic feature of the lentigo is linear (non-nested) melanocytic hyperplasia (hyperplasia restricted to the cell layer immediately above the basement membrane) that produces a hyperpigmented basal cell layer. So characteristic is this linear melanocytic hyperplasia that the term **lentiginous** is often used to describe similar patterns of cellular proliferation within the basal cell layer in melanocytic tumors, such as in lentiginous nevi and in certain melanomas (termed **acral lentiginous melanomas**). Elongation and thinning of the rete ridges are also commonly seen in a lentigo. In contrast to ordinary lentigo (lentigo simplex) a variant termed **solar or actinic lentigo** occurs in sun-damaged skin in older adults and is associated with subtle alteration in keratinocyte maturation.

MELANOCYTIC NEVUS (PIGMENTED NEVUS, MOLE)

Most of us have at least a few moles and probably regard them as mundane and uninteresting. It may be surprising to learn, then, that moles or nevi represent one of the most diverse, dynamic, and biologically intriguing tumors of the skin! Strictly speaking, the term *nevus* denotes any congenital lesion of the skin (e.g., birthmark). *Melanocytic nevus,* however, refers to any congenital or acquired neoplasm of melanocytes, and hence is somewhat of a misnomer.

In clinical appearance, common acquired melanocytic nevi are *tan to brown, uniformly pigmented, small (usually <6 mm across), solid regions of relatively flat (macules) to elevated skin (papules) with well-defined, rounded borders* (Figs. 25–4*A* and 25–5*A*). There are numerous clinical and histologic types of melanocytic nevi, and the clinical appearance may be variable. Table 25–1 provides a comparative summary of salient clinical and histologic features of the more commonly encountered forms of melanocytic nevi.

Morphology. Melanocytic nevi are initially formed by melanocytes that have been transformed from highly dendritic single cells normally interspersed among basal keratinocytes to round cells that grow in aggregates, or "nests," along the dermoepidermal junction (see Fig. 25–4*B*). Langerhans cells, the other type of dendritic cell within the epidermis, are unrelated to melanocytic nevi. Nuclei of nevus cells are uniform and rounded in contour, contain inconspicuous nucleoli, and show little or no mitotic activity. Such lesions are believed to represent an early developmental stage in melanocytic nevi and are called **junctional nevi.** Eventually, most junctional nevi grow into the underlying dermis as nests or cords of cells (Fig. 25–5*B*) **(compound nevi);** in older lesions, the epidermal nests may be lost entirely to form pure **intradermal nevi.** Clinically, compound and dermal nevi are often more elevated than junctional nevi.

Progressive growth of nevus cells from the dermoepidermal junction into the underlying dermis is accompanied by a process termed **maturation.** Whereas less mature, more superficial nevus cells are larger, tend to produce melanin, and grow in nests, more mature, deeper nevus cells are smaller, produce little or no pigment, and grow in cords. The most mature nevus cells may be found at the deepest extent of lesions, where they often acquire fusiform contours and grow in fascicles resembling neural tissue. This striking metamorphosis correlates with enzymatic changes (progressive loss of tyrosinase activity and acquisition of cholinesterase activity in deeper, nonpigmented, nervelike nevus cells). **This sequence of maturation of individual nevus cells is of diagnostic importance in distinguishing some benign nevi from melanomas, which usually show little or no maturation.**

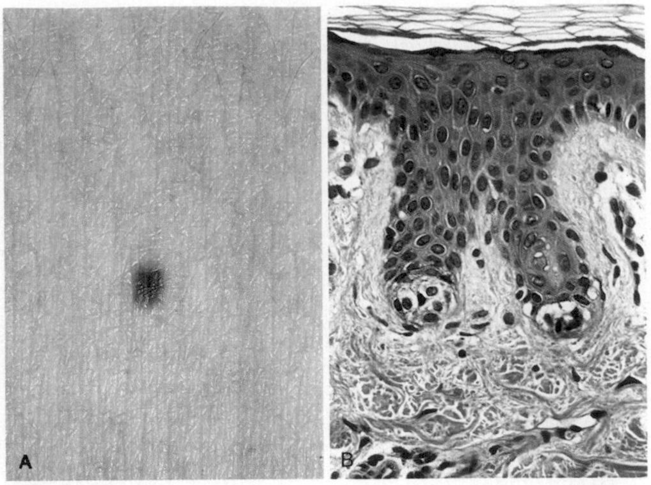

FIGURE 25–4 Nevocellular nevus, junctional type. *A,* In clinical appearance, lesions are small, relatively flat, symmetric, and uniform. *B,* On histologic examination, junctional nevi are characterized by rounded nests of nevus cells originating at the tips of rete ridges along the dermoepidermal junction.

Although melanocytic nevi are common, their clinical and histologic diversity necessitates thorough knowledge of their appearance and natural evolution, lest they become confused with other skin conditions, notably malignant melanoma. The biologic importance of some nevi, however, resides in their

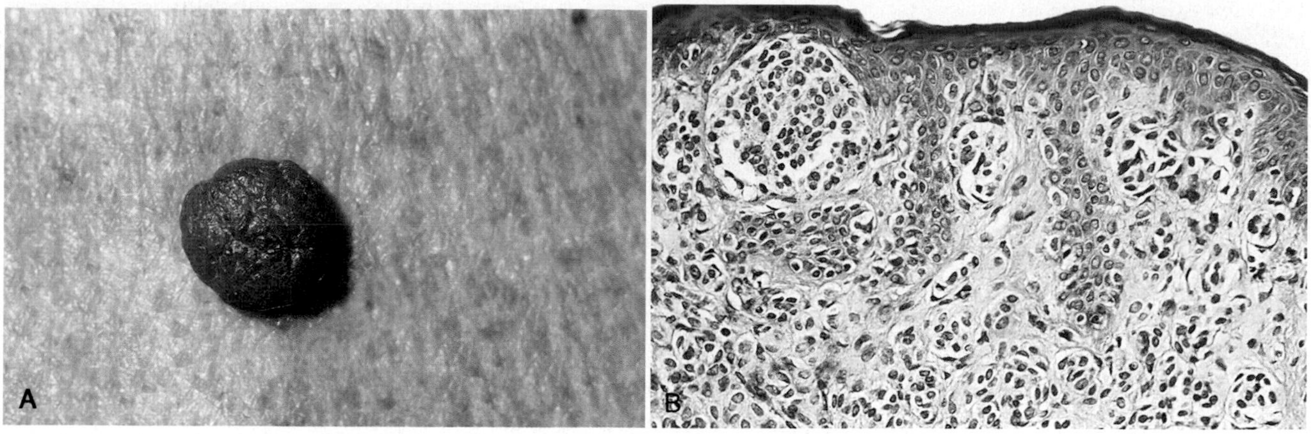

FIGURE 25–5 Nevocellular nevus, compound type. In contrast to the junctional nevus, the compound nevus *(A)* is more raised and dome shaped. The symmetry and uniform pigment distribution suggest a benign process. Histologically *(B)*, compound nevi combine the features of junctional nevi (intraepidermal nevus cell nests) with nests and cords of nevus cells in the underlying dermis.

recent recognition as an important model of tumor progression (dysplastic nevi and the heritable melanoma syndrome).

DYSPLASTIC NEVI

The association of melanocytic nevi with malignant melanoma was made more than 175 years ago,[10] although it was not until 1978 that a true precursor of malignant melanoma was described in detail. In 1978, Clark and colleagues[11] detailed the characteristics of lesions they termed BK moles (a name derived from the first letters of the last names of the initial two families studied).

Clinically, BK moles—or dysplastic nevi, as they are frequently called—are *larger than most acquired nevi (often >5 mm across) and may occur as hundreds of lesions on the body surface* (Fig. 25–6*A*, inset). They are *flat macules, slightly raised plaques with a "pebbly" surface, or target-like lesions with a darker raised center and irregular flat periphery.* They usually show variability in pigmentation (variegation) and borders that are irregular in contour. Unlike ordinary moles, dysplastic nevi have a tendency to occur on non–sun-exposed as well as on sun-exposed body surfaces. Dysplastic nevi have been documented in multiple members of families prone to the development of malignant melanoma *(the heritable melanoma syndrome).*[12] In these cases, genetic analyses have demonstrated the trait to be inherited as an autosomal dominant.[13,14] (See discussion under Molecular Genetics of Skin Cancers.) Transitions from these lesions to early melanoma have actually been documented clinically and histologically within a period as short as several weeks. However, most dysplastic nevi are clinically stable lesions. Dysplastic nevi may also occur as isolated lesions not associated with the heritable melanoma syndrome, in which case the risk of malignant change appears to be low.

Morphology. On histologic examination (see Fig. 25–6*A,B*), dysplastic nevi consist of compound nevi with both architectural and cytologic evidence of abnormal growth. **Nevus cell nests within the epidermis may be enlarged and exhibit abnormal fusion or coalescence with adjacent nests. As part of this**

TABLE 25–1 Variant Forms of Nevocellular Nevi

Nevus Variant	Diagnostic Architectural Features	Diagnostic Cytologic Features	Clinical Significance
Congenital nevus	Deep dermal and sometimes subcutaneous growth around adnexa, neurovascular bundles, and blood vessel walls	Identical to ordinary acquired nevi	Present at birth; large variants have increased melanoma risk
Blue nevus	Non-nested dermal infiltration, often with associated fibrosis	Highly dendritic, heavily pigmented nevus cells	Black-blue nodule; often confused with melanoma clinically
Spindle and epithelioid cell nevus (Spitz nevus)	Fascicular growth	Large, plump cells with pink-blue cytoplasm; fusiform cells	Common in children; red-pink nodule; often confused with hemangioma clinically
Halo nevus	Lymphocytic infiltration surrounding nevus cells	Identical to ordinary acquired nevi	Host immune response against nevus cells and surrounding normal melanocytes
Dysplastic nevus	Large, coalescent intraepidermal nests	Cytologic atypia	Potential precursor of malignant melanoma

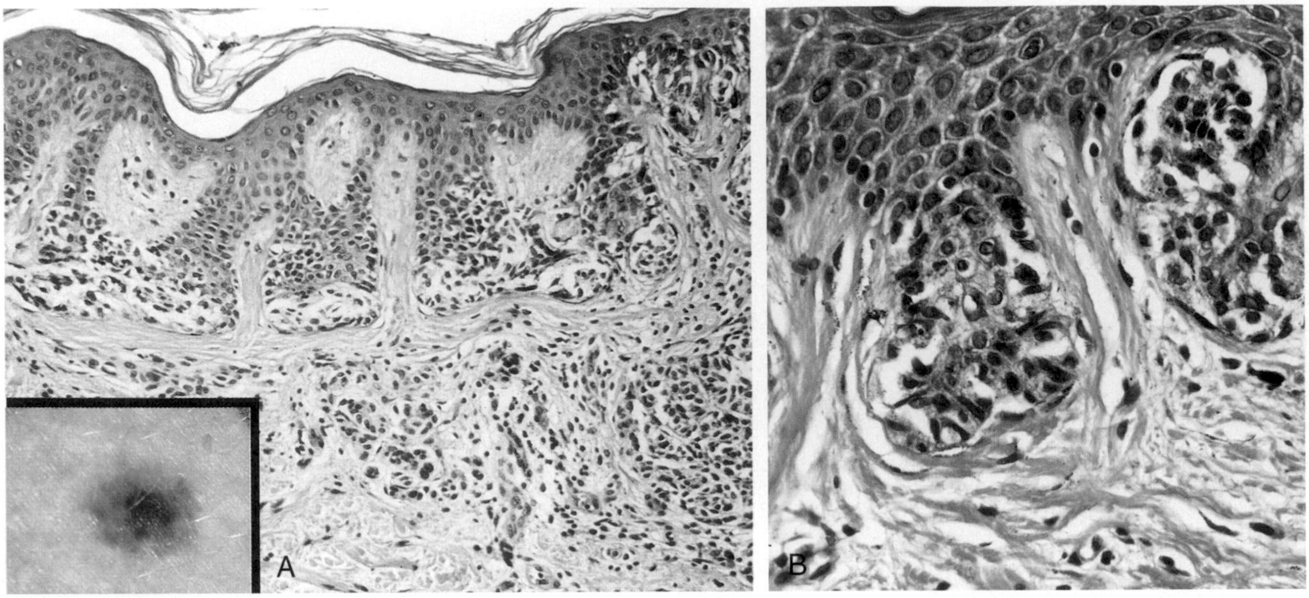

FIGURE 25–6 Dysplastic nevus. *A,* The lesion often has a compound nevus component (right side of scanning field) and an asymmetric "shoulder" composed of a junctional nevus component (left side of scanning field). The former correlates clinically with the more pigmented and raised central zone and the latter with the less pigmented, flat peripheral rim *(inset). B,* An important feature is the presence of cytologic atypia (irregularly shaped, dark-staining nuclei) at high magnification. The dermis underlying the atypical cells characteristically shows linear, or lamellar, fibrosis.

process, single nevus cells begin to replace the normal basal cell layer along the dermoepidermal junction, producing so-called lentiginous hyperplasia. Cytologic atypia consisting of irregular, often angulated, nuclear contours and hyperchromasia is frequently observed (see Fig. 25–6*B*). Associated alterations also occur in the superficial dermis. These consist of a usually sparse lymphocytic infiltrate, loss of melanin from presumably destroyed nevus cells, phagocytosis of this pigment by dermal macrophages (melanin pigment incontinence), and a peculiar linear fibrosis surrounding the epidermal rete ridges that are involved by the nevus. All of these features assist in the histologic recognition of a dysplastic nevus.

Several lines of evidence support the concept that some *dysplastic nevi are precursors of malignant melanoma.* In one study,[15] it was shown that in a large number of families prone to the development of melanoma, more than 5% of family members developed melanoma during an 8-year follow-up period, and new melanomas occurred only in individuals with dysplastic nevi. From this database, it was concluded that the actuarial probability of persons with the dysplastic nevus syndrome developing melanoma is 56% at age 59 years! Dysplastic nevi also demonstrate expression of some abnormal cell-surface antigens,[16] karyotypic abnormalities,[17] and in vitro vulnerability to the mutagenic effects of UV light.[18]

Clark and associates[19] have proposed steps whereby benign nevi may undergo aberrant differentiation to become dysplastic and eventually become metastasizing malignant tumors (Fig. 25–7). Parallels may be found in neoplasia involving other organ systems, and thus dysplastic nevi represent a general model of tumor progression.

MALIGNANT MELANOMA

Malignant melanoma is a relatively common neoplasm that not long ago was considered almost uniformly deadly. The great preponderance of melanomas arises in the skin; other sites of origin include the oral and anogenital mucosal surfaces, esophagus, meninges, and notably the eye. The following comments apply to cutaneous melanomas. Intraocular melanomas are discussed in Chapter 29.

Today, as a result of increased public awareness of the earliest signs of skin melanomas, most are cured surgically.[20] Nonetheless, the incidence of these lesions is on the rise, necessitating vigorous surveillance for their development.

As with epithelial malignant neoplasms of the skin, *sunlight appears to play an important role in the development of skin malignant melanoma.* For example, men commonly develop this tumor on the upper back, whereas women have a relatively high incidence on both the back and the legs. Lightly pigmented individuals are at higher risk for the development of melanoma than are darkly pigmented individuals. Sunlight, however, does not seem to be the only predisposing factor, and the presence of a pre-existing nevus (e.g., a dysplastic nevus), hereditary factors, or even exposure to certain carcinogens (as in the case of experimental melanomas in rodent models) may play a role in lesion development and evolution.[21]

Clinical Features. Malignant melanoma of the skin is usually asymptomatic, although itching may be an early manifestation. The majority of lesions are *greater than 10 mm in diameter.* The most important clinical sign of the disease is *change in color, size, or shape in a pigmented lesion.* Unlike benign (nondysplastic) nevi, melanomas exhibit striking *variations in pigmentation,* appearing in shades of black, brown, red, dark blue, and gray (Fig. 25–8*A*). On occasion, zones of white or flesh-colored hypopigmentation are also present. The *borders of melanomas are not smooth, round, and uniform,* as

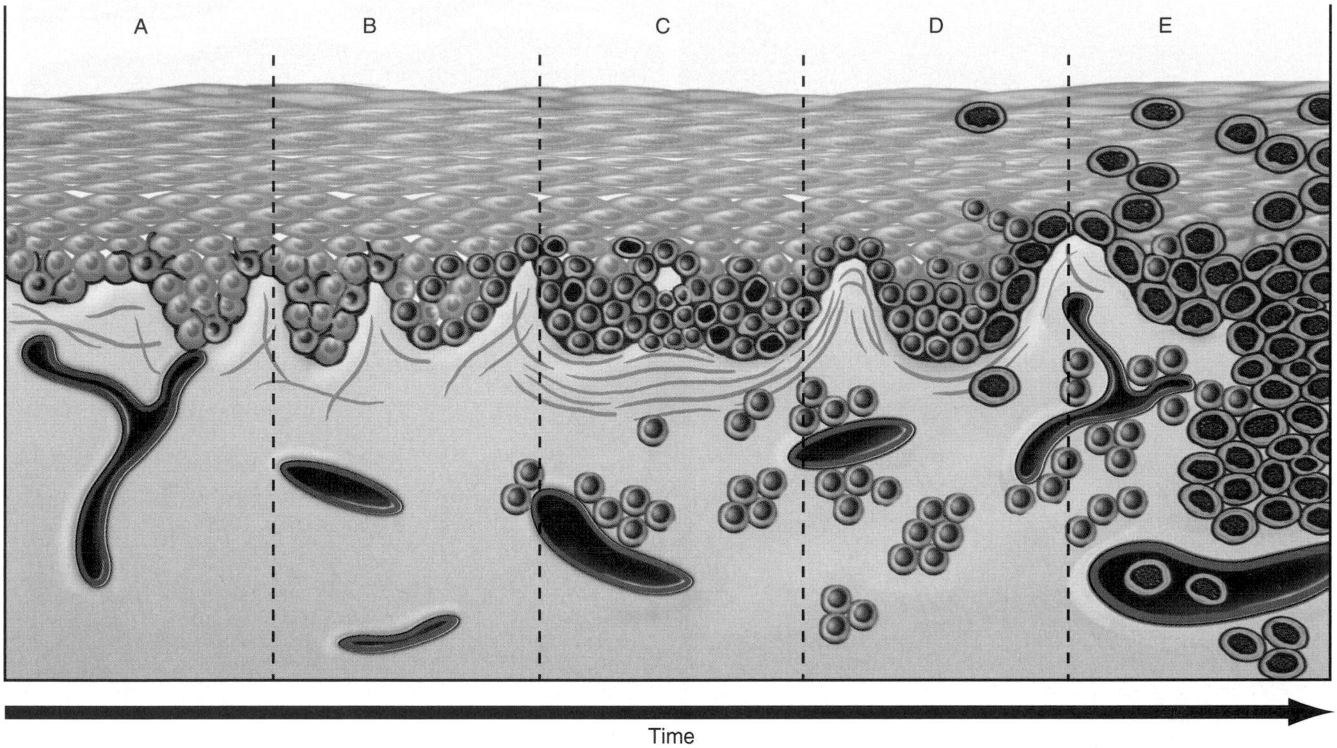

FIGURE 25–7 Steps of tumor progression in dysplastic nevi. *A,* Lentiginous melanocytic hyperplasia. *B,* Lentiginous junctional nevus. *C,* Lentiginous compound nevus with abnormal architectural and cytologic features (dysplastic nevus). *D,* Early melanoma, or radial growth phase melanoma (large dark cells in epidermis). *E,* Advanced melanoma (vertical growth phase) with malignant spread into the dermis and vessels.

in nevocellular nevi, but irregular and often "notched." In summary, the *clinical warning signs of melanoma are* (1) enlargement of a pre-existing mole, (2) itching or pain in a pre-existing mole, (3) development of a new pigmented lesion during adult life, (4) irregularity of the borders of a pigmented lesion, and (5) variegation of color within a pigmented lesion.

Growth Patterns and Morphology. Central to understanding the complicated histology of malignant melanoma is the concept of **radial and vertical growth.** Simply stated, radial growth indicates the tendency of a melanoma to grow horizontally within the epidermal and superficial dermal layers, often for a prolonged time (Fig. 25–8*B*). During this stage of growth, melanoma cells do not have the capacity to metastasize. Specific types of radial growth phase melanoma include lentigo maligna, superficial spreading, and acral/mucosal lentiginous. These are defined on the basis of architectural and cytologic features of growth within the epidermal layer as well as biologic behavior. For example, lentigo maligna radial growth typically occurs on sun-damaged facial skin of the elderly and may continue for as long as several decades before the tumor develops the capacity to metastasize. With time, the pattern of growth assumes a vertical component, and the melanoma now grows downward into the deeper dermal layers as an expansile mass lacking cellular maturation, without a tendency for the cells to become smaller as they descend into the reticular dermis (Fig. 25–8*C*). **This event is heralded clinically by the development of a nodule in the relatively flat radial growth phase and correlates with the emergence of a clone of cells with true metastatic potential.** Interestingly, the probability of metastasis in such lesions may be predicted by simply measuring in millimeters the depth of invasion of this vertical growth phase nodule below the granular cell layer of the overlying epidermis.[21] Prediction of clinical outcome has been refined further by taking into account factors such as number of mitoses and degree of infiltrative lymphocytic response within the tumor nodule.[22]

Individual melanoma cells are usually considerably larger than nevus cells. They contain large nuclei with irregular contours, having chromatin characteristically clumped at the periphery of the nuclear membrane and prominent red (eosinophilic) nucleoli (Fig. 25–8*D*). These cells proliferate as poorly formed nests or as individual cells at all levels of the epidermis (see Fig. 25–8*B*) in the radial phase of growth and, in the dermis, as expansile, balloon-like nodules in the vertical phase of growth (see Fig. 25–8*C*). **The nature and extent of the vertical growth phase determine the biologic behavior of malignant melanoma,** and thus it is important to observe and record vertical growth phase parameters in a pathology report.

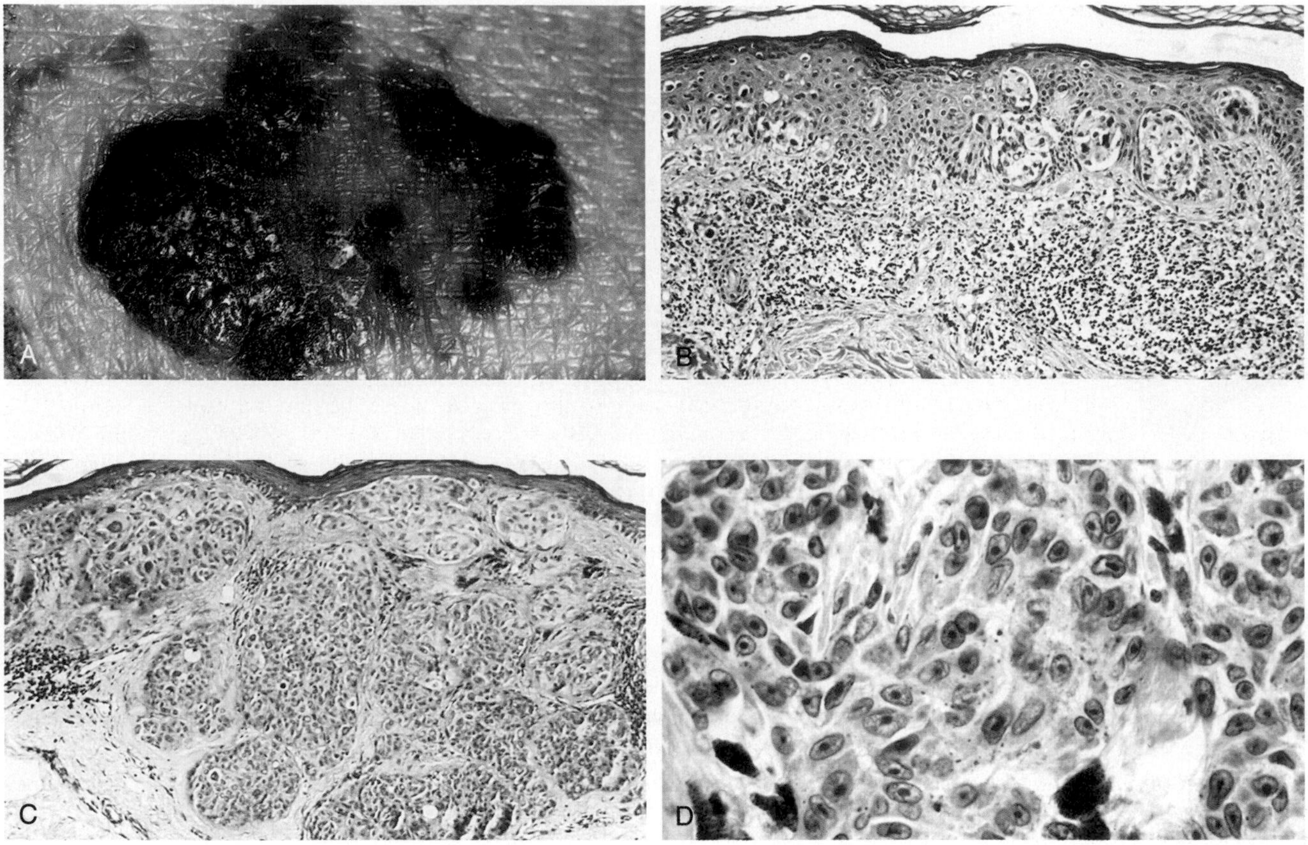

FIGURE 25–8 Malignant melanoma. *A,* In clinical appearance, lesions are irregular in contour and pigmentation. Macular areas correlate with the radial growth phase, while raised areas usually correspond to nodular aggregates of malignant cells in the vertical phase of growth. *B,* Radial growth phase of malignant melanoma, showing irregular nested and single-cell growth of melanoma cells within the epidermis and an underlying inflammatory response within the dermis. *C,* Photomicrograph of lesion in the vertical phase of growth, demonstrating nodular aggregates of infiltrating cells. *D,* High-power view of malignant melanoma cells.

Diagnostic Criteria and Prognostic Attributes. While most nevi and melanomas are clearly separable according to reproducible diagnostic criteria, a minority of lesions exhibit hybrid features that defy definitive classification as entirely benign or potentially malignant.[23] These lesions occupy a gray zone where morphologic characteristics may be insufficient to determine prognosis with accuracy. Such melanocytic proliferations have been termed *melanocytic tumors of uncertain malignant potential (MELTUMP).*[24] Such descriptive names underscore the limits of morphology in predicting outcome for these rare lesions and signify to the clinician the importance of excision to minimize local recurrence as well as of frequent follow-up.

For the majority of melanomas that have entered vertical growth, histologic and clinical attributes that permit prediction of outcome have been defined based on studies of large numbers of patients. One model that has received widespread attention over the past decade involves assessment of prognosis based on application of multiple variables to a given lesion.[25] These variables are (1) measurement of tumor *depth* in millimeters, (2) number of tumor cell *mitoses* per square millimeter, (3) evidence of an *immune response* to the superficial (radial) growth component (termed *regression*), (4) presence and degree of *tumor infiltrating lymphocytes* (TILs) at the base of the deep (vertical) growth component, (5) gender, and (6) location (central body or extremity). Determinants of a more *favorable prognosis* in this model include tumor depth of less than 1.7 mm, absence or low numbers of mitoses, presence of a brisk TIL response, absence of regression, female gender, and location on extremity skin. In a study by the American Joint Committee on Cancer, tumor thickness and presence or absence of ulceration, in addition to clinical stage, were found to be of prognostic significance.[26] *Because melanomas evolve over time from entirely curable lesions to tumors with progressive potential for metastasis as they enlarge and invade more deeply, early and complete excision is critical to minimizing the likelihood of systemic dissemination.*

The pathogenesis of melanomas is discussed later.

Benign Epithelial Tumors

Benign epithelial neoplasms are common and usually biologically inconsequential, although they may represent significant sources of psychologic discomfort for the patient. These tumors, derived from the keratinizing stratified squamous epithelium of the epidermis and hair follicles (keratinocytes) and the ductular epithelium of cutaneous glands, may recapitulate the cell layers from which they arise. They are often confused clinically with malignancy, particularly when they are pigmented or inflamed, and histologic examination of a biopsy specimen is frequently required to establish a definitive diagnosis. In rare instances they can be part of specific syndromes associated with potentially life-threatening visceral malignancies (e.g., multiple trichilemmomas as in Cowden syndrome or multiple, benign or malignant sebaceous neoplasms as in Muir-Torre syndrome). Precise diagnosis of epithelial tumors in these instances may facilitate recognition of a syndrome and implementation of appropriate intervention and follow-up.

SEBORRHEIC KERATOSES

These common epidermal tumors occur most frequently in middle-aged or older individuals. They arise spontaneously and may become particularly numerous on the trunk, although the extremities, head, and neck may also be involved. In people of color, multiple small lesions on the face are termed *dermatosis papulosa nigra.*

Seborrheic keratoses have characteristic clinical features. They appear as round, flat, coinlike, waxy plaques that vary in diameter from millimeters to several centimeters (Fig. 25–9*A*). They are uniformly tan to dark brown and usually show a velvety to granular surface. Lesions may give the impression that they are "stuck on" and may be easily peeled off. Inspection with a hand lens will usually reveal small, round, porelike ostia impacted with keratin, a feature helpful in differentiating these pigmented lesions from melanomas.

Morphology. On histologic examination, these neoplasms are exophytic and demarcated sharply from the adjacent epidermis. They are composed of sheets of small cells that most resemble basal cells of the normal epidermis (Fig. 25–9*B*). Variable melanin pigmentation is present within these basaloid cells, accounting for the brown coloration clinically. Exuberant keratin production (hyperkeratosis) occurs at the surface of seborrheic keratoses, and small keratin-filled cysts (horn cysts) and invaginations of keratin into the main tumor mass (invagination cysts) are characteristic features. Interestingly, when seborrheic keratoses become irritated and inflamed, they undergo squamous differentiation[27] and are characterized by foci of "whorling" squamous cells resembling eddy currents in a stream. A biologic explanation for this intriguing phenomenon awaits discovery. When seborrheic keratoses involve the epithelium of hair follicles, they may grow in an endophytic (downward) fashion, and they generally also show the effects of inflammation; such lesions are termed **inverted follicular keratoses.**

Seborrheic keratoses may occur explosively in large numbers, as part of a paraneoplastic syndrome *(Leser-Trélat sign).* Transforming growth factor-α produced by tumor cells is thought to contribute to the development of such lesions.[28]

ACANTHOSIS NIGRICANS

Acanthosis nigricans is used to describe thickened (*acanthosis* = hyperplasia of the stratum spinosum of the epidermis), hyperpigmented zones of skin often with a "velvet-like" texture involving most commonly the flexural areas (axillae, skin folds of the neck, groin, and anogenital regions). *It is an important cutaneous marker for associated benign and malignant conditions* and, accordingly, is divided into two types.[29] The *benign type,* which constitutes about 80% of all cases, develops gradually and usually occurs in childhood or during puberty. It may occur (1) as an autosomal dominant trait with variable penetrance, (2) in association with obesity or

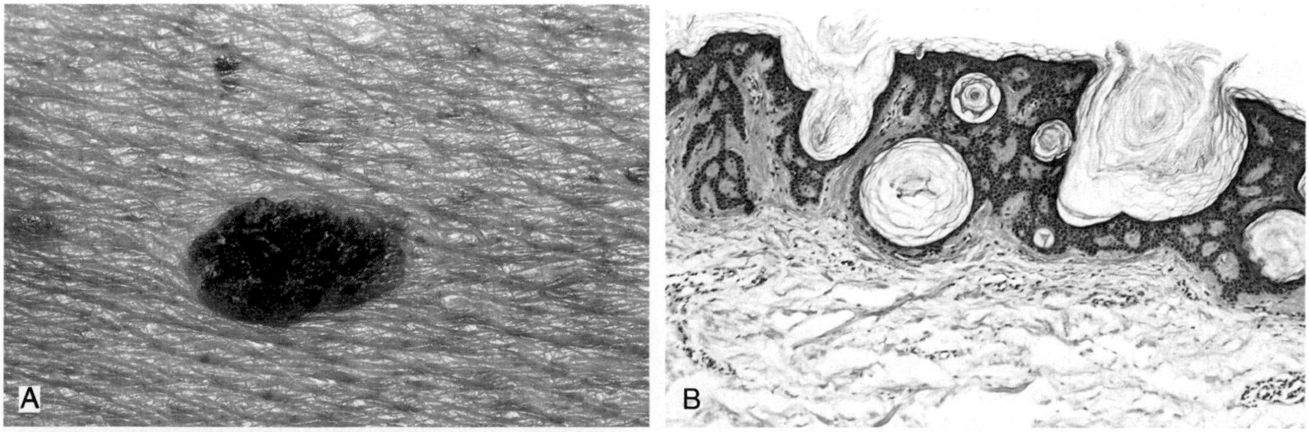

FIGURE 25–9 Seborrheic keratosis. *A,* A well-demarcated coinlike pigmented lesion containing dark keratin-filled surface plugs is composed histologically of proliferations of basaloid cells with formation of prominent keratin-filled "horn" cysts *(B),* some of which communicate with the surface (pseudo-horn cysts) and correlate with the plugs observed clinically.

endocrine abnormalities (particularly with pituitary and pineal tumors and with diabetes), and (3) as part of a number of rare congenital syndromes. As with seborrheic keratoses, acanthosis nigricans may result from abnormal production of epidermal growth-promoting factors by a variety of tumors. This occurrence may account for many instances of the *malignant type,* in which lesions arise in middle-aged and older individuals, often in association with an underlying gastrointestinal adenocarcinoma.

Morphology. All forms of acanthosis nigricans have similar histologic features. The epidermis and underlying enlarged dermal papillae undulate sharply to form numerous repeating peaks and valleys. Variable hyperplasia may be seen, along with hyperkeratosis and slight basal cell layer hyperpigmentation (but no melanocytic hyperplasia).

Because lesions of acanthosis nigricans may precede clinical symptoms and signs of the underlying disorder, knowledge and recognition of this entity may be of great diagnostic importance in early recognition of covert systemic disease.

FIBROEPITHELIAL POLYP

The fibroepithelial polyp has many names (acrochordon, squamous papilloma, skin tag) and is one of the most common cutaneous lesions. It is generally detected as an incidental finding in middle-aged and older individuals on the neck, trunk, face, and intertriginous areas as a soft, flesh-colored, baglike tumor attached to the skin surface by a small, often slender stalk. Rarely, fibroepithelial polyps, along with tumors differentiating toward perifollicular mesenchyme, are part of a syndrome called Birt-Hogg-Dubé syndrome.

Morphology. On histologic examination, these tumors are merely fibrovascular cores covered by benign squamous epithelium. It is not uncommon to discover ischemic necrosis in histologic sections (the result of torsion that produced the pain and swelling that may precipitate their removal).

Fibroepithelial polyps are usually biologically inconsequential, although they have been associated with diabetes and intestinal polyposis. It is of interest that along with melanocytic nevi and hemangiomas, they often become more numerous or prominent during pregnancy. The pathogenesis of this is unclear but may be related to hormonal stimulation.

EPITHELIAL CYST (WEN)

Epithelial cysts are common lesions formed by the invagination and cystic expansion of the epidermis or of the epithelium forming the hair follicle. The lay term, *wen,* derives from the Anglo-Saxon *wenn,* meaning a lump or tumor. These cysts are filled with keratin and variable amounts of lipid-containing debris derived from sebaceous secretions. Clinically, they are dermal or subcutaneous, well-circumscribed, firm, and often moveable nodules. When large, they may be dome shaped and flesh colored and often become painful on traumatic rupture.

Morphology. Epithelial cysts are divided into several histologic types according to the structural components of their walls. The **epidermal inclusion cyst** has a wall nearly identical to the epidermis and is filled with laminated strands of keratin. **Pilar** or **trichilemmal cysts** have a wall that resembles follicular epithelium, without a granular cell layer and filled by a more homogeneous mixture of keratin and lipid. The **dermoid cyst** is similar to the epidermal inclusion cyst, but it also shows multiple appendages (such as small hair follicles) budding outward from its wall. Finally, **steatocystoma multiplex** constitutes a curious cyst with a wall resembling the sebaceous gland duct, and from which numerous compressed sebaceous lobules originate. The importance of recognition of this cyst derives from the often dominantly heritable nature of the lesion.

ADNEXAL (APPENDAGE) TUMORS

There are literally hundreds of benign neoplasms arising from cutaneous appendages.[30] Although some show no aggressive behavior and remain localized, they may be confused with certain types of cutaneous cancers (e.g., basal cell carcinoma). Certain appendage tumors are associated with Mendelian patterns of inheritance and occur as multiple disfiguring lesions. In some instances, these lesions serve as markers for internal malignancy, as in the case of multiple trichilemmomas and breast carcinoma of Cowden syndrome.[31] Selected examples are provided here to illustrate neoplasms of hair follicles, eccrine glands, and apocrine glands.

Appendage tumors are often clinically nondescript, flesh-colored solitary or multiple papules and nodules. Some have a predisposition for occurrence on specific body surfaces. For example, the *eccrine poroma* occurs predominantly on the palms and soles. The *cylindroma,* an appendage tumor with apocrine differentiation, usually occurs on the forehead and scalp (Fig. 25–10*A*), where coalescence of nodules with time may produce a hatlike growth, hence the name *turban tumor.* These lesions may be dominantly inherited and first appear early in life. *Syringomas,* lesions of eccrine differentiation, in comparison, usually occur as multiple, small, tan papules in the vicinity of the lower eyelids. *Trichoepitheliomas,* showing follicular differentiation, are dominantly inherited when they are seen as multiple, semitransparent, dome-shaped papules that involve the face, scalp, neck, and upper trunk (Fig. 25–10*C*).

Morphology. The **cylindroma** is composed of islands of cells resembling those of the normal epidermal or adnexal basal cell layer (basaloid cells). These islands fit together like pieces of a jigsaw puzzle within a fibrous dermal matrix (Fig. 25–10*B*). The **trichoepithelioma** is a proliferation of basaloid cells that forms primitive structures resembling hair follicles (Fig. 25–10*D*). **Mixed tumor (chondroid syringoma)** is composed of variably dilated sweat gland–like ducts surrounded by a blue-gray matrix with features of true cartilage (Fig. 25–11*A*). The **trichilemmoma** is a local-

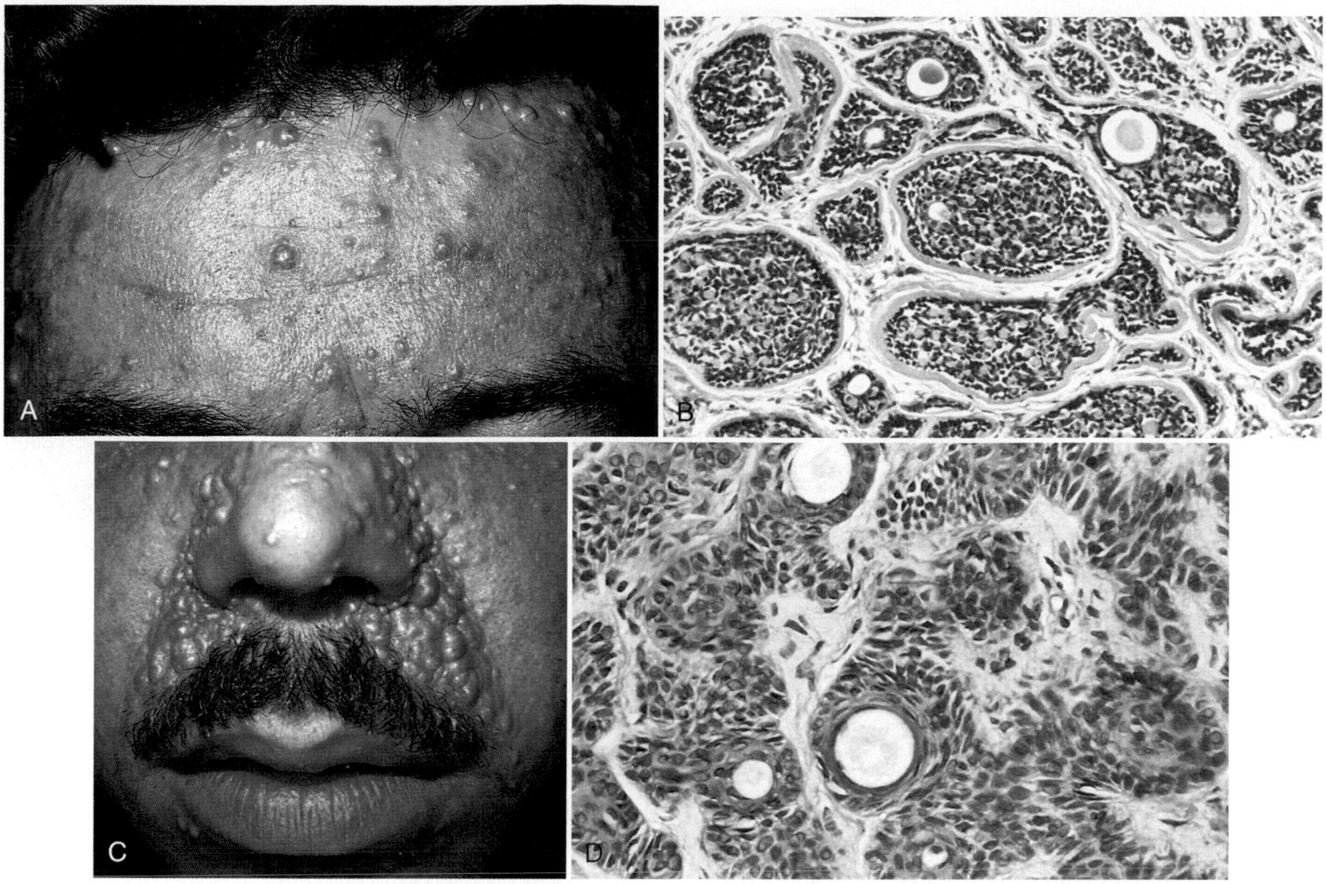

FIGURE 25–10 Adnexal tumors. The clinical appearance is often nondescript (*A* shows multiple cylindromas and *C* shows multiple trichoepitheliomas). *B*, On histologic examination, the cylindroma is composed of islands of basaloid cells containing occasional ducts and seemingly fitting together like pieces of a jigsaw puzzle. *D*, Trichoepithelioma is composed of buds of basaloid cells that resemble primitive hair follicles. Here the small ductlike structures are actually keratin-filled microcysts.

ized proliferation of pale pink, glassy cells that resembles the uppermost portion of the hair follicle (infundibulum) (Fig. 25–11*B*). **Hidradenoma papilliferum** is composed of ducts lined by apocrine-type cells that show characteristic decapitation secretion and a fibrous stroma (Fig. 25–11*C*). Table 25–2 summarizes common adnexal tumors according to histologic features that recapitulate mature adnexal counterparts.

Although most appendage tumors are benign, malignant variants do exist. *Sebaceous carcinoma,* for example, arises from the meibomian glands of the eyelid and may follow an aggressive biologic course with systemic metastases. *Eccrine* and *apocrine carcinomas* are often confused with metastatic adenocarcinomas to the skin because of their tendency for abortive gland formation.

KERATOACANTHOMA

Keratoacanthoma is a rapidly developing neoplasm that clinically and histologically may mimic well-differentiated squamous cell carcinoma. Often it will heal spontaneously, without treatment! Men are more often affected than women, and lesions most frequently affect sun-exposed skin of whites older than age 50 years.[32]

Keratoacanthomas appear clinically as flesh-colored, dome-shaped nodules with a central, keratin-filled plug, imparting a crater-like topography (Fig. 25–12*A*). Lesions range in size from 1 cm to several centimeters across and have a predilection for facial skin, including the cheeks, nose, and ears, and the dorsa of the hands.

Morphology. Keratoacanthomas are characterized histologically by a central, keratin-filled crater surrounded by proliferating epithelial cells that extend upward in a liplike fashion over the sides of the crater and downward into the dermis as irregular tongues (Fig. 25–12*B*). This epithelium is composed of enlarged cells showing evidence of reactive cytologic atypia. These cells have a characteristically "glassy" eosinophilic cytoplasm (Fig. 25–12*C*) and produce keratin abruptly (without the development of an intervening granular cell layer). This mode of keratinization is analogous to that of the normal hair follicle and is similar to that seen in the pilar cyst described earlier, giving rise to speculation that the keratoacan-

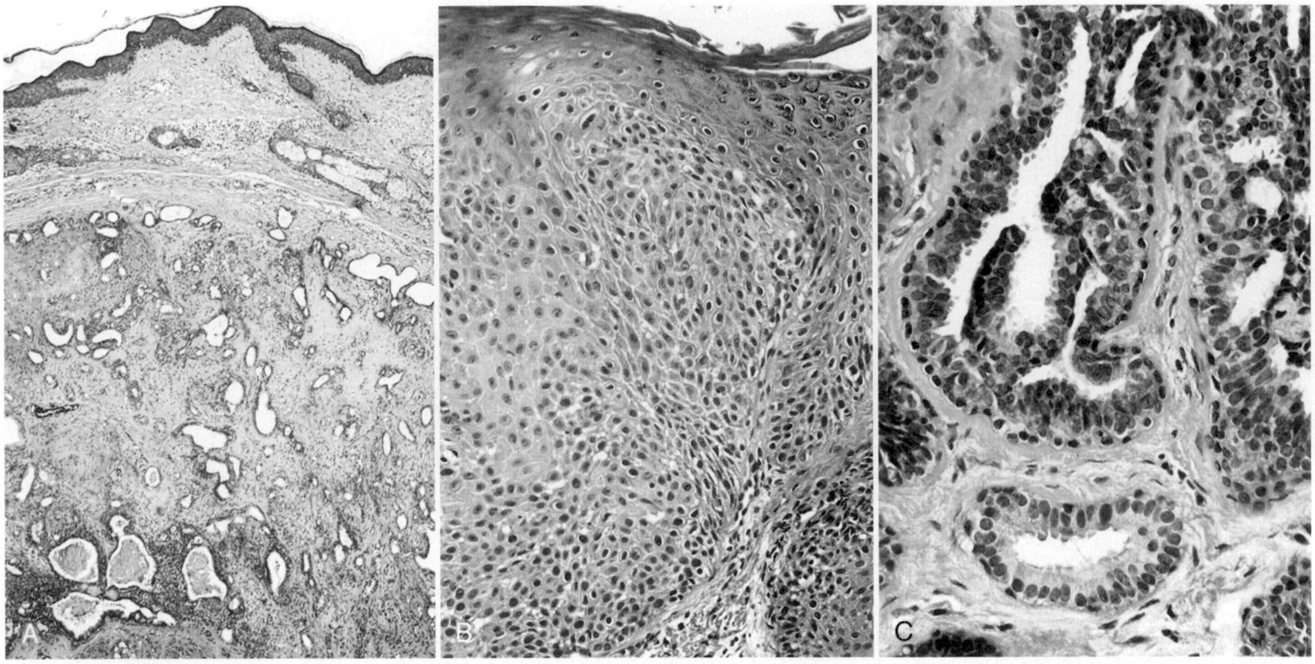

FIGURE 25–11 Adnexal tumors. *A,* Mixed tumor (chondroid syringoma). *B,* Trichilemmoma. *C,* Hidradenoma papilliferum.

thoma is a neoplasm of follicular epithelium. The early tumor infiltrates into the collagen and elastic fibers and entraps them. Little, if any, host inflammatory response is present during this rapidly proliferative phase, but as the lesion evolves, there is some stromal response that is fibrotic and contains numerous inflammatory cells.

There is growing belief that keratoacanthomas may represent a form of squamous cell carcinoma that regresses as a consequence of interactions with host tissues that fail to support inexorable growth. It is presently unclear whether this relates to factors in the host (e.g., immune response) or inherent to the tumor (e.g., expression of angiogenesis or cell-cycle inhibitors). Like most squamous cell carcinomas, the majority of keratoacanthomas have mutations in the *p53* gene.[33]

Premalignant and Malignant Epidermal Tumors

ACTINIC KERATOSIS

Before the development of overt malignancy of the epidermis, a series of progressively dysplastic changes occur, a phenomenon analogous to the atypia that precedes carcinoma of the squamous mucosa of the uterine cervix (Chapter 22). Because this dysplasia is usually the result of chronic exposure to sunlight and is associated with build-up of excess keratin, these lesions are called *actinic keratoses.* As would be expected, they occur with particularly high incidence in lightly pigmented individuals. Exposure to ionizing radiation, hydrocarbons, and arsenicals may induce similar lesions.

Actinic keratoses are usually less than 1 cm in diameter; are tan-brown, red, or skin-colored; and have a rough, sandpaper-like consistency. Some lesions may produce so much keratin that a "cutaneous horn" develops (Fig. 25–13*A*). Such horns may become so prominent that they actually resemble the

TABLE 25–2 Common Adnexal Tumors

Adnexal Tumors	Mature Counterpart	Histologic Features	Clinical Significance
Trichoepithelioma Trichofolliculoma	Hair follicle	Hair matrix, outer root sheath differentiation	Multiple trichoepitheliomas, dominant inheritance
Sebaceous adenoma Sebaceous epithelioma	Sebaceous gland	Cytoplasmic lipid vacuoles	Association with internal malignancy
Syringocystadenoma papilliferum	Apocrine gland	Apocrine type ("decapitation") secretion	May develop in mixed epidermal-adnexal hamartomas of face and scalp termed *nevus sebaceus*
Syringoma	Eccrine gland	Eccrine ducts lined by membranous eosinophilic cuticles; tadpole-like epithelial structures	May be confused with basal cell carcinoma clinically

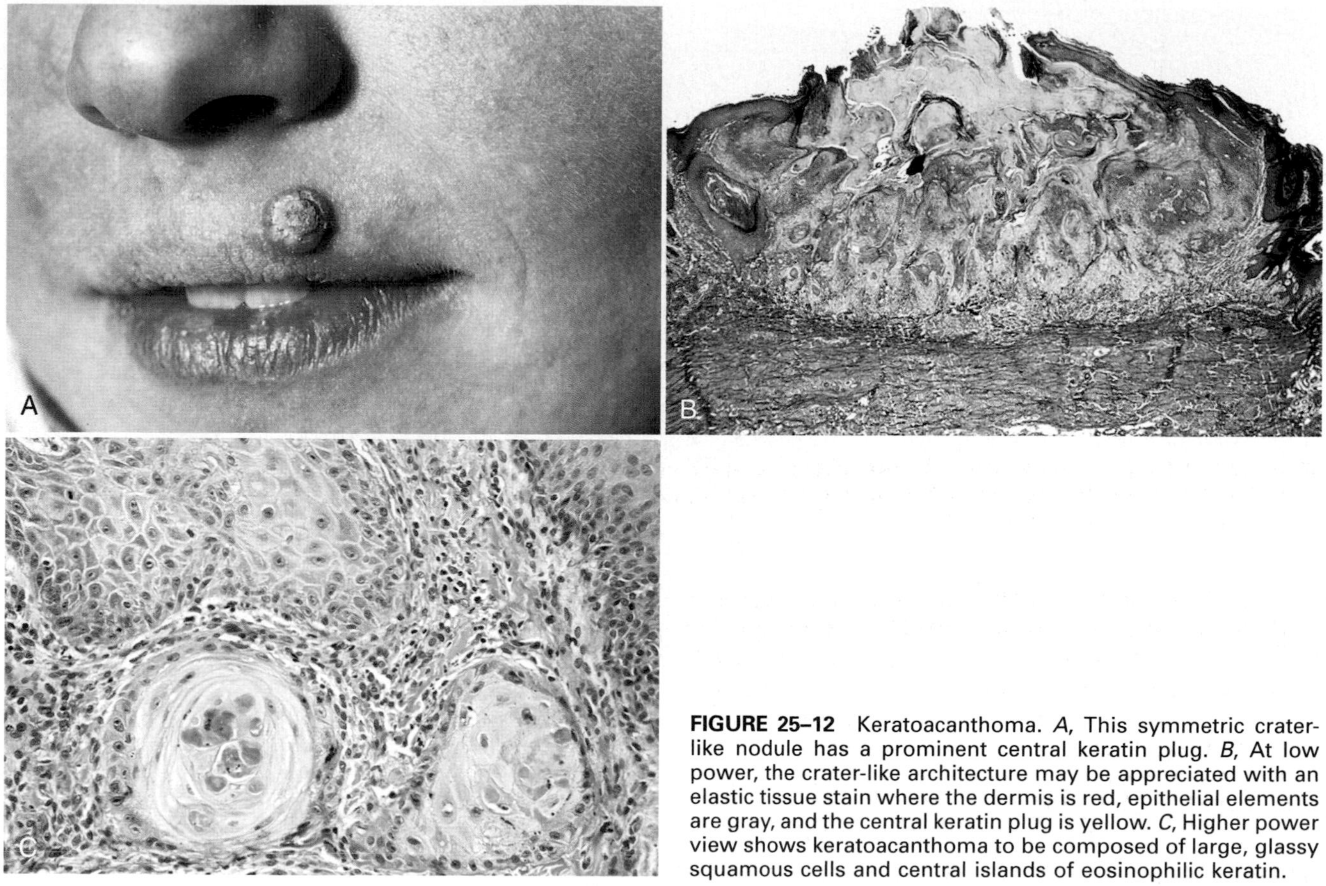

FIGURE 25–12 Keratoacanthoma. *A,* This symmetric crater-like nodule has a prominent central keratin plug. *B,* At low power, the crater-like architecture may be appreciated with an elastic tissue stain where the dermis is red, epithelial elements are gray, and the central keratin plug is yellow. *C,* Higher power view shows keratoacanthoma to be composed of large, glassy squamous cells and central islands of eosinophilic keratin.

horns of animals! Skin sites commonly exposed to sun (face, arms, dorsum of hands) are most frequently affected. The lips may also develop similar lesions (termed *actinic cheilitis*).

Morphology. Cytologic atypia is seen in the lowermost layers of the epidermis and may be associated with hyperplasia of basal cells (Fig. 25–13*B*) or, alternatively, with early atrophy that results in diffuse thinning of the epidermal surface of the lesion. The atypical basal cells usually have evidence of dyskeratosis with pink or reddish cytoplasm. Also, intercellular bridges are present, in contrast to basal cell carcinoma, in which the cytoplasm is usually basophilic and the cells lack intercellular bridges identifiable by light microscopy. The dermis contains thickened, blue-gray elastic fibers (elastosis), a probable result of abnormal dermal elastic fiber synthesis by sun-damaged fibroblasts[34] within the superficial dermis. The stratum corneum is thickened, and unlike in normal skin, nuclei in the cells in this layer are often retained (a pattern termed **parakeratosis**).

Whether all actinic keratoses would lead to skin cancer (usually squamous cell carcinoma), if given enough time, is conjectural. Many believe that certain lesions may regress or remain stable during a normal life span. However, enough do become malignant to warrant local eradication of these potential precursor lesions. This can usually be accomplished by gentle curettage, freezing, or topical application of chemotherapeutic agents.

SQUAMOUS CELL CARCINOMA

Squamous cell carcinoma is the second most common tumor arising on sun-exposed sites in older people, exceeded only by basal cell carcinoma. Except for lesions on the lower legs, these tumors have a higher incidence in men than in women. Exposure to sunlight is the major predisposing factor; others include industrial carcinogens (tars and oils), chronic ulcers and draining osteomyelitis, old burn scars, ingestion of arsenicals, ionizing radiation, and (in the oral cavity) tobacco and betel nut chewing.

The most commonly accepted exogenous cause of squamous cell carcinoma is exposure to UV light with subsequent DNA damage. Individuals who are immunosuppressed as a result of chemotherapy or organ transplantation, or who have xeroderma pigmentosum (Chapter 7), are at increased risk for developing neoplasms.[35] A considerable proportion of these are squamous cell carcinomas. Sunlight, in addition to its effect on DNA, also seems to have a direct and, at least, a tran-

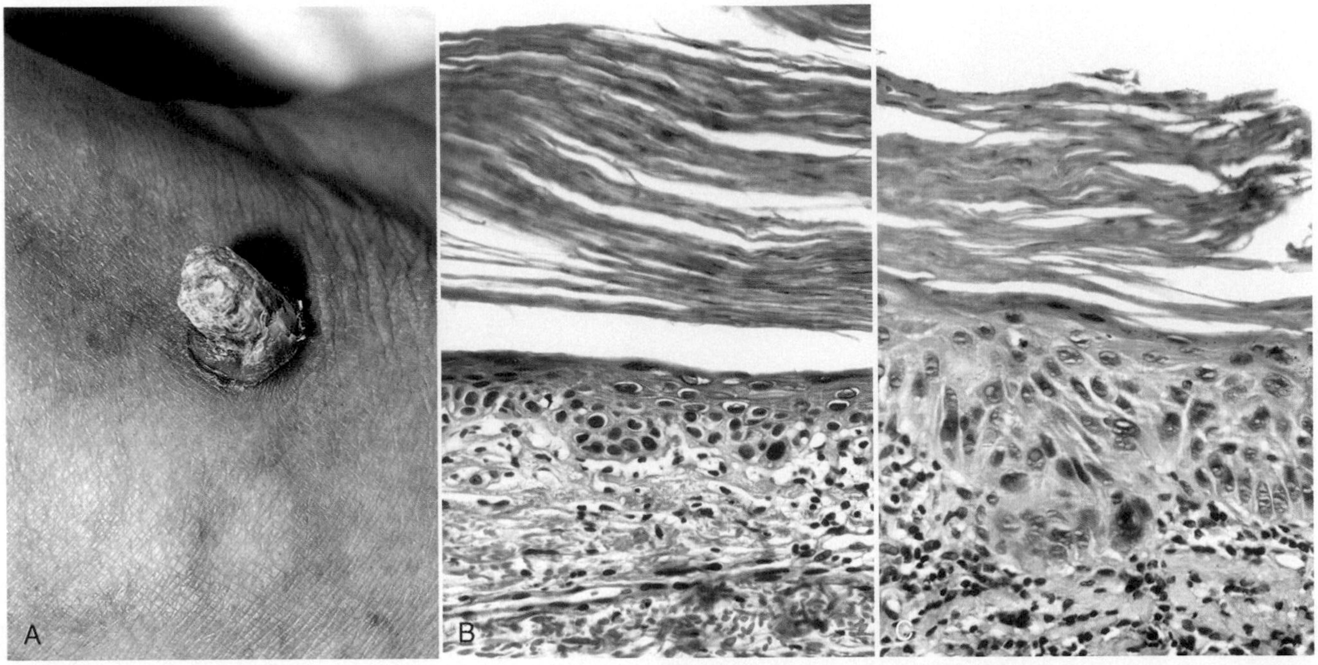

FIGURE 25–13 Actinic keratosis. *A*, Excessive scale formation in this lesion has produced a "cutaneous horn." *B*, Basal cell layer atypia is associated with marked hyperkeratosis and parakeratosis. *C*, Progression to full-thickness nuclear atypia, with or without the presence of superficial epidermal maturation, heralds the development of early squamous cell carcinoma in situ.

sient immunosuppressive effect on skin by affecting the normal surveillance function of antigen-presenting Langerhans cells in the epidermis.[36,37] DNA sequences of certain viruses (e.g., human papillomavirus [HPV] type 36) have been detected in potential precursors of squamous cell carcinoma, suggesting a role for these agents in the evolution of certain, but not all,[38] cutaneous epithelial neoplasms. Finally, certain chemical agents appear to have direct mutagenic effects by producing DNA adducts with subsequent oncogene activation.[39] (See Molecular Genetics of Skin Cancers for additional details).

Morphology. Squamous cell carcinomas that have not invaded through the basement membrane of the dermoepidermal junction (termed **in situ carcinoma**) appear as sharply defined, red, scaling plaques. More advanced, invasive lesions are nodular, show variable keratin production appreciated clinically as hyperkeratosis, and may ulcerate (Fig. 25–14*A*). Well-differentiated lesions may be indistinguishable from keratoacanthoma. When the oral mucosa is involved, a zone of white thickening may be seen, an appearance caused by a variety of disorders and referred to clinically as **leukoplakia**.

Unlike actinic keratoses, squamous cell carcinoma in situ is characterized by cells with atypical (enlarged and hyperchromatic) nuclei at **all levels** of the epidermis. When these cells break through the basement membrane, the process has become invasive. Invasive squamous cell carcinoma (Fig. 25–14*B,C*) exhibits variable differentiation, ranging from tumors formed by polygonal squamous cells, arranged in orderly lobules and exhibiting numerous large zones of keratinization, to neoplasms formed by highly anaplastic, rounded cells with foci of necrosis and only abortive, single-cell keratinization (dyskeratosis). These latter tumors may be so poorly differentiated that electron microscopy for the detection of keratinocyte intercellular attachment sites (desmosomes) or reaction of tissue with antibodies to keratin or epithelial membrane–associated antigens may be necessary to definitively establish cell lineage.

Invasive squamous cell carcinomas are usually discovered while they are small and resectable; less than 5% have metastases to regional nodes, and these lesions are generally deeply invasive.

BASAL CELL CARCINOMA

Basal cell carcinomas are common, slow-growing tumors that rarely metastasize. They have a tendency to occur at sites subject to chronic sun exposure and in lightly pigmented people. As with squamous cell carcinoma, the incidence of basal cell carcinoma rises sharply with immunosuppression and in patients with inherited defects in DNA repair (e.g., xeroderma pigmentosum; Chapter 7).

These tumors present clinically as *pearly papules often containing prominent, dilated subepidermal blood vessels (telangiectasias)* (Fig. 25–15*A*). Some tumors contain melanin and, thus, appear similar to melanocytic nevi or melanomas. Advanced lesions may ulcerate, and extensive local invasion of bone or facial sinuses may occur after many years of neglect or in unusually aggressive tumors, explaining the past designation *rodent ulcers.* One common and important variant, the superficial basal cell carcinoma, presents as an erythematous, occasionally pigmented plaque that may resemble early forms of malignant melanoma. Careful inspection usually reveals characteristic pearly papules at the periphery of the plaque.

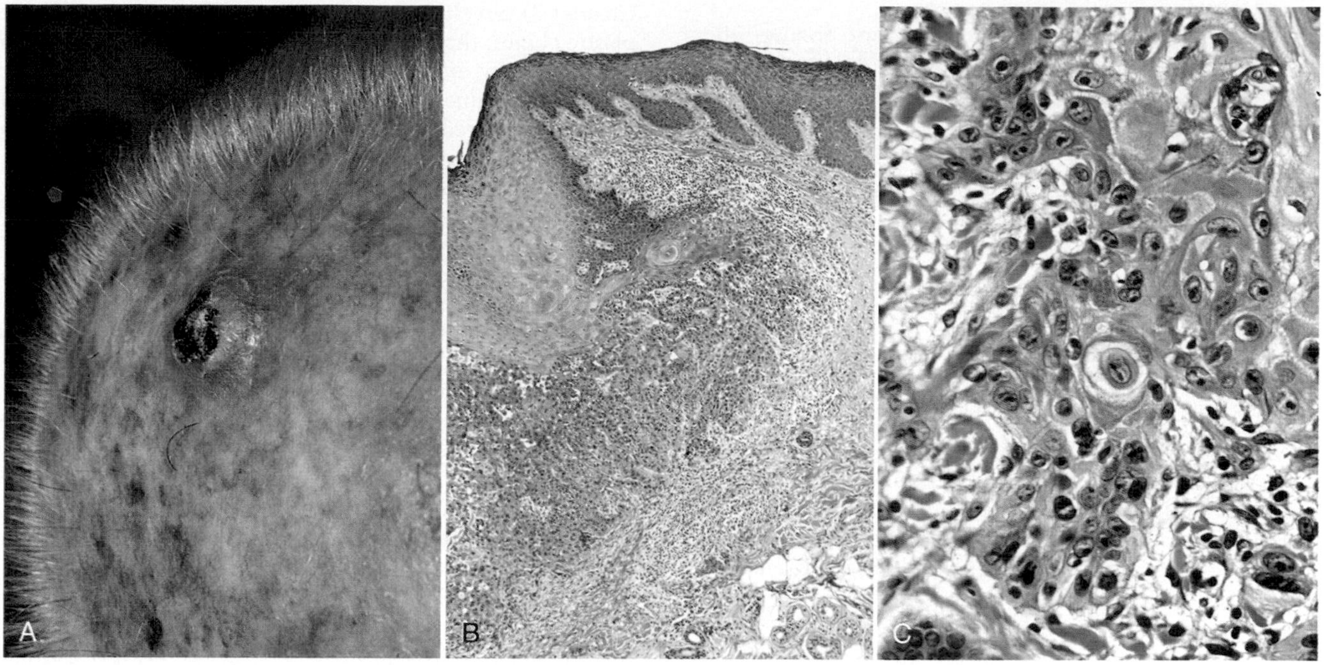

FIGURE 25–14 Invasive squamous cell carcinoma. *A*, Lesions are often nodular and ulcerated. *B*, Tongues of atypical squamous epithelium have transgressed the basement membrane, invading deeply into the dermis. *C*, Invasive tumor cells exhibit enlarged nuclei with angulated contours and prominent nucleoli.

Morphology. On histologic examination, tumor cells resemble those in the normal basal cell layer of the epidermis. They arise from the epidermis or follicular epithelium and do not occur on mucosal surfaces. Two patterns are seen: **multifocal growths** originating from the epidermis and extending over several square centimeters or more of skin surface (multifocal superficial type) and **nodular lesions** growing downward deeply into the dermis as cords and islands of variably basophilic cells with hyperchromatic nuclei, embedded in a mucinous matrix, and often surrounded by many fibroblasts and lym-

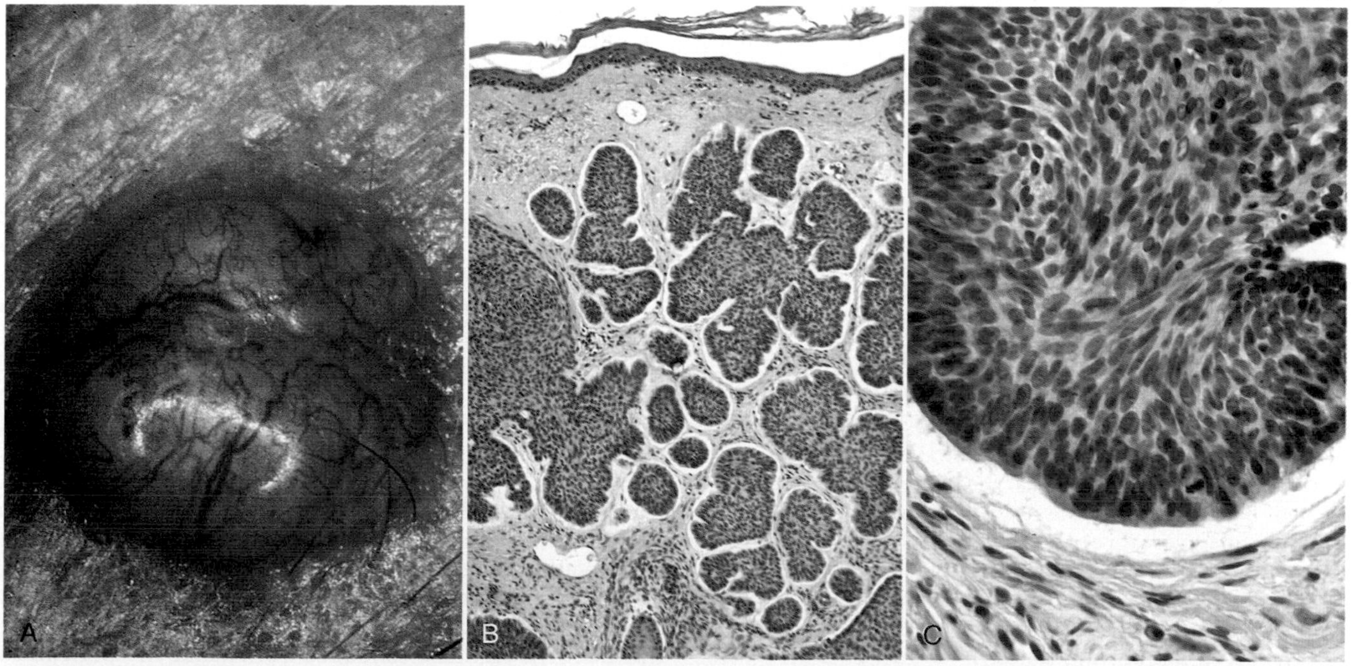

FIGURE 25–15 Basal cell carcinoma. Pearly, telangiectatic nodules *(A)* are composed of nests of basaloid cells within the dermis *(B)* that are often separated from the adjacent stroma by thin clefts *(C)*.

phocytes (Fig. 25–15*B*). The cells forming the periphery of the tumor cell islands tend to be arranged radially with their long axes in approximately parallel alignment (palisading). The stroma shrinks away from the epithelial tumor nests (Fig. 25–15*C*), creating clefts or separation artifacts that assist in differentiating basal cell carcinomas from certain appendage tumors also characterized by proliferation of basaloid cells (e.g., trichoepithelioma).

Basal Cell Nevus Syndrome. This rare, dominantly inherited syndrome[40] is associated with the development of numerous basal cell carcinomas in early life and with abnormalities of bone, nervous system, eyes, and reproductive organs. The molecular genetics of this rare yet informative condition are described below under Molecular Genetics of Skin Cancers.

MERKEL CELL CARCINOMA

This rare neoplasm is derived from the infrequent and functionally obscure Merkel cell of the epidermis, a neural crest–derived cell putatively important for tactile sensation in lower animals.[41] Lesions may clinically present as ulcerated nodules and thus resemble eroded basal cell carcinoma or relatively nonpigmented (amelanotic) forms of malignant melanoma. These tumors are capable of metastasis and are potentially lethal. They are composed of small, round malignant cells containing neurosecretory-type cytoplasmic granules. The tumor cells also share some features with epithelial cells, expressing a type of keratin (cytokeratin 20) within their cytoplasm. Pathologists must be aware of this rare primary skin tumor since it may closely resemble metastatic small cell carcinoma from lung or certain lymphomas that spread to the dermis.

MOLECULAR GENETICS OF SKIN CANCERS

The study of skin tumors requires understanding of morphologic and molecular alterations, as well as the interactions between genetic and environmental factors. No other organ is so constantly exposed to environmental hazards as the skin; as a consequence, the skin is the tissue most commonly affected by neoplasms. Basal cell carcinoma is the most common invasive cancer in humans, with nearly 1 million estimated cases per year in the United States.[42] The incidence of malignant melanoma, once a rare tumor, has risen almost exponentially. This increase is larger than for any other tumor, with the exception of lung cancer in women.[43] Although the immune system and various genetic repair mechanisms (see Chapter 7) can eliminate the vast majority of potentially neoplastic clones, the cumulative effects of sunlight (mostly but not exclusively of UVB), in combination with genetic factors (i.e., skin pigmentation, some rare inherited mutations, and familial predispositions) act eventually to cause nonmelanoma tumors and melanomas.

Much has been learned from rare hereditary cancer syndromes with high incidence of skin tumors (Table 25–3).[44] Although uncommon, these syndromes have provided important insights into the molecular pathogenesis of sporadic nonmelanoma skin tumors and melanomas.

Nevoid Basal Cell Carcinoma Syndrome (NBCCS) and Sporadic Basal Cell Carcinomas. Also known as *basal cell nevus syndrome* or *Gorlin syndrome,*[45] this is an autosomal dominant disorder characterized by multiple basal cell carcinomas. Most of these tumors develop before age 20 and are accompanied by various other conditions. These include other tumors (especially medulloblastomas and ovarian fibromas), odontogenic keratocysts, pits of the palms and soles, and generalized overgrowth. Multiple systemic manifestations such as intracranial calcification, cleft lip and palate, abnormal segmentation of the vertebra, and rib anomalies (bifid, fused, missing, splayed ribs) may also be present.[46] With an estimated incidence of 1 in 56,000, this rare syndrome has helped to elucidate the molecular genetics of basal cell carcinoma, not only of the hereditary form, but also of the sporadic type that occurs frequently in the general population.[47]

The gene for NBCCS, located on chromosome 9q22.3, is known as *PTCH,* and it is the human homologue of the *Drosophila* developmental gene known as *patched.*[48] The pathogenesis of basal cell carcinomas in NBCCS fits the "two-hit" hypothesis originally proposed by Knudson for familial retinoblastoma (see Chapter 7). Patients with NBCCS are born with a germ-line mutation in one of the *PTCH* alleles; the second mutation involves the inactivation of the normal homologue either by environmental mutagens or random genetic rearrangement. In sporadic basal cell carcinomas both copies of *PTCH* are altered by the latter mechanisms.

The *PTCH* gene encodes a receptor for the protein product of the *sonic hedgehog gene (SHH),* a member of the hedgehog *(HH)* family of genes that determine polarity during embryonic development[49] (Fig. 25–16). The PTCH protein forms a receptor complex with another transmembrane protein, known as SMO (for "smoothened").[50] In the absence of its ligand, SHH, PTCH inactivates SMO and keeps it from transducing a downstream signal. Binding of SHH to PTCH releases the suppression of SMO, causing the up-regulation of hedgehog target genes through a signal cascade that involves the GLI1 transcription factor (Fig. 25–16). Experimental work in mice has shown that animals with defects in the *PTCH* signaling pathway, including overexpression of GLI1, develop skin tumors resembling basal cell carcinomas.[51] In NBCCS, the constitutive absence of functional *PTCH* causes uninhibited activation of SMO, leading to the development of basal cell carcinoma.

Mutations of genes belonging to the *PTCH* signaling pathway are also important for the development of the common sporadic form of basal cell carcinoma, as documented by the inactivation of *PTCH* and the presence of *SMO* activating mutations in these skin neoplasms.[52,53] *PTCH*

TABLE 25–3 A Survey of Familial Cancer Syndromes with Cutaneous Manifestations[44]

Disease	Inheritance	Chromosomal Location	Gene/Protein	Function/Manifestation
Ataxia–telangiectasia	AR	11q22.3	*AT*/AT[†]	DNA repair after radiation injury; p53 signaling/neurologic and vascular lesions
Nevoid basal cell carcinoma syndrome	AD	9q22.3	*PTCH*//PTCH	Developmental gene/multiple basal cell carcinomas; jaw cysts, etc.
Cowden syndrome	AD	10q23	*PTEN, MMAC1*/PTEN, TEP1, MMAC1	Lipid/protein phosphatase/benign follicular appendage tumors (trichilemmomas); internal adenocarcinoma
Familial melanoma syndrome	AD	9p21	*CDKN2*/p16INK4 *CDKN2*/p14ARF	Inhibits CDKs from phosphorylating Rb, thus arresting cell cycle/melanoma Binds MDM2 and thus, preserves p53/melanoma
Muir-Torre syndrome	AD	2p22	*hMSH2*/hMSH2	Involved in DNA mismatch repair/benign and malignant sebaceous tumors; internal adenocarcinoma
Neurofibromatosis I	AD	17q11.2	*NF1*/neurofibromin	Negatively regulates Ras family of signal molecules/neurofibromas
Neurofibromatosis II	AD	22q12.2	*NF2*/merlin	Integrates cytoskeletal signaling/neurofibromas and acoustic neuromas
Tuberous sclerosis	AD	9q34 16p13.3	*TSC1*/hamartin *TSC2*/tuberin	Interacts with tuberin; function unknown Interacts with hamartin; may regulate ras proteins/angiofibromas, mental retardation
Xeroderma pigmentosum	AR	9q22 and others	*XPA*/XPA and others	Nucleotide excision repair/melanoma and nonmelanoma skin cancers

AD, Autosomal dominant; AR, autosomal recessive.
[†]By convention, genes are italicized and proteins are not italicized.

mutations are found in approximately 30% of sporadic basal cell carcinomas, and of these, about one-third have mutations (C to T transitions) that are considered to be the hallmark of UV damage. Mutations in *p53* occur in 40% to 60% of basal cell carcinomas, and 60% of these have such a "UV signature."[54] Xeroderma pigmentosum, a disorder of DNA repair, presents a striking example of the connection between sun exposure and defects in *PTCH* and *p53*.[55] In these tumors, the frequency of mutations in *PTCH* and *p53* are, respectively, 90% and 40%, and the majority of these bear the UV signature.

In summary, mutations of PTCH are the cause of NBCCS. In sporadic basal cell carcinomas there are frequent mutations in PTCH and p53, most mutations being the product of unrepaired DNA damage by UV light.

Squamous Cell Carcinoma. By contrast to basal cell carcinomas, there is no inherited single gene defect associated with squamous cell carcinomas. Thus, most studies of the molecular genetics of squamous cell carcinoma have examined defects in sporadic tumors and their precursors (actinic keratoses), and the relationships between these defects and sun exposure.[56] The incidence of mutations in *p53* in Caucasian patients with actinic keratoses is high, suggesting that sunlight causes alterations at the early stages of carcinogenesis.[57] However it is not known whether lesions with *p53* mutations are more likely to progress to carcinomas than lesions without the mutation. The immediate effects of UV light on *p53* are positive, involving its induction, resulting in cell-cycle arrest in G_1 to permit DNA repair, or elimination by apoptosis of the damaged cells that are beyond repair (see Chapter 7). When this protective function of *p53* is lost because of unrepaired UV-induced damage of the gene through production of pyrimidine dimers,[58] continuous division of the mutant cells is favored. Such mutations are found in some but not all invasive squamous cell carcinomas. Unlike basal cell carcinomas, aneuploidy is very common in squamous cell carcinomas, and loss of heterozygosity involving chromosomes 3, 9, and 17 occurs in approximately 30% of cases. With the exception of the *p53* locus on chromosome 17, putative tumor suppressor genes localized in the other chromosomes have not been identified.

HPV types 5 and 8, among others (see Chapter 7), are involved in the molecular pathogenesis of a rare condition, epidermodysplasia verruciformis, associated with formation of numerous cutaneous squamous cell carcinomas. A decreased immune response also seems to play a role, since this condition may be found in severely immunosuppressed individuals.[59]

Melanomas. It is estimated that 10% to 15% of melanomas arise in a familial setting.[60] This was first observed in families whose members have large numbers of dysplastic nevi. As already mentioned, some dysplastic nevi develop into melanoma, as in the familial BK mole syndrome, also known as *dysplastic nevus syndrome, familial atypical multiple mole–melanoma syndrome,* or simply *familial melanoma syndrome* (FMS). Unlike NBCCS, which has a clear Mendelian mode of inheritance, FMS does not display distinct and predictable inherited phenotypic abnormalities.[44] The situation is even more complex because not all familial melanomas develop in the setting of multiple dysplastic nevi; conversely, melanomas can occur in patients with multiple sporadic dysplastic nevi. To complicate matters, there is no complete agreement about the histopathologic criteria for the diagnosis of dysplastic nevi.[61–63]

The main locus associated with familial predisposition to melanomas has been mapped to chromosome 9p21[64] and it encodes *p16INK4A* (also known as cyclin-dependent kinase inhibitor 2, or *CDNK2*). It is frequently deleted in melanomas.[65,66] As you may recall from the discussions of the cell cycle, lack of functional p16INK4A leads to unrestricted phosphorylation of RB, release of E2F, and uncontrolled cell growth. *p16INK4A* is the most commonly mutated gene in familial melanoma, in one study affecting 92% of melanoma patients from families with FMS.[67] Mutation is present in approximately 20% of melanomas in familial cases without FMS,[68] suggesting that additional genes may be involved in the familial predisposition to melanomas. Although the role of *p16INK4A* as a melanoma susceptibility gene is firmly established, less is known about its role in sporadic melanomas. Only about 10% of primary sporadic melanomas have mutations of this gene,[58] and loss of the gene has been considered to be a late event in melanoma progression.[69]

The *p16INK4A* locus is unique in that it encodes two different gene products by simply shifting the reading frame. Besides p16INK4A, it also encodes a protein, p14ARF (see Chapter 7). Like p16INK4A, p14ARF is an inhibitor of cell growth, albeit by a different mechanism. p14ARF inhibits MDM2, which binds p53 and targets it for destruction via the ubiquitin pathway.[70] Thus, by binding to MDM2, p14ARF preserves p53 function. Few cases of melanoma have been reported that involve p14ARF.[71,72]

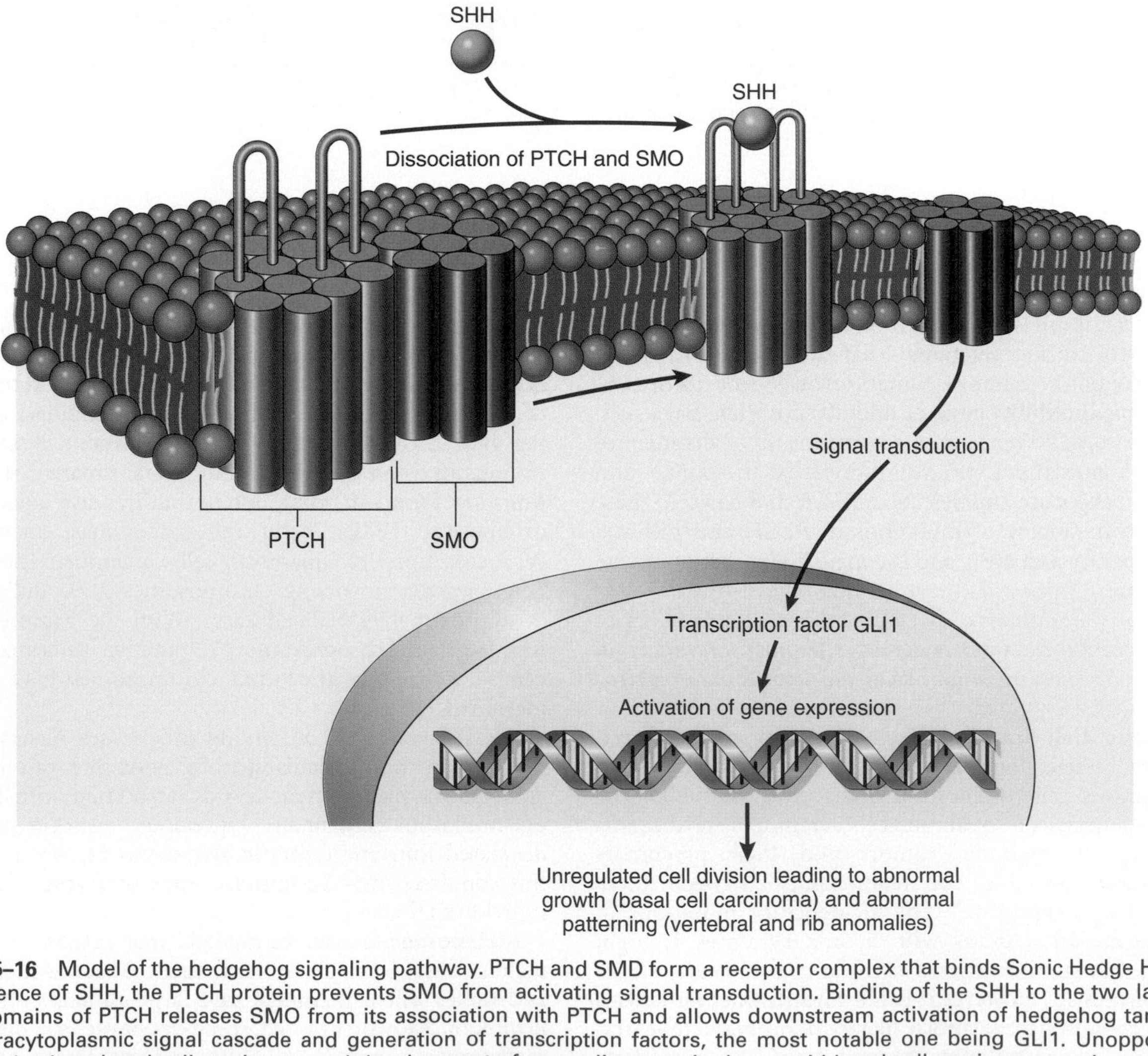

FIGURE 25–16 Model of the hedgehog signaling pathway. PTCH and SMD form a receptor complex that binds Sonic Hedge Hog (SHH). In the absence of SHH, the PTCH protein prevents SMO from activating signal transduction. Binding of the SHH to the two large extracellular domains of PTCH releases SMO from its association with PTCH and allows downstream activation of hedgehog target genes via an intracytoplasmic signal cascade and generation of transcription factors, the most notable one being GLI1. Unopposed gene expression leads to basal cell carcinoma and development of anomalies seen in the nevoid basal cell carcinoma syndrome (NBCCS). Perturbations of this pathway are also important in sporadic forms of basal cell carcinoma.

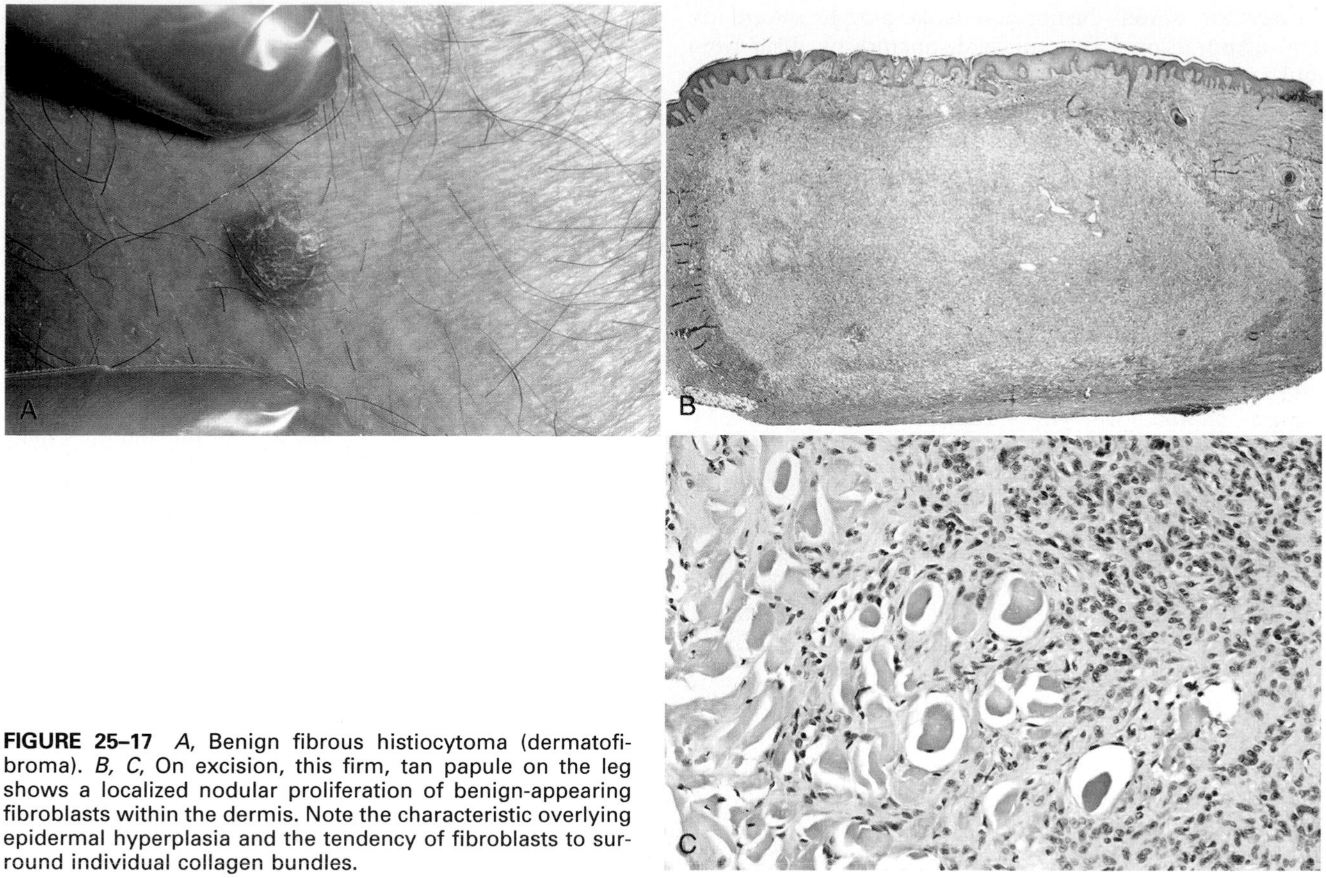

FIGURE 25–17 *A,* Benign fibrous histiocytoma (dermatofibroma). *B, C,* On excision, this firm, tan papule on the leg shows a localized nodular proliferation of benign-appearing fibroblasts within the dermis. Note the characteristic overlying epidermal hyperplasia and the tendency of fibroblasts to surround individual collagen bundles.

Many other genes are probably involved in the pathogenesis of melanoma; among them two, *CDK4* and *BRAF*, are worthy of special mention. *CDK4* may function as a melanoma susceptibility gene, as mutations of this gene occur in familial melanomas, although at a low frequency.[73] Recently, mutations in *BRAF* were identified in 60% to 70% of melanomas and in an equally large proportion of melanocytic nevi.[74,75] BRAF protein (one of the isoforms of RAF) is a component of the RAS/RAF/MAP kinase signal transduction pathway, discussed in Chapters 3 and 7. Early-stage melanomas in radial growth phase exhibit a low frequency of *BRAF* mutations, whereas late-stage melanomas in vertical growth phase have a higher frequency of *BRAF* mutations. This suggests that changes in the RAS/RAF/MAP kinase pathway are late events associated with tumor progression.[76] However, the high incidence of *BRAF* mutations in nevi demonstrate that BRAF activation alone may be insufficient for the development of melanoma.[75]

Tumors of the Dermis

The dermis is composed of a variety of different cellular elements, including smooth muscle, pericytes, fibroblasts, neural tissue, and endothelium. All of these components can give rise to neoplasia within the skin, but many of these tumors also arise in soft tissues and viscera (e.g., leiomyosarcoma) or occur as part of a syndrome primarily affecting another organ system (e.g., as with cutaneous neurofibromas in neurofibromatosis). In this section, therefore, we consider only representative dermal neoplasms that arise primarily in the skin, have unique characteristics in the skin, or have not been presented in other chapters.

BENIGN FIBROUS HISTIOCYTOMA (DERMATOFIBROMA)

Benign fibrous histiocytoma refers to a heterogeneous family of morphologically and histogenetically related benign dermal neoplasms of fibroblasts and histiocytes. (They are also discussed with the soft tissue tumors in Chapter 26.) These tumors are usually seen in adults and often occur on the legs of young to middle-aged women. Their biologic behavior is indolent, and they should not be confused with the unrelated malignant fibrous histiocytoma, which arises de novo in skin and in extracutaneous sites and often has an aggressive clinical course.

On gross inspection, these neoplasms are firm, tan to brown papules (Fig. 25–17*A*). Lesions are asymptomatic or tender, and their size may increase and decrease slightly over time. Although the majority of lesions are less than 1 cm in diameter, actively growing lesions may reach several centimeters in diameter; with time, they often become flattened. The tendency for fibrous histiocytomas to dimple inward on lateral compression is helpful in distinguishing them from nodular melanomas, which protrude when they are similarly manipulated.

Morphology. The most common form of fibrous histiocytoma is referred to as a **dermatofibroma.** These tumors are formed by benign, spindle-shaped fibroblasts arranged in a well-defined, nonencapsulated mass within the mid-dermis (Fig. 25–17*B, C*). Extension of these cells into the subcutaneous fat is frequently observed. The majority of cases demonstrate a peculiar form of overlying epidermal hyperplasia, characterized by downward elongation of hyperpigmented rete ridges ("dirty fingers" pattern). Although foamy histiocytes (macrophages) may be seen in dermatofibromas, they are generally not conspicuous, but certain variants are composed predominantly of these foamy histiocytes and a small number of fibroblasts. Finally, variants containing numerous blood vessels and deposits of hemosiderin may be encountered.

The histogenesis of fibrous histiocytomas remains a mystery. Many cases have a history of antecedent trauma, suggesting an abnormal response to injury and inflammation,[77,78] perhaps analogous to the deposition of increased amounts of altered collagen in a hypertrophic scar or keloid. Many of the cells that form dermatofibromas express coagulation factor XIIIa. These common yet curious tumors appear to be composed partially of factor XIIIa-positive dermal dendrocytes, described as normal dermal constituents at the beginning of this chapter.

DERMATOFIBROSARCOMA PROTUBERANS

Dermatofibrosarcoma protuberans is best regarded as a well-differentiated, primary fibrosarcoma of the skin. These tumors are slow growing, and although they are locally aggressive, they rarely metastasize.

Clinically, they are firm, solid nodules that arise most frequently on the trunk. They often develop as aggregated "protuberant" tumors within a firm (indurated) plaque that may ulcerate.

Morphology. On microscopic examination, these neoplasms are cellular, composed of fibroblasts arranged radially, reminiscent of blades of a pinwheel, a pattern referred to as **storiform.** Mitoses are usually present but are not as numerous as in a moderately or poorly differentiated fibrosarcoma (see section on soft tissue tumors in Chapter 26). In contrast to that in dermatofibroma, the overlying epidermis is generally thinned. Deep extension from the dermis into subcutaneous fat, producing a characteristic "honeycomb" pattern, is frequently present, hindering attempts at complete surgical removal.

XANTHOMAS

Xanthomas are tumor-like collections of foamy histiocytes within the dermis. They may be associated with familial (Chapter 5) or acquired disorders resulting in hyperlipidemia, with lymphoproliferative malignant neoplasms, or with no underlying disorder.

On the basis of clinical appearance, xanthomas are divided into five types. Identification of these types may provide important clinical markers of the underlying hyperlipoproteinemia.[79] *Eruptive xanthomas* occur as sudden showers of yellow papules that wax and wane according to variations in plasma triglyceride and lipid content. They occur on the buttocks, posterior thighs, knees, and elbows. *Tuberous* and *tendinous xanthomas* occur as yellow nodules; the latter frequently are found on the Achilles tendon and the extensor tendons of the fingers. *Plane xanthomas* (associated with primary biliary cirrhosis) are linear yellow lesions in the skin folds, especially the palmar creases. *Xanthelasma* (without lipid abnormality) refers to soft yellow plaques on the eyelids.

Morphology. All types are characterized histologically by dermal accumulation of benign-appearing histiocytes (macrophages) with abundant, finely vacuolated (foamy) cytoplasm. Cholesterol (free and esterified), phospholipids, and triglycerides are present within cells. The cellularity of the infiltrate is variable, and with the exception of xanthelasma, lesions may also be surrounded by inflammatory cells and fibrosis about the central zone of lipid-laden cells.

DERMAL VASCULAR TUMORS

Benign vascular neoplasms (capillary and cavernous hemangiomas), malformations (nevus flammeus or port-wine stain), multifocal angioproliferative lesions (Kaposi sarcoma, bacillary angiomatosis), vascularized variants of other tumors (e.g., the sclerosing hemangioma variant of benign fibrous histiocytoma), and malignant vascular tumors (angiosarcomas) are frequently encountered in the skin. Most are discussed in Chapter 11. The capillary hemangioma is by far the most commonly encountered form of cutaneous hemangioma. It appears clinically either in childhood (strawberry hemangioma) or with advancing age, as discrete, deeply erythematous papules. In adults, lesions may slowly enlarge and occasionally undergo thrombosis, whereas in young children, they usually regress by fibrosis.

Morphology. Cutaneous hemangiomas must be differentiated from dermal vascular hyperplasia (as may occur in venous stasis), reactive vascular proliferations (as in pyogenic granulomas), unregulated multifocal vascular proliferations (as seen in Kaposi sarcoma), and vascular malignant tumors (angiosarcoma). Typically, hemangiomas are represented histologically by well-formed, blood-filled vascular spaces lined by benign endothelial cells within the superficial and sometimes deep dermis.

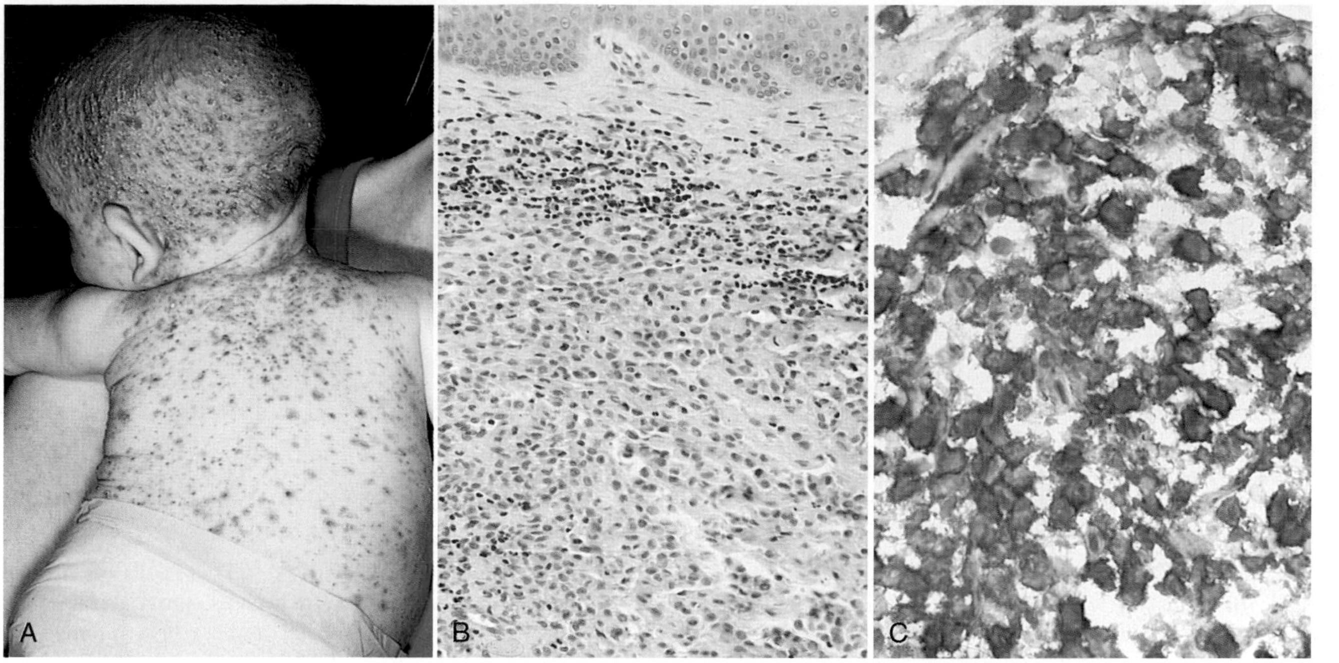

FIGURE 25–18 Langerhans cell histiocytosis. *A*, Lesions may appear clinically as papules and nodules or, as in this case, as erythematous scaling plaques mimicking the infantile form of seborrheic dermatitis. *B*, Dermal infiltration by bland mononuclear cells with infolded nuclei presents a nonspecific histologic pattern. *C*, Immunohistochemical demonstration of CD1a antigen confirms the origin of these mononuclear cells from Langerhans cells.

Tumors of Cellular Immigrants to the Skin

Aside from tumors that arise directly from epidermal and dermal cells, several proliferative disorders of the skin involve primarily cells whose progenitors have arisen elsewhere but that exhibit a peculiar homing to the cutaneous microenvironment. Examples of such cells are epidermal Langerhans cells, which arise from precursors in the bone marrow and, in their mature form, traffic freely from skin to regional lymph nodes by way of dermal lymphatics; T lymphocytes that are normally in residence in low numbers in the dermis and epidermis; and dermal mast cells derived from marrow precursors. The proliferative lesions discussed in this section—namely, Langerhans cell histiocytosis, cutaneous T-cell lymphoma (CTCL), and mastocytosis—are primary cutaneous disorders that arise from these three cell types, respectively.

LANGERHANS CELL HISTIOCYTOSIS

Langerhans cell histiocytosis, once called *histiocytosis X,* is described in detail in Chapter 14. In the skin, this condition presents in multiple forms, including solitary or multiple lesions ranging from papules to nodules to scaling erythematous plaques that in infants may resemble seborrheic dermatitis (Fig. 25–18*A*).

Morphology of Skin Lesions. Langerhans cell histiocytosis involving the skin has several histologic patterns, all of which may show marked infiltration of the skin. The first is that of a diffuse dermal infiltrate of large, round to ovoid cells with pale pink cytoplasm containing indented, often bland nuclei (Fig. 25–18*B*). A second pattern consists of a clustering of similar cells into small aggregates that resemble granulomas. The third is characterized by a dermal infiltrate of cells with foamy, xanthoma-like cytoplasm. Variable numbers of eosinophils may also be observed, particularly with the first pattern. Because these patterns are not specific, special immunohistochemical methods to identify cell-surface markers common to Langerhans cells (such as CD1a antigen),[80] may be necessary to establish a definitive histologic diagnosis (Fig. 25–18*C*). In addition, ultrastructural identification of specific organelles (Birbeck granules), characteristic of the epidermal Langerhans cells from which Langerhans cell histiocytosis is believed to originate is also helpful (see Fig. 14–37, Chapter 14).

MYCOSIS FUNGOIDES (CUTANEOUS T-CELL LYMPHOMA)

Cutaneous T-cell lymphoma (CTCL) represents a spectrum of lymphoproliferative disorders affecting the skin (see also Chapter 14). Two different clinical types of malignant T-cell disorders were originally recognized: *mycosis fungoides*, a chronic proliferative process; and a nodular eruptive variant, *mycosis fungoides d'emblée*. It is now known that a variety of presentations of T-cell lymphoma occur, including mycosis fungoides, the eruptive nodular type, and an adult T-cell leukemia/lymphoma type. The latter disorder may have a rapidly progressive downhill course.

Mycosis fungoides is the T-cell lymphoproliferative disorder that arises primarily in the skin and that may evolve

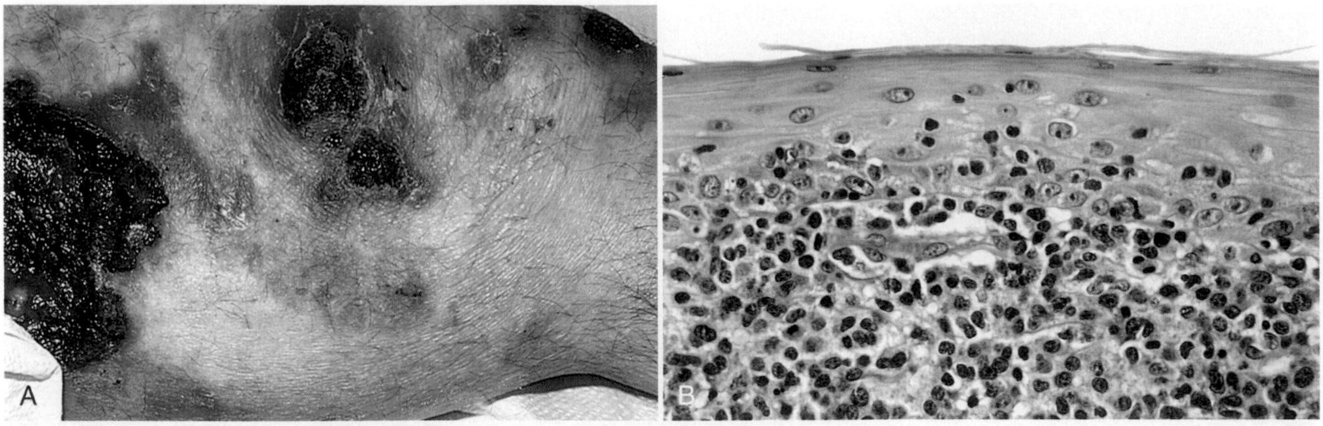

FIGURE 25–19 Cutaneous T-cell lymphoma. The histologic correlate of ill-defined, erythematous, often scaling, and occasionally ulcerated plaques *(A)* is an infiltrate of atypical lymphocytes that show a tendency to accumulate beneath the epidermal layer *(B)* and to invade the epidermis as small microabscesses.

into generalized lymphoma.[81] Most affected individuals have disease that remains localized to the skin for many years; a minority have rapid systemic dissemination. This condition may occur at any age, but most commonly it afflicts persons older than age 40.

Clinically, lesions of the mycosis fungoides type of CTCL include scaly, red-brown patches; raised, scaling plaques that may even be confused with psoriasis; and fungating nodules. Eczema-like lesions typify early stages of disease when obvious visceral or nodal spread has not occurred. Raised, indurated, irregularly outlined, erythematous plaques may then supervene. Development of multiple, large (up to 10 cm or more in diameter), red-brown nodules correlates with systemic spreading. Sometimes plaques and nodules ulcerate, as depicted in Figure 25–19*A*. Lesions may affect numerous body surfaces, including the trunk, extremities, face, and scalp. In some individuals, seeding of the blood by malignant T cells is accompanied by diffuse erythema and scaling of the entire body surface (erythroderma), a condition known as *Sézary syndrome* (Chapter 14).

Morphology. The histological hallmark of CTCL of the mycosis fungoides type is the presence of the **Sézary-Lutzner cells.** These are T-helper cells (CD4 positive) that characteristically form bandlike aggregates within the superficial dermis (Fig. 25–19*B*) and invade the epidermis as single cells and small clusters **(Pautrier microabscesses).** These cells have markedly infolded nuclear membranes, imparting a hyperconvoluted or cerebriform contour. Although patches and plaques show pronounced epidermal infiltration by Sézary-Lutzner cells (epidermotropism), in more advanced nodular lesions the malignant T cells often lose this epidermotropic tendency, grow deeply into the dermis, and eventually seed lymphatics and the peripheral circulation.

As described in Chapters 7 and 14, HTLV-1 may cause certain forms of T-cell lymphoma (e.g., adult T-cell leukemia/lymphoma).[82] CTCL also may have an infectious causation, although a definitive organism has not been identified. The proliferating cells in CTCL are clonal populations of lymphocytes of the CD4 subset.[83] These cells often express aberrant cell-surface antigens as well as clonal T-cell receptor gene rearrangements. Detection of these features may be of diagnostic assistance in difficult cases.

Topical therapy with steroids or UV light is often employed for early lesions of CTCL, whereas more aggressive systemic chemotherapy is indicated for advanced disease.

MASTOCYTOSIS

The term *mastocytosis* refers to a spectrum of rare disorders characterized by increased numbers of mast cells in the skin and, in some instances, in other organs. A localized cutaneous form of the disease that affects predominantly children and accounts for more than 50% of all cases is termed *urticaria pigmentosa.* These lesions are multiple, although solitary mastocytomas may also occur, usually shortly after birth. About 10% of patients with mast cell disease have overt systemic mastocytosis, with mast cell infiltration of many organs. These individuals are often adults, and unlike the case with localized cutaneous disease, the prognosis may be poor.

The clinical picture of mastocytosis is highly variable. In urticaria pigmentosa, lesions are multiple and widely distributed, consisting of round to oval, red-brown, nonscaling papules and small plaques. Solitary mastocytomas present as one or several pink to tan-brown nodules that may be pruritic or exhibit blister formation (Fig. 25–20*A*). In systemic mastocytosis, skin lesions similar to those of urticaria pigmentosa are accompanied by mast cell infiltration of bone marrow, liver, spleen, and lymph nodes. Many of the signs and symptoms of mastocytosis are due to the effects of histamine, heparin, and other substances released as a result of degranulation. *Darier sign* refers to a localized area of dermal edema and erythema (wheal) that occurs when lesion skin is rubbed. *Dermatographism* refers to an area of dermal edema resembling a hive that occurs in normal skin as a result of localized stroking with a pointed instrument. In systemic disease, all of the following may be seen: pruritus and flushing triggered by certain foods, temperature changes, alcohol, and certain drugs (morphine, codeine, aspirin); watery nasal discharge (rhinorrhea); rarely, gastrointestinal or nasal bleeding, possibly due to the anticoagulant effects of heparin; and bone pain as a result of osteoblastic and osteoclastic involvement.

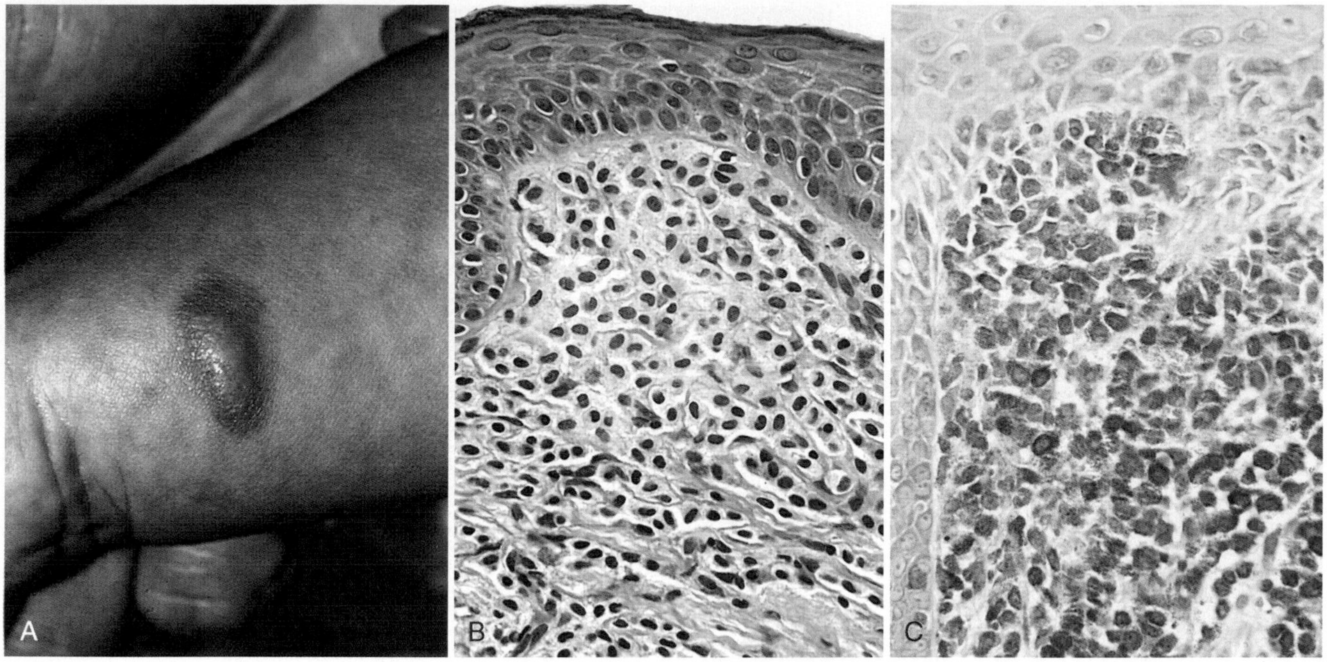

FIGURE 25–20 Mastocytosis. *A,* Solitary mastocytoma in a 1-year-old child. *B,* By routine histology, numerous ovoid cells with uniform, centrally located nuclei are observed in the dermis. *C,* Giemsa staining reveals purple, "metachromatic" granules within the cytoplasm of the cells.

Morphology. The histologic picture in urticaria pigmentosa or solitary mastocytoma varies from a subtle increase in the numbers of spindle-shaped and stellate mast cells around superficial dermal blood vessels, to large numbers of tightly packed, round to oval mast cells in the upper to mid-dermis (Fig. 25–20*B*). Variable fibrosis, edema, and small numbers of eosinophils may also be present. Mast cells may be difficult to differentiate from lymphocytes in routine, H&E-stained sections, and special metachromatic stains (toluidine blue or Giemsa) must be used to visualize their granules (Fig. 25–20*C*). Even with these stains, extensive degranulation may result in failure to detect these cells by light microscopy, and ultrastructural analysis must then be performed.

Pathogenesis. The pathogenesis of at least some cases of mastocytosis now appears to involve a clonal proliferation of mast cells containing a point mutation of the *c-KIT* proto-oncogene. The mutation causes activation of a receptor tyrosine kinase expressed by mast cells (and hematopoietic stem cells) that is involved in their growth and differentiation.[84] Although some clonal proliferations of mast cells have features of true neoplasia, the cells remain subject to phenotypic modifications in differing tissue microenvironments.[85] Such heterogeneity has resulted in the previous misconception that the disorder is exclusively a hyperplasia of mast cells.

Disorders of Epidermal Maturation

ICHTHYOSIS

Of the numerous disorders that impair epidermal maturation, ichthyosis is perhaps one of the most striking. The term is derived from the Greek root *ichthy-*, meaning fishy, and accordingly, this group of genetically inherited disorders is associated with excessive keratin build-up (hyperkeratosis) that results clinically in fishlike scales (Fig. 25–21*A*). Most ichthyoses become apparent either at or around the time of birth. Acquired (noninherited) variants exist; in the acquired vulgaris type in adults, there is an association with lymphoid and visceral malignant neoplasms. The clinical types of ichthyosis vary according to the mode of inheritance, histology, and clinical features; the primary categories include ichthyosis vulgaris (autosomal dominant or acquired), congenital ichthyosiform erythroderma (autosomal recessive), lamellar ichthyosis (autosomal recessive), and X-linked ichthyosis.

Morphology. The general histology of all forms of ichthyosis is often subtle build-up of compacted stratum corneum, with loss of the normal basketweave pattern seen in this layer when it involves hair-bearing skin (Fig. 25–21*B*). There is generally little or no inflammation, and subtle associated variations in the thickness of the epidermis and the stratum granulosum, along with the clinical picture, assist in assigning the correct diagnostic subclassification.

Pathogenesis. The primary abnormality in some forms of ichthyosis may reside in defective mechanisms of desquamation, leading to retention of abnormally formed scale. For example, in X-linked ichthyosis, affected homozygotes demonstrate a deficiency in steroid sulfatase, an enzyme important for the removal of proadhesive cholesterol sulfate secreted into the intercellular spaces along with adhesive organelles called *Odland bodies,* or *membrane-coating granules.* Accumulation of this nondegraded cholesterol sulfate results in persistent cell-to-cell adhesion within the stratum corneum, hindering the desquamation process. Compare this

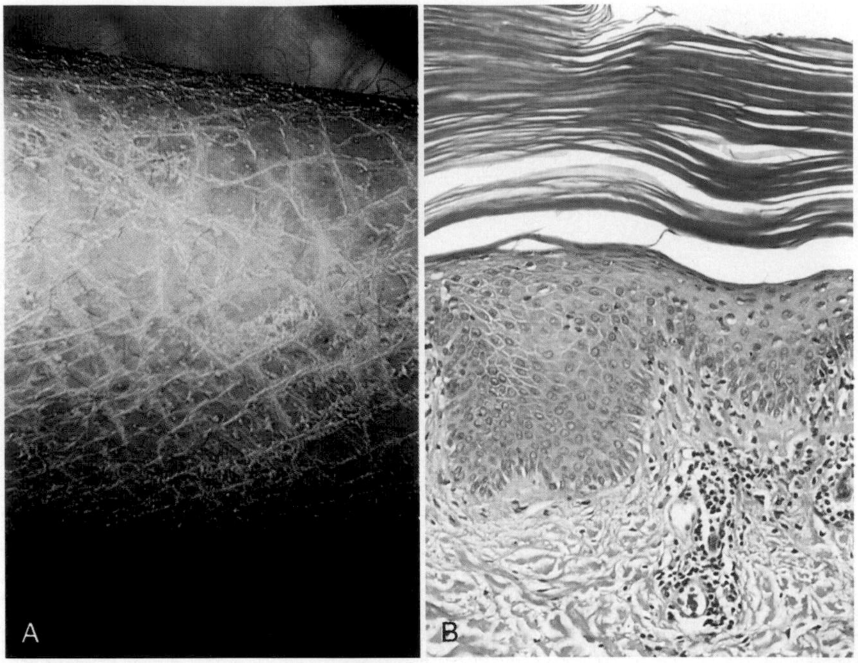

FIGURE 25–21 Ichthyosis. Note prominent fish-like scales *(A)* and compacted stratum corneum *(B)*.

with pemphigus vulgaris (see later), in which dramatically different lesions form as a consequence of *decreased* cell-to-cell adhesion.

Acute Inflammatory Dermatoses

Inflammatory dermatoses are usually mediated by local or systemic immunologic factors, although the causes for many remain a mystery. Literally thousands of specific inflammatory dermatoses exist. In general, acute lesions last from days to weeks and are characterized by inflammation (often marked by mononuclear cells, not neutrophils), edema, and epidermal, vascular, or subcutaneous injury in some. Chronic lesions, on the other hand, persist for months to years and often show significant components of altered epidermal growth (atrophy or hyperplasia) or dermal fibrosis. The lesions discussed here are selected as examples of the more commonly encountered dermatoses within the acute category.

URTICARIA

Urticaria (hives) is a common disorder of the skin characterized by localized mast cell degranulation and resultant dermal microvascular hyperpermeability, culminating in pruritic edematous plaques called *wheals*. Angioedema is closely related to urticaria and is characterized by deeper edema of both the dermis and the subcutaneous fat.

Urticaria most often occurs between ages 20 and 40, although all age groups are susceptible. Individual lesions develop and fade within hours (usually <24 hours), and episodes may last for days or persist for months. Lesions vary from small, pruritic papules to large edematous plaques (Fig. 25–22). Individual lesions may coalesce to form annular, linear, or arciform configurations. Sites of predilection for urticarial eruptions include any area exposed to pressure, such as the trunk, distal extremities, and ears. Persistent episodes of urticaria may simply be the result of inability to eliminate the causative antigen or may herald underlying disease (e.g., collagen vascular disorders, Hodgkin disease). In the majority of cases, no underlying cause can be identified.

Morphology. The histologic features of urticaria may be so subtle that many biopsy specimens at first resemble normal skin. There is usually a sparse superficial perivenular infiltrate consisting of mononuclear cells and rare neutrophils. Eosinophils may also be present. Collagen bundles are more widely spaced than in normal skin, a result of superficial dermal edema fluid that does not stain in routinely prepared tissue (Fig. 25–23). Superficial lymphatic channels are dilated in an attempt to accommodate this transudated edema fluid. Epidermal changes are typically not present.

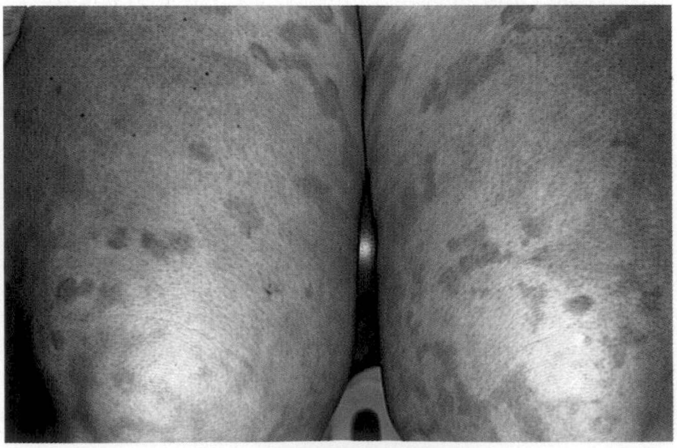

FIGURE 25–22 Urticaria. Clinically, there are erythematous, edematous, often circular plaques covered by a normal epidermal surface.

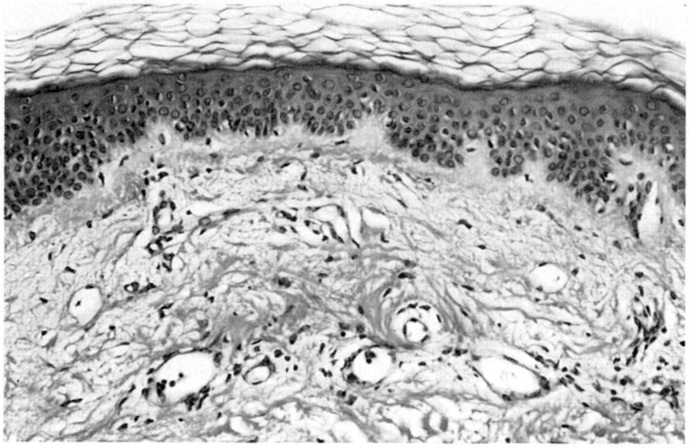

FIGURE 25–23 Urticaria. Histologically, there is superficial dermal edema and dilated lymphatic and blood-filled vascular spaces. The edema is manifested by widening of spaces that separate the collagen bundles.

Pathogenesis. In most cases, urticaria results from antigen-induced release of vasoactive mediators from mast cell granules through sensitization with specific immunoglobulin E (IgE) antibodies. This *IgE-dependent* degranulation can follow exposure to a number of antigens (pollens, foods, drugs, insect venom) and specifically results from bridging of mast cell-bound IgE molecules by multivalent ligand, as discussed in Chapter 6. *IgE-independent* urticaria may result from substances that in certain individuals directly incite the degranulation of mast cells, such as opiates, certain antibiotics, curare, and radiographic contrast media. Another cause of IgE-independent urticaria is exposure to chemicals, such as aspirin, that suppress prostaglandin synthesis from arachidonic acid. Hereditary angioneurotic edema (Chapter 6) is caused by an inherited deficiency of C1 inhibitor that results in uncontrolled activation of the early components of the complement system and production of vasoactive mediators (*complement-mediated urticaria*).[86]

ACUTE ECZEMATOUS DERMATITIS

Eczema is a clinical term that embraces a number of pathogenetically different conditions. All are characterized by red, papulovesicular, oozing, and crusted lesions early on that, with persistence, develop into raised, scaling plaques. In time, acute spongiotic dermatitis may evolve to a more chronic form in which epidermal hyperplasia and excessive scale, rather than blistering, dominate the clinical and histologic picture (Fig. 25–24). Clinical differences permit classification of eczematous dermatitis into the following categories: (1) allergic contact dermatitis, (2) atopic dermatitis, (3) drug-related eczematous dermatitis, (4) photoeczematous dermatitis, and (5) primary irritant dermatitis (Table 25–4).

The Greek word *eczema,* meaning "to boil over," vividly describes the clinical appearance of acute eczematous der-

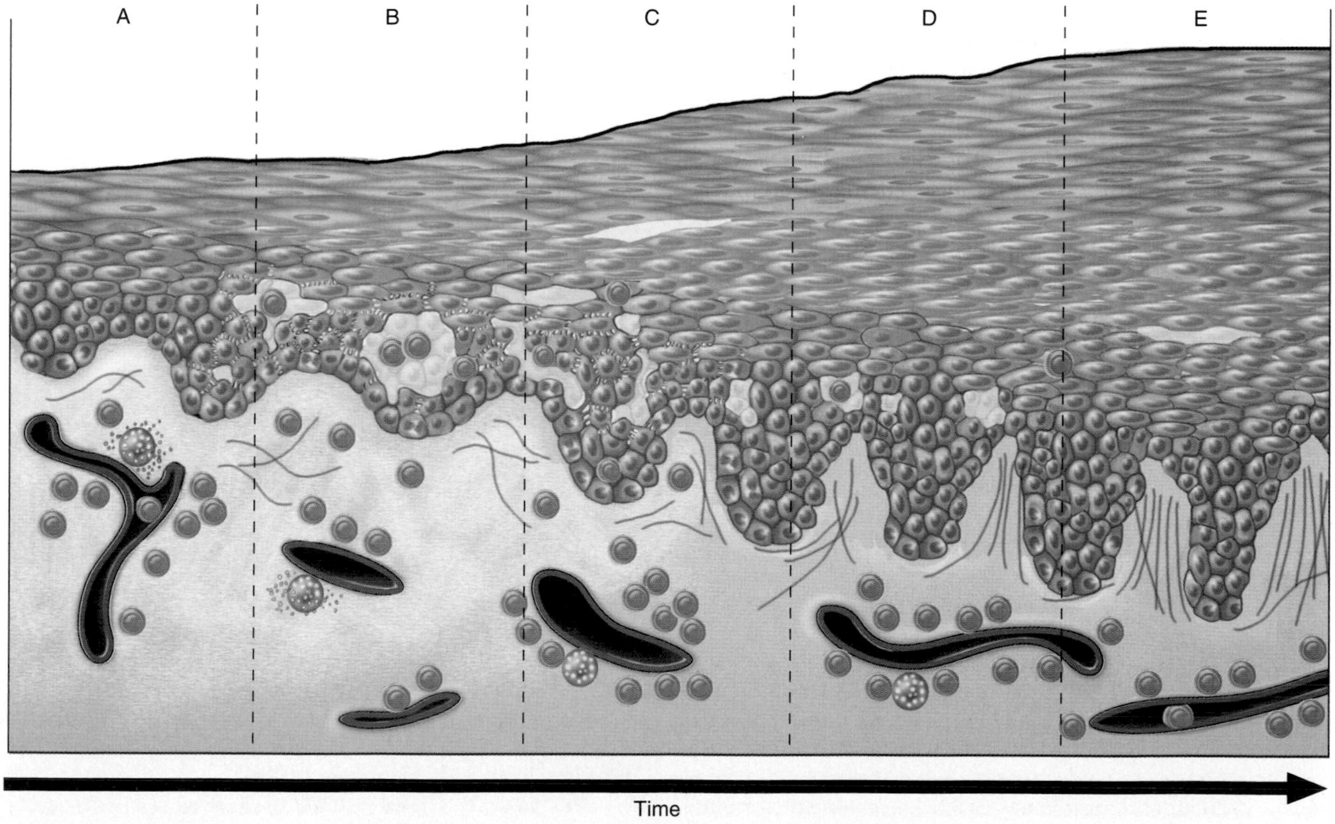

FIGURE 25–24 Stages of eczema development. *A,* Initial dermal edema and perivascular infiltration by inflammatory cells is followed within 24 to 48 hours by epidermal spongiosis and microvesicle formation *(B). C,* Abnormal scale, including parakeratosis, follows, along with progressive epidermal hyperplasia *(D)* and hyperkeratosis *(E)* as the lesion enters into a more chronic stage.

TABLE 25–4 Classification of Eczematous Dermatitis

Type	Cause or Pathogenesis	Histology*	Clinical Features
Contact dermatitis	Topically applied antigens	Spongiotic dermatitis	Marked itching, burning, or both; requires antecedent exposure
Atopic dermatitis	Unknown; may be heritable	Spongiotic dermatitis	Erythematous plaques in flexural areas; family history of eczema, hay fever, or asthma
Drug-related eczematous dermatitis	Systemically administered antigens or haptens (e.g. penicillin)	Spongiotic dermatitis; infiltrate often deeper with abundant eosinophils	Temporal relationship to drug administration; remits with cessation of drug
Eczematous insect bite reaction	Locally injected antigen or toxin	Spongiotic dermatitis; wedge-shaped infiltrate; many eosinophils	Papules, nodules, and plaques with vesicles; may be linear when multiple
Photoeczematous eruption	Ultraviolet light	Spongiotic dermatitis; infiltrate that diminishes gradually with depth	Occurs at sites of sun exposure; may require associated exposure to systemic or topical antigen; photopatch testing may help in diagnosis
Primary irritant dermatitis	Repeated trauma or chemical irritants (as in detergent)	Spongiotic dermatitis in early stages; acanthosis predominates in later stages	Localized mechanical or chemical irritants (nonimmunologic)

*All types, with time, may develop chronic changes, with prominent acanthosis of the epidermal layer.

matitis. The most obvious example is an acute contact reaction to topical antigens such as poison ivy, characterized by pruritic, edematous, oozing plaques, often containing small and large blisters (vesicles and bullae) (Fig. 25–25*A*). Such lesions are prone to bacterial superinfection, which produces a yellow crust (impetiginization). With time, persistent lesions become less "wet" (fail to ooze or form vesicles) and become progressively scaly (hyperkeratotic) as the epidermis thickens (acanthosis).

Pathogenesis. This has been well studied in dermatitis due to contact hypersensitivity (e.g., poison ivy dermatitis). Initially, antigens at the epidermal surface are taken up by dendritic Langerhans cells, which then migrate by way of dermal lymphatics to draining lymph nodes (Fig. 25–26). Here, antigens, now processed by the Langerhans cell, are presented to naive CD4 T cells, which are activated and develop into effector and memory cells (Chapter 6). On antigen re-exposure, these memory T cells migrate to affected skin sites, where they release cytokines and factors that recruit the numerous inflammatory cells responsible for the clinical lesion of spongiotic dermatitis.

An early event in the genesis of T-cell recruitment to the challenge site is local cytokine release in the vicinity of dermal postcapillary venules.[87,88] This results in endothelial activation, a phenomenon whereby endothelial cells become enlarged and express molecules on their plasma membranes that promote adhesion of circulating memory T lymphocytes. Once these memory T cells enter the site of antigen challenge through activated microvessels, they elaborate a potent array of lymphokines that recruits of large numbers of inflammatory cells to the site of antigen contact. This process occurs within 24 hours and accounts for the initial erythema and pruritus that characterize cutaneous delayed hypersensitivity in the acute, spongiotic phase.

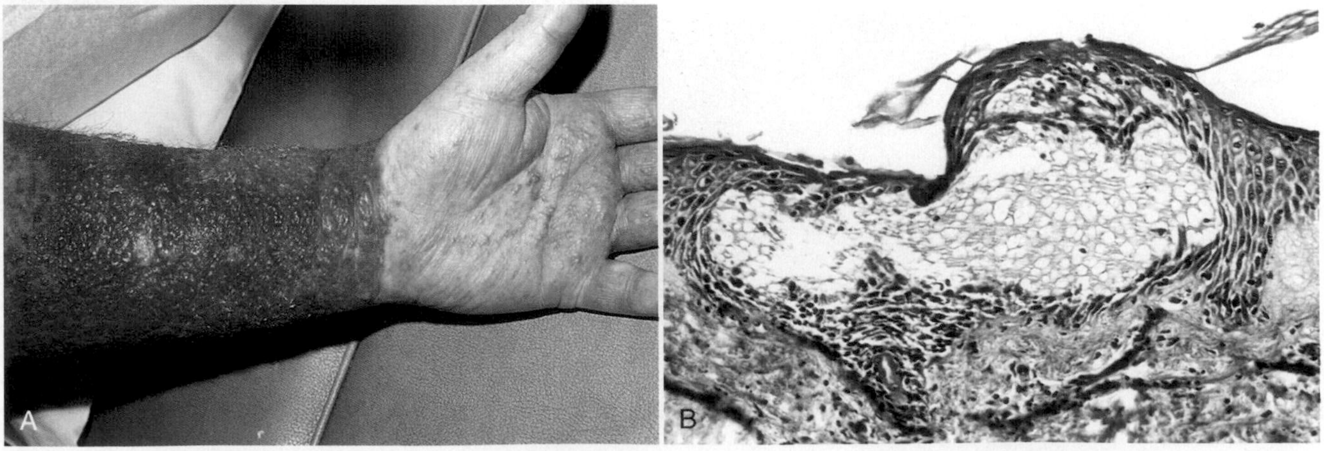

FIGURE 25–25 Eczematous dermatitis. *A*, In an acute allergic contact dermatitis, numerous vesicles appear at the site of antigen exposure (in this case, laundry detergent that persisted in clothing). *B*, Histologically, intercellular edema produces widened intercellular spaces within the epidermis, eventually resulting in small, fluid-filled intraepidermal vesicles.

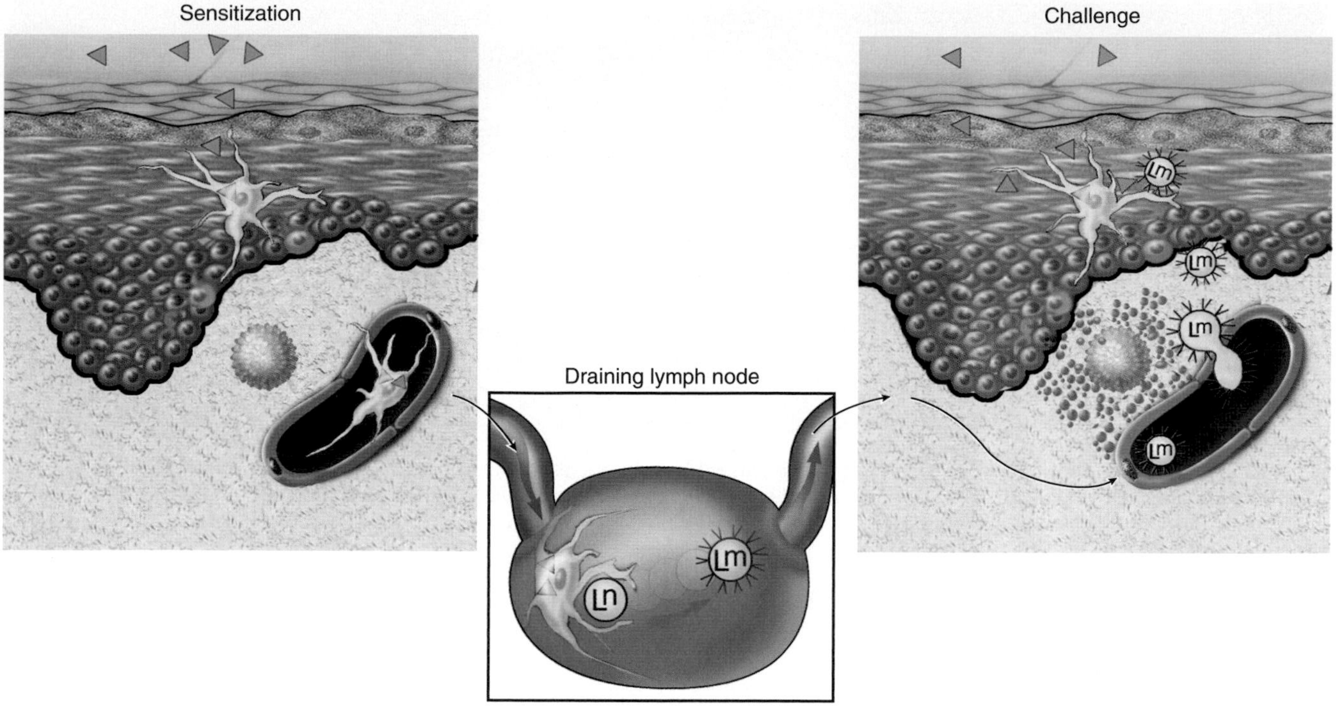

FIGURE 25–26 Schematic diagram of mechanisms of allergic contact dermatitis. ▲, antigen; Ln, naive T lymphocyte; Lm, memory T lymphocyte.

The ability of skin to develop contact hypersensitivity depends in part on the structural and functional integrity of Langerhans cells within the epidermis. Chronic exposure to UV light is injurious to epidermal Langerhans cells, although those sequestered within the protected environment of the upper portion of hair follicles remain unaffected.[87,89] Other factors that modulate Langerhans cell function include neuropeptides released from nerve endings that terminate near to the Langerhans cell body.[90,91] This interaction has intriguing implications concerning the potential role of the nervous system in the development and severity of certain forms of dermatitis.

Morphology. Spongiosis—the accumulation of edema fluid within the intercellular spaces of the epidermis—characterizes acute eczematous dermatitis, hence the synonym spongiotic dermatitis. Whereas edema is localized to the perivascular spaces of the superficial dermis in urticaria, edema seeps into the intercellular spaces of the epidermis in spongiotic dermatitis, splaying apart keratinocytes located primarily in the stratum spinosum. Intercellular bridges appear prominent, giving a spongy appearance to the epidermis. Mechanical shearing of intercellular attachment sites (desmosomes) and cell membranes by progressive accumulation of intercellular fluid may result in the formation of intraepidermal vesicles (see Fig. 25–25*B*).

During the earliest stages of the evolution of spongiotic dermatitis, there is a superficial, perivascular, lymphocytic infiltrate associated with papillary dermal edema and mast cell degranulation. The pattern and composition of this infiltrate may provide clues to the underlying cause.[92] For example, spongiotic dermatitis resulting from systemic antigens, such as those related to ingestion of certain drugs, will show a lymphocytic infiltrate, often containing eosinophils, and extending around deep as well as superficial dermal vessels. Spongiotic dermatitis resulting from surface contact with antigens tends to produce an inflammatory reaction that preferentially affects the more superficial dermal layer.

ERYTHEMA MULTIFORME

Erythema multiforme is an uncommon, self-limited disorder that appears to be a hypersensitivity reaction to certain infections and drugs. Erythema multiforme is a prototype of a cytotoxic reaction pattern (one typified by extensive epithelial cell degeneration and death). This disorder affects individuals of any age and is associated with the following conditions: (1) infections such as herpes simplex, mycoplasmal infections, histoplasmosis, coccidioidomycosis, typhoid, and leprosy, among others; (2) administration of certain drugs (sulfonamides, penicillin, barbiturates, salicylates, hydantoins, and antimalarials); (3) malignant disease (carcinomas and lymphomas); and (4) collagen vascular diseases (lupus erythematosus, dermatomyositis, and periarteritis nodosa).

Patients present clinically with an array of "multiform" lesions, including macules, papules, vesicles, and bullae as well as the characteristic target lesion consisting of a red macule or papule with a pale, vesicular, or eroded center (Fig. 25–27*A*). Although lesions may be widely distributed, symmetric involvement of the extremities frequently occurs. An extensive and symptomatic febrile form of the disease, which is often but not exclusively seen in children, is called the *Stevens-*

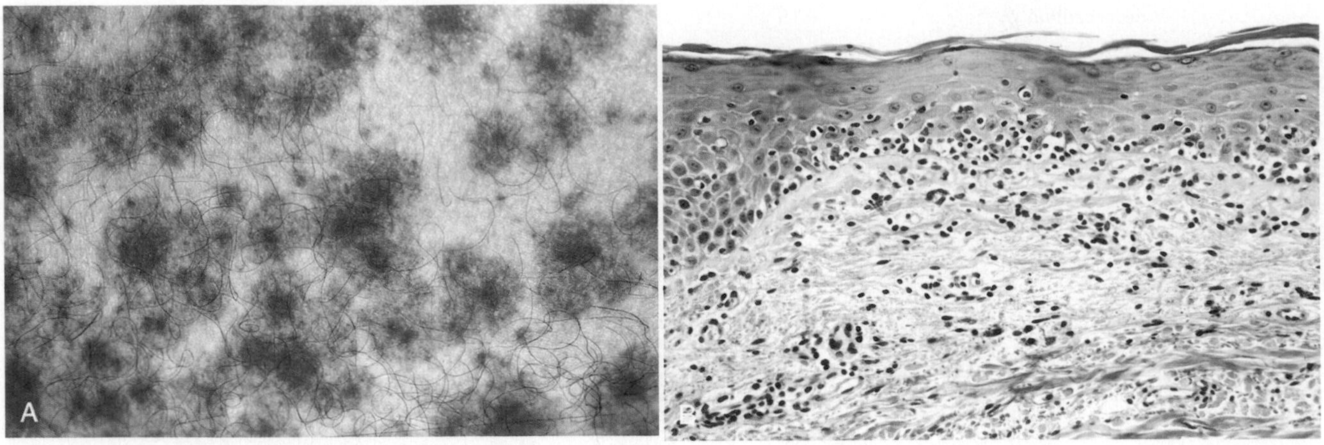

FIGURE 25–27 Erythema multiforme. *A*, The target-like clinical lesions consist of a central blister or zone of epidermal necrosis surrounded by macular erythema. *B*, Early lesions show lymphocytes collecting along the dermal epidermal junction where basal keratinocytes have begun to become vacuolated.

Johnson syndrome. Typically, erosions and hemorrhagic crusts involve the lips and oral mucosa, although the conjunctiva, urethra, and genital and perianal areas may also be affected. Infection of involved areas may result in life-threatening sepsis. Another variant, termed *toxic epidermal necrolysis,* results in diffuse necrosis and sloughing of cutaneous and mucosal epithelial surfaces, producing a clinical situation analogous to an extensive burn.

Morphology. On histologic examination, early lesions show a superficial perivascular, lymphocytic infiltrate associated with dermal edema and accumulation of lymphocytes along the dermoepidermal junction, where they are intimately associated with degenerating and necrotic keratinocytes (Fig. 25–27*B*). With time, there is upward migration of lymphocytes into the epidermis. Discrete and confluent zones of epidermal necrosis occur with concomitant blister formation. Epidermal sloughing leads to shallow erosions. The **target lesion** exhibits central necrosis surrounded by a rim of perivenular inflammation.

Pathogenesis. Erythema multiforme has immunologic similarities to other conditions characterized by epidermal cell injury (e.g., acute graft-versus-host disease change to [GVHD],[93] skin allograft rejection,[94] and fixed drug eruptions[95]). In all these conditions, epithelial cells are killed by CD8+ cytotoxic T lymphocytes (CTLs). The precise target antigens within the epidermis that are recognized by CTLs in erythema multiforme remain unknown. Based on studies of histologically similar acute forms of cytotoxic dermatitis, such as acute GVHD, there is growing evidence that the basal cells that reside at the very tips of epidermal rete ridges may preferentially undergo apoptosis.[96,97]

Chronic Inflammatory Dermatoses

This category focuses on those persistent inflammatory skin disorders that exhibit their most characteristic clinical and histologic features for many months to years. Unlike the normal cutaneous surface, the skin surface in some chronic inflammatory dermatoses is roughened as a result of excessive or abnormal scale formation and shedding. However, not all scaling lesions are inflammatory—witness the hereditary ichthyoses with fishlike scales as the result of some defect in the adhesive properties of cells in the stratum corneum.

PSORIASIS

Psoriasis is a common chronic inflammatory dermatosis affecting as many as 1% to 2% of people in the United States. Persons of all ages may develop the disease. Psoriasis is sometimes associated with arthritis, myopathy, enteropathy, spondylitic joint disease, or the acquired immunodeficiency syndrome. Psoriatic arthritis may be mild or may produce severe deformities resembling the joint changes seen in rheumatoid arthritis.

Clinically, psoriasis most frequently affects the *skin of the elbows, knees, scalp, lumbosacral areas, intergluteal cleft, and glans penis.* The most typical lesion is a well-demarcated, pink to *salmon-colored plaque* covered by loosely adherent scales that are characteristically *silver-white in color* (Fig. 25–28). Variations exist, with some lesions occurring in annular, linear, gyrate, or serpiginous configurations. Psoriasis can be one cause of total body erythema and scaling known as *erythroderma. Nail changes*[98] occur in 30% of cases of psoriasis and consist of yellow-brown discoloration (often likened to an oil slick), with pitting, dimpling, separation of the nail plate from the underlying bed (onycholysis), thickening, and crumbling. In the rare variant called *pustular psoriasis,* multiple small pustules form on erythematous plaques. This type of psoriasis is either benign and localized (hands and feet) or generalized and life-threatening, with associated fever, leukocytosis, arthralgia, diffuse cutaneous and mucosal pustules, secondary infection, and electrolyte disturbances.

Morphology. Established lesions of psoriasis have a characteristic histologic picture. Increased epidermal cell turnover results in marked epidermal thickening (acanthosis), with regular downward elongation of the rete ridges (Fig. 25–29). Mitotic figures are easily identified well above the basal cell layer, where mitotic activity is confined in normal skin. **The stratum granulosum is thinned or absent, and extensive over-**

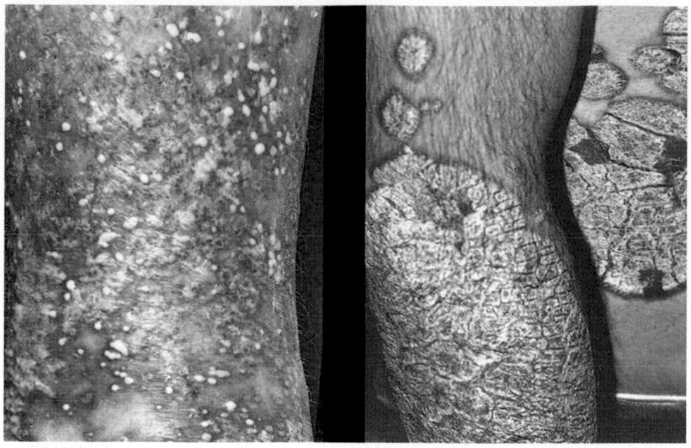

FIGURE 25–28 Clinical evolution of psoriasis. Early and eruptive lesions may be dominated by signs of inflammation and erythema *(left).* Established, chronic lesions demonstrate erythema surmounted by characteristic silver-white scale *(right).* Rarely, the early inflammatory phase predominates throughout the course of the disease (pustular psoriasis).

lying parakeratotic scale is seen. Typical of psoriatic plaques is thinning of the portion of the epidermal cell layer that overlies the tips of dermal papillae (suprapapillary plates) and dilated, tortuous blood vessels within these papillae. This constellation of changes results in abnormal proximity of dermal vessels within the dermal papillae to the overlying parakeratotic scale, and it accounts for the characteristic clinical phenomenon of multiple, minute, bleeding points when the scale is lifted from the plaque **(Auspitz sign).** Neutrophils form small aggregates within slightly spongiotic foci of the superficial epidermis **(spongiform pustules)** and within the parakeratotic stratum corneum **(Munro microabscesses).** In pustular psoriasis, larger abscess-like accumulations of neutrophils are present directly beneath the stratum corneum.

Pathogenesis. Psoriasis is a T cell-mediated disease that involves increased keratinocyte proliferation along with inflammation and angiogenesis.[99] There is a strong association between psoriasis and HLA-C, particularly with the HLA-

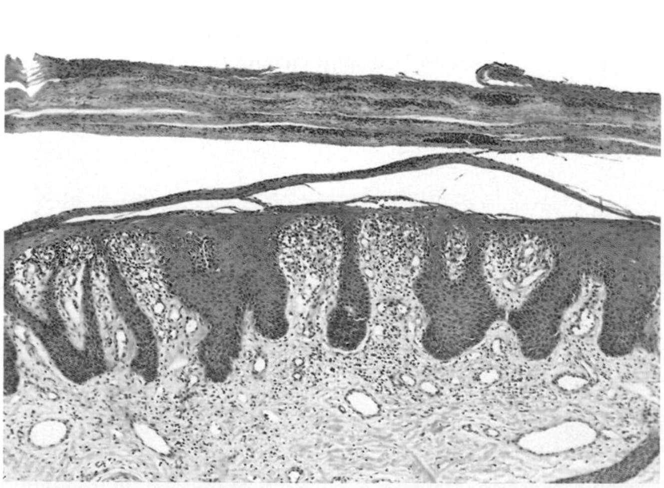

FIGURE 25–29 Psoriasis. Histologically, established lesions demonstrate marked epidermal hyperplasia, parakeratotic scale, and, importantly, minute microabscesses of neutrophils within the superficial epidermal layers.

Cw*0602 allele. About two-thirds of patients carry this allele; homozygotes for HLA-Cw*0602 have a 2.5-fold higher risk of developing psoriasis than heterozygotes. Nevertheless, only 10% of carriers develop psoriasis, indicating that other genes interact with HLA-Cw0602 in causing disease susceptibility.[100] It is likely that CD4+ T cells initiate the disease by interacting with antigen-presenting cells in the skin, providing signals for the activation of CD8+ T cells in the epidermis. The interactions between CD4+ T cells, CD8+ T cells, dendritic cells and keratinocytes give rise to a cytokine "soup" dominated by T_H1 type cytokines such as IL-12, IFN-γ and TNF. The infiltrated lymphocytes also produce growth factors for keratinocytes. There is much evidence that, as with rheumatoid arthritis, TNF is a major mediator in the pathogenesis of psoriasis.[101] Much higher levels of TNF are found in lesional skin, when compared to normal skin; more importantly, TNF-antagonists provide significant improvement in patients with psoriasis. As with many other autoimmune diseases, the antigen that triggers the immune response remains elusive.

SEBORRHEIC DERMATITIS

Seborrheic dermatitis is a chronic inflammatory dermatosis even more common than psoriasis. It classically involves the regions with a high density of sebaceous glands, such as the scalp, forehead (especially the glabella), external auditory canal, retroauricular area, nasolabial folds, and the presternal area. However, it is important to note that seborrheic dermatitis is not a disease of the sebaceous glands. The individual lesions are macules and papules on an erythematous-yellow, often greasy base, typically in association with extensive scaling and crusting. Fissures may also be present, particularly behind the ears. Dandruff is the common clinical expression of seborrheic dermatitis of the scalp. In infants, seborrheic dermatitis presents as cradle cap but can also be part of a disorder known as *Leiner disease,* in which the condition is generalized and associated with diarrhea and failure to thrive. A severe and difficult to treat form of seborrheic dermatitis is seen in human immunodeficiency virus (HIV)-infected individuals.[102] In this setting, it affects up to 83% of patients, in contrast to an incidence of 1% to 3% in the general population.

Morphology. Lesions of seborrheic dermatitis share histologic features with both spongiotic dermatitis and psoriasis, with earlier lesions being more spongiotic and latter ones more acanthotic. Typically mounds of parakeratosis containing neutrophils and serum are present at the ostia of hair follicles (so-called *follicular lipping*). A superficial perivascular inflammatory infiltrate generally consists of an admixture of lymphocytes and neutrophils. With HIV infection, apoptotic keratinocytes and plasma cells may also be present.[103]

The etiology of seborrheic dermatitis is unknown. However, therapeutic studies with ketoconazole, an antifungal agent, suggest that the lipophilic yeast *Malassezia furfur,* which is associated with tinea versicolor, may play a pivotal role.[104] That the sebum is also involved is supported by clinical observations of patients with parkinsonism, who typically show increased sebum production and an increased incidence of seborrheic dermatitis.[105] Indeed, once treated with levodopa, the oiliness of the skin decreases and the seborrheic dermatitis improves. However, because other conditions associated with increased sebaceous activity (e.g., acne) are not necessarily associated with seborrheic dermatitis, sebum production is unlikely to be the sole or primary factor in the pathogenesis of seborrheic dermatitis.

LICHEN PLANUS

"Pruritic, purple, polygonal papules" are the presenting signs of this disorder of the skin and mucous membranes. Lichen planus is self-limiting and generally resolves spontaneously 1 to 2 years after onset, often leaving zones of postinflammatory hyperpigmentation. Oral lesions may persist for years. Malignant degeneration has been noted to occur in chronic mucosal and paramucosal lesions of lichen planus, although the direct pathogenetic relationship has not been shown.[106]

Cutaneous lesions consist of itchy, violaceous, flat-topped papules that may coalesce focally to form plaques (Fig. 25–30*A*). These papules are often highlighted by white dots or lines called *Wickham striae,* representing the clinical correlates of zones of hypergranulosis that typify lesions histologically. In darkly pigmented individuals, lesions may acquire a dark brown color due to loss of melanin pigmentation into the dermis as the basal cell layer is destroyed. Multiple lesions are characteristic and are symmetrically distributed, particularly on the extremities, often about the wrists and elbows, and on the glans penis. In 70% of cases, oral lesions are present as white, reticulated, or netlike areas involving the mucosa. As in psoriasis, the Koebner phenomenon may be seen in lichen planus.

Morphology. Lichen planus is characterized histologically by a dense, continuous infiltrate of lymphocytes along the dermoepidermal junction (Fig. 25–30*B*). The lymphocytes are intimately associated with basal keratinocytes, which show degeneration, necrosis, and a resemblance in size and contour to more mature cells of the stratum spinosum (squamatization). A consequence of this destructive infiltration of lymphocytes is a redefinition of the normal, smoothly undulating configuration of the dermoepidermal interface to a more angulated zigzag contour (saw-toothing). Anucleate, necrotic basal cells may become incorporated into the inflamed papillary dermis, where they are referred to as **colloid** or **Civatte bodies.** Although characteristic of lichen planus, these bodies may be detected in any chronic dermatitis where basal keratinocytes are injured and destroyed. Although this destructive relationship between lymphocytes and epidermal cells bears some similarities to that in erythema multiforme, lichen planus shows changes of chronicity, namely, epidermal hyperplasia (or rarely atrophy) and thickening of the granular cell layer and stratum corneum (hypergranulosis and hyperkeratosis, respectively). Lichen planus preferentially affecting the epithelium of hair follicles is referred to as **lichen planopilaris.**

The pathogenesis of lichen planus is not known. It is plausible that lesions are caused by cell-mediated immune reactions secondary to release of antigens at the levels of the basal cell layer and the dermoepidermal junction. Supporting this notion are data indicating that infiltrates of primarily T lymphocytes associated with hyperplasia of Langerhans cells are characteristics of lesion formation and evolution.[107]

LUPUS ERYTHEMATOSUS

The manifestations of systemic lupus erythematosus (SLE) are described in detail in Chapter 6. There is also a localized, cutaneous form of lupus erythematosus, with no associated systemic manifestations, called *discoid lupus erythematosus (DLE).* Patients who present with DLE usually do not go on to develop systemic disease. However, more than one-third of patients with SLE may exhibit, during their course, lesions that are clinically and histologically indistinguishable from those of the discoid type. Thus, it is often impossible to distinguish patients with SLE from those with DLE on the basis of clinical and histologic inspection of skin lesions alone.

Cutaneous lesions usually consist of either poorly defined malar erythema (typically seen in systemic disease) or large, sharply demarcated erythematous scaling plaques (Fig. 25–31*A*). These "discoid" plaques may occur in either pure cutaneous lupus erythematosus or SLE. Cutaneous manifestations of lupus erythematosus may develop or worsen with sun exposure. The epidermal surface of lesions is shiny or

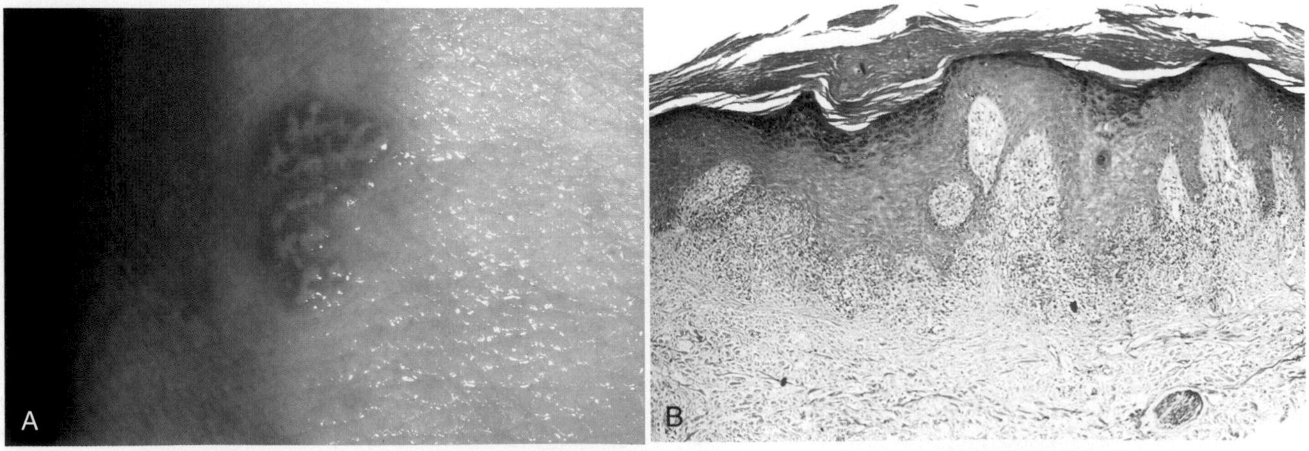

FIGURE 25–30 Lichen planus. *A,* A solitary lesion of lichen planus (glistening surface is due to application of mineral oil, rendering the scale transparent). This flat-topped pink-purple, polygonal papule shows prominent Wickham striae that are more easily appreciated through the transparent scale. *B,* Biopsy of one of the lesions demonstrates the bandlike infiltrate of lymphocytes at the dermoepidermal junction and pointed rete ridges (saw-toothing; compare with Fig. 25–1).

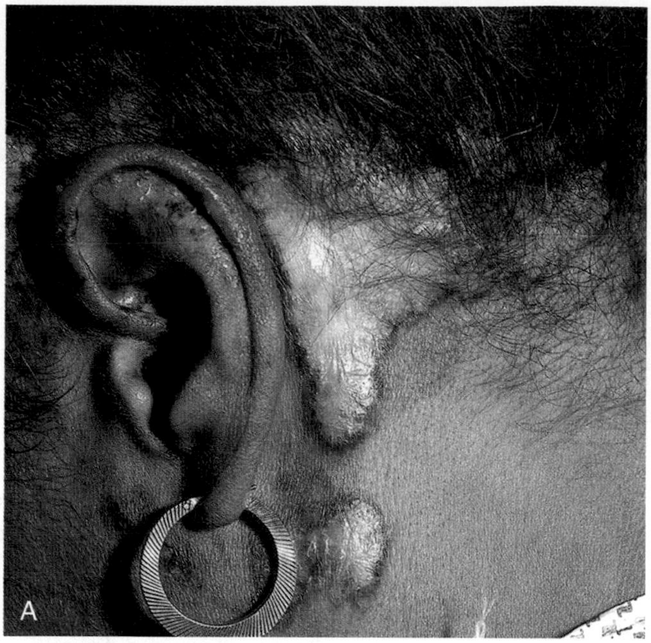

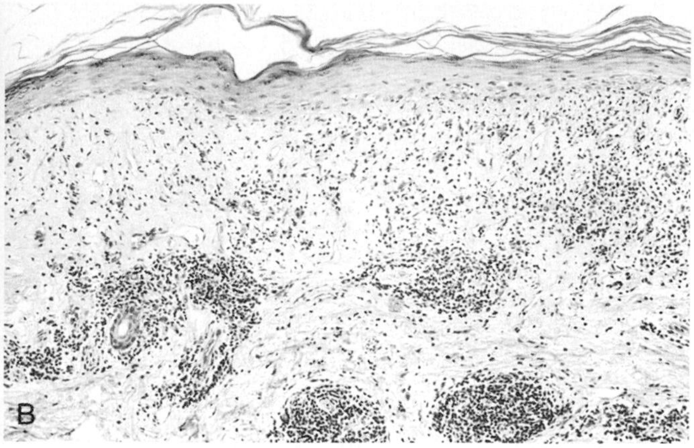

FIGURE 25–31 Lupus erythematosus. *A*, These chronic plaques show a thinned and glistening (atrophic) epidermis, areas where dilated and tortuous dermal vessels are apparent, and central hypopigmentation surrounded by peripheral hyperpigmentation. Note areas of early hair loss due to follicular involvement. *B*, There is an infiltrate of lymphocytes within the superficial and deep dermis, marked thinning of the epidermis with loss of normal rete ridges, and hyperkeratosis.

scaly, and lateral compression often produces wrinkling, a sign of epidermal atrophy. Through this thinned epidermis, dilated and tortuous blood vessels (telangiectasia) and small zones of hypopigmentation and hyperpigmentation may be seen. Small, keratotic plugs in follicular ostia may be observed with a hand lens.

Morphology. Lesions of DLE are characterized histologically by an infiltrate of lymphocytes along the dermoepidermal or the dermal–follicular epithelial junction, or both (Fig. 25–31*B*). Deep perivascular and periappendageal (e.g., around sweat glands) infiltrates are also observed, and preferential infiltration of subcutaneous fat is called **lupus profundus.** The basal cell layer generally shows diffuse vacuolization. The epidermal layer is markedly thinned or atrophied, with loss of the normal rete ridge pattern. Variable hyperkeratosis is present on the epidermal surface. Involved hair follicles may also show epithelial atrophy, and their infundibula are frequently dilated and plugged with keratin. Periodic acid-Schiff (PAS) stain of established lesions reveals marked thickening of the epidermal basement membrane zone, and **direct immunofluorescence shows a characteristic granular band of immunoglobulin and complement along the dermoepidermal and dermal–follicular junctions (so-called lupus band test**[108]**)** (Fig. 25–32). Such bands are typically seen in lesional skin but not normal skin in DLE and in both lesional and normal skin in many cases of SLE.

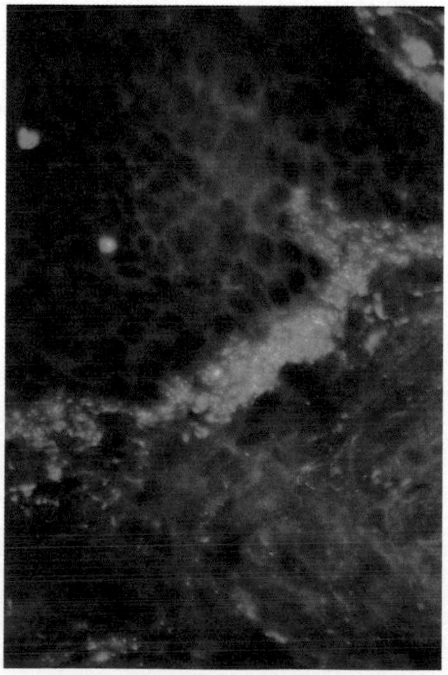

FIGURE 25–32 Granular deposits of immunoglobulin (here IgG) and complement at the dermoepidermal junction constitute a positive "band test" in lupus erythematosus.

The immunopathogenesis of lupus erythematosus is discussed in Chapter 6. In the skin, humoral mechanisms of injury may involve both formation and deposition of immune complexes and complement components C5b to C9 (membrane attack complex)[109] at the dermoepithelial junction.

Blistering (Bullous) Diseases

Although vesicles and bullae (blisters) occur as secondary phenomena in a number of unrelated conditions (e.g., herpesvirus infection, spongiotic dermatitis, erythema multiforme, and thermal burns), there exists a group of disorders in which blisters are the primary and most distinctive features. These bullous diseases, as they are called, produce visually dramatic clinical lesions and in some instances (e.g., pemphigus vulgaris) are uniformly fatal if untreated. Blisters can occur at multiple levels within the skin (Fig. 25–33), and assessment of these levels is essential to formulating an accurate histologic diagnosis.

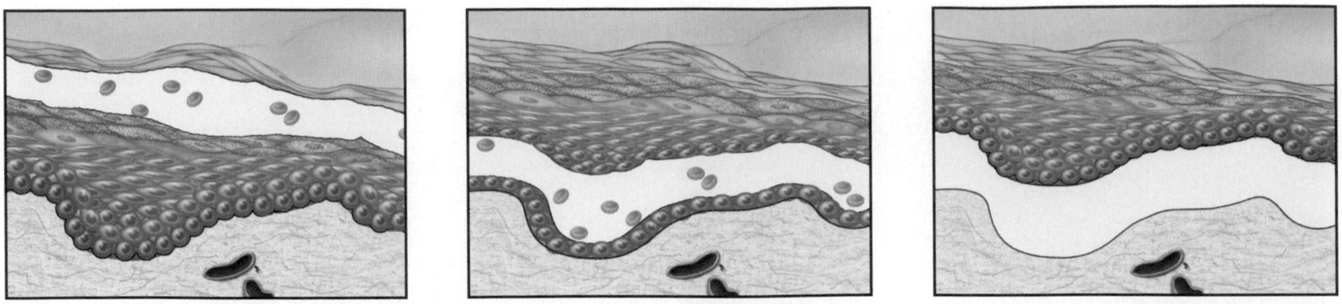

FIGURE 25–33 Schematic representation of sites of blister formation. *A,* In a subcorneal blister, the stratum corneum forms the roof of the bulla (as in impetigo or pemphigus foliaceus). *B,* In a suprabasal blister, a portion of the epidermis including the stratum corneum forms the roof (as in pemphigus vulgaris). *C,* In a subepidermal blister, the entire epidermis separates from the dermis (as in bullous pemphigoid and dermatitis herpetiformis).

PEMPHIGUS

Pemphigus is an autoimmune blistering disorder resulting from loss of the integrity of normal intercellular attachments within the epidermis and mucosal epithelium.[110] Although rare, its clinical consequences without treatment may be life-threatening, and its pathobiology provides important insight into the molecular mechanisms of keratinocyte adhesion. The majority of individuals who develop pemphigus are in the fourth to sixth decades of life, and men and women are affected equally. There are four clinical and pathologic variants: (1) pemphigus vulgaris, (2) pemphigus vegetans, (3) pemphigus foliaceus, and (4) pemphigus erythematosus.

Pemphigus vulgaris, by far the most common type (accounting for more than 80% of cases worldwide), involves the mucosa and skin, especially on the scalp, face, axilla, groin, trunk, and points of pressure. It may present as oral ulcers that persist sometimes for months before skin involvement appears. Primary lesions are superficial vesicles and bullae that rupture easily, leaving shallow erosions covered with dried serum and crust (Fig. 25–34*A*). *Pemphigus vegetans* is a rare form that usually presents not with blisters but with large, moist, verrucous (wartlike), vegetating plaques studded with pustules on the groin, axillae, and flexural surfaces. *Pemphigus foliaceus* is a more benign form that occurs in an epidemic form in South America as well as in isolated cases in other countries. Sites of predilection are the scalp, face, chest, and back, and the mucous membranes are only rarely affected. Bullae are so superficial that only zones of erythema and crusting, sites of previous blister rupture, are usually present on physical examination. *Pemphigus erythematosus* is considered to be a localized, less severe form of pemphigus foliaceus that may selectively involve the malar area of the face in a lupus erythematosus–like fashion.

Morphology. The common denominator, histologically, in all forms of pemphigus is **acantholysis.** This term implies dissolution, or lysis, of the intercellular adhesion sites within a squamous epithelial surface. Acantholytic cells that are no longer attached to other epithelial cells lose their polyhedral shape and characteristically become rounded. In pemphigus vulgaris and pemphigus vegetans, acantholysis selectively involves the layer of cells immediately above the basal cell layer. (The vegetans variant has considerable overlying epidermal hyperplasia.) The **suprabasal acantholytic blister** that forms is characteristic of pemphigus vulgaris (Fig. 25–34*B*). The single layer of intact basal cells that forms the blister base has been likened to a row of tombstones. In pemphigus foliaceus, a blister forms by similar mechanisms but, unlike the case with pemphigus vulgaris, selectively

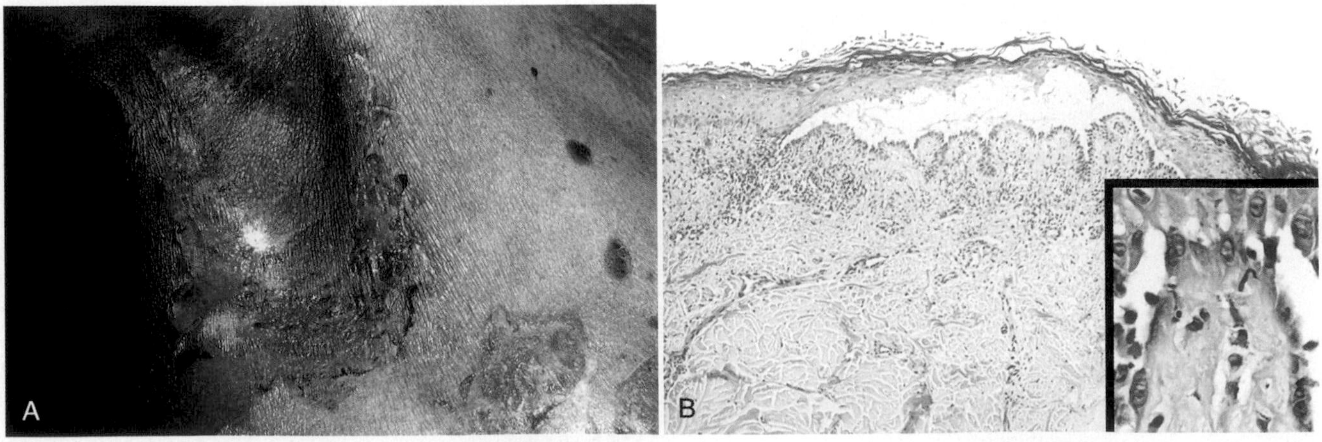

FIGURE 25–34 Pemphigus vulgaris. *A,* Eroded plaques are formed on rupture of confluent, thin-roofed bullae, here affecting axillary skin. *B,* Suprabasal acantholysis results in an intraepidermal blister in which rounded (acantholytic) epidermal cells are identified *(inset).*

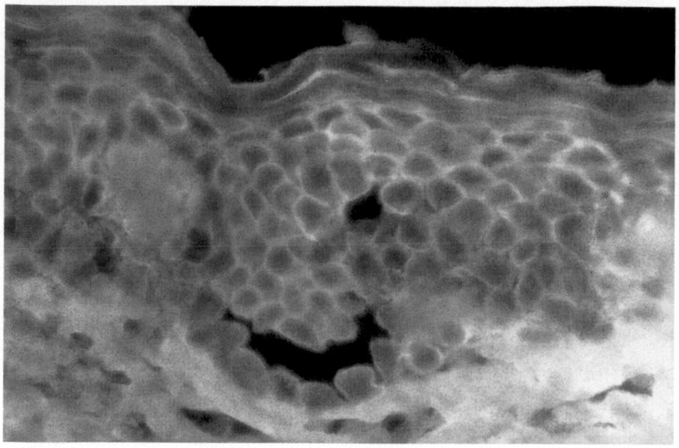

FIGURE 25–35 Direct immunofluorescence of pemphigus vulgaris. There is deposition of immunoglobulin along the plasma membranes of epidermal keratinocytes in a fishnet-like pattern. Also note the early suprabasal separation due to loss of cell-to-cell adhesion (acantholysis).

involves the superficial epidermis at the level of the stratum granulosum. Variable superficial dermal infiltration by lymphocytes, histiocytes, and eosinophils accompanies all forms of pemphigus.

Pathogenesis. Sera from patients with pemphigus contain antibodies (IgG) to intercellular cement substance of skin and mucous membranes.[111] This phenomenon is the basis for direct and indirect diagnostic immunofluorescence testing of skin and serum, respectively. Lesional sites show a characteristic netlike pattern of intercellular IgG deposits localized to sites of developed or incipient acantholysis (Fig. 25–35). It is now known that the antibody in pemphigus vulgaris reacts with desmoglein 3, a component of the desmosomes that appear to bind keratinocytes together. When the gene for desmoglein 3 is disrupted in genetically engineered mice, suprabasal blisters akin to pemphigus develop owing to lack of desmosome adhesion. This suggests a direct role for pemphigus autoantibodies in interfering with the function of this protein.[112] Some of the acantholytic process may also be the consequence of synthesis and liberation of a serine protease (plasminogen activator) by epidermal cells, an event that is triggered by the pemphigus antibody.[113,114] The relevant antibody in pemphigus foliaceus reacts with desmoglein 1, which is expressed in the uppermost epidermal layers, thus correlating with the characteristic subcorneal plane of blister formation in this variant.[115]

BULLOUS PEMPHIGOID

Originally considered to be a form of pemphigus, bullous pemphigoid has been recognized for almost four decades as a distinct and relatively common autoimmune, vesiculobullous disease. Generally affecting elderly individuals, bullous pemphigoid shows a wide range of clinical presentations, with localized to generalized cutaneous lesions and, albeit less often than in pemphigus vulgaris, involvement of mucosal surfaces.

Clinically, lesions are tense bullae, filled with clear fluid, on normal or erythematous skin (Fig. 25–36*A*). Lesions are usually up to 2 cm in diameter, but occasionally may reach 4 to 8 cm in diameter. The bullae do not rupture as easily as do the blisters seen in pemphigus and, if uncomplicated by infection, heal without scarring. Sites of occurrence include the inner aspects of the thighs, flexor surfaces of the forearms, axillae, groin, and lower abdomen. Oral involvement is present in 10% to 15% of patients, usually after the development of cutaneous lesions. Some patients may present with urticarial plaques, with extreme associated pruritus.

Morphology. The separation of bullous pemphigoid from pemphigus, establishing the former as a distinctive entity, was based on the seminal observation that pemphigoid resulted from a **subepidermal, nonacantholytic** blister.[116] Early lesions show a superficial and sometimes deep perivascular infiltrate of lymphocytes and variable numbers of eosinophils, occasional neutrophils, superficial dermal edema, and associated basal cell layer vacuolization (Fig. 25–36*B*). Eosinophils showing degranulation are typically detected directly beneath the epidermal basal cell layer. The vacuolated basal cell layer eventually gives rise to a fluid-filled blister.

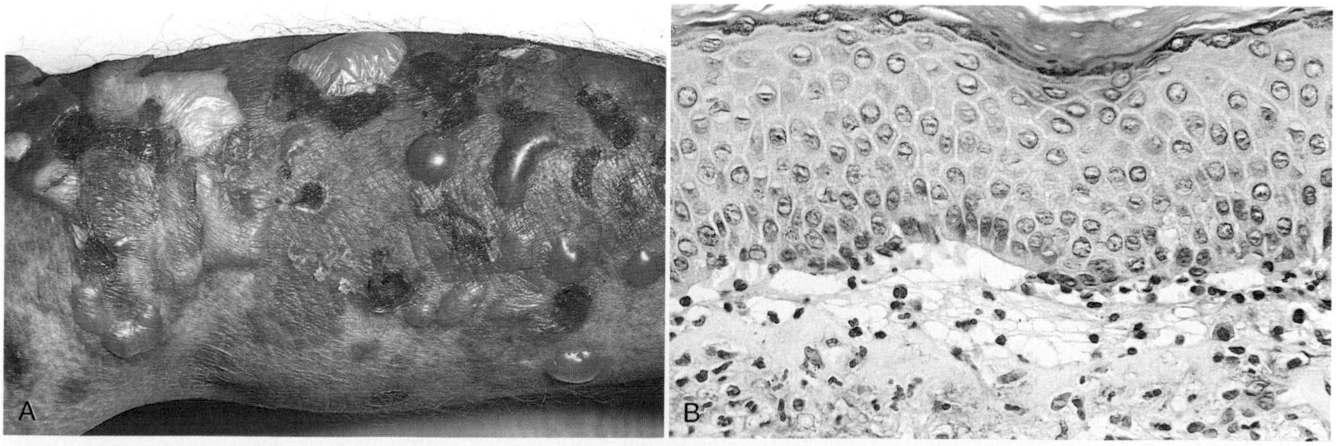

FIGURE 25–36 Bullous pemphigoid. Clinical bullae *(A)* result from basal cell layer vacuolization, producing a subepidermal blister *(B)*. Histopathology of the edge of an early lesion showing the onset of epidermal separation from the underlying dermis. Eosinophils, as well as lymphocytes and occasional neutrophils, may be intimately associated with basal cell layer destruction, creating the subepidermal cleft.

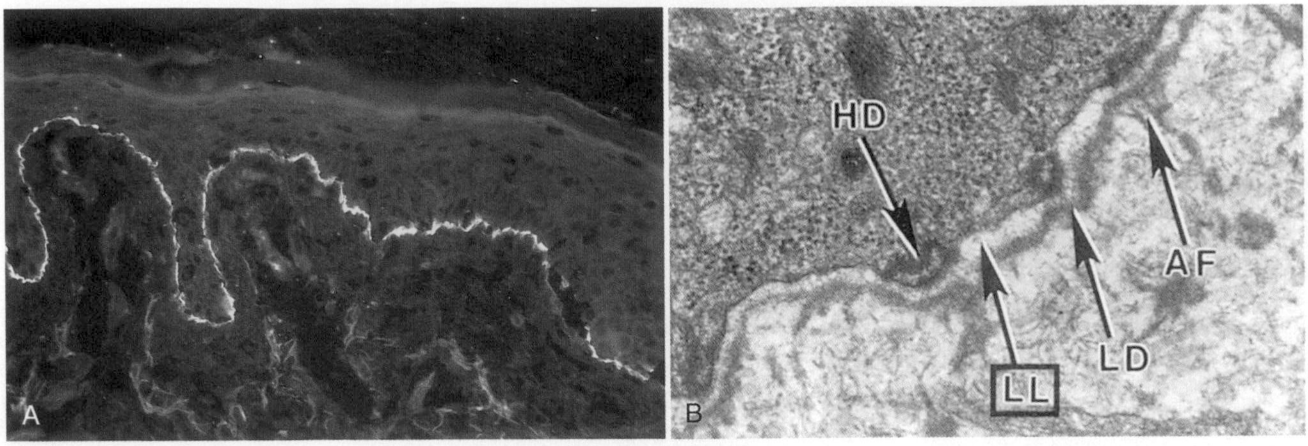

FIGURE 25–37 *A*, Linear deposition of complement along the dermoepidermal junction in bullous pemphigoid; the pattern has been likened to ribbon candy. *B*, Bullous pemphigoid antigen is located in the lowermost portion of the basal cell cytoplasm in association with hemidesmosomes (HD), with blister formation affecting the lamina lucida (LL) of the basement membrane zone. LD, lamina densa; AF, anchoring fibrils.

Pathogenesis. Bullous pemphigoid is caused by antibodies directed against proteins at the dermal-epidermal junction. There is *linear* zone deposition of immunoglobulin and complement (Fig. 25–37*A*) at this site[117] (recall that the pattern for lupus erythematosus is similar, but granular in character). Ultrastructural studies have shown that circulating antibody reacts with antigen present in the basal cell–basement membrane attachment plaques (hemidesmosomes) (Fig. 25–37*B*). The actual blister develops at the level of a narrow clear zone (lamina lucida) of the epidermal basement membrane that separates the underlying lamina densa from the plasma membrane of the basal cells. The antigens present at these sites have been named bullous pemphigoid antigens 1 and 2, and they are now recognized as normal constituents of the hemidesmosomes that bind basal cells at the dermoepidermal junction. In bullous pemphigoid, it is likely that the generation of autoantibodies to these basement membrane components results in the fixation of complement and subsequent tissue injury at this site through locally recruited neutrophils[118] and eosinophils. Degranulating eosinophils are often associated with necrosis of basal keratinocytes possibly related to the liberation of major basic protein from the eosinophil granule.

DERMATITIS HERPETIFORMIS

Dermatitis herpetiformis[119] is a rare and fascinating entity characterized by papules, vesicles, and occasional bullae on an erythematous, often urticarial base. Males tend to be affected more frequently than are females, and the age at onset is often in the third and fourth decades, although the disease has been known to develop at any age after weaning. A major association is with celiac disease (Chapter 17); both the vesicular dermatosis and the enteropathy respond to a diet free of gluten.

The urticarial plaques and vesicles of dermatitis herpetiformis are extremely pruritic. They characteristically occur bilaterally and symmetrically, involving preferentially the extensor surfaces, elbows, knees, upper back, and buttocks. Vesicles are frequently grouped, as are those of true herpesvirus, and hence the name herpetiformis (Fig. 25–38*A*).

Morphology. The early lesions of dermatitis herpetiformis are histologically characteristic. Fibrin and neutrophils accumulate selectively at the **tips of dermal papillae,** forming small microabscesses (Fig.

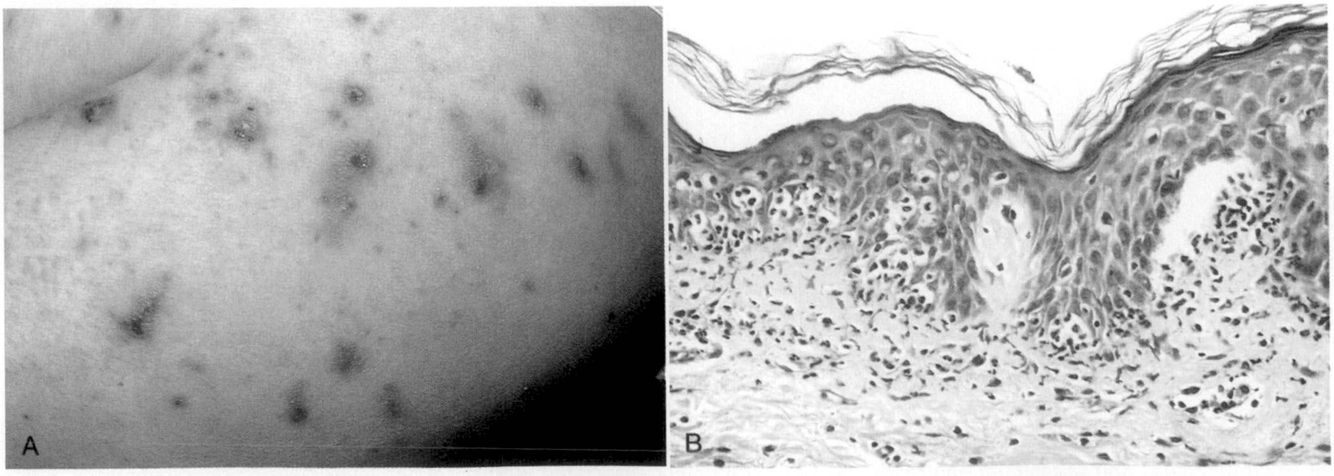

FIGURE 25–38 Dermatitis herpetiformis. *A*, Clinical lesions consist of intact and eroded erythematous blisters that are often grouped together. *B*, Histologically, neutrophilic microabscesses selectively involve the dermal papilla.

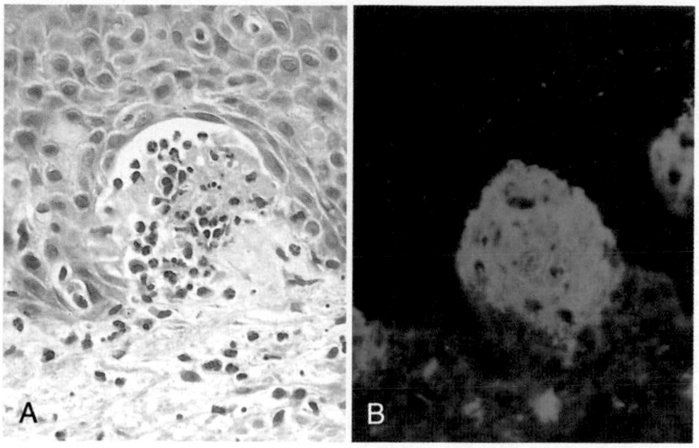

FIGURE 25–39 Dermatitis herpetiformis. *A,* Papillary dermal microabscesses are associated with zones of dermoepidermal cleavage that eventually coalesce to form a clinical blister. *B,* By direct immunofluorescence, these abscesses are rich in IgA and fibrin deposits.

25–38*B*). The basal cells overlying these microabscesses show vacuolization, and minute zones of dermoepidermal separation (microscopic blisters) may occur at the tips of involved papillae (Fig. 25–39*A*). In time, these zones coalesce to form a true subepidermal blister. Eosinophils may occur in the infiltrates of older lesions, creating confusion with the histologic picture of bullous pemphigoid. Attention to the early alterations at the blister edge, however, usually allows separation of these two disorders. By direct immunofluorescence, dermatitis herpetiformis shows granular deposits of **IgA** selectively localized in the tips of dermal papillae, where they are deposited on anchoring fibrils (Fig. 25–39*B*).

Pathogenesis. This disease results from formation of antibodies against gliadin, a protein found in the gluten fraction of wheat. Patients with dermatitis herpetiformis may develop antibodies of the IgA and IgG classes to gliadin and reticulin, a component of the anchoring fibrils that tether the epidermal basement membrane to the superficial dermis. In addition, individuals with certain histocompatibility types (HLA-B8 and HLA-DRw3) are particularly prone to this disease. It is thus thought that genetically predisposed persons may develop IgA antibodies to components of dietary gluten and that these antibodies (or immune complexes) then cross-react with or are deposited in the dermal papillae of the skin, resulting in clinical disease. Some individuals with dermatitis herpetiformis and enteropathy respond to a gluten-free diet (as with celiac disease).[120]

NONINFLAMMATORY BLISTERING DISEASES: EPIDERMOLYSIS BULLOSA, PORPHYRIA

To this point, we have discussed inflammatory blistering diseases. However, some primary disorders characterized by vesicles and bullae are not mediated by inflammatory mechanisms. Two such diseases are *epidermolysis bullosa* and *porphyria.*

Epidermolysis bullosa constitutes a group of disorders unified by the common link of blisters that develop at sites of pressure, rubbing, or trauma, at or soon after birth. In the *simplex type,* for example, degeneration of the basal cell layer of the epidermis results in clinical bullae. This form of the disease is caused by mutations in the genes encoding keratins 14 and 5.[121] In the *junctional type,* blisters occur in otherwise histologically normal skin at precisely the level of the lamina lucida (Fig. 25–40). In the scarring *dystrophic types,* blisters develop beneath the lamina densa, in association with rudimentary or defective anchoring fibrils. Dystrophic epidermolysis bullosa is an inherited disease resulting from mutations in the *COL 7A1* gene that encodes type VII collagen[122] (see Chapter 3). The histologic changes are so subtle that electron microscopy may be required to differentiate among these types in clinically ambiguous settings.

Porphyria refers to a group of uncommon inborn or acquired disturbances of porphyrin metabolism. Porphyrins are pigments normally present in hemoglobin, myoglobin, and cytochromes. The classification of porphyrias is based on both clinical and biochemical features. The five major types are (1) congenital erythropoietic porphyria, (2) erythrohepatic protoporphyria, (3) acute intermittent porphyria, (4) porphyria cutanea tarda, and (5) mixed porphyria. Cutaneous manifestations consist of urticaria and vesicles that heal with scarring and that are exacerbated by exposure to sunlight. The primary alterations by light microscopy are a *subepidermal vesicle* (Fig. 25–41) *with associated marked thickening of*

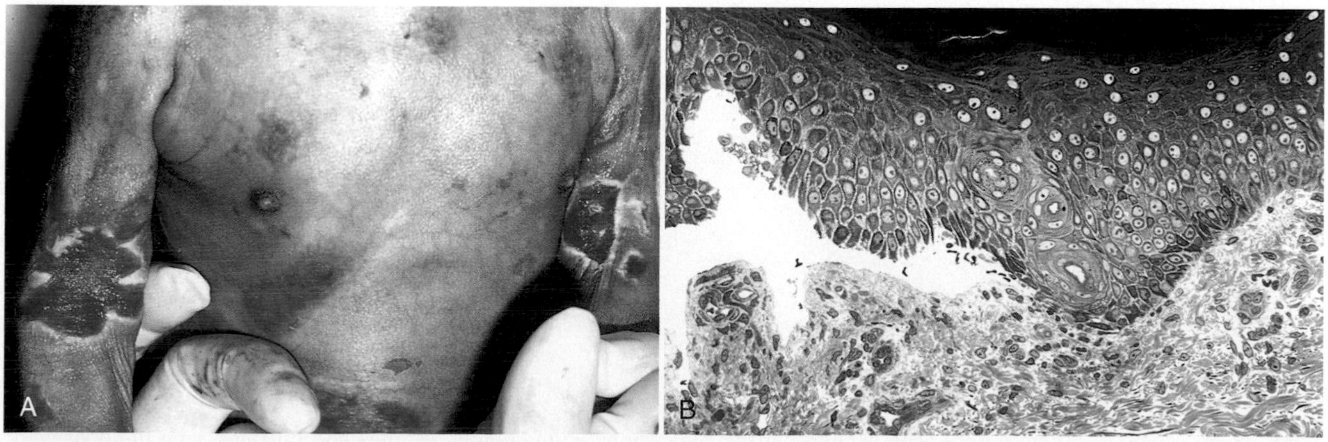

FIGURE 25–40 Epidermolysis bullosa. *A,* Junctional epidermolysis bullosa showing typical erosions in flexural creases. *B,* A noninflammatory subepidermal blister in this case has formed at the level of the lamina lucida (Giemsa-stained section).

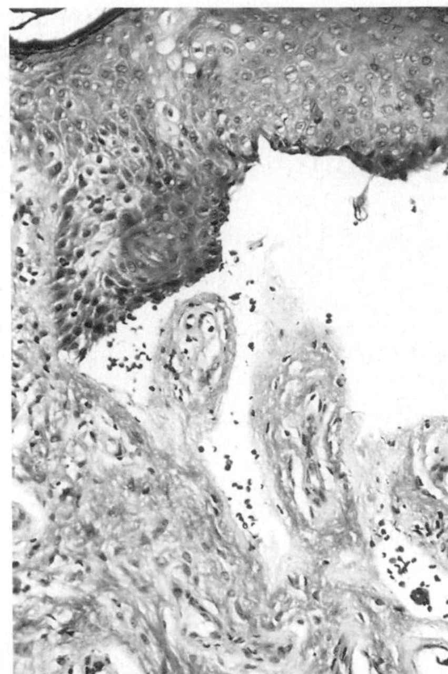

FIGURE 25–41 Porphyria. A noninflammatory blister is forming at the dermoepidermal junction; note the seemingly rigid dermal papillae at the base that contain the altered superficial vessels.

the walls of superficial dermal vessels. The pathogenesis of these alterations is not well understood, although serum proteins, including immunoglobulins, typically form glassy deposits in the walls of superficial dermal microvessels.

Disorders of Epidermal Appendages

ACNE VULGARIS

Virtually universal in the middle to late teenage years, acne vulgaris affects both males and females, although males tend to have more severe disease. Acne is seen in all races, but is usually milder in people of Asian descent. Acne vulgaris in adolescents is believed to occur as a result of physiologic hormonal variations and alterations in hair follicle maturation. The clinical features of acne may be induced or exacerbated by drugs (corticosteroids, adrenocorticotropic hormone, testosterone, gonadotropins, contraceptives, trimethadione, iodides, and bromides), occupational contactants (cutting oils, chlorinated hydrocarbons, and coal tars), and occlusive conditions such as heavy clothing and tropical climates. Some families seem to be particularly affected by acne, suggesting a heritable factor.

Acne is divided into noninflammatory and inflammatory types, although the types may coexist. The former consists of open and closed comedones. *Open comedones* are small follicular papules containing a central black keratin plug. This color is the result of oxidation of melanin pigment (not dirt). *Closed comedones* are follicular papules without a visible central plug. Because the keratin plug is trapped beneath the epidermal surface, these lesions are potential sources of follicular rupture and inflammation. Inflammatory acne is characterized by erythematous papules, nodules, and pustules (Fig. 25–42*A*). Severe variants (e.g., acne conglobata) result in sinus tract formation and physical scarring, in addition to the emotional scars.

Morphology. Four key components contribute to the development of acne: (1) changes in keratinization of the lower portion of the follicular infundibulum with the development of a keratin plug blocking outflow of sebum to the skin surface; (2) increase in size of sebaceous glands with puberty or increased activity due to hormonal stimulation; (3) lipase-synthesizing bacteria *(Propionibacterium acnes)* colonizing the upper and midportion of the hair follicle, converting lipids within sebum to pro-inflammatory fatty acids; and (4) induction of inflammation in the follicle associated with release of cytotoxic and chemotactic factors. Depending on the stage of the disease, open or closed comedones, papules, pustules, or deep inflammatory nodules may develop (see Fig. 25–42*A*). Open comedones have large, patulous orifices, whereas those of closed comedones are identifiable only microscopically. Variable lymphohistiocytic infiltrates are present in and around affected follicles, and extensive acute and chronic inflammation accompanies follicular rupture. Dermal abscesses may form in association with rupture (Fig. 25–42*B*), and gradual resolution, often with scarring, ensues.[123]

Pathogenesis. The pathogenesis of acne is incompletely understood. Endocrine factors have been implicated (especially androgens) because castrated persons never develop the

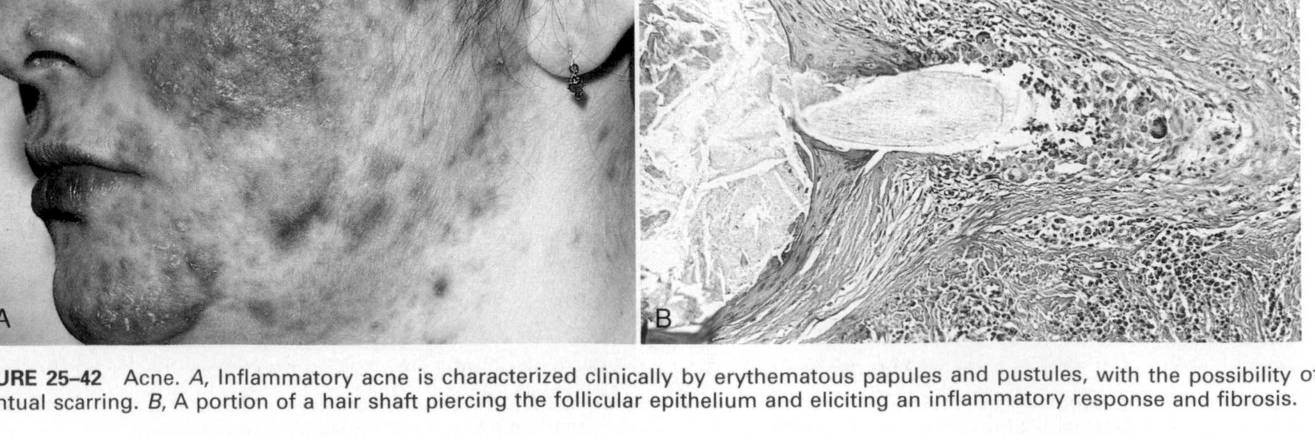

FIGURE 25–42 Acne. *A*, Inflammatory acne is characterized clinically by erythematous papules and pustules, with the possibility of eventual scarring. *B*, A portion of a hair shaft piercing the follicular epithelium and eliciting an inflammatory response and fibrosis.

condition. However, these do not appear to be the sole or primary cause.[124] It has been postulated that bacterial lipases of *Propionibacterium acnes* break down sebaceous oils, liberating highly irritating fatty acids and resulting in the earliest inflammatory phases of acne.[125] Inhibition of lipase production is a rationale for administration of antibiotics to patients with inflammatory acne.[126] The synthetic vitamin A derivative 13-*cis*-retinoic acid (isotretinoin) has brought about remarkable clinical improvement in some cases of severe acne.[127]

Panniculitis

ERYTHEMA NODOSUM AND ERYTHEMA INDURATUM

Panniculitis is an inflammatory reaction in the subcutaneous fat that may affect (1) principally the connective tissue septa separating lobules of fat or (2) predominantly the lobules of fat themselves. *Erythema nodosum* is the most common form of panniculitis and usually has an acute presentation. Its occurrence is often associated with infections (beta-hemolytic streptococcal infection, tuberculosis and, less commonly, coccidioidomycosis, histoplasmosis, and leprosy), drug administration (sulfonamides, oral contraceptives), sarcoidosis, inflammatory bowel disease, and certain malignant neoplasms, but many times a cause cannot be identified. Many types of panniculitis have a subacute to chronic course.

Panniculitis often involves the lower legs. Erythema nodosum presents as poorly defined, exquisitely tender, erythematous plaques and nodules that may be better felt than seen. Fever and malaise may accompany the cutaneous signs. Over the course of weeks, lesions usually flatten and become bruise-like, leaving no residual clinical scars, while new lesions develop. Biopsy of a deep wedge of tissue is usually required to establish a definitive diagnosis.

Erythema induratum is an uncommon type of panniculitis that affects primarily adolescents and menopausal women. Although the cause is not known, most observers today regard this disorder as the result of a primary vasculitis affecting deep vessels supplying lobules of the subcutis, with subsequent necrosis and inflammation within the fat. Erythema induratum presents as an erythematous, slightly tender nodule that usually goes on to ulcerate. Originally considered a hypersensitivity response to tuberculosis, erythema induratum today most commonly occurs without an associated underlying disease.

Morphology. The histopathology of **erythema nodosum** is distinctive. In early lesions, widening of the connective tissue septa is due to edema, fibrin exudation, and neutrophilic infiltration. Later, infiltration by lymphocytes, histiocytes, multinucleated giant cells, and occasional eosinophils is associated with septal fibrosis. Vasculitis is not present. In **erythema induratum**, on the other hand, granulomatous inflammation and zones of caseous necrosis involve the fat lobule. Early lesions show necrotizing vasculitis affecting small to medium-sized arteries and veins in the deep dermis and subcutis.

Erythema nodosum and erythema induratum are but two examples among the many types of panniculitis. *Weber-Christian disease (relapsing febrile nodular panniculitis)* is a rare form of lobular, nonvasculitic panniculitis seen in children and adults. It is marked by crops of erythematous plaques or nodules, predominantly on the lower extremities, created by deep-seated foci of inflammation with aggregates of foamy histiocytes admixed with lymphocytes, neutrophils, and giant cells. *Factitial panniculitis* is a form of secondary panniculitis caused by self-inflicted trauma or injection of foreign or toxic substances. *Deep mycotic infections* in immunocompromised individuals may produce histologic changes that mimic primary panniculitis. Finally, disorders such as *lupus erythematosus* may occasionally have deep inflammatory components with associated panniculitis.

Infection and Infestation

Although the skin is a protective organ, it frequently succumbs to the attack of microorganisms, parasites, and insects. We have already discussed the possible role of bacteria in the pathogenesis of common acne, and the dermatoses resulting from viruses are too numerous to list. In the setting of the immunocompromised patient, ordinarily trivial cutaneous infections may be life-threatening.

Many disorders, such as herpes simplex and herpes zoster, the viral exanthems, and deep fungal infections, are discussed in Chapter 8. In addition, immune reactions in skin provoked by infectious agents, such as the annular erythema termed erythema chronicum migrans, a harbinger of Lyme disease, are also discussed in Chapter 8. Here we address a representative sampling of common infections and infestations whose primary clinical manifestations are in the skin.

VERRUCAE (WARTS)

Verrucae are common lesions of children and adolescents, although they may be encountered at any age. They are caused by human papillomaviruses. Transmission of disease usually involves direct contact between individuals or autoinoculation. Verrucae are generally self-limited, regressing spontaneously within 6 months to 2 years.

The classification of verrucae is based largely on clinical morphology and location. *Verruca vulgaris* is the most common type of wart. The lesions of verruca vulgaris occur anywhere but most frequently on the hands, particularly on the dorsal surfaces and periungual areas, where they appear as gray-white to tan, flat to convex, 0.1- to 1-cm papules with a rough, pebble-like surface (Fig. 25–43*A*). *Verruca plana,* or *flat wart,* is common on the face or the dorsal surfaces of the hands. The warts are slightly elevated, flat, smooth, tan papules that are generally smaller than verruca vulgaris. *Verruca plantaris* and *verruca palmaris* occur on the soles and palms, respectively. Rough, scaly lesions may reach 1 to 2 cm in diameter, coalesce, and be confused with ordinary calluses. *Condyloma acuminatum (venereal wart)* occurs on the penis, female genitalia, urethra, perianal areas, and rectum. Venereal warts appear as soft, tan, cauliflower-like masses that in occasional cases reach many centimeters in diameter.

Morphology. Histologic features common to verrucae include epidermal hyperplasia that is often undulant in character (so-called verrucous or papillomatous epidermal hyperplasia; Fig. 25–43*B*)

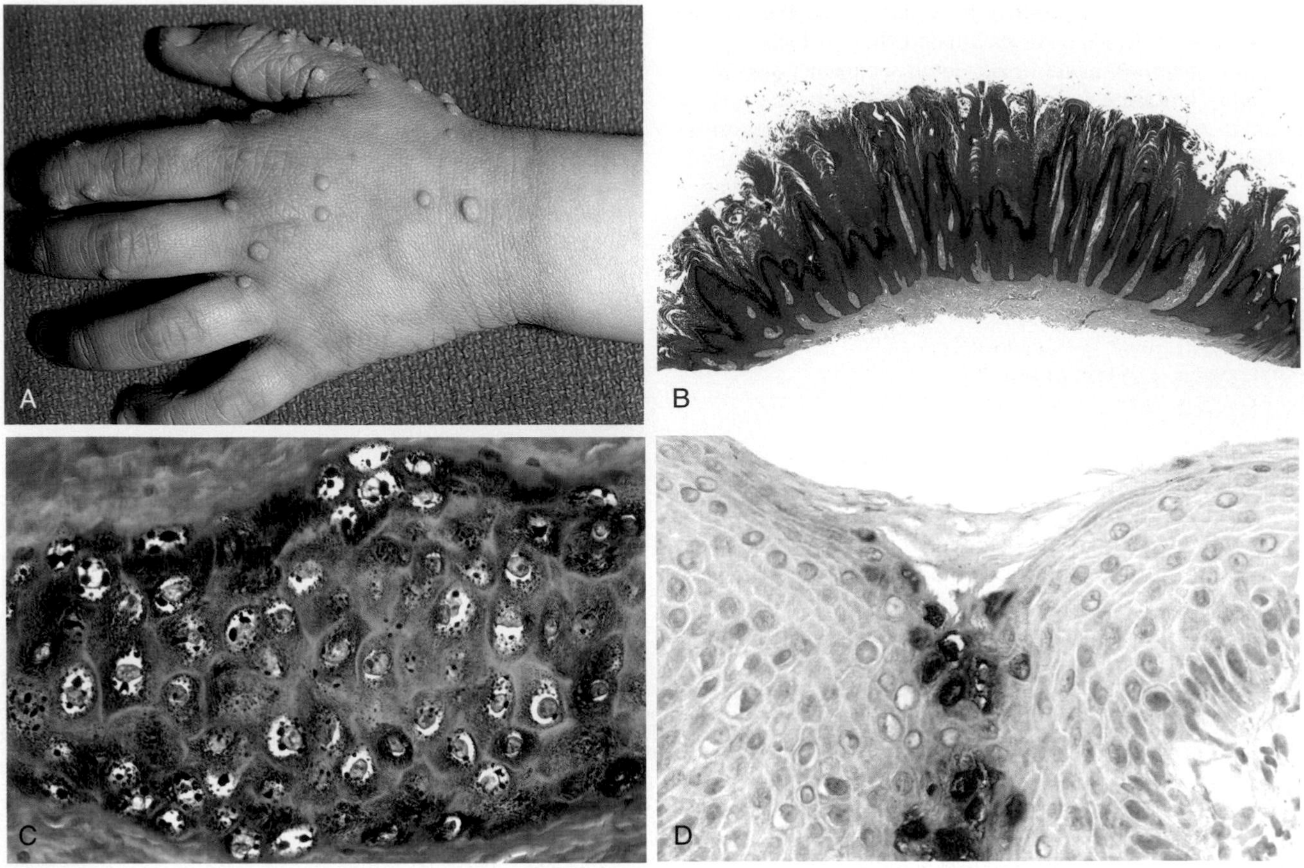

FIGURE 25–43 Verruca vulgaris. *A,* Multiple papules with rough pebble-like surfaces. *B* (low power) and *C* (high power), histology of the lesions show papillomatous epidermal hyperplasia and cytopathic alterations that include nuclear pallor and prominent keratohyaline granules. *D,* In situ hybridization showing viral DNA within epidermal cells.

and cytoplasmic vacuolization (koilocytosis) that preferentially involves the more superficial epidermal layers, producing halos of pallor surrounding infected nuclei. Electron microscopy of these zones reveals numerous viral particles within nuclei. Infected cells may also demonstrate prominent and apparently condensed keratohyaline granules and jagged eosinophilic intracytoplasmic keratin aggregates as a result of viral cytopathic effects (Fig. 25–43*C*). These cellular alterations are not as prominent in condylomas; hence, their diagnosis is based primarily on hyperplastic papillary architecture containing wedge-shaped zones of koilocytosis.

Pathogenesis. It is now recognized that the clinically different types of warts just described result not solely because of the anatomically different sites in which they arise but also as a consequence of distinct types of HPV. More than 150 types of papillomavirus have been identified, many of them capable of producing warts in humans. The virus can be identified by molecular hybridization (Fig. 25–43*D*) and polymerase chain reaction (PCR). For example, anogenital warts are caused predominantly by HPV types 6 and 11. In contrast, there is a tendency for lesions induced by HPV type 16 to show some degree of dysplasia.[128] HPV type 16 has also been associated with in situ squamous cell carcinoma of the genitalia and with *bowenoid papulosis* (genital lesions of young adults with the histology of carcinoma in situ but with a biologic course of spontaneous regression).[129] These findings are consistent with previous observations of the association of HPV types 16 and 18 with carcinomas of the uterine cervix[130] (Chapter 22). The potential relationship of papillomavirus to carcinoma is reinforced by the rare heritable condition termed *epidermodysplasia verruciformis.* In this disorder, patients develop multiple flat warts, some of which evolve to become invasive squamous cell carcinomas. The genomes of HPV types 5 and 8 have been detected in some of these cutaneous tumors.[131] Thus, the types of papillomavirus differ not only in the morphology of the lesions they produce but also in their oncogenic potential (Chapter 7).

MOLLUSCUM CONTAGIOSUM

Molluscum contagiosum is a common, self-limited viral disease of the skin caused by a poxvirus. The virus is characteristically brick shaped, has a dumbbell-shaped DNA core, and measures 300 nm in maximal dimension, and thus represents the largest pathogenic poxvirus in humans and one of the largest viruses in nature. Infection is usually spread by direct contact, particularly among children and young adults.

Clinically, multiple lesions may occur on the skin and mucous membranes, with a predilection for the trunk and anogenital areas. Individual lesions are firm, often pruritic, pink to skin-colored umbilicated papules generally ranging in diameter from 0.2 to 0.4 cm. Rarely, "giant" forms occur measuring up to 2 cm in diameter. A curd-like material can be expressed from the central umbilication. Smearing this material onto a glass slide and staining with Giemsa reagent often shows diagnostic molluscum bodies.

Morphology. On microscopic examination, lesions show cuplike verrucous epidermal hyperplasia. The diagnostically specific structure is the molluscum body, which occurs as a large (up to 35 μm), ellipsoid, homogeneous, cytoplasmic inclusion in cells of the stratum granulosum and the stratum corneum (Fig. 25–44). In the H&E stain, these inclusions are eosinophilic in the blue-purple stratum granulosum and acquire a pale blue hue in the red stratum corneum. Numerous virions are present within molluscum bodies.

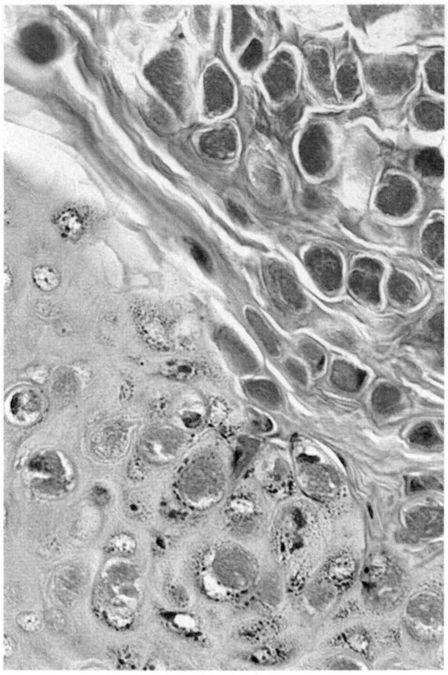

FIGURE 25–44 Molluscum contagiosum. A focus of verrucous epidermal hyperplasia contains numerous cells with ellipsoid cytoplasmic inclusions (molluscum bodies) within the stratum granulosum and stratum corneum.

IMPETIGO

Impetigo is a common superficial bacterial infection of the skin. It is highly contagious and is frequently seen in otherwise healthy children as well as occasionally in adults in poor health. Two forms exist, classically referred to as impetigo contagiosa and impetigo bullosa; they differ from each other simply by the size of the pustules. Over the past decade, a remarkable shift in the etiologic agent has been observed. Whereas in the past impetigo contagiosa was almost exclusively caused by group A beta-hemolytic streptococci and impetigo bullosa by *Staphylococcus aureus,* all cases of impetigo nowadays tend to be caused by the latter.[132,133]

The infection usually involves exposed skin, particularly that of the face and hands. Initially it is an erythematous macule, but multiple small pustules rapidly supervene. As pustules break, shallow erosions form, covered with drying serum, giving the characteristic clinical appearance of *honey-colored crust.* If the crust is not removed, new lesions form about the periphery and extensive epidermal damage may ensue. A bullous form of impetigo occurs in children.

Morphology. The characteristic microscopic feature of impetigo is accumulation of neutrophils beneath the stratum corneum, often with the formation of a subcorneal pustule. Special stains reveal the presence of bacteria in these foci. Nonspecific, reactive epidermal alterations and superficial dermal inflammation accompany these findings. Rupture of pustules results in superficial layering of serum, neutrophils, and cellular debris to form the characteristic crust. Blistering lesions may show accumulation of fluid and neutrophils beneath the stratum corneum.

It is of interest that the pathogenesis of blister formation in impetigo (as well as in staphylococcal scalded skin syndrome) is related to bacterial production of a toxin that specifically cleaves the desmoglein 1 molecule responsible for cell-to-cell adhesion within the uppermost epidermal layers[134] (recall that in pemphigus foliaceus, which also exhibits a similar plane of blister formation, desmoglein 1 is compromised not by a toxin but by an autoantibody).

SUPERFICIAL FUNGAL INFECTIONS

As opposed to deep fungal infections of the skin, where the dermis or sub-cutis is primarily involved, superficial fungal infections of the skin are confined to the stratum corneum, and are caused primarily by dermatophytes. These organisms grow in the soil and on animals and produce a number of diverse and characteristic clinical lesions.

Tinea capitis usually occurs in children and is only rarely seen in infants and adults. It is a dermatophytosis of the scalp characterized by asymptomatic, often hairless patches of skin associated with mild erythema, crust formation, and scale. *Tinea barbae* is a dermatophyte infection of the beard area that affects adult men; it is a relatively uncommon disorder. *Tinea corporis,* on the other hand, is a common superficial fungal infection of the body surface that affects persons of all ages, but particularly children. Predisposing factors include excessive heat and humidity, exposure to infected animals, and chronic dermatophytosis of the feet or nails. The most common type of tinea corporis is an expanding, round, slightly erythematous plaque with an elevated scaling border (Fig. 25–45*A*). *Tinea cruris* occurs most frequently in the inguinal areas of obese men during warm weather. Heat, friction, and maceration all predispose to its development. The infection usually first appears on the upper inner thighs, with gradual extension of moist, red patches that have raised, scaling borders. *Tinea pedis (athlete's foot)* affects 30% to 40% of the population at some time in their lives. There is diffuse erythema and scaling, often initially localized to the web spaces. Most of the inflammatory tissue reaction, however, has recently been shown to be the result of bacterial superinfection and not directly related to the primary dermatophytosis.[135] Spread to or primary infection of the nails is referred to as *onychomycosis.* This produces discoloration, thickening, and deformity of the nail plate. *Tinea versicolor* usually occurs on the upper trunk and is highly distinctive in appearance. Caused by *Malassezia furfur,* a yeast rather than a dermato-

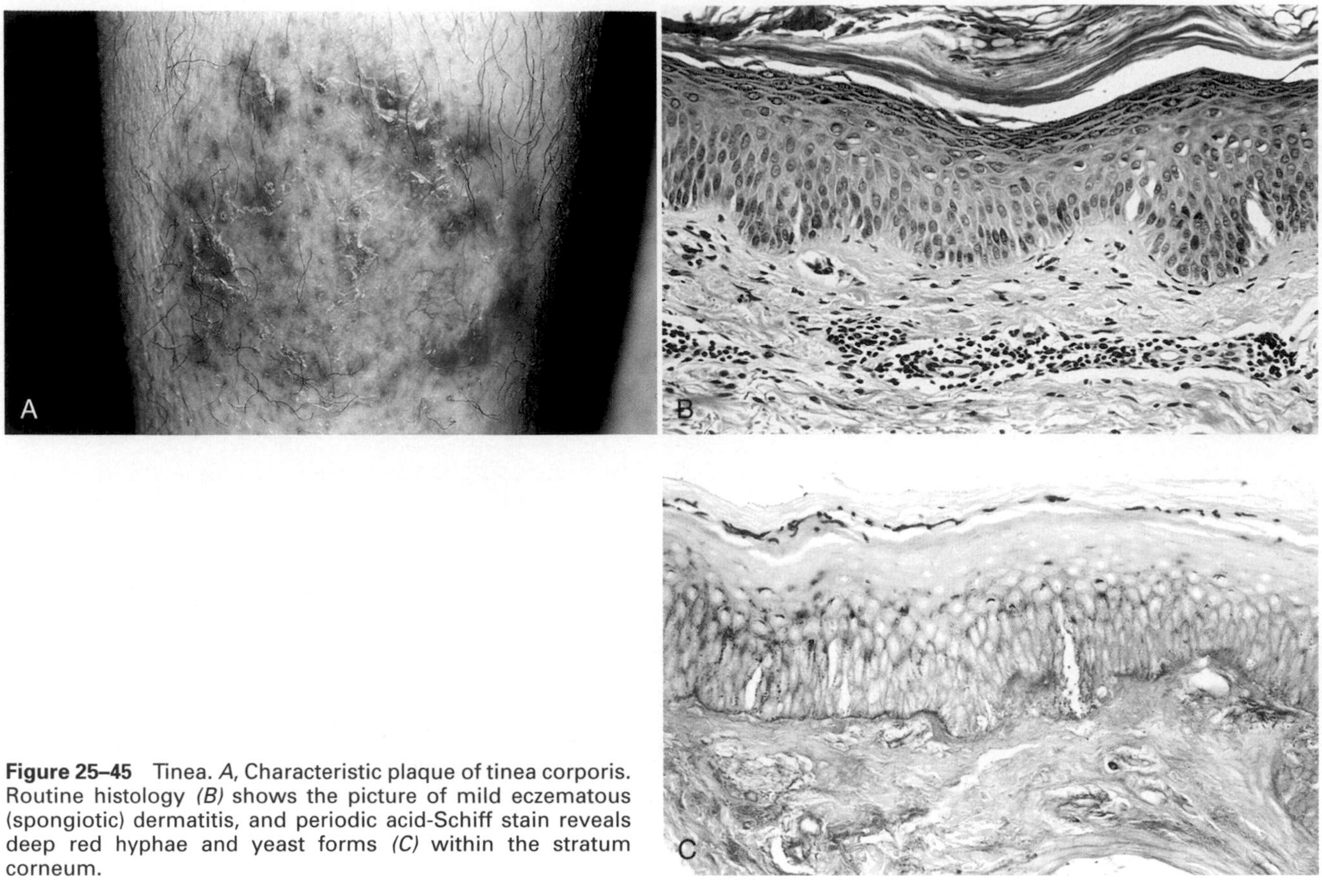

Figure 25–45 Tinea. *A*, Characteristic plaque of tinea corporis. Routine histology *(B)* shows the picture of mild eczematous (spongiotic) dermatitis, and periodic acid-Schiff stain reveals deep red hyphae and yeast forms *(C)* within the stratum corneum.

phyte, the lesions consist of groups of macules of all sizes, lighter or darker than surrounding skin, with a fine peripheral scale.

Morphology. The histologic features of all dermatophytoses are variable, depending on the antigenic properties of the organism, the corresponding host response, and the degree of bacterial superinfection. The histology may take the form of a mild eczematous dermatitis (Fig. 25–45*B*). Fungal cell walls, rich in mucopolysaccharides, stain bright pink to red with PAS stain. They are present in the anucleate cornified layer of lesional skin, hair, or nails (Fig. 25–45*C*), and scraping of these areas and subsequent culture of organisms will usually produce colonies that permit definitive classification of the offending species.

ARTHROPOD BITES, STINGS, AND INFESTATIONS

Arthropods are ubiquitous, and we all are susceptible to the bites, stings, and other discomforts they cause. The arthropods include *Arachnida* (spiders, scorpions, ticks, and mites), *Insecta* (lice, bedbugs, bees, wasps, fleas, flies, and mosquitoes), and *Chilopoda* (centipedes). All can cause skin lesions, but there is a wide variability in clinical patterns of reaction. Some persons suffer minimal symptoms, others considerable discomfort, and some may die as a consequence of a bite or sting. Arthropods can produce lesions in several ways: (1) by direct irritant effects of insect parts or secretions; (2) by immediate or delayed hypersensitivity responses (including an anaphylactic reaction) to retained or injected body parts or secretions; (3) by specific effects of venoms (e.g., the black widow spider venom produces severe cramps and excruciating pain; the brown recluse spider venom contains potent enzymes that produce tissue necrosis); and (4) by serving as vectors for secondary invaders, such as viruses, bacteria, rickettsiae, and parasites.

Macroscopically, arthropod bites may be urticarial or inflamed papules and nodules, sometimes with ulceration. Individual lesions may last for several weeks. In the case of the tick bite caused by *Ixodes dammini*, the vector for the spirochete that causes Lyme disease (Chapter 8), a characteristic expanding, erythematous plaque (erythema chronicum migrans) develops. Such extensive necrosis may result from the bite of the brown recluse spider that radical surgical excision of the involved area is necessary. *Pediculosis* is caused by the head louse, crab louse, and body louse. The disease is pruritic, and the louse, or its eggs, attached to hair shafts can usually be seen with the unaided eye (Fig. 25–46*A*). In pediculosis of the scalp, impetigo and enlarged cervical lymph nodes may be frequent complications, especially in children. The pubic louse may be transmitted through sexual contact. Infection with the body louse (vagabond's disease) is usually characterized by areas of hyperpigmentation and scratch marks (excoriations). *Scabies* is a contagious, pruritic dermatosis

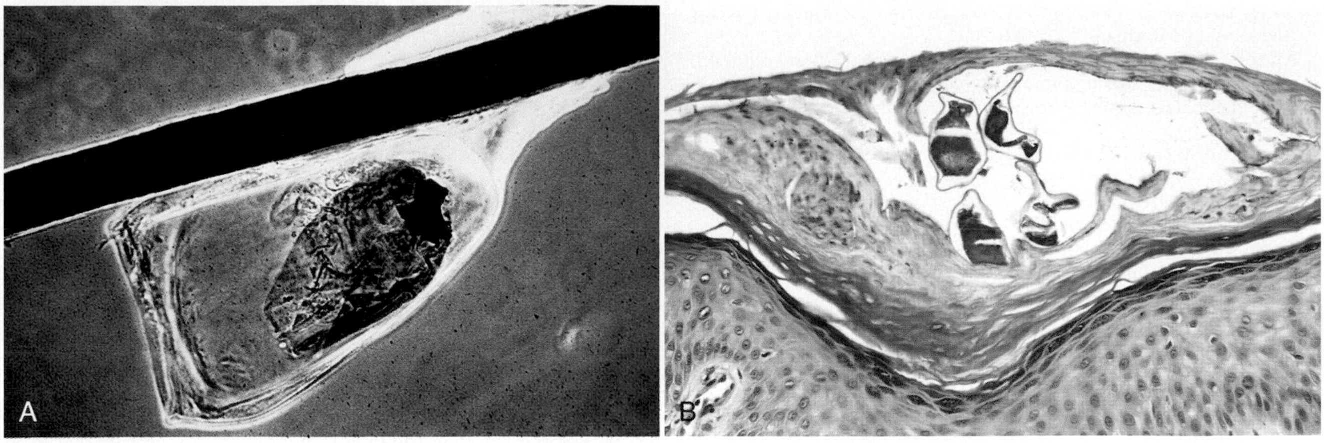

FIGURE 25–46 *A*, Pediculosis. Egg case (nit) of head louse attached to hair shaft. *B*, Portions of a scabies mite within a burrow involving the stratum corneum.

caused by the mite *Sarcoptes scabiei.* The female mite burrows under the stratum corneum (Fig. 25–46*B*), producing burrows (linear, poorly defined streaks, 0.2 to 0.6 cm in length) on the interdigital skin, palms, wrists, periareolar skin of women, and genital skin of men.

Morphology. The histologic picture of arthropod bites is highly varied. The classic lesion shows a wedge-shaped perivascular infiltrate of lymphocytes, histiocytes, and eosinophils within the dermis. There may be a central zone of exceedingly focal epidermal necrosis, directly under which birefringent insect mouthparts may be found (the site of the bite is called the *punctum*). In some bites, a primarily urticarial reaction is seen histologically, whereas in others the inflammatory infiltrate is so florid and dense that it may superficially resemble a cutaneous lymphoma. Spongiosis, resulting in intraepidermal blisters, is present in some biopsy specimens, and in certain settings, insect bites even resemble bullous pemphigoid.

Careful correlation with a clinical history of exposure to insects and the clinical finding of clustered or linear lesions facilitate the clinicopathologic diagnosis.

REFERENCES

1. Virchow R: Cellular Pathology. London, John Churchill, 1860, p 33.
2. Williams IR, Kupper TS: Immunity at the surface: homeostatic mechanisms of the skin immune system. Life Sci 58:1485, 1996.
3. Murphy GF: The secret of "NIN," a novel neural immunological network potentially integral to immunologic function in human skin. In Nickoloff BJ (ed): Mast Cells, Macrophages and Dendritic Cells in Skin Disease. Boca Raton, FL, CRC Press, 1993, pp 227–244.
4. Johnson KO: The roles and functions of cutaneous mechanoreptors. Curr Opin Neurobiol 11:455, 2001.
5. Lavker RM, et al: Hair follicle stem cells. J Investig Dermatol Symp Proc 8:28, 2003.
6. Deguchi M, et al: 12E2: a cloned murine dermal cell with features of dermal dendrocytes and capacity to produce pathologic changes resembling early Kaposi's sarcoma Am J Pathol 163:1817, 2003.
7. Fishman P, et al: Autoantibodies to tyrosinase: the bridge between melanoma and vitiligo. Cancer 79:1461, 1997.
8. Le Poole IC, et al: Presence of T cells and macrophages in inflammatory vitiligo skin parallels melanocyte disappearance. Am J Pathol 148:1219, 1996.
9. Mandelcorn-Monson RL, et al: Cytotoxic T lymphocyte reactivity to gp100, MelanA/MART-1, and tyrosinase, in HLA-A2-positive vitiligo patients. J Invest Dermatol 121:550, 2003.
10. Norris W: A case of fungoid disease. Edinburgh Med Surg J 16:562, 1820.
11. Clark WH Jr, et al: Origin of familial malignant melanomas from heritable melanotic lesions: the BK mole syndrome. Arch Dermatol 114:732, 1978.
12. Kamb A, Herlyn M: Malignant melanoma. In Vogelstein B, Kinzler K (eds.): The Genetic Basis of Human Cancer, New York, McGraw-Hill, 2002, pp 515–525.
13. Greene MH: Genetics of cutaneous melanoma and nevi [review]. Mayo Clin Proc 72:467, 1997.
14. Monzon J, et al: *CDKN2A* mutations in multiple primary melanomas. N Engl J Med 338:879, 1998.
15. Greene MH, et al: The high risk of melanoma in melanoma prone families with dysplastic nevi. Ann Intern Med 102:458, 1985.
16. van Duinen CM, et al: The distribution of cellular adhesion molecules in pigmented skin lesions. Cancer 73:2131, 1994.
17. Hussein MR, Wood GS: Molecular aspects of melanocytic dysplastic nevi. J Mol Diagn 4:71, 2002.
18. Shannon JA, Kefford RF, Mann GJ: Responses to ultraviolet-B in cell lines from hereditary melanoma kindreds. Melanoma Res 11:1, 2001.
19. Clark WH, et al: A study of tumor progression: the precursor lesions of superficial spreading and nodular melanoma. Hum Pathol 15:1147, 1985.
20. Crowson AN, et al: The precursors of malignant melanoma. Recent Results Cancer Res 160:75, 2002.
21. Weedon D: Lentigines, nevi, and melanomas. In Weedon D: Skin Pathology, 2nd ed. Edinburgh, Churchill Livingstone, 2002, pp 803–858.
22. Breslow A: Prognosis in cutaneous melanoma: tumor thickness as a guide to treatment. Pathol Annu 15:1, 1980.
23. Kim JC, Murphy GF: Dysplastic melanocytic nevi and prognostically indeterminate nevomelanocytic proliferations ("PINM Tumors"), In Clinics in Laboratory Medicine, Philadelphia, WB Saunders, 2000, pp 691–712.
24. Elder DE, Murphy GF: Melanocytic tumors of the skin. In Rosai J, Sobin LH (eds.): Atlas of Tumor Pathology, Third Series, Fascicle 1. Washington, DC, Armed Forces Institute of Pathology, 1991, pp. 183–185.
25. Clark WH Jr, et al: Model predicting survival in stage I melanoma based on tumor progression. J Natl Cancer Inst 81:1893, 1989.
26. Balch CM, et al: Final version of the American Joint Committee on Cancer staging system for cutaneous melanoma. Clin Oncol 15:3635, 2001.
27. Chen M, et al: Acantholytic variant of seborrheic keratosis. J Cutan Pathol 17:27, 1990.
28. Ellis DL, et al: Melanoma, growth factors, acanthosis nigricans, the sign of Leser-Trélat, and multiple acrochordons. A possible role for alpha-transforming growth factor in cutaneous paraneoplastic syndromes. N Engl J Med 317:1582, 1987.

29. Torley D, Bellus GA, Munro CS: Genes, growth factors and acanthosis nigricans. Br J Dermatol 147:1096, 2002.
30. Murphy GF, Elder D: Non-melanocytic tumors of the skin. In Rosai J, Sobin LH (eds.): Atlas of Tumor Pathology, Third Series, Fascicle 1. Washington, DC, Armed Forces Institute of Pathology, 1991, pp 61–154.
31. Hanssen AM, Fryns JP: Cowden syndrome. J Med Genet 32:117, 1995.
32. LeBoit PE: Can we understand keratoacanthoma? Am J Dermatopathol 24:116, 2002.
33. Perez MI, et al: *P53* oncoprotein expression and gene mutations in some keratoacanthomas. Arch Dermatol 133:189, 1997.
34. Matsumura Y, Ananthaswamy HN: Short-term and long-term cellular and molecular events following UV irradiation of skin: implications for molecular medicine. Expert Rev Mol Med 4:1, 2002.
35. Penn I: Neoplastic consequences of transplantation and chemotherapy. Cancer Detect Prev 1 (suppl):149, 1987.
36. Duthie MS, Kimber I, Norval M: The effects of ultraviolet radiation on the human immune system. Br J Dermatol 140:995, 1999.
37. Beissert S, Schwarz T: Mechanisms involved in ultraviolet light-induced immunosuppression. J Investig Dermatol Symp Proc 4:61, 1999.
38. Lu S, et al: No evidence of human papillomavirus DNA in actinic keratosis. Arch Dermatol Res 287:649, 1995.
39. Green CL, Khavari PA: Targets for molecular therapy of skin cancer. Semin Cancer Biol 14:63, 2004.
40. Bale AE: The nevoid basal cell carcinoma syndrome: genetics and mechanism of carcinogenesis. Cancer Invest 15:180, 1997.
41. Al-Ghazal SK, et al: Merkel cell carcinoma of the skin. Br J Plast Surg 49:491, 1996.
42. Miller DL, Weinstock MA: Nonmelanoma skin cancer in the United States: incidence. J Am Acad Dermatol 30:774, 1994.
43. Ries LAG, et al: SEER Cancer Statistics Review, 1993–1997. Bethesda, MD, National Cancer Institute, 2000.
44. Tsao H: Update on familial cancer syndromes and the skin. J Am Acad Dermatol 42:939, 2000.
45. Gorlin RJ, Goltz RW: Multiple nevoid basal-cell epithelioma, jaw cysts and bifid rib: a syndrome. N Engl J Med 262:908, 1962.
46. Mirowski GW, et al: Nevoid basal cell carcinoma syndrome. J Am Acad Dermatol 43:1092, 2000.
47. Rees J: Skin cancer. In B Vogelstein,KW Kinzler: The Genetic Basis of Human Cancer, New York, McGraw-Hill, 2002, pp 539–548.
48. Hahn H, et al: Mutations of the human homologue of *Drosophila* patched in the nevoid basal cell carcinoma syndrome. Cell 85:841, 1996.
49. Bonifas JM, et al: Activation of expression of hedgehog target genes in basal cell carcinoma. J Invest Dermatol 116:739, 2001.
50. Cohen MM, Jr: The hedgehog signaling network. Am J Med Genet 123A:5, 2003.
51. Nilsson M, et al: Induction of basal cell carcinomas and trichoepitheliomas in mice overexpressing GLI1. Proc Natl Acad Sci U S A 97:3438, 2000.
52. Bale AE, Yu K-P: The hedgehog pathway and basal cell carcinomas. Hum Mol Genet 10:757, 2001.
53. Kim MY, et al: Mutations of the *p53* and *PTCH* gene in basal cell carcinomas: UV mutation signature and strand bias. J Dermatol Sci 29:1, 2002.
54. Lacour JP: Carcinogenesis of basal cell carcinomas: genetics and molecular mechanisms. Br J Dermatol 146 (Suppl) 61:17, 2002.
55. D'Errico M, et al: UV mutation signature in tumor suppressor genes involved in skin carcinogenesis in xeroderma pigmentosum patients. Oncogene 19:463, 2000.
56. Einspahr JG, Bowden GT, Alberts DS: Skin cancer chemoprevention: strategies to save our skin. Recent Results Cancer Res 163:151, 2003.
57. Ortonne JP: From actinic keratosis to squamous cell carcinoma. Br J Dermatol 146 (Suppl) 61:20, 2002.
58. Soenge H, Ananthaswamy HN: Mechanisms of induction of skin cancer by UV radiation. Frontiers Biosci 2:538, 1997.
59. Majewski S, et al: Epidermodysplasia verruciformis. Immunological and nonimmunological surveillance mechanisms: role in tumor progression. Clin Dermatol 15:321, 1997.
60. Chin L: The genetics of malignant melanoma: lessons from mouse and man. Nat Rev Cancer 3:559, 2003.
61. Hayward NK: Genetics of melanoma predisposition. Oncogene 22:3053, 2003.
62. Piepkorn M: Melanoma genetics: an update with focus on the *CDKN2A(p16)/ARF* tumor suppressors. J Am Acad Dermatol 42:705, 2000.
63. Chin L, et al: Malignant melanoma: modern black plague and genetic black box. GenesDevelop 12:3467, 1998.
64. Cannon-Albright LA, et al: Assignment of a locus for familial melanoma, MLM, to chromosome 9p13-p22. Science 258:1148, 1992.
65. Kannengiesser C, et al: CDKN2A as a uveal and cutaneous melanoma susceptibility gene. Genes Chromosomes Cancer 38:265, 2003.
66. Sharpless NE, Chin L: The *INK4/ARF* locus and melanoma. Oncogene 22:3092, 2003.
67. Hussussian CJ, et al: Germline *p16* mutations in familial melanoma. Nature Genet 8:15, 1994.
68. Houghton AN, Polsky D: Focus on melanoma. Cancer Cell 2:275, 2002.
69. Pavey SJ, et al: Loss of *p16* expression is associated with histological features of melanoma invasion. Melanoma Res 12:539, 2002.
70. Pomerantz J, et al: The *INK4a* tumor suppressor gene product, p19ARF, interacts with MDM2 and neutralizes MDM2's inhibition of *p53.* Cell 92:713, 1998.
71. Rizos H, et al: A melanoma-associated germline mutation in exon 1 β inactivates p14ARF. Oncogene 20:5543, 2001.
72. Randerson-Moor JA, et al: A germline deletion of *p14ARF* but not *CDKN2A* in a melanoma-neural system tumour syndrome family. Hum Mol Genet 10:55, 2001.
73. Soufir N, et al: Prevalence of *p16* and *CDK4* germline mutations in 48 melanoma-prone families in France. The French Familial Melanoma Study Group. Hum Mol Genet 7:209, 1998.
74. Davies H, et al: Mutations of the *BRAF* gene in human cancer. Nature 417:949, 2002.
75. Pollock PM, et al: High frequency of *BRAF* mutations in nevi. Nat Genet 33:19, 2002.
76. Dong J, et al: *BRAF* oncogenic mutations correlate with progression rather than initiation of human melanoma. Cancer Res 63:3883, 2003.
77. Calonje E: Is cutaneous benign fibrous histiocytoma dermatofibroma a reactive inflammatory process or a neoplasm? Histopathology 37:278, 2000.
78. Zegler BG, et al: Dermatofibroma (fibrous histiocytoma): an inflammatory or neoplastic disorder? Histopathology 38:379, 2001.
79. Lever WF, Schaumburg-Lever G: Histopathology of the Skin. Philadelphia, JB Lippincott, 1997, p 593.
80. Laman JD, et al: Langerhans-cell histiocytosis 'insight into DC biology'. Trends Immunol 24:190, 2003.
81. Berger CL, Edelson RL: Current concepts of the immunobiology and immunotherapy of cutaneous T cell lymphoma: insights gained through cross-talk between the clinic and the bench. Leuk Lymphoma 44:1697, 2003.
82. Uchiyama T: Human T cell leukemia virus type I (HTLV-1) and human disease. Ann Rev Immunol 15:15, 1997.
83. Bakels V, et al: Immunophenotyping and gene rearrangement analysis provide additional criteria to differentiate between cutaneous T-cell lymphomas and pseudo-T-cell lymphomas. Am J Pathol 150:1941, 1997.
84. Longley BJ, et al: Somatic c-*KIT* activating mutation in urticaria pigmentosa and aggressive mastocytosis: establishment of clonality in a human mast cell neoplasm. Nat Genet 12:312, 1996.
85. Longley BJ, et al: Chronically *KIT*-stimulated clonally derived human mast cells show heterogeneity in different tissue microenvironments. J Invest Dermatol 108:792, 1997.
86. Nettis E, et al: Clinical and aetiological aspects in urticaria and angio-oedema. Br J Dermatol 148:501, 2003.
87. Schon MP, Zollner TM, Boehncke WH: The molecular basis of lymphocyte recruitment to the skin: clues for pathogenesis and selective therapies of inflammatory disorders. J Invest Dermatol 121:951, 2003.
88. Haas N, Hermes B, Henz BM: Adhesion molecules and cellular infiltrate: histology of urticaria. J Investig Dermatol Symp Proc 6:137, 2001.
89. Murphy GF, et al: Topical tretinoin replenishes CD1a-positive epidermal Langerhans cells in chronically photodamaged human skin. J Cutan Pathol 25:30,1998.
90. Steinhoff M, et al: Modern aspects of cutaneous neurogenic inflammation. Arch Dermatol 139:1479, 2003.

91. Egan CL, et al: Characterization of unmyelinated axons uniting epidermal and dermal immune cells in primate and murine skin. J Cutan Pathol 25:20, 1998.
92. Murphy GF, et al: Reaction patterns in the skin and special dermatologic techniques. In Moschella S (ed): Dermatology. Philadelphia, WB Saunders, 1984, p 104.
93. Sackstein R, Messina JL, Elfenbein GJ: In vitro adherence of lymphocytes to dermal endothelium under shear stress: implications in pathobiology and steroid therapy of acute cutaneous GVHD. Blood 101:771, 2003.
94. Binet I, Wood KJ: In vivo models of inflammation: immune rejection and skin transplantation in vivo. Methods Mol Biol 225:239, 2003.
95. Murphy GF, et al: Cytotoxic T lymphocytes and phenotypically abnormal epidermal dendritic cells in fixed cutaneous eruptions. Hum Pathol 16:1264, 1985.
96. Gilliam A, et al: Apoptosis is the predominant form of epithelial target cell injury in acute experimental graft-versus-host disease. J Invest Dermatol 107:377, 1996.
97. Kim JC, et al: Novel expression of vascular cell adhesion molecule-1 (CD106) by squamous epithelium in experimental acute graft-versus-host disease. Am J Pathol 161:763, 2002.
98. de Jong EM: Psoriasis of the nails associated with disability in a large number of patients: results of a recent interview with 1,728 patients. Dermatology 193:300, 1996.
99. Gudjonsson JE, et al: Immunopathogenic mechanisms in psoriasis. Clin Exp Immunol 135:1, 2004.
100. Bowcock AM, Cookson WO: The genetics of psoriasis, psoriatic arthritis and atopic dermatitis. Hum Mol Genet 13 (Suppl 1):R43, 2004.
101. Kreuger G, Callis K: Potential of tumor necrosis factor inhibitors in psoriasis and psoriatic arthritis. Arch Dermatol 140:218, 2004.
102. Schechtman RC, et al: HIV and *Malassezia* yeasts: a quantitative study of patients presenting with seborrheic dermatitis. Br J Dermatol 133:694, 1995.
103. Gupta A, Bluhm R: Seborrheic dermatitis. J Eur Acad Dermatol Venereol 18:13, 2004.
104. Hay RJ, Graham-Brown RA: Dandruff and seborrheic dermatitis: causes and management. Clin Exp Dermatol 22:3, 1997.
105. Fischer M, et al: Skin function and skin disorders in Parkinson's disease. J Neural Transm 108:205, 2001.
106. Franck JM, Young AW Jr: Squamous cell carcinoma in situ arising within lichen planus of the vulva. Dermatol Surg 21:890, 1995.
107. Iijima W, et al: Infiltrating CD8+ T cells in oral lichen planus predominantly express CCR5 and CXCR3 and carry respective chemokine ligands RANTES/CCL5 and IP-10/CXCL10 in their cytolytic granules: a potential self-recruiting mechanism. Am J Pathol 163:261, 2003.
108. Maddison PJ: Is it SLE? Best Pract Res Clin Rheumatol 16:167, 2002.
109. Boumpas DT, et al: Systemic lupus erythematosus: emerging concepts. Part 2: Dermatologic and joint disease, the antiphospholipid antibody syndrome, pregnancy and hormonal therapy, morbidity and mortality, and pathogenesis. Ann Intern Med 123:42, 1995.
110. Hashimoto T: Recent advances in the study of the pathophysiology of pemphigus. Arch Dermatol Res 295 (Suppl 1):S2, 2003.
111. Hacker-Foegen MK, et al: Pathogenicity and epitope characteristics of anti-desmoglein-1 from pemphigus foliaceus patients expressing only IgG1 autoantibodies. J Invest Dermatol 121:1373, 2003.
112. Koch PJ, et al: Targeted disruption of the pemphigus vulgaris antigen (desmoglein 3) gene in mice causes loss of keratinocyte cell adhesion with a phenotype similar to pemphigus vulgaris. J Cell Biol 137:1091, 1997.
113. Xue W, Hashimoto K, Toi Y: Functional involvement of urokinase-type plasminogen activator receptor in pemphigus acantholysis. J Cutan Pathol 25:469, 1998.
114. Seishima M, et al: Pemphigus IgG induces expression of urokinase plasminogen activator receptor on the cell surface of cultured keratinocytes. J Invest Dermatol 10:650, 1997.
115. Hanakawa Y, et al: Expression of desmoglein 1 compensates for genetic loss of desmoglein 3 in keratinocyte adhesion. J Invest Dermatol 119:27, 2002.
116. Yeh SW, et al: Blistering disorders: diagnosis and treatment. Dermatol Ther 16:214, 2003.
117. Imber MJ, et al: The immunopathology of bullous pemphigoid. In Ahmed AR (ed): Clinics in Dermatology-Bullous Pemphigoid. Philadelphia, JB Lippincott, 1987, p 81.
118. Liu Z, et al: A major role for neutrophils in experimental bullous pemphigoid. J Clin Invest 100:1256, 1997.
119. Duhring L: Dermatitis herpetiformis. JAMA 250:212, 1983.
120. Bickle K, Roark TR, Hsu S: Autoimmune bullous dermatoses: a review. Am Fam Physician 65: 1861, 2002.
121. Mitsuhashi Y, Hashimoto I: Genetic abnormalities and clinical classification of epidermolysis bullosa. Arch Dermatol Res 295:529, 2003.
122. Mallipeddi R, et al: Dilemmas in distinguishing between dominant and recessive forms of dystrophic epidermolysis bullosa. Br J Dermatol 149:810, 2003.
123. Harper JC, Thiboutot DM: Pathogenesis of acne: recent research advances. Adv Dermatol 19:1–10, 2003.
124. Walton S, et al: Clinical, ultrasound and hormonal markers of androgenicity in acne vulgaris. Br J Dermatol 133:249, 1995.
125. Leyden JJ: New understandings of the pathogenesis of acne. J Am Acad Dermatol 32(pt 3):S15, 1995.
126. Miskin JE, et al: Propionibacterium acnes, a resident of lipid-rich human skin, produces a 33 kDa extracellular lipase encoded by gehA. Microbiology 143:1745, 1997.
127. Berson DS, Shalita AR: The treatment of acne: the role of combination therapies. J Am Acad Dermatol 32(pt 3):S31, 1995.
128. de Villiers EM: Papillomavirus and HPV typing. Clin Dermatol 15:199, 1997.
129. Hart WR: Vulvar intraepithelial neoplasia: historical aspects and current status. Int J Gynecol Pathol 20:16, 2001.
130. Majewski S, Jablonska S: Human papillomavirus-associated tumors of the skin and mucosa. J Am Acad Dermatol 36(pt 1):659, 1997.
131. Harris AJ, et al: A novel human papillomavirus identified in epidermodysplasia verruciformis. Br J Dermatol 136:587, 1997.
132. Sadick NS: Current aspects of bacterial infections of the skin. Dermatol Clin 15:341, 1997.
133. Darmstadt GL, Lane AT: Impetigo: an overview. Pediatr Dermatol 11:293, 1994.
134. Hanakawa Y, et al: Molecular mechanisms of blister formation in bullous impetigo and staphylococcal scalded skin syndrome. J Clin Invest 110:53, 2002.
135. Leyden JJ, Aly R: Tinea pedis. Semin Dermatol 12:280, 1993.

CHAPTER 26

Bones, Joints, and Soft Tissue Tumors

Andrew E. Rosenberg, MD

BONES

BONE MODELING AND REMODELING

BONE GROWTH AND DEVELOPMENT

DEVELOPMENTAL (GENETIC) AND ACQUIRED ABNORMALITIES IN BONE CELLS, MATRIX, AND STRUCTURE

Malformations and Diseases Caused by Defects in Nuclear Proteins and Transcription Factors

Diseases Caused by Defects in Hormones and Signal Transduction Mechanisms

Diseases Associated with Defects in Extracellular Structural Proteins

Type 1 Collagen Diseases (Osteogenesis Imperfecta)

Types 2, 10, and 11 Collagen Diseases

Diseases Associated with Defects in Folding and Degradation of Macromolecules

Mucopolysaccharidoses

Diseases Associated with Defects in Metabolic Pathways (Enzymes, Ion Channels, and Transporters)

Osteopetrosis

Diseases Associated with Decreased Bone Mass

Osteoporosis

Diseases Caused by Osteoclast Dysfunction

Paget Disease (Osteitis Deformans)

Diseases Associated with Abnormal Mineral Homeostasis

Rickets and Osteomalacia

Hyperparathyroidism

Renal Osteodystrophy

FRACTURES

OSTEONECROSIS (AVASCULAR NECROSIS)

INFECTIONS—OSTEOMYELITIS

Pyogenic Osteomyelitis

Tuberculous Osteomyelitis

Skeletal Syphilis

BONE TUMORS AND TUMOR-LIKE LESIONS

Bone-Forming Tumors

Osteoma

Osteoid Osteoma and Osteoblastoma

Osteosarcoma

Cartilage-Forming Tumors

Osteochondroma

Chondromas

Chondroblastoma

Chondromyxoid Fibroma

Chondrosarcoma

Fibrous and Fibro-Osseous Tumors

Fibrous Cortical Defect and Nonossifying Fibroma

Fibrous Dysplasia

Fibrosarcoma and Malignant Fibrous Histiocytoma

MISCELLANEOUS TUMORS

Ewing Sarcoma and Primitive Neuroectodermal Tumor (PNET)

Giant Cell Tumor

Metastatic Disease

JOINTS

ARTHRITIS

Osteoarthritis

Rheumatoid Arthritis

Juvenile Rheumatoid Arthritis

Seronegative Spondyloarthropathies
Ankylosing Spondyloarthritis
Reactive Arthritis
Psoriatic Arthritis
Infectious Arthritis
Suppurative Arthritis
Tuberculous Arthritis
Lyme Arthritis
Viral Arthritis
Gout and Gouty Arthritis
Calcium Pyrophosphate Crystal Deposition Disease (Pseudogout)
TUMORS AND TUMOR-LIKE LESIONS
Ganglion and Synovial Cyst
Pigmented Villonodular Synovitis and Giant Cell Tumor of Tendon Sheath
■ SOFT TISSUE TUMORS AND TUMOR-LIKE LESIONS
PATHOGENESIS AND GENERAL FEATURES
FATTY TUMORS
Lipoma
Liposarcoma
FIBROUS TUMORS AND TUMOR-LIKE LESIONS
Reactive Pseudosarcomatous Proliferations
Nodular Fasciitis
Myositis Ossificans
Fibromatoses
Superficial Fibromatosis (Palmar, Plantar, and Penile Fibromatoses)
Deep-Seated Fibromatosis (Desmoid Tumors)
Fibrosarcoma
FIBROHISTIOCYTIC TUMORS
Benign Fibrous Histiocytoma (Dermatofibroma)
Malignant Fibrous Histiocytoma
TUMORS OF SKELETAL MUSCLE
Rhabdomyosarcoma
TUMORS OF SMOOTH MUSCLE
Leiomyoma
Leiomyosarcoma
SYNOVIAL SARCOMA

BONES

Normal

The skeletal system is as vital to life as any organ system because of its essential roles in mechanical support and mineral homeostasis. Importantly, the skeleton also houses the hematopoietic elements, protects viscera, and determines body size and shape. The skeletal system is composed of 206 bones that vary in size and shape (tubular, flat, cuboid). The bones are interconnected by a variety of joints that allow for a wide range of movement while maintaining structural stability.

Bone is a type of connective tissue, and it is unique because it is one of the few tissues that normally undergo mineralization. Biochemically, it is defined by its distinctive admixture of inorganic elements (65%) and organic matrix (35%). The inorganic component, calcium hydroxyapatite $[10Ca{:}6(PO_4){:}(OH)_2]$, is the mineral that gives bone strength and hardness, and is the storehouse for 99% of the body's calcium, 85% of the body's phosphorus, and 65% of the body's sodium and magnesium. The formation of hydroxyapatite crystal in bone is a phase transformation from liquid to solid analogous to the conversion of water to ice. The process involves the initiation and induction of mineralization by the organic matrix and it is tightly regulated by numerous factors.[1] The rate of mineralization can vary, but normally there is a 12- to 15-day lag time between the formation of the matrix and its mineralization. Bone that is unmineralized is known as *osteoid.*

The organic component includes the cells of bone and the proteins of the matrix. The bone-forming cells include the osteoprogenitor cells, osteoblasts, and osteocytes. The generation and stimulation of these cells are regulated by cytokines and growth factors such as bone morphogenic proteins (BMPs), fibroblast growth factor (FGF), platelet-derived growth factor (PDGF), insulin-like growth factor, and transforming growth factor-β (TGF-β).[2]

- *Osteoprogenitor* cells are pluripotent mesenchymal stem cells that are located in the vicinity of all bony surfaces. When appropriately stimulated by growth factors such as bone morphogenic proteins, which are members of the TGF-β superfamily, they undergo cell division and produce offspring that differentiate into osteoblasts. The process of osteoblastic differentiation is initiated and governed by the transcription factor core binding factor a1, which activates osteoblast-specific gene expression.[3] The generation of osteoblasts from osteoprogenitor cells is vital to growth, remodeling, and repair of bone throughout life.
- *Osteoblasts and surface lining cells* are located on the surface of bone and synthesize, transport, and arrange

the many proteins of matrix detailed later (Fig. 26–1). They also initiate the process of mineralization. Osteoblasts express cell-surface receptors that bind many hormones (parathyroid hormone [PTH], vitamin D, and estrogen), cytokines, growth factors, and extracellular matrix proteins. Recently, the hormone leptin and low-density lipoprotein receptor-related protein 5 have been shown to play an important role in determining osteoblastic activity, and they may represent evidence of central nervous system and cell-autonomous control of bone mass, respectively.[4–6] Metabolically active osteoblasts have a life span of approximately 3 months and then either undergo apoptosis, become surrounded by matrix and transform into *osteocytes,* or become quiescent, flattened, bone surface–lining cells.

- *Osteocytes* are more numerous than any other bone-forming cell and outnumber osteoblasts by about 10:1. Although encased by bone, they communicate with each other and with surface cells via an intricate network of tunnels through the matrix known as *canaliculi.* The osteocytic cell processes traverse the canaliculi, and their contacts along gap junctions allow the transfer of surface membrane potentials and substrates. The large number of osteocytic processes and their distribution throughout bone tissue enable them to be the key cells in several biologic processes. Studies have shown that this network may be important in controlling the second-to-second fluctuations in serum calcium and phosphorus levels by altering the concentration of these minerals in the local extracellular fluid compartment. Osteocytes also can detect mechanical forces and translate them into biologic activity, including the release of chemical mediators by signal transduction pathways, which activate second messengers such as cyclic adenosine monophosphate (cAMP).[7]
- The *osteoclast* is the cell responsible for bone resorption. It is derived from hematopoietic progenitor cells that also give rise to monocytes and macrophages. Information regarding the molecular regulation of osteoclast formation in humans is limited. In mice, a number of transcription factors, including PU.1 and Fos, are essential for developing an osteoclast phenotype.[8] The cytokines and growth factors crucial for osteoclast differentiation and maturation in humans include interleukin (IL)-1, IL-3, IL-6, IL-11, tumor necrosis factor (TNF), granulocyte-macrophage colony-stimulating factor (GM-CSF), and macrophage colony-stimulating factor (M-CSF).[9] These factors work by either stimulating osteoclast progenitor cells or participating in a paracrine system in which osteoblasts and marrow stromal cells play a central role. This paracrine system is essential to bone metabolism, and its mediators include the molecules RANK (Receptor Activator for Nuclear factor κB), RANK ligand (RANKL), and osteoprotegerin (OPG).[9,10] RANK is a member of the TNF family of receptors expressed mainly on cells of macrophage/monocytic lineage such as preosteoclasts. When this receptor binds its specific ligand (RANKL) through cell-to-cell contact, osteoclastogenesis is initiated. RANKL is produced by and expressed on the cell membranes of osteoblasts and marrow stromal cells; its major role in bone metabolism is stimulation of osteoclast formation, fusion, differentiation, activation, and survival. The actions of RANKL can be blocked by another member of the TNF family of receptors, osteoprotegrin (OPG), which is a soluble protein produced by a number of tissues, including bone, hematopoietic marrow cells, and immune cells. OPG inhibits osteoclastogenesis by acting as a decoy receptor that binds to RANKL, thus preventing the interaction of RANK with RANKL. Therefore, interplay between bone cells and these molecules permits osteoblasts and stromal cells to control osteoclast development[10] (Fig. 26–2). This ensures the tight coupling of bone formation and resorption vital to the success of the skeletal system, and provides a mechanism for a wide variety of biologic mediators (hormones, cytokines, growth factors) to influence the homeostasis of bone tissue.

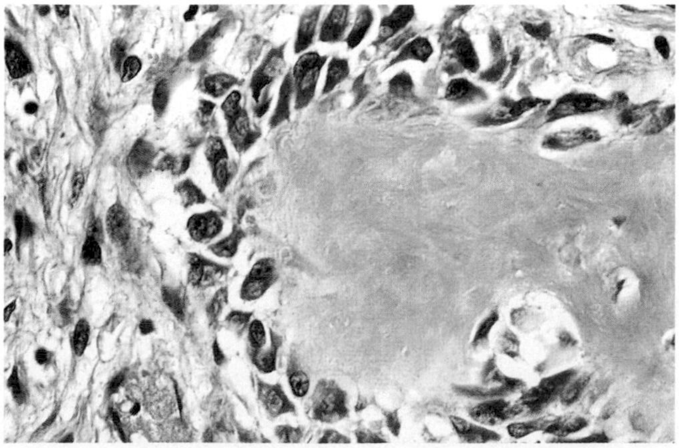

FIGURE 26–1 Active osteoblasts synthesizing bone matrix. The surrounding spindle cells represent osteoprogenitor cells.

Mature multinucleated osteoclasts (containing 6 to 12 nuclei) form from fusion of circulating mononuclear precursors and have a limited life span (approximately 2 weeks). They are intimately related to the bone surface (Fig. 26–3), where their activity is initiated by binding to matrix adhesion proteins. The scalloped *resorption pits* they produce, and frequently reside in, are known as *Howship lacunae.* The portion of the osteoclast cell membrane overlying the resorption surface is modified by numerous villous extensions, known as the *ruffled border,* which serve to increase the membrane surface area. The plasmalemma bordering this region is specialized and forms a seal with the underlying bone, preventing leakage of digestion products. This self-contained extracellular space is analogous to a secondary lysosome, and the osteoclast acidifies it with a hydrogen pump system that solubilizes the mineral. The osteoclast also releases into this space a multitude of enzymes that help disassemble the matrix proteins into amino acids and liberate and activate growth factors, cytokines, and enzymes (such as collagenase), which have been previously deposited and bound to the matrix by osteoblasts. *Thus, as bone is broken down to its elemental units, substances are released into the microenvironment that initiate its renewal* (Fig. 26–4).

- The *proteins of bone* include type 1 collagen and a family of noncollagenous proteins that are derived mainly from osteoblasts. Type 1 collagen forms the backbone of matrix and accounts for 90% of the weight of the organic component. Osteoblasts deposit collagen either in a random weave known as *woven bone* or in an orderly layered manner designated

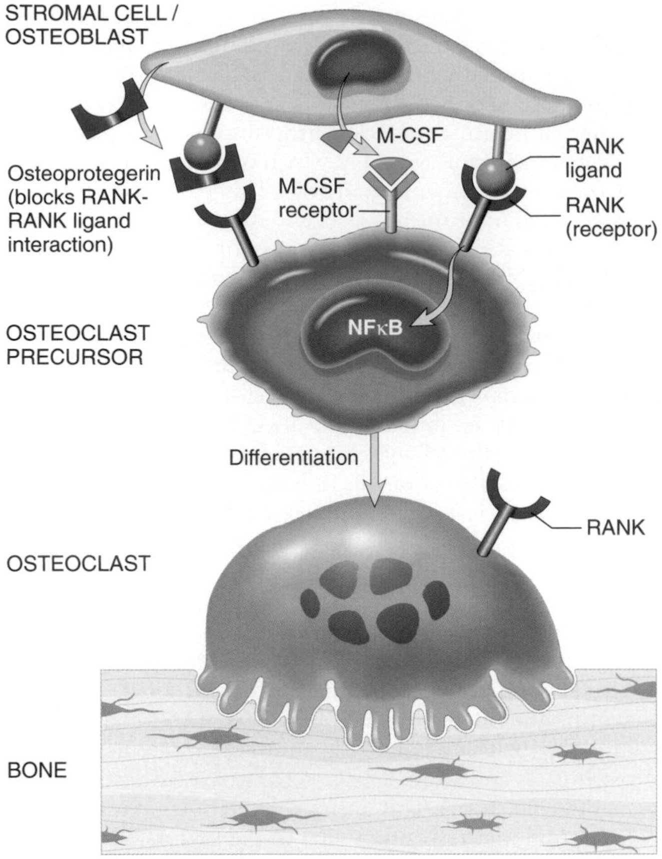

FIGURE 26–2 Paracrine molecular mechanisms that regulate osteoclast formation and function. Osteoclasts are derived from the same stem cells that produce macrophages. Osteoblast/stromal cell membrane–associated RANK ligand (RANKL) binds to its receptor RANK located on the cell surface of osteoclast precursors. This interaction in the background of macrophage colony-stimulating factor (M-CSF) causes the precursor cells to produce functional osteoclasts. Stromal cells also secrete osteoprotegerin (OPG) which acts as a decoy receptor for RANKL, preventing it from binding the RANK receptor on osteoclast precursors. Consequently OPG prevents bone resorption by inhibiting osteoclast differentiation.

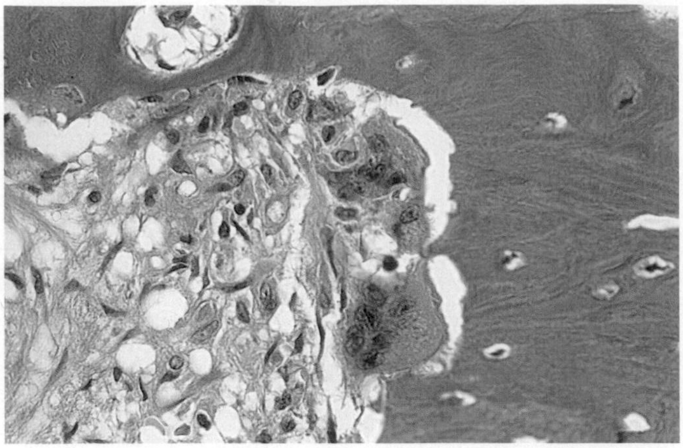

FIGURE 26–3 Two osteoclasts resorbing bone.

lamellar bone (Fig. 26–5). Normally, woven bone is seen in the fetal skeleton and is formed at growth plates. Its advantages are that it is produced quickly and resists forces equally from all directions. The presence of woven bone in the adult is always indicative of a pathologic state; however, it is not diagnostic of a particular disease. For instance, in circumstances requiring rapid reparative stability, such as a fracture, woven bone is produced. It is also formed around sites of infection and composes the matrix of bone-forming tumors. *Lamellar bone, which gradually replaces woven bone during growth, is deposited much more slowly and is stronger than woven bone.* There are four different types of lamellar bone. Three are present only in the cortex—circumferential, concentric, and interstitial (Fig. 26–6). The fourth type, trabecular lamellae, composes the bone trabeculae in which the lamellae are oriented parallel to the long axis of the trabeculum.

The noncollagenous proteins of bone are bound to the matrix and grouped according to their function as adhesion proteins, calcium-binding proteins, mineralization proteins, enzymes, cytokines, and growth factors (Table 26–1).[11] Of these, only osteocalcin is unique to bone. It is used as a sensitive and specific serum marker for osteoblast activity. Cytokines and growth factors control bone cell proliferation, maturation, and metabolism.[12] They serve an important messenger function in translating mechanical and metabolic signals into local bone cell activity and eventual skeletal adaptation. In this fashion the skeleton is uniquely able to change its structure in response to new physical forces; witness the repositioning of teeth by the forces of braces.

Bone Modeling and Remodeling

Osteoblasts and osteoclasts act in coordination and are considered the functional unit of bone known as the *basic multicellular unit* (BMU). The processes of bone formation and resorption are tightly coupled, and their balance determines skeletal mass at any point in time.[13] As the skeleton grows and enlarges (modeling), bone formation predominates. Once the skeleton has reached maturity, the breakdown and renewal of bone that are responsible for skeletal maintenance is called *remodeling* and is likely initiated at sites experiencing fatigue and microdamage. In adults, approximately 1 million BMUs are active at one time, and they *remodel*, or replace, 10% of the skeleton annually.

Peak bone mass is achieved in early adulthood after the cessation of modeling, and it is determined by a variety of factors, including the type of vitamin D receptor inherited, state of nutrition, level of physical activity, age, and hormonal status. Beginning in the fourth decade, however, the amount of bone resorbed by the BMUs exceeds that which has been formed, resulting in a steady decrease in skeletal mass. Eventually, this results in senescent osteoporosis, which is exacerbated in women by the rapid bone loss that occurs during the decade following menopause (postmenopausal osteoporosis).

Bone Growth and Development

The blueprint for skeletal morphogenesis is encoded in the *Homeobox genes*. Homeobox genes are a large family that encodes transcriptional regulators essential for growth and differentiation. Their expression occurs in a specific orderly and temporal sequence; in the skeletal system, their expression produces localized cellular condensations of prim-

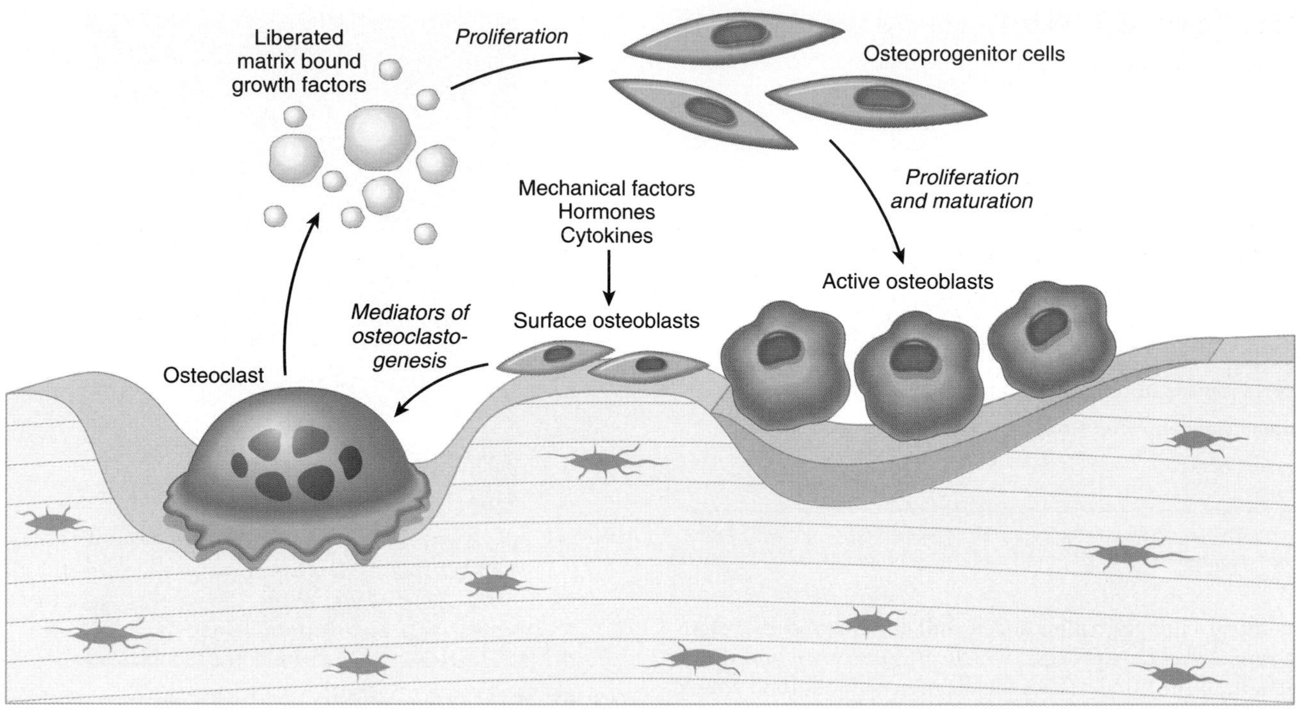

FIGURE 26–4 Bone resorption and formation are coupled processes that are controlled by systemic factors and local cytokines and growth factors, some of which are deposited in the bone matrix. Cytokines, growth factors, and signal-transducing molecules are key in the communication between osteoblasts and osteoclasts.

itive mesenchyme at the sites of future bones. These are the earliest precursors of bone and as such are vital to the formation of the skeleton.[13] The mesenchymal cells of the condensations are derived from the cranial neural crest (cranial facial skeleton), paraxial mesoderm (axial skeleton), and the lateral plate mesoderm (appendicular skeleton). Shortly after being formed, the mesenchymal cells in the condensations differentiate into chondrocytes and osteoblasts and manufacture cartilage and bone, respectively. Most bones are first formed as a cartilage model or anlage. Subsequently, around the eighth week of gestation, the process of *enchondral ossification* begins, and the cartilage in the center of the anlage undergoes

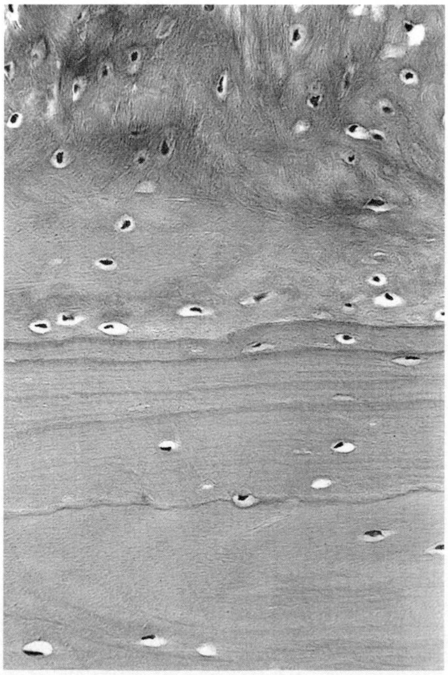

FIGURE 26–5 Woven bone *(top)* deposited on the surface of pre-existing lamellar bone *(bottom).*

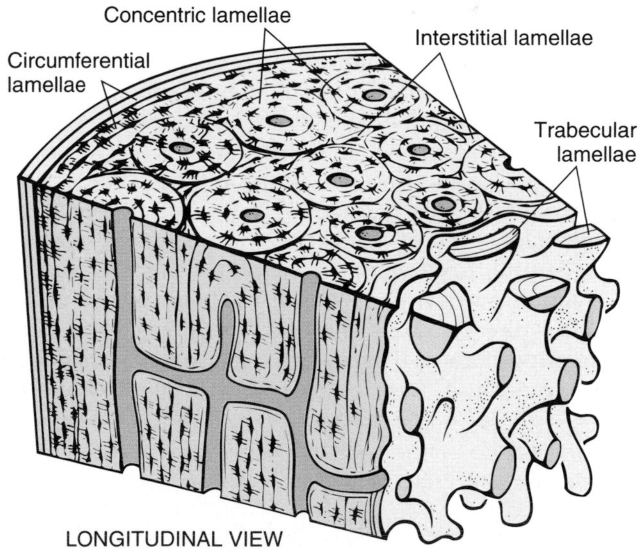

FIGURE 26–6 The schematic of normal bone structure reveals the subperiosteal and endosteal circumferential lamellae, concentric lamellae about vascular cores creating haversian systems, and the interstitial lamellae that fill the spaces in between the haversian systems. The trabecular lamellae extend from the endosteal surface. The individual lamellae are punctuated by osteocytic lacunae with their finely ramifying and interconnecting canals, which contain cell processes.

TABLE 26–1 Proteins of Bone Matrix

Osteoblast-Derived Proteins	
Type 1 collagen	
Cell adhesion proteins	
	Osteopontin, fibronectin, thrombospondin
Calcium-binding proteins	
	Osteonectin, bone sialoprotein
Proteins involved in mineralization	
	Osteocalcin
Enzymes	
	Collagenase, alkaline phosphatase
Growth factors	
	IGF-1, TGF-β, PDGF
Cytokines	
	Prostaglandins, IL-1, IL-6, RANKL
Proteins Concentrated from Serum	
β_2-microglobulin	
Albumin	

IGF, insulin-like growth factor; TGF, transforming growth factor; PDGF, platelet-derived growth factor; IL, interleukin; RANKL, RANK ligand.

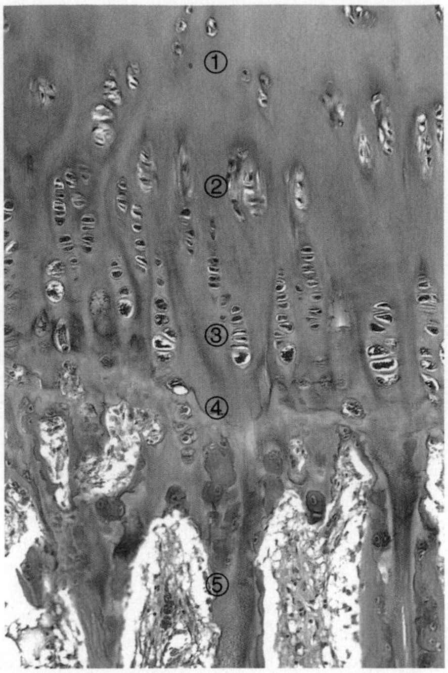

FIGURE 26–7 Active growth plate with ongoing enchondral ossification. *1,* Reserve zone. *2,* Zone of proliferation. *3,* Zone of hypertrophy. *4,* Zone of mineralization. *5,* Primary spongiosa.

degradative changes, mineralizes, and is removed by osteoclast-type cells. This process, which progresses up and down the length of the bone, allows for the ingrowth of blood vessels and osteoprogenitor cells that provide the bone-forming cells. Concurrently, the periosteum in the midshaft of the anlage produces osteoblasts that deposit the beginnings of the cortex. This region is known as the *primary center of ossification.* In the epiphyses, a similar sequence of events leading to the removal of cartilage occurs *(secondary center of ossification)* such that a plate of the cartilage model becomes entrapped between the expanding centers of ossification; this structure is known as the *physis,* or *growth plate* (Fig. 26–7). The chondrocytes within the growth plate undergo a series of events, including proliferation, growth, maturation, and necrosis. Important regulators of this sequence of chondrocyte growth and maturation are the *Indian hedgehog* gene and parathyroid hormone (PTH)–related protein (PTHRP).[5,9] Eventually, the cartilage matrix mineralizes and this acts as a signal for its resorption by osteoclasts; however, remnant struts persist and act as scaffolding for the deposition of bone on their surfaces. These structures, composed of a core of cartilage covered by a layer of bone, are known as *primary spongiosa.* The process of enchondral ossification also occurs at the base of articular cartilage, and by this mechanism bones increase in length and articular surfaces increase in diameter. In contrast, bones derived from *intramembranous formation,* such as the cranium and portions of the clavicles, are formed by osteoblasts directly from a fibrous layer of tissue derived from mesenchyme. Because bone tissue is made only by osteoblasts, the enlargement of bones is achieved only by the deposition of new bone on a pre-existing surface. This mechanism of *appositional growth* is key to understanding the facets of bone growth and modeling.

Pathology

The skeletal system is susceptible to circulatory, inflammatory, neoplastic, metabolic, and congenital disorders, similar to the other organ systems of the body. The complexity of its growth, development, and maintenance, and its relationships with other organ systems make the skeletal system unusually vulnerable to adverse influences. Not surprisingly, primary and secondary diseases of bone are varied and numerous.

Developmental (Genetic) and Acquired Abnormalities in Bone Cells, Matrix, and Structure

Developmental abnormalities of the skeleton are complex, variable, frequently genetically based, and first become manifest during the earliest stages of bone formation. In contrast, many of the acquired diseases are usually detected in adulthood.[12] Developmental anomalies resulting from localized problems in the migration of mesenchymal cells and their formation of condensations are known as *dysostoses.* They are usually limited to defined embryologic structures and may result from mutations in certain transcription factors (*Homeobox* genes). Mutations in the regulators of skeletal organogenesis, such as cellular signaling mechanisms (e.g., growth factors and their receptors), and matrix components (e.g., types 1 and 2 collagen), affect cartilage and bone tissues globally, and these disorders are known as *dysplasias*[12–15] (Chapter 10). Currently, the molecular–pathogenetic classification of genetic disorders is based on the functional properties of the involved gene or protein and includes: (1) defects in nuclear proteins and transcription factors, (2) defects in hormones and signal transduction mechanisms, (3) defects in extracellular structural proteins, (4) defects in folding and degradation of molecules, (5) defects in oncogenes and tumor suppressor genes, (6) defects in metabolic pathways (enzymes, ion channels transporters), and (7) defects in RNA and DNA processing and metabolism.[16] More than 200 different developmental disorders have been defined, some of which are listed in Table 26–2; their manifestations vary greatly and range from simple loss of a phalanx to fatal widespread deformities.

MALFORMATIONS AND DISEASES CAUSED BY DEFECTS IN NUCLEAR PROTEINS AND TRANSCRIPTION FACTORS

Congenital malformations or dysostoses of bone are relatively uncommon. The more simple anomalies include failure of development of a bone (e.g., congenital absence of a phalanx, rib, or clavicle), the formation of extra bones (supernumerary ribs or digits), the fusion of two adjacent digits (syndactyly), or the development of long, spider-like digits. Some of these result from defects in the formation of the mesenchymal condensations and their differentiation into the cartilage anlage. They are caused by genetic alterations that affect transcription factors, especially those coded for by the Homeobox genes, and certain cytokines.[12] An example of a defect in mesenchymal condensation is a mutation in the homeobox HOXD-13 transcription factor, which produces an extra digit between the third and fourth fingers as well as some degree of syndactyly.[13] Anomalies that affect the skull and vertebral column, such as *craniorachischisis* (failure of closure of the spinal column and skull), are frequently of great clinical importance. This defect produces a persistent opening through which the meninges and central nervous system herniate to produce a meningomyelocele or meningoencephalocele (Chapter 28).

DISEASES CAUSED BY DEFECTS IN HORMONES AND SIGNAL TRANSDUCTION MECHANISMS

Achondroplasia is the most common disease of the growth plate and is a major cause of dwarfism. Achondroplasia is an example of a disease that is caused by a defect in paracrine cell signaling, and it manifests as a reduction in the proliferation of the chondrocytes in the growth plate. Patients with this disorder have a point mutation (usually Arg for Gly375) in the gene that codes for FGF receptor 3 (FGFR3), which is located on the short arm of chromosome 4.[12] In the normal growth plate, activation of FGFR3 *inhibits* cartilage proliferation; in achondroplasia the mutation causes the receptor to be in a state of constant activation, thereby suppressing growth.

Achondroplasia is an autosomal dominant disorder; however, approximately 80% of cases represent new spontaneous mutations. Affected individuals have shortened proximal extremities, a trunk of relatively normal length, and an enlarged head with bulging forehead and conspicuous depression of the root of the nose. The skeletal abnormalities are usually not associated with changes in longevity, intelligence, or reproductive status.

Morphology. The histologic abnormalities in achondroplasia can be found in the growth plates. The zones of proliferation and hypertrophy are narrowed and disorganized and contain clusters of large chondrocytes instead of well-formed columns. At the base of the growth plate, there is premature deposition of horizontal struts of bone that seals the plate and prevents further growth. Appositional intramembranous bone formation is not disrupted; therefore the cortices form normally and appear thickened in relation to the short length of the bone.

Thanatophoric dwarfism is the most common lethal form of dwarfism and affects about 1 in every 20,000 live births. It is also caused by a mutation in FGFR3 that is either a missense mutation or a point mutation that is different from that in achondroplasia.[12] The affected patients have micromelic shortening of the limbs, frontal bossing with relative macrocephaly, a small chest cavity, and a bell-shaped abdomen. The underdeveloped thoracic cavity leads to respiratory insufficiency, and the patients frequently die at birth or soon after. The histologic changes in the growth plate show diminished proliferation of chondrocytes and poor columnization in the zone of proliferation.

DISEASES ASSOCIATED WITH DEFECTS IN EXTRACELLULAR STRUCTURAL PROTEINS

Many of the organic components of bone matrix have been only recently identified, and their interactions are far more complex than originally imagined. Therefore, this field of skeletal pathology is still in its early stages of discovery. Examples of the potential importance of abnormalities in bone matrix are the diseases associated with deranged metabolism of collagen. These result from mutations in the genes that code for the collagens that are important in bone and cartilage, including types 1, 2, 9, 10, and 11 (Chapter 3). Their clinical manifestations are variable and range from lethal disease to premature osteoarthritis.

Type 1 Collagen Diseases (Osteogenesis Imperfecta)

Osteogenesis imperfecta is a group of phenotypically related disorders that are caused by deficiencies in the synthesis of type 1 collagen. Although osteogenesis imperfecta, or brittle bone disease, has prominent skeletal manifestations, other anatomic structures rich in type I collagen, such as joints, eyes, ears, skin, and teeth, are affected as well. The genetic defects in osteogenesis imperfecta reside in mutations in the genes that code for the $\alpha1$ and $\alpha2$ chains of the collagen molecule,[17] and common ones are inherited in an autosomal dominant fashion. Mutations resulting in the production of qualitatively normal collagen that is synthesized in decreased amounts are associated with mild skeletal abnormalities. More severe or lethal phenotypes result from genetic defects producing abnormal polypeptide chains that cannot assemble into a triple helix configuration, which is required for functional collagen molecules.

Morphologically, *the basic abnormality in all forms of osteogenesis imperfecta is too little bone,* resulting in a type of osteoporosis with marked cortical thinning and attenuation of trabeculae. The clinical expression of osteogenesis imperfecta constitutes a spectrum of disorders that are all marked by extreme skeletal fragility. Four major subtypes have been rec-

TABLE 26–2 Molecular Genetics of Diseases of the Skeleton

Human Disorder	Gene Mutation	Affected Molecule	Phenotype
Defects in Transcription Factors Producing Abnormalities in Mesenchymal Condensation and Related Cell Differentiation			
Synpolydactyly	HOXD-13	Transcription factor	Extra digit with fusion
Waardenburg syndrome	PAX-3	Transcription factor	Hearing loss, abnormal pigmentation, craniofacial abnormalities
Greig syndrome	GL13	Transcription factor	Synpolydactyly, craniofacial abnormalities
Campomelic dysplasia	SOX9	Transcription factor	Sex reversal, abnormal skeletal development
Oligodontia	PAX9	Transcription factor	Congenital absence of teeth
Nail-patella syndrome	LMX1B	Transcription factor	Hypoplastic nails, hypoplastic or aplastic patellae, dislocated radial head, progressive nephropathy
Holt-Oram syndrome	TBX5	Transcription factor	Congenital abnormalities, forelimb anomalies
Ulnar-mammary syndrome	TBX3	Transcription factor	Hypoplasia or absent ulna, 3rd–5th digits, breast, and teeth, delayed puberty
Cleidocranial dysplasia	CBFA1	Transcription factor	Abnormal clavicles, wormian bones, supernumerary teeth
Defects in Extracellular Structural Proteins			
Osteogenesis imperfecta types 1–4	COL1A1 COL1A2	Type 1 collagen	Bone fragility, hearing loss, blue sclerae Dentinogenesis imperfecta
Achondrogenesis II	COL2A1	Type 2 collagen	Short trunk, severely shortened extremities, relatively enlarged cranium, flattened face
Hypochondrogenesis	COL2A1		Short trunk, shortened extremities, relatively enlarged cranium, flattened face
Stickler syndrome	COL2A1	Type 2 collagen	Myopia, retinal detachment, hearing loss, flattened face, premature osteoarthritis
Multiple epiphyseal dysplasia	COL9A2	Type 9 collagen	Short or normal stature, small epiphyses, early onset osteoarthritis
Schmid metaphyseal chondrodysplasia	COL10A1	Type 10 collagen	Mild short stature, bowing of lower extremities, coxa vara, metaphyseal flaring
Defects in Hormones and Signal Transduction Mechanisms Producing Abnormal Proliferation or Maturation of Chondrocytes and Osteoblasts			
Brachydactyly type C	CDMP1	Signaling molecule	Shortened metacarpals and phalanges
Jansen metaphyseal chondroplasia	PTHrp receptor	Receptor	Short bowed limbs, clinodactyly, facial abnormalities, hypercalcemia, hypophosphatemia
Achondroplasia	FGFR3	Receptor	Short stature, rhizomelic shortening of limbs, frontal bossing, midface deficiency
Hypochondroplasia	FGFR3	Receptor	Disproportionate short stature, micromelia, relative macrocephaly
Thanatophoric dwarfism	FGFR3	Receptor	Severe limb shortening and bowing, frontal bossing, depressed nasal bridge
Crouzon syndrome	FGFR2	Receptor	Craniosynostosis

Adapted from Mundlos S, Olsen BR: Heritable diseases of the skeleton. Part I: Molecular insights into skeletal development—transcription factors and signaling pathways. Faseb J 11:125–132, 1997; Mundlos S, Olsen BR: Heritable diseases of the skeleton. Part II: Molecular insights into skeletal development—matrix components and their homeostasis. Faseb J 11:227–233, 1997; Superti-Furga A, Bonafe L, Rimoin DL: Molecular-pathogenetic classification of genetic disorders of the skeleton. Am J Med Genet 106:282–293, 2001.

ognized (Table 26–3). The *type II variant* is at one end of the spectrum and is uniformly fatal in utero or during the perinatal period. It is characterized by extraordinary bone fragility with multiple fractures occurring when the fetus is still within the womb (Fig. 26–8). In contrast, the *type I form,* which is more often due to an acquired rather than an inherited mutation, permits a normal life span but with an increased number of fractures during childhood that decrease in frequency after puberty. Other findings include *blue sclerae* caused by a decrease in collagen content, making the sclera translucent and allowing partial visualization of the underlying choroid; *hearing loss* related to both a sensorineural deficit and impaired conduction owing to abnormalities in the bones of the middle and inner ear; and *dental imperfections* (small, misshapen, and blue-yellow teeth) secondary to a deficiency in dentin. In some variants, the skeleton fails to model properly, and there are persistent foci of hypercellular woven bone.[18] New and less well-characterized variants are still being identified. The recognition of particular variants and their modes of inheritance is important in genetic counseling.

Types 2, 10, and 11 Collagen Diseases

Types 2, 10, and 11 collagens are important structural components of hyaline cartilage. Mutations that result in their abnormal metabolism, although uncommon, produce a spectrum of disorders ranging from those that are fatal to those compatible with life but associated with early destruction of joints (see Table 26–2). More than 30 mutations have been identified in the type 2 collagen gene, and all have affected the triple helical component of the molecule. In severe disorders, the type 2 collagen molecules are not secreted by the chondrocytes, and insufficient bone formation occurs. In the milder phenotypes, a nonfunctioning or null collagen gene

TABLE 26–3 Osteogenesis Imperfecta

	Subtype	Inheritance	Collagen Defect	Major Clinical Features
OI I	Postnatal fractures, blue sclerae	Autosomal dominant	Decreased synthesis pro-α1(1) chain Abnormal pro-α1(1) or pro-α2(1) chains	Compatible with survival Normal stature Skeletal fragility Dentinogenesis imperfecta Hearing impairment Joint laxity Blue sclerae
OI II	Perinatal lethal	Most autosomal recessive Some autosomal dominant ?New mutations	Abnormally short pro-α1(1) chain Unstable triple helix Abnormal or insufficient pro-α2(1)	Death in utero or within days of birth Skeletal deformity with excessive fragility and multiple fractures Blue sclerae
OI III	Progressive deforming	Autosomal dominant (75%) Autosomal recessive (25%)	Altered structure of pro-peptides of pro-α2(1) Impaired formation of triple helix	Compatible with survival Growth retardation Multiple fractures Progressive kyphoscoliosis Blue sclerae at birth that become white Hearing impairment Dentinogenesis imperfecta
OI IV	Postnatal fractures, normal sclerae	Autosomal dominant	Short pro-α2(1) chain Unstable triple helix	Compatible with survival Moderate skeletal fragility Short stature Sometimes dentinogenesis imperfecta

OI, osteogenesis imperfecta.

allele is formed, leading to a reduced content of type 2 collagen in the cartilage.[12]

DISEASES ASSOCIATED WITH DEFECTS IN FOLDING AND DEGRADATION OF MACROMOLECULES

Mucopolysaccharidoses

The mucopolysaccharidoses, as discussed in Chapter 5, are a group of lysosomal storage diseases caused by deficiencies in the enzymes that degrade dermatan sulfate, heparan sulfate, and keratan sulfate. The implicated enzymes are mainly acid hydrolases. Mesenchymal cells, especially chondrocytes, play an important role in the metabolism of extracellular matrix mucopolysaccharides and therefore are most severely affected. Consequently, many of the skeletal manifestations of the mucopolysaccharidoses result from abnormalities in hyaline cartilage, including the cartilage anlage, growth plates, costal cartilages, and articular surfaces. It is not surprising therefore that patients with mucopolysaccharidoses are frequently of short stature and have chest wall abnormalities and malformed bones.

DISEASES ASSOCIATED WITH DEFECTS IN METABOLIC PATHWAYS (ENZYMES, ION CHANNELS, AND TRANSPORTERS)

Osteopetrosis

Osteopetrosis refers to a group of rare genetic diseases that are characterized by reduced osteoclast bone resorption, resulting in diffuse symmetric skeletal sclerosis (Fig. 26–9). The term *osteopetrosis* was coined because of the stonelike quality of the bones; however, the bones are abnormally brittle and fracture like a piece of chalk. Osteopetrosis, which is also known as *marble bone disease* and *Albers-Schönberg disease,* is classified into variants based on both the mode of inheritance and the clinical findings. The autosomal recessive malignant type and the autosomal dominant benign type are the most common variants.

Pathogenesis. Four types of osteopetrosis have been identified: infantile malignant osteopetrosis, type II carbonic anhydrase deficiency, and autosomal-dominant types I and II. However, the precise nature of the osteoclast dysfunction in many cases remains unknown. An example of a form of the disease in which the molecular mechanism is understood is the variant associated with *carbonic anhydrase II* deficiency.[19] Carbonic anhydrase II is required by osteoclasts and renal tubular cells to excrete hydrogen ions and acidify their environment. The absence of this enzyme prevents osteoclasts from acidifying the resorption pit and solubilizing the hydroxyapatite crystals and also blocks the acidification of urine by renal tubular cells. In another form of the disease, a mutation in the *ClC-7* chloride channel gene causes osteoclast dysfunction by interfering with the chloride channel that is important in the proton pump of the H^+-ATPase located on the osteoclast ruffled border. Consequently, osteoclasts cannot acidify the resorption pit, thus preventing the digestion of bone.[20] In mice, osteopetrosis can also be caused by targeted mutations in the genes coding for M-CSF, *c-src,* RANK, and OPG.[19] It is possible that some of these genes will be linked to the human disease.

Morphology. The morphologic changes of osteopetrosis are explained by deficient osteoclast activity. Grossly the bones lack a medullary canal, and the

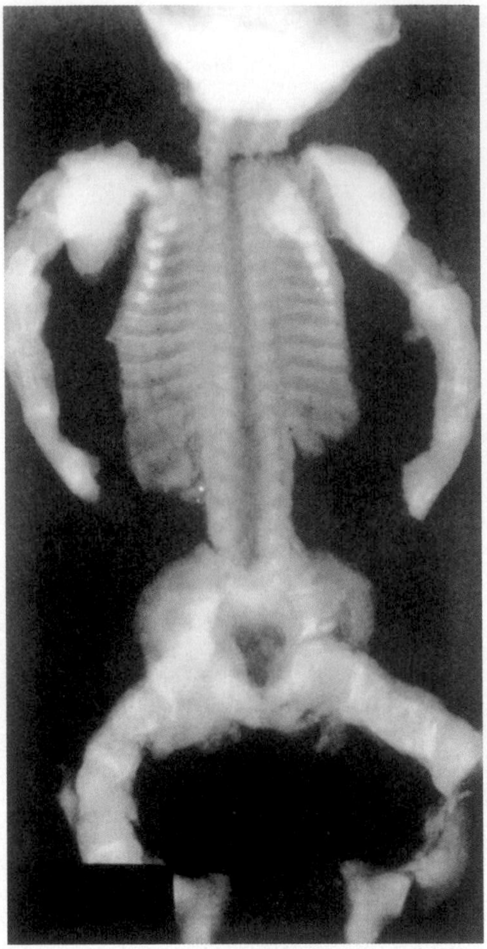

FIGURE 26–8 Skeletal radiograph of a fetus with lethal type II osteogenesis imperfecta. Note the numerous fractures of virtually all bones, resulting in accordion-like shortening of the limbs.

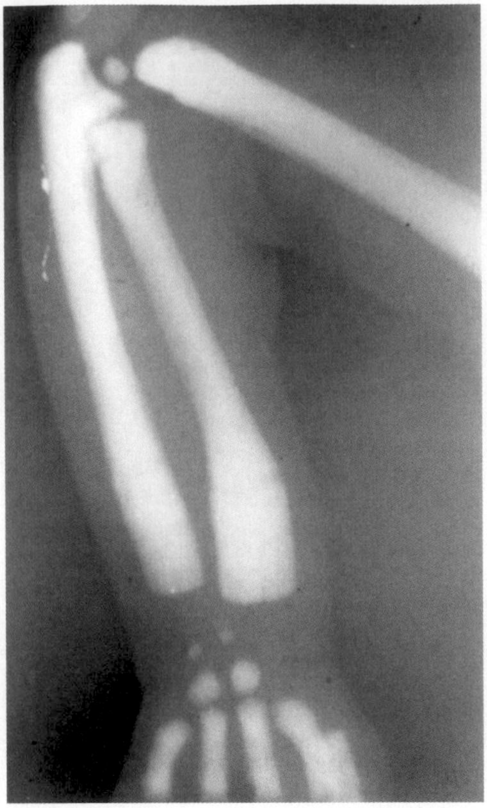

FIGURE 26–9 Radiograph of the upper extremity in a patient with osteopetrosis. The bones are diffusely sclerotic, and the distal metaphyses of the ulna and radius are poorly formed (Erlenmeyer flask deformity).

ends of long bones are bulbous (Erlenmeyer flask deformity) and misshapen. The neural foramina are small and compress exiting nerves. The primary spongiosa, which is normally removed during growth, persists and fills the medullary cavity, leaving no room for the hematopoietic marrow and preventing the formation of mature trabeculae (Fig. 26–10). Bone that forms is not remodeled and tends to be woven in architecture. In the end, these intrinsic abnormalities cause the bone to be brittle. Histologically, the number of osteoclasts may be normal, increased, or decreased depending on the underlying mechanism of the disease.

Clinical Features. Infantile malignant osteopetrosis is autosomal recessive and usually becomes evident in utero or soon after birth. Fracture, anemia, and hydrocephaly are often seen, resulting in postpartum mortality. Patients who survive into their infancy have cranial nerve problems (optic atrophy, deafness, and facial paralysis) and repeated, often fatal, infections because of decreased hematopoiesis resulting from the reduced marrow space. Patients develop extramedullary hematopoiesis, which causes prominent hepatosplenomegaly. The autosomal dominant benign form may not be detected until adolescence or adulthood, when it is discovered on x-rays performed because of repeated fractures. These patients may also have milder cranial nerve deficits and anemia.

Because osteoclasts are derived from marrow monocyte precursors, bone marrow transplants provide affected patients with progenitor cells that can produce normal functioning osteoclasts. Follow-up studies in patients who have received transplants have shown reversal of many of the skeletal abnormalities.

DISEASES ASSOCIATED WITH DECREASED BONE MASS

Osteoporosis

Osteoporosis is a disease characterized by increased porosity of the skeleton resulting from reduced bone mass. The associated structural changes predispose the bone to fracture. The disorder may be localized to a certain bone or region, as in *disuse osteoporosis of a limb,* or may involve the entire skeleton, as a manifestation of a *metabolic bone disease.* Generalized osteoporosis may be primary, or secondary to a large variety of conditions (Table 26–4).

The most common forms of osteoporosis are senile and postmenopausal osteoporosis. In these disorders, the critical loss of bone mass makes the skeleton vulnerable to fractures. It is estimated that 1 million Americans experience a significant

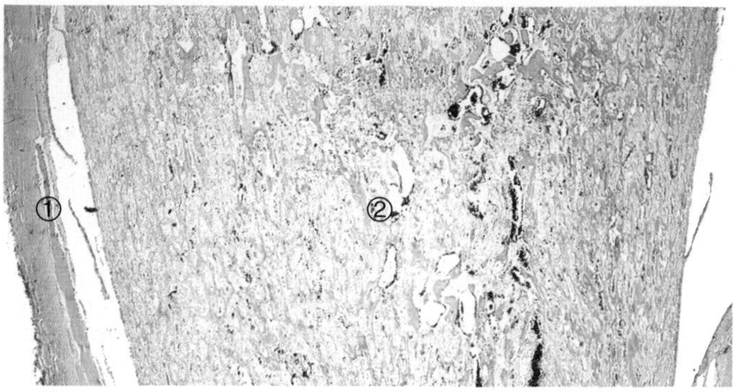

FIGURE 26–10 Section of proximal tibial diaphysis from a fetus with osteopetrosis. The cortex *(1)* is being formed, and the medullary cavity *(2)* is abnormally filled with primary spongiosa replacing the hematopoietic elements.

fragility fracture each year at a cost of over $14 billion. Effective treatment and prevention are imperative. The following discussion relates largely to these dominant forms of osteoporosis.

Pathogenesis. Peak bone mass is achieved during young adulthood. Its magnitude is determined largely by hereditary factors, especially the vitamin D receptor allele that is expressed, as well as the genes for collagen 1A1, estrogen receptor, and insulin-like growth factor 1 and its binding protein.[21] Physical activity, muscle strength, diet, and hormonal state, however, all contribute. Once maximal skeletal mass is attained, after the third or fourth decade a small deficit in bone formation accrues with every resorption and formation cycle of each basic muticellular unit. Accordingly, age-related bone loss, which may average 0.7% per year, is a normal and predictable biologic phenomenon, similar to the graying of hair. Both sexes are affected equally and whites more so than blacks. Differences in the peak skeletal mass in men versus women and in blacks versus whites may partially explain why certain populations are prone to develop this disorder.

Although much remains unknown, recent advances in elucidating the molecular biology of bone have provided intriguing new hypotheses in the pathogenesis of osteoporosis (Fig. 26–11):

- *Age-related changes* in bone cells and matrix have a strong impact on bone metabolism. Osteoblasts from elderly individuals have reduced replicative and biosynthetic potential when compared with osteoblasts from younger individuals.[22] Also, proteins bound to the extracellular matrix (such as growth factors, which are mitogenic to osteoprogenitor cells and stimulate osteoblastic synthetic activity) lose their biologic potency over time. The end result is a skeleton populated by bone-forming cells that have a diminished capacity to make bone. This form of osteoporosis, also known as *senile osteoporosis,* is categorized as a *low turnover variant.*
- *Reduced physical activity* increases the rate of bone loss in experimental animals and humans because mechanical forces are important stimuli for normal bone remodeling. The bone loss seen in an immobilized or paralyzed extremity, the reduction of skeletal mass observed in astronauts subjected to a gravity-free environment for prolonged periods, and the higher bone density in athletes as compared with nonathletes all support a role for physical activity in preventing bone loss. The type of exercise is important because load magnitude influences bone density more than the number of load cycles. Because muscle contraction is the dominant source of skeletal loading, it is logical that resistance exercises such as weight training are more effective stimuli for increasing bone mass than repetitive endurance activities such as jogging. Certainly the decreased physical activity that is associated with aging contributes to senile osteoporosis.
- *Genetic factors are also important,* as noted previously. The type of vitamin D receptor molecule that is inherited accounts for approximately 75% of the maximal peak mass achieved. Polymorphism in the vitamin D receptor molecule is associated with either a higher or lower maximal bone mass. Calcium deficiency, increased PTH levels, and reduced levels of vitamin D also may play a role in the development of senile osteoporosis.

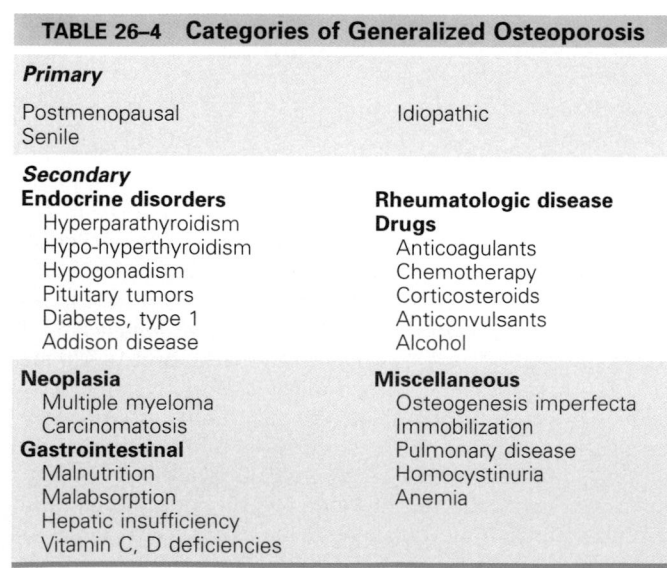

TABLE 26–4 Categories of Generalized Osteoporosis

Primary	
Postmenopausal	Idiopathic
Senile	
Secondary	
Endocrine disorders	**Rheumatologic disease**
Hyperparathyroidism	**Drugs**
Hypo-hyperthyroidism	Anticoagulants
Hypogonadism	Chemotherapy
Pituitary tumors	Corticosteroids
Diabetes, type 1	Anticonvulsants
Addison disease	Alcohol
Neoplasia	**Miscellaneous**
Multiple myeloma	Osteogenesis imperfecta
Carcinomatosis	Immobilization
Gastrointestinal	Pulmonary disease
Malnutrition	Homocystinuria
Malabsorption	Anemia
Hepatic insufficiency	
Vitamin C, D deficiencies	

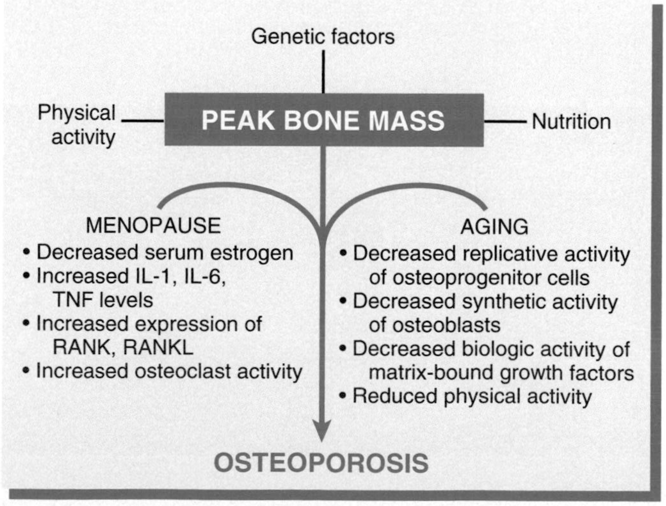

FIGURE 26–11 Pathophysiology of postmenopausal and senile osteoporosis (see text).

- The body's calcium *nutritional state* is important. It has been shown that adolescent girls (but not boys) have insufficient calcium intake in the diet. This calcium deficiency occurs during a period of rapid bone growth, stunting the peak bone mass ultimately achieved; thus, these individuals are at greater risk of developing osteoporosis.
- *Hormonal influences.* In the decade after menopause, yearly reductions in bone mass may reach up to 2% of cortical bone and 9% of cancellous bone. Women may lose as much as 35% of their cortical bone and 50% of their trabecular bone within the 30 to 40 years after menopause. It is thus no surprise that 1 out of every 2 women suffers an osteoporotic fracture, in contrast to 1 in 40 men. *Postmenopausal osteoporosis* is characterized by a hormone-dependent acceleration of bone loss that occurs during the decade after menopause. *Estrogen deficiency plays the major role in this phenomenon, and estrogen replacement at menopause is protective against bone loss.* The effects of estrogen on bone mass are mediated by cytokines. Decreased estrogen levels result in increased secretion of IL-1, IL-6, and TNF by blood monocytes and bone marrow cells.[23] These cytokines are potent stimulators of osteoclast recruitment and activity; they act, in part, by increasing the levels of RANK and RANKL and diminishing the quantity of OPG. Compensatory osteoblastic activity occurs, but it does not keep pace, leading to what is classified as a *high turnover form* of osteoporosis.

The secondary causes of osteoporosis are manifold and some are acquiring increased importance. An example is the potentially severe osteoporosis and increase in fracture risk associated with prolonged glucocorticoid therapy. In this setting, the osteoporosis develops rapidly and is dose and duration dependent. Glucocorticoids diminish bone mass by increasing bone resorption and reducing bone formation on both cortical and trabecular surfaces. Accordingly, strategies that prevent bone loss, such as the administration of biphosphonates, should be considered in all high-risk individuals beginning long-term steroid therapy.

Morphology. The entire skeleton is affected in postmenopausal and senile osteoporosis (Fig. 26–12), but certain regions tend to be more severely involved than others. In **postmenopausal** osteoporosis, the increase in osteoclast activity affects mainly bones or portions of bones that have increased surface area, such as the cancellous compartment of vertebral bodies. The osteoporotic trabeculae are thinned and lose their interconnections, leading to progressive microfractures and eventual vertebral collapse. In senile osteoporosis, the osteoporotic cortex is thinned by subperiosteal and endosteal resorption and the haversian systems are widened. In severe cases, the haversian systems are so enlarged that the cortex mimics cancellous bone. The bone that remains is of normal composition.

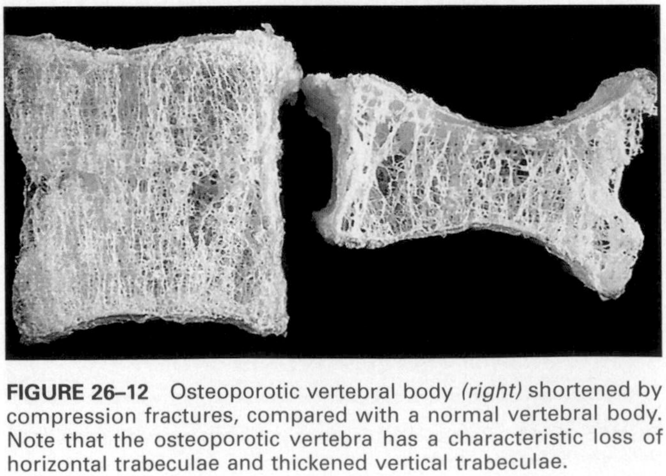

FIGURE 26–12 Osteoporotic vertebral body *(right)* shortened by compression fractures, compared with a normal vertebral body. Note that the osteoporotic vertebra has a characteristic loss of horizontal trabeculae and thickened vertical trabeculae.

Clinical Course. The clinical manifestations of structural failure of the skeleton depend on which bones are involved. Vertebral fractures that frequently occur in the thoracic and lumbar regions are painful. Multilevel fractures can cause significant loss of height and various deformities, including lumbar lordosis and kyphoscoliosis. Complications of overt fractures of the femoral neck, pelvis, or spine, such as pulmonary embolism and pneumonia, are frequent and result in 40,000 to 50,000 deaths per year.

Osteoporosis cannot be reliably detected in plain radiographs until 30% to 40% of the bone mass is lost, and measurement of blood levels of calcium, phosphorus, and alkaline phosphatase is not diagnostic. Osteoporosis is thus a difficult condition to diagnose accurately since it remains asymptomatic until skeletal fragility is well advanced. Currently the best procedures that accurately estimate the amount of bone loss, aside from biopsy, are specialized radiographic imaging techniques, such as dual-energy absorptiometry and quantitative computed tomography, which measure bone density.

The prevention and treatment of senile and postmenopausal osteoporosis include exercise, appropriate calcium and vitamin D intake, and pharmacologic agents, including estrogen replacing agents, bisphosphonates, and recombinant PTH. The latter increases skeletal mass by stimulating the formation of bone in amounts greater than that which is resorbed.[21]

DISEASES CAUSED BY OSTEOCLAST DYSFUNCTION

Paget Disease (Osteitis Deformans)

This unique skeletal disease can be characterized as a *collage of matrix madness.* At the outset, Paget disease is marked by regions of furious osteoclastic bone resorption, which is followed by a period of hectic bone formation, and then finally the bone cell activity becomes markedly diminished. *This repetitive and overlapping sequence forms the basis for dividing Paget disease into (1) an initial osteolytic stage, followed by (2) a mixed osteoclastic–osteoblastic stage, which ends with a predominance of osteoblastic activity and evolves ultimately into (3) a burnt-out quiescent osteosclerotic stage* (Fig. 26–13). The net effect of this process is a *gain in bone mass;* however, the newly formed bone is disordered and architecturally unsound.

Paget disease usually begins during mid-adulthood and becomes progressively more common thereafter. An intriguing aspect is the striking variation in prevalence both within certain countries and throughout the world. Paget disease is relatively common in whites in England, France, Austria,

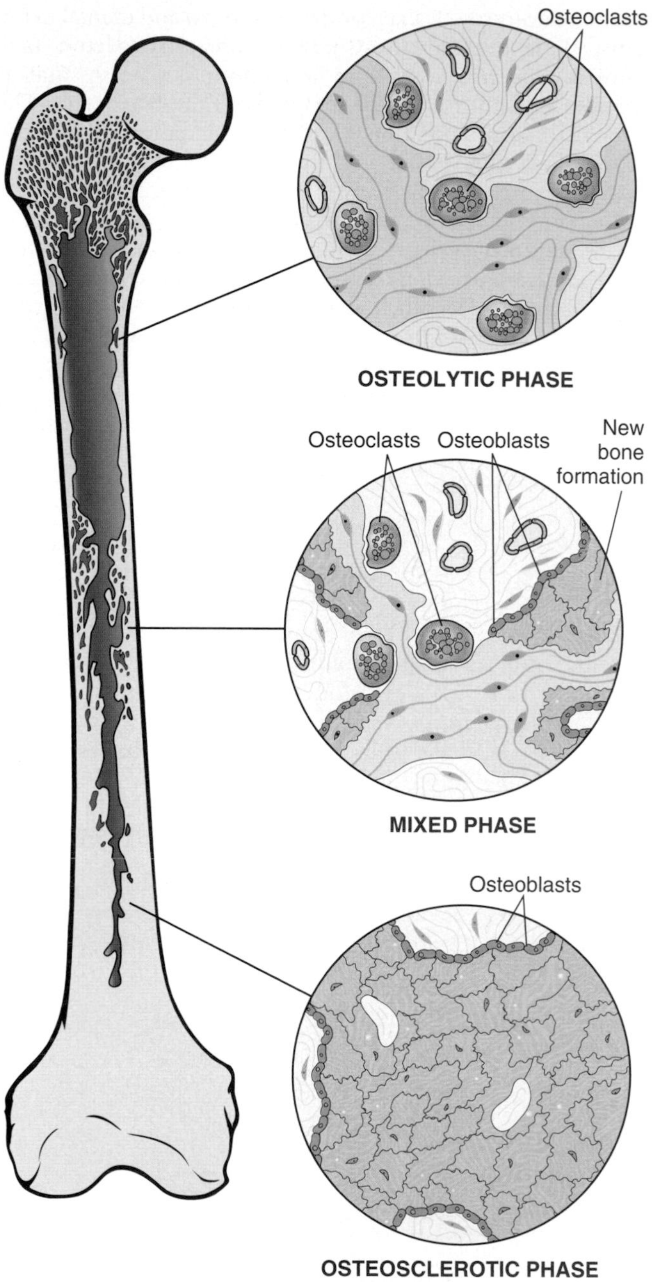

FIGURE 26–13 Diagrammatic representation of Paget disease of bone, demonstrating the three phases in the evolution of the disease.

regions of Germany, Australia, New Zealand, and the United States. The exact incidence is hard to determine because most affected individuals are asymptomatic, but it is estimated to affect 5% to 11% of the adult populations in these countries. In contrast, Paget disease is rare in the native populations of Scandinavia, China, Japan, and Africa.

Pathogenesis. When Sir James Paget first described this condition in 1876, he attributed the skeletal changes to an inflammatory process, hence the term *osteitis deformans.* It is ironic that after numerous subsequent hypotheses were proposed, Paget may be finally proven correct. Current evidence suggests a slow virus infection by a *paramyxovirus* as the cause of Paget disease. This likens it to other slow virus diseases, such as subacute sclerosing leukoencephalitis, produced by the same family of viruses (Chapter 28). Viral particles resembling the nucleocapsids of paramyxovirus have been seen in the cytoplasm and nuclei of osteoclasts, and immunologic analyses have identified antigens associated with both the measles and respiratory syncytial viruses (both paramyxoviruses) in osteoclasts from affected sites. Additionally, measles virus nucleocapsid transcripts have been identified in bone cells from pagetic tissue.[24] Viruses such as the paramyxovirus can induce the secretion of IL-6 from infected cells. This cytokine, as well as M-CSF, are produced in large amounts in pagetic bone; they are potent stimulators of osteoclast recruitment and resorptive activity. Intriguing as these observations may be, to date no infectious virus has been isolated from affected tissue.

There is some evidence that osteoclasts are abnormal in this disease, and hyperresponsive to activating agents such as vitamin D and RANKL.[24] Additionally, Paget disease has a hereditary component, as it has a high incidence within families and its predisposition has been linked to a locus on chromosome 18q.[25]

Morphology. Paget disease is a focal process with remarkable variation in its stage of development in separate sites. The histologic hallmark is the **mosaic pattern** of lamellar bone. This pattern, which is likened to a jigsaw puzzle, is produced by prominent cement lines that anneal haphazardly oriented units of lamellar bone (Fig. 26–14). In the initial lytic phase, there are waves of osteoclastic activity and numerous resorption pits. The osteoclasts are abnormally large and have many more than the normal 10 to 12 nuclei; sometimes 100 nuclei are present. Osteoclasts persist in the mixed phase, but now many of the bone surfaces are lined by prominent osteoblasts. The marrow adjacent to the bone-forming surface is replaced by loose connective tissue that contains osteoprogenitor cells and numerous blood vessels, which transport nutrients and catabolites to and from these metabolically active sites. The newly formed bone may be woven or lamellar, but eventually all of it is remodeled into lamellar bone. As the mosaic pattern unfolds and the cell activity decreases, the periosseous

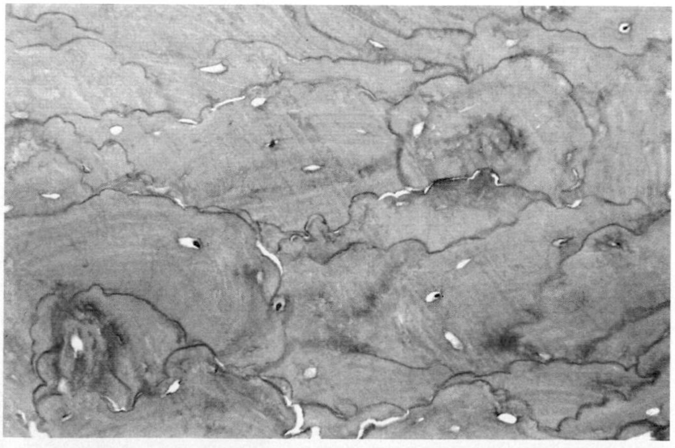

FIGURE 26–14 Mosaic pattern of lamellar bone pathognomonic of Paget disease.

fibrovascular tissue recedes and is replaced by normal marrow. In the end, the bone becomes a caricature of itself: larger than normal and composed of coarsely thickened trabeculae (Fig. 26–15) and cortices that are soft and porous and lack structural stability. These aspects make the bones vulnerable to deformation under stress; consequently, they fracture easily.

Clinical Course. Clinical findings are extremely variable and depend on the extent and site of the disease. Most cases are mild and are discovered as an incidental radiographic finding. Paget disease can, however, produce a variety of skeletal, neuromuscular, and cardiovascular complications.

The diagnosis can frequently be made from the radiographic findings. Pagetic bone is typically enlarged with thick, coarsened cortices and cancellous bone (Fig. 26–15). Many patients exhibit an elevated serum level of alkaline phosphatase and increased urinary excretion of hydroxyproline.

Paget disease occurs in one or more bones. It is monostotic (tibia, ilium, femur, skull, vertebra, and humerus) in about 15% of cases and polyostotic (pelvis, spine, and skull) in the remainder. The axial skeleton or proximal femur is involved in up to 80% of cases. Even though no bone is immune, involvement of the ribs, fibula, and small bones of the hands and feet is unusual.

Pain is the most common problem and is localized to the affected bone. It is caused by a combination of microfractures and bone overgrowth that compresses spinal and cranial nerve roots. Bone overgrowth in the craniofacial skeleton may produce *leontiasis ossea* and a cranium so heavy that it becomes difficult for the patient to hold the head erect. The weakened pagetic bone may lead to invagination of the base of the skull *(platybasia)* and compression of the posterior fossa structures. Weight bearing causes anterior bowing of the femora and tibiae and distorts the femoral heads, resulting in the development of *severe secondary osteoarthritis. Chalkstick-type* fractures are the next most common complication and usually occur in the long bones of the lower extremities. Compression fractures of the spine result in spinal cord injury and the development of kyphoses. The hypervascularity of pagetic bone warms the overlying skin; in severe polyostotic disease the increased blood flow behaves as an arteriovenous shunt leading to high-output heart failure or exacerbation of underlying cardiac disease.

A variety of tumor and tumor-like conditions develop in pagetic bone. The benign lesions include giant cell tumor, giant cell reparative granuloma, and extraosseous masses of hematopoiesis. The most dreaded complication is the development of sarcoma, which occurs in 0.7% to 0.9% of all patients with Paget disease but increases to 5% to 10% in those patients with severe polyostotic disease.[26] The sarcomas are usually osteosarcoma, malignant fibrous histiocytoma, or chondrosarcoma, and they arise in the long bones, pelvis, skull, and spine. In the absence of malignant transformation, Paget disease is usually not a serious or life-threatening disease. Most patients have mild symptoms that are readily suppressed by calcitonin and bisphosphonates.

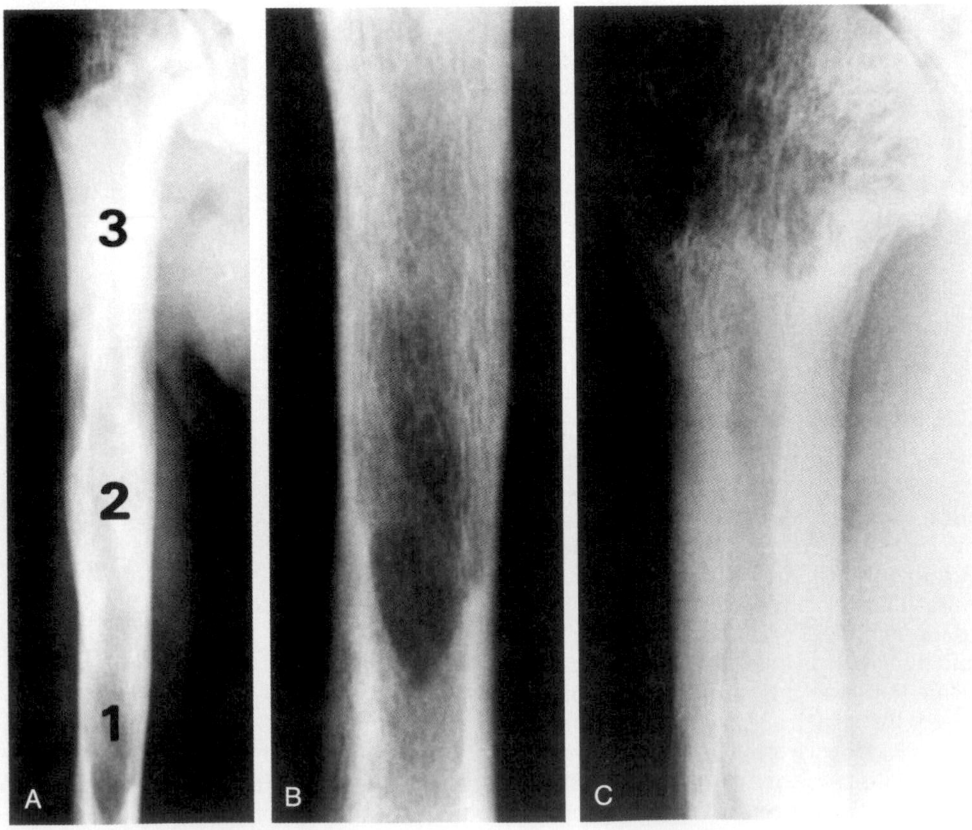

FIGURE 26–15 Paget disease of the humerus. *A,* The three sequential stages: *(1)* lytic, *(2)* mixed, and *(3)* sclerotic. *B,* Area 1, the lytic stage, is seen in close-up. Area 2, the mixed stage *(upper portion of B)* reveals central and endosteal cortical resorption and replacement by less compact new bone. *C,* Area 3, the sclerotic stage, with irregular thickening of both cortical and trabecular bone. (From Maldague B, Malghem J: Dynamic radiologic pattern of Paget's disease of bone. Clin Orthop 217:127, 1987.)

DISEASES ASSOCIATED WITH ABNORMAL MINERAL HOMEOSTASIS

Rickets and Osteomalacia

Rickets and osteomalacia represent a group of diseases of divergent causes that are characterized by a defect in matrix mineralization, most often related to a lack of vitamin D or some disturbance in its metabolism. The term *rickets* refers to the disorder in children in which deranged bone growth produces distinctive skeletal deformities. In the adult, the disorder is called *osteomalacia* because the bone that forms during the remodeling process is undemineralized. This results in osteopenia and predisposition to insufficiency fractures. Rickets and osteomalacia are discussed in Chapter 9.

Hyperparathyroidism

Hyperparathyroidism is classified into primary and secondary types, as discussed in Chapter 24. Primary hyperparathyroidism results from autonomous hyperplasia or a tumor, usually an adenoma, of the parathyroid gland, whereas secondary hyperparathyroidism is commonly caused by prolonged states of hypocalcemia resulting in compensatory hypersecretion of PTH. Whatever the basis, the increased PTH levels are detected by receptors on osteoblasts, which then release molecules that stimulate osteoclast activity. Thus, through a chain of signals, the skeletal manifestations of hyperparathyroidism are caused by unabated osteoclastic bone resorption. The following points should be noted:

- Similar to all metabolic bone disease, the entire skeleton is affected in hyperparathyroidism, even though some sites are more severely affected than others.
- The anatomic changes of severe hyperparathyroidism, known as *osteitis fibrosa cystica*, are now rarely encountered because hyperparathyroidism is currently being diagnosed and treated at an early stage.
- Secondary hyperparathyroidism is usually not as severe or as prolonged as primary hyperparathyroidism; hence, the skeletal abnormalities tend to be milder.

Morphology. For unknown reasons, the increased osteoclast activity in hyperparathyroidism affects cortical bone (subperiosteal, osteonal, and endosteal surfaces) more severely than cancellous bone. Subperiosteal resorption produces thinned cortices and the loss of the lamina dura around the teeth. The x-ray pattern, which is virtually diagnostic of hyperparathyroidism, is most frequently identified along the radial aspect of the middle phalanges of the index and middle fingers. Characteristic of hyperparathyroidism are cortical cutting cones composed of a spearhead arrangement of osteoclasts that bore along and enlarge haversian and Volkmann canals. In cancellous bone, osteoclasts tunnel into and dissect centrally along the length of the trabeculae, creating the appearance of railroad tracks and producing what is known as **dissecting osteitis** (Fig. 26–16). The correlative radiographic finding is a decrease in bone density, or osteopenia. Since bone resorption and formation are coupled processes, it is not surprising that osteoblast activity is also increased in hyperparathyroidism. In the regions of bone cell activity, the marrow spaces around the affected surfaces are replaced by fibrovascular tissue.

The bone loss predisposes to microfractures and secondary hemorrhages that elicit an influx of multinucleated macrophages and an ingrowth of reparative fibrous tissue, creating a mass of reactive tissue known as a **brown tumor** (Fig. 26–17). The brown color is the result of the vascularity, hemorrhage, and hemosiderin deposition; it is not uncommon for the lesions to undergo cystic degeneration. The combined picture of increased bone cell activity, peritrabecular fibrosis, and cystic brown tumors is the hallmark of severe hyperparathyroidism and is known as **generalized osteitis fibrosa cystica (von Recklinghausen disease of bone).**

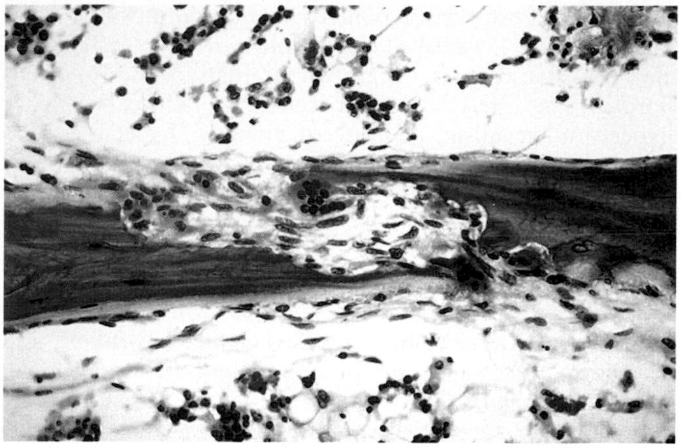

FIGURE 26–16 Hyperparathyroidism with osteoclasts boring into the center of the trabeculum (dissecting osteitis).

The decrease in bone mass predisposes to fractures, deformities caused by the stress of weight bearing, and joint pain and dysfunction as the lines of normal weight bearing are altered. Control of the hyperparathyroidism allows the bony changes to regress significantly or disappear completely.

Renal Osteodystrophy

The term *renal osteodystrophy* is used to describe collectively all of the skeletal changes of chronic renal disease, including

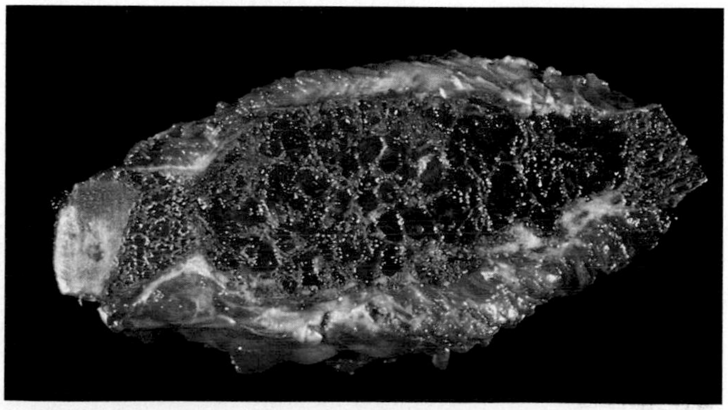

FIGURE 26–17 Resected rib, harboring an expansile brown tumor adjacent to the costal cartilage.

(1) increased osteoclastic bone resorption mimicking osteitis fibrosa cystica, (2) delayed matrix mineralization (osteomalacia), (3) osteosclerosis, (4) growth retardation, and (5) osteoporosis. The interrelation between renal failure, secondary hyperparathyroidism, and altered vitamin D metabolism is well recognized, and as advances in medical technology have prolonged the lives of patients with renal diseases, their impact on skeletal homeostasis has assumed greater clinical importance.

The bone disorders in patients with end-stage renal failure are divided into two major types.[27] *High-turnover osteodystrophy* is characterized by increased bone resorption and formation, with the former predominating. In contrast, *low-turnover* or *aplastic disease* is manifested by adynamic bone (little osteoclastic and osteoblastic activity) and, less commonly, osteomalacia. Many patients have a mixed pattern of disease.

Pathogenesis. The pathogenesis of the mix of skeletal lesions can be summarized as follows:

- Chronic renal failure results in *phosphate retention* and hyperphosphatemia.
- Hyperphosphatemia, in turn, induces *secondary hyperparathyroidism* because phosphate regulates PTH secretion.
- Hypocalcemia develops as the levels of vitamin D, or 1,25-dihydroxyvitamin D_3 (1,25-$[OH]_2D_3$) fall because of decreased conversion from the vitamin D metabolite 25-$(OH)D_3$ by damaged kidneys; inhibition of the renal hydroxylase involved in the conversion of 25-$(OH)D_3$ to the more active metabolite 1,25-$(OH)D_3$ by the high levels of phosphorus; and reduced intestinal absorption of calcium because of low levels of 1,25-$(OH)_2D_3$.
- PTH secretion markedly increases at all levels of serum calcium. 1,25-$(OH)_2D_3$ suppresses PTH gene expression and secretion; in renal failure, there is a decrease in the binding of 1,25-$(OH)_2D_3$ to parathyroid cells; and there is decreased degradation and excretion of PTH because of compromised renal function.
- The resultant *secondary hyperparathyroidism* produces increased osteoclast activity.
- *Metabolic acidosis* associated with renal failure stimulates bone resorption and the release of calcium hydroxyapatite from the matrix.
- Other factors that are important in the genesis of renal osteodystrophy are iron accumulation in bone and aluminum deposition at the site of mineralization. *Aluminum deposition*, in particular, has received a great deal of attention because of its iatrogenic origin. The sources of the aluminum include dialysis solutions prepared from water with a high aluminum content and oral aluminum-containing phosphate binders. Aluminum interferes with the deposition of calcium hydroxyapatite and hence promotes osteomalacia. Aluminum is not only toxic to bone but also has been implicated as the cause of dialysis encephalopathy and microcytic anemia in patients with chronic renal failure.
- Another complication seen in association with renal osteodystrophy is the deposition of masses of *amyloid* in bone and periarticular structures. The amyloid is formed from β_2-microglobulin, which is increased in the serum of patients who undergo long-term hemodialysis (Chapter 6).

Fractures

Traumatic and nontraumatic fractures are some of the most common pathologic conditions affecting bone. Fractures are classified as *complete* or *incomplete; closed (simple),* when the overlying tissue is intact; *compound,* when the fracture site *communicates* with the skin surface; *comminuted,* when the bone is splintered; or *displaced,* when the ends of the bone at the fracture site are not aligned. If the break occurs in bone already altered by a disease process, it is described as a *pathologic fracture.* A *stress fracture* is a slowly developing fracture that follows a period of increased physical activity in which the bone is subjected to new repetitive loads—as in sports training or marching in military boot camp.

Bone is unique in its ability to repair itself; it can completely reconstitute itself by reactivating processes that normally occur during embryogenesis. Bone repair is a highly regulated process that can be separated into overlapping histologic, biochemical, and biomechanical stages. The completion of each stage initiates the next stage, and this is accomplished by a series of interactions and communications among the various cells and proteins located in the healing zone.

- Immediately after fracture, rupture of blood vessels results in a hematoma, which fills the fracture gap and surrounds the area of bone injury. The clotted blood provides a fibrin mesh, which helps seal off the fracture site and at the same time creates a framework for the influx of inflammatory cells and ingrowth of fibroblasts and new capillary vessels. Simultaneously, degranulated platelets and migrating inflammatory cells release PDGF, TGF-β, FGF, and other cytokines, which activate the osteoprogenitor cells in the periosteum, medullary cavity, and surrounding soft tissues and stimulate the production of osteoclastic and osteoblastic activity.[28] Thus, by the end of the first week, the hematoma is organizing, the adjacent tissue is being modulated for future matrix production, and the fractured ends of the bones are being remodeled. This fusiform and predominantly uncalcified tissue—called *soft tissue callus or procallus*—provides some anchorage between the ends of the fractured bones but offers no structural rigidity for weight bearing.
- Subsequently, the activated osteoprogenitor cells deposit subperiosteal trabeculae of woven bone that are oriented perpendicular to the cortical axis and within the medullary cavity. In some cases the activated mesenchymal cells in the soft tissues and bone surrounding the fracture line also differentiate into chondroblasts that make fibrocartilage and hyaline cartilage. In an uncomplicated fracture, the repair tissue reaches its maximal girth at the end of the second or third week, which helps stabilize the fracture site, but it is not yet strong enough for weight bearing. The newly formed cartilage along the fracture line undergoes enchondral ossification, such as normally occurs at the growth plate, forming a network of bone that connects to the reactive trabeculae deposited elsewhere in the medullary cavity and beneath the periosteum. In this fashion, the fractured ends are bridged by a *bony callus,* and as it mineralizes, the stiffness and strength of the callus increase to the point that controlled weight bearing can be tolerated (Fig. 26–18).
- In the early stages of callus formation, an excess of fibrous tissue, cartilage, and bone is produced. If the bones are not

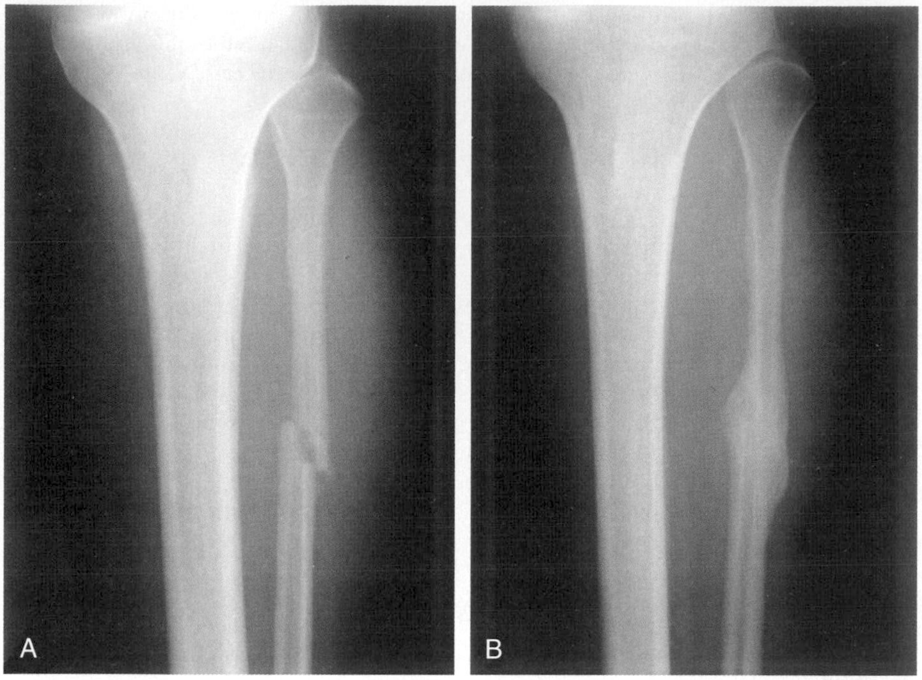

FIGURE 26–18 *A,* Recent fracture of the fibula. *B,* Marked callus formation 6 weeks later. (Courtesy of Dr. Barbara Weissman, Brigham and Women's Hospital, Boston, MA.)

perfectly aligned, the volume of callus is greatest in the concave portion of the fracture site. As the callus matures and transmits weight-bearing forces, the portions that are not physically stressed are resorbed, and in this manner the callus is reduced in size until the shape and outline of the fractured bone has been reestablished. The medullary cavity is also restored, and after this has been completed it may be impossible to demonstrate the site of previous injury.

The sequence of events in the healing of a fracture can be easily impeded or even blocked. Displaced and comminuted fractures frequently result in some deformity. The devitalized fragments of splintered bone require resorption, and this delays healing, enlarges the callus, and requires extremely long periods of remodeling so that in essence there is a permanent abnormality. Inadequate immobilization permits constant movement at the fracture site so that the normal constituents of callus do not form. Consequently the callus may be composed mainly of fibrous tissue and cartilage, perpetuating the instability and resulting in delayed union and nonunion. If a nonunion allows for too much motion along the fracture gap, the central portion of the callus undergoes cystic degeneration, and the luminal surface can actually become lined by synovial-like cells, creating a false joint, or *pseudoarthrosis.* In the setting of a nonunion or pseudoarthrosis, the normal healing process can be re-instituted if the interposed soft tissues are removed and the fracture site stabilized. A serious obstacle to healing is *infection* of the fracture site, which is a risk in comminuted and open fractures. The infection must be eradicated before bony union can be achieved. Bone repair can also be derailed by inadequate levels of calcium or phosphorus, vitamin deficiencies, systemic infection, diabetes, and vascular insufficiency.

Generally, with children and young adults, in whom most fractures are uncomplicated, practically perfect reconstitution can be anticipated. In older age groups, in whom fractures tend to occur on a background of some other disease (e.g., osteoporosis and osteomalacia), repair is less optimal and often requires mechanical methods of immobilization to facilitate healing.

Osteonecrosis (Avascular Necrosis)

Infarction of bone and marrow is a relatively common event and can occur in the medullary cavity of the metaphysis or diaphysis and the subchondral region of the epiphysis. *All forms of bone necrosis result from ischemia.* The mechanisms that produce ischemia are varied, however, and include (1) mechanical vascular interruption (fracture), (2) corticosteroids, (3) thrombosis and embolism (nitrogen bubbles in dysbarism) (Chapter 9), (4) vessel injury (secondary to vasculitis, radiation therapy), (5) increased intraosseous pressure with vascular compression, and (6) venous hypertension.[29] Although the disease states associated with bone infarcts are diverse (Table 26–5), in many cases the cause of necrosis is uncertain. Aside from fracture, most cases of bone necrosis are either idiopathic or follow corticosteroid administration. The

TABLE 26–5 Disorders Associated with Osteonecrosis

Idiopathic	Pregnancy
Trauma	Gaucher disease
Corticosteroid administration	Sickle cell and other anemias
Infection	Alcohol abuse
Dysbarism	Chronic pancreatitis
Radiation therapy	Tumors
Connective tissue disorders	Epiphyseal disorders

pathophysiology underlying steroid-induced bone infarcts is obscure. The infarcts follow high-dose steroid therapy for short periods, long-term administration of smaller doses, and even intra-articular injections.

Morphology. The pathologic features of bone necrosis are the same regardless of the cause. In medullary infarcts, the necrosis is geographic and involves the cancellous bone and marrow. The cortex is usually not affected because of its collateral blood flow. In subchondral infarcts, necrosis involves a triangular or wedge-shaped segment of tissue that has the subchondral bone plate as its base and the center of the epiphysis as its apex. The overlying articular cartilage remains viable because it receives nutrition from the synovial fluid. The dead bone, recognized by its empty lacunae, is surrounded by necrotic adipocytes that frequently rupture, releasing their fatty acids, which bind calcium and form insoluble calcium soaps that may remain for life. In the healing response, osteoclasts resorb the necrotic trabeculae; however, those that remain act as scaffolding for the deposition of new living bone in a process known as **creeping substitution.** In subchondral infarcts, the pace of creeping substitution is too slow to be effective so there is eventual collapse of the necrotic cancellous bone and distortion, fracture, and even sloughing of the articular cartilage (Fig. 26–19).

Clinical Course. The symptoms depend on the location and extent of infarction. Typically, subchondral infarcts cause chronic pain that is initially associated only with physical activity but then becomes progressively more constant as secondary changes supervene. In contrast, medullary infarcts are clinically silent except for large ones occurring in Gaucher disease, dysbarism, and hemoglobinopathies. Medullary infarcts usually remain stable over time and rarely are the site of malignant transformation. Subchondral infarcts, however, often collapse and may predispose to severe, secondary osteoarthritis. More than 10% of the 500,000 joint replacements performed annually in the United States are for treatment of the complications of osteonecrosis.

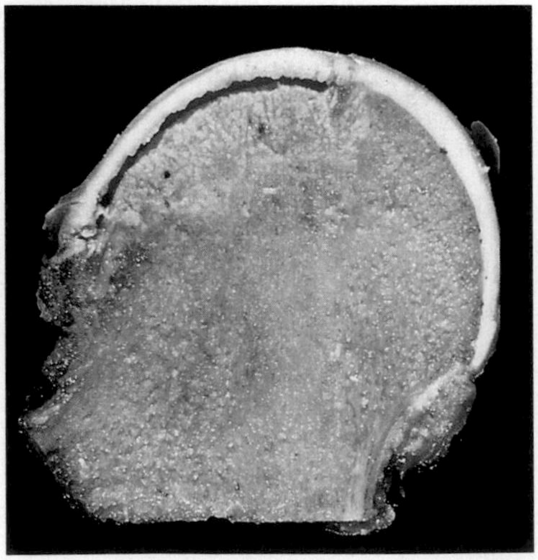

FIGURE 26–19 Femoral head with a subchondral, wedge-shaped pale yellow area of osteonecrosis. The space between the overlying articular cartilage and bone is caused by trabecular compression fractures without repair.

Infections—Osteomyelitis

Osteomyelitis denotes inflammation of bone and marrow, and the common use of the term virtually always implies infection. Osteomyelitis may be a complication of any systemic infection but frequently manifests as a primary solitary focus of disease. All types of organisms, including viruses, parasites, fungi, and bacteria, can produce osteomyelitis, but infections caused by certain pyogenic bacteria and mycobacteria are the most common. Currently in the United States, unusual infections in third world immigrants and opportunistic infections in immunosuppressed patients have made the diagnosis and treatment of osteomyelitis ever more challenging.

PYOGENIC OSTEOMYELITIS

Pyogenic osteomyelitis is almost always caused by bacteria. Organisms may reach the bone by (1) hematogenous spread, (2) extension from a contiguous site, and (3) direct implantation. Most cases of osteomyelitis are hematogenous in origin and develop in the long bones or vertebral bodies in otherwise healthy individuals.[30] The initiating bacteremia may follow trivial occurrences, such as occult injury to the intestinal mucosa during defecation, vigorous chewing of hard foods, or minor infections of the skin.

Staphylococcus aureus is responsible for 80% to 90% of the cases of pyogenic osteomyelitis in which an organism is recovered. Its propensity to infect bone may be related to the fact that it expresses receptors for bone matrix components such as collagen, thereby facilitating its adherence to bone tissue.[31] *Escherichia coli, Pseudomonas,* and *Klebsiella* are more frequently isolated from patients with genitourinary tract infections or those who are intravenous drug abusers. Mixed bacterial infections are seen in the setting of direct spread or inoculation of organisms during surgery or open fractures. In the neonatal period, *Haemophilus influenzae* and group B streptococci are frequent pathogens; patients with sickle cell disease, for unknown reasons, are predisposed to *Salmonella* infection. In almost 50% of cases, no organisms can be isolated.

The location of the lesions within specific bones is influenced by the vascular circulation, which varies with age. In the neonate, the metaphyseal vessels penetrate the growth plate, resulting in frequent infection of the metaphysis, epiphysis, or both. In children, localization of microorganisms in the metaphysis is typical. After growth plate closure, the metaphyseal vessels reunite with their epiphyseal counterparts and provide a route for the bacteria to seed the epiphyses and subchondral regions in the adult.

Morphology. The morphologic changes in osteomyelitis depend on the stage (acute, subacute, or chronic) and location of the infection. Once localized in bone, the bacteria proliferate and induce an acute inflammatory reaction and cause cell death. The entrapped bone undergoes necrosis within the first

48 hours, and the bacteria and inflammation spread within the shaft of the bone and may percolate throughout the haversian systems to reach the periosteum. In children, the periosteum is loosely attached to the cortex; therefore, sizable **subperiosteal** abscesses may form, which can trek for long distances along the bone surface. Lifting of the periosteum further impairs the blood supply to the affected region, and both suppurative and ischemic injury may cause segmental bone necrosis; the dead piece of bone is known as the **sequestrum.** Rupture of the periosteum leads to an abscess in the surrounding soft tissue and the eventual formation of a **draining sinus.** Sometimes the sequestrum crumbles and forms free foreign bodies that pass through the sinus tract.

In infants, but uncommonly in adults, epiphyseal infection spreads through the articular surface or along capsular and tendoligamentous insertions into a joint, to produce septic or suppurative arthritis, sometimes causing extensive destruction of the articular cartilage and permanent disability. An analogous process involves the vertebrae, in which the infection destroys the hyaline cartilage end plate and intervertebral discs and spreads into adjacent vertebrae.

Over time, the host response develops, and after the first week of infection chronic inflammatory cells become more numerous. The release of cytokines from leukocytes stimulates osteoclastic bone resorption, ingrowth of fibrous tissue, and the deposition of reactive bone in the periphery. Reactive woven or lamellar bone may be deposited, and when it forms a sleeve of living tissue around a segment of devitalized bone, it is known as an **involucrum** (Fig. 26–20). Several morphologic variants of osteomyelitis have been given eponyms because of their distinguishing features: **Brodie abscess** is a small intraosseous abscess that frequently involves the cortex and is walled off by reactive bone; **sclerosing osteomyelitis of Garré** typically develops in the jaw and is associated with extensive new bone formation that obscures much of the underlying osseous structure.

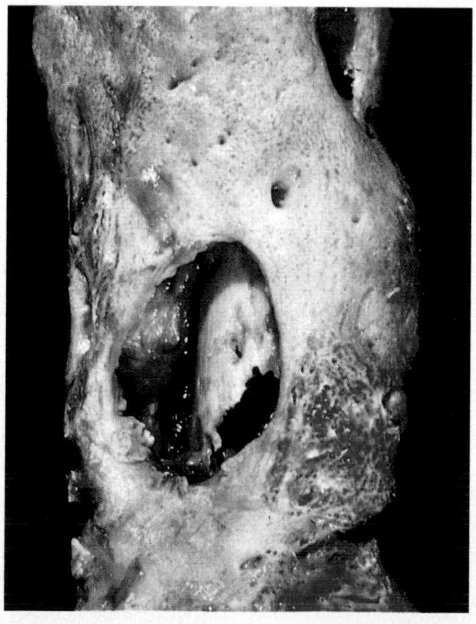

FIGURE 26–20 Resected femur in a patient with draining osteomyelitis. The drainage tract in the subperiosteal shell of viable new bone (involucrum) reveals the inner native necrotic cortex (sequestrum).

Clinical Course. Clinically, hematogenous osteomyelitis may manifest as an acute systemic illness with malaise, fever, chills, leukocytosis, and throbbing pain, often intense, over the affected region. The presentation may be subtler with only unexplained fever, particularly in infants, or only localized pain in the absence of fever in the adult. The diagnosis can be strongly suggested by the characteristic x-ray findings of a lytic focus of bone destruction surrounded by a zone of sclerosis. In many untreated cases, blood cultures are positive, but biopsy and bone cultures are required to identify the pathogen in most instances. The combination of antibiotics and surgical drainage is usually curative. In 5% to 25% of cases, acute osteomyelitis fails to resolve and persists as chronic infection. Chronicity may develop when there is delay in diagnosis, extensive bone necrosis, abbreviated antibiotic therapy, inadequate surgical debridement, and weakened host defenses. Acute flare-ups may mark the clinical course of chronic infection; they are usually spontaneous, have no obvious cause, and may occur after years of dormancy. Other complications of chronic osteomyelitis include pathologic fracture, secondary amyloidosis, endocarditis, sepsis, development of squamous cell carcinoma in the sinus tract, and rarely sarcoma in the infected bone.

TUBERCULOUS OSTEOMYELITIS

A resurgence of tuberculous osteomyelitis is occurring in industrialized nations, attributed to the influx of immigrants from third world countries and the greater numbers of immunosuppressed people (Chapter 8). In developing countries, the affected individuals are usually adolescents or young adults, whereas in the indigenous population of the United States, the victims tend to be older, except for those who are immunosuppressed. From 1% to 3% of patients with pulmonary or extrapulmonary tuberculosis have osseous infection.

Morphology. The organisms are usually blood borne and originate from a focus of active visceral disease. Direct extension (e.g., from a pulmonary focus into a rib or from tracheobronchial nodes into adjacent vertebrae) or spread via draining lymphatics may also occur. The bony infection is usually solitary and in some cases may be the only manifestation of tuberculosis. Similar to the more common pulmonary form, it may fester for years before being recognized. In patients with acquired immunodeficiency syndrome, the bone infection is frequently multifocal.

The spine (especially the thoracic and lumbar vertebrae), is the most common site of skeletal involvement, followed by the knees and hips. Tuberculous osteomyelitis tends to be more destructive and resistant to control than pyogenic osteomyelitis. The infection spreads through large areas of the medullary cavity and causes extensive necrosis. In the spine **(Pott disease),** the infection breaks through intervertebral discs to involve multiple vertebrae and extends into the soft tissues, forming abscesses.

Typically, patients present with pain on motion, localized tenderness, low-grade fevers, chills, and weight loss. Rarely, patients may complain of an inguinal mass, which represents a cold fluctuant psoas abscess. Severe destruction of vertebrae frequently results in permanent compression fractures that produce severe scoliotic or kyphotic deformities and neurologic deficits secondary to spinal cord and nerve compression. Other complications of tuberculous osteomyelitis include tuberculous arthritis, sinus tract formation, and amyloidosis.

SKELETAL SYPHILIS

Both syphilis *(Treponema pallidum)* and yaws *(Treponema pertenue)* can involve bone. Currently, syphilis is experiencing resurgence; however, bone involvement remains infrequent because the disease is readily diagnosed and treated before this complication develops.

In congenital syphilis, the bone lesions begin to appear about the fifth month of gestation and are fully developed at birth. The spirochetes tend to localize in areas of active enchondral ossification (osteochondritis) and in the periosteum (periostitis). In acquired syphilis, bone disease may begin early in the tertiary stage, which usually is seen 2 to 5 years after the initial infection. The bones most frequently involved are those of the nose, palate, skull, and extremities, especially the long tubular bones such as the tibia. The syphilitic *saber shin* is produced by massive reactive periosteal bone deposition on the medial and anterior surfaces of the tibia.

Morphology. The histology of congenital syphilitic bone infection is characterized by edematous granulation tissue containing numerous plasma cells and necrotic bone. This type of response is also seen in acquired syphilis. Gummata also occur in the acquired disease. The spirochetes can be demonstrated in the inflammatory tissue with special silver stains.

Bone Tumors and Tumor-Like Lesions

Bone tumors are diverse in their gross and morphologic features and range in their biologic potential from the innocuous to the rapidly fatal. This diversity makes it critical to accurately diagnose and stage tumors, and treat them appropriately, so that the patients can not only survive, but also maintain optimal function of the affected body parts.

Most bone tumors are classified according to the normal cell or tissue of origin. Lesions that do not have normal tissue counterparts are grouped according to their distinct clinicopathologic features (Table 26–6). Overall, matrix-producing and fibrous tumors are the most common, and among the benign tumors, osteochondroma and fibrous cortical defect are most frequent. Excluding malignant neoplasms of marrow origin (myeloma, lymphoma, and leukemia), osteosarcoma is the most common primary cancer of bone, followed by chondrosarcoma and Ewing sarcoma.

The precise incidence of different bone tumors is not known because many benign lesions are not biopsied. Benign tumors outnumber their malignant counterparts, however, by at least several hundredfold. Benign tumors have their greatest frequency within the first three decades of life, whereas in the elderly a bone tumor is likely to be malignant. In the United States, about 2,100 new cases of bone sarcoma are

TABLE 26–6 Classification of Primary Tumors Involving Bones

Histologic Type	Benign	Malignant
Hematopoietic (40%)		Myeloma Malignant lymphoma
Chondrogenic (22%)	Osteochondroma Chondroma Chondroblastoma Chondromyxoid fibroma	Chondrosarcoma Dedifferentiated chondrosarcoma Mesenchymal chondrosarcoma
Osteogenic (19%)	Osteoid osteoma Osteoblastoma	Osteosarcoma
Unknown origin (10%)	Giant cell tumor	Ewing tumor Giant cell tumor Adamantinoma
Histiocytic origin	Fibrous histiocytoma	Malignant fibrous histiocytoma
Fibrogenic	Metaphyseal fibrous defect (fibroma)	Desmoplastic fibroma Fibrosarcoma
Notochordal		Chordoma
Vascular	Hemangioma	Hemangioendothelioma Hemangiopericytoma
Lipogenic	Lipoma	Liposarcoma
Neurogenic	Neurilemmoma	

Data on percentage of each type from Unni KK: Dahlin's Bone Tumors, 5th ed. Philadelphia, Lippincott-Raven, 1996, p 4; by permission of Mayo Foundation.

diagnosed annually, and approximately 1,300 deaths from bone sarcoma occur each year.

As a group these neoplasms affect all ages and arise in virtually every bone, but most develop during the first several decades of life and have a propensity to originate in the long bones of the extremities. However, specific types of tumors target certain age groups and anatomic sites.[32] For instance, most osteosarcomas occur during adolescence, and about half of them arise in the metaphysis around the knee, either in the distal femur or proximal tibia. These are the sites of greatest skeletal growth activity. In contrast, chondrosarcomas tend to develop during mid- to late adulthood and frequently involve the trunk, limb girdles, and proximal long bones. Chondroblastomas and giant cell tumors almost always arise in the epiphysis of long bones; by comparison, Ewing sarcoma, osteofibrous dysplasia, and adamantinoma most often are centered in the diaphysis. Thus, the location of a tumor provides important diagnostic information.

Although the cause of most bone tumors is unknown, genetic alterations similar to those that occur in other tumors clearly play a role. For instance, bone sarcomas occur in the Li-Fraumeni and hereditary retinoblastoma cancer syndromes, which are linked to mutations in *p53* and *RB* (Chapter 7). Bone infarcts, chronic osteomyelitis, Paget disease, radiation, and metal prostheses are also associated with an increased incidence of bone neoplasia. Such secondary neoplasms, however, account for only a small fraction of all skeletal tumors.

Clinically, bone tumors present in various ways. The more common benign lesions are frequently asymptomatic and are detected as incidental findings. Many tumors, however, produce pain or are noticed as a slow-growing mass. Sometimes, the first hint of a tumor's presence is a sudden pathologic fracture. Radiographic analysis plays an important role in diagnosing these lesions. In addition to providing the exact location and extent of the tumor, imaging studies can detect features that help limit diagnostic possibilities and give clues to the aggressiveness of the tumor. Ultimately, in most instances, biopsy and histologic study are necessary. In addition to classifying the tumor, histologic grade must also be determined in most primary malignancies. *The histologic grade has been shown to be the most important prognostic feature of a bone sarcoma* and is a key component of the major staging systems of bone neoplasms.

BONE-FORMING TUMORS

Common to all these neoplasms is the production of bone by the neoplastic cells. The tumor bone is usually deposited as woven trabeculae (except in osteomas) and is variably mineralized.

Osteoma

Osteomas are bosselated, round to oval sessile tumors that project from the subperiosteal or endosteal surfaces of the cortex. Subperiosteal osteomas most often arise on or inside the skull and facial bones. They are usually solitary and are detected in middle-aged adults. Multiple osteomas are seen in the setting of *Gardner syndrome* (Chapter 17). They are composed of woven and lamellar bone that is frequently deposited in a cortical pattern with haversian-like systems. Some variants contain a component of trabecular bone in which the intertrabecular spaces are filled with hematopoietic marrow. Histologically the reactive bone induced by infection, trauma, or hemangiomas may simulate an osteoma and should be considered in the differential diagnosis.

Osteomas are generally slow-growing tumors of little clinical significance except when they cause obstruction of a sinus cavity, impinge on the brain or eye, interfere with function of the oral cavity, or produce cosmetic problems. Osteomas do not transform into osteosarcoma.

Osteoid Osteoma and Osteoblastoma

Osteoid osteoma and *osteoblastoma* are terms used to describe benign bone tumors that have identical histologic features but that differ in size, sites of origin, and symptoms. *Osteoid osteomas* are, by definition, less than 2 cm in greatest dimension and usually occur in patients in their teens and twenties. Seventy-five per cent of patients are under age 25, and men outnumber women 2:1. Osteoid osteomas can arise in any bone but have a predilection for the appendicular skeleton. Fifty percent of cases involve the femur or tibia, where they commonly arise in the cortex and less frequently within the medullary cavity. Osteoid osteomas are painful lesions. The pain, which is caused by excess prostaglandin E_2 produced by the proliferating osteoblasts, is severe in relation to the small size of the lesion, is characteristically nocturnal, and is dramatically relieved by aspirin.[33] *Osteoblastoma* differs from osteoid osteoma in that it more frequently involves the spine; the pain is dull, achy, and not responsive to salicylates; and it does not induce a marked bony reaction.

Morphology. Grossly, both osteoid osteoma and osteoblastoma are round to oval masses of hemorrhagic gritty tan tissue. Histologically, they are well circumscribed and composed of a morass of randomly interconnecting trabeculae of woven bone prominently rimmed by osteoblasts (Fig. 26–21). The stroma surrounding the tumor bone consists of loose connective tissue that contains many dilated and congested capillaries. The relatively small size and well-defined margins of these tumors in combination

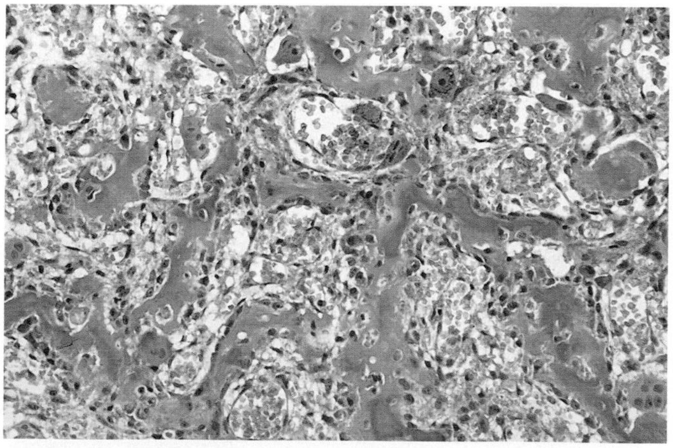

FIGURE 26–21 Osteoid osteoma composed of haphazardly interconnecting trabeculae of woven bone that are rimmed by prominent osteoblasts. The intertrabecular spaces are filled by vascular loose connective tissue.

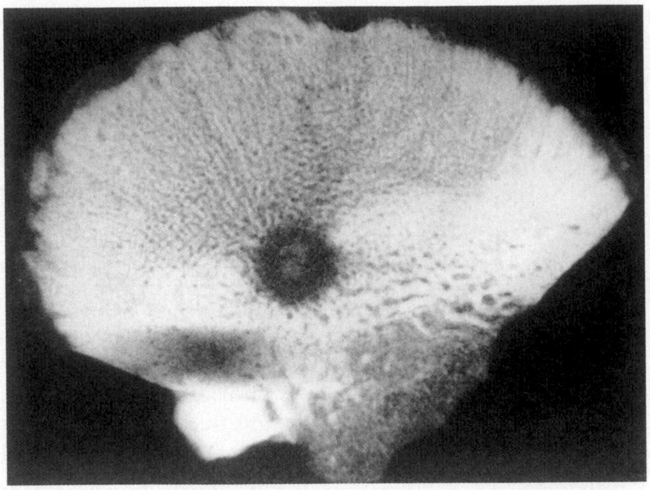

FIGURE 26–22 Specimen radiograph of intracortical osteoid osteoma. The round radiolucency with central mineralization represents the lesion and is surrounded by abundant reactive bone that has massively thickened the cortex.

with the benign cytologic features of the neoplastic osteoblasts helps distinguish them from osteosarcoma. Osteoid osteomas, especially those that arise beneath the periosteum, usually elicit a tremendous amount of reactive bone formation that encircles the lesion. The actual tumor, known as the **nidus,** manifests radiographically as a small round lucency that is variably mineralized (Fig. 26–22).[33]

Osteoid osteoma and osteoblastoma are readily treated by conservative surgery; if not entirely excised, they can recur. The possibility of malignant transformation is remote except when treated with radiation, which promotes this dreaded complication.

Osteosarcoma

Osteosarcoma is defined as a malignant mesenchymal tumor in which the cancerous cells produce bone matrix. It is the most common primary malignant tumor of bone, exclusive of myeloma and lymphoma, and accounts for approximately 20% of primary bone cancers. Osteosarcoma occurs in all age groups but has a bimodal age distribution; 75% occur in patients younger than age 20. The smaller second peak occurs in the elderly, who frequently suffer from conditions known to be associated with the development of osteosarcoma —Paget disease, bone infarcts, and prior irradiation. Overall, men are more commonly affected than women (1.6:1). The tumors usually arise in the metaphyseal region of the long bones of the extremities, and almost 60% occur about the knee (Fig. 26–23). Any bone may be involved, however, and in persons over age 25, the incidence in flat bones and long bones is almost equal.

Pathogenesis. Genetic mutations are fundamental to the development of osteosarcoma. Patients with hereditary retinoblastomas have up to 1,000 times greater risk of subsequently developing osteosarcoma, attributed to germ-line mutations in the *RB* gene. Loss of heterozygosity, structural rearrangements, or point mutations in the *RB* gene are also present in 60% to 70% of sporadic tumors. Abnormalities in genes that regulate cell cycling, such as *p53, CDK4, p16, INK4A, CYCLIN D1,* and *MDM2* have also been implicated in the genesis of nonhereditary osteosarcomas (Chapter 7).[34] It is also noteworthy that many osteosarcomas develop at sites of greatest bone growth, where bone cell mitotic activity is at its peak. It is not surprising that large dog breeds such as St. Bernards and Great Danes have a high incidence of this type of tumor.

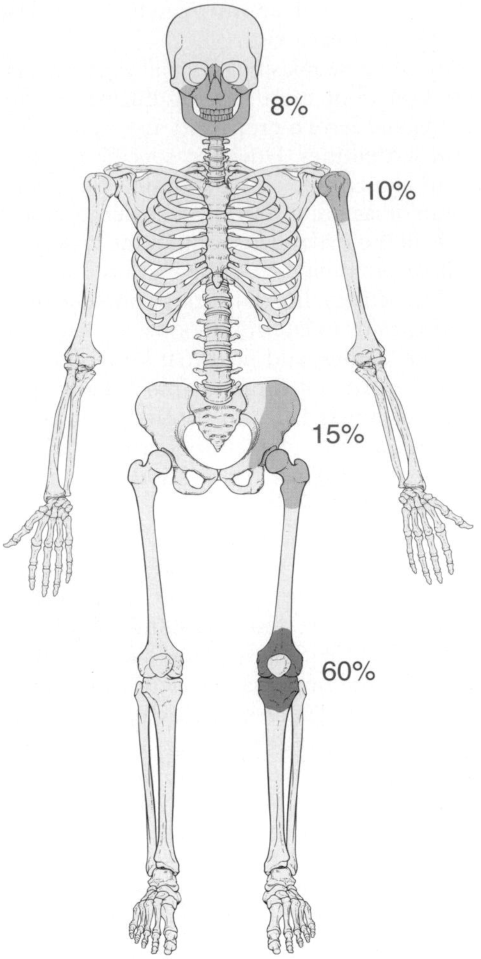

FIGURE 26–23 Major sites of origin of osteosarcomas. The numbers are approximate percentages.

Morphology. Several subtypes of osteosarcoma are recognized and are grouped according to:

- The anatomic portion of the bone from which they arise (intramedullary, intracortical, or surface)
- Degree of differentiation
- Multicentricity (synchronous, metachronous)
- Primary (underlying bone is unremarkable) or secondary (e.g., osteosarcoma associated with pre-existing disorders such as benign tumors, Paget disease, bone infarcts, previous irradiation)

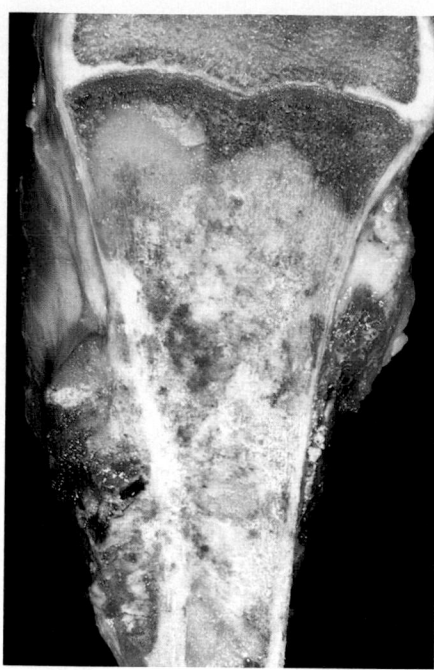

FIGURE 26–24 Osteosarcoma of the upper end of the tibia. The tan-white tumor fills most of the medullary cavity of the metaphysis and proximal diaphysis. It has infiltrated through the cortex, lifted the periosteum, and formed soft tissue masses on both sides of the bone.

- Histologic variants (osteoblastic, chondroblastic, fibroblastic, telangiectatic, small cell, and giant cell).[35]

The most common subtype is osteosarcoma that arises in the metaphysis of long bones; is primary, solitary, intramedullary, and poorly differentiated; and produces a predominantly bony matrix.

Grossly, osteosarcomas are bulky tumors that are gritty, gray-white, and often contain areas of hemorrhage and cystic degeneration (Fig. 26–24). The tumors frequently destroy the surrounding cortices and produce soft tissue masses. They spread extensively in the medullary canal, infiltrating and replacing the marrow surrounding the pre-existing bone trabeculae. Infrequently, they penetrate the epiphyseal plate or enter the joint. When joint invasion occurs, the tumor grows into it along tendinoligamentous structures or through the attachment site of the joint capsule. The tumor cells vary in size and shape and frequently have large hyperchromatic nuclei. Bizarre tumor giant cells are common, as are mitoses. **The formation of bone by the tumor cells is characteristic of osteosarcoma** (Fig. 26–25). The neoplastic bone has a coarse, lacelike architecture but is also deposited in broad sheets or as primitive trabeculae. Other matrices, including cartilage or fibrous tissue, may be present in varying amounts. When malignant cartilage is abundant, the tumor is called **chondroblastic osteosarcoma**. Vascular invasion is usually conspicuous, and up to 50% to 60% of an individual tumor may demonstrate spontaneous necrosis.

Clinical Course. Osteosarcomas typically present as painful and progressively enlarging masses. Sometimes a sudden fracture of the bone is the first symptom. Radiographs of the primary tumor usually show a large, destructive, mixed lytic and blastic mass that has permeative margins (Fig. 26–26). The tumor frequently breaks through the cortex and lifts the periosteum, resulting in reactive periosteal bone formation. The triangular shadow between the cortex and raised ends of periosteum is known radiographically as *Codman*

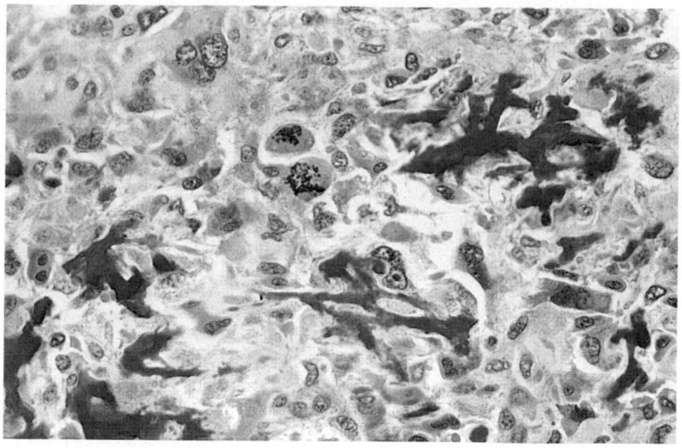

FIGURE 26–25 Osteosarcoma. Coarse, lacelike pattern of neoplastic bone produced by anaplastic malignant tumor cells. Note the mitotic figures.

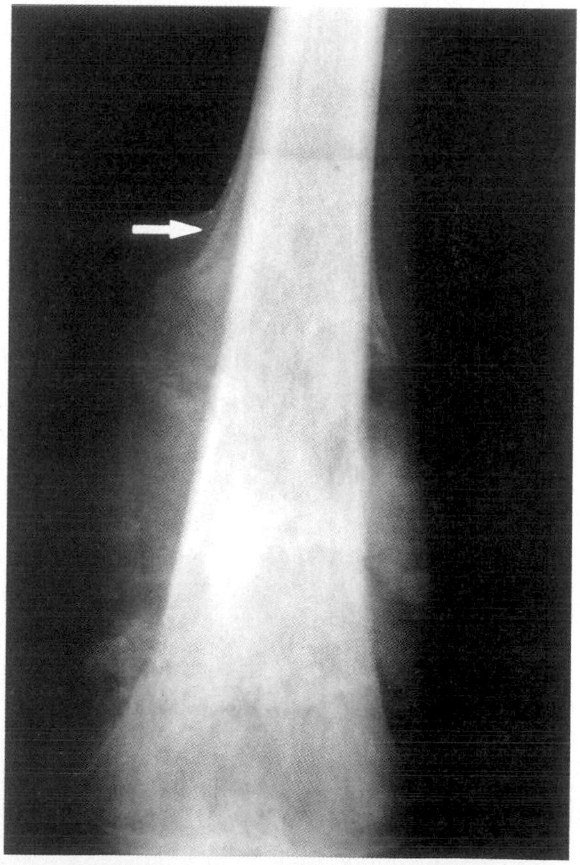

FIGURE 26–26 Distal femoral osteosarcoma with prominent bone formation extending into the soft tissues. The periosteum, which has been lifted, has laid down a proximal triangular shell of reactive bone known as a Codman triangle *(arrow)*.

triangle and is characteristic but not diagnostic of this tumor. These aggressive neoplasms spread through the bloodstream, and at the time of diagnosis, approximately 10% to 20% of patients have demonstrable pulmonary metastases. In those who die of the neoplasm, 90% have metastases to the lungs, bones, brain, and elsewhere.

Advances in treatment have substantially improved the prognosis of osteosarcoma. Long-term survival is 60% to 70%, compared with previous rates of 25%.[36] Standard treatment now includes chemotherapy and limb-salvage therapy.

CARTILAGE-FORMING TUMORS

Cartilage tumors are characterized by the formation of hyaline or myxoid cartilage; fibrocartilage and elastic cartilage are rare components. As in most types of bone tumors, benign cartilage tumors are much more common than malignant ones.

Osteochondroma

Osteochondroma, also known as an *exostosis,* is a benign cartilage-capped outgrowth that is attached to the underlying skeleton by a bony stalk. It is a relatively common lesion and can be solitary or multiple. Multiple osteochondromas occur in *multiple hereditary exostosis,* which is an autosomal dominant hereditary disease. Inactivation of both copies of the *EXT* gene in growth plate chondrocytes has been implicated in the pathogenesis of both sporadic and hereditary osteochondromas. This finding and other molecular genetic studies support the concept that osteochondromas are neoplasms (Fig. 26–27). Solitary osteochondromas are usually first diagnosed in late adolescence and early adulthood, but multiple osteochondromas become apparent during childhood. For unknown reasons, men are affected three times more often than women. Osteochondromas develop only in bones of endochondral origin and arise from the metaphysis near the growth plate of long tubular bones, especially about the knee. Occasionally, they develop from bones of the pelvis, scapula, and ribs, and in these sites they are frequently sessile and have short stalks. Rarely, these benign lesions involve the short tubular bones of the hands and feet.

Morphology. Osteochondromas are mushroom shaped and range in size from 1 to 20 cm. The cap is composed of benign hyaline cartilage varying in thickness and is covered peripherally by perichondrium. The cartilage has the appearance of disorganized growth plate and undergoes enchondral ossification, with the newly made bone forming the inner portion of the head and stalk. The cortex of the stalk merges with the cortex of the host bone so that the medullary cavity of the osteochondroma and bone are in continuity.

Clinically, osteochondromas present as slow-growing masses, which can be painful if they impinge on a nerve or if the stalk is fractured. In many cases, they are detected as an incidental finding. In multiple hereditary exostosis, the underlying bones may be bowed and shortened, reflecting an associated disturbance in epiphyseal growth. Osteochondromas usually stop growing at the time of growth plate closure. Rarely (<1% of cases), they give rise to a chondrosarcoma or some other type of sarcoma. The risk of this complication is substantially higher in patients with the hereditary syndrome.

Chondroma

Chondromas are benign tumors of hyaline cartilage. They may arise within the medullary cavity, where they are known as *enchondromas,* or on the surface of bone, where they are called *subperiosteal* or *juxtacortical chondromas.* Enchondromas are the most common of the intraosseous cartilage tumors, and are usually diagnosed in patients between age 20 and 50.

Enchondromas are usually solitary and are located in the metaphyseal region of tubular bones, the favored sites being the short tubular bones of the hands and feet.[34] The syndrome of multiple enchondromas, or enchondromatosis, is known as *Ollier disease.* If the enchondromatosis is associated with soft tissue hemangiomas, the disorder is called *Maffucci syndrome.* Chondromas are thought to develop from rests of growth plate cartilage that subsequently proliferate and slowly enlarge. Consistent with this theory is the observation that these tumors arise mainly in bones that develop from enchondral ossification. However, a more recent idea is that chon-

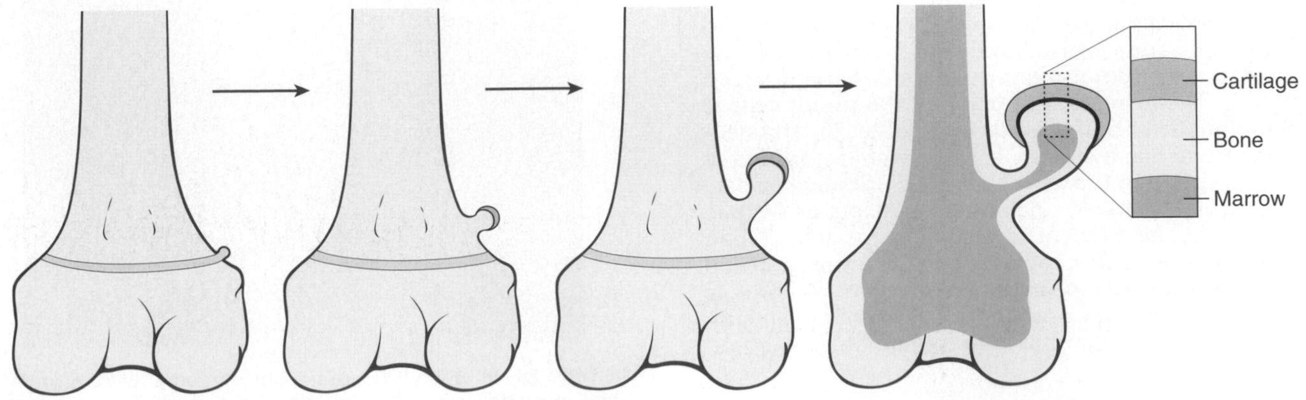

FIGURE 26–27 Schematic of the development over time of an osteochondroma, beginning with an outgrowth from the epiphyseal cartilage.

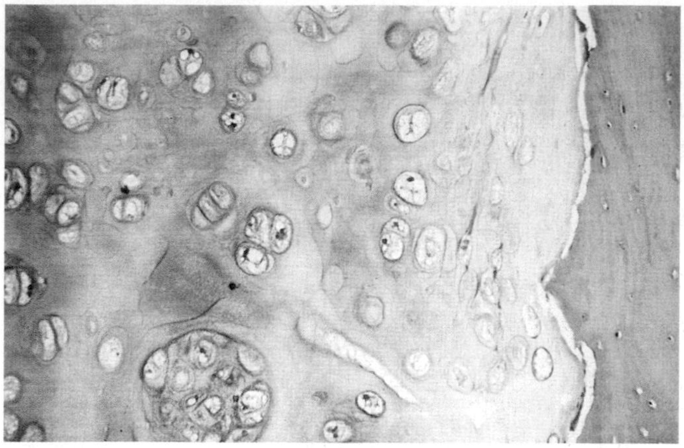

FIGURE 26–28 Enchondroma with a nodule of hyaline cartilage encased by a thin layer of reactive bone.

dromas develop from genetic alterations in mesenchymal stem cells.

Morphology. Enchondromas are usually smaller than 3 cm and grossly are gray-blue, translucent, and have a nodular configuration. Microscopically the nodules of cartilage are well circumscribed and have a hyaline matrix, and the neoplastic chondrocytes that reside in lacunae are cytologically benign (Fig. 26–28). At the periphery of the nodules, the cartilage undergoes enchondral ossification, and the center frequently calcifies and dies. The chondromas in Ollier disease and Maffucci syndrome may demonstrate a greater degree of cellularity and cytologic atypia and may be difficult to distinguish from chondrosarcoma.

Most enchondromas are asymptomatic and are detected as incidental findings. Occasionally, they are painful and cause pathologic fracture. The cartilage tumors in enchondromatosis may be numerous and large, producing severe deformities. The radiographic features are characteristic, as the unmineralized nodules of cartilage produce well-circumscribed oval lucencies that are surrounded by a thin rim of radiodense bone *(O ring sign)*. If the matrix calcifies, it is detected as irregular opacities. The nodules scallop the endosteum, and in long bones they do not result in complete cortical destruction (Fig. 26–29). The growth potential of chondromas is limited, and most remain stable. They may recur if incompletely excised surgically. Solitary chondromas rarely undergo sarcomatous transformation, but those associated with enchondromatoses do so more frequently. Patients with Maffucci syndrome are also at risk of developing other types of malignancies, including ovarian carcinomas and brain gliomas.

Chondroblastoma

Chondroblastoma is a rare benign tumor that accounts for less than 1% of primary bone tumors. It usually occurs in young patients in their teens with a male-to-female ratio of 2:1. Most arise near the knee. Less common sites such as the pelvis and ribs are affected in older patients. Chondroblastoma has a striking predilection for epiphyses and apophyses (epiphyseal equivalents, i.e., iliac crest).[37]

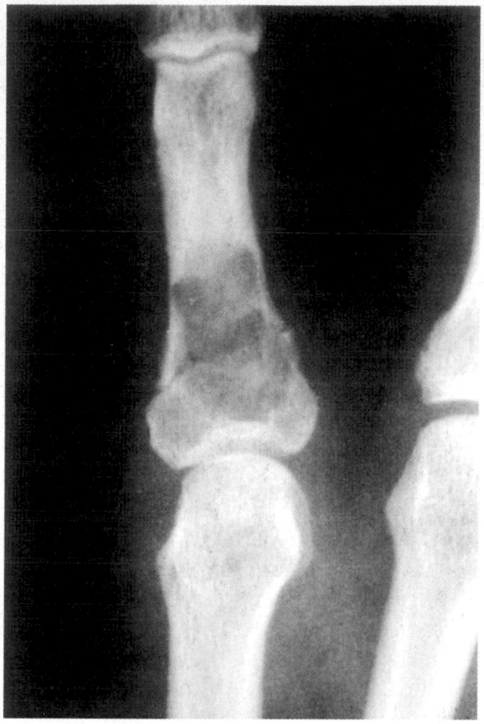

FIGURE 26–29 Enchondroma of the phalanx with a pathologic fracture. The radiolucent nodules of hyaline cartilage scallop the endosteal surface.

Morphology. The tumor is cellular and is composed of sheets of compact polyhedral chondroblasts that have well-defined cytoplasmic borders, moderate amounts of pink cytoplasm, and nuclei that are hyperlobulated with longitudinal grooves (Fig. 26–30). Mitotic activity and necrosis are frequently present. The tumor cells are surrounded by scant amounts of hyaline matrix that is deposited in a lacelike configuration; nodules of well-formed hyaline cartilage are distinctly uncommon. When the matrix calcifies, it produces a characteristic chicken-wire pattern of mineralization (see Fig. 26–30). Scattered through the

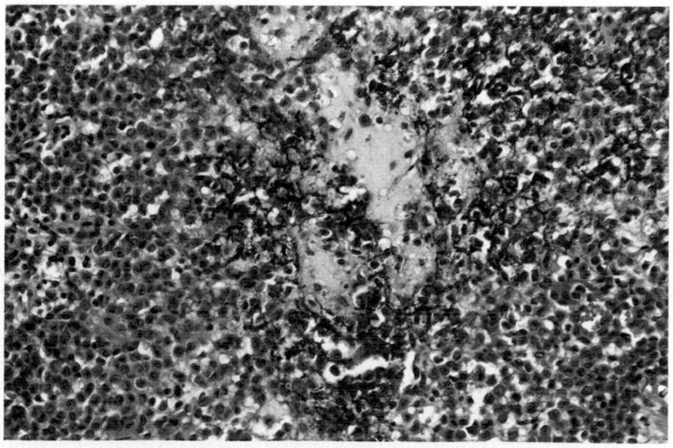

FIGURE 26–30 Chondroblastoma with scant mineralized matrix surrounding chondroblasts in a chicken wire-like fashion.

lesion are non-neoplastic osteoclast-type giant cells. Occasionally the tumors undergo prominent hemorrhagic cystic degeneration.

Chondroblastomas are usually painful, and because of their location near a joint they also cause effusions and restrict joint mobility. Radiographically, they produce a well-defined geographic lucency that commonly has spotty calcifications. Recurrences are not uncommon after surgical excision or curettage. Distant metastases, e.g., to the lungs, are rare, and usually occur after lesions have undergone prior pathologic fracture or repeated curettage. Apparently, in these circumstances, the tumor cells are pushed into ruptured vessels, giving them access to the systemic circulation.

Chondromyxoid Fibroma

Chondromyxoid fibroma is the rarest of cartilage tumors and because of its varied morphology can be mistaken for sarcoma. It affects patients in their teens and twenties, with a definite male preponderance. The tumors most frequently arise in the metaphysis of long tubular bones; however, they may involve virtually any bone of the body.

Morphology. The tumors range from 3 to 8 cm in greatest dimension and are well-circumscribed, solid, and glistening tan-gray. Microscopically, there are nodules of poorly formed hyaline cartilage and myxoid tissue delineated by fibrous septae. The cellularity varies; the areas of greatest cellularity are at the periphery of the nodules. In the cartilaginous regions, the tumor cells are situated in lacunae; however, in the myxoid areas, the cells are stellate, and their delicate cell processes extend through the mucinous ground substance and approach or contact neighboring cells (Fig. 26–31). In contrast to other benign cartilage tumors, the neoplastic cells in chondromyxoid fibroma show varying degrees of cytologic atypia, including the presence of large hyperchromatic nuclei. Other findings include small foci of calcification of the cartilaginous matrix and scattered non-neoplastic, osteoclast-type giant cells.[38]

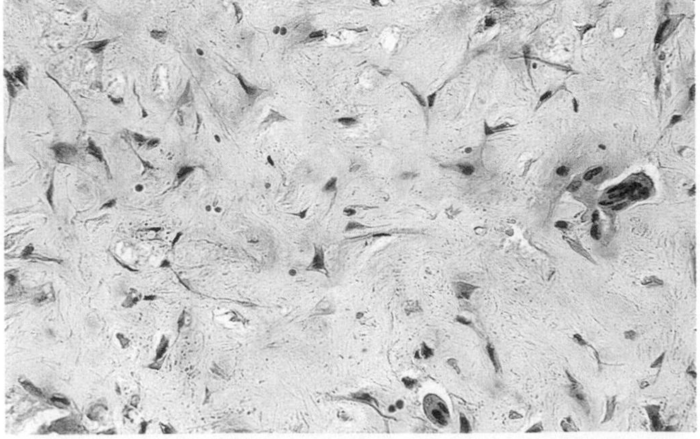

FIGURE 26–31 Chondromyxoid fibroma with prominent stellate and spindle cells surrounded by myxoid matrix. Occasional osteoclast-type giant cells are also present.

Patients with chondromyxoid fibroma usually complain of localized dull, achy pain. In most instances, x-rays demonstrate an eccentric geographic lucency that is well delineated from the adjacent bone by a rim of sclerosis. Occasionally the tumor expands the overlying cortex. The treatment of choice is simple curettage, and even though the tumors may recur, they do not pose a threat for malignant transformation or metastasis.

Chondrosarcoma

Chondrosarcomas comprise a group of tumors with a broad spectrum of clinical and pathologic findings. The feature common to all of them is the production of neoplastic cartilage. Chondrosarcoma is subclassified according to site as *intramedullary* and *juxtacortical*, and histologically as *conventional (hyaline and/or myxoid), clear cell, dedifferentiated,* and *mesenchymal* variants.

Chondrosarcoma of the skeleton is about half as frequent as osteosarcoma and is the second most common malignant matrix-producing tumor of bone. Patients with chondrosarcoma are usually age 40 or older. The clear cell and especially the mesenchymal variants occur in younger patients, in their teens or twenties. The tumor affects men twice as frequently as women and has no race predilection. Although a significant number of conventional chondrosarcomas arise in association with a pre-existing enchondroma, few develop within an osteochondroma, chondroblastoma, or fibrous dysplasia or in the setting of Paget disease.

Morphology. Conventional chondrosarcoma is composed of malignant hyaline and myxoid cartilage. The large bulky tumors are made up of nodules of gray-white, somewhat translucent glistening tissue (Fig. 26–32). In predominantly myxoid variants, the tumors are viscous and gelatinous and the matrix oozes from the cut surface. Spotty calcifications are typically present, and central necrosis may create cystic spaces. The adjacent cortex is thickened or eroded, and the tumor grows with broad pushing fronts into the surrounding soft tissue. The malignant cartilage infiltrates the marrow space and surrounds pre-existing bony trabeculae. The tumors vary in degree of cellularity, cytologic atypia, and mitotic activity (Fig. 26–33). Low-grade, or grade 1 lesions demonstrate mild hypercellularity, and the chondrocytes have plump vesicular nuclei with small nucleoli. Binucleate cells are sparse, and mitotic figures are difficult to find. Portions of the matrix frequently mineralize, and the cartilage may undergo enchondral ossification. By contrast, grade 3 chondrosarcomas are characterized by marked hypercellularity and extreme pleomorphism with bizarre tumor giant cells and mitoses. Pure grade 3 chondrosarcomas are uncommon. Such malignant cartilage is more frequently a component of **chondroblastic osteosarcoma** (described earlier).

Approximately 10% of conventional low-grade chondrosarcomas have a second high-grade component that has the morphology of a poorly differentiated sarcoma, such as malignant fibrous histiocytoma, fibrosarcoma, or osteosarcoma; this combination defines **dedifferentiated chondrosarcomas.** The hallmark of **clear cell chondrosarcoma** is

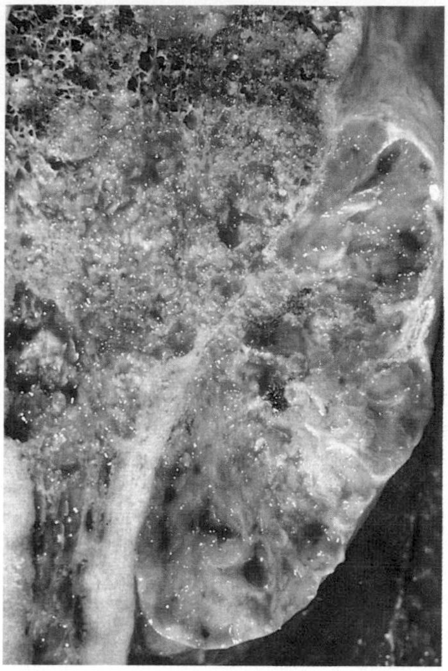

FIGURE 26–32 Chondrosarcoma with lobules of hyaline and myxoid cartilage permeating throughout the medullary cavity, growing through the cortex, and forming a relatively well-circumscribed soft tissue mass.

sheets of large malignant chondrocytes that have abundant clear cytoplasm, numerous osteoclast-type giant cells, and intralesional reactive bone formation. The last-mentioned aspect often causes confusion with osteosarcoma. **Mesenchymal chondrosarcoma** is composed of islands of well-differentiated hyaline cartilage surrounded by sheets of small round cells, which can mimic Ewing sarcoma.

Chondrosarcomas commonly arise in the central portions of the skeleton, including the pelvis, shoulder, and ribs. The clear cell variant is unique in that it originates in the epiphyses of long tubular bones. *In contrast to enchondroma, chondrosarcoma rarely involves the distal extremities.* These tumors usually present as painful, progressively enlarging masses. The nodular growth pattern of the cartilage produces prominent endosteal scalloping radiographically. The calcified matrix appears as foci of flocculent density. The more radiolucent the tumor, the greater the likelihood it is high grade. A slow-growing, low-grade tumor causes reactive thickening of the cortex, whereas a more aggressive high-grade neoplasm destroys the cortex and forms a soft tissue mass. There is a direct correlation between the grade and the biologic behavior of the tumor.[39] Fortunately, most conventional chondrosarcomas are indolent and fall into the range of grade 1 and grade 2. In one analysis, the 5-year survival rates were 90%, 81%, and 43% for grades 1 through 3, respectively. None of the grade 1 tumors metastasized, whereas 70% of the grade 3 tumors disseminated. Another prognostic feature is size. Tumors greater than 10 cm behave significantly more aggressively than smaller tumors. When chondrosarcomas metastasize, they spread preferentially to the lungs and skeleton. The treatment of conventional chondrosarcoma is wide surgical excision. The mesenchymal and dedifferentiated tumors are additionally treated with chemotherapy, because of their aggressive clinical course.

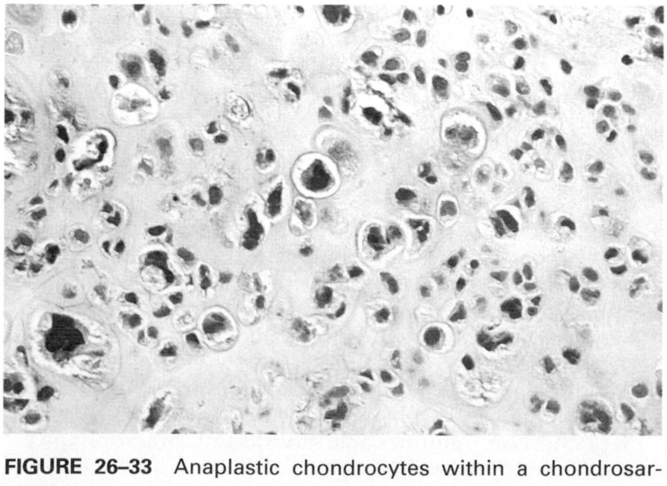

FIGURE 26–33 Anaplastic chondrocytes within a chondrosarcoma.

FIBROUS AND FIBRO-OSSEOUS TUMORS

Tumors composed solely or predominantly of fibrous elements are diverse and include some of the most common lesions of the skeleton.

Fibrous Cortical Defect and Nonossifying Fibroma

Fibrous cortical defects are extremely common, found in 30% to 50% of all children older than age 2 years. They are believed to be developmental defects rather than neoplasms. The vast majority arise eccentrically in the metaphysis of the distal femur and proximal tibia, and almost one half are bilateral or multiple. Often, they are small, about 0.5 cm in diameter. Those that grow to 5 or 6 cm in size develop into *nonossifying fibromas* and are usually not detected until adolescence.

Morphology. Both fibrous cortical defects and nonossifying fibromas produce elongated, sharply demarcated radiolucencies that are surrounded by a thin zone of sclerosis (Fig. 26–34). They consist of gray and yellow-brown tissue and are cellular lesions composed of fibroblasts and histiocytes (activated macrophages). The cytologically benign fibroblasts are frequently arranged in a storiform (pinwheel) pattern, and the histiocytes are either multinucleated giant cells or clusters of foamy macrophages (Fig. 26–35).

Fibrous cortical defects are asymptomatic and are usually detected on x-ray as an incidental finding. The vast majority have limited growth potential and undergo spontaneous resolution within several years, being replaced by normal cortical bone. The few that progressively enlarge into nonossifying fibromas may present with pathologic fracture or require biopsy and curettage to exclude other types of tumors.

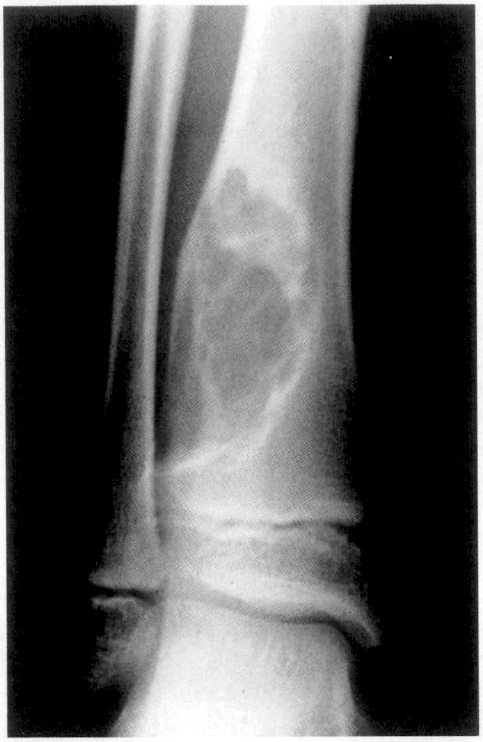

FIGURE 26–34 Nonossifying fibroma of the distal tibial metaphysis, producing an eccentric lobulated radiolucency surrounded by a sclerotic margin.

Fibrous Dysplasia

Fibrous dysplasia is a benign tumor that has been likened to a localized developmental arrest; all of the components of normal bone are present, but they do not differentiate into their mature structures. The lesions appear in three distinctive but sometimes overlapping clinical patterns: (1) involvement of a single bone (monostotic); (2) involvement of multiple, but never all, bones (polyostotic); and (3) polyostotic disease, associated with café au lait skin pigmentations and endocrine abnormalities, especially precocious puberty. The skeletal, skin and endocrine lesions result from a somatic (not hereditary) mutation occurring during embryogenesis that involves the gene that codes for a guanine nucleotide–binding protein (G-protein). The G-protein normally couples receptors to the effector enzyme adenylyl cyclase, and the mutation results in constitutive activation of the enzyme so that excess production of cAMP occurs, leading to hyperfunction of cells in the involved tissues.[40]

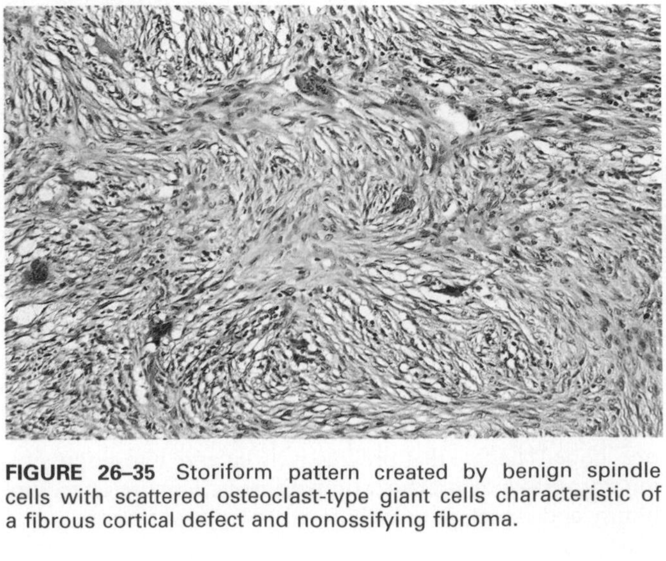

FIGURE 26–35 Storiform pattern created by benign spindle cells with scattered osteoclast-type giant cells characteristic of a fibrous cortical defect and nonossifying fibroma.

Monostotic fibrous dysplasia accounts for 70% of all cases. It occurs equally in boys and girls, usually in early adolescence, and often stops growing at the time of growth plate closure. The ribs, femur, tibia, jawbones, calvaria, and humerus are most commonly affected, in descending order of frequency. The lesion is asymptomatic and usually discovered incidentally. Fibrous dysplasia can cause marked enlargement and distortion of bone, so that if the craniofacial skeleton is involved, disfigurement, sometimes severe, can occur. Monostotic disease does not evolve into the polyostotic form.

Polyostotic fibrous dysplasia without endocrine dysfunction accounts for 27% of all cases. It manifests at a slightly earlier age than the monostotic type and may continue to cause problems into adulthood. The bones affected, in descending order of frequency, are the femur, skull, tibia, humerus, ribs, fibula, radius, ulna, mandible, and vertebrae. Craniofacial involvement is present in 50% of patients who have a moderate number of bones affected and in 100% of patients with extensive skeletal disease. All forms of polyostotic disease have a propensity to involve the shoulder and pelvic girdles, resulting in severe, sometimes crippling, deformities (e.g., shepherd-crook deformity of the proximal femur) and spontaneous and often recurrent fractures.

Polyostotic fibrous dysplasia associated with café au lait skin pigmentation and endocrinopathies is known as the *McCune-Albright syndrome* and accounts for 3% of all cases. The endocrinopathies include sexual precocity, hyperthyroidism, pituitary adenomas that secrete growth hormone, and primary adrenal hyperplasia. The severity of manifestations in McCune-Albright syndrome depends on the number and cell types that harbor the mutation in the G-protein. The most common clinical presentation is precocious sexual development, and in this setting girls are affected more often than boys. The bone lesions are often unilateral, and the skin pigmentation is usually limited to the same side of the body. The cutaneous macules are classically large; are dark to café au lait; have irregular serpiginous borders (coastline of Maine); and are found primarily on the neck, chest, back, shoulder, and pelvic region.

Morphology. Grossly the lesions of fibrous dysplasia are well-circumscribed, are intramedullary, and vary greatly in size. Larger lesions expand and distort the bone. The lesional tissue is tan-white and gritty and is composed of curvilinear trabeculae of woven bone surrounded by a moderately cellular fibroblastic proliferation. The shapes of the trabeculae mimic Chinese characters, and the bone lacks osteoblastic rimming (Fig. 26–36). Nodules of hyaline cartilage with the appearance of disorganized growth plate are also present in approximately 20% of cases. Cystic degeneration, hemorrhage, and foamy macrophages are other common findings.

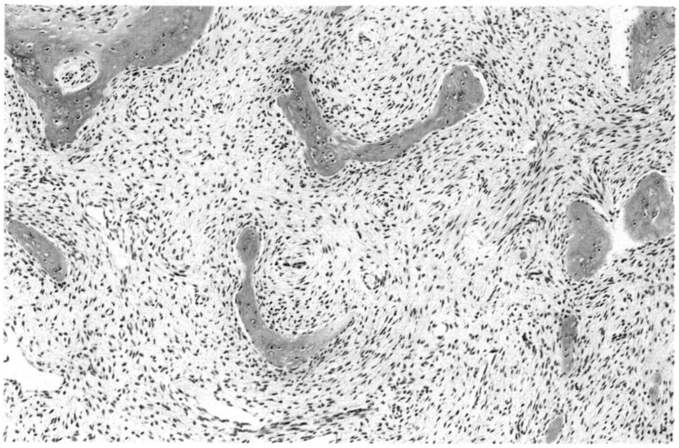

FIGURE 26–36 Fibrous dysplasia composed of curvilinear trabeculae of woven bone that lack conspicuous osteoblastic rimming and arise in a background of fibrous tissue.

Clinical Course. The natural history of fibrous dysplasia is variable and depends on the extent of skeletal involvement. Patients with monostotic disease usually have minimal symptoms. The lesion is readily diagnosed by x-ray because of its typical ground-glass appearance and well-defined margins. Lesions that fracture or cause significant symptoms are readily cured by conservative surgery. Polyostotic involvement is frequently associated with progressive disease, and the earlier the age at diagnosis, the more likely are severe skeletal complications, such as recurring fractures, long bone deformities, and distorting involvement of the craniofacial bones. A rare complication, usually in the setting of polyostotic involvement, is malignant transformation of a lesion into a sarcoma, such as osteosarcoma, or malignant fibrous histiocytoma. The risk of this occurrence is increased if the lesion has been irradiated.

Fibrosarcoma and Malignant Fibrous Histiocytoma

Fibrosarcoma and malignant fibrous histiocytoma are fibroblastic collagen-producing sarcomas of bone. They have overlapping clinical, radiographic, and pathologic features, and somewhat arbitrary morphologic criteria are used to distinguish them. They occur at any age, but most affect the middle-aged and elderly. Fibrosarcoma has a nearly equal sex distribution, whereas malignant fibrous histiocytoma occurs more frequently in men. Both sarcomas usually arise de novo; however, a minority are secondary tumors and develop in preexisting benign tumors, bone infarcts, pagetic bone, and previously irradiated tissue.

Morphology. Grossly, these tumors are large, hemorrhagic, tan-white masses that destroy the underlying bone and frequently extend into the soft tissues. Fibrosarcoma is composed of malignant fibroblasts arranged in a herringbone pattern. The level of differentiation determines the amount of collagen produced and the degree of cytologic atypia. Bizarre multinucleated cells are not common, and most fibrosarcomas have the appearance of a low- to intermediate-grade malignancy. Malignant fibrous histiocytoma consists of a background of spindled fibroblasts arranged in a storiform pattern admixed with large, ovoid, bizarre multinucleated tumor giant cells. Morphologically, some tumor cells resemble neoplastic histiocytes; however, the evidence shows they are actually fibroblasts. Malignant fibrous histiocytoma of bone is generally a high-grade pleomorphic tumor.[41]

Fibrosarcoma and malignant fibrous histiocytoma present as enlarging painful masses that usually arise in the metaphyses of long bones and pelvic flat bones. Pathologic fracture is a frequent complication. Radiographically, they are permeative and lytic and often extend into the adjacent soft tissue. The prognosis of these two sarcomas depends on their grade; high-grade tumors have a poor prognosis.

Miscellaneous Tumors

EWING SARCOMA AND PRIMITIVE NEUROECTODERMAL TUMOR (PNET)

Ewing sarcoma and PNET are primary malignant *small round cell tumors* of bone and soft tissue (Chapter 10). They have long posed difficult diagnostic problems because their neoplastic cells resemble those of lymphoma, rhabdomyosarcoma, neuroblastoma, and oat cell carcinoma. Current evidence indicates that both Ewing sarcoma and PNET have a similar neural phenotype and, because they share an identical chromosome translocation, they should be viewed as the same tumor, differing only in their degree of neural differentiation. Tumors that demonstrate neural differentiation by light microscopy, immunohistochemistry, or electron microscopy have been traditionally labeled PNETs, and those that are undifferentiated by these analyses have been diagnosed as Ewing sarcoma.

Ewing sarcoma and PNET account for approximately 6% to 10% of primary malignant bone tumors and follow osteosarcoma as the second most common group of bone sarcomas in children. Of all bone sarcomas, Ewing sarcoma has the youngest average age at presentation, as most patients are 10 to 15 years old, and approximately 80% are younger than age 20 years. Boys are affected slightly more frequently than girls, and there is a striking predilection for whites; blacks are rarely afflicted. In approximately 85% of Ewing sarcomas and PNETs, there is a t(11;22)(q24;q12) translocation; in 5% to 10% of cases, the translocation is t(21;21)(q21;q12); and in less than 1% of tumors, a t(7;22)(q22;12) translocation is present (see Table 26–9). In all cases there is fusion of the EWS gene on 22q12 to a member of the ETS family of transcription factor, mainly FLT1. Evidence suggests that the most common fusion gene *(EWS-FLI1)* generated from the t(11;22) translocation acts as a dominant oncogene, and the resultant chimeric protein acts as a constitutively active transcription factor that stimulates cell proliferation.[42]

Morphology. Arising in the medullary cavity, Ewing sarcoma and PNET usually invade the cortex and periosteum, producing a soft tissue mass. The tumor is tan-white and frequently contains areas of hemor-

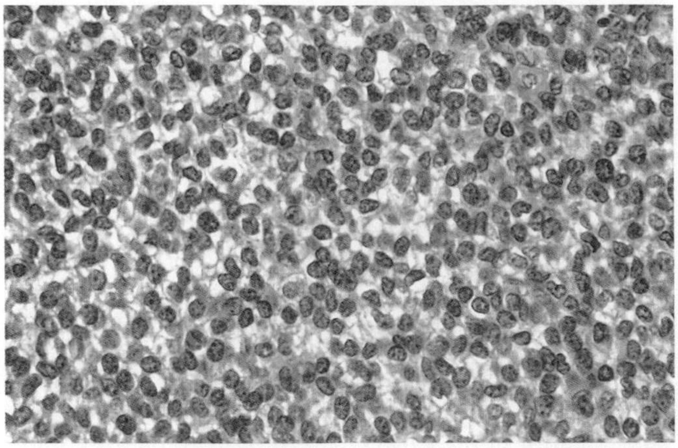

FIGURE 26–37 Ewing sarcoma composed of sheets of small round cells with small amounts of clear cytoplasm.

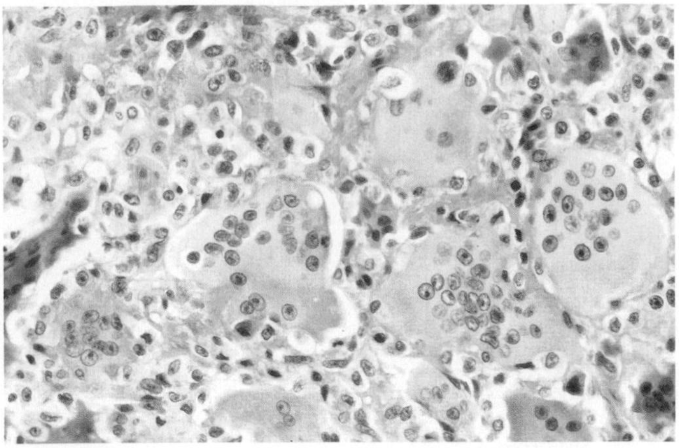

FIGURE 26–38 Benign giant cell tumor illustrating an abundance of multinucleated giant cells with background mononuclear stromal cells.

rhage and necrosis. It is composed of sheets of uniform small, round cells that are slightly larger than lymphocytes (Fig. 26–37). They have scant cytoplasm, which may appear clear because it is rich in glycogen. The presence of Homer-Wright rosettes (where the tumor cells are arranged in a circle about a central fibrillary space) is indicative of neural differentiation. Although the tumor contains fibrous septae, there is generally little stroma. Necrosis may be prominent, and there are relatively few mitotic figures in relation to the dense cellularity of the tumor.

Ewing sarcoma and PNET usually arise in the diaphyses of long tubular bones, especially the femur and the flat bones of the pelvis. They present as painful enlarging masses, and the affected site is frequently tender, warm, and swollen. Some patients have systemic findings, including fever, ele-vated sedimentation rate, anemia, and leukocytosis, which mimic infection. Plain x-rays show a destructive lytic tumor that has permeative margins and extension into the surrounding soft tissues. The characteristic periosteal reaction produces layers of reactive bone deposited in an onionskin fashion.

The treatment of Ewing sarcoma and PNET includes chemotherapy and surgical excision with or without radiation. The advent of effective chemotherapy has dramatically improved the prognosis from a dismal 5% to 15% to a 75% 5-year survival; at least 50% are long-term cures.

GIANT CELL TUMOR

Giant cell tumor is so named because it contains a profusion of multinucleated osteoclast-type giant cells, giving rise to the synonym *osteoclastoma.* Giant cell tumor is a relatively uncommon benign but locally aggressive neoplasm. It usually arises in patients in their twenties to forties. Giant cell tumors are believed to have a monocyte–macrophage lineage,[43] and the giant cells are believed to form via fusion of the mononuclear cells.

Morphology. These tumors are large and red-brown and frequently undergo cystic degeneration. They are composed of uniform oval mononuclear cells that have indistinct cell membranes and appear to grow in a syncytium. The mononuclear cells are the proliferating component of the tumor, and mitoses are frequent. Scattered within this background are numerous osteoclast-type giant cells having 100 or more nuclei that have identical features to those of the mononuclear cells (Fig. 26–38). Necrosis, hemorrhage, hemosiderin deposition, and reactive bone formation are common secondary features. The histologic differential diagnosis includes other giant cell lesions, such as the brown tumor seen in hyperparathyroidism, giant cell reparative granuloma, chondroblastoma, and pigmented villonodular synovitis. The morphologic identity between the nuclei of the stromal cells and those of the giant cells helps distinguish giant cell tumor from these other lesions.

Clinical Course. Giant cell tumors in adults involve both the epiphyses and the metaphyses, but in adolescents they are confined proximally by the growth plate and are limited to the metaphysis. The majority of giant cell tumors arise around the knee (distal femur and proximal tibia), but virtually any bone may be involved. The location of these tumors in the ends of bones near joints frequently causes patients to complain of arthritic symptoms. Occasionally, they present as pathologic fractures. Most are solitary; however, multiple or multicentric tumors do occur, especially in the distal extremities. Radiographically, giant cell tumors are large, purely lytic, and eccentric, and erode into the subchondral bone plate (Fig. 26–39). The overlying cortex is frequently destroyed, producing a bulging soft tissue mass delineated by a thin shell of reactive bone. The margins with the adjacent bone are fairly circumscribed but seldom sclerotic. The biologic unpredictability of these neoplasms complicates their management. Conservative surgery such as curettage is associated with a 40% to 60% recurrence rate. Up to 4% metastasize to the lungs. The metastatic deposits have the same morphology as the primary tumor. Sarcomatous transformation of a giant cell tumor, either de novo or after previous treatment, is a rare event.

METASTATIC DISEASE

Metastatic tumors are the most common form of skeletal malignancy. The pathways of spread include (1) direct exten-

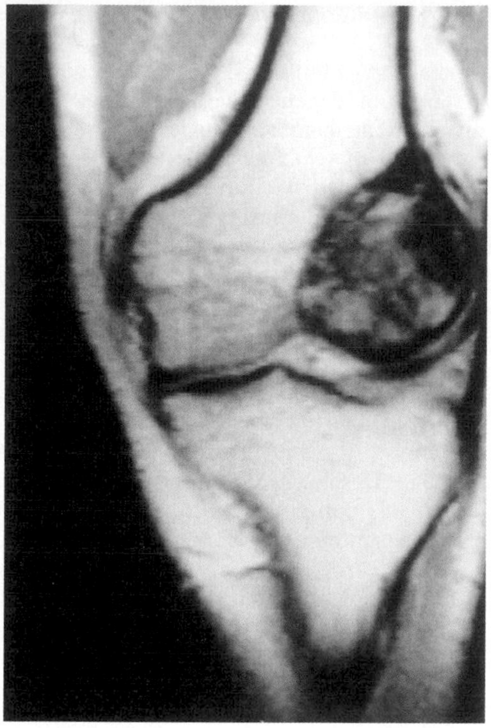

FIGURE 26–39 Magnetic resonance image of a giant cell tumor that replaces most of the femoral condyle and extends to the subchondral bone plate.

sion, (2) lymphatic or hematogenous dissemination, and (3) intraspinal seeding (Batson plexus of veins). Any cancer can spread to bone, but in adults, more than 75% of skeletal metastases originate from cancers of the prostate, breast, kidney, and lung. In children, metastases to bone originate from neuroblastoma, Wilms tumor, osteosarcoma, Ewing sarcoma, and rhabdomyosarcoma.

Skeletal metastases are typically multifocal; however, carcinomas of the kidney and thyroid are notorious for producing solitary lesions. The metastases may occur in any bone, but most involve the axial skeleton (vertebral column, pelvis, ribs, skull, sternum), proximal femur, and humerus, in descending order of frequency. The red marrow in these areas with its rich capillary network, slow blood flow, and nutrient environment facilitates implantation and growth of the tumor cells. Metastases to the small bones of the hands and feet are uncommon and usually originate in cancers of the lung, kidney, or colon.

The radiographic manifestations of metastases may be purely lytic, purely blastic, or mixed lytic and blastic. In lytic lesions, the metastatic cells secrete substances such as prostaglandins, interleukins, and PTHRP, which stimulate osteoclastic bone resorption; the tumor cells themselves do not directly resorb bone. Carcinomas of the kidney, lung, and gastrointestinal tract and malignant melanoma produce this type of bone destruction. Similarly, metastases that elicit a sclerotic response, particularly prostate adenocarcinoma, do so by stimulating osteoblastic bone formation. Most metastases induce a mixed lytic and blastic reaction.

JOINTS

Normal

Joints are constructed to provide both movement and mechanical support. Their anatomy is directly related to their function, and they are classified as solid (nonsynovial) and cavitated (synovial). The solid joints, known as *synarthroses,* provide structural integrity and allow for minimal movement. They lack a joint space and are grouped according to the type of connective tissue (fibrous tissue or cartilage) that bridges the ends of the bones; fibrous synarthroses include the cranial sutures and the bonds between roots of teeth and the jawbones; cartilaginous synarthroses (synchondroses) are represented by the symphyses (manubriosternalis and pubic). *Synovial joints,* in contrast, have a joint space that allows for a wide range of motion. Situated between the ends of bones formed via enchondral ossification, they are strengthened by a dense fibrous capsule reinforced by ligaments and muscles. The boundary of the joint space is formed by the synovial membrane, which is firmly anchored to the underlying capsule. Its contour is smooth except near the osseous insertion, where it is thrown into numerous villous folds. The surface lining of cubioidal cells, or synoviocytes, is one to four cell layers deep. These cells are not present over the cartilage surfaces. Traditionally, they are segregated into type A cells (macrophage-like), which are phagocytic and synthesize hyaluronic acid, and type B cells (fibroblast-like), which produce various proteins. The type A and B cells are now best considered one cell population that alters its phenotype according to functional demands. The synovial lining lacks a basement membrane and merges with the underlying loose connective tissue stroma, which is generally very vascular. The absence of a basement membrane allows for quick exchange between blood and synovial fluid. The clear, viscous synovial fluid is a filtrate of plasma containing hyaluronic acid that acts as a lubricant and provides nutrition for the articular hyaline cartilage.

Hyaline cartilage is a unique connective tissue ideally suited to serve as an elastic shock absorber and wear-resistant surface. It lacks a blood supply and does not have lymphatic drainage or innervation. Adult articular cartilage varies in thickness from 2 to 4 mm and is thickest at the periphery of concave surfaces and in the central portions of convex surfaces. Hyaline cartilage is composed of type 2 collagen, water, proteoglycans, and chondrocytes, each of which has specific functions. The collagen fibers are arranged in arches so that near the surface they are horizontal in orientation—this allows the cartilage to resist tensile stresses and transmit vertical loads. The water and proteoglycans give hyaline cartilage its turgor and elasticity and play an important role in limiting friction. The chondrocytes synthesize the matrix as well as enzymatically digest it, with the half-life of the different components ranging from weeks (proteoglycans) to years (type 2 collagen). Matrix turnover is carefully controlled as chondrocytes secrete the degradative enzymes in an inactive form and enrich the matrix with enzyme inhibitors. Diseases that destroy articular cartilage do so by activating the catabolic enzymes and decreasing the production of inhibitors, thereby accelerating the rate of matrix breakdown. The chondrocytes react by increasing matrix production; however, the response is usually inadequate. Cytokines such as IL-1 and TNF trigger the degradative process, and their sources include chondrocytes, synoviocytes, fibroblasts, and inflammatory cells. Destruction of articular cartilage by indigenous cells is an important mechanism in many joint diseases.

Pathology

Arthritis

OSTEOARTHRITIS

Osteoarthritis, also called *degenerative joint disease,* is the most common type of joint disease and is one of the most disabling conditions in developed nations. *It is characterized by the progressive erosion of articular cartilage.* It is estimated that over $33 billion are spent annually in the United States for its treatment and for lost days of work. The term *osteoarthritis* implies an inflammatory disease. However, although inflammatory cells may be present, osteoarthritis is considered to be an intrinsic disease of articular cartilage in which biochemical and metabolic alterations result in its breakdown.

In the great majority of instances, osteoarthritis appears insidiously, without apparent initiating cause, as an aging phenomenon (idiopathic or primary osteoarthritis). In these cases, the disease usually affects few joints (oligoarticular) but may be generalized. In about 5% of cases, osteoarthritis may appear in younger individuals having some predisposing condition, such as previous macrotraumatic or repeated microtraumatic injuries to a joint, a congenital developmental deformity of a joint(s), or some underlying systemic disease such as diabetes, ochronosis, hemochromatosis, or marked obesity. In these settings, the disease is called *secondary osteoarthritis* and often involves one or several predisposed joints—witness the shoulder or elbow involvements in baseball players and knees in basketball players. Gender has some influence on distribution. The knees and hands are more commonly affected in women and the hips in men.

Pathogenesis. As mentioned earlier, articular cartilage is the major target of degenerative changes in osteoarthritis. Normal articular cartilage is strategically located at the ends of bones to perform two functions: (1) bathed in synovial fluid, it ensures virtually friction-free movements within the joint; and (2) in weight-bearing joints, it spreads the load across the joint surface in a manner that allows the underlying bones to absorb shock and weight without being crushed. These functions require the cartilage to be elastic (i.e., to regain normal architecture after being compressed) and for it to have unusually high tensile strength. These attributes are provided by the two major components of the cartilage: a special type of collagen (type II) and proteoglycans, both secreted by chondrocytes. As is the case with adult bones, articular cartilage is not static; it undergoes turnover in which "worn out" matrix components are degraded and replaced. This balance is maintained by chondrocytes, which not only synthesize the matrix but also secrete matrix-degrading enzymes. Thus, the health of the chondrocytes and their ability to maintain the essential properties of the cartilage matrix determine joint integrity.[44] In osteoarthritis, this process is disturbed by a variety of influences.

Perhaps the most important of these influences are *aging and mechanical effects.* Although osteoarthritis is not exclusively a wear-and-tear process, there is little doubt that mechanical stresses on the joint play a major role in its development. Evidence for this includes the increasing frequency of osteoarthritis with advancing age; its occurrence in weight-bearing joints; and an increase in the frequency of the disease in conditions that predispose the joints to abnormal mechanical stresses, such as obesity and previous joint deformity.

Genetic factors also appear to play a role in susceptibility to osteoarthritis, particularly in cases involving the hands and hips. The specific gene or genes responsible for this have not been identified, although linkage to chromosomes 2 and 11 has been suggested in some cases. The risk of osteoarthritis is increased in direct proportion to bone density, and high levels of estrogens have also been associated with an increased risk of the disease. The overall role played by hormones in the pathogenesis of osteoarthritis remains unclear, however.

Osteoarthritis is characterized by significant changes in both the composition and the mechanical properties of cartilage. Early in the course of the disease, the degenerating cartilage contains increased water and a decreased concentration of proteoglycans compared with healthy cartilage. In addition, there appears to be a weakening of the collagen network, presumably caused by decreased local synthesis of type II collagen, and increased breakdown of preexisting collagen. The levels of certain molecular messengers, including IL-1, TNF and nitric oxide, are increased in osteoarthritic cartilage and appear to be responsible for some of these changes in the composition of the cartilage. Apoptosis is also increased, likely responsible for a decrease in the number of functional chondrocytes. In aggregate, these changes tend to reduce the tensile strength and the resilience of the articular cartilage. In response to these regressive changes, chondrocytes in the deeper layers proliferate and attempt to "repair" the damage by producing new collagen and proteoglycans. Although these reparative changes are initially able to keep pace with the deterioration of cartilage, molecular signals causing chondrocyte loss and changes in the extracellular matrix, as noted earlier, eventually predominate. Factors responsible for this shift from a reparative to a predominantly degenerative picture remain poorly understood.

Morphology. In the early stages of osteoarthritis, the chondrocytes proliferate. This process is accompanied by biochemical changes as the water content of the matrix increases and the concentration of proteoglycans decreases. Subsequently, vertical and horizontal fibrillation and cracking of the matrix occur as the superficial layers of the cartilage are degraded. Gross examination at this stage reveals a granular articular surface that is softer than normal. Eventually, full-thickness portions of the cartilage are sloughed, and the exposed subchondral bone plate becomes the new articular surface. Friction smoothes and burnishes the exposed bone, giving it the appearance of polished ivory **(bone eburnation)** (Fig. 26–40). Concurrently, there is rebuttressing and sclerosis of the underlying cancellous bone. Small fractures through the articulating bone are common, and the dislodged pieces of cartilage and subchondral bone tumble into the joint, forming loose bodies **(joint mice)**. The fracture gaps allow synovial fluid to be forced into the subchondral regions in a one-way, ball-valve–like mechanism. The loculated fluid collection increases in size, forming fibrous walled cysts. Mushroom-shaped osteophytes (bony outgrowths) develop at the margins of the articular surface and are capped by fibrocartilage and hyaline cartilage that gradually ossify. The synovium shows minor alterations in comparison to the destruction of the articular surface and is congested and fibrotic and may have scattered chronic inflammatory cells. In severe disease, a fibrous synovial pannus covers the peripheral portions of the articular surface.

Clinical Course. Osteoarthritis is an insidious disease. Patients with primary disease are usually asymptomatic until they are in their fifties. If a young patient has significant manifestations of osteoarthritis, a search for some underlying cause should be made. Characteristic symptoms include deep, achy pain that worsens with use; morning stiffness; crepitus; and limitation of range of movement. Impingement on spinal foramina by osteophytes results in cervical and lumbar nerve root compression with radicular pain, muscle spasms, muscle atrophy, and neurologic deficits. Typically, only one or a few joints are involved, except in the uncommon generalized variant. The joints commonly involved include the hips, knees, lower lumbar and cervical vertebrae, proximal and distal interphalangeal joints of the fingers, first carpometacarpal joints, and first tarsometatarsal joints of the feet (Fig. 26–41). Characteristic in women, but not in men, are *Heberden nodes* in the fingers, representing prominent osteophytes at the distal interphalangeal joints. The wrists, elbows, and shoulders are usually spared. There are still no satisfactory means of preventing primary osteoarthritis, and there are no methods for halting its progression. The disease may stabilize for years at any stage but more often is slowly progressive over the remaining years of life; osteoarthritis is second only to cardiovascular diseases in causing long-term disability.

RHEUMATOID ARTHRITIS

Rheumatoid arthritis (RA) is a chronic systemic inflammatory disorder that may affect many tissues and organs—skin, blood vessels, heart, lungs, and muscles—but principally attacks the joints, producing a nonsuppurative proliferative and inflammatory synovitis that often progresses to destruction of the articular cartilage and ankylosis of the joints. Although the cause of RA remains unknown, autoimmunity plays a pivotal role in its chronicity and progression.

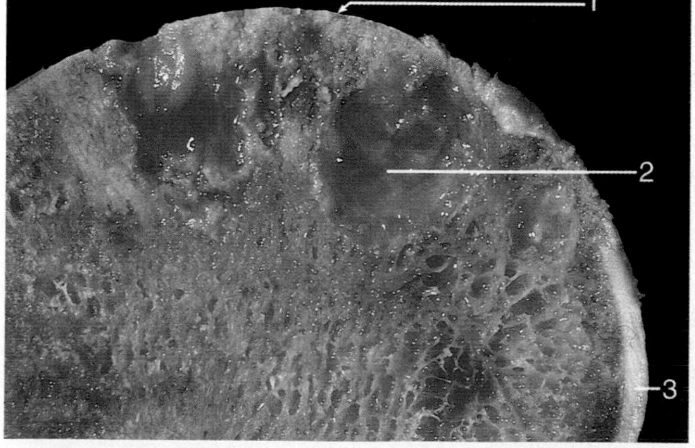

FIGURE 26–40 Severe osteoarthritis with small islands of residual articular cartilage next to exposed subchondral bone. *1,* Eburnated articular surface. *2,* Subchondral cyst. *3,* Residual articular cartilage.

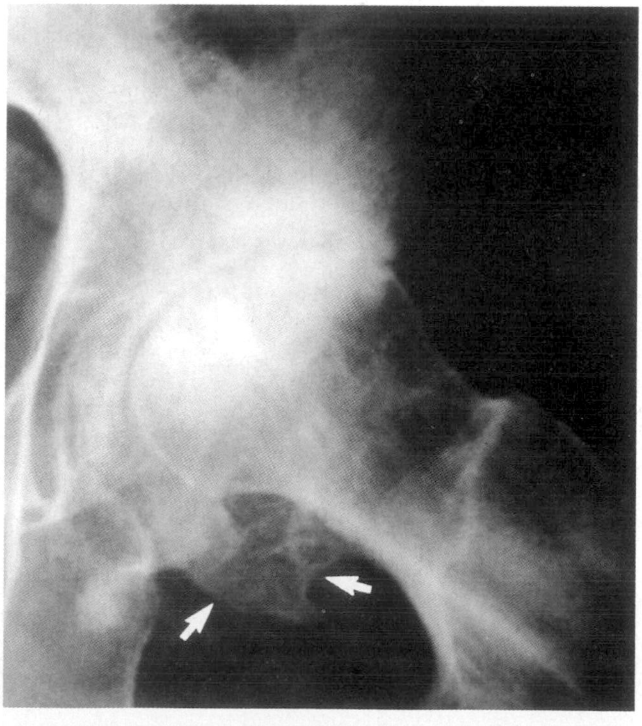

FIGURE 26–41 Severe osteoarthritis of the hip. The joint space is narrowed, and there is subchondral sclerosis with scattered oval radiolucent cysts and peripheral osteophyte lipping *(arrows)*.

About 1% of the world's population is afflicted by RA, women two to three times more often than men. It is most common in those age 40 to 70, but no age is immune. We first consider the morphology as a background to discuss pathogenesis.

Morphology

Joints. RA causes a broad spectrum of morphologic alterations; the most severe are manifested in the joints. Initially the synovium becomes grossly edematous, thickened, and hyperplastic, transforming its smooth contour to one covered by delicate and bulbous fronds (Fig. 26–42). The characteristic histologic features include (1) infiltration of synovial stroma by dense perivascular inflammatory cells, consisting of B cells and CD4+ helper T cells (often forming lymphoid follicles), plasma cells, and macrophages; (2) increased vascularity owing to vasodilation and angiogenesis, with superficial hemosiderin deposits; (3) aggregation of organizing fibrin covering portions of the synovium and floating in the joint space as rice bodies; (4) accumulation of neutrophils in the synovial fluid and along the surface of synovium but usually not deep in the synovial stroma; (5) osteoclastic activity in underlying bone, allowing the synovium to penetrate into the bone forming juxta-articular erosions, subchondral cysts, and osteoporosis; and (6) **pannus** formation—the pannus is a mass of synovium and synovial stroma consisting of inflammatory cells, granulation tissue, and fibroblasts, which grows over the articular cartilage and causes its erosion. In time, after the cartilage has been destroyed, the pannus bridges the apposing bones, forming a fibrous ankylosis, which eventually ossifies, ultimately resulting in bony ankylosis. Inflammation in the tendons, ligaments, and occasionally the adjacent skeletal muscle frequently accompanies the arthritis.

Skin. **Rheumatoid nodules** are the most common cutaneous lesions in RA. They occur in approximately 25% of patients, usually those with severe disease, and arise in regions of the skin that are subjected to pressure, including the ulnar aspect of the forearm, elbows, occiput, and lumbosacral area. Less commonly, they form in the lungs, spleen, pericardium, myocardium, heart valves, aorta, and other viscera. Rheumatoid nodules are firm, nontender, and round to oval; in the skin, they arise in the subcutaneous tissue. Microscopically, they have a central zone of fibrinoid necrosis surrounded by a prominent rim of epithelioid histiocytes and numerous lymphocytes and plasma cells (Fig. 26–43).

Blood Vessels. Patients with severe erosive disease, rheumatoid nodules, and high titers of rheumatoid factor are at risk of developing vasculitic syndromes (Chapter 11). Rheumatoid vasculitis is a potentially catastrophic complication of RA, particularly when it affects vital organs. The involvement of medium to small arteries is similar to that occurring in polyarteritis nodosa except that in RA the kidneys are not involved. Frequently, segments of small arteries such as **vasa nervorum** and **digital arteries** are obstructed by an obliterating endarteritis, resulting in peripheral neuropathy, ulcers, and gangrene. Leukocytoclastic venulitis produces purpura, cutaneous ulcers, and nail bed infarction.

Pathogenesis. It is believed that *RA is an autoimmune disease triggered by exposure of a genetically susceptible host to an unknown arthritogenic antigen.* It is the continuing autoim-

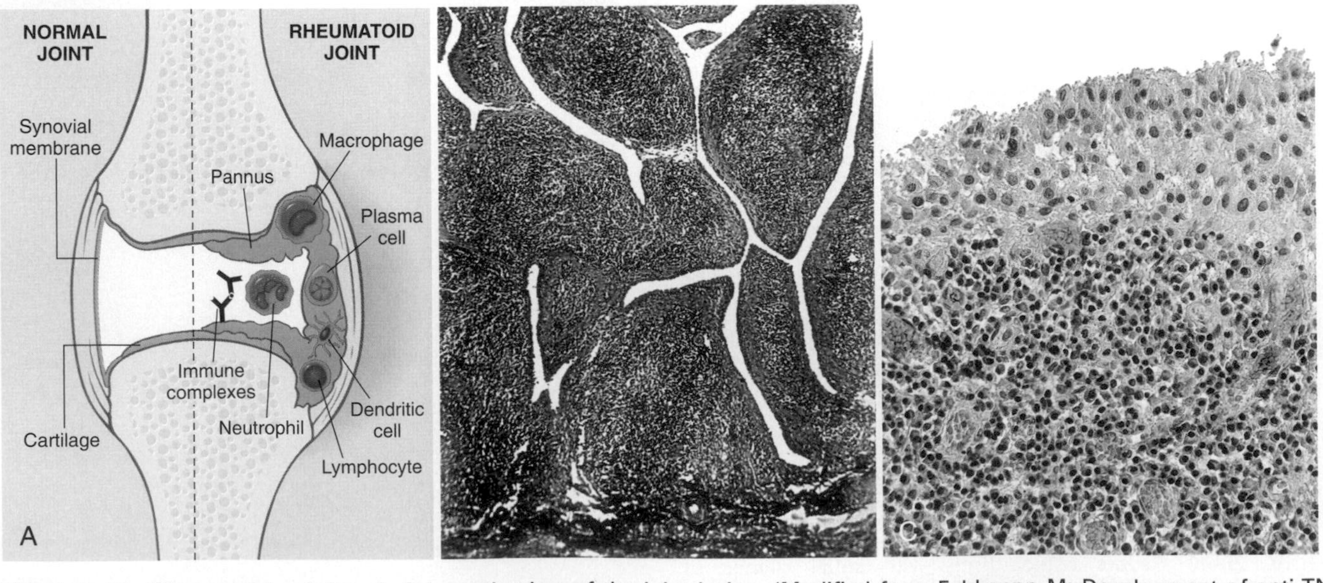

FIGURE 26–42 Rheumatoid arthritis. *A,* Schematic view of the joint lesion. (Modified from Feldmann M: Development of anti-TNF therapy for rheumatoid arthritis. Nat Rev Immunol 2:364, 2002.) *B,* Low magnification reveals marked synovial hypertrophy with formation of villi. *C,* At higher magnification, subsynovial tissue containing a dense lymphoid aggregate is seen.

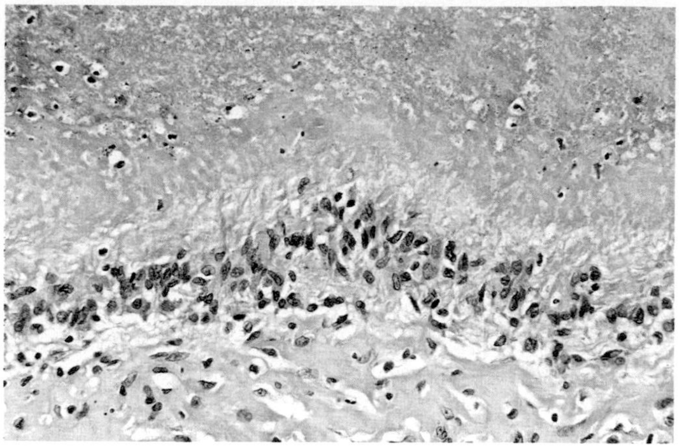

FIGURE 26–43 Subcutaneous rheumatoid nodule with an area of necrosis *(top)* surrounded by a palisade of macrophages and scattered chronic inflammatory cells.

mune reaction, with activation of CD4+ helper T cells and other lymphocytes, and the local release of inflammatory mediators and cytokines that ultimately destroys the joint[45,46] (Fig. 26–44). Therefore, the key considerations in the pathogenesis of the disease are (1) the nature of the autoimmune reaction, (2) the mediators of tissue injury, (3) genetic susceptibility, and (4) the arthritogenic antigen(s). We discuss what is known about each of these.

- The *autoimmune reaction* in RA consists of activated CD4+ T cells, and probably B lymphocytes, as well. The target antigens of these lymphocytes, and how they are initially activated, are still unknown. The T cells apparently function mainly by stimulating other cells in the joint to produce cytokines that are central mediators of the synovial reaction (see below). Although the contribution of autoreactive B cells has been an issue of controversy, there is increasing evidence that immune complex deposition may also play some role in the joint destruction.
- Perhaps the major advances in our understanding of the disease have been a better appreciation of the actual *mediators of joint injury*. Cytokines are believed to play a pivotal role, and the most important of these cytokines are *TNF and IL-1*. Both are probably produced by macrophages and synovial lining cells that are activated by the T cells in the joint. TNF and IL-1, in turn, stimulate synovial cells to proliferate and produce various mediators of inflammation (such as prostaglandins), and matrix metalloproteinases that contribute to cartilage destruction. Activated T cells and synovial fibroblasts also produce RANKL, which activates osteoclasts and promotes bone destruction. Thus, a chain of events is set up that leads to progressive joint damage. The hyperplastic synovium rich in inflammatory cells becomes adherent to and grows over the articular

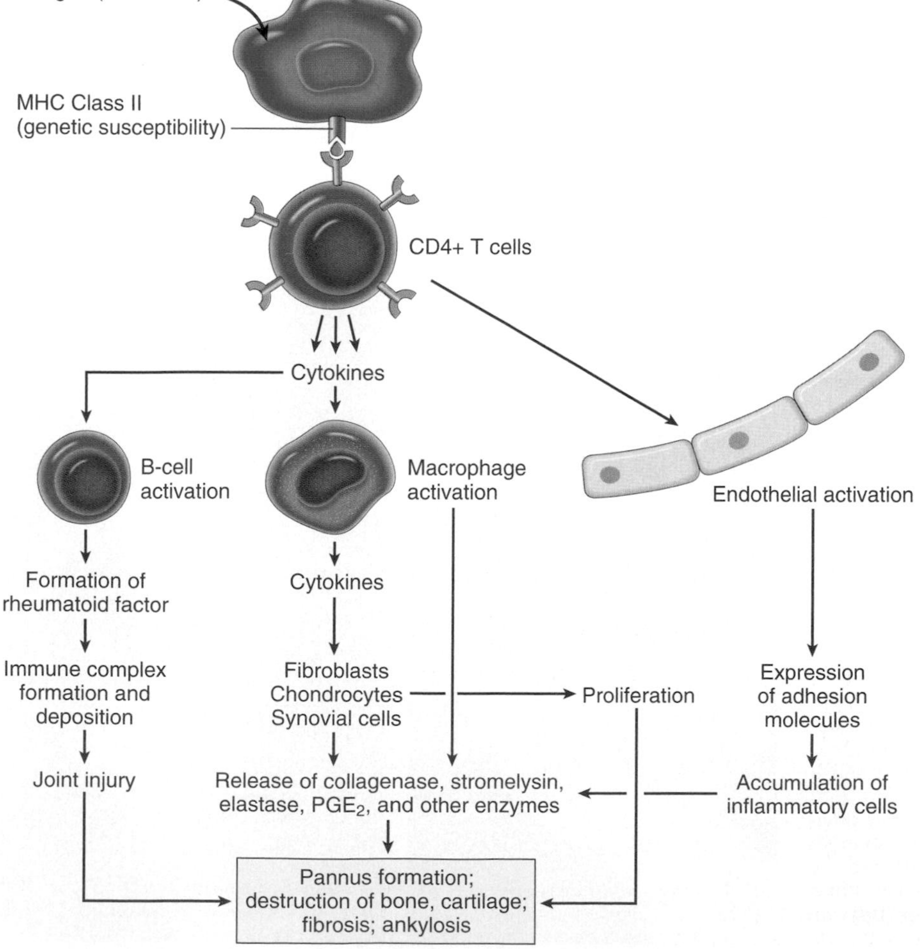

FIGURE 26–44 Immunopathogenesis of rheumatoid arthritis.

surface, forming a pannus, and stimulates resorption of the adjacent cartilage. *In the end, the pannus produces sustained, irreversible cartilage destruction and erosion of subchondral bone.*[47] The realization of the important roles of TNF and IL-1 is the basis for the successful use of anticytokine therapy, especially against TNF.

- *Genetic susceptibility* is a significant component of the development of RA.[48] There is a high rate of concordance between monozygotic twins and a well-defined familial predisposition. Multiple gene loci are believed to be responsible for susceptibility to the disease, but most of these have not been identified yet. One susceptibility gene that is known is in the class II HLA locus, and specifically a region of four amino acids loated in the antigen-binding cleft that is shared in the HLA DRB1*0401 and *0404 alleles. This HLA-DR allele may bind and display the arthritogenic antigen to T cells, although there is no formal evidence in support of this idea.
- The *antigens* that trigger autoimmunity and perpetuate the reaction are not known. There has been great interest in exploring microbial antigens as the initiating triggers, but no firm evidence has definitively identified a microbial organism as an etiologic agent in rheumatoid arthritis.[49]

Clinical Course. The clinical course of RA is variable. The disease begins slowly and insidiously in more than half of patients. Initially, there is malaise, fatigue, and generalized musculoskeletal pain, after which the joints become clearly involved. Approximately 10% of patients have an acute onset with severe symptoms and polyarticular involvement developing more rapidly. The pattern of joint involvement varies, but generally the small joints are affected before the larger ones. Symptoms usually develop in the small bones of the hands (metacarpophalangeal (MCP) and proximal interphalangeal (PIP) joints) and feet (metatarsophalangeal (MTP) and interphalangeal (IP) joints) followed by the wrists, ankles, elbows, and knees. The cervical spine may also be involved, but the hips are usually involved only later in the disease, if at all, and the lumbosacral region is typically spared.

The involved joints are swollen, warm, painful, and particularly stiff on arising or following inactivity. The disease course may be slow or rapid and fluctuates over a period of years, with the greatest damage occurring during the first 4 or 5 years. Approximately 20% of patients enjoy periods of partial or complete remission, but the symptoms inevitably return and can involve previously unaffected joints.

The radiographic hallmarks are juxta-articular osteopenia and bone erosions with narrowing of the joint space from loss of articular cartilage (Fig. 26–45). Destruction of tendons, ligaments, and joint capsules contribute to characteristic deformities, including radial deviation of the wrist, ulnar deviation of the fingers, and flexion-hyperextension abnormalities of the fingers (swan neck, boutonnière). The end result is deformed joints that have no stability and minimal or no range of motion. Large synovial cysts, such as the Baker cyst in the posterior knee, may develop as the increased intra-articular pressure causes outpouchings of the synovium.

No specific laboratory tests are diagnostic of RA. Many patients have serum rheumatoid factor, an IgM antibody reactive with the Fc portions of the patients' own IgG, but this may not be present throughout the course of the disease and also appears in many other conditions. Analysis of synovial fluid indicates a nonspecific inflammatory arthritis with neutrophils, high protein content, and low mucin content. The diagnosis is made primarily on the clinical features and includes the presence of four of the following criteria: (1) morning stiffness, (2) arthritis in three or more joint areas, (3) arthritis of typical hand joints, (4) symmetric arthritis, (5) rheumatoid nodules, (6) serum rheumatoid factor, and (7) typical radiographic changes.

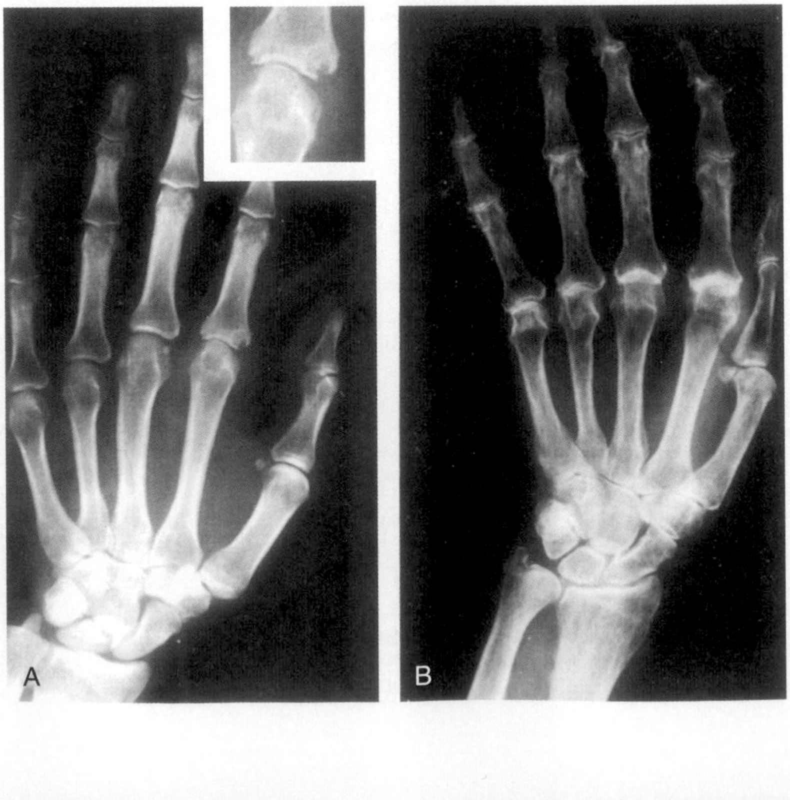

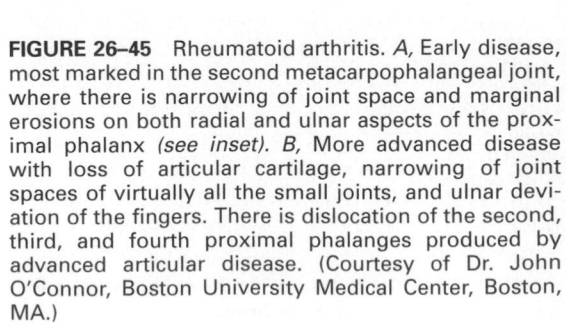

FIGURE 26–45 Rheumatoid arthritis. *A,* Early disease, most marked in the second metacarpophalangeal joint, where there is narrowing of joint space and marginal erosions on both radial and ulnar aspects of the proximal phalanx *(see inset). B,* More advanced disease with loss of articular cartilage, narrowing of joint spaces of virtually all the small joints, and ulnar deviation of the fingers. There is dislocation of the second, third, and fourth proximal phalanges produced by advanced articular disease. (Courtesy of Dr. John O'Connor, Boston University Medical Center, Boston, MA.)

It is difficult to predict the natural history of the disease in individuals. Fortunate patients have a mild onset and few sequelae. Most, however, have progressive disease for life. Overall, life expectancy is reduced by a mean of three to seven years. The fatalities are usually due to the complication of RA, such as systemic amyloidosis and vasculitis, which can involve vessels of all sizes including the aorta, or to iatrogenic effects of therapy—in particular, gastrointestinal bleeding related to long-term use of anti-inflammatory drugs (aspirin, nonsteroidal anti-inflammatory drugs) and infections associated with chronic steroid use, treatment with cytokine antagonists, and the underlying disease itself. The recent advent of *TNF antagonists* (anti-TNF antibody and soluble TNF receptor) has had a dramatic effect on the progression and symptoms of the disease in a substantial proportion of patients.[50]

JUVENILE RHEUMATOID ARTHRITIS

Juvenile rheumatoid arthritis (JRA) is one of the more common connective tissue diseases and affects 30,000 to 50,000 children in the United States. It is a heterogeneous group of chronic arthritides that is a major cause of functional disability.[51] JRA is classified into oligoarticular (<5 joints involved), polyarticular (5 or more joints involved), and systemic variants. By definition, it begins before age 16 (most patients are diagnosed during early childhood), and the arthritis must be present for a minimum duration of 6 weeks. There is a 2:1 female predominance except in the subgroup that has systemic onset, in which the sexes are equally affected.

JRA differs from RA in adults in the following ways: (1) oligoarthritis is more common, (2) systemic onset is more frequent, (3) large joints are affected more often than small joints, (4) rheumatoid nodules and rheumatoid factor are usually absent, and (5) antinuclear antibody seropositivity is common. Pathogenetic factors, similar to those in RA, include genetic association with particular HLA haplotypes (DRB1); mycobacterial, bacterial, or viral infection; abnormal immunoregulation with the prevalence of activated CD4+ T cells within involved joints; and cytokine production.[51] The morphologic changes in joint pathology are similar to those seen in adult RA.

Commonly targeted joints are the knees, wrists, elbows, and ankles. They become warm and swollen and are often involved symmetrically. Pericarditis, myocarditis, pulmonary fibrosis, glomerulonephritis, uveitis, and growth retardation are potential extra-articular manifestations. A systemic onset may begin rather abruptly, associated with high spiking fevers, migratory and transient skin rash, hepatosplenomegaly, and serositis. Long-term studies of patients with JRA show that one third to one half of patients have active disease when followed for at least 10 years.

SERONEGATIVE SPONDYLOARTHROPATHIES

The seronegative spondyloarthropathies are a group of diseases that develop in genetically predisposed individuals and are initiated by environmental factors, especially prior infections or exposures. The manifestations are immune mediated and may be triggered by a T-cell response to unknown antigens. Clinically, the diseases produce inflammatory peripheral or axial arthritis and inflammation of tendinous attachment. The seronegative spondyloarthropathies include *ankylosing spondylitis, reactive arthritis (Reiter syndrome and enteritis-associated arthritis), psoriatic arthritis, and arthritis associated with inflammatory bowel disease* (ulcerative colitis, Crohn disease). They share overlapping clinical features, and many are associated with HLA-B27 and a triggering infection.

Ankylosing Spondyloarthritis

Also known as *rheumatoid spondylitis* and *Marie-Strümpell disease,* ankylosing spondyloarthritis is a chronic inflammatory joint disease of axial joints, especially the sacroiliac joints. It usually becomes symptomatic in the second and third decades of life, and men are affected two to three times more frequently than woman. Approximately 90% of affected individuals are HLA-B27 positive; however, certain HLA-B27 subtypes are not associated with disease susceptibility. Analogous to RA, this immunogenetic phenotype may predispose to the activation of T cells and antibodies that react with joint elements.[52] Histologically, there is a chronic synovitis with destruction of articular cartilage and bony ankylosis, especially in the sacroiliac and apophyseal joints (between tuberosities and processes). Inflammation of tendinoligamentous insertion sites leads to their ossification, producing bony outgrowths, which compound the fibrous and bony ankylosis, and results in severe spinal immobility. The patients characteristically present with low back pain, which frequently follows a chronic progressive course. Involvement of peripheral joints, such as the hips, knees, and shoulders, occurs in at least one third of patients. Fracture of the spine, uveitis, aortitis, and amyloidosis are other recognized complications.

Reactive Arthritis

Reactive arthritis is defined as an episode of noninfectious arthritis of the appendicular skeleton that occurs within one month of a primary infection localized elsewhere in the body. Most of the infections are centered in the genitourinary system (*Chlamydia*) and the gastrointesintinal tract (*Shigella, Salmonella, Yersinia, Campylobacter*). *The triad of arthritis, nongonococcal urethritis or cervicitis, and conjunctivitis is called Reiter syndrome,* but most patients with reactive arthritis do not have these defining symptoms. Most cases of reactive arthritis are associated with genitourinary infection; it typically affects individuals in their twenties or thirties, more than 80% are positive for HLA-B27, and a very small percentage of patients are infected with HIV. The evidence suggests that the disease is caused by an autoimmune reaction initiated by prior infection; the organisms associated with enteric infections have lipopolysaccharide as a major component in their outer cell membrane, and their derived antigens stimulate an array of immunologic responses.[53] Arthritic symptoms usually develop within several weeks of the inciting bout of urethritis or diarrhea. Joint stiffness and low back pain are common early symptoms. The ankles, knees, and feet are affected most often, frequently in an asymmetric pattern. Synovitis of a digital tendon sheath produces the sausage finger or toe and ossification of tendoligamentous insertion sites leads to calcaneal spurs and bony outgrowths. Patients with severe chronic disease have involvement of the spine that is indistinguishable from ankylosing spondylitis. Extraarticular involvement manifests as inflammatory balanitis, conjunctivitis, cardiac conduction abnormalities, and aortic regurgitation. The episodes of arthritis usually wax and wane over a period of several weeks to six months. Almost 50% of patients have recurrent arthritis, tendinitis, fasciitis, and lumbosacral back pain that can cause significant functional disability.

Psoriatic Arthritis

Psoriatic arthritis affects more than 10% of patients with psoriasis. The disease manifests itself between ages 30 and 50. The joint symptoms usually develop slowly but are acute in onset in one-third of patients. The patterns of joint involvement are diverse. The distal interphalangeal joints of the hands and feet are first affected in an asymmetric distribution in more than 50% of patients. The large joints such as the ankles, knees, hips, and wrists may be involved as well.[54] Inflammation of the digital tendon sheaths produces the sausage finger. Sacroiliac and spinal disease occurs in 20% to 40% of patients. Aside from conjunctivitis and iritis, extra-articular manifestations are uncommon and are similar in scope to those of the other seronegative spondyloarthropathies. Histologically, psoriatic arthritis is similar to RA. Psoriatic arthritis, however, is usually not as severe, remissions are more frequent, and joint destruction is less frequent.

INFECTIOUS ARTHRITIS

Microorganisms of all types can lodge in joints during hematogenous dissemination. Articular structures can also become infected by direct inoculation or from contiguous spread from a soft tissue abscess or focus of osteomyelitis. Infectious arthritis is potentially serious because it can cause rapid destruction of the joint and produce permanent deformities.

Suppurative Arthritis

Bacterial infections almost always cause an acute suppurative arthritis. The bacteria usually seed the joint during an episode of bacteremia; however, in neonates, there is an increased incidence of contiguous spread from underlying epiphyseal osteomyelitis. The most common organisms are gonococcus, *Staphylococcus, Streptococcus, Haemophilus influenzae,* and gram-negative bacilli (*E. coli, Salmonella, Pseudomonas,* and others). *H. influenzae* arthritis predominates in children under age 2 years, *S. aureus* is the main causative agent in older children and adults, and gonococcus is prevalent during late adolescence and young adulthood. Individuals with sickle cell disease are prone to infection with *Salmonella* at any age. These joint infections affect both sexes equally, except for gonococcal arthritis, which is seen mainly in sexually active women. Predisposing conditions include immune deficiencies (congenital and acquired), debilitating illness, joint trauma, chronic arthritis of any cause, and intravenous drug abuse.

The classic presentation is the sudden development of an acutely painful, hot, and swollen joint that has a restricted range of motion. Systemic findings of fever, leukocytosis, and elevated sedimentation rate are common. In disseminated gonococcal infection, the symptoms are more subacute. In 90% of nongonococcal cases, the infection involves only a single joint, usually the knee followed in frequency by the hip, shoulder, elbow, wrist, and sternoclavicular joints. Axial articulations are more commonly involved in drug addicts. Prompt recognition and effective therapy prevent rapid joint destruction.

Tuberculous Arthritis

Tuberculous arthritis (Chapter 8) is a chronic progressive monoarticular disease that occurs in all age groups, especially adults. It usually develops as a complication of adjoining osteomyelitis or after hematogenous dissemination from a visceral (usually pulmonary) site of infection. Onset is insidious and causes gradual progressive pain. Systemic symptoms may or may not be present. Mycobacterial seeding of the joint induces the formation of confluent granulomas with central caseous necrosis. The affected synovium may grow as a pannus over the articular cartilage and erode into bone along the joint margins. Chronic disease results in severe destruction with fibrous ankylosis and obliteration of the joint space. The weight-bearing joints are usually affected, especially the hips, knees, and ankles, in descending order of frequency.

Lyme Arthritis

Lyme arthritis is caused by infection with the spirochete *Borrelia burgdorferi,* which is transmitted by the ticks of the *Ixodes ricinus* complex. The initial infection of the skin is followed within several days or weeks by dissemination of the organism to other sites, especially the joints (Chapter 8).

Approximately 60% to 80% of untreated patients with Lyme disease develop joint symptoms within a few weeks to 2 years after the onset of the disease. The arthritis is the dominant feature of late disease; it tends to be remitting and migratory and primarily involves large joints, especially the knees, shoulders, elbows, and ankles, in descending order of frequency. Usually one or two joints are affected at a time, and the attacks last for a few weeks to months with periods of remission. Infected synovium takes the form of a chronic papillary synovitis with synoviocyte hyperplasia, fibrin deposition, mononuclear cell infiltrates (especially helper/inducer T cells), and onionskin thickening of arterial walls. The morphology in severe cases can closely resemble that of RA. Silver stains may reveal small numbers of organisms in the vicinity of blood vessels in approximately 25% of cases. Chronic arthritis with pannus formation resulting in permanent deformities develops in approximately 10% of patients. The arthritis may be caused by immune responses against *Borrelia* antigens (such as OspA) that cross-react with proteins in the joints.[55]

Viral Arthritis

Arthritis can occur in the setting of a variety of viral infections, including parvovirus B19, rubella, and hepatitis C virus. The clinical manifestations of the arthritis are variable and range from acute to subacute symptoms. It is unclear whether the joint symptoms are caused by direct infection of the joint by the virus or whether the viral infection generates an autoimmune reaction, as seen in other forms of reactive arthritides.[56] The possible role of viruses in the generation of chronic joint diseases such as RA has been previously discussed. A variety of different rheumatic conditions, including reactive arthritis, psoriatic arthritis, and septic arthritis, have developed in patients infected with HIV. The pathogenesis of some of these forms of HIV-associated chronic arthritis is suspected of being similar to that of RA. The new effective therapies for HIV may ameliorate their severity.

GOUT AND GOUTY ARTHRITIS

Articular crystal deposits are associated with a variety of acute and chronic joint disorders. Endogenous crystals shown to be pathogenic include monosodium urate (gout), calcium pyrophosphate dihydrate, and basic calcium phosphate (hydroxyapatite). Exogenous crystals, such as corticosteroid ester crystals, talcum, polyethylene, and methyl methacrylate, may also induce joint disease. Silicone, polyethylene, and methyl methacrylate are used in prosthetic joints, and their debris, which accumulates with long use and wear, may result in local arthritis and failure of the prosthesis. Endogenous and exogenous crystals produce disease by triggering the cascade that results in cytokine-mediated cartilage destruction. Here we discuss the two most important crystal arthropathies: gout, caused by urates, and pseudogout, caused by calcium pyrophosphate.

Gout is the common end point of a group of disorders that produce hyperuricemia. It is marked by transient attacks of *acute arthritis* initiated by crystallization of urates within and about joints, leading eventually to *chronic gouty arthritis* and the deposition of masses of urates in joints and other sites, creating *tophi.* Tophi consist of large aggregates of urate crystals and the surrounding inflammatory reaction. Most, but not all, patients with chronic gout also develop urate nephropathy. Although hyperuricemia is a sine qua non for the development of gout, it is not the sole determinant. More than 10% of the population of the Western hemisphere has hyperuricemia, but gout develops in less than 0.5% of the population. A plasma urate level above 7 mg/dL is considered elevated because it exceeds the saturation value for urate at normal body temperature and blood pH. The various conditions producing hyperuricemia and gout (Table 26–7) are divided into those that produce primary gout, in which the basic metabolic defect is unknown or gout is the main manifestation of a known defect, and those that produce secondary gout, in which the cause of the hyperuricemia is known or gout is not the main clinical dysfunction.

Pathogenesis. Uric acid is the end product of purine metabolism. Two pathways are involved in purine synthesis:[57] (1) a de novo pathway in which purines are synthesized from nonpurine precursors, and (2) a salvage pathway in which free purine bases derived from the breakdown of nucleic acids of endogenous or exogenous origin are recaptured (salvaged) (Fig. 26–46). The enzyme hypoxanthine guanine phosphoribosyl transferase (HGPRT) is involved in the salvage pathway. A deficiency of this enzyme leads to increased synthesis of purine nucleotides through the de novo pathway and hence increased production of uric acid. A complete lack of HGPRT occurs in the uncommon X-linked *Lesch-Nyhan syndrome,* seen only in males and characterized by hyperuricemia, severe neurologic deficits with mental retardation, self-mutilation,

TABLE 26–7 Classification of Gout

Clinical Category	Metabolic Defect
Primary Gout (90% of cases)	
Enzyme defects unknown (85%–90% of primary gout)	■ Overproduction of uric acid Normal excretion (majority) Increased excretion (minority) Underexcretion of uric acid with normal production
Known enzyme defects—e.g., partial HGPRT deficiency (rare)	■ Overproduction of uric acid
Secondary Gout (10% of cases)	
Associated with increased nucleic acid turnover—e.g., leukemias	■ Overproduction of uric acid with increased urinary excretion
Chronic renal disease	■ Reduced excretion of uric acid with normal production
Inborn errors of metabolism—e.g., complete HGPRT deficiency (Lesch-Nyhan syndrome)	■ Overproduction of uric acid with increased urinary excretion

HGPRT, hypoxanthine guanine phosphoribosyl transferase.

and in some cases gouty arthritis. Less severe deficiencies of the enzyme may also induce hyperuricemia and gouty arthritis with only mild neurologic deficits, but together these causes of gout are uncommon. The great majority of cases of gout are primary, in which the metabolic defect underlying the increased levels of uric acid is unknown.

As stated earlier, hyperuricemia does not necessarily lead to gouty arthritis. Many factors contribute to the conversion of asymptomatic hyperuricemia into primary gout, including the following:

- *Age* of the individual and duration of the hyperuricemia are factors. Gout rarely appears before 20 to 30 years of hyperuricemia.
- *Genetic predisposition* is another factor. In addition to the well-defined X-linked abnormalities of HGPRT, primary gout follows multifactorial inheritance and runs in families.
- Heavy *alcohol* consumption predisposes to attacks of gouty arthritis.
- *Obesity* increases the risk of asymptomatic gout.
- Certain *drugs* (e.g., thiazides) predispose to the development of gout.
- *Lead toxicity* increases the tendency to develop saturnine gout (Chapter 9).

Central to the pathogenesis of the arthritis is precipitation of monosodium urate crystals into the joints (Fig. 26–47). Synovial fluid is a poorer solvent for monosodium urate than plasma, and so with hyperuricemia the urates in the joint fluid become supersaturated, particularly in the peripheral joints (ankle), which may have temperatures as low as 20°C. With prolonged hyperuricemia, crystals and microtophi of urates develop in the synovium and in the joint cartilage. Some unknown event, possibly trauma, then initiates release of crystals into the synovial fluid, which begins a cascade of events. The released crystals are chemotactic to leukocytes and also activate com-

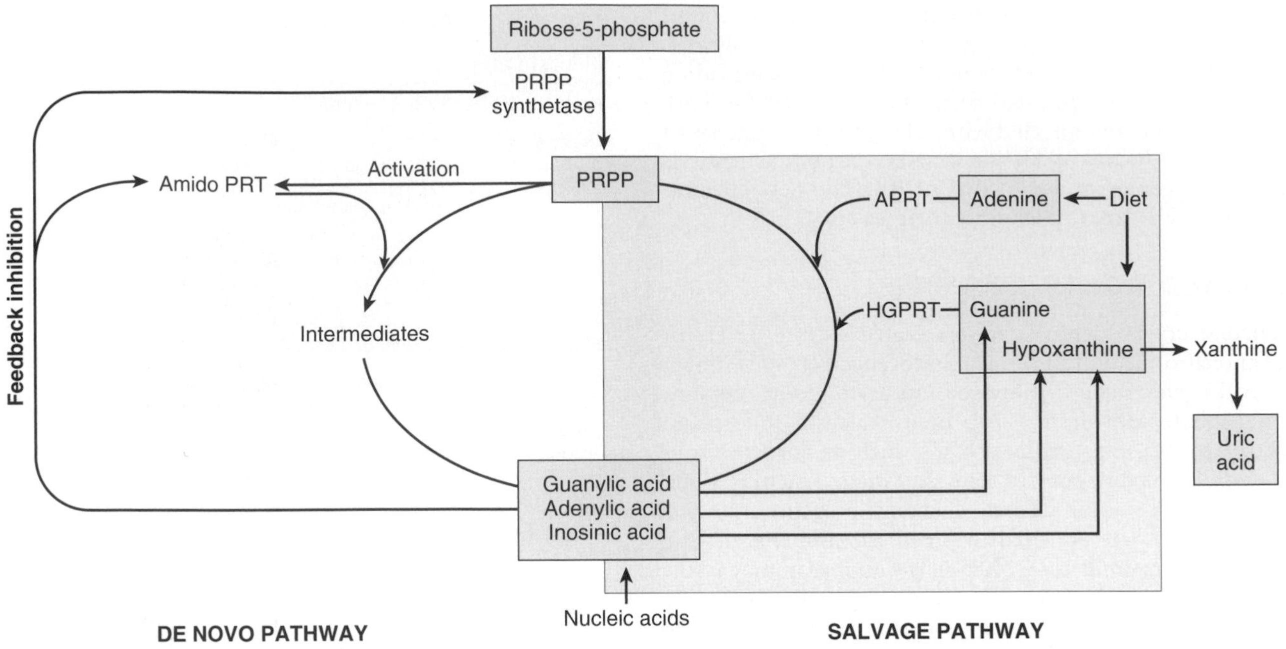

FIGURE 26–46 Purine metabolism. The conversion of PRPP to purine nucleotides is catalyzed by amido PRT in the de novo pathway and by APRT and HGPRT in the salvage pathway. APRT, amido-phosphoribosyltransferase; HGPRT, hypoxanthine-guanine phosphoribosyltransferase; PRPP, phosphoribosyl pyrophosphate; PRT, phosphoribosyltransferase.

plement, with the generation of C3a and C5a, leading to the accumulation of neutrophils and macrophages in the joints and synovial membranes. The production of chemokines by monocytes and fibroblasts also increases the flow of neutrophils into the involved joint.[58] Phagocytosis of crystals induces release of toxic free radicals and leukotrienes (LTB_4). Activated neutrophils release destructive lysosomal enzymes, and the macrophages and synoviocytes secrete a variety of mediators, which further intensify the inflammatory reaction and augment the injury to the articular structures. Activation of Hageman factor pours fuel onto the fire. Thus comes about an acute arthritis, which typically remits (days to weeks) even if untreated. A scheme of these events is shown in Figure 26–47.

Repeated attacks of acute arthritis lead eventually to chronic arthritis and the formation of tophi in the inflamed synovial membranes and periarticular tissue as well as elsewhere. In time, severe damage to the cartilage and the function of the joints develops. It is not known why the chronic arthritis is asymptomatic for intervals of days to months, even though synovial crystals are undoubtedly present in abundance in the joints.

Morphology. The distinctive morphologic changes in gout are (1) acute arthritis, (2) chronic tophaceous arthritis, (3) tophi in various sites, and sometimes (4) gouty nephropathy. **Acute arthritis** is characterized by a dense neutrophilic infiltrate that permeates the synovium and synovial fluid. The monosodium urate crystals are frequently found in the cytoplasm of the neutrophils and are arranged in small clusters in the synovium. They are long, slender, and needle shaped and are negatively birefringent. The synovium is edematous and congested and also contains scattered lymphocytes, plasma cells, and macrophages. When the episode of crystallization abates and the crystals are resolubilized, the acute attack remits.

Chronic tophaceous arthritis evolves from the repetitive precipitation of urate crystals during acute attacks. The urates may heavily encrust the articular surfaces and form visible deposits in the synovium (Fig. 26–48). The synovium becomes hyperplastic, fibrotic, and thickened by inflammatory cells and forms a pannus that destroys the underlying cartilage, leading to juxta-articular bone erosions. In severe cases, fibrous or bony ankylosis ensues, resulting in partial to complete loss of joint function.

Tophi are the pathognomonic hallmark of gout. They are formed by large aggregations of urate crystals surrounded by an intense inflammatory reaction of macrophages, lymphocytes, and large foreign body giant cells, which may have completely or partially engulfed masses of crystals (Fig. 26–49). Tophi may appear in the articular cartilage of joints and in the periarticular ligaments, tendons, and soft tissues, including the olecranon and patellar bursae, Achilles tendons, and ear lobes. Less frequently, they may occur in the kidneys, nasal cartilages, skin of the fingertips, palms, or soles as well as elsewhere. Superficial tophi can lead to large ulcerations of the overlying skin.

Gouty nephropathy (Chapter 20) refers to the renal disorder associated with the deposition of monosodium urate crystals in the renal medullary interstitium, sometimes forming tophi, intratubular precipitations, or free uric acid crystals, and the production of uric acid renal stones. Secondary complications, such as pyelonephritis, may ensue, particularly when the urates induce some urinary obstruction.

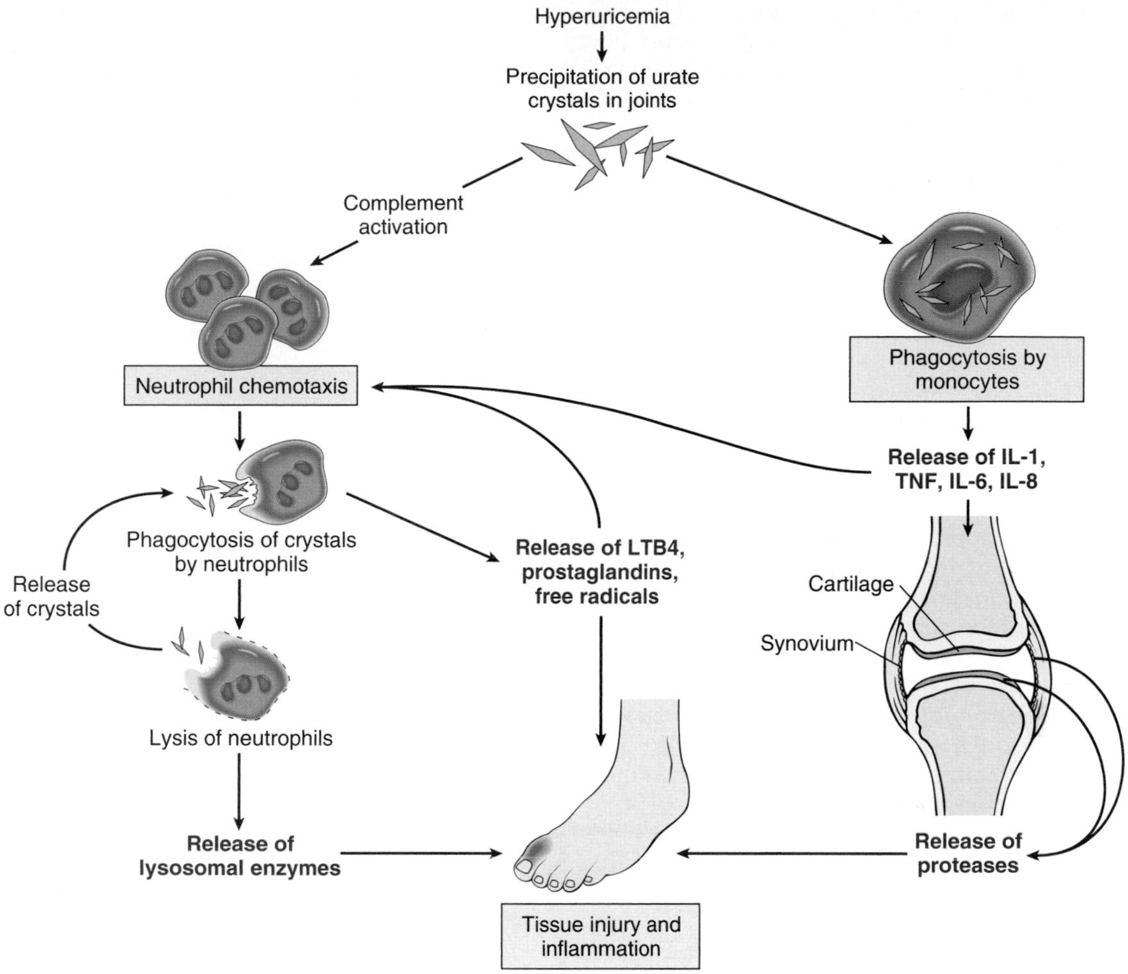

FIGURE 26–47 Pathogenesis of acute gouty arthritis.

Clinical Course. The natural history of gout is said to pass through four stages: (1) asymptomatic hyperuricemia, (2) acute gouty arthritis, (3) intercritical gout, and (4) chronic tophaceous gout. *Asymptomatic hyperuricemia* appears around puberty in males and after the menopause in females. After a long interval of years, *acute arthritis* appears in the form of the sudden onset of excruciating joint pain associated with localized hyperemia, warmth, and exquisite tenderness. Yet constitutional symptoms are uncommon, except possibly mild fever. The vast majority of first attacks are monarticular; 50% occur in the first metatarsophalangeal joint. About 90% of patients experience acute attacks in the following locations

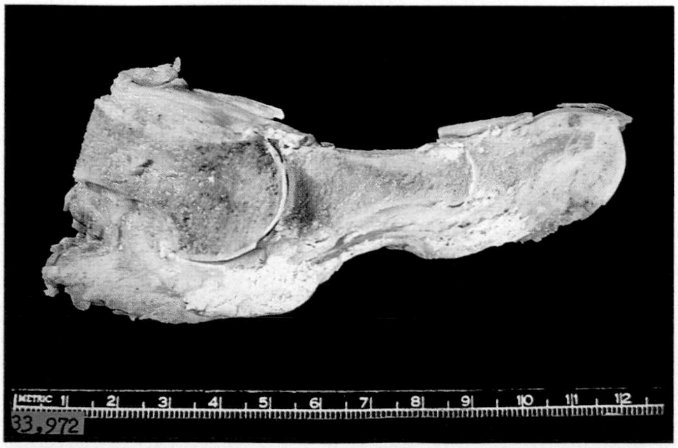

FIGURE 26–48 Amputated great toe with white tophi involving the joint and soft tissues.

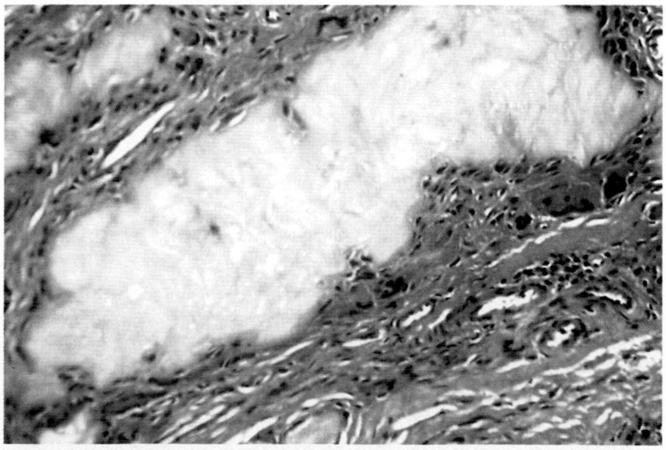

FIGURE 26–49 Photomicrograph of a gouty tophus. An aggregate of dissolved urate crystals is surrounded by reactive fibroblasts, mononuclear inflammatory cells, and giant cells.

(in descending order of frequency): insteps, ankles, heels, knees, wrists, fingers, and elbows. Untreated, acute gouty arthritis may last for hours to weeks, but gradually there is complete resolution and the patient enters an *asymptomatic intercritical period.* Although some patients never have another attack, most experience a second acute episode within months to a few years. In the absence of appropriate therapy, the attacks recur at shorter intervals and frequently become polyarticular. Eventually, over the span of years, symptoms fail to resolve completely with the development of disabling *chronic tophaceous gout.* On average, it takes about 12 years between the initial acute attack and the development of chronic tophaceous arthritis. At this stage, x-rays show characteristic juxta-articular bone erosion caused by the crystal deposits and loss of the joint space. Progression leads to severe crippling disease.

Cardiovascular disease, including atherosclerosis and hypertension, is common in patients with gout. Renal manifestations sometimes appear in the form of renal colic associated with the passage of gravel and stones and may proceed to chronic gouty nephropathy. About 20% of those with chronic gout die of renal failure. The diagnosis of gout should not be delayed because numerous drugs are available to abort or prevent acute attacks of arthritis and mobilize tophaceous deposits. Their use is important because many aspects of the disease are related to the duration and severity of the hyperuricemia. Generally, gout does not materially shorten the life span, but it may impair quality of life.

CALCIUM PYROPHOSPHATE CRYSTAL DEPOSITION DISEASE (PSEUDOGOUT)

Calcium pyrophosphate crystal deposition disease (CPPD), also known as *pseudogout* and *chondrocalcinosis,* is one of the more common disorders associated with intra-articular crystal formation. It usually occurs in individuals over age 50 and becomes more common with increasing age, rising to a prevalence of 30% to 60% in those age 85 or older. The sexes and races are equally affected. CPPD is divided into sporadic (idiopathic), hereditary, and secondary types. In the hereditary variant, the crystals develop relatively early in life and are associated with severe osteoarthritis. The autosomal dominant form of the disease has been shown to be related to a mutation in the *ANKH* gene, which encodes a transmembrane inorganic pyrophosphate transport channel.[59] The secondary form is associated with various disorders, including previous joint damage, hyperparathyroidism, hemochromatosis, hypomagnesemia, hypothyroidism, ochronosis, and diabetes. The conditions leading to crystal formation are not entirely known but include altered activity of the matrix enzymes that produce and degrade pyrophosphate, resulting in its accumulation and eventual crystallization with calcium.

Morphology. The crystals first develop in the articular matrix, menisci, and intervertebral discs, and as the deposits enlarge, they may rupture and seed the joint. Once released into the joint they elicit the production of chemokines such as IL-8, which helps produce an inflammatory infiltrate rich in neutrophils.

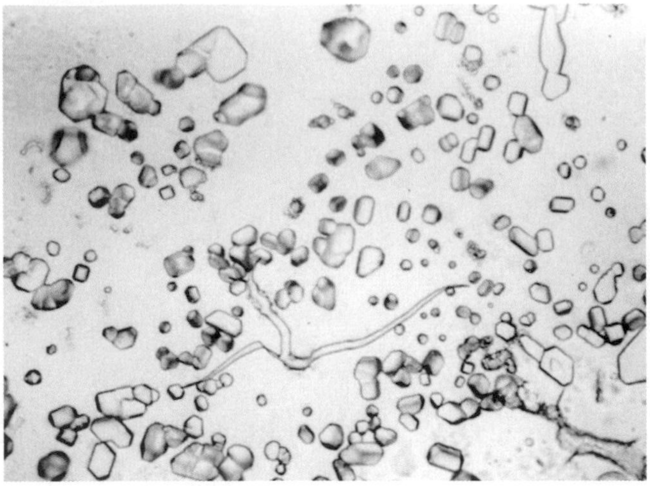

FIGURE 26–50 Smear preparation of synovial fluid containing calcium pyrophosphate crystals.

Neutrophils are thought to produce damage through the release of oxygen metabolites, catabolic enzymes, and cytokines, calling forth the more chronic reactions associated with macrophages and fibrosis.[58] The crystals form chalky white friable deposits, which are seen histologically in stained preparations as oval blue-purple aggregates. Individual crystals are generally 0.5 to 5 μm in greatest dimension, are weakly birefringent, and have geometric shapes (Fig. 26–50). Rarely the crystals are deposited in masslike aggregates simulating tophi.

CPPD is frequently asymptomatic; however, it is a great simulator because it produces acute, subacute, or chronic arthritis that may mimic other disorders, such as osteoarthritis or RA. The joint involvement may last from several days to weeks and may be monarticular or polyarticular; the knees, followed by the wrists, elbows, shoulders, and ankles, are most commonly affected. Ultimately, approximately 50% of patients experience significant joint damage. Therapy is supportive; no known treatment prevents or retards crystal formation.

Tumors and Tumor-Like Lesions

Reactive tumor-like lesions, such as ganglions, synovial cysts, and osteochondral loose bodies, commonly involve joints and tendon sheaths. They usually result from trauma or degenerative processes and are much more common than neoplasms. Primary neoplasms are unusual and tend to recapitulate the cells and tissue types (synovial membrane, fat, blood vessels, fibrous tissue, and cartilage) native to joints and related structures. Benign tumors are much more frequent than their malignant counterparts, which are rare and are discussed with the soft tissue tumors.

GANGLION AND SYNOVIAL CYST

A *ganglion* is a small (1 to 1.5 cm) cyst that is almost always located near a joint capsule or tendon sheath. A common location is around the joints of the wrist, where it appears as a firm, fluctuant, pea-sized translucent nodule. It arises as a result of cystic or myxoid degeneration of connective tissue; hence the cyst wall lacks a true cell lining. The lesion may be multilocular and enlarges through coalescence of adjacent areas of myxoid change. The fluid that fills the cyst is similar to synovial fluid; however, there is no communication with the joint space.

Herniation of synovium through a joint capsule or massive enlargement of a bursa may produce a *synovial cyst.* A well-recognized example is the synovial cyst that forms in the popliteal space in the setting of RA (Baker cyst). The synovial lining may be hyperplastic and contain inflammatory cells and fibrin but is otherwise unremarkable.

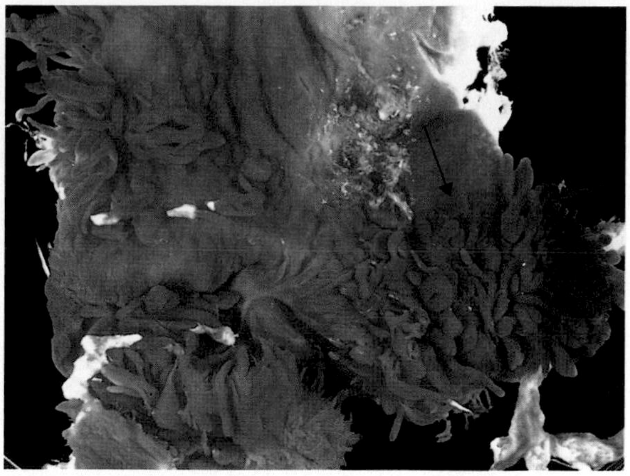

FIGURE 26–51 Excised synovium with fronds and nodules typical of pigmented villonodular synovitis (PVNS) *(arrow).*

PIGMENTED VILLONODULAR SYNOVITIS AND GIANT CELL TUMOR OF TENDON SHEATH

Villonodular synovitis is the term for several closely related benign neoplasms that develop in the synovial lining of joints, tendon sheaths, and bursae. They were previously considered reactive synovial proliferations (hence the designation *synovitis*); however, cytogenetic studies have demonstrated consistent chromosomal aberrations in these lesions, indicating that they arise from a clonal proliferation of cells and are neoplastic.[60] The prototypes of these tumors are *pigmented villonodular synovitis* (PVNS), which involves the synovium of a joint, and *giant cell tumor of tendon sheath* (GCT), which is also known as *localized nodular tenosynovitis.* Whereas PVNS tends to involve one or more joints diffusely, GCT usually occurs as a discrete nodule on a tendon sheath. Both PVNS and GCT usually arise in the twenties to forties and affect the sexes equally.

Morphology. Grossly, the lesions of PVNS and GCT are both red-brown to mottled orange-yellow. In PVNS, the normally smooth joint synovium, most often of the knee, is converted into a tangled mat by red-brown folds, finger-like projections, and nodules (Fig. 26–51). In contrast, GCT is localized and well circumscribed and resembles a small walnut. The tumor cells in both lesions are polyhedral, moderately sized, and resemble synoviocytes (Fig. 26–52). In PVNS, they spread along the surface and infiltrate the subsynovial compartment. In GCT, the cells grow in a solid nodular aggregate that may be attached to the synovium by a pedicle. Other frequent findings in both lesions include hemosiderin deposits, foamy macrophages, multinucleated giant cells, and zones of sclerosis.

PVNS usually presents as a monoarticular arthritis that affects the knee in 80% of cases, followed in frequency by the hip, ankle, and calcaneocuboid joints. Patients typically complain of pain, locking, and recurrent swelling. Tumor progression limits the range of movement of the joint and causes it to become stiff and firm. Sometimes a palpable mass can be appreciated. Aggressive tumors erode into adjacent bones and soft tissues, causing confusion with other types of neoplasia. In contrast, GCT manifests as a solitary, slow-growing, painless mass that frequently involves the tendon sheaths along the wrists and fingers; it is the most common mesenchymal neoplasm of the hand. Cortical erosion of adjacent bone occurs in approximately 15% of cases. Surgery is the recommended treatment for both lesions; PVNS has a significant recurrence rate because it is difficult to excise, and GCT often recurs locally.

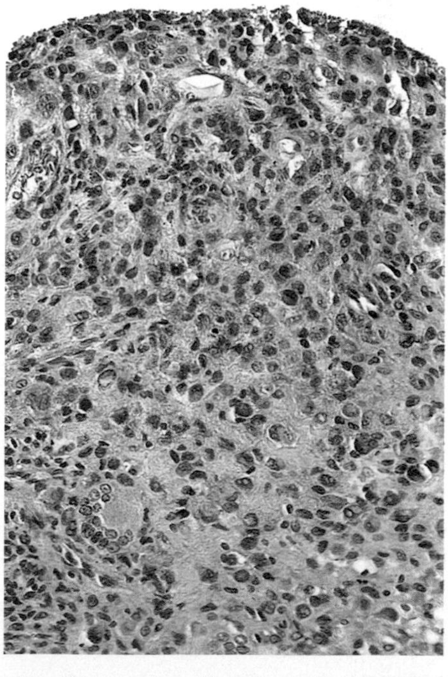

FIGURE 26–52 Sheets of proliferating cells in PVNS bulging the synovial lining.

SOFT TISSUE TUMORS AND TUMOR-LIKE LESIONS

Soft tissue tumors are defined as mesenchymal proliferations that occur in the extraskeletal, nonepithelial tissues of the body, excluding the viscera, coverings of the brain, and lymphoreticular system. They are classified according to the tissue they *recapitulate* (muscle, fat, fibrous tissue, vessels, and nerves; Table 26–8). Some soft tissue tumors have no normal tissue counterpart but have consistent clinicopathologic features warranting their designation as distinct entities. The true frequency of soft tissue tumors is difficult to estimate because most benign lesions are not removed. A conservative estimate is that benign tumors outnumber their malignant counterparts by a ratio of at least 100:1. In the United States, little more than 8000 sarcomas are diagnosed annually (0.8% of invasive malignancies), yet they are responsible for 2% of all cancer deaths, reflecting their lethal nature.

TABLE 26–8 Soft Tissue Tumors

■ ***Tumors of adipose tissue***
Lipomas
Liposarcoma
■ ***Tumors and tumor-like lesions of fibrous tissue***
Nodular fasciitis
Fibromatoses
Superficial fibromatoses
Deep fibromatoses
Fibrosarcoma
■ ***Fibrohistiocytic tumors***
Fibrous histiocytoma
Dermatofibrosarcoma protuberans
Malignant fibrous histiocytoma
■ ***Tumors of skeletal muscle***
Rhabdomyoma
Rhabdomyosarcoma
■ ***Tumors of smooth muscle***
Leiomyoma
Smooth muscle tumors of uncertain malignant potential
Leiomyosarcoma
■ ***Vascular tumors***
Hemangioma
Lymphangioma
Hemangioendothelioma
Hemangiopericytoma
Angiosarcoma
■ ***Peripheral nerve tumors***
Neurofibroma
Schwannoma
Granular cell tumor
Malignant peripheral nerve sheath tumors
■ ***Tumors of uncertain histogenesis***
Synovial sarcoma
Alveolar soft part sarcoma
Epithelioid sarcoma

Pathogenesis and General Features

The cause of most soft tissue tumors is unknown. There are documented associations, however, between radiation therapy and rare instances in which chemical burns, thermal burns, or trauma were associated with subsequent development of a sarcoma. Exposure to phenoxyherbicides and chlorophenols has also been implicated in some cases. Kaposi sarcoma is causally associated with the human herpesvirus 8; however, viruses are probably not important in the pathogenesis of most sarcomas. The majority of soft tissue tumors occur sporadically, but a small minority is associated with genetic syndromes, the most notable of which are neurofibromatosis type 1 (neurofibroma, malignant schwannoma), Gardner syndrome (fibromatosis), Li-Fraumeni syndrome (soft tissue sarcoma), and Osler-Weber-Rendu syndrome (telangiectasia). Cytogenetic and molecular analyses of soft tissue tumors have provided significant insight into their biology. Specific chromosomal abnormalities and genetic derangements can not only be used as diagnostic markers, but also provide important clues about the genesis of the neoplasms.[60] For example, many of the mutations target oncogenes that encode transcription factors or cell-cycle regulators, and their dysfunction results in uncontrolled cell proliferation (Table 26–9).

Soft tissue tumors may arise in any location, although approximately 40% occur in the lower extremities, especially the thigh; 20% in the upper extremities; 10% in the head and neck; and 30% in the trunk and retroperitoneum. Regarding sarcomas, males are affected more frequently than females (1.4:1), and the incidence generally increases with age. Fifteen per cent arise in children; they constitute the fourth most common malignancy in this age group, following brain tumors, hematopoietic cancers, and Wilms tumor in frequency. Specific sarcomas tend to appear in certain age groups (e.g., rhabdomyosarcoma in children, synovial sarcoma in young adulthood, and liposarcoma and malignant fibrous histiocytoma in mid- to late adult life).

Several features of soft tissue tumors influence their prognosis:

- Accurate histologic classification contributes significantly to establishing the prognosis of a sarcoma. Important diagnostic features are cell morphology and architectural arrangement (Tables 26–10 and 26–11). Often these features are not sufficient to distinguish one sarcoma

TABLE 26–9 Chromosomal and Genetic Abnormalities in Soft Tissue Sarcomas

Tumor	Cytogenetic Abnormality	Genetic Abnormality
Extraosseous Ewing sarcoma and primitive neuroectodermal tumor	t(11:22)(q24;q12)	FLI-1-EWS fusion gene
	t(21:22)(q22;q12)	ERG-EWS fusion gene
	t(7;22)(q22;q12)	ETV1-EWS fusion gene
Liposarcoma—myxoid and round cell type	t(12:16)(q13;p11)	CHOP/TLS fusion gene
Synovial sarcoma	t(x;18)(p11;q11)	SYT-SSX fusion gene
Rhabdomyosarcoma—alveolar type	t(2;13)(q35;q14)	PAX3-FKHR fusion gene
	t(1;13)(p36;q14)	PAX7-FKHR fusion gene
Extraskeletal myxoid chondrosarcoma	t(9;22)(q22;q12)	CHN-EWS fusion gene
Desmoplastic small round cell tumor	t(11;22)(p13;q12)	EWS-WT1 fusion gene
Clear cell sarcoma	t(12;22)(q13;q12)	EWS-ATF1 fusion gene
Dermatofibrosarcoma protuberans	t(17:22)(q22;q15)	COLA1-PDGFB fusion gene
Alveolar soft part sarcoma	t(X;17)(p11.2;q25)	TFE3-ASPL fusion gene
Congenital fibrosarcoma	t(12;15)(p13;q23)	ETV6-NTRK3 fusion gene

from another, particularly with poorly differentiated aggressive tumors. Great reliance must, therefore, be placed on immunohistochemistry, electron microscopy, cytogenetics, and molecular genetics.

- Whatever the type, the *grade* of a soft tissue sarcoma is important for predicting its behavior. Grading, usually I to III, is based largely on the degree of differentiation, the average number of mitoses per high-power field, cellularity, pleomorphism, and an estimate of the extent of necrosis (presumably a reflection of rate of growth). Mitotic activity and extent of necrosis are thought to be particularly significant. The size, depth, and stage of the tumor also provide important diagnostic and prognostic information.[61]
- Staging helps determine the prognosis and chance of successful excision of a tumor. Several staging systems are utilized in treating sarcomas.
- In general, tumors arising in superficial locations (e.g., skin and subcutis) have a better prognosis than deep-seated lesions. In patients with deep-seated, high-grade sarcomas, metastatic disease develops in 80% of those with a tumor larger than 20 cm and 30% of those with a tumor larger than 5 cm. Overall the 10-year survival rate for sarcomas is approximately 40%.

TABLE 26–10 Morphology of Cells in Soft Tissue Tumors

Cell Type	Features	Tumor Type
Spindle cell	Rod-shaped, long axis twice as great as short axis	Fibrous, fibrohistiocytic, smooth muscle, Schwann cell
Small round cell	Size of a lymphocyte with little cytoplasm	Rhabdomyosarcoma, primitive neuroectodermal tumor
Epithelioid	Polyhedral with abundant cytoplasm, nucleus is centrally located	Smooth muscle, Schwann cell endothelial, epithelioid sarcoma

TABLE 26–11 Architectural Patterns in Soft Tissue Tumors

Pattern	Tumor Type
Fascicles of eosinophilic spindle cells intersecting at right angles	Smooth muscle
Short fascicles of spindle cells radiating from a central point (like spokes on a wheel)—storiform	Fibrohistiocytic
Nuclei arranged in columns—palisading	Schwann cell
Herringbone	Fibrosarcoma
Mixture of fascicles of spindle cells and groups of epithelioid cells—biphasic	Synovial sarcoma

With this brief background, we now turn to the individual tumors and tumor-like lesions. Some of the soft tissue tumors are presented elsewhere—tumors of peripheral nerve (Chapter 27); and tumors of vascular origin, including Kaposi sarcoma (Chapter 11).

Fatty Tumors

LIPOMA

Benign tumors of fat, known as *lipomas,* are the most common soft tissue tumor of adulthood. They are subclassified according to particular morphologic features as conventional lipoma, fibrolipoma, angiolipoma, spindle cell lipoma, myelolipoma, and pleomorphic lipoma. Some of the variants have characteristic chromosomal abnormalities; for example, conventional lipomas often show rearrangements of 12q14-15, 6p, and 13q, and spindle cell and pleomorphic lipomas have rearrangements of 16q and 13q.

Morphology. The conventional lipoma, the most common subtype, is a well-encapsulated mass of mature adipocytes that varies considerably in size. It arises in the subcutis of the proximal extremities and trunk, most frequently during mid-adulthood. Infrequently, lipomas are large, intramuscular, and poorly circumscribed. Histologically, they consist of mature white fat cells with no pleomorphism.

Lipomas are soft, mobile, and painless (except angiolipoma) and are usually cured by simple excision.

LIPOSARCOMA

Liposarcomas are one of the most common sarcomas of adulthood and appear in those in their forties to sixties; they are uncommon in children. They usually arise in the deep soft tissues of the proximal extremities and retroperitoneum and are notorious for developing into large tumors.

Morphology. Histologically, liposarcomas can be divided into well-differentiated, myxoid, round cell, and pleomorphic variants. The cells in well-differentiated liposarcomas are readily recognized as lipocytes. In the other variants, most of the tumor cells are not obviously adipogenic, but some cells indicative of fatty differentiation are almost always present. These cells are known as **lipoblasts;** they mimic fetal fat cells and contain round clear cytoplasmic vacuoles of lipid that scallop the nucleus (Fig. 26–53). The myxoid and round cell variant of liposarcoma has a t(12;16) chromosomal abnormality in most cases (Table 26–9).

The well-differentiated variant is relatively indolent, the myxoid type is intermediate in its malignant behavior, and the round cell and pleomorphic variants usually are aggressive and frequently metastasize. All types of liposarcoma recur locally and often repeatedly unless adequately excised.

Fibrous Tumors and Tumor-Like Lesions

REACTIVE PSEUDOSARCOMATOUS PROLIFERATIONS

Reactive pseudosarcomatous proliferations are non-neoplastic lesions that either develop in response to some form of local trauma (physical or ischemic) or are idiopathic. They are composed of plump reactive fibroblasts or related mesenchymal cells. Clinically, they are alarming because they develop suddenly and grow rapidly; histologically, they cause concern because they mimic sarcomas owing to their hypercellularity, mitotic activity, and a primitive appearance. Representative of this family of lesions are *nodular fasciitis* and *myositis ossificans.*

Nodular Fasciitis

Nodular fasciitis, also known as *infiltrative or pseudosarcomatous fasciitis,* is the most common of the reactive pseudosarcomas. It most often occurs in adults on the volar aspect of the forearm, followed in order of frequency by the chest and back. Patients typically present with a several-week history of a solitary, rapidly growing, and sometimes painful mass. Preceding trauma is noted in only 10% to 15% of cases.

Morphology. Nodular fasciitis lesions arise in the deep dermis, subcutis, or muscle. Grossly the lesion is several centimeters in greatest dimension, is nodular in configuration, and has poorly defined margins. By light microscopy, nodular fasciitis is richly cellular and consists of plump, immature-appearing fibroblasts arranged randomly (simulating cells growing in tissue culture) or in short intersecting fascicles (Fig. 26–54). The cells vary in size and shape (spindle to stellate) and have conspicuous nucleoli and abundant mitotic figures. Frequently the stroma is myxoid and contains lymphocytes and extravasated red blood cells. The histologic differential is extensive, but important lesions that should be excluded are fibromatosis and spindle cell sarcomas. Because nodular fasciitis is reactive, the lesion rarely recurs after excision.

Other pseudosarcomas related to nodular fasciitis are *proliferative fasciitis* and *proliferative myositis.* These lesions occur in slightly older patients and develop in the trunk or proximal extremities. The proliferating fibroblasts are often large and round, have prominent nucleoli, and resemble ganglion cells. Ischemic fasciitis, affecting debilitated and bed-ridden individuals, and localized massive lymphedema that develops in the morbidly obese are additional reactive processes that can be confused with various types of sarcomas.

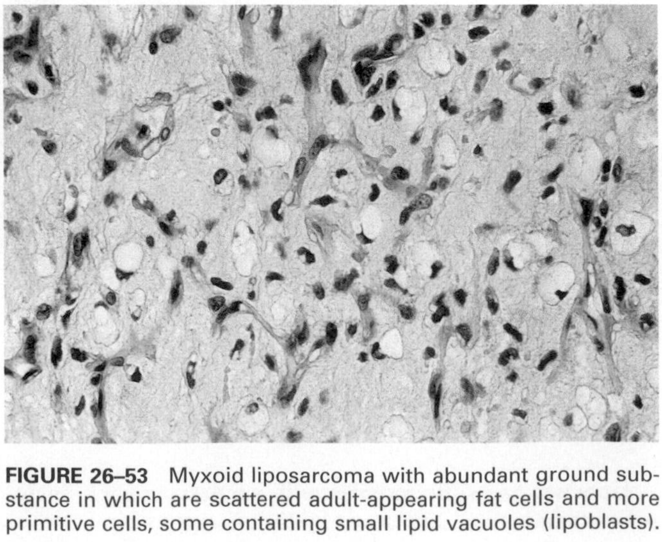

FIGURE 26–53 Myxoid liposarcoma with abundant ground substance in which are scattered adult-appearing fat cells and more primitive cells, some containing small lipid vacuoles (lipoblasts).

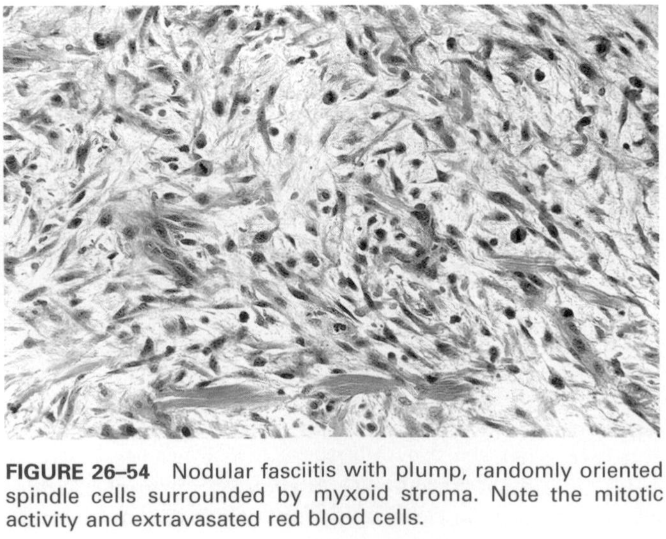

FIGURE 26–54 Nodular fasciitis with plump, randomly oriented spindle cells surrounded by myxoid stroma. Note the mitotic activity and extravasated red blood cells.

Myositis Ossificans

Myositis ossificans is distinguished from the other fibroblastic proliferations by the presence of *metaplastic bone.* It usually develops in athletic adolescents and young adults and follows an episode of trauma in more than 50% of cases. The lesion typically arises in the musculature of the proximal extremities. The clinical findings are related to its stage of development; in the early phase, the involved area is swollen and painful, and within several weeks, it becomes more circumscribed and firm. Eventually, it evolves into a painless, hard, well-demarcated mass.

Morphology. Grossly, the usual lesions are 3 to 6 cm in greatest dimension. Most are well delineated and have soft, glistening centers and a firm, gritty periphery. The microscopic findings vary according to the age of the lesion; in the earliest phase, the lesion is the most cellular and consists of plump, elongated fibroblast-like cells simulating nodular fasciitis (see earlier). Morphologic zonation begins within 3 weeks; the center retains its population of fibroblasts; however, it merges with an adjacent intermediate zone that contains osteoblasts, which deposit ill-defined trabeculae of woven bone. The most peripheral zone contains well-formed, mineralized trabeculae that closely resemble cancellous bone. Frequently, skeletal muscle fibers and regenerating muscle giant cells are trapped within the margins. Eventually the entire lesion ossifies, and the intertrabecular spaces become filled with bone marrow. The mature lesion is completely ossified.

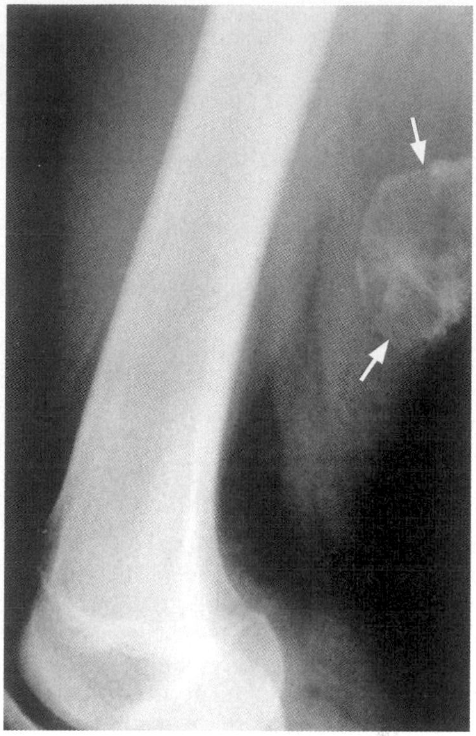

FIGURE 26–55 Peripherally mineralized myositis ossificans (*arrows*) involving the posterior thigh.

The radiographic findings parallel the morphologic progression. Initially the x-rays may show only soft tissue fullness, but at about 3 weeks, patchy flocculent radiodensities form in the periphery. The radiodensities become more extensive with time and slowly encroach on the radiolucent center (Fig. 26–55). Myositis ossificans must be distinguished from extraskeletal osteosarcoma. The latter usually occurs in elderly patients, the proliferating cells are cytologically malignant, and the tumor lacks the zonation of myositis ossificans. To be noted, the most peripheral regions of osteosarcoma are the most cellular and primitive, which is the reverse of myositis ossificans. Simple excision of myositis ossificans is usually curative.

FIBROMATOSES

Superficial Fibromatosis (Palmar, Plantar, and Penile Fibromatoses)

Palmar, plantar, and penile fibromatoses, more bothersome than serious lesions, constitute a small group of superficial fibromatoses. They are characterized by nodular or poorly defined broad fascicles of mature-appearing fibroblasts surrounded by abundant dense collagen. Immunohistochemical and ultrastructural studies indicate that many of these cells are *myofibroblasts.* Several nonrandom karyotypic abnormalities have been described in these tumors (e.g., trisomy 3 and 8), but their significance is still unclear.[62] Regardless, the superficial fibromatoses are genetically distinct from their deep-seated counterparts.

In the palmar variant *(Dupuytren contracture),* there is irregular or nodular thickening of the palmar fascia either unilaterally or bilaterally (50%). Over a span of years, attachment to the overlying skin causes puckering and dimpling. At the same time, a slowly progressive flexion contracture develops, mainly of the fourth and fifth fingers of the hand. Essentially similar changes are seen with *plantar fibromatosis,* except that flexion contractures are uncommon and bilateral involvement is infrequent. In *penile fibromatosis (Peyronie disease),* a palpable induration or mass appears usually on the dorsolateral aspect of the penis. It may cause eventually abnormal curvature of the shaft or constriction of the urethra, or both.

All forms of superficial fibromatosis affect males more frequently than females. In about 20% to 25% of cases, the palmar and plantar fibromatoses stabilize and do not progress, in some instances resolving spontaneously. Some recur after excision, particularly the plantar variant.

Deep-Seated Fibromatosis (Desmoid Tumors)

Biologically, deep-seated fibromatoses lie in the borderland between nonaggressive fibrous tumors and low-grade fibrosarcomas. On the one hand, they commonly present as large, infiltrative masses that frequently recur after incomplete excision; on the other hand, they are composed of banal well-differentiated fibroblasts that do not metastasize. They may occur at any age but are most frequent in the teens to thirties. Desmoids are divided into *extra-abdominal, abdominal, and intra-abdominal,* but all have essentially similar gross and microscopic features. Extra-abdominal desmoids occur in men and women with equal frequency and arise principally in the musculature of the shoulder, chest wall, back, and thigh. Abdominal desmoids generally arise in the musculoaponeurotic structures of the anterior abdominal wall in women during or after pregnancy. Intra-abdominal desmoids tend to occur in the mesentery or pelvic walls, often in patients having familial adenomatous polyposis (Gardner syndrome) (Chapter 17). Mutations in the *APC* or β-catenin genes are present in the majority of these tumors and likely play an important role in their genesis, irrespective of whether or not the patients have underlying Gardner syndrome.

Morphology. These tumors occur as gray-white, firm, poorly demarcated masses varying from 1 to 15 cm in greatest diameter. They are rubbery and tough and infiltrate surrounding structures. Histologically deep-seated fibromatosis is composed of plump fibroblasts arranged in broad sweeping fascicles that infiltrate to the adjacent tissue (Fig. 26–56). Mitoses are usually infrequent. Regenerating muscle cells, when trapped within these lesions, may take on the appearance of multinucleated giant cells.

In addition to their possibly being disfiguring or disabling, desmoids are occasionally painful. Although curable by adequate excision, they frequently recur when incompletely removed. Some tumors have responded to treatment with tamoxifen, and in other cases chemotherapy or irradiation has been effective. The rare reports of metastasis of a desmoid must be interpreted as misdiagnosis of fibrosarcoma.

FIBROSARCOMA

Fibrosarcomas are rare but may occur anywhere in the body, most commonly in the retroperitoneum, the thigh, the knee, and the distal extremities. Many tumors previously considered fibrosarcoma have been reclassified as aggressive fibromatosis (desmoid), malignant fibrous histiocytoma, malignant peripheral nerve sheath tumors, or synovial sarcomas.

Morphology. Typically, these neoplasms are unencapsulated, infiltrative, soft, fish-flesh masses often having areas of hemorrhage and necrosis. Better-differentiated lesions may appear deceptively encapsulated. Histologic examination discloses all degrees of differentiation, from slowly growing tumors that closely resemble cellular fibromatosis sometimes having spindled cells growing in a herringbone fashion (Fig. 26–57) to highly cellular neoplasms dominated by architectural disarray, pleomorphism, frequent mitoses, and areas of necrosis.

Because true fibrosarcomas are frequently classified as some other type of sarcoma, data on their properties are variable. They are aggressive tumors, however, recurring in more than 50% of the cases and metastasizing in more than 25%.

Fibrohistiocytic Tumors

Fibrohistiocytic tumors contain cellular elements that resemble both fibroblasts and histiocytes. Originally, they were believed to be neoplasms of histiocytes (the name pathologists often use for activated macrophages), but studies suggest that the phenotype of the neoplastic cells most closely resembles that of fibroblasts. Thus, the term *fibrohistiocytic* should be viewed as descriptive in nature and not one that connotes histogenetic origin.

BENIGN FIBROUS HISTIOCYTOMA (DERMATOFIBROMA)

Benign fibrous histiocytoma is a relatively common lesion that usually occurs in the dermis and subcutis. It is painless and slow growing and most often presents in mid-adult life as a firm, small (up to 1 cm) mobile nodule.

Morphology. Most benign fibrous histiocytomas consist of a proliferation of bland spindle cells arranged in a storiform pattern. These tumors have infiltrative margins; common secondary findings include the presence of foam cells, hemosiderin deposits, multinucleated giant cells, and hyperplasia of the overlying epidermis. They most frequently arise

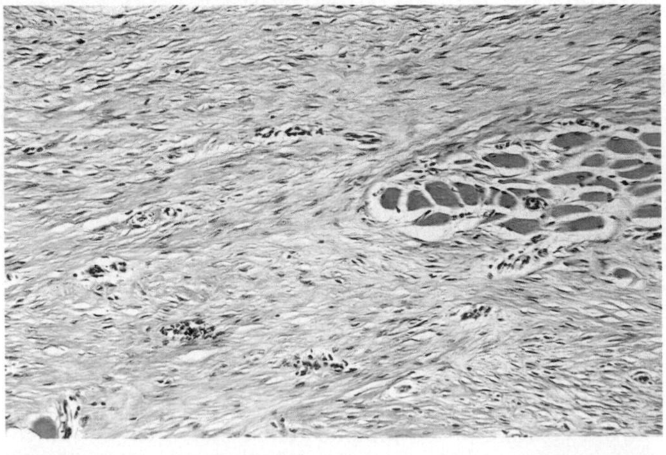

FIGURE 26–56 Fibromatosis infiltrating between skeletal muscle cells.

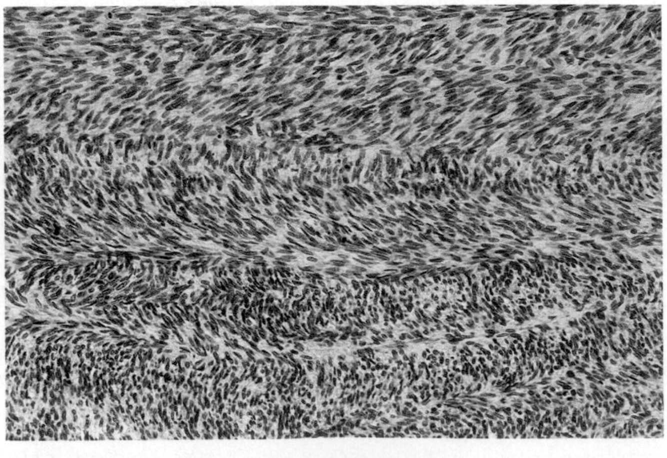

FIGURE 26–57 Fibrosarcoma composed of malignant spindle cells arranged in a herringbone pattern.

in the dermis where they are known as **dermatofibromas.** Other types of benign fibrohistiocytic tumors include juvenile xanthogranuloma, epithelioid histiocytoma, and reticulohistiocytoma. Adequate treatment is simple excision.

MALIGNANT FIBROUS HISTIOCYTOMA

Malignant fibrous histiocytoma refers to a group of related soft tissue sarcomas characterized by considerable cytologic pleomorphism, the presence of bizarre multinucleate cells, and storiform architecture. Despite the name, which was originally based on tissue culture characteristics of the neoplastic cells, the phenotype of the tumors is fibroblastic and not histiocytic. Importantly, pleomorphic variants of liposarcoma, leiomyosarcoma, and rhabdomyosarcoma can resemble malignant fibrous histiocytoma, and ancillary studies may be necessary to distinguish among them. Malignant fibrous histiocytoma usually arises in the musculature of the proximal extremities and the retroperitoneum. Cutaneous variants have also been called *atypical fibroxanthomas*.

Morphology. These tumors are usually large (5 to 20 cm), gray-white unencapsulated masses but often appear deceptively circumscribed. Malignant fibrous histiocytomas have been categorized into **storiform-pleomorphic, myxoid, inflammatory, giant cell,** and **angiomatoid** variants based on their histologic features. The storiform–pleomorphic type is the most common and as the name indicates is composed of malignant spindle cells oriented in a storiform pattern with scattered, large round pleomorphic cells (Fig. 26–58).

Most variants of malignant fibrous histiocytoma, except for the angiomatoid type, are aggressive, recur unless widely excised, and have a metastatic rate of 30% to 50%. However, cutaneous tumors rarely disseminate; the angiomatoid variant is also indolent and in contrast to the other types occurs in adolescents and young adults.

Tumors of Skeletal Muscle

Skeletal muscle neoplasms, in contrast to other groups of tumors, are almost all malignant. The benign variant, rhabdomyoma, is distinctly rare. The so-called *cardiac rhabdomyoma* is probably hamartomatous in origin and is discussed in Chapter 12.

RHABDOMYOSARCOMA

Rhabdomyosarcoma, the most common soft tissue sarcoma of childhood and adolescence, usually appears before age 20. They may arise in any anatomic location, but most occur in the head and neck or genitourinary tract, where there is little, if any, skeletal muscle as a normal constituent. Only in the extremities do they appear in relation to skeletal muscle.

Much interest has been focused on the cytogenic abnormalities in rhabdomyosarcoma:[63] t(2;13)(q35;14) and, less commonly, t(1;13)(q36;q14) translocations have been found in most cases. In the more common t(2;13), the *PAX3* gene on chromosome 2 fuses with the *FKHR* gene on chromosome 13. Interestingly, the *PAX3* gene functions upstream of genes that control skeletal muscle differentiation. Thus, it is proposed that the pathogenesis of the tumor involves dysregulation of muscle differentiation by the chimeric PAX3-FKHR protein.

Morphology. Rhabdomyosarcoma is histologically subclassified into the **embryonal, alveolar,** and **pleomorphic** variants.[64] The rhabdomyoblast—the diagnostic cell in all types—contains eccentric eosinophilic granular cytoplasm rich in thick and thin filaments. The rhabdomyoblasts may be round or elongate; the latter are known as **tadpole or strap cells** and may contain cross-striations visible by light microscopy (Fig. 26–59). Ultrastructurally, rhabdomyoblasts contain sarcomeres, and immunohistochemically they stain with antibodies to the myogenic markers desmin, MYOD1, and myogenin.

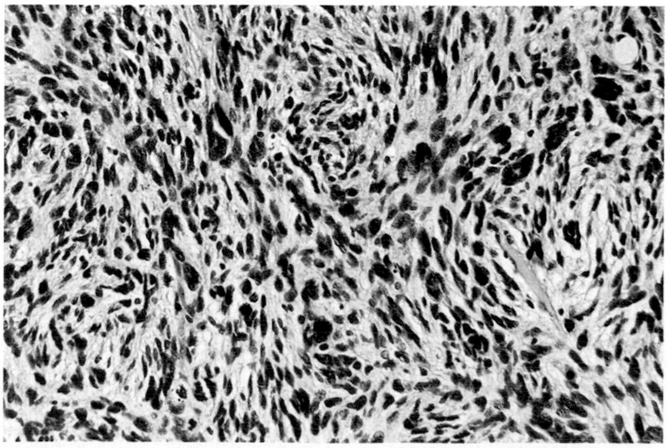

FIGURE 26–58 Malignant fibrous histiocytoma revealing fascicles of plump spindle cells in a swirling (storiform) pattern, typical but not pathognomonic of this neoplasm. (Courtesy of Dr. J. Corson, Brigham and Women's Hospital, Boston, MA.)

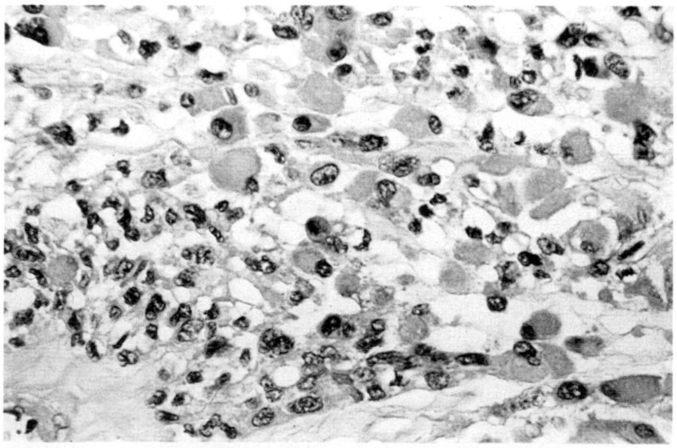

FIGURE 26–59 Rhabdomyosarcoma composed of malignant small round cells. The rhabdomyoblasts are large and round and have abundant eosinophilic cytoplasm; no cross-striations are evident.

Embryonal rhabdomyosarcoma is the most common type, accounting for 66% of rhabdomyosarcomas. It includes the **sarcoma botryoides** described in Chapter 22 and spindle cell variants. The tumor occurs in children under age 10 years and typically arises in the nasal cavity, orbit, middle ear, prostate, and paratesticular region. This variant of rhabdomyosarcoma commonly has allelic loss of chromosome 11p15.5 as its major genomic abnormality.[64] The sarcoma botryoides subtype develops in the walls of hollow, mucosa-lined structures, such as the nasopharynx, common bile duct, bladder, and vagina.

Most embryonal rhabdomyosarcomas present as a soft gray infiltrative mass. The tumor cells mimic skeletal muscle cells at various stages of embryogenesis and consist of sheets of both malignant round and spindled cells in a variably myxoid stroma. Sarcoma botryoides grows in a polypoid fashion, producing the appearance of a cluster of grapes protruding into a hollow structure such as the bladder or vagina. Where the tumor abuts the mucosa of an organ, it forms a submucosal zone of hypercellularity known as the **cambium layer.** Rhabdomyoblasts with visible cross-striations may be present.

Alveolar rhabdomyosarcoma is most common in early to mid-adolescence and usually arises in the deep musculature of the extremities. Histologically the tumor is traversed by a network of fibrous septae that divide the cells into clusters or aggregates; as the central cells degenerate and drop out, a crude resemblance to pulmonary alveolae is created (Fig. 26–60). The tumor cells are moderate in size, and many have little cytoplasm. Those in the center of the aggregates are discohesive while those at the periphery adhere to the septae. Cells with cross-striations are identified in about 25% of cases. Cytogenetic studies have shown that this variant of rhabdomyosarcoma has a t(2;13) or t(1;13) chromosomal translocation.[63]

Pleomorphic rhabdomyosarcoma is characterized by numerous large, sometimes multinucleated, bizarre eosinophilic tumor cells. This variant is rare, has a tendency to arise in the deep soft tissue of adults and, as noted earlier, can resemble malignant fibrous histiocytoma histologically.

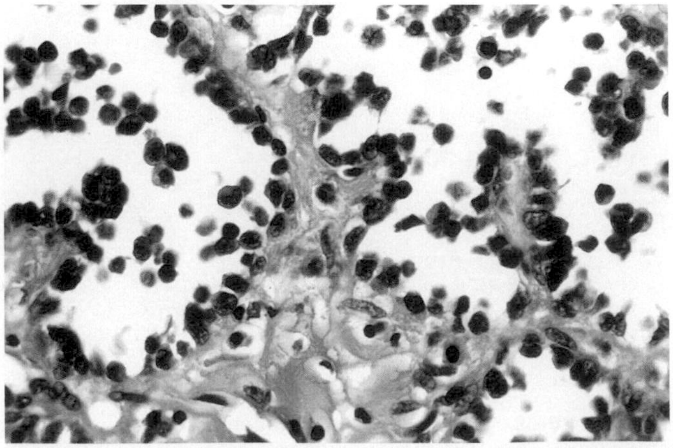

FIGURE 26–60 Alveolar rhabdomyosarcoma with numerous spaces lined by tumor cells.

Rhabdomyosarcomas are aggressive neoplasms and are usually treated with a combination of surgery and chemotherapy with or without radiation. The histologic variant and location of the tumor influence survival. The botryoid subtype has the best prognosis, followed by the embryonal, pleomorphic, and alveolar variants. Overall, approximately 65% of children are cured of their disease, but adults fare less well.

Tumors of Smooth Muscle

LEIOMYOMA

Leiomyomas, the benign smooth muscle tumors, often arise in the uterus where they represent the most common neoplasm in women (Chapter 22). Leiomyomas may also arise in the erector pili muscles found in the skin, nipples, scrotum, and labia (genital leiomyomas) and less frequently develop in the deep soft tissues. Those arising in the erector muscles *(pilar leiomyomas)* are frequently multiple and painful. The tendency to develop multiple lesions is thought to be hereditary and transmitted as an autosomal dominant trait. In whatever setting, these lesions tend to occur in adolescence and early adult life.

They are usually not larger than 1 to 2 cm in greatest dimension and are composed of fascicles of spindle cells that tend to intersect each other at right angles. The tumor cells have blunt-ended, elongated nuclei and show minimal atypia and few mitotic figures. Solitary lesions are easily cured; however, they may be so numerous that complete surgical removal is impractical.

LEIOMYOSARCOMA

Leiomyosarcomas account for 10% to 20% of soft tissue sarcomas. They occur in adults and afflict women more frequently than men. Most develop in the skin and deep soft tissues of the extremities and retroperitoneum.

Morphology. Leiomyosarcomas present as painless firm masses. Retroperitoneal tumors may be large and bulky and cause abdominal symptoms. Histologically, they are characterized by malignant spindle cells that have cigar-shaped nuclei arranged in interweaving fascicles. Morphologic variants include tumors with a prominent myxoid stroma and others with epithelioid cells. Ultrastructurally, malignant smooth muscle cells contain bundles of thin filaments with dense bodies and pinocytotic vesicles, and individual cells are surrounded by basal lamina. Immunohistochemically, they stain with antibodies to vimentin, actin, smooth muscle actin, and desmin.

Treatment depends on the size, location, and grade of the tumor. Superficial or cutaneous leiomyosarcomas are usually small and have a good prognosis, whereas those of the retroperitoneum are large, cannot be entirely excised, and cause death by both local extension and metastatic spread.

Synovial Sarcoma

Synovial sarcoma is so named because it was once believed to recapitulate synovium, but the cell of origin is still unclear. In addition, although the term *synovial sarcoma* implies an origin from the joint linings, less than 10% are intra-articular. Synovial sarcomas account for approximately 10% of all soft tissue sarcomas and rank as the fourth most common sarcoma. Most occur in patients in their twenties to forties. The majority develop in the deep soft tissue in the vicinity of the large joints of the extremities, and about 60% to 70% involve the lower extremities, especially around the knee and thigh. Patients usually present with a deep-seated mass that has been noted for several years. Uncommonly, these tumors occur in the head and neck or the different viscera.

Morphology. The histologic hallmark of biphasic synovial sarcoma is the dual line of differentiation of the tumor cells (i.e., epithelial-like and spindle cells). Despite the mimicry of synovium, the tumor cells do not have the features of synoviocytes. The epithelial cells are cuboidal to columnar and form glands or grow in solid cords or aggregates. The spindle cells are arranged in densely cellular fascicles that surround the epithelial cells (Fig. 26–61). Many synovial sarcomas are *monophasic* in that they are composed of only spindled cells or, rarely, epithelial cells. Lesions composed solely of spindled cells are easily mistaken for fibrosarcomas or malignant peripheral nerve sheath tumors. A characteristic feature when present is calcified concretions that can sometimes be detected radiographically. Immunohistochemistry is helpful in identifying these tumors, since the tumor cells yield positive reactions for keratin and epithelial membrane antigen, differentiating these tumors from most other sarcomas.

Most synovial sarcomas show a characteristic chromosomal translocation t(x;18) producing *SYT-SSX1* or *-SSX2* fusion genes.[60] The normal *SYT* gene encodes a transcription factor and evidence suggests that the *SSX1* and *SSX2* genes produce proteins that are transcription inhibitors. The specific type of

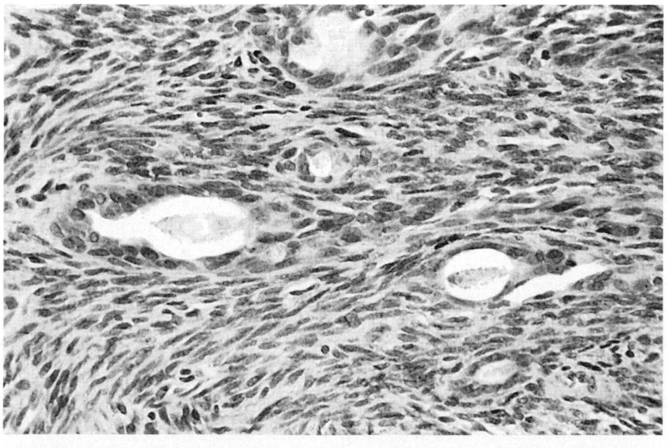

FIGURE 26–61 Synovial sarcoma revealing the classic biphasic spindle cell and glandular-like histologic appearance.

translocation in synovial sarcoma has been shown to be related to prognosis.

Synovial sarcomas are treated aggressively with limb-sparing therapy and frequently chemotherapy. The 5-year survival rate varies from 25% to 62%, and only 11% to 30% live for 10 years or longer. Common sites of metastases are the lung, skeleton, and occasionally the regional lymph nodes.

REFERENCES

1. Glimcher MJ, ed: Metabolic Bone Disease and Clinical Related Disorders, 2nd ed. Philadelphia: WB Saunders, 1990.
2. Manolagas SC: Birth and death of bone cells: basic regulatory mechanisms and implications for the pathogenesis and treatment of osteoporosis. Endocr Rev 21:115, 2000.
3. Ducy P, Schinke T, Karsenty G: The osteoblast: a sophisticated fibroblast under central surveillance. Science 289:1501, 2000.
4. Patel MS, Karsenty G: Regulation of bone formation and vision by LRP5. N Engl J Med 346:1572, 2002.
5. Wagner EF, Karsenty G: Genetic control of skeletal development. Curr Opin Genet Dev 11:527, 2001.
6. Harada S, Rodan GA: Control of osteoblast function and regulation of bone mass. Nature 423:349, 2003.
7. Turner CH, et al: Do bone cells behave like a neuronal network? Calcif Tissue Int 70:435, 2002.
8. Teitelbaum SL: Bone resorption by osteoclasts. Science 289:1504, 2000.
9. Boyle WJ, Simonet WS, Lacey DL: Osteoclast differentiation and activation. Nature 423:337, 2003.
10. Lars ET, Boyle WJ, Penninger JM: RANK-L and RANK: T cells, bone loss and mammalian evolution. Ann Rev Immunol 20:795, 2002.
11. Young MF, et al: Structure, expression, and regulation of the major noncollagenous matrix proteins of bone. Clin Orthop 281:275, 1992.
12. Raisz LG: Physiology and pathophysiology of bone remodeling. Clin Chem 45:1353, 1999.
13. Olsen BR, Reginato AM, Wang W: Bone development. Annu Rev Cell Dev Biol 16:191, 2000.
14. Mundlos S, Olsen BR: Heritable diseases of the skeleton. Part I: Molecular insights into skeletal development—transcription factors and signaling pathways. FASEB J 11:125, 1997.
15. Mundlos S, Olsen BR: Heritable diseases of the skeleton. Part II: Molecular insights into skeletal development—matrix components and their homeostasis. FASEB J 11:227, 1997.
16. Superti-Furga A, Bonafe L, Rimoin DL: Molecular–pathogenetic classification of genetic disorders of the skeleton. Am J Med Genet 106:282, 2001.
17. Cole WG: Advances in osteogenesis imperfecta. Clin Orthop 401:6, 2002.
18. Bullough PG, Davidson DD, Lorenzo JC: The morbid anatomy of the skeleton in osteogenesis imperfecta. Clin Orthop 159:42, 1981.
19. de Vernejoul MC, Besichow O: Human osteopetrosis and other sclerosing disorders: recent genetic developments. Calcified Tiss Int 69:1, 2002.
20. Kornak U, et al:. Loss of the ClC-7 chloride channel leads to osteopetrosis in mice and man. Cell 104:205, 2001.
21. Tuck SP, Francis RM: Osteoporosis. Postgrad Med J 78:526, 2002.
22. Mosekilde L: Mechanisms of age-related bone loss. Novartis Found Symp 235:150, 2001.
23. Kenny AM, Prestwood KM: Osteoporosis. Pathogenesis, diagnosis, and treatment in older adults. Rheum Dis Clin North Am 26:569, 2000.
24. Reddy SV, et al: Paget's disease of bone: a disease of osteoclast. Rev Endocr Metab Disord 2:195, 2001.
25. Leach RJ, Singer FR, Roodman G: The genetics of Paget's disease of the bone. J Clinical Endocrin Metab 86:24, 2001.
26. Hadjipavlou AG, Gaitanis IN, Kontakis GM: Paget's disease of the bone and its management. J Bone Joint Surg Br 84:160, 2002.
27. Gonzalez EA, Martin KJ: Renal osteodystrophy. Rev Endocr Metab Disord 2:187, 2001.
28. Khan SN, Bostrom MP, Lane JM: Bone growth factors. Orthop Clin North Am 31:375, 2000.
29. Saucacos PN, Urbaniak JR: Osteonecrosis. Clin Orthop 386:2, 2001.
30. Lew DP, Waldvogel FA: Osteomyelitis. N Engl J Med 336:999, 1997.
31. Cunningham R, Cockayne A, Humphreys H: Clinical and molecular aspects of the pathogenesis of *Staphylococcus aureus* bone and joint infections. J Med Microbiol 44:157, 1996.

32. Senac MO, Jr., Isaacs H, Gwinn JL: Primary lesions of bone in the 1st decade of life: retrospective survey of biopsy results. Radiology 160:491, 1986.
33. Klein MH, Shankman S: Osteoid osteoma: radiologic and pathologic correlation. Skeletal Radiol 21:23, 1992.
34. Ragland BD, et al: Cytogenetics and molecular biology of osteosarcoma. Lab Invest 82:365, 2002.
35. Unni KK, Dahlin DC: Osteosarcoma: pathology and classification. Semin Roentgenol 24:143, 1989.
36. Bielack SS, et al: Prognostic factors in high-grade osteosarcoma of the extremities or trunk: an analysis of 1,702 patients treated on neoadjuvant cooperative osteosarcoma study group protocols. J Clin Oncol 20:776, 2002.
37. Ramappa AJ, et al: Chondroblastoma of bone. J Bone Joint Surg Am 82-A:1140, 2000.
38. Zillmer DA, Dorfman HD: Chondromyxoid fibroma of bone: thirty-six cases with clinicopathologic correlation. Hum Pathol 20:952, 1989.
39. Lee FY, et al: Chondrosarcoma of bone: an assessment of outcome. J Bone Joint Surg Am 81:326, 1999.
40. Weinstein LS, Chen M, Liu J: Gs(α) mutations and imprinting defects in human disease. Ann NY Acad Sci 968:173, 2002.
41. Papagelopoulos PJ, et al: Clinicopathologic features, diagnosis, and treatment of malignant fibrous histiocytoma of bone. Orthopedics 23:59, 2000.
42. Arvand A, Denny CT: Biology of *EWS/ETS* fusions in Ewing's family tumors. Oncogene 20:5747, 2001.
43. Meideiros LJ, et al: Giant cells and mononuclear cells of giant cell tumor of bone resemble histiocytes. Appl Immunohistochem 1:115, 1993.
44. Aigner T, McKenna L: Molecular pathology and pathobiology of osteoarthritic cartilage. Cell Mol Life Sci 59:5, 2002.
45. Firestein GS: Evolving concepts of rheumatoid arthritis. Nature 423:356, 2003.
46. Lee DM, Weinblatt ME: Rheumatoid arthritis. Lancet 358:903, 2001.
47. Gravallese EM, Goldring SR: Cellular mechanisms and the role of cytokines in bone erosions in rheumatoid arthritis. Arthritis Rheum 43:2143, 2000.
48. Gregersen PK: Teasing apart the complex genetics of human autoimmunity: lesions from rheumatoid arthritis. Clin Immunol 107:1, 2003.
49. Hyrich KL, Inman RD: Infectious agents in chronic rheumatic diseases. Curr Opin Rheumatol 13:300, 2001.
50. Feldmann M: Development of anti-TNF therapy for rheumatoid arthritis. Nat Rev Immunol 2:364, 2002.
51. Schneider R, Passo MH: Juvenile rheumatoid arthritis. Rheum Dis Clin North Am 28:503, 2002.
52. Sieper J, et al: Ankylosing spondylitis: an overview. Ann Rheum Dis 61 (suppl 3):III8, 2002.
53. Granfors K: Host–microbe interaction in HLA-B27–associated diseases. Ann Med 29:153, 1997.
54. Gross M: Molecular recognition. Crystallographic antibodies. Nature 373:105, 1995.
55. Steere AC: Lyme disease. N Engl J Med 345:115, 2001.
56. Ytterberg SR: Viral arthritis. Curr Opin Rheumatol 11:275, 1999.
57. German DC, Holmes EW: Hyperuricemia and gout. Med Clin North Am 70:419, 1986.
58. Morgan MP, McCarthy GM: Signaling mechanisms involved in crystal-induced tissue damage. Curr Opin Rheumatol 14:292, 2002.
59. Timms AE, et al: Genetic studies of disorders of calcium crystal deposition. Rheumatology (Oxford) 41:725, 2002.
60. Sandberg AA: Cytogenetics and molecular genetics of bone and soft-tissue tumors. Am J Med Genet 115:189, 2002.
61. Oliveira AM, Nascimento AG: Grading in soft tissue tumors: principles and problems. Skeletal Radiol 30:543, 2001.
62. De Wever I, et al: Cytogenetic, clinical, and morphologic correlations in 78 cases of fibromatosis: a report from the CHAMP Study Group. Chromosomes and Morphology. Mod Pathol 13:1080, 2000.
63. Xia SJ, Pressey JG, Barr FG: Molecular pathogenesis of rhabdomyosarcoma. Cancer Biol Ther 1:97, 2002.
64. Malogolowkin MH, Ortega JA: Rhabdomyosarcoma of childhood. Pediatr Ann 17:251, 1988.

CHAPTER 27

Peripheral Nerve and Skeletal Muscle

Douglas C. Anthony, MD, PhD •
Matthew P. Frosch, MD, PhD • Umberto De Girolami, MD

Normal Peripheral Nerve
Normal Skeletal Muscle

GENERAL REACTIONS OF THE MOTOR UNIT

Segmental Demyelination
Axonal Degeneration and Muscle Fiber Atrophy
Nerve Regeneration and Reinnervation of Muscle
Reactions of the Muscle Fiber

DISEASES OF PERIPHERAL NERVE

Inflammatory Neuropathies
Immune-Mediated Neuropathies
Infectious Polyneuropathies
Leprosy
Diphtheria
Varicella-Zoster Virus
Hereditary Neuropathies
Hereditary Motor and Sensory Neuropathy Type I
Other Hereditary Motor and Sensory Neuropathies
Acquired Metabolic and Toxic Neuropathies
Peripheral Neuropathy in Adult-Onset Diabetes Mellitus
Metabolic and Nutritional Peripheral Neuropathies
Neuropathies Associated with Malignancy
Toxic Neuropathies
Traumatic Neuropathies
Tumors of Peripheral Nerve

DISEASES OF SKELETAL MUSCLE

Denervation Atrophy
Spinal Muscular Atrophy (Infantile Motor Neuron Disease)
Muscular Dystrophies
X-Linked Muscular Dystrophy (Duchenne Muscular Dystrophy and Becker Muscular Dystrophy)
Autosomal Muscular Dystrophies
Myotonic Dystrophy
Ion Channel Myopathies (Channelopathies)
Congenital Myopathies
Myopathies Associated with Inborn Errors of Metabolism
Lipid Myopathies
Mitochondrial Myopathies (Oxidative Phosphorylation Diseases)
Inflammatory Myopathies
Noninfectious Inflammatory Myopathies
Toxic Myopathies
Thyrotoxic Myopathy
Ethanol Myopathy
Drug-Induced Myopathies
Diseases of the Neuromuscular Junction
Myasthenia Gravis
Lambert-Eaton Myasthenic Syndrome
Tumors of Skeletal Muscle

Normal

The functional unit of the neuromuscular system is the *motor unit,* which consists of (1) a *lower motor neuron* in the anterior horn of the spinal cord or cranial nerve motor nucleus in the brain stem, (2) the *axon* of that neuron, and (3) the multiple *muscle fibers* it innervates (Fig. 27–1). Lower motor neurons are distributed in the anterior horns of the spinal cord in columns or groups; they are arranged somatotopically so that cells lying medially innervate proximal muscles and those lying laterally supply the distal musculature. The number of muscle fibers within each unit varies considerably. Muscles with highly refined movements, such as the extrinsic muscles of the eye, have a high neuron-to-muscle-fiber ratio (1:10); those with relatively coarse and stereotyped movements, such as calf muscles, have a much lower ratio (1:1800).[1]

NORMAL PERIPHERAL NERVE

The principal structural component of peripheral nerve is the *nerve fiber* (an axon with its Schwann cells and myelin sheath). A nerve consists of numerous fibers that are grouped into fascicles by connective tissue sheaths. *Myelinated* and *unmyelinated* nerve fibers are intermingled within the fascicle (Fig. 27–2). In the sural nerve, the nerve that is most commonly examined by biopsy and a relatively pure sensory nerve, myelinated fibers range between 2 and 16 μm in diameter and have a bimodal distribution; the smaller axons, which average 4 μm, are about twice as numerous as the larger axons, which average 11 μm.[2] Peripheral nervous system (PNS) axons are myelinated in segments (*internodes*) separated by *nodes of Ranvier*. A single Schwann cell supplies the myelin sheath for each internode. The thickness of the myelin sheath is directly proportional to the diameter of the axon,[3] and the larger the axon diameter, the longer is the internodal distance. Myelin in the PNS is similar in overall lipid and protein composition to central nervous system (CNS) myelin; however, PNS myelin contains a higher proportion of sphingomyelins and glycoproteins. Some myelin proteins are specific to PNS myelin; others are shared with CNS myelin. Myelin protein zero (MPZ) is the major protein, making up over 50% of PNS myelin protein. MPZ is a transmembrane protein, which functions in the compaction of apposing lipid bilayers of myelin.[4] Myelin basic protein is the second most abundant protein; it is located topographically on the internal surface of bilayers at the major dense line of myelin. Peripheral myelin protein 22 (PMP22) is a 22-kDa transmembrane protein located in com-

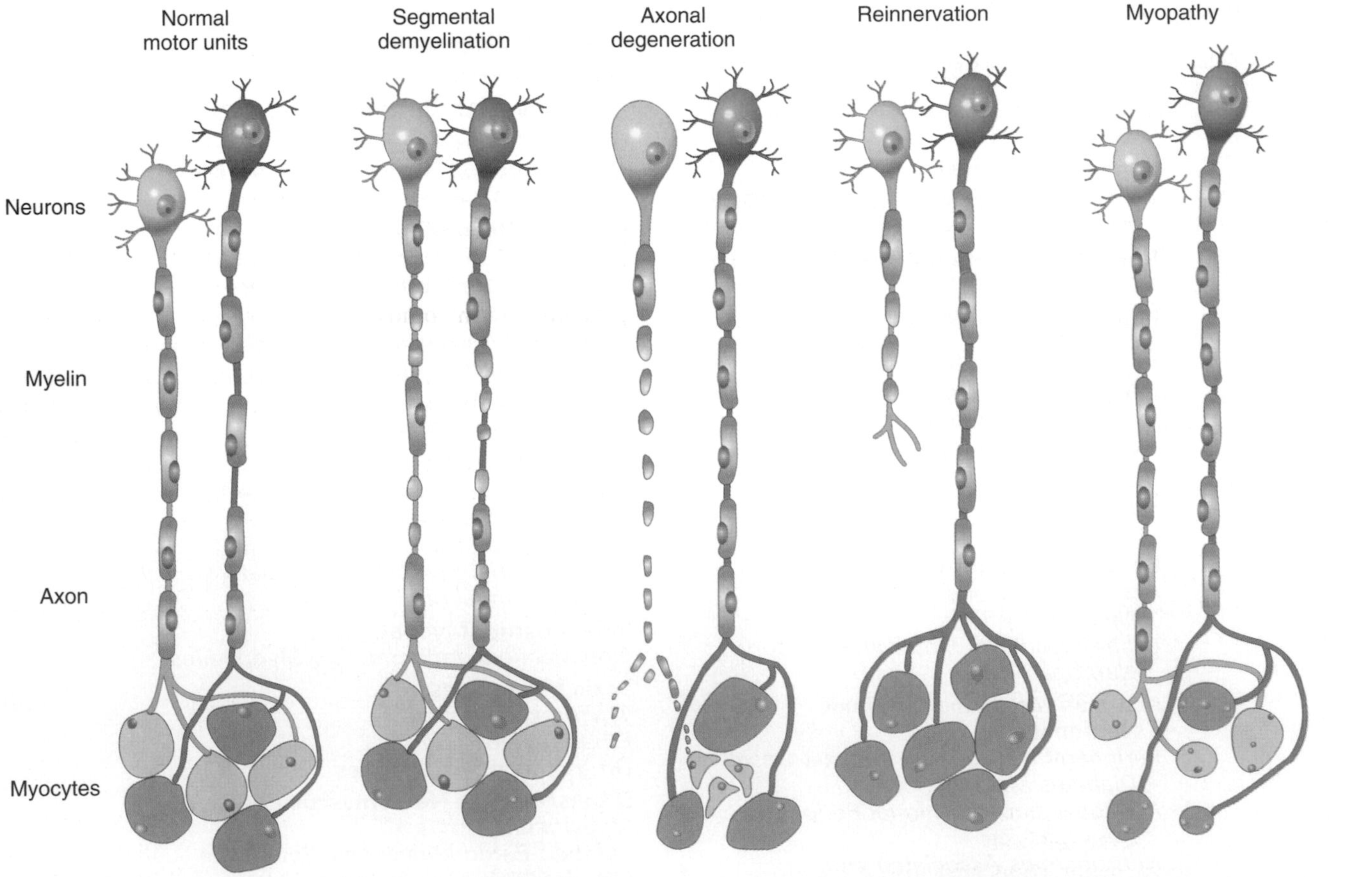

FIGURE 27–1 Normal and abnormal motor units. *Normal motor units*: Two adjacent motor units are shown. *Segmental demyelination:* Random internodes of myelin are injured and are remyelinated by multiple Schwann cells, while the axon and myocytes remain intact. *Axonal degeneration:* The axon and its myelin sheath undergo anterograde degeneration (shown for the green neuron), with resulting denervation atrophy of the myocytes within its motor unit. *Reinnervation of muscle:* Sprouting of adjacent (red) uninjured motor axons leads to fiber type grouping of myocytes, while the injured axon attempts axonal sprouting. *Myopathy:* Scattered myocytes of adjacent motor units are small (degenerated or regenerated), whereas the neurons and nerve fibers are normal.

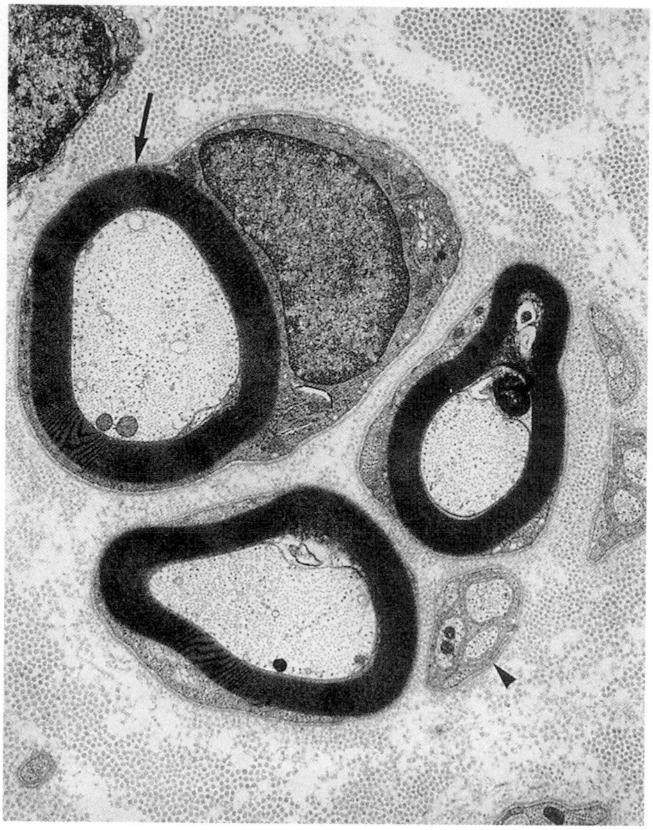

FIGURE 27–2 Electron micrograph of myelinated *(arrow)* and unmyelinated *(arrowhead)* fibers in human sural nerve. One Schwann cell nucleus is present.

pacted myelin. The periaxin gene encodes two proteins that are involved in the maintenance of myelin.[5] Early growth response 2 is a transcription factor that regulates the expression of these myelin proteins and is essential for the maintenance of myelin.[6]

Unmyelinated axons, which are far more numerous than myelinated axons, range in size from 0.2 to 3 μm. The cytoplasm of one Schwann cell envelops, and isolates from each other, a variable number of unmyelinated fibers (5 to 20 axons in humans). The Schwann cells associated with either myelinated or unmyelinated fibers have pale oval nuclei with an even chromatin distribution and an elongated bipolar cell body. By electron microscopy, Schwann cells have a basement membrane, unlike neighboring endoneurial fibroblasts and histiocytes.

Peripheral axons contain organelles and cytoskeletal structures, including microfilaments, neurofilaments, microtubules, mitochondria, vesicles, smooth endoplasmic reticulum, and lysosomes. Dense-core granules and coated vesicles are located in the nerve terminals. Protein synthesis does not occur in the axon. Instead, axoplasmic flow delivers proteins and other substances synthesized in the perikaryon down the axon.[7,8] A retrograde transport system serves as a feedback system for the cell body.

There are three major connective tissue components of peripheral nerve: the *epineurium*, which encloses the entire nerve; the *perineurium*, a multilayered concentric connective tissue sheath that encloses each fascicle; and the *endoneurium*, which surrounds individual nerve fibers. The nerve microenvironment is regulated by the *perineurial barrier* (formed by the tight junctions between perineurial cells), the *blood-nerve barrier*,[9] and the *nerve–cerebrospinal fluid* (CSF) barrier. Endoneurial capillaries derive from the vasa nervorum, and their endothelial cells form tight junctions to establish the blood-nerve barrier. This barrier has been found to be relatively less competent within nerve roots, dorsal root ganglia, and autonomic ganglia than along the rest of the nerve. The nerve-CSF barrier is formed by the tight junctions between the cells that form the outer layer of the arachnoid membrane. These cells fuse with the perineurium of the roots and cranial nerves as they leave the subarachnoid space. The motor and sensory fibers, which are separated within anterior and posterior roots, intermingle within the mixed sensorimotor nerves that exit the spinal canal.

NORMAL SKELETAL MUSCLE

Skeletal muscle fibers (*muscle fibers, myocytes*) are syncytia derived from the fusion of a contiguous column of individual embryonic cells and are therefore multinucleated. The multiple nuclei normally are located just beneath the plasma membrane (*sarcolemma*) of the myocyte. Transverse sections of muscle demonstrate the subsarcolemmal position of the nucleus in most fibers. Under normal circumstances, one nucleus in 3% to 5% of muscle fibers may be located within the interior of the muscle fiber;[10] these "internalized" nuclei occur more often in some pathologic conditions. *Satellite cells*, a stem cell population, are located adjacent to the sarcolemma and are covered by basement membrane, which encircles the entire muscle fiber.

Most of the cytoplasm of muscle fibers is filled with *myofilaments*, which form the contractile apparatus of the *myofibrils* (Fig. 27–3). A myofibril consists of identical repeating units (*sarcomeres*) composed of interlaced, longitudinally directed thin filaments (actin) and thick filaments (myosin) and perpendicularly disposed *Z-bands* (primarily α-actinin). The myofibrils interact with the sarcolemma through a series of proteins. Actin binds to dystrophin, a subsarcolemmal cytoskeletal protein, which forms an interface with the extracellular matrix through a complex of transmembrane proteins, known as the dystroglycan and sarcoglycan complexes (or dystrophin-associated proteins).[11] The T-tubule system, involved in calcium release during excitation, is an invagination of the sarcolemmal membrane into the interior of the cell. The T system runs parallel to the Z-bands, accompanied on each side by sarcoplasmic reticulum, which stores calcium, to be released during contraction. Between the myofibrils is the myocyte cytoplasm (sarcoplasm), which accounts for 40% of the volume of the fiber and contains myoglobin, glycogen, mitochondria, lysosomes, and lipid vacuoles.

Adult muscle fibers on transverse section are polygonal; in infancy, fibers tend to be round, as are those of the extrinsic eye muscles and some facial muscles in adults. The cross-sectional diameter of individual fibers varies, depending on the individual's age, the specific muscle, and the functional status of the fiber. In humans, two major types of fibers, *type 1* and *type 2*, have been defined on the basis of histochemistry and physiology (Table 27–1). Type 1 fibers are high in myoglobin and oxidative enzymes and have many mitochondria, in keeping with their ability to perform tonic contraction; operationally, they are most often defined by their dark staining for adenosine triphosphatase (ATPase) at pH 4.2 but light

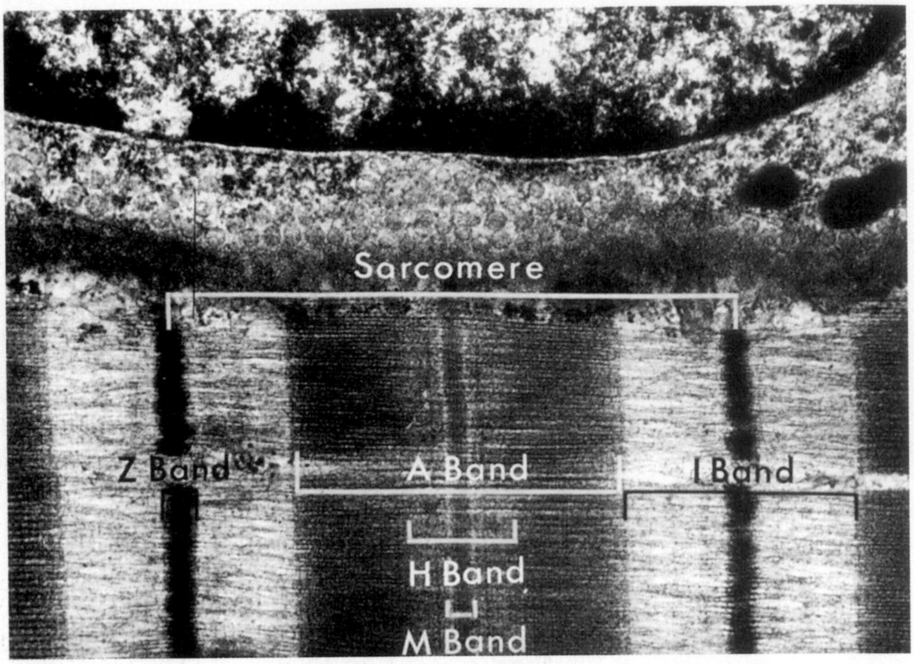

FIGURE 27–3 Electron micrograph of skeletal muscle in the longitudinal plane. A nucleus is located at the top of the illustration and the sarcomeres of two myofibrils are located below. The principal components of the sarcomere are identified, creating the pattern of cross-striations. (From Bloom W, Fawcett DW: A Textbook of Histology, 11th ed. Philadelphia, WB Saunders, 1986.)

staining at pH 9.4. Type 2 fibers are rich in glycolytic enzymes and are involved in rapid phasic contractions; they are dark staining on ATPase stain performed at pH 9.4 but light staining at pH 4.2. *Since the motor neuron determines fiber types, all fibers of a single unit are of the same type.* The fibers of a single motor unit are distributed across the muscle, giving rise to a checkerboard pattern of alternating fiber types, as is demonstrated especially well with staining for ATPase (Fig. 27–4*A*). Normally, there is some variability in the relative abundance of type 1 and type 2 fibers among different muscles.[12] The mnemonic "*one* (type 1 fiber) *slow* (twitch) *fat* (lipid-rich) *red* (appearance) *ox* (oxidative)" is useful to keep the physiology and histochemistry of the fiber types in mind.

Muscle spindles are fusiform structures that respond to stretch in muscles and have a role in maintaining tone. They consist of specialized muscle and nerve fibers, delimited by a connective tissue capsule.

The connective tissue sheath of muscles includes the *endomysium*, which surrounds individual muscle fibers; the *perimysium*, which groups muscle fibers into primary and secondary bundles (fasciculi); and the *epimysium*, which envelops single muscles or large groups of fibers.

TABLE 27–1 Muscle Fiber Types

	Type 1	Type 2
Action	Sustained force	Sudden movements
Strength	Weight-bearing	Purposeful motion
Enzyme content	NADH dark staining ATPase at pH 4.2, dark staining ATPase at pH 9.4, light staining	NADH light staining ATPase at pH 4.2, light staining ATPase at pH 9.4, dark staining
Lipids	Abundant	Scant
Glycogen	Scant	Abundant
Ultrastructure	Many mitochondria Wide Z-band	Few mitochondria Narrow Z-band
Physiology	Slow-twitch	Fast-twitch
Color	Red	White
Prototype	Soleus (pigeon)	Pectoral (pigeon)

Pathology

General Reactions of the Motor Unit

The two main responses of peripheral nerve to injury are based on the target of the insult: either the Schwann cell or the axon. Diseases that affect primarily the Schwann cell lead to a loss of myelin, referred to as *segmental demyelination*. In contrast, primary involvement of the neuron and its axon leads to axonal degeneration. In some diseases, axonal degeneration may be followed by *axonal regeneration* and *reinnervation* of muscle. The two principal pathologic processes seen in skeletal muscle are denervation atrophy, which follows loss of axons, and those due to a primary abnormality of the muscle fiber itself, referred to as *myopathy*. We now consider the general features of these processes.

SEGMENTAL DEMYELINATION

Segmental demyelination occurs when there is dysfunction of the Schwann cell (as in Guillain–Barré Syndrome) or damage to the myelin sheath (e.g., in hereditary motor and sensory neuropathy); there is no primary abnormality of the axon. The process affects some Schwann cells and their corresponding internodes while sparing others (see Fig. 27–1). The disintegrating myelin is engulfed initially by Schwann cells

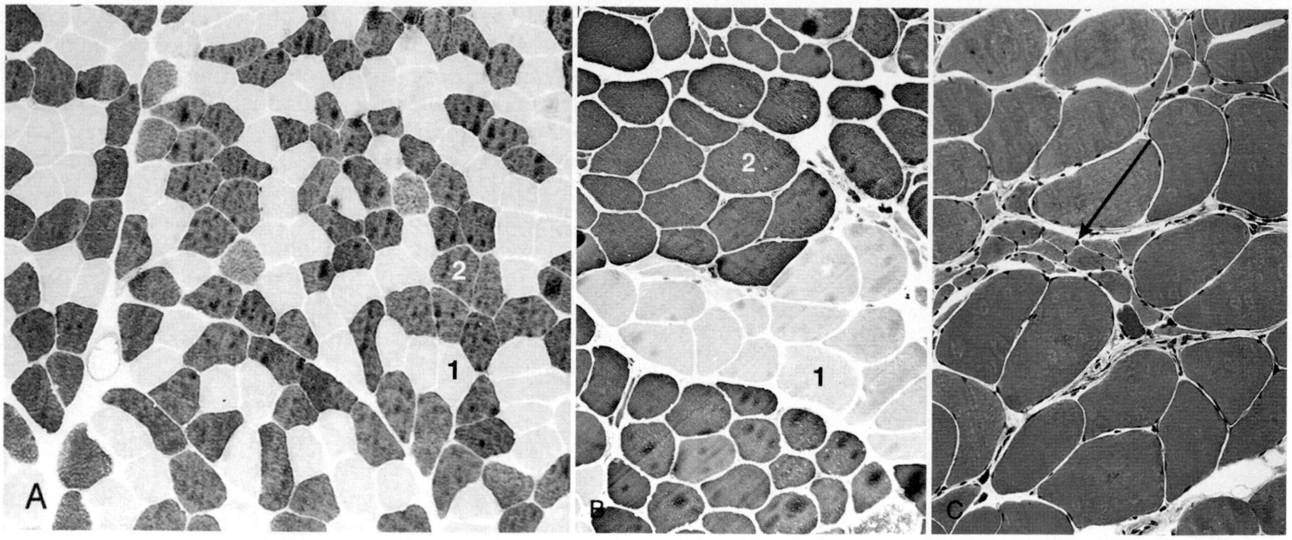

FIGURE 27–4 *A,* ATPase histochemical staining, at pH 9.4, of normal muscle showing checkerboard distribution of intermingled type 1 *(light)* and type 2 *(dark)* fibers. *B,* In contrast, fibers of either histochemical type are grouped together after reinnervation of muscle. *C,* A cluster of atrophic fibers (group atrophy) in the center *(arrow).*

and later by macrophages. The denuded axon provides a stimulus for remyelination. A population of cells within the endoneurium has the capacity to replace injured Schwann cells. These cells proliferate and encircle the axon and, in time, remyelinate the denuded portion.[13] Newly formed myelinated internodes are shorter than normal, however, and several are required to bridge the demyelinated region (see Fig. 27–1). The new myelin sheath is also thin in proportion to the diameter of the axon.

With sequential episodes of demyelination and remyelination, there is an accumulation of tiers of Schwann cell processes that, on transverse section, appear as concentric layers of Schwann cell cytoplasm and redundant basement membrane surrounding a thinly myelinated axon (*onion bulbs*) (Fig. 27–5). In time, many chronic demyelinating neuropathies give way to axonal injury. The specific conditions giving rise to such demyelination are described later.

AXONAL DEGENERATION AND MUSCLE FIBER ATROPHY

Axonal degeneration is the result of primary destruction of the axon, with secondary disintegration of its myelin sheath. Damage to the axon may be due either to a focal event occurring at some point along the length of the nerve (such as trauma or ischemia) or to a more generalized abnormality affecting the neuron cell body (*neuronopathy*) or its axon (*axonopathy*). When axonal injury occurs as the result of a focal lesion, such as traumatic transection of a nerve, the distal portion of the fiber undergoes *wallerian degeneration* (Fig. 27–6). Within a day, the axon begins to break down, and the affected Schwann cells begin to catabolize myelin and later engulf axon fragments, forming small oval compartments (*myelin ovoids*). Macrophages are recruited into the area and participate in the phagocytosis of axonal and myelin-derived debris.[14] The stump of the proximal portion of the severed nerve shows degenerative changes involving only the most distal two or three internodes and then undergoes regenerative activity. In the slowly evolving neuronopathies or axonopathies, evidence of axonal degeneration is scant because only a few fibers are actively degenerating at any given time.

When axonal degeneration occurs, the muscle fibers within the affected motor unit lose their neural input and undergo

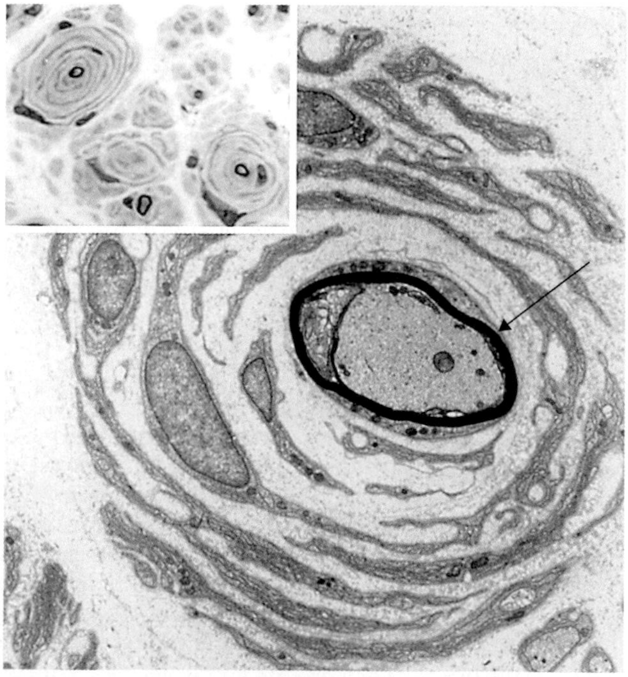

FIGURE 27–5 Electron micrograph of a single, thinly myelinated axon *(arrow)* surrounded by concentrically arranged Schwann cells, forming an onion bulb. (Courtesy of G. Richard Dickersin, MD, from Diagnostic Electron Microscopy: A Text-Atlas. New York, Igaku-Shoin Medical Publishers, 2000, p. 984.) *Inset,* Light microscopic appearance of an onion bulb neuropathy, characterized by "onion bulbs" surrounding axons.

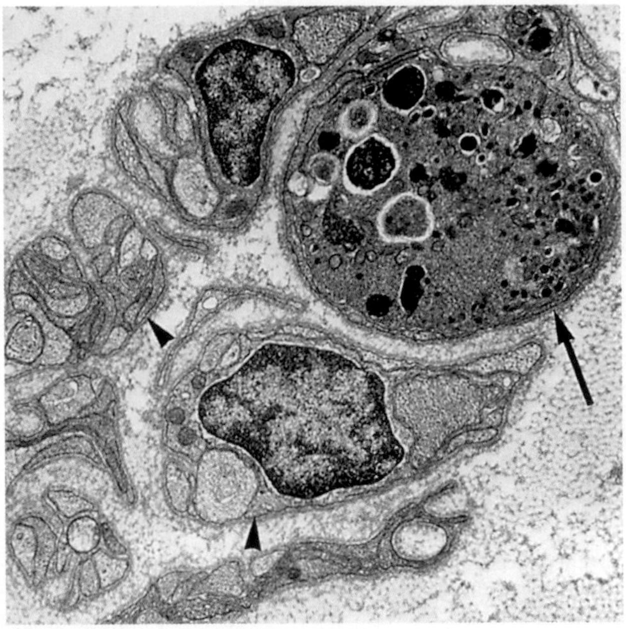

FIGURE 27–6 Electron micrograph of a degenerating axon *(arrow)* adjacent to several intact unmyelinated fibers *(arrowheads)*. The axon is markedly distended and contains numerous degenerating organelles and dense bodies.

denervation atrophy. Denervation of muscle leads to breakdown of myosin and actin,[15] with a decrease in cell size and resorption of myofibrils, but cells remain viable. In cross-section, the atrophic fibers are smaller than normal and have a roughly triangular shape ("angulated"). There is also cytoskeletal reorganization of some muscle cells, which results in a rounded zone of disorganized filaments in the center of the fiber (*target fiber*).

Type-specific atrophy is characteristic of some disease states. Type 2 fiber atrophy is a relatively common finding and is associated with inactivity or disuse. This type of "disuse atrophy" may occur after fracture of a limb and application of a plaster cast, in pyramidal tract degeneration, or in neurodegenerative diseases.

NERVE REGENERATION AND REINNERVATION OF MUSCLE

The proximal stumps of degenerated axons sprout and elongate, and they may develop new growth cones during the process of axonal regeneration. These growth cones use the Schwann cells vacated by the degenerated axons to guide them. The presence of multiple closely aggregated, thinly myelinated small-caliber axons is evidence of regeneration (*regenerating cluster*). This regrowth of axons is a slow process, apparently limited by the rate of the slow component of axonal transport, the movement of tubulin, actin, and intermediate filaments, on the order of 1 mm per day.[16] In spite of its slow pace, axonal regeneration accounts for some of the potential for functional recovery after peripheral axonal injury.

Reinnervation of the atrophic muscle fibers within an injured motor unit occurs when the axons belonging to an unaffected neighboring motor unit extend sprouts to reinnervate the denervated myocytes and incorporate them into the healthy motor unit. The number of muscle fibers within the healthy reinnervating motor unit will thus be increased. Furthermore, since muscle fiber type is imparted by the innervating neuron, the newly adopted reinnervated fibers assume the fiber type of their neighboring new siblings. The result of reinnervation is the loss of the checkerboard pattern and the occurrence of a patch of contiguous myocytes having the same histochemical type (*type grouping*) (see Fig. 27–4*B*). *Group atrophy* ensues when a type group in turn becomes denervated because it is affected in the course of disease progression (see Fig. 27–4*C*).

REACTIONS OF THE MUSCLE FIBER

Although a wide spectrum of diseases may affect muscle, the number of pathologic reactions of myocytes is relatively limited.[17] The following pathologic changes may be seen in myopathies as well as in diseases in which the pathogenesis involves factors outside of the muscle and only secondarily involves the muscle cells. The most common forms of reaction include the following:

- *Segmental necrosis*, destruction of a portion of the length of a myocyte, may be followed by *myophagocytosis* as macrophages infiltrate the region. The loss of muscle fibers in time leads to extensive deposition of collagen and fatty infiltration.
- *Vacuolation, alterations in structural proteins or organelles, and accumulation of intracytoplasmic deposits* may be seen in many diseases.
- *Regeneration* occurs when peripherally located satellite cells proliferate and reconstitute the destroyed portion of the fiber. The regenerating portion of the muscle fiber has large internalized nuclei and prominent nucleoli, and the cytoplasm, laden with RNA, is basophilic.
- Fiber *hypertrophy* occurs in response to increased load, either in the setting of exercise or in pathologic conditions in which muscle fibers are injured. Large fibers may divide along a segment (*muscle fiber splitting*) so that in cross-section, a single large fiber contains a cell membrane traversing its diameter, often with adjacent nuclei.

Diseases of Peripheral Nerve

Peripheral nerve is susceptible to the same wide range of categories of disease (inflammatory, traumatic, metabolic, toxic, genetic, neoplastic) as are other tissues. The pattern of disease, however, reflects the unique structure and function of nerves.

INFLAMMATORY NEUROPATHIES

These diseases are characterized by inflammatory cell infiltrates in peripheral nerves, roots, and sensory and autonomic ganglia. In some, an infectious agent elicits the inflammatory responses; in others, immune mechanisms are presumed to be the primary cause of the inflammation.

Immune-Mediated Neuropathies

Guillain-Barré Syndrome (Acute Inflammatory Demyelinating Polyradiculoneuropathy)

Guillain-Barré syndrome is a life-threatening disease of the peripheral nervous system, with an overall annual incidence of one to three cases per 100,000 persons in the United States.[18] The disease is characterized clinically by weakness beginning in the distal limbs but rapidly advancing to affect proximal muscle function ("ascending paralysis"), and histologically by inflammation and demyelination of spinal nerve roots and peripheral nerves (radiculoneuropathy).

Pathogenesis. Approximately two-thirds of cases are preceded by an acute, influenza-like illness from which the patient has recovered by the time the neuropathy becomes symptomatic. Infections with *Campylobacter jejuni*, cytomegalovirus, Epstein-Barr virus, and *Mycoplasma pneumoniae* have been shown to have a significant epidemiologic association with Guillain-Barré syndrome.[18] There has been no consistent demonstration of an infectious agent in peripheral nerves in these patients, and an immunological reaction is now generally favored as the underlying cause.[18–20] A similar inflammatory disease of peripheral nerves can be induced in experimental animals by immunization with peripheral nerve myelin or its components. A T cell–mediated immune response ensues, accompanied by segmental demyelination induced by activated macrophages. Transfer of these T cells to a naive animal results in comparable lesions.[21,22] Moreover, lymphocytes from patients with Guillain-Barré syndrome have been shown to produce demyelination in tissue cultures of myelinated nerve fibers. Circulating antibodies may also play a part,[22] and plasmapheresis is reported to be an effective treatment.

Morphology. The dominant histopathologic finding is **inflammation of peripheral nerve,** manifested as perivenular and endoneurial infiltration by lymphocytes, macrophages, and a few plasma cells. The invading inflammatory cells vary in number from a sparse seeding of the perivenous spaces to large collections of mononuclear cells disseminated throughout the entire nerve. Segmental demyelination affecting peripheral nerves is the primary lesion, but damage to axons is also characteristic, particularly when the disease is severe. Electron microscopy has identified an early effect on myelin sheaths. The cytoplasmic processes of macrophages penetrate the basement membrane of Schwann cells, particularly in the vicinity of the nodes of Ranvier, and extend between the myelin lamellae, stripping away the myelin sheath from the axon. Ultimately, the remnants of the myelin sheath are engulfed by the macrophages. Remyelination follows the demyelination.

Inflammatory foci and demyelination are widely distributed throughout the peripheral nervous system, although their intensity is variable. The most intense inflammatory reaction is often localized in spinal and cranial motor roots and the adjacent parts of the spinal and cranial nerves.

Clinical Course. The clinical picture is dominated by the ascending paralysis. Deep tendon reflexes disappear early in the process; although sensory involvement can often be detected, it is less troublesome than the weakness. The nerve conduction velocity is slowed because of the multifocal destruction of myelin segments involving many axons within a nerve; there is elevation of the CSF protein due to inflammation and altered permeability of the microcirculation within the spinal roots as they traverse the subarachnoid space. Inflammatory cells are contained within the roots, however, and there is little to no CSF pleocytosis. Many patients spend weeks in hospital intensive-care units before recovering normal function. With improved respiratory care and support, the mortality rate has fallen from 25% in the past but is still considerable, with some 2% to 5% dying of respiratory paralysis, autonomic instability, cardiac arrest, and the complications of treatment.[18]

Chronic Inflammatory Demyelinating Polyradiculoneuropathy

In some patients, inflammatory demyelinating polyradiculoneuropathy, instead of occurring as an acute illness as in Guillain-Barré syndrome, follows a subacute or chronic course, usually with relapses and remissions over the period of several years.[20,23] In these cases, there is often a symmetric, mixed sensorimotor polyneuropathy, although some patients have predominantly sensory or motor impairment. Clinical remissions may occur with steroid treatment and plasmapheresis. Biopsies of sural nerves show evidence of recurrent demyelination and remyelination with well-developed onion bulb structures.[23]

INFECTIOUS POLYNEUROPATHIES

Many infectious processes affect peripheral nerve. Here, we briefly review the changes in leprosy, diphtheria, and varicella-zoster because they cause unique and specific pathologic changes in nerves (see also in Chapter 8).

Leprosy

There is peripheral nerve involvement in both lepromatous and tuberculoid leprosy (discussed in Chapter 8). In lepromatous leprosy, Schwann cells are often invaded by *Mycobacterium leprae*, which proliferates and eventually infects other cells. There is evidence of segmental demyelination and remyelination and loss of both myelinated and unmyelinated axons. As the infection advances, endoneurial fibrosis and multilayered thickening of the perineurial sheaths occur. Patients develop a symmetric polyneuropathy that prominently involves pain fibers; the resulting loss of sensation contributes to injury since the patient is rendered unaware of injurious stimuli and damaged tissues. Thus, large traumatic ulcers may develop in the extremities. Tuberculoid leprosy shows evidence of active cell-mediated immune response to *M. leprae*, with nodular granulomatous inflammation situated in the dermis. The inflammation injures cutaneous nerves in the vicinity; axons, Schwann cells, and myelin are lost, and there is fibrosis of the perineurium and endoneurium. In tuberculoid leprosy, patients have much more localized nerve involvement.

Diphtheria

Peripheral nerve involvement results from the effects of the diphtheria exotoxin and begins with paresthesias and weakness; early loss of proprioception and vibratory sensation is common.[24] The earliest changes are seen in the sensory ganglia, where the incomplete blood-nerve barrier allows entry of the toxin. There is selective demyelination of axons that extends into adjacent anterior and posterior roots as well as into mixed sensorimotor nerves. The mechanism of action of diphtheria toxin was described in Chapter 8.

Varicella-Zoster Virus

Varicella-zoster virus (VZV) is one of the most common viral infections of the peripheral nervous system. Latent infection of neurons in the sensory ganglia of the spinal cord and brain stem follows chickenpox, and reactivation leads to a painful, vesicular skin eruption in the distribution of sensory dermatomes (*shingles*), most frequently thoracic or trigeminal. The virus may be transported along the sensory nerves to the skin, where it establishes an active infection of epidermal cells. In a small proportion of patients, weakness is also apparent in the same distribution. Although the factors that give rise to reactivation are not fully understood, decreased cell-mediated immunity is of major importance in some cases.[25]

Affected ganglia show neuronal destruction and loss, usually accompanied by abundant mononuclear inflammatory infiltrates; regional necrosis with hemorrhage may also be found. Peripheral nerve shows axonal degeneration after the death of the sensory neurons. Focal destruction of the large motor neurons of the anterior horns or cranial nerve motor nuclei may be seen at the corresponding levels. Intranuclear inclusions generally are not found in the peripheral nervous system.

HEREDITARY NEUROPATHIES

This is a group of heterogeneous, typically progressive, and often disabling syndromes that affect peripheral nerves. The genetic and molecular basis of many of the hereditary peripheral neuropathies is being elucidated,[26,27] and as they are further defined, adjustments in the current classification scheme can be anticipated. They can be divided into several groups:

- *Hereditary motor and sensory neuropathies* (HMSN): The most common form of hereditary neuropathies, these disorders affect both strength and sensation (sensorimotor neuropathies). *They present as a spectrum of disorders, all caused by mutations in genes whose products are involved in the formation and maintenance of myelin.* Different mutations within the same gene may give rise to diseases with varying clinical features.
- *Hereditary sensory and autonomic neuropathies* (HSAN): Symptoms in HSAN are usually limited to numbness, pain, and autonomic dysfunction such as orthostatic hypotension (Table 27–2).
- *Familial amyloid polyneuropathies* (FAP): These are hereditary peripheral neuropathies characterized by the deposition of amyloid within the peripheral nervous system. Most kindreds exhibit mutations of the *transthyretin* gene, located on chromosome 18q11.2–q12.1. Their clinical presentation is similar to that of HSAN. The amyloid fibrils are composed of transthyretin (Chapter 1), a protein involved in serum binding and transport of thyroid hormone.
- *Peripheral neuropathy accompanying inherited metabolic disorders*: Several hereditary metabolic disorders are accompanied by prominent peripheral neuropathy during the course of the disease; the molecular basis and the clinicopathologic characteristics of some of these are presented in Table 27–3.

The pathologic findings of many of the hereditary neuropathies are those of an axonal neuropathy. Fiber loss is the most prominent finding.

Hereditary Motor and Sensory Neuropathy Type I

The most common hereditary peripheral neuropathy, *Charcot-Marie-Tooth (CMT) disease, hypertrophic form (HMSN I)*, usually presents in childhood or early adulthood. A characteristic progressive muscular atrophy of the calf seen in these patients gives rise to the common clinical term *peroneal muscular atrophy*. Patients may be asymptomatic, but when they present, it is often with symptoms such as distal muscle weakness, atrophy of the calf, or secondary orthopedic problems of the foot (such as *pes cavus*).

Molecular Genetics. The disease is genetically heterogeneous. In most pedigrees (known as HMSN IA or CMT1A), there is a duplication of a large region of chromosome 17p11.2–p12, resulting in "segmental trisomy" of the duplicated region. The duplicated segment includes the gene for

TABLE 27–2 Hereditary Sensory and Autonomic Neuropathies

Disease and Inheritance	Gene and Locus	Clinical and Pathologic Findings
HSAN I; autosomal-dominant	Serine palmitoyl transferase, long-chain base, subunit 1 (SPTLC1) gene; 9q22.1–q22.3	Predominantly sensory neuropathy, presenting in young adults; axonal degeneration (mostly myelinated fibers)
HSAN II; autosomal-recessive (some cases are sporadic)	Unknown	Predominantly sensory neuropathy, presenting in infancy; axonal degeneration (mostly myelinated fibers)
HSAN III (Riley-Day syndrome; familial dysautonomia; most often in Jewish children); autosomal-recessive	Inhibitor of kappa light polypeptide gene enhancer in B cells, kinase complex-associated protein (IKBKAP or IKAP) gene; 9q31–q33	Predominantly autonomic neuropathy, presenting in infancy; axonal degeneration (mostly unmyelinated fibers); atrophy and loss of sensory and autonomic ganglion cells

TABLE 27–3 Hereditary Neuropathies Accompanying Inherited Metabolic Disease

Disease	Metabolic Defect	Inheritance	Clinical Findings	Pathologic Findings
Adrenoleukodystrophy	ATP-binding cassette, or ABC, transporter protein, subfamily D, member 1 (ALD protein, or ABCD1) gene; Xq28	X-linked; 4% of female carriers are symptomatic	Mixed motor and sensory neuropathy, adrenal insufficiency, spastic paraplegia; onset between 10 and 20 years for males with leukodystrophy, between 20 and 40 years for females with myeloneuropathy	Segmental demyelination, with onion bulbs; axonal degeneration (myelinated and unmyelinated); electron microscopy; linear inclusions in Schwann cells
Familial amyloid polyneuropathies	Transthyretin (TTR) gene (rarely other genes); 18q11.2–q12.1	Autosomal-dominant	Sensory and autonomic dysfunction; age at onset varies with site of mutation	Amyloid deposits in vessel walls and connective tissue with axonal degeneration
Porphyria, acute intermittent (AIP) or variegate coproporphyria	Enzymes involved in heme synthesis (acute intermittent porphyria —porphobilinogen deaminase deficiency; 11q24.1–q24.2)	Autosomal-dominant	Acute episodes of neurologic dysfunction, psychiatric disturbances, abdominal pain, seizures, proximal weakness, autonomic dysfunction; attacks may be precipitated by drugs	Acute and chronic axonal degeneration; regenerating clusters
Refsum disease	Peroxisomal enzyme phytanoyl CoA α-hydroxylase (PAHX) gene; 10pter–p11.2	Autosomal-recessive	Mixed motor and sensory neuropathy with palpable nerves; ataxia, night blindness, retinitis pigmentosa, ichthyosis; age at onset before 20 years (a genetically distinct infantile form also exists)	Severe onion bulb formation

peripheral myelin protein 22 (PMP22), but whether the disease is caused by overexpression of PMP22, by gene dosage effect,[28,29] or by duplication of other adjacent genes is not clear. A separate genetic locus on chromosome 1 involves myelin protein zero (MPZ) but produces an identical clinical phenotype (HMSN IB).[26] A third set of pedigrees shows linkage to chromosome 16p, and is associated with mutations in a gene whose product is involved in protein degradation pathways.[30] In addition, some pedigrees are associated with mutations in the gene for the gap junction protein connexin-32, which is located on the X chromosome.[31]

Morphology. CMT1 is a demyelinating neuropathy, both by nerve conduction velocity studies and pathologically. Histologic examination shows the consequences of repetitive demyelination and remyelination, with multiple onion bulbs, more pronounced in distal nerves than in proximal nerves (see Fig. 27–5). The axon is often present in the center of the onion bulb, and the myelin sheath is usually thin or absent. The redundant layers of Schwann cell hyperplasia surrounding individual axons are associated with enlargement of individual peripheral nerves that may be individually palpable, which has led to the term **hypertrophic neuropathy**. In the longitudinal plane, individual segments of the axon may show evidence of segmental demyelination. Autopsy studies of affected individuals have shown degeneration of the posterior columns of the spinal cord.

Clinical Course. The disorder is usually autosomal-dominant, and although it is slowly progressive, the disability of sensorimotor deficits and associated orthopedic problems such as pes cavus are usually limited in severity, and a normal life span is typical. The relationship between the molecular events and the observed peripheral nerve pathology is not well understood.

Other Hereditary Motor and Sensory Neuropathies

HMSN II

This is a neuronal form of autosomal-dominant Charcot-Marie-Tooth disease that presents with signs and symptoms similar to those of HMSN I, although nerve enlargement is not seen and the disease presents at a slightly later age. This form is less common than HMSN I, and in some families (designated CMT2A), it is linked to chromosome 1p35–p36.[26] Additional, less common loci have been linked to forms CMT 2B to 2G.[26] Nerve biopsy specimens in this disorder show loss of myelinated axons as the predominant finding. Segmental demyelination of internodes is infrequent. These findings suggest that the site of primary cellular dysfunction is the axon or neuron.

Dejerine-Sottas Disease (HMSN III)

Dejerine-Sottas disease is a slowly progressive, autosomal-recessive disorder that begins in early childhood, manifested by delay in developmental milestones, such as the acquisition of motor skills. In contrast to HMSN I and HMSN II, in which muscular atrophy is limited to the leg, both trunk and limb muscles are involved in Dejerine-Sottas disease. On physical examination, *enlarged peripheral nerves* can be detected by inspection and palpation. The deep tendon reflexes are depressed or absent, and nerve conduction velocity is slowed. HMSN III is genetically heterogeneous, and arises from distinct mutations in the same myelin-associated genes that are mutated in HMSN I. These include genes encoding peripheral myelin protein 22 (PMP22), myelin protein zero (MPZ), periaxin (PRX), and early growth response 2 (EGR2).[32–34] Morphologically, the size of individual peripheral nerve fascicles is increased, often dramatically, with abundant onion bulb formation as well as segmental demyelination. There is usually evidence of axonal loss, and the axons that remain are often of diminished caliber. These findings are most severe in the distal portions of the peripheral nervous system; however, autopsy studies have shown that similar findings may be present in spinal roots.

Other less common forms of HMSN are characterized by additional neurologic and ophthalmologic abnormalities, such as retinitis pigmentosa and deafness.

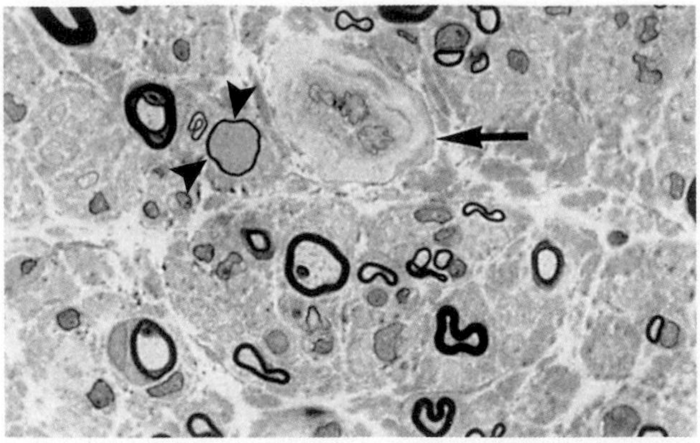

FIGURE 27–7 Diabetic neuropathy with marked loss of myelinated fibers, a thinly myelinated fiber *(arrowheads)*, and thickening of endoneurial vessel wall *(arrow)*.

ACQUIRED METABOLIC AND TOXIC NEUROPATHIES

Functional and structural changes in peripheral nerve develop in response to various metabolic alterations—either from endogenous disorders or from exogenous agents. The most common of these processes are discussed here.

Peripheral Neuropathy in Adult-Onset Diabetes Mellitus

The prevalence of peripheral neuropathy in patients with diabetes mellitus depends on the duration of the disease, with up to 50% of diabetic patients having peripheral neuropathy clinically after 25 years of diabetes and nearly 100% having conduction abnormalities electrophysiologically.[35] Several distinct clinicopathologic patterns of diabetes-related peripheral nerve abnormalities have been recognized (Chapter 24). They are categorized as *distal symmetric sensory or sensorimotor neuropathy*, *autonomic neuropathy*, and *focal or multifocal asymmetric neuropathy*. Individuals may develop any combination of these lesions; in fact, the first two (sensorimotor and autonomic) are often found together.

Morphology. In patients with a distal symmetric sensorimotor neuropathy, the predominant pathologic finding is an axonal neuropathy. As with other chronic axonal neuropathies, there is often some segmental demyelination. There is a relative loss of small myelinated fibers and of unmyelinated fibers, but large fibers are also affected. Endoneurial arterioles show thickening, hyalinization, and intense periodic acid–Schiff (PAS) positivity in their walls and extensive reduplication of the basement membrane[36] (Fig. 27–7). Whether the lesions are due to ischemia[37] or metabolic derangement is unclear.

Clinical Course. The most common peripheral neuropathy is the symmetric neuropathy that involves distal sensory and motor nerves. Patients with the neuropathy develop decreased sensation in the distal extremities with less evident motor abnormalities. The loss of pain sensation can result in the development of ulcers that heal poorly because of the diffuse vascular injury in diabetes, and are a major cause of morbidity. Another manifestation of diabetic neuropathy is *dysfunction of the autonomic nervous system*; this affects 20% to 40% of diabetics, nearly always in association with a distal sensorimotor neuropathy.[38] Some patients, especially elderly adults with a long history of diabetes, develop a peripheral neuropathy that manifests itself as a disorder of single individual peripheral or cranial (oculomotor nerve) nerves (*mononeuropathy*), or of several individual nerves in an asymmetric distribution (*multiple mononeuropathy or mononeuropathy multiplex*). The pathogenesis of mononeuropathies in adult-onset diabetes is thought to involve vascular insufficiency, creating ischemic injury of the peripheral nerve.[38]

Metabolic and Nutritional Peripheral Neuropathies

As many as 65% of patients with renal failure have clinical evidence of peripheral neuropathy before dialysis (*uremic neuropathy*). This is typically a distal, symmetric neuropathy that may be asymptomatic or may be associated with muscle cramps, distal dysesthesias, and diminished deep tendon reflexes. In these patients, axonal degeneration is the primary event, with degenerating fibers and fiber loss; occasionally, there is secondary demyelination. Regeneration and recovery are common after dialysis.

Peripheral neuropathy can also develop in patients with chronic liver disease, chronic respiratory insufficiency, and thyroid dysfunction. *Thiamine deficiency* is characterized by axonal neuropathy, a clinical condition termed *neuropathic beriberi*. Axonal neuropathies also occur with deficiencies of vitamins B_{12} (cobalamin), B_6 (pyridoxine), and E (α-tocopherol). Excessive chronic consumption of ethyl alcohol often leads to axonal neuropathy. There is a strong contribution of associated dietary deficiency, and patients often have signs of thiamine deficiency. Ethyl alcohol may have a direct toxic effect on peripheral nerve, as some patients have alcoholic neuropathy in spite of adequate thiamine nutritional status.[39]

Neuropathies Associated with Malignancy

Direct infiltration or compression of peripheral nerves by tumor is a common cause of mononeuropathy and may be the presenting symptom of cancer. These neuropathies include *brachial plexopathy* from neoplasms of the apex of the lung, *obturator palsy* from pelvic malignant neoplasms, and *cranial nerve palsies* from intracranial tumors and tumors of the base of the skull. A *polyradiculopathy* involving the lower extremity may develop when the cauda equina is involved by meningeal carcinomatosis.

A diffuse, symmetric peripheral neuropathy may occur in patients with a distant carcinoma and is considered a remote, or *paraneoplastic,* effect (Chapters 7 and 28). The most common type is a sensorimotor neuropathy characterized by weakness and sensory deficits that are often more pronounced in the lower extremities and that progress during months to years.[40] The neuropathy is most frequently associated with small cell carcinoma of the lung; as many as 2% to 5% of patients with lung cancer may have clinical evidence of peripheral neuropathy. Patients with the less frequent pure sensory neuropathy present with numbness and paresthesias that may precede the identification of the malignant neoplasm by 6 to 15 months. An immunologic mechanism for the neuropathy has been suggested on the basis of the presence of inflammatory infiltrates within the dorsal root ganglia and the identification of a circulating polyclonal immunoglobulin G antibody (anti-Hu) in such patients. The antibody, which binds a 35- to 38-kDa RNA-binding protein[41] expressed by neurons and the tumor,[42] is thought to give rise to the paraneoplastic syndrome. In keeping with this, the severity of clinical symptoms correlates with antibody titer.[40]

Paraneoplastic neuropathy may also develop in patients with plasma cell dyscrasias in one of two ways. The first is through the deposition of light-chain (AL type) amyloid in peripheral nerves (Chapter 6). The second is independent of the presence or deposition of amyloid and may be related to the binding of monoclonal immunoglobulin to myelin-associated glycoprotein.[43]

Toxic Neuropathies

Peripheral neuropathies can occur after exposure to industrial or environmental chemicals, biologic toxins, or therapeutic drugs.[44] Prominent among the environmental chemicals are heavy metals, including lead and arsenic (Chapter 9). In addition, many organic compounds are known to be neurotoxic.

TRAUMATIC NEUROPATHIES

Peripheral nerves are commonly injured in the course of trauma. *Lacerations* result from cutting injuries and can complicate fractures when a sharp fragment of bone lacerates the nerve. *Avulsions* occur when tension is applied to a peripheral nerve, often as the result of a force applied to one of the limbs. The direct severance of nerves is associated with hemorrhage, and there is transection of the connective tissue planes. Regeneration of peripheral nerve axons does occur, albeit slowly. Regrowth may be complicated by discontinuity between the proximal and distal portions of the nerve sheath as well as by the misalignment of individual fascicles. Axons, even in the absence of correctly positioned distal segments, may continue to grow, resulting in a mass of tangled axonal processes known as a *traumatic neuroma (pseudoneuroma or amputation neuroma).* Within this mass, small bundles of axons appear randomly oriented; each, however, is surrounded by organized layers containing Schwann cells, fibroblasts, and perineurial cells (Fig. 27–8).

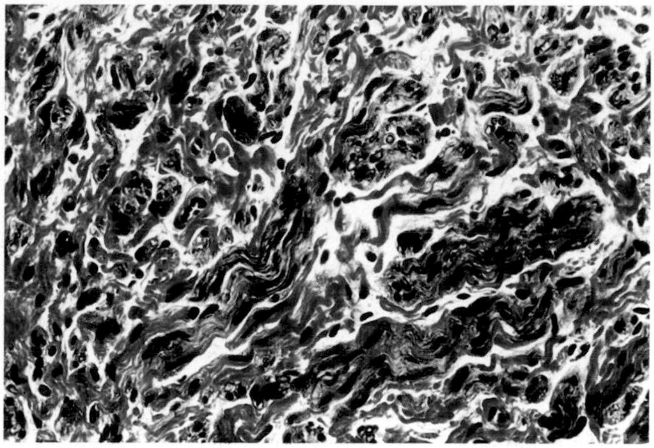

FIGURE 27–8 Traumatic neuroma showing disordered orientation of nerve fiber bundles *(purple)* intermixed with connective tissue *(blue).*

Compression neuropathy (entrapment neuropathy) occurs when a peripheral nerve is compressed, often within an anatomic compartment. *Carpal tunnel syndrome* is the most common entrapment neuropathy and results from compression of the median nerve at the level of the wrist within the compartment delimited by the transverse carpal ligament. Women are more commonly affected than men, and the problem is frequently bilateral. The disorder may be observed with any condition that causes decreased available space within the carpal tunnel, such as tissue edema, but common predisposing factors include pregnancy, inflammatory arthritis, hypothyroidism, amyloidosis (especially that related to β_2-microglobulin deposition in renal dialysis patients), acromegaly, diabetes mellitus, and excessive repetitive motions of the wrist.[45] Symptoms are limited to dysfunction of the median nerve, including numbness and paresthesias of the tips of the thumb and first two digits. Additional compression neuropathies include involvement of the ulnar nerve at the level of the elbow, the peroneal nerve at the level of the knee, and the radial nerve in the upper arm as seen after sleeping with the arm improperly positioned ("Saturday night palsy"). Another form of compression neuropathy is found in the foot, affecting the interdigital nerve at intermetatarsal sites. This problem, which occurs more often in women than in men, leads to foot pain (metatarsalgia). The histologic findings of the lesion (*Morton neuroma*) include evidence of chronic compression injury.

TUMORS OF PERIPHERAL NERVE

Both benign and malignant tumors can be derived from elements of the nerve sheath. These are discussed with tumors of the central nervous system (Chapter 28).

Diseases of Skeletal Muscle

DENERVATION ATROPHY

Neurogenic atrophy of muscle is caused by any process that affects the anterior horn cell or its axon in the peripheral nervous system. The response of muscle to denervation and the histologic changes associated with reinnervation are described earlier.

Spinal Muscular Atrophy (Infantile Motor Neuron Disease)

Motor neuron diseases are progressive neurologic illnesses that selectively affect the anterior horn cells in the spinal cord and cranial nerve motor neurons, resulting in their loss. Motor neuron diseases in adults are discussed in Chapter 28. Spinal muscular atrophy (SMA) is a distinctive group of autosomal-recessive motor neuron diseases that begin in childhood or adolescence. SMA is discussed here because the disease is commonly considered with the childhood myopathies and because the pathologic findings in skeletal muscle are characteristic.

Genetics. All forms of SMA are associated with a locus on chromosome 5 that harbors the survival motor neuron gene (*SMN1*). Homozygous deletions of *SMN1* (or less commonly, intragenic mutations) occur in over 90% of patients with SMA,[46,47] and contiguous deletion of the nearby neuronal apoptosis inhibitory protein gene (*NAIP*) may be associated with a severe clinical phenotype.[48] The SMN gene product contains a Tudor homology region (a highly conserved motif involved in RNA processing), which is thought to be involved in spliceosome function, including removal of introns from pre-mRNA.[47]

Morphology. The typical histologic finding in muscle is large numbers of atrophic fibers, often only a few micrometers in diameter (Fig. 27–9). This is unlike the groups of angulated atrophic fibers seen in denervation atrophy of muscle in adults. In SMA, the muscle fiber atrophy often involves an entire fascicle, and is called **panfascicular atrophy.** There are also scattered large fibers that are two to four times normal size.

Clinical Course. The most common form of spinal muscular atrophy, Werdnig-Hoffmann disease (SMA type 1), has its onset at birth or within the first 4 months of life and usually leads to death within the first 3 years of life. The other two forms (SMA 2 and SMA 3) present at later ages, either in early childhood (between 3 and 15 months of age in SMA 2) or in later childhood (after 2 years of age in SMA 3). The clinical progression is related to the subtype, with shorter survival (more than 4 years) in the earlier-onset form (SMA 2) than in patients with SMA 3, who often survive into adulthood.

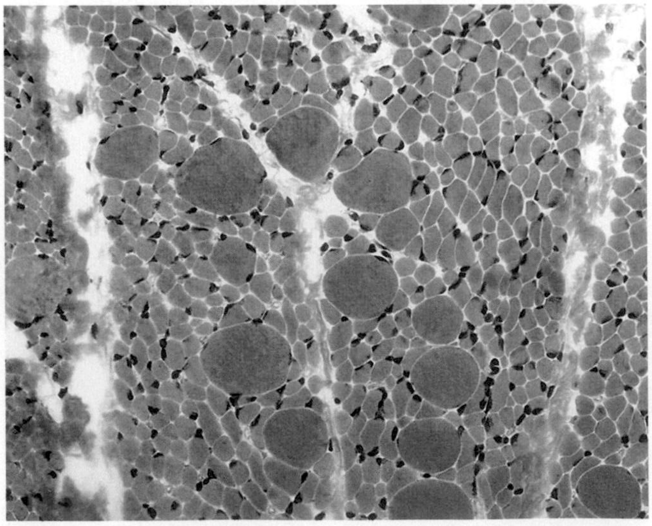

FIGURE 27–9 Spinal muscular atrophy with groups of atrophic muscle fibers resulting from denervation atrophy of muscle in early childhood.

MUSCULAR DYSTROPHIES

The muscular dystrophies are a heterogeneous group of inherited disorders, often beginning in childhood, that are characterized clinically by progressive muscle weakness and wasting. Histologically, the advanced cases are characterized by the replacement of muscle fibers by fibrofatty tissue. This feature distinguishes dystrophies from myopathies (described later), which also present with muscle weakness.

X-Linked Muscular Dystrophy (Duchenne Muscular Dystrophy and Becker Muscular Dystrophy)

The two most common forms of muscular dystrophy are X-linked: *Duchenne muscular dystrophy* (DMD) and *Becker muscular dystrophy* (BMD). DMD is the most severe and the most common form of muscular dystrophy, with an incidence of about 1 per 3500 live male births.[49] DMD becomes clinically manifest by the age of 5 years, with weakness leading to wheelchair dependence by 10 to 12 years of age, and progresses relentlessly until death by the early twenties. Although BMD involves the same genetic locus, it is less common and much less severe than DMD.

Pathogenesis and Genetics. DMD and BMD are caused by abnormalities in a gene that is located in the Xp21 region and encodes a 427-kDa protein termed *dystrophin*. Deletions appear to represent a large proportion of the genetic abnormalities, with frameshift and point mutations accounting for the rest.[11] Approximately two-thirds of the cases are familial, and the remainder represent new mutations. In the affected families, females are carriers; they are clinically asymptomatic but often have elevated serum creatine kinase and show minimal histologic abnormalities on muscle biopsy. Female carriers are at risk for developing dilated cardiomyopathy later in life.

Dystrophin is a cytoplasmic protein located adjacent to the sarcolemmal membrane in myocytes (Fig. 27–10). The dystrophin molecule concentrates at the plasma membrane over Z-bands, where it forms a strong mechanical link to cytoplasmic actin. Thus, *dystrophin and the dystrophin-associated protein complex form an interface between the intracellular contractile apparatus and the extracellular connective tissue matrix.* The role of this complex of proteins in transferring the force of contraction to connective tissue has been proposed to be the basis for the myocyte degeneration that occurs in the absence of dystrophin[50] or various other proteins that interact with dystrophin (see later). Muscle biopsy specimens from patients with DMD show minimal evidence of dystrophin by both staining and Western blot analysis.[50] BMD patients, who also have mutations in the dystrophin gene, have diminished amounts of dystrophin, usually of an abnormal molecular weight, reflecting mutations that allow synthesis of the protein (Fig. 27–11*B*).

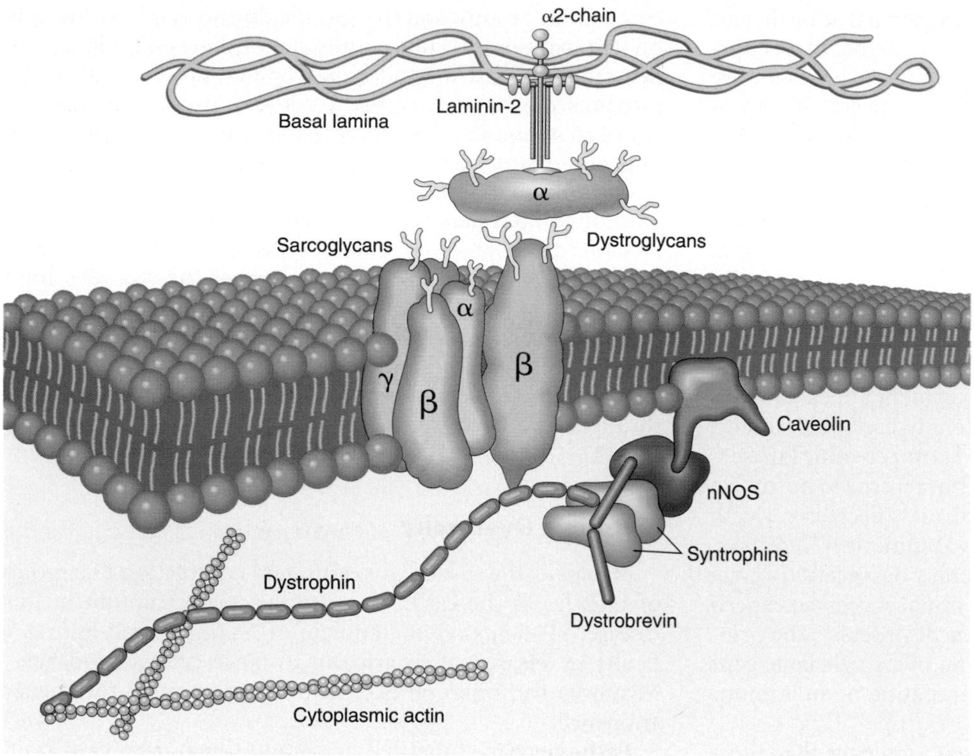

FIGURE 27–10 Diagram showing the relationship between the cell membrane (sarcolemma) and the sarcolemmal associated proteins. Dystrophin, an intracellular protein, forms an interface between the cytoskeletal proteins and a group of transmembrane proteins, the dystroglycans and the sarcoglycans. These transmembrane proteins have interactions with the extracellular matrix, including the laminin proteins. Dystrophin also interacts with dystrobrevin and the syntrophins, which form a link with neuronal-type nitric oxide synthetase (nNOS) and caveolin. Mutations in dystrophin are associated with the X-linked muscular dystrophies, mutations in caveolin and the sarcoglycan proteins with the autosomal limb girdle muscular dystrophies, and mutations in the α2-laminin (merosin) with a form of congenital muscular dystrophy.

Morphology. Histopathologic abnormalities common to DMD and BMD include (1) **variation in fiber size** (diameter) due to the presence of both small and enlarged fibers, sometimes with fiber splitting; (2) **increased numbers of internalized nuclei** (beyond the normal range of 3% to 5%); (3) **degeneration, necrosis, and phagocytosis of muscle fibers;** (4) **regeneration of muscle fibers;** and (5) **proliferation of endomysial connective tissue** (Fig. 27–11*A*). DMD cases also often show enlarged, rounded, hyaline fibers that have lost their normal cross-striations, believed to be hypercontracted fibers; this finding is rare in BMD. Both type 1 and type 2 fibers are involved, and no alterations in the proportion or distribution of fiber types are evident. Histochemical reactions sometimes fail to identify distinct fiber types in DMD. In later stages, **the muscles eventually become almost totally replaced by fat and connective tissue**. Cardiac involvement, when present, consists of interstitial fibrosis, more prominent in the subendocardial layers. Despite the clinical evidence of CNS dysfunction in DMD, no consistent neuropathologic abnormalities have been described.

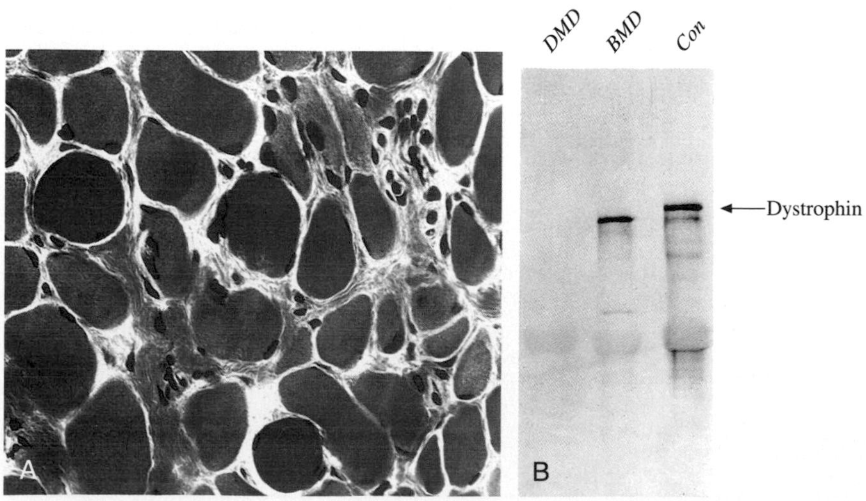

FIGURE 27–11 *A,* Duchenne muscular dystrophy (DMD) showing variation in muscle fiber size, increased endomysial connective tissue, and regenerating fibers *(blue hue)*. *B,* Western blot showing absence of dystrophin in DMD and altered dystrophin size in Becker muscular dystrophy (BMD) compared with control (Con). (Courtesy of Dr. L. Kunkel, Children's Hospital, Boston, MA.)

Clinical Course. Boys with DMD are normal at birth, and early motor milestones are met on time. Walking, however, is often delayed, and the first indications of muscle weakness are clumsiness and inability to keep up with peers. Weakness begins in the pelvic girdle muscles and then extends to the shoulder girdle. Enlargement of the calf muscles associated with weakness, a phenomenon termed *pseudohypertrophy*, is an important clinical finding. The increased muscle bulk is caused initially by an increase in the size of the muscle fibers and then, as the muscle atrophies, by an increase in fat and connective tissue. Pathologic changes are also found in the heart, and patients may develop heart failure or arrhythmias. Although there are no well-established structural abnormalities of the central nervous system, cognitive impairment appears to be a component of the disease and is severe enough in some patients to be considered mental retardation.[51] Serum creatine kinase is elevated during the first decade of life but returns to normal in the later stages of the disease, as muscle mass decreases. Death results from respiratory insufficiency, pulmonary infection, and cardiac decompensation. Gene therapy has received a great deal of attention in DMD, with some initial success in experimental animals with genetically similar disorders.[50] The principal obstacle has been the introduction of a single large gene targeted into all muscle cells without initiation of an immune response to the new gene product.

Boys with BMD develop symptoms at a later age than those with DMD. The onset occurs in later childhood or in adolescence, and it is accompanied by a slower and more variable rate of progression, although there is considerable variation between pedigrees. Many patients have a nearly normal life span. Cardiac disease is frequently seen in these patients.

Autosomal Muscular Dystrophies

Other forms of muscular dystrophy share many features of DMD and BMD but have distinct clinical and pathologic characteristics. Some of these muscular dystrophics affect specific muscle groups, and the specific diagnosis is based largely on the pattern of clinical muscle weakness (Table 27–4). Several autosomal muscular dystrophies, however, affect the proximal musculature of the trunk and limbs, similar to the X-linked muscular dystrophies, and are termed *limb girdle muscular dystrophies.*

Limb girdle muscular dystrophies are inherited in either an autosomal-dominant (type 1) or an autosomal-recessive (type 2) pattern (Table 27–5). Six subtypes of the dominant dystrophies (1A to 1F) and ten subtypes of the recessive limb girdle dystrophies (2A to 2J) have been identified. Mutations of the *sarcoglycan complex of proteins* have been identified in four of the limb girdle muscular dystrophies[52] (2C, 2D, 2E, and 2F). These membrane proteins interact with dystrophin through another transmembrane protein, β-dystroglycan (Fig. 27–10).

Myotonic Dystrophy

Myotonia, the sustained involuntary contraction of a group of muscles, is the cardinal neuromuscular symptom in this disease.[53] Patients often complain of "stiffness" and have difficulty in releasing their grip, for instance, after a handshake. Myotonia can often be elicited by percussion of the thenar eminence.

Pathogenesis. Inherited as an autosomal-dominant trait, the disease tends to increase in severity and appear at a younger age in succeeding generations, a phenomenon termed *anticipation*. Myotonic dystrophy is associated with a trinucleotide CTG repeat expansion on chromosome 19q13.2–13.3. This expansion affects the mRNA for the dystrophila myotonia-protein kinase (DMPK).[54] In normal subjects, fewer than 30 repeats are present; disease develops with expansion of this repeat, and in severely affected individuals, several thousand repeats may be present.[54] The mutation is not stable within a pedigree; with each generation, more repeats accumulate, and this appears to correspond to the clin-

TABLE 27–4 Other Muscular Dystrophies

Disease and Inheritance	Gene and Locus	Clinical Findings	Pathologic Findings
Facioscapulohumeral muscular dystrophy; autosomal-dominant	Type 1A—deletion of variable number of 3.3-kB subunits of a tandemly arranged repeat (D4Z4) on 4q35 Type 1B (FSHMD1B)—locus unknown	Variable age at onset (most commonly 10–30 years); Weakness of muscles of face, neck, and shoulder girdle	Dystrophic myopathy, but also often including inflammatory infiltrates of muscle.
Oculopharyngeal muscular dystrophy; autosomal-dominant	Poly(A)-binding protein-2 (PABP2) gene; 14q11.2–q13	Onset in midadult life; ptosis and weakness of extraocular muscles; difficulty in swallowing	Dystrophic myopathy, but often including rimmed vacuoles in type 1 fibers
Emery-Dreifuss muscular dystrophy; X-linked (mostly)	Emerin (EMD1) gene; Xq28	Variable onset (most commonly 10–20 years); prominent contractures, especially of elbows and ankles	Mild myopathic changes; absent emerin by immunohistochemistry
Congenital muscular dystrophies; autosomal-recessive (Also called muscular dystrophy, congenital, subtypes MDC1A, MDC1B, MDC1C)	Type 1A (merosin-deficient type)—laminin α2 (merosin) gene; 6q22-q23 Type 1B—locus at 1q42; gene unknown Type 1C; fukutin-related protein gene; 19q13.3	Neonatal hypotonia, respiratory insufficiency, delayed motor milestones	Variable fiber size and extensive endomysial fibrosis

TABLE 27–5 Limb Girdle Muscular Dystrophies

Type	Inheritance	Locus	Gene	Clinicopathologic Features
1A	Autosomal-dominant	5q31	Myotilin	Onset in adult life with slow progression of limb weakness, but sparing of facial muscles; dysarthric speech
1B	Autosomal-dominant	1q21	Lamin A/C	Onset before the age of 20 years in lower limbs, progression during many years with cardiac involvement
1C	Autosomal-dominant	3p25	Caveolin-3 (M-caveolin)	Onset before the age of 20, clinically similar to type 1B
1D	Autosomal-dominant	7p	Unknown	Limb girdle muscle weakness, adult onset
2A	Autosomal-recessive	15q15.1–21.1	Calpain 3	Onset in late childhood to middle age; slow progression during 20–30 years
2B	Autosomal-recessive	2p13.3–q13.1	Dysferlin	Mild clinical course with onset in early adulthood
2C	Autosomal-recessive	13q12	γ-Sarcoglycan	Severe weakness during childhood, rapid progression; dystrophic myopathy on muscle biopsy
2D	Autosomal-recessive	17q21	α-Sarcoglycan (adhalin)	Severe weakness during childhood, rapid progression; dystrophic myopathy on muscle biopsy
2E	Autosomal-recessive	4q12	β-Sarcoglycan	Onset in early childhood, with Duchenne-like clinical course
2F	Autosomal-recessive	5q33	δ-Sarcoglycan	Early onset and severe myopathy; dystrophic myopathy on muscle biopsy
2G	Autosomal-recessive	17q11–q12	Telethonin	Distal weakness with limb-girdle weakness in late childhood to adulthood; rimmed vacuoles in muscle cells
2H	Autosomal-recessive	9q31–q34.1	Tripartite motif-containing protein 32 (TRIM32)	Limb-girdle and facial weakness with onset in childhood, mild, slowly progressive course

ical feature of anticipation. Expansion of the trinucleotide repeat influences the eventual level of protein product.

The pathologic features of the disease relate only in part to altered DMPK function. RNA that contains trinucleotide repeat expansions can directly affect splicing of other RNAs, including those for the ClC-1 chloride channel.[55] A second form of myotonic dystrophy is associated with untranslated CCTG expansion in a gene called *ZNF9* on chromosome 3.[56]

Morphology. Skeletal muscle may show variation in fiber size. In addition, there is a striking increase in the number of internal nuclei, which on longitudinal section may form conspicuous chains. Another well-recognized abnormality is the **ring fiber**, with a subsarcolemmal band of cytoplasm that appears distinct from the center of the fiber. The rim contains myofibrils that are oriented circumferentially around the longitudinally oriented fibrils in the rest of the fiber. The ring fiber may be associated with an irregular mass of sarcoplasm **(sarcoplasmic mass)** extending outward from the ring. These sarcoplasmic masses stain blue with hematoxylin and eosin, red with Gomori trichrome, and intensely blue with the nicotinamide adenine dinucleotide-tetrazolium reductase (NADH-TR) histochemical reaction. Histochemical techniques have demonstrated a relative atrophy of type 1 fibers early in the course of the disease in some cases. Of all the dystrophies, only myotonic dystrophy shows pathologic changes in the intrafusal fibers of muscle spindles, with fiber splitting, necrosis, and regeneration.

Clinical Course. The disease often presents in late childhood with abnormalities in gait secondary to weakness of foot dorsiflexors and subsequently progresses to weakness of the hand intrinsic muscles and wrist extensors. Atrophy of muscles of the face and ptosis ensue, leading to the typical facial appearance. Cataracts, which are present in virtually every patient, may be detected early in the course of the disease with slit-lamp examination. Other associated abnormalities include frontal balding, gonadal atrophy, cardiomyopathy, smooth muscle involvement, decreased plasma immunoglobulin G, and an abnormal glucose tolerance test response. Dementia has been reported in some cases.

ION CHANNEL MYOPATHIES (CHANNELOPATHIES)

The *ion channel myopathies*, or channelopathies, are a group of familial diseases characterized clinically by myotonia, relapsing episodes of hypotonic paralysis (induced by vigorous exercise, cold, or a high-carbohydrate meal), or both. Hypotonia variants associated with elevated, depressed, or normal serum potassium levels at the time of the attack are called *hyperkalemic, hypokalemic, and normokalemic periodic paralysis*, respectively.

Pathogenesis. As their name indicates, at the molecular level these diseases are caused by mutations in genes that encode ion channels.[57,58] Hyperkalemic periodic paralysis results from mutations in the gene that encodes a skeletal muscle sodium channel protein (SCN4A), which regulates the entry of sodium into muscle during contraction. The gene for hypokalemic periodic paralysis encodes a voltage-gated calcium channel.

TABLE 27–6 Congenital Myopathies

Disease and Inheritance	Gene and Locus	Clinical Findings	Pathologic Findings
Central core disease; autosomal-dominant	Ryanodine receptor-1 (RYR1) gene; 19q13.1	Early-onset hypotonia and nonprogressive weakness; associated skeletal deformities; may develop malignant hyperthermia	Cytoplasmic cores are lightly eosinophilic and distinct from surrounding sarcoplasm; Found only in type 1 fibers, which usually predominate, best seen on NADH stain
Nemaline myopathy; autosomal-dominant or autosomal-recessive	Autosomal-dominant (NEM1)—Tropomyosin 3 (TPM3) gene; Autosomal-recessive (NEM2)—nebulin (NEB) gene; 2q22 Autosomal-dominant or recessive—skeletal muscle actin, α chain (ACTA1) gene; 1q42.1	Weakness, hypotonia, and delayed motor development in childhood; may also be seen in adults; usually nonprogressive; involves proximal limb muscles most severely; skeletal abnormalities may be present	Aggregates of subsarcolemmal spindle-shaped particles *(nemaline rods)*; occur predominantly in type 1 fibers; derived from Z-band material (α-actinin) and best seen on modified Gomori stain
Myotubular (centronuclear) myopathy; X-linked (MTM1), autosomal-recessive, or autosomal-dominant	X-linked—myotubularin (MTM1) gene; Xq28 Autosomal-dominant—myogenic factor 6 (MYF6) gene; 12q21 Autosomal-recessive—locus and gene unknown	X-linked form presents in infancy with prominent hypotonia and poor prognosis; autosomal forms have limb weakness and are slowly progressive; autosomal-recessive form is intermediate in severity and prognosis	Abundance of centrally located nuclei involving the majority of muscle fibers; central nuclei are usually confined to type 1 fibers, which are small in diameter, but can occur in both fiber types

Malignant hyperpyrexia (malignant hyperthermia) is a rare clinical syndrome characterized by a dramatic hypermetabolic state (tachycardia, tachypnea, muscle spasms, and later hyperpyrexia) triggered by the induction of anesthesia, usually with halogenated inhalational agents and succinylcholine. The clinical syndrome may also occur in predisposed individuals with hereditary muscle diseases, including congenital myopathies, dystrophinopathies, and metabolic myopathies. The only reliable method of diagnosis is contraction of biopsied muscle on exposure to anesthetic. Mutations in different genes have been identified in families with susceptibility to malignant hyperthermia, including genes encoding a voltage-gated calcium channel (lq32), an L-type voltage-dependent calcium channel (7q21–q22), and a ryanodine receptor (19q13.1).[59]

CONGENITAL MYOPATHIES

The congenital myopathies are a group of disorders defined largely on the basis of the pathologic findings within muscle.[60] Most of these conditions share common clinical features, including onset in early life, nonprogressive or slowly progressive course, proximal or generalized muscle weakness, and hypotonia. Those affected at birth or in early infancy may present as "floppy babies" because of hypotonia or may have severe joint contractures (*arthrogryposis*); however, both hypotonia and arthrogryposis may also be caused by other neuromuscular dysfunction.

The best-characterized congenital myopathies are listed in Table 27–6. Figure 27–12 shows the structural characteristics

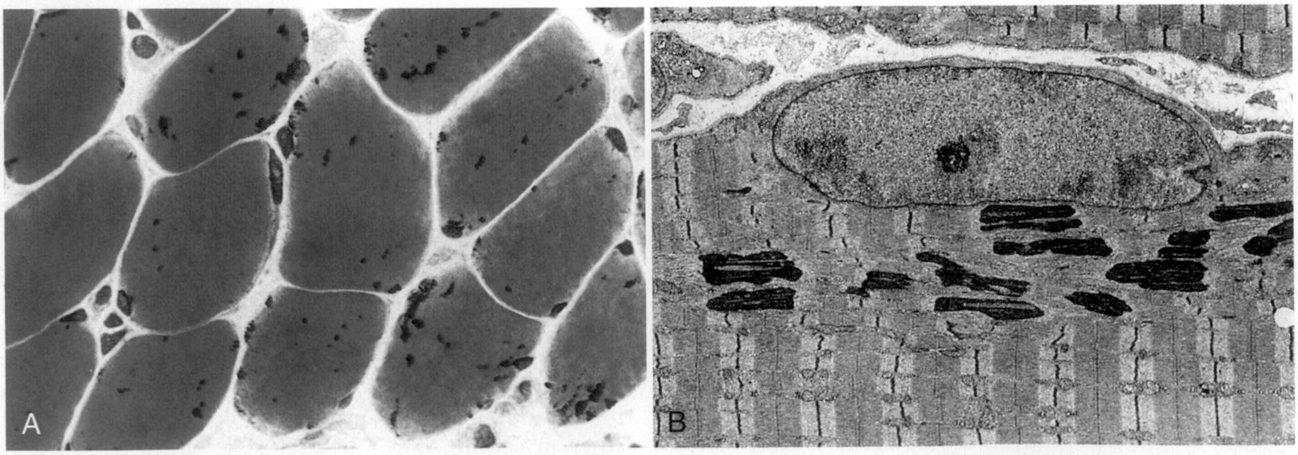

FIGURE 27–12 *A*, Nemaline myopathy with numerous rod-shaped, intracytoplasmic inclusions *(dark purple structures)*. *B*, Electron micrograph of subsarcolemmal nemaline bodies, showing material of Z-band density.

of nemaline ("rod body") myopathy, one of the most distinctive types.

MYOPATHIES ASSOCIATED WITH INBORN ERRORS OF METABOLISM

Many of the myopathies associated with metabolic disease are found in the setting of disorders of glycogen synthesis and degradation (Chapter 5). Combinations of clinical, pathologic, and molecular information are used to arrive at a specific diagnosis.[61] Myopathies can also result from disorders of mitochondrial function.

Lipid Myopathies

Abnormalities of the carnitine transport system or deficiencies of the mitochondrial dehydrogenase enzyme systems can lead to the accumulation of lipid droplets within muscle (lipid myopathies).[62] To undergo β-oxidation, cytoplasmic fatty acyl coenzyme A (acyl-CoA) esters are (1) transesterified with carnitine through the action of an outer membrane carnitine palmitoyltransferase (CPT I), (2) transported across the inner mitochondrial membrane, (3) re-esterified to acyl-CoA esters by an inner membrane mitochondrial CPT (CPT II), and (4) catabolized to acetyl-CoA units by the acyl-CoA dehydrogenases. In different patients with lipid myopathy, the defect may involve carnitine, acyl-CoA dehydrogenase, or CPT enzymes.[63,64]

Morphology. In all of these lipid myopathies, the principal morphologic characteristic is accumulation of lipid within myocytes.[62] The myofibrils are separated by vacuoles that stain with oil red O or Sudan black and have the typical appearance of lipid by electron microscopy. The vacuoles occur predominantly in type 1 fibers, and they are dispersed diffusely throughout the fiber.

Mitochondrial Myopathies (Oxidative Phosphorylation Diseases)

Approximately one-fifth of the proteins involved in mitochondrial oxidative phosphorylation are encoded by the mitochondrial genome (mtDNA); additionally, this circular genome encodes 22 mitochondrial-specific tRNAs and 2 rRNA species.[66,67] The remainder of the mitochondrial enzyme complexes are encoded in the nuclear genome. Mutations in both nuclear and mitochondrial genes cause the so-called *mitochondrial myopathies.* Diseases that involve the mtDNA show maternal inheritance, since only the oocyte contributes mitochondria to the embryo. There is a high mutation rate for mtDNA compared with nuclear DNA.[68] The mitochondrial diseases may present in young adulthood and manifest with proximal muscle weakness, sometimes with severe involvement of the muscles that move the eyes (external ophthalmoplegia). The weakness may be accompanied by other neurologic symptoms, lactic acidosis, and cardiomyopathy, so this group of disorders is sometimes classified as mitochondrial encephalomyopathies (Chapter 28).

Morphology. The most consistent pathologic finding in skeletal muscle is aggregates of abnormal mitochondria that are demonstrable only by special techniques.[67,69,70] These occur under the subsarcolemma in early stages; but with severe involvement, they may extend throughout the fiber. The abnormal mitochondria impart a blotchy red appearance to the muscle fiber on the modified Gomori trichrome stain. Since they are also associated with distortion of the myofibrils, the muscle fiber contour becomes irregular on cross-section, and the descriptive term **ragged red fibers** has been applied to them (Fig. 27–13*A*).[67] The electron microscopic appearance is often distinctive: There are increased numbers of, and abnormalities in, the shape and size of mitochondria, some of which contain paracrystalline **parking lot inclusions** or alterations in the structure of cristae[67,69] (Fig. 27–13*B*). Cytochrome oxidase activity can be determined in muscle biopsy specimens using histochemistry, and cytochrome oxidase negative fibers may be present in a number of mitochondrial myopathies.

Clinical Course and Genetics. The relationship between clinical course in the mitochondrial disorders and the genetic alterations is not entirely clear; however, three general categories have been defined.[69] One set of mutations consists of

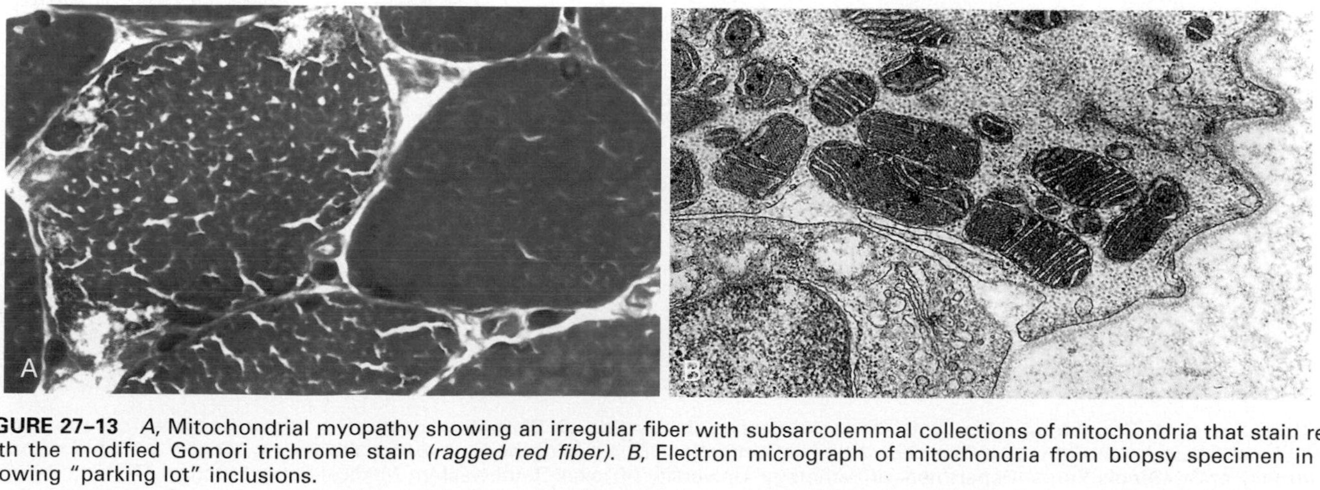

FIGURE 27–13 *A,* Mitochondrial myopathy showing an irregular fiber with subsarcolemmal collections of mitochondria that stain red with the modified Gomori trichrome stain *(ragged red fiber). B,* Electron micrograph of mitochondria from biopsy specimen in *A* showing "parking lot" inclusions.

point mutations in mtDNA. These disorders tend to show a maternal pattern of inheritance, and some examples include myoclonic epilepsy with ragged red fibers (MERRF), Leber hereditary optic neuropathy (LHON), and mitochondrial encephalomyopathy with lactic acidosis and strokelike episodes (MELAS). A second set of mutations involves *genes encoded by nuclear DNA* and shows autosomal-dominant or autosomal-recessive inheritance. Some cases of subacute necrotizing encephalopathy (Leigh syndrome), exertional myoglobinuria, and infantile X-linked cardioskeletal myopathy (Barth syndrome) are due to mutations in nuclear DNA. The final subset of mitochondrial myopathies is caused by *deletions or duplications of mtDNA*. Examples include chronic progressive external ophthalmoplegia, characterized by a myopathy with prominent weakness of external ocular movements. Kearns-Sayre syndrome, another myopathy in this group, is also characterized by ophthalmoplegia but, in addition, includes pigmentary degeneration of the retina and complete heart block.[67]

INFLAMMATORY MYOPATHIES

There are three subgroups of inflammatory muscle diseases: infectious, noninfectious inflammatory, and systemic inflammatory diseases that involve muscle along with other organs. Infectious myositis (Chapter 8) and systemic inflammatory diseases (Chapter 6) are discussed elsewhere.

Noninfectious Inflammatory Myopathies

Noninfectious inflammatory myopathies are a heterogeneous group of disorders that are probably immunologically mediated and are characterized by injury and inflammation of skeletal muscle. Three relatively distinct disorders, *dermatomyositis, polymyositis*, and *inclusion body myositis*, are included in this category.[62,71] These may occur as an isolated myopathy or as one component of an immune-mediated systemic disease, particularly systemic sclerosis (Chapter 6). The clinical features of each disorder are presented first to facilitate discussion of pathogenesis and morphologic changes.

Dermatomyositis. As the name implies, patients with dermatomyositis have an inflammatory disorder of the skin as well as skeletal muscle. It is characterized by a distinctive skin rash that may accompany or precede the onset of muscle disease. The *classic rash takes the form of a lilac or heliotrope discoloration of the upper eyelids with periorbital edema* (Fig. 27–14*A*). It is often accompanied by a scaling erythematous eruption or dusky red patches over the knuckles, elbows, and knees (Grotton lesions). *Muscle weakness* is slow in onset, is bilaterally symmetric, is often accompanied by myalgias, and *typically affects the proximal muscles first*. As a result, tasks such as getting up from a chair and climbing steps become increasingly difficult. Fine movements controlled by distal muscles are affected only late in the disease. Dysphagia resulting from involvement of oropharyngeal and esophageal muscles occurs in one-third of the patients. Extramuscular manifestations, including interstitial lung disease, vasculitis, and myocarditis, may be present in some cases. Compared to the normal population, patients with dermatomyositis have a higher risk of developing visceral cancers. According to several studies, nearly 40% of adult patients with dermatomyositis have cancer.[72]

Juvenile dermatomyositis has a similar onset of rash and muscle weakness but more often is accompanied by abdominal pain and involvement of the gastrointestinal tract. Mucosal ulceration, hemorrhage, and perforation may occur as the

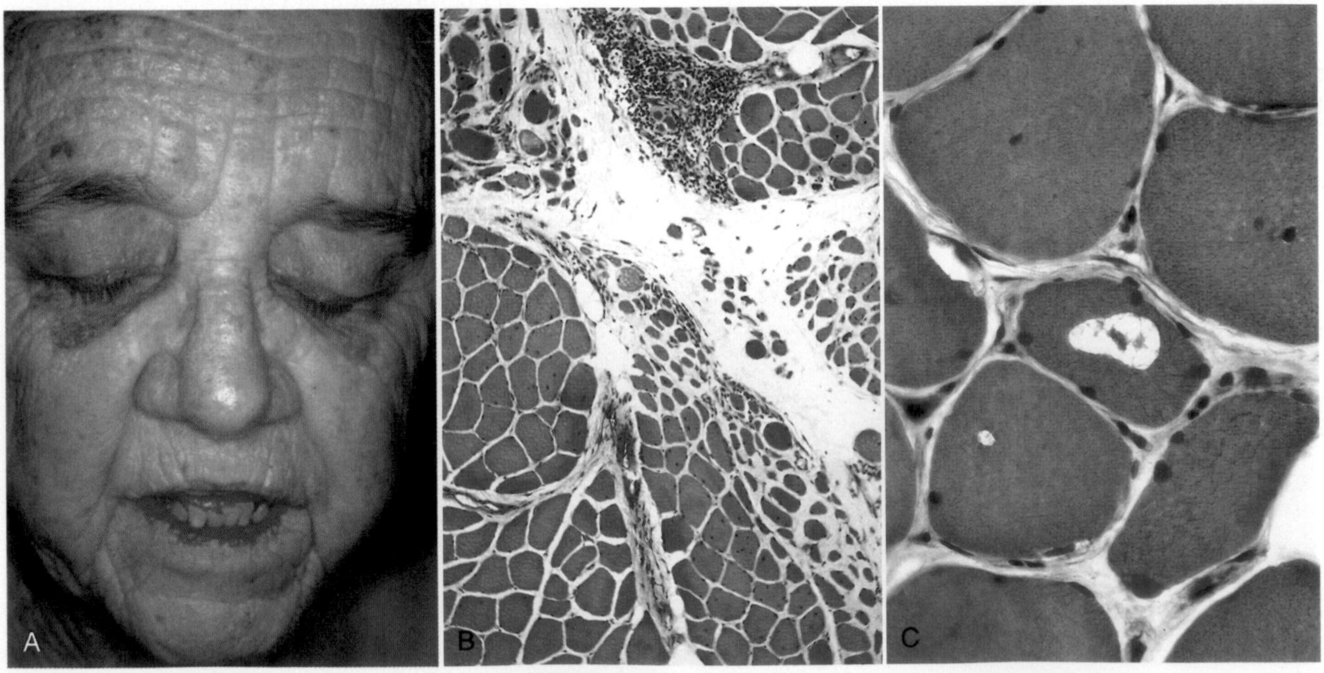

FIGURE 27–14 *A*, Dermatomyositis. Note the rash affecting the eyelids. *B*, Dermatomyositis. The histologic appearance of muscle shows perifascicular atrophy of muscle fibers and inflammation. *C*, Inclusion body myositis showing a vacuole within a myocyte. (Courtesy of Dr. Dennis Burns, Department of Pathology, University of Texas Southwestern Medical School, Dallas, TX.)

result of the dermatomyositis-associated vasculopathy. Calcinosis, which is uncommon in adult dermatomyositis, occurs in one third of patients with juvenile dermatomyositis.[71,73]

Polymyositis. In this inflammatory myopathy, the pattern of symmetric proximal muscle involvement is similar to that seen in dermatomyositis. *It differs from dermatomyositis by the lack of cutaneous involvement and its occurrence mainly in adults.* Similar to dermatomyositis, there may be inflammatory involvement of heart, lungs, and blood vessels.

Inclusion Body Myositis. In contrast with the other two entities, inclusion body myositis begins with the *involvement of distal muscles*, especially extensors of the knee (quadriceps) and flexors of the wrists and fingers. Furthermore, the weakness may be *asymmetric.* It is an insidiously developing disorder that typically affects individuals over the age of 50 years. Most cases are sporadic, but familial cases have been recognized as "inclusion body myopathy."[74]

Etiology and Pathogenesis. The cause of inflammatory myopathies is unknown, but the tissue injury seems to be mediated by immunologic mechanisms.[62,71] In dermatomyositis, capillaries seem to be the principal targets. The microvasculature is attacked by antibodies and complement, resulting in foci of ischemic myocyte necrosis. The deposition of antibodies and complement in capillaries precedes inflammation and destruction of muscle fibers. B cells and CD4+ T cells are present within the muscle, but there is a paucity of lymphocytes within the areas of myofiber injury. The perifascicular distribution of myocyte injury also suggests a vascular pathogenesis.

In contrast, polymyositis appears to be caused by cell-mediated injury of myocytes. CD8+ cytotoxic T cells and macrophages are seen near damaged muscle fibers, and the expression of HLA class I and class II molecules is increased on the sarcolemma of normal fibers. Similar to other immune-mediated diseases, ANAs are present in a variable number of cases, regardless of the clinical category (Chapter 6). The specificities of autoantibodies are quite varied, but those directed against tRNA synthetases seem to be more or less specific for inflammatory myopathies.

The pathogenesis of inclusion body myositis is less clear. As in polymyositis, CD8+ cytotoxic T cells are found in the muscle, but in contrast to the other two forms of myositis, immunosuppressive therapy is not beneficial. Intracellular deposits of β-amyloid protein, amyloid β-pleated sheet fibrils, and hyperphosphorylated Tau protein are features in common with Alzheimer disease that have drawn attention to a possible relationship to aging. Abnormalities of protein folding have received some attention in inclusion body myopathy,[74] as have similar deposits of amyloid fibrils in Alzheimer disease.[75] The hereditary forms of inclusion body myopathy have a similar morphology but result from genetic mutations. The autosomal-recessive form is caused by mutations in the GNE gene (encoding UDP-*N*-acetylglucosamine-2 epimerase/*N*-acetylmannosamine kinase), and the autosomal-dominant form is caused by mutations in the gene encoding myosin heavy chain IIa.[74] The role of these mutations in the pathogenesis of inclusion body myopathy is unclear.

Morphology. The histologic features of the individual forms of myositis are quite distinctive and are described separately.

Dermatomyositis. The inflammatory infiltrates in dermatomyositis are located predominantly around small blood vessels and in the perimysial connective tissue. Typically, groups of atrophic fibers are particularly prominent at the periphery of fascicles. This "perifascicular atrophy" is sufficient for diagnosis, even if the inflammation is mild or absent (Fig. 27–14*B*). The perifascicular atrophy is most likely related to a relative state of hypoperfusion of the periphery of muscle fascicles. Quantitative analyses reveal a dramatic reduction in the intramuscular capillaries, believed to result from vascular endothelial injury and fibrosis. Necrotic muscle fibers and regeneration may also be seen throughout the fascicle, as in polymyositis.

Polymyositis. In this condition, the inflammatory cells are found in the endomysium. CD8+ lymphocytes and other lymphoid cells surround and invade healthy muscle fibers. Both necrotic and regenerating muscle fibers are scattered throughout the fascicle, without the perifascicular atrophy seen in dermatomyositis. There is no evidence of vascular injury in polymyositis.

Inclusion Body Myositis. The diagnostic finding in inclusion body myositis is the presence of rimmed vacuoles (Fig. 27–14*C*). The vacuoles are present within myocytes, and they are highlighted by basophilic granules at their periphery. In addition, the vacuolated fibers may also contain amyloid deposits that reveal typical staining with Congo Red. Under the electron microscope, tubular and filamentous inclusions are seen in the cytoplasm and the nucleus, and they are composed of β-amyloid or hyperphosphorylated tau.[76] The pattern of the inflammatory cell infiltrate is similar to that seen in polymyositis.

The diagnosis of myositis is based on clinical symptoms, electromyography (EMG), elevated creatinine kinase in serum, and biopsy. EMG is particularly informative in inflammatory myopathies, with mixed neurogenic and myopathic findings suggestive of inflammatory myopathy. As might be expected, muscle injury is associated with elevated serum levels of creatine kinase. Biopsy is required for definitive diagnosis. Immunosuppressive therapy is beneficial in adult and juvenile dermatomyositis and in polymyositis.

TOXIC MYOPATHIES

Thyrotoxic Myopathy

Thyrotoxic myopathy presents most commonly as an acute or chronic proximal muscle weakness that may precede the onset of other signs of thyroid dysfunction. *Exophthalmic ophthalmoplegia* is characterized by swelling of the eyelids, edema of the conjunctiva, and diplopia. In *hypothyroidism*, there may be cramping or aching of muscles, and movements and reflexes are slowed. Findings include fiber atrophy, an increased number of internal nuclei, glycogen aggregates, and, occasionally, deposition of mucopolysaccharides in the connective tissue.

In thyrotoxic myopathy, there is myofiber necrosis, regeneration, and interstitial lymphocytosis. In chronic thyrotoxic myopathy, there may be only slight variability of muscle fiber size, mitochondrial hypertrophy, and focal myofibril degeneration; fatty infiltration of muscle is seen in severe cases. Exophthalmic ophthalmoplegia is limited to the extraocular muscles, which may be edematous and enlarged. Another muscle disease associated with thyroid dysfunction is *thyrotoxic periodic paralysis*, which is characterized by episodic weakness that is often accompanied by hypokalemia. Males are affected four times more often than are females, with a high incidence in individuals of Japanese descent.

Ethanol Myopathy

Binge drinking of alcohol is known to produce an acute toxic syndrome of rhabdomyolysis with accompanying myoglobinuria, which may lead to renal failure. Clinically, the patient may acutely develop pain that is either generalized or confined to a single muscle group. Some patients have a complicated clinicopathologic syndrome consisting of proximal muscle weakness with electrophysiologic evidence of myopathy superimposed on alcoholic neuropathy. On histologic examination, there is swelling of myocytes, with fiber necrosis, myophagocytosis, and regeneration. There may also be evidence of denervation.

Drug-Induced Myopathies

Proximal muscle weakness and atrophy can occur as a result of the deleterious effects of steroids on muscle, whether in Cushing syndrome or during therapeutic administration of steroids, a condition known as *steroid myopathy*. The severity of clinical disability is variable and not directly related to the steroid level or the therapeutic regimen. It is characterized by muscle fiber atrophy, predominantly affecting type 2 fibers.[76] When the myopathy is severe, there may be a bimodal distribution of fiber sizes, with type 1 fibers of nearly normal caliber and markedly atrophic type 2 fibers. Electron microscopy has shown dilation of the sarcoplasmic reticulum and thickening of the basal laminae.

Chloroquine, originally used in the treatment of malaria but subsequently used in other clinical settings, can produce a proximal myopathy in humans. The most prominent finding in chloroquine myopathy is the presence of vacuoles within myocytes. Two types of vacuoles have been described: autophagic membrane-bound vacuoles containing membranous debris and curvilinear bodies with short curved membranous structures with alternating light and dark zones. Vacuoles can be seen in as many as 50% of the myocytes, most commonly type 1 fibers, and with progression, myocyte necrosis may develop. A similar vacuolar myopathy occurs in some patients treated with hydrochloroquine.[77]

DISEASES OF THE NEUROMUSCULAR JUNCTION

Myasthenia Gravis

Now recognized as one of the best-defined forms of autoimmune disease, myasthenia gravis is a muscle disease caused by immune-mediated loss of acetylcholine receptors and having characteristic temporal and anatomic patterns as well as drug responses. The disease has a prevalence of about 3 in 100,000 persons.[78] When arising before age 40 years, it is most commonly seen in women, but there is equal occurrence between the sexes in older patients. Thymic hyperplasia is found in 65% and thymoma in 15% of patients. Analysis of neuromuscular transmission in myasthenia gravis shows a decrease in the number of muscle acetylcholine receptors (AChRs), and circulating antibodies to the AChR are present in nearly all patients with myasthenia gravis.[79,80] The disease can be passively transferred to animals with serum from affected patients.

Morphology. By light microscopic examination, muscle biopsy specimens from patients with myasthenia are usually unrevealing. In severe cases, disuse changes with type 2 fiber atrophy may be found. The postsynaptic membrane is simplified, with loss of AChRs from the region of the synapse. Immune complexes as well as the membrane attack complex of the complement cascade (C5–Cq) can be found along the postsynaptic membrane as well.

Pathogenesis. In most cases, the autoantibodies against the AChR lead to loss of functional AChRs at the neuromuscular junction by: (1) fixing complement and causing direct injury to the post-synaptic membrane, (2) increasing the internalization and degradation of the receptors, and (3) inhibiting binding and function of ACh. Electrophysiologic studies are notable for decrement in motor responses with repeated stimulation; nerve conduction study findings are normal. Sensory as well as autonomic functions are not affected. Despite the evidence that anti-AChR antibodies play a critical pathogenic role in the disease, there is not always a correlation between antibody levels and neurologic deficit. Interestingly, in light of the immune-mediated etiology of the disease, thymic abnormalities are common in these patients, but the precise link with autoimmunity to AChRs is uncertain. Regardless of the pattern of thymic pathology, most patients show improvement after thymectomy.

Clinical Course. Typically, weakness begins with extraocular muscles; drooping eyelids (ptosis) and double vision (diplopia) cause the patient to seek medical attention. However, the initial symptoms may include generalized weakness. The weakness fluctuates, with alterations occurring during days, hours, or even minutes, and intercurrent medical conditions can lead to exacerbations of the weakness. Patients show improvement in strength in response to administration of anticholinesterase agents. This remains a most useful test on clinical examination.[84] Respiratory compromise was a major cause of mortality in the past; 95% of patients now survive more than 5 years after diagnosis because of improved methods of treatment and better ventilatory support. Effective forms of treatment include anticholinesterase drugs, prednisone, plasmapheresis, and resection of thymoma if it is present.[81]

Lambert-Eaton Myasthenic Syndrome

Lambert-Eaton myasthenic syndrome is a disease of the neuromuscular junction that is distinct from myasthenia gravis. It usually develops as a paraneoplastic process, most commonly with small cell carcinoma of the lung (60% of cases), although it can occur in the absence of underlying malignant disease. Patients develop proximal muscle weakness along with autonomic dysfunction. Unlike in myasthenia gravis, no clinical improvement is found upon administration of acetylcholine agents, and electrophysiologic studies show evidence of enhanced neurotransmission with repetitive stimulation. These clinical features allow this disorder to be distinguished from myasthenia gravis.

The content of acetylcholine is normal in neuromuscular junction synaptic vesicles, and the postsynaptic membrane is normally responsive to acetylcholine, but fewer vesicles are released in response to each presynaptic action potential. Some patients have antibodies that recognize presynaptic PQ-type voltage-gated calcium channels, and a similar disease can be transferred to animals with these antibodies.[82,83] This suggests that autoimmunity to the calcium channel causes the disease.

TUMORS OF SKELETAL MUSCLE

Skeletal muscle tumors are discussed with other soft tissue tumors (Chapter 26).

REFERENCES

1. Victor M, Ropper AH: Adams and Victor's Principles of Neurology, 7th ed. New York, McGraw-Hill, 2001, p 1465.
2. Pamphelt R, Sjarif A: Is quantitation necessary for assessment of sural nerve biopsies? Muscle & Nerve 27:562, 2003.
3. Bosboom WM, et al: Diagnostic value of sural nerve demyelination in chronic inflammatory demyelinating polyneuropathy. Brain 124:2427, 2001.
4. Hof PR, et al: The cellular components of nervous tissue. In Zigmond MJ, et al (eds): Fundamental Neuroscience. San Diego, Academic Press, 1999, p 56.
5. Gillespie CS, et al: Peripheral demyelination and neuropathic pain behavior in periaxin-deficient mice. Neuron 26:523, 2000.
6. Nagarajan R, et al: EGR2 mutations in inherited neuropathies dominant-negatively inhibit myelin gene expression. Neuron 30:35568, 2001.
7. Schnapp BJ: Trafficking of signaling modules by kinesin motors. J Cell Sci 116:2125, 2003.
8. Miller FD, Kaplan DR: On Trk for retrograde signaling. Neuron 32:767, 2001.
9. Smith CE, et al: Development of the blood-nerve barrier in neonatal rats. Microsurgery 21:290, 2001.
10. De Girolami U, Beggs AH: Skeletal muscle. In Silverberg SG, et al (eds): Principles and Practice of Surgical Pathology and Cytopathology. New York, Churchill Livingstone, 1997, p. 943.
11. Dalkilic J, Kunkel LM: Muscular dystrophies: genes to pathogenesis. Curr Opin Genet Dev 13:23, 2003.
12. Carpenter S, Karpati G: Pathology of Skeletal Muscle, 2nd ed. Oxford, England, Oxford University Press, 2001, p 41.
13. DeVries GH: Schwann cell proliferation. In Dyck PJ, et al (eds): Peripheral Neuropathy. Philadelphia, WB Saunders, 1993, p 290.
14. Mueller M, et al: Rapid response of identified resident endoneurial macrophages to nerve injury. Am J Pathol 159:2187, 2001.
15. Gomes MD, et al: Atrogin-1, a muscle-specific F-box protein highly expressed during muscle atrophy. Proc Natl Acad Sci U S A 98:14440, 2001.
16. Shah JV, Cleveland DW: Slow axonal transport: fast motors in the slow lane. Curr Opin Cell Biol 14:58, 2002.
17. Carpenter S, Karpati G: Pathology of Skeletal Muscle, 2nd ed. Oxford, England, Oxford University Press, 2001, p 662.
18. Govoni V, Granieri E: Epidemiology of the Guillain-Barré syndrome. Curr Opin Neurol 14:605, 2001.
19. Winer JB: Guillain Barré syndrome. Mol Pathol 54:381, 2001.
20. Kieseier BC, Hartung HP: Therapeutic strategies in the Guillain-Barré syndrome. Sem Neurol 23:159, 2003.
21. Stienekemeier M: Vaccination, prevention, and treatment of experimental autoimmune neuritis (EAN) by an oligomerized T cell epitope. Proc Nat Acad Sci 98:13872, 2001.
22. Hartung HP, et al: Progress in Guillain-Barré syndrome. Curr Opin Neurol 14:597, 2001.
23. Said G: Chronic inflammatory demyelinative polyneuropathy. J Neurol 249:245, 2002.
24. Piradov MA: Diphtheritic polyneuropathy: clinical analysis of severe forms. Arch Neurol 58:1438, 2001.
25. Kleinschmidt-DeMasters BK, Gilden DH: Varicella-zoster virus infections of the nervous system: clinical and pathologic correlates. Arch Pathol Lab Med 125:770, 2001.
26. Reilly MM: Classification of the hereditary motor and sensory neuropathies. Curr Opin Neurol 13:561, 2000.
27. Vallat JM: Dominantly inherited peripheral neuropathies. J Neuropath Exp Neurol 62:699, 2003.
28. Robaglia-Schlupp A, et al: PMP22 overexpression causes dysmyelination in mice. Brain 125:2213, 2002.
29. Norreel JC, et al: Close relationship between motor impairments and loss of functional motoneurons in a Charcot-Marie-Tooth type 1A model. Neurosci 116:695, 2003.
30. Street VA, et al: Mutation of a putative protein degradation gene LITAF/SIMPLE in Charcot-Marie-Tooth disease. Neurology 60:22, 2003.
31. Abrams CK: Pathogenesis of X-linked Charcot-Marie-Tooth disease: differential effects of two mutations in connexin 32. J Neurosci 23:10548, 2003.
32. Plante-Bordeneuve V, Said G: Dejerine-Sottas disease and hereditary demyelinating polyneuropathy of infancy. Muscle & Nerve 26:608, 2002.
33. Boerkoel CF, et al: EGR2 mutation R359W causes a spectrum of Dejerine-Sottas neuropathy. Neurogenetics 3:153, 2001.
34. Boerkoel CF, et al: Periaxin mutations cause recessive Dejerine-Sottas neuropathy. Am J Hum Genet 68:325, 2001.
35. Bertora P: Prevalence of subclinical neuropathy in diabetic patients: assessment by study of conduction velocity distribution within motor and sensory nerve fibres. J Neurol 245:81, 1998.
36. Thrainsdottir S: Endoneurial capillary abnormalities presage deterioration of glucose tolerance and accompany peripheral neuropathy in man. Diabetes 52:2615, 2003.
37. Dyck PJ, Giannini C: Pathologic alterations in the diabetic neuropathies of humans: a review. J Neuropathol Exp Neurol 55:1181, 1996.
38. Richardson EP, De Girolami U: Pathology of the Peripheral Nerve. Philadelphia, WB Saunders, 1995, p 78.
39. Koike H, et al: Alcoholic neuropathy is clinicopathologically distinct from thiamine-deficiency neuropathy. Ann Neurol 54:19, 2003.
40. Rauer S, et al: Quantification of circulating anti-Hu antibody in serial samples from patients with paraneoplastic neurological syndromes: possible correlation of antibody concentration and course of neurological syndromes. J Neurol 249:285, 2002.
41. Musunuru K, Darnell RB: Paraneoplastic neurologic disease antigens: RNA-binding proteins and signaling proteins in neuronal degeneration. Annu Rev Neurosci 24:239, 2001.
42. Hughes R, et al: Carcinoma and the peripheral nervous system. J Neurol 243:371, 1996.
43. Steck AJ, et al: Paraproteinaemic neuropathies. Brain Pathol 9:361, 1999.
44. Spencer PS, Schaumburg HH: Experimental and Clinical Neurotoxicology, 2nd ed. New York, Oxford University Press, 2000, p 1310
45. Katz JN, Simmons BP: Carpal tunnel syndrome. New Engl J Med 346:1807, 2002.
46. Martin Y, et al: Genetic study of SMA patients without homozygous SMN1 deletions: identification of compound heterozygotes and characterisation of novel intragenic SMN1 mutations. Hum Genet 110:257, 2002.
47. Crawford TO: Spinal muscular atrophies. In Jones HR, DeVivo DC, Darras BT (eds): Neuromuscular Disorders of Infancy, Childhood, and Adolescence. Amsterdam, Butterworth Heinemann. 2003, p 145.
48. Zatkova A, et al: Analysis of the SMN and NAIP genes in Slovak spinal muscular atrophy patients. Hum Hered 50:171, 2000.
49. Darras BT, et al: Dystrophinopathies. In Jones HR, et al (eds): Neuromuscular Disorders of Infancy, Childhood, and Adolescence. A Clinician's Approach. Philadelphia, Elsevier Science, Inc., 2003, p. 649.
50. Burton EA, Davies KE: Muscular dystrophy: reason for optimism. Cell 108:5, 2002.
51. Anderson JL: Brain function in Duchenne muscular dystrophy. Brain 125:4, 2002.

52. Zatz M, et al: The 10 autosomal-recessive limb-girdle muscular dystrophies. Neuromuscular Disorders 13:532, 2003.
53. Mankodi A, Thornton CA: Myotonic syndromes. Curr Opin Neurol. 15:545, 2002.
54. Meola G: Clinical and genetic heterogeneity in myotonic dystrophies. Muscle Nerve 23:1789, 2000.
55. Mankodi A, et al: Expanded CUG repeats trigger aberrant splicing of ClC-1 chloride channel pre-mRNA and hyperexcitability of skeletal muscle in myotonic dystrophy. Mol Cell 10:35, 2002.
56. Liquori CL, et al: Myotonic dystrophy type 2 caused by a CCTG expansion in nitron 1 of ZNF9. Science 293:864, 2001.
57. Tawil R, et al: Channelopathies. In Pulst SM (ed): Neurogenetics. New York, Oxford University Press, 2000, p 45.
58. Davies NP, Hanna MG: The skeletal muscle channelopathies: distinct entities and overlapping syndromes. Curr Opin Neurol 16:559, 2003.
59. McCarthy TV, et al: Ryanodine receptor mutations in malignant hyperthermia and central core disease. Hum Mutat 15:410, 2000.
60. Tubridy N, et al: Congenital myopathies and congenital muscular dystrophies. Curr Opin Neurol 14:575, 2001.
61. Vladutiu GD: Laboratory diagnosis of metabolic myopathies. Muscle Nerve 25:649, 2002.
62. Weller RO, et al: Diseases of muscle. In Graham DI, Lantos PL (eds): Greenfield's Neuropathology, Vol 2, 7th ed. London, Oxford University Press, 2002, p 667
63. Roe CR, Ding J: Mitochondrial fatty acid oxidation disorders. In Scriver CR, et al (eds): The Metabolic and Molecular Bases of Inherited Disease, 8th ed. New York, McGraw-Hill, 2001, p 2297.
64. Lahjouji K, et al: Carnitine transport by organic cation transporters and systemic carnitine deficiency. Mol Genet Metab 73:287, 2001.
65. Bodman M, et al: Medium-chain acyl coenzyme A dehydrogenase deficiency: occurrence in an infant and his father. Arch Neurol 58:811, 2001.
66. DiMauro S, Schon EA: Mitochondrial respiratory-chain diseases. N Engl J Med 348:2656, 2003.
67. Shoffner JM: Oxidative phosphorylation diseases. In Scriver CR, et al (eds): The Metabolic and Molecular Bases of Inherited Disease, 8th ed. New York, McGraw-Hill, 2001, p 2367.
68. Wallace DC, et al: Mitochondria and neuro-ophthalmologic diseases. In Scriver CR, et al (eds): The Metabolic and Molecular Bases of Inherited Disease, 8th ed. New York, McGraw-Hill, 2001, p 2425.
69. Vogel H: Mitochondrial myopathies and the role of the pathologist in the molecular era. J Neuropathol Exp Neurol 60:217, 2001.
70. Oldfors A, Tulinius M: Mitochondrial encephalomyopathies. J Neuropathol Exp Neurol. 62:217, 2003.
71. Dalakas MC, Hohlfeld R: Polymyositis and dermatomyositis. Lancet 362:971, 2003.
72. Buchbinder R, et al: Incidence of malignant disease in biopsy-proven inflammatory myopathy. Ann Intern Med 134:1087, 2001.
73. Ramanan AV, Feldman RM: Clinical outcomes in juvenile dermatomyositis. Curr Opin Rheumatol 14:658, 2002.
74. Askanas V, Engel WK: Inclusion-body myositis and myopathies: different etiologies, possibly similar pathogenetic mechanisms. Curr Opin Neurol 15:525, 2002.
75. Ellis RJ, Pinheiro TJJ: Danger: misfolding proteins. Nature 416:483, 2002.
76. Kanda F, et al: Steroid myopathy: pathogenesis and effects of growth hormone and insulin-like growth factor-I administration. Hormone Res 56 (suppl 1):24, 2001.
77. Stein M, et al: Hydroxychloroquine neuromyotoxicity. J Rheum 27:2927, 2000.
78. Poulas K, et al: Equal male and female incidence of myasthenia gravis. Neurol 54:1202, 2000.
79. Ricny J, et al: Determination of anti-acetylcholine receptor antibodies in myasthenic patients by use of time-resolved fluorescence. Clin Chem 48:549, 2002.
80. Palace J, et al: Myasthenia gravis: diagnostic and management dilemmas. Curr Opin Neurol 14:583, 2001.
81. Younger DS, Raksadawan N: Medical therapies in myasthenia gravis. Chest Surg Clin North Am 11:329, 2001.
82. Pascuzzi RM: Myasthenia gravis and Lambert-Eaton syndrome. Ther Apher 6:57, 2002.
83. Pinto A, et al: The action of Lambert-Eaton myasthenic syndrome immunoglobulin G on cloned human voltage-gated calcium channels. Muscle Nerve 25:715, 2002.

CHAPTER 28

The Central Nervous System

Matthew P. Frosch, MD, PhD • Douglas C. Anthony, MD, PhD • Umberto De Girolami, MD

NEURONS

GLIA

Astrocytes

Oligodendrocytes

Ependymal Cells

Microglia

CELLULAR PATHOLOGY OF THE CENTRAL NERVOUS SYSTEM

Reactions of Neurons to Injury

Reactions of Astrocytes to Injury

CEREBRAL EDEMA, RAISED INTRACRANIAL PRESSURE AND HERNIATION, AND HYDROCEPHALUS

Cerebral Edema

Raised Intracranial Pressure and Herniation

Hydrocephalus

MALFORMATIONS AND DEVELOPMENTAL DISEASES

Neural Tube Defects

Forebrain Anomalies

Posterior Fossa Anomalies

Syringomyelia and Hydromyelia

PERINATAL BRAIN INJURY

TRAUMA

Skull Fractures

Parenchymal Injuries

Concussion

Direct Parenchymal Injury

Diffuse Axonal Injury

Traumatic Vascular Injury

Epidural Hematoma

Subdural Hematoma

Sequelae of Brain Trauma

Spinal Cord Trauma

CEREBROVASCULAR DISEASES

Hypoxia, Ischemia, and Infarction

Hypotension, Hypoperfusion, and Low-Flow States (Global Cerebral Ischemia)

Infarction from Obstruction of Local Blood Supply (Focal Cerebral Ischemia)

Intracranial Hemorrhage

Intracerebral (Intraparenchymal) Hemorrhage

Subarachnoid Hemorrhage and Ruptured Saccular Aneurysms

Vascular Malformations

Hypertensive Cerebrovascular Disease

Lacunar Infarcts

Slit Hemorrhages

Hypertensive Encephalopathy

INFECTIONS

Acute Meningitis

Acute Pyogenic (Bacterial) Meningitis

Acute Aseptic (Viral) Meningitis

Acute Focal Suppurative Infections

Brain Abscess

Subdural Empyema

Extradural Abscess

Chronic Bacterial Meningoencephalitis

Tuberculosis

Neurosyphilis

Neuroborreliosis (Lyme Disease)

Viral Meningoencephalitis

Arthropod-Borne Viral Encephalitis

Herpes Simplex Virus Type 1 (HSV-1)

Herpes Simplex Virus Type 2 (HSV-2)

Varicella-Zoster Virus (Herpes Zoster)

Cytomegalovirus

Poliomyelitis

Rabies

Human Immunodeficiency Virus

Progressive Multifocal Leukoencephalopathy
Subacute Sclerosing Panencephalitis
Fungal Meningoencephalitis
Other Infectious Diseases of the Nervous System
TRANSMISSIBLE SPONGIFORM ENCEPHALOPATHIES (PRION DISEASES)
DEMYELINATING DISEASES
Multiple Sclerosis
Multiple Sclerosis Variants
Acute Disseminated Encephalomyelitis and Acute Necrotizing Hemorrhagic Encephalomyelitis
Other Diseases with Demyelination
DEGENERATIVE DISEASES
Degenerative Diseases Affecting the Cerebral Cortex
Alzheimer Disease
Frontotemporal Dementias
Frontotemporal Dementia with Parkinsonism Linked to Chromosome 17 (FTD(P)-17)
Pick Disease
Progressive Supranuclear Palsy
Corticobasal Degeneration (CBD)
Frontotemporal Dementias Without Tau Pathology
Vascular Dementia
Degenerative Diseases of Basal Ganglia and Brainstem
Parkinsonism
Parkinson Disease
Multiple System Atrophy
Huntington Disease
Spinocerebellar Degenerations
Spinocerebellar Ataxias
Degenerative Diseases Affecting Motor Neurons
Amyotrophic Lateral Sclerosis (Motor Neuron Disease)
Bulbospinal Atrophy (Kennedy Syndrome)
Spinal Muscular Atrophy
GENETIC METABOLIC DISEASES
Leukodystrophies
Krabbe Disease
Metachromatic Leukodystrophy
Adrenoleukodystrophy
Pelizaeus-Merzbacher Disease
Canavan Disease
Mitochondrial Encephalomyopathies
Leigh Syndrome (Subacute Necrotizing Encephalopathy)
Other Mitochondrial Encephalomyopathies
TOXIC AND ACQUIRED METABOLIC DISEASES
Vitamin Deficiencies
Thiamine (Vitamin B_1) Deficiency
Vitamin B_{12} Deficiency
Neurologic Sequelae of Metabolic Disturbances
Hypoglycemia
Hyperglycemia
Hepatic Encephalopathy
Toxic Disorders
Carbon Monoxide
Methanol
Ethanol
Radiation
TUMORS
Gliomas
Astrocytoma
Oligodendroglioma
Ependymoma and Related Paraventricular Mass Lesions
Neuronal Tumors
Ganglion Cell Tumors
Other Tumors with Glial and Neuronal Components
Tumors with Only Neuronal Elements
Poorly Differentiated Neoplasms
Medulloblastoma
Atypical Teratoid/Rhabdoid Tumor (AT/RT)
Other Parenchymal Tumors
Primary CNS Lymphoma
Germ Cell Tumors
Pineal Parenchymal Tumors
Meningiomas
Metastatic Tumors
Paraneoplastic Syndromes
Peripheral Nerve Sheath Tumors
Schwannoma
Neurofibroma
Malignant Peripheral Nerve Sheath Tumor (Malignant Schwannoma)
Familial Tumor Syndromes
Neurofibromatosis Type 1 (NF1)
Neurofibromatosis Type 2 (NF2)
Tuberous Sclerosis
Von Hippel-Lindau Disease

The human central nervous system (CNS) is an enormously complex tissue serving the organism as a processing center linking information between the outside world and the body. The principal functional unit of the CNS is the neuron; the best estimates are that there are about 10^{11} neurons in the human brain. Neurons, although similar in many ways to other cells in the body, are unique in their ability to receive, store, and transmit information. Neurons differ greatly from one another in many important properties: their functional roles (e.g., sensory, motor, autonomic), the distribution of their connections, the neurotransmitters they use for synaptic transmission, their metabolic requirements, and their levels of electrical activity at a given moment. A set of neurons, not necessarily clustered together in a region of the brain, may thus be singled out for destruction in a pathologic condition—*selective vulnerability*—because it shares one or more of these properties. Furthermore, and of particular importance in medicine, most mature neurons are postmitotic cells that are incapable of cell division, so destruction of even a small number of neurons responsible for a specific function may leave the patient with a severe clinical neurologic deficit. Stem cell populations have been described in several areas of the brain and represent a potential mechanism for repair after injury.[1] In comparison to other organ systems of the body, the nervous system has several unique anatomic and physiologic characteristics: the protective bony enclosure of the skull and spinal column that contains it, a specialized system of autoregulation of cerebral blood flow, metabolic substrate requirements, the absence of a conventional lymphatic system, a special cerebrospinal fluid (CSF) circulation, limited immunologic surveillance, and distinctive responses to injury and wound healing. As a result of these special characteristics, the CNS is vulnerable to unique pathologic processes, and the reactions of CNS tissue to injury differ considerably from those encountered elsewhere.[2,3]

Normal Cells

The principal cells of the CNS are neurons, glia, and the cells that compose the meninges and blood vessels.

Neurons

In the CNS, neurons are topographically organized either as aggregates (nuclei, ganglia) or as elongated columns or layers (such as the intermediolateral gray column of the spinal cord or the six-layered cerebral cortex).[4] Functional domains are located in many of these anatomically defined regions (such as the hypoglossal nucleus of the medulla for motor fibers of the twelfth cranial nerve; calcarine cortex of the occipital lobe for primary visual cortex). In addition, as a further dimension of anatomic-functional specificity, some cortical and subcortical neurons and their projections are arranged somatotopically (such as motor and sensory homunculi).[5] Neurons vary considerably in structure and size throughout the nervous system and within a given brain region. With conventional histologic preparations, an anterior horn neuron in the spinal cord has a cell body (perikaryon) that is about 50 μm wide, a relatively large and somewhat eccentrically placed nucleus, a prominent nucleolus, and abundant Nissl substance; the nucleus of a granule cell neuron of the cerebellar cortex is about 10 μm across, and its perikaryon and nucleolus are not readily visible by light microscopy. Electron microscopic study reveals further variability among neurons in cytoplasmic content and the shape of the cells and their processes.[6] Characteristic ultrastructural features common to many neurons include microtubules, neurofilaments, prominent Golgi apparatus and rough endoplasmic reticulum, and synaptic specializations. Despite these shared structures, axon length may vary greatly (hundreds of microns for interneurons versus a meter for an upper motor neuron). Immunohistochemical markers for neurons and their processes commonly used in diagnostic work include neurofilament protein, NeuN, and synaptophysin.[7]

Glia

Glial cells are derived from neuroectoderm (macroglia: astrocytes, oligodendrocytes, ependyma) or from bone marrow (microglia). Glial cells have important structural and metabolic interactions with neurons and their dendritic and axonal processes; they also have a primary role in a wide range of normal functions and reactions to injury, including inflammation, repair, fluid balance, and energy metabolism. The size and shape of the nucleus helps in the light microscopic distinction of one glial cell type from another, as their cytoplasmic processes are often not apparent on H&E preparations and can be demonstrated only with the use of metallic impregnation, immunohistochemical, or electron microscopic methods. *Astrocytes* typically have round to oval nuclei (10 μm wide) with evenly dispersed, pale chromatin; *oligodendrocytes* have a denser, more homogeneous chromatin in a rounder and smaller nucleus (8 μm); and *microglia* have an elongated, irregularly shaped nucleus (5 to 10 μm) with clumped chromatin. *Ependymal cells,* on the other hand, do have visible cytoplasm; seen with H & E, they are columnar epithelial-like cells with a ciliated/microvillous border facing the ventricular surface with pale, vesiculated nuclei (each about 8 μm) located at the abluminal end of the cell.

ASTROCYTES

This glial cell is found throughout the CNS in both gray and white matter. *Protoplasmic* astrocytes occur mainly in the gray matter; *fibrous* astrocytes occur in white and gray matter. The cell derives its name from its star-shaped appearance, which is imparted by the multipolar, branching cytoplasmic processes that emanate from the cell body containing the characteristic cytoplasmic intermediate filament protein called glial fibrillary acidic protein (GFAP). These are seen well in tissue sections only with metallic impregnation techniques (e.g., the Golgi method) (Fig. 28–1*A*) or immunohistochemical preparations (Fig. 28–1*B*). The filaments are either aggregated in fascicles (in protoplasmic astrocytes) or dispersed diffusely throughout the cytoplasm (in fibrous astrocytes). Some astrocytic processes are directed toward neurons and their processes and synapses, where they are believed to act as metabolic buffers or detoxifiers, suppliers of nutrients, and electrical insulators. Others surround capillaries or extend to the subpial and subependymal zones, where they contribute to barrier functions controlling the flow of macromolecules between the blood, the CSF, and the brain. Astrocytes are also the principal cells responsible for repair and scar formation in the brain. Fibroblasts, which have a major role in wound healing elsewhere, are located mainly around large CNS blood vessels and in the meninges; they participate in wound healing only to a limited extent (primarily in the organization of subdural hematomas and the formation of abscess cavities).

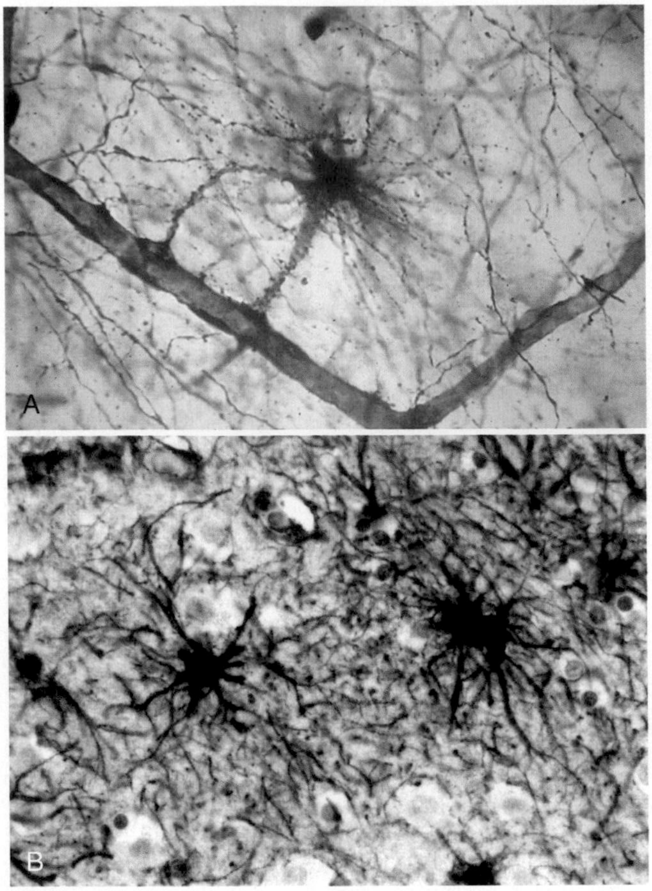

FIGURE 28–1 *A*, Astrocytes and their processes. Some processes extend toward blood vessels (Golgi). *B*, Immunoperoxidase staining for glial fibrillary acidic protein shows astrocytic perinuclear cytoplasm and well-developed processes (*brown*). (Courtesy of Dr. J. Corbo, Brigham and Women's Hospital, Boston, MA.)

OLIGODENDROCYTES

Oligodendroglial cytoplasmic processes wrap around the axons of neurons to form myelin in a manner analogous to the Schwann cells of the peripheral nervous system. Unlike Schwann cells, which form the myelin of a single internode, each oligodendrocyte myelinates numerous internodes on multiple axons. In routine sections, oligodendroglia are recognizable by their small, rounded, lymphocyte-like nuclei, often in linear arrays. Injury to oligodendroglial cells is a feature of acquired demyelinating disorders (e.g., multiple sclerosis); it is also seen in the leukodystrophies. Oligodendroglial nuclei may harbor viral inclusions in progressive multifocal leukoencephalopathy.

EPENDYMAL CELLS

Ependymal cells line the ventricular system. They are closely related to the cuboidal cells comprising the choroid plexus. Disruption of ependymal cells is often associated with a local proliferation of subependymal astrocytes to produce small irregularities on the ventricular surfaces termed *ependymal granulations*. Certain infectious agents, particularly cytomegalovirus, may produce extensive ependymal injury, and viral inclusions may be seen within ependymal cells.

MICROGLIA

Microglia are mesoderm-derived cells whose primary function is to serve as a fixed macrophage system in the CNS. They express many surface markers in common with peripheral monocytes/macrophages (such as CR3 and CD68). They respond to injury by (1) proliferation; (2) developing elongated nuclei (*rod cells*), as in neurosyphilis; (3) forming aggregates about small foci of tissue necrosis (*microglial nodules*); or (4) congregating around cell bodies of dying neurons (*neuronophagia*). In addition to resident microglia, blood-derived macrophages are the principal phagocytic cells present in inflammatory foci.[8–10]

Pathology

Cellular Pathology of the Central Nervous System

The tissues of the CNS undergo fairly stereotyped changes in response to diverse types of injury.

REACTIONS OF NEURONS TO INJURY

There are several well-characterized forms of pathologic reaction of neurons, the main ones being neuronal degeneration and cell death and reactions associated with repair after injury. Neuronal death occurs either as programmed cell death (apoptosis), as when there is elimination of sets of neurons during the course of fetal brain development, or as acute or slowly progressive cell injury culminating in necrosis.

- *Acute neuronal injury (red neuron)* refers to a spectrum of changes that accompany acute CNS hypoxia/ischemia or other acute insults that ultimately lead to death of the cell (see Fig. 28–13*B*). Red neurons are evident with hematoxylin and eosin (H & E) preparations at about 12 to 24 hours after an irreversible hypoxic/ischemic insult. The morphologic features consist of shrinkage of the cell body, pyknosis of the nucleus, disappearance of the nucleolus, and loss of Nissl substance, with intense eosinophilia of the cytoplasm. Often, the nucleus assumes the angulated shape of the shrunken perikaryon. Experimental studies have defined even earlier (4 to 8 hours) structural changes that accompany irreversible neuronal injury, consisting of small vacuoles within the cell body;[11] these are difficult to detect in human brain tissue examined at postmortem.
- *Subacute and chronic neuronal injury ("degeneration")* refers to situations leading to neuronal death occurring as a result of a progressive disease process of some duration, as is seen in certain slowly evolving neurologic diseases (such as amyotrophic lateral sclerosis). The characteristic histologic feature is cell loss, often selectively involving functionally related systems of neurons, and reactive gliosis. When the process is at an early stage, the cell loss is difficult to detect; the associated reactive glial changes are often the best indicator of the pathologic process. Neuronal *transsynaptic degeneration* is seen when there is a destructive process that interrupts the majority of the afferent

input to a group of neurons, such as the degeneration of sets of lateral geniculate neurons after eye enucleation.

■ *Axonal reaction* refers to the reaction within the cell body that attends *regeneration* of the axon; it has been extensively studied in motor neurons following nerve injury in experimental animals.[12] In the anterior horn cells of the spinal cord, axonal reaction occurs when motor axons are cut or seriously damaged. This reparative process is associated with increased protein synthesis, and its most important effect is axonal sprouting. Morphologic changes visible in the perikaryon include enlargement and rounding up of the cell body, peripheral displacement of the nucleus, enlargement of the nucleolus, and dispersion of Nissl substance from the center to the periphery of the cell (*central chromatolysis*). Degenerative changes in an injured axon occur over the course of time, involving the distal regions of the axon (see Chapter 27).

■ Neuronal damage may be associated with a wide range of subcellular alterations in the neuronal organelles and cytoskeleton. *Neuronal inclusions* may occur as a manifestation of aging, when there are intracytoplasmic accumulations of complex lipids (*lipofuscin*), proteins, or carbohydrates. Abnormal cytoplasmic deposition of complex lipids and other substances also occurs in genetically determined disorders of metabolism in which substrates or intermediates accumulate (Chapter 5). In these conditions, the neuronal cell body becomes greatly swollen at first because of the intracytoplasmic accumulation of the abnormal metabolite, and the process culminates in death of the cell. Viral infection can lead to abnormal intranuclear inclusions, as seen in herpetic infection (Cowdry body), cytoplasmic inclusions, as seen in rabies (Negri body), or both nucleus and cytoplasm (cytomegalovirus).

■ Some degenerative diseases of the CNS are associated with neuronal intracytoplasmic inclusions, such as *neurofibrillary tangles* of Alzheimer disease and *Lewy bodies* of Parkinson disease; others cause abnormal vacuolization of the perikaryon and neuronal cell processes in the neuropil (Creutzfeldt-Jakob disease). (Table 28–1). These aggregates are highly resistant to degradation, contain proteins with altered conformation, and may result from mutations in proteins that affect protein folding, ubiquitination, and intracellular trafficking (see discussion of protein folding in Chapter 1). They may be referred to as *proteinopathies*.

REACTIONS OF ASTROCYTES TO INJURY

The cellular pathology of astrocytes may be subdivided into reactive responses that accompany the cells' proliferation (*gliosis*) and the sets of reactions to injury that lead to their death. In addition, morphologically diverse intracellular inclusions and deposits are seen in injured astrocytes.

■ *Gliosis* is the most important histopathologic indicator of CNS injury, regardless of etiology. Astrocytes participate in this process by undergoing both hypertrophy and hyperplasia. The nucleus enlarges and becomes vesicular, and the nucleolus is prominent. The previously scant cytoplasm expands to a bright pink, somewhat irregular swath around an eccentric nucleus, from which emerge numerous stout, ramifying processes (*gemistocytic astrocyte*). Immunohistochemistry for glial fibrillary acidic protein (GFAP) splendidly demonstrates the extraordinary metamorphosis. In long-standing lesions, the nuclei become small and dark and lie in a dense net of processes. These cell processes, *glial "fibrils,"* are not true extracellular fibers. Proliferation of astrocytes residing between the molecular and granule cell layers of the cerebellum is a regular accompaniment of anoxic injury and other conditions associated with death of Purkinje cells, termed *Bergmann gliosis*.

■ *Cellular swelling*, or swelling of the astrocyte cytoplasm, occurs regularly in acute insults when there is a failure of the cell's pump systems, as occurs in hypoxia, hypoglycemia, and toxic injuries.[13]

■ *Rosenthal fibers* are thick, elongated, brightly eosinophilic structures that are somewhat irregular in contour and occur within astrocytic processes. Ultrastructurally, they exhibit dense osmiophilic deposits that contain two heat-shock proteins (αB-crystallin and hsp27) and ubiquitin. Rosenthal fibers are typically found in regions of long-standing gliosis; they are also characteristic of cerebellar pilocytic astrocytoma (see later), as well as the reactive brain adjacent to craniopharyngioma or syrinx cavities. In *Alexander*

TABLE 28–1 Neurodegenerative Diseases Associated with Aggregated Proteins

Disease	Protein	Normal Structure	Aggregate/Inclusion	Location
Transmissible spongiform encephalopathies (Prion disease) (see Fig. 28–31)	Prion protein (PrP)	α-Helix and random coil	β-pleated sheet, proteinase K-resistant	Extracellular
Alzheimer disease (see Fig. 28–35*C*)	Amyloid precursor protein (APP)	α-Helix and random coil	β-pleated sheet, amyloid (fragment of APP)	Extracellular
Tauopathies and Alzheimer disease	Tau (microtubule binding protein)	3 and 4 repeat isoforms	Hyperphosphorylated aggregated protein	Intracellular
Parkinson disease (see Fig. 28–37*C*)	α-Synuclein	Random coil, repeats	Aggregated, Lewy bodies	Cytoplasmic
Multiple system atrophy	α-Synuclein	Random coil, repeats	Aggregated, Glial cytoplasmic inclusions	Cytoplasmic
Huntington disease	Huntingtin	Trinucleotide repeats	Insoluble aggregates	Nuclear
Spinocerebellar ataxias	Ataxins	Trinucleotide repeats	Insoluble aggregates	Nuclear

Modified from Welch WJ, Gambetti P: Chaperoning brain diseases. Nature 392:23–24, 1998.

disease, a leukodystrophy due to a mutation in the gene for GFAP,[14] abundant Rosenthal fibers are found in periventricular, perivascular, and subpial locations.

- *Corpora amylacea,* or polyglucosan bodies, are round, faintly basophilic, periodic acid–Schiff (PAS)–positive, concentrically lamellated structures ranging between 5 and 50 μm in diameter and located wherever there are astrocytic end processes, especially in the subpial and perivascular zones. Although consisting primarily of glycosaminoglycan polymers, they also contain heat-shock proteins and ubiquitin. They represent a degenerative change in the astrocyte, and they occur in increasing numbers with advancing age and in a rare condition called *adult polyglucosan body disease.* The *Lafora bodies* that are seen in the cytoplasm of neurons (as well as hepatocytes, myocytes, and other cells) in myoclonic epilepsy (Lafora body myoclonus with epilepsy) are of similar structure and biochemical composition.
- *Glial cytoplasmic inclusions* consisting of silver-positive meshes of 20- to 40-nm intermediate filaments that contain the protein α-synuclein[15] are characteristic of a number of CNS degenerative diseases, collectively known as multiple system atrophy.[16]
- The *Alzheimer type II astrocyte* is a gray matter astrocyte with a large (two to three times normal) nucleus, pale-staining central chromatin, an intranuclear glycogen droplet, and a prominent nuclear membrane and nucleolus. Despite its name, it is unrelated to Alzheimer disease; rather, it occurs especially in patients with long-standing hyperammonemia due to chronic liver disease, Wilson disease, or hereditary metabolic disorders of the urea cycle.

Cerebral Edema, Raised Intracranial Pressure and Herniation, and Hydrocephalus

The brain and spinal cord exist within a rigid compartment defined by the skull, vertebral bodies, and dura mater. The advantage of housing as vital and delicate a structure as the CNS in a protective environment is obvious. On the other hand, such rigid confines provide little room for brain parenchymal expansion in disease states. A number of disorders may upset the delicate balance between brain volume and the fixed boundaries of the intracranial vault. These conditions include generalized brain edema, hydrocephalus, and focally expanding mass lesions.

CEREBRAL EDEMA

Cerebral edema or, more precisely, brain parenchymal edema may arise in the setting of a number of diseases. Two principal types are recognized:

- *Vasogenic edema* occurs when the integrity of the normal blood-brain barrier is disrupted and increased vascular permeability occurs, allowing fluid to escape from the intravascular compartment predominantly into the intercellular spaces of the brain. The paucity of conventional lymphatics and the close apposition of cell processes of neurons and glia in the brain greatly impairs the resorption of excess extracellular fluid. Vasogenic edema may be either localized, as when it results from abnormally permeable vessels adjacent to inflammatory disease or neoplasms, or generalized.
- *Cytotoxic edema,* in contrast, implies an increase in intracellular fluid secondary to neuronal, glial or endothelial cell membrane injury, as might be encountered in a patient with a generalized hypoxic/ischemic insult or with some intoxications.

In practice, conditions associated with generalized edema often have elements of both vasogenic and cytotoxic edema.

Interstitial edema (hydrocephalic edema) occurs especially around the lateral ventricles when there is an abnormal flow of fluid from the intraventricular CSF across the ependymal lining to the periventricular white matter in a setting of increased intraventricular pressure.

Morphology. The edematous brain is softer than normal and often appears to "overfill" the cranial vault. In generalized edema, the gyri are flattened, the intervening sulci are narrowed, and the ventricular cavities are compressed. As the brain expands, herniation may occur.

RAISED INTRACRANIAL PRESSURE AND HERNIATION

Raised intracranial pressure is an increase in mean CSF pressure above 200 mm water with the patient recumbent. It occurs when the volume of brain tissue increases beyond the limit permitted by compression of veins and displacement of CSF. Most cases are associated with a mass effect, either diffuse, as in generalized brain edema, or focal, as with tumors, abscesses, or hemorrhages. Because the cranial vault is subdivided by rigid dural folds (the falx and tentorium), a focal expansion of the brain causes it to be displaced in relation to these partitions. If the expansion is sufficiently severe, a *herniation* of the brain will occur (Fig. 28–2).

- *Subfalcine (cingulate) herniation* occurs when unilateral or asymmetric expansion of a cerebral hemisphere displaces the cingulate gyrus under the falx cerebri. This may be associated with compression of branches of the anterior cerebral artery.
- *Transtentorial (uncinate, mesial temporal) herniation* occurs when the medial aspect of the temporal lobe is compressed against the free margin of the tentorium cerebelli. With increasing displacement of the temporal lobe, the third cranial nerve is compromised, resulting in pupillary dilation and impairment of ocular movements on the side of the lesion. The posterior cerebral artery may also be compressed, resulting in ischemic injury to the territory supplied by that vessel, including the primary visual cortex. When the extent of herniation is large enough, the contralateral cerebral peduncle may be compressed, resulting in hemiparesis ipsilateral to the side of the herniation; the changes in the peduncle in this setting are known as *Kernohan's notch.* Progression of transtentorial herniation is often accompanied by hemorrhagic lesions in the midbrain and pons, termed *secondary brainstem,* or *Duret, hemorrhages* (Fig. 28–3). These linear or flame-shaped lesions usually occur in the midline and paramedian regions and

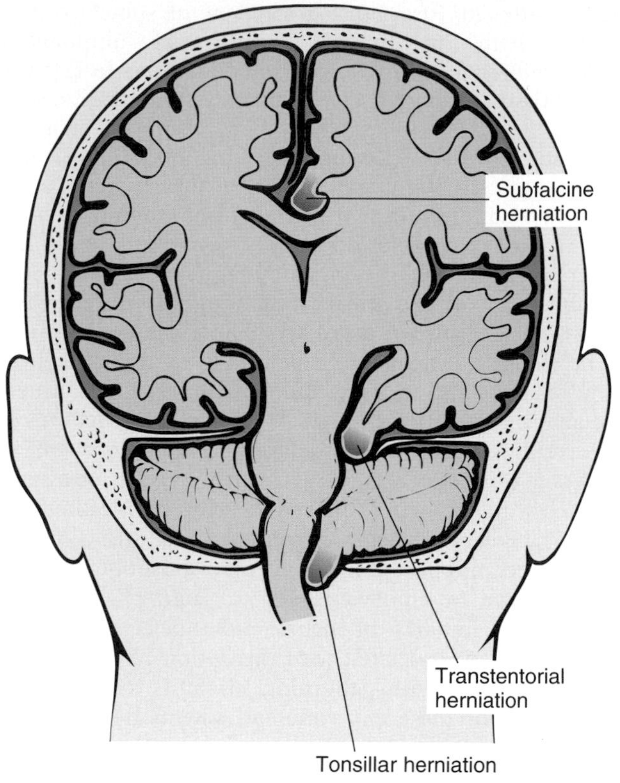

FIGURE 28–2 Major herniations of the brain: subfalcine, transtentorial, and tonsillar. (Adapted from Fishman RA: Brain edema. N Engl J Med 293:706, 1975. Copyright © 1975, Massachusetts Medical Society. All rights reserved.)

are believed to be due to tearing of penetrating veins and arteries supplying the upper brainstem.

- *Tonsillar herniation* refers to displacement of the cerebellar tonsils through the foramen magnum. This pattern of herniation is life-threatening because it causes brainstem compression and compromises vital respiratory and cardiac centers in the medulla oblongata.

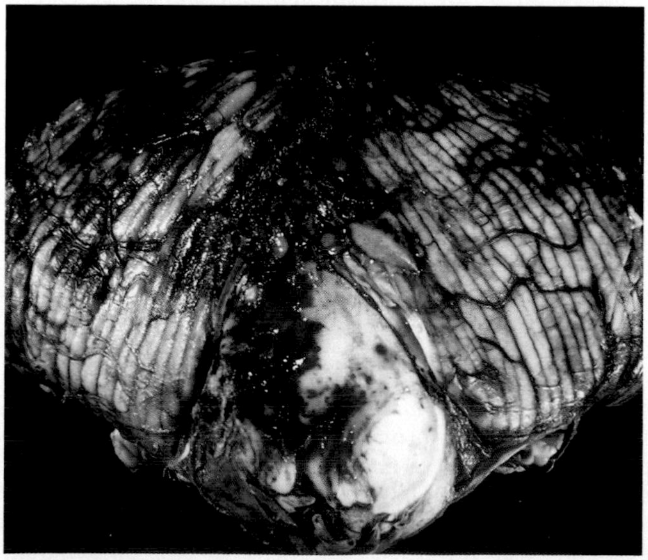

FIGURE 28–3 Duret hemorrhage involving the brainstem at the junction of the pons and midbrain.

HYDROCEPHALUS

In the normal brain, CSF is produced by the choroid plexus within the lateral and fourth ventricles. The CSF normally circulates through the ventricular system and enters the cisterna magna at the base of the brain stem through the foramina of Luschka and Magendie. Subarachnoid CSF bathes the superior cerebral convexities and is absorbed by the arachnoid granulations.[17] *Hydrocephalus* refers to the accumulation of excessive CSF within the ventricular system. Most cases occur as a consequence of impaired flow and resorption of CSF; in rare instances (e.g., tumors of the choroid plexus), overproduction of CSF may be responsible. Whatever its cause, an increased volume of CSF within the ventricles expands them and can cause an elevation in intracranial pressure.

When hydrocephalus develops before closure of the cranial sutures, there is enlargement of the head, manifested by an increase in head circumference. Hydrocephalus developing after fusion of the sutures, in contrast, is associated with expansion of the ventricles and increased intracranial pressure, without a change in head circumference (Fig. 28–4). If a portion of the ventricular system is enlarged because of excess CSF, as may occur because of a mass in the third ventricle, the pattern is called *noncommunicating hydrocephalus*. In contrast, in *communicating hydrocephalus*, there is enlargement of the entire ventricular system.

The term *hydrocephalus ex vacuo* refers to dilation of the ventricular system with a compensatory increase in CSF volume secondary to a loss of brain parenchyma.

Malformations and Developmental Diseases

The incidence of developmental disability, including mental retardation, cerebral palsy, neural tube defects, and other forms, has been estimated at 1% to 2%,[18] with high incidences seen in some populations such as those with multiple birth defects.[19] Prenatal or perinatal insults may either cause failure of normal CNS development or result in tissue destruction. The anatomic pattern of the malformation reflects the stage of formation of the brain at the time of injury.[20] Although the pathogenesis and etiology of CNS malformations are largely unknown, both genetic and environmental factors clearly play a role and have been the topic of intensive research in recent years, as was detailed in Chapter 10. Signaling molecules and homeotic and other genes control body patterning, and such genes are expressed in a regulated fashion during the segmental development of the CNS.[21–24] Finally, many toxic compounds and infectious agents are known to have teratogenic effects in humans and experimental animals (Chapter 9).

NEURAL TUBE DEFECTS

Failure of a portion of the neural tube to close, or reopening of a region of the tube after successful closure, may lead to one of several malformations. All are characterized by abnormalities involving some combination of neural tissue, menginges, and overlying bone or soft tissues. Collectively, neural tube defects account for most CNS malformations.

Anencephaly is a malformation of the anterior end of the neural tube, with absence of the brain and calvarium. It occurs

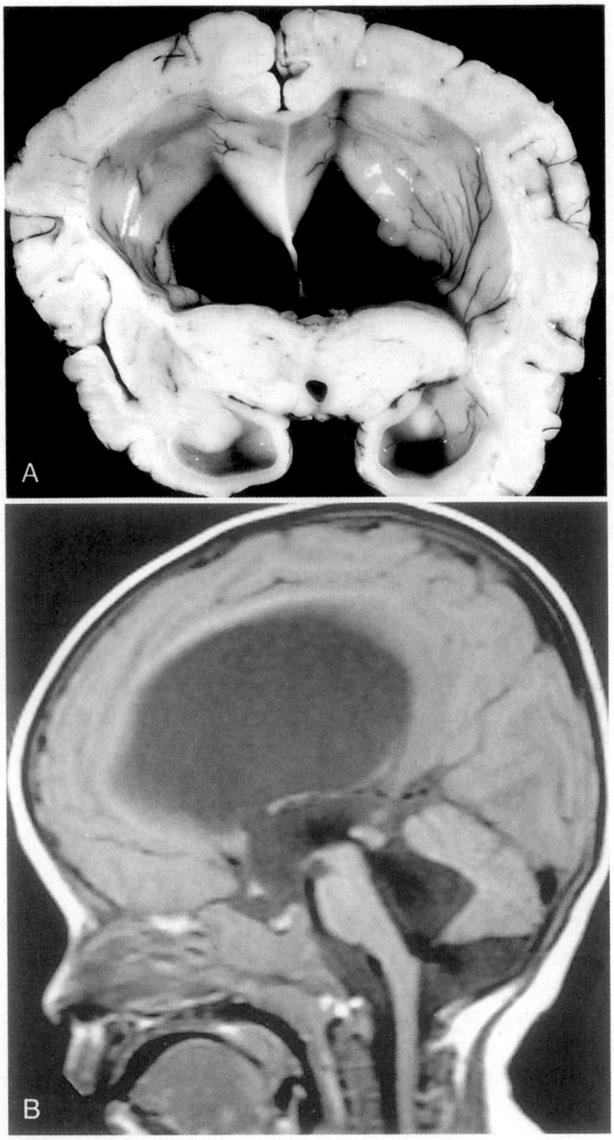

FIGURE 28–4 *A*, Hydrocephalus. Dilated lateral ventricles seen in a coronal section through the midthalamus. *B*, Midsagittal plane T1-weighted magnetic resonance image of a child with communicating hydrocephalus, involving all ventricles. (*B*, courtesy of Dr. P. Barnes, Stanford University Medical Center, CA.)

in 1 to 5 per 1000 live births, more commonly in females, and is thought to develop at approximately 28 days of gestation. Forebrain development is disrupted and all that remains in its place is the *area cerebrovasculosa*, a flattened remnant of disorganized brain tissue with admixed ependyma, choroid plexus, and meningothelial cells. The posterior fossa structures may be spared, depending on the extent of the skull deficit; descending tracts associated with disrupted structures are, as expected, absent.

An *encephalocele* is a diverticulum of malformed CNS tissue extending through a defect in the cranium. It most often occurs in the occipital region or in the posterior fossa.

The most common forms of neural tube defects in newborns involve the spinal cord and are caused by a failure of closure or reopening of the caudal portions of the neural tube. *Spinal dysraphism* or *spina bifida* may be an asymptomatic bony defect (spina bifida occulta) or a severe malformation with a flattened, disorganized segment of spinal cord, associated with an overlying meningeal outpouching. *Myelomeningocele* (or meningomyelocele) refers to extension of CNS tissue through a defect in the vertebral column; the term *meningocele* applies when there is only a meningeal extrusion. Clinical neurologic dysfunction is most often related to the structural abnormality of the cord itself and to superimposed infection that extends from the thin, overlying skin. Myelomeningoceles occur most commonly in the lumbosacral region, and the patient manifests clinical deficits referable to motor and sensory function in the lower extremities as well as disturbances of bowel and bladder control.

The etiology of neural tube defects is unknown; their frequency varies widely among different ethnic groups. Antenatal diagnosis has been facilitated by new imaging methods and the screening of maternal blood samples for evidence of elevated α-fetoprotein. The overall recurrence rate for a neural tube defect in subsequent pregnancies has been estimated at 4% to 5%. Folate deficiency during the initial weeks of gestation has been implicated as a risk factor, possibly interacting with maternal or embryonic genetic factors.[25–27] Although many mouse models of neural tube defects have been described, often associated with disruption of transcription factors associated with patterning, attempts to find human counterparts of these experimental systems have not been successful to date.[28,29]

FOREBRAIN ANOMALIES

Polymicrogyria is characterized by a loss of the normal external contour of the cerebral convolutions, which appear small, unusually numerous, and irregularly formed. The gray matter is composed of four layers (or fewer), with entrapment of apparent meningeal tissue at points of fusion of what would otherwise be the cortical surface. Animal studies suggest that polymicrogyria can be induced by localized tissue injury during the time of neuronal migration.

The volume of brain may be abnormally large (*megalencephaly*) or small (*microencephaly*). Microencephaly, by far the more common of the two, can occur in a wide range of clinical settings, including chromosome abnormalities, fetal alcohol syndrome, and human immunodeficiency virus 1 (HIV-1) infection acquired in utero. Alterations in cell proliferation have been shown, in mice, to be associated with alterations in the volume of cerebral cortex.[35] A reduction in the number of neurons that reach the neocortex is postulated, and this leads to a simplification of the gyral folding. This can range from a noticeable decrease in the number of gyri to total absence, leaving a smooth-surfaced brain, *lissencephaly (agyria)*. In the Miller-Dieker syndrome (seizures, mental retardation, and lissencephaly) about 90% of patients have a deletion in chromosome 17p13.3. The involved gene has been termed *LIS1*; it is normally expressed in the CNS but is absent in the disorder.[30,31] Abnormal gyral patterns are also found in chondrodysplasias; *thanatophoric dwarfism* is a lethal form characterized by abnormally large and hyperconvoluted temporal lobes and skeletal anomalies (micromelia, and chest and skull deformities).

The migration of neurons, from the germinal matrix (the periventricular region of neuronal and glial proliferation) through the deeper structures to reach their final destinations in the cerebral cortex, is a complicated process that can go awry. There are critical interactions between Cajal-Retzius cells (a population of cells at the surface of the developing cortex[32]) and migrating neurons through diffusible molecules, as well as intracellular signaling pathways in the migrating population. Mutations in genes for proteins involved in these interactions have been identified as the basis for many forms of migrational disorders.[33,34] Stranded clusters of neurons (*neuronal heterotopias*) may be found strewn along the path of migration, either as large conglomerates or as small clusters within the white matter.

Holoprosencephaly is a spectrum of malformations characterized by incomplete separation of the cerebral hemispheres across the midline (Fig. 28–5). Severe forms manifest midline facial abnormalities, including cyclopia; less severe variants (arrhinencephaly) show absence of the olfactory cranial nerves and related structures. Intrauterine diagnosis of severe forms by ultrasound examination is now possible. Holoprosencephaly is associated with trisomy 13 (rarely, with trisomy 18), and there is an increased incidence in the offspring of diabetic mothers. Mutations in the human *Sonic hedgehog* gene or functional alterations in the protein (a member of a family of secreted proteins synthesized by the notochord and neural plate during induction) have been shown in some cases of holoprosencephaly.[36,37]

In *agenesis of the corpus callosum*, a relatively common malformation, there is an absence of the white matter bundles that carry cortical projections from one hemisphere to the other (Fig. 28–6). Radiologic imaging studies show misshapen lateral ventricles ("bat-wing" deformity); on coronal whole-mount sections of the brain, bundles of anteroposteriorly oriented white matter can be demonstrated. Agenesis of the corpus callosum can be found in patients with mental retardation or in clinically normal individuals. It can be present in isolation or can be associated with a wide range of other malformations. It represents the major structural abnormality in Aicardi syndrome, an X-linked syndrome that is lethal in males, in which it is associated with chorioretinal defects and seizures. Unlike patients with surgical callosal section who show clinical evidence of hemispheric disconnection, patients with this malformation can be shown to have only minimal deficits even with neuropsychologic testing. The malformation may be complete or partial; in the latter case, the caudal portion of the callosum is absent, and a lipoma sometimes occupies the defect.

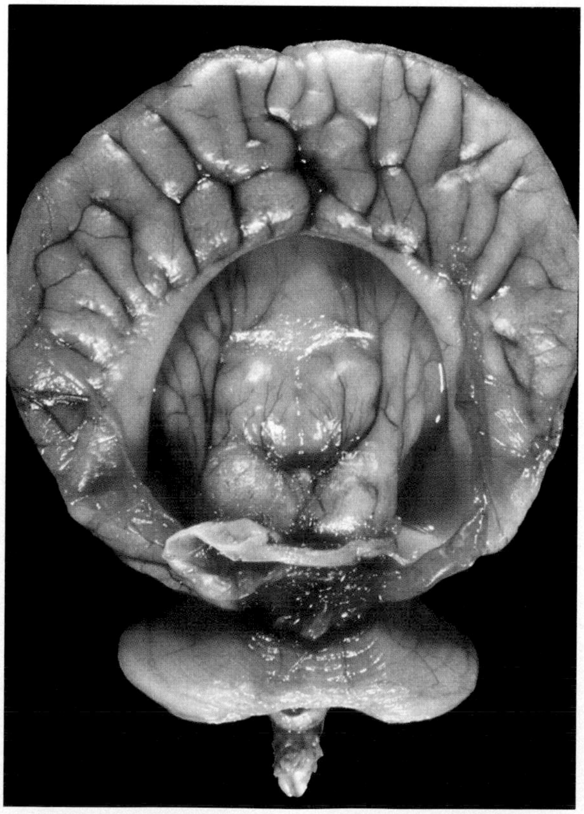

FIGURE 28–5 Holoprosencephaly (severe alobar form). View of the dorsal surface showing a lack of separation of cerebral hemispheres, a single ventricle, and fused basal ganglia.

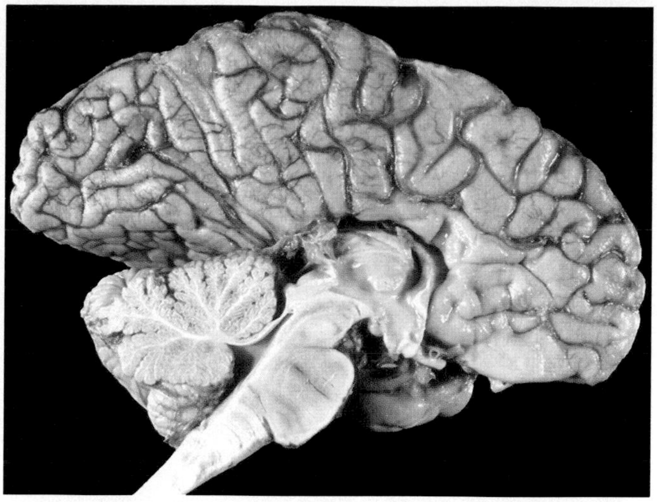

FIGURE 28–6 Agenesis of the corpus callosum. The midsagittal view of the left hemisphere shows the lack of a corpus callosum and cingulate gyrus above the third ventricle.

POSTERIOR FOSSA ANOMALIES

The *Arnold-Chiari malformation* (Chiari type II malformation) consists of a small posterior fossa, a misshapen midline cerebellum with downward extension of vermis through the foramen magnum (Fig. 28–7), and, almost invariably, hydrocephalus and a lumbar myelomeningocele. Other associated changes may include caudal displacement of the medulla, malformation of the tectum, aqueductal stenosis, cerebral heterotopias, and hydromyelia (see later). In the *Chiari I malformation*, low-lying cerebellar tonsils extend down into the vertebral canal and may cause symptoms referable to obstruction of CSF flow and medullary compression that are amenable to neurosurgical intervention.

The *Dandy-Walker malformation* is characterized by an enlarged posterior fossa. The cerebellar vermis is absent or present only in rudimentary form in its anterior portion. In its place is a large midline cyst that is lined by ependyma and is contiguous with leptomeninges on its outer surface. This cyst represents the expanded, roofless fourth ventricle in the absence of a normally formed vermis. Dysplasias of brain stem nuclei are commonly found in association with Dandy-Walker malformation.

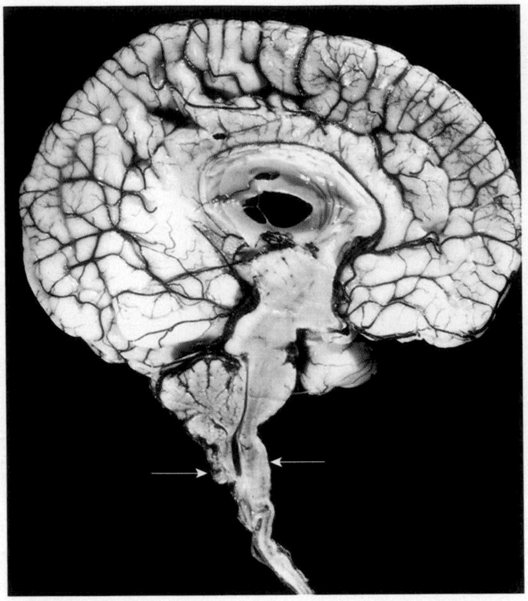

FIGURE 28–7 Arnold-Chiari malformation. Midsagittal section showing small posterior fossa contents, downward displacement of the cerebellar vermis, and deformity of the medulla (arrows indicate the approximate level of the foramen magnum).

SYRINGOMYELIA AND HYDROMYELIA

These are disorders characterized by a discontinuous multisegmental or confluent expansion of the ependyma-lined central canal of the cord (*hydromyelia*) or by the formation of a fluid-filled cleftlike cavity in the inner portion of the cord (*syringomyelia, syrinx*). These lesions are associated with destruction of the adjacent gray and white matter and are surrounded by a dense feltwork of reactive gliosis. The cervical spinal cord is most often affected, and the slitlike cavity may extend into the brainstem (*syringobulbia*). Associated anomalies of the spinal column are common (vertebral fusions, scoliosis, platybasia).

Syringomyelia may be associated with the Chiari I malformation; it may also occur in association with intraspinal tumors or following traumatic injury. In general, the histologic appearance of the lesions is comparable in all these conditions. The disease generally becomes manifest in the second or third decade of life. The distinctive initial clinical symptoms and signs of a syrinx are progressive evolution of dissociated sensory loss of pain and temperature sensation in the upper extremities due to early involvement of the crossing anterior spinal commissural fibers, with retention of position sense and absence of motor deficits.

Perinatal Brain Injury

A variety of exogenous factors may injure the developing brain. Injuries that occur early in gestation may destroy brain tissue without evoking the usual "reactive" changes in the parenchyma and may be difficult to distinguish from malformations. Brain injury occurring in the perinatal period is an important cause of childhood neurologic disability.

The broad clinical term *cerebral palsy* refers to a nonprogressive neurologic motor deficit characterized by spasticity, dystonia, ataxia/athetosis, and paresis attributable to insults occurring during the prenatal and perinatal periods.[38] Signs and symptoms may not be apparent at birth and only later declare themselves as development proceeds. Postmortem examinations of children with this syndrome have shown a wide range of neuropathologic findings, including destructive lesions traced to remote events that may have caused hemorrhage and infarction.[39]

In premature infants, there is an increased risk of *intraparenchymal hemorrhage* within the germinal matrix, often near the junction between the thalamus and the caudate nucleus. Hemorrhages may remain localized or extend into the ventricular system and thence to the subarachnoid space, sometimes leading to hydrocephalus.

Infarcts may occur in the supratentorial periventricular white matter (*periventricular leukomalacia*), especially in premature babies. These are chalky yellow plaques consisting of discrete regions of white matter necrosis and mineralization (Fig. 28–8). When both gray and white matter are involved by extensive ischemic damage, large destructive cystic lesions develop throughout the hemispheres; this condition is termed *multicystic encephalopathy*.

In perinatal ischemic lesions of the cerebral cortex, the depths of sulci bear the brunt of injury and result in thinned-out, gliotic gyri (*ulegyria*). The basal ganglia and thalamus may also suffer ischemic injury, with patchy neuronal loss and reactive gliosis. Later, with the development of myelination, aberrant and irregular myelin formation gives rise to a marble-like appearance of the deep nuclei: *status marmoratus.* Because the lesions are in the caudate, putamen and thalamus, choreoathetosis and related movement disorders are important clinical sequelae.

Trauma

The anatomic location of the lesion and the limited capacity of the brain for functional repair are two factors of great significance in CNS trauma. Injury of several cubic centimeters of brain parenchyma may be clinically silent (e.g., in the frontal lobe), severely disabling (in the spinal cord), or fatal (in the brainstem).

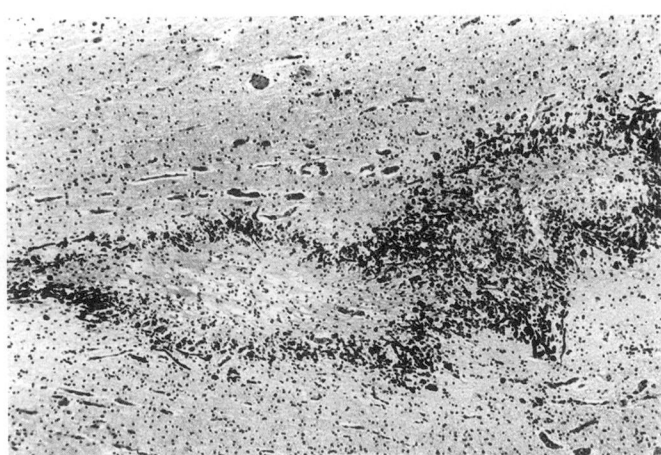

FIGURE 28–8 Periventricular leukomalacia. Central focus of white matter necrosis with a peripheral rim of mineralized axonal processes (staining blue).

The magnitude and distribution of a traumatic brain lesion depend on the shape of the object causing the trauma, the force of impact, and whether the head is in motion at the time of injury. A blow to the head may be *penetrating* or *blunt*; it may cause either an *open* or a *closed injury*. Severe brain damage can occur in the absence of external signs of head injury; conversely, severe lacerations and even skull fractures do not necessarily indicate damage to the underlying brain. The physical forces associated with head injury may result in *skull fractures*, *parenchymal injury*, and *vascular injury*; all three can coexist.[40,41]

SKULL FRACTURES

The kinetic energy that causes a fracture is dissipated at a fused suture; fractures that cross sutures are termed *diastatic*. With multiple points of impact or repeated blows to the head, the fracture lines of subsequent injuries do not extend across fracture lines of prior injury. A fracture in which bone is displaced into the cranial cavity by a distance greater than the thickness of the bone is called a *displaced skull fracture*. The thickness of the cranial bones varies; therefore, their resistance to fracture differs greatly. Also, the relative incidence of fractures among skull bones is related to the pattern of falls. When an individual falls while awake, such as might occur when stepping off a ladder, the site of impact is often in the occipital portion of the skull; in contrast, a fall that follows loss of consciousness, as might follow a syncopal attack, commonly results in a frontal impact. Basal skull fractures typically follow an impact to the occiput or sides of the head rather than a blow to the vertex; these fractures are difficult to detect at postmortem examination and require careful removal of the dura, which normally is tightly adherent to the base of the skull. Symptoms referable to the lower cranial nerves or the cervicomedullary region, and the presence of orbital or mastoid hematomas distant from the point of impact, raise the clinical suspicion of a basal skull fracture. CSF discharge from the nose or ear and infection (meningitis) may follow.

PARENCHYMAL INJURIES

Concussion

Concussion is a clinical syndrome of alteration of consciousness secondary to head injury typically brought about by a change in the momentum of the head (movement of the head arrested by a rigid surface). The characteristic neurologic picture includes instantaneous onset of transient neurologic dysfunction, including loss of consciousness, temporary respiratory arrest, and loss of reflexes.[3] Although neurologic recovery is complete, amnesia for the event persists. Postconcussive neuropsychiatric syndromes are well recognized. The pathogenesis of the sudden disruption of nervous activity is unknown, but biochemical and physiologic abnormalities occur, such as depolarization due to excitatory amino acid–mediated ionic fluxes across cell membranes, depletion of mitochondrial adenosine triphosphate (ATP), and alterations in vascular permeability. Patients who die after a postconcussive syndrome may show evidence of direct parenchymal injury, but in others, there is no evidence of damage.

Direct Parenchymal Injury

Contusion and *laceration* are lesions associated with direct parenchymal injury of the brain, either through transmission of kinetic energy to the brain and bruising analogous to what is seen in soft tissues (contusion) or by penetration of an object and tearing of tissue (laceration). As with any other organ, a blow to the surface of the brain, transmitted through the skull, leads to rapid tissue displacement, disruption of vascular channels, and subsequent hemorrhage, tissue injury, and edema (Figs. 28–9 and 28–10). The crests of gyri are most susceptible, whereas the cerebral cortex along the sulci is less vulnerable. The most common locations where contusions occur correspond to the most frequent sites of direct impact and to regions of the brain that overlie a rough and irregular inner skull surface, such as the frontal lobes along the orbital gyri, and the temporal lobes. Contusions are less frequent over the occipital lobes, brainstem, and cerebellum unless these sites are adjacent to a skull fracture (*fracture contusions*).

A patient who suffers a blow to the head may develop a cerebral injury at the point of contact (a *coup* injury) or damage to the brain surface diametrically opposite to it (a *contrecoup* injury). Both coup and contrecoup lesions are contusions. Since their macroscopic and microscopic appearance is indistinguishable, the distinction between them is based on forensic identification of the point of impact and the circumstances attending the incident. In general, if the head is immobile at the time of trauma, only a coup injury is found. When the head is mobile, there may be coup lesions beneath the site of impact and also contrecoup lesions. Whereas the coup lesion is caused by the force of direct impact between the brain and skull at the site of impact, the contrecoup contusion is thought to develop when the brain strikes the opposite inner surface of the skull after sudden deceleration.

Morphology. Contusions, when seen on cross-section, are wedge-shaped, with the broad base spanning the surface and centered on the point of impact (Fig. 28–9*B*). The histologic appearance of contusions is independent of the type of trauma. In the earliest stages, there is evidence of edema and hemorrhage, which is often pericapillary. During the next few hours, the extravasation of blood extends throughout the involved tissue, across the width of the cerebral cortex, and into the white matter and subarachnoid space. Morphologic evidence of injury in the neuronal cell body (pyknosis of the nucleus, eosinophilia of the cytoplasm, disintegration of the cell) takes about 24 hours to appear, although functional brain injury occurs earlier. Axonal swellings develop in the vicinity of damaged neurons or at great distances away. The inflammatory response to the injured tissue follows its usual course, with the appearance of neutrophils followed by macrophages. Old traumatic lesions on the surface of the brain have a characteristic macroscopic appearance: They are depressed, retracted, yellowish brown patches involving the crests of gyri most commonly located at the sites of contrecoup lesions (inferior frontal cortex, temporal and occipital poles). The term *plaque jaune* is applied to these lesions, as seen on the inferior frontal surface of the brain in Fig. 28–9*C*; they can be foci of clinical seizure discharges. More extensive hemorrhagic

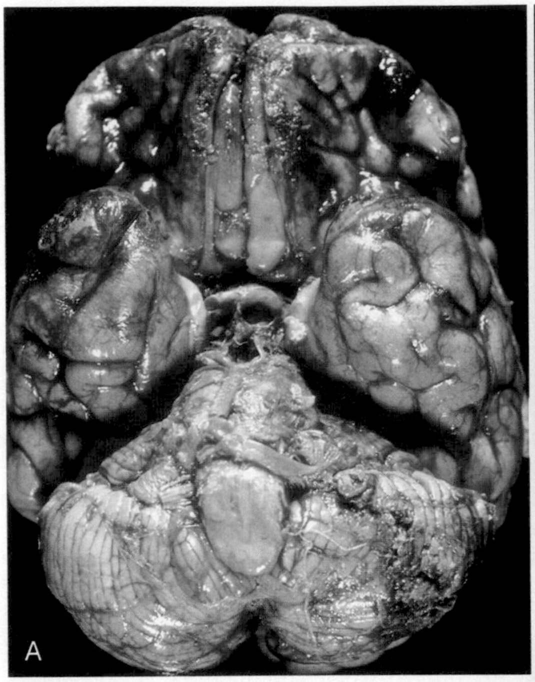

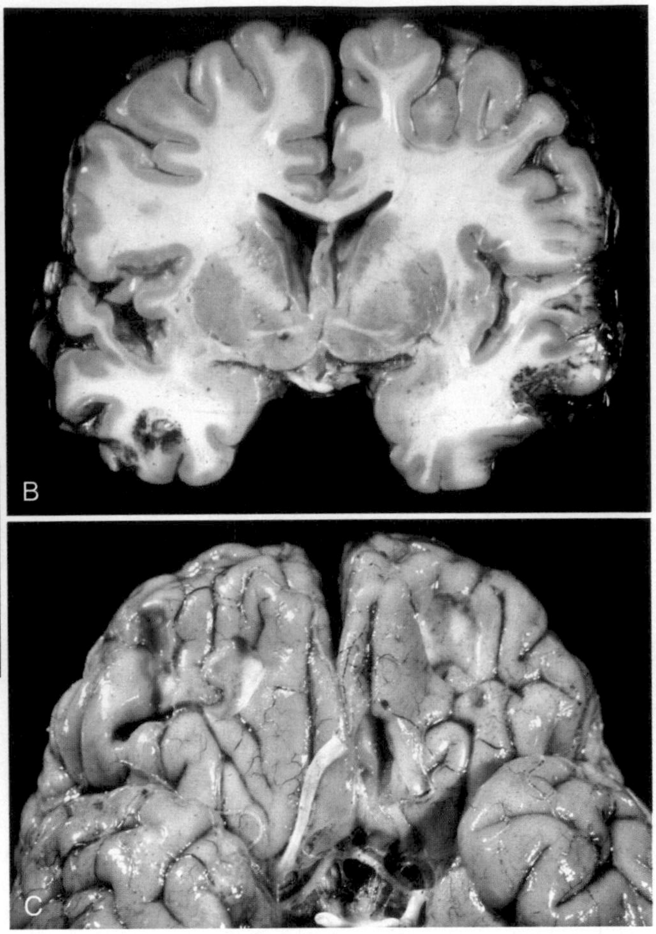

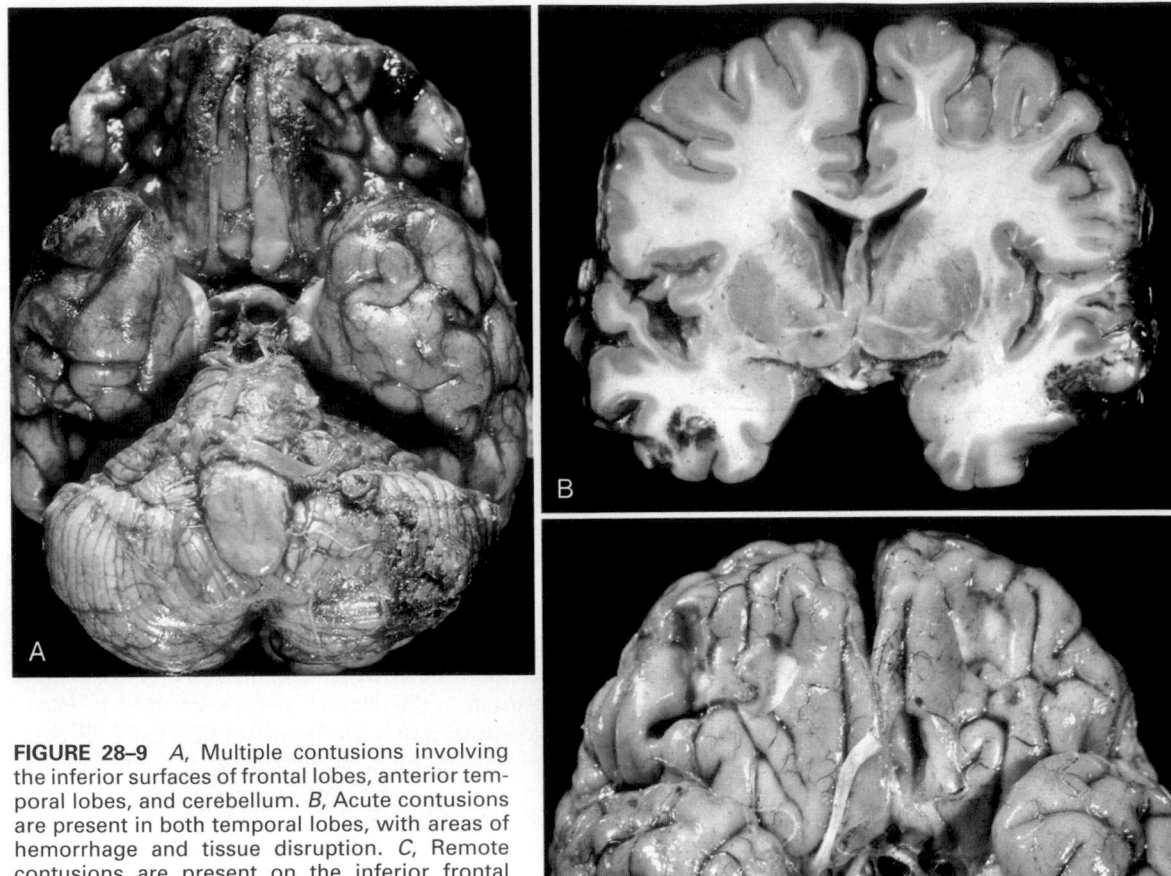

FIGURE 28–9 *A*, Multiple contusions involving the inferior surfaces of frontal lobes, anterior temporal lobes, and cerebellum. *B*, Acute contusions are present in both temporal lobes, with areas of hemorrhage and tissue disruption. *C*, Remote contusions are present on the inferior frontal surface of this brain, with a yellow color (associated with the term *plaque jaune*).

regions of brain trauma give rise to larger cavitated lesions, which can resemble remote infarcts. In sites of old contusions, gliosis and residual hemosiderin-laden macrophages predominate.

Sudden impacts that result in violent posterior or lateral hyperextension of the neck (as occurs when a pedestrian is struck from the rear by a vehicle) may actually avulse the pons from the medulla or the medulla from the cervical cord, causing instantaneous death.

Diffuse Axonal Injury

The surface of the brain is not the only region of damage in traumatic injury, although it is often the most affected. The deep centroaxial white matter regions—in the supratentorial compartment, particularly the corpus callosum, paraventricular and hippocampal areas and the brainstem along the cerebral peduncles, brachium conjunctivum, superior colliculi, and deep reticular formation—may also be involved. The microscopic findings include axonal swelling, indicative of *diffuse axonal injury*, and focal hemorrhagic lesions. Angular acceleration alone, in the absence of impact, can cause diffuse axonal injury as well as hemorrhage. As many as 50% of patients who develop coma shortly after trauma, even without cerebral contusions, are believed to have white matter damage and diffuse axonal injury. The most widely accepted explanation for diffuse axonal injury is that mechanical forces damage the integrity of the axon at the node of Ranvier, with subsequent alterations in axoplasmic flow.[42]

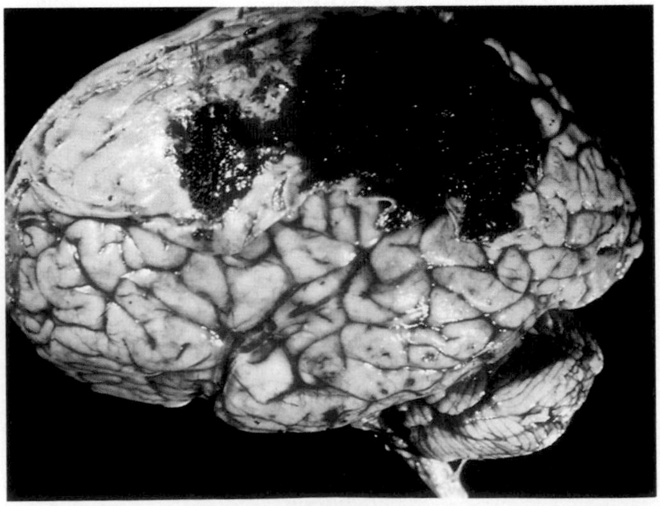

FIGURE 28–10 Epidural hematoma covering a portion of the dura. Multiple small contusions are seen in the temporal lobe. (Courtesy of Dr. Raymond D. Adams, Massachusetts General Hospital, Boston, MA.)

Morphology. The histopathology of diffuse axonal injury is characterized by the wide but often asymmetric distribution of axonal swellings that appear within hours of the injury and may persist for much longer. These are best demonstrated with silver impregnation techniques or with immunoperoxidase stains for Aβ protein.[43,44] Later, there are increased numbers of microglia in related areas of cerebral cortex and, subsequently, degeneration of the involved fiber tracts.

TRAUMATIC VASCULAR INJURY

Vascular injury is a frequent component of CNS trauma and results from direct trauma and disruption of the vessel wall, leading to hemorrhage. Depending on the anatomic position of the ruptured vessel, hemorrhage will occur in any of several compartments (sometimes in combination): *epidural*, *subdural*, *subarachnoid*, and *intraparenchymal* (Fig. 28–11). In the cavernous sinus, a traumatic tear of the carotid artery leads to the formation of an arteriovenous fistula.

Epidural Hematoma

The epidural space is a potential space, as the dura is closely applied to the internal surface of the skull and is fused with the periosteum. Vessels that course within the dura, most importantly the middle meningeal artery, are vulnerable to injury, particularly with skull fractures. Trauma to the skull, especially in the region of the temporal bone, can lead to laceration of this artery if the fracture lines cross the course of the vessel. In children, in whom the skull is deformable, a temporary displacement of the skull bones leading to laceration of a vessel can occur in the absence of a skull fracture.

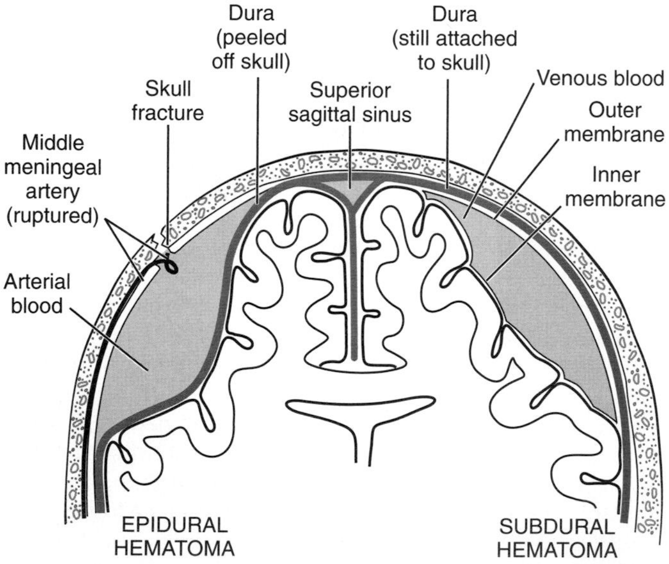

FIGURE 28–11 Epidural hematoma *(left)* in which rupture of a meningeal artery, usually associated with a skull fracture, leads to accumulation of arterial blood between the dura and the skull. In a subdural hematoma *(right)*, damage to bridging veins between the brain and the superior sagittal sinus leads to the accumulation of blood between the dura and the arachnoid.

Once a vessel has been torn, the accumulation of blood under arterial pressure can cause separation of the dura from the inner surface of the skull. The expanding hematoma has a smooth inner contour that compresses the brain surface (Fig. 28–10). Clinically, patients can be lucid for several hours between the moment of trauma and the development of neurologic signs. An epidural hematoma may expand rapidly and is a neurosurgical emergency requiring prompt drainage.

Subdural Hematoma

The space beneath the inner surface of the dura mater and the outer arachnoid layer of the leptomeninges is also a potential space. *Bridging veins* travel from the surface of the convexities of the cerebral hemispheres through the subarachnoid space and the subdural space to empty with dural vessels into the superior sagittal sinus. Similar anatomic relationships exist with other dural sinuses. These vessels are particularly prone to tearing along their course through the subdural space; they are the source of bleeding in most cases of subdural hematoma. The most commonly accepted mechanism of damage postulates that the brain, floating freely in its bath of CSF, can move within the skull, but the venous sinuses are fixed. The displacement of the brain that occurs in trauma can tear the veins at the point where they penetrate the dura. In elderly patients with brain atrophy, the bridging veins are stretched out and the brain has additional space for movement, hence the increased rate of subdural hematomas in these patients, even after relatively minor head trauma. Infants are also susceptible to subdural hematomas because their bridging veins are thin-walled.

Morphology. On macroscopic examination, the **acute subdural hematoma** appears as a collection of freshly clotted blood along the contour of the brain surface, without extension into the depths of sulci. The underlying brain is flattened, and the subarachnoid space is often clear. Typically, venous bleeding is self-limited; breakdown and organization of the hematoma take place in time. The organization of subdural hematomas typically occurs in the following sequence:

- Lysis of the clot (about 1 week)
- Growth of fibroblasts from the dural surface into the hematoma (2 weeks)
- Early development of hyalinized connective tissue (1 to 3 months)

A macroscopic characteristic of an organized hematoma is that the lesion is firmly attached by fibrous tissue only to the inner surface of the dura and is not at all adherent to the underlying smooth arachnoid, which does not contribute to its formation (Fig. 28–12). The lesion can eventually retract as the granulation tissue matures, until there may be only a thin layer of reactive connective tissue ("subdural membranes"). A common finding in subdural hematomas, however, is the occurrence of multiple episodes of rebleeding (**chronic subdural hematomas**), presumably from the thin-walled vessels of the granulation tissue. The risk of rebleeding is greatest in the first few months after the initial hemorrhage. The treatment of

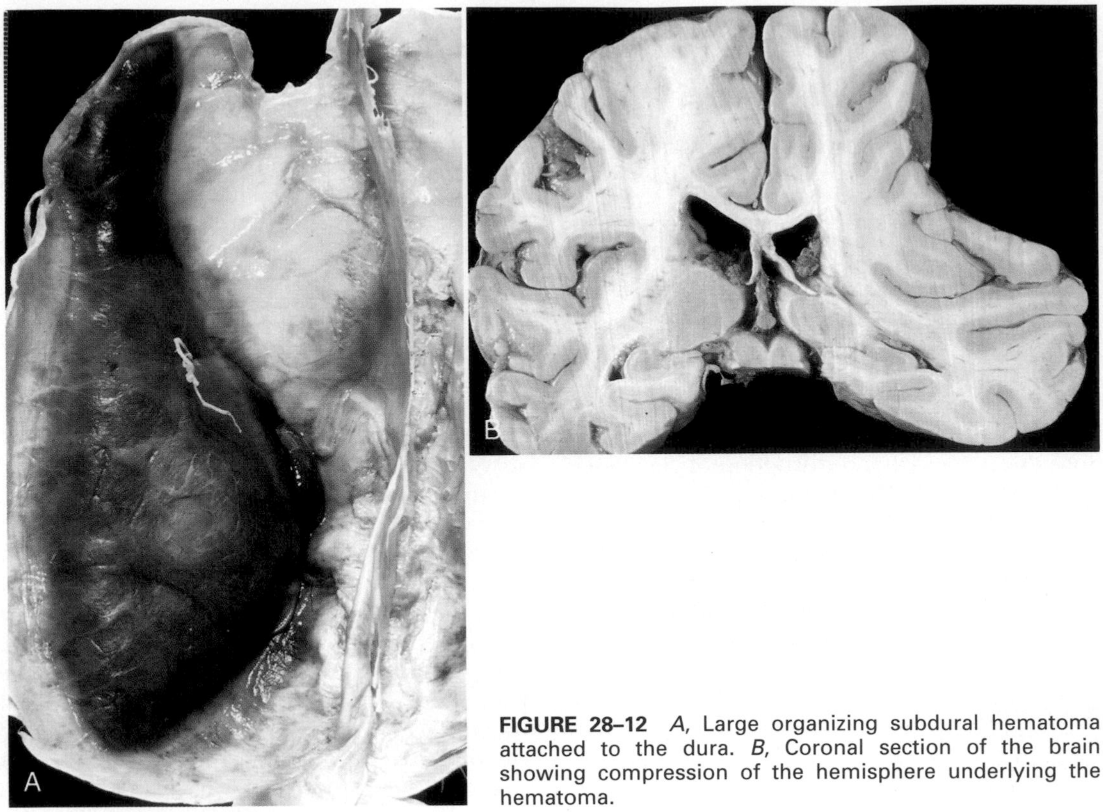

FIGURE 28–12 *A*, Large organizing subdural hematoma attached to the dura. *B*, Coronal section of the brain showing compression of the hemisphere underlying the hematoma.

subdural hematomas is to remove the organized blood and associated organizing tissue.

Subarachnoid and intraparenchymal hemorrhages most often occur concomitantly in the setting of brain trauma with superficial contusions and lacerations. Spät-apoplexie (delayed posttraumatic hemorrhage) is a syndrome of sudden, deep intracerebral hemorrhage that follows even minor head trauma by an interval of 1 to 2 weeks.

Clinical Features. Subdural hematomas most often become manifest within the first 48 hours after injury. They are most common over the lateral aspects of the cerebral hemispheres and are bilateral in about 10% of cases. Neurologic signs commonly observed are attributable to the pressure exerted on the adjacent brain. There may be focal signs, but often the clinical manifestations are nonlocalizing and include headache and confusion. In time, there may be slowly progressive neurologic deterioration, but acute decompensation is rare.

SEQUELAE OF BRAIN TRAUMA

The broad range of neurologic syndromes that become manifest months or years after brain trauma of any cause have gained increasing notice in the context of legal medicine and litigation involving issues of compensation of victims in the work force and the military services. *Posttraumatic hydrocephalus* is largely due to obstruction of CSF resorption from hemorrhage into the subarachnoid spaces. *Posttraumatic dementia* and the *punch-drunk syndrome* (dementia pugilistica) follow repeated head trauma during a protracted period; the neuropathologic findings include hydrocephalus, thinning of the corpus callosum, diffuse axonal injury, neurofibrillary tangles (mainly in the medial temporal areas), and diffuse Aβ-positive plaques (see the section on Alzheimer disease). Other important sequelae of brain trauma include posttraumatic epilepsy, brain tumors (meningioma), infectious diseases, and psychiatric disorders.[3]

SPINAL CORD TRAUMA

The spinal cord, normally protected within the bony vertebral canal, is vulnerable to trauma from its skeletal encasement. Most injuries that damage the cord are associated with displacement of the vertebral column, either rapid and temporary or persistent. The level of cord injury determines the extent of neurologic manifestations: Lesions involving the thoracic vertebrae or below can lead to paraplegia; cervical lesions result in quadriplegia; and those above C-4 can, in addition, lead to respiratory compromise from paralysis of the diaphragm. Segmental damage to the descending and ascending white matter tracts isolates the distal spinal cord from its cortical connections with the cerebrum and brainstem; this interruption, rather than the segmental gray matter damage that may occur at the level of the impact, causes the principal clinical deficits. Besides traumatic tissue disruption, progression and extension of the lesion occur secondary to vascular injury/ischemia and excitotoxicity.[45,46]

Morphology. The histologic changes of traumatic injury of the spinal cord are similar to those found at other sites in the CNS. At the level of injury, the acute phase consists of hemorrhage, necrosis, and axonal swelling in the surrounding white matter. The lesion tapers above and below the level of injury. In time, the central necrotic lesion becomes cystic and gliotic; cord sections above and below the lesion show secondary ascending and descending wallerian degeneration, respectively, involving the long white matter tracts affected at the site of trauma.

Cerebrovascular Diseases

Cerebrovascular disease is the third leading cause of death (after heart disease and cancer) in the United States; it is also the most prevalent neurologic disorder in terms of both morbidity and mortality. The term *cerebrovascular disease* denotes any abnormality of the brain caused by a pathologic process of blood vessels. Cerebrovascular diseases, from the clinical point of view, include three major categories: thrombosis, embolism, and hemorrhage; this operational division is useful especially because the management of patients differs greatly in each group. "Stroke" is the clinical designation that applies to all these conditions, particularly when symptoms begin acutely.[3,47] From the standpoint of pathophysiology and pathologic anatomy, it is convenient to consider cerebrovascular disease as two processes:

- Hypoxia, ischemia, and infarction resulting from impairment of blood supply and oxygenation of CNS tissue
- Hemorrhage resulting from rupture of CNS vessels

Some forms of hypertensive cerebrovascular disease combine aspects of both and are discussed separately. The most common cerebrovascular disorders are thrombosis secondary to atherosclerosis, embolism, hypertensive intraparenchymal hemorrhage, and ruptured aneurysm.

HYPOXIA, ISCHEMIA, AND INFARCTION

The brain requires a constant supply of glucose and oxygen, which is delivered by the circulation. Although the brain accounts for only 1% to 2% of body weight, it receives 15% of the resting cardiac output and accounts for 20% of the total body oxygen consumption. Cerebral blood flow, normally about 50 mL per minute for each 100 gm of tissue (with considerable regional variations between white and gray matter and among different portions of the gray matter), remains constant over a wide range of blood pressure and intracranial pressure because of autoregulation of vascular resistance. The brain is a highly aerobic tissue, with oxygen rather than metabolic substrate serving as the limiting substance. The brain may be deprived of oxygen by any of several mechanisms: *functional hypoxia* in a setting of a low partial pressure of oxygen (pO_2), impaired oxygen-carrying capacity of the blood, or inhibition of oxygen use by tissue; or *ischemia*, either transient or permanent, after interruption of the normal circulatory flow. Cessation of blood flow can result from a reduction in perfusion pressure, as in hypotension, or secondary to small- or large-vessel obstruction, or both.

When blood flow to a portion of the brain is reduced, the survival of the tissue at risk depends on a number of modifying factors: the availability of collateral circulation, the duration of ischemia, and the magnitude and rapidity of the reduction of flow. These factors will determine, in turn, the precise anatomic site and size of the lesion and, consequently, the clinical deficit. Two principal types of acute ischemic injury are recognized:

- *Global cerebral ischemia* (ischemic/hypoxic encephalopathy) occurs when there is a generalized reduction of cerebral perfusion, such as in cardiac arrest, shock, and severe hypotension.
- *Focal cerebral ischemia* follows reduction or cessation of blood flow to a localized area of the brain due to large-vessel disease (such as embolic or thrombotic arterial occlusion, often in a setting of atherosclerosis) or to small-vessel disease (such as vasculitis or occlusion secondary to arteriosclerotic lesions seen in hypertension).

Hypotension, Hypoperfusion, and Low-Flow States (Global Cerebral Ischemia)

The clinical outcome of a severe hypotensive episode that produces *global cerebral ischemia (diffuse hypoxic/ischemic encephalopathy)* varies with the severity of the insult. In mild cases, there may be only a transient postischemic confusional state, with eventual complete recovery and no irreversible tissue damage. On the other hand, irreversible damage to CNS tissue does occur in some patients who suffer mild or transient global ischemic insults. There is a hierarchy of CNS cells that show preferential susceptibility. Neurons are the most sensitive cells, although glial cells (oligodendrocytes and astrocytes) are also vulnerable. There is also great variability in the susceptibility of different populations of neurons in different regions of the CNS (*selective vulnerability*); this is based in part on differences in regional cerebral blood flow and cellular metabolic requirements. In severe global cerebral ischemia, widespread neuronal death, irrespective of regional vulnerability, occurs. Patients who survive in this state often remain severely impaired neurologically and deeply comatose (persistent vegetative state). Other patients meet the current clinical criteria for "brain death," including persistent evidence of diffuse cortical injury (isoelectric, or "flat," electroencephalogram) as well as brainstem damage, including absent reflexes and respiratory drive, and absent cerebral perfusion. When patients with this pervasive form of injury are maintained on mechanical ventilation, the brain gradually undergoes an autolytic process, leading to soft disintegrated tissue that does not fix well in formalin and stains poorly with dyes—so-called "respirator brain."

Morphology. In the setting of global ischemia, the brain is swollen, the gyri are widened, and the sulci are narrowed. The cut surface shows poor demarcation between gray and white matter. The histopathologic changes that attend irreversible ischemic injury (infarction) are grouped into three categories. **Early changes,** occurring 12 to 24 hours after the insult, include acute neuronal cell change (red neurons; Figs. 28–13*A* and 28–13*B*) characterized at first by microvacuolization, then eosinophilia of the neuronal cytoplasm, and later nuclear pyknosis and karyorrhexis. Similar acute changes occur somewhat later in

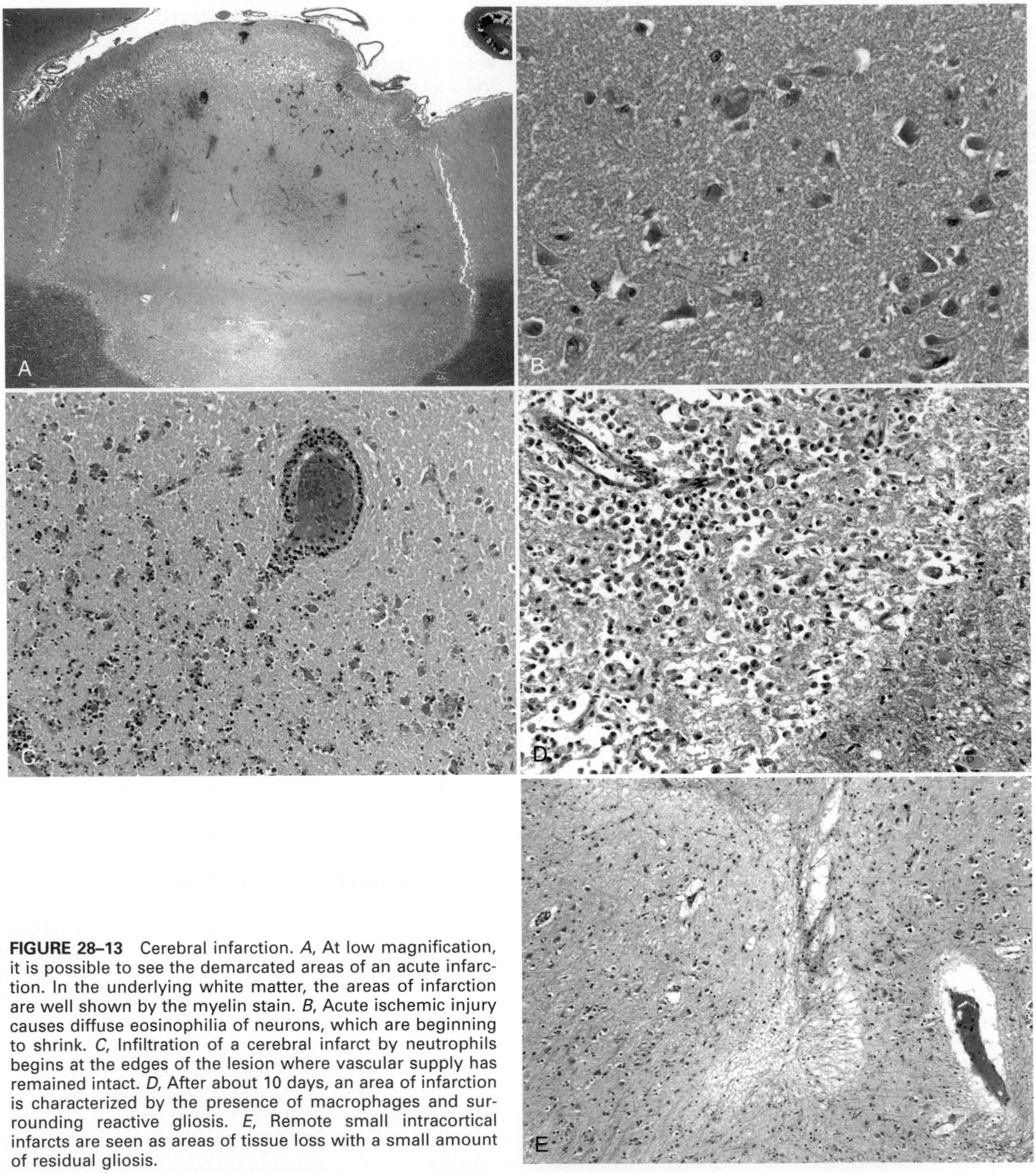

FIGURE 28–13 Cerebral infarction. *A*, At low magnification, it is possible to see the demarcated areas of an acute infarction. In the underlying white matter, the areas of infarction are well shown by the myelin stain. *B*, Acute ischemic injury causes diffuse eosinophilia of neurons, which are beginning to shrink. *C*, Infiltration of a cerebral infarct by neutrophils begins at the edges of the lesion where vascular supply has remained intact. *D*, After about 10 days, an area of infarction is characterized by the presence of macrophages and surrounding reactive gliosis. *E*, Remote small intracortical infarcts are seen as areas of tissue loss with a small amount of residual gliosis.

astrocytes and oligodendroglia. Pyramidal cells of the Sommer sector (CA1) of the hippocampus, Purkinje cells of the cerebellum, and pyramidal neurons in the neocortex are the most susceptible to global ischemia of short duration. After the acute injury, the reaction to tissue damage begins with infiltration by neutrophils (Fig. 28–13*C*). **Subacute changes,** occurring at 24 hours to 2 weeks, include necrosis of tissue, influx of macrophages, vascular proliferation, and reactive gliosis (Fig. 28–13*D*). **Repair,** seen after approximately 2 weeks, is characterized by eventual removal of all necrotic tissue, loss of normally organized CNS structure, and gliosis (Fig. 28–13*E*). In the cerebral cortex, the neuronal loss and gliosis produce an uneven destruction of the neocortex, with preservation of some layers and involvement of others, a pattern termed *pseudolaminar necrosis*.

Border zone ("watershed") infarcts are wedge-shaped areas of infarction that occur in the regions of the brain and spinal cord that lie at the most distal fields of arterial irrigation. In the cerebral hemispheres, the border zone between the anterior and the middle cerebral artery distributions is at greatest risk. Damage to this region produces a sickle-shaped band of necrosis over the cerebral convexity a few centimeters lateral to the interhemispheric fissure. Border zone infarcts are usually seen after hypotensive episodes.

Infarction from Obstruction of Local Blood Supply (Focal Cerebral Ischemia)

Cerebral arterial occlusion may lead to focal ischemia and ultimately, if it is sustained, to infarction of a specific region of CNS tissue within the territory of distribution of the compromised vessel. The size, location, and shape of the infarct and the extent of tissue damage that results from focal cerebral ischemia brought about by occlusion of a blood vessel are determined by the *modifying factors* mentioned earlier, the most important being the adequacy of collateral flow. The major source of collateral flow is the circle of Willis (supplemented by the external carotid-ophthalmic pathway). Partial and inconstant reinforcement is available over the surface of the brain for the distal branches of the anterior, middle, and posterior cerebral arteries through cortical-leptomeningeal anastomoses. In contrast, there is little if any collateral flow for the deep penetrating vessels supplying structures such as the thalamus, basal ganglia, and deep white matter.

The biochemical changes that attend the cellular reactions in ischemia are discussed in Chapter 1. There are, however, several special responses to ischemia in the central nervous system.[2] Excitatory amino acid neurotransmitters, such as glutamate, are released during ischemia and may cause cell damage by overstimulation and persistent opening of specific membrane channels including *N*-methyl-D-aspartate and kainate receptors. This may cause cell death through an uncontrolled influx of calcium ions or through the neurotransmitter and potential toxin nitric oxide. Inhibitors of these ion channels or of nitric oxide synthase protect against the effects of cerebral ischemia in some experimental models and may have therapeutic potential in humans.[48]

Occlusive vascular disease of severity sufficient to lead to cerebral infarction may be due to *in situ thrombosis* or *embolization* from a distant source; the pathology of these conditions is discussed in Chapters 4 and 11.

The majority of thrombotic occlusions are due to atherosclerosis. The most common sites of primary thrombosis causing cerebral infarction are the carotid bifurcation, the origin of the middle cerebral artery, and either end of the basilar artery.[49] The evolution of arterial stenosis varies from progressive narrowing of the lumen and thrombosis, which may be accompanied by anterograde extension, to fragmentation and distal embolization. Another important aspect of occlusive cerebrovascular disease is its frequent association with systemic diseases such as hypertension and diabetes.

A variety of inflammatory processes that involve blood vessels may lead to luminal compromise and cerebral infarcts.[50] In years past, *arteritis* of small and large vessels was found most commonly in association with syphilis and tuberculosis; infectious vasculitis is now more commonly seen in the setting of immunosuppression and opportunistic infection (such as toxoplasmosis, aspergillosis, and CMV encephalitis). Polyarteritis nodosa and other collagen-vascular diseases may involve cerebral vessels and cause single or multiple infarcts throughout the brain. *Primary angiitis of the central nervous system* is an inflammatory disorder that involves multiple small to medium-sized parenchymal and subarachnoid vessels and is characterized by chronic inflammation, multinucleated giant cells, and destruction of the vessel wall.[51] The granuloma formation associated with the giant cells in many cases underlies the alternative name for the disease: granulomatous angiitis of the nervous system. Affected individuals manifest a diffuse encephalopathic or multifocal clinical picture, often with cognitive dysfunction; patients improve with steroid and immunosuppressive treatment. Other conditions that may cause thrombosis and infarction (and intracranial hemorrhage) include hematologic disease with hypercoagulable states, dissecting aneurysm of extracranial arteries in the neck vessels supplying the brain, and drug abuse (amphetamines, heroin, cocaine).

Cerebral autosomal-dominant arteriopathy with subcortical infarcts and leukoencephalopathy (CADASIL) is a rare hereditary form of stroke caused by mutations in the *Notch3* gene.[52,53] The disease is characterized clinically by recurrent strokes (usually infarcts, less often hemorrhages) and dementia. Histopathologic study has shown abnormalities of white matter and leptomeningeal arteries (also involving non-CNS vessels) consisting of concentric thickening of the media and adventitia. Basophilic, PAS-positive granules, which appear as osmiophilic compact deposits of granular material by electron microscopy, have been consistently detected in the walls of affected vessels, with loss of smooth muscle cells. The diagnosis can be made through the identification of these deposits in other tissues, such as skin or muscle biopsies. Many of the *Notch3* mutations add or remove Cys residues from the EGF repeats of the extracellular domain of the protein. The underlying mechanism linking the mutations to disease remains unclear; possibilities include altered processing of this protein,[54] altered signaling,[55] or protein aggregation.[56]

Cerebral amyloid angiopathy (CAA) is a condition in which amyloidogenic peptides, nearly always the same one found in Alzheimer disease ($A\beta_{40}$; see the discussion below), deposit in the walls of medium- and small-caliber meningeal and cortical vessels. This deposition can result in weakening of the vessel wall and risk of hemorrhage.[57] There is an effect of apoE genotype on the risk of recurrence of hemorrhage from sporadic CAA, the presence of either an ε2 or ε4 allele increasing the risk of rebleeding.[58] This is of note since there is also an interaction between apoE genotype and Alzheimer disease. A mutation in the precursor protein for the $A\beta_{40}$ peptide (amyloid precursor protein, APP) causes a familial form of CAA, termed *hereditary cerebral hemorrhage with amyloidosis, Dutch type*. Another peptide that can be found in a similar disorder is derived from cystatin C (a secreted inhibitor of cysteine proteases), which causes the syndrome of *hereditary cerebral hemorrhage with amyloidosis, Icelandic type*.

Embolism to the brain occurs from a wide range of origins. Cardiac mural thrombi are among the most common sources; myocardial infarct, valvular disease, and atrial fibrillation are important predisposing factors. Next in importance are thromboemboli arising in arteries, most often originating over atheromatous plaques within the carotid arteries. Other sources of emboli include paradoxical emboli, particularly in children with cardiac anomalies; emboli associated with cardiac surgery; and emboli of other material (tumor, fat, or air). The territory of distribution of the middle cerebral artery—the direct extension of the internal carotid artery—is most frequently affected by embolic infarction; the incidence is about equal in the two hemispheres. Emboli tend to lodge where blood vessels branch or in areas of pre-existing luminal stenosis. In many cases, the site of occlusion cannot be identified at postmortem examination, perhaps because the embolus has lysed by the time the tissue is examined. "Shower embolization," as in fat embolism, may occur after fractures; affected patients manifest generalized cerebral dysfunction with disturbances of higher cortical function and consciousness, often without localizing signs. Widespread hemorrhagic lesions involving the white matter are characteristic of embolization of bone marrow after trauma (Fig. 28–14).

Infarcts are subdivided into two broad groups based on their macroscopic and corresponding radiologic appearance (Fig. 28–15). *Hemorrhagic (red) infarction*, characterized macroscopically by multiple, sometimes confluent, petechial hemorrhages, is typically associated with embolic events (Figs.

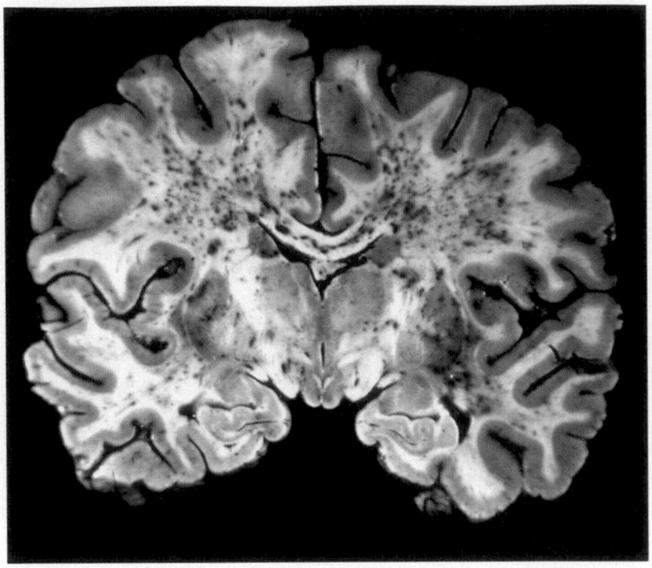

FIGURE 28–14 Widespread white matter hemorrhages are characteristic of bone marrow embolization.

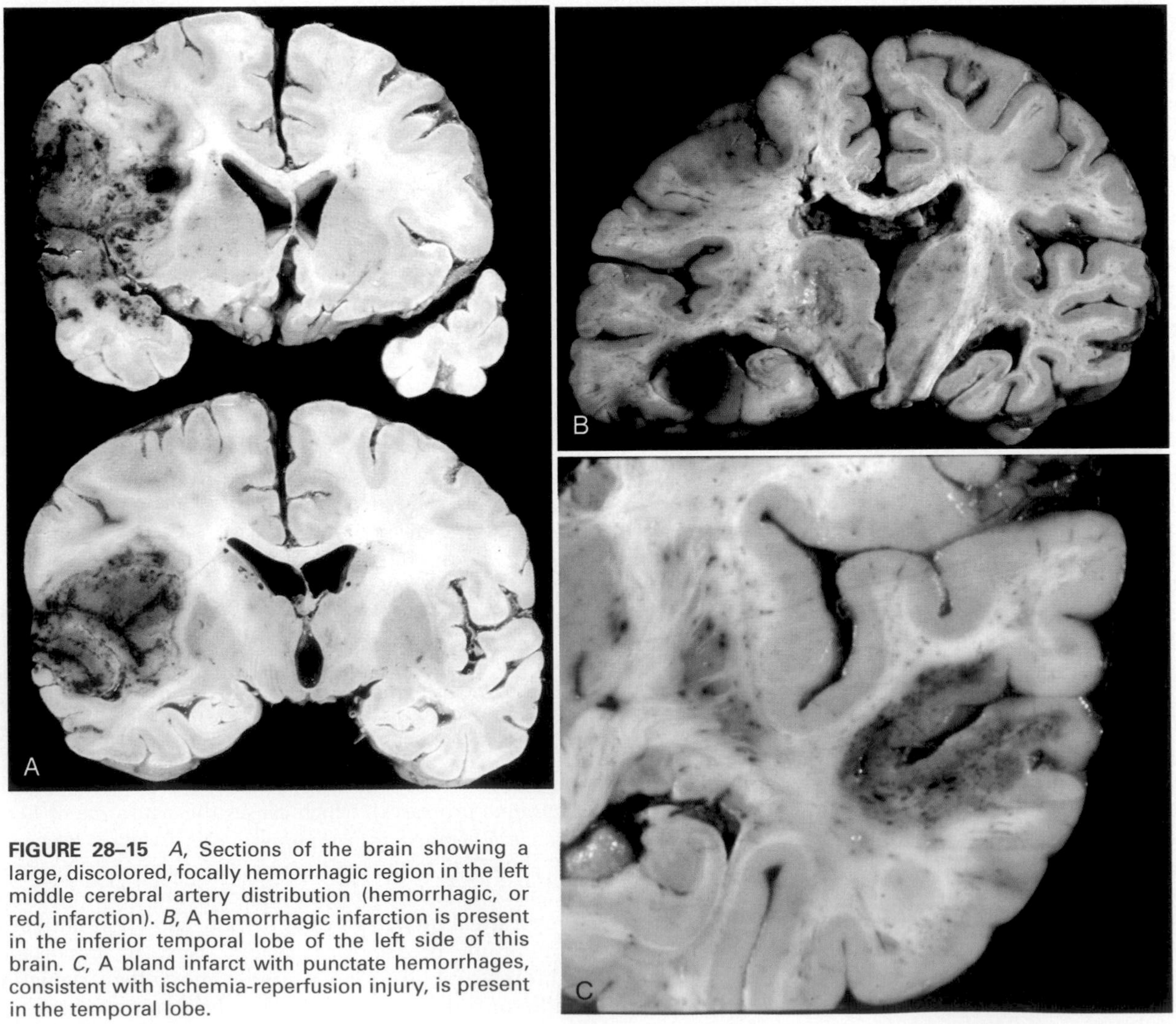

FIGURE 28–15 *A*, Sections of the brain showing a large, discolored, focally hemorrhagic region in the left middle cerebral artery distribution (hemorrhagic, or red, infarction). *B*, A hemorrhagic infarction is present in the inferior temporal lobe of the left side of this brain. *C*, A bland infarct with punctate hemorrhages, consistent with ischemia-reperfusion injury, is present in the temporal lobe.

28–15*A* and 28–15*B*). The hemorrhage is presumed to be secondary to reperfusion of damaged vessels and tissue, either through collaterals or directly after dissolution of intravascular occlusive material. In contrast, *nonhemorrhagic (pale, bland, anemic) infarcts* are usually associated with thrombosis (Fig. 28–15*C*). The clinical management of patients with these two types of infarcts differs greatly: For obvious reasons, anticoagulation may be used in cases of thrombosis but is contraindicated in hemorrhagic infarcts.

Morphology. The macroscopic appearance of a **nonhemorrhagic infarct** changes with time. During the first 6 hours of irreversible injury, little can be observed. By 48 hours, the tissue becomes pale, soft, and swollen, and the corticomedullary junction becomes indistinct. From 2 to 10 days, the brain becomes gelatinous and friable, and the previously ill-defined boundary between normal and abnormal tissue becomes more distinct as edema resolves in the adjacent tissue that has survived. From 10 days to 3 weeks, the tissue liquefies, eventually leaving a fluid-filled cavity lined by dark gray tissue, which gradually expands as dead tissue is removed (Fig. 28–16).

On microscopic examination, the tissue reaction evolves along the following sequence: *After the first 12 hours,* ischemic neuronal change (red neurons; see earlier) and both cytotoxic and vasogenic edema predominate. There is loss of the usual tinctorial characteristics of white and gray matter structures. Endothelial and glial cells, mainly astrocytes, swell, and myelinated fibers begin to disintegrate. *Up to 48 hours,* neutrophilic emigration progressively increases and then falls off. Phagocytic cells derived from circulating monocytes and activated microglia are evident at 48 hours and become the predominant cell type in the ensuing *2 to 3 weeks.* The macrophages become stuffed with the products of myelin breakdown or blood and may persist in the lesion for months to years. As the process of liquefaction and phagocytosis proceeds, astrocytes at the edges of the lesion progressively enlarge, divide, and develop a prominent network of protoplasmic extensions. Reactive astrocytes can be seen as early as *1 week* after the insult.

After several months, the striking astrocytic nuclear and cytoplasmic enlargement recedes. In the wall of the cavity, astrocyte processes form a dense feltwork of glial fibers admixed with new capillaries and a few perivascular connective tissue fibers. In the cerebral cortex, the cavity is delimited from the meninges and subarachnoid space by a gliotic layer of tissue, derived from the molecular layer of the cortex. The pia and arachnoid are not affected and do not contribute to the healing process.

The microscopic picture and evolution of **hemorrhagic infarction** parallel ischemic infarction, with the addition of blood extravasation and resorption. In patients receiving anticoagulant treatment, hemorrhagic infarcts may be associated with extensive intracerebral hematomas. Venous infarcts are often hemorrhagic, and may occur after thrombotic occlusion of the superior sagittal sinus or other sinuses or occlusion of the deep cerebral veins. Carcinoma, localized infections, and other conditions leading to a hypercoagulable state place patients at risk for venous thrombosis.

Incomplete infarction occurs in focal cerebral ischemia when there is selective necrosis of neurons with relative preservation of glia and supporting tissues; it is reproduced in experimental animals by transient and incomplete focal ischemia and reperfusion.[59,60]

Spinal cord infarction may be seen in the setting of hypoperfusion or as a consequence of interruption of the feeding tributaries derived from the aorta. Occlusion of the anterior spinal artery is rarer and may occur as a result of embolism or vasculitis.

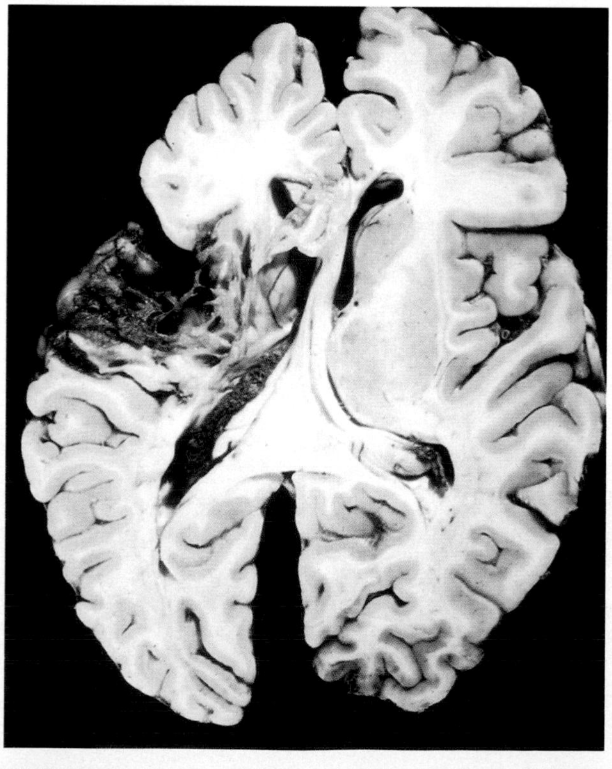

FIGURE 28–16 Old cystic infarct. Destruction of cortex and surrounding gliosis.

Clinical Features. The area of the brain that is affected determines whether the patient remains asymptomatic or develops a hemiplegia, a sensory deficit, blindness, aphasia, or some other deficit. The deficit evolves over time, and the outcome either is fatal or is characterized by some degree of slow improvement during a period of months. Genetic risk factors for stroke are currently being elucidated, but the nature of the relevant genes and their links with the underlying mechanisms of infarction are unknown.[61]

INTRACRANIAL HEMORRHAGE

Hemorrhages may occur at any site within the CNS. In some instances, they may be a secondary phenomenon occurring, for example, within infarcts in arterial border zones or in infarcts caused by only partial or transient vascular obstruction. Primary hemorrhages within the epidural or subdural space are typically related to trauma and were discussed earlier with traumatic lesions. Hemorrhages within the brain parenchyma and subarachnoid space, in contrast, are often a manifestation of underlying cerebrovascular disease, although trauma may also cause hemorrhage in these sites.

Intracerebral (Intraparenchymal) Hemorrhage

Spontaneous (nontraumatic) intraparenchymal hemorrhages occur most commonly in middle to late adult life, with a peak incidence at about age 60 years. Most are caused by rupture of a small intraparenchymal vessel. *Hypertension is the most common underlying cause of primary brain parenchymal hemorrhage,* accounting for more than 50% of clinically significant hemorrhages. Conversely, brain hemorrhage accounts for roughly 15% of deaths among patients with chronic hypertension. Hypertension causes a number of abnormalities in vessel walls, including accelerated atherosclerosis in larger arteries; hyaline arteriolosclerosis in smaller vessels; and, in severe cases, proliferative changes and frank necrosis of arterioles. Arteriolar walls affected by hyaline change are presumably weaker than are normal vessels and are therefore more vulnerable to rupture. In some instances, chronic hypertension is associated with the development of minute aneurysms, termed *Charcot-Bouchard microaneurysms,* which may be the site of rupture. Charcot-Bouchard aneurysms, not to be confused with saccular aneurysms of larger intracranial vessels, occur in vessels that are less than 300 μm in diameter, most commonly within the basal ganglia. In addition to hypertension, other local and systemic factors may cause or contribute to nontraumatic hemorrhage, including systemic coagulation disorders, open heart surgery, neoplasms, amyloid angiopathy, vasculitis, fusiform aneurysms, and vascular malformations.

Morphology. Hypertensive intraparenchymal hemorrhage may originate in the putamen (50% to 60% of cases), thalamus, pons, cerebellar hemispheres (rarely), and other regions of the brain (Fig. 28–17). When the hemorrhages occur in the basal ganglia and thalamus, they are designated **ganglionic hemorrhages** to distinguish them from those that occur in the lobes of the cerebral hemispheres, which are called **lobar hemorrhages.** Acute hemorrhages of either type are characterized by extravasation of blood with compression of the adjacent parenchyma. Old hemorrhages show an area of cavitary destruction of brain with a rim of brownish discoloration. On microscopic examination, the early lesion consists of a central core of clotted blood surrounded by a rim of brain tissue showing anoxic neuronal and glial changes as well as edema. Eventually, the edema resolves, pigment- and lipid-laden macrophages appear, and proliferation of reactive astrocytes is seen at the periphery of the lesion. The cellular events then follow the same time course that is observed after cerebral infarction.

Lobar hemorrhages[62] may arise in the setting of hemorrhagic diathesis, neoplasms, drug abuse, infectious and noninfectious vasculitis, and **cerebral amyloid angiopathy**.

Clinical Features. Intracerebral hemorrhage can be clinically devastating when it affects large portions of the brain and extends into the ventricular system, or it can affect small regions and either be clinically silent or evolve like an infarct. Over weeks or months, there is a gradual resolution of the hematoma, sometimes with considerable clinical improvement. Again, the location of the bleed will determine the clinical manifestations.

Subarachnoid Hemorrhage and Ruptured Saccular Aneurysms

The most frequent cause of clinically significant subarachnoid hemorrhage is rupture of a *saccular (berry) aneurysm.* Subarachnoid hemorrhage may also result from extension of a traumatic hematoma, rupture of a hypertensive intracerebral hemorrhage into the ventricular system, vascular malformation, hematologic disturbances, and tumors.

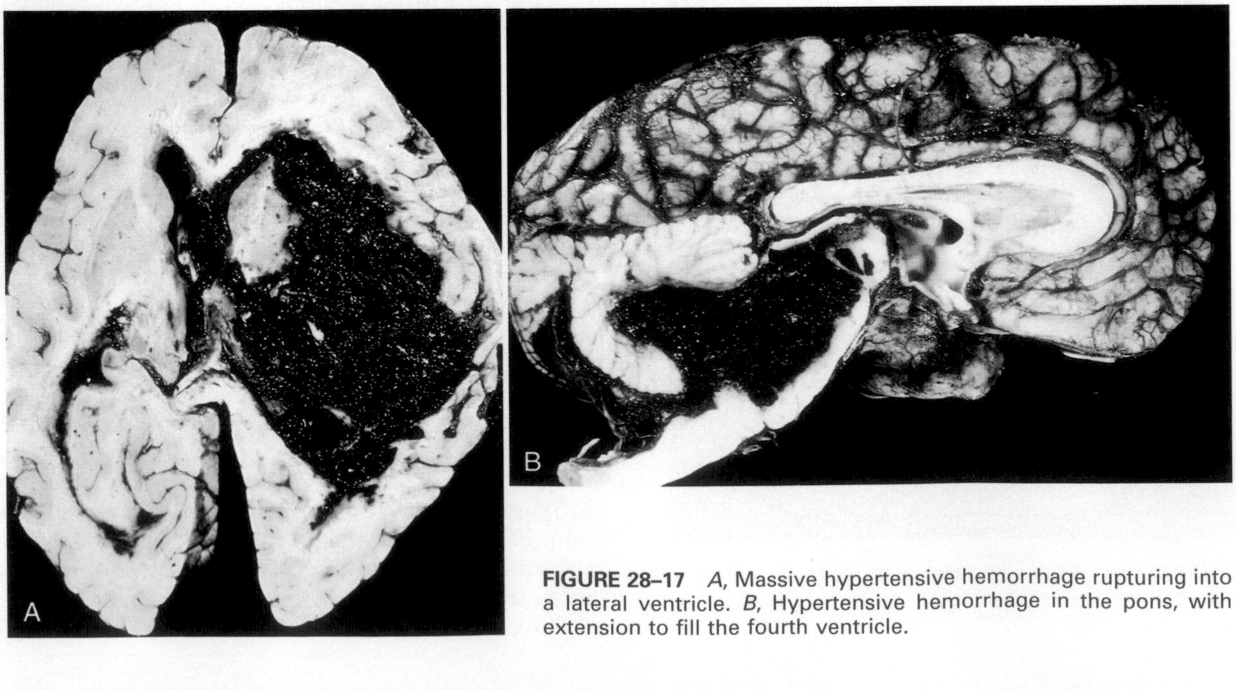

FIGURE 28–17 *A,* Massive hypertensive hemorrhage rupturing into a lateral ventricle. *B,* Hypertensive hemorrhage in the pons, with extension to fill the fourth ventricle.

Saccular (berry) aneurysm (congenital aneurysm) is the most common type of intracranial aneurysm.[63] Other, rarer, types of aneurysms include atherosclerotic (fusiform; mostly of the basilar artery), mycotic, traumatic, and dissecting aneurysms. These latter three, like saccular aneurysms, are most often found in the anterior circulation. They usually present with cerebral infarction rather than subarachnoid hemorrhage.

Saccular aneurysms, ruptured and unruptured, are found in about 2% of postmortem examinations; a somewhat lower figure is reported from radiologic clinics.[64] About 90% of saccular aneurysms occur in the anterior circulation and are found near major arterial branch points (Fig. 28–18); multiple aneurysms exist in 20% to 30% of cases in autopsy series.

Pathogenesis of Saccular Aneurysms. The etiology of saccular aneurysms is unknown. Although the majority occur sporadically, genetic factors may be important in their pathogenesis. There is an increased risk of occurrence among patients with certain heritable disorders (such as autosomal-dominant polycystic kidney disease, vascular type Ehlers-Danlos syndrome [type IV], neurofibromatosis type 1, and Marfan syndrome) and with fibromuscular dysplasia of extracranial arteries and coarctation of the aorta. Cigarette smoking and hypertension (estimated to be present in 54% of these patients) are accepted predisposing factors for the development of saccular aneurysms. Although they are sometimes referred to as congenital, the aneurysms are not present at birth but develop over time owing to the underlying defect in the media of the vessel.

Morphology. An unruptured saccular aneurysm is a thin-walled outpouching at an arterial branch point along the circle of Willis or a major vessel just beyond. Saccular aneurysms measure a few millimeters to 2 or 3 cm in diameter and have a bright red, shiny surface and a thin, translucent wall (Fig. 28–19). Demonstration of the site of rupture requires careful dissection and removal of blood in the unfixed brain. Atheromatous plaques, calcification, or thrombotic occlusion of the sac may be found in the wall or lumen of the aneurysm. Brownish discoloration of the adjacent brain and meninges is evidence of prior hemorrhage. The neck of the aneurysm may be either wide or narrow. Rupture usually occurs at the apex of the sac with extravasation of blood into the subarachnoid space, the substance of the brain, or both. The arterial wall adjacent to the neck of the aneurysm often shows some intimal thickening and gradual attenuation of the media as it approaches the neck. At the neck of the aneurysm, the muscular wall and intimal elastic lamina stop short and are absent from the aneurysm sac itself. The sac is made up of thickened hyalinized intima. The adventitia covering the sac is continuous with that of the parent artery.

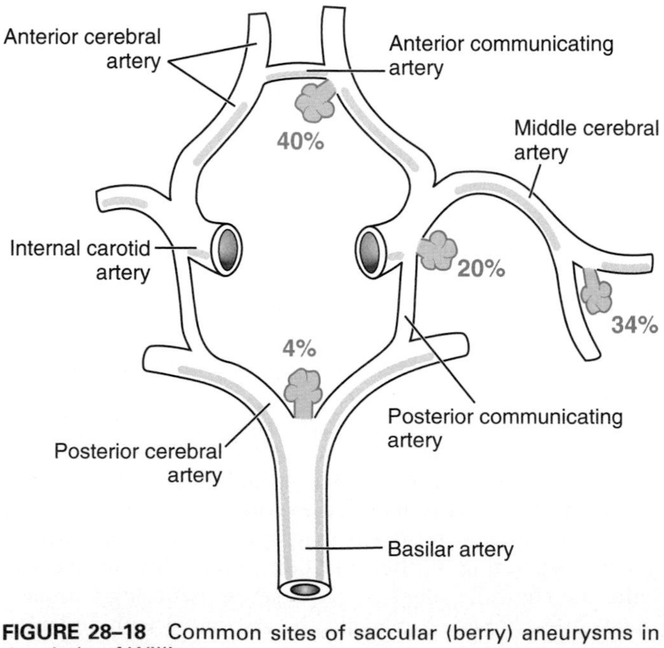

FIGURE 28–18 Common sites of saccular (berry) aneurysms in the circle of Willis.

Clinical Features. Rupture of an aneurysm with clinically significant subarachnoid hemorrhage is most frequent in the fifth decade and is slightly more frequent in females. When estimated across the range of aneurysm sizes, there is a roughly 1.3% per year rate of bleeding, although the probability of rupture increases with the size of the lesion.[65] Aneurysms greater than 10 mm in diameter have a roughly 50% risk of bleeding per year. Rupture may occur at any time but in about one-third of cases it is associated with acute increases in intracranial pressure, such as with straining at stool or sexual orgasm. Blood under arterial pressure is forced into the subarachnoid space, and patients are stricken with a sudden, excruciating headache, typically "the worst headache I've ever had," and rapidly lose consciousness. Between 25% and 50% of patients die with the first rupture, but most patients who survive improve and recover consciousness in minutes. Rebleeding is common in survivors, and it is currently not possible to predict in which patients rebleeding will occur. With each episode of bleeding, the prognosis is worse.

The clinical consequences of blood in the subarachnoid space can be separated into acute events, occurring in the hours to days after the hemorrhage, and late sequelae associated with the healing process. In the early post-subarachnoid hemorrhage period, regardless of the etiology of the hemorrhage, there is an increased risk of injury from vasospasm involving vessels other than those originally injured. This vasospasm can lead to additional ischemic injury. This problem is of greatest significance in cases of basal subarachnoid hemorrhage, in which vasospasm can involve major vessels of the circle of Willis. Various mediators have been proposed to play a role in this reactive process; some data suggest a vasoconstrictive effect of endothelin-1 acting from the adventitial side, associated with a reduced level of the vasodilator NO.[66] In the healing phase of subarachnoid hemorrhage, meningeal fibrosis and scarring occur, sometimes leading to obstruction of CSF flow as well as interruption of the normal pathways of CSF resorption.

Vascular Malformations

Vascular malformations of the brain are classified into four principal groups: arteriovenous malformations, cavernous angiomas, capillary telangiectasias, and venous angiomas.

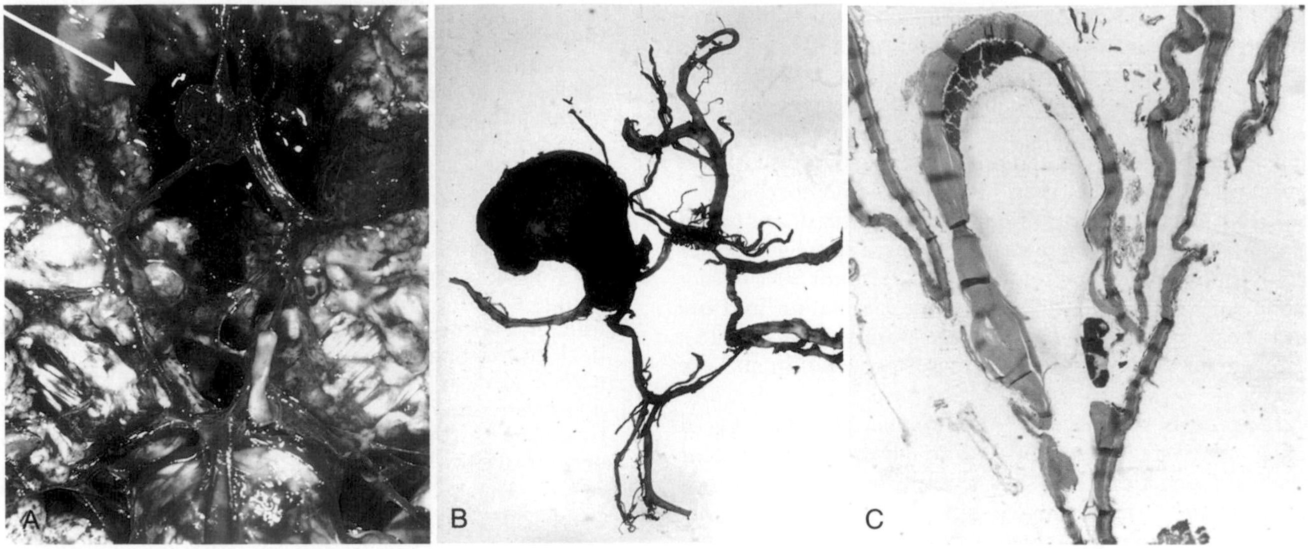

FIGURE 28–19 *A*, View of the base of the brain, dissected to show the circle of Willis with an aneurysm of the anterior cerebral artery *(arrow)*. *B*, Dissected circle of Willis to show large aneurysm. *C*, Section through a saccular aneurysm showing the hyalinized fibrous vessel wall (H & E).

Morphology. Arteriovenous malformations involve vessels in the subarachnoid space extending into brain parenchyma or may occur exclusively within the brain. In macroscopic appearance, they resemble a tangled network of wormlike vascular channels and have a prominent, pulsatile arteriovenous shunt with high blood flow through the malformation. On microscopic examination, they are composed of greatly enlarged blood vessels separated by gliotic tissue, often with evidence of prior hemorrhage. Some vessels can be recognized as arteries with duplication and fragmentation of the internal elastic lamina, while others show marked thickening or partial replacement of the media by hyalinized connective tissue.

Cavernous hemangiomas consist of greatly distended, loosely organized vascular channels with thin, collagenized walls and are devoid of intervening nervous tissue (thus distinguishing them from capillary telangiectasias). They occur most often in the cerebellum, pons, and subcortical regions, in decreasing order of frequency, and have a low flow without arteriovenous shunting. Foci of old hemorrhage, infarction, and calcification frequently surround the abnormal vessels. **Capillary telangiectasias** are microscopic foci of dilated, thin-walled vascular channels separated by relatively normal brain parenchyma and occurring most frequently in the pons. **Venous angiomas** (varices) consist of aggregates of ectatic venous channels. **Foix-Alajouanine disease** (angiodysgenetic necrotizing myelopathy) is a venous angiomatous malformation of the spinal cord and overlying meninges associated with ischemic myelomalacia and slowly progressive neurologic symptoms most often referable to the lumbosacral cord.

Clinical Features. Arteriovenous malformations are the most common type of clinically significant vascular malformation. Males are affected twice as frequently as females, and the lesion is often recognized clinically between the ages of 10 and 30 years, presenting as a seizure disorder, an intracerebral hemorrhage, or a subarachnoid hemorrhage. The most common site is the territory of the middle cerebral artery, particularly its posterior branches, but arteriovenous malformations may occur anywhere along the midbrain, cerebellum, or spinal cord. Large arteriovenous malformations occurring in the newborn period can lead to congestive heart failure because of shunt effects, especially if the malformation involves the vein of Galen.

HYPERTENSIVE CEREBROVASCULAR DISEASE

The most important effects of hypertension on the brain include massive hypertensive intracerebral hemorrhage (discussed earlier), lacunar infarcts and slit hemorrhages, and hypertensive encephalopathy. Atherosclerosis and diabetes are frequently associated diseases.

Lacunar Infarcts

Hypertension affects the deep penetrating arteries and arterioles that supply the basal ganglia and hemispheric white matter as well as the brainstem. These cerebral vessels develop *arteriolar sclerosis* and may become occluded; the structural changes are similar to those described in the systemic vessels of hypertensive patients (Chapter 11). An important clinical and pathologic outcome of CNS arterial lesions is the development of single or multiple, small, cavitary infarcts—*lacunes*, or lacunar state (*état lacunaire*) (Fig. 28–20). These are lakelike spaces, less than 15 mm wide, which occur in the lenticular nucleus, thalamus, internal capsule, deep white matter, caudate nucleus, and pons, in descending order of frequency. On microscopic examination, they consist of cavities of tissue loss with scattered fat-laden macrophages and surrounding gliosis. Depending on their location in the CNS, lacunes can either be clinically silent or cause severe neurologic impairment. Affected vessels may also be associated with widening

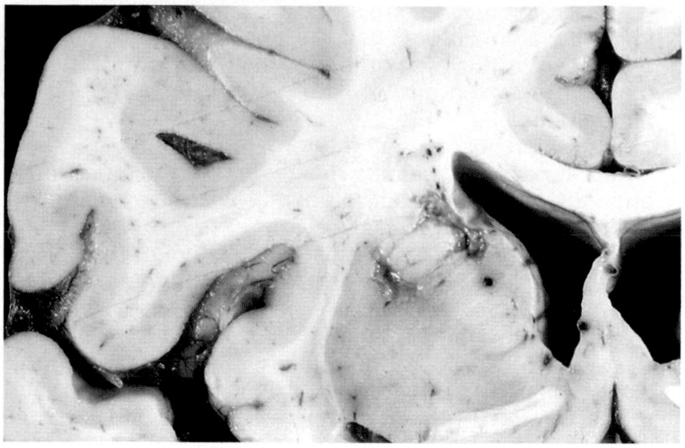

FIGURE 28–20 Lacunar infarcts in the caudate and putamen.

of the perivascular spaces but without tissue infarction (*état criblé*).

Slit Hemorrhages

Hypertension also gives rise to rupture of the small-caliber penetrating vessels and the development of small hemorrhages. In time, these hemorrhages resorb, leaving behind a slitlike cavity (*slit hemorrhage*) surrounded by brownish discoloration; on microscopic examination, slit hemorrhages show focal tissue destruction, pigment-laden macrophages, and gliosis.

Hypertensive Encephalopathy

Acute hypertensive encephalopathy is a clinicopathologic syndrome arising in a hypertensive patient characterized by diffuse cerebral dysfunction, including headaches, confusion, vomiting, and convulsions, sometimes leading to coma. Rapid therapeutic intervention to reduce the accompanying increased intracranial pressure is required, as the syndrome often does not remit spontaneously. Patients coming to postmortem examination may show an edematous brain with or without transtentorial or tonsillar herniation. Petechiae and fibrinoid necrosis of arterioles in the gray and white matter may be seen microscopically.

Patients who, over the course of many months and years, suffer multiple, bilateral, gray matter (cortex, thalamus, basal ganglia) and white matter (centrum semiovale) infarcts may develop a distinctive clinical syndrome characterized by dementia, gait abnormalities, and pseudobulbar signs, often with superimposed focal neurologic deficits. The syndrome, generally referred to as *vascular (multi-infarct) dementia*, is caused by multifocal vascular disease, consisting largely of (1) cerebral atherosclerosis, (2) vessel thrombosis or embolization from carotid vessels or from the heart, or (3) cerebral arteriolar sclerosis from chronic hypertension. When the pattern of injury preferentially involves large areas of the subcortical white matter with myelin and axon loss, the disorder is referred to as *Binswanger disease*; this distribution of vascular white matter injury needs to be distinguished clinically and radiologically from other diseases that affect the hemispheral white matter.

Infections

General aspects of the pathology of infectious agents, including pathogenetic mechanisms involving the CNS, are discussed in Chapter 8. To briefly recapitulate here, there are four principal routes by which infectious microbes enter the nervous system.[2,3] *Hematogenous spread* is the most common means of entry; infectious agents ordinarily enter through the arterial circulation, but retrograde venous spread can occur through anastomotic connections between veins of the face and cerebral circulation. *Direct implantation* of microorganisms is almost invariably traumatic; rarely, it is iatrogenic, as when microbes are introduced with a lumbar puncture needle, or is associated with congenital malformations (such as meningomyelocele). *Local extension* occurs secondary to an established infection in an air sinus, most often the mastoid or frontal; an infected tooth; or a surgical site in the cranium or spine causing osteomyelitis, bone erosion, and propagation of the infection into the CNS. The fourth pathway is through the *peripheral nervous system* into the CNS, as occurs with certain viruses, such as rabies and herpes zoster. Damage to nervous tissue may be the consequence of direct injury of neurons or glia by the infectious agent or may occur indirectly through the elaboration of microbial toxins, destructive effects of the inflammatory response, or the result of immune-mediated mechanisms.[67]

ACUTE MENINGITIS

Meningitis refers to an inflammatory process of the leptomeninges and CSF within the subarachnoid space. *Meningoencephalitis* refers to inflammation of the meninges and brain parenchyma. Meningitis is usually caused by an infection, but *chemical meningitis* may also occur in response to a nonbacterial irritant introduced into the subarachnoid space. Infiltration of the subarachnoid space by carcinoma is referred to as *meningeal carcinomatosis* (sometimes called carcinomatous meningitis) and by lymphoma as *meningeal lymphomatosis.* Infectious meningitis is broadly classified into *acute pyogenic* (usually bacterial meningitis), *aseptic* (usually acute viral meningitis), and *chronic* (usually tuberculous, spirochetal, or cryptococcal) on the basis of the characteristics of inflammatory exudate on CSF examination and the clinical evolution of the illness.

Acute Pyogenic (Bacterial) Meningitis

The microorganisms that cause acute pyogenic meningitis vary with the age of the patient.[68,69] In neonates, the organisms include *Escherichia coli* and the group B streptococci;[70] at the other extreme of life, *Streptococcus pneumoniae* and *Listeria monocytogenes* are more common.[71] Among adolescents and in young adults, *Neisseria meningitidis* is the most common pathogen, with clusters of cases representing frequent public health concerns.[72] The introduction of immunization against *Haemophilus influenzae* has markedly reduced the incidence of meningitis associated with this organism in the developed world;[73] the population that was previously at highest risk (infants) now has a much lower risk of meningitis, with *S. pneumoniae* being the most prevalent organism.

Patients typically show systemic signs of infection superimposed on clinical evidence of meningeal irritation and neurologic impairment, including headache, photophobia, irritability, clouding of consciousness, and neck stiffness. *A spinal tap yields cloudy or frankly purulent CSF, under increased pressure, with as many as 90,000 neutrophils/mm³, a raised protein level, and a markedly reduced glucose content.* Bacteria may be seen on a smear or can be cultured, sometimes a few hours before the neutrophils appear. Untreated, pyogenic meningitis can be fatal. The Waterhouse-Friderichsen syndrome results from meningitis-associated septicemia with hemorrhagic infarction of the adrenal glands and cutaneous petechiae. It is particularly common with meningococcal and pneumococcal meningitis. Effective antimicrobial agents markedly reduce mortality associated with meningitis.[74] In the immunosuppressed patient, purulent meningitis may be caused by other agents, such as *Klebsiella* or an anaerobic organism, and may have an atypical course and uncharacteristic CSF findings, all of which make the diagnosis more difficult.

Morphology. The normally clear CSF is cloudy and sometimes frankly purulent. In acute meningitis, an exudate is evident within the leptomeninges over the surface of the brain (Fig. 28–21). The meningeal vessels are engorged and stand out prominently. The location of the exudate varies; in *H. influenzae* meningitis, for example, it is usually basal, whereas in pneumococcal meningitis, it is often densest over the cerebral convexities near the sagittal sinus. From the areas of greatest accumulation, tracts of pus can be followed along blood vessels on the surface of the brain. When the meningitis is fulminant, the inflammation may extend to the ventricles, producing ventriculitis.

On microscopic examination, neutrophils fill the entire subarachnoid space in severely affected areas and are found predominantly around the leptomeningeal blood vessels in less severe cases. In untreated meningitis, Gram stain reveals varying numbers of the causative organism, although they are frequently not demonstrable in treated cases. In fulminant meningitis, the inflammatory cells infiltrate the walls of the leptomeningeal veins with potential extension of the inflammatory infiltrate into the substance of the brain (focal cerebritis). Phlebitis may also lead to venous occlusion and hemorrhagic infarction of the underlying brain.

Leptomeningeal fibrosis and consequent hydrocephalus may follow pyogenic meningitis, although if it is treated early, there may be little remaining evidence of the infection. In some infections, particularly in pneumococcal meningitis, large quantities of the capsular polysaccharide of the organism produce a particularly gelatinous exudate that encourages arachnoid fibrosis, **chronic adhesive arachnoiditis.**

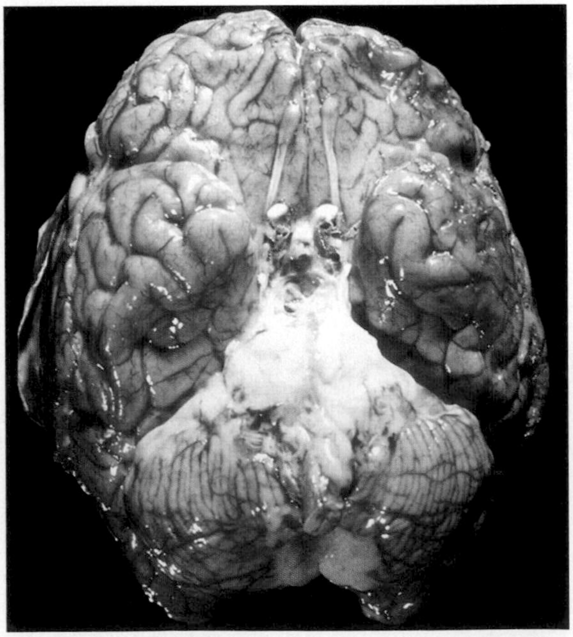

FIGURE 28–21 Pyogenic meningitis. A thick layer of suppurative exudate covers the brain stem and cerebellum and thickens the leptomeninges. (From Golden JA, Louis DN: Images in clinical medicine: Acute bacterial meningitis. N Engl J Med 333:364, 1994.)

Acute Aseptic (Viral) Meningitis

Aseptic meningitis is a misnomer, but it is a clinical term referring to the absence of recognizable organisms in an illness with meningeal irritation, fever, and alterations of consciousness of relatively acute onset. The disease is generally of viral, and rarely of bacterial or other etiology. The clinical course is less fulminant than that of pyogenic meningitis, and the CSF findings also differ between the two conditions. *In aseptic meningitis, there is a lymphocytic pleocytosis, the protein elevation is only moderate, and the sugar content is nearly always normal.* The viral aseptic meningitides are usually self-limiting and are treated symptomatically. In approximately 70% of cases, a pathogen can be identified, most commonly an enterovirus. Echovirus, coxsackievirus, and nonparalytic poliomyelitis are responsible for up to 80% of these cases.

Morphology. There are no distinctive macroscopic characteristics except for brain swelling, seen in some instances. Pathologic material is limited, however, because recovery of patients is the rule. On microscopic examination, there is either no abnormality or a mild to moderate infiltration of the leptomeninges with lymphocytes.

A true noninfectious process has been associated with some classes of medications, including NSAIDs and antibiotics; this entity has been termed *drug-induced aseptic meningitis.*[75] An aseptic meningitis-like picture may also develop subsequent to rupture of an epidermoid cyst into the subarachnoid space or the introduction of a chemical irritant ("chemical" meningitis). In these cases, the CSF is sterile, there is pleocytosis with neutrophils and a raised protein level, but the sugar content is usually normal.

ACUTE FOCAL SUPPURATIVE INFECTIONS

Brain Abscess

Brain abscesses may arise by direct implantation of organisms, local extension from adjacent foci (mastoiditis, paranasal sinusitis), or hematogenous spread (usually from a primary site in the heart, lungs, or distal bones or after tooth extraction). Predisposing conditions include *acute bacterial endocarditis*, which tends to produce multiple abscesses; *cyanotic congenital heart disease,* in which there is a right-to-left shunt and loss of pulmonary filtration of organisms; and *chronic pulmonary sepsis*, as can be seen with bronchiectasis. Streptococci and staphylococci are the most common offending organisms identified in nonimmunosuppressed populations.[76,77]

Morphology. On macroscopic examination, abscesses are discrete lesions with central liquefactive necrosis, a surrounding fibrous capsule, and edema (Fig. 28–22). The most common brain regions that are affected, in descending order of frequency, are the frontal lobe, the parietal lobe, and the cerebellum. On microscopic examination, there is exuberant granulation tissue with neovascularization around the necrosis that is responsible for the marked vasogenic edema. The collagen of the capsule is produced by fibroblasts derived from the walls of blood vessels. Outside the fibrous capsule is a zone of reactive gliosis with numerous gemistocytic astrocytes.

Cerebral abscesses are destructive lesions, and patients almost invariably present clinically with progressive focal deficits in addition to the general signs of raised intracranial pressure. *The CSF is under increased pressure; the white cell count and protein level are raised but the sugar content is normal.* A systemic or local source of infection may be apparent, or a small systemic focus may have ceased to be symptomatic. The increased intracranial pressure and progressive herniation can be fatal, and abscess rupture can lead to ventriculitis, meningitis, and venous sinus thrombosis. With surgery and antibiotics, the otherwise high mortality rate can be reduced to less than 10%.

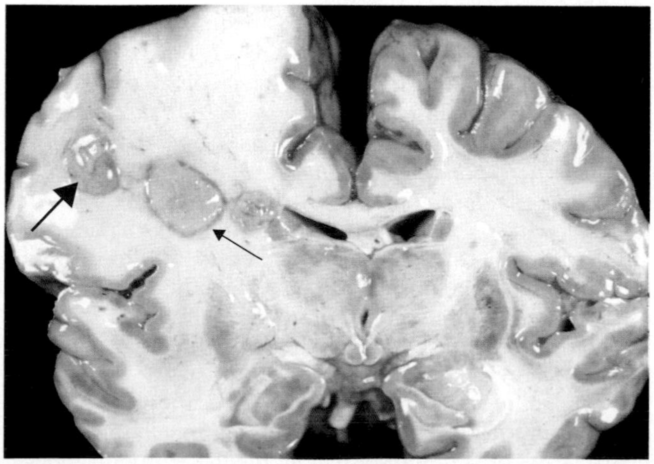

FIGURE 28–22 Frontal abscesses (*arrows*).

Subdural Empyema

Bacterial or occasionally fungal infection of the skull bones or air sinuses can spread to the subdural space and produce a subdural empyema. The underlying arachnoid and subarachnoid spaces are usually unaffected, but a large subdural empyema may produce a mass effect. Further, a thrombophlebitis may develop in the bridging veins that cross the subdural space, resulting in venous occlusion and infarction of the brain. With treatment, including surgical drainage, resolution of the empyema occurs from the dural side, and if it is complete, a thickened dura may be the only residual finding. Symptoms include those referable to the source of the infection. In addition, most patients are febrile, with headache and neck stiffness, and, if untreated, may develop focal neurologic signs, lethargy, and coma. The CSF profile is similar to that seen in brain abscesses, because both are parameningeal infectious processes. If diagnosis and treatment are prompt, complete recovery is usual.

Extradural Abscess

Extradural abscess, commonly associated with osteomyelitis, often arises from an adjacent focus of infection, such as sinusitis or a surgical procedure. When the process occurs in the spinal epidural space, it may cause spinal cord compression and constitute a neurosurgical emergency.

CHRONIC BACTERIAL MENINGOENCEPHALITIS

Tuberculosis

Patients with tuberculous meningitis usually have symptoms of headache, malaise, mental confusion, and vomiting. There is only a moderate CSF pleocytosis made up of mononuclear cells or a mixture of polymorphonuclear and mononuclear cells; the protein level is elevated, often strikingly so; and the glucose content typically is moderately reduced or normal.

Morphology. On macroscopic examination, the subarachnoid space contains a gelatinous or fibrinous exudate, most often at the base of the brain, obliterating the cisterns and encasing cranial nerves. There may be discrete, white granules scattered over the leptomeninges. The most common pattern of involvement is a diffuse **meningoencephalitis.**[78] On microscopic examination, there are mixtures of lymphocytes, plasma cells, and macrophages. Florid cases show well-formed granulomas, often with caseous necrosis and giant cells. Arteries running through the subarachnoid space may show **obliterative endarteritis** with inflammatory infiltrates in their walls and marked intimal thickening. Organisms can often be seen with acid-fast stains. The infectious process may spread to the choroid plexuses and ependymal surface, traveling through the CSF. In cases of long-standing duration, a dense, fibrous adhesive arachnoiditis may develop, most conspicuous around the base of the brain.

Another manifestation of the disease is the development of a single (or often multiple) well-circumscribed intraparenchymal mass **(tuberculoma),** which may be associated with meningitis. A tuberculoma may be up to several centimeters in diameter, causing significant mass effect. On microscopic examination, there is usually a central core of caseous necrosis surrounded by a typical tuberculous granulomatous reaction; calcification may occur in inactive lesions.

Clinical Features. The most serious complications of chronic tuberculous meningitis are arachnoid fibrosis, which may produce hydrocephalus, and obliterative endarteritis, which may produce arterial occlusion and infarction of underlying brain. Because the process involves the spinal cord subarachnoid space, spinal roots may also be affected.

Infection by *Mycobacterium tuberculosis* in patients with acquired immunodeficiency syndrome (AIDS) is often similar to that in non-AIDS patients, but there may be less host reaction. HIV-positive patients are also at risk for infection by *M. avium-intracellulare*, usually in the setting of disseminated infection.[79] When this occurs, the lesions may consist of confluent sheets of macrophages filled with organisms, and minimal granulomatous reaction.

Neurosyphilis

Neurosyphilis is the tertiary stage of syphilis and occurs in only about 10% of patients with untreated infection.[69] The major forms are meningovascular neurosyphilis, paretic neurosyphilis, and tabes dorsalis.

Morphology. Meningovascular neurosyphilis is a chronic meningitis involving the base of the brain and, variably, also the cerebral convexities and the spinal leptomeninges. In addition, there may be an associated obliterative endarteritis (Heubner arteritis) accompanied by a distinctive perivascular inflammatory reaction rich in plasma cells and lymphocytes. Cerebral gummas (plasma cell–rich mass lesions) may also occur in relation to meninges and extending into the cerebral hemispheres, diencephalon, or spinal cord.

Paretic neurosyphilis is caused by invasion of the brain by *Treponema pallidum* and is clinically manifested as insidious but progressive loss of mental and physical functions with mood alterations (including delusions of grandeur), terminating in severe dementia **(general paresis of the insane)**. On microscopic examination, inflammatory lesions are associated with parenchymal damage in the cerebral cortex (particularly the frontal lobe but also affecting other areas of the isocortex) characterized by loss of neurons with proliferations of microglia (rod cells), gliosis, and iron deposits demonstrable with the Prussian blue stain (perivascularly and in the neuropil, presumably from damage to the microcirculation). The spirochetes can be, at times, demonstrated in tissue sections. There is often an associated hydrocephalus with damage to the ependymal lining and proliferation of subependymal glia, called **granular ependymitis.**

Tabes dorsalis is the result of damage by the spirochete to the sensory nerves in the dorsal roots, which produces impaired joint position sense and resultant ataxia (locomotor ataxia); loss of pain sensation, leading to skin and joint damage (Charcot joints); other sensory disturbances, particularly the characteristic "lightning pains"; and absence of deep tendon reflexes. On microscopic examination, there is loss of both axons and myelin in the dorsal roots, with pallor and atrophy in the dorsal columns of the spinal cord. Organisms are not demonstrable in the cord lesions.

Although these three forms of expression of neurosyphilis have been described separately, patients often show incomplete or mixed pictures, notably the combination of tabes dorsalis and general paresis (taboparesis).

Patients with HIV infection are at increased risk for neurosyphilis, and the rate of progression and severity of the disease appear to be accelerated, presumably related to the impaired cell-mediated immunity. CNS involvement by *T. pallidum* in this setting may be manifested as asymptomatic infection, acute syphilitic meningitis, meningovascular syphilis, and, rarely, direct parenchymal invasion of the brain.

Neuroborreliosis (Lyme Disease)

Lyme disease is caused by the spirochete *Borrelia burgdorferi*, transmitted by various species of *Ixodes* tick; involvement of the nervous system is referred to as neuroborreliosis. Neurologic symptoms are highly variable and include aseptic meningitis, facial nerve palsies, mild encephalopathy, and polyneuropathies.[80–82] The rare cases that have come to autopsy have shown a focal proliferation of microglial cells in the brain as well as scattered organisms (identified by Dieterle stain) in the extracellular spaces. Other findings include granulomas and vasculitis.

VIRAL MENINGOENCEPHALITIS

Viral encephalitis is a parenchymal infection of the brain almost invariably associated with meningeal inflammation *(meningoencephalitis)* and sometimes with simultaneous involvement of the spinal cord *(encephalomyelitis).*[83–85] *The most characteristic histologic features of viral encephalitis are perivascular and parenchymal mononuclear cell infiltrates (lymphocytes, plasma cells, and macrophages), glial cell reactions (including the formation of microglial nodules), and neuronophagia* (Fig. 28–23). Direct indications of viral infection are the presence of viral inclusion bodies and, most important, the identification of viral pathogens by ultrastructural, immunocytochemical, and molecular methods.

The phenomenon of nervous system *tropism* that characterizes some viral encephalitides is particularly noteworthy; there are pathogenic viruses that infect specific cell types (such as oligodendrocytes), while others preferentially involve particular areas of the brain (such as medial temporal lobes or the limbic system). The capacity of some viruses for *latency* is especially important in neurologic disease (see the discussion

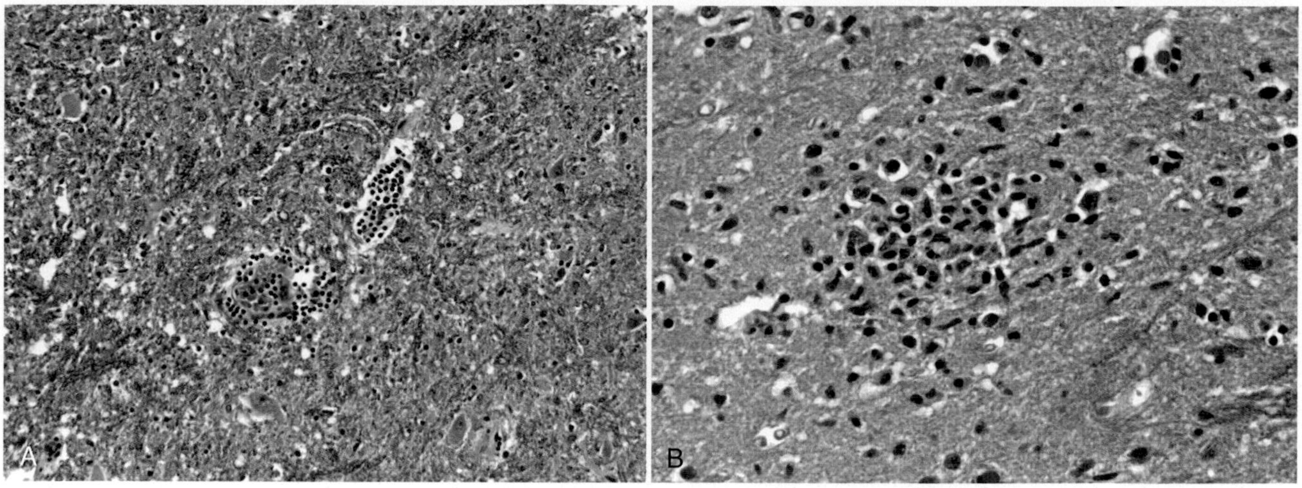

FIGURE 28–23 Characteristic findings of viral meningitis include perivascular cuffs of lymphocytes *(A)* and microglial nodules *(B)*.

of herpes zoster later in this chapter). Systemic viral infections in the absence of direct evidence of viral penetration into the CNS may be followed by an *immune-mediated disease*, such as perivenous demyelination (see later, acute disseminated encephalomyelitis). Intrauterine viral infection may cause *congenital malformations*, as occurs with rubella. A slowly progressive degenerative disease syndrome may follow many years after a viral illness; an example is *postencephalitic parkinsonism* after the viral influenza epidemic that occurred during and after the First World War.[86]

Arthropod-Borne Viral Encephalitis

Arboviruses are an important cause of epidemic encephalitis, especially in tropical regions of the world, and they are capable of causing serious morbidity and high mortality. In the Western hemisphere, the most important types are Eastern and Western equine, Venezuelan, St. Louis, and La Crosse; elsewhere in the world, pathogenic arboviruses include Japanese B (Far East), Murray Valley (Australia and New Guinea), and tick-borne (Russia and Eastern Europe).[83] In the United States, West Nile virus has recently emerged as a pathogen, with associated public health concerns.[87] All have animal hosts and mosquito vectors, except for the tick-borne type. Clinically, affected patients develop generalized neurologic deficits, such as seizures, confusion, delirium, and stupor or coma, and often focal signs, such as reflex asymmetry and ocular palsies. *The CSF is usually colorless but with a slightly elevated pressure and, initially, a neutrophilic pleocytosis that rapidly converts to lymphocytes; the protein level is elevated, but sugar content is normal.*

Morphology. The encephalitides caused by various arboviruses differ in epidemiology and prognosis, but the histopathologic picture is similar among them, except for variations in the severity and extent of the lesions within the CNS. Characteristically, there is a lymphocytic meningoencephalitis (sometimes with neutrophils) with a tendency for inflammatory cells to accumulate perivascularly. Multiple foci of necrosis of gray and white matter are found; in particular, there is evidence of single-cell neuronal necrosis with phagocytosis of the debris **(neuronophagia).** Viral antigens can be detected in neurons by immunoperoxidase staining. In severe cases, there may be a necrotizing vasculitis with associated focal hemorrhages. Some cases have predominantly cortical involvement, whereas in others, the basal ganglia bear the brunt of the disease, as can be demonstrated with neuroradiographic studies.[88]

Herpes Simplex Virus Type 1 (HSV-1)

HSV-1 produces an encephalitis that occurs in any age group but is most common in children and young adults. Only about 10% of the patients have a history of prior herpes. The most commonly observed clinical presenting symptoms in herpes encephalitis are alterations in mood, memory, and behavior. PCR-based methods for virus detection in CSF samples have increased the ease of diagnosis and the recognition of a subset of patients with less severe disease.[89]

Morphology. This encephalitis starts in, and most severely involves, the inferior and medial regions of the temporal lobes and the orbital gyri of the frontal lobes (Fig. 28–24). The infection is necrotizing and often hemorrhagic in the most severely affected regions. Perivascular inflammatory infiltrates are usually present, and Cowdry type A intranuclear viral inclusion bodies may be found in both neurons and glia. In patients with slowly evolving HSV-1 encephalitis, there is more diffuse involvement of the brain.

Antiviral agents now provide effective treatment in many cases, with a significant reduction in the mortality rate. In some individuals, HSV-1 encephalitis follows a subacute course with clinical manifestations (weakness, lethargy, ataxia, seizures) that evolve during a more protracted period (4 to 6 weeks).

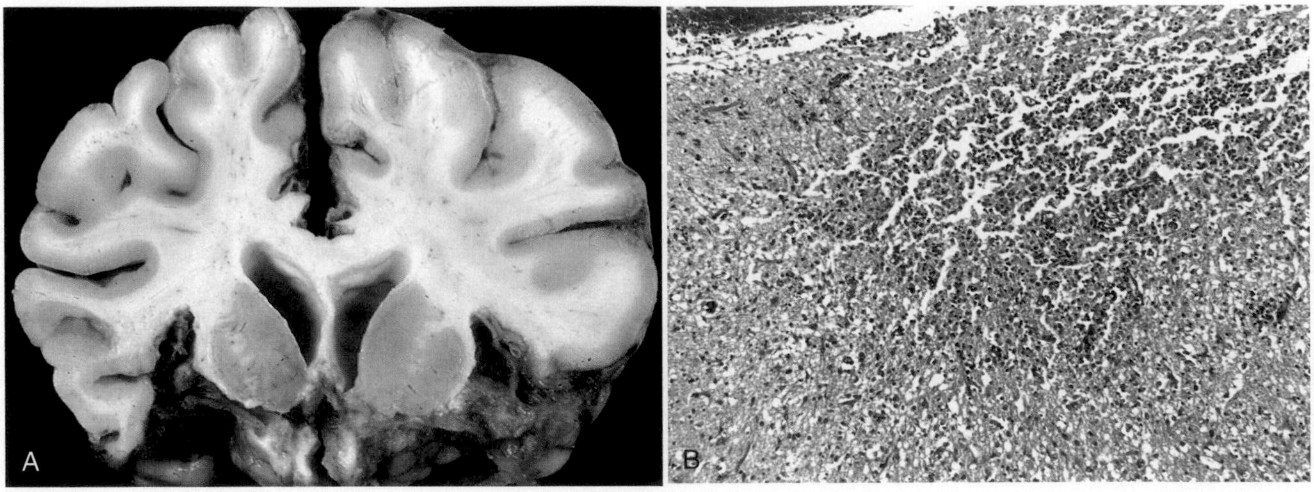

FIGURE 28–24 *A*, Herpes encephalitis showing extensive destruction of inferior frontal and anterior temporal lobes. (Courtesy of Dr. T.W. Smith, University of Massachusetts Medical School, Worcester, MA.) *B*, Necrotizing inflammatory process characterizes the acute herpes encephalitis.

Herpes Simplex Virus Type 2 (HSV-2)

HSV-2 also infects the nervous system and usually manifests in adults as a meningitis. A generalized and usually severe encephalitis develops in as many as 50% of neonates born by vaginal delivery to women with active *primary* HSV genital infections. The dependence on route of delivery indicates that the infection is acquired during passage through the birth canal rather than transplacentally. HSV-1 causes a similar encephalitis in neonates. In AIDS patients, HSV-2 may cause an acute, hemorrhagic, necrotizing encephalitis.

Varicella-Zoster Virus (Herpes Zoster)

Primary varicella infection presents as one of the childhood exanthems (chickenpox), ordinarily without any evidence of neurologic involvement. Reactivation in adults (commonly called "shingles") usually manifests as a painful, vesicular skin eruption in a single or limited dermatomal distribution.

Herpes zoster reactivation is usually a self-limited process, but there may be a persistent postherpetic neuralgia syndrome in up to 10% of patients. Overt CNS involvement with herpes zoster is much rarer but can be more severe. Herpes zoster has been associated with a granulomatous arteritis; immunocytochemical and electron microscopic evidence of viral involvement has been obtained in a few of these cases. In immunosuppressed patients, herpes zoster may cause an acute *encephalitis* with numerous sharply circumscribed lesions characterized by demyelination followed by necrosis. Inclusion bodies can be found in glia and neurons. Varicella-zoster virus infection accounts for about 12% of all systemic herpesvirus infections in patients with AIDS.

Cytomegalovirus

This infection of the nervous system occurs in fetuses and immunosuppressed individuals. The outcome of infection in utero is periventricular necrosis that produces severe brain destruction followed later by microcephaly with periventricular calcification. Cytomegalovirus (CMV) is the most common opportunistic viral pathogen in patients with AIDS, affecting the CNS in 15% to 20% of cases.[90]

Morphology. In the immunosuppressed individual, the most common pattern of involvement is that of a subacute encephalitis, which may be associated with CMV inclusion-bearing cells (see Fig. 8–13). Although any type of cell within the CNS (neurons, glia, ependyma, endothelium) can be infected by CMV, there is a tendency for the virus to localize in the paraventricular subependymal regions of the brain. This results in a severe hemorrhagic necrotizing ventriculoencephalitis and a choroid plexitis. The virus can also attack the lower spinal cord and roots, producing a painful radiculoneuritis. Prominent cytomegalic cells with intranuclear and intracytoplasmic inclusions can be readily identified by conventional light microscopy, immunocytochemistry, and in situ hybridization. These latter two techniques have also shown that normal-appearing, noncytomegalic cells at the edges of the lesions may contain virus.

Poliomyelitis

Poliovirus is a member of the picorna group of enteroviruses. While paralytic poliomyelitis has been effectively eradicated by vaccination in many parts of the world, there are still many regions where it remains a problem. In nonimmunized individuals, poliovirus infection causes a subclinical or mild gastroenteritis. In a small fraction of the vulnerable population, however, it secondarily invades the nervous system.

Morphology. Acute cases show mononuclear cell perivascular cuffs and neuronophagia of the anterior horn motor neurons of the spinal cord. In situ reverse transcriptase-polymerase chain reaction has shown poliovirus RNA in anterior horn cell motor neurons.[91] The inflammatory reaction is usually confined to the anterior horns but may extend into the posterior horns, and the damage is occasionally severe enough to produce cavitation. The motor cranial nuclei are sometimes involved. Postmortem examination in long-term survivors of symptomatic poliomyelitis shows loss of neurons and long-standing gliosis in the affected anterior horns of the spinal cord, some residual inflammation, atrophy of the anterior (motor) spinal roots, and neurogenic atrophy of denervated muscle.[92]

Clinical Features. CNS infection manifests initially with meningeal irritation and a CSF picture of aseptic meningitis. The disease may progress no further or advance to involve the spinal cord. When the disease affects the spinal cord with loss of motor neurons, it produces a flaccid paralysis with muscle wasting and hyporeflexia in the corresponding region of the body—the permanent neurologic residue of poliomyelitis. In the acute disease, death can occur from paralysis of the respiratory muscles, and a myocarditis sometimes complicates the clinical course. Permanent cranial nerve (bulbar) weakness is rare, as is any evidence of encephalitis, but severe respiratory compromise is an important cause of long-term morbidity.

A late neurologic syndrome can develop in patients affected by poliomyelitis who had been stable during intervening years (*postpolio syndrome*). This syndrome, which typically develops 25 to 35 years after the resolution of the initial illness, is characterized by progressive weakness associated with decreased muscle mass and pain, and has an unclear pathogenesis.[93]

Rabies

Rabies is a severe encephalitis transmitted to humans by the bite of a rabid animal, a dog or various wild animals that form natural reservoirs. Exposure to bats, even without a known bite, has also been identified as a risk factor for developing infection, although transmission appears to be limited to certain bat species.[94]

Morphology. On macroscopic examination, the brain shows intense edema and vascular congestion. On microscopic examination, there is widespread neuronal degeneration and an inflammatory reaction that is most severe in the rhombencephalon (midbrain, and floor of the fourth ventricle, particularly in the medulla). The basal ganglia, spinal cord, and dorsal root ganglia may also be involved. Negri bodies, the pathognomonic microscopic finding, are cytoplasmic, round to oval, eosinophilic inclusions that can be found in pyramidal neurons of the hippocampus and Purkinje cells of the cerebellum, sites usually devoid of inflammation (Fig. 28–25).[95] The presence of rabies virus can be detected within Negri bodies by ultrastructural and immunohistochemical examination.

Clinical Features. Since the virus enters the CNS by ascending along the peripheral nerves from the wound site, the incubation period (commonly between 1 and 3 months) depends on the distance between the wound and the brain. The disease manifests initially with nonspecific symptoms of malaise, headache, and fever, but the conjunction of these symptoms with local paresthesias around the wound is diagnostic. As the infection advances, the patient exhibits extraordinary CNS excitability; the slightest touch is painful, with violent motor responses progressing to convulsions. Contracture of the pharyngeal musculature on swallowing produces foaming at the mouth, which may create an aversion to swallowing even water (hydrophobia). There is meningismus and, as the disease progresses, flaccid paralysis. Periods of alternating mania and stupor progress to coma and death from respiratory center failure.

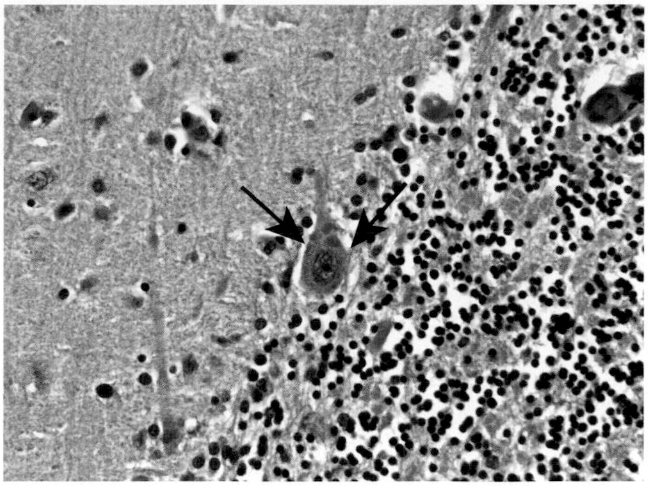

FIGURE 28–25 The diagnostic histologic finding in rabies is the eosinophilic Negri body, as seen here in a Purkinje cell *(arrows)*.

Human Immunodeficiency Virus

As many as 60% of patients with AIDS develop neurologic dysfunction during the course of their illness; in some, it dominates the clinical picture until death. (See Chapter 6 for a discussion of the epidemiology and pathogenesis of AIDS.) In the first 15 years or so after recognition of the disease, neuropathologic changes were demonstrated at postmortem examination in as many as 80% to 90% of cases. In recent years, with the introduction of highly active antiretroviral therapy, these figures have dropped dramatically.[79] The changes described include direct or indirect effects of HIV, opportunistic infection, and primary CNS lymphoma (Chapter 14).[96]

HIV aseptic meningitis occurs within 1 to 2 weeks of seroconversion in about 10% of patients; antibodies to HIV can be demonstrated, and the virus can be isolated from the CSF. The few neuropathologic studies of the early and acute phases of symptomatic or asymptomatic HIV invasion of the nervous system have shown a mild lymphocytic meningitis, perivascular inflammation, and some myelin loss in the hemispheres.

HIV Meningoencephalitis (Subacute Encephalitis)

Patients affected with this remarkable neurologic disorder can manifest clinically with dementia referred to as AIDS-dementia complex (ADC). The dementia begins insidiously, with mental slowing, memory loss, and mood disturbances, such as apathy and depression. Motor abnormalities, ataxia, bladder and bowel incontinence, and seizures can also be present. Radiologic imaging of the brain may be normal or may show some diffuse cortical atrophy, focal abnormalities of the cerebral white matter, and ventricular dilation.[96]

Morphology. The brains of individuals with HIV encephalitis with or without dementia show comparable findings. On macroscopic examination, the meninges are clear, and there is some ventricular dilation with sulcal widening but normal cortical thickness. The process is best characterized microscopically as a chronic inflammatory reaction with widely distributed infiltrates of **microglial nodules,** sometimes with associated foci of tissue necrosis and reactive gliosis (Fig. 28–26). The microglial nodules are also found in the vicinity of small blood vessels, which show abnormally prominent endothelial cells and perivascular foamy or pigment-laden macrophages. These changes occur especially in the subcortical white matter, diencephalon, and brainstem. An important component of the microglial nodule is the macrophage-derived **multinucleated giant cell.** In some cases, there is also a disorder of white matter characterized by multifocal or diffuse areas of myelin pallor with associated axonal swellings and gliosis.

HIV can be detected in CD4-positive mononuclear and multinucleated macrophages and microglia by immunoperoxidase and molecular methods. HIV infection has been reported in retinal and cerebral endothelial cells and astrocytes in some studies. It appears likely that neurons and oligodendrocytes are not directly infected by HIV, and damage to these cells occurs indirectly through the release of toxic cytokines and alterations of the blood-brain barrier. The pathogenesis of the dementing illness has not been fully elucidated (see the discussion in Chapter 6).

Vacuolar Myelopathy

This disorder of the spinal cord is found in 20% to 30% of patients with AIDS in the United States, less often in Europe. The histopathologic findings resemble those of subacute combined degeneration, though serum levels of vitamin B_{12} are normal. The pathogenesis of the lesion is unknown; it does not appear to be caused directly by HIV, and virus is not present within the lesions.

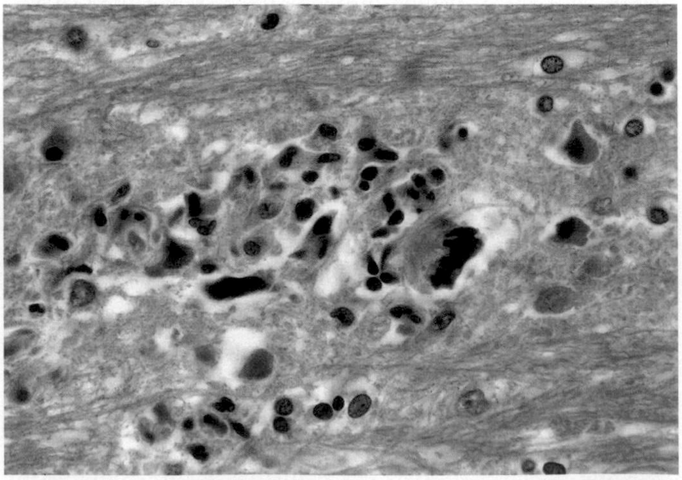

FIGURE 28–26 HIV encephalitis. Note the microglial nodule and multinucleated giant cells.

Of related interest is the condition known as *tropical spastic paraparesis* or HTLV-1–associated myelopathy (HAM), which occurs in several countries in the Caribbean, along the Indian Ocean, in Japan, and in South America. Some cases show a severe lymphocytic meningomyelitis unlike that seen in vacuolar myelopathy. Virologic studies and polymerase chain reaction data have implicated another retrovirus: human T-cell lymphotrophic virus 1 (HTLV-1).

AIDS-Associated Myopathy and Peripheral Neuropathy

Inflammatory myopathy has been the most often described skeletal muscle disorder in patients with HIV infection. The disease is characterized by the subacute onset of proximal weakness, sometimes pain, and elevated levels of serum creatine kinase. The histologic findings include muscle fiber necrosis and phagocytosis, interstitial infiltration with HIV-positive macrophages, and, in a few cases, cytoplasmic bodies and nemaline rods. An acute, toxic, reversible myopathy with "ragged red" fibers and myoglobulinuria may also develop in patients treated with zidovudine (AZT).

The most commonly reported clinical syndromes of peripheral neuropathy include acute and chronic inflammatory demyelinating polyneuropathy, distal symmetric polyneuropathy, polyradiculopathy, mononeuritis multiplex, and, rarely, sensory neuropathy due to ganglioneuronitis. The histopathologic findings that are observed in most of these cases include segmental demyelination, axonal degeneration, and epineurial and endoneurial mononuclear cell inflammation.

AIDS in Children

Neurologic disease was common in children with congenital AIDS, occurring in 15% to 30% of infants born to seropositive mothers; the incidence of the disease has decreased dramatically with the introduction of multidrug antiretroviral therapy. Clinical manifestations of neurologic dysfunction are evident by the first years of life and include microcephaly with mental retardation and motor developmental delay with spasticity of limbs. The most frequent morphologic abnormality is calcification of the large and small vessels and parenchyma within the basal ganglia and deep cerebral white matter. There is also loss of hemispheric myelin or delay in myelination; multinucleated giant cells and microglial nodules are also observed in many cases. HIV is present in brain tissue. Opportunistic infections of the CNS, including toxoplasmosis, CMV infection, progressive multifocal leukoencephalopathy, and cryptococcal meningitis, are relatively rare in infants and children with AIDS compared with adults.

Progressive Multifocal Leukoencephalopathy

Progressive multifocal leukoencephalopathy (PML) is a viral encephalitis caused by the JC polyomavirus; because the virus preferentially infects oligodendrocytes, demyelination is its principal pathologic effect. The disease occurs almost invariably in immunosuppressed individuals in various clinical settings, including chronic lymphoproliferative or myeloproliferative illnesses, immunosuppressive chemotherapy, granulomatous diseases, and AIDS.[97] Although the incidence of PML appears to be decreasing in HIV-infected individuals with the advent of newer antiretroviral therapies,[98] there may be direct interaction between HIV and JC viruses within cells.[99]

No clinical disease has been associated with primary infection by the JC virus, but about 65% of normal people have serologic evidence of exposure to the virus by the age of 14 years. It is though that PML results from the reactivation of virus as a result of immunosuppression.[100] Clinically, patients develop focal and relentlessly progressive neurologic symptoms and signs, and both computed tomography (CT) and magnetic resonance imaging (MRI) scans show extensive, often multifocal lesions in the hemispheric or cerebellar white matter.

Morphology. The lesions consist of patches of irregular, ill-defined destruction of the white matter ranging in size from millimeters to extensive involvement of an entire lobe of the brain (Fig. 28–27). The cerebrum, the brainstem, the cerebellum, and occasionally the spinal cord can be involved. On microscopic examination, the typical lesion consists of a patch of demyelination, most often in a subcortical location, in the center of which are scattered lipid-laden macrophages and a reduced number of axons. At the edge of the lesion are greatly enlarged oligodendrocyte nuclei whose chromatin is replaced by glassy amphophilic viral inclusion. These oligodendrocytes can be shown to contain viral antigens by immunohistochemistry (Fig. 28–27*B*), viral genome by in situ hybridization, and viral nucleocapsids by electron microscopy. Within the lesions, there may be bizarre giant astrocytes with irregular, hyperchromatic, sometimes multiple nuclei. Reactive fibrillary astrocytes are scattered among the bizarre forms.

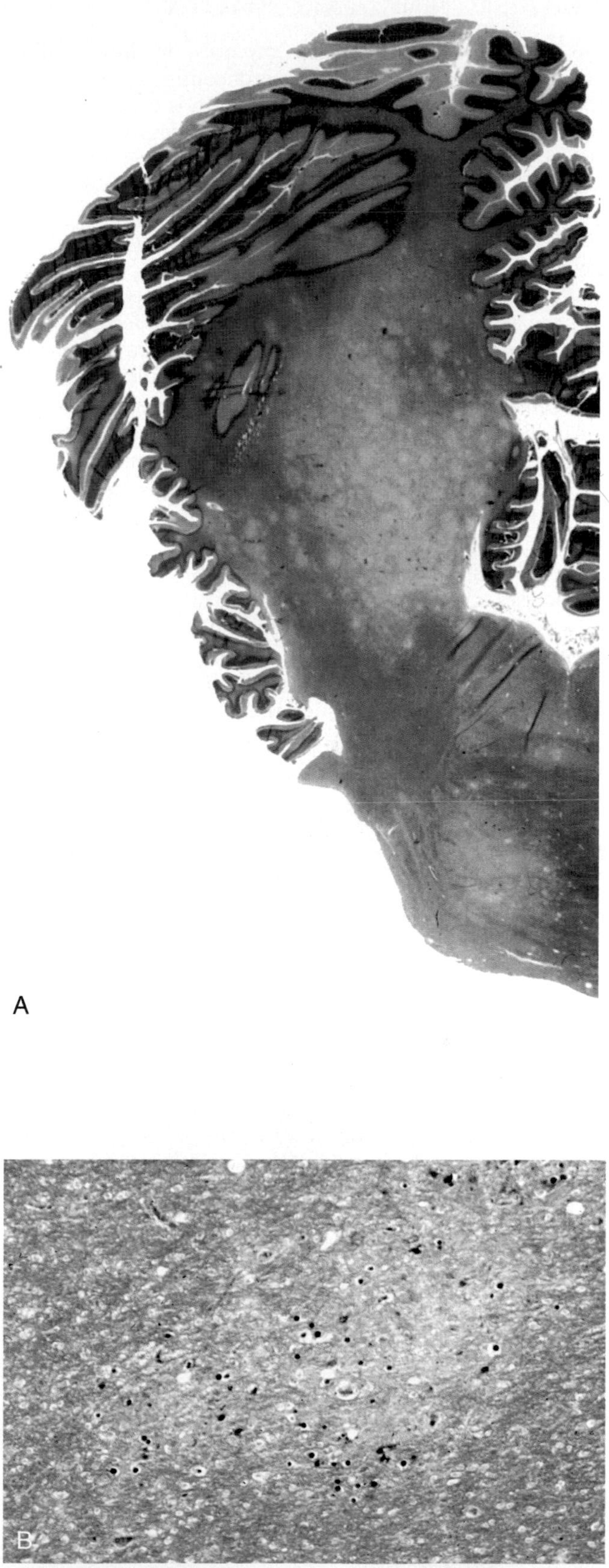

FIGURE 28–27 Progressive multifocal leukoencephalopathy. *A*, Section stained for myelin showing irregular, poorly defined areas of demyelination, which become confluent in places. *B*, Enlarged oligodendrocyte nuclei stained for viral antigens surround an area of early myelin loss.

Subacute Sclerosing Panencephalitis

Subacute sclerosing panencephalitis (SSPE) is a rare progressive clinical syndrome characterized by cognitive decline, spasticity of limbs, and seizures. It occurs in children or young adults, months or years after an initial, early-age acute infection with measles. This disease is thought to represent persistent, but nonproductive, infection of the CNS by an altered measles virus; changes in several viral genes have been associated with the disease. On microscopic examination, there are widespread gliosis and myelin degeneration; viral inclusions, largely within the nuclei, of oligodendrocytes and neurons; variable inflammation of white and gray matter; and neurofibrillary tangles.[101] Ultrastructural study shows that the inclusions contain nucleocapsids characteristic of measles, and immunohistochemistry for measles virus antigen is positive. With widespread measles vaccination programs, the disease seems to have largely disappeared. However, there are still cases being reported around the world.

FUNGAL MENINGOENCEPHALITIS

As with the systemic deep mycoses, in industrialized nations, fungal disease of the CNS is encountered primarily in immunocompromised patients. The brain is usually involved only late in the disease, when there is widespread hematogenous dissemination of the fungus, most often *Candida albicans, Mucor, Aspergillus fumigatus,* and *Cryptococcus neoformans.* In endemic areas, pathogens such as *Histoplasma capsulatum, Coccidioides immitis,* and *Blastomyces dermatitidis* may involve the CNS after a primary pulmonary or cutaneous infection; again, this often follows immunosuppression.[102]

There are three main patterns of fungal infection in the CNS: chronic meningitis, vasculitis, and parenchymal invasion. Vasculitis is most frequently seen with *Mucor* and *Aspergillus,* both of which have a marked predilection for invasion of blood vessel walls, but it occasionally occurs with other organisms, such as *Candida.* The resultant vascular thrombosis produces infarction that is often strikingly hemorrhagic and that subsequently becomes septic from ingrowth of the causative fungus.

Parenchymal invasion, usually in the form of granulomas or abscesses, can occur with most of the fungi and often coexists with meningitis. The most commonly encountered fungi invading the brain are *Candida* and *Cryptococcus. Candida* usually produces multiple microabscesses, with or without granuloma formation. Although most fungi invade the brain by hematogenous dissemination, direct extension may also occur, particularly with *Mucor,* most commonly in diabetics with ketoacidosis.

Cryptococcal meningitis, observed now with increasing frequency in association with AIDS, may be fulminant and fatal in as little as 2 weeks or indolent, evolving over months or years. The CSF may have few cells but a high concentration of protein. The mucoid encapsulated yeasts can be visualized in the CSF by India ink preparations and in tissue sections by PAS and mucicarmine as well as silver stains.

Morphology. With cryptococcal infection, the brain shows a chronic meningitis affecting the basal leptomeninges, which are opaque and thickened by reactive connective tissue and may obstruct the outflow of CSF from the foramina of Luschka and Magendie, giving rise to hydrocephalus. Sections of the brain disclose a gelatinous material within the subarachnoid space and small cysts within the parenchyma ("soap bubbles"), which are especially prominent in the basal ganglia in the distribution of the lenticulostriate arteries (Fig. 28–28*A*). Parenchymal lesions consist of aggregates of organisms within expanded perivascular (Virchow-Robin) spaces associated with minimal or absent inflammation or gliosis (Fig. 28–28*B*). The meningeal infiltrates consist of chronic inflammatory cells and fibroblasts admixed with cryptococci. Well-formed granulomas are not seen ordinarily; in some cases, however, there is a marked chronic inflammatory and granulomatous reaction similar to that seen with *M. tuberculosis.*

OTHER INFECTIOUS DISEASES OF THE NERVOUS SYSTEM

Protozoal diseases (including malaria, toxoplasmosis, amebiasis, and trypanosomiasis), rickettsial infections (such as typhus and Rocky Mountain spotted fever), and metazoal diseases (especially cysticercosis and echinococcosis) may also involve the CNS and are discussed in Chapter 8.

Cerebral toxoplasmosis has assumed greater importance with the AIDS epidemic.[103] Infection of the brain by *Toxoplasma gondii* is one of the most common causes of neurologic symptoms and morbidity in patients with AIDS. The average incidence of CNS infection in most clinical and autopsy series ranges from 4% to 30%. The clinical symptoms are subacute, evolving during a 1- or 2-week period, and may

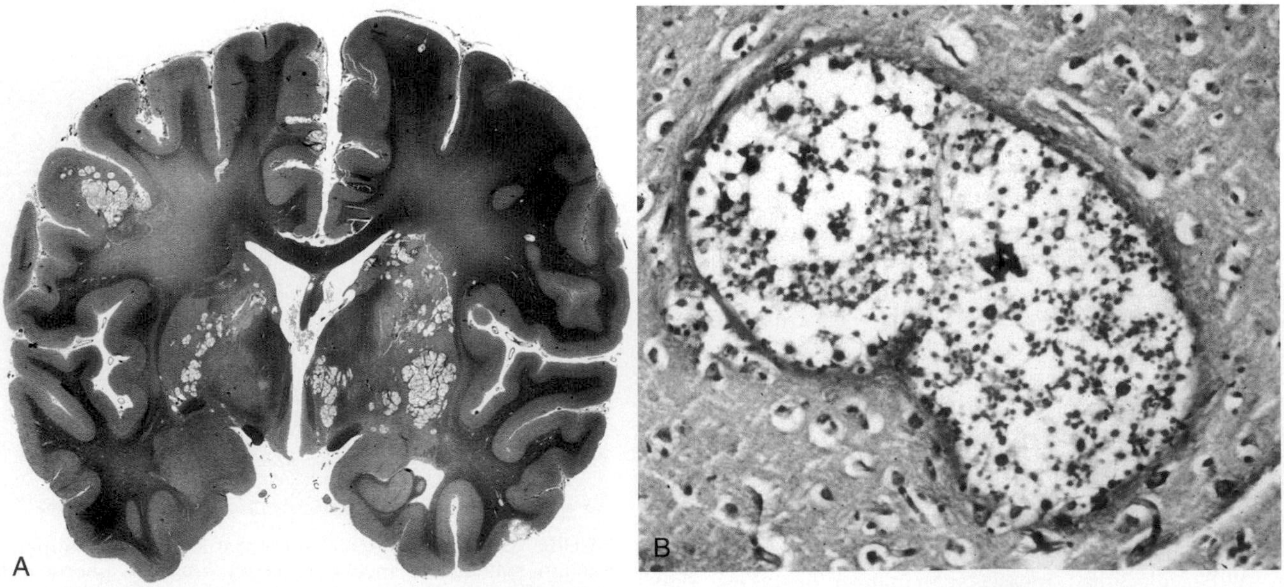

FIGURE 28–28 Cryptococcal infection. *A,* Whole brain section showing the numerous areas of tissue destruction associated with the spread of organisms in the perivascular spaces. *B,* At higher magnification, it is possible to see the cryptococci in the lesions.

be both focal and diffuse. CT and MRI studies may show multiple ring-enhancing lesions; however, this radiographic appearance is not pathognomonic, since similar findings may be associated with CNS lymphoma, tuberculosis, and fungal infections.

Morphology. In toxoplasmosis of the CNS, the brain shows abscesses, frequently multiple, most involving the cerebral cortex (near the gray-white junction) and deep gray nuclei, less often the cerebellum and brainstem, and rarely the spinal cord (Fig. 28–29*A*). Acute lesions consist of central foci of necrosis with variable petechiae surrounded by acute and chronic inflammation, macrophage infiltration, and vascular proliferation. Both free tachyzoites (Fig. 28–29*B*) and encysted bradyzoites (Fig. 28–29*C*) may be found at the periphery of the necrotic foci. The organisms are usually seen on routine H & E or Giemsa stains, but they can be more easily recognized by immunocytochemical methods. The blood vessels in the vicinity of these lesions may show marked intimal proliferation or even frank vasculitis with fibrinoid necrosis and thrombosis. After treatment, the lesions consist of large, well-demarcated areas of coagulation necrosis surrounded by lipid-laden macrophages. Cysts and free tachyzoites can also be found adjacent to these lesions but may be considerably reduced in number or absent if therapy has been effective. Chronic lesions consist of small cystic spaces containing small numbers of lipid- and hemosiderin-laden macrophages with surrounding gliosis. Organisms are difficult to detect in these older lesions.

Like CMV encephalitis, toxoplasmosis may also occur in the fetus. Primary maternal infection with toxoplasmosis, particularly if it occurs early in the pregnancy, may be followed by a cerebritis in the fetus, with the production of multifocal cerebral necrotizing lesions that may calcify, producing severe damage to the developing brain.

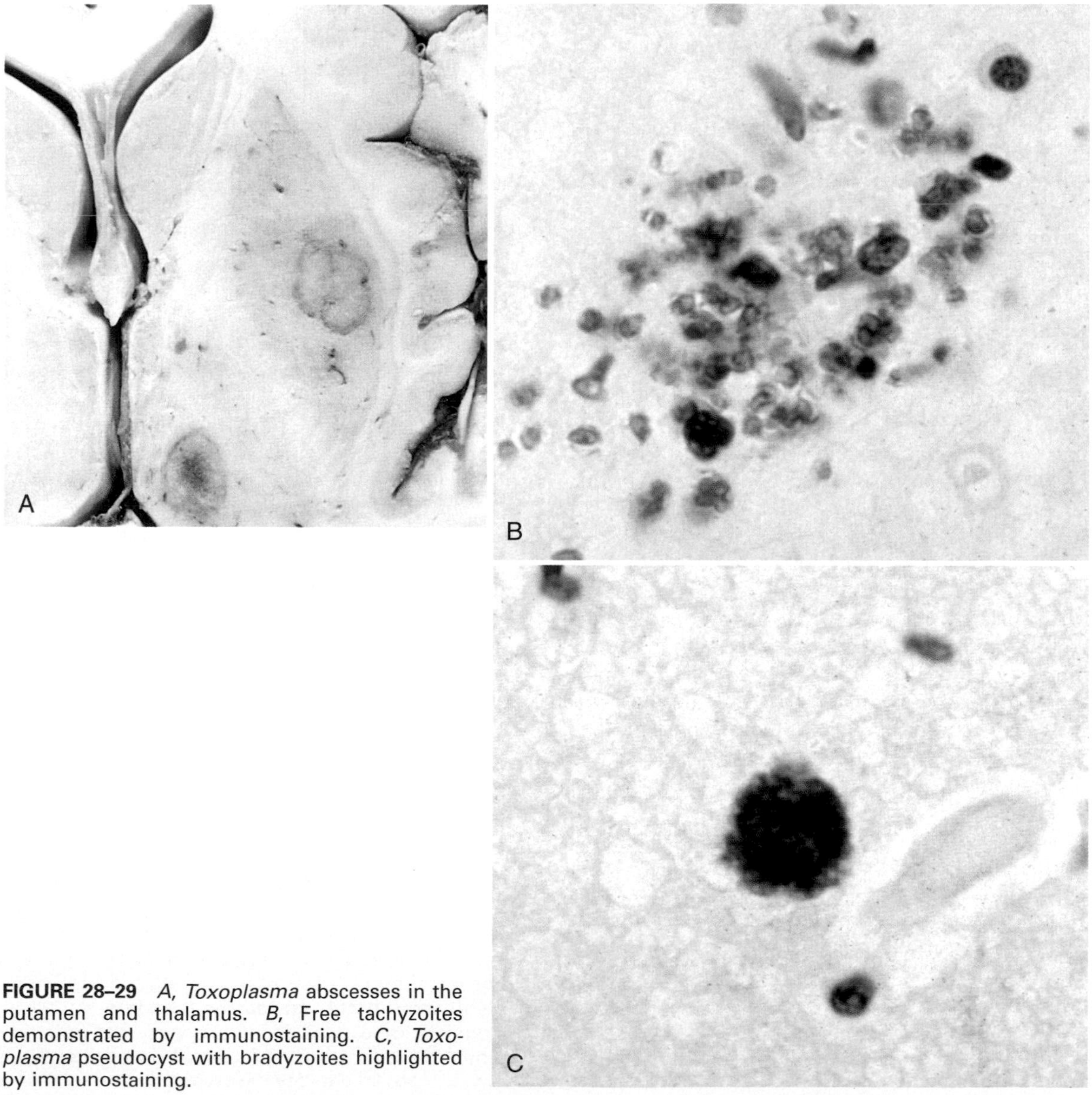

FIGURE 28–29 *A*, *Toxoplasma* abscesses in the putamen and thalamus. *B*, Free tachyzoites demonstrated by immunostaining. *C*, *Toxoplasma* pseudocyst with bradyzoites highlighted by immunostaining.

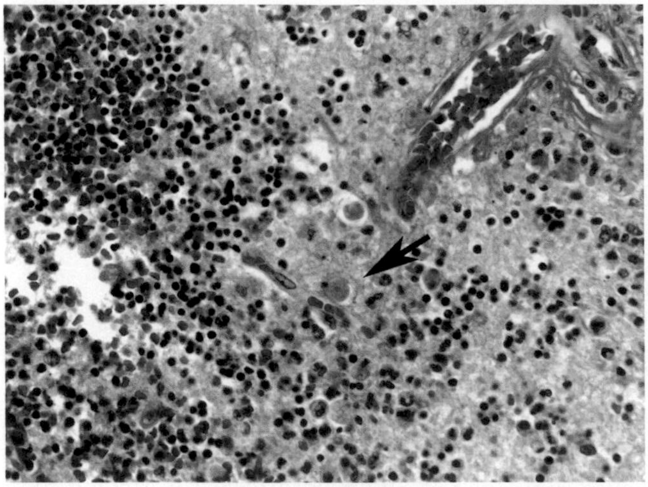

FIGURE 28–30 Necrotizing amoebic meningoencephalitis involving the cerebellum *(organism highlighted by arrow).*

A rapidly fatal necrotizing encephalitis occurs with infection with *Naegleria* species, and a chronic granulomatous meningoencephalitis has been associated with infection with *Acanthamoeba.*[104] The amoebae may sometimes be difficult to distinguish from histiocytes (Fig. 28–30). Methenamine silver or PAS stains are helpful in visualizing the organisms, although definitive identification ultimately depends on combined immunofluorescence studies, morphology, culture, and molecular methods.

Transmissible Spongiform Encephalopathies (Prion Diseases)

This group of diseases—which includes Creutzfeldt-Jakob disease (CJD), Gerstmann-Sträussler-Scheinker syndrome (GSS), fatal familial insomnia, and kuru in humans; scrapie in sheep and goats; mink transmissible encephalopathy; chronic wasting disease of deer and elk; and bovine spongiform encephalopathy (BSE)—share an etiologic basis that distinguishes them from other neurodegenerative and infectious diseases.[105,106] While differences exist among these disorders, they are all associated with abnormal forms of a specific protein, termed prion protein (PrP), and are both infectious and transmissible. As the name implies, they are predominantly characterized by "spongiform change" caused by intracellular vacuoles in neurons and glia. Clinically, most of these patients develop progressive dementia. The most common clinical presentation is CJD. The sporadic form occurs with an annual incidence of approximately 1 case per 1,000,000 population and accounts for about 90% of cases of CJD; familial and transmitted forms make up the rest.

Pathogenesis and Molecular Genetics. PrP is a 30-kDa normal cellular protein present in neurons. Disease occurs when the prion protein undergoes a conformational change from its normal α-helix–containing isoform (PrP^{c}) to an abnormal β-pleated sheet isoform, usually termed either PrP^{sc} (for *sc*rapie) or PrP^{res} (for protease *res*istant) (see Table 28–1). Associated with the conformational change, the prion protein acquires relative resistance to digestion with proteases, such as proteinase K. The conformational change resulting in PrP^{sc} may occur spontaneously at an extremely low rate (resulting in sporadic cases) or at a higher rate if various mutations are present in PrP^{c}, such as occurs in familial forms of CJD and in GSS and fatal familial insomnia. PrP^{sc}, independent of the means by which it originates, then facilitates, in a cooperative fashion, comparable transformation of other PrP^{c} molecules (Fig. 28–31*A*). The infectious nature of PrP^{sc} molecules comes from this ability to disrupt the integrity of normal cellular components through conformational changes (Fig. 28–31*A*). Material prepared from sporadic cases of CJD or from the related familial disorders has been demonstrated to be infectious when it is inoculated into appropriate animal hosts.

The ability to transmit the disease through inoculation with PrP^{sc} has revealed several important aspects of the pathologic process: (1) PrP^{sc} from one species is more effective at transmitting disease to the same species than to others; (2) this effect is dependent only on the host PrP^{c}, as has been shown in experiments with transgenic mice; and (3) engineered absence of a host *PRNP* gene (see below) renders an animal resistant to infection by PrP^{sc}. When administered peripherally, infectivity of PrP^{sc} requires a functional lymphoid system, particularly follicular dendritic cells in the spleen.[107]

A gene on chromosome 20, termed *PRNP*, codes for PrP^{c} protein. It has a single exon coding for the entire open reading frame and shows a high degree of conservation across species. Studies of the *PRNP* gene from cases of familial forms of these diseases have revealed interesting similarities and differences among them, which may shed some light on their variable clinical expression. In cases of familial CJD and GSS, a wide variety of disease-causing mutations have been identified. For example, in certain families with CJD and fatal familial insomnia, the disease is linked to a point mutation (D178N) in the *PRNP* gene (Fig. 28–31*B*). In addition, various polymorphisms have been found in the *PRNP* gene; of these, the Met/Val polymorphism at codon 129 has been found to influence disease pattern. The combination of Met at codon 129 in the same allele as the D178N mutation results in fatal familial insomnia, while a Val at codon 129 results in CJD.[108] Other influences of the codon 129 polymorphism have been observed in sporadic CJD: individuals who are homozygous at codon 129 for either Met or Val are over-represented among cases of CJD compared to the general population, suggesting that heterozygosity at codon 129 is protective against development of the disease. Interestingly, this protection also applies against iatrogenic CJD.

Accumulation of PrP^{sc} in neural tissue appears to be the cause of the pathology in these diseases, but how this material causes the development of cytoplasmic vacuoles and eventual neuronal death is still unknown. Western blotting of tissue extracts after partial digestion with proteinase K allows diagnostic detection of PrP^{sc}.[109]

Morphology. The progression of the dementia in CJD is usually so rapid that there is little if any macroscopic evidence of brain atrophy. On microscopic examination, the pathognomonic finding is a **spongiform** transformation of the cerebral cortex and, often, deep gray matter structures (caudate, putamen); this consists of a multifocal process that results in the uneven formation of small, apparently empty,

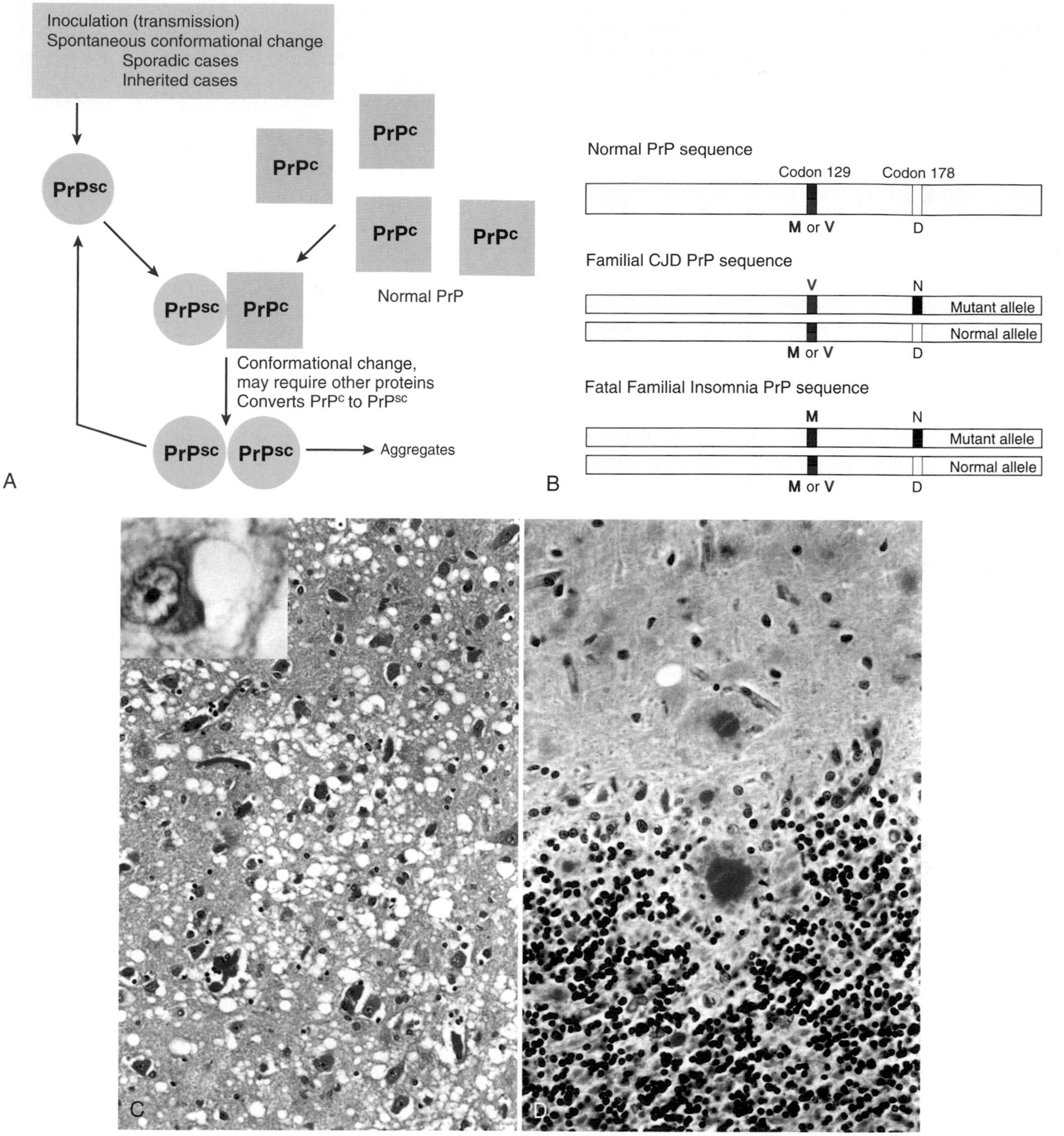

FIGURE 28–31 Mechanism and pathology of prion disease. *A*, Proposed mechanism for the conversion of PrP^{c} through protein-protein interactions. The initiating molecules of PrP^{sc} may arise through inoculation (as in directly transmitted cases) or through an extremely low-rate spontaneous conformational change. The effect of the mutations in PrP (see *B*) is to increase the rate of the conformational change once PrP^{sc} is able to recruit and convert other molecules of PrP^{c} into the abnormal form of the protein. Although the model is drawn with no other proteins involved, it is possible that other proteins play critical roles in the conversion of Prp^{c} to PrP^{sc}. *B*, The basic structure of the PrP protein with important sites of mutation (codon 178) and disease-associated polymorphism (codon 129). In normal individuals, codon 178 encodes Asp (D), and codon 129 encodes either Met (M) or Val (V). In some familial forms of disease, the mutation changes codon 178 to Asn (D178N). When the allele containing the D178N mutation also has a Val at codon 129, the patient develops Creutzfeldt-Jakob disease (CJD). In contrast, when the D178N allele has Met at codon 129, the clinical disorder is fatal familial insomnia. *C*, Histology of CJD showing spongiform change in the cerebral cortex. *Inset*, High magnification of neuron with vacuoles. *D*, Cerebellar cortex showing *kuru plaques* (periodic acid-Schiff [PAS] stain) representing aggregated PrP^{sc}.

microscopic vacuoles of varying sizes within the neuropil and sometimes in the perikaryon of neurons (Fig. 28–31*C*). In advanced cases, there is severe neuronal loss, reactive gliosis, and sometimes expansion of the vacuolated areas into cystlike spaces ("status spongiosus"). No inflammatory infiltrate is present. Electron microscopy shows the vacuoles to be intracytoplasmic and membrane-bound in neuronal processes. **Kuru plaques** are extracellular deposits of aggregated abnormal protein; they are Congo red–positive as well as PAS-positive and occur in the cerebellum in cases of GSS (Fig. 28–31*D*); they are present in abundance in the cerebral cortex in cases of variant CJD. In all forms of prion disease, immunohistochemical staining demonstrates the presence of proteinase-K–resistant PrP^{sc} in tissue.

Creutzfeldt-Jakob Disease

CJD is a rare but well-characterized disease that manifests clinically as a rapidly progressive dementia. It is primarily sporadic (about 85% of cases) in its occurrence, with a worldwide annual incidence of about 1 per million; familial forms also exist. The disease has a peak incidence in the seventh decade. There are well-established cases of iatrogenic transmission, notably by corneal transplantation, deep implantation electrodes, and contaminated preparations of human growth hormone. The clinical picture is usually typical, with the initial subtle changes in memory and behavior followed by a rapidly progressive dementia, often with pronounced involuntary jerking muscle contractions on sudden stimulation (startle myoclonus). Signs of cerebellar dysfunction, usually manifested as ataxia, are present in a minority of patients. The disease is uniformly fatal, with an average duration of only 7 months, although a few patients have survived for several years. These cases exhibit extensive atrophy of involved gray matter.

Variant Creutzfeldt-Jakob Disease (vCJD)

Starting in 1995, a series of cases with a CJD-like illness came to medical attention in the United Kingdom.[110] These new cases were different from typical examples of CJD in several important respects: The disease affected young adults, behavioral disorders figured prominently in the early stages of the disease, and the neurologic syndrome progressed more slowly than in patients with other forms of CJD. The neuropathologic findings and molecular features of these new cases were similar to those of CJD, suggesting a close relationship between the two illnesses. Pathologically, vCJD is characterized by the presence of extensive cortical plaques with a surrounding halo of spongiform change.[111] No alterations in the *PRNP* gene were found in any of these patients, and all cases studied have been found to be Met/Met homozygotes at codon 129. Several lines of evidence have served to link vCJD and bovine spongiform encephalopathy[112,113] and have raised serious public health issues.[114,115] While the extent of the population at risk for vCJD is uncertain, recent estimates have suggested that the overall size of the epidemic may be limited to hundreds or thousands of cases.[116,117]

Gerstmann-Sträussler-Scheinker Syndrome

GSS syndrome is an inherited disease with mutations of the *PRNP* gene that typically begins with a chronic cerebellar ataxia, followed by a progressive dementia. The clinical course is usually slower than that of CJD, with progression to death several years after the onset of symptoms. In addition to the pathologic features of a spongiform encephalopathy, GSS is often marked by numerous plaques of PrP^{sc} as well as neurofibrillary tangles.

Fatal Familial Insomnia

Fatal familial insomnia is named, in part, for the sleep disturbances that characterize its initial stages.[118] In the course of the illness, which typically lasts fewer than 3 years, patients develop other neurologic signs, such as ataxia, autonomic disturbances, stupor, and finally coma. A noninherited form of the disorder (fatal sporadic insomnia) has also been described.[119]

Morphology. Unlike other prion diseases, fatal familial insomnia does not show spongiform pathology. Instead, the most striking alteration is neuronal loss and reactive gliosis in the anterior ventral and dorsomedial nuclei of the thalamus; neuronal loss is also prominent in the inferior olivary nuclei. Proteinase-K–resistant PrP^{sc} can be detected by immunostaining or Western blotting.

Demyelinating Diseases

Demyelinating diseases of the CNS are acquired conditions characterized by preferential damage to myelin, with relative preservation of axons. The clinical deficits are due to the effect of myelin loss on the transmission of electrical impulses along axons. The natural history of demyelinating diseases is determined, in part, by the limited capacity of the CNS to regenerate normal myelin and by the degree of secondary damage to axons that occurs as the disease runs its course.

Other disease processes can involve myelin. In progressive multifocal leukoencephalopathy, JC virus infection of oligodendrocytes results in loss of myelin (see the section on infections). In addition, there are inherited disorders that affect myelin synthesis and turnover. These disorders are termed *leukodystrophies* and are discussed with metabolic disorders.

MULTIPLE SCLEROSIS

Multiple sclerosis (MS) is *an autoimmune demyelinating disorder characterized by distinct episodes of neurologic deficits, separated in time, attributable to white matter lesions that are separated in space.* It is the most common of the demyelinating disorders, having a prevalence of approximately 1 per 1,000 persons in most of the United States and Europe. The disease becomes clinically apparent at any age, although onset in childhood or after age 50 years is relatively rare. Women are affected twice as often as are men. In most patients with MS, the clinical course of the illness evolves as relapsing and remitting episodes of neurologic deficit during variable intervals of time (weeks to months to years), followed by gradual, partial recovery of neurologic function. The frequency of relapses tends to decrease during the course of time, but there is a steady neurologic deterioration in most patients.

Pathogenesis. The lesions of MS are caused by a cellular immune response that is inappropriately directed against the components of the myelin sheath. The likelihood of developing this autoimmune process is influenced by genetic and environmental factors (Chapter 6). The risk of developing MS is 15-fold higher when the disease is present in a first-degree relative and even an order of magnitude greater for monozygotic twins (although the concordance rate remains below 50%).[120] Genetic linkage of MS susceptibility to the DR2 extended haplotype of the major histocompatibility complex is also well established. The molecular basis for the influence of this particular haplotype on the risk of developing MS is unknown; other genetic loci are involved as well.[121] While many studies in the past have focused on a relationship between latitude and the risk of MS, it is now clear that the basis for these phenomena was actually the effect of genetic differences between populations confounded with patterns of migration.

Given the prominence of chronic inflammatory cells within and around MS plaques, immune mechanisms that underlie the destruction of myelin have been the focus of much investigation. The available evidence indicates that the disease is initiated by CD4+ T_H1 T cells that react against self myelin antigens and secrete cytokines, such as IFN-γ, that activate macrophages. The demyelination is caused by these activated macrophages and their injurious products.[122,123] The infiltrate in plaques and surrounding regions of the brain consists of T cells (mainly CD4+, some CD8+) and macrophages. Antibodies are also frequently present; their role in demyelination is less clear. How the autoimmune reaction is initiated is also not understood; as in other autoimmune disorders (Chapter 6), microbial triggers and a number of susceptibility genes are thought to play a role.[124,125] Experimental allergic encephalomyelitis (EAE) is an animal model of MS in which demyelination and inflammation occur after immunization of animals with myelin proteins. The experimental disorder can be passively transferred to other animals with T_H1 cells that recognize these myelin antigens. Based on the growing understanding of the pathogenesis of the disease, therapies are being developed that modulate or inhibit T_H1 responses and block the recruitment of T cells into the brain.[126]

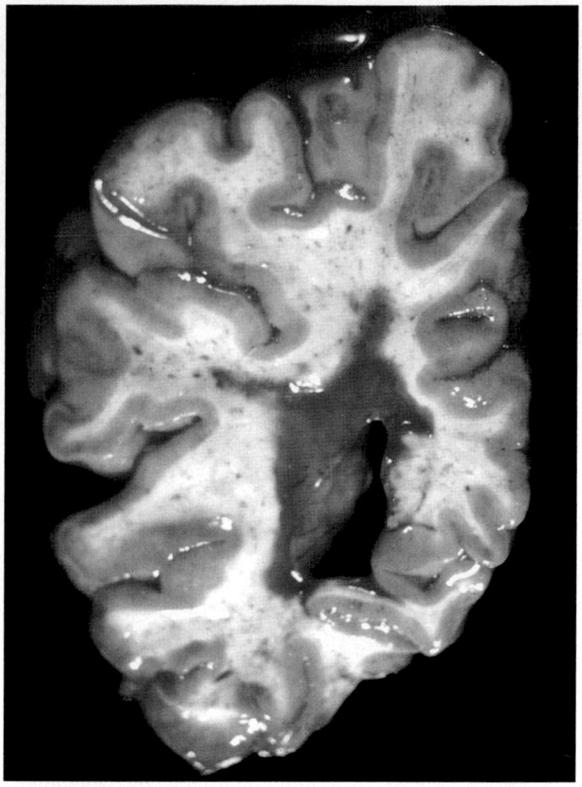

FIGURE 28–32 Multiple sclerosis. Section of fresh brain showing brown plaque around occipital horn of the lateral ventricle.

Morphology. Since MS is a white matter disease and gray matter covers much of the surface of the hemispheres, macroscopic examination of the outer aspect of the cerebral gyri is unremarkable. On the other hand, evidence of the disease may be found on the surface of the brainstem (e.g., basis pontis) or along the spinal cord, where myelinated fiber tracts course superficially; here lesions appear as multiple, well-circumscribed, somewhat depressed, glassy, gray-tan, irregularly shaped **plaques,** both on external examination and on section (Fig. 28–32). In the fresh state, these have firmer consistency than the surrounding white matter **(sclerosis)**. Plaques can be found throughout the white matter of the neuraxis; they may also extend into the gray matter structures, as these have myelinated fibers running through them, although their recognition within these regions is more difficult. The size of lesions varies considerably, from small foci that are recognizable only at microscopic examination to confluent plaques that involve large portions of the centrum semiovale. Plaques commonly occur beside the lateral ventricles and may be demonstrated to follow the course of paraventricular veins when the surface of the ventricle is inspected en face. They are also frequent in the optic nerves and chiasm, brain stem ascending and descending fiber tracts, cerebellum, and spinal cord.

The lesions have sharply defined borders at the microscopic level (Fig. 28–33*A*). In an **active plaque,** there is evidence of ongoing myelin breakdown with abundant macrophages containing lipid-rich, PAS-positive debris. Inflammatory cells, including both lymphocytes and monocytes, are present, mostly as perivascular cuffs, especially at the outer edge of the lesion (Fig. 28–33*B*). Small active lesions are often centered on small veins. Within a plaque, there is relative preservation of axons and depletion of oligodendrocytes. In time, astrocytes undergo reactive changes. As lesions become quiescent, there is a diminution of the inflammatory cell infiltrate and of macrophages. Within the center of an **inactive plaque,** little to no myelin is found, and there is a reduction in the number of oligodendrocyte nuclei; instead, astrocytic proliferation and gliosis are prominent. Axons in old gliotic plaques show severe depletion of myelin and are also greatly diminished in number (Fig. 28–33*C*).

In some MS plaques (**shadow plaques**), the border between normal and affected white matter is not sharply circumscribed. In this type of lesion, some abnormally thinned-out myelin sheaths can be demonstrated, especially at the outer edges. This phenomenon has been interpreted either as evidence of partial and incomplete myelin loss or as remyelination by surviving oligodendrocytes. Abnormally myelinated fibers have also been observed at the edges of typical plaques. Although these histologic

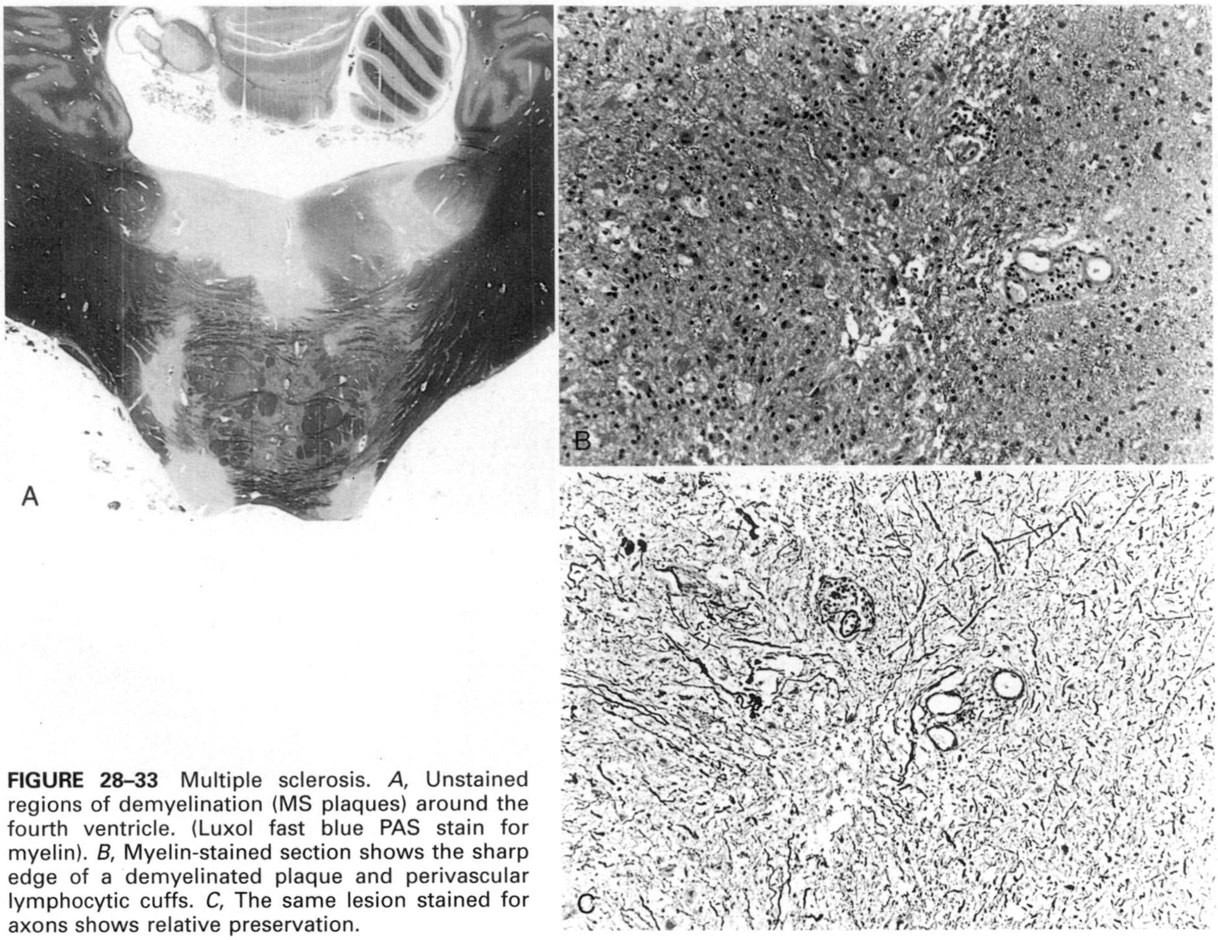

FIGURE 28–33 Multiple sclerosis. *A*, Unstained regions of demyelination (MS plaques) around the fourth ventricle. (Luxol fast blue PAS stain for myelin). *B*, Myelin-stained section shows the sharp edge of a demyelinated plaque and perivascular lymphocytic cuffs. *C*, The same lesion stained for axons shows relative preservation.

findings suggest a limited potential for remyelination in the CNS, the remaining axons within most MS plaques remain unmyelinated. The pathologic findings are remarkably similar regardless of the clinical tempo of disease progression. Autopsy studies and radiologic studies using MRI have demonstrated that subclinical forms of the disease exist and that some plaques may be clinically silent even in symptomatic patients.

Several studies have suggested recently that active plaques can also be grouped into four patterns: those that are sharply demarcated and centered on blood vessels, either with (pattern I) or without (pattern II) deposition of immunoglobulin and complement, and those that are less well demarcated and are not centered on vessels (patterns III and IV). These latter two are distinguished by the distribution of oligodendrocyte apoptosis (III: widespread; IV: central only). There are also differences in the severity of myelin protein loss between these patterns and in the degree of remyelination present. Autopsy studies have shown that only one pair of patterns (I/II or III/IV) is present in a given individual, suggesting that these may reflect distinct mechanisms rather than different stages of lesion.[127–129]

Clinical Features. Although MS lesions can occur anywhere in the CNS and, as a consequence, may induce a wide range of clinical manifestations, certain patterns of neurologic symptoms and signs are commonly observed. Unilateral visual impairment during the course of a few days, due to involvement of the optic nerve (*optic neuritis, retrobulbar neuritis*), is a frequent initial manifestation of MS. However, only some patients (10% to 50%, depending on the population studied) with optic neuritis go on to develop MS. Involvement of the brainstem produces cranial nerve signs, ataxia, nystagmus, and internuclear ophthalmoplegia from interruption of the fibers of the medial longitudinal fasciculus. Spinal cord lesions give rise to motor and sensory impairment of trunk and limbs, spasticity, and difficulties with the voluntary control of bladder function.

Examination of the CSF in MS patients shows a mildly elevated protein level, and in one third of cases, there is moderate pleocytosis. The proportion of gamma globulin is increased, and most MS patients show *oligoclonal bands.* This increase in CSF immunoglobulin is the result of proliferation of B cells within the nervous system; the target epitopes of these antibodies are widely variable.

MULTIPLE SCLEROSIS VARIANTS

Some individuals, especially Asians, develop a demyelinating disease similar to MS with presenting symptoms of bilateral optic neuritis and prominent spinal cord involvement. This disease is referred to as *neuromyelitis optica* or *Devic disease.* It may be rapidly and relentlessly progressive (in approximately 20% of cases), follow a relapsing-remitting course, or manifest as a single episode without subsequent relapses. The lesions in Devic disease are similar in histologic appearance to MS, although they are considerably more destructive, and gray matter involvement of the spinal cord can be striking. Another variant, *acute MS (Marburg form)*, tends to occur in young individuals and is characterized clinically by a fulminant course during a period of several months. On pathologic examination, the plaques are large and numerous, and there is widespread destruction of myelin with some axonal loss.

ACUTE DISSEMINATED ENCEPHALOMYELITIS AND ACUTE NECROTIZING HEMORRHAGIC ENCEPHALOMYELITIS

Acute disseminated encephalomyelitis (ADEM, perivenous encephalomyelitis) is a monophasic demyelinating disease that follows either a viral infection or, rarely, a viral immunization. Symptoms typically develop a week or two after the antecedent infection and include evidence of diffuse brain involvement with headache, lethargy, and coma rather than focal findings, as seen in MS. Symptoms progress rapidly, with a fatal outcome in as many as 20% of cases; in the remaining patients, there is complete recovery.

Acute necrotizing hemorrhagic encephalomyelitis (ANHE, acute hemorrhagic leukoencephalitis of Weston Hurst) is a fulminant syndrome of CNS demyelination, typically affecting young adults and children. The illness is almost invariably preceded by a recent episode of upper respiratory infection; sometimes, it is due to *Mycoplasma pneumoniae*, but often it is of indeterminate cause. The disease is fatal in many patients, but some have survived with minimal residual symptoms.

Morphology. In ADEM, macroscopic examination of the brain shows only grayish discoloration around white matter vessels. On microscopic examination, myelin loss with relative preservation of axons can be found throughout the white matter. In the early stages of the disease, polymorphonuclear leukocytes can be found within the lesions; later, mononuclear infiltrates predominate. The breakdown of myelin is associated with the accumulation of lipid-laden macrophages.

ANHE shows histologic similarities with ADEM, including perivenular distribution of demyelination and widespread dissemination throughout the CNS (sometimes with extensive confluence of lesions). However, the lesions are much more devastating than those of ADEM and include destruction of small blood vessels, disseminated necrosis of white and gray matter with acute hemorrhage, fibrin deposition, abundant neutrophils, and scattered lymphocytes recognizable in less severely damaged areas and in foci of demyelination.

The lesions of ADEM are similar to those induced by immunization of animals with myelin components or with early rabies vaccines that had been prepared from brains of infected animals. This has suggested that ADEM may represent an acute autoimmune reaction to myelin and that ANHE may represent a hyperacute variant, although no inciting antigens have been identified.

OTHER DISEASES WITH DEMYELINATION

Central pontine myelinolysis is characterized by loss of myelin (with relative preservation of axons and neuronal cell bodies) in a roughly symmetric pattern involving the basis pontis and portions of the pontine tegmentum but sparing the periventricular and subpial regions. Lesions may be found more rostrally; it is extremely rare for the process to extend below the pontomedullary junction. Extrapontine lesions occur in the supratentorial compartment, with similar appearance and apparent etiology. The condition is believed to be caused by rapid correction of hyponatremia;[130] however, alternative pathogenetic hypotheses attribute the disorder to extreme serum hyperosmolarity or other metabolic imbalance. The clinical presentation of central pontine myelinolysis is that of a rapidly evolving quadriplegia; radiologic imaging studies localize the lesion to the basis pontis. It occurs in a variety of clinical settings, including alcoholism, severe electrolyte or osmolar imbalance, and orthotopic liver transplantation.[131,132]

Marchiafava-Bignami disease is a rare disorder of myelin characterized by relatively symmetric damage to the myelin of central fibers of the corpus callosum and anterior commissure.

Degenerative Diseases

These are diseases of gray matter characterized principally by the progressive loss of neurons with associated secondary changes in white matter tracts. Two other general characteristics bring them together as a group. First, the pattern of neuronal loss is selective, affecting one or more groups of neurons while leaving others intact. Second, the diseases arise without any clear inciting event in patients without previous neurologic deficits. The neuropathologic findings observed in the degenerative diseases differ greatly; in some, there are intracellular abnormalities with some degree of specificity (e.g., Lewy bodies, neurofibrillary tangles), while in others, there is only loss of the affected neurons. It is convenient to group the degenerative diseases according to the anatomic regions of the CNS that are primarily affected. Some degenerative diseases have prominent involvement of the cerebral cortex, such as Alzheimer disease; others are more restricted to subcortical areas and may present with movement disorders such as tremors and dyskinesias. As genetic and molecular studies of these diseases have progressed, there has been recognition of shared features across many of the disorders.[133]

A common theme among the neurodegenerative disorders is the development of protein aggregates that are resistant to normal cellular mechanisms of degradation through the ubiquitin-proteasome system. These aggregates can be recognized histologically as inclusions, which often form the diagnostic hallmarks of these different diseases. The basis for aggregation varies across diseases. For example, it may be directly related to an intrinsic feature of a mutated protein (e.g., expanded polyglutamine repeat in Huntington disease), a feature of a peptide derived from a larger precursor protein (e.g., Aβ in Alzheimer disease), or an unexplained alteration of a normal cellular protein (e.g., α-synuclein in sporadic Parkinson disease). The aggregated proteins are generally cytotoxic, but the mechanisms by which protein aggregation is linked to cell death may be different in these various diseases.

DEGENERATIVE DISEASES AFFECTING THE CEREBRAL CORTEX

The major cortical degenerative disease is Alzheimer disease, and its principal clinical manifestation is *dementia*, that is, progressive loss of cognitive function independent of the state of attention. There are many other causes of dementia, including the various forms of frontotemporal dementia, vascular disease (multi-infarct dementia), dementia with Lewy bodies (considered later in the context of Parkinson disease, the other Lewy body disorder), Creutzfeldt-Jakob disease, and neurosyphilis (both considered earlier). These diseases also involve subcortical structures, but many of the clinical symptoms are related to the changes in the cerebral cortex. Regardless of etiology, dementia is not part of normal aging and always represents a pathologic process.

Alzheimer Disease

Alzheimer disease (AD) is the most common cause of dementia in the elderly. The disease usually becomes clinically apparent as insidious impairment of higher intellectual function, with alterations in mood and behavior. Later, progressive disorientation, memory loss, and aphasia indicate severe cortical dysfunction, and eventually, in 5 to 10 years, the patient becomes profoundly disabled, mute, and immobile. Patients rarely become symptomatic before 50 years of age, but the incidence of the disease rises with age, and the prevalence roughly doubles every five years, starting from a level of 1% for the 60- to 64-year-old population and reaching 40% or more for the 85- to 89-year-old cohort.[134–137] This progressive increase in the incidence of the disease with age has given rise to major medical, social, and economic problems in countries with a growing number of elderly individuals. Most cases are sporadic, although at least 5% to 10% of cases are familial. Pathologic changes identical to those observed in Alzheimer disease occur in almost all individuals with trisomy 21 who survive beyond 45 years, and a decline in cognition can be clinically demonstrated in many. Although pathologic examination of brain tissue remains necessary for the definitive diagnosis of Alzheimer disease, the combination of clinical assessment and modern radiologic methods allows accurate diagnosis in 80% to 90% of cases.

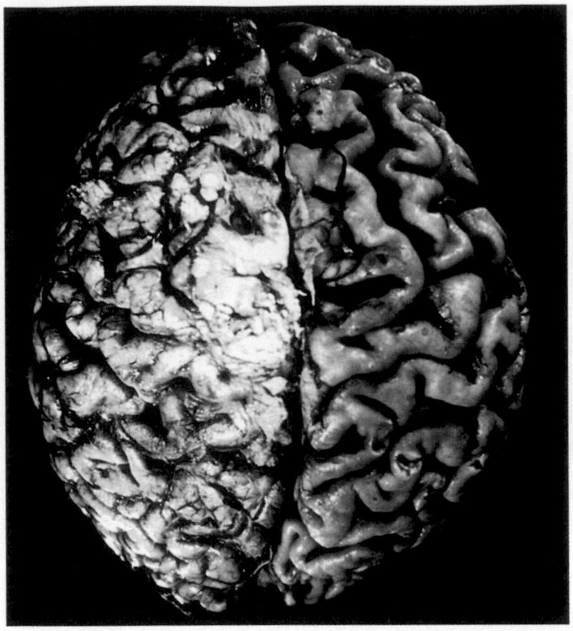

FIGURE 28–34 Alzheimer disease with cortical atrophy most evident on the right, where meninges have been removed. (Courtesy of Dr. E.P. Richardson, Jr., Massachusetts General Hospital, Boston, MA.)

Morphology. Macroscopic examination of the brain shows a variable degree of **cortical atrophy** with widening of the cerebral sulci that is most pronounced in the frontal, temporal, and parietal lobes. With significant atrophy, there is compensatory ventricular enlargement (hydrocephalus ex vacuo) secondary to loss of parenchyma (Fig. 28–34). The major microscopic abnormalities of Alzheimer disease are **neuritic (senile) plaques, neurofibrillary tangles, and amyloid angiopathy.** All of these may be present to a lesser extent in the brains of elderly nondemented individuals. The diagnosis of Alzheimer disease is based on a combination of clinical and pathologic features. Several different diagnostic methods have been proposed, which include evaluation of different regions of the brain and various methods for estimating the frequency of plaques and tangles.[138–142] There is a fairly constant pattern of progression of involvement of brain regions: Pathologic changes (specifically plaques, tangles, and the associated neuronal loss and glial reaction) are evident earliest in the entorhinal cortex, then spread through the hippocampal formation and isocortex, and then extend into the neocortex.[138,139,143]

Neuritic plaques are focal, spherical collections of dilated, tortuous, silver-staining neuritic processes (dystrophic neurites) often around a central amyloid core, which may be surrounded by clear halo (Fig. 28–35*A*). Neuritic plaques range in size from 20 to 200 μm in diameter; microglial cells and reactive astrocytes are present at their periphery. Plaques can be found in the hippocampus and amygdala as well as in the neocortex, although there is usually relative sparing of primary motor and sensory cortices (this also applies to neurofibrillary tangles). Plaques can also be found in the corresponding regions of the brains of aged, nonhuman primates. The dystrophic neurites contain paired helical filaments as well as synaptic vesicles and abnormal mitochondria. The amyloid core, which can be stained by Congo red, contains several abnormal proteins. The dominant component of the plaque core is **Aβ**, a peptide derived through specific processing events from a larger molecule, amyloid precursor protein (APP). The two dominant species of Aβ, called $A\beta_{40}$ and $A\beta_{42}$, share an N-terminus and differ in length by two amino acids. Other proteins are present in plaques in lesser abundance, including components of the complement cascade, proinflammatory cytokines, α1-antichymotrypsin, and apolipoproteins.

Immunostaining for Aβ demonstrates the existence, in some patients, of amyloid peptide deposits in

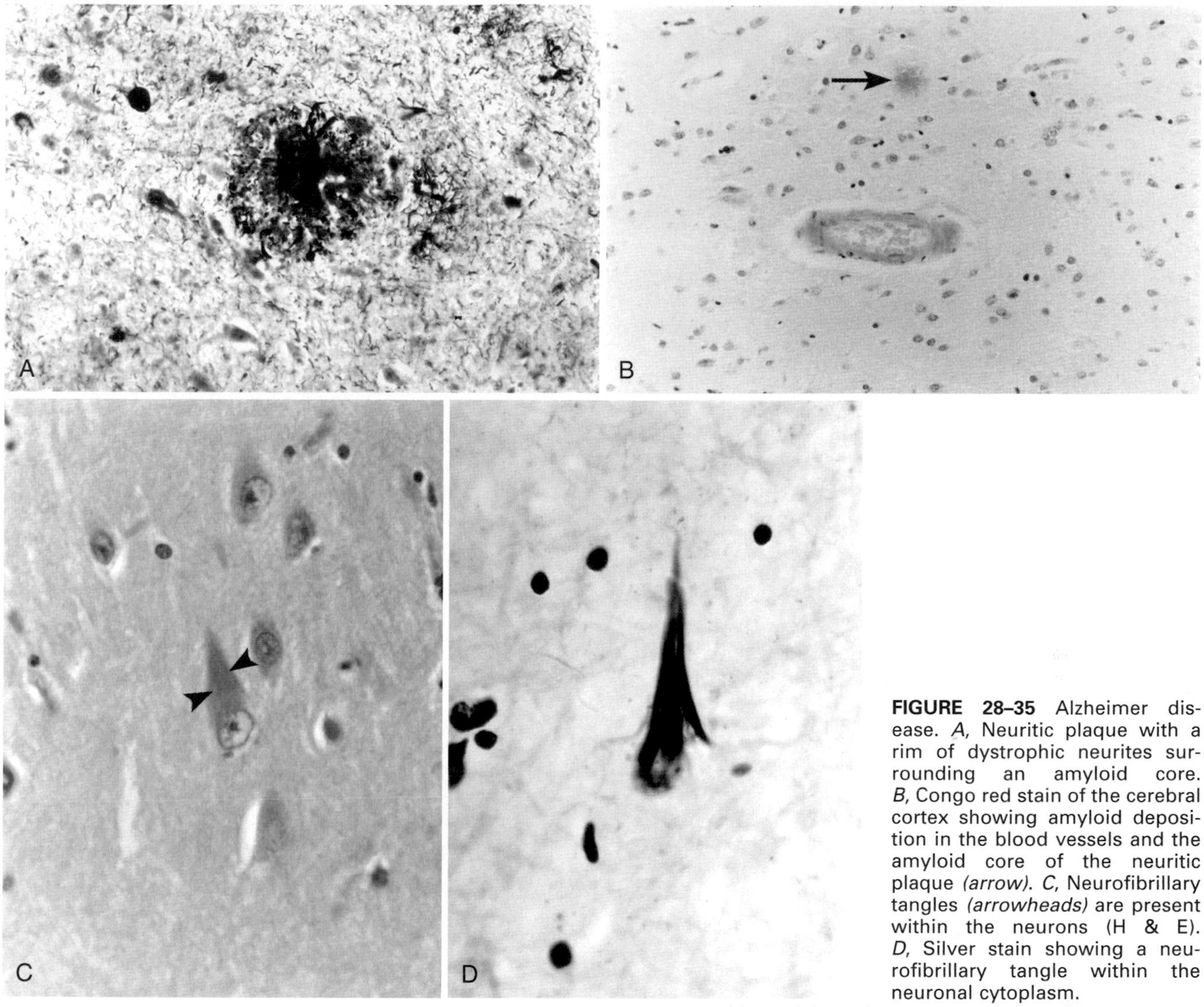

FIGURE 28–35 Alzheimer disease. *A,* Neuritic plaque with a rim of dystrophic neurites surrounding an amyloid core. *B,* Congo red stain of the cerebral cortex showing amyloid deposition in the blood vessels and the amyloid core of the neuritic plaque *(arrow)*. *C,* Neurofibrillary tangles *(arrowheads)* are present within the neurons (H & E). *D,* Silver stain showing a neurofibrillary tangle within the neuronal cytoplasm.

lesions lacking the surrounding neuritic reaction. These lesions, termed **diffuse plaques,** are found in superficial portions of cerebral cortex as well as in basal ganglia and cerebellar cortex. Diffuse plaques appear to represent an early stage of plaque development, based primarily on studies of brains from individuals with trisomy 21.[144] In some brain regions (cerebellar cortex and striatum), they persist as a major manifestation of the disease. They may be present in the brains of individuals with other clear-cut findings of Alzheimer disease or in isolation. While neuritic plaques contain both $A\beta_{40}$ and $A\beta_{42}$, diffuse plaques are predominantly made up of $A\beta_{42}$.[145,146]

Neurofibrillary tangles are bundles of filaments in the cytoplasm of the neurons that displace or encircle the nucleus. In pyramidal neurons, they often have an elongated "flame" shape; in rounder cells, the basket weave of fibers around the nucleus takes on a rounded contour ("globose" tangles). Neurofibrillary tangles are visible as basophilic fibrillary structures with H & E staining but are dramatically demonstrated by silver (Bielschowsky) staining (Figs. 28–35*B* and 28–35*C*). They are commonly found in cortical neurons, especially in the entorhinal cortex, as well as in other sites such as pyramidal cells of the hippocampus, the amygdala, the basal forebrain, and the raphe nuclei. Neurofibrillary tangles are insoluble and apparently resistant to clearance in vivo, thus remaining visible in tissue sections as "ghost" or "tombstone" tangles long after the death of the parent neuron.

Ultrastructurally, neurofibrillary tangles are composed predominantly of paired helical filaments along with some straight filaments that appear to have a comparable composition. A major component of paired helical filaments is abnormally hyperphosphorylated forms of the protein **tau**, an axonal microtubule-associated protein that enhances microtubule assembly. Other antigens include MAP2 (another microtubule-associated protein) and ubiquitin. Tangles are not specific to Alzheimer disease, being found in other diseases as well. Paired helical filaments are also found in the dystrophic neurites that form the outer portions of neuritic plaques and in axons coursing through the affected gray matter as **neuropil threads.**

Cerebral amyloid angiopathy (CAA) is an almost invariable accompaniment of Alzheimer disease; however, it can also be found in brains of individuals without Alzheimer disease (Fig. 28–35*D*). Vascular amyloid is predominantly $A\beta_{40}$, as is also true when CAA occurs without AD.

Granulovacuolar degeneration is the formation of small (~5 µm in diameter), clear intraneuronal cytoplasmic vacuoles, each of which contains an argyrophilic granule. While it occurs with normal aging, it is most commonly found in great abundance in hippocampus and olfactory bulb in Alzheimer disease. **Hirano bodies**, found especially in Alzheimer disease, are elongated, glassy, eosinophilic bodies consisting of paracrystalline arrays of beaded filaments, with actin as their major component. They are found most commonly within hippocampal pyramidal cells.

Pathogenesis and Molecular Genetics. The pathogenesis of Alzheimer disease as well as the temporal and pathophysiologic relationships between the different morphologic changes described are being intensively investigated. There remains disagreement regarding the best correlate of dementia in patients with Alzheimer disease. The number of neurofibrillary tangles correlates better with the degree of dementia than does the number of neuritic plaques. Biochemical markers that have been correlated with the degree of dementia include loss of choline acetyltransferase, synaptophysin immunoreactivity, and amyloid burden. Although not assessed by standard histologic methods, the best correlation of severity of dementia appears to be with loss of synapses. The insights from familial forms of AD have suggested, however, that *Aβ is a critical molecule in the pathogenesis of this dementia.*

Current understanding of the principal events in the pathogenesis of AD is centered on the properties of Aβ. This peptide aggregates readily, forms β-pleated sheets and binds Congo red, is relatively resistant to degradation, elicits a response from astrocytes and microglia, and can be directly neurotoxic. The Aβ peptides are derived through processing of APP. APP is a protein of uncertain cellular function that is synthesized with a single transmembrane domain and expressed on the cell surface (Fig. 28–36). A soluble form of APP can be released from the cell surface by proteolytic cleavage, by an enzymatic activity termed α-secretase; at least three distinct enzymes have been shown to have α-secretase activity. Molecules of APP that have undergone this cleavage cannot give rise to the Aβ fragment (see Fig. 28–36). However, surface APP can also be endocytosed and may then undergo processing to generate Aβ peptides that are less soluble and tend to aggregate into amyloid fibrils. These are generated through cleavage at a site N-terminal to the start of the transmembrane domain by an

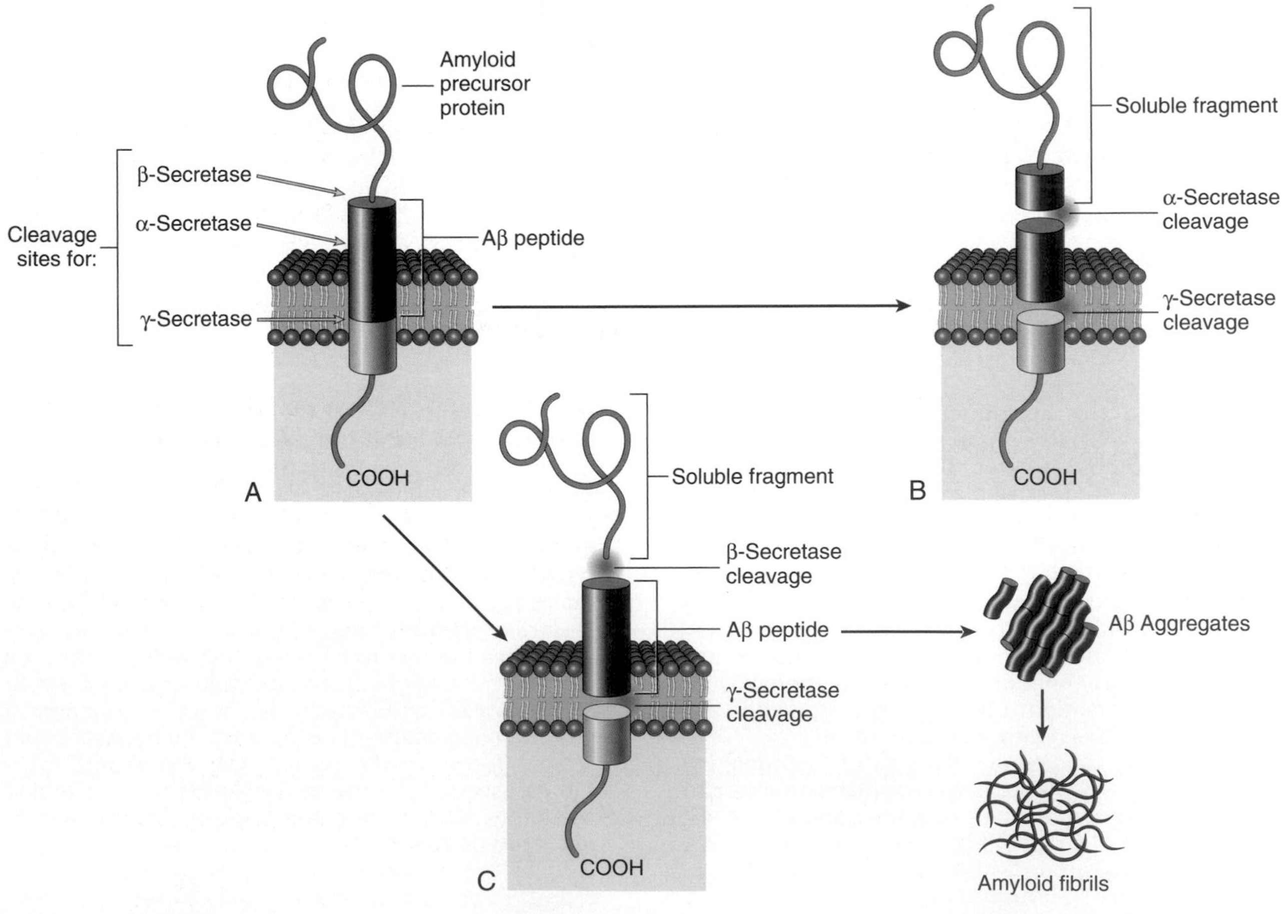

FIGURE 28–36 Mechanism of amyloid generation in Alzheimer disease. Amyloid precursor protein (APP) is a transmembrane protein, with potential cleavage sites for three distinct enzymes (α-, β- and γ-secretases) as shown in *A*. The Aβ domain extends from the extracellular side of the protein into the transmembrane domain. When APP is cleaved by α-secretase (*B*), subsequent cleavage by γ-secretase does not yield Aβ. In contrast, cleavage by β-secretase followed by γ-secretase (*C*) results in production of Aβ, which can then aggregate and form fibrils. In either pathway, intramembranous cleavage by γ-secretase follows cleavage at a site located closer to the N-terminus of the protein.

enzyme called β-secretase (BACE-1) and cleavage within the transmembrane domain by γ-secretase. This process is constitutively active in cells, and γ-secretase appears to perform other important intramembranous proteolysis events, including cleavage of Notch, a cell fate–determining molecule. The cleavage of Notch results in release into the cell of a portion of the molecule that is involved in cell signaling and transcriptional regulation.[147] Both by inference and by direct experimentation, it has been suggested that a similar function can be attributed to a fragment of the C-terminal portion of APP that is generated by the same cleavages that generate Aβ.[148]

Several gene loci have been identified for familial Alzheimer disease (Table 28–2). The first of these was the gene for APP on chromosome 21. The pathogenic mutations in the APP gene all result in increased generation of Aβ. Furthermore, the development of Alzheimer disease in individuals with trisomy 21 has been related to a gene dosage effect with increased production of APP and subsequently Aβ. Two other genetic loci linked to early-onset familial Alzheimer disease have been identified on chromosomes 14 and 1; these probably account for the majority of early-onset familial Alzheimer disease pedigrees. The genes on these two chromosomes encode highly related intracellular proteins, presenilin-1 (PS1) and presenilin-2 (PS2). Even before these genes were cloned, it was recognized that the cellular phenotype of these mutations was an increased level of Aβ generation, particularly $A\beta_{42}$. It has now become clear from studies of knockout mice, from directed mutatagenesis of PS1 and PS2, from pharmacologic studies, and from biochemical purifications that the presenilins are a component of γ-secretase and possibly are the portion of a multiprotein complex containing the active proteolytic site.[149] Thus, the genetic evidence strongly supports the notion that the underlying pathogenetic event in AD is the accumulation of Aβ.

Distinct from these loci in which mutations cause Alzheimer disease, one allele (ε4) of the apolipoprotein E (ApoE) gene on chromosome 19 increases the risk of Alzheimer disease and lowers the age at onset of the disease.[150] Individuals with the ε4 allele are overrepresented in populations of patients with Alzheimer disease compared with control populations, and their Aβ burden in the brain is larger. ApoE can bind Aβ and is present in plaques, but how this allele increases the risk for Alzheimer disease has not been established. Other genetic loci involved in AD risk have been identified, including loci on chromosome 12, in or near the α_2-macroglobulin gene, and on chromosome 10.[151,152]

How Aβ is related to the neurodegeneration of AD, how it is linked to the other pathologic features of AD such as tangles and abnormal hyperphosphorylation of tau, and what controls the stereotypic pattern of involvement of brain regions and the pattern of progression all remain open questions. There are various lines of evidence indicating that the small aggregates of Aβ as well as larger fibrils are directly neurotoxic and can elicit various cellular responses, including oxidative damage and alterations in calcium homeostasis. In addition, the reactions of other cell types in the brain influence the disease. There is evidence that the inflammatory response that accompanies Aβ deposition may have both protective effects (through assisting clearance of the aggregated peptide) and injurious effects.[153–156]

Clinical Features. The progression of Alzheimer disease is slow but relentless, with a symptomatic course often running more than 10 years. Initial symptoms are forgetfulness and other memory disturbances; with progression of the disease, other symptoms emerge, including language deficits, loss of mathematical skills, and loss of learned motor skills. In the final stages of Alzheimer disease, patients may become incontinent, mute, and unable to walk. Intercurrent disease, often pneumonia, is usually the terminal event in these individuals. While biomarkers for AD are still unavailable, there are indicators that structural imaging can suggest which individuals are at increased risk of progressing from a mild memory disturbance to a diagnosis of probable AD.[157]

Frontotemporal Dementias

These are a group of disorders that were first gathered under a single broad term because they shared clinical features (progressive deterioration of language and changes in personality) that corresponded to degeneration and atrophy of temporal and frontal lobes. These entities have recently been better understood through a combination of immunohistochemical and biochemical studies as well as genetic insights.[158,159]

Frontotemporal Dementia with Parkinsonism Linked to Chromosome 17 (FTD(P)-17)

As the name implies, this is a genetically determined disorder in which the clinical syndrome of a frontotemporal dementia is often accompanied by parkinsonian symptoms. In these families, the disease has been mapped to chromosome 17; in particular, it has been linked to a variety of mutations

TABLE 28–2 Genetics of Alzheimer Disease

Chromosome	Gene	Mutations/Alleles	Consequences
21	Amyloid precursor protein (*APP*)	• Single missense mutations Double missense mutation Trisomy 21 (gene dosage effect)	• Early-onset FAD Increased Aβ production
14	Presenilin-1 (*PS1*)	• Missense mutations Splice site mutations	• Early-onset FAD Increased Aβ production
1	Presenilin-2 (*PS2*)	• Missense mutations	• Early-onset FAD Increased Aβ production
19	Apolipoprotein E (*ApoE*)	• Allele ε4	• Increased *risk* of development of AD Decreased age at onset of AD

AD, Alzheimer disease; FAD, familial Alzheimer disease.

in the *tau* gene. Tau is a microtubule binding protein that has numerous sites of potential phosphorylation and exists in six splice forms as the result of alternative splicing of exons 2, 3 and 10.[160] The protein contains either three or four copies of the microtubule binding domain depending on whether exon 10 is included (4 repeat tau) or not (3 repeat tau).

Morphology. There is evidence of atrophy of frontal and temporal lobes in various combinations and to various degrees. The pattern of atrophy can often be predicted in part by the clinical symptomatology. The atrophic regions of cortex are marked by neuronal loss and gliosis as well as the presence of tau-containing neurofibrillary tangles. These tangles may contain either 4 repeat tau or a mixture of 3 and 4 repeat tau, depending on the underlying genetic basis for the disease. Nigral degeneration may also occur. Inclusions can also be found in glial cells in some forms of the disease.

Pathogenesis and Molecular Genetics. The study of families with frontotemporal dementia led to the recognition that in some, but not all, pedigrees, there is linkage to mutations in the *tau* gene. The mutations fall into several broad categories: coding region mutations and intronic mutations that affect the splicing of exon 10.[161] The intronic mutations result in increased production of 4 repeat forms of tau. Coding region mutations appear to have several different consequences, including alterations in the interaction of tau with microtubules (mutations in exon 10 will change this interaction only for 4 repeat tau) and altering the intrinsic tendency to aggregate.

Pick Disease

Pick disease (lobar atrophy) is a rare, distinct, progressive dementia characterized clinically by early onset of behavioral changes together with alterations in personality (frontal lobe signs) and language disturbances (temporal lobe signs).[162] While most cases of Pick disease are sporadic, there have been some familial forms identified and linked to mutations in *tau*.

Morphology. The brain invariably shows a pronounced, frequently asymmetric, atrophy of the frontal and temporal lobes with conspicuous sparing of the posterior two thirds of the superior temporal gyrus and only rare involvement of either the parietal or occipital lobe. The atrophy can be severe, reducing the gyri to a thin wafer ("knife-edge" appearance). This pattern of **lobar atrophy** is often prominent enough to distinguish Pick disease from Alzheimer disease on macroscopic examination. In addition to the localized cortical atrophy, there may also be bilateral atrophy of the caudate nucleus and putamen.

On microscopic examination, neuronal loss is most severe in the outer three layers of the cortex. Some of the surviving neurons show a characteristic swelling (**Pick cells**) or contain **Pick bodies,** which are cytoplasmic, round to oval, filamentous inclusions that are only weakly basophilic but stain strongly with silver methods. Ultrastructurally, these are composed of straight filaments, vesiculated endoplasmic reticulum, and paired helical filaments that are immunocytochemically similar to those found in Alzheimer disease and contain 3 repeat tau. Unlike the neurofibrillary tangles of Alzheimer disease, Pick bodies do not survive the death of their host neuron and do not remain as markers of the disease.

Progressive Supranuclear Palsy (PSP)

This is an illness characterized clinically by truncal rigidity with dysequilibrium and nuchal dystonia; pseudobulbar palsy and abnormal speech; ocular disturbances, including vertical gaze palsy progressing to difficulty with all eye movements; and mild progressive dementia in most patients. The onset of the disease is usually between the fifth and seventh decades, and males are affected approximately twice as frequently as are females. The disease is often fatal within 5 to 7 years of onset.

Morphology. There is widespread neuronal loss in the globus pallidus, subthalamic nucleus, substantia nigra, colliculi, periaqueductal gray matter, and dentate nucleus of the cerebellum. Globose neurofibrillary tangles are found in these affected regions, in neurons as well as in glia. Ultrastructural analysis reveals 15-nm straight filaments that are composed of 4 repeat tau.

Mutations in *tau* have not been found in PSP. Analysis of the *tau* gene has shown that there is an extended haplotype (a series of polymorphic markers spread out along the gene that are in complete linkage disequilibrium; that is, recombination events do not appear to occur between the sites). Of the two haplotypes, one of them is strongly overrepresented in PSP patients.[163] How this haplotype influences the risk of PSP is unknown.

Corticobasal Degeneration (CBD)

This is a disease of the elderly, with considerable clinical and neuropathologic heterogeneity. The extrapyramidal signs and symptoms result in this disorder's also being grouped with syndromes of basal ganglia dysfunction.

Morphology. On macroscopic examination, there is cortical atrophy, mainly of the motor, premotor, and anterior parietal lobes. The regions of cortex show severe loss of neurons, gliosis, and *"ballooned" neurons* (neuronal achromasia) that can be highlighted with immunocytochemical methods for phosphorylated neurofilaments. Tau immunoreactivity has been found in astrocytes ("tufted astrocytes"), oligodendrocytes ("coiled bodies"), basal ganglionic neurons, and, variably, cortical neurons.[164,165] Clusters of tau-positive processes around an astrocyte ("astrocytic plaques") and the presence of tau-positive threads in gray and white matter may be the most specific pathologic findings of CBD.[166] The substantia nigra and locus ceruleus show loss of pigmented neurons, neuronal achromasia, and tangles. Similar to

PSP, the tau deposits in CBD contain predominantly 4 repeat tau. Recently proposed consensus diagnostic criteria for CBD focus on the presence of tau-positive inclusions in neurons and glia of the cortex and striatum, including astrocytic plaques, associated with neuronal loss from substantia nigra and cortex.[167]

Clinical Features. The disease is characterized by extrapyramidal rigidity, asymmetric motor disturbances (jerking movements of limbs: "alien hand"), and sensory cortical dysfunction (apraxias, disorders of language); cognitive decline occurs, and may be prominent in some cases.[168,169] The same extended *tau* haplotype is linked to CBD as to PSP.[170] Although tau deposits are a hallmark of CBD, it is rare to find CBD pathology in individuals with mutations in the *tau* gene.[171]

Frontotemporal Dementias Without Tau Pathology

Some cases with clinical and pathologic findings involving these brain regions do not show evidence of Tau deposition. Some cases with this pattern are found in association with motor neuron disease (see below); in this setting, Tau-negative, ubiquitin-positive inclusions can be found in superficial cortical layers in temporal and frontal lobe and in the dentate gyrus. This pattern of pathology is termed *motor neuron disease inclusion dementia.* It has also been described in the absence of ALS-like pathology. Other cases show no specific inclusions but rather have cortical atrophy and some thalamic gliosis. This pattern of injury has been termed dementia lacking distinctive histology (DLDH).[172] With time and increased biochemical and molecular investigations, these unusual entities are likely to be reclassified.

Vascular Dementia

It is now clear from autopsy studies of individuals who were carefully studied during life that various types of vascular injury to the brain can result in dementia.[173] Some individuals with a rapidly progressive cognitive decline have vasculitis (discussed above) and will often show improvement with treatment. Among the irreversible disorders, several specific entities have been identified, which can be separated in part by their clinical course (typically a stepwise progression rather than a gradual decline) and imaging features. Various etiologies include small areas of infarction (granular atrophy from cortical microinfarcts, multiple lacunar infarcts, cortical laminar necrosis associated with reduced perfusion/oxygenation) and diffuse white matter injury (Binswanger disease, CADASIL). Additionally, dementia has been associated with so-called strategic infarcts, which are usually embolic and involve brain regions such as the hippocampus, dorsomedial thalamus, or frontal cortex including cingulate gyrus. Many individuals, in fact, will demonstrate a combination of pathologic changes. There is also an interaction between vascular injury and other dementing disorders, such as AD. It has been found that patients with vascular changes above a certain threshold have a lower burden of plaques and tangles for their level of cognitive impairment than do those without vascular-based cerebral pathology.[174]

DEGENERATIVE DISEASES OF BASAL GANGLIA AND BRAINSTEM

Diseases affecting these regions of the brain are frequently associated with movement disorders, including rigidity, abnormal posturing, and chorea. In general, they can be categorized as manifesting either a reduction of voluntary movement or an abundance of involuntary movement. The basal ganglia and especially the nigrostriatal pathway play an important role in the system of positive and negative regulatory synaptic pathways that serve to modulate feedback from the thalamus to the motor cortex. The most important disorders in this group are those associated with parkinsonism and Huntington chorea.

Parkinsonism

Parkinsonism is a clinical syndrome characterized by diminished facial expression, stooped posture, slowness of voluntary movement, festinating gait (progressively shortened, accelerated steps), rigidity, and a "pill-rolling" tremor. This type of motor disturbance is seen in a number of conditions that have in common damage to the nigrostriatal dopaminergic system. Parkinsonism may also be induced by drugs that affect this system, particularly dopamine antagonists and toxins. The principal diseases to be discussed here that involve the nigrostriatal system are as follows:

- Parkinson disease (PD)
- Multiple system atrophy, a disorder that may have parkinsonism as a prominent symptom (clinical presentation as striatonigral degeneration) as well as other symptoms (cerebellar ataxia and autonomic dysfunction)
- Postencephalitic parkinsonism, which was observed in the wake of the influenza pandemic that occurred between 1914 and 1918 and is now vanishingly rare
- Progressive supranuclear palsy (PSP) and corticobasal degeneration (CBD), which are movement disorders that may also exhibit cognitive impairment; they share some pathologic and genetic features with each other and with other tauopathies (see the discussion above in the section on frontotemporal dementias).

Parkinson Disease

This diagnosis is made in patients with progressive parkinsonism in the absence of a toxic or other known underlying etiology. Familial forms with autosomal-dominant or autosomal-recessive inheritance exist. Although these make up a limited number of cases, they have contributed to our understanding of the pathogenesis of the disease. In addition to the movement disorder, there are other, less well-characterized changes in mental function, which may include dementia, in a subset of individuals with PD.

Morphology. On pathologic examination, the typical macroscopic findings are **pallor of the substantia nigra** (Fig. 28–37) and locus ceruleus. On microscopic examination, there is loss of the pigmented, catecholaminergic neurons in these regions associated with gliosis. Lewy bodies (Fig. 28–37*C*) may be found in some of the remaining neurons.

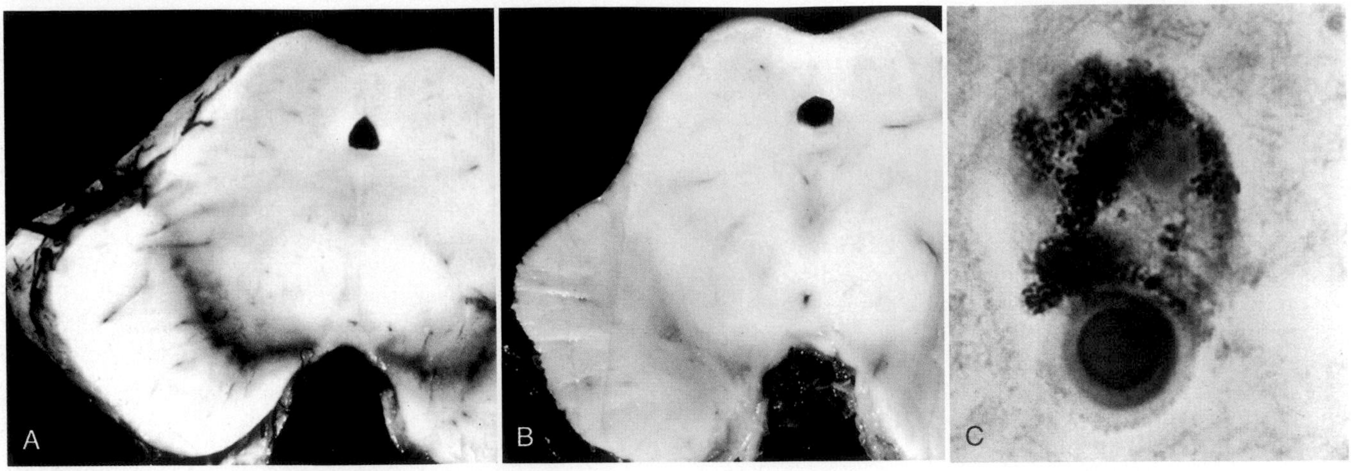

FIGURE 28–37 Parkinson disease (PD). *A*, Normal substantia nigra. *B*, Depigmented substantia nigra in idiopathic PD. *C*, Lewy bodies in a substantia nigra neuron stain bright pink. (*C*, courtesy of Dr. R. Kim, V.A. Medical Center, Long Beach, CA.)

These are single or multiple, cytoplasmic, eosinophilic, round to elongated inclusions that often have a dense core surrounded by a pale halo. Ultrastructurally, Lewy bodies are composed of fine filaments, densely packed in the core but loose at the rim. These filaments are composed of α-synuclein, as was realized after the gene for this protein was linked to familial PD; neurofilament antigens, parkin, and ubiquitin are also present in the Lewy body.[175] Lewy bodies may also be found in the cholinergic cells of the basal nucleus of Meynert, which is depleted of neurons (particularly in patients with abnormal mental function), as well as in other brainstem nuclei.

Pathogenesis and Molecular Genetics. The dopaminergic neurons of the substantia nigra project to the striatum, and their degeneration in Parkinson disease is associated with a reduction in the striatal dopamine content. The severity of the motor syndrome is proportional to the dopamine deficiency, which can, at least in part, be corrected by replacement therapy with L-DOPA (the immediate precursor of dopamine). Treatment does not, however, reverse the morphologic changes or arrest the progress of the disease; and with progression, drug therapy tends to become less effective, and symptoms become more difficult to manage.

An acute parkinsonian syndrome and destruction of neurons in the substantia nigra follows exposure to MPTP (1-methyl-4-phenyl-1,2,3,6-tetrahydropyridine), a contaminant in the illicit synthesis of psychoactive meperidine analogs. Action by monoamine oxidase B is required for the toxicity of MPTP. The use of this toxin in experimental animals has proved highly useful in studies of therapeutic interventions for PD, including transplantation.[176] Epidemiologic evidence has also suggested that pesticide exposure may increase the risk of PD,[177] while caffeine and nicotine may be protective.[178–180]

Studies of PD took a major step forward when the gene encoding α-synuclein, an abundant lipid-binding protein associated with synapses, was identified as the basis for an inherited autosomal-dominant form of PD, prompting the recognition that it was a major component of the Lewy body.[181,182] To date, a few mutations (A53T, A30P, and E46K) have been characterized as causal for PD.[183–185] However, only rare cases of PD have mutations in α-synuclein. Families with autosomal dominant PD and genomic triplication of the region containing the gene for α-synuclein (as well as flanking genes) have been found.[186,187] This suggests that gene dosage may also be related to PD, similar to the relationship between AD and trisomy 21. A second gene, encoding the protein parkin, was linked with a juvenile autosomal recessive form of PD.[188] Alterations including deletions and nonsense and missense mutations resulting in loss of parkin functions have been found in various families. These mutations are most prevalent in the population of young-onset PD patients.[189] The pathology of parkin-linked PD is similar to that of α-synuclein–linked or sporadic PD except for the absence of Lewy bodies in most but not all cases.[190–192] Parkin functions as an E3 ubiquitin ligase, with α-synuclein as one of its substrates.[193] A third genetic locus connected with PD encodes the deubiquitination enzyme UCH-L1. The mutant protein (I93M) has decreased activity and is linked with inherited PD in a single family.[194] It has also been suggested that this enzyme can catalyze the reverse reaction as well.[195] Another locus for autosomal recessive Parkinson disease has been mapped to the gene for a multifunctional protein, DJ-1, that is expressed mainly in astrocytes in the brain.[196–198] Thus, the genetics of PD have begun to explain the presence of the diagnostic inclusions and to suggest a link between altered protein degradation and the disease. Numerous other genetic loci are linked to Parkinson disease but the relevant genes remain to be mapped; their identification will undoubtedly lead to additional insights into the disease.

Clinical Features. About 10% to 15% of patients with PD develop dementia, with increasing incidence with advancing age. Characteristic features of this disorder include a fluctuating course, hallucinations, and prominent frontal signs. While many affected individuals also have pathologic evidence of Alzheimer disease (or, less frequently, other degenerative diseases associated with cognitive changes), the dementia in others is attributed to widely disseminated Lewy bodies that are less distinct but still demonstrable by immunohistochemistry for ubiquitin and α-synuclein, particularly in the cerebral cortex but also involving the amygdala and brainstem neurons.[199] Similar pathology, with this distribution of cortical Lewy bodies, can also be found in individuals with symptoms of dementia as their primary complaint—this is the disorder recognized as *dementia with Lewy bodies* (DLB). The relationship between DLB and PD with subsequent development of dementia remains to be clarified.

Symptomatic response to L-DOPA therapy is one of the features, in addition to clinical signs and symptoms, that support a diagnosis of PD. While L-DOPA therapy is often extremely effective in symptomatic treatment, it does not significantly alter the intrinsically progressive nature of the disease. Over time, L-DOPA becomes less able to help the patient through symptomatic relief and begins to lead to fluctuations in motor function on its own. As a result, there has been a search for alternative therapies that might alter the disease course. Given the well-characterized biochemical defect in PD, therapy through neural transplantation has been attempted. Clinical improvement has been reported in patients with PD or MPTP-induced Parkinson disease treated with stereotactic implants of fetal mesencephalic tissue into the striatum.[200] Other current neurosurgical approaches to this disease include the strategic placement of lesions elsewhere in the extrapyramidal system to compensate for the loss of nigrostriatal function.[201] Strategic placement of stimulating electrodes (deep brain stimulation) can also provide relief of motor symptoms of PD.[202]

Multiple System Atrophy

While the designation *multiple system atrophy* (MSA) originally applied to a wide spectrum of neurodegenerative disorders affecting multiple neural "systems," it is now used to describe a group of disorders characterized by the presence of glial cytoplasmic inclusions (GCIs), typically within the cytoplasm of oligodendrocytes.[203] With recognition of GCIs, the three clinicopathologic entities of striatonigral degeneration, Shy-Drager syndrome, and olivopontocerebellar atrophy were gathered into a single pathologic category.[204] Subsequently, the identification of α-synuclein as the major component of the inclusions has resulted in this disorder being considered as a synucleinopathy.[205] Unlike PD, with which it shares the feature of α-synuclein–containing inclusions, no mutations in the gene for this synaptic protein have been found in cases of MSA.

Morphology. On macroscopic examination, there is typically atrophy of the cerebellum, including the cerebellar peduncles, pons (especially the basis pontis), medulla (especially the inferior olive), substantia nigra, and striatum (especially putamen). These brain regions show evidence of neuronal loss as well as variable numbers of neuronal cytoplasmic and nuclear inclusions.

The shared diagnostic feature of these disorders, the cytoplasmic inclusions, were originally demonstrated with silver impregnation methods and by immunostaining have been shown to contain α-synuclein[206] as well as ubiquitin and αB-crystallin. Tau may be present in the inclusions but is not hyperphosphorylated as compared with other diseases marked by tau inclusions.[207] The inclusions are ultrastructurally distinct from those found in other neurodegenerative diseases and are composed primarily of 20- to 40-nm tubules. Similar inclusions may also be found in the cytoplasm of neurons, sometimes in neuronal and glial nuclei, and in axons. It appears that glial cytoplasmic inclusions can occur in the absence of neuronal loss, suggesting that they may represent a primary pathologic event.[208]

Clinical Features. The two principal symptoms of MSA are parkinsonism and autonomic dysfunction, particularly orthostatic hypotension. When these are present in relative isolation, the syndromes may be referred to as striatonigral degeneration and Shy-Drager syndrome, respectively. Presentation as an isolated ataxic disorder with cerebellar dysfunction (olivopontocerebellar atrophy) is much rarer. In general, patients have clinical signs and symptoms that represent a combination of these entities, corresponding to a combination of anatomic sites of pathology. Parkinsonism (akinesia and rigidity) can be related to the degree of cell loss from the substantia nigra and striatum; ataxia with changes in the circuits involving the pons, cerebellum, and inferior olive; and autonomic symptoms with cell loss from the catecholaminergic nuclei of the medulla and the intermediolateral cell column of the spinal cord.

Huntington Disease

Huntington disease (HD) is an inherited autosomal-dominant disease characterized clinically by progressive movement disorders and dementia and histologically by degeneration of striatal neurons. The movement disorder chorea consists of jerky, hyperkinetic, sometimes dystonic movements affecting all parts of the body; patients may later develop parkinsonism with bradykinesia and rigidity. The disease is relentlessly progressive, with an average course of about 15 years to death.

Morphology. On macroscopic examination, the brain is small and shows striking atrophy of the caudate nucleus and, less dramatically, the putamen (Fig. 28–38). The globus pallidus may be atrophied secondarily, and the lateral and third ventricles are dilated. Atrophy is frequently also seen in the frontal

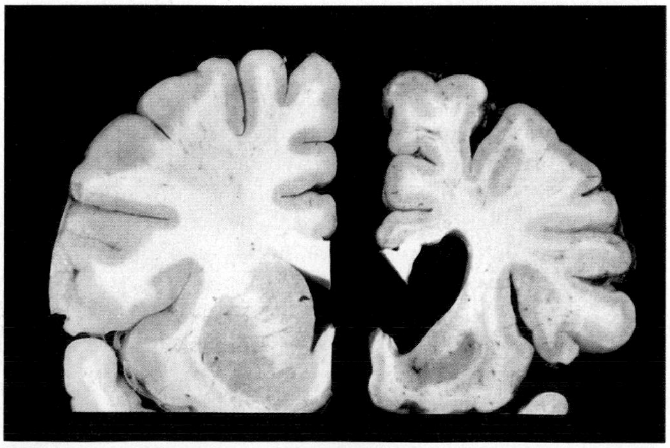

FIGURE 28–38 Huntington disease (HD). Normal hemisphere on the left compared with the hemisphere with HD on the right showing atrophy of the striatum and ventricular dilation. (Courtesy of Dr. J.-P. Vonsattel, Columbia University, New York, NY.)

lobe, less often in the parietal lobe, and occasionally in the entire cortex.

On microscopic examination, there is severe loss of striatal neurons; the most dramatic changes are found in the caudate nucleus, especially in the tail and portions nearer the ventricle. The putamen is less involved. Pathologic abnormalities develop in a medial-to-lateral direction in the caudate and from dorsal to ventral in the putamen. The nucleus accumbens is the best preserved structure. Both the large and small neurons are affected, but loss of the small neurons generally precedes that of the large. The medium-sized, spiny neurons that use GABA as their neurotransmitter, along with enkephalin, dynorphin, and substance P, are especially affected. Two populations of neurons are relatively spared in the disease: the diaphorase-positive neurons that contain nitric oxide synthase and the large cholinesterase-positive neurons; both appear to serve as local interneurons. There is also fibrillary gliosis that is more extensive than in the usual reaction to neuronal loss. There is a direct relationship between the degree of degeneration in the striatum and the severity of clinical symptoms.[209]

Pathogenesis and Molecular Genetics. The functional significance of the loss of medium spiny striatal neurons is to dysregulate the basal ganglia circuitry that modulates motor output. The loss of the striatal inhibitory output to the external portion of the globus pallidus results in increased inhibitory input to the subthalamic nucleus. This inhibition of the subthalamic nucleus prevents it from exerting its regulatory effects on motor activity and thus leads to choreoathetosis. The structural basis of the cognitive changes associated with the disease remains unclear, although there is evidence of neuronal loss from cerebral cortex as well.

The *HD* gene, located on 4p16.3, encodes a predicted protein, called *huntingtin*, of 348-kD molecular mass.[210] The coding region of the gene contains a polymorphic CAG trinucleotide repeat encoding a polyglutamine region of the protein. Normal *HD* genes contain 6 to 35 copies of the repeat; in disease-causing genes, the number of repeats is increased. The disease is thus an example of the "trinucleotide repeat disorders" discussed in Chapter 5. There is strong genotype-phenotype correlation, in the sense that the larger the number of repeats, the earlier the onset of the disease, although other genetic modifiers play a role.[211] Repeat expansions occur during spermatogenesis, and paternal transmission is associated with early onset in the next generation (anticipation; Chapter 5). Newly occurring mutations are uncommon, and most apparently sporadic cases can be related to errors in paternal identification or the death of a parent before expression of the disease. Some unaffected fathers have expanded repeats that are further expanded during transmission to their children.

The biologic function of huntingtin and how mutations cause disease remain unknown but are the focus of much study.[212] The protein is clearly essential, as targeted gene disruption in the mouse has demonstrated an early embryonic lethal phenotype. In tissue from HD patients, both wild-type and mutant protein are present. The expanded polyglutamine repeat results in protein aggregation and formation of intranuclear inclusions.[213] There are potential interactions between aggregated huntingtin and pathways involved in protein turnover, oxidative injury, and glutamate toxicity. Additionally, huntingtin with expanded polyglutamine repeats may alter transcription.[214,215]

Clinical Features. The age at onset is most commonly in the fourth and fifth decades and is related to the length of the CAG repeat in the *HD* gene. Motor symptoms often precede the cognitive impairment. The movement disorder of HD is choreiform, with increased and involuntary jerky movements of all parts of the body; writhing movements of the extremities are typical. Early symptoms of higher cortical dysfunction include forgetfulness and thought and affective disorders, but there is progression to a severe dementia. HD patients have an increased risk of suicide, with intercurrent infection being the most common natural cause of death. Given the ability to screen for disease-causing mutations and the devastating nature of the disease, HD is often the focal point of discussion of ethical issues in genetic diagnosis.

SPINOCEREBELLAR DEGENERATIONS

This group of diseases affects, to a variable extent, the cerebellar cortex, spinal cord, peripheral nerves, and other regions of the neuraxis. The clinical spectrum includes cerebellar and sensory ataxia, spasticity, and sensorimotor peripheral neuropathy. This is a clinically heterogeneous group of illnesses that include several distinct diseases; these can be distinguished on the basis of their patterns of inheritance, age at onset, and pattern of signs and symptoms. Degeneration of neurons, without distinctive histopathologic changes, occurs in the affected areas and is associated with mild gliosis. Genetic analysis continues to redefine and subclassify these illnesses.[133]

Spinocerebellar Ataxias

This is a group of genetically distinct diseases characterized by signs and symptoms referable to the cerebellum (progressive ataxia), brainstem, spinal cord, and peripheral nerves, as well as other brain regions in different subtypes. Pathologically, they are characterized by neuronal loss from the affected areas with secondary degeneration of white matter tracts. The clinically identified spinocerebellar ataxias can be separated on the basis of inheritance pattern into autosomal dominant and recessive types; the genetic understanding of this large and diverse group of diseases continues to evolve (Table 28–3).[216,217] Among dominantly inherited forms, there are many that are associated with trinucleotide (or larger) repeat expansion. In those forms in which there is expansion of a CAG repeat encoding polyglutamine tract (SCA1-3,6,7,17), neuronal intranuclear inclusions containing the abnormal protein can be found, similar to Huntington disease. As with HD, these forms of spinocerebellar ataxia show correlation between the degree of repeat expansion and age of onset. All but SCA6 also show anticipation, with expansion of the repeat length during gametogenesis. Curiously, SCA6 shares its genetic locus with another cerebellar disorder—episodic ataxia type 2 (EA-2)—which is associated with point mutations. The other form of episodic ataxia (EA-1) is also a channelopathy, being caused by mutations in the delayed rectifier potassium channel subunit Kv1.1.

TABLE 28–3 Spinocerebellar Ataxias

Disease	Chromosome	Gene Product	Inheritance	Mutation
SCA1	6p23	ataxin-1	AD	CAG in coding region
SCA2	12q24.1	ataxin-2	AD	CAG in coding region
SCA3	14q21	ataxin-3	AD	CAG in coding region
SCA4	16q22.1	?	AD	?
SCA5	11	?	AD	?
SCA6	19p13.1–2	α_{1A} voltage-dependent calcium channel subunit	AD	CAG in coding region
SCA7	3p21.1–p12	ataxin7	AD	CAG in coding region
SCA8	13q21	?	AD	Untranslated CTG repeat on antisense strand
SCA10	22q13	ataxin-10	AD	Intronic ATTTC repeat
SCA11	15q14–21	?	AD	
SCA12	5q31	protein phosphatase 2A	AD	CAG in 5′ UTR region
SCA13	19q13	?	AD	?
SCA14	19q13.4	?	AD	?
SCA15	3pter–24.2	?	AD	?
SCA16	8q22.24	?	AD	?
SCA17	6q27	TATA-binding protein	AD	CAG in coding region
FA	9q13–21	frataxin-1	AR	Intronic GAA repeat
Ataxia-telangiectasia	11q22–23	ATM	AR	Point mutations

Friedreich Ataxia

This is an autosomal-recessive progressive illness, generally beginning in the first decade of life with gait ataxia, followed by hand clumsiness and dysarthria. Deep tendon reflexes are depressed or absent, but an extensor plantar reflex is typically present. Joint position and vibratory sense are impaired, and there is sometimes loss of pain and temperature sensation and light touch. Most patients develop pes cavus and kyphoscoliosis. There is a high incidence of cardiac disease with arrhythmias and congestive heart failure. Concomitant diabetes is found in about 10% of patients. Most patients become wheelchair-bound within about 5 years of onset; the cause of death is intercurrent pulmonary infections and cardiac disease.

The gene for Friedreich ataxia has been mapped to chromosome 9q13, and in most cases, there is a GAA trinucleotide repeat expansion in the first intron of a gene encoding a protein named *frataxin*.[218] Affected individuals inherit abnormal forms of the *frataxin* gene from both parents and have extremely low levels of the protein. In some cases of Friedreich ataxia, one of the mutant alleles harbors a missense or nonsense mutation. Frataxin undergoes processing and ends up in the inner mitochondrial membrane, where it has been suggested to play a role in regulation of iron levels.[219,220] Because of the need for this metal in many of the complexes of the oxidative phosphorylation chain, mutations in frataxin have been suggested to result in generalized mitochondrial dysfunction. Thus, Friedreich ataxia shares biologic features with other spinocerebellar ataxias (anatomic distribution of pathology, trinucleotide repeat expansion) and the mitochondrial encephalopathies.

Morphology. The spinal cord shows loss of axons and gliosis in the posterior columns, the distal portions of corticospinal tracts, and the spinocerebellar tracts. There is degeneration of neurons in the spinal cord (Clarke column), the brainstem (cranial nerve nuclei VIII, X, and XII), the cerebellum (dentate nucleus and the Purkinje cells of the superior vermis), and to some extent the Betz cells of the motor cortex. Large dorsal root ganglion neurons are also decreased in number; their large myelinated axons, traveling first in the dorsal roots and then in dorsal columns, therefore undergo secondary degeneration. The heart is enlarged and may have pericardial adhesions. Multifocal destruction of myocardial fibers with inflammation and fibrosis is detectable in about half the patients who come to autopsy examination.

Ataxia-Telangiectasia

Ataxia-telangiectasia (Chapter 7) is an autosomal-recessive disorder characterized by an ataxic-dyskinetic syndrome beginning in early childhood, caused by neuronal degeneration predominantly in the cerebellum, the subsequent development of telangiectasias in the conjunctiva and skin, and immunodeficiency. Cells from patients with the disease show increased sensitivity to x-ray-induced chromosome abnormalities; these cells continue to replicate damaged DNA rather than stopping to allow repair or apoptosis. The ataxia-telangiectasia locus on chromosome 11q22–23 has been identified as a large gene, *ATM*, that encodes a protein with a kinase domain; the protein orchestrates the cellular response to double-stranded DNA breaks.[221,222] The carrier frequency of ataxia-telangiectasia has been estimated at 1%; in these individuals, the mutated ataxia-telangiectasia allele may underlie an increased risk of cancer, specifically breast cancer.

Morphology. The abnormalities are predominantly in the cerebellum, with loss of Purkinje and granule cells; there is also degeneration of the dorsal columns, spinocerebellar tracts, and anterior horn cells and a peripheral neuropathy. Telangiectatic lesions have been reported in the CNS as well as in the conjunctiva and skin of the face, neck, and arms. The nuclei of cells in many organs (e.g., Schwann cells in dorsal root ganglia and peripheral nerves, endothelial cells, pituicytes) show a bizarre enlargement of the cell nucleus to two to five times normal size and are referred to as amphicytes. The lymph nodes, thymus, and gonads are hypoplastic.

Clinical Features. The disease relentlessly progresses to death early in the second decade. Patients first come to medical attention because of recurrent sinopulmonary infections and unsteadiness in walking. Later on, speech is noted to become dysarthric, and eye movement abnormalities develop. Many affected individuals develop lymphoid malignant disease (T-cell leukemia, T-cell lymphoma); gliomas and carcinomas have been reported in some.

DEGENERATIVE DISEASES AFFECTING MOTOR NEURONS

These are a group of inherited or sporadic diseases that, in variable degrees of severity, affect:

- *Lower motor neurons* in the anterior horns of the spinal cord
- *Lower motor neurons* in certain cranial nerve motor nuclei (V, VII, IX, XII) but not those that control eye movements (III, IV, VI)
- *Upper motor neurons* (Betz cells) in the motor cortex

The disorders occur in all age groups, and the course of the illness is extremely variable, ranging from slowly progressive or nonprogressive to rapidly progressive and fatal in a period of months or a few years. Denervation of muscles from loss of lower motor neurons and their axons results in muscular atrophy, weakness, and fasciculations; the corresponding histologic changes in nerve and muscle are discussed in Chapter 27. The clinical manifestations include paresis, hyperreflexia, spasticity, and extensor plantar responses (Babinski sign). Sensory systems and cognitive functions are unaffected, but types with dementia do occur.

Amyotrophic Lateral Sclerosis (Motor Neuron Disease)

Amytrophic lateral sclerosis (ALS) is characterized by neuronal muscle atrophy (amyotrophy) and hyperreflexia due to loss of lower motor neurons in the anterior horns of the spinal cord and upper motor neurons that project in corticospinal tracts, respectively.[223] The disease affects men slightly more frequently than women and becomes clinically manifest in the fifth decade or later. Five per cent to 10% of cases are familial, mostly with autosomal-dominant inheritance.[224]

Pathogenesis. The etiology and pathogenesis of amyotrophic lateral sclerosis are unknown. For a subset of the familial cases, the genetic locus has been mapped to the copper-zinc superoxide dismutase gene (*SOD1*) on chromosome 21.[225] A wide variety of missense mutations have been identified that appear to generate an adverse gain-of-function phenotype. Among the mutations, the A4V mutation is the most common (approaching 50% of cases), is associated with a rapid course, and rarely has upper motor neuron signs.[226,227] A recessive locus on chromosome 2 has been mapped to a gene encoding a protein termed alsin that has structural homology to proteins involved in GTPase regulation.[228,229] Other genetic loci for ALS have been mapped but not yet cloned. There is also evidence of roles of glutamate toxicity and protein nitration in the development of ALS pathology.[224] The basis for the selective involvement of motor neurons remains uncertain.

Morphology. On macroscopic examination, the anterior roots of the spinal cord are thin; the precentral gyrus may be atrophic in especially severe cases. Microscopic examination demonstrates a reduction in the number of anterior horn neurons throughout the length of the spinal cord with associated reactive gliosis and loss of anterior root myelinated fibers. Similar findings are found with involvement of the hypoglossal, ambiguus, and motor trigeminal cranial nerve nuclei. Remaining neurons often contain Bunina bodies: PAS-positive cytoplasmic inclusions that appear to be remnant of autophagic vacuoles. Skeletal muscles innervated by the degenerated lower motor neurons show neurogenic atrophy. Destruction of the upper motor neurons leads to degeneration of myelin in the corticospinal tracts, resulting in pale staining that is particularly evident at the lower segmental levels but traceable throughout the corticospinal system with special studies (Fig. 28–39).

Clinical Features. Early symptoms include asymmetric weakness of the hands, manifested as dropping objects and difficulty in performing fine motor tasks, and cramping and

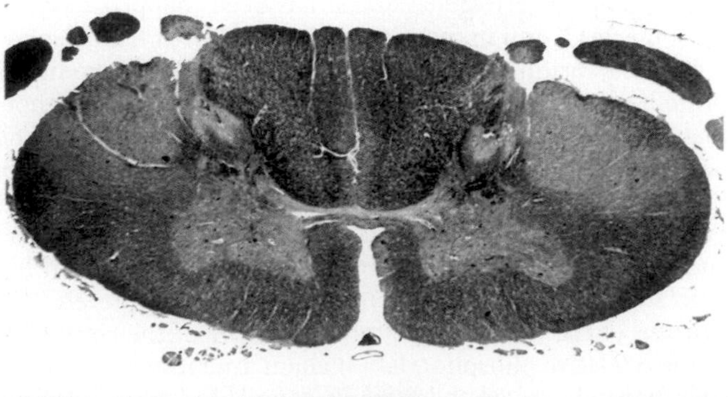

FIGURE 28–39 Amyotrophic lateral sclerosis. Spinal cord showing loss of myelinated fibers (lack of stain) in corticospinal tracts. The anterior roots are smaller than the posterior roots.

spasticity of the arms and legs. As the disease progresses, muscle strength and bulk diminish, and involuntary contractions of individual motor units, termed fasciculations, occur. The disease eventually involves the respiratory muscles, leading to recurrent bouts of pulmonary infection. The severity of involvement of the upper and lower motor neurons is variable; the term *progressive muscular atrophy* applies to those relatively uncommon cases in which lower motor neuron involvement predominates. In some patients, degeneration of the lower brainstem cranial motor nuclei occurs early and progresses rapidly, a pattern referred to as *progressive bulbar palsy* or *bulbar amyotrophic lateral sclerosis*. In these individuals, abnormalities of deglutition and phonation dominate, and the clinical course is inexorable during a 1- or 2-year period. Familial cases develop symptoms earlier than most sporadic cases do, but the clinical course is comparable.

Bulbospinal Atrophy (Kennedy Syndrome)

This X-linked adult-onset disease is characterized by distal limb amyotrophy and bulbar signs such as atrophy and fasciculations of the tongue and dysphagia. Affected individuals manifest androgen insensitivity with gynecomastia, testicular atrophy, and oligospermia. On microscopic examination, there is degeneration of lower motor neurons in the spinal cord and brainstem. The gene defect is expansion of a CAG/polyglutamine repeat in the androgen receptor (40 to 60 for affected individuals as opposed to 11 to 33 for the normal allele); nuclear inclusions containing aggregated androgen receptor can be found.[230] There is no anticipation with this disorder, and there is not a strong correlation between the size of the expansion and severity of clinical phenotype.[231]

Spinal Muscular Atrophy

This group of diseases affects mainly the lower motor neurons in children. As in ALS, there is a selective loss of anterior horn cells and atrophy of anterior spinal roots. It includes several entities with distinct clinical courses (Chapter 27).

Genetic Metabolic Diseases

A subset of genetic metabolic diseases affects the nervous system preferentially and will be discussed here; other metabolic diseases are covered elsewhere in this book. Many of these disorders express themselves in children who are normal at birth but who begin to miss developmental milestones during infancy and childhood.

- *Neuronal storage diseases* are mostly autosomal-recessive diseases caused by a deficiency of a specific enzyme involved in the catabolism of sphingolipids, mucopolysaccharides, or mucolipids. They are often characterized by the accumulation of the substrate of the enzyme within the lysosomes of neurons, leading to neuronal death. Cortical neuronal involvement leads to loss of cognitive function and may also cause seizures. The relationship between the accumulated material and cell injury and death is usually unclear.
- *Leukodystrophies* show a selective involvement of myelin (either abnormal synthesis or turnover), and generally exhibit no neuronal storage defects. Some of these disorders involve lysosomal enzymes; others affect peroxisomal enzymes. Diffuse involvement of white matter leads to deterioration in motor skills, spasticity, hypotonia, or ataxia. Although most are autosomal-recessive disorders, adrenoleukodystrophy, an X-linked disease, is a notable exception. Subtypes, or variants, are recognized for many of these disorders. These variants frequently follow the principle that the earlier the age at onset, the more severe the clinical course.
- *Mitochondrial encephalomyopathies* are a group of disorders of oxidative phosphorylation, usually resulting from mutations in the mitochondrial genome. They typically involve gray matter as well as skeletal muscle (Chapter 27).

LEUKODYSTROPHIES

Krabbe Disease

This disease is an autosomal-recessive leukodystrophy resulting from a deficiency of *galactocerebroside β-galactosidase (galactosylceramidase)*, the enzyme required for the catabolism of galactocerebroside to ceramide and galactose.[232] Over 40 different mutations have been found in the gene encoding this enzyme, which is located on chromosome 14q31. While some accumulation of galactocerebroside may occur, this is not the direct toxic agent in this disease. Instead, it appears that an alternative catabolic pathway removes a fatty acid from this molecule, generating galactosylsphingosine, which is a cytotoxic compound that could cause oligodendrocyte injury.

The clinical course is rapidly progressive, with onset of symptoms often between the ages of 3 and 6 months. Survival beyond 2 years of age is uncommon. The clinical symptoms are dominated by motor signs, including stiffness and weakness, with gradually worsening difficulties in feeding. The brain shows loss of myelin and oligodendrocytes in the CNS and a similar process in peripheral nerves. Neurons and axons are relatively spared. A unique feature of Krabbe disease is the aggregation of macrophages filled with cerebroside, forming multinucleated cells (*globoid cells*), around blood vessels.

Metachromatic Leukodystrophy

This disorder is transmitted in an autosomal-recessive pattern and results from a deficiency of the lysosomal enzyme *arylsulfatase A*. This enzyme, present in a variety of tissues, cleaves the sulfate from sulfate-containing lipids (sulfatides), the first step in their degradation. Enzyme deficiency leads to an accumulation of the sulfatides, especially cerebroside sulfate; how this leads to myelin breakdown is not known. The gene for arylsulfatase A has been localized to chromosome 22q, and a wide range of mutations have been described.

Recognized clinical subtypes of the disorder include a late infantile form (the most common), a juvenile form, and an adult form. The two forms with childhood onset often present with motor symptoms and progress gradually, leading to death in 5 to 10 years. In the adult form, psychiatric or cognitive symptoms are the usual initial complaint, with motor symptoms coming later, and the disease has a slower course than in the infantile form. Five allelic and two nonallelic forms are now recognized, with onset from childhood to adulthood corresponding to mutations that lead to decreased synthesis or activity of the enzyme. Although there is no known cure,

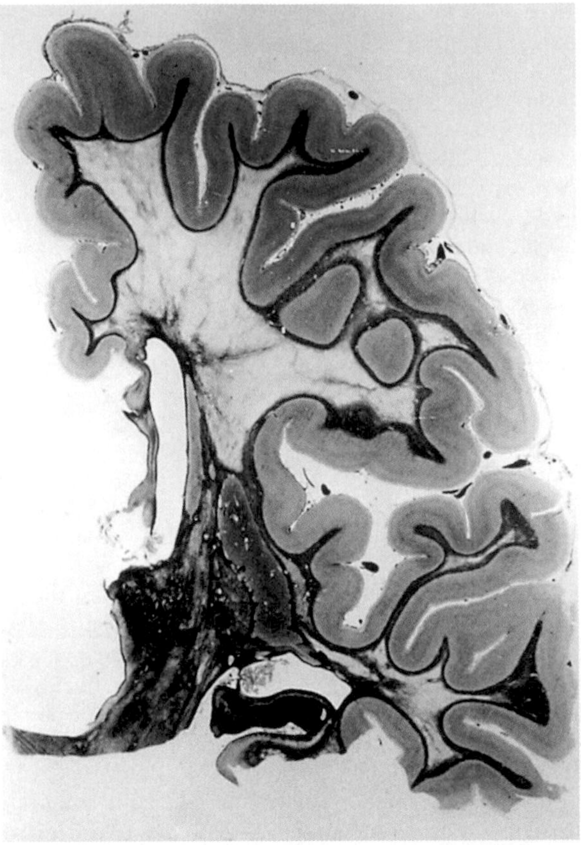

FIGURE 28–40 Metachromatic leukodystrophy. Demyelination is extensive. The subcortical fibers in the cerebral hemisphere are spared (Luxol fast blue PAS stain for myelin).

promising results have recently been achieved with bone marrow transplantation.

The most striking histologic finding is demyelination with resulting gliosis (Fig. 28–40). Macrophages with vacuolated cytoplasm are scattered throughout the white matter. The membrane-bound vacuoles contain complex crystalloid structures composed of sulfatides; when bound to certain dyes such as toluidine blue, sulfatides shift the absorbance spectrum of the dye, a property called *metachromasia.* Similar changes in peripheral nerve are observed. The detection of metachromatic material in the urine is also a sensitive method of establishing the diagnosis.

Adrenoleukodystrophy

This disorder, which has several clinically and genetically distinct forms, is a progressive disease with symptoms referable to myelin loss from the CNS and peripheral nerves as well as adrenal insufficiency. In general, forms with earlier onset have a more rapid course. The X-linked form usually presents in the early school years with neurologic symptoms and adrenal insufficiency and is rapidly progressive and fatal. In individuals with later onset, the course is more protracted; when it develops in adults, it is usually a slowly progressive disorder with predominantly peripheral nerve involvement developing over a period of decades. The disease is associated with mutations in the *ALD* gene on chromosome Xq28, which encodes a member of the ATP-binding cassette transporter family of proteins. However, there is little correlation between clinical course and the underlying mutations. The disease is characterized by the inability to properly catabolize very-long-chain fatty acids (VLCFA) within peroxisomes, with elevated levels of VLCFA in serum. There is loss of myelin, with relative preservation of the subcortical U fibers, accompanied by gliosis and lymphocytic inflammation. Atrophy of the adrenal cortex is present, and VLCFA accumulation can be seen in remaining cells.

Pelizaeus-Merzbacher Disease

This is an X-linked, invariably fatal, leukodystrophy beginning either in early childhood or just after birth, and characterized by slowly progressive signs and symptoms resulting from widespread white matter dysfunction.[233] Patients present with pendular eye movements, hypotonia, choreoathetosis, and pyramidal signs early in the disease, followed later by spasticity, dementia, and ataxia. The disease has been shown to arise in most cases from defects in a gene on the X chromosome that encodes proteolipid protein (PLP), a major protein of CNS myelin.[234] Although myelin is nearly completely lost in the cerebral hemispheres, patches may remain, giving a "tigroid" appearance to tissue sections stained for myelin.

Canavan Disease

The disease is characterized by megalocephaly, severe mental deficits, blindness, and signs and symptoms of white matter injury beginning in early infancy and relentlessly progressing to death by 18 months of age. Autopsy studies have shown spongy degeneration of the white matter, particularly affecting subcortical U fibers and Alzheimer type II astrocytes in the gray matter. Aspartoacylase activity is deficient in affected individuals, and point mutations and deletions in the gene for aspartylacylase, located on chromosome 17pter-p13, underlie this autosomal-recessive disease.[235] The function of N-acetylaspartic acid, which accumulates when this enzyme is mutated, and its relationship to myelin are not known.

MITOCHONDRIAL ENCEPHALOMYOPATHIES

Although many of the inherited disorders of mitochondrial oxidative phosphorylation present as muscle diseases (Chapter 27), some of them involve the central nervous system either as a primary target or in addition to skeletal muscle.[236,237] While these disorders are typically associated with a specific class of mutation, there remains some genetic heterogeneity within otherwise well-defined clinicopathologic entities.[238,239]

Leigh Syndrome (Subacute Necrotizing Encephalopathy)

This disease of early childhood is characterized by lactic acidemia, arrest of psychomotor development, feeding problems, seizures, extraocular palsies, and weakness with hypotonia. Death usually occurs within 1 to 2 years. On histologic examination, there are multifocal, moderately symmetric regions of destruction of brain tissue with a spongiform appearance and proliferation of blood vessels. The areas that are most commonly affected include the periventricular gray matter of the midbrain, the tegmentum of the pons, and the periventricular regions of the thalamus and hypothalamus. Most cases are inherited in an autosomal-recessive pattern and show decreased activity of complex IV (cytochrome c oxidase) of mitochondrial oxidative phosphorylation.[240] Most often, the mutation affects a protein that is required for assembly of this complex of oxidative phosphorylation, rather than a structural component of the complex.[241] Other cases with comparable clinical and pathologic features have been linked to deficits in other complexes of the respiratory chain as well as mtDNA tRNA mutations.[239] Interestingly, a point mutation in the mitochondrial gene for ATPase 6 subunit of complex V (T8993G) can cause a maternally inherited form of Leigh syndrome; in this form, heteroplasmy results in mitochondria with this mutation being nearly the only kind present.[242] When there is a higher degree of heteroplasmy with normal mitochondria, the disease takes on a different clinical and pathologic appearance, as *neuropathy, ataxia, and retinitis pigmentosa* (NARP).

Other Mitochondrial Encephalomyopathies

Myoclonic epilepsy and ragged red fibers (MERRF) is a maternally transmitted disease in which patients have myoclonus, a seizure disorder, and evidence of a myopathy (Chapter 27). Ataxia, associated with evidence of neuronal loss from the cerebellar system (including inferior olive in the medulla, cerebellar cortex, and outflow nuclei), is also a common component. Two common mutations involve the mitochondrial tRNA, affecting protein synthesis within mitochodria.

Mitochondrial encephalomyopathy, lactic acidosis, and stroke-like episodes (MELAS) is another syndrome caused by mitochondrial abnormalities, in which children have acute episodes of neurologic dysfunction, cognitive changes, and evidence of muscle involvement with weakness and lactic acidosis. The stroke-like episodes that give the syndrome its name are often reversible deficits that do not correspond well to specific vascular territories. Pathologically, areas of infarction are observed, often with vascular proliferation and focal calcification. This syndrome is associated with mutations involving a different mitochondrial tRNA. Metabolic abnormalities are present in cerebral vessels, which may underlie the stroke-like episodes.[243]

Kearns-Sayre syndrome (KSS) ("ophthalmoplegia plus") is a sporadic disorder, associated with a large mtDNA deletion/rearrangement.[244] The disorder may present with cerebellar ataxia in addition to the progressive external ophthalmoplegia, pigmentary retinopathy, and cardiac conduction defects. Pathologically, there is spongiform change in gray and white matter, with neuronal loss most evident in the cerebellum.

Toxic and Acquired Metabolic Diseases

Toxic and acquired metabolic diseases are relatively common causes of neurologic illnesses. These diseases were discussed in Chapter 9, and only aspects that are relevant to CNS pathology are discussed here.

VITAMIN DEFICIENCIES

Thiamine (Vitamin B_1) Deficiency

As was discussed in Chapter 9, thiamine deficiency may result in the slowly evolving clinical disorder *beriberi.* In certain patients, thiamine deficiency may also lead to the development of psychotic symptoms or ophthalmoplegia that begin abruptly, a syndrome termed *Wernicke encephalopathy.* The acute stages, if unrecognized and untreated, may be followed by a prolonged and largely irreversible condition, *Korsakoff syndrome,* characterized clinically by memory disturbances and confabulation. Because the two syndromes are closely linked, the term *Wernicke-Korsakoff syndrome* is often applied. The syndrome is particularly common in the setting of chronic alcoholism, but it may also be encountered in patients with thiamine deficiency resulting from gastric disorders, including carcinoma, chronic gastritis, or persistent vomiting. Treatment with vitamin B_1 may reverse manifestations of Wernicke syndrome.

Morphology. Wernicke encephalopathy is characterized by foci of hemorrhage and necrosis, particularly in the mammillary bodies but also adjacent to the ventricle, especially the third and fourth ventricles. Early lesions show dilated capillaries with prominent endothelial cells. Subsequently, the capillaries leak red cells into the interstitium, producing hemorrhagic areas that are easily detectable macroscopically. With time, there is infiltration of macrophages and development of a cystic space with hemosiderin-laden macrophages as a permanent sign of the process. These chronic hemosiderin-laden lesions predominate in patients with Korsakoff syndrome. Lesions in the medial dorsal nucleus of the thalamus appear to be the best correlate of the memory disturbance and confabulation.

Vitamin B_{12} Deficiency

Deficiency of vitamin B_{12} often causes anemia (Chapter 13), but its most severe and potentially irreversible effects are related to nervous system lesions. The neurologic symptoms may present in the course of a few weeks, initially with slight ataxia and numbness and tingling in the lower extremities, but may progress rapidly to include spastic weakness of the lower extremities. Complete paraplegia may occur, usually only later in the course of the disease. With prompt vitamin replacement therapy, clinical improvement occurs; however, if complete paraplegia has developed, recovery is poor. On microscopic examination, vitamin B_{12} deficiency leads to a swelling of myelin layers, producing vacuoles that begin segmentally at the midthoracic level of the spinal cord in the early stages. With time, axons in both the ascending tracts of the posterior columns and the descending pyramidal tracts degenerate. While isolated involvement of descending or ascending tracts may be observed in a variety of spinal cord diseases, the combined degeneration of both ascending and descending tracts of the spinal cord is characteristic of vitamin B_{12} deficiency and has led to the designation of the disorder as *subacute combined degeneration of the spinal cord.*

NEUROLOGIC SEQUELAE OF METABOLIC DISTURBANCES

Hypoglycemia

Since the brain requires glucose and oxygen for its energy production, the cellular effects of diminished glucose resemble those of oxygen deprivation, as described earlier. Some regions of the brain are more sensitive to hypoglycemia than are others. Glucose deprivation initially leads to selective injury to large pyramidal neurons of the cerebral cortex, which, if it is severely involved, may result in pseudolaminar necrosis of the cortex, predominantly involving layers III to V. The hippocampus is also vulnerable to glucose depletion, as it is to hypoxia, and may show a dramatic loss of pyramidal neurons in Sommer sector (area CA1 of the hippocampus). Purkinje cells of the cerebellum are also vulnerable to hypoglycemia, although to a lesser extent than to hypoxia. If the level and duration of hypoglycemia are of sufficient severity, there may be widespread injury to many areas of the brain.

Hyperglycemia

Hyperglycemia is most commonly found in the setting of inadequately controlled diabetes mellitus and can be associated with either ketoacidosis or hyperosmolar coma. The patient becomes dehydrated and develops confusion, stupor, and eventually coma. The fluid depletion must be corrected gradually; otherwise, severe cerebral edema may follow.

Hepatic Encephalopathy

The pathogenesis of hepatic encephalopathy or hepatic coma is discussed in Chapter 18. The cellular response in the CNS is predominantly glial. *Alzheimer type II changes* are evident in the cortex and basal ganglia and other subcortical gray matter regions.

TOXIC DISORDERS

Cellular and tissue injury from toxic agents is discussed in Chapter 1. Aspects of several important toxic disorders that are of unique neurologic importance are discussed here.

Carbon Monoxide

Many of the pathologic findings that follow acute carbon monoxide exposure are the result of hypoxia. Thus, selective injury of the neurons of layers III and V of the cerebral cortex, Sommer sector of the hippocampus, and Purkinje cells is the recognized consequence of carbon monoxide exposure. Bilateral necrosis of the globus pallidus may also occur, and is more common in carbon monoxide–induced hypoxia than in hypoxia from other causes. Demyelination of white matter tracts may be a later event.

Methanol

The pathologic findings of methanol toxicity are seen in the retina, where degeneration of retinal ganglion cells may cause blindness. Selective bilateral putamenal necrosis and focal white matter necrosis also occur when the exposure is severe. There is some evidence that formate, a major metabolite of methanol, may play a role in the retinal toxicity.

Ethanol

The effects of acute ethanol intoxication are reversible, but chronic alcohol abuse is associated with a variety of neurologic sequelae, including Wernicke-Korsakoff syndrome, considered above. The "toxic" effects of chronic alcohol intake may be either direct effects of ethanol or secondary nutritional deficits. Cerebellar dysfunction occurs in about 1% of chronic alcoholics, associated with a clinical syndrome of truncal ataxia, unsteady gait, and nystagmus. The histologic changes are atrophy and loss of granule cells predominantly in the anterior vermis (Fig. 28–41). In advanced cases, there is loss of Purkinje cells and proliferation of the adjacent astrocytes (*Bergmann gliosis*) between the depleted granular cell layer and the molecular layer of the cerebellum. The fetal alcohol syndrome is discussed in Chapter 10.

Radiation

Delayed effects of radiation present with rapidly evolving symptoms of an intracranial mass, including headaches, nausea, vomiting, and papilledema that may develop months to years after irradiation.[245] The pathologic findings consist of large areas of coagulative necrosis with adjacent edema. The typical lesion is restricted to white matter, and all elements within the area undergo necrosis, including astrocytes, axons, oligodendrocytes, and blood vessels. Adjacent to the area of coagulative necrosis, proteinaceous spheroids may be identified, and blood vessels exhibit thickened walls with intramural fibrin-like material. Radiation can also induce tumors, which are usually are not seen until years after radiation therapy and include poorly differentiated sarcomas, gliomas, and meningiomas.

Combined Methotrexate and Radiation-Induced Injury

Methotrexate toxicity most commonly develops when the drug has been administered in association with radiotherapy, either together or at separate times. The interval between the inciting events and the onset of symptoms varies considerably but may be as long as months. Symptoms often begin with drowsiness, ataxia, and confusion, and may progress rapidly. While some patients recover function after the initial onset of symptoms, others may become comatose; rarely, methotrexate neurotoxicity may be responsible for the patient's death.

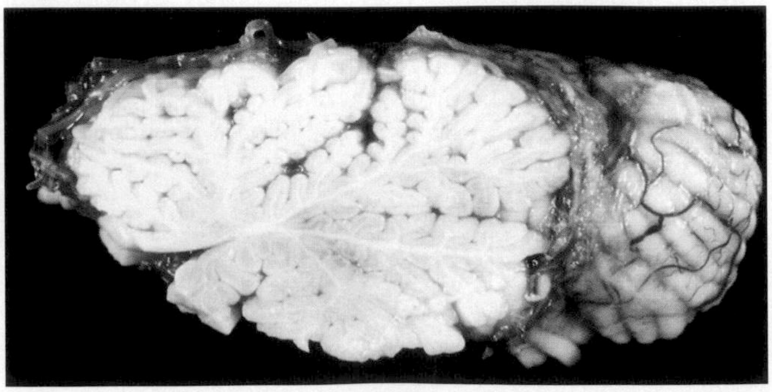

FIGURE 28–41 Alcoholic cerebellar degeneration. The anterior portion of the vermis *(upper portion of figure)* is atrophic with widened spaces between the folia.

The mechanisms of these delayed effects of methotrexate are unclear.

The pathologic basis of the symptoms are focal areas of coagulative necrosis within white matter, often adjacent to the lateral ventricles but at times distributed throughout the white matter or in the brainstem. Surrounding axons are often dilated and form axonal spheroids. Axons and cell bodies in the vicinity of the lesions undergo dystrophic mineralization, and there is adjacent gliosis.

Tumors

The annual incidence of tumors of the CNS ranges from 10 to 17 per 100,000 persons for intracranial tumors and 1 to 2 per 100,000 persons for intraspinal tumors; about half to three-quarters are primary tumors, and the rest are metastatic. Tumors of the CNS account for 20% of all cancers of childhood. Seventy per cent of childhood CNS tumors arise in the posterior fossa; a comparable number of tumors in adults arise within the cerebral hemispheres above the tentorium.[246–251]

Tumors of the nervous system have several unique characteristics that set them apart from neoplastic processes elsewhere in the body. First, the distinction between benign and malignant lesions is less evident in the CNS than in other organs. Some glial tumors with histologic features of a benign neoplasm, including low mitotic rate, cellular uniformity, and slow growth, may infiltrate large regions of the brain, thereby leading to serious clinical deficits and poor prognosis. Second, the ability to surgically resect infiltrating glial neoplasms without compromising neurologic function is limited. Third, the anatomic site of the neoplasm can have lethal consequences irrespective of histologic classification; for example, a benign meningioma, by compressing the medulla, can cause cardiorespiratory arrest. Finally, the pattern of spread of primary CNS neoplasms differs from that of other tumors: Even the most highly malignant gliomas rarely metastasize outside the CNS. The subarachnoid space provides a pathway for spread, so seeding along the brain and spinal cord can occur in highly anaplastic as well as in well-differentiated neoplasms that extend into the CSF pathways.

The four major classes of brain tumors are:

- Gliomas
- Neuronal tumors
- Poorly differentiated neoplasms
- Meningiomas

GLIOMAS

Gliomas, derived from glial cells, include *astrocytomas*, *oligodendrogliomas*, and *ependymomas*.

Astrocytoma

Several different categories of tumors derived from astrocytes are recognized, including fibrillary astrocytoma, glioblastoma, pilocytic astrocytoma, and pleomorphic xanthoastrocytoma as well as rarer types. These have characteristic histologic features, distribution within the brain, age groups typically affected, and clinical course.

Fibrillary (Diffuse) Astrocytomas and Glioblastoma

These account for about 80% of adult primary brain tumors. Usually found in the cerebral hemispheres, they may also occur in the cerebellum, brainstem, or spinal cord, most often in the fourth through sixth decades. The most common presenting signs and symptoms are seizures, headaches, and focal neurologic deficits related to the anatomic site of involvement. Fibrillary astrocytomas show a spectrum of histologic differentiation that correlates well with clinical course and outcome.

Morphology. Among the diffuse fibrillary astrocytomas, tumors can be well differentiated (astrocytoma) or less differentiated (higher-grade), ranging from **anaplastic astrocytoma** to **glioblastoma.** The macroscopic appearance of diffuse fibrillary astrocytoma is that of a poorly defined, gray, infiltrative tumor that expands and distorts the invaded brain (Fig. 28–42). These tumors range in size from a few centimeters to enormous lesions that replace an entire hemisphere. The cut surface of the tumor is either firm or soft and gelatinous; cystic degeneration may be seen. In glioblastoma, variation in the gross appearance of the tumor from region to region is characteristic (Fig. 28–43). Some areas are firm and white, others are soft and yellow (the result of tissue necrosis), and yet others show regions of cystic degeneration and hemorrhage. The tumor may appear well demarcated from the surrounding brain tissue, but infiltration beyond the outer margins is always present.

Radiologic studies show mass effect as well as changes in the brain adjacent to the tumor, such as edema. High-grade astrocytomas have abnormal vessels that are "leaky" and are therefore demonstrable when contrast media are injected into the venous system.

On microscopic examination, **well-differentiated fibrillary astrocytomas** are characterized by a mild to moderate increase in the number of glial cell nuclei, somewhat variable nuclear pleomorphism, and an intervening feltwork of fine, GFAP-positive astrocytic cell processes that give the background a fibrillary appearance. The transition between neoplastic and normal tissue is indistinct, and tumor cells can be seen infiltrating normal tissue at some distance from the main lesion. **Anaplastic astrocytomas** show regions that are more densely cellular and have greater nuclear pleomorphism from well-differentiated fibrillary astrocytoma; mitotically active cells are often observed.

The term **gemistocytic astrocytoma** is used for tumors in which the predominant neoplastic astrocyte shows a brightly eosinophilic cell body from which emanate abundant, stout processes.

Glioblastoma (previously called *glioblastoma multiforme*) has a histologic appearance similar to anaplastic astrocytoma with the additional features of *necrosis* and *vascular or endothelial cell proliferation*, each of which often has a stereotypic appearance. Necrosis in glioblastoma, often in a serpentine pattern, occurs in areas of hypercellularity with highly malignant tumor cells crowded along the edges of the necrotic regions, producing a histologic pattern

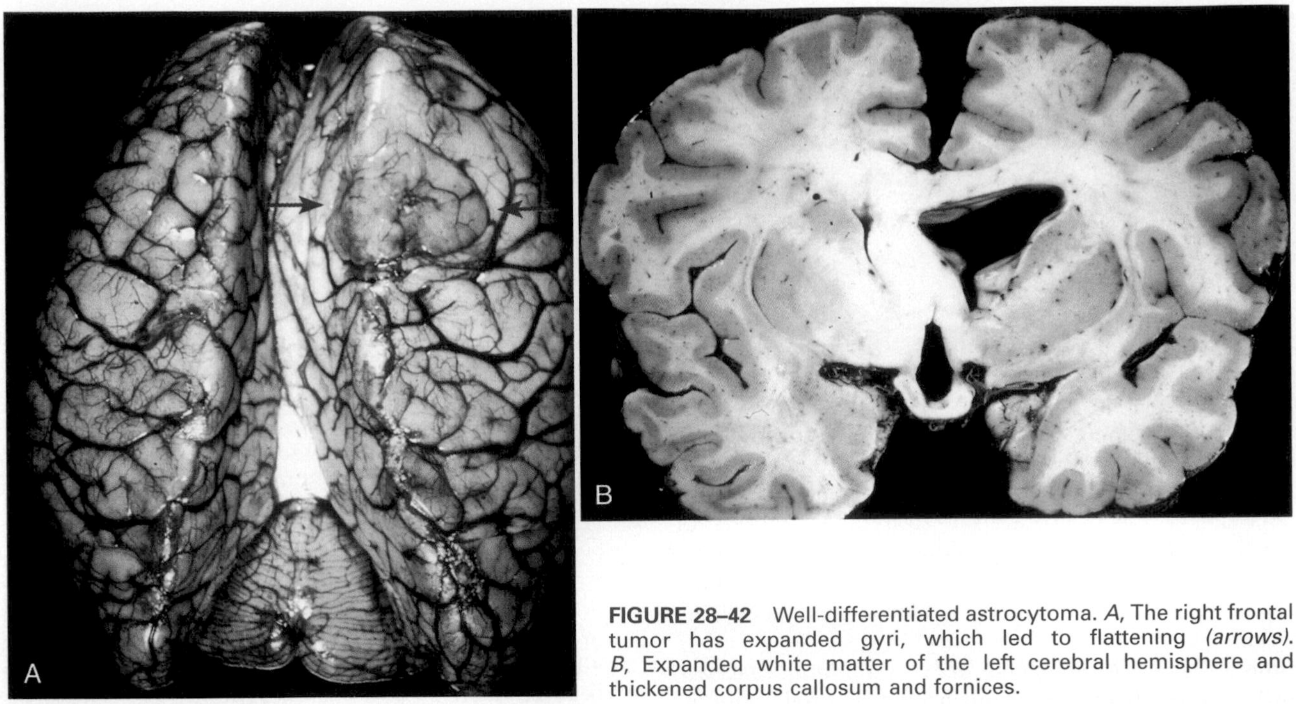

FIGURE 28–42 Well-differentiated astrocytoma. *A,* The right frontal tumor has expanded gyri, which led to flattening *(arrows)*. *B,* Expanded white matter of the left cerebral hemisphere and thickened corpus callosum and fornices.

referred to as **pseudopalisading** (Fig. 28–44). Vascular cell proliferation is characterized by tufts of piled-up vascular cells that bulge into the vascular lumen; the minimal criterion for this feature of glioblastoma is a double layer of endothelial cells. When vascular cell proliferation is extreme, the tuft forms a ball-like structure, the **glomeruloid body** (Fig. 28–44). Vascular endothelial cell growth factor (VEGF), produced by malignant astrocytes, perhaps in response to hypoxia, contributes to this distinctive form of vascular change.

In the condition called **gliomatosis cerebri,** multiple regions of the brain, in some cases the entire brain, are infiltrated by neoplastic astrocytes.

Grading schemes for fibrillary astrocytomas have clinical utility in predicting prognosis and in fashioning treatment options. Currently, clinical protocols and trials are based on the World Health Organization (WHO) grading scheme, which considers tumors to be one of four grades based on

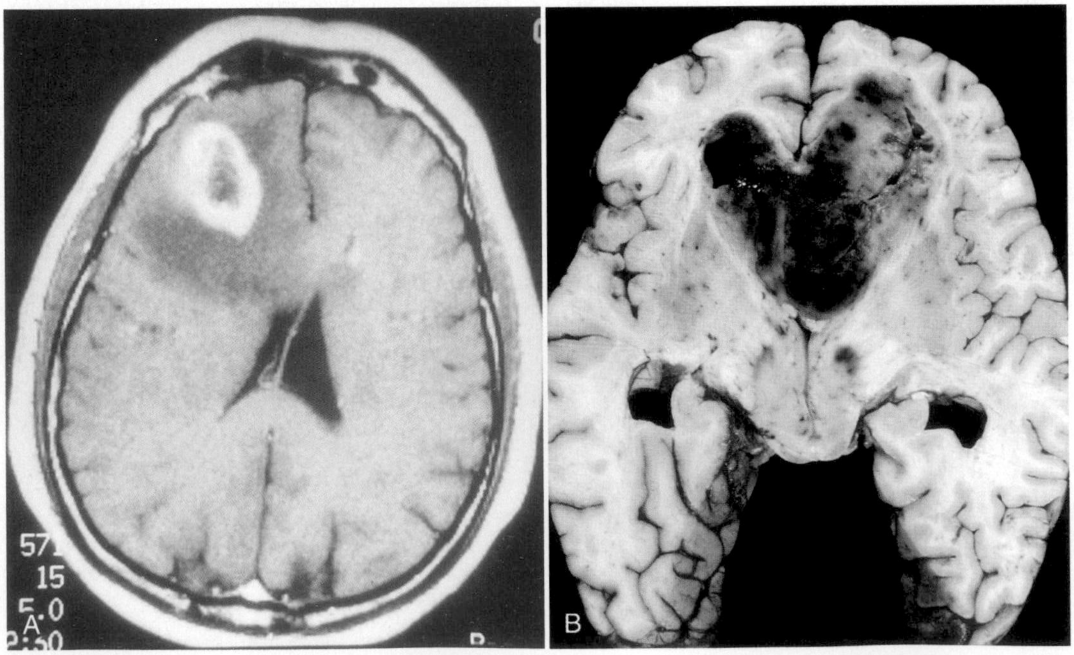

FIGURE 28–43 *A,* Computed tomographic (CT) scan of a large tumor in the cerebral hemisphere showing signal enhancement with contrast material and pronounced peritumoral edema. *B,* Glioblastoma multiforme appearing as a necrotic, hemorrhagic, infiltrating mass.

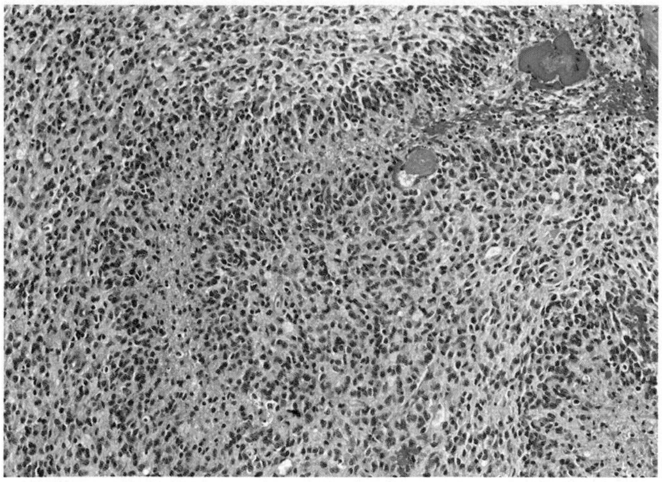

FIGURE 28–44 Glioblastoma. Foci of necrosis with pseudopalisading of malignant nuclei.

their biologic behavior, ranging from grade I to grade IV. To ensure that all involved in a patient's care are aware of the grading system being used, tumor grade is expressed in the format "x/IV." For diffuse fibrillary astrocytomas, the most recent WHO scheme separates these tumors into well-differentiated astrocytoma (grade II/IV), anaplastic astrocytoma (III/IV), and glioblastoma (IV/IV).[247–252] Since the range of cellular anaplasia and presence of other histologic features of high grade can be extremely variable from one region of the neoplasm to another, a single small biopsy specimen might not be representative of the tumor.

Molecular Genetics. Genetic alterations have been observed to be correlated with the progression of astrocytic tumors from low to high grade, which is part of the natural course of the disease in many patients.[253] Among the alterations that are most commonly found in the low-grade astrocytomas are inactivation of p53 and overexpression of PDGF-A and its receptor. The transition to higher-grade astrocytoma is associated with additional disruption of tumor-suppressor genes, the *RB* gene, the *p16/CDKNZA* gene, and a putative tumor suppressor on chromosome 19q.

It was recognized well before advances in genetic analyses that there were two distinct clinical histories that could be associated with glioblastoma: a short, rapidly progressive disease arising without a preexisting low-grade tumor, typically in older individuals (*primary glioblastoma*), and a disease of comparable clinical course that arose in younger patients with a previously diagnosed lower-grade astrocytoma (*secondary glioblastoma*). With the advent of genetic characterization of glioblastoma, it became clear that secondary glioblastomas shared *p53* mutations that characterized low-grade gliomas, while primary glioblastomas were characterized by amplification of the epidermal growth factor receptor (*EGFR*) gene. In addition to these two changes, there are certain other genetic alterations that mark the two pathways to glioblastoma: *PDGF-A* amplification in secondary glioblastomas and *MDM2* overexpression, *p16* deletion, or *PTEN* mutation in primary glioblastoma. Despite the genetic distinctions, it remains uncertain whether survival after diagnosis is different in these groups.[254–256] There is, however, a correlation between the presence of small cells in glioblastoma and *EGFR* amplification.[257]

Clinical Features. The presenting symptoms of astrocytomas depend, in part, on the location of the tumor and its rate of growth. Astrocytomas have a tendency to become more anaplastic with time. With well-differentiated astrocytomas, the symptoms may remain static or progress only slowly over a number of years, with a mean survival of more than 5 years. Eventually, however, patients usually have more rapid clinical deterioration that is generally correlated with the appearance of anaplastic features and more rapid growth of the tumor. The prognosis for patients with glioblastoma is very poor. With current treatment, consisting of resection when feasible together with radiotherapy and chemotherapy, the mean length of survival after diagnosis is only 8 to 10 months; fewer than 10% of patients are alive after 2 years. Survival is substantially shorter in older patients.

Pilocytic Astrocytoma

Pilocytic astrocytomas are distinguished from the other types by their pathologic appearance and relatively benign behavior. They typically occur in children and young adults and are usually located in the cerebellum but may also appear in the floor and walls of the third ventricle, the optic nerves, and occasionally the cerebral hemispheres.

Morphology. On macroscopic examination, a pilocytic astrocytoma is often cystic, with a mural nodule in the wall of the cyst (Fig. 28–45); if solid, it may be well circumscribed or, less frequently, infiltrative. On microscopic examination, the tumor is composed of bipolar cells with long, thin "hairlike" processes that are GFAP-positive; Rosenthal fibers, eosinophilic granular bodies, and microcysts are often present. An increase in the number of blood vessels, often with thickened walls or vascular cell proliferation, is seen but does not imply an unfavorable prognosis; necrosis and mitoses are uncommon. Unlike diffuse fibrillary astrocytomas of any grade, pilocytic astrocytomas have a narrow infiltrative border with the surrounding brain.

These tumors grow very slowly, are considered as WHO grade I/IV, and, in the cerebellum particularly, may be treated by resection. Symptomatic recurrence from incompletely resected lesions is often associated with cyst enlargement rather than growth of the solid component. Tumors that extend into the hypothalamic region from the optic tract can

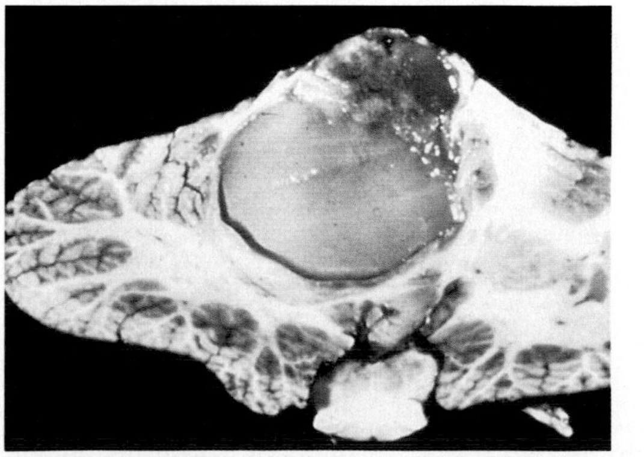

FIGURE 28–45 Pilocytic astrocytoma in the cerebellum with a nodule of tumor in a cyst.

have a more difficult clinical course because of location. The histologic separation of these tumors from other astrocytomas is supported by genetic studies; these have shown that pilocytic astrocytomas rarely have *p53* mutations or other changes found in diffuse fibrillary astrocytomas.

Pleomorphic Xanthoastrocytoma

This is a tumor that occurs most often relatively superficially in the temporal lobe of children and young adults, usually with a history of seizures. On microscopic examination, the tumor consists of neoplastic, occasionally bizarre, astrocytes, which are sometimes lipidized. The degree of nuclear atypia can be extreme and may suggest a high-grade astrocytoma, but the presence of abundant reticulin deposits, relative circumscription, and chronic inflammatory cell infiltrates along with an absence of necrosis and mitotic activity will redirect the pathologist toward the diagnosis. This is usually a low-grade tumor (WHO grade II/IV), with a survival rate estimated at 80% at 5 years. Necrosis and mitotic activity are markers of a more anaplastic form, with a correspondingly more aggressive course.[258]

Brainstem Glioma

A clinical subgroup of astrocytomas, brainstem gliomas occur mostly in the first two decades of life and make up about 20% of primary brain tumors in this age group. Several distinct anatomic patterns have been defined in the pediatric age group, with differences in clinical course: intrinsic pontine gliomas (the most common, with an aggressive course and short survival); tumors, often exophytic, arising in the cervicomedullary junction region (with a less aggressive course); and tectal gliomas (with an even more benign course and which are rarely biopsied).[259] Among the rarer brainstem gliomas affecting adults, most are intrinsic pontine gliomas. These can be separated into low-grade diffuse fibrillary astrocytomas and glioblastoma, with the expected differences in clinical course and survival.[260]

Oligodendroglioma

These tumors constitute 5% to 15% of gliomas and are most common in the fourth and fifth decades. Patients may have had several years of neurologic complaints, often including seizures. The lesions are found mostly in the cerebral hemispheres, with a predilection for white matter.

Morphology. On macroscopic examination, oligodendrogliomas are well-circumscribed, gelatinous, gray masses, often with cysts, focal hemorrhage, and calcification. On microscopic examination, the tumors are composed of sheets of regular cells with spherical nuclei containing finely granular chromatin (similar to normal oligodendrocytes) surrounded by a clear halo of cytoplasm. The tumor typically contains a delicate network of anastomosing capillaries. Calcification, present in as many as 90% of these tumors, ranges from microscopic foci to massive depositions. As the tumor cells infiltrate cerebral cortex, there is often formation of secondary structures, particularly with perineuronal satellitosis. Mitotic activity is usually very difficult to detect, and labeling indices are low. Oligodendrogliomas are considered to be WHO grade II/IV lesions.

Anaplastic oligodendrogliomas (WHO grade III/IV) are characterized by increased cell density, with nuclear anaplasia, increased mitotic activity, and necrosis. These changes can often be found in nodules within an otherwise grade II/IV oligodendroglioma. Also often present in these higher-grade lesions are discrete round cells with cytoplasmic GFAP and nuclei that resemble the other elements of the tumor. These microgemistocytes differ from gemistocytic astrocytes because they lack abundant processes; the intermediate filaments are restricted to a small lump of cytoplasm.

Molecular Genetics. The underlying genetic processes for oligodendroglial tumors, along with their histologic appearance, distinguishes them from astrocytic tumors. The most common genetic alterations in oligodendrogliomas are loss of heterozygosity for chromosomes 1p and 19q. The specific tumor suppressor loci that are involved in the generation of these tumors remain unknown. Additional genetic alterations tend to accumulate with progression to anaplastic oligodendroglioma. The more common of these include loss of 9p, loss of 10q, and mutation in *CDKN2A*. In addition to implications for the biology of the tumors, the study of molecular alterations in anaplastic oligodendrogliomas has also had direct clinical impact in planning treatment. Tumors with loss of 1p and 19q but without other alterations have a consistent and long-lasting response to therapy (chemotherapy and radiation). Those with additional genetic changes have a shorter-lived response, and those without loss of 1p and 19q appear to be refractory to these therapies.[261,262]

Clinical Features. In general, patients with oligodendrogliomas have a better prognosis than do patients with astrocytomas. Current treatment with surgery, chemotherapy, and radiotherapy has yielded an average survival of 5 to 10 years. Patients with anaplastic oligodendroglioma have a worse prognosis, although there are subgroups of tumors, as defined by genetic alterations, that respond well to therapy.

The terms *oligoastrocytoma* and *anaplastic oligoastrocytoma* have been employed to designate neoplasms consisting of distinct regions of oligodendroglioma and astrocytoma of appropriate grade. The diagnostic criteria for these entities remain controversial; genetic analysis has not clarified the issue, as tumors with these histologic descriptors can be found that share alterations with either astrocytomas or oligodendrogliomas. The idea that these tumors are not a true mixture is supported by the observation that the genetic changes are usually of one type or another (1p/19q vs. p53/chr17).[263–265]

Ependymoma and Related Paraventricular Mass Lesions

Ependymomas most often arise next to the ependyma-lined ventricular system, including the oft-obliterated central canal of the spinal cord. In the first two decades of life, they typically occur near the fourth ventricle and constitute 5% to 10% of the primary brain tumors in this age group. In adults, the spinal cord is their most common location; tumors in this site are particularly frequent in the setting of neurofibromatosis type 2 (see below).

Morphology. In the fourth ventricle, ependymomas are typically solid or papillary masses extending from the floor of the ventricle (Fig. 28–46*A*). Although they are often better demarcated from adjacent brain than are astrocytomas, their proximity to the vital pontine and medullary nuclei usually makes complete extirpation impossible. In the intraspinal tumors, this sharp demarcation sometimes makes total removal feasible. On microscopic examination, ependymomas are composed of cells with regular, round to oval nuclei with abundant granular chromatin. Between the nuclei, there is a variably dense fibrillary background. Tumor cells may form gland-like round or elongated structures (rosettes, canals) that resemble the embryologic ependymal canal, with long, delicate processes extending into a lumen (Fig. 28–46*B*); more frequently present are **perivascular pseudorosettes** (Fig. 28–46*B*) in which tumor cells are arranged around vessels with an intervening zone consisting of thin ependymal processes directed toward the wall of the vessel. GFAP expression is found in most ependymomas. While most ependymomas are well differentiated and behave as WHO grade II/IV lesions, anaplastic ependymomas occur with increased cell density, high mitotic rates, areas of necrosis, and less evident ependymal differentiation. These lesions are more aggressive (WHO grade III/IV).

Myxopapillary ependymomas are distinct but related lesions that occur in the filum terminale of the spinal cord and contain papillary elements in a myxoid background, admixed with ependymoma-like cells. Cuboidal cells, sometimes with clear cytoplasm, are arranged around papillary cores containing connective tissue and blood vessels. The myxoid areas contain neutral and acidic mucopolysaccharides. Prognosis depends on completeness of surgical resection; if the tumor has extended into the subarachnoid space and surrounded the roots of the cauda equina, recurrence is likely.

Molecular Genetics. Because of the association of spinal ependymomas with neurofibromatosis type 2, the *NF2* gene on chromosome 22 has been examined as a candidate locus for alterations in ependymomas. Interestingly, it appears that alterations at this site may be involved in the pathogenesis of ependymomas in the spinal cord but not at other sites.[266] Ependymomas do not appear to share the genetic alterations that are found in other gliomas, such as mutations in *p53*.

Clinical Features. Posterior fossa ependymomas often manifest with hydrocephalus secondary to progressive obstruction of the fourth ventricle rather than invasion of the pons or medulla. Prognosis is poor despite the slow growth of the tumor and the usual lack of histologic evidence of anaplasia. Because of the relationship of ependymomas to the ventricular system, CSF dissemination is a common occurrence. An average survival of about 4 years after surgery and radiotherapy has been reported. The clinical outcome for completely resected supratentorial and spinal ependymomas is better.

Several other tumors occur either immediately below the ependymal lining of the ventricle or in association with the other cell type that forms the walls of the ventricular system: choroid plexus. With the exception of the rare choroid plexus carcinoma, these are benign to low-grade lesions; however, their location may cause clinical problems.

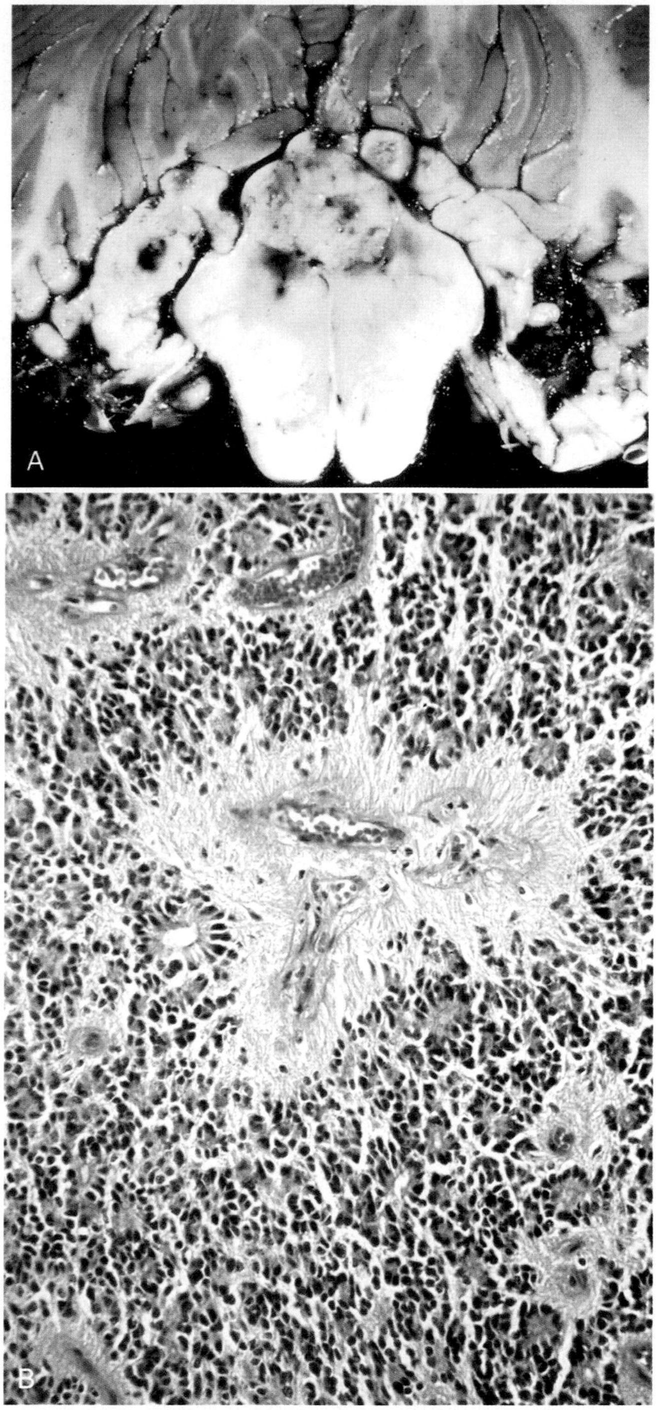

FIGURE 28–46 Ependymoma. *A*, Tumor growing into the fourth ventricle, distorting, compressing, and infiltrating surrounding structures. *B*, Microscopic appearance of ependymoma.

- *Subependymomas* are solid, sometimes calcified, slow-growing nodules attached to the ventricular lining and protruding into the ventricle. They are usually asymptomatic and are incidental findings at autopsy, but if they are sufficiently large or strategically located, they may cause hydrocephalus. They are most often found in the lateral and fourth ventricles and there, as is the case with other fourth ventricular tumors, are difficult for the neurosurgeon to remove. They have a characteristic microscopic appearance, with clumps of ependymal-appearing nuclei scattered in a dense, fine, glial fibrillar background.

- *Choroid plexus papillomas* can occur anywhere along the choroid plexus and are most common in children, in whom they are most often found in the lateral ventricles. In adults, they are more often found in the fourth ventricle. These tumors almost exactly recapitulate the structure of the normal choroid plexus and are markedly papillary growths. The papillae have connective tissue stalks covered with a cuboidal or columnar epithelium. Clinically, choroid plexus papillomas usually present with hydrocephalus due to obstruction of the ventricular system by tumor or to overproduction of CSF. There are rare cases of *choroid plexus carcinoma*; the histologic appearance of these lesions closely resembles that of adenocarcinoma. They are usually found in children and may be associated with Li-Fraumeni syndrome; in adults, they need to be differentiated from the much more common metastatic carcinoma.
- *Colloid cyst of the third ventricle* is a non-neoplastic lesion that most often occurs in young adults. The cyst is attached to the roof of the third ventricle, thereby being capable of obstructing one or both of the foramina of Monro and, as a result, causing noncommunicating hydrocephalus, which may be rapidly fatal. Headache, sometimes positional, is an important clinical symptom. The cyst has a thin, fibrous capsule and a lining of low to flat cuboidal epithelium; it contains gelatinous, proteinaceous material.

NEURONAL TUMORS

Ganglion Cell Tumors

Several types of CNS tumors contain mature-appearing neurons (*ganglion cells*); these may constitute the entire population of the lesion (*gangliocytomas*). More commonly, there is an admixture with a glial neoplasm, and the lesion is termed a *ganglioglioma*. Most of these tumors are slow growing, but the glial component occasionally becomes frankly anaplastic, and the disease then progresses rapidly. Lesions that contain mixtures of neuronal and glial elements often present as a seizure disorder; surgical resection of the tumor is usually effective in controlling the seizures.

Morphology. Gangliocytomas are well-circumscribed masses with focal calcification and small cysts usually found in the floor of the third ventricle, the hypothalamus, or the temporal lobe. On microscopic examination, the neoplastic ganglion cells are present as clumps of cells separated by a relatively acellular stroma. The **ganglioglioma** has a macroscopic appearance similar to that of a glioma of comparable grade. It is most commonly found in the temporal lobe and may often have a cystic component. The neoplastic ganglion cells are irregularly clustered and have apparently random orientation of neurites. Binucleate forms are frequent. The neoplastic neurons can often be detected with the use of immunohistochemical reactions for neuronal proteins, neurofilaments, and synaptophysin. These tumors are usually considered as WHO grade I to II/IV lesions. Anaplastic gangliogliomas also occur, and behave as grade III/IV lesions.

Another recently recognized entity, which contains both glial and neuronal elements and can be considered a variant of ganglioglioma, is **papillary glioneuronal tumor.**[267] In this low-grade lesion, the glial cells often form a single cell layer on stalks of blood vessels (pseudopapillae), while the neuronal elements are more solid.

Other Tumors with Glial and Neuronal Components

Dysembryoplastic neuroepithelial tumor (DNT) is a distinctive, low-grade tumor of childhood that often presents as a seizure disorder, showing slow growth and a relatively good prognosis after surgical extirpation.[268,269] These lesions are typically located in the superficial temporal lobe, although other cortical sites are seen. There is often attenuation of the overlying skull, suggesting that the lesion has been present for a long time. Sites outside of the cerebral hemisphere are distinctly less common.

Morphology. This mixed glial-neuronal tumor is characterized by a **"specific glioneuronal element"** that consists of small, round cells with features of neurons that are arranged in columns around central cores of processes. These typically form multiple discrete intracortical nodules that have a myxoid background. There are well-differentiated "floating neurons" that sit in the pools of mucopolysaccharide-rich fluid of the myxoid background. The larger neurons and the small, round cells of the specific element express neuronal markers and do not show evidence of glial differentiation. In contrast to ganglioglioma, binucleate and other dysplastic neuronal forms are not part of this tumor. Surrounding the nodules, several different patterns are observed. There is often evidence of focal cortical dysplasia, with misplacing of cortical layers with maloriented neurons. Elements of neoplastic glia may also be part of the picture in DNT; lesions that show both the specific element and a glial component are termed **complex.** These components of the tumor are typically astrocytic and may resemble other types of low-grade glioma.

Tumors with Only Neuronal Elements

Cerebral neuroblastomas are rare neoplasms that occur in the hemispheres of children and show highly aggressive clinical behavior. On microscopic examination, they resemble peripheral neuroblastomas (Chapter 10), being composed of small, undifferentiated cells with characteristic Homer Wright rosettes. In contrast, *central neurocytoma* typically is a low-grade neuronal neoplasm found within and adjacent to the ventricular system (most commonly the lateral or third ventricles), characterized by evenly spaced, round, uniform nuclei and often islands of neuropil. Although in pattern and shape the cells resemble oligodendroglioma, ultrastructural and immunohistochemical studies reveal the neuronal lineage of the tumor cells.

POORLY DIFFERENTIATED NEOPLASMS

Some tumors, although of neuroectodermal origin, express few if any of the phenotypic markers of mature cells of the nervous system and are described as poorly differentiated, or embryonal, meaning that they retain cellular features of primitive, undifferentiated cells. The most common is the *medulloblastoma*, which accounts for 20% of the brain tumors in children.

Medulloblastoma

This tumor occurs predominantly in children and exclusively in the cerebellum. Neuronal and glial markers may be expressed, but the tumor is often largely undifferentiated.

Morphology. In children, medulloblastomas are located in the midline of the cerebellum (Fig. 28–47*A*), but lateral locations are more often found in adults. Rapid growth may occlude the flow of CSF, leading to hydrocephalus. The tumor is often well circumscribed, gray, and friable and may be seen extending to the surface of the cerebellar folia and involving the leptomeninges (Fig. 28–47*B*). On microscopic examination, medulloblastoma is usually extremely cellular, with sheets of anaplastic cells (Fig. 28–47*C*). Individual tumor cells are small, with little cytoplasm and hyperchromatic nuclei that are frequently elongated or crescent shaped. Mitoses are abundant, and markers of cellular proliferation, such as Ki-67, are detected in a high percentage of the cells. The tumor has the potential to express neuronal (neurosecretory granules or Homer Wright rosettes, as occur in neuroblastoma; Chapter 10) and glial (GFAP) phenotypes. The **desmoplastic variant** is characterized by areas of stromal response with collagen and reticulin deposition and nodules of cells forming "pale islands" that have more neuropil and lack the reticulin deposition.

At the edges of the main tumor mass, medulloblastoma cells have a propensity to form linear chains of cells infiltrating through cerebellar cortex to aggregate beneath the pia, penetrate the pia, and seed into the subarachnoid space. Dissemination through the CSF is a common complication, presenting as nodular masses elsewhere in the CNS, including metastases to the cauda equina that are sometimes termed "drop" metastases because of their direct route of dissemination through the CSF.

Tumors of similar histology and poor degree of differentiation can be found elsewhere in the nervous system; while most fall into other specific categories (e.g., pineoblastoma), there can be lesions in the cerebral hemispheres that strongly resemble medulloblastomas. These lesions are referred to by some as supratentorial primitive neuroectodermal tumors (PNET—an unfortunate acronym, since it leads to confusion with the peripheral lesion that shares a genetic alteration with Ewing sarcoma).

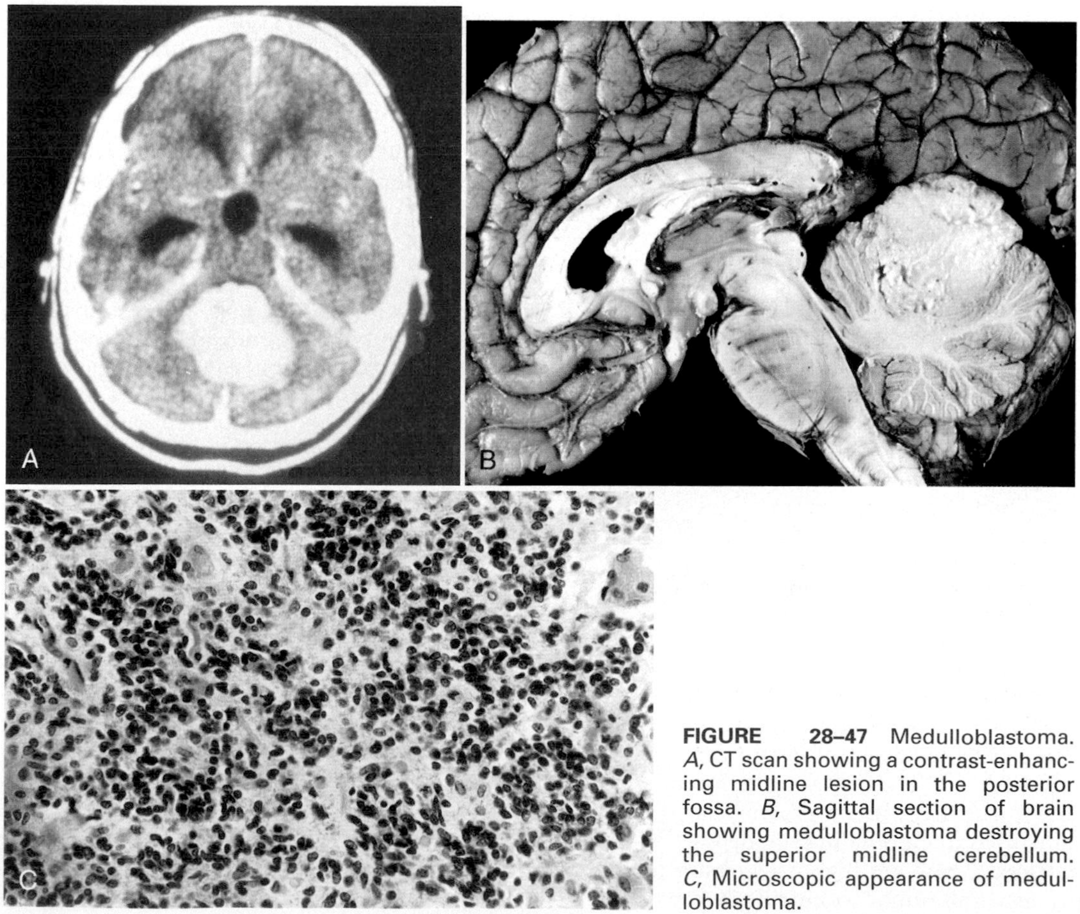

FIGURE 28–47 Medulloblastoma. *A,* CT scan showing a contrast-enhancing midline lesion in the posterior fossa. *B,* Sagittal section of brain showing medulloblastoma destroying the superior midline cerebellum. *C,* Microscopic appearance of medulloblastoma.

Molecular Genetics. The most common genetic alteration is loss of material from the short arm of chromosome 17. This often occurs in the setting of an abnormal chromosome derived from duplication of the long arm of chromosome 17 (isochromosome 17q or i(17q)). The identity of the tumor suppressor gene that is lost from chromosome 17 is not clear; although the *p53* gene is located on this chromosome, it does not appear to be the relevant gene. A variety of other genetic alterations have been found in medulloblastomas, including in the Sonic hedgehog/patched pathway (involved in control of normal proliferation of cerebellar granule cells), the Wnt signaling pathway (including APC and β-catenin), and others. Tumors that have increased levels of neurotrophin receptor *trkC* have a better clinical outcome.[270] Microarray analysis has recently demonstrated that there are distinct patterns of gene expression that are found in classic, compared to desmoplastic, medulloblastomas, and that patterns of expression can be used to stratify tumors according to clinical outcome.[271]

Clinical Features. The tumor is highly malignant, and the prognosis for untreated patients is dismal; however, it is an exquisitely radiosensitive tumor. Prognosis is also related to the amount of tumor resected, with better survival rates following complete resection. In addition, radiation of the brain and spinal cord decreases the likelihood of recurrence. With total excision and radiation, the 5-year survival rate may be as high as 75%.

Atypical Teratoid/Rhabdoid Tumor (AT/RT)

This is a recently recognized highly malignant tumor of young children.[272] The lesions are found in the posterior fossa and supratentorial compartments in nearly equal proportion. The histologic component of rhabdoid cells, resembling those of a rhabdomyosarcoma, is the defining characteristic of the lesion.

Morphology. AT/RT tumors tend to be large, with a soft consistency and spread along the surface of the brain. The rhabdoid cells have eosinophilic cytoplasm with sharp cell borders and eccentrically located nuclei. When these cells are smaller, the cytoplasm can take on the elongated appearance that mimics a rhabdomyosarcoma cell. The cytoplasm of the rhabdoid cell contains intermediate filaments and is immunoreactive for epithelial membrane antigen and vimentin. Some other markers that may be positive include smooth muscle actin and keratins. Other muscle markers such as desmin and myoglobin are not present. These cells are rarely a majority of the tumor; instead, islands of tumor with this pattern of differentiation are mixed with a small cell component, as well as other histologic patterns (including mesenchymal and epithelial). Mitotic activity is extremely prominent.

Molecular Genetics. One of the distinguishing features that allowed this lesion to be recognized as a separate entity was the frequent (>90%) evidence of loss of genetic material from chromosome 22.[273,274] The relevant gene has been shown to be *hSNF5/INI1*, which encodes a protein that is part of a large complex involved in chromatin remodeling.[275]

Clinical Features. These are highly aggressive tumors of the very young, nearly all tumors occurring before the age of 5 and most patients living less than a year after diagnosis.

OTHER PARENCHYMAL TUMORS

Primary CNS Lymphoma

Primary CNS lymphoma (PCNSL) accounts for 2% of extranodal lymphomas and 1% of intracranial tumors. It is the most common CNS neoplasm in immunosuppressed patients, including those with AIDS and immunosuppression after transplantation. Various epidemiologic studies have indicated an increase in the incidence of PCNSL, even in populations without immunosuppression.[276,277] In nonimmunosuppressed populations, the age spectrum is relatively wide, and the frequency increases after 60 years of age.

The term *primary* emphasizes the distinction between these lesions and secondary involvement of the CNS by non-Hodgkin lymphoma arising elsewhere in the body (Chapter 14). Patients with primary brain lymphoma often have multiple sites of tumor within the brain parenchyma; nodal, bone marrow, or extranodal involvement outside of the CNS is a rare and late complication. Conversely, non-Hodgkin lymphoma arising outside the CNS rarely involves the brain parenchyma; involvement of the nervous system, when it occurs in non-Hodgkin lymphoma, is manifested by the presence of malignant cells within the CSF and around intradural nerve roots and occasionally by the infiltration of superficial areas of the cerebrum or spinal cord by malignant cells.

The majority of primary brain lymphomas are of B-cell origin. In immunosuppressed patients, all the neoplasms appear to contain Epstein-Barr virus genomes within the transformed B cells. Regardless of the clinical context in which it occurs, primary brain lymphoma is an aggressive disease with relatively poor response to chemotherapy compared with peripheral lymphomas. Angiotropic lymphoma (intravascular lymphoma) often involves the brain along with other regions of the body. The occlusion of small vessels with malignant cells can result in widespread microscopic infarcts.

Morphology. Lesions are frequently multiple and often involve deep gray matter as well as white matter and cortex. Periventricular spread is common. The tumors are relatively well defined in comparison with glial neoplasms but are not as discrete as metastases and often show extensive areas of central necrosis. The tumors are nearly always high-grade lymphomas (Chapter 14), most commonly large cell lymphomas, although other histologic types can be observed. Within lesions, malignant cells infiltrate the parenchyma of the brain and accumulate around blood vessels. Reticulin stains demonstrate that the infiltrating cells are separated from one another by silver-staining material; this pattern, referred to as hooping, is characteristic of primary brain lymphoma. A benign mixed T- and B-cell infiltrate, which often contains a plasmacytic component, can also be found adjacent to lesions. When biopsies are obtained after partial treatment with high-dose steroids, this reactive component may be all that is identified.

Germ Cell Tumors

Primary brain germ cell tumors occur along the midline, most commonly in the pineal and the suprasellar regions. They account for 0.2% to 1% of brain tumors in people of European descent but up to 10% in Japanese people. They are a tumor of the young, with 90% occurring during the first two decades. Germ cell tumors, particularly teratomas, are among the more common tumors that present as congenital tumor. Germ cell tumors in the pineal region show a strong male predominance, which is not seen in suprasellar lesions.

It is not clear whether these tumors arise by the transformation of an otherwise normal resident population of germ cells, of a developmentally derived ectopic rest of germ cells, or of germ cells that migrated into the CNS late in development. Regardless of these uncertainties, germ cell tumors share many features with their counterparts in the gonads. In contrast to lymphomas, however, CNS involvement by a gonadal germ cell tumor is not uncommon; thus, the presence of a non-CNS primary must be excluded before a diagnosis of primary germ cell tumor is made. The histologic classification of brain germ cell tumors is similar to that used in the testis (Chapter 21), but the tumor that is histologically similar to the seminoma in the testis is referred to as germinoma in the CNS. The responses to radiotherapy and chemotherapy roughly parallel those of similar histologic lesions at other sites. However, since the tumor frequently extends into the CSF, it can disseminate widely along the surface of the brain and within the ventricular system, complicating therapy.

Pineal Parenchymal Tumors

These lesions arise from the specialized cells of the pineal gland (pineocytes) that have features of neuronal differentiation. The tumors range in histologic appearance from well-differentiated lesions (*pineocytomas*) with areas of neuropil—tumor cells with small, round nuclei and no evidence of mitoses or necrosis—to high-grade tumors (*pineoblastomas*) of densely packed small cells with necrosis and frequent mitotic figures and little light microscopic evidence of neuronal differentiation. The highly aggressive pineoblastoma commonly spreads throughout the CSF space, is more commonly found in children, and may occur in patients with bilateral retinoblastoma, associated with mutations in *RB*.

Gliomas are also found in the pineal region, arising from the glial stroma of the gland. Low-grade gliomas at this site can be difficult to distinguish in a small biopsy from the glial reaction that can accompany non-neoplastic pineal region cysts.

MENINGIOMAS

Meningiomas are predominantly benign tumors of adults, usually attached to the dura, that arise from the meningothelial cell of the arachnoid. Meningiomas may be found along any of the external surfaces of the brain as well as within the ventricular system, where they arise from the stromal arachnoid cells of the choroid plexus.

Morphology. Meningiomas are usually rounded masses with a well-defined dural base that compress underlying brain but are easily separated from it (Fig. 28–48*A*). Extension into the overlying bone may be present. The surface of the mass is usually encapsulated with thin, fibrous tissue and may have a bosselated or polypoid appearance. Another characteristic growth pattern is the **en plaque** variant, in which the tumor spreads in a sheetlike fashion along the surface of the dura. This form is commonly associated with hyperostotic reactive changes in the overlying bone. The lesions range from firm and fibrous to finely gritty, or they may be extremely calcified with psammoma bodies. Gross evidence of necrosis or extensive hemorrhage is not present.

Most meningiomas are considered grade I/IV by the WHO classification scheme, having a relatively low risk of recurrence or aggressive growth.[240] Various histologic patterns can be observed in these low-grade lesions and carry no prognostic significance. These include **syncytial,** appropriately named for the whorled clusters of cells that sit in tight groups without visible cell membranes; **fibroblastic,** with elongated cells and abundant collagen deposition between them; **transitional,** which share features of the syncytial and fibroblastic types; **psammomatous,** with numerous psammoma bodies, apparently forming from calcification of the syncytial nests of meningothelial cells (Fig. 28–48*B*); **secretory,** with PAS-positive intracytoplasmic droplets and intracellular lumens by electron microscopy; and **microcystic,** with a loose, spongy appearance. Xanthomatous degeneration, metaplasia (often osseous), and moderate nuclear pleomorphism are common in meningiomas but have no prognostic significance.

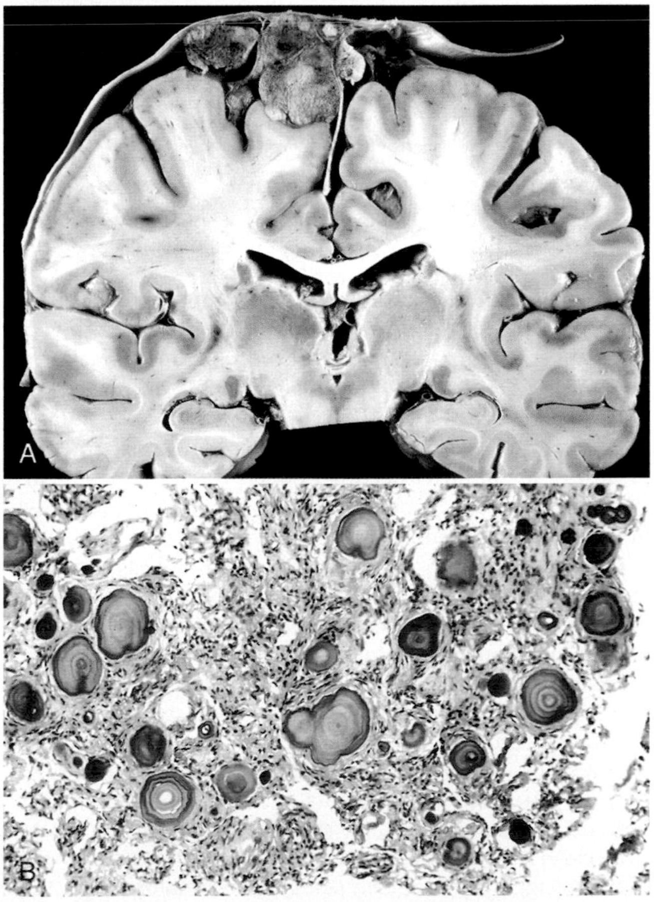

FIGURE 28–48 *A,* Parasagittal multilobular meningioma attached to the dura with compression of underlying brain. *B,* Meningioma with a whorled pattern of cell growth and psammoma bodies.

Atypical meningiomas (WHO grade II/IV) are lesions with a higher rate of recurrence and more aggressive local growth that may require therapy in addition to surgery. The diagnostic criteria for this category of meningioma require either a mitotic index of four or more mitoses per 10 high power fields or three or more of the atypical features (increased cellularity, small cells with a high nuclear:cytoplasmic ratio, prominent nucleoli, patternless growth, or necrosis). Certain histologic patterns (clear cell and chordoid) are also considered to be grade II/IV because of their more aggressive behavior.

Anaplastic (malignant) meningioma (WHO grade III/IV) is a highly aggressive tumor that has the overall appearance of a high-grade sarcoma, although there is usually some histologic evidence that indicates a meningothelial cell origin. Mitotic rates are often extremely high (>20 mitoses per 10 high power fields). Certain histologic subtypes of meningioma are also considered to be WHO grade III/IV tumors. **Papillary** meningioma (with pleomorphic cells arranged around fibrovascular cores) and **rhabdoid** meningioma (with sheets of tumor cells with hyaline eosinophilic cytoplasm containing intermediate filaments) both have a high propensity to recur.

While most meningiomas are easily separable from the brain even if they displace it, some tumors infiltrate the brain. This can occur with broad, pushing edges or as single cells. The presence of brain invasion is associated with increased risk of recurrence but does not alter the histologic grade of the lesion.

Meningiomas are commonly immunoreactive for epithelial membrane antigen, in contrast to other tumors arising in this region, although the higher the grade, the less prominent this may be. Keratin is restricted to lesions with the secretory pattern, and these tumors are also positive for carcinoembryonic antigen.

Molecular Genetics. The most common cytogenetic abnormality is loss of chromosome 22, especially the long arm (22q). The deletions include the region of 22q12 that harbors the *NF2* gene (see later). Indeed, 50% to 60% of meningiomas not associated with neurofibromatosis type 2 have mutations in the *NF2* gene; the majority of these mutations are predicted to result in absence of functional protein. These genetic abnormalities are more common in meningiomas with fibroblastic or transitional histologic appearance.[278]

Clinical Features. Meningiomas are usually slow-growing lesions that present either with vague nonlocalizing symptoms or with focal findings referable to compression of underlying brain. Common sites of involvement include the parasagittal aspect of the brain convexity, dura over the lateral convexity, wing of the sphenoid, olfactory groove, sella turcica, and foramen magnum. They are uncommon in children and show a moderate (3:2) female predominance, although the ratio becomes 10:1 among patients with spinal meningiomas. Lesions are usually solitary, and their presence at multiple sites, especially in association with acoustic neuromas or glial tumors, suggests a diagnosis of neurofibromatosis type 2. The tumors often express progesterone receptors, and rapid growth during pregnancy has been reported. While WHO grade is a strong predictor of clinical course, proliferation index as assessed by MIB-1 labeling is an independent factor among grade I/IV meningiomas.

METASTATIC TUMORS

Metastatic lesions, mostly carcinomas, account for approximately a quarter to half of intracranial tumors in hospital patients. The five most common primary sites are lung, breast, skin (melanoma), kidney, and gastrointestinal tract, accounting for about 80% of all metastases. Some rare tumors (e.g., choriocarcinoma) have a high likelihood of metastasizing to the brain, whereas other, more common tumors (e.g., prostatic carcinoma) almost never do even when they are metastatic to adjacent bone and dura. The meninges are also a frequent site of involvement by metastatic disease. Metastatic tumors present clinically as mass lesions and may occasionally be the first manifestation of the cancer.

Morphology. On macroscopic examination, intraparenchymal metastases form sharply demarcated masses, often at the gray matter–white matter junction, usually surrounded by a zone of edema. The boundary between tumor and brain parenchyma is well defined microscopically as well; melanoma is one tumor that does not always follow this rule. Nodules of tumor, often with central areas of necrosis, are surrounded by reactive gliosis. Meningeal carcinomatosis, with tumor nodules studding the surface of the brain, spinal cord, and intradural nerve roots, is associated particularly with small cell carcinoma and adenocarcinoma of the lung and carcinoma of the breast.

PARANEOPLASTIC SYNDROMES

In addition to the direct and localized effects produced by metastases, *paraneoplastic syndromes* may involve the peripheral and central nervous systems, sometimes even preceding the clinical recognition of the malignant neoplasm.[279] The most common tumor causing paraneoplastic syndromes is small cell carcinoma of the lung (Table 28–4). These syndromes share the findings of a paraneoplastic encephalomyelitis with the specific clinical syndromes reflecting the distribution of the pathologic burden in the brain:

- *Paraneoplastic cerebellar degeneration,* in which typical morphologic findings include destruction of Purkinje cells, gliosis, and a mild inflammatory infiltrate.
- *Limbic encephalitis* is characterized by subacute dementia. The pathologic findings are most striking in the anterior and medial portions of the temporal lobe and resemble an infectious process, with perivascular inflammatory cuffs, microglial nodules, some neuronal loss, and gliosis. A comparable process involving the brainstem can be seen in isolation or together with limbic system involvement.
- *Subacute sensory neuropathy* may be found in association with limbic encephalitis or in isolation. It is marked by loss of sensory neurons from dorsal root ganglia, again in association with inflammation.
- *Eye movement disorders,* most commonly opsoclonus, may be found, often in association with other evidence of cerebellar and brainstem dysfunction. In children, this is

TABLE 28–4 Paraneoplastic Syndromes

Syndrome	Target	Tumor	Antigen
Subacute cerebellar degeneration	Purkinje cells	Hodgkin lymphoma Breast, GYN SCLC, neuroblastoma	Tr Yo Hu
Limbic encephalitis; brainstem encephalitis	Various neurons in mesial temporal lobe, brainstem	SCLC, neuroblastoma Testicular, others	Hu Ma
Subacute sensory neuropathy	Dorsal root ganglion neurons	SCLC, neuroblastoma	Hu
Opsoclonus myoclonus	Unknown (presumed brain stem)	Neuroblastoma, Breast	Ri
Retinal degeneration	Photoreceptors	SCLC	Recoverin
Stiff-man syndrome	Spinal interneurons	Breast	Amphiphysin
Lambert-Eaton myasthenic syndrome	Presynaptic terminals at neuromuscular junction	SCLC	Presynaptic calcium channel

SCLC, Small cell lung carcinoma.

most commonly associated with neuroblastoma and is found along with myoclonus.

The major underlying mechanism of these diseases involves the systemic development of an immune response against tumor antigens that can cross-react with antigens in the central or peripheral nervous systems.[280,281] The relationship among the underlying malignant process, the clinical features, and the antigens underlying the syndrome are complex. Some tumor types are associated with multiple types of autoantibodies, and the same antibodies can be present in different clinical syndromes. What allows these antibodies access to the nervous system and how this immune response to intracellular proteins (for the most part) elicits disease remain unanswered questions. There may also be a component of T cell–mediated neuronal injury in some settings.[282]

PERIPHERAL NERVE SHEATH TUMORS

These tumors arise from cells of the peripheral nerve, including Schwann cells, perineurial cells, and fibroblasts. Many express Schwann cell characteristics, including the presence of S-100 antigen as well as the potential for melanocytic differentiation. As nerves exit the brain and spinal cord, there is a transition between myelination by oligodendrocytes and myelination by Schwann cells. This occurs within several millimeters of the substance of the brain; thus, peripheral nerve tumors can arise within the dura and may cause changes in adjacent brain or spinal cord. Tumors of comparable histogenesis and biologic behavior also arise along the peripheral course of nerves.

Schwannoma

These benign tumors arise from the neural crest–derived Schwann cell and are associated with neurofibromatosis type 2. Symptoms are referable to local compression of the involved nerve or to compression of adjacent structures (such as brain stem or spinal cord). Sporadic schwannomas are associated with mutations in the *NF2* gene on chromosome 22; there is usually absence of the *NF2* gene product by Western blotting or immunostaining, even if there is no evidence of a mutation in the gene.[283]

Morphology. Schwannomas are well-circumscribed, encapsulated masses that are attached to the nerve but can be separated from it (Fig. 28–49*A*). Tumors form firm, gray masses but may also have areas of cystic and xanthomatous change. On microscopic examination, tumors show a mixture of two growth patterns (Fig. 28–49*B*). In the **Antoni A** pattern of growth, elongated cells with cytoplasmic processes are arranged in fascicles in areas of moderate to high cellularity with little stromal matrix; the "nuclear-free zones" of processes that lie between the regions of nuclear palisading are termed Verocay bodies. In the **Antoni B** pattern of growth, the tumor is less densely cellular with a loose meshwork of cells along with microcysts and myxoid changes. In both areas, the cytology of the individual cells is similar, with elongated cell shape and regular oval nuclei. Electron microscopy shows basement membrane deposits encasing single cells and long-spacing collagen. Because the lesion displaces the nerve of origin as it grows, silver stains or immunostains for neurofilament proteins demonstrate that axons are largely excluded from the tumor, although they may become entrapped in the capsule. The Schwann cell origin of these tumors is borne out by their S-100 immunoreactivity. A variety of degenerative changes may be found in schwannomas, including nuclear pleomorphism, xanthomatous change, and vascular hyalinization. Malignant change is extremely rare in schwannomas, although local recurrence can follow incomplete resection.

Clinical Features. Within the cranial vault, the most common location of schwannomas is in the cerebellopontine angle, where they are attached to the vestibular branch of the eighth nerve (Fig. 28–49). Patients often present with tinnitus and hearing loss, and the tumor is often referred to as an acoustic neuroma, although it is more accurately called a vestibular schwannoma. Elsewhere within the dura, sensory nerves are preferentially involved, including branches of the trigeminal nerve and dorsal roots. When extradural, schwannomas are most commonly found in association with large nerve trunks, where motor and sensory modalities are intermixed.

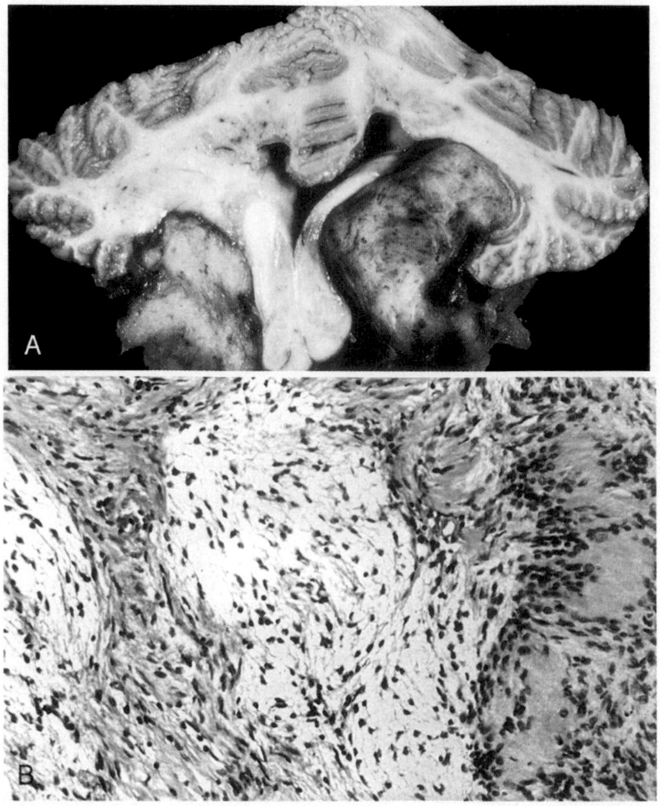

FIGURE 28–49 Schwannoma. *A,* Bilateral eighth nerve schwannomas. (Courtesy of Dr. K.M. Earle.) *B,* Tumor showing cellular areas (Antoni A), including Verocay bodies *(far right)*, as well as looser, myxoid regions (Antoni B).

Neurofibroma

Two histologically, and perhaps biologically, distinct lesions have been termed *neurofibromas*. The most common form occurs in the skin (*cutaneous neurofibroma*) or in peripheral nerve (*solitary neurofibroma*). These arise sporadically or in association with neurofibromatosis type 1 (see later). The skin lesions are evident as nodules, sometimes with overlying hyperpigmentation; they may grow to be large and become pedunculated. The risk of malignant transformation from these tumors is extremely small, and cosmetic concerns are their major morbidity.

The second type is the *plexiform neurofibroma*, which is considered by some to occur only in patients with neurofibromatosis type 1. Plexiform neurofibromas arising in individuals with NF1 show loss of the wild-type copy of the *NF1* gene.[284] A major concern in the care of these patients is the difficulty in surgical removal of these plexiform tumors when they involve major nerve trunks, since they have a significant potential for malignant transformation.

Morphology

Cutaneous Neurofibroma. Present in the dermis and subcutaneous fat, these well-delineated but unencapsulated masses are composed of spindle cells. Although they are not invasive, the adnexal structures are sometimes enwrapped by the edges of the lesion. The stroma of these tumors is highly collagenized and contains little myxoid material. Lesions within peripheral nerves are of identical histologic appearance.

Plexiform Neurofibroma. These tumors may arise anywhere along a nerve, although the large nerve trunk is the most common site. They are frequently multiple. At the site of each lesion, the nerve is irregularly expanded, as each of its fascicles is infiltrated by the neoplasm. Unlike the case with schwannomas, it is not possible to separate the lesion from the nerve. The proximal and distal extremes of the tumor may have poorly defined margins, as fingers of tumor and individual neoplastic cells insert themselves between the nerve fibers. On microscopic examination, the lesion has a loose, myxoid background with a low cellularity. A number of cell phenotypes are present, including Schwann cells with typical elongated nuclei and extensions of pink cytoplasm, larger multipolar fibroblastic cells, and a sprinkling of inflammatory cells, often including mast cells. Although the myxoid appearance dominates the picture, there are often areas of collagen bundles, which have a "shredded carrot" appearance. In contrast to schwannomas, axons can be demonstrated within the tumor. Various ultrastructural and immunohistochemical studies have identified the neoplastic cells as showing markers of diverse lineages, including Schwann cells, perineurial cells, and fibroblasts.

Malignant Peripheral Nerve Sheath Tumor (MPNST, Malignant Schwannoma)

MPNSTs are highly malignant sarcomas that are locally invasive, frequently leading to multiple recurrences and eventual metastatic spread. Despite their name, these tumors do not arise from malignant degeneration of schwannomas. Instead, they arise de novo or from transformation of a plexiform neurofibroma and therefore are strongly associated with neurofibromatosis type 1. These tumors may also follow radiation therapy. Genetic alterations in MPNSTs include mutations of the *NF1* gene; since this alteration is also found in benign plexiform neurofibromas, additional genetic alterations must be involved. There is evidence for involvement of *p53* and *p16*, as well as probably other loci.[285,286]

Morphology. The lesions are poorly defined tumor masses with frequent infiltration along the axis of the parent nerve as well as invasion of adjacent soft tissues. Associated with the malignant nature of the neoplasm, necrosis is commonly present. On microscopic examination, a wide range of histologic findings can be encountered. Patterns reminiscent of fibrosarcoma or malignant fibrous histiocytoma may be found. In other areas, the tumor cells resemble Schwann cells, with elongated nuclei and prominent bipolar processes. Fascicle formation may be present. Mitoses, necrosis, and extreme nuclear anaplasia are common. Some but not all malignant peripheral nerve sheath tumors are immunoreactive for S-100 protein. In addition to the basic appearance of these tumors, a wide variety of "divergent" histologic patterns may be admixed, including epithelial structures, rhabdomyoblastic differentiation (termed **Triton tumors**), cartilage, and even bone. **Epithelioid malignant**

schwannomas are aggressive variants derived from nerve sheaths and contain tumor cells having visible cell borders and epithelial type nests. They are immunoreactive for S-100 but not for keratin, the latter differentiating them from epithelial tumors.

FAMILIAL TUMOR SYNDROMES

These are a group of inherited diseases characterized by the development of hamartomas and neoplasms throughout the body with particular involvement of the nervous system. Many of the disorders are inherited in an autosomal-dominant pattern and have been linked to tumor-suppressor genes. Symptoms are referable in part to the location of hamartomas or neoplasms; some patients are severely retarded, and seizure disorders are a serious problem in others.

Neurofibromatosis Type 1 (NF1)

This autosomal-dominant disorder is characterized by neurofibromas (plexiform and solitary), gliomas of the optic nerve, pigmented nodules of the iris (*Lisch nodules*), and cutaneous hyperpigmented macules (*café au lait spots*). It is one of the more common genetic disorders, having a frequency of 1 in 3000. Except for plexiform neurofibromas, the tumors that occur in NF1 are histologically comparable to those that occur sporadically. In patients with NF1, there is a propensity for the neurofibromas to undergo malignant degeneration at a higher rate than that observed for comparable tumors in the general population. This is especially true for plexiform neurofibromas.

The *NF1* gene, located at 17q11.2, has been identified and encodes a protein termed *neurofibromin.*[287,288] The protein contains a region homologous to the RAS family of GTPase-activating proteins, and it is presumed that neurofibromin plays a role in regulating signal transduction. The protein is widely expressed, the highest levels being found in neural tissue. The *NF1* gene is a tumor-suppressor gene, based on evidence of loss of heterozygosity in tumors from NF1 patients. A variety of mutations involving the *NF1* gene have been detected, and there do not appear to be specific "hot spots" for changes. The clinical phenotype does not correlate with the type or location of the *NF1* mutation. The course of the disease is highly variable; some individuals who carry a mutated gene have no symptoms, while others develop progressive disease with spinal deformities, disfiguring lesions, and compression of vital structures, including the spinal cord.

Neurofibromatosis Type 2 (NF2)

This is an autosomal-dominant disorder in which patients develop a range of tumors, most commonly bilateral VIII nerve schwannomas and multiple meningiomas. Gliomas, typically ependymomas of the spinal cord, also occur in these patients. Many individuals with NF2 also have non-neoplastic lesions, which include nodular ingrowth of Schwann cells into the spinal cord (schwannosis), meningioangiomatosis (a proliferation of meningeal cells and blood vessels that grows into the brain), and glial hamartia (microscopic nodular collections of glial cells at abnormal locations, often in the superficial and deep layers of cerebral cortex). This disorder is much less common than NF1, having a frequency of 1 in 40,000 to 50,000.

The *NF2* gene is located on chromosome 22q12, and the gene product, merlin, shows structural similarity to a series of cytoskeletal proteins.[289,290] The protein is widely distributed throughout tissues, and its function remains uncertain. There is some correlation between the type of mutation and clinical symptoms, with nonsense mutations usually causing a more severe phenotype than missense mutations.[291] As was mentioned previously, the *NF2* gene is commonly mutated in sporadic meningiomas and schwannomas as well.

Tuberous Sclerosis

Tuberous sclerosis is an autosomal-dominant syndrome characterized by the development of hamartomas and benign neoplasms involving the brain and other tissues. Hamartomas within the CNS occur as cortical tubers and subependymal hamartomas. Elsewhere in the body, lesions include renal angiomyolipomas, retinal glial hamartomas, and pulmonary lesions and cardiac rhabdomyomas. Cysts may be found at various sites, including the liver, kidneys, and pancreas. Cutaneous lesions include angiofibromas, leathery thickenings in localized patches (shagreen patches), hypopigmented areas (ash-leaf patches), and subungual fibromas. Genetic analysis is rendered complex because there are patients who are obligate carriers of the gene but have no evidence of the disease. Several distinct genetic loci have been identified at which mutations can cause tuberous sclerosis; however, the clinical and pathologic features caused by these different genes are indistinguishable. One tuberous sclerosis locus (*TSC1*) is found on chromosome 9q34, where it encodes a protein of unknown function (hamartin).[292] The more commonly mutated tuberous sclerosis locus (*TSC2*) is found on chromosome 16p13.3 and encodes a protein (tuberin) with homology to a GTPase-activating protein.[293] The inability to distinguish between these two loci based on clinical or pathologic features may be because these proteins interact directly with each other.[294,295] The complex containing these proteins may play a role in regulating cell proliferation.[296]

Morphology. Cortical hamartomas of tuberous sclerosis are firm areas of the cortex that, in contrast to the softer adjacent cortex, have been likened to potatoes, hence the appellation "tubers." These hamartomas are composed of haphazardly arranged neurons that lack the normal laminar organization of neocortex. In addition, some large cells express phenotypes intermediate between glia and neurons, with intermediate filaments of both neuronal (neurofilament) and glial (GFAP) types. Interestingly, these cells often stain for both tuberin and hamartin.[297] These cells have large vesicular nuclei with nucleoli, resembling neurons, and abundant eosinophilic cytoplasm like gemistocytic astrocytes. Similar hamartomatous features are present in the subependymal nodules, where the large astrocyte-like cells cluster beneath the ventricular surface. These multiple droplike masses that bulge into the ventricular system gave rise to the term "candle-guttering." In subependymal areas, a tumor unique to tuberous sclerosis (subependymal giant cell astrocytoma) occurs.

Treatment is symptomatic, including anticonvulsant therapy for control of seizures.

Von Hippel-Lindau Disease

This is an autosomal-dominant disease in which affected individuals develop tumors (capillary hemangioblastomas) within the cerebellar hemispheres, the retina, and, less commonly, the brainstem and spinal cord. Patients may also have cysts involving the pancreas, liver, and kidneys and have a propensity to develop renal cell carcinoma of the kidney (Chapter 20). The disease frequency is 1 in 30,000 to 40,000.

The gene for von Hippel-Lindau disease, a tumor-suppressor gene, is located on chromosome 3p25–26 and encodes a protein (pVHL) that appears to play a role in regulating several aspects of cellular function. The protein can serve as a component of a complex that functions in the ubiquitination pathway, contributing to protein degradation.[298] One of the targets of the complex containing pVHL is hypoxia-induced factor 1 (HIF-1), a transcription factor involved in regulation of expression of VEGF.[299] This link may explain the vascular component of various VHL-associated tumors. Other roles for pVHL in regulation of cell cycle proteins have been found as well.[300] Missense mutations, but not other types of mutations, are highly likely to result in a phenotype that includes, in addition to the vascular tumors, adrenal pheochromocytoma.

Morphology. The cerebellar capillary hemangioblastoma, the principal neurologic manifestation of the disease, is a highly vascular neoplasm that occurs as a mural nodule associated with a large fluid-filled cyst. On microscopic examination, the lesion consists of a mixture of variable proportions of capillary-size or somewhat larger thin-walled vessels with intervening stromal cells of uncertain histogenesis characterized by vacuolated, lightly PAS-positive, lipid-rich cytoplasm and indefinite immunohistochemical phenotype.

Therapy is directed at the symptomatic neoplasms, including resection of the cerebellar hemangioblastomas and laser therapy for retinal hemangioblastomas. Partial nephrectomy is performed for renal carcinomas when these malignant neoplasms are bilateral. Approximately 10% of hemangioblastomas are associated with polycythemia; the tumor has been shown to be a source of erythropoietin in these cases, although the cell of origin of the growth factor is not known.

REFERENCES

1. Gage FH: Mammalian neural stem cells. Science 287:1433, 2000.
2. Graham D, Lantos P (eds): Greenfield's Neuropathology. London, Arnold, 2002.
3. Victor M, Ropper AH, Adams RD: Adams & Victor's Principles of Neurology. New York, McGraw-Hill, 2000.
4. Parent A: Carpenter's Human Neuroanatomy. Baltimore, Williams and Wilkins, 1996.
5. Mountcastle V: The columnar organization of the neocortex. Brain 120:701, 1997.
6. Peters A, Palay S, Webster H: The Fine Structure of the Nervous System: Neurons and Their Supporting Cells. Philadelphia, WB Saunders, 1991.
7. Cáccamo D, Rubinstein L: Tumors: application of immunohistochemical methods. In Garcia J (ed): Neuropathology: The Diagnostic Approach. St. Louis, Mosby, 1997, p 193.
8. Hickey WF: Basic principles of immunological surveillance of the normal central nervous system. Glia 36:118, 2001.
9. Hickey WF, Kimura H: Perivascular microglial cells of the CNS are bone-marrow derived and present antigen in vivo. Science 239:290, 1988.
10. Keane R, Hickey WF (eds): Immunology of the Nervous System. New York, Oxford University Press, 1997.
11. Garcia J, Mena H: Vascular diseases. In Garcia J (ed): Neuropathology: The Diagnostic Approach, St. Louis, Mosby, 1997, p 263.
12. Koliatsos V, Price D, Axotomy as an experimental model of neuronal injury and cell death. Brain Pathol 6:447, 1996.
13. Norenberg M: Astrocyte responses to CNS injury. J Neuropathol Exp Neurol 53:213–220, 1994.
14. Brenner M, et al: Mutations in GFAP, encoding glial fribrillary acidic protein, are associated with Alexander disease. Nat Genet 27:117, 2001.
15. Wakabayashi K, et al, Alpha-synuclein immunoreactivity in glial cytoplasmic inclusions in multiple system atrophy. Neurosci Lett 249:180, 1998.
16. Chin S-M, Goldman J: Glial inclusions in CNS degenerative disease. J Neuropathol Exp Neurol 55:499, 1996.
17. Laterra J, Goldstein W: Ventricular organization of cerebrospinal fluid: blood-brain barrier, brain edema, and hydrocephalus. In Kandel ER, Schwartz JH, Jessell TM (eds): Principles of Neural Science. Elsevier, New York, 2000, p 1288.
18. Yeargin-Allsopp M, Boyle C: Overview: The epidemiology of neurodevelopmental disorders. Ment Retard Dev Disabil Res Rev 8:113, 2002.
19. Kirby R: Co-occurrence of developmental disabilities with birth defects. Ment Retard Dev Disabil Res Rev 8:182, 2002.
20. Norman M, et al: Congenital Malformations of the Brain: Pathological, Embryological, Clinical, Radiological and Genetic Aspects. New York, Oxford University Press. 1995, p 452.
21. Rubenstein J, et al: Regionalization of the prosencephalic neural plate. Annu Rev Neurosci 21:445, 1998.
22. Friede RL: Developmental Neuropathology. Berlin, Springer-Verlag, 1989.
23. Kammermeier L, Reichert H: Common developmental genetic mechanisms for patterning invertebrate and vertebrate brains. Brain Res Bull 55:675, 2001.
24. Trainor P, Krumlauf R: Patterning the cranial neural crest: hindbrain segmentation and Hox gene plasticity. Nat Rev Neurosci 1:116, 2000.
25. Lucock M: Folic acid: nutritional biochemistry, molecular biology, and role in disease processes. Mol Genet Metab 71:121, 2000.
26. Lucock M, et al: An examination of polymorphic genes and folate metabolism in mothers affected by a spina bifida pregnancy. Mol Genet Metab 73:322, 2001.
27. Moyers S, Bailey L: Fetal malformations and folate metabolism: review of recent evidence. Nutr Rev 59:215, 2001.
28. Gelineau-van Waes J, Finnell R: Genetics of neural tube defects. Semin Pediatr Neurol 8:160, 2001.
29. Volcik, K, et al: Testing for genetic associations in a spina bifida population: analysis of the HOX gene family and human candidate gene regions implicated by mouse models of neural tube defects. Am J Med Genet 110:203, 2002.
30. Dobyns W: Lissencephaly and other genetic disorders of neuronal migration: 1995 update. Neuropediatrics 26:132, 1995.
31. Mizuguchi M, et al: Lissencephaly gene product. Localization in the central nervous system and loss of immunoreactivity in Miller-Dieker syndrome. Am J Pathol 147:1142, 1995.
32. Fairen A, Morante-Oria J, Frassoni C: The surface of the developing cerebral cortex: still special cells one century later. Prog Brain Res 136:281, 2002.
33. Ross ME, Walsh CA: Human brain malformations and their lessons for neuronal migration. Annu Rev Neurosci 24:1041, 2001.
34. Monuki E.S, Walsh CA: Mechanisms of cerebral cortical patterning in mice and humans. Nat Neurosci 4:S1199, 2001.
35. Chenn A, Walsh CA: Regulation of cerebral cortical size by control of cell cycle exit in neural precursors. Science 297:365, 2002.
36. Roessler E: Mutations in the human Sonic hedgehog gene cause holoprosencephaly. Nat Genet 14:357, 1996.
37. Cohen MJ, Shiota K: Teratogenesis of holoprosencephaly. Am J Med Genet 109:1, 2002.
38. Volpe J: Neurology of the Newborn. Philadelphia, Saunders, 2001.
39. Kinney H, Armstrong D: Perinatal neuropathology. In Graham D, Lantos P (eds): Greenfield's Neuropathology. London, Arnold, 2002, p 519.

40. Graham D, et al: The nature, distribution and causes of traumatic brain injury. Brain Pathol 5:397, 1995.
41. Leestma J: Forensic neuropathology. In Garcia J (ed): Neuropathology: The Diagnostic Approach. St. Louis, Mosby, 1997, p 475.
42. Povlishock J, Jenkins L: Are the pathobiological changes evoked by traumatic brain injury immediate and irreversible? Brain Pathol 5:415, 1995.
43. Gleckman A, et al: Optic nerve damage in shaken baby syndrome: detection by beta-amyloid precursor protein immunohistochemistry. Arch Pathol Lab Med 124:251, 2000.
44. Stone J, Singleton R, Povlishock JT: Antibodies to the C-terminus of the beta-amyloid precursor protein (APP): a site specific marker for the detection of traumatic axonal injury. Brain Res 871:288, 2000.
45. Tator C, Koyanagi I: Vascular mechanisms in the pathophysiology of human spinal cord injury. J Neurosurg 86:483, 1997.
46. De Girolami U, Frosch M, Tator C: Regional neuropathology: disease of the spinal cord and vertebral column. In: Graham D, Lantos P (eds): Greenfield's Neuropathology. London, Arnold, 2002, p 1063.
47. Lo EH, Dalkara T, Moskowitz MA: Mechanisms, challenges, and opportunities in stroke. Nat Rev Neurosci 4:399, 2003.
48. Gladstone DJ, et al: Toward wisdom from failure: lessons from neuroprotective stroke trials and new therapeutic directions. Stroke 33:2123, 2002.
49. Stehbens W, Lie J (eds): Vascular Pathology. London, Chapman & Hall, 1995.
50. Lie J: Classification and histopathologic spectrum of central nervous system vasculitis. Neurol Clin 15:805, 1997.
51. Siva A: Vasculitis of the nervous system. J Neurol 248:451, 2001.
52. Joutel A, et al: Notch3 mutations in CADASIL, a hereditary adult-onset condition causing stroke and dementia. Nature 383:707 1996.
53. Dichgans M: CADASIL: a monogenic condition causing stroke and subcortical vascular dementia. Cerebrovasc Dis 13:S37, 2002.
54. Karlström H, et al: A CADASIL-mutated Notch 3 receptor exhibits impaired intracellular trafficking and maturation but normal ligand-induced signaling. Proc Natl Acad Sci U S A 99:17119, 2002.
55. Joutel A, et al: Pathogenic mutations associated with cerebral autosomal dominant arteriopathy with subcortical infarcts and leukoencephalopathy differentially affect Jagged 1 binding and Notch 3 activity via the RBP/JK signaling pathway. Am J Human Genet 74:338, 2004.
56. Donahue CP, Kosik KS: Distribution pattern of Notch 3 mutations suggests a gain-of-function mechanism for CADASIL. Genomics 83:59, 2004.
57. Greenberg S: Cerebral amyloid angiopathy: prospects for clinical diagnosis and treatment. Neurology 51:690, 1998.
58. O'Donnell H, et al: Apolipoprotein E genotype and the risk of recurrent lobar intracerebral hemorrhage. N Engl J Med 342:240, 2000.
59. De Girolami U, Crowell R, Marcoux F: Selective necrosis and total necrosis in focal cerebral ischemia: neuropathologic observations on experimental middle cerebral artery occlusion in the macaque monkey. J Neuropathol Exp Neurol 43:57, 1984.
60. Garcia J, et al: Ischemic stroke and incomplete infarction. Stroke 27:761, 1996.
61. Gretasdottir S, et al: The gene encoding phosphodiesterase 4D confers risk of ischemic stroke. Nat Genet 35:131, 2003.
62. Molinari GF: Lobar hemorrhages: Where do they come from? How did they get there? Stroke 24:523, 1993.
63. Schievink W: Intracranial aneurysms. N Engl J Med 336:28–40, 1997.
64. Winn H, et al: Prevalence of asymptomatic incidental aneurysms: review of 4568 arteriograms. J Neurosurg 96:43, 2002.
65. Juvela S, Porras M, Poussa K: Natural history of unruptured intracranial aneurysms: probability of and risk factors for aneurysm rupture. J Neurosurg 93:379, 2000.
66. Sobey C, Faraci F: Subarachnoid haemorrhage: what happens to the cerebral arteries? Clin Exp Pharm Physiol 25:867, 1997.
67. Quan N, Herkenham M, Connecting cytokines and brain: a review of current issues. Histol Histopathol 17:273, 2002.
68. Durand ML, et al: Acute bacterial meningitis in adults: review of 493 episodes. N Engl J Med 328:21, 1993.
69. Gray F: Bacterial infections. Brain Pathol 7:629, 1997.
70. Pong A, Bradley J: Bacterial meningitis and the newborn infant. Infect Dis Clin North Am 13:711, 1999.
71. Choi C: Bacterial meningitis in aging adults. Clin Infect Dis 33:1380, 2001.
72. Booy R, Kroll J: Bacterial meningitis and meningococcal infection. Curr Opin Pediatr 10:13, 1998.
73. Schuchat A, et al: Bacterial meningitis in the United States in 1995. N Engl J Med 337:970, 1997.
74. Quagliarello V, Scheid W: Treatment of bacterial meningitis. N Engl J Med 336:708, 1997.
75. Moris G, Garcia-Monco J: The challenge of drug-induced aseptic meningitis. Arch Int Med 159:1185, 1999.
76. Chun CH, et al: Brain abscess: a study of 45 consecutive cases. Medicine 65:415, 1986.
77. Calfee D, Wispelwey B: Brain abscess. Semin Neurol 20:353, 2000.
78. Thwaites G, et al: Tuberculous meningitis. J Neurol Neurosurg Psychiatry 68:289, 2000.
79. Jellinger K, et al: Neuropathology and general autopsy findings in AIDS during the last 15 years. Acta Neuropathol 100:213, 2000.
80. Garcia-Monco JC, Benach J: Lyme neuroborreliosis. Ann Neurol 37:691, 1995.
81. Logigian EL, Kaplan RF, Steere AC: Chronic neurologic manifestations of Lyme disease. N Engl J Med 323:1438. 1990.
82. Coyle P, Schutzer S: Neurologic aspects of Lyme disease. Med Clinic North Am 86:261–284, 2002.
83. Esiri M: Viruses and rickettsiae. Brain Pathol 7:695, 1997.
84. Redington J, Tyler K: Viral infections of the nervous system, 2002: update on diagnosis and treatment. Arch Neurol 59:712, 2002.
85. Whitley R, Gnann J: Viral encephalitis: familiar infections and emerging pathogens. Lancet 359:507, 2002.
86. Taubenberger J, et al: Initial genetic characterization of the 1918 "Spanish" influenza virus. Science 275:1793. 1997.
87. Roehrig J, et al: The emergence of West Nile virus in North America: ecology, epidemiology, and surveillance. Curr Top Microbiol Immunol 267:223, 2002.
88. Deresiewicz R, et al: Clinical and neuroradiographic manifestation of eastern equine encephalitis. N Engl J Med 336:1867, 1997.
89. Kleinschmidt-DeMasters B, DeBiasi R, Tyler KL: Polymerase chain reaction as a diagnostic adjunct in herpesvirus infections of the nervous system. Brain Pathol 11:452, 2001.
90. Morgello S, et al: Cytomegalovirus encephalitis in patients with acquired immunodeficiency syndrome. Hum Pathol 18:289, 1987.
91. Isaacson S, et al: Cellular localization of poliovirus RNA in the spinal cord during acute paralytic poliomyelitis. Ann N Y Acad Sci 753:194, 1995.
92. Kaminski H, et al: Spinal cord histopathology in long-term survivors of poliomyelitis. Muscle Nerve 18:1208, 1995.
93. Dalakas M: The post-polio syndrome as an evolved clinical entity: definition and clinical description. Ann N Y Acad Sci 753:68, 1995.
94. Noah D, et al: Epidemiology of human rabies in the United States, 1980 to 1996. Ann Internal Med 128:992, 1998.
95. Mrak R, Young L: Rabies encephalitis in humans: pathology, pathogenesis and pathophysiology. J Neuropathol Exp Neurol 53:1, 1994.
96. De Girolami U, et al: Neuropathology of AIDS and pathogenetic considerations. In Worsmer G (ed): AIDS and Other Manifestations of HIV Infection. San Diego, Academic Press, 2004.
97. Hou J, Major E: Progressive multifocal leukoencephalopathy: JC virus induced demyelination in the immune compromised host. J Neurovirol 6 (suppl 2):S98, 2000.
98. Neuenburg JK, et al: HIV-related neuropathology, 1985 to 1999: rising prevalence of HIV encephalopathy in the era of highly active antiretroviral therapy. J Acquir Immune Defic Syndr Hum Retrovirol 31:171, 2002.
99. Berger J, et al: Epidemiological evidence and molecular basis of interactions between HIV and JC virus. J Neurovirol 7:329, 2001.
100. Sabath B, Major E: Traffic of JC virus from sites of initial infection to the brain: the path to progressive multifocal leukoencephalopathy. J Infect Dis 186:S180, 2002.
101. Allen I, et al: The significance of measles virus antigen and genome distribution in the CNS in SSPE for mechanisms of viral spread and demyelination. J Neuropathol Exp Neurol 55:471, 1996.
102. Chimelli L, Mahler-Araújo B: Fungal infections. Brain Pathol 7:613, 1997.
103. Porter SB, Sande MA: Toxoplasmosis of the central nervous system in the acquired immunodeficiency syndrome. N Eng J Med 327:1643, 1992.
104. Martinez A, Visvesvara G: Free-living, amphizoic and opportunistic amebas. Brain Pathol 7:583, 1997.
105. Prusiner SB: Shattuck lecture: neurodegenerative diseases and prions. N Engl J Med 344:1516, 2001.

106. Jackson GS, Collinge J: The molecular pathology of CJD: old and new variants. Mol Pathol 54:393, 2001.
107. Montrasio F, et al: Impaired prion replication in spleens of mice lacking functional follicular dendritic cells. Science 288:1257, 2000.
108. Goldfarb L, et al: Fatal familial insomnia and familial Creutzfeldt-Jakob disease: disease phenotype determined by a DNA polymorphism. Science 258:806, 1992.
109. Parchi P, et al: Classification of sporadic Creutzfeldt-Jakob disease based on molecular and phenotypic analysis of 300 subjects. Ann Neurol 46:224, 1999.
110. Will R, et al: A new variant of Creutzfeldt-Jakob disease in the UK. Lancet 374:921, 1996.
111. Ironside J: Pathology of variant Creutzfeldt-Jakob disease. Arch Virol Suppl 143, 2000.
112. Hill A, et al: The same prion strain causes vCJD and BSE. Nature 389:448, 1997.
113. Bruce M, et al: Transmissions to mice indicate that 'new variant' CJD is caused by the BSE agent. Nature 389:498, 1997.
114. Prusiner S: Prion diseases and the BSE crisis. Science 278:245, 1997.
115. Foster P: Prions and blood products. Ann Med 32:501, 2000.
116. Valleron A, et al: Estimation of epidemic size and incubation time based on age characteristics of vCJD in the United Kingdom. Science 294:1726, 2001.
117. Huillard d'Aignaux J, Cousens S, Smith P: Predictability of the UK variant Creutzfeldt-Jakob disease epidemic. Science 294:1729, 2001.
118. Gambetti P, et al: Fatal familial insomnia and familial Creutzfeldt-Jakob disease: clinical, pathological and molecular features. Brain Pathol 5:43, 1995.
119. Mastrianni J, et al: Prion protein conformation in a patient with sporadic fatal insomnia. N Engl J Med 340:1630, 1999.
120. Sadovnick A: The genetics of multiple sclerosis. Clin Neurol Neurosurg 104:199, 2002.
121. Dyment, D, et al: Genetic susceptibility to MS: a second stage analysis in Canadian MS families. Neurogenetics 3:145, 2001.
122. O'Connor K, Bar-Or A, Hafler D: The neuroimmunology of multiple sclerosis: possible roles of T and B lymphocytes in immunopathogenesis. J Clin Immunol 21:81, 2001.
123. Wingerchuk DM, Lucchinetti CF, Noseworthy JH: Multiple sclerosis: current pathophysiological concepts. Lab Invest 81:263, 2001.
124. Martin R, et al: Molecular mimicry and antigen-specific T cell responses in multiple sclerosis and chronic CNS Lyme disease. J Autoimmun 16:187, 2001.
125. Baranzini SE, Oksenberg JR, Hauser SL: New insights into the genetics of multiple sclerosis. J Rehabil Res Dev 39:201, 2002.
126. Steinman L, et al: Multiple sclerosis: deeper understanding of its pathogenesis reveals new targets for therapy. Annu Rev Neurosci 25:491, 2002.
127. Lucchinetti C, et al: Distinct patterns of multiple sclerosis pathology indicates heterogeneity on pathogenesis. Brain Pathol 6:259, 1996.
128. Lucchinetti C, et al: Heterogeneity of multiple sclerosis lesions: implications for the pathogenesis of demyelination. Ann Neurol 47:707, 2000.
129. Wingerchuk D, Lucchinetti C, Noseworthy J: Multiple sclerosis: current pathophysiological concepts. Lab Invest 81:263, 2001.
130. Kleinschmidt-DeMasters BK, Norenberg MD Rapid correction of hyponatremia causes demyelination: relation to central pontine myelinolysis. Science 211:1068, 1981.
131. Lampl C, Yazdi K: Central pontine myelinolysis. Eur Neurol 47:3, 2002.
132. Brown W: Osmotic demyelination disorders: central pontine and extrapontine myelinolysis. Curr Opin Neurol 13:691, 2001.
133. Dickson DW: Neurodegeneration: the molecular pathology of dementia and movement disorders. ISN Neuropath Press, Basel, 2003.
134. Evans DA, et al: Prevalence of Alzheimer's disease in a community population of older persons: higher than previously reported. JAMA 262:2551, 1989.
135. Gao S, et al: The relationships between age, sex, and the incidence of dementia and alzheimer disease: a meta-analysis. Arch Gen Psychiatry 55:809, 1998.
136. von Strauss E, et al: Aging and the occurrence of dementia: findings from a population-based cohort with a large sample of nonagenarians. Arch Neurol 56:587, 1999.
137. Cummings J, Cole G: Alzheimer disease. JAMA 287:2335, 2002.
138. Braak H, Braak E: Frequency of stages of Alzheimer-related lesions in different age categories. Neurobiol Aging 18:351, 1997.
139. Braak H, Braak E: Neuropathological staging of Alzheimer-related changes. Acta Neuropathol (Berl) 82:239, 1991.
140. Mirra S, et al: The consortium to establish a registry for Alzheimer's disease (CERAD). Part II: standardization of the neuropathologic assessment of Alzheimer's disease. Neurology 41:479, 1991.
141. Mirra SM, Hart MN, Terry RD: Making the diagnosis of Alzheimer's disease. Arch Pathol Lab Med 117:131, 1993.
142. National Institute on Aging and Reagan Institute Working Group on Diagnostic Criteria for the Neuropathological Assessment of Alzheimer's Disease: Consensus recommendations for the postmortem diagnosis of Alzheimer's disease. Neurobiol Aging 18:S1, 1997.
143. Thal D, et al: Phases of A beta-deposition in the human brain and its relevance for the development of AD. Neurology 58:1791, 2002.
144. Lemere C, et al: Sequence of deposition of heterogeneous amyloid beta-peptides and Apo E in Down syndrome: implications for initial events in amyloid plaque formation. Neurobiol Dis 3:16, 1996.
145. Iwatsubo T, et al: Visualization of A beta 42(43) and A beta 40 in senile plaques with end-specific A beta monoclonals: evidence that an initially deposited species is A beta 42(43). Neuron 13:45, 1994.
146. Iwatsubo T, et al: Amyloid beta protein (Abeta) deposition: Abeta42(43) precedes Abeta40 in Down syndrome. Ann Neurol 37:294, 1995.
147. Mumm J, Kopan R: Notch signaling: from the outside in. Dev Biol 228:151, 2000.
148. Selkoe D: Presenilin, Notch, and the genesis and treatment of Alzheimer's disease. Proc Natl Acad Sci U S A 98:11039, 2001.
149. Selkoe D: Alzheimer's disease: genes, proteins, and therapy. Phys Rev 81:741, 2001.
150. Strittmatter W, et al: Apolipoprotein E: high avidity binding to beta-amyloid and increased frequency of type 4 allele in late-onset familial Alzheimer disease. Proc Natl Acad Sci U S A 90:1977, 1993.
151. Blacker D, et al: Alpha-2 macroglobulin is genetically associated with Alzheimer disease. Nat Genet 19:357, 1998.
152. Bertram L, et al: Evidence for genetic linkage of Alzheimer's disease to chromosome 10q. Science 290:2302, 2000.
153. Zandi PJ, Breitner J: Do NSAIDs prevent Alzheimer's disease? And, if so, why? The epidemiological evidence. Neurobiol Aging 22:811, 2001.
154. McGeer P, McGeer E: Inflammation, autotoxicity and Alzheimer disease. Neurobiol Aging 22:799, 2001.
155. in t' Veld B, et al: Nonsteroidal antiinflammatory drugs and the risk of Alzheimer's disease. N Engl J Med 345:1515, 2001.
156. Weggen S, et al: A subset of NSAIDs lower amyloidogenic Abeta42 independently of cyclooxygenase activity. Nature 414:212, 2001.
157. Killiany R, et al: Use of structural magnetic resonance imaging to predict who will get Alzheimer's disease. Ann Neurol 47:430, 2000.
158. Yoshiyama Y, Lee V-Y, Trojanowski J: Frontotemporal dementia and tauopathy. Curr Neurol Neurosci Rep 1:413, 2001.
159. McKann G, et al: Clinical and pathological diagnosis of frontotemporal dementia: Report of the Work Group on Frontotemporal Dementia and Pick's Disease. Arch Neurol 58:1803, 2001.
160. Buee L, et al: Tau protein isoforms, phosphorylation and role in neurodegenerative disorders. Brain Res Rev 33:95, 2000.
161. Lee V.-Y, Goedert M, Trojanowski J: Neurodegenerative tauopathies. Ann Rev Neurosci 24:1121, 2001.
162. Dickson D: Neuropathology of Pick's disease. Neurology 56 (suppl 4):S16, 2001.
163. Baker M, et al: Association of an extended haplotype in the tau gene with progressive supranuclear palsy. Hum Mol Genet 8:711, 1999.
164. Feany M, Dickson D: Widespread cytoskeletal pathology characterizes corticobasal degeneration. Am J Pathol 146:1388, 1995.
165. Feany M, Mattiace L, Dickson D: Neuropathologic overlap of progressive supranuclear palsy, Pick's disease and corticobasal degeneration. J Neuropathol Exp Neurol 55:53, 1996.
166. Dickson D, et al: Cytoskeletal pathology in non-Alzheimer degenerative dementia: new lesions in diffuse Lewy body disease, Pick's disease, and corticobasal degeneration. J Neural Transm Suppl 47:31, 1996.
167. Dickson DW, et al: Office of Rare Diseases neuropathologic criteria for corticobasal degeneration. J Neuropathol Exp Neurol 61:935, 2002.
168. Rebeiz J, Kolodny E, Richardson EJ: Corticodentatonigral degeneration with neuronal achromasia. Arch Neurol 18:20, 1968.
169. Schneider J, et al: Corticobasal degeneration: neuropathologic and clinical heterogeneity. Neurology 48:959, 1997.
170. Di Maria E, et al: Corticobasal degeneration shares a common genetic background with progressive supranuclear palsy. Ann Neurol 47:374, 2000.

171. Mirra S, et al: Tau pathology in a family with dementia and a P301L mutation in tau. J Neuropath Exp Neurol 58:335, 1999.
172. Knopman D, et al: Dementia lacking distinctive histologic features: a common non-Alzheimer degenerative dementia. Neurology 40:251, 1990.
173. Vinters H, et al: Neuopathologic substrates of ischemic vascular dementia. J Neuropath Exp Neurol 59:931, 2000.
174. Snowdon D, et al: Brain infarction and the clinical expression of Alzheimer disease: the nun study. JAMA 277:813, 1997.
175. Schlossmacher M, et al: Parkin localizes to the Lewy bodies of Parkinson disease and dementia with Lewy bodies. Am J Pathol 160:1655, 2002.
176. Bergman H, Deuschl G: Pathophysiology of Parkinson's disease: from clinical neurology to basic neuroscience and back. Mov Disord 17:S28, 2002.
177. Le Couteur D, et al: Pesticides and Parkinson's disease. Biomed Pharmacother 53:122–130, 1999.
178. Chen J, et al: Neuroprotection by caffeine and A(2A) adenosine receptor inactivation in a model of Parkinson's disease. J Neurosci 21:RC143, 2001.
179. Ross G, Petrovitch H: Current evidence for neuroprotective effects of nicotine and caffeine against Parkinson's disease. Drugs Aging 18:797, 2001.
180. Tanner C, et al: Smoking and Parkinson's disease in twins. Neurology 58:581, 2002.
181. Goedert M: Alpha-synuclein and neurodegenerative diseases. Nat Rev Neurosci 2:492, 2001.
182. Lotharius J, et al: Effect of mutant alpha-synuclein on dopamine homeostasis in a new human mesencephalic cell line. J Biol Chem 277:38884, 2002.
183. Polymeropoulos M.H, et al: Mutation in the alpha-synuclein gene identified in families with Parkinson's disease. Science 276:2045, 1997.
184. Kruger R, et al: Ala30Pro mutation in the gene encoding alpha-synuclein in Parkinson's disease. Nat Genet 18:106, 1988.
185. Zarranz JJ, et al: The new mutation, E46K, of α-synuclein causes Parkinson and Levy body dementia. Ann Neurol 55:164, 2004.
186. Singleton AB, et al: α-synuclein locus triplication causes Parkinson's disease. Science 302:841, 2003.
187. Farrer M, et al: Comparison of kindreds with parkinsonism and α-synuclein genomic multiplications. Ann Neurol 55:174, 2004.
188. Kitada T, et al: Mutations in the parkin gene cause autosomal recessive juvenile parkinsonism. Nature 392:605, 1988.
189. Lucking C.B, et al: Association between early-onset Parkinson's disease and mutations in the parkin gene: French Parkinson's Disease Genetics Study Group. New Engl J Med 342:1560, 2000.
190. Hayashi S, et al: An autopsy case of autosomal-recessive juvenile parkinsonism with a homozygous exon 4 deletion in the parkin gene. Mov Disord 15:884, 2000.
191. van de Warrenburg BP, et al: Clinical and pathologic abnormalities in a family with parkinsonism and parkin gene mutations. Neurology 56:555, 2001.
192. Farrer M, et al: Lewy bodies and parkinsonism in families with parkin mutations. Ann Neurol 50:293, 2001.
193. Shimura H, et al: Ubiquitination of a new form of alpha-synuclein by parkin from human brain: implications for Parkinson's disease. Science 293:263, 2001.
194. Leroy E, et al: The ubiquitin pathway in Parkinson's disease. Nature 395:451, 1998.
195. Liu Y, et al: The UCH-L1 gene encodes two opposing enzymatic activities that affect alpha-synuclein degradation and Parkinson's disease susceptibility. Cell 111:209, 2002.
196. Bonifati V, et al: Mutations in the DJ-1 gene associated with autosomal recessive early-onset parkinsonism. Science 299:526, 2003.
197. Bonifati V, Oostra BA, Heutink P: Linking DJ-1 to neurodegeneration offers novel insights for understanding the pathogenesis of Parkinson's disease. J Mol Med Jan 8, 2004 (epub ahead of print).
198. Bandopadhyay R, et al: The expression of DJ-1 (PARK7) in normal human CNS and idiopathic Parkinson's disease. Brain 127:420, 2004.
199. McKeith I, et al: Consensus guidelines for the clinical and pathologic diagnosis of dementia with Lewy bodies (DLB): report of the consortium on DLB international workshop. Neurology 47:1113, 1996.
200. Freed C, et al: Transplantation of embryonic dopamine neurons for severe Parkinson's disease. N Engl J Med 344:710, 2001.
201. Lozano A, Lang A: Pallidotomy for Parkinson's disease. Adv Neurol 86:413, 2001.
202. Olanow C, Brin M, Obeso J: The role of deep brain stimulation as a surgical treatment for Parkinson's disease. Neurology 55:S60, 2000.
203. Papp M, Kahn J, Lantos P: Glial cytoplasmic inclusions in the CNS of patients with multiple system atrophy (striatonigral degeneration, olivopontocerebellar atrophy, Shy-Drager syndrome). J Neurol Sci 94:79, 1989.
204. Burn J, Jaros E: Multiple system atrophy: cellular and molecular pathology. Mol Pathol 54:419, 2001.
205. Duda J, Lee V-Y, Trojanowski J: Neuropathology of synuclein aggregates: new insights into mechanisms of neurodegenerative diseases. J Neurosci Res 61:121, 2000.
206. Spillantini M, et al: Filamentous alpha-synuclein inclusions link multiple system atrophy with Parkinson's disease and dementia with Lewy bodies. Neurosci Lett 251:205, 1988.
207. Cairns N, et al: Tau protein in the glial cytoplasmic inclusions of multiple system atrophy can be distinguished from abnormal tau in Alzheimer's disease. Neurosci Lett 230:49, 1997.
208. Papp M, Lantos P: The distribution of oligodendroglial inclusions in multiple system atrophy and its relevance to clinical symptomatology. Brain 271:235, 1994.
209. Richardson E: Huntington's disease: some recent neuropathological studies. Neuropathol Appl Neurobiol 16:451, 1990.
210. The Huntington's Disease Collaborative Research Group: A novel gene containing a trinucleotide repeat that is expanded and unstable on Huntington's disease chromosomes. Cell 72:971, 1993.
211. Snell R, et al: Relationship between trinucleotide repeat expansion and phenotypic variation in Huntington's disease. Nat Genet 4:393, 1993.
212. Davies S, Ramsden D: Huntington's disease. Mol Pathol 54:409, 2001.
213. DiFiglia M, et al: Aggregation of huntingtin in neuronal intranuclear inclusions and dystrophic neurites in brain. Science 277:1990, 1997.
214. Nucifora FJ, et al: Interference by huntingtin and atrophin-1 with cbp-mediated transcription leading to cellular toxicity. Science 291:2423, 2001.
215. Dunah A, et al: Sp1 and TAFII130 transcriptional activity disrupted in early Huntington's disease. Science 296:2238, 2002.
216. Klockgether T, et al: The molecular biology of the autosomal-dominant cerebellar ataxias. Mov Dis 15:604, 2000.
217. Perlman S: Spinocerebellar degenerations: an update. Curr Neurol Neurosci Rep 2:331, 2002.
218. Campuzano V, et al: Friedreich's ataxia: autosomal recessive disease caused by an intronic GAA triplet repeat expansion. Science 271:1423, 1996.
219. Babcock M, et al: Regulation of mitochondrial iron accumulation by Yfh1p, a putative homolog of frataxin. Science 276:1709, 1997.
220. Branda S, et al: Yeast and human frataxin are processed to mature form in two sequential steps by the mitochondrial processing peptidase. J Biol Chem 274:22763, 1999.
221. Shiloh Y: ATM (ataxia telangiectasia mutated): expanding roles in the DNA damage response and cellular homeostasis. Biochem Soc Trans 29:661, 2001.
222. Rotman G, Shiloh Y: ATM: from gene to function. Hum Mol Genet 7:1555, 1998.
223. Mitsumoto H, Chad D, Pioro E: Amyotrophic Lateral Sclerosis. Philadelphia, FA Davis, 1998.
224. Hand C, Rouleau G: Familial amyotrophic lateral sclerosis. Muscle Nerve 25:135, 2002.
225. Rosen D, et al: Mutations in Cu/Zn superoxide dismutase gene are associated with familial amyotrophic lateral sclerosis. Nature 362:59, 1993.
226. Cudkowicz M, et al: Epidemiology of mutations in superoxide dismutase in amyotrophic lateral sclerosis. Ann Neurol 41:210, 1997.
227. Cudkowicz M, et al: Limited corticospinal tract involvement in amyotrophic lateral sclerosis subjects with the A4V mutation in the copper/zinc superoxide dismutase gene. Ann Neurol 43:703, 1998.
228. Yang Y, et al: The gene encoding alsin, a protein with three guanine-nucleotide exchange factor domains, is mutated in a form of recessive amyotrophic lateral sclerosis. Nat Genet 29:160, 2001.
229. Hadano S, et al: A gene encoding a putative GTPase regulator is mutated in familial amyotrophic lateral sclerosis 2. Nat Genet 29:166, 2001.
230. Li M, et al: Nuclear inclusions of the androgen receptor protein in spinal and bulbar muscular atrophy. Ann Neurol 44:249, 1998.
231. Amato A, et al: Kennedy's disease: a clinicopathologic correlation with mutations in the androgen receptor gene. Neurology 43:791, 1993.
232. Wenger D, et al: Krabbe disease: genetic aspects and progress towards therapy. Molec Gen Metab 70:1, 2000.

233. Koeppen AH, Robitaille Y: Pelizaeus-Merzbacher disease. J Neuropathol Exp Neurol 61:747, 2002.
234. Sistermans E, et al: Duplication of the proteolipid protein gene is the major cause of Pelizaeus-Merzbacher disease. Neurology 50:1749, 1998.
235. Kaul R, et al: Cloning of the human aspartoacylase cDNA and a common mutation in Canavan disease. Nat Genet 5:118, 1993.
236. Leonard J, Schapira A: Mitochondrial respiratory chain disorders Part I: mitochondrial DNA defects. Lancet 355:299, 2000.
237. Leonard J, Schapira A: Mitochondrial respiratory chain disorders. Part II: neurodegenerative disorders and nuclear gene defects. Lancet 355:389, 2000.
238. Tanji K, et al: Neuropathological features of mitochondrial disorders. Semin Cell Dev Biol 12:429, 2001.
239. Di Donato S: Disorders related to mitochondrial membranes: pathology of the respiratory chain and neurodegeneration. J Inherit Metab Dis 23:247, 2000.
240. DiMauro S, Servidei S, Zeviani M: Cytochrome c oxidase deficiency in Leigh syndrome. Ann Neurol 22:498, 1987.
241. Tiranti V, Jaksch M, Hofmann S: Loss-of-function mutations of SURF-1 are specifically associated with Leigh syndrome with cytochrome c oxidase deficiency. Ann Neurol 46:161, 1999.
242. Tatuch Y, et al: Heteroplasmic mtDNA mutation (T->G) at 8993 can cause Leigh disease when the percentage of abnormal mtDNA is high. Am J Hum Genet 50:852, 1992.
243. Tanji K, et al: Cytochrome c oxidase deficiency in the microvasculature of MELAS-3243 brains. Ann Neurol 44:458, 1998.
244. Zeviani M, et al: Deletions of mitochondrial DNA in Kearns-Sayre syndrome. Neurology 38:1339, 1988.
245. Schultheiss T, et al: Radiation response of the central nervous system. Int J Radiat Oncol Biol Phys 31:1093, 1995.
246. Russell DS, Rubinstein LJ: Pathology of Tumors of the Nervous System. Baltimore, Williams & Wilkins, 1989.
247. Kleihues P, Cavanee W (eds): Pathology and Genetics of Tumours of the Nervous System: World Health Organizaiton Classification of Tumors. Lyon, France, IARC Press, 2000.
248. Burger P, Scheithauer B, Vogel F: Surgical Pathology of the Nervous System and its Coverings. New York, Churchill Livingstone, 2002.
249. Lantos P, et al: Tumours of the nervous system. In Graham D, Lantos P (eds): Greenfield's Neuropathology. London, Arnold, 2002, p 767.
250. Ironside J, et al: Diagnostic Pathology of Nervous System Tumours. London, Churchill Livingstone, 2002.
251. Bigner D, McLendon R, Bruner J (eds): Russell and Rubinstein's Pathology of Tumors of the Nervous System. Arnold, London, 1998.
252. Kleihues P, et al: The WHO classification of tumors of the nervous system. J Neuropathol Exp Neurol 61:215, 2002.
253. Louis D: A molecular genetic model of astrocytoma histopathology. Brain Pathol 7:755, 1997.
254. von Deimling A, et al: Subsets of glioblastoma multiforme defined by molecular genetic analysis. Brain Pathol 3:19–26. 1997.
255. Watanabe K, et al: Overexpression of the EGF receptor and p53 mutations are mutually exclusive in the evolution of primary and secondary glioblastomas. Brain Pathol 6:217, 1996.
256. Kleihues P, Ohgaki H: Primary and secondary glioblastoma: from concept to clinical diagnosis. Neuro-oncol 1:44, 1999.
257. Burger P, et al: Small cell architecture: a histological equivalent of EGFR amplification in glioblastoma multiforme? J Neuropathol Exp Neurol 60:1099, 2001.
258. Giannini C, et al: Pleomorphic xanthoastrocytoma: what do we really know about it? Cancer 85:2033, 1999.
259. Freeman C, Farmer J: Pediatric brain stem gliomas: a review. Int J Radiat Oncol Biol Phys 40:265, 1998.
260. Guillamo J-S, et al: Brainstem gliomas in adults: prognostic factors and classification. Brain 124:2528, 2001.
261. Cairncross J, et al: Specific genetic predictors of chemotherapeutic response and survival in patients with anaplastic oligodendrogliomas. J Natl Cancer Inst 90:1473, 1998.
262. Ino Y, et al: Molecular subtypes of anaplastic oligodendroglioma: implications for patient management at diagnosis. Clin Cancer Res 7:839, 2001.
263. Reifenberger J, et al: Molecular genetic analysis of oligodendroglial tumors shows preferential allelic deletions on 19q and 1p. Am J Pathol 145:1175, 1994.
264. Maintz D, et al: Molecular genetic evidence for subtypes of oligoastrocytomas. J Neuropathol Exp Neurol 56:1098, 1997.
265. Ueki K, et al: Correlation of histology and molecular genetic analysis of 1p, 19q, 10q, TP53, EGFR, CDK4, and CDKN2A in 91 astrocytic and oligodendroglial tumors. Clin Cancer Res 8:196, 2002.
266. Ebert C, et al: Molecular genetic analysis of ependymal tumors. NF2 mutations and chromosome 22q loss occur preferentially in intramedullary spinal ependymomas. Am J Pathol 155:627, 1999.
267. Komori T, et al: Papillary glioneuronal tumor: a new variant of mixed neuronal-glial neoplasm. Am J Surg Pathol 22:1171, 1998.
268. Stanescu Cosson R, et al: Dysembryoplastic neuroepithelial tumors: CT, MR findings and imaging follow-up: a study of 53 cases. J Neuroradiol 28:230, 2001.
269. Daumas-Duport C, et al: Dysembryoplastic neuroepithelial tumor: a surgically curable tumor of young patients with intractable partial seizures. Report of thirty-nine cases. Neurosurgery 23:545, 1988.
270. Segal R, et al: Expression of the neurotrophin receptor TRKC is linked to a favorable outcome in medulloblastoma. Proc Natl Acad Sci U S A 91:12867, 1994.
271. Pomeroy S, et al: Prediction of central nervous system embryonal tumour outcome based on gene expression. Nature 415:436, 2002.
272. Rorke L, Packer R, Biegel J: Central nervous system atypical teratoid/rhabdoid tumors of infancy and childhood: definition of an entity. J Neurosurg 85:56 1996.
273. Biegel J, et al: Narrowing the critical region for a rhabdoid tumor locus in 22q11. Genes Chromosomes Cancer 16:94, 1996.
274. Biegel J, et al: Germ-line and acquired mutations of INI1 in atypical teratoid and rhabdoid tumors. Cancer Res 59:74, 1999.
275. Uno K, et al: Aberrations of the hSNF5/INI1 gene are restricted to malignant rhabdoid tumors or atypical teratoid/rhabdoid tumors in pediatric solid tumors. Genes Chromosomes Cancer 34:33, 2002.
276. Hao D, et al: Is primary CNS lymphoma really becoming more common?: a population-based study of incidence, clinicopathological features and outcomes in Alberta from 1975 to 1996. Ann Oncol 10:65, 1999.
277. Corn B, et al: Will primary central nervous system lymphoma be the most frequent brain tumor diagnosed in the year 2000? Cancer 79:2409, 1997.
278. Wellenreuther R, et al: Analysis of the neurofibromatosis 2 gene reveals molecular variants of meningioma. Am J Pathol 146:827, 1995.
279. Rosenfeld M, Dalmau J: The clinical spectrum and pathogenesis of paraneoplastic disorders of the central nervous system. Hematol Oncol Clin North Am 15:1109, 2001.
280. Rudnicki S, Dalmau J: Paraneoplastic syndromes of the spinal cord, nerve, and muscle. Muscle Nerve 23:1800, 2000.
281. Posner J, Dalmau J: Paraneoplastic syndromes of the nervous system. Clin Chem Lab Med 38:117, 2000.
282. Voltz R, et al: T-cell receptor analysis in anti-Hu associated paraneoplastic encephalomyelitis. Neurology 51:1146, 1998.
283. Huynh D, et al: Immunohistochemical detection of schwannomin and neurofibromin in vestibular schwannomas, ependymomas and meningiomas. J Neuropathol Exp Neurol 56:382, 1997.
284. Serra E, et al: Confirmation of the double-hit model for the NF1 gene in benign neurofibromas. Am J Hum Genet 61:512, 1997.
285. Neilsen G, et al: Malignant transformation of neurofibromas in neurofibromatosis 1 is associated with CDKN2A/p16 inactivation. Am J Pathol 155:1879, 1999.
286. Birindelli S, et al: Rb and TP53 pathway alterations in sporadic and NF1-related malignant peripheral nerve sheath tumors. Lab Invest 81:833, 2001.
287. North K: Neurofibromatosis type 1. Am J Med Genet 97:119, 2000.
288. Korf B: Diagnosis and management of neurofibromatosis type 1. Curr Neurol Neurosci Rep 1:162, 2001.
289. Gusella J, et al: Merlin: the neurofibromatosis 2 tumor suppressor. Biochim Biophys Acta 1423:M29, 1999.
290. Bretscher A, Edwards K, Fehon R: ERM proteins and merlin: integrators at the cell cortex. Nat Rev Mol Cell Biol 3:586, 2002.
291. Merel P, et al: Screening for germ-line mutations in the NF2 gene. Genes Chromosomes Cancer 12:117, 1995.
292. van Slegtenhorst M, et al: Identification of the tuberous sclerosis gene TSC1 in chromosome 9q34. Science 277:805, 1997.
293. The European Chromosome 16 Tuberous Sclerosis Consortium: identification and characterization of the tuberous sclerosis gene on chromosome 16. Cell 75:1305, 1993.
294. Plank T, Yeung R, Henske E: Hamartin, the product of the tuberous sclerosis 1 (TSC1) gene, interacts with tuberin and appears to be localized to cytoplasmic vesicles. Cancer Res 58:4766, 1998.

295. Cheadle J, et al: Molecular genetic advances in tuberous sclerosis. Hum Genet 107:97, 2000.
296. Hengstschlager M, et al: Tuberous sclerosis gene products in proliferation control. Mutat Res 488:233, 2001.
297. Johnson M, et al: Co-localization of TSC1 and TSC2 gene products in tubers of patients with tuberous sclerosis. Brain Pathol 9:45, 1999.
298. Iwai K, et al: Identification of the von Hippel-Lindau tumor-suppressor protein as part of an active E3 ubiquitin ligase complex. Proc Natl Acad Sci U S A 96:12436, 1999.
299. Maxwell PH, et al: The tumour suppressor protein VHL targets hypoxia-inducible factors for oxygen-dependent proteolysis. Nature 399:271, 1999.
300. Pause A, et al: The von Hippel-Lindau tumor suppressor gene is required for cell cycle exit upon serum withdrawal. Proc Natl Acad Sci U S A 95:993, 1998.

CHAPTER 29

The Eye

Robert Folberg, MD

ORBIT

Functional Anatomy and Proptosis

Thyroid Ophthalmopathy (Graves Disease)

Other Orbital Inflammatory Conditions

Neoplasms

EYELID

Functional Anatomy

Neoplasms

CONJUNCTIVA

Functional Anatomy

Conjunctival Scarring

Pinguecula and Pterygium

Neoplasms

SCLERA

CORNEA

Functional Anatomy

Keratitis and Ulcers

Corneal Degenerations and Dystrophies

Band Keratopathies

Keratoconus

Fuchs Endothelial Dystrophy

Stromal Dystrophies

ANTERIOR SEGMENT

Functional Anatomy

Cataract

The Anterior Segment and Glaucoma

Endophthalmitis and Panophthalmitis

UVEA

Uveitis

Neoplasms

Uveal Nevi and Melanomas

RETINA AND VITREOUS

Functional Anatomy

Retinal Detachment

Retinal Vascular Disease

Hypertension

Diabetes Mellitus

Retinopathy of Prematurity (Retrolental Fibroplasia)

Sickle Retinopathy, Retinal Vasculitis, Radiation Retinopathy

Retinal Artery and Vein Occlusions

Age-Related Macular Degeneration (ARMD)

Other Retinal Degenerations

Retinitis Pigmentosa

Retinitis

Retinal Neoplasms

Retinoblastoma

Retinal Lymphoma

OPTIC NERVE

Anterior Ischemic Optic Neuropathy

Papilledema

Glaucomatous Optic Nerve Damage

Other Optic Neuropathies

Optic Neuritis

THE END-STAGE EYE: PHTHISIS BULBI

Although this chapter comes at the end of the book, it is not least important. Vision is a major quality-of-life issue for individuals. In the mid-1960s and again in the mid-1970s, the Gallup Organization polled Americans and asked the following question: "Which disease do you fear most?" Before the public awareness of AIDS and Alzheimer disease, the most feared disease among Americans was cancer. The second most feared disease was blindness. So great is the fear of blindness that even today, patients often tell their physicians, "Doctor, I'd rather be dead than be blind!"

In general, diseases that produce loss of vision do not attract as much of our attention as do many of the conditions described in this book that are life-threatening. Typically, loss of vision is enacted in the theater of the mundane. Age-related macular degeneration (ARMD) is the most common cause of irreversible visual loss in the United States. ARMD is not life-threatening and most patients do not even suffer from a total loss of vision—an immersion into total darkness. The pathology is quantitatively and qualitatively unspectacular: Small scars develop in the macula. But consider the effect of these tiny scars perhaps in a retired schoolteacher with ARMD. The small macular scars make it impossible for her to see anything clearly in the central portion of her vision. She looks directly at her life-long companion, her spouse, and cannot see his face. She cannot read a book or newspaper or look up telephone numbers. She, who raised children, had a career, and was the model of independence, can no longer drive a car and must ask people to take her where she wishes to go: true, her life is not threatened by the small scars in the macula of her eyes, but the quality of her life declines as she is sapped of the common joys she—and most of us—take for granted until they are lost.

To study the eye, one needs to comprehend all that has come before. For example, the pathology of the eyelids builds on knowledge of dermatopathology (Chapter 25), and the pathology of the retina and optic nerve extends what was learned in Chapter 28 about the brain and central nervous system. But the study of ocular pathology does not merely repeat what has been presented thus far. The eye provides the only site in which a physician may visualize a variety of pathophysiologic disturbances in the microcirculation ranging from arteriosclerosis to angiogenesis in a clinical setting. Although there are conditions that are unique to the eye (such as cataract and glaucoma), many ocular conditions share similarities with disease processes elsewhere in the body that are modified by the unique structure and function of the eye (Fig. 29–1). Moreover, the eye has much to teach us about important mechanisms of disease that extend far beyond the visual system. For example, the tumor suppressor gene, *RB*, was described in retinoblastoma,[1] a quite uncommon ocular tumor of infants and very young children, but the discovery of *RB* opened an important pathway to the understanding of how cellular replication is regulated.

This chapter is organized on the basis of ocular anatomy. The discussion of each region of the eye begins with anatomical and functional considerations, and their impact on the understanding of ocular diseases.

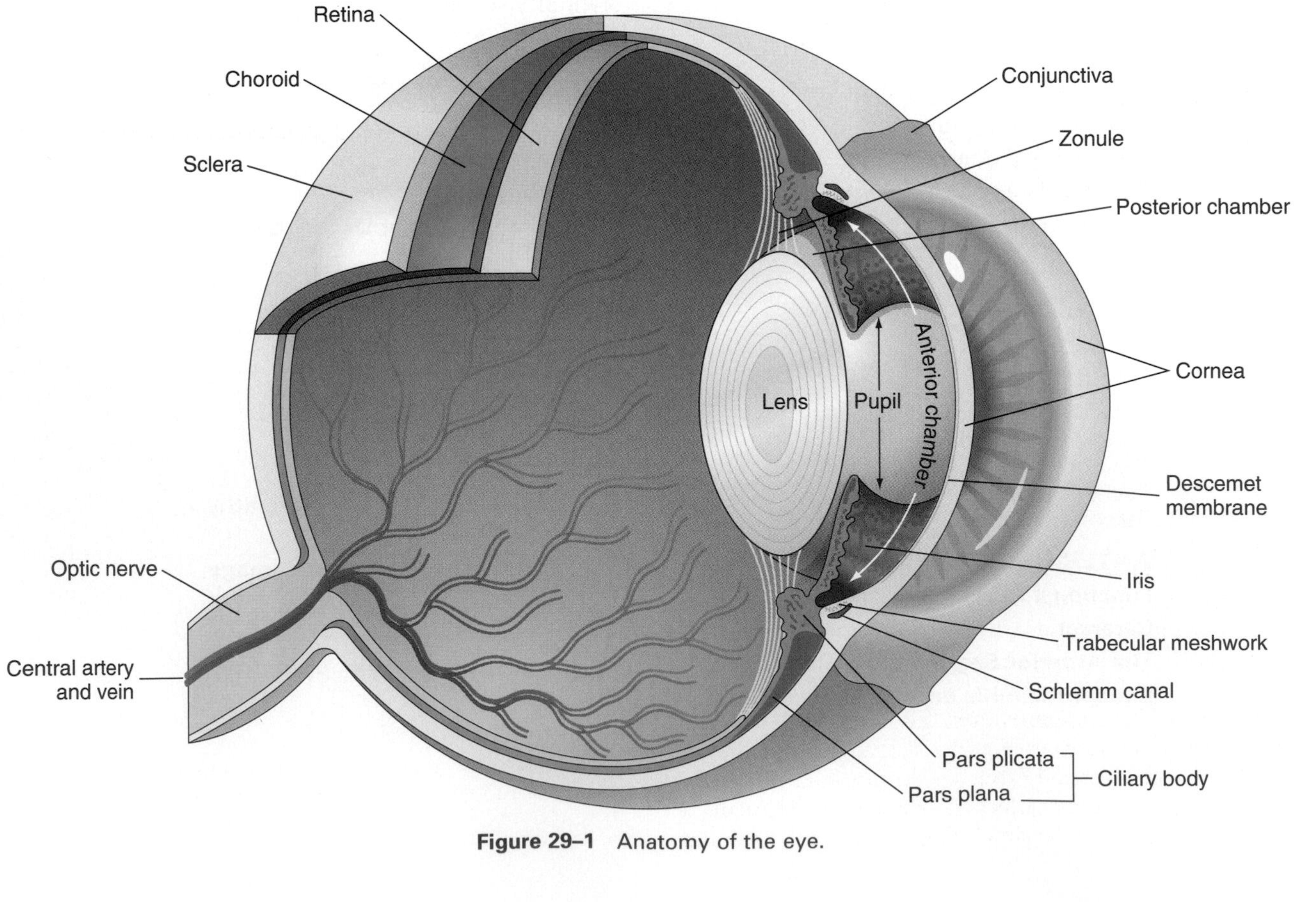

Figure 29–1 Anatomy of the eye.

Orbit

FUNCTIONAL ANATOMY AND PROPTOSIS

The orbit is a compartment that is closed medially, laterally, and posteriorly. Any disease process that increases orbital contents results in the forward displacement of the eye, *proptosis*. Aside from the obvious cosmetic concerns, the proptotic eye might not be covered completely by the eyelids, and the tear film might not be distributed evenly across the cornea. Corneal exposure is painful and can predispose to corneal infection. Proptosis may be axial (directly forward) or positional. For example, any enlargement of the lacrimal gland from inflammation (e.g., *sarcoid*) or neoplasm (e.g., *lymphoma* or epithelial neoplasm such as *pleomorphic adenoma* or *adenoid cystic carcinoma*) produces a proptosis that displaces the eye inferiorly and medially because the lacrimal gland is positioned superotemporally within the orbit.

Masses contained within the cone formed by the horizontal rectus muscles generate axial proptosis: the eye bulges straight forward. The two most common primary tumors of the optic nerve (a tract of the central nervous system and not a peripheral nerve), *glioma* and *meningioma*, produce axial proptosis because the optic nerve is positioned within the muscle cone. The orbital contents are subject to the same disease processes that affect other tissues. Representative inflammatory conditions and neoplasms of the orbit are discussed briefly next.

THYROID OPHTHALMOPATHY (GRAVES DISEASE)

In the chapter on endocrine disorders (Chapter 24), it was noted that axial proptosis is an important clinical manifestation of Graves disease. Proptosis is caused by the accumulation of extracellular matrix proteins and variable degrees of fibrosis in the rectus muscles (Fig. 29–2). The development of thyroid ophthalmopathy may be independent of the status of thyroid function.[2]

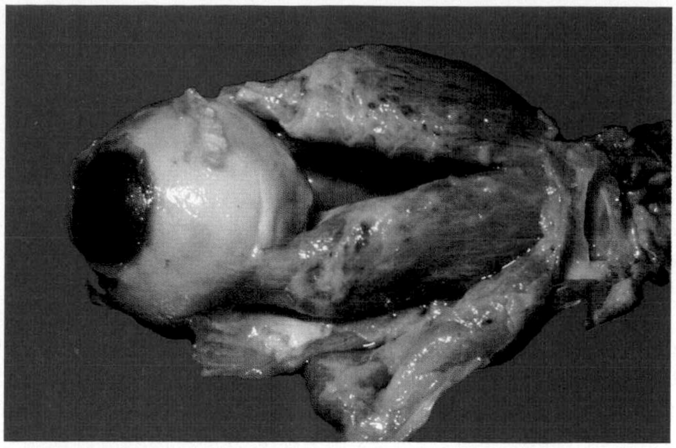

Figure 29–2 The extraocular muscles are greatly distended in this postmortem dissection of tissues from a patient with thyroid (Graves) ophthalmopathy. Note that the tendons of the muscles are spared involvement. (Courtesy of Dr. Ralph C. Eagle Jr, Wills Eye Hospital, Philadelphia, PA.)

OTHER ORBITAL INFLAMMATORY CONDITIONS

The floor of the orbit is the roof of the maxillary sinus, and the medial wall of the orbit—the lamina papyracea—separates the orbit from the ethmoidal sinuses. Thus, uncontrolled sinus infection may spread to the orbit either acutely (orbital *cellulitis*) or as part of a fungal infection (*Mucormycosis*) in immunosuppressed patients, in ketoacidosis in diabetic patients, and, rarely, in patients without any predisposition. Systemic conditions such as *Wegener granulomatosis* (Chapter 11) may present first in the orbit and may be confined to the orbit for prolonged periods of time.[3] Alternatively, Wegener granulomatosis may involve the orbit secondarily by means of primary sinus involvement.

Idiopathic orbital inflammation, also known as orbital inflammatory pseudotumor (Fig. 29–3), is another inflammatory condition affecting the orbit. This condition may be unilateral or bilateral and may affect all orbital tissue elements or may be confined to the lacrimal gland (*sclerosing dacryoadenitis*), the extraocular muscles (*orbital myositis*), or the Tenon's capsule, the fascial layer that wraps around the eye (*posterior scleritis*). In long-term follow-up, a subset of patients with idiopathic orbital inflammation may show evidence of systemic vasculitis or other forms of connective tissue diseases.

Morphology. Idiopathic orbital inflammation is characterized histologically by chronic inflammation and variable degrees of fibrosis. The inflammatory infiltrate typically includes lymphocytes and plasma cells and possibly eosinophils. Germinal centers, when present, may raise the suspicion of a reactive lymphoid hyperplasia. Elements of vasculitis, when present, are suggestive of an underlying systemic vasculitis. The presence of necrotic collagen along with

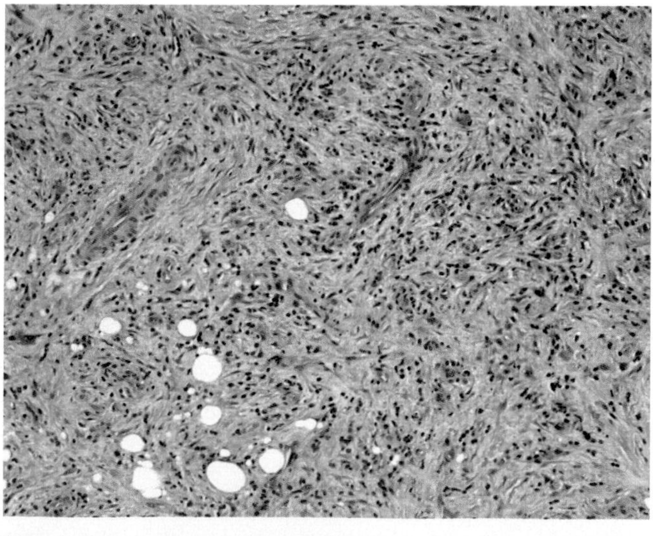

Figure 29–3 In idiopathic orbital inflammation (orbital inflammatory pseudotumor), the orbital fat is replaced by fibrosis. Note the chronic inflammation, accompanied in this case by eosinophils.

vasculitis should raise the suspicion of Wegener granulomatosis. Idiopathic orbital inflammation is typically confined to the orbit but may develop concomitantly with sclerosing inflammation in the retroperitoneum, the mediastinum, and the thyroid.

NEOPLASMS

The most frequently encountered primary neoplasms of the orbit are vascular in origin: the capillary hemangioma of infancy and early childhood and the lymphangioma (both of which are unencapsulated) and the encapsulated cavernous hemangioma found typically in adults. These are described in other chapters. Only a handful of orbital masses are encapsulated (e.g., pleomorphic adenoma of the lacrimal gland, dermoid cyst, neurilemmoma), and the recognition of encapsulation on imaging studies allows the surgeon to anticipate pathologic findings.

Malignant lymphoma, like idiopathic orbital inflammation, may affect the entire orbit or may be confined to compartments of the orbit such as the lacrimal gland. Orbital lymphomas are classified according to the histologic classification systems used for lymph nodes (Chapter 14).

Primary orbital malignancies may arise from any of the orbital tissues and are classified according to the scheme used for the parent tissue. For example, the lacrimal gland may be considered a minor salivary gland, and tumors of the lacrimal gland are classified as salivary gland tumors are classified.

Metastases to the orbit may present with distinctive signs and symptoms that point to the origin of the tumor. For example, metastatic prostatic carcinoma may present clinically like idiopathic orbital inflammation; metastatic neuroblastoma and Wilms tumor—richly vascular neoplasms—may produce characteristic periocular ecchymoses. Neoplasms may also invade from the sinuses into the orbit.

Eyelid

FUNCTIONAL ANATOMY

The eyelid is a composite of skin externally and a mucosa (the conjunctiva) on the surface apposed to the eye (Fig. 29–4). Aside from covering and protecting the eye, elements within the eyelid generate critical components of the tear film. Accessory lacrimal glands are embedded above the fibrous tarsus of the eyelid (and are also located in the conjunctival fornix). Eccrine and apocrine glands (glands of Moll) populate the eyelid. The sebaceous glands (Zeis glands associated with the eyelash and the Meibomian glands embedded within the eyelid fibrous tarsus) generate the lipid layer of the tear film, which helps to retard evaporation of tears. If the drainage system of the sebaceous glands is obstructed by chronic inflammation at the eyelid margin (*blepharitis*) or, less commonly, by neoplasm, then lipid may extravasate into surrounding tissue and provoke a granulomatous response: a lipogranuloma, or *chalazion*.

NEOPLASMS

The most common malignancy of the eyelid is basal cell carcinoma. In several studies, however, the second most common malignancy is sebaceous carcinoma, not squamous cell carcinoma. Surprisingly, primary melanomas of the eyelid skin are extremely rare. Regardless of histogenesis, eyelid neoplasms may distort tissue and prevent the eyelids from closing completely. Exposure of the cornea is not only painful, but also might predispose the patient to corneal ulceration. Therefore, prompt treatment of locally invasive basal cell carcinomas, which are typically not a threat to the patient's life, is imperative to preserve vision. *Basal cell carcinoma has a distinct predilection for the lower eyelid and the medial canthus.*

Sebaceous carcinoma may form a local tumefaction and thus mimic *chalazion* or may diffusely thicken the eyelid. This neoplasm may also mimic inflammatory processes such as

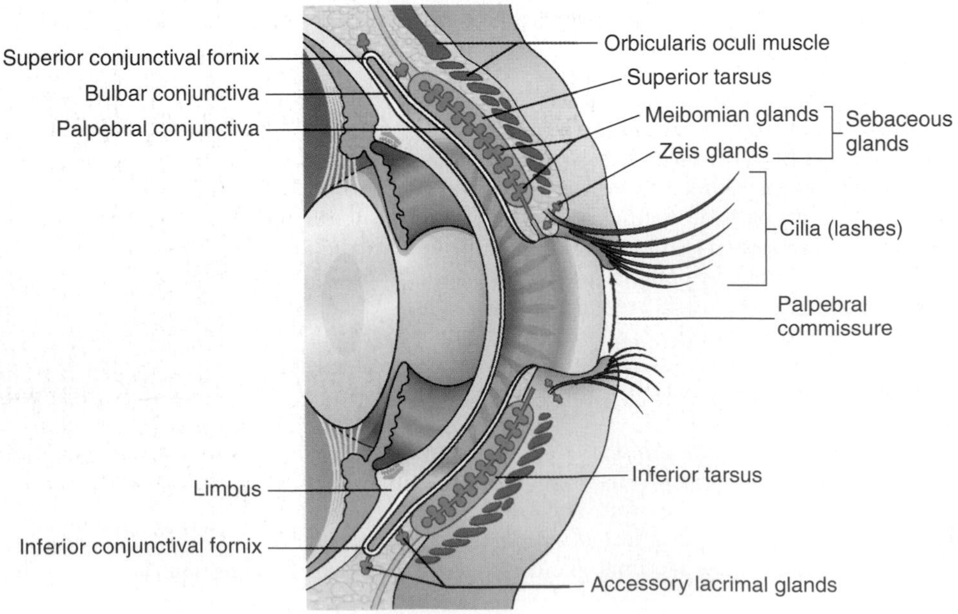

Figure 29–4 Anatomy of the conjunctiva and eyelids.

blepharitis or *ocular cicatricial pemphigoid* because of intraepithelial spread resembling that seen in Paget disease of the nipple (Chapter 23) or vulva. Sebaceous carcinoma tends to spread first to the parotid and submandibular nodes. The overall mortality rate may be as high as 22%.[4]

Morphology. In moderately differentiated or well-differentiated sebaceous carcinoma, vacuolization of the cytoplasm is present and helps in the diagnosis. This cancer may, however, mimic a variety of other malignancies histologically, including even basal cell carcinoma, and establishing the correct diagnosis can be difficult. Pagetoid spread (Fig. 29–5) may mimic Bowenoid actinic keratosis in the eyelid and carcinoma in situ in the conjunctiva. Sebaceous carcinoma may spread through the conjunctival epithelium and the epidermis to the lacrimal drainage system and the nasopharynx. It may also extend into the lacrimal gland ductules and thereby into the main lacrimal gland.

In patients with AIDS, *Kaposi sarcoma* may develop in either the eyelid or the conjunctiva. In the eyelid, the lesion may appear clinically to have a purple hue because the vascular lesion is embedded in the dermis, but in the thin mucous membrane of the conjunctiva, Kaposi sarcoma appears bright red and may be confused clinically with a subconjunctival hemorrhage. It may be possible to distinguish Kaposi sarcoma from subconjunctival hemorrhage, since subconjunctival hemorrhages are clinically flat but the conjunctival Kaposi sarcoma typically thickens the conjunctiva.

Conjunctiva

FUNCTIONAL ANATOMY

The conjunctiva is divided into topologic zones (see Fig. 29–4), each with distinctive histologic features and responses to disease. The conjunctiva lining the interior of the eyelid, the *palpebral conjunctiva*, is tightly tethered to the tarsus and may respond to inflammation by being thrown into minute papillary folds in allergic conjunctivitis and bacterial infectious conjunctivitis. The conjunctiva in the *fornix* is a pseudostratified columnar epithelium rich in goblet cells. The fornix also contains accessory lacrimal tissue, and the ductules of the main lacrimal gland pierce through the conjunctiva in the fornix superiorly and laterally. The lymphoid population of the conjunctiva is most noticeable in the fornix, and *in viral conjunctivitis, lymphoid follicles may enlarge sufficiently to be visualized clinically by* slit-lamp examination. *Granulomas* associated with systemic sarcoidosis may be detected in the conjunctival fornix, and the yield of granulomas from a nondirected conjunctival biopsy in patients suspected of sarcoid may be as high as 50%.[5] Primary lymphoma of the conjunctiva (typically of the mucosa-associated lymphoid tissue type) is most likely to develop in the fornix. The *bulbar conjunctiva*—the conjunctiva that covers the surface of the eye—is a nonkeratinizing stratified squamous epithelium. Goblet cells decrease in concentration from the fornix to the limbus.

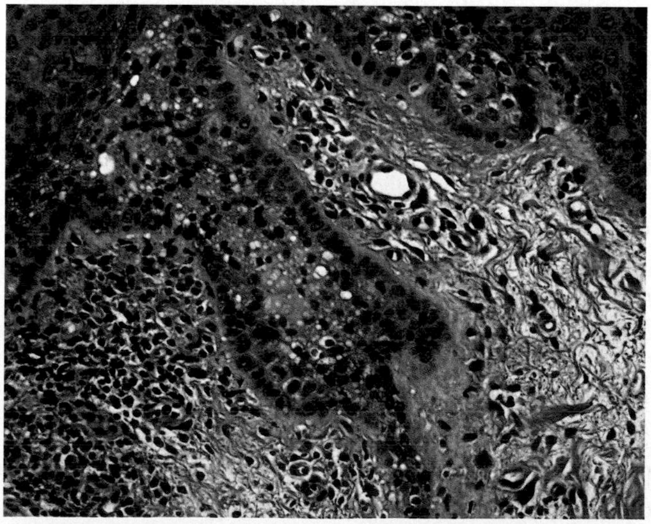

Figure 29–5 Pagetoid spread of sebaceous carcinoma. Neoplastic cells with foamy cytoplasm are detected within the epidermis. Invasive sebaceous carcinoma was identified elsewhere in this biopsy sample.

The junction of the sclera and cornea is termed the *limbus*; the epithelium of the limbus contains epithelial stem cells that are capable of differentiating into conjunctival epithelium (which may contain goblet cells) or corneal epithelium (devoid of goblet cells). The transdifferentiation of limbal stem cells may be influenced by the subepithelial connective tissue of the conjunctiva and cornea.

The conjunctiva, like the eyelid, is richly invested with lymphatic channels. Neoplasms arising in the eyelid and conjunctiva tend to spread to regional lymph nodes (parotid and submandibular node groups).

CONJUNCTIVAL SCARRING

Many cases of bacterial or viral conjunctivitis cause redness and itching but most heal without sequelae. However, infection with *Chlamydia trachomatis (trachoma)* may produce significant conjunctival scarring. Conjunctival scarring is also seen after exposure of the ocular surface to caustic alkalis or as a sequela to ocular cicatricial *pemphigoid* (Chapter 25). A reduction in the number of goblet cells due to conjunctival scarring leads to a decrease in surface mucin, which is essential for the adherence of the aqueous component of tears to the corneal epithelium. Thus, even if the aqueous component of the tear film is adequate, the patient will suffer from a dry eye, a condition that, when severe, can be painful and can predispose to corneal opacification and ulceration. More commonly, however, dry eye results from a deficiency in the aqueous component of the tear film generated by the accessory lacrimal gland embedded within the eyelid and fornix.

The conjunctiva may be scarred iatrogenically through reaction to drugs or as a consequence of surgery. In other parts of the body, cancer surgery requires excision of the lesion with a margin of normal tissue to ensure complete removal. However, the surgical excision of large amounts of even diseased conjunctiva can remove large populations of goblet cells or compromise lacrimal gland ductules that traverse the conjunctiva. Thus, excision of a conjunctival neoplasm or a precursor lesion may leave the patient with a painful dry eye that can compromise vision. Therefore, it is reasonable for surgeons to remove the invasive components of conjunctival neoplasms and to treat the intraepithelial components with tissue-sparing modalities such as cryotherapy or topical chemotherapy delivered as eyedrops.

PINGUECULA AND PTERYGIUM

Both pinguecula and pterygium appear as submucosal elevations on the conjuctiva. They result from actinic damage, and are therefore located in the sun-exposed regions of the conjunctiva (i.e., in the fissure between both the upper and lower eyelids—the interpalpebral fissure). Pterygium typically originates in the conjunctiva astride the limbus. It is formed by a submucosal growth *of fibrovascular connective tissue that migrates onto the cornea*, dissecting into the plane occupied normally by Bowman's layer. Pterygium does not cross the pupillary axis and, aside from the possible induction of mild astigmatism, does not pose a threat to vision. These lesions are commonly excised to relieve patients of the white blemish over the surface of the eye, which may be mildly irritating and cosmetically unacceptable. Although most pterygia are entirely benign, it is worthwhile submitting the excised tissue to the pathologist for examination because, on occasion, precursors of actinic-induced neoplasms—squamous cell carcinoma and melanoma—are detected in these lesions.

Pinguecula, which, like pterygium, appears astride the limbus, is a small, yellowish submucosal elevation. Although the *pinguecula does not invade the cornea as pterygium* does, the presence of a focal conjunctival elevation near the limbus can result in an uneven distribution of the tear film over the adjacent cornea. As a consequence of focal dehydration, a saucer-like depression in the corneal tissue—a *dellen*—may develop. The yellow color of the pinguecula originates not from the accumulation of lipid, as one might expect, but rather from the accumulation of focal zones of sun-damaged collagen with elastic-like properties: *solar elastosis*. On occasion, pinguecula may become inflamed secondary to a foreign body granulomatous reaction against the elastotic collagen: *actinic granuloma*.

NEOPLASMS

Both squamous neoplasms and melanocytic neoplasms and their precursors tend to develop at the limbus. Conjunctival squamous cell carcinoma may be preceded by intraepithelial neoplastic changes analogous to those seen in the evolution of cervical squamous cell carcinoma. In the conjunctiva, the spectrum of changes from mild dysplasia through carcinoma in situ is also designated as *CIN*, which in this context designates *conjunctival intraepithelial neoplasia*. Squamous papillomas and conjunctival intraepithelial neoplasia may be associated with the presence of human papillomavirus types 16 and 18.[6] Although conjunctival squamous cell carcinoma tends to follow an indolent course, *mucoepidermoid carcinoma* of the conjunctiva (reflecting the ability of conjunctival stem cells to differentiate into squamous epithelium and goblet cells) follows a much more aggressive course.

Conjunctival nevi are encountered commonly in clinical practice but seldom invade the cornea or appear in the fornix or over the palpebral conjunctiva.[7] Pigmented lesions in these zones of the conjunctiva most likely represent melanomas or melanoma precursors. Compound nevi of the conjunctiva characteristically contain subepithelial cysts lined by surface epithelium (Figs. 29–6*A* and *B*). In late childhood or adolescence, conjunctival nevi may acquire an inflammatory component rich in lymphocytes, plasma cells, and eosinophils. The resultant *inflamed juvenile nevus* is completely benign and not associated with vitiligo or halo nevus.

Conjunctival melanomas are unilateral neoplasms, typically affecting fair-complexioned individuals in middle age[8] (Figs. 29–6*C* and *D*). Most cases of conjunctival melanoma develop through a phase of intraepithelial growth termed *primary acquired melanosis with atypia*, which is roughly analogous to *melanoma in situ* but does not correspond neatly to the radial growth phase of cutaneous melanoma. Between 50% and 90% of patients with incompletely treated primary acquired melanosis with atypia will develop conjunctival melanoma; the best treatment of conjunctival melanoma is its prevention through extirpation of its precursor lesion. The lesions tend to spread first to the parotid or submandibular lymph nodes. The mortality rate for conjunctival melanoma is 25%.

Sclera

The sclera is relatively deficient in both blood vessels and fibroblasts; hence, wounds and surgical incisions of the sclera tend to heal poorly. The sclera is physiologically thin at the limbus, behind the insertion of the rectus muscles, and around the insertion of the optic nerve. Therefore, it is prone to rupture in these locations from blunt trauma. Immune complex deposits within the sclera, such as in *rheumatoid arthritis*, may produce a necrotizing *scleritis*.

The sclera may appear "blue" in a variety of conditions. It may become thin following episodes of scleritis, and the normally brown color of the uvea may appear blue clinically because of the optical Tyndall effect. In eyes with exceptionally high intraocular pressure, the sclera may become thin, and because this zone of scleral ectasia is lined by uveal tissue, the resulting lesion, known as a *staphyloma*, also appears blue clinically. The sclera may appear blue in osteogenesis imperfecta. Finally, the sclera may appear blue because of a heavily pigmented congenital nevus of the underlying uvea, a condition known as *congenital melanosis oculi*. When accompanied by periocular cutaneous pigmentation, this condition is known as *nevus of Ota*.

Cornea

FUNCTIONAL ANATOMY

The cornea and its overlying tear film—and not the lens—make up the major refractive surface of the eye (Fig. 29–7). Parenthetically, myopia typically develops because the eye is too long for its refractive power, and hyperopia results from an eye that is too short. The popularity of procedures such as laser-assisted in situ keratomileusis (LASIK) to sculpt the cornea and change its refractive properties attests to the importance of corneal shape in contributing to the refractive power of the eye.

Anteriorly, the cornea is covered by *epithelium* that rests on a basement membrane. *Bowman's layer*, situated just beneath the epithelial basement membrane, is acellular and forms an

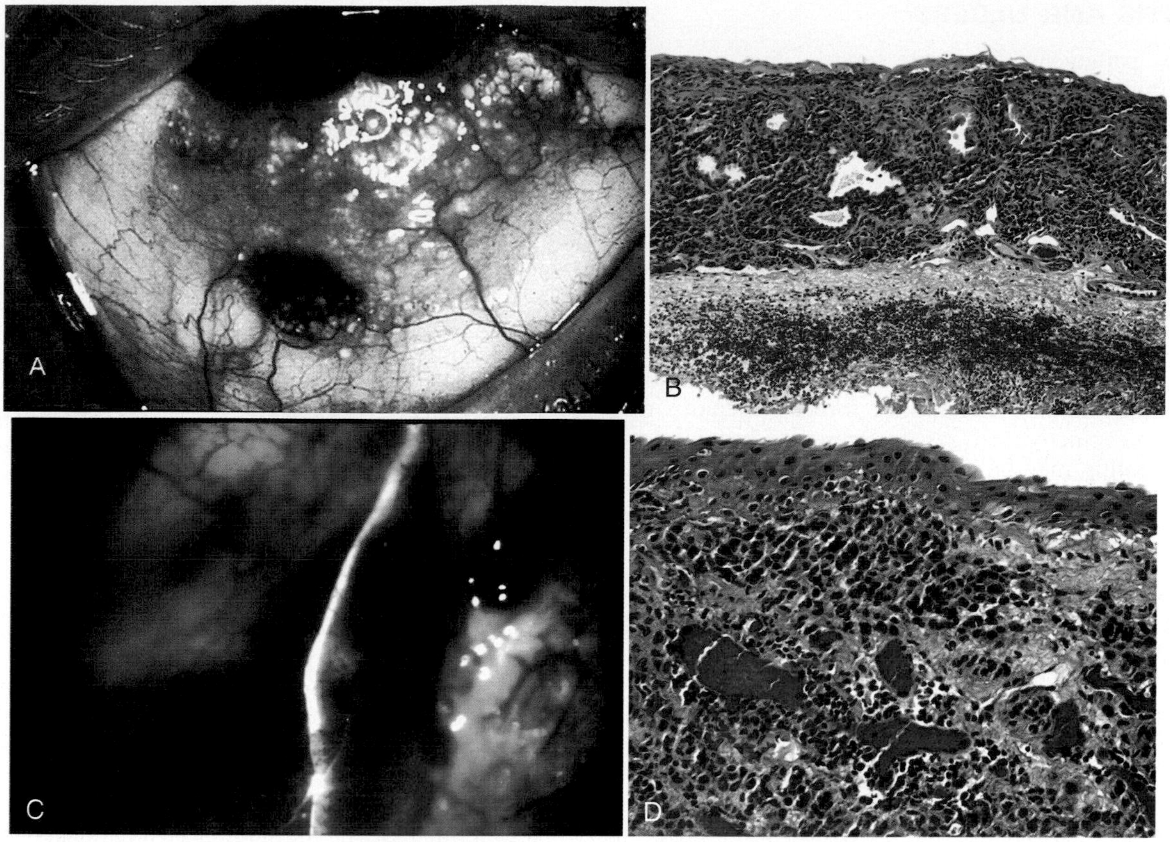

Figure 29–6 *A, B,* Cystic compound nevus of the conjunctiva. (From Folberg R, Jakobiec FA, Bernardino VB, Iwamoto T: Benign conjunctival melanocytic lesions: clinicopathologic features. Ophthalmology 96:436–461, 1989.) *C, D,* Conjunctival malignant melanoma. In *C,* note the deflection of the beam of the slit lamp over the surface of the lesion, indicative of invasion.

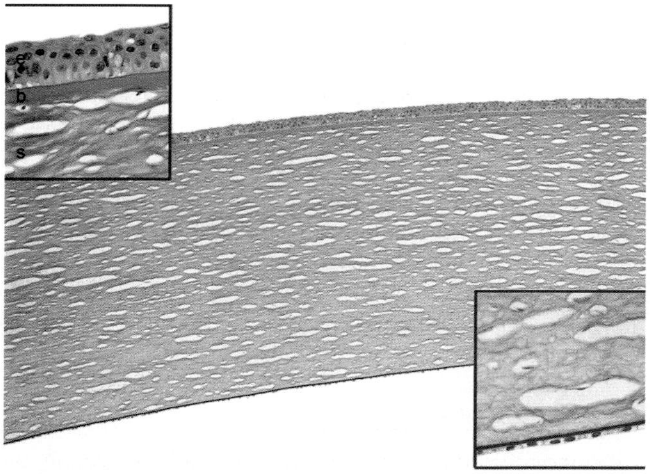

Figure 29–7 Normal corneal microarchitecture. The corneal tissue is stained by periodic acid–Schiff (PAS) to highlight basement membranes. The inset at the upper left is a high magnification of the anterior layers of the cornea: the epithelium *(e),* Bowman's layer *(b),* and the stroma *(s).* A very thin PAS-positive basement membrane separates the epithelium from Bowman's layer. Note that Bowman's layer is acellular. The inset at the lower right is a high magnification of the PAS-positive Descemet membrane and the corneal endothelium. The "holes" in the stroma are artifactitious spaces between parallel collagenous stromal lamellae.

efficient barrier against the penetration of malignant cells from the epithelium into the underlying stroma.

The *corneal stroma* lacks blood vessels and lymphatics, a feature that contributes not only to the transparency of the cornea, but also to high rate of success of corneal transplantation. Indeed, nonimmunologic graft failure (associated with loss of endothelial cells and subsequent corneal edema) is seen more commonly than is immunologic graft rejection. The risk of corneal graft rejection increases with stromal vascularization and inflammation. A precise alignment of collagen in the corneal stroma also contributes to transparency. Scarring and edema both disrupt the spatial alignment of stromal collagen and contribute to corneal opacification. Scars may result from trauma or inflammation. Normally, the corneal stroma is in a state of relative deturgescence (dehydration), maintained in large part by active pumping of fluid from the stroma back into the anterior chamber by the corneal endothelium.

The corneal *endothelium* is derived from neural crest and is not related to vascular endothelium. It rests on its basement membrane, Descemet membrane. A decrease in endothelial cells or a malfunction of endothelium results in stromal edema, which may be complicated by bullous separation of the epithelium (*bullous keratopathy*). *Descemet membrane* increases in thickness with age. It is the site of copper deposition in the Kayser-Fleischer ring of Wilson disease (Chapter 18).

KERATITIS AND ULCERS

Various pathogens—bacterial, fungal, viral (especially herpes simplex and herpes zoster), and protozoal (Acanthamoeba) may cause corneal ulceration. In all forms of keratitis, dissolution of the corneal stroma may be accelerated by activation of collagenases within corneal epithelium and stromal fibroblasts (also known as keratocytes). Exudate and cells leaking from iris and ciliary body vessels into the anterior chamber may be visible by slit-lamp examination and may accumulate in sufficient quantity to become visible even by a penlight examination (*hypopyon*). Although the corneal ulcer may be infectious, the hypopyon seldom contains organisms and is an example par excellence of the vascular response to acute inflammation. The specific forms of keratitis may have certain distinctive features. For example, chronic herpes simplex keratitis may be associated with a granulomatous reaction to Descemet's membrane (Fig. 29–8).

CORNEAL DEGENERATIONS AND DYSTROPHIES

Ophthalmologists have traditionally divided many corneal disorders into degenerations and dystrophies. Corneal degenerations may be either unilateral or bilateral and are typically non-familial. By contrast, corneal dystrophies are typically bilateral and are hereditary. Corneal dystrophies may affect selective corneal layers (e.g., *Reis-Bückler dystrophy* affects Bowman's layer, and *posterior polymorphous dystrophy* affects the endothelium), or the changes may be distributed throughout multiple layers.

Band Keratopathies

Two types of band keratopathy serve as examples of corneal degenerations. *Calcific band keratopathy* is characterized by deposition of calcium in Bowman's layer. This condition may complicate chronic uveitis, especially in patients with chronic juvenile rheumatoid arthritis. *Actinic band keratopathy* develops in patients who are exposed chronically to high levels of ultraviolet light. In this condition, extensive solar elastosis develops in the superficial layers of corneal collagen in the sun-exposed interpalpebral fissure, hence the horizontally distributed band of pathology. Similar to pinguecula, the sun-damaged collagen of the cornea appears clinically to be yellow to the point that this condition is sometimes erroneously called "oil-droplet keratopathy."

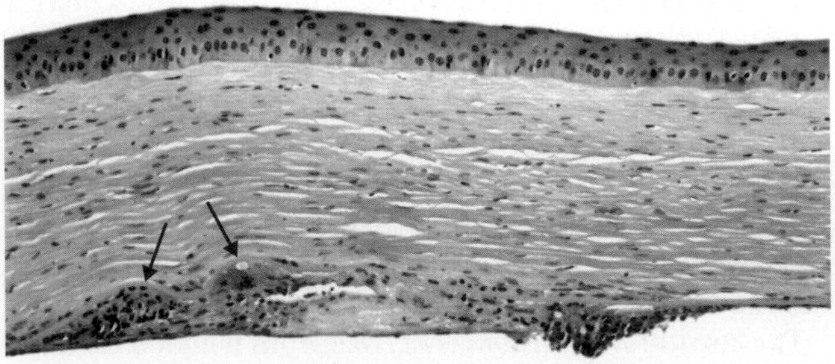

Figure 29–8 Chronic herpes simplex keratitis. The cornea is thin and scarred (note the increased number of fibroblast nuclei). Granulomatous reaction to Descemet's membrane, illustrated in this photomicrograph (*arrows*), is a histologic hallmark or chronic herpes simplex keratitis.

Keratoconus

With an incidence of 1 in 2000, *keratoconus* is a rather common disorder. It is characterized by progressive thinning and ectasia of the cornea without evidence of inflammation or vascularization. Such thinning results in a cornea that has a conical rather than spherical shape. This abnormal shape generates irregular astigmatism that is difficult to correct with spectacles. Rigid contact lenses generate a smooth, spherical surface to the cornea and may provide refractive relief for keratoconus patients. Patients whose vision cannot be corrected with spectacles or contact lenses are excellent candidates for corneal transplantation, which has a high degree of success in this condition. The etiology of keratoconus is unknown. Unlike many degenerations, it is typically bilateral, and in some patients, there is an association between keratoconus, Down syndrome and Marfan syndrome, as well as with atopic disorders. Activation of collagenases, gelatinases, and matrix-metalloproteinases has been implicated in the pathogenesis of this condition.

Morphology. Thinning of the cornea with breaks in Bowman's layer are the histologic hallmarks of keratoconus (Fig. 29–9). In some patients, Descemet's membrane may rupture precipitously, allowing the aqueous humor in the anterior chamber to gain access to the corneal stroma. The sudden effusion of aqueous humor through a gap in Descemet's membrane—corneal **hydrops**—may also cause the vision to worsen suddenly. An episode of hydrops may be followed by corneal scarring that can also contribute to visual loss. Acute corneal hydrops can complicate Descemet's membrane ruptures that develop secondary to extraordinary elevations of intraocular pressure in **infantile glaucoma (Haab's striae)** or following the now uncommon obstetrical forceps injury to the eye.

Fuchs Endothelial Dystrophy

This condition, one of several dystrophies affecting the endothelium is one of the principal indications for corneal transplantation in the United States. The two major clinical manifestations of Fuchs endothelial dystrophy—*stromal edema and bullous keratopathy*—are both related to a primary loss of endothelial cells. Early in the course of the disease, endothelial cells produce droplike deposits of abnormal basement membrane material (*guttata*) that resemble the fetal component of Descemet's membrane ultrastructurally. Guttata can be visualized clinically by slit-lamp examination. With disease progression, there is a decrease in the total number of endothelial cells, and the residual cells are inca-

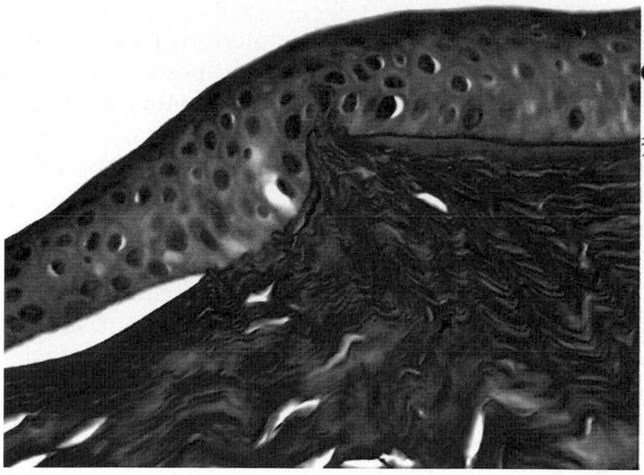

Figure 29–9 Keratoconus. This high-magnification photomicrograph captures the epithelium, Bowman's layer, and the superficial layers of the corneal stroma; the posterior layers of the stroma, Descemet's membrane, and the endothelium are not included. The tissue section is stained by periodic acid–Schiff to highlight the epithelial basement membrane (ebm), which is intact. Bowman's layer (bl), situated between the epithelial basement membrane and the stroma (s), is not a basement membrane. By tracing Bowman's layer from the right side of the photomicrograph toward the center, one notices a discontinuity in this layer, diagnostic of keratoconus. The epithelial separation just to the left of the Bowman's layer break resulted from an episode of corneal hydrops, secondary to a break in Descemet's membrane (not shown).

pable of maintaining stromal deturgescence. Consequently, the stroma becomes edematous and thickens; it acquires a ground-glass appearance clinically, and vision is blurred (Fig. 29–10). Because of chronic edema, the stroma may eventually become vascularized.

With increasing stromal edema, the epithelium undergoes hydropic change, and the detachment of the epithelium from the Bowman's layer produces epithelial bullae that may eventually rupture. Fibrous connective tissue may be deposited between the epithelium and Bowman's layer (*degenerative pannus*) either by ingrowth from the limbus or perhaps through fibrous metaplasia of the corneal epithelium.

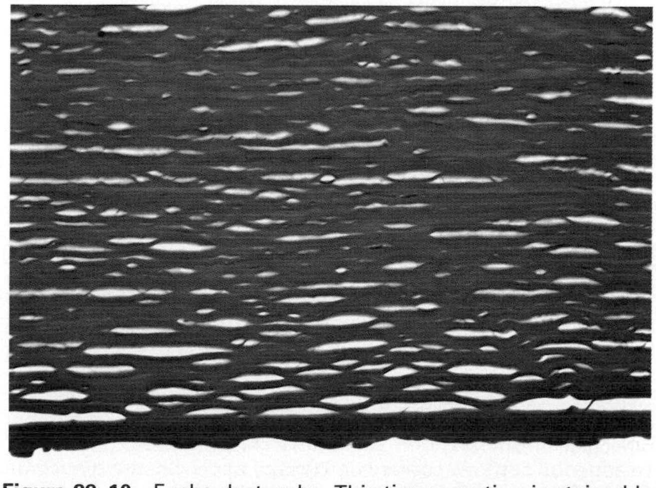

Figure 29–10 Fuchs dystrophy. This tissue section is stained by periodic acid–Schiff to highlight the Descemet's membrane, which is thick. Numerous droplike excrescences—guttata—protrude downward from Descemet's membrane. Endothelial cell nuclei are not seen. Epithelial bullae, not shown in this micrograph, were present, reflecting corneal edema.

Although the signs and symptoms of Fuchs dystrophy (blurring and loss of vision) first manifest themselves in late middle age, ultrastructural evidence suggests that the endothelium and Descemet's membrane are abnormal even in young, asymptomatic patients with this disorder. Therefore, asymptomatic patients with Fuchs dystrophy may develop frank corneal edema following intraocular surgery such as cataract extraction with implantation of a prosthetic intraocular lens; the loss of even a minimal number of endothelial cells during surgery may tip the balance and lead to corneal edema. On occasion, the number of endothelial cells may decrease following cataract surgery even in patients who do not have early forms of Fuchs dystrophy, and the condition is then known as *pseudophakic bullous keratopathy*.

Stromal Dystrophies

There are a large number of dystrophies that affect the corneal stroma principally. Although the clinical manifestations of these conditions may emerge in childhood, they typically come to attention in young adulthood and may be progressive.

In these conditions, the stromal deposits generate discrete opacities in the corneal stroma, which may eventually compromise vision. Deposits in the vicinity of the epithelium, its basement membrane, and Bowman's layer may result in painful epithelial erosions. Scarring in the vicinity of Bowman's layer may generate an irregular corneal surface, further compromising vision. *Macular corneal dystrophy* is so named because early in the disease, small nummular (macular) deposits of keratan sulfate distribute in the corneal stroma. Later in the course of this autosomal-recessive dystrophy, keratan sulfate is distributed diffusely throughout the stroma and may affect the endothelium.

Until recently, the stromal dystrophies were classified on the basis of clinical appearance. However, the identification of specific mutations responsible for various dystrophies is generating a new molecular classification of these disorders.[9] For example, three stromal dystrophies, each with autosomal-dominant inheritance, had been classified separately by the shape of discrete stromal deposits: needle-shaped deposits of amyloid were classified as one form of *lattice dystrophy*, chunky deposits of hyalin were classified as *granular dystrophy*, and combinations of these opacities in the same patient were classified as *Avellino dystrophy* (named for the location of the first families discovered with this condition). The development of each of these three disorders has now been attributed to defects in the gene encoding β-keratoepithelin.

In conclusion, it should be noted that the division of corneal diseases into dystrophies and degenerations might not be entirely accurate. For example, there are bilateral inherited conditions in which amyloid is deposited beneath the epithelium (*gelatinous drop dystrophy*) or, more typically, in the corneal stroma. The depositions in the cornea may be without systemic manifestations (such as in *lattice corneal dystrophy*) or may be accompanied by conditions such as peripheral neuropathies (*Meratoja syndrome*). However, amyloid may also be deposited focally deep within the cornea of elderly patients in a condition known as *polymorphic amyloid degeneration*. Although this condition is grouped with degenerations, patients have been reported to have bilateral corneal opacities, and there are examples of this disorder in siblings, an observation that suggests that this disorder might indeed be hereditary.

Anterior Segment

FUNCTIONAL ANATOMY

The eye can be divided conceptually and anatomically into two compartments: the anterior segment (which includes the cornea, anterior chamber, posterior chamber, iris, and lens) and the posterior pole (the remainder of the eye). In understanding the pathophysiology of the eye, it is helpful to consider the tissues that contribute to the anterior segment as a functional unit.

The anterior chamber is bounded anteriorly by the cornea, laterally by the trabecular meshwork, and posteriorly by the iris (Fig. 29–11). Aqueous humor, formed by the pars plicata of the ciliary body, enters the posterior chamber, bathes the lens, and circulates through the pupil to gain access to the anterior chamber.

The lens is a closed epithelial system; the basement membrane of the lens epithelium (known as the lens capsule) totally envelops the lens. Thus, the lens epithelium does not exfoliate like the epidermis or a mucosal epithelium. Instead, the lens epithelium and its derivative fibers accumulate within the confines of the enveloping lens capsule, thus "infoliating." With aging, therefore, the size of the lens increases. Neoplasms of the lens have not been described.

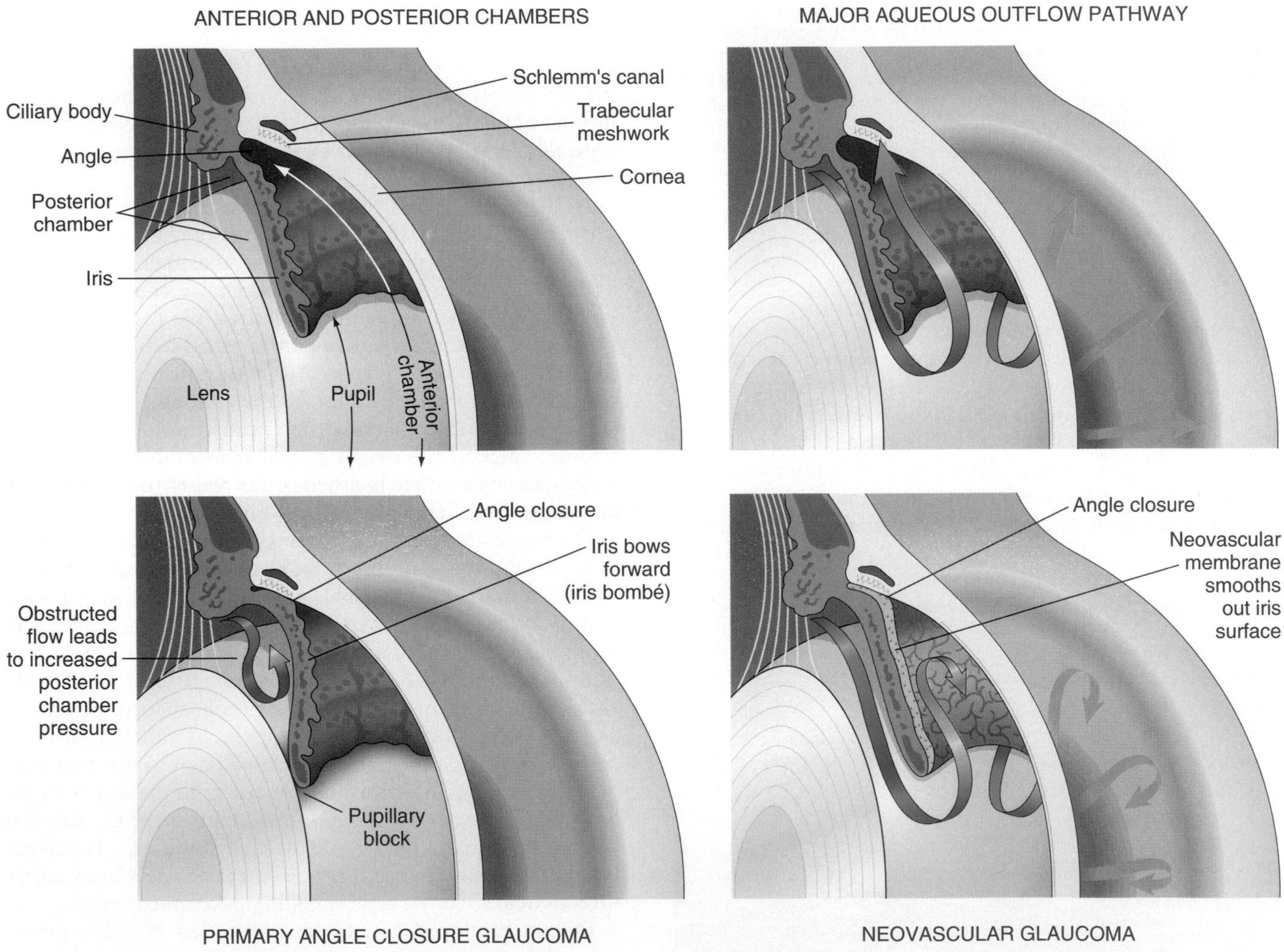

Figure 29–11 *Upper left,* The normal eye. Note that the surface of the iris is highly textured with crypts and folds. *Upper right,* The normal flow of aqueous humor. Aqueous humor, produced in the posterior chamber, flows through the pupil into the anterior chamber. The major pathway for the egress of aqueous humor is through the trabecular meshwork, into Schlemm's canal. Minor outflow pathways (uveoscleral and iris, not depicted) contribute to a limited extent to aqueous outflow. *Lower left,* Primary angle closure glaucoma. In anatomically predisposed eyes, transient apposition of the iris at the pupillary margin to the lens blocks the passage of aqueous humor from the posterior chamber to the anterior chamber. Pressure builds in the posterior chamber, bowing the iris forward (iris bombé) and occluding the trabecular meshwork. *Lower right,* A neovascular membrane has grown over the surface of the iris, smoothing the iris folds and crypts. Myofibroblasts within the neovascular membrane cause the membrane to contract and to become apposed to the trabecular meshwork (peripheral anterior synechiae). Outflow of aqueous humor is blocked, and the intraocular pressure becomes elevated.

CATARACT

The term *cataract* describes lenticular opacities that may be congenital or acquired. Systemic diseases (such as galactosemia, diabetes mellitus, Wilson disease, and atopic dermatitis), drugs (especially corticosteroids), radiation, trauma, and many intraocular disorders are associated with cataract. Age-related cataract typically results from opacification of the lens nucleus (*nuclear sclerosis*). The accumulation of urochrome pigment may render the lens nucleus brown, thus distorting the patient's perception of blue color (the predominance of yellow hues in Rembrandt's paintings later in life might have been a consequence of nuclear sclerotic cataracts). Other physical changes in the lens may generate opacities. For example, the lens cortex may liquefy. Migration of the lens epithelium posterior to the lens equator may result in *posterior subcapsular cataract* secondary to enlargement of abnormally positioned lens epithelium. The technique that is most commonly used to remove opacified lenses extracts the lens contents, leaving the lens capsule intact (extracapsular cataract extraction). A prosthetic intraocular lens may be inserted into the eye. Residual lens epithelial cells may migrate over the lens capsule, contributing to opacification of the capsule and reduction in vision after surgery.

Inflammatory reactions to lens material may develop as the result of the exposure of intact lens cortex by rupture of the lens capsule (either by trauma or as part of cataract extraction). It has been suggested that antigen-antibody complexes develop to lens cortical material, especially in the presence of *Propionibacterium acnes* as an adjuvant, generating a *lens-induced uveitis*.

Occasionally, the lens cortex may liquefy nearly entirely, a condition known as hypermature or *Morgagnian cataract*. High-molecular-weight proteins from liquefied lens cortex may leak through the lens capsule (*phacolysis*). This phacolytic protein—either free or contained within macrophages—may clog the trabecular meshwork and contribute to elevation in intraocular pressure and optic nerve damage; phacolytic glaucoma is an example of secondary open angle glaucoma.

THE ANTERIOR SEGMENT AND GLAUCOMA

The term *glaucoma* refers to a collection of diseases characterized by distinctive changes in the visual field and in the cup of the optic nerve. Most of the glaucomas are associated with elevated intraocular pressure, although some patients with normal intraocular pressure may develop characteristic optic nerve and visual field changes (*normal* or *low-tension glaucoma*). The relationship between intraocular pressure and optic nerve damage is discussed later in the section on the optic nerve.

To understand the *pathophysiology of glaucoma*, it is useful to consider the formation and drainage of aqueous humor. As Figure 29–11 illustrates, aqueous humor is produced in the ciliary body and passes from the posterior chamber through the pupil into the anterior chamber. Although there are multiple pathways for the egress of fluid from the anterior chamber, most of the aqueous humor drains through the trabecular meshwork, situated in the angle formed by the intersection between the corneal periphery and the anterior surface of the iris. With this background, glaucoma may be classified into two major categories. In *open angle glaucoma*, the aqueous humor has complete physical access to the trabecular meshwork, and the elevation in intraocular pressure results from an increased resistance to aqueous outflow in the open angle. In *angle closure glaucoma*, the peripheral zone of the iris adheres to the trabecular meshwork and physically impedes the egress of aqueous from the eye. Both open angle and angle closure glaucoma may be subclassified into *primary* and *secondary* types.

In *primary open angle glaucoma*, the most common form of glaucoma, the angle is open, and few changes are apparent structurally. Mutations in the *GLC1A* gene (also known as the trabecular meshwork inducible glucocorticoid response gene, or TIGR, located on chromosome 1) have been associated with a subset of patients with juvenile and adult primary open angle glaucoma.[10] The function of the gene product, myocilin, is unknown. Myocilin is distributed not only in the trabecular meshwork and other anterior segment tissues, but also within the optic nerve,[11] suggesting that the pathogenesis of optic nerve damage in open angle glaucoma may be complex.

There are multiple causes of *secondary open angle glaucoma*. Particulate material such as high-molecular-weight lens proteins in phacolysis, senescent red blood cells after trauma (*ghost cell glaucoma*), iris pigment epithelial granules (*pigmentary glaucoma*), fragments of oxytalan fibers (*exfoliation glaucoma*), and necrotic tumors (*melanomalytic glaucoma*) may clog the trabecular meshwork in the presence of an open angle. Elevations in the pressure on the surface of the eye (episcleral venous pressure) in the presence of an open angle contribute to other types of secondary open angle glaucoma. This type of glaucoma is associated with surface ocular vascular malformations seen in *Sturge-Weber syndrome* or as a consequence of arterialization of the episcleral veins following a spontaneous or traumatic carotid-cavernous fistula.

Primary angle closure glaucoma typically develops in eyes with shallow anterior chambers, often found in patients with hyperopia. Transient apposition of the pupillary margin of the iris to the anterior surface of the lens may result in obstruction to the flow of aqueous humor through the pupillary aperture (*pupillary block*). Continued production of aqueous humor by the ciliary body thus elevates pressure in the posterior chamber and may bow the iris periphery forward (*iris bombé*), apposing it to the trabecular meshwork. These anatomic changes provoke a dramatic elevation in intraocular pressure (see Fig. 29–11). Since the crystalline lens is avascular and the lens epithelium receives its nutrition from the aqueous humor, unremitting elevation in intraocular pressure in primary angle closure glaucoma can damage the lens epithelium. This leads to minute anterior subcapsular opacities that are visible by slit-lamp examination (*glaukomflecken*). Although the patient might have a normal complement of healthy corneal endothelial cells, sustained elevated intraocular pressure can produce corneal edema and bullous keratopathy.

There are many causes of *secondary angle closure glaucoma*. Contraction of various types of pathologic membranes that form over the surface of the iris can draw the iris over the trabecular meshwork, occluding aqueous outflow. For example, chronic retinal ischemia is associated with the up-regulation of vascular endothelial growth factor (VEGF) and other pro-angiogenic factors. The appearance of VEGF in the aqueous humor is thought to induce the development of thin, clinically transparent fibrovascular membranes over the surface of the iris. Contraction of myofibroblastic elements in these membranes leads to occlusion of the trabecular meshwork by the iris: *neovascular glaucoma* (see Fig. 29–11). Necrotic tumors, especially retinoblastomas, can also induce iris neovascularization and glaucoma. Abnormal corneal endothelium may migrate over the trabecular meshwork and onto the surface of the iris in a group of disorders known collectively as the *iridocorneal endothelial syndrome*. Contraction of this abnormal endothelial membrane is another cause of secondary angle closure glaucoma. Following intraocular surgery or penetrating trauma to the anterior segment, conjunctival or corneal epithelium may grow through the wound and into the anterior chamber, and the contraction of these *epithelial downgrowth* membranes may yet cause secondary angle closure glaucoma. The development of secondary angle closure glaucoma may be unrelated to iris membranes; for example, tumors in the ciliary body can mechanically compress the iris onto the trabecular meshwork, closing off the major pathway of aqueous outflow.

The discussion of glaucomatous optic nerve damage continues in a later section of this chapter dedicated to the pathology of the optic nerve.

ENDOPHTHALMITIS AND PANOPHTHALMITIS

Anterior segment inflammation can develop as a consequence of such diverse etiologies as blunt trauma to the eye (*traumatic iridocyclitis*), corneal infections, and inflammation originating within the uvea: uveitis. The purpose of this section is to describe the final common pathways of anterior segment inflammation and to discuss briefly acute suppurative inflammation that extends to encompass the entire eye: endophthalmitis and panophthalmitis.

In intraocular inflammation, vessels in the ciliary body and iris become leaky, allowing cells and exudate to accumulate in the anterior chamber. These changes can be visualized with the slit lamp; at times, the inflammatory cells may adhere to the corneal endothelium, forming clinically visible *keratic precipitates*. The size and shape of these precipitates can provide clues to the underlying cause of the inflammation. For example, aggregates of macrophages on the endothelium in sarcoid produce characteristic "mutton-fat" keratic precipitates.

Just as pleural exudate in acute bronchopneumonia can lead to adhesions between the visceral and parietal pleura, the presence of exudate in the anterior chamber can facilitate the formation of adhesions between the iris and the trabecular meshwork or cornea (*anterior synechiae*) or adhesions between the iris and anterior surface of the lens (*posterior synechiae*). Anterior synechiae can lead to elevation in intraocular pressure and optic nerve damage. Prolonged contact between the iris and the anterior surface of the lens can deprive lens epithelium of contact with aqueous humor and can induce fibrous metaplasia of the lens epithelium: *anterior subcapsular cataract* (Fig. 29–12). The pharmacologic induction of pupillary dilation and cycloplegia in patients with intraocular inflammation is intended in part to prevent the formation of synechiae and the sequelae that develop as a consequence of these adhesions.

Although inflammation confined to the anterior segment is technically intraocular inflammation, the term *endophthalmitis* is not applied clinically unless there is inflammation within the vitreous humor. The retina lines the vitreous cavity, and suppurative inflammation in the vitreous humor (*endophthalmitis*) is poorly tolerated by the retina; after only a few hours of exposure to acute inflammation, the function of the retina may be irreversibly damaged. Endophthalmitis is classified as *exogenous* (originating in the environment and gaining access to the interior of the eye through a wound) or *endogenous* (delivered to the eye hematogenously). The term *panophthalmitis* is applied to inflammation within the eye that involves the retina, choroid, and sclera and extends into the orbit (Fig. 29–13). The accumulation of inflammatory exudate and cells within the orbit may produce proptosis of the inflamed eye.

Uvea

Together with the iris, the choroid and ciliary body constitute the uvea. The choroid is among the most richly vascularized sites in the body. As in the retina, there are no lymphatics within the uvea.

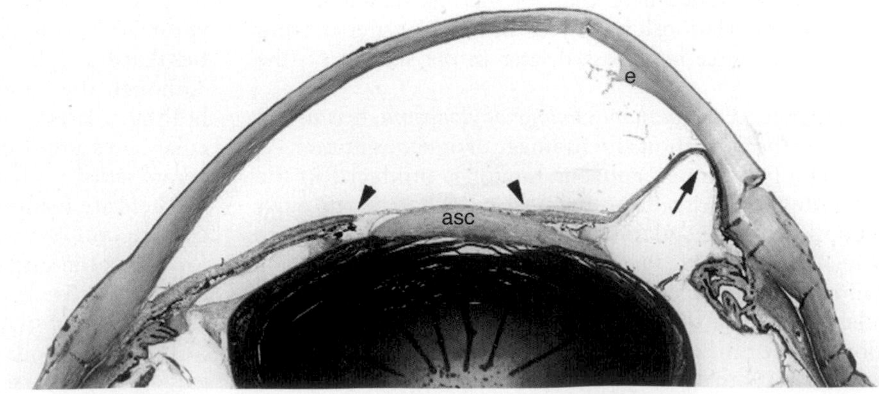

Figure 29–12 Sequelae of anterior segment inflammation. This eye was removed for complications of chronic corneal inflammation (which cannot be discerned at this magnification). The exudate (e) present in the anterior chamber would have been visualized at the slit lamp as an optical "flare." The iris is adherent focally to the cornea, obstructing the trabecular meshwork (anterior synechia, *arrow*), and adheres to the lens (posterior synechiae, *arrowheads*). An anterior subcapsular cataract (asc) has formed. The radial folds in the lens are artifacts.

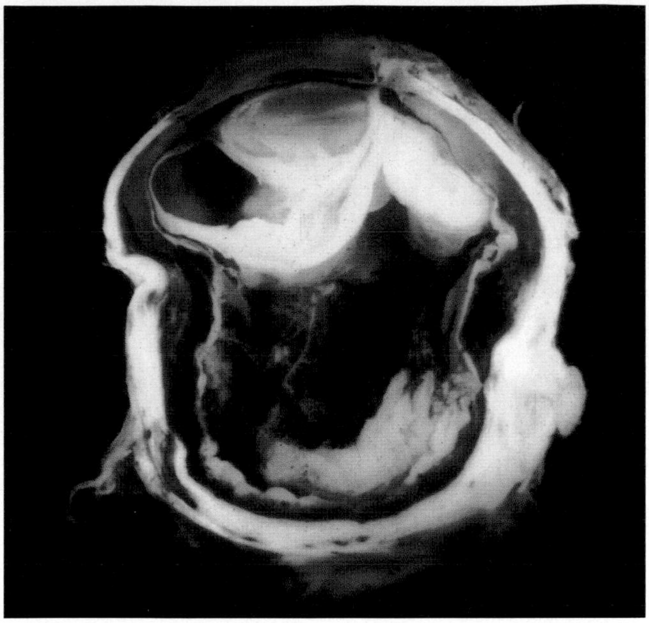

Figure 29–13 Exogenous panophthalmitis. This eye was removed after a foreign body injury. Note the suppurative inflammation behind the lens and drawn up to the right of the lens to the cornea, the site of the wound. The central portion of the vitreous humor was extracted surgically (by vitrectomy). Note the adhesions to the surface of the eye at the eight o'clock position, indicating that the intraocular inflammation has spread through the sclera into the orbit: panophthalmitis. (From Folberg R: The Eye. In Spencer WH (ed.) Ophthalmic Pathology—An Atlas and Textbook (4th Edition). Philadelphia, WB Saunders, 1985.)

UVEITIS

Technically, the term *uveitis* can be applied to any type of inflammation in one or more of the tissues that comprise the uvea. Thus, the iritis that develops after blunt trauma to the eye or that accompanies a corneal ulcer is technically a form of uveitis. However, in clinical practice, the term *uveitis* is restricted to a diverse group of chronic diseases that may either be components of a systemic process or localized to the eye. Uveal inflammation may be manifest principally in the anterior segment (e.g., in *juvenile rheumatoid arthritis*) or may affect both the anterior and posterior segments. The complications of chronic anterior segment inflammation were discussed earlier; the remainder of this discussion therefore focuses on the effects of uveal inflammation on the posterior segment of the eye. As will be described briefly, uveitis is frequently accompanied by retinal pathology. Uveitis may be caused by infectious agents (e.g. *pneumocystis carnii*), may be idiopathic (e.g. sarcoidosis), or may be autoimmune in origin (sympathetic ophthalmia). Some examples are described below.

Granulomatous uveitis is a common complication of sarcoidosis (Chapter 15). In the anterior segment, it gives rise to an exudate that evolves into "mutton-fat" keratic precipitates described earlier. In the posterior segment, sarcoid may involve the choroid and retina. Thus, granulomas may be seen in the choroid. Retinal pathology is characterized by perivascular inflammation; this is responsible for the well-known ophthalmoscopic sign of "candle wax drippings." Conjunctival biopsy may be used to detect granulomatous inflammation and confirm the diagnosis of ocular sarcoid.

Numerous infectious processes may affect the choroid or the retina. Inflammation in one compartment is typically associated with inflammation in the other. Retinal *toxoplasmosis* is usually accompanied by uveitis and even scleritis. Patients with AIDS who are immunocompromised may develop cytomegalovirus retinitis and exotic forms of uveal infection such as pneumocystis or *Mycobacterium avium* choroiditis.[12,13]

Sympathetic ophthalmia is an example of noninfectious uveitis limited to the eye. This condition is characterized by bilateral granulomatous inflammation typically affecting all components of the uvea: a panuveitis. Sympathetic ophthalmia, which blinded young Louis Braille, may complicate a penetrating injury of the eye. In the injured eye, retinal antigens sequestered from the immune system may gain access to lymphatics in the conjunctiva and thus set up a delayed hypersensitivity reaction that affects not only the injured eye, but also the contralateral, noninjured eye.[14] The condition may develop from 2 weeks to many years after injury. Enucleation of a blind eye (which can be the sympathizing eye rather than the directly injured eye) may yield diagnostic findings. Sympathetic ophthalmia is treated by the administration of systemic immunosuppressive agents.

Morphology. Sympathetic ophthalmia is characterized by diffuse granulomatous inflammation of the uvea (choroid, ciliary body, and iris). Plasma cells are typically absent, but eosinophils may be identified in the infiltrate (Fig. 29–14).

NEOPLASMS

The most common intraocular malignancy of adults is metastasis to the uvea, typically to the choroid. The appearance of metastases to the eye is suggestive of extremely short survival, and treatment of ocular metastases is usually palliative and delivered by radiation therapy.

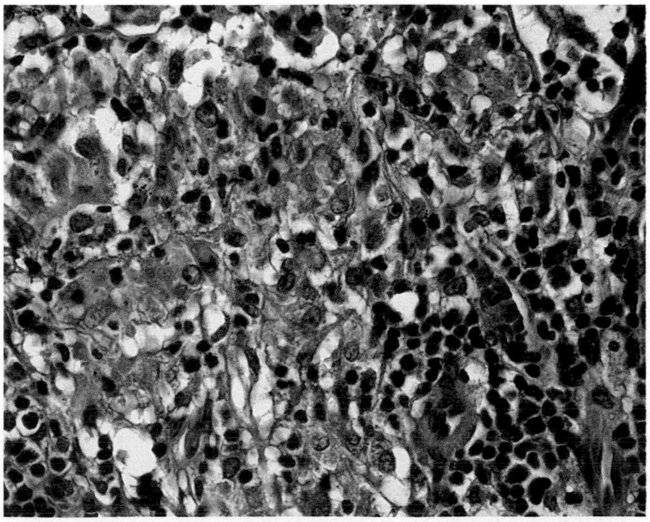

Figure 29–14 Sympathetic ophthalmia. The granulomatous inflammation depicted here was identified diffusely throughout the uvea. The uveal granulomas may contain melanin pigment and may be accompanied by eosinophils.

Uveal Nevi and Melanomas

Uveal melanoma is the most common primary intraocular malignancy of adults. Although it was formerly thought to be rather rare (7 per million per year), the incidence of this tumor increases with age and by the seventh decade, the incidence is more than 20 per million per year. Unlike cutaneous melanoma, the occurrence of uveal melanoma has remained stable over many years.[15] Although some experts have implicated excessive childhood exposure to ultraviolet radiation, the link between ultraviolet light and uveal melanoma is not nearly as clear as it is for cutaneous melanoma. It is therefore reasonable to conclude that the etiology of uveal melanoma is unresolved at this time. Uveal nevi, especially choroidal nevi, are rather common, affecting an estimated 10% of the Caucasian population. The progression of a uveal nevus to melanoma is therefore likely to be an exceptionally uncommon event.

There are no lymphatics within the eye; hence, uveal melanomas, with very rare exception, spread exclusively by a hematogenous route (the only exception being the rare case of melanoma that spreads through the sclera and invades the conjunctiva, thereby gaining access to conjunctival lymphatics). Most uveal melanomas spread first to the liver, thereby providing an excellent example of organ-specific metastasis. Although the 5-year survival rate is approximately 80%,[16] the cumulative melanoma mortality rate is 40% at 10 years, increasing 1% per year thereafter.[17] Examples of metastases appearing many years after treatment are well known, making uveal melanoma a prime candidate for the investigation of tumor dormancy.

Morphology. Histologically, uveal melanomas may contain two types of cells, spindle and epithelioid, in various proportions (Fig. 29–15). Spindle cells are fusiform in shape and have little atypia, whereas epithelioid cells are spherical and have greater cytologic atypicality. Melanomas situated exclusively in the iris tend to follow a relatively indolent course, whereas melanomas of the ciliary body and choroid are more aggressive. The prognosis of choroidal and ciliary body melanomas is classically related to size (in contrast to cutaneous melanoma, the lateral extent of the tumor rather than tumor depth is the size dimension related to adverse outcome), cell type (tumors containing epithelioid cells have a worse prognosis than do those containing exclusively spindle cells), and proliferative index. In contrast to cutaneous melanomas, large numbers of tumor-infiltrating lymphocytes are associated with an adverse outcome.[18] Extraocular extension is related to poor prognosis. Monosomy 3 and trisomy 8 are seen with consistency in uveal melanomas of a poor prognosis.[19] The presence histologically of looping patterns rich in laminin that surround packets of tumor cells is also associated with an adverse outcome. These patterns, which are not blood vessels, connect to blood vessels and serve as extravascular conduits for the transport of plasma and possibly blood.[20,21] Laminin-rich extravascular patterns have also been identified in cutaneous melanoma, ovarian carcinoma, inflammatory breast cancer, prostate cancer, and some soft tissue sarcomas. In vitro studies and examinations of human tissues suggest that these patterns are formed by aggressive tumor cells in a process termed **vasculogenic mimicry.**[20,20a]

Uveal melanomas can have an adverse effect on vision, producing changes ranging from retinal detachment to glaucoma. It has recently been shown that there appears to be no difference in survival between tumors treated by removal of the eye (enucleation) and those treated by radiation treatment. It should be noted that patients treated by radiation and other vision-sparing modalities are treated without ever having tissue examined by a pathologist. There is currently no effective treatment for metastatic uveal melanoma.

Retina and Vitreous

FUNCTIONAL ANATOMY

The neurosensory retina, like the optic nerve, is an embryologic derivative of the diencephalon. The retina therefore responds to injury by means of gliosis. As in the brain, there are no lymphatics. The architecture of the retina explains the ophthalmoscopic appearance of a variety of ocular disorders. Hemorrhages in the nerve fiber layer of the retina are oriented horizontally and appear ophthalmoscopically as streaks or "flames"; the external retinal layers are oriented perpendicular to the retinal surface, and hemorrhages in these outer layers appear as dots (cross-sections of cylinders). Exudates tend to accumulate in the outer plexiform layer of the retina, especially in the macula (Fig. 29–16).

The retinal pigment epithelium, like the retina, is derived embryologically from the primary optic vesicle, an outpouching of the brain. Separation of the neurosensory retina from the retinal pigment epithelium defines a *retinal detachment.* The retinal pigment epithelium (RPE) plays an important role physiologically in the maintenance of the outer segments of the photoreceptors. Disturbances in the RPE-photoreceptor interface may play important roles in hereditary retinal degenerations such as *retinitis pigmentosa.*

The adult vitreous humor is avascular. Incomplete regression of fetal vasculature running through the vitreous humor can produce significant pathology as a retrolental mass (*persistent hyperplastic primary vitreous*). The vitreous humor can be opacified by hemorrhage from trauma or retinal neovascularization. Calcium soaps may accumulate as particulate debris in the vitreous humor. This condition, *asteroid hyalosis,* so named because reflections from these opacities reflect the light of the ophthalmoscope to resemble astronomical bodies of light; these opacities typically do not reduce vision. On the other hand, deposits of amyloid in the vitreous humor can significantly reduce vision.

With age, the vitreous humor may liquefy and even collapse, creating the visual sensation of "floaters." Also, with aging, the posterior face of the vitreous humor—the posterior hyaloid—may separate from the neurosensory retina (*posterior vitreous detachment*). The relationship between the posterior hyaloid and the neurosensory retina plays a key role in the pathogenesis of retinal neovascularization and in some forms of retinal detachment.

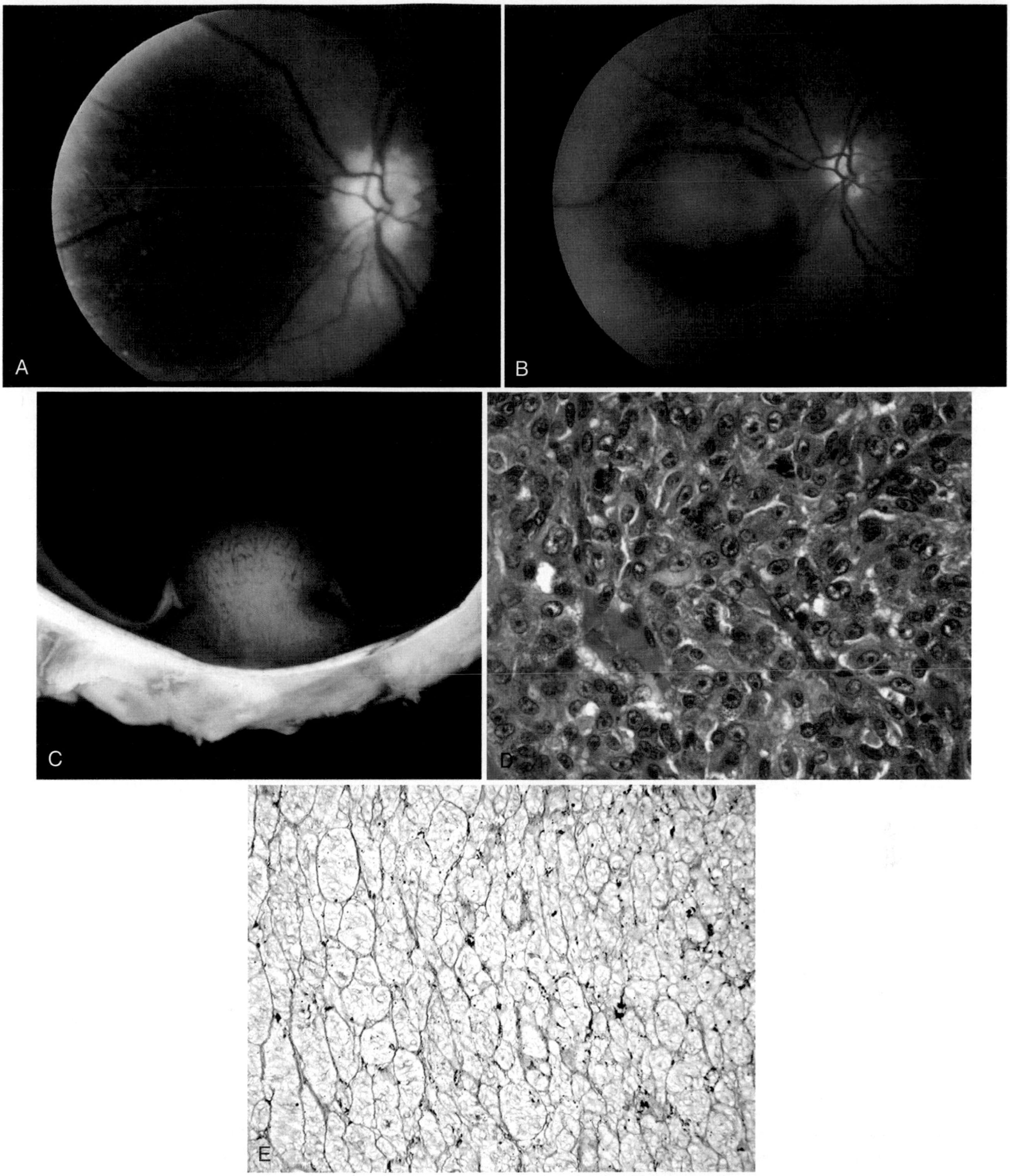

Figure 29–15 Uveal melanoma. *A*, Fundus photograph from a patient with a relatively flat pigmented lesion of the choroid near the optic disc. *B*, Fundus photograph of the same patient several years later; the tumor has grown and has ruptured through Bruch's membrane. *C*, Gross photograph of a choroidal melanoma that has ruptured Bruch's membrane. The overlying retina is detached. *D*, Epithelioid melanoma cells are associated with an adverse outcome. *E*, Patterns rich in laminin (that are periodic acid–Schiff positive) surround aggregates of melanoma cells; these patterns form a "fluid-conducting meshwork" in uveal melanoma and are associated with an adverse outcome. (*A* to *C* from Folberg R: Pathology of the eye—an interactive CD-ROM program. Philadelphia, Mosby, 1996; *E* from Maniotis AJ, Chen X, Garcia C, et al: Control of melanoma morphogenesis, endothelial survival, and perfusion by extracellular matrix. *Lab Invest* 82(8):1031–1043, 2002.)

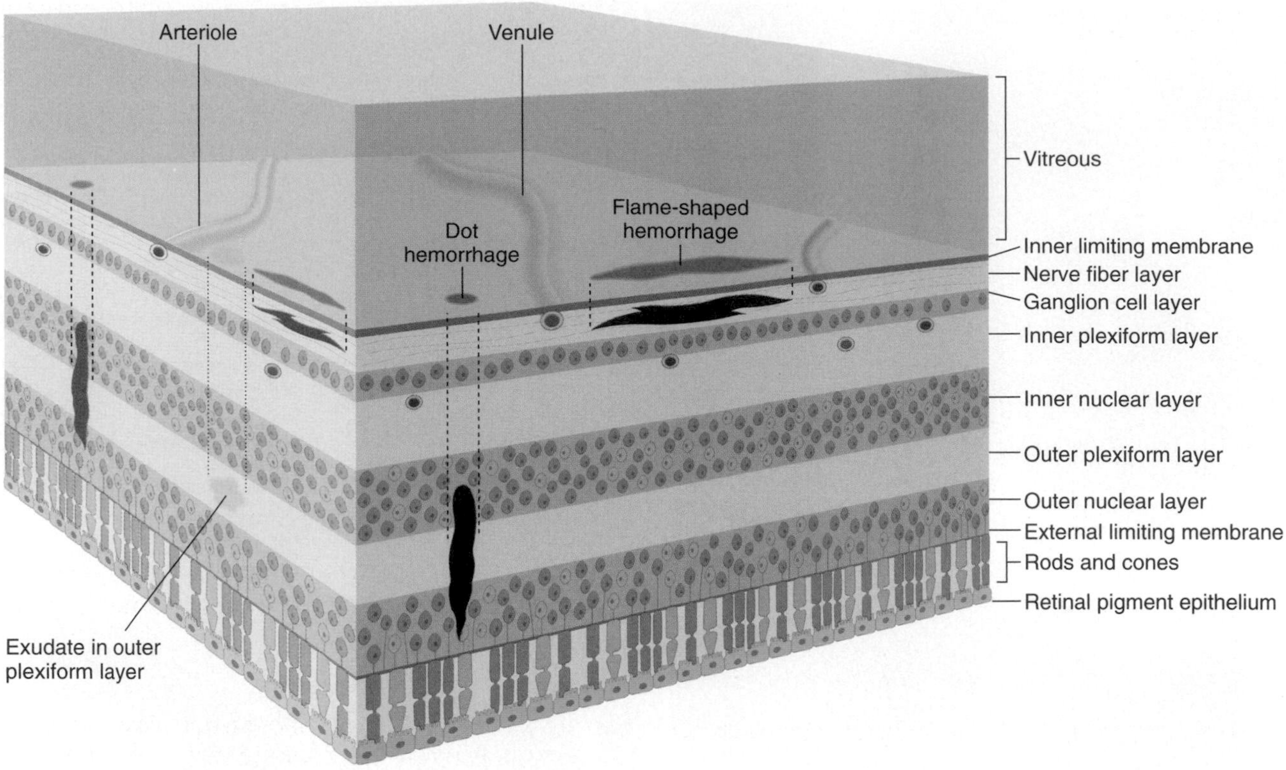

Figure 29–16 Clinicopathologic correlations of retinal hemorrhages and exudates. The location of the hemorrhage within the retina determines its appearance by ophthalmoscopy. The retinal nerve fiber layer is oriented parallel to the internal limiting membrane, and hemorrhages of this layer appear to be flame-shaped ophthalmoscopically. The deeper retinal layers are oriented perpendicular to the internal limiting membrane and hemorrhages in this location appear as cross-sections of a cylinder or "dot" hemorrhages. Exudates that originate from leaky retinal vessels accumulate in the outer plexiform layer.

RETINAL DETACHMENT

Retinal detachment (separation of the neurosensory retina from the retinal pigment epithelium) is broadly classified by etiology based on the presence or absence of a break in the retina. *Rhegmatogenous retinal detachment* is associated with a full-thickness retinal defect. Retinal tears may develop after the vitreous collapses structurally, and the posterior hyaloid exerts traction on points of abnormally strong adhesion to the retinal internal limiting membrane. Liquefied vitreous humor then seeps through the tear and gains access to the potential space between the neurosensory retina and the retinal pigment epithelium (Fig. 29–17). Reattachment of the retina to the retinal pigment epithelium generally involves relief of vitreous traction through indenting the sclera by a variety of surgical procedures. This may be accomplished by the application of strips of silicon to the surface of the eye (scleral buckling) and possibly by excision of vitreous material (vitrectomy). Rhegmatogenous retinal detachment may be complicated by *proliferative vitreoretinopathy*, the formation of epiretinal or subretinal membranes by retinal glial cells (Müller cells) or retinal pigment epithelial cells.

Non-rhegmatogenous retinal detachment, (retinal detachment without retinal break), may complicate retinal vascular disorders associated with significant exudation and any condition that damages the RPE and permits fluid to leak from the choroidal circulation beneath the retina. Retinal detachments associated with choroidal tumors and malignant hypertension, as was mentioned above, are examples of non-rhegmatogenous retinal detachment.

Chronic retinal detachment, regardless of etiology, may be complicated by loss of photoreceptor outer segments, gliosis, and the development of microcystic spaces within the detached retina.

RETINAL VASCULAR DISEASE

Hypertension

Normally, the thin walls of retinal arterioles permit a direct visualization of the circulating blood column by ophthalmoscopy. In retinal arteriolosclerosis, the thickened arteriolar wall changes the ophthalmic perception of circulating blood: Vessels may appear narrowed, and the color of the blood column may change from bright red to copper and to silver depending on the degree of vascular wall thickness (Fig. 29–18*A*). Retinal arterioles and veins share a common adventitial sheath. Therefore, in pronounced retinal arteriolosclerosis, the arteriole may compress the vein at points where both vessels cross (Fig. 29–18*B*). Venous stasis distal to arteriolar-venous crossing may precipitate occlusions of the retinal vein branches.

In malignant hypertension, vessels in the retina and choroid may be damaged. Damage to choroidal vessels may produce focal choroidal infarcts, seen clinically as *Elschnig's spots.* Damage to the choriocapillaris, the internal layer of the choroidal vasculature, may, in turn, damage the overlying retinal pigment epithelium and permit exudate to accumulate in the potential space between the neurosensory retina and the retinal pigment epithelium, thereby producing a

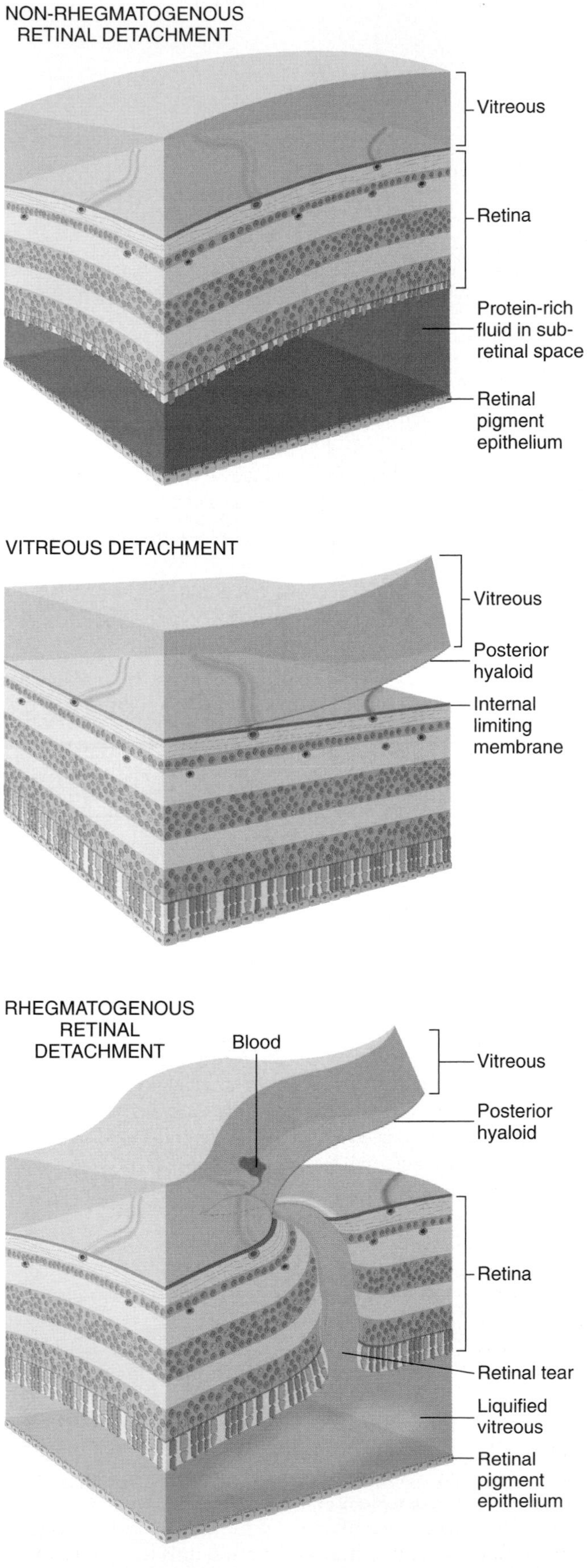

Figure 29–17 Retinal detachment is defined as the separation of the neurosensory retina from the retinal pigment epithelium. Retinal detachments are classified broadly into non-rhegmatogenous (without a retinal break) and rhegmatogenous (with a retinal break) types. *Top,* In non-rhegmatogenous retinal detachment, the subretinal space is filled with protein-rich exudate. Note in this sketch that the outer segments of the photoreceptors are missing. This indicates a chronic retinal detachment, a finding that can be seen in both non-rhegmatogenous and rhegmatogenous detachments. *Middle,* Posterior vitreous detachment involves the separation of the posterior hyaloid from the internal limiting membrane of the retina and is a normal occurrence in the aging eye. *Bottom,* If, during a posterior vitreous detachment, the posterior hyaloid does not separate cleanly from the internal limiting membrane of the retina, the vitreous humor will exert traction on the retina which will be torn at this point. Liquefied vitreous humor seeps through the retinal defect, and the retina is separated from the retinal pigment epithelium. Note in this sketch that the photoreceptor outer segments are intact, suggesting that an acute detachment is being illustrated.

retinal detachment. Exudate from damaged retinal arterioles typically accumulates in the outer plexiform layer of the retina (Fig. 29–18*A*). The ophthalmoscopic finding of a macular star—a spokelike arrangement of exudate in the macula in malignant hypertension—results from exudate accumulating in the outer plexiform layer of the macula that is oriented obliquely rather than perpendicular to the retinal surface.

Occlusion of retinal arterioles may produce infarcts of the nerve fiber layer of the retina (axons of the retinal ganglion cell layer populate the nerve fiber layer). Axoplasmic transport in the nerve fiber layer is interrupted at the point of axonal damage, and accumulation of mitochondria at the swollen ends of damaged axons creates the histologic illusion of cells (*cytoid bodies*). Collections of cytoid bodies populate the nerve fiber layer infarct, seen ophthalmoscopically as "cotton-wool spots" (Fig. 29–19). Although nerve fiber layer infarcts are described here in the context of hypertension, they may be detected in a variety of retinal occlusive vasculopathies. For example, retinal nerve fiber layer infarcts may develop in AIDS patients secondary to a retinal vasculopathy that is similar to the vasculopathy that may develop in the brain in this condition.

Diabetes Mellitus

The eye is profoundly affected by diabetes mellitus. The effects of hyperglycemia on the lens and iris have already been mentioned. Thickening of the basement membrane of the epithelium of the pars plicata of the ciliary body is a reliable histologic marker of diabetes mellitus in the eye (Fig. 29–20) and is reminiscent of similar changes in glomerular mesangium. This discussion focuses on the retinal microangiopathy associated with diabetes mellitus, a prototype for the consideration of other retinal microangiopathies.

The retinal vasculopathy of diabetes mellitus may be classified into *background (preproliferative) diabetic retinopathy* and *proliferative diabetic retinopathy.*[22]

Background (preproliferative) diabetic retinopathy includes a spectrum of changes ranging from structural and functional

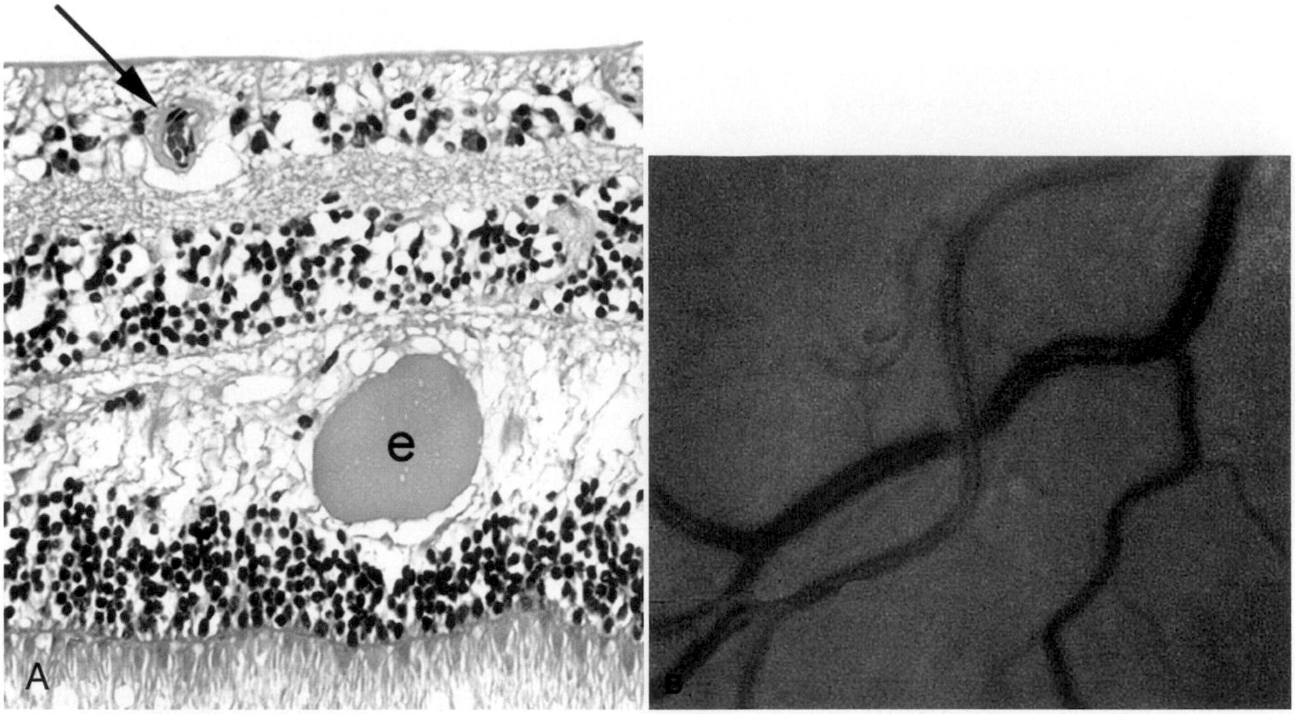

Figure 29–18 The retina in hypertension. *A,* The wall of the retinal arteriole *(arrow)* is thick. Note the exudate (e) in the retinal outer plexiform layer. *B,* The fundus in hypertension. The diameter of the arterioles is reduced, and the color of the blood column appears to be less saturated (copper wire–like). The retinal venule is compressed at a point where the artery and vein cross. If the wall of the vessel were thicker still, the degree of red color would diminish such that the vessels might appear clinically to have a "silver-wire" appearance. In this fundus photograph, note that the vein is compressed where the sclerotic arteriole crosses over it. (*B,* courtesy of Dr. Thomas A. Weingeist, Department of Ophthalmology & Visual Science, University of Iowa, Iowa City, IA.)

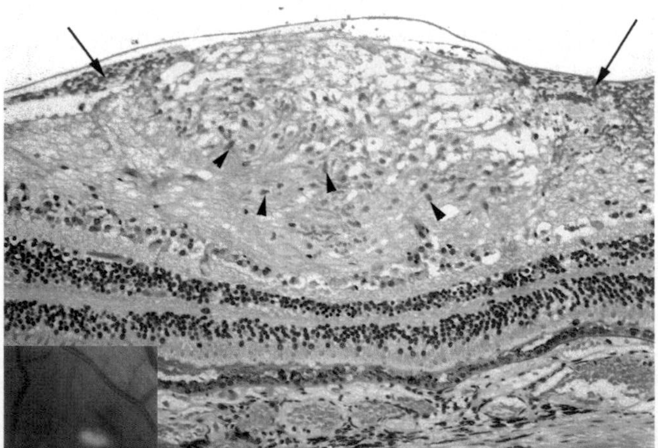

Figure 29–19 Nerve fiber layer infarct. A "cotton-wool spot" is illustrated in the inset, adjacent to a flame-shaped (nerve fiber layer) hemorrhage. The histology of a cotton-wool spot—an infarct of the nerve fiber layer of the retina—is illustrated in the photomicrograph. A focal swelling of the nerve fiber layer is occupied by numerous red to pink cytoid bodies *(arrowheads),* bulbous ends of severed axons. Hemorrhage *(arrows)* surrounding the nerve fiber layer infarct as illustrated here is a variable and inconsistent finding. (The fundus photo courtesy of Dr. Thomas A. Weingeist, Department of Ophthalmology & Visual Science, University of Iowa, Iowa City, IA.)

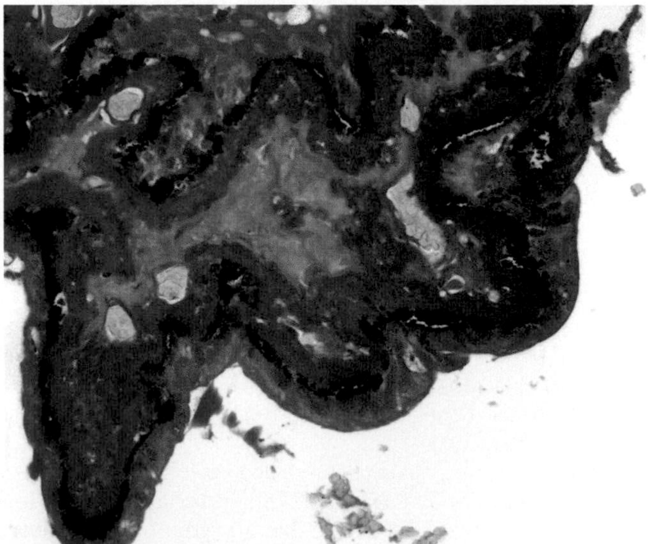

Figure 29–20 The ciliary body in chronic diabetes mellitus, periodic acid–Schiff stain. Note the massive thickening of the basement membrane of the ciliary body epithelia, reminiscent of changes in the mesangium of the renal glomerulus.

abnormalities of angiogenesis located within the retina (i.e., confined beneath the internal limiting membrane of the retina). As with all diabetic microangiopathy in general, the *basement membrane of retinal blood vessels is thickened*. In addition, the number of pericytes relative to endothelial cells diminishes. *Microaneurysms* are an important manifestation of diabetic microangiopathy. They are typically smaller than the resolution of direct ophthalmoscopes, and findings that are customarily described as microaneurysms by ophthalmoscopy may in fact be retinal microhemorrhages. Structural changes in the retinal microcirculation have been associated with a physiologic breakdown in the blood-retinal barrier. Thus, the retinal microcirculation in diabetics may be exceptionally leaky, giving rise to *macular edema*, a common cause of visual loss in these patients. The vascular changes may also produce *hemorrhagic exudates* that accumulate in the outer plexiform layer and may be visualized ophthalmoscopically. Although the retinal microcirculation is often hyperpermeable, it is also subject to the effects of micro-occlusion. Both vascular incompetence and vascular micro-occlusions may be visualized clinically after intravenous injection of fluorescein.

Nonperfusion of the retina due to the microcirculatory change described above is associated with up-regulation of VEGF and retinal angiogenesis.[23,24] The development of intraretinal angiogenesis—new vessels confined within the retina beneath the internal limiting membrane—may be included with lesions termed *intraretinal microangiopathy*.

Clinically, *proliferative diabetic retinopathy* is defined by the appearance of new vessels that sprout from existing vessels—angiogenic vessels—on the surface of either the optic nerve head, which is termed *neovascularization of the disc*, or the surface of the retina, which is designated by the somewhat nebulous term *neovascularization elsewhere*. It is worth emphasizing that the term *retinal neovascularization* is not applied either clinically or pathologically unless the newly formed vessels breach the internal limiting membrane of the retina. The quantity and location of retinal neovascularization guide the ophthalmologist in the treatment of proliferative diabetic retinopathy. The web of newly formed vessels is called a *neovascular membrane* both clinically and histopathologically. It is composed of angiogenic vessels with or without a substantial supportive fibrous or glial stroma (Fig. 29–21).

If the vitreous humor has not detached and the posterior hyaloid is intact, neovascular membranes extend along the potential plane between the retinal internal limiting membrane and the posterior hyaloid. Thus, the separation of the vitreous humor from the internal limiting membrane of the retina (*posterior vitreous detachment*) after retinal neovascularization may precipitate massive hemorrhage from the disrupted neovascular membrane. Organization of the retinal neovascular membrane may wrinkle the retina, disrupting the orientation of retinal photoreceptors and producing visual distortion, and may exert traction on the retina, separating it from the retinal pigment epithelium (retinal detachment). *Traction retinal detachment* may begin as a non-rhegmatogenous detachment, but severe traction may tear the retina and result in a traction-induced rhegmatogenous detachment.

Retinal neovascularization may be accompanied by the development of a neovascular membrane on the iris surface, presumably secondary to increased levels of VEGF in the aqueous humor.[25] Contraction of the iris neovascular membrane may lead to adhesions between the iris and trabecular meshwork (anterior synechiae), thus occluding a major pathway for aqueous outflow and thereby contributing to elevation of the intraocular pressure (*neovascular glaucoma*). Ablating nonperfused retina by laser photocoagulation or cryopexy triggers regression of both retinal and iris neovascularization.

Retinopathy of Prematurity (Retrolental Fibroplasia)

At term, the nasal (medial) aspect of the retina is vascularized, but the temporal (lateral) aspect of the retinal periphery is incompletely vascularized. In premature or low-birth-weight infants treated with oxygen, the immature retinal vessels in the temporal retinal periphery may constrict, rendering the retinal tissue distal to this zone ischemic. Retinal ischemia may result in up-regulation of proangiogenic factors such as VEGF, and lead to retinal angiogenesis.[26] Contraction of a peripheral retinal neovascular membrane may result in "dragging" of the temporal aspect of the retina toward the temporal peripheral zone such that the macula (situated temporal to the optic nerve) is displaced laterally. With significant contraction, the retina may detach. There is some evidence that retinopathy of prematurity develops in genetically susceptible infants.

Sickle Retinopathy, Retinal Vasculitis, Radiation Retinopathy

Sickle retinopathy has been divided into two types by terminology that is roughly parallel to that used for diabetic retinopathy: nonproliferative (intraretinal angiopathic changes) and proliferative (retinal neovascularization). The final common pathway in both types is vascular occlusion.[27] As oxygen tension drops within the erythrocytes of affected patients in the retinal periphery, the red cells deform, causing microvascular occlusions. In the nonproliferative form (which has been observed in patients with sickle disease, SS disease, sickle-thalassemia, and hemoglobin SC), *vascular occlusions* are thought to contribute to preretinal, intraretinal, and subretinal hemorrhages. The resolution of these hemorrhages may give rise to a variety of ophthalmoscopically visible changes, including *salmon patches*, *iridescent spots*, and *black sunburst lesions*. Organization of preretinal hemorrhage may result in retinal traction and *retinal detachment*. Vascular occlusions may also contribute to angiogenesis secondary to up-regulation of both VEGF and bFGF.[28] This can give rise to florid zones of retinal neovascularization in the periphery that are described clinically as "sea-fans." Pigment epithelial derived factor (PEDF) may inhibit angiogenesis in this condition and may contribute to the regression of sea-fans.[29]

The final common pathway of "retinal vasculopathy–occlusion–ischemia–up-regulation of angiogenic factors" may be associated with neovascularization in a variety of clinical settings such as peripheral retinal vasculitis, and in radiation used to treat intraocular tumors. The feature common to these conditions is damage to retinal vessels, producing zones of retinal ischemia that drive retinal angiogenesis and its complications, hemorrhage and traction.

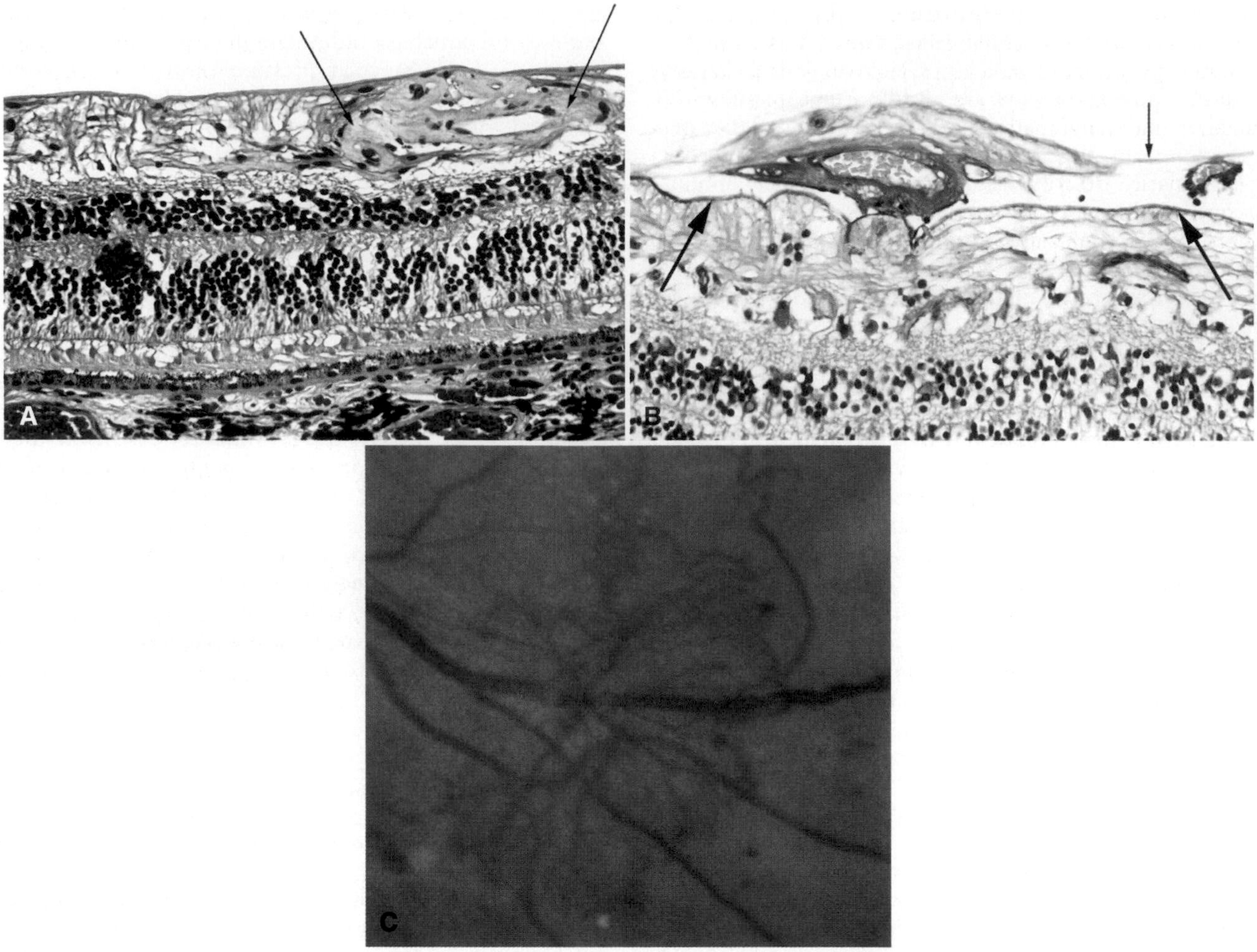

Figure 29–21 The retina in diabetes mellitus. *A*, Note the tangle of abnormal vessels just beneath the internal limiting membrane of the retina on the right half of the photomicrograph *(between arrows)*. This is an example of intraretinal angiogenesis known as intraretinal microangiopathy (IRMA). Note the retinal hemorrhage in the outer plexiform layer in the left half of this photomicrograph. Ophthalmoscopically, this outer retinal layer hemorrhage would appear as a "dot" hemorrhage. Finally, note that there are only two well-defined layers of retinal nuclei: the outer nuclear layer and the inner nuclear layer. The ganglion cell layer is absent, and the nerve fiber layer—the axons of the ganglion cells—is also absent. The rarefied space beneath internal limiting membrane to the left of the focus of IRMA consists largely of elements of retinal glial (Müller) cells. Absence of the ganglion cell and nerve fiber layers is a hallmark of glaucoma. The chronic diabetes mellitus in this patient was complicated by the development of iris neovascularization and secondary angle closure glaucoma (neovascular glaucoma). *B*, In this histologic section, stained by periodic acid–Schiff, the internal limiting membrane is noted by the long, thick arrows and the posterior hyaloid of the vitreous by the thin, short arrows. Note the vessels in the potential space between these two landmarks. The vessels to the left of the short arrow are invested with a fibrous-glial stroma and would appear ophthalmoscopically as a white neovascular membrane. However, the thin-walled vessel to the right of the short arrow is not invested with a connective tissue stroma and would appear ophthalmoscopically as merely a very thin vessel. A posterior vitreous detachment in an eye such as this might exert traction on these new vessels and precipitate a massive vitreous hemorrhage. *C*, Ophthalmoscopic view of retinal neovascularization (known clinically as neovascularization "elsewhere" in contrast with neovascularization of the optic disc). Note the blush of thin-walled vessels that are not accompanied by a fibrous stroma (analogous to the thin walled vessel in *B*). Even without a connective tissue stroma, this qualifies clinically as a neovascular membrane and is reminiscent of the appearance of experimental angiogenesis on a chick chorioallantoic membrane.

Retinal Artery and Vein Occlusions

The central or branch retinal arteries may be occluded by disorders that affect the vessels in general. For example, the lumen of the central retinal artery may be narrowed significantly by atherosclerosis, thus predisposing to thrombosis. Emboli to the central retinal artery may originate from thrombi in the heart or on ulcerated atheromatous plaques in the carotid arteries. Fragments of atherosclerotic plaques may lodge within the retinal circulation (*Hollenhorst plaques*). Total occlusion of a branch retinal artery may produce a segmental infarct of the retina. With sudden cessation of blood supply, the retina (an embryologic derivative of brain tissue) swells and acutely becomes optically opaque. By ophthalmoscopy, the fundus in the affected area appears white instead of red or orange because the retinal opacity blocks the view of the richly vascular choroid.

Total occlusion of the central retinal artery may produce a *diffuse infarct* of the retina. Following an acute occlusion, the retina appears relatively opaque by ophthalmoscopy. The fovea and foveola are physiologically thin; therefore, the normal orange-red of the choroid is not only visible but highlighted by the surrounding opaque retina—the origin of the *cherry-red spot* of the central retinal artery occlusion. The cherry-red spots seen in rare storage diseases such as *Tay-Sachs* and *Niemann-Pick* disease also have their basis in the anatomic variations of the macula. The storage material accumulates in retinal ganglion cells: The ganglion cell layer of the macula surrounding the fovea is thick, but there are no ganglion cells in the center of the macula, the fovea. Thus, the fovea is relatively transparent to the underlying choroidal vasculature but is rimmed by relatively opaque retina, the result of storage material accumulating in the perifoveal macular ganglion cells (Fig. 29–22).

Retinal arterial occlusions are typically sudden events; therefore, they are not often complicated by prolonged ischemia to allow for up-regulation of proangiogenic factors. Hence, retinal arterial occlusions are seldom complicated by either retinal or iris neovascularization.

The term *retinal vein occlusion* describes at least two different pathogenic mechanisms: with or without ischemia.[30] In ischemic retinal vein occlusion, VEGF and other proangiogenic factors are up-regulated in the retina, leading to neovascularization of the retina and surface of the optic nerve head as well as neovascularization of the iris and subsequent angle closure glaucoma.[31] Nonischemic retinal vein occlusion may be complicated by hemorrhages, exudates, and macular edema but is seldom complicated by retinal or iris neovascularization.

AGE-RELATED MACULAR DEGENERATION (ARMD)

This chapter began with a description of the visual impairment experienced by a patient with age-related macular degeneration, the most common cause of irreversible visual morbidity in the United States. It may be worthwhile to review this description in the context of the information that follows. From the name of this disorder, it is clear that advancing age is a risk factor. The etiology of this condition is unclear, having been attributed to a variety of environmental exposures, including smoking, nutritional factors, and vascular pathology such as atherosclerosis and hypertension.[32] Suffice it to say that no specific patterns of inheritance can be identified in the typical patient with ARMD. By contrast, well-established forms of hereditary macular degenerations typically appear in younger patients, and specific genes have been associated with these conditions. There are important phenotypic differences between many of the hereditary maculopathies and ARMD as well.[33]

To understand the pathogenesis of ARMD, it is important to appreciate the existence of a structural and functional unit composed of the retinal pigment epithelium, Bruch's membrane (which contains the basement membrane of the retinal pigment epithelium), and the innermost layer of the choroidal vasculature, the choriocapillaris. Disturbance in any component of this "unit" affects the health of the overlying photoreceptors, producing visual loss.

It is commonplace to describe ARMD as either *atrophic* (dry) or *exudative* (wet). *Atrophic* ARMD is identified ophthalmoscopically by diffuse or discrete deposits in Bruch's membrane (drusen) and geographic atrophy of the retinal pigment epithelium. Approximately 10% to 20% of patients with *atrophic* ARMD develop choroidal neovascular membranes, the hallmark of *exudative* ARMD. Considerable attention is being devoted to identifying the characteristics that predict the development of choroidal neovascularization because the loss of vision is substantially more severe in these patients.

Choroidal neovascularization is defined by the presence of angiogenic vessels that presumably originate from the choriocapillaris and penetrate through Bruch's membrane beneath the retinal pigment epithelium (Fig. 29–23). This neovascular membrane may also penetrate the retinal pigment epithelium and become situated directly beneath the neurosensory retina. The vessels in this membrane may leak, and the exuded blood may be organized by retinal pigment epithelial cells into macular scars. Occasionally, hemorrhage from these neovascular membranes may be massive, leading to the localized suffusion of blood that may be mistaken clinically

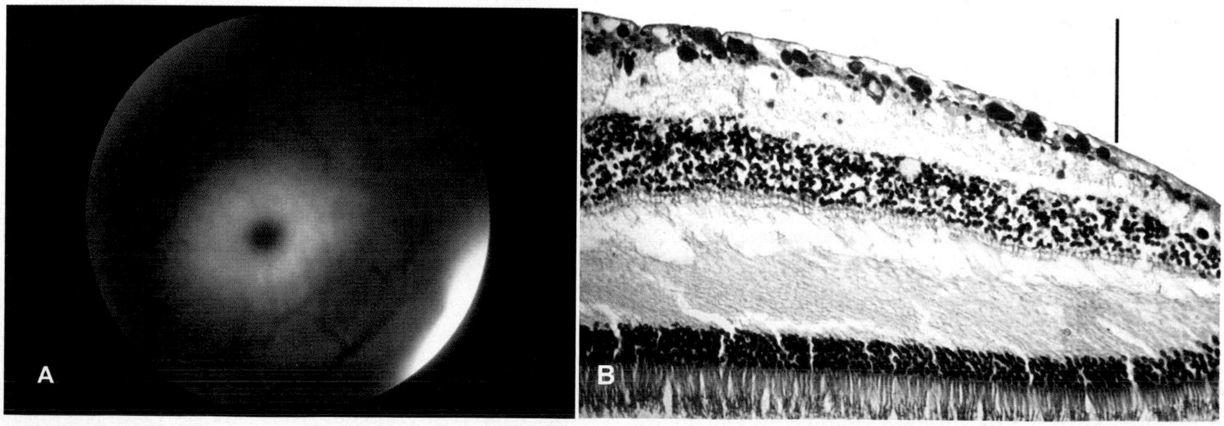

Figure 29–22 The cherry-red spot in Tay-Sachs disease. *A*, Fundus photograph of the cherry-red spot in Tay-Sachs disease. *B*, Photomicrograph of the macula in a patient with Tay-Sachs disease, stained with periodic acid–Schiff to highlight the accumulation of ganglioside material in the retinal ganglion cells. The presence of ganglion cells filled with gangliosides outside the fovea blocks the transmission of the normal orange-red color of the choroid, but absence of ganglion cells within the fovea (to the right of the vertical bar) permits the normal orange-red color to be visualized, accounting for the so-called cherry-red spot. (*A* courtesy of Dr. Thomas A. Weingeist, Department of Ophthalmology & Visual Science, University of Iowa, Iowa City, IA; *B* originates from the teaching collection of the Armed Forces Institute of Pathology.)

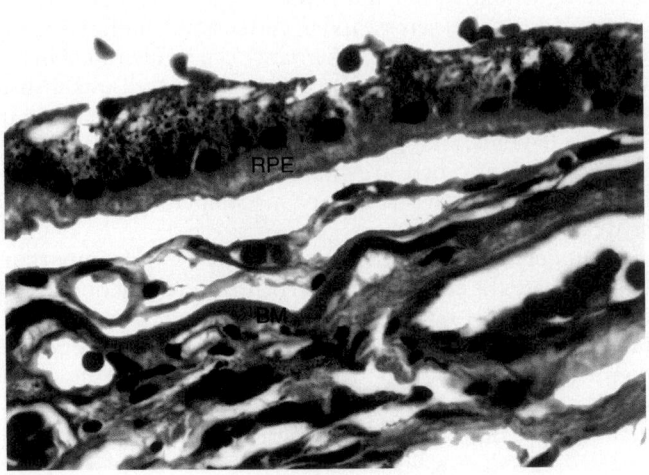

Figure 29–23 Age-related macular degeneration. A neovascular membrane is positioned between the retinal pigment epithelium (RPE) and Bruch's membrane (BM). Note the blue discoloration of Bruch's membrane to the right of the label, indicating focal calcification.

for an intraocular neoplasm, or may produce diffuse vitreous hemorrhage.

Choroidal neovascular membranes may develop in conditions that are unrelated to age, such as pathological myopia (Fuchs' spot), following traumatic disruption of Bruch's membrane, angioid streaks, or an immunologic response to systemic histoplasmosis (presumed ocular histoplasmosis syndrome).

OTHER RETINAL DEGENERATIONS

Many other forms of degeneration not related to age may affect the retina. These conditions may be caused, for example, by exogenous factors such as drugs (e.g., *chloroquine retinopathy*). Cancer patients may also develop symptoms of night blindness, photopsia (flashes of light), and compromise of the visual field. The symptoms associated with *cancer-associated retinopathy* and *melanoma-associated retinopathy*[34] result from the production of autoantibodies to the tumor that cross-react with corresponding epitopes within the retina. The symptoms associated with these paraneoplastic retinopathies mimic the symptoms of patients with inherited retinal degenerations such as retinitis pigmentosa. This is described next.

Retinitis Pigmentosa

The term *"retinitis" pigmentosa* is an unfortunate relic that is used to describe a collection of inherited retinal disorders that were, in the past, incorrectly presumed to be inflammatory. The conditions that are grouped under the rubric of retinitis pigmentosa are fairly common and have an incidence of 1 in 3600. They may be inherited as X-linked recessive, autosomal recessive, and autosomal dominant (the age of onset correlates with the inheritance pattern with autosomal dominant retinitis pigmentosa appearing later in life). Retinitis pigmentosa may be part of a syndrome such as *Refsum disease* or may develop in isolation (nonsystemic retinitis pigmentosa).

Retinitis pigmentosa has attracted considerable interest because the various forms of this condition have been linked to mutations in genes whose products are important for vision. Such mutations may affect genes that regulate the functions of either the photoreceptor cells or the retinal pigment epithelium. These include genes that regulate the visual cascade and visual cycle, structural genes (transpanins), transcription factors, retinal catabolic pathways, and mitochondrial metabolism.[35] *Typically, both rods and cones are lost to apoptosis*, although in varying proportions. Loss of rods may lead to early *night blindness* and constricted visual fields. As cones are lost, *central visual acuity* may be affected as well. Clinically, retinal atrophy is accompanied by constriction of retinal vessels and optic nerve head atrophy ("waxy pallor" of the optic disk) and the accumulation of retinal pigment around blood vessels, thus accounting for the "pigmentosa" in the disease's name. The electoretinogram reveals abnormalities characteristic of this disease.

RETINITIS

A variety of pathogens can contribute to the development of infectious retinitis. For example, *Candida* may disseminate to the retina hematogenously, especially in the setting of intravenous drug abuse or in systemic candidemia from other causes. Hematogenous dissemination of pathogens to the retina typically results in multiple retinal abscesses. As was mentioned previously, cytomegalovirus retinitis is an important cause of visual morbidity in immunocompromised patients, especially those with AIDS.

RETINAL NEOPLASMS

Retinoblastoma

Retinoblastoma is the most common primary intraocular malignancy of children. The molecular genetics of retinoblastoma has been discussed in detail (Chapter 7). Although the name *retinoblastoma* might suggest origin from a primitive retinal cell that is capable of differentiation into both glial and neuronal cells, it is now clear that the cell of origin of retinoblastoma is neuronal. Prognosis is adversely affected by extraocular extension and invasion along the optic nerve and possibly by choroidal invasion. Recall that in approximately 40% of cases, retinoblastoma occurs in individuals who inherit a germ-line mutation of one *RB* allele. Retinoblastomas arising in the context of germ line mutations not only may be bilateral, but also may be associated with pinealoblastoma (so-called "trilateral" retinoblastoma), which is associated with a dismal outcome.[36]

Morphology. The pathology of retinoblastoma of both hereditary and sporadic types is identical. Tumors may contain both undifferentiated and differentiated elements. The former appear as collections of small, round cells with hyperchromatic nuclei. In well-differentiated tumors there are Flexner-Wintersteiner rosettes and fleurettes reflecting photoreceptor differentiation. It should be noted, however, that the degree of tumor differentiation does not appear to be associated with the prognosis. As can be noted in Figure 29–24, viable tumor cells are found encircling tumor blood vessels with zones of necrosis typically

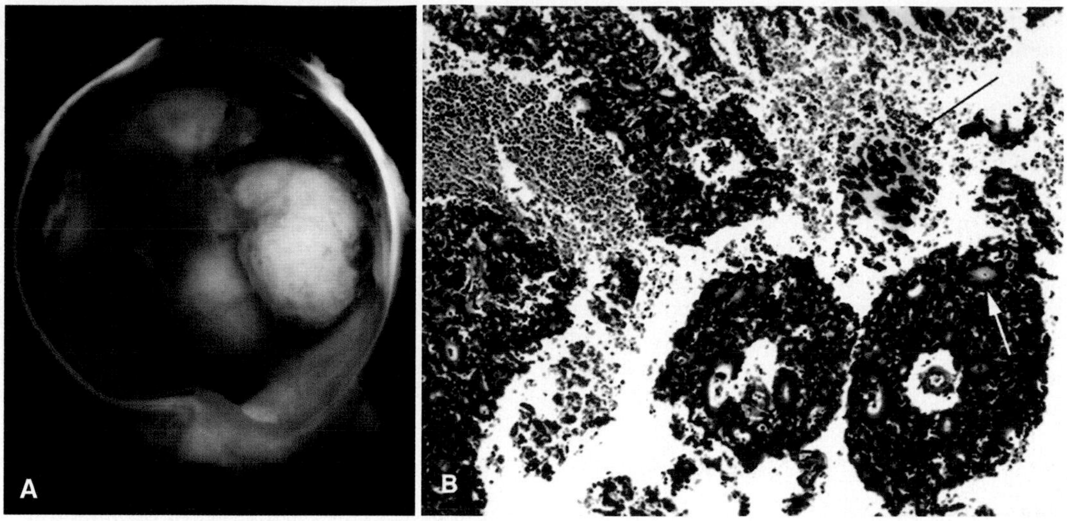

Figure 29–24 Retinoblastoma. *A,* Gross photograph of retinoblastoma. *B,* Tumor cells appear viable when in proximity to blood vessels, but necrosis is seen as the distance from the vessel increases. Dystrophic calcification *(dark arrow)* is present in the zones of tumor necrosis. Flexner-Wintersteiner rosettes—arrangements of a single layer of tumor cells around an apparent "lumen"—are seen throughout the tumor, and one such rosette is indicated by the white arrow.

found in relatively avascular areas. This illustrates graphically the dependence of retinoblastoma on its blood supply. Focal zones of dystrophic calcification are characteristic of retinoblastoma.

In an effort to preserve vision and eradicate the tumor, many ophthalmic oncologists now attempt to reduce tumor burden by administration of chemotherapy; after chemoreduction, tumors may be obliterated by laser treatment or cryopexy. Retinoblastoma tends to spread to the brain and bone marrow and seldom disseminates to the lungs. A benign variant of retinoblastoma—retinocytoma—has been reported.[37] The appearance of retinoblastoma in one eye and retinocytoma in the other eye is characteristic of heritable retinoblastoma.

Retinal Lymphoma

There are two distinctive profiles of intraocular lymphoma. Systemic lymphoma tends to involve the uvea (iris, ciliary body, and choroid). By contrast, primary retinal lymphoma is analogous to primary large cell lymphoma of the brain; therefore, it involves the two retinal layers derived from brain: the neurosensory retina and the retinal pigment epithelium. The underlying choroid is typically filled with a cytologically benign lymphoid infiltrate. Primary intraocular lymphoma tends to occur in older patients and may mimic uveitis clinically. The diagnosis depends on a demonstration of lymphoma cells in vitreous aspirates.

Optic Nerve

As a sensory tract of the central nervous system, the optic nerve is surrounded by meninges, and cerebrospinal fluid circulates around the nerve. The pathology of the optic nerve is similar to the pathology of the brain. For example, the most common primary neoplasms of the optic nerve are glioma (typically *pilocytic astrocytomas*) and meningioma.

ANTERIOR ISCHEMIC OPTIC NEUROPATHY

There are striking similarities between stroke and a condition known in ophthalmic terminology as *anterior ischemic optic neuropathy* (AION).[38] As used clinically, the term *AION* comprises a spectrum of injuries to the optic nerve varying from ischemia to infarction. Thus, transient partial interruptions in blood flow to the optic nerve may produce episodes of transient loss of vision, whereas total interruption in blood flow may produce an optic nerve infarct, either segmental or total. Zones of relative ischemia may surround segmental infarcts of the optic nerve. Optic nerve function in these poorly perfused but not infarcted zones may recover. The optic nerve does not regenerate, and visual loss from infarction is permanent.

Interruption in the blood supply to the optic nerve may result from inflammation of the vessels that supply the optic nerve, known as *arteritic AION*, or from embolic or thrombotic events, known as *nonarteritic AION*. Bilateral total infarcts of the optic nerve resulting in total blindness have been reported in temporal arteritis (arteritic AION), adding urgency to the treatment of this condition with high doses of corticosteroids.

PAPILLEDEMA

Edema of the head of the optic nerve may develop as a consequence of compression of the nerve (as in a primary neoplasm of the optic nerve) or from elevations of cerebrospinal fluid pressure surrounding the nerve. Elevation in intracranial pressure is transmitted to the optic nerve by the cerebrospinal fluid circulating around the nerve. The concentric increase in pressure not only contributes to venous stasis at the nerve head, but also contributes to stasis in axoplasmic transport, leading to nerve head swelling.[39,40] Swelling of the optic nerve head in elevated intracranial pressure is typically bilateral (unless the patient has experienced previous unilateral optic atrophy) and is commonly termed *papilledema*. Typically, acute papilledema from increased intracranial pressure is not associated with visual loss. Ophthalmoscopically, the optic nerve head in papilledema is swollen but hyperemic; by contrast, the optic nerve head in the relatively acute phases of anterior ischemic optic neuropathy appears swollen but pale because of decreased nerve perfusion (Fig. 29–25). In papilledema secondary to increased intracranial pressure, the optic nerve may remain congested for a prolonged period of time; by contrast, the appearance of the optic nerve in acute ischemic optic neuropathy evolves into a very pale disc clinically, reflecting optic atrophy.

GLAUCOMATOUS OPTIC NERVE DAMAGE

As discussed previously, the majority of patients with glaucoma have elevated intraocular pressure. However, there is a small group that develops the visual field and optic nerve changes typical of glaucoma with normal intraocular pressure: so-called *normal-tension glaucoma*. Interestingly, mutations in the optineurin gene are seen in patients with normal-tension glaucoma but are not seen in patients with primary open angle glaucoma, in which pressure is elevated chronically.[41] Conversely, some patients with elevated intraocular pressure who are followed over long periods of time never develop visual field changes or optic nerve cupping. Therefore, it is clear that whatever the mechanism of damage to the retinal ganglion cell—the axons of which populate the optic nerve—there is a spectrum of neuronal susceptibility to the effects of elevated intraocular pressure. Therefore, significant research is now directed toward understanding mechanisms by which the optic nerve axons may be protected from injury.[42,43]

Morphology. Characteristically, there is a diffuse loss of ganglion cells and thinning of the retinal nerve fiber layer (Fig. 29–26). These changes are more than a histologic curiosity because the technique of optical coherence tomography permits measurement of nerve fiber layer thickness in patients. In advanced cases, the optic nerve is both cupped and atrophic. Glaucoma might well be the only condition in which optic atrophy is accompanied by cupping.

Elevated intraocular pressure in infants and children can lead to diffuse enlargement of the eye (**buphthalmos**) or enlargement of the cornea (**megalocornea**). Several gene mutations have been associated with the development of infantile glaucoma, but the mechanisms by which these genes produce glaucoma is unclear. After the eye reaches its adult size, prolonged elevation of intraocular pressure may lead to focal thinning of the sclera, and uveal tissue may line ectatic sclera (**staphyloma**). In adults, the cornea may become edematous, and degenerative pannus may form.

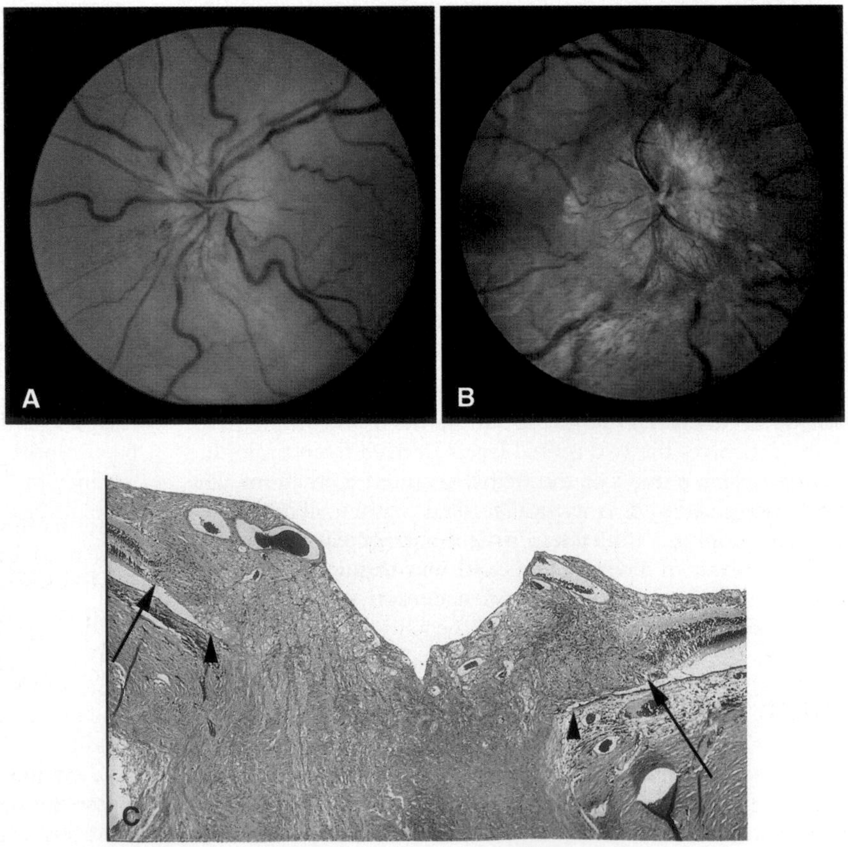

Figure 29–25 The optic nerve in anterior ischemic optic neuropathy (AION) and papilledema. *A*, In the relatively acute phases of AION, the optic nerve may be swollen, but it is relatively pale because of decreased perfusion. *B*, In papilledema secondary to increased intracranial pressure, the optic nerve is typically swollen and hyperemic. *C*, Normally, the termination of Bruch's membrane *(arrowhead)* is aligned with the beginning of the neurosensory retina, as indicated by the presence of stratified nuclei *(arrow)*, but in papilledema, the optic nerve is swollen, and the retina is displaced laterally. This is the histologic explanation for the blurred margins of the optic nerve head seen clinically in this condition. (*A* and *B* courtesy of Dr. Sohan S. Hayreh, Department of Ophthalmology & Visual Science, University of Iowa, Iowa City, IA; *C* originates from the teaching collection of the Armed Forces Institute of Pathology.)

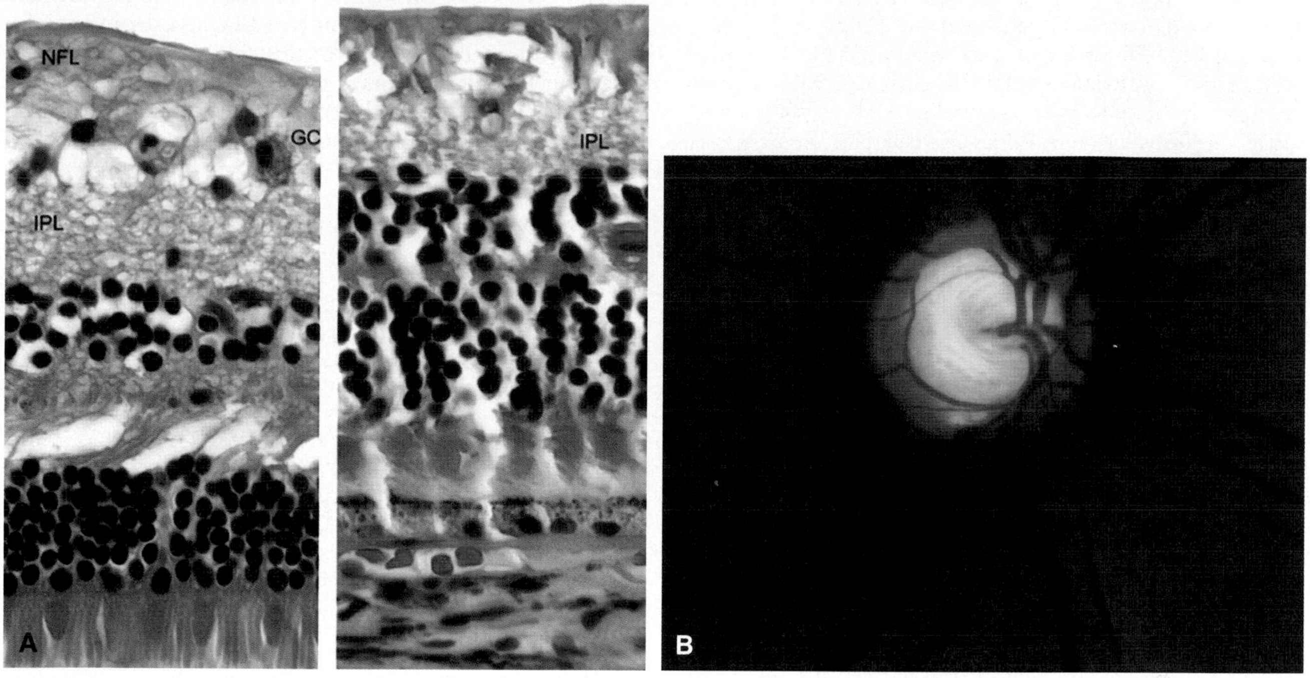

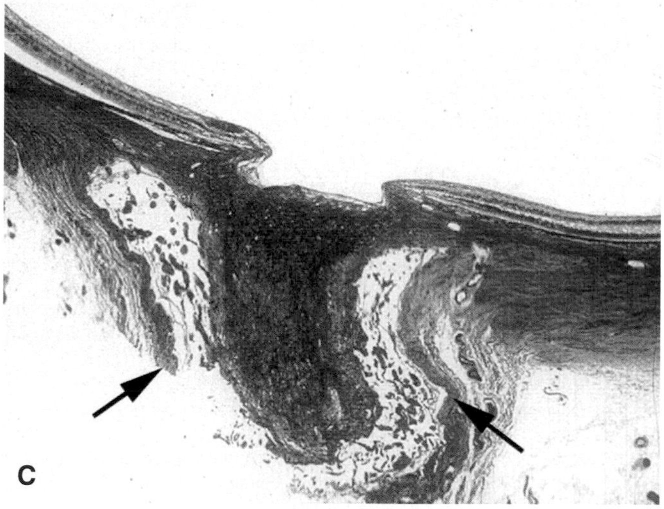

Figure 29–26 The retina and optic nerve in glaucoma. *A*, The normal retina is illustrated in the left panel, and the retina in long-standing glaucoma is in the right panel. Both pictures were taken at the same magnification. Note that the full thickness of the glaucomatous retina is captured (right), whereas only a portion of the normal retina (left) can be seen—a reflection of the thinning of the retina in glaucoma. In the glaucomatous retina, the areas corresponding to the nerve fiber layer (NFL) and ganglion cell layer (GC) are atrophic; the inner plexiform layer (IPL) is labeled for a point of reference. *B*, Glaucomatous optic nerve cupping results, in part, from loss of retinal ganglion cells, the axons of which populate the optic nerve. *C*, The arrows point to the dura of the optic nerve. Notice the wide subdural space, a result of atrophy of the substance of the optic nerve. The degree of cupping on the surface of the nerve is striking in this eye, which was removed because of complications of long-standing glaucoma.

OTHER OPTIC NEUROPATHIES

Optic neuropathy may be inherited (as in Leber hereditary optic neuropathy) or may be secondary to nutritional deficiencies (as in so-called tobacco-alcohol amblyopia) or toxins such as methanol. Patients may experience a severe visual disability if fibers in the optic nerve degenerate, especially if the central visual acuity is lost owing to degeneration of the nerve fibers that originate from the macula.

The predilection for Leber's hereditary optic neuropathy (LHON) to develop in young men is explained by inheritance of mitochondrial gene mutations (Chapter 5). It is possible that these mutations provide for a genetic susceptibility to a variety of environmental exposures that constitute the final trigger for optic nerve degeneration.[44] Studies of an epidemic of blindness in Cuba affecting 50,000 patients suggested acquired impairment of mitochondrial function through exposure to toxins, low folate, and high formic acid levels. These patients developed a syndrome that is phenotypically similar to LHON. The factor common to these optic neuropathies—inherited or acquired—appears to be a derangement in mitochondrial function. Since neuronal health is dependent on axoplasmic transport of mitochondria, mitochondrial dysfunctions give rise to neurologic disorders.[45]

OPTIC NEURITIS

Many unrelated conditions have historically been grouped under the heading of optic neuritis. Unfortunately, the term itself suggests optic nerve inflammation, which might not

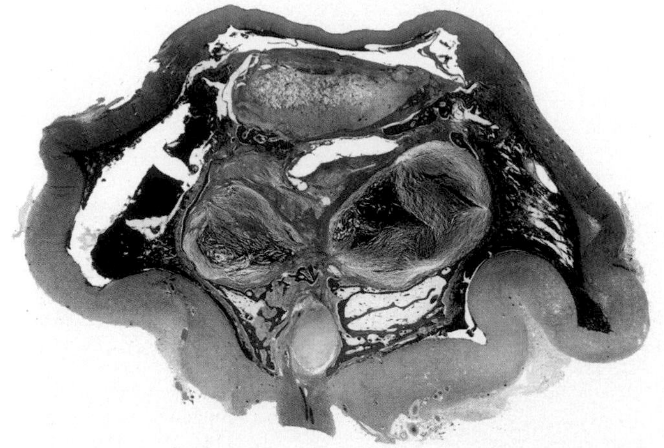

Figure 29–27 Phthisis bulbi. The eye is small and internally disorganized. The tension exerted on this hypotonic eye by the extraocular muscles contributes to a square rather than round shape. Note the atrophic optic nerve and the presence of intraocular bone posteriorly and anteriorly.

accurately describe the pathophysiologic changes. In common clinical usage, the term *optic neuritis* is used to describe a loss of vision secondary to demyelinization of the optic nerve. One of the most important causes of optic neuritis is multiple sclerosis (Chapter 28). Indeed, optic neuritis may be the first manifestation of this disease. Recent evidence indicates that the 10-year risk of developing multiple sclerosis after the first attack of optic neuritis increases if the patient has concomitant evidence of brain lesions as detected by magnetic resonance imaging. However, even when brain lesions are detectable, the risk of progression to multiple sclerosis is only 40%.[46] Patients with a single episode of optic nerve demyelinization may recover vision and remain systemically disease free.

The End-Stage Eye: Phthisis Bulbi

Trauma, intraocular inflammation, chronic retinal detachment, and many other conditions may give rise to an eye that is both small (atrophic) and internally disorganized: *phthisis bulbi*. Congenitally small eyes—hypoplastic or *microphthalmic* eyes—are generally not disorganized internally.

Morphology. Phthisical eyes typically feature the following changes: the presence of exudate or blood in the potential space between the ciliary body and sclera and the choroid and sclera (**ciliochoroidal effusion**), the presence of a membrane extending across the eye from one aspect of the ciliary body to the other (**cyclitic membrane**); chronic retinal detachment; optic nerve atrophy; the presence of intraocular bone, which is thought by many to originate from **osseous metaplasia** of the retinal pigment epithelium; and a thickened sclera, especially posteriorly. Ciliochoroidal effusion is typically associated with the physiologic state of low intraocular pressure (**hypotony**). The normal pull of the extraocular muscles on a hypotonous eye may render the appearance of the eye as square rather than round (Fig. 29–27).

Acknowledgments. The author is very grateful to Dr. Amy Y. Lin, Fellow in Ophthalmic Pathology in the Department of Pathology, University of Illinois at Chicago, for her assistance in assembling illustrations for this chapter. The author is also extremely grateful for input from Dr. Richard K. Parrish from the Department of Ophthalmology & Visual Science, Bascom-Palmer Eye Institute, University of Miami, for many helpful suggestions and comments.

REFERENCES

1. Friend SH, Bernards R, Rogelj S, et al: A human DNA segment with properties of the gene that predisposes to retinoblastoma and osteosarcoma. Nature 323:643–646, 1986.
2. Hatton MP, Rubin PA: The pathophysiology of thyroid-associated ophthalmopathy. Ophthalmol Clin North Am 15:113–119, 2002.
3. Perry SR, Rootman J, White VA: The clinical and pathologic constellation of Wegener granulomatosis of the orbit. Ophthalmology 104:683–694, 1997.
4. Rao NA, Hidayat AA, McLean IW, Zimmerman LE: Sebaceous carcinomas of the ocular adnexa: a clinicopathologic study of 104 cases, with five-year follow-up data. Hum Pathol 13:113–122, 1982.
5. Nichols CW, Eagle RC Jr, Yanoff M, Menocal NG: Conjunctival biopsy as an aid in the evaluation of the patient with suspected sarcoidosis. Ophthalmology 87:287–291, 1980.
6. Scott IU, Karp CL, Nuovo GJ: Human papillomavirus 16 and 18 expression in conjunctival intraepithelial neoplasia. Ophthalmology 109:542–547, 2002.
7. Folberg,R, Jakobiec FA, Bernardino VB Jr, Iwamoto T: Benign conjunctival melanocytic lesions: clinicopathologic features. Ophthalmology 96:436–461, 1989.
8. Jakobiec FA, Folberg R, Iwamoto T: Clinicopathologic characteristics of premalignant and malignant melanocytic lesions of the conjunctiva. Ophthalmology 96:147–166, 1989.
9. Klintworth, GK: The molecular genetics of the corneal dystrophies: current status. Front Biosci 8:D687–D713, 2003.
10. Stone EM, Fingert JH, Alward WL, et al: Identification of a gene that causes primary open angle glaucoma. Science 275:668–670, 1997.
11. Swiderski RE, Ross JL, Fingert JH, et al: Localization of MYOC transcripts in human eye and optic nerve by in situ hybridization. Invest Ophthalmol Vis Sci 41:3420–3428, 2000.
12. Kuo I, Rao NA: Ocular disease in AIDS. Springer Semin Immunopathol 21:161–177, 1999.
13. Zamir E, Hudson H, Ober RR, et al: Massive mycobacterial choroiditis during highly active antiretroviral therapy: another immune-recovery uveitis? Ophthalmology 109:2144–2148, 2002.
14. Boyd SR, Young S, Lightman S: Immunopathology of the noninfectious posterior and intermediate uveitides. Surv Ophthalmol 46:209–233, 2001.
15. Singh AD, Topham A: Incidence of uveal melanoma in the United States: 1973–1997. Ophthalmology 110:956–961, 2003.
16. Singh AD, Topham A: Survival rates with uveal melanoma in the United States: 1973–1997. Ophthalmology 110:962–965, 2003.
17. Seddon JM, Albert DM, Lavin PT, Robinson N: A prognostic factor study of disease-free interval and survival following enucleation for uveal melanoma. Arch Ophthalmol 101:1894–1899, 1983.
18. Folberg R, Salomao D, Grossniklaus HE, Proia AD, Rao NA, Cameron JD: Recommendations for the reporting of tissues removed as part of the surgical treatment of common malignancies of the eye and its adnexa: the Association of Directors of Anatomic and Surgical Pathology. Hum Pathol 34:114–118, 2003.
19. Aalto Y, Eriksson L, Seregard S, Larsson O, Knuutila S: Concomitant loss of chromosome 3 and whole arm losses and gains of chromosome 1, 6, or 8 in metastasizing primary uveal melanoma. Invest Ophthalmol Vis Sci 42:313–317, 2001.
20. Maniotis AJ, Chen X, Garcia C, et al: Control of melanoma morphogenesis, endothelial survival, and perfusion by extracellular matrix. Lab Invest 82:1031–1043, 2002.
20a. Folberg R, Maniotis AJ: Vasculogenic mimicry. ARMIS (in press), 2004.
21. Clarijs R, Otte-Holler I, Ruiter DJ, de Waal RM. Presence of a fluid-conducting meshwork in xenografted cutaneous and primary human uveal melanoma. Invest Ophthalmol Vis Sci 43:912–918, 2002.

22. Frank RN: Diabetic retinopathy. N Engl J Med 350:48–58, 2004.
23. Pe'er J, Folberg R, Itin A, Gnessin H, Hemo I, Keshet E: Upregulated expression of vascular endothelial growth factor in proliferative diabetic retinopathy. Br J Ophthalmol 80:241–245, 1996.
24. Tolentino MJ, McLeod DS, Taomoto M, Otsuji T, Adamis AP, Lutty GA: Pathologic features of vascular endothelial growth factor-induced retinopathy in the nonhuman primate. Am J Ophthalmol 133:373–385, 2002.
25. Pe'er J, Shweiki D, Itin A, Hemo I, Gnessin H, Keshet E: Hypoxia-induced expression of vascular endothelial growth factor by retinal cells is a common factor in neovascularizing ocular diseases. Lab Invest 72:638–645, 1995.
26. Mechoulam H, Pierce E: Retinopathy of prematurity: molecular pathology and therapeutic strategies. Am J Pharmacogenomics 3:261–277, 2003.
27. Romayananda N, Goldberg MF: Histopathology of sickle cell retinopathy. Trans Am Acad Ophthalmol Otolaryngol 77:652–676, 1973.
28. Cao J, Mathews MK, McLeod DS, Merges C, Hjelmeland LM, Lutty GA: Angiogenic factors in human proliferative sickle cell retinopathy. Br J Ophthalmol 83:838–846, 1999.
29. Kim SY, Mocanu C, McLeod DS, et al: Expression of pigment epithelium-derived factor (PEDF) and vascular endothelial growth factor (VEGF) in sickle cell retina and choroid. Exp Eye Res 77:433–445, 2003.
30. Hayreh SS: So-called "central retinal vein occlusion." Part I: Pathogenesis, terminology, clinical features. Ophthalmologica 172:1–13, 1976.
31. Pe'er J, Folberg R, Itin A, Gnessin H, Hemo I, Keshet E: Vascular endothelial growth factor upregulation in human central retinal vein occlusion. Ophthalmology 105:412–416, 1998.
32. Hyman L, Neborsky R: Risk factors for age-related macular degeneration: an update. Curr Opin Ophthalmol 13:171–175, 2002;
33. Bird AC: The Bowman lecture: towards an understanding of age-related macular disease. Eye 17:457–466, 2003.
34. Pfohler C, Haus A, Palmowski A, et al: Melanoma-associated retinopathy: high frequency of subclinical findings in patients with melanoma. Br J Dermatol 149:74–78, 2003.
35. Rivolta C, Sharon D, DeAngelis MM, Dryja TP: Retinitis pigmentosa and allied diseases: numerous diseases, genes, and inheritance patterns. Hum Mol Genet 11:1219–1227, 2002.
36. Marcus DM, Brooks SE, Leff G, et al: Trilateral retinoblastoma: insights into histogenesis and management. Surv Ophthalmol 43:59–70, 1998.
37. Margo C, Hidayat A, Kopelman J, Zimmerman LE: Retinocytoma: a benign variant of retinoblastoma. Arch Ophthalmol 101:1519–1531, 1983.
38. Hayreh SS: Anterior ischemic optic neuropathy. Clin Neurosci 4:251–263, 1997.
39. Tso MO, Hayreh SS: Optic disc edema in raised intracranial pressure. Part IV: axoplasmic transport in experimental papilledema. Arch Ophthalmol 95:1458–1462, 1977.
40. Tso MO, Hayreh SS: Optic disc edema in raised intracranial pressure. Part IV: axoplasmic transport in experimental papilledema. Arch Ophthalmol 95:1458–1462, 1977.
41. Wiggs JL, Auguste J, Allingham RR, et al: Lack of association of mutations in optineurin with disease in patients with adult-onset primary open-angle glaucoma. Arch Ophthalmol 121:1181–1183, 2003.
42. Wax MB, Tezel G: Neurobiology of glaucomatous optic neuropathy: diverse cellular events in neurodegeneration and neuroprotection. Mol Neurobiol 26:45–55, 2002.
43. Schwartz M: Neurodegeneration and neuroprotection in glaucoma: development of a therapeutic neuroprotective vaccine: the Friedenwald lecture. Invest Ophthalmol Vis Sci 44:1407–1411, 2003.
44. Howell N: Leber hereditary optic neuropathy: respiratory chain dysfunction and degeneration of the optic nerve. Vision Res 38:1495–1504, 1998.
45. Sadun A: Acquired mitochondrial impairment as a cause of optic nerve disease. Trans Am Ophthalmol Soc 96:881–923, 1998.
46. Beck RW, Trobe JD, Moke PS, et al: High- and low-risk profiles for the development of multiple sclerosis within 10 years after optic neuritis: experience of the optic neuritis treatment trial. Arch Ophthalmol 121:944–949, 2003.

Index

Note: Page numbers followed by f indicate figures; those followed by t indicate tables; those followed by b indicate boxed material.

A

AA (arachidonic acid), 68
AA (arachidonic acid) metabolites, in inflammation, 57, 61, 68–70, 68t, 69f, 70f
AA (amyloid-associated) protein, 259, 260, 260t
Abdominal abscesses, 393
Abdominal aortic aneurysm (AAA), 531–532, 531f
  inflammatory, 531
  mycotic, 531
  rupture of, 532
Aß fragments, 1388, 1388f, 1389
Aß (ß-amyloid) protein, 259, 260, 260t
Abetalipoproteinemia, 846
ABL oncogene, 295t, 297, 314
ABO incompatibility, 485
Abortion, spontaneous, 1105
ABPA (allergic bronchopulmonary aspergillosis), 400, 727–728
Abrasion, 443, 443f
Abscess(es), 393
  abdominal, 393
  Bartholin, 393, 1065
  brain, 1371, 1371f
  Brodie, 1291
  crypt, 848, 850, 850f
  defined, 77
  extradural, 1371
  liver, 902
    amebic, 839
  lung, 747t, 753, 753f
    due to pneumonia, 750
    pyemic, 753, 753f
    staphylococcal, 373, 373f
  micro-
    Munro, 1257
    Pautrier, 1250
  pancreatic, 944
  perinephric, 999
  recurrent subareolar, 1125, 1125f
  ring, 596
  subcutaneous bacterial, 78f
  subperiosteal, 1291
  tubo-ovarian, 393, 1064
Absidia, 400
Acanthamoeba spp, 351t, 1380
Acantholysis, 1230, 1260, 1260f, 1261f
Acantholytic blister, suprabasal, 1260, 1260f
Acanthosis, 1230
Acanthosis nigricans, 1237–1238
  paraneoplastic, 334t, 335
Acetaldehyde, in alcoholic liver disease, 906
Acetaminophen (Tylenol)
  adverse effects of, 428
  cell injury due to, 25–26
Acetylaminofluorene, 322
Acetylcholine receptors (AChRs), in myasthenia gravis, 1344
Acetyl-glyceryl-ether-phosphorylcholine (AGEPC), 70
Acetylsalicylic acid. *See* Aspirin.
Achalasia, 800–801, 801f
Achondrogenesis II, 1280t
Achondroplasia, 1280t
Acid aerosols, as air pollutants, 429, 429t
Acid hydrolases, 159
Acid maltase deficiency, 167
Acid phosphatase deficiency, 161t
Acid proteases, 73
Acid-fast stain, 361t
Acidic fibroblast growth factor (aFGF), 95t, 96
Acinar cell(s), 940, 940f
Acinar cell carcinoma, of pancreas, 951
Acinic cell tumor, of salivary gland, 794
Acinus(i)
  of liver, 878
  of lung, 712
  pancreatic, 940, 940f
Acne vulgaris, 1264–1265, 1264f
Acoustic neuroma, 1411
Acquired immunodeficiency syndrome (AIDS), 245–258
  Addison disease in, 1216
  B-cell lymphomas in, 257–258, 326
  central nervous system involvement in, 253, 258
  clinical features of, 255–258, 255t, 257f
  cytomegalovirus in, 256, 367–368
  diarrhea in, 841
  epidemiology of, 245–246
  etiology of, 246–248, 247f
  in children, 1376
  infections with, 361
  Kaposi sarcoma in, 256–257, 257f, 548–549, 550
  life cycle of HIV in, 248–253, 249f–252f, 252t
  major abnormalities of immune function in, 252, 252t
  mechanism of T-cell immunodeficiency in, 250–252, 251f
  meningitis due to, 1375
  meningoencephalitis due to, 1375–1376, 1376f
  morphology of, 258
  Mycobacterium avium-intracellulare complex in, 256, 386, 387f, 1372
Acquired immunodeficiency syndrome (AIDS) *(Continued)*
  myocarditis in, 608
  myopathy due to, 1376
  natural history of, 253–255, 254f, 255t
  nephropathy associated with, 984
  oral manifestations of, 778t
  pathogenesis of, 248, 248f
  perinatal, 355
  peripheral neuropathy due to, 1376
  pneumonia with, 756
  pulmonary disease with, 756
  sexual transmission of, 356t
  thrombocytopenia in, 652
  transmission of, 245–246
  tuberculosis with, 256, 384, 1372
  vacuolar myelopathy in, 1376
  white cell neoplasia with, 667
Acral lentiginous melanomas, 1232
Acrodermatitis enteropathica, 461, 461f
Acromegaly, 1161
ACTH. *See* Adrenocorticotropic hormone (ACTH).
α-Actin, 106f
Actin filaments, abnormalities of, 34
Actinic band keratopathy, 1428
Actinic cheilitis, 1242
Actinic granuloma, 1426
Actinic keratosis, 1240–1242, 1241f
Actinic lentigo, 1231
Actinomycetaceae, 349t
Activation-induced cell death, 224f, 225
Acute alveolar injury. *See* Acute respiratory distress syndrome (ARDS).
Acute chest syndrome, in sickle cell disease, 631
Acute coronary syndromes. *See* Ischemic heart disease (IHD); Myocardial infarction (MI).
Acute disseminated encephalomyelitis (ADEM), 1385
Acute erosive hemorrhagic gastritis, 813, 813f
Acute fatty liver of pregnancy (AFLP), 920
Acute gastric ulceration, 819–820, 820f
Acute hemorrhagic leukoencephalitis of Weston Hurst, 1385
Acute intermittent porphyria (AIP), 1333t
Acute lung injury, 714–716, 714t, 715f, 715t, 717f
Acute lymphoblastic leukemia/lymphoma (ALL), 670–673, 671t
  clinical features of, 671t, 672–673
  genetic and other markers of, 500t, 671t, 672
  immunophenotype of, 672
  morphology of, 670–672, 672f

Acute lymphoblastic leukemia/lymphoma (ALL) *(Continued)*
oncogenes in, 314t
prognosis for, 673
progression of polycythemia vera to, 699–700
Acute monocytic leukemia, 694f
Acute myelogenous leukemia (AML), 666, 691, 692–695
chromosomal abnormalities in, 693
classification of, 692, 693t
clinical features of, 693–694
immunophenotype of, 693
morphology of, 692, 694f
oncogenes in, 314t
pathophysiology of, 692
prognosis for, 694–695
progression of myelodysplastic syndromes to, 695–696
Acute myocardial infarction. *See* Myocardial infarction (MI).
Acute necrotizing hemorrhagic encephalomyelitis (ANHE), 1385
Acute phase response, 84–85
Acute promyelocytic leukemia, 692, 694f
Acute radiation syndrome, 437, 438t, 439
Acute respiratory distress syndrome (ARDS), 715–716
clinical course of, 716
due to amniotic fluid embolism, 137
etiology of, 715, 715t
morphology of, 715, 715f
pathogenesis of, 85, 142f, 715–716, 717f
Acute tubular necrosis (ATN), 993–996
clinical course of, 995–996
due to shock, 142
etiology of, 993
ischemic, 993–995, 994f, 995f
morphology of, 994–995, 995f
nephrotoxic, 993, 995, 995f
pathogenesis of, 993–994, 994f
Acute-phase proteins, 84
Acylating agents, as carcinogens, 321t
AD. *See* Alzheimer disease (AD).
ADA (adenosine deaminase) deficiency, 241f, 244
ADAM(s), 111
ADAM-33 gene, in asthma, 724
ADAMTS 13, 1010
ADAMTS 13 deficiency, 653
ADC (AIDS-dementia complex), 1375–1376, 1376f
ADCC (antibody-dependent cellular cytotoxicity), 201, 210
Addison, Thomas, 1215
Addison disease, 1215–1216, 1216f
Additives, to food, 446–447
ADEM (acute disseminated encephalomyelitis), 1385
Adenocarcinoma, 271
endometrial, 1087, 1087f
of anal canal, 870
of bladder, 1032
of breast. *See* Breast carcinoma.
of cervix, 1078f
of colon. *See* Colorectal carcinoma.
of esophagus, 808–809, 809f
of fallopian tubes, 1091
of gallbladder, 935f
of kidney, 1016–1018, 1017f, 1018f
of lung, 759, 760–762, 761f, 762f, 769f
of ovaries, 1095, 1095f, 1098
of pancreas, 951
of prostate, 1050–1056, 1052f–1054f
of small intestine, 857
of vagina, 1071, 1071f
Adenohypophysis, 1157–1158, 1157f
Adenoid cystic carcinoma, of salivary gland, 793–794, 794f
Adenoma(s)
ACTH-producing, 1208
adrenocortical, 1208, 1209, 1210, 1212f, 1217
colonic, 858, 858f, 859–861, 860f, 861f
corticotroph cell, 1162
defined, 270
FSH-producing, 1162
gastric, 821, 822f
gonadotroph, 1162
growth hormone, 1161–1162
Hürthle cell, 1176, 1176f
lactational, 1127
lactotroph, 1160–1161, 1161f
LH-producing, 1162
liver cell, 922–923, 923f
mammosomatotroph, 1161
micro-
ACTH-producing, 1208
pancreatic, in MEN-1, 1222
pituitary, 1159
nephrogenic, 1028
null cell, 1162
of biliary tract, 934
of small intestine, 857, 857f
oxyphil, 1185
parathyroid, 1185–1186, 1185f, 1186f
pedunculated, 860f
pituitary, 1158–1162
ACTH-producing, 1208
classification of, 1158–1159, 1158t
clinical course of, 1160
corticotroph cell, 1162
diagnosis of, 1159
functional *vs.* silent, 1158
genetic abnormalities in, 1159, 1159f
gonadotroph, 1162
growth hormone (somatotroph cell), 1161–1162
hormone-negative, 1158–1159, 1162
lactotroph, 1160–1161, 1161f
mammosomatotroph, 1161
micro- *vs.* macro-, 1159
morphology of, 1160, 1160f
nonfunctioning, 1158, 1160f, 1162
null cell, 1162
prolactinomas as, 1160–1161, 1161f
thyrotroph, 1162
with MEN type 1, 1159
pleomorphic, 271
of salivary gland, 791–792, 792f
renal papillary, 1015
sebaceous, 1240t
sessile, 861f
somatotroph cell, 1161–1162
thyroid, 1175–1177
clinical features of, 1177
follicular, 1175–1177, 1176f, 1181f
morphology of, 274f, 1176–1177, 1176f
pathogenesis of, 1176
thyrotroph, 1162
tubular, 860–861, 860f
tubulovillous, 860, 861
villous, 860, 861, 861f
Adenoma-carcinoma sequence, 862
Adenomatoid tumors
of fallopian tubes, 1091
paratesticular, 1040
Adenomatous polyp(s), of colon, 858, 858f, 859–861, 860f, 861f
Adenomatous polyposis, familial, 284–285, 861–862, 862f, 1151
Adenomatous polyposis coli *(APC)* gene, 287t
in colorectal carcinoma, 317–318, 317f, 339, 339t, 863, 863f
Adenomatous polyposis coli *(APC)* gene *(Continued)*
in familial adenomatous polyposis, 284–285
Adenomyosis
of endometrial tissue, 1083, 1083f
of gallbladder, 934
Adenosarcomas, endometrial, 1088–1089
Adenosine 3,′5′-cyclic monophosphate (cAMP), 98f, 100
Adenosine deaminase (ADA) deficiency, 241f, 244
Adenosine triphosphate (ATP), cell injury due to depletion of, 14–15, 14f
Adenosis
of breast, 1127
sclerosing, 1128, 1128f
complex, 1128, 1129f
vaginal, 1071
Adenosquamous carcinoma
of cervix, 1078
of pancreas, 951
Adenoviruses, 347t, 348f
enteric, 833, 833t
ADH (alcohol dehydrogenase), 422, 422f
ADH (antidiuretic hormone), 1158
syndrome of inappropriate secretion of, 1163
ADH (atypical ductal hyperplasia), 1129, 1130f
Adhesins, 358
Adhesion molecules, 54–56, 54t, 55b, 56f, 57
Adhesions, intestinal, 856, 856f
Adhesive glycoproteins, in extracellular matrix, 103f, 104–105, 106f
Adipokines, and insulin resistance, 1196, 1196f
Adiponectin, and insulin resistance, 1196, 1196f
Adiposity signals, 463f
Adnexa, of skin, 1228f
tumors of, 1238–1240, 1239f, 1240t
ADPKD (autosomal-dominant polycystic kidney disease), 962–964, 962t, 964f, 965f
Adrenal adenoma, 1208, 1209, 1210, 1212f
Adrenal androgens, 1211–1212, 1213f
Adrenal carcinoma, 1217–1218, 1217f
androgen-secreting, 1212
Cushing syndrome due to, 1208, 1209
Adrenal cortex, 1207–1218. *See also under* Adrenocortical.
normal anatomy and physiology of, 1207
Adrenal crisis, 1214, 1214t
Adrenal cysts, 1218
Adrenal effects, of shock, 142
Adrenal glands, 1207–1223
amyloidosis of, 263
normal anatomy and physiology of, 1207
primary neoplasms of, 1208
Adrenal hemorrhage, massive, 1214–1215, 1215f
Adrenal hyperplasia, congenital, 1212–1214
Adrenal hypoplasia congenital (AHC), 1216
Adrenal incidentaloma, 1218
Adrenal medulla, 1218–1221
neuroblastoma of, 1221
normal anatomy and physiology of, 1207, 1218, 1219f
pheochromocytoma of, 1219–1221, 1219t, 1220f
Adrenal metastases, Addison disease due to, 1216
Adrenal myelolipomas, 1218
Adrenal neuroblastoma, 501, 501f
Adrenal virilism, nonclassic or late-onset, 1213
Adrenaline, 1218
Adrenalitis, autoimmune, 1215–1216, 1216f
Adrenocortical adenomas, 1208, 1209, 1210, 1212f, 1217
Adrenocortical carcinoma, 1217–1218, 1217f
androgen-secreting, 1212
Cushing syndrome due to, 1208, 1209

Adrenocortical hyperfunction, 1207–1214
due to adrenogenital syndromes, 1211–1214, 1213f
due to hypercortisolism (Cushing syndrome), 1207–1210, 1208f, 1209t
due to primary hyperaldosteronism, 1210–1211, 1211f, 1212f
Adrenocortical hyperplasia, primary
Cushing syndrome due to, 1208–1209
hyperaldosteronism due to, 1210, 1212f
Adrenocortical insufficiency, 1214–1217
due to Waterhouse-Friderichsen syndrome, 1214–1215, 1215f
primary
acute, 1214, 1214t
chronic, 1215–1216, 1216f
secondary, 1214t, 1216–1217
Adrenocortical neoplasm(s), 1217–1218, 1217f, 1218f
androgen excess due to, 1211–1212
Cushing syndrome due to, 1208, 1209
hyperaldosteronism due to, 1210
Adrenocorticotropic hormone (ACTH)
ectopic secretion, 1209, 1210
excess production of, 1162
primary hypersecretion of, 1208
Adrenocorticotropic hormone (ACTH) deficiency, adrenocortical insufficiency due to, 1216–1217
Adrenocorticotropic hormone (ACTH)-producing microadenoma, 1208
Adrenogenital syndrome(s), 1211–1214, 1213f
simple virilizing, without salt wasting, 1213
Adrenoleukodystrophy, 1216, 1333t, 1398
Adrenomedullary dysplasia, 1214
Adriamycin (doxorubicin), myocardial disease due to, 609–610
Adult polycystic kidney disease, 962–964, 962t, 964f, 965f
Adult polyglucosan body disease, 1352
Adult respiratory distress syndrome (ARDS)
clinical course of, 716
due to amniotic fluid embolism, 137
etiology of, 715, 715t
morphology of, 715, 715f
pathogenesis of, 85, 142f, 715–716, 717f
Adult T-cell leukemia/lymphoma, 671t, 685
Adult-onset medullary cystic disease, 962t, 966
Advanced glycation end products (AGEs), 42
in diabetes mellitus, 1198, 1198t, 1204
Adventitia, of blood vessel, 512, 512f
Adverse drug reactions, 426, 426t
genetically determined, 154
aFGF (acidic fibroblast growth factor), 95t, 96
Aflatoxin(s)
and hepatocellular carcinoma, 924
in *Aspergillus* infection, 400
Aflatoxin B1, and hepatocellular carcinoma, 321, 322, 436
AFLP (acute fatty liver of pregnancy), 920
AFP (alpha-fetoprotein), 330, 338, 339t
in germ cell tumors, 1045–1046
African tick fever, 396t
African trypanosomiasis, 405, 405f
African-Americans, breast cancer in, 1132
AGA (appropriate for gestational age), 476
Agammaglobulinemia of Bruton, X-linked, 240–242, 241f
Age, and cancer, 284, 286t, 287t
of breast, 1131
AGE(s) (advanced glycation end products), 42
in diabetes mellitus, 1198, 1198t, 1204
Agenesis, 472
Agent Orange, 435
AGEPC (acetyl-glyceryl-ether-phosphorylcholine), 70
Age-related macular degeneration (ARMD), 1422, 1441–1442, 1442f
atrophic *vs.* exudative, 1441
Age-related osteoporosis, 1283, 1283f
Aggregometer, 655
Aggressive fibromatoses, 115
Aging
atrophy due to, 9
effects on heart of, 558–559, 559t
genes that influence, 43
Agouti-related peptide (AgRP), 463f, 464b
Agranulocytosis, 662–663
in hypersensitivity, 210
oral manifestations of, 778t
Agricultural hazards, 434–435, 434t
Agyria, 1354
AHC (adrenal hypoplasia congenital), 1216
AHO (Albright hereditary osteodystrophy), pseudohypoparathyroidism in, 1189
AIB1 gene, in pancreatic cancer, 950, 950t
AIDS. *See* Acquired immunodeficiency syndrome (AIDS).
AIDS enteropathy, 841
AIDS indicator diseases, 253
AIDS-dementia complex (ADC), 1375–1376, 1376f
AIF (apoptosis inducing factor), 30, 30f
AION (anterior ischemic optic neuropathy), 1443
nonarteritic, 1443
AIP (acute intermittent porphyria), 1333t
Air blast, 446
Air embolism, 137
Air pollution
and lung cancer, 758
indoor, 430, 430t
outdoor, 428–430, 428t, 429t
Air quality standards, 428, 428t
Air-conditioner lung, 739
AIRE (autoimmune regulator), 224
AIRE (autoimmune regulator) gene, 224, 226, 1188, 1215–1216
Airspace enlargement, with fibrosis, 719
Airway(s), upper, 783–787, 783f, 785f, 787f
Airway disease, 717–728, 718t
asthma as, 718t, 723–727, 724f, 725f, 727f
bronchiectasis as, 718t, 727–728, 728f
bronchiolitis as, 718t, 722
chronic bronchitis as, 718t, 722–723, 723f
emphysema as, 717–722, 718f–721f, 718t, 721t
of small airways, 718t, 722
restrictive pulmonary disease *vs.*, 716–717
Airway remodeling, in asthma, 724
AJC (American Joint Committee) on Cancer Staging, 335
Akt, 99
AKT2 gene, in pancreatic cancer, 950, 950t
AL (amyloid light chain) protein, 259–260, 260t
Alagille syndrome, 916
Albers-Schönberg disease, 1281–1282, 1282f, 1283f
Albinism, 153
Albright hereditary osteodystrophy (AHO), pseudohypoparathyroidism in, 1189
Alcohol abuse, 421–424, 422f, 422t, 423f
and malnutrition, 447
thiamine deficiency in, 456
Alcohol dehydrogenase (ADH), 422, 422f
Alcohol use
and cancer, 284
of breast, 1132
and peptic ulcer disease, 818
congenital anomalies due to, 422t, 424, 473
ethanol myopathy due to, 1344
Alcoholic cardiomyopathy, 423, 603
Alcoholic cerebellar degeneration, 1400, 1400f
Alcoholic cirrhosis, 423
and other alcoholic liver disease, 904, 904f
clinical features of, 907
hemochromatosis in, 909
morphology of, 423, 423f, 905–906, 906f
Alcoholic hepatitis
acute, 423, 423f
clinical features of, 907
interrelation with other liver disease of, 904, 904f
morphology of, 905, 905f
Alcoholic hyalin, 34, 34f
Alcoholic hyalin bodies, 423
Alcoholic liver disease, 422t, 423, 423f, 904–907, 904f–906f
Alcoholic pancreatitis, 943–944
Alcoholism, 421–424, 422f, 422t, 423f
and malnutrition, 447
thiamine deficiency in, 456
ALD gene, 1398
Aldehyde dehydrogenase (ALDH), 422, 422f
Aldose reductase, in diabetes mellitus, 1198
Aldosterone metabolism, and hypertension, 528
Aldosterone-producing adenomas, 1210, 1212f
Aldosteronism
glucocorticoid-remediable, 1210
idiopathic, 1210
primary, 1210–1211, 1211f, 1212f
secondary, 121, 1210
Alexander disease, 1351–1352
Alginate, 379, 493
ALH (atypical lobular hyperplasia), 1129, 1130f
"Alien hand," 1391
Alimentary system. *See* Gastrointestinal tract.
Alimentary tract, in systemic sclerosis, 238
Aliphatic hydrocarbons, 431
ALK gene, in anaplastic large cell lymphoma, 684, 685
Alkaline phosphatase, in cholestasis, 888
Alkaptonuria, 39, 167–168
Alkylating agents, as carcinogens, 321t, 322
ALL. *See* Acute lymphoblastic leukemia/lymphoma (ALL).
Allergens, 206, 206f, 208
Allergic asthma, 724–726, 725f
Allergic bronchopulmonary aspergillosis (ABPA), 400, 727–728
Allergic contact dermatitis, 1254f, 1255, 1255f
Allergic gastroenteropathy, 816
Allergic granulomatosis and angiitis, 537t, 541
Allergic rhinitis, 783
Allergy, 206
atopic, 210
All-*trans*-retinal, in vision, 451
All-*trans*-retinoic acid, and congenital anomalies, 475
α cell(s), 1189
glucagon production in, 1191f
α chemokines, 71
Alpha granules, in hemostasis, 126
Alpha particles, 436
α-cell tumors, 1207
Alpha-fetoprotein (AFP), 330, 338, 339t
in germ cell tumors, 1045–1046
α-globin, in α-thalassemia, 635
α-group viruses, 365
α-helical transmembrane receptors, 56, 58–59, 58f
α-toxin, 371–372, 393
Alport syndrome, 988, 988f
ALS (amyotrophic lateral sclerosis), 1396, 1396f
ALTE (apparent life-threatening event), 496
Alternative pathway, of complement activation, 64, 66b
Aluminum deposition, renal osteodystrophy due to, 1288

Alveolar bone, 774f
Alveolar damage, diffuse. *See* Acute respiratory distress syndrome (ARDS).
Alveolar ducts, 712
Alveolar epithelium, 713
Alveolar injury, acute. *See* Acute respiratory distress syndrome (ARDS).
Alveolar macrophages, 713
Alveolar rhabdomyosarcoma, 1322, 1322f
Alveolar sacs, 712
Alveolar walls, microscopic structure of, 712–713, 712f
Alzheimer disease (AD), 1386–1389
  aggregated proteins in, 1351t
  cerebral amyloid angiopathy in, 1388
  clinical features of, 1389
  cortical atrophy in, 1386, 1386f
  Down syndrome and, 176
  epidemiology of, 1386
  familial, 1389, 1389t
  granulovacuolar degeneration in, 1388
  Hirano bodies in, 1388
  morphology of, 1386–1388, 1386f, 1387f
  neuritic plaques in, 1386–1387, 1387f
  neurofibrillary tangles in, 34, 1351, 1387, 1387f
  pathogenesis and molecular genetics of, 1388–1389, 1388f, 1389t
Alzheimer type II astrocyte, 1352
Amastigotes, 403–404
Amebapore, 839
Amebiasis, 839–840, 839f
Amebic dysentery, 834, 839–840, 839f
Amebic liver abscesses, 839
Amebic meningoencephalitis, necrotizing, 1380, 1380f
Ameloblastoma, 782
Amenorrhea
  due to anorexia nervosa, 449
  in Turner syndrome, 180
American Heart Association, classification of atherosclerotic lesions by, 517, 518f
American Joint Committee (AJC) on Cancer Staging, 335
Ames test, 320
Amides, as carcinogens, 321t, 322
Aminoaciduria, in galactosemia, 489
AML. *See* Acute myelogenous leukemia (AML).
Amnion nodosum, 472
Amniotic bands, 470–471, 471f
Amniotic fluid embolism, 137
Amoebic. *See* Amebic.
Amphetamines, abuse of, 425–426
Amphiboles, in asbestos-related diseases, 735
Amphiregulin, 505
Ampulla of Vater, 928
  adenoma of, 857, 857f
Amputation neuroma, 1335
Amylin, 1196
Amyloid, 259
  chemical nature of, 259–260
  deposits of, 259, 259f
  endocrine, 261–262
  of aging, 262
  physical nature of, 259, 259f
  renal osteodystrophy due to, 1288
  structure of, 259f
Amyloid degeneration, polymorphic, of corneal, 1430
Amyloid deposits, in medullary carcinoma of thyroid, 1182, 1182f
Amyloid light chain (AL) protein, 259–260, 260t
Amyloid precursor protein (APP), 1388–1389, 1388f, 1389t
Amyloid transthyretin (ATTR), 260, 260t, 261
Amyloid-associated (AA) protein, 259, 260, 260t
Amyloidosis, 258–264
  bleeding disorders due to, 650
  cardiac, 263, 264, 264f
  classification of, 260–262, 260t
  clinical correlation with, 264
  diagnosis of, 259, 259f, 263, 264
  gastrointestinal, 263–264
  glomerular lesions in, 992
  hemodialysis-associated, 261
  hereditary cerebral hemorrhage with, 1363
  hereditary dyscrasias with, 260–261
  heredofamilial, 260, 261, 262
  immunocyte-associated, 678
  in multiple myeloma, 680, 1005
  isolated atrial, 610
  localized, 260, 260t, 261
  morphology of, 263–264, 263f, 264f
  myocardial disease due to, 610
  of tongue, 264
  pathogenesis of, 262, 262f
  primary, 260–261, 678
  prognosis for, 264
  proteins in, 39
  secondary, 84, 260, 261
  senile
    cardiac, 262, 610
    systemic, 262
  systemic (generalized), 260, 260t
    reactive, 261
    senile, 262
Amyotrophic lateral sclerosis (ALS), 1396–1397, 1396f
ANA(s) (antinuclear antibodies)
  in Sjögren syndrome, 229t, 235
  in systemic lupus erythematosus, 227, 228, 228t, 229t, 230, 234
  in systemic sclerosis, 229t, 237
Anaerobic bacteria, 393–394, 394f
Anaerobic glycolysis, 15
Anal canal
  carcinoma of, 866, 870
  tumors of, 869–870
Analgesic nephropathy, 428, 1003–1004, 1003f, 1004t
Anaphase lag, 173
Anaphylactic reaction, cell injury due to, 13
Anaphylactic shock, 139
Anaphylatoxins, 64, 207
Anaphylaxis, systemic, 209–210
Anaplasia, 272, 273–275, 274f, 275f, 336
  in Wilms tumor, 506, 506f
Anaplasma phagocytophila, 395, 396t
Anaplastic carcinoma, of thyroid gland, 1178, 1183
Anaplastic large cell lymphoma, 671t, 684–685, 685f
Anasarca, 120, 562
Anastomosis, 531, 552
ANCAs (antineutrophil cytoplasmic antibodies)
  in pauci-immune crescentic glomerulonephritis, 977
  vasculitis due to, 212t, 535–536
ANCAs (antineutrophil cytoplasmic antibodies)-associated vasculitides, 535–536
Ancylostoma duodenale, 838
Androblastomas
  ovarian, 1103, 1104f
  testicular, 1046
Androgen(s), adrenal, 1211–1212, 1213f
Androgen insensitivity syndrome, 181
Androgen receptor *(AR)* gene, in prostate cancer, 1051
Androstenedione, 1211
Anemia(s), 622–649
  aplastic, 647–648, 647f, 647t, 648f
    oral manifestations of, 778t
Anemia(s) *(Continued)*
  classification of, 623, 623t
  clinical features of, 623
  defined, 622–623
  due to chronic liver failure, 649
  due to diffuse liver disease, 649
  Fanconi, 307, 308f, 647
  hemolytic, 623t, 624–638
    classification of, 625
    clinical manifestations of, 624
    due to trauma to red cells, 638, 638f
    etiology of, 624
    features of, 624
    immuno- (autoimmune), 210, 212t, 636–638, 637t
    in glucose-6-phosphate dehydrogenase deficiency, 627–628, 627f, 628f
    in hereditary spherocytosis, 625–627, 626f, 627f
    in paroxysmal nocturnal hemoglobinuria, 636, 636f
    in thalassemia syndromes, 632–636, 632f, 633f, 634t, 635f
    microangiopathic, 638, 638f
    morphology of, 625, 625f
    pathogenesis of, 624–625, 624f
  in fetal hydrops, 485–486
  iron deficiency, 643–646, 643t, 644f–646f
  megaloblastic, 638–643, 639f, 640t
  myelophthisic, 648–649
  of blood loss, 623–624, 645
  of chronic disease, 646
  of diminished erythropoiesis, 623t, 638–649
  of folate deficiency, 640t, 642–643, 642f
  paraneoplastic, 334t
  pernicious, 212t, 639–642, 640f, 640t, 641f
  pure red cell aplasia as, 648
  sickle cell, 628–632
    alterations in structural proteins in, 154
    clinical course of, 631–632
    genetic basis for, 150, 628
    impaired hepatic circulation in, 918
    infections with, 360
    morphology of, 630, 631f
    pathogenesis of, 628–630, 629f, 630f
    thrombus formation in, 131
Anemic infarction, 1364f, 1365, 1365f
Anencephaly, 1353–1354
Anergy, 224f, 225
Aneuploidy, 173
Aneurysm(s), 530–532
  aortic
    abdominal, 531–532, 531f
    causes of, 531
    thoracic, 532
  Charcot-Bouchard, 1366
  defined, 131, 530
  false (pseudo-), 530f, 531, 584
  fusiform, 531
  mycotic, 134, 534, 542
  saccular (berry), 531, 1366–1367, 1367f, 1368f
    in polycystic kidney disease, 964
    ruptured, 1366–1367
  syphilitic (luetic), 532
  true, 530–531, 530f
  ventricular, after myocardial infarction, 586
Aneurysmal dilation, in atherosclerosis, 520
ANF (atrial natriuretic factor), in cardiac hypertrophy, 8
Angelman syndrome, 186–187, 186f
Angiitis
  allergic granulomatosis and, 537t, 541
  of central nervous system, 1363
Angina, Ludwig, 778t

Angina pectoris, 572, 575, 575t
Prinzmetal (variant), 575
stable (typical), 575
unstable (crescendo), 575
Angioblasts, 107, 108, 515
Angiodysgenetic necrotizing myelopathy, 1368
Angiodysplasia, of intestines, 854
Angioedema, hereditary, 245
Angiofibroma, nasopharyngeal, 784
Angiogenesis, 107–109, 515
ECM proteins as regulators of, 109
from endothelial precursor cells, 108, 108f
from pre-existing vessels, 108, 108f
growth factors and receptors in, 109, 109t
in inflammation, 51f, 52
sustained, in cancer, 289, 309, 310f
vascular endothelial growth factor in, 96
Angiogenic switch, 309
Angioimmunoblastic T-cell lymphoma, 671t
Angioma(s), 545–547, 546f
spider, in hepatic failure, 882
venous, of brain, 1368
Angiomatosis, 545
bacillary, 548, 548f
encephalotrigeminal, 547
Angiomyolipoma, of kidney, 1015
Angiopathy, cerebral amyloid, 1363, 1366, 1388
Angioplasty, balloon, 551, 552f
Angiopoietins, 109
Angiosarcoma(s), 550–551, 550f
cardiac, 614
hepatic, 923
of breast, 1151
Angiotensin I and II, in blood pressure regulation, 527, 527f
Angiotensinogen, in blood pressure regulation, 527, 527f, 529f
Angiotensinogen gene, 191
ANHE (acute necrotizing hemorrhagic encephalomyelitis), 1385
Animal toxins, 435–436, 435t
ANKH gene, 1314
Ankylosing spondylitis, and HLA-B27, 205, 205t
Ankylosing spondyloarthritis, 1309
Ankyrin, in hereditary spherocytosis, 625, 626f
Anopheles mosquito, 401
Anorectal canal
carcinoma of, 866, 870
tumors of, 869–870
Anorexia, in cancer, 333
Anorexia nervosa, 449
Anorexigenic neuropeptides, 464b
Anovulatory cycle, dysfunctional uterine bleeding due to, 1081–1082, 1082f
ANP (atrial natriuretic peptide), 557
Anterior chamber, of eye, 1422f, 1430, 1430f
Anterior ischemic optic neuropathy (AION), 1443
nonarteritic, 1443
Anterior pituitary, 1157–1158, 1157f
Anterior segment, of eye, 1430–1432
and glaucoma, 1431–1432
cataract in, 1431
endophthalmitis and panophthalmitis of, 1432, 1432f, 1433f
functional anatomy of, 1430, 1430f
Anterior synechiae, 1432
Anthracosis, 39, 733
Anthrax, 345, 375–376, 376f
cutaneous, 375
gastrointestinal, 375
inhalational, 375, 376, 376f
Antibiotic-associated colitis, 836, 837–838, 837f
Antibody(ies)
antireceptor, 210, 211f
antitumor effect of, 331
Antibody(ies) *(Continued)*
in adaptive immunity, 194f
to glomerular cells, 970–971
Antibody deficiency, infections with, 360
Antibody probes, 361t
Antibody-dependent cellular cytotoxicity (ADCC), 201, 210
Antibody-mediated cellular dysfunction, 210, 211f
Antibody-mediated glomerular injury, 968–971, 968t, 969f
Antibody-mediated graft rejection, 219–220
Antibody-mediated hypersensitivity, 205, 206t, 210, 211f, 212t
Antibody-secreting cells, 199
Anticentromere antibody, in systemic sclerosis, 238
Anticipation
in fragile-X syndrome, 183
in myotonic dystrophy, 1338
Anticoagulant effects, of endothelium, 125, 126f
Antidiuretic hormone (ADH), 1158
syndrome of inappropriate secretion of, 1163
paraneoplastic, 334t
Antiendothelial cell antibodies, in vasculitides, 536
Antifibrinolytic effects, of endothelium, 126
Anti-GBM antibody—induced nephritis, 968, 969f, 976–977
Antigen(s), 194, 210
exogenous *vs.* endogenous, 211
processing and recognition of, 204, 204f
self-, 223
tumor, 328–330, 329f
Antigen masking, 331
Antigen sequestration, 225
Antigenic drift, 751
Antigenic shift, 752
Antigen-presenting cells (APCs), 196f, 197, 198f
Antineutrophil cytoplasmic antibodies (ANCAs)
in pauci-immune crescentic glomerulonephritis, 977
vasculitis due to, 212t, 535–536
Antineutrophil cytoplasmic antibodies (ANCAs)-associated vasculitides, 535–536
Antinuclear antibodies (ANAs)
in Sjögren syndrome, 229t, 235
in systemic lupus erythematosus, 227, 228, 228t, 229t, 230, 234
in systemic sclerosis, 229t, 237
Antioxidant, vitamin E as, 455
Antioxidant enzymes, 17–18, 17f
Antioxidant mechanisms, 74
Antiphospholipid antibodies, in systemic lupus erythematosus, 229
Antiphospholipid antibody syndrome, 132
hemolytic-uremic syndrome due to, 1010
secondary, 229
α-Antiplasmin, 130f
Antiplatelet effects, of endothelium, 125
Antiproteases, 73, 313
Antireceptor antibodies, 210, 211f
Anti-Scl70, in systemic sclerosis, 238
Antithrombin III, in hemostasis, 125, 126f, 130
Antithrombotic properties, of endothelium, 125, 125f, 126f
Antithyroid agents, 1165–1166
Antitreponemal antibody tests, 390
α_1-Antitrypsin (α_1-AT), 911
in emphysema, 719–720, 720f
α_1-Antitrypsin (α_1-AT) deficiency, 911–912, 912f
α_2-Antitrypsin (α_2-AT) deficiency
genetic basis for, 153
protein folding in, 38
Anti—TSH receptor autoantibodies, 1168
Antitumor effector mechanisms, 330–331
Antral glands, 810
Antrum, of stomach, 810, 810f
Anus, imperforate, 830
Aorta
aging effect on, 559t
anatomy and physiology of, 512–513
coarctation of, 564t, 570–571, 571f
"double-barreled," 533
Aortic aneurysms
abdominal, 531–532, 531f
inflammatory, 531
mycotic, 531
rupture of, 532
causes of, 531
thoracic, 532
Aortic dilation, in Marfan syndrome, 155
Aortic dissection, 532–534, 533f, 534f
Aortic insufficiency, 589
Aortic regurgitation, 589t
Aortic stenosis, 589t
acquired, 590
and atresia, 564t, 571
calcific, 590–591, 590f
of congenitally bicuspid valve, 590f, 591
senile, 590
supravalvular, 571
valvular, 571
Aortic valve, 558, 558f
infective endocarditis of, 597f
Aortic valve sclerosis, 590
Aorticosympathetic paraganglia, 1218, 1219f
Aortitis
giant cell, 536
syphilitic, 532
Aortocoronary bypass, 553
Apaf-1 (apoptosis activating factor-1), 30
APC(s) (antigen-presenting cells), 196f, 197, 198f
APC (adenomatous polyposis coli) gene, 287t
in colorectal carcinoma, 317–318, 317f, 339, 339t, 863, 863f
in familial adenomatous polyposis, 284–285
APC/ß-catenin gene, 300t, 304, 304f
APC/ß-catenin pathway, in colorectal carcinoma, 863, 863f
APECED (autoimmune polyendocrinopathy, candidiasis, and ectodermal dystrophy), 1215–1216
Apgar, Virginia, 479
Apgar score, 479, 479t
Aphthous ulcers, 776, 776f
in Crohn disease, 847, 847f, 848
Aplasia, 472
Aplastic anemia, 647–648, 647f, 647t, 648f
oral manifestations of, 778t
Aplastic crises
in hereditary spherocytosis, 627
in sickle cell disease, 631
Apocrine cysts, 1127, 1127f
Apoprotein E (ApoE) gene, 1389, 1389t
Apoptosis, 5, 11, 11f, 26–32
after growth factor deprivation, 31
biochemical features of, 27–28, 28f
causes of, 26–27
cytotoxic T-lymphocyte—stimulated, 31–32
defined, 5, 26
DNA damage—mediated, 31
dysregulated, 31–32
evasion of, in cancer, 289, 306
examples of, 31–32
execution phase of, 30–31
extrinsic (death receptor—initiated) pathway in, 28–29, 29f, 30f
features of, 13t
genes that regulate, 294f, 295t
in autoimmune disorders, 32

Apoptosis *(Continued)*
in cancer, 32
in hepatitis, 899, 900f, 901f
in HIV infection, 251–252
in neurodegenerative diseases, 32
in pathologic conditions, 26–27
in phagocytosis, 61
in physiologic situations, 26
in tissue homeostasis, 89, 89f
intrinsic (mitochondrial) pathway in, 29–30, 29f, 30f
mechanisms of, 28–31, 29f, 30f
morphologic features of, 27, 27f, 28f
of cytotoxic T lymphocytes, 331
of liver, 880
p53 gene in, 31, 302, 303, 303f
removal of dead cells in, 31
TNF-induced, 31
ultrastructural changes in, 13f
viruses and, 357
Apoptosis activating factor-1 (Apaf-1), 30
Apoptosis inducing factor (AIF), 30, 30f
Apoptotic bodies, 27
APP (amyloid precursor protein), 1388–1389, 1388f, 1389t
Apparent life-threatening event (ALTE), 496
Appendage tumors, of skin, 1238–1240, 1239f, 1240t
Appendicitis, 870–871, 871f
Appendix, 870–872
normal anatomy of, 870
tumors of, 871–872, 872f
carcinoid, 867
Appositional growth, 1278
Appropriate for gestational age (AGA), 476
APS1 (autoimmune polyendocrine syndrome type 1), 1188, 1215–1216
Aqueous humor, 1430, 1430f
AR (androgen receptor) gene, in prostate cancer, 1051
Arachidonic acid, in immediate hypersensitivity, 208, 208f
Arachidonic acid (AA), 68
Arachidonic acid (AA) metabolites, in inflammation, 57, 61, 68–70, 68t, 69f, 70f
Arachnodactyly, congenital contractural, 154
Arachnoiditis, chronic adhesive, 1370
Arboviruses, 347t
encephalitis due to, 1373
Arcuate arteries, 956
Arcuate nucleus, hypoplasia of, in sudden infant death syndrome, 496, 497
ARDS. *See* Acute respiratory distress syndrome (ARDS).
Area cerebrovasculosa, 1354
Ariboflavinosis, 457
Aristolochic acid, nephropathy due to, 1004
ARMD (age-related macular degeneration), 1422, 1441–1442, 1442f
atrophic *vs.* exudative, 1441
Arnold-Chiari malformation, 1355, 1356f
Aromatic amines, as carcinogens, 321t, 322
Aromatic hydrocarbons, 431
as carcinogens, 321t, 322
polycyclic, 431–432
Aromatic hydroxylation, of toxicant, 420f
ARPKD (autosomal-recessive polycystic kidney disease), 962t, 964–965, 965f
Arrhythmia(s)
after myocardial infarction, 584
due to mitral valve prolapse, 592
due to myocardial ischemia, 577
sudden cardiac death due to, 587
Arrhythmogenic right ventricular cardiomyopathy, 604, 604f
Arsenic
as carcinogen, 285t, 323
exposure to, 432t
Arterial dissection, 531, 532–534, 533f, 534f
Arterial embolism, ischemic bowel disease due to, 852
Arterial spider, 547–548
Arterial thrombosis, 132–133, 134, 135
ischemic bowel disease due to, 852, 852f
Arteriolar sclerosis, cerebral, 1368
Arterioles, anatomy and physiology of, 512, 513
Arteriolitis, necrotizing, 530
Arteriolosclerosis, 516
hyaline
in benign nephrosclerosis, 1006, 1007f
in diabetes, 1200, 1200f, 1201
in hypertension, 529–530, 530f
hyperplastic, 529, 530, 530f
malignant, 1008
Arteriopathy
graft, 615–616, 615f
plexogenic pulmonary, 744–745
Arteriosclerosis, 515–516
graft coronary, 615–616, 615f
Arteriovenous fistulas, 515
Arteriovenous malformations, of brain, 1368
Arteritis
giant cell (temporal), 536–538, 537f, 537t
Heubner, 1372
microscopic, 537t, 539f, 540–541
of central nervous system, 1363
Takayasu, 537t, 538–540, 538f
Artery(ies)
anatomy and physiology of, 512–513, 512f
ectatic, 513
elastic, 512–513
muscular, 512, 513
types of, 512
Arthritis, 1304–1314
chronic tophaceous, 1313, 1313f
due to rheumatic fever, 594
gouty, 1311–1314, 1312f, 1313f
in systemic lupus erythematosus, 228t
infectious, 542, 542f, 1310–1311
Lyme, 393, 1310
osteo-, 1304–1305, 1305f
due to Paget disease, 1286
obesity and, 465
secondary, 1304
pathogenesis of, 214
psoriatic, 1310
reactive, 212t, 1309–1310
rheumatoid, 1305–1309
amyloidosis with, 261
clinical course of, 1307–1309, 1308f
immune system in, 235
juvenile, 1309
uveitis in, 1433
morphology of, 1306, 1306f, 1307f
pathogenesis of, 1305–1307, 1308f
pulmonary involvement in, 731
T cell—mediated hypersensitivity in, 215t
suppurative, 1310
tuberculous, 1310
viral, 1310–1311
Arthrochalasia, 156, 156t
Arthrogryposis, 1340
Arthropod bites, 1268–1269, 1269f
Arthropod-borne viral encephalitis, 1373
Arthus reaction, 212t, 215
Artificial valves, complications of, 600–601, 600f, 600t
Arylamine exposure, and bladder carcinoma, 1032
Arylsulfatase A deficiency, 1397
Asbestos, as carcinogen, 285t, 322–323, 758, 768
Asbestos bodies, 736, 736f, 768
Asbestos fibers, as air pollutant, 430, 430t
Asbestos plaque, 736, 736f, 768
Asbestosis, 735–737, 736f
Asbestos-related diseases, 735–737, 736f
Ascaris lumbricoides, 351, 353, 838
Ascending infections, perinatal, 480
Aschoff bodies, 593, 594f, 595f
Ascites, 120, 884
chylous, 545
in right-sided heart failure, 563
Ascorbic acid, 458–459, 460f
ASD. *See* Atrial septal defect (ASD).
Aspartylglycosaminuria, 161t
Aspergilloma, 400
Aspergillosis, 399–400, 400f
allergic bronchopulmonary, 400, 727–728
invasive, 400, 400f
Aspergillus, 399–400, 400f
Aspergillus fumigatus, 400
meningoencephalitis due to, 1378
Aspiration pneumonia, 747t, 752
Aspirin
adverse effects of, 428
and colon cancer, 865
bleeding disorders related to, 653
peptic ulcer disease due to, 818
Aspirin toxicity, chronic, 428
Aspirin-sensitive asthma, 726
Asteroid hyalosis, 1434
Asthma, 718t, 723–727
atopic (allergic), 724–726, 725f
classification of, 723
clinical course of, 726–727
clinical manifestations of, 723
drug-induced, 726
immediate hypersensitivity and, 209
morphology of, 726, 727f
nonatopic (nonreaginic), 726
occupational, 726
pathogenesis of, 723–726, 724f, 725f
Asthmatic chronic bronchitis, 722
Astrocyte(s), 1349, 1350f
Alzheimer type II, 1352
fibrous, 1349
gemistocytic, 1351
protoplasmic, 1349
reactions to injury of, 1351–1352
tufted, 1390
Astrocytoma(s), 1401–1404
anaplastic, 1401
fibrillary (diffuse), 1401–1403, 1402f
gemistocytic, 1401
oligo-, 1404
pilocytic, 1403–1404, 1403f
pleomorphic xantho-, 1404
Astrogliosis, in sudden infant death syndrome, 496
Astroviruses, gastroenteritis due to, 833, 833t
α_1-AT (α_1-antitrypsin), 911
in emphysema, 719–720, 720f
α_1-AT (α_1-antitrypsin) deficiency, 911–912, 912f
α_2-AT (α_2-antitrypsin) deficiency
genetic basis for, 153
protein folding in, 38
Ataxia(s)
Friedreich, 1395, 1395t
spinocerebellar, 184t, 1394–1396, 1395t
aggregated proteins in, 1351t
Ataxia-telangiectasia
clinical features of, 1396
cutaneous manifestations of, 1245t
genetic basis for, 43, 307, 1395–1396, 1395t
morphology of, 1396

Ataxia-telangiectasia mutated *(ATM)* gene, 292t, 307
and breast cancer, 1134
and DNA repair, 308f, 1396
p53 and, 302
Ataxin, 1395t
Atelectasis, 713–714, 714f
compression, 714, 714f
contraction, 714, 714f
in neonatal respiratory distress syndrome, 481, 482, 482f
resorption, 714, 714f
Atheroemboli, 519
Atheroembolic renal disease, 1011, 1011f
Atherogenesis, 516f, 521–524, 522f, 525f
diet and, 465
Atheroma(s), 516, 517–519, 518f, 519f
Atheromatous plaques, 516, 517–519, 518f, 519f
rupture of, 573, 573f, 576
Atherosclerosis (ATH), 516–525
and ischemic heart disease, 572–575, 573f, 574f, 575t
cerebral infarction due to, 1363
cholesterol and cholesterol esters in, 37
classification of, 517, 518f
clinical features of, 516
clinical significance of, 516–517, 516f, 517f
complications of, 516f, 525
diet and, 465
epidemiology and risk factors for, 520–521, 520f, 520t
fatty streaks in, 516, 516f, 517f
in diabetes, 1200, 1200f, 1201, 1204, 1204f
in systemic lupus erythematosus, 234
infection and, 524
inflammation in, 79, 523, 574
morphology of, 516f, 517–520, 518f, 519f
natural history of, 516f
oligoclonality of lesions in, 524
pathogenesis of, 516f, 521–524, 522f, 525f
prevention of, 524
thrombosis due to, 135, 519
Atherosclerotic ischemic renal disease, 1011
Atherosis, of uterine vessels, in toxemia of pregnancy, 1109, 1110f
Athlete's foot, 1267
ATM (ataxia-telangiectasia mutated) gene, 292t, 307
and breast cancer, 1134
and DNA repair, 308f, 1396
p53 and, 302
Atmospheric pressure, injuries related to changes in, 446
ATN. *See* Acute tubular necrosis (ATN).
Atopic asthma, 724–726, 725f
Atopic dermatitis, 1254t
Atopy, 209, 210
ATP (adenosine triphosphate), cell injury due to depletion of, 14–15, 14f
ATP7B gene, 910
Atresia, 472
Atrial myxoma, 613–614, 613f
Atrial natriuretic factor (ANF), in cardiac hypertrophy, 8
Atrial (A-type) natriuretic peptide (ANP), 557
Atrial septal defect (ASD), 567–568, 567f
clinical course of, 568
defined, 567
frequency of, 564t
genetic basis for, 565
morphology of, 567–568
primum, 567
secundum, 567
Atrioventricular (AV) canal defect, complete, 564t, 567f, 568–569
Atrioventricular (AV) node, 557
Atrioventricular septal defect (AVSD), 564t, 567f, 568–569
Atrioventricular (AV) valves, 558
Atrophy, 5, 9–10
brown, 10
causes of, 9
cellular changes associated with, 10
defined, 4, 9
denervation, 9
mechanisms of, 10
of disuse, 9, 1330
pathologic, 9
physiologic, 9, 9f
senile, 9
AT/RT (atypical teratoid/rhabdoid tumor), 1408
ATTR (amyloid transthyretin), 260, 260t, 261
A-type (atrial) natriuretic peptide (ANP), 557
Atypical ductal hyperplasia (ADH), 1129, 1130f
Atypical lobular hyperplasia (ALH), 1129, 1130f
Atypical teratoid/rhabdoid tumor (AT/RT), 1408
Auer rods, in acute myelogenous leukemia, 692, 694f
Auerbach plexus, 799, 830
Auspitz sign, 1257
Autoantibodies
in diabetes, 1194
in systemic lupus erythematosus, 230
Autoantibody model, of warm antibody immunohemolytic anemia, 637
Autocatalytic reaction, 25
Autocoids, 68
Autocrine effect, of cytokines, 202
Autocrine loop, 97
Autocrine signaling, 97, 97f
Autoimmune adrenalitis, 1215–1216, 1216f
Autoimmune cholangitis, 903
Autoimmune disorder(s), 223–240
apoptosis in, 32
chronic inflammation due to, 79
criteria for, 223
etiology of, 223
examples of, 223t
generalized, 223
immunologic tolerance and, 223–226, 224f
infections and, 226–227, 226f, 227f
inflammatory myopathies as, 229t, 239
lupus erythematosus as. *See* Lupus erythematosus.
mechanisms of, 226–227, 226f, 227f
mixed connective tissue disease as, 239
organ-specific, 223
pathogenesis of, 226–227, 226f, 227f
polyarteritis nodosa and other vasculitides as, 239–240
rheumatoid arthritis as, 235
Sjögren syndrome as, 229t, 235–237, 236f
susceptibility genes in, 226, 226f
systemic sclerosis (scleroderma) as, 229t, 237–239, 237f, 238f
Autoimmune gastritis, 814, 815, 816, 824
Autoimmune hemolytic anemia, 210, 212t
Autoimmune hepatitis, 903
Autoimmune hypothyroidism, 1168
Autoimmune lymphoproliferative syndrome, 225
Autoimmune polyendocrine syndrome type 1 (APS1), 1188, 1215–1216
Autoimmune polyendocrine syndrome type 2 (APS2), 1216
Autoimmune polyendocrinopathy, candidiasis, and ectodermal dystrophy (APECED), 1215–1216
Autoimmune reaction, in rheumatoid arthritis, 1307
Autoimmune regulator (AIRE), 224
Autoimmune regulator *(AIRE)* gene, 224, 226, 1188, 1215–1216
Autoimmune thrombocytopenic purpura, 212t
Autoimmunity, 79
Autoinducer peptides, 358
Autologous saphenous vein graft, 551
Autolysis, 21
Autophagic vacuoles, 10, 32, 32f
Autophagolysosome, 32
Autophagy, 32, 32f, 159
Autoregulation, of blood pressure, 527, 527f
Autosomal dominant disorders, 150–151, 151t
Autosomal dominant inherited cancer syndromes, 284–285, 287t
Autosomal muscular dystrophies, 1338, 1338t, 1339t
Autosomal recessive disorders, 151, 151t
Autosomal-dominant polycystic kidney disease (ADPKD), 962–964, 962t, 964f, 965f
Autosomal-recessive polycystic kidney disease (ARPKD), 962t, 964–965, 965f
Autosomes, cytogenetic disorders involving, 175–178
Autosplenectomy, in sickle cell disease, 630, 631f
AV. *See* Atrioventricular (AV).
Avascular necrosis, 1289–1290, 1289t, 1290f
Avellino dystrophy, 1429
Avery, Oswald, 344
Avitaminosis A, 451, 452f
Avulsions, 1335
Axillary nodes, metastasis to, 280, 280f
Axon, 1349
regeneration of, 1351
Axonal degeneration, 1326f, 1328, 1329–1330, 1330f
Axonal injury, diffuse, of brain, 1358–1359
Axonal processes, in skin, 1228–1229
Axonal reaction, 1351
Axonopathy, 1329
Azo dyes, as carcinogens, 321t, 322
Azoospermia, in cystic fibrosis, 494
Azotemia, 960
postrenal, 960
prerenal, 960
due to heart failure, 563
Azurophil granules, 73, 73f

B

B cells (B lymphocytes)
in HIV infection, 253
in immune system, 194f, 196f, 198–199, 199f
marginal zone, 662
hyperplasia of, 666
monocytoid, 666
B ring, 800
B7-1, 198, 198f
B7-2, 198, 198f
Babesia bovis, 351t
Babesia microti, 351t, 403
Babesiosis, 403, 403f
BACE-1 (ß-secretase), 1388, 1388f
Bacillary angiomatosis, 548, 548f
Bacillary dysentery, 834–835
Bacillary peliosis, 548
Bacillus anthracis, 375–376, 376f
Backward failure, 560
Bacteremia, 84
Bacteria, 348–349, 349t
adherence to host cells by, 358
anaerobic, 393–394, 394f
enteropathogenic, 353
flesh-eating, 373
gram-negative, 348, 349t, 350f, 377–381
gram-positive, 348, 350f, 371–376

Bacteria *(Continued)*
morphology of, 348, 350f
normal, 348–349
obligate intracellular, 394–397, 395f, 396t, 397f
pyogenic, 77
virulence of, 358
Bacterial adhesion, 833–834
Bacterial endocarditis, 595–598
acute *vs.* subacute, 596
brain abscess due to, 1371
clinical features of, 596–598
diagnostic criteria for, 596–598, 598t
due to mitral valve prolapse, 592
etiology and pathogenesis of, 596
glomerular lesions in, 990
morphology of, 596, 597f
of prosthetic valve, 601
thromboembolism due to, 133
Bacterial enterocolitis, 832–838, 834t, 836f, 837f
Bacterial enterotoxins, 834
Bacterial infection(s), 371–397
abscesses as, 393
agents for, 346t, 348–349, 349t, 350f
anaerobic, 393–394, 394f
anthrax as, 375–376, 376f
chancroid as, 380
chlamydial, 346t, 349–351, 394–395
clostridial, 393–394, 394f
contagious childhood, 349t
diphtheria as, 374–375, 374f
gram-negative, 377–381
gram-positive, 371–376
granuloma inguinale as, 380–381
leprosy as, 387–388, 388f
listeriosis as, 375
Lyme disease as, 392–393, 392f
mechanisms of, 358–359
myco-, 381–388, 382f–388f
neisserial, 377–378, 378f
obligate intracellular, 394–397, 395f, 396t, 397f
of gastrointestinal tract, 353
of liver, 902
plague as, 379–380
relapsing fever as, 391–392
rickettsial, 346t, 349–351, 395–397, 395f, 396t, 397f
sexually transmitted, 356t
staphylococcal, 371–373, 372f, 373f
streptococcal, 373–374, 374f
syphilis as, 388–391, 388f–391f
tuberculosis as, 381–386, 382f–386f
whooping cough as, 378, 379f
with *Mycobacterium avium-intracellulare* complex, 386, 387f
with nocardia, 376, 376f
with *Pseudomonas,* 378–379, 379f
with spirochetes, 388–393, 388f–392f
Bacterial invasion, 834
Bacterial meningoencephalitis, 1371–1372
Bacterial overgrowth syndrome, 838
malabsorption due to, 843
Bacterial peritonitis, 872–873
Bacterial replication, 834
Bacterial toxins, 358–359
Bactericidal permeability increasing protein (BPI), 61
Bacteriophages, 348
Bacteroides fragilis, 393
BAGE proteins, 330
Balanced reciprocal translocation, 174–175, 174f
Balanitis, 398
Balanoposthitis, 1035
Balantidium coli, 351t
Balloon angioplasty, 551, 552f
Ballooned neurons, 1390
Ballooning, 1230
of fused cells in HIV infection, 251
Ballooning degeneration, of liver, 880
in hepatitis, 898, 900f
Band 3, in hereditary spherocytosis, 625, 626f
Band 4.2, in hereditary spherocytosis, 625, 626f
Band keratopathies, 1428
Banti syndrome, 917–918
Barbiturates
abuse of, 424–425
induction of smooth endoplasmic reticulum due to, 33, 33f
Bare lymphocyte syndrome, 244
Barr body, 178
Barrett esophagus, 804–805, 805f
adenocarcinoma arising from, 808–809, 809f
Barrett metaplasia, 10, 10f
Barth syndrome, 1342
Bartholin abscess, 393, 1065
Bartholin cyst, 1065
Bartonella henselae, 548
Bartonella quintana, 548
Bartonella spp, 548
Bartter syndrome, 529f
Basal cell(s), in skin, 1228f
Basal cell carcinoma (BCC)
nevoid, 1244–1245, 1245t, 1246f
of eyelid, 1424
of skin, 1242–1244, 1243f
of vulva, 1068, 1069f
Basal cell nevus syndrome, 1244–1245, 1245t, 1246f
Basal ganglia, degenerative diseases of, 1391–1394, 1392f, 1393f
Basal keratin, in breast carcinoma, 1136b, 1137b
Basement membrane (BM), 103, 103f
glomerular. *See* Glomerular basement membrane (GBM).
Basement membrane thickening, in glomerulonephritis, 967
Basic fibroblast growth factor (bFGF), 95t, 96, 294, 309
Basic multicellular unit (BMU), 1276
Basophil(s)
in immediate hypersensitivity, 207, 208
origin and differentiation of, 621f
Basophilia, 664t
Basophilic degeneration, 559
Basophilic leukocytosis, 664t
"Bat-wing" deformity, 1355
BAX gene, 303, 303f, 306
BCC. *See* Basal cell carcinoma (BCC).
B-cell antigen receptor, 198–199, 199f
B-cell lymphoma(s)
AIDS-related, 257–258, 326
gastrointestinal, 868–869
large
body cavity, 677
diffuse, 671t, 676–677, 676f, 677f
immunodeficiency-associated, 677
B-cell neoplasm(s)
peripheral, 673–683
Burkitt lymphoma as, 671t, 677–678, 678f
chronic lymphocytic leukemia as, 673–674, 674f
classification of, 671t
diffuse large B-cell lymphoma as, 671t, 676–677, 676f, 677f
follicular lymphoma as, 671t, 674–676, 675f, 676f
hairy cell leukemia as, 671t, 683, 684f
lymphoplasmacytic lymphoma as, 681–682, 681f
mantle cell lymphoma as, 671t, 682–683, 682f
B-cell neoplasm(s) *(Continued)*
marginal zone lymphoma as, 671t, 683
of plasma cells, 671t, 678–681, 679f, 680f
small lymphocytic lymphoma as, 671t, 673–674, 674f
precursor, 670–673, 671t, 672f
B-cell tyrosine kinase (Btk), 240, 241f
BCL2 oncogene, 295t, 306, 314
in follicular lymphoma, 675
BCL2 protein, 29–30, 30f
in follicular lymphoma, 675, 676f
BCL6 gene, in diffuse large B-cell lymphoma, 676
BCR-ABL protein, 297, 315
in chronic myelogenous leukemia, 697, 697f, 698
BDNF (brain-derived neurotrophic factor), in sudden infant death syndrome, 497
Becker muscular dystrophy (BMD), 1336–1338, 1337f
Beckwith-Wiedemann syndrome, 505
Becquerel (Bq), 436
Bellini duct carcinoma, 1017
Bence Jones proteins, 261, 678, 680
Bence Jones proteinuria, 1005, 1006
Bence Jones tubular casts, 1006, 1006f
Bends, 137, 446
Benign fibrous histiocytoma, 1247–1248, 1247f
Benign prostatic hyperplasia (BPH), 7, 1048–1050, 1049f
Benign recurrent intrahepatic cholestasis (BRIC), 889
Benign tumors, vascular, 545–548, 545t
Benzene, 431
cancer due to, 285t
Benzo[a]pyrene, 418, 420f, 432
Berger disease, 975t, 986–988, 987f
Bergmann gliosis, 1351, 1400
Beriberi, 457, 457f, 1399
neuropathic, 1334
Bernard-Soulier syndrome, 126, 653
Berry aneurysm, 531, 1366–1367, 1367f, 1368f
in polycystic kidney disease, 964
ruptured, 1366–1367
Beryllium
cancer due to, 285t
exposure to, 432t
ß cell(s), 1189
insulin production in, 1191, 1191f
ß cell destruction, in diabetes, 1193–1194, 1193f, 1200
ß chemokines, 71
Beta particles, 436
$ß_1$ integrins, 55b
$ß_2$ integrins, 55b
ß-amyloid (Aß) protein, 259, 260, 260t
Beta-carotene, in cancer prevention, 466
ß-cell dysfunction, in diabetes, 1196–1197
ß-cell tumors, 1205–1206, 1206f
ß-globin, in ß-thalassemia, 632, 632f, 633, 633f
ß-group viruses, lymphotropic, 365
ß-hemolytic streptococci, immune response to, 359
ß-myosin heavy chain (ß-MHC) gene, in hypertrophic cardiomyopathy, 605f, 606
ß-toxin, 372
Bezoars, 820, 820f
bFGF (basic fibroblast growth factor), 95t, 96, 294, 309
BH_4 (tetrahydrobiopterin), 488
Bicarbonate secretion, by gastric mucosa, 811
BID, 306
Bile, storage of, 927
Bile acids, 886–887
Bile canaliculi, 878, 879f

Bile duct(s), 878, 879f
  common, 928
    agenesis of, 928
  congenital anomalies of, 928
  extrahepatic
    carcinoma of, 935
    disorders of, 933–934, 934f
Bile ductules, 878, 879f
Bile formation, 885–887, 886f
Bile lakes, 889
Bile peritonitis, 936
Bile plugs, in hepatitis, 898–899, 900f
Bile salts, 886
Biliary atresia, 928, 933–934, 934f
Biliary cirrhosis
  in cystic fibrosis, 493, 495
  primary, 913t, 914–915, 914f
  secondary, 913–914, 913t, 914f
Biliary excretory function, evaluation of, 881t
Biliary stricture, 936
Biliary tract, 927–936
  congenital anomalies of, 928, 928f
  normal structure of, 927–928, 928f
  tumors of, 934–935, 935f
Biliary tract disease, intrahepatic, 913–916, 913t, 914f–916f
Biliary tree
  anomalies of, 915–916, 916f
  iatrogenic injury to, 935–936
Bilirubin, 41
  in jaundice, 887–888, 887t, 888t
  metabolism and elimination of, 885–887, 886f
  unconjugated *vs.* conjugated, 887
Biliverdin, 886f
BIM, 225
Binge eating, 449
Binswanger disease, 1369
Bioaccumulation, of toxic chemical, 419
Bioaerosols, as air pollutant, 430, 430t
Biogenic amines, in immediate hypersensitivity, 208
Bioinformatics, 146
Biologic effective dose, 417
Biologically active agents, production of, 147
Biomethylation, of inorganic mercury, 418–419, 421f
Bioprostheses, 600, 600f
Biopsy
  bone marrow, 622
    for aplastic anemia, 648, 648f
  breast, 1132
  cervical, 1079
  endomyocardial, 601
  for diagnosis of cancer, 336
  of sentinel lymph nodes, 280
Bioptome, 601
Bioterrorism agents, 345–346, 346t, 375
Biotin, 450t
Birbeck granules, 701, 702f
Bird fancier's disease, 739
Birth defects. *See* Congenital anomaly(ies).
Birth injuries, 479–480
Birth weight, 476–479
Bishop, Michael, 293
Bisphenol-A, 432
"Bite cells," 628, 628f
Bitot spots, 451, 452f
BK moles, 1233–1234, 1234f, 1245–1246
Black Death, 379–380
"Black fever," 404, 404f
Bladder, 1026–1034
  anatomy and physiology of, 1024
  congenital anomalies of, 1026, 1026f
  diverticula of, 1026
  exstrophy of, 1026, 1026f
  inflammations of, 1027–1028, 1028f
Bladder *(Continued)*
  metaplastic lesions of, 1028
  obstruction of, 1033–1034, 1033f
  radiation effect on, 440–441
Bladder carcinoma
  adeno-, 1032
  clinical course of, 1032–1033
  epidemiology and pathogenesis of, 1032
  in situ, 1029, 1030–1031, 1031f
  papillary, 1029, 1029f, 1029t, 1030, 1030f
  signet-ring cell, 1032
  squamous cell, 1031–1032
  staging of, 1031, 1031t
  treatment for, 1033
  urothelial, 1029–1031, 1029f–1031f, 1029t, 1031t
Bladder tumors, 1028–1033, 1029t
  adenocarcinomas as, 1032
  clinical course of, 1032–1033
  epidemiology and pathogenesis of, 1032
  mesenchymal, 1033
  secondary, 1033
  squamous cell carcinomas as, 1031–1032
  urothelial (transitional cell), 1028–1031, 1029f–1031f, 1029t, 1031t
Bland infarction, 1364f, 1365, 1365f
Blast injury, 446
Blastoconidia, of *Candida,* 398, 398f
Blastomyces dermatidis, pneumonia due to, 754, 755, 755f
Blastomycosis, 754, 755, 755f
Bleeding, anemia due to, 623–624
Bleeding diathesis, 123
  due to vitamin K deficiency, 456
Bleeding disorder(s), 649–658
  due to abnormalities in clotting factors, 653–656, 654f
  due to defective platelet functions, 653
  due to disseminated intravascular coagulation, 656–658, 657t, 658f
  due to thrombocytopenia, 650–653, 651t
  due to vessel wall abnormalities, 650
Bleeding time, 649
Blepharitis, 1424
Blister, 1229
Blistering diseases, 1259–1264, 1260f–1264f
BLM helicase, 307
Blood
  formed elements of, 620
  oxygen content of, and infarction, 139
Blood alcohol level, 421–422
Blood cells, normal development of, 620–622, 621f
Blood flow
  in inflammation, 49, 50, 50f
  in thrombosis, 131, 131f
  laminar *vs.* turbulent, 131
Blood glucose
  in diabetes, 1190
  in regulation of insulin release, 1191, 1192f
Blood loss, anemias of, 623–624, 645
Blood pressure, regulation of, 526–528, 527f
Blood supply, to heart, 557–558
Blood transfusion, transmission of HIV via, 245, 246
Blood vessels
  amyloid infiltration of, 650
  development, growth, and remodeling of, 514–515
  normal anatomy of, 512–513, 512f
  of kidney, 956
  radiation effect on, 439–440, 440f
  response to injury of, 515, 515f
Blood-brain barrier, 1327
Bloodstream expression sites, 405
Bloom syndrome, 307
Blue bloaters, 721
Blue nevus, 1233t
Blue sclerae, 1280, 1281t, 1426
"Blueberry muffin baby," 502
BM (basement membrane), 103, 103f
  glomerular. *See* Glomerular basement membrane (GBM).
BMD (Becker muscular dystrophy), 1336–1338, 1337f
BMI1 gene, 278
BMPR2 (bone morphogenetic protein receptor type 2), in pulmonary hypertension, 743–744, 744f
BMU (basic multicellular unit), 1276
Body cavity large cell lymphoma, 677
Body mass index (BMI), 461, 462, 462t, 464b
Boil, 372
Bone(s), 1273–1303
  fractures of, 1288–1289, 1289f
  growth and development of, 1276–1278, 1278f
    abnormalities in, 1278–1288, 1280t
    and rickets, 453, 454f
  heterotopic, 41
  lamellar, 1275–1276, 1277f
    mosaic pattern of, 1285–1286, 1285f
  marble, 1281–1282, 1282f, 1283f
  modeling and remodeling of, 1276
  normal anatomy and physiology of, 1274–1276, 1275f–1277f, 1278t
  proteins of, 1275–1276, 1278t
  vitamin D effect on, 453, 453f
  woven, 1275–1276, 1277f
Bone cells, abnormalities in, 1278–1288
Bone disorder(s)
  due to abnormal mineral homeostasis, 1287–1288, 1287f
  due to collagen diseases, 1279–1281, 1281t, 1282f
  due to defects in extracellular structural proteins, 1279–1281, 1280t, 1281t, 1282f
  due to defects in folding and degradation of macromolecules, 1281
  due to defects in hormones, 1279, 1280t
  due to defects in metabolic pathways, 1281–1282, 1282f, 1283f
  due to defects in nuclear proteins, 1279
  due to defects in signal transduction mechanisms, 1279, 1280t
  due to defects in transcription factors, 1279, 1280t
  due to developmental abnormalities, 1278–1288, 1280t
  due to hyperparathyroidism, 1287, 1287f
  due to infections, 1290–1292, 1291f
  due to osteoclast dysfunction, 1284–1286, 1285f, 1286f
  genetic basis for, 1278–1279, 1280t
  mucopolysaccharidoses as, 1281
  osteogenesis imperfecta as, 1279–1280, 1280t, 1281t, 1282f
  osteomalacia as, 1287
  osteomyelitis as
    pyogenic, 1290–1291, 1291f
    tuberculous, 1291–1292
  osteonecrosis (avascular necrosis) as, 1289–1290, 1289t, 1290f
  osteopetrosis as, 1281–1282, 1282f, 1283f
  osteoporosis as, 1282–1284, 1283f, 1283t, 1284f
  Paget disease (osteitis deformans) as, 1284–1286, 1285f, 1286f
  renal osteodystrophy as, 1287–1288
  rickets as, 453–455, 454f, 454t, 455f, 1287
  skeletal syphilis as, 1292
Bone eburnation, 1305, 1305f

Bone marrow
  anatomy of, 622
  in ariboflavinosis, 457
  in malnutrition, 449
  sarcoidosis of, 738
Bone marrow biopsy, 622
  for aplastic anemia, 648, 648f
Bone marrow embolization, 1364, 1364f
Bone marrow stem cells, 92–93, 94f
Bone marrow stromal cells, 92, 94f
Bone marrow suppression, due to leukocyte defects, 62
Bone marrow transplantation
  hepatic complications of, 921
  infections with, 361
  rejection of, 222–223
Bone mass
  decreased, 1282–1284, 1283f, 1283t, 1284f
  peak, 1276, 1283, 1283f
Bone matrix, 1274
  abnormalities in, 1278–1288
Bone morphogenetic protein receptor type 2 (BMPR2), in pulmonary hypertension, 743–744, 744f
Bone resorption, 1275, 1276f, 1277f
Bone tissue, hypercalcemia due to destruction of, 41–42
Bone tumor(s), 1292–1303
  bone-forming, 1293–1296, 1293f–1295f
  cartilage-forming, 1296–1299, 1296f–1299f
  chondroblastoma as, 1297–1298, 1297f
  chondroma as, 1296–1297, 1297f
  chondrosarcoma as, 1298–1299, 1299f
  classification of, 1292, 1292t
  clinical presentation of, 1293
  epidemiology of, 1292–1293
  Ewing sarcoma as, 1301–1302, 1302f
  fibroma as
    chondromyxoid, 1298, 1298f
    nonossifying, 1299, 1300f
  fibrosarcoma as, 1301
  fibrous and fibro-osseous, 1299–1301, 1300f, 1301f
  fibrous cortical defect as, 1299, 1300f
  fibrous dysplasia as, 1300–1301, 1301f
  genetic basis for, 1293
  giant cell tumor (osteoclastoma) as, 1302, 1302f, 1303f
  malignant fibrous histiocytoma as, 1301
  metastatic, 1302–1303
  osteoblastoma as, 1293–1294
  osteochondroma as, 1296, 1296f
  osteoma as, 1293
    osteoid, 1293–1294, 1293f, 1294f
  osteosarcoma as, 1294–1296, 1294f, 1295f
  primitive neuroectodermal tumor as, 1301–1302
Bone-forming tumor(s), 1293–1296, 1293f–1295f
Bony callus, 1288–1289, 1289f
Border zone infarcts, 1362–1363
Bordetella pertussis, 353, 378, 379f
Bordetella virulence gene *(bvg),* 378
Borrelia burgdorferi, 350f, 392–393
  arthritis due to, 1310
  immune evasion by, 359–360
  myocarditis due to, 608
  neuroborreliosis due to, 1372
Borrelia recurrentis, 359, 391
Botanical agents, 434t
Botulism, 393–394
Botulism toxin (Botox), 393–394
Boutonneuse fever, 396t
Bovine spongiform encephalopathy (BSE), 346
Bowel. *See* Large intestine; Small intestine.
Bowel infarction, 851–854, 852f, 853f
Bowen disease, 1036, 1036f
Bowenoid papulosis, 1036, 1266
Bowing, of legs, 455, 455f
BPD (bronchopulmonary dysplasia), 482, 483
BPH (benign prostatic hyperplasia), 7, 1048–1050, 1049f
BPI (bactericidal permeability increasing protein), 61
Bq (becquerel), 436
Brachial plexopathy, 1334
Brachydactyly type C, 1280t
Brachytherapy, for prostate cancer, 1055
Bradykinin, 65, 68, 74t
BRAF oncogene, 295t, 296
  in melanoma, 1247
  in thyroid carcinoma, 1177, 1178
Brain. *See also* Central nervous system (CNS).
  concussion of, 1357
  contusion of, 1357–1358, 1358f
  effects of shock on, 141
  in heart failure
    left-sided, 563
    right-sided, 563
  in malnutrition, 449
  in Wilson disease, 911
  laceration of, 1357
  neurogenesis in, 94
  of preterm infant, 479
  respirator, 1361
  vascular malformations of, 1367–1368
Brain abscess, 1371, 1371f
"Brain death," 1361
Brain herniation, 122, 1352–1353, 1353f
Brain injury
  coup *vs.* contrecoup, 1357
  open *vs.* closed, 1357
  parenchymal, 1357–1359, 1360f
  perinatal, 1356, 1356f
  sequelae of, 1360
  vascular, 1359–1360, 1359f, 1360f
Brain (B-type) natriuretic peptide, 557
Brain-derived neurotrophic factor (BDNF), in sudden infant death syndrome, 497
Brainstem, degenerative diseases of, 1391–1394, 1392f, 1393f
Brainstem encephalitis, paraneoplastic, 1410, 1411t
Brainstem glioma, 1404
Brainstem hemorrhage, secondary, 1353–1354, 1354f
Branchial cyst, 788–789
Branchiomeric paraganglia, 1218, 1219f
BRCA1 gene, 287t, 300t, 307–308
  and DNA repair, 308f
  DNA methylation and, 315
  in breast cancer, 1133–1134, 1133t
    and nongenetic factors, 286
    male, 1152
  in ovarian cancer, 1093
BRCA2 gene, 287t, 300t, 307–308
  and DNA repair, 308f
  in breast cancer, 1133–1134, 1133t
    and nongenetic factors, 286
    male, 1152
  in ovarian cancer, 1093
  in pancreatic cancer, 949f, 950, 950t
BRCA3 gene, 1134–1135
"Bread-and-butter" pericarditis, due to rheumatic fever, 593, 595f
Breast(s), 1119–1152
  adenosis of, 1127
    sclerosing, 1128, 1128f
      complex, 1128, 1129f
  benign epithelial lesions of, 1126–1129, 1127f–1130f, 1130t
  calcifications in, 1123t, 1124
Breast(s) *(Continued)*
  cysts of, 1127, 1127f
  densities in, 1123t, 1124
  developmental disorders of, 1122
  epithelial hyperplasia of, 1128, 1128f
  fibroadenoma of, 278f, 1149–1150, 1149f, 1150f
  fibrocystic changes of, 1127, 1127f
  fibromatosis of, 1151
  fibrosis of, 1127
  fibrous tumors of, 1151
  gynecomastia of, 1151–1152, 1152f
  inflammations of, 1124–1126, 1125f, 1126f
  lactational adenomas of, 1127
  life cycle changes in, 1120–1121, 1121f
  lymphomas of, 1151
  male, 1151–1152, 1152f
  metastasis to, 1151
  nonproliferative changes in, 1127, 1127f, 1130t
  normal anatomy of, 1120, 1120f, 1121f
  papillomas of, 1128–1129, 1129f
  phyllodes tumor of, 1150, 1150f
  proliferative changes in
    with atypia, 1129, 1130t
    without atypia, 1127–1129, 1128f, 1129f, 1130t
  pseudoangiomatous stromal hyperplasia of, 1151
  radiation effect on, 441, 441f
  sarcomas of, 1150–1151
  stromal tumors of, 1149–1151, 1149f, 1150f
  supernumerary, 1122
Breast augmentation, 1122
Breast biopsies, and breast cancer, 1132
Breast carcinoma, 1129–1149
  basal-like, 1136b, 1137b
  classification of, 1138–1146, 1143t
  clinical presentation of, 1123t
  DNA content in, 1148
  ductal (intraductal)
    in situ, 1123t, 1130t, 1135, 1139–1141, 1139f–1141f
    invasive, 279f, 1142–1144, 1143f, 1144f
  epidemiology of, 1129–1133, 1130t, 1131f
  estrogen and progesterone receptors in, 1147–1148, 1148f
  estrogen receptor—negative, 1136b, 1138
  estrogen receptor—positive, 1136b, 1137b, 1138
  etiology and pathogenesis of, 1133–1138
  first-degree relatives with, 1132
  gene expression profiling of, 315, 316b, 1135, 1136b–1137b, 1148
  genetic predisposition to, 286, 1133–1135, 1133t
  grading of, 1147
  HER2-positive, 1136b, 1137b
  in males, 1152
  in situ, 1138–1142, 1139f–1142f, 1143t
    ductal, 1123t, 1130t, 1135, 1139–1141, 1139f–1141f
    lobular, 1123t, 1130t, 1141–1142, 1142f
  inflammatory, 1142, 1147
  invasive (infiltrating), 1123t, 1142–1145, 1143t
    ductal, 279f, 1142–1144, 1143f, 1144f
    lobular, 1144–1145, 1144f
  lobular
    in situ, 1123t, 1130t, 1141–1142, 1142f
    invasive, 1144–1145, 1144f
  locally advanced, 1147
  lymphatic spread of, 279–280, 280f
  lymphedema due to, 121–122
  lymphovascular invasion in, 1148
  mammographic screening for, 1123–1124, 1123t, 1124f, 1131

Breast carcinoma *(Continued)*
mechanisms of carcinogenesis for, 1135–1138, 1138f
medullary, 1145, 1145f
metaplastic, 1146
metastatic, 1146–1147
mucinous (colloid), 1145–1146, 1145f
of contralateral breast, 1132
oral contraceptives and, 427
papillary
in situ, 1140, 1141f
invasive, 1146
prognostic and predictive factors for, 1146–1149, 1148f
proliferative rate in, 1148
radiation exposure and, 441
risk factors for, 1131–1133, 1135
sporadic, 1135
therapy for, 1148–1149
tubular, 1146, 1146f
tumor size in, 1147
with lymph node metastases, 1123t
Breast disease, clinical presentation of, 1122–1124, 1123f, 1123t, 1124f
Breast implants, 1122
Breast lesions, anatomical locations of common, 1120f
Breast masses, 1123, 1124f
Breast pain, 1122–1123
Breast reconstruction, 1122
Breast tissue, accessory axillary, 1122
Breast-feeding, and breast cancer, 1132
Brenner tumor, 1098, 1099f
BRIC (benign recurrent intrahepatic cholestasis), 889
Bridging fibrosis, in hepatitis, 899, 900f
Bridging necrosis, of liver, 880
in hepatitis, 899, 900f
Bridging veins, 1359
Brill-Zinsser disease, 396t
Broad-spectrum inhibitors, 70
Brodie abscess, 1291
Bronchial carcinoids, 764–765, 764f
Bronchiectasis, 718t, 727–728, 728f
in cystic fibrosis, 495, 728f
saccular, 728
Bronchioles, 712
Bronchiolitis, 718t, 722
due to influenza, 752
Bronchiolitis obliterans, 722
in lung transplant patients, 757, 757f
Bronchiolitis obliterans organizing pneumonia, 731, 732f
Bronchiolitis-associated interstitial lung disease, 740–741
Bronchioloalveolar carcinoma, 760, 761–762, 762f
Bronchitis, chronic, 722–723, 723t
emphysema *vs.*, 721t
Bronchogenic cyst, 713, 799
Bronchopneumonia, 749, 749f, 750
herpes, 366
Bronchopulmonary dysplasia (BPD), 482, 483
Bronchopulmonary sequestration, 713
Bronchospasm, 723
Bronchus(i), 712
Brown atrophy, 10, 559
Brown induration, 715
Brown tumors, 1186, 1287, 1287f
Brugia malayi, 410
Bruise, 40
Brunn nests, 1028
Brunner glands, 829
Brush border, 829
BSE (bovine spongiform encephalopathy), 346
Btk (B-cell tyrosine kinase), 240, 241f
B-type natriuretic peptide, 557
Buboes, 380
Bubonic plague, 380
Budd-Chiari syndrome, 699, 919, 919f
Buerger disease, 539f, 542
Buffalo hump, 1209
Bulbar amyotrophic lateral sclerosis, 1397
Bulbar palsy, progressive, 1397
Bulbospinal atrophy, 184t, 1397
Bulimia, 449
Bulla, 1229
Bullet wounds, 444, 444f
Bullous diseases, 1259–1264, 1260f–1264f
Bullous impetigo, 372, 1260f
Bullous keratopathy, 1427
in Fuchs endothelial dystrophy, 1428
pseudophakic, 1429
Bullous pemphigoid, 1260f–1262f, 1261–1262
oral manifestations of, 778t
Bundle of His, 557
Buphthalmos, 1444
Burkholderia cepacia, 379, 494, 495
Burkitt lymphoma, 677–678
cell of origin of, 671t
chromosomal translocation and oncogenes for, 298t, 314, 314t, 671t, 677
clinical features of, 671t, 678
Epstein-Barr virus and, 326, 326f, 677–678
genetic and other markers of, 500t
immunophenotype of, 677
morphology of, 677, 678f
Burn(s)
first-degree, 445
fourth-degree, 444
full-thickness, 444, 445
infections with, 361
partial-thickness, 444–445
second-degree, 445
thermal, 444–445
third-degree, 444
Burnet, Macfarlane, 328
bvg (*Bordetella* virulence gene), 378
BVGS, 378
Byler disease, 889
Byler syndrome, 889

C

C cells, 1166
C chemokines, 72
C1, in inflammation, 64
C1 inhibitor (C1INH), 66b, 67b
C1 inhibitor (C1INH) deficiency, 245
C1q, in systemic lupus erythematosus, 229–230
C2, in systemic lupus erythematosus, 229
C2 deficiency, 67b, 244
C2 kinin, 67b
C3, in inflammation, 64–65, 66b
C3 convertase, 64, 66b
C3 deficiency, 67b, 244
C3 nephritic factor (C3NeF), 985, 987f
C3a
in antibody-mediated hypersensitivity, 210
in inflammation, 64, 68, 74t
in systemic immune complex disease, 213
C3b
in antibody-mediated hypersensitivity, 210
in inflammation, 64
C4, in systemic lupus erythematosus, 229
C4 deficiency, 67b
C4a
in antibody-mediated hypersensitivity, 210
in inflammation, 64
C4b, in antibody-mediated hypersensitivity, 210
C5, in inflammation, 64–65, 66b
C5 convertase, 64, 66b
C5 deficiency, 245
C5a
in antibody-mediated hypersensitivity, 210
in inflammation, 64, 68, 74t
in systemic immune complex disease, 213
C5b, in inflammation, 64
C5b-C9, in glomerulonephritis, 972
C6 deficiency, 245
C7 deficiency, 245
C8 deficiency, 245
C9 deficiency, 245
C282Y mutation, 908
Ca^{2+}. *See* Calcium (Ca^{2+}).
CA-15-3, 339t
CA-19-9, 330, 339t
CA-125, 330, 339, 339t
CAA (cerebral amyloid angiopathy), 1363, 1366, 1388
c-ABL oncogene, 297
Cachexia, 9, 448
due to cancer, 333
in ß-thalassemia, 634
CAD. *See* Coronary artery disease (CAD).
CADASIL (cerebral autosomal-dominant arteriopathy with subcortical infarcts and leukoencephalopathy), 1363
Cadherins, 104, 105, 305–306, 311
Cadmium
cancer due to, 285t
exposure to, 432t, 433
Café au lait macules, in neurofibromatosis, 169, 1412
CagA (cytotoxin-associated antigen) gene, 328
in peptic ulcer disease, 818
CAH (congenital adrenal hyperplasia), 1212–1214
Caisson disease, 137, 446
Cajal-Retzius cells, 1355
Calcific band keratopathy, 1428
Calcification(s)
dystrophic, 22, 41, 41f
in breast, 1123t, 1124
metastatic, 41–42
of atheroma, 518
of fatty acid residues, 24
of prosthetic valve, 600f
pathologic, 5, 41–42, 41f
valvular degeneration due to, 589–591, 590f
Calciphylaxis, 1188
Calcitonin, 1166
as tumor marker, 339t
in medullary carcinoma of thyroid, 1182, 1182f
Calcium (Ca^{2+})
and osteoporosis, 1284
intracellular influx of, 15–16, 16f
milk of, 1127
Calcium absorption, vitamin D and, 453, 453f
Calcium homeostasis, loss of, 15–16, 16f
Calcium hydroxyapatite, in bone, 1274
Calcium ions, in coagulation cascade, 128, 128f, 129f
Calcium oxalate stones, 1014, 1014t
Calcium pyrophosphate crystal deposition disease (CPPD), 1314, 1314f
Calcium signals, 100
Calcium soaps, 24
Calcium-sensing receptor *(CASR)* gene, 1185
Calciviruses, gastroenteritis due to, 833, 833t
Calculus(i)
renal, 960, 1014–1015, 1014t, 1015f
staghorn, 1014
ureteral, 1025t
CALLA (common acute lymphoblastic leukemia antigen), 330
Call-Exner bodies, 1102, 1102f

Callus
bony, 1288–1289, 1289f
soft tissue, 1288
Caloric deficiency, 448
Calpain 3, 1339t
Calymmatobacterium granulomatis, 356t, 380–381
Calyx(ces), major and minor, 956
Cambium layer, 1322
cAMP (adenosine 3,'5'-cyclic monophosphate), 98f, 100
Campomelic dysplasia, 1280t
CAMPs (cationic antimicrobial peptides), 360
Campylobacter, 353, 356t
Campylobacter enterocolitis, 835, 837
Campylobacter jejuni, 835, 837
CAMs (cell adhesion molecules), in extracellular matrix, 103f, 104–105, 106f
Canaliculi, 1275
Canals of Hering, 878, 879f
liver stem cells in, 93, 93f
Canavan disease, 1398
c-ANCA (cytoplasmic antineutrophil cytoplasmic antibodies), 535
in pauci-immune crescentic glomerulonephritis, 977
Cancer. *See also* Neoplasm(s); Tumor(s).
age and, 284, 286t, 287t
apoptosis in, 32
cachexia due to, 333
chemoprevention of, 466
chronic inflammation and, 287
defective DNA repair in, 285, 287t, 288, 289, 306–308, 308t
defined, 270
dissemination of, 279–281, 280f
via hematogenous spread, 280–281, 280f
via lymphatic spread, 279–280, 280f
via seeding of body cavities and surfaces, 279, 280f
effect on host of, 332–335, 334t
epidemiology of, 270, 281–288
essential alterations for transformation to, 289, 290f
ethanol and, 424
evasion of apoptosis in, 289, 306
familial, 286–287, 287t
genetic predisposition to, 284–286, 287t, 338
geographic and environmental factors in, 283–284, 284f, 285t
grading and staging of, 335
in infants and children, 499–506, 500t
incidence of, 282–283, 282f, 283f
insensitivity to growth inhibitory signals in, 289, 298–306, 300t, 301f–304f
laboratory diagnosis of, 335–339, 336f, 337f, 339t
limitless replicative potential of, 289, 308–309, 308f
local and hormonal effects of, 332–333
local invasion by, 278–279, 278f, 279f, 289, 311–313, 312f
metastasis of. *See* Metastasis(es).
molecular basis of, 288–315
mortality rates from, 282–283, 282f, 283f
nonhereditary predisposing conditions for, 286–288
obesity and, 284, 465, 465t
occupational, 283, 285t
oncogenes in, 292–298, 294f, 295t, 297f–299f
paraneoplastic syndromes due to, 333–335, 334t
polypoid, 271
precancerous conditions and, 287–288
self-sufficiency in growth signals in, 289, 292–298, 294f, 295t, 297f–299f
Cancer. *See also* Neoplasm(s); Tumor(s) *(Continued)*
sustained angiogenesis in, 289, 309, 310f
tumor markers for, 338–339, 339t
Cancer cell(s)
chromosomal changes in, 314–315
epigenetic changes in, 315
gene amplification in, 315
molecular profiles of, 315, 316b, 317f
Cancer cell lineages, 278
Cancer immunoediting, 328
Cancer stem cells, 278
Cancer suppressor genes, 294f
Cancer-associated genes, dysregulation of, 314–315, 316b, 317f
Cancer-associated retinopathy, 1442
Candida albicans, 352, 397
Candida endocarditis, 399
Candida esophagitis, 398
Candida infection
meningoencephalitis due to, 1378
of female genital tract, 1063, 1063t
of gastrointestinal tract, 353
Candida vaginitis, 398
"Candidate gene" approach, 146, 147f
Candidiasis, 397–399, 398f
chronic mucocutaneous, 398–399
cutaneous, 398
esophagitis due to, 806
in AIDS, 256
invasive, 399
oral, 777
Canker sores, 776, 776f
Cannabinoids, abuse of, 424t, 426
Capillary(ies), anatomy and physiology of, 513
Capillary hemangioma, 498f, 546, 546f
cutaneous, 1248
lobular, 547
Capillary lymphangioma, 547
Capillary telangiectasias, of brain, 1368
Capsular drops, 992
Caput succedaneum, 480
Carbamates, 434t, 435
Carbaryl (Sevin), 435
Carbon, accumulations of, 39
Carbon monoxide
as air pollutant, 428t, 430, 430t
in tobacco smoke, 419
Carbon monoxide toxicity, neurologic effects of, 1400
Carbon tetrachloride (CCl_4), 431
cell injury due to, 25, 25f, 26f
Carbonic anhydrase II deficiency, osteopetrosis due to, 1281
Carboxyhemoglobin, 431
Carbuncle, 372–373
Carcinoembryonic antigen (CEA), 330, 338, 339t
Carcinogen(s)
chemical, 320–321, 321t, 322–323
in tobacco smoke, 419, 419t
metabolic activation of, 320
naturally occurring, 321t, 322
ultimate, 320, 322
Carcinogenesis
chemical, 319–323, 320f, 321f, 321t
initiation and promotion phases of, 319–322, 320f, 321f
multistep, 288–289, 315–318, 317f, 318f
of breast carcinoma, 1135–1138, 1138f
of ionizing radiation, 323–324, 438
promotion of, 321–322
radiation, 323–324
stromal microenvironment and, 313
viral and microbial, 324–328, 325f, 326f
Carcinoid heart disease, 599–600, 599f
Carcinoid syndrome, 334t, 868, 868t
Carcinoid tumors
bronchial, 764–765, 764f
gastric, 827
gastrointestinal, 866–868, 867f, 868t
ovarian, 1100
pancreatic, 1207
strumal, 1100
Carcinoma, 271
adeno-. *See* Adenocarcinoma.
adenoid cystic, of salivary gland, 793–794, 794f
adenosquamous
of cervix, 1078
of pancreas, 951
adrenocortical, 1217–1218, 1217f
androgen-secreting, 1212
Cushing syndrome due to, 1208, 1209
basal cell
nevoid, 1244–1245, 1245t, 1246f
of eyelid, 1424
of skin, 1242–1244, 1243f
of vulva, 1068, 1069f
bladder. *See* Bladder carcinoma.
breast. *See* Breast carcinoma.
cervical. *See* Cervical carcinoma.
cholangio-, 926–927, 926f
chorio-
gestational, 1112–1113, 1113f
ovarian, 1101–1102
testicular, 1041, 1043–1044, 1044f
clear cell
of endometrium, 1088
of ovaries, 1098
of vagina, 1071, 1071f
colorectal. *See* Colorectal carcinoma.
embryonal, 1041, 1043, 1043f
infantile, 1043
endometrial, 1086–1088, 1087f
endometrioid, 1087–1088, 1097–1098
esophageal, 806–809, 807f–809f, 807t
fibrolamellar, of liver, 925, 925f, 926
gastric. *See* Gastric carcinoma.
hepatocellular. *See* Hepatocellular carcinoma (HCC).
invasive, 275
laryngeal, 786, 787f
lung. *See* Lung carcinoma.
Merkel cell, 1244
mucoepidermoid
of conjunctiva, 1426
of salivary gland, 793, 794f
nasopharyngeal, 785, 785f
neuroendocrine, of cervix, 1078f
of anal canal, 870
of cecum, 865, 865f
of ear, 788
of extrahepatic bile ducts, 935
of eyelid, 1424–1425, 1425f
of gallbladder, 934–935, 935f
of penis, 1036–1037, 1036f, 1037f
of ureter, 1025, 1025f
of urethra, 1034, 1034f
of vagina, 1071, 1071f
of vulva, 1067–1068, 1069f
ovarian, 1095, 1095f, 1096f, 1098, 1099
pancreatic. *See* Pancreatic carcinoma.
papillary
of breast
in situ, 1140, 1141f
invasive, 1146
of kidney, 1016, 1017, 1017f, 1018, 1018f
of thyroid gland, 1177–1180, 1179f, 1179t
serous, of endometrium, 1087, 1088
transitional cell
of renal pelvis, 1004
of ureter, 1025, 1025f

Carcinoma *(Continued)*
parathyroid, 1186
periampullary, 935
pituitary, 1162
renal cell, 1016–1018, 1017f, 1018f
sebaceous, of eyelid, 1424–1425, 1425f
serous
of endometrium, 1087, 1088
of ovaries, 1096, 1096f
signet-ring cell
gastric, 825, 825f
of bladder, 1032
squamous cell. *See* Squamous cell carcinoma (SCC).
thymic, 707, 708
thyroid. *See* Thyroid carcinoma.
urothelial
in situ, 1029, 1030–1031, 1031f
of prostate, 1056
of renal pelvis, 1018–1019, 1019f
papillary, 1029, 1029f, 1029t, 1030, 1030f
verrucous
of penis, 1037
of vulva, 1068, 1069f
Carcinoma ex pleomorphic adenoma, of salivary gland, 792
Carcinoma in situ (CIS), 275, 275f, 279
of breast, 1138–1142, 1139f–1142f, 1143t
ductal, 1123t, 1130t, 1135, 1139–1141, 1139f–1141f
lobular, 1123t, 1130t, 1141–1142, 1142f
of penis, 1036, 1036f
of skin, 1242
urothelial, 1029, 1030–1031, 1031f
Carcinoma-associated fibroblasts, 313
Carcinosarcomas, endometrial, 1088, 1089f
Cardia, of stomach, 810, 810f
Cardia glands, 810
Cardiac. *See also* Heart.
Cardiac amyloidosis, 263, 264, 264f
Cardiac cirrhosis, 563, 883
Cardiac death, sudden, 575t, 577, 586–587
Cardiac disease, in Down syndrome, 176
Cardiac dysfunction, principles of, 559–563, 561f, 562f
Cardiac effects, of shock, 141–142
Cardiac hypertrophy, 7–9, 8f, 560–562, 561f, 562f
Cardiac murmurs, 589
Cardiac muscle, regeneration of, 91, 94
Cardiac myocytes, 556–557, 556f
Cardiac output, in blood pressure regulation, 526, 527f
Cardiac rupture syndromes, 584–585, 585f
Cardiac sclerosis, 563, 918
Cardiac tamponade, 611
Cardiac thrombosis, 132–133, 133f, 135
Cardiac transplantation, 615–616, 615f
Cardiac valves, 558, 558f
aging effect on, 559, 559t
artificial, complications of, 600–601, 600f, 600t
Cardiogenic shock, 139, 140t, 584
Cardiomegaly, 556
Cardiomyopathy(ies), 601–611
alcoholic, 423, 603
arrhythmogenic right ventricular, 604, 604f
catecholamine, 1221
causes of, 601, 602t
classification of, 601, 601f, 602t
defined, 601
diagnosis of, 601
dilated (congestive), 601, 602–604
arrhythmogenic right ventricular, 604, 604f
clinical features of, 604
etiology of, 602, 602t
Cardiomyopathy(ies) *(Continued)*
idiopathic, 602
morphology of, 601f, 602–603, 603f
pathogenesis of, 603–604, 606, 607f
thyrotoxic, 1166
due to adriamycin and other drugs, 609–610
due to amyloidosis, 610
due to catecholamines, 610
due to hyperthyroidism and hypothyroidism, 610–611
due to iron overload, 610
hypertrophic, 601, 604–606
clinical features of, 606
etiology of, 602t
morphology of, 601f, 605–606, 605f
pathogenesis of, 604f, 606, 607f
idiopathic, 601
ischemic, 586, 601
myocarditis form of, 608–609, 608t, 609f
peripartum (pregnancy-associated), 603
restrictive, 601, 601f, 602t, 606–607
Cardiovascular collapse. *See* Shock.
Cardiovascular disease
hormone replacement therapy and, 428
in diabetes, 1200, 1200f, 1201, 1204, 1204f
oral contraceptives and, 427
Cardiovascular lesions, in Marfan syndrome, 155
Cardiovascular system
alcohol effect on, 422t, 423
in systemic lupus erythematosus, 233–234, 234f
occupational exposures and, 431t
Carditis, rheumatic, 594–595
Caretaker genes, 318, 318f
Caries, 774–775
Carney syndrome, 614
Caroli disease, 916, 916f
Carotid body tumor, 789–790, 789f, 1221
Carpal tunnel syndrome, 1335
Carroll, James, 344
CART (cocaine and amphetamine-related transcript), 463f, 464b
Cartilage, hyaline, 1304
Cartilage-forming tumors, 1296–1299, 1296f–1299f
Caruncle, urethral, 1034
Caseation, in tuberculosis, 384, 384f–386f, 385
Caspases, in apoptosis, 27, 29, 29f, 30–31, 30f
CASR (calcium-sensing receptor) gene, 1185
Cast nephropathy, 1005, 1006, 1006f
Catabolism, 464b
lysosomal, 32–33, 32f
Catalase, 17, 74
Cataract(s), 1431
hypermature (Morgagnian), 1431
in diabetes, 1205
in galactosemia, 489
subcapsular
anterior, 1432, 1432f
posterior, 1431
Catecholamine(s), 1207, 1218
as tumor markers, 339t
myocardial disease due to, 610
Catecholamine cardiomyopathy, 1221
Catenin(s), 105, 312
ß-catenin gene, 295t, 300t, 304–305, 304f
Cationic antigens, in poststreptococcal glomerulonephritis, 974
Cationic antimicrobial peptides (CAMPs), 360
Cationic trypsinogen *(PRSS1)* gene, and pancreatitis, 942, 945
Cat-scratch disease, granulomatous inflammation in, 83t
Caveolin, 1337f, 1339t
Cavernous hemangiomas, 546–547, 546f
of brain, 1368
of liver, 922
Cavernous lymphangioma, 547
CBAVD (congenital bilateral absence of the vas deferens), in cystic fibrosis, 494, 495
CBD (corticobasal degeneration), 1390–1391
CBF1α, in acute myelogenous leukemia, 692
CBF1ß, in acute myelogenous leukemia, 692
C-C chemokines, 71, 202
C-cell hyperplasia, 1182
CCl_4 (carbon tetrachloride), 431
cell injury due to, 25, 25f, 26f
CCR5, in human immunodeficiency virus, 248, 249, 249f
CCR7, in breast cancer, 313
CD. *See* Crohn disease (CD).
CD3 proteins, 197, 198f
CD4, 197–198, 198f
CD4+ T cells, 198, 198f
in asthma, 723, 724f
in atherosclerosis, 523
in human immunodeficiency virus, 248, 248f, 249–252, 251f, 254–255, 254f, 255t
in transplant rejection, 218–219, 219f, 220
recognition of tumor antigens by, 328
viruses and, 360
CD8, 197–198
CD8+ T cells, 198
in atherosclerosis, 523
in human immunodeficiency virus, 254, 254f, 255
in transplant rejection, 218–219, 219f, 220
recognition of tumor antigens by, 328, 329f
viruses and, 360
CD10, 330
CD11a-cCD18, 55b
CD16, 201
CD20, 330
CD21, 199, 199f
CD28, 198, 198f
CD31, 53f, 54t
CD34, 55b
CD40, 199
CD44, in neuroblastoma, 504
CD44 adhesion molecule, 313
CD49a-hCD29, 55b
CD56, 201
CD59, 66b
CD62E, 54, 54t, 55b
CD62L, 55b
CD62P, 54, 54t, 55b
CD80, 198, 198f
CD86, 198, 198f
Cdc 25, in cell cycle, 290
CDH1 gene, in gastric carcinoma, 824
CDK(s). *See* Cyclin-dependent kinase(s) (CDKs).
CDK1 oncogene, 292t
CDK2 oncogene, 292t
CDK4 oncogene, 292t, 295t, 298, 300
in melanoma, 1247
CDNK2 gene. *See p16INK4a* gene.
CEA (carcinoembryonic antigen), 330, 338, 339t
Cecum
anatomy of, 828
carcinoma of, 865, 865f
ced genes, 28
Ceiling effect, 417, 417f
Celiac disease, 843–844, 843f
Celiac sprue, 843–844, 843f
Cell adhesion molecules (CAMs), in extracellular matrix, 103f, 104–105, 106f
Cell adhesion proteins, in extracellular matrix, 103f, 104–105, 106f
Cell aging, 5, 42–44, 42f–44f

Cell body, of neuron, 1349
Cell cycle, 90, 90f, 100–101, 289–292
  checkpoints of, 292
  cyclin D and RB phosphorylation in, 289–290, 290f, 291f
  inhibitors of, 290–292, 292t
  progression beyond G_1/S restriction point of, 290
Cell death, 5, 5f
  activation-induced, 224f, 225
  programmed, 26
  stages in evolution of, 11, 11f, 19
Cell deletion, in proliferating cell populations, 26
Cell growth
  defects in proteins that regulate, 168–169
  signaling mechanisms in, 97–100, 97f–99f
Cell injury, 5, 5f, 5t
  causes of, 11–14
  cellular and biochemical sites of damage in, 14, 14f
  chemical, 12–13, 25–26, 25f, 26f
  due to accumulation of oxygen-derived free radicals, 14f, 16–18, 17f
  due to ATP depletion, 14–15, 14f
  due to defects in membrane permeability, 14f, 18–19, 18f
  due to genetic derangements, 13
  due to immunologic reactions, 13
  due to infectious agents, 13
  due to influx of intracellular calcium and loss of calcium homeostasis, 14f, 15–16, 16f
  due to mitochondrial damage, 14f, 15, 15f
  due to nutritional imbalances, 13–14
  due to oxygen deprivation, 11–12
  due to physical agents, 12
  examples of, 23–26, 24f–26f
  factors in, 14
  hypoxic, 11–12, 23
  ischemia-reperfusion, 23, 24–25
  ischemic, 11–12, 23–24, 24f
  mechanisms of, 14–19, 14f
  morphologic changes in, 12f, 19–22, 19f–23f
  overview of, 11, 11f–13f, 13t
  reversible *vs.* irreversible, 5, 11, 11f, 19
    ischemic, 23–24, 24f
    morphologic changes in, 12f, 19–22, 19f–23f
Cell proliferation, 89–90, 89f, 293
Cell replication, regulation of, 100–101
Cell shrinkage, in apoptosis, 27
Cell swelling, 15, 19–20, 20f
Cell-cycle checkpoint kinase *(CHEK2)* gene
  and DNA repair, 308, 308f
  in breast cancer, 1134
Cell-mediated hypersensitivity, 205, 206t, 215–218, 215f–217f, 215t
Cell-mediated immunity, in glomerulonephritis, 971
Cellular adaptation(s), 4, 5f, 5t
  atrophy as, 4, 5, 9–10, 9f
  hyperplasia as, 4, 5, 6–7
  hypertrophy as, 4, 5, 7–9, 8f
  metaplasia as, 5, 10–11, 10f
  of growth and differentiation, 5–11
Cellular aging, 5, 42–44, 42f–44f
Cellular energy metabolism, alteration in, 15
Cellular oncogene (*c-onc)*, 293
Cellular proteins, overexpressed or aberrantly expressed, 329–330
Cellular responses, to stress and noxious stimuli, 4–5, 5f, 5t
Cellular senescence, 42–43, 43f, 44f
Cellular swelling, 15, 19–20, 20f, 1351
Cellulitis
  clostridial, 394, 394f
  orbital, 1423
Celsus, 49
Cementum, 774, 774f
Central core disease, 1340t
Central nervous system (CNS), 1347–1414
  angiitis of, 1363
  cellular pathology of, 1350–1352, 1351t
  cerebral edema of, 1352
  cerebrovascular disease(s) of, 1361–1369
    hypertensive, 1368–1369, 1369f
    hypoxia, ischemia, and infarction as, 1361–1365, 1362f, 1364f, 1365f
    intracranial hemorrhage as, 1365–1368, 1366f–1368f
  degenerative diseases of, 1385–1397
    affecting cerebral cortex, 1386–1391, 1386f–1388f, 1389t
    affecting motor neurons, 1396–1397, 1396f
    aggregated proteins in, 1351, 1351t
    of basal ganglia and brain stem, 1391–1394, 1392f, 1393f
    spinocerebellar, 1394–1396, 1395t
  demyelinating diseases of, 1382–1385, 1383f, 1384f
  hydrocephalus of, 1353, 1354f
  in HIV infection, 253, 258
  in infectious mononucleosis, 370
  in pernicious anemia, 642
  in systemic lupus erythematosus, 233
  malformations and developmental diseases of, 1353–1356, 1355f, 1356f
  metabolic diseases of
    genetic, 1397–1399, 1398f
    toxic and acquired, 1399–1401, 1400f
  normal cells of, 1348–1350, 1349f
  paraneoplastic disorders of, 334t
  perinatal injury of, 1356, 1356f
  radiation effect on, 441
  raised intracranial pressure and herniation of, 1352–1353, 1353f
  transmissible spongiform encephalopathies (prion diseases) of, 1351t, 1380–1382, 1381f
Central nervous system (CNS) infection(s), 1369–1380
  acute focal suppurative, 1371, 1371f
  acute meningitis as, 1369–1370, 1370f
  meningoencephalitis as
    chronic bacterial, 1371–1372
    fungal, 1378, 1378f
    necrotizing amoebic, 1380, 1380f
    viral, 1372–1377, 1373f–1377f
  pathogenesis of, 1369
  toxoplasmosis as, 1378–1379, 1378f, 1379f
  viral, 347t
Central nervous system (CNS) trauma, 1356–1361
  parenchymal injuries due to, 1357–1359, 1360f
  sequelae of, 1360
  skull fractures due to, 1357
  spinal cord, 1360–1361
  vascular injuries due to, 1359–1360, 1359f, 1360f
Central nervous system (CNS) tumor(s), 1401–1414
  characteristics of, 1401
  epidemiology of, 1401
  familial syndromes of, 1413–1414
  gliomas as, 1401–1406, 1402f, 1403f, 1405f
  meningiomas as, 1409–1410, 1409f
  metastatic, 1410
  neuronal, 1406
Central nervous system (CNS) tumor(s) *(Continued)*
  paraneoplastic syndromes with, 1410–1411, 1411t
  parenchymal, 1408–1409
  peripheral nerve sheath, 1411–1413, 1412f
  poorly differentiated, 1407–1408, 1407f
Central neurocytoma, 1406
Central pontine myelinolysis, 1385
Central tolerance, 223–225, 224f
Centric fusion, 174f, 175
Centrilobular necrosis, 880
  due to fulminant hepatitis, 901
  due to right-sided heart failure, 563
  impaired hepatic circulation due to, 918, 918f
Centroblasts, 665, 675, 675f
Centrocytes, 665, 675, 675f
Centronuclear myopathy, 1340t
Cephalhematoma, 480
Cephalic phase, of gastric acid secretion, 811
Cerebellar degeneration
  alcoholic, 1400, 1400f
  paraneoplastic, 1410, 1411t
Cerebral abscess, 1371, 1371f
Cerebral amyloid angiopathy (CAA), 1363, 1366, 1388
Cerebral autosomal-dominant arteriopathy with subcortical infarcts and leukoencephalopathy (CADASIL), 1363
Cerebral cortex, degenerative diseases affecting, 1386–1391, 1386f–1388f, 1389t
Cerebral edema, 1352
Cerebral embolism, 1363–1364, 1364f
Cerebral gummas, 1372
Cerebral hemorrhage
  due to trauma, 1360
  hereditary, with amyloidosis, 1363
  in premature infants, 1356
  spontaneous, 1366, 1366f
Cerebral hypoxia, 1361–1365, 1362f, 1364f, 1365f
Cerebral infarction, 1361–1365, 1362f
  hemorrhagic (red), 1364–1365, 1364f
  incomplete, 1365
  nonhemorrhagic (pale, bland, anemic), 1365, 1365f
Cerebral ischemia, 1361–1365
  focal, 1361, 1363–1365, 1364f, 1365f
  global, 1361–1363, 1362f
Cerebral neuroblastomas, 1406
Cerebral palsy, 1356
Cerebral thrombosis, 1363–1364
Cerebral toxoplasmosis, 1378–1379, 1378f, 1379f
Cerebrospinal fluid (CSF), in meningitis, 1370
Cerebrovascular disease(s), 1361–1369. *See also* Stroke.
  defined, 1361
  hypertensive, 1368–1369, 1369f
  hypoxia, ischemia, and infarction as, 1361–1365, 1362f, 1364f, 1365f
  intracranial hemorrhage as, 1365–1368, 1366f–1368f
Ceruloplasmin, 74, 910
Cervical biopsy, 1079
Cervical carcinoma, 1073–1079
  clinical course and management of, 1078–1079, 1079f
  epidemiology of, 1073–1074
  human papillomavirus and, 324, 1074–1075, 1074f, 1076, 1076f, 1078–1079, 1079f
  morphology of, 1077–1078, 1078f
  pathogenesis of, 1074–1075, 1074f
  risk factors for, 284
  squamous cell, 1076–1077
  staging of, 1077

Cervical intraepithelial neoplasia (CIN), 1074f–1077f, 1075–1076, 1078–1079
Cervical transformation zone, 1081–1082, 1082f, 1083f
Cervicitis, 1072–1073, 1073f
Cervicovaginal smear
  malignant cells in, 336f
  metaplasia in, 336f
Cervix, 1072–1079
  anatomy of, 1081–1082, 1082f, 1083f
  inflammations of, 1072–1073, 1073f
  intraepithelial and invasive squamous neoplasia of, 1073–1079, 1074f–1079f
Cestodes, 406–407, 407f
  enterocolitis due to, 839
CFM1 (cystic fibrosis modifier locus), 492
c-*FMS*, 295
c-*FOS*, 100, 101f, 102
CFTR (cystic fibrosis transmembrane conductance regulator) gene
  in cystic fibrosis, 490–492, 490f–492f, 495
  in pancreatitis, 945
CFUs (colony-forming units), 620
Chagas disease, 405–406
  achalasia in, 801
  acute, 406
  chronic, 406
  megacolon in, 831
  morphology of, 406
  myocarditis due to, 608, 609, 609f
  pathogenesis of, 405–406
Chain terminator mutations, in ß-thalassemia, 632, 632f
Chalazion, 1424
Chalkstick-type fractures, 1286
Chancre
  in African trypanosomiasis, 405
  in syphilis, 389, 390, 390f
  soft, 380
Chancroid, 380
Channelopathies, 1339–1340
Chaperones, in protein folding, 37–38, 37f
Charcot-Bouchard microaneurysms, 1366
Charcot-Marie-Tooth (CMT) disease, 1332–1333
Checkpoints, cell-cycle, 100–101, 292
Chédiak-Higashi syndrome, 61–62, 62t
Cheilitis, actinic, 1242
Cheilosis, 457
CHEK2 (cell-cycle checkpoint kinase) gene
  and DNA repair, 308, 308f
  in breast cancer, 1134
Chemical agents
  aplastic anemia due to, 647, 647t
  cell injury due to, 12–13, 25–26, 25f, 26f
  congenital anomalies due to, 473
Chemical carcinogen(s), 320–321, 321t, 322–323
Chemical carcinogenesis, 319–323, 320f, 321f, 321t
Chemical esophagitis, 805–806
"Chemical" meningitis, 1370
Chemoattractants, 56–57
Chemodectomas, 1221
Chemokines
  in delayed type hypersensitivity, 217
  in glomerulonephritis, 972
  in human immunodeficiency virus, 248–249, 249f
  in immediate hypersensitivity, 209
  in immunity, 202
  in inflammation, 53f, 54, 71–72, 74t
  in leukocyte movement, 202
  in metastasis, 313
  in pancreatitis, 946
Chemoprevention, of cancer, 466
Chemotactic agents, 56–57
Chemotaxis, in inflammation, 56–57, 58f
Chemotherapeutic agents
  apoptosis due to, 26, 31
  myocardial disease due to, 609–610
  white cell neoplasia due to, 667
Chenodeoxycholic acid, 886
Cherry-red spot, 161, 1441, 1441f
CHF (congestive heart failure), 560–563
  edema due to, 120–121, 121f, 122
Chiari malformation
  type I, 1355
  type II, 1355, 1356f
Chickenpox, 368, 368f, 1374
Chief cells, 811, 1184, 1185, 1186f
Child(ren)
  AIDS in, 245, 1376
  causes of death in, 470, 470t
  iron deficiency anemia in, 645
  lead exposure in, 433
  radiation effect on, 439
  tumors in, 498–506
    benign, 498–499, 498f, 499f
    malignant, 499–506, 500t
      incidence and types of, 499–500, 500t
      neuroblastic, 500–504, 501f, 502f, 503t, 504f
      Wilms, 504–506, 505f, 506f
Childhood polycystic kidney disease, 962t, 964–965, 965f
Childhood retinoblastoma, 284
Chimerism, mixed, 221
Chinese herbs nephropathy, 1004
Chitotriosidase, in Gaucher disease, 164–165
Chlamydia trachomatis
  conjunctival scarring due to, 1425
  genital infection with, 394–395
    female, 350, 356t, 395, 1063t
    male, 356t, 395
  life cycle of, 394
  perinatal, 355
  transmission of, 355
Chlamydiae, 346t, 349–350, 394–395
Chlamydiae pneumoniae, and atherosclerosis, 524
Chlordane, 435
Chlorofluorocarbons, 441
Chloroform, 431
Chloromas, 694
Chloroquine myopathy, 1344
Chloroquine retinopathy, 1442
Chokes, 137, 446
Cholangiocarcinoma, 926–927, 926f
Cholangitis, 933
  ascending, 902, 913, 933
  autoimmune, 903
  primary sclerosing, 913t, 915, 915f
  suppurative, 933
Cholecystitis, 931–933
  acute, 931–932
    acalculous, 931, 932
    calculous, 931, 931f, 932
  chronic, 932–933, 932f
  gangrenous, 932
  hormone replacement therapy and, 428
  xanthogranulomatous, 933
Cholecystokinin, 940–941
Choledochal cysts, 934
Choledocholithiasis, 933
Cholelithiasis, 928–931
  and pancreatitis, 942
  clinical features of, 931
  epidemiology of, 928–929
  morphology of, 930–931, 930f, 931f
  obesity and, 465
  pathogenesis of, 929–930, 930f
  risk factors for, 929, 929t
Cholera, 835–836, 836f
Cholera toxin, 834, 835–836, 836f
Cholestasis, 888–890
  clinical presentation of, 888
  in hepatitis, 898–899, 900f
  intrahepatic, 889
    benign recurrent, 889
    familial, 889–890, 890t
    of pregnancy, 921
  laboratory findings in, 888–889
  morphology of, 889, 889f
  neonatal, 912–913, 912t
Cholesteatomas, 788
Cholesterol
  in atherosclerosis, 523, 525f
  in familial hypercholesterolemia, 156–158, 157f, 158f
  intracellular accumulation of, 37, 37f
Cholesterol emboli, 135, 519
Cholesterol esters, intracellular accumulation of, 37, 37f
Cholesterol stones, 928, 929, 929t, 930, 930f
Cholesterolosis, 37, 37f, 930
Cholic acid, 886
Chondroblastic osteosarcoma, 1295
Chondroblastoma, 1297–1298, 1297f
Chondrocalcinosis, 1314, 1314f
Chondrocytes, 1304
Chondrodysplasia, Schmid metaphyseal, 1280t
Chondroid syringoma, 1238, 1239f
Chondroma(s), 270, 1296–1297, 1297f
  subperiosteal or juxtacortical, 1296
Chondromyxoid fibroma, 1298, 1298f
Chondroplasia, Jansen metaphyseal, 1280t
Chondrosarcoma, 1298–1299, 1299f
  clear cell, 1298–1299
  dedifferentiated, 1298
  mesenchymal, 1299
Chordae tendineae, 558
Chorioamnionitis, 477, 480, 1106, 1108f
Choriocarcinoma
  gestational, 1112–1113, 1113f
  ovarian, 1101–1102
  testicular, 1041, 1043–1044, 1044f
Choristoma, 272, 498
Choroid, 1422f
Choroid plexus papillomas, 1406
Choroidal neovascularization, 1441–1442, 1442f
Christmas disease, 656
Chromaffin cells, 1218
Chromatin condensation, in apoptosis, 27, 27f
Chromatolysis, central, 1351
Chromium
  as carcinogen, 285t, 323
  exposure to, 432t, 433–434
Chromophobe renal carcinoma, 1016–1017, 1018
Chromosomal abnormalities, fetal growth restriction due to, 477
Chromosomal changes, in cancer cells, 314–315
Chromosomal syndromes, 472
Chromosomal translocations, 174–175, 174f
  in cancer cells, 314–315
  molecular diagnosis of, 337
  white cell neoplasia due to, 667
Chromosome(s), 170–171
  marker, 337
  normal complement of, 173
  ring, 174, 174f
Chromosome 1p loss, in neuroblastoma, 503–504, 503t
Chromosome 17q gain, in neuroblastoma, 503, 503t
Chromosome 22q11.2 deletion syndrome, 172f, 176–178

Chromosome analysis
postnatal, 187–188
prenatal, 187
Chromosome mutations. *See* Cytogenetic disorder(s).
Chromosome-breakage syndromes, 174
Chronic bronchitis, 722–723, 723t
emphysema *vs.*, 721t
Chronic disease, anemia of, 646
Chronic ischemic heart disease (CIHD), 586
Chronic lymphocytic leukemia (CLL), 673–674, 673f, 674f
Chronic myelogenous leukemia (CML), 697–698, 697f, 698f
chromosomal translocation and oncogenes for, 298t, 314–315, 314t
Chronic myeloproliferative disorders, 666–667, 691, 696–701
Chronic obstructive pulmonary disease (COPD), 717–728, 718t
asthma as, 718t, 723–727, 724f, 725f, 727f
bronchiectasis as, 718t, 727–728, 728f
bronchiolitis as, 718t, 722
chronic bronchitis as, 718t, 722–723, 723f
emphysema as, 717–722, 718f–721f, 718t, 721t
of small airways, 718t, 722
restrictive pulmonary disease *vs.*, 716–717
Chrysotiles, in asbestos-related diseases, 735
Churg-Strauss syndrome, 537t, 541
Chvostek sign, 1188
Chylocele, of tunica vaginalis, 1047
Chylopericardium, 545
Chylothorax, 545, 767
Chylous ascites, 545
Cicatricial pemphigoid, ocular, 1425
CID (cytomegalic inclusion disease), 367
Cigarette smoking, 419–421
and atherosclerosis, 521
and cancer, 284, 419–421
bladder, 1032
lung, 758, 759
pancreatic, 950
and chronic bronchitis, 722
and emphysema, 719, 720
and peptic ulcer disease, 421, 818
and thromboangiitis obliterans (Buerger disease), 542
benzo[a]pyrene from, 432
carcinogens in, 419, 419t
congenital anomalies due to, 473
diffuse interstitial lung disease due to, 740–741, 740f
environmental tobacco smoke due to, 421
mortality due to, 419, 421t
passive, 421
Ciguatera poisoning, 435–436
Ciguatoxin, 435–436
CIHD (chronic ischemic heart disease), 586
Ciliary body, of eye, 1422f, 1430f
in diabetes mellitus, 1437, 1438f
Ciliary dyskinesia, primary, 727
Ciliochoroidal effusion, 1446
CIN (cervical intraepithelial neoplasia), 1074f–1077f, 1075–1076, 1078–1079
Cingulate herniation, 1352, 1353f
Cip/Kip inhibitors, 291f, 292, 292f
Circulating immune complex nephritis, 970, 971f
Circulatory status, and wound healing, 114
Circumferential lamellae, 1276, 1277f
Cirrhosis, 882–883
alcoholic, 423
and other alcoholic liver disease, 904, 904f
clinical features of, 907
hemochromatosis in, 909
morphology of, 423, 423f, 905–906, 906f
Cirrhosis *(Continued)*
biliary
in cystic fibrosis, 493, 495
primary, 913t, 914–915, 914f
secondary, 913–914, 913t, 914f
cardiac, 563, 883
classification of, 883
clinical features of, 882, 883
cryptogenic, 883, 899
defined, 882
due to hepatitis, 899, 901f
etiology of, 883
in Wilson disease, 911
Laennec, 906
pathogenesis of, 883, 884f
portal hypertension due to, 884, 885f
postnecrotic, 899
CIS. *See* Carcinoma in situ (CIS).
11-*cis*-retinal, 451
13-*cis*-retinoic acid, in cancer prevention, 466
Civatte bodies, 1258
CJD (Creutzfeldt-Jakob disease), 346, 1351, 1382
variant, 1382
c-*JUN*, 100, 101f, 102
c-KIT
in gastrointestinal stomal tumors, 827
in stromal tumors, 296
c-KIT ligand, 622
CK-MB (creatinine kinase—MB fraction), 584
Class I MHC—restricted cells, 204
Class II MHC—restricted cells, 204
Classical pathway, of complement activation, 64, 66b
ClC-1 chloride channel gene, in myotonic dystrophy, 1339
ClC-7 chloride channel gene, in osteopetrosis, 1281
Clear cell adenocarcinoma, of ovaries, 1098
Clear cell carcinoma
of endometrium, 1088
of kidney, 1016, 1017–1018, 1017f, 1018f
of vagina, 1071, 1071f
Clear cell chondrosarcoma, 1298–1299
Cleft lip, 471f, 474
Cleft palate, 471f, 474
Cleidocranial dysplasia, 1280t
Clinical manifestations, defined, 4
Clinical significance, 4
Clofibrate, and gallstones, 929
Cloning, 146, 147f
therapeutic, 91, 92f
Clostridial cellulitis, 394, 394f
Clostridial gas gangrene, 393, 394
Clostridial infections, 349t, 393–394, 394f
Clostridium botulinum, 359, 393
Clostridium difficile, 393, 394
immune evasion by, 359
pseudomembranous colitis due to, 836, 837–838, 837f
Clostridium perfringens, 362, 393, 394f, 837
Clostridium septicum, 393
Clostridium sordellii, 350f
Clostridium tetani, 359, 393
Clotting factor deficiencies, 653–656, 654f
Clotting system, in inflammation, 65–68, 67f
Clumping factor, 371
c-MET, 96, 294, 295
CML (chronic myelogenous leukemia), 697–698, 697f, 698f
chromosomal translocation and oncogenes for, 298t, 314–315, 314t
CMT (Charcot-Marie-Tooth) disease, 1332–1333
CMV. *See* Cytomegalovirus (CMV).
c-*MYC* oncogene
amplification of, 315
in Burkitt lymphoma, 314, 326, 677
c-*MYC* oncogene *(Continued)*
in gene transcription, 100
in liver regeneration, 101f, 102
tumors associated with, 295t
CNS. *See* Central nervous system (CNS).
Coagulation, disseminated intravascular, 135, 656–658
clinical course of, 658
etiology and pathogenesis of, 656–657, 657t, 658f
impaired hepatic circulation in, 918
in toxemia of pregnancy, 1106, 1107–1108, 1109f
morphology of, 657–658
paraneoplastic, 335
tumor necrosis factor and, 85, 657
Coagulation cascade, 125f, 127–130, 128f, 129f
Coagulation factor V mutation, 188–189, 188f
Coagulation pathway
extrinsic, 128, 128f
intrinsic, 127, 128, 128f
Coagulation system, in glomerulonephritis, 972
Coagulopathy
consumption, 135
in hepatic failure, 882
Coal dust, accumulations of, 39
Coal macules, 733
Coal nodules, 733
Coal workers' pneumoconiosis (CWP), 39, 733–734, 734f
Coarctation, of aorta, 564t, 570–571, 571f
Cobalamin. *See* Vitamin B_{12}.
Cobalophilins, 639
Cobalt, exposure to, 432t, 433
Cocaine
abuse of, 425, 425f
myocardial disease due to, 610
Cocaine and amphetamine-related transcript (CART), 463f, 464b
Coccidioides immitis, pneumonia due to, 754, 755, 756f
Coccidioidomycosis, 754, 755, 756f
Codeine, abuse of, 426
Codman triangle, 1295–1296, 1295f
Codominance, 150
Cofactor, in coagulation cascade, 128, 129f
Cohnheim, Julius, 49
Coiled bodies, 1390
Coin lesion, 765
COL4A5 gene, 988
Cold agglutinin immunohemolytic anemia, 637, 637t
Cold hemolysin hemolytic anemia, 637–638, 637t
Cold sores, 366, 777
Colitis
antibiotic-associated, 836, 837–838, 837f
collagenous, 840–841
cytomegalovirus, 368
diversion, 841–842
lymphocytic, 840–841
neutropenic, 841
pseudomembranous, 836, 837–838, 837f
ulcerative, 849–851
and carcinoma, 850–851
clinical features of, 851, 851t
diagnosis of, 847
epidemiology of, 849
etiology and pathogenesis of, 846
genetic susceptibility to, 846
morphology of, 849–851, 849f, 850f
T-cells in, 847
Collagen(s)
basement membrane, 104t
fibrillar (interstitial), 104, 104f
in bone, 1275

Collagen(s) *(Continued)*
in cirrhosis, 883
in extracellular matrix, 103f, 104, 104t, 105f
Collagen defect, in Ehlers-Danlos syndromes, 155
Collagen diseases, 1279–1281, 1281t, 1282f
Collagen vascular diseases, pulmonary involvement in, 731–732
Collagenases, 111
Collagenous colitis, 840–841
Collapsing glomerulopathy, 983
Collar-button lesion, 765
Collateral circulation, 558
and infarction, 139
Collecting duct carcinoma, 1017, 1018
Colloid bodies, 1258
Colloid carcinoma
of breast, 1145–1146, 1145f
of prostate, 1056
Colloid cyst, of third ventricle, 1406
Colloid osmotic pressure, reduced, edema due to, 120f, 120t, 121
Colon, 828–870
adenomas of, 858, 858f, 859–861, 860f, 861f
anatomy of, 828
congenital anomalies of, 830–831
diverticular disease of, 854–855, 855f
enterocolitis of, 831–842
idiopathic inflammatory bowel disease of, 846–851, 847f–850f, 851t
immune system of, 829–830
incarceration of, 856
mucosa of, 828f, 829
neuromuscular function of, 830
obstruction of, 855–856, 855t, 856f
papilloma of, 270f
polyps of, 271, 271f, 857–859, 858f, 859f
strangulation of, 856
tumors of, 857–870, 857t
vascular disorders of, 851–854, 852f, 853f
vasculature of, 828
Colon cancer. *See* Colorectal carcinoma.
Colonic diverticula, 854–855, 855f
Colony-forming units (CFUs), 620
Colony-stimulating factor(s) (CSFs), 202
Colony-stimulating factor-1 (CSF-1), oncogene for, 295, 295t
Colorectal carcinoma, 862–866
adenomatous polyps and, 860, 861
carcinogenesis of, 862–864, 863f
clinical features of, 866
diet and, 466, 864–865
epidemiology of, 856, 864
hereditary nonpolyposis, 285, 306–307, 862, 864
gastric carcinoma in, 824
metastatic, 280f
molecular model for evolution of, 317–318, 317f
morphology of, 274f, 865–866, 865f, 866f
pathogenesis and etiology of, 864–865
prognosis for, 866
TNM classification of, 866, 866f
ulcerative colitis and, 850–851
Columnar absorptive cells, 828f, 829
Coma, hyperosmolar nonketotic, 1202
Comedocarcinoma, 1139, 1139f
Comedones, 1264
Common acute lymphoblastic leukemia antigen (CALLA), 330
Common bile duct, 928
agenesis of, 928
Common cold, 783
Common variable immunodeficiency, 242
Comparative genomic hybridization, 337
Compensatory growth, 101
Compensatory hyperinflation, 721
Complement deficiencies, in systemic lupus erythematosus, 229–230
Complement pathway
alternative, in glomerulonephritis, 971, 985, 987f
in ischemia-reperfusion injury, 24–25
Complement proteins, in innate immunity, 194, 194f
Complement receptor(s), 199
Complement receptor type 1 (CR1), 59
Complement system
activation of, 64, 66b
disorders of, 66b–67b
genetic deficiencies of, 244–245
in immediate hypersensitivity, 207
in inflammation, 59, 64–65, 65f, 66b–67b, 68
in systemic immune complex disease, 213, 213f
Complement-mediated inflammation, 210, 211f
Complement-mediated phagocytosis, 210, 211f
Complement-mediated urticaria, 1253
Complete androgen insensitivity syndrome, 181
Complex sclerosing lesion, of breast, 1128, 1129f
Compound nevi, 1232, 1233f
Compression atelectasis, 714, 714f
Compression neuropathy, 1335
conc (cellular oncogene), 293
Concentric hypertrophy, 561, 561f
Concentric lamellae, 1276, 1277f
Concretio cordis, 612
Concussion, 1357
Conduction disturbances, after myocardial infarction, 584
Condyloma, of esophagus, 806
Condyloma acuminatum, 1265
of penis, 1035–1036, 1035f, 1036f
of vulva, 1067, 1067f
Confined placental mosaicism, 477, 478f
Congenital adrenal hyperplasia (CAH), 1212–1214
Congenital aganglionic megacolon, 830–831
Congenital anomaly(ies), 470–476
causes of, 472–474, 473t, 474t
definitions related to, 470–472, 471f, 472f
frequency of common, 474t
major, 470
of biliary tract, 928
of bladder, 1026, 1026f
of breast, 1122
of esophagus, 799–800, 800f
of kidney, 961
of lung, 713
of pancreas, 941
of penis, 1035
of small and large intestines, 830–831, 830f
of spleen, 705
of stomach, 812–816, 813f, 814t, 815f, 816f
of testes, 1037–1038, 1038f
of thyroid gland, 1183
of ureters, 1024–1025
of vagina, 1070–1071
pathogenesis of, 474–476, 475f, 476f
sequence of, 471–472, 472f
syndrome of, 472
vascular, 515
Congenital bilateral absence of the vas deferens (CBAVD), in cystic fibrosis, 494, 495
Congenital contractural arachnodactyly, 154
Congenital disorders, 147
Congenital heart disease, 564–571
aortic stenosis and atresia as, 564t, 571
atrial septal defect as, 564t, 565, 567–568, 567f
atrioventricular septal defect as, 564t, 567f, 568–569
Congenital heart disease *(Continued)*
causing left-to-right shunts, 566–569, 567f, 568f
causing right-to-left shunts, 566, 569–570, 569f, 570f
clinical features of, 566–567
coarctation of aorta as, 564t, 570–571, 571f
cyanotic, 566, 569, 569f
brain abscess due to, 1371
etiology and pathogenesis of, 565
genetics of, 565–566, 566f
in Turner syndrome, 179–180
incidence of, 564–565, 564t
obstructive, 567, 570–571, 571f
patent ductus arteriosus as, 564t, 567f, 568
pulmonary stenosis and atresia as, 564t, 571
tetralogy of Fallot as, 564t, 565, 569, 569f
total anomalous pulmonary venous connection as, 564t, 570
transposition of great arteries as, 564t, 569–570, 569f, 570f
tricuspid atresia as, 564t, 570
truncus arteriosus as, 564t, 565, 570
ventricular septal defect as, 564t, 565, 567f, 568, 569f
Congenital hepatic fibrosis, 916, 916f, 965
Congenital infection, with cytomegalovirus, 366, 367
Congenital melanosis oculi, 1426
Congenital muscular dystrophy, 1338t
Congenital myopathies, 1340–1341, 1340f, 1340t
Congenital nevus, 1233t
Congenital pulmonary airway malformation (CPAM), 713
Congenital syphilis, 389, 391
Congenital-infantile fibrosarcomas, 499
Congestion, 122–123, 123f
chronic passive, 122
of liver, 122–123, 123f
hepatic
acute, 122
chronic passive, 122–123, 123f
pulmonary
acute, 122
chronic, 122
Congestion stage, of lobar pneumonia, 750
Congestive heart failure (CHF), 560–563
edema due to, 120–121, 121f, 122
Conidia, 351
Conjunctiva, 1425–1426
bulbar, 1424f, 1425
functional anatomy of, 1422f, 1424f, 1425
Kaposi sarcoma of, 1425
neoplasms of, 1425–1426, 1427f
palpebral, 1424f, 1425
pinguecula and pterygium of, 1426
scarring of, 1425–1426
Conjunctival fornices, 1424f, 1425
Conjunctival intraepithelial neoplasia, 1426
Conjunctival melanomas, 1426, 1427f
Conjunctival nevi, 1426, 1427f
Conjunctival scarring, 1425–1426
Conjunctivitis, viral, 1425
Connective tissue defects, in Ehlers-Danlos syndromes, 155
Connective tissue disease, mixed, 239
Connective tissue growth factor (CTGF), 95t
Connective tissue metaplasia, 11
Constrictive pericarditis, due to radiation exposure, 440
Consumer Products Safety Commission, 416
Consumption coagulopathy, 135
Contact dermatitis, 217, 217f, 1254f, 1254t, 1255, 1255f
Contact inhibition, 105
Contact skin sensitivity, 215

Contaminants, of food, 446–447
Continuously dividing tissues, 90, 90f
Contractile dysfunction, after myocardial infarction, 584
Contraction atelectasis, 714, 714f
Contraction band(s), myocardial necrosis with, 581
Contraction band necrosis, 142
Contractural arachnodactyly, congenital, 154
Contracture, 113f, 115
Contrecoup injury, 1357
Contusion, 443–444, 443f
of brain, 1357–1358, 1358f
Coombs antiglobulin test, for immunohemolytic anemias, 636–637
COP (cryptogenic organizing pneumonia), 731, 732f
COPD. *See* Chronic obstructive pulmonary disease (COPD).
Copper, 461t
accumulation of, 880, 910–911
Coproporphyria, variegate, 1333t
Cor pulmonale, 563, 588, 588f
acute, 742
disorders predisposing to, 588t
due to pulmonary thromboembolism, 136
in cystic fibrosis, 495
Cords of Billroth, 702–703
Cornea, 1426–1430
functional anatomy of, 1422f, 1426–1427, 1427f, 1430f
keratitis and ulcers of, 1428, 1428f
Corneal degenerations, 1428, 1429f
Corneal dystrophies, 1428–1430, 1429f
Corneal endothelium, 1427
Corneal hydrops, 1428
Corneal lesions, due to herpes simplex virus, 366
Corneal stroma, 1427
Corneal ulcer(s), 1428
due to vitamin A deficiency, 451, 452f
Coronary arteries, 557–558
aging effect on, 559t
epicardial, 557
Coronary arteriosclerosis, graft, 615–616, 615f
Coronary artery bypass graft surgery, 553
Coronary artery disease (CAD). *See also* Ischemic heart disease (IHD).
clinicopathologic effects of, 525
epidemiology and risk factors for, 520–521, 520f, 520t
in systemic lupus erythematosus, 234
obesity and, 465
pathogenesis of, 572–575, 573f, 574f, 575t
Coronary artery occlusion, myocardial infarction due to, 576–577, 577f, 578f
Coronary heart disease. *See* Coronary artery disease (CAD); Ischemic heart disease (IHD).
Coronary stents, 551, 552f
Coronary thrombus, 573f, 574
Coronavirus, 347t
Corpora amylacea, 1352
Corpus, of stomach, 810, 810f
Corpus callosum, agenesis of, 1355, 1355f
Corpus luteum, 1081
Cortical atrophy, in Alzheimer disease, 1386, 1386f
Cortical müllerian inclusion cyst, 1095, 1095f
Cortical stromal hyperplasia, 1092
Corticobasal degeneration (CBD), 1390–1391
Corticosteroids, peptic ulcer disease due to, 818
Corticotroph(s), 1157
Corticotroph cell adenomas, 1162
Corticotroph cell hyperplasia, 1208
Corticotropin releasing hormone (CRH)-producing tumor, 1208
Corynebacterium diphtheriae, 374
myocarditis due to, 608
Costimulators, 198, 225
Costochondral junction, 454f
scorbutic, 459, 460f
Cot death, 495–497, 496t
"Cotton-wool spots," 1437, 1438f
Coup injury, 1357
Cowden syndrome
and breast cancer, 1134
cutaneous manifestations of, 1245t
gastrointestinal manifestations of, 859
Cowdry body, 1351
COX-1 (cyclooxygenase 1), 68, 69
COX-2 (cyclooxygenase 2), 68, 69
and cancer, 287
colorectal, 318
COX-2 (cyclooxygenase 2) inhibitors, 70
Coxsackievirus, 347t
myocarditis due to, 608
CPAM (congenital pulmonary airway malformation), 713
C-peptide, 1191
CPPD (calcium pyrophosphate crystal deposition disease), 1314, 1314f
CR1 (complement receptor type 1), 59
CRABP (cytoplasmic/cellular retinoic acid—binding protein), 475, 476f
"Crack," 425
Cranial nerve palsies, 1334
Craniopharyngiomas, 1164
Craniotabes, 455
CRBP (cytoplasmic retinol-binding protein), 476f
C-reactive protein (CRP), 84
in atherosclerosis, 574
in innate immunity, 194
in myocardial infarction, 584
Creatinine kinase—MB fraction (CK-MB), 584
Creeping substitution, 1290
Crescent formation, in glomerulonephritis, 967, 977–978, 977f
Crescentic glomerulonephritis, 967t, 975t, 976–978, 977f, 977t, 978f
CREST syndrome, 229t, 237, 238, 239
Cretinism, 1168
Creutzfeldt-Jakob disease (CJD), 346, 1351, 1382
variant, 1382
CRH (corticotropin releasing hormone)-producing tumor, 1208
Crib death, 495–497, 496t
Crigler-Najjar syndrome, 887–888, 888t
Crohn disease (CD), 847–849
clinical features of, 848–849, 851t
diagnosis of, 847
epidemiology of, 847
etiology and pathogenesis of, 846
genetic susceptibility to, 846
morphology of, 847–848, 847f–849f
T-cells in, 847
Cronkhite-Canada syndrome, 859
Crooke hyaline change, 1209
Cross-linking, of collagen, 104, 105f
Croup, 786
Crouzon syndrome, 1280t
CRP. *See* C-reactive protein (CRP).
Cryoglobulinemia, essential mixed, glomerular lesions in, 993
Crypt abscess, 848, 850, 850f
Crypt cell, 908, 909f
Cryptococcal meningitis, 1378, 1378f
Cryptococcosis, 399, 399f
in AIDS, 256
Cryptococcus neoformans, 399
Cryptogenic organizing pneumonia (COP), 731, 732f
Cryptorchidism, 1037–1038, 1038f
Cryptosporidia, 353
Cryptosporidium spp, 351t
Crypts of Lieberkühn, 828–829, 828f
CSF (cerebrospinal fluid), in meningitis, 1370
CSF-1 (colony-stimulating factor-1), oncogene for, 295, 295t
CSFs (colony-stimulating factors), 202
CTGF (connective tissue growth factor), 95t
CTL(s). *See* Cytotoxic T lymphocytes (CTLs).
CTLA-4, 225, 226
C-type lectins, 55b
Cunninghamella, 400
Curling ulcers, 819
Curschmann spirals, 726
Cushing disease, 1208
Cushing syndrome, 1207–1210
ACTH-independent (adrenal), 1208, 1208f
bleeding disorders due to, 650
clinical course of, 1209–1210, 1209t
iatrogenic, 1208f
morphology of, 1209
paraneoplastic, 333, 334t, 1208f
pathogenesis of, 1162, 1207–1209
pituitary, 1208f, 1210
Cushing ulcers, 819–820
Cutaneous appendages, 1228f
tumors of, 1238–1240, 1239f, 1240t
Cutaneous horn, 1240–1242, 1241f
Cutaneous T-cell lymphoma, 1249–1250, 1250f
Cutaneous wound healing, 111–115
by first intention, 111–113, 112f
by second intention, 112f, 113, 113f
complications of, 114–115, 115f
factors influencing, 114, 114t
growth factors and cytokines in, 111t
phases of, 111, 111f
strength of, 113–114
summary of, 114
CWP (coal workers' pneumoconiosis), 39, 733–734, 734f
CX_3C chemokines, 72
C-X-C chemokines, 71, 202
CXCR4
in breast cancer, 313
in human immunodeficiency virus, 248, 249
Cyanide poisoning, 25
Cyanotic congenital heart disease, 566, 569, 569f
brain abscess due to, 1371
Cycasin, 435
Cyclin(s), 100
protooncogenes for, 295t, 298
Cyclin A—CDK2 complex, in cell cycle, 290
Cyclin B—CDK1 complex, in cell cycle, 290
Cyclin D, in cell cycle, 289, 290f, 291f
Cyclin D oncogene, 295t, 298, 300
in squamous cell carcinoma, 780, 781f
CYCLIN D1 gene, 298, 314, 315
Cyclin D—CDK4 complex
in cell cycle, 289, 290f, 291f
in retinoblastoma, 300, 302f, 305
Cyclin E oncogene, 295t
Cyclin E—CDK2 complex, 290, 302f
Cyclin-dependent kinase(s) (CDKs), 100
in cell cycle, 289–292, 290f, 291f
protooncogenes for, 295t, 298
Cyclin-dependent kinase (CDK) inhibitor(s), 100
in cell cycle, 290–292, 291f, 292t
Cyclin-dependent kinase inhibitor 2 *(CDNK2)* gene. *See p16INK4a* gene.
Cyclitic membrane, 1446
Cyclooxygenase(s), 68–69, 69f
Cyclooxygenase 1 (COX-1), 68, 69

Cyclooxygenase 2 (COX-2), 68, 69
and cancer, 287
colorectal, 318
Cyclooxygenase 2 (COX-2) inhibitors, 70
Cyclooxygenase inhibitors, 70
Cyclophosphamide (Cytoxan)
and bladder carcinoma, 1032
myocardial disease due to, 610
Cyclosporine, with transplant, 220
Cylindrical papilloma, 784
Cylindroma, 1238, 1239f
CYP1A1 gene, 320, 417, 759
CYP11B1 gene, 1210
CYP11B2 gene, 1210
CYP21A pseudogene, 1213
CYP21B gene, 1213
Cyst(s)
adrenal, 1218
apocrine, 1127, 1127f
Bartholin, 1065
branchial, 788–789
bronchogenic, 713, 799
choledochal, 934
colloid, of third ventricle, 1406
cortical müllerian inclusion, 1095, 1095f
cysticercus, 407, 407f
dentigerous, 782
dermoid
of skin, 1238
ovarian, 272, 272f, 1099–1100, 1100f
endometriotic, 1084f
epidermal inclusion, 1238
epithelial, 1238
follicular, 1092
foregut, 713
ganglion, 1315
Gartner duct, 1060, 1070
luteal, 1092
lymphoepithelial, 788–789
mesenteric, 873
multilocular, 407
odontogenic, 782, 782t
of breast, 1127, 1127f
of esophagus, congenital, 799
of fallopian tubes, 1091
of thyroid gland, 1177
ovarian, 1092–1093, 1093f
dermoid, 272, 272f, 1099–1100, 1100f
pancreatic
congenital, 946–947
neoplastic, 947–948, 948f, 949f
pseudo-, 947, 947f
paratubal, 1091
periapical, 782
pilar, 1238
Rathke cleft, 1163
renal, 962–966, 962t
synovial, 1315
thymic, 706
thyroglossal duct, 1183
thyroglossal tract, 789
trichilemmal, 1238
urachal, 1026
Cystadenocarcinoma
mucinous, of appendix, 872, 872f
of ovaries, 1095–1097, 1095f–1097f
Cystadenofibroma, of ovaries, 1098
Cystadenoma(s), 270
mucinous, of appendix, 871, 872
of ovaries, 1095–1097, 1095f–1097f
of pancreas
mucinous, 947, 948f
serous, 947, 948f
papillary, 271
Cystic disease, of kidney, 962–966, 962t, 963f–966f
Cystic fibrosis, 489–495
bronchiectasis in, 495, 728f
classic, 492
clinical course of, 494–495, 494t
diagnosis of, 494t, 495
epidemiology of, 489–490
gene for, 490–492, 490f–492f
genetic and environmental modifiers in, 492–493
genotype-phenotype correlations in, 491–492, 492f, 493
infections with, 360
morphology of, 493–494, 493f
mutation in, 149f
nonclassic or atypical, 492
prognosis for, 495
protein folding in, 38
Pseudomonas aeruginosa in, 379, 493, 494, 495
transport system defects in, 154
Cystic fibrosis modifier locus (CFM1), 492
Cystic fibrosis transmembrane conductance regulator *(CFTR)* gene
in cystic fibrosis, 490–492, 490f–492f, 495
in pancreatitis, 945
Cystic follicles, 1092
Cystic hygroma(s), 484f, 486, 547
in Turner syndrome, 179
Cystic medial degeneration, in aortic dissection, 533, 534f
Cystic medionecrosis, 155
Cystic renal dysplasia, 962, 963f
Cystic teratoma, 272, 272f
Cysticercosis, 406–407, 407f
Cysticercus cyst, 407, 407f
Cystine stones, 1014, 1014t
Cystitis, 1027–1028
acute, 1027
chronic, 1027
eosinophilic, 1027
follicular, 1027
hemorrhagic, 1027
interstitial, 1027
polypoid, 1028
suppurative, 1027
with malacoplakia, 1027–1028, 1028f
Cystitis cystica, 1028
Cystitis cystica et glandularis, 1028
Cystitis glandularis, 1028
Cystocele, 1024
Cytochrome c
in apoptosis, 30, 30f
leakage into cytosol of, 15
Cytochrome P-450, in alcoholic liver disease, 906
Cytochrome P-450 enzymes, 417
Cytochrome P-450—dependent monooxygenases, 320, 418
Cytogenetic disorder(s), 173–181, 174f
chromosome 22q11.2 deletion syndrome as, 172f, 176–178
Down syndrome (trisomy 21) as, 175–176, 175f, 177f
hermaphroditism and pseudohermaphroditism as, 181
involving autosomes, 175–178
involving sex chromosomes, 178–181
Klinefelter syndrome as, 179
other trisomies as, 176, 177f
Turner syndrome as, 178, 179–180, 180f, 181f
Cytoid bodies, 1437, 1438f
Cytokines
and hematopoiesis, 202
and lymphocyte growth, activation, and differentiation, 202
and lymphocyte movement, 202
as growth factors, 97
general properties of, 202–203
Cytokines *(Continued)*
in asthma, 726
in cirrhosis, 884f
in diabetes, 1194
in glomerulonephritis, 972
in immediate hypersensitivity, 209
in immune system, 198, 202–203
in inflammation, 53f, 54, 56f, 57, 70–71, 71f, 74t, 202
in rheumatoid arthritis, 1307
in septic shock, 140, 141f, 142f
in wound healing, 111t
Cytologic smears, 336
Cytomegalic inclusion disease (CID), 367
Cytomegalovirus (CMV), 347t, 366–368
and atherosclerosis, 524
congenital anomalies due to, 473
congenital infection with, 366, 367
encephalitis due to, 1374
esophagitis due to, 806
immune evasion by, 359, 367
in AIDS, 256, 367–368
in immunosuppressed individuals, 367–368
morphology of, 367, 367f
perinatal infection with, 367
transmission of, 366–367
Cytomegalovirus colitis, 368
Cytomegalovirus mononucleosis, 367
Cytomegalovirus pneumonitis, 368
Cytomegalovirus retinitis, 368
Cytoplasmic antineutrophil cytoplasmic antibodies (c-ANCA), 535
in pauci-immune crescentic glomerulonephritis, 977
Cytoplasmic blebs, 13f, 20f, 23, 27
Cytoplasmic retinol-binding protein (CRBP), 476f
Cytoplasmic/cellular retinoic acid—binding protein (CRABP), 475, 476f
Cytoskeletal abnormalities, 18, 34, 34f
Cytoskeleton, 34
Cytostatic drugs, 11
Cytotoxic anticancer drugs, apoptosis due to, 26, 31
Cytotoxic edema, 1352
Cytotoxic release, in phagocytosis, 61
Cytotoxic T lymphocytes (CTLs), 198
antitumor effect of, 330
apoptosis of, 331
cell death induced by, 26, 31–32
hepatitis B virus and, 369
in cell-mediated hypersensitivity, 217–218
recognition of tumor antigens by, 328, 329f
Cytotoxicity, antibody-dependent cell-mediated, 201
Cytotoxin(s), 834
Cytotoxin-associated antigen *(CagA)* gene, 328
in peptic ulcer disease, 818
Cytoxan (cyclophosphamide)
and bladder carcinoma, 1032
myocardial disease due to, 610

D

D1 cells, 1189
Dacryoadenitis, sclerosing, 1423
DAD (diffuse alveolar damage). *See* Acute respiratory distress syndrome (ARDS).
DAD-R gene, 1041
DAF (decay-accelerating factor), 405
Dandy-Walker malformation, 1355
Dane particle, 892, 896
Darier sign, 1250
DC(s). *See* Dendritic cells (DCs).
DCIS. *See* Ductal carcinoma in situ (DCIS).
DCM. *See* Dilated cardiomyopathy (DCM).
DDE, 434–435

D-dimer, 130
DDT, 434–435
De Quervain thyroiditis, 1170–1171, 1171f
Dead cells, removal of, 31
Deafness, eighth nerve, in syphilis, 391
Death domain, 29, 30f
Death receptor—initiated pathway, in apoptosis, 28–29, 29f, 30f
Decay-accelerating factor (DAF), 405
Decompression disease/sickness, 137, 446
Decoy receptor, 1184
Deep venous thrombosis
  clinical correlations of, 134–135
  edema due to, 120
  thrombophlebitis and phlebothrombosis due to, 544
Deep-seated fibromatosis, 1319–1320, 1320f
Deer tick, 392, 392f
Defective DNA repair syndromes, 285, 287t, 288, 289, 306–308, 308f
Defensins
  in phagocytosis, 61
  in small intestinal mucosa, 829
Deformations, 471
Degenerative diseases, 1385–1397
  affecting cerebral cortex, 1386–1391, 1386f–1388f, 1389t
  affecting motor neurons, 1396–1397, 1396f
  aggregated proteins in, 1351, 1351t
  characteristics of, 1385–1386
  of basal ganglia and brain stem, 1391–1394, 1392f, 1393f
  of central nervous system, 1385–1397
    affecting cerebral cortex, 1386–1391, 1386f–1388f, 1389t
    affecting motor neurons, 1396–1397, 1396f
    aggregated proteins in, 1351, 1351t
    of basal ganglia and brain stem, 1391–1394, 1392f, 1393f
    spinocerebellar, 1394–1396, 1395t
  of joint, 1304–1305, 1305f
  spinocerebellar, 1394–1396, 1395t
Dehydroepiandrosterone, 1211
Dejerine-Sottas disease, 1333–1334
Delayed type hypersensitivity, 79, 215, 215f–217f, 216–217
Deletions, 147, 149, 149f, 174, 174f
Dellen, 1426
Delta agent, 347t, 891t, 895–896, 896t, 897f
Delta antigen, 896
δ cell(s), 1189
  somatostatin production in, 1191f
δ granules (dense bodies), in hemostasis, 126, 127
δ-cell tumors, 1207
δ-toxin, 372
Dementia(s)
  Alzheimer. *See* Alzheimer disease (AD).
  defined, 1386
  due to niacin deficiency, 458
  frontotemporal, 1389–1391
  hormone replacement therapy and, 428
  motor neuron disease inclusion, 1391
  posttraumatic, 1360
  vascular (multi-infarct), 1369, 1391
Dementia lacking distinctive histology (DLDH), 1391
Dementia pugilistica, 1360
Dementia with Lewy bodies (DLB), 1393
Demyelinating diseases, 1382–1385, 1383f, 1384f
Demyelination, segmental, 1326f, 1328–1329, 1329f
Dendritic cells (DCs)
  in HIV infection, 252–253, 258
  in immune system, 199–201, 200f
  in Langerhans histiocytosis, 701
Dendrocytes, in skin, 1228f, 1229
Denervation atrophy, 9, 1330, 1335–1336, 1336f
Dengue virus, 347t
Dense bodies (δ granules), in hemostasis, 126, 127
Dense-deposit disease, 971, 975t, 984, 985, 986f
Dental caries, 774–775
Dental imperfections, in osteogenesis imperfecta, 1280
Dental plaque, 775
Dentatorubral-pallidoluysian atrophy, 184t
Dentigerous cyst, 782
Dentin, 774, 774f
Denys-Drash syndrome, 504–505
Deoxyribonucleic acid. *See* DNA.
Dermatitis
  atopic, 1254t
  contact, 217, 217f, 1254f, 1254t, 1255, 1255f
  due to niacin deficiency, 458, 458f
  eczematous, 1253–1255, 1253f–1255f, 1254t
  in ariboflavinosis, 457
  irritant, 1254t
  radiation, 440, 440f
  seborrheic, 1257–1258
  spongiotic, 1254f, 1255
Dermatitis herpetiformis, 1260f, 1262–1263, 1262f, 1263f
Dermatofibroma, 1247–1248, 1247f, 1320–1321
Dermatofibrosarcoma protuberans, 1248
Dermatographism, 1250
Dermatologic disorders. *See* Skin disorder(s).
Dermatomyositis, 1342–1343, 1342f
  paraneoplastic, 334t
Dermatophytes, 351, 352
Dermatophytoses, 1267–1268, 1268f
Dermatosis(es), inflammatory
  acute, 1252–1256, 1252f–1256f, 1254t
  chronic, 1256–1259, 1257f–1259f
Dermatosis papulosa nigra, 1237
Dermatosparaxis, 156, 156t
Dermis, 1228f, 1229f
  tumors of, 1247–1248, 1247f
Dermoid cyst(s)
  of skin, 1238
  ovarian, 272, 272f, 1099–1100, 1100f
Descemet membrane, 1422f, 1427, 1427f
Desmoid tumors, 115, 1319–1320, 1320f
Desmoplasia, 270
Desmoplastic response, 950
Desmoplastic small round cell tumor, 873
Desmosomes, 105
Desquamative interstitial pneumonia (DIP), 729, 740, 740f
Destruction complex, 304f
Development
  embryonic, 474, 475f
  fibroblast growth factor in, 96
Developmental abnormalities
  of bone, 1278–1288, 1280t
  of central nervous system, 1353–1356, 1355f, 1356f
Developmental plasticity, 92
Devic disease, 1384–1385
DHT (dihydrotestosterone), in benign prostatic hyperplasia, 1048–1049, 1049f
Diabesity, 1205
Diabetes insipidus, 1162, 1163–1164
Diabetes mellitus (DM), 1189–1205
  advanced glycation end products in, 1198, 1198t
  and atherosclerosis, 521
  as autoimmune disease, 223
  classification of, 1190, 1190t
  clinical features of, 1202–1205, 1203f, 1204f, 1204t
  complications of, 1204–1205
Diabetes mellitus (DM) *(Continued)*
    morphology of, 1199–1201, 1199f–1202f
    pathogenesis of, 1197–1199, 1198t
  diagnosis of, 1190
  due to insulin gene or insulin receptor mutations, 1197
  epidemiology of, 1189–1190
  glycogen in, 39
  insulin-resistant, 212t
  macrovascular disease in, 1197, 1200, 1200f
  maternal, congenital anomalies due to, 473–474
  maturity-onset, of the young, 1197
  microvascular disease in, 1197, 1200–1201, 1201f
  mitochondrial, 1197
  monogenic forms of, 1197
  morphology of, 1199–1201, 1199f–1202f
  normal insulin physiology and, 1190–1192, 1191f–1193f
  obesity and, 462
  papillary necrosis in, 998, 1004t
  pathogenesis of, 1192–1199
  polyol pathway in, 1198–1199
  protein kinase C in, 1198
  pyelonephritis with, 999
  retina in, 1437–1439, 1438f, 1440f
  T cell—mediated hypersensitivity in, 215t
  type 1
    ß-cell destruction in, 1193–1194, 1193f
    clinical features of, 1202–1205, 1203f, 1204t
    defined, 1190, 1190t
    environmental factors in, 1194
    genetic susceptibility to, 1194, 1204t
    honeymoon period for, 1202
    infections and, 1194
    pathogenesis of, 1192–1194, 1193f, 1204t
  type 2
    ß-cell dysfunction in, 1196–1197
    clinical features of, 1202–1204, 1204t
    complications of, 1204–1205
    defined, 1190, 1190t
    genetic susceptibility to, 1194–1195, 1204t
    insulin resistance in, 1195–1196, 1195f, 1196f
    obesity and, 1195–1196, 1196f, 1202, 1204
    pathogenesis of, 1194–1197, 1195f, 1196f, 1204t
Diabetic glomerulosclerosis, 990–992, 991f, 992f
Diabetic ketoacidosis (DKA), 1202
Diabetic microangiopathy, 1197, 1200–1201, 1201f
Diabetic nephropathy, 990–992
  clinical features of, 992, 1204–1205
  epidemiology of, 990–991
  morphology of, 991–992, 991f, 992f, 1201, 1201f, 1202f
  pathogenesis of, 991
Diabetic neuropathy, 1201, 1205, 1334, 1334f
Diabetic retinopathy, 1437–1439, 1438f, 1440f
  background (preproliferative), 1437–1439
  epidemiology of, 1205
  proliferative, 1439
Diacylglycerol, 99
Diagonals, 557
Dialysis, in chronic glomerulonephritis, 989
Dialysis-associated cystic disease, 966
Diapedesis, of leukocytes, 53, 53f, 54–56, 57f
Diaper rash, 398
Diaphragmatic hernia, 812
Diarrhea, 831–832, 832t
  defined, 831
  due to AIDS, 841, 841f
  due to deranged motility, 832, 832t
  due to malabsorption, 832, 832t
  due to niacin deficiency, 458

Diarrhea *(Continued)*
exudative, 832, 832t
in AIDS, 256
osmotic, 832, 832t
secretory, 832, 832t
traveler's, 832
with transplantation, 841, 841f
Diastole, 557
Diastolic dysfunction, 560
Diathesis(es)
hemorrhagic (bleeding), 123, 649–658
due to abnormalities in clotting factors, 653–656, 654f
due to defective platelet functions, 653
due to disseminated intravascular coagulation, 656–658, 657t, 658f
due to thrombocytopenia, 650–653, 651t
due to vessel wall abnormalities, 650
due to vitamin K deficiency, 456
thrombotic, acquired, 131–132, 132f
DIC. *See* Disseminated intravascular coagulation (DIC).
Diet. *See also* Nutrition.
and breast cancer, 1132
and colorectal carcinoma, 864–865
and gastric carcinoma, 823–824
and systemic diseases, 465–466
for phenylketonuria, 487, 488
in cancer prevention, 466
Dietary fiber, 466
Differentiation
cellular adaptations of, 5–11
in neoplasia, 272–276, 274f, 275f
in tissue homeostasis, 89, 89f
terminal, 89
Differentiation antigens, 330
Diffuse alveolar damage (DAD). *See* Acute respiratory distress syndrome (ARDS).
Diffuse axonal injury, of brain, 1358–1359
Diffuse cortical necrosis, 1011–1012, 1012f
Diffuse hyperplasia of the islets, 1206
Diffuse hypoxic/ischemic encephalopathy, 1361–1363, 1362f
Diffuse interstitial disease(s), 728–741, 729t
cryptogenic organizing pneumonia as, 731, 732f
due to complications of therapies, 737, 737t
fibrosing, 729–737
granulomatous, 737–739, 738f, 739f
hypersensitivity pneumonitis as, 739, 739f
idiopathic pulmonary fibrosis as, 729–731, 730f, 731f
interstitial pneumonia as
desquamative, 740, 740f
nonspecific, 731, 732f
obstructive *vs.*, 716–717
pneumoconioses as, 732–737, 733t, 734f–736f
pulmonary alveolar proteinosis as, 741, 741f
pulmonary eosinophilia as, 740
pulmonary involvement in collagen vascular diseases as, 731–732
respiratory bronchiolitis—associated, 740–741
sarcoidosis as, 737–739, 738f, 739f
smoking-related, 740–741, 740f
Diffuse large B-cell lymphoma (DLBCL), 671t, 676–677, 676f, 677f
Diffuse mesangial sclerosis
in Denys-Drash syndrome, 504
in diabetes, 1201
Diffuse nuclear staining, 228
DiGeorge syndrome, 178, 243
congenital heart disease in, 565
genetic basis for, 241f, 243, 565
partial, 243
thymic hypoplasia or aplasia in, 565, 706
Digestive system. *See* Gastrointestinal tract.
Digital arteries, in rheumatoid arthritis, 1306
Dihydropteridine reductase, 488
Dihydropteridine synthetase, 488
Dihydrotestosterone (DHT), in benign prostatic hyperplasia, 1048–1049, 1049f
1,25-Dihydroxyvitamin D_3 (1,25-$[OH]_2D_3$) deficiency, renal osteodystrophy due to, 1288
Dilantin (phenytoin) ingestion, oral manifestations of, 778t
Dilated cardiomyopathy (DCM), 601, 602–604
arrhythmogenic right ventricular, 604, 604f
clinical features of, 604
etiology of, 602, 602t
idiopathic, 602
morphology of, 601f, 602–603, 603f
pathogenesis of, 603–604, 606, 607f
thyrotoxic, 1166
Dimerization, of receptors, 98, 99f
DIP (desquamative interstitial pneumonia), 729, 740, 740f
Diphtheria, 374–375, 374f
oral manifestations of, 778t
peripheral neuropathy in, 1332
Diphtheritic myocarditis, 608
Diphyllobothrium latum, 353, 407, 839
Direct cell toxicity, 215, 215f
Direct gene diagnosis, 188–189, 188f, 189f
Disaccharidase deficiency, 844–845
Discoid lupus erythematosus (DLE), 1258–1259, 1259f
Discoid rash, in systemic lupus erythematosus, 228t
Disintegrin, 111
Disruptions, 470–471, 471f
Dissecting osteitis, 1287, 1287f
Dissection
aortic, 532–534, 533f, 534f
arterial, 531
Disseminated intravascular coagulation (DIC), 135, 656–658
clinical course of, 658
etiology and pathogenesis of, 656–657, 657t, 658f
impaired hepatic circulation in, 918
in toxemia of pregnancy, 1106, 1107–1108, 1109f
morphology of, 657–658
paraneoplastic, 335
tumor necrosis factor and, 85, 657
Disseminated peritoneal leiomyomatosis, 1090
Disuse atrophy, 9, 1330
Divalent metal transporter 1 (DMT1), 644
Diversion colitis, 841–842
Diverticulosis, 854, 855f
Diverticulum(a)
colonic, 854–855, 855f
defined, 802, 854
epiphrenic, 801f, 802
false *vs.* true, 802
Meckel, 830, 830f, 854
of bladder, 1026
traction, 802
ureteral, 1024
Zenker, 801f, 802
DJ-1, in Parkinson disease, 1392
DKA (diabetic ketoacidosis), 1202
DLB (dementia with Lewy bodies), 1393
DLBCL (diffuse large B-cell lymphoma), 671t, 676–677, 676f, 677f
DLDH (dementia lacking distinctive histology), 1391
DLE (discoid lupus erythematosus), 1258–1259, 1259f
DM. *See* Diabetes mellitus (DM).
DMD (Duchenne muscular dystrophy), 1336–1338, 1337f
DMPK (dystrophica myotonia-protein kinase), 1338–1339
DMT1 (divalent metal transporter 1), 644
DNA
breakdown of, in apoptosis, 27, 28f
damage to, apoptosis due to, 31
mitochondrial, 185, 185f
DNA content, in breast carcinoma, 1148
DNA gene chips, 316b
DNA methylation, silencing of tumor suppressor genes by, 315
DNA microarrays, 316b, 317f, 338
DNA mismatch repair genes, in colorectal cancer, 864
DNA probes, 361t
DNA repair, defective, 285, 287t, 288, 289, 306–308, 308f
DNA repair genes, 294f
DNA topoisomerase I, in systemic sclerosis, 238
DNA viruses, oncogenic, 324–327, 325f, 326f
DNT (dysembryoplastic neuroepithelial tumor), 1406
Döhle bodies, 665, 665f
Dominant negative allele, 151, 154
Donovanosis, 380–381
Dose-response curve, for chemical toxicity, 417, 417f
Double minutes (dms), 315
Down syndrome, 175–176, 175f, 177f, 472
Doxorubicin (Adriamycin), myocardial disease due to, 609–610
DPC4 gene, 305
Draining sinus, in osteomyelitis, 1291
Drug(s)
aplastic anemia due to, 647, 647t
cell injury due to, 13, 25–26
congenital anomalies due to, 473
hemolysis due to, 628
lysosomal diseases due to, 33
Drug abuse, 424–426, 424t, 425f
Drug reactions
adverse, 426, 426t
antibody-mediated cell destruction in, 210
bleeding disorders due to, 650
genetically determined, 154
vasculitides due to, 535
Drug toxicity, after bone marrow transplantation, 921
Drug-induced agranulocytosis, 663
Drug-induced aseptic meningitis, 1370
Drug-induced asthma, 726
Drug-induced interstitial nephritis, 1002–1004, 1002f, 1003f, 1004t
Drug-induced intestinal injury, 841
Drug-induced liver disease, 903–907, 903t
Drug-induced lung diseases, 737, 737t
Drug-induced lupus erythematosus, 229t, 235
Drug-induced myopathies, 1344
Drug-induced neutropenia, 663
Drug-induced thrombocytopenia, 652
Drug-related eczematous dermatitis, 1254t
Dubin-Johnson syndrome, 888, 888f, 888t
Duchenne muscular dystrophy (DMD), 1336–1338, 1337f
Duct hyperplasia, atypical, 1129, 1130f
Duct obstruction, apoptosis due to, 26
Duct of Santorini, 939, 940f
Duct of Wirsung, 939, 940f
Ductal carcinoma in situ (DCIS), 1139–1141
clinical presentation of, 1123t
comedo, 1139, 1139f
cribriform, 1140, 1140f
management of, 1140

Ductal carcinoma in situ (DCIS) *(Continued)*
mechanisms of carcinogenesis for, 1135
micropapillary, 1140, 1141f
morphology of, 1139–1140, 1139f–1141f
natural history of, 1140
noncomedo, 1140, 1140f, 1141f
papillary, 1140, 1141f
prognosis for, 1140–1141
risk modifiers for, 1130t
solid, 1140, 1140f
Ductal hyperplasia, atypical, 1129, 1130f
Ductal sex, 181
Ducts of Luschka, 928
Ductular reaction, 880
Ductus arteriosus, patent, 564t, 567f, 568
coarctation of aorta with, 571, 571f
Duke criteria, for infective endocarditis, 598, 598t
Duncan disease, 371
Duodenal ulcer, 78f, 819f
Duodenum, anatomy of, 828
Dupuytren contracture, 1319
Dürck granulomas, 403
Duret hemorrhages, 1353–1354, 1354f
Dutcher bodies, 680, 681
Dwarf tapeworm, 839
Dwarfism
pituitary, 1163
thanatophoric, 1280t, 1354
Dyscrasias, hereditary, with amyloidosis, 260–261
Dysembryoplastic neuroepithelial tumor (DNT), 1406
Dysentery, 831–832, 833
amebic, 834, 839–840, 839f
bacillary, 834–835
Dysferlin, 1339t
Dysfunctional uterine bleeding, 1081–1083, 1081t, 1082f
Dysgerminoma, 1041, 1101, 1101f
Dyskeratosis, 1230
Dyslipidemias, in diabetes, 1204
Dysmorphogenesis, 471f
Dysostoses, 1278
Dysphagia, 799
Dysplasias, 275–276, 275f, 472, 1278
Dysplastic nevus, 1233–1234, 1233t, 1234f, 1245–1246
Dyspnea, in left-sided heart failure, 562
paroxysmal nocturnal, 563
Dystrobrevin, 1337f
Dystroglycans, 1327, 1337f
Dystrophic calcification, 22
Dystrophica myotonia-protein kinase (DMPK), 1338–1339
Dystrophin, 1336, 1337f
Dystrophin-associated proteins, 1327

E

E2F transcription factor, in cell cycle, 289
E2F/DP1/RB complex, in cell cycle, 289, 291f
E6 protein, of human papillomavirus, 324–325, 325f
E7 protein, of human papillomavirus, 324–325, 325f
Ears, 787–788
EB (elementary body), of *Chlamydia trachomatis,* 394
EBNA-2 gene, 325
EBV. *See* Epstein-Barr virus (EBV).
EC(s) (endothelial cells)
anatomy and physiology of, 513–514, 514f, 514t
in atherosclerosis, 522–523, 525f
E-cadherin gene, 300t, 305–306
and extracellular matrix, 311
E-cadherin gene *(Continued)*
in *APC*/ß-catenin pathway, 304f
in breast carcinoma, 1136b, 1137b
in gastric carcinoma, 824
Ecchymoses, 123
in immune thrombocytopenic purpura, 652
Eccrine poroma, 1238
Echinococcus granulosus, 406, 407
Echinococcus multilocularis, 407
Echinococcus spp, 351, 353
ECL (enterochromaffin-like) cells, 811
Eclampsia, 920, 920f, 1106–1110
clinical course of, 1110
impaired hepatic circulation in, 918
morphology of, 1109–1110, 1110f
pathogenesis of, 1107–1108, 1109f
ECM. *See* Extracellular matrix (ECM).
Ecstasy, 426
Ecthyma gangrenosum, 379
Ectocervix, 1081
Ectoparasites, 352
Ectopia lentis, 154–155
Ectopic hormones, 276, 333, 339t
Ectopic pregnancy, 1105, 1106f
Eczema, 1253–1255, 1253f–1255f, 1254t
immunodeficiency with thrombocytopenia and, 244
Eczema herpeticum, 366
Eczematous dermatitis, 1253–1255, 1253f–1255f, 1254t
Edema, 120–122
cardiac, 120–121, 121f, 122
cerebral, 1352
clinical correlation of, 122
cytotoxic, 1352
defined, 49, 119, 120
due to increased hydrostatic pressure, 120–121, 120f, 120t
due to inflammation, 120t
due to lymphatic obstruction, 120t, 121–122
due to reduced plasma osmotic pressure (hypoproteinemia), 120f, 120t, 121
due to renal dysfunction, 122
due to sodium retention, 120t, 122
hereditary angioneurotic, 67b
in inflammation, 49, 50, 50f
in nephrotic syndrome, 978
morphology of, 122
of brain, 122
pathophysiologic categories of, 120, 120f, 120t
periorbital, 122
pulmonary, 122, 714–715, 714t
due to microvascular injury, 714t, 715
hemodynamic (cardiogenic), 714–715, 714t
in left-sided heart failure, 562
in sudden infant death syndrome, 496
simple orthostatic, 543
stromal, in Fuchs endothelial dystrophy, 1428, 1429
subcutaneous, 122
vasogenic, 1352
Edema factor (EF), of anthrax, 375, 376f
Edwards syndrome, 176, 177f
Effector molecules, 98–99, 99f
Effector T cells, 194f
Effusion, 76, 77f
EGF (epidermal growth factor), 95–96, 95t
in scar formation, 110
oncogene for, 295t
EGFR (epidermal growth factor receptor), 95, 96
in colorectal cancer, 318
EGFR (epidermal growth factor receptor) gene, 295t, 296
in glioblastoma, 1403
EGFR oncogene, 295t, 296
EHEC (enterohemorrhagic *E. coli),* 834, 838
Ehlers-Danlos syndrome (EDS), 152, 155–156, 156t
bleeding disorders due to, 650
Ehrlich, Paul, 49, 328
Ehrlichia chaffeensis, 395, 396t
Ehrlichia ewengii, 396t
Ehrlichiosis, 350, 395, 395f
granulocytic, 396t
monocytic, 396t
Eicosanoids, in inflammation, 68–70, 68t, 69f, 70f
EIEC (enteroinvasive *E. coli),* 834, 838
Eighth nerve deafness, in syphilis, 391
EIN (endometrial intraepithelial neoplasia), 1085–1086, 1086f
ELAM-1 (endothelial leukocyte adhesion molecule-1), 54, 54t, 55b
Elastic fibers, in extracellular matrix, 104
Elastin, in extracellular matrix, 103f, 104
Electrical injuries, 446
Electromagnetic fields, 442
Electromagnetic radiation
ionizing, 436–441, 436t, 438t, 439f–441f
nonionizing, 436, 436t, 442
ultraviolet, 436t, 441–442, 441t, 442f
Electromechanical dissociation, due to pulmonary embolism, 743
Elementary body (EB), of *Chlamydia trachomatis,* 394
Elephantiasis, 410, 410f
Elschnig's spots, 1436
Embolism, 135–137
air, 137
amniotic fluid, 137
cerebral, 1363–1364, 1364f
defined, 119
due to infective endocarditis, 596
fat, 136–137, 137f
paradoxical, 566
pulmonary, 136, 136f, 742, 742f, 743
due to deep venous thrombosis, 544
hormone replacement therapy and, 427–428
oral contraceptives and, 427
Embolization, bone marrow, 1364, 1364f
Embolus(i), 132, 135
athero-, 519
cholesterol, 135, 519
myocardial infarction due to, 576
paradoxical, 136, 576
saddle, 136
Embryogenesis, programmed destruction of cells during, 26
Embryonal carcinoma, 1041, 1043, 1043f
infantile, 1043
Embryonal rhabdomyosarcoma
of bladder, 1033
of skeletal muscle, 1322
of vagina, 1071–1072, 1072f
Embryonic development, 474, 475f
Embryonic stem cells (ES), 91, 92f
Embryopathy
retinoic acid, 474, 475, 476f
rubella, 473
Emery-Dreifuss muscular dystrophy, 1338t
Emphysema, 717–722
bullous, 721, 721f
centriacinar (centrilobular), 718, 718f, 719f
due to coal workers' pneumoconiosis, 734
chronic bronchitis *vs.,* 721t
clinical course of, 721
compensatory hyperinflation, 721
distal acinar (paraseptal), 719
incidence of, 719
interstitial, 721–722
irregular, 719

Emphysema *(Continued)*
morphology of, 720–721
obstructive overinflation, 721
panacinar (panlobular), 718–719, 718f, 719f, 720–721
pathogenesis of, 719–720, 720f, 723
types of, 717–719, 721–722
Empty sella syndrome, 1163
Empyema
of gallbladder, 932
of lung, 750, 766t, 767
of sinus, 784
subdural, 1371
tuberculous, 386
ENaC (epithelial sodium channel), in cystic fibrosis, 490, 491f
Enamel, 774, 774f
Encephalitis
herpes, 1373–1374, 1374f
HIV, 1375–1376, 1376f
measles inclusion body, 363
mumps, 364
paraneoplastic limbic (brainstem), 1410, 1411t
viral, 1372
arthropod-borne, 1373
Encephalocele, 1354
Encephalomyelitis
acute disseminated (perivenous), 1385
acute necrotizing hemorrhagic, 1385
viral, 1372
Encephalomyopathies, mitochondrial, 1397, 1398–1399
Encephalopathy(ies)
diffuse hypoxic/ischemic, 1361–1363, 1362f
hepatic, 882, 899, 1400
hypertensive, 1369
hypoxic, due to heart failure, 563
ischemic, 141
multicystic, 1356
spongiform, 346
transmissible, 1351t, 1380–1382, 1381f
subacute necrotizing, 1342, 1398
Wernicke, 457, 457f, 1399
Encephalotrigeminal angiomatosis, 547
Enchondral ossification, 1277–1278, 1278f
Enchondromas, 1296–1297, 1297f
Enchondromatosis, 1296
Endarteritis, obliterative, due to tuberculosis, 1371
Endemic relapsing fever, 391
Endocardial fibroelastosis, 607–608
Endocarditis
acute, 596
Candida, 399
infective (bacterial), 595–598
acute *vs.* subacute, 596
brain abscess due to, 1371
clinical features of, 596–598
diagnostic criteria for, 596–598, 598t
due to mitral valve prolapse, 592
etiology and pathogenesis of, 596
glomerular lesions in, 990
morphology of, 596, 597f
of prosthetic valve, 601
thromboembolism due to, 133
Libman-Sacks, 133, 234, 234f, 597f, 598–599
nonbacterial thrombotic, 133, 597f, 598, 599f
paraneoplastic, 334t, 335
of systemic lupus erythematosus, 133, 234, 234f, 597f, 598–599
prosthetic valve, 596
subacute, 596
verrucous (fungal), 133, 596
in systemic lupus erythematosus, 234, 234f
Endocervical glands, 1081
Endocervical polyps, 1073.1073f
Endocervix, 1081
Endocrine atypia, 1186
Endocrine cells
of intestine, 829
of stomach, 811
Endocrine effects
of cytokines, 202
of obesity, 465t
Endocrine signaling, 97f, 98
Endocrine stimulation, atrophy due to loss of, 9
Endocrine system, 1155–1224
adrenal glands in, 1207–1223
pancreas in, 1189–1207
parathyroid glands in, 1183–1189
pineal gland in, 1223–1224
pituitary gland in, 1156–1164
thyroid gland in, 1164–1183
Endocrine therapy, for prostate cancer, 1056
Endocrinopathies, paraneoplastic, 333–334, 334t
Endocytosis, 32, 32f
Endodermal sinus tumor
ovarian, 1101, 1101f
testicular, 1043
Endolymphatic stromal myosis, 1089
Endometrial adenocarcinoma, 1087, 1087f
Endometrial adenosarcomas, 1088–1089
Endometrial carcinoma, 1086–1088, 1087f
and breast cancer, 1132
hormone replacement therapy and, 427
Endometrial carcinosarcomas, 1088, 1089f
Endometrial hyperplasia, 7, 1085–1086, 1086f
Endometrial intraepithelial neoplasia (EIN), 1085–1086, 1086f
Endometrial polyps, 1085
Endometrial stromal sarcoma, 1089f
Endometrial stromal tumors, 1089, 1089f
Endometrioid carcinoma, 1087–1088, 1097–1098
Endometrioid tumors, of ovaries, 1097–1098
Endometriosis, 1083–1084, 1084f
Endometriotic cyst, 1084f
Endometritis, chronic, 1083
Endometrium, 1079–1089
endometriosis and adenomyosis of, 1083–1084, 1083f, 1084f
functional disorders of, 1081–1083, 1081t, 1082f
hyperplasia of, 1085–1086, 1086f
in menstrual cycle, 1080–1081, 1080f, 1081f
inflammation of, 1083
malignant tumors of, 1086–1089, 1087f, 1089f
menopausal and postmenopausal changes in, 1082–1083
oral contraceptive effect on, 1082
Endomyocardial biopsies, 601
Endomyocardial fibrosis, 607
Endomyocarditis, Loeffler, 607
Endomysium, 1328
Endoneurium, 1327
Endonucleases, 16
Endophthalmitis, 1432, 1432f
Endoplasmic reticulum (ER)
dilation of, in cell injury, 20, 20f
smooth, induction (hypertrophy) of, 33, 33f
Endoplasmic reticulum (ER) stress
apoptosis due to, 26
due to unfolded or misfolded proteins, 38
Endosalpingiosis, 1095
Endostreptosin, in poststreptococcal glomerulonephritis, 974
Endothelial activation, 71, 514, 514f
Endothelial cells (ECs)
anatomy and physiology of, 513–514, 514f, 514t
in atherosclerosis, 522–523, 525f
Endothelial dysfunction, 514
Endothelial gaps, in inflammation, 50–52, 51f
Endothelial injury
disseminated intravascular coagulation due to, 656
in atherosclerosis, 522–523, 525f
in thrombosis, 130–131, 131f
in thrombotic microangiopathies, 1010
Endothelial leukocyte adhesion molecule-1 (ELAM-1), 54, 54t, 55b
Endothelial nitric oxide synthase (eNOS), 72, 72f
Endothelial precursor cells (EPCs), angiogenesis from, 107, 108, 108f
Endothelin, in hemostasis, 124
Endothelitis, 220
Endothelium, in hemostasis, 124–126, 126f
Endotoxic shock, 139, 140
Endotoxins, bacterial, 358
Endovascular stents, 551, 552f
End-stage renal disease, 961
Energy balance, 462, 463f
eNOS (endothelial nitric oxide synthase), 72, 72f
Entamoeba histolytica, 839–840
clinical features of, 840
forms of, 351, 351t
morphology of, 839, 839f
necrotizing inflammation due to, 362
pathogenesis of, 839
transmission and dissemination of, 353, 355
Enteritis
eosinophilic, 816
radiation, 841
regional, 847
Enterobacteriaceae, 350f
Enterobiasis, 838–839
Enterobius vermicularis, 838–839
Enterochromaffin cells, 1189
Enterochromaffin-like (ECL) cells, 811
Enterococcus faecalis, 373
Enterococcus faecium, 373
Enterocolitis, 831–842
antibiotic-associated (pseudomembranous), 836, 837–838, 837f
bacterial, 832–838, 834t, 836f, 837f
Campylobacter, 835, 837
collagenous and lymphocytic, 840–841
diarrhea and dysentery in, 831–832, 832t
diversion, 841–842
due to drug-induced intestinal injury, 841
in AIDS patients, 841
in bacterial overgrowth syndrome, 838
in solitary rectal ulcer syndrome, 842
infectious, 832–841
necrotizing, 483, 483f, 840
neutropenic, 841
parasitic, 838–840, 839f, 840f
radiation, 841
Salmonella, 834, 835, 836–837
Shigella, 834–835, 836, 837f
viral gastroenteritis as, 832–833, 833t
with transplantation, 841, 841f
Enteroendocrine cells, 811
Enterohemorrhagic *E. coli* (EHEC), 834, 838
Enterohepatic circulation, 887
Enteroinvasive *E. coli* (EIEC), 834, 838
Enteropathic infections, bacterial, 349t
Enteropathogenic bacteria, 353
Enteropathogenic *E. coli* (EPEC), 838
Enteropathy
AIDS, 841
gluten-sensitive, 843–844, 843f
hemorrhagic, due to shock, 142
protein-losing, 821
in Crohn disease, 849
Enterotoxigenic *E. coli* (ETEC), 834, 838

Enterotoxins, bacterial, 834
Entrapment neuropathy, 1335
env gene, in human immunodeficiency virus, 247, 247f
Environment, and disease, 415–419, 416t, 417f, 418f
Environmental agents, white cell neoplasia due to, 667
Environmental causes, of congenital anomalies, 473–474, 473t
Environmental diseases
  epidemiology of, 416, 416t
  prevention of, 416–417
  recognition of, 416–417, 416t
Environmental exposures, 416
  personal, 419–426
  therapeutic, 426–428, 426t, 427t
  to air pollution
    indoor, 430, 430t
    outdoor, 428–430, 428t, 429t
  to natural toxins, 435–436, 435t
  to physical environment, 442–446, 443f, 443t, 444f
  to radiation, 436–442
    ionizing, 436–441, 436t, 438t, 439f–441f
    nonionizing, 436, 436t, 442
    ultraviolet, 441–442, 441t, 442f
Environmental factors
  in cancer, 283–284, 285t
  in hypertension, 528f, 529
  in systemic lupus erythematosus, 230
Environmental hazard(s)
  air pollution as
    indoor, 430, 430t
    outdoor, 428–430, 428t, 429t
  alcohol abuse as, 421–424, 422f, 422t, 423f
  drug abuse as, 424–426, 424t, 425f
  in physical environment, 442–446, 443f, 443t, 444f
  mechanisms of toxicity of, 417–419, 417f, 418f, 420f–421f
  natural toxins as, 435–436, 435t
  personal, 419–426
  radiation as, 436–442
    ionizing, 436–441, 436t, 438t, 439f–441f
    nonionizing, 436, 436t, 442
    ultraviolet, 441–442, 441t, 442f
  regulatory agencies for, 416
  therapeutic drugs as, 426–428, 426t, 427t
  tobacco use as, 419–421, 419t, 421t
Environmental Protection Agency, 416
Environmental tobacco smoke (ETS), 421
Environmental toxins, and breast cancer, 1133
Enzyme(s)
  in coagulation cascade, 127, 129f
  in immediate hypersensitivity, 208
Enzyme defect(s), 152–153, 153f, 158–168
  alkaptonuria due to, 167–168
  bone disorders due to, 1281–1282, 1282f, 1283f
  Gaucher disease due to, 161t, 163–165, 164f
  glycogen storage diseases due to, 165–167, 166f, 167f, 168t
  lysosomal storage diseases due to, 153, 158–165, 159f, 160f, 161t
  mucopolysaccharidoses due to, 161t, 165
  Niemann-Pick disease due to, 161t, 163, 163f
  Tay-Sachs disease due to, 160–161, 161t, 162f
Eosinophil(s)
  in chronic inflammation, 82, 82f
  in immediate hypersensitivity, 209
  origin and differentiation of, 621f
Eosinophilia, 664, 664t
  due to inflammation, 84
  in necrosis, 21, 21f
  pulmonary, 740
Eosinophilic enteritis, 816
Eosinophilic gastritis, 816
Eosinophilic granuloma, 701, 702
  of stomach, 822, 822f
Eosinophilic leukocytosis, 664, 664t
Eotaxin, 71
EPCs (endothelial precursor cells), angiogenesis from, 107, 108, 108f
EPEC (enteropathogenic *E. coli)*, 838
Ependymal cells, 1349, 1350
Ependymal granulations, 1350
Ependymitis, granular, 1372
Ependymoma(s), 1404–1405, 1405f
  myxopapillary, 1405
  sub-, 1405–1406
Ephelis, 1231
Epicardial coronary arteries, 557
  aging effect on, 559t
Epidemic(s), of influenza, 751
Epidemic relapsing fever, 391
Epidermal appendages, disorders of, 1264–1265, 1264f
Epidermal growth factor (EGF), 95–96, 95t
  in scar formation, 110
  oncogene for, 295t
Epidermal growth factor receptor (EGFR), 95, 96
  in colorectal cancer, 318
Epidermal growth factor receptor *(EGFR)* gene, 295t, 296
  in glioblastoma, 1403
Epidermal inclusion cyst, 1238
Epidermal maturation, disorders of, 1251–1252, 1252f
Epidermal stem cells, 93f
Epidermal tumor(s), premalignant and malignant, 1240–1247
  actinic keratosis as, 1240–1242, 1241f
  basal cell carcinoma as, 1242–1244, 1243f
  Merkel cell carcinoma as, 1244
  molecular genetics of, 1244–1247, 1245t, 1246f
  squamous cell carcinoma as, 1242, 1243f
Epidermis, 1228f, 1229f
Epidermodysplasia verruciformis, 1266
Epidermolysis bullosa, 1263, 1263f
Epididymis, inflammations of, 1039–1040, 1039f
Epididymitis, 1039, 1039f
Epidural hematoma, 1358f, 1359, 1359f
Epigenetic changes, in cancer cells, 315
Epilepsy, myoclonic, with ragged red fibers, 1342, 1399
Epimysium, 1328
Epinephrine, 1218
  in diabetic ketoacidosis, 1202
Epineurium, 1327
Epiphrenic diverticulum, 801f, 802
Epiphyseal dysplasia, multiple, 1280t
Epispadias, 1035
Epithelial barrier, of gastric mucosa, 811
Epithelial cell injury, in glomerulonephritis, 971, 972f
Epithelial cyst, 1238
Epithelial downgrowth membranes, 1432
Epithelial hyperplasia, of breast, 1128, 1128f
Epithelial skin tumors, benign, 1237–1240, 1237f, 1239f, 1240t, 1241f
Epithelial sodium channel (ENaC), in cystic fibrosis, 490, 491f
Epithelial tissue, renewal of, 94
Epithelioid cells, 216, 216f, 362
Epithelioid hemangioendothelioma, 550
Epithelioma, sebaceous, 1240t
Epitope spreading, 227
Epoxidation, of toxicant, 420f
Epstein-Barr virus (EBV), 347t, 369–371
  in AIDS-related B-cell lymphomas, 258
  in Burkitt lymphoma, 326, 326f, 677–678
  in carcinogenesis, 325–327, 326f
  in Hodgkin lymphoma, 690
  in immunodeficiency-associated large B-cell lymphoma, 677
  latency genes for, 370
  morphology of, 348f, 370–371, 370f
  pathogenesis of, 369–370, 369f
  white cell neoplasia due to, 667
Epulis, giant cell, of oral cavity, 776
ER. *See* Endoplasmic reticulum (ER).
ERB-B1 oncogene, 96, 295t, 296
ERB-B2 oncogene, 295t, 296, 315
ERK, 99f
Erlenmeyer flask deformity, 1282, 1282f
Erosion, 1230
Erysipelas, 373, 374f
Erythema chronicum migrans, 392, 1268
Erythema induratum, 1265
Erythema marginatum, due to rheumatic fever, 593
Erythema multiforme, 1255–1256, 1256f
  oral manifestations of, 778t
Erythema nodosum, 1265
Erythroblastosis fetalis, 210, 486, 487f
Erythrocyte(s)
  hemolytic anemia resulting from trauma to, 638, 638f
  in hemostatic plugs, 127
  origin and differentiation of, 621f
Erythrocyte sedimentation rate (ESR), 84
Erythrocytosis, 649, 649t
Erythroderma, 1256
Erythroid progenitors, in hemolytic anemia, 625, 625f
Erythroplakia, of oral cavity, 778–780, 779f
Erythroplasia of Queyrat, 1036
Erythropoiesis, anemias of diminished, 623t, 638–649
Erythropoietin receptor, mutations in, 649
ES (embryonic stem cells), 91, 92f
Escherichia coli
  adherence to host cell by, 358
  enteroadherent, 838
  enterohemorrhagic, 834, 838
  enteroinvasive, 834, 838
  enteropathogenic, 838
  enterotoxigenic, 834, 838
  immune invasion by, 360
  in abscesses, 393
  in bronchoalveolar lavage specimen, 350f
  meningitis due to, 1369
  transmission and dissemination of, 353
Escherichia coli strain O157:H7
  enterocolitis due to, 834, 838
  hemolytic-uremic syndrome due to, 653
E-selectin, 53f, 54, 54t, 55b
Esophageal atresia, 800, 800f
Esophageal carcinoma, 806–809, 807f–809f, 807t
Esophageal mucosal webs, 800
Esophageal rings, 800
Esophageal stenosis, 800
Esophageal varices, 802–803, 803f
Esophageal webs, 800
Esophagitis, 803–806
  Candida, 398
  herpes, 366
  infectious and chemical, 805–806
  reflux, 804, 804f
Esophagus, 798–809
  agenesis of, 800
  Barrett, 804–805, 805f
    adenocarcinoma arising from, 808–809, 809f

Esophagus (Continued)
congenital anomalies of, 799–800, 800f
ectopic tissue rests in, 799
inflammation of, 803–806, 804f, 805f
lesions associated with motor dysfunction of, 800–802, 801f, 802f
normal anatomy and physiology of, 798–799
symptoms of pathology of, 799
tumors of, 806–809, 807f–809f, 807t
Espundia, 404
ESR (erythrocyte sedimentation rate), 84
Essential thrombocytosis, 700, 700f
Esthesioneuroblastomas, 785
Estrogen, and gallstones, 929
Estrogen deficiency, and osteoporosis, 1284
Estrogen exposure, and breast cancer, 1132
Estrogen receptor(s), in breast carcinoma, 1147, 1148f
Estrogen receptor (ER)-negative carcinomas, 1136b, 1147
Estrogen receptor (ER)-positive carcinomas, 1136b, 1137b, 1138
État lunaire, 1368
ETEC (enterotoxigenic *E. coli),* 834, 838
Ethanol
abuse of, 421–424, 422f, 422t
neurologic effects of, 1400, 1400f
Ethanol myopathy, 1344
Ethylene glycol, 424
Ethylene oxide, cancer due to, 285t
Etiology, defined, 4
ETS (environmental tobacco smoke), 421
Euploidy, 173
Ewing sarcoma (ES), 1301–1302
epidemiology of, 1301
genetic and other markers of, 500t
genetic basis for, 1301
molecular diagnosis of, 337
morphology of, 1301–1302, 1302f
oncogenes in, 314t, 315
Ewing sarcoma *(EWS)* gene, 315
EWS-FLI 1 protein, 315
Excoriation, 1230
Execution phase, of apoptosis, 30–31
Exercise
and breast cancer, 1132
and osteoporosis, 1283
Exertional myoglobinuria, 1342
Exocytosis, 32f, 1230
in phagocytosis, 61
Exophthalmic ophthalmoplegia, 1343
Exophthalmos, in Graves disease, 1167f, 1173
Exostosis, 1296, 1296f
multiple hereditary, 1296
Exotoxins, bacterial, 358, 359
Expanded-polytetrafluoroethylene graft, 551–552
Exstrophy, of bladder, 1026, 1026f
EXT genes, in osteochondroma, 1296
External elastic lamina, 512, 512f
External os, 1081, 1083f
Extra-adrenal paraganglia, 1218, 1219f
tumors of, 1221
Extracellular matrix (ECM), 4, 103–106
and carcinogenesis, 313
cell adhesion proteins in, 103f, 104–105, 106f
collagen in, 103f, 104, 104t, 105f
damage to, 89
elastin, fibrillin, and elastic fibers in, 103f, 104
in inflammation, 53f
invasion of, 311–313, 312f
major components of, 103–106, 103f
other adhesive glycoproteins in, 105
proteoglycans and hyaluronic acid in, 103f, 106
Extracellular matrix (ECM) deposition, and scar formation, 110
Extracellular matrix (ECM) proteins, as regulators of angiogenesis, 109
Extracellular structural proteins, bone disorders due to defects in, 1279–1281, 1280t, 1281t, 1282f
Extradural abscess, 1371
Extralobar sequestrations, 713
Extramedullary hematopoiesis, in sudden infant death syndrome, 496
Extranodal marginal zone lymphomas, 671t, 683
Extravasation, of plasma fluid and proteins, in inflammation, 49, 50–53, 50f–52f
Extrinsic pathway, in apoptosis, 28–29, 29f, 30f
Exuberant granulation, 115
Exudate
defined, 49
fibrinous, 76, 77f
in edema, 120
retinal, 1434, 1436f
Exudation, defined, 49
Eye(s), 1421–1446
anatomy of, 1422f
anterior segment of, 1430–1432, 1430f, 1432f, 1433f
conjunctiva of, 1422f, 1424f, 1425–1426, 1427f
cornea of, 1426–1430, 1427f–1429f
end-stage, 1446, 1446f
microphthalmic, 1446
optic nerve of, 1422f, 1443–1446, 1444f, 1445f
orbit of, 1423–1424, 1423f
radiation effect on, 441
retina of, 1434–1443
sclera of, 1422f, 1426
uvea of, 1432–1434, 1433f, 1435f
vitamin A effect on, 451, 452f
vitreous of, 1434
Eye involvement
in ariboflavinosis, 457
in sarcoidosis, 738
in Wilson disease, 911
Eye movement disorders, paraneoplastic, 1411, 1411t
Eyelashes, 1424f
Eyelid(s), 1424–1425, 1424f, 1425f

F

FAB classification, of acute myelogenous leukemias, 692, 693t
Fabry disease, 161t
Facioscapulohumeral muscular dystrophy, 1338t
Factor D deficiency, 244
Factor V mutation, 131
Factor VIII deficiency, 655–656
Factor VIII-vWF complex deficiencies, 654–655, 654f
Factor IX deficiency, 656
FADD (Fas-associated death domain), 29, 30f
Fallopian tubes, 1091
anatomy of, 1081
False aneurysm, 584
Familial adenomatous polyposis (FAP), 284–285, 861–862, 862f, 1151
Familial amyloid polyneuropathies (FAP), 1332, 1333t
Familial atypical multiple mole—melanoma syndrome, 1246
Familial cancers, 285–286
Familial disorders, 147
Familial hypercholesterolemia, 154, 156–158, 157f–159f
Familial hypocalciuric hypercalcemia (FHH), 1185
Familial intrahepatic cholestasis, 889–890, 890t
Familial juvenile nephronophthisis, 962t
Familial Mediterranean fever, 261
Familial medullary thyroid cancer, 1223
Familial melanoma syndrome (FMS), 287, 1245t, 1246
Familial mental retardation protein (FMRP), 183, 184f
Familial mental retardation-1 *(FMR-1)* gene, 149, 182, 183
Familial polyposis syndrome, 284–285, 861–862, 862f, 1151
Familial tumor syndromes, of central nervous system, 1413–1414
FANCD1 gene, 308
Fanconi anemia, 307, 308f, 647
FAP (familial adenomatous polyposis), 284–285, 861–862, 862f, 1151
FAP (familial amyloid polyneuropathies), 1332, 1333t
Farmer's lung, 739
Fas gene, in autoimmunity, 226
Fas protein, in apoptosis, 29, 29f, 30f
Fas-associated death domain (FADD), 29, 30f
Fasciitis
nodular (infiltrative, pseudosarcomatous), 1318, 1318f
proliferative, 1318
Fas-Fas ligand system, 225
Fat embolism, 136–137, 137f
Fat necrosis, of breast, 1126
Fatal familial insomnia, 1382
Fatty acid residues, calcification of, 24
Fatty change, 19–20, 35–36
in liver, 36f, 423
in hepatitis, 900f
Fatty liver, 904, 904f
clinical features of, 907
due to carbon tetrachloride poisoning, 25, 25f, 26f
in cystic fibrosis, 493
in hepatitis, 899
in kwashiorkor, 448
in Wilson disease, 911
mechanisms of, 36, 36f, 896
morphology of, 905, 905f
nonalcoholic, 907–908
of pregnancy, 920
Fatty streaks, 516, 516f, 517f
Fatty tumors, 1317–1318, 1318f
Favism, 628
FBN1 gene, 154, 155
FBN2 gene, 154
Fc receptor—mediated inflammation, 210, 211f
Fc receptor—mediated phagocytosis, 210, 211f
FcγRI, 59
FDA (Food and Drug Administration), 416
Feathery degeneration, of liver, 880
Fecal-oral route, 355
Feedback inhibition, 1156
Feet. *See* Foot.
Felons, 373
Female genital tract, 1059–1114
anatomy of, 1061–1062, 1061f–1063f
cervix in, 1072–1079
inflammations of, 1072–1073, 1073f
intraepithelial and invasive squamous neoplasia of, 1073–1079, 1074f–1079f
embryology of, 1060–1061, 1061f
endometrium in, 1079–1089
endometriosis and adenomyosis of, 1083–1084, 1083f, 1084f
functional disorders of, 1081–1083, 1081t, 1082f
hyperplasia of, 1085–1086, 1086f
in menstrual cycle, 1080–1081, 1080f, 1081f
inflammation of, 1083

Female genital tract *(Continued)*
malignant tumors of, 1086–1089, 1087f, 1089f
polyps of, 1085
fallopian tubes in, 1091
gestational and placental disorders of, 1104–1114
gestational trophoblastic disease as, 1110–1114, 1110t, 1111f–1114f
of early pregnancy, 1105, 1106f
of late pregnancy, 1105–1110, 1106f–1110f
infections of, 1062–1065, 1063t, 1064f
myometrium in, 1079, 1089–1090, 1090f, 1091f
ovaries in, 1092–1104
non-neoplastic and functional cysts of, 1092–1093, 1092f
tumors of, 1093–1104
classification of, 1093, 1093t, 1094f
frequency data for, 1094t
germ cell, 1099–1102, 1099f–1101f
metastatic, 1104
of Müllerian epithelium, 1094–1099, 1095f–1099f
sex cord—stromal, 1102–1104, 1102f–1104f
vagina in, 1070–1072, 1071f, 1072f
vulva in, 1065–1070
Bartholin cyst of, 1065
neoplasms of, 1066–1070, 1067f–1070f
non-neoplastic epithelial disorders of, 1065–1066, 1066f
vestibulitis of, 1065
Female pseudohermaphroditism, 181
Feminization disorders, 1211–1214, 1213f
Fenestrations, in blood vessels, 512
Fenton reaction, 16, 17f
Ferritin, 39, 644, 645f
Ferruginous bodies, in asbestosis, 736
Fetal alcohol syndrome, 422t, 424, 473
Fetal development, 474, 475f
Fetal factors, fetal growth restriction due to, 477
Fetal growth restriction (FGR), 477–478, 478f
Fetal hemoglobin (HbF), 628, 629
Fetal hydrops, 484–487, 484f, 634t, 636
causes of, 484, 484t
immune, 484, 485–486, 485f
nonimmune, 484, 486–487, 486f, 487f
Fetal infection, fetal growth restriction due to, 477
Fetor hepaticus, 881–882
Fetus, lung maturation in, 478, 479f
Fever(s)
African tick, 396t
black, 404
Boutonneuse, 396t
due to inflammation, 84
in tuberculosis, 384
Pontiac, 749
relapsing, 391–392
rheumatic, 212t, 359, 373, 593–595
scarlet, 374
oral manifestations of, 778t
spotted, 395
Japanese, 396t
Rocky Mountain, 350, 395, 396–397, 396t, 397f
typhus, 396
viral hemorrhagic, 347t, 365
Fever blisters, 366
FFAs (free fatty acids), and insulin resistance, 1195–1196, 1196f
FGF. *See* Fibroblast growth factor (FGF).
FGR (fetal growth restriction), 477–478, 478f
FH_4 (tetrahydrofolate) derivatives, 642, 642f
FHH (familial hypocalciuric hypercalcemia), 1185
Fiber, in diet, 466
Fibrillae, 358
Fibrillary glomerulonephritis, 992
Fibrillin, in extracellular matrix, 103f, 104
Fibrillin-1, in Marfan syndrome, 154
Fibrin
in hemostasis, 124, 125f, 127, 128f–130f, 130
in inflammation, 53f
Fibrin caps, 992
Fibrin degradation products, 68, 127, 130, 130f
Fibrin split products (FSPs), 68, 127, 130, 130f
Fibrinogen, 84
in hemostasis, 127, 128f, 129f
Fibrinoid necrosis, 214, 214f
in malignant hypertension, 1007, 1008, 1008f
Fibrinolytic cascade, 126f, 130, 130f
Fibrinolytic effects, of endothelium, 125
Fibrinolytic system, 68
Fibroadenoma, 278f, 1149–1150, 1149f, 1150f
Fibroblast(s)
carcinoma-associated, 313
in scar formation, 110
in skin, 1228f
migration and proliferation of, 110
Fibroblast growth factor (FGF), 95t, 96
acidic, 95t, 96
and congenital anomalies, 474
basic, 95t, 96, 294, 309
in scar formation, 110
oncogenes for, 294, 295t
Fibroblast growth factor-7 (FGF-7), 95t
Fibrocystic changes, 1127, 1127f
Fibrocystin, 964–965
Fibroelastic hyperplasia, in benign nephrosclerosis, 1016
Fibroelastoma, cardiac papillary, 614
Fibroelastosis, endocardial, 607–608
Fibroepithelial polyp, 1238
of ureter, 1025
Fibrohistiocytic tumors, 1320–1321, 1321f
Fibroids, 1089–1090, 1090f
Fibrolamellar carcinoma, of liver, 925, 925f, 926
Fibroma, 270
chondromyxoid, 1298, 1298f
dermato-, 1320–1321
irritation, of oral cavity, 775, 775f
nonossifying, 1299, 1300f
peripheral ossifying, of oral cavity, 775–776
renal, 1015
Fibroma-thecomas, 1103, 1103f
Fibromatosis(es), 1319–1320, 1320f
aggressive, 115
deep-seated, 1319–1320, 1320f
in infants and children, 499
of breast, 1151
superficial (palmar, plantar, and penile), 1319
Fibromuscular dysplasia, in renal artery stenosis, 1009, 1009f
Fibronectin, 104–105, 106f
in inflammation, 53f
Fibro-osseous tumors, 1299–1301, 1300f, 1301f
Fibroplasia, retrolental, 1439
Fibrosa, 558, 558f
Fibrosarcoma
congenital-infantile, 499
of bone, 1301
of soft tissue, 1320, 1320f
Fibrosing pulmonary disease(s), 729–737
cryptogenic organizing pneumonia as, 731, 732f
due to complications of therapies, 737, 737t
idiopathic pulmonary fibrosis as, 729–731, 730f, 731f
Fibrosing pulmonary disease(s) *(Continued)*
nonspecific interstitial pneumonia as, 731, 732f
pneumoconioses as, 732–737, 733t, 734f–736f
pulmonary involvement in collagen vascular diseases as, 731–732
Fibrosing strictures, in Crohn disease, 849
Fibrosis, 115
airspace enlargement with, 719
congenital hepatic, 916, 916f
due to inflammation
acute, 75–76, 75f
chronic, 80f, 81f, 116f
due to ionizing radiation, 437
healing by, 75–76, 75f, 107
in alcoholic hepatitis, 905
leptomeningeal, 1370, 1370f
of breast, 1127
of liver, 880–881
"onion-skin," 915, 915f
Fibrous capsule, of tumor, 278, 278f
Fibrous cortical defect, 1299, 1300f
Fibrous dysplasia, 1300–1301, 1301f
monostotic, 1300
polyostotic, 1300
Fibrous histiocytoma
benign, 1247–1248, 1247f, 1320–1321
malignant, 1301, 1321, 1321f
Fibrous proliferative lesions, of oral cavity, 775–776, 775f, 776f
Fibrous tumors
in infants and children, 499
of bone, 1299–1301, 1300f, 1301f
of breast, 1151
of soft tissue, 1318–1320, 1318f–1320f
Fibrovascular polyps, of esophagus, 806
Fibroxanthomas, atypical, 1321
"Field effect," 758
Fifth disease, during pregnancy, 480
Filariasis
lymphatic, 409–410, 410f
lymphedema due to, 121
Filopodia, of leukocytes, 57, 58f
Filtration slits, of glomerulus, 958, 958f
Fimbriae, 358
Fine-needle aspiration, of tumors, 336
First intention, healing by, 111–113, 112f
FISH (fluorescence in situ hybridization), 171–173, 172f, 173f
Fish oil, 70
Fish tapeworm, 839
Fistula(s)
arteriovenous, 515
of bladder, 1026
tracheoesophageal, 800, 800f
FKHR gene, in rhabdomyosarcoma, 1321
Flagella, 348, 350f
Flame cells, 405, 680
Flashover, 446
Flatworms, 839
Flavin, 457
Flavin-containing monooxygenase (FMO) system, 418, 420f
Flesh-eating bacteria, 373
FLIP protein, 29
"Floaters," 1434
Flow cytometry, 338
FLT3, in acute promyelocytic leukemia, 692
flt3-ligand, 621f, 622
Fluid conservation, in shock, 141
Fluid homeostasis, 119
Fluorescence in situ hybridization (FISH), 171–173, 172f, 173f
Fluorescence patterns, 228
Fluorescent treponemal antibody absorption tests (FTA-Abs), 390

Fluoride, 461t
FMO (flavin-containing monooxygenase) system, 418, 420f
FMR-1 (familial mental retardation-1) gene, 149, 182, 183
FMRP (familial mental retardation protein), 183, 184f
FMS (familial melanoma syndrome), 287, 1245t, 1246
FMS oncogene, 295, 295t
Foam cells
  in Alport syndrome, 988
  in atherosclerosis, 523, 525f
  in Niemann-Pick disease, 163, 163f
Focal adhesion complexes, 105, 106f
Focal necrosis, of liver, 880
Focal nodular hyperplasia, of liver, 922
Focal segmental glomerulosclerosis (FSGS), 973, 982–984
  classification and types of, 982–983
  clinical course of, 21t, 984
  glomerular pathology in, 973, 973f, 975t
  morphology of, 983, 983f
  pathogenesis of, 21t, 982–984
  with pyelonephritis, 1002
α-Fodrin, in Sjögren syndrome, 235
Foix-Alajouanine disease, 1368
Folate, 450t, 459
Folate deficiency, 640t, 642–643, 642f
Folic acid antagonists, 643
Folic acid deficiency, 640t, 642–643, 642f
Follicle stimulating hormone (FSH)-producing adenomas, 1162
Follicular carcinoma, of thyroid gland, 1177, 1180–1181, 1180f, 1181f
Follicular cysts, 1092
Follicular dendritic cells, 200–201
  in HIV infection, 253, 258
Follicular hyperplasia, 665–666, 666f
  in AIDS, 258
Follicular lopping, 1257
Follicular lymphoma, 671t, 674–676, 675f, 676f
  oncogenes in, 314, 314t
Folliculitis, 398
Food and Drug Administration (FDA), 416
Food poisoning, 832–838, 834t, 836f, 837f
Food safety, 446–447
Foot
  athlete's, 1267
  trench, 446
Foot processes, of glomerulus, 957f–959f, 958, 959
  in minimal change disease, 982, 982f
Foramen ovale, patent, 567
Forebrain anomalies, 1354–1355, 1355f
Foregut cysts, 713
Foreign bodies, and wound healing, 114
Formaldehyde, as air pollutant, 430, 430t
Forward failure, 560
Fossil fuels, 428, 432
Foveolar compartment, of gastric mucosa, 810, 810f
Fracture(s), 1288–1289, 1289f
  chalkstick-type, 1286
  closed, 1288
  comminuted, 1288
  healing of, 1288–1289, 1289f
  pathologic, 1288
  skull, 1357
    basal, 1357
    diastatic, 1357
    displaced, 1357
  stress, 1288
  types of, 1288
Fracture contusions, of brain, 1357
Fragile site, 182
Fragile-X syndrome, 149, 181–183, 182f, 189f
Frameshift mutations, 147, 148f, 149
Frank-Starling mechanism, 557, 560
Frataxin, 1395, 1395t
Freckle, 1231
Free fatty acids (FFAs), and insulin resistance, 1195–1196, 1196f
Free radicals, oxygen-derived
  accumulation of, 14f, 16–17, 17f
  in chemical injury, 25
  in inflammation, 73–74, 74t
  in ischemia-reperfusion injury, 24
  removal of, 17–18
Friedreich ataxia, 184t, 1395, 1395t
Frizzled (FRZ) receptors, 304
Frontal bossing, 455
Frontotemporal dementias, 1389–1391
FSGS. *See* Focal segmental glomerulosclerosis (FSGS).
FSH (follicle stimulating hormone)-producing adenomas, 1162
FSPs (fibrin split products), 68, 127, 130, 130f
FTA-Abs (fluorescent treponemal antibody absorption tests), 390
Fuchs endothelial dystrophy, 1428–1429, 1429f
Fucosidosis, 161t
Full mutations, 183, 189f
Fumigants, 434t
Functional cloning, 146, 147f
Functional derangements, defined, 4
Functional regurgitation, 589
Fundic gland(s), 810, 811
Fundic gland polyps, 821–822
Fundus, of stomach, 810, 810f
Fungal infection(s), 397–401
  agents of, 346t, 351
  aspergillosis as, 399–400, 400f
  candidiasis as, 397–399, 398f
  cryptococcosis as, 399, 399f
  due to molds, 399–401, 400f, 401f
  due to yeasts, 397–399, 398f, 399f
  of gastrointestinal tract, 353
  of oral cavity, 777
  of skin, 1267–1268, 1268f
  zygomycosis as, 400–401, 401f
Fungal meningoencephalitis, 1378, 1378f
Fungicides, 434, 434t
Funisitis, 477, 480, 1106
Furuncle, 372
Fusobacterium necrophorum, 393

G

G banding, 170, 171f
G (gastrin-producing) cells, 811
G-protein(s), 98f, 99–100
G-protein mutations, in pituitary adenoma, 1159, 1159f
G-protein—coupled receptors (GPCRs), seven transmembrane, 56, 58–59, 58f, 98f, 99–100
G_0 stage, of cell cycle, 90, 90f, 100
G_1 stage, of cell cycle, 90, 90f, 100
G_2 stage, of cell cycle, 90, 90f
G6PD (glucose-6-phosphate dehydrogenase) deficiency, 627–628, 627f, 628f
  adverse reactions to drugs in, 154
  genetic basis for, 152
GAD (glutamic acid decarboxylase), 1193
GADD45 gene, 302, 303f
gag gene, in human immunodeficiency virus, 247, 247f
GAGE proteins, 330
GAGs (glycosaminoglycans), 106
Gain of function mutations, 151
Galactitol, 488, 489
Galactocerebroside ß-galactosidase deficiency, 1397
Galactokinase, 488, 489f
Galactose-1-phosphate, 488, 489
Galactose-1-phosphate uridyl transferase (GALT), 488, 489, 489f
Galactosemia, 488–489, 489f
Galactosylceramidase deficiency, 1397
Gallbladder
  aberrant locations of, 928
  absence of, 928
  adenomyosis of, 934
  bilobed, 928
  carcinoma of, 934–935, 935f
  cholecystitis of, 931–933, 931f, 932f
  cholelithiasis of, 928–931, 929t, 930f, 931f
  congenital anomalies of, 928
  disorders of, 928–933
  duplication of, 928
  empyema of, 932
  folded fundus of, 928
  hydrops of, 933
  normal structure of, 927–928, 928f
  phrygian cap of, 928, 928f
  porcelain, 933
  "strawberry," 931
Gallbladder stasis, 929
Gallstone(s), 928–931
  and pancreatitis, 942
  cholesterol, 928, 929, 929t, 930, 930f
  clinical features of, 931
  epidemiology of, 928–929
  morphology of, 930–931, 930f, 931f
  obesity and, 465
  pathogenesis of, 929–930, 930f
  pigment, 928, 929–930, 929t, 931f
  risk factors for, 929, 929t
Gallstone ileus, 931
GALT (galactose-1-phosphate uridyl transferase), 488, 489, 489f
Gametocytes, 401, 402f
γ chemokines, 72
Gamma rays, exposure to, 436t
α-group viruses, 365
β-toxin, 372
Ganglia, 1349
Gangliocytomas, 1406
Ganglioglioma, 1406
Ganglion cell(s)
  in neuroblastic tumors, 501
  in Tay-Sachs disease, 162f
Ganglion cell tumors, 1406
Ganglion cyst, 1315
Ganglioneuroblastoma, 501
Ganglioneuroma(s), 501, 502f
  in MEN-2B, 1222
Ganglionic hemorrhages, 1376
Ganglioside $G_{D2,}$ in melanoma, 330
Ganglioside $G_{D3,}$ in melanoma, 330
Ganglioside $G_{M2,}$ in melanoma, 330
Gangliosidoses, 160–161, 161t, 162f
Gangliosidosis, GM1, 160–161, 161t, 162f
Gangrene
  gas, 393, 394
  of lower extremities, in diabetes, 1200
  wet, 22
Gangrenous cholecystitis, 932
GANTs (gastrointestinal autonomic nerve tumors), 826
GAP, 99f
Gap junctions, 557
GAPs (GTPase-activating proteins), 296
Gardner syndrome, 862
  multiple osteomas in, 1293
Garlic, 466
Garrod, Archibald, 487
Gartner duct, 1060, 1061f
Gartner duct cysts, 1060, 1070

Gas gangrene, 393, 394
Gasoline, exposure to, 431
Gastrectomy, and gastric carcinoma, 824
Gastric. *See also* Stomach.
Gastric adenoma, 821, 822f
Gastric antral vascular ectasia, 816
Gastric carcinoid tumors, 827
Gastric carcinoma, 822–826
  classification of, 823, 823t, 824–825, 824f, 825f
  clinical features of, 826
  epidemiology of, 822–823
  growth patterns of, 824f, 825
  Helicobacter pylori and, 327–328
  intestinal *vs.* diffuse, 823, 825, 825f
  location of, 824
  morphology of, 824–826, 824f, 825f
  pathogenesis of, 823–824, 823t
Gastric dilation, 820
Gastric foveolae, 810
Gastric gland(s), 810, 811
Gastric gland hyperplasia, 821
Gastric heterotopia, 812
Gastric lipomas, 827
Gastric lymphoma, 826, 826f
  Helicobacter pylori and, 327–328
Gastric mucosa
  anatomy of, 810–811, 810f
  physiology of, 811–812
Gastric neuroendocrine cell tumors, 827
Gastric phase, of gastric acid secretion, 811
Gastric pits, 810
Gastric polyps, 821–822, 822f
Gastric rupture, 820
Gastric ulceration, acute, 819–820, 820f
Gastric ulcers, 818
Gastric varices, 821
Gastrinoma(s), 1206–1207
  in MEN-1, 1222
Gastrinoma triangle, 1206
Gastrin-producing (G) cells, 811
Gastritis, 812–816
  acute, 812–813, 813f
    erosive hemorrhagic, 813, 813f
  alcoholic, 423
  autoimmune, 814, 815, 816, 824
  chronic, 813–816, 814t, 815f
    atrophic, in pernicious anemia, 641
    in peptic ulcer disease, 819
  defined, 812
  eosinophilic, 816
  granulomatous, 816
  lymphocytic, 816
Gastroenteritis, viral, 832–833, 833t
Gastroenteropathy
  allergic, 816
  protein-losing, 821
    in Crohn disease, 849
Gastroesophageal reflux disease (GERD), 804, 804f
Gastrointestinal. *See also under* Intestinal.
Gastrointestinal autonomic nerve tumors (GANTs), 826
Gastrointestinal effects
  of obesity, 465t
  of shock, 142
Gastrointestinal stomal tumor (GIST), 826–827, 827f
Gastrointestinal tract, 797–873
  alcohol effect on, 422t, 423
  amyloidosis of, 263–264
  appendix in, 870–872, 871f, 872f
  barriers to infection in, 352–353
  esophagus in, 798–809
    congenital anomalies of, 799–800, 800f
    inflammation of, 803–806, 804f, 805f
Gastrointestinal tract *(Continued)*
    lesions associated with motor dysfunction of, 800–802, 801f, 802f
    normal anatomy and physiology of, 798–799
    symptoms of pathology of, 799
    tumors of, 806–809, 807f–809f, 807t
    varices of, 802–803, 803f
  in pernicious anemia, 642
  occupational exposures and, 431t
  peritoneum in, 872–873
  radiation effect on, 441
  small and large intestines in, 828–870
    congenital anomalies of, 830–831, 830f
    diverticular disease of, 854–855, 855f
    endocrine cells of, 829
    enterocolitis of, 831–842
    hereditary syndromes of, 858t, 861–862, 862f
    idiopathic inflammatory bowel disease of, 846–851, 847f–850f, 851t
    immune system of, 829–830
    lymphoma as, 868–869
    malabsorption syndromes of, 842–846, 842t, 843f, 845f
    mesenchymal, 869
    mucosa of, 828–829, 828f
    neuromuscular function of, 830
    obstruction of, 855–856, 855t, 856f
    tumors of, 856–870, 857t
    vascular disorders of, 851–854, 852f, 853f
    vasculature of, 828
  stomach in, 810–827
    bezoars of, 820, 820f
    congenital anomalies of, 812–816, 813f, 814t, 815f, 816f
    dilation of, 820
    hypertrophic gastropathy of, 820–821, 821f
    normal anatomy of, 810–811, 810f
    peptic ulcer disease of, 816–820, 817f, 819f, 819t, 820f
    physiology of gastric mucosa of, 811–812
    rupture of, 820
    tumors of, 821–827, 822f, 823t, 824f–827f
    varices of, 821
  viral infections of, 347t
Gastropathy
  hypertrophic, 820–821, 821f
  hypertrophic-hypersecretory, 821
  reactive, 816, 816f
Gatekeeper genes, 318, 318f
Gaucher cells, 164, 164f
Gaucher disease, 161t, 163–165, 164f
GBM. *See* Glomerular basement membrane (GBM).
GCIs (glial cytoplasmic inclusions), 1352, 1393
G-CSF (granulocyte colony-stimulating factor), 621f
GCT (giant cell tumor), 1302, 1302f, 1303f
  of tendon sheath, 1315
GDNF (glial-derived neurotrophic factor), 1222
Gelatinases, 111
Gelatinous drop dystrophy, 1429
Gene amplification, in cancer cells, 315
Gene arrays, 1136b–1137b
Gene chips, 1136b
Gene expression profiling, 315, 316b
  for breast carcinoma, 315, 316b, 1135, 1136b–1137b, 1148
Gene expression signatures, 315, 316b
Gene mutations, 147
  congenital anomalies due to, 473
Gene therapy, 147
General paresis of the insane, 1372
Genetic causes, of congenital anomalies, 472–473, 473t
Genetic derangements, cell injury due to, 13
Genetic disorder(s), 145–191
  adverse reactions to drugs due to, 154
  alkaptonuria as, 167–168
  alterations in structure, function, or quantity of nonenzyme proteins as, 154
  Angelman syndrome as, 186–187, 186f
  autosomal dominant, 150–151, 151t
  autosomal recessive, 151, 151t
  chromosome 22q11.2 deletion syndrome, 172f, 176–178
  cyto-, 147, 173–181, 174f
    involving autosomes, 175–178
    involving sex chromosomes, 178–181
  defects in receptors and transport systems as, 154
  diagnosis of, 147, 187–191, 188f–190f
  Down syndrome (trisomy 21) as, 175–176, 175f, 177f
  due to defects in proteins that regulate cell growth, 168–169
  due to defects in receptor proteins, 156–158, 157f, 158f
  due to defects in structural proteins, 154–156, 156t
  due to enzyme defects, 152–153, 153f, 158–168
  due to genomic imprinting, 185–187, 186f
  Ehlers-Danlos syndromes as, 152, 155–156, 156t
  epidemiology of, 146
  familial hypercholesterolemia as, 154, 156–158, 157f–159f
  fragile-X syndrome as, 149, 181–183, 182f, 189f
  Gaucher disease as, 161t, 163–165, 164f
  glycogen storage diseases as, 165–167, 166f, 167f, 168t
  gonadal mosaicism as, 187
  hermaphroditism and pseudohermaphroditism as, 181
  Klinefelter syndrome as, 179
  Leber hereditary optic neuropathy as, 185, 185f
  lysosomal storage diseases as, 153, 158–165, 159f, 160f, 161t
  Marfan syndrome as, 154–155
  mendelian (single-gene), 149–169
    biochemical and molecular basis of, 152–154, 153f, 153t
    transmission patterns of, 150–152, 151t, 152t
  mucopolysaccharidoses as, 165
  multifactorial, 149, 169–170, 170t
  mutations as, 147–149, 148f, 149f
    in mitochondrial genes, 185, 185f
    triplet-repeat, 181–184, 182f
  neurofibromatosis as, 168–169
  Niemann-Pick disease as, 161t, 163, 163f
  other trisomies as, 176, 177f
  Prader-Willi syndrome as, 186–187, 186f
  single-gene disorders with nonclassic inheritance as, 181–187
  Tay-Sachs disease as, 148f, 160–161, 162f
  Turner syndrome as, 178, 179–180, 180f, 181f
  with unstable nucleotide repeats, 183–184, 184f, 184t, 185f
  X-linked, 152, 152t
Genetic factors
  in hypertension, 528, 528f
  in systemic lupus erythematosus, 229–230
Genetic heterogeneity, 150
Genetic instability, induced, 438
Genetic predisposition, to cancer, 284–286, 287t, 338
Genetic profile, 314

Genetic sex, 181
Genetic signature, 314
Genital chlamydia, 394–395
Genital herpes, 366, 1062–1063, 1063t
Genital sex, 181
Genital tract. *See* Female genital tract; Male genital tract.
Genital ulcer(s), due to chancroid, 380
Genitourinary effects, of obesity, 465t
Genome mutations, 147
Genomic imprinting, 185–187, 186f, 315
in Wilms tumor, 505
Genomic instability, in cancer cells, 306–308, 308f
Genomics, 146
Genotoxic stress, 31
Geographic factors, in cancer, 283, 284f
GERD (gastroesophageal reflux disease), 804, 804f
Germ cell tumor(s)
biologic markers for, 1045–1046
intratubular, 1041
ovarian, 1099–1102
choriocarcinoma as, 1101–1102
classification of, 1093t
dysgerminoma as, 1101, 1101f
endodermal sinus (yolk sac), 1101, 1101f
epidemiology of, 1094f
histogenesis and interrelationships of, 1099f
teratomas as, 1099–1100, 1100f, 1101f
primary brain, 1408–1409
testicular, 1040–1046, 1041t
choriocarcinoma as, 1041, 1043–1044, 1044f
clinical features of, 1045–1046
embryonal carcinoma as, 1041, 1043, 1043f
mixed, 1045
nonseminomatous, 1041, 1045
seminoma as, 1041–1042, 1042f, 1045
spermatocytic, 1042
teratoma as, 1044, 1044f, 1045f
yolk sac, 1041, 1043
Germ line mosaicism, 187
Germinal centers, of lymph nodes, 662
Germinal matrix hemorrhage, in preterm infants, 484
Germinomas, 1223
Germ-line mutations, in colorectal cancer, 864
Gerstmann-Sträussler-Scheinker syndrome, 1382
Gestational age, 476–479
Gestational choriocarcinoma, 1112–1113, 1113f
Gestational disorder(s), 1104–1114
gestational trophoblastic disease as, 1110–1114, 1110t, 1111f–1114f
of early pregnancy, 1105, 1106f
of late pregnancy, 1105–1110, 1106f–1110f
Gestational trophoblastic disease, 1110–1114, 1110t, 1111f–1114f
GFAP (glial fibrillary acidic protein), 1349, 1350f, 1351
GH (growth hormone) adenomas, 1161–1162
Ghon complex, 384, 384f
Ghon focus, 384
Ghrelin, in energy balance, 462, 463f
Giant cell(s), 83, 83f
in anaplasia, 274
in HIV infection, 251, 251f
Giant cell aortitis, 536
Giant cell arteritis, 536–538, 537f, 537t
Giant cell epulis, of oral cavity, 776
Giant cell myocarditis, 608–609, 609f
Giant cell tumor (GCT), 1302, 1302f, 1303f
of tendon sheath, 1315
Giant granules, 62
Giardia lamblia, 840, 840f
forms of, 351, 351t
transmission and dissemination of, 352, 353
Giardiasis, 840, 840f
Giardins, 840
Giemsa stain, 361t
Gigantism, 1161
Gilbert syndrome, 888, 888t
Gingiva, 774f
Gingivitis, 775
Gingivostomatitis, 366
herpetic, 776–777
GIST (gastrointestinal stomal tumor), 826–827, 827f
Gitelman syndrome, 529f
GL13 gene, 473
Glands of Moll, 1424
Glandular compartment, of gastric mucosa, 810, 810f
Glanzmann thrombasthenia, 127, 653
Glaucoma, 1431–1432
angle closure, 1430f, 1431–1432
defined, 1431
exfoliation, 1431
ghost cell, 1431
in diabetes, 1205
infantile, 1428
low-tension, 1431
melanomalytic, 1431
neovascular, 1430f, 1432
normal-tension, 1431, 1444, 1445f
open angle, 1431
pigmentary, 1431
Glaukomflecken, 1431
GLC1A gene, in glaucoma, 1431
Gleason system, for grading of prostate cancer, 1053
Glia, 1349
Gliadin, 843
Glial cytoplasmic inclusions (GCIs), 1352, 1393
Glial "fibril(s)," 1351
Glial fibrillary acidic protein (GFAP), 1349, 1350f, 1351
Glial-derived neurotrophic factor (GDNF), 1222
Glioblastoma(s), 1401–1402, 1403f
EGFR expression in, 296
primary *vs.* secondary, 1403
Glioma(s), 1401–1406
astrocytoma as, 1401–1404, 1402f, 1403f
brainstem, 1404
choroid plexus papillomas as, 1406
colloid cyst of third ventricle as, 1406
ependymoma as, 1404–1405, 1405f
hypothalamic, 1164
metastasis of, 279
oligodendro-, 1404
pineal, 1409
subependymomas as, 1405–1406
Gliomatosis cerebri, 1402
Glioneuronal element, specific, 1406
Glioneuronal tumor, papillary, 1406
Gliosis, 1351
Bergmann, 1351, 1400
Glomangioma, 547
Glomerular barrier function, 959
Glomerular basement membrane (GBM), 956–958, 957f–959f
in Alport syndrome, 988
in diabetic nephropathy, 991, 991f
in glomerulonephritis
membranoproliferative, 984, 985f, 986f
rapidly progressive, 978, 978f
thickening of, 967
thin, 989
Glomerular cells
antibodies to, 970–971
in glomerulonephritis, 972
Glomerular disease(s), 966–993
clinical manifestations of, 967, 967t
focal segmental glomerulosclerosis as, 973, 973f, 975t, 982–984, 983f
glomerulonephritis as. *See* Glomerulonephritis(ides).
hereditary syndromes of isolated hematuria as, 988–989, 988f
histologic alterations in, 967–968
IgA nephropathy as, 975t, 986–988, 987f, 990
mechanisms of progression in, 972–973, 973f, 974f
membranous glomerulopathy as, 975t, 979–981, 980f
minimal change disease as, 975t, 981–982, 981f, 982f
nephrotic syndrome as, 960, 967t, 978–979, 979t
pathogenesis of, 968–972, 968t, 969f, 971f, 972f, 975t
primary, 966–967, 967t, 975t
secondary, 966, 967t
with systemic diseases, 990–993, 991f, 992f
Glomerular filtration, normal, 959
Glomerular filtration rate, in blood pressure regulation, 528
Glomerular injury
immune mechanisms of, 968–971, 968t, 969f, 971f
mediators of, 971–972, 972f
pathogenesis of, 968–972, 968t, 969f, 971f, 972f, 975t
Glomerular syndromes, 967, 967t
Glomeruloid body, 1402, 1403f
Glomerulonephritis, poststreptococcal, 359
Glomerulonephritis(ides), 214
acute, 212t, 973–976, 976f
proliferative, 974–976, 976f
basement membrane thickening in, 967
cell-mediated immunity in, 971
chronic, 975t, 989–990, 989f
crescent formation in, 967, 977–978, 977f
diffuse changes in, 968
epithelial cell injury in, 971, 972f
fibrillary, 992
focal changes in, 968
global changes in, 968
histologic alterations in, 967–968
hyalinization and sclerosis in, 967–968
hypercellularity in, 967
immunotactoid, 992
lupus, 990
membranous, 231–232
mesangial, 231
proliferative
diffuse, 231, 232f
focal, 231, 231f
mechanisms of progression in, 972–973, 973f, 974f
membranoproliferative, 971, 975t, 984–985, 985f–987f
mesangial changes in, 968
postinfectious, 976
poststreptococcal, 212t, 359, 974–976, 975t, 976f
primary, 966–967, 967t, 975t
rapidly progressive (crescentic), 967t, 975t, 976–978, 977f, 977t, 978f
segmental changes in, 968
Glomerulopathy(ies)
collapsing, 983
immunotactoid, 992

Glomerulopathy(ies) *(Continued)*
membranous, 975t, 979–981, 980f
primary, 966–967, 967t, 975t
Glomerulosclerosis
diabetic, 990–992, 991f, 992f
focal segmental, 973, 982–984
classification and types of, 982–983
clinical course of, 21t, 984
glomerular pathology in, 973, 973f, 975t
morphology of, 983, 983f
pathogenesis of, 21t, 982–984
with pyelonephritis, 1002
in diabetes, 1201, 1202f
nodular, 991–992
Glomerulus(i), 956–959, 957f–959f
Glomus tumor, 547
Glossitis, 457, 776
atrophic, in pernicious anemia, 642
Glucagon
in glucose homeostasis, 1191
production of, 1191f
Glucagonomas, 1207
Glucocerebrosides, in Gaucher disease, 163–164
Glucocorticoids, 70, 1207
Glucokinase, in maturity-onset diabetes of the young, 1197
Glucose
in diabetes, 1190
in regulation of insulin release, 1191, 1192f
Glucose homeostasis, 1191
Glucose tolerance, impaired, 1190
Glucose uptake, insulin and, 1191–1192, 1192f
Glucose-6-phosphate dehydrogenase (G6PD) deficiency, 627–628, 627f, 628f
adverse reactions to drugs in, 154
genetic basis for, 152
Glucose-transporting protein (GLUT-2), 1191, 1192f
α-Glucosidase deficiency, 167
Glucotoxicity, 1196
Glucuronidation, of naphthylamine, 418, 421f
Glutamic acid decarboxylase (GAD), 1193
γ-Glutamyl transpeptidase, in cholestasis, 888
Glutathione (GSH)
in diabetes mellitus, 1198–1199
in metabolism of toxicant, 417, 418
Glutathione conjugation, of vinyl chloride, 419, 421f
Glutathione peroxidase, 18, 74
Glutathione S-transferase, 320, 417
Glutathione S-transferase (GSTP1) gene promotor, hypermethylation of, in prostate cancer, 1051
Gluten-sensitive enteropathy, 843–844, 843f
Glycan-bearing cell adhesion molecule-1 (GlyCAM-1), 54t, 55b
Glycogen
intracellular accumulation of, 39
metabolism of, 165–166, 166f
Glycogen storage diseases, 39, 161, 165–167
hepatic type, 166–167, 167f, 168t
miscellaneous, 167
myopathic type, 167, 167f, 168t
Glycogen stores, depletion of, 15
Glycogenosis(es), 39, 161, 165–167, 166f
hepatic type, 166–167, 167f, 168t
miscellaneous, 167
myopathic type, 167, 167f, 168t
Glycolipids, altered cell-surface, 330
Glycolysis, anaerobic, 15
Glycolytic pathway, 15
Glycoproteins
adhesive, in extracellular matrix, 103f, 104–105, 106f
altered cell-surface, 330
Glycosaminoglycans (GAGs), 106
Glycosuria, in diabetes, 1202, 1202f
Glycosyl phosphatidyl inositol (GPI), in paroxysmal nocturnal hemoglobinuria, 636, 636f
GM1 gangliosidosis, 160–161, 161t, 162f
GM-CSF (granulocyte-macrophage colony-stimulating factor), 209, 621f, 633
in pulmonary alveolar proteinosis, 741
GNAS1 gene, in pseudohypoparathyroidism, 1188–1189
Goblet cells, 829
Goiter(s)
colloid, 1174
diffuse nontoxic (simple), 1173–1174
dyshormonogenetic, 1168
endemic, 1174
intrathoracic, 1175
multinodular, 1173–1175, 1175f
plunging, 1175
sporadic, 1174
Goitrogens, 1165–1166, 1174
Golgi apparatus, synthesis of lysosomal enzymes in, 159, 159f
Gonadal dysgenesis, in Denys-Drash syndrome, 504
Gonadal mosaicism, 187
Gonadal sex, 181
Gonadoblastoma, 505
ovarian, 1104
testicular, 1046
Gonadotroph(s), 1158
Gonadotroph adenomas, 1162
Gonococcal infection, pelvic inflammatory disease due to, 1064–1065
Gonococci, 378f
Gonorrhea, 350f, 377–378, 378f
of epididymis, 1039
Goodpasture syndrome, 212t, 223, 745–746
glomerular lesions in, 968, 975t, 977, 978, 993
pulmonary hemorrhage in, 746
Gorlin syndrome, 1244–1245, 1245t, 1246f
Gout, 1311–1314, 1311t, 1312f
chronic tophaceous, 1314
pseudo-, 1314, 1314f
due to hemochromatosis, 910
Gouty arthritis, 1311–1314, 1312f, 1313f
Gouty nephropathy, 1313
gp63, 404
GPCRs (G-protein—coupled receptors), seven transmembrane, 56, 58–59, 58f, 98f, 99–100
GPI (glycosyl phosphatidyl inositol), in paroxysmal nocturnal hemoglobinuria, 636, 636f
Graafian follicle, 1081
Grading, of tumors, 335
Graft arteriopathy, 615–616, 615f
Graft rejection. *See* Transplant rejection.
Graft-*versus*-host disease (GVHD), 222–223
esophagitis due to, 806
gastritis due to, 816
of intestines, 841, 841f
of liver, 921
Graft-*versus*-leukemia effect, 223
Gram stain, 361t
Gram-negative bacillus, granulomatous inflammation due to, 83t
Gram-negative bacteria, 348, 349t, 350f, 377–381
Gram-positive bacteria, 348, 350f, 371–376
Granular corneal dystrophy, 1429
Granular ependymitis, 1372
Granulation, exuberant, 115
Granulation tissue, 107, 107f, 110
in healing by first intention, 112, 112f
in healing by second intention, 113, 113f
inadequate formation of, 114
Granulocyte colony-stimulating factor (G-CSF), 621f
Granulocyte-macrophage colony-stimulating factor (GM-CSF), 209, 621f, 633
in pulmonary alveolar proteinosis, 741
Granulocytic sarcomas, 694
Granulocytopenia, 662
Granuloma(s)
actinic, 1426
eosinophilic, 701, 702
of stomach, 822, 822f
foreign body, 83
immune, 83
in cell-mediated hypersensitivity, 216, 216f, 217f
in conjunctival fornix, 1425
in tuberculosis, 382, 384
lethal midline, 686, 784
malarial (Dürck), 403
noncaseating
in Crohn disease, 848, 848f
in sarcoidosis, 738, 738f
of oral cavity
peripheral giant cell, 776
pyogenic, 775, 776f
periapical, 782
peripheral giant cell, of oral cavity, 776
pyogenic, 546f, 547
of oral cavity, 775, 776f
Granuloma gravidarum, 547
Granuloma inguinale, 380–381
Granulomatosis
allergic, and angiitis, 537t, 541
lymphomatoid, 542
Wegener, 541–542
clinical features of, 537t, 541–542
glomerular lesions in, 993
morphology of, 539f, 541
orbit in, 1423
pathogenesis of, 541
pulmonary hemorrhage in, 746–747
Granulomatous disease(s)
chronic, 62, 62t
pulmonary, 737–739, 738f, 739f
Granulomatous gastritis, 816
Granulomatous mastitis, 1126
Granulomatous reaction, 79, 82–83, 83f, 83t
Granulosa cell tumors, 1102–1103, 1102f
Granulosa-theca cell tumors, 1102–1103, 1102f
Granulovacuolar degeneration, 1388
Granzyme(s), 218
Granzyme A, in systemic sclerosis, 237
Granzyme B, 31
Graves disease, 212t, 1172–1173
clinical course of, 1173
clinical findings in, 1172
Hashimoto thyroiditis with, 1172
morphology of, 1173, 1173f
ophthalmopathy in, 1167f, 1172, 1173
pathogenesis of, 1172–1173
pretibial myxedema in, 1172, 1173
proptosis in, 1423, 1423f
treatment of, 1173
Gray (Gy), 436
Gray hepatization stage, of lobar pneumonia, 750, 750f
GRB-2, 99
Greig syndrome, 1280t
Grotton lesions, 1342
Ground glass hepatocytes, 898, 900f
Ground glass nuclei, in thyroid carcinoma, 1178, 1179f
Ground-glass picture, 481
Group atrophy, 1329f, 1330
Group B streptococci, meningitis due to, 1369
Growth, cellular adaptations of, 5–11

Growth factor(s), 95–97, 95t
  apoptosis after deprivation of, 31
  in wound healing, 111t
  protooncogenes for, 293–294, 295t
Growth factor receptors, protooncogenes for, 294–296, 295t
Growth fraction, 276
Growth hormone (GH) adenomas, 1161–1162
Growth inhibitory signals, insensitivity to, in cancer, 289, 298–306, 300t, 301f–304f
Growth plate, 1278, 1278f
Growth rates, of tumors, 276–277, 277f, 278f
Growth signals, self-sufficiency in, in cancer, 289, 292–298, 294f, 295t, 297f–299f
GSH. *See* glutathione (GSH).
GSTM1 deficiency, 418
GSTP1 (glutathione S-transferase) gene promotor, hypermethylation of, in prostate cancer, 1051
Guanosine triphosphatase (GTPase)-activating proteins (GAPs), 296
Guanosine triphosphate (GTP)—binding protein, oncogene for, 295t
Guanosine triphosphate (GTP) proteins. *See* G protein(s).
Guillain-Barré syndrome, 1331
  T cell—mediated hypersensitivity in, 215t
Gull, William, 1168
Gull disease, 1168–1169
Gummas, 389, 391, 391f
  cerebral, 1372
Gunshot wounds, 444, 444f
Guttata, in Fuchs endothelial dystrophy, 1428, 1429f
GVHD. *See* Graft-*versus*-host disease (GVHD).
Gy (gray), 436
Gynecologic effects, of obesity, 465t
Gynecomastia, 1151–1152, 1152f

H

H_2O_2. *See* Hydrogen peroxide (H_2O_2).
HA (hyaluronic acid), in extracellular matrix, 103f, 106
Haab's striae, 1428
HACEK group, infective endocarditis due to, 596
Haemophilus, immune invasion by, 360
Haemophilus ducreyi, 356t, 380
Haemophilus influenzae, 353
  meningitis due to, 1369, 1370
  pneumonia due to, 748
Hageman factor
  activation of, 65, 67f, 68
  in coagulation cascade, 128f
Hair follicles, 1228f, 1229
"Hairballs," 820, 820f
Hairy cell leukemia (HCL), 671t, 683, 684f
Hairy leukoplakia, of oral cavity, 777–778
Hallmark cells, 684.685f
Hallucinogens, 424t, 426
Halo nevus, 1233t
Halogenation, 61
HAM (HTLV-1-associated myelopathy), 1376
Hamartin, 1413
Hamartoma(s), 272
  in infancy and childhood, 498
  multiple, 1134
  of lung, 765
  renal, 1015
Hamartomatous polyps, 859, 859f
Hand(s), "alien," 1391
Hand-foot-genital syndrome, 475
Hand-Schuller-Christian disease, 701, 702
Hansen's disease, 387–388, 388f
Haploid number, 173
Haploinsufficiency, 288
"Happy puppets," 186
Hapten model, of warm antibody immunohemolytic anemia, 637
Hard metal disease, 433
Harrison's groove, 455
Hashimoto thyroiditis, 1169–1170, 1170f
  with Graves disease, 1172
Hashitoxicosis, 1170, 1172
Hassall corpuscles, 706
HAV (hepatitis A virus), 347t, 890–891, 891f, 891t
Haw River syndrome, 184t
Hay fever, 783
Hazardous waste sites, common chemicals at, 416t
HbA (hemoglobin A), in ß-thalassemia, 632, 633
HbC (hemoglobin C), 629
HbF (fetal hemoglobin), 628, 629
HbH (hemoglobin H) disease, 634t, 636
HbS. *See* Hemoglobin S (HbS).
HbSC disease, 629
HBV. *See* Hepatitis B virus (HBV).
HBx protein, 327
HCC. *See* Hepatocellular carcinoma (HCC).
HCG (human chorionic gonadotropin)
  as tumor marker, 338, 339t
  in germ cell tumors, 1045–1046
HCL (hairy cell leukemia), 671t, 683, 684f
HCM. *See* Hypertrophic cardiomyopathy (HCM).
HCV. *See* Hepatitis C virus (HCV).
HD. *See* Huntington disease (HD).
HD gene, 1394
HDL (high-density lipoprotein), and atherosclerosis, 521
HDM2, 302
HDV (hepatitis D virus), 347t, 891t, 895–896, 896f, 897f
Head and neck squamous cell carcinoma (HNSCC), 780–781, 781f
Head injury
  open *vs.* closed, 1357
  parenchymal, 1357–1359, 1360f
  perinatal, 1356, 1356f
  sequelae of, 1360
  vascular, 1359–1360, 1359f, 1360f
Healing, 88–89, 88f, 107
  cutaneous wound, 111–115
    by first intention, 111–113, 112f
    by second intention, 112f, 113, 113f
    complications of, 114–115, 115f
    factors influencing, 114, 114t
    growth factors and cytokines in, 111t
    phases of, 111, 111f
    strength of, 113–114
    summary of, 114
  of fracture, 1288–1289, 1289f
Hearing loss, in osteogenesis imperfecta, 1280
Heart. *See also under* Cardiac.
  aging effect on, 558–559, 559t
  amyloidosis of, 263, 264, 264f
  blood supply to, 557–558
  dilation of, 556
  effects of shock on, 141–142
  hypertrophy of, 556
  in systemic sclerosis, 239
  lipid droplets in, 36
  myocardium of, 556–557, 556f
  myxedema, 611
  normal weight and size of, 556
  radiation effect on, 440, 440f
Heart attack. *See* Myocardial infarction (MI).
Heart disease, 564–615
  cardiomyopathy(ies) as, 601–611
    causes of, 601, 602t
    diagnosis of, 601
Heart disease *(Continued)*
    dilated, 601, 601f, 602–604, 602t, 603f, 604f
    due to adriamycin and other drugs, 609–610
    due to amyloidosis, 610
    due to catecholamines, 610
    due to hyperthyroidism and hypothyroidism, 610–611
    due to iron overload, 610
    hypertrophic, 601, 601f, 602t, 604–606, 605f, 607f
    myocarditis form of, 608–609, 608t, 609f
    restrictive, 601, 601f, 602t, 606–608
  congenital, 564–571
    aortic stenosis and atresia as, 564t, 571
    atrial septal defect as, 564t, 565, 567–568, 567f
    atrioventricular septal defect as, 564t, 567f, 568–569
    causing left-to-right shunts, 566–569, 567f, 568f
    causing right-to-left shunts, 566, 569–570, 569f, 570f
    clinical features of, 566–567
    coarctation of aorta as, 564t, 570–571, 571f
    cyanotic, 566, 569, 569f
      brain abscess due to, 1371
    etiology and pathogenesis of, 565
    genetics of, 565–566, 566f
    incidence of, 564–565, 564t
    obstructive, 567, 570–571, 571f
    patent ductus arteriosus as, 564t, 567f, 568
    pulmonary stenosis and atresia as, 564t, 571
    tetralogy of Fallot as, 564t, 565, 569, 569f
    total anomalous pulmonary venous connection as, 564t, 570
    transposition of great arteries as, 564t, 569–570, 569f, 570f
    tricuspid atresia as, 564t, 570
    truncus arteriosus as, 564t, 565, 570
    ventricular septal defect as, 564t, 565, 567f, 568, 569f
  hypertensive, 587–588
    pulmonary (right-sided), 588, 588f, 588t
    systemic (left-sided), 587–588, 587f
  ischemic, 571–587
    angina pectoris as, 572, 575, 575t
    chronic, 586
    clinical manifestations of, 572
    defined, 571–572
    epidemiology and risk factors for, 520–521, 520f, 520t, 572
    myocardial infarction as, 575–586
      clinical features of, 582–584
      consequences and complications of, 584–586, 585f
      defined, 572, 575
      incidence and risk factors for, 576
      infarct modification by reperfusion in, 581–582, 583f
      morphology of, 577–581, 579f, 579t, 580f, 582f
      pathogenesis of, 573, 573f, 575t, 576–577, 577f, 577t, 578f
      transmural *vs.* subendocardial, 575–576, 575t
    pathogenesis of, 572–575, 573f, 574f, 575t
    reversible *vs.* irreversible, 577, 579f, 582f
    sudden cardiac death as, 575t, 577, 586–587
  neoplastic, 613–615, 613f, 614t
  pericardial, 611–612, 611t, 612f
  rheumatic, 135, 593–595, 594f, 595f, 597f
  rheumatoid, 613
  valvular, 588–601
    calcific degeneration as, 589–591, 590f
    carcinoid, 599–600, 599f

Heart disease *(Continued)*
due to complications of artificial valves, 600–601, 600f, 600t
etiology of, 589, 589t
infective endocarditis as, 595–598, 597f, 598t
isolated *vs.* combined, 589
mitral valve prolapse as, 591–592, 592f
noninfected vegetations as, 598–599, 599f
Heart failure, 560–563
congestive, 560–563
edema due to, 120–121, 121f, 122
left-sided, 562–563
right-sided, 563
Heart failure cells, 122, 562
Heart murmurs, 589
Heart transplantation, 221, 615–616, 615f
Heart valves, 558, 558f
aging effect on, 559, 559t
artificial, complications of, 600–601, 600f, 600t
Heartburn, 799
Heat cramps, 445
Heat exhaustion, 445
Heat stroke, 445
Heat-labile (LT) toxin, 834
Heat-shock proteins, 38
Heat-stable (ST) toxin, 834
Heavy-chain disease, 678
Heberden nodes, 1305
Hedgehog *(HH)* genes, 306, 1244
Heinz bodies, 628, 628f
Helicobacter heilmannii, 814
Helicobacter pylori
in carcinogenesis, 327–328
in chronic gastritis, 813–814, 814t, 815, 815f, 816
in gastric carcinoma, 823
in gastric lymphoma, 826
in peptic ulcer disease, 817–818, 819
HELLP syndrome, 920
Helminth(s), 346t, 351–352, 353
Helminthic infections, of liver, 902
Helper T cells, 198, 199
in asthma, 723, 724f
in hypersensitivity
delayed, 216, 217f
immediate, 207–208, 207f
in tuberculosis, 381–382
Hemangioblast, 108
Hemangioendothelioma, 550
Hemangioma(s), 545–547, 546f
capillary, 498f, 546, 546f
cutaneous, 1248
lobular, 547
cavernous, 546–547, 546f
of brain, 1368
of liver, 922
in infancy, 498, 498f
juvenile, 498f, 546, 546f
Hemangiopericytoma, 551
Hemangiosarcoma, 550
Hemarthrosis(es), 123, 655–656
Hematemesis, due to esophageal disease, 799
Hematocele, of tunica vaginalis, 1047
Hematocrit, 623
reference ranges for, 623t
Hematogenous spread, 280–281, 280f
Hematologic disorder(s), 622–658
anemia(s) as, 622–649
aplastic, 647–648, 647f, 647t, 648f
classification of, 623, 623t
clinical features of, 623
defined, 622–623
due to chronic liver failure, 649
due to diffuse liver disease, 649
Hematologic disorder(s) *(Continued)*
hemolytic, 623t, 624–638
classification of, 625
clinical manifestations of, 624
due to trauma to red cells, 638, 638f
etiology of, 624
features of, 624
immuno-, 210, 212t, 636–638, 637t
in glucose-6-phosphate dehydrogenase deficiency, 627–628, 627f, 628f
in hereditary spherocytosis, 625–627, 626f, 627f
in paroxysmal nocturnal hemoglobinuria, 636, 636f
in sickle cell disease, 628–632, 629f–631f
in thalassemia syndromes, 632–636, 632f, 633f, 634t, 635f
microangiopathic, 638, 638f
morphology of, 625, 625f
pathogenesis of, 624–625, 624f
iron deficiency, 643–646, 643t, 644f–646f
megaloblastic, 638–643, 639f, 640t
myelophthisic, 648–649
of blood loss, 623–624
of chronic disease, 646
of diminished erythropoiesis, 623t, 638–649
of folate deficiency, 640t, 642–643, 642f
pernicious, 639–642, 640f, 640t, 641f
pure red cell aplasia as, 648
hemorrhagic diatheses as, 649–658
due to abnormalities in clotting factors, 653–656, 654f
due to defective platelet functions, 653
due to disseminated intravascular coagulation, 656–658, 657t, 658f
due to thrombocytopenia, 650–653, 651t
due to vessel wall abnormalities, 650
in systemic lupus erythematosus, 228t
polycythemia as, 649, 649t
Hematologic infections, perinatal, 480, 480f
Hematologic manifestations, of cancer, 334t, 335
Hematoma(s), 123
dissecting, 531, 532–534, 533f, 534f
epidural, 1358f, 1359, 1359f
pulsating, 530f, 531
subdural, 1359–1360, 1359f, 1360f
Hematopoiesis, 620–622, 621f
cytokines that stimulate, 202
fibroblast growth factor in, 96
Hematopoietic cell transplants, rejection of, 222–223
Hematopoietic cells, origin and differentiation of, 620–622, 621f
Hematopoietic disorders, systemic viral infections with, 347t
Hematopoietic stem cells (HSCs), 92
Hematopoietic system, occupational exposures and, 431t
Hematuria
asymptomatic, 960, 967t
benign familial, 989
hereditary syndromes of isolated, 988–989, 988f
Heme, 885, 886f
Heme iron, 644, 645f
Hemizygosity, 152
Hemochromatosis, 908–910
clinical features of, 910
epidemiology of, 908
hereditary, 205, 908, 910
morphology of, 41, 909–910, 910f
pathogenesis of, 908–909, 909f
secondary, 908–909, 908t
Hemodialysis-associated amyloidosis, 261
Hemodynamic disorder(s), 119–143
disseminated intravascular coagulation as, 135
edema as, 119, 120–122, 120f, 120t, 121f
embolism as, 119, 135–137, 136f, 137f
hemorrhage as, 119, 123–124, 123f
hyperemia and congestion as, 122–123, 123f
infarction as, 119, 137–139, 138f, 139f
shock as, 119, 139–143, 140t, 141f, 142f
thrombosis as, 119, 130–135, 131f, 132t, 133f–135f
Hemoglobin
fetal, 628, 629
mean cell (corpuscular), 623, 623t
reference ranges for, 623t
Hemoglobin A (HbA), in ß-thalassemia, 632, 633
Hemoglobin Barts, 636
Hemoglobin C (HbC), 629
Hemoglobin concentration, mean cell, 623, 623t
Hemoglobin H (HbH) disease, 634t, 636
Hemoglobin S (HbS)
and resistance to *Plasmodium,* 402
in sickle cell disease
diagnosis of, 632
partial expression of, 150
pathogenesis of, 628, 629, 630f
Hemoglobinopathy(ies)
alterations in structural proteins in, 154
hereditary, 628
Hemoglobinuria, paroxysmal
cold, 637–638, 637t
nocturnal, 67b, 245, 636, 636f
Hemolysis
extravascular, 624–625, 624f
intravascular, 624
Hemolytic anemia(s), 623t, 624–638
classification of, 625
clinical manifestations of, 624
due to trauma to red cells, 638, 638f
etiology of, 624
features of, 624
immuno- (autoimmune), 210, 212t, 636–638.637t
in glucose-6-phosphate dehydrogenase deficiency, 627–628, 627f, 628f
in hereditary spherocytosis, 625–627, 626f, 627f
in paroxysmal nocturnal hemoglobinuria, 636, 636f
in sickle cell disease. *See* Sickle cell disease.
in thalassemia syndromes, 632–636, 632f, 633f, 634t, 635f
microangiopathic, 638, 638f
morphology of, 625, 625f
pathogenesis of, 624–625, 624f
Hemolytic crises, in hereditary spherocytosis, 627
Hemolytic disease of the newborn, 887
Hemolytic-uremic syndrome (HUS), 1009–1011
adult, 1009, 1010–1011
classic (childhood), 1009, 1010
familial, 1011
hemolytic anemia due to, 638, 638f
thrombotic microangiopathy due to, 652, 653, 1009–1011
Hemopericardium, 123, 611
Hemoperitoneum, 123
Hemophilia A, 655–656
Hemophilia B, 656
Hemoptysis, in tuberculosis, 384, 385
Hemorrhage(s), 119, 123–124, 123f
anemia due to, 623–624
due to scurvy, 459
Duret, 1353–1354, 1354f
ganglionic, 1376

Hemorrhage(s) *(Continued)*
germinal matrix—intraventricular, in preterm infants, 484
hereditary cerebral, with amyloidosis, 1363
hypertensive, 1366, 1366f
into atheromatous plaques, 519
intracerebral (intraparenchymal)
due to trauma, 1360
hereditary, with amyloidosis, 1363
in premature infants, 1356
spontaneous, 1366, 1366f
intracranial, 1365–1368, 1366f–1368f
as birth injury, 480
lobar, 1376
pinpoint, in immune thrombocytopenic purpura, 652
pulmonary, 742–743, 742f, 745–747, 746f
retinal, 1434, 1436f, 1440f
secondary brainstem, 1353–1354, 1354f
slit, 1369
splinter, 598
subarachnoid, 1360, 1366–1367, 1366f
subungual, 598
Hemorrhagic diathesis(es), 123, 649–658
due to abnormalities in clotting factors, 653–656, 654f
due to defective platelet functions, 653
due to disseminated intravascular coagulation, 656–658, 657t, 658f
due to thrombocytopenia, 650–653, 651t
due to vessel wall abnormalities, 650
due to vitamin K deficiency, 456
Hemorrhagic enteropathy, due to shock, 142
Hemorrhagic fevers, 347t
Hemorrhagic infarction, 1364–1365, 1364f
Hemorrhagic pleuritis, 766t, 767
Hemorrhagic shock, 124, 139, 140t
Hemorrhoids, 544, 854
Hemosiderin, 39
intracellular accumulation of, 39–41, 40f
Hemosiderin deposits, in hemochromatosis, 909
Hemosiderin granules, 39, 40f, 644
Hemosiderosis, 40–41
idiopathic pulmonary, 746
Hemostasis, 124–130
coagulation cascade in, 125f, 127–130, 128f, 129f
endothelium in, 124–126, 126f
platelets in, 125f, 126–127, 127f
primary, 124, 125f
secondary, 124, 125f
sequence of events in, 124, 125f
tests of, 649–650
Hemostatic plug, 124, 125f, 127
Hemothorax, 123, 767
Henoch-Schönlein purpura, 650, 986–987, 990
Hepacivirus, 894
Hepadnaviridae, 892
Hepar lobatum, 391, 391f
Heparin-induced thrombocytopenia (HIT), 132, 652
Heparin-like molecules, in hemostasis, 125, 126f
Hepatectomy, partial, liver regeneration after, 101–103, 101f, 102f
Hepatic. *See also* Liver.
Hepatic angiosarcomas, 550
Hepatic artery, 879f
Hepatic artery compromise, 917, 917f
Hepatic circulatory disorders, 917–920, 917f–919f
Hepatic complications, of organ or bone marrow transplantation, 921
Hepatic congestion
acute, 122
chronic passive, 122–123, 123f
Hepatic duct, agenesis of, 928
Hepatic effects, of shock, 142
Hepatic encephalopathy, 882, 899, 1400
Hepatic failure, 881–882
fulminant, 899–902, 902f
Hepatic fibrosis, congenital, 916, 916f, 965
Hepatic forms, of glycogen storage disease, 166–167, 167f, 168t
Hepatic injury, patterns of, 880–881, 881t
Hepatic necrosis, due to acetaminophen, 428
Hepatic neoplasm(s), 922–927
angiosarcoma as, 923
benign, 47f, 922–923
cavernous hemangiomas as, 922
cholangiocarcinoma as, 926–927, 926f
hepatoblastoma as, 923
hepatocellular carcinomas as, 923, 924–926, 925f
liver cell adenomas as, 922–923, 923f
malignant, 923–927, 923f, 925f–927f
metastatic, 927, 927f
Hepatic steatosis, 904, 904f, 1377–1378
clinical features of, 907
due to carbon tetrachloride poisoning, 25, 25f, 26f
in cystic fibrosis, 493
in kwashiorkor, 448
in Wilson disease, 911
mechanisms of, 36, 36f, 906
morphology of, 905, 905f
nonalcoholic, 907–908
obesity and, 465
of pregnancy, 920
Hepatic vein(s), terminal, 878, 879f
Hepatic vein thrombosis, 919, 919f
Hepatitis, 890–902
acute, 897–899, 899t, 900f, 901f
alcoholic, 423, 423f
alcoholic
acute, 423, 423f
clinical features of, 907
interrelation with other liver disease of, 904, 904f
morphology of, 905, 905f
autoimmune, 903
"carriers" of, 898
chronic, 898, 899, 900f, 901f
clinicopathologic syndromes of, 897–902
defined, 880
fulminant, 899–902, 902f
herpes, 366
icteric phase of, 898
in Wilson disease, 911
interface, 880, 899
preicteric phase of, 898
steato-, 907–908
viral, 890–902, 891t
Hepatitis A virus (HAV), 347t, 890–891, 891f, 891t
Hepatitis B virus (HBV), 347t, 891–894, 891t
acute infection with, 900f
and hepatitis D virus, 895–896, 896f
and hepatocellular carcinoma, 327, 924–925
"carriers" of, 898
chronic productive infection with, 369
epidemiology of, 891–892
immune response to, 359
mutant strains of, 893
outcomes of, 891, 892f
pathogenesis of, 892–893
serologic diagnosis of, 893–894, 893f
sexual transmission of, 356t
transmission of, 892
virology of, 892, 893f
Hepatitis C virus (HCV), 347t, 891t, 894–895
and hepatocellular carcinoma, 327
chronic infection with, 901f
Hepatitis C virus (HCV) *(Continued)*
epidemiology of, 894
mutations of, 894–895
potential outcomes of, 894, 894f
serologic diagnosis of, 895, 895f
transmission of, 894
virology of, 894–895, 895f
Hepatitis D (delta) virus (HDV), 347t, 891t, 895–896, 896f, 897f
Hepatitis E virus (HEV), 347t, 891t, 896–897
Hepatitis G virus (HGV), 891t, 897
Hepatoblastoma, 923
Hepatocavopathy, obliterative, 919
Hepatocellular carcinoma (HCC), 923, 924–926
aflatoxin B1 and, 321
clinical features of, 926
epidemiology of, 924
fibrolamellar, 925, 925f, 926
hepatitis B virus and, 327, 924–925
hepatitis C virus and, 327
metastasis of, 925–926
morphology of, 925–926, 925f
pathogenesis of, 924
Hepatocyte(s), 878, 879f
centrilobular and periportal, 878
ground glass, 898, 900f
Hepatocyte function, evaluation of, 881t
Hepatocyte growth factor (HGF), 95t, 96
in liver regeneration, 102, 103
oncogene for, 294, 295t
Hepatocyte integrity, evaluation of, 881t
Hepatocyte necrosis, 880
Hepatoma, 272
Hepatomegaly
congestive, 563
in cystic fibrosis, 495
in galactosemia, 489
Hepatorenal syndrome, 882, 883
Hepatovirus, 890
Hepcidin, 644–645
HER-2/neu oncogene, 96, 296
in breast cancer, 1136b, 1137b, 1144, 1147–1148, 1148f
in ovarian cancer, 1093
in Paget disease, 1140
in prostate cancer, 1051
Herbal medicines, adverse effects of, 426, 427t
Herbicides, 434, 434t, 435
Herceptin (trastuzumab), 1148
Hereditary angioneurotic edema, 67b
Hereditary cerebral hemorrhage with amyloidosis, 1363
Hereditary disorders, 147
Hereditary dyscrasias, with amyloidosis, 260–261
Hereditary hemochromatosis, 205
Hereditary hemoglobinopathy, 628
Hereditary hemorrhagic telangiectasia, 548, 650
Hereditary motor and sensory neuropathies (HMSN), 1332–1334
Hereditary nephritis, 988–989, 988f
Hereditary neuropathies, 1332–1334, 1332t, 1333t
Hereditary nonpolyposis colorectal cancer (HNPCC), 285, 306–307, 862, 864
gastric carcinoma in, 824
Hereditary sensory and autonomic neuropathies (HSAN), 1332, 1332t
Hereditary spherocytosis (HS), 625–627, 626f, 627f
Heredofamilial congenital lymphedema, 545
Heritable melanoma syndrome, 1233
Hermaphroditism, 181
Hernia
diaphragmatic, 812
hiatal, 801–802, 801f
inguinal, 856f

Hernia *(Continued)*
intestinal, 855–856, 856f
umbilical, 856f
Herniation
external, 855
internal, 856
of brain, 122, 1352–1353, 1353f
subfalcine (cingulate), 1352, 1353f
tonsillar, 1354, 1354f
transtentorial (uncinate, mesial temporal), 1353–1354, 1354f
Heroin abuse, 426
Herpes bronchopneumonia, 366
Herpes encephalitis, 1373–1374, 1374f
Herpes epithelial keratitis, 366
Herpes esophagitis, 366
Herpes hepatitis, 366
Herpes labialis, 777
Herpes simplex keratitis, 1428, 1428f
Herpes simplex virus (HSV), 365–366, 366f
in AIDS, 256
sexual transmission of, 356t
Herpes simplex virus 1 (HSV-1), 347t, 365–366
encephalitis due to, 1373, 1374f
Herpes simplex virus 2 (HSV-2), 347t, 365–366
encephalitis due to, 1374
Herpes simplex virus (HSV) inclusion bodies, 366, 366f
Herpes simplex virus (HSV) infection
of female genital tract, 1062–1063, 1063t
of oral cavity, 776–777
Herpes stromal keratitis, 366
Herpes zoster, 368, 368f
encephalitis due to, 1374
Herpesvirus(es)
esophagitis due to, 806
Kaposi sarcoma
in body cavity large cell lymphoma, 667, 677
in Kaposi sarcoma, 256–257, 257f, 366, 549–550
Herpesvirus blister, 362f
Herpesvirus infections, 365–368, 366f–368f
Herpetic gingivostomatitis, 776–777
Herpetic stomatitis, recurrent, 777
5-HETE, 69, 69f
Heterocyclic aromatic hydrocarbons, as carcinogens, 321t
Heterophagy, 32, 32f, 159
Heterotopia(s), 498
neuronal, 1355
Heterotypic interaction, 104
Heterozygosity, loss of, 299
Heubner arteritis, 1372
HEV (hepatitis E virus), 347t, 891t, 896–897
Hexosaminidase α-subunit deficiency, 160–161, 161t, 162f
Heymann nephritis, 968–970, 969f
HFE gene, 205, 645, 908, 909f
HGF (hepatocyte growth factor), 95t, 96
in liver regeneration, 102, 103
oncogene for, 294, 295t
HGF oncogene, 295t
HGPRT (hypoxanthine guanine phosphoribosyl transferase) deficiency, and gout, 1311, 1312f
HGV (hepatitis G virus), 891t, 897
HH (Hedgehog) genes, 306, 1244
HHD (hypertensive heart disease), 587–588
pulmonary (right-sided), 588, 588f, 588t
systemic (left-sided), 587–588, 587f
HHV-8 (human herpesvirus 8)
in body cavity large cell lymphoma, 667, 677
in Kaposi sarcoma, 256–257, 257f, 366, 549–550
Hiatal hernia, 801–802, 801f
Hibernating myocardium, 582
Hidradenitis suppurativa, 373
Hidradenoma, papillary, of vulva, 1067
Hidradenoma papilliferum, 1239f, 1240
Hierarchical clustering, 316b
HIF-1 (hypoxia-induced factor 1), 309
HIF-1α (hypoxia-induced factor 1α), 74
High-altitude illness, 446
High-density lipoprotein (HDL), and atherosclerosis, 521
Hill, John, 319
Hilus cell(s), 1081
Hilus cell tumors, 1103–1104
Hirano bodies, 1388
Hirschsprung disease, 830–831
Histamine
in asthma, 726
in inflammation, 63–64, 74t
Histiocytes, sea-blue, 698
Histiocytoma, fibrous
benign, 1247–1248, 1247f, 1320–1321
malignant, 1301, 1321, 1321f
Histiocytosis(es), 667
Langerhans cell, 701–702, 702f, 1249, 1249f
sinus, 666
Histiocytosis X, 701–702, 702f, 1247–1248, 1247f
Histocompatibility molecules, structure and function of, 203–205, 203f, 204f, 205t
Histone deacetylase, in cell cycle, 289, 291f
Histoplasma capsulatum
meningoencephalitis due to, 1378
pneumonia due to, 754–755, 754f
Histoplasmosis, 754–755, 754f
HIT (heparin-induced thrombocytopenia), 132, 652
HIV. *See* Human immunodeficiency virus (HIV).
Hives, 1252–1253, 1252f, 1253f
HL. *See* Hodgkin lymphoma (HL).
HLA complex. *See* Human leukocyte antigen (HLA) complex.
HLA-B27, and ankylosing spondylitis, 205, 205t
HLA-D region, 204
hMSH1 gene, in colorectal cancer, 864
hMSH2 gene, in colorectal cancer, 864
HMSN (hereditary motor and sensory neuropathies), 1332–1334
HNPCC (hereditary nonpolyposis colorectal cancer), 285, 306–307, 862, 864
gastric carcinoma in, 824
HNSCC (head and neck squamous cell carcinoma), 780–781, 781f
Hodgkin lymphoma (HL), 686–690
classification of, 671t, 686, 688t
clinical course of, 690, 691t
etiology and pathogenesis of, 690, 691f
lymphocyte depletion type of, 688t, 689
lymphocyte predominance type of, 688t, 689–690, 689f
lymphocyte-rich type of, 688–689, 688t
mixed cellularity type of, 688, 688t, 689f
morphology of, 686–690
nodular sclerosis type of, 687–688, 688t, 689f
non-Hodgkin lymphoma *vs.*, 668, 686, 690, 691t
Reed-Sternberg cells in, 686–687, 687f, 690, 691f
spread of, 670
staging of, 687, 688t
Hollenhorst plaques, 1440
Holoprosencephaly, 473, 1355, 1355f
Holt-Oram syndrome, 565, 1280t
Homeobox *(HOX)* genes, 475, 476f, 1276–1277, 1278
Homeostasis, 4, 5f
normal fluid, 119
Homer-Wright pseudorosettes, 501
Homicide, mortality rates for, 443t
Homing, of tumor cells, 313
Homocysteine, in thrombosis, 131
Homocystinuria, and atherosclerosis, 521
Homogeneous nuclear staining, 228
Homogeneous staining regions (HSRs), 315
Homogentisic acid, 39
in alkaptonuria, 167–168
Homogentisic oxidase, in alkaptonuria, 167
Homologous recombination, inherited diseases with defects in DNA repair by, 307–308, 308f
Homotypic interaction, 104
Honeycomb fibrosis, 730
Hookworms, 353, 838
Hormonal effects, of cancer, 332–333
Hormone(s)
and wound healing, 114
classification of, 1156
defects in, bone disorders due to, 1279, 1280t
defined, 1156
ectopic, 276, 333, 339t
Hormone replacement therapy (HRT), adverse effects of, 427–428
Hormone-dependent involution, 26
Horn, cutaneous, 1240–1242, 1241f
Horner syndrome, with lung cancer, 764
Horseshoe kidney, 961
Host barriers, to infection, 352–353
Host defense, against tumors, 328–332, 329f, 332f
Host immunity
and infection, 359
injurious effects of, 359
Host resistance, vitamin A in, 451
Howell-Jolly bodies, 627f
Howship lacunae, 1275
HOX (Homeobox) genes, 475, 476f, 1276–1277, 1278
hPMS1 gene, in colorectal cancer, 864
hPMS2 gene, in colorectal cancer, 864
HPV. *See* Human papillomavirus (HPV).
H-RAS oncogene, 295t, 296
HRT (hormone replacement therapy), adverse effects of, 427–428
HS (hereditary spherocytosis), 625–627, 626f, 627f
HSAN (hereditary sensory and autonomic neuropathies), 1332, 1332t
HSCs (hematopoietic stem cells), 92
hSNF5/INI1, 1408
HSRs (homogeneous staining regions), 315
HST-1 oncogene, 294, 295t
HSV. *See* Herpes simplex virus (HSV).
5-HT (5-hydroxytryptamine)
in carcinoid syndrome, 868
in inflammation, 64
HTLV-1 (human T-cell leukemia virus type 1), 327, 347t, 667, 685
HTLV-1 (human T-cell leukemia virus type 1)-associated myelopathy (HAM), 1376
Human adjuvant disease, 1122
Human androgen receptor gene (HUMARA), 288
Human biologically active agents, production of, 147
Human chorionic gonadotropin (HCG)
as tumor marker, 338, 339t
in germ cell tumors, 1045–1046
Human herpesvirus 8 (HHV-8)
in body cavity large cell lymphoma, 667, 677
in Kaposi sarcoma, 256–257, 257f, 366, 549–550
Human immunodeficiency virus (HIV), 245–258, 347t

Human immunodeficiency virus (HIV) *(Continued)*
Addison disease with, 1216
B-cell lymphomas in, 257–258, 326
clinical features of, 255–258, 255t, 257f
CNS involvement in, 253, 258
cytomegalovirus with, 256, 367–368
diarrhea in, 841
epidemiology of, 245–246
etiology of, 246–248, 247f
in children, 1376
infections with, 361
Kaposi sarcoma in, 256–257, 257f, 548–549, 550
life cycle of, 248–253, 249f–252f, 252t
major abnormalities of immune function in, 252, 252t
mechanism of T-cell immunodeficiency in, 250–252, 251f
meningitis due to, 1375
meningoencephalitis due to, 1375–1376, 1376f
morphology of, 258
M-tropic and T-tropic strains of, 249
Mycobacterium avium-intracellulare complex in, 256, 386, 387f, 1372
myocarditis in, 608
myopathy due to, 1376
natural history of, 253–255, 254f, 255t
nephropathy associated with, 984
oral manifestations of, 778t
pathogenesis of, 248, 248f
perinatal, 355
peripheral neuropathy due to, 1376
pneumonia with, 756
pulmonary disease with, 756
structure of, 246–248, 247f
thrombocytopenia in, 652
transmission of, 245–246
sexual, 356t
tuberculosis with, 256, 384, 1372
vacuolar myelopathy in, 1376
white cell neoplasia with, 667
Human immunodeficiency virus (HIV)-associated thrombocytopenia, 652
Human leukocyte antigen (HLA) complex
and disease association, 205, 205f
in autoimmunity, 226
in diabetes, 1194
in Sjögren syndrome, 235
in systemic lupus erythematosus, 229
in transplant rejection, 218, 219–220, 221, 222
structure and function of, 203–204, 203f, 204f
Human papillomavirus (HPV), 347t, 356t, 371
carcinogenesis of, 324–325, 325f
carcinoma of penis due to, 1037
cervical cancer due to, 1074–1075, 1074f, 1076, 1076f, 1078–1079, 1079f
condyloma acuminatum due to, 1035–1036, 1036f, 1067
of female genital tract, 1063t
vulvar carcinoma due to, 1067–1068, 1068f, 1069f
warts due to, 1266
Human T-cell leukemia virus type 1 (HTLV-1), 327, 347t, 667, 685
Human T-cell leukemia virus type 1 (HTLV-1)-associated myelopathy (HAM), 1376
HUMARA (human androgen receptor gene), 288
Humidifier lung, 739
Hunner ulcer, 1027
Hunter, John, 49
Hunter syndrome, 161t, 165
Huntingtin, 1394
Huntington disease (HD), 1393–1394
aggregated proteins in, 1351t
Huntington disease (HD) *(Continued)*
clinical features of, 1394
morphology of, 1393, 1393f
pathogenesis and molecular genetics of, 183, 184t, 1393–1394
Hurler syndrome, 161t, 165
Hürthle cell(s), 1169, 1170f
in follicular thyroid carcinoma, 1181
Hürthle cell adenoma, 1176, 1176f
HUS. *See* Hemolytic-uremic syndrome (HUS).
Hutchinson teeth, 391
Hyalin
alcoholic, 34, 34f
extracellular, 39
Hyaline arteriolosclerosis
in benign nephrosclerosis, 1006, 1007f
in diabetes, 1200, 1200f
in hypertension, 529–530, 530f
Hyaline cartilage, 1304
Hyaline change, 39
Hyaline deposits, intracellular, 39
Hyaline membrane(s), in acute respiratory distress syndrome, 715, 715f
Hyaline membrane disease, 481–483, 481f, 482f
Hyalinization, in glomerulonephritis, 967–968, 989
Hyalinizing trabecular tumors, 1180
Hyalinosis, in glomerulonephritis, 967–968
Hyalosis, asteroid, 1434
Hyaluronic acid (HA, hyaluronan, hyaluronate), in extracellular matrix, 103f, 106
Hydatid disease, 406, 407
Hydatidiform mole, 1110–1112, 1110t, 1111f, 1112f
Hydatids of Morgagni, 1091
Hydrocarbons
aliphatic, 431
aromatic, 431
polycyclic, 431–432
Hydrocele, of tunica vaginalis, 1047
Hydrocephalus, 1354, 1355f
communicating, 1354, 1355f
noncommunicating, 1354
posttraumatic, 1360
Hydrocephalus ex vacuo, 1353
Hydrochloric acid, gastric secretion of, 811
Hydrogen peroxide (H_2O_2)
in cell injury, 16, 17f
in inflammation, 73
in phagocytosis, 60, 60f, 61
Hydromyelia, 1356
Hydronephrosis, 1013–1014, 1013f
Hydropericardium, 120
Hydroperitoneum, 120
Hydropic change, 20
Hydropic swelling, 1230
Hydrops
corneal, 1428
of gallbladder, 933
Hydrops fetalis, 484–487, 484f, 634t, 636
causes of, 484, 484t
immune, 484, 485–486, 485f
nonimmune, 484, 486–487, 486f, 487f
Hydrosalpinx, 1064
Hydrostatic pressure, increased, edema due to, 120–121, 120f, 120t
Hydrothorax, 120, 767
Hydroureter, 1024–1025
Hydroxyl ions (OH)
in cell injury, 16, 17f
in inflammation, 73
21-Hydroxylase deficiency, 205, 1212–1214, 1213f
14-Hydroxyretinol, 451
3ß-Hydroxysteroid dehydrogenase deficiency, 890
5-Hydroxytryptamine (5-HT)
in carcinoid syndrome, 868
in inflammation, 64
25-Hydroxyvitamin D, 452
Hygromas, cystic, 484f, 486, 547
Hymenolepis nana, 839
Hyperadrenalism, 1207–1214
due to adrenogenital syndromes, 1211–1214, 1213f
due to hypercortisolism (Cushing syndrome), 1207–1210, 1208f, 1209t
due to primary hyperaldosteronism, 1210–1211, 1211f, 1212f
Hyperaldosteronism
glucocorticoid-remediable, 1210
idiopathic, 1210
primary, 1210–1211, 1211f, 1212f
secondary, 121, 1210
Hyperammonemia, in hepatic failure, 881
Hyperbilirubinemia
hereditary, 887–888, 888t
predominantly conjugated, 887t
predominantly unconjugated, 887t
Hypercalcemia
and calcium oxalate stones, 1014
and nephrocalcinosis, 1005
asymptomatic, 1186–1187
causes of, 41–42, 1187t
due to hyperparathyroidism, 1185, 1186–1187
familial hypocalciuric, 1185
metastatic calcification with, 41–42
of malignancy, 333–334, 334t, 1184
parathyroid hormone and, 1184
Hypercalciuria, and calcium oxalate stones, 1014
Hypercellularity, in glomerulonephritis, 967
Hypercholesterolemia
familial, 154, 156–158, 157f–159f
protein folding in, 38
in atherosclerosis, 521, 523, 525f
Hyperchromatic nucleus, 274
Hypercoagulability, in thrombosis, 131–132, 131f, 132t
Hypercoagulable state, in systemic lupus erythematosus, 229
Hypercortisolism, 1162, 1207–1210, 1208f, 1209t
Hyperemia, 122–123, 123f
Hyperglycemia, neurologic sequelae of, 1400
Hypergranulosis, 1230
Hyperhomocysteinemia, 131
Hyper-IgM syndrome, 241f, 242–243
Hyperinflation, compensatory, 721
Hyperinsulinemia, obesity and, 462
Hyperinsulinism, 1205–1206, 1206f
Hyperkalemic periodic paralysis, 1339
Hyperkeratosis, 1230
Hyperlipidemia
in atherosclerosis, 521, 523, 525f
in nephrotic syndrome, 978–979
Hypermetabolic state, with burns, 445
Hypernephroma, 1016
Hyperopia, 1426
Hyperorthokeratosis, 1252f
Hyperosmolar nonketotic coma, 1202
Hyperostosis, 1161
Hyperparathyroidism, 1184–1188
asymptomatic, 1186–1187
bone disorders due to, 1287, 1287f, 1288
brown tumors of, 1186
clinical course of, 1186–1187, 1187f
epidemiology of, 1185
in MEN-1, 1185, 1221
morphology of, 1185–1186, 1186f
pathogenesis of, 1185, 1185f
primary, 1185–1187, 1185f–1187f, 1187t
secondary, 1187–1188

Hyperparathyroidism *(Continued)*
symptomatic, 1187
tertiary, 1188
Hyperphenylalaninemia, benign, 488
Hyperphosphatemia, bone disease due to, 1288
Hyperpituitarism, 1158–1162
Hyperplasia, 5, 6–7, 472
benign prostatic, 7
compensatory, 6
defined, 4, 6
endometrial, 7
hormonal, 6
mechanisms of, 6–7
pathologic, 7
physiologic, 6–7
Hyperplastic arteriolosclerosis, 529, 530, 530f
Hyperplastic polyps, 858–859, 858f, 859f
Hyperprolactinemia, 1160–1161, 1163
Hyperpyrexia, malignant, 1340
Hypersensitivity myocarditis, 608, 609f
Hypersensitivity pneumonitis, 739, 739f
Hypersensitivity reactions, 205–223
antibody-mediated (type II), 205, 206t, 210, 211f, 212t
cell-mediated (type IV), 205, 206t, 215–218, 215f–217f, 215t
classification of, 205–206, 206t
defined, 205
delayed type, 79, 215, 215f–217f, 216–217
immediate (type I), 205, 206–210, 206f, 206t, 208f, 209t
immune complex—mediated (type III), 205, 206t, 210–215, 212t, 213f, 214f
systemic anaphylaxis as, 209–210
transplant rejection as, 218–223, 219f–221f
Hypersensitivity vasculitis, 535, 537t, 539f, 540–541
Hypersplenism, 704
thrombocytopenia in, 651
Hypertension, 525–530
accelerated, 526, 1007–1008, 1008f
alcoholic, 423
and atherosclerosis, 521
arterial, 526
causes of, 526, 526t
defined, 525, 526
environmental factors in, 528f, 529
essential (idiopathic), 526, 528–529, 528f, 529f
genetic factors in, 528, 528f
in diabetes, 1204
in diabetic nephropathy, 992
in systemic sclerosis, 239
in toxemia of pregnancy, 1108, 1109f
malignant, 526, 1007–1008, 1008f
morphology of, 529–530
obesity and, 465
pathogenesis of, 526–529, 527f–530f
portal, 883–885, 885f
esophageal varices due to, 802–803, 803f
idiopathic, 918
pulmonary, 743–745, 744f, 745f
in systemic sclerosis, 239
renovascular, 526
retina in, 1436–1437, 1438f
secondary, 526t, 1007t
sodium metabolism and, 527f–529f, 528
types of, 1007t
vascular pathology in, 529–530, 530f
with pheochromocytoma, 1221
Hypertensive cerebrovascular disease, 1368–1369, 1369f
Hypertensive encephalopathy, 1369
Hypertensive heart disease (HHD), 587–588
pulmonary (right-sided), 588, 588f, 588t
systemic (left-sided), 587–588, 587f
Hypertensive intraparenchymal hemorrhage, 1366, 1366f
Hyperthecosis, stomal, 1092
Hyperthermia, 445
malignant, 1340
Hyperthyroidism, 212t, 1166–1167
apathetic, 1167
clinical course of, 1166–1167, 1167f
disorders associated with, 1166t
in Graves disease, 212t, 1166f, 1172–1173, 1173f
proptosis in, 1423, 1423f
myocardial disease due to, 610–611
Hypertriglyceridemia, obesity and, 465
Hypertrophic cardiomyopathy (HCM), 601, 604–606
clinical features of, 606
etiology of, 602t
morphology of, 601f, 605–606, 605f
pathogenesis of, 605f, 606, 607f
Hypertrophic gastropathy, 820–821, 821f
Hypertrophic neuropathy, 1333
Hypertrophic osteoarthropathy, paraneoplastic, 334t, 335
Hypertrophic-hypersecretory gastropathy, 821
Hypertrophy, 5, 7–9, 472
defined, 4, 7
of cardiac muscle, 7–9, 8f
of skeletal muscle, 7
of smooth endoplasmic reticulum, 33, 33f
of uterus during pregnancy, 7
Hyperuricemia, and gout, 1311–1313, 1312f
Hyperuricosuric calcium nephrolithiasis, 1014
Hyperviscosity syndromes, 682
thrombus formation in, 131
Hyphae, 351
Hypnozoites, 401
Hypoadrenalism
primary, 1214, 1214t
secondary, 1214t, 1216–1217
Hypoalbuminemia
in hepatic failure, 881
in nephrotic syndrome, 978
Hypocalcemia, due to vitamin D deficiency, 453
Hypochondrogenesis, 1280t
Hypochondroplasia, 1280t
Hypochromia, 632
Hypocitraturia, and calcium oxalate stones, 1014
Hypoglycemia, neurologic sequelae of, 1400
Hyponatremia, in SIADH, 1163
Hypoparathyroidism, 1188
pseudo-, 1188–1189
Hypopituitarism, 1158, 1162–1163
Hypoplasia, 472
Hypoplastic left heart syndrome, 571
Hypoproteinemia, edema due to, 120t, 121
Hypopyon, 1428
Hypospadias, 1035
Hypothalamic suprasellar tumors, 1164
Hypothalamus, in energy balance, 462, 463f, 464b
Hypothalamus-pituitary-thyroid axis, homeostasis in, 1165f
Hypothermia, 445–446
Hypothyroidism, 1167–1169
autoimmune, 1168
causes of, 1167–1168, 1167t
goitrous, 1167, 1168, 1173, 1175
myocardial disease due to, 610–611
primary, 1167–1168
secondary, 1168
tertiary, 1168
thyroprivic, 1167
toxic myopathies in, 1343–1344
Hypotony, in phthisis bulbi, 1446
Hypotrophy, 472
Hypoventilation syndrome, obesity and, 465
Hypovitaminosis B_6, 450t, 458
Hypovitaminosis C, 450t, 458–459, 460f
Hypovitaminosis D, 450t, 453–455, 453f–455f, 454t
Hypovitaminosis E, 450t, 455–456
Hypovitaminosis K, 450t, 456
Hypovolemic shock, 124, 139, 140t
Hypoxanthine guanine phosphoribosyl transferase (HGPRT) deficiency, and gout, 1311, 1312f
Hypoxia
and infarction, 139
and inflammation, 74
and *p53* gene, 303
cell injury due to, 11–12, 23
cerebral, 1361–1365, 1362f, 1364f, 1365f
defined, 11, 23
Hypoxia-induced factor 1 (HIF-1), 309
Hypoxia-induced factor 1α (HIF-1α), 74
Hypoxic encephalopathy, due to heart failure, 563
Hypoxic/ischemic encephalopathy, diffuse, 1361–1363, 1362f

I

Iatrogenic injury, to biliary tree, 935–936
IBD. *See* Inflammatory bowel disease (IBD).
ICAM-1 (intercellular adhesion molecule 1), 53f, 54, 54t
ICAT (isotope-coding affinity tags), 316b
I-cell disease, 161t
Ichthyosis, 1251–1252, 1252f
Icterus, 885, 887
Idiogram, 172f
Idiopathic hypertrophic subaortic stenosis. *See* Hypertrophic cardiomyopathy (HCM).
Idiopathic pulmonary fibrosis (IPF), 729–731, 730f, 731f
Idiopathic pulmonary hemosiderosis, 746
Idiopathic retroperitoneal fibrosis, 873
IDL (intermediate-density lipoprotein), 157
IE. *See* Infective endocarditis (IE).
IFN-γ. *See* Interferon-γ (IFN-γ).
IgA (immunoglobulin A) deficiency, 240, 242
IgA (immunoglobulin A) nephropathy, 975t, 986–988, 987f, 990
IgD (immunoglobulin D), 198, 199f
IgE (immunoglobulin E) antibodies, in immediate hypersensitivity, 207, 207f
IgE (immunoglobulin E)-dependent urticaria, 1253
IgE (immunoglobulin E)-independent urticaria, 1253
IGF-1 (insulin-like growth factor-1), 95t
in neonatal respiratory distress syndrome, 482
IGF-1 (insulin-like growth factor-1) receptor, 43
IGF-2 (insulin-like growth factor-2), in Wilms tumor, 505
IgM (immunoglobulin M), 198, 199f
IGT (impaired glucose tolerance), 1190
IHD. *See* Ischemic heart disease (IHD).
IL. *See* Interleukin(s) (IL).
Ileitis, terminal, 847
Ileocecal junction, carcinoid tumor at, 867f
Ileum
anatomy of, 828
carcinoid tumors of, 866
Ileus
gallstone, 931
meconium, in cystic fibrosis, 493, 494
Imatinib mesylate, 297
Immediate early gene response, 102
Immediate sustained response, 52
Immersion blast, 446
Immotile cilia syndrome, 34

Immune complex(es)
glomerular injury due to, 968–970, 968t, 969f, 971f, 977
in systemic lupus erythematosus, 230
in vasculitides, 214f, 535
Immune complex—mediated hypersensitivity, 205, 206t, 210–215, 212t, 213f, 214f
Immune disorder(s), 205–264
auto-, 223–240, 223t
chronic discoid lupus erythematosus as, 235
drug-induced lupus erythematosus as, 229t, 235
immunologic tolerance and, 223–226, 224f
inflammatory myopathies as, 229t, 239
mechanisms of, 226–227, 226f, 227f
mixed connective tissue disease as, 239
polyarteritis nodosa and other vasculitides as, 239–240
rheumatoid arthritis as, 235
Sjögren syndrome as, 229t, 235–237, 236f
subacute cutaneous lupus erythematosus as, 235
systemic lupus erythematosus. *See* Systemic lupus erythematosus (SLE).
systemic sclerosis (scleroderma) as, 229t, 237–239, 237f, 238f
hypersensitivity reactions as, 205–223
antibody-mediated (type II), 205, 206t, 210, 211f, 212t
cell-mediated (type IV), 205, 206t, 215–218, 215f–217f, 215t
classification of, 205–206, 206t
delayed type, 215, 215f–217f, 216–217
immediate (type I), 205, 206–210, 206f, 206t, 208f, 209t
immune complex—mediated (type III), 205, 206t, 210–215, 212t, 213f, 214f
systemic anaphylaxis as, 209–210
transplant rejection as, 218–223, 219f–221f
immunologic deficiency syndromes as. *See* Immunologic deficiency syndromes.
in Down syndrome, 176
Immune evasion, by microbes, 359–360, 359t, 360f
Immune inflammation, 217
Immune mechanisms, of glomerular injury, 968–971, 968t, 969f, 971f
Immune response, apoptosis in, 26, 28f
Immune surveillance, 328, 331–332, 332f
Immune system
cells and tissue of, 196–202, 196f–201f
general features of, 194–205
Immune thrombocytopenic purpura (ITP), 651–652
Immune-mediated neuropathies, 1331
Immunity
adaptive (acquired, specific), 194, 194f, 196, 196f
cell-mediated (cellular), 196, 196f
humoral, 196, 196f
innate (natural, native), 194–196, 194f, 195b
tumor, 328–332, 329f, 332f
Immunocompromised host, pneumonia in, 747t, 755–756, 756t
Immunodeficiency syndromes. *See* Immunologic deficiency syndromes.
Immunodeficiency-associated large B-cell lymphoma, 677
Immunoediting, cancer, 328
Immunoglobulin(s), 199, 199f
as tumor markers, 339t
thyroid-stimulating, 1172
TSH-binding inhibitor, 1172
Immunoglobulin A (IgA) deficiency, 240, 242
Immunoglobulin A (IgA) nephropathy, 975t, 986–988, 987f, 990
Immunoglobulin D (IgD), 198, 199f
Immunoglobulin E (IgE) antibodies, in immediate hypersensitivity, 207, 207f
Immunoglobulin E (IgE)-dependent urticaria, 1253
Immunoglobulin E (IgE)-independent urticaria, 1253
Immunoglobulin family cell adhesion molecules, 104
Immunoglobulin M (IgM), 198, 199f
Immunohemolytic anemia, 210, 212t, 636–638, 637t
Immunohistochemistry, 336–337, 337f
Immunologic deficiency syndromes, 240–258
acquired, 245–258
clinical features of, 255–258, 255t, 257f
epidemiology of, 245–246
etiology of, 246–248, 247f
infections with, 361
life cycle of HIV in, 248–253, 249f–252f, 252t
morphology of, 258
natural history of, 253–255, 254f, 255t
pathogenesis of, 248, 248f
common variable, 242
DiGeorge syndrome (thymic hypoplasia) as, 241f, 243
genetic deficiencies of complement system as, 244–245
hyper-IgM syndrome as, 241f, 242–243
isolated IgA, 240, 242
primary, 240–245, 240t, 241f
severe combined, 241f, 243–244
with thrombocytopenia and eczema (Wiskott-Aldrich syndrome), 244
X-linked agammaglobulinemia of Bruton as, 240–242, 241f
Immunologic factors, in systemic lupus erythematosus, 228t, 230
Immunologic reactions, cell injury due to, 13
Immunologic tolerance, 223–226, 224f
Immunoproliferative small-intestinal disease (IPSID), 869
Immunosuppressed individuals
cancer in, 331–332, 332f
cytomegalovirus in, 367–368
infections in, 360–361
fungal, 351
Immunosuppression, 331
Immunosuppression-associated Kaposi sarcoma, 549
Immunosuppressive therapy, with transplant, 220–221
Immunotactoid glomerulopathy, 992
Impaired glucose tolerance (IGT), 1190
Imperforate anus, 830
Impetiginization, 1254
Impetigo, 1267
bullous, 372, 1260f
Implantation theory, of endometriosis, 1083, 1084
Imprinting, genomic, 185–187, 186f
Inborn errors of metabolism, 487–489, 487t, 488f, 489f
myopathies associated with, 1341–1342, 1341f
thyroid, 1168
Incarceration, 856
Incidentaloma, adrenal, 1218
Incision, laceration *vs.*, 443
Incisura angularis, 810
Inclusion bodies, 347
cytomegalovirus, 367f
herpes simplex virus, 366, 366f
Inclusion body myositis, 1343
Indian hedgehog gene, 1278
Indirect DNA diagnosis, 189–191, 190f
Indoor air pollution, 430, 430t
Induced genetic instability, 438
Inducible nitric oxide synthase (iNOS), 72, 72f
Induction, of smooth endoplasmic reticulum, 33, 33f
Industrial exposures, 430–434, 431t, 432t, 433f
and lung cancer, 758
Industry, air pollution from, 429
Infant(s)
birthweight and gestational age of, 476–479, 478f, 479f, 479t
causes of death in, 470, 470t
iron deficiency anemia in, 645
necrotizing enterocolitis in, 483, 483f
tumors in, 498–506
benign, 498–499, 498f, 499f
malignant, 499–506, 500t
incidence and types of, 499–500, 500t
neuroblastic, 500–504, 501f, 502f, 503t, 504f
Wilms, 504–506, 505f, 506f
Infant mortality rate, 469–470
Infantile embryonal carcinoma, 1043
Infantile glaucoma, 1428
Infantile motor neuron disease, 1336, 1336f
Infantile X-linked cardioskeletal myopathy, 1342
Infarct(s)
border zone ("watershed"), 1362–1363
lacunar, 1368–1369, 1369f
of Zahn, 918
retinal, 1437, 1438f
strategic, 1391
Infarction, 137–139
bland, 138
bowel, 851–854, 852f, 853f
causes of, 137–138
cerebral, 1361–1365, 1362f
hemorrhagic (red), 1364–1365, 1364f
incomplete, 1365
nonhemorrhagic (pale, bland, anemic), 1365, 1365f
defined, 119, 135, 137
factors influencing development of, 139
liver, 917, 917f
morphology of, 138, 138f, 139f
myocardial. *See* Myocardial infarction (MI).
pulmonary, 742–743, 742f
red (hemorrhagic), 138, 138f
cerebral, 1364–1365, 1364f
septic, 138
pulmonary, 742
spinal cord, 1365
white (anemic), 138, 138f
Infection(s)
Addison disease due to, 1216
and atherosclerosis, 524
and autoimmune disorders, 226–227, 226f, 227f
and chronic bronchitis, 722
and diabetes, 1194
and wound healing, 114
bacterial, 371–397
abscesses as, 393
agents for, 346t, 348–349, 349t, 350f
anaerobic, 393–394, 394f
anthrax as, 375–376, 376f
chancroid as, 380
chlamydial, 346t, 349–351, 394–395
clostridial, 393–394, 394f
contagious childhood, 349t
diphtheria as, 374–375, 374f
gram-negative, 377–381
gram-positive, 371–376
granuloma inguinale as, 380–381

Infection(s) *(Continued)*
leprosy as, 387–388, 388f
listeriosis as, 375
Lyme disease as, 392–393, 392f
mechanisms of, 358–359
myco-, 381–388, 382f–388f
neisserial, 377–378, 378f
obligate intracellular, 394–397, 395f, 396t, 397f
of gastrointestinal tract, 353
of liver, 902
plague as, 379–380
relapsing fever as, 391–392
rickettsial, 346t, 349–351, 395–397, 395f, 396t, 397f
sexually transmitted, 356t
staphylococcal, 371–373, 372f, 373f
streptococcal, 373–374, 374f
syphilis as, 388–391, 388f–391f
tuberculosis as, 381–386, 382f–386f
whooping cough as, 378, 379f
with *Mycobacterium avium-intracellulare* complex, 386, 387f
with nocardia, 376, 376f
with *Pseudomonas*, 378–379, 379f
with spirochetes, 388–393, 388f–392f
bleeding disorders due to, 650
due to agranulocytosis, 663
fetal, 477
glomerulonephritis after, 976
hemolysis due to, 628
host barriers to, 352–353
host immunity and, 359
in immunodeficiencies, 240, 240t
in immunosuppressed hosts, 360–361
inflammatory responses to, 361–363, 362f, 363f
intrauterine, 477
mycologic, 397–401
agents of, 346t, 351
aspergillosis as, 399–400, 400f
candidiasis as, 397–399, 398f
cryptococcosis as, 399, 399f
due to molds, 399–401, 400f, 401f
due to yeasts, 397–399, 398f, 399f
of gastrointestinal tract, 353
of oral cavity, 777
of skin, 1267–1268, 1268f
zygomycosis as, 400–401, 401f
of bone, 1290–1292, 1291f
of central nervous system, 1369–1380
acute focal suppurative, 1371, 1371f
acute meningitis as, 1369–1370, 1370f
meningoencephalitis as
chronic bacterial, 1371–1372
fungal, 1378, 1378f
necrotizing amoebic, 1380, 1380f
viral, 1372–1377, 1373f–1377f
pathogenesis of, 1369
toxoplasmosis as, 1378–1379, 1378f, 1379f
viral, 347t
of female genital tract, 1062–1065, 1063t, 1064f
of fracture, 1289
of liver, 890–902
of oral cavity, 776–777
opportunistic
in AIDS, 255–256, 255t
of lungs, 353
parasitic, 401–411
African trypanosomiasis as, 406, 406f
babesiosis as, 403, 403f
Chagas disease as, 406–407
leishmaniasis as, 403–405, 404f
lymphatic filariasis as, 409–410, 410f
malaria as, 401–403, 402f, 403f

Infection(s) *(Continued)*
metazoal, 406–411, 407f–411f
onchocerciasis as, 410–411, 411f
protozoal, 346t, 351, 351t, 401–406, 402f–405f
schistosomiasis as, 408–409, 408f, 409f
strongyloidiasis as, 406, 407f
trichinosis as, 407–408, 408f
with tapeworms, 406–407, 407f
perinatal, 480–481, 480f
peritoneal, 872–873
placental, 1106, 1108f
pulmonary, 747–756, 747t
aspiration pneumonia as, 747t, 752
barriers to, 353
chronic pneumonia as, 747t, 753–755, 754f–756f
community-acquired pneumonia as
acute, 747t, 748–751, 749f, 750f
atypical, 747t, 751–752
in lung transplant patients, 757
lung abscess as, 747t, 753, 753f
necrotizing pneumonia as, 747t
nosocomial pneumonia as, 747t, 752
pneumonia in immunocompromised host as, 747t, 755–756, 756t
severe acute respiratory syndrome (SARS) as, 752
viral, 347t
with HIV, 756
sexually transmitted, 355–356, 356t
skin, 1265–1268, 1266f–1268f
superficial fungal, 1267–1268, 1268f
transcervical, 480
transplacental, 480, 480f
urinary tract, 353, 960
pyelonephritis and, 996–998, 997f, 998f
viral, 363–371
agents for, 346t, 347–348, 347t, 348f
chronic latent, 365–368, 366f–368f
chronic productive, 368–369
hemorrhagic fevers as, 365
latency of, 1372–1373
measles as, 363–364, 364f
mechanism of, 356–357
mumps as, 364, 364f
transforming, 369–371, 369f, 370f
transient, 363–365, 364f
with cytomegalovirus, 366–368, 367f
with Epstein-Barr virus, 369–371, 369f, 370f
with hepatitis B virus, 369
with herpes simplex virus, 365–366, 366f
with human papillomavirus, 371
with poliovirus, 364
with varicella-zoster virus, 368, 368f
with West Nile virus, 364–365
with burns, 445
with splenomegaly, 704
zoonotic, 349t, 355
Infectious agents
bacteria as, 346t, 348–349, 349t, 350f
bacteriophages as, 348
categories of, 346–352, 346t
cell injury due to, 13
chlamydiae as, 346t, 349–351
diagnosis of, 361, 361t
ectoparasites as, 352
fungi as, 346t, 351
helminths as, 346t, 351–352
immune evasion by, 359–360, 360f
mechanism of disease caused by, 356–359, 357f
mycoplasmas as, 346t, 349–351
plasmids as, 348
prions as, 346–347

Infectious agents *(Continued)*
protozoa as, 346t, 351, 351t
rickettsiae as, 346t, 349–351
transmission and dissemination of, 352–356, 354f, 356t
transposons as, 348
viruses as, 346t, 347–348, 347t, 348f
Infectious arthritis, 542, 542f, 1310–1311
Infectious disease(s), 343–411
abscesses as, 393
African trypanosomiasis as, 406, 406f
anthrax as, 375–376, 376f
aspergillosis as, 399–400, 400f
babesiosis as, 403, 403f
candidiasis as, 397–399, 398f
Chagas disease as, 406–407
chancroid as, 380
chlamydial, 346t, 349–351, 394–395
clostridial, 393–394, 394f
cryptococcosis as, 399, 399f
cysticercosis as, 406–407, 407f
diphtheria as, 374–375, 374f
granuloma inguinale as, 380–381
history of study of, 344–345
hydatid disease as, 406–407
in bioterrorism, 345–346, 346t
leishmaniasis as, 403–405, 404f
leprosy as, 387–388, 388f
listeriosis as, 375
Lyme disease as, 392–393, 392f
lymphatic filariasis as, 409–410, 410f
malaria as, 401–403, 402f, 403f
measles as, 363–364, 364f
mumps as, 364, 364f
neisserial, 377–378, 378f
new and emerging, 345, 345t
onchocerciasis as, 410–411, 411f
pathogenesis of, 344–363
plague as, 379–380
poliovirus as, 364
relapsing fever as, 391–392
rickettsial, 346t, 349–351, 395–397, 395f, 396t, 397f
schistosomiasis as, 408–409, 408f, 409f
staphylococcal, 371–373, 372f, 373f
streptococcal, 373–374, 374f
strongyloidiasis as, 406, 407f
syphilis as, 388–391, 388f–391f
trichinosis as, 407–408, 408f
tuberculosis as, 381–386, 382f–386f
viral hemorrhagic fevers as, 365
whooping cough as, 378, 379f
zygomycosis as, 400–401, 401f
Infectious enterocolitis, 832–841
bacterial, 832–838, 834t, 836f, 837f
necrotizing, 840
parasitic, 838–840, 839f, 840f
viral, 832–833, 833t
Infectious esophagitis, 805–806
Infectious mononucleosis, 326, 369–371, 369f, 370f
oral manifestations of, 778t
Infectious polyneuropathies, 1331–1332
Infectious rhinitis, 783
Infective endocarditis (IE), 595–598
acute *vs.* subacute, 596
brain abscess due to, 1371
clinical features of, 596–598
diagnostic criteria for, 596–598, 598t
due to mitral valve prolapse, 592
etiology and pathogenesis of, 596
morphology of, 596, 597f
of prosthetic valve, 601
thromboembolism due to, 133
Inferior conjunctival fornix, 1424f, 1425
Inferior tarsus, 1424f

Inferior vena cava thrombosis, 919
Inferior vena caval syndrome, 544
Infertility, in cystic fibrosis, 494, 495
Infestations, skin, 1268–1269, 1269f
Infiltrative fasciitis, 1318, 1318f
Infiltrative ophthalmopathy, in Graves disease, 1172
Inflamed juvenile nevus, 1426
Inflammation(s), 47–85
  acute, 49–78
    apoptosis in, 26
    cellular events in, 53–62, 53f
    chemotaxis in, 56–57, 58f
    defects in leukocyte function in, 61–62, 62t
    defined, 49
    leukocyte activation in, 57–59, 58f
    leukocyte adhesion and transmigration in, 54–56, 54t, 55b, 56f, 57f
    manifestations of, 49, 50f
    morphologic patterns of, 76–77, 77f, 78f
    outcomes of, 75–76, 75f, 76f
    phagocytosis in, 59–61, 60f
    release of leukocyte products and leukocyte-induced tissue injury in, 61, 61t
    stimuli for, 49–50
    summary of, 77–78
    termination of, 49, 62–63
    vascular changes in, 50–53, 51f, 52f
  cells and tissues involved in, 48–49, 48f
  chemical mediator(s) of, 63–75, 63f, 74t, 76t
    arachidonic acid metabolites (prostaglandins, leukotrienes, and lipoxins) as, 68–70, 68t, 69f, 70f
    clotting system as, 65–68, 67f
    complement system as, 59, 64–65, 65f, 66b–67b
    cytokines and chemokines as, 54, 56f, 70–72, 71f, 202
    histamine as, 63–64
    kinin system as, 65, 67f
    lysosomal constituents of leukocytes as, 73, 73f
    neuropeptides as, 74
    nitric oxide as, 60f, 61, 72–73, 72f
    oxygen-derived free radicals as, 73–74
    plasma proteins as, 64–68
    platelet-activating factor as, 70
    serotonin as, 64
    vasoactive amines as, 63–64, 64f
  chronic, 78–84
    and cancer, 287
    causes of, 79
    defined, 49, 78
    due to infection, 363, 363f
    eosinophils in, 82, 82f
    fibrosis in, 115, 116f
    mononuclear cell infiltration in, 79–81, 79f–81f, 362, 362f
  complement- and Fc receptor—mediated, 210, 211f
  cytopathic-cytoproliferative, 362, 362f
  due to infarction, 138
  fibrinous, 76–77, 77f
  functions of, 48
  general features of, 48–49, 48f
  granulomatous, 79, 82–83, 83f, 83t, 216, 362
  harmful effects of, 48
  healing by fibrosis of, 75–76, 75f
  historical highlights on, 49
  immune, 217
  immune complex—mediated, 213, 213f
  in atherosclerosis, 79, 523, 574
  in ischemia-reperfusion injury, 24
  intracellular accumulation of cholesterol due to, 37
Inflammation(s) *(Continued)*
  lymphatics in, 83–84
  lymphocytes in, 81–82, 82f
  mast cells in, 82
  morphologic features of, 79–81
  nasal, 783–784, 783f
  necrotizing, 362–363
    due to *Pseudomonas,* 379
  of bladder, 1027–1028, 1028f
  of breast, 1124–1126, 1125f, 1126f
  of ears, 788
  of endometrium, 1083
  of fallopian tubes, 1091
  of larynx, 786
  of liver, 880, 890–902
  of nasopharynx, 784
  of penis, 1035
  of peritoneum, 872–873
  of salivary gland, 790, 791f
  of thyroid gland, 1169–1172, 1170f, 1171f
  of ureters, 1025, 1025f
  of urethra, 1034
  orbital, 1423–1424, 1423f
  placental, 1106, 1108f
  progression to, 75f, 76
  purulent, 49, 77, 78f
  resolution of, 75, 75f, 76f
  serous, 76, 77f
  suppurative (polymorphonuclear), 77, 78f, 361–362, 362f
  systemic effects of, 84–85
  ulcers due to, 77, 78f
Inflammatory bowel disease (IBD), 846–851
  Crohn disease as, 846, 847–849, 847f–849f, 851t
  diagnosis of, 847
  etiology and pathogenesis of, 846–847
  genetic susceptibility to, 846
  role of intestinal flora in, 846
  T-cells in, 846–847
  ulcerative colitis as, 846, 847, 849–851, 849f, 850f, 851t
Inflammatory carcinoma, of breast, 1142, 1147
Inflammatory demyelinating polyradiculoneuropathy
  acute, 1331
  chronic, 1331
Inflammatory dermatoses
  acute, 1252–1256, 1252f–1256f, 1254t
  chronic, 1256–1259, 1257f–1259f
Inflammatory fibroid polyp, of stomach, 822, 822f
Inflammatory myofibroblastic tumor, of lung, 765
Inflammatory myopathies, 229t, 239, 1342–1343, 1342f
Inflammatory neuropathies, 1330–1331
Inflammatory polyp
  of biliary tract, 934
  of esophagus, 806
  of stomach, 822, 822f
Inflammatory proliferations, of white cells and nodes, 663–666, 664f–666f, 664t
Inflammatory pseudotumor, of esophagus, 806
Inflammatory responses, to infection, 361–363, 362f, 363f
Inflammatory vascular disease, 534–542
  Churg-Strauss syndrome as, 537t, 541
  classification of, 535, 535t, 536, 536f, 537t
  giant cell (temporal) arteritis as, 536–538, 537f
  infectious arthritis as, 542, 542f
  Kawasaki disease (mucocutaneous lymph node syndrome) as, 540
  leukocytoclastic vasculitis as, 539f, 540–541
  pathogenesis of, 535–536, 535t
Inflammatory vascular disease *(Continued)*
  polyarteritis nodosa as, 539f, 540
  Takayasu arteritis as, 538–540, 538f
  thromboangiitis obliterans (Buerger disease) as, 539f, 542
  vasculitis with other disorders as, 542, 542f
  Wegener granulomatosis as, 539f, 541–542
Influenza, 751–752
Influenza virus(es), 347t, 353, 359
Infrared radiation, exposure to, 436t
Inguinal hernia, 856f
Inhalation injury, with burns, 445
Initiation, of carcinogenesis, 319–321, 320f, 321f, 321t
Initiators, in carcinogenesis, 319–321, 320f, 321f, 321t
Injurious stimuli, apoptosis due to, 26
Injury(ies), 442–446
  acute lung, 714–716, 714t, 715f, 715t, 717f
  birth, 479–480
  cellular responses to, 4–5, 5f, 5t
  due to mechanical force, 443–444, 443f, 444f
  electrical, 446
  hepatic, 880–881, 881t
  mortality rates for, 443t
  related to changes in atmospheric pressure, 446
  subcellular responses to, 5, 32–34, 32f–34f
  thermal, 444–446
INK4a/ARF locus, 292t, 305
Inlet patch, 799
iNOS (inducible nitric oxide synthase), 72, 72f
Inositol triphosphate (IP_3), 98f, 99, 100
Insane, general paresis of the, 1372
Insect bites and stings, 1268–1269, 1269f
  eczematous reaction to, 1254t
Insecticides, 323, 434–435, 434t
Insertion(s), 147, 149
Insertional mutagenesis, 293
Insomnia, fatal familial, 1382
Insulin
  actions of, 1191–1192, 1192f, 1193f
  in energy balance, 462, 463f
  in glucose homeostasis, 1191
  normal physiology of, 1190–1192, 1191f–1193f
  synthesis of, 1191
Insulin gene, diabetes due to, 1197
Insulin receptor, 1192, 1193f
  genetic defects of, 1195
Insulin receptor mutations, diabetes due to, 1197
Insulin release, regulation of, 1191, 1191f, 1192f
Insulin resistance, 1195–1196, 1195f, 1196f
  obesity and, 462
Insulin signaling pathways, 1192, 1193f
  genetic defects of, 1195
Insulin-like growth factor-1 (IGF-1), 95t
  in neonatal respiratory distress syndrome, 482
Insulin-like growth factor-1 (IGF-1) receptor, 43
Insulin-like growth factor-2 (IGF-2), in Wilms tumor, 505
Insulinoma(s), 1205–1206, 1206f
  in MEN-1, 1222
Insulitis, 1193, 1199, 1200f
INT-2 oncogene, 294, 295t
Integrins
  as regulators of angiogenesis, 109
  in cell replication, 100
  in extracellular matrix, 104–105, 106f
  in inflammatory response, 53f, 54, 54t, 55b
  in tumor cell invasion, 312
Intercalated disks, 557
Intercellular adhesion molecule 1 (ICAM-1), 53f, 54, 54t
Interdigitating dendritic cells, 199–200
Interface hepatitis, 880, 899

Interferon(s), 95t
in immunity, 202
viruses and, 360
Interferon-γ (IFN-γ), 59
in delayed type hypersensitivity, 217, 217f
in immunity, 202
in tuberculosis, 382
Interleukin(s) (IL), 95t, 202
Interleukin-1 (IL-1)
in immediate hypersensitivity, 209
in immunity, 202
in inflammation, 53f, 54, 56f, 71, 71f, 74t
in rheumatoid arthritis, 1307
in scar formation, 110
in septic shock, 140, 141f
Interleukin-1 (IL-1) receptor associated kinase (IRAK), 195b
Interleukin-2 (IL-2)
in autoimmunity, 226
in delayed type hypersensitivity, 217, 217f
in immune system, 198, 202
Interleukin-3 (IL-3), in immediate hypersensitivity, 207f, 209
Interleukin-4 (IL-4)
in immediate hypersensitivity, 208, 209
in immune system, 202
Interleukin-5 (IL-5)
in immediate hypersensitivity, 207f, 208, 209
in immune system, 202
Interleukin-6 (IL-6)
in immediate hypersensitivity, 209
in immunity, 202
in liver regeneration, 102
in septic shock, 141f, 142f
Interleukin-8 (IL-8), in septic shock, 141f, 142f
Interleukin-12 (IL-12)
in delayed type hypersensitivity, 216, 217f
in immunity, 202
Interleukin-13 (IL-13)
in immediate hypersensitivity, 208
in scar formation, 110
Interleukin-15 (IL-15), in immunity, 202
Interlobar arteries, 956
Intermediate filaments, abnormalities of, 34, 34f
Intermediate-density lipoprotein (IDL), 157
Internal elastic lamina, 512, 512f
Internalins, 375
Internodes, 1326
Interstitial cell tumors, 1046
Interstitial collagenases, 111
Interstitial disease, diffuse. *See* Diffuse interstitial disease(s).
Interstitial fluid pressure, increased, in edema, 120, 120f
Interstitial keratitis, in syphilis, 391
Interstitial lamellae, 1276, 1277f
Interstitial matrix, 103, 103f
Interstitial nephritis, 236, 996–1004
acute, 996
causes of, 996t
chronic, 996
drug- and toxin-induced, 1002–1004, 1002f, 1003f, 1004t
in multiple melanoma, 1005–1006, 1005t, 1006f
nephrocalcinosis as, 1005
pyelonephritis as, 994–1002
acute, 998–1000, 998f, 999f
and urinary tract infection, 996–998, 997f, 998f
chronic, 1000–1002, 1001f
secondary, 996
urate nephropathy as, 1004–1005, 1005f
Intertrigo, 398
Intervillositis, 1108f
Intestinal. *See also under* Gastrointestinal.
Intestinal adhesions, 856, 856f
Intestinal flora, in inflammatory bowel disease, 846
Intestinal ischemia, in necrotizing enterocolitis, 483
Intestinal metaplasia, 815
Intestinal obstruction, 855–856, 855t, 856f
Intestinal phase, of gastric acid secretion, 811
Intestinal pseudo-obstruction, 855t
Intestinal stem cells, 93f
Intestinalization, in pernicious anemia, 642
Intestine. *See* Large intestine; Small intestine.
Intima, of blood vessel, 512, 512f
Intimal hyperplasia, 515
Intimal thickening, 515, 515f
Intracellular accumulation(s), 5, 34–41
categories of, 34–35
mechanisms of, 35, 35f
of glycogen, 39
of hyaline, 39
of lipids, 35–37, 36f, 37f
of pigments, 39–41, 40f
of proteins, 37–39, 37f, 38f
Intracerebral hemorrhage
due to trauma, 1360
hereditary, with amyloidosis, 1363
in premature infants, 1356
spontaneous, 1366, 1366f
Intracranial berry aneurysms, 531, 1366–1367, 1367f, 1368f
in polycystic kidney disease, 964
ruptured, 1366–1367
Intracranial hemorrhage, 1365–1368, 1366f–1368f
as birth injury, 480
Intracranial pressure, raised, 1352–1353, 1353f
Intradermal nevi, 1232
Intraductal papillary mucinous neoplasms (IPMNs), 947–948, 949f
Intraductal papilloma, 1128–1129, 1129f
Intraepithelial lymphocytes, in intestines, 829
Intrahepatic biliary tract disease, 913–916, 913t, 914f–916f
Intralobar sequestrations, 713
Intramembranous formation, 1278
Intramural arteries, 557
Intraparenchymal hemorrhage
due to trauma, 1360
hereditary, with amyloidosis, 1363
in premature infants, 1356
spontaneous, 1366, 1366f
Intrarenal reflux, 998
Intrarenal vasoconstriction, 994
Intraretinal microangiopathy (IRMA), 1439, 1440f
Intratubular germ cell neoplasia (ITGCN), 1041
Intrauterine development, 474, 475f
Intrauterine growth restriction (IUGR), 477–478, 478f, 1110
Intrauterine infection, 477
Intravagal paraganglia, 1218, 1219f
Intraventricular hemorrhage, in preterm infants, 484
Intrinsic factor, 811
in vitamin B_{12} metabolism, 639, 640f
Intrinsic pathway, in apoptosis, 29–30, 29f, 30f
Intussusception, 830, 856, 856f
Invasive mole, 1112, 1112f
Inversions, 174, 174f
Inverted follicular keratoses, 1237
Inverted papillomas
of bladder, 1030
sinonasal, 784, 785f
Involucrum, 1291, 1291f
Iodides, as antithyroid agents, 1166
Iodine, 461t
as antithyroid agent, 1166
Ion channel(s), defects in, bone disorders due to, 1281–1282, 1282f, 1283f
Ion channel myopathies, 1339–1340
Ionizing radiation, 436–441
as carcinogen, 323–324, 438
cellular effects of, 437–438, 438t
clinical manifestations of, 436t, 439–441, 439f–441f
IP_3 (inositol triphosphate), 98f, 99, 100
IPF (idiopathic pulmonary fibrosis), 729–731, 730f, 731f
IPMNs (intraductal papillary mucinous neoplasms), 947–948, 949f
IPSID (immunoproliferative small-intestinal disease), 869
IRAK (IL-1 receptor associated kinase), 195b
Iridocorneal endothelial syndrome, 1432
Iridocyclitis, traumatic, 1432
Iris, 1422f, 1430f
Iris bombé, 1430f, 1431
IRMA (intraretinal microangiopathy), 1439, 1440f
Iron
accumulation in liver of, 880
deficiency in, 461t
functions of, 461t
impaired absorption of, 645
increased requirement for, 645
intracellular accumulation of, 39–41, 40f
Iron deficiency anemia, 643–646, 646f
Iron metabolism, 643–645, 643t, 644f, 645f
Iron overload
in hemochromatosis, 908–910, 908t, 909f, 910f
in ß-thalassemia, 634, 635
myocardial disease due to, 610
Iron-binding capacity, total, 644
Irritant dermatitis, 1254t
Irritation fibroma, of oral cavity, 775, 775f
Ischemia
atrophy due to, 9, 9f
cerebral, 1361–1365
focal, 1361, 1363–1365, 1364f, 1365f
global, 1361–1363, 1362f
defined, 11
Ischemia-reperfusion injury, 23, 24–25
Ischemic bowel disease, 851–854, 852f, 853f
Ischemic cardiomyopathy, 586
Ischemic coagulative necrosis
due to infarction, 138
of liver, 880
Ischemic encephalopathy, 141
Ischemic heart disease (IHD), 571–587
angina pectoris as, 572, 575, 575t
chronic, 586
clinical manifestations of, 572
defined, 571–572
epidemiology and risk factors for, 520–521, 520f, 520t, 572
myocardial infarction as, 575–586
atherosclerotic plaque rupture in, 573, 573f
clinical features of, 582–584
consequences and complications of, 584–586, 585f
coronary artery pathology in, 575t
defined, 572, 575
incidence and risk factors for, 576
infarct modification by reperfusion in, 581–582, 583f
morphology of, 577–581, 579f, 579t, 580f, 582f
pathogenesis of, 576–577, 577f, 577t, 578f
transmural *vs.* subendocardial, 575–576, 575t

Ischemic heart disease (IHD) *(Continued)*
pathogenesis of, 572–575, 573f, 574f, 575t
reversible *vs.* irreversible, 577, 579t, 582f
sudden cardiac death as, 575t, 577, 586–587
Ischemic injury, 11–12, 23–24, 24f
Islet amyloidosis, 1196
Islet cell tumors, 1205–1207, 1206f
Islets of Langerhans, 940, 1189
diffuse hyperplasia of the, 1206
in diabetes, 1200, 1204t
insulin production in, 1191, 1191f
Isochromosomes, 174, 174f
Isospora belli, 351t
Isotope-coding affinity tags (ICAT), 316b
Isotype switching, 243
ITGCN (intratubular germ cell neoplasia), 1041
ITP (immune thrombocytopenic purpura), 651–652
IUGR (intrauterine growth restriction), 477–478, 478f, 1110
Ixodes dammini, 1268
Ixodes deer tick, 392, 392f

J

Jak3, 244
Jansen metaphyseal chondroplasia, 1280t
Janus kinases (JAKs), 98f, 99
Japanese spotted fever, 396t
Jaundice, 885–888
causes of, 887, 887t
defined, 885
in fetal hydrops, 485–486
in hepatitis, 898
neonatal, 887
pathophysiology of, 887–888
physiologic, 479
JC virus, 347t, 357
Jejunum, anatomy of, 828
Joint(s), 1303–1315
arthritis of, 1304–1314
ankylosing spondylo-, 1309
chronic tophaceous, 1313, 1313f
gouty, 1311–1314, 1312f, 1313f
infectious, 1310–1311
Lyme, 1310
osteo-, 1304–1305, 1305f
psoriatic, 1310
reactive, 1309–1310
rheumatoid, 1305–1309, 1306f–1308f
juvenile, 1309
suppurative, 1310
tuberculous, 1310
viral, 1310–1311
calcium pyrophosphate crystal deposition disease of, 1314, 1314f
ganglion cyst of, 1315
giant cell tumor of tendon sheath of, 1315
gout of, 1311–1314, 1311t, 1312f
pseudo-, 1314, 1314f
in systemic lupus erythematosus, 233
normal anatomy of, 1303–1304
pigmented villonodular synovitis of, 1315, 1315f
seronegative spondyloarthropathies of, 1309–1310
synovial, 1303
synovial cyst of, 1315
tumors and tumor-like lesions of, 1314–1315
Joint disease, degenerative, 1304–1305, 1305f
Joint laxity
in Ehlers-Danlos syndromes, 155
in Marfan syndrome, 154
Joint mice, 1305
Junctional nevi, 1232
Juvenile gastric polyps, 822
Juvenile polyposis syndrome, 859
Juvenile rheumatoid arthritis (JRA), 1309
uveitis in, 1433
Juxtacrine signaling, 97–98
Juxtaglomerular apparatus, 959
Juxtaglomerular cells, 959

K

KAI1 gene, 313
in prostate cancer, 1051
Kala-azar, 404, 404f
Kallikreins, 65, 68
Kaposi sarcoma (KS), 548–550
chronic (classic, European), 548
clinical course of, 550
in AIDS, 256–257, 257f, 548–549, 550
lymphadenopathic (African, endemic), 548–549
morphology of, 549, 549f
of eyelid or conjunctiva, 1425
pathogenesis of, 549–550
transplant-associated (immunosuppression-associated), 549
Kaposi sarcoma herpesvirus (KSHV)
in body cavity large cell lymphoma, 667, 677
in Kaposi sarcoma, 256–257, 257f, 366, 549–550
Kaposi varicelliform eruption, 366
Kartagener syndrome, 34, 727, 784
Karyolysis, 12f, 21
Karyorrhexis, 12f, 21, 501
Karyotype, 170–173, 171f–173f
Karyotypic abnormalities
congenital anomalies due to, 472
in tumor cells, 314–315
Karyotyping, 170
spectral, 171, 173f, 337
Kawasaki disease, 537t, 540
Kayser-Fleischer rings, 911
Kearns-Sayre syndrome (KSS), 1342, 1399
Keloid, 115, 115f
Kennedy disease/syndrome, 184t, 1397
Keratic precipitates, 1432
Keratin, basal, in breast carcinoma, 1136b, 1137b
Keratinocyte(s), 1228, 1228f, 1229f
Keratinocyte growth factor (KGF), 95t
Keratitis, 1428, 1428f
herpes
epithelial, 366
stromal, 366
interstitial, in syphilis, 391
punctate, 411
Keratoacanthoma, 1240, 1241f
Keratoconjunctivitis sicca, 790
in Sjögren syndrome, 235, 236
Keratoconus, 1428, 1429f
Keratocyst, odontogenic, 782
Keratocytes, 1428
Keratomalacia, 451, 452f
Keratopathy(ies)
band, 1428
bullous, 1427
in Fuchs endothelial dystrophy, 1428
pseudophakic, 1429
Keratosis(es)
actinic, 1240–1242, 1241f
inverted follicular, 1237
para-, 1242
seborrheic, 1237, 1237f
Kerley's B lines, 562
Kernicterus, 486, 887
Kernohan's notch, 1353
Kerosene, 431
Keshan disease, 461
Ketoacidosis
diabetic, 1202
metabolic, 1202
Ketone bodies, 1202
Ketonemia, 1202
Ketonuria, 1202
KGF (keratinocyte growth factor), 95t
Kidney(s), 955–1021
agenesis of, 961
amyloidosis of, 263, 263f, 264
anatomy and physiology of, 956–959, 957f–959f
blood vessels of, 956
congenital anomalies of, 961
diseases of. *See* Renal disease(s).
ectopic, 961
effects of shock on, 142
horseshoe, 961
hypoplastic, 961
in blood pressure regulation, 527–528, 527f, 529f
in heart failure
left-sided, 563
right-sided, 563
in systemic lupus erythematosus, 231–233, 231f–233f
in systemic sclerosis, 238–239
in toxemia of pregnancy, 1109–1110
medullary sponge, 962t, 965
myeloma, 680
of preterm infants, 478–479
radiation effect on, 440–441
Kidney disease. *See* Renal disease(s).
Kidney grafts, rejection of, 218–222, 219f–221f
Kidney stones. *See* Nephrolithiasis.
Kidney transplant, rejection of, 218–222, 219f–221f
Kimmelstiel-Wilson disease, 991–992
in diabetes, 1201
Kinetoplast, 403
Kinin system, in inflammation, 65, 67f, 68
Kininogens, 65
KiSS gene, 313
KIT oncogene, 295t, 296
Klatskin tumors, 935
Klebsiella pneumoniae, 350f
pneumonia due to, 748
KLF6 gene, 300t, 306
Klinefelter syndrome, 179, 472, 1038
Knockout mice, 91
Koch, Robert, 344
Koebner phenomenon, 1257, 1258
Koebnerization, 1230
Koilocytosis, in condyloma acuminatum, 1067, 1067f
Koilocytotic atypia, 1067
Koilonychia, in anemia, 623
Korsakoff psychosis, 457, 457f
Korsakoff syndrome, 1399
Krabbe disease, 161t, 1397
K-RAS oncogene, 295t, 296
in colorectal cancer, 863, 863f
in pancreatic cancer, 949f, 950, 950t, 952
Krox20, in sudden infant death syndrome, 497
Krukenberg tumor, 826, 1104
KS. *See* Kaposi sarcoma (KS).
KSHV (Kaposi sarcoma herpesvirus)
in body cavity large cell lymphoma, 667, 677
in Kaposi sarcoma, 256–257, 257f, 366, 549–550
KSS (Kearns-Sayre syndrome), 1342, 1399
Kupffer cells, 878
in cirrhosis, 884f
in hepatitis, 899
Kuru, 346
Kuru plaques, 1382
Kwashiorkor, 448, 448f, 449, 449t
Kyphoscoliosis type, of Ehlers-Danlos syndromes, 155–156, 156t

L
Labile tissues, 90, 90f
Laceration, 443, 443f
of brain, 1357
of peripheral nerve, 1335
Lacis cells, 959
Lacrimal glands
accessory, 1424, 1424f
tumors of, 1424
Lactase deficiency, 844–845
Lactate dehydrogenase (LDH), in germ cell tumors, 1045
Lactation, 1121
Lactational adenomas, 1127
Lactic acid, accumulation of, 15
Lactic acidosis, in shock, 141
Lactiferous ducts, squamous metaplasia of, 1125, 1125f
Lactoferrin, in phagocytosis, 61
Lactotroph(s), 1157
Lactotroph adenomas, 1160–1161, 1161f
Lactotroph hyperplasia, 1161
Lacunar cells, 686, 687f
Lacunar infarcts, 1368–1369, 1369f
Lacunes, 1368
LAD (left anterior descending) coronary artery, 557
atherosclerosis of, 572
in myocardial infarction, 578
LAD1 (leukocyte adhesion deficiency type 1), 56, 61, 62t
LAD2 (leukocyte adhesion deficiency type 2), 56, 61, 62t
Laennec cirrhosis, 906
Lafora bodies, 1352
Lambert-Eaton myasthenic syndrome, 1344–1345
paraneoplastic, 1411t
with lung cancer, 764
Lambl excrescences, 559, 614
Lamellar bodies, 713
Lamellar bone, 1275–1276, 1277f
mosaic pattern of, 1285–1286, 1285f
Lamin A/C, 1339t
Lamina densa, of glomerulus, 956, 958f
Lamina papyracea, 1423
Lamina rara externa, of glomerulus, 956, 958f
Lamina rara interna, of glomerulus, 956, 958f
Laminar blood flow, 131
Laminin
in extracellular matrix, 103f, 105, 106f
in tumor cell invasion, 312
Langerhans cell(s), 199, 200f, 1228, 1228f
in contact dermatitis, 1255
Langerhans cell histiocytosis, 701–702, 702f, 1249, 1249f
Lanugo, in anorexia nervosa, 449
Large cell carcinoma, of lung, 759, 761f, 762
Large for gestational age (LGA), 476
Large granular lymphocytes. *See* Natural killer (NK) cells.
Large granular lymphocytic leukemia (LGL), 671t, 685–686
Large intestine, 828–870
adenomas of, 858, 858f, 859–861, 860f, 861f
anatomy of, 828
congenital anomalies of, 830–831
diverticular disease of, 854–855, 855f
enterocolitis of. *See* Enterocolitis.
idiopathic inflammatory bowel disease of, 846–851, 847f–850f, 851t
immune system of, 829–830
incarceration of, 856
mucosa of, 828f, 829
neuromuscular function of, 830
obstruction of, 855–856, 855t, 856f
Large intestine *(Continued)*
papilloma of, 270f
polyps of, 271, 271f, 857–859, 858f, 859f
strangulation of, 856
tumors of, 857–870, 857t
vascular disorders of, 851–854, 852f, 853f
vasculature of, 828
Laryngeal carcinoma, 786, 787f
Laryngitis, 786
Laryngotracheobronchitis, 786
due to influenza, 752
Larynx, 786–787
inflammations of, 786
reactive nodules of, 786
squamous papilloma and papillomatosis of, 786–787, 787f
Laser capture microdissection, 316b
Laser-assisted in situ keratomileusis (LASIK), 1426
Latency, of viral infections, 1372–1373
Latency-associated transcripts (LATs), 365
Latent membrane protein-1 (LMP-1), Epstein-Barr virus and, 325
Late-phase reaction, 206, 206f
LATS (long-acting thyroid stimulator), 1172
Lattice corneal dystrophy, 1429
LBP (lipopolysaccharide-binding protein), 195b
LCIS (lobular carcinoma in situ), 1123t, 1130t, 1141–1142, 1142f
LCX (left circumflex) coronary artery, 557
atherosclerosis of, 572
in myocardial infarction, 578
LDH (lactate dehydrogenase), in germ cell tumors, 1045
LDL. *See* Low-density lipoprotein (LDL).
L-DOPA, for Parkinson disease, 1393
LE (lupus erythematosus) bodies, 230
Lead, exposure to, 428t, 432–433, 432t, 433f
Leber hereditary optic neuropathy (LHON), 185, 185f, 1342, 1445
Lectin(s)
C-type, 55b
mannose-binding, in cystic fibrosis, 492
Lectin pathway, of complement activation, 64, 66b
Left anterior descending (LAD) coronary artery, 557
atherosclerosis of, 572
in myocardial infarction, 578
Left circumflex (LCX) coronary artery, 557
atherosclerosis of, 572
in myocardial infarction, 578
Left ventricular hypertrophy, 561, 561f, 562
Left ventricular remodeling, 560
Left-sided heart failure, 562–563
Left-to-right shunts, 566–569, 567f, 568f
Leg(s), bowing of, 455, 455f
Legionella pneumophila, pneumonia due to, 749
Legionnaires disease, 749
Leiden mutation, 131
Leigh syndrome, 1342, 1398–1399
Leiner disease, 1257
Leiomyoma(s), 1322
benign metastasizing, 1090
genital, 1322
of esophagus, 806
pilar, 1322
uterine, 274f, 281f, 1089–1090, 1090f
Leiomyomatosis, disseminated peritoneal, 1090
Leiomyosarcoma(s), 1322
uterine, 281f, 1090, 1091f
Leishmania aethiopica, 404
Leishmania braziliensis, 404
Leishmania chagasi, 404
Leishmania donovani, 351t, 404, 404f
Leishmania major, 404
Leishmania spp, 351, 403–405
Leishmaniasis, 403–405, 404f
cutaneous, 404
diffuse, 405
mucocutaneous, 404
visceral, 404, 404f
Lemierre syndrome, 393
Length polymorphisms, 190, 190f
Lens, 1422f, 1430, 1430f
cataract of, 1431
nuclear sclerosis of, 1431
Lens capsule, 1430
Lens-induced uveitis, 1431
Lentiginous, defined, 1230
Lentigo (lentigines), 1231, 1232
solar or actinic, 1232
Leontiasis ossea, 1286
Lepidic cells, 613
Lepromin, 387
Leprosy, 387–388, 388f
granulomatous inflammation in, 83t
lepromatous, 387–388, 388f
peripheral neuropathy in, 1331
tuberculoid, 387, 388f
Leptin
and insulin resistance, 1196, 1196f
in bone formation, 1275
in energy balance, 462, 463f, 464b
Leptin-melanocortin circuit, 462, 463f, 464b
Leptomeningeal fibrosis, 1370, 1370f
LES. *See* Lower esophageal sphincter (LES).
Lesch-Nyhan syndrome, 1311
genetic basis for, 153
Leser-Trélat sign, 1237
Lesion-protected areas, in atherosclerosis, 522
LET (linear energy transfer), 437
Lethal factor (LF), of anthrax, 375, 376f
Lethal midline granuloma, 686, 784
Letterer-Siwe syndrome, 701–702
Leukemia
acute lymphoblastic, 670–673, 671t, 672f
clinical features of, 671t, 672–673
genetic and other markers of, 500t, 671t, 672
immunophenotype of, 672
morphology of, 670–672, 672f
oncogenes in, 314t
prognosis for, 673
progression of polycythemia vera to, 699–700
acute myelogenous, 666, 691, 692–695
chromosomal abnormalities in, 693
classification of, 692, 693t
clinical features of, 693–694
immunophenotype of, 693
morphology of, 692, 694f
oncogenes in, 314t
pathophysiology of, 692
prognosis for, 694–695
progression of myelodysplastic syndromes to, 695–696
acute promyelocytic, 692, 694f
adult T-cell, 671t, 685
chronic lymphocytic, 673–674, 673f, 674f
chronic myelogenous, 697–698, 697f, 698f
chromosomal translocation and oncogenes for, 298t, 314–315, 314t
defined, 667
Down syndrome and, 176
hairy cell, 671t, 683, 684f
immunohistochemistry of, 337
infections with, 361
lymphocytic
chronic, 673–674, 673f, 674f
large granular, 671t, 685–686
lymphoma *vs.,* 667–668

Leukemia *(Continued)*
monocytic
acute, 694f
oral manifestations of, 778t
oral manifestations of, 778t
plasma cell, 680
Leukemia cutis, 694
Leukemoid reactions, 84, 665
Leukocyte(s)
in hemostatic plugs, 127
in inflammation
activation of, 57–59, 58f
adhesion and transmigration of, 53, 53f, 54–56, 54t, 55b, 56f, 57f
chemotaxis of, 53f, 56–57
emigration and accumulation of, 49, 50, 50f, 53–57, 53f
extravasation of, 53–59
lysosomal constituents of, 73, 73f
margination of, 53
rolling of, 53, 53f
Leukocyte adhesion deficiency type 1 (LAD1), 56, 61, 62t
Leukocyte adhesion deficiency type 2 (LAD2), 56, 61, 62t
Leukocyte adhesion molecules, 54–56, 54t, 55b, 56f, 57
Leukocyte function, defects in, 61–62, 62t
Leukocyte function-associated antigen-1 (LFA-1), 55b
Leukocyte products, release of, 61
Leukocyte-dependent injury, in inflammation, 51f, 52
Leukocyte-induced tissue injury, 61, 61t
Leukocytoclastic vasculitis, 537t, 539f, 540–541
Leukocytosis, 663–665, 664f, 664t, 665f
due to blood loss, 624
in inflammation, 84–85
Leukodystrophy(ies), 1382, 1397–1398
adreno-, 1398
metachromatic, 161t, 1397–1398, 1398f
Leukoencephalitis, acute hemorrhagic, of Weston Hurst, 1385
Leukoencephalopathy
cerebral autosomal-dominant arteriopathy with subcortical infarcts and, 1363
progressive multifocal, 1376–1377, 1377f
Leukoerythroblastosis, 701
Leukoerythroplakia, speckled, 779
Leukomalacia, periventricular, 1356, 1356f
Leukopenia, 84–85, 662–663
Leukoplakia, 1242
of oral cavity, 778–780, 779f
hairy, 777–778
of vulva, 1065–1066, 1066f
Leukotriene(s)
in asthma, 726
in immediate hypersensitivity, 208, 208f
in inflammation, 68, 69, 69f, 70f
Leukotriene A_4 (LTA_4), 69f, 70f
Leukotriene B_4 (LTB_4), 69, 69f, 70f, 74t
Leukotriene C_4 (LTC_4), 69, 69f, 70f, 74t
Leukotriene D_4 (LTD_4), 69, 69f, 74t
Leukotriene E_4 (LTE_4), 69, 69f, 74t
Lewis, Thomas, 49
Lewy bodies
dementia with, 1393
in Parkinson disease, 1351, 1391–1392, 1392f
Leydig cell tumors
ovarian, 1103–1104
testicular, 1046
LF (lethal factor), of anthrax, 375, 376f
LFA-1 (leukocyte function-associated antigen-1), 55b
LGA (large for gestational age), 476
L&H (lymphohistiocytic variants), 687, 687f
LH (luteinizing hormone)-producing adenomas, 1162
LHON (Leber hereditary optic neuropathy), 185, 185f, 1342, 1445
LHRH (luteinizing hormone—releasing hormone) agonists, for prostate cancer, 1056
Libman-Sacks endocarditis, 133, 234, 234f, 597f, 598–599
Lice, 1268, 1269f
Lichen planopilaris, 1258
Lichen planus, 1258, 1258f
oral manifestations of, 778t
Lichen sclerosus, of vulva, 1065–1066, 1066f
Lichen simplex chronicus, of vulva, 1066, 1066f
Lichenification, 1230
Liddle syndrome, 528, 529f
Lifestyle factors, and atherosclerosis, 521
Li-Fraumeni syndrome, 285, 302
Ligand(s), 97
Light-chain deposition disease, glomerular lesions in, 993, 1006
Lightning marks, 446
Limb girdle muscular dystrophies, 1338, 1339t
Limbic encephalitis, paraneoplastic, 1410, 1411t
Limbus, 1424f, 1425
Limit dextrin, 165
Limiting plate, 878
Lindane, 435
Linear energy transfer (LET), 437
Lines of Zahn, 133
Lingual thyroid, 1164–1165
Linitis plastica, 824f, 825, 827
Linkage analysis, 189–191, 190f
Linoleic acid, 68
Lipid(s)
in atherosclerosis, 523, 525f
intracellular accumulation of, 35–37, 36f, 37f
Lipid A, 140
Lipid breakdown products, defects in membrane permeability due to, 18
Lipid droplets, in heart, 36
Lipid myopathies, 1341
Lipid peroxidation, of membranes, 16, 17f
Lipiduria, in nephrotic syndrome, 978–979
Lipoblasts, 1318, 1318f
Lipochrome, 39, 40f, 42
Lipodystrophy, partial, 985
Lipofuscin, 39, 40f, 42
as neuronal inclusion, 1351
Lipofuscin pigment granules, 10, 32–33, 32f
Lipogranuloma, of eyelid, 1424
Lipoid nephrosis, 975t, 981–982, 981f, 982f
Lipoma(s), 1317
cardiac, 614
gastric, 827
gastrointestinal, 869
paratesticular, 1040
pedunculated, of esophagus, 806
subcutaneous, 332
Lipophilic toxicants, metabolism of, 417–418, 418f
Lipophosphoglycan, 404
Lipopolysaccharide(s) (LPS)
and toll-like receptors, 195b
bacterial, 358
in septic shock, 140–141, 141f, 142f
Lipopolysaccharide-binding protein (LBP), 195b
Lipoprotein(s), in atherosclerosis, 523, 525f
Lipoprotein Lp(a), and atherosclerosis, 521
Liposarcoma, 1318, 1318f
"Lipostat," 462
Lipoteichoic acids, 358
Lipotoxicity, 1196
Lipoxin(s), in inflammation, 68, 69–70, 69f, 70f
Lipoxin A_4 (LXA_4), 69, 69f
Lipoxin B_4 (LXB_4), 69, 69f
Lipoxygenase(s), 68, 69, 69f
5-Lipoxygenase (5-LO), 69
Lipoxygenase inhibitors, 70
Liquefactive necrosis, after infarction, 138
Lisch nodules, 1413
in neurofibromatosis, 169
Lissencephaly, 1354
Listeria monocytogenes, 358, 375
meningitis due to, 1369
Listeriosis, 375
Liver, 877–927. *See also under* Hepatic.
amyloidosis of, 263
apoptosis of, 880
degeneration of, 880
ballooning, 880, 898, 900f
feathery, 880
effects of shock on, 142
fatty, 904, 904f
clinical features of, 907
due to carbon tetrachloride poisoning, 25, 25f, 26f
in cystic fibrosis, 493
in hepatitis, 899
in kwashiorkor, 448
in Wilson disease, 911
mechanisms of, 36, 36f, 906
morphology of, 905, 905f
nonalcoholic, 907–908
of pregnancy, 920
fibrosis of, 880–881
in cystic fibrosis, 493, 495
in infectious mononucleosis, 370
in malnutrition, 449
in right-sided heart failure, 563
in syphilis, 391, 391f
in toxemia of pregnancy, 1109
inflammation of, 880
intracellular accumulation in, 880
lobes of, 878
lobules of, 878
metastasis to, 280–281, 280f
necrosis of, 880
in Wilson disease, 911
normal structure of, 878, 879f
nutmeg, 122, 123f, 918, 918f
of preterm infant, 479
passive congestion of, 918
sarcoidosis of, 738
segments of, 878
zones of, 879f
Liver abscess(es), 902
amebic, 839
Liver allografts, nonimmunologic damage to, 921
Liver cancer, hepatitis B virus and, 327
Liver cell adenomas, 922–923, 922f
Liver disease
alcoholic, 422t, 423, 423f, 904–907, 904f–906f
α_1-antitrypsin deficiency as, 911–912, 912f
bacterial infections as, 902
cholestasis as, 888–890, 889f, 890t
neonatal, 912–913, 912t
circulatory, 917–920, 917f–919f
cirrhosis as. *See* Cirrhosis.
clinical consequences of, 881t
diffuse, anemia due to, 649
drug- and toxin-induced, 903–907, 903t
epidemiology of, 880
general features of, 879–890
helminthic infections as, 902
hemochromatosis as, 908–910, 908t, 909f, 910f
hepatitis as. *See* Hepatitis.
jaundice as, 885–888, 886f, 887t, 888f, 888t
laboratory evaluation of, 881t

Liver disease *(Continued)*
metabolic, 907–913
neoplastic, 922–927, 922f, 923f, 925f–927f
parasitic infections as, 902
polycystic, 915–916, 916f, 964
portal hypertension as, 883–885, 885f
pregnancy-associated, 920–921, 920f
Wilson disease as, 910–911
Liver infarct, 917, 917f
Liver regeneration, 101–103, 101f, 102f, 880
after fulminant hepatitis, 901
Liver stem cells, 93–94, 93f
Liver toxicity, after bone marrow transplantation, 921
Liver transplantation, 221
rejection of, 921
Liver tumors. *See also* Hepatocellular carcinoma (HCC).
oral contraceptives and, 427
LKB1 gene, and breast cancer, 1134
LKB1/STK11 gene, in pancreatic cancer, 950, 950t
L-MYC oncogene, 295t, 298, 315
5-LO (5-lipoxygenase), 69
Lobar atrophy, 1390
Lobar hemorrhages, 1376
Lobular carcinoma in situ (LCIS), 1123t, 1130t, 1141–1142, 1142f
Lobular hyperplasia, atypical, 1129, 1130f
Localized nodular tenosynovitis, 1315
Lockjaw, 393
Loeffler endomyocarditis, 607
Long-acting thyroid stimulator (LATS), 1172
Lordosis, due to rickets, 455
Loss of function mutations, 150–151
Loss of heterozygosity (LOH), 299
in breast carcinoma, 1135
Low-density lipoprotein (LDL)
in atherosclerosis, 521, 523, 525f
in familial hypercholesterolemia, 156–158, 157f, 158f
Low-density lipoprotein (LDL) receptor, 157, 157f–159f, 158
Low-density lipoprotein (LDL) receptor—related protein 5, 1275
Lower esophageal sphincter (LES)
achalasia of, 800–801, 801f
anatomy and physiology of, 798, 799
diverticula of, 802
in hiatal hernia, 801f, 802
Lower extremities, gangrene of, in diabetes, 1200
LPS. *See* Lipopolysaccharide(s) (LPS).
LSD (lysergic acid diethylamide), 426
L-selectin, 55b
LT (heat-labile) toxin, 834
LTA_4 (leukotriene A_4), 69f, 70f
LTB_4 (leukotriene B_4), 69, 69f, 70f, 74t
LTC_4 (leukotriene C_4), 69, 69f, 70f, 74t
LTD_4 (leukotriene D_4), 69, 69f, 74t
LTE_4 (leukotriene E_4), 69, 69f, 74t
Ludwig angina, 778t
Luetic aneurysms, 532
Luetic aortitis, 532
Lumbar lordosis, due to rickets, 455
Luminal tubule obstruction, 994
Lung(s), 711–770. *See also under* Pulmonary; Respiratory.
atelectasis of, 713–714, 714f
congenital anomalies of, 713
farmer's, 739
humidifier or air-conditioner, 739
in cystic fibrosis, 493, 493f, 494, 495
in left-sided heart failure, 562–563
in syphilis, 391
in systemic lupus erythematosus, 234
in systemic sclerosis, 239
Lung(s) *(Continued)*
normal anatomy and physiology of, 712–713, 712f
of preterm infants, 478, 479f, 481–483, 481f, 482f
pigeon breeder's, 739
radiation effect on, 440
shock, 142. *See also* Acute respiratory distress syndrome (ARDS).
zygomycosis of, 401
Lung abscess, 747t, 753, 753f
due to pneumonia, 750
primary cryptogenic, 753
pyemic, 753, 753f
staphylococcal, 373, 373f
Lung carcinoma, 757–764
adeno-, 759, 760–762, 761f, 762f, 769f
asbestosis and, 736
bronchioloalveolar, 760, 761–762, 762f
cigarette smoking and, 419–420, 419t, 421t
classification of, 759, 759t
clinical course of, 763, 763t
combined, 762
epidemiology of, 757
etiology and pathogenesis of, 757–759
extension of, 760
large cell, 759, 761f, 762
metastatic, 760
molecular genetics of, 758–759
morphology of, 759–762, 759f–762f
non—small cell, 758, 759
paraneoplastic syndromes with, 763–764
precursor lesions for, 759
secondary pathology due to, 762
silicosis and, 735
small cell, 758, 759, 761f, 762
Cushing syndrome due to, 1209
squamous cell, 759–760, 759f–761f
staging of, 762–763, 763t
Lung disease. *See* Pulmonary disease(s).
Lung injury, acute, 714–716, 714t, 715f, 715t, 717f
Lung surfactant, in innate immunity, 194–196
Lung transplantation, 221, 756–757, 757f
Lung tumor(s), 757–766
carcinoid, 764–765, 764f
carcinomas as. *See* Lung carcinoma.
hamartoma as, 765
inflammatory myofibroblastic, 765
metastatic, 765–766, 766f
miscellaneous, 765, 765t
neuroendocrine, 764–765, 764f
Lunula, 558
Lupus anticoagulant(s), 229
Lupus anticoagulant syndrome, 132
Lupus erythematosus
discoid, 1258–1259, 1259f
chronic, 235
drug-induced, 229t, 235
subacute cutaneous, 235
systemic, 223, 227–235
clinical and pathologic manifestations of, 230–234, 231f–234f, 231t
clinical course of, 234–235
clinical presentation of, 227, 228t
diagnostic criteria for, 227, 228t
endocarditis of, 133, 234, 234f, 597f, 598–599
epidemiology of, 227
etiology and pathogenesis of, 227–230, 229t, 230f
morphology of, 230–234, 231f–234f, 231t
pulmonary involvement in, 731
vasculitis in, 542, 542f
Lupus erythematosus (LE) bodies, 230
Lupus nephritis, 990
Lupus nephritis *(Continued)*
membranous, 231–232
mesangial, 231
proliferative
diffuse, 231, 232f
focal, 231, 231f
Lupus profundus, 1259
Luteal cysts, 1092
Luteal phase, inadequate, dysfunctional uterine bleeding due to, 1082
Luteinizing hormone (LH)-producing adenomas, 1162
Luteinizing hormone—releasing hormone (LHRH) agonists, for prostate cancer, 1056
Luteoma, pregnancy, 1104
LVI (lymphovascular invasion), in breast carcinoma, 1148
LXA_4 (lipoxin A_4), 69, 69f
LXB_4 (lipoxin B_4), 69, 69f
Lyell's disease, 373
Lyme arthritis, 393, 1310
Lyme disease, 392–393
epidemiology of, 392
erythema chronicum migrans due to, 392, 1268
immune evasion by, 359–360
morphology of, 350f, 393
myocarditis in, 608
neuroborreliosis due to, 1362
pathogenesis of, 392–393
transmission of, 392, 392f
Lymph node(s), 196, 197f
in infectious mononucleosis, 370
in sarcoidosis, 738
in Sjögren syndrome, 236–237
normal anatomy and pathology of, 662
sentinel, 280
Lymph node metastases, of breast cancer, 1146–1147
Lymphadenitis, 84
acute, 545
due to tuberculosis, 386
nonspecific
acute, 665
chronic, 665–666, 666f
reactive (inflammatory), 84
Lymphangiectasis, in infants and children, 498, 499
Lymphangioma(s)
capillary, 547
cavernous, 547
in infants and children, 498–499
Lymphangioma circumscriptum, 547
Lymphangiosarcoma, 550–551
Lymphangitis, 84, 544–545
Lymphatic dissemination theory, of endometriosis, 1083, 1084f
Lymphatic filariasis, 409–410, 410f
Lymphatic obstruction, edema due to, 120t, 121–122
Lymphatic spread, 279–280, 280f
Lymphatic tumors, in infants and children, 498–499
Lymphatics, 513
in inflammation, 83–84
Lymphedema, 120t, 121–122, 545
heredofamilial congenital, 545
obstructive, 545
primary, 545
Lymphedema praecox, 545
Lymphocyte(s)
atypical, in infectious mononucleosis, 370, 370f
B. *See* B cells (B lymphocytes).
bare, 244
chemokines and, 202

Lymphocyte(s) *(Continued)*
cytokines and, 202
elimination of potentially harmful self-reactive, 26
in chronic inflammation, 81–82, 82f
in immune system, 194f, 196–199, 196f–199f
intraepithelial, in intestines, 829
large granular. *See* Natural killer (NK) cells.
T. *See* T cell(s) (T lymphocytes).
Lymphocytic colitis, 840–841
Lymphocytic gastritis, 816
Lymphocytic mastopathy, 1126
Lymphocytosis, 84, 664t
in infectious mononucleosis, 370
Lymphoepithelial cyst, 788–789
Lymphoepithelioma, 785, 785f
Lymphogranuloma venereum, 395
Lymphohistiocytic variants (L&H cells), 687, 687f
Lymphoid aggregates, in hepatitis, 899, 901f
Lymphoid differentiation, 620
Lymphoid hyperplasia, paracortical, 666
Lymphoid neoplasm(s), 666, 667–690
acute lymphoblastic leukemia/lymphoma as, 670–673, 671t, 672f
adult T-cell leukemia/lymphoma as, 671t, 685
amyloidosis as, 678
anaplastic large cell lymphoma as, 671t, 684–685, 685f
Burkitt lymphoma as, 671t, 677–678, 678f
chronic lymphocytic leukemia as, 673–674, 673f, 674f
definitions and classifications of, 667–670, 668t, 669f, 670t, 671t
diffuse large B-cell lymphoma as, 671t, 676–677, 676f, 677f
follicular lymphoma as, 671t, 674–676, 675f, 676f
hairy cell leukemia as, 671t, 683, 684f
heavy-chain disease as, 678
Hodgkin lymphoma as, 686–690
important principles relevant to, 668–669
large granular lymphocytic leukemia as, 671t, 685–686
lymphoplasmacytic lymphoma as, 681–682, 681f
mantle cell lymphoma as, 671t, 682–683, 682f
marginal zone lymphomas as, 671t, 683
monoclonal gammopathy of undetermined significance as, 679, 681
multiple myeloma as, 671t, 678, 679–681, 679f, 680f
mycosis fungoides as, 671t, 685
origin of, 669, 669f
pathogenesis of, 667
peripheral B-cell, 673–683
peripheral T-cell and NK-cell, 684–686, 684f, 685f
peripheral T-cell lymphoma, unspecified, as, 684, 684f
plasma cell, 668, 671t, 678–681, 679f, 680f
plasmacytoma as, 671t, 681
precursor B- and T-cell, 670–673, 671t, 672f
Sézary syndrome as, 671t, 685
sinonasal NK/T-cell lymphoma as, 686
small lymphocytic lymphoma as, 671t, 673–674, 673f, 674f
solitary myeloma as, 681
Waldenström macroglobulinemia as, 678
Lymphoid organogenesis, 82
Lymphoid tissue, 620
in intestines, 829
Lymphoma(s)
acute lymphoblastic, 670–673, 671t, 672f
progression of polycythemia vera to, 699–700

Lymphoma(s) *(Continued)*
AIDS-related, 257–258, 326
anaplastic large cell, 671t, 684–685, 685f
B-cell
AIDS-related, 257–258, 327
diffuse large, 671t, 676–677, 676f, 677f
immunodeficiency-associated large, 677
body cavity large cell, 677
Burkitt, 677–678
cell of origin of, 671t
chromosomal translocation and oncogenes for, 298t, 300t, 314, 671t, 677
clinical features of, 671t, 678
Epstein-Barr virus and, 326, 326f, 677–678
genetic and other markers of, 500t
immunophenotype of, 677
morphology of, 677, 678f
defined, 667
follicular, 671t, 674–676, 675f, 676f
oncogenes in, 314, 314t
gastric, 826, 826f
Helicobacter pylori and, 327–328
gastrointestinal, 868–869
Hodgkin, 686–690
classification of, 671t, 686, 688t
clinical course of, 690, 691t
etiology and pathogenesis of, 690, 691f
lymphocyte depletion type of, 688t, 689
lymphocyte predominance type of, 688t, 689–690, 689f
lymphocyte-rich type of, 688–689, 688t
mixed cellularity type of, 688, 688t, 689f
morphology of, 686–690
nodular sclerosis type of, 687–688, 688t, 689f
non-Hodgkin lymphoma *vs.*, 668, 686, 690, 691t
Reed-Sternberg cells in, 686–687, 687f, 690, 691f
spread of, 670
staging of, 687, 688t
immunohistochemistry of, 337
leukemia *vs.*, 667–668
lymphoblastic, 500t
acute, 670–673, 671t, 672f
lymphoplasmacytic, 681–682, 681f
MALT, 683, 826, 868–869
Helicobacter pylori and, 328, 826
morphology of, 826, 826f
pathogenesis of, 868–869
mantle cell, 671t, 682–683, 682f
oncogenes in, 314, 314t
marginal zone, 328, 671t, 683
Mediterranean, 869
non-Hodgkin, 668
Hodgkin lymphoma *vs.*, 668, 686, 690, 691t
of breast, 1151
of prostate, 1056
orbital, 1424
primary CNS, 1408
retinal, 1443
sinonasal NK/T-cell, 686
small lymphocytic, 671t, 673–674, 673f, 674f
T-cell
adult, 671t, 685
angioimmunoblastic, 671t
cutaneous, 1249–1250, 1250f
peripheral, unspecified, 684, 684f
sinonasal, 686
testicular, 1046
Lymphomatoid granulomatosis, 542
Lymphopenia, 662
Lymphoplasmacytic lymphoma, 681–682, 681f
Lymphoproliferative syndrome, X-linked, 331, 371

Lymphotoxin, 71, 202
in delayed type hypersensitivity, 217
Lymphotropic ß-group viruses, 365
Lymphovascular invasion (LVI), in breast carcinoma, 1148
Lyon hypothesis, 178
Lysergic acid diethylamide (LSD), 426
Lysosomal catabolism, 32–33, 32f
Lysosomal constituents, of leukocytes, in inflammation, 73, 73f
Lysosomal diseases, acquired or drug-induced (iatrogenic), 33
Lysosomal enzymes, 158–160, 159f
in phagocytosis, 61
Lysosomal membranes, injury to, 18–19
Lysosomal storage diseases, 33, 153, 158–165, 159f, 160f, 161t
Lysosomes, 10, 158
primary and secondary, 32–33, 32f
Lysozyme, in phagocytosis, 61
Lytic necrosis, of liver, 880

M

M (membranous) cells, 352, 829
M component, 678
M protein, 358, 373, 680, 680f, 681
MAC (*Mycobacterium avium-intracellulare* complex), 386, 387f
in AIDS, 256, 386, 387f, 1372
MacCallum's plaques, 593
Machado-Joseph disease, 184t
Macroadenomas, pituitary, 1159
Macroglobulinemia, Waldenström, 678
Macromastia, 1122
Macromolecules, bone disorders due to defects in folding and degradation of, 1281
Macroovalocytes, 638
Macrophage(s)
alveolar, 713
antitumor effect of, 331
in atherosclerosis, 523, 525f
in glomerulonephritis, 972
in HIV infection, 252
in immune system, 199
in inflammation, 53f, 57, 62, 76f, 79–81, 79f–82f
in scar formation, 110
in tuberculosis, 381
origin and differentiation of, 621f
smokers,' 740, 741
tingible-body, 665, 666f
Macrophage aggregates, in hepatitis, 899, 900f
Macrophage colony-stimulating factor (M-CSF), 621f
Macrophage inflammatory protein-1α (MIP-1α), 71, 209
Macrophage inflammatory protein-1ß (MIP-1ß), 209
Macropolymorphonuclear cells, 638
Macrovascular disease, in diabetes mellitus, 1197, 1200, 1200f
Macula, cherry-red spot in, 161, 1441, 1441f
Macular corneal dystrophy, 1429
Macular degeneration, age-related, 1422, 1441–1442, 1442f
atrophic *vs.* exudative, 1441
Macule, 1229
Mad cow disease, 346
MadCAM-1 (mucosal addressin cell adhesion molecule-1), 55b
Maffucci syndrome, 1296
MAGE (melanoma antigen) proteins, 329–330
MAGE-1, 331
Magnesium ammonium phosphate stones, 1014, 1014t

Major basic protein
in chronic inflammation, 82
in phagocytosis, 61
Major calyces, 956
Major histocompatibility complex (MHC) molecules
and disease association, 205, 205f
classes of, 203–204, 203f
in autoimmunity, 226
in diabetes, 1194
in systemic lupus erythematosus, 229
in transplant rejection, 218
natural killer cells and, 201
structure and function of, 203–204, 203f, 204f
T lymphocytes and, 196–197, 198, 198f, 204
viruses and, 360, 360f
Malabsorption, diarrhea due to, 832, 832t
Malabsorption syndromes, 842–846, 842t, 843f, 845f
Malacoplakia, 1027–1028, 1028f
Malar rash, in systemic lupus erythematosus, 228t
Malaria, 359, 401–403, 402f, 403f
malignant cerebral, 403, 403f
Malarial granulomas, 403
Malassezia furfur
in seborrheic dermatitis, 1257
tinea versicolor due to, 1268
Male breast, 1151–1152, 1152f
Male genital tract, 1034–1056
penis in, 1034–1037, 1035f–1037f
prostate in, 1047–1056
benign enlargement of, 1048–1050, 1049f
inflammations of, 1047–1048
normal anatomy of, 1047, 1047f
tumors of, 1050–1056, 1052f–1054f
testis and epididymis in, 1037–1047
congenital anomalies of, 1037–1038, 1038f
inflammations of, 1039–1040, 1039f
regressive changes of, 1038–1039
tumors of, 1040–1046, 1041t, 1042f–1045f
vascular disturbances of, 1040, 1040f
tunica vaginalis in, 1047
Male pseudohermaphroditism, 181
Malformation(s), 470, 471f
of central nervous system, 1353–1356, 1355f, 1356f
Malformation syndrome, 471f
Malignancy(ies)
hypercalcemia of, 333–334, 334t, 1184
neuropathies with, 1334–1335
of white cells, 666–702
etiology and pathogenesis of, 667
histiocytoses as, 667, 701–702, 702f
lymphoid, 666, 667–690, 668t, 669f, 670t
myeloid, 666–667, 690–701
Malignant arteriosclerosis, 1008
Malignant fibrous histiocytoma, 1301
Malignant hyperpyrexia, 1340
Malignant hypertension, 1007–1008, 1008f
Malignant hyperthermia, 1340
Malignant melanoma. *See* Melanoma(s).
Malignant mixed tumor, of salivary gland, 792
Malignant nephrosclerosis, 1007–1008, 1008f
Malignant peripheral nerve sheath tumor (MPNST), 1412–1413
Malignant transformation, essential alterations for, 289, 290f
Malignant vascular tumors, 545t, 550–551
Mallory bodies, 34, 34f, 423, 905, 905f
Mallory-Weiss tear, 801f, 802
Malnutrition
atrophy due to, 9
causes of, 447
in developing countries, 447
in United States, 447
Malnutrition *(Continued)*
primary, 447
protein-energy, 447–449, 448f, 449t
secondary or conditional, 447, 448–449, 449t
MALT (mucosa-associated lymphoid tissue), 328, 352
MALT (mucosa-associated lymphoid tissue) lymphoma (MALToma), 683, 826, 868–869
Helicobacter pylori and, 328, 826
morphology of, 826, 826f
pathogenesis of, 868–869
Mammalian Toll-like receptor protein 4, 140
Mammary duct ectasia, 1126, 1126f
Mammographic screening, 1123–1124, 1123t, 1124f, 1131
Mammosomatotroph adenomas, 1161
Manganese, 461t
Mannose receptor, 58f, 59, 60f
Mannose-binding lectin
in cystic fibrosis, 492
in innate immunity, 194
Mannosidosis, 161t
Mantle cell lymphoma, 671t, 682–683, 682f
oncogenes in, 314, 314t
Mantoux test, 381
Manufactured mineral fibers, as air pollutant, 430, 430t
MAP kinase, 99f
MAP kinase (mitogen-activated protein kinase), 98f, 99, 99f
MAP kinase kinase, 99f
MAP kinase kinase kinase, 99f
MAP2 (microtubule-associated protein 2), 1387
MAPCs (multipotent adult progenitor cells), 92–93
MAPK (mitogen-activated protein kinase) pathway, in insulin metabolism, 1192, 1193f
MAPKKs (mitogen-activated protein kinase kinases), in anthrax, 375–376
Marasmus, 448, 449, 449t
atrophy due to, 9
Marble bone disease, 1281–1282, 1282f, 1283f
Marburg form, of multiple sclerosis, 1385
Marchiafava-Bignami disease, 1385
Marfan syndrome, 154–155
aortic dissection in, 532–534, 533f, 534f
Marfanoid habitus, in MEN-2B, 1222
Marginal zone B cells, 662
Marginal zone B-cell hyperplasia, 666
Marginal zone lymphomas, 328, 671t, 683
Margination, of leukocytes, 53
Marie-Strümpell disease, 1309
Marijuana, 426
Marker chromosomes, 337
Marrow hyperplasia, in megaloblastic anemia, 639
Massive macronodular adrenocortical disease (MMAD), 1208
Massive necrosis, of liver, 880
Masson bodies, 732f
Mast cells
in immediate hypersensitivity, 206–207, 207f, 208f, 209, 209t
in inflammation, 62, 64f, 82
in skin, 1228f, 1229f
Mastectomy, bilateral prophylactic, 1133
Mastitis, 1125
granulomatous, 1126
periductal, 1125, 1125f
Mastocytosis, 1250–1251, 1251f
Mastopathy, lymphocytic, 1126
Masugi nephritis, 968, 969f
Maternal age, and Down syndrome, 176
Maternal factors, fetal growth restriction due to, 478
Maternal imprinting, 186
Maternal-fetal transmission, 355
Matricellular proteins, as regulators of angiogenesis, 109
Matrix metalloproteinases (MMPs)
in abdominal aortic aneurysm, 532
in angiogenesis, 109
in scar formation, 110–111, 110f
in tumor cell invasion, 312–313
membrane-bound, 111
Matrix vesicles, 41
Maturation, of nevus, 1232
Maturity-onset diabetes of the young (MODY), 1197
Mazzotti reaction, 411
MC4R (melanocortin 4 receptor), 463f, 464b
McArdle syndrome, 168t
McCune-Albright syndrome, 1300
MCH (melanin-concentrating hormone), 463f, 464b
MCHC (mean cell/corpuscular hemoglobin concentration), 623, 623t
in sickle cell disease, 629
MCKD1 gene, 966
MCKD2 gene, 966
MCP-1 (monocyte chemoattractant protein), 71
in atherosclerosis, 523
M-CSF (macrophage colony-stimulating factor), 621f
MD2, 195b
MDM2, in glioblastoma, 1403
MDMA, 426
MDS (myelodysplastic syndromes), 666, 691, 695–696, 696f
Mean cell hemoglobin, 623, 623t
Mean cell hemoglobin concentration (MCHC), 623, 623t
in sickle cell disease, 629
Mean cell volume, 623, 623t
Mean corpuscular hemoglobin concentration (MCHC), 623, 623t
in sickle cell disease, 629
Measles, 347t, 363–364, 364f
"black," 363
oral manifestations of, 778t
Measles inclusion body encephalitis, 363
Mechanical factors, and wound healing, 114
Mechanical force, trauma due to, 443–444, 443f, 444f
Mechanical triggers, for myocardial hypertrophy, 8
Meckel diverticulum, 830, 830f, 854
Meconium ileus, in cystic fibrosis, 493, 494
Media, of blood vessel, 512, 512f
Medial degeneration, in aortic dissection, 533, 534f
Median lobe hypertrophy, of prostate, 1049
Mediastinal fibrosis, due to radiation exposure, 440f
Mediastinal tumors, 765, 765t
Mediastinopericarditis, 612
adhesive, 612
Mediterranean fever, familial, 261
Mediterranean lymphoma, 869
Medullary carcinoma
of breast, 1145, 1145f
of thyroid gland, 1178, 1182–1183, 1182f
in MEN-2A, 1222
Medullary cystic disease, 965–966, 966f
adult-onset, 962t, 966
Medullary sponge kidney, 962t, 965
Medulloblastoma, 1407–1408
clinical features of, 1407
desmoplastic variant of, 1407
molecular genetics of, 500t, 1407
morphology of, 1406–1407, 1407f

Megacolon
congenital aganglionic, 830–831
toxic, 831, 849, 850f
Megakaryocytes, pawn ball, 695, 696f
Megalencephaly, 1354
Megalin, 970
Megaloblast(s), 638–639, 639f
Megaloblastic anemia, 638–643, 639f, 640t
Megaloblastoid maturation, in myelodysplastic syndromes, 695
Megalocornea, 1444
Megaloureter, 1024–1025
Megamitochondria, 33
Meibomian glands, 1424, 1424f
Meissner plexus, 830
MEK, 99f
Melanin, 39, 1228
Melanin pigment incontinence, 1231
Melanin-concentrating hormone (MCH), 463f, 464b
Melanocortin 4 receptor (MC4R), 463f, 464b
Melanocytes, 1228, 1228f
disorders of, 1230–1236, 1231f–1236f, 1233f
α-Melanocyte-stimulating hormone (α-MSH), 463f, 464b
Melanocytic nevus, 1232–1233, 1232f, 1233f, 1233t
Melanocytic tumors of uncertain malignant potential (MELTUMP), 1236
Melanoma(s), 272, 1234–1236, 1236f
acral lentiginous, 1232
clinical features of, 1234–1235, 1236f
conjunctival, 1426, 1427f
diagnostic criteria for, 1235–1236
dysplastic nevi and, 1233–1234, 1234f, 1235f
familial, 286, 1245t, 1246
glycolipids in, 330
growth patterns and morphology of, 1235, 1236f
heritable, 1233
molecular genetics of, 1245–1247
of eyelid, 1424
of vulva, 1070, 1070f
prognosis for, 1236
uveal, 1434, 1435f
Melanoma antigen (MAGE) proteins, 329–330
Melanoma-associated retinopathy, 1442
Melanosis, primary acquired, with atypia, of conjunctiva, 1426
Melanosis oculi, congenital, 1426
Melanotic pigmentation, of oral cavity, 778t
MELAS (mitochondrial encephalomyopathy with lactic acidosis and stroke-like episodes), 1342, 1399
Melasma, 1231–1232
MELTUMP (melanocytic tumors of uncertain malignant potential), 1236
Membrane inhibitor of reactive lysis, 66b
Membrane permeability, cell injury due to defects in, 14f, 18–19, 18f
Membrane-coating granules, 1251
Membranoproliferative glomerulonephritis (MPGN), 971, 975t, 984–985, 985f–987f
Membranous (M) cells, 352, 829
Membranous glomerulopathy, 975t, 979–981, 980f
Membranous nephropathy, 975t, 979–981, 980f
MEN syndrome. *See* Multiple endocrine neoplasia (MEN) syndrome.
Menarche, age at, and breast cancer, 1131–1132
Mendelian disorder(s), 149–169
adverse reactions to drugs due to, 154
alkaptonuria as, 167–168
alterations in structure, function, or quantity of nonenzyme proteins as, 154
autosomal dominant, 150–151, 151t
Mendelian disorder(s) *(Continued)*
autosomal recessive, 151, 151t
biochemical and molecular basis of, 152–154, 153t
defects in receptors and transport systems as, 154
due to defects in proteins that regulate cell growth, 168–169
due to defects in receptor proteins, 156–158, 157f, 158f
due to defects in structural proteins, 154–156, 156t
due to enzyme defects, 152–153, 153f, 158–168
Ehlers-Danlos syndromes as, 155–156, 156t
familial hypercholesterolemia as, 156–158, 157f–159f
Gaucher disease as, 163–165, 164f
glycogen storage diseases as, 165–167, 166f, 167f, 168t
lysosomal storage diseases as, 158–165, 159f, 160f, 161t
Marfan syndrome as, 154–155
mucopolysaccharidoses as, 165
neurofibromatosis, 168–169
Niemann-Pick disease as, 163, 163f
Tay-Sachs disease as, 148f, 160–161, 162f
transmission patterns of, 150–152, 151t, 152t
X-linked, 152, 152t
Ménétrier disease, 820, 821, 824
Meningioma(s), 1409–1410, 1409f
anaplastic (malignant), 1410
atypical, 1410
en plaque variant of, 1409
fibroblastic, 1409
microcystic, 1409
papillary, 1410
psammomatous, 1409
rhabdoid, 1410
secretory, 1409
syncytial, 1409
transitional, 1409
Meningitis
acute, 1369–1370, 1370f
aseptic (viral), 1370
pyogenic (bacterial), 1369–1370, 1370f
"chemical," 1370
cryptococcal, 1378, 1378f
drug-induced, 1370
due to HIV, 1375
due to listeriosis, 375
tuberculous, 383, 386, 1371–1372
viral, 1373f
Meningoencephalitis
chronic bacterial, 1371–1372
fungal, 1378, 1378f
HIV, 1375–1376, 1376f
Lyme disease, 350f
necrotizing amoebic, 1380, 1380f
viral, 1372–1377, 1373f–1377f
Meningomyelocele, 1354
Menopausal changes, in endometrium, 1082–1083
Menopause, osteoporosis after, 1283f, 1284
Menstrual cycle, 1082
anovulatory, 1081–1082, 1082f
breast changes during, 1121, 1121f
endometrium in, 1080–1081, 1080f, 1081f
Mental retardation
due to trisomy 21 (Down syndrome), 175–176
in Angelman syndrome, 186
in fragile-X syndrome, 182
in Prader-Willi syndrome, 186
Meratoja syndrome, 1429
Mercuric chloride poisoning, 25
Mercury
exposure to, 432t
metabolism of, 418–419, 421f
Merkel cell(s), 1228f, 1229
Merkel cell carcinoma, 1244
Merlin, 305
Merosin, 1337f
Merozoites, 401, 402f
MERRF (myoclonic epilepsy with ragged red fibers), 1342, 1399
Mesangial cells, 957f, 958–959
in glomerulonephritis, 972
Mesangial matrix, of glomerulus, 957f, 958–959
Mesangial sclerosis, in diabetic nephropathy, 991, 992f
Mescaline, 426
Mesenchymal tumors, 869–870
of bladder, 1033
of prostate, 1056
Mesenteric cysts, 873
Mesial temporal herniation, 1353–1354, 1354f
Mesonephric duct, 1060, 1061f
Mesothelioma(s), 873
asbestosis and, 736
benign, 768
malignant, 768–770, 768f, 769f
of fallopian tubes, 1091
peritoneal, 769
Metabolic acidosis, renal osteodystrophy due to, 1288
Metabolic disease(s)
hereditary neuropathies with, 1332, 1333t
of nervous system
genetic, 1397–1399, 1398f
toxic and acquired, 1399–1401, 1400f
Metabolic disturbances, neurologic sequelae of, 1400
Metabolic effects, of obesity, 465t
Metabolic ketoacidosis, 1202
Metabolic liver disease, 907–913
α_1-antitrypsin deficiency as, 911–912, 912f
hemochromatosis as, 908–910, 908t, 909f, 910f
neonatal cholestasis as, 912–913, 912t
nonalcoholic fatty liver and steatohepatitis as, 907–908
Wilson disease as, 910–911
Metabolic neuropathies, acquired, 1334–1335, 1334f
Metabolic pathways, bone disorders due to defects in, 1281–1282, 1282f, 1283f
Metabolic status, and wound healing, 114
Metabolism, inborn errors of, 487–489, 487t, 488f, 489f
myopathies associated with, 1341–1342, 1341f
thyroid, 1168
Metachromasia, 1398
Metachromatic granules, 207
Metachromatic leukodystrophy, 161t, 1397–1398, 1398f
Metal(s), occupational and environmental exposure to, 432–434, 432t, 433f
Metalloproteinase(s), matrix. *See* Matrix metalloproteinase(s) (MMPs).
Metalloproteinase-domain family, 111
Metaphyseal chondrodysplasia, Schmid, 1280t
Metaphyseal chondroplasia, Jansen, 1280t
Metaplasia, 5, 10–11
Barrett, 10, 10f
columnar to squamous, 10, 10f
connective tissue, 11
defined, 10
in cervicovaginal smear, 336f
intestinal, 815
mechanisms of, 11
squamous to columnar, 10, 10f

Metaplastic carcinoma, of breast, 1146
Metaplastic lesions, of bladder, 1028
Metaplastic theory, of endometriosis, 1083
Metastasis(es), 279–281, 280f, 281t
  adrenal, Addison disease due to, 1216
  determining site of origin of, 337
    cardiac, 614–615
  hepatic, 927, 927f
  malignant transformation and, 289
  molecular mechanisms of, 309–310, 311f, 313
  of breast carcinoma, 280f, 1146–1147
  of hepatocellular carcinoma, 925–926
  of lung carcinoma, 760
  of neuroblastoma, 502
  of prostate cancer, 1051–1052, 1052f
  osteolytic, 1184
  pathways of spread of, 279–281
  skeletal, 1302–1303
  to breast, 1151
  to central nervous system, 1410
  to liver, 280f
  to lung, 765–766, 766f
  to orbit, 1424
  to ovaries, 1104
  to stomach, 827
  to uvea, 1433
Metastasis signature, 310, 311f
Metastatic cascade, 309, 311f
Metazoa, 406–411
Metchnikoff, Elie, 49
Methanol toxicity, 424
  neurologic effects of, 1400
Methotrexate toxicity, 1400–1401
Methyl isocyanate, 429
1-Methyl-4-phenyl-1,2,3,6-tetrahydropyridine (MPTP), parkinsonism due to, 1392, 1393
Methylcobalamin, 641, 641f
Methylene chloride, 431
Methylmalonic acid, 641
Methylmercury, exposure to, 419
N^5-Methyltetrahydrofolic acid (N^5-methyl FH_4), 641, 641f
MGUS (monoclonal gammopathy of undetermined significance), 679, 681
MHATP (microhemagglutination assay for *T. pallidum* antibodies), 390
MHC molecules. *See* Major histocompatibility complex (MHC) molecules.
MI. *See* Myocardial infarction (MI).
Mice, knockout, 91
Michaelis-Gutmann bodies, 1027, 1028f
Microabscesses
  Munro, 1257
  Pautrier, 1250
Microadenoma(s)
  ACTH-producing, 1208
  pancreatic, in MEN-1, 1222
  pituitary, 1159
Microalbuminuria, in diabetes, 991, 992, 1205
Microaneurysms, Charcot-Bouchard, 1366
Microangiopathic hemolytic anemia, 638, 638f
Microangiopathy(ies)
  diabetic, 1197, 1200–1201, 1201f
  intraretinal, 1439, 1440f
  thrombotic, 652–653, 1009–1011, 1010f
Microarray technologies, 1136b–1137b
Microbes
  immune evasion by, 359–360, 359t, 360f
  release from body of, 354f, 355
  spread and dissemination of, 354–355, 354f
Microbial carcinogenesis, 321t, 322, 324–328, 325f, 326f
Microbicidal activity, defects in, 62
Microencephaly, 1354
Microglia, 1349, 1350
Microglial nodules, 1350
ß₂-Microglobulin, 203, 203f
  in amyloidosis, 260
Microhemagglutination assay for *T. pallidum* antibodies (MHATP), 390
Microorganisms, mechanism of disease caused by, 356–359, 357f
Microsatellite(s), 307
Microsatellite instability, 307
  in colorectal cancer, 864
Microscopic polyangiitis, 537t, 539f, 540–541
Microscopic polyarteritis, 537t, 539f, 540–541
  glomerular lesions in, 993
Microtubule(s), abnormalities of, 34
Microtubule-associated protein 2 (MAP2), 1387
Microvascular disease
  in diabetes mellitus, 1197, 1200–1201, 1201f
  in systemic sclerosis, 237
Microvilli, intestinal, 829
Microwaves, exposure to, 436t
Midline malignant reticulosis, 686
Midzonal necrosis, of liver, 880
Migratory thrombophlebitis, 135, 334t, 335, 544
  in pancreatic cancer, 951
Mikulicz syndrome, 236
Milk of calcium, 1127
Milkline remnants, 1122
Miller-Dieker syndrome, 1354
Milroy disease, 545
Mineral deficiencies, 459–461, 461t
Mineral homeostasis, bone disorders due to abnormal, 1287–1288, 1287f
Mineral oil, 431
Mineralocorticoids, 1207
Minimal change disease, 975t, 981–982, 981f, 982f
Minimal residue disease, 337–338
Minor calyces, 956
MIP-1α (macrophage inflammatory protein-1α), 71, 209
MIP-1ß (macrophage inflammatory protein-1ß), 209
Misfolded proteins
  endoplasmic reticulum stress due to, 38
  in amyloidosis, 262
Mismatch errors, 306
Missense mutations, 148
Mitochondrial alterations, in cell injury, 20, 20f, 33, 33f
Mitochondrial damage, cell injury due to, 14f, 15, 15f
Mitochondrial diabetes, 1197
Mitochondrial DNA (mtDNA), 185, 185f
Mitochondrial dysfunction, 18
Mitochondrial encephalomyopathy(ies), 1397, 1398–1399
Mitochondrial encephalomyopathy with lactic acidosis and stroke-like episodes (MELAS), 1342, 1398–1399
Mitochondrial genes, mutations in, 185, 185f
Mitochondrial myopathies, 33, 1341–1342, 1341f
Mitochondrial permeability transition (MPT), 15, 15f, 24, 30f
Mitogen-activated protein kinase (MAP kinase), 98f, 99, 99f
Mitogen-activated protein kinase kinases (MAPKKs), in anthrax, 375–376
Mitogen-activated protein kinase (MAPK) pathway, in insulin metabolism, 1192, 1193f
Mitogillin, 400
Mitosis(es), in malignant tumors, 274, 275f
Mitotic figures, in malignant tumors, 274, 275, 275f
Mitral annular calcification, 590f, 591
Mitral apparatus, 558
Mitral insufficiency, 589
  due to mitral valve prolapse, 592
Mitral regurgitation, 589t
Mitral stenosis, 589, 589t
  due to rheumatic heart disease, 593, 594f
  thrombus formation in, 131
Mitral valve, 558
  infective endocarditis of, 597f
  myxomatous degeneration of, 591–592, 592f
Mitral valve disease, 589t
Mitral valve lesions, in Marfan syndrome, 155
Mitral valve prolapse, 591–592, 592f
  in polycystic kidney disease, 964
Mixed chimerism, 221
Mixed connective tissue disease, 239
Mixed tumors, 271
  of salivary gland, 271, 271f, 791–792, 792f
  of skin, 1238, 1239f
  of testes, 1045
MKK4 gene, in pancreatic cancer, 950, 950t
ML (mucolipidoses), 161t
MLH1 gene, 287t, 307, 315
MLL gene, 315
MMAD (massive macronodular adrenocortical disease), 1208
MMPs. *See* Matrix metalloproteinases (MMPs).
MODY (maturity-onset diabetes of the young), 1197
Molds, 399–401, 400f, 401f
Mole(s), 1232–1233, 1232f, 1233f, 1233t
  BK, 1233–1234, 1234f, 1245–1246
  hydatidiform, 1110–1112, 1110t, 1111f, 1112f
  invasive, 1112, 1112f
Molecular basis, of human disease, 146–147, 147f
Molecular diagnosis, 187–191, 188f–190f
  of cancer, 337–338
Molecular mimicry, 227
Molecular portrait, 1136b
Molecular profiles, of cancer cells, 315, 316b, 317f
Molluscum contagiosum, 1266–1267, 1267f
Mönckeberg medial calcific sclerosis, 516
Monoblasts, in acute myelogenous leukemia, 692
Monoclonal gammopathy of undetermined significance (MGUS), 679, 681
Monoclonality, of tumors, 288, 288f
Monocyte(s)
  in atherosclerosis, 523
  in glomerulonephritis, 971–972
  in HIV infection, 252
  in inflammation, 57f
  origin and differentiation of, 621f
Monocyte chemoattractant protein (MCP-1), 71
  in atherosclerosis, 523
Monocytoid B cells, 666
Monocytosis, 664t
Mononeuropathy, 1334
Mononeuropathy multiplex, 1334
Mononuclear cell infiltration, in chronic inflammation, 79–81, 79f–81f, 362, 362f
Mononuclear phagocyte system, 79–80, 79f
Mononuclear variants, 686, 687f
Mononucleosis
  cytomegalovirus, 367
  infectious, 326, 369–371, 369f, 370f
    oral manifestations of, 778t
Monosodium urate crystals, in gout, 1311–1313, 1312f
Monosomy, 173
Monostotic fibrous dysplasia, 1300
Montezuma's revenge, 832
Montgomery tubercles, 1121
Moraxella catarrhalis, pneumonia due to, 748
Morgagnian cataract, 1431
Morphologic changes, 4
Morton neuroma, 1335

Mosaic pattern, of lamellar bone, 1285–1286, 1285f
Mosaicism, 173
confined placental, 477, 478f
gonadal, 187
Motor dysfunction, of esophagus, 800–802, 801f, 802f
Motor neuron(s), degenerative diseases affecting, 1396–1397, 1396f
Motor neuron disease, 1396–1397, 1396f
infantile, 1336, 1336f
Motor neuron disease inclusion dementia, 1391
Motor unit(s)
general reactions of, 1328–1330, 1329f, 1330f
normal and abnormal, 1326, 1326f
Mott cells, 405, 680
MPDs (myeloproliferative disorders), chronic, 666–667, 691, 696–701
MPGN (membranoproliferative glomerulonephritis), 971, 975t, 984–985, 985f–987f
MPNST (malignant peripheral nerve sheath tumor), 1412–1413
MPO (myeloperoxidase)
deficiency in, 62t
in phagocytosis, 60f, 61
MPS (mucopolysaccharidoses), 161t, 165, 1281
MPT (mitochondrial permeability transition), 15, 15f, 24, 30f
MPTP (1-methyl-4-phenyl-1,2,3,6-tetrahydropyridine), parkinsonism due to, 1392, 1393
MPZ (myelin protein zero), 1326
mRNA arrays, 1136b–1137b
MRP (multidrug resistance associated protein), in neuroblastoma, 504
MS. *See* Multiple sclerosis (MS).
MSA (multiple system atrophy), 1391, 1393
aggregated proteins in, 1351t
α-MSH (α-melanocyte-stimulating hormone), 463f, 464b
MSH2 gene, 287t, 307
MSH6 gene, 287t
in colorectal cancer, 864
mtDNA (mitochondrial DNA), 185, 185f
MUC-1, 330
Mucicarmine stain, 361t
Mucin(s), in carcinogenesis, 330
Mucin-like glycoproteins, 54, 54t
Mucinous carcinoma, of breast, 1145–1146, 1145f
Mucinous cystadenocarcinoma, of appendix, 872, 872f
Mucinous cystadenoma, of appendix, 871, 872
Mucinous cystic neoplasms, of pancreas, 947, 948f
Mucinous tumors, of ovaries, 1097, 1097f, 1098f
Mucocele
of appendix, 871, 872
of salivary gland, 790, 791f
of sinus, 784
Mucocutaneous lymph node syndrome, 537t, 540
Mucoepidermoid carcinoma
of conjunctiva, 1426
of salivary gland, 793, 794f
Mucolipidoses (ML), 161t
Mucopolysaccharidoses (MPS), 161t, 1651281
Mucor, 400
meningoencephalitis due to, 1378
Mucormycosis, 400–401, 401f
rhinocerebral, 401
Mucosa-associated lymphoid tissue (MALT), 328, 352
Mucosa-associated lymphoid tissue (MALT) lymphoma, 683, 826, 868–869
Mucosa-associated lymphoid tissue (MALT) lymphoma *(Continued)*
Helicobacter pylori and, 328, 826
morphology of, 826, 826f
pathogenesis of, 868–869
Mucosal addressin cell adhesion molecule-1 (MadCAM-1), 55b
Mucosal dendritic cells, in HIV infection, 252–253
Mucosal infarction, of bowel, 852f, 853, 853f
Mucous cells, of stomach, 810
Mucous neck cells, 810
Mucous plugs, in asthma, 726
Mucoviscidosis. *See* Cystic fibrosis.
Mucus secretion, by gastric mucosa, 811
Muir-Torre syndrome, cutaneous manifestations of, 1245t
Müllerian duct, 1060, 1061f
Müllerian epithelial tumors, 1093t, 1094–1099, 1094f–1099f
Müllerian inhibitory substance, 1037, 1060
Müllerian tubercle, 1060, 1061f
Multicystic encephalopathy, 1356
Multidrug resistance associated protein (MRP), in neuroblastoma, 504
Multifactorial causes, of congenital anomalies, 473t, 474
Multifactorial genetic disorders, 149, 169–170, 170t, 472
Multi-infarct dementia, 1369, 1391
Multilocular cysts, 407
Multinucleate polykaryons, in herpes simplex virus infections, 777
Multiorgan system failure, 140–141
Multiple chemical sensitivity syndrome, 430
Multiple endocrine neoplasia (MEN) syndrome, 1221–1223, 1222t
Multiple endocrine neoplasia type 1 (MEN-1), 1221–1222, 1222t
genetic basis for, 285, 287t
hyperparathyroidism in, 1185, 1221
with pituitary adenoma, 1159
Multiple endocrine neoplasia type 1 *(MEN1)* gene, 1222
Multiple endocrine neoplasia type 2 (MEN-2), 1222–1223, 1222t
genetic basis for, 285
thyroid carcinoma in, 1178, 1182.1183
with hyperparathyroidism, 1185
Multiple endocrine neoplasia type 2A (MEN-2A), 1222, 1222t
pheochromocytomas in, 1219, 1219t, 1222
Multiple endocrine neoplasia type 2B (MEN-2B), 1222–1223, 1222t
pheochromocytomas in, 1219, 1219t
Multiple epiphyseal dysplasia, 1280t
Multiple hamartoma syndrome, 1134
Multiple hereditary exostosis, 1296
Multiple mononeuropathy, 1334
Multiple myeloma, 679–681
amyloidosis with, 261
cell of origin in, 671t
clinical features of, 671t, 678, 680, 680f
diagnosis of, 681
etiology and pathogenesis of, 679
genetic basis of, 671t
morphology of, 679–680, 679f
prognosis for, 681
renal involvement in, 993, 1005–1006, 1005t, 1006f
Multiple sclerosis (MS), 1382–1385
clinical features of, 1384
morphology of, 1383–1384, 1383f, 1384f
pathogenesis of, 1382–1383
T cell—mediated hypersensitivity in, 215t
variants of, 1384–1385
Multiple sulfatase deficiency, 161t
Multiple system atrophy (MSA), 1391, 1393
aggregated proteins in, 1351t
Multipotent adult progenitor cells (MAPCs), 92–93
Mumps, 347t, 364
testicular involvement in, 1039
Mumps encephalitis, 364
Mumps orchitis, 364
Mumps parotitis, 364
Munro microabscesses, 1257
Mural infarction, of bowel, 852f, 853
Mural thrombus(i), 133, 133f
after myocardial infarction, 585f, 586
Murmurs, 589
Muscle(s)
hypertrophy of, 7
reinnervation of, 1326f, 1328, 1330
Muscle fiber(s), 1327–1328, 1328f, 1328t, 1329f
atrophy of, 1329–1330
hypertrophy of, 1330
reactions of, 1330
regeneration of, 1330
Muscle fiber splitting, 1330
Muscle involvement, in sarcoidosis, 738
Muscle spindles, 1328
Muscle tumors
skeletal, 1321–1322, 1321f, 1322f
smooth, 1322
Muscular atrophy
progressive, 1397
spinal, 1336, 1336f, 1397
Muscular dystrophy(ies), 1336–1339
autosomal, 1338, 1338t, 1339t
congenital, 1338t
Emery-Dreifuss, 1338t
facioscapulohumeral, 1338t
limb girdle, 1338, 1339t
myotonic, 1338–1339
oculopharyngeal, 1338t
X-linked (Duchenne and Becker), 1336–1338, 1337f
Musculoskeletal effects, of obesity, 465t
Musculoskeletal system, in systemic sclerosis, 238
Mutated genes, products of, 328
Mutations, 147–149, 148f, 149f
chromosome. *See* Cytogenetic disorder(s).
due to radiation exposure, 439
frameshift, 147, 148f, 149
full, 183, 189f
gain of function, 151
gene, 147
genome, 147
in cancer-causing genes, 289, 290f
in mitochondrial genes, 185, 185f
in ß-thalassemia, 632–633, 632f
loss of function, 150–151
missense, 148
nonsense, 148
point, 147, 148, 148f, 149f
pre-, 183, 189f
trinucleotide repeat, 149, 181–184, 182f
triplet-repeat, 149, 181–184, 182f
Mutator phenotype, 318
Myasthenia gravis, 212t, 1344
paraneoplastic, 334, 334t
MYB gene, in pancreatic cancer, 950, 950t
MYBP-C (myosin-binding protein C) gene, in hypertrophic cardiomyopathy, 605f, 606
MYC oncogene, 298, 306, 317
in pituitary adenoma, 1159
Mycobacterial infections, 349t, 381–388
immune response to, 359

Mycobacterium avium-intracellulare complex (MAC), 386, 387f
in AIDS, 256, 386, 387f, 1372
Mycobacterium leprae, 387, 1331
granulomatous inflammation due to, 83t
Mycobacterium tuberculosis, 381
and host defenses, 353, 358
granulomatous inflammation due to, 83t
immune response to, 359
in AIDS, 256, 384, 1372
in primary pulmonary tuberculosis, 382f
Mycologic infection(s), 397–401
agents for, 346t, 351
aspergillosis as, 399–400, 400f
candidiasis as, 397–399, 398f
cryptococcosis as, 399, 399f
due to molds, 399–401, 400f, 401f
due to yeasts, 397–399, 398f, 399f
of gastrointestinal tract, 353
of oral cavity, 777
of skin, 1267–1268, 1268f
zygomycosis as, 400–401, 401f
Mycoplasma(s), 346t, 349, 350–351
sexually transmitted, 356t
Mycoplasma infection, of female genital tract, 1064
Mycoplasma pneumoniae, 350–351, 353
pneumonia due to, 751
Mycosis fungoides, 671t, 685, 1249–1250, 1250f
Mycosis fungoides d'emblée, 1249
Mycotic aneurysm, 134, 531, 542
Mycotic infections, of female genital tract, 1063
Mycotoxins, 435, 435t
MyD88, 195b
Myelin basic protein, 1326
Myelin figures, 12f, 21, 23
Myelin ovoids, 1329
Myelin protein zero (MPZ), 1326
Myelin sheath, 1326
Myelinated nerve fibers, 1326–1327, 1327f
Myelinolysis, central pontine, 1385
Myelitis, transverse, 441
Myeloblast(s)
in acute myelogenous leukemia, 692, 694f
in myelodysplastic syndromes, 695
Myeloblastomas, 694
Myelodysplastic syndromes (MDS), 666, 691, 695–696, 696f
Myelofibrosis, 699, 700–701, 701f
Myeloid neoplasm(s), 666–667, 690–701
acute myelogenous leukemia as, 666, 691, 692–695, 693t, 694f
chronic myelogenous leukemia as, 697–698, 697f, 698f
chronic myeloproliferative disorders as, 666–667, 691, 696–701
essential thrombocytosis as, 700, 700f
myelodysplastic syndromes as, 666, 691, 695–696, 696f
polycythemia vera as, 699–700, 699f
primary myelofibrosis as, 700–701, 701f
Myeloid tissue, 620
Myelolipomas, adrenal, 1218
Myeloma
multiple (plasma cell). *See* Multiple myeloma.
solitary, 678, 681
Myeloma kidney, 680
Myelomeningocele, 1354
Myelopathy
angiodysgenetic necrotizing, 1368
vacuolar, in AIDS, 1376
Myeloperoxidase (MPO)
deficiency in, 62t
in phagocytosis, 60f, 61
Myelophthisic anemia, 648–649
Myeloproliferative disorders (MPDs), chronic, 666–667, 691, 696–701
Myelotoxins, 647, 647t
Myenteric plexus, 830
Myocardial disease
due to Adriamycin and other drugs, 609–610
due to amyloidosis, 610
due to catecholamines, 610
due to hyperthyroidism and hypothyroidism, 610–611
due to iron overload, 610
Myocardial fibrosis, in systemic sclerosis, 239
Myocardial hypertrophy, 7–9, 8f
Myocardial infarct, 578f, 579, 579f
expansion of, 585f, 586
extension of, 581, 586
healing of, 580–581, 580f
reperfusion of, 581–582, 583f
Myocardial infarction (MI), 575–586
and atherosclerosis, 521
atherosclerotic plaque rupture in, 573, 573f
clinical features of, 582–584
consequences and complications of, 584–586, 585f
coronary artery pathology in, 575t
defined, 572, 575
diet and, 466
in diabetes, 1200
incidence and risk factors for, 576
infarct modification by reperfusion in, 581–582, 583f
morphology of, 577–581, 579f, 579t, 580f, 582f
pathogenesis of, 576–577, 577f, 577t, 578f
prognosis after, 586
reversible *vs.* irreversible changes in, 577, 579t, 582f
silent, 582
temporal sequence of, 579–581, 579t, 580f, 582f
thrombus formation in, 131
transmural *vs.* subendocardial, 575–576, 575t
Myocardial irritability, after myocardial infarction, 584
Myocardial ischemia. *See* Ischemic heart disease (IHD).
Myocardial necrosis, 580, 580f, 581, 583f
with contraction bands, 581
Myocardial rupture, 584–585, 585f
Myocardial stunning, 581, 582, 583f
Myocarditis, 601, 608–609
clinical features of, 609
dilated cardiomyopathy due to, 603
diphtheritic, 608
etiology and pathogenesis of, 608, 608t
giant cell, 608–609, 609f
hypersensitivity, 608, 609f
in AIDS, 608
in systemic lupus erythematosus, 233
lymphocytic, 609f
morphology of, 608–609
of Chagas disease, 405–406, 608, 609, 609f
rheumatic, 594–595
Myocardium, 556–557, 556f
aging effect on, 559, 559t
ischemic necrosis of, 21f
Myocilin, 1431
Myoclonic epilepsy with ragged red fibers (MERRF), 1342, 1399
Myocytes, 1327–1328, 1328f, 1328t, 1329f
cardiac, 556–557, 556f
Myocytolysis, 580
Myofibrils, 1327, 1328f
Myofibroblast(s), 1319
in healing by second intention, 113
Myofibroblastic tumor, inflammatory, of lung, 765
Myofibromatoses, in infants and children, 499
Myofilaments, 1327
Myoglobinuria, exertional, 1342
Myometrium, 1079
tumors of, 1089–1090, 1090f, 1091f
Myonecrosis, in clostridial gas gangrene, 394
Myopathic forms, of glycogen storage disease, 167, 168t
Myopathy(ies), 1326f, 1328
AIDS-associated, 1376
associated with inborn errors of metabolism, 1341–1342, 1341f
congenital, 1340–1341, 1340f, 1340t
drug-induced, 1344
ethanol, 1344
infantile X-linked cardioskeletal, 1342
inflammatory, 229t, 239, 1342–1343, 1342f
ion channel, 1339–1340
lipid, 1341
mitochondrial, 1341–1342, 1341f
myotubular (centronuclear), 1340t
nemaline, 1340f, 1340t
steroid, 1344
thyroid, 1166
thyrotoxic, 1343–1344
toxic, 1343–1344
Myopericarditis, 611
Myophagocytosis, 1330
Myopia, 1426
Myosin-binding protein C *(MYBP-C)* gene, in hypertrophic cardiomyopathy, 605f, 606
Myositis
inclusion body, 1343
orbital, 1423
proliferative, 1318
Myositis ossificans, 11, 1319, 1319f
Myotilin, 1339t
Myotonia, 1338
Myotonic dystrophy, 184t, 1338–1339
Myotubular myopathy, 1340t
Myxedema, 1168–1169
pretibial, 1172, 1173
Myxedema heart, 611
Myxoma, cardiac, 613–614, 613f
Myxomatous degeneration, of mitral valve, 591–592, 592f

N

NAATs (nucleic acid amplification tests), 361t
NAD (nicotinamide adenine dinucleotide), 458
NADP (nicotinamide adenine dinucleotide phosphate), 458
NADPH (nicotinamide adenine dinucleotide phosphate)—cytochrome P-450 reductase, 418, 420f
NADPH (nicotinamide adenine dinucleotide phosphate) oxidase, in phagocytosis, 60–61, 60f
Naegleria fowleri, 351t
Naegleria spp, necrotizing amoebic encephalitis due to, 1379, 1379f
NAFL (nonalcoholic fatty liver disease), 907–908
Nailfold capillary loops, in systemic sclerosis, 237
Nail-patella syndrome, 1280t
NAIP (neuronal apoptosis inhibitory protein) gene, 1336
Na^+K^+-ATPase, ouabain-sensitive, reduced activity of, 15
ß-Naphthylamine, 322
2-Naphthylamine, metabolism of, 420f, 421f
Napkin-ring constrictions, of bowel, 865, 865f
Narcotics, abuse of, 424t, 426

NARP (neuropathy, ataxia, and retinitis pigmentosa), 1399
Nasal inflammations, 783–784, 783f
Nasal polyps, 783, 783f
Nasal tumors, 784–785, 785f
NASH (nonalcoholic steatohepatitis), 907–908
Nasopharyngeal angiofibroma, 784
Nasopharyngeal carcinoma, 785, 785f
  Epstein-Barr virus and, 326–327
Nasopharynx, 784
National Ambient Air Quality Standards, 428, 428t
Natriuretic factors, in blood pressure regulation, 528
Natural killer (NK) cells
  antitumor effect of, 330–331
  in immune system, 194, 194f, 201–202, 201f
  origin and differentiation of, 621f
Natural toxins, 435–436, 435t
Naxos syndrome, 604
NBCCS (nevoid basal cell carcinoma syndrome), 1244–1245, 1245t, 1246f
NBTE (nonbacterial thrombotic endocarditis), 597f, 598, 599f
NEC (necrotizing enterocolitis), 483, 483f, 840
Necator duodenale, 838
Neck, 788–790, 789f
Neck webbing, in Turner syndrome, 179
Necrolysis, toxic epidermal, 373
Necrosis, 5, 11, 11f
  acute tubular, 993–996, 994f, 995f
  and inflammation, 74
  avascular, 1289–1290, 1289t, 1290f
  caseous, 21, 22, 22f
  defined, 21
  diffuse cortical, 1011–1012, 1012f
  examples of, 23–26, 24f–26f
  fat, 21, 22, 23f
  features of, 13t
  fibrinoid, 214, 214f
    in malignant hypertension, 1007, 1008, 1008f
  gangrenous, 22
  in anaplastic tumors, 275
  intracellular accumulation of cholesterol due to, 37
  ischemic, 21f
    coagulative, 21–22, 21f, 22f
      due to infarction, 138
      of liver, 880
  liquefactive, 21, 22, 22f
    after infarction, 138
  morphologic changes in, 12f, 21–22, 21f–23f
  of liver, 880
    in hepatitis, 899, 900f
  papillary, 1004, 1004t
    in acute pyelonephritis, 998, 999f, 1000
    in analgesic nephropathy, 1003, 1003f.1004t
    in sickle cell disease nephropathy, 1011
  segmental, 1330
  ultrastructural changes in, 13f
Necrotizing amoebic meningoencephalitis, 1380, 1380f
Necrotizing arteriolitis, 530
Necrotizing encephalopathy, subacute, 1398
Necrotizing enterocolitis (NEC), 483, 483f, 840
Necrotizing lesions, of nose and upper airways, 784
nef gene, in human immunodeficiency virus, 247, 247f
Negri body, 1351
Neisseria, immune evasion by, 360
Neisseria gonorrhoeae, 350f, 356t, 377–378
  of female genital tract, 1063t
  pili of, 358, 377–378, 378f
  transmission of, 355
Neisseria meningitidis, 377, 378
  meningitis due to, 1369
Neisserial infections, 377–378
Nelson syndrome, 1162
Nemaline myopathy, 1340f, 1340t
Nematodes, enterocolitis due to, 838–839
Neointima, 515, 515f, 553
Neonatal cholestasis, 912–913, 912t
Neonatal jaundice, 887
Neonatal respiratory distress syndrome, 481–483, 481f, 482f
Neonate. *See* Newborn.
Neoplasia, 269–339. *See also* Cancer; Tumor(s).
  defined, 270
Neoplasm(s). *See also* Cancer; Tumor(s).
  defined, 270
  of conjunctiva, 1425–1426, 1427f
  of eyelid, 1424–1425, 1425f
  of orbit, 1424
  of thyroid gland, 1175–1183
  of uvea, 1433–1434, 1435f
  retinal, 1442–1443, 1443f
  salivary gland, 790–795, 791t
  splenic, 705
Neoplastic heart disease, 613–615, 613f, 614t
Neoplastic proliferations, of white cells, 666–702
  etiology and pathogenesis of, 667
  histiocytoses as, 667, 701–702, 702f
  lymphoid, 666, 667–690, 668t, 669f, 670t
  myeloid, 666–667, 690–701
Neovascular membrane
  in age-related macular degeneration, 1441–1442, 1442f
  in diabetic retinopathy, 1439, 1440f
Neovascularization, 96, 107–109, 108f, 109t
  retinal, 1439, 1440f
Nephrin, 981, 983
Nephritic syndrome, acute, 960, 967t
Nephritis
  anti-GBM antibody—induced (Masugi, nephrotoxic), 968, 969f, 976–977
  circulating immune complex, 970, 971f
  hereditary, 988–989, 988f
  Heymann, 968–970, 969f
  lupus, 990
    membranous, 231–232
    mesangial, 231
    proliferative
      diffuse, 231, 232f
      focal, 231, 231f
  tubulointerstitial, 236, 996–1004
    acute, 996
    causes of, 996t
    chronic, 996
    drug- and toxin-induced, 1002–1004, 1002f, 1003f, 1004t
    in multiple melanoma, 1005–1006, 1005t, 1006f
    nephrocalcinosis as, 1005
    pyelonephritis as, 994–1002
      acute, 998–1000, 998f, 999f
      and urinary tract infection, 996–998, 997f, 998f
      chronic, 1000–1002, 1001f
    secondary, 996
  urate nephropathy as, 1004–1005, 1005f
Nephrocalcinosis, hypercalcemia and, 1005
Nephrogenic adenoma, 1028
Nephrogenic metaplasia, 1028
Nephrogenic rests, 505
Nephrolithiasis, 1014–1015
  cause and pathogenesis of, 1014–1015, 1014t
  clinical manifestations of, 960, 1015
  hyperuricosuric calcium, 1014
  in hyperparathyroidism, 1186, 1187
Nephrolithiasis *(Continued)*
  in hyperuricemia, 1005
  morphology of, 1015, 1015f
Nephronophthisis, familial juvenile, 962t, 966
Nephronophthisis—medullary cystic disease complex, 965–966, 966f
Nephropathy
  analgesic, 428, 1003–1004, 1003f, 1004t
  cast, 1005, 1006, 1006f
  Chinese herbs, 1004
  diabetic, 990–992
    clinical features of, 992, 1204–1205
    epidemiology of, 990–991
    morphology of, 991–992, 991f, 992f, 1201, 1201f, 1202f
    pathogenesis of, 991
  gouty, 1313
  HIV-associated, 984
  IgA, 975t, 986–988, 987f, 990
  in Denys-Drash syndrome, 504
  membranous, 975t, 979–981, 980f
  NSAID-associated, 1004
  polyoma virus, 1000, 1000f
  reflux, 1000, 1001f
  sickle cell disease, 1011
  urate, 1004–1005, 1005f
Nephrosclerosis
  accelerated, 1007–1008
  benign, 1006–1007, 1007f
  in diabetes, 1201, 1202f
  malignant, 1007–1008, 1008f
Nephrosis, lipoid, 975t, 981–982, 981f, 982f
Nephrotic syndrome, 960, 978–979
  causes of, 979, 979t
  edema due to, 121, 122
  manifestations of, 967t, 978
  paraneoplastic, 334t
  pathophysiology of, 978–979
Nephrotoxic nephritis, 968, 969f
NER (nucleotide excision repair), 307
NER pathway, 323
Nerve fiber(s), 1326
  myelinated and unmyelinated, 1326, 1327f
Nerve regeneration, 1330
Nerve—cerebrospinal fluid (CSF) barrier, 1327
Nervous system
  alcohol effect on, 422t, 423
  central. *See* Central nervous system (CNS).
  occupational exposures and, 431t
  peripheral. *See* Peripheral nervous system.
Nervous system tropism, 1372
Nesidioblastosis, 1206
Nestin, 94
Neural crest abnormalities, cardiac defects related to, 565, 566f
Neural end organs, in skin, 1228–1229
Neural precursor cells, 94
Neural stem cells, 94
Neural tube defects, 1353–1354
Neuritic plaques, 1386–1387, 1386f
Neuritis
  optic, 1445–1446
    in multiple sclerosis, 1384
  retrobulbar, in multiple sclerosis, 1384
Neuroblastic tumors, 500–504, 501f, 502f, 503t, 504f
Neuroblastoma(s), 500–504
  cerebral, 1406
  clinical course and prognostic features of, 502–504, 503t, 504f
  diagnostic features of, 500t
  genetic markers for, 500t
  morphology of, 501–502, 501f
  of adrenal medulla, 1221
  olfactory, 785
  staging of, 502

Neuroborreliosis, 1372
Neurocytoma, central, 1406
Neurodegenerative disorders, 1385–1397
  affecting cerebral cortex, 1386–1391, 1386f–1388f, 1389t
  affecting motor neurons, 1396–1397, 1396f
  aggregated proteins in, 1351, 1351t
  characteristics of, 1385–1386
  of basal ganglia and brain stem, 1391–1394, 1392f, 1393f
  spinocerebellar, 1394–1395, 1395t
Neuroendocrine carcinoma, of cervix, 1078f
Neuroendocrine cell tumors, gastric, 827
Neuroendocrine proliferations and tumors, of lung, 764–765, 764f
Neuroepithelial tumor, dysembryoplastic, 1406
Neurofibrillary tangles, 34, 1351, 1387, 1387f
Neurofibroma(s), 169, 1412
  cutaneous, 169, 1412
  plexiform, 169, 1412
  solitary, 1412
  subcutaneous, 169
Neurofibromatosis(es), 168–169
  cutaneous manifestations of, 1245t
Neurofibromatosis type 1 (NF1), 305, 1413
Neurofibromatosis type 1 (*NF-1*) gene, 169, 287t, 296, 300t, 305, 1413
Neurofibromatosis type 2 (NF2), 305, 1413
Neurofibromatosis type 2 (*NF-2*) gene, 169, 287t, 300t, 305, 1413
  in schwannoma, 1411
Neurofibromin, 1413
Neurogenesis, 94
Neurogenic shock, 139
Neurogenin 3 (Ngn3), 1189
Neurohumoral mechanisms, in shock, 141
Neurohypophysis, 1158
  syndromes of, 1163–1164
Neurokinin A, 74
Neurologic disorder, in systemic lupus erythematosus, 228t
Neurologic effects, of obesity, 465t
Neurologic sequelae, of metabolic disturbances, 1400
Neuroma(s)
  acoustic, 1411
  amputation, 1335
  in MEN-2B, 1222
  Morton, 1335
  pseudo-, 1335
  traumatic, 1335
Neuromuscular junction, diseases of, 1344–1345
Neuromyelitis optica, 1384–1385
Neuromyopathic neoplastic syndromes, 334–335, 334t
Neuron(s), 1348–1349
  ballooned, 1390
  reactions to injury of, 1350–1352
  red, 1350
  regeneration of, 91, 94
  subacute and chronic, 1350–1351
Neuronal apoptosis inhibitory protein *(NAIP)* gene, 1336
Neuronal degeneration, 1350–1351
  transsynaptic, 1350–1351
Neuronal heterotopias, 1355
Neuronal inclusions, 1351, 1351t
Neuronal injury, acute, 1350
Neuronal nitric oxide synthase (nNOS), 72
Neuronal storage diseases, 1397
Neuronal tumors, 1406
Neuronopathy, 1329
Neuronophagia, 1350, 1373
Neuron-specific enolase, as tumor marker, 339t
Neuropathic beriberi, 1334
Neuropathy, ataxia, and retinitis pigmentosa (NARP), 1399
Neuropathy(ies), 1330–1335
  acquired metabolic and toxic, 1334–1335, 1334f
  AIDS-associated peripheral, 1376
  compression, 1335
  diabetic, 1201, 1205, 1334, 1334f
  entrapment, 1335
  hereditary, 1332–1334, 1332t, 1333t
    motor and sensory, 1332–1334
    sensory and autonomic, 1332
  hypertrophic, 1333
  immune-mediated, 1331
  infectious, 1331–1332
  inflammatory, 1330–1331
  optic, 1445
    anterior ischemic, 1443, 1444f
      nonarteritic, 1443
    Leber hereditary, 185, 185f, 1342, 1445
  paraneoplastic, 1335
    subacute sensory, 1410, 1411t
  traumatic, 1335
  uremic, 1334
  with malignancy, 1334–1335
Neuropeptide(s), in inflammation, 74
Neuropeptide Y (NPY), 463f, 464b
Neuropil, 501
Neuropil threads, 1387
Neurosecretory granules, in skin, 1228f
Neurosyphilis, 389, 391, 1372
  meningovascular, 1372
  paretic, 1372
Neurotoxins, bacterial, 359
Neurotrophic factor receptors, oncogene for, 295t
Neurotrophic tyrosine kinase receptor 1 *(NTRK1)* gene, in thyroid carcinoma, 1177, 1178
Neutral proteases, 73
Neutropenia, 662–663
Neutropenic colitis, 841
Neutrophil(s)
  in glomerulonephritis, 971–972
  in inflammation, 56, 57f
  in megaloblastic anemia, 638, 639f
  reactive changes in, 665, 665f
Neutrophil elastase, 73
Neutrophil emigration, in inflammation, 49, 50f
Neutrophil granules, 73, 73f
Neutrophilia, 84
Neutrophilic leukocytosis, 664f, 664t
Neutrophilic reaction, in alcoholic hepatitis, 905
Nevocellular nevus, 1233f
Nevoid basal cell carcinoma syndrome (NBCCS), 1244–1245, 1245t, 1246f
Nevus(i)
  basal cell, 1244–1245, 1245t, 1246f
  blue, 1233t
  compound, 1232, 1233f
  congenital, 1233t
  conjunctival, 1426, 1427f
  dysplastic, 1233–1234, 1233t, 1234f, 1245–1246
  halo, 1233t
  inflamed juvenile, 1426
  intradermal, 1232
  junctional, 1232
  melanocytic (pigmented), 1232–1233, 1232f, 1233f, 1233t
  nevocellular, 1233f
  spindle and epithelioid cell (Spitz), 1233t
  uveal, 1434
Nevus flammeus, 547
Nevus of Ota, 1426
Newborn
  evaluation of, 479, 479t
  hemolytic disease of, 887
NF1 (neurofibromatosis type 1), 305, 1412–1413
NF-1 (neurofibromatosis type 1) gene, 169, 287t, 296, 300t, 305, 1413
NF2 (neurofibromatosis type 2), 305, 1413
NF-2 (neurofibromatosis type 2) gene, 169, 287t, 300t, 305, 1413
  in schwannoma, 1411
NF-$_F$B. *See* Nuclear factor $_F$B (NF-$_F$B).
Ngn3 (neurogenin 3), 1189
NGU (nongonococcal urethritis), 394–395
NHL (non-Hodgkin lymphoma), 668. *See also* Lymphoma(s).
  Hodgkin lymphoma *vs.*, 668, 686, 690, 691t
Niacin, 450t, 458, 458f
Niches, stem-cell, 92, 93f
Nickel, exposure to, 432t, 434
Nickel compounds, cancer due to, 285t
Nicotinamide, 458
Nicotinamide adenine dinucleotide (NAD), 458
Nicotinamide adenine dinucleotide phosphate (NADP), 458
Nicotinamide adenine dinucleotide phosphate (NADPH)—cytochrome P-450 reductase, 418, 420f
Nicotinamide adenine dinucleotide phosphate (NADPH) oxidase, in phagocytosis, 60–61, 60f
Nicotine
  abuse of, 424t
  exposure to, 419
  metabolism of, 420f
Nicotinic acid, 458
Niemann-Pick disease, 161t, 163, 163f
  cherry-red spot in, 1441
  type C, 37
Night sweats, in tuberculosis, 384
Nipple(s)
  Paget disease of, 1140, 1141f
  supernumerary, 1122
Nipple discharge, 1123, 1124f
Nipple inversion, congenital, 1122
Nitric oxide (NO), 16
  in inflammation, 60f, 61, 72–73, 72f, 74t
  in septic shock, 142f
  in sickle cell disease, 630
  in tuberculosis, 382
  inhibition of platelet aggregation by, 126, 127f
Nitric oxide synthase (NOS), 72
Nitrogen dioxide, as air pollutant, 428t–430t, 429, 430
Nitrosamines, as carcinogens, 322
NK cells. *See* Natural killer (NK) cells.
NKG2D receptors, 201
NK-T cells, 197
NK/T-cell lymphoma, sinonasal, 686
NKX2.5, in congenital heart disease, 565
NM23 gene, 313
N-MYC oncogene, 295t, 298, 299f, 315
  in neuroblastoma, 503, 503t, 504, 504f
nNOS (neuronal nitric oxide synthase), 72
NO. *See* Nitric oxide (NO).
Nocardia, 376, 377f
Nocardia asteroides, 376, 377f
Nocardia brasiliensis, 376
NOD2 gene, in Crohn disease, 846
Nodes of Ranvier, 1326
Nodular fasciitis, 1318, 1318f
Nodular glomerulosclerosis, 991–992
  in diabetes, 1201
Nodular hyperplasias, of liver, 922, 922f
Nodule(s), 1229
  Lisch, 1413
  microglial, 1350

Nodule(s) *(Continued)*
of Arantius, 558
solitary thyroid, 1175
vocal cord (singers'), 786
Nonalcoholic fatty liver disease (NAFL), 907–908
Nonalcoholic steatohepatitis (NASH), 907–908
Nonbacterial thrombotic endocarditis (NBTE), 597f, 598, 599f
Noncaseating granulomas, in Crohn disease, 848, 848f
Noncomedo ductal carcinoma in situ, 1140, 1140f, 1141f
Nondisjunction, 173
Nondividing tissues, 90f, 91
Nonenzyme proteins, alterations in structure, function, or quantity of, 154
Nongonococcal urethritis (NGU), 394–395
Nongranular cells, 959
Nonheme iron, 644, 645f
Nonhemorrhagic infarction, 1364f, 1365, 1365f
Non-Hodgkin lymphoma (NHL), 668. *See also* Lymphoma(s).
Hodgkin lymphoma *vs.*, 668, 686, 690, 691t
Nonionizing radiation, 436, 436t, 442
Nonossifying fibroma, 1299, 1300f
Nonproliferative breast changes, 1127, 1127f, 1130t
Nonseminomatous germ cell tumors (NSGCT), 1041, 1045
Nonsense mutation, 148
Non—small cell carcinoma, of lung, 758, 759
Nonspecific interstitial pneumonia (NSIP), 731
Nonsteroidal anti-inflammatory drugs (NSAIDs), 70
and colon cancer, 865
bleeding disorders related to, 653
intestinal injury due to, 841
nephropathy associated with, 1004
peptic ulcer disease due to, 818
Nonstreptococcal acute glomerulonephritis, 976
Nonthrombocytopenic purpuras, 650
Nontreponemal antibody tests, 390
Norepinephrine, 1218
Normocytes, in hemolytic anemia, 625, 625f
North Asia tick typhus, 396t
Norwalk agent, 347t
Norwalk virus, gastroenteritis due to, 833, 833t
NOS (nitric oxide synthase), 72
Nose
inflammations of, 783–784, 783f
tumors of, 784–785, 785f
Noxious stimuli, cellular responses to, 4–5, 5f, 5t
NPH1 gene, 966
NPH2 gene, 966
NPH3 gene, 966
NPHS1 gene, 983–984
NPHS2 gene, 984
NPY (neuropeptide Y), 463f, 464b
NPY/AgRP neurons, 463f, 464b
NRAMP1 gene, 381, 382f
N-RAS oncogene, 295t, 296
in thyroid carcinoma, 1177
NSAIDs. *See* Nonsteroidal anti-inflammatory drugs (NSAIDs).
NSGCT (nonseminomatous germ cell tumors), 1041, 1045
NSIP (nonspecific interstitial pneumonia), 731
NTRK1 (neurotrophic tyrosine kinase receptor 1) gene, in thyroid carcinoma, 1177, 1178
Nuclear alterations, in cell injury, 20, 20f
Nuclear budding abnormalities, in myelodysplastic syndromes, 695
Nuclear changes, in necrosis, 21
Nuclear factor $_{\kappa}$B (NF-$_{\kappa}$B)
in acute respiratory distress syndrome, 716
in human immunodeficiency virus, 250
in immunity, 194, 195b
receptor activator for, 1184, 1275, 1276f
Nuclear factor $_{\kappa}$B (NF-$_{\kappa}$B) ligand, receptor activator for, 1184, 1275, 1276f
in rheumatoid arthritis, 1307
Nuclear morphology, abnormal, 274, 275f
Nuclear proteins, bone disorders due to defects in, 1279
Nuclear regulatory proteins, oncogene for, 295t
Nuclear sclerosis, of lens, 1431
Nucleic acid amplification tests (NAATs), 361t
Nucleolar pattern, 228
Nucleotide excision repair (NER), 307
Nucleotide repeats, unstable, 183–184, 184f, 184t, 185f
Nucleus(i), 1349
Null cell adenomas, 1162
Nutmeg liver, 122, 123f, 918, 918f
Nutrition. *See also* Diet.
and disease, 446–466
and wound healing, 114
Nutritional deficiency(ies), 447–461
causes of, 447
due to anorexia nervosa and bulimia, 449
in developing nations, 447
in primary malnutrition, 447
in secondary or conditional malnutrition, 447, 448–449, 449t
in United States, 447
of minerals, 459–461, 461t
of vitamins, 450–459, 450t
protein-energy malnutrition as, 447–449, 448f, 449t
Nutritional imbalances, cell injury due to, 13–14

O

O ring sign, 1297
O_2^-. *See* Superoxide anion radical (O_2^-).
OB gene, 464b
Obesity, 461–465
and cancer, 284, 465, 465t
breast, 1132
and diabetes, 1195–1196, 1196f, 1202, 1204
and insulin resistance, 1195–1196, 1196f
central or visceral, 462
epidemiology of, 461
etiology of, 462, 463f, 464b
genetic basis for, 464b
measurement of, 461–462, 462t
medical complications of, 462–465, 465t
Obligate intracellular bacteria, 394–397, 395f, 396t, 397f
Obliterative endarteritis, due to tuberculosis, 1371
Obliterative fibrous pleuritis, due to tuberculosis, 386
Obliterative hepatocavopathy, 919
Obstructive congenital heart defects, 567, 570–571, 571f
Obstructive overinflation, 721
Obstructive uropathy
of bladder, 1033–1034, 1033f
of kidney, 960, 1012–1014, 1013f
papillary necrosis in, 998, 1004t
Obturator palsy, 1334
Obtuse marginals, 557
Occupational asthma, 726
Occupational cancer, 283, 285t
Occupational diseases
epidemiology of, 416, 416t
prevention of, 416–417
recognition of, 416–417, 416t
Occupational hazard(s)
agricultural, 434–435, 434t
industrial, 430–434, 431t, 432t, 433f
mechanisms of toxicity of, 417–419, 417f, 418f, 420f–421f
regulatory agencies for, 416
Occupational Safety and Health Administration, 416
Ochronosis, 39, 167–168
Ocular changes, in Marfan syndrome, 154–155
Ocular cicatricial pemphigoid, 1425
Oculopharyngeal muscular dystrophy, 1338t
Odland bodies, 1251
Odontogenic cysts, 782, 782t
Odontogenic keratocyst (OKC), 782
Odontogenic tumors, 782, 782t
Odontoma, 782
OGTT (oral glucose tolerance test), 1190
OH (hydroxyl ions)
in cell injury, 16, 17f
in inflammation, 73
1,25-$(OH)_2$D, 452–453, 453f
1,25-$(OH)_2D_3$ deficiency, renal osteodystrophy due to, 1288
25(OH)D, 452
OKC (odontogenic keratocyst), 782
Olfactory neuroblastomas, 785
Oligoastrocytoma, 1404
anaplastic, 1404
Oligoclonal bands, in multiple sclerosis, 1384
Oligodendrocytes, 1349, 1350
Oligodendroglioma, 1404
anaplastic, 1404
Oligodontia, 1280t
Oligohydramnios sequence, 471–472, 472f
Ollier disease, 1296
Onchocerca volvulus, 410–411, 411f
Onchocerciasis, 410–411, 411f
Onchocercoma, 411
Oncocytoma, of kidney, 1015–1016
Oncofetal antigens, 330
Oncogenes, 100, 292–298
activated by translocation, 314t
cellular, 293
defined, 292
for cyclins and cyclin-dependent kinases, 295t, 298
for growth factor(s), 293–294, 295t
for growth factor receptors, 294–296, 295t
for nonreceptor-associated tyrosine kinase, 295t, 297, 298f
for transcription factors, 295t, 297–298, 299f
nomenclature for, 293
products of mutated, 328
signal-transducing, 295t, 296–297, 297f
transduction of, 293
viral, 293
white cell neoplasia due to, 667
Oncogenesis
of breast carcinoma, 1135–1138, 1138f
two-hit hypothesis of, 299, 301f
Oncology, defined, 270
Oncoproteins, 293, 295t
cyclins and cyclin-dependent kinases as, 295t, 298
growth factor receptors as, 294–296, 295t
growth factors as, 293–294, 295t
nonreceptor-associated tyrosine kinase as, 295t, 297, 298f
signal-transducing, 295t, 296–297, 297f
transcription factors as, 295t, 297–298, 299f
Onion bulbs, 1329, 1329f
"Onion-skin fibrosis," 915, 915f
Onion-skinning, 1008
Onycholysis, 1230
Onychomycosis, 398, 1267

OPA genes, 378
OPG (osteoprotegerin), 1184, 1275, 1276f
Ophthalmologic effects, of obesity, 465t
Ophthalmopathy
  infiltrative, in Graves disease, 1172
  thyroid, 1166, 1167f, 1423, 1423f
Ophthalmoplegia
  chronic progressive external, 1342
  exophthalmic, 1343
Ophthalmoplegia plus, 1399
Opioid narcotics, abuse of, 424t, 426
Opportunistic infections
  in AIDS, 255–256, 255t
  of lungs, 353
Opsoclonus, paraneoplastic, 1411, 1411t
Opsonin(s), 59
Opsonin receptors, 59
Opsonization, 59
  by antibody, 210, 211f
Optic nerve, 1422f, 1443–1446
  papilledema of, 1443–1444, 1444f
Optic neuritis, 1445–1446
  in multiple sclerosis, 1384
Optic neuropathy(ies), 1445
  anterior ischemic, 1443, 1444f
    nonarteritic, 1443
  Leber hereditary, 185, 185f, 1342, 1445
Oral cancer, 780–781, 781f
Oral candidiasis, 777
Oral cavity, 774–782
  infections of, 776–777
  inflammatory/reactive lesions of, 775–776, 775f, 776f
  manifestations of systemic disease in, 777–778, 778t
  odontogenic cysts and tumors of, 782, 782t
  teeth and supporting structure of, 774–775, 774f
  tumors and precancerous lesions of, 778–781, 779f, 781f
Oral contraceptives
  adverse effects of, 427
  endometrial changes due to, 1082
Oral glucose tolerance test (OGTT), 1190
Oral ulcers, in systemic lupus erythematosus, 228t
Oraxins A and B, 463f, 464b
Oraxogenic neuropeptides, 464b
Orbicularis oculi muscle, 1424f
Orbit, 1423–1424, 1423f
Orbital cellulitis, 1423
Orbital inflammation, idiopathic, 1423–1424, 1423f
Orbital inflammatory pseudotumor, 1423–1424, 1423f
Orbital myositis, 1423
Orbital preadipocyte fibroblasts, in Graves disease, 1172
Orchitis
  granulomatous (autoimmune), 1039
  mumps, 364
  non-specific, 1039
Organ transplantation. *See* Transplantation.
Organization
  in inflammation, 76, 77, 89
  of thrombi, 134, 134f
Organochlorines, 434t, 435
Organogenesis, 474, 475f
Organophosphates, 434t, 435
Organs of Zuckerkandl, 1218
Orienta tsutsugamushi, 395, 396t
Ormond disease, 873
Orphan Annie eye nuclei, in thyroid carcinoma, 1178, 1179f
Orthopnea, in left-sided heart failure, 562–563
Orthostatic edema, simple, 543
Osler nodes, 598
Osler-Weber-Rendu disease, 548
Osmotic lysis, in hereditary spherocytosis, 627
Osseous metaplasia, of retinal pigment epithelium, 1446
Ossification
  enchondral, 1277–1278, 1278f
  primary and secondary centers of, 1278
Osteitic fibrosa cystica, 1287
Osteitis, dissecting, 1287, 1287f
Osteitis deformans, 1284–1286, 1285f, 1286f
Osteitis fibrosa cystica, in hyperparathyroidism, 1186
Osteoarthritis, 1304–1305, 1305f
  due to Paget disease, 1286
  obesity and, 465
  secondary, 1304
Osteoarthropathy, paraneoplastic hypertrophic, 334t, 335
Osteoblast(s), 1274–1275, 1275f, 1276, 1277f
Osteoblastoma, 1293–1294
Osteocalcin, 1276
Osteochondritis, syphilitic, 391
Osteochondroma, 1296, 1296f
Osteoclast(s), 1275, 1276, 1276f, 1277f
  dysfunction of, 1284–1286, 1285f, 1286f
Osteoclast differentiation factor, 1184
Osteoclastoma, 1302, 1302f, 1303f
Osteocytes, 1275
Osteodystrophy
  Albright hereditary, pseudohypoparathyroidism in, 1189
  renal, 1287–1288
Osteogenesis imperfecta, 1279–1280, 1280t, 1281t, 1282f
Osteoid, 1274
Osteoid osteoma, 1293–1294, 1293f, 1294f
Osteolytic metastases, 1184
Osteoma, 270, 1293
Osteomalacia, 453–455, 454f, 454t, 1287
Osteomyelitis
  pyogenic, 1290–1291, 1291f
  sclerosing, of Garré, 1291
  tuberculous, 1291–1292
Osteonecrosis, 1289–1290, 1289t, 1290f
Osteonectin, 105
Osteopenia, 455
Osteopetrosis, 1281–1282, 1282f, 1283f
Osteopontin, 105
Osteoporosis, 455, 1282–1284, 1283f, 1283t, 1284f
Osteoprogenitor cells, 1274, 1275f, 1277f
Osteoprotegerin (OPG), 1184, 1275, 1276f
Osteosarcoma, 1294–1296, 1294f, 1295f
  chondroblastic, 1295, 1298
Otitis media, 788
Otosclerosis, 788
Ouabain-sensitive $Na^{+}K^{+}$-ATPase, reduced activity of, 15
Outdoor air pollution, 428–430, 428t, 429t
Oval cells, 93–94, 93f
Ovarian carcinoid, 1100
Ovarian carcinoma
  clear cell adenocarcinoma, 1098
  clinical course, detection, and prevention of, 1099
  cystadeno-, 1095, 1095f, 1096f
  epidemiology of, 1093
  genetic predisposition to, 286
  risk factors for, 1093
  serous, 1096, 1096f
Ovarian cystic teratoma, 272, 272f
Ovarian disease, polycystic, 1092–1093, 1093f
Ovarian tumor(s), 1093–1104
  bilateral, 1093, 1094t
  Brenner, 1098, 1099f
Ovarian tumor(s) *(Continued)*
  choriocarcinoma as, 1101–1102
  classification of, 1093, 1093t, 1094f
  cystadenofibroma as, 1098
  cystadenomas and cystadenocarcinomas as, 1095–1097, 1095f–1097f
  dysgerminoma as, 1101, 1101f
  endodermal sinus (yolk sac), 1101, 1101f
  endometrioid, 1097–1098
  epidemiology of, 1093
  frequency data for, 1094t
  germ cell, 1093t, 1094f, 1099–1102, 1099f–1101f
  gonadoblastoma as, 1104
  granulosa-theca cell, 1102–1103, 1102f
  hilus cell, 1103–1104
  Leydig cell, 1103–1104
  metastatic, 1094f, 1104
  mucinous, 1097, 1097f, 1098f
  of Müllerian epithelium, 1093t, 1094–1099, 1094f–1099f
  pregnancy luteoma as, 1104
  risk factors for, 1093
  serous, 1095–1097, 1095f, 1096f
  Sertoli-Leydig cell (androblastomas), 1103, 1104f
  sex cord—stromal, 1093t, 1094f, 1102–1104, 1102f–1104f
  teratomas as, 1099–1100, 1100f, 1101f
  thecoma-fibromas as, 1103, 1103f
Ovary(ies), 1092–1104
  anatomy of, 1081, 1081f
  cysts of
    cortical müllerian inclusion, 1095, 1095f
    non-neoplastic and functional, 1092–1093, 1092f
  radiation effect on, 441
  streak, 180
Overinflation, obstructive, 721
Overweight, and cancer, 284
Ovotestes, 181
Oxidant-antioxidant imbalance, in emphysema, 720, 720f
Oxidative damage, 42, 43
Oxidative modification, of proteins, 16–17
Oxidative phosphorylation, 14–15, 14f
Oxidative phosphorylation diseases, 1341–1342, 1341f
Oxidative stress, 14f, 16–18, 17f
Oxygen, singlet, 17f
Oxygen content, of blood, and infarction, 139
Oxygen deprivation, cell injury due to, 11–12
Oxygen toxicity, 482
Oxygen-derived free radicals
  accumulation of, 14f, 16–17, 17f
  in chemical injury, 25
  in inflammation, 73–74, 74t
  in ischemia-reperfusion injury, 24
  removal of, 17–18
Oxyntic glands, 810, 811
Oxyphil adenomas, 1185
Oxyphil cells, 1184
Oxytocin, 1158
Oxyuriasis vermicularis, 870
Ozone
  as air pollutant, 428t, 429, 429t
  depletion of, 441

P

P pilus, 358
p6, in human immunodeficiency virus, 247f
p14, in human immunodeficiency virus, 247f
p14ARF, 291f, 292, 302, 315
  in melanoma, 1246
p15, in human immunodeficiency virus, 247f
p16 CDKNZA, in pancreatic cancer, 950, 950t

p16 gene, in glioblastoma, 1403
p16INK4a gene
as tumor suppressor gene, 286, 300t, 305, 315
in cervical cancer, 1076, 1076f
in melanoma, 287t, 1246
in regulating cell cycle, 291f, 292, 292t
in retinoblastoma, 300
p17, in human immunodeficiency virus, 247, 247f
p19, in human immunodeficiency virus, 247f
p19ARF, 292t
p21 gene, 291f, 292, 292t, 302, 303f
p23, in human immunodeficiency virus, 247f
p24, in human immunodeficiency virus, 247f
p27, 291f, 292, 292t
p53 gene
and angiogenesis, 309
and human papillomavirus, 325, 325f
and transcription factors, 100
as guardian of the genome, 302–303, 303f
as tumor marker, 339, 339t
growth-inhibiting effects of, 302
hypoxia and, 303
in apoptosis, 31, 302, 303, 303f, 306
in breast cancer, 1134
in cell-cycle checkpoints, 292, 292t, 302–303, 303f
in colorectal cancer, 317, 317f, 318, 863f, 864
in glioblastoma, 1403
in pancreatic cancer, 949f, 950, 950t
Li-Fraumeni syndrome due to, 285, 302
mutations in, 302, 320
P57, 292
p73 gene, 303
PA (plasminogen activator), 68, 130
PAF. *See* Platelet-activating factor (PAF).
Paget, James, 1285
Paget cells, 1140, 1141f
Paget disease
extramammary, 1068–1069, 1069f
of bone, 1284–1286, 1285f, 1286f
of nipple, 1140, 1141f
Pain, breast, 1122–1123
Pain crises, in sickle cell disease, 631
Paired Homeobox genes. *See PAX* genes.
PAIs (plasminogen activator inhibitors), 126, 130, 130f
Pale infarction, 1364f, 1365, 1365f
Palmar erythema, in hepatic failure, 882
Palmar fibromatosis, 1319
Palpation thyroiditis, 1171–1172
Palpebral commissure, 1424f
Palsy
progressive bulbar, 1397
progressive supranuclear, 1390, 1391
PAN (polyarteritis nodosa), 212t, 239–240, 537t, 539f, 540
P-ANCA (perinuclear antineutrophil cytoplasmic antibodies), 535
in pauci-immune crescentic glomerulonephritis, 977
Pancarditis, 593
Pancolitis, 849
Pancreas, 939–952
agenesis of, 941
annular, 941
congenital anomalies of, 941
congenital cysts of, 946–947
cystic neoplasms of, 947–948, 948f, 949f
ectopic, 941
embryonic development of, 939
endocrine, 940, 1189–1207
exocrine, 939–940
in cystic fibrosis, 493, 493f, 494
in diabetes mellitus, 1189–1205
Pancreas *(Continued)*
multihormonal tumors of, 1207
mumps effect on, 364
normal anatomy and physiology of, 939–941, 940f, 1189
Pancreas divisum, 941
Pancreatic abscess, 944
Pancreatic carcinoid tumors, 1207
Pancreatic carcinoma, 948–952
clinical features of, 951–952
epidemiology of, 948, 950
etiology of, 950
familial clustering of, 950, 951t
molecular basis for, 949–950, 950t
morphology of, 950–951, 951f
pathogenesis of, 950
precursors to, 949, 949f
Pancreatic cysts
congenital, 946–947
neoplastic, 947–948, 948f, 949f
pseudo-, 945, 947, 947f
Pancreatic ducts, 939, 940f
obstruction of, 943, 945
Pancreatic endocrine neoplasms, 1205–1207, 1206f
Pancreatic enzymes, 941
in pancreatitis, 943, 944f
Pancreatic fibrosis, in hemochromatosis, 909, 910
Pancreatic heterotopia, 812
Pancreatic insufficiency
in cystic fibrosis, 494, 495
malabsorption due to, 843
Pancreatic intraepithelial neoplasias (PanINs), 949, 949f
Pancreatic microadenomas, in MEN-1, 1222
Pancreatic polypeptide (PP) cells, 1189
Pancreatic polypeptide (PP)—secreting endocrine tumors, 1207
Pancreatic pseudocysts, 945, 947, 947f
Pancreatitis, 941–946
acute, 942–945, 942t, 943f–945f
hemorrhagic, peritonitis due to, 872
interstitial, 942, 943f
necrotizing, 942–943, 943f
alcoholic, 943–944
chronic, 942, 945–946, 945f, 946f
hemorrhagic, 943
peritonitis due to, 872
hereditary, 942, 945
in cystic fibrosis, 494–495
tropical, 945
Pancreatoblastoma, 952
Pancytopenia, oral manifestations of, 778t
Pandemics, of influenza, 751–752
Panencephalitis, subacute sclerosing, 363, 1377
Paneth cells, 829
Panfascicular atrophy, 1336
PanINs (pancreatic intraepithelial neoplasias), 949, 949f
Panniculitis, 1265
factitious, 1265
relapsing febrile nodular, 1265
Pannus, 1306
degenerative, in Fuchs endothelial dystrophy, 1429
Panophthalmitis, 1432, 1433f
Pantothenic acid, 450t
PAP (pulmonary alveolar proteinosis), 741, 741f
Pap smears, 336
Papanicolaou smear, 1075, 1077f, 1078
Papillae
in esophagus, 799
renal, 956
Papillary adenoma, renal, 1015
Papillary carcinoma
of breast
in situ, 1140, 1141f
invasive, 1146
of kidney, 1016, 1017, 1017f, 1018, 1018f
of thyroid gland, 1177–1180, 1179f, 1179t
serous, of endometrium, 1087, 1088
transitional cell
of renal pelvis, 1004
of ureter, 1025, 1025f
Papillary cystadenoma(s), 271
of ovaries, 1095, 1096f
Papillary cystadenoma lymphomatosum, 792–793, 793f
Papillary fibroelastoma, cardiac, 614
Papillary glioneuronal tumor, 1406
Papillary hidradenoma, of vulva, 1067
Papillary muscle dysfunction, after myocardial infarction, 586
Papillary muscle rupture, after myocardial infarction, 584–585, 585f
Papillary necrosis, 1004, 1004t
in acute pyelonephritis, 998, 999f, 1000
in analgesic nephropathy, 1003, 1003f, 1004t
in sickle cell disease nephropathy, 1011
Papillary serous carcinoma, of endometrium, 1087, 1088
Papillary transitional cell carcinoma
of renal pelvis, 1004
of ureter, 1025, 1025f
Papillary urothelial neoplasms of low malignant potential (PUNLMP), 1030
Papilledema, of optic nerve, 1443–1444, 1444f
Papilloma(s), 270, 270f
choroid plexus, 1406
inverted
of bladder, 1030
sinonasal, 784, 785f
of bladder, 1030, 1030f
of breast, 1128–1129, 1129f
sinonasal, 784–785, 785f
squamous
esophageal, 806
laryngeal, 786–787, 787f
Papillomatosis, 1230
laryngeal, 787
Papillomavirus, human. *See* Human papillomavirus (HPV).
Papule, 1229
Papulosis, bowenoid, 1036, 1266
PAR(s) (protease-activated receptors), 65–67, 67f
in coagulation cascade, 128
Paracentric inversion, 174, 174f
Paracortical lymphoid hyperplasia, 666
Paracrine effect, of cytokines, 202
Paracrine signaling, 97–98, 97f
Paradoxical embolism, 566, 576
Parafollicular cells, 1166
Paragangliomas, 789–790, 789f, 1221
nonchromaffin, 789
Paraganglion system, 1218, 1219f
Parakeratosis, 1230, 1242
Paramyxovirus, 348f
Paraneoplastic cerebellar degeneration, 1410, 1411t
Paraneoplastic neuropathy, 1335
Paraneoplastic syndromes, 333–335, 334t
of central nervous system, 1410–1411, 1411t
with lung cancer, 763–764
Paraparesis, tropical spastic, 327, 1376
Paraphimosis, 1035
Paraquat, metabolism of, 420f
Parasitic enterocolitis, 838–840, 839f, 840f
Parasitic infection(s), 401–411
African trypanosomiasis as, 406, 406f
babesiosis as, 403, 403f

Parasitic infection(s) *(Continued)*
Chagas disease as, 406–407
leishmaniasis as, 403–405, 404f
lymphatic filariasis as, 409–410, 410f
malaria as, 401–403, 402f, 403f
metazoal, 406–411, 407f–411f
of liver, 902
onchocerciasis as, 410–411, 411f
protozoal, 346t, 351, 351t, 401–406, 402f–405f
schistosomiasis as, 408–409, 408f, 409f
strongyloidiasis as, 406, 407f
trichinosis as, 407–408, 408f
with tapeworms, 406–407, 407f
Paratesticular tumors, 1040
Parathyroid adenoma(s), 1185–1186, 1185f, 1186f
Parathyroid adenoma 1 *(PRAD1)* gene, 1185
Parathyroid carcinomas, 1186
Parathyroid glands, 1183–1189
hyperparathyroidism of, 1184–1188, 1185f–1187f, 1187t
hypoparathyroidism of, 1188
pseudo-, 1188–1189
normal anatomy and physiology of, 1183–1184
Parathyroid hormone (PTH), 1184
and hypercalcemia, 41, 1187, 1187t
in bone disease, 1287, 1287f, 1288
in calcium absorption, 453, 453f
Parathyroid hormone receptor (PTH-R), 333
Parathyroid hormone (PTH)-related protein (PTHRP), 1184, 1278
in hypercalcemia of malignancy, 333–334
Parathyroid hormone (PTH)-related protein receptor (PTHRP-R), 333, 335
Parathyroid hyperplasia, 1185, 1185f, 1186
in MEN-2A, 1222
Paratubal cysts, 1091
Parenchyma, of tumors, 270
Parenchymal injuries, of brain, 1357–1359, 1360f
Parenchymal tumors, of central nervous system, 1408–1409
Parietal cells, of stomach, 810–811
Parkin, 1392
Parking lot inclusions, 1341, 1341f
Parkinson disease (PD), 1391–1393
aggregated proteins in, 1351t
clinical features of, 1392–1393
Lewy bodies in, 1351, 1391–1392, 1392f
morphology of, 1391–1392, 1392f
pathogenesis and molecular genetics of, 1392
treatment for, 1393
Parkinsonism, 1391
frontotemporal dementia with, 1389–1390
postencephalitic, 1373, 1391
Paronychia, 373, 398
Parotid gland, mixed tumor of, 271f
Parotitis, mumps, 364
Paroxysmal cold hemoglobinuria, 637–638, 637t
Paroxysmal nocturnal dyspnea, in left-sided heart failure, 563
Paroxysmal nocturnal hemoglobinuria (PNH), 67b, 245, 636, 636f
Pars plana, of eye, 1422f
Pars plicata, of eye, 1422f
Partial lipodystrophy, 985
Partial thromboplastin time (PTT), 649–650
Particulate radiation, 436
Particulates (PM_{10}), as air pollutants, 428t, 429–430, 429t
Parvovirus, 347t
Parvovirus B19, during pregnancy, 480, 480f
PASH (pseudoangiomatous stromal hyperplasia), 1151
Passive smoking, 421
Pasteur, Louis, 344
Patau syndrome, 176, 177f, 472
Patch, 1229
Patched *(PTCH)* gene, 287t, 306, 1244–1245, 1246f
Patent ductus arteriosus (PDA), 564t, 567f, 568
coarctation of aorta with, 571, 571f
Patent foramen ovale, 567
Paternal imprinting, 186
Paterson-Kelly syndrome, 776
Pathogenesis, defined, 4
Pathogenicity islands, 358
Pathologic hypertrophy, 562
Pathology, defined, 4
Pauci-immune crescentic glomerulonephritis, 977
Pautrier microabscesses, 1250
Pavementing, 53
Pawn ball megakaryocytes, 695, 696f
PAX genes, 476
PAX3 gene, in rhabdomyosarcoma, 1321
PAX6 gene, 504
PAX8 gene, mutations in, 1168
PAX8-PPARγ1 fusion gene, in thyroid carcinoma, 1177
Paxillin, 105
PC1, 464b
PCBs (polychlorinated biphenyls), 435
PCNSL (primary CNS lymphoma), 1408
PCOD (polycystic ovarian disease), 1092–1093, 1093f
PCP (phencyclidine), 426
PCP (phencyclidine)-like drugs, abuse of, 424t
PCR (polymerase chain reaction) analysis, 188, 188f, 189f
of cancer, 337
of infectious agents, 361
PD. *See* Parkinson disease (PD).
PDA (patent ductus arteriosus), 564t, 567f, 568
coarctation of aorta with, 571, 571f
PDGF. *See* Platelet-derived growth factor (PDGF).
Peau d'orange appearance, 122
PECAM-1 (platelet endothelial cell adhesion molecule), 53f, 54t, 56
Pedicels, of glomerulus, 957f–959f, 958, 959
Pediculosis, 352, 1268, 1269f
Pedunculated lipomas, of esophagus, 806
Pelger-Hüet cells, pseudo-, in myelodysplastic syndromes, 695, 696f
Peliosis, bacillary, 548
Peliosis hepatis, 918–919
Pelizaeus-Merzbacher disease, 1398
Pellagra, 458, 458f
Pelvic inflammatory disease (PID), 1064–1065, 1064f
Pelvis, renal, 956
PEM (protein-energy malnutrition), 447–449, 448f, 449t
Pemphigoid
bullous, 1260f–1261f, 1260f–1262
oral manifestations of, 778t
ocular cicatricial, 1425
Pemphigus, 1260–1261, 1260f, 1261f
oral manifestations of, 778t
Pemphigus erythematosus, 1260
Pemphigus foliaceus, 1260–1261, 1260f
Pemphigus vegetans, 1260
Pemphigus vulgaris, 212t, 1260, 1260f, 1261f
Pendred syndrome, 1168
Penetrance, reduced, 150
Penile fibromatosis, 1319
Penis, 1034–1037
congenital anomalies of, 1035
inflammations of, 1035
tumors of, 1035–1037, 1035f1037f
Pepsin, 811
Pepsinogen I and II, 811
Peptic ulcer disease, 816–820
clinical features of, 819, 819f
complications of, 819, 819t
epidemiology of, 817
in Zollinger-Ellison syndrome, 1206–1207
morphology of, 818–819, 819f
pathogenesis of, 817–818, 817f
sites of, 816–817
stress ulcers in, 819–820, 820f
Peptostreptococcus spp, 393
Perchloroethylene, 431
Percutaneous transluminal coronary angioplasty (PTCA), 551
Perforins, 31, 218
Perfusion, 557
Periadrenal brown fat, in sudden infant death syndrome, 496
Periampullary carcinomas, 935
Periapical cyst, 782
Periapical granuloma, 782
Periaxin gene, 1327
Pericardial disease, 611–612, 611t, 612f
Pericardial effusion, 611
Pericardial friction rub, 612
Pericardial space, in right-sided heart failure, 563
Pericarditis, 611–612
acute, 611–612
adhesive, 612
after myocardial infarction, 585, 585f
caseous, 612
causes of, 611t
chronic (healed), 611, 612
constrictive, 89, 612
due to radiation exposure, 440
due to rheumatic fever, 593, 595f
fibrinous and serofibrinous, 76, 77f, 611–612
hemorrhagic, 612
in systemic lupus erythematosus, 233
in systemic sclerosis, 239
mediastino-, 612
adhesive, 612
purulent or suppurative, 612, 612f
serous, 611
Pericentric inversion, 174, 174f
Periductal mastitis, 1125, 1125f
Periendothelial cells, 108
Perifascicular atrophy, 1343
Perikaryon, 1349
Perimysium, 1328
Perinatal brain injury, 1356, 1356f
Perinatal infection(s), 480–481, 480f
with cytomegalovirus, 367
Perinephric abscess, 999
Perineural barrier, 1327
Perineurium, 1327
Perinuclear antineutrophil cytoplasmic antibodies (P-ANCA), 535
in pauci-immune crescentic glomerulonephritis, 977
Periodic acid-Schiff stain, 361t
Periodontal ligament, 774, 774f
Periodontitis, 775
Periostitis, syphilitic, 391
Peripheral B-cell neoplasm(s), 673–683
Burkitt lymphoma as, 671t, 677–678, 678f
chronic lymphocytic leukemia as, 673–674, 674f
classification of, 671t
diffuse large B-cell lymphoma as, 671t, 676–677, 676f, 677f
follicular lymphoma as, 671t, 674–676, 675f, 676f
hairy cell leukemia as, 671t, 683, 684f

Peripheral B-cell neoplasm(s) *(Continued)*
lymphoplasmacytic lymphoma as, 681–682, 681f
mantle cell lymphoma as, 671t, 682–683, 682f
marginal zone lymphoma as, 671t, 683
of plasma cells, 671t, 678–681, 679f, 680f
small lymphocytic lymphoma as, 671t, 673–674, 674f
Peripheral giant cell granuloma, of oral cavity, 776
Peripheral myelin protein 22 (PMP22), 1326–1327
Peripheral nerve(s), normal anatomy and physiology of, 1326–1327, 1327f
Peripheral nerve sheath tumors, 1411–1412, 1412f
malignant, 1412–1413
Peripheral nervous system disorder(s), 1330–1335
acquired metabolic and toxic, 1334–1335, 1334f
hereditary, 1332–1334, 1332t, 1333t
immune-mediated, 1331
infectious, 1331–1332
inflammatory, 1330–1331
neoplastic, 1335
paraneoplastic, 334t
traumatic, 1335
Peripheral neuroectodermal tumor (PNET), 500t, 1301–1302
Peripheral neuropathy
AIDS-associated, 1376
T cell—mediated hypersensitivity in, 215t
Peripheral ossifying fibroma, of oral cavity, 775–776
Peripheral staining, 228
Peripheral T-cell lymphoma, unspecified, 684, 684f
Peripheral T-cell neoplasm(s), 671t, 684–686, 684f, 685f
Peripheral tolerance, 224f, 225–226
Peripheral vascular resistance, in blood pressure regulation, 527, 527f
Peripheral vasoconstriction, in shock, 141
Periportal fibrosis, in hepatitis, 899, 900f
Periportal necrosis, 880
in hepatitis, 899f
Perisinusoidal stellate cells, 878
in cirrhosis, 883, 884f
Peritoneal cavity, seeding of, 279, 280f
Peritoneal infection, 872–873
Peritoneal mesotheliomas, 769
Peritoneum, 872–873
inflammation of, 872–873
tumors of, 873
Peritonitis, 872–873
adhesions due to, 856
bacterial, 872–873
bile, 936
Peritubular vascular network, 956
Perivascular pseudorosettes, 1405, 1405f
Perivenous encephalomyelitis, 1385
Periventricular leukomalacia, 1356, 1356f
Permanent tissues, 90f, 91
Permissible exposure level, 417
Pernicious anemia, 212t, 639–642, 640f, 640t, 641f
Peroneal muscular atrophy, 1332
Peroxidase-dependent cooxidation, 418, 420f
Peroxidase-positive granules, in acute myelogenous leukemia, 692
Peroxisome proliferator—activated receptor gamma (PPARγ), and insulin resistance, 1196, 1196f
Peroxisome proliferator—activated receptors (PPARs), 100
Persistent hyperplastic primary vitreous, 1434
Personal exposure(s), 419–426
to alcohol, 421–424, 422f, 422t, 423f
to drugs, 424–426, 424t, 425f
to tobacco, 419–421, 419t, 421t
Pertussis, 378, 379f
Pesticides, 323, 434–435, 434t
Petechiae, 123, 124f
in immune thrombocytopenic purpura, 652
in sudden infant death syndrome, 496
Petroleum products, 431
Peutz-Jeghers polyps, 822, 859, 859f
Peutz-Jeghers syndrome, 859, 862
and breast cancer, 1134
Peyer patches, 829
Peyronie disease, 1319
PfEMP1, 402
PFIC-1 (progressive familial intrahepatic cholestasis 1), 889
PFIC-2 (progressive familial intrahepatic cholestasis 2), 889
PFIC-3 (progressive familial intrahepatic cholestasis 3), 889–890
PGE_2 (prostaglandin E_2), 68, 69, 69f
$PGF_{2\alpha}$ (prostaglandin $F_{2\alpha}$), 68, 69, 69f
PGG_2 (prostaglandin G_2), 69f
PGH_2 (prostaglandin H_2), 69f
PGI_2 (prostaglandin I_2), 68, 69, 69f
Ph. *See* Philadelphia chromosome (Ph).
Phacolysis, 1431
Phagocytes, in innate immunity, 194, 194f
Phagocytic recognition, breakdown of, 27–28
Phagocytosis, 32, 32f
by antibody, 210, 211f
complement- and Fc receptor—mediated, 210, 211f
complement system in, 64
discovery of, 49
engulfment in, 59, 60f
frustrated, 61
in inflammation, 59–61, 60f, 76f
killing and degradation in, 59–61, 60f
of apoptotic cells or cell bodies, 27
recognition and attachment in, 59, 60f
splenic, 703
Phagolysosomes, 32, 32f, 59, 60f
defects in function of, 61–62
Phagosome, 59, 60f
Pharmacogenetics, 154
Pharmacogenomics, 426
Pharyngitis, 784
streptococcal, 373–374
Phencyclidine (PCP), 426
Phencyclidine (PCP)-like drugs, abuse of, 424t
Phenotypic sex, 181
Phenylalanine hydroxylase system, 488, 488f
Phenylketonuria (PKU), 487–488, 488f
Phenytoin (Dilantin) ingestion, oral manifestations of, 778t
Pheochromocytoma, 1219–1221, 1219t, 1220f
Philadelphia chromosome (Ph)
gene fusion in, 314–315
in acute lymphoblastic leukemia, 672, 673
in chronic myelogenous leukemia, 696, 697, 697f
Phimosis, 1035
Phlebosclerosis, 544
Phlebothrombosis, 132, 134–135, 544
Phlegmasia alba dolens, 544
Phosphatidyl inositol glycan A (PIGA), in paroxysmal nocturnal hemoglobinuria, 636
Phosphatidylinositol-3 kinase (PI-3K)
in chemotaxis, 56
in insulin signaling pathway, 1192, 1193f
in signal transduction, 98f, 99, 99f
Phosphatidylserine, in apoptosis, 27
Phospholipase(s), 15–16, 69f
Phospholipase A_2 (PLA_2), 68
Phospholipase Cγ (PLCγ), 56, 98f, 99, 99f
Phospholipid(s), membrane, loss of, 18
Phospholipid complexes, in hemostasis, 127, 128
Photochemical reactions, air pollution from, 429
Photoeczematous eruption, 1254t
Photosensitivity, in systemic lupus erythematosus, 228t
Phrygian cap, of gallbladder, 928, 928f
Phthalate esters, 432
Phthisis bulbi, 1446, 1446f
Phycomycosis, 400–401, 401f
Phyllodes tumor, 1150, 1150f
Physical activity, and osteoporosis, 1283
Physical agents, cell injury due to, 12
Physical environment, hazards of, 442–446, 443f, 443t, 444f
Physiologic hypertrophy, 562
Physiologic jaundice of the newborn, 887
Physis, 1278, 1278f
Phytobezoars, 820
Phytotoxins, 435, 435t
PI-3K. *See* Phosphatidylinositol-3 kinase (PI-3K).
Pick bodies, 1390
Pick cells, 1390
Pick disease, 1390
Pickwickian syndrome, 465
PID (pelvic inflammatory disease), 1064–1065, 1064f
PIGA (phosphatidyl inositol glycan A), in paroxysmal nocturnal hemoglobinuria, 636
Pigeon breast deformity, 455
Pigeon breeder's lung, 739
Pigment(s)
defined, 39
endogenous, 39–40, 40f
exogenous, 39
intracellular accumulation of, 39–41, 40f
Pigment stones, 928, 929–930, 929t, 931f
Pigmentation disorders, 1230–1236, 1231f–1236f, 1233f
Pigmented nevus, 1232–1233, 1232f, 1233f, 1233t
Pigmented villonodular synovitis (PVNS), 1315, 1315f
Pilar cyst, 1238
Pilar leiomyomas, 1322
Pili, 348, 358
"Pill-rolling" tremor, 1391
PiMM phenotype
emphysema with, 719
in α_1-antitrypsin deficiency, 911
PIN (prostatic intraepithelial neoplasia), high-grade, 1053
Pineal gland, 1223–1224
Pineal parenchymal tumors, 1409
Pinealomas, 1223–1224
Pineoblastomas, 1223, 1409
Pineocytes, 1223, 1409
Pineocytomas, 1223–1224, 1409
Pineocytomatous pseudorosettes, 1223
Pinguecula, 1426
Pink puffers, 721
Pinna, tumors of, 788
Pinocytosis, 32
Pinpoint hemorrhages, in immune thrombocytopenic purpura, 652
Pinta, 388
Pinworms, 838–839
Pipe-stem fibrosis, 409, 409f
Pituitary adenomas, 1158–1162
ACTH-producing, 1208
classification of, 1158–1159, 1158t
clinical course of, 1160

Pituitary adenomas *(Continued)*
corticotroph cell, 1162
diagnosis of, 1159
functional *vs.* silent, 1158
genetic abnormalities in, 1159, 1159f
gonadotroph, 1162
growth hormone (somatotroph cell), 1161–1162
hormone-negative, 1158–1159, 1162
lactotroph, 1160–1161, 1161f
mammosomatotroph, 1161
micro- *vs.* macro-, 1159
morphology of, 1160, 1160f
nonfunctioning, 1158, 1160f, 1162
null cell, 1162
prolactinomas as, 1160–1161, 1161f
thyrotroph, 1162
with MEN type 1, 1159
Pituitary apoplexy, 1158, 1160, 1162, 1163
Pituitary carcinomas, 1162
Pituitary dwarfism, 1163
Pituitary gland, 1156–1164
amyloidosis of, 263
anterior, 1157–1158, 1157f
hyperpituitarism of, 1158–1162
hypopituitarism of, 1158, 1162–1163
hypothalamic suprasellar tumors and, 1164
in Cushing syndrome, 1209
ischemic necrosis of, 1163
local mass effects of, 1158
normal anatomy and physiology of, 1156–1158, 1157f
posterior, 1158
syndromes of, 1163–1164
"Pituitary stone," 1160
PiZZ phenotype
emphysema with, 719
in α_1-antitrypsin deficiency, 911
PKC (protein kinase C)
in diabetes mellitus, 1198
in signal transduction, 99
PKD. *See* Polycystic kidney disease (PKD).
PKD1 gene, 963, 964
PKD2 gene, 963, 964
PKHD1 gene, in polycystic kidney disease, 964
PKU (phenylketonuria), 487–488, 488f
PLA_2 (phospholipase A_2), 68
Placenta(s)
anatomy of, 1107f
in toxemia of pregnancy, 1109
inflammations and infections of, 1106, 1108f
twin, 1106, 1108f
Placenta accreta, 1105–1106
Placental factors, fetal growth restriction due to, 477, 478f
Placental ischemia, 1107, 1109f
Placental membranes, premature rupture of, 477
Placental site trophoblastic tumor (PSTT), 1114, 1114f
Placental-fetal route, 355
Placentitis, 1106
Plague, 379–380
Plant products, as carcinogens, 321t, 322
Plantar fibromatosis, 1319
Plaque(s)
asbestos, 736, 736f, 768
atheromatous (atherosclerotic, fibrous, fibrofatty, lipid, fibrolipid), 516, 517–519, 518f, 519f
rupture of, 573, 573f, 576
defined, 1229
dental, 775
Hollenhorst, 1440
in Kaposi sarcoma, 549, 549f
in multiple sclerosis, 1383–1384, 1383f, 1384f
kuru, 1380
Plaque(s) *(Continued)*
MacCallum's, 593
neuritic (senile), 1386–1387, 1386f
shadow, 1383
"soldier's," 612
Plaque jaune, 1357, 1358f
Plasma cell(s), 199
in chronic inflammation, 81–82
origin and differentiation of, 621f
Plasma cell dyscrasias, glomerular lesions in, 993
Plasma cell leukemia, 680
Plasma cell myeloma. *See* Multiple myeloma.
Plasma cell neoplasms, 668, 671t, 678–681, 679f, 680f
Plasma exchange, for Goodpasture syndrome, 746
Plasma membrane alterations, in cell injury, 20, 20f
Plasma membrane energy-dependent sodium pump, reduced activity of, 15
Plasma osmotic pressure, edema due to reduced, 120f, 120t, 121
Plasma proteins, in inflammation, 64–68
Plasmablasts, 679–680
Plasmacytomas, 671t, 678, 681
sinonasal, 785
Plasmids, 348
Plasmin, 68, 130, 130f
Plasminogen, 68, 130, 130f
Plasminogen activator (PA), 68, 130
Plasminogen activator inhibitors (PAIs), 126, 130, 130f
Plasmodium falciparum, 401–403, 402f, 403f
Plasmodium malariae, 401
Plasmodium ovale, 401
Plasmodium spp, 351, 351t, 401–403
Plasmodium vivax, 401, 402
Plastic(s), exposure to, 432
Plasticity, developmental, 92
Platelet(s)
in glomerulonephritis, 972
in hemostasis, 125f, 126–127, 127f
origin and differentiation of, 621f
sequestration of, 651
Platelet adhesiveness, in diabetes, 1204
Platelet aggregation, 124, 125f, 127, 127f
in thrombotic microangiopathies, 1010
Platelet contraction, 127
Platelet count(s), 649
bleeding related to reduced, 650–653, 651t
Platelet effects, of endothelium, 126
Platelet endothelial cell adhesion molecule (PECAM-1), 53f, 54t, 56
Platelet functions, defective, bleeding disorders related to, 653
Platelet-activating factor (PAF)
in asthma, 726
in immediate hypersensitivity, 208–209, 208f
in inflammation, 70, 74t
in necrotizing enterocolitis, 483
in septic shock, 142f
Platelet-derived growth factor (PDGF), 95t, 96
in angiogenesis, 109
in atherosclerosis, 525f
in scar formation, 110
Platelet-derived growth factor A (PDGF-A), in glioblastoma, 1403
Platelet-derived growth factor-ß chain (PDGF-ß chain), oncogene for, 293, 295t
Platelet-derived growth factor receptor-α (PDGFRA), in gastrointestinal stomal tumors, 827
Platelet-derived growth factor receptor *(PDGF-R)* gene, 295t
Platybasia, 1286
PLCγ (phospholipase Cγ), 56, 98f, 99, 99f
Pleiotropism, 150
Pleomorphic adenoma, 271
of salivary gland, 791–792, 792f
Pleomorphic rhabdomyosarcoma, 1322
Pleomorphism, 273, 274f
Pleura, 766–770
Pleural effusions, 766–767, 766t
in right-sided heart failure, 563
in systemic lupus erythematosus, 234
in tuberculosis, 386
inflammatory, 766–767, 766t
noninflammatory, 766t, 767
Pleural plaques, due to asbestos exposure, 736, 736f, 768
Pleural tumors, 768–770, 768f, 769f
Pleuritic pain, in tuberculosis, 384
Pleuritis, 750
hemorrhagic, 766t, 767
in systemic lupus erythematosus, 234
obliterative fibrous, due to tuberculosis, 386
serofibrinous, 766, 766t
suppurative, 766t, 767
Plexogenic pulmonary arteriopathy, 744–745
PLP (proteolipid protein), 1398
Plummer syndrome, 1175
Plummer-Vinson syndrome, 645, 776
PM_{10} (particulates), as air pollutants, 428t, 429–430, 429t
PML (progressive multifocal leukoencephalopathy), 1376–1377, 1377f
PML (promyelocytic leukemia), acute, 692, 694f
PMP22 (peripheral myelin protein 22), 1326–1327
PMS gene, 307
PMS2 gene, 307
PNET (primitive neuroectodermal tumor), 500t, 1301–1302
Pneumatosis intestinalis, 483, 483f
Pneumococcal pneumonia, 362f
Pneumoconiosis(es), 732–737
asbestosis as, 735–737, 736f
classification of, 733t
coal workers,' 39, 733–734, 734f
pathogenesis of, 732–733
silicosis as, 734–735, 735f
Pneumocystis carinii pneumonia, 756
Pneumocytes, 713
Pneumolysin, 373
Pneumonia(s), 350f
aspiration, 747t, 752
bacterial, 748–751, 749f, 750f
broncho-, 749, 749f, 750
chronic, 747t, 753–755, 754f–756f
community-acquired
acute, 747t, 748–751, 749f, 750f
atypical, 747t, 751–752
cryptogenic (bronchiolitis obliterans) organizing, 731, 732f
Haemophilus influenzae, 748
in immunocompromised host, 747t, 755–756, 756t
interstitial
acute, 716
desquamative, 729, 740, 740f
nonspecific, 731
usual, 729, 731f
Klebsiella pneumoniae, 748
Legionella pneumophila, 749
lobar, 749–750, 749f
Moraxella catarrhalis, 748
mycoplasmal, 751
necrotizing, 747t
nosocomial, 747t, 752
organization of exudates in, 750, 750f
pneumococcal, 362f, 748
Pneumocystis carinii, 756

Pneumonia(s) *(Continued)*
Pseudomonas, 379, 748–749
Staphylococcus aureus, 748
Streptococcus pneumoniae, 748
viral, 751–752
Pneumonia alba, 391
Pneumonic plague, 380
Pneumonitis
cytomegalovirus, 368
hypersensitivity, 739, 739f
radiation, 440, 737
Pneumothorax, 714, 767–768
spontaneous idiopathic, 767
tension, 714, 768
PNH (paroxysmal nocturnal hemoglobinuria), 67b, 245, 636, 636f
Podocin, 984
Podocytes, of glomerulus, 957f–959f, 958, 959
Point mutations, 147, 148, 148f, 149f
Poisons. *See* Toxin(s).
pol gene, in human immunodeficiency virus, 247, 247f
Polarity, loss of, in malignant tumors, 274
Poliomyelitis, 364
encephalitis due to, 1374–1375
Poliovirus, 347t, 359, 364
Polyangiitis, microscopic, 537t, 539f, 540–541
Polyarteritis, microscopic, 537t, 539f, 540–541
glomerular lesions in, 993
Polyarteritis nodosa (PAN), 212t, 239–240, 537t, 539f, 540
Polychlorinated biphenyls (PCBs), 435
Polycyclic aromatic hydrocarbons, 431–432
as carcinogens, 321t, 322
Polycystic kidney disease (PKD)
autosomal-dominant (adult), 962–964, 962t, 964f, 965f
autosomal-recessive (childhood), 962t, 964–965, 965f
bile duct anomalies and, 916, 916f
Polycystic liver disease, 915–916, 916f, 964
Polycystic ovarian disease (PCOD), 1092–1093, 1093f
Polycystin-1, 963
Polycystin-2, 963
Polycythemia, 649, 649t
paraneoplastic, 334t
Polycythemia vera, 649, 699–700, 699f
Polydactyly, 471f, 473
Polydipsia, in diabetes, 1202, 1202f
Polydystrophy, pseudo-Hurler, 161t
Polyglucosan bodies, 1352
Polyglutamine diseases, 184
Polykaryons, multinucleate, in herpes simplex virus infections, 777
Polymer(s), exposure to, 432
Polymerase chain reaction (PCR) analysis, 188, 188f, 189f
of cancer, 337
of infectious agents, 361
Polymicrogyria, 1354
Polymorphic amyloid degeneration, of corneal, 1430
Polymorphic reticulosis, 784
Polymorphisms, 150
length, 190, 190f
restriction fragment, 189–190, 190f
single nucleotide, 146, 190–191
site, 189
Polymorphonuclear leukocyte(s), origin and differentiation of, 621f
Polymyositis, 1343
Polyneuropathy(ies)
familial amyloid, 1332, 1333t
infectious, 1331–1332
Polyol pathway, in diabetes mellitus, 1198–1199
Polyoma virus nephropathy, 1000, 1000f
Polyostotic fibrous dysplasia, 1300
Polyp(s), 271, 271f
adenomatous, of colon, 858, 858f, 859–861, 860f, 861f
endocervical, 1073.1073f
endometrial, 1085
fibroepithelial, 1238
of ureter, 1025
fibrovascular, of esophagus, 806
fundic gland, 821–822
gastric, 821–822, 822f
juvenile, 822
hamartomatous, 859, 859f
hyperplastic, 858–859, 858f, 859f
inflammatory
of biliary tract, 934
of esophagus, 806
of stomach, 822, 822f
juvenile
gastric, 822
of colon, 859
nasal, 783, 783f
of colon, 857–859, 858f, 859f
pedunculated, 857, 858f
Peutz-Jeghers, 822, 859, 859f
pseudo-, in ulcerative colitis, 849, 849f, 850f
retention, 859
sessile, 857, 858f
sinonasal, in cystic fibrosis, 495
vocal cord, 786
Polyphagia, in diabetes, 1202
Polypoid cancer, 271
Polyposis, familial adenomatous, 284–285, 861–862, 862f, 1151
Polyradiculoneuropathy, inflammatory demyelinating
acute, 1331
chronic, 1331
Polyradiculopathy, 1334–1335
Polyuria, in diabetes, 1202, 1202f
POMC (pro-opiomelanocortin)
in lung cancer, 333
in obesity, 463f, 464b
POMC/CART neurons, 463f, 464b
Pompe disease, 161t, 167, 167f, 168t
Pontiac fever, 749
"Popcorn cell," 689, 689f
Pores of Kohn, 713, 721
Pork tapeworm, 839
Poroma, eccrine, 1238
Porphyria, 1263–1264, 1264f
acute intermittent, 1333t
Porphyromonas spp, 393
Porta hepatis, 878
Portal hypertension, 883–885, 885f
esophageal varices due to, 802–803, 803f
idiopathic, 918
Portal tracts, 878, 879f
Portal vein, 879f
obstruction of, 917–918
Portal vein thrombosis, 917–918
splenomegaly due to, 704
Portosystemic shunts, 884–885
Port-wine stains, 498, 547
Positional cloning, 146, 147f
Postconcussive syndrome, 1357
Postencephalitic parkinsonism, 1373, 1391
Posterior chamber, of eye, 1422f, 1430f
Posterior fossa anomalies, 1355, 1356f
Posterior pituitary, 1158
syndromes of, 1163–1164
Posterior polymorphous dystrophy, 1428
Posterior scleritis, 1423
Posterior synechiae, 1432
Posterior vitreous detachment, 1434, 1439
Postinfectious glomerulonephritis, 976
Postinfectious sprue, 844
Postmenopausal changes, in endometrium, 1082–1083
Postmenopausal osteoporosis, 1283f, 1284
Postnatal chromosome analysis, 187–188
Postoperative events, obesity and, 465t
Postpartum changes, in breast, 1121
Postpartum renal failure, 1011
Postpartum thyroiditis, 1171
Postpolio syndrome, 1375
Poststreptococcal glomerulonephritis, 212t, 359, 974–976, 975t, 976f
Postterm infants, 476
Posttraumatic dementia, 1360
Posttraumatic hydrocephalus, 1360
Pott, Percival, 282, 319
Pott disease, 386, 1291
Potter sequence, 471–472, 472f
Pouch of Douglas, 828
Power plants, air pollution from, 429
Poxviruses, 359
PP (pancreatic polypeptide) cells, 1189
PP (pancreatic polypeptide)—secreting endocrine tumors, 1207
PPAR(s) (peroxisome proliferator—activated receptors), 100
PPARγ (peroxisome proliferator—activated receptor gamma), and insulin resistance, 1196, 1196f
PPD (purified protein derivative), 381
PPNAD (primary pigmented nodular adrenal disease), 1208–1209
PPROM (preterm premature rupture of placental membranes), 477
PRAD (parathyroid adenoma 1) gene, 1185
Prader-Willi syndrome, 186–187, 186f
Precancerous conditions, 287–288
Preconditioning, 582
Precursor B- and T-cell neoplasms, 670–673, 671t, 672f
Preeclampsia, 920, 1106–1110
clinical course of, 1110
fetal growth restriction due to, 478
morphology of, 1109–1110, 1110f
pathogenesis of, 1106–1107, 1109f
Pregnancy
age at full-term, and breast cancer, 1132
breast changes during, 1121, 1121f
cardiomyopathy in, 603
cigarette smoking during, 420–421
cocaine use during, 425
disorder(s) of, 1105–1114
early, 1105, 1106f
gestational trophoblastic disease as, 1110–1114, 1110t, 1111f–1114f
late, 1105–1110, 1106f–1110f
ectopic, 1105, 1106f
folate during, 459
hemolytic-uremic syndrome in, 1011
hepatic disease associated with, 920–921, 920f
hypertrophy of uterus during, 7, 7f
intrauterine growth restriction during, 1110
lead exposure during, 433
listeriosis during, 375
phenylketonuria during, 487–488
pyelonephritis during, 999
radiation exposure during, 436, 439
rubella during, 355
sexually transmitted infections during, 355–356
theca lutein hyperplasia of, 1092–1093
toxemia of, 1106–1110, 1109f, 1110f
fetal growth restriction due to, 478
Treponema pallidum during, 355
Pregnancy luteoma, 1104

"Pregnancy tumor," 778t
Prekallikrein, 65
Premature infants. *See* Preterm infants.
Premature rupture of placental membranes (PROM), 477
Prematurity, 476–478
  retinopathy of, 482
Premutations, 183, 189f
Prenatal chromosome analysis, 187
Preprocollagen, 104
Prerenal azotemia, due to heart failure, 563
Presenilin-1 (PS1), 1389, 1389t
Presenilin-2 (PS2), 1389, 1389t
Pressure, atrophy due to, 9
Pressure-overload hypertrophy, 561, 561f
Preterm infants, 476–478
  germinal matrix—intraventricular hemorrhage in, 484
  immaturity of organ systems in, 478–479, 479f
  necrotizing enterocolitis in, 483, 483f
  retinopathy in, 482
Preterm premature rupture of placental membranes (PPROM), 477
Pretibial myxedema, 1172, 1173
Prevotella spp, 393
Primary CNS lymphoma (PCNSL), 1408
Primary cortical hyperplasia, 1208–1209
Primary follicles, of lymph nodes, 662
Primary irritant dermatitis, 1254t
Primary pigmented nodular adrenal disease (PPNAD), 1208–1209
Primary spongiosa, 1278, 1278f
Primary union, 111–113, 112f
Primitive embryonal tumor, 1223
Primitive neuroectodermal tumor (PNET), 500t, 1301–1302
Prinzmetal angina, 575
Prion(s), 346–347
Prion diseases, 1351t, 1380–1382, 1381f
Prion protein (PrP), 260, 346–347, 1380, 1381f
PRKAR1 gene, 614
PRNP gene, 1380
Procallus, 1288
Procarcinogens, 320
Procoagulant effects, of endothelium, 126, 126f
Procollagen, 104, 105f
Progesterone receptors, in breast carcinoma, 1147, 1148f
Proglottids, 839
Prognathism, 1161
Programmed cell death, 26
Progressive bulbar palsy, 1397
Progressive familial intrahepatic cholestasis 1 (PFIC-1), 889
Progressive familial intrahepatic cholestasis 2 (PFIC-2), 889
Progressive familial intrahepatic cholestasis 3 (PFIC-3), 889–890
Progressive massive fibrosis (PMF), in coal workers' pneumoconiosis, 734, 734f
Progressive multifocal leukoencephalopathy (PML), 1376–1377, 1377f
Progressive muscular atrophy, 1397
Progressive supranuclear palsy (PSP), 1390, 1391
Prolactinemia, 1160–1161, 1163
Prolactinomas, 1160–1161, 1161f
Proliferation centers, 673
Proliferative breast changes
  with atypia, 1129, 1130t
  without atypia, 1127–1129, 1128f, 1129f, 1130t
Proliferative fasciitis, 1318
Proliferative myositis, 1318
Proliferative rate, in breast carcinoma, 1148
Proliferative vitreoretinopathy, 1436
Prolymphocytes, 673, 673f, 674
Prolymphocytic transformation, 674
PROM (premature rupture of placental membranes), 477
Promastigote, 403
Promoter(s), in carcinogenesis, 319–320, 320f, 321–322, 321f, 323
Promoter region mutations, in ß-thalassemia, 632, 632f
Promotion, of carcinogenesis, 319–320, 320f, 321–322, 321f, 323
Promyelocytic leukemia (PML), acute, 692, 694f
Pro-opiomelanocortin (POMC)
  in lung cancer, 333
  in obesity, 463f, 464b
Propagation, 17
Properdin deficiency, 244
Propionate, 641
Propionibacterium acnes, 1264–1265
Proptosis, 1423, 1423f
Propylthiouracil, 1165–1166
Prostacyclin, 68, 69f
Prostaglandin(s), in inflammation, 68, 69, 69f, 70f, 74t
Prostaglandin D_2 (PGD_2), 68, 69, 69f
  in asthma, 726
  in immediate hypersensitivity, 208, 208f
Prostaglandin E_2 (PGE_2), 68, 69, 69f
Prostaglandin $F_{2\alpha}$ ($PGF_{2\alpha}$), 68, 69, 69f
Prostaglandin G_2 (PGG_2), 69f
Prostaglandin H_2 (PGH_2), 69f
Prostaglandin I_2 (PGI_2), 68, 69, 69f
  inhibition of platelet aggregation by, 126, 127f
Prostaglandin synthesis, by gastric mucosa, 811
Prostaglandin-H synthase, 418
Prostate, 1047–1056
  benign enlargement of, 1048–1050, 1049f
  inflammations of, 1047–1048
  normal anatomy of, 1047, 1047f
  transurethral resection of, 1050
  tumor(s) of, 1050–1056, 1052f–1054f
  zones of, 1047, 1047f
Prostate acid phosphatase, as tumor marker, 339t
Prostate cancer, 1050–1056
  clinical course of, 1054–1056
  etiology of, 1051
  grading and staging of, 1053–1054, 1054f
  incidence of, 1050–1051
  metastatic, 1051–1052, 1052f
  morphology of, 1051–1053, 1052f, 1053f
  spread of, 1051–1052
  stromal microenvironment and, 313
Prostatectomy, radical, 1055
Prostate-specific antigen (PSA), 338, 339t, 1054–1056
Prostate-specific membrane antigen (PSMA), 338, 339t
Prostatic hyperplasia, benign, 1048–1050, 1049f
Prostatic intraepithelial neoplasia (PIN), high-grade, 1053
Prostatitis, 1047–1048
Prosthetic valve(s), complications of, 600–601, 600f, 600t
Prosthetic valve endocarditis, 596
Protease(s), 16, 312
Protease-activated receptors (PARs), 65–67, 67f
  in coagulation cascade, 128
Protease-antiprotease theory, of emphysema, 719–720, 720f
Proteasome, 10
Protective antigen, of anthrax, 375, 376f
Protein(s)
  aggregation of abnormal, 39
  heat-shock, 38
  intracellular accumulation of, 37–39, 37f, 38f
Protein(s) *(Continued)*
  oxidative modification of, 16–17
  unfolded, 15
Protein C, in hemostasis, 125, 130
Protein cleavage, in apoptosis, 27
Protein compartments, somatic and visceral, 448
Protein deficiency, 448
Protein F, 358
Protein folding, 37–38, 37f
Protein kinase B, 99
Protein kinase C (PKC)
  in diabetes mellitus, 1198
  in signal transduction, 99
Protein phosphatase, in cell cycle, 290
Protein reabsorption droplets, in proximal renal tubules, 37, 37f
Protein S, in coagulation cascade, 130
Protein synthesis, reduction in, 15
Protein-aggregation diseases, 39
Proteinases, as regulators of angiogenesis, 109
Protein-calorie malnutrition, atrophy due to, 9
Protein-energy malnutrition (PEM), 447–449, 448f, 449t
Protein—iron complex, 644
Protein-losing gastroenteropathy, 821
  in Crohn disease, 849
Proteinopathies, 39
Proteinosis, pulmonary alveolar, 741, 741f
Proteinuria, 960, 967t
  Bence Jones, 1005, 1006
  in diabetic nephropathy, 990–991
  in nephrotic syndrome, 978
  in sickle cell disease nephropathy, 1011
Proteoglycans
  in extracellular matrix, 103f, 106
  in immediate hypersensitivity, 208
Proteolipid protein (PLP), 1398
Proteomics, 146, 316b, 338
Prothrombin, 65
  in coagulation cascade, 129f
Prothrombin gene mutation, 131
Prothrombin time (PT), 649
Prothrombotic properties, of endothelium, 126, 126f
Proton pump, in gastric acid secretion, 811
Protooncogenes, 100
  defined, 292
  discovery of, 293
  dominance in, 288
  for cyclins and cyclin-dependent kinases, 295t, 298
  for growth factor receptors, 294–296, 295t
  for growth factors, 293–294, 295t
  for nonreceptor-associated tyrosine kinase, 295t, 297, 298f
  for transcription factors, 295t, 297–298, 299f
  functions of proteins encoded by, 293
  insertional mutagenesis of, 293
  localization and functions of, 293, 294f
  nomenclature for, 293
  overexpression of
    due to gene amplification, 315
    translocation-induced, 314–315
  signal-transducing, 295t, 296–297, 297f
Protozoa, intestinal, 353
Protozoal infection(s), 401–406
  African trypanosomiasis due to, 405
  agents for, 346t, 351, 351t
  babesiosis due to, 403, 403f
  Chagas disease due to, 405–406
  leishmaniasis due to, 403–406, 404f
  malaria due to, 401–403, 402f
  sexually transmitted, 356t
Proud flesh, 115
Proximal renal tubules, reabsorption droplets in, 37, 37f

Proximal tubular cells, 959
PrP (prion protein), 260, 346–347, 1380, 1381f
PRSS1 (cationic trypsinogen) gene, and pancreatitis, 942, 945
Pruritus, due to cholestasis, 888
PS1 (presenilin-1), 1389, 1389t
PS2 (presenilin-2), 1389, 1389t
PSA (prostate-specific antigen), 338, 339t, 1054–1056
Psammoma bodies, 41
  in thyroid carcinoma, 1178, 1180
P-selectin, 53f, 54, 54t, 55b, 56f
  in hemostasis, 127
Pseudoaneurysms, 530f, 531, 584
Pseudoangiomatous stromal hyperplasia (PASH), 1151
Pseudoarthrosis, 1289
Pseudocysts, pancreatic, 945, 947, 947f
Pseudoepitheliomatous hyperplasia, 380
Pseudogene, 1213
Pseudogout, 1314, 1314f
  due to hemochromatosis, 910
Pseudohermaphroditism, 181
Pseudo-Hurler polydystrophy, 161t
Pseudohypertrophy, 1338
Pseudohyphae, of *Candida,* 398, 398f
Pseudohypoparathyroidism, 1188–1189
Pseudomembranous colitis, 836, 837–838, 837f
Pseudomonas aeruginosa, 352, 353, 378–379
  in cystic fibrosis, 379, 493, 494, 495
Pseudomonas infection, 378–379, 379f
Pseudomonas pneumonia, 379, 748–749
Pseudomonas vasculitis, 379f
Pseudomyxoma peritonei, 279, 872, 1097, 1098f
Pseudoneuroma, 1335
Pseudo-obstruction, intestinal, 855t
Pseudopalisading pattern, 1402, 1403f
Pseudo-Pelger-Hüet cells, in myelodysplastic syndromes, 695, 696f
Pseudophakic bullous keratopathy, 1429
Pseudopolyps, in ulcerative colitis, 849, 849f, 850f
Pseudopseudohypoparathyroidism, 1189
Pseudorosettes
  perivascular, 1405, 1405f
  pineocytomatous, 1223
Pseudosarcomatous fasciitis, 1318, 1318f
Pseudotumor, inflammatory, of esophagus, 806
Psilocybin, 426
PSMA (prostate-specific membrane antigen), 338, 339t
Psoriasis, 1256–1257, 1257f
  pustular, 1256
Psoriatic arthritis, 1310
PSP (progressive supranuclear palsy), 1390, 1391
PSTT (placental site trophoblastic tumor), 1114, 1114f
Psychomotor stimulants, abuse of, 424t, 425–426
Psychosis, Korsakoff, 457, 457f
PT (prothrombin time), 649
PTCA (percutaneous transluminal coronary angioplasty), 551
PTCH (patched) gene, 287t, 306, 1244–1245, 1246f
PTEN gene, 300t, 305
  in breast cancer, 1134
  in endometrial hyperplasia, 1085, 1086f
  in glioblastoma, 1403
  in prostate cancer, 1051
Pteroylmonoglutamic acid deficiency, 640t, 642–643, 642f
Pterygium, 1426
PTH. *See* Parathyroid hormone (PTH).
PTHRP. *See* Parathyroid hormone (PTH)-related protein (PTHRP).
PTT (partial thromboplastin time), 649–650
Pulmonary. *See also under* Lung(s); Respiratory.
Pulmonary abscess, 747t, 753, 753f
  due to pneumonia, 750
  primary cryptogenic, 753
  pyemic, 753, 753f
  staphylococcal, 373, 373f
Pulmonary airway malformation, congenital, 713
Pulmonary alveolar proteinosis (PAP), 741, 741f
Pulmonary arteriopathy, plexogenic, 744–745
Pulmonary atresia, 564t, 571
Pulmonary congestion
  acute, 122
  chronic, 122
Pulmonary disease(s)
  diffuse interstitial (infiltrative, restrictive), 728–741, 729t, 730f
    cryptogenic organizing pneumonia as, 731, 732f
    desquamative interstitial pneumonia as, 740, 740f
    due to complications of therapies, 737, 737t
    fibrosing, 729–737
    granulomatous, 737–739, 738f, 739f
    hypersensitivity pneumonitis as, 739, 739f
    idiopathic pulmonary fibrosis as, 729–731, 730f, 731f
    nonspecific interstitial pneumonia as, 731, 732f
    obstructive *vs.,* 716–717
    pneumoconioses as, 732–737, 733t, 734f–736f
    pulmonary alveolar proteinosis as, 741, 741f
    pulmonary eosinophilia as, 740
    pulmonary involvement in collagen vascular diseases as, 731–732
    respiratory bronchiolitis—associated, 740–741
    sarcoidosis as, 737–739, 738f, 739f
    smoking-related, 740–741, 740f
  drug-induced, 737, 737t
  infectious, 747–756, 747t
    aspiration pneumonia as, 747t, 752
    chronic pneumonia as, 747t, 753–755, 754f–756f
    community-acquired acute pneumonias as, 747t, 748–751, 749f, 750f
    community-acquired atypical pneumonia as, 747t, 751–752
    in lung transplant patients, 757
    lung abscess as, 747t, 753, 753f
    necrotizing pneumonia as, 747t
    nosocomial pneumonia as, 747t, 752
    pneumonia in immunocompromised host as, 747t, 755–756, 756t
    severe acute respiratory syndrome (SARS) as, 752
    with HIV infection, 756
  obstructive, 717–728, 718t
    asthma as, 718t, 723–727, 724f, 725f, 727f
    bronchiectasis as, 718t, 727–728, 728f
    bronchiolitis as, 718t, 722
    chronic, 717–728, 718t
    chronic bronchitis as, 718t, 722–723, 723f
    emphysema as, 717–722, 718f–721f, 718t, 721t
    restrictive *vs.,* 716–717
    small airway disease as, 718t, 722
  of vascular origin, 742–747
    diffuse pulmonary hemorrhage syndromes as, 745–747, 746f
    Goodpasture syndrome as, 745–746
    idiopathic pulmonary hemosiderosis as, 746
Pulmonary disease(s) *(Continued)*
    pulmonary embolism, hemorrhage, and infarction as, 742–743, 742f
    pulmonary hypertension as, 743–745, 744f, 745f
    Wegener granulomatosis as, 746–747
  radiation-induced, 737
Pulmonary edema, 122, 714–715, 714t
  due to microvascular injury, 714t, 715
  hemodynamic (cardiogenic), 714–715, 714t
  in left-sided heart failure, 562
  in sudden infant death syndrome, 496
Pulmonary embolism, 136, 136f, 742, 742f, 743
  due to deep venous thrombosis, 544
  hormone replacement therapy and, 427–428
  oral contraceptives and, 427
Pulmonary eosinophilia, 740
Pulmonary fibrosis, idiopathic, 729–731, 730f, 731f
Pulmonary hemorrhage, 742–743, 742f, 745–747, 746f
Pulmonary hemosiderosis, idiopathic, 746
Pulmonary hypertension, 743–745, 744f, 745f
  in systemic sclerosis, 239
Pulmonary hypoplasia, 713
Pulmonary infarct, 742–743, 742f
Pulmonary infection(s), 747–756, 747t
  aspiration pneumonia as, 747t, 752
  barriers to, 353
  chronic pneumonia as, 747t, 753–755, 754f–756f
  community-acquired pneumonia as
    acute, 747t, 748–751, 749f, 750f
    atypical, 747t, 751–752
  in lung transplant patients, 757
  lung abscess as, 747t, 753, 753f
  necrotizing pneumonia as, 747t
  nosocomial pneumonia as, 747t, 752
  pneumonia in immunocompromised host as, 747t, 755–756, 756t
  severe acute respiratory syndrome (SARS) as, 752
  viral, 347t
  with HIV infection, 756
Pulmonary interstitium, 713
Pulmonary involvement, in collagen vascular diseases, 731–732
Pulmonary lobule, 712
Pulmonary sepsis, chronic, brain abscess due to, 1371
Pulmonary sequestration, 799
Pulmonary stenosis, 564t, 571
Pulmonary surfactant, 713
  in neonatal respiratory distress syndrome, 481–482
Pulmonary thromboembolism, 136, 136f
Pulmonary valve, 558
Pulmonary venous connection, total anomalous, 564t, 570
Pulp chamber, 774, 774f
Pulseless disease, 537
Punch-drunk syndrome, 1360
Punctate keratitis, 411
Punctum, 1269
PUNLMP (papillary urothelial neoplasms of low malignant potential), 1030
Pupil, 1422f, 1430f
Pupillary block, 1431
Pure red cell aplasia, 648
Purified protein derivative (PPD), 381
Purpura(s), 123
  Henoch-Schönlein, 650, 986–987, 990
  nonthrombocytopenic, 650
  thrombocytopenic
    autoimmune, 212t

Purpura(s) *(Continued)*
immune, 651–652
thrombotic, 652–653, 1009–1010, 1011
Pus, defined, 22, 49
Pustular psoriasis, 1256
Pustule, 1229
PVNS (pigmented villonodular synovitis), 1315, 1315f
Pyelonephritis
acute, 996, 998–1000, 999f, 1000f
and urinary tract infection, 996–998, 997f, 998f
chronic, 996, 1000–1002, 1001f
drug- and toxin-induced, 1002–1004, 1002f, 1003f, 1003t
in diabetes, 1201
xanthogranulomatous, 1001
Pyknosis, 12f, 20f, 21
Pylephlebitis, 704
Pyloric glands, 810
Pyloric sphincter, 810, 810f
Pyloric stenosis, 812
Pyogenic bacteria, 77
Pyogenic cocci, 349t
Pyogenic granuloma, 546f, 547
of oral cavity, 775, 776f
Pyogenic osteomyelitis, 1290–1291, 1291f
Pyonephrosis, 998–999
Pyridoxine, 450t, 458
Pyrogens, 84
exogenous *vs.* endogenous, 84
Pyuria, 999

Q

Q fever, 350
Queensland tick typhus, 396t
"Quick-frozen section," 336
Quiescent tissues, 90–91, 90f
Quinsy sore throat, 374

R

RA. *See* Rheumatoid arthritis (RA).
Rabies, encephalitis due to, 1375, 1375f
Rachitic rosary, 455
Racial differences, in breast cancer, 1132
Rad, 436
RAD51, 308, 308f
Radar, exposure to, 436t
Radial scar, of breast, 1128, 1129f
Radiation
ionizing, 436–441, 436t, 438t, 439f–441f
nonionizing, 436, 436t, 442
particulate, 436
ultraviolet, 436t, 441–442, 441t, 442f
Radiation carcinogenesis, 323–324
Radiation dermatitis, 440, 440f
Radiation enteritis, 841
Radiation enterocolitis, 841
Radiation exposure
and breast cancer, 1132
and lung cancer, 758
and thyroid carcinoma, 324, 1175, 1178
apoptosis due to, 26, 31
congenital anomalies due to, 473
neurologic effects of, 1400
Radiation injury, 436–442
acute, 437, 438t, 439
cellular mechanisms of, 437–438, 438t
delayed, 437, 438t, 439
Radiation pneumonitis, 440, 737
Radiation retinopathy, 1439
Radiation sickness, 437, 438t, 439
Radiation therapy
and bladder carcinoma, 1032
aplastic anemia due to, 647
effects of, 439
Radiation therapy *(Continued)*
for prostate cancer, 1055
white cell neoplasia due to, 667
Radiation-induced lung diseases, 737
Radio waves, exposure to, 436t
Radioisotopes, 436
Radiotherapy. *See* Radiation therapy.
Radon
as air pollutant, 430, 430t
cancer due to, 285t
RAF, 99f
RAGE proteins, 330
Ragged red fibers, 1341, 1341f, 1342, 1399
RANK (receptor activator for nuclear factor $_{F}$B), 1184, 1275, 1276f
RANKL (receptor activator for nuclear factor $_{F}$B ligand), 1184, 1275, 1276f
in rheumatoid arthritis, 1307
RANTES, 71
Rapid plasma reagin (RPR) test, 390
Rapidly progressive glomerulonephritis (RPGN), 967t, 975t, 976–978, 977f, 977t, 978f
RARα (retinoic acid receptor-α), in acute promyelocytic leukemia, 692
RAR (retinoic acid receptor), 475, 476f
RAREs (retinoic acid response elements), 475, 476f
RAS oncogene
as tumor marker, 339, 339t
in colorectal cancer, 317, 317f
in multistep carcinogenesis, 317, 317f
in pituitary adenoma, 1159
in signal transduction, 99, 99f, 295t, 296–297, 305
in thyroid carcinoma, 1177, 1180
model for action of, 297f
mutations in, 320–321
overexpression of growth factors due to, 293
Rathke cleft cyst, 1163
Raynaud phenomenon, 542–543, 543f
in systemic sclerosis, 239
RB (reticulate body), of *Chlamydia trachomatis*, 394
RB phosphorylation, in cell cycle, 289–290, 291f, 301
RB pocket, 300
RB (retinoblastoma susceptibility) protein, 100
RB tumor suppressor gene, 284, 299–302, 300t, 301f, 302f
RB1 gene, in pancreatic cancer, 950t
RBCs. *See* Red blood cell(s) (RBCs).
RBE (relative biologic effectiveness), 437
R-binders, 639
RBP (retinol-binding protein), 476f
RCA (right coronary artery), 557
atherosclerosis of, 572
in myocardial infarction, 578
RDS. *See* Respiratory distress syndrome (RDS).
Reabsorption droplets, in proximal renal tubules, 37, 37f
Reactive arthritis, 212t, 1309–1310
Reactive gastropathy, 816, 816f
Reactive nodules, of larynx, 786
Reactive oxygen intermediates (ROIs), in phagocytosis, 59–61, 60f
Reactive oxygen species, 14f, 16–17, 17f
defects in membrane permeability due to, 18
removal of, 17–18
Reactive proliferations
of white cells and nodes, 663–666, 664f–666f, 664t
pseudosarcomatous, 1318–1319, 1318f, 1319f
REAL (Revised European-American Classification of Lymphoid Neoplasms), 668
Recanalization, of thrombi, 134, 134f
Receptor(s), 97
defects in, 154
dimerization of, 98, 99f
in signal transduction, 98–100, 98f, 99f
seven transmembrane G-protein—coupled, 98f, 99–100
steroid hormone, 100
with intrinsic tyrosine kinase activity, 98–99, 98f, 99f
without intrinsic tyrosine kinase activity, 98f, 99
Receptor activator for nuclear factor $_{F}$B (RANK), 1184, 1275, 1276f
Receptor activator for nuclear factor $_{F}$B ligand (RANKL), 1184, 1275, 1276f
in rheumatoid arthritis, 1307
Receptor proteins, defects in, 156–158, 157f, 158f
Rectal ulcer, solitary, 842
Rectum
carcinoid tumors of, 867
vasculature of, 828
Red blood cell(s) (RBCs)
hemolytic anemia resulting from trauma to, 638, 638f
origin and differentiation of, 621f
reference ranges for, 623t
Red blood cell (RBC) distribution width, 623, 623t
Red cell aplasia, pure, 648
Red cell count, reference ranges for, 623t
Red hepatization stage, of lobar pneumonia, 750, 750f
Red infarction, 1364–1365, 1364f
Red neuron, 1350
Red pulp, of spleen, 702–703, 703f
Reduced penetrance, 150
Reed, Walter, 344
Reed-Sternberg cells, 686–687, 687f, 690, 691f
Reflux esophagitis, 804, 804f
Reflux nephropathy, 1000, 1001f
Refsum disease, 1442
Regenerating cluster, 1330
Regeneration, 48, 88, 88f, 89
mechanisms of, 101–103, 101f, 102f
of axon, 1351
of liver, 880
of muscle fiber, 1330
Regional enteritis, 847
Regional hemorrhagic fever viruses, 347t
Regression, of melanoma, 1236
Regulatory T cells, suppression by, 224f, 225
Regurgitation
during feeding, in phagocytosis, 61
functional, 589
Regurgitation/implantation theory, of endometriosis, 1083, 1084, 1084f
Reid index, 722
Reinnervation, 1326f, 1328, 1330
Reis-Buckler dystrophy, 1428
Reiter syndrome, 835, 1309
Rejection vasculitis, 220, 221f
Relapsing fever, 391–392
Relative biologic effectiveness (RBE), 437
Rem, 437
Renal ablation focal segmental glomerulosclerosis, 984
Renal arteriosclerosis, in diabetes, 1201
Renal artery, 956
Renal artery stenosis, 1008–1009, 1009f
Renal atherosclerosis, in diabetes, 1201
Renal calculi, 960, 1014–1015, 1014t, 1015f
Renal cell carcinoma, 1016–1018, 1017f, 1018f
Renal columns of Bertin, 956
Renal cortex, 956
Renal cysts, simple, 962t, 966

Renal disease(s), 960–1019
calculi as, 1014–1015, 1014t, 1015f
clinical manifestations of, 960–961, 961t
cystic, 962–966, 962t, 963f–966f
edema due to, 122
end-stage, 961
epidemiology of, 960
glomerular, 966–993
acute glomerulonephritis as, 973–976, 976f
chronic glomerulonephritis as, 975t, 989–990, 989f
clinical manifestations of, 967, 967t
focal segmental glomerulosclerosis as, 973, 973f, 974t, 982–984, 983f
hereditary syndromes of isolated hematuria as, 988–989, 988f
histologic alterations in, 967–968
IgA nephropathy as, 975t, 986–988, 987f, 990
mechanisms of progression in, 972–973, 973f, 974f
membranoproliferative glomerulonephritis as, 975t, 984–985, 985f, 986f
membranous glomerulopathy as, 975t, 979–981, 980f
minimal change disease as, 975t, 981–982, 981f, 982f
nephrotic syndrome as, 960, 967t, 978–979, 979t
pathogenesis of, 968–972, 968t, 969f, 971f, 972f, 975t
primary, 966–967, 967t, 975t
rapidly progressive (crescentic) glomerulonephritis as, 967t, 975t, 976–978, 977f, 977t, 978f
secondary, 966, 967t
with systemic diseases, 990–993, 991f, 992f
in systemic lupus erythematosus, 228t
neoplastic, 1015–1019
benign, 1015–1016
malignant, 1016–1019, 1017f–1019f
of blood vessels, 1006–1012
accelerated nephrosclerosis as, 1007–1008
atheroembolic, 1011, 1011f
atherosclerotic ischemic, 1011
benign nephrosclerosis as, 1006–1007, 1007f
diffuse cortical necrosis as, 1011–1012, 1012f
malignant hypertension as, 1007–1008, 1008f
renal artery stenosis as, 1008–1009, 1009f
renal infarcts as, 1012
sickle cell disease nephropathy as, 1011
thrombotic microangiopathies as, 1009–1011, 1010f
of tubules and interstitium, 960, 993–1006
acute tubular necrosis as, 993–996, 994f, 995f
hypercalcemia and nephrocalcinosis as, 1005
in multiple myeloma, 1005–1006, 1006t
tubulointerstitial nephritis as, 996–1004, 996t, 997f–1003f, 1004t
urate nephropathy as, 1004–1005, 1005f
polycystic
adult, 962–964, 962t, 964f, 965f
bile duct anomalies and, 916, 916f
childhood, 962t, 964–965, 965f
urinary tract obstruction as, 960, 1012–1014, 1013f
Renal dysplasia, cystic, 962, 963f
Renal effects, of shock, 142
Renal failure
acute, 960–961
chronic, 960, 961, 961t, 967t
Renal failure *(Continued)*
anemia due to, 649
hypercalcemia due to, 42
hyperparathyroidism due to, 1187–1188
postpartum, 1011
Renal fibroma, 1015
Renal hamartoma, 1015
Renal hypoplasia, 961
Renal infarcts, 1012
Renal insufficiency, 961
Renal interstitium, 959
disorders of, 996–1006
Renal medulla, 956
cystic diseases of, 962t, 965–966, 966f
Renal osteodystrophy, 1287–1288
Renal papillary adenoma, 1015
Renal pelvis, 956
transitional papillary carcinoma of, 1004
urothelial carcinomas of, 1018–1019, 1019f
Renal pyramids, 956
Renal reserve, diminished, 961
Renal stones. *See* Nephrolithiasis.
Renal transplant, rejection of, 218–222, 219f–221f
Renal tubular defect(s), 960, 993–1006
acute tubular necrosis as, 993–996, 994f, 995f
hypercalcemia and nephrocalcinosis as, 1005
in multiple myeloma, 1005–1006, 1006t
tubulointerstitial nephritis as, 996–1004, 996t, 997f–1003f, 1004t
urate nephropathy as, 1004–1005, 1005f
Renal tubules, thyroidization of, 1001
Renal tumors, 1015–1019
benign, 1015–1016
malignant, 1016–1019, 1017f–1019f
Renal-retinal dysplasia, 966
Rendu-Osler-Weber syndrome, oral manifestations of, 778t
Renin-angiotensin system, in blood pressure regulation, 527, 527f, 529f
Renomedullary interstitial cell tumor, 1015
Renovascular hypertension, 526
Repair, 107–116
angiogenesis in, 107–109, 108f, 109t
by fibrosis, 115, 116f
by healing, 88–89, 107
cutaneous wound, 111–115
by first intention, 111–113, 112f
by second intention, 112f, 113, 113f
complications of, 114–115, 115f
factors influencing, 114, 114t
phases of, 111, 111f
strength of, 113–114
summary of, 114
by regeneration, 88, 89
factors influencing, 107
general features of, 107
granulation tissue in, 107, 107f
overview of, 116, 116f
scar formation in, 110–111, 110f
Reperfusion, of myocardial infarct, 581–582, 583f
Reperfusion injury
in ischemic bowel disease, 852
in myocardial infarction, 581
Replication error phenotype, 307
Replicative senescence, 42–43, 43f, 44f, 308
Reproductive system. *See also* Female genital tract; Male genital tract.
alcohol effect on, 422t, 424
occupational exposures and, 431t
Residual bodies, 10, 32, 32f
Resistin, and insulin resistance, 1196, 1196f
Resolution stage, of lobar pneumonia, 750
Resolvins, 70
Resorption atelectasis, 714, 714f
Resorption pits, 1275
"Respirator brain," 1361
Respiratory. *See also under* Lung(s); Pulmonary.
Respiratory bronchioles, 712
Respiratory bronchiolitis—associated interstitial lung disease, 740–741
Respiratory distress syndrome (RDS)
acute (adult), 715–716
clinical course of, 716
due to amniotic fluid embolism, 137
etiology of, 715, 715t
morphology of, 715, 715f
pathogenesis of, 85, 142f, 715–716, 717f
neonatal, 481–483, 481f, 482f
Respiratory effects, of obesity, 465t
Respiratory route, of transmission, 355
Respiratory syncytial virus, 347t
Respiratory system, occupational exposures and, 431t
Respiratory tract infection(s). *See* Pulmonary infection(s).
Response to injury hypothesis, 521–522, 522f
Restitution, in gastric mucosal barrier, 811
Restriction fragment length polymorphisms (RFLPs), 189–190, 190f
Restriction point, 100
Restrictocin, 400
RET oncogene, 285, 287t, 294–295, 295t
in Hirschsprung disease, 831
in MEN-2A, 1222
in thyroid carcinoma, 1177, 1178, 1182, 1183
Rete ovarii, 1081
Retention polyps, 859
Reticular hyperplasia, 666
Reticulate body (RB), of *Chlamydia trachomatis,* 394
Reticulocyte count
reference range for, 623t
with blood loss, 624
Reticulocytosis, in peripheral blood, in hemolytic anemia, 625
Reticuloendothelial system, 79, 79f
Reticulosis
midline malignant, 686
polymorphic, 784
Retina, 1434–1443
functional anatomy of, 1422f, 1434, 1436f
in age-related macular degeneration, 1422, 1441–1442, 1442f
in diabetes mellitus. *See* Retinopathy, diabetic.
in hypertension, 1436–1437, 1438f
retrolental fibroplasia of, 1439
Retinal, 450, 451, 451f
Retinal artery, occlusions of, 1440–1441, 1441f
Retinal degeneration, paraneoplastic, 1411t
Retinal detachment, 1434, 1436, 1437f
non-rhegmatogenous, 1436, 1437f
rhegmatogenous, 1436, 1437f
traction, 1439
Retinal exudate, 1434, 1436f
Retinal hemorrhage, 1434, 1436f, 1440f
Retinal infarct, 1437, 1438f
Retinal lymphoma, 1443
Retinal neoplasms, 1442–1443, 1443f
Retinal neovascularization, 1439, 1440f
Retinal pigment epithelium (RPE), 1434, 1436f
osseous metaplasia of, 1446
Retinal tears, 1436, 1437f
Retinal toxoplasmosis, 1433
Retinal vascular disease, 1436–1441
Retinal vasculitis, 1439
Retinal vein, occlusions of, 1441
Retinitis, 1442
cytomegalovirus, 368
Retinitis pigmentosa, 1434, 1442

Retinoblastoma, 1442–1443
  genetic and other markers for, 500t
  morphology of, 1442–1443, 1443f
  pathogenesis of, 299–302, 301f, 302f
  trilateral, 1442
Retinoblastoma susceptibility (RB) protein, 100
Retinocytoma, 1443
Retinoic acid, 450, 451f
  and congenital anomalies, 474, 475, 476f
Retinoic acid "differentiation therapy," for acute myelogenous leukemia, 695
Retinoic acid embryopathy, 474, 475, 476f
Retinoic acid receptor(s) (RAR, RXR), 475, 476f
Retinoic acid receptor-α (RARα), in acute promyelocytic leukemia, 692
Retinoic acid response elements (RAREs), 475, 476f
Retinoic acid—binding protein, cytoplasmic/cellular, 475, 476f
Retinoids, 450, 451f
Retinol, 450, 451, 451f
Retinol-binding protein (RBP), 476f
Retinopathy
  cancer-associated, 1442
  chloroquine, 1442
  diabetic, 1437–1439, 1438f, 1440f
    background (preproliferative), 1437–1439
    epidemiology of, 1205
    proliferative, 1439
  melanoma-associated, 1442
  of prematurity, 482
  radiation, 1439
  sickle, 1439
Retinyl palmitate, in cancer prevention, 466
ret/PTC fusion gene, in thyroid carcinoma, 1178, 1179, 1180
Retrobulbar neuritic, in multiple sclerosis, 1384
Retrolental fibroplasia, 482
Retroperitoneal fibrosis
  idiopathic, 873
  sclerosing, 1026
Retroperitonitis, sclerosing, 873
Retroviral syndrome, acute, 253
Retroviruses, acute transforming, 293
rev gene, in human immunodeficiency virus, 247, 247f
Revised European-American Classification of Lymphoid Neoplasms (REAL), 668
Reye syndrome, 905
RF (rheumatic fever), 212t, 359, 373, 593–595
RFLPs (restriction fragment length polymorphisms), 189–190, 190f
Rh incompatibility, 485, 485f
Rhabdomyoma, cardiac, 614
Rhabdomyosarcoma, 1321–1322
  alveolar, 1322, 1322f
  embryonal
    of bladder, 1033
    of skeletal muscle, 1322
    of vagina, 1071–1072, 1072f
  genetic and other markers for, 500t
  morphology of, 274f, 1321–1322, 1321f, 1322f
  pleomorphic, 1322
RHD (rheumatic heart disease), 135, 593–595, 594f, 595f, 597f
Rheumatic fever (RF), 212t, 359, 373, 593–595
Rheumatic heart disease (RHD), 135, 593–595, 594f, 595f, 597f
Rheumatoid arthritis (RA), 1305–1309
  amyloidosis with, 261
  clinical course of, 1307–1309, 1308f
  immune system in, 235
  juvenile, 1309
    uveitis in, 1433
  morphology of, 1306, 1306f, 1307f
  pathogenesis of, 1305–1307, 1308f
Rheumatoid arthritis (RA) *(Continued)*
  pulmonary involvement in, 731
  T cell—mediated hypersensitivity in, 215t
Rheumatoid factor, 1307
  in Sjögren syndrome, 235
Rheumatoid nodules, 1306, 1307f
Rheumatoid spondylitis, 1309
Rheumatoid vasculitis, 542
Rhinitis
  allergic, 783
  chronic, 783
  infectious, 783
Rhinovirus(es), 347t, 353, 357, 359
Rhizopus, 400
Riboflavin, 450t, 457
Richter syndrome, 674
Rickets, 453–455, 454f, 454t, 455f, 1287
Rickettsia africae, 396t
Rickettsia akari, 396t
Rickettsia australis, 396t
Rickettsia conorii, 396t
Rickettsia felis, 396t
Rickettsia japonica, 396t
Rickettsia prowazekii, 395, 396t
Rickettsia ricketsii, 395, 396t
Rickettsia sibirica, 396t
Rickettsia typhi, 396t
Rickettsiae, 346t, 349–350, 395–397, 395f, 396t, 397f
Rickettsialpox, 396t
Riedel thyroiditis, 1171
Right coronary artery (RCA), 557
  atherosclerosis of, 572
  in myocardial infarction, 578
Right dominant circulation, 557
Right ventricular cardiomyopathy, arrhythmogenic, 604, 604f
Right ventricular dysplasia, arrhythmogenic, 604, 604f
Right ventricular infarction, after myocardial infarction, 585–586
Right-sided heart failure, 563
Right-to-left shunts, 566, 569–570, 569f, 570f
Rim staining, 228
Ring abscess, 596
Ring chromosome, 174, 174f
Ring fiber, 1339
Ringed sideroblasts, in myelodysplastic syndromes, 695, 696f
Ristocetin agglutination test, 654–655
Ritter disease, 373
RNA viruses, oncogenic, 327
Robertsonian translocation, 174f, 175
Rocky Mountain spotted fever (RMSF), 350, 395, 396–397, 396t, 397f
Rod cells, 1350
Rodent ulcers, 279, 1242
Rodenticides, 434t, 435
Roentgen, 436
ROIs (reactive oxygen intermediates), in phagocytosis, 59–61, 60f
Rokitansky-Aschoff sinuses, 928, 933
Rolling, of leukocytes, 53, 53f
Rosenthal fibers, 1351–1352
Ross, Ronald, 344
Rotavirus, 347t, 348f
  gastroenteritis due to, 832–833, 833t
Roth spots, 598
Rotor syndrome, 888, 888t
Rouleaux formation, 84, 680
Rous, F. Peyton, 344
RPE (retinal pigment epithelium), 1434, 1436f
  osseous metaplasia of, 1446
RPGN (rapidly progressive glomerulonephritis), 967t, 975t, 976–978, 977f, 977t, 978f
RPR (rapid plasma reagin) test, 390
Rubber, exposure to, 432
Rubella, 347t
  during pregnancy, 355, 473
Rubella embryopathy, 473
Rubeola, 347t, 363–364, 364f
Ruffled border, 1275
Rugae, of gastric wall, 810
Russell bodies, 37, 680, 681
RXR (retinoic acid receptor), 475, 476f

S

SA (sinoatrial) node, 557
SAA (serum amyloid—associated) protein, 84, 260, 262
Saccular aneurysm, 531, 1366–1367, 1367f, 1368f
  in polycystic kidney disease, 964
  ruptured, 1366–1367
Sacrococcygeal teratomas, 499, 499f
Saddle embolus, 136
Sago spleen, 263
Salicylism, 428
Salivary gland(s), 790–795
  in cystic fibrosis, 493
  in Sjögren syndrome, 236, 236f
  inflammation of, 790, 791f
  sarcoidosis of, 738
Salivary gland neoplasm(s), 790–795, 791t
  acinic cell tumor as, 794
  adenoid cystic carcinoma as, 793–794, 794f
  mucoepidermoid carcinoma as, 793, 794f
  pleomorphic adenoma as, 791–792, 792f
  Warthin tumor as, 792–793, 793f
Salivary gland origin, mixed tumors of, 271, 271f
Salmonella, 353, 358
Salmonella enteritidis, 835
Salmonella enterocolitis, 834, 835, 836–837
Salmonella paratyphi, 836
Salmonella typhi, 353, 355, 359, 835, 836–837
Salmonella typhimurium, 835, 836
Salmonellosis, 835
Salpingitis
  suppurative, 1064, 1091
  tuberculous, 1091
Salpingo-oophoritis, 1064, 1064f
Salt-wasting syndrome, 1212, 1213
Sandhoff disease, 161t
SAP gene, 331, 371
Saphenous vein graft, autologous, 551
Sapporo-like viruses, gastroenteritis due to, 833, 833t
Sarcoglycans, 1327, 1337f, 1338, 1339t
Sarcoidosis, 737–739, 738f, 739f
Sarcolemma, 1327
Sarcoma(s), 271
  angio-, 550–551, 550f
    cardiac, 614
    hepatic, 923
    of breast, 1151
  carcino-, endometrial, 1088, 1089f
  cardiac, 614
  chondro-, 1298–1299, 1299f
    clear cell, 1298–1299
    dedifferentiated, 1298
    mesenchymal, 1299
  due to Paget disease, 1286
  endometrial, 1088–1089, 1089f
  Ewing, 1301–1302
    epidemiology of, 1301
    genetic and other markers of, 500t
    genetic basis for, 1301
    molecular diagnosis of, 337
    morphology of, 1301–1302, 1302f
    oncogenes in, 314t, 315
  fibro-
    congenital-infantile, 499

Sarcoma(s) *(Continued)*
of bone, 1301
of soft tissue, 1320, 1320f
granulocytic, 694
Kaposi, 548–550
chronic (classic, European), 548
clinical course of, 550
in AIDS, 256–257, 257f
lymphadenopathic (African, endemic), 548–549
morphology of, 549, 549f
of eyelid or conjunctiva, 1425
pathogenesis of, 549–550
transplant-associated (immunosuppression-associated), 549
leiomyo-, 1090, 1091f
lipo-, 1318, 1318f
of bladder, 1033
of breast, 1150–1151
osteo-, 1294–1296, 1294f, 1295f
chondroblastic, 1295, 1298
rhabdomyo-, 1321–1322, 1321f, 1322f
soft-tissue, chromosomal and genetic abnormalities in, 1316, 1317t
synovial, 1323, 1323f
Sarcoma botryoides, 1322
of bladder, 1033
of vagina, 1071–1072, 1072f
Sarcomere, 557, 1327, 1328f
Sarcoplasmic mass, 1339
Sarcoptes scabiei, 1269
SARS (severe acute respiratory syndrome), 752
Satellite cells, 91, 94, 1327
"Saturday night palsy," 1335
Saxitoxin, 436
SCA (senile cardiac amyloidosis), 610
Scabies, 352, 1268–1269
Scale, 1230
Scar, radial, of breast, 1128, 1129f
Scar formation, 89, 107, 110–111, 110f
after infarction, 138, 139f
due to infection, 363, 363f
hypertrophic, 115
in inflammatory response, 48
Scarlet fever, 374
oral manifestations of, 778t
Scatter factor, 95t, 96
Scavenger receptors, 59, 60f
in atherosclerosis, 523, 525f
SCC. *See* Squamous cell carcinoma (SCC).
SCD (sudden cardiac death), 575t, 577, 586–587
SCF (stem cell factor), 621f, 622
SCF (stem cell factor) receptor, oncogene for, 295t
Schatzki ring, 800
Schiller-Duval bodies, 1043, 1101, 1101f
Schilling test, 642
Schistosoma haematobium, 363f, 408, 409
and bladder carcinoma, 1032
Schistosoma japonicum, 408, 409, 409f
Schistosoma larvae, 352
Schistosoma mansoni, 360, 408, 409, 409f
Schistosoma mekongi, 408
Schistosomiasis, 408–409, 408f, 409f
Schizont, 401, 402f
Schlemm canal, 1422f, 1430f
Schmid metaphyseal chondrodysplasia, 1280t
Schwann cells, 1326, 1327, 1327f
in neuroblastoma, 501–502
in neurofibromatosis, 169
Schwannian stroma, 501
Schwannoma, 1411, 1412f
Antoni A and B patterns of, 1411, 1412f
malignant, 1412–1413
epithelioid, 1412–1413
SCID (severe combined immunodeficiency), 241f, 243–244
Sclera(e), 1422f, 1426
blue, 1280, 1281t, 1426
Scleral buckling, 1436
Scleritis, posterior, 1423
Scleroderma, 229t, 237–239, 237f, 238f
Sclerosing adenosis, of breast, 1128, 1129f
Sclerosing cholangitis, primary, 913t, 915, 915f
Sclerosing dacryoadenitis, 1423
Sclerosing osteomyelitis of Garré, 1291
Sclerosing retroperitoneal fibrosis, 1026
Sclerosing retroperitonitis, 873
Sclerosis, in glomerulonephritis, 967–968
Scolex, 839
Scorbutic changes, 459, 460f
Scrofula, 386
Scurvy, 458–459, 460f
bleeding disorders due to, 650
Sea-blue histiocytes, 698
Sebaceous adenoma, 1240t
Sebaceous carcinoma, of eyelid, 1424–1425, 1425f
Sebaceous epithelioma, 1240t
Sebaceous glands, 1228f
of eye, 1424, 1424f
Seborrheic dermatitis, 1257–1258
Seborrheic keratosis(es), 1237, 1237f
Second intention, healing by, 112f, 113, 113f
Second messengers, 100
Second signals, 198, 225
Secondary union, 112f, 113, 113f
α-Secretase, 1388f, 1389
ß-Secretase (BACE-1), 1388f, 1389
Secreted protein acidic and rich in cysteine (SPARC), 105
Secretin, 940
Sedative-hypnotics, abuse of, 424–425, 424t
Seeding, of body cavities and surfaces, 279, 280f
Segmental demyelination, 1326f, 1328–1329, 1329f
Segmental necrosis, 1330
Selectins, 53f, 54, 54t, 55b, 56f, 104
Selective estrogen receptor modulators (SERMs), for prevention of breast cancer, 1133
Selective vulnerability, 1349, 1361
Selenium, 461, 461t
Self-antigens, 223, 225
Self-MHC molecules, 204
Self-reactive B cells, 225
Self-reactive T cells, 224, 225
Self-tolerance, 223
Semilunar valves, 558
Seminoma, 272, 1041–1042, 1042f
anaplastic, 1042
spermatocytic, 1042
vs. nonseminomatous germ cell tumor, 1045
Senescence, replicative, 42–43, 43f, 44f, 308
Senile atrophy, 9
Senile cardiac amyloidosis (SCA), 610
Senile osteoporosis, 1283, 1283f
Senile plaques, 1386–1387, 1386f
Sensory neuropathy, paraneoplastic subacute, 1410, 1411t
Sentinel lymph node, 280
Sepsis, 85
perinatal, 480–481
Septal perforators, 557
Septal veins, 879f
Septal venules, 878
Septic infarcts, 596
Septic shock, 85, 139–141, 140t, 141f, 142f
Septicemic plague, 380
Sequestration, bronchopulmonary, 713
Sequestration crises, in sickle cell disease, 631
Sequestrum, 1291, 1291f
Serine protease inhibitor, Kazal type 1 *(SPINK1)* gene, and pancreatitis, 942, 945
SERMs (selective estrogen receptor modulators), for prevention of breast cancer, 1133
Serofibrinous pleuritis, 766, 766t
Seronegative spondyloarthropathies, 1309–1310
Serositis, in systemic lupus erythematosus, 228t
Serotonin
in carcinoid syndrome, 868
in inflammation, 64, 74t
Serous carcinoma, of endometrium, 1087, 1088
Serous cystadenocarcinomas, of ovaries, 1095, 1095f, 1096f
Serous tumors, of ovaries, 1095–1097, 1095f, 1096f
Sertoli cell tumors
ovarian, 1103, 1104f
testicular, 1046
Serum amyloid—associated (SAA) protein, 84, 260, 262
Serum sickness, 212, 212t, 214
Seven transmembrane G-protein—coupled receptors, 98f, 99–100
Severe acute respiratory syndrome (SARS), 752
Severe combined immunodeficiency (SCID), 241f, 243–244
Sevin (carbaryl), 435
Sex chromosomes, cytogenetic disorders involving, 178–181
Sex cord—stromal tumors
ovarian, 1093t, 1094f, 1102–1104, 1102f–1104f
testicular, 1046
Sex hormones, and systemic lupus erythematosus, 230
Sex steroids, 1207
Sex-linked disorders, 152
Sexual differentiation, disorders of, 1211–1214, 1213f
Sexually transmitted infections (STIs), 355–356, 356t
Sézary syndrome, 671t, 685, 1250
Sézary-Lutzner cells, 1250
SGA (small for gestational age), 476
SH2D1A gene, 371
Shadow plaques, 1383
Sheehan syndrome, 1163
SHH (Sonic hedgehog) gene, 473, 1244, 1246f, 1355
Shiga toxin, 834, 835
Shiga-like toxins, 834
Shigella, 352, 353, 355, 356t, 358
Shigella bacillary dysentery, 834–835, 836, 837f
Shigella boydii, 834
Shigella dysenteriae, 834
Shigella enterocolitis, 834–835, 836, 837f
Shigella flexneri, 834, 835
Shigella sonnei, 834
Shigellosis, 834–835
Shingles, 368, 368f, 1332, 1374
Shock, 139–143
anaphylactic, 139
cardiogenic, 139, 140t, 584
clinical course of, 142–143
endotoxic, 139, 140
hemorrhagic (hypovolemic), 124, 139, 140t
morphology of, 141–142
neurogenic, 139
pathogenesis of, 119
septic, 85, 139–141, 140t, 141f, 142f
stages of, 141
types of, 139, 140t
Shock lung, 142. *See also* Acute respiratory distress syndrome (ARDS).
Short stature Homeobox *(SHOX)* gene, 180, 181f

SIADH (syndrome of inappropriate antidiuretic hormone secretion), 1163
paraneoplastic, 334t
Sialadenitis, 790, 791f
Sialolithiasis, 790
Sialyl-Lewis X, 54t, 56
Sicca syndrome, 235
Sick building syndrome, 430
Sickle cell disease, 628–632
alterations in structural proteins in, 154
clinical course of, 631–632
genetic basis for, 150, 628
impaired hepatic circulation in, 918
infections with, 360
morphology of, 630, 631f
papillary necrosis in, 1004t
pathogenesis of, 628–630, 629f, 630f
thrombus formation in, 131
Sickle cell disease nephropathy, 1011
Sickle cell trait, 150
and resistance to *Plasmodium,* 402
Sickle retinopathy, 1439
Sideroblasts, ringed, in myelodysplastic syndromes, 695, 696f
Siderophages, 562
Sidestream smoke, 421
SIDS (sudden infant death syndrome), 495–497, 496t
Sievert (Sv), 437
Sigmoid colon, anatomy of, 828
Sigmoid septum, 559
Signal transducers and activation of transcription (STATs), 98f, 99
Signal transduction mechanisms, bone disorders due to defects in, 1279, 1280t
Signal transduction pathways, 98–100, 98f, 99f
Signaling mechanisms, in cell growth, 97–100, 97f–99f
Signal-transducing genes, 295t, 296–297, 297f
Signet-ring cell carcinoma
gastric, 825, 825f
of bladder, 1032
Silicone breast implants, 1122
Silicosis, 79, 734–735, 735f
Silver stains, 361t
SIM1, 464b
Singers' nodules, 786
Single nucleotide polymorphism (SNP), 146, 190–191
Sinoatrial (SA) node, 557
Sinonasal NK/T-cell lymphoma, 686
Sinonasal papillomas, 784–785, 785f
Sinonasal polyps, in cystic fibrosis, 495
Sinus(es)
draining, in osteomyelitis, 1291
tumors of, 784–785, 785f
Sinus histiocytosis, 666
Sinus venosus defects, 567
Sinusitis, 784
Sinusoid(s), 878, 879f
Sinusoidal obstruction syndrome, 919–920, 919f
Sipple syndrome. *See* Multiple endocrine neoplasia type 2A (MEN-2A).
SIRS (systemic inflammatory response syndrome), 84–85
SIS protooncogene, 293, 295t
Sister Mary Joseph nodule, 826
Site polymorphisms, 189
Sjögren syndrome, 229t, 235–237, 236f
Skeletal abnormalities, in Marfan syndrome, 154
Skeletal changes, due to scurvy, 459, 460f
Skeletal muscle(s)
alcohol effect on, 422t, 424
congenital myopathies of, 1340–1341, 1340f, 1340t
denervation atrophy of, 1335–1336, 1336f
Skeletal muscle(s) *(Continued)*
diseases of, 1335–1345
inflammatory myopathies of, 1342–1343, 1342f
ion channel myopathies of, 1339–1340
muscular dystrophies of, 1336–1339, 1337f, 1338t, 1339t
myopathies associated with inborn errors of metabolism of, 1341–1342, 1341f
normal anatomy and physiology of, 1327–1328, 1328f, 1328t, 1329f
regeneration of, 91, 94
toxic myopathies of, 1343–1344
tumors of, 1321–1322, 1321f, 1322f
Skin, 1227–1269
barriers to infection in, 352
hyperextensibility of, in Ehlers-Danlos syndromes, 155
in systemic lupus erythematosus, 233, 233f
in systemic sclerosis, 238, 238f
normal anatomy of, 1228–1229, 1228f, 1229f
occupational exposures and, 431t
premature aging of, 442
radiation effect on, 440, 440f
Skin cancer
basal cell carcinoma as, 1242–1244, 1243f
dermatofibrosarcoma protuberans as, 1248
malignant melanoma as, 1234–1236, 1235f, 1236f
Merkel cell carcinoma as, 1244
molecular genetics of, 1244–1247, 1245t, 1246f
mycosis fungoides (cutaneous T-cell lymphoma) as, 1249–1250, 1250f
squamous cell carcinoma as, 1242, 1243f
Skin damage, due to ultraviolet radiation, 442, 442f
Skin disorder(s)
acanthosis nigricans as, 1237–1238
acne vulgaris as, 1264–1265, 1264f
arthropod bites, stings, and infestations as, 1268–1269, 1269f
blistering (bullous), 1259–1264, 1260f–1264f
bullous pemphigoid as, 1261–1262, 1261f, 1262f
dermatitis herpetiformis as, 1262–1263, 1262f, 1263f
eczema as, 1253–1255, 1253f–1255f, 1254t
epidermolysis bullosa as, 1263, 1263f
epithelial cyst as, 1238
erythema multiforme as, 1255–1256, 1256f
fibroepithelial polyp as, 1238
freckle (ephelis) as, 1231
ichthyosis as, 1251–1252, 1252f
impetigo as, 1267
infections as, 1265–1268, 1266f–1268f
superficial fungal, 1267–1268, 1268f
inflammatory dermatoses as
acute, 1252–1256, 1252f–1256f, 1254t
chronic, 1256–1259, 1257f–1259f
keratoacanthoma as, 1240, 1241f
keratoses as
actinic, 1240–1242, 1241f
seborrheic, 1237, 1237f
Langerhans cell histiocytosis as, 1249, 1249f
lentigo as, 1232
lichen planus as, 1258, 1258f
lupus erythematosus as, 1258–1259, 1259f
macroscopic terms related to, 1229–1230
mastocytosis as, 1250–1251, 1251f
melasma as, 1231–1232
microscopic terms related to, 1230
molluscum contagiosum as, 1266–1267, 1267f
nevi as
dysplastic, 1233–1234, 1234f
Skin disorder(s) *(Continued)*
melanocytic (pigmented), 1232–1233, 1232f, 1233f, 1233t
of epidermal appendages, 1264–1265, 1264f
of epidermal maturation, 1251–1252, 1252f
of pigmentation and melanocytes, 1230–1236, 1231f–1236f, 1233f
panniculitis as, 1265
paraneoplastic, 334t, 335
pemphigus as, 1260–1261, 1260f, 1261f
porphyria as, 1263–1264
psoriasis as, 1256–1257, 1257f
seborrheic dermatitis as, 1257–1258
urticaria as, 1252–1253, 1252f, 1253f
verrucae (warts) as, 1265–1266, 1266f
vitiligo as, 1230, 1231f
xanthomas as, 1248
due to cholestasis, 888
Skin eruptions, systemic viral infections with, 347t
Skin lesions, in sarcoidosis, 738
Skin pigmentation
disorders of, 1230–1236, 1231f–1236f, 1233f
in hemochromatosis, 910
Skin tumor(s)
adnexal (appendage), 1238–1240, 1239f, 1240t
benign epithelial, 1237–1240, 1237f, 1239f, 1240t, 1241f
benign fibrous histiocytoma (dermatofibroma) as, 1247–1248, 1247f
dermal vascular, 1248
of cellular immigrants, 1249–1251, 1249f–1251f
of dermis, 1247–1248, 1247f
premalignant and malignant epidermal, 1240–1247, 1241f, 1243f, 1245t, 1246f
"Skip" lesions, in Crohn disease, 847, 849f
Skull fractures, 1357
basal, 1357
diastatic, 1357
displaced, 1357
SLE. *See* Systemic lupus erythematosus (SLE).
Slit hemorrhages, 1369
SLL (small lymphocytic lymphoma), 671t, 673–674, 673f, 674f
Slow transforming viruses, 293
Sm (Smith) antigen, 228, 229t, 234
SMA (spinal muscular atrophy), 1336, 1336f, 1397
SMAD2 gene, 300t, 305, 317
in colorectal cancer, 863–864
SMAD4 gene, 300t, 305, 317
in colorectal cancer, 863–864
in pancreatic cancer, 949f, 950, 950t
Smads, 96
Small airway disease, 718t, 722
Small cell carcinoma, of lung, 758, 759, 761f, 762
Cushing syndrome due to, 1209
Small for gestational age (SGA), 476
Small intestine, 828–870
adenocarcinoma of, 857
adenomas of, 857, 857f
anatomy of, 828
atresia and stenosis of, 830
bacterial overgrowth syndrome of, 838
congenital anomalies of, 830, 830f
enterocolitis of. *See* Enterocolitis.
immune system of, 829–830
in malnutrition, 449
malabsorption syndromes of, 842–846, 842t, 843f, 845f
mucosa of, 828–829, 828f
neuromuscular function of, 830
obstruction of, 855–856, 855t, 856f
tumors of, 856–857, 857f, 857t

Small intestine *(Continued)*
vascular disorders of, 851–854, 852f, 853f
vasculature of, 828
Small lymphocytic lymphoma (SLL), 671t, 673–674, 673f, 674f
Small round blue cell tumors, 337, 500, 501
Smallpox, 345–346
SMCs (smooth muscle cells)
in atherosclerosis, 523–524, 525f
of vascular wall, 513, 514
Smegma, 1035
Smelters, air pollution from, 429
Smith (Sm) antigen, 228, 229t, 234
SMN1 (survival motor neuron) gene, 1336
SMO protein, 1245, 1246f
Smokers' macrophages, 740, 741
Smoking. *See* Cigarette smoking.
Smooth muscle, tumors of, 1322
Smooth muscle cells (SMCs)
in atherosclerosis, 523–524, 525f
of vascular wall, 513, 514
Smudge cells, 673, 674f
SNP (single nucleotide polymorphism), 146, 190–191
SOD (superoxide dismutase), 17, 74
SOD1 gene, in amyotrophic lateral sclerosis, 1396
Sodium metabolism, and hypertension, 527f–529f, 528
Sodium pump, plasma membrane energy-dependent, reduced activity of, 15
Sodium retention, edema due to, 120t, 122
Soft tissue callus, 1288
Soft tissue tumor(s), 1316–1323
chromosomal and genetic abnormalities in, 1316, 1317t
classification of, 1316–1317, 1316t, 1317t
defined, 1316
fatty, 1317–1318, 1318f
fibrohistiocytic, 1320–1321, 1321f
fibromatosis as, 1319–1320, 1320f
fibrosarcoma as, 1320, 1320f
fibrous, 1318–1320, 1318f1320f
general features of, 1316–1317, 1317t
grading of, 1317
leiomyoma as, 1322
leiomyosarcoma as, 1322
lipoma as, 1317
liposarcoma as, 1318, 1318f
myositis ossificans as, 1319, 1319f
nodular fasciitis as, 1318, 1318f
of skeletal muscle, 1321–1322, 1321f, 1322f
of smooth muscle, 1322
pathogenesis of, 1316, 1317t
reactive pseudosarcomatous proliferations of, 1318–1319, 1318f, 1319f
rhabdomyosarcoma as, 1321–1322, 1321f, 1322f
synovial sarcoma as, 1323, 1323f
Solar elastosis, 442, 442f, 1426
Solar lentigo, 1231
"Soldier's plaque," 612
Solid organ transplant, rejection of, 222
Solid-pseudopapillary tumor, of pancreas, 948
Solitary rectal ulcer syndrome, 842
Solitary thyroid nodule, 1175
Somatic protein compartment, 448
Somatostatinomas, 1207
Somatotroph(s), 1157
Somatotroph cell adenomas, 1161–1162
Sonic hedgehog *(SHH)* gene, 473, 1244, 1246f, 1355
SOS, 99
Space of Disse, in cirrhosis, 883, 884f
SPARC (secreted protein acidic and rich in cysteine), 105
Spät-apoplexie, 1360
Specific atrial granules, 557
"Specific glioneuronal element," 1406
Specific granules, 73, 73f
Speckled leukoerythroplakia, 779
Speckled pattern, of nuclear fluorescence, 228
Spectral karyotyping, 171, 173f, 337
Spectrin, in hereditary spherocytosis, 625, 626f
Spermatic cord
and paratesticular tumors, 1040
twisting of, 1040, 1040f
Spermatocele, 1047
Spermatocytic seminoma, 1042
Spherocytes, 625–627, 626f, 627f, 674f
Spherocytosis, hereditary, 625–627, 626f, 627f
Sphingolipidoses, 161t
Spider angiomas, in hepatic failure, 882
Spider telangiectasia, 547–548
Spina bifida, 1354
Spinal cord, subacute combined degeneration of, 1399
Spinal cord infarction, 1365
Spinal cord trauma, 1360–1361
Spinal dysraphism, 1354
Spinal muscular atrophy (SMA), 1336, 1336f, 1397
Spindle and epithelioid cell nevus, 1233t
SPINK1 (serine protease inhibitor, Kazal type 1) gene, and pancreatitis, 942, 945
Spinobulbar muscular atrophy, 184t, 1396
Spinocerebellar ataxias, 184t, 1394–1396, 1395t
aggregated proteins in, 1351t
Spinocerebellar degenerations, 1394–1396, 1395t
Spiral valves of Heister, 928
Spirochetes, 388–393
Spironolactone bodies, 1210
Spitz nevus, 1233t
Spleen, 702–705
accessory, 705
amyloidosis of, 263
complete absence of, 705
congenital anomalies of, 705
in infectious mononucleosis, 370
in sickle cell disease, 630, 631f
in systemic lupus erythematosus, 234
lardaceous, 263
miliary tuberculosis of, 386f
neoplasms of, 705
normal anatomy and physiology of, 702–703, 703f
pathology of, 703–705, 704t, 705f
rupture of, 705
sago, 263
sarcoidosis of, 738
Splenic cords, 702–703
Splenic infarcts, 705, 705f
Spleniculi, 705
Splenitis, nonspecific acute, 704
Splenomegaly, 703–705, 705f
congestive, 563, 704–705
disorders associated with, 704t
due to portal hypertension, 885
thrombocytopenia in, 651
Splicing mutations, in ß-thalassemia, 632–633, 632f
Splinter hemorrhages, 598
Spondylitis, rheumatoid, 1309
Spondyloarthritis, ankylosing, 1309
Spondyloarthropathies, seronegative, 1309–1310
Spongiform encephalopathies, 346
transmissible, 1351t, 1380–1382, 1381f
Spongiform pustules, 1257
Spongiform transformation, 1380
Spongiosa, 558, 558f
primary, 1278, 1278f
Spongiosis, 1230, 1254f, 1255
Spongiotic dermatitis, 1254f, 1255
Spontaneous abortion, 1105
Sporozoites, 401, 402f
Spotted fevers, 395
Spotty necrosis, of liver, 880
Sprue
celiac, 843–844, 843f
tropical (postinfectious), 844
Squamous cell carcinoma (SCC), 271, 275f
molecular genetics of, 1245
of anal canal, 870
of bladder, 1031–1032
of cervix, 1076–1077
of conjunctiva, 1426
of esophagus, 806–808, 807f, 807t, 808f
of head and neck, 780–781, 781f
of lung, 759–760, 759f–761f
of penis, 1036–1037, 1037f
of skin, 1242, 1243f
of vagina, 1071
Squamous epithelial cells, 1228, 1228f, 1229f
Squamous metaplasia
due to vitamin A deficiency, 451, 452f
of bladder, 1028
of lactiferous ducts, 1125, 1125f
Squamous papillomas
esophageal, 806
laryngeal, 786–787, 787f
SSPE (subacute sclerosing panencephalitis), 363, 1377
SSX1 gene, in synovial sarcoma, 1323
SSX2 gene, in synovial sarcoma, 1323
ST (heat-stable) toxin, 834
Stable tissues, 90–91, 90f
Staggers, 446
Staghorn calculi, 1014
Staging, of tumors, 335
Staphylococcal enterotoxins, 834
Staphylococcal infections, 371–373, 372f, 373f
Staphylococcal lung abscess, 373, 373f
Staphylococcal scalded skin syndrome, 372, 373
Staphylococcus aureus, 371–373
immune invasion by, 360
infective endocarditis due to, 596
morphology of, 350f, 372–373
pathogenesis of, 371–372
pneumonia due to, 748
pyogenic osteomyelitis due to, 1291
superantigens made by, 359
virulence of, 358
Staphylococcus epidermidis, 352
prosthetic valve endocarditis due to, 596
Staphylococcus spp, in respiratory tract, 353
Staphyloma, 1426, 1444
"Starry sky" pattern, 677
Stasis, 131
STAT(s) (signal transducers and activation of transcription), 98f, 99
Statins, 521
Status asthmaticus, 723, 726
Status marmoratus, 1356
Status spongiosus, 1382
Steatocystoma multiplex, 1238
Steatohepatitis. *See* Steatosis, hepatic.
Steatorrhea, 842
Steatosis, 35–36, 36f
hepatic, 904, 904f, 907–908
clinical features of, 907
due to carbon tetrachloride poisoning, 25, 25f, 26f
in cystic fibrosis, 493
in hepatitis, 899
in kwashiorkor, 448
in Wilson disease, 911
mechanisms of, 36, 36f, 906
morphology of, 905, 905f

Steatosis *(Continued)*
nonalcoholic, 907–908
obesity and, 465
of pregnancy, 920
macrovesicular, 880
microvesicular, 880
Steel factor receptor, oncogene for, 295t
Stein-Leventhal syndrome, 1092–1093, 1093f
Stellate cells, 878
in cirrhosis, 883, 884f
Stem cell(s), 91–95
adult, 91–93, 93f, 94f
bone marrow, 92–93, 94f, 622
cancer, 278
committed, 620
embryonic, 91, 92f
epidermal, 93f
hematopoietic, 92
homing of, 622
in cell proliferation, 89, 89f
in hyperplasia, 7
in tissue homeostasis, 93–95
intestinal, 93f
lineage-restricted, 622
liver, 93–94, 93f
lymphoid, 621f
myeloid, 621f
neural, 94
niches for, 92, 93f
pluripotent, 620, 621f
properties of, 622
tissue, 91, 93
transdifferentiation of, 92, 94f
Stem cell dysfunction, 622
Stem cell factor (SCF), 621f, 622
Stem cell factor (SCF) receptor, oncogene for, 295t
Stents, endovascular, 551, 552f
Stercoral ulcers, 831
Steroid myopathy, 1344
Stevens-Johnson syndrome, 778t, 1255–1256
Stewart-Treves syndrome, 1151
Stickler syndrome, 1280t
Stiff-man syndrome, paraneoplastic, 1411t
Stimulants, abuse of, 424t, 425–426
STIs (sexually transmitted infections), 355–356, 356t
Stomach, 810–827. *See also under* Gastric.
antrum of, 810, 810f
bezoars of, 820, 820f
body (corpus) of, 810, 810f
cardia of, 810, 810f
congenital anomalies of, 812–816, 813f, 814t, 815f, 816f
dilation of, 820
fundus of, 810, 810f
greater curvature of, 810
hypertrophic gastropathy of, 820–821, 821f
incisura angularis of, 810
lesser curvature of, 810
normal anatomy of, 810–811, 810f
peptic ulcer disease of, 816–820, 817f, 819f, 819t, 820f
physiology of gastric mucosa of, 811–812
pyloric sphincter of, 810, 810f
rupture of, 820
tumors of, 821–827, 822f, 823t, 824f–827f
varices of, 821
watermelon, 816
Stomach cancer. *See* Gastric carcinoma.
Stomatitis, recurrent herpetic, 777
Storage pool disorders, 653
Storiform pattern, 1248
Strangulation, of large intestine, 856
Strap cells, 1321
Strategic infarcts, 1391
Stratum corneum, 1228f
Streak ovaries, 180
Streptococcal infection(s), 373–374, 374f
glomerulonephritis after, 212t, 359, 974–976, 975t, 976f
Streptococcal pharyngitis, 373–374
Streptococci, group B, meningitis due to, 1369
Streptococcus, immune invasion by, 360
Streptococcus agalactiae, 373, 393
Streptococcus mutans, 373
Streptococcus pneumoniae, 373, 374
immune evasion by, 359
meningitis due to, 1369
morphology of, 350f
pathogenesis of, 373
pneumonia due to, 353, 748
Streptococcus pyogenes, 358, 359, 372, 373, 374
Streptococcus viridans, infective endocarditis due to, 596
Stress
and peptic ulcer disease, 818
cellular responses to, 4–5, 5f, 5t
Stress fracture, 1288
Stress ulcers, 819–820, 820f
Stricture(s)
biliary, 936
fibrosing, in Crohn disease, 849
Stroke, 1361. *See also* Cerebrovascular disease(s).
and atherosclerosis, 521
due to mitral valve prolapse, 592
heat, 445
obesity and, 465
Stromal cells, bone marrow, 92, 94f
Stromal dystrophies, of cornea, 1429–1430
Stromal edema, in Fuchs endothelial dystrophy, 1428, 1429
Stromal hyperplasia, cortical, 1092
Stromal hyperthecosis, 1092
Stromal microenvironment, and carcinogenesis, 313
Stromal nodule, endometrial, 1089
Stromal sarcoma, endometrial, 1089, 1089f
Stromal tumors
endometrial, 1089, 1089f
of breast, 1149–1151, 1149f, 1150f
Stromata, of tumors, 270
Stromelysins, 111
Strongyloides, 838
Strongyloides stercoralis, 352, 406, 407f
Strongyloidiasis, 406, 407f
Structural proteins, defects in, 154–156, 156t
Struma lymphomatosa, 1169
Struma ovarii, 1100
Strumal carcinoid, 1100
Struvite stones, 1014, 1014t
Stunned myocardium, 581, 582, 583f
Sturge-Weber syndrome, 547
glaucoma in, 1431
pheochromocytomas in, 1219, 1219t
Subacute necrotizing encephalopathy, 1398
Subacute sclerosing panencephalitis (SSPE), 363, 1377
Subaortic stenosis, 571
idiopathic hypertrophic. *See* Hypertrophic cardiomyopathy (HCM).
Subarachnoid hemorrhage, 1360, 1366–1367, 1366f
Subareolar abscess, recurrent, 1125, 1125f
Subcellular responses, to injury, 5, 32–34, 32f–34f
Subcutaneous tissues, in right-sided heart failure, 563
Subdural empyema, 1371
Subdural hematoma, 1359–1360, 1359f, 1360f
Subependymal hemorrhage, in preterm infants, 484
Subependymomas, 1405–1406
Subepidermal nonacantholytic blister, 1261
Subfalcine herniation, 1352, 1353f
Submassive necrosis, of liver, 880
Subperiosteal abscesses, 1291
Substance abuse
of alcohol, 421–424, 422f, 422t, 423f
of drugs, 424–426, 424t, 425f
Substance P, 74
Substantia nigra, in Parkinson disease, 1391, 1392f
Substitution, 147
Substrate
accumulation of, 152–153
in coagulation cascade, 127, 129f
Subungual hemorrhages, 598
Sudden cardiac death (SCD), 575t, 577, 586–587
Sudden infant death syndrome (SIDS), 495–497, 496t
Suicide, mortality rates for, 443t
Sulfatase deficiency, multiple, 161t
Sulfatidoses, 161t
Sulfur dioxide, as air pollutant, 428t, 429, 429t
Sunlight, and malignant melanoma, 1234
Superantigens, 141, 359, 372
Superficial fibromatosis, 1319
Superior conjunctival fornix, 1424f, 1425
Superior tarsus, 1424f
Superior vena caval syndrome, 544, 615
due to lung carcinoma, 762
Superoxide anion radical ($O_2^{\cdot}$), 16, 17f
in inflammation, 73
in ischemia-reperfusion injury, 24
Superoxide dismutase (SOD), 17, 74
Suppurative arthritis, 1310
Suprabasal acantholytic blister, 1260, 1260f
Supranuclear palsy, progressive, 1390, 1391
Surface lining cells, 1274–1275
Surfactant, 713
in neonatal respiratory distress syndrome, 481–482
Survival motor neuron *(SMN1)* gene, 1336
Susceptibility genes, 226, 226f
Sv (sievert), 437
Sweat ducts, in cystic fibrosis, 490, 491f
Sweat glands, 1228f, 1229
Sweat test, 495
Sydenham chorea, due to rheumatic fever, 593
Sympathetic ophthalmia, 1433
Synarthroses, 1303
Synchondroses, 1303
Syncytia, in HIV infection, 251, 251f
Syncytiotrophoblasts, in seminoma, 1042
Syndactyly, 471f, 473
Syndrome of inappropriate antidiuretic hormone secretion (SIADH), 1163
paraneoplastic, 334t
Syndrome X, 465
Synovial cyst, 1315
Synovial joints, 1303
Synovial membrane, 1303
Synovial sarcoma, 1323, 1323f
Synovitis
in hemochromatosis, 910
pigmented villonodular, 1315, 1315f
Synpolydactyly, 475, 1280t
Syntrophins, 1337f
α-Synuclein, in Parkinson disease, 1392
Syphilis, 388–391
cardiovascular, 389, 390
congenital, 389, 391
during pregnancy, 355
epidemiology of, 388
false-positive test results for, 229
granulomatous inflammation in, 83t
in dermis, 362f

Syphilis *(Continued)*
morphology of, 390–391, 390f, 391f
neuro-, 389, 391, 1372
meningovascular, 1372
paretic, 1372
of epididymis and testes, 1040
organism of, 388, 388f
pathogenesis of, 391
primary, 389, 389f, 390, 390f
secondary, 389, 389f, 390
serologic tests for, 390
skeletal, 1292
tertiary, 389, 389f, 390–391, 391f
benign, 389, 391, 391f
transmission of, 388
Syphilitic aneurysms, 532
Syphilitic aortitis, 532
Syphilitic osteochondritis, 391
Syphilitic periostitis, 391
Syringocystadenoma papilliferum, 1240t
Syringoma, 1238, 1240t
chondroid, 1238, 1239f
Syringomyelia, 1356
Systemic inflammatory response syndrome (SIRS), 84–85
Systemic lupus erythematosus (SLE), 223, 227–235
clinical and pathologic manifestations of, 230–234, 231f–234f, 231t
clinical course of, 234–235
clinical presentation of, 227, 228t
diagnostic criteria for, 227, 228t
endocarditis of, 133, 234, 234f, 597f, 598–599
epidemiology of, 227
etiology and pathogenesis of, 227–230, 229t, 230f
morphology of, 230–234, 231f–234f, 231t
pulmonary involvement in, 731
vasculitis in, 542, 542f
Systemic sclerosis, 229t, 237–239, 237f, 238f
Systole, 557
Systolic dysfunction, 560
SYT gene, in synovial sarcoma, 1323

T

T cell(s) (T lymphocytes)
cytotoxic, 198
antitumor effect of, 330
apoptosis of, 331
cell death induced by, 26, 31–32
hepatitis B virus and, 369
in cell-mediated hypersensitivity, 217–218
recognition of tumor antigens by, 328, 329f
effector, 194f
helper, 198, 199
in asthma, 723, 724f
in hypersensitivity
delayed, 216, 217f
immediate, 207–208, 207f
in tuberculosis, 381–382
in atherosclerosis, 523
in immune system, 194f, 196–198, 196f–198f
in inflammatory bowel disease, 846, 847
origin and differentiation of, 621f
T cell—mediated cytolysis, 215f
T cell—mediated cytotoxicity, 217–218
T cell—mediated graft rejection, 218–219, 219f
T cell—mediated hypersensitivity, 215–218, 215f–217f, 215t
T_3 (triiodothyronine), 1165, 1165f
T_3 (triiodothyronine) toxicosis, 1167
T_4 (thyroxine), 1165, 1165f
Tabes dorsalis, 1372
Taboparesis, 1372
TACE, 111
Tachycardia, in shock, 141
Tadpole cells, 1321
Taenia saginata, 407
Taenia solium, 406–407, 839
Tailpipe emissions, 428
Takayasu arteritis, 537t, 538–540, 538f
Talin, 105, 106f
Tamm-Horsfall protein, 995
Tamoxifen, for prevention of breast cancer, 1133
Tanning, 441–442
Tapeworms, 359, 406–407, 407f, 839
TAPVC (total anomalous pulmonary venous connection), 564t, 570
Target cells, in thalassemia major, 634
Target fiber, 1330
Target lesion, in erythema multiforme, 1256
Target lesions, in aspergillosis, 400, 400f
Targeted therapy, 296–297
Tarsus
inferior, 1424f
superior, 1424f
tat gene, in HIV, 247, 247f
Tattooing, 39
Tau gene, 1387, 1389–1390
Tauopathies, 1351t
TAX gene, in T-cell leukemia, 327
Tay-Sachs disease, 148f, 160–161, 161t, 162f
cherry-red spot in, 161, 1441, 1441f
T-bet, in asthma, 724
TBG (thyroxine-binding globulin), 1165
TBII (TSH-binding inhibitor immunoglobulins), 1172
TBX5, in congenital heart disease, 565
TCDD exposure, 435
T-cell acute lymphoblastic leukemia, oncogenes in, 314t
T-cell granular lymphocytic leukemia, 671t, 685–686
T-cell immunodeficiency, in HIV infection, 250–252, 251f
T-cell leukemia, adult, 671t, 685
T-cell lymphoma
adult, 671t, 685
angioimmunoblastic, 671t
cutaneous, 1249–1250, 1250f
gastrointestinal, 869
peripheral, unspecified, 684, 684f
sinonasal, 686
T-cell neoplasm(s)
peripheral, 671t, 684–686, 684f, 685f
precursor, 670–673, 671t, 672f
T-cell receptor (TCR), 196–197, 198f
TcF, 304f
TDLU (terminal duct lobular unit), 1120, 1121f
Teeth, 774–775, 774f
decay of, 774–775
Hutchinson, 391
Telangiectasia(s)
capillary, of brain, 1368
hereditary hemorrhagic, 548, 650
spider, 547–548
Telangiectasis, 547
Telethonin, 1339t
Telomerase, 43, 44f, 308–309
in colorectal cancer, 864
in neuroblastoma, 504
Telomere(s), 43, 44f, 308
Telomere shortening, 43, 308–309, 308f
Telomeric reverse transcriptase (TERT), 864
Temporal arteritis, 536–538, 537f, 537t
Tenacin, 105
Tendon sheath, giant cell tumor of, 1315
Tenosynovitis, localized nodular, 1315
Tension pneumothorax, 714, 768
Teratocarcinoma, 1045
Teratogens, 474
Teratoid/rhabdoid tumor, atypical, 1408
Teratoma, 271–272
ovarian, 1099–1100, 1101f
immature malignant, 1100, 1101
mature cystic, 272, 272f, 1099–1100, 1100f
monodermal or specialized, 1100
sacrococcygeal, 499, 499f
testicular, 1044, 1044f, 1045f
Terminal bronchioles, 712
Terminal duct lobular unit (TDLU), 1120, 1121f
Terminal ileitis, 847
TERT (telomeric reverse transcriptase), 864
Testicles. *See* Testis(es).
Testicular atrophy, 1038, 1038f
Testicular feminization, 181
Testicular torsion, 1040, 1040f
Testicular tumor(s), 1040–1046
biologic markers for, 1045–1046
choriocarcinoma as, 1041, 1043–1044, 1044f
classification of, 1041t
clinical features of, 1045–1046
embryonal carcinoma as, 1041, 1043, 1043f
germ cell, 1040–1046, 1041t
gonadoblastoma as, 1046
Leydig (interstitial) cell, 1046
lymphoma as, 1046
mixed, 1045
nonseminomatous, 1041, 1045
of sex cord—gonadal stroma, 1046
seminoma as, 1041–1042, 1042f, 1045
spermatocytic, 1042
Sertoli cell (androblastoma), 1046
staging of, 1045
teratoma as, 1044, 1044f, 1045f
therapy and prognosis for, 1046
yolk sac, 1041, 1043
Testis(es), 1037–1047
congenital anomalies of, 1037–1038, 1038f
in hemochromatosis, 910
in mumps, 1039
in syphilis, 1040
inflammations of, 1039–1040, 1039f
radiation effect on, 441
regressive changes of, 1038–1039
tuberculosis of, 1039
undescended, 1037–1038, 1038f
vascular disturbances of, 1040, 1040f
Tetany, due to hypoparathyroidism, 1188
Tetradecanoyl phorbol-13 acetate (TPA), 322
Tetrahydrobiopterin (BH_4), 488
Δ^9-Tetrahydrocannabinol (THC), 426
Tetrahydrofolate (FH_4) derivatives, 642, 642f
Tetralogy of Fallot, 564t, 565, 569, 569f
TFPI (tissue factor pathway inhibitor), 85, 126f, 130
TGA (transposition of the great arteries), 564t, 569–570, 569f, 570f
TGF. *See* Transforming growth factor (TGF).
TGI (thyroid growth-stimulating immunoglobulins), 1172
T_H1. *See* T-helper-1 (T_H1).
T_H2. *See* T-helper-2 (T_H2).
α-Thalassemia(s), 634t, 635–636
silent carrier state of, 634t, 635
ß-Thalassemia(s), 632–635
clinical syndromes of, 634–635, 634t, 635f
molecular pathogenesis of, 632–634, 632f, 633f
morphology of, 634–635, 635f
Thalassemia intermedia, 634, 634t
Thalassemia major, 634–635, 634t, 635f
Thalassemia minor, 635, 645, 645t
Thalassemia syndromes, 632–636, 632f, 633f, 634t, 635f
alterations in structural proteins in, 154
α-Thalassemia trait, 634t, 635–636
ß-Thalassemia trait, 634

Thalidomide, congenital anomalies due to, 473
Thanatophoric dwarfism, 1280t, 1354
THC (Δ^9-tetrahydrocannabinol), 426
Theca lutein hyperplasia of pregnancy, 1092–1093
Thecoma-fibromas, 1103, 1103f
T-helper-1 (T_H1), 198
in asthma, 723, 724f
in delayed hypersensitivity, 216, 217f
in tuberculosis, 381–382
T-helper-2 (T_H2), 198
in asthma, 723, 724f
in immediate hypersensitivity, 207–208, 207f
Therapeutic cloning, 91, 92f
Therapy-related myelodysplastic syndromes (t-MDS), 695
Thermal burns, 444–445
Thermal injuries, 444–446
Thiamine, 450t, 456–457, 457f
Thiamine deficiency
neurologic manifestations of, 1399
peripheral neuropathy due to, 1334
Thiazolidinediones (TZDs), and insulin resistance, 1196, 1196f
Thin basement membrane disease, 989
Thin filaments, abnormalities of, 34
Third ventricle, colloid cyst of, 1406
Thomas, Lewis, 328
Threshold dose, 417, 417f
Threshold limit value, 417
Thrombasthenia, Glanzmann, 127, 653
Thrombin, 65, 68
in coagulation cascade, 127, 128–129, 128f, 129f
in normal hemostasis, 124, 125f, 126f
Thromboangiitis obliterans, 539f, 542
Thrombocytopenia(s), 210
alloimmune, 650–651
autoimmune, 650
bleeding related to, 650–653, 651t
drug-induced, 652
heparin-induced, 132, 652
HIV-associated, 652
immunodeficiency with eczema and, 244
petechiae due to, 123
Thrombocytopenic purpura
autoimmune, 212t
immune, 651–652
thrombotic, 652–653, 1009–1010, 1011
Thrombocytosis
due to blood loss, 624
essential, 700, 700f
Thromboembolism, 135
after myocardial infarction, 586
pulmonary, 136, 136f
systemic, 136
Thrombomodulin, 85
in disseminated intravascular coagulation, 656
in hemostasis, 125, 126f
Thrombophlebitis, 544
migratory, 135, 334t, 335, 544
in pancreatic cancer, 951
Thromboplastin time, partial, 649–650
Thrombosis, 130–135
arterial, 132–133, 134, 135
cardiac, 132–133, 133f, 135
cerebral, 1363–1364
clinical correlations of, 134–135
defined, 119
fate of thrombus in, 133–134, 134f, 135f
hepatic vein, 919, 919f
inferior vena cava, 919
morphology of, 132–133, 133f
of atheromatous plaques, 519
of prosthetic valve, 600f, 601
pathogenesis of, 130–132, 131f, 132t
Thrombosis *(Continued)*
venous. *See* Venous thrombosis.
Virchow triad in, 130–132, 131f, 132t
Thrombospondins, 105
in apoptosis, 27
Thrombotic diatheses, acquired, 131–132, 132f
Thrombotic microangiopathies, 652–653, 1009–1011, 1010f
Thrombotic thrombocytopenic purpura (TTP), 652–653, 1009–1010, 1011
Thromboxane(s), 68–69, 69f
Thromboxane A_2 (TXA_2), 68–69, 69f
in platelet aggregation, 127
Thrombus(i), 125f
coronary, 573f, 574
fate of, 133–134, 134f, 135f
mural, 133, 133f
on heart valves, 133
red (stasis), 133
Thrush, 398, 777
Thymic aplasia, 706
Thymic carcinoma, 707, 708
Thymic cysts, 706
Thymic follicular hyperplasia, 706
Thymic hyperplasia, 706–707
Thymic hypoplasia, 241f, 243, 706
Thymomas, 707–708, 707f
Thymus gland, 706–708, 707f
radiation effect on, 439f
Thyroglossal duct cyst, 1183
Thyroglossal tract cyst, 789
Thyroid adenomas, 1175–1177
clinical features of, 1177
follicular, 1175–1177, 1176f, 1181f
morphology of, 274f, 1176–1177, 1176f
pathogenesis of, 1176
Thyroid autonomy, 1165, 1176
Thyroid carcinoma, 1177–1183
anaplastic, 1178, 1183
epidemiology of, 1175
follicular, 1177, 1180–1181, 1180f, 1181f
medullary, 1178, 1182–1183, 1182f
familial, 1223
papillary, 1177–1180, 1179f, 1179t
pathogenesis of, 1177–1178
radiation exposure and, 324, 1175, 1178
Thyroid gland, 1164–1183
agenesis of, 1168
amyloidosis of, 263
congenital anomalies of, 1183
cysts of, 1177
diffuse and multinodular goiters of, 1173–1175, 1175f
Graves disease of, 1172–1173, 1173f
hyperthyroidism of, 1166–1167, 1166t, 1167f
hypoplasia of, 1168
hypothyroidism of, 1167–1169, 1167t
inflammation of, 1169–1172, 1170f, 1171f
lingual, 1164–1165
neoplasms of, 1175–1183
normal anatomy and physiology of, 1164–1166, 1165f
Thyroid growth-stimulating immunoglobulins (TGI), 1172
Thyroid hormone(s), 1165, 1165f
Thyroid hormone receptor (TR), 1165, 1165f
mutations in, 1168
Thyroid hormone resistance syndrome, 1168
Thyroid hormone response elements (TREs), 1165, 1165f
Thyroid metabolism, inborn errors of, 1168
Thyroid myopathy, 1166
Thyroid nodule(s)
cold *vs.* hot, 1177
solitary, 1175
Thyroid ophthalmopathy, 1166, 1167f, 1423, 1423f
Thyroid storm, 1167
Thyroid tissue, ectopic, 1164–1165
Thyroid transcription factor-2 (TTF-2), mutations in, 1168
Thyroiditis, 1169–1172
De Quervain, 1170–1171, 1171f
granulomatous, 1170–1171, 1171f
Hashimoto, 1169–1170, 1170f
with Graves disease, 1172
infectious, 1169
lymphocytic
chronic, 1169–1170, 1170f
subacute, 1171–1172
painless, 1171–1172
palpation, 1171–1172
postpartum, 1171
Riedel, 1171
silent, 1171–1172
subacute, 1170–1171, 1171f
lymphocytic, 1171–1172
Thyroidization, of renal tubules, 1001
Thyroid-stimulating hormone (TSH), 1165, 1165f
in hyperthyroidism, 1167
in hypothyroidism, 1168, 1169
Thyroid-stimulating hormone (TSH)-binding inhibitor immunoglobulins (TBII), 1172
Thyroid-stimulating hormone (TSH)-producing adenomas, 1162
Thyroid-stimulating hormone (TSH) receptor
in thyroid adenoma, 1176
mutations in, 1168
Thyroid-stimulating immunoglobulin (TSI), 1172
Thyrotoxic dilated cardiomyopathy, 1166, 1166t
Thyrotoxic myopathy, 1343–1344
Thyrotoxic periodic paralysis, 1344
Thyrotoxicosis, 1166, 1166t
Thyrotroph(s), 1157
Thyrotroph adenomas, 1162
Thyrotropin, 1165, 1165f
Thyrotropin-releasing hormone (TRH), 1165f
deficiency in, 1168
Thyrotropin-releasing hormone (TRH) stimulation test, 1167
Thyroxine (T_4), 1165, 1165f
Thyroxine-binding globulin (TBG), 1165
Tick(s), deer, 392, 392f
Tick bites, 1268
T-ICs (tumor-initiating cells), 278
Tie2, 109
Tigered effect, 36
TIGR (trabecular meshwork inducible glucocorticoid response) gene, 1431
TIMP (tissue inhibitor of metalloproteinases), 110f, 111
in abdominal aortic aneurysm, 532
Tinea, 351
Tinea barbae, 1267
Tinea capitis, 1267
Tinea corporis, 1267, 1268f
Tinea cruris, 1267
Tinea pedis, 1267
Tinea versicolor, 1267–1268
Tingible bodies, 665, 666f
TIR (Toll/IL-1 receptor) domain, 195b
Tissue(s)
continuously dividing (labile), 90, 90f
nondividing (permanent), 90f, 91
quiescent (stable), 90–91, 90f
Tissue arrays, 338
Tissue factor, in hemostasis, 124, 125f, 126, 128
Tissue factor pathway inhibitor (TFPI), 85, 126f, 130

Tissue homeostasis, stem cells in, 93–95
Tissue inhibitor of metalloproteinases (TIMP), 110f, 111
  in abdominal aortic aneurysm, 532
Tissue plasminogen activator (tPA), in hemostasis, 124, 125, 125f, 130, 130f
Tissue regeneration, mechanisms of, 101–103, 101f, 102f
Tissue remodeling, 110–111, 110f
Tissue stem cells, 91, 93
Tissue tropism, 356–357
Tissue-proliferative activity, 90–91, 90f
TLR(s) (Toll-like receptors), 58, 58f
  in innate immunity, 194, 195b
TLR-4 (Toll-like receptor protein 4), 140
t-MDS (therapy-related myelodysplastic syndromes), 695
TNF. *See* Tumor necrosis factor (TNF).
TnI (troponin-I), 583
TNM System, 335
TnT (troponin-T), 583
  in hypertrophic cardiomyopathy, 605f, 606
Tobacco use. *See* Cigarette smoking.
Tocopherol(s), 455
α-Tocopherol, 455
Tocotrienols, 455
Tolerance, immunologic, 223–226, 224f
Toll/IL-1 receptor (TIR) domain, 195b
Toll-like receptor(s) (TLRs), 58, 58f
  in innate immunity, 194, 195b
Toll-like receptor protein 4 (TLR-4), 140
Toluene, 431
Tongue, amyloid of, 264
Tonsillar herniation, 1354, 1354f
Tonsillitis, 784
  follicular, 784
Tooth decay, 774–775
Tophaceous arthritis, chronic, 1313, 1313f
Tophaceous gout, chronic, 1314
Tophus(i), 1311, 1313, 1313f
TORCH infections, prenatal, 477, 480
Torsion, testicular, 1040, 1040f
Total anomalous pulmonary venous connection (TAPVC), 564t, 570
Toxemia of pregnancy, 1106–1110, 1109f, 1110f
  fetal growth restriction due to, 478
Toxic agents, neurologic sequelae of, 1400, 1400f
Toxic epidermal necrolysis, 373, 1256
Toxic granulations, 665, 665f
Toxic megacolon, 831, 849, 850f
Toxic myopathies, 1343–1344
Toxic neuropathies, 1335
  acquired, 1334–1335, 1334f
Toxic shock syndrome (TSS), 141, 359, 372
Toxic shock syndrome (TSS) toxin-1, 141
Toxicants, absorption and distribution of, 417, 417f
Toxicity
  defined, 417
  mechanisms of, 417–419, 417f, 418f, 420f–421f
Toxicology, 417
Toxin(s)
  animal, 435–436, 435t
  bacterial, 358–359
  cell injury due to, 25
  natural, 435–436, 435t
Toxin-induced liver disease, 903–907, 903t
Toxocara canis, 351
Toxoplasma gondii, 351, 351t
  in AIDS, 256
Toxoplasmosis
  cerebral, 1378–1379, 1378f, 1379f
  retinal, 1433
TPA (tetradecanoyl phorbol-13 acetate), 322
tPA (tissue plasminogen activator), in hemostasis, 124, 125, 125f, 130, 130f
TR (thyroid hormone receptor), 1165, 1165f
  mutations in, 1168
Trabecular lamellae, 1276, 1277f
Trabecular meshwork, of eye, 1422f, 1430f
Trabecular meshwork inducible glucocorticoid response *(TIGR)* gene, 1431
Trace elements, 459–461, 461t
Tracheoesophageal fistula, 800, 800f
Trachoma, conjunctival scarring due to, 1425
Traction diverticulum, 802
TRAF-6 (TNF-receptor associated factor-6), 195b
Transcervical infections, 480
Transcobalamin II, 639
Transcription factors, 100
  bone disorders due to defects in, 1279, 1280t
  in cancer cells, 315
  protooncogenes for, 295t, 297–298, 299f
Transcription-mediated amplification, 361
Transcytosis, increased, in inflammation, 51f, 52
Transdifferentiation, of stem cells, 92, 94f
Transduction, of oncogenes, 293
Transferrin, 74, 644, 644f, 645f
Transforming growth factor (TGF), and congenital anomalies, 474
Transforming growth factor-α (TGF-α), 95–96, 95t
  in liver regeneration, 102, 103
  oncogene for, 293–294, 295t
Transforming growth factor-ß (TGF-ß), 95t, 96–97
  in angiogenesis, 109
  in immunity, 202
  in scar formation, 110
  inhibition of cellular proliferation by, 300
Transforming growth factor-α *(TGFα)* oncogene, 295t
Transforming growth factor-ß (TGF-ß) pathway, 305
Transforming growth factor-ß (TGF-ß) receptor gene, 300t, 305
Transforming growth factor-ß receptor genes *(TGFß-R1* and *TGFß-R2),* in pancreatic cancer, 950, 950t
Transforming infections, 369–371, 369f, 370f
Transfusion(s), thrombocytopenia due to, 651
Transfusion reactions, 210
Transitional cell carcinoma, of ureter, 1025, 1025f
Transitional cell tumors, of bladder, 1028–1031, 1029f–1031f, 1029t, 1031t
Transitional papillary carcinoma, of renal pelvis, 1004
Translocations, 174–175, 174f
  in cancer cells, 314–315
  molecular diagnosis of, 337
  white cell neoplasia due to, 667
Transmembrane receptors, seven α-helical, 56, 58–59, 58f
Transmigration, of leukocytes, 53, 53f, 54–56, 57f
Transmissible spongiform encephalopathies, 1351t, 1380–1382, 1381f
Transmitting males, 183
Transmural infarction, of bowel, 852–853, 852f
Transplacental infections, 480, 480f
Transplant rejection, 218–223
  acute, 220
    cellular, 220, 220f
    humoral, 220, 221f
  antibody-mediated, 219–220
  cellular, 218–219, 219f
  chronic, 221, 221f
Transplant rejection *(Continued)*
  hematopoietic cell, 222–223
  humoral, 219
  hyperacute, 219, 220
  kidney, 218–222, 219f–221f
  morphology of, 220–221, 220f, 221f
  of other solid organs, 222
  prevention of, 221–222
  T cell—mediated, 218–219, 219f
Transplant-associated Kaposi sarcoma, 549
Transplantation
  cardiac, 615–616, 615f
  diarrhea with, 841, 841f
  hepatic complications of, 921
  lung, 221, 756–757, 757f
Transport systems, defects in, 154
Transporters, bone disorders due to defects in, 1281–1282, 1282f, 1283f
Transposition of the great arteries (TGA), 564t, 569–570, 569f, 570f
Transposons, 348
Transrectal ultrasonography (TRUS), of prostate cancer, 1054
Transtentorial herniation, 1353–1354, 1354f
Transthyretin (TTR), 260, 261
Transudate
  defined, 49
  in edema, 120
Transurethral resection of the prostate (TURP), 1050
Transverse myelitis, 441
Trastuzumab (Herceptin), 1148
Trauma, 442–446
  due to mechanical force, 443–444, 443f, 444f
  electrical, 446
  mortality rates for, 443t
  related to changes in atmospheric pressure, 446
  thermal, 444–446
  to central nervous system, 1356–1361
    parenchymal injuries due to, 1357–1359, 1360f
    sequelae of, 1360
    skull fractures due to, 1357
    spinal cord, 1360–1361
    vascular injuries due to, 1359–1360, 1359f, 1360f
Traumatic neuroma, 1335, 1335f
Traumatic neuropathies, 1335, 1335f
Traveler's diarrhea, 832
TRE(s) (thyroid hormone response elements), 1165, 1165f
"Trench foot," 446
Treponema pallidum, 388, 388f, 391
  during pregnancy, 355
  granulomatous inflammation due to, 83t
  neurosyphilis due to, 1372
  skeletal syphilis due to, 1292
Treponema pertenue, skeletal syphilis due to, 1292
Treponemal antibody tests, 390
Treponemal infections, 349t
TRH (thyrotropin-releasing hormone), 1165f
  deficiency in, 1168
TRH (thyrotropin-releasing hormone) stimulation test, 1167
Trichilemmal cyst, 1238
Trichilemmoma, 1239f, 1240, 1240t
Trichinella, 359
Trichinella spiralis, 353, 407–408, 408f
Trichinosis, 407–408, 408f
Trichobezoars, 820, 820f
Trichoepithelioma, 1238, 1239f, 1240t
Trichomonas vaginalis, 351, 351t, 356t, 1063, 1063t
Trichuris trichiura, 839

Tricuspid atresia, 564t, 570
Tricuspid valve, 558
Triglycerides, intracellular accumulation of, 35–36, 36f
Trigone, 1024
Triiodothyronine (T_3), 1165, 1165f
Triiodothyronine (T_3) toxicosis, 1167
TRIM32, 1339t
Trinucleotide repeat mutations, 149, 181–184, 182f
Triphenyltetrazolium chloride (TTC) stain, of myocardial infarct, 579, 579f
Triple stones, 1014, 1014t
Triplet-repeat mutations, 149, 181–184, 182f
Trisomy(ies), 173, 176
Trisomy 13, 176, 177f, 471f, 472
Trisomy 18, 176, 177f
Trisomy 21, 175–176, 175f, 177f, 472
Trisomy 22, 173f
Triton tumors, 1412
TRK-A, in neuroblastoma, 504
Tropheryma whippelii, 844
Trophic triggers, for myocardial hypertrophy, 8
Trophoblastic disease, gestational, 1110–1114, 1110t, 1111f–1114f
Trophoblastic tumor, placental site, 1114, 1114f
Trophozoites, 401, 402f
Tropical sore, 404
Tropical spastic paraparesis, 327, 1376
Tropical sprue, 844
Tropism, nervous system, 1372
α-Tropomyosin gene, in hypertrophic cardiomyopathy, 605f, 606
Troponin-I (TnI), 583
Troponin-T (TnT), 583
  in hypertrophic cardiomyopathy, 605f, 606
Trousseau phenomenon (sign, syndrome), 135, 334t, 335, 544
  in hypocalcemia, 1188
  in pancreatic cancer, 951
Truncus arteriosus, 564t, 565, 570
TRUS (transrectal ultrasonography), of prostate cancer, 1054
Trypanosoma brucei gambiense, 405
Trypanosoma brucei rhodesiense, 405
Trypanosoma cruzi, 351t, 405–406
  achalasia due to, 801
  immune evasion by, 359
  myocarditis due to, 608
Trypanosoma spp, 351, 351t
Trypanosomiasis
  African, 405, 405f
  American, 405–406
Trypsin, 943, 945
Trypsinogen, 943
TSC1 gene, 1413
TSC2 gene, 1413
TSH. *See* Thyroid-stimulating hormone (TSH).
TSI (thyroid-stimulating immunoglobulin), 1172
TSS (toxic shock syndrome), 141, 359, 372
TSS (toxic shock syndrome) toxin-1, 141
TTC (triphenyltetrazolium chloride) stain, of myocardial infarct, 579, 579f
TTF-2 (thyroid transcription factor-2), mutations in, 1168
TTP (thrombotic thrombocytopenic purpura), 652–653, 1009–1010, 1011
TTR (transthyretin), 260, 261
T-tubule system, 1327
Tubal pregnancy, 1105, 1106f
Tufted astrocytes, 1390
Tuberculin reaction, 216
Tuberculin test, 381
Tuberculoid leprosy, 387, 388f
Tuberculoma, 1372
Tuberculosis, 381–386
  Addison disease due to, 1216
  clinical features of, 383–384, 383f
  diagnosis of, 381, 384
  endobronchial, endotracheal, and laryngeal, 386
  epidemiology of, 381
  granulomatous inflammation in, 83t
  in AIDS, 256, 384, 1372
  intestinal, 386
  isolated-organ, 386
  lymphadenitis, 386
  miliary, 383
    pulmonary, 385–386
    systemic, 386, 386f
  morphology of, 384–386, 384f–386f
  "nonreactive," 385f
  of epididymis and testes, 1039
  pathogenesis of, 381–382, 382f
  primary, 381–382, 382f–385f, 383, 384
    progressive, 383, 383f
    pulmonary, 384, 384f
  pulmonary
    primary, 384, 384f
    progressive, 385–386
    secondary, 385–386, 386f
  secondary, 383–384, 383f, 385, 386f
    pulmonary, 385–386, 386f
  silicosis and, 735
Tuberculous arthritis, 1310
Tuberculous empyema, 386
Tuberculous meningitis, 383, 386, 1371–1372
Tuberculous osteomyelitis, 1291–1292
Tuberculous salpingitis, 1091
Tuberin, 1413
Tuberous sclerosis, 1413–1414
  angiomyolipoma in, 1015
  cutaneous manifestations of, 1245t
Tubo-ovarian abscess, 393, 1064
Tubular adenomas, 860–861, 860f
Tubular carcinoma, of breast, 1146, 1146f
Tubular necrosis, acute. *See* Acute tubular necrosis (ATN).
Tubules, of glomerulus, 959
Tubulitis, 1002
Tubuloglomerular feedback, 994
Tubulointerstitial disease, 960, 993–1006
  acute tubular necrosis as, 993–996, 994f, 995f
  hypercalcemia and nephrocalcinosis as, 1005
  in multiple myeloma, 1005–1006, 1006t
  tubulointerstitial nephritis as, 996–1004, 996t, 997f–1003f, 1004t
  urate nephropathy as, 1004–1005, 1005f
Tubulointerstitial fibrosis, 973, 974f
Tubulointerstitial nephritis, 236, 996–1004
  acute, 996
  causes of, 996t
  chronic, 996
  drug- and toxin-induced, 1002–1004, 1002f, 1003f, 1004t
  in multiple melanoma, 1005–1006, 1005t, 1006f
  nephrocalcinosis as, 1005
  pyelonephritis as, 994–1002
    acute, 998–1000, 998f, 999f
    and urinary tract infection, 996–998, 997f, 998f
    chronic, 1000–1002, 1001f
  secondary, 996
  urate nephropathy as, 1004–1005, 1005f
Tubulovillous adenomas, 860, 861
Tufted astrocytes, 1390
Tumor(s). *See also* Cancer; Neoplasia; Neoplasm(s).
  benign, 270–271, 270f, 271f, 273t, 281f, 281t
    in infants and children, 498–499, 498f, 499f
Tumor(s). *See also* Cancer; Neoplasia; Neoplasm(s) *(Continued)*
  bone. *See* Bone tumor(s).
  cardiac, 613–615, 613f, 614t
  carotid body, 789–790, 789f
  cell death in, 26
  clinical features of, 332–339, 334t, 336f, 337f, 339t
  components of, 270
  defined, 270
  effect on host of, 332–335, 334t
  esophageal, 806–809, 807f–809f, 807t
  grading and staging of, 335
  growth of, 272–281
    differentiation and anaplasia in, 272–276, 274f, 275f
    rates of, 276–277, 277f, 278f
  heterogeneity of, 319
  host defense against, 328–332, 329f, 332f
  in infants and children, 498–506
    benign, 498–499, 498f, 499f
    malignant, 499–506, 500t
      incidence and types of, 499–500, 500t
      neuroblastic, 500–504, 501f, 502f, 503t, 504f
      Wilms, 504–506, 505f, 506f
  local invasion by, 278–279, 278f, 279f, 312–313, 313f
  malignant, 271–272, 271f, 272f, 273t, 281f, 281t
    in infants and children, 499–506, 500t
    undifferentiated, 336–337, 337f
  mesenchymal, 869–870
  metastasis of. *See* Metastasis(es).
  mixed, 271
    of salivary gland origin, 271, 271f
  monoclonality of, 288, 288f
  nomenclature for, 270–272, 273t
  odontogenic, 782, 782t
  of anal canal, 869–870
  of appendix, 871–872, 872f
  of biliary tract, 934–935, 935f
  of bladder, 1028–1033, 1029f–1031f, 1029t, 1031t
  of central nervous system. *See* Central nervous system (CNS) tumor(s).
  of ear, 788
  of fallopian tubes, 1091
  of joints, 1314–1315, 1315f
  of large intestine, 857–870, 857t
  of lung. *See* Lung tumor(s).
  of oral cavity, 778–781, 779f, 781f
  of penis, 1035–1037, 1035f1037f
  of peripheral nerve, 1335
  of peritoneum, 873
  of prostate, 1050–1056, 1052f–1054f
  of small intestine, 856–857, 857f, 857t
  of stomach, 821–827, 822f, 823t, 824f–827f
  of ureters, 1025, 1025f
  of urethra, 1034, 1034f
  of vulva, 1066–1070, 1067f–1070f
  ovarian. *See* Ovarian tumor(s).
  paratesticular, 1040
  pleural, 768–770, 768f, 769f
  renal, 1015–1019
    benign, 1015–1016
    malignant, 1016–1019, 1017f–1019f
  soft tissue. *See* Soft tissue tumor(s).
  testicular. *See* Testicular tumor(s).
  vascular. *See* Vascular tumors and tumor-like conditions.
  Warthin, 792–793, 793f
Tumor antigens, 328–330, 329f
Tumor cell(s)
  chromosomal changes in, 314–315
  epigenetic changes in, 315

Tumor cell(s) *(Continued)*
gene amplification in, 315
molecular profiles of, 315, 316b, 317f
vascular dissemination and homing of, 313
Tumor cell invasion, 278–279, 278f, 279f, 312–313, 312f
Tumor giant cells, 274
Tumor immunity, 328–332, 329f, 332f
Tumor markers, 338–339, 339t
Tumor necrosis factor (TNF)
in cachexia, 333
in delayed type hypersensitivity, 217, 217f
in disseminated intravascular coagulation, 85, 657
in immediate hypersensitivity, 209
in immunity, 202
in inflammation, 53f, 54, 56f, 71, 71f, 74t
in liver regeneration, 102–103
in rheumatoid arthritis, 1307
in scar formation, 110
in septic shock, 140, 141f
in wound healing, 95t
Tumor necrosis factor-α (TNF-α)
in atherosclerosis, 522
in immunity, 202
Tumor necrosis factor-ß (TNF-ß), in immunity, 202
Tumor necrosis factor (TNF) antagonists, 1308
Tumor necrosis factor (TNF)-converting enzyme, 111
Tumor necrosis factor (TNF)-receptor (TNF-R) associated factor-6 (TRAF-6), 195b
Tumor necrosis factor receptor type 1 (TNFR1), in apoptosis, 29, 29f, 31
Tumor progression, 288–289, 319
Tumor suppressor gene(s), 288, 298–306, 300t
products of, 328
RB, 284, 299–302, 300t, 301f, 302f
silencing by DNA methylation of, 315
Tumor-associated antigens, 328
Tumor-forming amyloid, of tongue, 264
Tumor-initiating cells (T-ICs), 278
Tumorlets, of lung, 764
Tumor-specific antigens, 328
Tumor-specific transplantation antigens, 328–329
Tungsten carbide, exposure to, 432t, 433
Tunica vaginalis, lesions of, 1047
Turban tumor, 1238
Turbulence, 131
Turbulent blood flow, 131
Turcot syndrome, 862
Turista, 832
Turner syndrome, 178, 179–180, 180f, 181f, 472
TURP (transurethral resection of the prostate), 1050
Turpentine, 431
Twin-twin transfusion, 1106, 1108f
Two-hit hypothesis, of oncogenesis, 299, 301f
TXA_2 (thromboxane A_2), 68–69, 69f
in platelet aggregation, 127
Tylenol (acetaminophen)
adverse effects of, 428
cell injury due to, 25–26
Typhlitis, 841
Typhoid fever, 835
Typhoid nodule, 837
Typhus
epidemic, 350, 395, 396, 396t, 397f
murine, 396t
scrub, 350, 395, 396, 396t
tick
North Asia, 396t
Queensland, 396t
Typhus fever, 396
Tyrosinase, as tumor antigen, 329
Tyrosine kinase, nonreceptor-associated, protooncogenes for, 295t, 297, 298f
Tyrosine kinase activity, intrinsic
receptors with, 98–99, 98f, 99f
receptors without, 98f, 99
Tyvelose, 408
Tzanck test, 777
TZDs (thiazolidinediones), and insulin resistance, 1196, 1196f

U

UBE3A, 187
Ubiquitin, 1387
Ubiquitin-proteasome pathway, 10, 289
UC. *See* Ulcerative colitis (UC).
UCH-L1, in Parkinson disease, 1392
UDP-galactose, 489, 489f
UDP-glucuronosyltransferase (UGT1A1), 885–886, 887–888, 888t
UES (upper esophageal sphincter)
anatomy and physiology of, 798
diverticula of, 802
UGT1 gene, 885–886
UICC (Union Internationale Contre Cancer), 335
UIP (usual interstitial pneumonia), 729, 731f
Ulcer(s), 77, 78f
aphthous, 776, 776f
in Crohn disease, 847, 847f, 848
corneal, 1428
due to vitamin A deficiency, 451, 452f
Curling, 819
Cushing, 819–820
duodenal, 78f, 819f
gastric, 818
genital, due to chancroid, 380
Hunner, 1027
oral, in systemic lupus erythematosus, 228t
peptic. *See* Peptic ulcer disease.
rodent, 279, 1242
solitary rectal, 842
stercoral, 831
stress, 819–820, 820f
varicose, 134
Ulceration
acute gastric, 819–820, 820f
defined, 1230
of wound, 114
Ulcerative colitis (UC), 849–851
and carcinoma, 850–851
clinical features of, 851, 851t
diagnosis of, 847
epidemiology of, 849
etiology and pathogenesis of, 846
genetic susceptibility to, 846
morphology of, 849–851, 849f, 850f
T-cells in, 847
Ulegyria, 1356
Ulnar-mammary syndrome, 1280t
Ultrastructural changes, of cell injury, 20, 20f
Ultraviolet A (UVA), 441–442, 441t
Ultraviolet B (UVB), 441–442, 441t
Ultraviolet C (UVC), 441, 441t
Ultraviolet (UV) radiation, 441–442
acute and delayed effects of, 436t, 441–442, 441t, 442f
and systemic lupus erythematosus, 230, 233
as carcinogen, 323
Ultraviolet response pathway, 442
Umbilical hernia, 856f
Umbrella cells, 1024
Uncinate herniation, 1353–1354, 1354f
Unfolded protein response, 15, 26, 38
Union Internationale Contre Cancer (UICC), 335
Uniparental disomy, 186
Unmyelinated nerve fibers, 1326, 1327, 1327f
Unstable nucleotide repeats, 183–184, 184f, 184t, 185f
u-PA (urokinase-like plasminogen activator), 130, 130f
Upper airways, 783–787, 783f, 785f, 787f
Upper esophageal sphincter (UES)
anatomy and physiology of, 798
diverticula of, 802
Urachal cysts, 1026
Urachus, persistent, 1026
Uranium, and lung cancer, 758
Urate crystals, in gout, 1311–1313, 1312f
Urate nephropathy, 1004–1005, 1005f
Ureaplasma, 350, 351
Ureaplasma urealyticum, 356t
Uremia, 960
bleeding disorders related to, 653
systemic manifestations of, 961t
Uremic complications, of chronic glomerulonephritis, 989–990
Uremic medullary cystic disease, 966f
Uremic neuropathy, 1334
Ureter(s), 1024–1026
anatomy and physiology of, 1024
congenital anomalies of, 1024–1025
diverticula of, 1024
double, 1024
hydro-, 1024–1025
inflammations of, 1025, 1025f
megalo-, 1024–1025
obstructive lesions of, 1025–1026, 1025t
tumors and tumor-like lesions of, 1025, 1025f
Ureteritis, 1025, 1025f
Ureteritis cystica, 1025, 1025f
Ureteritis follicularis, 1025
Ureteropelvic junction obstruction, 1024
Urethra
inflammations of, 1034
tumors and tumor-like lesions of, 1034, 1034f
Urethral caruncle, 1034
Urethritis, 1034
nongonococcal, 394–395
Uric acid stones, 1005, 1014, 1014t
Urinary bladder. *See* Bladder.
Urinary system, occupational exposures and, 431t
Urinary tract infection (UTI), 353, 960
Urinary tract obstruction, 960, 1012–1014, 1013f
papillary necrosis in, 998, 1004t
Urinary tract stones, in hyperparathyroidism, 1186, 1187
Urogenital sinus, 1060, 1061f
Urogenital tract, barriers to infection in, 353
Urokinase-like plasminogen activator (u-PA), 130, 130f
Urolithiasis, 960, 1014–1015, 1014t, 1015f
Uroplakins, 1024
Urothelial carcinoma
in situ, 1029, 1030–1031, 1031f
of prostate, 1056
of renal pelvis, 1018–1019, 1019f
papillary, 1029, 1029f, 1029t, 1030, 1030f
Urothelial tumors, 1028–1031, 1029f–1031f, 1029t, 1031t
Urothelium, 1024
Urticaria, 1252–1253, 1252f, 1253f
Urticaria pigmentosa, 1250
Usual interstitial pneumonia (UIP), 729, 731f
Uterine bleeding, dysfunctional, 1081–1083, 1081t, 1082f
Uterine constraint, 471
Uterine leiomyomas, 1089–1090, 1090f
Uterine vessels, atherosis of, in toxemia of pregnancy, 1109, 1110f

Uteroplacental insufficiency, fetal growth restriction due to, 477
Uterus
anatomy of, 1081–1082, 1082f, 1083f
hypertrophy of, during pregnancy, 7, 7f
leiomyoma of, 274f
UTI (urinary tract infection), 353, 960
pyelonephritis and, 996–998, 997f, 998f
UV. *See* Ultraviolet (UV).
Uvea, 1432–1434, 1433f, 1435f
neoplasms of, 1433–1434, 1435f
Uveal melanoma, 1434, 1435f
Uveal nevi, 1434
Uveitis, 1433, 1433f
granulomatous, 1433
lens-induced, 1431

V

VacA gene, 328
Vaccinia virus, 347t
Vacuolar degeneration, 20
Vacuolar myelopathy, in AIDS, 1376
Vacuolating toxin (VacA), in peptic ulcer disease, 818
Vacuolation, 1330
Vacuoles, autophagic, 10
Vacuolization, 1230
Vagina, 1070–1072
atresia and total absence of, 1070
congenital anomalies of, 1070–1071
premalignant and malignant neoplasms of, 1071–1072, 1071f, 1072f
septate, 1070
Vaginal adenosis, 1071
Vaginal intraepithelial neoplasia, 1071
Vaginal portio, 1081, 1083f
Vaginitis, *Candida,* 398
Valvular abnormalities, in systemic lupus erythematosus, 234, 234f
Valvular degeneration, due to calcification, 589–591, 590f
Valvular heart disease, 588–601
calcific degeneration as, 589–591, 590f
carcinoid, 599–600, 599f
due to complications of artificial valves, 600–601, 600f, 600t
etiology of, 589, 589t
infective endocarditis as, 595–598, 597f, 598t
isolated *vs.* combined, 589
mitral valve prolapse as, 591–592, 592f
noninfected vegetations as, 598–599, 599f
rheumatic, 593–595, 594f, 595f
Valvular insufficiency, 589
Valvular regurgitation, functional, 589
Valvular stenosis, 588–589
Valvulitis, rheumatic, 594f
Variable expressivity, 150
Variant Creutzfeldt-Jakob disease (vCJD), 346, 1382
Variant surface glycoprotein (VSG), 405
Varicella-zoster virus (VZV), 347t, 368, 368f
encephalitis due to, 1374
peripheral neuropathy in, 1332
Varices
esophageal, 802–803, 803f
gastric, 821
Varicocele, 1047
Varicose ulcers, 134
Varicose veins, 543–544, 543f
Variegate coproporphyria, 1333t
Varmus, Harold, 293
Vas deferens, congenital bilateral absence of, in cystic fibrosis, 494, 495
Vasa nervorum, in rheumatoid arthritis, 1306
Vasa vasorum, 512
Vascular cell adhesion molecule 1 (VCAM-1), 54, 54t, 55b
in atherosclerosis, 522
Vascular changes, in inflammation, 50–53, 51f, 52f
Vascular dementia, 1369, 1391
Vascular dilation, in inflammation, 49, 50f
Vascular disease(s), 515–551
aneurysms and dissections as, 530–534, 530f, 531f, 533f, 534f
arteriosclerosis as, 515–516
arteriovenous fistulas as, 515
atherosclerosis as, 516–525
classification of, 517, 518f
clinical features of, 516
clinical significance of, 516–517, 516f, 517f
complications of, 516f, 525
epidemiology and risk factors for, 520–521, 520f, 520t
fatty streaks in, 516, 517f
morphology of, 516f, 517–520, 518f, 519f
natural history of, 516f
pathogenesis of, 516f, 521–524, 522f, 525f
prevention of, 524
congenital anomalies as, 515
hypertension as, 525–530
accelerated (malignant), 526
causes of, 526, 526t
essential (idiopathic), 526, 528–529, 528f, 529f
morphology of, 529–530
pathogenesis of, 526–529, 527f–530f
secondary, 526t
inflammatory, 534–542
Churg-Strauss syndrome as, 537t, 541
classification of, 535, 535t, 536, 536f, 537t
giant cell (temporal) arteritis as, 536–538, 537f, 537t
infectious arthritis as, 542, 542f
Kawasaki disease (mucocutaneous lymph node syndrome) as, 537t, 540
leukocytoclastic vasculitis as, 537t, 539f, 540–541
pathogenesis of, 535–536, 535t
polyarteritis nodosa as, 537t, 539f, 540
Takayasu arteritis as, 537t, 538–540, 538f
thromboangiitis obliterans (Buerger disease) as, 539f, 542
vasculitis with other disorders as, 542, 542f
Wegener granulomatosis as, 537t, 539f, 541–542
lymphangitis and lymphedema as, 544–545
of intestines, 851–854, 852f, 853f
pulmonary, 742–747
diffuse pulmonary hemorrhage syndromes as, 745–747, 746f
Goodpasture syndrome as, 745–746
idiopathic pulmonary hemosiderosis as, 746
pulmonary embolism, hemorrhage, and infarction as, 742–743, 742f
pulmonary hypertension as, 743–745, 744f, 745f
Wegener granulomatosis as, 746–747
Raynaud phenomenon as, 542–543, 543f
renal, 1006–1012
accelerated nephrosclerosis as, 1007–1008
atheroembolic, 1011, 1011f
atherosclerotic, 1011
benign nephrosclerosis as, 1006–1007, 1007f
diffuse cortical necrosis as, 1011–1012, 1012f
malignant hypertension as, 1007–1008, 1008f
renal artery stenosis as, 1008–1009, 1009f
Vascular disease(s) *(Continued)*
renal infarcts as, 1012
sickle cell nephropathy as, 1011
thrombotic microangiopathies as, 1009–1011, 1010f
superior and inferior vena caval syndromes as, 544
thrombophlebitis and phlebothrombosis as, 544
tumors and tumor-like conditions as, 545–551
angiosarcoma as, 550–551, 550f
bacillary angiomatosis as, 548, 548f
benign, 545–548, 545t
glomus, 547
hemangioendothelioma as, 550
hemangioma as, 545–547, 546f
hemangiopericytoma as, 551
intermediate-grade (borderline, low-grade malignant), 545t, 548–550
Kaposi sarcoma as, 548–550, 549f
lymphangioma as, 547
malignant, 545t, 550–551
vascular ectasias as, 547–548
varicose veins as, 543–544, 543f
Vascular dissemination, of tumor cells, 313
Vascular dissemination theory, of endometriosis, 1083, 1084f
Vascular disturbances, of testes, 1040, 1040f
Vascular ectasias, 547–548
Vascular endothelial growth factor (VEGF), 95t, 96
in angiogenesis, 109, 109t, 309–310
in neonatal respiratory distress syndrome, 482
in scar formation, 110
Vascular endothelium
anatomy and physiology of, 513–514, 514f, 514t
in atherosclerosis, 522–523, 525f
Vascular engorgement, in sudden infant death syndrome, 496
Vascular injury(ies)
of brain, 1359–1360, 1359f, 1360f
response to, 515, 515f
Vascular intervention(s), 551–553, 552f
Vascular leakage, in inflammation, 49, 50–53, 50f–52f
Vascular malformations, of brain, 1367–1368
Vascular manifestations, of cancer, 334t, 335
Vascular pathology, in hypertension, 529–530, 530f
Vascular permeability, increased, in inflammation, 49, 50–53, 50f–52f
Vascular phenomena, complement system in, 64
Vascular replacement, 551–553, 552f
Vascular smooth muscle cells, 513, 514
in atherosclerosis, 523–524, 525f
Vascular supply, and infarction, 139
Vascular tumors and tumor-like conditions, 545–551
angiosarcoma as, 550–551, 550f
bacillary angiomatosis as, 548, 548f
benign, 545–548, 545t
glomus, 547
hemangioendothelioma as, 550
hemangioma as, 545–547, 546f
hemangiopericytoma as, 551
intermediate-grade (borderline, low-grade malignant), 545t, 548–550
Kaposi sarcoma as, 548–550, 549f
lymphangioma as, 547
malignant, 545t, 550–551
of dermis, 1248
vascular ectasias as, 547–548
Vascular type, of Ehlers-Danlos syndromes, 156, 156t

Vascular wall(s), 512, 512f
cells of, 513–514, 514f, 514t
development, growth, and remodeling of, 514–515
response to injury of, 515, 515f
Vasculitis(ides), 534–542
ANCA-associated, 212t, 535–536
antiendothelial cell antibodies in, 536
Churg-Strauss syndrome as, 537t, 541
classification of, 535, 535t, 536, 536f, 537t
clinical manifestations of, 534
defined, 214, 534
giant cell (temporal) arteritis as, 536–538, 537f, 537t
hypersensitivity, 535, 537t, 539f, 540–541
immune complex, 214f, 535
infectious arthritis as, 542, 542f
Kawasaki disease (mucocutaneous lymph node syndrome) as, 537t, 540
large vessel, 536f, 537t
leukocytoclastic, 537t, 539f, 540–541
lupus, 542, 542f
medium-sized vessel, 536f, 537t
noninfectious necrotizing, 239–240
pathogenesis of, 535–536, 535t
polyarteritis nodosa as, 537t, 539f, 540
Pseudomonas, 379f
purpura due to, 123
rejection, 220, 221f
retinal, 1439
rheumatoid, 542
small vessel, 535, 536f, 537t
systemic necrotizing, 534–535
Takayasu arteritis as, 537t, 538–540, 538f
thromboangiitis obliterans (Buerger disease) as, 539f, 542
thrombus formation due to, 130
Wegener granulomatosis as, 537t, 539f, 541–542
Vasculogenesis, 96, 107, 514–515
Vasculogenic mimicry, 309, 1434
Vasoactive amines, in inflammation, 63–64, 64f
Vasoactive intestinal polypeptide (VIP), 1189
Vasoconstriction, 513
and hypertension, 529
in ischemic heart disease, 574–575
in shock, 141
intrarenal, 994
Vasodilation, 513
in inflammation, 49, 50, 50f
Vasogenic edema, 1352
Vaso-occlusive crises, in sickle cell disease, 631
Vasopressin, 1158
Vasospasm, myocardial infarction due to, 576
VCAM-1 (vascular cell adhesion molecule 1), 54, 54t, 55b
in atherosclerosis, 522
vCJD (variant Creutzfeldt-Jakob disease), 346, 1382
VDRL (Venereal Disease Research Laboratory) test, 390
Vectors, 355
Vegetations, 133
in infective endocarditis, 596, 597f
VEGF. *See* Vascular endothelial growth factor (VEGF).
Vein(s)
anatomy and physiology of, 512, 512f, 513
bridging, 1359
varicose, 543–544, 543f
Velocardiofacial syndrome, 178
Venereal Disease Research Laboratory (VDRL) test, 390
Venereal wart, 1265
Veno-occlusive disease, hepatic, 919–920, 919f
Venous angiomas, of brain, 1368
Venous stasis, 131
Venous thrombosis
clinical correlations of, 134–135
hormone replacement therapy and, 427–428
ischemic bowel disease due to, 852
morphology of, 132, 133
obesity and, 465
oral contraceptives and, 427
paraneoplastic, 334t, 335
superficial, 134–135
thrombophlebitis and phlebothrombosis due to, 544
Ventricular aneurysm, after myocardial infarction, 586
Ventricular remodeling, 586
left, 560
Ventricular septal defect (VSD), 568
after myocardial infarction, 584
genetic basis for, 565
incidence of, 564t
morphology of, 568, 569f
shunt through, 567, 567f
Ventricular septum, rupture of, after myocardial infarction, 584–585, 585f
Ventricularis, 558, 558f
Venules
collecting, 513
formation of endothelial gaps in, in inflammation, 50–52, 51f
postcapillary, 513
Verocytotoxins, in hemolytic-uremic syndrome, 1010
Verruca(e), 1265–1266, 1266f
Verruca palmaris, 1265
Verruca plana, 1265
Verruca plantaris, 1265
Verruca vulgaris, 1265, 1266f
Verrucous carcinoma
of penis, 1037
of vulva, 1068, 1069f
Very late activation (VLA) molecules, 55b
Very-long-chain fatty acids (VLCFA), in adrenoleukodystrophy, 1398
Very-low-density lipoproteins (VLDL), 157, 157f
Vesicle, 1229
Vesicoureteral reflux, 997–998, 997f, 998f, 1000, 1001f, 1026
Vessel wall abnormalities, bleeding disorders caused by, 650
Vestibular schwannoma, 1411
Vestibulitis, vulvar, 1065
VHFs (viral hemorrhagic fevers), 347t, 365
VHL disease. *See* von Hippel-Lindau (VHL) disease.
VHL (von Hippel Lindau) gene, 299, 305, 315, 1414
Vibrio cholerae, 352, 353, 834, 835, 837
vif gene, in human immunodeficiency virus, 247, 247f
Villitis, 1106
Villous adenomas, 860, 861, 861f
Villus(i), intestinal, 828–829, 828f
VIN (vulvar intraepithelial neoplasia), 1067–1068, 1068f
Vinculin, 105, 106f
Vinyl chloride
as carcinogen, 285t, 323
metabolism of, 421f
occupational exposure to, 432
VIP (vasoactive intestinal polypeptide), 1189
VIPomas, 1207
Viral arthritis, 1310–1311
Viral carcinogenesis, 324–328, 325f, 326f
Viral encephalitis, 1372
arthropod-borne, 1373
Viral encephalomyelitis, 1372
Viral gastroenteritis, 832–833, 833t
Viral hemorrhagic fevers (VHFs), 347t, 365
Viral infection(s), 363–371
agents for, 346t, 347–348, 347t, 348f
cell injury in, 26
chronic latent, 365–368, 366f–368f
chronic productive, 368–369
congenital anomalies due to, 473
digestive, 347t
hemorrhagic fevers as, 347t, 365
latency of, 359, 1372–1373
measles as, 363–364, 364f
mechanism of, 356–357, 357f
mumps as, 364, 364f
of central nervous system, 347t
respiratory, 347t
sexually transmitted, 356t
transforming, 369–371, 369f, 370f
transient, 363–365, 364f
warty growths due to, 347t
with arbovirus, 347t
with cytomegalovirus, 366–368, 367f
with Epstein-Barr virus, 369–371, 369f, 370f
with hematopoietic disorders, 347t
with hepatitis B virus, 369
with herpes simplex virus, 365–366, 366f
with human papillomavirus, 371
with poliovirus, 364
with skin eruptions, 347t
with varicella-zoster virus, 368, 368f
with West Nile virus, 364–365
Viral latency, 359, 1372–1373
Viral meningitis, 1373f
Viral meningoencephalitis, 1372–1377, 1373f–1377f
Viral oncogenes (v-*onc*), 293
tumor antigens produced by, 330
Viral receptors, 356–357, 357f
Virchow, Rudolf, 49, 1228
Virchow node, metastasis of gastric carcinoma to, 825–826
Virchow triad, in thrombosis, 130–132, 131f, 132t
Virilization disorders, 1211–1214, 1213f
Virulence, bacterial, 358
Virulence factors, 358
Virus(es), 347–348, 347t
slow transforming, 293
structure of, 348f
Visceral epithelial cells, of glomerulus, 957f–959f, 958, 959
in minimal change disease, 981–982, 982f
Visceral paraganglia, 1218
Visceral protein compartment, 448
Viscous metamorphosis, 127
Visible light, exposure to, 436t
Vision, vitamin A in, 451, 452f
Vitamin(s), fat soluble and water soluble, 450, 450t
Vitamin A, 450–452
functions of, 450t, 451
in cancer prevention, 466
metabolism of, 450–451, 451f
toxicity of, 451–452
Vitamin A deficiency, 451, 452f
and congenital anomalies, 474, 476f
Vitamin B_1, 450t
Vitamin B_1 deficiency, neurologic manifestations of, 1399
Vitamin B_6, 450t, 458
Vitamin B_{12}
biochemical functions of, 450t, 641, 641f
normal metabolism of, 639–640, 640f
Vitamin B_{12} deficiency, 450t, 639–642
as antibody-mediated disease, 212t, 641
clinical course of, 642

Vitamin B_{12} deficiency *(Continued)*
etiology of, 639, 640–641, 640t
incidence of, 641
morphology of, 642
neurologic manifestations of, 1399
pathogenesis of, 641
Vitamin C, 450t, 458–459, 460f
Vitamin D, 452–455
and osteoporosis, 1283
functions of, 450t, 452–453, 453f
metabolism of, 452, 453f
sources of, 452
Vitamin D deficiency, 450t, 453–455, 453f–455f, 454t
renal osteodystrophy due to, 1288
Vitamin deficiencies, 450–459, 450t
neurologic manifestations of, 1399
Vitamin D—related disorders, hypercalcemia due to, 42
Vitamin E, 450t, 455–456
Vitamin K, 450t, 456
Vitiligo, 1230, 1231f
Vitrectomy, 1436
Vitreoretinopathy, proliferative, 1436
Vitreous detachment, 1434, 1437f, 1439
Vitreous humor, 1434, 1436f
persistent hyperplastic primary, 1434
VLA (very late activation) molecules, 55b
VLCFA (very-long-chain fatty acids), in adrenoleukodystrophy, 1397–1398
VLDL (very-low-density lipoproteins), 157, 157f
Vocal cord nodules, 786
Vocal cord polyps, 786
Volatile organic compounds (VOCs), 431
Volume-overload hypertrophy, 561
Volvulus, 856, 856f
von Gierke disease, 168t
von Hippel Lindau *(VHL)* gene, 299, 305, 315, 1414
von Hippel-Lindau (VHL) disease, 947, 1414
cavernous hemangiomas in, 547
pheochromocytomas in, 1219, 1219t
renal cell carcinoma in, 1016
von Meyenburg complexes, 915, 916, 916f
von Pirquet, Clemens, 212
von Recklinghausen disease, 168–169
of bone, 1287
pheochromocytomas in, 1219t
von Willebrand disease, 126, 655
von Willebrand factor (vWF)
deficiencies in, 654–655, 654f
in hemostasis, 125f, 126, 126f, 127f
in vascular endothelial cells, 513
von Willebrand factor (vWF) metalloprotease deficiency, 653
v*onc* (viral oncogenes), 293
tumor antigens produced by, 330
vpr gene, in HIV, 247, 247f
vpu gene, in HIV, 247, 247f
VSD. *See* Ventricular septal defect (VSD).
VSG (variant surface glycoprotein), 405
Vulnerability, selective, 1349, 1361
Vulva, 1065–1070
Bartholin cyst of, 1065
neoplasms of, 1066–1070, 1067f–1070f
non-neoplastic epithelial disorders of, 1065–1066, 1066f
Vulvar carcinoma, 1067–1068, 1069f
Vulvar intraepithelial neoplasia (VIN), 1067–1068, 1068f
Vulvar vestibulitis, 1065
Vulvodynia, 1065
vWF. *See* von Willebrand factor (vWF).
VZV (varicella-zoster virus), 347t, 368, 368f
encephalitis due to, 1374
peripheral neuropathy in, 1332

W

Waardenburg syndrome, 1280t
WAGR syndrome, 504
Waldenström macroglobulinemia, 678
Wallerian degeneration, 1329, 1330f
Warm antibody immunohemolytic anemia, 637, 637t
Wart(s), 1265–1266, 1266f
flat, 1265
venereal, 1265
Warthin tumor, 792–793, 793f
Warthin-Finkeldey cells, 364, 364f
WASP (Wiskott-Aldrich syndrome protein), 244
Waste incinerators, air pollution from, 429
Water retention, edema due to, 122
Water-clear cells, 1186, 1188
Waterhouse-Friderichsen syndrome, 1214–1215, 1215f, 1370
Watermelon stomach, 816
"Watershed" infarcts, 1362–1363
Watery diarrhea, hypokalemia, achlorhydria (WDHA) syndrome, 1207
Weber-Christian disease, 1265
Wegener granulomatosis (WG), 541–542
clinical features of, 537t, 541–542
glomerular lesions in, 993
morphology of, 539f, 541
orbit in, 1423
pathogenesis of, 541
pulmonary hemorrhage in, 746–747
Weibel-Palade bodies, 54, 56f, 513
Wen, 1238
Wermer's syndrome. *See* Multiple endocrine neoplasia type 1 (MEN-1).
Werner syndrome, 42, 43, 43f
Wernicke encephalopathy, 457, 457f, 1399
Wernicke syndrome, 423
Wernicke-Korsakoff syndrome, 457, 457f, 1399, 1400
West Nile virus, 364–365, 1373
WG. *See* Wegener granulomatosis (WG).
Wheals, 1229, 1252
Whipple, George, 844
Whipple disease, 844, 845f
Whipworm, 839
White blood cell(s)
decreased number of, 662–663
neoplastic proliferations of, 666–702
etiology and pathogenesis of, 667
histiocytoses as, 667, 701–702, 702f
lymphoid, 666, 667–690, 668t, 669f, 670t
myeloid, 666–667, 690–701
normal anatomy and physiology of, 662
reactive (inflammatory) proliferations of, 663–665, 664f, 664t, 665f
WHO (World Health Organization) classification
of acute myelogenous leukemias, 692, 693t
of lymphoid neoplasms, 668, 668t
Whole-body irradiation
aplastic anemia due to, 647
effects of, 439, 439f
Whooping cough, 378, 379f
Wickham striae, 1258, 1258f
Williams syndrome, 571
Wilms tumor, 504–506
clinical features of, 506
epidemiology of, 504
gene for, 305
genetic and other markers for, 500t
morphology of, 505–506, 505f, 506f
nephrogenic rests and, 505
pathogenesis and genetics of, 504–505
prognosis for, 506
Wilms tumor—associated gene 1 *(WT1)*, 300t, 305, 504, 505
Wilms tumor—associated gene 2 *(WT2)*, 505
Wilson disease, 910–911
Wire loop lesion, 232, 232f, 233f
Wiskott-Aldrich syndrome, 34, 244
Wiskott-Aldrich syndrome protein (WASP), 244
WNT signal transduction, oncogene for, 295t
WNT signaling pathway, 105, 304, 305f
Wolbachia, 410, 411
Wolffian duct, 1081
Wolman disease, 161t
Wood smoke, as air pollutant, 430, 430t
World Health Organization (WHO) classification
of acute myelogenous leukemias, 692, 693t
of lymphoid neoplasms, 668, 668t
Wound(s), gunshot, 444, 444f
Wound contraction, 112f, 113, 115
Wound contracture, 113f, 115
Wound dehiscence, 114
Wound healing, 88–89, 88f, 111–115
by first intention, 111–113, 112f
by second intention, 112f, 113, 113f
complications of, 114–115, 115f
factors influencing, 114, 114t
growth factors and cytokines in, 111t
phases of, 111, 111f
summary of, 114
Wound repair, fibroblast growth factor in, 96
Wound strength, 113–114
Woven bone, 1275–1276, 1277f
WT1 (Wilms tumor—associated gene 1), 300t, 305, 504, 505
WT2 (Wilms tumor—associated gene 2), 505
Wuchereria bancrofti, 409

X

X chromatin, 178
X chromosome, 178, 181
banding pattern of, 172f
X inactivation, random, 288f
Xanthelasma, 1248
Xanthoastrocytoma, pleomorphic, 1404
Xanthogranulomatous cholecystitis, 933
Xanthogranulomatous pyelonephritis, 1001
Xanthomas, 37, 1248
due to cholestasis, 888
Xenobiotic metabolisms, 417–418, 418f, 420f–421f
Xeroderma pigmentosum
cutaneous manifestations of, 1245t
DNA repair genes in, 307, 323
Xerophthalmia, 451
Xerosis, 451
Xerostomia, 790
in Sjögren syndrome, 235, 236
X-inactivation, 178
Xist, 178
X-linked agammaglobulinemia of Bruton, 240–242, 241f
X-linked disorders, 152, 152t
X-linked hyper-IgM syndrome, 199
X-linked lymphoproliferative syndrome (XLP), 331, 371
X-linked muscular dystrophy, 1336–1338, 1337f
X-linked severe combined immunodeficiency, 241f, 243–244
X-rays
as carcinogens, 323–324
exposure to, 436t
Xylene, 431

Y

Y chromosome, 178, 181
Yaws, 388

Yaws *(Continued)*
skeletal, 1292
Yeast infections, 397–399, 398f, 399f
of female genital tract, 1063
Yellow fever virus, 347t
Yersinia enterocolitica, 379–380, 834, 837
Yersinia pestis, 379–380
Yersinia pseudotuberculosis, 380, 837
Yolk sac tumor
ovarian, 1101, 1101f
testicular, 1041, 1043
Yop virulon, 380

Z
Z-bands, 1327
Zeis glands, 1424, 1424f
Zellballen
in carotid body tumor, 789, 789f
in pheochromocytoma, 1220, 1220f
Zenker diverticulum, 801f, 802
ζ proteins, 197
Zinc, 461, 461f, 461t
ZNF9 gene, 1339
Zollinger-Ellison syndrome, 1206–1207
Zollinger-Ellison syndrome *(Continued)*
gastric carcinoids in, 868
hypertrophic gastropathy in, 821
in MEN-1, 1222
peptic ulcers in, 818
Zonula adherens, 105
Zonule, of eye, 1422f
Zoonotic infections, 349t, 355
Zuska disease, 1125, 1125f
Zygomycosis, 400–401, 401f
Zymogen granules, 940